2014 DRAFT

ICD-10-PCS Code Book

Anne B. Casto, RHIA, CCS

Consulting Editor

AHIMA

American Health Information
Management Association®

ISBN: 978-1-58426-090-5
AHIMA Product No.: AC222013

AHIMA Staff:
Jessica Block, MA, Assistant Editor
Angie Comfort, RHIT, CDIP, CCS, Director, HIM Practice Excellence
Melanie A. Endicott, MBA/HCM, RHIA, CDIP, CCS, CCS-P, Director, HIM Practice Excellence
Jason O. Malley, Vice President, Business and Innovation
Pamela Woolf, Managing Editor

For more information about AHIMA Press publications, including updates, visit http://www.ahima.org/publications/updates.aspx

American Health Information Management Association
233 North Michigan Avenue, 21st Floor
Chicago, Illinois 60601-5809
ahima.org

Contents

About the Consulting Editor

Anne B. Casto, RHIA, CCS, is the president of Casto Consulting, LLC. Casto Consulting, LLC is a consulting firm that provides services to hospitals and other healthcare stakeholders primarily in the areas of reimbursement and coding. Casto Consulting, LLC specializes in linking coding and billing practices to positive revenue cycle outcomes. Additionally, the firm provides guidance to consulting firms, healthcare organizations and healthcare insurers regarding reimbursement methodologies and Medicare regulations.

Prior to founding the firm Anne was the program manager of the HIMS Division at The Ohio State University School of Allied Medical Professions. Ms. Casto taught healthcare reimbursement, ICD-9-CM coding and CPT coding courses for several years. Additionally, Ms. Casto was responsible for curriculum revisions in the areas of chargemaster management, clinical data management and healthcare reimbursement.

Additionally, Ms. Casto was the vice president of clinical information for Cleverley & Associates where she worked very closely with APC regulations and guidelines, preparing hospitals for the implementation of the Medicare OPPS. Ms. Casto was also the clinical information product manager for CHIPS/Ingenix. She joined CHIPS/Ingenix in 1998 and spent the majority of her time developing coding compliance products for the inpatient and outpatient settings.

Ms. Casto has been responsible for inpatient and outpatient coding activities in several large hospitals including Mt. Sinai Medical Center (NYC), Beth Israel Medical Center (NYC), and The Ohio State University. She has worked extensively with CMI, quality measures, physician documentation, and coding accuracy efforts at these facilities.

Ms. Casto received her degree in Health Information Management at The Ohio State University in 1995. She received her Certified Coding Specialist credential in 1998 from the American Health Information Management Association. Ms. Casto is the co-author of an AHIMA published text book entitled *Principles of Healthcare Reimbursement*. Additionally, Ms. Casto was a contributing author to the published AHIMA books: *Severity DRGs and Reimbursement; A MS-DRG Primer* and *Effective Management of Coding Services*. Most recently Ms. Casto authored the AHIMA published text entitled *The CDM Handbook*.

Ms. Casto received the AHIMA Legacy Award, part of the FORE Triumph Awards, in 2007 which honors a significant contribution to the knowledge base of the HIM field through an insightful publication. Additionally, Ms. Casto was honored with the Ohio Health Information Management Association's Distinguished Member Award in 2008 and the Ohio Health Information Management Association's Professional Achievement Award in 2011.

Acknowledgments

Many thanks to my family for their support during this project. Thanks to Dr. Susan White, The Ohio State University; your data manipulation skills are second to none. Thanks to Drew Beverick for providing valuable insight from the students perspective. I thank the reviewers for their thoughtful comments and suggestions. And special thanks to Pamela Woolf, for her never-ending support; you made this project one of the most fulfilling experiences of my career.

ICD-10-PCS Overview

The International Classification of Diseases, Tenth Revision, Procedure Coding System (ICD-10-PCS) was created to accompany the World Health Organization's (WHO) ICD-10 diagnosis classification. This coding system was developed to replace ICD-9-CM procedure codes for reporting inpatient procedures. Unlike the ICD-9-CM classification, ICD-10-PCS was designed to enable each code to have a standard structure and be very descriptive, and yet flexible enough to accommodate future needs.

History of ICD-10-PCS

The WHO has maintained the International Classification of Diseases (ICD) for recording cause of death since 1893. It has updated the ICD periodically to reflect new discoveries in epidemiology and changes in medical understanding of disease. The International Classification of Diseases Tenth Revision (ICD-10), published in 1992, is the latest revision of the ICD. The WHO authorized the National Center for Health Statistics (NCHS) to develop a clinical modification of ICD-10 for use in the United States. This version of ICD-10 is called ICD-10-CM, and is intended to replace the previous US clinical modification, ICD-9-CM, that has been in use since 1979. ICD-9-CM contains a procedure classification; ICD-10-CM does not.

The Centers for Medicare and Medicaid Services (CMS), the agency responsible for maintaining the inpatient procedure code set in the United States, contracted with 3M Health Information Systems in 1993 to design and then develop a procedure classification system to replace Volume 3 of ICD-9-CM. ICD-10-PCS is the result. ICD-10-PCS was initially released in 1998. It has been updated annually since that time.

ICD-9-CM Volume 3 Compared with ICD-10-PCS

With ICD-10 implementation, the US clinical modification of the ICD will not include a procedure classification based on the same principles of organization as the diagnosis classification. Instead, a separate procedure coding system has been developed to meet the rigorous and varied demands that are made of coded data in the healthcare industry. This represents a significant step toward building a health information infrastructure that functions optimally in the electronic age. The following information highlights some of the basic differences between ICD-9-CM Volume 3 and ICD-10-PCS:

ICD-9-CM Volume 3

- Follows ICD structure (designed for diagnosis coding)
- Codes available as a fixed/finite set in list form
- Codes are numeric
- Codes are three or four digits long

ICD-10-PCS

- Designed and developed to meet healthcare needs for a procedure code system
- Codes constructed from flexible code components (values) using tables
- Codes are alphanumeric
- All codes are seven characters long

ICD-10-PCS Design

ICD-10-PCS is fundamentally different from ICD-9-CM in its structure, organization, and capabilities. It was designed and developed to adhere to recommendations made by the National Committee on Vital and Health Statistics (NCVHS). It also incorporates input from a wide range of organizations, individual physicians, healthcare professionals, and researchers. Several structural attributes were recommended for a new procedure coding system. These attributes include a multiaxial structure, completeness, and expandability.

Multiaxial Structure

The key attribute that provides the framework for all other structural attributes is multiaxial code structure. *Multiaxial code structure* makes it possible for the ICD-10-PCS to be complete, expandable, and provide a high degree of flexibility and functionality.

ICD-10-PCS codes are composed of seven characters. Each character represents a category of information that can be specified about the procedure performed. A character defines both the category of information and its physical position in the code. A character's position can be understood as a semi-independent axis of classification that allows different specific values to be inserted into that space, and whose physical position remains stable. Within a defined code range, a character retains the general meaning that it confers on any value in that position.

Completeness

Completeness is considered a key structural attribute for a new procedure coding system. The specific recommendation for completeness included that a unique code be available for each significant procedure, that each code retain its unique definition, and that codes that have been deleted are not reused.

In Volume 3 of ICD-9-CM, procedures performed on many different body parts using different approaches or devices may be assigned to the same procedure code. In ICD-10-PCS, a unique code is constructed for every significantly different procedure.

Within each section, a character defines a consistent component of a code, and contains all applicable values for that character. The values define individual expressions (Open, Percutaneous) of the character's general meaning (approach) that are then used to construct unique procedure codes. Because all approaches by which a procedure is performed are assigned a separate approach value, every procedure which uses a different approach will have its own unique code. This is true of the other characters as well. The same procedure performed on a different body part has its own unique code; the same procedure performed using a different device has its own unique code, and so on.

Because ICD-10-PCS codes are constructed of individual values rather than lists of fixed codes and text descriptions, the unique, stable definition of a code in the system is retained. New values may be added to the system to represent a specific new approach or device or qualifier, but whole codes by design cannot be given new meanings and reused.

Expandability

Expandability was also recommended as a key structural attribute. The specific recommendation for expandability included that the system be capable of accommodating new procedures and technology and that these new codes could be added to the system without disrupting the existing structure.

ICD-10-PCS is designed to be easily updated as new codes are required for new procedures and new techniques. Changes to ICD-10-PCS can all be made within the existing structure because whole codes are not added. Instead, a new value for a character can be added to the system as needed. Likewise, an existing value for a character can be added to a table(s) in the system.

ICD-10-PCS Additional Characteristics

ICD-10-PCS possesses several additional characteristics in response to government and industry recommendations. These characteristics are

- Standardized terminology within the coding system
- Standardized level of specificity
- No diagnostic information
- No explicit "not otherwise specified" (NOS) code options
- Limited use of "not elsewhere classified" (NEC) code options

Standardized Terminology

Words commonly used in clinical vocabularies may have multiple meanings. This can cause confusion and result in inaccurate data. ICD-10-PCS is standardized and self-contained. Characters and values used in the system are defined in the system. For example, the word *excision* is used to describe a wide variety of surgical procedures. In ICD-10-PCS, the word *excision* describes a single, precise surgical objective, defined as "cutting out or off, without replacement, a portion of a body part."

No Eponyms or Common Procedure Names

The terminology used in ICD-10-PCS is standardized to provide precise and stable definitions of all procedures performed. This standardized terminology is used in all ICD-10-PCS code descriptions. As a result, ICD-10-PCS code descriptions do not include eponyms or common procedure names. Two examples from ICD-9-CM are

22.61, Excision of lesion of maxillary sinus with Caldwell-Luc approach

51.10, Endoscopic retrograde cholangiopancreatography [ERCP]

In ICD-10-PCS, physicians' names are not included in a code description, nor are procedures identified by common terms or acronyms such as appendectomy or CABG. Instead, such procedures are coded to the root operation that accurately identifies the objective of the procedure.

The procedures described in the preceding paragraph by ICD-9-CM codes are coded in ICD-10-PCS according to the root operation that matches the objective of the procedure. Here, the ICD-10-PCS equivalents would be Excision and Inspection, respectively. By relying on the universal objectives defined in root operations rather than eponyms or specific procedure titles that change or become obsolete, ICD-10-PCS preserves the capacity to define past, present, and future procedures accurately using stable terminology in the form of characters and values.

No Combination Codes

With rare exceptions, ICD-10-PCS does not define multiple procedures with one code. This is to preserve standardized terminology and consistency across the system. Procedures that are typically performed together but are distinct procedures may be defined by a single *combination code* in ICD-9-CM. An example of a combination code in ICD-9-CM is 28.3, Tonsillectomy with adenoidectomy.

A procedure that meets the reporting criteria for a separate procedure is coded separately in ICD-10-PCS. This allows the system to respond to changes in technology and medical practice with the maximum degree of stability and flexibility.

Standardized Level of Specificity

In ICD-9-CM, one code with its description and includes notes may encompass a vast number of procedure variations while another code defines a single specific procedure. ICD-10-PCS provides a standardized level of specificity for each code, so each code represents a single procedure variation.

The ICD-9-CM code 39.31, Suture of artery, does not specify the artery, whereas the code range 38.40–38.49, Resection of artery with replacement, provides a fourth-digit subclassification for specifying the artery by anatomical region (Thoracic, Abdominal, etc.). In ICD-10-PCS, the codes identifying all artery suture and artery replacement procedures possess the same degree of specificity. The ICD-9-CM examples above coded to their ICD-10-PCS equivalents would use the same artery body part values in all codes identifying the respective procedures.

In general, ICD-10-PCS code descriptions are much more specific than their ICD-9-CM counterparts, but sometimes an ICD-10-PCS code description is actually less specific. In most cases this is because the ICD-9-CM code contains diagnosis information. The standardized level of code specificity in ICD-10-PCS cannot always take account of these fluctuations in ICD-9-CM level of specificity. Instead, ICD-10-PCS provides a standardized level of specificity that can be predicted across the system.

Diagnosis Information Excluded

Another key feature of ICD-10-PCS is that information pertaining to a diagnosis is excluded from the code descriptions. ICD-9-CM often contains information about the diagnosis in its procedure codes. Adding diagnosis information limits the flexibility and functionality of a procedure coding system. It has the effect of placing a code "off limits" because the diagnosis in the medical record does not match the diagnosis in the procedure code description. The code cannot be used even though the procedural part of the code description precisely matches the procedure performed. Diagnosis information is not contained in any ICD-10-PCS code. The diagnosis codes, not the procedure codes, will specify the reason the procedure is performed.

NOS Code Options Restricted

ICD-9-CM often designates codes as "unspecified" or "not otherwise specified" (NOS) codes. By contrast, the standardized level of specificity designed into ICD-10-PCS restricts the use of broadly applicable NOS or unspecified code options in the system. A minimal level of specificity is required to construct a valid code.

Limited NEC Code Options

ICD-9-CM often designates codes as "not elsewhere classified" (NEC) or "other specified" versions of a procedure throughout the code set. NEC options are also provided in ICD-10-PCS, but only for specific, limited use.

In the Medical and Surgical section, two significant NEC options are the root operation value Q, Repair, and the device value Y, Other Device. The root operation Repair is a true NEC value. It is used only when the procedure performed is not one of the other root operations in the Medical and Surgical section. Other Device, on the other hand, is intended to be used to temporarily define new devices that do not have a specific value assigned, until one can be added to the system. No categories of medical or surgical devices are permanently classified to Other Device.

ICD-10-PCS Code Structure

Undergirding ICD-10-PCS is a logical, consistent structure that informs the system as a whole, down to the level of a single code. This means the process of constructing codes in ICD-10-PCS is also logical and consistent: the spaces of the code, called *characters* are filled with individual letters and numbers, called *values*.

Characters

All codes in ICD-10-PCS are seven characters long. Each character in the seven-character code represents an aspect of the procedure. The following are two examples of the code structure: one from the Medical and Surgical section and one from the Ancillary section.

Medical and Surgical Code Structure

Character 1	Character 2	Character 3	Character 4	Character 5	Character 6	Character 7
Section	Body System	Operation	Body Part	Approach	Device	Qualifier

Imaging Section Code Structure

Character 1	Character 2	Character 3	Character 4	Character 5	Character 6	Character 7
Section	Body System	Type	Body Part	Contrast	Qualifier	Qualifier

An ICD-10-PCS code is best understood as the result of a process rather than as an isolated, fixed quantity. The process consists of assigning values from among the valid choices for that part of the system, according to the rules governing the construction of codes.

Values

One of 34 possible values can be assigned to each character in a code: the numbers 0 through 9 and the alphabet (except the letters I and O, because they are easily confused with the numbers 1 and 0). A finished code looks like this: 02103D4.

This code is derived by choosing a specific value for each of the seven characters. Based on details about the procedure performed, values for each character specifying the section, body system, root operation, body part, approach, device, and qualifier are assigned. Because the definition of each character is a function of its physical position in the code, the same value placed in a different position in the code means something different. The value 0 in the first character means something different than 0 in the second character, or 0 in the third character, and so on.

Code Structure Example

The following example defines each character using the code 0LB50ZZ, Excision of right lower arm and wrist tendon, Open approach. This example comes from the Medical and Surgical section of ICD-10-PCS.

Character 1: Section

The first character in the code determines the broad procedure category, or section, where the code is found. In this example, the section is Medical and Surgical. 0 is the value that represents Medical and Surgical in the first character.

Character 1	Character 2	Character 3	Character 4	Character 5	Character 6	Character 7
Section	Body System	Root Operation	Body Part	Approach	Device	Qualifier
0						

Character 2: Body System

The second character defines the body system—the general physiological system or anatomical region involved. Examples of body systems include Lower Arteries, Central Nervous System, and Respiratory System. In this example, the body system is Tendons, represented by the value L.

Character 1	Character 2	Character 3	Character 4	Character 5	Character 6	Character 7
Section	**Body System**	Root Operation	Body Part	Approach	Device	Qualifier
0	**L**					

Character 3: Root Operation

The third character defines the root operation, or the objective of the procedure. Some examples of root operations are Bypass, Drainage, and Reattachment. In this example code, the root operation is Excision. When used in the third character of the code, the value B represents Excision.

Character 1	Character 2	Character 3	Character 4	Character 5	Character 6	Character 7
Section	Body System	**Root Operation**	Body Part	Approach	Device	Qualifier
0	L	**B**				

Character 4: Body Part

The fourth character defines the body part or specific anatomical site where the procedure was performed. The body system (second character) provides only a general indication of the procedure site. The body part and body system values together provide a precise description of the procedure site. Examples of body parts are Kidney, Tonsils, and Thymus. In this example, the body part value is 5, Lower Arm and Wrist, Right. When the second character is L, the value 5 when used in the fourth character of the code represents the right lower arm and wrist tendon.

Character 1	Character 2	Character 3	Character 4	Character 5	Character 6	Character 7
Section	Body System	Root Operation	**Body Part**	Approach	Device	Qualifier
0	L	B	**5**			

Character 5: Approach

The fifth character defines the approach, or the technique used to reach the procedure site. Seven different approach values are used in the Medical and Surgical section to define the approach. Examples of approaches include Open and Percutaneous Endoscopic. In this example code, the approach is Open and is represented by the value 0.

Character 1	Character 2	Character 3	Character 4	Character 5	Character 6	Character 7
Section	Body System	Root Operation	Body Part	**Approach**	Device	Qualifier
0	L	B	5	**0**		

Character 6: Device

Depending on the procedure performed, there may be a device left in place at the end of the procedure. The sixth character defines the device. Device values fall into four basic categories:

- Grafts and Prostheses
- Implants
- Simple or Mechanical Appliances
- Electronic Appliances

In this example, there is no device used in the procedure. The value Z is used to represent No Device, as shown here:

Character 1	Character 2	Character 3	Character 4	Character 5	Character 6	Character 7
Section	Body System	Operation	Body Part	Approach	**Device**	Qualifier
0	L	B	5	0	**Z**	

Character 7: Qualifier

The seventh character defines a qualifier for the code. A qualifier specifies an additional attribute of the procedure, if applicable. Examples of qualifiers include Diagnostic and Stereotactic. Qualifier choices vary depending on the previous values selected. In this example, there is no specific qualifier applicable to this procedure, so the value is No Qualifier, represented by the letter Z.

Character 1	Character 2	Character 3	Character 4	Character 5	Character 6	Character 7
Section	Body System	Operation	Body Part	Approach	Device	**Qualifier**
0	L	B	5	0	Z	**Z**

0LB50ZZ is the complete specification of the procedure "Excision of right lower arm and wrist tendon, Open approach."

ICD-10-PCS Organization and Official Conventions

The *ICD-10-PCS Code Book, 2014 Draft* is based on the official draft of the International Classification of Diseases, Tenth Revision, Procedure Classification System, issued by the US Department of Health and Human Services (HHS) and CMS. This book is consistent with the content of the government's version of ICD-10-PCS and follows the official conventions.

Index

The Alphabetic Index is provided to assist the user with locating the appropriate table to construct procedure codes. Each table contains all the information required to construct valid procedure codes. Coders should not code from the PCS Index alone; the PCS code tables should always be consulted before assigning a PCS procedure code.

Main Terms

Main terms in the Alphabetic Index reflect the root operations, third character, of procedures. The Index includes not only root operation terms, but also other common procedural terms, anatomical sites, and device terms. The main terms are listed alphabetically. After the coder has located the correct main term and subterm in the Alphabetic Index, he or she is provided with the first three to four digits of the procedure code. The coder should then move to the Tables section of the code book and locate the appropriate table to complete the code construction. Even if the entire seven-digit code is provided in the Index, the coder should still reference the Tables to ensure the correct PCS code has been constructed.

See Reference

Common procedure terms are often listed with the *see* reference. The coder is instructed to follow the reference provided in order to locate the appropriate table to construct the code. For example, the *see* reference is present for the main term Colectomy. The Index excerpt is as follows:

Colectomy

   see Excision, Gastrointestinal System 0DB

   see Resection, Gastrointestinal System 0DT

In this example, the coder should review the definition of the root operations Excision and Resection to determine which is consistent with the medical record documentation. The coder should then proceed to the corresponding table as suggested by the *see* reference.

Use Reference

Anatomical site terms and device terms are often listed with the *use* reference. The coder is instructed to follow the reference provided in order to locate the appropriate main term for the procedure in question. For example, the *use* reference is present for the main term Inferior rectus muscle. The Index excerpt is as follows:

Inferior rectus muscle

   use Muscle, Extraocular, Left

   use Muscle, Extraocular, Right

In this example, the coder should identify the root operation for the procedure, and then look for the subterm that identifies the body part indicated in the *use* reference. For example, the procedure is excision of the inferior rectus muscle. The coder would locate the main term Excision. The Index excerpt is as follows:

Excision

   Muscle

      Extraocular

         Left 08BM

         Right 08BL

In this example, the coder knows that the Code Table 08B is the correct table because the previous review of the *use* reference identified that the inferior rectus muscle is and extraocular muscle. The coder can now proceed to the 08B Table to finish constructing the PCS code.

   In addition to the *use* reference, the coder may also consult appendix D for Body Part Table or appendix E for the Device Table.

Code Tables

ICD-10-PCS contains 16 sections of Code Tables, represented by the numbers 0 through 9 and the letters B through D and F through H. The Tables are organized by general type of procedure. The three main sections of tables include:

1. **Medical and Surgical section**

   • Medical and Surgical (first character 0)

2. **Medical and Surgical Related sections**
   - Obstetrics (first character 1)
   - Placement (first character 2)
   - Administration (first character 3)
   - Measurement and Monitoring (first character 4)
   - Extracorporeal Assistance and Performance (first character 5)
   - Extracorporeal Therapies (first character 6)
   - Osteopathic (first character 7)
   - Other Procedures (first character 8)
   - Chiropractic (first character 9)

3. **Ancillary sections**
   - Imaging (first character B)
   - Nuclear Medicine (first character C)
   - Radiation Therapy (first character D)
   - Physical Rehabilitation and Diagnostic Audiology (first character F)
   - Mental Health (first character G)
   - Substance Abuse (first character H)

Each code table is defined by the first three characters of the PCS code. Each of these characters is displayed above the table. The table consists of all the options for characters 4 through 7. The root operation or root type, character 3, is present along with its official definition. Table 097 is provided here as an example of the table structure.

0 Medical and Surgical

9 Ear, Nose, Sinus

7 Dilation, Expanding an orifice or the lumen of a tubular body part

Body Part Character 4	Approach Character 5	Device Character 6	Qualifier Character 7
F Eustachian Tube, Right G Eustachian Tube, Left	0 Open 7 Via Natural or Artificial Opening 8 Via Natural or Artificial Opening Endoscopic	D Intraluminal Device Z No Device	Z No Qualifier
F Eustachian Tube, Right G Eustachian Tube, Left	3 Percutaneous 4 Percutaneous Endoscopic	Z No Device	Z No Qualifier

There can be multiple rows within the table for the first three characters, so the coder must carefully review all the applicable rows. Additionally, a table may cover multiple pages. Therefore, the coder must continue to review the code table options until the end of the table is reached to ensure the correct PCS code has been constructed.

Code Listing

Code Listings for the Medical and Surgical and Obstetrics sections are included in this manual to assist coders with ensuring that the intended code has been selected for reporting. The Code Listings are presented in alphanumeric order. Within the Code Listing, several additional conventions are included to assist coders with navigating the Medicare Code Editor (MCE) edits, official coding guidelines, and other reporting requirements such as the Inpatient Prospective Payment System (IPPS) Hospital-Acquired Conditions (HACs) related codes. The Code Listings are combined with the Tables section of the code book. In the Medical and Surgical section, the Code Listing appears after each body system. For the Obstetrics section, the Code Listing appears at the end of the section.

ICD-10-PCS Additional Conventions

The use of symbols has been added to this code book to alert the user to Medicare reimbursement logic and edits that are impacted by procedure coding. Some codes may be included in multiple reimbursement issues and, therefore, may have more than one symbol. For a quick reference review, the legend at the bottom of each page of the Code Listing (Medical/Surgical section and Obstetrics section) as well as the inside cover of the code book. The symbols are described in detail here.

Medicare Code Edits

Hospital inpatient Medicare claims paid under the IPPS are processed through the MCE prior to payment by the Medicare administrative contractor (MAC). The code edits are intended to ensure that all claims processed by the MAC are accurate and complete. Medicare has released an ICD-10 version of the MCE v30 and is provided to the general public as a tool to assist in the implementation of ICD-10-CM/PCS. The information in this manual is based on the MCE v30.

Several of the MCE edits pertain to procedures. We have included identification of the codes included in these edits in this manual to assist users with preparing accurate and complete claims. The MCE edits included in this manual:

- Sex conflict
- Medicare non-covered procedures
- Medicare limited coverage procedures

Note: It is important to remember these edits are Medicare edits and may not apply to other third-party payers claim processing.

Sex Conflict Edit

The sex conflict edit is activated when the sex of the patient and the type of procedure performed does not match. The following symbols are used to identify female-only and male-only procedures.

♀ Female-only procedure: This symbol appears to the left of the applicable code in the code listing.

♂ Male-only procedure: This symbol appears to the left of the applicable code in the code listing.

Medicare Non-covered Procedure

Medicare does not reimburse for all ICD-10-PCS procedures. There are some procedures that are never reimbursed, and there are some procedures that are only reimbursed when certain specified diagnosis codes are also included on the claim. Non-covered procedures are designated by a red hexagon symbol ⬡ located next to the code description for the applicable code. If there is conditional logic for the non-coverage, it is provided to the right of the red hexagon.

Medicare Limited Coverage Procedures

For certain procedures whose medical complexity and serious nature incur extraordinary associated costs, Medicare limits coverage to a portion of the cost. The limited coverage edit indicates this type of limited coverage. Limited coverage procedures are designated by a yellow hexagon symbol ⬡ located next to the code description for the applicable code. If there is conditional logic for the limited coverage, it is provided to the right of the yellow hexagon.

MS-DRG Procedure Designations

The MS-DRG system is utilized within the IPPS to determine the unadjusted reimbursement amount for Medicare hospital inpatient claims. The MS-DRG Definitions Manual includes the logic for MS-DRG refinement and selection as well as logic based on the IPPS final rules released each August. CMS has released an ICD-10-CM/PCS version of the MS-DRG v30. The information in this manual is based on the MS-DRG v30. *Note:* It is important to remember that these edits are Medicare edits and may not apply to other third-party payers claim processing.

Non-Operating Room Procedures

Within the MS-DRG logic, CMS designates which procedures are operating room (OR) procedures and which procedures are non-OR procedures. Non-OR procedures do not impact the MS-DRG assignment; in the basic sense they do not covert medical MS-DRGs to surgical MS-DRGs. Once an encounter is determined as "surgical" specified OR procedures are utilized to refine the final MS-DRG assignment. Throughout the Medical and Surgical and Obstetrics sections, non-OR procedures are indicated with a purple dot ●. The purple dot symbol is located to the left of the applicable code in the code listing.

Hospital-Acquired Conditions Related Procedures

As part of the Medicare Value-Based Purchasing program, CMS has implemented a Paying for Value program entitled Hospital-Acquired Conditions (HACs). This program is designed to reduce reimbursements to facilities where value of the medical or surgical has been comprised due to preventable conditions. The HAC program identifies diagnosis and procedure codes that when reported as "not present on admission" activate the HAC reduced reimbursement logic. In this manual, the HAC-associated procedures are identified with an orange rectangle ▮HAC▮ with HAC. The orange rectangle is located below the code description in the code listing. If there is conditional logic for the procedure code, it is included to the right of the orange rectangle.

Combination Codes Required

Within the MS-DRG logic CMS has designated codes that must be reported with specified other codes in order to fully report a complete procedure. For such procedures, such as simultaneous pancreas and kidney transplants, if the correct combination of codes is not reported, the desired MS-DRG will not be calculated for the encounter. Combination codes are identified with a green box with a plus sign in the middle ➕. The green box with a code-specific note is located below the code description for applicable code in the code listing.

ICD-10-PCS Draft Coding Guidelines

The ICD-10-PCS Draft Coding Guidelines are presented throughout this manual. The Conventions and Selection of Principal Procedure sections are presented in the front of the manual prior to the start of the Alphabetical Index. The Medical and Surgical Section Guidelines are presented after the Introduction of the Medical and Surgical section. The Obstetric Section Guidelines are presented after the Introduction of the Obstetrics section.

Throughout the Code Listings, applicable guidelines are identified via an instruction note in order to remind users to reference the coding guidelines prior to code reporting. The instruction note *Review Coding Guideline...* followed by the guideline reference number is included after the section header for applicable sections or after the code description for applicable codes. It is imperative to review the ICD-10-PCS draft coding guidelines to ensure the procedure code being reported is accurate and complete.

ICD-10-PCS Official Guidelines for Coding and Reporting 2014

The Centers for Medicare and Medicaid Services (CMS) and the National Center for Health Statistics (NCHS), two departments within the US federal government's Department of Health and Human Services (HHS) provide the following guidelines for coding and reporting using the International Classification of Diseases, 10th Revision, Procedure Coding System (ICD-10-PCS). These guidelines should be used as a companion document to the official version of the ICD-10-PCS as published on the CMS website. The ICD-10-PCS is a procedure classification published by the United States for classifying procedures performed in hospital inpatient health care settings.

These guidelines have been approved by the four organizations that make up the Cooperating Parties for the ICD-10-PCS: the American Hospital Association (AHA), the American Health Information Management Association (AHIMA), CMS, and NCHS.

These guidelines are a set of rules that have been developed to accompany and complement the official conventions and instructions provided within the ICD-10-PCS itself. The instructions and conventions of the classification take precedence over guidelines. These guidelines are based on the coding and sequencing instructions in the Tables, Index, and Definitions of ICD-10-PCS, but provide additional instruction. Adherence to these guidelines when assigning ICD-10-PCS procedure codes is required under the Health Insurance Portability and Accountability Act (HIPAA). The procedure codes have been adopted under HIPAA for hospital inpatient healthcare settings. A joint effort between the healthcare provider and the coder is essential to achieve complete and accurate documentation, code assignment, and reporting of diagnoses and procedures. These guidelines have been developed to assist both the healthcare provider and the coder in identifying those procedures that are to be reported. The importance of consistent, complete documentation in the medical record cannot be overemphasized. Without such documentation, accurate coding cannot be achieved.

Conventions

A1. ICD-10-PCS codes are composed of seven characters. Each character is an axis of classification that specifies information about the procedure performed. Within a defined code range, a character specifies the same type of information in that axis of classification.

Example: The fifth axis of classification specifies the approach in sections 0 through 4 and 7 through 9 of the system.

A2. One of 34 possible values can be assigned to each axis of classification in the seven-character code: they are the numbers 0 through 9 and the alphabet (except the letters I and O because they are easily confused with the numbers 1 and 0). The number of unique values used in an axis of classification differs as needed.

Example: Where the fifth axis of classification specifies the approach, seven different approach values are currently used to specify the approach.

A3. The valid values for an axis of classification can be added to as needed.

Example: If a significantly distinct type of device is used in a new procedure, a new device value can be added to the system.

A4. As with words in their context, the meaning of any single value is a combination of its axis of classification and any preceding values on which it may be dependent.

Example: The meaning of a body part value in the Medical and Surgical section is always dependent on the body system value. The body part value 0 in the Central Nervous body system specifies Brain and the body part value 0 in the Peripheral Nervous body system specifies Cervical Plexus.

A5. As the system is expanded to become increasingly detailed, more values will depend on preceding values for their meaning.

Example: In the Lower Joints body system, the device value 3 in the root operation Insertion specifies Infusion Device and the device value 3 in the root operation Replacement specifies Ceramic Synthetic Substitute.

A6. The purpose of the Alphabetic Index is to locate the appropriate table that contains all information necessary to construct a procedure code. The PCS Tables should always be consulted to find the most appropriate valid code.

A7. It is not required to consult the Index first before proceeding to the tables to complete the code. A valid code may be chosen directly from the Tables.

A8. All seven characters must be specified to be a valid code. If the documentation is incomplete for coding purposes, the physician should be queried for the necessary information.

A9. Within a PCS Table, valid codes include all combinations of choices in characters 4 through 7 contained in the same row of the table. In the example below, 0JHT3VZ is a valid code, and 0JHW3VZ is *not* a valid code.

Section:	0	Medical and Surgical
Body System:	**J**	**Subcutaneous Tissue and Fascia**
Operation:	**H**	**Insertion:** Putting in a nonbiological appliance that monitors, assists, performs, or prevents a physiological function but does not physically take the place of a body part

Body Part (4ᵗʰ)	Approach (5ᵗʰ)	Device (6ᵗʰ)	Qualifier (7ᵗʰ)
S Subcutaneous Tissue and Fascia, Head and Neck V Subcutaneous Tissue and Fascia, Upper Extremity W Subcutaneous Tissue and Fascia, Lower Extremity	0 Open 3 Percutaneous	1 Radioactive Element 3 Infusion Device	Z No Qualifier
T Subcutaneous Tissue and Fascia, Trunk	0 Open 3 Percutaneous	1 Radioactive Element 3 Infusion Device V Infusion Pump	Z No Qualifier

A10. "And," when used in a code description, means "and/or."

Example: Lower Arm and Wrist Muscle means lower arm and/or wrist muscle.

A11. Many of the terms used to construct PCS codes are defined within the system. It is the coder's responsibility to determine what the documentation in the medical record equates to in the PCS definitions. The physician is not expected to use the terms used in PCS code descriptions, nor is the coder required to query the physician when the correlation between the documentation and the defined PCS terms is clear.

Example: When the physician documents "partial resection" the coder can independently correlate "partial resection" to the root operation Excision without querying the physician for clarification.

Selection of Principal Procedure

The following instructions should be applied in the selection of principal procedure and clarification on the importance of the relation to the principal diagnosis when more than one procedure is performed:

1. Procedure performed for definitive treatment of both principal diagnosis and secondary diagnosis

    a. Sequence procedure performed for definitive treatment most related to principal diagnosis as principal procedure.

2. Procedure performed for definitive treatment and diagnostic procedures performed for both principal diagnosis and secondary diagnosis

    a. Sequence procedure performed for definitive treatment most related to principal diagnosis as principal procedure

3. A diagnostic procedure was performed for the principal diagnosis and a procedure is performed for definitive treatment of a secondary diagnosis.

    a. Sequence diagnostic procedure as principal procedure, since the procedure most related to the principal diagnosis takes precedence.

4. No procedures performed that are related to principal diagnosis; procedures performed for definitive treatment and diagnostic procedures were performed for secondary diagnosis

    a. Sequence procedure performed for definitive treatment of secondary diagnosis as principal procedure, since there are no procedures (definitive or nondefinitive treatment) related to principal diagnosis.

3

3f (Aortic) Bioprosthesis valve
use Zooplastic Tissue in Heart and Great Vessels

A

Abdominal aortic plexus
use Nerve, Abdominal Sympathetic
Abdominal esophagus
use Esophagus, Lower
Abdominohysterectomy
see Excision, Uterus 0UB9
see Resection, Uterus 0UT9
Abdominoplasty
see Alteration, Abdominal Wall 0W0F
see Repair, Abdominal Wall 0WQF
see Supplement, Abdominal Wall 0WUF
Abductor hallucis muscle
use Muscle, Foot, Right
use Muscle, Foot, Left
AbioCor® Total Replacement Heart
use Synthetic Substitute
Ablation
see Destruction
Abortion
Products of Conception 10A0
Abortifacient 10A07ZX
Laminaria 10A07ZW
Vacuum 10A07Z6
Abrasion
see Extraction
Accessory cephalic vein
use Vein, Cephalic, Right
use Vein, Cephalic, Left
Accessory obturator nerve
use Nerve, Lumbar Plexus
Accessory phrenic nerve
use Nerve, Phrenic
Accessory spleen
use Spleen
Acellular Hydrated Dermis
use Nonautologous Tissue Substitute
Acetabulectomy
see Excision, Lower Bones 0QB
see Resection, Lower Bones 0QT
Acetabulofemoral joint
use Joint, Hip, Right
use Joint, Hip, Left
Acetabuloplasty
see Repair, Lower Bones 0QQ
see Replacement, Lower Bones 0QR
see Supplement, Lower Bones 0QU
Achilles tendon
use Tendon, Lower Leg, Left
use Tendon, Lower Leg, Right
Achillorrhaphy
see Repair, Tendons 0LQ
Achillotenotomy, achillotomy
see Division, Tendons 0L8
see Drainage, Tendons 0L9
Acromioclavicular ligament
use Bursa and Ligament, Shoulder, Right
use Bursa and Ligament, Shoulder, Left
Acromion (process)
use Scapula, Left
use Scapula, Right
Acromionectomy
see Excision, Upper Joints 0RB
see Resection, Upper Joints 0RT
Acromioplasty
see Repair, Upper Joints 0RQ
see Replacement, Upper Joints 0RR
see Supplement, Upper Joints 0RU
Activa PC neurostimulator
use Stimulator Generator, Multiple Array in 0JH
Activa RC neurostimulator
use Stimulator Generator, Multiple Array Rechargeable in 0JH
Activa SC neurostimulator
use Stimulator Generator, Single Array in 0JH
Activities of Daily Living Assessment F02
Activities of Daily Living Treatment F08

ACUITY™ Steerable Lead
use Cardiac Lead, Defibrillator in 02H
use Cardiac Lead, Pacemaker in 02H
Acupuncture
Breast
Anesthesia 8E0H300
No Qualifier 8E0H30Z
Integumentary System
Anesthesia 8E0H300
No Qualifier 8E0H30Z
Adductor brevis muscle
use Muscle, Upper Leg, Left
use Muscle, Upper Leg, Right
Adductor hallucis muscle
use Muscle, Foot, Left
use Muscle, Foot, Right
Adductor longus muscle
use Muscle, Upper Leg, Right
use Muscle, Upper Leg, Left
Adductor magnus muscle
use Muscle, Upper Leg, Right
use Muscle, Upper Leg, Left
Adenohypophysis
use Gland, Pituitary
Adenoidectomy
see Excision, Adenoids 0CBQ
see Resection, Adenoids 0CTQ
Adenoidotomy
see Drainage, Adenoids 0C9Q
Adhesiolysis
see Release
Administration
Blood products
see Transfusion
Other substance
see Introduction of substance in or on
Adrenalectomy
see Excision, Endocrine System 0GB
see Resection, Endocrine System 0GT
Adrenalorrhaphy
see Repair, Endocrine System 0GQ
Adrenalotomy
see Drainage, Endocrine System 0G9
Advancement
see Reposition
see Transfer
Alar ligament of axis
use Bursa and Ligament, Head and Neck
Alimentation
see Introduction of substance in or on
Alteration
Abdominal Wall 0W0F
Ankle Region
Left 0Y0L
Right 0Y0K
Arm
Lower
Left 0X0F
Right 0X0D
Upper
Left 0X09
Right 0X08
Axilla
Left 0X05
Right 0X04
Back
Lower 0W0L
Upper 0W0K
Breast
Bilateral 0H0V
Left 0H0U
Right 0H0T
Buttock
Left 0Y01
Right 0Y00
Chest Wall 0W08
Ear
Bilateral 0902
Left 0901
Right 0900
Elbow Region
Left 0X0C
Right 0X0B

Alteration *(continued)*
Extremity
Lower
Left 0Y0B
Right 0Y09
Upper
Left 0X07
Right 0X06
Eyelid
Lower
Left 080R
Right 080Q
Upper
Left 080P
Right 080N
Face 0W02
Head 0W00
Jaw
Lower 0W05
Upper 0W04
Knee Region
Left 0Y0G
Right 0Y0F
Leg
Lower
Left 0Y0J
Right 0Y0H
Upper
Left 0Y0D
Right 0Y0C
Lip
Lower 0C01X
Upper 0C00X
Neck 0W06
Nose 090K
Perineum
Female 0W0N
Male 0W0M
Shoulder Region
Left 0X03
Right 0X02
Subcutaneous Tissue and Fascia
Abdomen 0J08
Back 0J07
Buttock 0J09
Chest 0J06
Face 0J01
Lower Arm
Left 0J0H
Right 0J0G
Lower Leg
Left 0J0P
Right 0J0N
Neck
Anterior 0J04
Posterior 0J05
Upper Arm
Left 0J0F
Right 0J0D
Upper Leg
Left 0J0M
Right 0J0L
Wrist Region
Left 0X0H
Right 0X0G
Alveolar process of mandible
use Mandible, Left
use Mandible, Right
Alveolar process of maxilla
use Maxilla, Right
use Maxilla, Left
Alveolectomy
see Excision, Head and Facial Bones 0NB
see Resection, Head and Facial Bones 0NT
Alveoloplasty
see Repair, Head and Facial Bones 0NQ
see Replacement, Head and Facial Bones 0NR
see Supplement, Head and Facial Bones 0NU
Alveolotomy
see Division, Head and Facial Bones 0N8
see Drainage, Head and Facial Bones 0N9
Ambulatory cardiac monitoring 4A12X45
Amniocentesis
see Drainage, Products of Conception 1090

Amnioinfusion
  see Introduction of substance in or on, Products of
    Conception 3E0E
Amnioscopy 10J08ZZ
Amniotomy
  see Drainage, Products of Conception 1090
AMPLATZER® Muscular VSD Occluder
  use Synthetic Substitute
Amputation
  see Detachment
AMS 800® Urinary Control System
  use Artificial Sphincter in Urinary System
Anal orifice
  use Anus
Analog radiography
  see Plain Radiography
Analog radiology
  see Plain Radiography
Anastomosis
  see Bypass
Anatomical snuffbox
  use Muscle, Lower Arm and Wrist, Left
  use Muscle, Lower Arm and Wrist, Right
AneuRx® AAA Advantage®
  use Intraluminal Device
Angiectomy
  see Excision, Heart and Great Vessels 02B
  see Excision, Upper Arteries 03B
  see Excision, Lower Arteries 04B
  see Excision, Upper Veins 05B
  see Excision, Lower Veins 06B
Angiocardiography
  Combined right and left heart
    see Fluoroscopy, Heart, Right and Left B216
  Left Heart
    see Fluoroscopy, Heart, Left B215
  Right Heart
    see Fluoroscopy, Heart, Right B214
  SPY
    see Fluoroscopy, Heart B21
Angiography
  see Plain Radiography, Heart B20
  see Fluoroscopy, Heart B21
Angioplasty
  see Dilation, Heart and Great Vessels 027
  see Repair, Heart and Great Vessels 02Q
  see Replacement, Heart and Great Vessels 02R
  see Dilation, Upper Arteries 037
  see Repair, Upper Arteries 03Q
  see Replacement, Upper Arteries 03R
  see Dilation, Lower Arteries 047
  see Repair, Lower Arteries 04Q
  see Replacement, Lower Arteries 04R
  see Supplement, Heart and Great Vessels 02U
  see Supplement, Upper Arteries 03U
  see Supplement, Lower Arteries 04U
Angiorrhaphy
  see Repair, Heart and Great Vessels 02Q
  see Repair, Upper Arteries 03Q
  see Repair, Lower Arteries 04Q
Angioscopy
  02JY4ZZ
  03JY4ZZ
  04JY4ZZ
Angiotripsy
  see Occlusion, Upper Arteries 03L
  see Occlusion, Lower Arteries 04L
Angular artery
  use Artery, Face
Angular vein
  use Vein, Face, Left
  use Vein, Face, Right
Annular ligament
  use Bursa and Ligament, Elbow, Left
  use Bursa and Ligament, Elbow, Right
Annuloplasty
  see Repair, Heart and Great Vessels 02Q
  see Supplement, Heart and Great Vessels
    02U
Annuloplasty ring
  use Synthetic Substitute
Anoplasty
  see Repair, Anus 0DQQ
  see Supplement, Anus 0DUQ
Anorectal junction
  use Rectum
Anoscopy 0DJD8ZZ
Ansa cervicalis
  use Nerve, Cervical Plexus
Antabuse therapy HZ93ZZZ
Antebrachial fascia
  use Subcutaneous Tissue and Fascia, Lower Arm, Left
  use Subcutaneous Tissue and Fascia, Lower Arm,
    Right

Anterior (pectoral) lymph node
  use Lymphatic, Axillary, Right
  use Lymphatic, Axillary, Left
Anterior cerebral artery
  use Artery, Intracranial
Anterior cerebral vein
  use Vein, Intracranial
Anterior choroidal artery
  use Artery, Intracranial
Anterior circumflex humeral artery
  use Artery, Axillary, Left
  use Artery, Axillary, Right
Anterior communicating artery
  use Artery, Intracranial
Anterior cruciate ligament (ACL)
  use Bursa and Ligament, Knee, Left
  use Bursa and Ligament, Knee, Right
Anterior crural nerve
  use Nerve, Femoral
Anterior facial vein
  use Vein, Face, Left
  use Vein, Face, Right
Anterior intercostal artery
  use Artery, Internal Mammary, Right
  use Artery, Internal Mammary, Left
Anterior interosseous nerve
  use Nerve, Median
Anterior lateral malleolar artery
  use Artery, Anterior Tibial, Right
  use Artery, Anterior Tibial, Left
Anterior lingual gland
  use Gland, Minor Salivary
Anterior medial malleolar artery
  use Artery, Anterior Tibial, Right
  use Artery, Anterior Tibial, Left
Anterior spinal artery
  use Artery, Vertebral, Right
  use Artery, Vertebral, Left
Anterior tibial recurrent artery
  use Artery, Anterior Tibial, Right
  use Artery, Anterior Tibial, Left
Anterior ulnar recurrent artery
  use Artery, Ulnar, Right
  use Artery, Ulnar, Left
Anterior vagal trunk
  use Nerve, Vagus
Anterior vertebral muscle
  use Muscle, Neck, Left
  use Muscle, Neck, Right
Antihelix
  use Ear, External, Right
  use Ear, External, Left
  use Ear, External, Bilateral
Antitragus
  use Ear, External, Bilateral
  use Ear, External, Right
  use Ear, External, Left
Antrostomy
  see Drainage, Ear, Nose, Sinus 099
Antrotomy
  see Drainage, Ear, Nose, Sinus 099
Antrum of Highmore
  use Sinus, Maxillary, Left
  use Sinus, Maxillary, Right
Aortic annulus
  use Valve, Aortic
Aortic arch
  use Aorta, Thoracic
Aortic intercostal artery
  use Aorta, Thoracic
Aortography
  see Plain Radiography, Upper Arteries B30
  see Fluoroscopy, Upper Arteries B31
  see Plain Radiography, Lower Arteries B40
  see Fluoroscopy, Lower Arteries B41
Aortoplasty
  see Repair, Aorta, Thoracic 02QW
  see Replacement, Aorta, Thoracic 02RW
  see Supplement, Aorta, Thoracic 02UW
  see Repair, Aorta, Abdominal 04Q0
  see Replacement, Aorta, Abdominal 04R0
  see Supplement, Aorta, Abdominal 04U0
Apical (subclavicular) lymph node
  use Lymphatic, Axillary, Left
  use Lymphatic, Axillary, Right
Apneustic center
  use Pons
Appendectomy
  see Excision, Appendix 0DBJ
  see Resection, Appendix 0DTJ
Appendicolysis
  see Release, Appendix 0DNJ
Appendicotomy
  see Drainage, Appendix 0D9J

Application
  see Introduction of substance in or on
Aquaperesis 6A550Z3
Aqueduct of Sylvius
  use Cerebral Ventricle
Aqueous humour
  use Anterior Chamber, Right
  use Anterior Chamber, Left
Arachnoid mater
  use Spinal Meninges
  use Cerebral Meninges
Arcuate artery
  use Artery, Foot, Left
  use Artery, Foot, Right
Areola
  use Nipple, Left
  use Nipple, Right
AROM (artificial rupture of membranes) 10907ZC
Arterial canal (duct)
  use Artery, Pulmonary, Left
Arterial pulse tracing
  see Measurement, Arterial 4A03
Arteriectomy
  see Excision, Heart and Great Vessels 02B
  see Excision, Upper Arteries 03B
  see Excision, Lower Arteries 04B
Arteriography
  see Plain Radiography, Heart B20
  see Fluoroscopy, Heart B21
  see Plain Radiography, Upper Arteries B30
  see Fluoroscopy, Upper Arteries B31
  see Plain Radiography, Lower Arteries B40
  see Fluoroscopy, Lower Arteries B41
Arterioplasty
  see Repair, Heart and Great Vessels 02Q
  see Replacement, Heart and Great Vessels 02R
  see Repair, Upper Arteries 03Q
  see Replacement, Upper Arteries 03R
  see Repair, Lower Arteries 04Q
  see Replacement, Lower Arteries 04R
  see Supplement, Upper Arteries 03U
  see Supplement, Lower Arteries 04U
  see Supplement, Heart and Great Vessels 02U
Arteriorrhaphy
  see Repair, Heart and Great Vessels 02Q
  see Repair, Upper Arteries 03Q
  see Repair, Lower Arteries 04Q
Arterioscopy
  02JY4ZZ
  03JY4ZZ
  04JY4ZZ
Arthrectomy
  see Excision, Upper Joints 0RB
  see Resection, Upper Joints 0RT
  see Excision, Lower Joints 0SB
  see Resection, Lower Joints 0ST
Arthrocentesis
  see Drainage, Upper Joints 0R9
  see Drainage, Lower Joints 0S9
Arthrodesis
  see Fusion, Upper Joints 0RG
  see Fusion, Lower Joints 0SG
Arthrography
  see Plain Radiography, Skull and Facial Bones
    BN0
  see Plain Radiography, Non-Axial Upper Bones
    BP0
  see Plain Radiography, Non-Axial Lower Bones
    BQ0
Arthrolysis
  see Release, Upper Joints 0RN
  see Release, Lower Joints 0SN
Arthropexy
  see Repair, Upper Joints 0RQ
  see Reposition, Upper Joints 0RS
  see Repair, Lower Joints 0SQ
  see Reposition, Lower Joints 0SS
Arthroplasty
  see Repair, Upper Joints 0RQ
  see Replacement, Upper Joints 0RR
  see Repair, Lower Joints 0SQ
  see Replacement, Lower Joints 0SR
  see Supplement, Lower Joints 0SU
  see Supplement, Upper Joints 0RU
Arthroscopy
  see Inspection, Upper Joints 0RJ
  see Inspection, Lower Joints 0SJ
Arthrotomy
  see Drainage, Upper Joints 0R9
  see Drainage, Lower Joints 0S9
Artificial anal sphincter (AAS)
  use Artificial Sphincter in Gastrointestinal System
Artificial bowel sphincter (neosphincter)
  use Artificial Sphincter in Gastrointestinal System

Beam Radiation *(continued)*
    Femur DP09
        Intraoperative DP093Z0
    Fibula DP0B
        Intraoperative DP0B3Z0
    Gallbladder DF01
        Intraoperative DF013Z0
    Gland
        Adrenal DG02
            Intraoperative DG023Z0
        Parathyroid DG04
            Intraoperative DG043Z0
        Pituitary DG00
            Intraoperative DG003Z0
        Thyroid DG05
            Intraoperative DG053Z0
    Glands
        Salivary D906
        Intraoperative D9063Z0
    Head and Neck DW01
        Intraoperative DW013Z0
    Hemibody DW04
        Intraoperative DW043Z0
    Humerus DP06
        Intraoperative DP063Z0
    Hypopharynx D903
        Intraoperative D9033Z0
    Ileum DD04
        Intraoperative DD043Z0
    Jejunum DD03
        Intraoperative DD033Z0
    Kidney DT00
        Intraoperative DT003Z0
    Larynx D90B
        Intraoperative D90B3Z0
    Liver DF00
        Intraoperative DF003Z0
    Lung DB02
        Intraoperative DB023Z0
    Lymphatics
        Abdomen D706
            Intraoperative D7063Z0
        Axillary D704
            Intraoperative D7043Z0
        Inguinal D708
            Intraoperative D7083Z0
        Neck D703
            Intraoperative D7033Z0
        Pelvis D707
            Intraoperative D7073Z0
        Thorax D705
            Intraoperative D7053Z0
    Mandible DP03
        Intraoperative DP033Z0
    Maxilla DP02
        Intraoperative DP023Z0
    Mediastinum DB06
        Intraoperative DB063Z0
    Mouth D904
        Intraoperative D9043Z0
    Nasopharynx D90D
        Intraoperative D90D3Z0
    Neck and Head DW01
        Intraoperative DW013Z0
    Nerve
        Peripheral D007
        Intraoperative D0073Z0
    Nose D901
        Intraoperative D9013Z0
    Oropharynx D90F
        Intraoperative D90F3Z0
    Ovary DU00
        Intraoperative DU003Z0
    Palate
        Hard D908
            Intraoperative D9083Z0
        Soft D909
            Intraoperative D9093Z0
    Pancreas DF03
        Intraoperative DF033Z0
    Parathyroid Gland DG04
        Intraoperative DG043Z0
    Pelvic Bones DP08
        Intraoperative DP083Z0
    Pelvic Region DW06
        Intraoperative DW063Z0
    Pineal Body DG01
        Intraoperative DG013Z0
    Pituitary Gland DG00
        Intraoperative DG003Z0
    Pleura DB05
        Intraoperative DB053Z0
    Prostate DV00
        Intraoperative DV003Z0

Beam Radiation *(continued)*
    Radius DP07
        Intraoperative DP073Z0
    Rectum DD07
        Intraoperative DD073Z0
    Rib DP05
        Intraoperative DP053Z0
    Sinuses D907
        Intraoperative D9073Z0
    Skin
        Abdomen DH08
            Intraoperative DH083Z0
        Arm DH04
            Intraoperative DH043Z0
        Back DH07
            Intraoperative DH073Z0
        Buttock DH09
            Intraoperative DH093Z0
        Chest DH06
            Intraoperative DH063Z0
        Face DH02
            Intraoperative DH023Z0
        Leg DH0B
            Intraoperative DH0B3Z0
        Neck DH03
            Intraoperative DH033Z0
    Skull DP00
        Intraoperative DP003Z0
    Spinal Cord D006
        Intraoperative D0063Z0
    Spleen D702
        Intraoperative D7023Z0
    Sternum DP04
        Intraoperative DP043Z0
    Stomach DD01
        Intraoperative DD013Z0
    Testis DV01
        Intraoperative DV013Z0
    Thymus D701
        Intraoperative D7013Z0
    Thyroid Gland DG05
        Intraoperative DG053Z0
    Tibia DP0B
        Intraoperative DP0B3Z0
    Tongue D905
        Intraoperative D9053Z0
    Trachea DB00
        Intraoperative DB003Z0
    Ulna DP07
        Intraoperative DP073Z0
    Ureter DT01
        Intraoperative DT013Z0
    Urethra DT03
        Intraoperative DT033Z0
    Uterus DU02
        Intraoperative DU023Z0
    Whole Body DW05
        Intraoperative DW053Z0

Berlin Heart Ventricular Assist Device
    use Implantable Heart Assist System in Heart and Great
        Vessels

Biceps brachii muscle
    use Muscle, Upper Arm, Right
    use Muscle, Upper Arm, Left

Biceps femoris muscle
    use Muscle, Upper Leg, Right
    use Muscle, Upper Leg, Left

Bicipital aponeurosis
    use Subcutaneous Tissue and Fascia, Lower Arm, Left
    use Subcutaneous Tissue and Fascia, Lower Arm,
        Right

Bicuspid valve
    use Valve, Mitral

Bililite therapy
    see Ultraviolet Light Therapy, Skin 6A80

Bioactive embolization coil(s)
    use Intraluminal Device, Bioactive in Upper
        Arteries

Biofeedback GZC9ZZZ

Biopsy
    see Drainage with qualifier Diagnostic
    see Excision with qualifier Diagnostic
    Bone Marrow
        see Extraction with qualifier Diagnostic

BiPAP
    see Assistance, Respiratory 5A09

Bisection
    see Division

Biventricular external heart assist system
    use External Heart Assist System in Heart and Great
        Vessels

Blepharectomy
    see Excision, Eye 08B
    see Resection, Eye 08T

Blepharoplasty
    see Repair, Eye 08Q
    see Replacement, Eye 08R
    see Supplement, Eye 08U
    see Reposition, Eye 08S

Blepharorrhaphy
    see Repair, Eye 08Q

Blepharotomy
    see Drainage, Eye 089

Block, Nerve, anesthetic injection 3E0T3CZ

Blood glucose monitoring system
    use Monitoring Device

Blood pressure
    see Measurement, Arterial 4A03

BMR (basal metabolic rate)
    see Measurement, Physiological Systems 4A0Z

Body of femur
    use Femoral Shaft, Right
    use Femoral Shaft, Left

Body of fibula
    use Fibula, Right
    use Fibula, Left

Bone anchored hearing device
    use Hearing Device, Bone Conduction in 09H
    use Hearing Device in Head and Facial Bones

Bone bank bone graft
    use Nonautologous Tissue Substitute

Bone Growth Stimulator
    Insertion of device in
        Bone
            Facial 0NHW
            Lower 0QHY
            Nasal 0NHB
            Upper 0PHY
        Skull 0NH0
    Removal of device from
        Bone
            Facial 0NPW
            Lower 0QPY
            Nasal 0NPB
            Upper 0PPY
        Skull 0NP0
    Revision of device in
        Bone
            Facial 0NWW
            Lower 0QWY
            Nasal 0NWB
            Upper 0PWY
        Skull 0NW0

Bone marrow transplant
    see Transfusion

Bone screw (interlocking)(lag)(pedicle)(recessed)
    use Internal Fixation Device in Head and Facial Bones
    use Internal Fixation Device in Upper Bones
    use Internal Fixation Device in Lower Bones

Bony labyrinth
    use Ear, Inner, Left
    use Ear, Inner, Right

Bony orbit
    use Orbit, Right
    use Orbit, Left

Bony vestibule
    use Ear, Inner, Right
    use Ear, Inner, Left

Botallo's duct
    use Artery, Pulmonary, Left

Bovine pericardial valve
    use Zooplastic Tissue in Heart and Great Vessels

Bovine pericardium graft
    use Zooplastic Tissue in Heart and Great Vessels

BP (blood pressure)
    see Measurement, Arterial 4A03

Brachial (lateral) lymph node
    use Lymphatic, Axillary, Left
    use Lymphatic, Axillary, Right

Brachialis muscle
    use Muscle, Upper Arm, Right
    use Muscle, Upper Arm, Left

Brachiocephalic artery
    use Artery, Innominate

Brachiocephalic trunk
    use Artery, Innominate

Brachiocephalic vein
    use Vein, Innominate, Right
    use Vein, Innominate, Left

Brachioradialis muscle
    use Muscle, Lower Arm and Wrist, Right
    use Muscle, Lower Arm and Wrist, Left

Brachytherapy
    Abdomen DW13
    Adrenal Gland DG12
    Bile Ducts DF12
    Bladder DT12
    Bone Marrow D710

Bypass *(continued)*
  Vein *(continued)*
    Hypogastric *(continued)*
      Right 061H
    Inferior Mesenteric 0616
    Innominate
      Left 0514
      Right 0513
    Internal Jugular
      Left 051N
      Right 051M
    Intracranial 051L
    Lesser Saphenous
      Left 061S
      Right 061R
    Portal 0618
    Renal
      Left 061B
      Right 0619
    Splenic 0611
    Subclavian
      Left 0516
      Right 0515
    Superior Mesenteric 0615
    Vertebral
      Left 051S
      Right 051R
    Vena Cava
      Inferior 0610
      Superior 021V
  Ventricle
    Left 021L
    Right 021K
Bypass, cardiopulmonary 5A1221Z

C

Caesarean section
  see Extraction, Products of Conception 10D0
Calcaneocuboid joint
  use Joint, Tarsal, Left
  use Joint, Tarsal, Right
Calcaneocuboid ligament
  use Bursa and Ligament, Foot, Right
  use Bursa and Ligament, Foot, Left
Calcaneofibular ligament
  use Bursa and Ligament, Ankle, Left
  use Bursa and Ligament, Ankle, Right
Calcaneus
  use Tarsal, Right
  use Tarsal, Left
Cannulation
  see Bypass
  see Dilation
  see Drainage
  see Irrigation
Canthorrhaphy
  see Repair, Eye 08Q
Canthotomy
  see Release, Eye 08N
Capitate bone
  use Carpal, Left
  use Carpal, Right
Capsulectomy, lens
  see Excision, Eye 08B
Capsulorrhaphy, joint
  see Repair, Upper Joints 0RQ
  see Repair, Lower Joints
    0SQ
Cardia
  use Esophagogastric Junction
Cardiac contractility modulation lead
  use Cardiac Lead in Heart and Great Vessels
Cardiac event recorder
  use Monitoring Device
Cardiac Lead
  Defibrillator
    Atrium
      Left 02H7
      Right 02H6
    Pericardium 02HN
    Vein, Coronary 02H4
    Ventricle
      Left 02HL
      Right 02HK
  Insertion of device in
    Atrium
      Left 02H7Z
      Right 02H6
    Pericardium 02HN
    Vein, Coronary 02H4
    Ventricle
      Left 02HL
      Right 02HK

Cardiac Lead *(continued)*
  Pacemaker
    Atrium
      Left 02H7
      Right 02H6
    Pericardium 02HN
    Vein, Coronary 02H4
    Ventricle
      Left 02HL
      Right 02HK
  Removal of device from, Heart 02PA
  Revision of device in, Heart 02WA
Cardiac plexus
  use Nerve, Thoracic Sympathetic
Cardiac Resynchronization Defibrillator Pulse Generator
  Abdomen 0JH8
  Chest 0JH6
Cardiac Resynchronization Pacemaker Pulse Generator
  Abdomen 0JH8
  Chest 0JH6
Cardiac resynchronization therapy (CRT) lead
  use Cardiac Lead, Pacemaker in 02H
  use Cardiac Lead, Defibrillator in 02H
Cardiac Rhythm Related Device
  Insertion of device in
    Abdomen 0JH8
    Chest 0JH6
  Removal of device from, Subcutaneous Tissue and Fascia, Trunk 0JPT
  Revision of device in, Subcutaneous Tissue and Fascia, Trunk 0JWT
Cardiocentesis
  see Drainage, Pericardial Cavity 0W9D
Cardioesophageal junction
  use Esophagogastric Junction
Cardiolysis
  see Release, Heart and Great Vessels 02N
CardioMEMS® pressure sensor
  use Monitoring Device, Pressure Sensor in 02H
Cardiomyotomy
  see Division, Esophagogastric Junction 0D84
Cardioplegia
  see Introduction of substance in or on, Heart 3E08
Cardiorrhaphy
  see Repair, Heart and Great Vessels 02Q
Cardioversion 5A2204Z
Caregiver Training F0FZ
Caroticotympanic artery
  use Artery, Internal Carotid, Right
  use Artery, Internal Carotid, Left
Carotid (artery) sinus (baroreceptor) lead
  use Stimulator Lead in Upper Arteries
Carotid glomus
  use Carotid Bodies, Bilateral
  use Carotid Body, Right
  use Carotid Body, Left
Carotid sinus
  use Artery, Internal Carotid, Left
  use Artery, Internal Carotid, Right
Carotid sinus nerve
  use Nerve, Glossopharyngeal
Carotid WALLSTENT® Monorail® Endoprosthesis
  use Intraluminal Device
Carpectomy
  see Excision, Upper Bones 0PB
  see Resection, Upper Bones 0PT
Carpometacarpal (CMC) joint
  use Joint, Metacarpocarpal, Left
  use Joint, Metacarpocarpal, Right
Carpometacarpal ligament
  use Bursa and Ligament, Hand, Left
  use Bursa and Ligament, Hand, Right
Casting
  see Immobilization
CAT scan
  see Computerized Tomography (CT Scan)
Catheterization
  see Dilation
  see Drainage
  see Irrigation
  see Insertion of device in
  Heart
    see Measurement, Cardiac 4A02
  Umbilical vein, for infusion 06H033T
Cauda equina
  use Spinal Cord, Lumbar
Cauterization
  see Destruction
  see Repair
Cavernous plexus
  use Nerve, Head and Neck Sympathetic
Cecectomy
  see Excision, Cecum 0DBH
  see Resection, Cecum 0DTH

Cecocolostomy
  see Bypass, Gastrointestinal System 0D1
  see Drainage, Gastrointestinal System 0D9
Cecopexy
  see Repair, Cecum 0DQH
  see Reposition, Cecum 0DSH
Cecoplication
  see Restriction, Cecum 0DVH
Cecorrhaphy
  see Repair, Cecum 0DQH
Cecostomy
  see Bypass, Cecum 0D1H
  see Drainage, Cecum 0D9H
Cecotomy
  see Drainage, Cecum 0D9H
Celiac (solar) plexus
  use Nerve, Abdominal Sympathetic
Celiac ganglion
  use Nerve, Abdominal Sympathetic
Celiac lymph node
  use Lymphatic, Aortic
Celiac trunk
  use Artery, Celiac
Central axillary lymph node
  use Lymphatic, Axillary, Left
  use Lymphatic, Axillary, Right
Central venous pressure
  see Measurement, Venous 4A04
Centrimag® Blood Pump
  use Intraluminal Device
Cephalogram BN00ZZZ
Cerclage
  see Restriction
Cerebral aqueduct (Sylvius)
  use Cerebral Ventricle
Cerebrum
  use Brain
Cervical esophagus
  use Esophagus, Upper
Cervical facet joint
  use Joint, Cervical Vertebral
  use Joint, Cervical Vertebral, 2 or more
Cervical ganglion
  use Nerve, Head and Neck Sympathetic
Cervical interspinous ligament
  use Bursa and Ligament, Head and Neck
Cervical intertransverse ligament
  use Bursa and Ligament, Head and Neck
Cervical ligamentum flavum
  use Bursa and Ligament, Head and Neck
Cervical lymph node
  use Lymphatic, Neck, Right
  use Lymphatic, Neck, Left
Cervicectomy
  see Excision, Cervix 0UBC
  see Resection, Cervix
    0UTC
Cervicothoracic facet joint
  use Joint, Cervicothoracic Vertebral
Cesarean section
  see Extraction, Products of Conception 10D0
Change device in
  Abdominal Wall 0W2FX
  Back
    Lower 0W2LX
    Upper 0W2KX
  Bladder 0T2BX
  Bone
    Facial 0N2WX
    Lower 0Q2YX
    Nasal 0N2BX
    Upper 0P2YX
  Bone Marrow 072TX
  Brain 0020X
  Breast
    Left 0H2UX
    Right 0H2TX
  Bursa and Ligament
    Lower 0M2YX
    Upper 0M2XX
  Cavity, Cranial 0W21X
  Chest Wall 0W28X
  Cisterna Chyli 072LX
  Diaphragm 0B2TX
  Duct
    Hepatobiliary 0F2BX
    Pancreatic 0F2DX
  Ear
    Left 092JX
    Right 092HX
  Epididymis and Spermatic Cord 0V2MX
  Extremity
    Lower
      Left 0Y2BX
      Right 0Y29X

Change device in (continued)
  Extremity (continued)
    Upper
      Left 0X27X
      Right 0X26X
  Eye
    Left 0821X
    Right 0820X
  Face 0W22X
  Fallopian Tube 0U28X
  Gallbladder 0F24X
  Gland
    Adrenal 0G25X
    Endocrine 0G2SX
    Pituitary 0G20X
    Salivary 0C2AX
  Head 0W20X
  Intestinal Tract
    Lower 0D2DXUZ
    Upper 0D20XUZ
  Jaw
    Lower 0W25X
    Upper 0W24X
  Joint
    Lower 0S2YX
    Upper 0R2YX
  Kidney 0T25X
  Larynx 0C2SX
  Liver 0F20X
  Lung
    Left 0B2LX
    Right 0B2KX
  Lymphatic 072NX
    Thoracic Duct 072KX
  Mediastinum 0W2CX
  Mesentery 0D2VX
  Mouth and Throat 0C2YX
  Muscle
    Lower 0K2YX
    Upper 0K2XX
  Neck 0W26X
  Nerve
    Cranial 002EX
    Peripheral 012YX
  Nose 092KX
  Omentum 0D2UX
  Ovary 0U23X
  Pancreas 0F2GX
  Parathyroid Gland 0G2RX
  Pelvic Cavity 0W2JX
  Penis 0V2SX
  Pericardial Cavity 0W2DX
  Perineum
    Female 0W2NX
    Male 0W2MX
  Peritoneal Cavity 0W2GX
  Peritoneum 0D2WX
  Pineal Body 0G21X
  Pleura 0B2QX
  Pleural Cavity
    Left 0W2BX
    Right 0W29X
  Products of Conception 10207
  Prostate and Seminal Vesicles
    0V24X
  Retroperitoneum 0W2HX
  Scrotum and Tunica Vaginalis 0V28X
  Sinus 092YX
  Skin 0H2PX
  Skull 0N20X
  Spinal Canal 002UX
  Spleen 072PX
  Subcutaneous Tissue and Fascia
    Head and Neck 0J2SX
    Lower Extremity 0J2WX
    Trunk 0J2TX
    Upper Extremity 0J2VX
  Tendon
    Lower 0L2YX
    Upper 0L2XX
  Testis 0V2SX
  Thymus 072MX
  Thyroid Gland 0G2KX
  Trachea 0B21
  Tracheobronchial Tree 0B20X
  Ureter 0T29X
  Urethra 0T2DX
  Uterus and Cervix 0U2DXHZ
  Vagina and Cul-de-sac 0U2HXGZ
  Vas Deferens 0V2RX
  Vulva 0U2MX
Change device in or on
  Abdominal Wall 2W03X
  Anorectal 2Y03X5Z

Change device in or on (continued)
  Arm
    Lower
      Left 2W0DX
      Right 2W0CX
    Upper
      Left 2W0BX
      Right 2W0AX
  Back 2W05X
  Chest Wall 2W04X
  Ear 2Y02X5Z
  Extremity
    Lower
      Left 2W0MX
      Right 2W0LX
    Upper
      Left 2W09X
      Right 2W08X
  Face 2W01X
  Finger
    Left 2W0KX
    Right 2W0JX
  Foot
    Left 2W0TX
    Right 2W0SX
  Genital Tract, Female 2Y04X5Z
  Hand
    Left 2W0FX
    Right 2W0EX
  Head 2W00X
  Inguinal Region
    Left 2W07X
    Right 2W06X
  Leg
    Lower
      Left 2W0RX
      Right 2W0QX
    Upper
      Left 2W0PX
      Right 2W0NX
  Mouth and Pharynx 2Y00X5Z
  Nasal 2Y01X5Z
  Neck 2W02X
  Thumb
    Left 2W0HX
    Right 2W0GX
  Toe
    Left 2W0VX
    Right 2W0UX
  Urethra 2Y05X5Z
Chemoembolization
  see Introduction of substance in or on
Chemosurgery, Skin 3E00XTZ
Chemothalamectomy
  see Destruction, Thalamus 0059
Chemotherapy, Infusion for cancer
  see Introduction of substance in or on
Chest x-ray
  see Plain Radiography, Chest BW03
Chiropractic Manipulation
  Abdomen 9WB9X
  Cervical 9WB1X
  Extremities
    Lower 9WB6X
    Upper 9WB7X
  Head 9WB0X
  Lumbar 9WB3X
  Pelvis 9WB5X
  Rib Cage 9WB8X
  Sacrum 9WB4X
  Thoracic 9WB2X
Choana
  use Nasopharynx
Cholangiogram
  see Plain Radiography, Hepatobiliary System and
    Pancreas BF0
  see Fluoroscopy, Hepatobiliary System and Pancreas
    BF1
Cholecystectomy
  see Excision, Gallbladder 0FB4
  see Resection, Gallbladder 0FT4
Cholecystojejunostomy
  see Bypass, Hepatobiliary System and Pancreas 0F1
  see Drainage, Hepatobiliary System and
    Pancreas 0F9
Cholecystopexy
  see Repair, Gallbladder 0FQ4
  see Reposition, Gallbladder 0FS4
Cholecystoscopy 0FJ44ZZ
Cholecystostomy
  see Drainage, Gallbladder 0F94
  see Bypass, Gallbladder 0F14
Cholecystotomy
  see Drainage, Gallbladder 0F94

Choledochectomy
  see Excision, Hepatobiliary System and Pancreas 0FB
  see Resection, Hepatobiliary System and Pancreas 0FT
Choledocholithotomy
  see Extirpation, Duct, Common Bile 0FC9
Choledochoplasty
  see Repair, Hepatobiliary System and Pancreas 0FQ
  see Replacement, Hepatobiliary System and Pancreas
    0FR
  see Supplement, Hepatobiliary System and Pancreas
    0FU
Choledochoscopy 0FJB8ZZ
Choledochotomy
  see Drainage, Hepatobiliary System and Pancreas 0F9
Cholelithotomy
  see Extirpation, Hepatobiliary System and Pancreas 0FC
Chondrectomy
  see Excision, Upper Joints 0RB
  see Excision, Lower Joints 0SB
  Knee *see* Excision, Lower Joints 0SB
  Semilunar cartilage
    see Excision, Lower Joints 0SB
Chondroglossus muscle
  use Muscle, Tongue, Palate, Pharynx
Chorda tympani
  use Nerve, Facial
Chordotomy
  see Division, Central Nervous System 008
Choroid plexus
  use Cerebral Ventricle
Choroidectomy
  see Excision, Eye 08B
  see Resection, Eye 08T
Ciliary body
  use Eye, Right
  use Eye, Left
Ciliary ganglion
  use Nerve, Head and Neck Sympathetic
Circle of Willis
  use Artery, Intracranial
Circumflex iliac artery
  use Artery, Femoral, Right
  use Artery, Femoral, Left
Clamp and rod internal fixation system (CRIF)
  use Internal Fixation Device in Upper Bones
  use Internal Fixation Device in Lower Bones
Clamping
  see Occlusion
Claustrum
  use Basal Ganglia
Claviculectomy
  see Excision, Upper Bones 0PB
  see Resection, Upper Bones 0PT
Claviculotomy
  see Division, Upper Bones 0P8
  see Drainage, Upper Bones 0P9
Clipping, aneurysm
  see Restriction using Extraluminal Device
Clitorectomy, clitoridectomy
  see Excision, Clitoris 0UBJ
  see Resection, Clitoris 0UTJ
Closure
  see Occlusion
  see Repair
Clysis
  see Introduction of substance in or on
Coagulation
  see Destruction
CoAxia NeuroFlo catheter
  use Intraluminal Device
Cobalt/chromium head and polyethylene socket
  use Synthetic Substitute, Metal on Polyethylene in 0SR
Cobalt/chromium head and socket
  use Synthetic Substitute, Metal in 0SR
Coccygeal body
  use Coccygeal Glomus
Coccygeus muscle
  use Muscle, Trunk, Left
  use Muscle, Trunk, Right
Cochlea
  use Ear, Inner, Left
  use Ear, Inner, Right
Cochlear implant (CI), multiple channel (electrode)
  use Hearing Device, Multiple Channel Cochlear
    Prosthesis in 09H
Cochlear implant (CI), single channel (electrode)
  use Hearing Device, Single Channel Cochlear Prosthesis
    in 09H
Cochlear Implant Treatment F0BZ0
Cochlear nerve
  use Nerve, Acoustic
COGNIS® CRT-D
  use Cardiac Resynchronization Defibrillator Pulse
    Generator in 0JH

Colectomy
  see Excision, Gastrointestinal System 0DB
  see Resection, Gastrointestinal System 0DT
Collapse
  see Occlusion
Collection from
  Breast, Breast Milk 8E0HX62
  Indwelling Device
    Circulatory System
      Blood 8C02X6K
      Other Fluid 8C02X6L
    Nervous System
      Cerebrospinal Fluid 8C01X6J
      Other Fluid 8C01X6L
  Integumentary System, Breast Milk
    8E0HX62
  Reproductive System, Male, Sperm 8E0VX63
Colocentesis
  see Drainage, Gastrointestinal System 0D9
Colofixation
  see Repair, Gastrointestinal System 0DQ
  see Reposition, Gastrointestinal System 0DS
Cololysis
  see Release, Gastrointestinal System 0DN
Colonic Z-Stent®
  use Intraluminal Device
Colonoscopy 0DJD8ZZ
Colopexy
  see Repair, Gastrointestinal System 0DQ
  see Reposition, Gastrointestinal System 0DS
Coloplication
  see Restriction, Gastrointestinal System 0DV
Coloproctectomy
  see Excision, Gastrointestinal System 0DB
  see Resection, Gastrointestinal System 0DT
Coloproctostomy
  see Bypass, Gastrointestinal System 0D1
  see Drainage, Gastrointestinal System 0D9
Colopuncture
  see Drainage, Gastrointestinal System 0D9
Colorrhaphy
  see Repair, Gastrointestinal System 0DQ
Colostomy
  see Bypass, Gastrointestinal System 0D1
  see Drainage, Gastrointestinal System 0D9
Colpectomy
  see Excision, Vagina 0UBG
  see Resection, Vagina 0UTG
Colpocentesis
  see Drainage, Vagina 0U9G
Colpopexy
  see Repair, Vagina 0UQG
  see Reposition, Vagina 0USG
Colpoplasty
  see Repair, Vagina 0UQG
  see Supplement, Vagina 0UUG
Colporrhaphy
  see Repair, Vagina 0UQG
Colposcopy 0UJH8ZZ
Columella
  use Nose
Common digital vein
  use Vein, Foot, Right
  use Vein, Foot, Left
Common facial vein
  use Vein, Face, Left
  use Vein, Face, Right
Common fibular nerve
  use Nerve, Peroneal
Common hepatic artery
  use Artery, Hepatic
Common iliac (subaortic) lymph node
  use Lymphatic, Pelvis
Common interosseous artery
  use Artery, Ulnar, Left
  use Artery, Ulnar, Right
Common peroneal nerve
  use Nerve, Peroneal
Complete (SE) stent
  use Intraluminal Device
Compression
  see Restriction
  Abdominal Wall 2W13X
  Arm
    Lower
      Left 2W1DX
      Right 2W1CX
    Upper
      Left 2W1BX
      Right 2W1AX
  Back 2W15X
  Chest Wall 2W14X
  Extremity
    Lower
      Left 2W1MX
      Right 2W1LX

Compression *(continued)*
  Extremity *(continued)*
    Upper
      Left 2W19X
      Right 2W18X
  Face 2W11X
  Finger
    Left 2W1KX
    Right 2W1JX
  Foot
    Left 2W1TX
    Right 2W1SX
  Hand
    Left 2W1FX
    Right 2W1EX
  Head 2W10X
  Inguinal Region
    Left 2W17X
    Right 2W16X
  Leg
    Lower
      Left 2W1RX
      Right 2W1QX
    Upper
      Left 2W1PX
      Right 2W1NX
  Neck 2W12X
  Thumb
    Left 2W1HX
    Right 2W1GX
  Toe
    Left 2W1VX
    Right 2W1UX
Computer Assisted Procedure
  Extremity
    Lower
      No Qualifier 8E0YXBZ
      With Computerized Tomography 8E0YXBG
      With Fluoroscopy 8E0YXBF
      With Magnetic Resonance Imaging
        8E0YXBH
    Upper
      No Qualifier 8E0XXBZ
      With Computerized Tomography 8E0XXBG
      With Fluoroscopy 8E0XXBF
      With Magnetic Resonance Imaging
        8E0XXBH
  Head and Neck Region
    No Qualifier 8E09XBZ
    With Computerized Tomography
      8E09XBG
    With Fluoroscopy 8E09XBF
    With Magnetic Resonance Imaging 8E09XBH
  Trunk Region
    No Qualifier 8E0WXBZ
    With Computerized Tomography 8E0WXBG
    With Fluoroscopy 8E0WXBF
    With Magnetic Resonance Imaging 8E0WXBH
Computerized Tomography (CT Scan)
  Abdomen BW20
    Chest and Pelvis BW25
  Abdomen and Chest BW24
  Abdomen and Pelvis BW21
  Airway, Trachea BB2F
  Ankle
    Left BQ2H
    Right BQ2G
  Aorta
    Abdominal B420
      Intravascular Optical Coherence B420Z2Z
    Thoracic B320
      Intravascular Optical Coherence B320Z2Z
  Arm
    Left BP2F
    Right BP2E
  Artery
    Celiac B421
      Intravascular Optical Coherence B421Z2Z
    Common Carotid
      Bilateral B325
      Intravascular Optical Coherence B325Z2Z
    Coronary
      Bypass Graft
        Multiple B223
          Intravascular Optical Coherence
            B223Z2Z
        Multiple B221
          Intravascular Optical Coherence
            B221Z2Z
    Internal Carotid
      Bilateral B328
      Intravascular Optical Coherence B328Z2Z
    Intracranial B32R
      Intravascular Optical Coherence B32RZ2Z
    Lower Extremity
      Bilateral B42H

Computerized Tomography (CT Scan) *(continued)*
  Artery *(continued)*
    Lower Extremity *(continued)*
      Bilateral B42H *(continued)*
        Intravascular Optical Coherence
          B42HZ2Z
      Left B42G
        Intravascular Optical Coherence
          B42GZ2Z
      Right B42F
        Intravascular Optical Coherence
          B42FZ2Z
    Pelvic B42C
      Intravascular Optical Coherence
        B42CZ2Z
    Pulmonary
      Left B32T
        Intravascular Optical Coherence
          B32TZ2Z
      Right B32S
        Intravascular Optical Coherence
          B32SZ2Z
    Renal
      Bilateral B428
        Intravascular Optical Coherence
          B428Z2Z
      Transplant B42M
        Intravascular Optical Coherence
          B42MZ2Z
    Superior Mesenteric B424
      Intravascular Optical Coherence B424Z2Z
    Vertebral
      Bilateral B32G
      Intravascular Optical Coherence B32GZ2Z
  Bladder BT20
  Bone
    Facial BN25
    Temporal BN2F
  Brain B020
  Calcaneus
    Left BQ2K
    Right BQ2J
  Cerebral Ventricle B028
  Chest, Abdomen and Pelvis
    BW25
  Chest and Abdomen BW24
  Cisterna B027
  Clavicle
    Left BP25
    Right BP24
  Coccyx BR2F
  Colon BD24
  Ear B920
  Elbow
    Left BP2H
    Right BP2G
  Extremity
    Lower
      Left BQ2S
      Right BQ2R
    Upper
      Bilateral BP2V
      Left BP2U
      Right BP2T
  Eye
    Bilateral B827
    Left B826
    Right B825
  Femur
    Left BQ24
    Right BQ23
  Fibula
    Left BQ2C
    Right BQ2B
  Finger
    Left BP2S
    Right BP2R
  Foot
    Left BQ2M
    Right BQ2L
  Forearm
    Left BP2K
    Right BP2J
  Gland
    Adrenal, Bilateral BG22
    Parathyroid BG23
    Parotid, Bilateral B926
    Salivary, Bilateral B92D
    Submandibular, Bilateral B929
    Thyroid BG24
  Hand
    Left BP2P
    Right BP2N
  Hands and Wrists, Bilateral BP2Q
  Head BW28
  Head and Neck BW29

Continuous Negative Airway Pressure *(continued)*
Less than 24 Consecutive Hours, Ventilation
5A09359
Continuous Positive Airway Pressure
24-96 Consecutive Hours, Ventilation 5A09457
Greater than 96 Consecutive Hours, Ventilation
5A09557
Less than 24 Consecutive Hours, Ventilation 5A09357
Contraceptive Device
Change device in, Uterus and Cervix 0U2DXHZ
Insertion of device in
Cervix 0UHC
Subcutaneous Tissue and Fascia
Abdomen 0JH8
Chest 0JH6
Lower Arm
Left 0JHH
Right 0JHG
Lower Leg
Left 0JHP
Right 0JHN
Upper Arm
Left 0JHF
Right 0JHD
Upper Leg
Left 0JHM
Right 0JHL
Uterus 0UH9
Removal of device from
Subcutaneous Tissue and Fascia
Lower Extremity 0JPW
Trunk 0JPT
Upper Extremity 0JPV
Uterus and Cervix 0UPD
Revision of device in
Subcutaneous Tissue and Fascia
Lower Extremity 0JWW
Trunk 0JWT
Upper Extremity 0JWV
Uterus and Cervix 0UWD
Contractility Modulation Device
Abdomen 0JH8
Chest 0JH6
Control postprocedural bleeding in
Abdominal Wall 0W3F
Ankle Region
Left 0Y3L
Right 0Y3K
Arm
Lower
Left 0X3F
Right 0X3D
Upper
Left 0X39
Right 0X38
Axilla
Left 0X35
Right 0X34
Back
Lower 0W3L
Upper 0W3K
Buttock
Left 0Y31
Right 0Y30
Cavity, Cranial 0W31
Chest Wall 0W38
Elbow Region
Left 0X3C
Right 0X3B
Extremity
Lower
Left 0Y3B
Right 0Y39
Upper
Left 0X37
Right 0X36
Face 0W32
Femoral Region
Left 0Y38
Right 0Y37
Foot
Left 0Y3N
Right 0Y3M
Gastrointestinal Tract 0W3P
Genitourinary Tract 0W3R
Hand
Left 0X3K
Right 0X3J
Head 0W30
Inguinal Region
Left 0Y36
Right 0Y35
Jaw
Lower 0W35
Upper 0W34

Control postprocedural bleeding in *(continued)*
Knee Region
Left 0Y3G
Right 0Y3F
Leg
Lower
Left 0Y3J
Right 0Y3H
Upper
Left 0Y3D
Right 0Y3C
Mediastinum 0W3C
Neck 0W36
Oral Cavity and Throat 0W33
Pelvic Cavity 0W3J
Pericardial Cavity 0W3D
Perineum
Female 0W3N
Male 0W3M
Peritoneal Cavity 0W3G
Pleural Cavity
Left 0W3B
Right 0W39
Respiratory Tract 0W3Q
Retroperitoneum 0W3H
Shoulder Region
Left 0X33
Right 0X32
Wrist Region
Left 0X3H
Right 0X3G
Conus arteriosus
use Ventricle, Right
Conus medullaris
use Spinal Cord, Lumbar
Conversion
Cardiac rhythm 5A2204Z
Gastrostomy to jejunostomy feeding device
see Insertion of device in, Jejunum 0DHA
Coracoacromial ligament
use Bursa and Ligament, Shoulder, Right
use Bursa and Ligament, Shoulder, Left
Coracobrachialis muscle
use Muscle, Upper Arm, Left
use Muscle, Upper Arm, Right
Coracoclavicular ligament
use Bursa and Ligament, Shoulder, Left
use Bursa and Ligament, Shoulder, Right
Coracohumeral ligament
use Bursa and Ligament, Shoulder, Left
use Bursa and Ligament, Shoulder, Right
Coracoid process
use Scapula, Right
use Scapula, Left
Cordotomy
see Division, Central Nervous System 008
Core needle biopsy
see Excision with qualifier Diagnostic
CoreValve transcatheter aortic valve
use Zooplastic Tissue in Heart and
Great Vessels
Cormet Hip Resurfacing System
use Resurfacing Device in Lower Joints
Corniculate cartilage
use Larynx
CoRoent® XL
use Interbody Fusion Device in Lower Joints
Coronary arteriography
see Plain Radiography, Heart B20
see Fluoroscopy, Heart B21
Corox (OTW) Bipolar Lead
use Cardiac Lead, Pacemaker in 02H
use Cardiac Lead, Defibrillator in 02H
Corpus callosum
use Brain
Corpus cavernosum
use Penis
Corpus spongiosum
use Penis
Corpus striatum
use Basal Ganglia
Corrugator supercilii muscle
use Muscle, Facial
Cortical strip neurostimulator lead
use Neurostimulator Lead in
Central Nervous System
Costatectomy
see Excision, Upper Bones 0PB
see Resection, Upper Bones 0PT
Costectomy
see Excision, Upper Bones 0PB
see Resection, Upper Bones 0PT
Costocervical trunk
use Artery, Subclavian, Left
use Artery, Subclavian, Right

Costochondrectomy
see Excision, Upper Bones 0PB
see Resection, Upper Bones 0PT
Costoclavicular ligament
use Bursa and Ligament, Shoulder, Left
use Bursa and Ligament, Shoulder, Right
Costosternoplasty
see Repair, Upper Bones 0PQ
see Replacement, Upper Bones 0PR
see Supplement, Upper Bones 0PU
Costotomy
see Division, Upper Bones 0P8
see Drainage, Upper Bones 0P9
Costotransverse joint
use Joint, Thoracic Vertebral
use Joint, Thoracic Vertebral, 2 to 7
use Joint, Thoracic Vertebral, 8 or more
Costotransverse ligament
use Bursa and Ligament, Thorax, Right
use Bursa and Ligament, Thorax, Left
Costovertebral joint
use Joint, Thoracic Vertebral, 8 or more
use Joint, Thoracic Vertebral, 2 to 7
use Joint, Thoracic Vertebral
Costoxiphoid ligament
use Bursa and Ligament, Thorax, Right
use Bursa and Ligament, Thorax, Left
Counseling
Family, for substance abuse, Other Family Counseling
HZ63ZZZ
Group
12-Step HZ43ZZZ
Behavioral HZ41ZZZ
Cognitive HZ40ZZZ
Cognitive-Behavioral HZ42ZZZ
Confrontational HZ48ZZZ
Continuing Care HZ49ZZZ
Infectious Disease
Post-Test HZ4CZZZ
Pre-Test HZ4CZZZ
Interpersonal HZ44ZZZ
Motivational Enhancement HZ47ZZZ
Psychoeducation HZ46ZZZ
Spiritual HZ4BZZZ
Vocational HZ45ZZZ
Individual
12-Step HZ33ZZZ
Behavioral HZ31ZZZ
Cognitive HZ30ZZZ
Cognitive-Behavioral HZ32ZZZ
Confrontational HZ38ZZZ
Continuing Care HZ39ZZZ
Infectious Disease
Post-Test HZ3CZZZ
Pre-Test HZ3CZZZ
Interpersonal HZ34ZZZ
Motivational Enhancement
HZ37ZZZ
Psychoeducation HZ36ZZZ
Spiritual HZ3BZZZ
Vocational HZ35ZZZ
Mental Health Services
Educational GZ60ZZZ
Other Counseling GZ63ZZZ
Vocational GZ61ZZZ
Countershock, cardiac 5A2204Z
Cowper's (bulbourethral) gland
use Urethra
CPAP (continuous positive airway pressure)
see Assistance, Respiratory 5A09
Cranial dura mater
use Dura Mater
Cranial epidural space
use Epidural Space
Cranial subarachnoid space
use Subarachnoid Space
Cranial subdural space
use Subdural Space
Craniectomy
see Excision, Head and Facial Bones 0NB
see Resection, Head and Facial Bones 0NT
Cranioplasty
see Repair, Head and Facial Bones 0NQ
see Replacement, Head and Facial Bones
0NR
see Supplement, Head and Facial Bones 0NU
Craniotomy
see Drainage, Central Nervous System 009
see Division, Head and Facial Bones 0N8
see Drainage, Head and Facial Bones 0N9
Creation
Female 0W4N0
Male 0W4M0
Cremaster muscle
use Muscle, Perineum

Destruction

Destruction *(continued)*
  Artery *(continued)*
    Common Carotid
      Left 035J
      Right 035H
    Common Iliac
      Left 045D
      Right 045C
    External Carotid
      Left 035N
      Right 035M
    External Iliac
      Left 045J
      Right 045H
    Face 035R
    Femoral
      Left 045L
      Right 045K
    Foot
      Left 045W
      Right 045V
    Gastric 0452
    Hand
      Left 035F
      Right 035D
    Hepatic 0453
    Inferior Mesenteric 045B
    Innominate 0352
    Internal Carotid
      Left 035L
      Right 035K
    Internal Iliac
      Left 045F
      Right 045E
    Internal Mammary
      Left 0351
      Right 0350
    Intracranial 035G
    Lower 045Y
    Peroneal
      Left 045U
      Right 045T
    Popliteal
      Left 045N
      Right 045M
    Posterior Tibial
      Left 045S
      Right 045R
    Pulmonary
      Left 025R
      Right 025Q
    Pulmonary Trunk 025P
    Radial
      Left 035C
      Right 035B
    Renal
      Left 045A
      Right 0459
    Splenic 0454
    Subclavian
      Left 0354
      Right 0353
    Superior Mesenteric 0455
    Temporal
      Left 035T
      Right 035S
    Thyroid
      Left 035V
      Right 035U
    Ulnar
      Left 035A
      Right 0359
    Upper 035Y
    Vertebral
      Left 035Q
      Right 035P
  Atrium
    Left 0257
    Right 0256
  Auditory Ossicle
    Left 095A0ZZ
    Right 09590ZZ
  Basal Ganglia 0058
  Bladder 0T5B
  Bladder Neck 0T5C
  Bone
    Ethmoid
      Left 0N5G
      Right 0N5F
    Frontal
      Left 0N52
      Right 0N51
    Hyoid 0N5X
    Lacrimal
      Left 0N5J
      Right 0N5H

Destruction *(continued)*
  Bone *(continued)*
    Nasal 0N5B
    Occipital
      Left 0N58
      Right 0N57
    Palatine
      Left 0N5L
      Right 0N5K
    Parietal
      Left 0N54
      Right 0N53
    Pelvic
      Left 0Q53
      Right 0Q52
    Sphenoid
      Left 0N5D
      Right 0N5C
    Temporal
      Left 0N56
      Right 0N55
    Zygomatic
      Left 0N5N
      Right 0N5M
  Brain 0050
  Breast
    Bilateral 0H5V
    Left 0H5U
    Right 0H5T
  Bronchus
    Lingula 0B59
    Lower Lobe
      Left 0B5B
      Right 0B56
    Main
      Left 0B57
      Right 0B53
    Middle Lobe, Right 0B55
    Upper Lobe
      Left 0B58
      Right 0B54
  Buccal Mucosa 0C54
  Bursa and Ligament
    Abdomen
      Left 0M5J
      Right 0M5H
    Ankle
      Left 0M5R
      Right 0M5Q
    Elbow
      Left 0M54
      Right 0M53
    Foot
      Left 0M5T
      Right 0M5S
    Hand
      Left 0M58
      Right 0M57
    Head and Neck 0M50
    Hip
      Left 0M5M
      Right 0M5L
    Knee
      Left 0M5P
      Right 0M5N
    Lower Extremity
      Left 0M5W
      Right 0M5V
    Perineum 0M5K
    Shoulder
      Left 0M52
      Right 0M51
    Thorax
      Left 0M5G
      Right 0M5F
    Trunk
      Left 0M5D
      Right 0M5C
    Upper Extremity
      Left 0M5B
      Right 0M59
    Wrist
      Left 0M56
      Right 0M55
  Carina 0B52
  Carotid Bodies, Bilateral 0G58
  Carotid Body
    Left 0G56
    Right 0G57
  Carpal
    Left 0P5N
    Right 0P5M
  Cecum 0D5H
  Cerebellum 005C
  Cerebral Hemisphere 0057
  Cerebral Meninges 0051

Destruction *(continued)*
  Cerebral Ventricle 0056
  Cervix 0U5C
  Chordae Tendineae 0259
  Choroid
    Left 085B
    Right 085A
  Cisterna Chyli 075L
  Clavicle
    Left 0P5B
    Right 0P59
  Clitoris 0U5J
  Coccygeal Glomus 0G5B
  Coccyx 0Q5S
  Colon
    Ascending 0D5K
    Descending 0D5M
    Sigmoid 0D5N
    Transverse 0D5L
  Conduction Mechanism 0258
  Conjunctiva
    Left 085TXZZ
    Right 085SXZZ
  Cord
    Bilateral 0V5H
    Left 0V5G
    Right 0V5F
  Cornea
    Left 0859XZZ
    Right 0858XZZ
  Cul-de-sac 0U5F
  Diaphragm
    Left 0B5S
    Right 0B5R
  Disc
    Cervical Vertebral 0R53
    Cervicothoracic
      Vertebral 0R55
    Lumbar Vertebral 0S52
    Lumbosacral 0S54
    Thoracic Vertebral 0R59
    Thoracolumbar Vertebral 0R5B
  Duct
    Common Bile 0F59
    Cystic 0F58
    Hepatic
      Left 0F56
      Right 0F55
    Lacrimal
      Left 085Y
      Right 085X
    Pancreatic 0F5D
      Accessory 0F5F
    Parotid
      Left 0C5C
      Right 0C5B
  Duodenum 0D59
  Dura Mater 0052
  Ear
    External
      Left 0951
      Right 0950
    External Auditory Canal
      Left 0954
      Right 0953
    Inner
      Left 095E0ZZ
      Right 095D0ZZ
    Middle
      Left 09560ZZ
      Right 09550ZZ
  Endometrium 0U5B
  Epididymis
    Bilateral 0V5L
    Left 0V5K
    Right 0V5J
  Epiglottis 0C5R
  Esophagogastric Junction
    0D54
  Esophagus 0D55
    Lower 0D53
    Middle 0D52
    Upper 0D51
  Eustachian Tube
    Left 095G
    Right 095F
  Eye
    Left 0851XZZ
    Right 0850XZZ
  Eyelid
    Lower
      Left 085R
      Right 085Q
    Upper
      Left 085P
      Right 085N

Destruction (continued)

Nerve (continued)
Trochlear 005J
Ulnar 0154
Vagus 005Q
Nipple
Left 0H5X
Right 0H5W
Nose 095K
Omentum
Greater 0D5S
Lesser 0D5T
Orbit
Left 0N5Q
Right 0N5P
Ovary
Bilateral 0U52
Left 0U51
Right 0U50
Palate
Hard 0C52
Soft 0C53
Pancreas 0F5G
Para-aortic Body 0G59
Paraganglion Extremity 0G5F
Parathyroid Gland 0G5R
Inferior
Left 0G5P
Right 0G5N
Multiple 0G5Q
Superior
Left 0G5M
Right 0G5L
Patella
Left 0Q5F
Right 0Q5D
Penis 0V5S
Pericardium 025N
Peritoneum 0D5W
Phalanx
Finger
Left 0P5V
Right 0P5T
Thumb
Left 0P5S
Right 0P5R
Toe
Left 0Q5R
Right 0Q5Q
Pharynx 0C5M
Pineal Body 0G51
Pleura
Left 0B5P
Right 0B5N
Pons 005B
Prepuce 0V5T
Prostate 0V50
Radius
Left 0P5J
Right 0P5H
Rectum 0D5P
Retina
Left 085F3ZZ
Right 085E3ZZ
Retinal Vessel
Left 085H3ZZ
Right 085G3ZZ
Rib
Left 0P52
Right 0P51
Sacrum 0Q51
Scapula
Left 0P56
Right 0P55
Sclera
Left 0857XZZ
Right 0856XZZ
Scrotum 0V55
Septum
Atrial 0255
Nasal 095M
Ventricular 025M
Sinus
Accessory 095P
Ethmoid
Left 095V
Right 095U
Frontal
Left 095T
Right 095S
Mastoid
Left 095C
Right 095B
Maxillary
Left 095R
Right 095Q

Destruction (continued)

Sinus (continued)
Sphenoid
Left 095X
Right 095W
Skin
Abdomen 0H57XZ
Back 0H56XZ
Buttock 0H58XZ
Chest 0H55XZ
Ear
Left 0H53XZ
Right 0H52XZ
Face 0H51XZ
Foot
Left 0H5NXZ
Right 0H5MXZ
Genitalia 0H5AXZ
Hand
Left 0H5GXZ
Right 0H5FXZ
Lower Arm
Left 0H5EXZ
Right 0H5DXZ
Lower Leg
Left 0H5LXZ
Right 0H5KXZ
Neck 0H54XZ
Perineum 0H59XZ
Scalp 0H50XZ
Upper Arm
Left 0H5CXZ
Right 0H5BXZ
Upper Leg
Left 0H5JXZ
Right 0H5HXZ
Skull 0N50
Spinal Cord
Cervical 005W
Lumbar 005Y
Thoracic 005X
Spinal Meninges 005T
Spleen 075P
Sternum 0P50
Stomach 0D56
Pylorus 0D57
Subcutaneous Tissue and Fascia
Abdomen 0J58
Back 0J57
Buttock 0J59
Chest 0J56
Face 0J51
Foot
Left 0J5R
Right 0J5Q
Hand
Left 0J5K
Right 0J5J
Lower Arm
Left 0J5H
Right 0J5G
Lower Leg
Left 0J5P
Right 0J5N
Neck
Anterior 0J54
Posterior 0J55
Pelvic Region 0J5C
Perineum 0J5B
Scalp 0J50
Upper Arm
Left 0J5F
Right 0J5D
Upper Leg
Left 0J5M
Right 0J5L
Tarsal
Left 0Q5M
Right 0Q5L
Tendon
Abdomen
Left 0L5G
Right 0L5F
Ankle
Left 0L5T
Right 0L5S
Foot
Left 0L5W
Right 0L5V
Hand
Left 0L58
Right 0L57
Head and Neck 0L50
Hip
Left 0L5K
Right 0L5J

Destruction (continued)

Tendon (continued)
Knee
Left 0L5R
Right 0L5Q
Lower Arm and Wrist
Left 0L56
Right 0L55
Lower Leg
Left 0L5P
Right 0L5N
Perineum 0L5H
Shoulder
Left 0L52
Right 0L51
Thorax
Left 0L5D
Right 0L5C
Trunk
Left 0L5B
Right 0L59
Upper Arm
Left 0L54
Right 0L53
Upper Leg
Left 0L5M
Right 0L5L
Testis
Bilateral 0V5C
Left 0V5B
Right 0V59
Thalamus 0059
Thymus 075M
Thyroid Gland 0G5K
Left Lobe 0G5G
Right Lobe 0G5H
Tibia
Left 0Q5H
Right 0Q5G
Toe Nail 0H5RXZZ
Tongue 0C57
Tonsils 0C5P
Tooth
Lower 0C5X
Upper 0C5W
Trachea 0B51
Tunica Vaginalis
Left 0V57
Right 0V56
Turbinate, Nasal 095L
Tympanic Membrane
Left 0958
Right 0957
Ulna
Left 0P5L
Right 0P5K
Ureter
Left 0T57
Right 0T56
Urethra 0T5D
Uterine Supporting Structure 0U54
Uterus 0U59
Uvula 0C5N
Vagina 0U5G
Valve
Aortic 025F
Mitral 025G
Pulmonary 025H
Tricuspid 025J
Vas Deferens
Bilateral 0V5Q
Left 0V5P
Right 0V5N
Vein
Axillary
Left 0558
Right 0557
Azygos 0550
Basilic
Left 055C
Right 055B
Brachial
Left 055A
Right 0559
Cephalic
Left 055F
Right 055D
Colic 0657
Common Iliac
Left 065D
Right 065C
Coronary 0254
Esophageal 0653
External Iliac
Left 065G
Right 065F

Dilation (*continued*)
  Bronchus (*continued*)
    Main
      Left 0B77
      Right 0B73
    Middle Lobe, Right 0B75
    Upper Lobe
      Left 0B78
      Right 0B74
  Carina 0B72
  Cecum 0D7H
  Cervix 0U7C
  Colon
    Ascending 0D7K
    Descending 0D7M
    Sigmoid 0D7N
    Transverse 0D7L
  Duct
    Common Bile 0F79
    Cystic 0F78
    Hepatic
      Left 0F76
      Right 0F75
    Lacrimal
      Left 087Y
      Right 087X
    Pancreatic 0F7D
      Accessory 0F7F
    Parotid
      Left 0C7C
      Right 0C7B
  Duodenum 0D79
  Esophagogastric Junction 0D74
  Esophagus 0D75
    Lower 0D73
    Middle 0D72
    Upper 0D71
  Eustachian Tube
    Left 097G
    Right 097F
  Fallopian Tube
    Left 0U76
    Right 0U75
  Fallopian Tubes,
    Bilateral 0U77
  Hymen 0U7K
  Ileocecal Valve 0D7C
  Ileum 0D7B
  Intestine
    Large 0D7E
      Left 0D7G
      Right 0D7F
    Small 0D78
  Jejunum 0D7A
  Kidney Pelvis
    Left 0T74
    Right 0T73
  Larynx 0C7S
  Pharynx 0C7M
  Rectum 0D7P
  Stomach 0D76
    Pylorus 0D77
  Trachea 0B71
  Ureter
    Left 0T77
    Right 0T76
  Ureters, Bilateral 0T78
  Urethra 0T7D
  Uterus 0U79
  Vagina 0U7G
  Valve
    Aortic 027F
    Mitral 027G
    Pulmonary 027H
    Tricuspid 027J
  Vas Deferens
    Bilateral 0V7Q
    Left 0V7P
    Right 0V7N
  Vein
    Axillary
      Left 0578
      Right 0577
    Azygos 0570
    Basilic
      Left 057C
      Right 057B
    Brachial
      Left 057A
      Right 0579
    Cephalic
      Left 057F
      Right 057D
    Colic 0677

Dilation (*continued*)
  Vein (*continued*)
    Common Iliac
      Left 067D
      Right 067C
    Esophageal 0673
    External Iliac
      Left 067G
      Right 067F
    External Jugular
      Left 057Q
      Right 057P
    Face
      Left 057V
      Right 057T
    Femoral
      Left 067N
      Right 067M
    Foot
      Left 067V
      Right 067T
    Gastric 0672
    Greater Saphenous
      Left 067Q
      Right 067P
    Hand
      Left 057H
      Right 057G
    Hemiazygos 0571
    Hepatic 0674
    Hypogastric
      Left 067J
      Right 067H
    Inferior Mesenteric 0676
    Innominate
      Left 0574
      Right 0573
    Internal Jugular
      Left 057N
      Right 057M
    Intracranial 057L
    Lesser Saphenous
      Left 067S
      Right 067R
    Lower 067Y
    Portal 0678
    Pulmonary
      Left 027T
      Right 027S
    Renal
      Left 067B
      Right 0679
    Splenic 0671
    Subclavian
      Left 0576
      Right 0575
    Superior Mesenteric 0675
    Upper 057Y
    Vertebral
      Left 057S
      Right 057R
  Vena Cava
    Inferior 0670
    Superior 027V
  Ventricle, Right 027K
Direct Lateral Interbody Fusion (DLIF) device
  use Interbody Fusion Device in
  Lower Joints
Disarticulation
  see Detachment
Discectomy, diskectomy
  see Excision, Upper Joints 0RB
  see Resection, Upper Joints 0RT
  see Excision, Lower Joints 0SB
  see Resection, Lower Joints 0ST
Discography
  see Plain Radiography, Axial Skeleton, Except Skull and
    Facial Bones BR0
  see Fluoroscopy, Axial Skeleton, Except Skull and
    Facial Bones BR1
Distal humerus
  use Humeral Shaft, Right
  use Humeral Shaft, Left
Distal humerus, involving joint
  use Joint, Elbow, Right
  use Joint, Elbow, Left
Distal radioulnar joint
  use Joint, Wrist, Right
  use Joint, Wrist, Left
Diversion
  see Bypass
Diverticulectomy
  see Excision, Gastrointestinal
    System 0DB

Division
  Acetabulum
    Left 0Q85
    Right 0Q84
  Anal Sphincter 0D8R
  Basal Ganglia 0088
  Bladder Neck 0T8C
  Bone
    Ethmoid
      Left 0N8G
      Right 0N8F
    Frontal
      Left 0N82
      Right 0N81
    Hyoid 0N8X
    Lacrimal
      Left 0N8J
      Right 0N8H
    Nasal 0N8B
    Occipital
      Left 0N88
      Right 0N87
    Palatine
      Left 0N8L
      Right 0N8K
    Parietal
      Left 0N84
      Right 0N83
    Pelvic
      Left 0Q83
      Right 0Q82
    Sphenoid
      Left 0N8D
      Right 0N8C
    Temporal
      Left 0N86
      Right 0N85
    Zygomatic
      Left 0N8N
      Right 0N8M
  Brain 0080
  Bursa and Ligament
    Abdomen
      Left 0M8J
      Right 0M8H
    Ankle
      Left 0M8R
      Right 0M8Q
    Elbow
      Left 0M84
      Right 0M83
    Foot
      Left 0M8T
      Right 0M8S
    Hand
      Left 0M88
      Right 0M87
    Head and Neck 0M80
    Hip
      Left 0M8M
      Right 0M8L
    Knee
      Left 0M8P
      Right 0M8N
    Lower Extremity
      Left 0M8W
      Right 0M8V
    Perineum 0M8K
    Shoulder
      Left 0M82
      Right 0M81
    Thorax
      Left 0M8G
      Right 0M8F
    Trunk
      Left 0M8D
      Right 0M8C
    Upper Extremity
      Left 0M8B
      Right 0M89
    Wrist
      Left 0M86
      Right 0M85
  Carpal
    Left 0P8N
    Right 0P8M
  Cerebral Hemisphere 0087
  Chordae Tendineae 0289
  Clavicle
    Left 0P8B
    Right 0P89
  Coccyx 0Q8S
  Conduction Mechanism 0288
  Esophagogastric Junction 0D84

Division

Doppler study
   see Ultrasonography
Dorsal digital nerve
   use Nerve, Radial
Dorsal metacarpal vein
   use Vein, Hand, Left
   use Vein, Hand, Right
Dorsal metatarsal artery
   use Artery, Foot, Left
   use Artery, Foot, Right
Dorsal metatarsal vein
   use Vein, Foot, Right
   use Vein, Foot, Left
Dorsal scapular artery
   use Artery, Subclavian, Right
   use Artery, Subclavian, Left
Dorsal scapular nerve
   use Nerve, Brachial Plexus
Dorsal venous arch
   use Vein, Foot, Right
   use Vein, Foot, Left
Dorsalis pedis artery
   use Artery, Anterior Tibial, Right
   use Artery, Anterior Tibial, Left
Drainage
   Abdominal Wall 0W9F
   Acetabulum
      Left 0Q95
      Right 0Q94
   Adenoids 0C9Q
   Ampulla of Vater 0F9C
   Anal Sphincter 0D9R
   Ankle Region
      Left 0Y9L
      Right 0Y9K
   Anterior Chamber
      Left 0893
      Right 0892
   Anus 0D9Q
   Aorta, Abdominal 0490
   Aortic Body 0G9D
   Appendix 0D9J
   Arm
      Lower
         Left 0X9F
         Right 0X9D
      Upper
         Left 0X99
         Right 0X98
   Artery
      Anterior Tibial
         Left 049Q
         Right 049P
      Axillary
         Left 0396
         Right 0395
      Brachial
         Left 0398
         Right 0397
      Celiac 0491
      Colic
         Left 0497
         Middle 0498
         Right 0496
      Common Carotid
         Left 039J
         Right 039H
      Common Iliac
         Left 049D
         Right 049C
      External Carotid
         Left 039N
         Right 039M
      External Iliac
         Left 049J
         Right 049H
      Face 039R
      Femoral
         Left 049L
         Right 049K
      Foot
         Left 049W
         Right 049V
      Gastric 0492
      Hand
         Left 039F
         Right 039D
      Hepatic 0493
      Inferior Mesenteric 049B
      Innominate 0392
      Internal Carotid
         Left 039L
         Right 039K
      Internal Iliac
         Left 049F
         Right 049E

Drainage *(continued)*
   Artery *(continued)*
      Internal Mammary
         Left 0391
         Right 0390
      Intracranial 039G
      Lower 049Y
      Peroneal
         Left 049U
         Right 049T
      Popliteal
         Left 049N
         Right 049M
      Posterior Tibial
         Left 049S
         Right 049R
      Radial
         Left 039C
         Right 039B
      Renal
         Left 049A
         Right 0499
      Splenic 0494
      Subclavian
         Left 0394
         Right 0393
      Superior Mesenteric 0495
      Temporal
         Left 039T
         Right 039S
      Thyroid
         Left 039V
         Right 039U
      Ulnar
         Left 039A
         Right 0399
      Upper 039Y
      Vertebral
         Left 039Q
         Right 039P
   Auditory Ossicle
      Left 099A
      Right 0999
   Axilla
      Left 0X95
      Right 0X94
   Back
      Lower 0W9L
      Upper 0W9K
   Basal Ganglia 0098
   Bladder 0T9B
   Bladder Neck 0T9C
   Bone
      Ethmoid
         Left 0N9G
         Right 0N9F
      Frontal
         Left 0N92
         Right 0N91
      Hyoid 0N9X
      Lacrimal
         Left 0N9J
         Right 0N9H
      Nasal 0N9B
      Occipital
         Left 0N98
         Right 0N97
      Palatine
         Left 0N9L
         Right 0N9K
      Parietal
         Left 0N94
         Right 0N93
      Pelvic
         Left 0Q93
         Right 0Q92
      Sphenoid
         Left 0N9D
         Right 0N9C
      Temporal
         Left 0N96
         Right 0N95
      Zygomatic
         Left 0N9N
         Right 0N9M
   Bone Marrow 079T
   Brain 0090
   Breast
      Bilateral 0H9V
      Left 0H9U
      Right 0H9T
   Bronchus
      Lingula 0B99
      Lower Lobe
         Left 0B9B
         Right 0B96

Drainage *(continued)*
   Bronchus *(continued)*
      Main
         Left 0B97
         Right 0B93
      Middle Lobe, Right 0B95
      Upper Lobe
         Left 0B98
         Right 0B94
   Buccal Mucosa 0C94
   Bursa and Ligament
      Abdomen
         Left 0M9J
         Right 0M9H
      Ankle
         Left 0M9R
         Right 0M9Q
      Elbow
         Left 0M94
         Right 0M93
      Foot
         Left 0M9T
         Right 0M9S
      Hand
         Left 0M98
         Right 0M97
      Head and Neck 200M90
      Hip
         Left 0M9M
         Right 0M9L
      Knee
         Left 0M9P
         Right 0M9N
      Lower Extremity
         Left 0M9W
         Right 0M9V
      Perineum 0M9K
      Shoulder
         Left 0M92
         Right 0M91
      Thorax
         Left 0M9G
         Right 0M9F
      Trunk
         Left 0M9D
         Right 0M9C
      Upper Extremity
         Left 0M9B
         Right 0M99
      Wrist
         Left 0M96
         Right 0M95
   Buttock
      Left 0Y91
      Right 0Y90
   Carina 0B92
   Carotid Bodies, Bilateral 0G98
   Carotid Body
      Left 0G96
      Right 0G97
   Carpal
      Left 0P9N
      Right 0P9M
   Cavity, Cranial 0W91
   Cecum 0D9H
   Cerebellum 009C
   Cerebral Hemisphere 0097
   Cerebral Meninges 0091
   Cerebral Ventricle 0096
   Cervix 0U9C
   Chest Wall 0W98
   Choroid
      Left 089B
      Right 089A
   Cisterna Chyli 079L
   Clavicle
      Left 0P9B
      Right 0P99
   Clitoris 0U9J
   Coccygeal Glomus 0G9B
   Coccyx 0Q9S
   Colon
      Ascending 0D9K
      Descending 0D9M
      Sigmoid 0D9N
      Transverse 0D9L
   Conjunctiva
      Left 089T
      Right 089S
   Cord
      Bilateral 0V9H
      Left 0V9G
      Right 0V9F
   Cornea
      Left 0899
      Right 0898

Drainage

Drainage (continued)
  Lymphatic (continued)
    Neck
      Left 0792
      Right 0791
    Pelvis 079C
    Thoracic Duct 079K
    Thorax 0797
    Upper Extremity
      Left 0794
      Right 0793
  Mandible
    Left 0N9V
    Right 0N9T
  Maxilla
    Left 0N9S
    Right 0N9R
  Mediastinum 0W9C
  Medulla Oblongata 009D
  Mesentery 0D9V
  Metacarpal
    Left 0P9Q
    Right 0P9P
  Metatarsal
    Left 0Q9P
    Right 0Q9N
  Muscle
    Abdomen
      Left 0K9L
      Right 0K9K
    Extraocular
      Left 089M
      Right 089L
    Facial 0K91
    Foot
      Left 0K9W
      Right 0K9V
    Hand
      Left 0K9D
      Right 0K9C
    Head 0K90
    Hip
      Left 0K9P
      Right 0K9N
    Lower Arm and Wrist
      Left 0K9B
      Right 0K99
    Lower Leg
      Left 0K9T
      Right 0K9S
    Neck
      Left 0K93
      Right 0K92
    Perineum 0K9M
    Shoulder
      Left 0K96
      Right 0K95
    Thorax
      Left 0K9J
      Right 0K9H
    Tongue, Palate, Pharynx 0K94
    Trunk
      Left 0K9G
      Right 0K9F
    Upper Arm
      Left 0K98
      Right 0K97
    Upper Leg
      Left 0K9R
      Right 0K9Q
  Nasopharynx 099N
  Neck 0W96
  Nerve
    Abdominal Sympathetic 019M
    Abducens 009L
    Accessory 009R
    Acoustic 009N
    Brachial Plexus 0193
    Cervical 0191
    Cervical Plexus 0190
    Facial 009M
    Femoral 019D
    Glossopharyngeal 009P
    Head and Neck Sympathetic 019K
    Hypoglossal 009S
    Lumbar 019B
    Lumbar Plexus 0199
    Lumbar Sympathetic 019N
    Lumbosacral Plexus 019A
    Median 0195
    Oculomotor 009H
    Olfactory 009F

Drainage (continued)
  Nerve (continued)
    Optic 009G
    Peroneal 019H
    Phrenic 0192
    Pudendal 019C
    Radial 0196
    Sacral 019R
    Sacral Plexus 019Q
    Sacral Sympathetic 019P
    Sciatic 019F
    Thoracic 0198
    Thoracic Sympathetic 019L
    Tibial 019G
    Trigeminal 009K
    Trochlear 009J
    Ulnar 0194
    Vagus 009Q
  Nipple
    Left 0H9X
    Right 0H9W
  Nose 099K
  Omentum
    Greater 0D9S
    Lesser 0D9T
  Oral Cavity and Throat 0W93
  Orbit
    Left 0N9Q
    Right 0N9P
  Ovary
    Bilateral 0U92
    Left 0U91
    Right 0U90
  Palate
    Hard 0C92
    Soft 0C93
  Pancreas 0F9G
  Para-aortic Body 0G99
  Paraganglion Extremity 0G9F
  Parathyroid Gland 0G9R
    Inferior
      Left 0G9P
      Right 0G9N
    Multiple 0G9Q
    Superior
      Left 0G9M
      Right 0G9L
  Patella
    Left 0Q9F
    Right 0Q9D
  Pelvic Cavity 0W9J
  Penis 0V9S
  Pericardial Cavity 0W9D
  Perineum
    Female 0W9N
    Male 0W9M
  Peritoneal Cavity 0W9G
  Peritoneum 0D9W
  Phalanx
    Finger
      Left 0P9V
      Right 0P9T
    Thumb
      Left 0P9S
      Right 0P9R
    Toe
      Left 0Q9R
      Right 0Q9Q
  Pharynx 0C9M
  Pineal Body 0G91
  Pleura
    Left 0B9P
    Right 0B9N
  Pleural Cavity
    Left 0W9B
    Right 0W99
  Pons 009B
  Prepuce 0V9T
  Products of Conception
    Amniotic Fluid
      Diagnostic 1090
      Therapeutic 1090
    Fetal Blood 1090
    Fetal Cerebrospinal Fluid 1090
    Fetal Fluid, Other 1090
    Fluid, Other 1090
  Prostate 0V90
  Radius
    Left 0P9J
    Right 0P9H
  Rectum 0D9P
  Retina
    Left 089F
    Right 089E

Drainage (continued)
  Retinal Vessel
    Left 089H
    Right 089G
  Retroperitoneum 0W9H
  Rib
    Left 0P92
    Right 0P91
  Sacrum 0Q91
  Scapula
    Left 0P96
    Right 0P95
  Sclera
    Left 0897
    Right 0896
  Scrotum 0V95
  Septum, Nasal 099M
  Shoulder Region
    Left 0X93
    Right 0X92
  Sinus
    Accessory 099P
    Ethmoid
      Left 099V
      Right 099U
    Frontal
      Left 099T
      Right 099S
    Mastoid
      Left 099C
      Right 099B
    Maxillary
      Left 099R
      Right 099Q
    Sphenoid
      Left 099X
      Right 099W
  Skin
    Abdomen 0H97
    Back 0H96
    Buttock 0H98
    Chest 0H95
    Ear
      Left 0H93
      Right 0H92
    Face 0H91
    Foot
      Left 0H9N
      Right 0H9M
    Genitalia 0H9A
    Hand
      Left 0H9G
      Right 0H9F
    Lower Arm
      Left 0H9E
      Right 0H9D
    Lower Leg
      Left 0H9L
      Right 0H9K
    Neck 0H94
    Perineum 0H99
    Scalp 0H90
    Upper Arm
      Left 0H9C
      Right 0H9B
    Upper Leg
      Left 0H9J
      Right 0H9H
  Skull 0N90
  Spinal Canal 009U
  Spinal Cord
    Cervical 009W
    Lumbar 009Y
    Thoracic 009X
  Spinal Meninges 009T
  Spleen 079P
  Sternum 0P90
  Stomach 0D96
    Pylorus 0D97
  Subarachnoid Space 0095
  Subcutaneous Tissue and Fascia
    Abdomen 0J98
    Back 0J97
    Buttock 0J99
    Chest 0J96
    Face 0J91
    Foot
      Left 0J9R
      Right 0J9Q
    Hand
      Left 0J9K
      Right 0J9J

Duodenorrhaphy
 see Repair, Duodenum 0DQ9
Duodenostomy
 see Bypass, Duodenum 0D19
 see Drainage, Duodenum 0D99
Duodenotomy
 see Drainage, Duodenum 0D99
DuraHeart Left Ventricular Assist
 System
 use Implantable Heart Assist System in Heart and Great
 Vessels
Dural venous sinus
 use Vein, Intracranial
Durata® Defibrillation Lead
 use Cardiac Lead, Defibrillator in 02H
Dynesys® Dynamic Stabilization System
 use Spinal Stabilization Device, Pedicle-Based in 0RH
 use Spinal Stabilization Device, Pedicle-Based in 0SH

E

E-Luminexx™ (Biliary)(Vascular) Stent
 use Intraluminal Device
Earlobe
 use Ear, External, Left
 use Ear, External, Bilateral
 use Ear, External, Right
Echocardiogram
 see Ultrasonography, Heart B24
Echography
 see Ultrasonography
ECMO
 see Performance, Circulatory 5A15
EEG (electroencephalogram)
 see Measurement, Central Nervous 4A00
EGD (esophagogastroduodenoscopy) 0DJ08ZZ
Eighth cranial nerve
 use Nerve, Acoustic
Ejaculatory duct
 use Vas Deferens, Bilateral
 use Vas Deferens, Left
 use Vas Deferens, Right
 use Vas Deferens
EKG (electrocardiogram)
 see Measurement, Cardiac 4A02
Electrical bone growth stimulator (EBGS)
 use Bone Growth Stimulator in Head and
 Facial Bones
 use Bone Growth Stimulator in Upper Bones
 use Bone Growth Stimulator in Lower Bones
Electrical muscle stimulation (EMS) lead
 use Stimulator Lead in Muscles
Electrocautery
 Destruction
  see Destruction
 Repair
  see Repair
Electroconvulsive Therapy
 Bilateral-Multiple Seizure GZB3ZZZ
 Bilateral-Single Seizure GZB2ZZZ
 Electroconvulsive Therapy, Other
  GZB4ZZZ
 Unilateral-Multiple Seizure GZB1ZZZ
 Unilateral-Single Seizure GZB0ZZZ
Electroencephalogram (EEG)
 see Measurement, Central Nervous 4A00
Electromagnetic Therapy
 Central Nervous 6A22
 Urinary 6A21
Electronic muscle stimulator lead
 use Stimulator Lead in Muscles
Electrophysiologic stimulation (EPS)
 see Measurement, Cardiac 4A02
Electroshock therapy
 see Electroconvulsive Therapy
Elevation, bone fragments, skull
 see Reposition, Head and Facial Bones 0NS
Eleventh cranial nerve
 use Nerve, Accessory
Embolectomy
 see Extirpation
Embolization
 see Occlusion
 see Restriction
Embolization coil(s)
 use Intraluminal Device
EMG (electromyogram)
 see Measurement, Musculoskeletal 4A0F
Encephalon
 use Brain
Endarterectomy
 see Extirpation, Upper Arteries 03C
 see Extirpation, Lower Arteries 04C

Endeavor® (III)(IV) (Sprint) Zotarolimus-eluting
 Coronary Stent System
 use Intraluminal Device, Drug-eluting in Heart and
 Great Vessels
EndoSure® sensor
 use Monitoring Device, Pressure Sensor in 02H
ENDOTAK RELIANCE® (G) Defibrillation Lead
 use Cardiac Lead, Defibrillator in 02H
Endotracheal tube (cuffed)(double-lumen)
 use Intraluminal Device, Endotracheal Airway in
 Respiratory System
Endurant® Endovascular Stent Graft
 use Intraluminal Device
Enlargement
 see Dilation
 see Repair
EnRhythm
 use Pacemaker, Dual Chamber in 0JH
Enterorrhaphy
 see Repair, Gastrointestinal System 0DQ
Enterra gastric neurostimulator
 use Stimulator Generator, Multiple Array in 0JH
Enucleation
 Eyeball
  see Resection, Eye 08T
 Eyeball with prosthetic implant
  see Replacement, Eye 08R
Ependyma
 use Cerebral Ventricle
Epicel® cultured epidermal autograft
 use Autologous Tissue Substitute
Epic™ Stented Tissue Valve (aortic)
 use Zooplastic Tissue in Heart and Great
 Vessels
Epidermis
 use Skin
Epididymectomy
 see Excision, Male Reproductive System 0VB
 see Resection, Male Reproductive System 0VT
Epididymoplasty
 see Repair, Male Reproductive System 0VQ
 see Supplement, Male Reproductive System 0VU
Epididymorrhaphy
 see Repair, Male Reproductive System 0VQ
Epididymotomy
 see Drainage, Male Reproductive System 0V9
Epiphysiodesis
 see Fusion, Upper Joints 0RG
 see Fusion, Lower Joints 0SG
Epiploic foramen
 use Peritoneum
Epiretinal Visual Prosthesis
 use Epiretinal Visual Prosthesis in Eye
 Insertion of device in
  Left 08H105Z
  Right 08H005Z
Episiorrhaphy
 see Repair, Perineum, Female 0WQN
Episiotomy
 see Division, Perineum, Female 0W8N
Epithalamus
 use Thalamus
Epitrochlear lymph node
 use Lymphatic, Upper Extremity, Left
 use Lymphatic, Upper Extremity, Right
EPS (electrophysiologic stimulation)
 see Measurement, Cardiac 4A02
Eptifibatide, infusion
 see Introduction of Platelet Inhibitor
ERCP (endoscopic retrograde
 cholangiopancreatography)
 see Fluoroscopy, Hepatobiliary System and Pancreas BF1
Erector spinae muscle
 use Muscle, Trunk, Left
 use Muscle, Trunk, Right
Esophageal artery
 use Aorta, Thoracic
Esophageal obturator airway (EOA)
 use Intraluminal Device, Airway in Gastrointestinal
 System
Esophageal plexus
 use Nerve, Thoracic Sympathetic
Esophagectomy
 see Excision, Gastrointestinal System 0DB
 see Resection, Gastrointestinal System 0DT
Esophagocoloplasty
 see Repair, Gastrointestinal System 0DQ
 see Supplement, Gastrointestinal System 0DU
Esophagoenterostomy
 see Bypass, Gastrointestinal System 0D1
 see Drainage, Gastrointestinal System 0D9
Esophagoesophagostomy
 see Bypass, Gastrointestinal System 0D1
 see Drainage, Gastrointestinal System 0D9

Esophagogastrectomy
 see Excision, Gastrointestinal System 0DB
 see Resection, Gastrointestinal System 0DT
Esophagogastroduodenoscopy (EGD) 0DJ08ZZ
Esophagogastroplasty
 see Repair, Gastrointestinal System 0DQ
 see Supplement, Gastrointestinal
 System 0DU
Esophagogastroscopy 0DJ68ZZ
Esophagogastrostomy
 see Bypass, Gastrointestinal System 0D1
 see Drainage, Gastrointestinal System 0D9
Esophagojejunoplasty
 see Supplement, Gastrointestinal System 0DU
Esophagojejunostomy
 see Drainage, Gastrointestinal System 0D9
 see Bypass, Gastrointestinal System 0D1
Esophagomyotomy
 see Division, Esophagogastric Junction 0D84
Esophagoplasty
 see Repair, Gastrointestinal System 0DQ
 see Replacement, Esophagus 0DR5
 see Supplement, Gastrointestinal System 0DU
Esophagoplication
 see Restriction, Gastrointestinal System 0DV
Esophagorrhaphy
 see Repair, Gastrointestinal System 0DQ
Esophagoscopy 0DJ08ZZ
Esophagotomy
 see Drainage, Gastrointestinal System 0D9
Esteem® implantable hearing system
 use Hearing Device in Ear, Nose, Sinus
ESWL (extracorporeal shock wave lithotripsy)
 see Fragmentation
Ethmoidal air cell
 use Sinus, Ethmoid, Left
 use Sinus, Ethmoid, Right
Ethmoidectomy
 see Excision, Ear, Nose, Sinus 09B
 see Resection, Ear, Nose, Sinus 09T
 see Excision, Head and Facial Bones 0NB
 see Resection, Head and Facial Bones 0NT
Ethmoidotomy
 see Drainage, Ear, Nose, Sinus 099
Evacuation
 Hematoma
  see Extirpation
 Other Fluid
  see Drainage
Everolimus-eluting coronary stent
 use Intraluminal Device, Drug-eluting in Heart and
 Great Vessels
Evisceration
 Eyeball
  see Resection, Eye 08T
 Eyeball with prosthetic implant
  see Replacement, Eye 08R
Ex-PRESS™ mini glaucoma shunt
 use Synthetic Substitute
Examination
 see Inspection
Exchange
 see Change device in
Excision
 Abdominal Wall 0WBF
 Acetabulum
  Left 0QB5
  Right 0QB4
 Adenoids 0CBQ
 Ampulla of Vater 0FBC
 Anal Sphincter 0DBR
 Ankle Region
  Left 0YBL
  Right 0YBK
 Anus 0DBQ
 Aorta
  Abdominal 04B0
  Thoracic 02BW
 Aortic Body 0GBD
 Appendix 0DBJ
 Arm
  Lower
   Left 0XBF
   Right 0XBD
  Upper
   Left 0XB9
   Right 0XB8
 Artery
  Anterior Tibial
   Left 04BQ
   Right 04BP
  Axillary
   Left 03B6
   Right 03B5

Excision (continued)

Elbow Region
Left 0XBC
Right 0XBB
Epididymis
Bilateral 0VBL
Left 0VBK
Right 0VBJ
Epiglottis 0CBR
Esophagogastric Junction
0DB4
Esophagus 0DB5
Lower 0DB3
Middle 0DB2
Upper 0DB1
Eustachian Tube
Left 09BG
Right 09BF
Extremity
Lower
Left 0YBB
Right 0YB9
Upper
Left 0XB7
Right 0XB6
Eye
Left 08B1
Right 08B0
Eyelid
Lower
Left 08BR
Right 08BQ
Upper
Left 08BP
Right 08BN
Face 0WB2
Fallopian Tube
Left 0UB6
Right 0UB5
Fallopian Tubes, Bilateral 0UB7
Femoral Region
Left 0YB8
Right 0YB7
Femoral Shaft
Left 0QB9
Right 0QB8
Femur
Lower
Left 0QBC
Right 0QBB
Upper
Left 0QB7
Right 0QB6
Fibula
Left 0QBK
Right 0QBJ
Finger Nail 0HBQXZ
Foot
Left 0YBN
Right 0YBM
Gallbladder 0FB4
Gingiva
Lower 0CB6
Upper 0CB5
Gland
Adrenal
Bilateral 0GB4
Left 0GB2
Right 0GB3
Lacrimal
Left 08BW
Right 08BV
Minor Salivary 0CBJ
Parotid
Left 0CB9
Right 0CB8
Pituitary 0GB0
Sublingual
Left 0CBF
Right 0CBD
Submaxillary
Left 0CBH
Right 0CBG
Vestibular 0UBL
Glenoid Cavity
Left 0PB8
Right 0PB7
Glomus Jugulare 0GBC
Hand
Left 0XBK
Right 0XBJ
Head 0WB0
Humeral Head
Left 0PBD
Right 0PBC

Excision (continued)

Humeral Shaft
Left 0PBG
Right 0PBF
Hymen 0UBK
Hypothalamus 00BA
Ileocecal Valve 0DBC
Ileum 0DBB
Inguinal Region
Left 0YB6
Right 0YB5
Intestine
Large 0DBE
Left 0DBG
Right 0DBF
Small 0DB8
Iris
Left 08BD3Z
Right 08BC3Z
Jaw
Lower 0WB5
Upper 0WB4
Jejunum 0DBA
Joint
Acromioclavicular
Left 0RBH
Right 0RBG
Ankle
Left 0SBG
Right 0SBF
Carpal
Left 0RBR
Right 0RBQ
Cervical Vertebral 0RB1
Cervicothoracic Vertebral
0RB4
Coccygeal 0SB6
Elbow
Left 0RBM
Right 0RBL
Finger Phalangeal
Left 0RBX
Right 0RBW
Hip
Left 0SBB
Right 0SB9
Knee
Left 0SBD
Right 0SBC
Lumbar Vertebral 0SB0
Lumbosacral 0SB3
Metacarpocarpal
Left 0RBT
Right 0RBS
Metacarpophalangeal
Left 0RBV
Right 0RBU
Metatarsal-Phalangeal
Left 0SBN
Right 0SBM
Metatarsal-Tarsal
Left 0SBL
Right 0SBK
Occipital-cervical 0RB0
Sacrococcygeal 0SB5
Sacroiliac
Left 0SB8
Right 0SB7
Shoulder
Left 0RBK
Right 0RBJ
Sternoclavicular
Left 0RBF
Right 0RBE
Tarsal
Left 0SBJ
Right 0SBH
Temporomandibular
Left 0RBD
Right 0RBC
Thoracic Vertebral 0RB6
Thoracolumbar Vertebral
0RBA
Toe Phalangeal
Left 0SBQ
Right 0SBP
Wrist
Left 0RBP
Right 0RBN
Kidney
Left 0TB1
Right 0TB0
Kidney Pelvis
Left 0TB4
Right 0TB3

Excision (continued)

Knee Region
Left 0YBG
Right 0YBF
Larynx 0CBS
Leg
Lower
Left 0YBJ
Right 0YBH
Upper
Left 0YBD
Right 0YBC
Lens
Left 08BK3Z
Right 08BJ3Z
Lip
Lower 0CB1
Upper 0CB0
Liver 0FB0
Left Lobe 0FB2
Right Lobe 0FB1
Lung
Bilateral 0BBM
Left 0BBL
Lower Lobe
Left 0BBJ
Right 0BBF
Middle Lobe, Right
0BBD
Right 0BBK
Upper Lobe
Left 0BBG
Right 0BBC
Lung Lingula 0BBH
Lymphatic
Aortic 07BD
Axillary
Left 07B6
Right 07B5
Head 07B0
Inguinal
Left 07BJ
Right 07BH
Internal Mammary
Left 07B9
Right 07B8
Lower Extremity
Left 07BG
Right 07BF
Mesenteric 07BB
Neck
Left 07B2
Right 07B1
Pelvis 07BC
Thoracic Duct 07BK
Thorax 07B7
Upper Extremity
Left 07B4
Right 07B3
Mandible
Left 0NBV
Right 0NBT
Maxilla
Left 0NBS
Right 0NBR
Mediastinum 0WBC
Medulla Oblongata 00BD
Mesentery 0DBV
Metacarpal
Left 0PBQ
Right 0PBP
Metatarsal
Left 0QBP
Right 0QBN
Muscle
Abdomen
Left 0KBL
Right 0KBK
Extraocular
Left 08BM
Right 08BL
Facial 0KB1
Foot
Left 0KBW
Right 0KBV
Hand
Left 0KBD
Right 0KBC
Head 0KB0
Hip
Left 0KBP
Right 0KBN
Lower Arm and Wrist
Left 0KBB
Right 0KB9

Excision (*continued*)
  Tendon (*continued*)
    Upper Leg
      Left 0LBM
      Right 0LBL
  Testis
    Bilateral 0VBC
    Left 0VBB
    Right 0VB9
  Thalamus 00B9
  Thymus 07BM
  Thyroid Gland
    Left Lobe 0GBG
    Right Lobe 0GBH
  Tibia
    Left 0QBH
    Right 0QBG
  Toe Nail 0HBRXZ
  Tongue 0CB7
  Tonsils 0CBP
  Tooth
    Lower 0CBX
    Upper 0CBW
  Trachea 0BB1
  Tunica Vaginalis
    Left 0VB7
    Right 0VB6
  Turbinate, Nasal 09BL
  Tympanic Membrane
    Left 09B8
    Right 09B7
  Ulna
    Left 0PBL
    Right 0PBK
  Ureter
    Left 0TB7
    Right 0TB6
  Urethra 0TBD
  Uterine Supporting Structure 0UB4
  Uterus 0UB9
  Uvula 0CBN
  Vagina 0UBG
  Valve
    Aortic 02BF
    Mitral 02BG
    Pulmonary 02BH
    Tricuspid 02BJ
  Vas Deferens
    Bilateral 0VBQ
    Left 0VBP
    Right 0VBN
  Vein
    Axillary
      Left 05B8
      Right 05B7
    Azygos 05B0
    Basilic
      Left 05BC
      Right 05BB
    Brachial
      Left 05BA
      Right 05B9
    Cephalic
      Left 05BF
      Right 05BD
    Colic 06B7
    Common Iliac
      Left 06BD
      Right 06BC
    Coronary 02B4
    Esophageal 06B3
    External Iliac
      Left 06BG
      Right 06BF
    External Jugular
      Left 05BQ
      Right 05BP
    Face
      Left 05BV
      Right 05BT
    Femoral
      Left 06BN
      Right 06BM
    Foot
      Left 06BV
      Right 06BT
    Gastric 06B2
    Greater Saphenous
      Left 06BQ
      Right 06BP
    Hand
      Left 05BH
      Right 05BG
    Hemiazygos 05B1
    Hepatic 06B4

Excision (*continued*)
  Vein (*continued*)
    Hypogastric
      Left 06BJ
      Right 06BH
    Inferior Mesenteric 06B6
    Innominate
      Left 05B4
      Right 05B3
    Internal Jugular
      Left 05BN
      Right 05BM
    Intracranial 05BL
    Lesser Saphenous
      Left 06BS
      Right 06BR
    Lower 06BY
    Portal 06B8
    Pulmonary
      Left 02BT
      Right 02BS
    Renal
      Left 06BB
      Right 06B9
    Splenic 06B1
    Subclavian
      Left 05B6
      Right 05B5
    Superior Mesenteric 06B5
    Upper 05BY
    Vertebral
      Left 05BS
      Right 05BR
  Vena Cava
    Inferior 06B0
    Superior 02BV
  Ventricle
    Left 02BL
    Right 02BK
  Vertebra
    Cervical 0PB3
    Lumbar 0QB0
    Thoracic 0PB4
  Vesicle
    Bilateral 0VB3
    Left 0VB2
    Right 0VB1
  Vitreous
    Left 08B53Z
    Right 08B43Z
  Vocal Cord
    Left 0CBV
    Right 0CBT
  Vulva 0UBM
  Wrist Region
    Left 0XBH
    Right 0XBG

Exclusion, Left atrial appendage (LAA)
  see Occlusion, Atrium, Left 02L7
Exercise, rehabilitation
  see Motor Treatment, Rehabilitation F07
Exploration
  see Inspection
Express® (LD) Premounted Stent System
  use Intraluminal Device
Express® Biliary SD Monorail® Premounted Stent System
  use Intraluminal Device
Express® SD Renal Monorail® Premounted Stent System
  use Intraluminal Device
Extensor carpi radialis muscle
  use Muscle, Lower Arm and Wrist, Left
  use Muscle, Lower Arm and Wrist, Right
Extensor carpi ulnaris muscle
  use Muscle, Lower Arm and Wrist, Left
  use Muscle, Lower Arm and Wrist, Right
Extensor digitorum brevis muscle
  use Muscle, Foot, Right
  use Muscle, Foot, Left
Extensor digitorum longus muscle
  use Muscle, Lower Leg, Left
  use Muscle, Lower Leg, Right
Extensor hallucis brevis muscle
  use Muscle, Foot, Right
  use Muscle, Foot, Left
Extensor hallucis longus muscle
  use Muscle, Lower Leg, Right
  use Muscle, Lower Leg, Left
External anal sphincter
  use Anal Sphincter
External auditory meatus
  use Ear, External Auditory Canal, Left
  use Ear, External Auditory Canal, Right
External fixator
  use External Fixation Device in Head and Facial Bones

External fixator (*continued*)
  use External Fixation Device in Upper Bones
  use External Fixation Device in Lower Bones
  use External Fixation Device in Upper Joints
  use External Fixation Device in Lower Joints
External maxillary artery
  use Artery, Face
External naris
  use Nose
External oblique aponeurosis
  use Subcutaneous Tissue and Fascia, Trunk
External oblique muscle
  use Muscle, Abdomen, Left
  use Muscle, Abdomen, Right
External popliteal nerve
  use Nerve, Peroneal
External pudendal artery
  use Artery, Femoral, Right
  use Artery, Femoral, Left
External pudendal vein
  use Vein, Greater Saphenous, Right
  use Vein, Greater Saphenous, Left
External urethral sphincter
  use Urethra
Extirpation
  Acetabulum
    Left 0QC5
    Right 0QC4
  Adenoids 0CCQ
  Ampulla of Vater 0FCC
  Anal Sphincter 0DCR
  Anterior Chamber
    Left 08C3
    Right 08C2
  Anus 0DCQ
  Aorta
    Abdominal 04C0
    Thoracic 02CW
  Aortic Body 0GCD
  Appendix 0DCJ
  Artery
    Anterior Tibial
      Left 04CQ
      Right 04CP
    Axillary
      Left 03C6
      Right 03C5
    Brachial
      Left 03C8
      Right 03C7
    Celiac 04C1
    Colic
      Left 04C7
      Middle 04C8
      Right 04C6
    Common Carotid
      Left 03CJ
      Right 03CH
    Common Iliac
      Left 04CD
      Right 04CC
    Coronary
      Four or More Sites 02C3
      One Site 02C0
      Three Sites 02C2
      Two Sites 02C1
    External Carotid
      Left 03CN
      Right 03CM
    External Iliac
      Left 04CJ
      Right 04CH
    Face 03CR
    Femoral
      Left 04CL
      Right 04CK
    Foot
      Left 04CW
      Right 04CV
    Gastric 04C2
    Hand
      Left 03CF
      Right 03CD
    Hepatic 04C3
    Inferior Mesenteric 04CB
    Innominate 03C2
    Internal Carotid
      Left 03CL
      Right 03CK
    Internal Iliac
      Left 04CF
      Right 04CE
    Internal Mammary
      Left 03C1
      Right 03C0

Extirpation (*continued*)
Gland
  Adrenal
    Bilateral 0GC4
    Left 0GC2
    Right 0GC3
  Lacrimal
    Left 08CW
    Right 08CV
  Minor Salivary 0CCJ
  Parotid
    Left 0CC9
    Right 0CC8
  Pituitary 0GC0
  Sublingual
    Left 0CCF
    Right 0CCD
  Submaxillary
    Left 0CCH
    Right 0CCG
  Vestibular 0UCL
Glenoid Cavity
  Left 0PC8
  Right 0PC7
Glomus Jugulare 0GCC
Humeral Head
  Left 0PCD
  Right 0PCC
Humeral Shaft
  Left 0PCG
  Right 0PCF
Hymen 0UCK
Hypothalamus 00CA
Ileocecal Valve 0DCC
Ileum 0DCB
Intestine
  Large 0DCE
    Left 0DCG
    Right 0DCF
  Small 0DC8
Iris
  Left 08CD
  Right 08CC
Jejunum 0DCA
Joint
  Acromioclavicular
    Left 0RCH
    Right 0RCG
  Ankle
    Left 0SCG
    Right 0SCF
  Carpal
    Left 0RCR
    Right 0RCQ
  Cervical Vertebral 0RC1
  Cervicothoracic Vertebral 0RC4
  Coccygeal 0SC6
  Elbow
    Left 0RCM
    Right 0RCL
  Finger Phalangeal
    Left 0RCX
    Right 0RCW
  Hip
    Left 0SCB
    Right 0SC9
  Knee
    Left 0SCD
    Right 0SCC
  Lumbar Vertebral 0SC0
  Lumbosacral 0SC3
  Metacarpocarpal
    Left 0RCT
    Right 0RCS
  Metacarpophalangeal
    Left 0RCV
    Right 0RCU
  Metatarsal-Phalangeal
    Left 0SCN
    Right 0SCM
  Metatarsal-Tarsal
    Left 0SCL
    Right 0SCK
  Occipital-cervical 0RC0
  Sacrococcygeal 0SC5
  Sacroiliac
    Left 0SC8
    Right 0SC7
  Shoulder
    Left 0RCK
    Right 0RCJ
  Sternoclavicular
    Left 0RCF
    Right 0RCE

Extirpation (*continued*)
Joint (*continued*)
  Tarsal
    Left 0SCJ
    Right 0SCH
  Temporomandibular
    Left 0RCD
    Right 0RCC
  Thoracic Vertebral 0RC6
  Thoracolumbar Vertebral 0RCA
  Toe Phalangeal
    Left 0SCQ
    Right 0SCP
  Wrist
    Left 0RCP
    Right 0RCN
Kidney
  Left 0TC1
  Right 0TC0
Kidney Pelvis
  Left 0TC4
  Right 0TC3
Larynx 0CCS
Lens
  Left 08CK
  Right 08CJ
Lip
  Lower 0CC1
  Upper 0CC0
Liver 0FC0
  Left Lobe 0FC2
  Right Lobe 0FC1
Lung
  Bilateral 0BCM
  Left 0BCL
  Lower Lobe
    Left 0BCJ
    Right 0BCF
  Middle Lobe, Right 0BCD
  Right 0BCK
  Upper Lobe
    Left 0BCG
    Right 0BCC
Lung Lingula 0BCH
Lymphatic
  Aortic 07CD
  Axillary
    Left 07C6
    Right 07C5
  Head 07C0
  Inguinal
    Left 07CJ
    Right 07CH
  Internal Mammary
    Left 07C9
    Right 07C8
  Lower Extremity
    Left 07CG
    Right 07CF
  Mesenteric 07CB
  Neck
    Left 07C2
    Right 07C1
  Pelvis 07CC
  Thoracic Duct 07CK
  Thorax 07C7
  Upper Extremity
    Left 07C4
    Right 07C3
Mandible
  Left 0NCV
  Right 0NCT
Maxilla
  Left 0NCS
  Right 0NCR
Mediastinum 0WCC
Medulla Oblongata 00CD
Mesentery 0DCV
Metacarpal
  Left 0PCQ
  Right 0PCP
Metatarsal
  Left 0QCP
  Right 0QCN
Muscle
  Abdomen
    Left 0KCL
    Right 0KCK
  Extraocular
    Left 08CM
    Right 08CL
  Facial 0KC1

Extirpation (*continued*)
Muscle (*continued*)
  Foot
    Left 0KCW
    Right 0KCV
  Hand
    Left 0KCD
    Right 0KCC
  Head 0KC0
  Hip
    Left 0KCP
    Right 0KCN
  Lower Arm and Wrist
    Left 0KCB
    Right 0KC9
  Lower Leg
    Left 0KCT
    Right 0KCS
  Neck
    Left 0KC3
    Right 0KC2
  Papillary 02CD
  Perineum 0KCM
  Shoulder
    Left 0KC6
    Right 0KC5
  Thorax
    Left 0KCJ
    Right 0KCH
  Tongue, Palate, Pharynx 0KC4
  Trunk
    Left 0KCG
    Right 0KCF
  Upper Arm
    Left 0KC8
    Right 0KC7
  Upper Leg
    Left 0KCR
    Right 0KCQ
Nasopharynx 09CN
Nerve
  Abdominal Sympathetic 01CM
  Abducens 00CL
  Accessory 00CR
  Acoustic 00CN
  Brachial Plexus 01C3
  Cervical 01C1
  Cervical Plexus 01C0
  Facial 00CM
  Femoral 01CD
  Glossopharyngeal 00CP
  Head and Neck Sympathetic 01CK
  Hypoglossal 00CS
  Lumbar 01CB
  Lumbar Plexus 01C9
  Lumbar Sympathetic 01CN
  Lumbosacral Plexus 01CA
  Median 01C5
  Oculomotor 00CH
  Olfactory 00CF
  Optic 00CG
  Peroneal 01CH
  Phrenic 01C2
  Pudendal 01CC
  Radial 01C6
  Sacral 01CR
  Sacral Plexus 01CQ
  Sacral Sympathetic 01CP
  Sciatic 01CF
  Thoracic 01C8
  Thoracic Sympathetic 01CL
  Tibial 01CG
  Trigeminal 00CK
  Trochlear 00CJ
  Ulnar 01C4
  Vagus 00CQ
Nipple
  Left 0HCX
  Right 0HCW
Nose 09CK
Omentum
  Greater 0DCS
  Lesser 0DCT
Oral Cavity and Throat 0WC3
Orbit
  Left 0NCQ
  Right 0NCP
Ovary
  Bilateral 0UC2
  Left 0UC1
  Right 0UC0
Palate
  Hard 0CC2
  Soft 0CC3

Extirpation (continued)
  Vein (continued)
    Femoral
      Left 06CN
      Right 06CM
    Foot
      Left 06CV
      Right 06CT
    Gastric 06C2
    Greater Saphenous
      Left 06CQ
      Right 06CP
    Hand
      Left 05CH
      Right 05CG
    Hemiazygos 05C1
    Hepatic 06C4
    Hypogastric
      Left 06CJ
      Right 06CH
    Inferior Mesenteric 06C6
    Innominate
      Left 05C4
      Right 05C3
    Internal Jugular
      Left 05CN
      Right 05CM
    Intracranial 05CL
    Lesser Saphenous
      Left 06CS
      Right 06CR
    Lower 06CY
    Portal 06C8
    Pulmonary
      Left 02CT
      Right 02CS
    Renal
      Left 06CB
      Right 06C9
    Splenic 06C1
    Subclavian
      Left 05C6
      Right 05C5
    Superior Mesenteric
      06C5
    Upper 05CY
    Vertebral
      Left 05CS
      Right 05CR
  Vena Cava
    Inferior 06C0
    Superior 02CV
  Ventricle
    Left 02CL
    Right 02CK
  Vertebra
    Cervical 0PC3
    Lumbar 0QC0
    Thoracic 0PC4
  Vesicle
    Bilateral 0VC3
    Left 0VC2
    Right 0VC1
  Vitreous
    Left 08C5
    Right 08C4
  Vocal Cord
    Left 0CCV
    Right 0CCT
  Vulva 0UCM
Extracorporeal shock wave lithotripsy
  see Fragmentation
Extracranial-intracranial bypass (EC-IC)
  see Bypass, Upper Arteries 031
Extraction
  Auditory Ossicle
    Left 09DA0ZZ
    Right 09D90ZZ
  Bone Marrow
    Iliac 07DR
    Sternum 07DQ
    Vertebral 07DS
  Bursa and Ligament
    Abdomen
      Left 0MDJ
      Right 0MDH
    Ankle
      Left 0MDR
      Right 0MDQ
    Elbow
      Left 0MD4
      Right 0MD3
    Foot
      Left 0MDT
      Right 0MDS

Extraction (continued)
  Bursa and Ligament (continued)
    Hand
      Left 0MD8
      Right 0MD7
    Head and Neck 0MD0
    Hip
      Left 0MDM
      Right 0MDL
    Knee
      Left 0MDP
      Right 0MDN
    Lower Extremity
      Left 0MDW
      Right 0MDV
    Perineum 0MDK
    Shoulder
      Left 0MD2
      Right 0MD1
    Thorax
      Left 0MDG
      Right 0MDF
    Trunk
      Left 0MDD
      Right 0MDC
    Upper Extremity
      Left 0MDB
      Right 0MD9
    Wrist
      Left 0MD6
      Right 0MD5
  Cerebral Meninges 00D1
  Cornea
    Left 08D9XZ
    Right 08D8XZ
  Dura Mater 00D2
  Endometrium 0UDB
  Finger Nail 0HDQXZZ
  Hair 0HDSXZZ
  Kidney
    Left 0TD1
    Right 0TD0
  Lens
    Left 08DK3ZZ
    Right 08DJ3ZZ
  Nerve
    Abdominal Sympathetic
      01DM
    Abducens 00DL
    Accessory 00DR
    Acoustic 00DN
    Brachial Plexus 01D3
    Cervical 01D1
    Cervical Plexus 01D0
    Facial 00DM
    Femoral 01DD
    Glossopharyngeal 00DP
    Head and Neck Sympathetic
      01DK
    Hypoglossal 00DS
    Lumbar 01DB
    Lumbar Plexus 01D9
    Lumbar Sympathetic 01DN
    Lumbosacral Plexus 01DA
    Median 01D5
    Oculomotor 00DH
    Olfactory 00DF
    Optic 00DG
    Peroneal 01DH
    Phrenic 01D2
    Pudendal 01DC
    Radial 01D6
    Sacral 01DR
    Sacral Plexus 01DQ
    Sacral Sympathetic 01DP
    Sciatic 01DF
    Thoracic 01D8
    Thoracic Sympathetic
      01DL
    Tibial 01DG
    Trigeminal 00DK
    Trochlear 00DJ
    Ulnar 01D4
    Vagus 00DQ
  Ova 0UDN
  Pleura
    Left 0BDP
    Right 0BDN
  Products of Conception
    Classical 10D00Z0
    Ectopic 10D2
    Extraperitoneal 10D00Z2
    High Forceps 10D07Z5
    Internal Version 10D07Z7
    Low Cervical 10D00Z1

Extraction (continued)
  Products of Conception (continued)
    Low Forceps 10D07Z3
    Mid Forceps 10D07Z4
    Other 10D07Z8
    Retained 10D1
    Vacuum 10D07Z6
  Septum, Nasal 09DM
  Sinus
    Accessory 09DP
    Ethmoid
      Left 09DV
      Right 09DU
    Frontal
      Left 09DT
      Right 09DS
    Mastoid
      Left 09DC
      Right 09DB
    Maxillary
      Left 09DR
      Right 09DQ
    Sphenoid
      Left 09DX
      Right 09DW
  Skin
    Abdomen 0HD7XZZ
    Back 0HD6XZZ
    Buttock 0HD8XZZ
    Chest 0HD5XZZ
    Ear
      Left 0HD3XZZ
      Right 0HD2XZZ
    Face 0HD1XZZ
    Foot
      Left 0HDNXZZ
      Right 0HDMXZZ
    Genitalia 0HDAXZZ
    Hand
      Left 0HDGXZZ
      Right 0HDFXZZ
    Lower Arm
      Left 0HDEXZZ
      Right 0HDDXZZ
    Lower Leg
      Left 0HDLXZZ
      Right 0HDKXZZ
    Neck 0HD4XZZ
    Perineum 0HD9XZZ
    Scalp 0HD0XZZ
    Upper Arm
      Left 0HDCXZZ
      Right 0HDBXZZ
    Upper Leg
      Left 0HDJXZZ
      Right 0HDHXZZ
  Spinal Meninges 00DT
  Subcutaneous Tissue and Fascia
    Abdomen 0JD8
    Back 0JD7
    Buttock 0JD9
    Chest 0JD6
    Face 0JD1
    Foot
      Left 0JDR
      Right 0JDQ
    Hand
      Left 0JDK
      Right 0JDJ
    Lower Arm
      Left 0JDH
      Right 0JDG
    Lower Leg
      Left 0JDP
      Right 0JDN
    Neck
      Anterior 0JD4
      Posterior 0JD5
    Pelvic Region 0JDC
    Perineum 0JDB
    Scalp 0JD0
    Upper Arm
      Left 0JDF
      Right 0JDD
    Upper Leg
      Left 0JDM
      Right 0JDL
  Toe Nail 0HDRXZZ
  Tooth
    Lower 0CDXXZ
    Upper 0CDWXZ
  Turbinate, Nasal 09DL
  Tympanic Membrane
    Left 09D8
    Right 09D7

Fluoroscopy *(continued)*
  Artery *(continued)*
    Upper
      Other B31N
        Laser, Intraoperative B31N
      Upper Extremity
        Bilateral B31K
          Laser, Intraoperative B31K
        Left B31J
          Laser, Intraoperative B31J
        Right B31H
          Laser, Intraoperative B31H
      Vertebral
        Bilateral B31G
          Laser, Intraoperative B31G
        Left B31F
          Laser, Intraoperative B31F
        Right B31D
          Laser, Intraoperative B31D
  Bile Duct BF10
    Pancreatic Duct and Gallbladder BF14
  Bile Duct and Gallbladder BF13
  Biliary Duct BF11
  Bladder BT10
    Kidney and Ureter BT14
    Left BT1F
    Right BT1D
  Bladder and Urethra BT1B
  Bowel, Small BD1
  Calcaneus
    Left BQ1KZZZ
    Right BQ1JZZZ
  Clavicle
    Left BP15ZZZ
    Right BP14ZZZ
  Coccyx BR1F
  Colon BD14
  Corpora Cavernosa BV10
  Dialysis Fistula B51W
  Dialysis Shunt B51W
  Diaphragm BB16ZZZ
  Disc
    Cervical BR11
    Lumbar BR13
    Thoracic BR12
  Duodenum BD19
  Elbow
    Left BP1H
    Right BP1G
  Epiglottis B91G
  Esophagus BD11
  Extremity
    Lower BW1C
    Upper BW1J
  Facet Joint
    Cervical BR14
    Lumbar BR16
    Thoracic BR15
  Fallopian Tube
    Bilateral BU12
    Left BU11
    Right BU10
  Fallopian Tube and Uterus BU18
  Femur
    Left BQ14ZZZ
    Right BQ13ZZZ
  Finger
    Left BP1SZZZ
    Right BP1RZZZ
  Foot
    Left BQ1MZZZ
    Right BQ1LZZZ
  Forearm
    Left BP1KZZZ
    Right BP1JZZZ
  Gallbladder BF12
    Bile Duct and Pancreatic Duct BF14
  Gallbladder and Bile Duct BF13
  Gastrointestinal, Upper BD1
  Hand
    Left BP1PZZZ
    Right BP1NZZZ
  Head and Neck BW19
  Heart
    Left B215
    Right B214
    Right and Left B216
  Hip
    Left BQ11
    Right BQ10
  Humerus
    Left BP1BZZZ
    Right BP1AZZZ
  Ileal Diversion Loop BT1C
  Ileal Loop, Ureters and Kidney BT1G
  Intracranial Sinus B512

Fluoroscopy *(continued)*
  Joint
    Acromioclavicular, Bilateral BP13ZZZ
    Finger
      Left BP1D
      Right BP1C
    Foot
      Left BQ1Y
      Right BQ1X
    Hand
      Left BP1D
      Right BP1C
    Lumbosacral BR1B
    Sacroiliac BR1D
    Sternoclavicular
      Bilateral BP12ZZZ
      Left BP11ZZZ
      Right BP10ZZZ
    Temporomandibular
      Bilateral BN19
      Left BN18
      Right BN17
    Thoracolumbar BR18
    Toe
      Left BQ1Y
      Right BQ1X
  Kidney
    Bilateral BT13
    Ileal Loop and Ureter BT1G
    Left BT12
    Right BT11
    Ureter and Bladder BT14
      Left BT1F
      Right BT1D
  Knee
    Left BQ18
    Right BQ17
  Larynx B91J
  Leg
    Left BQ1FZZZ
    Right BQ1DZZZ
  Lung
    Bilateral BB14ZZZ
    Left BB13ZZZ
    Right BB12ZZZ
  Mediastinum BB1CZZZ
  Mouth BD1B
  Neck and Head BW19
  Oropharynx BD1B
  Pancreatic Duct BF1
    Gallbladder and Bile Duct BF14
  Patella
    Left BQ1WZZZ
    Right BQ1VZZZ
  Pelvis BR1C
  Pelvis and Abdomen BW11
  Pharynix B91G
  Ribs
    Left BP1YZZZ
    Right BP1XZZZ
  Sacrum BR1F
  Scapula
    Left BP17ZZZ
    Right BP16ZZZ
  Shoulder
    Left BP19
    Right BP18
  Sinus, Intracranial B512
  Spinal Cord B01B
  Spine
    Cervical BR10
    Lumbar BR19
    Thoracic BR17
    Whole BR1G
  Sternum BR1H
  Stomach BD12
  Toe
    Left BQ1QZZZ
    Right BQ1PZZZ
  Tracheobronchial Tree
    Bilateral BB19YZZ
    Left BB18YZZ
    Right BB17YZZ
  Ureter
    Ileal Loop and Kidney BT1G
    Kidney and Bladder BT14
      Left BT1F
      Right BT1D
    Left BT17
    Right BT16
  Urethra BT15
  Urethra and Bladder BT1B
  Uterus BU16
  Uterus and Fallopian Tube BU18
  Vagina BU19
  Vasa Vasorum BV18

Fluoroscopy *(continued)*
  Vein
    Cerebellar B511
    Cerebral B511
    Epidural B510
    Jugular
      Bilateral B515
      Left B514
      Right B513
    Lower Extremity
      Bilateral B51D
      Left B51C
      Right B51B
    Other B51V
    Pelvic (Iliac)
      Left B51G
      Right B51F
    Pelvic (Iliac) Bilateral B51H
    Portal B51T
    Pulmonary
      Bilateral B51S
      Left B51R
      Right B51Q
    Renal
      Bilateral B51L
      Left B51K
      Right B51J
    Spanchnic B51T
    Subclavian
      Left B517
      Right B516
    Upper Extremity
      Bilateral B51P
      Left B51N
      Right B51M
    Vena Cava
      Inferior B519
      Superior B518
    Wrist
      Left BP1M
      Right BP1L
Flushing
  see Irrigation
Foley catheter
  use Drainage Device
Foramen magnum
  use Bone, Occipital, Right
  use Bone, Occipital, Left
Foramen of Monro (intraventricular)
  use Cerebral Ventricle
Foreskin
  use Prepuce
Formula™ Balloon-Expandable Renal Stent System
  use Intraluminal Device
Fossa of Rosenmuller
  use Nasopharynx
Fourth cranial nerve
  use Nerve, Trochlear
Fourth ventricle
  use Cerebral Ventricle
Fovea
  use Retina, Right
  use Retina, Left
Fragmentation
  Ampulla of Vater 0FFC
  Anus 0DFQ
  Appendix 0DFJ
  Bladder 0TFB
  Bladder Neck 0TFC
  Bronchus
    Lingula 0BF9
    Lower Lobe
      Left 0BFB
      Right 0BF6
    Main
      Left 0BF7
      Right 0BF3
    Middle Lobe, Right 0BF5
    Upper Lobe
      Left 0BF8
      Right 0BF4
  Carina 0BF2
  Cavity, Cranial 0WF1
  Cecum 0DFH
  Cerebral Ventricle 00F6
  Colon
    Ascending 0DFK
    Descending 0DFM
    Sigmoid 0DFN
    Transverse 0DFL
  Duct
    Common Bile 0FF9
    Cystic 0FF8
    Hepatic
      Left 0FF6
      Right 0FF5

Glossectomy
  see Excision, Tongue 0CB7
  see Resection, Tongue 0CT7
Glossoepiglottic fold
  use Epiglottis
Glossopexy
  see Repair, Tongue 0CQ7
  see Reposition, Tongue 0CS7
Glossoplasty
  see Repair, Tongue 0CQ7
  see Replacement, Tongue 0CR7
  see Supplement, Tongue 0CU7
Glossorrhaphy
  see Repair, Tongue 0CQ7
Glossotomy
  see Drainage, Tongue 0C97
Glottis
  use Larynx
Gluteal Artery Perforator Flap
  Bilateral 0HRV079
  Left 0HRU079
  Right 0HRT079
Gluteal lymph node
  use Lymphatic, Pelvis
Gluteal vein
  use Vein, Hypogastric, Right
  use Vein, Hypogastric, Left
Gluteus maximus muscle
  use Muscle, Hip, Right
  use Muscle, Hip, Left
Gluteus medius muscle
  use Muscle, Hip, Right
  use Muscle, Hip, Left
Gluteus minimus muscle
  use Muscle, Hip, Left
  use Muscle, Hip, Right
GORE® DUALMESH®
  use Synthetic Substitute
Gracilis muscle
  use Muscle, Upper Leg, Left
  use Muscle, Upper Leg, Right
Graft
  see Replacement
  see Supplement
Great auricular nerve
  use Nerve, Cervical Plexus
Great cerebral vein
  use Vein, Intracranial
Great saphenous vein
  use Vein, Greater Saphenous, Left
  use Vein, Greater Saphenous, Right
Greater alar cartilage
  use Nose
Greater occipital nerve
  use Nerve, Cervical
Greater splanchnic nerve
  use Nerve, Thoracic Sympathetic
Greater superficial petrosal nerve
  use Nerve, Facial
Greater trochanter
  use Femur, Upper, Left
  use Femur, Upper, Right
Greater tuberosity
  use Humeral Head, Right
  use Humeral Head, Left
Greater vestibular (Bartholin's) gland
  use Gland, Vestibular
Greater wing
  use Bone, Sphenoid, Left
  use Bone, Sphenoid, Right
Guedel airway
  use Intraluminal Device, Airway in Mouth and Throat
Guidance, catheter placement
  EKG
    see Measurement, Physiological Systems 4A0
  Fluoroscopy
    see Fluoroscopy, Veins B51
  Ultrasound
    see Ultrasonography, Veins B54

H

Hallux
  use Toe, 1st, Right
  use Toe, 1st, Left
Hamate bone
  use Carpal, Right
  use Carpal, Left
Hancock Bioprosthesis (aortic) (mitral) valve
  use Zooplastic Tissue in Heart and Great Vessels
Hancock Bioprosthetic Valved Conduit
  use Zooplastic Tissue in Heart and Great Vessels
Harvesting, stem cells
  see Pheresis, Circulatory 6A55

Head of fibula
  use Fibula, Right
  use Fibula, Left
Hearing Aid Assessment F14Z
Hearing Assessment F13Z
Hearing Device
  Bone Conduction
    Left 09HE
    Right 09HD
  Insertion of device in
    Left 0NH6
    Right 0NH5
  Multiple Channel Cochlear Prosthesis
    Left 09HE
    Right 09HD
  Removal of device from, Skull 0NP0
  Revision of device in, Skull 0NW0
  Single Channel Cochlear Prosthesis
    Left 09HE
    Right 09HD
Hearing Treatment F09Z
Heart Assist System
  External
    Insertion of device in, Heart 02HA
    Removal of device from, Heart 02PA
    Revision of device in, Heart 02WA
  Implantable
    Insertion of device in, Heart 02HA
    Removal of device from, Heart 02PA
    Revision of device in, Heart 02WA
HeartMate II® Left Ventricular Assist Device (LVAD)
  use Implantable Heart Assist System in Heart and Great Vessels
HeartMate XVE® Left Ventricular Assist Device (LVAD)
  use Implantable Heart Assist System in Heart and Great Vessels
HeartMate® implantable heart assist system
  see Insertion of device in, Heart 02HA
Helix
  use Ear, External, Bilateral
  use Ear, External, Right
  use Ear, External, Left
Hemicolectomy
  see Resection, Gastrointestinal System 0DT
Hemicystectomy
  see Excision, Urinary System 0TB
Hemigastrectomy
  see Excision, Gastrointestinal System 0DB
Hemiglossectomy
  see Excision, Mouth and Throat 0CB
Hemilaminectomy
  see Excision, Upper Bones 0PB
  see Excision, Lower Bones 0QB
Hemilaryngectomy
  see Excision, Larynx 0CBS
Hemimandibulectomy
  see Excision, Head and Facial Bones 0NB
Hemimaxillectomy
  see Excision, Head and Facial Bones 0NB
Hemipylorectomy
  see Excision, Gastrointestinal System 0DB
Hemispherectomy
  see Excision, Central Nervous System 00B
  see Resection, Central Nervous System 00T
Hemithyroidectomy
  see Resection, Endocrine System 0GT
  see Excision, Endocrine System 0GB
Hemodialysis 5A1D00Z
Hepatectomy
  see Excision, Hepatobiliary System and Pancreas 0FB
  see Resection, Hepatobiliary System and Pancreas 0FT
Hepatic artery proper
  use Artery, Hepatic
Hepatic flexure
  use Colon, Ascending
Hepatic lymph node
  use Lymphatic, Aortic
Hepatic plexus
  use Nerve, Abdominal Sympathetic
Hepatic portal vein
  use Vein, Portal
Hepaticoduodenostomy
  see Bypass, Hepatobiliary System and Pancreas 0F1
  see Drainage, Hepatobiliary System and Pancreas 0F9
Hepaticotomy
  see Drainage, Hepatobiliary System and Pancreas 0F9
Hepatocholedochostomy
  see Drainage, Duct, Common Bile 0F99
Hepatogastric ligament
  use Omentum, Lesser
Hepatopancreatic ampulla
  use Ampulla of Vater

Hepatopexy
  see Repair, Hepatobiliary System and Pancreas 0FQ
  see Reposition, Hepatobiliary System and Pancreas 0FS
Hepatorrhaphy
  see Repair, Hepatobiliary System and Pancreas 0FQ
Hepatotomy
  see Drainage, Hepatobiliary System and Pancreas 0F9
Herniorrhaphy
  see Repair, Anatomical Regions, General 0WQ
  see Repair, Anatomical Regions, Lower Extremities 0YQ
  with synthetic substitute
  see Supplement, Anatomical Regions, General 0WU
  see Supplement, Anatomical Regions, Lower Extremities 0YU
Hip (joint) liner
  use Liner in Lower Joints
Holter monitoring 4A12X45
Holter valve ventricular shunt
  use Synthetic Substitute
Humeroradial joint
  use Joint, Elbow, Right
  use Joint, Elbow, Left
Humeroulnar joint
  use Joint, Elbow, Left
  use Joint, Elbow, Right
Humerus, distal
  use Humeral Shaft, Right
  use Humeral Shaft, Left
Hydrocelectomy
  see Excision, Male Reproductive System 0VB
Hydrotherapy
  Assisted exercise in pool
    see Motor Treatment, Rehabilitation F07
  Whirlpool
    see Activities of Daily Living Treatment, Rehabilitation F08
Hymenectomy
  see Excision, Hymen 0UBK
  see Resection, Hymen 0UTK
Hymenoplasty
  see Repair, Hymen 0UQK
  see Supplement, Hymen 0UUK
Hymenorrhaphy
  see Repair, Hymen 0UQK
Hymenotomy
  see Division, Hymen 0U8K
  see Drainage, Hymen 0U9K
Hyoglossus muscle
  use Muscle, Tongue, Palate, Pharynx
Hyoid artery
  use Artery, Thyroid, Right
  use Artery, Thyroid, Left
Hyperalimentation
  see Introduction of substance in or on
Hyperbaric oxygenation
  Decompression sickness treatment
    see Decompression, Circulatory 6A15
  Wound treatment
    see Assistance, Circulatory 5A05
Hyperthermia
  Radiation Therapy
    Abdomen DWY38ZZ
    Adrenal Gland DGY28ZZ
    Bile Ducts DFY28ZZ
    Bladder DTY28ZZ
    Bone, Other DPYC8ZZ
    Bone Marrow D7Y08ZZ
    Brain D0Y08ZZ
    Brain Stem D0Y18ZZ
    Breast
      Left DMY08ZZ
      Right DMY18ZZ
    Bronchus DBY18ZZ
    Cervix DUY18ZZ
    Chest DWY28ZZ
    Chest Wall DBY78ZZ
    Colon DDY58ZZ
    Diaphragm DBY88ZZ
    Duodenum DDY28ZZ
    Ear D9Y08ZZ
    Esophagus DDY08ZZ
    Eye D8Y08ZZ
    Femur DPY98ZZ
    Fibula DPYB8ZZ
    Gallbladder DFY18ZZ
    Gland
      Adrenal DGY28ZZ
      Parathyroid DGY48ZZ
      Pituitary DGY08ZZ
      Thyroid DGY58ZZ
    Glands, Salivary D9Y68ZZ
    Head and Neck DWY18ZZ
    Hemibody DWY48ZZ

Hyperthermia (continued)
  Radiation Therapy (continued)
    Humerus DPY68ZZ
    Hypopharynx D9Y38ZZ
    Ileum DDY48ZZ
    Jejunum DDY38ZZ
    Kidney DTY08ZZ
    Larynx D9YB8ZZ
    Liver DFY08ZZ
    Lung DBY28ZZ
    Lymphatics
      Abdomen D7Y68ZZ
      Axillary D7Y48ZZ
      Inguinal D7Y88ZZ
      Neck D7Y38ZZ
      Pelvis D7Y78ZZ
      Thorax D7Y58ZZ
    Mandible DPY38ZZ
    Maxilla DPY28ZZ
    Mediastinum DBY68ZZ
    Mouth D9Y48ZZ
    Nasopharynx D9YD8ZZ
    Neck and Head DWY18ZZ
    Nerve, Peripheral D0Y78ZZ
    Nose D9Y18ZZ
    Oropharynx D9YF8ZZ
    Ovary DUY08ZZ
    Palate
      Hard D9Y88ZZ
      Soft D9Y98ZZ
    Pancreas DFY38ZZ
    Parathyroid Gland DGY48ZZ
    Pelvic Bones DPY88ZZ
    Pelvic Region DWY68ZZ
    Pineal Body DGY18ZZ
    Pituitary Gland DGY08ZZ
    Pleura DBY58ZZ
    Prostate DVY08ZZ
    Radius DPY78ZZ
    Rectum DDY78ZZ
    Rib DPY58ZZ
    Sinuses D9Y78ZZ
    Skin
      Abdomen DHY88ZZ
      Arm DHY48ZZ
      Back DHY78ZZ
      Buttock DHY98ZZ
      Chest DHY68ZZ
      Face DHY28ZZ
      Leg DHYB8ZZ
      Neck DHY38ZZ
    Skull DPY08ZZ
    Spinal Cord D0Y68ZZ
    Spleen D7Y28ZZ
    Sternum DPY48ZZ
    Stomach DDY18ZZ
    Testis DVY18ZZ
    Thymus D7Y18ZZ
    Thyroid Gland DGY58ZZ
    Tibia DPYB8ZZ
    Tongue D9Y58ZZ
    Trachea DBY08ZZ
    Ulna DPY78ZZ
    Ureter DTY18ZZ
    Urethra DTY38ZZ
    Uterus DUY28ZZ
    Whole Body DWY58ZZ
  Whole Body 6A3Z
Hypnosis GZFZZZZ
Hypogastric artery
  use Artery, Internal Iliac, Right
  use Artery, Internal Iliac, Left
Hypopharynx
  use Pharynx
Hypophysectomy
  see Excision, Gland, Pituitary 0GB0
  see Resection, Gland, Pituitary 0GT0
Hypophysis
  use Gland, Pituitary
Hypothalamotomy
  see Destruction, Thalamus 0059
Hypothenar muscle
  use Muscle, Hand, Right
  use Muscle, Hand, Left
Hypothermia, Whole Body 6A4Z
Hysterectomy
  see Excision, Uterus 0UB9
  see Resection, Uterus 0UT9
Hysterolysis
  see Release, Uterus 0UN9
Hysteropexy
  see Repair, Uterus 0UQ9
  see Reposition, Uterus 0US9
Hysteroplasty
  see Repair, Uterus 0UQ9

Hysterorrhaphy
  see Repair, Uterus 0UQ9
Hysteroscopy 0UJD8ZZ
Hysterotomy
  see Drainage, Uterus 0U99
Hysterotrachelectomy
  see Resection, Uterus 0UT9
Hysterotracheloplasty
  see Repair, Uterus 0UQ9
Hysterotrachelorrhaphy
  see Repair, Uterus 0UQ9

I

IABP (Intra-aortic balloon pump)
  see Assistance, Cardiac 5A02
IAEMT (Intraoperative anesthetic effect monitoring and titration)
  see Monitoring, Central Nervous 4A10
Ileal artery
  use Artery, Superior Mesenteric
Ileectomy
  see Excision, Ileum 0DBB
  see Resection, Ileum 0DTB
Ileocolic artery
  use Artery, Superior Mesenteric
Ileocolic vein
  use Vein, Colic
Ileopexy
  see Repair, Ileum 0DQB
  see Reposition, Ileum 0DSB
Ileorrhaphy
  see Repair, Ileum 0DQB
Ileoscopy 0DJD8ZZ
Ileostomy
  see Bypass, Ileum 0D1B
  see Drainage, Ileum 0D9B
Ileotomy
  see Drainage, Ileum 0D9B
Ileoureterostomy
  see Bypass, Urinary System 0T1
Iliac crest
  use Bone, Pelvic, Left
  use Bone, Pelvic, Right
Iliac fascia
  use Subcutaneous Tissue and Fascia, Upper Leg, Left
  use Subcutaneous Tissue and Fascia, Upper Leg, Right
Iliac lymph node
  use Lymphatic, Pelvis
Iliacus muscle
  use Muscle, Hip, Right
  use Muscle, Hip, Left
Iliofemoral ligament
  use Bursa and Ligament, Hip, Left
  use Bursa and Ligament, Hip, Right
Iliohypogastric nerve
  use Nerve, Lumbar Plexus
Ilioinguinal nerve
  use Nerve, Lumbar Plexus
Iliolumbar artery
  use Artery, Internal Iliac, Left
  use Artery, Internal Iliac, Right
Iliolumbar ligament
  use Bursa and Ligament, Trunk, Left
  use Bursa and Ligament, Trunk, Right
Iliotibial tract (band)
  use Subcutaneous Tissue and Fascia, Upper Leg, Right
  use Subcutaneous Tissue and Fascia, Upper Leg, Left
Ilium
  use Bone, Pelvic, Left
  use Bone, Pelvic, Right
Ilizarov external fixator
  use External Fixation Device, Ring in 0PH
  use External Fixation Device, Ring in 0PS
  use External Fixation Device, Ring in 0QH
  use External Fixation Device, Ring in 0QS
Ilizarov-Vecklich device
  use External Fixation Device, Limb Lengthening in 0PH
  use External Fixation Device, Limb Lengthening in 0QH
Imaging, diagnostic
  see Plain Radiography
  see Fluoroscopy
  see Computerized Tomography (CT Scan)
  see Magnetic Resonance Imaging (MRI)
  see Ultrasonography
Immobilization
  Abdominal Wall 2W33X
  Arm
    Lower
      Left 2W3DX
      Right 2W3CX

Immobilization (continued)
  Arm (continued)
    Upper
      Left 2W3BX
      Right 2W3AX
  Back 2W35X
  Chest Wall 2W34X
  Extremity
    Lower
      Left 2W3MX
      Right 2W3LX
    Upper
      Left 2W39X
      Right 2W38X
  Face 2W31X
  Finger
    Left 2W3KX
    Right 2W3JX
  Foot
    Left 2W3TX
    Right 2W3SX
  Hand
    Left 2W3FX
    Right 2W3EX
  Head 2W30X
  Inguinal Region
    Left 2W37X
    Right 2W36X
  Leg
    Lower
      Left 2W3RX
      Right 2W3QX
    Upper
      Left 2W3PX
      Right 2W3NX
  Neck 2W32X
  Thumb
    Left 2W3H
    Right 2W3GX
  Toe
    Left 2W3VX
    Right 2W3UX
Immunization
  see Introduction of Serum, Toxoid, and Vaccine
Immunotherapy
  see Introduction of Immunotherapeutic Substance
Immunotherapy, antineoplastic
  Interferon
    see Introduction of Low-dose Interleukin-2
  Interleukin-2, high-dose
    see Introduction of High-dose Interleukin-2
  Interleukin-2, low-dose
    see Introduction of Low-dose Interleukin-2
  Monoclonal antibody
    see Introduction of Monoclonal Antibody
  Proleukin, high-dose
    see Introduction of High-dose Interleukin-2
  Proleukin, low-dose
    see Introduction of Low-dose Interleukin-2
Impella® (2.5)(5.0)(LD) cardiac assist device
  use Intraluminal Device
Impeller Pump
  Continuous, Output 5A0221D
  Intermittent, Output 5A0211D
Implantable cardioverter-defibrillator (ICD)
  use Defibrillator Generator in 0JH
Implantable drug infusion pump (anti-spasmodic) (chemotherapy)(pain)
  use Infusion Device, Pump in Subcutaneous Tissue and Fascia
Implantable glucose monitoring device
  use Monitoring Device
Implantable hemodynamic monitor (IHM)
  use Monitoring Device, Hemodynamic in 0JH
Implantable hemodynamic monitoring system (IHMS)
  use Monitoring Device, Hemodynamic in 0JH
Implantable Miniature Telescope™ (IMT)
  use Synthetic Substitute, Intraocular Telescope in 08R
Implantation
  see Insertion
  see Replacement
Implanted (venous)(access) port
  use Vascular Access Device, Reservoir in Subcutaneous Tissue and Fascia
IMV (intermittent mandatory ventilation)
  see Assistance, Respiratory 5A09
In Vitro Fertilization 8E0ZXY1
Incision, abscess
  see Drainage
Incudectomy
  see Excision, Ear, Nose, Sinus 09B
  see Resection, Ear, Nose, Sinus 09T
Incudopexy
  see Reposition, Ear, Nose, Sinus 09S
  see Repair, Ear, Nose, Sinus 09Q

Incus
    use Auditory Ossicle, Left
    use Auditory Ossicle, Right
Induction of labor
    Artificial rupture of membranes
        see Drainage, Pregnancy 109
    Oxytocin
        see Introduction of Hormone
InDura, intrathecal catheter (1P) (spinal)
    use Infusion Device
Inferior cardiac nerve
    use Nerve, Thoracic Sympathetic
Inferior cerebellar vein
    use Vein, Intracranial
Inferior cerebral vein
    use Vein, Intracranial
Inferior epigastric artery
    use Artery, External Iliac, Right
    use Artery, External Iliac, Left
Inferior epigastric lymph node
    use Lymphatic, Pelvis
Inferior genicular artery
    use Artery, Popliteal, Left
    use Artery, Popliteal, Right
Inferior gluteal artery
    use Artery, Internal Iliac, Right
    use Artery, Internal Iliac, Left
Inferior gluteal nerve
    use Nerve, Sacral Plexus
Inferior hypogastric plexus
    use Nerve, Abdominal Sympathetic
Inferior labial artery
    use Artery, Face
Inferior longitudinal muscle
    use Muscle, Tongue, Palate, Pharynx
Inferior mesenteric ganglion
    use Nerve, Abdominal Sympathetic
Inferior mesenteric lymph node
    use Lymphatic, Mesenteric
Inferior mesenteric plexus
    use Nerve, Abdominal Sympathetic
Inferior oblique muscle
    use Muscle, Extraocular, Right
    use Muscle, Extraocular, Left
Inferior pancreaticoduodenal artery
    use Artery, Superior Mesenteric
Inferior phrenic artery
    use Aorta, Abdominal
Inferior rectus muscle
    use Muscle, Extraocular, Right
    use Muscle, Extraocular, Left
Inferior suprarenal artery
    use Artery, Renal, Left
    use Artery, Renal, Right
Inferior tarsal plate
    use Eyelid, Lower, Right
    use Eyelid, Lower, Left
Inferior thyroid vein
    use Vein, Innominate, Left
    use Vein, Innominate, Right
Inferior tibiofibular joint
    use Joint, Ankle, Right
    use Joint, Ankle, Left
Inferior turbinate
    use Turbinate, Nasal
Inferior ulnar collateral artery
    use Artery, Brachial, Right
    use Artery, Brachial, Left
Inferior vesical artery
    use Artery, Internal Iliac, Right
    use Artery, Internal Iliac, Left
Infraauricular lymph node
    use Lymphatic, Head
Infraclavicular (deltopectoral) lymph node
    use Lymphatic, Upper Extremity, Left
    use Lymphatic, Upper Extremity, Right
Infrahyoid muscle
    use Muscle, Neck, Left
    use Muscle, Neck, Right
Infraparotid lymph node
    use Lymphatic, Head
Infraspinatus fascia
    use Subcutaneous Tissue and Fascia, Upper Arm, Right
    use Subcutaneous Tissue and Fascia, Upper Arm, Left
Infraspinatus muscle
    use Muscle, Shoulder, Right
    use Muscle, Shoulder, Left
Infundibulopelvic ligament
    use Uterine Supporting Structure
Infusion
    see Introduction of substance in or on
Infusion Device
    Insertion of device in
        Abdomen 0JH8
        Back 0JH7

Infusion Device *(continued)*
    Insertion of device in *(continued)*
        Chest 0JH6
        Lower Arm
            Left 0JHH
            Right 0JHG
        Lower Leg
            Left 0JHP
            Right 0JHN
        Trunk 0JHT
        Upper Arm
            Left 0JHF
            Right 0JHD
        Upper Leg
            Left 0JHM
            Right 0JHL
    Removal of device from
        Lower Extremity 0JPW
        Trunk 0JPT
        Upper Extremity 0JPV
    Revision of device in
        Lower Extremity 0JWW
        Trunk 0JWT
        Upper Extremity 0JWV
Infusion, glucarpidase
    Central vein 3E043GQ
    Peripheral vein 3E033GQ
Inguinal canal
    use Inguinal Region, Right
    use Inguinal Region, Left
    use Inguinal Region, Bilateral
Inguinal triangle
    use Inguinal Region, Right
    use Inguinal Region, Bilateral
    use Inguinal Region, Left
Injection
    see Introduction of substance in or on
Injection reservoir, port
    use Vascular Access Device, Reservoir in Subcutaneous
        Tissue and Fascia
Injection reservoir, pump
    use Infusion Device, Pump in Subcutaneous Tissue
        and Fascia
Insemination, artificial 3E0P7LZ
Insertion
    Antimicrobial envelope
        see Introduction of Anti-infective
    Aqueous drainage shunt
        see Bypass, Eye 081
        see Drainage, Eye 089
    Products of Conception 10H0
    Spinal Stabilization Device
        see Insertion of device in, Upper Joints 0RH
        see Insertion of device in, Lower Joints 0SH
Insertion of device in
    Abdominal Wall 0WHF
    Acetabulum
        Left 0QH5
        Right 0QH4
    Anal Sphincter 0DHR
    Ankle Region
        Left 0YHL
        Right 0YHK
    Anus 0DHQ
    Aorta
        Abdominal 04H0
        Thoracic 02HW
    Arm
        Lower
            Left 0XHF
            Right 0XHD
        Upper
            Left 0XH9
            Right 0XH8
    Artery
        Anterior Tibial
            Left 04HQ
            Right 04HP
        Axillary
            Left 03H6
            Right 03H5
        Brachial
            Left 03H8
            Right 03H7
        Celiac 04H1
        Colic
            Left 04H7
            Middle 04H8
            Right 04H6
        Common Carotid
            Left 03HJ
            Right 03HH
        Common Iliac
            Left 04HD
            Right 04HC

Insertion of device in *(continued)*
    Artery *(continued)*
        External Carotid
            Left 03HN
            Right 03HM
        External Iliac
            Left 04HJ
            Right 04HH
        Face 03HR
        Femoral
            Left 04HL
            Right 04HK
        Foot
            Left 04HW
            Right 04HV
        Gastric 04H2
        Hand
            Left 03HF
            Right 03HD
        Hepatic 04H3
        Inferior Mesenteric 04HB
        Innominate 03H2
        Internal Carotid
            Left 03HL
            Right 03HK
        Internal Iliac
            Left 04HF
            Right 04HE
        Internal Mammary
            Left 03H1
            Right 03H0
        Intracranial 03HG
        Lower 04HY
        Peroneal
            Left 04HU
            Right 04HT
        Popliteal
            Left 04HN
            Right 04HM
        Posterior Tibial
            Left 04HS
            Right 04HR
        Pulmonary
            Left 02HR
            Right 02HQ
        Pulmonary Trunk 02HP
        Radial
            Left 03HC
            Right 03HB
        Renal
            Left 04HA
            Right 04H9
        Splenic 04H4
        Subclavian
            Left 03H4
            Right 03H3
        Superior Mesenteric 04H5
        Temporal
            Left 03HT
            Right 03HS
        Thyroid
            Left 03HV
            Right 03HU
        Ulnar
            Left 03HA
            Right 03H9
        Upper 03HY
        Vertebral
            Left 03HQ
            Right 03HP
    Atrium
        Left 02H7
        Right 02H6
    Axilla
        Left 0XH5
        Right 0XH4
    Back
        Lower 0WHL
        Upper 0WHK
    Bladder 0THB
    Bladder Neck 0THC
    Bone
        Ethmoid
            Left 0NHG
            Right 0NHF
        Facial 0NHW
        Frontal
            Left 0NH2
            Right 0NH1
        Hyoid 0NHX
        Lacrimal
            Left 0NHJ
            Right 0NHH
        Lower 0QHY
        Nasal 0NHB

Insertion of device in (continued)
    Radius
        Left 0PHJ
        Right 0PHH
    Rectum 0DHP
    Respiratory Tract 0WHQ
    Retroperitoneum 0WHH
    Rib
        Left 0PH2
        Right 0PH1
    Sacrum 0QH1
    Scapula
        Left 0PH6
        Right 0PH5
    Scrotum and Tunica Vaginalis 0VH8
    Shoulder Region
        Left 0XH3
        Right 0XH2
    Skull 0NH0
    Spinal Canal 00HU
    Spinal Cord 00HV
    Spleen 07HP
    Sternum 0PH0
    Stomach 0DH6
    Subcutaneous Tissue and Fascia
        Abdomen 0JH8
        Back 0JH7
        Buttock 0JH9
        Chest 0JH6
        Face 0JH1
        Foot
            Left 0JHR
            Right 0JHQ
        Hand
            Left 0JHK
            Right 0JHJ
        Head and Neck 0JHS
        Lower Arm
            Left 0JHH
            Right 0JHG
        Lower Extremity 0JHW
        Lower Leg
            Left 0JHP
            Right 0JHN
        Neck
            Anterior 0JH4
            Posterior 0JH5
        Pelvic Region 0JHC
        Perineum 0JHB
        Scalp 0JH0
        Trunk 0JHT
        Upper Arm
            Left 0JHF
            Right 0JHD
        Upper Extremity 0JHV
        Upper Leg
            Left 0JHM
            Right 0JHL
    Tarsal
        Left 0QHM
        Right 0QHL
    Testis 0VHD
    Thymus 07HM
    Tibia
        Left 0QHH
        Right 0QHG
    Tongue 0CH7
    Trachea 0BH1
    Tracheobronchial Tree 0BH0
    Ulna
        Left 0PHL
        Right 0PHK
    Ureter 0TH9
    Urethra 0THD
    Uterus 0UH9
    Uterus and Cervix 0UHD
    Vagina 0UHG
    Vagina and Cul-de-sac
        0UHH
    Vas Deferens 0VHR
    Vein
        Axillary
            Left 05H8
            Right 05H7
        Azygos 05H0
        Basilic
            Left 05HC
            Right 05HB
        Brachial
            Left 05HA
            Right 05H9
        Cephalic
            Left 05HF
            Right 05HD
        Colic 06H7

Insertion of device in (continued)
    Vein (continued)
        Common Iliac
            Left 06HD
            Right 06HC
        Coronary 02H4
        Esophageal 06H3
        External Iliac
            Left 06HG
            Right 06HF
        External Jugular
            Left 05HQ
            Right 05HP
        Face
            Left 05HV
            Right 05HT
        Femoral
            Left 06HN
            Right 06HM
        Foot
            Left 06HV
            Right 06HT
        Gastric 06H2
        Greater Saphenous
            Left 06HQ
            Right 06HP
        Hand
            Left 05HH
            Right 05HG
        Hemiazygos 05H1
        Hepatic 06H4
        Hypogastric
            Left 06HJ
            Right 06HH
        Inferior Mesenteric 06H6
        Innominate
            Left 05H4
            Right 05H3
        Internal Jugular
            Left 05HN
            Right 05HM
        Intracranial 05HL
        Lesser Saphenous
            Left 06HS
            Right 06HR
        Lower 06HY
        Portal 06H8
        Pulmonary
            Left 02HT
            Right 02HS
        Renal
            Left 06HB
            Right 06H9
        Splenic 06H1
        Subclavian
            Left 05H6
            Right 05H5
        Superior Mesenteric
            06H5
        Upper 05HY
        Vertebral
            Left 05HS
            Right 05HR
    Vena Cava
        Inferior 06H0
        Superior 02HV
    Ventricle
        Left 02HL
        Right 02HK
    Vertebra
        Cervical 0PH3
        Lumbar 0QH0
        Thoracic 0PH4
    Wrist Region
        Left 0XHH
        Right 0XHG

Inspection
    Abdominal Wall
        0WJF
    Ankle Region
        Left 0YJL
        Right 0YJK
    Arm
        Lower
            Left 0XJF
            Right 0XJD
        Upper
            Left 0XJ9
            Right 0XJ8
    Artery
        Lower 04JY
        Upper 03JY
    Axilla
        Left 0XJ5
        Right 0XJ4

Inspection (continued)
    Back
        Lower 0WJL
        Upper 0WJK
    Bladder 0TJB
    Bone
        Facial 0NJW
        Lower 0QJY
        Nasal 0NJB
        Upper 0PJY
    Bone Marrow 07JT
    Brain 00J0
    Breast
        Left 0HJU
        Right 0HJT
    Bursa and Ligament
        Lower 0MJY
        Upper 0MJX
    Buttock
        Left 0YJ1
        Right 0YJ0
    Cavity, Cranial 0WJ1
    Chest Wall 0WJ8
    Cisterna Chyli 07JL
    Diaphragm 0BJT
    Disc
        Cervical Vertebral 0RJ3
        Cervicothoracic Vertebral 0RJ5
        Lumbar Vertebral 0SJ2
        Lumbosacral 0SJ4
        Thoracic Vertebral 0RJ9
        Thoracolumbar Vertebral
            0RJB
    Duct
        Hepatobiliary 0FJB
        Pancreatic 0FJD
    Ear
        Inner
            Left 09JE
            Right 09JD
        Left 09JJ
        Right 09JH
    Elbow Region
        Left 0XJC
        Right 0XJB
    Epididymis and Spermatic Cord
        0VJM
    Extremity
        Lower
            Left 0YJB
            Right 0YJ9
        Upper
            Left 0XJ7
            Right 0XJ6
    Eye
        Left 08J1XZZ
        Right 08J0XZZ
    Face 0WJ2
    Fallopian Tube 0UJ8
    Femoral Region
        Bilateral 0YJE
        Left 0YJ8
        Right 0YJ7
    Finger Nail 0HJQXZZ
    Foot
        Left 0YJN
        Right 0YJM
    Gallbladder 0FJ4
    Gastrointestinal Tract 0WJP
    Genitourinary Tract 0WJR
    Gland
        Adrenal 0GJ5
        Endocrine 0GJS
        Pituitary 0GJ0
        Salivary 0CJA
    Great Vessel 02JY
    Hand
        Left 0XJK
        Right 0XJJ
    Head 0WJ0
    Heart 02JA
    Inguinal Region
        Bilateral 0YJA
        Left 0YJ6
        Right 0YJ5
    Intestinal Tract
        Lower 0DJD
        Upper 0DJ0
    Jaw
        Lower 0WJ5
        Upper 0WJ4
    Joint
        Acromioclavicular
            Left 0RJH
            Right 0RJG

Interventricular septum
  use Septum, Ventricular
Intestinal lymphatic trunk
  use Cisterna Chyli
Intraluminal Device
  Airway
    Esophagus 0DH5
    Mouth and Throat 0CHY
    Nasopharynx 09HN
  Bioactive
    Occlusion
      Common Carotid
        Left 03LJ
        Right 03LH
      External Carotid
        Left 03LN
        Right 03LM
      Internal Carotid
        Left 03LL
        Right 03LK
      Intracranial 03LG
      Vertebral
        Left 03LQ
        Right 03LP
    Restriction
      Common Carotid
        Left 03VJ
        Right 03VH
      External Carotid
        Left 03VN
        Right 03VM
      Internal Carotid
        Left 03VL
        Right 03VK
      Intracranial 03VG
      Vertebral
        Left 03VQ
        Right 03VP
  Endobronchial Valve
    Lingula 0BH9
    Lower Lobe
      Left 0BHB
      Right 0BH6
    Main
      Left 0BH7
      Right 0BH3
    Middle Lobe, Right 0BH5
    Upper Lobe
      Left 0BH8
      Right 0BH4
  Endotracheal Airway
    Change device in, Trachea 0B21XEZ
    Insertion of device in, Trachea
      0BH1
  Pessary
    Change device in, Vagina and Cul-de-sac
      0U2HXGZ
    Insertion of device in
      Cul-de-sac 0UHF
      Vagina 0UHG
Intramedullary (IM) rod (nail)
  use Internal Fixation Device, Intramedullary in Upper
    Bones
  use Internal Fixation Device, Intramedullary in Lower
    Bones
Intramedullary skeletal kinetic distractor (ISKD)
  use Internal Fixation Device, Intramedullary in Upper
    Bones
  use Internal Fixation Device, Intramedullary in Lower
    Bones
Intraocular Telescope
  Left 08RK30Z
  Right 08RJ30Z
Intraoperative Radiation Therapy (IORT)
  Anus DDY8CZZ
  Bile Ducts DFY2CZZ
  Bladder DTY2CZZ
  Cervix DUY1CZZ
  Colon DDY5CZZ
  Duodenum DDY2CZZ
  Gallbladder DFY1CZZ
  Ileum DDY4CZZ
  Jejunum DDY3CZZ
  Kidney DTY0CZZ
  Larynx D9YBCZZ
  Liver DFY0CZZ
  Mouth D9Y4CZZ
  Nasopharynx D9YDCZZ
  Ovary DUY0CZZ
  Pancreas DFY3CZZ
  Pharynx D9YCCZZ
  Prostate DVY0CZZ
  Rectum DDY7CZZ
  Stomach DDY1CZZ
  Ureter DTY1CZZ

Intraoperative Radiation Therapy (IORT) *(continued)*
  Urethra DTY3CZZ
  Uterus DUY2CZZ
Intrauterine device (IUD)
  use Contraceptive Device in Female Reproductive
    System
Introduction of substance in or on
  Artery
    Central 3E06
      Analgesics 3E06
      Anesthetic, Intracirculatory 3E06
      Anti-infective 3E06
      Anti-inflammatory 3E06
      Antiarrhythmic 3E06
      Antineoplastic 3E06
      Destructive Agent 3E06
      Diagnostic Substance, Other 3E06
      Electrolytic Substance 3E06
      Hormone 3E06
      Hypnotics 3E06
      Immunotherapeutic 3E06
      Nutritional Substance 3E06
      Platelet Inhibitor 3E06
      Radioactive Substance 3E06
      Sedatives 3E06
      Serum 3E06
      Thrombolytic 3E06
      Toxoid 3E06
      Vaccine 3E06
      Vasopressor 3E06
      Water Balance Substance 3E06
    Coronary 3E07
      Diagnostic Substance, Other 3E07
      Platelet Inhibitor 3E07
      Thrombolytic 3E07
    Peripheral 3E05
      Analgesics 3E05
      Anesthetic, Intracirculatory 3E05
      Anti-infective 3E052
      Anti-inflammatory 3E05
      Antiarrhythmic 3E05
      Antineoplastic 3E05
      Destructive Agent 3E05
      Diagnostic Substance, Other 3E05
      Electrolytic Substance 3E05
      Hormone 3E05
      Hypnotics 3E05
      Immunotherapeutic 3E05
      Nutritional Substance 3E05
      Platelet Inhibitor 3E05
      Radioactive Substance 3E05
      Sedatives 3E05
      Serum 3E05
      Thrombolytic 3E05
      Toxoid 3E05
      Vaccine 3E05
      Vasopressor 3E05
      Water Balance Substance 3E05
  Biliary Tract 3E0J
    Analgesics 3E0J
    Anesthetic, Local 3E0J
    Anti-infective 3E0J
    Anti-inflammatory 3E0J
    Antineoplastic 3E0J
    Destructive Agent 3E0J
    Diagnostic Substance, Other 3E0J
    Electrolytic Substance 3E0J
    Gas 3E0J
    Hypnotics 3E0J
    Islet Cells, Pancreatic 3E0J
    Nutritional Substance 3E0J
    Radioactive Substance 3E0J
    Sedatives 3E0J
    Water Balance Substance 3E0J
  Bone 3E0V
    Analgesics 3E0V3NZ
    Anesthetic, Local 3E0V3BZ
    Anti-infective 3E0V32
    Anti-inflammatory 3E0V33Z
    Antineoplastic 3E0V30
    Destructive Agent 3E0V3TZ
    Diagnostic Substance, Other 3E0V3KZ
    Electrolytic Substance 3E0V37Z
    Hypnotics 3E0V3NZ
    Nutritional Substance 3E0V36Z
    Radioactive Substance 3E0V3HZ
    Sedatives 3E0V3NZ
    Water Balance Substance 3E0V37Z
  Bone Marrow 3E0A3GC
    Antineoplastic 3E0A30
  Brain 3E0Q3GC
    Analgesics 3E0Q3NZ
    Anesthetic, Local 3E0Q3BZ
    Anti-infective 3E0Q32
    Anti-inflammatory 3E0Q33Z

Introduction of substance in or on *(continued)*
  Brain 3E0Q3GC *(continued)*
    Antineoplastic 3E0Q
    Destructive Agent 3E0Q3TZ
    Diagnostic Substance, Other 3E0Q3KZ
    Electrolytic Substance 3E0Q37Z
    Gas 3E0Q
    Hypnotics 3E0Q3NZ
    Nutritional Substance 3E0Q36Z
    Radioactive Substance 3E0Q3HZ
    Sedatives 3E0Q3NZ
    Stem Cells
      Embryonic 3E0Q
      Somatic 3E0Q
    Water Balance Substance 3E0Q37Z
  Cranial Cavity 3E0Q3GC
    Analgesics 3E0Q3NZ
    Anesthetic, Local 3E0Q3BZ
    Anti-infective 3E0Q32
    Anti-inflammatory 3E0Q33Z
    Antineoplastic 3E0Q
    Destructive Agent 3E0Q3TZ
    Diagnostic Substance, Other 3E0Q3KZ
    Electrolytic Substance 3E0Q37Z
    Gas 3E0Q
    Hypnotics 3E0Q3NZ
    Nutritional Substance 3E0Q36Z
    Radioactive Substance 3E0Q3HZ
    Sedatives 3E0Q3NZ
    Stem Cells
      Embryonic 3E0Q
      Somatic 3E0Q
    Water Balance Substance 3E0Q37Z
  Ear 3E0B
    Analgesics 3E0B
    Anesthetic, Local 3E0B
    Anti-infective 3E0B
    Anti-inflammatory 3E0B
    Antineoplastic 3E0B
    Destructive Agent 3E0B
    Diagnostic Substance, Other 3E0B
    Hypnotics 3E0B
    Radioactive Substance 3E0B
    Sedatives 3E0B
  Epidural Space 3E0S3GC
    Analgesics 3E0S3NZ
    Anesthetic
      Local 3E0S3BZ
      Regional 3E0S3CZ
    Anti-infective 3E0S32
    Anti-inflammatory 3E0S33Z
    Antineoplastic 3E0S30
    Destructive Agent 3E0S3TZ
    Diagnostic Substance, Other 3E0S3KZ
    Electrolytic Substance 3E0S37Z
    Gas 3E0S
    Hypnotics 3E0S3NZ
    Nutritional Substance 3E0S36Z
    Radioactive Substance 3E0S3HZ
    Sedatives 3E0S3NZ
    Water Balance Substance 3E0S37Z
  Eye 3E0C
    Analgesics 3E0C
    Anesthetic, Local 3E0C
    Anti-infective 3E0C
    Anti-inflammatory 3E0C
    Antineoplastic 3E0C
    Destructive Agent 3E0C
    Diagnostic Substance, Other 3E0C
    Gas 3E0C
    Hypnotics 3E0C
    Pigment 3E0C
    Radioactive Substance 3E0C
    Sedatives 3E0C
  Gastrointestinal Tract
    Lower 3E0H
      Analgesics 3E0H
      Anesthetic, Local 3E0H
      Anti-infective 3E0H
      Anti-inflammatory 3E0H
      Antineoplastic 3E0H
      Destructive Agent 3E0H
      Diagnostic Substance, Other 3E0H
      Electrolytic Substance 3E0H
      Gas 3E0H
      Hypnotics 3E0H
      Nutritional Substance 3E0H
      Radioactive Substance 3E0H
      Sedatives 3E0H
      Water Balance Substance 3E0H
    Upper 3E0G
      Analgesics 3E0G
      Anesthetic, Local 3E0G
      Anti-infective 3E0G
      Anti-inflammatory 3E0G

Introduction of substance in or on (continued)
  Respiratory Tract 3E0F (continued)
    Antineoplastic 3E0F
    Destructive Agent 3E0F
    Diagnostic Substance, Other 3E0F
    Electrolytic Substance 3E0F
    Gas 3E0F
    Hypnotics 3E0F
    Nutritional Substance 3E0F
    Radioactive Substance 3E0F
    Sedatives 3E0F
    Water Balance Substance 3E0F
  Skin 3E00XGC
    Analgesics 3E00XNZ
    Anesthetic, Local 3E00XBZ
    Anti-infective 3E00X2
    Anti-inflammatory 3E00X3Z
    Antineoplastic 3E00X0
    Destructive Agent 3E00XTZ
    Diagnostic Substance, Other 3E00XKZ
    Hypnotics 3E00XNZ
    Pigment 3E00XMZ
    Sedatives 3E00XNZ
    Serum 3E00X4Z
    Toxoid 3E00X4Z
    Vaccine 3E00X4Z
  Spinal Canal 3E0R3GC
    Analgesics 3E0R3NZ
    Anesthetic
      Local 3E0R3BZ
      Regional 3E0R3CZ
    Anti-infective 3E0R32
    Anti-inflammatory 3E0R33Z
    Antineoplastic 3E0R30
    Destructive Agent 3E0R3TZ
    Diagnostic Substance, Other 3E0R3KZ
    Electrolytic Substance 3E0R37Z
    Gas 3E0R
    Hypnotics 3E0R3NZ
    Nutritional Substance 3E0R36Z
    Radioactive Substance 3E0R3HZ
    Sedatives 3E0R3NZ
    Stem Cells
      Embryonic 3E0R
      Somatic 3E0R
    Water Balance Substance 3E0R37Z
  Subcutaneous Tissue 3E013GC
    Analgesics 3E013NZ
    Anesthetic, Local 3E013BZ
    Anti-infective 3E01
    Anti-inflammatory 3E0133Z
    Antineoplastic 3E0130
    Destructive Agent 3E013TZ
    Diagnostic Substance, Other 3E013KZ
    Electrolytic Substance 3E0137Z
    Hormone 3E013V
    Hypnotics 3E013NZ
    Nutritional Substance 3E0136Z
    Radioactive Substance 3E013HZ
    Sedatives 3E013NZ
    Serum 3E0134Z
    Toxoid 3E0134Z
    Vaccine 3E0134Z
    Water Balance Substance 3E0137Z
  Vein
    Central 3E04
      Analgesics 3E04
      Anesthetic, Intracirculatory 3E04
      Anti-infective 3E04
      Anti-inflammatory 3E04
      Antiarrhythmic 3E04
      Antineoplastic 3E04
      Destructive Agent 3E04
      Diagnostic Substance, Other 3E04
      Electrolytic Substance 3E04
      Hormone 3E04
      Hypnotics 3E04
      Immunotherapeutic 3E04
      Nutritional Substance 3E04
      Platelet Inhibitor 3E04
      Radioactive Substance 3E04
      Sedatives 3E04
      Serum 3E04
      Thrombolytic 3E04
      Toxoid 3E04
      Vaccine 3E04
      Vasopressor 3E04
      Water Balance Substance 3E04
    Peripheral 3E03
      Analgesics 3E03
      Anesthetic, Intracirculatory 3E03
      Anti-infective 3E03
      Anti-inflammatory 3E03
      Antiarrhythmic 3E03
      Antineoplastic 3E03

Introduction of substance in or on (continued)
  Vein (continued)
    Peripheral 3E03 (continued)
      Destructive Agent 3E03
      Diagnostic Substance, Other 3E03
      Electrolytic Substance 3E03
      Hormone 3E03
      Hypnotics 3E03
      Immunotherapeutic 3E03
      Islet Cells, Pancreatic 3E03
      Nutritional Substance 3E03
      Platelet Inhibitor 3E03
      Radioactive Substance 3E03
      Sedatives 3E03
      Serum 3E03
      Thrombolytic 3E03
      Toxoid 3E03
      Vaccine 3E03
      Vasopressor 3E03
      Water Balance Substance 3E03

Intubation
  Airway
    see Insertion of device in, Trachea 0BH1
    see Insertion of device in, Mouth and Throat 0CHY
    see Insertion of device in, Esophagus 0DH5
  Drainage device
    see Drainage
  Feeding Device
    see Insertion of device in, Gastrointestinal System 0DH
IPPB (intermittent positive pressure breathing)
  see Assistance, Respiratory 5A09
Iridectomy
  see Excision, Eye 08B
  see Resection, Eye 08T
Iridoplasty
  see Repair, Eye 08Q
  see Replacement, Eye 08R
  see Supplement, Eye 08U
Iridotomy
  see Drainage, Eye 089
Irrigation
  Biliary Tract, Irrigating Substance 3E1J
  Brain, Irrigating Substance 3E1Q38Z
  Cranial Cavity, Irrigating Substance 3E1Q38Z
  Ear, Irrigating Substance 3E1B
  Epidural Space, Irrigating Substance 3E1S38Z
  Eye, Irrigating Substance 3E1C
  Gastrointestinal Tract
    Lower, Irrigating Substance 3E1H
    Upper, Irrigating Substance 3E1G
  Genitourinary Tract, Irrigating Substance 3E1K
  Irrigating Substance 3C1ZX8Z
  Joint, Irrigating Substance 3E1U38Z
  Mucous Membrane, Irrigating Substance 3E10
  Nose, Irrigating Substance 3E19
  Pancreatic Tract, Irrigating Substance 3E1J
  Pericardial Cavity, Irrigating Substance 3E1Y38Z
  Peritoneal Cavity
    Dialysate 3E1M39Z
    Irrigating Substance 3E1M38Z
  Pleural Cavity, Irrigating Substance 3E1L38Z
  Reproductive
    Female, Irrigating Substance 3E1P
    Male, Irrigating Substance 3E1N
  Respiratory Tract, Irrigating Substance 3E1F
  Skin, Irrigating Substance 3E10
  Spinal Canal, Irrigating Substance 3E1R38Z
Ischiatic nerve
  use Nerve, Sciatic
Ischiocavernosus muscle
  use Muscle, Perineum
Ischiofemoral ligament
  use Bursa and Ligament, Hip, Left
  use Bursa and Ligament, Hip, Right
Ischium
  use Bone, Pelvic, Right
  use Bone, Pelvic, Left
Isolation 8E0ZXY6
Isotope Administration, Whole Body DWY5G
Itrel (3)(4) neurostimulator
  use Stimulator Generator, Single Array in 0JH

J

Jejunal artery
  use Artery, Superior Mesenteric
Jejunectomy
  see Excision, Jejunum 0DBA
  see Resection, Jejunum 0DTA
Jejunocolostomy
  see Bypass, Gastrointestinal System 0D1
  see Drainage, Gastrointestinal System 0D9

Jejunopexy
  see Repair, Jejunum 0DQA
  see Reposition, Jejunum 0DSA
Jejunostomy
  see Bypass, Jejunum 0D1A
  see Drainage, Jejunum 0D9A
Jejunotomy
  see Drainage, Jejunum 0D9A
Joint fixation plate
  use Internal Fixation Device in Upper Joints
  use Internal Fixation Device in Lower Joints
Joint liner (insert)
  use Liner in Lower Joints
Joint spacer (antibiotic)
  use Spacer in Upper Joints
  use Spacer in Lower Joints
Jugular body
  use Glomus Jugulare
Jugular lymph node
  use Lymphatic, Neck, Left
  use Lymphatic, Neck, Right

K

Kappa
  use Pacemaker, Dual Chamber in 0JH
Keratectomy, kerectomy
  see Excision, Eye 08B
  see Resection, Eye 08T
Keratocentesis
  see Drainage, Eye 089
Keratoplasty
  see Repair, Eye 08Q
  see Replacement, Eye 08R
  see Supplement, Eye 08U
Keratotomy
  see Drainage, Eye 089
  see Repair, Eye 08Q
Kinetra® neurostimulator
  use Stimulator Generator, Multiple Array in 0JH
Kirschner wire (K-wire)
  use Internal Fixation Device in Head and Facial Bones
  use Internal Fixation Device in Upper Bones
  use Internal Fixation Device in Lower Bones
  use Internal Fixation Device in Upper Joints
  use Internal Fixation Device in Lower Joints
Knee (implant) insert
  use Liner in Lower Joints
KUB x-ray
  see Plain Radiography, Kidney, Ureter and Bladder BT04
Kuntscher nail
  use Internal Fixation Device, Intramedullary in Upper Bones
  use Internal Fixation Device, Intramedullary in Lower Bones

L

Labia majora
  use Vulva
Labia minora
  use Vulva
Labial gland
  use Lip, Upper
  use Lip, Lower
Labiectomy
  see Excision, Female Reproductive System 0UB
  see Resection, Female Reproductive System 0UT
Lacrimal canaliculus
  use Duct, Lacrimal, Left
  use Duct, Lacrimal, Right
Lacrimal punctum
  use Duct, Lacrimal, Right
  use Duct, Lacrimal, Left
Lacrimal sac
  use Duct, Lacrimal, Right
  use Duct, Lacrimal, Left
Laminectomy
  see Excision, Upper Bones 0PB
  see Excision, Lower Bones 0QB
Laminotomy
  see Drainage, Upper Joints 0R9
  see Drainage, Lower Joints 0S9
  see Release, Upper Joints 0RN
  see Release, Lower Joints 0SN
  see Release, Central Nervous System 00N
  see Release, Peripheral Nervous System 01N
LAP-BAND® adjustable gastric banding system
  use Extraluminal Device
Laparoscopy
  see Inspection

Laparotomy
  Drainage
    see Drainage, Peritoneal Cavity 0W9G
  Exploratory
    see Inspection, Peritoneal Cavity 0WJG
Laryngectomy
  see Excision, Larynx 0CBS
  see Resection, Larynx 0CTS
Laryngocentesis
  see Drainage, Larynx 0C9S
Laryngogram
  see Fluoroscopy, Larynx B91J
Laryngopexy
  see Repair, Larynx 0CQS
Laryngopharynx
  use Pharynx
Laryngoplasty
  see Repair, Larynx 0CQS
  see Replacement, Larynx 0CRS
  see Supplement, Larynx 0CUS
Laryngorrhaphy
  see Repair, Larynx 0CQS
Laryngoscopy 0CJS8ZZ
Laryngotomy
  see Drainage, Larynx 0C9S
Laser Interstitial Thermal Therapy
  Adrenal Gland DGY2KZZ
  Anus DDY8KZZ
  Bile Ducts DFY2KZZ
  Brain D0Y0KZZ
  Brain Stem D0Y1KZZ
  Breast
    Left DMY0KZZ
    Right DMY1KZZ
  Bronchus DBY1KZZ
  Chest Wall DBY7KZZ
  Colon DDY5KZZ
  Diaphragm DBY8KZZ
  Duodenum DDY2KZZ
  Esophagus DDY0KZZ
  Gallbladder DFY1KZZ
  Gland
    Adrenal DGY2KZZ
    Parathyroid DGY4KZZ
    Pituitary DGY0KZZ
    Thyroid DGY5KZZ
  Ileum DDY4KZZ
  Jejunum DDY3KZZ
  Liver DFY0KZZ
  Lung DBY2KZZ
  Mediastinum DBY6KZZ
  Nerve, Peripheral D0Y7KZZ
  Pancreas DFY3KZZ
  Parathyroid Gland DGY4KZZ
  Pineal Body DGY1KZZ
  Pituitary Gland DGY0KZZ
  Pleura DBY5KZZ
  Prostate DVY0KZZ
  Rectum DDY7KZZ
  Spinal Cord D0Y6KZZ
  Stomach DDY1KZZ
  Thyroid Gland DGY5KZZ
  Trachea DBY0KZZ
Lateral (brachial) lymph node
  use Lymphatic, Axillary, Left
  use Lymphatic, Axillary, Right
Lateral canthus
  use Eyelid, Upper, Right
  use Eyelid, Upper, Left
Lateral collateral ligament (LCL)
  use Bursa and Ligament, Knee, Right
  use Bursa and Ligament, Knee, Left
Lateral condyle of femur
  use Femur, Lower, Right
  use Femur, Lower, Left
Lateral condyle of tibia
  use Tibia, Left
  use Tibia, Right
Lateral cuneiform bone
  use Tarsal, Right
  use Tarsal, Left
Lateral epicondyle of femur
  use Femur, Lower, Left
  use Femur, Lower, Right
Lateral epicondyle of humerus
  use Humeral Shaft, Right
  use Humeral Shaft, Left
Lateral femoral cutaneous nerve
  use Nerve, Lumbar Plexus
Lateral malleolus
  use Fibula, Right
  use Fibula, Left
Lateral meniscus
  use Joint, Knee, Left
  use Joint, Knee, Right

Lateral nasal cartilage
  use Nose
Lateral plantar artery
  use Artery, Foot, Left
  use Artery, Foot, Right
Lateral plantar nerve
  use Nerve, Tibial
Lateral rectus muscle
  use Muscle, Extraocular, Left
  use Muscle, Extraocular, Right
Lateral sacral artery
  use Artery, Internal Iliac, Left
  use Artery, Internal Iliac, Right
Lateral sacral vein
  use Vein, Hypogastric, Left
  use Vein, Hypogastric, Right
Lateral sural cutaneous nerve
  use Nerve, Peroneal
Lateral tarsal artery
  use Artery, Foot, Right
  use Artery, Foot, Left
Lateral temporomandibular ligament
  use Bursa and Ligament, Head and
    Neck
Lateral thoracic artery
  use Artery, Axillary, Left
  use Artery, Axillary, Right
Latissimus dorsi muscle
  use Muscle, Trunk, Left
  use Muscle, Trunk, Right
Latissimus Dorsi Myocutaneous Flap
  Bilateral 0HRV075
  Left 0HRU075
  Right 0HRT075
Lavage
  see Irrigation
  bronchial alveolar, diagnostic
    see Drainage, Respiratory System
    0B9
Least splanchnic nerve
  use Nerve, Thoracic Sympathetic
Left ascending lumbar vein
  use Vein, Hemiazygos
Left atrioventricular valve
  use Valve, Mitral
Left auricular appendix
  use Atrium, Left
Left colic vein
  use Vein, Colic
Left coronary sulcus
  use Heart, Left
Left gastric artery
  use Artery, Gastric
Left gastroepiploic artery
  use Artery, Splenic
Left gastroepiploic vein
  use Vein, Splenic
Left inferior phrenic vein
  use Vein, Renal, Left
Left inferior pulmonary vein
  use Vein, Pulmonary, Left
Left jugular trunk
  use Lymphatic, Thoracic Duct
Left lateral ventricle
  use Cerebral Ventricle
Left ovarian vein
  use Vein, Renal, Left
Left second lumbar vein
  use Vein, Renal, Left
Left subclavian trunk
  use Lymphatic, Thoracic Duct
Left subcostal vein
  use Vein, Hemiazygos
Left superior pulmonary vein
  use Vein, Pulmonary, Left
Left suprarenal vein
  use Vein, Renal, Left
Left testicular vein
  use Vein, Renal, Left
Lengthening
  Bone, with device
    see Insertion of Limb Lengthening Device
  Muscle, by incision
    see Division, Muscles 0K8
  Tendon, by incision
    see Division, Tendons 0L8
Leptomeninges
  use Cerebral Meninges
  use Spinal Meninges
Lesser alar cartilage
  use Nose
Lesser occipital nerve
  use Nerve, Cervical Plexus
Lesser splanchnic nerve
  use Nerve, Thoracic Sympathetic

Lesser trochanter
  use Femur, Upper, Right
  use Femur, Upper, Left
Lesser tuberosity
  use Humeral Head, Left
  use Humeral Head, Right
Lesser wing
  use Bone, Sphenoid, Right
  use Bone, Sphenoid, Left
Leukopheresis, therapeutic
  see Pheresis, Circulatory 6A55
Levator anguli oris muscle
  use Muscle, Facial
Levator ani muscle
  use Muscle, Trunk, Left
  use Muscle, Trunk, Right
Levator labii superioris alaeque nasi muscle
  use Muscle, Facial
Levator labii superioris muscle
  use Muscle, Facial
Levator palpebrae superioris muscle
  use Eyelid, Upper, Left
  use Eyelid, Upper, Right
Levator scapulae muscle
  use Muscle, Neck, Left
  use Muscle, Neck, Right
Levator veli palatini muscle
  use Muscle, Tongue, Palate, Pharynx
Levatores costarum muscle
  use Muscle, Thorax, Left
  use Muscle, Thorax, Right
LifeStent® (Flexstar)(XL) Vascular Stent System
  use Intraluminal Device
Ligament of head of fibula
  use Bursa and Ligament, Knee, Right
  use Bursa and Ligament, Knee, Left
Ligament of the lateral malleolus
  use Bursa and Ligament, Ankle, Left
  use Bursa and Ligament, Ankle, Right
Ligamentum flavum
  use Bursa and Ligament, Trunk, Left
  use Bursa and Ligament, Trunk, Right
Ligation
  see Occlusion
Ligation, hemorrhoid
  see Occlusion, Lower Veins, Hemorrhoidal Plexus
Light Therapy GZJZZZZ
Liner
  Removal of device from
    Hip
      Left 0SPB09Z
      Right 0SP909Z
    Knee
      Left 0SPD09Z
      Right 0SPC09Z
  Revision of device in
    Hip
      Left 0SWB09Z
      Right 0SW909Z
    Knee
      Left 0SWD09Z
      Right 0SWC09Z
  Supplement
    Hip
      Left 0SUB09Z
        Acetabular Surface 0SUE09Z
        Femoral Surface 0SUS09Z
      Right 0SU909Z
        Acetabular Surface 0SUA09Z
        Femoral Surface 0SUR09Z
    Knee
      Left 0SUD09
        Femoral Surface 0SUU09Z
        Tibial Surface 0SUW09Z
      Right 0SUC09
        Femoral Surface 0SUT09Z
        Tibial Surface 0SUV09Z
Lingual artery
  use Artery, External Carotid, Right
  use Artery, External Carotid, Left
Lingual tonsil
  use Tongue
Lingulectomy, lung
  see Excision, Lung Lingula 0BBH
  see Resection, Lung Lingula 0BTH
Lithotripsy
  see Fragmentation
  with removal of fragments
    see Extirpation
LIVIAN™ CRT-D
  use Cardiac Resynchronization Defibrillator Pulse
    Generator in 0JH
Lobectomy
  see Excision, Central Nervous System 00B
  see Excision, Respiratory System 0BB

Lobectomy *(continued)*
  see Resection, Respiratory System 0BT
  see Excision, Hepatobiliary System and Pancreas 0FB
  see Resection, Hepatobiliary System and Pancreas 0FT
  see Excision, Endocrine System 0GB
  see Resection, Endocrine System 0GT
Lobotomy
  see Division, Brain 0080
Localization
  see Map
  see Imaging
Locus ceruleus
  use Pons
Long thoracic nerve
  use Nerve, Brachial Plexus
Loop ileostomy
  see Bypass, Ileum 0D1B
Loop recorder, implantable
  use Monitoring Device
Lower GI series
  see Fluoroscopy, Colon BD14
Lumbar artery
  use Aorta, Abdominal
Lumbar facet joint
  use Joint, Lumbar Vertebral, 2 or more
  use Joint, Lumbar Vertebral
Lumbar ganglion
  use Nerve, Lumbar Sympathetic
Lumbar lymph node
  use Lymphatic, Aortic
Lumbar lymphatic trunk
  use Cisterna Chyli
Lumbar splanchnic nerve
  use Nerve, Lumbar Sympathetic
Lumbosacral facet joint
  use Joint, Lumbosacral
Lumbosacral trunk
  use Nerve, Lumbar
Lumpectomy
  see Excision
Lunate bone
  use Carpal, Left
  use Carpal, Right
Lunotriquetral ligament
  use Bursa and Ligament, Hand, Left
  use Bursa and Ligament, Hand, Right
Lymphadenectomy
  see Excision, Lymphatic and Hemic Systems 07B
  see Resection, Lymphatic and Hemic Systems 07T
Lymphadenotomy
  see Drainage, Lymphatic and Hemic Systems 079
Lymphangiectomy
  see Excision, Lymphatic and Hemic Systems 07B
  see Resection, Lymphatic and Hemic Systems 07T
Lymphangiogram
  see Plain Radiography, Lymphatic System B70
Lymphangioplasty
  see Repair, Lymphatic and Hemic Systems 07Q
  see Supplement, Lymphatic and Hemic Systems 07U
Lymphangiorrhaphy
  see Repair, Lymphatic and Hemic Systems 07Q
Lymphangiotomy
  see Drainage, Lymphatic and Hemic Systems 079
Lysis
  see Release

M

Macula
  use Retina, Right
  use Retina, Left
Magnet extraction, ocular foreign body
  see Extirpation, Eye 08C
Magnetic Resonance Imaging (MRI)
  Abdomen BW30
  Ankle
    Left BQ3H
    Right BQ3G
  Aorta
    Abdominal B430
    Thoracic B330
  Arm
    Left BP3F
    Right BP3E
  Artery
    Celiac B431
    Cervico-Cerebral Arch B33Q
    Common Carotid, Bilateral B335
    Coronary
      Bypass Graft, Multiple B233
      Multiple B231
    Internal Carotid, Bilateral B338
    Intracranial B33R

Magnetic Resonance Imaging (MRI) *(continued)*
  Artery *(continued)*
    Lower Extremity
      Bilateral B43H
      Left B43G
      Right B43F
    Pelvic B43C
    Renal, Bilateral B438
    Spinal B33M
    Superior Mesenteric B434
    Upper Extremity
      Bilateral B33K
      Left B33J
      Right B33H
    Vertebral, Bilateral B33G
  Bladder BT30
  Brachial Plexus BW3P
  Brain B030
  Breast
    Bilateral BH32
    Left BH31
    Right BH30
  Calcaneus
    Left BQ3K
    Right BQ3J
  Chest BW33Y
  Coccyx BR3F
  Connective Tissue
    Lower Extremity BL31
    Upper Extremity BL30
  Corpora Cavernosa BV30
  Disc
    Cervical BR31
    Lumbar BR33
    Thoracic BR32
  Ear B930
  Elbow
    Left BP3H
    Right BP3G
  Eye
    Bilateral B837
    Left B836
    Right B835
  Femur
    Left BQ34
    Right BQ33
  Fetal Abdomen BY33
  Fetal Extremity BY35
  Fetal Head BY30
  Fetal Heart BY31
  Fetal Spine BY34
  Fetal Thorax BY32
  Fetus, Whole BY36
  Foot
    Left BQ3M
    Right BQ3L
  Forearm
    Left BP3K
    Right BP3J
  Gland
    Adrenal, Bilateral BG32
    Parathyroid BG33
    Parotid, Bilateral B936
    Salivary, Bilateral B93D
    Submandibular, Bilateral B939
    Thyroid BG34
  Head BW38
  Heart, Right and Left B236
  Hip
    Left BQ31
    Right BQ30
  Intracranial Sinus B532
  Joint
    Finger
      Left BP3D
      Right BP3C
    Hand
      Left BP3D
      Right BP3C
    Temporomandibular, Bilateral BN39
  Kidney
    Bilateral BT33
    Left BT32
    Right BT31
    Transplant BT39
  Knee
    Left BQ38
    Right BQ37
  Larynx B93J
  Leg
    Left BQ3F
    Right BQ3D
  Liver BF35
  Liver and Spleen BF36
  Lung Apices BB3G

Magnetic Resonance Imaging (MRI) *(continued)*
  Nasopharynx B93F
  Neck BW3F
  Nerve
    Acoustic B03C
    Brachial Plexus BW3P
  Oropharynx B93F
  Ovary
    Bilateral BU35
    Left BU34
    Right BU33
  Ovary and Uterus BU3C
  Pancreas BF37
  Patella
    Left BQ3W
    Right BQ3V
  Pelvic Region BW3G
  Pelvis BR3C
  Pituitary Gland B039
  Plexus, Brachial BW3P
  Prostate BV33
  Retroperitoneum BW3H
  Sacrum BR3F
  Scrotum BV34
  Sella Turcica B039
  Shoulder
    Left BP39
    Right BP38
  Sinus
    Intracranial B532
    Paranasal B932
  Spinal Cord B03B
  Spine
    Cervical BR30
    Lumbar BR39
    Thoracic BR37
  Spleen and Liver BF36
  Subcutaneous Tissue
    Abdomen BH3H
    Extremity
      Lower BH3J
      Upper BH3F
    Head BH3D
    Neck BH3D
    Pelvis BH3H
    Thorax BH3G
  Tendon
    Lower Extremity BL33
    Upper Extremity BL32
  Testicle
    Bilateral BV37
    Left BV36
    Right BV35
  Toe
    Left BQ3Q
    Right BQ3P
  Uterus BU36
    Pregnant BU3B
  Uterus and Ovary BU3C
  Vagina BU39
  Vein
    Cerebellar B531
    Cerebral B531
    Jugular, Bilateral B535
    Lower Extremity
      Bilateral B53D
      Left B53C
      Right B53B
    Other B53V
    Pelvic (Iliac) Bilateral B53H
    Portal B53T
    Pulmonary, Bilateral B53S
    Renal, Bilateral B53L
    Spanchnic B53T
    Upper Extremity
      Bilateral B53P
      Left B53N
      Right B53M
  Vena Cava
    Inferior B539
    Superior B538
  Wrist
    Left BP3M
    Right BP3L
Malleotomy
  see Drainage, Ear, Nose, Sinus 099
Malleus
  use Auditory Ossicle, Right
  use Auditory Ossicle, Left
Mammaplasty, mammoplasty
  see Alteration, Skin and Breast 0H0
  see Repair, Skin and Breast 0HQ
  see Replacement, Skin and Breast 0HR
  see Supplement, Skin and Breast 0HU

Meniscectomy
  see Excision, Lower Joints 0SB
  see Resection, Lower Joints 0ST
Mental foramen
  use Mandible, Left
  use Mandible, Right
Mentalis muscle
  use Muscle, Facial
Mentoplasty
  see Alteration, Jaw, Lower 0W05
Mesenterectomy
  see Excision, Mesentery 0DBV
Mesenteriorrhaphy, mesenterorrhaphy
  see Repair, Mesentery 0DQV
Mesenteriplication
  see Repair, Mesentery 0DQV
Mesoappendix
  use Mesentery
Mesocolon
  use Mesentery
Metacarpal ligament
  use Bursa and Ligament, Hand, Left
  use Bursa and Ligament, Hand, Right
Metacarpophalangeal ligament
  use Bursa and Ligament, Hand, Right
  use Bursa and Ligament, Hand, Left
Metatarsal ligament
  use Bursa and Ligament, Foot, Right
  use Bursa and Ligament, Foot, Left
Metatarsectomy
  see Excision, Lower Bones 0QB
  see Resection, Lower Bones 0QT
Metatarsophalangeal (MTP) joint
  use Joint, Metatarsal-Phalangeal, Left
  use Joint, Metatarsal-Phalangeal, Right
Metatarsophalangeal ligament
  use Bursa and Ligament, Foot, Right
  use Bursa and Ligament, Foot, Left
Metathalamus
  use Thalamus
Micro-Driver stent (RX) (OTW)
  use Intraluminal Device
MicroMed HeartAssist
  use Implantable Heart Assist System in Heart and Great
    Vessels
Micrus CERECYTE microcoil
  use Intraluminal Device, Bioactive in Upper Arteries
Midcarpal joint
  use Joint, Carpal, Right
  use Joint, Carpal, Left
Middle cardiac nerve
  use Nerve, Thoracic
    Sympathetic
Middle cerebral artery
  use Artery, Intracranial
Middle cerebral vein
  use Vein, Intracranial
Middle colic vein
  use Vein, Colic
Middle genicular artery
  use Artery, Popliteal, Left
  use Artery, Popliteal, Right
Middle hemorrhoidal vein
  use Vein, Hypogastric, Left
  use Vein, Hypogastric, Right
Middle rectal artery
  use Artery, Internal Iliac, Right
  use Artery, Internal Iliac, Left
Middle suprarenal artery
  use Aorta, Abdominal
Middle temporal artery
  use Artery, Temporal, Left
  use Artery, Temporal, Right
Middle turbinate
  use Turbinate, Nasal
MitraClip valve repair system
  use Synthetic Substitute
Mitral annulus
  use Valve, Mitral
Mitroflow® Aortic Pericardial Heart Valve
  use Zooplastic Tissue in Heart and Great Vessels
Mobilization, adhesions
  see Release
Molar gland
  use Buccal Mucosa
Monitoring
  Arterial
    Flow
      Coronary 4A13
      Peripheral 4A13
      Pulmonary 4A13
    Pressure
      Coronary 4A13
      Peripheral 4A13
      Pulmonary 4A13

Monitoring *(continued)*
  Arterial *(continued)*
    Pulse
      Coronary 4A13
      Peripheral 4A13
      Pulmonary 4A13
    Saturation, Peripheral 4A13
    Sound, Peripheral 4A13
  Cardiac
    Electrical Activity 4A12
      Ambulatory 4A12X45
      No Qualifier 4A12X4Z
    Output 4A12
    Rate 4A12
    Rhythm 4A12
    Sound 4A12
    Total Activity, Stress 4A12XM4
  Central Nervous
    Conductivity 4A10
    Electrical Activity
      Intraoperative 4A10
      No Qualifier 4A10
    Pressure 4A100BZ
      Intracranial 4A10
    Saturation, Intracranial 4A10
    Temperature, Intracranial 4A10
  Gastrointestinal
    Motility 4A1B
    Pressure 4A1B
    Secretion 4A1B
  Lymphatic
    Flow 4A16
    Pressure 4A16
  Peripheral Nervous
    Conductivity
      Motor 4A11
      Sensory 4A11
    Electrical Activity
      Intraoperative 4A11
      No Qualifier 4A11
  Products of Conception
    Cardiac
      Electrical Activity 4A1H
      Rate 4A1H
      Rhythm 4A1H
      Sound 4A1H
    Nervous
      Conductivity 4A1J
      Electrical Activity 4A1J
      Pressure 4A1J
  Respiratory
    Capacity 4A19
    Flow 4A19
    Rate 4A19
    Resistance 4A19
    Volume 4A19
  Sleep 4A1ZXQZ
  Temperature 4A1Z
  Urinary
    Contractility 4A1D73Z
    Flow 4A1D75Z
    Pressure 4A1D7BZ
    Resistance 4A1D7DZ
    Volume 4A1D7LZ
  Venous
    Flow
      Central 4A14
      Peripheral 4A14
      Portal 4A14
      Pulmonary 4A14
    Pressure
      Central 4A14
      Peripheral 4A14
      Portal 4A14
      Pulmonary 4A14
    Pulse
      Central 4A14
      Peripheral 4A14
      Portal 4A14
      Pulmonary 4A14
    Saturation
      Central 4A14
      Portal 4A14
      Pulmonary 4A14
Monitoring Device
  Abdomen 0JH8
  Chest 0JH6
Motor Function Assessment F01
Motor Treatment F07
MR Angiography
  see Magnetic Resonance Imaging (MRI), Heart B23
  see Magnetic Resonance Imaging (MRI), Upper
    Arteries B33
  see Magnetic Resonance Imaging (MRI), Lower
    Arteries B43

Multiple sleep latency test 4A0ZXQZ
Musculocutaneous nerve
  use Nerve, Brachial Plexus
Musculopexy
  see Repair, Muscles 0KQ
  see Reposition, Muscles 0KS
Musculophrenic artery
  use Artery, Internal Mammary, Left
  use Artery, Internal Mammary, Right
Musculoplasty
  see Repair, Muscles 0KQ
  see Supplement, Muscles 0KU
Musculorrhaphy
  see Repair, Muscles 0KQ
Musculospiral nerve
  use Nerve, Radial
Myectomy
  see Excision, Muscles 0KB
  see Resection, Muscles 0KT
Myelencephalon
  use Medulla Oblongata
Myelogram
  CT
      see Computerized Tomography (CT Scan), Central
        Nervous System B02
  MRI
      see Magnetic Resonance Imaging (MRI), Central
        Nervous System B03
Myenteric (Auerbach's) plexus
  use Nerve, Abdominal Sympathetic
Myomectomy
  see Excision, Female Reproductive System 0UB
Myometrium
  use Uterus
Myopexy
  see Repair, Muscles 0KQ
  see Reposition, Muscles 0KS
Myoplasty
  see Repair, Muscles 0KQ
  see Supplement, Muscles 0KU
Myorrhaphy
  see Repair, Muscles 0KQ
Myoscopy
  see Inspection, Muscles 0KJ
Myotomy
  see Division, Muscles 0K8
  see Drainage, Muscles 0K9
Myringectomy
  see Excision, Ear, Nose, Sinus 09B
  see Resection, Ear, Nose, Sinus 09T
Myringoplasty
  see Repair, Ear, Nose, Sinus 09Q
  see Replacement, Ear, Nose, Sinus 09R
  see Supplement, Ear, Nose, Sinus 09U
Myringostomy
  see Drainage, Ear, Nose, Sinus 099
Myringotomy
  see Drainage, Ear, Nose, Sinus 099

N

Nail bed
  use Finger Nail
  use Toe Nail
Nail plate
  use Finger Nail
  use Toe Nail
Narcosynthesis GZGZZZZ
Nasal cavity
  use Nose
Nasal concha
  use Turbinate, Nasal
Nasalis muscle
  use Muscle, Facial
Nasolacrimal duct
  use Duct, Lacrimal, Right
  use Duct, Lacrimal, Left
Nasopharyngeal airway (NPA)
  use Intraluminal Device, Airway in Ear, Nose, Sinus
Navicular bone
  use Tarsal, Left
  use Tarsal, Right
Near Infrared Spectroscopy, Circulatory System 8E023DZ
Neck of femur
  use Femur, Upper, Right
  use Femur, Upper, Left
Neck of humerus (anatomical)(surgical)
  use Humeral Head, Right
  use Humeral Head, Left
Nephrectomy
  see Excision, Urinary System 0TB
  see Resection, Urinary System 0TT
Nephrolithotomy
  see Extirpation, Urinary System 0TC

Occlusion *(continued)*
  Artery *(continued)*
    Ulnar
      Left 03LA
      Right 03L9
    Upper 03LY
    Vertebral
      Left 03LQ
      Right 03LP
  Atrium, Left 02L7
  Bladder 0TLB
  Bladder Neck 0TLC
  Bronchus
    Lingula 0BL9
    Lower Lobe
      Left 0BLB
      Right 0BL6
    Main
      Left 0BL7
      Right 0BL3
    Middle Lobe, Right 0BL5
    Upper Lobe
      Left 0BL8
      Right 0BL4
  Carina 0BL2
  Cecum 0DLH
  Cisterna Chyli 07LL
  Colon
    Ascending 0DLK
    Descending 0DLM
    Sigmoid 0DLN
    Transverse 0DLL
  Cord
    Bilateral 0VLH
    Left 0VLG
    Right 0VLF
  Cul-de-sac 0ULF
  Duct
    Common Bile 0FL9
    Cystic 0FL8
    Hepatic
      Left 0FL6
      Right 0FL5
    Lacrimal
      Left 08LY
      Right 08LX
    Pancreatic 0FLD
      Accessory 0FLF
    Parotid
      Left 0CLC
      Right 0CLB
  Duodenum 0DL9
  Esophagogastric Junction 0DL4
  Esophagus 0DL5
    Lower 0DL3
    Middle 0DL2
    Upper 0DL1
  Fallopian Tube
    Left 0UL6
    Right 0UL5
  Fallopian Tubes, Bilateral 0UL7
  Ileocecal Valve 0DLC
  Ileum 0DLB
  Intestine
    Large 0DLE
      Left 0DLG
      Right 0DLF
    Small 0DL8
  Jejunum 0DLA
  Kidney Pelvis
    Left 0TL4
    Right 0TL3
  Left atrial appendage (LAA)
    see Occlusion, Atrium, Left 02L7
  Lymphatic
    Aortic 07LD
    Axillary
      Left 07L6
      Right 07L5
    Head 07L0
    Inguinal
      Left 07LJ
      Right 07LH
    Internal Mammary
      Left 07L9
      Right 07L8
    Lower Extremity
      Left 07LG
      Right 07LF
    Mesenteric 07LB
    Neck
      Left 07L2
      Right 07L1
    Pelvis 07LC
    Thoracic Duct 07LK

Occlusion *(continued)*
  Lymphatic *(continued)*
    Thorax 07L7
    Upper Extremity
      Left 07L4
      Right 07L3
  Rectum 0DLP
  Stomach 0DL6
    Pylorus 0DL7
  Trachea 0BL1
  Ureter
    Left 0TL7
    Right 0TL6
  Urethra 0TLD
  Vagina 0ULG
  Vas Deferens
    Bilateral 0VLQ
    Left 0VLP
    Right 0VLN
  Vein
    Axillary
      Left 05L8
      Right 05L7
    Azygos 05L0
    Basilic
      Left 05LC
      Right 05LB
    Brachial
      Left 05LA
      Right 05L9
    Cephalic
      Left 05LF
      Right 05LD
    Colic 06L7
    Common Iliac
      Left 06LD
      Right 06LC
    Esophageal 06L3
    External Iliac
      Left 06LG
      Right 06LF
    External Jugular
      Left 05LQ
      Right 05LP
    Face
      Left 05LV
      Right 05LT
    Femoral
      Left 06LN
      Right 06LM
    Foot
      Left 06LV
      Right 06LT
    Gastric 06L2
    Greater Saphenous
      Left 06LQ
      Right 06LP
    Hand
      Left 05LH
      Right 05LG
    Hemiazygos 05L1
    Hepatic 06L4
    Hypogastric
      Left 06LJ
      Right 06LH
    Inferior Mesenteric 06L6
    Innominate
      Left 05L4
      Right 05L3
    Internal Jugular
      Left 05LN
      Right 05LM
    Intracranial 05LL
    Lesser Saphenous
      Left 06LS
      Right 06LR
    Lower 06LY
    Portal 06L8
    Pulmonary
      Left 02LT
      Right 02LS
    Renal
      Left 06LB
      Right 06L9
    Splenic 06L1
    Subclavian
      Left 05L6
      Right 05L5
    Superior Mesenteric 06L5
    Upper 05LY
    Vertebral
      Left 05LS
      Right 05LR

Occlusion *(continued)*
  Vena Cava
    Inferior 06L0
    Superior 02LV
Occupational therapy
  see Activities of Daily Living Treatment, Rehabilitation F08
Odentectomy
  see Excision, Mouth and Throat 0CB
  see Resection, Mouth and Throat 0CT
Olecranon bursa
  use Bursa and Ligament, Elbow, Left
  use Bursa and Ligament, Elbow, Right
Olecranon process
  use Ulna, Left
  use Ulna, Right
Olfactory bulb
  use Nerve, Olfactory
Omentectomy, omentumectomy
  see Excision, Gastrointestinal System 0DB
  see Resection, Gastrointestinal System 0DT
Omentofixation
  see Repair, Gastrointestinal System 0DQ
Omentoplasty
  see Repair, Gastrointestinal System 0DQ
  see Replacement, Gastrointestinal System 0DR
  see Supplement, Gastrointestinal System 0DU
Omentorrhaphy
  see Repair, Gastrointestinal System 0DQ
Omentotomy
  see Drainage, Gastrointestinal System 0D9
Onychectomy
  see Excision, Skin and Breast 0HB
  see Resection, Skin and Breast 0HT
Onychoplasty
  see Repair, Skin and Breast 0HQ
  see Replacement, Skin and Breast 0HR
Onychotomy
  see Drainage, Skin and Breast 0H9
Oophorectomy
  see Excision, Female Reproductive System 0UB
  see Resection, Female Reproductive System 0UT
Oophoropexy
  see Repair, Female Reproductive System 0UQ
  see Reposition, Female Reproductive System 0US
Oophoroplasty
  see Repair, Female Reproductive System 0UQ
  see Supplement, Female Reproductive System 0UU
Oophororrhaphy
  see Repair, Female Reproductive System 0UQ
Oophorostomy
  see Drainage, Female Reproductive System 0U9
Oophorotomy
  see Drainage, Female Reproductive System 0U9
  see Division, Female Reproductive System 0U8
Oophorrhaphy
  see Repair, Female Reproductive System 0UQ
Ophthalmic artery
  use Artery, Internal Carotid, Right
  use Artery, Internal Carotid, Left
Ophthalmic nerve
  use Nerve, Trigeminal
Ophthalmic vein
  use Vein, Intracranial
Opponensplasty
  Tendon replacement
    see Replacement, Tendons 0LR
  Tendon transfer
    see Transfer, Tendons 0LX
Optic chiasma
  use Nerve, Optic
Optic disc
  use Retina, Left
  use Retina, Right
Optic foramen
  use Bone, Sphenoid, Right
  use Bone, Sphenoid, Left
Optical coherence tomography, intravascular
  see Computerized Tomography (CT Scan)
Optimizer™ III implantable pulse generator
  use Contractility Modulation Device in 0JH
Orbicularis oculi muscle
  use Eyelid, Upper, Left
  use Eyelid, Upper, Right
Orbicularis oris muscle
  use Muscle, Facial
Orbital fascia
  use Subcutaneous Tissue and Fascia, Face
Orbital portion of ethmoid bone
  use Orbit, Left
  use Orbit, Right
Orbital portion of frontal bone
  use Orbit, Right
  use Orbit, Left

Parasternal lymph node
use Lymphatic, Thorax
Parathyroidectomy
see Excision, Endocrine System 0GB
see Resection, Endocrine System 0GT
Paratracheal lymph node
use Lymphatic, Thorax
Paraurethral (Skene's) gland
use Gland, Vestibular
Parenteral nutrition, total
see Introduction of Nutritional Substance
Parietal lobe
use Cerebral Hemisphere
Parotid lymph node
use Lymphatic, Head
Parotid plexus
use Nerve, Facial
Parotidectomy
see Excision, Mouth and Throat 0CB
see Resection, Mouth and Throat
0CT
Pars flaccida
use Tympanic Membrane, Right
use Tympanic Membrane, Left
Partial joint replacement
Hip
see Replacement, Lower Joints 0SR
Knee
see Replacement, Lower Joints 0SR
Shoulder
see Replacement, Upper Joints 0RR
Partially absorbable mesh
use Synthetic Substitute
Patch, blood, spinal 3E0S3GC
Patellapexy
see Repair, Lower Bones 0QQ
see Reposition, Lower Bones 0QS
Patellaplasty
see Repair, Lower Bones 0QQ
see Replacement, Lower Bones 0QR
see Supplement, Lower Bones 0QU
Patellar ligament
use Bursa and Ligament, Knee, Right
use Bursa and Ligament, Knee, Left
Patellar tendon
use Tendon, Knee, Left
use Tendon, Knee, Right
Patellectomy
see Excision, Lower Bones 0QB
see Resection, Lower Bones 0QT
Patellofemoral joint
use Joint, Knee, Right
use Joint, Knee, Left
use Joint, Knee, Right, Femoral Surface
use Joint, Knee, Left, Femoral Surface
Pectineus muscle
use Muscle, Upper Leg, Left
use Muscle, Upper Leg, Right
Pectoral (anterior) lymph node
use Lymphatic, Axillary, Right
use Lymphatic, Axillary, Left
Pectoral fascia
use Subcutaneous Tissue and Fascia, Chest
Pectoralis major muscle
use Muscle, Thorax, Left
use Muscle, Thorax, Right
Pectoralis minor muscle
use Muscle, Thorax, Right
use Muscle, Thorax, Left
Pedicle-based dynamic stabilization device
use Spinal Stabilization Device, Pedicle-Based
in 0RH
use Spinal Stabilization Device, Pedicle-Based
in 0SH
PEEP (positive end expiratory pressure)
see Assistance, Respiratory 5A09
PEG (percutaneous endoscopic gastrostomy) 0DH64UZ
PEJ (percutaneous endoscopic jejunostomy) 0DHA4UZ
Pelvic splanchnic nerve
use Nerve, Abdominal Sympathetic
use Nerve, Sacral Sympathetic
Penectomy
see Excision, Male Reproductive System 0VB
see Resection, Male Reproductive System 0VT
Penile urethra
use Urethra
**Percutaneous endoscopic gastrojejunostomy (PEG/J)
tube**
use Feeding Device in Gastrointestinal System
Percutaneous endoscopic gastrostomy (PEG) tube
use Feeding Device in Gastrointestinal System
Percutaneous nephrostomy catheter
use Drainage Device
Percutaneous transluminal coronary angioplasty (PTCA)
see Dilation, Heart and Great Vessels 027

Performance
Biliary
Multiple, Filtration 5A1C60Z
Single, Filtration 5A1C00Z
Cardiac
Continuous
Output 5A1221Z
Pacing 5A1223Z
Intermittent, Pacing 5A1213Z
Single, Output, Manual 5A12012
Circulatory, Continuous, Oxygenation, Membrane
5A15223
Respiratory
24-96 Consecutive Hours, Ventilation 5A1945Z
Greater than 96 Consecutive Hours, Ventilation
5A1955Z
Less than 24 Consecutive Hours, Ventilation
5A1935Z
Single, Ventilation, Nonmechanical5A19054
Urinary
Multiple, Filtration 5A1D60Z
Single, Filtration 5A1D00Z
Perfusion
see Introduction of substance in or on
Pericardiectomy
see Excision, Pericardium 02BN
see Resection, Pericardium 02TN
Pericardiocentesis
see Drainage, Pericardial Cavity 0W9D
Pericardiolysis
see Release, Pericardium 02NN
Pericardiophrenic artery
use Artery, Internal Mammary, Left
use Artery, Internal Mammary, Right
Pericardioplasty
see Repair, Pericardium 02QN
see Replacement, Pericardium 02RN
see Supplement, Pericardium 02UN
Pericardiorrhaphy
see Repair, Pericardium 02QN
Pericardiostomy
see Drainage, Pericardial Cavity 0W9D
Pericardiotomy
see Drainage, Pericardial Cavity 0W9D
Perimetrium
use Uterus
Peripheral parenteral nutrition
see Introduction of Nutritional Substance
Peripherally inserted central catheter (PICC)
use Infusion Device
Peritoneal dialysis 3E1M39Z
Peritoneocentesis
see Drainage, Peritoneum 0D9W
see Drainage, Peritoneal Cavity 0W9G
Peritoneoplasty
see Repair, Peritoneum 0DQW
see Replacement, Peritoneum 0DRW
see Supplement, Peritoneum 0DUW
Peritoneoscopy 0DJW4ZZ
Peritoneotomy
see Drainage, Peritoneum 0D9W
Peritoneumectomy
see Excision, Peritoneum 0DBW
Peroneus brevis muscle
use Muscle, Lower Leg, Left
use Muscle, Lower Leg, Right
Peroneus longus muscle
use Muscle, Lower Leg, Right
use Muscle, Lower Leg, Left
Pessary ring
use Intraluminal Device, Pessary in Female
Reproductive System
PET scan
see Positron Emission Tomographic (PET) Imaging
Petrous part of temporal bone
use Bone, Temporal, Right
use Bone, Temporal, Left
Phacoemulsification, lens
With IOL implant
see Replacement, Eye 08R
Without IOL implant
see Extraction, Eye 08D
Phalangectomy
see Excision, Upper Bones 0PB
see Resection, Upper Bones 0PT
see Excision, Lower Bones 0QB
see Resection, Lower Bones 0QT
Phallectomy
see Excision, Penis 0VBS
see Resection, Penis 0VTS
Phalloplasty
see Repair, Penis 0VQS
see Supplement, Penis 0VUS
Phallotomy
see Drainage, Penis 0V9S

Pharmacotherapy
Antabuse HZ93ZZZ
Bupropion HZ97ZZZ
Clonidine HZ96ZZZ
Levo-alpha-acetyl-methadol (LAAM) HZ92ZZZ
Methadone Maintenance HZ91ZZZ
Naloxone HZ95ZZZ
Naltrexone HZ94ZZZ
Nicotine Replacement HZ90ZZZ
Psychiatric Medication HZ98ZZZ
Replacement Medication, Other HZ99ZZZ
Pharyngeal constrictor muscle
use Muscle, Tongue, Palate, Pharynx
Pharyngeal plexus
use Nerve, Vagus
Pharyngeal recess
use Nasopharynx
Pharyngeal tonsil
use Adenoids
Pharyngogram
see Fluoroscopy, Pharynix B91G
Pharyngoplasty
see Repair, Mouth and Throat 0CQ
see Replacement, Mouth and Throat 0CR
see Supplement, Mouth and Throat 0CU
Pharyngorrhaphy
see Repair, Mouth and Throat 0CQ
Pharyngotomy
see Drainage, Mouth and Throat 0C9
Pharyngotympanic tube
use Eustachian Tube, Right
use Eustachian Tube, Left
Pheresis
Erythrocytes 6A55
Leukocytes 6A55
Plasma 6A55
Platelets 6A55
Stem Cells
Cord Blood 6A55
Hematopoietic 6A55
Phlebectomy
see Excision, Upper Veins 05B
see Extraction, Upper Veins 05D
see Excision, Lower Veins 06B
see Extraction, Lower Veins 06D
Phlebography
see Plain Radiography, Veins B50
Impedance 4A04X51
Phleborrhaphy
see Repair, Upper Veins 05Q
see Repair, Lower Veins 06Q
Phlebotomy
see Drainage, Upper Veins 059
see Drainage, Lower Veins 069
Photocoagulation
for Destruction
see Destruction
for Repair
see Repair
Photopheresis, therapeutic
see Phototherapy, Circulatory 6A65
Phototherapy
Circulatory 6A65
Skin 6A60
Phrenectomy, phrenoneurectomy
see Excision, Nerve, Phrenic 01B2
Phrenemphraxis
see Destruction, Nerve, Phrenic 0152
Phrenic nerve stimulator generator
use Stimulator Generator in Subcutaneous Tissue and
Fascia
Phrenic nerve stimulator lead
use Diaphragmatic Pacemaker Lead in Respiratory
System
Phreniclasis
see Destruction, Nerve, Phrenic 0152
Phrenicoexeresis
see Extraction, Nerve, Phrenic 01D2
Phrenicotomy
see Division, Nerve, Phrenic 0182
Phrenicotripsy
see Destruction, Nerve, Phrenic 0152
Phrenoplasty
see Repair, Respiratory System 0BQ
see Supplement, Respiratory System 0BU
Phrenotomy
see Drainage, Respiratory System 0B9
Physiatry
see Motor Treatment, Rehabilitation F07
Physical medicine
see Motor Treatment, Rehabilitation F07
Physical therapy
see Motor Treatment, Rehabilitation F07
PHYSIOMESH™ Flexible Composite Mesh
use Synthetic Substitute

Pia mater
  use Spinal Meninges
  use Cerebral Meninges
Pinealectomy
  see Excision, Pineal Body 0GB1
  see Resection, Pineal Body 0GT1
Pinealoscopy 0GJ14ZZ
Pinealotomy
  see Drainage, Pineal Body 0G91
Pinna
  use Ear, External, Left
  use Ear, External, Bilateral
  use Ear, External, Right
Pipeline™ Embolization device (PED)
  use Intraluminal Device
Piriform recess (sinus)
  use Pharynx
Piriformis muscle
  use Muscle, Hip, Left
  use Muscle, Hip, Right
Pisiform bone
  use Carpal, Left
  use Carpal, Right
Pisohamate ligament
  use Bursa and Ligament, Hand, Right
  use Bursa and Ligament, Hand, Left
Pisometacarpal ligament
  use Bursa and Ligament, Hand, Left
  use Bursa and Ligament, Hand, Right
Pituitectomy
  see Excision, Gland, Pituitary 0GB0
  see Resection, Gland, Pituitary 0GT0
Plain film radiology
  see Plain Radiography
Plain Radiography
  Abdomen BW00ZZZ
  Abdomen and Pelvis BW01ZZZ
  Abdominal Lymphatic
    Bilateral B701
    Unilateral B700
  Airway, Upper BB0DZZZ
  Ankle
    Left BQ0H
    Right BQ0G
  Aorta
    Abdominal B400
    Thoracic B300
    Thoraco-Abdominal B30P
  Aorta and Bilateral Lower Extremity Arteries B40D
  Arch
    Bilateral BN0DZZZ
    Left BN0CZZZ
    Right BN0BZZZ
  Arm
    Left BP0FZZZ
    Right BP0EZZZ
  Artery
    Brachiocephalic-Subclavian, Right B301
    Bronchial B30L
    Bypass Graft, Other B20F
    Cervico-Cerebral Arch B30Q
    Common Carotid
      Bilateral B305
      Left B304
      Right B303
    Coronary
      Bypass Graft
        Multiple B203
        Single B202
      Multiple B201
      Single B200
    External Carotid
      Bilateral B30C
      Left B30B
      Right B309
    Hepatic B402
    Inferior Mesenteric B405
    Intercostal B30L
    Internal Carotid
      Bilateral B308
      Left B307
      Right B306
    Internal Mammary Bypass Graft
      Left B208
      Right B207
    Intra-Abdominal, Other B40B
    Intracranial B30R
    Lower, Other B40J
    Lower Extremity
      Bilateral and Aorta B40D
      Left B40G
      Right B40F
    Lumbar B409
    Pelvic B40C

Plain Radiography (*continued*)
  Artery (*continued*)
    Pulmonary
      Left B30T
      Right B30S
    Renal
      Bilateral B408
      Left B407
      Right B406
      Transplant B40M
    Spinal B30M
    Splenic B403
    Subclavian, Left B302
    Superior Mesenteric B404
    Upper, Other B30N
    Upper Extremity
      Bilateral B30K
      Left B30J
      Right B30H
    Vertebral
      Bilateral B30G
      Left B30F
      Right B30D
  Bile Duct BF00
  Bile Duct and Gallbladder BF03
  Bladder BT00
    Kidney and Ureter BT04
  Bladder and Urethra BT0B
  Bone
    Facial BN05ZZZ
    Nasal BN04ZZZ
  Bones, Long, All BW0BZZZ
  Breast
    Bilateral BH02ZZZ
    Left BH01ZZZ
    Right BH00ZZZ
  Calcaneus
    Left BQ0KZZZ
    Right BQ0JZZZ
  Chest BW03ZZZ
  Clavicle
    Left BP05ZZZ
    Right BP04ZZZ
  Coccyx BR0FZZZ
  Corpora Cavernosa BV00
  Dialysis Fistula B50W
  Dialysis Shunt B50W
  Disc
    Cervical BR01
    Lumbar BR03
    Thoracic BR02
  Duct
    Lacrimal
      Bilateral B802
      Left B801
      Right B800
    Mammary
      Multiple
        Left BH06
        Right BH05
      Single
        Left BH04
        Right BH03
  Elbow
    Left BP0H
    Right BP0G
  Epididymis
    Left BV02
    Right BV01
  Extremity
    Lower BW0CZZZ
    Upper BW0JZZZ
  Eye
    Bilateral B807ZZZ
    Left B806ZZZ
    Right B805ZZZ
  Facet Joint
    Cervical BR04
    Lumbar BR06
    Thoracic BR05
  Fallopian Tube
    Bilateral BU02
    Left BU01
    Right BU00
  Fallopian Tube and Uterus BU08
  Femur
    Left, Densitometry BQ04ZZ1
    Right, Densitometry BQ03ZZ1
  Finger
    Left BP0SZZZ
    Right BP0RZZZ
  Foot
    Left BQ0MZZZ
    Right BQ0LZZZ

Plain Radiography (*continued*)
  Forearm
    Left BP0KZZZ
    Right BP0JZZZ
  Gallbladder and Bile Duct BF03
  Gland
    Parotid
      Bilateral B906
      Left B905
      Right B904
    Salivary
      Bilateral B90D
      Left B90C
      Right B90B
    Submandibular
      Bilateral B909
      Left B908
      Right B907
  Hand
    Left BP0PZZZ
    Right BP0NZZZ
  Heart
    Left B205
    Right B204
    Right and Left B206
  Hepatobiliary System, All BF0C
  Hip
    Left BQ01
      Densitometry BQ01ZZ1
    Right BQ00
      Densitometry BQ00ZZ1
  Humerus
    Left BP0BZZZ
    Right BP0AZZZ
  Ileal Diversion Loop BT0C
  Intracranial Sinus B502
  Joint
    Acromioclavicular, Bilateral BP03ZZZ
    Finger
      Left BP0D
      Right BP0C
    Foot
      Left BQ0Y
      Right BQ0X
    Hand
      Left BP0D
      Right BP0C
    Lumbosacral BR0BZZZ
    Sacroiliac BR0D
    Sternoclavicular
      Bilateral BP02ZZZ
      Left BP01ZZZ
      Right BP00ZZZ
    Temporomandibular
      Bilateral BN09
      Left BN08
      Right BN07
    Thoracolumbar BR08ZZZ
    Toe
      Left BQ0Y
      Right BQ0X
  Kidney
    Bilateral BT03
    Left BT02
    Right BT01
    Ureter and Bladder BT04
  Knee
    Left BQ08
    Right BQ07
  Leg
    Left BQ0FZZZ
    Right BQ0DZZZ
  Lymphatic
    Head B704
    Lower Extremity
      Bilateral B70B
      Left B709
      Right B708
    Neck B704
    Pelvic B70C
    Upper Extremity
      Bilateral B707
      Left B706
      Right B705
  Mandible BN06ZZZ
  Mastoid B90HZZZ
  Nasopharynx B90FZZZ
  Optic Foramina
    Left B804ZZZ
    Right B803ZZZ
  Orbit
    Bilateral BN03ZZZ
    Left BN02ZZZ
    Right BN01ZZZ

Plain Radiography (continued)
Oropharynx B90FZZZ
Patella
   Left BQ0WZZZ
   Right BQ0VZZZ
Pelvis BR0CZZZ
Pelvis and Abdomen BW01ZZZ
Prostate BV03
Retroperitoneal Lymphatic
   Bilateral B701
   Unilateral B700
Ribs
   Left BP0YZZZ
   Right BP0XZZZ
Sacrum BR0FZZZ
Scapula
   Left BP07ZZZ
   Right BP06ZZZ
Shoulder
   Left BP09
   Right BP08
Sinus
   Intracranial B502
   Paranasal B902ZZZ
Skull BN00ZZZ
Spinal Cord B00B
Spine
   Cervical, Densitometry BR00ZZ1
   Lumbar, Densitometry BR09ZZ1
   Thoracic, Densitometry BR07ZZ1
   Whole, Densitometry BR0GZZ1
Sternum BR0HZZZ
Teeth
   All BN0JZZZ
   Multiple BN0HZZZ
Testicle
   Left BV06
   Right BV05
Toe
   Left BQ0QZZZ
   Right BQ0PZZZ
Tooth, Single BN0GZZZ
Tracheobronchial Tree
   Bilateral BB09YZZ
   Left BB08Y
   Right BB07Y
Ureter
   Bilateral BT08
   Kidney and Bladder BT04
   Left BT07
   Right BT06
Urethra BT05
Urethra and Bladder BT0B
Uterus BU06
Uterus and Fallopian Tube BU08
Vagina BU09
Vasa Vasorum BV08
Vein
   Cerebellar B501
   Cerebral B501
   Epidural B500
   Jugular
      Bilateral B505
      Left B504
      Right B503
   Lower Extremity
      Bilateral B50D
      Left B50C
      Right B50B
   Other B50V
   Pelvic (Iliac)
      Left B50G
      Right B50F
   Pelvic (Iliac) Bilateral B50H
   Portal B50T
   Pulmonary
      Bilateral B50S
      Left B50R
      Right B50Q
   Renal
      Bilateral B50L
      Left B50K
      Right B50J
   Spanchnic B50T
   Subclavian
      Left B507
      Right B506
   Upper Extremity
      Bilateral B50P
      Left B50N
      Right B50M
Vena Cava
   Inferior B509
   Superior B508

Plain Radiography (continued)
Whole Body BW0KZZZ
   Infant BW0MZZZ
Whole Skeleton BW0LZZZ
Wrist
   Left BP0M
   Right BP0L
Planar Nuclear Medicine Imaging CP1
Abdomen CW10
Abdomen and Chest CW14
Abdomen and Pelvis CW11
Anatomical Regions, Multiple CW1YYZZ
Bladder, Kidneys and Ureters CT13
Bladder and Ureters CT1H
Blood C713
Bone Marrow C710
Brain C010
Breast CH1YYZZ
   Bilateral CH12
   Left CH11
   Right CH10
Bronchi and Lungs CB12
Central Nervous System C01YYZZ
Cerebrospinal Fluid C015
Chest CW13
Chest and Abdomen CW14
Chest and Neck CW16
Digestive System CD1YYZZ
Ducts, Lacrimal, Bilateral C819
Ear, Nose, Mouth and Throat C91YYZZ
Endocrine System CG1YYZZ
Extremity
   Lower CW1D
      Bilateral CP1F
      Left CP1D
      Right CP1C
   Upper CW1M
      Bilateral CP1B
      Left CP19
      Right CP18
Eye C81YYZZ
Gallbladder CF14
Gastrointestinal Tract CD17
   Upper CD15
Gland
   Adrenal, Bilateral CG14
   Parathyroid CG11
   Thyroid CG12
Glands, Salivary, Bilateral C91B
Head and Neck CW1B
Heart C21YYZZ
   Right and Left C216
Hepatobiliary System, All CF1C
Hepatobiliary System and Pancreas CF1YYZZ
Kidneys, Ureters and Bladder CT13
Liver CF15
Liver and Spleen CF16
Lungs and Bronchi CB12
Lymphatics
   Head C71J
   Head and Neck C715
   Lower Extremity C71P
   Neck C71K
   Pelvic C71D
   Trunk C71M
   Upper Chest C71L
   Upper Extremity C71N
Lymphatics and Hematologic System
   C71YYZZ
Musculoskeletal System, All CP1Z
Myocardium C21G
Neck and Chest CW16
Neck and Head CW1B
Pancreas and Hepatobiliary System
   CF1YYZZ
Pelvic Region CW1J
Pelvis CP16
Pelvis and Abdomen CW11
Pelvis and Spine CP17
Reproductive System, Male CV1YYZZ
Respiratory System CB1YYZZ
Skin CH1YYZZ
Skull CP11
Spine CP15
Spine and Pelvis CP17
Spleen C712
Spleen and Liver CF16
Subcutaneous Tissue CH1YYZZ
Testicles, Bilateral CV19
Thorax CP14
Ureters, Kidneys and Bladder
   CT13
Ureters and Bladder CT1H
Urinary System CT1YYZZ

Planar Nuclear Medicine Imaging CP1 (continued)
Veins C51YYZZ
   Central C51R
   Lower Extremity
      Bilateral C51D
      Left C51C
      Right C51B
   Upper Extremity
      Bilateral C51Q
      Left C51P
      Right C51N
Whole Body CW1N
Plantar digital vein
   use Vein, Foot, Right
   use Vein, Foot, Left
Plantar fascia (aponeurosis)
   use Subcutaneous Tissue and Fascia, Foot, Right
   use Subcutaneous Tissue and Fascia, Foot, Left
Plantar metatarsal vein
   use Vein, Foot, Right
   use Vein, Foot, Left
Plantar venous arch
   use Vein, Foot, Right
   use Vein, Foot, Left
Plaque Radiation
Abdomen DWY3FZZ
Adrenal Gland DGY2FZZ
Anus DDY8FZZ
Bile Ducts DFY2FZZ
Bladder DTY2FZZ
Bone, Other DPYCFZZ
Bone Marrow D7Y0FZZ
Brain D0Y0FZZ
Brain Stem D0Y1FZZ
Breast
   Left DMY0FZZ
   Right DMY1FZZ
Bronchus DBY1FZZ
Cervix DUY1FZZ
Chest DWY2FZZ
Chest Wall DBY7FZZ
Colon DDY5FZZ
Diaphragm DBY8FZZ
Duodenum DDY2FZZ
Ear D9Y0FZZ
Esophagus DDY0FZZ
Eye D8Y0FZZ
Femur DPY9FZZ
Fibula DPYBFZZ
Gallbladder DFY1FZZ
Gland
   Adrenal DGY2FZZ
   Parathyroid DGY4FZZ
   Pituitary DGY0FZZ
   Thyroid DGY5FZZ
Glands, Salivary D9Y6FZZ
Head and Neck DWY1FZZ
Hemibody DWY4FZZ
Humerus DPY6FZZ
Ileum DDY4FZZ
Jejunum DDY3FZZ
Kidney DTY0FZZ
Larynx D9YBFZZ
Liver DFY0FZZ
Lung DBY2FZZ
Lymphatics
   Abdomen D7Y6FZZ
   Axillary D7Y4FZZ
   Inguinal D7Y8FZZ
   Neck D7Y3FZZ
   Pelvis D7Y7FZZ
   Thorax D7Y5FZZ
Mandible DPY3FZZ
Maxilla DPY2FZZ
Mediastinum DBY6FZZ
Mouth D9Y4FZZ
Nasopharynx D9YDFZZ
Neck and Head DWY1FZZ
Nerve, Peripheral D0Y7FZZ
Nose D9Y1FZZ
Ovary DUY0FZZ
Palate
   Hard D9Y8FZZ
   Soft D9Y9FZZ
Pancreas DFY3FZZ
Parathyroid Gland DGY4FZZ
Pelvic Bones DPY8FZZ
Pelvic Region DWY6FZZ
Pharynx D9YCFZZ
Pineal Body DGY1FZZ
Pituitary Gland DGY0FZZ
Pleura DBY5FZZ
Prostate DVY0FZZ
Radius DPY7FZZ

PSV (pressure support ventilation)
　　see Performance, Respiratory 5A19
Psychoanalysis GZ54ZZZ
Psychological Tests
　　Cognitive Status GZ14ZZZ
　　Developmental GZ10ZZZ
　　Intellectual and Psychoeducational
　　　　GZ12ZZZ
　　Neurobehavioral Status GZ14ZZZ
　　Neuropsychological GZ13ZZZ
　　Personality and Behavioral GZ11ZZZ
Psychotherapy
　　Family, Mental Health Services GZ72ZZZ
　　Group
　　　　GZHZZZZ
　　　　Mental Health Services GZHZZZZ
　　Individual
　　see Psychotherapy, Individual, Mental Health Services
　　　　for substance abuse
　　　　　　12-Step HZ53ZZZ
　　　　　　Behavioral HZ51ZZZ
　　　　　　Cognitive HZ50ZZZ
　　　　　　Cognitive-Behavioral HZ52ZZZ
　　　　　　Confrontational HZ58ZZZ
　　　　　　Interactive HZ55ZZZ
　　　　　　Interpersonal HZ54ZZZ
　　　　　　Motivational Enhancement HZ57ZZZ
　　　　　　Psychoanalysis HZ5BZZZ
　　　　　　Psychodynamic HZ5CZZZ
　　　　　　Psychoeducation HZ56ZZZ
　　　　　　Psychophysiological HZ5DZZZ
　　　　　　Supportive HZ59ZZZ
　　　　Mental Health Services
　　　　　　Behavioral GZ51ZZZ
　　　　　　Cognitive GZ52ZZZ
　　　　　　Cognitive-Behavioral GZ58ZZZ
　　　　　　Interactive GZ50ZZZ
　　　　　　Interpersonal GZ53ZZZ
　　　　　　Psychoanalysis GZ54ZZZ
　　　　　　Psychodynamic GZ55ZZZ
　　　　　　Psychophysiological GZ59ZZZ
　　　　　　Supportive GZ56ZZZ
PTCA (percutaneous transluminal coronary angioplasty)
　　see Dilation, Heart and Great Vessels 027
Pterygoid muscle
　　use Muscle, Head
Pterygoid process
　　use Bone, Sphenoid, Right
　　use Bone, Sphenoid, Left
Pterygopalatine (sphenopalatine) ganglion
　　use Nerve, Head and Neck Sympathetic
Pubic ligament
　　use Bursa and Ligament, Trunk, Right
　　use Bursa and Ligament, Trunk, Left
Pubis
　　use Bone, Pelvic, Right
　　use Bone, Pelvic, Left
Pubofemoral ligament
　　use Bursa and Ligament, Hip, Left
　　use Bursa and Ligament, Hip, Right
Pudendal nerve
　　use Nerve, Sacral Plexus
Pull-through, rectal
　　see Resection, Rectum 0DTP
Pulmoaortic canal
　　use Artery, Pulmonary, Left
Pulmonary annulus
　　use Valve, Pulmonary
Pulmonary artery wedge monitoring
　　see Monitoring, Arterial 4A13
Pulmonary plexus
　　use Nerve, Vagus
　　use Nerve, Thoracic Sympathetic
Pulmonic valve
　　use Valve, Pulmonary
Pulpectomy
　　see Excision, Mouth and Throat 0CB
Pulverization
　　see Fragmentation
Pulvinar
　　use Thalamus
Pump reservoir
　　use Infusion Device, Pump in Subcutaneous Tissue
　　　　and Fascia
Punch biopsy
　　see Excision with qualifier Diagnostic
Puncture
　　see Drainage
Puncture, lumbar
　　see Drainage, Spinal Canal 009U
Pyelography
　　see Plain Radiography, Urinary System BT0
　　see Fluoroscopy, Urinary System BT1
Pyeloileostomy, urinary diversion
　　see Bypass, Urinary System 0T1

Pyeloplasty
　　see Repair, Urinary System 0TQ
　　see Replacement, Urinary System 0TR
　　see Supplement, Urinary System 0TU
Pyelorrhaphy
　　see Repair, Urinary System 0TQ
Pyeloscopy 0TJ58ZZ
Pyelostomy
　　see Drainage, Urinary System 0T9
　　see Bypass, Urinary System 0T1
Pyelotomy
　　see Drainage, Urinary System 0T9
Pylorectomy
　　see Excision, Stomach, Pylorus 0DB7
　　see Resection, Stomach, Pylorus 0DT7
Pyloric antrum
　　use Stomach, Pylorus
Pyloric canal
　　use Stomach, Pylorus
Pyloric sphincter
　　use Stomach, Pylorus
Pylorodiosis
　　see Dilation, Stomach, Pylorus 0D77
Pylorogastrectomy
　　see Excision, Gastrointestinal System 0DB
　　see Resection, Gastrointestinal System 0DT
Pyloroplasty
　　see Repair, Stomach, Pylorus 0DQ7
　　see Supplement, Stomach, Pylorus 0DU7
Pyloroscopy 0DJ68ZZ
Pylorotomy
　　see Drainage, Stomach, Pylorus 0D97
Pyramidalis muscle
　　use Muscle, Abdomen, Left
　　use Muscle, Abdomen, Right

Q

Quadrangular cartilage
　　use Septum, Nasal
Quadrant resection of breast
　　see Excision, Skin and Breast 0HB
Quadrate lobe
　　use Liver
Quadratus femoris muscle
　　use Muscle, Hip, Left
　　use Muscle, Hip, Right
Quadratus lumborum muscle
　　use Muscle, Trunk, Left
　　use Muscle, Trunk, Right
Quadratus plantae muscle
　　use Muscle, Foot, Left
　　use Muscle, Foot, Right
Quadriceps (femoris)
　　use Muscle, Upper Leg, Left
　　use Muscle, Upper Leg, Right
Quarantine 8E0ZXY6

R

Radial collateral carpal ligament
　　use Bursa and Ligament, Wrist, Right
　　use Bursa and Ligament, Wrist, Left
Radial collateral ligament
　　use Bursa and Ligament, Elbow, Left
　　use Bursa and Ligament, Elbow, Right
Radial notch
　　use Ulna, Left
　　use Ulna, Right
Radial recurrent artery
　　use Artery, Radial, Right
　　use Artery, Radial, Left
Radial vein
　　use Vein, Brachial, Right
　　use Vein, Brachial, Left
Radialis indicis
　　use Artery, Hand, Right
　　use Artery, Hand, Left
Radiation Therapy
　　see Beam Radiation
　　see Brachytherapy
Radiation treatment
　　see Radiation Oncology
Radiocarpal joint
　　use Joint, Wrist, Left
　　use Joint, Wrist, Right
Radiocarpal ligament
　　use Bursa and Ligament, Wrist,
　　　　Left
　　use Bursa and Ligament, Wrist, Right
Radiography
　　see Plain Radiography
Radiology, analog
　　see Plain Radiography

Radiology, diagnostic
　　see Imaging, Diagnostic
Radioulnar ligament
　　use Bursa and Ligament, Wrist, Right
　　use Bursa and Ligament, Wrist, Left
Range of motion testing
　　see Motor Function Assessment,
　　　　Rehabilitation F01
REALIZE® Adjustable Gastric Band
　　use Extraluminal Device
Reattachment
　　Abdominal Wall 0WMF0ZZ
　　Ampulla of Vater 0FMC
　　Ankle Region
　　　　Left 0YML0ZZ
　　　　Right 0YMK0ZZ
　　Arm
　　　　Lower
　　　　　　Left 0XMF0ZZ
　　　　　　Right 0XMD0ZZ
　　　　Upper
　　　　　　Left 0XM90ZZ
　　　　　　Right 0XM80ZZ
　　Axilla
　　　　Left 0XM50ZZ
　　　　Right 0XM40ZZ
　　Back
　　　　Lower 0WML0ZZ
　　　　Upper 0WMK0ZZ
　　Bladder 0TMB
　　Bladder Neck 0TMC
　　Breast
　　　　Bilateral 0HMVXZZ
　　　　Left 0HMUXZZ
　　　　Right 0HMTXZZ
　　Bronchus
　　　　Lingula 0BM90ZZ
　　　　Lower Lobe
　　　　　　Left 0BMB0ZZ
　　　　　　Right 0BM60ZZ
　　　　Main
　　　　　　Left 0BM70ZZ
　　　　　　Right 0BM30ZZ
　　　　Middle Lobe, Right 0BM50ZZ
　　　　Upper Lobe
　　　　　　Left 0BM80ZZ
　　　　　　Right 0BM40ZZ
　　Bursa and Ligament
　　　　Abdomen
　　　　　　Left 0MMJ
　　　　　　Right 0MMH
　　　　Ankle
　　　　　　Left 0MMR
　　　　　　Right 0MMQ
　　　　Elbow
　　　　　　Left 0MM4
　　　　　　Right 0MM3
　　　　Foot
　　　　　　Left 0MMT
　　　　　　Right 0MMS
　　　　Hand
　　　　　　Left 0MM8
　　　　　　Right 0MM7
　　　　Head and Neck 0MM0
　　　　Hip
　　　　　　Left 0MMM
　　　　　　Right 0MML
　　　　Knee
　　　　　　Left 0MMP
　　　　　　Right 0MMN
　　　　Lower Extremity
　　　　　　Left 0MMW
　　　　　　Right 0MMV
　　　　Perineum 0MMK
　　　　Shoulder
　　　　　　Left 0MM2
　　　　　　Right 0MM1
　　　　Thorax
　　　　　　Left 0MMG
　　　　　　Right 0MMF
　　　　Trunk
　　　　　　Left 0MMD
　　　　　　Right 0MMC
　　　　Upper Extremity
　　　　　　Left 0MMB
　　　　　　Right 0MM9
　　　　Wrist
　　　　　　Left 0MM6
　　　　　　Right 0MM5
　　Buttock
　　　　Left 0YM10ZZ
　　　　Right 0YM00ZZ
　　Carina 0BM20ZZ
　　Cecum 0DMH
　　Cervix 0UMC

Reattachment *(continued)*
   Thumb
      Left 0XMM0ZZ
      Right 0XML0ZZ
   Thyroid Gland
      Left Lobe 0GMG
      Right Lobe 0GMH
   Toe
      1st
         Left 0YMQ0ZZ
         Right 0YMP0ZZ
      2nd
         Left 0YMS0ZZ
         Right 0YMR0ZZ
      3rd
         Left 0YMU0ZZ
         Right 0YMT0ZZ
      4th
         Left 0YMW0ZZ
         Right 0YMV0ZZ
      5th
         Left 0YMY0ZZ
         Right 0YMX0ZZ
   Tongue 0CM70ZZ
   Tooth
      Lower 0CMX
      Upper 0CMW
   Trachea 0BM10ZZ
   Tunica Vaginalis
      Left 0VM7
      Right 0VM6
   Ureter
      Left 0TM7
      Right 0TM6
   Ureters, Bilateral 0TM8
   Urethra 0TMD
   Uterine Supporting Structure 0UM4
   Uterus 0UM9
   Uvula 0CMN0ZZ
   Vagina 0UMG
   Vulva 0UMMXZZ
   Wrist Region
      Left 0XMH0ZZ
      Right 0XMG0ZZ
Rebound HRD® (Hernia Repair Device)
   use Synthetic Substitute
Recession
   see Repair
   see Reposition
Reclosure, disrupted abdominal wall 0WQFXZZ
Reconstruction
   see Repair
   see Replacement
   see Supplement
Rectectomy
   see Excision, Rectum 0DBP
   see Resection, Rectum 0DTP
Rectocele repair
   see Repair, Subcutaneous Tissue and Fascia, Pelvic
      Region 0JQC
Rectopexy
   see Repair, Gastrointestinal System 0DQ
   see Reposition, Gastrointestinal System 0DS
Rectoplasty
   see Repair, Gastrointestinal System 0DQ
   see Supplement, Gastrointestinal System 0DU
Rectorrhaphy
   see Repair, Gastrointestinal System 0DQ
Rectoscopy 0DJD8ZZ
Rectosigmoid junction
   use Colon, Sigmoid
Rectosigmoidectomy
   see Excision, Gastrointestinal System 0DB
   see Resection, Gastrointestinal System 0DT
Rectostomy
   see Drainage, Rectum 0D9P
Rectotomy
   see Drainage, Rectum 0D9P
Rectus abdominis muscle
   use Muscle, Abdomen, Left
   use Muscle, Abdomen, Right
Rectus femoris muscle
   use Muscle, Upper Leg, Left
   use Muscle, Upper Leg, Right
Recurrent laryngeal nerve
   use Nerve, Vagus
Reduction
   Dislocation
      see Reposition
   Fracture
      see Reposition
   Intussusception, intestinal
      see Reposition, Gastrointestinal System 0DS
   Mammoplasty
      see Excision, Skin and Breast 0HB

Reduction *(continued)*
   Prolapse
      see Reposition
   Torsion
      see Reposition
   Volvulus, gastrointestinal
      see Reposition, Gastrointestinal System 0DS
Refusion
   see Fusion
Reimplantation
   see Reposition
   see Transfer
   see Reattachment
Reinforcement
   see Repair
   see Supplement
Relaxation, scar tissue
   see Release
Release
   Acetabulum
      Left 0QN5
      Right 0QN4
   Adenoids 0CNQ
   Ampulla of Vater 0FNC
   Anal Sphincter 0DNR
   Anterior Chamber
      Left 08N33ZZ
      Right 08N23ZZ
   Anus 0DNQ
   Aorta
      Abdominal 04N0
      Thoracic 02NW
   Aortic Body 0GND
   Appendix 0DNJ
   Artery
      Anterior Tibial
         Left 04NQ
         Right 04NP
      Axillary
         Left 03N6
         Right 03N5
      Brachial
         Left 03N8
         Right 03N7
      Celiac 04N1
      Colic
         Left 04N7
         Middle 04N8
         Right 04N6
      Common Carotid
         Left 03NJ
         Right 03NH
      Common Iliac
         Left 04ND
         Right 04NC
      External Carotid
         Left 03NN
         Right 03NM
      External Iliac
         Left 04NJ
         Right 04NH
      Face 03NR
      Femoral
         Left 04NL
         Right 04NK
      Foot
         Left 04NW
         Right 04NV
      Gastric 04N2
      Hand
         Left 03NF
         Right 03ND
      Hepatic 04N3
      Inferior Mesenteric 04NB
      Innominate 03N2
      Internal Carotid
         Left 03NL
         Right 03NK
      Internal Iliac
         Left 04NF
         Right 04NE
      Internal Mammary
         Left 03N1
         Right 03N0
      Intracranial 03NG
      Lower 04NY
      Peroneal
         Left 04NU
         Right 04NT
      Popliteal
         Left 04NN
         Right 04NM
      Posterior Tibial
         Left 04NS
         Right 04NR

Release *(continued)*
   Artery *(continued)*
      Pulmonary
         Left 02NR
         Right 02NQ
      Pulmonary Trunk 02NP
      Radial
         Left 03NC
         Right 03NB
      Renal
         Left 04NA
         Right 04N9
      Splenic 04N4
      Subclavian
         Left 03N4
         Right 03N3
      Superior Mesenteric 04N5
      Temporal
         Left 03NT
         Right 03NS
      Thyroid
         Left 03NV
         Right 03NU
      Ulnar
         Left 03NA
         Right 03N9
      Upper 03NY
      Vertebral
         Left 03NQ
         Right 03NP
   Atrium
      Left 02N7
      Right 02N6
   Auditory Ossicle
      Left 09NA0ZZ
      Right 09N90ZZ
   Basal Ganglia 00N8
   Bladder 0TNB
   Bladder Neck 0TNC
   Bone
      Ethmoid
         Left 0NNG
         Right 0NNF
      Frontal
         Left 0NN2
         Right 0NN1
      Hyoid 0NNX
      Lacrimal
         Left 0NNJ
         Right 0NNH
      Nasal 0NNB
      Occipital
         Left 0NN8
         Right 0NN7
      Palatine
         Left 0NNL
         Right 0NNK
      Parietal
         Left 0NN4
         Right 0NN3
      Pelvic
         Left 0QN3
         Right 0QN2
      Sphenoid
         Left 0NND
         Right 0NNC
      Temporal
         Left 0NN6
         Right 0NN5
      Zygomatic
         Left 0NNN
         Right 0NNM
   Brain 00N0
   Breast
      Bilateral 0HNV
      Left 0HNU
      Right 0HNT
   Bronchus
      Lingula 0BN9
      Lower Lobe
         Left 0BNB
         Right 0BN6
      Main
         Left 0BN7
         Right 0BN3
      Middle Lobe, Right
         0BN5
      Upper Lobe
         Left 0BN8
         Right 0BN4
   Buccal Mucosa 0CN4
   Bursa and Ligament
      Abdomen
         Left 0MNJ
         Right 0MNH

Release

Release

Release (*continued*)
Larynx 0CNS
Lens
  Left 08NK3ZZ
  Right 08NJ3ZZ
Lip
  Lower 0CN1
  Upper 0CN0
Liver 0FN0
  Left Lobe 0FN2
  Right Lobe 0FN1
Lung
  Bilateral 0BNM
  Left 0BNL
  Lower Lobe
    Left 0BNJ
    Right 0BNF
  Middle Lobe, Right
    0BND
  Right 0BNK
  Upper Lobe
    Left 0BNG
    Right 0BNC
Lung Lingula 0BNH
Lymphatic
  Aortic 07ND
  Axillary
    Left 07N6
    Right 07N5
  Head 07N0
  Inguinal
    Left 07NJ
    Right 07NH
  Internal Mammary
    Left 07N9
    Right 07N8
  Lower Extremity
    Left 07NG
    Right 07NF
  Mesenteric 07NB
  Neck
    Left 07N2
    Right 07N1
  Pelvis 07NC
  Thoracic Duct 07NK
  Thorax 07N7
  Upper Extremity
    Left 07N4
    Right 07N3
Mandible
  Left 0NNV
  Right 0NNT
Maxilla
  Left 0NNS
  Right 0NNR
Medulla Oblongata 00ND
Mesentery 0DNV
Metacarpal
  Left 0PNQ
  Right 0PNP
Metatarsal
  Left 0QNP
  Right 0QNN
Muscle
  Abdomen
    Left 0KNL
    Right 0KNK
  Extraocular
    Left 08NM
    Right 08NL
  Facial 0KN1
  Foot
    Left 0KNW
    Right 0KNV
  Hand
    Left 0KND
    Right 0KNC
  Head 0KN0
  Hip
    Left 0KNP
    Right 0KNN
  Lower Arm and Wrist
    Left 0KNB
    Right 0KN9
  Lower Leg
    Left 0KNT
    Right 0KNS
  Neck
    Left 0KN3
    Right 0KN2
  Papillary 02ND
  Perineum 0KNM
  Shoulder
    Left 0KN6
    Right 0KN5

Release (*continued*)
  Muscle (*continued*)
    Thorax
      Left 0KNJ
      Right 0KNH
    Tongue, Palate, Pharynx
      0KN4
    Trunk
      Left 0KNG
      Right 0KNF
    Upper Arm
      Left 0KN8
      Right 0KN7
    Upper Leg
      Left 0KNR
      Right 0KNQ
Nasopharynx 09NN
Nerve
  Abdominal Sympathetic 01NM
  Abducens 00NL
  Accessory 00NR
  Acoustic 00NN
  Brachial Plexus 01N3
  Cervical 01N1
  Cervical Plexus 01N0
  Facial 00NM
  Femoral 01ND
  Glossopharyngeal 00NP
  Head and Neck Sympathetic
    01NK
  Hypoglossal 00NS
  Lumbar 01NB
  Lumbar Plexus 01N9
  Lumbar Sympathetic 01NN
  Lumbosacral Plexus 01NA
  Median 01N5
  Oculomotor 00NH
  Olfactory 00NF
  Optic 00NG
  Peroneal 01NH
  Phrenic 01N2
  Pudendal 01NC
  Radial 01N6
  Sacral 01NR
  Sacral Plexus 01NQ
  Sacral Sympathetic 01NP
  Sciatic 01NF
  Thoracic 01N8
  Thoracic Sympathetic 01NL
  Tibial 01NG
  Trigeminal 00NK
  Trochlear 00NJ
  Ulnar 01N4
  Vagus 00NQ
Nipple
  Left 0HNX
  Right 0HNW
Nose 09NKZZ
Omentum
  Greater 0DNS
  Lesser 0DNT
Orbit
  Left 0NNQ
  Right 0NNP
Ovary
  Bilateral 0UN2
  Left 0UN1
  Right 0UN0
Palate
  Hard 0CN2
  Soft 0CN3
Pancreas 0FNG
Para-aortic Body 0GN9
Paraganglion Extremity 0GNF
Parathyroid Gland 0GNR
  Inferior
    Left 0GNP
    Right 0GNN
  Multiple 0GNQ
  Superior
    Left 0GNM
    Right 0GNL
Patella
  Left 0QNF
  Right 0QND
Penis 0VNSZZ
Pericardium 02NN
Peritoneum 0DNW
Phalanx
  Finger
    Left 0PNV
    Right 0PNT
  Thumb
    Left 0PNS
    Right 0PNR

Release (*continued*)
  Phalanx (*continued*)
    Toe
      Left 0QNR
      Right 0QNQ
Pharynx 0CNM
Pineal Body 0GN1
Pleura
  Left 0BNP
  Right 0BNN
Pons 00NB
Prepuce 0VNT
Prostate 0VN0
Radius
  Left 0PNJ
  Right 0PNH
Rectum 0DNP
Retina
  Left 08NF3ZZ
  Right 08NE3ZZ
Retinal Vessel
  Left 08NH3ZZ
  Right 08NG3ZZ
Rib
  Left 0PN2
  Right 0PN1
Sacrum 0QN1
Scapula
  Left 0PN6
  Right 0PN5
Sclera
  Left 08N7XZZ
  Right 08N6XZZ
Scrotum 0VN5
Septum
  Atrial 02N5
  Nasal 09NM
  Ventricular 02NM
Sinus
  Accessory 09NP
  Ethmoid
    Left 09NV
    Right 09NU
  Frontal
    Left 09NT
    Right 09NS
  Mastoid
    Left 09NC
    Right 09NB
  Maxillary
    Left 09NR
    Right 09NQ
  Sphenoid
    Left 09NX
    Right 09NW
Skin
  Abdomen 0HN7XZZ
  Back 0HN6XZZ
  Buttock 0HN8XZZ
  Chest 0HN5XZZ
  Ear
    Left 0HN3XZZ
    Right 0HN2XZZ
  Face 0HN1XZZ
  Foot
    Left 0HNNXZZ
    Right 0HNMXZZ
  Genitalia 0HNAXZZ
  Hand
    Left 0HNGXZZ
    Right 0HNFXZZ
  Lower Arm
    Left 0HNEXZZ
    Right 0HNDXZZ
  Lower Leg
    Left 0HNLXZZ
    Right 0HNKXZZ
  Neck 0HN4XZZ
  Perineum 0HN9XZZ
  Scalp 0HN0XZZ
  Upper Arm
    Left 0HNCXZZ
    Right 0HNBXZZ
  Upper Leg
    Left 0HNJXZZ
    Right 0HNHXZZ
Spinal Cord
  Cervical 00NW
  Lumbar 00NY
  Thoracic 00NX
Spinal Meninges 00NT
Spleen 07NP
Sternum 0PN0
Stomach 0DN6
  Pylorus 0DN7

Removal of device from *(continued)*

Artery
  Lower 04PY
  Upper 03PY
Back
  Lower 0WPL
  Upper 0WPK
Bladder 0TPB
Bone
  Facial 0NPW
  Lower 0QPY
  Nasal 0NPB
  Pelvic
    Left 0QP3
    Right 0QP2
  Upper 0PPY
Bone Marrow 07PT
Brain 00P0
Breast
  Left 0HPU
  Right 0HPT
Bursa and Ligament
  Lower 0MPY
  Upper 0MPX
Carpal
  Left 0PPN
  Right 0PPM
Cavity, Cranial 0WP1
Cerebral Ventricle 00P6
Chest Wall 0WP8
Cisterna Chyli 07PL
Clavicle
  Left 0PPB
  Right 0PP9
Coccyx 0QPS
Diaphragm 0BPT
Disc
  Cervical Vertebral 0RP3
  Cervicothoracic Vertebral 0RP5
  Lumbar Vertebral 0SP2
  Lumbosacral 0SP4
  Thoracic Vertebral 0RP9
  Thoracolumbar Vertebral 0RPB
Duct
  Hepatobiliary 0FPB
  Pancreatic 0FPD
Ear
  Inner
    Left 09PE
    Right 09PD
  Left 09PJ
  Right 09PH
Epididymis and Spermatic Cord 0VPM
Esophagus 0DP5
Extremity
  Lower
    Left 0YPB
    Right 0YP9
  Upper
    Left 0XP7
    Right 0XP6
Eye
  Left 08P1
  Right 08P0
Face 0WP2
Fallopian Tube 0UP8
Femoral Shaft
  Left 0QP9
  Right 0QP8
Femur
  Lower
    Left 0QPC
    Right 0QPB
  Upper
    Left 0QP7
    Right 0QP6
Fibula
  Left 0QPK
  Right 0QPJ
Finger Nail 0HPQX
Gallbladder 0FP4
Gastrointestinal Tract 0WPP
Genitourinary Tract 0WPR
Gland
  Adrenal 0GP5
  Endocrine 0GPS
  Pituitary 0GP0
  Salivary 0CPA
Glenoid Cavity
  Left 0PP8
  Right 0PP7
Great Vessel 02PY
Hair 0HPSX
Head 0WP0
Heart 02PA

Removal of device from *(continued)*

Humeral Head
  Left 0PPD
  Right 0PPC
Humeral Shaft
  Left 0PPG
  Right 0PPF
Intestinal Tract
  Lower 0DPD
  Upper 0DP0
Jaw
  Lower 0WP5
  Upper 0WP4
Joint
  Acromioclavicular
    Left 0RPH
    Right 0RPG
  Ankle
    Left 0SPG
    Right 0SPF
  Carpal
    Left 0RPR
    Right 0RPQ
  Cervical Vertebral 0RP1
  Cervicothoracic Vertebral
    0RP4
  Coccygeal 0SP6
  Elbow
    Left 0RPM
    Right 0RPL
  Finger Phalangeal
    Left 0RPX
    Right 0RPW
  Hip
    Left 0SPB
    Right 0SP9
  Knee
    Left 0SPD
    Right 0SPC
  Lumbar Vertebral 0SP0
  Lumbosacral 0SP3
  Metacarpocarpal
    Left 0RPT
    Right 0RPS
  Metacarpophalangeal
    Left 0RPV
    Right 0RPU
  Metatarsal-Phalangeal
    Left 0SPN
    Right 0SPM
  Metatarsal-Tarsal
    Left 0SPL
    Right 0SPK
  Occipital-cervical 0RP0
  Sacrococcygeal 0SP5
  Sacroiliac
    Left 0SP8
    Right 0SP7
  Shoulder
    Left 0RPK
    Right 0RPJ
  Sternoclavicular
    Left 0RPF
    Right 0RPE
  Tarsal
    Left 0SPJ
    Right 0SPH
  Temporomandibular
    Left 0RPD
    Right 0RPC
  Thoracic Vertebral 0RP6
  Thoracolumbar Vertebral
    0RPA
  Toe Phalangeal
    Left 0SPQ
    Right 0SPP
  Wrist
    Left 0RPP
    Right 0RPN
Kidney 0TP5
Larynx 0CPS
Lens
  Left 08PK3J
  Right 08PJ3J
Liver 0FP0
Lung
  Left 0BPL
  Right 0BPK
Lymphatic 07PN
  Thoracic Duct 07PK
Mediastinum 0WPC
Mesentery 0DPV
Metacarpal
  Left 0PPQ
  Right 0PPP

Removal of device from *(continued)*

Metatarsal
  Left 0QPP
  Right 0QPN
Mouth and Throat 0CPY
Muscle
  Extraocular
    Left 08PM
    Right 08PL
  Lower 0KPY
  Upper 0KPX
Neck 0WP6
Nerve
  Cranial 00PE
  Peripheral 01PY
Nose 09PK
Omentum 0DPU
Ovary 0UP3
Pancreas 0FPGZ
Parathyroid Gland 0GPR0
Patella
  Left 0QPF
  Right 0QPD
Pelvic Cavity 0WPJ
Penis 0VPS
Pericardial Cavity 0WPD
Perineum
  Female 0WPN
  Male 0WPM
Peritoneal Cavity 0WPG
Peritoneum 0DPW
Phalanx
  Finger
    Left 0PPV
    Right 0PPT
  Thumb
    Left 0PPS
    Right 0PPR
  Toe
    Left 0QPR
    Right 0QPQ
Pineal Body 0GP10
Pleura 0BPQ
Pleural Cavity
  Left 0WPB
  Right 0WP9
Products of Conception 10P0
Prostate and Seminal Vesicles
  0VP4
Radius
  Left 0PPJ
  Right 0PPH
Rectum 0DPP1
Respiratory Tract 0WPQZ
Retroperitoneum 0WPH
Rib
  Left 0PP2
  Right 0PP1
Sacrum 0QP1
Scapula
  Left 0PP6
  Right 0PP5
Scrotum and Tunica Vaginalis
  0VP8
Sinus 09PY0
Skin 0HPPX
Skull 0NP0
Spinal Canal 00PU
Spinal Cord 00PV
Spleen 07PP
Sternum 0PP0
Stomach 0DP6
Subcutaneous Tissue and Fascia
  Head and Neck 0JPS
  Lower Extremity 0JPW
  Trunk 0JPT
  Upper Extremity 0JPV
Tarsal
  Left 0QPM
  Right 0QPL
Tendon
  Lower 0LPY
  Upper 0LPX
Testis 0VPD
Thymus 07PM
Thyroid Gland 0GPK0
Tibia
  Left 0QPH
  Right 0QPG
Toe Nail 0HPRXZ
Trachea 0BP1
Tracheobronchial Tree 0BP0
Tympanic Membrane
  Left 09P80
  Right 09P70

Repair (*continued*)

Buttock
 Left 0YQ1
 Right 0YQ0
Carina 0BQ2
Carotid Bodies, Bilateral 0GQ8
Carotid Body
 Left 0GQ6
 Right 0GQ7
Carpal
 Left 0PQN
 Right 0PQM
Cecum 0DQH
Cerebellum 00QC
Cerebral Hemisphere 00Q7
Cerebral Meninges 00Q1
Cerebral Ventricle 00Q6
Cervix 0UQC
Chest Wall 0WQ8
Chordae Tendineae 02Q9
Choroid
 Left 08QB
 Right 08QA
Cisterna Chyli 07QL
Clavicle
 Left 0PQB
 Right 0PQ9
Clitoris 0UQJ
Coccygeal Glomus 0GQB
Coccyx 0QQS
Colon
 Ascending 0DQK
 Descending 0DQM
 Sigmoid 0DQN
 Transverse 0DQL
Conduction Mechanism 02Q8
Conjunctiva
 Left 08QTXZZ
 Right 08QSXZZ
Cord
 Bilateral 0VQH
 Left 0VQG
 Right 0VQF
Cornea
 Left 08Q9XZZ
 Right 08Q8XZZ
Cul-de-sac 0UQF
Diaphragm
 Left 0BQS
 Right 0BQR
Disc
 Cervical Vertebral 0RQ3
 Cervicothoracic Vertebral 0RQ5
 Lumbar Vertebral 0SQ2
 Lumbosacral 0SQ4
 Thoracic Vertebral 0RQ9
 Thoracolumbar Vertebral 0RQB
Duct
 Common Bile 0FQ9
 Cystic 0FQ8
 Hepatic
  Left 0FQ6
  Right 0FQ5
 Lacrimal
  Left 08QY
  Right 08QX
 Pancreatic 0FQD
  Accessory 0FQF
 Parotid
  Left 0CQC
  Right 0CQB
Duodenum 0DQ9
Dura Mater 00Q2
Ear
 External
  Bilateral 09Q2
  Left 09Q1
  Right 09Q0
 External Auditory Canal
  Left 09Q4
  Right 09Q3
 Inner
  Left 09QE0ZZ
  Right 09QD0ZZ
 Middle
  Left 09Q60ZZ
  Right 09Q50ZZ
Elbow Region
 Left 0XQC
 Right 0XQB
Epididymis
 Bilateral 0VQL
 Left 0VQK
 Right 0VQJ

Repair (*continued*)

Epiglottis 0CQR
Esophagogastric Junction 0DQ4
Esophagus 0DQ5
 Lower 0DQ3
 Middle 0DQ2
 Upper 0DQ1
Eustachian Tube
 Left 09QG
 Right 09QF
Extremity
 Lower
  Left 0YQB
  Right 0YQ9
 Upper
  Left 0XQ7
  Right 0XQ6
Eye
 Left 08Q1XZZ
 Right 08Q0XZZ
Eyelid
 Lower
  Left 08QR
  Right 08QQ
 Upper
  Left 08QP
  Right 08QN
Face 0WQ2
Fallopian Tube
 Left 0UQ6
 Right 0UQ5
Fallopian Tubes, Bilateral 0UQ7
Femoral Region
 Bilateral 0YQE
 Left 0YQ8
 Right 0YQ7
Femoral Shaft
 Left 0QQ9
 Right 0QQ8
Femur
 Lower
  Left 0QQC
  Right 0QQB
 Upper
  Left 0QQ7
  Right 0QQ6
Fibula
 Left 0QQK
 Right 0QQJ
Finger
 Index
  Left 0XQP
  Right 0XQN
 Little
  Left 0XQW
  Right 0XQV
 Middle
  Left 0XQR
  Right 0XQQ
 Ring
  Left 0XQT
  Right 0XQS
Finger Nail 0HQQXZZ
Foot
 Left 0YQN
 Right 0YQM
Gallbladder 0FQ4
Gingiva
 Lower 0CQ6
 Upper 0CQ5
Gland
 Adrenal
  Bilateral 0GQ4
  Left 0GQ2
  Right 0GQ3
 Lacrimal
  Left 08QW
  Right 08QV
 Minor Salivary 0CQJ
 Parotid
  Left 0CQ9
  Right 0CQ8
 Pituitary 0GQ0
 Sublingual
  Left 0CQF
  Right 0CQD
 Submaxillary
  Left 0CQH
  Right 0CQG
 Vestibular 0UQL
Glenoid Cavity
 Left 0PQ8
 Right 0PQ7
Glomus Jugulare 0GQC

Repair (*continued*)

Hand
 Left 0XQK
 Right 0XQJ
Head 0WQ0
Heart 02QA
 Left 02QC
 Right 02QB
Humeral Head
 Left 0PQD
 Right 0PQC
Humeral Shaft
 Left 0PQG
 Right 0PQF
Hymen 0UQK
Hypothalamus 00QA
Ileocecal Valve 0DQC
Ileum 0DQB
Inguinal Region
 Bilateral 0YQA
 Left 0YQ6
 Right 0YQ5
Intestine
 Large 0DQE
  Left 0DQG
  Right 0DQF
 Small 0DQ8
Iris
 Left 08QD3ZZ
 Right 08QC3ZZ
Jaw
 Lower 0WQ5
 Upper 0WQ4
Jejunum 0DQA
Joint
 Acromioclavicular
  Left 0RQH
  Right 0RQG
 Ankle
  Left 0SQG
  Right 0SQF
 Carpal
  Left 0RQR
  Right 0RQQ
 Cervical Vertebral 0RQ1
 Cervicothoracic Vertebral 0RQ4
 Coccygeal 0SQ6
 Elbow
  Left 0RQM
  Right 0RQL
 Finger Phalangeal
  Left 0RQX
  Right 0RQW
 Hip
  Left 0SQB
  Right 0SQ9
 Knee
  Left 0SQD
  Right 0SQC
 Lumbar Vertebral 0SQ0
 Lumbosacral 0SQ3
 Metacarpocarpal
  Left 0RQT
  Right 0RQS
 Metacarpophalangeal
  Left 0RQV
  Right 0RQU
 Metatarsal-Phalangeal
  Left 0SQN
  Right 0SQM
 Metatarsal-Tarsal
  Left 0SQL
  Right 0SQK
 Occipital-cervical 0RQ0
 Sacrococcygeal 0SQ5
 Sacroiliac
  Left 0SQ8
  Right 0SQ7
 Shoulder
  Left 0RQK
  Right 0RQJ
 Sternoclavicular
  Left 0RQF
  Right 0RQE
 Tarsal
  Left 0SQJ
  Right 0SQH
 Temporomandibular
  Left 0RQD
  Right 0RQC
 Thoracic Vertebral 0RQ6
 Thoracolumbar Vertebral 0RQA
 Toe Phalangeal
  Left 0SQQ
  Right 0SQP

Repair

Repair (continued)
  Skin (continued)
    Genitalia 0HQAXZZ
    Hand
      Left 0HQGXZZ
      Right 0HQFXZZ
    Lower Arm
      Left 0HQEXZZ
      Right 0HQDXZZ
    Lower Leg
      Left 0HQLXZZ
      Right 0HQKXZZ
    Neck 0HQ4XZZ
    Perineum 0HQ9XZZ
    Scalp 0HQ0XZZ
    Upper Arm
      Left 0HQCXZZ
      Right 0HQBXZZ
    Upper Leg
      Left 0HQJXZZ
      Right 0HQHXZZ
  Skull 0NQ0
  Spinal Cord
    Cervical 00QW
    Lumbar 00QY
    Thoracic 00QX
  Spinal Meninges 00QT
  Spleen 07QP
  Sternum 0PQ0
  Stomach 0DQ6
    Pylorus 0DQ7
  Subcutaneous Tissue and Fascia
    Abdomen 0JQ8
    Back 0JQ7
    Buttock 0JQ9
    Chest 0JQ6
    Face 0JQ1
    Foot
      Left 0JQR
      Right 0JQQ
    Hand
      Left 0JQK
      Right 0JQJ
    Lower Arm
      Left 0JQH
      Right 0JQG
    Lower Leg
      Left 0JQP
      Right 0JQN
    Neck
      Anterior 0JQ4
      Posterior 0JQ5
    Pelvic Region 0JQC
    Perineum 0JQB
    Scalp 0JQ0
    Upper Arm
      Left 0JQF
      Right 0JQD
    Upper Leg
      Left 0JQM
      Right 0JQL
  Tarsal
    Left 0QQM
    Right 0QQL
  Tendon
    Abdomen
      Left 0LQG
      Right 0LQF
    Ankle
      Left 0LQT
      Right 0LQS
    Foot
      Left 0LQW
      Right 0LQV
    Hand
      Left 0LQ8
      Right 0LQ7
    Head and Neck 0LQ0
    Hip
      Left 0LQK
      Right 0LQJ
    Knee
      Left 0LQR
      Right 0LQQ
    Lower Arm and Wrist
      Left 0LQ6
      Right 0LQ5
    Lower Leg
      Left 0LQP
      Right 0LQN
    Perineum 0LQH
    Shoulder
      Left 0LQ2
      Right 0LQ1

Repair (continued)
  Tendon (continued)
    Thorax
      Left 0LQD
      Right 0LQC
    Trunk
      Left 0LQB
      Right 0LQ9
    Upper Arm
      Left 0LQ4
      Right 0LQ3
    Upper Leg
      Left 0LQM
      Right 0LQL
  Testis
    Bilateral 0VQC
    Left 0VQB
    Right 0VQ9
  Thalamus 00Q9
  Thumb
    Left 0XQM
    Right 0XQL
  Thymus 07QM
  Thyroid Gland 0GQK
    Left Lobe 0GQG
    Right Lobe 0GQH
  Thyroid Gland Isthmus 0GQJ
  Tibia
    Left 0QQH
    Right 0QQG
  Toe
    1st
      Left 0YQQ
      Right 0YQP
    2nd
      Left 0YQS
      Right 0YQR
    3rd
      Left 0YQU
      Right 0YQT
    4th
      Left 0YQW
      Right 0YQV
    5th
      Left 0YQY
      Right 0YQX
  Toe Nail 0HQRXZZ
  Tongue 0CQ7
  Tonsils 0CQP
  Tooth
    Lower 0CQX
    Upper 0CQW
  Trachea 0BQ1
  Tunica Vaginalis
    Left 0VQ7
    Right 0VQ6
  Turbinate, Nasal 09QL
  Tympanic Membrane
    Left 09Q8
    Right 09Q7
  Ulna
    Left 0PQL
    Right 0PQK
  Ureter
    Left 0TQ7
    Right 0TQ6
  Urethra 0TQD
  Uterine Supporting Structure 0UQ4
  Uterus 0UQ9
  Uvula 0CQN
  Vagina 0UQG
  Valve
    Aortic 02QF
    Mitral 02QG
    Pulmonary 02QH
    Tricuspid 02QJ
  Vas Deferens
    Bilateral 0VQQ
    Left 0VQP
    Right 0VQN
  Vein
    Axillary
      Left 05Q8
      Right 05Q7
    Azygos 05Q0
    Basilic
      Left 05QC
      Right 05QB
    Brachial
      Left 05QA
      Right 05Q9
    Cephalic
      Left 05QF
      Right 05QD

Repair (continued)
  Vein (continued)
    Colic 06Q7
    Common Iliac
      Left 06QD
      Right 06QC
    Coronary 02Q4
    Esophageal 06Q3
    External Iliac
      Left 06QG
      Right 06QF
    External Jugular
      Left 05QQ
      Right 05QP
    Face
      Left 05QV
      Right 05QT
    Femoral
      Left 06QN
      Right 06QM
    Foot
      Left 06QV
      Right 06QT
    Gastric 06Q2
    Greater Saphenous
      Left 06QQ
      Right 06QP
    Hand
      Left 05QH
      Right 05QG
    Hemiazygos 05Q1
    Hepatic 06Q4
    Hypogastric
      Left 06QJ
      Right 06QH
    Inferior Mesenteric 06Q6
    Innominate
      Left 05Q4
      Right 05Q3
    Internal Jugular
      Left 05QN
      Right 05QM
    Intracranial 05QL
    Lesser Saphenous
      Left 06QS
      Right 06QR
    Lower 06QY
    Portal 06Q8
    Pulmonary
      Left 02QT
      Right 02QS
    Renal
      Left 06QB
      Right 06Q9
    Splenic 06Q1
    Subclavian
      Left 05Q6
      Right 05Q5
    Superior Mesenteric 06Q5
    Upper 05QY
    Vertebral
      Left 05QS
      Right 05QR
  Vena Cava
    Inferior 06Q0
    Superior 02QV
  Ventricle
    Left 02QL
    Right 02QK
  Vertebra
    Cervical 0PQ3
    Lumbar 0QQ0
    Thoracic 0PQ4
  Vesicle
    Bilateral 0VQ3
    Left 0VQ2
    Right 0VQ1
  Vitreous
    Left 08Q53ZZ
    Right 08Q43ZZ
  Vocal Cord
    Left 0CQV
    Right 0CQT
  Vulva 0UQM
  Wrist Region
    Left 0XQH
    Right 0XQG
Replacement
  Acetabulum
    Left 0QR5
    Right 0QR4
  Ampulla of Vater 0FRC
  Anal Sphincter 0DRR

Replacement

Replacement *(continued)*
    Joint *(continued)*
        Occipital-cervical 0RR00
        Sacrococcygeal 0SR50
        Sacroiliac
            Left 0SR80
            Right 0SR70
        Shoulder
            Left 0RRK
            Right 0RRJ
        Sternoclavicular
            Left 0RRF0
            Right 0RRE0
        Tarsal
            Left 0SRJ0
            Right 0SRH0
        Temporomandibular
            Left 0RRD0
            Right 0RRC0
        Thoracic Vertebral 0RR60
        Thoracolumbar Vertebral
            0RRA0
        Toe Phalangeal
            Left 0SRQ0
            Right 0SRP0
        Wrist
            Left 0RRP0
            Right 0RRN0
    Kidney Pelvis
        Left 0TR4
        Right 0TR3
    Larynx 0CRS
    Lens
        Left 08RK30Z
        Right 08RJ30Z
    Lip
        Lower 0CR1
        Upper 0CR0
    Mandible
        Left 0NRV
        Right 0NRT
    Maxilla
        Left 0NRS
        Right 0NRR
    Mesentery 0DRV
    Metacarpal
        Left 0PRQ
        Right 0PRP
    Metatarsal
        Left 0QRP
        Right 0QR
    Muscle, Papillary 02RD
    Nasopharynx 09RN
    Nipple
        Left 0HRX
        Right 0HRW
    Nose 09RK
    Omentum
        Greater 0DRS
        Lesser 0DRT
    Orbit
        Left 0NRQ
        Right 0NRP
    Palate
        Hard 0CR2
        Soft 0CR3
    Patella
        Left 0QRF
        Right 0QRD
    Pericardium 02RN
    Peritoneum 0DRW
    Phalanx
        Finger
            Left 0PRV
            Right 0PRT
        Thumb
            Left 0PRS
            Right 0PRR
        Toe
            Left 0QRR
            Right 0QRQ
    Pharynx 0CRM
    Radius
        Left 0PRJ
        Right 0PRH
    Retinal Vessel
        Left 08RH3
        Right 08RG3
    Rib
        Left 0PR2
        Right 0PR1
    Sacrum 0QR1
    Scapula
        Left 0PR6
        Right 0PR5

Replacement *(continued)*
    Sclera
        Left 08R7X
        Right 08R6X
    Septum
        Atrial 02R5
        Nasal 09RM
        Ventricular
            02RM
    Skin
        Abdomen 0HR7
        Back 0HR6
        Buttock 0HR8
        Chest 0HR5
        Ear
            Left 0HR3
            Right 0HR2
        Face 0HR1
        Foot
            Left 0HRN
            Right 0HRM
        Genitalia 0HRA
        Hand
            Left 0HRG
            Right 0HRF
        Lower Arm
            Left 0HRE
            Right 0HRD
        Lower Leg
            Left 0HRL
            Right 0HRK
        Neck 0HR4
        Perineum 0HR9
        Scalp 0HR0
        Upper Arm
            Left 0HRC
            Right 0HRB
        Upper Leg
            Left 0HRJ
            Right 0HRH
    Skull 0NR0
    Sternum 0PR0
    Subcutaneous Tissue and Fascia
        Abdomen 0JR8
        Back 0JR7
        Buttock 0JR9
        Chest 0JR6
        Face 0JR1
        Foot
            Left 0JRR
            Right 0JRQ
        Hand
            Left 0JRK
            Right 0JRJ
        Lower Arm
            Left 0JRH
            Right 0JRG
        Lower Leg
            Left 0JRP
            Right 0JRN
        Neck
            Anterior 0JR4
            Posterior 0JR5
        Pelvic Region 0JRC
        Perineum 0JRB
        Scalp 0JR0
        Upper Arm
            Left 0JRF
            Right 0JRD
        Upper Leg
            Left 0JRM
            Right 0JRL
    Tarsal
        Left 0QRM
        Right 0QRL
    Tendon
        Abdomen
            Left 0LRG
            Right 0LRF
        Ankle
            Left 0LRT
            Right 0LRS
        Foot
            Left 0LRW
            Right 0LRV
        Hand
            Left 0LR8
            Right 0LR7
        Head and Neck 0LR0
        Hip
            Left 0LRK
            Right 0LRJ
        Knee
            Left 0LRR
            Right 0LRQ

Replacement *(continued)*
    Tendon *(continued)*
        Lower Arm and Wrist
            Left 0LR6
            Right 0LR5
        Lower Leg
            Left 0LRP
            Right 0LRN
        Perineum 0LRH
        Shoulder
            Left 0LR2
            Right 0LR1
        Thorax
            Left 0LRD
            Right 0LRC
        Trunk
            Left 0LRB
            Right 0LR9
        Upper Arm
            Left 0LR4
            Right 0LR3
        Upper Leg
            Left 0LRM
            Right 0LRL
    Testis
        Bilateral 0VRC0J
        Left 0VRB0J
        Right 0VR90J
    Thumb
        Left 0XRM
        Right 0XRL
    Tibia
        Left 0QRH
        Right 0QRG
    Toe Nail 0HRRX
    Tongue 0CR7
    Tooth
        Lower 0CRX
        Upper 0CRW
    Turbinate, Nasal
        09RL
    Tympanic Membrane
        Left 09R8
        Right 09R7
    Ulna
        Left 0PRL
        Right 0PRK
    Ureter
        Left 0TR7
        Right 0TR6
    Urethra 0TRD
    Uvula 0CRN
    Valve
        Aortic 02RF
        Mitral 02RG
        Pulmonary 02RH
        Tricuspid 02RJ
    Vein
        Axillary
            Left 05R8
            Right 05R7
        Azygos 05R0
        Basilic
            Left 05RC
            Right 05RB
        Brachial
            Left 05RA
            Right 05R9
        Cephalic
            Left 05RF
            Right 05RD
        Colic 06R7
        Common Iliac
            Left 06RD
            Right 06RC
        Esophageal 06R3
        External Iliac
            Left 06RG
            Right 06RF
        External Jugular
            Left 05RQ
            Right 05RP
        Face
            Left 05RV
            Right 05RT
        Femoral
            Left 06RN
            Right 06RM
        Foot
            Left 06RV
            Right 06RT
        Gastric 06R2
        Greater Saphenous
            Left 06RQ
            Right 06RP

Replacement

Reposition (continued)

Duct
  Common Bile 0FS9
  Cystic 0FS8
  Hepatic
    Left 0FS6
    Right 0FS5
  Lacrimal
    Left 08SY
    Right 08SX
  Pancreatic 0FSD
    Accessory 0FSF
  Parotid
    Left 0CSC
    Right 0CSB
Duodenum 0DS9ZZ
Ear
  Bilateral 09S2ZZ
  Left 09S1ZZ
  Right 09S0ZZ
Epiglottis 0CSR
Esophagus 0DS5ZZ
Eustachian Tube
  Left 09SG
  Right 09SF
Eyelid
  Lower
    Left 08SR
    Right 08SQ
  Upper
    Left 08SP
    Right 08SN
Fallopian Tube
  Left 0US6
  Right 0US5
Fallopian Tubes, Bilateral
  0US7
Femoral Shaft
  Left 0QS9
  Right 0QS8
Femur
  Lower
    Left 0QSC
    Right 0QSB
  Upper
    Left 0QS7
    Right 0QS6
Fibula
  Left 0QSK
  Right 0QSJ
Gallbladder 0FS4
Gland
  Adrenal
    Left 0GS2
    Right 0GS3
  Lacrimal
    Left 08SW
    Right 08SV
Glenoid Cavity
  Left 0PS8
  Right 0PS7
Hair 0HSSXZZ
Humeral Head
  Left 0PSD
  Right 0PSC
Humeral Shaft
  Left 0PSG
  Right 0PSF
Ileum 0DSB
Iris
  Left 08SD3ZZ
  Right 08SC3ZZ
Jejunum 0DSAZZ
Joint
  Acromioclavicular
    Left 0RSHZ
    Right 0RSGZ
  Ankle
    Left 0SSG
    Right 0SSF
  Carpal
    Left 0RSR
    Right 0RSQ
  Cervical Vertebral 0RS1
  Cervicothoracic Vertebral 0RS4
  Coccygeal 0SS6
  Elbow
    Left 0RSM
    Right 0RSL
  Finger Phalangeal
    Left 0RSX
    Right 0RSW
  Hip
    Left 0SSB
    Right 0SS9

Reposition (continued)

Joint (continued)
  Knee
    Left 0SSD
    Right 0SSC
  Lumbar Vertebral 0SS0
  Lumbosacral 0SS3
  Metacarpocarpal
    Left 0RST
    Right 0RSS
  Metacarpophalangeal
    Left 0RSV
    Right 0RSU
  Metatarsal-Phalangeal
    Left 0SSN
    Right 0SSM
  Metatarsal-Tarsal
    Left 0SSL
    Right 0SSK
  Occipital-cervical 0RS0
  Sacrococcygeal 0SS5
  Sacroiliac
    Left 0SS8
    Right 0SS7
  Shoulder
    Left 0RSK
    Right 0RSJ
  Sternoclavicular
    Left 0RSF
    Right 0RSE
  Tarsal
    Left 0SSJ
    Right 0SSH
  Temporomandibular
    Left 0RSD
    Right 0RSC
  Thoracic Vertebral 0RS6
  Thoracolumbar Vertebral 0RSA
  Toe Phalangeal
    Left 0SSQ
    Right 0SSP
  Wrist
    Left 0RSP
    Right 0RSN
Kidney
  Left 0TS1
  Right 0TS0
Kidney Pelvis
  Left 0TS4
  Right 0TS3
Kidneys, Bilateral 0TS2
Lens
  Left 08SK3ZZ
  Right 08SJ3ZZ
Lip
  Lower 0CS1
  Upper 0CS0
Liver 0FS0
Lung
  Left 0BSL0ZZ
  Lower Lobe
    Left 0BSJ0ZZ
    Right 0BSF0ZZ
  Middle Lobe, Right 0BSD0ZZ
  Right 0BSK0ZZ
  Upper Lobe
    Left 0BSG0ZZ
    Right 0BSC0ZZ
Lung Lingula 0BSH0ZZ
Mandible
  Left 0NSV
  Right 0NST
Maxilla
  Left 0NSS
  Right 0NSR
Metacarpal
  Left 0PSQ
  Right 0PSP
Metatarsal
  Left 0QSP
  Right 0QSN
Muscle
  Abdomen
    Left 0KSL
    Right 0KSK
  Extraocular
    Left 08SM
    Right 08SL
  Facial 0KS1
  Foot
    Left 0KSW
    Right 0KSV
  Hand
    Left 0KSD
    Right 0KSC

Reposition (continued)

Muscle (continued)
  Head 0KS0
  Hip
    Left 0KSP
    Right 0KSN
  Lower Arm and Wrist
    Left 0KSB
    Right 0KS9
  Lower Leg
    Left 0KST
    Right 0KSS
  Neck
    Left 0KS3
    Right 0KS2
  Perineum 0KSM
  Shoulder
    Left 0KS6
    Right 0KS5
  Thorax
    Left 0KSJ
    Right 0KSH
  Tongue, Palate, Pharynx
    0KS4
  Trunk
    Left 0KSG
    Right 0KSF
  Upper Arm
    Left 0KS8
    Right 0KS7
  Upper Leg
    Left 0KSR
    Right 0KSQ
Nerve
  Abducens 00SL
  Accessory 00SR
  Acoustic 00SN
  Brachial Plexus 01S3
  Cervical 01S1
  Cervical Plexus 01S0
  Facial 00SM
  Femoral 01SD
  Glossopharyngeal 00SP
  Hypoglossal 00SS
  Lumbar 01SB
  Lumbar Plexus 01S9
  Lumbosacral Plexus
    01SA
  Median 01S5
  Oculomotor 00SH
  Olfactory 00SF
  Optic 00SG
  Peroneal 01SH
  Phrenic 01S2
  Pudendal 01SC
  Radial 01S6
  Sacral 01SR
  Sacral Plexus 01SQ
  Sciatic 01SF
  Thoracic 01S8
  Tibial 01SG
  Trigeminal 00SK
  Trochlear 00SJ
  Ulnar 01S4
  Vagus 00SQ
Nipple
  Left 0HSXXZZ
  Right 0HSWXZZ
Nose 09SK
Orbit
  Left 0NSQ
  Right 0NSP
Ovary
  Bilateral 0US2
  Left 0US1
  Right 0US0
Palate
  Hard 0CS2
  Soft 0CS3
Pancreas 0FSG
Parathyroid Gland 0GSR
  Inferior
    Left 0GSP
    Right 0GSN
  Multiple 0GSQ
  Superior
    Left 0GSM
    Right 0GSL
Patella
  Left 0QSF
  Right 0QSD
Phalanx
  Finger
    Left 0PSV
    Right 0PST

Resection

Resection *(continued)*
  Bursa and Ligament *(continued)*
    Knee
      Left 0MTP
      Right 0MTN
    Lower Extremity
      Left 0MTW
      Right 0MTV
    Perineum 0MTK
    Shoulder
      Left 0MT2
      Right 0MT1
    Thorax
      Left 0MTG
      Right 0MTF
    Trunk
      Left 0MTD
      Right 0MTC
    Upper Extremity
      Left 0MTB
      Right 0MT9
    Wrist
      Left 0MT6
      Right 0MT5
  Carina 0BT2
  Carotid Bodies, Bilateral 0GT8
  Carotid Body
    Left 0GT6
    Right 0GT7
  Carpal
    Left 0PTN0ZZ
    Right 0PTM0ZZ
  Cecum 0DTH
  Cerebral Hemisphere 00T7
  Cervix 0UTC
  Chordae Tendineae 02T9
  Cisterna Chyli 07TL
  Clavicle
    Left 0PTB0ZZ
    Right 0PT90ZZ
  Clitoris 0UTJ
  Coccygeal Glomus 0GTB
  Coccyx 0QTS0ZZ
  Colon
    Ascending 0DTK
    Descending 0DTM
    Sigmoid 0DTN
    Transverse 0DTL
  Conduction Mechanism 02T8
  Cord
    Bilateral 0VTH
    Left 0VTG
    Right 0VTF
  Cornea
    Left 08T9XZZ
    Right 08T8XZZ
  Cul-de-sac 0UTF
  Diaphragm
    Left 0BTS
    Right 0BTR
  Disc
    Cervical Vertebral 0RT30ZZ
    Cervicothoracic Vertebral 0RT50ZZ
    Lumbar Vertebral 0ST20ZZ
    Lumbosacral 0ST40ZZ
    Thoracic Vertebral 0RT90ZZ
    Thoracolumbar Vertebral 0RTB0ZZ
  Duct
    Common Bile 0FT9
    Cystic 0FT8
    Hepatic
      Left 0FT6
      Right 0FT5
    Lacrimal
      Left 08TY
      Right 08TX
    Pancreatic 0FTD
      Accessory 0FTF
    Parotid
      Left 0CTC0ZZ
      Right 0CTB0ZZ
  Duodenum 0DT9
  Ear
    External
      Left 09T1
      Right 09T0
    Inner
      Left 09TE0
      Right 09TD0
    Middle
      Left 09T60
      Right 09T50
  Epididymis
    Bilateral 0VTL
    Left 0VTK
    Right 0VTJ

Resection *(continued)*
  Epiglottis 0CTR
  Esophagogastric Junction 0DT4
  Esophagus 0DT5
    Lower 0DT3
    Middle 0DT2
    Upper 0DT1
  Eustachian Tube
    Left 09TG
    Right 09TF
  Eye
    Left 08T1XZZ
    Right 08T0XZZ
  Eyelid
    Lower
      Left 08TR
      Right 08TQ
    Upper
      Left 08TP
      Right 08TN
  Fallopian Tube
    Left 0UT6
    Right 0UT5
  Fallopian Tubes, Bilateral 0UT7
  Femoral Shaft
    Left 0QT90ZZ
    Right 0QT80ZZ
  Femur
    Lower
      Left 0QTC0ZZ
      Right 0QTB0ZZ
    Upper
      Left 0QT70ZZ
      Right 0QT60ZZ
  Fibula
    Left 0QTK0ZZ
    Right 0QTJ0ZZ
  Finger Nail 0HTQXZZ
  Gallbladder 0FT4
  Gland
    Adrenal
      Bilateral 0GT4
      Left 0GT2
      Right 0GT3
    Lacrimal
      Left 08TW
      Right 08TV
    Minor Salivary 0CTJ0ZZ
    Parotid
      Left 0CT90ZZ
      Right 0CT80ZZ
    Pituitary 0GT0
    Sublingual
      Left 0CTF0ZZ
      Right 0CTD0ZZ
    Submaxillary
      Left 0CTH0ZZ
      Right 0CTG0ZZ
    Vestibular 0UTL
  Glenoid Cavity
    Left 0PT80ZZ
    Right 0PT70ZZ
  Glomus Jugulare 0GTC
  Humeral Head
    Left 0PTD0ZZ
    Right 0PTC0ZZ
  Humeral Shaft
    Left 0PTG0ZZ
    Right 0PTF0ZZ
  Hymen 0UTK
  Ileocecal Valve 0DTC
  Ileum 0DTB
  Intestine
    Large 0DTE
      Left 0DTG
      Right 0DTF
    Small 0DT8
  Iris
    Left 08TD3ZZ
    Right 08TC3ZZ
  Jejunum 0DTA
  Joint
    Acromioclavicular
      Left 0RTH0ZZ
      Right 0RTG0ZZ
    Ankle
      Left 0STG0ZZ
      Right 0STF0ZZ
    Carpal
      Left 0RTR0ZZ
      Right 0RTQ0ZZ
    Cervicothoracic Vertebral 0RT40ZZ
    Coccygeal 0ST60ZZ
    Elbow
      Left 0RTM0ZZ
      Right 0RTL0ZZ

Resection *(continued)*
  Joint *(continued)*
    Finger Phalangeal
      Left 0RTX0ZZ
      Right 0RTW0ZZ
    Hip
      Left 0STB0ZZ
      Right 0ST90ZZ
    Knee
      Left 0STD0ZZ
      Right 0STC0ZZ
    Metacarpocarpal
      Left 0RTT0ZZ
      Right 0RTS0ZZ
    Metacarpophalangeal
      Left 0RTV0ZZ
      Right 0RTU0ZZ
    Metatarsal-Phalangeal
      Left 0STN0ZZ
      Right 0STM0ZZ
    Metatarsal-Tarsal
      Left 0STL0ZZ
      Right 0STK0ZZ
    Sacrococcygeal 0ST50ZZ
    Sacroiliac
      Left 0ST80ZZ
      Right 0ST70ZZ
    Shoulder
      Left 0RTK0ZZ
      Right 0RTJ0ZZ
    Sternoclavicular
      Left 0RTF0ZZ
      Right 0RTE0ZZ
    Tarsal
      Left 0STJ0ZZ
      Right 0STH0ZZ
    Temporomandibular
      Left 0RTD0ZZ
      Right 0RTC0ZZ
    Toe Phalangeal
      Left 0STQ0ZZ
      Right 0STP0ZZ
    Wrist
      Left 0RTP0ZZ
      Right 0RTN0ZZ
  Kidney
    Left 0TT1
    Right 0TT0
  Kidney Pelvis
    Left 0TT4
    Right 0TT3
  Kidneys, Bilateral 0TT2
  Larynx 0CTS
  Lens
    Left 08TK3ZZ
    Right 08TJ3ZZ
  Lip
    Lower 0CT1
    Upper 0CT0
  Liver 0FT0
    Left Lobe 0FT2
    Right Lobe 0FT1
  Lung
    Bilateral 0BTM
    Left 0BTL
    Lower Lobe
      Left 0BTJ
      Right 0BTF
    Middle Lobe, Right 0BTD
    Right 0BTK
    Upper Lobe
      Left 0BTG
      Right 0BTC
  Lung Lingula 0BTH
  Lymphatic
    Aortic 07TD
    Axillary
      Left 07T6
      Right 07T5
    Head 07T0
    Inguinal
      Left 07TJ
      Right 07TH
    Internal Mammary
      Left 07T9
      Right 07T8
    Lower Extremity
      Left 07TG
      Right 07TF
    Mesenteric 07TB
    Neck
      Left 07T2
      Right 07T1
    Pelvis 07TC
    Thoracic Duct 07TK
    Thorax 07T7

Restriction (continued)
Artery (continued)
External Carotid
Left 03VN
Right 03VM
External Iliac
Left 04VJ
Right 04VHZ
Face 03VR
Femoral
Left 04VL
Right 04VK
Foot
Left 04VW
Right 04VV
Gastric 04V2
Hand
Left 03VF
Right 03VD
Hepatic 04V3
Inferior Mesenteric 04VB
Innominate 03V2
Internal Carotid
Left 03VL
Right 03VK
Internal Iliac
Left 04VF
Right 04VE
Internal Mammary
Left 03V1
Right 03V0
Intracranial 03VG
Lower 04VY
Peroneal
Left 04VU
Right 04VT
Popliteal
Left 04VN
Right 04VM
Posterior Tibial
Left 04VS
Right 04VR
Pulmonary
Left 02VR
Right 02VQ
Pulmonary Trunk 02VP
Radial
Left 03VC
Right 03VB
Renal
Left 04VA
Right 04V9
Splenic 04V4
Subclavian
Left 03V4
Right 03V3
Superior Mesenteric 04V5
Temporal
Left 03VT
Right 03VS
Thyroid
Left 03VV
Right 03VU
Ulnar
Left 03VA
Right 03V9
Upper 03VY
Vertebral
Left 03VQ
Right 03VP
Bladder 0TVB
Bladder Neck 0TVC
Bronchus
Lingula 0BV9
Lower Lobe
Left 0BVB
Right 0BV6
Main
Left 0BV7
Right 0BV3
Middle Lobe, Right 0BV5
Upper Lobe
Left 0BV8
Right 0BV4
Carina 0BV2
Cecum 0DVH
Cervix 0UVC
Cisterna Chyli 07VL
Colon
Ascending 0DVK
Descending 0DVM
Sigmoid 0DVN
Transverse 0DVL
Duct
Common Bile 0FV9
Cystic 0FV8

Restriction (continued)
Duct (continued)
Hepatic
Left 0FV6
Right 0FV5
Lacrimal
Left 08VY
Right 08VX
Pancreatic 0FVD
Accessory 0FVF
Parotid
Left 0CVC
Right 0CVB
Duodenum 0DV9
Esophagogastric Junction
0DV4
Esophagus 0DV5
Lower 0DV3
Middle 0DV2
Upper 0DV1
Heart 02VA
Ileocecal Valve 0DVC
Ileum 0DVB
Intestine
Large 0DVE
Left 0DVG
Right 0DVF
Small 0DV8
Jejunum 0DVA
Kidney Pelvis
Left 0TV4
Right 0TV3
Lymphatic
Aortic 07VD
Axillary
Left 07V6
Right 07V5
Head 07V0
Inguinal
Left 07VJ
Right 07VH
Internal Mammary
Left 07V9
Right 07V8
Lower Extremity
Left 07VG
Right 07VF
Mesenteric 07VB
Neck
Left 07V2
Right 07V1
Pelvis 07VC
Thoracic Duct 07VK
Thorax 07V7
Upper Extremity
Left 07V4
Right 07V3
Rectum 0DVP
Stomach 0DV6
Pylorus 0DV7
Trachea 0BV1
Ureter
Left 0TV7
Right 0TV6
Urethra 0TVD
Vein
Axillary
Left 05V8
Right 05V7
Azygos 05V0
Basilic
Left 05VC
Right 05VB
Brachial
Left 05VA
Right 05V9
Cephalic
Left 05VF
Right 05VD
Colic 06V7Z
Common Iliac
Left 06VD
Right 06VC
Esophageal 06V3
External Iliac
Left 06VG
Right 06VF
External Jugular
Left 05VQ
Right 05VP
Face
Left 05VV
Right 05VT
Femoral
Left 06VN
Right 06VM

Restriction (continued)
Vein (continued)
Foot
Left 06VV
Right 06VT
Gastric 06V2
Greater Saphenous
Left 06VQ
Right 06VP
Hand
Left 05VH
Right 05VG
Hemiazygos 05V1
Hepatic 06V4
Hypogastric
Left 06VJ
Right 06VH
Inferior Mesenteric 06V6
Innominate
Left 05V4
Right 05V3
Internal Jugular
Left 05VN
Right 05VM
Intracranial 05VL
Lesser Saphenous
Left 06VS
Right 06VR
Lower 06VY
Portal 06V8
Pulmonary
Left 02VT
Right 02VS
Renal
Left 06VB
Right 06V9
Splenic 06V1
Subclavian
Left 05V6
Right 05V5
Superior Mesenteric 06V5
Upper 05VY
Vertebral
Left 05VS
Right 05VR
Vena Cava
Inferior 06V0
Superior 02VV
Resurfacing Device
Removal of device from
Left 0SPB0BZ
Right 0SP90BZ
Revision of device in
Left 0SWB0BZ
Right 0SW90BZ
Supplement
Left 0SUB0BZ
Acetabular Surface 0SUE0BZ
Femoral Surface 0SUS0BZ
Right 0SU90BZ
Acetabular Surface 0SUA0BZ
Femoral Surface 0SUR0BZ
Resuscitation
Cardiopulmonary
see Assistance, Cardiac 5A02
Cardioversion 5A2204Z
Defibrillation 5A2204Z
Endotracheal intubation
see Insertion of device in, Trachea 0BH1
External chest compression 5A12012
Pulmonary 5A19054
Resuture, Heart valve prosthesis
see Revision of device in, Heart and Great Vessels 02W
Retraining
Cardiac
see Motor Treatment, Rehabilitation F07
Vocational
see Activities of Daily Living Treatment,
Rehabilitation F08
Retrogasserian rhizotomy
see Division, Nerve, Trigeminal 008K
Retroperitoneal lymph node
use Lymphatic, Aortic
Retroperitoneal space
use Retroperitoneum
Retropharyngeal lymph node
use Lymphatic, Neck, Left
use Lymphatic, Neck, Right
Retropubic space
use Pelvic Cavity
Reveal (DX)(XT)
use Monitoring Device
Reverse total shoulder replacement
see Replacement, Upper Joints 0RR
Reverse® Shoulder Prosthesis
use Synthetic Substitute, Reverse Ball and Socket in 0RR

Revision of device in (continued)
  Tibia
    Left 0QWH
    Right 0QWG
  Toe Nail 0HWRX
  Trachea 0BW1F
  Tracheobronchial Tree 0BW0
  Tympanic Membrane
    Left 09W8
    Right 09W7
  Ulna
    Left 0PWL
    Right 0PWK
  Ureter 0TW9M
  Urethra 0TWD
  Uterus and Cervix 0UWD
  Vagina and Cul-de-sac 0UWH
  Valve
    Aortic 02WF
    Mitral 02WG
    Pulmonary 02WH
    Tricuspid 02WJ
  Vas Deferens 0VWR
  Vein
    Lower 06WY
    Upper 05WY
  Vertebra
    Cervical 0PW3
    Lumbar 0QW0
    Thoracic 0PW4
  Vulva 0UWM
Revo MRI™ SureScan® pacemaker
  use Pacemaker, Dual Chamber in 0JH
Rheos® System device
  use Cardiac Rhythm Related Device in Subcutaneous
    Tissue and Fascia
Rheos® System lead
  use Stimulator Lead in Upper Arteries
Rhinopharynx
  use Nasopharynx
Rhinoplasty
  see Alteration, Nose 090K
  see Repair, Nose 09QK
  see Replacement, Nose 09RK
  see Supplement, Nose 09UK
Rhinorrhaphy
  see Repair, Nose 09QK
Rhinoscopy 09JKXZZ
Rhizotomy
  see Division, Central Nervous System 008
  see Division, Peripheral Nervous System 018
Rhomboid major muscle
  use Muscle, Trunk, Left
  use Muscle, Trunk, Right
Rhomboid minor muscle
  use Muscle, Trunk, Right
  use Muscle, Trunk, Left
Rhythm electrocardiogram
  see Measurement, Cardiac 4A02
Rhytidectomy
  see Face lift
Right ascending lumbar vein
  use Vein, Azygos
Right atrioventricular valve
  use Valve, Tricuspid
Right auricular appendix
  use Atrium, Right
Right colic vein
  use Vein, Colic
Right coronary sulcus
  use Heart, Right
Right gastric artery
  use Artery, Gastric
Right gastroepiploic vein
  use Vein, Superior Mesenteric
Right inferior phrenic vein
  use Vena Cava, Inferior
Right inferior pulmonary vein
  use Vein, Pulmonary, Right
Right jugular trunk
  use Lymphatic, Neck, Right
Right lateral ventricle
  use Cerebral Ventricle
Right lymphatic duct
  use Lymphatic, Neck, Right
Right ovarian vein
  use Vena Cava, Inferior
Right second lumbar vein
  use Vena Cava, Inferior
Right subclavian trunk
  use Lymphatic, Neck, Right
Right subcostal vein
  use Vein, Azygos
Right superior pulmonary vein
  use Vein, Pulmonary, Right

Right suprarenal vein
  use Vena Cava, Inferior
Right testicular vein
  use Vena Cava, Inferior
Rima glottidis
  use Larynx
Risorius muscle
  use Muscle, Facial
RNS System lead
  use Neurostimulator Lead in Central Nervous System
RNS system neurostimulator generator
  use Neurostimulator Generator in Head and Facial
    Bones
Robotic Assisted Procedure
  Extremity
    Lower 8E0Y
    Upper 8E0X
  Head and Neck Region 8E09
  Trunk Region 8E0W
Rotation of fetal head
  Forceps 10S07ZZ
  Manual 10S0XZZ
Round ligament of uterus
  use Uterine Supporting Structure
Round window
  use Ear, Inner, Right
  use Ear, Inner, Left
Roux-en-Y operation
  see Bypass, Gastrointestinal System 0D1
  see Bypass, Hepatobiliary System and
    Pancreas 0F1
Rupture
  Adhesions
    see Release
  Fluid collection
    see Drainage

S

Sacral ganglion
  use Nerve, Sacral Sympathetic
Sacral lymph node
  use Lymphatic, Pelvis
Sacral nerve modulation (SNM) lead
  use Stimulator Lead in Urinary System
Sacral neuromodulation lead
  use Stimulator Lead in Urinary System
Sacral splanchnic nerve
  use Nerve, Sacral Sympathetic
Sacrectomy
  see Excision, Lower Bones 0QB
Sacrococcygeal ligament
  use Bursa and Ligament, Trunk, Right
  use Bursa and Ligament, Trunk, Left
Sacrococcygeal symphysis
  use Joint, Sacrococcygeal
Sacroiliac ligament
  use Bursa and Ligament, Trunk, Left
  use Bursa and Ligament, Trunk, Right
Sacrospinous ligament
  use Bursa and Ligament, Trunk, Left
  use Bursa and Ligament, Trunk, Right
Sacrotuberous ligament
  use Bursa and Ligament, Trunk, Left
  use Bursa and Ligament, Trunk, Right
Salpingectomy
  see Excision, Female Reproductive System 0UB
  see Resection, Female Reproductive System 0UT
Salpingolysis
  see Release, Female Reproductive System 0UN
Salpingopexy
  see Repair, Female Reproductive System 0UQ
  see Reposition, Female Reproductive System 0US
Salpingopharyngeus muscle
  use Muscle, Tongue, Palate, Pharynx
Salpingoplasty
  see Repair, Female Reproductive System 0UQ
  see Supplement, Female Reproductive System 0UU
Salpingorrhaphy
  see Repair, Female Reproductive System 0UQ
Salpingoscopy 0UJ88ZZ
Salpingostomy
  see Drainage, Female Reproductive System 0U9
Salpingotomy
  see Drainage, Female Reproductive System 0U9
Salpinx
  use Fallopian Tube, Left
  use Fallopian Tube, Right
SAPIEN transcatheter aortic valve
  use Zooplastic Tissue in Heart and Great Vessels
Sartorius muscle
  use Muscle, Upper Leg, Right
  use Muscle, Upper Leg, Left

Scalene muscle
  use Muscle, Neck, Right
  use Muscle, Neck, Left
Scan
  Computerized Tomography (CT)
    see Computerized Tomography (CT Scan)
  Radioisotope
    see Planar Nuclear Medicine Imaging
Scaphoid bone
  use Carpal, Left
  use Carpal, Right
Scapholunate ligament
  use Bursa and Ligament, Hand, Right
  use Bursa and Ligament, Hand, Left
Scaphotrapezium ligament
  use Bursa and Ligament, Hand, Right
  use Bursa and Ligament, Hand, Left
Scapulectomy
  see Excision, Upper Bones 0PB
  see Resection, Upper Bones 0PT
Scapulopexy
  see Repair, Upper Bones 0PQ
  see Reposition, Upper Bones 0PS
Scarpa's (vestibular) ganglion
  use Nerve, Acoustic
Sclerectomy
  see Excision, Eye 08B
Sclerotherapy, mechanical
  see Destruction
Sclerotomy
  see Drainage, Eye 089
Scrotectomy
  see Excision, Male Reproductive System 0VB
  see Resection, Male Reproductive System 0VT
Scrotoplasty
  see Repair, Male Reproductive System 0VQ
  see Supplement, Male Reproductive System 0VU
Scrotorrhaphy
  see Repair, Male Reproductive System 0VQ
Scrototomy
  see Drainage, Male Reproductive System 0V9
Sebaceous gland
  use Skin
Second cranial nerve
  use Nerve, Optic
Section, cesarean
  see Extraction, Pregnancy 10D
Secura (DR) (VR)
  use Defibrillator Generator in 0JH
Sella Turcica
  use Bone, Sphenoid, Right
  use Bone, Sphenoid, Left
Semicircular canal
  use Ear, Inner, Right
  use Ear, Inner, Left
Semimembranosus muscle
  use Muscle, Upper Leg, Left
  use Muscle, Upper Leg, Right
Semitendinosus muscle
  use Muscle, Upper Leg, Left
  use Muscle, Upper Leg, Right
Septal cartilage
  use Septum, Nasal
Septectomy
  see Excision, Heart and Great Vessels 02B
  see Resection, Heart and Great Vessels 02T
  see Excision, Ear, Nose, Sinus 09B
  see Resection, Ear, Nose, Sinus 09T
Septoplasty
  see Repair, Ear, Nose, Sinus 09Q
  see Replacement, Ear, Nose, Sinus 09R
  see Supplement, Ear, Nose, Sinus 09U
  see Reposition, Ear, Nose, Sinus 09S
  see Repair, Heart and Great Vessels 02Q
  see Replacement, Heart and Great
    Vessels 02R
  see Supplement, Heart and Great
    Vessels 02U
Septotomy
  see Drainage, Ear, Nose, Sinus 099
Sequestrectomy, bone
  see Extirpation
Serratus anterior muscle
  use Muscle, Thorax, Left
  use Muscle, Thorax, Right
Serratus posterior muscle
  use Muscle, Trunk, Left
  use Muscle, Trunk, Right
Seventh cranial nerve
  use Nerve, Facial
Sheffield hybrid external fixator
  use External Fixation Device, Hybrid in 0PH
  use External Fixation Device, Hybrid in 0PS
  use External Fixation Device, Hybrid in 0QH
  use External Fixation Device, Hybrid in 0QS

Spacer (continued)
   Revision of device in (continued)
      Shoulder
         Left 0RWK
         Right 0RWJ
      Sternoclavicular
         Left 0RWF
         Right 0RWE
      Tarsal
         Left 0SWJ
         Right 0SWH
      Temporomandibular
         Left 0RWD
         Right 0RWC
      Thoracic Vertebral 0RW6
      Thoracolumbar Vertebral 0RWA
      Toe Phalangeal
         Left 0SWQ
         Right 0SWP
      Wrist
         Left 0RWP
         Right 0RWN
Spectroscopy
   Intravascular 8E023DZ
   Near infrared 8E023DZ
Speech Assessment F00
Speech therapy
   see Speech Treatment, Rehabilitation F06
Speech Treatment F06
Sphenoidectomy
   see Excision, Ear, Nose, Sinus 09B
   see Resection, Ear, Nose, Sinus 09T
   see Excision, Head and Facial Bones 0NB
   see Resection, Head and Facial Bones 0NT
Sphenoidotomy
   see Drainage, Ear, Nose. Sinus 099
Sphenomandibular ligament
   use Bursa and Ligament, Head and Neck
Sphenopalatine (pterygopalatine) ganglion
   use Nerve, Head and Neck Sympathetic
Sphincterorrhaphy, anal
   see Repair, Anal Sphincter 0DQR
Sphincterotomy, anal
   see Drainage, Anal Sphincter 0D9R
   see Division, Anal Sphincter 0D8R
Spinal cord neurostimulator lead
   use Neurostimulator Lead in Central Nervous
      System
Spinal dura mater
   use Dura Mater
Spinal epidural space
   use Epidural Space
Spinal nerve, cervical
   use Nerve, Cervical
Spinal nerve, lumbar
   use Nerve, Lumbar
Spinal nerve, sacral
   use Nerve, Sacral
Spinal nerve, thoracic
   use Nerve, Thoracic
Spinal Stabilization Device
   Facet Replacement
      Cervical Vertebral 0RH1
      Cervicothoracic Vertebral 0RH4
      Lumbar Vertebral 0SH0
      Lumbosacral 0SH3
      Occipital-cervical 0RH0
      Thoracic Vertebral 0RH6
      Thoracolumbar Vertebral 0RHA
   Interspinous Process
      Cervical Vertebral 0RH1
      Cervicothoracic Vertebral 0RH4
      Lumbar Vertebral 0SH0
      Lumbosacral 0SH3
      Occipital-cervical 0RH0
      Thoracic Vertebral 0RH6
      Thoracolumbar Vertebral 0RHA
   Pedicle-Based
      Cervical Vertebral 0RH1
      Cervicothoracic Vertebral 0RH4
      Lumbar Vertebral 0SH0
      Lumbosacral 0SH3
      Occipital-cervical 0RH0
      Thoracic Vertebral 0RH6
      Thoracolumbar Vertebral 0RHA
Spinal subarachnoid space
   use Subarachnoid Space
Spinal subdural space
   use Subdural Space
Spinous process
   use Vertebra, Thoracic
   use Vertebra, Lumbar
   use Vertebra, Cervical
Spiral ganglion
   use Nerve, Acoustic

Spiration IBV™ Valve System
   use Intraluminal Device, Endobronchial Valve in
      Respiratory System
Splenectomy
   see Excision, Lymphatic and Hemic Systems 07B
   see Resection, Lymphatic and Hemic Systems 07T
Splenic flexure
   use Colon, Transverse
Splenic plexus
   use Nerve, Abdominal Sympathetic
Splenius capitis muscle
   use Muscle, Head
Splenius cervicis muscle
   use Muscle, Neck, Left
   use Muscle, Neck, Right
Splenolysis
   see Release, Lymphatic and Hemic Systems 07N
Splenopexy
   see Repair, Lymphatic and Hemic Systems 07Q
   see Reposition, Lymphatic and Hemic Systems 07S
Splenoplasty
   see Repair, Lymphatic and Hemic Systems 07Q
Splenorrhaphy
   see Repair, Lymphatic and Hemic Systems 07Q
Splenotomy
   see Drainage, Lymphatic and Hemic Systems 079
Splinting, musculoskeletal
   see Immobilization, Anatomical Regions 2W3
Stapedectomy
   see Excision, Ear, Nose, Sinus 09B
   see Resection, Ear, Nose, Sinus 09T
Stapediolysis
   see Release, Ear, Nose, Sinus 09N
Stapedioplasty
   see Repair, Ear, Nose, Sinus 09Q
   see Replacement, Ear, Nose, Sinus 09R
   see Supplement, Ear, Nose, Sinus 09U
Stapedotomy
   see **Drainage, Ear, Nose, Sinus** 099
Stapes
   use Auditory Ossicle, Right
   use Auditory Ossicle, Left
Stellate ganglion
   use Nerve, Head and Neck Sympathetic
Stensen's duct
   use Duct, Parotid, Right
   use Duct, Parotid, Left
Stent (angioplasty)(embolization)
   use Intraluminal Device
Stented tissue valve
   use Zooplastic Tissue in Heart and
      Great Vessels
Stereotactic Radiosurgery
   Gamma Beam
      Abdomen DW23JZZ
      Adrenal Gland DG22JZZ
      Bile Ducts DF22JZZ
      Bladder DT22JZZ
      Bone Marrow D720JZZ
      Brain D020JZZ
      Brain Stem D021JZZ
      Breast
         Left DM20JZZ
         Right DM21JZZ
      Bronchus DB21JZZ
      Cervix DU21JZZ
      Chest DW22JZZ
      Chest Wall DB27JZZ
      Colon DD25JZZ
      Diaphragm DB28JZZ
      Duodenum DD22JZZ
      Ear D920JZZ
      Esophagus DD20JZZ
      Eye D820JZZ
      Gallbladder DF21JZZ
      Gland
         Adrenal DG22JZZ
         Parathyroid DG24JZZ
         Pituitary DG20JZZ
         Thyroid DG25JZZ
      Glands, Salivary D926JZZ
      Head and Neck DW21JZZ
      Ileum DD24JZZ
      Jejunum DD23JZZ
      Kidney DT20JZZ
      Larynx D92BJZZ
      Liver DF20JZZ
      Lung DB22JZZ
      Lymphatics
         Abdomen D726JZZ
         Axillary D724JZZ
         Inguinal D728JZZ
         Neck D723JZZ
         Pelvis D727JZZ
         Thorax D725JZZ

Stereotactic Radiosurgery (continued)
   Gamma Beam (continued)
      Mediastinum DB26JZZ
      Mouth D924JZZ
      Nasopharynx D92DJZZ
      Neck and Head DW21JZZ
      Nerve, Peripheral D027JZZ
      Nose D921JZZ
      Ovary DU20JZZ
      Palate
         Hard D928JZZ
         Soft D929JZZ
      Pancreas DF23JZZ
      Parathyroid Gland DG24JZZ
      Pelvic Region DW26JZZ
      Pharynx D92CJZZ
      Pineal Body DG21JZZ
      Pituitary Gland DG20JZZ
      Pleura DB25JZZ
      Prostate DV20JZZ
      Rectum DD27JZZ
      Sinuses D927JZZ
      Spinal Cord D026JZZ
      Spleen D722JZZ
      Stomach DD21JZZ
      Testis DV21JZZ
      Thymus D721JZZ
      Thyroid Gland DG25JZZ
      Tongue D925JZZ
      Trachea DB20JZZ
      Ureter DT21JZZ
      Urethra DT23JZZ
      Uterus DU22JZZ
   Other Photon
      Abdomen DW23DZZ
      Adrenal Gland DG22DZZ
      Bile Ducts DF22DZZ
      Bladder DT22DZZ
      Bone Marrow D720DZZ
      Brain D020DZZ
      Brain Stem D021DZZ
      Breast
         Left DM20DZZ
         Right DM21DZZ
      Bronchus DB21DZZ
      Cervix DU21DZZ
      Chest DW22DZZ
      Chest Wall DB27DZZ
      Colon DD25DZZ
      Diaphragm DB28DZZ
      Duodenum DD22DZZ
      Ear D920DZZ
      Esophagus DD20DZZ
      Eye D820DZZ
      Gallbladder DF21DZZ
      Gland
         Adrenal DG22DZZ
         Parathyroid DG24DZZ
         Pituitary DG20DZZ
         Thyroid DG25DZZ
      Glands, Salivary D926DZZ
      Head and Neck DW21DZZ
      Ileum DD24DZZ
      Jejunum DD23DZZ
      Kidney DT20DZZ
      Larynx D92BDZZ
      Liver DF20DZZ
      Lung DB22DZZ
      Lymphatics
         Abdomen D726DZZ
         Axillary D724DZZ
         Inguinal D728DZZ
         Neck D723DZZ
         Pelvis D727DZZ
         Thorax D725DZZ
      Mediastinum DB26DZZ
      Mouth D924DZZ
      Nasopharynx D92DDZZ
      Neck and Head DW21DZZ
      Nerve, Peripheral D027DZZ
      Nose D921DZZ
      Ovary DU20DZZ
      Palate
         Hard D928DZZ
         Soft D929DZZ
      Pancreas DF23DZZ
      Parathyroid Gland DG24DZZ
      Pelvic Region DW26DZZ
      Pharynx D92CDZZ
      Pineal Body DG21DZZ
      Pituitary Gland DG20DZZ
      Pleura DB25DZZ
      Prostate DV20DZZ
      Rectum DD27DZZ
      Sinuses D927DZZ

Substance Abuse Treatment *(continued)*
  Counseling *(continued)*
    Individual *(continued)*
      Continuing Care HZ39ZZZ
      Infectious Disease
        Post-Test HZ3CZZZ
        Pre-Test HZ3CZZZ
      Interpersonal HZ34ZZZ
      Motivational Enhancement HZ37ZZZ
      Psychoeducation HZ36ZZZ
      Spiritual HZ3BZZZ
      Vocational HZ35ZZZ
  Detoxification Services, for substance abuse
    HZ2ZZZZ
  Medication Management
    Antabuse HZ83ZZZ
    Bupropion HZ87ZZZ
    Clonidine HZ86ZZZ
    Levo-alpha-acetyl-methadol (LAAM)
      HZ82ZZZ
    Methadone Maintenance HZ81ZZZ
    Naloxone HZ85ZZZ
    Naltrexone HZ84ZZZ
    Nicotine Replacement HZ80ZZZ
    Other Replacement Medication HZ89ZZZ
    Psychiatric Medication HZ88ZZZ
  Pharmacotherapy
    Antabuse HZ93ZZZ
    Bupropion HZ97ZZZ
    Clonidine HZ96ZZZ
    Levo-alpha-acetyl-methadol (LAAM)
      HZ92ZZZ
    Methadone Maintenance HZ91ZZZ
    Naloxone HZ95ZZZ
    Naltrexone HZ94ZZZ
    Nicotine Replacement HZ90ZZZ
    Psychiatric Medication HZ98ZZZ
    Replacement Medication, Other HZ99ZZZ
  Psychotherapy
    12-Step HZ53ZZZ
    Behavioral HZ51ZZZ
    Cognitive HZ50ZZZ
    Cognitive-Behavioral HZ52ZZZ
    Confrontational HZ58ZZZ
    Interactive HZ55ZZZ
    Interpersonal HZ54ZZZ
    Motivational Enhancement HZ57ZZZ
    Psychoanalysis HZ5BZZZ
    Psychodynamic HZ5CZZZ
    Psychoeducation HZ56ZZZ
    Psychophysiological HZ5DZZZ
    Supportive HZ59ZZZ
Substantia nigra
  use Basal Ganglia
Subtalar (talocalcaneal) joint
  use Joint, Tarsal, Right
  use Joint, Tarsal, Left
Subtalar ligament
  use Bursa and Ligament, Foot, Left
  use Bursa and Ligament, Foot, Right
Subthalamic nucleus
  use Basal Ganglia
Suction
  see Drainage
Suction curettage (D&C), nonobstetric
  see Extraction, Endometrium 0UDB
Suction curettage, obstetric post-delivery
  see Extraction, Products of Conception,
    Retained 10D1
Superficial circumflex iliac vein
  use Vein, Greater Saphenous, Right
  use Vein, Greater Saphenous, Left
Superficial epigastric artery
  use Artery, Femoral, Left
  use Artery, Femoral, Right
Superficial epigastric vein
  use Vein, Greater Saphenous, Right
  use Vein, Greater Saphenous, Left
Superficial Inferior Epigastric Artery Flap
  Bilateral 0HRV078
  Left 0HRU078
  Right 0HRT078
Superficial palmar arch
  use Artery, Hand, Left
  use Artery, Hand, Right
Superficial palmar venous arch
  use Vein, Hand, Left
  use Vein, Hand, Right
Superficial temporal artery
  use Artery, Temporal, Right
  use Artery, Temporal, Left
Superficial transverse perineal muscle
  use Muscle, Perineum
Superior cardiac nerve
  use Nerve, Thoracic Sympathetic

Superior cerebellar vein
  use Vein, Intracranial
Superior cerebral vein
  use Vein, Intracranial
Superior clunic (cluneal) nerve
  use Nerve, Lumbar
Superior epigastric artery
  use Artery, Internal Mammary, Right
  use Artery, Internal Mammary, Left
Superior genicular artery
  use Artery, Popliteal, Left
  use Artery, Popliteal, Right
Superior gluteal artery
  use Artery, Internal Iliac, Left
  use Artery, Internal Iliac, Right
Superior gluteal nerve
  use Nerve, Lumbar Plexus
Superior hypogastric plexus
  use Nerve, Abdominal Sympathetic
Superior labial artery
  use Artery, Face
Superior laryngeal artery
  use Artery, Thyroid, Left
  use Artery, Thyroid, Right
Superior laryngeal nerve
  use Nerve, Vagus
Superior longitudinal muscle
  use Muscle, Tongue, Palate,
    Pharynx
Superior mesenteric ganglion
  use Nerve, Abdominal Sympathetic
Superior mesenteric lymph node
  use Lymphatic, Mesenteric
Superior mesenteric plexus
  use Nerve, Abdominal Sympathetic
Superior oblique muscle
  use Muscle, Extraocular, Left
  use Muscle, Extraocular, Right
Superior olivary nucleus
  use Pons
Superior rectal artery
  use Artery, Inferior Mesenteric
Superior rectal vein
  use Vein, Inferior Mesenteric
Superior rectus muscle
  use Muscle, Extraocular, Left
  use Muscle, Extraocular, Right
Superior tarsal plate
  use Eyelid, Upper, Right
  use Eyelid, Upper, Left
Superior thoracic artery
  use Artery, Axillary, Left
  use Artery, Axillary, Right
Superior thyroid artery
  use Artery, Thyroid, Right
  use Artery, External Carotid, Right
  use Artery, Thyroid, Left
  use Artery, External Carotid, Left
Superior turbinate
  use Turbinate, Nasal
Superior ulnar collateral artery
  use Artery, Brachial, Right
  use Artery, Brachial, Left
Supplement
  Abdominal Wall 0WUF
  Acetabulum
    Left 0QU5
    Right 0QU4
  Ampulla of Vater 0FUC
  Anal Sphincter 0DUR
  Ankle Region
    Left 0YUL
    Right 0YUK
  Anus 0DUQ
  Aorta
    Abdominal 04U0
    Thoracic 02UW
  Arm
    Lower
      Left 0XUF
      Right 0XUD
    Upper
      Left 0XU9
      Right 0XU8
  Artery
    Anterior Tibial
      Left 04UQ
      Right 04UP
    Axillary
      Left 03U6
      Right 03U5
    Brachial
      Left 03U8
      Right 03U7
    Celiac 04U1

Supplement *(continued)*
  Artery *(continued)*
    Colic
      Left 04U7
      Middle 04U8
      Right 04U6
    Common Carotid
      Left 03UJ
      Right 03UH
    Common Iliac
      Left 04UD
      Right 04UC
    External Carotid
      Left 03UN
      Right 03UM
    External Iliac
      Left 04UJ
      Right 04UH
    Face 03UR
    Femoral
      Left 04UL
      Right 04UK
    Foot
      Left 04UW
      Right 04UV
    Gastric 04U2
    Hand
      Left 03UF
      Right 03UD
    Hepatic 04U3
    Inferior Mesenteric
      04UB
    Innominate 03U2
    Internal Carotid
      Left 03UL
      Right 03UK
    Internal Iliac
      Left 04UF
      Right 04UE
    Internal Mammary
      Left 03U1
      Right 03U0
    Intracranial 03UG
    Lower 04UY
    Peroneal
      Left 04UU
      Right 04UT
    Popliteal
      Left 04UN
      Right 04UM
    Posterior Tibial
      Left 04US
      Right 04UR
    Pulmonary
      Left 02UR
      Right 02UQ
    Pulmonary Trunk 02UP
    Radial
      Left 03UC
      Right 03UB
    Renal
      Left 04UA
      Right 04U9
    Splenic 04U4
    Subclavian
      Left 03U4
      Right 03U3
    Superior Mesenteric
      04U5
    Temporal
      Left 03UT
      Right 03US
    Thyroid
      Left 03UV
      Right 03UU
    Ulnar
      Left 03UA
      Right 03U9
    Upper 03UY
    Vertebral
      Left 03UQ
      Right 03UP
  Atrium
    Left 02U7
    Right 02U6
  Auditory Ossicle
    Left 09UA0
    Right 09U90
  Axilla
    Left 0XU5
    Right 0XU4
  Back
    Lower 0WUL
    Upper 0WUK
  Bladder 0TUB

Supplement *(continued)*
  Joint *(continued)*
    Hip
      Left 0SUB
        Acetabular Surface 0SUE
        Femoral Surface 0SUS
      Right 0SU9
        Acetabular Surface 0SUA
        Femoral Surface 0SUR
    Knee
      Left 0SUD
        Femoral Surface 0SUU09Z
        Tibial Surface 0SUW09Z
      Right 0SUC
        Femoral Surface 0SUT09Z
        Tibial Surface 0SUV09Z
    Lumbar Vertebral 0SU0
    Lumbosacral 0SU3
    Metacarpocarpal
      Left 0RUT
      Right 0RUS
    Metacarpophalangeal
      Left 0RUV
      Right 0RUU
    Metatarsal-Phalangeal
      Left 0SUN
      Right 0SUM
    Metatarsal-Tarsal
      Left 0SUL
      Right 0SUK
    Occipital-cervical 0RU0
    Sacrococcygeal 0SU5
    Sacroiliac
      Left 0SU8
      Right 0SU7
    Shoulder
      Left 0RUK
      Right 0RUJ
    Sternoclavicular
      Left 0RUF
      Right 0RUE
    Tarsal
      Left 0SUJ
      Right 0SUH
    Temporomandibular
      Left 0RUD
      Right 0RUC
    Thoracic Vertebral 0RU6
    Thoracolumbar Vertebral
      0RUA
    Toe Phalangeal
      Left 0SUQ
      Right 0SUP
    Wrist
      Left 0RUP
      Right 0RUN
  Kidney Pelvis
    Left 0TU4
    Right 0TU3
  Knee Region
    Left 0YUG
    Right 0YUF
  Larynx 0CUS
  Leg
    Lower
      Left 0YUJ
      Right 0YUH
    Upper
      Left 0YUD
      Right 0YUC
  Lip
    Lower 0CU1
    Upper 0CU0
  Lymphatic
    Aortic 07UD
    Axillary
      Left 07U6
      Right 07U5
    Head 07U0
    Inguinal
      Left 07UJ
      Right 07UH
    Internal Mammary
      Left 07U9
      Right 07U8
    Lower Extremity
      Left 07UG
      Right 07UF
    Mesenteric 07UB
    Neck
      Left 07U2
      Right 07U1
    Pelvis 07UC
    Thoracic Duct 07UK
    Thorax 07U7

Supplement *(continued)*
  Lymphatic *(continued)*
    Upper Extremity
      Left 07U4
      Right 07U3
  Mandible
    Left 0NUV
    Right 0NUT
  Maxilla
    Left 0NUS
    Right 0NUR
  Mediastinum 0WUC
  Mesentery 0DUV
  Metacarpal
    Left 0PUQ
    Right 0PUP
  Metatarsal
    Left 0QUP
    Right 0QUN
  Muscle
    Abdomen
      Left 0KUL
      Right 0KUK
    Extraocular
      Left 08UM
      Right 08UL
    Facial 0KU1
    Foot
      Left 0KUW
      Right 0KUV
    Hand
      Left 0KUD
      Right 0KUC
    Head 0KU0
    Hip
      Left 0KUP
      Right 0KUN
    Lower Arm and Wrist
      Left 0KUB
      Right 0KU9
    Lower Leg
      Left 0KUT
      Right 0KUS
    Neck
      Left 0KU3
      Right 0KU2
    Papillary 02UD
    Perineum 0KUM
    Shoulder
      Left 0KU6
      Right 0KU5
    Thorax
      Left 0KUJ
      Right 0KUH
    Tongue, Palate, Pharynx 0KU4
    Trunk
      Left 0KUG
      Right 0KUF
    Upper Arm
      Left 0KU8
      Right 0KU7
    Upper Leg
      Left 0KUR
      Right 0KUQ
  Nasopharynx 09UN
  Neck 0WU6
  Nerve
    Abducens 00UL
    Accessory 00UR
    Acoustic 00UN
    Cervical 01U1
    Facial 00UM
    Femoral 01UD
    Glossopharyngeal 00UP
    Hypoglossal 00US
    Lumbar 01UB
    Median 01U5
    Oculomotor 00UH
    Olfactory 00UF
    Optic 00UG
    Peroneal 01UH
    Phrenic 01U2
    Pudendal 01UC
    Radial 01U6
    Sacral 01UR
    Sciatic 01UF
    Thoracic 01U8
    Tibial 01UG
    Trigeminal 00UK
    Trochlear 00UJ
    Ulnar 01U4
    Vagus 00UQ
  Nipple
    Left 0HUX
    Right 0HUW

Supplement *(continued)*
  Nose 09UK
  Omentum
    Greater 0DUS
    Lesser 0DUT
  Orbit
    Left 0NUQ
    Right 0NUP
  Palate
    Hard 0CU2
    Soft 0CU3
  Patella
    Left 0QUF
    Right 0QUD
  Penis 0VUS
  Pericardium 02UN
  Perineum
    Female 0WUN
    Male 0WUM
  Peritoneum 0DUW
  Phalanx
    Finger
      Left 0PUV
      Right 0PUT
    Thumb
      Left 0PUS
      Right 0PUR
    Toe
      Left 0QUR
      Right 0QUQ
  Pharynx 0CUM
  Prepuce 0VUT
  Radius
    Left 0PUJ
    Right 0PUH
  Rectum 0DUP
  Retina
    Left 08UF
    Right 08UE
  Retinal Vessel
    Left 08UH
    Right 08UG
  Rib
    Left 0PU2
    Right 0PU1
  Sacrum 0QU1
  Scapula
    Left 0PU6
    Right 0PU5
  Scrotum 0VU5
  Septum
    Atrial 02U5
    Nasal 09UM
    Ventricular 02UM
  Shoulder Region
    Left 0XU3
    Right 0XU2
  Skull 0NU0
  Spinal Meninges 00UT
  Sternum 0PU0
  Stomach 0DU6
    Pylorus 0DU7
  Subcutaneous Tissue and Fascia
    Abdomen 0JU8
    Back 0JU7
    Buttock 0JU9
    Chest 0JU6
    Face 0JU1
    Foot
      Left 0JUR
      Right 0JUQ
    Hand
      Left 0JUK
      Right 0JUJ
    Lower Arm
      Left 0JUH
      Right 0JUG
    Lower Leg
      Left 0JUP
      Right 0JUN
    Neck
      Anterior 0JU4
      Posterior 0JU5
    Pelvic Region 0JUC
    Perineum 0JUB
    Scalp 0JU0
    Upper Arm
      Left 0JUF
      Right 0JUD
    Upper Leg
      Left 0JUM
      Right 0JUL
  Tarsal
    Left 0QUM
    Right 0QUL

T

Takedown
   Arteriovenous shunt
      see Removal of device from, Upper Arteries 03P
      Arteriovenous shunt, with creation of new shunt
   see Bypass, Upper Arteries 031
   Stoma
   see Repair
Talent® Converter
   use Intraluminal Device
Talent® Occluder
   use Intraluminal Device
Talent® Stent Graft (abdominal)(thoracic)
   use Intraluminal Device
Talocalcaneal (subtalar) joint
   use Joint, Tarsal, Left
   use Joint, Tarsal, Right
Talocalcaneal ligament
   use Bursa and Ligament, Foot, Left
   use Bursa and Ligament, Foot, Right
Talocalcaneonavicular joint
   use Joint, Tarsal, Right
   use Joint, Tarsal, Left
Talocalcaneonavicular ligament
   use Bursa and Ligament, Foot, Left
   use Bursa and Ligament, Foot, Right
Talocrural joint
   use Joint, Ankle, Right
   use Joint, Ankle, Left
Talofibular ligament
   use Bursa and Ligament, Ankle, Right
   use Bursa and Ligament, Ankle, Left
Talus bone
   use Tarsal, Right
   use Tarsal, Left
TandemHeart® System
   use External Heart Assist System in Heart and Great
      Vessels
Tarsectomy
   see Excision, Lower Bones 0QB
   see Resection, Lower Bones 0QT
Tarsometatarsal joint
   use Joint, Metatarsal-Tarsal, Right
   use Joint, Metatarsal-Tarsal, Left
Tarsometatarsal ligament
   use Bursa and Ligament, Foot, Right
   use Bursa and Ligament, Foot, Left
Tarsorrhaphy
   see Repair, Eye 08Q
Tattooing
   Cornea 3E0CXMZ
   Skin
   see Introduction of substance in or on, Skin 3E00
**TAXUS® Liberté® Paclitaxel-eluting Coronary Stent
   System**
   use Intraluminal Device, Drug-eluting in Heart and
      Great Vessels
TBNA (transbronchial needle aspiration)
   see Drainage, Respiratory System 0B9
Telemetry
   4A12X4Z
   Ambulatory 4A12X45
Temperature gradient study 4A0ZXKZ
Temporal lobe
   use Cerebral Hemisphere
Temporalis muscle
   use Muscle, Head
Temporoparietalis muscle
   use Muscle, Head
Tendolysis
   see Release, Tendons 0LN
Tendonectomy
   see Excision, Tendons 0LB
   see Resection, Tendons 0LT
Tendonoplasty, tenoplasty
   see Repair, Tendons 0LQ
   see Replacement, Tendons 0LR
   see Supplement, Tendons 0LU
Tendorrhaphy
   see Repair, Tendons 0LQ
Tendototomy
   see Division, Tendons 0L8
   see Drainage, Tendons 0L9
Tenectomy, tenonectomy
   see Excision, Tendons 0LB
   see Resection, Tendons 0LT
Tenolysis
   see Release, Tendons 0LN
Tenontorrhaphy
   see Repair, Tendons 0LQ
Tenontotomy
   see Division, Tendons 0L8
   see Drainage, Tendons 0L9

Tenorrhaphy
   see Repair, Tendons 0LQ
Tenosynovectomy
   see Excision, Tendons 0LB
   see Resection, Tendons 0LT
Tenotomy
   see Division, Tendons 0L8
   see Drainage, Tendons 0L9
Tensor fasciae latae muscle
   use Muscle, Hip, Left
   use Muscle, Hip, Right
Tensor veli palatini muscle
   use Muscle, Tongue, Palate, Pharynx
Tenth cranial nerve
   use Nerve, Vagus
Tentorium cerebelli
   use Dura Mater
Teres major muscle
   use Muscle, Shoulder, Left
   use Muscle, Shoulder, Right
Teres minor muscle
   use Muscle, Shoulder, Right
   use Muscle, Shoulder, Left
Termination of pregnancy
   Aspiration curettage 10A07ZZ
   Dilation and curettage 10A07ZZ
   Hysterotomy 10A00ZZ
   Intra-amniotic injection 10A03ZZ
   Laminaria 10A07ZW
   Vacuum 10A07Z6
Testectomy
   see Excision, Male Reproductive System 0VB
   see Resection, Male Reproductive System 0VT
Testicular artery
   use Aorta, Abdominal
Testing
   Glaucoma 4A07XBZ
   Hearing
      see Hearing Assessment, Diagnostic
         Audiology F13
   Mental health
      see Psychological Tests
   Muscle function, electromyography (EMG)
      see Measurement, Musculoskeletal 4A0F
   Muscle function, manual
      see Motor Function Assessment, Rehabilitation F01
   Neurophysiologic monitoring, intra-operative
      see Monitoring, Physiological Systems 4A1
   Range of motion
      see Motor Function Assessment, Rehabilitation
         F01
   Vestibular function
      see Vestibular Assessment, Diagnostic Audiology
         F15
Thalamectomy
   see Excision, Thalamus 00B9
Thalamotomy
   see Drainage, Thalamus 0099
Thenar muscle
   use Muscle, Hand, Right
   use Muscle, Hand, Left
Therapeutic Massage
   Musculoskeletal System 8E0KX1Z
   Reproductive System
      Prostate 8E0VX1C
      Rectum 8E0VX1D
Therapeutic occlusion coil(s)
   use Intraluminal Device
Thermography 4A0ZXKZ
Thermotherapy, prostate
   see Destruction, Prostate 0V50
Third cranial nerve
   use Nerve, Oculomotor
Third occipital nerve
   use Nerve, Cervical
Third ventricle
   use Cerebral Ventricle
Thoracectomy
   see Excision, Anatomical Regions, General 0WB
Thoracentesis
   see Drainage, Anatomical Regions, General 0W9
Thoracic aortic plexus
   use Nerve, Thoracic Sympathetic
Thoracic esophagus
   use Esophagus, Middle
Thoracic facet joint
   use Joint, Thoracic Vertebral, 2 to 7
   use Joint, Thoracic Vertebral, 8 or more
   use Joint, Thoracic Vertebral
Thoracic ganglion
   use Nerve, Thoracic Sympathetic
Thoracoacromial artery
   use Artery, Axillary, Right
   use Artery, Axillary, Left

Thoracocentesis
   see Drainage, Anatomical Regions, General 0W9
Thoracolumbar facet joint
   use Joint, Thoracolumbar Vertebral
Thoracoplasty
   see Repair, Anatomical Regions, General 0WQ
   see Supplement, Anatomical Regions, General 0WU
Thoracostomy tube
   use Drainage Device
Thoracostomy, for lung collapse
   see Drainage, Respiratory System 0B9
Thoracotomy
   see Drainage, Anatomical Regions, General 0W9
Thoratec IVAD (Implantable Ventricular Assist Device)
   use Implantable Heart Assist System in Heart and Great
      Vessels
Thoratec Paracorporeal Ventricular Assist Device
   use External Heart Assist System in Heart and Great
      Vessels
Thrombectomy
   see Extirpation
Thymectomy
   see Excision, Lymphatic and Hemic Systems 07B
   see Resection, Lymphatic and Hemic Systems 07T
Thymopexy
   see Repair, Lymphatic and Hemic Systems 07Q
   see Reposition, Lymphatic and Hemic
      Systems 07S
Thymus gland
   use Thymus
Thyroarytenoid muscle
   use Muscle, Neck, Right
   use Muscle, Neck, Left
Thyrocervical trunk
   use Artery, Thyroid, Right
   use Artery, Thyroid, Left
Thyroid cartilage
   use Larynx
Thyroidectomy
   see Excision, Endocrine System 0GB
   see Resection, Endocrine System 0GT
Thyroidorrhaphy
   see Repair, Endocrine System 0GQ
Thyroidoscopy 0GJK4ZZ
Thyroidotomy
   see Drainage, Endocrine System 0G9
Tibialis anterior muscle
   use Muscle, Lower Leg, Right
   use Muscle, Lower Leg, Left
Tibialis posterior muscle
   use Muscle, Lower Leg, Right
   use Muscle, Lower Leg, Left
Tibiofemoral joint
   use Joint, Knee, Right, Tibial Surface
   use Joint, Knee, Left, Tibial Surface
   use Joint, Knee, Right
   use Joint, Knee, Left
TigerPaw® system for closure of left atrial appendage
   use Extraluminal Device
Tissue bank graft
   use Nonautologous Tissue Substitute
Tissue Expander
   Insertion of device in
      Breast
         Bilateral 0HHV
         Left 0HHU
         Right 0HHT
      Nipple
         Left 0HHX
         Right 0HHW
      Subcutaneous Tissue and Fascia
         Abdomen 0JH8
         Back 0JH7
         Buttock 0JH9
         Chest 0JH6
         Face 0JH1
         Foot
            Left 0JHR
            Right 0JHQ
         Hand
            Left 0JHK
            Right 0JHJ
         Lower Arm
            Left 0JHH
            Right 0JHG
         Lower Leg
            Left 0JHP
            Right 0JHN
         Neck
            Anterior 0JH4
            Posterior 0JH5
         Pelvic Region 0JHC
         Perineum 0JHB
         Scalp 0JH0

Transfer (*continued*)
  Muscle (*continued*)
    Head 0KX0
    Hip
      Left 0KXP
      Right 0KXN
    Lower Arm and Wrist
      Left 0KXB
      Right 0KX9
    Lower Leg
      Left 0KXT
      Right 0KXS
    Neck
      Left 0KX3
      Right 0KX2
    Perineum 0KXM
    Shoulder
      Left 0KX6
      Right 0KX5
    Thorax
      Left 0KXJ
      Right 0KXH
    Tongue, Palate, Pharynx 0KX4
    Trunk
      Left 0KXG
      Right 0KXF
    Upper Arm
      Left 0KX8
      Right 0KX7
    Upper Leg
      Left 0KXR
      Right 0KXQ
  Nerve
    Abducens 00XL
    Accessory 00XR
    Acoustic 00XN
    Cervical 01X1
    Facial 00XM
    Femoral 01XD
    Glossopharyngeal 00XP
    Hypoglossal 00XS
    Lumbar 01XB
    Median 01X5
    Oculomotor 00XH
    Olfactory 00XF
    Optic 00XG
    Peroneal 01XH
    Phrenic 01X2
    Pudendal 01XC
    Radial 01X6
    Sciatic 01XF
    Thoracic 01X8
    Tibial 01XG
    Trigeminal 00XK
    Trochlear 00XJ
    Ulnar 01X4
    Vagus 00XQ
  Palate, Soft 0CX3
  Skin
    Abdomen 0HX7ZZ
    Back 0HX6XZZ
    Buttock 0HX8XZZ
    Chest 0HX5XZZ
    Ear
      Left 0HX3XZZ
      Right 0HX2XZZ
    Face 0HX1XZZ
    Foot
      Left 0HXNXZZ
      Right 0HXMXZZ
    Genitalia 0HXAXZZ
    Hand
      Left 0HXGXZZ
      Right 0HXFXZZ
    Lower Arm
      Left 0HXEXZZ
      Right 0HXDXZZ
    Lower Leg
      Left 0HXLXZZ
      Right 0HXKXZZ
    Neck 0HX4XZZ
    Perineum 0HX9XZZ
    Scalp 0HX0XZZ
    Upper Arm
      Left 0HXCXZZ
      Right 0HXBXZZ
    Upper Leg
      Left 0HXJXZZ
      Right 0HXHXZZ
  Stomach 0DX6
  Subcutaneous Tissue and Fascia
    Abdomen 0JX8
    Back 0JX7

Transfer (*continued*)
  Subcutaneous Tissue and Fascia (*continued*)
    Buttock 0JX9
    Chest 0JX6
    Face 0JX1
    Foot
      Left 0JXR
      Right 0JXQ
    Hand
      Left 0JXK
      Right 0JXJ
    Lower Arm
      Left 0JXH
      Right 0JXG
    Lower Leg
      Left 0JXP
      Right 0JXN
    Neck
      Anterior 0JX4
      Posterior 0JX5
    Pelvic Region 0JXC
    Perineum 0JXB
    Scalp 0JX0
    Upper Arm
      Left 0JXF
      Right 0JXD
    Upper Leg
      Left 0JXM
      Right 0JXL
  Tendon
    Abdomen
      Left 0LXG
      Right 0LXF
    Ankle
      Left 0LXT
      Right 0LXS
    Foot
      Left 0LXW
      Right 0LXV
    Hand
      Left 0LX8
      Right 0LX7
    Head and Neck 0LX0
    Hip
      Left 0LXK
      Right 0LXJ
    Knee
      Left 0LXR
      Right 0LXQ
    Lower Arm and Wrist
      Left 0LX6
      Right 0LX5
    Lower Leg
      Left 0LXP
      Right 0LXN
    Perineum 0LXH
    Shoulder
      Left 0LX2
      Right 0LX1
    Thorax
      Left 0LXD
      Right 0LXC
    Trunk
      Left 0LXB
      Right 0LX9
    Upper Arm
      Left 0LX4
      Right 0LX3
    Upper Leg
      Left 0LXM
      Right 0LXL
  Tongue 0CX7

Transfusion
  Artery
    Central
      Antihemophilic Factors 3026
      Blood
        Platelets 3026
        Red Cells 3026
          Frozen 3026
        White Cells 3026
        Whole 3026
      Bone Marrow 3026
      Factor IX 3026
      Fibrinogen 3026
      Globulin 3026
      Plasma
        Fresh 3026
        Frozen 3026
      Plasma Cryoprecipitate 3026
      Serum Albumin 3026
      Stem Cells
        Cord Blood 3026
        Hematopoietic 3026

Transfusion (*continued*)
  Artery (*continued*)
    Peripheral
      Antihemophilic Factors 3025
      Blood
        Platelets 3025
        Red Cells 3025
          Frozen 3025
        White Cells 3025
        Whole 3025
      Bone Marrow 3025
      Factor IX 3025
      Fibrinogen 3025
      Globulin 3025
      Plasma
        Fresh 3025
        Frozen 3025
      Plasma Cryoprecipitate 3025
      Serum Albumin 3025
      Stem Cells
        Cord Blood 3025
        Hematopoietic 3025
  Products of Conception
    Antihemophilic Factors 3027
    Blood
      Platelets 3027
      Red Cells 3027
        Frozen 3027
      White Cells 3027
      Whole 3027
    Factor IX 3027
    Fibrinogen 3027
    Globulin 3027
    Plasma
      Fresh 3027
      Frozen 3027
    Plasma Cryoprecipitate 3027
    Serum Albumin 3027
  Vein
    4-Factor Prothrombin Complex Concentrate 3028
    Central
      Antihemophilic Factors 3024
      Blood
        Platelets 3024
        Red Cells 3024
          Frozen 3024
        White Cells 3024
        Whole 3024
      Bone Marrow 3024
      Factor IX 3024
      Fibrinogen 3024
      Globulin 3024
      Plasma
        Fresh 3024
        Frozen 3024
      Plasma Cryoprecipitate 3024
      Serum Albumin 3024
      Stem Cells
        Cord Blood 3024
        Embryonic 3024
        Hematopoietic 3024
    Peripheral
      Antihemophilic Factors 3023
      Blood
        Platelets 3023
        Red Cells 3023
          Frozen 3023
        White Cells 3023
        Whole 3023
      Bone Marrow 3023
      Factor IX 3023
      Fibrinogen 3023
      Globulin 3023
      Plasma
        Fresh 3023
        Frozen 3023
      Plasma Cryoprecipitate 3023
      Serum Albumin 3023
      Stem Cells
        Cord Blood 3023X
        Embryonic 3023
        Hematopoietic 3023

Transplantation
  Esophagus 0DY50Z
  Heart 02YA0Z
  Intestine
    Large 0DYE0Z
    Small 0DY80Z
  Kidney
    Left 0TY10Z
    Right 0TY00Z
  Liver 0FY00Z
  Lung
    Bilateral 0BYM0Z
    Left 0BYL0Z

Ultrasonography *(continued)*
Heart with Aorta B24BYZZ
Intravascular B24BZZ3
Transesophageal B24BZZ4
Hepatobiliary System, All BF4CZZZ
Hip
Bilateral BQ42ZZZ
Left BQ41ZZZ
Right BQ40ZZZ
Kidney
and Bladder BT4JZZZ
Bilateral BT43ZZZ
Left BT42ZZZ
Right BT41ZZZ
Transplant BT49ZZZ
Knee
Bilateral BQ49ZZZ
Left BQ48ZZZ
Right BQ47ZZZ
Liver BF45ZZZ
Liver and Spleen BF46ZZZ
Mediastinum BB4CZZZ
Neck BW4FZZZ
Ovary
Bilateral BU45
Left BU44
Right BU43
Ovary and Uterus BU4C
Pancreas BF47ZZZ
Pelvic Region BW4GZZZ
Pelvis and Abdomen BW41ZZZ
Penis BV4BZZZ
Pericardium B24CYZZ
Intravascular B24CZZ3
Transesophageal B24CZZ4
Placenta BY48ZZZ
Pleura BB4BZZZ
Prostate and Seminal Vesicle BV49ZZZ
Rectum BD4CZZZ
Sacrum BR4FZZZ
Scrotum BV44ZZZ
Seminal Vesicle and Prostate BV49ZZZ
Shoulder
Left, Densitometry BP49ZZ1
Right, Densitometry BP48ZZ1
Spinal Cord B04BZZZ
Spine
Cervical BR40ZZZ
Lumbar BR49ZZZ
Thoracic BR47ZZZ
Spleen and Liver BF46ZZZ
Stomach BD42ZZZ
Tendon
Lower Extremity BL43ZZZ
Upper Extremity BL42ZZZ
Ureter
Bilateral BT48ZZZ
Left BT47ZZZ
Right BT46ZZZ
Urethra BT45ZZZ
Uterus BU46
Uterus and Ovary BU4C
Vein
Jugular
Left, Intravascular B544ZZ3
Right, Intravascular B543ZZ3
Lower Extremity
Bilateral, Intravascular B54DZZ3
Left, Intravascular B54CZZ3
Right, Intravascular B54BZZ3
Portal, Intravascular B54TZZ3
Renal
Bilateral, Intravascular B54LZZ3
Left, Intravascular B54KZZ3
Right, Intravascular B54JZZ3
Spanchnic, Intravascular B54TZZ3
Subclavian
Left, Intravascular B547ZZ3
Right, Intravascular B546ZZ3
Upper Extremity
Bilateral, Intravascular B54PZZ3
Left, Intravascular B54NZZ3
Right, Intravascular B54MZZ3
Vena Cava
Inferior, Intravascular B549ZZ3
Superior, Intravascular B548ZZ3
Wrist
Left, Densitometry BP4MZZ1
Right, Densitometry BP4LZZ1
Ultrasound bone healing system
use Bone Growth Stimulator in Upper Bones
use Bone Growth Stimulator in Head and Facial Bones
use Bone Growth Stimulator in Lower Bones
Ultrasound Therapy
Heart 6A75
No Qualifier 6A75

Ultrasound Therapy *(continued)*
Vessels
Head and Neck 6A75
Other 6A75
Peripheral 6A75
Ultraviolet Light Therapy, Skin 6A80
Umbilical artery
use Artery, Internal Iliac, Left
use Artery, Internal Iliac, Right
Uniplanar external fixator
use External Fixation Device, Monoplanar in 0PH
use External Fixation Device, Monoplanar in 0PS
use External Fixation Device, Monoplanar in 0QH
use External Fixation Device, Monoplanar in 0QS
Upper GI series
see Fluoroscopy, Gastrointestinal, Upper BD15
Ureteral orifice
use Ureter, Left
use Ureter
use Ureter, Right
use Ureters, Bilateral
Ureterectomy
see Excision, Urinary System 0TB
see Resection, Urinary System 0TT
Ureterocolostomy
see Bypass, Urinary System 0T1
Ureterocystostomy
see Bypass, Urinary System 0T1
Ureteroenterostomy
see Bypass, Urinary System 0T1
Ureteroileostomy
see Bypass, Urinary System 0T1
Ureterolithotomy
see Extirpation, Urinary System 0TC
Ureterolysis
see Release, Urinary System 0TN
Ureteroneocystostomy
see Bypass, Urinary System 0T1
see Reposition, Urinary System 0TS
Ureteropelvic junction (UPJ)
use Kidney Pelvis, Right
use Kidney Pelvis, Left
Ureteropexy
see Repair, Urinary System 0TQ
see Reposition, Urinary System 0TS
Ureteroplasty
see Repair, Urinary System 0TQ
see Replacement, Urinary System 0TR
see Supplement, Urinary System 0TU
Ureteroplication
see Restriction, Urinary System 0TV
Ureteropyelography
see Fluoroscopy, Urinary System BT1
Ureterorrhaphy
see Repair, Urinary System 0TQ
Ureteroscopy 0TJ98ZZ
Ureterostomy
see Bypass, Urinary System 0T1
see Drainage, Urinary System 0T9
Ureterotomy
see Drainage, Urinary System 0T9
Ureteroureterostomy
see Bypass, Urinary System 0T1
Ureterovesical orifice
use Ureter, Right
use Ureter, Left
use Ureters, Bilateral
use Ureter
Urethral catheterization, indwelling
0T9B70Z
Urethrectomy
see Excision, Urethra 0TBD
see Resection, Urethra 0TTD
Urethrolithotomy
see Extirpation, Urethra 0TCD
Urethrolysis
see Release, Urethra 0TND
Urethropexy
see Repair, Urethra 0TQD
see Reposition, Urethra 0TSD
Urethroplasty
see Repair, Urethra 0TQD
see Replacement, Urethra 0TRD
see Supplement, Urethra 0TUD
Urethrorrhaphy
see Repair, Urethra 0TQD
Urethroscopy 0TJD8ZZ
Urethrotomy
see Drainage, Urethra 0T9D
Urinary incontinence stimulator lead
use Stimulator Lead in Urinary System
Urography
see Fluoroscopy, Urinary System BT1
Uterine Artery
use Artery, Internal Iliac, Left
use Artery, Internal Iliac, Right

Uterine Artery *(continued)*
Left, Occlusion, Artery, Internal Iliac,
Left 04LF
Right, Occlusion, Artery, Internal Iliac,
Right 04LET
Uterine artery embolization (UAE)
see Occlusion, Lower Arteries 04L
Uterine cornu
use Uterus
Uterine tube
use Fallopian Tube, Left
use Fallopian Tube, Right
Uterine vein
use Vein, Hypogastric, Left
use Vein, Hypogastric, Right
Uvulectomy
see Excision, Uvula 0CBN
see Resection, Uvula 0CTN
Uvulorrhaphy
see Repair, Uvula 0CQN
Uvulotomy
see Drainage, Uvula 0C9N

V

Vaccination
see Introduction of Serum, Toxoid, and Vaccine
Vacuum extraction, obstetric 10D07Z6
Vaginal artery
use Artery, Internal Iliac, Right
use Artery, Internal Iliac, Left
Vaginal pessary
use Intraluminal Device, Pessary in Female
Reproductive System
Vaginal vein
use Vein, Hypogastric, Right
use Vein, Hypogastric, Left
Vaginectomy
see Excision, Vagina 0UBG
see Resection, Vagina 0UTG
Vaginofixation
see Repair, Vagina 0UQG
see Reposition, Vagina 0USG
Vaginoplasty
see Repair, Vagina 0UQG
see Supplement, Vagina 0UUG
Vaginorrhaphy
see Repair, Vagina 0UQG
Vaginoscopy 0UJH8ZZ
Vaginotomy
see Drainage, Female Reproductive System 0U9
Vagotomy
see Division, Nerve, Vagus 008Q
Valiant Thoracic Stent Graft
use Intraluminal Device
Valvotomy, valvulotomy
see Division, Heart and Great Vessels 028
see Release, Heart and Great Vessels 02N
Valvuloplasty
see Repair, Heart and Great Vessels 02Q
see Replacement, Heart and Great Vessels 02R
see Supplement, Heart and Great Vessels 02U
Vascular Access Device
Insertion of device in
Abdomen 0JH8
Chest 0JH6
Lower Arm
Left 0JHH
Right 0JHG
Lower Leg
Left 0JHP
Right 0JHN
Upper Arm
Left 0JHF
Right 0JHD
Upper Leg
Left 0JHM
Right 0JHL
Removal of device from
Lower Extremity 0JPW
Trunk 0JPT
Upper Extremity 0JPV
Reservoir
Insertion of device in
Abdomen 0JH8
Chest 0JH6
Lower Arm
Left 0JHH
Right 0JHG
Lower Leg
Left 0JHP
Right 0JHN
Upper Arm
Left 0JHF
Right 0JHD

Vascular Access Device *(continued)*
   Reservoir *(continued)*
     Insertion of device in *(continued)*
      Upper Leg
       Left 0JHM
       Right 0JHL
     Removal of device from
      Lower Extremity 0JPW
      Trunk 0JPT
      Upper Extremity 0JPV
     Revision of device in
      Lower Extremity 0JWW
      Trunk 0JWT
      Upper Extremity 0JWV
   Revision of device in
     Lower Extremity 0JWW
     Trunk 0JWT
     Upper Extremity 0JWV
Vasectomy
  see Excision, Male Reproductive System 0VB
Vasography
  see Plain Radiography, Male Reproductive System BV0
  see Fluoroscopy, Male Reproductive System BV1
Vasoligation
  see Occlusion, Male Reproductive System 0VL
Vasorrhaphy
  see Repair, Male Reproductive System 0VQ
Vasostomy
  see Bypass, Male Reproductive System 0V1
Vasotomy
  Drainage
  see Drainage, Male Reproductive System 0V9
  With ligation
  see Occlusion, Male Reproductive System 0VL
Vasovasostomy
  see Repair, Male Reproductive System 0VQ
Vastus intermedius muscle
  use Muscle, Upper Leg, Right
  use Muscle, Upper Leg, Left
Vastus lateralis muscle
  use Muscle, Upper Leg, Left
  use Muscle, Upper Leg, Right
Vastus medialis muscle
  use Muscle, Upper Leg, Right
  use Muscle, Upper Leg, Left
VCG (vectorcardiogram)
  see Measurement, Cardiac 4A02
Vectra® Vascular Access Graft
  use Vascular Access Device in Subcutaneous Tissue and Fascia
Venectomy
  see Excision, Upper Veins 05B
  see Excision, Lower Veins 06B
Venography
  see Plain Radiography, Veins B50
  see Fluoroscopy, Veins B51
Venorrhaphy
  see Repair, Upper Veins 05Q
  see Repair, Lower Veins 06Q
Venotripsy
  see Occlusion, Upper Veins 05L
  see Occlusion, Lower Veins 06L
Ventricular fold
  use Larynx
Ventriculoatriostomy
  see Bypass, Central Nervous System 001
Ventriculocisternostomy
  see Bypass, Central Nervous System 001
Ventriculogram, cardiac
  Combined left and right heart
   see Fluoroscopy, Heart, Right and Left B216
  Left ventricle
   see Fluoroscopy, Heart, Left B215
  Right ventricle
   see Fluoroscopy, Heart, Right B214
Ventriculopuncture, through previously implanted catheter 8C01X6J
Ventriculoscopy 00J04ZZ
Ventriculostomy
  External drainage
   see Drainage, Cerebral Ventricle 0096
  Internal shunt
   see Bypass, Cerebral Ventricle 0016

Ventriculovenostomy
  see Bypass, Cerebral Ventricle 0016
Ventrio™ Hernia Patch
  use Synthetic Substitute
VEP (visual evoked potential) 4A07X0Z
Vermiform appendix
  use Appendix
Vermilion border
  use Lip, Lower
  use Lip, Upper
Versa
  use Pacemaker, Dual Chamber in 0JH
Version, obstetric
  External 10S0XZZ
  Internal 10S07ZZ
Vertebral arch
  use Vertebra, Thoracic
  use Vertebra, Lumbar
  use Vertebra, Cervical
Vertebral canal
  use Spinal Canal
Vertebral foramen
  use Vertebra, Thoracic
  use Vertebra, Lumbar
  use Vertebra, Cervical
Vertebral lamina
  use Vertebra, Thoracic
  use Vertebra, Cervical
  use Vertebra, Lumbar
Vertebral pedicle
  use Vertebra, Lumbar
  use Vertebra, Thoracic
  use Vertebra, Cervical
Vesical vein
  use Vein, Hypogastric, Left
  use Vein, Hypogastric, Right
Vesicotomy
  see Drainage, Urinary System 0T9
Vesiculectomy
  see Excision, Male Reproductive System 0VB
  see Resection, Male Reproductive System 0VT
Vesiculogram, seminal
  see Plain Radiography, Male Reproductive System BV0
Vesiculotomy
  see Drainage, Male Reproductive System 0V9
Vestibular (Scarpa's) ganglion
  use Nerve, Acoustic
Vestibular Assessment F15Z
Vestibular nerve
  use Nerve, Acoustic
Vestibular Treatment F0C
Vestibulocochlear nerve
  use Nerve, Acoustic
Virchow's (supraclavicular) lymph node
  use Lymphatic, Neck, Left
  use Lymphatic, Neck, Right
Virtuoso (II) (DR) (VR)
  use Defibrillator Generator in 0JH
Vitrectomy
  see Excision, Eye 08B
  see Resection, Eye 08T
Vitreous body
  use Vitreous, Left
  use Vitreous, Right
Vocal fold
  use Vocal Cord, Left
  use Vocal Cord, Right
Vocational
  Assessment
  see Activities of Daily Living Assessment, Rehabilitation F02
  Retraining
  see Activities of Daily Living Treatment, Rehabilitation F08
Volar (palmar) digital vein
  use Vein, Hand, Left
  use Vein, Hand, Right
Volar (palmar) metacarpal vein
  use Vein, Hand, Right
  use Vein, Hand, Left
Vomer bone
  use Septum, Nasal

Vomer of nasal septum
  use Bone, Nasal
Vulvectomy
  see Excision, Female Reproductive System 0UB
  see Resection, Female Reproductive System 0UT

W

WALLSTENT® Endoprosthesis
  use Intraluminal Device
Washing
  see Irrigation
Wedge resection, pulmonary
  see Excision, Respiratory System 0BB
Window
  see Drainage
Wiring, dental 2W31X9Z

X

X-ray
  see Plain Radiography
X-STOP® Spacer
  use Spinal Stabilization Device, Interspinous Process in 0RH
  use Spinal Stabilization Device, Interspinous Process in 0SH
Xenograft
  use Zooplastic Tissue in Heart and Great Vessels
XIENCE V Everolimus Eluting Coronary Stent System
  use Intraluminal Device, Drug-eluting in Heart and Great Vessels
Xiphoid process
  use Sternum
XLIF® System
  use Interbody Fusion Device in Lower Joints

Y

Yoga Therapy 8E0ZXY4

Z

Z-plasty, skin for scar contracture
  see Release, Skin and Breast 0HN
Zenith Flex® AAA Endovascular Graft
  use Intraluminal Device
Zenith TX2® TAA Endovascular Graft
  use Intraluminal Device
Zenith Renu™ AAA Ancillary Graft
  use Intraluminal Device
Zilver® PTX® (paclitaxel) Drug-Eluting Peripheral Stent
  use Intraluminal Device, Drug-eluting in Upper Arteries
  use Intraluminal Device, Drug-eluting in Lower Arteries
Zimmer® NexGen® LPS Mobile Bearing Knee
  use Synthetic Substitute
Zimmer® NexGen® LPS-Flex Mobile Knee
  use Synthetic Substitute
Zonule of Zinn
  use Lens, Left
  use Lens, Right
Zotarolimus-eluting coronary stent
  use Intraluminal Device, Drug-eluting in Heart and Great Vessels
Zygomatic process of frontal bone
  use Bone, Frontal, Left
  use Bone, Frontal, Right
Zygomatic process of temporal bone
  use Bone, Temporal, Right
  use Bone, Temporal, Left
Zygomaticus muscle
  use Muscle, Facial Stimulator Generator–Superior mesenteric plexus Contact Radiation

Addenda 2014 ICD-10-PCS Index

A

Arytenoidopexy *see* Repair, Larynx 0CQS

B

Biopsy
  Bone Marrow *see* Extraction with qualifier
    Diagnostic

D

Denticulate ligament *use* **Spinal Meninges**

E

Epiretinal Visual Prosthesis
  use Epiretinal Visual Prosthesis in Eye
  Insertion of device in
    Left 08H105Z
    Right 08H005Z

F

Femoropatellar joint
  use Joint, Knee, Right, Femoral Surface
  use Joint, Knee, Left, Femoral Surface
Femorotibial joint
  use Joint, Knee, Right, Tibial Surface
  use Joint, Knee, Left, Tibial Surface

H

Hearing Device
  Insertion of device in
    Left 0NH6
    Right 0NH5
  Removal of device from, Skull 0NP0
  Revision of device in, Skull 0NW0
Hyperthermia
  Radiation Therapy
    Abdomen DWY38ZZ
    Adrenal Gland
      DGY28ZZ
    Bile Ducts DFY28ZZ
    Bladder DTY28ZZ
    Bone, Other DPYC8ZZ
    Bone Marrow D7Y08ZZ
    Brain D0Y08ZZ
    Brain Stem D0Y18ZZ
    Breast
      Left DMY08ZZ
      Right DMY18ZZ
    Bronchus DBY18ZZ
    Cervix DUY18ZZ
    Chest DWY28ZZ
    Chest Wall DBY78ZZ
    Colon DDY58ZZ
    Diaphragm DBY88ZZ
    Duodenum DDY28ZZ
    Ear D9Y08ZZ
    Esophagus DDY08ZZ
    Eye D8Y08ZZ
    Femur DPY98ZZ
    Fibula DPYB8ZZ
    Gallbladder DFY18ZZ
    Gland
      Adrenal DGY28ZZ
      Parathyroid DGY48ZZ

Hyperthermia *(continued)*
  Radiation Therapy *(continued)*
    Gland *(continued)*
      Pituitary DGY08ZZ
      Thyroid DGY58ZZ
    Glands, Salivary D9Y68ZZ
    Head and Neck DWY18ZZ
    Hemibody DWY48ZZ
    Humerus DPY68ZZ
    Hypopharynx D9Y38ZZ
    Ileum DDY48ZZ
    Jejunum DDY38ZZ
    Kidney DTY08ZZ
    Larynx D9YB8ZZ
    Liver DFY08ZZ
    Lung DBY28ZZ
    Lymphatics
      Abdomen D7Y68ZZ
      Axillary D7Y48ZZ
      Inguinal D7Y88ZZ
      Neck D7Y38ZZ
      Pelvis D7Y78ZZ
      Thorax D7Y58ZZ
    Mandible DPY38ZZ
    Maxilla DPY28ZZ
    Mediastinum DBY68ZZ
    Mouth D9Y48ZZ
    Nasopharynx D9YD8ZZ
    Neck and Head DWY18ZZ
    Nerve, Peripheral D0Y78ZZ
    Nose D9Y18ZZ
    Oropharynx D9YF8ZZ
    Ovary DUY08ZZ
    Palate
      Hard D9Y88ZZ
      Soft D9Y98ZZ
    Pancreas DFY38ZZ
    Parathyroid Gland DGY48ZZ
    Pelvic Bones DPY88ZZ
    Pelvic Region DWY68ZZ
    Pineal Body DGY18ZZ
    Pituitary Gland DGY08ZZ
    Pleura DBY58ZZ
    Prostate DVY08ZZ
    Radius DPY78ZZ
    Rectum DDY78ZZ
    Rib DPY58ZZ
    Sin*uses* D9Y78ZZ
    Skin
      Abdomen DHY88ZZ
      Arm DHY48ZZ
      Back DHY78ZZ
      Buttock DHY98ZZ
      Chest DHY68ZZ
      Face DHY28ZZ
      Leg DHYB8ZZ
      Neck DHY38ZZ
    Skull DPY08ZZ
    Spinal Cord D0Y68ZZ
    Spleen D7Y28ZZ
    Sternum DPY48ZZ
    Stomach DDY18ZZ
    Testis DVY18ZZ
    Thymus D7Y18ZZ
    Thyroid Gland DGY58ZZ
    Tibia DPYB8ZZ
    Tongue D9Y58ZZ
    Trachea DBY08ZZ
    Ulna DPY78ZZ
    Ureter DTY18ZZ
    Urethra DTY38ZZ
    Uterus DUY28ZZ
    Whole Body DWY58ZZ

I

Impella® (2.5)(5.0)(LD) cardiac assist device *use*
  Intraluminal Device
Insertion of device in
  Eye
    Left 08H1
    Right 08H0

L

Laminotomy
  see Release, Central Nervous System 00N
  see Release, Peripheral Nervous System 01N

M

MicroMed HeartAssist *use* **Implantable**
  Heart Assist System in Heart and
  Great Vessels

P

Patellofemoral joint
  use Joint, Knee, Right
  use Joint, Knee, Left
  use Joint, Knee, Right, Femoral Surface
  use Joint, Knee, Left, Femoral Surface
Pneumonectomy *see* Resection, Respiratory System 0BT

R

Radiation Therapy
  see Beam Radiation
  see Brachytherapy
Rectocele repair *see* Repair, Subcutaneous Tissue and
  Fascia, Pelvic Region 0JQC
Restriction
  Aorta
    Abdominal 04V0
    Thoracic 02VW

S

Spinal nerve, cervical *use* **Nerve, Cervical**
Spinal nerve, lumbar *use* **Nerve, Lumbar**
Spinal nerve, sacral *use* **Nerve, Sacral**
Spinal nerve, thoracic *use* **Nerve, Thoracic**

T

TandemHeart® System *use* **External Heart**
  Assist System in Heart and Great
  Vessels
Thoratec Paracorporeal Ventricular Assist Device *use*
  External Heart Assist System in Heart and
  Great Vessels
Tibiofemoral joint
  use Joint, Knee, Right, Tibial Surface
  use Joint, Knee, Left, Tibial Surface
  use Joint, Knee, Right
  use Joint, Knee, Left
Transfusion
  Vein
    4-Factor Prothrombin Complex Concentrate 3028

Medical and Surgical Section (0)

Within each section of ICD-10-PCS the characters have different meanings. The seven character meanings for the Medical and Surgical section are illustrated here through the procedure example of *Percutaneous needle core biopsy of the right kidney*.

Section	Body System	Root Operation	Body Part	Approach	Device	Qualifier
Med/Surg	Urinary	Excision	Kidney, Right	Percutaneous	None	Diagnostic
0	T	B	0	3	Z	X

Section (Character 1)

All Medical and Surgical procedure codes have a first character value of 0.

Body System (Character 2)

The alphanumeric character for the body system is placed in the second position. The following are the body systems applicable to the Medical and Surgical section.

Character Value	Character Value Description
0	Central Nervous System
1	Peripheral Nervous System
2	Heart and Great Vessels
3	Upper Arteries
4	Lower Arteries
5	Upper Veins
6	Lower Veins
7	Lymphatic and Hemic Systems
8	Eye
9	Ear, Nose, Sinus
B	Respiratory System
C	Mouth and Throat
D	Gastrointestinal System
F	Hepatobiliary System and Pancreas
G	Endocrine System
H	Skin and Breast
J	Subcutaneous Tissue and Fascia
K	Muscles
L	Tendons

Continued

Character Value	Character Value Description
M	Bursae and Ligaments
N	Head and Facial Bones
P	Upper Bones
Q	Lower Bones
R	Upper Joints
S	Lower Joints
T	Urinary System
U	Female Reproductive System
V	Male Reproductive System
W	Anatomical Regions, General
X	Anatomical Regions, Upper Extremities
Y	Anatomical Regions, Lower Extremities

Root Operations (Character 3)

The alphanumeric character value for root operations is placed in the third position. Listed below are the root operations applicable to the Medical and Surgical section with their associated meaning. Note that the root operation definitions for ICD-10-PCS may differ from the terms that coders currently use today with ICD-9-CM Volume 3.

Character Value	Root Operation	Root Operation Definition
0	Alteration	Modifying the anatomic structure of a body part without affecting the function of the body part
1	Bypass	Altering the route of passage of the contents of a tubular body part
2	Change	Taking out or off a device from a body part and putting back an identical or similar device in or on the same body part without cutting or puncturing the skin or a mucous membrane
3	Control	Stopping, or attempting to stop, postprocedural bleeding
4	Creation	Making a new genital structure that does not take over the function of a body part
5	Destruction	Physical eradication of all or a portion of a body part by the direct use of energy, force, or a destructive agent
6	Detachment	Cutting off all or a portion of the upper or lower extremities
7	Dilation	Expanding an orifice or the lumen of a tubular body part
8	Division	Cutting into a body part, without draining fluids and/or gases from the body part, in order to separate or transect a body part
9	Drainage	Taking or letting out fluids and/or gases from a body part
B	Excision	Cutting out or off, without replacement, a portion of a body part
C	Extirpation	Taking or cutting out solid matter from a body part
D	Extraction	Pulling or stripping out or off all or a portion of a body part by the use of force
F	Fragmentation	Breaking solid matter in a body part into pieces

Continued

Character Value	Root Operation	Root Operation Definition
G	Fusion	Joining together portions of an articular body part rendering the articular body part immobile
H	Insertion	Putting in a nonbiological appliance that monitors, assists, performs, or prevents a physiological function but does not physically take the place of a body part
J	Inspection	Visually and/or manually exploring a body part
K	Map	Locating the route of passage of electrical impulses and/or locating functional areas in a body part
L	Occlusion	Completely closing an orifice or the lumen of a tubular body part
M	Reattachment	Putting back in or on all or a portion of a separated body part to its normal location or other suitable location
N	Release	Freeing a body part from an abnormal physical constraint by cutting or by the use of force
P	Removal	Taking out or off a device from a body part
Q	Repair	Restoring, to the extent possible, a body part to its normal anatomic structure and function
R	Replacement	Putting in or on biological or synthetic material that physically takes the place and/or function of all or a portion of a body part
S	Reposition	Moving to its normal location, or other suitable location, all or a portion of a body part
T	Resection	Cutting out or off, without replacement, all of a body part
V	Restriction	Partially closing an orifice or the lumen of a tubular body part
W	Revision	Correcting, to the extent possible, a portion of a malfunctioning device or the position of a displaced device
U	Supplement	Putting in or on biological or synthetic material that physically reinforces and/or augments the function of a portion of a body part
X	Transfer	Moving, without taking out, all or a portion of a body part to another location to take over the function of all or a portion of a body part
Y	Transplantation	Putting in or on all or a portion of a living body part taken from another individual or animal to physically take the place and/or function of all or a portion of a similar body part

Body Part (Character 4)

For each body system the applicable body part character values will be available for procedure code construction. An example of a body part for this section is the Large Intestines.

Approach (Character 5)

The approach is the technique used to reach the procedure site. The following are the approach character values for the Medical and Surgical section with the associated definitions.

Character Value	Approach	Approach Definition
0	Open	Cutting through the skin or mucous membrane and any other body layers necessary to expose the site of the procedure
3	Percutaneous	Entry, by puncture or minor incision, of instrumentation through the skin or mucous membrane and any other body layers necessary to reach the site of the procedure
4	Percutaneous Endoscopic	Entry, by puncture or minor incision, of instrumentation through the skin or mucous membrane and any other body layers necessary to reach and visualize the site of the procedure

Continued

Character Value	Approach	Approach Definition
7	Via Natural or Artificial Opening	Entry of instrumentation through a natural or artificial external opening to reach the site of the procedure
8	Via Natural or Artificial Opening Endoscopic	Entry of instrumentation through a natural or artificial external opening to reach and visualize the site of the procedure
F	Via Natural or Artificial Opening Percutaneous Endoscopic	Entry of instrumentation through a natural or artificial external opening to reach and visualize the site of the procedure, and entry, by puncture or minor incision, of instrumentation through the skin or mucous membrane and any other body layers necessary to aid in the performance of the procedure
X	External	Procedures performed directly on the skin or mucous membrane and procedures performed indirectly by the application of external force through the skin or mucous membrane

Device (Character 6)

Depending on the procedure performed there may or may not be a device used. There are several types of devices included in the Medical and Surgical section that fall into one of the four following categories.

- Electronic Appliances
- Grafts and Prostheses
- Implants
- Simple or Mechanical Appliances

When a device is not utilized during the procedure, the character value of Z should be reported.

Qualifier (Character 7)

The qualifier represents an additional attribute for the procedure when applicable. In the preceding example of *Percutaneous needle core biopsy of the right kidney*, the qualifier of X was used to report that the biopsy procedure was diagnostic in nature. If there is no qualifier for a procedure, the Z character value should be reported.

Official Coding Guidelines for the Medical and Surgical Section

Medical and Surgical Section Guidelines (section 0)

B2. Body System

General guidelines

B2.1a The procedure codes in the general anatomical regions body systems should only be used when the procedure is performed on an anatomical region rather than a specific body part (e.g., root operations Control and Detachment, Drainage of a body cavity) or on the rare occasion when no information is available to support assignment of a code to a specific body part.

Example: Control of postoperative hemorrhage is coded to the root operation Control found in the general anatomical regions body systems.

B2.1b Where the general body part values "upper" and "lower" are provided as an option in the Upper Arteries, Lower Arteries, Upper Veins, Lower Veins, Muscles and Tendons body systems, "upper" or "lower "specifies body parts located above or below the diaphragm respectively.

Example: Vein body parts above the diaphragm are found in the Upper Veins body system; vein body parts below the diaphragm are found in the Lower Veins body system.

B3. Root Operation

General guidelines

B3.1a In order to determine the appropriate root operation, the full definition of the root operation as contained in the PCS Tables must be applied.

B3.1b Components of a procedure specified in the root operation definition and explanation are not coded separately. Procedural steps necessary to reach the operative site and close the operative site, including anastomosis of a tubular body part, are also not coded separately.

Example: Resection of a joint as part of a joint replacement procedure is included in the root operation definition of Replacement and is not coded separately. Laparotomy performed to reach the site of an open liver biopsy is not coded separately. In a resection of sigmoid colon with anastomosis of descending colon to rectum, the anastomosis is not coded separately.

Multiple procedures

B3.2 During the same operative episode, multiple procedures are coded if:

a. The same root operation is performed on different body parts as defined by distinct values of the body part character.

   Example: Diagnostic excision of liver and pancreas are coded separately.

b. The same root operation is repeated at different body sites that are included in the same body part value.

   Example: Excision of the sartorius muscle and excision of the gracilis muscle are both included in the upper leg muscle body part value, and multiple procedures are coded.

c. Multiple root operations with distinct objectives are performed on the same body part.

   Example: Destruction of sigmoid lesion and bypass of sigmoid colon are coded separately.

d. The intended root operation is attempted using one approach, but is converted to a different approach.

   Example: Laparoscopic cholecystectomy converted to an open cholecystectomy is coded as percutaneous endoscopic Inspection and open Resection.

Discontinued procedures

B3.3 If the intended procedure is discontinued, code the procedure to the root operation performed. If a procedure is discontinued before any other root operation is performed, code the root operation Inspection of the body part or anatomical region inspected.

Example: A planned aortic valve replacement procedure is discontinued after the initial thoracotomy and before any incision is made in the heart muscle, when the patient becomes hemodynamically unstable. This procedure is coded as an open Inspection of the mediastinum.

Biopsy procedures

B3.4a Biopsy procedures are coded using the root operations Excision, Extraction, or Drainage and the qualifier Diagnostic. The qualifier Diagnostic is used only for biopsies.

Example: Fine needle aspiration biopsy of lung is coded to the root operation Drainage with the qualifier Diagnostic. Biopsy of bone marrow is coded to the root operation Extraction with the qualifier Diagnostic. Lymph node sampling for biopsy is coded to the root operation Excision with the qualifier Diagnostic.

Biopsy followed by more definitive treatment

B3.4b If a diagnostic Excision, Extraction, or Drainage procedure (biopsy) is followed by a more definitive procedure, such as Destruction, Excision or Resection at the same procedure site, both the biopsy and the more definitive treatment are coded.

Example: Biopsy of breast followed by partial mastectomy at the same procedure site, both the biopsy and the partial mastectomy procedure are coded.

Overlapping body layers

B3.5 If the root operations Excision, Repair or Inspection are performed on overlapping layers of the musculoskeletal system, the body part specifying the deepest layer is coded.

Example: Excisional debridement that includes skin and subcutaneous tissue and muscle is coded to the muscle body part.

Bypass procedures

B3.6a Bypass procedures are coded by identifying the body part bypassed "from" and the body part bypassed "to." The fourth character body part specifies the body part bypassed from, and the qualifier specifies the body part bypassed to.

Example: Bypass from stomach to jejunum, stomach is the body part and jejunum is the qualifier.

B3.6b Coronary arteries are classified by number of distinct sites treated, rather than number of coronary arteries or anatomic name of a coronary artery (e.g., left anterior descending). Coronary artery bypass procedures are coded differently than other bypass procedures as described in the previous guideline. Rather than identifying the body part bypassed from, the body part identifies the number of coronary artery sites bypassed to, and the qualifier specifies the vessel bypassed from.

Example: Aortocoronary artery bypass of one site on the left anterior descending coronary artery and one site on the obtuse marginal coronary artery is classified in the body part axis of classification as two coronary artery sites and the qualifier specifies the aorta as the body part bypassed from.

B3.6c If multiple coronary artery sites are bypassed, a separate procedure is coded for each coronary artery site that uses a different device and/or qualifier.

Example: Aortocoronary artery bypass and internal mammary coronary artery bypass are coded separately.

Control vs. more definitive root operations

B3.7 The root operation Control is defined as, "Stopping, or attempting to stop, postprocedural bleeding." If an attempt to stop postprocedural bleeding is initially unsuccessful, and to stop the bleeding requires performing any of the definitive root operations Bypass, Detachment, Excision, Extraction, Reposition, Replacement, or Resection, then that root operation is coded instead of Control.

Example: Resection of spleen to stop postprocedural bleeding is coded to Resection instead of Control.

Excision vs. Resection

B3.8 PCS contains specific body parts for anatomical subdivisions of a body part, such as lobes of the lungs or liver and regions of the intestine. Resection of the specific body part is coded whenever all of the body part is cut out or off, rather than coding Excision of a less specific body part.

Example: Left upper lung lobectomy is coded to Resection of Upper Lung Lobe, Left rather than Excision of Lung, Left.

Excision for graft

B3.9 If an autograft is obtained from a different body part in order to complete the objective of the procedure, a separate procedure is coded.

Example: Coronary bypass with excision of saphenous vein graft, excision of saphenous vein is coded separately.

Fusion procedures of the spine

B3.10a The body part coded for a spinal vertebral joint(s) rendered immobile by a spinal fusion procedure is classified by the level of the spine (e.g. thoracic). There are distinct body part values for a single vertebral joint and for multiple vertebral joints at each spinal level.

Example: Body part values specify Lumbar Vertebral Joint, Lumbar Vertebral Joints, 2 or More and Lumbosacral Vertebral Joint.

B3.10b If multiple vertebral joints are fused, a separate procedure is coded for each vertebral joint that uses a different device and/or qualifier.

Example: Fusion of lumbar vertebral joint, posterior approach, anterior column and fusion of lumbar vertebral joint, posterior approach, posterior column are coded separately.

B3.10c Combinations of devices and materials are often used on a vertebral joint to render the joint immobile. When combinations of devices are used on the same vertebral joint, the device value coded for the procedure is as follows:

- If an interbody fusion device is used to render the joint immobile (alone or containing other material like bone graft), the procedure is coded with the device value Interbody Fusion Device
- If bone graft is the only device used to render the joint immobile, the procedure is coded with the device value Nonautologous Tissue Substitute or Autologous Tissue Substitute
- If a mixture of autologous and nonautologous bone graft (with or without biological or synthetic extenders or binders) is used to render the joint immobile, code the procedure with the device value Autologous Tissue Substitute

Examples: Fusion of a vertebral joint using a cage style interbody fusion device containing morsellized bone graft is coded to the device Interbody Fusion Device.

Fusion of a vertebral joint using a bone dowel interbody fusion device made of cadaver bone and packed with a mixture of local morsellized bone and demineralized bone matrix is coded to the device Interbody Fusion Device.

Fusion of a vertebral joint using both autologous bone graft and bone bank bone graft is coded to the device Autologous Tissue Substitute.

Inspection procedures

B3.11a Inspection of a body part(s) performed in order to achieve the objective of a procedure is not coded separately.

Example: Fiberoptic bronchoscopy performed for irrigation of bronchus, only the irrigation procedure is coded.

B3.11b If multiple tubular body parts are inspected, the most distal body part inspected is coded. If multiple non-tubular body parts in a region are inspected, the body part that specifies the entire area inspected is coded.

Example: Cystoureteroscopy with inspection of bladder and ureters is coded to the ureter body part value.

Exploratory laparotomy with general inspection of abdominal contents is coded to the peritoneal cavity body part value.

B3.11c When both an Inspection procedure and another procedure are performed on the same body part during the same episode, if the Inspection procedure is performed using a different approach than the other procedure, the Inspection procedure is coded separately.

Example: Endoscopic Inspection of the duodenum is coded separately when open Excision of the duodenum is performed during the same procedural episode.

Occlusion vs. Restriction for vessel embolization procedures

B3.12 If the objective of an embolization procedure is to completely close a vessel, the root operation Occlusion is coded. If the objective of an embolization procedure is to narrow the lumen of a vessel, the root operation Restriction is coded.

Examples: Tumor embolization is coded to the root operation Occlusion, because the objective of the procedure is to cut off the blood supply to the vessel.

Embolization of a cerebral aneurysm is coded to the root operation Restriction, because the objective of the procedure is not to close off the vessel entirely, but to narrow the lumen of the vessel at the site of the aneurysm where it is abnormally wide.

Release procedures

B3.13 In the root operation Release, the body part value coded is the body part being freed and not the tissue being manipulated or cut to free the body part.

Example: Lysis of intestinal adhesions is coded to the specific intestine body part value.

Release vs. Division

B3.14 If the sole objective of the procedure is freeing a body part without cutting the body part, the root operation is Release. If the sole objective of the procedure is separating or transecting a body part, the root operation is Division.

Example: Freeing a nerve root from surrounding scar tissue to relieve pain is coded to the root operation Release. Severing a nerve root to relieve pain is coded to the root operation Division.

Reposition for fracture treatment

B3.15 Reduction of a displaced fracture is coded to the root operation Reposition and the application of a cast or splint in conjunction with the Reposition procedure is not coded separately. Treatment of a nondisplaced fracture is coded to the procedure performed.

Example: Putting a pin in a nondisplaced fracture is coded to the root operation Insertion.

Casting of a nondisplaced fracture is coded to the root operation Immobilization in the Placement section.

Transplantation vs. Administration

B3.16 Putting in a mature and functioning living body part taken from another individual or animal is coded to the root operation Transplantation. Putting in autologous or nonautologous cells is coded to the Administration section.

Example: Putting in autologous or nonautologous bone marrow, pancreatic islet cells or stem cells is coded to the Administration section.

B4. Body Part

General guidelines

B4.1a If a procedure is performed on a portion of a body part that does not have a separate body part value, code the body part value corresponding to the whole body part.

Example: A procedure performed on the alveolar process of the mandible is coded to the mandible body part.

B4.1b If the prefix "peri" is combined with a body part to identify the site of the procedure, the procedure is coded to the body part named.

Example: A procedure site identified as perirenal is coded to the kidney body part.

Branches of body parts

B4.2 Where a specific branch of a body part does not have its own body part value in PCS, the body part is coded to the closest proximal branch that has a specific body part value.

Example: A procedure performed on the mandibular branch of the trigeminal nerve is coded to the trigeminal nerve body part value.

Bilateral body part values

B4.3 Bilateral body part values are available for a limited number of body parts. If the identical procedure is performed on contralateral body parts, and a bilateral body part value exists for that body part, a single procedure is coded using the bilateral body part value. If no bilateral body part value exists, each procedure is coded separately using the appropriate body part value.

Example: The identical procedure performed on both fallopian tubes is coded once using the body part value Fallopian Tube, Bilateral. The identical procedure performed on both knee joints is coded twice using the body part values Knee Joint, Right and Knee Joint, Left.

Coronary arteries

B4.4 The coronary arteries are classified as a single body part that is further specified by number of sites treated and not by name or number of arteries. Separate body part values are used to specify the number of sites treated when the same procedure is performed on multiple sites in the coronary arteries.

Examples: Angioplasty of two distinct sites in the left anterior descending coronary artery with placement of two stents is coded as Dilation of Coronary Arteries, Two Sites, with Intraluminal Device.

Angioplasty of two distinct sites in the left anterior descending coronary artery, one with stent placed and one without, is coded separately as Dilation of Coronary Artery, One Site with Intraluminal Device, and Dilation of Coronary Artery, One Site with no device.

Tendons, ligaments, bursae and fascia near a joint

B4.5 Procedures performed on tendons, ligaments, bursae and fascia supporting a joint are coded to the body part in the respective body system that is the focus of the procedure. Procedures performed on joint structures themselves are coded to the body part in the joint body systems.

Example: Repair of the anterior cruciate ligament of the knee is coded to the knee bursae and ligament body part in the bursae and ligaments body system. Knee arthroscopy with shaving of articular cartilage is coded to the knee joint body part in the Lower Joints body system.

Skin, subcutaneous tissue and fascia overlying a joint

B4.6 If a procedure is performed on the skin, subcutaneous tissue or fascia overlying a joint, the procedure is coded to the following body part:

- Shoulder is coded to Upper Arm
- Elbow is coded to Lower Arm
- Wrist is coded to Lower Arm
- Hip is coded to Upper Leg
- Knee is coded to Lower Leg
- Ankle is coded to Foot

Fingers and toes

B4.7 If a body system does not contain a separate body part value for fingers, procedures performed on the fingers are coded to the body part value for the hand. If a body system does not contain a separate body part value for toes, procedures performed on the toes are coded to the body part value for the foot.

Example: Excision of finger muscle is coded to one of the hand muscle body part values in the Muscles body system.

Upper and lower intestinal tract

B4.8 In the Gastrointestinal body system, the general body part values Upper Intestinal Tract and Lower Intestinal Tract are provided as an option for the root operations Change, Inspection, Removal and Revision. Upper Intestinal Tract includes the portion of the gastrointestinal tract from the esophagus down to and including the duodenum, and Lower Intestinal Tract includes the portion of the gastrointestinal tract from the jejunum down to and including the rectum and anus.

Example: In the root operation Change table, change of a device in the jejunum is coded using the body part Lower Intestinal Tract.

B5. Approach

Open approach with percutaneous endoscopic assistance

B5.2 Procedures performed using the open approach with percutaneous endoscopic assistance are coded to the approach Open.

Example: Laparoscopic-assisted sigmoidectomy is coded to the approach Open.

External approach

B5.3a Procedures performed within an orifice on structures that are visible without the aid of any instrumentation are coded to the approach External.

Example: Resection of tonsils is coded to the approach External.

B5.3b Procedures performed indirectly by the application of external force through the intervening body layers are coded to the approach External.

Example: Closed reduction of fracture is coded to the approach External.

Percutaneous procedure via device

B5.4 Procedures performed percutaneously via a device placed for the procedure are coded to the approach Percutaneous.

Example: Fragmentation of kidney stone performed via percutaneous nephrostomy is coded to the approach Percutaneous.

B6. Device

General guidelines

B6.1a A device is coded only if a device remains after the procedure is completed. If no device remains, the device value No Device is coded.

B6.1b Materials such as sutures, ligatures, radiological markers and temporary post-operative wound drains are considered integral to the performance of a procedure and are not coded as devices.

B6.1c Procedures performed on a device only and not on a body part are specified in the root operations Change, Irrigation, Removal and Revision, and are coded to the procedure performed.

Example: Irrigation of percutaneous nephrostomy tube is coded to the root operation Irrigation of indwelling device in the Administration section.

Drainage device

B6.2 A separate procedure to put in a drainage device is coded to the root operation Drainage with the device value Drainage Device.

Central Nervous System

Brain

Cranial Nerves

Central Nervous System Tables 001–00X

Section	0	**Medical and Surgical**
Body System	0	**Central Nervous System**
Operation	1	**Bypass:** Altering the route of passage of the contents of a tubular body part

Body Part (4th)	Approach (5th)	Device (6th)	Qualifier (7th)

6 Cerebral Ventricle	0 Open
	3 Percutaneous
		7 Autologous Tissue
		    Substitute
		J Synthetic Substitute
		K Nonautologous Tissue
		    Substitute
			0 Nasopharynx
			1 Mastoid Sinus
			2 Atrium
			3 Blood Vessel
			4 Pleural Cavity
			5 Intestine
			6 Peritoneal Cavity
			7 Urinary Tract
			8 Bone Marrow
			B Cerebral Cisterns

U Spinal Canal	0 Open
	3 Percutaneous
		7 Autologous Tissue
		    Substitute
		J Synthetic Substitute
		K Nonautologous Tissue
		    Substitute
			4 Pleural Cavity
			6 Peritoneal Cavity
			7 Urinary Tract
			9 Fallopian Tube

Section	0	**Medical and Surgical**
Body System	0	**Central Nervous System**
Operation	2	**Change:** Taking out or off a device from a body part and putting back an identical or similar device in or on the same body part without cutting or puncturing the skin or a mucous membrane

Body Part (4th)	Approach (5th)	Device (6th)	Qualifier (7th)
0 Brain E Cranial Nerve U Spinal Canal	X External	0 Drainage Device Y Other Device	Z No Qualifier

Section	0	Medical and Surgical
Body System	0	Central Nervous System
Operation	5	**Destruction:** Physical eradication of all or a portion of a body part by the direct use of energy, force, or a destructive agent

Body Part (4th)	Approach (5th)	Device (6th)	Qualifier (7th)
0 Brain 1 Cerebral Meninges 2 Dura Mater 6 Cerebral Ventricle 7 Cerebral Hemisphere 8 Basal Ganglia 9 Thalamus A Hypothalamus B Pons C Cerebellum D Medulla Oblongata F Olfactory Nerve G Optic Nerve H Oculomotor Nerve J Trochlear Nerve K Trigeminal Nerve L Abducens Nerve M Facial Nerve N Acoustic Nerve P Glossopharyngeal Nerve Q Vagus Nerve R Accessory Nerve S Hypoglossal Nerve T Spinal Meninges W Cervical Spinal Cord X Thoracic Spinal Cord Y Lumbar Spinal Cord	0 Open 3 Percutaneous 4 Percutaneous Endoscopic	Z No Device	Z No Qualifier

Section	0	Medical and Surgical
Body System	0	Central Nervous System
Operation	8	**Division:** Cutting into a body part, without draining fluids and/or gases from the body part, in order to separate or transect a body part

Body Part (4th)	Approach (5th)	Device (6th)	Qualifier (7th)
0 Brain 7 Cerebral Hemisphere 8 Basal Ganglia F Olfactory Nerve G Optic Nerve H Oculomotor Nerve J Trochlear Nerve K Trigeminal Nerve L Abducens Nerve M Facial Nerve N Acoustic Nerve P Glossopharyngeal Nerve Q Vagus Nerve R Accessory Nerve S Hypoglossal Nerve W Cervical Spinal Cord X Thoracic Spinal Cord Y Lumbar Spinal Cord	0 Open 3 Percutaneous 4 Percutaneous Endoscopic	Z No Device	Z No Qualifier

Section	0	**Medical and Surgical**
Body System	0	**Central Nervous System**
Operation	9	**Drainage:** Taking or letting out fluids and/or gases from a body part

Body Part (4ᵗʰ)	Approach (5ᵗʰ)	Device (6ᵗʰ)	Qualifier (7ᵗʰ)
0 Brain 1 Cerebral Meninges 2 Dura Mater 3 Epidural Space 4 Subdural Space 5 Subarachnoid Space 6 Cerebral Ventricle 7 Cerebral Hemisphere 8 Basal Ganglia 9 Thalamus A Hypothalamus B Pons C Cerebellum D Medulla Oblongata F Olfactory Nerve G Optic Nerve H Oculomotor Nerve J Trochlear Nerve K Trigeminal Nerve L Abducens Nerve M Facial Nerve N Acoustic Nerve P Glossopharyngeal Nerve Q Vagus Nerve R Accessory Nerve S Hypoglossal Nerve T Spinal Meninges U Spinal Canal W Cervical Spinal Cord X Thoracic Spinal Cord Y Lumbar Spinal Cord	0 Open 3 Percutaneous 4 Percutaneous Endoscopic	0 Drainage Device	Z No Qualifier
0 Brain 1 Cerebral Meninges 2 Dura Mater 3 Epidural Space 4 Subdural Space 5 Subarachnoid Space 6 Cerebral Ventricle 7 Cerebral Hemisphere 8 Basal Ganglia 9 Thalamus A Hypothalamus B Pons C Cerebellum D Medulla Oblongata F Olfactory Nerve G Optic Nerve H Oculomotor Nerve J Trochlear Nerve K Trigeminal Nerve L Abducens Nerve M Facial Nerve N Acoustic Nerve P Glossopharyngeal Nerve Q Vagus Nerve R Accessory Nerve S Hypoglossal Nerve T Spinal Meninges U Spinal Canal W Cervical Spinal Cord X Thoracic Spinal Cord Y Lumbar Spinal Cord	0 Open 3 Percutaneous 4 Percutaneous Endoscopic	Z No Device	X Diagnostic Z No Qualifier

Section	0	Medical and Surgical
Body System	0	Central Nervous System
Operation	B	Excision: Cutting out or off, without replacement, a portion of a body part

Body Part (4th)	Approach (5th)	Device (6th)	Qualifier (7th)
0 Brain	0 Open	Z No Device	X Diagnostic
1 Cerebral Meninges	3 Percutaneous		Z No Qualifier
2 Dura Mater	4 Percutaneous Endoscopic		
6 Cerebral Ventricle			
7 Cerebral Hemisphere			
8 Basal Ganglia			
9 Thalamus			
A Hypothalamus			
B Pons			
C Cerebellum			
D Medulla Oblongata			
F Olfactory Nerve			
G Optic Nerve			
H Oculomotor Nerve			
J Trochlear Nerve			
K Trigeminal Nerve			
L Abducens Nerve			
M Facial Nerve			
N Acoustic Nerve			
P Glossopharyngeal Nerve			
Q Vagus Nerve			
R Accessory Nerve			
S Hypoglossal Nerve			
T Spinal Meninges			
W Cervical Spinal Cord			
X Thoracic Spinal Cord			
Y Lumbar Spinal Cord			

Section	0	Medical and Surgical
Body System	0	Central Nervous System
Operation	C	**Extirpation:** Taking or cutting out solid matter from a body part

Body Part (4th)	Approach (5th)	Device (6th)	Qualifier (7th)
0 Brain	0 Open	Z No Device	Z No Qualifier
1 Cerebral Meninges	3 Percutaneous		
2 Dura Mater	4 Percutaneous Endoscopic		
3 Epidural Space			
4 Subdural Space			
5 Subarachnoid Space			
6 Cerebral Ventricle			
7 Cerebral Hemisphere			
8 Basal Ganglia			
9 Thalamus			
A Hypothalamus			
B Pons			
C Cerebellum			
D Medulla Oblongata			
F Olfactory Nerve			
G Optic Nerve			
H Oculomotor Nerve			
J Trochlear Nerve			
K Trigeminal Nerve			
L Abducens Nerve			
M Facial Nerve			
N Acoustic Nerve			
P Glossopharyngeal Nerve			
Q Vagus Nerve			
R Accessory Nerve			
S Hypoglossal Nerve			
T Spinal Meninges			
W Cervical Spinal Cord			
X Thoracic Spinal Cord			
Y Lumbar Spinal Cord			

Section	0	Medical and Surgical
Body System	0	Central Nervous System
Operation	D	**Extraction:** Pulling or stripping out or off all or a portion of a body part by the use of force

Body Part (4th)	Approach (5th)	Device (6th)	Qualifier (7th)
1 Cerebral Meninges	0 Open	Z No Device	Z No Qualifier
2 Dura Mater	3 Percutaneous		
F Olfactory Nerve	4 Percutaneous Endoscopic		
G Optic Nerve			
H Oculomotor Nerve			
J Trochlear Nerve			
K Trigeminal Nerve			
L Abducens Nerve			
M Facial Nerve			
N Acoustic Nerve			
P Glossopharyngeal Nerve			
Q Vagus Nerve			
R Accessory Nerve			
S Hypoglossal Nerve			
T Spinal Meninges			

Section	0	Medical and Surgical
Body System	0	Central Nervous System
Operation	F	Fragmentation: Breaking solid matter in a body part into pieces

Body Part (4th)	Approach (5th)	Device (6th)	Qualifier (7th)
3 Epidural Space 4 Subdural Space 5 Subarachnoid Space 6 Cerebral Ventricle U Spinal Canal	0 Open 3 Percutaneous 4 Percutaneous Endoscopic X External	Z No Device	Z No Qualifier

Section	0	Medical and Surgical
Body System	0	Central Nervous System
Operation	H	Insertion: Putting in a nonbiological appliance that monitors, assists, performs, or prevents a physiological function but does not physically take the place of a body part

Body Part (4th)	Approach (5th)	Device (6th)	Qualifier (7th)
0 Brain 6 Cerebral Ventricle E Cranial Nerve U Spinal Canal V Spinal Cord	0 Open 3 Percutaneous 4 Percutaneous Endoscopic	2 Monitoring Device 3 Infusion Device M Neurostimulator Lead	Z No Qualifier

Section	0	Medical and Surgical
Body System	0	Central Nervous System
Operation	J	Inspection: Visually and/or manually exploring a body part

Body Part (4th)	Approach (5th)	Device (6th)	Qualifier (7th)
0 Brain E Cranial Nerve U Spinal Canal V Spinal Cord	0 Open 3 Percutaneous 4 Percutaneous Endoscopic	Z No Device	Z No Qualifier

Section	0	Medical and Surgical
Body System	0	Central Nervous System
Operation	K	Map: Locating the route of passage of electrical impulses and/or locating functional areas in a body part

Body Part (4th)	Approach (5th)	Device (6th)	Qualifier (7th)
0 Brain 7 Cerebral Hemisphere 8 Basal Ganglia 9 Thalamus A Hypothalamus B Pons C Cerebellum D Medulla Oblongata	0 Open 3 Percutaneous 4 Percutaneous Endoscopic	Z No Device	Z No Qualifier

Section　　　　　0　　　Medical and Surgical
Body System　　　0　　　Central Nervous System
Operation　　　　N　　　Release: Freeing a body part from an abnormal physical constraint by cutting or by the use of force

Body Part (4th)	Approach (5th)	Device (6th)	Qualifier (7th)
0　Brain 1　Cerebral Meninges 2　Dura Mater 6　Cerebral Ventricle 7　Cerebral Hemisphere 8　Basal Ganglia 9　Thalamus A　Hypothalamus B　Pons C　Cerebellum D　Medulla Oblongata F　Olfactory Nerve G　Optic Nerve H　Oculomotor Nerve J　Trochlear Nerve K　Trigeminal Nerve L　Abducens Nerve M　Facial Nerve N　Acoustic Nerve P　Glossopharyngeal Nerve Q　Vagus Nerve R　Accessory Nerve S　Hypoglossal Nerve T　Spinal Meninges W　Cervical Spinal Cord X　Thoracic Spinal Cord Y　Lumbar Spinal Cord	0　Open 3　Percutaneous 4　Percutaneous Endoscopic	Z　No Device	Z　No Qualifier

Section　　　　　0　　　Medical and Surgical
Body System　　　0　　　Central Nervous System
Operation　　　　P　　　Removal: Taking out or off a device from a body part

Body Part (4th)	Approach (5th)	Device (6th)	Qualifier (7th)
0　Brain V　Spinal Cord	0　Open 3　Percutaneous 4　Percutaneous Endoscopic	0　Drainage Device 2　Monitoring Device 3　Infusion Device 7　Autologous Tissue Substitute J　Synthetic Substitute K　Nonautologous Tissue Substitute M　Neurostimulator Lead	Z　No Qualifier
0　Brain V　Spinal Cord	X　External	0　Drainage Device 2　Monitoring Device 3　Infusion Device M　Neurostimulator Lead	Z　No Qualifier
6　Cerebral Ventricle U　Spinal Canal	0　Open 3　Percutaneous 4　Percutaneous Endoscopic	0　Drainage Device 2　Monitoring Device 3　Infusion Device J　Synthetic Substitute M　Neurostimulator Lead	Z　No Qualifier
6　Cerebral Ventricle U　Spinal Canal	X　External	0　Drainage Device 2　Monitoring Device 3　Infusion Device M　Neurostimulator Lead	Z　No Qualifier

Continued

Section	0	Medical and Surgical
Body System	0	Central Nervous System
Operation	P	**Removal:** Taking out or off a device from a body part

00P *Continued*

Body Part (4th)	Approach (5th)	Device (6th)	Qualifier (7th)
E Cranial Nerve	0 Open 3 Percutaneous 4 Percutaneous Endoscopic	0 Drainage Device 2 Monitoring Device 3 Infusion Device 7 Autologous Tissue Substitute M Neurostimulator Lead	Z No Qualifier
E Cranial Nerve	X External	0 Drainage Device 2 Monitoring Device 3 Infusion Device M Neurostimulator Lead	Z No Qualifier

Section	0	Medical and Surgical
Body System	0	Central Nervous System
Operation	Q	**Repair:** Restoring, to the extent possible, a body part to its normal anatomic structure and function

Body Part (4th)	Approach (5th)	Device (6th)	Qualifier (7th)
0 Brain 1 Cerebral Meninges 2 Dura Mater 6 Cerebral Ventricle 7 Cerebral Hemisphere 8 Basal Ganglia 9 Thalamus A Hypothalamus B Pons C Cerebellum D Medulla Oblongata F Olfactory Nerve G Optic Nerve H Oculomotor Nerve J Trochlear Nerve K Trigeminal Nerve L Abducens Nerve M Facial Nerve N Acoustic Nerve P Glossopharyngeal Nerve Q Vagus Nerve R Accessory Nerve S Hypoglossal Nerve T Spinal Meninges W Cervical Spinal Cord X Thoracic Spinal Cord Y Lumbar Spinal Cord	0 Open 3 Percutaneous 4 Percutaneous Endoscopic	Z No Device	Z No Qualifier

Section	0	Medical and Surgical
Body System	0	Central Nervous System
Operation	S	**Reposition:** Moving to its normal location, or other suitable location, all or a portion of a body part

Body Part (4th)	Approach (5th)	Device (6th)	Qualifier (7th)
F Olfactory Nerve G Optic Nerve H Oculomotor Nerve J Trochlear Nerve K Trigeminal Nerve L Abducens Nerve M Facial Nerve N Acoustic Nerve P Glossopharyngeal Nerve Q Vagus Nerve R Accessory Nerve S Hypoglossal Nerve W Cervical Spinal Cord X Thoracic Spinal Cord Y Lumbar Spinal Cord	0 Open 3 Percutaneous 4 Percutaneous Endoscopic	Z No Device	Z No Qualifier

Section	0	Medical and Surgical
Body System	0	Central Nervous System
Operation	T	**Resection:** Cutting out or off, without replacement, all of a body part

Body Part (4th)	Approach (5th)	Device (6th)	Qualifier (7th)
7 Cerebral Hemisphere	0 Open 3 Percutaneous 4 Percutaneous Endoscopic	Z No Device	Z No Qualifier

Section	0	Medical and Surgical
Body System	0	Central Nervous System
Operation	U	**Supplement:** Putting in or on biological or synthetic material that physically reinforces and/or augments the function of a portion of a body part

Body Part (4th)	Approach (5th)	Device (6th)	Qualifier (7th)
1 Cerebral Meninges 2 Dura Mater T Spinal Meninges	0 Open 3 Percutaneous 4 Percutaneous Endoscopic	7 Autologous Tissue Substitute J Synthetic Substitute K Nonautologous Tissue Substitute	Z No Qualifier
F Olfactory Nerve G Optic Nerve H Oculomotor Nerve J Trochlear Nerve K Trigeminal Nerve L Abducens Nerve M Facial Nerve N Acoustic Nerve P Glossopharyngeal Nerve Q Vagus Nerve R Accessory Nerve S Hypoglossal Nerve	0 Open 3 Percutaneous 4 Percutaneous Endoscopic	7 Autologous Tissue Substitute	Z No Qualifier

Section	0	Medical and Surgical
Body System	0	Central Nervous System
Operation	W	Revision: Correcting, to the extent possible, a portion of a malfunctioning device or the position of a displaced device

Body Part (4th)	Approach (5th)	Device (6th)	Qualifier (7th)
0 Brain V Spinal Cord	0 Open 3 Percutaneous 4 Percutaneous Endoscopic X External	0 Drainage Device 2 Monitoring Device 3 Infusion Device 7 Autologous Tissue Substitute J Synthetic Substitute K Nonautologous Tissue Substitute M Neurostimulator Lead	Z No Qualifier
6 Cerebral Ventricle U Spinal Canal	0 Open 3 Percutaneous 4 Percutaneous Endoscopic X External	0 Drainage Device 2 Monitoring Device 3 Infusion Device J Synthetic Substitute M Neurostimulator Lead	Z No Qualifier
E Cranial Nerve	0 Open 3 Percutaneous 4 Percutaneous Endoscopic X External	0 Drainage Device 2 Monitoring Device 3 Infusion Device 7 Autologous Tissue Substitute M Neurostimulator Lead	Z No Qualifier

Section	0	Medical and Surgical
Body System	0	Central Nervous System
Operation	X	Transfer: Moving, without taking out, all or a portion of a body part to another location to take over the function of all or a portion of a body part

Body Part (4th)	Approach (5th)	Device (6th)	Qualifier (7th)
F Olfactory Nerve G Optic Nerve H Oculomotor Nerve J Trochlear Nerve K Trigeminal Nerve L Abducens Nerve M Facial Nerve N Acoustic Nerve P Glossopharyngeal Nerve Q Vagus Nerve R Accessory Nerve S Hypoglossal Nerve	0 Open 4 Percutaneous Endoscopic	Z No Device	F Olfactory Nerve G Optic Nerve H Oculomotor Nerve J Trochlear Nerve K Trigeminal Nerve L Abducens Nerve M Facial Nerve N Acoustic Nerve P Glossopharyngeal Nerve Q Vagus Nerve R Accessory Nerve S Hypoglossal Nerve

Central Nervous System Code Listing 001–00X

001 – Central Nervous System, Bypass

Review Coding Guideline B3.6a

0016070 Bypass Cerebral Ventricle to Nasopharynx with Autologous Tissue Substitute, Open Approach

0016071 Bypass Cerebral Ventricle to Mastoid Sinus with Autologous Tissue Substitute, Open Approach

0016072 Bypass Cerebral Ventricle to Atrium with Autologous Tissue Substitute, Open Approach

0016073 Bypass Cerebral Ventricle to Blood Vessel with Autologous Tissue Substitute, Open Approach

0016074 Bypass Cerebral Ventricle to Pleural Cavity with Autologous Tissue Substitute, Open Approach

0016075 Bypass Cerebral Ventricle to Intestine with Autologous Tissue Substitute, Open Approach

0016076 Bypass Cerebral Ventricle to Peritoneal Cavity with Autologous Tissue Substitute, Open Approach

0016077 Bypass Cerebral Ventricle to Urinary Tract with Autologous Tissue Substitute, Open Approach

0016078 Bypass Cerebral Ventricle to Bone Marrow with Autologous Tissue Substitute, Open Approach

001607B Bypass Cerebral Ventricle to Cerebral Cisterns with Autologous Tissue Substitute, Open Approach

00160J0 Bypass Cerebral Ventricle to Nasopharynx with Synthetic Substitute, Open Approach

00160J1 Bypass Cerebral Ventricle to Mastoid Sinus with Synthetic Substitute, Open Approach

00160J2 Bypass Cerebral Ventricle to Atrium with Synthetic Substitute, Open Approach

00160J3 Bypass Cerebral Ventricle to Blood Vessel with Synthetic Substitute, Open Approach

♀ Female-only   ♂ Male-only   ● Limited Coverage   ● Non-OR   HAC HAC-associated procedure   ● Non-covered procedures   ✚ Combination

00160J4	Bypass Cerebral Ventricle to Pleural Cavity with Synthetic Substitute, Open Approach
00160J5	Bypass Cerebral Ventricle to Intestine with Synthetic Substitute, Open Approach
00160J6	Bypass Cerebral Ventricle to Peritoneal Cavity with Synthetic Substitute, Open Approach
00160J7	Bypass Cerebral Ventricle to Urinary Tract with Synthetic Substitute, Open Approach
00160J8	Bypass Cerebral Ventricle to Bone Marrow with Synthetic Substitute, Open Approach
00160JB	Bypass Cerebral Ventricle to Cerebral Cisterns with Synthetic Substitute, Open Approach
00160K0	Bypass Cerebral Ventricle to Nasopharynx with Nonautologous Tissue Substitute, Open Approach
00160K1	Bypass Cerebral Ventricle to Mastoid Sinus with Nonautologous Tissue Substitute, Open Approach
00160K2	Bypass Cerebral Ventricle to Atrium with Nonautologous Tissue Substitute, Open Approach
00160K3	Bypass Cerebral Ventricle to Blood Vessel with Nonautologous Tissue Substitute, Open Approach
00160K4	Bypass Cerebral Ventricle to Pleural Cavity with Nonautologous Tissue Substitute, Open Approach
00160K5	Bypass Cerebral Ventricle to Intestine with Nonautologous Tissue Substitute, Open Approach
00160K6	Bypass Cerebral Ventricle to Peritoneal Cavity with Nonautologous Tissue Substitute, Open Approach
00160K7	Bypass Cerebral Ventricle to Urinary Tract with Nonautologous Tissue Substitute, Open Approach
00160K8	Bypass Cerebral Ventricle to Bone Marrow with Nonautologous Tissue Substitute, Open Approach
00160KB	Bypass Cerebral Ventricle to Cerebral Cisterns with Nonautologous Tissue Substitute, Open Approach
0016370	Bypass Cerebral Ventricle to Nasopharynx with Autologous Tissue Substitute, Percutaneous Approach
0016371	Bypass Cerebral Ventricle to Mastoid Sinus with Autologous Tissue Substitute, Percutaneous Approach
0016372	Bypass Cerebral Ventricle to Atrium with Autologous Tissue Substitute, Percutaneous Approach
0016373	Bypass Cerebral Ventricle to Blood Vessel with Autologous Tissue Substitute, Percutaneous Approach
0016374	Bypass Cerebral Ventricle to Pleural Cavity with Autologous Tissue Substitute, Percutaneous Approach
0016375	Bypass Cerebral Ventricle to Intestine with Autologous Tissue Substitute, Percutaneous Approach
0016376	Bypass Cerebral Ventricle to Peritoneal Cavity with Autologous Tissue Substitute, Percutaneous Approach
0016377	Bypass Cerebral Ventricle to Urinary Tract with Autologous Tissue Substitute, Percutaneous Approach
0016378	Bypass Cerebral Ventricle to Bone Marrow with Autologous Tissue Substitute, Percutaneous Approach
001637B	Bypass Cerebral Ventricle to Cerebral Cisterns with Autologous Tissue Substitute, Percutaneous Approach
00163J0	Bypass Cerebral Ventricle to Nasopharynx with Synthetic Substitute, Percutaneous Approach
00163J1	Bypass Cerebral Ventricle to Mastoid Sinus with Synthetic Substitute, Percutaneous Approach
00163J2	Bypass Cerebral Ventricle to Atrium with Synthetic Substitute, Percutaneous Approach
00163J3	Bypass Cerebral Ventricle to Blood Vessel with Synthetic Substitute, Percutaneous Approach
00163J4	Bypass Cerebral Ventricle to Pleural Cavity with Synthetic Substitute, Percutaneous Approach
00163J5	Bypass Cerebral Ventricle to Intestine with Synthetic Substitute, Percutaneous Approach
00163J6	Bypass Cerebral Ventricle to Peritoneal Cavity with Synthetic Substitute, Percutaneous Approach
00163J7	Bypass Cerebral Ventricle to Urinary Tract with Synthetic Substitute, Percutaneous Approach
00163J8	Bypass Cerebral Ventricle to Bone Marrow with Synthetic Substitute, Percutaneous Approach
00163JB	Bypass Cerebral Ventricle to Cerebral Cisterns with Synthetic Substitute, Percutaneous Approach
00163K0	Bypass Cerebral Ventricle to Nasopharynx with Nonautologous Tissue Substitute, Percutaneous Approach
00163K1	Bypass Cerebral Ventricle to Mastoid Sinus with Nonautologous Tissue Substitute, Percutaneous Approach
00163K2	Bypass Cerebral Ventricle to Atrium with Nonautologous Tissue Substitute, Percutaneous Approach
00163K3	Bypass Cerebral Ventricle to Blood Vessel with Nonautologous Tissue Substitute, Percutaneous Approach
00163K4	Bypass Cerebral Ventricle to Pleural Cavity with Nonautologous Tissue Substitute, Percutaneous Approach
00163K5	Bypass Cerebral Ventricle to Intestine with Nonautologous Tissue Substitute, Percutaneous Approach
00163K6	Bypass Cerebral Ventricle to Peritoneal Cavity with Nonautologous Tissue Substitute, Percutaneous Approach
00163K7	Bypass Cerebral Ventricle to Urinary Tract with Nonautologous Tissue Substitute, Percutaneous Approach
00163K8	Bypass Cerebral Ventricle to Bone Marrow with Nonautologous Tissue Substitute, Percutaneous Approach
00163KB	Bypass Cerebral Ventricle to Cerebral Cisterns with Nonautologous Tissue Substitute, Percutaneous Approach
001U074	Bypass Spinal Canal to Pleural Cavity with Autologous Tissue Substitute, Open Approach
001U076	Bypass Spinal Canal to Peritoneal Cavity with Autologous Tissue Substitute, Open Approach
001U077	Bypass Spinal Canal to Urinary Tract with Autologous Tissue Substitute, Open Approach
001U079	Bypass Spinal Canal to Fallopian Tube with Autologous Tissue Substitute, Open Approach
001U0J4	Bypass Spinal Canal to Pleural Cavity with Synthetic Substitute, Open Approach
001U0J6	Bypass Spinal Canal to Peritoneal Cavity with Synthetic Substitute, Open Approach
001U0J7	Bypass Spinal Canal to Urinary Tract with Synthetic Substitute, Open Approach
001U0J9	Bypass Spinal Canal to Fallopian Tube with Synthetic Substitute, Open Approach
001U0K4	Bypass Spinal Canal to Pleural Cavity with Nonautologous Tissue Substitute, Open Approach
001U0K6	Bypass Spinal Canal to Peritoneal Cavity with Nonautologous Tissue Substitute, Open Approach
001U0K7	Bypass Spinal Canal to Urinary Tract with Nonautologous Tissue Substitute, Open Approach
001U0K9	Bypass Spinal Canal to Fallopian Tube with Nonautologous Tissue Substitute, Open Approach
001U374	Bypass Spinal Canal to Pleural Cavity with Autologous Tissue Substitute, Percutaneous Approach
001U376	Bypass Spinal Canal to Peritoneal Cavity with Autologous Tissue Substitute, Percutaneous Approach
001U377	Bypass Spinal Canal to Urinary Tract with Autologous Tissue Substitute, Percutaneous Approach
001U379	Bypass Spinal Canal to Fallopian Tube with Autologous Tissue Substitute, Percutaneous Approach
001U3J4	Bypass Spinal Canal to Pleural Cavity with Synthetic Substitute, Percutaneous Approach
001U3J6	Bypass Spinal Canal to Peritoneal Cavity with Synthetic Substitute, Percutaneous Approach
001U3J7	Bypass Spinal Canal to Urinary Tract with Synthetic Substitute, Percutaneous Approach
001U3J9	Bypass Spinal Canal to Fallopian Tube with Synthetic Substitute, Percutaneous Approach
001U3K4	Bypass Spinal Canal to Pleural Cavity with Nonautologous Tissue Substitute, Percutaneous Approach
001U3K6	Bypass Spinal Canal to Peritoneal Cavity with Nonautologous Tissue Substitute, Percutaneous Approach
001U3K7	Bypass Spinal Canal to Urinary Tract with Nonautologous Tissue Substitute, Percutaneous Approach
001U3K9	Bypass Spinal Canal to Fallopian Tube with Nonautologous Tissue Substitute, Percutaneous Approach

002 – Central Nervous System, Change

Review Coding Guideline B6.1c

0020X0Z	Change Drainage Device in Brain, External Approach
0020XYZ	Change Other Device in Brain, External Approach
002EX0Z	Change Drainage Device in Cranial Nerve, External Approach
002EXYZ	Change Other Device in Cranial Nerve, External Approach
002UX0Z	Change Drainage Device in Spinal Canal, External Approach
002UXYZ	Change Other Device in Spinal Canal, External Approach

005 – Central Nervous System, Destruction

00500ZZ	Destruction of Brain, Open Approach
00503ZZ	Destruction of Brain, Percutaneous Approach
00504ZZ	Destruction of Brain, Percutaneous Endoscopic Approach
00510ZZ	Destruction of Cerebral Meninges, Open Approach
00513ZZ	Destruction of Cerebral Meninges, Percutaneous Approach
00514ZZ	Destruction of Cerebral Meninges, Percutaneous Endoscopic Approach
00520ZZ	Destruction of Dura Mater, Open Approach
00523ZZ	Destruction of Dura Mater, Percutaneous Approach
00524ZZ	Destruction of Dura Mater, Percutaneous Endoscopic Approach
00560ZZ	Destruction of Cerebral Ventricle, Open Approach
00563ZZ	Destruction of Cerebral Ventricle, Percutaneous Approach
00564ZZ	Destruction of Cerebral Ventricle, Percutaneous Endoscopic Approach
00570ZZ	Destruction of Cerebral Hemisphere, Open Approach
00573ZZ	Destruction of Cerebral Hemisphere, Percutaneous Approach
00574ZZ	Destruction of Cerebral Hemisphere, Percutaneous Endoscopic Approach
00580ZZ	Destruction of Basal Ganglia, Open Approach
00583ZZ	Destruction of Basal Ganglia, Percutaneous Approach
00584ZZ	Destruction of Basal Ganglia, Percutaneous Endoscopic Approach
00590ZZ	Destruction of Thalamus, Open Approach
00593ZZ	Destruction of Thalamus, Percutaneous Approach
00594ZZ	Destruction of Thalamus, Percutaneous Endoscopic Approach
005A0ZZ	Destruction of Hypothalamus, Open Approach
005A3ZZ	Destruction of Hypothalamus, Percutaneous Approach
005A4ZZ	Destruction of Hypothalamus, Percutaneous Endoscopic Approach
005B0ZZ	Destruction of Pons, Open Approach
005B3ZZ	Destruction of Pons, Percutaneous Approach
005B4ZZ	Destruction of Pons, Percutaneous Endoscopic Approach
005C0ZZ	Destruction of Cerebellum, Open Approach
005C3ZZ	Destruction of Cerebellum, Percutaneous Approach
005C4ZZ	Destruction of Cerebellum, Percutaneous Endoscopic Approach
005D0ZZ	Destruction of Medulla Oblongata, Open Approach
005D3ZZ	Destruction of Medulla Oblongata, Percutaneous Approach
005D4ZZ	Destruction of Medulla Oblongata, Percutaneous Endoscopic Approach
005F0ZZ	Destruction of Olfactory Nerve, Open Approach
005F3ZZ	Destruction of Olfactory Nerve, Percutaneous Approach
005F4ZZ	Destruction of Olfactory Nerve, Percutaneous Endoscopic Approach
005G0ZZ	Destruction of Optic Nerve, Open Approach
005G3ZZ	Destruction of Optic Nerve, Percutaneous Approach
005G4ZZ	Destruction of Optic Nerve, Percutaneous Endoscopic Approach
005H0ZZ	Destruction of Oculomotor Nerve, Open Approach
005H3ZZ	Destruction of Oculomotor Nerve, Percutaneous Approach
005H4ZZ	Destruction of Oculomotor Nerve, Percutaneous Endoscopic Approach
005J0ZZ	Destruction of Trochlear Nerve, Open Approach
005J3ZZ	Destruction of Trochlear Nerve, Percutaneous Approach
005J4ZZ	Destruction of Trochlear Nerve, Percutaneous Endoscopic Approach
005K0ZZ	Destruction of Trigeminal Nerve, Open Approach
005K3ZZ	Destruction of Trigeminal Nerve, Percutaneous Approach
005K4ZZ	Destruction of Trigeminal Nerve, Percutaneous Endoscopic Approach
005L0ZZ	Destruction of Abducens Nerve, Open Approach
005L3ZZ	Destruction of Abducens Nerve, Percutaneous Approach
005L4ZZ	Destruction of Abducens Nerve, Percutaneous Endoscopic Approach
005M0ZZ	Destruction of Facial Nerve, Open Approach
005M3ZZ	Destruction of Facial Nerve, Percutaneous Approach
005M4ZZ	Destruction of Facial Nerve, Percutaneous Endoscopic Approach
005N0ZZ	Destruction of Acoustic Nerve, Open Approach
005N3ZZ	Destruction of Acoustic Nerve, Percutaneous Approach
005N4ZZ	Destruction of Acoustic Nerve, Percutaneous Endoscopic Approach
005P0ZZ	Destruction of Glossopharyngeal Nerve, Open Approach
005P3ZZ	Destruction of Glossopharyngeal Nerve, Percutaneous Approach
005P4ZZ	Destruction of Glossopharyngeal Nerve, Percutaneous Endoscopic Approach
005Q0ZZ	Destruction of Vagus Nerve, Open Approach
005Q3ZZ	Destruction of Vagus Nerve, Percutaneous Approach
005Q4ZZ	Destruction of Vagus Nerve, Percutaneous Endoscopic Approach
005R0ZZ	Destruction of Accessory Nerve, Open Approach
005R3ZZ	Destruction of Accessory Nerve, Percutaneous Approach
005R4ZZ	Destruction of Accessory Nerve, Percutaneous Endoscopic Approach
005S0ZZ	Destruction of Hypoglossal Nerve, Open Approach
005S3ZZ	Destruction of Hypoglossal Nerve, Percutaneous Approach
005S4ZZ	Destruction of Hypoglossal Nerve, Percutaneous Endoscopic Approach
005T0ZZ	Destruction of Spinal Meninges, Open Approach
005T3ZZ	Destruction of Spinal Meninges, Percutaneous Approach
005T4ZZ	Destruction of Spinal Meninges, Percutaneous Endoscopic Approach
005W0ZZ	Destruction of Cervical Spinal Cord, Open Approach
005W3ZZ	Destruction of Cervical Spinal Cord, Percutaneous Approach
005W4ZZ	Destruction of Cervical Spinal Cord, Percutaneous Endoscopic Approach
005X0ZZ	Destruction of Thoracic Spinal Cord, Open Approach
005X3ZZ	Destruction of Thoracic Spinal Cord, Percutaneous Approach
005X4ZZ	Destruction of Thoracic Spinal Cord, Percutaneous Endoscopic Approach
005Y0ZZ	Destruction of Lumbar Spinal Cord, Open Approach
005Y3ZZ	Destruction of Lumbar Spinal Cord, Percutaneous Approach
005Y4ZZ	Destruction of Lumbar Spinal Cord, Percutaneous Endoscopic Approach

008 – Central Nervous System, Division

Review Coding Guideline B3.14

00800ZZ	Division of Brain, Open Approach
00803ZZ	Division of Brain, Percutaneous Approach
00804ZZ	Division of Brain, Percutaneous Endoscopic Approach
00870ZZ	Division of Cerebral Hemisphere, Open Approach
00873ZZ	Division of Cerebral Hemisphere, Percutaneous Approach
00874ZZ	Division of Cerebral Hemisphere, Percutaneous Endoscopic Approach
00880ZZ	Division of Basal Ganglia, Open Approach
00883ZZ	Division of Basal Ganglia, Percutaneous Approach
00884ZZ	Division of Basal Ganglia, Percutaneous Endoscopic Approach
008F0ZZ	Division of Olfactory Nerve, Open Approach
008F3ZZ	Division of Olfactory Nerve, Percutaneous Approach
008F4ZZ	Division of Olfactory Nerve, Percutaneous Endoscopic Approach
008G0ZZ	Division of Optic Nerve, Open Approach
008G3ZZ	Division of Optic Nerve, Percutaneous Approach
008G4ZZ	Division of Optic Nerve, Percutaneous Endoscopic Approach
008H0ZZ	Division of Oculomotor Nerve, Open Approach
008H3ZZ	Division of Oculomotor Nerve, Percutaneous Approach
008H4ZZ	Division of Oculomotor Nerve, Percutaneous Endoscopic Approach
008J0ZZ	Division of Trochlear Nerve, Open Approach
008J3ZZ	Division of Trochlear Nerve, Percutaneous Approach
008J4ZZ	Division of Trochlear Nerve, Percutaneous Endoscopic Approach

008K0ZZ	Division of Trigeminal Nerve, Open Approach
008K3ZZ	Division of Trigeminal Nerve, Percutaneous Approach
008K4ZZ	Division of Trigeminal Nerve, Percutaneous Endoscopic Approach
008L0ZZ	Division of Abducens Nerve, Open Approach
008L3ZZ	Division of Abducens Nerve, Percutaneous Approach
008L4ZZ	Division of Abducens Nerve, Percutaneous Endoscopic Approach
008M0ZZ	Division of Facial Nerve, Open Approach
008M3ZZ	Division of Facial Nerve, Percutaneous Approach
008M4ZZ	Division of Facial Nerve, Percutaneous Endoscopic Approach
008N0ZZ	Division of Acoustic Nerve, Open Approach
008N3ZZ	Division of Acoustic Nerve, Percutaneous Approach
008N4ZZ	Division of Acoustic Nerve, Percutaneous Endoscopic Approach
008P0ZZ	Division of Glossopharyngeal Nerve, Open Approach
008P3ZZ	Division of Glossopharyngeal Nerve, Percutaneous Approach
008P4ZZ	Division of Glossopharyngeal Nerve, Percutaneous Endoscopic Approach
008Q0ZZ	Division of Vagus Nerve, Open Approach
008Q3ZZ	Division of Vagus Nerve, Percutaneous Approach
008Q4ZZ	Division of Vagus Nerve, Percutaneous Endoscopic Approach
008R0ZZ	Division of Accessory Nerve, Open Approach
008R3ZZ	Division of Accessory Nerve, Percutaneous Approach
008R4ZZ	Division of Accessory Nerve, Percutaneous Endoscopic Approach
008S0ZZ	Division of Hypoglossal Nerve, Open Approach
008S3ZZ	Division of Hypoglossal Nerve, Percutaneous Approach
008S4ZZ	Division of Hypoglossal Nerve, Percutaneous Endoscopic Approach
008W0ZZ	Division of Cervical Spinal Cord, Open Approach
008W3ZZ	Division of Cervical Spinal Cord, Percutaneous Approach
008W4ZZ	Division of Cervical Spinal Cord, Percutaneous Endoscopic Approach
008X0ZZ	Division of Thoracic Spinal Cord, Open Approach
008X3ZZ	Division of Thoracic Spinal Cord, Percutaneous Approach
008X4ZZ	Division of Thoracic Spinal Cord, Percutaneous Endoscopic Approach
008Y0ZZ	Division of Lumbar Spinal Cord, Open Approach
008Y3ZZ	Division of Lumbar Spinal Cord, Percutaneous Approach
008Y4ZZ	Division of Lumbar Spinal Cord, Percutaneous Endoscopic Approach

009 – Central Nervous System, Drainage

Review Coding Guidelines B3.4a and B3.4b

Review Coding Guideline B6.2

009000Z	Drainage of Brain with Drainage Device, Open Approach
00900ZX	Drainage of Brain, Open Approach, Diagnostic
00900ZZ	Drainage of Brain, Open Approach
009030Z	Drainage of Brain with Drainage Device, Percutaneous Approach
00903ZX	Drainage of Brain, Percutaneous Approach, Diagnostic
00903ZZ	Drainage of Brain, Percutaneous Approach
009040Z	Drainage of Brain with Drainage Device, Percutaneous Endoscopic Approach
00904ZX	Drainage of Brain, Percutaneous Endoscopic Approach, Diagnostic
00904ZZ	Drainage of Brain, Percutaneous Endoscopic Approach
009100Z	Drainage of Cerebral Meninges with Drainage Device, Open Approach
00910ZX	Drainage of Cerebral Meninges, Open Approach, Diagnostic
00910ZZ	Drainage of Cerebral Meninges, Open Approach
009130Z	Drainage of Cerebral Meninges with Drainage Device, Percutaneous Approach
00913ZX	Drainage of Cerebral Meninges, Percutaneous Approach, Diagnostic
00913ZZ	Drainage of Cerebral Meninges, Percutaneous Approach
009140Z	Drainage of Cerebral Meninges with Drainage Device, Percutaneous Endoscopic Approach
00914ZX	Drainage of Cerebral Meninges, Percutaneous Endoscopic Approach, Diagnostic
00914ZZ	Drainage of Cerebral Meninges, Percutaneous Endoscopic Approach
009200Z	Drainage of Dura Mater with Drainage Device, Open Approach
00920ZX	Drainage of Dura Mater, Open Approach, Diagnostic
00920ZZ	Drainage of Dura Mater, Open Approach
009230Z	Drainage of Dura Mater with Drainage Device, Percutaneous Approach
00923ZX	Drainage of Dura Mater, Percutaneous Approach, Diagnostic
00923ZZ	Drainage of Dura Mater, Percutaneous Approach
009240Z	Drainage of Dura Mater with Drainage Device, Percutaneous Endoscopic Approach
00924ZX	Drainage of Dura Mater, Percutaneous Endoscopic Approach, Diagnostic
00924ZZ	Drainage of Dura Mater, Percutaneous Endoscopic Approach
009300Z	Drainage of Epidural Space with Drainage Device, Open Approach
00930ZX	Drainage of Epidural Space, Open Approach, Diagnostic
00930ZZ	Drainage of Epidural Space, Open Approach
009330Z	Drainage of Epidural Space with Drainage Device, Percutaneous Approach
00933ZX	Drainage of Epidural Space, Percutaneous Approach, Diagnostic
00933ZZ	Drainage of Epidural Space, Percutaneous Approach
009340Z	Drainage of Epidural Space with Drainage Device, Percutaneous Endoscopic Approach
00934ZX	Drainage of Epidural Space, Percutaneous Endoscopic Approach, Diagnostic
00934ZZ	Drainage of Epidural Space, Percutaneous Endoscopic Approach
009400Z	Drainage of Subdural Space with Drainage Device, Open Approach
00940ZX	Drainage of Subdural Space, Open Approach, Diagnostic
00940ZZ	Drainage of Subdural Space, Open Approach
009430Z	Drainage of Subdural Space with Drainage Device, Percutaneous Approach
00943ZX	Drainage of Subdural Space, Percutaneous Approach, Diagnostic
00943ZZ	Drainage of Subdural Space, Percutaneous Approach
009440Z	Drainage of Subdural Space with Drainage Device, Percutaneous Endoscopic Approach
00944ZX	Drainage of Subdural Space, Percutaneous Endoscopic Approach, Diagnostic
00944ZZ	Drainage of Subdural Space, Percutaneous Endoscopic Approach
009500Z	Drainage of Subarachnoid Space with Drainage Device, Open Approach
00950ZX	Drainage of Subarachnoid Space, Open Approach, Diagnostic
00950ZZ	Drainage of Subarachnoid Space, Open Approach
009530Z	Drainage of Subarachnoid Space with Drainage Device, Percutaneous Approach
00953ZX	Drainage of Subarachnoid Space, Percutaneous Approach, Diagnostic
00953ZZ	Drainage of Subarachnoid Space, Percutaneous Approach
009540Z	Drainage of Subarachnoid Space with Drainage Device, Percutaneous Endoscopic Approach
00954ZX	Drainage of Subarachnoid Space, Percutaneous Endoscopic Approach, Diagnostic
00954ZZ	Drainage of Subarachnoid Space, Percutaneous Endoscopic Approach
009600Z	Drainage of Cerebral Ventricle with Drainage Device, Open Approach
00960ZX	Drainage of Cerebral Ventricle, Open Approach, Diagnostic
00960ZZ	Drainage of Cerebral Ventricle, Open Approach
009630Z	Drainage of Cerebral Ventricle with Drainage Device, Percutaneous Approach
00963ZX	Drainage of Cerebral Ventricle, Percutaneous Approach, Diagnostic
00963ZZ	Drainage of Cerebral Ventricle, Percutaneous Approach
009640Z	Drainage of Cerebral Ventricle with Drainage Device, Percutaneous Endoscopic Approach
00964ZX	Drainage of Cerebral Ventricle, Percutaneous Endoscopic Approach, Diagnostic
00964ZZ	Drainage of Cerebral Ventricle, Percutaneous Endoscopic Approach
009700Z	Drainage of Cerebral Hemisphere with Drainage Device, Open Approach
00970ZX	Drainage of Cerebral Hemisphere, Open Approach, Diagnostic
00970ZZ	Drainage of Cerebral Hemisphere, Open Approach
009730Z	Drainage of Cerebral Hemisphere with Drainage Device, Percutaneous Approach
00973ZX	Drainage of Cerebral Hemisphere, Percutaneous Approach, Diagnostic

00973ZZ	Drainage of Cerebral Hemisphere, Percutaneous Approach
009740Z	Drainage of Cerebral Hemisphere with Drainage Device, Percutaneous Endoscopic Approach
00974ZX	Drainage of Cerebral Hemisphere, Percutaneous Endoscopic Approach, Diagnostic
00974ZZ	Drainage of Cerebral Hemisphere, Percutaneous Endoscopic Approach
009800Z	Drainage of Basal Ganglia with Drainage Device, Open Approach
00980ZX	Drainage of Basal Ganglia, Open Approach, Diagnostic
00980ZZ	Drainage of Basal Ganglia, Open Approach
009830Z	Drainage of Basal Ganglia with Drainage Device, Percutaneous Approach
00983ZX	Drainage of Basal Ganglia, Percutaneous Approach, Diagnostic
00983ZZ	Drainage of Basal Ganglia, Percutaneous Approach
009840Z	Drainage of Basal Ganglia with Drainage Device, Percutaneous Endoscopic Approach
00984ZX	Drainage of Basal Ganglia, Percutaneous Endoscopic Approach, Diagnostic
00984ZZ	Drainage of Basal Ganglia, Percutaneous Endoscopic Approach
009900Z	Drainage of Thalamus with Drainage Device, Open Approach
00990ZX	Drainage of Thalamus, Open Approach, Diagnostic
00990ZZ	Drainage of Thalamus, Open Approach
009930Z	Drainage of Thalamus with Drainage Device, Percutaneous Approach
00993ZX	Drainage of Thalamus, Percutaneous Approach, Diagnostic
00993ZZ	Drainage of Thalamus, Percutaneous Approach
009940Z	Drainage of Thalamus with Drainage Device, Percutaneous Endoscopic Approach
00994ZX	Drainage of Thalamus, Percutaneous Endoscopic Approach, Diagnostic
00994ZZ	Drainage of Thalamus, Percutaneous Endoscopic Approach
009A00Z	Drainage of Hypothalamus with Drainage Device, Open Approach
009A0ZX	Drainage of Hypothalamus, Open Approach, Diagnostic
009A0ZZ	Drainage of Hypothalamus, Open Approach
009A30Z	Drainage of Hypothalamus with Drainage Device, Percutaneous Approach
009A3ZX	Drainage of Hypothalamus, Percutaneous Approach, Diagnostic
009A3ZZ	Drainage of Hypothalamus, Percutaneous Approach
009A40Z	Drainage of Hypothalamus with Drainage Device, Percutaneous Endoscopic Approach
009A4ZX	Drainage of Hypothalamus, Percutaneous Endoscopic Approach, Diagnostic
009A4ZZ	Drainage of Hypothalamus, Percutaneous Endoscopic Approach
009B00Z	Drainage of Pons with Drainage Device, Open Approach
009B0ZX	Drainage of Pons, Open Approach, Diagnostic
009B0ZZ	Drainage of Pons, Open Approach
009B30Z	Drainage of Pons with Drainage Device, Percutaneous Approach
009B3ZX	Drainage of Pons, Percutaneous Approach, Diagnostic
009B3ZZ	Drainage of Pons, Percutaneous Approach
009B40Z	Drainage of Pons with Drainage Device, Percutaneous Endoscopic Approach
009B4ZX	Drainage of Pons, Percutaneous Endoscopic Approach, Diagnostic
009B4ZZ	Drainage of Pons, Percutaneous Endoscopic Approach
009C00Z	Drainage of Cerebellum with Drainage Device, Open Approach
009C0ZX	Drainage of Cerebellum, Open Approach, Diagnostic
009C0ZZ	Drainage of Cerebellum, Open Approach
009C30Z	Drainage of Cerebellum with Drainage Device, Percutaneous Approach
009C3ZX	Drainage of Cerebellum, Percutaneous Approach, Diagnostic
009C3ZZ	Drainage of Cerebellum, Percutaneous Approach
009C40Z	Drainage of Cerebellum with Drainage Device, Percutaneous Endoscopic Approach
009C4ZX	Drainage of Cerebellum, Percutaneous Endoscopic Approach, Diagnostic
009C4ZZ	Drainage of Cerebellum, Percutaneous Endoscopic Approach
009D00Z	Drainage of Medulla Oblongata with Drainage Device, Open Approach
009D0ZX	Drainage of Medulla Oblongata, Open Approach, Diagnostic
009D0ZZ	Drainage of Medulla Oblongata, Open Approach
009D30Z	Drainage of Medulla Oblongata with Drainage Device, Percutaneous Approach
009D3ZX	Drainage of Medulla Oblongata, Percutaneous Approach, Diagnostic
009D3ZZ	Drainage of Medulla Oblongata, Percutaneous Approach
009D40Z	Drainage of Medulla Oblongata with Drainage Device, Percutaneous Endoscopic Approach
009D4ZX	Drainage of Medulla Oblongata, Percutaneous Endoscopic Approach, Diagnostic
009D4ZZ	Drainage of Medulla Oblongata, Percutaneous Endoscopic Approach
009F00Z	Drainage of Olfactory Nerve with Drainage Device, Open Approach
009F0ZX	Drainage of Olfactory Nerve, Open Approach, Diagnostic
009F0ZZ	Drainage of Olfactory Nerve, Open Approach
009F30Z	Drainage of Olfactory Nerve with Drainage Device, Percutaneous Approach
009F3ZX	Drainage of Olfactory Nerve, Percutaneous Approach, Diagnostic
009F3ZZ	Drainage of Olfactory Nerve, Percutaneous Approach
009F40Z	Drainage of Olfactory Nerve with Drainage Device, Percutaneous Endoscopic Approach
009F4ZX	Drainage of Olfactory Nerve, Percutaneous Endoscopic Approach, Diagnostic
009F4ZZ	Drainage of Olfactory Nerve, Percutaneous Endoscopic Approach
009G00Z	Drainage of Optic Nerve with Drainage Device, Open Approach
009G0ZX	Drainage of Optic Nerve, Open Approach, Diagnostic
009G0ZZ	Drainage of Optic Nerve, Open Approach
009G30Z	Drainage of Optic Nerve with Drainage Device, Percutaneous Approach
009G3ZX	Drainage of Optic Nerve, Percutaneous Approach, Diagnostic
009G3ZZ	Drainage of Optic Nerve, Percutaneous Approach
009G40Z	Drainage of Optic Nerve with Drainage Device, Percutaneous Endoscopic Approach
009G4ZX	Drainage of Optic Nerve, Percutaneous Endoscopic Approach, Diagnostic
009G4ZZ	Drainage of Optic Nerve, Percutaneous Endoscopic Approach
009H00Z	Drainage of Oculomotor Nerve with Drainage Device, Open Approach
009H0ZX	Drainage of Oculomotor Nerve, Open Approach, Diagnostic
009H0ZZ	Drainage of Oculomotor Nerve, Open Approach
009H30Z	Drainage of Oculomotor Nerve with Drainage Device, Percutaneous Approach
009H3ZX	Drainage of Oculomotor Nerve, Percutaneous Approach, Diagnostic
009H3ZZ	Drainage of Oculomotor Nerve, Percutaneous Approach
009H40Z	Drainage of Oculomotor Nerve with Drainage Device, Percutaneous Endoscopic Approach
009H4ZX	Drainage of Oculomotor Nerve, Percutaneous Endoscopic Approach, Diagnostic
009H4ZZ	Drainage of Oculomotor Nerve, Percutaneous Endoscopic Approach
009J00Z	Drainage of Trochlear Nerve with Drainage Device, Open Approach
009J0ZX	Drainage of Trochlear Nerve, Open Approach, Diagnostic
009J0ZZ	Drainage of Trochlear Nerve, Open Approach
009J30Z	Drainage of Trochlear Nerve with Drainage Device, Percutaneous Approach
009J3ZX	Drainage of Trochlear Nerve, Percutaneous Approach, Diagnostic
009J3ZZ	Drainage of Trochlear Nerve, Percutaneous Approach
009J40Z	Drainage of Trochlear Nerve with Drainage Device, Percutaneous Endoscopic Approach
009J4ZX	Drainage of Trochlear Nerve, Percutaneous Endoscopic Approach, Diagnostic
009J4ZZ	Drainage of Trochlear Nerve, Percutaneous Endoscopic Approach
009K00Z	Drainage of Trigeminal Nerve with Drainage Device, Open Approach
009K0ZX	Drainage of Trigeminal Nerve, Open Approach, Diagnostic
009K0ZZ	Drainage of Trigeminal Nerve, Open Approach
009K30Z	Drainage of Trigeminal Nerve with Drainage Device, Percutaneous Approach
009K3ZX	Drainage of Trigeminal Nerve, Percutaneous Approach, Diagnostic
009K3ZZ	Drainage of Trigeminal Nerve, Percutaneous Approach
009K40Z	Drainage of Trigeminal Nerve with Drainage Device, Percutaneous Endoscopic Approach
009K4ZX	Drainage of Trigeminal Nerve, Percutaneous Endoscopic Approach, Diagnostic
009K4ZZ	Drainage of Trigeminal Nerve, Percutaneous Endoscopic Approach
009L00Z	Drainage of Abducens Nerve with Drainage Device, Open Approach
009L0ZX	Drainage of Abducens Nerve, Open Approach, Diagnostic
009L0ZZ	Drainage of Abducens Nerve, Open Approach
009L30Z	Drainage of Abducens Nerve with Drainage Device, Percutaneous Approach
009L3ZX	Drainage of Abducens Nerve, Percutaneous Approach, Diagnostic

♀ Female-only ♂ Male-only ● Limited Coverage ● Non-OR 🅷🅰🅲 HAC-associated procedure ⬣ Non-covered procedures ➕ Combination

009L3ZZ   Drainage of Abducens Nerve, Percutaneous Approach

009L40Z   Drainage of Abducens Nerve with Drainage Device, Percutaneous Endoscopic Approach

009L4ZX   Drainage of Abducens Nerve, Percutaneous Endoscopic Approach, Diagnostic

009L4ZZ   Drainage of Abducens Nerve, Percutaneous Endoscopic Approach

009M00Z   Drainage of Facial Nerve with Drainage Device, Open Approach

009M0ZX   Drainage of Facial Nerve, Open Approach, Diagnostic

009M0ZZ   Drainage of Facial Nerve, Open Approach

009M30Z   Drainage of Facial Nerve with Drainage Device, Percutaneous Approach

009M3ZX   Drainage of Facial Nerve, Percutaneous Approach, Diagnostic

009M3ZZ   Drainage of Facial Nerve, Percutaneous Approach

009M40Z   Drainage of Facial Nerve with Drainage Device, Percutaneous Endoscopic Approach

009M4ZX   Drainage of Facial Nerve, Percutaneous Endoscopic Approach, Diagnostic

009M4ZZ   Drainage of Facial Nerve, Percutaneous Endoscopic Approach

009N00Z   Drainage of Acoustic Nerve with Drainage Device, Open Approach

009N0ZX   Drainage of Acoustic Nerve, Open Approach, Diagnostic

009N0ZZ   Drainage of Acoustic Nerve, Open Approach

009N30Z   Drainage of Acoustic Nerve with Drainage Device, Percutaneous Approach

009N3ZX   Drainage of Acoustic Nerve, Percutaneous Approach, Diagnostic

009N3ZZ   Drainage of Acoustic Nerve, Percutaneous Approach

009N40Z   Drainage of Acoustic Nerve with Drainage Device, Percutaneous Endoscopic Approach

009N4ZX   Drainage of Acoustic Nerve, Percutaneous Endoscopic Approach, Diagnostic

009N4ZZ   Drainage of Acoustic Nerve, Percutaneous Endoscopic Approach

009P00Z   Drainage of Glossopharyngeal Nerve with Drainage Device, Open Approach

009P0ZX   Drainage of Glossopharyngeal Nerve, Open Approach, Diagnostic

009P0ZZ   Drainage of Glossopharyngeal Nerve, Open Approach

009P30Z   Drainage of Glossopharyngeal Nerve with Drainage Device, Percutaneous Approach

009P3ZX   Drainage of Glossopharyngeal Nerve, Percutaneous Approach, Diagnostic

009P3ZZ   Drainage of Glossopharyngeal Nerve, Percutaneous Approach

009P40Z   Drainage of Glossopharyngeal Nerve with Drainage Device, Percutaneous Endoscopic Approach

009P4ZX   Drainage of Glossopharyngeal Nerve, Percutaneous Endoscopic Approach, Diagnostic

009P4ZZ   Drainage of Glossopharyngeal Nerve, Percutaneous Endoscopic Approach

009Q00Z   Drainage of Vagus Nerve with Drainage Device, Open Approach

009Q0ZX   Drainage of Vagus Nerve, Open Approach, Diagnostic

009Q0ZZ   Drainage of Vagus Nerve, Open Approach

009Q30Z   Drainage of Vagus Nerve with Drainage Device, Percutaneous Approach

009Q3ZX   Drainage of Vagus Nerve, Percutaneous Approach, Diagnostic

009Q3ZZ   Drainage of Vagus Nerve, Percutaneous Approach

009Q40Z   Drainage of Vagus Nerve with Drainage Device, Percutaneous Endoscopic Approach

009Q4ZX   Drainage of Vagus Nerve, Percutaneous Endoscopic Approach, Diagnostic

009Q4ZZ   Drainage of Vagus Nerve, Percutaneous Endoscopic Approach

009R00Z   Drainage of Accessory Nerve with Drainage Device, Open Approach

009R0ZX   Drainage of Accessory Nerve, Open Approach, Diagnostic

009R0ZZ   Drainage of Accessory Nerve, Open Approach

009R30Z   Drainage of Accessory Nerve with Drainage Device, Percutaneous Approach

009R3ZX   Drainage of Accessory Nerve, Percutaneous Approach, Diagnostic

009R3ZZ   Drainage of Accessory Nerve, Percutaneous Approach

009R40Z   Drainage of Accessory Nerve with Drainage Device, Percutaneous Endoscopic Approach

009R4ZX   Drainage of Accessory Nerve, Percutaneous Endoscopic Approach, Diagnostic

009R4ZZ   Drainage of Accessory Nerve, Percutaneous Endoscopic Approach

009S00Z   Drainage of Hypoglossal Nerve with Drainage Device, Open Approach

009S0ZX   Drainage of Hypoglossal Nerve, Open Approach, Diagnostic

009S0ZZ   Drainage of Hypoglossal Nerve, Open Approach

009S30Z   Drainage of Hypoglossal Nerve with Drainage Device, Percutaneous Approach

009S3ZX   Drainage of Hypoglossal Nerve, Percutaneous Approach, Diagnostic

009S3ZZ   Drainage of Hypoglossal Nerve, Percutaneous Approach

009S40Z   Drainage of Hypoglossal Nerve with Drainage Device, Percutaneous Endoscopic Approach

009S4ZX   Drainage of Hypoglossal Nerve, Percutaneous Endoscopic Approach, Diagnostic

009S4ZZ   Drainage of Hypoglossal Nerve, Percutaneous Endoscopic Approach

009T00Z   Drainage of Spinal Meninges with Drainage Device, Open Approach

009T0ZX   Drainage of Spinal Meninges, Open Approach, Diagnostic

009T0ZZ   Drainage of Spinal Meninges, Open Approach

009T30Z   Drainage of Spinal Meninges with Drainage Device, Percutaneous Approach

009T3ZX   Drainage of Spinal Meninges, Percutaneous Approach, Diagnostic

009T3ZZ   Drainage of Spinal Meninges, Percutaneous Approach

009T40Z   Drainage of Spinal Meninges with Drainage Device, Percutaneous Endoscopic Approach

009T4ZX   Drainage of Spinal Meninges, Percutaneous Endoscopic Approach, Diagnostic

009T4ZZ   Drainage of Spinal Meninges, Percutaneous Endoscopic Approach

009U00Z   Drainage of Spinal Canal with Drainage Device, Open Approach

009U0ZX   Drainage of Spinal Canal, Open Approach, Diagnostic

009U0ZZ   Drainage of Spinal Canal, Open Approach

009U30Z   Drainage of Spinal Canal with Drainage Device, Percutaneous Approach

009U3ZX   Drainage of Spinal Canal, Percutaneous Approach, Diagnostic

009U3ZZ   Drainage of Spinal Canal, Percutaneous Approach

009U40Z   Drainage of Spinal Canal with Drainage Device, Percutaneous Endoscopic Approach

009U4ZX   Drainage of Spinal Canal, Percutaneous Endoscopic Approach, Diagnostic

009U4ZZ   Drainage of Spinal Canal, Percutaneous Endoscopic Approach

009W00Z   Drainage of Cervical Spinal Cord with Drainage Device, Open Approach

009W0ZX   Drainage of Cervical Spinal Cord, Open Approach, Diagnostic

009W0ZZ   Drainage of Cervical Spinal Cord, Open Approach

009W30Z   Drainage of Cervical Spinal Cord with Drainage Device, Percutaneous Approach

009W3ZX   Drainage of Cervical Spinal Cord, Percutaneous Approach, Diagnostic

009W3ZZ   Drainage of Cervical Spinal Cord, Percutaneous Approach

009W40Z   Drainage of Cervical Spinal Cord with Drainage Device, Percutaneous Endoscopic Approach

009W4ZX   Drainage of Cervical Spinal Cord, Percutaneous Endoscopic Approach, Diagnostic

009W4ZZ   Drainage of Cervical Spinal Cord, Percutaneous Endoscopic Approach

009X00Z   Drainage of Thoracic Spinal Cord with Drainage Device, Open Approach

009X0ZX   Drainage of Thoracic Spinal Cord, Open Approach, Diagnostic

009X0ZZ   Drainage of Thoracic Spinal Cord, Open Approach

009X30Z   Drainage of Thoracic Spinal Cord with Drainage Device, Percutaneous Approach

009X3ZX   Drainage of Thoracic Spinal Cord, Percutaneous Approach, Diagnostic

009X3ZZ   Drainage of Thoracic Spinal Cord, Percutaneous Approach

009X40Z   Drainage of Thoracic Spinal Cord with Drainage Device, Percutaneous Endoscopic Approach

009X4ZX   Drainage of Thoracic Spinal Cord, Percutaneous Endoscopic Approach, Diagnostic

009X4ZZ   Drainage of Thoracic Spinal Cord, Percutaneous Endoscopic Approach

009Y00Z   Drainage of Lumbar Spinal Cord with Drainage Device, Open Approach

009Y0ZX   Drainage of Lumbar Spinal Cord, Open Approach, Diagnostic

009Y0ZZ   Drainage of Lumbar Spinal Cord, Open Approach

009Y30Z   Drainage of Lumbar Spinal Cord with Drainage Device, Percutaneous Approach

009Y3ZX   Drainage of Lumbar Spinal Cord, Percutaneous Approach, Diagnostic

♀ Female-only   ♂ Male-only   ⬤ Limited Coverage   ● Non-OR   ᴴᴬᶜ HAC-associated procedure   ⬢ Non-covered procedures   ✚ Combination

009Y3ZZ	Drainage of Lumbar Spinal Cord, Percutaneous Approach
009Y40Z	Drainage of Lumbar Spinal Cord with Drainage Device, Percutaneous Endoscopic Approach

009Y4ZX	Drainage of Lumbar Spinal Cord, Percutaneous Endoscopic Approach, Diagnostic
009Y4ZZ	Drainage of Lumbar Spinal Cord, Percutaneous Endoscopic Approach

00B – Central Nervous System, Excision

Review Coding Guidelines B3.4a and B3.4b

Review Coding Guideline B3.8

00B00ZX	Excision of Brain, Open Approach, Diagnostic
00B00ZZ	Excision of Brain, Open Approach
00B03ZX	Excision of Brain, Percutaneous Approach, Diagnostic
00B03ZZ	Excision of Brain, Percutaneous Approach
00B04ZX	Excision of Brain, Percutaneous Endoscopic Approach, Diagnostic
00B04ZZ	Excision of Brain, Percutaneous Endoscopic Approach
00B10ZX	Excision of Cerebral Meninges, Open Approach, Diagnostic
00B10ZZ	Excision of Cerebral Meninges, Open Approach
00B13ZX	Excision of Cerebral Meninges, Percutaneous Approach, Diagnostic
00B13ZZ	Excision of Cerebral Meninges, Percutaneous Approach
00B14ZX	Excision of Cerebral Meninges, Percutaneous Endoscopic Approach, Diagnostic
00B14ZZ	Excision of Cerebral Meninges, Percutaneous Endoscopic Approach
00B20ZX	Excision of Dura Mater, Open Approach, Diagnostic
00B20ZZ	Excision of Dura Mater, Open Approach
00B23ZX	Excision of Dura Mater, Percutaneous Approach, Diagnostic
00B23ZZ	Excision of Dura Mater, Percutaneous Approach
00B24ZX	Excision of Dura Mater, Percutaneous Endoscopic Approach, Diagnostic
00B24ZZ	Excision of Dura Mater, Percutaneous Endoscopic Approach
00B60ZX	Excision of Cerebral Ventricle, Open Approach, Diagnostic
00B60ZZ	Excision of Cerebral Ventricle, Open Approach
00B63ZX	Excision of Cerebral Ventricle, Percutaneous Approach, Diagnostic
00B63ZZ	Excision of Cerebral Ventricle, Percutaneous Approach
00B64ZX	Excision of Cerebral Ventricle, Percutaneous Endoscopic Approach, Diagnostic
00B64ZZ	Excision of Cerebral Ventricle, Percutaneous Endoscopic Approach
00B70ZX	Excision of Cerebral Hemisphere, Open Approach, Diagnostic
00B70ZZ	Excision of Cerebral Hemisphere, Open Approach
00B73ZX	Excision of Cerebral Hemisphere, Percutaneous Approach, Diagnostic
00B73ZZ	Excision of Cerebral Hemisphere, Percutaneous Approach
00B74ZX	Excision of Cerebral Hemisphere, Percutaneous Endoscopic Approach, Diagnostic
00B74ZZ	Excision of Cerebral Hemisphere, Percutaneous Endoscopic Approach
00B80ZX	Excision of Basal Ganglia, Open Approach, Diagnostic
00B80ZZ	Excision of Basal Ganglia, Open Approach
00B83ZX	Excision of Basal Ganglia, Percutaneous Approach, Diagnostic
00B83ZZ	Excision of Basal Ganglia, Percutaneous Approach
00B84ZX	Excision of Basal Ganglia, Percutaneous Endoscopic Approach, Diagnostic
00B84ZZ	Excision of Basal Ganglia, Percutaneous Endoscopic Approach
00B90ZX	Excision of Thalamus, Open Approach, Diagnostic
00B90ZZ	Excision of Thalamus, Open Approach
00B93ZX	Excision of Thalamus, Percutaneous Approach, Diagnostic
00B93ZZ	Excision of Thalamus, Percutaneous Approach
00B94ZX	Excision of Thalamus, Percutaneous Endoscopic Approach, Diagnostic
00B94ZZ	Excision of Thalamus, Percutaneous Endoscopic Approach
00BA0ZX	Excision of Hypothalamus, Open Approach, Diagnostic
00BA0ZZ	Excision of Hypothalamus, Open Approach
00BA3ZX	Excision of Hypothalamus, Percutaneous Approach, Diagnostic
00BA3ZZ	Excision of Hypothalamus, Percutaneous Approach
00BA4ZX	Excision of Hypothalamus, Percutaneous Endoscopic Approach, Diagnostic
00BA4ZZ	Excision of Hypothalamus, Percutaneous Endoscopic Approach
00BB0ZX	Excision of Pons, Open Approach, Diagnostic
00BB0ZZ	Excision of Pons, Open Approach
00BB3ZX	Excision of Pons, Percutaneous Approach, Diagnostic
00BB3ZZ	Excision of Pons, Percutaneous Approach
00BB4ZX	Excision of Pons, Percutaneous Endoscopic Approach, Diagnostic
00BB4ZZ	Excision of Pons, Percutaneous Endoscopic Approach

00BC0ZX	Excision of Cerebellum, Open Approach, Diagnostic
00BC0ZZ	Excision of Cerebellum, Open Approach
00BC3ZX	Excision of Cerebellum, Percutaneous Approach, Diagnostic
00BC3ZZ	Excision of Cerebellum, Percutaneous Approach
00BC4ZX	Excision of Cerebellum, Percutaneous Endoscopic Approach, Diagnostic
00BC4ZZ	Excision of Cerebellum, Percutaneous Endoscopic Approach
00BD0ZX	Excision of Medulla Oblongata, Open Approach, Diagnostic
00BD0ZZ	Excision of Medulla Oblongata, Open Approach
00BD3ZX	Excision of Medulla Oblongata, Percutaneous Approach, Diagnostic
00BD3ZZ	Excision of Medulla Oblongata, Percutaneous Approach
00BD4ZX	Excision of Medulla Oblongata, Percutaneous Endoscopic Approach, Diagnostic
00BD4ZZ	Excision of Medulla Oblongata, Percutaneous Endoscopic Approach
00BF0ZX	Excision of Olfactory Nerve, Open Approach, Diagnostic
00BF0ZZ	Excision of Olfactory Nerve, Open Approach
00BF3ZX	Excision of Olfactory Nerve, Percutaneous Approach, Diagnostic
00BF3ZZ	Excision of Olfactory Nerve, Percutaneous Approach
00BF4ZX	Excision of Olfactory Nerve, Percutaneous Endoscopic Approach, Diagnostic
00BF4ZZ	Excision of Olfactory Nerve, Percutaneous Endoscopic Approach
00BG0ZX	Excision of Optic Nerve, Open Approach, Diagnostic
00BG0ZZ	Excision of Optic Nerve, Open Approach
00BG3ZX	Excision of Optic Nerve, Percutaneous Approach, Diagnostic
00BG3ZZ	Excision of Optic Nerve, Percutaneous Approach
00BG4ZX	Excision of Optic Nerve, Percutaneous Endoscopic Approach, Diagnostic
00BG4ZZ	Excision of Optic Nerve, Percutaneous Endoscopic Approach
00BH0ZX	Excision of Oculomotor Nerve, Open Approach, Diagnostic
00BH0ZZ	Excision of Oculomotor Nerve, Open Approach
00BH3ZX	Excision of Oculomotor Nerve, Percutaneous Approach, Diagnostic
00BH3ZZ	Excision of Oculomotor Nerve, Percutaneous Approach
00BH4ZX	Excision of Oculomotor Nerve, Percutaneous Endoscopic Approach, Diagnostic
00BH4ZZ	Excision of Oculomotor Nerve, Percutaneous Endoscopic Approach
00BJ0ZX	Excision of Trochlear Nerve, Open Approach, Diagnostic
00BJ0ZZ	Excision of Trochlear Nerve, Open Approach
00BJ3ZX	Excision of Trochlear Nerve, Percutaneous Approach, Diagnostic
00BJ3ZZ	Excision of Trochlear Nerve, Percutaneous Approach
00BJ4ZX	Excision of Trochlear Nerve, Percutaneous Endoscopic Approach, Diagnostic
00BJ4ZZ	Excision of Trochlear Nerve, Percutaneous Endoscopic Approach
00BK0ZX	Excision of Trigeminal Nerve, Open Approach, Diagnostic
00BK0ZZ	Excision of Trigeminal Nerve, Open Approach
00BK3ZX	Excision of Trigeminal Nerve, Percutaneous Approach, Diagnostic
00BK3ZZ	Excision of Trigeminal Nerve, Percutaneous Approach
00BK4ZX	Excision of Trigeminal Nerve, Percutaneous Endoscopic Approach, Diagnostic
00BK4ZZ	Excision of Trigeminal Nerve, Percutaneous Endoscopic Approach
00BL0ZX	Excision of Abducens Nerve, Open Approach, Diagnostic
00BL0ZZ	Excision of Abducens Nerve, Open Approach
00BL3ZX	Excision of Abducens Nerve, Percutaneous Approach, Diagnostic
00BL3ZZ	Excision of Abducens Nerve, Percutaneous Approach
00BL4ZX	Excision of Abducens Nerve, Percutaneous Endoscopic Approach, Diagnostic
00BL4ZZ	Excision of Abducens Nerve, Percutaneous Endoscopic Approach
00BM0ZX	Excision of Facial Nerve, Open Approach, Diagnostic
00BM0ZZ	Excision of Facial Nerve, Open Approach
00BM3ZX	Excision of Facial Nerve, Percutaneous Approach, Diagnostic
00BM3ZZ	Excision of Facial Nerve, Percutaneous Approach
00BM4ZX	Excision of Facial Nerve, Percutaneous Endoscopic Approach, Diagnostic
00BM4ZZ	Excision of Facial Nerve, Percutaneous Endoscopic Approach

00BN0ZX	Excision of Acoustic Nerve, Open Approach, Diagnostic
00BN0ZZ	Excision of Acoustic Nerve, Open Approach
00BN3ZX	Excision of Acoustic Nerve, Percutaneous Approach, Diagnostic
00BN3ZZ	Excision of Acoustic Nerve, Percutaneous Approach
00BN4ZX	Excision of Acoustic Nerve, Percutaneous Endoscopic Approach, Diagnostic
00BN4ZZ	Excision of Acoustic Nerve, Percutaneous Endoscopic Approach
00BP0ZX	Excision of Glossopharyngeal Nerve, Open Approach, Diagnostic
00BP0ZZ	Excision of Glossopharyngeal Nerve, Open Approach
00BP3ZX	Excision of Glossopharyngeal Nerve, Percutaneous Approach, Diagnostic
00BP3ZZ	Excision of Glossopharyngeal Nerve, Percutaneous Approach
00BP4ZX	Excision of Glossopharyngeal Nerve, Percutaneous Endoscopic Approach, Diagnostic
00BP4ZZ	Excision of Glossopharyngeal Nerve, Percutaneous Endoscopic Approach
00BQ0ZX	Excision of Vagus Nerve, Open Approach, Diagnostic
00BQ0ZZ	Excision of Vagus Nerve, Open Approach
00BQ3ZX	Excision of Vagus Nerve, Percutaneous Approach, Diagnostic
00BQ3ZZ	Excision of Vagus Nerve, Percutaneous Approach
00BQ4ZX	Excision of Vagus Nerve, Percutaneous Endoscopic Approach, Diagnostic
00BQ4ZZ	Excision of Vagus Nerve, Percutaneous Endoscopic Approach
00BR0ZX	Excision of Accessory Nerve, Open Approach, Diagnostic
00BR0ZZ	Excision of Accessory Nerve, Open Approach
00BR3ZX	Excision of Accessory Nerve, Percutaneous Approach, Diagnostic
00BR3ZZ	Excision of Accessory Nerve, Percutaneous Approach
00BR4ZX	Excision of Accessory Nerve, Percutaneous Endoscopic Approach, Diagnostic
00BR4ZZ	Excision of Accessory Nerve, Percutaneous Endoscopic Approach
00BS0ZX	Excision of Hypoglossal Nerve, Open Approach, Diagnostic
00BS0ZZ	Excision of Hypoglossal Nerve, Open Approach
00BS3ZX	Excision of Hypoglossal Nerve, Percutaneous Approach, Diagnostic
00BS3ZZ	Excision of Hypoglossal Nerve, Percutaneous Approach
00BS4ZX	Excision of Hypoglossal Nerve, Percutaneous Endoscopic Approach, Diagnostic
00BS4ZZ	Excision of Hypoglossal Nerve, Percutaneous Endoscopic Approach
00BT0ZX	Excision of Spinal Meninges, Open Approach, Diagnostic
00BT0ZZ	Excision of Spinal Meninges, Open Approach
00BT3ZX	Excision of Spinal Meninges, Percutaneous Approach, Diagnostic
00BT3ZZ	Excision of Spinal Meninges, Percutaneous Approach
00BT4ZX	Excision of Spinal Meninges, Percutaneous Endoscopic Approach, Diagnostic
00BT4ZZ	Excision of Spinal Meninges, Percutaneous Endoscopic Approach
00BW0ZX	Excision of Cervical Spinal Cord, Open Approach, Diagnostic
00BW0ZZ	Excision of Cervical Spinal Cord, Open Approach
00BW3ZX	Excision of Cervical Spinal Cord, Percutaneous Approach, Diagnostic
00BW3ZZ	Excision of Cervical Spinal Cord, Percutaneous Approach
00BW4ZX	Excision of Cervical Spinal Cord, Percutaneous Endoscopic Approach, Diagnostic
00BW4ZZ	Excision of Cervical Spinal Cord, Percutaneous Endoscopic Approach
00BX0ZX	Excision of Thoracic Spinal Cord, Open Approach, Diagnostic
00BX0ZZ	Excision of Thoracic Spinal Cord, Open Approach
00BX3ZX	Excision of Thoracic Spinal Cord, Percutaneous Approach, Diagnostic
00BX3ZZ	Excision of Thoracic Spinal Cord, Percutaneous Approach
00BX4ZX	Excision of Thoracic Spinal Cord, Percutaneous Endoscopic Approach, Diagnostic
00BX4ZZ	Excision of Thoracic Spinal Cord, Percutaneous Endoscopic Approach
00BY0ZX	Excision of Lumbar Spinal Cord, Open Approach, Diagnostic
00BY0ZZ	Excision of Lumbar Spinal Cord, Open Approach
00BY3ZX	Excision of Lumbar Spinal Cord, Percutaneous Approach, Diagnostic
00BY3ZZ	Excision of Lumbar Spinal Cord, Percutaneous Approach
00BY4ZX	Excision of Lumbar Spinal Cord, Percutaneous Endoscopic Approach, Diagnostic
00BY4ZZ	Excision of Lumbar Spinal Cord, Percutaneous Endoscopic Approach

00C – Central Nervous System, Extirpation

00C00ZZ	Extirpation of Matter from Brain, Open Approach
00C03ZZ	Extirpation of Matter from Brain, Percutaneous Approach
00C04ZZ	Extirpation of Matter from Brain, Percutaneous Endoscopic Approach
00C10ZZ	Extirpation of Matter from Cerebral Meninges, Open Approach
00C13ZZ	Extirpation of Matter from Cerebral Meninges, Percutaneous Approach
00C14ZZ	Extirpation of Matter from Cerebral Meninges, Percutaneous Endoscopic Approach
00C20ZZ	Extirpation of Matter from Dura Mater, Open Approach
00C23ZZ	Extirpation of Matter from Dura Mater, Percutaneous Approach
00C24ZZ	Extirpation of Matter from Dura Mater, Percutaneous Endoscopic Approach
00C30ZZ	Extirpation of Matter from Epidural Space, Open Approach
00C33ZZ	Extirpation of Matter from Epidural Space, Percutaneous Approach
00C34ZZ	Extirpation of Matter from Epidural Space, Percutaneous Endoscopic Approach
00C40ZZ	Extirpation of Matter from Subdural Space, Open Approach
00C43ZZ	Extirpation of Matter from Subdural Space, Percutaneous Approach
00C44ZZ	Extirpation of Matter from Subdural Space, Percutaneous Endoscopic Approach
00C50ZZ	Extirpation of Matter from Subarachnoid Space, Open Approach
00C53ZZ	Extirpation of Matter from Subarachnoid Space, Percutaneous Approach
00C54ZZ	Extirpation of Matter from Subarachnoid Space, Percutaneous Endoscopic Approach
00C60ZZ	Extirpation of Matter from Cerebral Ventricle, Open Approach
00C63ZZ	Extirpation of Matter from Cerebral Ventricle, Percutaneous Approach
00C64ZZ	Extirpation of Matter from Cerebral Ventricle, Percutaneous Endoscopic Approach
00C70ZZ	Extirpation of Matter from Cerebral Hemisphere, Open Approach
00C73ZZ	Extirpation of Matter from Cerebral Hemisphere, Percutaneous Approach
00C74ZZ	Extirpation of Matter from Cerebral Hemisphere, Percutaneous Endoscopic Approach
00C80ZZ	Extirpation of Matter from Basal Ganglia, Open Approach
00C83ZZ	Extirpation of Matter from Basal Ganglia, Percutaneous Approach
00C84ZZ	Extirpation of Matter from Basal Ganglia, Percutaneous Endoscopic Approach
00C90ZZ	Extirpation of Matter from Thalamus, Open Approach
00C93ZZ	Extirpation of Matter from Thalamus, Percutaneous Approach
00C94ZZ	Extirpation of Matter from Thalamus, Percutaneous Endoscopic Approach
00CA0ZZ	Extirpation of Matter from Hypothalamus, Open Approach
00CA3ZZ	Extirpation of Matter from Hypothalamus, Percutaneous Approach
00CA4ZZ	Extirpation of Matter from Hypothalamus, Percutaneous Endoscopic Approach
00CB0ZZ	Extirpation of Matter from Pons, Open Approach
00CB3ZZ	Extirpation of Matter from Pons, Percutaneous Approach
00CB4ZZ	Extirpation of Matter from Pons, Percutaneous Endoscopic Approach
00CC0ZZ	Extirpation of Matter from Cerebellum, Open Approach
00CC3ZZ	Extirpation of Matter from Cerebellum, Percutaneous Approach
00CC4ZZ	Extirpation of Matter from Cerebellum, Percutaneous Endoscopic Approach
00CD0ZZ	Extirpation of Matter from Medulla Oblongata, Open Approach
00CD3ZZ	Extirpation of Matter from Medulla Oblongata, Percutaneous Approach
00CD4ZZ	Extirpation of Matter from Medulla Oblongata, Percutaneous Endoscopic Approach
00CF0ZZ	Extirpation of Matter from Olfactory Nerve, Open Approach
00CF3ZZ	Extirpation of Matter from Olfactory Nerve, Percutaneous Approach
00CF4ZZ	Extirpation of Matter from Olfactory Nerve, Percutaneous Endoscopic Approach
00CG0ZZ	Extirpation of Matter from Optic Nerve, Open Approach
00CG3ZZ	Extirpation of Matter from Optic Nerve, Percutaneous Approach

♀ Female-only   ♂ Male-only   ● Limited Coverage   ● Non-OR   ᴴᴬᶜ HAC-associated procedure   ● Non-covered procedures   ✚ Combination

00CG4ZZ	Extirpation of Matter from Optic Nerve, Percutaneous Endoscopic Approach
00CH0ZZ	Extirpation of Matter from Oculomotor Nerve, Open Approach
00CH3ZZ	Extirpation of Matter from Oculomotor Nerve, Percutaneous Approach
00CH4ZZ	Extirpation of Matter from Oculomotor Nerve, Percutaneous Endoscopic Approach
00CJ0ZZ	Extirpation of Matter from Trochlear Nerve, Open Approach
00CJ3ZZ	Extirpation of Matter from Trochlear Nerve, Percutaneous Approach
00CJ4ZZ	Extirpation of Matter from Trochlear Nerve, Percutaneous Endoscopic Approach
00CK0ZZ	Extirpation of Matter from Trigeminal Nerve, Open Approach
00CK3ZZ	Extirpation of Matter from Trigeminal Nerve, Percutaneous Approach
00CK4ZZ	Extirpation of Matter from Trigeminal Nerve, Percutaneous Endoscopic Approach
00CL0ZZ	Extirpation of Matter from Abducens Nerve, Open Approach
00CL3ZZ	Extirpation of Matter from Abducens Nerve, Percutaneous Approach
00CL4ZZ	Extirpation of Matter from Abducens Nerve, Percutaneous Endoscopic Approach
00CM0ZZ	Extirpation of Matter from Facial Nerve, Open Approach
00CM3ZZ	Extirpation of Matter from Facial Nerve, Percutaneous Approach
00CM4ZZ	Extirpation of Matter from Facial Nerve, Percutaneous Endoscopic Approach
00CN0ZZ	Extirpation of Matter from Acoustic Nerve, Open Approach
00CN3ZZ	Extirpation of Matter from Acoustic Nerve, Percutaneous Approach
00CN4ZZ	Extirpation of Matter from Acoustic Nerve, Percutaneous Endoscopic Approach
00CP0ZZ	Extirpation of Matter from Glossopharyngeal Nerve, Open Approach
00CP3ZZ	Extirpation of Matter from Glossopharyngeal Nerve, Percutaneous Approach
00CP4ZZ	Extirpation of Matter from Glossopharyngeal Nerve, Percutaneous Endoscopic Approach
00CQ0ZZ	Extirpation of Matter from Vagus Nerve, Open Approach
00CQ3ZZ	Extirpation of Matter from Vagus Nerve, Percutaneous Approach
00CQ4ZZ	Extirpation of Matter from Vagus Nerve, Percutaneous Endoscopic Approach
00CR0ZZ	Extirpation of Matter from Accessory Nerve, Open Approach
00CR3ZZ	Extirpation of Matter from Accessory Nerve, Percutaneous Approach
00CR4ZZ	Extirpation of Matter from Accessory Nerve, Percutaneous Endoscopic Approach
00CS0ZZ	Extirpation of Matter from Hypoglossal Nerve, Open Approach
00CS3ZZ	Extirpation of Matter from Hypoglossal Nerve, Percutaneous Approach
00CS4ZZ	Extirpation of Matter from Hypoglossal Nerve, Percutaneous Endoscopic Approach
00CT0ZZ	Extirpation of Matter from Spinal Meninges, Open Approach
00CT3ZZ	Extirpation of Matter from Spinal Meninges, Percutaneous Approach
00CT4ZZ	Extirpation of Matter from Spinal Meninges, Percutaneous Endoscopic Approach
00CW0ZZ	Extirpation of Matter from Cervical Spinal Cord, Open Approach
00CW3ZZ	Extirpation of Matter from Cervical Spinal Cord, Percutaneous Approach
00CW4ZZ	Extirpation of Matter from Cervical Spinal Cord, Percutaneous Endoscopic Approach
00CX0ZZ	Extirpation of Matter from Thoracic Spinal Cord, Open Approach
00CX3ZZ	Extirpation of Matter from Thoracic Spinal Cord, Percutaneous Approach
00CX4ZZ	Extirpation of Matter from Thoracic Spinal Cord, Percutaneous Endoscopic Approach
00CY0ZZ	Extirpation of Matter from Lumbar Spinal Cord, Open Approach
00CY3ZZ	Extirpation of Matter from Lumbar Spinal Cord, Percutaneous Approach
00CY4ZZ	Extirpation of Matter from Lumbar Spinal Cord, Percutaneous Endoscopic Approach

00D – Central Nervous System, Extraction

00D10ZZ	Extraction of Cerebral Meninges, Open Approach
00D13ZZ	Extraction of Cerebral Meninges, Percutaneous Approach
00D14ZZ	Extraction of Cerebral Meninges, Percutaneous Endoscopic Approach
00D20ZZ	Extraction of Dura Mater, Open Approach
00D23ZZ	Extraction of Dura Mater, Percutaneous Approach
00D24ZZ	Extraction of Dura Mater, Percutaneous Endoscopic Approach
00DF0ZZ	Extraction of Olfactory Nerve, Open Approach
00DF3ZZ	Extraction of Olfactory Nerve, Percutaneous Approach
00DF4ZZ	Extraction of Olfactory Nerve, Percutaneous Endoscopic Approach
00DG0ZZ	Extraction of Optic Nerve, Open Approach
00DG3ZZ	Extraction of Optic Nerve, Percutaneous Approach
00DG4ZZ	Extraction of Optic Nerve, Percutaneous Endoscopic Approach
00DH0ZZ	Extraction of Oculomotor Nerve, Open Approach
00DH3ZZ	Extraction of Oculomotor Nerve, Percutaneous Approach
00DH4ZZ	Extraction of Oculomotor Nerve, Percutaneous Endoscopic Approach
00DJ0ZZ	Extraction of Trochlear Nerve, Open Approach
00DJ3ZZ	Extraction of Trochlear Nerve, Percutaneous Approach
00DJ4ZZ	Extraction of Trochlear Nerve, Percutaneous Endoscopic Approach
00DK0ZZ	Extraction of Trigeminal Nerve, Open Approach
00DK3ZZ	Extraction of Trigeminal Nerve, Percutaneous Approach
00DK4ZZ	Extraction of Trigeminal Nerve, Percutaneous Endoscopic Approach
00DL0ZZ	Extraction of Abducens Nerve, Open Approach
00DL3ZZ	Extraction of Abducens Nerve, Percutaneous Approach
00DL4ZZ	Extraction of Abducens Nerve, Percutaneous Endoscopic Approach
00DM0ZZ	Extraction of Facial Nerve, Open Approach
00DM3ZZ	Extraction of Facial Nerve, Percutaneous Approach
00DM4ZZ	Extraction of Facial Nerve, Percutaneous Endoscopic Approach
00DN0ZZ	Extraction of Acoustic Nerve, Open Approach
00DN3ZZ	Extraction of Acoustic Nerve, Percutaneous Approach
00DN4ZZ	Extraction of Acoustic Nerve, Percutaneous Endoscopic Approach
00DP0ZZ	Extraction of Glossopharyngeal Nerve, Open Approach
00DP3ZZ	Extraction of Glossopharyngeal Nerve, Percutaneous Approach
00DP4ZZ	Extraction of Glossopharyngeal Nerve, Percutaneous Endoscopic Approach
00DQ0ZZ	Extraction of Vagus Nerve, Open Approach
00DQ3ZZ	Extraction of Vagus Nerve, Percutaneous Approach
00DQ4ZZ	Extraction of Vagus Nerve, Percutaneous Endoscopic Approach
00DR0ZZ	Extraction of Accessory Nerve, Open Approach
00DR3ZZ	Extraction of Accessory Nerve, Percutaneous Approach
00DR4ZZ	Extraction of Accessory Nerve, Percutaneous Endoscopic Approach
00DS0ZZ	Extraction of Hypoglossal Nerve, Open Approach
00DS3ZZ	Extraction of Hypoglossal Nerve, Percutaneous Approach
00DS4ZZ	Extraction of Hypoglossal Nerve, Percutaneous Endoscopic Approach
00DT0ZZ	Extraction of Spinal Meninges, Open Approach
00DT3ZZ	Extraction of Spinal Meninges, Percutaneous Approach
00DT4ZZ	Extraction of Spinal Meninges, Percutaneous Endoscopic Approach

00F – Central Nervous System, Fragmentation

00F30ZZ	Fragmentation in Epidural Space, Open Approach
00F33ZZ	Fragmentation in Epidural Space, Percutaneous Approach
00F34ZZ	Fragmentation in Epidural Space, Percutaneous Endoscopic Approach
● 00F3XZZ	Fragmentation in Epidural Space, External Approach
00F40ZZ	Fragmentation in Subdural Space, Open Approach
00F43ZZ	Fragmentation in Subdural Space, Percutaneous Approach
00F44ZZ	Fragmentation in Subdural Space, Percutaneous Endoscopic Approach
● 00F4XZZ	Fragmentation in Subdural Space, External Approach
00F50ZZ	Fragmentation in Subarachnoid Space, Open Approach
00F53ZZ	Fragmentation in Subarachnoid Space, Percutaneous Approach
00F54ZZ	Fragmentation in Subarachnoid Space, Percutaneous Endoscopic Approach

◆ 00F5XZZ   Fragmentation in Subarachnoid Space, External Approach
00F60ZZ   Fragmentation in Cerebral Ventricle, Open Approach
00F63ZZ   Fragmentation in Cerebral Ventricle, Percutaneous Approach
00F64ZZ   Fragmentation in Cerebral Ventricle, Percutaneous Endoscopic Approach

◆ 00F6XZZ   Fragmentation in Cerebral Ventricle, External Approach
00FU0ZZ   Fragmentation in Spinal Canal, Open Approach
00FU3ZZ   Fragmentation in Spinal Canal, Percutaneous Approach
00FU4ZZ   Fragmentation in Spinal Canal, Percutaneous Endoscopic Approach
00FUXZZ   Fragmentation in Spinal Canal, External Approach

Review Coding Guideline B4.6

00H – Central Nervous System, Insertion

00H002Z   Insertion of Monitoring Device into Brain, Open Approach
00H003Z   Insertion of Infusion Device into Brain, Open Approach
00H00MZ   Insertion of Neurostimulator Lead into Brain, Open Approach
00H032Z   Insertion of Monitoring Device into Brain, Percutaneous Approach
00H033Z   Insertion of Infusion Device into Brain, Percutaneous Approach
00H03MZ   Insertion of Neurostimulator Lead into Brain, Percutaneous Approach
00H042Z   Insertion of Monitoring Device into Brain, Percutaneous Endoscopic Approach
00H043Z   Insertion of Infusion Device into Brain, Percutaneous Endoscopic Approach
00H04MZ   Insertion of Neurostimulator Lead into Brain, Percutaneous Endoscopic Approach
00H602Z   Insertion of Monitoring Device into Cerebral Ventricle, Open Approach
00H603Z   Insertion of Infusion Device into Cerebral Ventricle, Open Approach
00H60MZ   Insertion of Neurostimulator Lead into Cerebral Ventricle, Open Approach
00H632Z   Insertion of Monitoring Device into Cerebral Ventricle, Percutaneous Approach
00H633Z   Insertion of Infusion Device into Cerebral Ventricle, Percutaneous Approach
00H63MZ   Insertion of Neurostimulator Lead into Cerebral Ventricle, Percutaneous Approach
00H642Z   Insertion of Monitoring Device into Cerebral Ventricle, Percutaneous Endoscopic Approach
00H643Z   Insertion of Infusion Device into Cerebral Ventricle, Percutaneous Endoscopic Approach
00H64MZ   Insertion of Neurostimulator Lead into Cerebral Ventricle, Percutaneous Endoscopic Approach
00HE02Z   Insertion of Monitoring Device into Cranial Nerve, Open Approach
00HE03Z   Insertion of Infusion Device into Cranial Nerve, Open Approach
00HE0MZ   Insertion of Neurostimulator Lead into Cranial Nerve, Open Approach
00HE32Z   Insertion of Monitoring Device into Cranial Nerve, Percutaneous Approach
00HE33Z   Insertion of Infusion Device into Cranial Nerve, Percutaneous Approach

00HE3MZ   Insertion of Neurostimulator Lead into Cranial Nerve, Percutaneous Approach
00HE42Z   Insertion of Monitoring Device into Cranial Nerve, Percutaneous Endoscopic Approach
00HE43Z   Insertion of Infusion Device into Cranial Nerve, Percutaneous Endoscopic Approach
00HE4MZ   Insertion of Neurostimulator Lead into Cranial Nerve, Percutaneous Endoscopic Approach
00HU02Z   Insertion of Monitoring Device into Spinal Canal, Open Approach
00HU03Z   Insertion of Infusion Device into Spinal Canal, Open Approach
00HU0MZ   Insertion of Neurostimulator Lead into Spinal Canal, Open Approach
00HU32Z   Insertion of Monitoring Device into Spinal Canal, Percutaneous Approach
00HU33Z   Insertion of Infusion Device into Spinal Canal, Percutaneous Approach
00HU3MZ   Insertion of Neurostimulator Lead into Spinal Canal, Percutaneous Approach
00HU42Z   Insertion of Monitoring Device into Spinal Canal, Percutaneous Endoscopic Approach
00HU43Z   Insertion of Infusion Device into Spinal Canal, Percutaneous Endoscopic Approach
00HU4MZ   Insertion of Neurostimulator Lead into Spinal Canal, Percutaneous Endoscopic Approach
00HV02Z   Insertion of Monitoring Device into Spinal Cord, Open Approach
00HV03Z   Insertion of Infusion Device into Spinal Cord, Open Approach
00HV0MZ   Insertion of Neurostimulator Lead into Spinal Cord, Open Approach
00HV32Z   Insertion of Monitoring Device into Spinal Cord, Percutaneous Approach
00HV33Z   Insertion of Infusion Device into Spinal Cord, Percutaneous Approach
00HV3MZ   Insertion of Neurostimulator Lead into Spinal Cord, Percutaneous Approach
00HV42Z   Insertion of Monitoring Device into Spinal Cord, Percutaneous Endoscopic Approach
00HV43Z   Insertion of Infusion Device into Spinal Cord, Percutaneous Endoscopic Approach
00HV4MZ   Insertion of Neurostimulator Lead into Spinal Cord, Percutaneous Endoscopic Approach

00J – Central Nervous System, Inspection

Review Coding Guidelines B3.11a, B3.11b and B3.11c

00J00ZZ   Inspection of Brain, Open Approach
00J03ZZ   Inspection of Brain, Percutaneous Approach
00J04ZZ   Inspection of Brain, Percutaneous Endoscopic Approach
00JE0ZZ   Inspection of Cranial Nerve, Open Approach
00JE3ZZ   Inspection of Cranial Nerve, Percutaneous Approach
00JE4ZZ   Inspection of Cranial Nerve, Percutaneous Endoscopic Approach

00JU0ZZ   Inspection of Spinal Canal, Open Approach
00JU3ZZ   Inspection of Spinal Canal, Percutaneous Approach
00JU4ZZ   Inspection of Spinal Canal, Percutaneous Endoscopic Approach
00JV0ZZ   Inspection of Spinal Cord, Open Approach
00JV3ZZ   Inspection of Spinal Cord, Percutaneous Approach
00JV4ZZ   Inspection of Spinal Cord, Percutaneous Endoscopic Approach

00K – Central Nervous System, Map

00K00ZZ   Map Brain, Open Approach
00K03ZZ   Map Brain, Percutaneous Approach
00K04ZZ   Map Brain, Percutaneous Endoscopic Approach
00K70ZZ   Map Cerebral Hemisphere, Open Approach
00K73ZZ   Map Cerebral Hemisphere, Percutaneous Approach
00K74ZZ   Map Cerebral Hemisphere, Percutaneous Endoscopic Approach
00K80ZZ   Map Basal Ganglia, Open Approach
00K83ZZ   Map Basal Ganglia, Percutaneous Approach
00K84ZZ   Map Basal Ganglia, Percutaneous Endoscopic Approach
00K90ZZ   Map Thalamus, Open Approach

00K93ZZ   Map Thalamus, Percutaneous Approach
00K94ZZ   Map Thalamus, Percutaneous Endoscopic Approach
00KA0ZZ   Map Hypothalamus, Open Approach
00KA3ZZ   Map Hypothalamus, Percutaneous Approach
00KA4ZZ   Map Hypothalamus, Percutaneous Endoscopic Approach
00KB0ZZ   Map Pons, Open Approach
00KB3ZZ   Map Pons, Percutaneous Approach
00KB4ZZ   Map Pons, Percutaneous Endoscopic Approach
00KC0ZZ   Map Cerebellum, Open Approach
00KC3ZZ   Map Cerebellum, Percutaneous Approach

00KC4ZZ   Map Cerebellum, Percutaneous Endoscopic Approach
00KD0ZZ   Map Medulla Oblongata, Open Approach

00KD3ZZ   Map Medulla Oblongata, Percutaneous Approach
00KD4ZZ   Map Medulla Oblongata, Percutaneous Endoscopic Approach

00N – Central Nervous System, Release

Review Coding Guideline B3.13

Review Coding Guideline B3.14

00N00ZZ   Release Brain, Open Approach
00N03ZZ   Release Brain, Percutaneous Approach
00N04ZZ   Release Brain, Percutaneous Endoscopic Approach
00N10ZZ   Release Cerebral Meninges, Open Approach
00N13ZZ   Release Cerebral Meninges, Percutaneous Approach
00N14ZZ   Release Cerebral Meninges, Percutaneous Endoscopic Approach
00N20ZZ   Release Dura Mater, Open Approach
00N23ZZ   Release Dura Mater, Percutaneous Approach
00N24ZZ   Release Dura Mater, Percutaneous Endoscopic Approach
00N60ZZ   Release Cerebral Ventricle, Open Approach
00N63ZZ   Release Cerebral Ventricle, Percutaneous Approach
00N64ZZ   Release Cerebral Ventricle, Percutaneous Endoscopic Approach
00N70ZZ   Release Cerebral Hemisphere, Open Approach
00N73ZZ   Release Cerebral Hemisphere, Percutaneous Approach
00N74ZZ   Release Cerebral Hemisphere, Percutaneous Endoscopic Approach
00N80ZZ   Release Basal Ganglia, Open Approach
00N83ZZ   Release Basal Ganglia, Percutaneous Approach
00N84ZZ   Release Basal Ganglia, Percutaneous Endoscopic Approach
00N90ZZ   Release Thalamus, Open Approach
00N93ZZ   Release Thalamus, Percutaneous Approach
00N94ZZ   Release Thalamus, Percutaneous Endoscopic Approach
00NA0ZZ   Release Hypothalamus, Open Approach
00NA3ZZ   Release Hypothalamus, Percutaneous Approach
00NA4ZZ   Release Hypothalamus, Percutaneous Endoscopic Approach
00NB0ZZ   Release Pons, Open Approach
00NB3ZZ   Release Pons, Percutaneous Approach
00NB4ZZ   Release Pons, Percutaneous Endoscopic Approach
00NC0ZZ   Release Cerebellum, Open Approach
00NC3ZZ   Release Cerebellum, Percutaneous Approach
00NC4ZZ   Release Cerebellum, Percutaneous Endoscopic Approach
00ND0ZZ   Release Medulla Oblongata, Open Approach
00ND3ZZ   Release Medulla Oblongata, Percutaneous Approach
00ND4ZZ   Release Medulla Oblongata, Percutaneous Endoscopic Approach
00NF0ZZ   Release Olfactory Nerve, Open Approach
00NF3ZZ   Release Olfactory Nerve, Percutaneous Approach
00NF4ZZ   Release Olfactory Nerve, Percutaneous Endoscopic Approach
00NG0ZZ   Release Optic Nerve, Open Approach
00NG3ZZ   Release Optic Nerve, Percutaneous Approach
00NG4ZZ   Release Optic Nerve, Percutaneous Endoscopic Approach
00NH0ZZ   Release Oculomotor Nerve, Open Approach
00NH3ZZ   Release Oculomotor Nerve, Percutaneous Approach

00NH4ZZ   Release Oculomotor Nerve, Percutaneous Endoscopic Approach
00NJ0ZZ   Release Trochlear Nerve, Open Approach
00NJ3ZZ   Release Trochlear Nerve, Percutaneous Approach
00NJ4ZZ   Release Trochlear Nerve, Percutaneous Endoscopic Approach
00NK0ZZ   Release Trigeminal Nerve, Open Approach
00NK3ZZ   Release Trigeminal Nerve, Percutaneous Approach
00NK4ZZ   Release Trigeminal Nerve, Percutaneous Endoscopic Approach
00NL0ZZ   Release Abducens Nerve, Open Approach
00NL3ZZ   Release Abducens Nerve, Percutaneous Approach
00NL4ZZ   Release Abducens Nerve, Percutaneous Endoscopic Approach
00NM0ZZ   Release Facial Nerve, Open Approach
00NM3ZZ   Release Facial Nerve, Percutaneous Approach
00NM4ZZ   Release Facial Nerve, Percutaneous Endoscopic Approach
00NN0ZZ   Release Acoustic Nerve, Open Approach
00NN3ZZ   Release Acoustic Nerve, Percutaneous Approach
00NN4ZZ   Release Acoustic Nerve, Percutaneous Endoscopic Approach
00NP0ZZ   Release Glossopharyngeal Nerve, Open Approach
00NP3ZZ   Release Glossopharyngeal Nerve, Percutaneous Approach
00NP4ZZ   Release Glossopharyngeal Nerve, Percutaneous Endoscopic Approach
00NQ0ZZ   Release Vagus Nerve, Open Approach
00NQ3ZZ   Release Vagus Nerve, Percutaneous Approach
00NQ4ZZ   Release Vagus Nerve, Percutaneous Endoscopic Approach
00NR0ZZ   Release Accessory Nerve, Open Approach
00NR3ZZ   Release Accessory Nerve, Percutaneous Approach
00NR4ZZ   Release Accessory Nerve, Percutaneous Endoscopic Approach
00NS0ZZ   Release Hypoglossal Nerve, Open Approach
00NS3ZZ   Release Hypoglossal Nerve, Percutaneous Approach
00NS4ZZ   Release Hypoglossal Nerve, Percutaneous Endoscopic Approach
00NT0ZZ   Release Spinal Meninges, Open Approach
00NT3ZZ   Release Spinal Meninges, Percutaneous Approach
00NT4ZZ   Release Spinal Meninges, Percutaneous Endoscopic Approach
00NW0ZZ   Release Cervical Spinal Cord, Open Approach
00NW3ZZ   Release Cervical Spinal Cord, Percutaneous Approach
00NW4ZZ   Release Cervical Spinal Cord, Percutaneous Endoscopic Approach
00NX0ZZ   Release Thoracic Spinal Cord, Open Approach
00NX3ZZ   Release Thoracic Spinal Cord, Percutaneous Approach
00NX4ZZ   Release Thoracic Spinal Cord, Percutaneous Endoscopic Approach
00NY0ZZ   Release Lumbar Spinal Cord, Open Approach
00NY3ZZ   Release Lumbar Spinal Cord, Percutaneous Approach
00NY4ZZ   Release Lumbar Spinal Cord, Percutaneous Endoscopic Approach

00P – Central Nervous System, Removal

Review Coding Guideline B6.1c

00P000Z   Removal of Drainage Device from Brain, Open Approach
00P002Z   Removal of Monitoring Device from Brain, Open Approach
00P003Z   Removal of Infusion Device from Brain, Open Approach
00P007Z   Removal of Autologous Tissue Substitute from Brain, Open Approach
00P00JZ   Removal of Synthetic Substitute from Brain, Open Approach
00P00KZ   Removal of Nonautologous Tissue Substitute from Brain, Open Approach
00P00MZ   Removal of Neurostimulator Lead from Brain, Open Approach
00P030Z   Removal of Drainage Device from Brain, Percutaneous Approach
00P032Z   Removal of Monitoring Device from Brain, Percutaneous Approach
00P033Z   Removal of Infusion Device from Brain, Percutaneous Approach
00P037Z   Removal of Autologous Tissue Substitute from Brain, Percutaneous Approach
00P03JZ   Removal of Synthetic Substitute from Brain, Percutaneous Approach
00P03KZ   Removal of Nonautologous Tissue Substitute from Brain, Percutaneous Approach

00P03MZ   Removal of Neurostimulator Lead from Brain, Percutaneous Approach
00P040Z   Removal of Drainage Device from Brain, Percutaneous Endoscopic Approach
00P042Z   Removal of Monitoring Device from Brain, Percutaneous Endoscopic Approach
00P043Z   Removal of Infusion Device from Brain, Percutaneous Endoscopic Approach
00P047Z   Removal of Autologous Tissue Substitute from Brain, Percutaneous Endoscopic Approach
00P04JZ   Removal of Synthetic Substitute from Brain, Percutaneous Endoscopic Approach
00P04KZ   Removal of Nonautologous Tissue Substitute from Brain, Percutaneous Endoscopic Approach
00P04MZ   Removal of Neurostimulator Lead from Brain, Percutaneous Endoscopic Approach
00P0X0Z   Removal of Drainage Device from Brain, External Approach
00P0X2Z   Removal of Monitoring Device from Brain, External Approach
00P0X3Z   Removal of Infusion Device from Brain, External Approach

---

♀ Female-only   ♂ Male-only   ◐ Limited Coverage   ● Non-OR   🄷🄰🄲 HAC-associated procedure   ● Non-covered procedures   ➕ Combination

00P0XMZ	Removal of Neurostimulator Lead from Brain, External Approach
00P600Z	Removal of Drainage Device from Cerebral Ventricle, Open Approach
00P602Z	Removal of Monitoring Device from Cerebral Ventricle, Open Approach
00P603Z	Removal of Infusion Device from Cerebral Ventricle, Open Approach
00P60JZ	Removal of Synthetic Substitute from Cerebral Ventricle, Open Approach
00P60MZ	Removal of Neurostimulator Lead from Cerebral Ventricle, Open Approach
00P630Z	Removal of Drainage Device from Cerebral Ventricle, Percutaneous Approach
00P632Z	Removal of Monitoring Device from Cerebral Ventricle, Percutaneous Approach
00P633Z	Removal of Infusion Device from Cerebral Ventricle, Percutaneous Approach
00P63JZ	Removal of Synthetic Substitute from Cerebral Ventricle, Percutaneous Approach
00P63MZ	Removal of Neurostimulator Lead from Cerebral Ventricle, Percutaneous Approach
00P640Z	Removal of Drainage Device from Cerebral Ventricle, Percutaneous Endoscopic Approach
00P642Z	Removal of Monitoring Device from Cerebral Ventricle, Percutaneous Endoscopic Approach
00P643Z	Removal of Infusion Device from Cerebral Ventricle, Percutaneous Endoscopic Approach
00P64JZ	Removal of Synthetic Substitute from Cerebral Ventricle, Percutaneous Endoscopic Approach
00P64MZ	Removal of Neurostimulator Lead from Cerebral Ventricle, Percutaneous Endoscopic Approach
00P6X0Z	Removal of Drainage Device from Cerebral Ventricle, External Approach
00P6X2Z	Removal of Monitoring Device from Cerebral Ventricle, External Approach
00P6X3Z	Removal of Infusion Device from Cerebral Ventricle, External Approach
00P6XMZ	Removal of Neurostimulator Lead from Cerebral Ventricle, External Approach
00PE00Z	Removal of Drainage Device from Cranial Nerve, Open Approach
00PE02Z	Removal of Monitoring Device from Cranial Nerve, Open Approach
00PE03Z	Removal of Infusion Device from Cranial Nerve, Open Approach
00PE07Z	Removal of Autologous Tissue Substitute from Cranial Nerve, Open Approach
00PE0MZ	Removal of Neurostimulator Lead from Cranial Nerve, Open Approach
00PE30Z	Removal of Drainage Device from Cranial Nerve, Percutaneous Approach
00PE32Z	Removal of Monitoring Device from Cranial Nerve, Percutaneous Approach
00PE33Z	Removal of Infusion Device from Cranial Nerve, Percutaneous Approach
00PE37Z	Removal of Autologous Tissue Substitute from Cranial Nerve, Percutaneous Approach
00PE3MZ	Removal of Neurostimulator Lead from Cranial Nerve, Percutaneous Approach
00PE40Z	Removal of Drainage Device from Cranial Nerve, Percutaneous Endoscopic Approach
00PE42Z	Removal of Monitoring Device from Cranial Nerve, Percutaneous Endoscopic Approach
00PE43Z	Removal of Infusion Device from Cranial Nerve, Percutaneous Endoscopic Approach
00PE47Z	Removal of Autologous Tissue Substitute from Cranial Nerve, Percutaneous Endoscopic Approach
00PE4MZ	Removal of Neurostimulator Lead from Cranial Nerve, Percutaneous Endoscopic Approach
00PEX0Z	Removal of Drainage Device from Cranial Nerve, External Approach
00PEX2Z	Removal of Monitoring Device from Cranial Nerve, External Approach
00PEX3Z	Removal of Infusion Device from Cranial Nerve, External Approach
00PEXMZ	Removal of Neurostimulator Lead from Cranial Nerve, External Approach
00PU00Z	Removal of Drainage Device from Spinal Canal, Open Approach
00PU02Z	Removal of Monitoring Device from Spinal Canal, Open Approach
00PU03Z	Removal of Infusion Device from Spinal Canal, Open Approach
00PU0JZ	Removal of Synthetic Substitute from Spinal Canal, Open Approach
00PU0MZ	Removal of Neurostimulator Lead from Spinal Canal, Open Approach
00PU30Z	Removal of Drainage Device from Spinal Canal, Percutaneous Approach
00PU32Z	Removal of Monitoring Device from Spinal Canal, Percutaneous Approach
00PU33Z	Removal of Infusion Device from Spinal Canal, Percutaneous Approach
00PU3JZ	Removal of Synthetic Substitute from Spinal Canal, Percutaneous Approach
00PU3MZ	Removal of Neurostimulator Lead from Spinal Canal, Percutaneous Approach
00PU40Z	Removal of Drainage Device from Spinal Canal, Percutaneous Endoscopic Approach
00PU42Z	Removal of Monitoring Device from Spinal Canal, Percutaneous Endoscopic Approach
00PU43Z	Removal of Infusion Device from Spinal Canal, Percutaneous Endoscopic Approach
00PU4JZ	Removal of Synthetic Substitute from Spinal Canal, Percutaneous Endoscopic Approach
00PU4MZ	Removal of Neurostimulator Lead from Spinal Canal, Percutaneous Endoscopic Approach
00PUX0Z	Removal of Drainage Device from Spinal Canal, External Approach
00PUX2Z	Removal of Monitoring Device from Spinal Canal, External Approach
00PUX3Z	Removal of Infusion Device from Spinal Canal, External Approach
00PUXMZ	Removal of Neurostimulator Lead from Spinal Canal, External Approach
00PV00Z	Removal of Drainage Device from Spinal Cord, Open Approach
00PV02Z	Removal of Monitoring Device from Spinal Cord, Open Approach
00PV03Z	Removal of Infusion Device from Spinal Cord, Open Approach
00PV07Z	Removal of Autologous Tissue Substitute from Spinal Cord, Open Approach
00PV0JZ	Removal of Synthetic Substitute from Spinal Cord, Open Approach
00PV0KZ	Removal of Nonautologous Tissue Substitute from Spinal Cord, Open Approach
00PV0MZ	Removal of Neurostimulator Lead from Spinal Cord, Open Approach
00PV30Z	Removal of Drainage Device from Spinal Cord, Percutaneous Approach
00PV32Z	Removal of Monitoring Device from Spinal Cord, Percutaneous Approach
00PV33Z	Removal of Infusion Device from Spinal Cord, Percutaneous Approach
00PV37Z	Removal of Autologous Tissue Substitute from Spinal Cord, Percutaneous Approach
00PV3JZ	Removal of Synthetic Substitute from Spinal Cord, Percutaneous Approach
00PV3KZ	Removal of Nonautologous Tissue Substitute from Spinal Cord, Percutaneous Approach
00PV3MZ	Removal of Neurostimulator Lead from Spinal Cord, Percutaneous Approach
00PV40Z	Removal of Drainage Device from Spinal Cord, Percutaneous Endoscopic Approach
00PV42Z	Removal of Monitoring Device from Spinal Cord, Percutaneous Endoscopic Approach
00PV43Z	Removal of Infusion Device from Spinal Cord, Percutaneous Endoscopic Approach
00PV47Z	Removal of Autologous Tissue Substitute from Spinal Cord, Percutaneous Endoscopic Approach
00PV4JZ	Removal of Synthetic Substitute from Spinal Cord, Percutaneous Endoscopic Approach
00PV4KZ	Removal of Nonautologous Tissue Substitute from Spinal Cord, Percutaneous Endoscopic Approach
00PV4MZ	Removal of Neurostimulator Lead from Spinal Cord, Percutaneous Endoscopic Approach
00PVX0Z	Removal of Drainage Device from Spinal Cord, External Approach
00PVX2Z	Removal of Monitoring Device from Spinal Cord, External Approach
00PVX3Z	Removal of Infusion Device from Spinal Cord, External Approach
00PVXMZ	Removal of Neurostimulator Lead from Spinal Cord, External Approach

00Q – Central Nervous System, Repair

00Q00ZZ	Repair Brain, Open Approach
00Q03ZZ	Repair Brain, Percutaneous Approach
00Q04ZZ	Repair Brain, Percutaneous Endoscopic Approach
00Q10ZZ	Repair Cerebral Meninges, Open Approach
00Q13ZZ	Repair Cerebral Meninges, Percutaneous Approach
00Q14ZZ	Repair Cerebral Meninges, Percutaneous Endoscopic Approach
00Q20ZZ	Repair Dura Mater, Open Approach
00Q23ZZ	Repair Dura Mater, Percutaneous Approach
00Q24ZZ	Repair Dura Mater, Percutaneous Endoscopic Approach
00Q60ZZ	Repair Cerebral Ventricle, Open Approach
00Q63ZZ	Repair Cerebral Ventricle, Percutaneous Approach
00Q64ZZ	Repair Cerebral Ventricle, Percutaneous Endoscopic Approach
00Q70ZZ	Repair Cerebral Hemisphere, Open Approach
00Q73ZZ	Repair Cerebral Hemisphere, Percutaneous Approach
00Q74ZZ	Repair Cerebral Hemisphere, Percutaneous Endoscopic Approach
00Q80ZZ	Repair Basal Ganglia, Open Approach
00Q83ZZ	Repair Basal Ganglia, Percutaneous Approach
00Q84ZZ	Repair Basal Ganglia, Percutaneous Endoscopic Approach
00Q90ZZ	Repair Thalamus, Open Approach
00Q93ZZ	Repair Thalamus, Percutaneous Approach
00Q94ZZ	Repair Thalamus, Percutaneous Endoscopic Approach
00QA0ZZ	Repair Hypothalamus, Open Approach
00QA3ZZ	Repair Hypothalamus, Percutaneous Approach
00QA4ZZ	Repair Hypothalamus, Percutaneous Endoscopic Approach
00QB0ZZ	Repair Pons, Open Approach
00QB3ZZ	Repair Pons, Percutaneous Approach
00QB4ZZ	Repair Pons, Percutaneous Endoscopic Approach
00QC0ZZ	Repair Cerebellum, Open Approach
00QC3ZZ	Repair Cerebellum, Percutaneous Approach
00QC4ZZ	Repair Cerebellum, Percutaneous Endoscopic Approach
00QD0ZZ	Repair Medulla Oblongata, Open Approach
00QD3ZZ	Repair Medulla Oblongata, Percutaneous Approach
00QD4ZZ	Repair Medulla Oblongata, Percutaneous Endoscopic Approach
00QF0ZZ	Repair Olfactory Nerve, Open Approach
00QF3ZZ	Repair Olfactory Nerve, Percutaneous Approach
00QF4ZZ	Repair Olfactory Nerve, Percutaneous Endoscopic Approach
00QG0ZZ	Repair Optic Nerve, Open Approach
00QG3ZZ	Repair Optic Nerve, Percutaneous Approach
00QG4ZZ	Repair Optic Nerve, Percutaneous Endoscopic Approach
00QH0ZZ	Repair Oculomotor Nerve, Open Approach
00QH3ZZ	Repair Oculomotor Nerve, Percutaneous Approach
00QH4ZZ	Repair Oculomotor Nerve, Percutaneous Endoscopic Approach
00QJ0ZZ	Repair Trochlear Nerve, Open Approach
00QJ3ZZ	Repair Trochlear Nerve, Percutaneous Approach
00QJ4ZZ	Repair Trochlear Nerve, Percutaneous Endoscopic Approach
00QK0ZZ	Repair Trigeminal Nerve, Open Approach
00QK3ZZ	Repair Trigeminal Nerve, Percutaneous Approach
00QK4ZZ	Repair Trigeminal Nerve, Percutaneous Endoscopic Approach
00QL0ZZ	Repair Abducens Nerve, Open Approach
00QL3ZZ	Repair Abducens Nerve, Percutaneous Approach
00QL4ZZ	Repair Abducens Nerve, Percutaneous Endoscopic Approach
00QM0ZZ	Repair Facial Nerve, Open Approach
00QM3ZZ	Repair Facial Nerve, Percutaneous Approach
00QM4ZZ	Repair Facial Nerve, Percutaneous Endoscopic Approach
00QN0ZZ	Repair Acoustic Nerve, Open Approach
00QN3ZZ	Repair Acoustic Nerve, Percutaneous Approach
00QN4ZZ	Repair Acoustic Nerve, Percutaneous Endoscopic Approach
00QP0ZZ	Repair Glossopharyngeal Nerve, Open Approach
00QP3ZZ	Repair Glossopharyngeal Nerve, Percutaneous Approach
00QP4ZZ	Repair Glossopharyngeal Nerve, Percutaneous Endoscopic Approach
00QQ0ZZ	Repair Vagus Nerve, Open Approach
00QQ3ZZ	Repair Vagus Nerve, Percutaneous Approach
00QQ4ZZ	Repair Vagus Nerve, Percutaneous Endoscopic Approach
00QR0ZZ	Repair Accessory Nerve, Open Approach
00QR3ZZ	Repair Accessory Nerve, Percutaneous Approach
00QR4ZZ	Repair Accessory Nerve, Percutaneous Endoscopic Approach
00QS0ZZ	Repair Hypoglossal Nerve, Open Approach
00QS3ZZ	Repair Hypoglossal Nerve, Percutaneous Approach
00QS4ZZ	Repair Hypoglossal Nerve, Percutaneous Endoscopic Approach
00QT0ZZ	Repair Spinal Meninges, Open Approach
00QT3ZZ	Repair Spinal Meninges, Percutaneous Approach
00QT4ZZ	Repair Spinal Meninges, Percutaneous Endoscopic Approach
00QW0ZZ	Repair Cervical Spinal Cord, Open Approach
00QW3ZZ	Repair Cervical Spinal Cord, Percutaneous Approach
00QW4ZZ	Repair Cervical Spinal Cord, Percutaneous Endoscopic Approach
00QX0ZZ	Repair Thoracic Spinal Cord, Open Approach
00QX3ZZ	Repair Thoracic Spinal Cord, Percutaneous Approach
00QX4ZZ	Repair Thoracic Spinal Cord, Percutaneous Endoscopic Approach
00QY0ZZ	Repair Lumbar Spinal Cord, Open Approach
00QY3ZZ	Repair Lumbar Spinal Cord, Percutaneous Approach
00QY4ZZ	Repair Lumbar Spinal Cord, Percutaneous Endoscopic Approach

00S – Central Nervous System, Reposition

00SF0ZZ	Reposition Olfactory Nerve, Open Approach
00SF3ZZ	Reposition Olfactory Nerve, Percutaneous Approach
00SF4ZZ	Reposition Olfactory Nerve, Percutaneous Endoscopic Approach
00SG0ZZ	Reposition Optic Nerve, Open Approach
00SG3ZZ	Reposition Optic Nerve, Percutaneous Approach
00SG4ZZ	Reposition Optic Nerve, Percutaneous Endoscopic Approach
00SH0ZZ	Reposition Oculomotor Nerve, Open Approach
00SH3ZZ	Reposition Oculomotor Nerve, Percutaneous Approach
00SH4ZZ	Reposition Oculomotor Nerve, Percutaneous Endoscopic Approach
00SJ0ZZ	Reposition Trochlear Nerve, Open Approach
00SJ3ZZ	Reposition Trochlear Nerve, Percutaneous Approach
00SJ4ZZ	Reposition Trochlear Nerve, Percutaneous Endoscopic Approach
00SK0ZZ	Reposition Trigeminal Nerve, Open Approach
00SK3ZZ	Reposition Trigeminal Nerve, Percutaneous Approach
00SK4ZZ	Reposition Trigeminal Nerve, Percutaneous Endoscopic Approach
00SL0ZZ	Reposition Abducens Nerve, Open Approach
00SL3ZZ	Reposition Abducens Nerve, Percutaneous Approach
00SL4ZZ	Reposition Abducens Nerve, Percutaneous Endoscopic Approach
00SM0ZZ	Reposition Facial Nerve, Open Approach
00SM3ZZ	Reposition Facial Nerve, Percutaneous Approach
00SM4ZZ	Reposition Facial Nerve, Percutaneous Endoscopic Approach
00SN0ZZ	Reposition Acoustic Nerve, Open Approach
00SN3ZZ	Reposition Acoustic Nerve, Percutaneous Approach
00SN4ZZ	Reposition Acoustic Nerve, Percutaneous Endoscopic Approach
00SP0ZZ	Reposition Glossopharyngeal Nerve, Open Approach
00SP3ZZ	Reposition Glossopharyngeal Nerve, Percutaneous Approach
00SP4ZZ	Reposition Glossopharyngeal Nerve, Percutaneous Endoscopic Approach
00SQ0ZZ	Reposition Vagus Nerve, Open Approach
00SQ3ZZ	Reposition Vagus Nerve, Percutaneous Approach
00SQ4ZZ	Reposition Vagus Nerve, Percutaneous Endoscopic Approach
00SR0ZZ	Reposition Accessory Nerve, Open Approach
00SR3ZZ	Reposition Accessory Nerve, Percutaneous Approach
00SR4ZZ	Reposition Accessory Nerve, Percutaneous Endoscopic Approach
00SS0ZZ	Reposition Hypoglossal Nerve, Open Approach
00SS3ZZ	Reposition Hypoglossal Nerve, Percutaneous Approach
00SS4ZZ	Reposition Hypoglossal Nerve, Percutaneous Endoscopic Approach
00SW0ZZ	Reposition Cervical Spinal Cord, Open Approach
00SW3ZZ	Reposition Cervical Spinal Cord, Percutaneous Approach
00SW4ZZ	Reposition Cervical Spinal Cord, Percutaneous Endoscopic Approach
00SX0ZZ	Reposition Thoracic Spinal Cord, Open Approach
00SX3ZZ	Reposition Thoracic Spinal Cord, Percutaneous Approach
00SX4ZZ	Reposition Thoracic Spinal Cord, Percutaneous Endoscopic Approach
00SY0ZZ	Reposition Lumbar Spinal Cord, Open Approach
00SY3ZZ	Reposition Lumbar Spinal Cord, Percutaneous Approach
00SY4ZZ	Reposition Lumbar Spinal Cord, Percutaneous Endoscopic Approach

00T – Central Nervous System, Resection

Review Coding Guideline B3.8

00T70ZZ Resection of Cerebral Hemisphere, Open Approach
00T73ZZ Resection of Cerebral Hemisphere, Percutaneous Approach

00T74ZZ Resection of Cerebral Hemisphere, Percutaneous Endoscopic Approach

00U – Central Nervous System, Supplement

00U107Z Supplement Cerebral Meninges with Autologous Tissue Substitute, Open Approach
00U10JZ Supplement Cerebral Meninges with Synthetic Substitute, Open Approach
00U10KZ Supplement Cerebral Meninges with Nonautologous Tissue Substitute, Open Approach
00U137Z Supplement Cerebral Meninges with Autologous Tissue Substitute, Percutaneous Approach
00U13JZ Supplement Cerebral Meninges with Synthetic Substitute, Percutaneous Approach
00U13KZ Supplement Cerebral Meninges with Nonautologous Tissue Substitute, Percutaneous Approach
00U147Z Supplement Cerebral Meninges with Autologous Tissue Substitute, Percutaneous Endoscopic Approach
00U14JZ Supplement Cerebral Meninges with Synthetic Substitute, Percutaneous Endoscopic Approach
00U14KZ Supplement Cerebral Meninges with Nonautologous Tissue Substitute, Percutaneous Endoscopic Approach
00U207Z Supplement Dura Mater with Autologous Tissue Substitute, Open Approach
00U20JZ Supplement Dura Mater with Synthetic Substitute, Open Approach
00U20KZ Supplement Dura Mater with Nonautologous Tissue Substitute, Open Approach
00U237Z Supplement Dura Mater with Autologous Tissue Substitute, Percutaneous Approach
00U23JZ Supplement Dura Mater with Synthetic Substitute, Percutaneous Approach
00U23KZ Supplement Dura Mater with Nonautologous Tissue Substitute, Percutaneous Approach
00U247Z Supplement Dura Mater with Autologous Tissue Substitute, Percutaneous Endoscopic Approach
00U24JZ Supplement Dura Mater with Synthetic Substitute, Percutaneous Endoscopic Approach
00U24KZ Supplement Dura Mater with Nonautologous Tissue Substitute, Percutaneous Endoscopic Approach
00UF07Z Supplement Olfactory Nerve with Autologous Tissue Substitute, Open Approach
00UF37Z Supplement Olfactory Nerve with Autologous Tissue Substitute, Percutaneous Approach
00UF47Z Supplement Olfactory Nerve with Autologous Tissue Substitute, Percutaneous Endoscopic Approach
00UG07Z Supplement Optic Nerve with Autologous Tissue Substitute, Open Approach
00UG37Z Supplement Optic Nerve with Autologous Tissue Substitute, Percutaneous Approach
00UG47Z Supplement Optic Nerve with Autologous Tissue Substitute, Percutaneous Endoscopic Approach
00UH07Z Supplement Oculomotor Nerve with Autologous Tissue Substitute, Open Approach
00UH37Z Supplement Oculomotor Nerve with Autologous Tissue Substitute, Percutaneous Approach
00UH47Z Supplement Oculomotor Nerve with Autologous Tissue Substitute, Percutaneous Endoscopic Approach
00UJ07Z Supplement Trochlear Nerve with Autologous Tissue Substitute, Open Approach
00UJ37Z Supplement Trochlear Nerve with Autologous Tissue Substitute, Percutaneous Approach
00UJ47Z Supplement Trochlear Nerve with Autologous Tissue Substitute, Percutaneous Endoscopic Approach
00UK07Z Supplement Trigeminal Nerve with Autologous Tissue Substitute, Open Approach
00UK37Z Supplement Trigeminal Nerve with Autologous Tissue Substitute, Percutaneous Approach

00UK47Z Supplement Trigeminal Nerve with Autologous Tissue Substitute, Percutaneous Endoscopic Approach
00UL07Z Supplement Abducens Nerve with Autologous Tissue Substitute, Open Approach
00UL37Z Supplement Abducens Nerve with Autologous Tissue Substitute, Percutaneous Approach
00UL47Z Supplement Abducens Nerve with Autologous Tissue Substitute, Percutaneous Endoscopic Approach
00UM07Z Supplement Facial Nerve with Autologous Tissue Substitute, Open Approach
00UM37Z Supplement Facial Nerve with Autologous Tissue Substitute, Percutaneous Approach
00UM47Z Supplement Facial Nerve with Autologous Tissue Substitute, Percutaneous Endoscopic Approach
00UN07Z Supplement Acoustic Nerve with Autologous Tissue Substitute, Open Approach
00UN37Z Supplement Acoustic Nerve with Autologous Tissue Substitute, Percutaneous Approach
00UN47Z Supplement Acoustic Nerve with Autologous Tissue Substitute, Percutaneous Endoscopic Approach
00UP07Z Supplement Glossopharyngeal Nerve with Autologous Tissue Substitute, Open Approach
00UP37Z Supplement Glossopharyngeal Nerve with Autologous Tissue Substitute, Percutaneous Approach
00UP47Z Supplement Glossopharyngeal Nerve with Autologous Tissue Substitute, Percutaneous Endoscopic Approach
00UQ07Z Supplement Vagus Nerve with Autologous Tissue Substitute, Open Approach
00UQ37Z Supplement Vagus Nerve with Autologous Tissue Substitute, Percutaneous Approach
00UQ47Z Supplement Vagus Nerve with Autologous Tissue Substitute, Percutaneous Endoscopic Approach
00UR07Z Supplement Accessory Nerve with Autologous Tissue Substitute, Open Approach
00UR37Z Supplement Accessory Nerve with Autologous Tissue Substitute, Percutaneous Approach
00UR47Z Supplement Accessory Nerve with Autologous Tissue Substitute, Percutaneous Endoscopic Approach
00US07Z Supplement Hypoglossal Nerve with Autologous Tissue Substitute, Open Approach
00US37Z Supplement Hypoglossal Nerve with Autologous Tissue Substitute, Percutaneous Approach
00US47Z Supplement Hypoglossal Nerve with Autologous Tissue Substitute, Percutaneous Endoscopic Approach
00UT07Z Supplement Spinal Meninges with Autologous Tissue Substitute, Open Approach
00UT0JZ Supplement Spinal Meninges with Synthetic Substitute, Open Approach
00UT0KZ Supplement Spinal Meninges with Nonautologous Tissue Substitute, Open Approach
00UT37Z Supplement Spinal Meninges with Autologous Tissue Substitute, Percutaneous Approach
00UT3JZ Supplement Spinal Meninges with Synthetic Substitute, Percutaneous Approach
00UT3KZ Supplement Spinal Meninges with Nonautologous Tissue Substitute, Percutaneous Approach
00UT47Z Supplement Spinal Meninges with Autologous Tissue Substitute, Percutaneous Endoscopic Approach
00UT4JZ Supplement Spinal Meninges with Synthetic Substitute, Percutaneous Endoscopic Approach
00UT4KZ Supplement Spinal Meninges with Nonautologous Tissue Substitute, Percutaneous Endoscopic Approach

00W – Central Nervous System, Revision

Review Coding Guideline B6.1c

00W000Z Revision of Drainage Device in Brain, Open Approach
00W002Z Revision of Monitoring Device in Brain, Open Approach
00W003Z Revision of Infusion Device in Brain, Open Approach
00W007Z Revision of Autologous Tissue Substitute in Brain, Open Approach
00W00JZ Revision of Synthetic Substitute in Brain, Open Approach
00W00KZ Revision of Nonautologous Tissue Substitute in Brain, Open Approach
00W00MZ Revision of Neurostimulator Lead in Brain, Open Approach
00W030Z Revision of Drainage Device in Brain, Percutaneous Approach
00W032Z Revision of Monitoring Device in Brain, Percutaneous Approach
00W033Z Revision of Infusion Device in Brain, Percutaneous Approach
00W037Z Revision of Autologous Tissue Substitute in Brain, Percutaneous Approach
00W03JZ Revision of Synthetic Substitute in Brain, Percutaneous Approach
00W03KZ Revision of Nonautologous Tissue Substitute in Brain, Percutaneous Approach
00W03MZ Revision of Neurostimulator Lead in Brain, Percutaneous Approach
00W040Z Revision of Drainage Device in Brain, Percutaneous Endoscopic Approach
00W042Z Revision of Monitoring Device in Brain, Percutaneous Endoscopic Approach
00W043Z Revision of Infusion Device in Brain, Percutaneous Endoscopic Approach
00W047Z Revision of Autologous Tissue Substitute in Brain, Percutaneous Endoscopic Approach
00W04JZ Revision of Synthetic Substitute in Brain, Percutaneous Endoscopic Approach
00W04KZ Revision of Nonautologous Tissue Substitute in Brain, Percutaneous Endoscopic Approach
00W04MZ Revision of Neurostimulator Lead in Brain, Percutaneous Endoscopic Approach
00W0X0Z Revision of Drainage Device in Brain, External Approach
00W0X2Z Revision of Monitoring Device in Brain, External Approach
00W0X3Z Revision of Infusion Device in Brain, External Approach
00W0X7Z Revision of Autologous Tissue Substitute in Brain, External Approach
00W0XJZ Revision of Synthetic Substitute in Brain, External Approach
00W0XKZ Revision of Nonautologous Tissue Substitute in Brain, External Approach
00W0XMZ Revision of Neurostimulator Lead in Brain, External Approach
00W600Z Revision of Drainage Device in Cerebral Ventricle, Open Approach
00W602Z Revision of Monitoring Device in Cerebral Ventricle, Open Approach
00W603Z Revision of Infusion Device in Cerebral Ventricle, Open Approach
00W60JZ Revision of Synthetic Substitute in Cerebral Ventricle, Open Approach
00W60MZ Revision of Neurostimulator Lead in Cerebral Ventricle, Open Approach
00W630Z Revision of Drainage Device in Cerebral Ventricle, Percutaneous Approach
00W632Z Revision of Monitoring Device in Cerebral Ventricle, Percutaneous Approach
00W633Z Revision of Infusion Device in Cerebral Ventricle, Percutaneous Approach
00W63JZ Revision of Synthetic Substitute in Cerebral Ventricle, Percutaneous Approach
00W63MZ Revision of Neurostimulator Lead in Cerebral Ventricle, Percutaneous Approach
00W640Z Revision of Drainage Device in Cerebral Ventricle, Percutaneous Endoscopic Approach
00W642Z Revision of Monitoring Device in Cerebral Ventricle, Percutaneous Endoscopic Approach
00W643Z Revision of Infusion Device in Cerebral Ventricle, Percutaneous Endoscopic Approach
00W64JZ Revision of Synthetic Substitute in Cerebral Ventricle, Percutaneous Endoscopic Approach
00W64MZ Revision of Neurostimulator Lead in Cerebral Ventricle, Percutaneous Endoscopic Approach

00W6X0Z Revision of Drainage Device in Cerebral Ventricle, External Approach
00W6X2Z Revision of Monitoring Device in Cerebral Ventricle, External Approach
00W6X3Z Revision of Infusion Device in Cerebral Ventricle, External Approach
00W6XJZ Revision of Synthetic Substitute in Cerebral Ventricle, External Approach
00W6XMZ Revision of Neurostimulator Lead in Cerebral Ventricle, External Approach
00WE00Z Revision of Drainage Device in Cranial Nerve, Open Approach
00WE02Z Revision of Monitoring Device in Cranial Nerve, Open Approach
00WE03Z Revision of Infusion Device in Cranial Nerve, Open Approach
00WE07Z Revision of Autologous Tissue Substitute in Cranial Nerve, Open Approach
00WE0MZ Revision of Neurostimulator Lead in Cranial Nerve, Open Approach
00WE30Z Revision of Drainage Device in Cranial Nerve, Percutaneous Approach
00WE32Z Revision of Monitoring Device in Cranial Nerve, Percutaneous Approach
00WE33Z Revision of Infusion Device in Cranial Nerve, Percutaneous Approach
00WE37Z Revision of Autologous Tissue Substitute in Cranial Nerve, Percutaneous Approach
00WE3MZ Revision of Neurostimulator Lead in Cranial Nerve, Percutaneous Approach
00WE40Z Revision of Drainage Device in Cranial Nerve, Percutaneous Endoscopic Approach
00WE42Z Revision of Monitoring Device in Cranial Nerve, Percutaneous Endoscopic Approach
00WE43Z Revision of Infusion Device in Cranial Nerve, Percutaneous Endoscopic Approach
00WE47Z Revision of Autologous Tissue Substitute in Cranial Nerve, Percutaneous Endoscopic Approach
00WE4MZ Revision of Neurostimulator Lead in Cranial Nerve, Percutaneous Endoscopic Approach
00WEX0Z Revision of Drainage Device in Cranial Nerve, External Approach
00WEX2Z Revision of Monitoring Device in Cranial Nerve, External Approach
00WEX3Z Revision of Infusion Device in Cranial Nerve, External Approach
00WEX7Z Revision of Autologous Tissue Substitute in Cranial Nerve, External Approach
00WEXMZ Revision of Neurostimulator Lead in Cranial Nerve, External Approach
00WU00Z Revision of Drainage Device in Spinal Canal, Open Approach
00WU02Z Revision of Monitoring Device in Spinal Canal, Open Approach
00WU03Z Revision of Infusion Device in Spinal Canal, Open Approach
00WU0JZ Revision of Synthetic Substitute in Spinal Canal, Open Approach
00WU0MZ Revision of Neurostimulator Lead in Spinal Canal, Open Approach
00WU30Z Revision of Drainage Device in Spinal Canal, Percutaneous Approach
00WU32Z Revision of Monitoring Device in Spinal Canal, Percutaneous Approach
00WU33Z Revision of Infusion Device in Spinal Canal, Percutaneous Approach
00WU3JZ Revision of Synthetic Substitute in Spinal Canal, Percutaneous Approach
00WU3MZ Revision of Neurostimulator Lead in Spinal Canal, Percutaneous Approach
00WU40Z Revision of Drainage Device in Spinal Canal, Percutaneous Endoscopic Approach
00WU42Z Revision of Monitoring Device in Spinal Canal, Percutaneous Endoscopic Approach
00WU43Z Revision of Infusion Device in Spinal Canal, Percutaneous Endoscopic Approach
00WU4JZ Revision of Synthetic Substitute in Spinal Canal, Percutaneous Endoscopic Approach
00WU4MZ Revision of Neurostimulator Lead in Spinal Canal, Percutaneous Endoscopic Approach
00WUX0Z Revision of Drainage Device in Spinal Canal, External Approach

---

♀ Female-only   ♂ Male-only   ● Limited Coverage   ● Non-OR   HAC HAC-associated procedure   ● Non-covered procedures   ✚ Combination

00WUX2Z Revision of Monitoring Device in Spinal Canal, External Approach
00WUX3Z Revision of Infusion Device in Spinal Canal, External Approach
00WUXJZ Revision of Synthetic Substitute in Spinal Canal, External Approach
00WUXMZ Revision of Neurostimulator Lead in Spinal Canal, External Approach
00WV00Z Revision of Drainage Device in Spinal Cord, Open Approach
00WV02Z Revision of Monitoring Device in Spinal Cord, Open Approach
00WV03Z Revision of Infusion Device in Spinal Cord, Open Approach
00WV07Z Revision of Autologous Tissue Substitute in Spinal Cord, Open Approach
00WV0JZ Revision of Synthetic Substitute in Spinal Cord, Open Approach
00WV0KZ Revision of Nonautologous Tissue Substitute in Spinal Cord, Open Approach
00WV0MZ Revision of Neurostimulator Lead in Spinal Cord, Open Approach
00WV30Z Revision of Drainage Device in Spinal Cord, Percutaneous Approach
00WV32Z Revision of Monitoring Device in Spinal Cord, Percutaneous Approach
00WV33Z Revision of Infusion Device in Spinal Cord, Percutaneous Approach
00WV37Z Revision of Autologous Tissue Substitute in Spinal Cord, Percutaneous Approach
00WV3JZ Revision of Synthetic Substitute in Spinal Cord, Percutaneous Approach
00WV3KZ Revision of Nonautologous Tissue Substitute in Spinal Cord, Percutaneous Approach

00WV3MZ Revision of Neurostimulator Lead in Spinal Cord, Percutaneous Approach
00WV40Z Revision of Drainage Device in Spinal Cord, Percutaneous Endoscopic Approach
00WV42Z Revision of Monitoring Device in Spinal Cord, Percutaneous Endoscopic Approach
00WV43Z Revision of Infusion Device in Spinal Cord, Percutaneous Endoscopic Approach
00WV47Z Revision of Autologous Tissue Substitute in Spinal Cord, Percutaneous Endoscopic Approach
00WV4JZ Revision of Synthetic Substitute in Spinal Cord, Percutaneous Endoscopic Approach
00WV4KZ Revision of Nonautologous Tissue Substitute in Spinal Cord, Percutaneous Endoscopic Approach
00WV4MZ Revision of Neurostimulator Lead in Spinal Cord, Percutaneous Endoscopic Approach
00WVX0Z Revision of Drainage Device in Spinal Cord, External Approach
00WVX2Z Revision of Monitoring Device in Spinal Cord, External Approach
00WVX3Z Revision of Infusion Device in Spinal Cord, External Approach
00WVX7Z Revision of Autologous Tissue Substitute in Spinal Cord, External Approach
00WVXJZ Revision of Synthetic Substitute in Spinal Cord, External Approach
00WVXKZ Revision of Nonautologous Tissue Substitute in Spinal Cord, External Approach
00WVXMZ Revision of Neurostimulator Lead in Spinal Cord, External Approach

00X – Central Nervous System, Transfer

00XF0ZF Transfer Olfactory Nerve to Olfactory Nerve, Open Approach
00XF0ZG Transfer Olfactory Nerve to Optic Nerve, Open Approach
00XF0ZH Transfer Olfactory Nerve to Oculomotor Nerve, Open Approach
00XF0ZJ Transfer Olfactory Nerve to Trochlear Nerve, Open Approach
00XF0ZK Transfer Olfactory Nerve to Trigeminal Nerve, Open Approach
00XF0ZL Transfer Olfactory Nerve to Abducens Nerve, Open Approach
00XF0ZM Transfer Olfactory Nerve to Facial Nerve, Open Approach
00XF0ZN Transfer Olfactory Nerve to Acoustic Nerve, Open Approach
00XF0ZP Transfer Olfactory Nerve to Glossopharyngeal Nerve, Open Approach
00XF0ZQ Transfer Olfactory Nerve to Vagus Nerve, Open Approach
00XF0ZR Transfer Olfactory Nerve to Accessory Nerve, Open Approach
00XF0ZS Transfer Olfactory Nerve to Hypoglossal Nerve, Open Approach
00XF4ZF Transfer Olfactory Nerve to Olfactory Nerve, Percutaneous Endoscopic Approach
00XF4ZG Transfer Olfactory Nerve to Optic Nerve, Percutaneous Endoscopic Approach
00XF4ZH Transfer Olfactory Nerve to Oculomotor Nerve, Percutaneous Endoscopic Approach
00XF4ZJ Transfer Olfactory Nerve to Trochlear Nerve, Percutaneous Endoscopic Approach
00XF4ZK Transfer Olfactory Nerve to Trigeminal Nerve, Percutaneous Endoscopic Approach
00XF4ZL Transfer Olfactory Nerve to Abducens Nerve, Percutaneous Endoscopic Approach
00XF4ZM Transfer Olfactory Nerve to Facial Nerve, Percutaneous Endoscopic Approach
00XF4ZN Transfer Olfactory Nerve to Acoustic Nerve, Percutaneous Endoscopic Approach
00XF4ZP Transfer Olfactory Nerve to Glossopharyngeal Nerve, Percutaneous Endoscopic Approach
00XF4ZQ Transfer Olfactory Nerve to Vagus Nerve, Percutaneous Endoscopic Approach
00XF4ZR Transfer Olfactory Nerve to Accessory Nerve, Percutaneous Endoscopic Approach
00XF4ZS Transfer Olfactory Nerve to Hypoglossal Nerve, Percutaneous Endoscopic Approach
00XG0ZF Transfer Optic Nerve to Olfactory Nerve, Open Approach
00XG0ZG Transfer Optic Nerve to Optic Nerve, Open Approach
00XG0ZH Transfer Optic Nerve to Oculomotor Nerve, Open Approach
00XG0ZJ Transfer Optic Nerve to Trochlear Nerve, Open Approach

00XG0ZK Transfer Optic Nerve to Trigeminal Nerve, Open Approach
00XG0ZL Transfer Optic Nerve to Abducens Nerve, Open Approach
00XG0ZM Transfer Optic Nerve to Facial Nerve, Open Approach
00XG0ZN Transfer Optic Nerve to Acoustic Nerve, Open Approach
00XG0ZP Transfer Optic Nerve to Glossopharyngeal Nerve, Open Approach
00XG0ZQ Transfer Optic Nerve to Vagus Nerve, Open Approach
00XG0ZR Transfer Optic Nerve to Accessory Nerve, Open Approach
00XG0ZS Transfer Optic Nerve to Hypoglossal Nerve, Open Approach
00XG4ZF Transfer Optic Nerve to Olfactory Nerve, Percutaneous Endoscopic Approach
00XG4ZG Transfer Optic Nerve to Optic Nerve, Percutaneous Endoscopic Approach
00XG4ZH Transfer Optic Nerve to Oculomotor Nerve, Percutaneous Endoscopic Approach
00XG4ZJ Transfer Optic Nerve to Trochlear Nerve, Percutaneous Endoscopic Approach
00XG4ZK Transfer Optic Nerve to Trigeminal Nerve, Percutaneous Endoscopic Approach
00XG4ZL Transfer Optic Nerve to Abducens Nerve, Percutaneous Endoscopic Approach
00XG4ZM Transfer Optic Nerve to Facial Nerve, Percutaneous Endoscopic Approach
00XG4ZN Transfer Optic Nerve to Acoustic Nerve, Percutaneous Endoscopic Approach
00XG4ZP Transfer Optic Nerve to Glossopharyngeal Nerve, Percutaneous Endoscopic Approach
00XG4ZQ Transfer Optic Nerve to Vagus Nerve, Percutaneous Endoscopic Approach
00XG4ZR Transfer Optic Nerve to Accessory Nerve, Percutaneous Endoscopic Approach
00XG4ZS Transfer Optic Nerve to Hypoglossal Nerve, Percutaneous Endoscopic Approach
00XH0ZF Transfer Oculomotor Nerve to Olfactory Nerve, Open Approach
00XH0ZG Transfer Oculomotor Nerve to Optic Nerve, Open Approach
00XH0ZH Transfer Oculomotor Nerve to Oculomotor Nerve, Open Approach
00XH0ZJ Transfer Oculomotor Nerve to Trochlear Nerve, Open Approach
00XH0ZK Transfer Oculomotor Nerve to Trigeminal Nerve, Open Approach
00XH0ZL Transfer Oculomotor Nerve to Abducens Nerve, Open Approach
00XH0ZM Transfer Oculomotor Nerve to Facial Nerve, Open Approach
00XH0ZN Transfer Oculomotor Nerve to Acoustic Nerve, Open Approach

00XH0ZP Transfer Oculomotor Nerve to Glossopharyngeal Nerve, Open Approach

00XH0ZQ Transfer Oculomotor Nerve to Vagus Nerve, Open Approach

00XH0ZR Transfer Oculomotor Nerve to Accessory Nerve, Open Approach

00XH0ZS Transfer Oculomotor Nerve to Hypoglossal Nerve, Open Approach

00XH4ZF Transfer Oculomotor Nerve to Olfactory Nerve, Percutaneous Endoscopic Approach

00XH4ZG Transfer Oculomotor Nerve to Optic Nerve, Percutaneous Endoscopic Approach

00XH4ZH Transfer Oculomotor Nerve to Oculomotor Nerve, Percutaneous Endoscopic Approach

00XH4ZJ Transfer Oculomotor Nerve to Trochlear Nerve, Percutaneous Endoscopic Approach

00XH4ZK Transfer Oculomotor Nerve to Trigeminal Nerve, Percutaneous Endoscopic Approach

00XH4ZL Transfer Oculomotor Nerve to Abducens Nerve, Percutaneous Endoscopic Approach

00XH4ZM Transfer Oculomotor Nerve to Facial Nerve, Percutaneous Endoscopic Approach

00XH4ZN Transfer Oculomotor Nerve to Acoustic Nerve, Percutaneous Endoscopic Approach

00XH4ZP Transfer Oculomotor Nerve to Glossopharyngeal Nerve, Percutaneous Endoscopic Approach

00XH4ZQ Transfer Oculomotor Nerve to Vagus Nerve, Percutaneous Endoscopic Approach

00XH4ZR Transfer Oculomotor Nerve to Accessory Nerve, Percutaneous Endoscopic Approach

00XH4ZS Transfer Oculomotor Nerve to Hypoglossal Nerve, Percutaneous Endoscopic Approach

00XJ0ZF Transfer Trochlear Nerve to Olfactory Nerve, Open Approach

00XJ0ZG Transfer Trochlear Nerve to Optic Nerve, Open Approach

00XJ0ZH Transfer Trochlear Nerve to Oculomotor Nerve, Open Approach

00XJ0ZJ Transfer Trochlear Nerve to Trochlear Nerve, Open Approach

00XJ0ZK Transfer Trochlear Nerve to Trigeminal Nerve, Open Approach

00XJ0ZL Transfer Trochlear Nerve to Abducens Nerve, Open Approach

00XJ0ZM Transfer Trochlear Nerve to Facial Nerve, Open Approach

00XJ0ZN Transfer Trochlear Nerve to Acoustic Nerve, Open Approach

00XJ0ZP Transfer Trochlear Nerve to Glossopharyngeal Nerve, Open Approach

00XJ0ZQ Transfer Trochlear Nerve to Vagus Nerve, Open Approach

00XJ0ZR Transfer Trochlear Nerve to Accessory Nerve, Open Approach

00XJ0ZS Transfer Trochlear Nerve to Hypoglossal Nerve, Open Approach

00XJ4ZF Transfer Trochlear Nerve to Olfactory Nerve, Percutaneous Endoscopic Approach

00XJ4ZG Transfer Trochlear Nerve to Optic Nerve, Percutaneous Endoscopic Approach

00XJ4ZH Transfer Trochlear Nerve to Oculomotor Nerve, Percutaneous Endoscopic Approach

00XJ4ZJ Transfer Trochlear Nerve to Trochlear Nerve, Percutaneous Endoscopic Approach

00XJ4ZK Transfer Trochlear Nerve to Trigeminal Nerve, Percutaneous Endoscopic Approach

00XJ4ZL Transfer Trochlear Nerve to Abducens Nerve, Percutaneous Endoscopic Approach

00XJ4ZM Transfer Trochlear Nerve to Facial Nerve, Percutaneous Endoscopic Approach

00XJ4ZN Transfer Trochlear Nerve to Acoustic Nerve, Percutaneous Endoscopic Approach

00XJ4ZP Transfer Trochlear Nerve to Glossopharyngeal Nerve, Percutaneous Endoscopic Approach

00XJ4ZQ Transfer Trochlear Nerve to Vagus Nerve, Percutaneous Endoscopic Approach

00XJ4ZR Transfer Trochlear Nerve to Accessory Nerve, Percutaneous Endoscopic Approach

00XJ4ZS Transfer Trochlear Nerve to Hypoglossal Nerve, Percutaneous Endoscopic Approach

00XK0ZF Transfer Trigeminal Nerve to Olfactory Nerve, Open Approach

00XK0ZG Transfer Trigeminal Nerve to Optic Nerve, Open Approach

00XK0ZH Transfer Trigeminal Nerve to Oculomotor Nerve, Open Approach

00XK0ZJ Transfer Trigeminal Nerve to Trochlear Nerve, Open Approach

00XK0ZK Transfer Trigeminal Nerve to Trigeminal Nerve, Open Approach

00XK0ZL Transfer Trigeminal Nerve to Abducens Nerve, Open Approach

00XK0ZM Transfer Trigeminal Nerve to Facial Nerve, Open Approach

00XK0ZN Transfer Trigeminal Nerve to Acoustic Nerve, Open Approach

00XK0ZP Transfer Trigeminal Nerve to Glossopharyngeal Nerve, Open Approach

00XK0ZQ Transfer Trigeminal Nerve to Vagus Nerve, Open Approach

00XK0ZR Transfer Trigeminal Nerve to Accessory Nerve, Open Approach

00XK0ZS Transfer Trigeminal Nerve to Hypoglossal Nerve, Open Approach

00XK4ZF Transfer Trigeminal Nerve to Olfactory Nerve, Percutaneous Endoscopic Approach

00XK4ZG Transfer Trigeminal Nerve to Optic Nerve, Percutaneous Endoscopic Approach

00XK4ZH Transfer Trigeminal Nerve to Oculomotor Nerve, Percutaneous Endoscopic Approach

00XK4ZJ Transfer Trigeminal Nerve to Trochlear Nerve, Percutaneous Endoscopic Approach

00XK4ZK Transfer Trigeminal Nerve to Trigeminal Nerve, Percutaneous Endoscopic Approach

00XK4ZL Transfer Trigeminal Nerve to Abducens Nerve, Percutaneous Endoscopic Approach

00XK4ZM Transfer Trigeminal Nerve to Facial Nerve, Percutaneous Endoscopic Approach

00XK4ZN Transfer Trigeminal Nerve to Acoustic Nerve, Percutaneous Endoscopic Approach

00XK4ZP Transfer Trigeminal Nerve to Glossopharyngeal Nerve, Percutaneous Endoscopic Approach

00XK4ZQ Transfer Trigeminal Nerve to Vagus Nerve, Percutaneous Endoscopic Approach

00XK4ZR Transfer Trigeminal Nerve to Accessory Nerve, Percutaneous Endoscopic Approach

00XK4ZS Transfer Trigeminal Nerve to Hypoglossal Nerve, Percutaneous Endoscopic Approach

00XL0ZF Transfer Abducens Nerve to Olfactory Nerve, Open Approach

00XL0ZG Transfer Abducens Nerve to Optic Nerve, Open Approach

00XL0ZH Transfer Abducens Nerve to Oculomotor Nerve, Open Approach

00XL0ZJ Transfer Abducens Nerve to Trochlear Nerve, Open Approach

00XL0ZK Transfer Abducens Nerve to Trigeminal Nerve, Open Approach

00XL0ZL Transfer Abducens Nerve to Abducens Nerve, Open Approach

00XL0ZM Transfer Abducens Nerve to Facial Nerve, Open Approach

00XL0ZN Transfer Abducens Nerve to Acoustic Nerve, Open Approach

00XL0ZP Transfer Abducens Nerve to Glossopharyngeal Nerve, Open Approach

00XL0ZQ Transfer Abducens Nerve to Vagus Nerve, Open Approach

00XL0ZR Transfer Abducens Nerve to Accessory Nerve, Open Approach

00XL0ZS Transfer Abducens Nerve to Hypoglossal Nerve, Open Approach

00XL4ZF Transfer Abducens Nerve to Olfactory Nerve, Percutaneous Endoscopic Approach

00XL4ZG Transfer Abducens Nerve to Optic Nerve, Percutaneous Endoscopic Approach

00XL4ZH Transfer Abducens Nerve to Oculomotor Nerve, Percutaneous Endoscopic Approach

00XL4ZJ Transfer Abducens Nerve to Trochlear Nerve, Percutaneous Endoscopic Approach

00XL4ZK Transfer Abducens Nerve to Trigeminal Nerve, Percutaneous Endoscopic Approach

00XL4ZL Transfer Abducens Nerve to Abducens Nerve, Percutaneous Endoscopic Approach

00XL4ZM Transfer Abducens Nerve to Facial Nerve, Percutaneous Endoscopic Approach

00XL4ZN Transfer Abducens Nerve to Acoustic Nerve, Percutaneous Endoscopic Approach

00XL4ZP Transfer Abducens Nerve to Glossopharyngeal Nerve, Percutaneous Endoscopic Approach

00XL4ZQ Transfer Abducens Nerve to Vagus Nerve, Percutaneous Endoscopic Approach

00XL4ZR Transfer Abducens Nerve to Accessory Nerve, Percutaneous Endoscopic Approach

00XL4ZS Transfer Abducens Nerve to Hypoglossal Nerve, Percutaneous Endoscopic Approach

00XM0ZF Transfer Facial Nerve to Olfactory Nerve, Open Approach

00XM0ZG Transfer Facial Nerve to Optic Nerve, Open Approach

00XM0ZH Transfer Facial Nerve to Oculomotor Nerve, Open Approach

00XM0ZJ Transfer Facial Nerve to Trochlear Nerve, Open Approach

00XM0ZK Transfer Facial Nerve to Trigeminal Nerve, Open Approach

---

♀ Female-only   ♂ Male-only   ⬤ Limited Coverage   ⬤ Non-OR   🅷🅰🅲 HAC-associated procedure   ⬤ Non-covered procedures   ✚ Combination

00XM0ZL   Transfer Facial Nerve to Abducens Nerve, Open Approach
00XM0ZM   Transfer Facial Nerve to Facial Nerve, Open Approach
00XM0ZN   Transfer Facial Nerve to Acoustic Nerve, Open Approach
00XM0ZP   Transfer Facial Nerve to Glossopharyngeal Nerve, Open Approach
00XM0ZQ   Transfer Facial Nerve to Vagus Nerve, Open Approach
00XM0ZR   Transfer Facial Nerve to Accessory Nerve, Open Approach
00XM0ZS   Transfer Facial Nerve to Hypoglossal Nerve, Open Approach
00XM4ZF   Transfer Facial Nerve to Olfactory Nerve, Percutaneous Endoscopic Approach
00XM4ZG   Transfer Facial Nerve to Optic Nerve, Percutaneous Endoscopic Approach
00XM4ZH   Transfer Facial Nerve to Oculomotor Nerve, Percutaneous Endoscopic Approach
00XM4ZJ   Transfer Facial Nerve to Trochlear Nerve, Percutaneous Endoscopic Approach
00XM4ZK   Transfer Facial Nerve to Trigeminal Nerve, Percutaneous Endoscopic Approach
00XM4ZL   Transfer Facial Nerve to Abducens Nerve, Percutaneous Endoscopic Approach
00XM4ZM   Transfer Facial Nerve to Facial Nerve, Percutaneous Endoscopic Approach
00XM4ZN   Transfer Facial Nerve to Acoustic Nerve, Percutaneous Endoscopic Approach
00XM4ZP   Transfer Facial Nerve to Glossopharyngeal Nerve, Percutaneous Endoscopic Approach
00XM4ZQ   Transfer Facial Nerve to Vagus Nerve, Percutaneous Endoscopic Approach
00XM4ZR   Transfer Facial Nerve to Accessory Nerve, Percutaneous Endoscopic Approach
00XM4ZS   Transfer Facial Nerve to Hypoglossal Nerve, Percutaneous Endoscopic Approach
00XN0ZF   Transfer Acoustic Nerve to Olfactory Nerve, Open Approach
00XN0ZG   Transfer Acoustic Nerve to Optic Nerve, Open Approach
00XN0ZH   Transfer Acoustic Nerve to Oculomotor Nerve, Open Approach
00XN0ZJ   Transfer Acoustic Nerve to Trochlear Nerve, Open Approach
00XN0ZK   Transfer Acoustic Nerve to Trigeminal Nerve, Open Approach
00XN0ZL   Transfer Acoustic Nerve to Abducens Nerve, Open Approach
00XN0ZM   Transfer Acoustic Nerve to Facial Nerve, Open Approach
00XN0ZN   Transfer Acoustic Nerve to Acoustic Nerve, Open Approach
00XN0ZP   Transfer Acoustic Nerve to Glossopharyngeal Nerve, Open Approach
00XN0ZQ   Transfer Acoustic Nerve to Vagus Nerve, Open Approach
00XN0ZR   Transfer Acoustic Nerve to Accessory Nerve, Open Approach
00XN0ZS   Transfer Acoustic Nerve to Hypoglossal Nerve, Open Approach
00XN4ZF   Transfer Acoustic Nerve to Olfactory Nerve, Percutaneous Endoscopic Approach
00XN4ZG   Transfer Acoustic Nerve to Optic Nerve, Percutaneous Endoscopic Approach
00XN4ZH   Transfer Acoustic Nerve to Oculomotor Nerve, Percutaneous Endoscopic Approach
00XN4ZJ   Transfer Acoustic Nerve to Trochlear Nerve, Percutaneous Endoscopic Approach
00XN4ZK   Transfer Acoustic Nerve to Trigeminal Nerve, Percutaneous Endoscopic Approach
00XN4ZL   Transfer Acoustic Nerve to Abducens Nerve, Percutaneous Endoscopic Approach
00XN4ZM   Transfer Acoustic Nerve to Facial Nerve, Percutaneous Endoscopic Approach
00XN4ZN   Transfer Acoustic Nerve to Acoustic Nerve, Percutaneous Endoscopic Approach
00XN4ZP   Transfer Acoustic Nerve to Glossopharyngeal Nerve, Percutaneous Endoscopic Approach
00XN4ZQ   Transfer Acoustic Nerve to Vagus Nerve, Percutaneous Endoscopic Approach
00XN4ZR   Transfer Acoustic Nerve to Accessory Nerve, Percutaneous Endoscopic Approach
00XN4ZS   Transfer Acoustic Nerve to Hypoglossal Nerve, Percutaneous Endoscopic Approach
00XP0ZF   Transfer Glossopharyngeal Nerve to Olfactory Nerve, Open Approach
00XP0ZG   Transfer Glossopharyngeal Nerve to Optic Nerve, Open Approach
00XP0ZH   Transfer Glossopharyngeal Nerve to Oculomotor Nerve, Open Approach

00XP0ZJ   Transfer Glossopharyngeal Nerve to Trochlear Nerve, Open Approach
00XP0ZK   Transfer Glossopharyngeal Nerve to Trigeminal Nerve, Open Approach
00XP0ZL   Transfer Glossopharyngeal Nerve to Abducens Nerve, Open Approach
00XP0ZM   Transfer Glossopharyngeal Nerve to Facial Nerve, Open Approach
00XP0ZN   Transfer Glossopharyngeal Nerve to Acoustic Nerve, Open Approach
00XP0ZP   Transfer Glossopharyngeal Nerve to Glossopharyngeal Nerve, Open Approach
00XP0ZQ   Transfer Glossopharyngeal Nerve to Vagus Nerve, Open Approach
00XP0ZR   Transfer Glossopharyngeal Nerve to Accessory Nerve, Open Approach
00XP0ZS   Transfer Glossopharyngeal Nerve to Hypoglossal Nerve, Open Approach
00XP4ZF   Transfer Glossopharyngeal Nerve to Olfactory Nerve, Percutaneous Endoscopic Approach
00XP4ZG   Transfer Glossopharyngeal Nerve to Optic Nerve, Percutaneous Endoscopic Approach
00XP4ZH   Transfer Glossopharyngeal Nerve to Oculomotor Nerve, Percutaneous Endoscopic Approach
00XP4ZJ   Transfer Glossopharyngeal Nerve to Trochlear Nerve, Percutaneous Endoscopic Approach
00XP4ZK   Transfer Glossopharyngeal Nerve to Trigeminal Nerve, Percutaneous Endoscopic Approach
00XP4ZL   Transfer Glossopharyngeal Nerve to Abducens Nerve, Percutaneous Endoscopic Approach
00XP4ZM   Transfer Glossopharyngeal Nerve to Facial Nerve, Percutaneous Endoscopic Approach
00XP4ZN   Transfer Glossopharyngeal Nerve to Acoustic Nerve, Percutaneous Endoscopic Approach
00XP4ZP   Transfer Glossopharyngeal Nerve to Glossopharyngeal Nerve, Percutaneous Endoscopic Approach
00XP4ZQ   Transfer Glossopharyngeal Nerve to Vagus Nerve, Percutaneous Endoscopic Approach
00XP4ZR   Transfer Glossopharyngeal Nerve to Accessory Nerve, Percutaneous Endoscopic Approach
00XP4ZS   Transfer Glossopharyngeal Nerve to Hypoglossal Nerve, Percutaneous Endoscopic Approach
00XQ0ZF   Transfer Vagus Nerve to Olfactory Nerve, Open Approach
00XQ0ZG   Transfer Vagus Nerve to Optic Nerve, Open Approach
00XQ0ZH   Transfer Vagus Nerve to Oculomotor Nerve, Open Approach
00XQ0ZJ   Transfer Vagus Nerve to Trochlear Nerve, Open Approach
00XQ0ZK   Transfer Vagus Nerve to Trigeminal Nerve, Open Approach
00XQ0ZL   Transfer Vagus Nerve to Abducens Nerve, Open Approach
00XQ0ZM   Transfer Vagus Nerve to Facial Nerve, Open Approach
00XQ0ZN   Transfer Vagus Nerve to Acoustic Nerve, Open Approach
00XQ0ZP   Transfer Vagus Nerve to Glossopharyngeal Nerve, Open Approach
00XQ0ZQ   Transfer Vagus Nerve to Vagus Nerve, Open Approach
00XQ0ZR   Transfer Vagus Nerve to Accessory Nerve, Open Approach
00XQ0ZS   Transfer Vagus Nerve to Hypoglossal Nerve, Open Approach
00XQ4ZF   Transfer Vagus Nerve to Olfactory Nerve, Percutaneous Endoscopic Approach
00XQ4ZG   Transfer Vagus Nerve to Optic Nerve, Percutaneous Endoscopic Approach
00XQ4ZH   Transfer Vagus Nerve to Oculomotor Nerve, Percutaneous Endoscopic Approach
00XQ4ZJ   Transfer Vagus Nerve to Trochlear Nerve, Percutaneous Endoscopic Approach
00XQ4ZK   Transfer Vagus Nerve to Trigeminal Nerve, Percutaneous Endoscopic Approach
00XQ4ZL   Transfer Vagus Nerve to Abducens Nerve, Percutaneous Endoscopic Approach
00XQ4ZM   Transfer Vagus Nerve to Facial Nerve, Percutaneous Endoscopic Approach
00XQ4ZN   Transfer Vagus Nerve to Acoustic Nerve, Percutaneous Endoscopic Approach
00XQ4ZP   Transfer Vagus Nerve to Glossopharyngeal Nerve, Percutaneous Endoscopic Approach
00XQ4ZQ   Transfer Vagus Nerve to Vagus Nerve, Percutaneous Endoscopic Approach

00XQ4ZR Transfer Vagus Nerve to Accessory Nerve, Percutaneous Endoscopic Approach

00XQ4ZS Transfer Vagus Nerve to Hypoglossal Nerve, Percutaneous Endoscopic Approach

00XR0ZF Transfer Accessory Nerve to Olfactory Nerve, Open Approach

00XR0ZG Transfer Accessory Nerve to Optic Nerve, Open Approach

00XR0ZH Transfer Accessory Nerve to Oculomotor Nerve, Open Approach

00XR0ZJ Transfer Accessory Nerve to Trochlear Nerve, Open Approach

00XR0ZK Transfer Accessory Nerve to Trigeminal Nerve, Open Approach

00XR0ZL Transfer Accessory Nerve to Abducens Nerve, Open Approach

00XR0ZM Transfer Accessory Nerve to Facial Nerve, Open Approach

00XR0ZN Transfer Accessory Nerve to Acoustic Nerve, Open Approach

00XR0ZP Transfer Accessory Nerve to Glossopharyngeal Nerve, Open Approach

00XR0ZQ Transfer Accessory Nerve to Vagus Nerve, Open Approach

00XR0ZR Transfer Accessory Nerve to Accessory Nerve, Open Approach

00XR0ZS Transfer Accessory Nerve to Hypoglossal Nerve, Open Approach

00XR4ZF Transfer Accessory Nerve to Olfactory Nerve, Percutaneous Endoscopic Approach

00XR4ZG Transfer Accessory Nerve to Optic Nerve, Percutaneous Endoscopic Approach

00XR4ZH Transfer Accessory Nerve to Oculomotor Nerve, Percutaneous Endoscopic Approach

00XR4ZJ Transfer Accessory Nerve to Trochlear Nerve, Percutaneous Endoscopic Approach

00XR4ZK Transfer Accessory Nerve to Trigeminal Nerve, Percutaneous Endoscopic Approach

00XR4ZL Transfer Accessory Nerve to Abducens Nerve, Percutaneous Endoscopic Approach

00XR4ZM Transfer Accessory Nerve to Facial Nerve, Percutaneous Endoscopic Approach

00XR4ZN Transfer Accessory Nerve to Acoustic Nerve, Percutaneous Endoscopic Approach

00XR4ZP Transfer Accessory Nerve to Glossopharyngeal Nerve, Percutaneous Endoscopic Approach

00XR4ZQ Transfer Accessory Nerve to Vagus Nerve, Percutaneous Endoscopic Approach

00XR4ZR Transfer Accessory Nerve to Accessory Nerve, Percutaneous Endoscopic Approach

00XR4ZS Transfer Accessory Nerve to Hypoglossal Nerve, Percutaneous Endoscopic Approach

00XS0ZF Transfer Hypoglossal Nerve to Olfactory Nerve, Open Approach

00XS0ZG Transfer Hypoglossal Nerve to Optic Nerve, Open Approach

00XS0ZH Transfer Hypoglossal Nerve to Oculomotor Nerve, Open Approach

00XS0ZJ Transfer Hypoglossal Nerve to Trochlear Nerve, Open Approach

00XS0ZK Transfer Hypoglossal Nerve to Trigeminal Nerve, Open Approach

00XS0ZL Transfer Hypoglossal Nerve to Abducens Nerve, Open Approach

00XS0ZM Transfer Hypoglossal Nerve to Facial Nerve, Open Approach

00XS0ZN Transfer Hypoglossal Nerve to Acoustic Nerve, Open Approach

00XS0ZP Transfer Hypoglossal Nerve to Glossopharyngeal Nerve, Open Approach

00XS0ZQ Transfer Hypoglossal Nerve to Vagus Nerve, Open Approach

00XS0ZR Transfer Hypoglossal Nerve to Accessory Nerve, Open Approach

00XS0ZS Transfer Hypoglossal Nerve to Hypoglossal Nerve, Open Approach

00XS4ZF Transfer Hypoglossal Nerve to Olfactory Nerve, Percutaneous Endoscopic Approach

00XS4ZG Transfer Hypoglossal Nerve to Optic Nerve, Percutaneous Endoscopic Approach

00XS4ZH Transfer Hypoglossal Nerve to Oculomotor Nerve, Percutaneous Endoscopic Approach

00XS4ZJ Transfer Hypoglossal Nerve to Trochlear Nerve, Percutaneous Endoscopic Approach

00XS4ZK Transfer Hypoglossal Nerve to Trigeminal Nerve, Percutaneous Endoscopic Approach

00XS4ZL Transfer Hypoglossal Nerve to Abducens Nerve, Percutaneous Endoscopic Approach

00XS4ZM Transfer Hypoglossal Nerve to Facial Nerve, Percutaneous Endoscopic Approach

00XS4ZN Transfer Hypoglossal Nerve to Acoustic Nerve, Percutaneous Endoscopic Approach

00XS4ZP Transfer Hypoglossal Nerve to Glossopharyngeal Nerve, Percutaneous Endoscopic Approach

00XS4ZQ Transfer Hypoglossal Nerve to Vagus Nerve, Percutaneous Endoscopic Approach

Peripheral Nervous System

Peripheral Nervous System

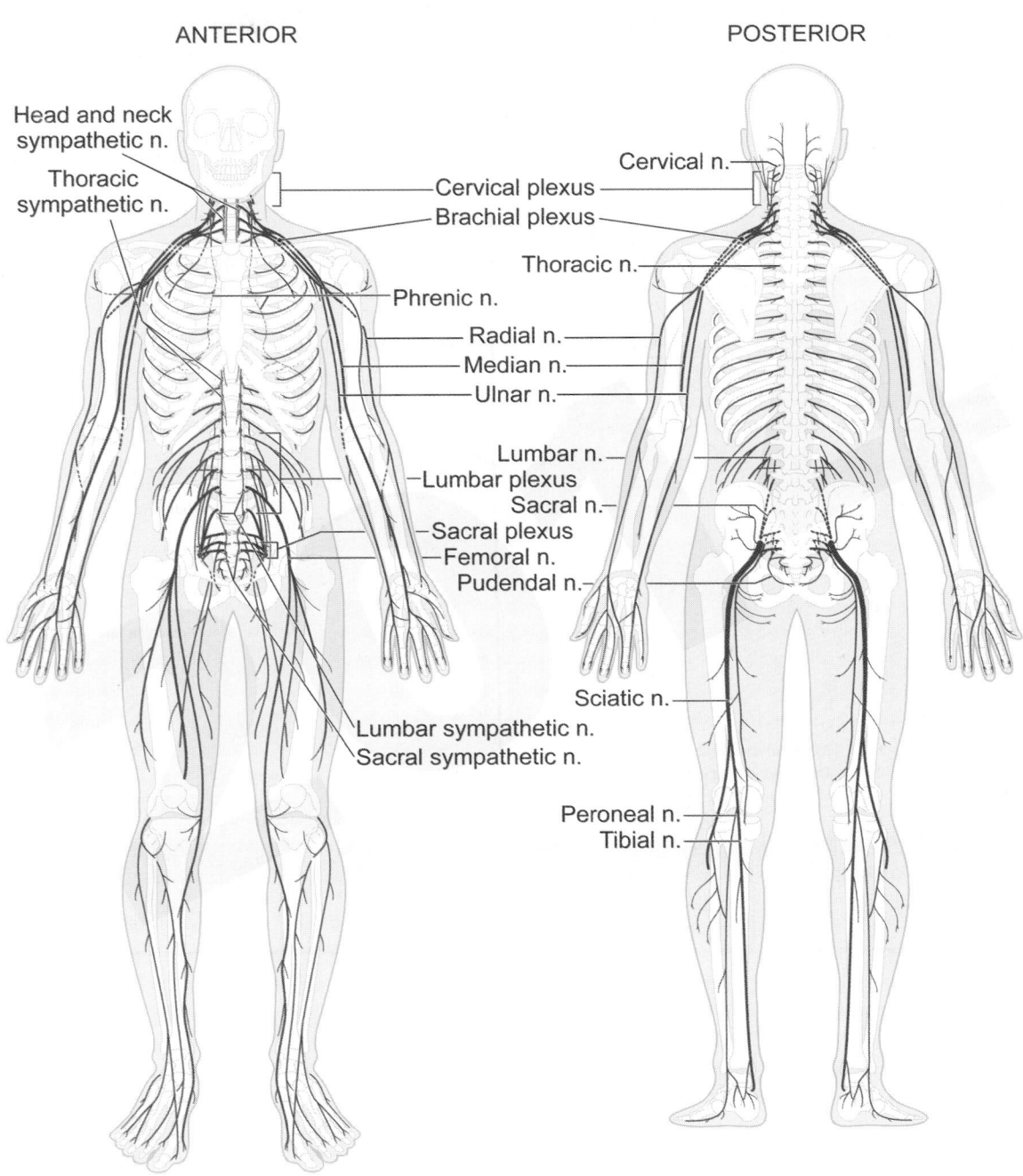

ANTERIOR

POSTERIOR

Head and neck sympathetic n.

Thoracic sympathetic n.

Cervical n.

Cervical plexus
Brachial plexus

Thoracic n.

Phrenic n.

Radial n.

Median n.

Ulnar n.

Lumbar n.
Lumbar plexus
Sacral n.
Sacral plexus
Femoral n.
Pudendal n.

Lumbar sympathetic n.
Sacral sympathetic n.

Sciatic n.

Peroneal n.
Tibial n.

Medical and Surgical Section (0)

012

Spinal Column

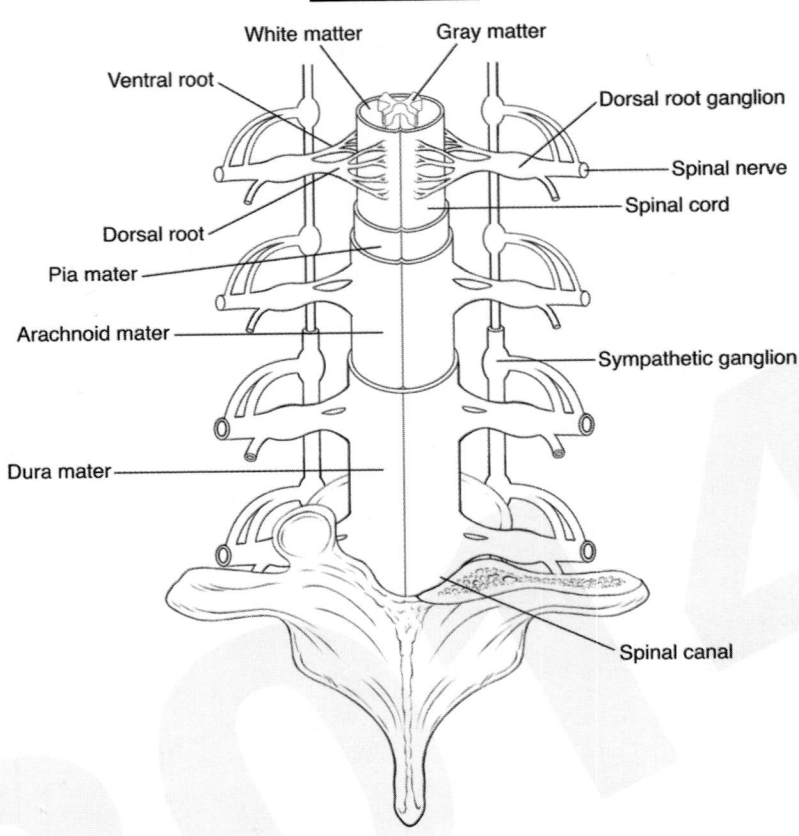

Spinal Column diagram labels: White matter, Gray matter, Ventral root, Dorsal root ganglion, Spinal nerve, Spinal cord, Dorsal root, Pia mater, Arachnoid mater, Sympathetic ganglion, Dura mater, Spinal canal

Peripheral Nervous System Tables 012–01X

Section	**0**	**Medical and Surgical**	
Body System	**1**	**Peripheral Nervous System**	
Operation	**2**	**Change:** Taking out or off a device from a body part and putting back an identical or similar device in or on the same body part without cutting or puncturing the skin or a mucous membrane	

Body Part (4ᵗʰ)	Approach (5ᵗʰ)	Device (6ᵗʰ)	Qualifier (7ᵗʰ)
Y Peripheral Nerve	**X** External	**0** Drainage Device **Y** Other Device	**Z** No Qualifier

Section	0	**Medical and Surgical**
Body System	1	**Peripheral Nervous System**
Operation	5	**Destruction:** Physical eradication of all or a portion of a body part by the direct use of energy, force, or a destructive agent

Body Part (4th)	Approach (5th)	Device (6th)	Qualifier (7th)
0 Cervical Plexus 1 Cervical Nerve 2 Phrenic Nerve 3 Brachial Plexus 4 Ulnar Nerve 5 Median Nerve 6 Radial Nerve 8 Thoracic Nerve 9 Lumbar Plexus A Lumbosacral Plexus B Lumbar Nerve C Pudendal Nerve D Femoral Nerve F Sciatic Nerve G Tibial Nerve H Peroneal Nerve K Head and Neck Sympathetic Nerve L Thoracic Sympathetic Nerve M Abdominal Sympathetic Nerve N Lumbar Sympathetic Nerve P Sacral Sympathetic Nerve Q Sacral Plexus R Sacral Nerve	0 Open 3 Percutaneous 4 Percutaneous Endoscopic	Z No Device	Z No Qualifier

Section	0	**Medical and Surgical**
Body System	1	**Peripheral Nervous System**
Operation	8	**Division:** Cutting into a body part, without draining fluids and/or gases from the body part, in order to separate or transect a body part

Body Part (4th)	Approach (5th)	Device (6th)	Qualifier (7th)
0 Cervical Plexus 1 Cervical Nerve 2 Phrenic Nerve 3 Brachial Plexus 4 Ulnar Nerve 5 Median Nerve 6 Radial Nerve 8 Thoracic Nerve 9 Lumbar Plexus A Lumbosacral Plexus B Lumbar Nerve C Pudendal Nerve D Femoral Nerve F Sciatic Nerve G Tibial Nerve H Peroneal Nerve K Head and Neck Sympathetic Nerve L Thoracic Sympathetic Nerve M Abdominal Sympathetic Nerve N Lumbar Sympathetic Nerve P Sacral Sympathetic Nerve Q Sacral Plexus R Sacral Nerve	0 Open 3 Percutaneous 4 Percutaneous Endoscopic	Z No Device	Z No Qualifier

Section	0	Medical and Surgical
Body System	1	Peripheral Nervous System
Operation	9	**Drainage:** Taking or letting out fluids and/or gases from a body part

Body Part (4th)	Approach (5th)	Device (6th)	Qualifier (7th)
0 Cervical Plexus 1 Cervical Nerve 2 Phrenic Nerve 3 Brachial Plexus 4 Ulnar Nerve 5 Median Nerve 6 Radial Nerve 8 Thoracic Nerve 9 Lumbar Plexus A Lumbosacral Plexus B Lumbar Nerve C Pudendal Nerve D Femoral Nerve F Sciatic Nerve G Tibial Nerve H Peroneal Nerve K Head and Neck Sympathetic Nerve L Thoracic Sympathetic Nerve M Abdominal Sympathetic Nerve N Lumbar Sympathetic Nerve P Sacral Sympathetic Nerve Q Sacral Plexus R Sacral Nerve	0 Open 3 Percutaneous 4 Percutaneous Endoscopic	0 Drainage Device	Z No Qualifier
0 Cervical Plexus 1 Cervical Nerve 2 Phrenic Nerve 3 Brachial Plexus 4 Ulnar Nerve 5 Median Nerve 6 Radial Nerve 8 Thoracic Nerve 9 Lumbar Plexus A Lumbosacral Plexus B Lumbar Nerve C Pudendal Nerve D Femoral Nerve F Sciatic Nerve G Tibial Nerve H Peroneal Nerve K Head and Neck Sympathetic Nerve L Thoracic Sympathetic Nerve M Abdominal Sympathetic Nerve N Lumbar Sympathetic Nerve P Sacral Sympathetic Nerve Q Sacral Plexus R Sacral Nerve	0 Open 3 Percutaneous 4 Percutaneous Endoscopic	Z No Device	X Diagnostic Z No Qualifier

Section   **0**   **Medical and Surgical**
Body System   **1**   **Peripheral Nervous System**
Operation   **B**   **Excision:** Cutting out or off, without replacement, a portion of a body part

Body Part (4th)	Approach (5th)	Device (6th)	Qualifier (7th)
0 Cervical Plexus 1 Cervical Nerve 2 Phrenic Nerve 3 Brachial Plexus 4 Ulnar Nerve 5 Median Nerve 6 Radial Nerve 8 Thoracic Nerve 9 Lumbar Plexus A Lumbosacral Plexus B Lumbar Nerve C Pudendal Nerve D Femoral Nerve F Sciatic Nerve G Tibial Nerve H Peroneal Nerve K Head and Neck Sympathetic Nerve L Thoracic Sympathetic Nerve M Abdominal Sympathetic Nerve N Lumbar Sympathetic Nerve P Sacral Sympathetic Nerve Q Sacral Plexus R Sacral Nerve	0 Open 3 Percutaneous 4 Percutaneous Endoscopic	Z No Device	X Diagnostic Z No Qualifier

Section   **0**   **Medical and Surgical**
Body System   **1**   **Peripheral Nervous System**
Operation   **C**   **Extirpation:** Taking or cutting out solid matter from a body part

Body Part (4th)	Approach (5th)	Device (6th)	Qualifier (7th)
0 Cervical Plexus 1 Cervical Nerve 2 Phrenic Nerve 3 Brachial Plexus 4 Ulnar Nerve 5 Median Nerve 6 Radial Nerve 8 Thoracic Nerve 9 Lumbar Plexus A Lumbosacral Plexus B Lumbar Nerve C Pudendal Nerve D Femoral Nerve F Sciatic Nerve G Tibial Nerve H Peroneal Nerve K Head and Neck Sympathetic Nerve L Thoracic Sympathetic Nerve M Abdominal Sympathetic Nerve N Lumbar Sympathetic Nerve P Sacral Sympathetic Nerve Q Sacral Plexus R Sacral Nerve	0 Open 3 Percutaneous 4 Percutaneous Endoscopic	Z No Device	Z No Qualifier

Section	0	Medical and Surgical
Body System	1	Peripheral Nervous System
Operation	D	**Extraction:** Pulling or stripping out or off all or a portion of a body part by the use of force

Body Part (4th)	Approach (5th)	Device (6th)	Qualifier (7th)
0 Cervical Plexus 1 Cervical Nerve 2 Phrenic Nerve 3 Brachial Plexus 4 Ulnar Nerve 5 Median Nerve 6 Radial Nerve 8 Thoracic Nerve 9 Lumbar Plexus A Lumbosacral Plexus B Lumbar Nerve C Pudendal Nerve D Femoral Nerve F Sciatic Nerve G Tibial Nerve H Peroneal Nerve K Head and Neck Sympathetic Nerve L Thoracic Sympathetic Nerve M Abdominal Sympathetic Nerve N Lumbar Sympathetic Nerve P Sacral Sympathetic Nerve Q Sacral Plexus R Sacral Nerve	0 Open 3 Percutaneous 4 Percutaneous Endoscopic	Z No Device	Z No Qualifier

Section	0	Medical and Surgical
Body System	1	Peripheral Nervous System
Operation	H	**Insertion:** Putting in a nonbiological appliance that monitors, assists, performs, or prevents a physiological function but does not physically take the place of a body part

Body Part (4th)	Approach (5th)	Device (6th)	Qualifier (7th)
Y Peripheral Nerve	0 Open 3 Percutaneous 4 Percutaneous Endoscopic	2 Monitoring Device M Neurostimulator Lead	Z No Qualifier

Section	0	Medical and Surgical
Body System	1	Peripheral Nervous System
Operation	J	**Inspection:** Visually and/or manually exploring a body part

Body Part (4th)	Approach (5th)	Device (6th)	Qualifier (7th)
Y Peripheral Nerve	0 Open 3 Percutaneous 4 Percutaneous Endoscopic	Z No Device	Z No Qualifier

Section	0	Medical and Surgical
Body System	1	Peripheral Nervous System
Operation	N	**Release:** Freeing a body part from an abnormal physical constraint by cutting or by the use of force

Body Part (4th)	Approach (5th)	Device (6th)	Qualifier (7th)
0 Cervical Plexus 1 Cervical Nerve 2 Phrenic Nerve 3 Brachial Plexus 4 Ulnar Nerve 5 Median Nerve 6 Radial Nerve 8 Thoracic Nerve 9 Lumbar Plexus A Lumbosacral Plexus B Lumbar Nerve C Pudendal Nerve D Femoral Nerve F Sciatic Nerve G Tibial Nerve H Peroneal Nerve K Head and Neck Sympathetic Nerve L Thoracic Sympathetic Nerve M Abdominal Sympathetic Nerve N Lumbar Sympathetic Nerve P Sacral Sympathetic Nerve Q Sacral Plexus R Sacral Nerve	0 Open 3 Percutaneous 4 Percutaneous Endoscopic	Z No Device	Z No Qualifier

Section	0	Medical and Surgical
Body System	1	Peripheral Nervous System
Operation	P	**Removal:** Taking out or off a device from a body part

Body Part (4th)	Approach (5th)	Device (6th)	Qualifier (7th)
Y Peripheral Nerve	0 Open 3 Percutaneous 4 Percutaneous Endoscopic	0 Drainage Device 2 Monitoring Device 7 Autologous Tissue Substitute M Neurostimulator Lead	Z No Qualifier
Y Peripheral Nerve	X External	0 Drainage Device 2 Monitoring Device M Neurostimulator Lead	Z No Qualifier

Section	0	Medical and Surgical
Body System	1	Peripheral Nervous System
Operation	Q	**Repair:** Restoring, to the extent possible, a body part to its normal anatomic structure and function

Body Part (4th)	Approach (5th)	Device (6th)	Qualifier (7th)
0 Cervical Plexus 1 Cervical Nerve 2 Phrenic Nerve 3 Brachial Plexus 4 Ulnar Nerve 5 Median Nerve 6 Radial Nerve 8 Thoracic Nerve 9 Lumbar Plexus A Lumbosacral Plexus B Lumbar Nerve C Pudendal Nerve D Femoral Nerve F Sciatic Nerve G Tibial Nerve H Peroneal Nerve K Head and Neck Sympathetic Nerve L Thoracic Sympathetic Nerve M Abdominal Sympathetic Nerve N Lumbar Sympathetic Nerve P Sacral Sympathetic Nerve Q Sacral Plexus R Sacral Nerve	0 Open 3 Percutaneous 4 Percutaneous Endoscopic	Z No Device	Z No Qualifier

Section	0	Medical and Surgical
Body System	1	Peripheral Nervous System
Operation	S	**Reposition:** Moving to its normal location, or other suitable location, all or a portion of a body part

Body Part (4th)	Approach (5th)	Device (6th)	Qualifier (7th)
0 Cervical Plexus 1 Cervical Nerve 2 Phrenic Nerve 3 Brachial Plexus 4 Ulnar Nerve 5 Median Nerve 6 Radial Nerve 8 Thoracic Nerve 9 Lumbar Plexus A Lumbosacral Plexus B Lumbar Nerve C Pudendal Nerve D Femoral Nerve F Sciatic Nerve G Tibial Nerve H Peroneal Nerve Q Sacral Plexus R Sacral Nerve	0 Open 3 Percutaneous 4 Percutaneous Endoscopic	Z No Device	Z No Qualifier

Section	0	Medical and Surgical
Body System	1	Peripheral Nervous System
Operation	U	**Supplement:** Putting in or on biological or synthetic material that physically reinforces and/or augments the function of a portion of a body part

Body Part (4th)	Approach (5th)	Device (6th)	Qualifier (7th)
1 Cervical Nerve 2 Phrenic Nerve 4 Ulnar Nerve 5 Median Nerve 6 Radial Nerve 8 Thoracic Nerve B Lumbar Nerve C Pudendal Nerve D Femoral Nerve F Sciatic Nerve G Tibial Nerve H Peroneal Nerve R Sacral Nerve	0 Open 3 Percutaneous 4 Percutaneous Endoscopic	7 Autologous Tissue Substitute	Z No Qualifier

Section	0	Medical and Surgical
Body System	1	Peripheral Nervous System
Operation	W	**Revision:** Correcting, to the extent possible, a portion of a malfunctioning device or the position of a displaced device

Body Part (4th)	Approach (5th)	Device (6th)	Qualifier (7th)
Y Peripheral Nerve	0 Open 3 Percutaneous 4 Percutaneous Endoscopic X External	0 Drainage Device 2 Monitoring Device 7 Autologous Tissue Substitute M Neurostimulator Lead	Z No Qualifier

Section	0	Medical and Surgical
Body System	1	Peripheral Nervous System
Operation	X	**Transfer:** Moving, without taking out, all or a portion of a body part to another location to take over the function of all or a portion of a body part

Body Part (4th)	Approach (5th)	Device (6th)	Qualifier (7th)
1 Cervical Nerve 2 Phrenic Nerve	0 Open 4 Percutaneous Endoscopic	Z No Device	1 Cervical Nerve 2 Phrenic Nerve
4 Ulnar Nerve 5 Median Nerve 6 Radial Nerve	0 Open 4 Percutaneous Endoscopic	Z No Device	4 Ulnar Nerve 5 Median Nerve 6 Radial Nerve
8 Thoracic Nerve	0 Open 4 Percutaneous Endoscopic	Z No Device	8 Thoracic Nerve
B Lumbar Nerve C Pudendal Nerve	0 Open 4 Percutaneous Endoscopic	Z No Device	B Lumbar Nerve C Perineal Nerve
D Femoral Nerve F Sciatic Nerve G Tibial Nerve H Peroneal Nerve	0 Open 4 Percutaneous Endoscopic	Z No Device	D Femoral Nerve F Sciatic Nerve G Tibial Nerve H Peroneal Nerve

Peripheral Nervous System Code Listing 012–01X

012 – Peripheral Nervous System, Change

Review Coding Guideline B6.1c

012YX0Z	Change Drainage Device in Peripheral Nerve, External Approach
012YXYZ	Change Other Device in Peripheral Nerve, External Approach

015 – Peripheral Nervous System, Destruction

01500ZZ	Destruction of Cervical Plexus, Open Approach
01503ZZ	Destruction of Cervical Plexus, Percutaneous Approach
01504ZZ	Destruction of Cervical Plexus, Percutaneous Endoscopic Approach
01510ZZ	Destruction of Cervical Nerve, Open Approach
01513ZZ	Destruction of Cervical Nerve, Percutaneous Approach
01514ZZ	Destruction of Cervical Nerve, Percutaneous Endoscopic Approach
01520ZZ	Destruction of Phrenic Nerve, Open Approach
01523ZZ	Destruction of Phrenic Nerve, Percutaneous Approach
01524ZZ	Destruction of Phrenic Nerve, Percutaneous Endoscopic Approach
01530ZZ	Destruction of Brachial Plexus, Open Approach
01533ZZ	Destruction of Brachial Plexus, Percutaneous Approach
01534ZZ	Destruction of Brachial Plexus, Percutaneous Endoscopic Approach
01540ZZ	Destruction of Ulnar Nerve, Open Approach
01543ZZ	Destruction of Ulnar Nerve, Percutaneous Approach
01544ZZ	Destruction of Ulnar Nerve, Percutaneous Endoscopic Approach
01550ZZ	Destruction of Median Nerve, Open Approach
01553ZZ	Destruction of Median Nerve, Percutaneous Approach
01554ZZ	Destruction of Median Nerve, Percutaneous Endoscopic Approach
01560ZZ	Destruction of Radial Nerve, Open Approach
01563ZZ	Destruction of Radial Nerve, Percutaneous Approach
01564ZZ	Destruction of Radial Nerve, Percutaneous Endoscopic Approach
01580ZZ	Destruction of Thoracic Nerve, Open Approach
01583ZZ	Destruction of Thoracic Nerve, Percutaneous Approach
01584ZZ	Destruction of Thoracic Nerve, Percutaneous Endoscopic Approach
01590ZZ	Destruction of Lumbar Plexus, Open Approach
01593ZZ	Destruction of Lumbar Plexus, Percutaneous Approach
01594ZZ	Destruction of Lumbar Plexus, Percutaneous Endoscopic Approach
015A0ZZ	Destruction of Lumbosacral Plexus, Open Approach
015A3ZZ	Destruction of Lumbosacral Plexus, Percutaneous Approach
015A4ZZ	Destruction of Lumbosacral Plexus, Percutaneous Endoscopic Approach
015B0ZZ	Destruction of Lumbar Nerve, Open Approach
015B3ZZ	Destruction of Lumbar Nerve, Percutaneous Approach
015B4ZZ	Destruction of Lumbar Nerve, Percutaneous Endoscopic Approach
015C0ZZ	Destruction of Pudendal Nerve, Open Approach
015C3ZZ	Destruction of Pudendal Nerve, Percutaneous Approach
015C4ZZ	Destruction of Pudendal Nerve, Percutaneous Endoscopic Approach
015D0ZZ	Destruction of Femoral Nerve, Open Approach
015D3ZZ	Destruction of Femoral Nerve, Percutaneous Approach
015D4ZZ	Destruction of Femoral Nerve, Percutaneous Endoscopic Approach
015F0ZZ	Destruction of Sciatic Nerve, Open Approach
015F3ZZ	Destruction of Sciatic Nerve, Percutaneous Approach
015F4ZZ	Destruction of Sciatic Nerve, Percutaneous Endoscopic Approach
015G0ZZ	Destruction of Tibial Nerve, Open Approach
015G3ZZ	Destruction of Tibial Nerve, Percutaneous Approach
015G4ZZ	Destruction of Tibial Nerve, Percutaneous Endoscopic Approach
015H0ZZ	Destruction of Peroneal Nerve, Open Approach
015H3ZZ	Destruction of Peroneal Nerve, Percutaneous Approach
015H4ZZ	Destruction of Peroneal Nerve, Percutaneous Endoscopic Approach
015K0ZZ	Destruction of Head and Neck Sympathetic Nerve, Open Approach
015K3ZZ	Destruction of Head and Neck Sympathetic Nerve, Percutaneous Approach
015K4ZZ	Destruction of Head and Neck Sympathetic Nerve, Percutaneous Endoscopic Approach
015L0ZZ	Destruction of Thoracic Sympathetic Nerve, Open Approach
015L3ZZ	Destruction of Thoracic Sympathetic Nerve, Percutaneous Approach
015L4ZZ	Destruction of Thoracic Sympathetic Nerve, Percutaneous Endoscopic Approach
015M0ZZ	Destruction of Abdominal Sympathetic Nerve, Open Approach
015M3ZZ	Destruction of Abdominal Sympathetic Nerve, Percutaneous Approach
015M4ZZ	Destruction of Abdominal Sympathetic Nerve, Percutaneous Endoscopic Approach
015N0ZZ	Destruction of Lumbar Sympathetic Nerve, Open Approach
015N3ZZ	Destruction of Lumbar Sympathetic Nerve, Percutaneous Approach
015N4ZZ	Destruction of Lumbar Sympathetic Nerve, Percutaneous Endoscopic Approach
015P0ZZ	Destruction of Sacral Sympathetic Nerve, Open Approach
015P3ZZ	Destruction of Sacral Sympathetic Nerve, Percutaneous Approach
015P4ZZ	Destruction of Sacral Sympathetic Nerve, Percutaneous Endoscopic Approach
015Q0ZZ	Destruction of Sacral Plexus, Open Approach
015Q3ZZ	Destruction of Sacral Plexus, Percutaneous Approach
015Q4ZZ	Destruction of Sacral Plexus, Percutaneous Endoscopic Approach
015R0ZZ	Destruction of Sacral Nerve, Open Approach
015R3ZZ	Destruction of Sacral Nerve, Percutaneous Approach
015R4ZZ	Destruction of Sacral Nerve, Percutaneous Endoscopic Approach

018 – Peripheral Nervous System, Division

Review Coding Guideline B3.14

01800ZZ	Division of Cervical Plexus, Open Approach
01803ZZ	Division of Cervical Plexus, Percutaneous Approach
01804ZZ	Division of Cervical Plexus, Percutaneous Endoscopic Approach
01810ZZ	Division of Cervical Nerve, Open Approach
01813ZZ	Division of Cervical Nerve, Percutaneous Approach
01814ZZ	Division of Cervical Nerve, Percutaneous Endoscopic Approach
01820ZZ	Division of Phrenic Nerve, Open Approach
01823ZZ	Division of Phrenic Nerve, Percutaneous Approach
01824ZZ	Division of Phrenic Nerve, Percutaneous Endoscopic Approach
01830ZZ	Division of Brachial Plexus, Open Approach
01833ZZ	Division of Brachial Plexus, Percutaneous Approach
01834ZZ	Division of Brachial Plexus, Percutaneous Endoscopic Approach
01840ZZ	Division of Ulnar Nerve, Open Approach
01843ZZ	Division of Ulnar Nerve, Percutaneous Approach
01844ZZ	Division of Ulnar Nerve, Percutaneous Endoscopic Approach
01850ZZ	Division of Median Nerve, Open Approach
01853ZZ	Division of Median Nerve, Percutaneous Approach
01854ZZ	Division of Median Nerve, Percutaneous Endoscopic Approach
01860ZZ	Division of Radial Nerve, Open Approach
01863ZZ	Division of Radial Nerve, Percutaneous Approach
01864ZZ	Division of Radial Nerve, Percutaneous Endoscopic Approach
01880ZZ	Division of Thoracic Nerve, Open Approach
01883ZZ	Division of Thoracic Nerve, Percutaneous Approach
01884ZZ	Division of Thoracic Nerve, Percutaneous Endoscopic Approach
01890ZZ	Division of Lumbar Plexus, Open Approach
01893ZZ	Division of Lumbar Plexus, Percutaneous Approach
01894ZZ	Division of Lumbar Plexus, Percutaneous Endoscopic Approach
018A0ZZ	Division of Lumbosacral Plexus, Open Approach
018A3ZZ	Division of Lumbosacral Plexus, Percutaneous Approach
018A4ZZ	Division of Lumbosacral Plexus, Percutaneous Endoscopic Approach
018B0ZZ	Division of Lumbar Nerve, Open Approach
018B3ZZ	Division of Lumbar Nerve, Percutaneous Approach
018B4ZZ	Division of Lumbar Nerve, Percutaneous Endoscopic Approach
018C0ZZ	Division of Pudendal Nerve, Open Approach
018C3ZZ	Division of Pudendal Nerve, Percutaneous Approach
018C4ZZ	Division of Pudendal Nerve, Percutaneous Endoscopic Approach
018D0ZZ	Division of Femoral Nerve, Open Approach
018D3ZZ	Division of Femoral Nerve, Percutaneous Approach
018D4ZZ	Division of Femoral Nerve, Percutaneous Endoscopic Approach

018F0ZZ	Division of Sciatic Nerve, Open Approach
018F3ZZ	Division of Sciatic Nerve, Percutaneous Approach
018F4ZZ	Division of Sciatic Nerve, Percutaneous Endoscopic Approach
018G0ZZ	Division of Tibial Nerve, Open Approach
018G3ZZ	Division of Tibial Nerve, Percutaneous Approach
018G4ZZ	Division of Tibial Nerve, Percutaneous Endoscopic Approach
018H0ZZ	Division of Peroneal Nerve, Open Approach
018H3ZZ	Division of Peroneal Nerve, Percutaneous Approach
018H4ZZ	Division of Peroneal Nerve, Percutaneous Endoscopic Approach
018K0ZZ	Division of Head and Neck Sympathetic Nerve, Open Approach
018K3ZZ	Division of Head and Neck Sympathetic Nerve, Percutaneous Approach
018K4ZZ	Division of Head and Neck Sympathetic Nerve, Percutaneous Endoscopic Approach
018L0ZZ	Division of Thoracic Sympathetic Nerve, Open Approach
018L3ZZ	Division of Thoracic Sympathetic Nerve, Percutaneous Approach
018L4ZZ	Division of Thoracic Sympathetic Nerve, Percutaneous Endoscopic Approach
018M0ZZ	Division of Abdominal Sympathetic Nerve, Open Approach
018M3ZZ	Division of Abdominal Sympathetic Nerve, Percutaneous Approach
018M4ZZ	Division of Abdominal Sympathetic Nerve, Percutaneous Endoscopic Approach
018N0ZZ	Division of Lumbar Sympathetic Nerve, Open Approach
018N3ZZ	Division of Lumbar Sympathetic Nerve, Percutaneous Approach
018N4ZZ	Division of Lumbar Sympathetic Nerve, Percutaneous Endoscopic Approach
018P0ZZ	Division of Sacral Sympathetic Nerve, Open Approach
018P3ZZ	Division of Sacral Sympathetic Nerve, Percutaneous Approach
018P4ZZ	Division of Sacral Sympathetic Nerve, Percutaneous Endoscopic Approach
018Q0ZZ	Division of Sacral Plexus, Open Approach
018Q3ZZ	Division of Sacral Plexus, Percutaneous Approach
018Q4ZZ	Division of Sacral Plexus, Percutaneous Endoscopic Approach
018R0ZZ	Division of Sacral Nerve, Open Approach
018R3ZZ	Division of Sacral Nerve, Percutaneous Approach
018R4ZZ	Division of Sacral Nerve, Percutaneous Endoscopic Approach

019 – Peripheral Nervous System, Drainage

Review Coding Guidelines B3.4a and B3.4b

Review Coding Guideline B6.2

019000Z	Drainage of Cervical Plexus with Drainage Device, Open Approach
01900ZX	Drainage of Cervical Plexus, Open Approach, Diagnostic
01900ZZ	Drainage of Cervical Plexus, Open Approach
019030Z	Drainage of Cervical Plexus with Drainage Device, Percutaneous Approach
01903ZX	Drainage of Cervical Plexus, Percutaneous Approach, Diagnostic
01903ZZ	Drainage of Cervical Plexus, Percutaneous Approach
019040Z	Drainage of Cervical Plexus with Drainage Device, Percutaneous Endoscopic Approach
01904ZX	Drainage of Cervical Plexus, Percutaneous Endoscopic Approach, Diagnostic
01904ZZ	Drainage of Cervical Plexus, Percutaneous Endoscopic Approach
019100Z	Drainage of Cervical Nerve with Drainage Device, Open Approach
01910ZX	Drainage of Cervical Nerve, Open Approach, Diagnostic
01910ZZ	Drainage of Cervical Nerve, Open Approach
019130Z	Drainage of Cervical Nerve with Drainage Device, Percutaneous Approach
01913ZX	Drainage of Cervical Nerve, Percutaneous Approach, Diagnostic
01913ZZ	Drainage of Cervical Nerve, Percutaneous Approach
019140Z	Drainage of Cervical Nerve with Drainage Device, Percutaneous Endoscopic Approach
01914ZX	Drainage of Cervical Nerve, Percutaneous Endoscopic Approach, Diagnostic
01914ZZ	Drainage of Cervical Nerve, Percutaneous Endoscopic Approach
019200Z	Drainage of Phrenic Nerve with Drainage Device, Open Approach
01920ZX	Drainage of Phrenic Nerve, Open Approach, Diagnostic
01920ZZ	Drainage of Phrenic Nerve, Open Approach
019230Z	Drainage of Phrenic Nerve with Drainage Device, Percutaneous Approach
01923ZX	Drainage of Phrenic Nerve, Percutaneous Approach, Diagnostic
01923ZZ	Drainage of Phrenic Nerve, Percutaneous Approach
019240Z	Drainage of Phrenic Nerve with Drainage Device, Percutaneous Endoscopic Approach
01924ZX	Drainage of Phrenic Nerve, Percutaneous Endoscopic Approach, Diagnostic
01924ZZ	Drainage of Phrenic Nerve, Percutaneous Endoscopic Approach
019300Z	Drainage of Brachial Plexus with Drainage Device, Open Approach
01930ZX	Drainage of Brachial Plexus, Open Approach, Diagnostic
01930ZZ	Drainage of Brachial Plexus, Open Approach
019330Z	Drainage of Brachial Plexus with Drainage Device, Percutaneous Approach
01933ZX	Drainage of Brachial Plexus, Percutaneous Approach, Diagnostic
01933ZZ	Drainage of Brachial Plexus, Percutaneous Approach
019340Z	Drainage of Brachial Plexus with Drainage Device, Percutaneous Endoscopic Approach
01934ZX	Drainage of Brachial Plexus, Percutaneous Endoscopic Approach, Diagnostic
01934ZZ	Drainage of Brachial Plexus, Percutaneous Endoscopic Approach
019400Z	Drainage of Ulnar Nerve with Drainage Device, Open Approach
01940ZX	Drainage of Ulnar Nerve, Open Approach, Diagnostic
01940ZZ	Drainage of Ulnar Nerve, Open Approach
019430Z	Drainage of Ulnar Nerve with Drainage Device, Percutaneous Approach
01943ZX	Drainage of Ulnar Nerve, Percutaneous Approach, Diagnostic
01943ZZ	Drainage of Ulnar Nerve, Percutaneous Approach
019440Z	Drainage of Ulnar Nerve with Drainage Device, Percutaneous Endoscopic Approach
01944ZX	Drainage of Ulnar Nerve, Percutaneous Endoscopic Approach, Diagnostic
01944ZZ	Drainage of Ulnar Nerve, Percutaneous Endoscopic Approach
019500Z	Drainage of Median Nerve with Drainage Device, Open Approach
01950ZX	Drainage of Median Nerve, Open Approach, Diagnostic
01950ZZ	Drainage of Median Nerve, Open Approach
019530Z	Drainage of Median Nerve with Drainage Device, Percutaneous Approach
01953ZX	Drainage of Median Nerve, Percutaneous Approach, Diagnostic
01953ZZ	Drainage of Median Nerve, Percutaneous Approach
019540Z	Drainage of Median Nerve with Drainage Device, Percutaneous Endoscopic Approach
01954ZX	Drainage of Median Nerve, Percutaneous Endoscopic Approach, Diagnostic
01954ZZ	Drainage of Median Nerve, Percutaneous Endoscopic Approach
019600Z	Drainage of Radial Nerve with Drainage Device, Open Approach
01960ZX	Drainage of Radial Nerve, Open Approach, Diagnostic
01960ZZ	Drainage of Radial Nerve, Open Approach
019630Z	Drainage of Radial Nerve with Drainage Device, Percutaneous Approach
01963ZX	Drainage of Radial Nerve, Percutaneous Approach, Diagnostic
01963ZZ	Drainage of Radial Nerve, Percutaneous Approach
019640Z	Drainage of Radial Nerve with Drainage Device, Percutaneous Endoscopic Approach
01964ZX	Drainage of Radial Nerve, Percutaneous Endoscopic Approach, Diagnostic
01964ZZ	Drainage of Radial Nerve, Percutaneous Endoscopic Approach
019800Z	Drainage of Thoracic Nerve with Drainage Device, Open Approach
01980ZX	Drainage of Thoracic Nerve, Open Approach, Diagnostic
01980ZZ	Drainage of Thoracic Nerve, Open Approach
019830Z	Drainage of Thoracic Nerve with Drainage Device, Percutaneous Approach
01983ZX	Drainage of Thoracic Nerve, Percutaneous Approach, Diagnostic
01983ZZ	Drainage of Thoracic Nerve, Percutaneous Approach
019840Z	Drainage of Thoracic Nerve with Drainage Device, Percutaneous Endoscopic Approach
01984ZX	Drainage of Thoracic Nerve, Percutaneous Endoscopic Approach, Diagnostic
01984ZZ	Drainage of Thoracic Nerve, Percutaneous Endoscopic Approach
019900Z	Drainage of Lumbar Plexus with Drainage Device, Open Approach
01990ZX	Drainage of Lumbar Plexus, Open Approach, Diagnostic

01990ZZ	Drainage of Lumbar Plexus, Open Approach
019930Z	Drainage of Lumbar Plexus with Drainage Device, Percutaneous Approach
01993ZX	Drainage of Lumbar Plexus, Percutaneous Approach, Diagnostic
01993ZZ	Drainage of Lumbar Plexus, Percutaneous Approach
019940Z	Drainage of Lumbar Plexus with Drainage Device, Percutaneous Endoscopic Approach
01994ZX	Drainage of Lumbar Plexus, Percutaneous Endoscopic Approach, Diagnostic
01994ZZ	Drainage of Lumbar Plexus, Percutaneous Endoscopic Approach
019A00Z	Drainage of Lumbosacral Plexus with Drainage Device, Open Approach
019A0ZX	Drainage of Lumbosacral Plexus, Open Approach, Diagnostic
019A0ZZ	Drainage of Lumbosacral Plexus, Open Approach
019A30Z	Drainage of Lumbosacral Plexus with Drainage Device, Percutaneous Approach
019A3ZX	Drainage of Lumbosacral Plexus, Percutaneous Approach, Diagnostic
019A3ZZ	Drainage of Lumbosacral Plexus, Percutaneous Approach
019A40Z	Drainage of Lumbosacral Plexus with Drainage Device, Percutaneous Endoscopic Approach
019A4ZX	Drainage of Lumbosacral Plexus, Percutaneous Endoscopic Approach, Diagnostic
019A4ZZ	Drainage of Lumbosacral Plexus, Percutaneous Endoscopic Approach
019B00Z	Drainage of Lumbar Nerve with Drainage Device, Open Approach
019B0ZX	Drainage of Lumbar Nerve, Open Approach, Diagnostic
019B0ZZ	Drainage of Lumbar Nerve, Open Approach
019B30Z	Drainage of Lumbar Nerve with Drainage Device, Percutaneous Approach
019B3ZX	Drainage of Lumbar Nerve, Percutaneous Approach, Diagnostic
019B3ZZ	Drainage of Lumbar Nerve, Percutaneous Approach
019B40Z	Drainage of Lumbar Nerve with Drainage Device, Percutaneous Endoscopic Approach
019B4ZX	Drainage of Lumbar Nerve, Percutaneous Endoscopic Approach, Diagnostic
019B4ZZ	Drainage of Lumbar Nerve, Percutaneous Endoscopic Approach
019C00Z	Drainage of Pudendal Nerve with Drainage Device, Open Approach
019C0ZX	Drainage of Pudendal Nerve, Open Approach, Diagnostic
019C0ZZ	Drainage of Pudendal Nerve, Open Approach
019C30Z	Drainage of Pudendal Nerve with Drainage Device, Percutaneous Approach
019C3ZX	Drainage of Pudendal Nerve, Percutaneous Approach, Diagnostic
019C3ZZ	Drainage of Pudendal Nerve, Percutaneous Approach
019C40Z	Drainage of Pudendal Nerve with Drainage Device, Percutaneous Endoscopic Approach
019C4ZX	Drainage of Pudendal Nerve, Percutaneous Endoscopic Approach, Diagnostic
019C4ZZ	Drainage of Pudendal Nerve, Percutaneous Endoscopic Approach
019D00Z	Drainage of Femoral Nerve with Drainage Device, Open Approach
019D0ZX	Drainage of Femoral Nerve, Open Approach, Diagnostic
019D0ZZ	Drainage of Femoral Nerve, Open Approach
019D30Z	Drainage of Femoral Nerve with Drainage Device, Percutaneous Approach
019D3ZX	Drainage of Femoral Nerve, Percutaneous Approach, Diagnostic
019D3ZZ	Drainage of Femoral Nerve, Percutaneous Approach
019D40Z	Drainage of Femoral Nerve with Drainage Device, Percutaneous Endoscopic Approach
019D4ZX	Drainage of Femoral Nerve, Percutaneous Endoscopic Approach, Diagnostic
019D4ZZ	Drainage of Femoral Nerve, Percutaneous Endoscopic Approach
019F00Z	Drainage of Sciatic Nerve with Drainage Device, Open Approach
019F0ZX	Drainage of Sciatic Nerve, Open Approach, Diagnostic
019F0ZZ	Drainage of Sciatic Nerve, Open Approach
019F30Z	Drainage of Sciatic Nerve with Drainage Device, Percutaneous Approach
019F3ZX	Drainage of Sciatic Nerve, Percutaneous Approach, Diagnostic
019F3ZZ	Drainage of Sciatic Nerve, Percutaneous Approach
019F40Z	Drainage of Sciatic Nerve with Drainage Device, Percutaneous Endoscopic Approach
019F4ZX	Drainage of Sciatic Nerve, Percutaneous Endoscopic Approach, Diagnostic
019F4ZZ	Drainage of Sciatic Nerve, Percutaneous Endoscopic Approach
019G00Z	Drainage of Tibial Nerve with Drainage Device, Open Approach
019G0ZX	Drainage of Tibial Nerve, Open Approach, Diagnostic
019G0ZZ	Drainage of Tibial Nerve, Open Approach
019G30Z	Drainage of Tibial Nerve with Drainage Device, Percutaneous Approach
019G3ZX	Drainage of Tibial Nerve, Percutaneous Approach, Diagnostic
019G3ZZ	Drainage of Tibial Nerve, Percutaneous Approach
019G40Z	Drainage of Tibial Nerve with Drainage Device, Percutaneous Endoscopic Approach
019G4ZX	Drainage of Tibial Nerve, Percutaneous Endoscopic Approach, Diagnostic
019G4ZZ	Drainage of Tibial Nerve, Percutaneous Endoscopic Approach
019H00Z	Drainage of Peroneal Nerve with Drainage Device, Open Approach
019H0ZX	Drainage of Peroneal Nerve, Open Approach, Diagnostic
019H0ZZ	Drainage of Peroneal Nerve, Open Approach
019H30Z	Drainage of Peroneal Nerve with Drainage Device, Percutaneous Approach
019H3ZX	Drainage of Peroneal Nerve, Percutaneous Approach, Diagnostic
019H3ZZ	Drainage of Peroneal Nerve, Percutaneous Approach
019H40Z	Drainage of Peroneal Nerve with Drainage Device, Percutaneous Endoscopic Approach
019H4ZX	Drainage of Peroneal Nerve, Percutaneous Endoscopic Approach, Diagnostic
019H4ZZ	Drainage of Peroneal Nerve, Percutaneous Endoscopic Approach
019K00Z	Drainage of Head and Neck Sympathetic Nerve with Drainage Device, Open Approach
019K0ZX	Drainage of Head and Neck Sympathetic Nerve, Open Approach, Diagnostic
019K0ZZ	Drainage of Head and Neck Sympathetic Nerve, Open Approach
019K30Z	Drainage of Head and Neck Sympathetic Nerve with Drainage Device, Percutaneous Approach
019K3ZX	Drainage of Head and Neck Sympathetic Nerve, Percutaneous Approach, Diagnostic
019K3ZZ	Drainage of Head and Neck Sympathetic Nerve, Percutaneous Approach
019K40Z	Drainage of Head and Neck Sympathetic Nerve with Drainage Device, Percutaneous Endoscopic Approach
019K4ZX	Drainage of Head and Neck Sympathetic Nerve, Percutaneous Endoscopic Approach, Diagnostic
019K4ZZ	Drainage of Head and Neck Sympathetic Nerve, Percutaneous Endoscopic Approach
019L00Z	Drainage of Thoracic Sympathetic Nerve with Drainage Device, Open Approach
019L0ZX	Drainage of Thoracic Sympathetic Nerve, Open Approach, Diagnostic
019L0ZZ	Drainage of Thoracic Sympathetic Nerve, Open Approach
019L30Z	Drainage of Thoracic Sympathetic Nerve with Drainage Device, Percutaneous Approach
019L3ZX	Drainage of Thoracic Sympathetic Nerve, Percutaneous Approach, Diagnostic
019L3ZZ	Drainage of Thoracic Sympathetic Nerve, Percutaneous Approach
019L40Z	Drainage of Thoracic Sympathetic Nerve with Drainage Device, Percutaneous Endoscopic Approach
019L4ZX	Drainage of Thoracic Sympathetic Nerve, Percutaneous Endoscopic Approach, Diagnostic
019L4ZZ	Drainage of Thoracic Sympathetic Nerve, Percutaneous Endoscopic Approach
019M00Z	Drainage of Abdominal Sympathetic Nerve with Drainage Device, Open Approach
019M0ZX	Drainage of Abdominal Sympathetic Nerve, Open Approach, Diagnostic
019M0ZZ	Drainage of Abdominal Sympathetic Nerve, Open Approach
019M30Z	Drainage of Abdominal Sympathetic Nerve with Drainage Device, Percutaneous Approach
019M3ZX	Drainage of Abdominal Sympathetic Nerve, Percutaneous Approach, Diagnostic
019M3ZZ	Drainage of Abdominal Sympathetic Nerve, Percutaneous Approach
019M40Z	Drainage of Abdominal Sympathetic Nerve with Drainage Device, Percutaneous Endoscopic Approach
019M4ZX	Drainage of Abdominal Sympathetic Nerve, Percutaneous Endoscopic Approach, Diagnostic
019M4ZZ	Drainage of Abdominal Sympathetic Nerve, Percutaneous Endoscopic Approach
019N00Z	Drainage of Lumbar Sympathetic Nerve with Drainage Device, Open Approach

019N0ZX	Drainage of Lumbar Sympathetic Nerve, Open Approach, Diagnostic
019N0ZZ	Drainage of Lumbar Sympathetic Nerve, Open Approach
019N30Z	Drainage of Lumbar Sympathetic Nerve with Drainage Device, Percutaneous Approach
019N3ZX	Drainage of Lumbar Sympathetic Nerve, Percutaneous Approach, Diagnostic
019N3ZZ	Drainage of Lumbar Sympathetic Nerve, Percutaneous Approach
019N40Z	Drainage of Lumbar Sympathetic Nerve with Drainage Device, Percutaneous Endoscopic Approach
019N4ZX	Drainage of Lumbar Sympathetic Nerve, Percutaneous Endoscopic Approach, Diagnostic
019N4ZZ	Drainage of Lumbar Sympathetic Nerve, Percutaneous Endoscopic Approach
019P00Z	Drainage of Sacral Sympathetic Nerve with Drainage Device, Open Approach
019P0ZX	Drainage of Sacral Sympathetic Nerve, Open Approach, Diagnostic
019P0ZZ	Drainage of Sacral Sympathetic Nerve, Open Approach
019P30Z	Drainage of Sacral Sympathetic Nerve with Drainage Device, Percutaneous Approach
019P3ZX	Drainage of Sacral Sympathetic Nerve, Percutaneous Approach, Diagnostic
019P3ZZ	Drainage of Sacral Sympathetic Nerve, Percutaneous Approach
019P40Z	Drainage of Sacral Sympathetic Nerve with Drainage Device, Percutaneous Endoscopic Approach
019P4ZX	Drainage of Sacral Sympathetic Nerve, Percutaneous Endoscopic Approach, Diagnostic
019P4ZZ	Drainage of Sacral Sympathetic Nerve, Percutaneous Endoscopic Approach
019Q00Z	Drainage of Sacral Plexus with Drainage Device, Open Approach
019Q0ZX	Drainage of Sacral Plexus, Open Approach, Diagnostic
019Q0ZZ	Drainage of Sacral Plexus, Open Approach
019Q30Z	Drainage of Sacral Plexus with Drainage Device, Percutaneous Approach
019Q3ZX	Drainage of Sacral Plexus, Percutaneous Approach, Diagnostic
019Q3ZZ	Drainage of Sacral Plexus, Percutaneous Approach
019Q40Z	Drainage of Sacral Plexus with Drainage Device, Percutaneous Endoscopic Approach
019Q4ZX	Drainage of Sacral Plexus, Percutaneous Endoscopic Approach, Diagnostic
019Q4ZZ	Drainage of Sacral Plexus, Percutaneous Endoscopic Approach
019R00Z	Drainage of Sacral Nerve with Drainage Device, Open Approach
019R0ZX	Drainage of Sacral Nerve, Open Approach, Diagnostic
019R0ZZ	Drainage of Sacral Nerve, Open Approach
019R30Z	Drainage of Sacral Nerve with Drainage Device, Percutaneous Approach
019R3ZX	Drainage of Sacral Nerve, Percutaneous Approach, Diagnostic
019R3ZZ	Drainage of Sacral Nerve, Percutaneous Approach
019R40Z	Drainage of Sacral Nerve with Drainage Device, Percutaneous Endoscopic Approach
019R4ZX	Drainage of Sacral Nerve, Percutaneous Endoscopic Approach, Diagnostic
019R4ZZ	Drainage of Sacral Nerve, Percutaneous Endoscopic Approach

01B – Peripheral Nervous System, Excision

Review Coding Guidelines B3.4a and B3.4b

Review Coding Guideline B3.8

01B00ZX	Excision of Cervical Plexus, Open Approach, Diagnostic
01B00ZZ	Excision of Cervical Plexus, Open Approach
01B03ZX	Excision of Cervical Plexus, Percutaneous Approach, Diagnostic
01B03ZZ	Excision of Cervical Plexus, Percutaneous Approach
01B04ZX	Excision of Cervical Plexus, Percutaneous Endoscopic Approach, Diagnostic
01B04ZZ	Excision of Cervical Plexus, Percutaneous Endoscopic Approach
01B10ZX	Excision of Cervical Nerve, Open Approach, Diagnostic
01B10ZZ	Excision of Cervical Nerve, Open Approach
01B13ZX	Excision of Cervical Nerve, Percutaneous Approach, Diagnostic
01B13ZZ	Excision of Cervical Nerve, Percutaneous Approach
01B14ZX	Excision of Cervical Nerve, Percutaneous Endoscopic Approach, Diagnostic
01B14ZZ	Excision of Cervical Nerve, Percutaneous Endoscopic Approach
01B20ZX	Excision of Phrenic Nerve, Open Approach, Diagnostic
01B20ZZ	Excision of Phrenic Nerve, Open Approach
01B23ZX	Excision of Phrenic Nerve, Percutaneous Approach, Diagnostic
01B23ZZ	Excision of Phrenic Nerve, Percutaneous Approach
01B24ZX	Excision of Phrenic Nerve, Percutaneous Endoscopic Approach, Diagnostic
01B24ZZ	Excision of Phrenic Nerve, Percutaneous Endoscopic Approach
01B30ZX	Excision of Brachial Plexus, Open Approach, Diagnostic
01B30ZZ	Excision of Brachial Plexus, Open Approach
01B33ZX	Excision of Brachial Plexus, Percutaneous Approach, Diagnostic
01B33ZZ	Excision of Brachial Plexus, Percutaneous Approach
01B34ZX	Excision of Brachial Plexus, Percutaneous Endoscopic Approach, Diagnostic
01B34ZZ	Excision of Brachial Plexus, Percutaneous Endoscopic Approach
01B40ZX	Excision of Ulnar Nerve, Open Approach, Diagnostic
01B40ZZ	Excision of Ulnar Nerve, Open Approach
01B43ZX	Excision of Ulnar Nerve, Percutaneous Approach, Diagnostic
01B43ZZ	Excision of Ulnar Nerve, Percutaneous Approach
01B44ZX	Excision of Ulnar Nerve, Percutaneous Endoscopic Approach, Diagnostic
01B44ZZ	Excision of Ulnar Nerve, Percutaneous Endoscopic Approach
01B50ZX	Excision of Median Nerve, Open Approach, Diagnostic
01B50ZZ	Excision of Median Nerve, Open Approach
01B53ZX	Excision of Median Nerve, Percutaneous Approach, Diagnostic
01B53ZZ	Excision of Median Nerve, Percutaneous Approach
01B54ZX	Excision of Median Nerve, Percutaneous Endoscopic Approach, Diagnostic
01B54ZZ	Excision of Median Nerve, Percutaneous Endoscopic Approach
01B60ZX	Excision of Radial Nerve, Open Approach, Diagnostic
01B60ZZ	Excision of Radial Nerve, Open Approach
01B63ZX	Excision of Radial Nerve, Percutaneous Approach, Diagnostic
01B63ZZ	Excision of Radial Nerve, Percutaneous Approach
01B64ZX	Excision of Radial Nerve, Percutaneous Endoscopic Approach, Diagnostic
01B64ZZ	Excision of Radial Nerve, Percutaneous Endoscopic Approach
01B80ZX	Excision of Thoracic Nerve, Open Approach, Diagnostic
01B80ZZ	Excision of Thoracic Nerve, Open Approach
01B83ZX	Excision of Thoracic Nerve, Percutaneous Approach, Diagnostic
01B83ZZ	Excision of Thoracic Nerve, Percutaneous Approach
01B84ZX	Excision of Thoracic Nerve, Percutaneous Endoscopic Approach, Diagnostic
01B84ZZ	Excision of Thoracic Nerve, Percutaneous Endoscopic Approach
01B90ZX	Excision of Lumbar Plexus, Open Approach, Diagnostic
01B90ZZ	Excision of Lumbar Plexus, Open Approach
01B93ZX	Excision of Lumbar Plexus, Percutaneous Approach, Diagnostic
01B93ZZ	Excision of Lumbar Plexus, Percutaneous Approach
01B94ZX	Excision of Lumbar Plexus, Percutaneous Endoscopic Approach, Diagnostic
01B94ZZ	Excision of Lumbar Plexus, Percutaneous Endoscopic Approach
01BA0ZX	Excision of Lumbosacral Plexus, Open Approach, Diagnostic
01BA0ZZ	Excision of Lumbosacral Plexus, Open Approach
01BA3ZX	Excision of Lumbosacral Plexus, Percutaneous Approach, Diagnostic
01BA3ZZ	Excision of Lumbosacral Plexus, Percutaneous Approach
01BA4ZX	Excision of Lumbosacral Plexus, Percutaneous Endoscopic Approach, Diagnostic
01BA4ZZ	Excision of Lumbosacral Plexus, Percutaneous Endoscopic Approach
01BB0ZX	Excision of Lumbar Nerve, Open Approach, Diagnostic
01BB0ZZ	Excision of Lumbar Nerve, Open Approach
01BB3ZX	Excision of Lumbar Nerve, Percutaneous Approach, Diagnostic
01BB3ZZ	Excision of Lumbar Nerve, Percutaneous Approach
01BB4ZX	Excision of Lumbar Nerve, Percutaneous Endoscopic Approach, Diagnostic

01BB4ZZ	Excision of Lumbar Nerve, Percutaneous Endoscopic Approach
01BC0ZX	Excision of Pudendal Nerve, Open Approach, Diagnostic
01BC0ZZ	Excision of Pudendal Nerve, Open Approach
01BC3ZX	Excision of Pudendal Nerve, Percutaneous Approach, Diagnostic
01BC3ZZ	Excision of Pudendal Nerve, Percutaneous Approach
01BC4ZX	Excision of Pudendal Nerve, Percutaneous Endoscopic Approach, Diagnostic
01BC4ZZ	Excision of Pudendal Nerve, Percutaneous Endoscopic Approach
01BD0ZX	Excision of Femoral Nerve, Open Approach, Diagnostic
01BD0ZZ	Excision of Femoral Nerve, Open Approach
01BD3ZX	Excision of Femoral Nerve, Percutaneous Approach, Diagnostic
01BD3ZZ	Excision of Femoral Nerve, Percutaneous Approach
01BD4ZX	Excision of Femoral Nerve, Percutaneous Endoscopic Approach, Diagnostic
01BD4ZZ	Excision of Femoral Nerve, Percutaneous Endoscopic Approach
01BF0ZX	Excision of Sciatic Nerve, Open Approach, Diagnostic
01BF0ZZ	Excision of Sciatic Nerve, Open Approach
01BF3ZX	Excision of Sciatic Nerve, Percutaneous Approach, Diagnostic
01BF3ZZ	Excision of Sciatic Nerve, Percutaneous Approach
01BF4ZX	Excision of Sciatic Nerve, Percutaneous Endoscopic Approach, Diagnostic
01BF4ZZ	Excision of Sciatic Nerve, Percutaneous Endoscopic Approach
01BG0ZX	Excision of Tibial Nerve, Open Approach, Diagnostic
01BG0ZZ	Excision of Tibial Nerve, Open Approach
01BG3ZX	Excision of Tibial Nerve, Percutaneous Approach, Diagnostic
01BG3ZZ	Excision of Tibial Nerve, Percutaneous Approach
01BG4ZX	Excision of Tibial Nerve, Percutaneous Endoscopic Approach, Diagnostic
01BG4ZZ	Excision of Tibial Nerve, Percutaneous Endoscopic Approach
01BH0ZX	Excision of Peroneal Nerve, Open Approach, Diagnostic
01BH0ZZ	Excision of Peroneal Nerve, Open Approach
01BH3ZX	Excision of Peroneal Nerve, Percutaneous Approach, Diagnostic
01BH3ZZ	Excision of Peroneal Nerve, Percutaneous Approach
01BH4ZX	Excision of Peroneal Nerve, Percutaneous Endoscopic Approach, Diagnostic
01BH4ZZ	Excision of Peroneal Nerve, Percutaneous Endoscopic Approach
01BK0ZX	Excision of Head and Neck Sympathetic Nerve, Open Approach, Diagnostic
01BK0ZZ	Excision of Head and Neck Sympathetic Nerve, Open Approach
01BK3ZX	Excision of Head and Neck Sympathetic Nerve, Percutaneous Approach, Diagnostic
01BK3ZZ	Excision of Head and Neck Sympathetic Nerve, Percutaneous Approach
01BK4ZX	Excision of Head and Neck Sympathetic Nerve, Percutaneous Endoscopic Approach, Diagnostic
01BK4ZZ	Excision of Head and Neck Sympathetic Nerve, Percutaneous Endoscopic Approach
01BL0ZX	Excision of Thoracic Sympathetic Nerve, Open Approach, Diagnostic
01BL0ZZ	Excision of Thoracic Sympathetic Nerve, Open Approach
01BL3ZX	Excision of Thoracic Sympathetic Nerve, Percutaneous Approach, Diagnostic
01BL3ZZ	Excision of Thoracic Sympathetic Nerve, Percutaneous Approach
01BL4ZX	Excision of Thoracic Sympathetic Nerve, Percutaneous Endoscopic Approach, Diagnostic
01BL4ZZ	Excision of Thoracic Sympathetic Nerve, Percutaneous Endoscopic Approach
01BM0ZX	Excision of Abdominal Sympathetic Nerve, Open Approach, Diagnostic
01BM0ZZ	Excision of Abdominal Sympathetic Nerve, Open Approach
01BM3ZX	Excision of Abdominal Sympathetic Nerve, Percutaneous Approach, Diagnostic
01BM3ZZ	Excision of Abdominal Sympathetic Nerve, Percutaneous Approach
01BM4ZX	Excision of Abdominal Sympathetic Nerve, Percutaneous Endoscopic Approach, Diagnostic
01BM4ZZ	Excision of Abdominal Sympathetic Nerve, Percutaneous Endoscopic Approach
01BN0ZX	Excision of Lumbar Sympathetic Nerve, Open Approach, Diagnostic
01BN0ZZ	Excision of Lumbar Sympathetic Nerve, Open Approach
01BN3ZX	Excision of Lumbar Sympathetic Nerve, Percutaneous Approach, Diagnostic
01BN3ZZ	Excision of Lumbar Sympathetic Nerve, Percutaneous Approach
01BN4ZX	Excision of Lumbar Sympathetic Nerve, Percutaneous Endoscopic Approach, Diagnostic
01BN4ZZ	Excision of Lumbar Sympathetic Nerve, Percutaneous Endoscopic Approach
01BP0ZX	Excision of Sacral Sympathetic Nerve, Open Approach, Diagnostic
01BP0ZZ	Excision of Sacral Sympathetic Nerve, Open Approach
01BP3ZX	Excision of Sacral Sympathetic Nerve, Percutaneous Approach, Diagnostic
01BP3ZZ	Excision of Sacral Sympathetic Nerve, Percutaneous Approach
01BP4ZX	Excision of Sacral Sympathetic Nerve, Percutaneous Endoscopic Approach, Diagnostic
01BP4ZZ	Excision of Sacral Sympathetic Nerve, Percutaneous Endoscopic Approach
01BQ0ZX	Excision of Sacral Plexus, Open Approach, Diagnostic
01BQ0ZZ	Excision of Sacral Plexus, Open Approach
01BQ3ZX	Excision of Sacral Plexus, Percutaneous Approach, Diagnostic
01BQ3ZZ	Excision of Sacral Plexus, Percutaneous Approach
01BQ4ZX	Excision of Sacral Plexus, Percutaneous Endoscopic Approach, Diagnostic
01BQ4ZZ	Excision of Sacral Plexus, Percutaneous Endoscopic Approach
01BR0ZX	Excision of Sacral Nerve, Open Approach, Diagnostic
01BR0ZZ	Excision of Sacral Nerve, Open Approach
01BR3ZX	Excision of Sacral Nerve, Percutaneous Approach, Diagnostic
01BR3ZZ	Excision of Sacral Nerve, Percutaneous Approach
01BR4ZX	Excision of Sacral Nerve, Percutaneous Endoscopic Approach, Diagnostic
01BR4ZZ	Excision of Sacral Nerve, Percutaneous Endoscopic Approach

01C – Peripheral Nervous System, Extirpation

01C00ZZ	Extirpation of Matter from Cervical Plexus, Open Approach
01C03ZZ	Extirpation of Matter from Cervical Plexus, Percutaneous Approach
01C04ZZ	Extirpation of Matter from Cervical Plexus, Percutaneous Endoscopic Approach
01C10ZZ	Extirpation of Matter from Cervical Nerve, Open Approach
01C13ZZ	Extirpation of Matter from Cervical Nerve, Percutaneous Approach
01C14ZZ	Extirpation of Matter from Cervical Nerve, Percutaneous Endoscopic Approach
01C20ZZ	Extirpation of Matter from Phrenic Nerve, Open Approach
01C23ZZ	Extirpation of Matter from Phrenic Nerve, Percutaneous Approach
01C24ZZ	Extirpation of Matter from Phrenic Nerve, Percutaneous Endoscopic Approach
01C30ZZ	Extirpation of Matter from Brachial Plexus, Open Approach
01C33ZZ	Extirpation of Matter from Brachial Plexus, Percutaneous Approach
01C34ZZ	Extirpation of Matter from Brachial Plexus, Percutaneous Endoscopic Approach
01C40ZZ	Extirpation of Matter from Ulnar Nerve, Open Approach
01C43ZZ	Extirpation of Matter from Ulnar Nerve, Percutaneous Approach
01C44ZZ	Extirpation of Matter from Ulnar Nerve, Percutaneous Endoscopic Approach
01C50ZZ	Extirpation of Matter from Median Nerve, Open Approach
01C53ZZ	Extirpation of Matter from Median Nerve, Percutaneous Approach
01C54ZZ	Extirpation of Matter from Median Nerve, Percutaneous Endoscopic Approach
01C60ZZ	Extirpation of Matter from Radial Nerve, Open Approach
01C63ZZ	Extirpation of Matter from Radial Nerve, Percutaneous Approach
01C64ZZ	Extirpation of Matter from Radial Nerve, Percutaneous Endoscopic Approach
01C80ZZ	Extirpation of Matter from Thoracic Nerve, Open Approach
01C83ZZ	Extirpation of Matter from Thoracic Nerve, Percutaneous Approach
01C84ZZ	Extirpation of Matter from Thoracic Nerve, Percutaneous Endoscopic Approach
01C90ZZ	Extirpation of Matter from Lumbar Plexus, Open Approach
01C93ZZ	Extirpation of Matter from Lumbar Plexus, Percutaneous Approach
01C94ZZ	Extirpation of Matter from Lumbar Plexus, Percutaneous Endoscopic Approach
01CA0ZZ	Extirpation of Matter from Lumbosacral Plexus, Open Approach
01CA3ZZ	Extirpation of Matter from Lumbosacral Plexus, Percutaneous Approach
01CA4ZZ	Extirpation of Matter from Lumbosacral Plexus, Percutaneous Endoscopic Approach
01CB0ZZ	Extirpation of Matter from Lumbar Nerve, Open Approach

---

♀ Female-only   ♂ Male-only   ● Limited Coverage   ● Non-OR   **HAC** HAC-associated procedure   ● Non-covered procedures   ✚ Combination

01CB3ZZ Extirpation of Matter from Lumbar Nerve, Percutaneous Approach
01CB4ZZ Extirpation of Matter from Lumbar Nerve, Percutaneous Endoscopic Approach
01CC0ZZ Extirpation of Matter from Pudendal Nerve, Open Approach
01CC3ZZ Extirpation of Matter from Pudendal Nerve, Percutaneous Approach
01CC4ZZ Extirpation of Matter from Pudendal Nerve, Percutaneous Endoscopic Approach
01CD0ZZ Extirpation of Matter from Femoral Nerve, Open Approach
01CD3ZZ Extirpation of Matter from Femoral Nerve, Percutaneous Approach
01CD4ZZ Extirpation of Matter from Femoral Nerve, Percutaneous Endoscopic Approach
01CF0ZZ Extirpation of Matter from Sciatic Nerve, Open Approach
01CF3ZZ Extirpation of Matter from Sciatic Nerve, Percutaneous Approach
01CF4ZZ Extirpation of Matter from Sciatic Nerve, Percutaneous Endoscopic Approach
01CG0ZZ Extirpation of Matter from Tibial Nerve, Open Approach
01CG3ZZ Extirpation of Matter from Tibial Nerve, Percutaneous Approach
01CG4ZZ Extirpation of Matter from Tibial Nerve, Percutaneous Endoscopic Approach
01CH0ZZ Extirpation of Matter from Peroneal Nerve, Open Approach
01CH3ZZ Extirpation of Matter from Peroneal Nerve, Percutaneous Approach
01CH4ZZ Extirpation of Matter from Peroneal Nerve, Percutaneous Endoscopic Approach
01CK0ZZ Extirpation of Matter from Head and Neck Sympathetic Nerve, Open Approach
01CK3ZZ Extirpation of Matter from Head and Neck Sympathetic Nerve, Percutaneous Approach
01CK4ZZ Extirpation of Matter from Head and Neck Sympathetic Nerve, Percutaneous Endoscopic Approach
01CL0ZZ Extirpation of Matter from Thoracic Sympathetic Nerve, Open Approach
01CL3ZZ Extirpation of Matter from Thoracic Sympathetic Nerve, Percutaneous Approach
01CL4ZZ Extirpation of Matter from Thoracic Sympathetic Nerve, Percutaneous Endoscopic Approach
01CM0ZZ Extirpation of Matter from Abdominal Sympathetic Nerve, Open Approach
01CM3ZZ Extirpation of Matter from Abdominal Sympathetic Nerve, Percutaneous Approach
01CM4ZZ Extirpation of Matter from Abdominal Sympathetic Nerve, Percutaneous Endoscopic Approach
01CN0ZZ Extirpation of Matter from Lumbar Sympathetic Nerve, Open Approach
01CN3ZZ Extirpation of Matter from Lumbar Sympathetic Nerve, Percutaneous Approach
01CN4ZZ Extirpation of Matter from Lumbar Sympathetic Nerve, Percutaneous Endoscopic Approach
01CP0ZZ Extirpation of Matter from Sacral Sympathetic Nerve, Open Approach
01CP3ZZ Extirpation of Matter from Sacral Sympathetic Nerve, Percutaneous Approach
01CP4ZZ Extirpation of Matter from Sacral Sympathetic Nerve, Percutaneous Endoscopic Approach
01CQ0ZZ Extirpation of Matter from Sacral Plexus, Open Approach
01CQ3ZZ Extirpation of Matter from Sacral Plexus, Percutaneous Approach
01CQ4ZZ Extirpation of Matter from Sacral Plexus, Percutaneous Endoscopic Approach
01CR0ZZ Extirpation of Matter from Sacral Nerve, Open Approach
01CR3ZZ Extirpation of Matter from Sacral Nerve, Percutaneous Approach
01CR4ZZ Extirpation of Matter from Sacral Nerve, Percutaneous Endoscopic Approach

01D – Peripheral Nervous System, Extraction

01D00ZZ Extraction of Cervical Plexus, Open Approach
01D03ZZ Extraction of Cervical Plexus, Percutaneous Approach
01D04ZZ Extraction of Cervical Plexus, Percutaneous Endoscopic Approach
01D10ZZ Extraction of Cervical Nerve, Open Approach
01D13ZZ Extraction of Cervical Nerve, Percutaneous Approach
01D14ZZ Extraction of Cervical Nerve, Percutaneous Endoscopic Approach
01D20ZZ Extraction of Phrenic Nerve, Open Approach
01D23ZZ Extraction of Phrenic Nerve, Percutaneous Approach
01D24ZZ Extraction of Phrenic Nerve, Percutaneous Endoscopic Approach
01D30ZZ Extraction of Brachial Plexus, Open Approach
01D33ZZ Extraction of Brachial Plexus, Percutaneous Approach
01D34ZZ Extraction of Brachial Plexus, Percutaneous Endoscopic Approach
01D40ZZ Extraction of Ulnar Nerve, Open Approach
01D43ZZ Extraction of Ulnar Nerve, Percutaneous Approach
01D44ZZ Extraction of Ulnar Nerve, Percutaneous Endoscopic Approach
01D50ZZ Extraction of Median Nerve, Open Approach
01D53ZZ Extraction of Median Nerve, Percutaneous Approach
01D54ZZ Extraction of Median Nerve, Percutaneous Endoscopic Approach
01D60ZZ Extraction of Radial Nerve, Open Approach
01D63ZZ Extraction of Radial Nerve, Percutaneous Approach
01D64ZZ Extraction of Radial Nerve, Percutaneous Endoscopic Approach
01D80ZZ Extraction of Thoracic Nerve, Open Approach
01D83ZZ Extraction of Thoracic Nerve, Percutaneous Approach
01D84ZZ Extraction of Thoracic Nerve, Percutaneous Endoscopic Approach
01D90ZZ Extraction of Lumbar Plexus, Open Approach
01D93ZZ Extraction of Lumbar Plexus, Percutaneous Approach
01D94ZZ Extraction of Lumbar Plexus, Percutaneous Endoscopic Approach
01DA0ZZ Extraction of Lumbosacral Plexus, Open Approach
01DA3ZZ Extraction of Lumbosacral Plexus, Percutaneous Approach
01DA4ZZ Extraction of Lumbosacral Plexus, Percutaneous Endoscopic Approach
01DB0ZZ Extraction of Lumbar Nerve, Open Approach
01DB3ZZ Extraction of Lumbar Nerve, Percutaneous Approach
01DB4ZZ Extraction of Lumbar Nerve, Percutaneous Endoscopic Approach
01DC0ZZ Extraction of Pudendal Nerve, Open Approach
01DC3ZZ Extraction of Pudendal Nerve, Percutaneous Approach
01DC4ZZ Extraction of Pudendal Nerve, Percutaneous Endoscopic Approach
01DD0ZZ Extraction of Femoral Nerve, Open Approach
01DD3ZZ Extraction of Femoral Nerve, Percutaneous Approach
01DD4ZZ Extraction of Femoral Nerve, Percutaneous Endoscopic Approach
01DF0ZZ Extraction of Sciatic Nerve, Open Approach
01DF3ZZ Extraction of Sciatic Nerve, Percutaneous Approach
01DF4ZZ Extraction of Sciatic Nerve, Percutaneous Endoscopic Approach
01DG0ZZ Extraction of Tibial Nerve, Open Approach
01DG3ZZ Extraction of Tibial Nerve, Percutaneous Approach
01DG4ZZ Extraction of Tibial Nerve, Percutaneous Endoscopic Approach
01DH0ZZ Extraction of Peroneal Nerve, Open Approach
01DH3ZZ Extraction of Peroneal Nerve, Percutaneous Approach
01DH4ZZ Extraction of Peroneal Nerve, Percutaneous Endoscopic Approach
01DK0ZZ Extraction of Head and Neck Sympathetic Nerve, Open Approach
01DK3ZZ Extraction of Head and Neck Sympathetic Nerve, Percutaneous Approach
01DK4ZZ Extraction of Head and Neck Sympathetic Nerve, Percutaneous Endoscopic Approach
01DL0ZZ Extraction of Thoracic Sympathetic Nerve, Open Approach
01DL3ZZ Extraction of Thoracic Sympathetic Nerve, Percutaneous Approach
01DL4ZZ Extraction of Thoracic Sympathetic Nerve, Percutaneous Endoscopic Approach
01DM0ZZ Extraction of Abdominal Sympathetic Nerve, Open Approach
01DM3ZZ Extraction of Abdominal Sympathetic Nerve, Percutaneous Approach
01DM4ZZ Extraction of Abdominal Sympathetic Nerve, Percutaneous Endoscopic Approach
01DN0ZZ Extraction of Lumbar Sympathetic Nerve, Open Approach
01DN3ZZ Extraction of Lumbar Sympathetic Nerve, Percutaneous Approach
01DN4ZZ Extraction of Lumbar Sympathetic Nerve, Percutaneous Endoscopic Approach
01DP0ZZ Extraction of Sacral Sympathetic Nerve, Open Approach
01DP3ZZ Extraction of Sacral Sympathetic Nerve, Percutaneous Approach
01DP4ZZ Extraction of Sacral Sympathetic Nerve, Percutaneous Endoscopic Approach
01DQ0ZZ Extraction of Sacral Plexus, Open Approach
01DQ3ZZ Extraction of Sacral Plexus, Percutaneous Approach
01DQ4ZZ Extraction of Sacral Plexus, Percutaneous Endoscopic Approach
01DR0ZZ Extraction of Sacral Nerve, Open Approach
01DR3ZZ Extraction of Sacral Nerve, Percutaneous Approach
01DR4ZZ Extraction of Sacral Nerve, Percutaneous Endoscopic Approach

01H – Peripheral Nervous System, Insertion

01HY02Z   Insertion of Monitoring Device into Peripheral Nerve, Open Approach

01HY0MZ   Insertion of Neurostimulator Lead into Peripheral Nerve, Open Approach

01HY32Z   Insertion of Monitoring Device into Peripheral Nerve, Percutaneous Approach

01HY3MZ   Insertion of Neurostimulator Lead into Peripheral Nerve, Percutaneous Approach

01HY42Z   Insertion of Monitoring Device into Peripheral Nerve, Percutaneous Endoscopic Approach

01HY4MZ   Insertion of Neurostimulator Lead into Peripheral Nerve, Percutaneous Endoscopic Approach

01J – Peripheral Nervous System, Inspection

Review Coding Guidelines B3.11a, B3.11b and B3.11c

01JY0ZZ   Inspection of Peripheral Nerve, Open Approach

01JY3ZZ   Inspection of Peripheral Nerve, Percutaneous Approach

01JY4ZZ   Inspection of Peripheral Nerve, Percutaneous Endoscopic Approach

01N – Peripheral Nervous System, Release

Review Coding Guideline B3.13

Review Coding Guideline B3.14

01N00ZZ   Release Cervical Plexus, Open Approach
01N03ZZ   Release Cervical Plexus, Percutaneous Approach
01N04ZZ   Release Cervical Plexus, Percutaneous Endoscopic Approach
01N10ZZ   Release Cervical Nerve, Open Approach
01N13ZZ   Release Cervical Nerve, Percutaneous Approach
01N14ZZ   Release Cervical Nerve, Percutaneous Endoscopic Approach
01N20ZZ   Release Phrenic Nerve, Open Approach
01N23ZZ   Release Phrenic Nerve, Percutaneous Approach
01N24ZZ   Release Phrenic Nerve, Percutaneous Endoscopic Approach
01N30ZZ   Release Brachial Plexus, Open Approach
01N33ZZ   Release Brachial Plexus, Percutaneous Approach
01N34ZZ   Release Brachial Plexus, Percutaneous Endoscopic Approach
01N40ZZ   Release Ulnar Nerve, Open Approach
01N43ZZ   Release Ulnar Nerve, Percutaneous Approach
01N44ZZ   Release Ulnar Nerve, Percutaneous Endoscopic Approach
01N50ZZ   Release Median Nerve, Open Approach
01N53ZZ   Release Median Nerve, Percutaneous Approach
01N54ZZ   Release Median Nerve, Percutaneous Endoscopic Approach
01N60ZZ   Release Radial Nerve, Open Approach
01N63ZZ   Release Radial Nerve, Percutaneous Approach
01N64ZZ   Release Radial Nerve, Percutaneous Endoscopic Approach
01N80ZZ   Release Thoracic Nerve, Open Approach
01N83ZZ   Release Thoracic Nerve, Percutaneous Approach
01N84ZZ   Release Thoracic Nerve, Percutaneous Endoscopic Approach
01N90ZZ   Release Lumbar Plexus, Open Approach
01N93ZZ   Release Lumbar Plexus, Percutaneous Approach
01N94ZZ   Release Lumbar Plexus, Percutaneous Endoscopic Approach
01NA0ZZ   Release Lumbosacral Plexus, Open Approach
01NA3ZZ   Release Lumbosacral Plexus, Percutaneous Approach
01NA4ZZ   Release Lumbosacral Plexus, Percutaneous Endoscopic Approach
01NB0ZZ   Release Lumbar Nerve, Open Approach
01NB3ZZ   Release Lumbar Nerve, Percutaneous Approach
01NB4ZZ   Release Lumbar Nerve, Percutaneous Endoscopic Approach
01NC0ZZ   Release Pudendal Nerve, Open Approach
01NC3ZZ   Release Pudendal Nerve, Percutaneous Approach
01NC4ZZ   Release Pudendal Nerve, Percutaneous Endoscopic Approach
01ND0ZZ   Release Femoral Nerve, Open Approach

01ND3ZZ   Release Femoral Nerve, Percutaneous Approach
01ND4ZZ   Release Femoral Nerve, Percutaneous Endoscopic Approach
01NF0ZZ   Release Sciatic Nerve, Open Approach
01NF3ZZ   Release Sciatic Nerve, Percutaneous Approach
01NF4ZZ   Release Sciatic Nerve, Percutaneous Endoscopic Approach
01NG0ZZ   Release Tibial Nerve, Open Approach
01NG3ZZ   Release Tibial Nerve, Percutaneous Approach
01NG4ZZ   Release Tibial Nerve, Percutaneous Endoscopic Approach
01NH0ZZ   Release Peroneal Nerve, Open Approach
01NH3ZZ   Release Peroneal Nerve, Percutaneous Approach
01NH4ZZ   Release Peroneal Nerve, Percutaneous Endoscopic Approach
01NK0ZZ   Release Head and Neck Sympathetic Nerve, Open Approach
01NK3ZZ   Release Head and Neck Sympathetic Nerve, Percutaneous Approach
01NK4ZZ   Release Head and Neck Sympathetic Nerve, Percutaneous Endoscopic Approach
01NL0ZZ   Release Thoracic Sympathetic Nerve, Open Approach
01NL3ZZ   Release Thoracic Sympathetic Nerve, Percutaneous Approach
01NL4ZZ   Release Thoracic Sympathetic Nerve, Percutaneous Endoscopic Approach
01NM0ZZ   Release Abdominal Sympathetic Nerve, Open Approach
01NM3ZZ   Release Abdominal Sympathetic Nerve, Percutaneous Approach
01NM4ZZ   Release Abdominal Sympathetic Nerve, Percutaneous Endoscopic Approach
01NN0ZZ   Release Lumbar Sympathetic Nerve, Open Approach
01NN3ZZ   Release Lumbar Sympathetic Nerve, Percutaneous Approach
01NN4ZZ   Release Lumbar Sympathetic Nerve, Percutaneous Endoscopic Approach
01NP0ZZ   Release Sacral Sympathetic Nerve, Open Approach
01NP3ZZ   Release Sacral Sympathetic Nerve, Percutaneous Approach
01NP4ZZ   Release Sacral Sympathetic Nerve, Percutaneous Endoscopic Approach
01NQ0ZZ   Release Sacral Plexus, Open Approach
01NQ3ZZ   Release Sacral Plexus, Percutaneous Approach
01NQ4ZZ   Release Sacral Plexus, Percutaneous Endoscopic Approach
01NR0ZZ   Release Sacral Nerve, Open Approach
01NR3ZZ   Release Sacral Nerve, Percutaneous Approach
01NR4ZZ   Release Sacral Nerve, Percutaneous Endoscopic Approach

01P – Peripheral Nervous System, Removal

Review Coding Guideline B6.1c

01PY00Z   Removal of Drainage Device from Peripheral Nerve, Open Approach

01PY02Z   Removal of Monitoring Device from Peripheral Nerve, Open Approach

01PY07Z   Removal of Autologous Tissue Substitute from Peripheral Nerve, Open Approach

01PY0MZ   Removal of Neurostimulator Lead from Peripheral Nerve, Open Approach

01PY30Z   Removal of Drainage Device from Peripheral Nerve, Percutaneous Approach

01PY32Z   Removal of Monitoring Device from Peripheral Nerve, Percutaneous Approach

01PY37Z   Removal of Autologous Tissue Substitute from Peripheral Nerve, Percutaneous Approach

01PY3MZ   Removal of Neurostimulator Lead from Peripheral Nerve, Percutaneous Approach

01PY40Z Removal of Drainage Device from Peripheral Nerve, Percutaneous Endoscopic Approach
01PY42Z Removal of Monitoring Device from Peripheral Nerve, Percutaneous Endoscopic Approach
01PY47Z Removal of Autologous Tissue Substitute from Peripheral Nerve, Percutaneous Endoscopic Approach
01PY4MZ Removal of Neurostimulator Lead from Peripheral Nerve, Percutaneous Endoscopic Approach

01PYX0Z Removal of Drainage Device from Peripheral Nerve, External Approach
01PYX2Z Removal of Monitoring Device from Peripheral Nerve, External Approach
01PYXMZ Removal of Neurostimulator Lead from Peripheral Nerve, External Approach

01Q – Peripheral Nervous System, Repair

01Q00ZZ Repair Cervical Plexus, Open Approach
01Q03ZZ Repair Cervical Plexus, Percutaneous Approach
01Q04ZZ Repair Cervical Plexus, Percutaneous Endoscopic Approach
01Q10ZZ Repair Cervical Nerve, Open Approach
01Q13ZZ Repair Cervical Nerve, Percutaneous Approach
01Q14ZZ Repair Cervical Nerve, Percutaneous Endoscopic Approach
01Q20ZZ Repair Phrenic Nerve, Open Approach
01Q23ZZ Repair Phrenic Nerve, Percutaneous Approach
01Q24ZZ Repair Phrenic Nerve, Percutaneous Endoscopic Approach
01Q30ZZ Repair Brachial Plexus, Open Approach
01Q33ZZ Repair Brachial Plexus, Percutaneous Approach
01Q34ZZ Repair Brachial Plexus, Percutaneous Endoscopic Approach
01Q40ZZ Repair Ulnar Nerve, Open Approach
01Q43ZZ Repair Ulnar Nerve, Percutaneous Approach
01Q44ZZ Repair Ulnar Nerve, Percutaneous Endoscopic Approach
01Q50ZZ Repair Median Nerve, Open Approach
01Q53ZZ Repair Median Nerve, Percutaneous Approach
01Q54ZZ Repair Median Nerve, Percutaneous Endoscopic Approach
01Q60ZZ Repair Radial Nerve, Open Approach
01Q63ZZ Repair Radial Nerve, Percutaneous Approach
01Q64ZZ Repair Radial Nerve, Percutaneous Endoscopic Approach
01Q80ZZ Repair Thoracic Nerve, Open Approach
01Q83ZZ Repair Thoracic Nerve, Percutaneous Approach
01Q84ZZ Repair Thoracic Nerve, Percutaneous Endoscopic Approach
01Q90ZZ Repair Lumbar Plexus, Open Approach
01Q93ZZ Repair Lumbar Plexus, Percutaneous Approach
01Q94ZZ Repair Lumbar Plexus, Percutaneous Endoscopic Approach
01QA0ZZ Repair Lumbosacral Plexus, Open Approach
01QA3ZZ Repair Lumbosacral Plexus, Percutaneous Approach
01QA4ZZ Repair Lumbosacral Plexus, Percutaneous Endoscopic Approach
01QB0ZZ Repair Lumbar Nerve, Open Approach
01QB3ZZ Repair Lumbar Nerve, Percutaneous Approach
01QB4ZZ Repair Lumbar Nerve, Percutaneous Endoscopic Approach
01QC0ZZ Repair Pudendal Nerve, Open Approach
01QC3ZZ Repair Pudendal Nerve, Percutaneous Approach
01QC4ZZ Repair Pudendal Nerve, Percutaneous Endoscopic Approach
01QD0ZZ Repair Femoral Nerve, Open Approach

01QD3ZZ Repair Femoral Nerve, Percutaneous Approach
01QD4ZZ Repair Femoral Nerve, Percutaneous Endoscopic Approach
01QF0ZZ Repair Sciatic Nerve, Open Approach
01QF3ZZ Repair Sciatic Nerve, Percutaneous Approach
01QF4ZZ Repair Sciatic Nerve, Percutaneous Endoscopic Approach
01QG0ZZ Repair Tibial Nerve, Open Approach
01QG3ZZ Repair Tibial Nerve, Percutaneous Approach
01QG4ZZ Repair Tibial Nerve, Percutaneous Endoscopic Approach
01QH0ZZ Repair Peroneal Nerve, Open Approach
01QH3ZZ Repair Peroneal Nerve, Percutaneous Approach
01QH4ZZ Repair Peroneal Nerve, Percutaneous Endoscopic Approach
01QK0ZZ Repair Head and Neck Sympathetic Nerve, Open Approach
01QK3ZZ Repair Head and Neck Sympathetic Nerve, Percutaneous Approach
01QK4ZZ Repair Head and Neck Sympathetic Nerve, Percutaneous Endoscopic Approach
01QL0ZZ Repair Thoracic Sympathetic Nerve, Open Approach
01QL3ZZ Repair Thoracic Sympathetic Nerve, Percutaneous Approach
01QL4ZZ Repair Thoracic Sympathetic Nerve, Percutaneous Endoscopic Approach
01QM0ZZ Repair Abdominal Sympathetic Nerve, Open Approach
01QM3ZZ Repair Abdominal Sympathetic Nerve, Percutaneous Approach
01QM4ZZ Repair Abdominal Sympathetic Nerve, Percutaneous Endoscopic Approach
01QN0ZZ Repair Lumbar Sympathetic Nerve, Open Approach
01QN3ZZ Repair Lumbar Sympathetic Nerve, Percutaneous Approach
01QN4ZZ Repair Lumbar Sympathetic Nerve, Percutaneous Endoscopic Approach
01QP0ZZ Repair Sacral Sympathetic Nerve, Open Approach
01QP3ZZ Repair Sacral Sympathetic Nerve, Percutaneous Approach
01QP4ZZ Repair Sacral Sympathetic Nerve, Percutaneous Endoscopic Approach
01QQ0ZZ Repair Sacral Plexus, Open Approach
01QQ3ZZ Repair Sacral Plexus, Percutaneous Approach
01QQ4ZZ Repair Sacral Plexus, Percutaneous Endoscopic Approach
01QR0ZZ Repair Sacral Nerve, Open Approach
01QR3ZZ Repair Sacral Nerve, Percutaneous Approach
01QR4ZZ Repair Sacral Nerve, Percutaneous Endoscopic Approach

01S – Peripheral Nervous System, Reposition

01S00ZZ Reposition Cervical Plexus, Open Approach
01S03ZZ Reposition Cervical Plexus, Percutaneous Approach
01S04ZZ Reposition Cervical Plexus, Percutaneous Endoscopic Approach
01S10ZZ Reposition Cervical Nerve, Open Approach
01S13ZZ Reposition Cervical Nerve, Percutaneous Approach
01S14ZZ Reposition Cervical Nerve, Percutaneous Endoscopic Approach
01S20ZZ Reposition Phrenic Nerve, Open Approach
01S23ZZ Reposition Phrenic Nerve, Percutaneous Approach
01S24ZZ Reposition Phrenic Nerve, Percutaneous Endoscopic Approach
01S30ZZ Reposition Brachial Plexus, Open Approach
01S33ZZ Reposition Brachial Plexus, Percutaneous Approach
01S34ZZ Reposition Brachial Plexus, Percutaneous Endoscopic Approach
01S40ZZ Reposition Ulnar Nerve, Open Approach
01S43ZZ Reposition Ulnar Nerve, Percutaneous Approach
01S44ZZ Reposition Ulnar Nerve, Percutaneous Endoscopic Approach
01S50ZZ Reposition Median Nerve, Open Approach
01S53ZZ Reposition Median Nerve, Percutaneous Approach
01S54ZZ Reposition Median Nerve, Percutaneous Endoscopic Approach
01S60ZZ Reposition Radial Nerve, Open Approach
01S63ZZ Reposition Radial Nerve, Percutaneous Approach
01S64ZZ Reposition Radial Nerve, Percutaneous Endoscopic Approach
01S80ZZ Reposition Thoracic Nerve, Open Approach

01S83ZZ Reposition Thoracic Nerve, Percutaneous Approach
01S84ZZ Reposition Thoracic Nerve, Percutaneous Endoscopic Approach
01S90ZZ Reposition Lumbar Plexus, Open Approach
01S93ZZ Reposition Lumbar Plexus, Percutaneous Approach
01S94ZZ Reposition Lumbar Plexus, Percutaneous Endoscopic Approach
01SA0ZZ Reposition Lumbosacral Plexus, Open Approach
01SA3ZZ Reposition Lumbosacral Plexus, Percutaneous Approach
01SA4ZZ Reposition Lumbosacral Plexus, Percutaneous Endoscopic Approach
01SB0ZZ Reposition Lumbar Nerve, Open Approach
01SB3ZZ Reposition Lumbar Nerve, Percutaneous Approach
01SB4ZZ Reposition Lumbar Nerve, Percutaneous Endoscopic Approach
01SC0ZZ Reposition Pudendal Nerve, Open Approach
01SC3ZZ Reposition Pudendal Nerve, Percutaneous Approach
01SC4ZZ Reposition Pudendal Nerve, Percutaneous Endoscopic Approach
01SD0ZZ Reposition Femoral Nerve, Open Approach
01SD3ZZ Reposition Femoral Nerve, Percutaneous Approach
01SD4ZZ Reposition Femoral Nerve, Percutaneous Endoscopic Approach
01SF0ZZ Reposition Sciatic Nerve, Open Approach
01SF3ZZ Reposition Sciatic Nerve, Percutaneous Approach
01SF4ZZ Reposition Sciatic Nerve, Percutaneous Endoscopic Approach
01SG0ZZ Reposition Tibial Nerve, Open Approach

01SG3ZZ	Reposition Tibial Nerve, Percutaneous Approach
01SG4ZZ	Reposition Tibial Nerve, Percutaneous Endoscopic Approach
01SH0ZZ	Reposition Peroneal Nerve, Open Approach
01SH3ZZ	Reposition Peroneal Nerve, Percutaneous Approach
01SH4ZZ	Reposition Peroneal Nerve, Percutaneous Endoscopic Approach
01SQ0ZZ	Reposition Sacral Plexus, Open Approach

01SQ3ZZ	Reposition Sacral Plexus, Percutaneous Approach
01SQ4ZZ	Reposition Sacral Plexus, Percutaneous Endoscopic Approach
01SR0ZZ	Reposition Sacral Nerve, Open Approach
01SR3ZZ	Reposition Sacral Nerve, Percutaneous Approach
01SR4ZZ	Reposition Sacral Nerve, Percutaneous Endoscopic Approach

01U – Peripheral Nervous System, Supplement

01U107Z	Supplement Cervical Nerve with Autologous Tissue Substitute, Open Approach
01U137Z	Supplement Cervical Nerve with Autologous Tissue Substitute, Percutaneous Approach
01U147Z	Supplement Cervical Nerve with Autologous Tissue Substitute, Percutaneous Endoscopic Approach
01U207Z	Supplement Phrenic Nerve with Autologous Tissue Substitute, Open Approach
01U237Z	Supplement Phrenic Nerve with Autologous Tissue Substitute, Percutaneous Approach
01U247Z	Supplement Phrenic Nerve with Autologous Tissue Substitute, Percutaneous Endoscopic Approach
01U407Z	Supplement Ulnar Nerve with Autologous Tissue Substitute, Open Approach
01U437Z	Supplement Ulnar Nerve with Autologous Tissue Substitute, Percutaneous Approach
01U447Z	Supplement Ulnar Nerve with Autologous Tissue Substitute, Percutaneous Endoscopic Approach
01U507Z	Supplement Median Nerve with Autologous Tissue Substitute, Open Approach
01U537Z	Supplement Median Nerve with Autologous Tissue Substitute, Percutaneous Approach
01U547Z	Supplement Median Nerve with Autologous Tissue Substitute, Percutaneous Endoscopic Approach
01U607Z	Supplement Radial Nerve with Autologous Tissue Substitute, Open Approach
01U637Z	Supplement Radial Nerve with Autologous Tissue Substitute, Percutaneous Approach
01U647Z	Supplement Radial Nerve with Autologous Tissue Substitute, Percutaneous Endoscopic Approach
01U807Z	Supplement Thoracic Nerve with Autologous Tissue Substitute, Open Approach
01U837Z	Supplement Thoracic Nerve with Autologous Tissue Substitute, Percutaneous Approach
01U847Z	Supplement Thoracic Nerve with Autologous Tissue Substitute, Percutaneous Endoscopic Approach
01UB07Z	Supplement Lumbar Nerve with Autologous Tissue Substitute, Open Approach
01UB37Z	Supplement Lumbar Nerve with Autologous Tissue Substitute, Percutaneous Approach

01UB47Z	Supplement Lumbar Nerve with Autologous Tissue Substitute, Percutaneous Endoscopic Approach
01UC07Z	Supplement Pudendal Nerve with Autologous Tissue Substitute, Open Approach
01UC37Z	Supplement Pudendal Nerve with Autologous Tissue Substitute, Percutaneous Approach
01UC47Z	Supplement Pudendal Nerve with Autologous Tissue Substitute, Percutaneous Endoscopic Approach
01UD07Z	Supplement Femoral Nerve with Autologous Tissue Substitute, Open Approach
01UD37Z	Supplement Femoral Nerve with Autologous Tissue Substitute, Percutaneous Approach
01UD47Z	Supplement Femoral Nerve with Autologous Tissue Substitute, Percutaneous Endoscopic Approach
01UF07Z	Supplement Sciatic Nerve with Autologous Tissue Substitute, Open Approach
01UF37Z	Supplement Sciatic Nerve with Autologous Tissue Substitute, Percutaneous Approach
01UF47Z	Supplement Sciatic Nerve with Autologous Tissue Substitute, Percutaneous Endoscopic Approach
01UG07Z	Supplement Tibial Nerve with Autologous Tissue Substitute, Open Approach
01UG37Z	Supplement Tibial Nerve with Autologous Tissue Substitute, Percutaneous Approach
01UG47Z	Supplement Tibial Nerve with Autologous Tissue Substitute, Percutaneous Endoscopic Approach
01UH07Z	Supplement Peroneal Nerve with Autologous Tissue Substitute, Open Approach
01UH37Z	Supplement Peroneal Nerve with Autologous Tissue Substitute, Percutaneous Approach
01UH47Z	Supplement Peroneal Nerve with Autologous Tissue Substitute, Percutaneous Endoscopic Approach
01UR07Z	Supplement Sacral Nerve with Autologous Tissue Substitute, Open Approach
01UR37Z	Supplement Sacral Nerve with Autologous Tissue Substitute, Percutaneous Approach
01UR47Z	Supplement Sacral Nerve with Autologous Tissue Substitute, Percutaneous Endoscopic Approach

01W – Peripheral Nervous System, Revision

Review Coding Guideline B6.1c

01WY00Z	Revision of Drainage Device in Peripheral Nerve, Open Approach
01WY02Z	Revision of Monitoring Device in Peripheral Nerve, Open Approach
01WY07Z	Revision of Autologous Tissue Substitute in Peripheral Nerve, Open Approach
01WY0MZ	Revision of Neurostimulator Lead in Peripheral Nerve, Open Approach
01WY30Z	Revision of Drainage Device in Peripheral Nerve, Percutaneous Approach
01WY32Z	Revision of Monitoring Device in Peripheral Nerve, Percutaneous Approach
01WY37Z	Revision of Autologous Tissue Substitute in Peripheral Nerve, Percutaneous Approach
01WY3MZ	Revision of Neurostimulator Lead in Peripheral Nerve, Percutaneous Approach

01WY40Z	Revision of Drainage Device in Peripheral Nerve, Percutaneous Endoscopic Approach
01WY42Z	Revision of Monitoring Device in Peripheral Nerve, Percutaneous Endoscopic Approach
01WY47Z	Revision of Autologous Tissue Substitute in Peripheral Nerve, Percutaneous Endoscopic Approach
01WY4MZ	Revision of Neurostimulator Lead in Peripheral Nerve, Percutaneous Endoscopic Approach
01WYX0Z	Revision of Drainage Device in Peripheral Nerve, External Approach
01WYX2Z	Revision of Monitoring Device in Peripheral Nerve, External Approach
01WYX7Z	Revision of Autologous Tissue Substitute in Peripheral Nerve, External Approach
01WYXMZ	Revision of Neurostimulator Lead in Peripheral Nerve, External Approach

♀ Female-only ♂ Male-only ● Limited Coverage ● Non-OR ▇ HAC-associated procedure ● Non-covered procedures ➕ Combination

01X – Peripheral Nervous System, Transfer

01X10Z1   Transfer Cervical Nerve to Cervical Nerve, Open Approach
01X10Z2   Transfer Cervical Nerve to Phrenic Nerve, Open Approach
01X14Z1   Transfer Cervical Nerve to Cervical Nerve, Percutaneous Endoscopic Approach
01X14Z2   Transfer Cervical Nerve to Phrenic Nerve, Percutaneous Endoscopic Approach
01X20Z1   Transfer Phrenic Nerve to Cervical Nerve, Open Approach
01X20Z2   Transfer Phrenic Nerve to Phrenic Nerve, Open Approach
01X24Z1   Transfer Phrenic Nerve to Cervical Nerve, Percutaneous Endoscopic Approach
01X24Z2   Transfer Phrenic Nerve to Phrenic Nerve, Percutaneous Endoscopic Approach
01X40Z4   Transfer Ulnar Nerve to Ulnar Nerve, Open Approach
01X40Z5   Transfer Ulnar Nerve to Median Nerve, Open Approach
01X40Z6   Transfer Ulnar Nerve to Radial Nerve, Open Approach
01X44Z4   Transfer Ulnar Nerve to Ulnar Nerve, Percutaneous Endoscopic Approach
01X44Z5   Transfer Ulnar Nerve to Median Nerve, Percutaneous Endoscopic Approach
01X44Z6   Transfer Ulnar Nerve to Radial Nerve, Percutaneous Endoscopic Approach
01X50Z4   Transfer Median Nerve to Ulnar Nerve, Open Approach
01X50Z5   Transfer Median Nerve to Median Nerve, Open Approach
01X50Z6   Transfer Median Nerve to Radial Nerve, Open Approach
01X54Z4   Transfer Median Nerve to Ulnar Nerve, Percutaneous Endoscopic Approach
01X54Z5   Transfer Median Nerve to Median Nerve, Percutaneous Endoscopic Approach
01X54Z6   Transfer Median Nerve to Radial Nerve, Percutaneous Endoscopic Approach
01X60Z4   Transfer Radial Nerve to Ulnar Nerve, Open Approach
01X60Z5   Transfer Radial Nerve to Median Nerve, Open Approach
01X60Z6   Transfer Radial Nerve to Radial Nerve, Open Approach
01X64Z4   Transfer Radial Nerve to Ulnar Nerve, Percutaneous Endoscopic Approach
01X64Z5   Transfer Radial Nerve to Median Nerve, Percutaneous Endoscopic Approach
01X64Z6   Transfer Radial Nerve to Radial Nerve, Percutaneous Endoscopic Approach
01X80Z8   Transfer Thoracic Nerve to Thoracic Nerve, Open Approach
01X84Z8   Transfer Thoracic Nerve to Thoracic Nerve, Percutaneous Endoscopic Approach
01XB0ZB   Transfer Lumbar Nerve to Lumbar Nerve, Open Approach
01XB0ZC   Transfer Lumbar Nerve to Perineal Nerve, Open Approach
01XB4ZB   Transfer Lumbar Nerve to Lumbar Nerve, Percutaneous Endoscopic Approach
01XB4ZC   Transfer Lumbar Nerve to Perineal Nerve, Percutaneous Endoscopic Approach
01XC0ZB   Transfer Pudendal Nerve to Lumbar Nerve, Open Approach
01XC0ZC   Transfer Pudendal Nerve to Perineal Nerve, Open Approach
01XC4ZB   Transfer Pudendal Nerve to Lumbar Nerve, Percutaneous Endoscopic Approach

01XC4ZC   Transfer Pudendal Nerve to Perineal Nerve, Percutaneous Endoscopic Approach
01XD0ZD   Transfer Femoral Nerve to Femoral Nerve, Open Approach
01XD0ZF   Transfer Femoral Nerve to Sciatic Nerve, Open Approach
01XD0ZG   Transfer Femoral Nerve to Tibial Nerve, Open Approach
01XD0ZH   Transfer Femoral Nerve to Peroneal Nerve, Open Approach
01XD4ZD   Transfer Femoral Nerve to Femoral Nerve, Percutaneous Endoscopic Approach
01XD4ZF   Transfer Femoral Nerve to Sciatic Nerve, Percutaneous Endoscopic Approach
01XD4ZG   Transfer Femoral Nerve to Tibial Nerve, Percutaneous Endoscopic Approach
01XD4ZH   Transfer Femoral Nerve to Peroneal Nerve, Percutaneous Endoscopic Approach
01XF0ZD   Transfer Sciatic Nerve to Femoral Nerve, Open Approach
01XF0ZF   Transfer Sciatic Nerve to Sciatic Nerve, Open Approach
01XF0ZG   Transfer Sciatic Nerve to Tibial Nerve, Open Approach
01XF0ZH   Transfer Sciatic Nerve to Peroneal Nerve, Open Approach
01XF4ZD   Transfer Sciatic Nerve to Femoral Nerve, Percutaneous Endoscopic Approach
01XF4ZF   Transfer Sciatic Nerve to Sciatic Nerve, Percutaneous Endoscopic Approach
01XF4ZG   Transfer Sciatic Nerve to Tibial Nerve, Percutaneous Endoscopic Approach
01XF4ZH   Transfer Sciatic Nerve to Peroneal Nerve, Percutaneous Endoscopic Approach
01XG0ZD   Transfer Tibial Nerve to Femoral Nerve, Open Approach
01XG0ZF   Transfer Tibial Nerve to Sciatic Nerve, Open Approach
01XG0ZG   Transfer Tibial Nerve to Tibial Nerve, Open Approach
01XG0ZH   Transfer Tibial Nerve to Peroneal Nerve, Open Approach
01XG4ZD   Transfer Tibial Nerve to Femoral Nerve, Percutaneous Endoscopic Approach
01XG4ZF   Transfer Tibial Nerve to Sciatic Nerve, Percutaneous Endoscopic Approach
01XG4ZG   Transfer Tibial Nerve to Tibial Nerve, Percutaneous Endoscopic Approach
01XG4ZH   Transfer Tibial Nerve to Peroneal Nerve, Percutaneous Endoscopic Approach
01XH0ZD   Transfer Peroneal Nerve to Femoral Nerve, Open Approach
01XH0ZF   Transfer Peroneal Nerve to Sciatic Nerve, Open Approach
01XH0ZG   Transfer Peroneal Nerve to Tibial Nerve, Open Approach
01XH0ZH   Transfer Peroneal Nerve to Peroneal Nerve, Open Approach
01XH4ZD   Transfer Peroneal Nerve to Femoral Nerve, Percutaneous Endoscopic Approach
01XH4ZF   Transfer Peroneal Nerve to Sciatic Nerve, Percutaneous Endoscopic Approach
01XH4ZG   Transfer Peroneal Nerve to Tibial Nerve, Percutaneous Endoscopic Approach
01XH4ZH   Transfer Peroneal Nerve to Peroneal Nerve, Percutaneous Endoscopic Approach

Heart and Great Vessels

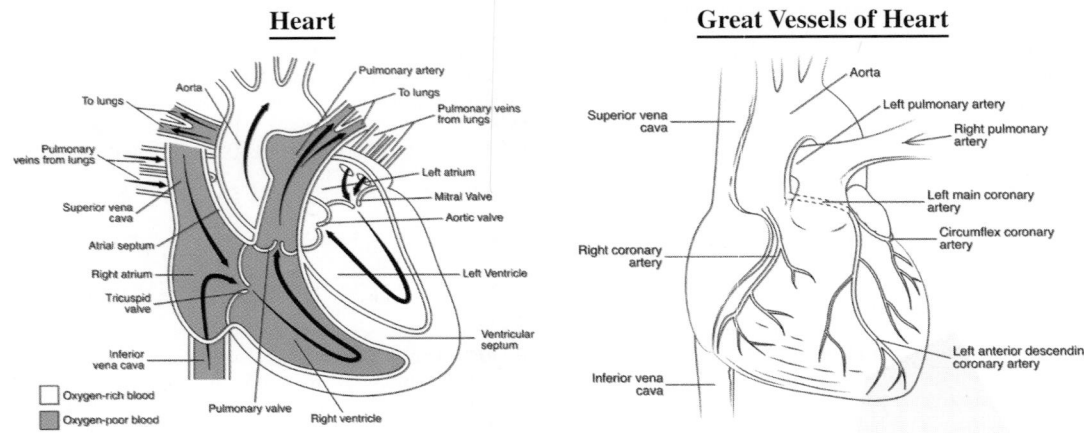

Heart

Great Vessels of Heart

Heart and Great Vessels Tables 021–02Y

Section	0	Medical and Surgical
Body System	2	Heart and Great Vessels
Operation	1	Bypass: Altering the route of passage of the contents of a tubular body part

021

Body Part (4th)	Approach (5th)	Device (6th)	Qualifier (7th)
0 Coronary Artery, One Site 1 Coronary Artery, Two Sites 2 Coronary Artery, Three Sites 3 Coronary Artery, Four or More Sites	0 Open	9 Autologous Venous Tissue A Autologous Arterial Tissue J Synthetic Substitute K Nonautologous Tissue Substitute	3 Coronary Artery 8 Internal Mammary, Right 9 Internal Mammary, Left C Thoracic Artery F Abdominal Artery W Aorta
0 Coronary Artery, One Site 1 Coronary Artery, Two Sites 2 Coronary Artery, Three Sites 3 Coronary Artery, Four or More Sites	0 Open	Z No Device	3 Coronary Artery 8 Internal Mammary, Right 9 Internal Mammary, Left C Thoracic Artery F Abdominal Artery
0 Coronary Artery, One Site 1 Coronary Artery, Two Sites 2 Coronary Artery, Three Sites 3 Coronary Artery, Four or More Sites	3 Percutaneous	4 Intraluminal Device, Drug-eluting D Intraluminal Device	4 Coronary Vein
0 Coronary Artery, One Site 1 Coronary Artery, Two Sites 2 Coronary Artery, Three Sites 3 Coronary Artery, Four or More Sites	4 Percutaneous Endoscopic	4 Intraluminal Device, Drug-eluting D Intraluminal Device	4 Coronary Vein
0 Coronary Artery, One Site 1 Coronary Artery, Two Sites 2 Coronary Artery, Three Sites 3 Coronary Artery, Four or More Sites	4 Percutaneous Endoscopic	9 Autologous Venous Tissue A Autologous Arterial Tissue J Synthetic Substitute K Nonautologous Tissue Substitute	3 Coronary Artery 8 Internal Mammary, Right 9 Internal Mammary, Left C Thoracic Artery F Abdominal Artery W Aorta
0 Coronary Artery, One Site 1 Coronary Artery, Two Sites 2 Coronary Artery, Three Sites 3 Coronary Artery, Four or More Sites	4 Percutaneous Endoscopic	Z No Device	3 Coronary Artery 8 Internal Mammary, Right 9 Internal Mammary, Left C Thoracic Artery F Abdominal Artery
6 Atrium, Right	0 Open 4 Percutaneous Endoscopic	9 Autologous Venous Tissue A Autologous Arterial Tissue J Synthetic Substitute K Nonautologous Tissue Substitute	P Pulmonary Trunk Q Pulmonary Artery, Right R Pulmonary Artery, Left

Continued

021 Continued

Section	0	**Medical and Surgical**
Body System	2	**Heart and Great Vessels**
Operation	1	**Bypass:** Altering the route of passage of the contents of a tubular body part

Body Part (4ᵗʰ)	Approach (5ᵗʰ)	Device (6ᵗʰ)	Qualifier (7ᵗʰ)
6 Atrium, Right	0 Open 4 Percutaneous Endoscopic	Z No Device	7 Atrium, Left P Pulmonary Trunk Q Pulmonary Artery, Right R Pulmonary Artery, Left

7 Atrium, Left
V Superior Vena Cava
	0 Open
	4 Percutaneous
	    Endoscopic
		9 Autologous Venous Tissue
		A Autologous Arterial Tissue
		J Synthetic Substitute
		K Nonautologous Tissue
		    Substitute
		Z No Device
			P Pulmonary Trunk
			Q Pulmonary Artery, Right
			R Pulmonary Artery, Left

K Ventricle, Right
L Ventricle, Left
	0 Open
	4 Percutaneous
	    Endoscopic
		9 Autologous Venous Tissue
		A Autologous Arterial Tissue
		J Synthetic Substitute
		K Nonautologous Tissue
		    Substitute
			P Pulmonary Trunk
			Q Pulmonary Artery, Right
			R Pulmonary Artery, Left

K Ventricle, Right L Ventricle, Left	0 Open 4 Percutaneous Endoscopic	Z No Device	5 Coronary Circulation 8 Internal Mammary, Right 9 Internal Mammary, Left C Thoracic Artery F Abdominal Artery P Pulmonary Trunk Q Pulmonary Artery, Right R Pulmonary Artery, Left W Aorta

W Thoracic Aorta	0 Open
	4 Percutaneous
	    Endoscopic
		9 Autologous Venous Tissue
		A Autologous Arterial Tissue
		J Synthetic Substitute
		K Nonautologous Tissue
		    Substitute
		Z No Device
			B Subclavian
			D Carotid
			P Pulmonary Trunk
			Q Pulmonary Artery, Right
			R Pulmonary Artery, Left

Section	0	**Medical and Surgical**
Body System	2	**Heart and Great Vessels**
Operation	5	**Destruction:** Physical eradication of all or a portion of a body part by the direct use of energy, force, or a destructive agent

Body Part (4ᵗʰ)	Approach (5ᵗʰ)	Device (6ᵗʰ)	Qualifier (7ᵗʰ)
4 Coronary Vein 5 Atrial Septum 6 Atrium, Right 8 Conduction Mechanism 9 Chordae Tendineae D Papillary Muscle F Aortic Valve G Mitral Valve H Pulmonary Valve J Tricuspid Valve K Ventricle, Right L Ventricle, Left M Ventricular Septum N Pericardium P Pulmonary Trunk Q Pulmonary Artery, Right R Pulmonary Artery, Left S Pulmonary Vein, Right T Pulmonary Vein, Left V Superior Vena Cava W Thoracic Aorta	0 Open 3 Percutaneous 4 Percutaneous Endoscopic	Z No Device	Z No Qualifier

Continued

025 *Continued*

Section	0	Medical and Surgical
Body System	2	Heart and Great Vessels
Operation	5	**Destruction:** Physical eradication of all or a portion of a body part by the direct use of energy, force, or a destructive agent

Body Part (4th)	Approach (5th)	Device (6th)	Qualifier (7th)
7 Atrium, Left	0 Open 3 Percutaneous 4 Percutaneous Endoscopic	Z No Device	K Left Atrial Appendage Z No Qualifier

Section	0	Medical and Surgical
Body System	2	Heart and Great Vessels
Operation	7	**Dilation:** Expanding an orifice or the lumen of a tubular body part

Body Part (4th)	Approach (5th)	Device (6th)	Qualifier (7th)
0 Coronary Artery, One Site 1 Coronary Artery, Two Sites 2 Coronary Artery, Three Sites 3 Coronary Artery, Four or More Sites	0 Open 3 Percutaneous 4 Percutaneous Endoscopic	4 Intraluminal Device, Drug-eluting D Intraluminal Device T Intraluminal Device, Radioactive Z No Device	6 Bifurcation Z No Qualifier
F Aortic Valve G Mitral Valve H Pulmonary Valve J Tricuspid Valve K Ventricle, Right P Pulmonary Trunk Q Pulmonary Artery, Right S Pulmonary Vein, Right T Pulmonary Vein, Left V Superior Vena Cava W Thoracic Aorta	0 Open 3 Percutaneous 4 Percutaneous Endoscopic	4 Intraluminal Device, Drug-eluting D Intraluminal Device Z No Device	Z No Qualifier
R Pulmonary Artery, Left	0 Open 3 Percutaneous 4 Percutaneous Endoscopic	4 Intraluminal Device, Drug-eluting D Intraluminal Device Z No Device	T Ductus Arteriosus Z No Qualifier

Section	0	Medical and Surgical
Body System	2	Heart and Great Vessels
Operation	8	**Division:** Cutting into a body part, without draining fluids and/or gases from the body part, in order to separate or transect a body part

Body Part (4th)	Approach (5th)	Device (6th)	Qualifier (7th)
8 Conduction Mechanism 9 Chordae Tendineae D Papillary Muscle	0 Open 3 Percutaneous 4 Percutaneous Endoscopic	Z No Device	Z No Qualifier

Section	0	Medical and Surgical
Body System	2	Heart and Great Vessels
Operation	B	**Excision:** Cutting out or off, without replacement, a portion of a body part

Body Part (4th)	Approach (5th)	Device (6th)	Qualifier (7th)
4 Coronary Vein 5 Atrial Septum 6 Atrium, Right 8 Conduction Mechanism 9 Chordae Tendineae D Papillary Muscle F Aortic Valve G Mitral Valve H Pulmonary Valve J Tricuspid Valve K Ventricle, Right L Ventricle, Left M Ventricular Septum N Pericardium P Pulmonary Trunk Q Pulmonary Artery, Right R Pulmonary Artery, Left S Pulmonary Vein, Right T Pulmonary Vein, Left V Superior Vena Cava W Thoracic Aorta	0 Open 3 Percutaneous 4 Percutaneous Endoscopic	Z No Device	X Diagnostic Z No Qualifier
7 Atrium, Left	0 Open 3 Percutaneous 4 Percutaneous Endoscopic	Z No Device	K Left Atrial Appendage X Diagnostic Z No Qualifier

Section	0	Medical and Surgical
Body System	2	Heart and Great Vessels
Operation	C	**Extirpation:** Taking or cutting out solid matter from a body part

Body Part (4th)	Approach (5th)	Device (6th)	Qualifier (7th)
0 Coronary Artery, One Site 1 Coronary Artery, Two Sites 2 Coronary Artery, Three Sites 3 Coronary Artery, Four or More Sites 4 Coronary Vein 5 Atrial Septum 6 Atrium, Right 7 Atrium, Left 8 Conduction Mechanism 9 Chordae Tendineae D Papillary Muscle F Aortic Valve G Mitral Valve H Pulmonary Valve J Tricuspid Valve K Ventricle, Right L Ventricle, Left M Ventricular Septum N Pericardium P Pulmonary Trunk Q Pulmonary Artery, Right R Pulmonary Artery, Left S Pulmonary Vein, Right T Pulmonary Vein, Left V Superior Vena Cava W Thoracic Aorta	0 Open 3 Percutaneous 4 Percutaneous Endoscopic	Z No Device	Z No Qualifier

Section	0	Medical and Surgical
Body System	2	Heart and Great Vessels
Operation	F	Fragmentation: Breaking solid matter in a body part into pieces

Body Part (4th)	Approach (5th)	Device (6th)	Qualifier (7th)
N Pericardium	0 Open 3 Percutaneous 4 Percutaneous Endoscopic X External	Z No Device	Z No Qualifier

Section	0	Medical and Surgical
Body System	2	Heart and Great Vessels
Operation	H	Insertion: Putting in a nonbiological appliance that monitors, assists, performs, or prevents a physiological function but does not physically take the place of a body part

Body Part (4th)	Approach (5th)	Device (6th)	Qualifier (7th)
4 Coronary Vein 6 Atrium, Right 7 Atrium, Left K Ventricle, Right L Ventricle, Left	0 Open 3 Percutaneous 4 Percutaneous Endoscopic	0 Monitoring Device, Pressure Sensor 2 Monitoring Device 3 Infusion Device D Intraluminal Device J Cardiac Lead, Pacemaker K Cardiac Lead, Defibrillator M Cardiac Lead	Z No Qualifier
A Heart	0 Open 3 Percutaneous 4 Percutaneous Endoscopic	Q Implantable Heart Assist System	Z No Qualifier
A Heart	0 Open 3 Percutaneous 4 Percutaneous Endoscopic	R External Heart Assist System	S Biventricular Z No Qualifier
N Pericardium	0 Open 3 Percutaneous 4 Percutaneous Endoscopic	0 Monitoring Device, Pressure Sensor 2 Monitoring Device J Cardiac Lead, Pacemaker K Cardiac Lead, Defibrillator M Cardiac Lead	Z No Qualifier
P Pulmonary Trunk Q Pulmonary Artery, Right R Pulmonary Artery, Left S Pulmonary Vein, Right T Pulmonary Vein, Left V Superior Vena Cava W Thoracic Aorta	0 Open 3 Percutaneous 4 Percutaneous Endoscopic	0 Monitoring Device, Pressure Sensor 2 Monitoring Device 3 Infusion Device D Intraluminal Device	Z No Qualifier

Section	0	Medical and Surgical
Body System	2	Heart and Great Vessels
Operation	J	Inspection: Visually and/or manually exploring a body part

Body Part (4th)	Approach (5th)	Device (6th)	Qualifier (7th)
A Heart Y Great Vessel	0 Open 3 Percutaneous 4 Percutaneous Endoscopic	Z No Device	Z No Qualifier

Section	0	Medical and Surgical
Body System	2	Heart and Great Vessels
Operation	K	Map: Locating the route of passage of electrical impulses and/or locating functional areas in a body part

Body Part (4ᵗʰ)	Approach (5ᵗʰ)	Device (6ᵗʰ)	Qualifier (7ᵗʰ)
8 Conduction Mechanism	0 Open 3 Percutaneous 4 Percutaneous Endoscopic	Z No Device	Z No Qualifier

Section	0	Medical and Surgical
Body System	2	Heart and Great Vessels
Operation	L	Occlusion: Completely closing an orifice or the lumen of a tubular body part

Body Part (4ᵗʰ)	Approach (5ᵗʰ)	Device (6ᵗʰ)	Qualifier (7ᵗʰ)
7 Atrium, Left	0 Open 3 Percutaneous 4 Percutaneous Endoscopic	C Extraluminal Device D Intraluminal Device Z No Device	K Left Atrial Appendage
R Pulmonary Artery, Left	0 Open 3 Percutaneous 4 Percutaneous Endoscopic	C Extraluminal Device D Intraluminal Device Z No Device	T Ductus Arteriosus
S Pulmonary Vein, Right T Pulmonary Vein, Left V Superior Vena Cava	0 Open 3 Percutaneous 4 Percutaneous Endoscopic	C Extraluminal Device D Intraluminal Device Z No Device	Z No Qualifier

Section	0	Medical and Surgical
Body System	2	Heart and Great Vessels
Operation	N	Release: Freeing a body part from an abnormal physical constraint by cutting or by the use of force

Body Part (4ᵗʰ)	Approach (5ᵗʰ)	Device (6ᵗʰ)	Qualifier (7ᵗʰ)
4 Coronary Vein 5 Atrial Septum 6 Atrium, Right 7 Atrium, Left 8 Conduction Mechanism 9 Chordae Tendineae D Papillary Muscle F Aortic Valve G Mitral Valve H Pulmonary Valve J Tricuspid Valve K Ventricle, Right L Ventricle, Left M Ventricular Septum N Pericardium P Pulmonary Trunk Q Pulmonary Artery, Right R Pulmonary Artery, Left S Pulmonary Vein, Right T Pulmonary Vein, Left V Superior Vena Cava W Thoracic Aorta	0 Open 3 Percutaneous 4 Percutaneous Endoscopic	Z No Device	Z No Qualifier

Section	**0**	**Medical and Surgical**
Body System	**2**	**Heart and Great Vessels**
Operation	**P**	**Removal:** Taking out or off a device from a body part

Body Part (4th)	Approach (5th)	Device (6th)	Qualifier (7th)
A Heart	0 Open 3 Percutaneous 4 Percutaneous Endoscopic	2 Monitoring Device 3 Infusion Device 7 Autologous Tissue Substitute 8 Zooplastic Tissue C Extraluminal Device D Intraluminal Device J Synthetic Substitute K Nonautologous Tissue Substitute M Cardiac Lead Q Implantable Heart Assist System R External Heart Assist System	Z No Qualifier
A Heart	X External	2 Monitoring Device 3 Infusion Device D Intraluminal Device M Cardiac Lead	Z No Qualifier
Y Great Vessel	0 Open 3 Percutaneous 4 Percutaneous Endoscopic	2 Monitoring Device 3 Infusion Device 7 Autologous Tissue Substitute 8 Zooplastic Tissue C Extraluminal Device D Intraluminal Device J Synthetic Substitute K Nonautologous Tissue Substitute	Z No Qualifier
Y Great Vessel	X External	2 Monitoring Device 3 Infusion Device D Intraluminal Device	Z No Qualifier

Section	0	**Medical and Surgical**
Body System	2	**Heart and Great Vessels**
Operation	Q	**Repair:** Restoring, to the extent possible, a body part to its normal anatomic structure and function

Body Part (4ᵗʰ)	Approach (5ᵗʰ)	Device (6ᵗʰ)	Qualifier (7ᵗʰ)
0 Coronary Artery, One Site 1 Coronary Artery, Two Sites 2 Coronary Artery, Three Sites 3 Coronary Artery, Four or More Sites 4 Coronary Vein 5 Atrial Septum 6 Atrium, Right 7 Atrium, Left 8 Conduction Mechanism 9 Chordae Tendineae A Heart B Heart, Right C Heart, Left D Papillary Muscle F Aortic Valve G Mitral Valve H Pulmonary Valve J Tricuspid Valve K Ventricle, Right L Ventricle, Left M Ventricular Septum N Pericardium P Pulmonary Trunk Q Pulmonary Artery, Right R Pulmonary Artery, Left S Pulmonary Vein, Right T Pulmonary Vein, Left V Superior Vena Cava W Thoracic Aorta	0 Open 3 Percutaneous 4 Percutaneous Endoscopic	Z No Device	Z No Qualifier

Section	0	**Medical and Surgical**
Body System	2	**Heart and Great Vessels**
Operation	R	**Replacement:** Putting in or on biological or synthetic material that physically takes the place and/or function of all or a portion of a body part

Body Part (4ᵗʰ)	Approach (5ᵗʰ)	Device (6ᵗʰ)	Qualifier (7ᵗʰ)
5 Atrial Septum 6 Atrium, Right 7 Atrium, Left 9 Chordae Tendineae D Papillary Muscle J Tricuspid Valve K Ventricle, Right L Ventricle, Left M Ventricular Septum N Pericardium P Pulmonary Trunk Q Pulmonary Artery, Right R Pulmonary Artery, Left S Pulmonary Vein, Right T Pulmonary Vein, Left V Superior Vena Cava W Thoracic Aorta	0 Open 4 Percutaneous Endoscopic	7 Autologous Tissue Substitute 8 Zooplastic Tissue J Synthetic Substitute K Nonautologous Tissue Substitute	Z No Qualifier
F Aortic Valve G Mitral Valve H Pulmonary Valve	0 Open 4 Percutaneous Endoscopic	7 Autologous Tissue Substitute 8 Zooplastic Tissue J Synthetic Substitute K Nonautologous Tissue Substitute	Z No Qualifier

Continued

Section	0	Medical and Surgical
Body System	2	Heart and Great Vessels
Operation	R	**Replacement:** Putting in or on biological or synthetic material that physically takes the place and/or function of all or a portion of a body part

Body Part (4th)	Approach (5th)	Device (6th)	Qualifier (7th)
F Aortic Valve G Mitral Valve H Pulmonary Valve	3 Percutaneous	7 Autologous Tissue Substitute 8 Zooplastic Tissue J Synthetic Substitute K Nonautologous Tissue Substitute	H Transapical Z No Qualifier

Section	0	Medical and Surgical
Body System	2	Heart and Great Vessels
Operation	S	**Reposition:** Moving to its normal location, or other suitable location, all or a portion of a body part

Body Part (4th)	Approach (5th)	Device (6th)	Qualifier (7th)
P Pulmonary Trunk Q Pulmonary Artery, Right R Pulmonary Artery, Left S Pulmonary Vein, Right T Pulmonary Vein, Left V Superior Vena Cava W Thoracic Aorta	0 Open	Z No Device	Z No Qualifier

Section	0	Medical and Surgical
Body System	2	Heart and Great Vessels
Operation	T	**Resection:** Cutting out or off, without replacement, all of a body part

Body Part (4th)	Approach (5th)	Device (6th)	Qualifier (7th)
5 Atrial Septum 8 Conduction Mechanism 9 Chordae Tendineae D Papillary Muscle H Pulmonary Valve M Ventricular Septum N Pericardium	0 Open 3 Percutaneous 4 Percutaneous Endoscopic	Z No Device	Z No Qualifier

Section	0	Medical and Surgical
Body System	2	Heart and Great Vessels
Operation	U	**Supplement:** Putting in or on biological or synthetic material that physically reinforces and/or augments the function of a portion of a body part

Body Part (4th)	Approach (5th)	Device (6th)	Qualifier (7th)
5 Atrial Septum 6 Atrium, Right 7 Atrium, Left 9 Chordae Tendineae A Heart D Papillary Muscle F Aortic Valve G Mitral Valve H Pulmonary Valve J Tricuspid Valve K Ventricle, Right L Ventricle, Left M Ventricular Septum N Pericardium P Pulmonary Trunk Q Pulmonary Artery, Right R Pulmonary Artery, Left S Pulmonary Vein, Right T Pulmonary Vein, Left V Superior Vena Cava W Thoracic Aorta	0 Open 3 Percutaneous 4 Percutaneous Endoscopic	7 Autologous Tissue Substitute 8 Zooplastic Tissue J Synthetic Substitute K Nonautologous Tissue Substitute	Z No Qualifier

Section	0	Medical and Surgical
Body System	2	Heart and Great Vessels
Operation	V	Restriction: Partially closing an orifice or the lumen of a tubular body part

Body Part (4th)	Approach (5th)	Device (6th)	Qualifier (7th)
A Heart	0 Open 3 Percutaneous 4 Percutaneous Endoscopic	C Extraluminal Device Z No Device	Z No Qualifier
P Pulmonary Trunk Q Pulmonary Artery, Right S Pulmonary Vein, Right T Pulmonary Vein, Left V Superior Vena Cava W Thoracic Aorta	0 Open 3 Percutaneous 4 Percutaneous Endoscopic	C Extraluminal Device D Intraluminal Device Z No Device	Z No Qualifier
R Pulmonary Artery, Left	0 Open 3 Percutaneous 4 Percutaneous Endoscopic	C Extraluminal Device D Intraluminal Device Z No Device	T Ductus Arteriosus Z No Qualifier

Section	0	Medical and Surgical
Body System	2	Heart and Great Vessels
Operation	W	Revision: Correcting, to the extent possible, a portion of a malfunctioning device or the position of a displaced device

Body Part (4th)	Approach (5th)	Device (6th)	Qualifier (7th)
5 Atrial Septum M Ventricular Septum	0 Open 4 Percutaneous Endoscopic	J Synthetic Substitute	Z No Qualifier
A Heart	0 Open 3 Percutaneous 4 Percutaneous Endoscopic X External	2 Monitoring Device 3 Infusion Device 7 Autologous Tissue Substitute 8 Zooplastic Tissue C Extraluminal Device D Intraluminal Device J Synthetic Substitute K Nonautologous Tissue Substitute M Cardiac Lead Q Implantable Heart Assist System R External Heart Assist System	Z No Qualifier
F Aortic Valve G Mitral Valve H Pulmonary Valve J Tricuspid Valve	0 Open 4 Percutaneous Endoscopic	7 Autologous Tissue Substitute 8 Zooplastic Tissue J Synthetic Substitute K Nonautologous Tissue Substitute	Z No Qualifier
Y Great Vessel	0 Open 3 Percutaneous 4 Percutaneous Endoscopic X External	2 Monitoring Device 3 Infusion Device 7 Autologous Tissue Substitute 8 Zooplastic Tissue C Extraluminal Device D Intraluminal Device J Synthetic Substitute K Nonautologous Tissue Substitute	Z No Qualifier

Section	0	Medical and Surgical
Body System	2	Heart and Great Vessels
Operation	Y	**Transplantation:** Putting in or on all or a portion of a living body part taken from another individual or animal to physically take the place and/or function of all or a portion of a similar body part

Body Part (4th)	Approach (5th)	Device (6th)	Qualifier (7th)
A Heart	0 Open	Z No Device	0 Allogeneic 1 Syngeneic 2 Zooplastic

Heart and Great Vessels Code Listing 021–02Y

021 – Heart and Great Vessels, Bypass

Review Coding Guideline B3.6a

For Bypass procedures involving the coronary arteries, review Coding Guidelines B3.6b and B3.6c

For Bypass procedures involving the coronary arteries, review Coding Guideline B4.4

0210093 Bypass Coronary Artery, One Site from Coronary Artery with Autologous Venous Tissue, Open Approach
HAC When reported with secondary diagnosis code J98.5

0210098 Bypass Coronary Artery, One Site from Right Internal Mammary with Autologous Venous Tissue, Open Approach
HAC When reported with secondary diagnosis code J98.5

0210099 Bypass Coronary Artery, One Site from Left Internal Mammary with Autologous Venous Tissue, Open Approach
HAC When reported with secondary diagnosis code J98.5

021009C Bypass Coronary Artery, One Site from Thoracic Artery with Autologous Venous Tissue, Open Approach
HAC When reported with secondary diagnosis code J98.5

021009F Bypass Coronary Artery, One Site from Abdominal Artery with Autologous Venous Tissue, Open Approach
HAC When reported with secondary diagnosis code J98.5

021009W Bypass Coronary Artery, One Site from Aorta with Autologous Venous Tissue, Open Approach
HAC When reported with secondary diagnosis code J98.5

02100A3 Bypass Coronary Artery, One Site from Coronary Artery with Autologous Arterial Tissue, Open Approach
HAC When reported with secondary diagnosis code J98.5

02100A8 Bypass Coronary Artery, One Site from Right Internal Mammary with Autologous Arterial Tissue, Open Approach
HAC When reported with secondary diagnosis code J98.5

02100A9 Bypass Coronary Artery, One Site from Left Internal Mammary with Autologous Arterial Tissue, Open Approach
HAC When reported with secondary diagnosis code J98.5

02100AC Bypass Coronary Artery, One Site from Thoracic Artery with Autologous Arterial Tissue, Open Approach
HAC When reported with secondary diagnosis code J98.5

02100AF Bypass Coronary Artery, One Site from Abdominal Artery with Autologous Arterial Tissue, Open Approach
HAC When reported with secondary diagnosis code J98.5

02100AW Bypass Coronary Artery, One Site from Aorta with Autologous Arterial Tissue, Open Approach
HAC When reported with secondary diagnosis code J98.5

02100J3 Bypass Coronary Artery, One Site from Coronary Artery with Synthetic Substitute, Open Approach
HAC When reported with secondary diagnosis code J98.5

02100J8 Bypass Coronary Artery, One Site from Right Internal Mammary with Synthetic Substitute, Open Approach
HAC When reported with secondary diagnosis code J98.5

02100J9 Bypass Coronary Artery, One Site from Left Internal Mammary with Synthetic Substitute, Open Approach
HAC When reported with secondary diagnosis code J98.5

02100JC Bypass Coronary Artery, One Site from Thoracic Artery with Synthetic Substitute, Open Approach
HAC When reported with secondary diagnosis code J98.5

02100JF Bypass Coronary Artery, One Site from Abdominal Artery with Synthetic Substitute, Open Approach
HAC When reported with secondary diagnosis code J98.5

02100JW Bypass Coronary Artery, One Site from Aorta with Synthetic Substitute, Open Approach
HAC When reported with secondary diagnosis code J98.5

02100K3 Bypass Coronary Artery, One Site from Coronary Artery with Nonautologous Tissue Substitute, Open Approach
HAC When reported with secondary diagnosis code J98.5

02100K8 Bypass Coronary Artery, One Site from Right Internal Mammary with Nonautologous Tissue Substitute, Open Approach
HAC When reported with secondary diagnosis code J98.5

02100K9 Bypass Coronary Artery, One Site from Left Internal Mammary with Nonautologous Tissue Substitute, Open Approach
HAC When reported with secondary diagnosis code J98.5

02100KC Bypass Coronary Artery, One Site from Thoracic Artery with Nonautologous Tissue Substitute, Open Approach
HAC When reported with secondary diagnosis code J98.5

02100KF Bypass Coronary Artery, One Site from Abdominal Artery with Nonautologous Tissue Substitute, Open Approach
HAC When reported with secondary diagnosis code J98.5

02100KW Bypass Coronary Artery, One Site from Aorta with Nonautologous Tissue Substitute, Open Approach
HAC When reported with secondary diagnosis code J98.5

02100Z3 Bypass Coronary Artery, One Site from Coronary Artery, Open Approach
HAC When reported with secondary diagnosis code J98.5

02100Z8 Bypass Coronary Artery, One Site from Right Internal Mammary, Open Approach
HAC When reported with secondary diagnosis code J98.5

02100Z9 Bypass Coronary Artery, One Site from Left Internal Mammary, Open Approach
HAC When reported with secondary diagnosis code J98.5

02100ZC Bypass Coronary Artery, One Site from Thoracic Artery, Open Approach
HAC When reported with secondary diagnosis code J98.5

02100ZF Bypass Coronary Artery, One Site from Abdominal Artery, Open Approach
HAC When reported with secondary diagnosis code J98.5

0210344 Bypass Coronary Artery, One Site from Coronary Vein with Drug-eluting Intraluminal Device, Percutaneous Approach

02103D4 Bypass Coronary Artery, One Site from Coronary Vein with Intraluminal Device, Percutaneous Approach

0210444 Bypass Coronary Artery, One Site from Coronary Vein with Drug-eluting Intraluminal Device, Percutaneous Endoscopic Approach

0210493 Bypass Coronary Artery, One Site from Coronary Artery with Autologous Venous Tissue, Percutaneous Endoscopic Approach
HAC When reported with secondary diagnosis code J98.5

0210498 Bypass Coronary Artery, One Site from Right Internal Mammary with Autologous Venous Tissue, Percutaneous Endoscopic Approach
HAC When reported with secondary diagnosis code J98.5

♀ Female-only   ♂ Male-only   ● Limited Coverage   ● Non-OR   HAC HAC-associated procedure   ● Non-covered procedures   + Combination

0210499 Bypass Coronary Artery, One Site from Left Internal Mammary with Autologous Venous Tissue, Percutaneous Endoscopic Approach
HAC When reported with secondary diagnosis code J98.5

021049C Bypass Coronary Artery, One Site from Thoracic Artery with Autologous Venous Tissue, Percutaneous Endoscopic Approach
HAC When reported with secondary diagnosis code J98.5

021049F Bypass Coronary Artery, One Site from Abdominal Artery with Autologous Venous Tissue, Percutaneous Endoscopic Approach
HAC When reported with secondary diagnosis code J98.5

021049W Bypass Coronary Artery, One Site from Aorta with Autologous Venous Tissue, Percutaneous Endoscopic Approach
HAC When reported with secondary diagnosis code J98.5

02104A3 Bypass Coronary Artery, One Site from Coronary Artery with Autologous Arterial Tissue, Percutaneous Endoscopic Approach
HAC When reported with secondary diagnosis code J98.5

02104A8 Bypass Coronary Artery, One Site from Right Internal Mammary with Autologous Arterial Tissue, Percutaneous Endoscopic Approach
HAC When reported with secondary diagnosis code J98.5

02104A9 Bypass Coronary Artery, One Site from Left Internal Mammary with Autologous Arterial Tissue, Percutaneous Endoscopic Approach
HAC When reported with secondary diagnosis code J98.5

02104AC Bypass Coronary Artery, One Site from Thoracic Artery with Autologous Arterial Tissue, Percutaneous Endoscopic Approach
HAC When reported with secondary diagnosis code J98.5

02104AF Bypass Coronary Artery, One Site from Abdominal Artery with Autologous Arterial Tissue, Percutaneous Endoscopic Approach
HAC When reported with secondary diagnosis code J98.5

02104AW Bypass Coronary Artery, One Site from Aorta with Autologous Arterial Tissue, Percutaneous Endoscopic Approach
HAC When reported with secondary diagnosis code J98.5

02104D4 Bypass Coronary Artery, One Site from Coronary Vein with Intraluminal Device, Percutaneous Endoscopic Approach
HAC When reported with secondary diagnosis code J98.5

02104J3 Bypass Coronary Artery, One Site from Coronary Artery with Synthetic Substitute, Percutaneous Endoscopic Approach
HAC When reported with secondary diagnosis code J98.5

02104J8 Bypass Coronary Artery, One Site from Right Internal Mammary with Synthetic Substitute, Percutaneous Endoscopic Approach
HAC When reported with secondary diagnosis code J98.5

02104J9 Bypass Coronary Artery, One Site from Left Internal Mammary with Synthetic Substitute, Percutaneous Endoscopic Approach
HAC When reported with secondary diagnosis code J98.5

02104JC Bypass Coronary Artery, One Site from Thoracic Artery with Synthetic Substitute, Percutaneous Endoscopic Approach
HAC When reported with secondary diagnosis code J98.5

02104JF Bypass Coronary Artery, One Site from Abdominal Artery with Synthetic Substitute, Percutaneous Endoscopic Approach
HAC When reported with secondary diagnosis code J98.5

02104JW Bypass Coronary Artery, One Site from Aorta with Synthetic Substitute, Percutaneous Endoscopic Approach
HAC When reported with secondary diagnosis code J98.5

02104K3 Bypass Coronary Artery, One Site from Coronary Artery with Nonautologous Tissue Substitute, Percutaneous Endoscopic Approach
HAC When reported with secondary diagnosis code J98.5

02104K8 Bypass Coronary Artery, One Site from Right Internal Mammary with Nonautologous Tissue Substitute, Percutaneous Endoscopic Approach
HAC When reported with secondary diagnosis code J98.5

02104K9 Bypass Coronary Artery, One Site from Left Internal Mammary with Nonautologous Tissue Substitute, Percutaneous Endoscopic Approach
HAC When reported with secondary diagnosis code J98.5

02104KC Bypass Coronary Artery, One Site from Thoracic Artery with Nonautologous Tissue Substitute, Percutaneous Endoscopic Approach
HAC When reported with secondary diagnosis code J98.5

02104KF Bypass Coronary Artery, One Site from Abdominal Artery with Nonautologous Tissue Substitute, Percutaneous Endoscopic Approach
HAC When reported with secondary diagnosis code J98.5

02104KW Bypass Coronary Artery, One Site from Aorta with Nonautologous Tissue Substitute, Percutaneous Endoscopic Approach
HAC When reported with secondary diagnosis code J98.5

02104Z3 Bypass Coronary Artery, One Site from Coronary Artery, Percutaneous Endoscopic Approach
HAC When reported with secondary diagnosis code J98.5

02104Z8 Bypass Coronary Artery, One Site from Right Internal Mammary, Percutaneous Endoscopic Approach
HAC When reported with secondary diagnosis code J98.5

02104Z9 Bypass Coronary Artery, One Site from Left Internal Mammary, Percutaneous Endoscopic Approach
HAC When reported with secondary diagnosis code J98.5

02104ZC Bypass Coronary Artery, One Site from Thoracic Artery, Percutaneous Endoscopic Approach
HAC When reported with secondary diagnosis code J98.5

02104ZF Bypass Coronary Artery, One Site from Abdominal Artery, Percutaneous Endoscopic Approach
HAC When reported with secondary diagnosis code J98.5

0211093 Bypass Coronary Artery, Two Sites from Coronary Artery with Autologous Venous Tissue, Open Approach
HAC When reported with secondary diagnosis code J98.5

0211098 Bypass Coronary Artery, Two Sites from Right Internal Mammary with Autologous Venous Tissue, Open Approach
HAC When reported with secondary diagnosis code J98.5

0211099 Bypass Coronary Artery, Two Sites from Left Internal Mammary with Autologous Venous Tissue, Open Approach
HAC When reported with secondary diagnosis code J98.5

021109C Bypass Coronary Artery, Two Sites from Thoracic Artery with Autologous Venous Tissue, Open Approach
HAC When reported with secondary diagnosis code J98.5

021109F Bypass Coronary Artery, Two Sites from Abdominal Artery with Autologous Venous Tissue, Open Approach
HAC When reported with secondary diagnosis code J98.5

021109W Bypass Coronary Artery, Two Sites from Aorta with Autologous Venous Tissue, Open Approach
HAC When reported with secondary diagnosis code J98.5

02110A3 Bypass Coronary Artery, Two Sites from Coronary Artery with Autologous Arterial Tissue, Open Approach
HAC When reported with secondary diagnosis code J98.5

02110A8 Bypass Coronary Artery, Two Sites from Right Internal Mammary with Autologous Arterial Tissue, Open Approach
HAC When reported with secondary diagnosis code J98.5

02110A9 Bypass Coronary Artery, Two Sites from Left Internal Mammary with Autologous Arterial Tissue, Open Approach
HAC When reported with secondary diagnosis code J98.5

02110AC Bypass Coronary Artery, Two Sites from Thoracic Artery with Autologous Arterial Tissue, Open Approach
HAC When reported with secondary diagnosis code J98.5

02110AF Bypass Coronary Artery, Two Sites from Abdominal Artery with Autologous Arterial Tissue, Open Approach
HAC When reported with secondary diagnosis code J98.5

02110AW Bypass Coronary Artery, Two Sites from Aorta with Autologous Arterial Tissue, Open Approach
HAC When reported with secondary diagnosis code J98.5

02110J3 Bypass Coronary Artery, Two Sites from Coronary Artery with Synthetic Substitute, Open Approach
HAC When reported with secondary diagnosis code J98.5

02110J8 Bypass Coronary Artery, Two Sites from Right Internal Mammary with Synthetic Substitute, Open Approach
HAC When reported with secondary diagnosis code J98.5

02110J9 Bypass Coronary Artery, Two Sites from Left Internal Mammary with Synthetic Substitute, Open Approach
HAC When reported with secondary diagnosis code J98.5

02110JC Bypass Coronary Artery, Two Sites from Thoracic Artery with Synthetic Substitute, Open Approach
HAC When reported with secondary diagnosis code J98.5

02110JF Bypass Coronary Artery, Two Sites from Abdominal Artery with Synthetic Substitute, Open Approach
HAC When reported with secondary diagnosis code J98.5

02110JW Bypass Coronary Artery, Two Sites from Aorta with Synthetic Substitute, Open Approach
HAC When reported with secondary diagnosis code J98.5

02110K3 Bypass Coronary Artery, Two Sites from Coronary Artery with Nonautologous Tissue Substitute, Open Approach
HAC When reported with secondary diagnosis code J98.5

02110K8 Bypass Coronary Artery, Two Sites from Right Internal Mammary with Nonautologous Tissue Substitute, Open Approach
HAC When reported with secondary diagnosis code J98.5

02110K9 Bypass Coronary Artery, Two Sites from Left Internal Mammary with Nonautologous Tissue Substitute, Open Approach
HAC When reported with secondary diagnosis code J98.5

02110KC Bypass Coronary Artery, Two Sites from Thoracic Artery with Nonautologous Tissue Substitute, Open Approach
HAC When reported with secondary diagnosis code J98.5

02110KF Bypass Coronary Artery, Two Sites from Abdominal Artery with Nonautologous Tissue Substitute, Open Approach
HAC When reported with secondary diagnosis code J98.5

02110KW Bypass Coronary Artery, Two Sites from Aorta with Nonautologous Tissue Substitute, Open Approach
HAC When reported with secondary diagnosis code J98.5

02110Z3 Bypass Coronary Artery, Two Sites from Coronary Artery, Open Approach
HAC When reported with secondary diagnosis code J98.5

02110Z8 Bypass Coronary Artery, Two Sites from Right Internal Mammary, Open Approach
HAC When reported with secondary diagnosis code J98.5

02110Z9 Bypass Coronary Artery, Two Sites from Left Internal Mammary, Open Approach
HAC When reported with secondary diagnosis code J98.5

02110ZC Bypass Coronary Artery, Two Sites from Thoracic Artery, Open Approach
HAC When reported with secondary diagnosis code J98.5

02110ZF Bypass Coronary Artery, Two Sites from Abdominal Artery, Open Approach
HAC When reported with secondary diagnosis code J98.5

0211344 Bypass Coronary Artery, Two Sites from Coronary Vein with Drug-eluting Intraluminal Device, Percutaneous Approach

02113D4 Bypass Coronary Artery, Two Sites from Coronary Vein with Intraluminal Device, Percutaneous Approach

0211444 Bypass Coronary Artery, Two Sites from Coronary Vein with Drug-eluting Intraluminal Device, Percutaneous Endoscopic Approach
HAC When reported with secondary diagnosis code J98.5

0211493 Bypass Coronary Artery, Two Sites from Coronary Artery with Autologous Venous Tissue, Percutaneous Endoscopic Approach
HAC When reported with secondary diagnosis code J98.5

0211498 Bypass Coronary Artery, Two Sites from Right Internal Mammary with Autologous Venous Tissue, Percutaneous Endoscopic Approach
HAC When reported with secondary diagnosis code J98.5

0211499 Bypass Coronary Artery, Two Sites from Left Internal Mammary with Autologous Venous Tissue, Percutaneous Endoscopic Approach
HAC When reported with secondary diagnosis code J98.5

021149C Bypass Coronary Artery, Two Sites from Thoracic Artery with Autologous Venous Tissue, Percutaneous Endoscopic Approach
HAC When reported with secondary diagnosis code J98.5

021149F Bypass Coronary Artery, Two Sites from Abdominal Artery with Autologous Venous Tissue, Percutaneous Endoscopic Approach
HAC When reported with secondary diagnosis code J98.5

021149W Bypass Coronary Artery, Two Sites from Aorta with Autologous Venous Tissue, Percutaneous Endoscopic Approach
HAC When reported with secondary diagnosis code J98.5

02114A3 Bypass Coronary Artery, Two Sites from Coronary Artery with Autologous Arterial Tissue, Percutaneous Endoscopic Approach
HAC When reported with secondary diagnosis code J98.5

02114A8 Bypass Coronary Artery, Two Sites from Right Internal Mammary with Autologous Arterial Tissue, Percutaneous Endoscopic Approach
HAC When reported with secondary diagnosis code J98.5

02114A9 Bypass Coronary Artery, Two Sites from Left Internal Mammary with Autologous Arterial Tissue, Percutaneous Endoscopic Approach
HAC When reported with secondary diagnosis code J98.5

02114AC Bypass Coronary Artery, Two Sites from Thoracic Artery with Autologous Arterial Tissue, Percutaneous Endoscopic Approach
HAC When reported with secondary diagnosis code J98.5

02114AF Bypass Coronary Artery, Two Sites from Abdominal Artery with Autologous Arterial Tissue, Percutaneous Endoscopic Approach
HAC When reported with secondary diagnosis code J98.5

02114AW Bypass Coronary Artery, Two Sites from Aorta with Autologous Arterial Tissue, Percutaneous Endoscopic Approach
HAC When reported with secondary diagnosis code J98.5

02114D4 Bypass Coronary Artery, Two Sites from Coronary Vein with Intraluminal Device, Percutaneous Endoscopic Approach

02114J3 Bypass Coronary Artery, Two Sites from Coronary Artery with Synthetic Substitute, Percutaneous Endoscopic Approach
HAC When reported with secondary diagnosis code J98.5

02114J8 Bypass Coronary Artery, Two Sites from Right Internal Mammary with Synthetic Substitute, Percutaneous Endoscopic Approach
HAC When reported with secondary diagnosis code J98.5

02114J9 Bypass Coronary Artery, Two Sites from Left Internal Mammary with Synthetic Substitute, Percutaneous Endoscopic Approach
HAC When reported with secondary diagnosis code J98.5

02114JC Bypass Coronary Artery, Two Sites from Thoracic Artery with Synthetic Substitute, Percutaneous Endoscopic Approach
HAC When reported with secondary diagnosis code J98.5

02114JF Bypass Coronary Artery, Two Sites from Abdominal Artery with Synthetic Substitute, Percutaneous Endoscopic Approach
HAC When reported with secondary diagnosis code J98.5

02114JW Bypass Coronary Artery, Two Sites from Aorta with Synthetic Substitute, Percutaneous Endoscopic Approach
HAC When reported with secondary diagnosis code J98.5

02114K3 Bypass Coronary Artery, Two Sites from Coronary Artery with Nonautologous Tissue Substitute, Percutaneous Endoscopic Approach
HAC When reported with secondary diagnosis code J98.5

02114K8 Bypass Coronary Artery, Two Sites from Right Internal Mammary with Nonautologous Tissue Substitute, Percutaneous Endoscopic Approach
HAC When reported with secondary diagnosis code J98.5

02114K9 Bypass Coronary Artery, Two Sites from Left Internal Mammary with Nonautologous Tissue Substitute, Percutaneous Endoscopic Approach
HAC When reported with secondary diagnosis code J98.5

02114KC Bypass Coronary Artery, Two Sites from Thoracic Artery with Nonautologous Tissue Substitute, Percutaneous Endoscopic Approach
HAC When reported with secondary diagnosis code J98.5

02114KF Bypass Coronary Artery, Two Sites from Abdominal Artery with Nonautologous Tissue Substitute, Percutaneous Endoscopic Approach
HAC When reported with secondary diagnosis code J98.5

02114KW Bypass Coronary Artery, Two Sites from Aorta with Nonautologous Tissue Substitute, Percutaneous Endoscopic Approach
HAC When reported with secondary diagnosis code J98.5

02114Z3 Bypass Coronary Artery, Two Sites from Coronary Artery, Percutaneous Endoscopic Approach
HAC When reported with secondary diagnosis code J98.5

02114Z8 Bypass Coronary Artery, Two Sites from Right Internal Mammary, Percutaneous Endoscopic Approach
HAC When reported with secondary diagnosis code J98.5

02114Z9 Bypass Coronary Artery, Two Sites from Left Internal Mammary, Percutaneous Endoscopic Approach
HAC When reported with secondary diagnosis code J98.5

02114ZC Bypass Coronary Artery, Two Sites from Thoracic Artery, Percutaneous Endoscopic Approach
HAC When reported with secondary diagnosis code J98.5

02114ZF Bypass Coronary Artery, Two Sites from Abdominal Artery, Percutaneous Endoscopic Approach
HAC When reported with secondary diagnosis code J98.5

0212093 Bypass Coronary Artery, Three Sites from Coronary Artery with Autologous Venous Tissue, Open Approach
HAC When reported with secondary diagnosis code J98.5

0212098 Bypass Coronary Artery, Three Sites from Right Internal Mammary with Autologous Venous Tissue, Open Approach
HAC When reported with secondary diagnosis code J98.5

0212099 Bypass Coronary Artery, Three Sites from Left Internal Mammary with Autologous Venous Tissue, Open Approach
HAC When reported with secondary diagnosis code J98.5

021209C Bypass Coronary Artery, Three Sites from Thoracic Artery with Autologous Venous Tissue, Open Approach
HAC When reported with secondary diagnosis code J98.5

021209F Bypass Coronary Artery, Three Sites from Abdominal Artery with Autologous Venous Tissue, Open Approach
HAC When reported with secondary diagnosis code J98.5

021209W Bypass Coronary Artery, Three Sites from Aorta with Autologous Venous Tissue, Open Approach
HAC When reported with secondary diagnosis code J98.5

02120A3 Bypass Coronary Artery, Three Sites from Coronary Artery with Autologous Arterial Tissue, Open Approach
HAC When reported with secondary diagnosis code J98.5

02120A8 Bypass Coronary Artery, Three Sites from Right Internal Mammary with Autologous Arterial Tissue, Open Approach
HAC When reported with secondary diagnosis code J98.5

02120A9 Bypass Coronary Artery, Three Sites from Left Internal Mammary with Autologous Arterial Tissue, Open Approach
HAC When reported with secondary diagnosis code J98.5

02120AC Bypass Coronary Artery, Three Sites from Thoracic Artery with Autologous Arterial Tissue, Open Approach
HAC When reported with secondary diagnosis code J98.5

02120AF Bypass Coronary Artery, Three Sites from Abdominal Artery with Autologous Arterial Tissue, Open Approach
HAC When reported with secondary diagnosis code J98.5

02120AW Bypass Coronary Artery, Three Sites from Aorta with Autologous Arterial Tissue, Open Approach
HAC When reported with secondary diagnosis code J98.5

02120J3 Bypass Coronary Artery, Three Sites from Coronary Artery with Synthetic Substitute, Open Approach
HAC When reported with secondary diagnosis code J98.5

02120J8 Bypass Coronary Artery, Three Sites from Right Internal Mammary with Synthetic Substitute, Open Approach
HAC When reported with secondary diagnosis code J98.5

02120J9 Bypass Coronary Artery, Three Sites from Left Internal Mammary with Synthetic Substitute, Open Approach
HAC When reported with secondary diagnosis code J98.5

02120JC Bypass Coronary Artery, Three Sites from Thoracic Artery with Synthetic Substitute, Open Approach
HAC When reported with secondary diagnosis code J98.5

02120JF Bypass Coronary Artery, Three Sites from Abdominal Artery with Synthetic Substitute, Open Approach
HAC When reported with secondary diagnosis code J98.5

02120JW Bypass Coronary Artery, Three Sites from Aorta with Synthetic Substitute, Open Approach
HAC When reported with secondary diagnosis code J98.5

02120K3 Bypass Coronary Artery, Three Sites from Coronary Artery with Nonautologous Tissue Substitute, Open Approach
HAC When reported with secondary diagnosis code J98.5

02120K8 Bypass Coronary Artery, Three Sites from Right Internal Mammary with Nonautologous Tissue Substitute, Open Approach
HAC When reported with secondary diagnosis code J98.5

02120K9 Bypass Coronary Artery, Three Sites from Left Internal Mammary with Nonautologous Tissue Substitute, Open Approach
HAC When reported with secondary diagnosis code J98.5

02120KC Bypass Coronary Artery, Three Sites from Thoracic Artery with Nonautologous Tissue Substitute, Open Approach
HAC When reported with secondary diagnosis code J98.5

02120KF Bypass Coronary Artery, Three Sites from Abdominal Artery with Nonautologous Tissue Substitute, Open Approach
HAC When reported with secondary diagnosis code J98.5

02120KW Bypass Coronary Artery, Three Sites from Aorta with Nonautologous Tissue Substitute, Open Approach
HAC When reported with secondary diagnosis code J98.5

02120Z3 Bypass Coronary Artery, Three Sites from Coronary Artery, Open Approach
HAC When reported with secondary diagnosis code J98.5

02120Z8 Bypass Coronary Artery, Three Sites from Right Internal Mammary, Open Approach
HAC When reported with secondary diagnosis code J98.5

02120Z9 Bypass Coronary Artery, Three Sites from Left Internal Mammary, Open Approach
HAC When reported with secondary diagnosis code J98.5

02120ZC Bypass Coronary Artery, Three Sites from Thoracic Artery, Open Approach
HAC When reported with secondary diagnosis code J98.5

02120ZF Bypass Coronary Artery, Three Sites from Abdominal Artery, Open Approach
HAC When reported with secondary diagnosis code J98.5

0212344 Bypass Coronary Artery, Three Sites from Coronary Vein with Drug-eluting Intraluminal Device, Percutaneous Approach

02123D4 Bypass Coronary Artery, Three Sites from Coronary Vein with Intraluminal Device, Percutaneous Approach

0212444 Bypass Coronary Artery, Three Sites from Coronary Vein with Drug-eluting Intraluminal Device, Percutaneous Endoscopic Approach

0212493 Bypass Coronary Artery, Three Sites from Coronary Artery with Autologous Venous Tissue, Percutaneous Endoscopic Approach

0212498 Bypass Coronary Artery, Three Sites from Right Internal Mammary with Autologous Venous Tissue, Percutaneous Endoscopic Approach
HAC When reported with secondary diagnosis code J98.5

0212499 Bypass Coronary Artery, Three Sites from Left Internal Mammary with Autologous Venous Tissue, Percutaneous Endoscopic Approach
HAC When reported with secondary diagnosis code J98.5

021249C Bypass Coronary Artery, Three Sites from Thoracic Artery with Autologous Venous Tissue, Percutaneous Endoscopic Approach
HAC When reported with secondary diagnosis code J98.5

021249F Bypass Coronary Artery, Three Sites from Abdominal Artery with Autologous Venous Tissue, Percutaneous Endoscopic Approach
HAC When reported with secondary diagnosis code J98.5

021249W Bypass Coronary Artery, Three Sites from Aorta with Autologous Venous Tissue, Percutaneous Endoscopic Approach
HAC When reported with secondary diagnosis code J98.5

02124A3 Bypass Coronary Artery, Three Sites from Coronary Artery with Autologous Arterial Tissue, Percutaneous Endoscopic Approach
HAC When reported with secondary diagnosis code J98.5

02124A8 Bypass Coronary Artery, Three Sites from Right Internal Mammary with Autologous Arterial Tissue, Percutaneous Endoscopic Approach
HAC When reported with secondary diagnosis code J98.5

02124A9 Bypass Coronary Artery, Three Sites from Left Internal Mammary with Autologous Arterial Tissue, Percutaneous Endoscopic Approach
HAC When reported with secondary diagnosis code J98.5

02124AC Bypass Coronary Artery, Three Sites from Thoracic Artery with Autologous Arterial Tissue, Percutaneous Endoscopic Approach
HAC When reported with secondary diagnosis code J98.5

02124AF Bypass Coronary Artery, Three Sites from Abdominal Artery with Autologous Arterial Tissue, Percutaneous Endoscopic Approach
HAC When reported with secondary diagnosis code J98.5

02124AW Bypass Coronary Artery, Three Sites from Aorta with Autologous Arterial Tissue, Percutaneous Endoscopic Approach
HAC When reported with secondary diagnosis code J98.5

02124D4 Bypass Coronary Artery, Three Sites from Coronary Vein with Intraluminal Device, Percutaneous Endoscopic Approach
HAC When reported with secondary diagnosis code J98.5

02124J3 Bypass Coronary Artery, Three Sites from Coronary Artery with Synthetic Substitute, Percutaneous Endoscopic Approach
HAC When reported with secondary diagnosis code J98.5

02124J8 Bypass Coronary Artery, Three Sites from Right Internal Mammary with Synthetic Substitute, Percutaneous Endoscopic Approach
HAC When reported with secondary diagnosis code J98.5

02124J9 Bypass Coronary Artery, Three Sites from Left Internal Mammary with Synthetic Substitute, Percutaneous Endoscopic Approach
HAC When reported with secondary diagnosis code J98.5

02124JC Bypass Coronary Artery, Three Sites from Thoracic Artery with Synthetic Substitute, Percutaneous Endoscopic Approach
HAC When reported with secondary diagnosis code J98.5

02124JF Bypass Coronary Artery, Three Sites from Abdominal Artery with Synthetic Substitute, Percutaneous Endoscopic Approach
HAC When reported with secondary diagnosis code J98.5

02124JW Bypass Coronary Artery, Three Sites from Aorta with Synthetic Substitute, Percutaneous Endoscopic Approach
HAC When reported with secondary diagnosis code J98.5

♀ Female-only   ♂ Male-only   ● Limited Coverage   ● Non-OR   HAC HAC-associated procedure   ● Non-covered procedures   ✚ Combination

02124K3 Bypass Coronary Artery, Three Sites from Coronary Artery with Nonautologous Tissue Substitute, Percutaneous Endoscopic Approach
HAC When reported with secondary diagnosis code J98.5

02124K8 Bypass Coronary Artery, Three Sites from Right Internal Mammary with Nonautologous Tissue Substitute, Percutaneous Endoscopic Approach
HAC When reported with secondary diagnosis code J98.5

02124K9 Bypass Coronary Artery, Three Sites from Left Internal Mammary with Nonautologous Tissue Substitute, Percutaneous Endoscopic Approach
HAC When reported with secondary diagnosis code J98.5

02124KC Bypass Coronary Artery, Three Sites from Thoracic Artery with Nonautologous Tissue Substitute, Percutaneous Endoscopic Approach
HAC When reported with secondary diagnosis code J98.5

02124KF Bypass Coronary Artery, Three Sites from Abdominal Artery with Nonautologous Tissue Substitute, Percutaneous Endoscopic Approach
HAC When reported with secondary diagnosis code J98.5

02124KW Bypass Coronary Artery, Three Sites from Aorta with Nonautologous Tissue Substitute, Percutaneous Endoscopic Approach
HAC When reported with secondary diagnosis code J98.5

02124Z3 Bypass Coronary Artery, Three Sites from Coronary Artery, Percutaneous Endoscopic Approach
HAC When reported with secondary diagnosis code J98.5

02124Z8 Bypass Coronary Artery, Three Sites from Right Internal Mammary, Percutaneous Endoscopic Approach
HAC When reported with secondary diagnosis code J98.5

02124Z9 Bypass Coronary Artery, Three Sites from Left Internal Mammary, Percutaneous Endoscopic Approach
HAC When reported with secondary diagnosis code J98.5

02124ZC Bypass Coronary Artery, Three Sites from Thoracic Artery, Percutaneous Endoscopic Approach
HAC When reported with secondary diagnosis code J98.5

02124ZF Bypass Coronary Artery, Three Sites from Abdominal Artery, Percutaneous Endoscopic Approach
HAC When reported with secondary diagnosis code J98.5

0213093 Bypass Coronary Artery, Four or More Sites from Coronary Artery with Autologous Venous Tissue, Open Approach
HAC When reported with secondary diagnosis code J98.5

0213098 Bypass Coronary Artery, Four or More Sites from Right Internal Mammary with Autologous Venous Tissue, Open Approach
HAC When reported with secondary diagnosis code J98.5

0213099 Bypass Coronary Artery, Four or More Sites from Left Internal Mammary with Autologous Venous Tissue, Open Approach
HAC When reported with secondary diagnosis code J98.5

021309C Bypass Coronary Artery, Four or More Sites from Thoracic Artery with Autologous Venous Tissue, Open Approach
HAC When reported with secondary diagnosis code J98.5

021309F Bypass Coronary Artery, Four or More Sites from Abdominal Artery with Autologous Venous Tissue, Open Approach
HAC When reported with secondary diagnosis code J98.5

021309W Bypass Coronary Artery, Four or More Sites from Aorta with Autologous Venous Tissue, Open Approach
HAC When reported with secondary diagnosis code J98.5

02130A3 Bypass Coronary Artery, Four or More Sites from Coronary Artery with Autologous Arterial Tissue, Open Approach
HAC When reported with secondary diagnosis code J98.5

02130A8 Bypass Coronary Artery, Four or More Sites from Right Internal Mammary with Autologous Arterial Tissue, Open Approach
HAC When reported with secondary diagnosis code J98.5

02130A9 Bypass Coronary Artery, Four or More Sites from Left Internal Mammary with Autologous Arterial Tissue, Open Approach
HAC When reported with secondary diagnosis code J98.5

02130AC Bypass Coronary Artery, Four or More Sites from Thoracic Artery with Autologous Arterial Tissue, Open Approach
HAC When reported with secondary diagnosis code J98.5

02130AF Bypass Coronary Artery, Four or More Sites from Abdominal Artery with Autologous Arterial Tissue, Open Approach
HAC When reported with secondary diagnosis code J98.5

02130AW Bypass Coronary Artery, Four or More Sites from Aorta with Autologous Arterial Tissue, Open Approach
HAC When reported with secondary diagnosis code J98.5

02130J3 Bypass Coronary Artery, Four or More Sites from Coronary Artery with Synthetic Substitute, Open Approach
HAC When reported with secondary diagnosis code J98.5

02130J8 Bypass Coronary Artery, Four or More Sites from Right Internal Mammary with Synthetic Substitute, Open Approach
HAC When reported with secondary diagnosis code J98.5

02130J9 Bypass Coronary Artery, Four or More Sites from Left Internal Mammary with Synthetic Substitute, Open Approach
HAC When reported with secondary diagnosis code J98.5

02130JC Bypass Coronary Artery, Four or More Sites from Thoracic Artery with Synthetic Substitute, Open Approach
HAC When reported with secondary diagnosis code J98.5

02130JF Bypass Coronary Artery, Four or More Sites from Abdominal Artery with Synthetic Substitute, Open Approach
HAC When reported with secondary diagnosis code J98.5

02130JW Bypass Coronary Artery, Four or More Sites from Aorta with Synthetic Substitute, Open Approach
HAC When reported with secondary diagnosis code J98.5

02130K3 Bypass Coronary Artery, Four or More Sites from Coronary Artery with Nonautologous Tissue Substitute, Open Approach
HAC When reported with secondary diagnosis code J98.5

02130K8 Bypass Coronary Artery, Four or More Sites from Right Internal Mammary with Nonautologous Tissue Substitute, Open Approach
HAC When reported with secondary diagnosis code J98.5

02130K9 Bypass Coronary Artery, Four or More Sites from Left Internal Mammary with Nonautologous Tissue Substitute, Open Approach
HAC When reported with secondary diagnosis code J98.5

02130KC Bypass Coronary Artery, Four or More Sites from Thoracic Artery with Nonautologous Tissue Substitute, Open Approach
HAC When reported with secondary diagnosis code J98.5

02130KF Bypass Coronary Artery, Four or More Sites from Abdominal Artery with Nonautologous Tissue Substitute, Open Approach
HAC When reported with secondary diagnosis code J98.5

02130KW Bypass Coronary Artery, Four or More Sites from Aorta with Nonautologous Tissue Substitute, Open Approach
HAC When reported with secondary diagnosis code J98.5

02130Z3 Bypass Coronary Artery, Four or More Sites from Coronary Artery, Open Approach
HAC When reported with secondary diagnosis code J98.5

02130Z8 Bypass Coronary Artery, Four or More Sites from Right Internal Mammary, Open Approach
HAC When reported with secondary diagnosis code J98.5

02130Z9 Bypass Coronary Artery, Four or More Sites from Left Internal Mammary, Open Approach
HAC When reported with secondary diagnosis code J98.5

02130ZC Bypass Coronary Artery, Four or More Sites from Thoracic Artery, Open Approach
HAC When reported with secondary diagnosis code J98.5

02130ZF Bypass Coronary Artery, Four or More Sites from Abdominal Artery, Open Approach
HAC When reported with secondary diagnosis code J98.5

0213344 Bypass Coronary Artery, Four or More Sites from Coronary Vein with Drug-eluting Intraluminal Device, Percutaneous Approach
HAC When reported with secondary diagnosis code J98.5

02133D4 Bypass Coronary Artery, Four or More Sites from Coronary Vein with Intraluminal Device, Percutaneous Approach
HAC When reported with secondary diagnosis code J98.5

0213444 Bypass Coronary Artery, Four or More Sites from Coronary Vein with Drug-eluting Intraluminal Device, Percutaneous Endoscopic Approach
HAC When reported with secondary diagnosis code J98.5

0213493 Bypass Coronary Artery, Four or More Sites from Coronary Artery with Autologous Venous Tissue, Percutaneous Endoscopic Approach
HAC When reported with secondary diagnosis code J98.5

0213498 Bypass Coronary Artery, Four or More Sites from Right Internal Mammary with Autologous Venous Tissue, Percutaneous Endoscopic Approach
HAC When reported with secondary diagnosis code J98.5

0213499 Bypass Coronary Artery, Four or More Sites from Left Internal Mammary with Autologous Venous Tissue, Percutaneous Endoscopic Approach
HAC When reported with secondary diagnosis code J98.5

♀ Female-only   ♂ Male-only   ◐ Limited Coverage   ● Non-OR   HAC HAC-associated procedure   ● Non-covered procedures   ✚ Combination

021349C Bypass Coronary Artery, Four or More Sites from Thoracic Artery with Autologous Venous Tissue, Percutaneous Endoscopic Approach
HAC When reported with secondary diagnosis code J98.5

021349F Bypass Coronary Artery, Four or More Sites from Abdominal Artery with Autologous Venous Tissue, Percutaneous Endoscopic Approach
HAC When reported with secondary diagnosis code J98.5

021349W Bypass Coronary Artery, Four or More Sites from Aorta with Autologous Venous Tissue, Percutaneous Endoscopic Approach
HAC When reported with secondary diagnosis code J98.5

02134A3 Bypass Coronary Artery, Four or More Sites from Coronary Artery with Autologous Arterial Tissue, Percutaneous Endoscopic Approach
HAC When reported with secondary diagnosis code J98.5

02134A8 Bypass Coronary Artery, Four or More Sites from Right Internal Mammary with Autologous Arterial Tissue, Percutaneous Endoscopic Approach
HAC When reported with secondary diagnosis code J98.5

02134A9 Bypass Coronary Artery, Four or More Sites from Left Internal Mammary with Autologous Arterial Tissue, Percutaneous Endoscopic Approach
HAC When reported with secondary diagnosis code J98.5

02134AC Bypass Coronary Artery, Four or More Sites from Thoracic Artery with Autologous Arterial Tissue, Percutaneous Endoscopic Approach
HAC When reported with secondary diagnosis code J98.5

02134AF Bypass Coronary Artery, Four or More Sites from Abdominal Artery with Autologous Arterial Tissue, Percutaneous Endoscopic Approach
HAC When reported with secondary diagnosis code J98.5

02134AW Bypass Coronary Artery, Four or More Sites from Aorta with Autologous Arterial Tissue, Percutaneous Endoscopic Approach
HAC When reported with secondary diagnosis code J98.5

02134D4 Bypass Coronary Artery, Four or More Sites from Coronary Vein with Intraluminal Device, Percutaneous Endoscopic Approach
HAC When reported with secondary diagnosis code J98.5

02134J3 Bypass Coronary Artery, Four or More Sites from Coronary Artery with Synthetic Substitute, Percutaneous Endoscopic Approach
HAC When reported with secondary diagnosis code J98.5

02134J8 Bypass Coronary Artery, Four or More Sites from Right Internal Mammary with Synthetic Substitute, Percutaneous Endoscopic Approach
HAC When reported with secondary diagnosis code J98.5

02134J9 Bypass Coronary Artery, Four or More Sites from Left Internal Mammary with Synthetic Substitute, Percutaneous Endoscopic Approach
HAC When reported with secondary diagnosis code J98.5

02134JC Bypass Coronary Artery, Four or More Sites from Thoracic Artery with Synthetic Substitute, Percutaneous Endoscopic Approach
HAC When reported with secondary diagnosis code J98.5

02134JF Bypass Coronary Artery, Four or More Sites from Abdominal Artery with Synthetic Substitute, Percutaneous Endoscopic Approach
HAC When reported with secondary diagnosis code J98.5

02134JW Bypass Coronary Artery, Four or More Sites from Aorta with Synthetic Substitute, Percutaneous Endoscopic Approach
HAC When reported with secondary diagnosis code J98.5

02134K3 Bypass Coronary Artery, Four or More Sites from Coronary Artery with Nonautologous Tissue Substitute, Percutaneous Endoscopic Approach
HAC When reported with secondary diagnosis code J98.5

02134K8 Bypass Coronary Artery, Four or More Sites from Right Internal Mammary with Nonautologous Tissue Substitute, Percutaneous Endoscopic Approach
HAC When reported with secondary diagnosis code J98.5

02134K9 Bypass Coronary Artery, Four or More Sites from Left Internal Mammary with Nonautologous Tissue Substitute, Percutaneous Endoscopic Approach
HAC When reported with secondary diagnosis code J98.5

02134KC Bypass Coronary Artery, Four or More Sites from Thoracic Artery with Nonautologous Tissue Substitute, Percutaneous Endoscopic Approach
HAC When reported with secondary diagnosis code J98.5

02134KF Bypass Coronary Artery, Four or More Sites from Abdominal Artery with Nonautologous Tissue Substitute, Percutaneous Endoscopic Approach
HAC When reported with secondary diagnosis code J98.5

02134KW Bypass Coronary Artery, Four or More Sites from Aorta with Nonautologous Tissue Substitute, Percutaneous Endoscopic Approach
HAC When reported with secondary diagnosis code J98.5

02134Z3 Bypass Coronary Artery, Four or More Sites from Coronary Artery, Percutaneous Endoscopic Approach
HAC When reported with secondary diagnosis code J98.5

02134Z8 Bypass Coronary Artery, Four or More Sites from Right Internal Mammary, Percutaneous Endoscopic Approach
HAC When reported with secondary diagnosis code J98.5

02134Z9 Bypass Coronary Artery, Four or More Sites from Left Internal Mammary, Percutaneous Endoscopic Approach
HAC When reported with secondary diagnosis code J98.5

02134ZC Bypass Coronary Artery, Four or More Sites from Thoracic Artery, Percutaneous Endoscopic Approach
HAC When reported with secondary diagnosis code J98.5

02134ZF Bypass Coronary Artery, Four or More Sites from Abdominal Artery, Percutaneous Endoscopic Approach
HAC When reported with secondary diagnosis code J98.5

021609P Bypass Right Atrium to Pulmonary Trunk with Autologous Venous Tissue, Open Approach

021609Q Bypass Right Atrium to Right Pulmonary Artery with Autologous Venous Tissue, Open Approach

021609R Bypass Right Atrium to Left Pulmonary Artery with Autologous Venous Tissue, Open Approach

02160AP Bypass Right Atrium to Pulmonary Trunk with Autologous Arterial Tissue, Open Approach

02160AQ Bypass Right Atrium to Right Pulmonary Artery with Autologous Arterial Tissue, Open Approach

02160AR Bypass Right Atrium to Left Pulmonary Artery with Autologous Arterial Tissue, Open Approach

02160JP Bypass Right Atrium to Pulmonary Trunk with Synthetic Substitute, Open Approach

02160JQ Bypass Right Atrium to Right Pulmonary Artery with Synthetic Substitute, Open Approach

02160JR Bypass Right Atrium to Left Pulmonary Artery with Synthetic Substitute, Open Approach

02160KP Bypass Right Atrium to Pulmonary Trunk with Nonautologous Tissue Substitute, Open Approach

02160KQ Bypass Right Atrium to Right Pulmonary Artery with Nonautologous Tissue Substitute, Open Approach

02160KR Bypass Right Atrium to Left Pulmonary Artery with Nonautologous Tissue Substitute, Open Approach

02160Z7 Bypass Right Atrium to Left Atrium, Open Approach

02160ZP Bypass Right Atrium to Pulmonary Trunk, Open Approach

02160ZQ Bypass Right Atrium to Right Pulmonary Artery, Open Approach

02160ZR Bypass Right Atrium to Left Pulmonary Artery, Open Approach

021649P Bypass Right Atrium to Pulmonary Trunk with Autologous Venous Tissue, Percutaneous Endoscopic Approach

021649Q Bypass Right Atrium to Right Pulmonary Artery with Autologous Venous Tissue, Percutaneous Endoscopic Approach

021649R Bypass Right Atrium to Left Pulmonary Artery with Autologous Venous Tissue, Percutaneous Endoscopic Approach

02164AP Bypass Right Atrium to Pulmonary Trunk with Autologous Arterial Tissue, Percutaneous Endoscopic Approach

02164AQ Bypass Right Atrium to Right Pulmonary Artery with Autologous Arterial Tissue, Percutaneous Endoscopic Approach

02164AR Bypass Right Atrium to Left Pulmonary Artery with Autologous Arterial Tissue, Percutaneous Endoscopic Approach

02164JP Bypass Right Atrium to Pulmonary Trunk with Synthetic Substitute, Percutaneous Endoscopic Approach

02164JQ Bypass Right Atrium to Right Pulmonary Artery with Synthetic Substitute, Percutaneous Endoscopic Approach

02164JR Bypass Right Atrium to Left Pulmonary Artery with Synthetic Substitute, Percutaneous Endoscopic Approach

02164KP Bypass Right Atrium to Pulmonary Trunk with Nonautologous Tissue Substitute, Percutaneous Endoscopic Approach

02164KQ Bypass Right Atrium to Right Pulmonary Artery with Nonautologous Tissue Substitute, Percutaneous Endoscopic Approach

02164KR Bypass Right Atrium to Left Pulmonary Artery with Nonautologous Tissue Substitute, Percutaneous Endoscopic Approach

02164Z7 Bypass Right Atrium to Left Atrium, Percutaneous Endoscopic Approach

---

♀ Female-only ♂ Male-only ● Limited Coverage ● Non-OR HAC HAC-associated procedure ● Non-covered procedures ✚ Combination

02164ZP Bypass Right Atrium to Pulmonary Trunk, Percutaneous Endoscopic Approach

02164ZQ Bypass Right Atrium to Right Pulmonary Artery, Percutaneous Endoscopic Approach

02164ZR Bypass Right Atrium to Left Pulmonary Artery, Percutaneous Endoscopic Approach

021709P Bypass Left Atrium to Pulmonary Trunk with Autologous Venous Tissue, Open Approach

021709Q Bypass Left Atrium to Right Pulmonary Artery with Autologous Venous Tissue, Open Approach

021709R Bypass Left Atrium to Left Pulmonary Artery with Autologous Venous Tissue, Open Approach

02170AP Bypass Left Atrium to Pulmonary Trunk with Autologous Arterial Tissue, Open Approach

02170AQ Bypass Left Atrium to Right Pulmonary Artery with Autologous Arterial Tissue, Open Approach

02170AR Bypass Left Atrium to Left Pulmonary Artery with Autologous Arterial Tissue, Open Approach

02170JP Bypass Left Atrium to Pulmonary Trunk with Synthetic Substitute, Open Approach

02170JQ Bypass Left Atrium to Right Pulmonary Artery with Synthetic Substitute, Open Approach

02170JR Bypass Left Atrium to Left Pulmonary Artery with Synthetic Substitute, Open Approach

02170KP Bypass Left Atrium to Pulmonary Trunk with Nonautologous Tissue Substitute, Open Approach

02170KQ Bypass Left Atrium to Right Pulmonary Artery with Nonautologous Tissue Substitute, Open Approach

02170KR Bypass Left Atrium to Left Pulmonary Artery with Nonautologous Tissue Substitute, Open Approach

02170ZP Bypass Left Atrium to Pulmonary Trunk, Open Approach

02170ZQ Bypass Left Atrium to Right Pulmonary Artery, Open Approach

02170ZR Bypass Left Atrium to Left Pulmonary Artery, Open Approach

021749P Bypass Left Atrium to Pulmonary Trunk with Autologous Venous Tissue, Percutaneous Endoscopic Approach

021749Q Bypass Left Atrium to Right Pulmonary Artery with Autologous Venous Tissue, Percutaneous Endoscopic Approach

021749R Bypass Left Atrium to Left Pulmonary Artery with Autologous Venous Tissue, Percutaneous Endoscopic Approach

02174AP Bypass Left Atrium to Pulmonary Trunk with Autologous Arterial Tissue, Percutaneous Endoscopic Approach

02174AQ Bypass Left Atrium to Right Pulmonary Artery with Autologous Arterial Tissue, Percutaneous Endoscopic Approach

02174AR Bypass Left Atrium to Left Pulmonary Artery with Autologous Arterial Tissue, Percutaneous Endoscopic Approach

02174JP Bypass Left Atrium to Pulmonary Trunk with Synthetic Substitute, Percutaneous Endoscopic Approach

02174JQ Bypass Left Atrium to Right Pulmonary Artery with Synthetic Substitute, Percutaneous Endoscopic Approach

02174JR Bypass Left Atrium to Left Pulmonary Artery with Synthetic Substitute, Percutaneous Endoscopic Approach

02174KP Bypass Left Atrium to Pulmonary Trunk with Nonautologous Tissue Substitute, Percutaneous Endoscopic Approach

02174KQ Bypass Left Atrium to Right Pulmonary Artery with Nonautologous Tissue Substitute, Percutaneous Endoscopic Approach

02174KR Bypass Left Atrium to Left Pulmonary Artery with Nonautologous Tissue Substitute, Percutaneous Endoscopic Approach

02174ZP Bypass Left Atrium to Pulmonary Trunk, Percutaneous Endoscopic Approach

02174ZQ Bypass Left Atrium to Right Pulmonary Artery, Percutaneous Endoscopic Approach

02174ZR Bypass Left Atrium to Left Pulmonary Artery, Percutaneous Endoscopic Approach

021K09P Bypass Right Ventricle to Pulmonary Trunk with Autologous Venous Tissue, Open Approach

021K09Q Bypass Right Ventricle to Right Pulmonary Artery with Autologous Venous Tissue, Open Approach

021K09R Bypass Right Ventricle to Left Pulmonary Artery with Autologous Venous Tissue, Open Approach

021K0AP Bypass Right Ventricle to Pulmonary Trunk with Autologous Arterial Tissue, Open Approach

021K0AQ Bypass Right Ventricle to Right Pulmonary Artery with Autologous Arterial Tissue, Open Approach

021K0AR Bypass Right Ventricle to Left Pulmonary Artery with Autologous Arterial Tissue, Open Approach

021K0JP Bypass Right Ventricle to Pulmonary Trunk with Synthetic Substitute, Open Approach

021K0JQ Bypass Right Ventricle to Right Pulmonary Artery with Synthetic Substitute, Open Approach

021K0JR Bypass Right Ventricle to Left Pulmonary Artery with Synthetic Substitute, Open Approach

021K0KP Bypass Right Ventricle to Pulmonary Trunk with Nonautologous Tissue Substitute, Open Approach

021K0KQ Bypass Right Ventricle to Right Pulmonary Artery with Nonautologous Tissue Substitute, Open Approach

021K0KR Bypass Right Ventricle to Left Pulmonary Artery with Nonautologous Tissue Substitute, Open Approach

021K0Z5 Bypass Right Ventricle to Coronary Circulation, Open Approach

021K0Z8 Bypass Right Ventricle to Right Internal Mammary, Open Approach

021K0Z9 Bypass Right Ventricle to Left Internal Mammary, Open Approach

021K0ZC Bypass Right Ventricle to Thoracic Artery, Open Approach

021K0ZF Bypass Right Ventricle to Abdominal Artery, Open Approach

021K0ZP Bypass Right Ventricle to Pulmonary Trunk, Open Approach

021K0ZQ Bypass Right Ventricle to Right Pulmonary Artery, Open Approach

021K0ZR Bypass Right Ventricle to Left Pulmonary Artery, Open Approach

021K0ZW Bypass Right Ventricle to Aorta, Open Approach

021K49P Bypass Right Ventricle to Pulmonary Trunk with Autologous Venous Tissue, Percutaneous Endoscopic Approach

021K49Q Bypass Right Ventricle to Right Pulmonary Artery with Autologous Venous Tissue, Percutaneous Endoscopic Approach

021K49R Bypass Right Ventricle to Left Pulmonary Artery with Autologous Venous Tissue, Percutaneous Endoscopic Approach

021K4AP Bypass Right Ventricle to Pulmonary Trunk with Autologous Arterial Tissue, Percutaneous Endoscopic Approach

021K4AQ Bypass Right Ventricle to Right Pulmonary Artery with Autologous Arterial Tissue, Percutaneous Endoscopic Approach

021K4AR Bypass Right Ventricle to Left Pulmonary Artery with Autologous Arterial Tissue, Percutaneous Endoscopic Approach

021K4JP Bypass Right Ventricle to Pulmonary Trunk with Synthetic Substitute, Percutaneous Endoscopic Approach

021K4JQ Bypass Right Ventricle to Right Pulmonary Artery with Synthetic Substitute, Percutaneous Endoscopic Approach

021K4JR Bypass Right Ventricle to Left Pulmonary Artery with Synthetic Substitute, Percutaneous Endoscopic Approach

021K4KP Bypass Right Ventricle to Pulmonary Trunk with Nonautologous Tissue Substitute, Percutaneous Endoscopic Approach

021K4KQ Bypass Right Ventricle to Right Pulmonary Artery with Nonautologous Tissue Substitute, Percutaneous Endoscopic Approach

021K4KR Bypass Right Ventricle to Left Pulmonary Artery with Nonautologous Tissue Substitute, Percutaneous Endoscopic Approach

021K4Z5 Bypass Right Ventricle to Coronary Circulation, Percutaneous Endoscopic Approach

021K4Z8 Bypass Right Ventricle to Right Internal Mammary, Percutaneous Endoscopic Approach

021K4Z9 Bypass Right Ventricle to Left Internal Mammary, Percutaneous Endoscopic Approach

021K4ZC Bypass Right Ventricle to Thoracic Artery, Percutaneous Endoscopic Approach

021K4ZF Bypass Right Ventricle to Abdominal Artery, Percutaneous Endoscopic Approach

021K4ZP Bypass Right Ventricle to Pulmonary Trunk, Percutaneous Endoscopic Approach

021K4ZQ Bypass Right Ventricle to Right Pulmonary Artery, Percutaneous Endoscopic Approach

021K4ZR Bypass Right Ventricle to Left Pulmonary Artery, Percutaneous Endoscopic Approach

021K4ZW Bypass Right Ventricle to Aorta, Percutaneous Endoscopic Approach

021L09P Bypass Left Ventricle to Pulmonary Trunk with Autologous Venous Tissue, Open Approach

021L09Q Bypass Left Ventricle to Right Pulmonary Artery with Autologous Venous Tissue, Open Approach

021L09R Bypass Left Ventricle to Left Pulmonary Artery with Autologous Venous Tissue, Open Approach

---

021L0AP Bypass Left Ventricle to Pulmonary Trunk with Autologous Arterial Tissue, Open Approach

021L0AQ Bypass Left Ventricle to Right Pulmonary Artery with Autologous Arterial Tissue, Open Approach

021L0AR Bypass Left Ventricle to Left Pulmonary Artery with Autologous Arterial Tissue, Open Approach

021L0JP Bypass Left Ventricle to Pulmonary Trunk with Synthetic Substitute, Open Approach

021L0JQ Bypass Left Ventricle to Right Pulmonary Artery with Synthetic Substitute, Open Approach

021L0JR Bypass Left Ventricle to Left Pulmonary Artery with Synthetic Substitute, Open Approach

021L0KP Bypass Left Ventricle to Pulmonary Trunk with Nonautologous Tissue Substitute, Open Approach

021L0KQ Bypass Left Ventricle to Right Pulmonary Artery with Nonautologous Tissue Substitute, Open Approach

021L0KR Bypass Left Ventricle to Left Pulmonary Artery with Nonautologous Tissue Substitute, Open Approach

021L0Z5 Bypass Left Ventricle to Coronary Circulation, Open Approach

021L0Z8 Bypass Left Ventricle to Right Internal Mammary, Open Approach

021L0Z9 Bypass Left Ventricle to Left Internal Mammary, Open Approach

021L0ZC Bypass Left Ventricle to Thoracic Artery, Open Approach

021L0ZF Bypass Left Ventricle to Abdominal Artery, Open Approach

021L0ZP Bypass Left Ventricle to Pulmonary Trunk, Open Approach

021L0ZQ Bypass Left Ventricle to Right Pulmonary Artery, Open Approach

021L0ZR Bypass Left Ventricle to Left Pulmonary Artery, Open Approach

021L0ZW Bypass Left Ventricle to Aorta, Open Approach

021L49P Bypass Left Ventricle to Pulmonary Trunk with Autologous Venous Tissue, Percutaneous Endoscopic Approach

021L49Q Bypass Left Ventricle to Right Pulmonary Artery with Autologous Venous Tissue, Percutaneous Endoscopic Approach

021L49R Bypass Left Ventricle to Left Pulmonary Artery with Autologous Venous Tissue, Percutaneous Endoscopic Approach

021L4AP Bypass Left Ventricle to Pulmonary Trunk with Autologous Arterial Tissue, Percutaneous Endoscopic Approach

021L4AQ Bypass Left Ventricle to Right Pulmonary Artery with Autologous Arterial Tissue, Percutaneous Endoscopic Approach

021L4AR Bypass Left Ventricle to Left Pulmonary Artery with Autologous Arterial Tissue, Percutaneous Endoscopic Approach

021L4JP Bypass Left Ventricle to Pulmonary Trunk with Synthetic Substitute, Percutaneous Endoscopic Approach

021L4JQ Bypass Left Ventricle to Right Pulmonary Artery with Synthetic Substitute, Percutaneous Endoscopic Approach

021L4JR Bypass Left Ventricle to Left Pulmonary Artery with Synthetic Substitute, Percutaneous Endoscopic Approach

021L4KP Bypass Left Ventricle to Pulmonary Trunk with Nonautologous Tissue Substitute, Percutaneous Endoscopic Approach

021L4KQ Bypass Left Ventricle to Right Pulmonary Artery with Nonautologous Tissue Substitute, Percutaneous Endoscopic Approach

021L4KR Bypass Left Ventricle to Left Pulmonary Artery with Nonautologous Tissue Substitute, Percutaneous Endoscopic Approach

021L4Z5 Bypass Left Ventricle to Coronary Circulation, Percutaneous Endoscopic Approach

021L4Z8 Bypass Left Ventricle to Right Internal Mammary, Percutaneous Endoscopic Approach

021L4Z9 Bypass Left Ventricle to Left Internal Mammary, Percutaneous Endoscopic Approach

021L4ZC Bypass Left Ventricle to Thoracic Artery, Percutaneous Endoscopic Approach

021L4ZF Bypass Left Ventricle to Abdominal Artery, Percutaneous Endoscopic Approach

021L4ZP Bypass Left Ventricle to Pulmonary Trunk, Percutaneous Endoscopic Approach

021L4ZQ Bypass Left Ventricle to Right Pulmonary Artery, Percutaneous Endoscopic Approach

021L4ZR Bypass Left Ventricle to Left Pulmonary Artery, Percutaneous Endoscopic Approach

021L4ZW Bypass Left Ventricle to Aorta, Percutaneous Endoscopic Approach

021V09P Bypass Superior Vena Cava to Pulmonary Trunk with Autologous Venous Tissue, Open Approach

021V09Q Bypass Superior Vena Cava to Right Pulmonary Artery with Autologous Venous Tissue, Open Approach

021V09R Bypass Superior Vena Cava to Left Pulmonary Artery with Autologous Venous Tissue, Open Approach

021V0AP Bypass Superior Vena Cava to Pulmonary Trunk with Autologous Arterial Tissue, Open Approach

021V0AQ Bypass Superior Vena Cava to Right Pulmonary Artery with Autologous Arterial Tissue, Open Approach

021V0AR Bypass Superior Vena Cava to Left Pulmonary Artery with Autologous Arterial Tissue, Open Approach

021V0JP Bypass Superior Vena Cava to Pulmonary Trunk with Synthetic Substitute, Open Approach

021V0JQ Bypass Superior Vena Cava to Right Pulmonary Artery with Synthetic Substitute, Open Approach

021V0JR Bypass Superior Vena Cava to Left Pulmonary Artery with Synthetic Substitute, Open Approach

021V0KP Bypass Superior Vena Cava to Pulmonary Trunk with Nonautologous Tissue Substitute, Open Approach

021V0KQ Bypass Superior Vena Cava to Right Pulmonary Artery with Nonautologous Tissue Substitute, Open Approach

021V0KR Bypass Superior Vena Cava to Left Pulmonary Artery with Nonautologous Tissue Substitute, Open Approach

021V0ZP Bypass Superior Vena Cava to Pulmonary Trunk, Open Approach

021V0ZQ Bypass Superior Vena Cava to Right Pulmonary Artery, Open Approach

021V0ZR Bypass Superior Vena Cava to Left Pulmonary Artery, Open Approach

021V49P Bypass Superior Vena Cava to Pulmonary Trunk with Autologous Venous Tissue, Percutaneous Endoscopic Approach

021V49Q Bypass Superior Vena Cava to Right Pulmonary Artery with Autologous Venous Tissue, Percutaneous Endoscopic Approach

021V49R Bypass Superior Vena Cava to Left Pulmonary Artery with Autologous Venous Tissue, Percutaneous Endoscopic Approach

021V4AP Bypass Superior Vena Cava to Pulmonary Trunk with Autologous Arterial Tissue, Percutaneous Endoscopic Approach

021V4AQ Bypass Superior Vena Cava to Right Pulmonary Artery with Autologous Arterial Tissue, Percutaneous Endoscopic Approach

021V4AR Bypass Superior Vena Cava to Left Pulmonary Artery with Autologous Arterial Tissue, Percutaneous Endoscopic Approach

021V4JP Bypass Superior Vena Cava to Pulmonary Trunk with Synthetic Substitute, Percutaneous Endoscopic Approach

021V4JQ Bypass Superior Vena Cava to Right Pulmonary Artery with Synthetic Substitute, Percutaneous Endoscopic Approach

021V4JR Bypass Superior Vena Cava to Left Pulmonary Artery with Synthetic Substitute, Percutaneous Endoscopic Approach

021V4KP Bypass Superior Vena Cava to Pulmonary Trunk with Nonautologous Tissue Substitute, Percutaneous Endoscopic Approach

021V4KQ Bypass Superior Vena Cava to Right Pulmonary Artery with Nonautologous Tissue Substitute, Percutaneous Endoscopic Approach

021V4KR Bypass Superior Vena Cava to Left Pulmonary Artery with Nonautologous Tissue Substitute, Percutaneous Endoscopic Approach

021V4ZP Bypass Superior Vena Cava to Pulmonary Trunk, Percutaneous Endoscopic Approach

021V4ZQ Bypass Superior Vena Cava to Right Pulmonary Artery, Percutaneous Endoscopic Approach

021V4ZR Bypass Superior Vena Cava to Left Pulmonary Artery, Percutaneous Endoscopic Approach

021W09B Bypass Thoracic Aorta to Subclavian with Autologous Venous Tissue, Open Approach

021W09D Bypass Thoracic Aorta to Carotid with Autologous Venous Tissue, Open Approach

021W09P Bypass Thoracic Aorta to Pulmonary Trunk with Autologous Venous Tissue, Open Approach

021W09Q Bypass Thoracic Aorta to Right Pulmonary Artery with Autologous Venous Tissue, Open Approach

021W09R Bypass Thoracic Aorta to Left Pulmonary Artery with Autologous Venous Tissue, Open Approach

021W0AB Bypass Thoracic Aorta to Subclavian with Autologous Arterial Tissue, Open Approach

021W0AD Bypass Thoracic Aorta to Carotid with Autologous Arterial Tissue, Open Approach

021W0AP Bypass Thoracic Aorta to Pulmonary Trunk with Autologous Arterial Tissue, Open Approach

021W0AQ Bypass Thoracic Aorta to Right Pulmonary Artery with Autologous Arterial Tissue, Open Approach

021W0AR Bypass Thoracic Aorta to Left Pulmonary Artery with Autologous Arterial Tissue, Open Approach

021W0JB Bypass Thoracic Aorta to Subclavian with Synthetic Substitute, Open Approach

021W0JD Bypass Thoracic Aorta to Carotid with Synthetic Substitute, Open Approach

021W0JP Bypass Thoracic Aorta to Pulmonary Trunk with Synthetic Substitute, Open Approach

021W0JQ Bypass Thoracic Aorta to Right Pulmonary Artery with Synthetic Substitute, Open Approach

021W0JR Bypass Thoracic Aorta to Left Pulmonary Artery with Synthetic Substitute, Open Approach

021W0KB Bypass Thoracic Aorta to Subclavian with Nonautologous Tissue Substitute, Open Approach

021W0KD Bypass Thoracic Aorta to Carotid with Nonautologous Tissue Substitute, Open Approach

021W0KP Bypass Thoracic Aorta to Pulmonary Trunk with Nonautologous Tissue Substitute, Open Approach

021W0KQ Bypass Thoracic Aorta to Right Pulmonary Artery with Nonautologous Tissue Substitute, Open Approach

021W0KR Bypass Thoracic Aorta to Left Pulmonary Artery with Nonautologous Tissue Substitute, Open Approach

021W0ZB Bypass Thoracic Aorta to Subclavian, Open Approach

021W0ZD Bypass Thoracic Aorta to Carotid, Open Approach

021W0ZP Bypass Thoracic Aorta to Pulmonary Trunk, Open Approach

021W0ZQ Bypass Thoracic Aorta to Right Pulmonary Artery, Open Approach

021W0ZR Bypass Thoracic Aorta to Left Pulmonary Artery, Open Approach

021W49B Bypass Thoracic Aorta to Subclavian with Autologous Venous Tissue, Percutaneous Endoscopic Approach

021W49D Bypass Thoracic Aorta to Carotid with Autologous Venous Tissue, Percutaneous Endoscopic Approach

021W49P Bypass Thoracic Aorta to Pulmonary Trunk with Autologous Venous Tissue, Percutaneous Endoscopic Approach

021W49Q Bypass Thoracic Aorta to Right Pulmonary Artery with Autologous Venous Tissue, Percutaneous Endoscopic Approach

021W49R Bypass Thoracic Aorta to Left Pulmonary Artery with Autologous Venous Tissue, Percutaneous Endoscopic Approach

021W4AB Bypass Thoracic Aorta to Subclavian with Autologous Arterial Tissue, Percutaneous Endoscopic Approach

021W4AD Bypass Thoracic Aorta to Carotid with Autologous Arterial Tissue, Percutaneous Endoscopic Approach

021W4AP Bypass Thoracic Aorta to Pulmonary Trunk with Autologous Arterial Tissue, Percutaneous Endoscopic Approach

021W4AQ Bypass Thoracic Aorta to Right Pulmonary Artery with Autologous Arterial Tissue, Percutaneous Endoscopic Approach

021W4AR Bypass Thoracic Aorta to Left Pulmonary Artery with Autologous Arterial Tissue, Percutaneous Endoscopic Approach

021W4JB Bypass Thoracic Aorta to Subclavian with Synthetic Substitute, Percutaneous Endoscopic Approach

021W4JD Bypass Thoracic Aorta to Carotid with Synthetic Substitute, Percutaneous Endoscopic Approach

021W4JP Bypass Thoracic Aorta to Pulmonary Trunk with Synthetic Substitute, Percutaneous Endoscopic Approach

021W4JQ Bypass Thoracic Aorta to Right Pulmonary Artery with Synthetic Substitute, Percutaneous Endoscopic Approach

021W4JR Bypass Thoracic Aorta to Left Pulmonary Artery with Synthetic Substitute, Percutaneous Endoscopic Approach

021W4KB Bypass Thoracic Aorta to Subclavian with Nonautologous Tissue Substitute, Percutaneous Endoscopic Approach

021W4KD Bypass Thoracic Aorta to Carotid with Nonautologous Tissue Substitute, Percutaneous Endoscopic Approach

021W4KP Bypass Thoracic Aorta to Pulmonary Trunk with Nonautologous Tissue Substitute, Percutaneous Endoscopic Approach

021W4KQ Bypass Thoracic Aorta to Right Pulmonary Artery with Nonautologous Tissue Substitute, Percutaneous Endoscopic Approach

021W4KR Bypass Thoracic Aorta to Left Pulmonary Artery with Nonautologous Tissue Substitute, Percutaneous Endoscopic Approach

021W4ZB Bypass Thoracic Aorta to Subclavian, Percutaneous Endoscopic Approach

021W4ZD Bypass Thoracic Aorta to Carotid, Percutaneous Endoscopic Approach

021W4ZP Bypass Thoracic Aorta to Pulmonary Trunk, Percutaneous Endoscopic Approach

021W4ZQ Bypass Thoracic Aorta to Right Pulmonary Artery, Percutaneous Endoscopic Approach

021W4ZR Bypass Thoracic Aorta to Left Pulmonary Artery, Percutaneous Endoscopic Approach

025 – Heart and Great Vessels, Destruction

02540ZZ Destruction of Coronary Vein, Open Approach

02543ZZ Destruction of Coronary Vein, Percutaneous Approach

02544ZZ Destruction of Coronary Vein, Percutaneous Endoscopic Approach

02550ZZ Destruction of Atrial Septum, Open Approach

02553ZZ Destruction of Atrial Septum, Percutaneous Approach

02554ZZ Destruction of Atrial Septum, Percutaneous Endoscopic Approach

02560ZZ Destruction of Right Atrium, Open Approach

02563ZZ Destruction of Right Atrium, Percutaneous Approach

02564ZZ Destruction of Right Atrium, Percutaneous Endoscopic Approach

● **02570ZK** Destruction of Left Atrial Appendage, Open Approach

02570ZZ Destruction of Left Atrium, Open Approach

● **02573ZK** Destruction of Left Atrial Appendage, Percutaneous Approach

02573ZZ Destruction of Left Atrium, Percutaneous Approach

● **02574ZK** Destruction of Left Atrial Appendage, Percutaneous Endoscopic Approach

02574ZZ Destruction of Left Atrium, Percutaneous Endoscopic Approach

02580ZZ Destruction of Conduction Mechanism, Open Approach

02583ZZ Destruction of Conduction Mechanism, Percutaneous Approach

02584ZZ Destruction of Conduction Mechanism, Percutaneous Endoscopic Approach

02590ZZ Destruction of Chordae Tendineae, Open Approach

02593ZZ Destruction of Chordae Tendineae, Percutaneous Approach

02594ZZ Destruction of Chordae Tendineae, Percutaneous Endoscopic Approach

025D0ZZ Destruction of Papillary Muscle, Open Approach

025D3ZZ Destruction of Papillary Muscle, Percutaneous Approach

025D4ZZ Destruction of Papillary Muscle, Percutaneous Endoscopic Approach

025F0ZZ Destruction of Aortic Valve, Open Approach

025F3ZZ Destruction of Aortic Valve, Percutaneous Approach

025F4ZZ Destruction of Aortic Valve, Percutaneous Endoscopic Approach

025G0ZZ Destruction of Mitral Valve, Open Approach

025G3ZZ Destruction of Mitral Valve, Percutaneous Approach

025G4ZZ Destruction of Mitral Valve, Percutaneous Endoscopic Approach

025H0ZZ Destruction of Pulmonary Valve, Open Approach

025H3ZZ Destruction of Pulmonary Valve, Percutaneous Approach

025H4ZZ Destruction of Pulmonary Valve, Percutaneous Endoscopic Approach

025J0ZZ Destruction of Tricuspid Valve, Open Approach

025J3ZZ Destruction of Tricuspid Valve, Percutaneous Approach

025J4ZZ Destruction of Tricuspid Valve, Percutaneous Endoscopic Approach

025K0ZZ Destruction of Right Ventricle, Open Approach

025K3ZZ Destruction of Right Ventricle, Percutaneous Approach

025K4ZZ Destruction of Right Ventricle, Percutaneous Endoscopic Approach

025L0ZZ Destruction of Left Ventricle, Open Approach

025L3ZZ Destruction of Left Ventricle, Percutaneous Approach

025L4ZZ Destruction of Left Ventricle, Percutaneous Endoscopic Approach

025M0ZZ Destruction of Ventricular Septum, Open Approach

025M3ZZ Destruction of Ventricular Septum, Percutaneous Approach

025M4ZZ Destruction of Ventricular Septum, Percutaneous Endoscopic Approach

025N0ZZ Destruction of Pericardium, Open Approach

025N3ZZ Destruction of Pericardium, Percutaneous Approach

025N4ZZ Destruction of Pericardium, Percutaneous Endoscopic Approach

025P0ZZ Destruction of Pulmonary Trunk, Open Approach

025P3ZZ Destruction of Pulmonary Trunk, Percutaneous Approach

025P4ZZ Destruction of Pulmonary Trunk, Percutaneous Endoscopic Approach

025Q0ZZ Destruction of Right Pulmonary Artery, Open Approach

025Q3ZZ Destruction of Right Pulmonary Artery, Percutaneous Approach

025Q4ZZ Destruction of Right Pulmonary Artery, Percutaneous Endoscopic Approach
025R0ZZ Destruction of Left Pulmonary Artery, Open Approach
025R3ZZ Destruction of Left Pulmonary Artery, Percutaneous Approach
025R4ZZ Destruction of Left Pulmonary Artery, Percutaneous Endoscopic Approach
025S0ZZ Destruction of Right Pulmonary Vein, Open Approach
025S3ZZ Destruction of Right Pulmonary Vein, Percutaneous Approach
025S4ZZ Destruction of Right Pulmonary Vein, Percutaneous Endoscopic Approach
025T0ZZ Destruction of Left Pulmonary Vein, Open Approach

025T3ZZ Destruction of Left Pulmonary Vein, Percutaneous Approach
025T4ZZ Destruction of Left Pulmonary Vein, Percutaneous Endoscopic Approach
025V0ZZ Destruction of Superior Vena Cava, Open Approach
025V3ZZ Destruction of Superior Vena Cava, Percutaneous Approach
025V4ZZ Destruction of Superior Vena Cava, Percutaneous Endoscopic Approach
025W0ZZ Destruction of Thoracic Aorta, Open Approach
025W3ZZ Destruction of Thoracic Aorta, Percutaneous Approach
025W4ZZ Destruction of Thoracic Aorta, Percutaneous Endoscopic Approach

027 – Heart and Great Vessels, Dilation

For Dilation procedures involving the coronary arteries, Review Coding Guideline B4.4

0270046 Dilation of Coronary Artery, One Site, Bifurcation, with Drug-eluting Intraluminal Device, Open Approach
027004Z Dilation of Coronary Artery, One Site with Drug-eluting Intraluminal Device, Open Approach
02700D6 Dilation of Coronary Artery, One Site, Bifurcation, with Intraluminal Device, Open Approach
02700DZ Dilation of Coronary Artery, One Site with Intraluminal Device, Open Approach
02700T6 Dilation of Coronary Artery, One Site, Bifurcation, with Radioactive Intraluminal Device, Open Approach
02700TZ Dilation of Coronary Artery, One Site with Radioactive Intraluminal Device, Open Approach
02700Z6 Dilation of Coronary Artery, One Site, Bifurcation, Open Approach
02700ZZ Dilation of Coronary Artery, One Site, Open Approach
0270346 Dilation of Coronary Artery, One Site, Bifurcation, with Drug-eluting Intraluminal Device, Percutaneous Approach
027034Z Dilation of Coronary Artery, One Site with Drug-eluting Intraluminal Device, Percutaneous Approach
02703D6 Dilation of Coronary Artery, One Site, Bifurcation, with Intraluminal Device, Percutaneous Approach
02703DZ Dilation of Coronary Artery, One Site with Intraluminal Device, Percutaneous Approach
02703T6 Dilation of Coronary Artery, One Site, Bifurcation, with Radioactive Intraluminal Device, Percutaneous Approach
02703TZ Dilation of Coronary Artery, One Site with Radioactive Intraluminal Device, Percutaneous Approach
02703Z6 Dilation of Coronary Artery, One Site, Bifurcation, Percutaneous Approach
02703ZZ Dilation of Coronary Artery, One Site, Percutaneous Approach
0270446 Dilation of Coronary Artery, One Site, Bifurcation, with Drug-eluting Intraluminal Device, Percutaneous Endoscopic Approach
027044Z Dilation of Coronary Artery, One Site with Drug-eluting Intraluminal Device, Percutaneous Endoscopic Approach
02704D6 Dilation of Coronary Artery, One Site, Bifurcation, with Intraluminal Device, Percutaneous Endoscopic Approach
02704DZ Dilation of Coronary Artery, One Site with Intraluminal Device, Percutaneous Endoscopic Approach
02704T6 Dilation of Coronary Artery, One Site, Bifurcation, with Radioactive Intraluminal Device, Percutaneous Endoscopic Approach
02704TZ Dilation of Coronary Artery, One Site with Radioactive Intraluminal Device, Percutaneous Endoscopic Approach
02704Z6 Dilation of Coronary Artery, One Site, Bifurcation, Percutaneous Endoscopic Approach
02704ZZ Dilation of Coronary Artery, One Site, Percutaneous Endoscopic Approach
0271046 Dilation of Coronary Artery, Two Sites, Bifurcation, with Drug-eluting Intraluminal Device, Open Approach
027104Z Dilation of Coronary Artery, Two Sites with Drug-eluting Intraluminal Device, Open Approach
02710D6 Dilation of Coronary Artery, Two Sites, Bifurcation, with Intraluminal Device, Open Approach
02710DZ Dilation of Coronary Artery, Two Sites with Intraluminal Device, Open Approach
02710T6 Dilation of Coronary Artery, Two Sites, Bifurcation, with Radioactive Intraluminal Device, Open Approach
02710TZ Dilation of Coronary Artery, Two Sites with Radioactive Intraluminal Device, Open Approach

02710Z6 Dilation of Coronary Artery, Two Sites, Bifurcation, Open Approach
02710ZZ Dilation of Coronary Artery, Two Sites, Open Approach
0271346 Dilation of Coronary Artery, Two Sites, Bifurcation, with Drug-eluting Intraluminal Device, Percutaneous Approach
027134Z Dilation of Coronary Artery, Two Sites with Drug-eluting Intraluminal Device, Percutaneous Approach
02713D6 Dilation of Coronary Artery, Two Sites, Bifurcation, with Intraluminal Device, Percutaneous Approach
02713DZ Dilation of Coronary Artery, Two Sites with Intraluminal Device, Percutaneous Approach
02713T6 Dilation of Coronary Artery, Two Sites, Bifurcation, with Radioactive Intraluminal Device, Percutaneous Approach
02713TZ Dilation of Coronary Artery, Two Sites with Radioactive Intraluminal Device, Percutaneous Approach
02713Z6 Dilation of Coronary Artery, Two Sites, Bifurcation, Percutaneous Approach
02713ZZ Dilation of Coronary Artery, Two Sites, Percutaneous Approach
0271446 Dilation of Coronary Artery, Two Sites, Bifurcation, with Drug-eluting Intraluminal Device, Percutaneous Endoscopic Approach
027144Z Dilation of Coronary Artery, Two Sites with Drug-eluting Intraluminal Device, Percutaneous Endoscopic Approach
02714D6 Dilation of Coronary Artery, Two Sites, Bifurcation, with Intraluminal Device, Percutaneous Endoscopic Approach
02714DZ Dilation of Coronary Artery, Two Sites with Intraluminal Device, Percutaneous Endoscopic Approach
02714T6 Dilation of Coronary Artery, Two Sites, Bifurcation, with Radioactive Intraluminal Device, Percutaneous Endoscopic Approach
02714TZ Dilation of Coronary Artery, Two Sites with Radioactive Intraluminal Device, Percutaneous Endoscopic Approach
02714Z6 Dilation of Coronary Artery, Two Sites, Bifurcation, Percutaneous Endoscopic Approach
02714ZZ Dilation of Coronary Artery, Two Sites, Percutaneous Endoscopic Approach
0272046 Dilation of Coronary Artery, Three Sites, Bifurcation, with Drug-eluting Intraluminal Device, Open Approach
027204Z Dilation of Coronary Artery, Three Sites with Drug-eluting Intraluminal Device, Open Approach
02720D6 Dilation of Coronary Artery, Three Sites, Bifurcation, with Intraluminal Device, Open Approach
02720DZ Dilation of Coronary Artery, Three Sites with Intraluminal Device, Open Approach
02720T6 Dilation of Coronary Artery, Three Sites, Bifurcation, with Radioactive Intraluminal Device, Open Approach
02720TZ Dilation of Coronary Artery, Three Sites with Radioactive Intraluminal Device, Open Approach
02720Z6 Dilation of Coronary Artery, Three Sites, Bifurcation, Open Approach
02720ZZ Dilation of Coronary Artery, Three Sites, Open Approach
0272346 Dilation of Coronary Artery, Three Sites, Bifurcation, with Drug-eluting Intraluminal Device, Percutaneous Approach
027234Z Dilation of Coronary Artery, Three Sites with Drug-eluting Intraluminal Device, Percutaneous Approach
02723D6 Dilation of Coronary Artery, Three Sites, Bifurcation, with Intraluminal Device, Percutaneous Approach
02723DZ Dilation of Coronary Artery, Three Sites with Intraluminal Device, Percutaneous Approach

---

♀ Female-only   ♂ Male-only   ● Limited Coverage   ● Non-OR   HAC HAC-associated procedure   ● Non-covered procedures   ✚ Combination

02723T6 Dilation of Coronary Artery, Three Sites, Bifurcation, with Radioactive Intraluminal Device, Percutaneous Approach

02723TZ Dilation of Coronary Artery, Three Sites with Radioactive Intraluminal Device, Percutaneous Approach

02723Z6 Dilation of Coronary Artery, Three Sites, Bifurcation, Percutaneous Approach

02723ZZ Dilation of Coronary Artery, Three Sites, Percutaneous Approach

0272446 Dilation of Coronary Artery, Three Sites, Bifurcation, with Drug-eluting Intraluminal Device, Percutaneous Endoscopic Approach

027244Z Dilation of Coronary Artery, Three Sites with Drug-eluting Intraluminal Device, Percutaneous Endoscopic Approach

02724D6 Dilation of Coronary Artery, Three Sites, Bifurcation, with Intraluminal Device, Percutaneous Endoscopic Approach

02724DZ Dilation of Coronary Artery, Three Sites with Intraluminal Device, Percutaneous Endoscopic Approach

02724T6 Dilation of Coronary Artery, Three Sites, Bifurcation, with Radioactive Intraluminal Device, Percutaneous Endoscopic Approach

02724TZ Dilation of Coronary Artery, Three Sites with Radioactive Intraluminal Device, Percutaneous Endoscopic Approach

02724Z6 Dilation of Coronary Artery, Three Sites, Bifurcation, Percutaneous Endoscopic Approach

02724ZZ Dilation of Coronary Artery, Three Sites, Percutaneous Endoscopic Approach

0273046 Dilation of Coronary Artery, Four or More Sites, Bifurcation, with Drug-eluting Intraluminal Device, Open Approach

027304Z Dilation of Coronary Artery, Four or More Sites with Drug-eluting Intraluminal Device, Open Approach

02730D6 Dilation of Coronary Artery, Four or More Sites, Bifurcation, with Intraluminal Device, Open Approach

02730DZ Dilation of Coronary Artery, Four or More Sites with Intraluminal Device, Open Approach

02730T6 Dilation of Coronary Artery, Four or More Sites, Bifurcation, with Radioactive Intraluminal Device, Open Approach

02730TZ Dilation of Coronary Artery, Four or More Sites with Radioactive Intraluminal Device, Open Approach

02730Z6 Dilation of Coronary Artery, Four or More Sites, Bifurcation, Open Approach

02730ZZ Dilation of Coronary Artery, Four or More Sites, Open Approach

0273346 Dilation of Coronary Artery, Four or More Sites, Bifurcation, with Drug-eluting Intraluminal Device, Percutaneous Approach

027334Z Dilation of Coronary Artery, Four or More Sites with Drug-eluting Intraluminal Device, Percutaneous Approach

02733D6 Dilation of Coronary Artery, Four or More Sites, Bifurcation, with Intraluminal Device, Percutaneous Approach

02733DZ Dilation of Coronary Artery, Four or More Sites with Intraluminal Device, Percutaneous Approach

02733T6 Dilation of Coronary Artery, Four or More Sites, Bifurcation, with Radioactive Intraluminal Device, Percutaneous Approach

02733TZ Dilation of Coronary Artery, Four or More Sites with Radioactive Intraluminal Device, Percutaneous Approach

02733Z6 Dilation of Coronary Artery, Four or More Sites, Bifurcation, Percutaneous Approach

02733ZZ Dilation of Coronary Artery, Four or More Sites, Percutaneous Approach

0273446 Dilation of Coronary Artery, Four or More Sites, Bifurcation, with Drug-eluting Intraluminal Device, Percutaneous Endoscopic Approach

027344Z Dilation of Coronary Artery, Four or More Sites with Drug-eluting Intraluminal Device, Percutaneous Endoscopic Approach

02734D6 Dilation of Coronary Artery, Four or More Sites, Bifurcation, with Intraluminal Device, Percutaneous Endoscopic Approach

02734DZ Dilation of Coronary Artery, Four or More Sites with Intraluminal Device, Percutaneous Endoscopic Approach

02734T6 Dilation of Coronary Artery, Four or More Sites, Bifurcation, with Radioactive Intraluminal Device, Percutaneous Endoscopic Approach

02734TZ Dilation of Coronary Artery, Four or More Sites with Radioactive Intraluminal Device, Percutaneous Endoscopic Approach

02734Z6 Dilation of Coronary Artery, Four or More Sites, Bifurcation, Percutaneous Endoscopic Approach

02734ZZ Dilation of Coronary Artery, Four or More Sites, Percutaneous Endoscopic Approach

027F04Z Dilation of Aortic Valve with Drug-eluting Intraluminal Device, Open Approach

027F0DZ Dilation of Aortic Valve with Intraluminal Device, Open Approach

027F0ZZ Dilation of Aortic Valve, Open Approach

027F34Z Dilation of Aortic Valve with Drug-eluting Intraluminal Device, Percutaneous Approach

027F3DZ Dilation of Aortic Valve with Intraluminal Device, Percutaneous Approach

027F3ZZ Dilation of Aortic Valve, Percutaneous Approach

027F44Z Dilation of Aortic Valve with Drug-eluting Intraluminal Device, Percutaneous Endoscopic Approach

027F4DZ Dilation of Aortic Valve with Intraluminal Device, Percutaneous Endoscopic Approach

027F4ZZ Dilation of Aortic Valve, Percutaneous Endoscopic Approach

027G04Z Dilation of Mitral Valve with Drug-eluting Intraluminal Device, Open Approach

027G0DZ Dilation of Mitral Valve with Intraluminal Device, Open Approach

027G0ZZ Dilation of Mitral Valve, Open Approach

027G34Z Dilation of Mitral Valve with Drug-eluting Intraluminal Device, Percutaneous Approach

027G3DZ Dilation of Mitral Valve with Intraluminal Device, Percutaneous Approach

027G3ZZ Dilation of Mitral Valve, Percutaneous Approach

027G44Z Dilation of Mitral Valve with Drug-eluting Intraluminal Device, Percutaneous Endoscopic Approach

027G4DZ Dilation of Mitral Valve with Intraluminal Device, Percutaneous Endoscopic Approach

027G4ZZ Dilation of Mitral Valve, Percutaneous Endoscopic Approach

027H04Z Dilation of Pulmonary Valve with Drug-eluting Intraluminal Device, Open Approach

027H0DZ Dilation of Pulmonary Valve with Intraluminal Device, Open Approach

027H0ZZ Dilation of Pulmonary Valve, Open Approach

027H34Z Dilation of Pulmonary Valve with Drug-eluting Intraluminal Device, Percutaneous Approach

027H3DZ Dilation of Pulmonary Valve with Intraluminal Device, Percutaneous Approach

027H3ZZ Dilation of Pulmonary Valve, Percutaneous Approach

027H44Z Dilation of Pulmonary Valve with Drug-eluting Intraluminal Device, Percutaneous Endoscopic Approach

027H4DZ Dilation of Pulmonary Valve with Intraluminal Device, Percutaneous Endoscopic Approach

027H4ZZ Dilation of Pulmonary Valve, Percutaneous Endoscopic Approach

027J04Z Dilation of Tricuspid Valve with Drug-eluting Intraluminal Device, Open Approach

027J0DZ Dilation of Tricuspid Valve with Intraluminal Device, Open Approach

027J0ZZ Dilation of Tricuspid Valve, Open Approach

027J34Z Dilation of Tricuspid Valve with Drug-eluting Intraluminal Device, Percutaneous Approach

027J3DZ Dilation of Tricuspid Valve with Intraluminal Device, Percutaneous Approach

027J3ZZ Dilation of Tricuspid Valve, Percutaneous Approach

027J44Z Dilation of Tricuspid Valve with Drug-eluting Intraluminal Device, Percutaneous Endoscopic Approach

027J4DZ Dilation of Tricuspid Valve with Intraluminal Device, Percutaneous Endoscopic Approach

027J4ZZ Dilation of Tricuspid Valve, Percutaneous Endoscopic Approach

027K04Z Dilation of Right Ventricle with Drug-eluting Intraluminal Device, Open Approach

027K0DZ Dilation of Right Ventricle with Intraluminal Device, Open Approach

027K0ZZ Dilation of Right Ventricle, Open Approach

027K34Z Dilation of Right Ventricle with Drug-eluting Intraluminal Device, Percutaneous Approach

027K3DZ Dilation of Right Ventricle with Intraluminal Device, Percutaneous Approach

027K3ZZ Dilation of Right Ventricle, Percutaneous Approach

027K44Z Dilation of Right Ventricle with Drug-eluting Intraluminal Device, Percutaneous Endoscopic Approach

027K4DZ Dilation of Right Ventricle with Intraluminal Device, Percutaneous Endoscopic Approach

027K4ZZ Dilation of Right Ventricle, Percutaneous Endoscopic Approach

027P04Z Dilation of Pulmonary Trunk with Drug-eluting Intraluminal Device, Open Approach

---

♀ Female-only ♂ Male-only ● Limited Coverage ● Non-OR ▨ HAC-associated procedure ● Non-covered procedures ＋ Combination

027P0DZ Dilation of Pulmonary Trunk with Intraluminal Device, Open Approach

027P0ZZ Dilation of Pulmonary Trunk, Open Approach

027P34Z Dilation of Pulmonary Trunk with Drug-eluting Intraluminal Device, Percutaneous Approach

027P3DZ Dilation of Pulmonary Trunk with Intraluminal Device, Percutaneous Approach

027P3ZZ Dilation of Pulmonary Trunk, Percutaneous Approach

027P44Z Dilation of Pulmonary Trunk with Drug-eluting Intraluminal Device, Percutaneous Endoscopic Approach

027P4DZ Dilation of Pulmonary Trunk with Intraluminal Device, Percutaneous Endoscopic Approach

027P4ZZ Dilation of Pulmonary Trunk, Percutaneous Endoscopic Approach

027Q04Z Dilation of Right Pulmonary Artery with Drug-eluting Intraluminal Device, Open Approach

027Q0DZ Dilation of Right Pulmonary Artery with Intraluminal Device, Open Approach

027Q0ZZ Dilation of Right Pulmonary Artery, Open Approach

027Q34Z Dilation of Right Pulmonary Artery with Drug-eluting Intraluminal Device, Percutaneous Approach

027Q3DZ Dilation of Right Pulmonary Artery with Intraluminal Device, Percutaneous Approach

027Q3ZZ Dilation of Right Pulmonary Artery, Percutaneous Approach

027Q44Z Dilation of Right Pulmonary Artery with Drug-eluting Intraluminal Device, Percutaneous Endoscopic Approach

027Q4DZ Dilation of Right Pulmonary Artery with Intraluminal Device, Percutaneous Endoscopic Approach

027Q4ZZ Dilation of Right Pulmonary Artery, Percutaneous Endoscopic Approach

027R04T Dilation of Ductus Arteriosus with Drug-eluting Intraluminal Device, Open Approach

027R04Z Dilation of Left Pulmonary Artery with Drug-eluting Intraluminal Device, Open Approach

027R0DT Dilation of Ductus Arteriosus with Intraluminal Device, Open Approach

027R0DZ Dilation of Left Pulmonary Artery with Intraluminal Device, Open Approach

027R0ZT Dilation of Ductus Arteriosus, Open Approach

027R0ZZ Dilation of Left Pulmonary Artery, Open Approach

027R34T Dilation of Ductus Arteriosus with Drug-eluting Intraluminal Device, Percutaneous Approach

027R34Z Dilation of Left Pulmonary Artery with Drug-eluting Intraluminal Device, Percutaneous Approach

027R3DT Dilation of Ductus Arteriosus with Intraluminal Device, Percutaneous Approach

027R3DZ Dilation of Left Pulmonary Artery with Intraluminal Device, Percutaneous Approach

027R3ZT Dilation of Ductus Arteriosus, Percutaneous Approach

027R3ZZ Dilation of Left Pulmonary Artery, Percutaneous Approach

027R44T Dilation of Ductus Arteriosus with Drug-eluting Intraluminal Device, Percutaneous Endoscopic Approach

027R44Z Dilation of Left Pulmonary Artery with Drug-eluting Intraluminal Device, Percutaneous Endoscopic Approach

027R4DT Dilation of Ductus Arteriosus with Intraluminal Device, Percutaneous Endoscopic Approach

027R4DZ Dilation of Left Pulmonary Artery with Intraluminal Device, Percutaneous Endoscopic Approach

027R4ZT Dilation of Ductus Arteriosus, Percutaneous Endoscopic Approach

027R4ZZ Dilation of Left Pulmonary Artery, Percutaneous Endoscopic Approach

027S04Z Dilation of Right Pulmonary Vein with Drug-eluting Intraluminal Device, Open Approach

027S0DZ Dilation of Right Pulmonary Vein with Intraluminal Device, Open Approach

027S0ZZ Dilation of Right Pulmonary Vein, Open Approach

027S34Z Dilation of Right Pulmonary Vein with Drug-eluting Intraluminal Device, Percutaneous Approach

027S3DZ Dilation of Right Pulmonary Vein with Intraluminal Device, Percutaneous Approach

027S3ZZ Dilation of Right Pulmonary Vein, Percutaneous Approach

027S44Z Dilation of Right Pulmonary Vein with Drug-eluting Intraluminal Device, Percutaneous Endoscopic Approach

027S4DZ Dilation of Right Pulmonary Vein with Intraluminal Device, Percutaneous Endoscopic Approach

027S4ZZ Dilation of Right Pulmonary Vein, Percutaneous Endoscopic Approach

027T04Z Dilation of Left Pulmonary Vein with Drug-eluting Intraluminal Device, Open Approach

027T0DZ Dilation of Left Pulmonary Vein with Intraluminal Device, Open Approach

027T0ZZ Dilation of Left Pulmonary Vein, Open Approach

027T34Z Dilation of Left Pulmonary Vein with Drug-eluting Intraluminal Device, Percutaneous Approach

027T3DZ Dilation of Left Pulmonary Vein with Intraluminal Device, Percutaneous Approach

027T3ZZ Dilation of Left Pulmonary Vein, Percutaneous Approach

027T44Z Dilation of Left Pulmonary Vein with Drug-eluting Intraluminal Device, Percutaneous Endoscopic Approach

027T4DZ Dilation of Left Pulmonary Vein with Intraluminal Device, Percutaneous Endoscopic Approach

027T4ZZ Dilation of Left Pulmonary Vein, Percutaneous Endoscopic Approach

027V04Z Dilation of Superior Vena Cava with Drug-eluting Intraluminal Device, Open Approach

027V0DZ Dilation of Superior Vena Cava with Intraluminal Device, Open Approach

027V0ZZ Dilation of Superior Vena Cava, Open Approach

027V34Z Dilation of Superior Vena Cava with Drug-eluting Intraluminal Device, Percutaneous Approach

027V3DZ Dilation of Superior Vena Cava with Intraluminal Device, Percutaneous Approach

027V3ZZ Dilation of Superior Vena Cava, Percutaneous Approach

027V44Z Dilation of Superior Vena Cava with Drug-eluting Intraluminal Device, Percutaneous Endoscopic Approach

027V4DZ Dilation of Superior Vena Cava with Intraluminal Device, Percutaneous Endoscopic Approach

027V4ZZ Dilation of Superior Vena Cava, Percutaneous Endoscopic Approach

027W04Z Dilation of Thoracic Aorta with Drug-eluting Intraluminal Device, Open Approach

027W0DZ Dilation of Thoracic Aorta with Intraluminal Device, Open Approach

027W0ZZ Dilation of Thoracic Aorta, Open Approach

027W34Z Dilation of Thoracic Aorta with Drug-eluting Intraluminal Device, Percutaneous Approach

027W3DZ Dilation of Thoracic Aorta with Intraluminal Device, Percutaneous Approach

027W3ZZ Dilation of Thoracic Aorta, Percutaneous Approach

027W44Z Dilation of Thoracic Aorta with Drug-eluting Intraluminal Device, Percutaneous Endoscopic Approach

027W4DZ Dilation of Thoracic Aorta with Intraluminal Device, Percutaneous Endoscopic Approach

027W4ZZ Dilation of Thoracic Aorta, Percutaneous Endoscopic Approach

028 – Heart and Great Vessels, Division

Review Coding Guideline B3.14

02880ZZ Division of Conduction Mechanism, Open Approach

02883ZZ Division of Conduction Mechanism, Percutaneous Approach

02884ZZ Division of Conduction Mechanism, Percutaneous Endoscopic Approach

02890ZZ Division of Chordae Tendineae, Open Approach

02893ZZ Division of Chordae Tendineae, Percutaneous Approach

♀ Female-only   ♂ Male-only   ● Limited Coverage   ● Non-OR   HAC HAC-associated procedure   ● Non-covered procedures   ✚ Combination

02894ZZ	Division of Chordae Tendineae, Percutaneous Endoscopic Approach
028D0ZZ	Division of Papillary Muscle, Open Approach

028D3ZZ	Division of Papillary Muscle, Percutaneous Approach
028D4ZZ	Division of Papillary Muscle, Percutaneous Endoscopic Approach

02B – Heart and Great Vessels, Excision

Review Coding Guidelines B3.4a and B3.4b

Review Coding Guideline B3.8

02B40ZX	Excision of Coronary Vein, Open Approach, Diagnostic
02B40ZZ	Excision of Coronary Vein, Open Approach
02B43ZX	Excision of Coronary Vein, Percutaneous Approach, Diagnostic
02B43ZZ	Excision of Coronary Vein, Percutaneous Approach
02B44ZX	Excision of Coronary Vein, Percutaneous Endoscopic Approach, Diagnostic
02B44ZZ	Excision of Coronary Vein, Percutaneous Endoscopic Approach
02B50ZX	Excision of Atrial Septum, Open Approach, Diagnostic
02B50ZZ	Excision of Atrial Septum, Open Approach
02B53ZX	Excision of Atrial Septum, Percutaneous Approach, Diagnostic
02B53ZZ	Excision of Atrial Septum, Percutaneous Approach
02B54ZX	Excision of Atrial Septum, Percutaneous Endoscopic Approach, Diagnostic
02B54ZZ	Excision of Atrial Septum, Percutaneous Endoscopic Approach
02B60ZX	Excision of Right Atrium, Open Approach, Diagnostic
02B60ZZ	Excision of Right Atrium, Open Approach
02B63ZX	Excision of Right Atrium, Percutaneous Approach, Diagnostic
02B63ZZ	Excision of Right Atrium, Percutaneous Approach
02B64ZX	Excision of Right Atrium, Percutaneous Endoscopic Approach, Diagnostic
02B64ZZ	Excision of Right Atrium, Percutaneous Endoscopic Approach
● 02B70ZK	Excision of Left Atrial Appendage, Open Approach
02B70ZX	Excision of Left Atrium, Open Approach, Diagnostic
02B70ZZ	Excision of Left Atrium, Open Approach
● 02B73ZK	Excision of Left Atrial Appendage, Percutaneous Approach
02B73ZX	Excision of Left Atrium, Percutaneous Approach, Diagnostic
02B73ZZ	Excision of Left Atrium, Percutaneous Approach
● 02B74ZK	Excision of Left Atrial Appendage, Percutaneous Endoscopic Approach
02B74ZX	Excision of Left Atrium, Percutaneous Endoscopic Approach, Diagnostic
02B74ZZ	Excision of Left Atrium, Percutaneous Endoscopic Approach
02B80ZX	Excision of Conduction Mechanism, Open Approach, Diagnostic
02B80ZZ	Excision of Conduction Mechanism, Open Approach
02B83ZX	Excision of Conduction Mechanism, Percutaneous Approach, Diagnostic
02B83ZZ	Excision of Conduction Mechanism, Percutaneous Approach
02B84ZX	Excision of Conduction Mechanism, Percutaneous Endoscopic Approach, Diagnostic
02B84ZZ	Excision of Conduction Mechanism, Percutaneous Endoscopic Approach
02B90ZX	Excision of Chordae Tendineae, Open Approach, Diagnostic
02B90ZZ	Excision of Chordae Tendineae, Open Approach
02B93ZX	Excision of Chordae Tendineae, Percutaneous Approach, Diagnostic
02B93ZZ	Excision of Chordae Tendineae, Percutaneous Approach
02B94ZX	Excision of Chordae Tendineae, Percutaneous Endoscopic Approach, Diagnostic
02B94ZZ	Excision of Chordae Tendineae, Percutaneous Endoscopic Approach
02BD0ZX	Excision of Papillary Muscle, Open Approach, Diagnostic
02BD0ZZ	Excision of Papillary Muscle, Open Approach
02BD3ZX	Excision of Papillary Muscle, Percutaneous Approach, Diagnostic
02BD3ZZ	Excision of Papillary Muscle, Percutaneous Approach
02BD4ZX	Excision of Papillary Muscle, Percutaneous Endoscopic Approach, Diagnostic
02BD4ZZ	Excision of Papillary Muscle, Percutaneous Endoscopic Approach
02BF0ZX	Excision of Aortic Valve, Open Approach, Diagnostic
02BF0ZZ	Excision of Aortic Valve, Open Approach
02BF3ZX	Excision of Aortic Valve, Percutaneous Approach, Diagnostic
02BF3ZZ	Excision of Aortic Valve, Percutaneous Approach
02BF4ZX	Excision of Aortic Valve, Percutaneous Endoscopic Approach, Diagnostic
02BF4ZZ	Excision of Aortic Valve, Percutaneous Endoscopic Approach
02BG0ZX	Excision of Mitral Valve, Open Approach, Diagnostic
02BG0ZZ	Excision of Mitral Valve, Open Approach

02BG3ZX	Excision of Mitral Valve, Percutaneous Approach, Diagnostic
02BG3ZZ	Excision of Mitral Valve, Percutaneous Approach
02BG4ZX	Excision of Mitral Valve, Percutaneous Endoscopic Approach, Diagnostic
02BG4ZZ	Excision of Mitral Valve, Percutaneous Endoscopic Approach
02BH0ZX	Excision of Pulmonary Valve, Open Approach, Diagnostic
02BH0ZZ	Excision of Pulmonary Valve, Open Approach
02BH3ZX	Excision of Pulmonary Valve, Percutaneous Approach, Diagnostic
02BH3ZZ	Excision of Pulmonary Valve, Percutaneous Approach
02BH4ZX	Excision of Pulmonary Valve, Percutaneous Endoscopic Approach, Diagnostic
02BH4ZZ	Excision of Pulmonary Valve, Percutaneous Endoscopic Approach
02BJ0ZX	Excision of Tricuspid Valve, Open Approach, Diagnostic
02BJ0ZZ	Excision of Tricuspid Valve, Open Approach
02BJ3ZX	Excision of Tricuspid Valve, Percutaneous Approach, Diagnostic
02BJ3ZZ	Excision of Tricuspid Valve, Percutaneous Approach
02BJ4ZX	Excision of Tricuspid Valve, Percutaneous Endoscopic Approach, Diagnostic
02BJ4ZZ	Excision of Tricuspid Valve, Percutaneous Endoscopic Approach
02BK0ZX	Excision of Right Ventricle, Open Approach, Diagnostic
⬣ 02BK0ZZ	Excision of Right Ventricle, Open Approach
02BK3ZX	Excision of Right Ventricle, Percutaneous Approach, Diagnostic
⬣ 02BK3ZZ	Excision of Right Ventricle, Percutaneous Approach
02BK4ZX	Excision of Right Ventricle, Percutaneous Endoscopic Approach, Diagnostic
⬣ 02BK4ZZ	Excision of Right Ventricle, Percutaneous Endoscopic Approach
02BL0ZX	Excision of Left Ventricle, Open Approach, Diagnostic
⬣ 02BL0ZZ	Excision of Left Ventricle, Open Approach
02BL3ZX	Excision of Left Ventricle, Percutaneous Approach, Diagnostic
⬣ 02BL3ZZ	Excision of Left Ventricle, Percutaneous Approach
02BL4ZX	Excision of Left Ventricle, Percutaneous Endoscopic Approach, Diagnostic
⬣ 02BL4ZZ	Excision of Left Ventricle, Percutaneous Endoscopic Approach
02BM0ZX	Excision of Ventricular Septum, Open Approach, Diagnostic
02BM0ZZ	Excision of Ventricular Septum, Open Approach
02BM3ZX	Excision of Ventricular Septum, Percutaneous Approach, Diagnostic
02BM3ZZ	Excision of Ventricular Septum, Percutaneous Approach
02BM4ZX	Excision of Ventricular Septum, Percutaneous Endoscopic Approach, Diagnostic
02BM4ZZ	Excision of Ventricular Septum, Percutaneous Endoscopic Approach
02BN0ZX	Excision of Pericardium, Open Approach, Diagnostic
02BN0ZZ	Excision of Pericardium, Open Approach
02BN3ZX	Excision of Pericardium, Percutaneous Approach, Diagnostic
02BN3ZZ	Excision of Pericardium, Percutaneous Approach
02BN4ZX	Excision of Pericardium, Percutaneous Endoscopic Approach, Diagnostic
02BN4ZZ	Excision of Pericardium, Percutaneous Endoscopic Approach
02BP0ZX	Excision of Pulmonary Trunk, Open Approach, Diagnostic
02BP0ZZ	Excision of Pulmonary Trunk, Open Approach
02BP3ZX	Excision of Pulmonary Trunk, Percutaneous Approach, Diagnostic
02BP3ZZ	Excision of Pulmonary Trunk, Percutaneous Approach
02BP4ZX	Excision of Pulmonary Trunk, Percutaneous Endoscopic Approach, Diagnostic
02BP4ZZ	Excision of Pulmonary Trunk, Percutaneous Endoscopic Approach
02BQ0ZX	Excision of Right Pulmonary Artery, Open Approach, Diagnostic
02BQ0ZZ	Excision of Right Pulmonary Artery, Open Approach
02BQ3ZX	Excision of Right Pulmonary Artery, Percutaneous Approach, Diagnostic
02BQ3ZZ	Excision of Right Pulmonary Artery, Percutaneous Approach
02BQ4ZX	Excision of Right Pulmonary Artery, Percutaneous Endoscopic Approach, Diagnostic
02BQ4ZZ	Excision of Right Pulmonary Artery, Percutaneous Endoscopic Approach

♀ Female-only   ♂ Male-only   ● Limited Coverage   ● Non-OR   ▨ HAC-associated procedure   ⬣ Non-covered procedures   ✚ Combination

02BR0ZX	Excision of Left Pulmonary Artery, Open Approach, Diagnostic
02BR0ZZ	Excision of Left Pulmonary Artery, Open Approach
02BR3ZX	Excision of Left Pulmonary Artery, Percutaneous Approach, Diagnostic
02BR3ZZ	Excision of Left Pulmonary Artery, Percutaneous Approach
02BR4ZX	Excision of Left Pulmonary Artery, Percutaneous Endoscopic Approach, Diagnostic
02BR4ZZ	Excision of Left Pulmonary Artery, Percutaneous Endoscopic Approach
02BS0ZX	Excision of Right Pulmonary Vein, Open Approach, Diagnostic
02BS0ZZ	Excision of Right Pulmonary Vein, Open Approach
02BS3ZX	Excision of Right Pulmonary Vein, Percutaneous Approach, Diagnostic
02BS3ZZ	Excision of Right Pulmonary Vein, Percutaneous Approach
02BS4ZX	Excision of Right Pulmonary Vein, Percutaneous Endoscopic Approach, Diagnostic
02BS4ZZ	Excision of Right Pulmonary Vein, Percutaneous Endoscopic Approach
02BT0ZX	Excision of Left Pulmonary Vein, Open Approach, Diagnostic
02BT0ZZ	Excision of Left Pulmonary Vein, Open Approach
02BT3ZX	Excision of Left Pulmonary Vein, Percutaneous Approach, Diagnostic
02BT3ZZ	Excision of Left Pulmonary Vein, Percutaneous Approach
02BT4ZX	Excision of Left Pulmonary Vein, Percutaneous Endoscopic Approach, Diagnostic
02BT4ZZ	Excision of Left Pulmonary Vein, Percutaneous Endoscopic Approach
02BV0ZX	Excision of Superior Vena Cava, Open Approach, Diagnostic
02BV0ZZ	Excision of Superior Vena Cava, Open Approach
02BV3ZX	Excision of Superior Vena Cava, Percutaneous Approach, Diagnostic
02BV3ZZ	Excision of Superior Vena Cava, Percutaneous Approach
02BV4ZX	Excision of Superior Vena Cava, Percutaneous Endoscopic Approach, Diagnostic
02BV4ZZ	Excision of Superior Vena Cava, Percutaneous Endoscopic Approach
02BW0ZX	Excision of Thoracic Aorta, Open Approach, Diagnostic
02BW0ZZ	Excision of Thoracic Aorta, Open Approach
02BW3ZX	Excision of Thoracic Aorta, Percutaneous Approach, Diagnostic
02BW3ZZ	Excision of Thoracic Aorta, Percutaneous Approach
02BW4ZX	Excision of Thoracic Aorta, Percutaneous Endoscopic Approach, Diagnostic
02BW4ZZ	Excision of Thoracic Aorta, Percutaneous Endoscopic Approach

02C – Heart and Great Vessels, Extirpation

For Extirpation procedures involving coronary arteries, Review Coding Guideline B4.4

02C00ZZ	Extirpation of Matter from Coronary Artery, One Site, Open Approach
02C03ZZ	Extirpation of Matter from Coronary Artery, One Site, Percutaneous Approach
02C04ZZ	Extirpation of Matter from Coronary Artery, One Site, Percutaneous Endoscopic Approach
02C10ZZ	Extirpation of Matter from Coronary Artery, Two Sites, Open Approach
02C13ZZ	Extirpation of Matter from Coronary Artery, Two Sites, Percutaneous Approach
02C14ZZ	Extirpation of Matter from Coronary Artery, Two Sites, Percutaneous Endoscopic Approach
02C20ZZ	Extirpation of Matter from Coronary Artery, Three Sites, Open Approach
02C23ZZ	Extirpation of Matter from Coronary Artery, Three Sites, Percutaneous Approach
02C24ZZ	Extirpation of Matter from Coronary Artery, Three Sites, Percutaneous Endoscopic Approach
02C30ZZ	Extirpation of Matter from Coronary Artery, Four or More Sites, Open Approach
02C33ZZ	Extirpation of Matter from Coronary Artery, Four or More Sites, Percutaneous Approach
02C34ZZ	Extirpation of Matter from Coronary Artery, Four or More Sites, Percutaneous Endoscopic Approach
02C40ZZ	Extirpation of Matter from Coronary Vein, Open Approach
02C43ZZ	Extirpation of Matter from Coronary Vein, Percutaneous Approach
02C44ZZ	Extirpation of Matter from Coronary Vein, Percutaneous Endoscopic Approach
02C50ZZ	Extirpation of Matter from Atrial Septum, Open Approach
02C53ZZ	Extirpation of Matter from Atrial Septum, Percutaneous Approach
02C54ZZ	Extirpation of Matter from Atrial Septum, Percutaneous Endoscopic Approach
02C60ZZ	Extirpation of Matter from Right Atrium, Open Approach
02C63ZZ	Extirpation of Matter from Right Atrium, Percutaneous Approach
02C64ZZ	Extirpation of Matter from Right Atrium, Percutaneous Endoscopic Approach
02C70ZZ	Extirpation of Matter from Left Atrium, Open Approach
02C73ZZ	Extirpation of Matter from Left Atrium, Percutaneous Approach
02C74ZZ	Extirpation of Matter from Left Atrium, Percutaneous Endoscopic Approach
02C80ZZ	Extirpation of Matter from Conduction Mechanism, Open Approach
02C83ZZ	Extirpation of Matter from Conduction Mechanism, Percutaneous Approach
02C84ZZ	Extirpation of Matter from Conduction Mechanism, Percutaneous Endoscopic Approach
02C90ZZ	Extirpation of Matter from Chordae Tendineae, Open Approach
02C93ZZ	Extirpation of Matter from Chordae Tendineae, Percutaneous Approach
02C94ZZ	Extirpation of Matter from Chordae Tendineae, Percutaneous Endoscopic Approach
02CD0ZZ	Extirpation of Matter from Papillary Muscle, Open Approach
02CD3ZZ	Extirpation of Matter from Papillary Muscle, Percutaneous Approach
02CD4ZZ	Extirpation of Matter from Papillary Muscle, Percutaneous Endoscopic Approach
02CF0ZZ	Extirpation of Matter from Aortic Valve, Open Approach
02CF3ZZ	Extirpation of Matter from Aortic Valve, Percutaneous Approach
02CF4ZZ	Extirpation of Matter from Aortic Valve, Percutaneous Endoscopic Approach
02CG0ZZ	Extirpation of Matter from Mitral Valve, Open Approach
02CG3ZZ	Extirpation of Matter from Mitral Valve, Percutaneous Approach
02CG4ZZ	Extirpation of Matter from Mitral Valve, Percutaneous Endoscopic Approach
02CH0ZZ	Extirpation of Matter from Pulmonary Valve, Open Approach
02CH3ZZ	Extirpation of Matter from Pulmonary Valve, Percutaneous Approach
02CH4ZZ	Extirpation of Matter from Pulmonary Valve, Percutaneous Endoscopic Approach
02CJ0ZZ	Extirpation of Matter from Tricuspid Valve, Open Approach
02CJ3ZZ	Extirpation of Matter from Tricuspid Valve, Percutaneous Approach
02CJ4ZZ	Extirpation of Matter from Tricuspid Valve, Percutaneous Endoscopic Approach
02CK0ZZ	Extirpation of Matter from Right Ventricle, Open Approach
02CK3ZZ	Extirpation of Matter from Right Ventricle, Percutaneous Approach
02CK4ZZ	Extirpation of Matter from Right Ventricle, Percutaneous Endoscopic Approach
02CL0ZZ	Extirpation of Matter from Left Ventricle, Open Approach
02CL3ZZ	Extirpation of Matter from Left Ventricle, Percutaneous Approach
02CL4ZZ	Extirpation of Matter from Left Ventricle, Percutaneous Endoscopic Approach
02CM0ZZ	Extirpation of Matter from Ventricular Septum, Open Approach
02CM3ZZ	Extirpation of Matter from Ventricular Septum, Percutaneous Approach
02CM4ZZ	Extirpation of Matter from Ventricular Septum, Percutaneous Endoscopic Approach
02CN0ZZ	Extirpation of Matter from Pericardium, Open Approach
02CN3ZZ	Extirpation of Matter from Pericardium, Percutaneous Approach
02CN4ZZ	Extirpation of Matter from Pericardium, Percutaneous Endoscopic Approach
02CP0ZZ	Extirpation of Matter from Pulmonary Trunk, Open Approach

♀ Female-only   ♂ Male-only   ◐ Limited Coverage   ● Non-OR   ▨ HAC-associated procedure   ⬣ Non-covered procedures   ✚ Combination

02CP3ZZ	Extirpation of Matter from Pulmonary Trunk, Percutaneous Approach
02CP4ZZ	Extirpation of Matter from Pulmonary Trunk, Percutaneous Endoscopic Approach
02CQ0ZZ	Extirpation of Matter from Right Pulmonary Artery, Open Approach
02CQ3ZZ	Extirpation of Matter from Right Pulmonary Artery, Percutaneous Approach
02CQ4ZZ	Extirpation of Matter from Right Pulmonary Artery, Percutaneous Endoscopic Approach
02CR0ZZ	Extirpation of Matter from Left Pulmonary Artery, Open Approach
02CR3ZZ	Extirpation of Matter from Left Pulmonary Artery, Percutaneous Approach
02CR4ZZ	Extirpation of Matter from Left Pulmonary Artery, Percutaneous Endoscopic Approach
02CS0ZZ	Extirpation of Matter from Right Pulmonary Vein, Open Approach
02CS3ZZ	Extirpation of Matter from Right Pulmonary Vein, Percutaneous Approach
02CS4ZZ	Extirpation of Matter from Right Pulmonary Vein, Percutaneous Endoscopic Approach
02CT0ZZ	Extirpation of Matter from Left Pulmonary Vein, Open Approach
02CT3ZZ	Extirpation of Matter from Left Pulmonary Vein, Percutaneous Approach
02CT4ZZ	Extirpation of Matter from Left Pulmonary Vein, Percutaneous Endoscopic Approach
02CV0ZZ	Extirpation of Matter from Superior Vena Cava, Open Approach
02CV3ZZ	Extirpation of Matter from Superior Vena Cava, Percutaneous Approach
02CV4ZZ	Extirpation of Matter from Superior Vena Cava, Percutaneous Endoscopic Approach
02CW0ZZ	Extirpation of Matter from Thoracic Aorta, Open Approach
02CW3ZZ	Extirpation of Matter from Thoracic Aorta, Percutaneous Approach
02CW4ZZ	Extirpation of Matter from Thoracic Aorta, Percutaneous Endoscopic Approach

02F – Heart and Great Vessels, Fragmentation

02FN0ZZ	Fragmentation in Pericardium, Open Approach
02FN3ZZ	Fragmentation in Pericardium, Percutaneous Approach
02FN4ZZ	Fragmentation in Pericardium, Percutaneous Endoscopic Approach
● **02FNXZZ**	Fragmentation in Pericardium, External Approach

02H – Heart and Great Vessels, Insertion

02H400Z	Insertion of Pressure Sensor Monitoring Device into Coronary Vein, Open Approach
02H402Z	Insertion of Monitoring Device into Coronary Vein, Open Approach
02H403Z	Insertion of Infusion Device into Coronary Vein, Open Approach
02H40DZ	Insertion of Intraluminal Device into Coronary Vein, Open Approach
02H40JZ	Insertion of Pacemaker Lead into Coronary Vein, Open Approach
✚	Lead device when reported with an Insertion of a pacemaker device or cardiac rhythm related device (6th character 4, 5, 6 or P) into the chest or abdomen subcutaneous tissue and fascia. *See table 0JH to construct the Insertion code.* When a device is replaced, also report the Removal of a cardiac rhythm related device (6th character P) from the trunk subcutaneous tissue and fascia. *See table 0JP to construct the Removal code.*
02H40KZ	Insertion of Defibrillator Lead into Coronary Vein, Open Approach
02H40MZ	Insertion of Cardiac Lead into Coronary Vein, Open Approach
✚	Lead device when reported with an Insertion of a pacemaker device or cardiac rhythm related device (6th character 4, 5, 6 or P) into the chest or abdomen subcutaneous tissue and fascia. *See table 0JH to construct the Insertion code.* When a device is replaced, also report the Removal of a cardiac rhythm related device (6th character P) from the trunk subcutaneous tissue and fascia. *See table 0JP to construct the Removal code.*
02H430Z	Insertion of Pressure Sensor Monitoring Device into Coronary Vein, Percutaneous Approach
02H432Z	Insertion of Monitoring Device into Coronary Vein, Percutaneous Approach
02H433Z	Insertion of Infusion Device into Coronary Vein, Percutaneous Approach
02H43DZ	Insertion of Intraluminal Device into Coronary Vein, Percutaneous Approach
02H43JZ	Insertion of Pacemaker Lead into Coronary Vein, Percutaneous Approach
ᴴᴬᶜ	With a secondary diagnosis code of K68.11, T81.4XXA, T82.6XXA, T82.7XXA
02H43KZ	Insertion of Defibrillator Lead into Coronary Vein, Percutaneous Approach
ᴴᴬᶜ	With a secondary diagnosis code of K68.11, T81.4XXA, T82.6XXA, T82.7XXA
02H43MZ	Insertion of Cardiac Lead into Coronary Vein, Percutaneous Approach
ᴴᴬᶜ	With a secondary diagnosis code of K68.11, T81.4XXA, T82.6XXA, T82.7XXA
02H440Z	Insertion of Pressure Sensor Monitoring Device into Coronary Vein, Percutaneous Endoscopic Approach
02H442Z	Insertion of Monitoring Device into Coronary Vein, Percutaneous Endoscopic Approach
02H443Z	Insertion of Infusion Device into Coronary Vein, Percutaneous Endoscopic Approach
02H44DZ	Insertion of Intraluminal Device into Coronary Vein, Percutaneous Endoscopic Approach
02H44JZ	Insertion of Pacemaker Lead into Coronary Vein, Percutaneous Endoscopic Approach
✚	Lead device when reported with an Insertion of a pacemaker device or cardiac rhythm related device (6th character 4, 5, 6 or P) into the chest or abdomen subcutaneous tissue and fascia. *See table 0JH to construct the Insertion code.* When a device is replaced, also report the Removal of a cardiac rhythm related device (6th character P) from the trunk subcutaneous tissue and fascia. *See table 0JP to construct the Removal code.*
02H44KZ	Insertion of Defibrillator Lead into Coronary Vein, Percutaneous Endoscopic Approach
02H44MZ	Insertion of Cardiac Lead into Coronary Vein, Percutaneous Endoscopic Approach
✚	Lead device when reported with an Insertion of a pacemaker device or cardiac rhythm related device (6th character 4, 5, 6 or P) into the chest or abdomen subcutaneous tissue and fascia. *See table 0JH to construct the Insertion code.* When a device is replaced, also report the Removal of a cardiac rhythm related device (6th character P) from the trunk subcutaneous tissue and fascia. *See table 0JP to construct the Removal code.*
02H600Z	Insertion of Pressure Sensor Monitoring Device into Right Atrium, Open Approach
02H602Z	Insertion of Monitoring Device into Right Atrium, Open Approach
02H603Z	Insertion of Infusion Device into Right Atrium, Open Approach
02H60DZ	Insertion of Intraluminal Device into Right Atrium, Open Approach
02H60JZ	Insertion of Pacemaker Lead into Right Atrium, Open Approach
✚	Lead device when reported with an Insertion of a pacemaker device or cardiac rhythm related device (6th character 4, 5, 6 or P) into the chest or abdomen subcutaneous tissue and fascia. *See table 0JH to construct the Insertion code.* When a device is replaced, also report the Removal of a cardiac rhythm related device (6th character P) from the trunk subcutaneous tissue and fascia. *See table 0JP to construct the Removal code.*
02H60KZ	Insertion of Defibrillator Lead into Right Atrium, Open Approach
02H60MZ	Insertion of Cardiac Lead into Right Atrium, Open Approach
✚	Lead device when reported with an Insertion of a pacemaker device or cardiac rhythm related device (6th character 4, 5, 6 or P) into the chest or abdomen subcutaneous tissue and fascia. *See table 0JH to construct the Insertion code.* When a device is replaced, also report the Removal of a cardiac rhythm related device (6th character P) from the trunk subcutaneous tissue and fascia. *See table 0JP to construct the Removal code.*
02H630Z	Insertion of Pressure Sensor Monitoring Device into Right Atrium, Percutaneous Approach
02H632Z	Insertion of Monitoring Device into Right Atrium, Percutaneous Approach

02H633Z   Insertion of Infusion Device into Right Atrium, Percutaneous Approach

02H63DZ   Insertion of Intraluminal Device into Right Atrium, Percutaneous Approach

● **02H63JZ**   Insertion of Pacemaker Lead into Right Atrium, Percutaneous Approach

HAC   With a secondary diagnosis code of K68.11, T81.4XXA, T82.6XXA, T82.7XXA

⊞   Lead device when reported with an Insertion of a pacemaker device or cardiac rhythm related device (6th character 4, 5, 6 or P) into the chest or abdomen subcutaneous tissue and fascia. *See table 0JH to construct the Insertion code.* When a device is replaced, also report the removal of a cardiac rhythm related device (6th character P) from the trunk subcutaneous tissue and fascia. *See table 0JP to construct the Removal code.* When a cardiac lead is replaced, also report the removal of cardiac lead (6th character M) from the heart. *See table 02P to construct the Removal code.*

02H63KZ   Insertion of Defibrillator Lead into Right Atrium, Percutaneous Approach

02H63MZ   Insertion of Cardiac Lead into Right Atrium, Percutaneous Approach

⊞   Lead device when reported with an Insertion of a pacemaker device or cardiac rhythm related device (6th character 4, 5, 6 or P) into the chest or abdomen subcutaneous tissue and fascia. *See table 0JH to construct the Insertion code.* When a device is replaced, also report the Removal of a cardiac rhythm related device (6th character P) from the trunk subcutaneous tissue and fascia. *See table 0JP to construct the Removal code.*

HAC   With a secondary diagnosis code of K68.11, T81.4XXA, T82.6XXA, T82.7XXA

02H640Z   Insertion of Pressure Sensor Monitoring Device into Right Atrium, Percutaneous Endoscopic Approach

02H642Z   Insertion of Monitoring Device into Right Atrium, Percutaneous Endoscopic Approach

02H643Z   Insertion of Infusion Device into Right Atrium, Percutaneous Endoscopic Approach

02H64DZ   Insertion of Intraluminal Device into Right Atrium, Percutaneous Endoscopic Approach

02H64JZ   Insertion of Pacemaker Lead into Right Atrium, Percutaneous Endoscopic Approach

⊞   Lead device when reported with an Insertion of a pacemaker device or cardiac rhythm related device (6th character 4, 5, 6 or P) into the chest or abdomen subcutaneous tissue and fascia. *See table 0JH to construct the Insertion code.* When a device is replaced, also report the Removal of a cardiac rhythm related device (6th character P) from the trunk subcutaneous tissue and fascia. *See table 0JP to construct the Removal code.*

02H64KZ   Insertion of Defibrillator Lead into Right Atrium, Percutaneous Endoscopic Approach

02H64MZ   Insertion of Cardiac Lead into Right Atrium, Percutaneous Endoscopic Approach

⊞   Lead device when reported with an Insertion of a pacemaker device or cardiac rhythm related device (6th character 4, 5, 6 or P) into the chest or abdomen subcutaneous tissue and fascia. *See table 0JH to construct the Insertion code.* When a device is replaced, also report the Removal of a cardiac rhythm related device (6th character P) from the trunk subcutaneous tissue and fascia. *See table 0JP to construct the Removal code.*

02H700Z   Insertion of Pressure Sensor Monitoring Device into Left Atrium, Open Approach

02H702Z   Insertion of Monitoring Device into Left Atrium, Open Approach

02H703Z   Insertion of Infusion Device into Left Atrium, Open Approach

02H70DZ   Insertion of Intraluminal Device into Left Atrium, Open Approach

02H70JZ   Insertion of Pacemaker Lead into Left Atrium, Open Approach

⊞   Lead device when reported with an Insertion of a pacemaker device or cardiac rhythm related device (6th character 4, 5, 6 or P) into the chest or abdomen subcutaneous tissue and fascia. *See table 0JH to construct the Insertion code.* When a device is replaced, also report the Removal of a cardiac rhythm related device (6th character P) from the trunk subcutaneous tissue and fascia. *See table 0JP to construct the Removal code.*

02H70KZ   Insertion of Defibrillator Lead into Left Atrium, Open Approach

02H70MZ   Insertion of Cardiac Lead into Left Atrium, Open Approach

⊞   Lead device when reported with an Insertion of a pacemaker device or cardiac rhythm related device (6th character 4, 5, 6 or P) into the chest or abdomen subcutaneous tissue and fascia. *See table 0JH to construct the Insertion code.* When a device is replaced, also report the Removal of a cardiac rhythm related device (6th character P) from the trunk subcutaneous tissue and fascia. *See table 0JP to construct the Removal code.*

02H730Z   Insertion of Pressure Sensor Monitoring Device into Left Atrium, Percutaneous Approach

02H732Z   Insertion of Monitoring Device into Left Atrium, Percutaneous Approach

02H733Z   Insertion of Infusion Device into Left Atrium, Percutaneous Approach

02H73DZ   Insertion of Intraluminal Device into Left Atrium, Percutaneous Approach

● **02H73JZ**   Insertion of Pacemaker Lead into Left Atrium, Percutaneous Approach

HAC   With a secondary diagnosis code of K68.11, T81.4XXA, T82.6XXA, T82.7XXA

⊞   Lead device when reported with an Insertion of a pacemaker device or cardiac rhythm related device (6th character 4, 5, 6 or P) into the chest or abdomen subcutaneous tissue and fascia. *See table 0JH to construct the Insertion code.* When a device is replaced, also report the removal of a cardiac rhythm related device (6th character P) from the trunk subcutaneous tissue and fascia. *See table 0JP to construct the Removal code.* When a cardiac lead is replaced, also report the removal of cardiac lead (6th character M) from the heart. *See table 02P to construct the Removal code.*

02H73KZ   Insertion of Defibrillator Lead into Left Atrium, Percutaneous Approach

02H73MZ   Insertion of Cardiac Lead into Left Atrium, Percutaneous Approach

HAC   With a secondary diagnosis code of K68.11, T81.4XXA, T82.6XXA, T82.7XXA

⊞   Lead device when reported with an Insertion of a pacemaker device or cardiac rhythm related device (6th character 4, 5, 6 or P) into the chest or abdomen subcutaneous tissue and fascia. *See table 0JH to construct the Insertion code.* When a device is replaced, also report the Removal of a cardiac rhythm related device (6th character P) from the trunk subcutaneous tissue and fascia. *See table 0JP to construct the Removal code.*

02H740Z   Insertion of Pressure Sensor Monitoring Device into Left Atrium, Percutaneous Endoscopic Approach

02H742Z   Insertion of Monitoring Device into Left Atrium, Percutaneous Endoscopic Approach

02H743Z   Insertion of Infusion Device into Left Atrium, Percutaneous Endoscopic Approach

02H74DZ   Insertion of Intraluminal Device into Left Atrium, Percutaneous Endoscopic Approach

02H74JZ   Insertion of Pacemaker Lead into Left Atrium, Percutaneous Endoscopic Approach

⊞   Lead device when reported with an Insertion of a pacemaker device or cardiac rhythm related device (6th character 4, 5, 6 or P) into the chest or abdomen subcutaneous tissue and fascia. *See table 0JH to construct the Insertion code.* When a device is replaced, also report the Removal of a cardiac rhythm related device (6th character P) from the trunk subcutaneous tissue and fascia. *See table 0JP to construct the Removal code.*

02H74KZ   Insertion of Defibrillator Lead into Left Atrium, Percutaneous Endoscopic Approach

02H74MZ   Insertion of Cardiac Lead into Left Atrium, Percutaneous Endoscopic Approach

⊞   Lead device when reported with an Insertion of a pacemaker device or cardiac rhythm related device (6th character 4, 5, 6 or P) into the chest or abdomen subcutaneous tissue and fascia. *See table 0JH to construct the Insertion code.* When a device is replaced, also report the Removal of a cardiac rhythm related device (6th character P) from the trunk subcutaneous tissue and fascia. *See table 0JP to construct the Removal code.*

02HA0QZ Insertion of Implantable Heart Assist System into Heart, Open Approach

02HA0RS Insertion of Biventricular External Heart Assist System into Heart, Open Approach
+ Heart assist system replacement when reported with a removal of an external heart assist system (6th character R) from the heart. *See table 02P to construct the Removal code.*

02HA0RZ Insertion of External Heart Assist System into Heart, Open Approach
+ Heart assist system replacement when reported with a removal of an external heart assist system (6th character R) from the heart. See table 02P to construct the Removal code.

02HA3QZ Insertion of Implantable Heart Assist System into Heart, Percutaneous Approach

02HA3RS Insertion of Biventricular External Heart Assist System into Heart, Percutaneous Approach
+ Heart assist system replacement when reported with a removal of an external heart assist system (6th character R) from the heart. *See table 02P to construct the Removal code.*

02HA3RZ Insertion of External Heart Assist System into Heart, Percutaneous Approach
+ Heart assist system replacement when reported with a removal of an external heart assist system (6th character R) from the heart. *See table 02P to construct the Removal code.*

02HA4QZ Insertion of Implantable Heart Assist System into Heart, Percutaneous Endoscopic Approach

02HA4RS Insertion of Biventricular External Heart Assist System into Heart, Percutaneous Endoscopic Approach
+ Heart assist system replacement when reported with a removal of an external heart assist system (6th character R) from the heart. *See table 02P to construct the Removal code.*

02HA4RZ Insertion of External Heart Assist System into Heart, Percutaneous Endoscopic Approach
+ Heart assist system replacement when reported with a removal of an external heart assist system (6th character R) from the heart. *See table 02P to construct the Removal code.*

02HK00Z Insertion of Pressure Sensor Monitoring Device into Right Ventricle, Open Approach
+ Intracardiac lead device when reported with an Insertion of a hemodynamic monitoring device (6th character 0) into the chest or abdomen sucutaneous tissue and fascia. *See table 0JH to construct the Insertion code.*

02HK02Z Insertion of Monitoring Device into Right Ventricle, Open Approach
+ Intracardiac lead device when reported with an Insertion of a hemodynamic monitoring device (6th character 0) into the chest or abdomen sucutaneous tissue and fascia. *See table 0JH to construct the Insertion code.*

02HK03Z Insertion of Infusion Device into Right Ventricle, Open Approach

02HK0DZ Insertion of Intraluminal Device into Right Ventricle, Open Approach

02HK0JZ Insertion of Pacemaker Lead into Right Ventricle, Open Approach
+ Lead device when reported with an Insertion of a pacemaker device or cardiac rhythm related device (6th character 4, 5, 6 or P) into the chest or abdomen subcutaneous tissue and fascia. *See table 0JH to construct the Insertion code.* When a device is replaced, also report the Removal of a cardiac rhythm related device (6th character P) from the trunk subcutaneous tissue and fascia. *See table 0JP to construct the Removal code.*

02HK0KZ Insertion of Defibrillator Lead into Right Ventricle, Open Approach

02HK0MZ Insertion of Cardiac Lead into Right Ventricle, Open Approach
+ Lead device when reported with an Insertion of a pacemaker device or cardiac rhythm related device (6th character 4, 5, 6 or P) into the chest or abdomen subcutaneous tissue and fascia. *See table 0JH to construct the Insertion code.* When a device is replaced, also report the Removal of a cardiac rhythm related device (6th character P) from the trunk subcutaneous tissue and fascia. *See table 0JP to construct the Removal code.*

02HK30Z Insertion of Pressure Sensor Monitoring Device into Right Ventricle, Percutaneous Approach
+ Intracardiac lead device when reported with an Insertion of a hemodynamic monitoring device (6th character 0) into the chest or abdomen sucutaneous tissue and fascia. *See table 0JH to construct the Insertion code.*

02HK32Z Insertion of Monitoring Device into Right Ventricle, Percutaneous Approach
+ Intracardiac lead device when reported with an Insertion of a hemodynamic monitoring device (6th character 0) into the chest or abdomen sucutaneous tissue and fascia. *See table 0JH to construct the Insertion code.*

02HK33Z Insertion of Infusion Device into Right Ventricle, Percutaneous Approach

02HK3DZ Insertion of Intraluminal Device into Right Ventricle, Percutaneous Approach

02HK3JZ Insertion of Pacemaker Lead into Right Ventricle, Percutaneous Approach
HAC With a secondary diagnosis code of K68.11, T81.4XXA, T82.6XXA, T82.7XXA
+ Lead device when reported with an Insertion of a pacemaker device or cardiac rhythm related device (6th character 4, 5, 6 or P) into the chest or abdomen subcutaneous tissue and fascia. *See table 0JH to construct the Insertion code.* When a device is replaced, also report the removal of a cardiac rhythm related device (6th character P) from the trunk subcutaneous tissue and fascia. *See table 0JP to construct the Removal code.* When a cardiac lead is replaced, also report the removal of cardiac lead (6th character M) from the heart. *See table 02P to construct the Removal code.*

02HK3KZ Insertion of Defibrillator Lead into Right Ventricle, Percutaneous Approach

02HK3MZ Insertion of Cardiac Lead into Right Ventricle, Percutaneous Approach
+ Lead device when reported with an Insertion of a pacemaker device or cardiac rhythm related device (6th character 4, 5, 6 or P) into the chest or abdomen subcutaneous tissue and fascia. *See table 0JH to construct the Insertion code.* When a device is replaced, also report the Removal of a cardiac rhythm related device (6th character P) from the trunk subcutaneous tissue and fascia. *See table 0JP to construct the Removal code.*

02HK40Z Insertion of Pressure Sensor Monitoring Device into Right Ventricle, Percutaneous Endoscopic Approach
+ Intracardiac lead device when reported with an Insertion of a hemodynamic monitoring device (6th character 0) into the chest or abdomen sucutaneous tissue and fascia. *See table 0JH to construct the Insertion code.*

02HK42Z Insertion of Monitoring Device into Right Ventricle, Percutaneous Endoscopic Approach
+ Intracardiac lead device when reported with an Insertion of a hemodynamic monitoring device (6th character 0) into the chest or abdomen sucutaneous tissue and fascia. *See table 0JH to construct the Insertion code.*

02HK43Z Insertion of Infusion Device into Right Ventricle, Percutaneous Endoscopic Approach

02HK4DZ Insertion of Intraluminal Device into Right Ventricle, Percutaneous Endoscopic Approach

02HK4JZ Insertion of Pacemaker Lead into Right Ventricle, Percutaneous Endoscopic Approach
+ Lead device when reported with an Insertion of a pacemaker device or cardiac rhythm related device (6th character 4, 5, 6 or P) into the chest or abdomen subcutaneous tissue and fascia. *See table 0JH to construct the Insertion code.* When a device is replaced, also report the Removal of a cardiac rhythm related device (6th character P) from the trunk subcutaneous tissue and fascia. *See table 0JP to construct the Removal code.*

02HK4KZ Insertion of Defibrillator Lead into Right Ventricle, Percutaneous Endoscopic Approach

02HK4MZ Insertion of Cardiac Lead into Right Ventricle, Percutaneous Endoscopic Approach
+ Lead device when reported with an Insertion of a pacemaker device or cardiac rhythm related device (6th character 4, 5, 6 or P) into the chest or abdomen subcutaneous tissue and fascia. *See table 0JH to construct the Insertion code.* When a device is replaced, also report the Removal of a cardiac rhythm related device (6th character P) from the trunk subcutaneous tissue and fascia. *See table 0JP to construct the Removal code.*

02HL00Z Insertion of Pressure Sensor Monitoring Device into Left Ventricle, Open Approach

02HL02Z Insertion of Monitoring Device into Left Ventricle, Open Approach

02HL03Z Insertion of Infusion Device into Left Ventricle, Open Approach

02HL0DZ Insertion of Intraluminal Device into Left Ventricle, Open Approach

02HL0JZ Insertion of Pacemaker Lead into Left Ventricle, Open Approach

 ⊞ Lead device when reported with an Insertion of a pacemaker device or cardiac rhythm related device (6th character 4, 5, 6 or P) into the chest or abdomen subcutaneous tissue and fascia. *See table 0JH to construct the Insertion code.* When a device is replaced, also report the Removal of a cardiac rhythm related device (6th character P) from the trunk subcutaneous tissue and fascia. *See table 0JP to construct the Removal code.*

02HL0KZ Insertion of Defibrillator Lead into Left Ventricle, Open Approach

02HL0MZ Insertion of Cardiac Lead into Left Ventricle, Open Approach

 ⊞ Lead device when reported with an Insertion of a pacemaker device or cardiac rhythm related device (6th character 4, 5, 6 or P) into the chest or abdomen subcutaneous tissue and fascia. *See table 0JH to construct the Insertion code.* When a device is replaced, also report the Removal of a cardiac rhythm related device (6th character P) from the trunk subcutaneous tissue and fascia. *See table 0JP to construct the Removal code.*

02HL30Z Insertion of Pressure Sensor Monitoring Device into Left Ventricle, Percutaneous Approach

02HL32Z Insertion of Monitoring Device into Left Ventricle, Percutaneous Approach

02HL33Z Insertion of Infusion Device into Left Ventricle, Percutaneous Approach

02HL3DZ Insertion of Intraluminal Device into Left Ventricle, Percutaneous Approach

● **02HL3JZ** Insertion of Pacemaker Lead into Left Ventricle, Percutaneous Approach

 HAC With a secondary diagnosis code of K68.11, T81.4XXA, T82.6XXA, T82.7XXA

 ⊞ Lead device when reported with an Insertion of a pacemaker device or cardiac rhythm related device (6th character 4, 5, 6 or P) into the chest or abdomen subcutaneous tissue and fascia. *See table 0JH to construct the Insertion code.* When a device is replaced, also report the removal of a cardiac rhythm related device (6th character P) from the trunk subcutaneous tissue and fascia. *See table 0JP to construct the Removal code.* When a cardiac lead is replaced, also report the removal of cardiac lead (6th character M) from the heart. *See table 02P to construct the Removal code.*

02HL3KZ Insertion of Defibrillator Lead into Left Ventricle, Percutaneous Approach

02HL3MZ Insertion of Cardiac Lead into Left Ventricle, Percutaneous Approach

 ⊞ Lead device when reported with an Insertion of a pacemaker device or cardiac rhythm related device (6th character 4, 5, 6 or P) into the chest or abdomen subcutaneous tissue and fascia. *See table 0JH to construct the Insertion code.* When a device is replaced, also report the Removal of a cardiac rhythm related device (6th character P) from the trunk subcutaneous tissue and fascia. *See table 0JP to construct the Removal code.*

02HL40Z Insertion of Pressure Sensor Monitoring Device into Left Ventricle, Percutaneous Endoscopic Approach

02HL42Z Insertion of Monitoring Device into Left Ventricle, Percutaneous Endoscopic Approach

02HL43Z Insertion of Infusion Device into Left Ventricle, Percutaneous Endoscopic Approach

02HL4DZ Insertion of Intraluminal Device into Left Ventricle, Percutaneous Endoscopic Approach

02HL4JZ Insertion of Pacemaker Lead into Left Ventricle, Percutaneous Endoscopic Approach

 ⊞ Lead device when reported with an Insertion of a pacemaker device or cardiac rhythm related device (6th character 4, 5, 6 or P) into the chest or abdomen subcutaneous tissue and fascia. *See table 0JH to construct the Insertion code.* When a device is replaced, also report the Removal of a cardiac rhythm related device (6th character P) from the trunk subcutaneous tissue and fascia. *See table 0JP to construct the Removal code.*

02HL4KZ Insertion of Defibrillator Lead into Left Ventricle, Percutaneous Endoscopic Approach

02HL4MZ Insertion of Cardiac Lead into Left Ventricle, Percutaneous Endoscopic Approach

 ⊞ Lead device when reported with an Insertion of a pacemaker device or cardiac rhythm related device (6th character 4, 5, 6 or P) into the chest or abdomen subcutaneous tissue and fascia. *See table 0JH to construct the Insertion code.* When a device is replaced, also report the Removal of a cardiac rhythm related device (6th character P) from the trunk subcutaneous tissue and fascia. *See table 0JP to construct the Removal code.*

02HN00Z Insertion of Pressure Sensor Monitoring Device into Pericardium, Open Approach

02HN02Z Insertion of Monitoring Device into Pericardium, Open Approach

02HN0JZ Insertion of Pacemaker Lead into Pericardium, Open Approach

 HAC With a secondary diagnosis code of K68.11, T81.4XXA, T82.6XXA, T82.7XXA

 ⊞ Lead device when reported with an Insertion of a pacemaker device or cardiac rhythm related device (6th character 4, 5, 6 or P) into the chest or abdomen subcutaneous tissue and fascia. *See table 0JH to construct the Insertion code.* When a device is replaced, also report the Removal of a cardiac rhythm related device (6th character P) from the trunk subcutaneous tissue and fascia. *See table 0JP to construct the Removal code.*

02HN0KZ Insertion of Defibrillator Lead into Pericardium, Open Approach

02HN0MZ Insertion of Cardiac Lead into Pericardium, Open Approach

 HAC With a secondary diagnosis code of K68.11, T81.4XXA, T82.6XXA, T82.7XXA

 ⊞ Lead device when reported with an Insertion of a pacemaker device or cardiac rhythm related device (6th character 4, 5, 6 or P) into the chest or abdomen subcutaneous tissue and fascia. *See table 0JH to construct the Insertion code.* When a device is replaced, also report the Removal of a cardiac rhythm related device (6th character P) from the trunk subcutaneous tissue and fascia. *See table 0JP to construct the Removal code.*

02HN30Z Insertion of Pressure Sensor Monitoring Device into Pericardium, Percutaneous Approach

02HN32Z Insertion of Monitoring Device into Pericardium, Percutaneous Approach

02HN3JZ Insertion of Pacemaker Lead into Pericardium, Percutaneous Approach

 HAC With a secondary diagnosis code of K68.11, T81.4XXA, T82.6XXA, T82.7XXA

 ⊞ Lead device when reported with an Insertion of a pacemaker device or cardiac rhythm related device (6th character 4, 5, 6 or P) into the chest or abdomen subcutaneous tissue and fascia. *See table 0JH to construct the Insertion code.* When a device is replaced, also report the Removal of a cardiac rhythm related device (6th character P) from the trunk subcutaneous tissue and fascia. *See table 0JP to construct the Removal code.*

02HN3KZ Insertion of Defibrillator Lead into Pericardium, Percutaneous Approach

02HN3MZ Insertion of Cardiac Lead into Pericardium, Percutaneous Approach

 HAC With a secondary diagnosis code of K68.11, T81.4XXA, T82.6XXA, T82.7XXA

 ⊞ Lead device when reported with an Insertion of a pacemaker device or cardiac rhythm related device (6th character 4, 5, 6 or P) into the chest or abdomen subcutaneous tissue and fascia. *See table 0JH to construct the Insertion code.* When a device is replaced, also report the Removal of a cardiac rhythm related device (6th character P) from the trunk subcutaneous tissue and fascia. *See table 0JP to construct the Removal code.*

02HN40Z Insertion of Pressure Sensor Monitoring Device into Pericardium, Percutaneous Endoscopic Approach

02HN42Z Insertion of Monitoring Device into Pericardium, Percutaneous Endoscopic Approach

02HN4JZ Insertion of Pacemaker Lead into Pericardium, Percutaneous Endoscopic Approach

 HAC With a secondary diagnosis code of K68.11, T81.4XXA, T82.6XXA, T82.7XXA

 ⊞ Lead device when reported with an Insertion of a pacemaker device or cardiac rhythm related device (6th character 4, 5, 6 or P) into the chest or abdomen subcutaneous tissue and fascia. *See table 0JH to construct the Insertion code.* When a device is replaced, also report the Removal of a cardiac rhythm related device (6th character P) from the trunk subcutaneous tissue and fascia. *See table 0JP to construct the Removal code.*

♀ Female-only   ♂ Male-only   ◯ Limited Coverage   ● Non-OR   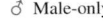 HAC-associated procedure   ⬤ Non-covered procedures   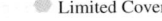 ⊞ Combination

02HN4KZ Insertion of Defibrillator Lead into Pericardium, Percutaneous Endoscopic Approach

02HN4MZ Insertion of Cardiac Lead into Pericardium, Percutaneous Endoscopic Approach

⬛ With a secondary diagnosis code of K68.11, T81.4XXA, T82.6XXA, T82.7XXA

➕ Lead device when reported with an Insertion of a pacemaker device or cardiac rhythm related device (6th character 4, 5, 6 or P) into the chest or abdomen subcutaneous tissue and fascia. *See table 0JH to construct the Insertion code.* When a device is replaced, also report the Removal of a cardiac rhythm related device (6th character P) from the trunk subcutaneous tissue and fascia. *See table 0JP to construct the Removal code.*

02HP00Z Insertion of Pressure Sensor Monitoring Device into Pulmonary Trunk, Open Approach

02HP02Z Insertion of Monitoring Device into Pulmonary Trunk, Open Approach

02HP03Z Insertion of Infusion Device into Pulmonary Trunk, Open Approach

02HP0DZ Insertion of Intraluminal Device into Pulmonary Trunk, Open Approach

02HP30Z Insertion of Pressure Sensor Monitoring Device into Pulmonary Trunk, Percutaneous Approach

02HP32Z Insertion of Monitoring Device into Pulmonary Trunk, Percutaneous Approach

02HP33Z Insertion of Infusion Device into Pulmonary Trunk, Percutaneous Approach

02HP3DZ Insertion of Intraluminal Device into Pulmonary Trunk, Percutaneous Approach

02HP40Z Insertion of Pressure Sensor Monitoring Device into Pulmonary Trunk, Percutaneous Endoscopic Approach

02HP42Z Insertion of Monitoring Device into Pulmonary Trunk, Percutaneous Endoscopic Approach

02HP43Z Insertion of Infusion Device into Pulmonary Trunk, Percutaneous Endoscopic Approach

02HP4DZ Insertion of Intraluminal Device into Pulmonary Trunk, Percutaneous Endoscopic Approach

02HQ00Z Insertion of Pressure Sensor Monitoring Device into Right Pulmonary Artery, Open Approach

02HQ02Z Insertion of Monitoring Device into Right Pulmonary Artery, Open Approach

02HQ03Z Insertion of Infusion Device into Right Pulmonary Artery, Open Approach

02HQ0DZ Insertion of Intraluminal Device into Right Pulmonary Artery, Open Approach

02HQ30Z Insertion of Pressure Sensor Monitoring Device into Right Pulmonary Artery, Percutaneous Approach

02HQ32Z Insertion of Monitoring Device into Right Pulmonary Artery, Percutaneous Approach

02HQ33Z Insertion of Infusion Device into Right Pulmonary Artery, Percutaneous Approach

02HQ3DZ Insertion of Intraluminal Device into Right Pulmonary Artery, Percutaneous Approach

02HQ40Z Insertion of Pressure Sensor Monitoring Device into Right Pulmonary Artery, Percutaneous Endoscopic Approach

02HQ42Z Insertion of Monitoring Device into Right Pulmonary Artery, Percutaneous Endoscopic Approach

02HQ43Z Insertion of Infusion Device into Right Pulmonary Artery, Percutaneous Endoscopic Approach

02HQ4DZ Insertion of Intraluminal Device into Right Pulmonary Artery, Percutaneous Endoscopic Approach

02HR00Z Insertion of Pressure Sensor Monitoring Device into Left Pulmonary Artery, Open Approach

02HR02Z Insertion of Monitoring Device into Left Pulmonary Artery, Open Approach

02HR03Z Insertion of Infusion Device into Left Pulmonary Artery, Open Approach

02HR0DZ Insertion of Intraluminal Device into Left Pulmonary Artery, Open Approach

02HR30Z Insertion of Pressure Sensor Monitoring Device into Left Pulmonary Artery, Percutaneous Approach

02HR32Z Insertion of Monitoring Device into Left Pulmonary Artery, Percutaneous Approach

02HR33Z Insertion of Infusion Device into Left Pulmonary Artery, Percutaneous Approach

02HR3DZ Insertion of Intraluminal Device into Left Pulmonary Artery, Percutaneous Approach

02HR40Z Insertion of Pressure Sensor Monitoring Device into Left Pulmonary Artery, Percutaneous Endoscopic Approach

02HR42Z Insertion of Monitoring Device into Left Pulmonary Artery, Percutaneous Endoscopic Approach

02HR43Z Insertion of Infusion Device into Left Pulmonary Artery, Percutaneous Endoscopic Approach

02HR4DZ Insertion of Intraluminal Device into Left Pulmonary Artery, Percutaneous Endoscopic Approach

02HS00Z Insertion of Pressure Sensor Monitoring Device into Right Pulmonary Vein, Open Approach

02HS02Z Insertion of Monitoring Device into Right Pulmonary Vein, Open Approach

02HS03Z Insertion of Infusion Device into Right Pulmonary Vein, Open Approach

02HS0DZ Insertion of Intraluminal Device into Right Pulmonary Vein, Open Approach

02HS30Z Insertion of Pressure Sensor Monitoring Device into Right Pulmonary Vein, Percutaneous Approach

02HS32Z Insertion of Monitoring Device into Right Pulmonary Vein, Percutaneous Approach

02HS33Z Insertion of Infusion Device into Right Pulmonary Vein, Percutaneous Approach

02HS3DZ Insertion of Intraluminal Device into Right Pulmonary Vein, Percutaneous Approach

02HS40Z Insertion of Pressure Sensor Monitoring Device into Right Pulmonary Vein, Percutaneous Endoscopic Approach

02HS42Z Insertion of Monitoring Device into Right Pulmonary Vein, Percutaneous Endoscopic Approach

02HS43Z Insertion of Infusion Device into Right Pulmonary Vein, Percutaneous Endoscopic Approach

02HS4DZ Insertion of Intraluminal Device into Right Pulmonary Vein, Percutaneous Endoscopic Approach

02HT00Z Insertion of Pressure Sensor Monitoring Device into Left Pulmonary Vein, Open Approach

02HT02Z Insertion of Monitoring Device into Left Pulmonary Vein, Open Approach

02HT03Z Insertion of Infusion Device into Left Pulmonary Vein, Open Approach

02HT0DZ Insertion of Intraluminal Device into Left Pulmonary Vein, Open Approach

02HT30Z Insertion of Pressure Sensor Monitoring Device into Left Pulmonary Vein, Percutaneous Approach

02HT32Z Insertion of Monitoring Device into Left Pulmonary Vein, Percutaneous Approach

02HT33Z Insertion of Infusion Device into Left Pulmonary Vein, Percutaneous Approach

02HT3DZ Insertion of Intraluminal Device into Left Pulmonary Vein, Percutaneous Approach

02HT40Z Insertion of Pressure Sensor Monitoring Device into Left Pulmonary Vein, Percutaneous Endoscopic Approach

02HT42Z Insertion of Monitoring Device into Left Pulmonary Vein, Percutaneous Endoscopic Approach

02HT43Z Insertion of Infusion Device into Left Pulmonary Vein, Percutaneous Endoscopic Approach

02HT4DZ Insertion of Intraluminal Device into Left Pulmonary Vein, Percutaneous Endoscopic Approach

02HV00Z Insertion of Pressure Sensor Monitoring Device into Superior Vena Cava, Open Approach

02HV02Z Insertion of Monitoring Device into Superior Vena Cava, Open Approach

02HV03Z Insertion of Infusion Device into Superior Vena Cava, Open Approach

02HV0DZ Insertion of Intraluminal Device into Superior Vena Cava, Open Approach

02HV30Z Insertion of Pressure Sensor Monitoring Device into Superior Vena Cava, Percutaneous Approach

02HV32Z Insertion of Monitoring Device into Superior Vena Cava, Percutaneous Approach

02HV33Z Insertion of Infusion Device into Superior Vena Cava, Percutaneous Approach

02HV3DZ Insertion of Intraluminal Device into Superior Vena Cava, Percutaneous Approach

---

♀ Female-only   ♂ Male-only   ⬤ Limited Coverage   ⬤ Non-OR   🔲 HAC-associated procedure   ⬤ Non-covered procedures   ➕ Combination

02HV40Z   Insertion of Pressure Sensor Monitoring Device into Superior Vena Cava, Percutaneous Endoscopic Approach

02HV42Z   Insertion of Monitoring Device into Superior Vena Cava, Percutaneous Endoscopic Approach

02HV43Z   Insertion of Infusion Device into Superior Vena Cava, Percutaneous Endoscopic Approach

02HV4DZ   Insertion of Intraluminal Device into Superior Vena Cava, Percutaneous Endoscopic Approach

02HW00Z   Insertion of Pressure Sensor Monitoring Device into Thoracic Aorta, Open Approach

02HW02Z   Insertion of Monitoring Device into Thoracic Aorta, Open Approach

02HW03Z   Insertion of Infusion Device into Thoracic Aorta, Open Approach

02HW0DZ   Insertion of Intraluminal Device into Thoracic Aorta, Open Approach

02HW30Z   Insertion of Pressure Sensor Monitoring Device into Thoracic Aorta, Percutaneous Approach

02HW32Z   Insertion of Monitoring Device into Thoracic Aorta, Percutaneous Approach

02HW33Z   Insertion of Infusion Device into Thoracic Aorta, Percutaneous Approach

02HW3DZ   Insertion of Intraluminal Device into Thoracic Aorta, Percutaneous Approach

02J – Heart and Great Vessels, Inspection

Review Coding Guidelines B3.11a, B3.11b and B3.11c

02JA0ZZ   Inspection of Heart, Open Approach
02JA3ZZ   Inspection of Heart, Percutaneous Approach
02JA4ZZ   Inspection of Heart, Percutaneous Endoscopic Approach

02JY0ZZ   Inspection of Great Vessel, Open Approach
02JY3ZZ   Inspection of Great Vessel, Percutaneous Approach
02JY4ZZ   Inspection of Great Vessel, Percutaneous Endoscopic Approach

02K – Heart and Great Vessels, Map

● **02K80ZZ**   Map Conduction Mechanism, Open Approach
● **02K83ZZ**   Map Conduction Mechanism, Percutaneous Approach

● **02K84ZZ**   Map Conduction Mechanism, Percutaneous Endoscopic Approach

02L – Heart and Great Vessels, Occlusion

● **02L70CK**   Occlusion of Left Atrial Appendage with Extraluminal Device, Open Approach
● **02L70DK**   Occlusion of Left Atrial Appendage with Intraluminal Device, Open Approach
● **02L70ZK**   Occlusion of Left Atrial Appendage, Open Approach
● **02L73CK**   Occlusion of Left Atrial Appendage with Extraluminal Device, Percutaneous Approach
● **02L73DK**   Occlusion of Left Atrial Appendage with Intraluminal Device, Percutaneous Approach
● **02L73ZK**   Occlusion of Left Atrial Appendage, Percutaneous Approach
● **02L74CK**   Occlusion of Left Atrial Appendage with Extraluminal Device, Percutaneous Endoscopic Approach
● **02L74DK**   Occlusion of Left Atrial Appendage with Intraluminal Device, Percutaneous Endoscopic Approach
● **02L74ZK**   Occlusion of Left Atrial Appendage, Percutaneous Endoscopic Approach
02LR0CT   Occlusion of Ductus Arteriosus with Extraluminal Device, Open Approach
02LR0DT   Occlusion of Ductus Arteriosus with Intraluminal Device, Open Approach
02LR0ZT   Occlusion of Ductus Arteriosus, Open Approach
02LR3CT   Occlusion of Ductus Arteriosus with Extraluminal Device, Percutaneous Approach
02LR3DT   Occlusion of Ductus Arteriosus with Intraluminal Device, Percutaneous Approach
02LR3ZT   Occlusion of Ductus Arteriosus, Percutaneous Approach
02LR4CT   Occlusion of Ductus Arteriosus with Extraluminal Device, Percutaneous Endoscopic Approach
02LR4DT   Occlusion of Ductus Arteriosus with Intraluminal Device, Percutaneous Endoscopic Approach
02LR4ZT   Occlusion of Ductus Arteriosus, Percutaneous Endoscopic Approach
02LS0CZ   Occlusion of Right Pulmonary Vein with Extraluminal Device, Open Approach
02LS0DZ   Occlusion of Right Pulmonary Vein with Intraluminal Device, Open Approach
02LS0ZZ   Occlusion of Right Pulmonary Vein, Open Approach
02LS3CZ   Occlusion of Right Pulmonary Vein with Extraluminal Device, Percutaneous Approach
02LS3DZ   Occlusion of Right Pulmonary Vein with Intraluminal Device, Percutaneous Approach

02LS3ZZ   Occlusion of Right Pulmonary Vein, Percutaneous Approach
02LS4CZ   Occlusion of Right Pulmonary Vein with Extraluminal Device, Percutaneous Endoscopic Approach
02LS4DZ   Occlusion of Right Pulmonary Vein with Intraluminal Device, Percutaneous Endoscopic Approach
02LS4ZZ   Occlusion of Right Pulmonary Vein, Percutaneous Endoscopic Approach
02LT0CZ   Occlusion of Left Pulmonary Vein with Extraluminal Device, Open Approach
02LT0DZ   Occlusion of Left Pulmonary Vein with Intraluminal Device, Open Approach
02LT0ZZ   Occlusion of Left Pulmonary Vein, Open Approach
02LT3CZ   Occlusion of Left Pulmonary Vein with Extraluminal Device, Percutaneous Approach
02LT3DZ   Occlusion of Left Pulmonary Vein with Intraluminal Device, Percutaneous Approach
02LT3ZZ   Occlusion of Left Pulmonary Vein, Percutaneous Approach
02LT4CZ   Occlusion of Left Pulmonary Vein with Extraluminal Device, Percutaneous Endoscopic Approach
02LT4DZ   Occlusion of Left Pulmonary Vein with Intraluminal Device, Percutaneous Endoscopic Approach
02LT4ZZ   Occlusion of Left Pulmonary Vein, Percutaneous Endoscopic Approach
02LV0CZ   Occlusion of Superior Vena Cava with Extraluminal Device, Open Approach
02LV0DZ   Occlusion of Superior Vena Cava with Intraluminal Device, Open Approach
02LV0ZZ   Occlusion of Superior Vena Cava, Open Approach
02LV3CZ   Occlusion of Superior Vena Cava with Extraluminal Device, Percutaneous Approach
02LV3DZ   Occlusion of Superior Vena Cava with Intraluminal Device, Percutaneous Approach
02LV3ZZ   Occlusion of Superior Vena Cava, Percutaneous Approach
02LV4CZ   Occlusion of Superior Vena Cava with Extraluminal Device, Percutaneous Endoscopic Approach
02LV4DZ   Occlusion of Superior Vena Cava with Intraluminal Device, Percutaneous Endoscopic Approach
02LV4ZZ   Occlusion of Superior Vena Cava, Percutaneous Endoscopic Approach

02N – Heart and Great Vessels, Release

Review Coding Guideline B3.13

Review Coding Guideline B3.14

02N40ZZ	Release Coronary Vein, Open Approach
02N43ZZ	Release Coronary Vein, Percutaneous Approach
02N44ZZ	Release Coronary Vein, Percutaneous Endoscopic Approach
02N50ZZ	Release Atrial Septum, Open Approach
02N53ZZ	Release Atrial Septum, Percutaneous Approach
02N54ZZ	Release Atrial Septum, Percutaneous Endoscopic Approach
02N60ZZ	Release Right Atrium, Open Approach
02N63ZZ	Release Right Atrium, Percutaneous Approach
02N64ZZ	Release Right Atrium, Percutaneous Endoscopic Approach
02N70ZZ	Release Left Atrium, Open Approach
02N73ZZ	Release Left Atrium, Percutaneous Approach
02N74ZZ	Release Left Atrium, Percutaneous Endoscopic Approach
02N80ZZ	Release Conduction Mechanism, Open Approach
02N83ZZ	Release Conduction Mechanism, Percutaneous Approach
02N84ZZ	Release Conduction Mechanism, Percutaneous Endoscopic Approach
02N90ZZ	Release Chordae Tendineae, Open Approach
02N93ZZ	Release Chordae Tendineae, Percutaneous Approach
02N94ZZ	Release Chordae Tendineae, Percutaneous Endoscopic Approach
02ND0ZZ	Release Papillary Muscle, Open Approach
02ND3ZZ	Release Papillary Muscle, Percutaneous Approach
02ND4ZZ	Release Papillary Muscle, Percutaneous Endoscopic Approach
02NF0ZZ	Release Aortic Valve, Open Approach
02NF3ZZ	Release Aortic Valve, Percutaneous Approach
02NF4ZZ	Release Aortic Valve, Percutaneous Endoscopic Approach
02NG0ZZ	Release Mitral Valve, Open Approach
02NG3ZZ	Release Mitral Valve, Percutaneous Approach
02NG4ZZ	Release Mitral Valve, Percutaneous Endoscopic Approach
02NH0ZZ	Release Pulmonary Valve, Open Approach
02NH3ZZ	Release Pulmonary Valve, Percutaneous Approach
02NH4ZZ	Release Pulmonary Valve, Percutaneous Endoscopic Approach
02NJ0ZZ	Release Tricuspid Valve, Open Approach
02NJ3ZZ	Release Tricuspid Valve, Percutaneous Approach
02NJ4ZZ	Release Tricuspid Valve, Percutaneous Endoscopic Approach

02NK0ZZ	Release Right Ventricle, Open Approach
02NK3ZZ	Release Right Ventricle, Percutaneous Approach
02NK4ZZ	Release Right Ventricle, Percutaneous Endoscopic Approach
02NL0ZZ	Release Left Ventricle, Open Approach
02NL3ZZ	Release Left Ventricle, Percutaneous Approach
02NL4ZZ	Release Left Ventricle, Percutaneous Endoscopic Approach
02NM0ZZ	Release Ventricular Septum, Open Approach
02NM3ZZ	Release Ventricular Septum, Percutaneous Approach
02NM4ZZ	Release Ventricular Septum, Percutaneous Endoscopic Approach
02NN0ZZ	Release Pericardium, Open Approach
02NN3ZZ	Release Pericardium, Percutaneous Approach
02NN4ZZ	Release Pericardium, Percutaneous Endoscopic Approach
02NP0ZZ	Release Pulmonary Trunk, Open Approach
02NP3ZZ	Release Pulmonary Trunk, Percutaneous Approach
02NP4ZZ	Release Pulmonary Trunk, Percutaneous Endoscopic Approach
02NQ0ZZ	Release Right Pulmonary Artery, Open Approach
02NQ3ZZ	Release Right Pulmonary Artery, Percutaneous Approach
02NQ4ZZ	Release Right Pulmonary Artery, Percutaneous Endoscopic Approach
02NR0ZZ	Release Left Pulmonary Artery, Open Approach
02NR3ZZ	Release Left Pulmonary Artery, Percutaneous Approach
02NR4ZZ	Release Left Pulmonary Artery, Percutaneous Endoscopic Approach
02NS0ZZ	Release Right Pulmonary Vein, Open Approach
02NS3ZZ	Release Right Pulmonary Vein, Percutaneous Approach
02NS4ZZ	Release Right Pulmonary Vein, Percutaneous Endoscopic Approach
02NT0ZZ	Release Left Pulmonary Vein, Open Approach
02NT3ZZ	Release Left Pulmonary Vein, Percutaneous Approach
02NT4ZZ	Release Left Pulmonary Vein, Percutaneous Endoscopic Approach
02NV0ZZ	Release Superior Vena Cava, Open Approach
02NV3ZZ	Release Superior Vena Cava, Percutaneous Approach
02NV4ZZ	Release Superior Vena Cava, Percutaneous Endoscopic Approach
02NW0ZZ	Release Thoracic Aorta, Open Approach
02NW3ZZ	Release Thoracic Aorta, Percutaneous Approach
02NW4ZZ	Release Thoracic Aorta, Percutaneous Endoscopic Approach

02P – Heart and Great Vessels, Removal

Review Coding Guideline B6.1c

02PA02Z	Removal of Monitoring Device from Heart, Open Approach
02PA03Z	Removal of Infusion Device from Heart, Open Approach
02PA07Z	Removal of Autologous Tissue Substitute from Heart, Open Approach
02PA08Z	Removal of Zooplastic Tissue from Heart, Open Approach
02PA0CZ	Removal of Extraluminal Device from Heart, Open Approach
02PA0DZ	Removal of Intraluminal Device from Heart, Open Approach
02PA0JZ	Removal of Synthetic Substitute from Heart, Open Approach
02PA0KZ	Removal of Nonautologous Tissue Substitute from Heart, Open Approach
02PA0MZ	Removal of Cardiac Lead from Heart, Open Approach
HAC	With a secondary diagnosis code of K68.11, T81.4XXA, T82.6XXA, T82.7XXA
02PA0QZ	Removal of Implantable Heart Assist System from Heart, Open Approach
02PA0RZ	Removal of External Heart Assist System from Heart, Open Approach
02PA32Z	Removal of Monitoring Device from Heart, Percutaneous Approach
02PA33Z	Removal of Infusion Device from Heart, Percutaneous Approach
02PA37Z	Removal of Autologous Tissue Substitute from Heart, Percutaneous Approach
02PA38Z	Removal of Zooplastic Tissue from Heart, Percutaneous Approach
02PA3CZ	Removal of Extraluminal Device from Heart, Percutaneous Approach
02PA3DZ	Removal of Intraluminal Device from Heart, Percutaneous Approach
02PA3JZ	Removal of Synthetic Substitute from Heart, Percutaneous Approach
02PA3KZ	Removal of Nonautologous Tissue Substitute from Heart, Percutaneous Approach

02PA3MZ	Removal of Cardiac Lead from Heart, Percutaneous Approach
HAC	With a secondary diagnosis code of K68.11, T81.4XXA, T82.6XXA, T82.7XXA
02PA3QZ	Removal of Implantable Heart Assist System from Heart, Percutaneous Approach
02PA3RZ	Removal of External Heart Assist System from Heart, Percutaneous Approach
02PA42Z	Removal of Monitoring Device from Heart, Percutaneous Endoscopic Approach
02PA43Z	Removal of Infusion Device from Heart, Percutaneous Endoscopic Approach
02PA47Z	Removal of Autologous Tissue Substitute from Heart, Percutaneous Endoscopic Approach
02PA48Z	Removal of Zooplastic Tissue from Heart, Percutaneous Endoscopic Approach
02PA4CZ	Removal of Extraluminal Device from Heart, Percutaneous Endoscopic Approach
02PA4DZ	Removal of Intraluminal Device from Heart, Percutaneous Endoscopic Approach
02PA4JZ	Removal of Synthetic Substitute from Heart, Percutaneous Endoscopic Approach
02PA4KZ	Removal of Nonautologous Tissue Substitute from Heart, Percutaneous Endoscopic Approach
02PA4MZ	Removal of Cardiac Lead from Heart, Percutaneous Endoscopic Approach
HAC	With a secondary diagnosis code of K68.11, T81.4XXA, T82.6XXA, T82.7XXA
02PA4QZ	Removal of Implantable Heart Assist System from Heart, Percutaneous Endoscopic Approach

---

♀ Female-only   ♂ Male-only   ⬤ Limited Coverage   ● Non-OR   HAC HAC-associated procedure   ● Non-covered procedures   ✚ Combination

02PA4RZ Removal of External Heart Assist System from Heart, Percutaneous Endoscopic Approach
02PAX2Z Removal of Monitoring Device from Heart, External Approach
02PAX3Z Removal of Infusion Device from Heart, External Approach
02PAXDZ Removal of Intraluminal Device from Heart, External Approach
02PAXMZ Removal of Cardiac Lead from Heart, External Approach
> **HAC** With a secondary diagnosis code of K68.11, T81.4XXA, T82.6XXA, T82.7XXA
02PY02Z Removal of Monitoring Device from Great Vessel, Open Approach
02PY03Z Removal of Infusion Device from Great Vessel, Open Approach
02PY07Z Removal of Autologous Tissue Substitute from Great Vessel, Open Approach
02PY08Z Removal of Zooplastic Tissue from Great Vessel, Open Approach
02PY0CZ Removal of Extraluminal Device from Great Vessel, Open Approach
02PY0DZ Removal of Intraluminal Device from Great Vessel, Open Approach
02PY0JZ Removal of Synthetic Substitute from Great Vessel, Open Approach
02PY0KZ Removal of Nonautologous Tissue Substitute from Great Vessel, Open Approach
02PY32Z Removal of Monitoring Device from Great Vessel, Percutaneous Approach
02PY33Z Removal of Infusion Device from Great Vessel, Percutaneous Approach
02PY37Z Removal of Autologous Tissue Substitute from Great Vessel, Percutaneous Approach
02PY38Z Removal of Zooplastic Tissue from Great Vessel, Percutaneous Approach
02PY3CZ Removal of Extraluminal Device from Great Vessel, Percutaneous Approach

02PY3DZ Removal of Intraluminal Device from Great Vessel, Percutaneous Approach
02PY3JZ Removal of Synthetic Substitute from Great Vessel, Percutaneous Approach
02PY3KZ Removal of Nonautologous Tissue Substitute from Great Vessel, Percutaneous Approach
02PY42Z Removal of Monitoring Device from Great Vessel, Percutaneous Endoscopic Approach
02PY43Z Removal of Infusion Device from Great Vessel, Percutaneous Endoscopic Approach
02PY47Z Removal of Autologous Tissue Substitute from Great Vessel, Percutaneous Endoscopic Approach
02PY48Z Removal of Zooplastic Tissue from Great Vessel, Percutaneous Endoscopic Approach
02PY4CZ Removal of Extraluminal Device from Great Vessel, Percutaneous Endoscopic Approach
02PY4DZ Removal of Intraluminal Device from Great Vessel, Percutaneous Endoscopic Approach
02PY4JZ Removal of Synthetic Substitute from Great Vessel, Percutaneous Endoscopic Approach
02PY4KZ Removal of Nonautologous Tissue Substitute from Great Vessel, Percutaneous Endoscopic Approach
02PYX2Z Removal of Monitoring Device from Great Vessel, External Approach
02PYX3Z Removal of Infusion Device from Great Vessel, External Approach
02PYXDZ Removal of Intraluminal Device from Great Vessel, External Approach

02Q – Heart and Great Vessels, Repair

For Repair of coronary arteries, Review Coding Guideline B4.4

02Q00ZZ Repair Coronary Artery, One Site, Open Approach
02Q03ZZ Repair Coronary Artery, One Site, Percutaneous Approach
02Q04ZZ Repair Coronary Artery, One Site, Percutaneous Endoscopic Approach
02Q10ZZ Repair Coronary Artery, Two Sites, Open Approach
02Q13ZZ Repair Coronary Artery, Two Sites, Percutaneous Approach
02Q14ZZ Repair Coronary Artery, Two Sites, Percutaneous Endoscopic Approach
02Q20ZZ Repair Coronary Artery, Three Sites, Open Approach
02Q23ZZ Repair Coronary Artery, Three Sites, Percutaneous Approach
02Q24ZZ Repair Coronary Artery, Three Sites, Percutaneous Endoscopic Approach
02Q30ZZ Repair Coronary Artery, Four or More Sites, Open Approach
02Q33ZZ Repair Coronary Artery, Four or More Sites, Percutaneous Approach
02Q34ZZ Repair Coronary Artery, Four or More Sites, Percutaneous Endoscopic Approach
02Q40ZZ Repair Coronary Vein, Open Approach
02Q43ZZ Repair Coronary Vein, Percutaneous Approach
02Q44ZZ Repair Coronary Vein, Percutaneous Endoscopic Approach
02Q50ZZ Repair Atrial Septum, Open Approach
02Q53ZZ Repair Atrial Septum, Percutaneous Approach
02Q54ZZ Repair Atrial Septum, Percutaneous Endoscopic Approach
02Q60ZZ Repair Right Atrium, Open Approach
02Q63ZZ Repair Right Atrium, Percutaneous Approach
02Q64ZZ Repair Right Atrium, Percutaneous Endoscopic Approach
02Q70ZZ Repair Left Atrium, Open Approach
02Q73ZZ Repair Left Atrium, Percutaneous Approach
02Q74ZZ Repair Left Atrium, Percutaneous Endoscopic Approach
02Q80ZZ Repair Conduction Mechanism, Open Approach
02Q83ZZ Repair Conduction Mechanism, Percutaneous Approach
02Q84ZZ Repair Conduction Mechanism, Percutaneous Endoscopic Approach
02Q90ZZ Repair Chordae Tendineae, Open Approach
02Q93ZZ Repair Chordae Tendineae, Percutaneous Approach
02Q94ZZ Repair Chordae Tendineae, Percutaneous Endoscopic Approach
02QA0ZZ Repair Heart, Open Approach
02QA3ZZ Repair Heart, Percutaneous Approach
02QA4ZZ Repair Heart, Percutaneous Endoscopic Approach

02QB0ZZ Repair Right Heart, Open Approach
02QB3ZZ Repair Right Heart, Percutaneous Approach
02QB4ZZ Repair Right Heart, Percutaneous Endoscopic Approach
02QC0ZZ Repair Left Heart, Open Approach
02QC3ZZ Repair Left Heart, Percutaneous Approach
02QC4ZZ Repair Left Heart, Percutaneous Endoscopic Approach
02QD0ZZ Repair Papillary Muscle, Open Approach
02QD3ZZ Repair Papillary Muscle, Percutaneous Approach
02QD4ZZ Repair Papillary Muscle, Percutaneous Endoscopic Approach
02QF0ZZ Repair Aortic Valve, Open Approach
02QF3ZZ Repair Aortic Valve, Percutaneous Approach
02QF4ZZ Repair Aortic Valve, Percutaneous Endoscopic Approach
02QG0ZZ Repair Mitral Valve, Open Approach
02QG3ZZ Repair Mitral Valve, Percutaneous Approach
02QG4ZZ Repair Mitral Valve, Percutaneous Endoscopic Approach
02QH0ZZ Repair Pulmonary Valve, Open Approach
02QH3ZZ Repair Pulmonary Valve, Percutaneous Approach
02QH4ZZ Repair Pulmonary Valve, Percutaneous Endoscopic Approach
02QJ0ZZ Repair Tricuspid Valve, Open Approach
02QJ3ZZ Repair Tricuspid Valve, Percutaneous Approach
02QJ4ZZ Repair Tricuspid Valve, Percutaneous Endoscopic Approach
02QK0ZZ Repair Right Ventricle, Open Approach
02QK3ZZ Repair Right Ventricle, Percutaneous Approach
02QK4ZZ Repair Right Ventricle, Percutaneous Endoscopic Approach
02QL0ZZ Repair Left Ventricle, Open Approach
02QL3ZZ Repair Left Ventricle, Percutaneous Approach
02QL4ZZ Repair Left Ventricle, Percutaneous Endoscopic Approach
02QM0ZZ Repair Ventricular Septum, Open Approach
02QM3ZZ Repair Ventricular Septum, Percutaneous Approach
02QM4ZZ Repair Ventricular Septum, Percutaneous Endoscopic Approach
02QN0ZZ Repair Pericardium, Open Approach
02QN3ZZ Repair Pericardium, Percutaneous Approach
02QN4ZZ Repair Pericardium, Percutaneous Endoscopic Approach
02QP0ZZ Repair Pulmonary Trunk, Open Approach
02QP3ZZ Repair Pulmonary Trunk, Percutaneous Approach
02QP4ZZ Repair Pulmonary Trunk, Percutaneous Endoscopic Approach
02QQ0ZZ Repair Right Pulmonary Artery, Open Approach
02QQ3ZZ Repair Right Pulmonary Artery, Percutaneous Approach

02QQ4ZZ	Repair Right Pulmonary Artery, Percutaneous Endoscopic Approach
02QR0ZZ	Repair Left Pulmonary Artery, Open Approach
02QR3ZZ	Repair Left Pulmonary Artery, Percutaneous Approach
02QR4ZZ	Repair Left Pulmonary Artery, Percutaneous Endoscopic Approach
02QS0ZZ	Repair Right Pulmonary Vein, Open Approach
02QS3ZZ	Repair Right Pulmonary Vein, Percutaneous Approach
02QS4ZZ	Repair Right Pulmonary Vein, Percutaneous Endoscopic Approach
02QT0ZZ	Repair Left Pulmonary Vein, Open Approach

02QT3ZZ	Repair Left Pulmonary Vein, Percutaneous Approach
02QT4ZZ	Repair Left Pulmonary Vein, Percutaneous Endoscopic Approach
02QV0ZZ	Repair Superior Vena Cava, Open Approach
02QV3ZZ	Repair Superior Vena Cava, Percutaneous Approach
02QV4ZZ	Repair Superior Vena Cava, Percutaneous Endoscopic Approach
02QW0ZZ	Repair Thoracic Aorta, Open Approach
02QW3ZZ	Repair Thoracic Aorta, Percutaneous Approach
02QW4ZZ	Repair Thoracic Aorta, Percutaneous Endoscopic Approach

02R – Heart and Great Vessels, Replacement

02R507Z	Replacement of Atrial Septum with Autologous Tissue Substitute, Open Approach
02R508Z	Replacement of Atrial Septum with Zooplastic Tissue, Open Approach
02R50JZ	Replacement of Atrial Septum with Synthetic Substitute, Open Approach
02R50KZ	Replacement of Atrial Septum with Nonautologous Tissue Substitute, Open Approach
02R547Z	Replacement of Atrial Septum with Autologous Tissue Substitute, Percutaneous Endoscopic Approach
02R548Z	Replacement of Atrial Septum with Zooplastic Tissue, Percutaneous Endoscopic Approach
02R54JZ	Replacement of Atrial Septum with Synthetic Substitute, Percutaneous Endoscopic Approach
02R54KZ	Replacement of Atrial Septum with Nonautologous Tissue Substitute, Percutaneous Endoscopic Approach
02R607Z	Replacement of Right Atrium with Autologous Tissue Substitute, Open Approach
02R608Z	Replacement of Right Atrium with Zooplastic Tissue, Open Approach
02R60JZ	Replacement of Right Atrium with Synthetic Substitute, Open Approach
02R60KZ	Replacement of Right Atrium with Nonautologous Tissue Substitute, Open Approach
02R647Z	Replacement of Right Atrium with Autologous Tissue Substitute, Percutaneous Endoscopic Approach
02R648Z	Replacement of Right Atrium with Zooplastic Tissue, Percutaneous Endoscopic Approach
02R64JZ	Replacement of Right Atrium with Synthetic Substitute, Percutaneous Endoscopic Approach
02R64KZ	Replacement of Right Atrium with Nonautologous Tissue Substitute, Percutaneous Endoscopic Approach
02R707Z	Replacement of Left Atrium with Autologous Tissue Substitute, Open Approach
02R708Z	Replacement of Left Atrium with Zooplastic Tissue, Open Approach
02R70JZ	Replacement of Left Atrium with Synthetic Substitute, Open Approach
02R70KZ	Replacement of Left Atrium with Nonautologous Tissue Substitute, Open Approach
02R747Z	Replacement of Left Atrium with Autologous Tissue Substitute, Percutaneous Endoscopic Approach
02R748Z	Replacement of Left Atrium with Zooplastic Tissue, Percutaneous Endoscopic Approach
02R74JZ	Replacement of Left Atrium with Synthetic Substitute, Percutaneous Endoscopic Approach
02R74KZ	Replacement of Left Atrium with Nonautologous Tissue Substitute, Percutaneous Endoscopic Approach
02R907Z	Replacement of Chordae Tendineae with Autologous Tissue Substitute, Open Approach
02R908Z	Replacement of Chordae Tendineae with Zooplastic Tissue, Open Approach
02R90JZ	Replacement of Chordae Tendineae with Synthetic Substitute, Open Approach
02R90KZ	Replacement of Chordae Tendineae with Nonautologous Tissue Substitute, Open Approach
02R947Z	Replacement of Chordae Tendineae with Autologous Tissue Substitute, Percutaneous Endoscopic Approach
02R948Z	Replacement of Chordae Tendineae with Zooplastic Tissue, Percutaneous Endoscopic Approach
02R94JZ	Replacement of Chordae Tendineae with Synthetic Substitute, Percutaneous Endoscopic Approach
02R94KZ	Replacement of Chordae Tendineae with Nonautologous Tissue Substitute, Percutaneous Endoscopic Approach

02RD07Z	Replacement of Papillary Muscle with Autologous Tissue Substitute, Open Approach
02RD08Z	Replacement of Papillary Muscle with Zooplastic Tissue, Open Approach
02RD0JZ	Replacement of Papillary Muscle with Synthetic Substitute, Open Approach
02RD0KZ	Replacement of Papillary Muscle with Nonautologous Tissue Substitute, Open Approach
02RD47Z	Replacement of Papillary Muscle with Autologous Tissue Substitute, Percutaneous Endoscopic Approach
02RD48Z	Replacement of Papillary Muscle with Zooplastic Tissue, Percutaneous Endoscopic Approach
02RD4JZ	Replacement of Papillary Muscle with Synthetic Substitute, Percutaneous Endoscopic Approach
02RD4KZ	Replacement of Papillary Muscle with Nonautologous Tissue Substitute, Percutaneous Endoscopic Approach
02RF07Z	Replacement of Aortic Valve with Autologous Tissue Substitute, Open Approach
02RF08Z	Replacement of Aortic Valve with Zooplastic Tissue, Open Approach
02RF0JZ	Replacement of Aortic Valve with Synthetic Substitute, Open Approach
02RF0KZ	Replacement of Aortic Valve with Nonautologous Tissue Substitute, Open Approach
02RF37H	Replacement of Aortic Valve with Autologous Tissue Substitute, Transapical, Percutaneous Approach
02RF37Z	Replacement of Aortic Valve with Autologous Tissue Substitute, Percutaneous Approach
02RF38H	Replacement of Aortic Valve with Zooplastic Tissue, Transapical, Percutaneous Approach
02RF38Z	Replacement of Aortic Valve with Zooplastic Tissue, Percutaneous Approach
02RF3JH	Replacement of Aortic Valve with Synthetic Substitute, Transapical, Percutaneous Approach
02RF3JZ	Replacement of Aortic Valve with Synthetic Substitute, Percutaneous Approach
02RF3KH	Replacement of Aortic Valve with Nonautologous Tissue Substitute, Transapical, Percutaneous Approach
02RF3KZ	Replacement of Aortic Valve with Nonautologous Tissue Substitute, Percutaneous Approach
02RF47Z	Replacement of Aortic Valve with Autologous Tissue Substitute, Percutaneous Endoscopic Approach
02RF48Z	Replacement of Aortic Valve with Zooplastic Tissue, Percutaneous Endoscopic Approach
02RF4JZ	Replacement of Aortic Valve with Synthetic Substitute, Percutaneous Endoscopic Approach
02RF4KZ	Replacement of Aortic Valve with Nonautologous Tissue Substitute, Percutaneous Endoscopic Approach
02RG07Z	Replacement of Mitral Valve with Autologous Tissue Substitute, Open Approach
02RG08Z	Replacement of Mitral Valve with Zooplastic Tissue, Open Approach
02RG0JZ	Replacement of Mitral Valve with Synthetic Substitute, Open Approach
02RG0KZ	Replacement of Mitral Valve with Nonautologous Tissue Substitute, Open Approach
02RG37H	Replacement of Mitral Valve with Autologous Tissue Substitute, Transapical, Percutaneous Approach
02RG37Z	Replacement of Mitral Valve with Autologous Tissue Substitute, Percutaneous Approach
02RG38H	Replacement of Mitral Valve with Zooplastic Tissue, Transapical, Percutaneous Approach

02RG38Z Replacement of Mitral Valve with Zooplastic Tissue, Percutaneous Approach

02RG3JH Replacement of Mitral Valve with Synthetic Substitute, Transapical, Percutaneous Approach

02RG3JZ Replacement of Mitral Valve with Synthetic Substitute, Percutaneous Approach

02RG3KH Replacement of Mitral Valve with Nonautologous Tissue Substitute, Transapical, Percutaneous Approach

02RG3KZ Replacement of Mitral Valve with Nonautologous Tissue Substitute, Percutaneous Approach

02RG47Z Replacement of Mitral Valve with Autologous Tissue Substitute, Percutaneous Endoscopic Approach

02RG48Z Replacement of Mitral Valve with Zooplastic Tissue, Percutaneous Endoscopic Approach

02RG4JZ Replacement of Mitral Valve with Synthetic Substitute, Percutaneous Endoscopic Approach

02RG4KZ Replacement of Mitral Valve with Nonautologous Tissue Substitute, Percutaneous Endoscopic Approach

02RH07Z Replacement of Pulmonary Valve with Autologous Tissue Substitute, Open Approach

02RH08Z Replacement of Pulmonary Valve with Zooplastic Tissue, Open Approach

02RH0JZ Replacement of Pulmonary Valve with Synthetic Substitute, Open Approach

02RH0KZ Replacement of Pulmonary Valve with Nonautologous Tissue Substitute, Open Approach

02RH37H Replacement of Pulmonary Valve with Autologous Tissue Substitute, Transapical, Percutaneous Approach

02RH37Z Replacement of Pulmonary Valve with Autologous Tissue Substitute, Percutaneous Approach

02RH38H Replacement of Pulmonary Valve with Zooplastic Tissue, Transapical, Percutaneous Approach

02RH38Z Replacement of Pulmonary Valve with Zooplastic Tissue, Percutaneous Approach

02RH3JH Replacement of Pulmonary Valve with Synthetic Substitute, Transapical, Percutaneous Approach

02RH3JZ Replacement of Pulmonary Valve with Synthetic Substitute, Percutaneous Approach

02RH3KH Replacement of Pulmonary Valve with Nonautologous Tissue Substitute, Transapical, Percutaneous Approach

02RH3KZ Replacement of Pulmonary Valve with Nonautologous Tissue Substitute, Percutaneous Approach

02RH47Z Replacement of Pulmonary Valve with Autologous Tissue Substitute, Percutaneous Endoscopic Approach

02RH48Z Replacement of Pulmonary Valve with Zooplastic Tissue, Percutaneous Endoscopic Approach

02RH4JZ Replacement of Pulmonary Valve with Synthetic Substitute, Percutaneous Endoscopic Approach

02RH4KZ Replacement of Pulmonary Valve with Nonautologous Tissue Substitute, Percutaneous Endoscopic Approach

02RJ07Z Replacement of Tricuspid Valve with Autologous Tissue Substitute, Open Approach

02RJ08Z Replacement of Tricuspid Valve with Zooplastic Tissue, Open Approach

02RJ0JZ Replacement of Tricuspid Valve with Synthetic Substitute, Open Approach

02RJ0KZ Replacement of Tricuspid Valve with Nonautologous Tissue Substitute, Open Approach

02RJ47Z Replacement of Tricuspid Valve with Autologous Tissue Substitute, Percutaneous Endoscopic Approach

02RJ48Z Replacement of Tricuspid Valve with Zooplastic Tissue, Percutaneous Endoscopic Approach

02RJ4JZ Replacement of Tricuspid Valve with Synthetic Substitute, Percutaneous Endoscopic Approach

02RJ4KZ Replacement of Tricuspid Valve with Nonautologous Tissue Substitute, Percutaneous Endoscopic Approach

02RK07Z Replacement of Right Ventricle with Autologous Tissue Substitute, Open Approach

02RK08Z Replacement of Right Ventricle with Zooplastic Tissue, Open Approach

02RK0JZ Replacement of Right Ventricle with Synthetic Substitute, Open Approach
    ○ *When reported with 02RL0JZ and diagnosis code Z00.6*

02RK0KZ Replacement of Right Ventricle with Nonautologous Tissue Substitute, Open Approach

02RK47Z Replacement of Right Ventricle with Autologous Tissue Substitute, Percutaneous Endoscopic Approach

02RK48Z Replacement of Right Ventricle with Zooplastic Tissue, Percutaneous Endoscopic Approach

02RK4JZ Replacement of Right Ventricle with Synthetic Substitute, Percutaneous Endoscopic Approach

02RK4KZ Replacement of Right Ventricle with Nonautologous Tissue Substitute, Percutaneous Endoscopic Approach

02RL07Z Replacement of Left Ventricle with Autologous Tissue Substitute, Open Approach

02RL08Z Replacement of Left Ventricle with Zooplastic Tissue, Open Approach

02RL0JZ Replacement of Left Ventricle with Synthetic Substitute, Open Approach
    ○ *When reported with 02RK0JZ and diagnosis code Z00.6*

02RL0KZ Replacement of Left Ventricle with Nonautologous Tissue Substitute, Open Approach

02RL47Z Replacement of Left Ventricle with Autologous Tissue Substitute, Percutaneous Endoscopic Approach

02RL48Z Replacement of Left Ventricle with Zooplastic Tissue, Percutaneous Endoscopic Approach

02RL4JZ Replacement of Left Ventricle with Synthetic Substitute, Percutaneous Endoscopic Approach

02RL4KZ Replacement of Left Ventricle with Nonautologous Tissue Substitute, Percutaneous Endoscopic Approach

02RM07Z Replacement of Ventricular Septum with Autologous Tissue Substitute, Open Approach

02RM08Z Replacement of Ventricular Septum with Zooplastic Tissue, Open Approach

02RM0JZ Replacement of Ventricular Septum with Synthetic Substitute, Open Approach

02RM0KZ Replacement of Ventricular Septum with Nonautologous Tissue Substitute, Open Approach

02RM47Z Replacement of Ventricular Septum with Autologous Tissue Substitute, Percutaneous Endoscopic Approach

02RM48Z Replacement of Ventricular Septum with Zooplastic Tissue, Percutaneous Endoscopic Approach

02RM4JZ Replacement of Ventricular Septum with Synthetic Substitute, Percutaneous Endoscopic Approach

02RM4KZ Replacement of Ventricular Septum with Nonautologous Tissue Substitute, Percutaneous Endoscopic Approach

02RN07Z Replacement of Pericardium with Autologous Tissue Substitute, Open Approach

02RN08Z Replacement of Pericardium with Zooplastic Tissue, Open Approach

02RN0JZ Replacement of Pericardium with Synthetic Substitute, Open Approach

02RN0KZ Replacement of Pericardium with Nonautologous Tissue Substitute, Open Approach

02RN47Z Replacement of Pericardium with Autologous Tissue Substitute, Percutaneous Endoscopic Approach

02RN48Z Replacement of Pericardium with Zooplastic Tissue, Percutaneous Endoscopic Approach

02RN4JZ Replacement of Pericardium with Synthetic Substitute, Percutaneous Endoscopic Approach

02RN4KZ Replacement of Pericardium with Nonautologous Tissue Substitute, Percutaneous Endoscopic Approach

02RP07Z Replacement of Pulmonary Trunk with Autologous Tissue Substitute, Open Approach

02RP08Z Replacement of Pulmonary Trunk with Zooplastic Tissue, Open Approach

02RP0JZ Replacement of Pulmonary Trunk with Synthetic Substitute, Open Approach

02RP0KZ Replacement of Pulmonary Trunk with Nonautologous Tissue Substitute, Open Approach

02RP47Z Replacement of Pulmonary Trunk with Autologous Tissue Substitute, Percutaneous Endoscopic Approach

02RP48Z Replacement of Pulmonary Trunk with Zooplastic Tissue, Percutaneous Endoscopic Approach

02RP4JZ Replacement of Pulmonary Trunk with Synthetic Substitute, Percutaneous Endoscopic Approach

---

♀ Female-only   ♂ Male-only   ○ Limited Coverage   ● Non-OR   🅷🅰🅲 HAC-associated procedure   ● Non-covered procedures   ➕ Combination

02RP4KZ Replacement of Pulmonary Trunk with Nonautologous Tissue Substitute, Percutaneous Endoscopic Approach

02RQ07Z Replacement of Right Pulmonary Artery with Autologous Tissue Substitute, Open Approach

02RQ08Z Replacement of Right Pulmonary Artery with Zooplastic Tissue, Open Approach

02RQ0JZ Replacement of Right Pulmonary Artery with Synthetic Substitute, Open Approach

02RQ0KZ Replacement of Right Pulmonary Artery with Nonautologous Tissue Substitute, Open Approach

02RQ47Z Replacement of Right Pulmonary Artery with Autologous Tissue Substitute, Percutaneous Endoscopic Approach

02RQ48Z Replacement of Right Pulmonary Artery with Zooplastic Tissue, Percutaneous Endoscopic Approach

02RQ4JZ Replacement of Right Pulmonary Artery with Synthetic Substitute, Percutaneous Endoscopic Approach

02RQ4KZ Replacement of Right Pulmonary Artery with Nonautologous Tissue Substitute, Percutaneous Endoscopic Approach

02RR07Z Replacement of Left Pulmonary Artery with Autologous Tissue Substitute, Open Approach

02RR08Z Replacement of Left Pulmonary Artery with Zooplastic Tissue, Open Approach

02RR0JZ Replacement of Left Pulmonary Artery with Synthetic Substitute, Open Approach

02RR0KZ Replacement of Left Pulmonary Artery with Nonautologous Tissue Substitute, Open Approach

02RR47Z Replacement of Left Pulmonary Artery with Autologous Tissue Substitute, Percutaneous Endoscopic Approach

02RR48Z Replacement of Left Pulmonary Artery with Zooplastic Tissue, Percutaneous Endoscopic Approach

02RR4JZ Replacement of Left Pulmonary Artery with Synthetic Substitute, Percutaneous Endoscopic Approach

02RR4KZ Replacement of Left Pulmonary Artery with Nonautologous Tissue Substitute, Percutaneous Endoscopic Approach

02RS07Z Replacement of Right Pulmonary Vein with Autologous Tissue Substitute, Open Approach

02RS08Z Replacement of Right Pulmonary Vein with Zooplastic Tissue, Open Approach

02RS0JZ Replacement of Right Pulmonary Vein with Synthetic Substitute, Open Approach

02RS0KZ Replacement of Right Pulmonary Vein with Nonautologous Tissue Substitute, Open Approach

02RS47Z Replacement of Right Pulmonary Vein with Autologous Tissue Substitute, Percutaneous Endoscopic Approach

02RS48Z Replacement of Right Pulmonary Vein with Zooplastic Tissue, Percutaneous Endoscopic Approach

02RS4JZ Replacement of Right Pulmonary Vein with Synthetic Substitute, Percutaneous Endoscopic Approach

02RS4KZ Replacement of Right Pulmonary Vein with Nonautologous Tissue Substitute, Percutaneous Endoscopic Approach

02RT07Z Replacement of Left Pulmonary Vein with Autologous Tissue Substitute, Open Approach

02RT08Z Replacement of Left Pulmonary Vein with Zooplastic Tissue, Open Approach

02RT0JZ Replacement of Left Pulmonary Vein with Synthetic Substitute, Open Approach

02RT0KZ Replacement of Left Pulmonary Vein with Nonautologous Tissue Substitute, Open Approach

02RT47Z Replacement of Left Pulmonary Vein with Autologous Tissue Substitute, Percutaneous Endoscopic Approach

02RT48Z Replacement of Left Pulmonary Vein with Zooplastic Tissue, Percutaneous Endoscopic Approach

02RT4JZ Replacement of Left Pulmonary Vein with Synthetic Substitute, Percutaneous Endoscopic Approach

02RT4KZ Replacement of Left Pulmonary Vein with Nonautologous Tissue Substitute, Percutaneous Endoscopic Approach

02RV07Z Replacement of Superior Vena Cava with Autologous Tissue Substitute, Open Approach

02RV08Z Replacement of Superior Vena Cava with Zooplastic Tissue, Open Approach

02RV0JZ Replacement of Superior Vena Cava with Synthetic Substitute, Open Approach

02RV0KZ Replacement of Superior Vena Cava with Nonautologous Tissue Substitute, Open Approach

02RV47Z Replacement of Superior Vena Cava with Autologous Tissue Substitute, Percutaneous Endoscopic Approach

02RV48Z Replacement of Superior Vena Cava with Zooplastic Tissue, Percutaneous Endoscopic Approach

02RV4JZ Replacement of Superior Vena Cava with Synthetic Substitute, Percutaneous Endoscopic Approach

02RV4KZ Replacement of Superior Vena Cava with Nonautologous Tissue Substitute, Percutaneous Endoscopic Approach

02RW07Z Replacement of Thoracic Aorta with Autologous Tissue Substitute, Open Approach

02RW08Z Replacement of Thoracic Aorta with Zooplastic Tissue, Open Approach

02RW0JZ Replacement of Thoracic Aorta with Synthetic Substitute, Open Approach

02RW0KZ Replacement of Thoracic Aorta with Nonautologous Tissue Substitute, Open Approach

02RW47Z Replacement of Thoracic Aorta with Autologous Tissue Substitute, Percutaneous Endoscopic Approach

02RW48Z Replacement of Thoracic Aorta with Zooplastic Tissue, Percutaneous Endoscopic Approach

02RW4JZ Replacement of Thoracic Aorta with Synthetic Substitute, Percutaneous Endoscopic Approach

02RW4KZ Replacement of Thoracic Aorta with Nonautologous Tissue Substitute, Percutaneous Endoscopic Approach

02S – Heart and Great Vessels, Reposition

02SP0ZZ Reposition Pulmonary Trunk, Open Approach
02SQ0ZZ Reposition Right Pulmonary Artery, Open Approach
02SR0ZZ Reposition Left Pulmonary Artery, Open Approach
02SS0ZZ Reposition Right Pulmonary Vein, Open Approach
02ST0ZZ Reposition Left Pulmonary Vein, Open Approach
02SV0ZZ Reposition Superior Vena Cava, Open Approach
02SW0ZZ Reposition Thoracic Aorta, Open Approach

02T – Heart and Great Vessels, Resection

Review Coding Guideline B3.8

02T50ZZ Resection of Atrial Septum, Open Approach
02T53ZZ Resection of Atrial Septum, Percutaneous Approach
02T54ZZ Resection of Atrial Septum, Percutaneous Endoscopic Approach
02T80ZZ Resection of Conduction Mechanism, Open Approach
02T83ZZ Resection of Conduction Mechanism, Percutaneous Approach
02T84ZZ Resection of Conduction Mechanism, Percutaneous Endoscopic Approach
02T90ZZ Resection of Chordae Tendineae, Open Approach
02T93ZZ Resection of Chordae Tendineae, Percutaneous Approach

02T94ZZ Resection of Chordae Tendineae, Percutaneous Endoscopic Approach
02TD0ZZ Resection of Papillary Muscle, Open Approach
02TD3ZZ Resection of Papillary Muscle, Percutaneous Approach
02TD4ZZ Resection of Papillary Muscle, Percutaneous Endoscopic Approach
02TH0ZZ Resection of Pulmonary Valve, Open Approach
02TH3ZZ Resection of Pulmonary Valve, Percutaneous Approach
02TH4ZZ Resection of Pulmonary Valve, Percutaneous Endoscopic Approach
02TM0ZZ Resection of Ventricular Septum, Open Approach
02TM3ZZ Resection of Ventricular Septum, Percutaneous Approach

02TM4ZZ Resection of Ventricular Septum, Percutaneous Endoscopic Approach

02TN0ZZ Resection of Pericardium, Open Approach

02TN3ZZ Resection of Pericardium, Percutaneous Approach

02TN4ZZ Resection of Pericardium, Percutaneous Endoscopic Approach

02U – Heart and Great Vessels, Supplement

02U507Z Supplement Atrial Septum with Autologous Tissue Substitute, Open Approach

02U508Z Supplement Atrial Septum with Zooplastic Tissue, Open Approach

02U50JZ Supplement Atrial Septum with Synthetic Substitute, Open Approach

02U50KZ Supplement Atrial Septum with Nonautologous Tissue Substitute, Open Approach

02U537Z Supplement Atrial Septum with Autologous Tissue Substitute, Percutaneous Approach

02U538Z Supplement Atrial Septum with Zooplastic Tissue, Percutaneous Approach

02U53JZ Supplement Atrial Septum with Synthetic Substitute, Percutaneous Approach

02U53KZ Supplement Atrial Septum with Nonautologous Tissue Substitute, Percutaneous Approach

02U547Z Supplement Atrial Septum with Autologous Tissue Substitute, Percutaneous Endoscopic Approach

02U548Z Supplement Atrial Septum with Zooplastic Tissue, Percutaneous Endoscopic Approach

02U54JZ Supplement Atrial Septum with Synthetic Substitute, Percutaneous Endoscopic Approach

02U54KZ Supplement Atrial Septum with Nonautologous Tissue Substitute, Percutaneous Endoscopic Approach

02U607Z Supplement Right Atrium with Autologous Tissue Substitute, Open Approach

02U608Z Supplement Right Atrium with Zooplastic Tissue, Open Approach

02U60JZ Supplement Right Atrium with Synthetic Substitute, Open Approach

02U60KZ Supplement Right Atrium with Nonautologous Tissue Substitute, Open Approach

02U637Z Supplement Right Atrium with Autologous Tissue Substitute, Percutaneous Approach

02U638Z Supplement Right Atrium with Zooplastic Tissue, Percutaneous Approach

02U63JZ Supplement Right Atrium with Synthetic Substitute, Percutaneous Approach

02U63KZ Supplement Right Atrium with Nonautologous Tissue Substitute, Percutaneous Approach

02U647Z Supplement Right Atrium with Autologous Tissue Substitute, Percutaneous Endoscopic Approach

02U648Z Supplement Right Atrium with Zooplastic Tissue, Percutaneous Endoscopic Approach

02U64JZ Supplement Right Atrium with Synthetic Substitute, Percutaneous Endoscopic Approach

02U64KZ Supplement Right Atrium with Nonautologous Tissue Substitute, Percutaneous Endoscopic Approach

02U707Z Supplement Left Atrium with Autologous Tissue Substitute, Open Approach

02U708Z Supplement Left Atrium with Zooplastic Tissue, Open Approach

02U70JZ Supplement Left Atrium with Synthetic Substitute, Open Approach

02U70KZ Supplement Left Atrium with Nonautologous Tissue Substitute, Open Approach

02U737Z Supplement Left Atrium with Autologous Tissue Substitute, Percutaneous Approach

02U738Z Supplement Left Atrium with Zooplastic Tissue, Percutaneous Approach

● **02U73JZ** Supplement Left Atrium with Synthetic Substitute, Percutaneous Approach

02U73KZ Supplement Left Atrium with Nonautologous Tissue Substitute, Percutaneous Approach

02U747Z Supplement Left Atrium with Autologous Tissue Substitute, Percutaneous Endoscopic Approach

02U748Z Supplement Left Atrium with Zooplastic Tissue, Percutaneous Endoscopic Approach

● **02U74JZ** Supplement Left Atrium with Synthetic Substitute, Percutaneous Endoscopic Approach

02U74KZ Supplement Left Atrium with Nonautologous Tissue Substitute, Percutaneous Endoscopic Approach

02U907Z Supplement Chordae Tendineae with Autologous Tissue Substitute, Open Approach

02U908Z Supplement Chordae Tendineae with Zooplastic Tissue, Open Approach

02U90JZ Supplement Chordae Tendineae with Synthetic Substitute, Open Approach

02U90KZ Supplement Chordae Tendineae with Nonautologous Tissue Substitute, Open Approach

02U937Z Supplement Chordae Tendineae with Autologous Tissue Substitute, Percutaneous Approach

02U938Z Supplement Chordae Tendineae with Zooplastic Tissue, Percutaneous Approach

02U93JZ Supplement Chordae Tendineae with Synthetic Substitute, Percutaneous Approach

02U93KZ Supplement Chordae Tendineae with Nonautologous Tissue Substitute, Percutaneous Approach

02U947Z Supplement Chordae Tendineae with Autologous Tissue Substitute, Percutaneous Endoscopic Approach

02U948Z Supplement Chordae Tendineae with Zooplastic Tissue, Percutaneous Endoscopic Approach

02U94JZ Supplement Chordae Tendineae with Synthetic Substitute, Percutaneous Endoscopic Approach

02U94KZ Supplement Chordae Tendineae with Nonautologous Tissue Substitute, Percutaneous Endoscopic Approach

02UA07Z Supplement Heart with Autologous Tissue Substitute, Open Approach

02UA08Z Supplement Heart with Zooplastic Tissue, Open Approach

02UA0JZ Supplement Heart with Synthetic Substitute, Open Approach

02UA0KZ Supplement Heart with Nonautologous Tissue Substitute, Open Approach

02UA37Z Supplement Heart with Autologous Tissue Substitute, Percutaneous Approach

02UA38Z Supplement Heart with Zooplastic Tissue, Percutaneous Approach

02UA3JZ Supplement Heart with Synthetic Substitute, Percutaneous Approach

02UA3KZ Supplement Heart with Nonautologous Tissue Substitute, Percutaneous Approach

02UA47Z Supplement Heart with Autologous Tissue Substitute, Percutaneous Endoscopic Approach

02UA48Z Supplement Heart with Zooplastic Tissue, Percutaneous Endoscopic Approach

02UA4JZ Supplement Heart with Synthetic Substitute, Percutaneous Endoscopic Approach

02UA4KZ Supplement Heart with Nonautologous Tissue Substitute, Percutaneous Endoscopic Approach

02UD07Z Supplement Papillary Muscle with Autologous Tissue Substitute, Open Approach

02UD08Z Supplement Papillary Muscle with Zooplastic Tissue, Open Approach

02UD0JZ Supplement Papillary Muscle with Synthetic Substitute, Open Approach

02UD0KZ Supplement Papillary Muscle with Nonautologous Tissue Substitute, Open Approach

02UD37Z Supplement Papillary Muscle with Autologous Tissue Substitute, Percutaneous Approach

02UD38Z Supplement Papillary Muscle with Zooplastic Tissue, Percutaneous Approach

02UD3JZ Supplement Papillary Muscle with Synthetic Substitute, Percutaneous Approach

02UD3KZ Supplement Papillary Muscle with Nonautologous Tissue Substitute, Percutaneous Approach

02UD47Z Supplement Papillary Muscle with Autologous Tissue Substitute, Percutaneous Endoscopic Approach

02UD48Z Supplement Papillary Muscle with Zooplastic Tissue, Percutaneous Endoscopic Approach

02UD4JZ Supplement Papillary Muscle with Synthetic Substitute, Percutaneous Endoscopic Approach

02UD4KZ Supplement Papillary Muscle with Nonautologous Tissue Substitute, Percutaneous Endoscopic Approach

02UF07Z Supplement Aortic Valve with Autologous Tissue Substitute, Open Approach

02UF08Z Supplement Aortic Valve with Zooplastic Tissue, Open Approach

02UF0JZ Supplement Aortic Valve with Synthetic Substitute, Open Approach

02UF0KZ Supplement Aortic Valve with Nonautologous Tissue Substitute, Open Approach

02UF37Z Supplement Aortic Valve with Autologous Tissue Substitute, Percutaneous Approach

02UF38Z Supplement Aortic Valve with Zooplastic Tissue, Percutaneous Approach

02UF3JZ Supplement Aortic Valve with Synthetic Substitute, Percutaneous Approach

02UF3KZ Supplement Aortic Valve with Nonautologous Tissue Substitute, Percutaneous Approach

02UF47Z Supplement Aortic Valve with Autologous Tissue Substitute, Percutaneous Endoscopic Approach

02UF48Z Supplement Aortic Valve with Zooplastic Tissue, Percutaneous Endoscopic Approach

02UF4JZ Supplement Aortic Valve with Synthetic Substitute, Percutaneous Endoscopic Approach

02UF4KZ Supplement Aortic Valve with Nonautologous Tissue Substitute, Percutaneous Endoscopic Approach

02UG07Z Supplement Mitral Valve with Autologous Tissue Substitute, Open Approach

02UG08Z Supplement Mitral Valve with Zooplastic Tissue, Open Approach

02UG0JZ Supplement Mitral Valve with Synthetic Substitute, Open Approach

02UG0KZ Supplement Mitral Valve with Nonautologous Tissue Substitute, Open Approach

02UG37Z Supplement Mitral Valve with Autologous Tissue Substitute, Percutaneous Approach

02UG38Z Supplement Mitral Valve with Zooplastic Tissue, Percutaneous Approach

02UG3JZ Supplement Mitral Valve with Synthetic Substitute, Percutaneous Approach

02UG3KZ Supplement Mitral Valve with Nonautologous Tissue Substitute, Percutaneous Approach

02UG47Z Supplement Mitral Valve with Autologous Tissue Substitute, Percutaneous Endoscopic Approach

02UG48Z Supplement Mitral Valve with Zooplastic Tissue, Percutaneous Endoscopic Approach

02UG4JZ Supplement Mitral Valve with Synthetic Substitute, Percutaneous Endoscopic Approach

02UG4KZ Supplement Mitral Valve with Nonautologous Tissue Substitute, Percutaneous Endoscopic Approach

02UH07Z Supplement Pulmonary Valve with Autologous Tissue Substitute, Open Approach

02UH08Z Supplement Pulmonary Valve with Zooplastic Tissue, Open Approach

02UH0JZ Supplement Pulmonary Valve with Synthetic Substitute, Open Approach

02UH0KZ Supplement Pulmonary Valve with Nonautologous Tissue Substitute, Open Approach

02UH37Z Supplement Pulmonary Valve with Autologous Tissue Substitute, Percutaneous Approach

02UH38Z Supplement Pulmonary Valve with Zooplastic Tissue, Percutaneous Approach

02UH3JZ Supplement Pulmonary Valve with Synthetic Substitute, Percutaneous Approach

02UH3KZ Supplement Pulmonary Valve with Nonautologous Tissue Substitute, Percutaneous Approach

02UH47Z Supplement Pulmonary Valve with Autologous Tissue Substitute, Percutaneous Endoscopic Approach

02UH48Z Supplement Pulmonary Valve with Zooplastic Tissue, Percutaneous Endoscopic Approach

02UH4JZ Supplement Pulmonary Valve with Synthetic Substitute, Percutaneous Endoscopic Approach

02UH4KZ Supplement Pulmonary Valve with Nonautologous Tissue Substitute, Percutaneous Endoscopic Approach

02UJ07Z Supplement Tricuspid Valve with Autologous Tissue Substitute, Open Approach

02UJ08Z Supplement Tricuspid Valve with Zooplastic Tissue, Open Approach

02UJ0JZ Supplement Tricuspid Valve with Synthetic Substitute, Open Approach

02UJ0KZ Supplement Tricuspid Valve with Nonautologous Tissue Substitute, Open Approach

02UJ37Z Supplement Tricuspid Valve with Autologous Tissue Substitute, Percutaneous Approach

02UJ38Z Supplement Tricuspid Valve with Zooplastic Tissue, Percutaneous Approach

02UJ3JZ Supplement Tricuspid Valve with Synthetic Substitute, Percutaneous Approach

02UJ3KZ Supplement Tricuspid Valve with Nonautologous Tissue Substitute, Percutaneous Approach

02UJ47Z Supplement Tricuspid Valve with Autologous Tissue Substitute, Percutaneous Endoscopic Approach

02UJ48Z Supplement Tricuspid Valve with Zooplastic Tissue, Percutaneous Endoscopic Approach

02UJ4JZ Supplement Tricuspid Valve with Synthetic Substitute, Percutaneous Endoscopic Approach

02UJ4KZ Supplement Tricuspid Valve with Nonautologous Tissue Substitute, Percutaneous Endoscopic Approach

02UK07Z Supplement Right Ventricle with Autologous Tissue Substitute, Open Approach

02UK08Z Supplement Right Ventricle with Zooplastic Tissue, Open Approach

02UK0JZ Supplement Right Ventricle with Synthetic Substitute, Open Approach

02UK0KZ Supplement Right Ventricle with Nonautologous Tissue Substitute, Open Approach

02UK37Z Supplement Right Ventricle with Autologous Tissue Substitute, Percutaneous Approach

02UK38Z Supplement Right Ventricle with Zooplastic Tissue, Percutaneous Approach

02UK3JZ Supplement Right Ventricle with Synthetic Substitute, Percutaneous Approach

02UK3KZ Supplement Right Ventricle with Nonautologous Tissue Substitute, Percutaneous Approach

02UK47Z Supplement Right Ventricle with Autologous Tissue Substitute, Percutaneous Endoscopic Approach

02UK48Z Supplement Right Ventricle with Zooplastic Tissue, Percutaneous Endoscopic Approach

02UK4JZ Supplement Right Ventricle with Synthetic Substitute, Percutaneous Endoscopic Approach

02UK4KZ Supplement Right Ventricle with Nonautologous Tissue Substitute, Percutaneous Endoscopic Approach

02UL07Z Supplement Left Ventricle with Autologous Tissue Substitute, Open Approach

02UL08Z Supplement Left Ventricle with Zooplastic Tissue, Open Approach

02UL0JZ Supplement Left Ventricle with Synthetic Substitute, Open Approach

02UL0KZ Supplement Left Ventricle with Nonautologous Tissue Substitute, Open Approach

02UL37Z Supplement Left Ventricle with Autologous Tissue Substitute, Percutaneous Approach

02UL38Z Supplement Left Ventricle with Zooplastic Tissue, Percutaneous Approach

02UL3JZ Supplement Left Ventricle with Synthetic Substitute, Percutaneous Approach

02UL3KZ Supplement Left Ventricle with Nonautologous Tissue Substitute, Percutaneous Approach

02UL47Z Supplement Left Ventricle with Autologous Tissue Substitute, Percutaneous Endoscopic Approach

02UL48Z Supplement Left Ventricle with Zooplastic Tissue, Percutaneous Endoscopic Approach

02UL4JZ Supplement Left Ventricle with Synthetic Substitute, Percutaneous Endoscopic Approach

02UL4KZ Supplement Left Ventricle with Nonautologous Tissue Substitute, Percutaneous Endoscopic Approach

02UM07Z Supplement Ventricular Septum with Autologous Tissue Substitute, Open Approach

02UM08Z Supplement Ventricular Septum with Zooplastic Tissue, Open Approach

02UM0JZ Supplement Ventricular Septum with Synthetic Substitute, Open Approach

02UM0KZ Supplement Ventricular Septum with Nonautologous Tissue Substitute, Open Approach

02UM37Z Supplement Ventricular Septum with Autologous Tissue Substitute, Percutaneous Approach

02UM38Z Supplement Ventricular Septum with Zooplastic Tissue, Percutaneous Approach

02UM3JZ Supplement Ventricular Septum with Synthetic Substitute, Percutaneous Approach

02UM3KZ Supplement Ventricular Septum with Nonautologous Tissue Substitute, Percutaneous Approach

02UM47Z Supplement Ventricular Septum with Autologous Tissue Substitute, Percutaneous Endoscopic Approach

02UM48Z Supplement Ventricular Septum with Zooplastic Tissue, Percutaneous Endoscopic Approach

02UM4JZ Supplement Ventricular Septum with Synthetic Substitute, Percutaneous Endoscopic Approach

02UM4KZ Supplement Ventricular Septum with Nonautologous Tissue Substitute, Percutaneous Endoscopic Approach

02UN07Z Supplement Pericardium with Autologous Tissue Substitute, Open Approach

02UN08Z Supplement Pericardium with Zooplastic Tissue, Open Approach

02UN0JZ Supplement Pericardium with Synthetic Substitute, Open Approach

02UN0KZ Supplement Pericardium with Nonautologous Tissue Substitute, Open Approach

02UN37Z Supplement Pericardium with Autologous Tissue Substitute, Percutaneous Approach

02UN38Z Supplement Pericardium with Zooplastic Tissue, Percutaneous Approach

02UN3JZ Supplement Pericardium with Synthetic Substitute, Percutaneous Approach

02UN3KZ Supplement Pericardium with Nonautologous Tissue Substitute, Percutaneous Approach

02UN47Z Supplement Pericardium with Autologous Tissue Substitute, Percutaneous Endoscopic Approach

02UN48Z Supplement Pericardium with Zooplastic Tissue, Percutaneous Endoscopic Approach

02UN4JZ Supplement Pericardium with Synthetic Substitute, Percutaneous Endoscopic Approach

02UN4KZ Supplement Pericardium with Nonautologous Tissue Substitute, Percutaneous Endoscopic Approach

02UP07Z Supplement Pulmonary Trunk with Autologous Tissue Substitute, Open Approach

02UP08Z Supplement Pulmonary Trunk with Zooplastic Tissue, Open Approach

02UP0JZ Supplement Pulmonary Trunk with Synthetic Substitute, Open Approach

02UP0KZ Supplement Pulmonary Trunk with Nonautologous Tissue Substitute, Open Approach

02UP37Z Supplement Pulmonary Trunk with Autologous Tissue Substitute, Percutaneous Approach

02UP38Z Supplement Pulmonary Trunk with Zooplastic Tissue, Percutaneous Approach

02UP3JZ Supplement Pulmonary Trunk with Synthetic Substitute, Percutaneous Approach

02UP3KZ Supplement Pulmonary Trunk with Nonautologous Tissue Substitute, Percutaneous Approach

02UP47Z Supplement Pulmonary Trunk with Autologous Tissue Substitute, Percutaneous Endoscopic Approach

02UP48Z Supplement Pulmonary Trunk with Zooplastic Tissue, Percutaneous Endoscopic Approach

02UP4JZ Supplement Pulmonary Trunk with Synthetic Substitute, Percutaneous Endoscopic Approach

02UP4KZ Supplement Pulmonary Trunk with Nonautologous Tissue Substitute, Percutaneous Endoscopic Approach

02UQ07Z Supplement Right Pulmonary Artery with Autologous Tissue Substitute, Open Approach

02UQ08Z Supplement Right Pulmonary Artery with Zooplastic Tissue, Open Approach

02UQ0JZ Supplement Right Pulmonary Artery with Synthetic Substitute, Open Approach

02UQ0KZ Supplement Right Pulmonary Artery with Nonautologous Tissue Substitute, Open Approach

02UQ37Z Supplement Right Pulmonary Artery with Autologous Tissue Substitute, Percutaneous Approach

02UQ38Z Supplement Right Pulmonary Artery with Zooplastic Tissue, Percutaneous Approach

02UQ3JZ Supplement Right Pulmonary Artery with Synthetic Substitute, Percutaneous Approach

02UQ3KZ Supplement Right Pulmonary Artery with Nonautologous Tissue Substitute, Percutaneous Approach

02UQ47Z Supplement Right Pulmonary Artery with Autologous Tissue Substitute, Percutaneous Endoscopic Approach

02UQ48Z Supplement Right Pulmonary Artery with Zooplastic Tissue, Percutaneous Endoscopic Approach

02UQ4JZ Supplement Right Pulmonary Artery with Synthetic Substitute, Percutaneous Endoscopic Approach

02UQ4KZ Supplement Right Pulmonary Artery with Nonautologous Tissue Substitute, Percutaneous Endoscopic Approach

02UR07Z Supplement Left Pulmonary Artery with Autologous Tissue Substitute, Open Approach

02UR08Z Supplement Left Pulmonary Artery with Zooplastic Tissue, Open Approach

02UR0JZ Supplement Left Pulmonary Artery with Synthetic Substitute, Open Approach

02UR0KZ Supplement Left Pulmonary Artery with Nonautologous Tissue Substitute, Open Approach

02UR37Z Supplement Left Pulmonary Artery with Autologous Tissue Substitute, Percutaneous Approach

02UR38Z Supplement Left Pulmonary Artery with Zooplastic Tissue, Percutaneous Approach

02UR3JZ Supplement Left Pulmonary Artery with Synthetic Substitute, Percutaneous Approach

02UR3KZ Supplement Left Pulmonary Artery with Nonautologous Tissue Substitute, Percutaneous Approach

02UR47Z Supplement Left Pulmonary Artery with Autologous Tissue Substitute, Percutaneous Endoscopic Approach

02UR48Z Supplement Left Pulmonary Artery with Zooplastic Tissue, Percutaneous Endoscopic Approach

02UR4JZ Supplement Left Pulmonary Artery with Synthetic Substitute, Percutaneous Endoscopic Approach

02UR4KZ Supplement Left Pulmonary Artery with Nonautologous Tissue Substitute, Percutaneous Endoscopic Approach

02US07Z Supplement Right Pulmonary Vein with Autologous Tissue Substitute, Open Approach

02US08Z Supplement Right Pulmonary Vein with Zooplastic Tissue, Open Approach

02US0JZ Supplement Right Pulmonary Vein with Synthetic Substitute, Open Approach

02US0KZ Supplement Right Pulmonary Vein with Nonautologous Tissue Substitute, Open Approach

02US37Z Supplement Right Pulmonary Vein with Autologous Tissue Substitute, Percutaneous Approach

02US38Z Supplement Right Pulmonary Vein with Zooplastic Tissue, Percutaneous Approach

02US3JZ Supplement Right Pulmonary Vein with Synthetic Substitute, Percutaneous Approach

02US3KZ Supplement Right Pulmonary Vein with Nonautologous Tissue Substitute, Percutaneous Approach

02US47Z Supplement Right Pulmonary Vein with Autologous Tissue Substitute, Percutaneous Endoscopic Approach

02US48Z Supplement Right Pulmonary Vein with Zooplastic Tissue, Percutaneous Endoscopic Approach

02US4JZ Supplement Right Pulmonary Vein with Synthetic Substitute, Percutaneous Endoscopic Approach

02US4KZ Supplement Right Pulmonary Vein with Nonautologous Tissue Substitute, Percutaneous Endoscopic Approach

02UT07Z Supplement Left Pulmonary Vein with Autologous Tissue Substitute, Open Approach

02UT08Z Supplement Left Pulmonary Vein with Zooplastic Tissue, Open Approach

02UT0JZ Supplement Left Pulmonary Vein with Synthetic Substitute, Open Approach

02UT0KZ Supplement Left Pulmonary Vein with Nonautologous Tissue Substitute, Open Approach

02UT37Z Supplement Left Pulmonary Vein with Autologous Tissue Substitute, Percutaneous Approach

02UT38Z Supplement Left Pulmonary Vein with Zooplastic Tissue, Percutaneous Approach

02UT3JZ Supplement Left Pulmonary Vein with Synthetic Substitute, Percutaneous Approach

02UT3KZ Supplement Left Pulmonary Vein with Nonautologous Tissue Substitute, Percutaneous Approach

02UT47Z Supplement Left Pulmonary Vein with Autologous Tissue Substitute, Percutaneous Endoscopic Approach

02UT48Z Supplement Left Pulmonary Vein with Zooplastic Tissue, Percutaneous Endoscopic Approach

02UT4JZ Supplement Left Pulmonary Vein with Synthetic Substitute, Percutaneous Endoscopic Approach

02UT4KZ Supplement Left Pulmonary Vein with Nonautologous Tissue Substitute, Percutaneous Endoscopic Approach

02UV07Z Supplement Superior Vena Cava with Autologous Tissue Substitute, Open Approach

02UV08Z Supplement Superior Vena Cava with Zooplastic Tissue, Open Approach

02UV0JZ Supplement Superior Vena Cava with Synthetic Substitute, Open Approach

02UV0KZ Supplement Superior Vena Cava with Nonautologous Tissue Substitute, Open Approach

02UV37Z Supplement Superior Vena Cava with Autologous Tissue Substitute, Percutaneous Approach

02UV38Z Supplement Superior Vena Cava with Zooplastic Tissue, Percutaneous Approach

02UV3JZ Supplement Superior Vena Cava with Synthetic Substitute, Percutaneous Approach

02UV3KZ Supplement Superior Vena Cava with Nonautologous Tissue Substitute, Percutaneous Approach

02UV47Z Supplement Superior Vena Cava with Autologous Tissue Substitute, Percutaneous Endoscopic Approach

02UV48Z Supplement Superior Vena Cava with Zooplastic Tissue, Percutaneous Endoscopic Approach

02UV4JZ Supplement Superior Vena Cava with Synthetic Substitute, Percutaneous Endoscopic Approach

02UV4KZ Supplement Superior Vena Cava with Nonautologous Tissue Substitute, Percutaneous Endoscopic Approach

02UW07Z Supplement Thoracic Aorta with Autologous Tissue Substitute, Open Approach

02UW08Z Supplement Thoracic Aorta with Zooplastic Tissue, Open Approach

02UW0JZ Supplement Thoracic Aorta with Synthetic Substitute, Open Approach

02UW0KZ Supplement Thoracic Aorta with Nonautologous Tissue Substitute, Open Approach

02UW37Z Supplement Thoracic Aorta with Autologous Tissue Substitute, Percutaneous Approach

02UW38Z Supplement Thoracic Aorta with Zooplastic Tissue, Percutaneous Approach

02UW3JZ Supplement Thoracic Aorta with Synthetic Substitute, Percutaneous Approach

02UW3KZ Supplement Thoracic Aorta with Nonautologous Tissue Substitute, Percutaneous Approach

02UW47Z Supplement Thoracic Aorta with Autologous Tissue Substitute, Percutaneous Endoscopic Approach

02UW48Z Supplement Thoracic Aorta with Zooplastic Tissue, Percutaneous Endoscopic Approach

02UW4JZ Supplement Thoracic Aorta with Synthetic Substitute, Percutaneous Endoscopic Approach

02UW4KZ Supplement Thoracic Aorta with Nonautologous Tissue Substitute, Percutaneous Endoscopic Approach

02V – Heart and Great Vessels, Restriction

02VA0CZ Restriction of Heart with Extraluminal Device, Open Approach

02VA0ZZ Restriction of Heart, Open Approach

02VA3CZ Restriction of Heart with Extraluminal Device, Percutaneous Approach

02VA3ZZ Restriction of Heart, Percutaneous Approach

02VA4CZ Restriction of Heart with Extraluminal Device, Percutaneous Endoscopic Approach

02VA4ZZ Restriction of Heart, Percutaneous Endoscopic Approach

02VP0CZ Restriction of Pulmonary Trunk with Extraluminal Device, Open Approach

02VP0DZ Restriction of Pulmonary Trunk with Intraluminal Device, Open Approach

02VP0ZZ Restriction of Pulmonary Trunk, Open Approach

02VP3CZ Restriction of Pulmonary Trunk with Extraluminal Device, Percutaneous Approach

02VP3DZ Restriction of Pulmonary Trunk with Intraluminal Device, Percutaneous Approach

02VP3ZZ Restriction of Pulmonary Trunk, Percutaneous Approach

02VP4CZ Restriction of Pulmonary Trunk with Extraluminal Device, Percutaneous Endoscopic Approach

02VP4DZ Restriction of Pulmonary Trunk with Intraluminal Device, Percutaneous Endoscopic Approach

02VP4ZZ Restriction of Pulmonary Trunk, Percutaneous Endoscopic Approach

02VQ0CZ Restriction of Right Pulmonary Artery with Extraluminal Device, Open Approach

02VQ0DZ Restriction of Right Pulmonary Artery with Intraluminal Device, Open Approach

02VQ0ZZ Restriction of Right Pulmonary Artery, Open Approach

02VQ3CZ Restriction of Right Pulmonary Artery with Extraluminal Device, Percutaneous Approach

02VQ3DZ Restriction of Right Pulmonary Artery with Intraluminal Device, Percutaneous Approach

02VQ3ZZ Restriction of Right Pulmonary Artery, Percutaneous Approach

02VQ4CZ Restriction of Right Pulmonary Artery with Extraluminal Device, Percutaneous Endoscopic Approach

02VQ4DZ Restriction of Right Pulmonary Artery with Intraluminal Device, Percutaneous Endoscopic Approach

02VQ4ZZ Restriction of Right Pulmonary Artery, Percutaneous Endoscopic Approach

02VR0CT Restriction of Ductus Arteriosus with Extraluminal Device, Open Approach

02VR0CZ Restriction of Left Pulmonary Artery with Extraluminal Device, Open Approach

02VR0DT Restriction of Ductus Arteriosus with Intraluminal Device, Open Approach

02VR0DZ Restriction of Left Pulmonary Artery with Intraluminal Device, Open Approach

02VR0ZT Restriction of Ductus Arteriosus, Open Approach

02VR0ZZ Restriction of Left Pulmonary Artery, Open Approach

02VR3CT Restriction of Ductus Arteriosus with Extraluminal Device, Percutaneous Approach

02VR3CZ Restriction of Left Pulmonary Artery with Extraluminal Device, Percutaneous Approach

02VR3DT Restriction of Ductus Arteriosus with Intraluminal Device, Percutaneous Approach

02VR3DZ Restriction of Left Pulmonary Artery with Intraluminal Device, Percutaneous Approach

02VR3ZT Restriction of Ductus Arteriosus, Percutaneous Approach

02VR3ZZ Restriction of Left Pulmonary Artery, Percutaneous Approach

02VR4CT Restriction of Ductus Arteriosus with Extraluminal Device, Percutaneous Endoscopic Approach

02VR4CZ Restriction of Left Pulmonary Artery with Extraluminal Device, Percutaneous Endoscopic Approach

02VR4DT Restriction of Ductus Arteriosus with Intraluminal Device, Percutaneous Endoscopic Approach

02VR4DZ Restriction of Left Pulmonary Artery with Intraluminal Device, Percutaneous Endoscopic Approach

02VR4ZT Restriction of Ductus Arteriosus, Percutaneous Endoscopic Approach

02VR4ZZ Restriction of Left Pulmonary Artery, Percutaneous Endoscopic Approach

02VS0CZ Restriction of Right Pulmonary Vein with Extraluminal Device, Open Approach

02VS0DZ Restriction of Right Pulmonary Vein with Intraluminal Device, Open Approach

02VS0ZZ Restriction of Right Pulmonary Vein, Open Approach

02VS3CZ Restriction of Right Pulmonary Vein with Extraluminal Device, Percutaneous Approach

02VS3DZ Restriction of Right Pulmonary Vein with Intraluminal Device, Percutaneous Approach

02VS3ZZ Restriction of Right Pulmonary Vein, Percutaneous Approach

02VS4CZ Restriction of Right Pulmonary Vein with Extraluminal Device, Percutaneous Endoscopic Approach

02VS4DZ Restriction of Right Pulmonary Vein with Intraluminal Device, Percutaneous Endoscopic Approach

02VS4ZZ Restriction of Right Pulmonary Vein, Percutaneous Endoscopic Approach

02VT0CZ Restriction of Left Pulmonary Vein with Extraluminal Device, Open Approach

02VT0DZ Restriction of Left Pulmonary Vein with Intraluminal Device, Open Approach

02VT0ZZ Restriction of Left Pulmonary Vein, Open Approach

02VT3CZ Restriction of Left Pulmonary Vein with Extraluminal Device, Percutaneous Approach

02VT3DZ Restriction of Left Pulmonary Vein with Intraluminal Device, Percutaneous Approach

02VT3ZZ Restriction of Left Pulmonary Vein, Percutaneous Approach

02VT4CZ Restriction of Left Pulmonary Vein with Extraluminal Device, Percutaneous Endoscopic Approach

02VT4DZ Restriction of Left Pulmonary Vein with Intraluminal Device, Percutaneous Endoscopic Approach

02VT4ZZ Restriction of Left Pulmonary Vein, Percutaneous Endoscopic Approach

02VV0CZ Restriction of Superior Vena Cava with Extraluminal Device, Open Approach

02VV0DZ Restriction of Superior Vena Cava with Intraluminal Device, Open Approach

02VV0ZZ Restriction of Superior Vena Cava, Open Approach

02VV3CZ Restriction of Superior Vena Cava with Extraluminal Device, Percutaneous Approach

02VV3DZ Restriction of Superior Vena Cava with Intraluminal Device, Percutaneous Approach

02VV3ZZ Restriction of Superior Vena Cava, Percutaneous Approach

02VV4CZ Restriction of Superior Vena Cava with Extraluminal Device, Percutaneous Endoscopic Approach

02VV4DZ Restriction of Superior Vena Cava with Intraluminal Device, Percutaneous Endoscopic Approach

02VV4ZZ Restriction of Superior Vena Cava, Percutaneous Endoscopic Approach

02VW0CZ Restriction of Thoracic Aorta with Extraluminal Device, Open Approach

02VW0DZ Restriction of Thoracic Aorta with Intraluminal Device, Open Approach

02VW0ZZ Restriction of Thoracic Aorta, Open Approach

02VW3CZ Restriction of Thoracic Aorta with Extraluminal Device, Percutaneous Approach

02VW3DZ Restriction of Thoracic Aorta with Intraluminal Device, Percutaneous Approach

02VW3ZZ Restriction of Thoracic Aorta, Percutaneous Approach

02VW4CZ Restriction of Thoracic Aorta with Extraluminal Device, Percutaneous Endoscopic Approach

02VW4DZ Restriction of Thoracic Aorta with Intraluminal Device, Percutaneous Endoscopic Approach

02VW4ZZ Restriction of Thoracic Aorta, Percutaneous Endoscopic Approach

02W – Heart and Great Vessels, Revision

Review Coding Guideline B6.1c

02W50JZ Revision of Synthetic Substitute in Atrial Septum, Open Approach

02W54JZ Revision of Synthetic Substitute in Atrial Septum, Percutaneous Endoscopic Approach

02WA02Z Revision of Monitoring Device in Heart, Open Approach

02WA03Z Revision of Infusion Device in Heart, Open Approach

02WA07Z Revision of Autologous Tissue Substitute in Heart, Open Approach

02WA08Z Revision of Zooplastic Tissue in Heart, Open Approach

02WA0CZ Revision of Extraluminal Device in Heart, Open Approach

02WA0DZ Revision of Intraluminal Device in Heart, Open Approach

⬢ **02WA0JZ** Revision of Synthetic Substitute in Heart, Open Approach

02WA0KZ Revision of Nonautologous Tissue Substitute in Heart, Open Approach

02WA0MZ Revision of Cardiac Lead in Heart, Open Approach
  HAC With a secondary diagnosis code of K68.11, T81.4XXA, T82.6XXA, T82.7XXA

⬢ **02WA0QZ** Revision of Implantable Heart Assist System in Heart, Open Approach
  ➕ Heart assist system replacement when reported with a removal of an external heart assist system (6th character R) from the heart. *See table 02P to construct the Removal code.*

02WA0RZ Revision of External Heart Assist System in Heart, Open Approach
  ➕ Heart assist system replacement when reported with a removal of an external heart assist system (6th character R) from the heart. *See table 02P to construct the Removal code.*

02WA32Z Revision of Monitoring Device in Heart, Percutaneous Approach

02WA33Z Revision of Infusion Device in Heart, Percutaneous Approach

02WA37Z Revision of Autologous Tissue Substitute in Heart, Percutaneous Approach

02WA38Z Revision of Zooplastic Tissue in Heart, Percutaneous Approach

02WA3CZ Revision of Extraluminal Device in Heart, Percutaneous Approach

02WA3DZ Revision of Intraluminal Device in Heart, Percutaneous Approach

02WA3JZ Revision of Synthetic Substitute in Heart, Percutaneous Approach

02WA3KZ Revision of Nonautologous Tissue Substitute in Heart, Percutaneous Approach

02WA3MZ Revision of Cardiac Lead in Heart, Percutaneous Approach
  HAC With a secondary diagnosis code of K68.11, T81.4XXA, T82.6XXA, T82.7XXA

⬢ **02WA3QZ** Revision of Implantable Heart Assist System in Heart, Percutaneous Approach
  ➕ Heart assist system replacement when reported with a removal of an external heart assist system (6th character R) from the heart. *See table 02P to construct the Removal code.*

02WA3RZ Revision of External Heart Assist System in Heart, Percutaneous Approach
  ➕ Heart assist system replacement when reported with a removal of an external heart assist system (6th character R) from the heart. *See table 02P to construct the Removal code.*

02WA42Z Revision of Monitoring Device in Heart, Percutaneous Endoscopic Approach

02WA43Z Revision of Infusion Device in Heart, Percutaneous Endoscopic Approach

02WA47Z Revision of Autologous Tissue Substitute in Heart, Percutaneous Endoscopic Approach

02WA48Z Revision of Zooplastic Tissue in Heart, Percutaneous Endoscopic Approach

02WA4CZ Revision of Extraluminal Device in Heart, Percutaneous Endoscopic Approach

02WA4DZ Revision of Intraluminal Device in Heart, Percutaneous Endoscopic Approach

02WA4JZ Revision of Synthetic Substitute in Heart, Percutaneous Endoscopic Approach

02WA4KZ Revision of Nonautologous Tissue Substitute in Heart, Percutaneous Endoscopic Approach

02WA4MZ Revision of Cardiac Lead in Heart, Percutaneous Endoscopic Approach

  ᴴᴬᶜ With a secondary diagnosis code of K68.11, T81.4XXA, T82.6XXA, T82.7XXA

⬤ **02WA4QZ** Revision of Implantable Heart Assist System in Heart, Percutaneous Endoscopic Approach

  ➕ Heart assist system replacement when reported with a removal of an external heart assist system (6th character R) from the heart. *See table 02P to construct the Removal code.*

02WA4RZ Revision of External Heart Assist System in Heart, Percutaneous Endoscopic Approach

  ➕ Heart assist system replacement when reported with a removal of an external heart assist system (6th character R) from the heart. *See table 02P to construct the Removal code.*

02WAX2Z Revision of Monitoring Device in Heart, External Approach

02WAX3Z Revision of Infusion Device in Heart, External Approach

02WAX7Z Revision of Autologous Tissue Substitute in Heart, External Approach

02WAX8Z Revision of Zooplastic Tissue in Heart, External Approach

02WAXCZ Revision of Extraluminal Device in Heart, External Approach

02WAXDZ Revision of Intraluminal Device in Heart, External Approach

02WAXJZ Revision of Synthetic Substitute in Heart, External Approach

02WAXKZ Revision of Nonautologous Tissue Substitute in Heart, External Approach

02WAXMZ Revision of Cardiac Lead in Heart, External Approach

02WAXQZ Revision of Implantable Heart Assist System in Heart, External Approach

02WAXRZ Revision of External Heart Assist System in Heart, External Approach

02WF07Z Revision of Autologous Tissue Substitute in Aortic Valve, Open Approach

02WF08Z Revision of Zooplastic Tissue in Aortic Valve, Open Approach

02WF0JZ Revision of Synthetic Substitute in Aortic Valve, Open Approach

02WF0KZ Revision of Nonautologous Tissue Substitute in Aortic Valve, Open Approach

02WF47Z Revision of Autologous Tissue Substitute in Aortic Valve, Percutaneous Endoscopic Approach

02WF48Z Revision of Zooplastic Tissue in Aortic Valve, Percutaneous Endoscopic Approach

02WF4JZ Revision of Synthetic Substitute in Aortic Valve, Percutaneous Endoscopic Approach

02WF4KZ Revision of Nonautologous Tissue Substitute in Aortic Valve, Percutaneous Endoscopic Approach

02WG07Z Revision of Autologous Tissue Substitute in Mitral Valve, Open Approach

02WG08Z Revision of Zooplastic Tissue in Mitral Valve, Open Approach

02WG0JZ Revision of Synthetic Substitute in Mitral Valve, Open Approach

02WG0KZ Revision of Nonautologous Tissue Substitute in Mitral Valve, Open Approach

02WG47Z Revision of Autologous Tissue Substitute in Mitral Valve, Percutaneous Endoscopic Approach

02WG48Z Revision of Zooplastic Tissue in Mitral Valve, Percutaneous Endoscopic Approach

02WG4JZ Revision of Synthetic Substitute in Mitral Valve, Percutaneous Endoscopic Approach

02WG4KZ Revision of Nonautologous Tissue Substitute in Mitral Valve, Percutaneous Endoscopic Approach

02WH07Z Revision of Autologous Tissue Substitute in Pulmonary Valve, Open Approach

02WH08Z Revision of Zooplastic Tissue in Pulmonary Valve, Open Approach

02WH0JZ Revision of Synthetic Substitute in Pulmonary Valve, Open Approach

02WH0KZ Revision of Nonautologous Tissue Substitute in Pulmonary Valve, Open Approach

02WH47Z Revision of Autologous Tissue Substitute in Pulmonary Valve, Percutaneous Endoscopic Approach

02WH48Z Revision of Zooplastic Tissue in Pulmonary Valve, Percutaneous Endoscopic Approach

02WH4JZ Revision of Synthetic Substitute in Pulmonary Valve, Percutaneous Endoscopic Approach

02WH4KZ Revision of Nonautologous Tissue Substitute in Pulmonary Valve, Percutaneous Endoscopic Approach

02WJ07Z Revision of Autologous Tissue Substitute in Tricuspid Valve, Open Approach

02WJ08Z Revision of Zooplastic Tissue in Tricuspid Valve, Open Approach

02WJ0JZ Revision of Synthetic Substitute in Tricuspid Valve, Open Approach

02WJ0KZ Revision of Nonautologous Tissue Substitute in Tricuspid Valve, Open Approach

02WJ47Z Revision of Autologous Tissue Substitute in Tricuspid Valve, Percutaneous Endoscopic Approach

02WJ48Z Revision of Zooplastic Tissue in Tricuspid Valve, Percutaneous Endoscopic Approach

02WJ4JZ Revision of Synthetic Substitute in Tricuspid Valve, Percutaneous Endoscopic Approach

02WJ4KZ Revision of Nonautologous Tissue Substitute in Tricuspid Valve, Percutaneous Endoscopic Approach

02WM0JZ Revision of Synthetic Substitute in Ventricular Septum, Open Approach

02WM4JZ Revision of Synthetic Substitute in Ventricular Septum, Percutaneous Endoscopic Approach

02WY02Z Revision of Monitoring Device in Great Vessel, Open Approach

02WY03Z Revision of Infusion Device in Great Vessel, Open Approach

02WY07Z Revision of Autologous Tissue Substitute in Great Vessel, Open Approach

02WY08Z Revision of Zooplastic Tissue in Great Vessel, Open Approach

02WY0CZ Revision of Extraluminal Device in Great Vessel, Open Approach

02WY0DZ Revision of Intraluminal Device in Great Vessel, Open Approach

02WY0JZ Revision of Synthetic Substitute in Great Vessel, Open Approach

02WY0KZ Revision of Nonautologous Tissue Substitute in Great Vessel, Open Approach

02WY32Z Revision of Monitoring Device in Great Vessel, Percutaneous Approach

02WY33Z Revision of Infusion Device in Great Vessel, Percutaneous Approach

02WY37Z Revision of Autologous Tissue Substitute in Great Vessel, Percutaneous Approach

02WY38Z Revision of Zooplastic Tissue in Great Vessel, Percutaneous Approach

02WY3CZ Revision of Extraluminal Device in Great Vessel, Percutaneous Approach

02WY3DZ Revision of Intraluminal Device in Great Vessel, Percutaneous Approach

02WY3JZ Revision of Synthetic Substitute in Great Vessel, Percutaneous Approach

02WY3KZ Revision of Nonautologous Tissue Substitute in Great Vessel, Percutaneous Approach

02WY42Z Revision of Monitoring Device in Great Vessel, Percutaneous Endoscopic Approach

02WY43Z Revision of Infusion Device in Great Vessel, Percutaneous Endoscopic Approach

02WY47Z Revision of Autologous Tissue Substitute in Great Vessel, Percutaneous Endoscopic Approach

02WY48Z Revision of Zooplastic Tissue in Great Vessel, Percutaneous Endoscopic Approach

02WY4CZ Revision of Extraluminal Device in Great Vessel, Percutaneous Endoscopic Approach

02WY4DZ Revision of Intraluminal Device in Great Vessel, Percutaneous Endoscopic Approach

02WY4JZ Revision of Synthetic Substitute in Great Vessel, Percutaneous Endoscopic Approach

02WY4KZ Revision of Nonautologous Tissue Substitute in Great Vessel, Percutaneous Endoscopic Approach

02WYX2Z Revision of Monitoring Device in Great Vessel, External Approach

02WYX3Z Revision of Infusion Device in Great Vessel, External Approach

02WYX7Z Revision of Autologous Tissue Substitute in Great Vessel, External Approach

02WYX8Z Revision of Zooplastic Tissue in Great Vessel, External Approach

02WYXCZ Revision of Extraluminal Device in Great Vessel, External Approach

02WYXDZ Revision of Intraluminal Device in Great Vessel, External
Approach

02WYXJZ Revision of Synthetic Substitute in Great Vessel, External Approach

02WYXKZ Revision of Nonautologous Tissue Substitute in Great Vessel,
External Approach

02Y – Heart and Great Vessels, Transplantation

Review Coding Guideline B3.16

02YA0Z0 Transplantation of Heart, Allogeneic, Open Approach

02YA0Z1 Transplantation of Heart, Syngeneic, Open Approach

02YA0Z2 Transplantation of Heart, Zooplastic, Open Approach

Upper Arteries

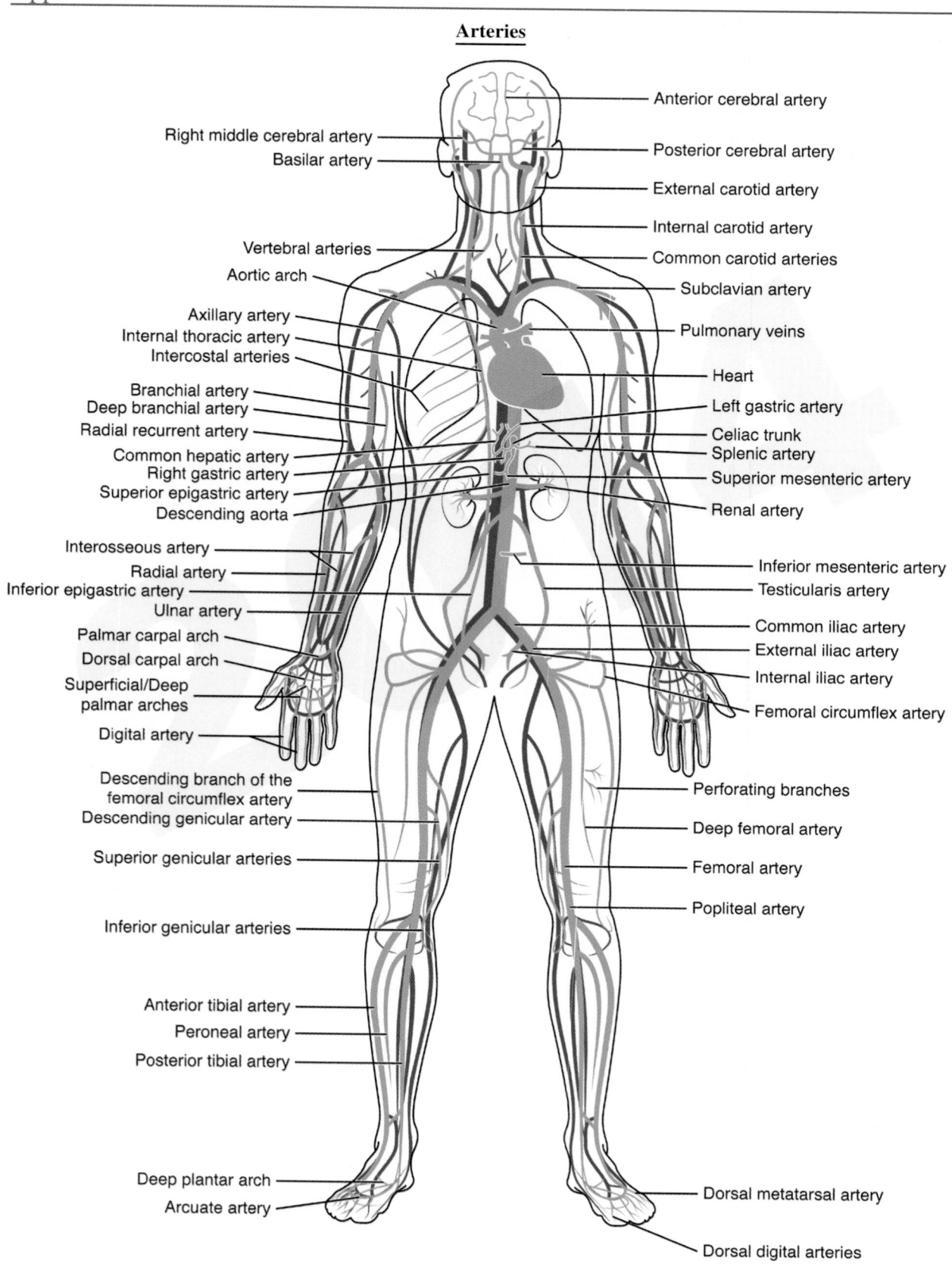

Arteries

Anterior cerebral artery

Right middle cerebral artery

Posterior cerebral artery

Basilar artery

External carotid artery

Internal carotid artery

Vertebral arteries

Common carotid arteries

Aortic arch

Subclavian artery

Axillary artery

Pulmonary veins

Internal thoracic artery

Intercostal arteries

Heart

Branchial artery

Left gastric artery

Deep branchial artery

Radial recurrent artery

Celiac trunk

Common hepatic artery

Splenic artery

Right gastric artery

Superior mesenteric artery

Superior epigastric artery

Renal artery

Descending aorta

Interosseous artery

Radial artery

Inferior mesenteric artery

Inferior epigastric artery

Testicularis artery

Ulnar artery

Palmar carpal arch

Common iliac artery

Dorsal carpal arch

External iliac artery

Superficial/Deep palmar arches

Internal iliac artery

Femoral circumflex artery

Digital artery

Descending branch of the femoral circumflex artery

Perforating branches

Descending genicular artery

Deep femoral artery

Superior genicular arteries

Femoral artery

Popliteal artery

Inferior genicular arteries

Anterior tibial artery

Peroneal artery

Posterior tibial artery

Deep plantar arch

Dorsal metatarsal artery

Arcuate artery

Dorsal digital arteries

Upper Arteries Tables 031–03W

Section	0	**Medical and Surgical**
Body System	3	**Upper Arteries**
Operation	1	**Bypass:** Altering the route of passage of the contents of a tubular body part

Body Part (4th)	Approach (5th)	Device (6th)	Qualifier (7th)
2 Innominate Artery 5 Axillary Artery, Right 6 Axillary Artery, Left	0 Open	9 Autologous Venous Tissue A Autologous Arterial Tissue J Synthetic Substitute K Nonautologous Tissue Substitute Z No Device	0 Upper Arm Artery, Right 1 Upper Arm Artery, Left 2 Upper Arm Artery, Bilateral 3 Lower Arm Artery, Right 4 Lower Arm Artery, Left 5 Lower Arm Artery, Bilateral 6 Upper Leg Artery, Right 7 Upper Leg Artery, Left 8 Upper Leg Artery, Bilateral 9 Lower Leg Artery, Right B Lower Leg Artery, Left C Lower Leg Artery, Bilateral D Upper Arm Vein F Lower Arm Vein J Extracranial Artery, Right K Extracranial Artery, Left
3 Subclavian Artery, Right 4 Subclavian Artery, Left	0 Open	9 Autologous Venous Tissue A Autologous Arterial Tissue J Synthetic Substitute K Nonautologous Tissue Substitute Z No Device	0 Upper Arm Artery, Right 1 Upper Arm Artery, Left 2 Upper Arm Artery, Bilateral 3 Lower Arm Artery, Right 4 Lower Arm Artery, Left 5 Lower Arm Artery, Bilateral 6 Upper Leg Artery, Right 7 Upper Leg Artery, Left 8 Upper Leg Artery, Bilateral 9 Lower Leg Artery, Right B Lower Leg Artery, Left C Lower Leg Artery, Bilateral D Upper Arm Vein F Lower Arm Vein J Extracranial Artery, Right K Extracranial Artery, Left M Pulmonary Artery, Right N Pulmonary Artery, Left
7 Brachial Artery, Right	0 Open	9 Autologous Venous Tissue A Autologous Arterial Tissue J Synthetic Substitute K Nonautologous Tissue Substitute Z No Device	0 Upper Arm Artery, Right 3 Lower Arm Artery, Right D Upper Arm Vein F Lower Arm Vein
8 Brachial Artery, Left	0 Open	9 Autologous Venous Tissue A Autologous Arterial Tissue J Synthetic Substitute K Nonautologous Tissue Substitute Z No Device	1 Upper Arm Artery, Left 4 Lower Arm Artery, Left D Upper Arm Vein F Lower Arm Vein

Continued

Medical and Surgical Section (0)

031

Section	0	Medical and Surgica
Body System	3	Upper Arteries
Operation	1	Bypass: Altering the route of passage of the contents of a tubular body part

Body Part (4th)	Approach (5th)	Device (6th)	Qualifier (7th)
9 Ulnar Artery, Right B Radial Artery, Right	0 Open	9 Autologous Venous Tissue A Autologous Arterial Tissue J Synthetic Substitute K Nonautologous Tissue Substitute Z No Device	3 Lower Arm Artery, Right F Lower Arm Vein
A Ulnar Artery, Left C Radial Artery, Left	0 Open	9 Autologous Venous Tissue A Autologous Arterial Tissue J Synthetic Substitute K Nonautologous Tissue Substitute Z No Device	4 Lower Arm Artery, Left F Lower Arm Vein
G Intracranial Artery S Temporal Artery, Right T Temporal Artery, Left	0 Open	9 Autologous Venous Tissue A Autologous Arterial Tissue J Synthetic Substitute K Nonautologous Tissue Substitute Z No Device	G Intracranial Artery
H Common Carotid Artery, Right	0 Open	9 Autologous Venous Tissue A Autologous Arterial Tissue J Synthetic Substitute K Nonautologous Tissue Substitute Z No Device	G Intracranial Artery J Extracranial Artery, Right
J Common Carotid Artery, Left	0 Open	9 Autologous Venous Tissue A Autologous Arterial Tissue J Synthetic Substitute K Nonautologous Tissue Substitute Z No Device	G Intracranial Artery K Extracranial Artery, Left
K Internal Carotid Artery, Right M External Carotid Artery, Right	0 Open	9 Autologous Venous Tissue A Autologous Arterial Tissue J Synthetic Substitute K Nonautologous Tissue Substitute Z No Device	J Extracranial Artery, Right
L Internal Carotid Artery, Left N External Carotid Artery, Left	0 Open	9 Autologous Venous Tissue A Autologous Arterial Tissue J Synthetic Substitute K Nonautologous Tissue Substitute Z No Device	K Extracranial Artery, Left

Section	0	**Medical and Surgical**
Body System	3	**Upper Arteries**
Operation	5	**Destruction:** Physical eradication of all or a portion of a body part by the direct use of energy, force, or a destructive agent

Body Part (4th)	Approach (5th)	Device (6th)	Qualifier (7th)
0 Internal Mammary Artery, Right	0 Open	Z No Device	Z No Qualifier
1 Internal Mammary Artery, Left	3 Percutaneous		
2 Innominate Artery	4 Percutaneous Endoscopic		
3 Subclavian Artery, Right			
4 Subclavian Artery, Left			
5 Axillary Artery, Right			
6 Axillary Artery, Left			
7 Brachial Artery, Right			
8 Brachial Artery, Left			
9 Ulnar Artery, Right			
A Ulnar Artery, Left			
B Radial Artery, Right			
C Radial Artery, Left			
D Hand Artery, Right			
F Hand Artery, Left			
G Intracranial Artery			
H Common Carotid Artery, Right			
J Common Carotid Artery, Left			
K Internal Carotid Artery, Right			
L Internal Carotid Artery, Left			
M External Carotid Artery, Right			
N External Carotid Artery, Left			
P Vertebral Artery, Right			
Q Vertebral Artery, Left			
R Face Artery			
S Temporal Artery, Right			
T Temporal Artery, Left			
U Thyroid Artery, Right			
V Thyroid Artery, Left			
Y Upper Artery			

Section	0	Medical and Surgical
Body System	3	Upper Arteries
Operation	7	**Dilation:** Expanding an orifice or the lumen of a tubular body part

Body Part (4th)	Approach (5th)	Device (6th)	Qualifier (7th)
0 Internal Mammary Artery, Right **1** Internal Mammary Artery, Left **2** Innominate Artery **3** Subclavian Artery, Right **4** Subclavian Artery, Left **5** Axillary Artery, Right **6** Axillary Artery, Left **7** Brachial Artery, Right **8** Brachial Artery, Left **9** Ulnar Artery, Right **A** Ulnar Artery, Left **B** Radial Artery, Right **C** Radial Artery, Left **D** Hand Artery, Right **F** Hand Artery, Left **G** Intracranial Artery **H** Common Carotid Artery, Right **J** Common Carotid Artery, Left **K** Internal Carotid Artery, Right **L** Internal Carotid Artery, Left **M** External Carotid Artery, Right **N** External Carotid Artery, Left **P** Vertebral Artery, Right **Q** Vertebral Artery, Left **R** Face Artery **S** Temporal Artery, Right **T** Temporal Artery, Left **U** Thyroid Artery, Right **V** Thyroid Artery, Left **Y** Upper Artery	**0** Open **3** Percutaneous **4** Percutaneous Endoscopic	**4** Intraluminal Device, Drug-eluting **D** Intraluminal Device **Z** No Device	**Z** No Qualifier

Section	0	**Medical and Surgical**
Body System	3	**Upper Arteries**
Operation	9	**Drainage:** Taking or letting out fluids and/or gases from a body part

Body Part (4th)	Approach (5th)	Device (6th)	Qualifier (7th)
0 Internal Mammary Artery, Right 1 Internal Mammary Artery, Left 2 Innominate Artery 3 Subclavian Artery, Right 4 Subclavian Artery, Left 5 Axillary Artery, Right 6 Axillary Artery, Left 7 Brachial Artery, Right 8 Brachial Artery, Left 9 Ulnar Artery, Right A Ulnar Artery, Left B Radial Artery, Right C Radial Artery, Left D Hand Artery, Right F Hand Artery, Left G Intracranial Artery H Common Carotid Artery, Right J Common Carotid Artery, Left K Internal Carotid Artery, Right L Internal Carotid Artery, Left M External Carotid Artery, Right N External Carotid Artery, Left P Vertebral Artery, Right Q Vertebral Artery, Left R Face Artery S Temporal Artery, Right T Temporal Artery, Left U Thyroid Artery, Right V Thyroid Artery, Left Y Upper Artery	0 Open 3 Percutaneous 4 Percutaneous Endoscopic	0 Drainage Device	Z No Qualifier
0 Internal Mammary Artery, Right 1 Internal Mammary Artery, Left 2 Innominate Artery 3 Subclavian Artery, Right 4 Subclavian Artery, Left 5 Axillary Artery, Right 6 Axillary Artery, Left 7 Brachial Artery, Right 8 Brachial Artery, Left 9 Ulnar Artery, Right A Ulnar Artery, Left B Radial Artery, Right C Radial Artery, Left D Hand Artery, Right F Hand Artery, Left G Intracranial Artery H Common Carotid Artery, Right J Common Carotid Artery, Left K Internal Carotid Artery, Right L Internal Carotid Artery, Left M External Carotid Artery, Right N External Carotid Artery, Left P Vertebral Artery, Right Q Vertebral Artery, Left R Face Artery S Temporal Artery, Right T Temporal Artery, Left U Thyroid Artery, Right V Thyroid Artery, Left Y Upper Artery	0 Open 3 Percutaneous 4 Percutaneous Endoscopic	Z No Device	X Diagnostic Z No Qualifier

Section	0	Medical and Surgical
Body System	3	Upper Arteries
Operation	B	Excision: Cutting out or off, without replacement, a portion of a body part

Body Part (4th)	Approach (5th)	Device (6th)	Qualifier (7th)
0 Internal Mammary Artery, Right	0 Open	Z No Device	X Diagnostic
1 Internal Mammary Artery, Left	3 Percutaneous		Z No Qualifier
2 Innominate Artery	4 Percutaneous Endoscopic		
3 Subclavian Artery, Right			
4 Subclavian Artery, Left			
5 Axillary Artery, Right			
6 Axillary Artery, Left			
7 Brachial Artery, Right			
8 Brachial Artery, Left			
9 Ulnar Artery, Right			
A Ulnar Artery, Left			
B Radial Artery, Right			
C Radial Artery, Left			
D Hand Artery, Right			
F Hand Artery, Left			
G Intracranial Artery			
H Common Carotid Artery, Right			
J Common Carotid Artery, Left			
K Internal Carotid Artery, Right			
L Internal Carotid Artery, Left			
M External Carotid Artery, Right			
N External Carotid Artery, Left			
P Vertebral Artery, Right			
Q Vertebral Artery, Left			
R Face Artery			
S Temporal Artery, Right			
T Temporal Artery, Left			
U Thyroid Artery, Right			
V Thyroid Artery, Left			
Y Upper Artery			

Section	0	Medical and Surgical
Body System	3	Upper Arteries
Operation	C	**Extirpation:** Taking or cutting out solid matter from a body part

Body Part (4th)	Approach (5th)	Device (6th)	Qualifier (7th)
0 Internal Mammary Artery, Right	0 Open	Z No Device	Z No Qualifier
1 Internal Mammary Artery, Left	3 Percutaneous		
2 Innominate Artery	4 Percutaneous Endoscopic		
3 Subclavian Artery, Right			
4 Subclavian Artery, Left			
5 Axillary Artery, Right			
6 Axillary Artery, Left			
7 Brachial Artery, Right			
8 Brachial Artery, Left			
9 Ulnar Artery, Right			
A Ulnar Artery, Left			
B Radial Artery, Right			
C Radial Artery, Left			
D Hand Artery, Right			
F Hand Artery, Left			
G Intracranial Artery			
H Common Carotid Artery, Right			
J Common Carotid Artery, Left			
K Internal Carotid Artery, Right			
L Internal Carotid Artery, Left			
M External Carotid Artery, Right			
N External Carotid Artery, Left			
P Vertebral Artery, Right			
Q Vertebral Artery, Left			
R Face Artery			
S Temporal Artery, Right			
T Temporal Artery, Left			
U Thyroid Artery, Right			
V Thyroid Artery, Left			
Y Upper Artery			

Section	0	Medical and Surgical
Body System	3	Upper Arteries
Operation	H	Insertion: Putting in a nonbiological appliance that monitors, assists, performs, or prevents a physiological function but does not physically take the place of a body part

Body Part (4th)	Approach (5th)	Device (6th)	Qualifier (7th)
0 Internal Mammary Artery, Right 1 Internal Mammary Artery, Left 2 Innominate Artery 3 Subclavian Artery, Right 4 Subclavian Artery, Left 5 Axillary Artery, Right 6 Axillary Artery, Left 7 Brachial Artery, Right 8 Brachial Artery, Left 9 Ulnar Artery, Right A Ulnar Artery, Left B Radial Artery, Right C Radial Artery, Left D Hand Artery, Right F Hand Artery, Left G Intracranial Artery H Common Carotid Artery, Right J Common Carotid Artery, Left M External Carotid Artery, Right N External Carotid Artery, Left P Vertebral Artery, Right Q Vertebral Artery, Left R Face Artery S Temporal Artery, Right T Temporal Artery, Left U Thyroid Artery, Right V Thyroid Artery, Left	0 Open 3 Percutaneous 4 Percutaneous Endoscopic	3 Infusion Device D Intraluminal Device	Z No Qualifier
K Internal Carotid Artery, Right L Internal Carotid Artery, Left	0 Open 3 Percutaneous 4 Percutaneous Endoscopic	3 Infusion Device D Intraluminal Device M Stimulator Lead	Z No Qualifier
Y Upper Artery	0 Open 3 Percutaneous 4 Percutaneous Endoscopic	2 Monitoring Device 3 Infusion Device D Intraluminal Device	Z No Qualifier

Section	0	Medical and Surgical
Body System	3	Upper Arteries
Operation	J	Inspection: Visually and/or manually exploring a body part

Body Part (4th)	Approach (5th)	Device (6th)	Qualifier (7th)
Y Upper Artery	0 Open 3 Percutaneous 4 Percutaneous Endoscopic X External	Z No Device	Z No Qualifier

Section	0	Medical and Surgical
Body System	3	Upper Arteries
Operation	L	Occlusion: Completely closing an orifice or the lumen of a tubular body part

Body Part (4th)	Approach (5th)	Device (6th)	Qualifier (7th)
0 Internal Mammary Artery, Right 1 Internal Mammary Artery, Left 2 Innominate Artery 3 Subclavian Artery, Right 4 Subclavian Artery, Left 5 Axillary Artery, Right 6 Axillary Artery, Left 7 Brachial Artery, Right 8 Brachial Artery, Left 9 Ulnar Artery, Right A Ulnar Artery, Left B Radial Artery, Right C Radial Artery, Left D Hand Artery, Right F Hand Artery, Left R Face Artery S Temporal Artery, Right T Temporal Artery, Left U Thyroid Artery, Right V Thyroid Artery, Left Y Upper Artery	0 Open 3 Percutaneous 4 Percutaneous Endoscopic	C Extraluminal Device D Intraluminal Device Z No Device	Z No Qualifier
G Intracranial Artery H Common Carotid Artery, Right J Common Carotid Artery, Left K Internal Carotid Artery, Right L Internal Carotid Artery, Left M External Carotid Artery, Right N External Carotid Artery, Left P Vertebral Artery, Right Q Vertebral Artery, Left	0 Open 3 Percutaneous 4 Percutaneous Endoscopic	B Intraluminal Device, Bioactive C Extraluminal Device D Intraluminal Device Z No Device	Z No Qualifier

Section	0	Medical and Surgical
Body System	3	Upper Arteries
Operation	N	**Release:** Freeing a body part from an abnormal physical constraint by cutting or by the use of force

Body Part (4th)	Approach (5th)	Device (6th)	Qualifier (7th)
0 Internal Mammary Artery, Right 1 Internal Mammary Artery, Left 2 Innominate Artery 3 Subclavian Artery, Right 4 Subclavian Artery, Left 5 Axillary Artery, Right 6 Axillary Artery, Left 7 Brachial Artery, Right 8 Brachial Artery, Left 9 Ulnar Artery, Right A Ulnar Artery, Left B Radial Artery, Right C Radial Artery, Left D Hand Artery, Right F Hand Artery, Left G Intracranial Artery H Common Carotid Artery, Right J Common Carotid Artery, Left K Internal Carotid Artery, Right L Internal Carotid Artery, Left M External Carotid Artery, Right N External Carotid Artery, Left P Vertebral Artery, Right Q Vertebral Artery, Left R Face Artery S Temporal Artery, Right T Temporal Artery, Left U Thyroid Artery, Right V Thyroid Artery, Left Y Upper Artery	0 Open 3 Percutaneous 4 Percutaneous Endoscopic	Z No Device	Z No Qualifier

Section	0	Medical and Surgical
Body System	3	Upper Arteries
Operation	P	**Removal:** Taking out or off a device from a body part

Body Part (4th)	Approach (5th)	Device (6th)	Qualifier (7th)
Y Upper Artery	0 Open 3 Percutaneous 4 Percutaneous Endoscopic	0 Drainage Device 2 Monitoring Device 3 Infusion Device 7 Autologous Tissue Substitute C Extraluminal Device D Intraluminal Device J Synthetic Substitute K Nonautologous Tissue Substitute M Stimulator Lead	Z No Qualifier
Y Upper Artery	X External	0 Drainage Device 2 Monitoring Device 3 Infusion Device D Intraluminal Device M Stimulator Lead	Z No Qualifier

Section	0	Medical and Surgical
Body System	3	Upper Arteries
Operation	Q	**Repair:** Restoring, to the extent possible, a body part to its normal anatomic structure and function

Body Part (4th)	Approach (5th)	Device (6th)	Qualifier (7th)
0 Internal Mammary Artery, Right	0 Open	Z No Device	Z No Qualifier
1 Internal Mammary Artery, Left	3 Percutaneous		
2 Innominate Artery	4 Percutaneous Endoscopic		
3 Subclavian Artery, Right			
4 Subclavian Artery, Left			
5 Axillary Artery, Right			
6 Axillary Artery, Left			
7 Brachial Artery, Right			
8 Brachial Artery, Left			
9 Ulnar Artery, Right			
A Ulnar Artery, Left			
B Radial Artery, Right			
C Radial Artery, Left			
D Hand Artery, Right			
F Hand Artery, Left			
G Intracranial Artery			
H Common Carotid Artery, Right			
J Common Carotid Artery, Left			
K Internal Carotid Artery, Right			
L Internal Carotid Artery, Left			
M External Carotid Artery, Right			
N External Carotid Artery, Left			
P Vertebral Artery, Right			
Q Vertebral Artery, Left			
R Face Artery			
S Temporal Artery, Right			
T Temporal Artery, Left			
U Thyroid Artery, Right			
V Thyroid Artery, Left			
Y Upper Artery			

Section	0	Medical and Surgical
Body System	3	Upper Arteries
Operation	R	**Replacement:** Putting in or on biological or synthetic material that physically takes the place and/or function of all or a portion of a body part

Body Part (4th)	Approach (5th)	Device (6th)	Qualifier (7th)
0 Internal Mammary Artery, Right 1 Internal Mammary Artery, Left 2 Innominate Artery 3 Subclavian Artery, Right 4 Subclavian Artery, Left 5 Axillary Artery, Right 6 Axillary Artery, Left 7 Brachial Artery, Right 8 Brachial Artery, Left 9 Ulnar Artery, Right A Ulnar Artery, Left B Radial Artery, Right C Radial Artery, Left D Hand Artery, Right F Hand Artery, Left G Intracranial Artery H Common Carotid Artery, Right J Common Carotid Artery, Left K Internal Carotid Artery, Right L Internal Carotid Artery, Left M External Carotid Artery, Right N External Carotid Artery, Left P Vertebral Artery, Right Q Vertebral Artery, Left R Face Artery S Temporal Artery, Right T Temporal Artery, Left U Thyroid Artery, Right V Thyroid Artery, Left Y Upper Artery	0 Open 4 Percutaneous Endoscopic	7 Autologous Tissue Substitute J Synthetic Substitute K Nonautologous Tissue Substitute	Z No Qualifier

Section	0	**Medical and Surgical**
Body System	3	**Upper Arteries**
Operation	S	**Reposition:** Moving to its normal location, or other suitable location, all or a portion of a body part

Body Part (4th)	Approach (5th)	Device (6th)	Qualifier (7th)
0 Internal Mammary Artery, Right **1** Internal Mammary Artery, Left **2** Innominate Artery **3** Subclavian Artery, Right **4** Subclavian Artery, Left **5** Axillary Artery, Right **6** Axillary Artery, Left **7** Brachial Artery, Right **8** Brachial Artery, Left **9** Ulnar Artery, Right **A** Ulnar Artery, Left **B** Radial Artery, Right **C** Radial Artery, Left **D** Hand Artery, Right **F** Hand Artery, Left **G** Intracranial Artery **H** Common Carotid Artery, Right **J** Common Carotid Artery, Left **K** Internal Carotid Artery, Right **L** Internal Carotid Artery, Left **M** External Carotid Artery, Right **N** External Carotid Artery, Left **P** Vertebral Artery, Right **Q** Vertebral Artery, Left **R** Face Artery **S** Temporal Artery, Right **T** Temporal Artery, Left **U** Thyroid Artery, Right **V** Thyroid Artery, Left **Y** Upper Artery	**0** Open **3** Percutaneous **4** Percutaneous Endoscopic	**Z** No Device	**Z** No Qualifier

Section	0	**Medical and Surgical**
Body System	3	**Upper Arteries**
Operation	U	**Supplement:** Putting in or on biological or synthetic material that physically reinforces and/or augments the function of a portion of a body part

Body Part (4th)	Approach (5th)	Device (6th)	Qualifier (7th)
0 Internal Mammary Artery, Right **1** Internal Mammary Artery, Left **2** Innominate Artery **3** Subclavian Artery, Right **4** Subclavian Artery, Left **5** Axillary Artery, Right **6** Axillary Artery, Left **7** Brachial Artery, Right **8** Brachial Artery, Left **9** Ulnar Artery, Right **A** Ulnar Artery, Left **B** Radial Artery, Right **C** Radial Artery, Left **D** Hand Artery, Right **F** Hand Artery, Left **G** Intracranial Artery **H** Common Carotid Artery, Right **J** Common Carotid Artery, Left **K** Internal Carotid Artery, Right **L** Internal Carotid Artery, Left **M** External Carotid Artery, Right	**0** Open **3** Percutaneous **4** Percutaneous Endoscopic	**7** Autologous Tissue Substitute **J** Synthetic Substitute **K** Nonautologous Tissue Substitute	**Z** No Qualifier

Continued

Section	0	Medical and Surgical
Body System	3	Upper Arteries
Operation	U	**Supplement:** Putting in or on biological or synthetic material that physically reinforces and/or augments the function of a portion of a body part

Body Part (4th)	Approach (5th)	Device (6th)	Qualifier (7th)
N External Carotid Artery, Left P Vertebral Artery, Right Q Vertebral Artery, Left R Face Artery S Temporal Artery, Right T Temporal Artery, Left U Thyroid Artery, Right V Thyroid Artery, Left Y Upper Artery			

Section	0	Medical and Surgical
Body System	3	Upper Arteries
Operation	V	**Restriction:** Partially closing an orifice or the lumen of a tubular body part

Body Part (4th)	Approach (5th)	Device (6th)	Qualifier (7th)
0 Internal Mammary Artery, Right 1 Internal Mammary Artery, Left 2 Innominate Artery 3 Subclavian Artery, Right 4 Subclavian Artery, Left 5 Axillary Artery, Right 6 Axillary Artery, Left 7 Brachial Artery, Right 8 Brachial Artery, Left 9 Ulnar Artery, Right A Ulnar Artery, Left B Radial Artery, Right C Radial Artery, Left D Hand Artery, Right F Hand Artery, Left R Face Artery S Temporal Artery, Right T Temporal Artery, Left U Thyroid Artery, Right V Thyroid Artery, Left Y Upper Artery	0 Open 3 Percutaneous 4 Percutaneous Endoscopic	C Extraluminal Device D Intraluminal Device Z No Device	Z No Qualifier
G Intracranial Artery H Common Carotid Artery, Right J Common Carotid Artery, Left K Internal Carotid Artery, Right L Internal Carotid Artery, Left M External Carotid Artery, Right N External Carotid Artery, Left P Vertebral Artery, Right Q Vertebral Artery, Left	0 Open 3 Percutaneous 4 Percutaneous Endoscopic	B Intraluminal Device, Bioactive C Extraluminal Device D Intraluminal Device Z No Device	Z No Qualifier

Section	0	Medical and Surgical
Body System	3	Upper Arteries
Operation	W	**Revision:** Correcting, to the extent possible, a portion of a malfunctioning device or the position of a displaced device

Body Part (4th)	Approach (5th)	Device (6th)	Qualifier (7th)
Y Upper Artery	0 Open 3 Percutaneous 4 Percutaneous Endoscopic X External	0 Drainage Device 2 Monitoring Device 3 Infusion Device 7 Autologous Tissue Substitute C Extraluminal Device D Intraluminal Device J Synthetic Substitute K Nonautologous Tissue Substitute M Stimulator Lead	Z No Qualifier

Upper Arteries Code Listing 031–03W

031 – Upper Arteries, Bypass

Review Coding Guideline B3.6a

0312090 Bypass Innominate Artery to Right Upper Arm Artery with Autologous Venous Tissue, Open Approach

0312091 Bypass Innominate Artery to Left Upper Arm Artery with Autologous Venous Tissue, Open Approach

0312092 Bypass Innominate Artery to Bilateral Upper Arm Artery with Autologous Venous Tissue, Open Approach

0312093 Bypass Innominate Artery to Right Lower Arm Artery with Autologous Venous Tissue, Open Approach

0312094 Bypass Innominate Artery to Left Lower Arm Artery with Autologous Venous Tissue, Open Approach

0312095 Bypass Innominate Artery to Bilateral Lower Arm Artery with Autologous Venous Tissue, Open Approach

0312096 Bypass Innominate Artery to Right Upper Leg Artery with Autologous Venous Tissue, Open Approach

0312097 Bypass Innominate Artery to Left Upper Leg Artery with Autologous Venous Tissue, Open Approach

0312098 Bypass Innominate Artery to Bilateral Upper Leg Artery with Autologous Venous Tissue, Open Approach

0312099 Bypass Innominate Artery to Right Lower Leg Artery with Autologous Venous Tissue, Open Approach

031209B Bypass Innominate Artery to Left Lower Leg Artery with Autologous Venous Tissue, Open Approach

031209C Bypass Innominate Artery to Bilateral Lower Leg Artery with Autologous Venous Tissue, Open Approach

031209D Bypass Innominate Artery to Upper Arm Vein with Autologous Venous Tissue, Open Approach

031209F Bypass Innominate Artery to Lower Arm Vein with Autologous Venous Tissue, Open Approach

031209J Bypass Innominate Artery to Right Extracranial Artery with Autologous Venous Tissue, Open Approach

031209K Bypass Innominate Artery to Left Extracranial Artery with Autologous Venous Tissue, Open Approach

03120A0 Bypass Innominate Artery to Right Upper Arm Artery with Autologous Arterial Tissue, Open Approach

03120A1 Bypass Innominate Artery to Left Upper Arm Artery with Autologous Arterial Tissue, Open Approach

03120A2 Bypass Innominate Artery to Bilateral Upper Arm Artery with Autologous Arterial Tissue, Open Approach

03120A3 Bypass Innominate Artery to Right Lower Arm Artery with Autologous Arterial Tissue, Open Approach

03120A4 Bypass Innominate Artery to Left Lower Arm Artery with Autologous Arterial Tissue, Open Approach

03120A5 Bypass Innominate Artery to Bilateral Lower Arm Artery with Autologous Arterial Tissue, Open Approach

03120A6 Bypass Innominate Artery to Right Upper Leg Artery with Autologous Arterial Tissue, Open Approach

03120A7 Bypass Innominate Artery to Left Upper Leg Artery with Autologous Arterial Tissue, Open Approach

03120A8 Bypass Innominate Artery to Bilateral Upper Leg Artery with Autologous Arterial Tissue, Open Approach

03120A9 Bypass Innominate Artery to Right Lower Leg Artery with Autologous Arterial Tissue, Open Approach

03120AB Bypass Innominate Artery to Left Lower Leg Artery with Autologous Arterial Tissue, Open Approach

03120AC Bypass Innominate Artery to Bilateral Lower Leg Artery with Autologous Arterial Tissue, Open Approach

03120AD Bypass Innominate Artery to Upper Arm Vein with Autologous Arterial Tissue, Open Approach

03120AF Bypass Innominate Artery to Lower Arm Vein with Autologous Arterial Tissue, Open Approach

03120AJ Bypass Innominate Artery to Right Extracranial Artery with Autologous Arterial Tissue, Open Approach

03120AK Bypass Innominate Artery to Left Extracranial Artery with Autologous Arterial Tissue, Open Approach

03120J0 Bypass Innominate Artery to Right Upper Arm Artery with Synthetic Substitute, Open Approach

03120J1 Bypass Innominate Artery to Left Upper Arm Artery with Synthetic Substitute, Open Approach

03120J2 Bypass Innominate Artery to Bilateral Upper Arm Artery with Synthetic Substitute, Open Approach

03120J3 Bypass Innominate Artery to Right Lower Arm Artery with Synthetic Substitute, Open Approach

03120J4 Bypass Innominate Artery to Left Lower Arm Artery with Synthetic Substitute, Open Approach

03120J5 Bypass Innominate Artery to Bilateral Lower Arm Artery with Synthetic Substitute, Open Approach

03120J6 Bypass Innominate Artery to Right Upper Leg Artery with Synthetic Substitute, Open Approach

03120J7 Bypass Innominate Artery to Left Upper Leg Artery with Synthetic Substitute, Open Approach

03120J8 Bypass Innominate Artery to Bilateral Upper Leg Artery with Synthetic Substitute, Open Approach

03120J9 Bypass Innominate Artery to Right Lower Leg Artery with Synthetic Substitute, Open Approach

03120JB Bypass Innominate Artery to Left Lower Leg Artery with Synthetic Substitute, Open Approach

03120JC Bypass Innominate Artery to Bilateral Lower Leg Artery with Synthetic Substitute, Open Approach

03120JD Bypass Innominate Artery to Upper Arm Vein with Synthetic Substitute, Open Approach

03120JF Bypass Innominate Artery to Lower Arm Vein with Synthetic Substitute, Open Approach

03120JJ Bypass Innominate Artery to Right Extracranial Artery with Synthetic Substitute, Open Approach

03120JK Bypass Innominate Artery to Left Extracranial Artery with Synthetic Substitute, Open Approach

03120K0 Bypass Innominate Artery to Right Upper Arm Artery with Nonautologous Tissue Substitute, Open Approach

03120K1 Bypass Innominate Artery to Left Upper Arm Artery with Nonautologous Tissue Substitute, Open Approach

03120K2 Bypass Innominate Artery to Bilateral Upper Arm Artery with Nonautologous Tissue Substitute, Open Approach

03120K3 Bypass Innominate Artery to Right Lower Arm Artery with Nonautologous Tissue Substitute, Open Approach

03120K4 Bypass Innominate Artery to Left Lower Arm Artery with Nonautologous Tissue Substitute, Open Approach

03120K5 Bypass Innominate Artery to Bilateral Lower Arm Artery with Nonautologous Tissue Substitute, Open Approach

03120K6 Bypass Innominate Artery to Right Upper Leg Artery with Nonautologous Tissue Substitute, Open Approach

03120K7 Bypass Innominate Artery to Left Upper Leg Artery with Nonautologous Tissue Substitute, Open Approach

03120K8 Bypass Innominate Artery to Bilateral Upper Leg Artery with Nonautologous Tissue Substitute, Open Approach

03120K9 Bypass Innominate Artery to Right Lower Leg Artery with Nonautologous Tissue Substitute, Open Approach

03120KB Bypass Innominate Artery to Left Lower Leg Artery with Nonautologous Tissue Substitute, Open Approach

03120KC Bypass Innominate Artery to Bilateral Lower Leg Artery with Nonautologous Tissue Substitute, Open Approach

03120KD Bypass Innominate Artery to Upper Arm Vein with Nonautologous Tissue Substitute, Open Approach

03120KF Bypass Innominate Artery to Lower Arm Vein with Nonautologous Tissue Substitute, Open Approach

03120KJ Bypass Innominate Artery to Right Extracranial Artery with Nonautologous Tissue Substitute, Open Approach

03120KK Bypass Innominate Artery to Left Extracranial Artery with Nonautologous Tissue Substitute, Open Approach

03120Z0 Bypass Innominate Artery to Right Upper Arm Artery, Open Approach

03120Z1 Bypass Innominate Artery to Left Upper Arm Artery, Open Approach

03120Z2 Bypass Innominate Artery to Bilateral Upper Arm Artery, Open Approach

03120Z3 Bypass Innominate Artery to Right Lower Arm Artery, Open Approach

03120Z4 Bypass Innominate Artery to Left Lower Arm Artery, Open Approach

03120Z5 Bypass Innominate Artery to Bilateral Lower Arm Artery, Open Approach

03120Z6 Bypass Innominate Artery to Right Upper Leg Artery, Open Approach

03120Z7 Bypass Innominate Artery to Left Upper Leg Artery, Open Approach

03120Z8 Bypass Innominate Artery to Bilateral Upper Leg Artery, Open Approach

03120Z9 Bypass Innominate Artery to Right Lower Leg Artery, Open Approach

03120ZB Bypass Innominate Artery to Left Lower Leg Artery, Open Approach

03120ZC Bypass Innominate Artery to Bilateral Lower Leg Artery, Open Approach

03120ZD Bypass Innominate Artery to Upper Arm Vein, Open Approach

03120ZF Bypass Innominate Artery to Lower Arm Vein, Open Approach

03120ZJ Bypass Innominate Artery to Right Extracranial Artery, Open Approach

03120ZK Bypass Innominate Artery to Left Extracranial Artery, Open Approach

0313090 Bypass Right Subclavian Artery to Right Upper Arm Artery with Autologous Venous Tissue, Open Approach

0313091 Bypass Right Subclavian Artery to Left Upper Arm Artery with Autologous Venous Tissue, Open Approach

0313092 Bypass Right Subclavian Artery to Bilateral Upper Arm Artery with Autologous Venous Tissue, Open Approach

0313093 Bypass Right Subclavian Artery to Right Lower Arm Artery with Autologous Venous Tissue, Open Approach

0313094 Bypass Right Subclavian Artery to Left Lower Arm Artery with Autologous Venous Tissue, Open Approach

0313095 Bypass Right Subclavian Artery to Bilateral Lower Arm Artery with Autologous Venous Tissue, Open Approach

0313096 Bypass Right Subclavian Artery to Right Upper Leg Artery with Autologous Venous Tissue, Open Approach

0313097 Bypass Right Subclavian Artery to Left Upper Leg Artery with Autologous Venous Tissue, Open Approach

0313098 Bypass Right Subclavian Artery to Bilateral Upper Leg Artery with Autologous Venous Tissue, Open Approach

0313099 Bypass Right Subclavian Artery to Right Lower Leg Artery with Autologous Venous Tissue, Open Approach

031309B Bypass Right Subclavian Artery to Left Lower Leg Artery with Autologous Venous Tissue, Open Approach

031309C Bypass Right Subclavian Artery to Bilateral Lower Leg Artery with Autologous Venous Tissue, Open Approach

031309D Bypass Right Subclavian Artery to Upper Arm Vein with Autologous Venous Tissue, Open Approach

031309F Bypass Right Subclavian Artery to Lower Arm Vein with Autologous Venous Tissue, Open Approach

031309J Bypass Right Subclavian Artery to Right Extracranial Artery with Autologous Venous Tissue, Open Approach

031309K Bypass Right Subclavian Artery to Left Extracranial Artery with Autologous Venous Tissue, Open Approach

031309M Bypass Right Subclavian Artery to Right Pulmonary Artery with Autologous Venous Tissue, Open Approach

031309N Bypass Right Subclavian Artery to Left Pulmonary Artery with Autologous Venous Tissue, Open Approach

03130A0 Bypass Right Subclavian Artery to Right Upper Arm Artery with Autologous Arterial Tissue, Open Approach

03130A1 Bypass Right Subclavian Artery to Left Upper Arm Artery with Autologous Arterial Tissue, Open Approach

03130A2 Bypass Right Subclavian Artery to Bilateral Upper Arm Artery with Autologous Arterial Tissue, Open Approach

03130A3 Bypass Right Subclavian Artery to Right Lower Arm Artery with Autologous Arterial Tissue, Open Approach

03130A4 Bypass Right Subclavian Artery to Left Lower Arm Artery with Autologous Arterial Tissue, Open Approach

03130A5 Bypass Right Subclavian Artery to Bilateral Lower Arm Artery with Autologous Arterial Tissue, Open Approach

03130A6 Bypass Right Subclavian Artery to Right Upper Leg Artery with Autologous Arterial Tissue, Open Approach

03130A7 Bypass Right Subclavian Artery to Left Upper Leg Artery with Autologous Arterial Tissue, Open Approach

03130A8 Bypass Right Subclavian Artery to Bilateral Upper Leg Artery with Autologous Arterial Tissue, Open Approach

03130A9 Bypass Right Subclavian Artery to Right Lower Leg Artery with Autologous Arterial Tissue, Open Approach

03130AB Bypass Right Subclavian Artery to Left Lower Leg Artery with Autologous Arterial Tissue, Open Approach

03130AC Bypass Right Subclavian Artery to Bilateral Lower Leg Artery with Autologous Arterial Tissue, Open Approach

03130AD Bypass Right Subclavian Artery to Upper Arm Vein with Autologous Arterial Tissue, Open Approach

03130AF Bypass Right Subclavian Artery to Lower Arm Vein with Autologous Arterial Tissue, Open Approach

03130AJ Bypass Right Subclavian Artery to Right Extracranial Artery with Autologous Arterial Tissue, Open Approach

03130AK Bypass Right Subclavian Artery to Left Extracranial Artery with Autologous Arterial Tissue, Open Approach

03130AM Bypass Right Subclavian Artery to Right Pulmonary Artery with Autologous Arterial Tissue, Open Approach

03130AN Bypass Right Subclavian Artery to Left Pulmonary Artery with Autologous Arterial Tissue, Open Approach

03130J0 Bypass Right Subclavian Artery to Right Upper Arm Artery with Synthetic Substitute, Open Approach

03130J1 Bypass Right Subclavian Artery to Left Upper Arm Artery with Synthetic Substitute, Open Approach

03130J2 Bypass Right Subclavian Artery to Bilateral Upper Arm Artery with Synthetic Substitute, Open Approach

03130J3 Bypass Right Subclavian Artery to Right Lower Arm Artery with Synthetic Substitute, Open Approach

03130J4 Bypass Right Subclavian Artery to Left Lower Arm Artery with Synthetic Substitute, Open Approach

03130J5 Bypass Right Subclavian Artery to Bilateral Lower Arm Artery with Synthetic Substitute, Open Approach

03130J6 Bypass Right Subclavian Artery to Right Upper Leg Artery with Synthetic Substitute, Open Approach

03130J7 Bypass Right Subclavian Artery to Left Upper Leg Artery with Synthetic Substitute, Open Approach

03130J8 Bypass Right Subclavian Artery to Bilateral Upper Leg Artery with Synthetic Substitute, Open Approach

03130J9 Bypass Right Subclavian Artery to Right Lower Leg Artery with Synthetic Substitute, Open Approach

03130JB Bypass Right Subclavian Artery to Left Lower Leg Artery with Synthetic Substitute, Open Approach

03130JC Bypass Right Subclavian Artery to Bilateral Lower Leg Artery with Synthetic Substitute, Open Approach

03130JD Bypass Right Subclavian Artery to Upper Arm Vein with Synthetic Substitute, Open Approach

03130JF Bypass Right Subclavian Artery to Lower Arm Vein with Synthetic Substitute, Open Approach

03130JJ Bypass Right Subclavian Artery to Right Extracranial Artery with Synthetic Substitute, Open Approach

03130JK Bypass Right Subclavian Artery to Left Extracranial Artery with Synthetic Substitute, Open Approach

03130JM Bypass Right Subclavian Artery to Right Pulmonary Artery with Synthetic Substitute, Open Approach

03130JN Bypass Right Subclavian Artery to Left Pulmonary Artery with Synthetic Substitute, Open Approach

03130K0 Bypass Right Subclavian Artery to Right Upper Arm Artery with Nonautologous Tissue Substitute, Open Approach

03130K1 Bypass Right Subclavian Artery to Left Upper Arm Artery with Nonautologous Tissue Substitute, Open Approach

03130K2 Bypass Right Subclavian Artery to Bilateral Upper Arm Artery with Nonautologous Tissue Substitute, Open Approach

03130K3 Bypass Right Subclavian Artery to Right Lower Arm Artery with Nonautologous Tissue Substitute, Open Approach

03130K4 Bypass Right Subclavian Artery to Left Lower Arm Artery with Nonautologous Tissue Substitute, Open Approach

03130K5 Bypass Right Subclavian Artery to Bilateral Lower Arm Artery with Nonautologous Tissue Substitute, Open Approach

03130K6 Bypass Right Subclavian Artery to Right Upper Leg Artery with Nonautologous Tissue Substitute, Open Approach

03130K7 Bypass Right Subclavian Artery to Left Upper Leg Artery with Nonautologous Tissue Substitute, Open Approach

03130K8 Bypass Right Subclavian Artery to Bilateral Upper Leg Artery with Nonautologous Tissue Substitute, Open Approach

03130K9 Bypass Right Subclavian Artery to Right Lower Leg Artery with Nonautologous Tissue Substitute, Open Approach

03130KB Bypass Right Subclavian Artery to Left Lower Leg Artery with Nonautologous Tissue Substitute, Open Approach

03130KC Bypass Right Subclavian Artery to Bilateral Lower Leg Artery with Nonautologous Tissue Substitute, Open Approach

03130KD Bypass Right Subclavian Artery to Upper Arm Vein with Nonautologous Tissue Substitute, Open Approach

03130KF Bypass Right Subclavian Artery to Lower Arm Vein with Nonautologous Tissue Substitute, Open Approach

03130KJ Bypass Right Subclavian Artery to Right Extracranial Artery with Nonautologous Tissue Substitute, Open Approach

03130KK Bypass Right Subclavian Artery to Left Extracranial Artery with Nonautologous Tissue Substitute, Open Approach

03130KM Bypass Right Subclavian Artery to Right Pulmonary Artery with Nonautologous Tissue Substitute, Open Approach

03130KN Bypass Right Subclavian Artery to Left Pulmonary Artery with Nonautologous Tissue Substitute, Open Approach

03130Z0 Bypass Right Subclavian Artery to Right Upper Arm Artery, Open Approach

03130Z1 Bypass Right Subclavian Artery to Left Upper Arm Artery, Open Approach

03130Z2 Bypass Right Subclavian Artery to Bilateral Upper Arm Artery, Open Approach

03130Z3 Bypass Right Subclavian Artery to Right Lower Arm Artery, Open Approach

03130Z4 Bypass Right Subclavian Artery to Left Lower Arm Artery, Open Approach

03130Z5 Bypass Right Subclavian Artery to Bilateral Lower Arm Artery, Open Approach

03130Z6 Bypass Right Subclavian Artery to Right Upper Leg Artery, Open Approach

03130Z7 Bypass Right Subclavian Artery to Left Upper Leg Artery, Open Approach

03130Z8 Bypass Right Subclavian Artery to Bilateral Upper Leg Artery, Open Approach

03130Z9 Bypass Right Subclavian Artery to Right Lower Leg Artery, Open Approach

03130ZB Bypass Right Subclavian Artery to Left Lower Leg Artery, Open Approach

03130ZC Bypass Right Subclavian Artery to Bilateral Lower Leg Artery, Open Approach

03130ZD Bypass Right Subclavian Artery to Upper Arm Vein, Open Approach

03130ZF Bypass Right Subclavian Artery to Lower Arm Vein, Open Approach

03130ZJ Bypass Right Subclavian Artery to Right Extracranial Artery, Open Approach

03130ZK Bypass Right Subclavian Artery to Left Extracranial Artery, Open Approach

03130ZM Bypass Right Subclavian Artery to Right Pulmonary Artery, Open Approach

03130ZN Bypass Right Subclavian Artery to Left Pulmonary Artery, Open Approach

0314090 Bypass Left Subclavian Artery to Right Upper Arm Artery with Autologous Venous Tissue, Open Approach

0314091 Bypass Left Subclavian Artery to Left Upper Arm Artery with Autologous Venous Tissue, Open Approach

0314092 Bypass Left Subclavian Artery to Bilateral Upper Arm Artery with Autologous Venous Tissue, Open Approach

0314093 Bypass Left Subclavian Artery to Right Lower Arm Artery with Autologous Venous Tissue, Open Approach

0314094 Bypass Left Subclavian Artery to Left Lower Arm Artery with Autologous Venous Tissue, Open Approach

0314095 Bypass Left Subclavian Artery to Bilateral Lower Arm Artery with Autologous Venous Tissue, Open Approach

0314096 Bypass Left Subclavian Artery to Right Upper Leg Artery with Autologous Venous Tissue, Open Approach

0314097 Bypass Left Subclavian Artery to Left Upper Leg Artery with Autologous Venous Tissue, Open Approach

0314098 Bypass Left Subclavian Artery to Bilateral Upper Leg Artery with Autologous Venous Tissue, Open Approach

0314099 Bypass Left Subclavian Artery to Right Lower Leg Artery with Autologous Venous Tissue, Open Approach

031409B Bypass Left Subclavian Artery to Left Lower Leg Artery with Autologous Venous Tissue, Open Approach

031409C Bypass Left Subclavian Artery to Bilateral Lower Leg Artery with Autologous Venous Tissue, Open Approach

031409D Bypass Left Subclavian Artery to Upper Arm Vein with Autologous Venous Tissue, Open Approach

031409F Bypass Left Subclavian Artery to Lower Arm Vein with Autologous Venous Tissue, Open Approach

031409J Bypass Left Subclavian Artery to Right Extracranial Artery with Autologous Venous Tissue, Open Approach

031409K Bypass Left Subclavian Artery to Left Extracranial Artery with Autologous Venous Tissue, Open Approach

031409M Bypass Left Subclavian Artery to Right Pulmonary Artery with Autologous Venous Tissue, Open Approach

031409N Bypass Left Subclavian Artery to Left Pulmonary Artery with Autologous Venous Tissue, Open Approach

03140A0 Bypass Left Subclavian Artery to Right Upper Arm Artery with Autologous Arterial Tissue, Open Approach

03140A1 Bypass Left Subclavian Artery to Left Upper Arm Artery with Autologous Arterial Tissue, Open Approach

03140A2 Bypass Left Subclavian Artery to Bilateral Upper Arm Artery with Autologous Arterial Tissue, Open Approach

03140A3 Bypass Left Subclavian Artery to Right Lower Arm Artery with Autologous Arterial Tissue, Open Approach

03140A4 Bypass Left Subclavian Artery to Left Lower Arm Artery with Autologous Arterial Tissue, Open Approach

03140A5 Bypass Left Subclavian Artery to Bilateral Lower Arm Artery with Autologous Arterial Tissue, Open Approach

03140A6 Bypass Left Subclavian Artery to Right Upper Leg Artery with Autologous Arterial Tissue, Open Approach

03140A7 Bypass Left Subclavian Artery to Left Upper Leg Artery with Autologous Arterial Tissue, Open Approach

03140A8 Bypass Left Subclavian Artery to Bilateral Upper Leg Artery with Autologous Arterial Tissue, Open Approach

03140A9 Bypass Left Subclavian Artery to Right Lower Leg Artery with Autologous Arterial Tissue, Open Approach

03140AB Bypass Left Subclavian Artery to Left Lower Leg Artery with Autologous Arterial Tissue, Open Approach

03140AC Bypass Left Subclavian Artery to Bilateral Lower Leg Artery with Autologous Arterial Tissue, Open Approach

03140AD Bypass Left Subclavian Artery to Upper Arm Vein with Autologous Arterial Tissue, Open Approach

03140AF Bypass Left Subclavian Artery to Lower Arm Vein with Autologous Arterial Tissue, Open Approach

03140AJ Bypass Left Subclavian Artery to Right Extracranial Artery with Autologous Arterial Tissue, Open Approach

03140AK Bypass Left Subclavian Artery to Left Extracranial Artery with Autologous Arterial Tissue, Open Approach

03140AM Bypass Left Subclavian Artery to Right Pulmonary Artery with Autologous Arterial Tissue, Open Approach

03140AN Bypass Left Subclavian Artery to Left Pulmonary Artery with Autologous Arterial Tissue, Open Approach

03140J0 Bypass Left Subclavian Artery to Right Upper Arm Artery with Synthetic Substitute, Open Approach

03140J1 Bypass Left Subclavian Artery to Left Upper Arm Artery with Synthetic Substitute, Open Approach

03140J2 Bypass Left Subclavian Artery to Bilateral Upper Arm Artery with Synthetic Substitute, Open Approach

03140J3 Bypass Left Subclavian Artery to Right Lower Arm Artery with Synthetic Substitute, Open Approach

03140J4 Bypass Left Subclavian Artery to Left Lower Arm Artery with Synthetic Substitute, Open Approach

03140J5 Bypass Left Subclavian Artery to Bilateral Lower Arm Artery with Synthetic Substitute, Open Approach

03140J6 Bypass Left Subclavian Artery to Right Upper Leg Artery with Synthetic Substitute, Open Approach

03140J7 Bypass Left Subclavian Artery to Left Upper Leg Artery with Synthetic Substitute, Open Approach

03140J8 Bypass Left Subclavian Artery to Bilateral Upper Leg Artery with Synthetic Substitute, Open Approach

03140J9 Bypass Left Subclavian Artery to Right Lower Leg Artery with Synthetic Substitute, Open Approach

03140JB Bypass Left Subclavian Artery to Left Lower Leg Artery with Synthetic Substitute, Open Approach

---

♀ Female-only   ♂ Male-only   ⬤ Limited Coverage   ● Non-OR   🅷🅰🅲 HAC-associated procedure   ⬤ Non-covered procedures   ➕ Combination

03140JC   Bypass Left Subclavian Artery to Bilateral Lower Leg Artery with Synthetic Substitute, Open Approach

03140JD   Bypass Left Subclavian Artery to Upper Arm Vein with Synthetic Substitute, Open Approach

03140JF   Bypass Left Subclavian Artery to Lower Arm Vein with Synthetic Substitute, Open Approach

03140JJ   Bypass Left Subclavian Artery to Right Extracranial Artery with Synthetic Substitute, Open Approach

03140JK   Bypass Left Subclavian Artery to Left Extracranial Artery with Synthetic Substitute, Open Approach

03140JM   Bypass Left Subclavian Artery to Right Pulmonary Artery with Synthetic Substitute, Open Approach

03140JN   Bypass Left Subclavian Artery to Left Pulmonary Artery with Synthetic Substitute, Open Approach

03140K0   Bypass Left Subclavian Artery to Right Upper Arm Artery with Nonautologous Tissue Substitute, Open Approach

03140K1   Bypass Left Subclavian Artery to Left Upper Arm Artery with Nonautologous Tissue Substitute, Open Approach

03140K2   Bypass Left Subclavian Artery to Bilateral Upper Arm Artery with Nonautologous Tissue Substitute, Open Approach

03140K3   Bypass Left Subclavian Artery to Right Lower Arm Artery with Nonautologous Tissue Substitute, Open Approach

03140K4   Bypass Left Subclavian Artery to Left Lower Arm Artery with Nonautologous Tissue Substitute, Open Approach

03140K5   Bypass Left Subclavian Artery to Bilateral Lower Arm Artery with Nonautologous Tissue Substitute, Open Approach

03140K6   Bypass Left Subclavian Artery to Right Upper Leg Artery with Nonautologous Tissue Substitute, Open Approach

03140K7   Bypass Left Subclavian Artery to Left Upper Leg Artery with Nonautologous Tissue Substitute, Open Approach

03140K8   Bypass Left Subclavian Artery to Bilateral Upper Leg Artery with Nonautologous Tissue Substitute, Open Approach

03140K9   Bypass Left Subclavian Artery to Right Lower Leg Artery with Nonautologous Tissue Substitute, Open Approach

03140KB   Bypass Left Subclavian Artery to Left Lower Leg Artery with Nonautologous Tissue Substitute, Open Approach

03140KC   Bypass Left Subclavian Artery to Bilateral Lower Leg Artery with Nonautologous Tissue Substitute, Open Approach

03140KD   Bypass Left Subclavian Artery to Upper Arm Vein with Nonautologous Tissue Substitute, Open Approach

03140KF   Bypass Left Subclavian Artery to Lower Arm Vein with Nonautologous Tissue Substitute, Open Approach

03140KJ   Bypass Left Subclavian Artery to Right Extracranial Artery with Nonautologous Tissue Substitute, Open Approach

03140KK   Bypass Left Subclavian Artery to Left Extracranial Artery with Nonautologous Tissue Substitute, Open Approach

03140KM   Bypass Left Subclavian Artery to Right Pulmonary Artery with Nonautologous Tissue Substitute, Open Approach

03140KN   Bypass Left Subclavian Artery to Left Pulmonary Artery with Nonautologous Tissue Substitute, Open Approach

03140Z0   Bypass Left Subclavian Artery to Right Upper Arm Artery, Open Approach

03140Z1   Bypass Left Subclavian Artery to Left Upper Arm Artery, Open Approach

03140Z2   Bypass Left Subclavian Artery to Bilateral Upper Arm Artery, Open Approach

03140Z3   Bypass Left Subclavian Artery to Right Lower Arm Artery, Open Approach

03140Z4   Bypass Left Subclavian Artery to Left Lower Arm Artery, Open Approach

03140Z5   Bypass Left Subclavian Artery to Bilateral Lower Arm Artery, Open Approach

03140Z6   Bypass Left Subclavian Artery to Right Upper Leg Artery, Open Approach

03140Z7   Bypass Left Subclavian Artery to Left Upper Leg Artery, Open Approach

03140Z8   Bypass Left Subclavian Artery to Bilateral Upper Leg Artery, Open Approach

03140Z9   Bypass Left Subclavian Artery to Right Lower Leg Artery, Open Approach

03140ZB   Bypass Left Subclavian Artery to Left Lower Leg Artery, Open Approach

03140ZC   Bypass Left Subclavian Artery to Bilateral Lower Leg Artery, Open Approach

03140ZD   Bypass Left Subclavian Artery to Upper Arm Vein, Open Approach

03140ZF   Bypass Left Subclavian Artery to Lower Arm Vein, Open Approach

03140ZJ   Bypass Left Subclavian Artery to Right Extracranial Artery, Open Approach

03140ZK   Bypass Left Subclavian Artery to Left Extracranial Artery, Open Approach

03140ZM   Bypass Left Subclavian Artery to Right Pulmonary Artery, Open Approach

03140ZN   Bypass Left Subclavian Artery to Left Pulmonary Artery, Open Approach

0315090   Bypass Right Axillary Artery to Right Upper Arm Artery with Autologous Venous Tissue, Open Approach

0315091   Bypass Right Axillary Artery to Left Upper Arm Artery with Autologous Venous Tissue, Open Approach

0315092   Bypass Right Axillary Artery to Bilateral Upper Arm Artery with Autologous Venous Tissue, Open Approach

0315093   Bypass Right Axillary Artery to Right Lower Arm Artery with Autologous Venous Tissue, Open Approach

0315094   Bypass Right Axillary Artery to Left Lower Arm Artery with Autologous Venous Tissue, Open Approach

0315095   Bypass Right Axillary Artery to Bilateral Lower Arm Artery with Autologous Venous Tissue, Open Approach

0315096   Bypass Right Axillary Artery to Right Upper Leg Artery with Autologous Venous Tissue, Open Approach

0315097   Bypass Right Axillary Artery to Left Upper Leg Artery with Autologous Venous Tissue, Open Approach

0315098   Bypass Right Axillary Artery to Bilateral Upper Leg Artery with Autologous Venous Tissue, Open Approach

0315099   Bypass Right Axillary Artery to Right Lower Leg Artery with Autologous Venous Tissue, Open Approach

031509B   Bypass Right Axillary Artery to Left Lower Leg Artery with Autologous Venous Tissue, Open Approach

031509C   Bypass Right Axillary Artery to Bilateral Lower Leg Artery with Autologous Venous Tissue, Open Approach

031509D   Bypass Right Axillary Artery to Upper Arm Vein with Autologous Venous Tissue, Open Approach

031509F   Bypass Right Axillary Artery to Lower Arm Vein with Autologous Venous Tissue, Open Approach

031509J   Bypass Right Axillary Artery to Right Extracranial Artery with Autologous Venous Tissue, Open Approach

031509K   Bypass Right Axillary Artery to Left Extracranial Artery with Autologous Venous Tissue, Open Approach

03150A0   Bypass Right Axillary Artery to Right Upper Arm Artery with Autologous Arterial Tissue, Open Approach

03150A1   Bypass Right Axillary Artery to Left Upper Arm Artery with Autologous Arterial Tissue, Open Approach

03150A2   Bypass Right Axillary Artery to Bilateral Upper Arm Artery with Autologous Arterial Tissue, Open Approach

03150A3   Bypass Right Axillary Artery to Right Lower Arm Artery with Autologous Arterial Tissue, Open Approach

03150A4   Bypass Right Axillary Artery to Left Lower Arm Artery with Autologous Arterial Tissue, Open Approach

03150A5   Bypass Right Axillary Artery to Bilateral Lower Arm Artery with Autologous Arterial Tissue, Open Approach

03150A6   Bypass Right Axillary Artery to Right Upper Leg Artery with Autologous Arterial Tissue, Open Approach

03150A7   Bypass Right Axillary Artery to Left Upper Leg Artery with Autologous Arterial Tissue, Open Approach

03150A8   Bypass Right Axillary Artery to Bilateral Upper Leg Artery with Autologous Arterial Tissue, Open Approach

03150A9   Bypass Right Axillary Artery to Right Lower Leg Artery with Autologous Arterial Tissue, Open Approach

03150AB   Bypass Right Axillary Artery to Left Lower Leg Artery with Autologous Arterial Tissue, Open Approach

03150AC   Bypass Right Axillary Artery to Bilateral Lower Leg Artery with Autologous Arterial Tissue, Open Approach

03150AD   Bypass Right Axillary Artery to Upper Arm Vein with Autologous Arterial Tissue, Open Approach

03150AF   Bypass Right Axillary Artery to Lower Arm Vein with Autologous Arterial Tissue, Open Approach

03150AJ   Bypass Right Axillary Artery to Right Extracranial Artery with Autologous Arterial Tissue, Open Approach

03150AK   Bypass Right Axillary Artery to Left Extracranial Artery with Autologous Arterial Tissue, Open Approach

03150J0 Bypass Right Axillary Artery to Right Upper Arm Artery with Synthetic Substitute, Open Approach

03150J1 Bypass Right Axillary Artery to Left Upper Arm Artery with Synthetic Substitute, Open Approach

03150J2 Bypass Right Axillary Artery to Bilateral Upper Arm Artery with Synthetic Substitute, Open Approach

03150J3 Bypass Right Axillary Artery to Right Lower Arm Artery with Synthetic Substitute, Open Approach

03150J4 Bypass Right Axillary Artery to Left Lower Arm Artery with Synthetic Substitute, Open Approach

03150J5 Bypass Right Axillary Artery to Bilateral Lower Arm Artery with Synthetic Substitute, Open Approach

03150J6 Bypass Right Axillary Artery to Right Upper Leg Artery with Synthetic Substitute, Open Approach

03150J7 Bypass Right Axillary Artery to Left Upper Leg Artery with Synthetic Substitute, Open Approach

03150J8 Bypass Right Axillary Artery to Bilateral Upper Leg Artery with Synthetic Substitute, Open Approach

03150J9 Bypass Right Axillary Artery to Right Lower Leg Artery with Synthetic Substitute, Open Approach

03150JB Bypass Right Axillary Artery to Left Lower Leg Artery with Synthetic Substitute, Open Approach

03150JC Bypass Right Axillary Artery to Bilateral Lower Leg Artery with Synthetic Substitute, Open Approach

03150JD Bypass Right Axillary Artery to Upper Arm Vein with Synthetic Substitute, Open Approach

03150JF Bypass Right Axillary Artery to Lower Arm Vein with Synthetic Substitute, Open Approach

03150JJ Bypass Right Axillary Artery to Right Extracranial Artery with Synthetic Substitute, Open Approach

03150JK Bypass Right Axillary Artery to Left Extracranial Artery with Synthetic Substitute, Open Approach

03150K0 Bypass Right Axillary Artery to Right Upper Arm Artery with Nonautologous Tissue Substitute, Open Approach

03150K1 Bypass Right Axillary Artery to Left Upper Arm Artery with Nonautologous Tissue Substitute, Open Approach

03150K2 Bypass Right Axillary Artery to Bilateral Upper Arm Artery with Nonautologous Tissue Substitute, Open Approach

03150K3 Bypass Right Axillary Artery to Right Lower Arm Artery with Nonautologous Tissue Substitute, Open Approach

03150K4 Bypass Right Axillary Artery to Left Lower Arm Artery with Nonautologous Tissue Substitute, Open Approach

03150K5 Bypass Right Axillary Artery to Bilateral Lower Arm Artery with Nonautologous Tissue Substitute, Open Approach

03150K6 Bypass Right Axillary Artery to Right Upper Leg Artery with Nonautologous Tissue Substitute, Open Approach

03150K7 Bypass Right Axillary Artery to Left Upper Leg Artery with Nonautologous Tissue Substitute, Open Approach

03150K8 Bypass Right Axillary Artery to Bilateral Upper Leg Artery with Nonautologous Tissue Substitute, Open Approach

03150K9 Bypass Right Axillary Artery to Right Lower Leg Artery with Nonautologous Tissue Substitute, Open Approach

03150KB Bypass Right Axillary Artery to Left Lower Leg Artery with Nonautologous Tissue Substitute, Open Approach

03150KC Bypass Right Axillary Artery to Bilateral Lower Leg Artery with Nonautologous Tissue Substitute, Open Approach

03150KD Bypass Right Axillary Artery to Upper Arm Vein with Nonautologous Tissue Substitute, Open Approach

03150KF Bypass Right Axillary Artery to Lower Arm Vein with Nonautologous Tissue Substitute, Open Approach

03150KJ Bypass Right Axillary Artery to Right Extracranial Artery with Nonautologous Tissue Substitute, Open Approach

03150KK Bypass Right Axillary Artery to Left Extracranial Artery with Nonautologous Tissue Substitute, Open Approach

03150Z0 Bypass Right Axillary Artery to Right Upper Arm Artery, Open Approach

03150Z1 Bypass Right Axillary Artery to Left Upper Arm Artery, Open Approach

03150Z2 Bypass Right Axillary Artery to Bilateral Upper Arm Artery, Open Approach

03150Z3 Bypass Right Axillary Artery to Right Lower Arm Artery, Open Approach

03150Z4 Bypass Right Axillary Artery to Left Lower Arm Artery, Open Approach

03150Z5 Bypass Right Axillary Artery to Bilateral Lower Arm Artery, Open Approach

03150Z6 Bypass Right Axillary Artery to Right Upper Leg Artery, Open Approach

03150Z7 Bypass Right Axillary Artery to Left Upper Leg Artery, Open Approach

03150Z8 Bypass Right Axillary Artery to Bilateral Upper Leg Artery, Open Approach

03150Z9 Bypass Right Axillary Artery to Right Lower Leg Artery, Open Approach

03150ZB Bypass Right Axillary Artery to Left Lower Leg Artery, Open Approach

03150ZC Bypass Right Axillary Artery to Bilateral Lower Leg Artery, Open Approach

03150ZD Bypass Right Axillary Artery to Upper Arm Vein, Open Approach

03150ZF Bypass Right Axillary Artery to Lower Arm Vein, Open Approach

03150ZJ Bypass Right Axillary Artery to Right Extracranial Artery, Open Approach

03150ZK Bypass Right Axillary Artery to Left Extracranial Artery, Open Approach

0316090 Bypass Left Axillary Artery to Right Upper Arm Artery with Autologous Venous Tissue, Open Approach

0316091 Bypass Left Axillary Artery to Left Upper Arm Artery with Autologous Venous Tissue, Open Approach

0316092 Bypass Left Axillary Artery to Bilateral Upper Arm Artery with Autologous Venous Tissue, Open Approach

0316093 Bypass Left Axillary Artery to Right Lower Arm Artery with Autologous Venous Tissue, Open Approach

0316094 Bypass Left Axillary Artery to Left Lower Arm Artery with Autologous Venous Tissue, Open Approach

0316095 Bypass Left Axillary Artery to Bilateral Lower Arm Artery with Autologous Venous Tissue, Open Approach

0316096 Bypass Left Axillary Artery to Right Upper Leg Artery with Autologous Venous Tissue, Open Approach

0316097 Bypass Left Axillary Artery to Left Upper Leg Artery with Autologous Venous Tissue, Open Approach

0316098 Bypass Left Axillary Artery to Bilateral Upper Leg Artery with Autologous Venous Tissue, Open Approach

0316099 Bypass Left Axillary Artery to Right Lower Leg Artery with Autologous Venous Tissue, Open Approach

031609B Bypass Left Axillary Artery to Left Lower Leg Artery with Autologous Venous Tissue, Open Approach

031609C Bypass Left Axillary Artery to Bilateral Lower Leg Artery with Autologous Venous Tissue, Open Approach

031609D Bypass Left Axillary Artery to Upper Arm Vein with Autologous Venous Tissue, Open Approach

031609F Bypass Left Axillary Artery to Lower Arm Vein with Autologous Venous Tissue, Open Approach

031609J Bypass Left Axillary Artery to Right Extracranial Artery with Autologous Venous Tissue, Open Approach

031609K Bypass Left Axillary Artery to Left Extracranial Artery with Autologous Venous Tissue, Open Approach

03160A0 Bypass Left Axillary Artery to Right Upper Arm Artery with Autologous Arterial Tissue, Open Approach

03160A1 Bypass Left Axillary Artery to Left Upper Arm Artery with Autologous Arterial Tissue, Open Approach

03160A2 Bypass Left Axillary Artery to Bilateral Upper Arm Artery with Autologous Arterial Tissue, Open Approach

03160A3 Bypass Left Axillary Artery to Right Lower Arm Artery with Autologous Arterial Tissue, Open Approach

03160A4 Bypass Left Axillary Artery to Left Lower Arm Artery with Autologous Arterial Tissue, Open Approach

03160A5 Bypass Left Axillary Artery to Bilateral Lower Arm Artery with Autologous Arterial Tissue, Open Approach

03160A6 Bypass Left Axillary Artery to Right Upper Leg Artery with Autologous Arterial Tissue, Open Approach

03160A7 Bypass Left Axillary Artery to Left Upper Leg Artery with Autologous Arterial Tissue, Open Approach

03160A8 Bypass Left Axillary Artery to Bilateral Upper Leg Artery with Autologous Arterial Tissue, Open Approach

03160A9 Bypass Left Axillary Artery to Right Lower Leg Artery with Autologous Arterial Tissue, Open Approach

03160AB Bypass Left Axillary Artery to Left Lower Leg Artery with Autologous Arterial Tissue, Open Approach

03160AC Bypass Left Axillary Artery to Bilateral Lower Leg Artery with Autologous Arterial Tissue, Open Approach

03160AD Bypass Left Axillary Artery to Upper Arm Vein with Autologous Arterial Tissue, Open Approach

03160AF Bypass Left Axillary Artery to Lower Arm Vein with Autologous Arterial Tissue, Open Approach

03160AJ Bypass Left Axillary Artery to Right Extracranial Artery with Autologous Arterial Tissue, Open Approach

03160AK Bypass Left Axillary Artery to Left Extracranial Artery with Autologous Arterial Tissue, Open Approach

03160J0 Bypass Left Axillary Artery to Right Upper Arm Artery with Synthetic Substitute, Open Approach

03160J1 Bypass Left Axillary Artery to Left Upper Arm Artery with Synthetic Substitute, Open Approach

03160J2 Bypass Left Axillary Artery to Bilateral Upper Arm Artery with Synthetic Substitute, Open Approach

03160J3 Bypass Left Axillary Artery to Right Lower Arm Artery with Synthetic Substitute, Open Approach

03160J4 Bypass Left Axillary Artery to Left Lower Arm Artery with Synthetic Substitute, Open Approach

03160J5 Bypass Left Axillary Artery to Bilateral Lower Arm Artery with Synthetic Substitute, Open Approach

03160J6 Bypass Left Axillary Artery to Right Upper Leg Artery with Synthetic Substitute, Open Approach

03160J7 Bypass Left Axillary Artery to Left Upper Leg Artery with Synthetic Substitute, Open Approach

03160J8 Bypass Left Axillary Artery to Bilateral Upper Leg Artery with Synthetic Substitute, Open Approach

03160J9 Bypass Left Axillary Artery to Right Lower Leg Artery with Synthetic Substitute, Open Approach

03160JB Bypass Left Axillary Artery to Left Lower Leg Artery with Synthetic Substitute, Open Approach

03160JC Bypass Left Axillary Artery to Bilateral Lower Leg Artery with Synthetic Substitute, Open Approach

03160JD Bypass Left Axillary Artery to Upper Arm Vein with Synthetic Substitute, Open Approach

03160JF Bypass Left Axillary Artery to Lower Arm Vein with Synthetic Substitute, Open Approach

03160JJ Bypass Left Axillary Artery to Right Extracranial Artery with Synthetic Substitute, Open Approach

03160JK Bypass Left Axillary Artery to Left Extracranial Artery with Synthetic Substitute, Open Approach

03160K0 Bypass Left Axillary Artery to Right Upper Arm Artery with Nonautologous Tissue Substitute, Open Approach

03160K1 Bypass Left Axillary Artery to Left Upper Arm Artery with Nonautologous Tissue Substitute, Open Approach

03160K2 Bypass Left Axillary Artery to Bilateral Upper Arm Artery with Nonautologous Tissue Substitute, Open Approach

03160K3 Bypass Left Axillary Artery to Right Lower Arm Artery with Nonautologous Tissue Substitute, Open Approach

03160K4 Bypass Left Axillary Artery to Left Lower Arm Artery with Nonautologous Tissue Substitute, Open Approach

03160K5 Bypass Left Axillary Artery to Bilateral Lower Arm Artery with Nonautologous Tissue Substitute, Open Approach

03160K6 Bypass Left Axillary Artery to Right Upper Leg Artery with Nonautologous Tissue Substitute, Open Approach

03160K7 Bypass Left Axillary Artery to Left Upper Leg Artery with Nonautologous Tissue Substitute, Open Approach

03160K8 Bypass Left Axillary Artery to Bilateral Upper Leg Artery with Nonautologous Tissue Substitute, Open Approach

03160K9 Bypass Left Axillary Artery to Right Lower Leg Artery with Nonautologous Tissue Substitute, Open Approach

03160KB Bypass Left Axillary Artery to Left Lower Leg Artery with Nonautologous Tissue Substitute, Open Approach

03160KC Bypass Left Axillary Artery to Bilateral Lower Leg Artery with Nonautologous Tissue Substitute, Open Approach

03160KD Bypass Left Axillary Artery to Upper Arm Vein with Nonautologous Tissue Substitute, Open Approach

03160KF Bypass Left Axillary Artery to Lower Arm Vein with Nonautologous Tissue Substitute, Open Approach

03160KJ Bypass Left Axillary Artery to Right Extracranial Artery with Nonautologous Tissue Substitute, Open Approach

03160KK Bypass Left Axillary Artery to Left Extracranial Artery with Nonautologous Tissue Substitute, Open Approach

03160Z0 Bypass Left Axillary Artery to Right Upper Arm Artery, Open Approach

03160Z1 Bypass Left Axillary Artery to Left Upper Arm Artery, Open Approach

03160Z2 Bypass Left Axillary Artery to Bilateral Upper Arm Artery, Open Approach

03160Z3 Bypass Left Axillary Artery to Right Lower Arm Artery, Open Approach

03160Z4 Bypass Left Axillary Artery to Left Lower Arm Artery, Open Approach

03160Z5 Bypass Left Axillary Artery to Bilateral Lower Arm Artery, Open Approach

03160Z6 Bypass Left Axillary Artery to Right Upper Leg Artery, Open Approach

03160Z7 Bypass Left Axillary Artery to Left Upper Leg Artery, Open Approach

03160Z8 Bypass Left Axillary Artery to Bilateral Upper Leg Artery, Open Approach

03160Z9 Bypass Left Axillary Artery to Right Lower Leg Artery, Open Approach

03160ZB Bypass Left Axillary Artery to Left Lower Leg Artery, Open Approach

03160ZC Bypass Left Axillary Artery to Bilateral Lower Leg Artery, Open Approach

03160ZD Bypass Left Axillary Artery to Upper Arm Vein, Open Approach

03160ZF Bypass Left Axillary Artery to Lower Arm Vein, Open Approach

03160ZJ Bypass Left Axillary Artery to Right Extracranial Artery, Open Approach

03160ZK Bypass Left Axillary Artery to Left Extracranial Artery, Open Approach

0317090 Bypass Right Brachial Artery to Right Upper Arm Artery with Autologous Venous Tissue, Open Approach

0317093 Bypass Right Brachial Artery to Right Lower Arm Artery with Autologous Venous Tissue, Open Approach

031709D Bypass Right Brachial Artery to Upper Arm Vein with Autologous Venous Tissue, Open Approach

031709F Bypass Right Brachial Artery to Lower Arm Vein with Autologous Venous Tissue, Open Approach

03170A0 Bypass Right Brachial Artery to Right Upper Arm Artery with Autologous Arterial Tissue, Open Approach

03170A3 Bypass Right Brachial Artery to Right Lower Arm Artery with Autologous Arterial Tissue, Open Approach

03170AD Bypass Right Brachial Artery to Upper Arm Vein with Autologous Arterial Tissue, Open Approach

03170AF Bypass Right Brachial Artery to Lower Arm Vein with Autologous Arterial Tissue, Open Approach

03170J0 Bypass Right Brachial Artery to Right Upper Arm Artery with Synthetic Substitute, Open Approach

03170J3 Bypass Right Brachial Artery to Right Lower Arm Artery with Synthetic Substitute, Open Approach

03170JD Bypass Right Brachial Artery to Upper Arm Vein with Synthetic Substitute, Open Approach

03170JF Bypass Right Brachial Artery to Lower Arm Vein with Synthetic Substitute, Open Approach

03170K0 Bypass Right Brachial Artery to Right Upper Arm Artery with Nonautologous Tissue Substitute, Open Approach

03170K3 Bypass Right Brachial Artery to Right Lower Arm Artery with Nonautologous Tissue Substitute, Open Approach

03170KD Bypass Right Brachial Artery to Upper Arm Vein with Nonautologous Tissue Substitute, Open Approach

03170KF Bypass Right Brachial Artery to Lower Arm Vein with Nonautologous Tissue Substitute, Open Approach

03170Z0 Bypass Right Brachial Artery to Right Upper Arm Artery, Open Approach

03170Z3 Bypass Right Brachial Artery to Right Lower Arm Artery, Open Approach

03170ZD Bypass Right Brachial Artery to Upper Arm Vein, Open Approach

03170ZF Bypass Right Brachial Artery to Lower Arm Vein, Open Approach

0318091 Bypass Left Brachial Artery to Left Upper Arm Artery with Autologous Venous Tissue, Open Approach

0318094 Bypass Left Brachial Artery to Left Lower Arm Artery with Autologous Venous Tissue, Open Approach

031809D Bypass Left Brachial Artery to Upper Arm Vein with Autologous Venous Tissue, Open Approach

031809F Bypass Left Brachial Artery to Lower Arm Vein with Autologous Venous Tissue, Open Approach

03180A1 Bypass Left Brachial Artery to Left Upper Arm Artery with Autologous Arterial Tissue, Open Approach

03180A4 Bypass Left Brachial Artery to Left Lower Arm Artery with Autologous Arterial Tissue, Open Approach

03180AD Bypass Left Brachial Artery to Upper Arm Vein with Autologous Arterial Tissue, Open Approach

03180AF Bypass Left Brachial Artery to Lower Arm Vein with Autologous Arterial Tissue, Open Approach

03180J1 Bypass Left Brachial Artery to Left Upper Arm Artery with Synthetic Substitute, Open Approach

03180J4 Bypass Left Brachial Artery to Left Lower Arm Artery with Synthetic Substitute, Open Approach

03180JD Bypass Left Brachial Artery to Upper Arm Vein with Synthetic Substitute, Open Approach

03180JF Bypass Left Brachial Artery to Lower Arm Vein with Synthetic Substitute, Open Approach

03180K1 Bypass Left Brachial Artery to Left Upper Arm Artery with Nonautologous Tissue Substitute, Open Approach

03180K4 Bypass Left Brachial Artery to Left Lower Arm Artery with Nonautologous Tissue Substitute, Open Approach

03180KD Bypass Left Brachial Artery to Upper Arm Vein with Nonautologous Tissue Substitute, Open Approach

03180KF Bypass Left Brachial Artery to Lower Arm Vein with Nonautologous Tissue Substitute, Open Approach

03180Z1 Bypass Left Brachial Artery to Left Upper Arm Artery, Open Approach

03180Z4 Bypass Left Brachial Artery to Left Lower Arm Artery, Open Approach

03180ZD Bypass Left Brachial Artery to Upper Arm Vein, Open Approach

03180ZF Bypass Left Brachial Artery to Lower Arm Vein, Open Approach

0319093 Bypass Right Ulnar Artery to Right Lower Arm Artery with Autologous Venous Tissue, Open Approach

031909F Bypass Right Ulnar Artery to Lower Arm Vein with Autologous Venous Tissue, Open Approach

03190A3 Bypass Right Ulnar Artery to Right Lower Arm Artery with Autologous Arterial Tissue, Open Approach

03190AF Bypass Right Ulnar Artery to Lower Arm Vein with Autologous Arterial Tissue, Open Approach

03190J3 Bypass Right Ulnar Artery to Right Lower Arm Artery with Synthetic Substitute, Open Approach

03190JF Bypass Right Ulnar Artery to Lower Arm Vein with Synthetic Substitute, Open Approach

03190K3 Bypass Right Ulnar Artery to Right Lower Arm Artery with Nonautologous Tissue Substitute, Open Approach

03190KF Bypass Right Ulnar Artery to Lower Arm Vein with Nonautologous Tissue Substitute, Open Approach

03190Z3 Bypass Right Ulnar Artery to Right Lower Arm Artery, Open Approach

03190ZF Bypass Right Ulnar Artery to Lower Arm Vein, Open Approach

031A094 Bypass Left Ulnar Artery to Left Lower Arm Artery with Autologous Venous Tissue, Open Approach

031A09F Bypass Left Ulnar Artery to Lower Arm Vein with Autologous Venous Tissue, Open Approach

031A0A4 Bypass Left Ulnar Artery to Left Lower Arm Artery with Autologous Arterial Tissue, Open Approach

031A0AF Bypass Left Ulnar Artery to Lower Arm Vein with Autologous Arterial Tissue, Open Approach

031A0J4 Bypass Left Ulnar Artery to Left Lower Arm Artery with Synthetic Substitute, Open Approach

031A0JF Bypass Left Ulnar Artery to Lower Arm Vein with Synthetic Substitute, Open Approach

031A0K4 Bypass Left Ulnar Artery to Left Lower Arm Artery with Nonautologous Tissue Substitute, Open Approach

031A0KF Bypass Left Ulnar Artery to Lower Arm Vein with Nonautologous Tissue Substitute, Open Approach

031A0Z4 Bypass Left Ulnar Artery to Left Lower Arm Artery, Open Approach

031A0ZF Bypass Left Ulnar Artery to Lower Arm Vein, Open Approach

031B093 Bypass Right Radial Artery to Right Lower Arm Artery with Autologous Venous Tissue, Open Approach

031B09F Bypass Right Radial Artery to Lower Arm Vein with Autologous Venous Tissue, Open Approach

031B0A3 Bypass Right Radial Artery to Right Lower Arm Artery with Autologous Arterial Tissue, Open Approach

031B0AF Bypass Right Radial Artery to Lower Arm Vein with Autologous Arterial Tissue, Open Approach

031B0J3 Bypass Right Radial Artery to Right Lower Arm Artery with Synthetic Substitute, Open Approach

031B0JF Bypass Right Radial Artery to Lower Arm Vein with Synthetic Substitute, Open Approach

031B0K3 Bypass Right Radial Artery to Right Lower Arm Artery with Nonautologous Tissue Substitute, Open Approach

031B0KF Bypass Right Radial Artery to Lower Arm Vein with Nonautologous Tissue Substitute, Open Approach

031B0Z3 Bypass Right Radial Artery to Right Lower Arm Artery, Open Approach

031B0ZF Bypass Right Radial Artery to Lower Arm Vein, Open Approach

031C094 Bypass Left Radial Artery to Left Lower Arm Artery with Autologous Venous Tissue, Open Approach

031C09F Bypass Left Radial Artery to Lower Arm Vein with Autologous Venous Tissue, Open Approach

031C0A4 Bypass Left Radial Artery to Left Lower Arm Artery with Autologous Arterial Tissue, Open Approach

031C0AF Bypass Left Radial Artery to Lower Arm Vein with Autologous Arterial Tissue, Open Approach

031C0J4 Bypass Left Radial Artery to Left Lower Arm Artery with Synthetic Substitute, Open Approach

031C0JF Bypass Left Radial Artery to Lower Arm Vein with Synthetic Substitute, Open Approach

031C0K4 Bypass Left Radial Artery to Left Lower Arm Artery with Nonautologous Tissue Substitute, Open Approach

031C0KF Bypass Left Radial Artery to Lower Arm Vein with Nonautologous Tissue Substitute, Open Approach

031C0Z4 Bypass Left Radial Artery to Left Lower Arm Artery, Open Approach

031C0ZF Bypass Left Radial Artery to Lower Arm Vein, Open Approach

031G09G Bypass Intracranial Artery to Intracranial Artery with Autologous Venous Tissue, Open Approach

031G0AG Bypass Intracranial Artery to Intracranial Artery with Autologous Arterial Tissue, Open Approach

031G0JG Bypass Intracranial Artery to Intracranial Artery with Synthetic Substitute, Open Approach

031G0KG Bypass Intracranial Artery to Intracranial Artery with Nonautologous Tissue Substitute, Open Approach

031G0ZG Bypass Intracranial Artery to Intracranial Artery, Open Approach

031H09G Bypass Right Common Carotid Artery to Intracranial Artery with Autologous Venous Tissue, Open Approach

⬣ **031H09J** Bypass Right Common Carotid Artery to Right Extracranial Artery with Autologous Venous Tissue, Open Approach

031H0AG Bypass Right Common Carotid Artery to Intracranial Artery with Autologous Arterial Tissue, Open Approach

⬣ **031H0AJ** Bypass Right Common Carotid Artery to Right Extracranial Artery with Autologous Arterial Tissue, Open Approach

031H0JG Bypass Right Common Carotid Artery to Intracranial Artery with Synthetic Substitute, Open Approach

⬣ **031H0JJ** Bypass Right Common Carotid Artery to Right Extracranial Artery with Synthetic Substitute, Open Approach

031H0KG Bypass Right Common Carotid Artery to Intracranial Artery with Nonautologous Tissue Substitute, Open Approach

⬣ **031H0KJ** Bypass Right Common Carotid Artery to Right Extracranial Artery with Nonautologous Tissue Substitute, Open Approach

031H0ZG Bypass Right Common Carotid Artery to Intracranial Artery, Open Approach

⬣ **031H0ZJ** Bypass Right Common Carotid Artery to Right Extracranial Artery, Open Approach

031J09G Bypass Left Common Carotid Artery to Intracranial Artery with Autologous Venous Tissue, Open Approach

⬣ **031J09K** Bypass Left Common Carotid Artery to Left Extracranial Artery with Autologous Venous Tissue, Open Approach

031J0AG Bypass Left Common Carotid Artery to Intracranial Artery with Autologous Arterial Tissue, Open Approach

⬣ **031J0AK** Bypass Left Common Carotid Artery to Left Extracranial Artery with Autologous Arterial Tissue, Open Approach

031J0JG Bypass Left Common Carotid Artery to Intracranial Artery with Synthetic Substitute, Open Approach

⬣ **031J0JK** Bypass Left Common Carotid Artery to Left Extracranial Artery with Synthetic Substitute, Open Approach

---

♀ Female-only   ♂ Male-only   ◐ Limited Coverage   ● Non-OR   🅷🅰🅲 HAC-associated procedure   ⬣ Non-covered procedures   ➕ Combination

⬟ 031J0KG   Bypass Left Common Carotid Artery to Intracranial Artery with Nonautologous Tissue Substitute, Open Approach

⬟ 031J0KK   Bypass Left Common Carotid Artery to Left Extracranial Artery with Nonautologous Tissue Substitute, Open Approach

031J0ZG   Bypass Left Common Carotid Artery to Intracranial Artery, Open Approach

⬟ 031J0ZK   Bypass Left Common Carotid Artery to Left Extracranial Artery, Open Approach

⬟ 031K09J   Bypass Right Internal Carotid Artery to Right Extracranial Artery with Autologous Venous Tissue, Open Approach

⬟ 031K0AJ   Bypass Right Internal Carotid Artery to Right Extracranial Artery with Autologous Arterial Tissue, Open Approach

⬟ 031K0JJ   Bypass Right Internal Carotid Artery to Right Extracranial Artery with Synthetic Substitute, Open Approach

⬟ 031K0KJ   Bypass Right Internal Carotid Artery to Right Extracranial Artery with Nonautologous Tissue Substitute, Open Approach

⬟ 031K0ZJ   Bypass Right Internal Carotid Artery to Right Extracranial Artery, Open Approach

⬟ 031L09K   Bypass Left Internal Carotid Artery to Left Extracranial Artery with Autologous Venous Tissue, Open Approach

⬟ 031L0AK   Bypass Left Internal Carotid Artery to Left Extracranial Artery with Autologous Arterial Tissue, Open Approach

⬟ 031L0JK   Bypass Left Internal Carotid Artery to Left Extracranial Artery with Synthetic Substitute, Open Approach

⬟ 031L0KK   Bypass Left Internal Carotid Artery to Left Extracranial Artery with Nonautologous Tissue Substitute, Open Approach

⬟ 031L0ZK   Bypass Left Internal Carotid Artery to Left Extracranial Artery, Open Approach

⬟ 031M09J   Bypass Right External Carotid Artery to Right Extracranial Artery with Autologous Venous Tissue, Open Approach

⬟ 031M0AJ   Bypass Right External Carotid Artery to Right Extracranial Artery with Autologous Arterial Tissue, Open Approach

⬟ 031M0JJ   Bypass Right External Carotid Artery to Right Extracranial Artery with Synthetic Substitute, Open Approach

⬟ 031M0KJ   Bypass Right External Carotid Artery to Right Extracranial Artery with Nonautologous Tissue Substitute, Open Approach

⬟ 031M0ZJ   Bypass Right External Carotid Artery to Right Extracranial Artery, Open Approach

⬟ 031N09K   Bypass Left External Carotid Artery to Left Extracranial Artery with Autologous Venous Tissue, Open Approach

⬟ 031N0AK   Bypass Left External Carotid Artery to Left Extracranial Artery with Autologous Arterial Tissue, Open Approach

⬟ 031N0JK   Bypass Left External Carotid Artery to Left Extracranial Artery with Synthetic Substitute, Open Approach

⬟ 031N0KK   Bypass Left External Carotid Artery to Left Extracranial Artery with Nonautologous Tissue Substitute, Open Approach

⬟ 031N0ZK   Bypass Left External Carotid Artery to Left Extracranial Artery, Open Approach

⬟ 031S09G   Bypass Right Temporal Artery to Intracranial Artery with Autologous Venous Tissue, Open Approach

⬟ 031S0AG   Bypass Right Temporal Artery to Intracranial Artery with Autologous Arterial Tissue, Open Approach

⬟ 031S0JG   Bypass Right Temporal Artery to Intracranial Artery with Synthetic Substitute, Open Approach

⬟ 031S0KG   Bypass Right Temporal Artery to Intracranial Artery with Nonautologous Tissue Substitute, Open Approach

⬟ 031S0ZG   Bypass Right Temporal Artery to Intracranial Artery, Open Approach

⬟ 031T09G   Bypass Left Temporal Artery to Intracranial Artery with Autologous Venous Tissue, Open Approach

⬟ 031T0AG   Bypass Left Temporal Artery to Intracranial Artery with Autologous Arterial Tissue, Open Approach

⬟ 031T0JG   Bypass Left Temporal Artery to Intracranial Artery with Synthetic Substitute, Open Approach

⬟ 031T0KG   Bypass Left Temporal Artery to Intracranial Artery with Nonautologous Tissue Substitute, Open Approach

⬟ 031T0ZG   Bypass Left Temporal Artery to Intracranial Artery, Open Approach

035 – Upper Arteries, Destruction

03500ZZ   Destruction of Right Internal Mammary Artery, Open Approach

03503ZZ   Destruction of Right Internal Mammary Artery, Percutaneous Approach

03504ZZ   Destruction of Right Internal Mammary Artery, Percutaneous Endoscopic Approach

03510ZZ   Destruction of Left Internal Mammary Artery, Open Approach

03513ZZ   Destruction of Left Internal Mammary Artery, Percutaneous Approach

03514ZZ   Destruction of Left Internal Mammary Artery, Percutaneous Endoscopic Approach

03520ZZ   Destruction of Innominate Artery, Open Approach

03523ZZ   Destruction of Innominate Artery, Percutaneous Approach

03524ZZ   Destruction of Innominate Artery, Percutaneous Endoscopic Approach

03530ZZ   Destruction of Right Subclavian Artery, Open Approach

03533ZZ   Destruction of Right Subclavian Artery, Percutaneous Approach

03534ZZ   Destruction of Right Subclavian Artery, Percutaneous Endoscopic Approach

03540ZZ   Destruction of Left Subclavian Artery, Open Approach

03543ZZ   Destruction of Left Subclavian Artery, Percutaneous Approach

03544ZZ   Destruction of Left Subclavian Artery, Percutaneous Endoscopic Approach

03550ZZ   Destruction of Right Axillary Artery, Open Approach

03553ZZ   Destruction of Right Axillary Artery, Percutaneous Approach

03554ZZ   Destruction of Right Axillary Artery, Percutaneous Endoscopic Approach

03560ZZ   Destruction of Left Axillary Artery, Open Approach

03563ZZ   Destruction of Left Axillary Artery, Percutaneous Approach

03564ZZ   Destruction of Left Axillary Artery, Percutaneous Endoscopic Approach

03570ZZ   Destruction of Right Brachial Artery, Open Approach

03573ZZ   Destruction of Right Brachial Artery, Percutaneous Approach

03574ZZ   Destruction of Right Brachial Artery, Percutaneous Endoscopic Approach

03580ZZ   Destruction of Left Brachial Artery, Open Approach

03583ZZ   Destruction of Left Brachial Artery, Percutaneous Approach

03584ZZ   Destruction of Left Brachial Artery, Percutaneous Endoscopic Approach

03590ZZ   Destruction of Right Ulnar Artery, Open Approach

03593ZZ   Destruction of Right Ulnar Artery, Percutaneous Approach

03594ZZ   Destruction of Right Ulnar Artery, Percutaneous Endoscopic Approach

035A0ZZ   Destruction of Left Ulnar Artery, Open Approach

035A3ZZ   Destruction of Left Ulnar Artery, Percutaneous Approach

035A4ZZ   Destruction of Left Ulnar Artery, Percutaneous Endoscopic Approach

035B0ZZ   Destruction of Right Radial Artery, Open Approach

035B3ZZ   Destruction of Right Radial Artery, Percutaneous Approach

035B4ZZ   Destruction of Right Radial Artery, Percutaneous Endoscopic Approach

035C0ZZ   Destruction of Left Radial Artery, Open Approach

035C3ZZ   Destruction of Left Radial Artery, Percutaneous Approach

035C4ZZ   Destruction of Left Radial Artery, Percutaneous Endoscopic Approach

035D0ZZ   Destruction of Right Hand Artery, Open Approach

035D3ZZ   Destruction of Right Hand Artery, Percutaneous Approach

035D4ZZ   Destruction of Right Hand Artery, Percutaneous Endoscopic Approach

035F0ZZ   Destruction of Left Hand Artery, Open Approach

035F3ZZ   Destruction of Left Hand Artery, Percutaneous Approach

035F4ZZ   Destruction of Left Hand Artery, Percutaneous Endoscopic Approach

035G0ZZ   Destruction of Intracranial Artery, Open Approach

035G3ZZ   Destruction of Intracranial Artery, Percutaneous Approach

035G4ZZ   Destruction of Intracranial Artery, Percutaneous Endoscopic Approach

035H0ZZ   Destruction of Right Common Carotid Artery, Open Approach

035H3ZZ   Destruction of Right Common Carotid Artery, Percutaneous Approach

035H4ZZ   Destruction of Right Common Carotid Artery, Percutaneous Endoscopic Approach

035J0ZZ   Destruction of Left Common Carotid Artery, Open Approach

035J3ZZ Destruction of Left Common Carotid Artery, Percutaneous Approach

035J4ZZ Destruction of Left Common Carotid Artery, Percutaneous Endoscopic Approach

035K0ZZ Destruction of Right Internal Carotid Artery, Open Approach

035K3ZZ Destruction of Right Internal Carotid Artery, Percutaneous Approach

035K4ZZ Destruction of Right Internal Carotid Artery, Percutaneous Endoscopic Approach

035L0ZZ Destruction of Left Internal Carotid Artery, Open Approach

035L3ZZ Destruction of Left Internal Carotid Artery, Percutaneous Approach

035L4ZZ Destruction of Left Internal Carotid Artery, Percutaneous Endoscopic Approach

035M0ZZ Destruction of Right External Carotid Artery, Open Approach

035M3ZZ Destruction of Right External Carotid Artery, Percutaneous Approach

035M4ZZ Destruction of Right External Carotid Artery, Percutaneous Endoscopic Approach

035N0ZZ Destruction of Left External Carotid Artery, Open Approach

035N3ZZ Destruction of Left External Carotid Artery, Percutaneous Approach

035N4ZZ Destruction of Left External Carotid Artery, Percutaneous Endoscopic Approach

035P0ZZ Destruction of Right Vertebral Artery, Open Approach

035P3ZZ Destruction of Right Vertebral Artery, Percutaneous Approach

035P4ZZ Destruction of Right Vertebral Artery, Percutaneous Endoscopic Approach

035Q0ZZ Destruction of Left Vertebral Artery, Open Approach

035Q3ZZ Destruction of Left Vertebral Artery, Percutaneous Approach

035Q4ZZ Destruction of Left Vertebral Artery, Percutaneous Endoscopic Approach

035R0ZZ Destruction of Face Artery, Open Approach

035R3ZZ Destruction of Face Artery, Percutaneous Approach

035R4ZZ Destruction of Face Artery, Percutaneous Endoscopic Approach

035S0ZZ Destruction of Right Temporal Artery, Open Approach

035S3ZZ Destruction of Right Temporal Artery, Percutaneous Approach

035S4ZZ Destruction of Right Temporal Artery, Percutaneous Endoscopic Approach

035T0ZZ Destruction of Left Temporal Artery, Open Approach

035T3ZZ Destruction of Left Temporal Artery, Percutaneous Approach

035T4ZZ Destruction of Left Temporal Artery, Percutaneous Endoscopic Approach

035U0ZZ Destruction of Right Thyroid Artery, Open Approach

035U3ZZ Destruction of Right Thyroid Artery, Percutaneous Approach

035U4ZZ Destruction of Right Thyroid Artery, Percutaneous Endoscopic Approach

035V0ZZ Destruction of Left Thyroid Artery, Open Approach

035V3ZZ Destruction of Left Thyroid Artery, Percutaneous Approach

035V4ZZ Destruction of Left Thyroid Artery, Percutaneous Endoscopic Approach

035Y0ZZ Destruction of Upper Artery, Open Approach

035Y3ZZ Destruction of Upper Artery, Percutaneous Approach

035Y4ZZ Destruction of Upper Artery, Percutaneous Endoscopic Approach

037 – Upper Arteries, Dilation

037004Z Dilation of Right Internal Mammary Artery with Drug-eluting Intraluminal Device, Open Approach

03700DZ Dilation of Right Internal Mammary Artery with Intraluminal Device, Open Approach

03700ZZ Dilation of Right Internal Mammary Artery, Open Approach

037034Z Dilation of Right Internal Mammary Artery with Drug-eluting Intraluminal Device, Percutaneous Approach

03703DZ Dilation of Right Internal Mammary Artery with Intraluminal Device, Percutaneous Approach

03703ZZ Dilation of Right Internal Mammary Artery, Percutaneous Approach

037044Z Dilation of Right Internal Mammary Artery with Drug-eluting Intraluminal Device, Percutaneous Endoscopic Approach

03704DZ Dilation of Right Internal Mammary Artery with Intraluminal Device, Percutaneous Endoscopic Approach

03704ZZ Dilation of Right Internal Mammary Artery, Percutaneous Endoscopic Approach

037104Z Dilation of Left Internal Mammary Artery with Drug-eluting Intraluminal Device, Open Approach

03710DZ Dilation of Left Internal Mammary Artery with Intraluminal Device, Open Approach

03710ZZ Dilation of Left Internal Mammary Artery, Open Approach

037134Z Dilation of Left Internal Mammary Artery with Drug-eluting Intraluminal Device, Percutaneous Approach

03713DZ Dilation of Left Internal Mammary Artery with Intraluminal Device, Percutaneous Approach

03713ZZ Dilation of Left Internal Mammary Artery, Percutaneous Approach

037144Z Dilation of Left Internal Mammary Artery with Drug-eluting Intraluminal Device, Percutaneous Endoscopic Approach

03714DZ Dilation of Left Internal Mammary Artery with Intraluminal Device, Percutaneous Endoscopic Approach

03714ZZ Dilation of Left Internal Mammary Artery, Percutaneous Endoscopic Approach

037204Z Dilation of Innominate Artery with Drug-eluting Intraluminal Device, Open Approach

03720DZ Dilation of Innominate Artery with Intraluminal Device, Open Approach

03720ZZ Dilation of Innominate Artery, Open Approach

037234Z Dilation of Innominate Artery with Drug-eluting Intraluminal Device, Percutaneous Approach

03723DZ Dilation of Innominate Artery with Intraluminal Device, Percutaneous Approach

03723ZZ Dilation of Innominate Artery, Percutaneous Approach

037244Z Dilation of Innominate Artery with Drug-eluting Intraluminal Device, Percutaneous Endoscopic Approach

03724DZ Dilation of Innominate Artery with Intraluminal Device, Percutaneous Endoscopic Approach

03724ZZ Dilation of Innominate Artery, Percutaneous Endoscopic Approach

037304Z Dilation of Right Subclavian Artery with Drug-eluting Intraluminal Device, Open Approach

03730DZ Dilation of Right Subclavian Artery with Intraluminal Device, Open Approach

03730ZZ Dilation of Right Subclavian Artery, Open Approach

037334Z Dilation of Right Subclavian Artery with Drug-eluting Intraluminal Device, Percutaneous Approach

03733DZ Dilation of Right Subclavian Artery with Intraluminal Device, Percutaneous Approach

03733ZZ Dilation of Right Subclavian Artery, Percutaneous Approach

037344Z Dilation of Right Subclavian Artery with Drug-eluting Intraluminal Device, Percutaneous Endoscopic Approach

03734DZ Dilation of Right Subclavian Artery with Intraluminal Device, Percutaneous Endoscopic Approach

03734ZZ Dilation of Right Subclavian Artery, Percutaneous Endoscopic Approach

037404Z Dilation of Left Subclavian Artery with Drug-eluting Intraluminal Device, Open Approach

03740DZ Dilation of Left Subclavian Artery with Intraluminal Device, Open Approach

03740ZZ Dilation of Left Subclavian Artery, Open Approach

037434Z Dilation of Left Subclavian Artery with Drug-eluting Intraluminal Device, Percutaneous Approach

03743DZ Dilation of Left Subclavian Artery with Intraluminal Device, Percutaneous Approach

03743ZZ Dilation of Left Subclavian Artery, Percutaneous Approach

037444Z Dilation of Left Subclavian Artery with Drug-eluting Intraluminal Device, Percutaneous Endoscopic Approach

03744DZ Dilation of Left Subclavian Artery with Intraluminal Device, Percutaneous Endoscopic Approach

03744ZZ Dilation of Left Subclavian Artery, Percutaneous Endoscopic Approach

037504Z Dilation of Right Axillary Artery with Drug-eluting Intraluminal Device, Open Approach

03750DZ Dilation of Right Axillary Artery with Intraluminal Device, Open Approach

03750ZZ Dilation of Right Axillary Artery, Open Approach

037534Z Dilation of Right Axillary Artery with Drug-eluting Intraluminal Device, Percutaneous Approach

03753DZ Dilation of Right Axillary Artery with Intraluminal Device, Percutaneous Approach

03753ZZ Dilation of Right Axillary Artery, Percutaneous Approach

037544Z	Dilation of Right Axillary Artery with Drug-eluting Intraluminal Device, Percutaneous Endoscopic Approach
03754DZ	Dilation of Right Axillary Artery with Intraluminal Device, Percutaneous Endoscopic Approach
03754ZZ	Dilation of Right Axillary Artery, Percutaneous Endoscopic Approach
037604Z	Dilation of Left Axillary Artery with Drug-eluting Intraluminal Device, Open Approach
03760DZ	Dilation of Left Axillary Artery with Intraluminal Device, Open Approach
03760ZZ	Dilation of Left Axillary Artery, Open Approach
037634Z	Dilation of Left Axillary Artery with Drug-eluting Intraluminal Device, Percutaneous Approach
03763DZ	Dilation of Left Axillary Artery with Intraluminal Device, Percutaneous Approach
03763ZZ	Dilation of Left Axillary Artery, Percutaneous Approach
037644Z	Dilation of Left Axillary Artery with Drug-eluting Intraluminal Device, Percutaneous Endoscopic Approach
03764DZ	Dilation of Left Axillary Artery with Intraluminal Device, Percutaneous Endoscopic Approach
03764ZZ	Dilation of Left Axillary Artery, Percutaneous Endoscopic Approach
037704Z	Dilation of Right Brachial Artery with Drug-eluting Intraluminal Device, Open Approach
03770DZ	Dilation of Right Brachial Artery with Intraluminal Device, Open Approach
03770ZZ	Dilation of Right Brachial Artery, Open Approach
037734Z	Dilation of Right Brachial Artery with Drug-eluting Intraluminal Device, Percutaneous Approach
03773DZ	Dilation of Right Brachial Artery with Intraluminal Device, Percutaneous Approach
03773ZZ	Dilation of Right Brachial Artery, Percutaneous Approach
037744Z	Dilation of Right Brachial Artery with Drug-eluting Intraluminal Device, Percutaneous Endoscopic Approach
03774DZ	Dilation of Right Brachial Artery with Intraluminal Device, Percutaneous Endoscopic Approach
03774ZZ	Dilation of Right Brachial Artery, Percutaneous Endoscopic Approach
037804Z	Dilation of Left Brachial Artery with Drug-eluting Intraluminal Device, Open Approach
03780DZ	Dilation of Left Brachial Artery with Intraluminal Device, Open Approach
03780ZZ	Dilation of Left Brachial Artery, Open Approach
037834Z	Dilation of Left Brachial Artery with Drug-eluting Intraluminal Device, Percutaneous Approach
03783DZ	Dilation of Left Brachial Artery with Intraluminal Device, Percutaneous Approach
03783ZZ	Dilation of Left Brachial Artery, Percutaneous Approach
037844Z	Dilation of Left Brachial Artery with Drug-eluting Intraluminal Device, Percutaneous Endoscopic Approach
03784DZ	Dilation of Left Brachial Artery with Intraluminal Device, Percutaneous Endoscopic Approach
03784ZZ	Dilation of Left Brachial Artery, Percutaneous Endoscopic Approach
037904Z	Dilation of Right Ulnar Artery with Drug-eluting Intraluminal Device, Open Approach
03790DZ	Dilation of Right Ulnar Artery with Intraluminal Device, Open Approach
03790ZZ	Dilation of Right Ulnar Artery, Open Approach
037934Z	Dilation of Right Ulnar Artery with Drug-eluting Intraluminal Device, Percutaneous Approach
03793DZ	Dilation of Right Ulnar Artery with Intraluminal Device, Percutaneous Approach
03793ZZ	Dilation of Right Ulnar Artery, Percutaneous Approach
037944Z	Dilation of Right Ulnar Artery with Drug-eluting Intraluminal Device, Percutaneous Endoscopic Approach
03794DZ	Dilation of Right Ulnar Artery with Intraluminal Device, Percutaneous Endoscopic Approach
03794ZZ	Dilation of Right Ulnar Artery, Percutaneous Endoscopic Approach
037A04Z	Dilation of Left Ulnar Artery with Drug-eluting Intraluminal Device, Open Approach
037A0DZ	Dilation of Left Ulnar Artery with Intraluminal Device, Open Approach
037A0ZZ	Dilation of Left Ulnar Artery, Open Approach
037A34Z	Dilation of Left Ulnar Artery with Drug-eluting Intraluminal Device, Percutaneous Approach
037A3DZ	Dilation of Left Ulnar Artery with Intraluminal Device, Percutaneous Approach
037A3ZZ	Dilation of Left Ulnar Artery, Percutaneous Approach
037A44Z	Dilation of Left Ulnar Artery with Drug-eluting Intraluminal Device, Percutaneous Endoscopic Approach
037A4DZ	Dilation of Left Ulnar Artery with Intraluminal Device, Percutaneous Endoscopic Approach
037A4ZZ	Dilation of Left Ulnar Artery, Percutaneous Endoscopic Approach
037B04Z	Dilation of Right Radial Artery with Drug-eluting Intraluminal Device, Open Approach
037B0DZ	Dilation of Right Radial Artery with Intraluminal Device, Open Approach
037B0ZZ	Dilation of Right Radial Artery, Open Approach
037B34Z	Dilation of Right Radial Artery with Drug-eluting Intraluminal Device, Percutaneous Approach
037B3DZ	Dilation of Right Radial Artery with Intraluminal Device, Percutaneous Approach
037B3ZZ	Dilation of Right Radial Artery, Percutaneous Approach
037B44Z	Dilation of Right Radial Artery with Drug-eluting Intraluminal Device, Percutaneous Endoscopic Approach
037B4DZ	Dilation of Right Radial Artery with Intraluminal Device, Percutaneous Endoscopic Approach
037B4ZZ	Dilation of Right Radial Artery, Percutaneous Endoscopic Approach
037C04Z	Dilation of Left Radial Artery with Drug-eluting Intraluminal Device, Open Approach
037C0DZ	Dilation of Left Radial Artery with Intraluminal Device, Open Approach
037C0ZZ	Dilation of Left Radial Artery, Open Approach
037C34Z	Dilation of Left Radial Artery with Drug-eluting Intraluminal Device, Percutaneous Approach
037C3DZ	Dilation of Left Radial Artery with Intraluminal Device, Percutaneous Approach
037C3ZZ	Dilation of Left Radial Artery, Percutaneous Approach
037C44Z	Dilation of Left Radial Artery with Drug-eluting Intraluminal Device, Percutaneous Endoscopic Approach
037C4DZ	Dilation of Left Radial Artery with Intraluminal Device, Percutaneous Endoscopic Approach
037C4ZZ	Dilation of Left Radial Artery, Percutaneous Endoscopic Approach
037D04Z	Dilation of Right Hand Artery with Drug-eluting Intraluminal Device, Open Approach
037D0DZ	Dilation of Right Hand Artery with Intraluminal Device, Open Approach
037D0ZZ	Dilation of Right Hand Artery, Open Approach
037D34Z	Dilation of Right Hand Artery with Drug-eluting Intraluminal Device, Percutaneous Approach
037D3DZ	Dilation of Right Hand Artery with Intraluminal Device, Percutaneous Approach
037D3ZZ	Dilation of Right Hand Artery, Percutaneous Approach
037D44Z	Dilation of Right Hand Artery with Drug-eluting Intraluminal Device, Percutaneous Endoscopic Approach
037D4DZ	Dilation of Right Hand Artery with Intraluminal Device, Percutaneous Endoscopic Approach
037D4ZZ	Dilation of Right Hand Artery, Percutaneous Endoscopic Approach
037F04Z	Dilation of Left Hand Artery with Drug-eluting Intraluminal Device, Open Approach
037F0DZ	Dilation of Left Hand Artery with Intraluminal Device, Open Approach
037F0ZZ	Dilation of Left Hand Artery, Open Approach
037F34Z	Dilation of Left Hand Artery with Drug-eluting Intraluminal Device, Percutaneous Approach
037F3DZ	Dilation of Left Hand Artery with Intraluminal Device, Percutaneous Approach
037F3ZZ	Dilation of Left Hand Artery, Percutaneous Approach
037F44Z	Dilation of Left Hand Artery with Drug-eluting Intraluminal Device, Percutaneous Endoscopic Approach
037F4DZ	Dilation of Left Hand Artery with Intraluminal Device, Percutaneous Endoscopic Approach
037F4ZZ	Dilation of Left Hand Artery, Percutaneous Endoscopic Approach
037G04Z	Dilation of Intracranial Artery with Drug-eluting Intraluminal Device, Open Approach
037G0DZ	Dilation of Intracranial Artery with Intraluminal Device, Open Approach
037G0ZZ	Dilation of Intracranial Artery, Open Approach
037G34Z	Dilation of Intracranial Artery with Drug-eluting Intraluminal Device, Percutaneous Approach

037G3DZ Dilation of Intracranial Artery with Intraluminal Device, Percutaneous Approach

● **037G3ZZ** Dilation of Intracranial Artery, Percutaneous Approach

037G44Z Dilation of Intracranial Artery with Drug-eluting Intraluminal Device, Percutaneous Endoscopic Approach

037G4DZ Dilation of Intracranial Artery with Intraluminal Device, Percutaneous Endoscopic Approach

● **037G4ZZ** Dilation of Intracranial Artery, Percutaneous Endoscopic Approach

037H04Z Dilation of Right Common Carotid Artery with Drug-eluting Intraluminal Device, Open Approach

037H0DZ Dilation of Right Common Carotid Artery with Intraluminal Device, Open Approach

037H0ZZ Dilation of Right Common Carotid Artery, Open Approach

037H34Z Dilation of Right Common Carotid Artery with Drug-eluting Intraluminal Device, Percutaneous Approach

037H3DZ Dilation of Right Common Carotid Artery with Intraluminal Device, Percutaneous Approach

037H3ZZ Dilation of Right Common Carotid Artery, Percutaneous Approach

037H44Z Dilation of Right Common Carotid Artery with Drug-eluting Intraluminal Device, Percutaneous Endoscopic Approach

037H4DZ Dilation of Right Common Carotid Artery with Intraluminal Device, Percutaneous Endoscopic Approach

037H4ZZ Dilation of Right Common Carotid Artery, Percutaneous Endoscopic Approach

037J04Z Dilation of Left Common Carotid Artery with Drug-eluting Intraluminal Device, Open Approach

037J0DZ Dilation of Left Common Carotid Artery with Intraluminal Device, Open Approach

037J0ZZ Dilation of Left Common Carotid Artery, Open Approach

037J34Z Dilation of Left Common Carotid Artery with Drug-eluting Intraluminal Device, Percutaneous Approach

037J3DZ Dilation of Left Common Carotid Artery with Intraluminal Device, Percutaneous Approach

037J3ZZ Dilation of Left Common Carotid Artery, Percutaneous Approach

037J44Z Dilation of Left Common Carotid Artery with Drug-eluting Intraluminal Device, Percutaneous Endoscopic Approach

037J4DZ Dilation of Left Common Carotid Artery with Intraluminal Device, Percutaneous Endoscopic Approach

037J4ZZ Dilation of Left Common Carotid Artery, Percutaneous Endoscopic Approach

037K04Z Dilation of Right Internal Carotid Artery with Drug-eluting Intraluminal Device, Open Approach

037K0DZ Dilation of Right Internal Carotid Artery with Intraluminal Device, Open Approach

037K0ZZ Dilation of Right Internal Carotid Artery, Open Approach

037K34Z Dilation of Right Internal Carotid Artery with Drug-eluting Intraluminal Device, Percutaneous Approach

037K3DZ Dilation of Right Internal Carotid Artery with Intraluminal Device, Percutaneous Approach

037K3ZZ Dilation of Right Internal Carotid Artery, Percutaneous Approach

037K44Z Dilation of Right Internal Carotid Artery with Drug-eluting Intraluminal Device, Percutaneous Endoscopic Approach

037K4DZ Dilation of Right Internal Carotid Artery with Intraluminal Device, Percutaneous Endoscopic Approach

037K4ZZ Dilation of Right Internal Carotid Artery, Percutaneous Endoscopic Approach

037L04Z Dilation of Left Internal Carotid Artery with Drug-eluting Intraluminal Device, Open Approach

037L0DZ Dilation of Left Internal Carotid Artery with Intraluminal Device, Open Approach

037L0ZZ Dilation of Left Internal Carotid Artery, Open Approach

037L34Z Dilation of Left Internal Carotid Artery with Drug-eluting Intraluminal Device, Percutaneous Approach

037L3DZ Dilation of Left Internal Carotid Artery with Intraluminal Device, Percutaneous Approach

037L3ZZ Dilation of Left Internal Carotid Artery, Percutaneous Approach

037L44Z Dilation of Left Internal Carotid Artery with Drug-eluting Intraluminal Device, Percutaneous Endoscopic Approach

037L4DZ Dilation of Left Internal Carotid Artery with Intraluminal Device, Percutaneous Endoscopic Approach

037L4ZZ Dilation of Left Internal Carotid Artery, Percutaneous Endoscopic Approach

037M04Z Dilation of Right External Carotid Artery with Drug-eluting Intraluminal Device, Open Approach

037M0DZ Dilation of Right External Carotid Artery with Intraluminal Device, Open Approach

037M0ZZ Dilation of Right External Carotid Artery, Open Approach

037M34Z Dilation of Right External Carotid Artery with Drug-eluting Intraluminal Device, Percutaneous Approach

037M3DZ Dilation of Right External Carotid Artery with Intraluminal Device, Percutaneous Approach

037M3ZZ Dilation of Right External Carotid Artery, Percutaneous Approach

037M44Z Dilation of Right External Carotid Artery with Drug-eluting Intraluminal Device, Percutaneous Endoscopic Approach

037M4DZ Dilation of Right External Carotid Artery with Intraluminal Device, Percutaneous Endoscopic Approach

037M4ZZ Dilation of Right External Carotid Artery, Percutaneous Endoscopic Approach

037N04Z Dilation of Left External Carotid Artery with Drug-eluting Intraluminal Device, Open Approach

037N0DZ Dilation of Left External Carotid Artery with Intraluminal Device, Open Approach

037N0ZZ Dilation of Left External Carotid Artery, Open Approach

037N34Z Dilation of Left External Carotid Artery with Drug-eluting Intraluminal Device, Percutaneous Approach

037N3DZ Dilation of Left External Carotid Artery with Intraluminal Device, Percutaneous Approach

037N3ZZ Dilation of Left External Carotid Artery, Percutaneous Approach

037N44Z Dilation of Left External Carotid Artery with Drug-eluting Intraluminal Device, Percutaneous Endoscopic Approach

037N4DZ Dilation of Left External Carotid Artery with Intraluminal Device, Percutaneous Endoscopic Approach

037N4ZZ Dilation of Left External Carotid Artery, Percutaneous Endoscopic Approach

037P04Z Dilation of Right Vertebral Artery with Drug-eluting Intraluminal Device, Open Approach

037P0DZ Dilation of Right Vertebral Artery with Intraluminal Device, Open Approach

037P0ZZ Dilation of Right Vertebral Artery, Open Approach

037P34Z Dilation of Right Vertebral Artery with Drug-eluting Intraluminal Device, Percutaneous Approach

037P3DZ Dilation of Right Vertebral Artery with Intraluminal Device, Percutaneous Approach

037P3ZZ Dilation of Right Vertebral Artery, Percutaneous Approach

037P44Z Dilation of Right Vertebral Artery with Drug-eluting Intraluminal Device, Percutaneous Endoscopic Approach

037P4DZ Dilation of Right Vertebral Artery with Intraluminal Device, Percutaneous Endoscopic Approach

037P4ZZ Dilation of Right Vertebral Artery, Percutaneous Endoscopic Approach

037Q04Z Dilation of Left Vertebral Artery with Drug-eluting Intraluminal Device, Open Approach

037Q0DZ Dilation of Left Vertebral Artery with Intraluminal Device, Open Approach

037Q0ZZ Dilation of Left Vertebral Artery, Open Approach

037Q34Z Dilation of Left Vertebral Artery with Drug-eluting Intraluminal Device, Percutaneous Approach

037Q3DZ Dilation of Left Vertebral Artery with Intraluminal Device, Percutaneous Approach

037Q3ZZ Dilation of Left Vertebral Artery, Percutaneous Approach

037Q44Z Dilation of Left Vertebral Artery with Drug-eluting Intraluminal Device, Percutaneous Endoscopic Approach

037Q4DZ Dilation of Left Vertebral Artery with Intraluminal Device, Percutaneous Endoscopic Approach

037Q4ZZ Dilation of Left Vertebral Artery, Percutaneous Endoscopic Approach

037R04Z Dilation of Face Artery with Drug-eluting Intraluminal Device, Open Approach

037R0DZ Dilation of Face Artery with Intraluminal Device, Open Approach

037R0ZZ Dilation of Face Artery, Open Approach

037R34Z Dilation of Face Artery with Drug-eluting Intraluminal Device, Percutaneous Approach

037R3DZ Dilation of Face Artery with Intraluminal Device, Percutaneous Approach

037R3ZZ Dilation of Face Artery, Percutaneous Approach

037R44Z Dilation of Face Artery with Drug-eluting Intraluminal Device, Percutaneous Endoscopic Approach

037R4DZ Dilation of Face Artery with Intraluminal Device, Percutaneous Endoscopic Approach

---

♀ Female-only   ♂ Male-only   ● Limited Coverage   ● Non-OR   **HAC** HAC-associated procedure   ● Non-covered procedures   ✚ Combination

037R4ZZ   Dilation of Face Artery, Percutaneous Endoscopic Approach

037S04Z   Dilation of Right Temporal Artery with Drug-eluting Intraluminal Device, Open Approach

037S0DZ   Dilation of Right Temporal Artery with Intraluminal Device, Open Approach

037S0ZZ   Dilation of Right Temporal Artery, Open Approach

037S34Z   Dilation of Right Temporal Artery with Drug-eluting Intraluminal Device, Percutaneous Approach

037S3DZ   Dilation of Right Temporal Artery with Intraluminal Device, Percutaneous Approach

037S3ZZ   Dilation of Right Temporal Artery, Percutaneous Approach

037S44Z   Dilation of Right Temporal Artery with Drug-eluting Intraluminal Device, Percutaneous Endoscopic Approach

037S4DZ   Dilation of Right Temporal Artery with Intraluminal Device, Percutaneous Endoscopic Approach

037S4ZZ   Dilation of Right Temporal Artery, Percutaneous Endoscopic Approach

037T04Z   Dilation of Left Temporal Artery with Drug-eluting Intraluminal Device, Open Approach

037T0DZ   Dilation of Left Temporal Artery with Intraluminal Device, Open Approach

037T0ZZ   Dilation of Left Temporal Artery, Open Approach

037T34Z   Dilation of Left Temporal Artery with Drug-eluting Intraluminal Device, Percutaneous Approach

037T3DZ   Dilation of Left Temporal Artery with Intraluminal Device, Percutaneous Approach

037T3ZZ   Dilation of Left Temporal Artery, Percutaneous Approach

037T44Z   Dilation of Left Temporal Artery with Drug-eluting Intraluminal Device, Percutaneous Endoscopic Approach

037T4DZ   Dilation of Left Temporal Artery with Intraluminal Device, Percutaneous Endoscopic Approach

037T4ZZ   Dilation of Left Temporal Artery, Percutaneous Endoscopic Approach

037U04Z   Dilation of Right Thyroid Artery with Drug-eluting Intraluminal Device, Open Approach

037U0DZ   Dilation of Right Thyroid Artery with Intraluminal Device, Open Approach

037U0ZZ   Dilation of Right Thyroid Artery, Open Approach

037U34Z   Dilation of Right Thyroid Artery with Drug-eluting Intraluminal Device, Percutaneous Approach

037U3DZ   Dilation of Right Thyroid Artery with Intraluminal Device, Percutaneous Approach

037U3ZZ   Dilation of Right Thyroid Artery, Percutaneous Approach

037U44Z   Dilation of Right Thyroid Artery with Drug-eluting Intraluminal Device, Percutaneous Endoscopic Approach

037U4DZ   Dilation of Right Thyroid Artery with Intraluminal Device, Percutaneous Endoscopic Approach

037U4ZZ   Dilation of Right Thyroid Artery, Percutaneous Endoscopic Approach

037V04Z   Dilation of Left Thyroid Artery with Drug-eluting Intraluminal Device, Open Approach

037V0DZ   Dilation of Left Thyroid Artery with Intraluminal Device, Open Approach

037V0ZZ   Dilation of Left Thyroid Artery, Open Approach

037V34Z   Dilation of Left Thyroid Artery with Drug-eluting Intraluminal Device, Percutaneous Approach

037V3DZ   Dilation of Left Thyroid Artery with Intraluminal Device, Percutaneous Approach

037V3ZZ   Dilation of Left Thyroid Artery, Percutaneous Approach

037V44Z   Dilation of Left Thyroid Artery with Drug-eluting Intraluminal Device, Percutaneous Endoscopic Approach

037V4DZ   Dilation of Left Thyroid Artery with Intraluminal Device, Percutaneous Endoscopic Approach

037V4ZZ   Dilation of Left Thyroid Artery, Percutaneous Endoscopic Approach

037Y04Z   Dilation of Upper Artery with Drug-eluting Intraluminal Device, Open Approach

037Y0DZ   Dilation of Upper Artery with Intraluminal Device, Open Approach

037Y0ZZ   Dilation of Upper Artery, Open Approach

037Y34Z   Dilation of Upper Artery with Drug-eluting Intraluminal Device, Percutaneous Approach

037Y3DZ   Dilation of Upper Artery with Intraluminal Device, Percutaneous Approach

037Y3ZZ   Dilation of Upper Artery, Percutaneous Approach

037Y44Z   Dilation of Upper Artery with Drug-eluting Intraluminal Device, Percutaneous Endoscopic Approach

037Y4DZ   Dilation of Upper Artery with Intraluminal Device, Percutaneous Endoscopic Approach

037Y4ZZ   Dilation of Upper Artery, Percutaneous Endoscopic Approach

039 – Upper Arteries, Drainage

Review Coding Guidelines B3.4a and B3.4b

Review Coding Guideline B6.2

039000Z   Drainage of Right Internal Mammary Artery with Drainage Device, Open Approach

03900ZX   Drainage of Right Internal Mammary Artery, Open Approach, Diagnostic

03900ZZ   Drainage of Right Internal Mammary Artery, Open Approach

039030Z   Drainage of Right Internal Mammary Artery with Drainage Device, Percutaneous Approach

03903ZX   Drainage of Right Internal Mammary Artery, Percutaneous Approach, Diagnostic

03903ZZ   Drainage of Right Internal Mammary Artery, Percutaneous Approach

039040Z   Drainage of Right Internal Mammary Artery with Drainage Device, Percutaneous Endoscopic Approach

03904ZX   Drainage of Right Internal Mammary Artery, Percutaneous Endoscopic Approach, Diagnostic

03904ZZ   Drainage of Right Internal Mammary Artery, Percutaneous Endoscopic Approach

039100Z   Drainage of Left Internal Mammary Artery with Drainage Device, Open Approach

03910ZX   Drainage of Left Internal Mammary Artery, Open Approach, Diagnostic

03910ZZ   Drainage of Left Internal Mammary Artery, Open Approach

039130Z   Drainage of Left Internal Mammary Artery with Drainage Device, Percutaneous Approach

03913ZX   Drainage of Left Internal Mammary Artery, Percutaneous Approach, Diagnostic

03913ZZ   Drainage of Left Internal Mammary Artery, Percutaneous Approach

039140Z   Drainage of Left Internal Mammary Artery with Drainage Device, Percutaneous Endoscopic Approach

03914ZX   Drainage of Left Internal Mammary Artery, Percutaneous Endoscopic Approach, Diagnostic

03914ZZ   Drainage of Left Internal Mammary Artery, Percutaneous Endoscopic Approach

039200Z   Drainage of Innominate Artery with Drainage Device, Open Approach

03920ZX   Drainage of Innominate Artery, Open Approach, Diagnostic

03920ZZ   Drainage of Innominate Artery, Open Approach

039230Z   Drainage of Innominate Artery with Drainage Device, Percutaneous Approach

03923ZX   Drainage of Innominate Artery, Percutaneous Approach, Diagnostic

03923ZZ   Drainage of Innominate Artery, Percutaneous Approach

039240Z   Drainage of Innominate Artery with Drainage Device, Percutaneous Endoscopic Approach

03924ZX   Drainage of Innominate Artery, Percutaneous Endoscopic Approach, Diagnostic

03924ZZ   Drainage of Innominate Artery, Percutaneous Endoscopic Approach

039300Z   Drainage of Right Subclavian Artery with Drainage Device, Open Approach

03930ZX   Drainage of Right Subclavian Artery, Open Approach, Diagnostic

03930ZZ   Drainage of Right Subclavian Artery, Open Approach

039330Z   Drainage of Right Subclavian Artery with Drainage Device, Percutaneous Approach

03933ZX   Drainage of Right Subclavian Artery, Percutaneous Approach, Diagnostic

03933ZZ   Drainage of Right Subclavian Artery, Percutaneous Approach

039340Z   Drainage of Right Subclavian Artery with Drainage Device, Percutaneous Endoscopic Approach

03934ZX   Drainage of Right Subclavian Artery, Percutaneous Endoscopic Approach, Diagnostic

03934ZZ   Drainage of Right Subclavian Artery, Percutaneous Endoscopic Approach

039400Z   Drainage of Left Subclavian Artery with Drainage Device, Open Approach

03940ZX   Drainage of Left Subclavian Artery, Open Approach, Diagnostic

03940ZZ   Drainage of Left Subclavian Artery, Open Approach

039430Z   Drainage of Left Subclavian Artery with Drainage Device, Percutaneous Approach

03943ZX   Drainage of Left Subclavian Artery, Percutaneous Approach, Diagnostic

03943ZZ   Drainage of Left Subclavian Artery, Percutaneous Approach

039440Z   Drainage of Left Subclavian Artery with Drainage Device, Percutaneous Endoscopic Approach

03944ZX   Drainage of Left Subclavian Artery, Percutaneous Endoscopic Approach, Diagnostic

03944ZZ   Drainage of Left Subclavian Artery, Percutaneous Endoscopic Approach

039500Z   Drainage of Right Axillary Artery with Drainage Device, Open Approach

03950ZX   Drainage of Right Axillary Artery, Open Approach, Diagnostic

03950ZZ   Drainage of Right Axillary Artery, Open Approach

039530Z   Drainage of Right Axillary Artery with Drainage Device, Percutaneous Approach

03953ZX   Drainage of Right Axillary Artery, Percutaneous Approach, Diagnostic

03953ZZ   Drainage of Right Axillary Artery, Percutaneous Approach

039540Z   Drainage of Right Axillary Artery with Drainage Device, Percutaneous Endoscopic Approach

03954ZX   Drainage of Right Axillary Artery, Percutaneous Endoscopic Approach, Diagnostic

03954ZZ   Drainage of Right Axillary Artery, Percutaneous Endoscopic Approach

039600Z   Drainage of Left Axillary Artery with Drainage Device, Open Approach

03960ZX   Drainage of Left Axillary Artery, Open Approach, Diagnostic

03960ZZ   Drainage of Left Axillary Artery, Open Approach

039630Z   Drainage of Left Axillary Artery with Drainage Device, Percutaneous Approach

03963ZX   Drainage of Left Axillary Artery, Percutaneous Approach, Diagnostic

03963ZZ   Drainage of Left Axillary Artery, Percutaneous Approach

039640Z   Drainage of Left Axillary Artery with Drainage Device, Percutaneous Endoscopic Approach

03964ZX   Drainage of Left Axillary Artery, Percutaneous Endoscopic Approach, Diagnostic

03964ZZ   Drainage of Left Axillary Artery, Percutaneous Endoscopic Approach

039700Z   Drainage of Right Brachial Artery with Drainage Device, Open Approach

03970ZX   Drainage of Right Brachial Artery, Open Approach, Diagnostic

03970ZZ   Drainage of Right Brachial Artery, Open Approach

039730Z   Drainage of Right Brachial Artery with Drainage Device, Percutaneous Approach

03973ZX   Drainage of Right Brachial Artery, Percutaneous Approach, Diagnostic

03973ZZ   Drainage of Right Brachial Artery, Percutaneous Approach

039740Z   Drainage of Right Brachial Artery with Drainage Device, Percutaneous Endoscopic Approach

03974ZX   Drainage of Right Brachial Artery, Percutaneous Endoscopic Approach, Diagnostic

03974ZZ   Drainage of Right Brachial Artery, Percutaneous Endoscopic Approach

039800Z   Drainage of Left Brachial Artery with Drainage Device, Open Approach

03980ZX   Drainage of Left Brachial Artery, Open Approach, Diagnostic

03980ZZ   Drainage of Left Brachial Artery, Open Approach

039830Z   Drainage of Left Brachial Artery with Drainage Device, Percutaneous Approach

03983ZX   Drainage of Left Brachial Artery, Percutaneous Approach, Diagnostic

03983ZZ   Drainage of Left Brachial Artery, Percutaneous Approach

039840Z   Drainage of Left Brachial Artery with Drainage Device, Percutaneous Endoscopic Approach

03984ZX   Drainage of Left Brachial Artery, Percutaneous Endoscopic Approach, Diagnostic

03984ZZ   Drainage of Left Brachial Artery, Percutaneous Endoscopic Approach

039900Z   Drainage of Right Ulnar Artery with Drainage Device, Open Approach

03990ZX   Drainage of Right Ulnar Artery, Open Approach, Diagnostic

03990ZZ   Drainage of Right Ulnar Artery, Open Approach

039930Z   Drainage of Right Ulnar Artery with Drainage Device, Percutaneous Approach

03993ZX   Drainage of Right Ulnar Artery, Percutaneous Approach, Diagnostic

03993ZZ   Drainage of Right Ulnar Artery, Percutaneous Approach

039940Z   Drainage of Right Ulnar Artery with Drainage Device, Percutaneous Endoscopic Approach

03994ZX   Drainage of Right Ulnar Artery, Percutaneous Endoscopic Approach, Diagnostic

03994ZZ   Drainage of Right Ulnar Artery, Percutaneous Endoscopic Approach

039A00Z   Drainage of Left Ulnar Artery with Drainage Device, Open Approach

039A0ZX   Drainage of Left Ulnar Artery, Open Approach, Diagnostic

039A0ZZ   Drainage of Left Ulnar Artery, Open Approach

039A30Z   Drainage of Left Ulnar Artery with Drainage Device, Percutaneous Approach

039A3ZX   Drainage of Left Ulnar Artery, Percutaneous Approach, Diagnostic

039A3ZZ   Drainage of Left Ulnar Artery, Percutaneous Approach

039A40Z   Drainage of Left Ulnar Artery with Drainage Device, Percutaneous Endoscopic Approach

039A4ZX   Drainage of Left Ulnar Artery, Percutaneous Endoscopic Approach, Diagnostic

039A4ZZ   Drainage of Left Ulnar Artery, Percutaneous Endoscopic Approach

039B00Z   Drainage of Right Radial Artery with Drainage Device, Open Approach

039B0ZX   Drainage of Right Radial Artery, Open Approach, Diagnostic

039B0ZZ   Drainage of Right Radial Artery, Open Approach

039B30Z   Drainage of Right Radial Artery with Drainage Device, Percutaneous Approach

039B3ZX   Drainage of Right Radial Artery, Percutaneous Approach, Diagnostic

039B3ZZ   Drainage of Right Radial Artery, Percutaneous Approach

039B40Z   Drainage of Right Radial Artery with Drainage Device, Percutaneous Endoscopic Approach

039B4ZX   Drainage of Right Radial Artery, Percutaneous Endoscopic Approach, Diagnostic

039B4ZZ   Drainage of Right Radial Artery, Percutaneous Endoscopic Approach

039C00Z   Drainage of Left Radial Artery with Drainage Device, Open Approach

039C0ZX   Drainage of Left Radial Artery, Open Approach, Diagnostic

039C0ZZ   Drainage of Left Radial Artery, Open Approach

039C30Z   Drainage of Left Radial Artery with Drainage Device, Percutaneous Approach

039C3ZX   Drainage of Left Radial Artery, Percutaneous Approach, Diagnostic

039C3ZZ   Drainage of Left Radial Artery, Percutaneous Approach

039C40Z   Drainage of Left Radial Artery with Drainage Device, Percutaneous Endoscopic Approach

039C4ZX   Drainage of Left Radial Artery, Percutaneous Endoscopic Approach, Diagnostic

039C4ZZ   Drainage of Left Radial Artery, Percutaneous Endoscopic Approach

039D00Z   Drainage of Right Hand Artery with Drainage Device, Open Approach

039D0ZX   Drainage of Right Hand Artery, Open Approach, Diagnostic

039D0ZZ   Drainage of Right Hand Artery, Open Approach

039D30Z   Drainage of Right Hand Artery with Drainage Device, Percutaneous Approach

039D3ZX   Drainage of Right Hand Artery, Percutaneous Approach, Diagnostic

039D3ZZ   Drainage of Right Hand Artery, Percutaneous Approach

039D40Z   Drainage of Right Hand Artery with Drainage Device, Percutaneous Endoscopic Approach

039D4ZX   Drainage of Right Hand Artery, Percutaneous Endoscopic Approach, Diagnostic

039D4ZZ   Drainage of Right Hand Artery, Percutaneous Endoscopic Approach

039F00Z   Drainage of Left Hand Artery with Drainage Device, Open Approach

039F0ZX Drainage of Left Hand Artery, Open Approach, Diagnostic
039F0ZZ Drainage of Left Hand Artery, Open Approach
039F30Z Drainage of Left Hand Artery with Drainage Device, Percutaneous Approach
039F3ZX Drainage of Left Hand Artery, Percutaneous Approach, Diagnostic
039F3ZZ Drainage of Left Hand Artery, Percutaneous Approach
039F40Z Drainage of Left Hand Artery with Drainage Device, Percutaneous Endoscopic Approach
039F4ZX Drainage of Left Hand Artery, Percutaneous Endoscopic Approach, Diagnostic
039F4ZZ Drainage of Left Hand Artery, Percutaneous Endoscopic Approach
039G00Z Drainage of Intracranial Artery with Drainage Device, Open Approach
039G0ZX Drainage of Intracranial Artery, Open Approach, Diagnostic
039G0ZZ Drainage of Intracranial Artery, Open Approach
039G30Z Drainage of Intracranial Artery with Drainage Device, Percutaneous Approach
039G3ZX Drainage of Intracranial Artery, Percutaneous Approach, Diagnostic
039G3ZZ Drainage of Intracranial Artery, Percutaneous Approach
039G40Z Drainage of Intracranial Artery with Drainage Device, Percutaneous Endoscopic Approach
039G4ZX Drainage of Intracranial Artery, Percutaneous Endoscopic Approach, Diagnostic
039G4ZZ Drainage of Intracranial Artery, Percutaneous Endoscopic Approach
039H00Z Drainage of Right Common Carotid Artery with Drainage Device, Open Approach
039H0ZX Drainage of Right Common Carotid Artery, Open Approach, Diagnostic
039H0ZZ Drainage of Right Common Carotid Artery, Open Approach
039H30Z Drainage of Right Common Carotid Artery with Drainage Device, Percutaneous Approach
039H3ZX Drainage of Right Common Carotid Artery, Percutaneous Approach, Diagnostic
039H3ZZ Drainage of Right Common Carotid Artery, Percutaneous Approach
039H40Z Drainage of Right Common Carotid Artery with Drainage Device, Percutaneous Endoscopic Approach
039H4ZX Drainage of Right Common Carotid Artery, Percutaneous Endoscopic Approach, Diagnostic
039H4ZZ Drainage of Right Common Carotid Artery, Percutaneous Endoscopic Approach
039J00Z Drainage of Left Common Carotid Artery with Drainage Device, Open Approach
039J0ZX Drainage of Left Common Carotid Artery, Open Approach, Diagnostic
039J0ZZ Drainage of Left Common Carotid Artery, Open Approach
039J30Z Drainage of Left Common Carotid Artery with Drainage Device, Percutaneous Approach
039J3ZX Drainage of Left Common Carotid Artery, Percutaneous Approach, Diagnostic
039J3ZZ Drainage of Left Common Carotid Artery, Percutaneous Approach
039J40Z Drainage of Left Common Carotid Artery with Drainage Device, Percutaneous Endoscopic Approach
039J4ZX Drainage of Left Common Carotid Artery, Percutaneous Endoscopic Approach, Diagnostic
039J4ZZ Drainage of Left Common Carotid Artery, Percutaneous Endoscopic Approach
039K00Z Drainage of Right Internal Carotid Artery with Drainage Device, Open Approach
039K0ZX Drainage of Right Internal Carotid Artery, Open Approach, Diagnostic
039K0ZZ Drainage of Right Internal Carotid Artery, Open Approach
039K30Z Drainage of Right Internal Carotid Artery with Drainage Device, Percutaneous Approach
039K3ZX Drainage of Right Internal Carotid Artery, Percutaneous Approach, Diagnostic
039K3ZZ Drainage of Right Internal Carotid Artery, Percutaneous Approach
039K40Z Drainage of Right Internal Carotid Artery with Drainage Device, Percutaneous Endoscopic Approach
039K4ZX Drainage of Right Internal Carotid Artery, Percutaneous Endoscopic Approach, Diagnostic
039K4ZZ Drainage of Right Internal Carotid Artery, Percutaneous Endoscopic Approach

039L00Z Drainage of Left Internal Carotid Artery with Drainage Device, Open Approach
039L0ZX Drainage of Left Internal Carotid Artery, Open Approach, Diagnostic
039L0ZZ Drainage of Left Internal Carotid Artery, Open Approach
039L30Z Drainage of Left Internal Carotid Artery with Drainage Device, Percutaneous Approach
039L3ZX Drainage of Left Internal Carotid Artery, Percutaneous Approach, Diagnostic
039L3ZZ Drainage of Left Internal Carotid Artery, Percutaneous Approach
039L40Z Drainage of Left Internal Carotid Artery with Drainage Device, Percutaneous Endoscopic Approach
039L4ZX Drainage of Left Internal Carotid Artery, Percutaneous Endoscopic Approach, Diagnostic
039L4ZZ Drainage of Left Internal Carotid Artery, Percutaneous Endoscopic Approach
039M00Z Drainage of Right External Carotid Artery with Drainage Device, Open Approach
039M0ZX Drainage of Right External Carotid Artery, Open Approach, Diagnostic
039M0ZZ Drainage of Right External Carotid Artery, Open Approach
039M30Z Drainage of Right External Carotid Artery with Drainage Device, Percutaneous Approach
039M3ZX Drainage of Right External Carotid Artery, Percutaneous Approach, Diagnostic
039M3ZZ Drainage of Right External Carotid Artery, Percutaneous Approach
039M40Z Drainage of Right External Carotid Artery with Drainage Device, Percutaneous Endoscopic Approach
039M4ZX Drainage of Right External Carotid Artery, Percutaneous Endoscopic Approach, Diagnostic
039M4ZZ Drainage of Right External Carotid Artery, Percutaneous Endoscopic Approach
039N00Z Drainage of Left External Carotid Artery with Drainage Device, Open Approach
039N0ZX Drainage of Left External Carotid Artery, Open Approach, Diagnostic
039N0ZZ Drainage of Left External Carotid Artery, Open Approach
039N30Z Drainage of Left External Carotid Artery with Drainage Device, Percutaneous Approach
039N3ZX Drainage of Left External Carotid Artery, Percutaneous Approach, Diagnostic
039N3ZZ Drainage of Left External Carotid Artery, Percutaneous Approach
039N40Z Drainage of Left External Carotid Artery with Drainage Device, Percutaneous Endoscopic Approach
039N4ZX Drainage of Left External Carotid Artery, Percutaneous Endoscopic Approach, Diagnostic
039N4ZZ Drainage of Left External Carotid Artery, Percutaneous Endoscopic Approach
039P00Z Drainage of Right Vertebral Artery with Drainage Device, Open Approach
039P0ZX Drainage of Right Vertebral Artery, Open Approach, Diagnostic
039P0ZZ Drainage of Right Vertebral Artery, Open Approach
039P30Z Drainage of Right Vertebral Artery with Drainage Device, Percutaneous Approach
039P3ZX Drainage of Right Vertebral Artery, Percutaneous Approach, Diagnostic
039P3ZZ Drainage of Right Vertebral Artery, Percutaneous Approach
039P40Z Drainage of Right Vertebral Artery with Drainage Device, Percutaneous Endoscopic Approach
039P4ZX Drainage of Right Vertebral Artery, Percutaneous Endoscopic Approach, Diagnostic
039P4ZZ Drainage of Right Vertebral Artery, Percutaneous Endoscopic Approach
039Q00Z Drainage of Left Vertebral Artery with Drainage Device, Open Approach
039Q0ZX Drainage of Left Vertebral Artery, Open Approach, Diagnostic
039Q0ZZ Drainage of Left Vertebral Artery, Open Approach
039Q30Z Drainage of Left Vertebral Artery with Drainage Device, Percutaneous Approach
039Q3ZX Drainage of Left Vertebral Artery, Percutaneous Approach, Diagnostic
039Q3ZZ Drainage of Left Vertebral Artery, Percutaneous Approach
039Q40Z Drainage of Left Vertebral Artery with Drainage Device, Percutaneous Endoscopic Approach

039Q4ZX	Drainage of Left Vertebral Artery, Percutaneous Endoscopic Approach, Diagnostic
039Q4ZZ	Drainage of Left Vertebral Artery, Percutaneous Endoscopic Approach
039R00Z	Drainage of Face Artery with Drainage Device, Open Approach
039R0ZX	Drainage of Face Artery, Open Approach, Diagnostic
039R0ZZ	Drainage of Face Artery, Open Approach
039R30Z	Drainage of Face Artery with Drainage Device, Percutaneous Approach
039R3ZX	Drainage of Face Artery, Percutaneous Approach, Diagnostic
039R3ZZ	Drainage of Face Artery, Percutaneous Approach
039R40Z	Drainage of Face Artery with Drainage Device, Percutaneous Endoscopic Approach
039R4ZX	Drainage of Face Artery, Percutaneous Endoscopic Approach, Diagnostic
039R4ZZ	Drainage of Face Artery, Percutaneous Endoscopic Approach
039S00Z	Drainage of Right Temporal Artery with Drainage Device, Open Approach
039S0ZX	Drainage of Right Temporal Artery, Open Approach, Diagnostic
039S0ZZ	Drainage of Right Temporal Artery, Open Approach
039S30Z	Drainage of Right Temporal Artery with Drainage Device, Percutaneous Approach
039S3ZX	Drainage of Right Temporal Artery, Percutaneous Approach, Diagnostic
039S3ZZ	Drainage of Right Temporal Artery, Percutaneous Approach
039S40Z	Drainage of Right Temporal Artery with Drainage Device, Percutaneous Endoscopic Approach
039S4ZX	Drainage of Right Temporal Artery, Percutaneous Endoscopic Approach, Diagnostic
039S4ZZ	Drainage of Right Temporal Artery, Percutaneous Endoscopic Approach
039T00Z	Drainage of Left Temporal Artery with Drainage Device, Open Approach
039T0ZX	Drainage of Left Temporal Artery, Open Approach, Diagnostic
039T0ZZ	Drainage of Left Temporal Artery, Open Approach
039T30Z	Drainage of Left Temporal Artery with Drainage Device, Percutaneous Approach
039T3ZX	Drainage of Left Temporal Artery, Percutaneous Approach, Diagnostic
039T3ZZ	Drainage of Left Temporal Artery, Percutaneous Approach
039T40Z	Drainage of Left Temporal Artery with Drainage Device, Percutaneous Endoscopic Approach
039T4ZX	Drainage of Left Temporal Artery, Percutaneous Endoscopic Approach, Diagnostic
039T4ZZ	Drainage of Left Temporal Artery, Percutaneous Endoscopic Approach
039U00Z	Drainage of Right Thyroid Artery with Drainage Device, Open Approach
039U0ZX	Drainage of Right Thyroid Artery, Open Approach, Diagnostic
039U0ZZ	Drainage of Right Thyroid Artery, Open Approach
039U30Z	Drainage of Right Thyroid Artery with Drainage Device, Percutaneous Approach
039U3ZX	Drainage of Right Thyroid Artery, Percutaneous Approach, Diagnostic
039U3ZZ	Drainage of Right Thyroid Artery, Percutaneous Approach
039U40Z	Drainage of Right Thyroid Artery with Drainage Device, Percutaneous Endoscopic Approach
039U4ZX	Drainage of Right Thyroid Artery, Percutaneous Endoscopic Approach, Diagnostic
039U4ZZ	Drainage of Right Thyroid Artery, Percutaneous Endoscopic Approach
039V00Z	Drainage of Left Thyroid Artery with Drainage Device, Open Approach
039V0ZX	Drainage of Left Thyroid Artery, Open Approach, Diagnostic
039V0ZZ	Drainage of Left Thyroid Artery, Open Approach
039V30Z	Drainage of Left Thyroid Artery with Drainage Device, Percutaneous Approach
039V3ZX	Drainage of Left Thyroid Artery, Percutaneous Approach, Diagnostic
039V3ZZ	Drainage of Left Thyroid Artery, Percutaneous Approach
039V40Z	Drainage of Left Thyroid Artery with Drainage Device, Percutaneous Endoscopic Approach
039V4ZX	Drainage of Left Thyroid Artery, Percutaneous Endoscopic Approach, Diagnostic
039V4ZZ	Drainage of Left Thyroid Artery, Percutaneous Endoscopic Approach
039Y00Z	Drainage of Upper Artery with Drainage Device, Open Approach
039Y0ZX	Drainage of Upper Artery, Open Approach, Diagnostic
039Y0ZZ	Drainage of Upper Artery, Open Approach
039Y30Z	Drainage of Upper Artery with Drainage Device, Percutaneous Approach
039Y3ZX	Drainage of Upper Artery, Percutaneous Approach, Diagnostic
039Y3ZZ	Drainage of Upper Artery, Percutaneous Approach
039Y40Z	Drainage of Upper Artery with Drainage Device, Percutaneous Endoscopic Approach
039Y4ZX	Drainage of Upper Artery, Percutaneous Endoscopic Approach, Diagnostic
039Y4ZZ	Drainage of Upper Artery, Percutaneous Endoscopic Approach

03B – Upper Arteries, Excision

Review Coding Guidelines B3.4a and B3.4b

Review Coding Guideline B3.8

03B00ZX	Excision of Right Internal Mammary Artery, Open Approach, Diagnostic
03B00ZZ	Excision of Right Internal Mammary Artery, Open Approach
03B03ZX	Excision of Right Internal Mammary Artery, Percutaneous Approach, Diagnostic
03B03ZZ	Excision of Right Internal Mammary Artery, Percutaneous Approach
03B04ZX	Excision of Right Internal Mammary Artery, Percutaneous Endoscopic Approach, Diagnostic
03B04ZZ	Excision of Right Internal Mammary Artery, Percutaneous Endoscopic Approach
03B10ZX	Excision of Left Internal Mammary Artery, Open Approach, Diagnostic
03B10ZZ	Excision of Left Internal Mammary Artery, Open Approach
03B13ZX	Excision of Left Internal Mammary Artery, Percutaneous Approach, Diagnostic
03B13ZZ	Excision of Left Internal Mammary Artery, Percutaneous Approach
03B14ZX	Excision of Left Internal Mammary Artery, Percutaneous Endoscopic Approach, Diagnostic
03B14ZZ	Excision of Left Internal Mammary Artery, Percutaneous Endoscopic Approach
03B20ZX	Excision of Innominate Artery, Open Approach, Diagnostic
03B20ZZ	Excision of Innominate Artery, Open Approach
03B23ZX	Excision of Innominate Artery, Percutaneous Approach, Diagnostic
03B23ZZ	Excision of Innominate Artery, Percutaneous Approach
03B24ZX	Excision of Innominate Artery, Percutaneous Endoscopic Approach, Diagnostic
03B24ZZ	Excision of Innominate Artery, Percutaneous Endoscopic Approach
03B30ZX	Excision of Right Subclavian Artery, Open Approach, Diagnostic
03B30ZZ	Excision of Right Subclavian Artery, Open Approach
03B33ZX	Excision of Right Subclavian Artery, Percutaneous Approach, Diagnostic
03B33ZZ	Excision of Right Subclavian Artery, Percutaneous Approach
03B34ZX	Excision of Right Subclavian Artery, Percutaneous Endoscopic Approach, Diagnostic
03B34ZZ	Excision of Right Subclavian Artery, Percutaneous Endoscopic Approach
03B40ZX	Excision of Left Subclavian Artery, Open Approach, Diagnostic
03B40ZZ	Excision of Left Subclavian Artery, Open Approach
03B43ZX	Excision of Left Subclavian Artery, Percutaneous Approach, Diagnostic
03B43ZZ	Excision of Left Subclavian Artery, Percutaneous Approach
03B44ZX	Excision of Left Subclavian Artery, Percutaneous Endoscopic Approach, Diagnostic

♀ Female-only   ♂ Male-only   ● Limited Coverage   ● Non-OR   🅷🅰🅲 HAC-associated procedure   ⬡ Non-covered procedures   ➕ Combination

03B44ZZ	Excision of Left Subclavian Artery, Percutaneous Endoscopic Approach
03B50ZX	Excision of Right Axillary Artery, Open Approach, Diagnostic
03B50ZZ	Excision of Right Axillary Artery, Open Approach
03B53ZX	Excision of Right Axillary Artery, Percutaneous Approach, Diagnostic
03B53ZZ	Excision of Right Axillary Artery, Percutaneous Approach
03B54ZX	Excision of Right Axillary Artery, Percutaneous Endoscopic Approach, Diagnostic
03B54ZZ	Excision of Right Axillary Artery, Percutaneous Endoscopic Approach
03B60ZX	Excision of Left Axillary Artery, Open Approach, Diagnostic
03B60ZZ	Excision of Left Axillary Artery, Open Approach
03B63ZX	Excision of Left Axillary Artery, Percutaneous Approach, Diagnostic
03B63ZZ	Excision of Left Axillary Artery, Percutaneous Approach
03B64ZX	Excision of Left Axillary Artery, Percutaneous Endoscopic Approach, Diagnostic
03B64ZZ	Excision of Left Axillary Artery, Percutaneous Endoscopic Approach
03B70ZX	Excision of Right Brachial Artery, Open Approach, Diagnostic
03B70ZZ	Excision of Right Brachial Artery, Open Approach
03B73ZX	Excision of Right Brachial Artery, Percutaneous Approach, Diagnostic
03B73ZZ	Excision of Right Brachial Artery, Percutaneous Approach
03B74ZX	Excision of Right Brachial Artery, Percutaneous Endoscopic Approach, Diagnostic
03B74ZZ	Excision of Right Brachial Artery, Percutaneous Endoscopic Approach
03B80ZX	Excision of Left Brachial Artery, Open Approach, Diagnostic
03B80ZZ	Excision of Left Brachial Artery, Open Approach
03B83ZX	Excision of Left Brachial Artery, Percutaneous Approach, Diagnostic
03B83ZZ	Excision of Left Brachial Artery, Percutaneous Approach
03B84ZX	Excision of Left Brachial Artery, Percutaneous Endoscopic Approach, Diagnostic
03B84ZZ	Excision of Left Brachial Artery, Percutaneous Endoscopic Approach
03B90ZX	Excision of Right Ulnar Artery, Open Approach, Diagnostic
03B90ZZ	Excision of Right Ulnar Artery, Open Approach
03B93ZX	Excision of Right Ulnar Artery, Percutaneous Approach, Diagnostic
03B93ZZ	Excision of Right Ulnar Artery, Percutaneous Approach
03B94ZX	Excision of Right Ulnar Artery, Percutaneous Endoscopic Approach, Diagnostic
03B94ZZ	Excision of Right Ulnar Artery, Percutaneous Endoscopic Approach
03BA0ZX	Excision of Left Ulnar Artery, Open Approach, Diagnostic
03BA0ZZ	Excision of Left Ulnar Artery, Open Approach
03BA3ZX	Excision of Left Ulnar Artery, Percutaneous Approach, Diagnostic
03BA3ZZ	Excision of Left Ulnar Artery, Percutaneous Approach
03BA4ZX	Excision of Left Ulnar Artery, Percutaneous Endoscopic Approach, Diagnostic
03BA4ZZ	Excision of Left Ulnar Artery, Percutaneous Endoscopic Approach
03BB0ZX	Excision of Right Radial Artery, Open Approach, Diagnostic
03BB0ZZ	Excision of Right Radial Artery, Open Approach
03BB3ZX	Excision of Right Radial Artery, Percutaneous Approach, Diagnostic
03BB3ZZ	Excision of Right Radial Artery, Percutaneous Approach
03BB4ZX	Excision of Right Radial Artery, Percutaneous Endoscopic Approach, Diagnostic
03BB4ZZ	Excision of Right Radial Artery, Percutaneous Endoscopic Approach
03BC0ZX	Excision of Left Radial Artery, Open Approach, Diagnostic
03BC0ZZ	Excision of Left Radial Artery, Open Approach
03BC3ZX	Excision of Left Radial Artery, Percutaneous Approach, Diagnostic
03BC3ZZ	Excision of Left Radial Artery, Percutaneous Approach
03BC4ZX	Excision of Left Radial Artery, Percutaneous Endoscopic Approach, Diagnostic
03BC4ZZ	Excision of Left Radial Artery, Percutaneous Endoscopic Approach
03BD0ZX	Excision of Right Hand Artery, Open Approach, Diagnostic
03BD0ZZ	Excision of Right Hand Artery, Open Approach
03BD3ZX	Excision of Right Hand Artery, Percutaneous Approach, Diagnostic
03BD3ZZ	Excision of Right Hand Artery, Percutaneous Approach
03BD4ZX	Excision of Right Hand Artery, Percutaneous Endoscopic Approach, Diagnostic
03BD4ZZ	Excision of Right Hand Artery, Percutaneous Endoscopic Approach
03BF0ZX	Excision of Left Hand Artery, Open Approach, Diagnostic
03BF0ZZ	Excision of Left Hand Artery, Open Approach
03BF3ZX	Excision of Left Hand Artery, Percutaneous Approach, Diagnostic
03BF3ZZ	Excision of Left Hand Artery, Percutaneous Approach
03BF4ZX	Excision of Left Hand Artery, Percutaneous Endoscopic Approach, Diagnostic
03BF4ZZ	Excision of Left Hand Artery, Percutaneous Endoscopic Approach
03BG0ZX	Excision of Intracranial Artery, Open Approach, Diagnostic
03BG0ZZ	Excision of Intracranial Artery, Open Approach
03BG3ZX	Excision of Intracranial Artery, Percutaneous Approach, Diagnostic
03BG3ZZ	Excision of Intracranial Artery, Percutaneous Approach
03BG4ZX	Excision of Intracranial Artery, Percutaneous Endoscopic Approach, Diagnostic
03BG4ZZ	Excision of Intracranial Artery, Percutaneous Endoscopic Approach
03BH0ZX	Excision of Right Common Carotid Artery, Open Approach, Diagnostic
03BH0ZZ	Excision of Right Common Carotid Artery, Open Approach
03BH3ZX	Excision of Right Common Carotid Artery, Percutaneous Approach, Diagnostic
03BH3ZZ	Excision of Right Common Carotid Artery, Percutaneous Approach
03BH4ZX	Excision of Right Common Carotid Artery, Percutaneous Endoscopic Approach, Diagnostic
03BH4ZZ	Excision of Right Common Carotid Artery, Percutaneous Endoscopic Approach
03BJ0ZX	Excision of Left Common Carotid Artery, Open Approach, Diagnostic
03BJ0ZZ	Excision of Left Common Carotid Artery, Open Approach
03BJ3ZX	Excision of Left Common Carotid Artery, Percutaneous Approach, Diagnostic
03BJ3ZZ	Excision of Left Common Carotid Artery, Percutaneous Approach
03BJ4ZX	Excision of Left Common Carotid Artery, Percutaneous Endoscopic Approach, Diagnostic
03BJ4ZZ	Excision of Left Common Carotid Artery, Percutaneous Endoscopic Approach
03BK0ZX	Excision of Right Internal Carotid Artery, Open Approach, Diagnostic
03BK0ZZ	Excision of Right Internal Carotid Artery, Open Approach
03BK3ZX	Excision of Right Internal Carotid Artery, Percutaneous Approach, Diagnostic
03BK3ZZ	Excision of Right Internal Carotid Artery, Percutaneous Approach
03BK4ZX	Excision of Right Internal Carotid Artery, Percutaneous Endoscopic Approach, Diagnostic
03BK4ZZ	Excision of Right Internal Carotid Artery, Percutaneous Endoscopic Approach
03BL0ZX	Excision of Left Internal Carotid Artery, Open Approach, Diagnostic
03BL0ZZ	Excision of Left Internal Carotid Artery, Open Approach
03BL3ZX	Excision of Left Internal Carotid Artery, Percutaneous Approach, Diagnostic
03BL3ZZ	Excision of Left Internal Carotid Artery, Percutaneous Approach
03BL4ZX	Excision of Left Internal Carotid Artery, Percutaneous Endoscopic Approach, Diagnostic
03BL4ZZ	Excision of Left Internal Carotid Artery, Percutaneous Endoscopic Approach
03BM0ZX	Excision of Right External Carotid Artery, Open Approach, Diagnostic
03BM0ZZ	Excision of Right External Carotid Artery, Open Approach
03BM3ZX	Excision of Right External Carotid Artery, Percutaneous Approach, Diagnostic
03BM3ZZ	Excision of Right External Carotid Artery, Percutaneous Approach
03BM4ZX	Excision of Right External Carotid Artery, Percutaneous Endoscopic Approach, Diagnostic
03BM4ZZ	Excision of Right External Carotid Artery, Percutaneous Endoscopic Approach
03BN0ZX	Excision of Left External Carotid Artery, Open Approach, Diagnostic
03BN0ZZ	Excision of Left External Carotid Artery, Open Approach
03BN3ZX	Excision of Left External Carotid Artery, Percutaneous Approach, Diagnostic
03BN3ZZ	Excision of Left External Carotid Artery, Percutaneous Approach
03BN4ZX	Excision of Left External Carotid Artery, Percutaneous Endoscopic Approach, Diagnostic
03BN4ZZ	Excision of Left External Carotid Artery, Percutaneous Endoscopic Approach

03BP0ZX Excision of Right Vertebral Artery, Open Approach, Diagnostic
03BP0ZZ Excision of Right Vertebral Artery, Open Approach
03BP3ZX Excision of Right Vertebral Artery, Percutaneous Approach, Diagnostic
03BP3ZZ Excision of Right Vertebral Artery, Percutaneous Approach
03BP4ZX Excision of Right Vertebral Artery, Percutaneous Endoscopic Approach, Diagnostic
03BP4ZZ Excision of Right Vertebral Artery, Percutaneous Endoscopic Approach
03BQ0ZX Excision of Left Vertebral Artery, Open Approach, Diagnostic
03BQ0ZZ Excision of Left Vertebral Artery, Open Approach
03BQ3ZX Excision of Left Vertebral Artery, Percutaneous Approach, Diagnostic
03BQ3ZZ Excision of Left Vertebral Artery, Percutaneous Approach
03BQ4ZX Excision of Left Vertebral Artery, Percutaneous Endoscopic Approach, Diagnostic
03BQ4ZZ Excision of Left Vertebral Artery, Percutaneous Endoscopic Approach
03BR0ZX Excision of Face Artery, Open Approach, Diagnostic
03BR0ZZ Excision of Face Artery, Open Approach
03BR3ZX Excision of Face Artery, Percutaneous Approach, Diagnostic
03BR3ZZ Excision of Face Artery, Percutaneous Approach
03BR4ZX Excision of Face Artery, Percutaneous Endoscopic Approach, Diagnostic
03BR4ZZ Excision of Face Artery, Percutaneous Endoscopic Approach
03BS0ZX Excision of Right Temporal Artery, Open Approach, Diagnostic
03BS0ZZ Excision of Right Temporal Artery, Open Approach
03BS3ZX Excision of Right Temporal Artery, Percutaneous Approach, Diagnostic
03BS3ZZ Excision of Right Temporal Artery, Percutaneous Approach
03BS4ZX Excision of Right Temporal Artery, Percutaneous Endoscopic Approach, Diagnostic
03BS4ZZ Excision of Right Temporal Artery, Percutaneous Endoscopic Approach

03BT0ZX Excision of Left Temporal Artery, Open Approach, Diagnostic
03BT0ZZ Excision of Left Temporal Artery, Open Approach
03BT3ZX Excision of Left Temporal Artery, Percutaneous Approach, Diagnostic
03BT3ZZ Excision of Left Temporal Artery, Percutaneous Approach
03BT4ZX Excision of Left Temporal Artery, Percutaneous Endoscopic Approach, Diagnostic
03BT4ZZ Excision of Left Temporal Artery, Percutaneous Endoscopic Approach
03BU0ZX Excision of Right Thyroid Artery, Open Approach, Diagnostic
03BU0ZZ Excision of Right Thyroid Artery, Open Approach
03BU3ZX Excision of Right Thyroid Artery, Percutaneous Approach, Diagnostic
03BU3ZZ Excision of Right Thyroid Artery, Percutaneous Approach
03BU4ZX Excision of Right Thyroid Artery, Percutaneous Endoscopic Approach, Diagnostic
03BU4ZZ Excision of Right Thyroid Artery, Percutaneous Endoscopic Approach
03BV0ZX Excision of Left Thyroid Artery, Open Approach, Diagnostic
03BV0ZZ Excision of Left Thyroid Artery, Open Approach
03BV3ZX Excision of Left Thyroid Artery, Percutaneous Approach, Diagnostic
03BV3ZZ Excision of Left Thyroid Artery, Percutaneous Approach
03BV4ZX Excision of Left Thyroid Artery, Percutaneous Endoscopic Approach, Diagnostic
03BV4ZZ Excision of Left Thyroid Artery, Percutaneous Endoscopic Approach
03BY0ZX Excision of Upper Artery, Open Approach, Diagnostic
03BY0ZZ Excision of Upper Artery, Open Approach
03BY3ZX Excision of Upper Artery, Percutaneous Approach, Diagnostic
03BY3ZZ Excision of Upper Artery, Percutaneous Approach
03BY4ZX Excision of Upper Artery, Percutaneous Endoscopic Approach, Diagnostic
03BY4ZZ Excision of Upper Artery, Percutaneous Endoscopic Approach

03C – Upper Arteries, Extirpation

03C00ZZ Extirpation of Matter from Right Internal Mammary Artery, Open Approach
03C03ZZ Extirpation of Matter from Right Internal Mammary Artery, Percutaneous Approach
03C04ZZ Extirpation of Matter from Right Internal Mammary Artery, Percutaneous Endoscopic Approach
03C10ZZ Extirpation of Matter from Left Internal Mammary Artery, Open Approach
03C13ZZ Extirpation of Matter from Left Internal Mammary Artery, Percutaneous Approach
03C14ZZ Extirpation of Matter from Left Internal Mammary Artery, Percutaneous Endoscopic Approach
03C20ZZ Extirpation of Matter from Innominate Artery, Open Approach
03C23ZZ Extirpation of Matter from Innominate Artery, Percutaneous Approach
03C24ZZ Extirpation of Matter from Innominate Artery, Percutaneous Endoscopic Approach
03C30ZZ Extirpation of Matter from Right Subclavian Artery, Open Approach
03C33ZZ Extirpation of Matter from Right Subclavian Artery, Percutaneous Approach
03C34ZZ Extirpation of Matter from Right Subclavian Artery, Percutaneous Endoscopic Approach
03C40ZZ Extirpation of Matter from Left Subclavian Artery, Open Approach
03C43ZZ Extirpation of Matter from Left Subclavian Artery, Percutaneous Approach
03C44ZZ Extirpation of Matter from Left Subclavian Artery, Percutaneous Endoscopic Approach
03C50ZZ Extirpation of Matter from Right Axillary Artery, Open Approach
03C53ZZ Extirpation of Matter from Right Axillary Artery, Percutaneous Approach
03C54ZZ Extirpation of Matter from Right Axillary Artery, Percutaneous Endoscopic Approach
03C60ZZ Extirpation of Matter from Left Axillary Artery, Open Approach
03C63ZZ Extirpation of Matter from Left Axillary Artery, Percutaneous Approach

03C64ZZ Extirpation of Matter from Left Axillary Artery, Percutaneous Endoscopic Approach
03C70ZZ Extirpation of Matter from Right Brachial Artery, Open Approach
03C73ZZ Extirpation of Matter from Right Brachial Artery, Percutaneous Approach
03C74ZZ Extirpation of Matter from Right Brachial Artery, Percutaneous Endoscopic Approach
03C80ZZ Extirpation of Matter from Left Brachial Artery, Open Approach
03C83ZZ Extirpation of Matter from Left Brachial Artery, Percutaneous Approach
03C84ZZ Extirpation of Matter from Left Brachial Artery, Percutaneous Endoscopic Approach
03C90ZZ Extirpation of Matter from Right Ulnar Artery, Open Approach
03C93ZZ Extirpation of Matter from Right Ulnar Artery, Percutaneous Approach
03C94ZZ Extirpation of Matter from Right Ulnar Artery, Percutaneous Endoscopic Approach
03CA0ZZ Extirpation of Matter from Left Ulnar Artery, Open Approach
03CA3ZZ Extirpation of Matter from Left Ulnar Artery, Percutaneous Approach
03CA4ZZ Extirpation of Matter from Left Ulnar Artery, Percutaneous Endoscopic Approach
03CB0ZZ Extirpation of Matter from Right Radial Artery, Open Approach
03CB3ZZ Extirpation of Matter from Right Radial Artery, Percutaneous Approach
03CB4ZZ Extirpation of Matter from Right Radial Artery, Percutaneous Endoscopic Approach
03CC0ZZ Extirpation of Matter from Left Radial Artery, Open Approach
03CC3ZZ Extirpation of Matter from Left Radial Artery, Percutaneous Approach
03CC4ZZ Extirpation of Matter from Left Radial Artery, Percutaneous Endoscopic Approach
03CD0ZZ Extirpation of Matter from Right Hand Artery, Open Approach
03CD3ZZ Extirpation of Matter from Right Hand Artery, Percutaneous Approach

---

♀ Female-only   ♂ Male-only   ⬤ Limited Coverage   ● Non-OR   ▨ HAC-associated procedure   ⬤ Non-covered procedures   ➕ Combination

03CD4ZZ Extirpation of Matter from Right Hand Artery, Percutaneous Endoscopic Approach

03CF0ZZ Extirpation of Matter from Left Hand Artery, Open Approach

03CF3ZZ Extirpation of Matter from Left Hand Artery, Percutaneous Approach

03CF4ZZ Extirpation of Matter from Left Hand Artery, Percutaneous Endoscopic Approach

03CG0ZZ Extirpation of Matter from Intracranial Artery, Open Approach

⬤ **03CG3ZZ** Extirpation of Matter from Intracranial Artery, Percutaneous Approach

⬤ **03CG4ZZ** Extirpation of Matter from Intracranial Artery, Percutaneous Endoscopic Approach

03CH0ZZ Extirpation of Matter from Right Common Carotid Artery, Open Approach

03CH3ZZ Extirpation of Matter from Right Common Carotid Artery, Percutaneous Approach

03CH4ZZ Extirpation of Matter from Right Common Carotid Artery, Percutaneous Endoscopic Approach

03CJ0ZZ Extirpation of Matter from Left Common Carotid Artery, Open Approach

03CJ3ZZ Extirpation of Matter from Left Common Carotid Artery, Percutaneous Approach

03CJ4ZZ Extirpation of Matter from Left Common Carotid Artery, Percutaneous Endoscopic Approach

03CK0ZZ Extirpation of Matter from Right Internal Carotid Artery, Open Approach

03CK3ZZ Extirpation of Matter from Right Internal Carotid Artery, Percutaneous Approach

03CK4ZZ Extirpation of Matter from Right Internal Carotid Artery, Percutaneous Endoscopic Approach

03CL0ZZ Extirpation of Matter from Left Internal Carotid Artery, Open Approach

03CL3ZZ Extirpation of Matter from Left Internal Carotid Artery, Percutaneous Approach

03CL4ZZ Extirpation of Matter from Left Internal Carotid Artery, Percutaneous Endoscopic Approach

03CM0ZZ Extirpation of Matter from Right External Carotid Artery, Open Approach

03CM3ZZ Extirpation of Matter from Right External Carotid Artery, Percutaneous Approach

03CM4ZZ Extirpation of Matter from Right External Carotid Artery, Percutaneous Endoscopic Approach

03CN0ZZ Extirpation of Matter from Left External Carotid Artery, Open Approach

03CN3ZZ Extirpation of Matter from Left External Carotid Artery, Percutaneous Approach

03CN4ZZ Extirpation of Matter from Left External Carotid Artery, Percutaneous Endoscopic Approach

03CP0ZZ Extirpation of Matter from Right Vertebral Artery, Open Approach

03CP3ZZ Extirpation of Matter from Right Vertebral Artery, Percutaneous Approach

03CP4ZZ Extirpation of Matter from Right Vertebral Artery, Percutaneous Endoscopic Approach

03CQ0ZZ Extirpation of Matter from Left Vertebral Artery, Open Approach

03CQ3ZZ Extirpation of Matter from Left Vertebral Artery, Percutaneous Approach

03CQ4ZZ Extirpation of Matter from Left Vertebral Artery, Percutaneous Endoscopic Approach

03CR0ZZ Extirpation of Matter from Face Artery, Open Approach

03CR3ZZ Extirpation of Matter from Face Artery, Percutaneous Approach

03CR4ZZ Extirpation of Matter from Face Artery, Percutaneous Endoscopic Approach

03CS0ZZ Extirpation of Matter from Right Temporal Artery, Open Approach

03CS3ZZ Extirpation of Matter from Right Temporal Artery, Percutaneous Approach

03CS4ZZ Extirpation of Matter from Right Temporal Artery, Percutaneous Endoscopic Approach

03CT0ZZ Extirpation of Matter from Left Temporal Artery, Open Approach

03CT3ZZ Extirpation of Matter from Left Temporal Artery, Percutaneous Approach

03CT4ZZ Extirpation of Matter from Left Temporal Artery, Percutaneous Endoscopic Approach

03CU0ZZ Extirpation of Matter from Right Thyroid Artery, Open Approach

03CU3ZZ Extirpation of Matter from Right Thyroid Artery, Percutaneous Approach

03CU4ZZ Extirpation of Matter from Right Thyroid Artery, Percutaneous Endoscopic Approach

03CV0ZZ Extirpation of Matter from Left Thyroid Artery, Open Approach

03CV3ZZ Extirpation of Matter from Left Thyroid Artery, Percutaneous Approach

03CV4ZZ Extirpation of Matter from Left Thyroid Artery, Percutaneous Endoscopic Approach

03CY0ZZ Extirpation of Matter from Upper Artery, Open Approach

03CY3ZZ Extirpation of Matter from Upper Artery, Percutaneous Approach

03CY4ZZ Extirpation of Matter from Upper Artery, Percutaneous Endoscopic Approach

03H – Upper Arteries, Insertion

03H003Z Insertion of Infusion Device into Right Internal Mammary Artery, Open Approach

03H00DZ Insertion of Intraluminal Device into Right Internal Mammary Artery, Open Approach

03H033Z Insertion of Infusion Device into Right Internal Mammary Artery, Percutaneous Approach

03H03DZ Insertion of Intraluminal Device into Right Internal Mammary Artery, Percutaneous Approach

03H043Z Insertion of Infusion Device into Right Internal Mammary Artery, Percutaneous Endoscopic Approach

03H04DZ Insertion of Intraluminal Device into Right Internal Mammary Artery, Percutaneous Endoscopic Approach

03H103Z Insertion of Infusion Device into Left Internal Mammary Artery, Open Approach

03H10DZ Insertion of Intraluminal Device into Left Internal Mammary Artery, Open Approach

03H133Z Insertion of Infusion Device into Left Internal Mammary Artery, Percutaneous Approach

03H13DZ Insertion of Intraluminal Device into Left Internal Mammary Artery, Percutaneous Approach

03H143Z Insertion of Infusion Device into Left Internal Mammary Artery, Percutaneous Endoscopic Approach

03H14DZ Insertion of Intraluminal Device into Left Internal Mammary Artery, Percutaneous Endoscopic Approach

03H203Z Insertion of Infusion Device into Innominate Artery, Open Approach

03H20DZ Insertion of Intraluminal Device into Innominate Artery, Open Approach

03H233Z Insertion of Infusion Device into Innominate Artery, Percutaneous Approach

03H23DZ Insertion of Intraluminal Device into Innominate Artery, Percutaneous Approach

03H243Z Insertion of Infusion Device into Innominate Artery, Percutaneous Endoscopic Approach

03H24DZ Insertion of Intraluminal Device into Innominate Artery, Percutaneous Endoscopic Approach

03H303Z Insertion of Infusion Device into Right Subclavian Artery, Open Approach

03H30DZ Insertion of Intraluminal Device into Right Subclavian Artery, Open Approach

03H333Z Insertion of Infusion Device into Right Subclavian Artery, Percutaneous Approach

03H33DZ Insertion of Intraluminal Device into Right Subclavian Artery, Percutaneous Approach

03H343Z Insertion of Infusion Device into Right Subclavian Artery, Percutaneous Endoscopic Approach

03H34DZ Insertion of Intraluminal Device into Right Subclavian Artery, Percutaneous Endoscopic Approach

03H403Z Insertion of Infusion Device into Left Subclavian Artery, Open Approach

03H40DZ Insertion of Intraluminal Device into Left Subclavian Artery, Open Approach

03H433Z   Insertion of Infusion Device into Left Subclavian Artery, Percutaneous Approach

03H43DZ   Insertion of Intraluminal Device into Left Subclavian Artery, Percutaneous Approach

03H443Z   Insertion of Infusion Device into Left Subclavian Artery, Percutaneous Endoscopic Approach

03H44DZ   Insertion of Intraluminal Device into Left Subclavian Artery, Percutaneous Endoscopic Approach

03H503Z   Insertion of Infusion Device into Right Axillary Artery, Open Approach

03H50DZ   Insertion of Intraluminal Device into Right Axillary Artery, Open Approach

03H533Z   Insertion of Infusion Device into Right Axillary Artery, Percutaneous Approach

03H53DZ   Insertion of Intraluminal Device into Right Axillary Artery, Percutaneous Approach

03H543Z   Insertion of Infusion Device into Right Axillary Artery, Percutaneous Endoscopic Approach

03H54DZ   Insertion of Intraluminal Device into Right Axillary Artery, Percutaneous Endoscopic Approach

03H603Z   Insertion of Infusion Device into Left Axillary Artery, Open Approach

03H60DZ   Insertion of Intraluminal Device into Left Axillary Artery, Open Approach

03H633Z   Insertion of Infusion Device into Left Axillary Artery, Percutaneous Approach

03H63DZ   Insertion of Intraluminal Device into Left Axillary Artery, Percutaneous Approach

03H643Z   Insertion of Infusion Device into Left Axillary Artery, Percutaneous Endoscopic Approach

03H64DZ   Insertion of Intraluminal Device into Left Axillary Artery, Percutaneous Endoscopic Approach

03H703Z   Insertion of Infusion Device into Right Brachial Artery, Open Approach

03H70DZ   Insertion of Intraluminal Device into Right Brachial Artery, Open Approach

03H733Z   Insertion of Infusion Device into Right Brachial Artery, Percutaneous Approach

03H73DZ   Insertion of Intraluminal Device into Right Brachial Artery, Percutaneous Approach

03H743Z   Insertion of Infusion Device into Right Brachial Artery, Percutaneous Endoscopic Approach

03H74DZ   Insertion of Intraluminal Device into Right Brachial Artery, Percutaneous Endoscopic Approach

03H803Z   Insertion of Infusion Device into Left Brachial Artery, Open Approach

03H80DZ   Insertion of Intraluminal Device into Left Brachial Artery, Open Approach

03H833Z   Insertion of Infusion Device into Left Brachial Artery, Percutaneous Approach

03H83DZ   Insertion of Intraluminal Device into Left Brachial Artery, Percutaneous Approach

03H843Z   Insertion of Infusion Device into Left Brachial Artery, Percutaneous Endoscopic Approach

03H84DZ   Insertion of Intraluminal Device into Left Brachial Artery, Percutaneous Endoscopic Approach

03H903Z   Insertion of Infusion Device into Right Ulnar Artery, Open Approach

03H90DZ   Insertion of Intraluminal Device into Right Ulnar Artery, Open Approach

03H933Z   Insertion of Infusion Device into Right Ulnar Artery, Percutaneous Approach

03H93DZ   Insertion of Intraluminal Device into Right Ulnar Artery, Percutaneous Approach

03H943Z   Insertion of Infusion Device into Right Ulnar Artery, Percutaneous Endoscopic Approach

03H94DZ   Insertion of Intraluminal Device into Right Ulnar Artery, Percutaneous Endoscopic Approach

03HA03Z   Insertion of Infusion Device into Left Ulnar Artery, Open Approach

03HA0DZ   Insertion of Intraluminal Device into Left Ulnar Artery, Open Approach

03HA33Z   Insertion of Infusion Device into Left Ulnar Artery, Percutaneous Approach

03HA3DZ   Insertion of Intraluminal Device into Left Ulnar Artery, Percutaneous Approach

03HA43Z   Insertion of Infusion Device into Left Ulnar Artery, Percutaneous Endoscopic Approach

03HA4DZ   Insertion of Intraluminal Device into Left Ulnar Artery, Percutaneous Endoscopic Approach

03HB03Z   Insertion of Infusion Device into Right Radial Artery, Open Approach

03HB0DZ   Insertion of Intraluminal Device into Right Radial Artery, Open Approach

03HB33Z   Insertion of Infusion Device into Right Radial Artery, Percutaneous Approach

03HB3DZ   Insertion of Intraluminal Device into Right Radial Artery, Percutaneous Approach

03HB43Z   Insertion of Infusion Device into Right Radial Artery, Percutaneous Endoscopic Approach

03HB4DZ   Insertion of Intraluminal Device into Right Radial Artery, Percutaneous Endoscopic Approach

03HC03Z   Insertion of Infusion Device into Left Radial Artery, Open Approach

03HC0DZ   Insertion of Intraluminal Device into Left Radial Artery, Open Approach

03HC33Z   Insertion of Infusion Device into Left Radial Artery, Percutaneous Approach

03HC3DZ   Insertion of Intraluminal Device into Left Radial Artery, Percutaneous Approach

03HC43Z   Insertion of Infusion Device into Left Radial Artery, Percutaneous Endoscopic Approach

03HC4DZ   Insertion of Intraluminal Device into Left Radial Artery, Percutaneous Endoscopic Approach

03HD03Z   Insertion of Infusion Device into Right Hand Artery, Open Approach

03HD0DZ   Insertion of Intraluminal Device into Right Hand Artery, Open Approach

03HD33Z   Insertion of Infusion Device into Right Hand Artery, Percutaneous Approach

03HD3DZ   Insertion of Intraluminal Device into Right Hand Artery, Percutaneous Approach

03HD43Z   Insertion of Infusion Device into Right Hand Artery, Percutaneous Endoscopic Approach

03HD4DZ   Insertion of Intraluminal Device into Right Hand Artery, Percutaneous Endoscopic Approach

03HF03Z   Insertion of Infusion Device into Left Hand Artery, Open Approach

03HF0DZ   Insertion of Intraluminal Device into Left Hand Artery, Open Approach

03HF33Z   Insertion of Infusion Device into Left Hand Artery, Percutaneous Approach

03HF3DZ   Insertion of Intraluminal Device into Left Hand Artery, Percutaneous Approach

03HF43Z   Insertion of Infusion Device into Left Hand Artery, Percutaneous Endoscopic Approach

03HF4DZ   Insertion of Intraluminal Device into Left Hand Artery, Percutaneous Endoscopic Approach

03HG03Z   Insertion of Infusion Device into Intracranial Artery, Open Approach

03HG0DZ   Insertion of Intraluminal Device into Intracranial Artery, Open Approach

03HG33Z   Insertion of Infusion Device into Intracranial Artery, Percutaneous Approach

03HG3DZ   Insertion of Intraluminal Device into Intracranial Artery, Percutaneous Approach

03HG43Z   Insertion of Infusion Device into Intracranial Artery, Percutaneous Endoscopic Approach

03HG4DZ   Insertion of Intraluminal Device into Intracranial Artery, Percutaneous Endoscopic Approach

03HH03Z   Insertion of Infusion Device into Right Common Carotid Artery, Open Approach

03HH0DZ   Insertion of Intraluminal Device into Right Common Carotid Artery, Open Approach

03HH33Z   Insertion of Infusion Device into Right Common Carotid Artery, Percutaneous Approach

03HH3DZ   Insertion of Intraluminal Device into Right Common Carotid Artery, Percutaneous Approach

03HH43Z   Insertion of Infusion Device into Right Common Carotid Artery, Percutaneous Endoscopic Approach

03HH4DZ Insertion of Intraluminal Device into Right Common Carotid Artery, Percutaneous Endoscopic Approach

03HJ03Z Insertion of Infusion Device into Left Common Carotid Artery, Open Approach

03HJ0DZ Insertion of Intraluminal Device into Left Common Carotid Artery, Open Approach

03HJ33Z Insertion of Infusion Device into Left Common Carotid Artery, Percutaneous Approach

03HJ3DZ Insertion of Intraluminal Device into Left Common Carotid Artery, Percutaneous Approach

03HJ43Z Insertion of Infusion Device into Left Common Carotid Artery, Percutaneous Endoscopic Approach

03HJ4DZ Insertion of Intraluminal Device into Left Common Carotid Artery, Percutaneous Endoscopic Approach

03HK03Z Insertion of Infusion Device into Right Internal Carotid Artery, Open Approach

03HK0DZ Insertion of Intraluminal Device into Right Internal Carotid Artery, Open Approach

03HK0MZ Insertion of Stimulator Lead into Right Internal Carotid Artery, Open Approach

03HK33Z Insertion of Infusion Device into Right Internal Carotid Artery, Percutaneous Approach

03HK3DZ Insertion of Intraluminal Device into Right Internal Carotid Artery, Percutaneous Approach

03HK3MZ Insertion of Stimulator Lead into Right Internal Carotid Artery, Percutaneous Approach

03HK43Z Insertion of Infusion Device into Right Internal Carotid Artery, Percutaneous Endoscopic Approach

03HK4DZ Insertion of Intraluminal Device into Right Internal Carotid Artery, Percutaneous Endoscopic Approach

03HK4MZ Insertion of Stimulator Lead into Right Internal Carotid Artery, Percutaneous Endoscopic Approach

03HL03Z Insertion of Infusion Device into Left Internal Carotid Artery, Open Approach

03HL0DZ Insertion of Intraluminal Device into Left Internal Carotid Artery, Open Approach

03HL0MZ Insertion of Stimulator Lead into Left Internal Carotid Artery, Open Approach

03HL33Z Insertion of Infusion Device into Left Internal Carotid Artery, Percutaneous Approach

03HL3DZ Insertion of Intraluminal Device into Left Internal Carotid Artery, Percutaneous Approach

03HL3MZ Insertion of Stimulator Lead into Left Internal Carotid Artery, Percutaneous Approach

03HL43Z Insertion of Infusion Device into Left Internal Carotid Artery, Percutaneous Endoscopic Approach

03HL4DZ Insertion of Intraluminal Device into Left Internal Carotid Artery, Percutaneous Endoscopic Approach

03HL4MZ Insertion of Stimulator Lead into Left Internal Carotid Artery, Percutaneous Endoscopic Approach

03HM03Z Insertion of Infusion Device into Right External Carotid Artery, Open Approach

03HM0DZ Insertion of Intraluminal Device into Right External Carotid Artery, Open Approach

03HM33Z Insertion of Infusion Device into Right External Carotid Artery, Percutaneous Approach

03HM3DZ Insertion of Intraluminal Device into Right External Carotid Artery, Percutaneous Approach

03HM43Z Insertion of Infusion Device into Right External Carotid Artery, Percutaneous Endoscopic Approach

03HM4DZ Insertion of Intraluminal Device into Right External Carotid Artery, Percutaneous Endoscopic Approach

03HN03Z Insertion of Infusion Device into Left External Carotid Artery, Open Approach

03HN0DZ Insertion of Intraluminal Device into Left External Carotid Artery, Open Approach

03HN33Z Insertion of Infusion Device into Left External Carotid Artery, Percutaneous Approach

03HN3DZ Insertion of Intraluminal Device into Left External Carotid Artery, Percutaneous Approach

03HN43Z Insertion of Infusion Device into Left External Carotid Artery, Percutaneous Endoscopic Approach

03HN4DZ Insertion of Intraluminal Device into Left External Carotid Artery, Percutaneous Endoscopic Approach

03HP03Z Insertion of Infusion Device into Right Vertebral Artery, Open Approach

03HP0DZ Insertion of Intraluminal Device into Right Vertebral Artery, Open Approach

03HP33Z Insertion of Infusion Device into Right Vertebral Artery, Percutaneous Approach

03HP3DZ Insertion of Intraluminal Device into Right Vertebral Artery, Percutaneous Approach

03HP43Z Insertion of Infusion Device into Right Vertebral Artery, Percutaneous Endoscopic Approach

03HP4DZ Insertion of Intraluminal Device into Right Vertebral Artery, Percutaneous Endoscopic Approach

03HQ03Z Insertion of Infusion Device into Left Vertebral Artery, Open Approach

03HQ0DZ Insertion of Intraluminal Device into Left Vertebral Artery, Open Approach

03HQ33Z Insertion of Infusion Device into Left Vertebral Artery, Percutaneous Approach

03HQ3DZ Insertion of Intraluminal Device into Left Vertebral Artery, Percutaneous Approach

03HQ43Z Insertion of Infusion Device into Left Vertebral Artery, Percutaneous Endoscopic Approach

03HQ4DZ Insertion of Intraluminal Device into Left Vertebral Artery, Percutaneous Endoscopic Approach

03HR03Z Insertion of Infusion Device into Face Artery, Open Approach

03HR0DZ Insertion of Intraluminal Device into Face Artery, Open Approach

03HR33Z Insertion of Infusion Device into Face Artery, Percutaneous Approach

03HR3DZ Insertion of Intraluminal Device into Face Artery, Percutaneous Approach

03HR43Z Insertion of Infusion Device into Face Artery, Percutaneous Endoscopic Approach

03HR4DZ Insertion of Intraluminal Device into Face Artery, Percutaneous Endoscopic Approach

03HS03Z Insertion of Infusion Device into Right Temporal Artery, Open Approach

03HS0DZ Insertion of Intraluminal Device into Right Temporal Artery, Open Approach

03HS33Z Insertion of Infusion Device into Right Temporal Artery, Percutaneous Approach

03HS3DZ Insertion of Intraluminal Device into Right Temporal Artery, Percutaneous Approach

03HS43Z Insertion of Infusion Device into Right Temporal Artery, Percutaneous Endoscopic Approach

03HS4DZ Insertion of Intraluminal Device into Right Temporal Artery, Percutaneous Endoscopic Approach

03HT03Z Insertion of Infusion Device into Left Temporal Artery, Open Approach

03HT0DZ Insertion of Intraluminal Device into Left Temporal Artery, Open Approach

03HT33Z Insertion of Infusion Device into Left Temporal Artery, Percutaneous Approach

03HT3DZ Insertion of Intraluminal Device into Left Temporal Artery, Percutaneous Approach

03HT43Z Insertion of Infusion Device into Left Temporal Artery, Percutaneous Endoscopic Approach

03HT4DZ Insertion of Intraluminal Device into Left Temporal Artery, Percutaneous Endoscopic Approach

03HU03Z Insertion of Infusion Device into Right Thyroid Artery, Open Approach

03HU0DZ Insertion of Intraluminal Device into Right Thyroid Artery, Open Approach

03HU33Z Insertion of Infusion Device into Right Thyroid Artery, Percutaneous Approach

03HU3DZ Insertion of Intraluminal Device into Right Thyroid Artery, Percutaneous Approach

03HU43Z Insertion of Infusion Device into Right Thyroid Artery, Percutaneous Endoscopic Approach

03HU4DZ Insertion of Intraluminal Device into Right Thyroid Artery, Percutaneous Endoscopic Approach

03HV03Z Insertion of Infusion Device into Left Thyroid Artery, Open Approach

03HV0DZ Insertion of Intraluminal Device into Left Thyroid Artery, Open Approach

03HV33Z Insertion of Infusion Device into Left Thyroid Artery, Percutaneous Approach

03HV3DZ Insertion of Intraluminal Device into Left Thyroid Artery, Percutaneous Approach

03HV43Z   Insertion of Infusion Device into Left Thyroid Artery, Percutaneous Endoscopic Approach

03HV4DZ   Insertion of Intraluminal Device into Left Thyroid Artery, Percutaneous Endoscopic Approach

03HY02Z   Insertion of Monitoring Device into Upper Artery, Open Approach

03HY03Z   Insertion of Infusion Device into Upper Artery, Open Approach

03HY0DZ   Insertion of Intraluminal Device into Upper Artery, Open Approach

03HY32Z   Insertion of Monitoring Device into Upper Artery, Percutaneous Approach

03HY33Z   Insertion of Infusion Device into Upper Artery, Percutaneous Approach

03HY3DZ   Insertion of Intraluminal Device into Upper Artery, Percutaneous Approach

03HY42Z   Insertion of Monitoring Device into Upper Artery, Percutaneous Endoscopic Approach

03HY43Z   Insertion of Infusion Device into Upper Artery, Percutaneous Endoscopic Approach

03HY4DZ   Insertion of Intraluminal Device into Upper Artery, Percutaneous Endoscopic Approach

03J – Upper Arteries, Inspection

Review Coding Guidelines B3.11a, B3.11b and B3.11c

03JY0ZZ   Inspection of Upper Artery, Open Approach

03JY3ZZ   Inspection of Upper Artery, Percutaneous Approach

03JY4ZZ   Inspection of Upper Artery, Percutaneous Endoscopic Approach

03JYXZZ   Inspection of Upper Artery, External Approach

03L – Upper Arteries, Occlusion

Review Coding Guideline B3.12

03L00CZ   Occlusion of Right Internal Mammary Artery with Extraluminal Device, Open Approach

03L00DZ   Occlusion of Right Internal Mammary Artery with Intraluminal Device, Open Approach

03L00ZZ   Occlusion of Right Internal Mammary Artery, Open Approach

03L03CZ   Occlusion of Right Internal Mammary Artery with Extraluminal Device, Percutaneous Approach

03L03DZ   Occlusion of Right Internal Mammary Artery with Intraluminal Device, Percutaneous Approach

03L03ZZ   Occlusion of Right Internal Mammary Artery, Percutaneous Approach

03L04CZ   Occlusion of Right Internal Mammary Artery with Extraluminal Device, Percutaneous Endoscopic Approach

03L04DZ   Occlusion of Right Internal Mammary Artery with Intraluminal Device, Percutaneous Endoscopic Approach

03L04ZZ   Occlusion of Right Internal Mammary Artery, Percutaneous Endoscopic Approach

03L10CZ   Occlusion of Left Internal Mammary Artery with Extraluminal Device, Open Approach

03L10DZ   Occlusion of Left Internal Mammary Artery with Intraluminal Device, Open Approach

03L10ZZ   Occlusion of Left Internal Mammary Artery, Open Approach

03L13CZ   Occlusion of Left Internal Mammary Artery with Extraluminal Device, Percutaneous Approach

03L13DZ   Occlusion of Left Internal Mammary Artery with Intraluminal Device, Percutaneous Approach

03L13ZZ   Occlusion of Left Internal Mammary Artery, Percutaneous Approach

03L14CZ   Occlusion of Left Internal Mammary Artery with Extraluminal Device, Percutaneous Endoscopic Approach

03L14DZ   Occlusion of Left Internal Mammary Artery with Intraluminal Device, Percutaneous Endoscopic Approach

03L14ZZ   Occlusion of Left Internal Mammary Artery, Percutaneous Endoscopic Approach

03L20CZ   Occlusion of Innominate Artery with Extraluminal Device, Open Approach

03L20DZ   Occlusion of Innominate Artery with Intraluminal Device, Open Approach

03L20ZZ   Occlusion of Innominate Artery, Open Approach

03L23CZ   Occlusion of Innominate Artery with Extraluminal Device, Percutaneous Approach

03L23DZ   Occlusion of Innominate Artery with Intraluminal Device, Percutaneous Approach

03L23ZZ   Occlusion of Innominate Artery, Percutaneous Approach

03L24CZ   Occlusion of Innominate Artery with Extraluminal Device, Percutaneous Endoscopic Approach

03L24DZ   Occlusion of Innominate Artery with Intraluminal Device, Percutaneous Endoscopic Approach

03L24ZZ   Occlusion of Innominate Artery, Percutaneous Endoscopic Approach

03L30CZ   Occlusion of Right Subclavian Artery with Extraluminal Device, Open Approach

03L30DZ   Occlusion of Right Subclavian Artery with Intraluminal Device, Open Approach

03L30ZZ   Occlusion of Right Subclavian Artery, Open Approach

03L33CZ   Occlusion of Right Subclavian Artery with Extraluminal Device, Percutaneous Approach

03L33DZ   Occlusion of Right Subclavian Artery with Intraluminal Device, Percutaneous Approach

03L33ZZ   Occlusion of Right Subclavian Artery, Percutaneous Approach

03L34CZ   Occlusion of Right Subclavian Artery with Extraluminal Device, Percutaneous Endoscopic Approach

03L34DZ   Occlusion of Right Subclavian Artery with Intraluminal Device, Percutaneous Endoscopic Approach

03L34ZZ   Occlusion of Right Subclavian Artery, Percutaneous Endoscopic Approach

03L40CZ   Occlusion of Left Subclavian Artery with Extraluminal Device, Open Approach

03L40DZ   Occlusion of Left Subclavian Artery with Intraluminal Device, Open Approach

03L40ZZ   Occlusion of Left Subclavian Artery, Open Approach

03L43CZ   Occlusion of Left Subclavian Artery with Extraluminal Device, Percutaneous Approach

03L43DZ   Occlusion of Left Subclavian Artery with Intraluminal Device, Percutaneous Approach

03L43ZZ   Occlusion of Left Subclavian Artery, Percutaneous Approach

03L44CZ   Occlusion of Left Subclavian Artery with Extraluminal Device, Percutaneous Endoscopic Approach

03L44DZ   Occlusion of Left Subclavian Artery with Intraluminal Device, Percutaneous Endoscopic Approach

03L44ZZ   Occlusion of Left Subclavian Artery, Percutaneous Endoscopic Approach

03L50CZ   Occlusion of Right Axillary Artery with Extraluminal Device, Open Approach

03L50DZ   Occlusion of Right Axillary Artery with Intraluminal Device, Open Approach

03L50ZZ   Occlusion of Right Axillary Artery, Open Approach

03L53CZ   Occlusion of Right Axillary Artery with Extraluminal Device, Percutaneous Approach

03L53DZ   Occlusion of Right Axillary Artery with Intraluminal Device, Percutaneous Approach

03L53ZZ   Occlusion of Right Axillary Artery, Percutaneous Approach

03L54CZ   Occlusion of Right Axillary Artery with Extraluminal Device, Percutaneous Endoscopic Approach

03L54DZ   Occlusion of Right Axillary Artery with Intraluminal Device, Percutaneous Endoscopic Approach

03L54ZZ   Occlusion of Right Axillary Artery, Percutaneous Endoscopic Approach

03L60CZ   Occlusion of Left Axillary Artery with Extraluminal Device, Open Approach

03L60DZ   Occlusion of Left Axillary Artery with Intraluminal Device, Open Approach

03L60ZZ   Occlusion of Left Axillary Artery, Open Approach

03L63CZ   Occlusion of Left Axillary Artery with Extraluminal Device, Percutaneous Approach

03L63DZ Occlusion of Left Axillary Artery with Intraluminal Device, Percutaneous Approach

03L63ZZ Occlusion of Left Axillary Artery, Percutaneous Approach

03L64CZ Occlusion of Left Axillary Artery with Extraluminal Device, Percutaneous Endoscopic Approach

03L64DZ Occlusion of Left Axillary Artery with Intraluminal Device, Percutaneous Endoscopic Approach

03L64ZZ Occlusion of Left Axillary Artery, Percutaneous Endoscopic Approach

03L70CZ Occlusion of Right Brachial Artery with Extraluminal Device, Open Approach

03L70DZ Occlusion of Right Brachial Artery with Intraluminal Device, Open Approach

03L70ZZ Occlusion of Right Brachial Artery, Open Approach

03L73CZ Occlusion of Right Brachial Artery with Extraluminal Device, Percutaneous Approach

03L73DZ Occlusion of Right Brachial Artery with Intraluminal Device, Percutaneous Approach

03L73ZZ Occlusion of Right Brachial Artery, Percutaneous Approach

03L74CZ Occlusion of Right Brachial Artery with Extraluminal Device, Percutaneous Endoscopic Approach

03L74DZ Occlusion of Right Brachial Artery with Intraluminal Device, Percutaneous Endoscopic Approach

03L74ZZ Occlusion of Right Brachial Artery, Percutaneous Endoscopic Approach

03L80CZ Occlusion of Left Brachial Artery with Extraluminal Device, Open Approach

03L80DZ Occlusion of Left Brachial Artery with Intraluminal Device, Open Approach

03L80ZZ Occlusion of Left Brachial Artery, Open Approach

03L83CZ Occlusion of Left Brachial Artery with Extraluminal Device, Percutaneous Approach

03L83DZ Occlusion of Left Brachial Artery with Intraluminal Device, Percutaneous Approach

03L83ZZ Occlusion of Left Brachial Artery, Percutaneous Approach

03L84CZ Occlusion of Left Brachial Artery with Extraluminal Device, Percutaneous Endoscopic Approach

03L84DZ Occlusion of Left Brachial Artery with Intraluminal Device, Percutaneous Endoscopic Approach

03L84ZZ Occlusion of Left Brachial Artery, Percutaneous Endoscopic Approach

03L90CZ Occlusion of Right Ulnar Artery with Extraluminal Device, Open Approach

03L90DZ Occlusion of Right Ulnar Artery with Intraluminal Device, Open Approach

03L90ZZ Occlusion of Right Ulnar Artery, Open Approach

03L93CZ Occlusion of Right Ulnar Artery with Extraluminal Device, Percutaneous Approach

03L93DZ Occlusion of Right Ulnar Artery with Intraluminal Device, Percutaneous Approach

03L93ZZ Occlusion of Right Ulnar Artery, Percutaneous Approach

03L94CZ Occlusion of Right Ulnar Artery with Extraluminal Device, Percutaneous Endoscopic Approach

03L94DZ Occlusion of Right Ulnar Artery with Intraluminal Device, Percutaneous Endoscopic Approach

03L94ZZ Occlusion of Right Ulnar Artery, Percutaneous Endoscopic Approach

03LA0CZ Occlusion of Left Ulnar Artery with Extraluminal Device, Open Approach

03LA0DZ Occlusion of Left Ulnar Artery with Intraluminal Device, Open Approach

03LA0ZZ Occlusion of Left Ulnar Artery, Open Approach

03LA3CZ Occlusion of Left Ulnar Artery with Extraluminal Device, Percutaneous Approach

03LA3DZ Occlusion of Left Ulnar Artery with Intraluminal Device, Percutaneous Approach

03LA3ZZ Occlusion of Left Ulnar Artery, Percutaneous Approach

03LA4CZ Occlusion of Left Ulnar Artery with Extraluminal Device, Percutaneous Endoscopic Approach

03LA4DZ Occlusion of Left Ulnar Artery with Intraluminal Device, Percutaneous Endoscopic Approach

03LA4ZZ Occlusion of Left Ulnar Artery, Percutaneous Endoscopic Approach

03LB0CZ Occlusion of Right Radial Artery with Extraluminal Device, Open Approach

03LB0DZ Occlusion of Right Radial Artery with Intraluminal Device, Open Approach

03LB0ZZ Occlusion of Right Radial Artery, Open Approach

03LB3CZ Occlusion of Right Radial Artery with Extraluminal Device, Percutaneous Approach

03LB3DZ Occlusion of Right Radial Artery with Intraluminal Device, Percutaneous Approach

03LB3ZZ Occlusion of Right Radial Artery, Percutaneous Approach

03LB4CZ Occlusion of Right Radial Artery with Extraluminal Device, Percutaneous Endoscopic Approach

03LB4DZ Occlusion of Right Radial Artery with Intraluminal Device, Percutaneous Endoscopic Approach

03LB4ZZ Occlusion of Right Radial Artery, Percutaneous Endoscopic Approach

03LC0CZ Occlusion of Left Radial Artery with Extraluminal Device, Open Approach

03LC0DZ Occlusion of Left Radial Artery with Intraluminal Device, Open Approach

03LC0ZZ Occlusion of Left Radial Artery, Open Approach

03LC3CZ Occlusion of Left Radial Artery with Extraluminal Device, Percutaneous Approach

03LC3DZ Occlusion of Left Radial Artery with Intraluminal Device, Percutaneous Approach

03LC3ZZ Occlusion of Left Radial Artery, Percutaneous Approach

03LC4CZ Occlusion of Left Radial Artery with Extraluminal Device, Percutaneous Endoscopic Approach

03LC4DZ Occlusion of Left Radial Artery with Intraluminal Device, Percutaneous Endoscopic Approach

03LC4ZZ Occlusion of Left Radial Artery, Percutaneous Endoscopic Approach

03LD0CZ Occlusion of Right Hand Artery with Extraluminal Device, Open Approach

03LD0DZ Occlusion of Right Hand Artery with Intraluminal Device, Open Approach

03LD0ZZ Occlusion of Right Hand Artery, Open Approach

03LD3CZ Occlusion of Right Hand Artery with Extraluminal Device, Percutaneous Approach

03LD3DZ Occlusion of Right Hand Artery with Intraluminal Device, Percutaneous Approach

03LD3ZZ Occlusion of Right Hand Artery, Percutaneous Approach

03LD4CZ Occlusion of Right Hand Artery with Extraluminal Device, Percutaneous Endoscopic Approach

03LD4DZ Occlusion of Right Hand Artery with Intraluminal Device, Percutaneous Endoscopic Approach

03LD4ZZ Occlusion of Right Hand Artery, Percutaneous Endoscopic Approach

03LF0CZ Occlusion of Left Hand Artery with Extraluminal Device, Open Approach

03LF0DZ Occlusion of Left Hand Artery with Intraluminal Device, Open Approach

03LF0ZZ Occlusion of Left Hand Artery, Open Approach

03LF3CZ Occlusion of Left Hand Artery with Extraluminal Device, Percutaneous Approach

03LF3DZ Occlusion of Left Hand Artery with Intraluminal Device, Percutaneous Approach

03LF3ZZ Occlusion of Left Hand Artery, Percutaneous Approach

03LF4CZ Occlusion of Left Hand Artery with Extraluminal Device, Percutaneous Endoscopic Approach

03LF4DZ Occlusion of Left Hand Artery with Intraluminal Device, Percutaneous Endoscopic Approach

03LF4ZZ Occlusion of Left Hand Artery, Percutaneous Endoscopic Approach

03LG0BZ Occlusion of Intracranial Artery with Bioactive Intraluminal Device, Open Approach

03LG0CZ Occlusion of Intracranial Artery with Extraluminal Device, Open Approach

03LG0DZ Occlusion of Intracranial Artery with Intraluminal Device, Open Approach

03LG0ZZ Occlusion of Intracranial Artery, Open Approach

03LG3BZ Occlusion of Intracranial Artery with Bioactive Intraluminal Device, Percutaneous Approach

03LG3CZ Occlusion of Intracranial Artery with Extraluminal Device, Percutaneous Approach

03LG3DZ Occlusion of Intracranial Artery with Intraluminal Device, Percutaneous Approach

03LG3ZZ Occlusion of Intracranial Artery, Percutaneous Approach

03LG4BZ Occlusion of Intracranial Artery with Bioactive Intraluminal Device, Percutaneous Endoscopic Approach

03LG4CZ Occlusion of Intracranial Artery with Extraluminal Device, Percutaneous Endoscopic Approach

03LG4DZ Occlusion of Intracranial Artery with Intraluminal Device, Percutaneous Endoscopic Approach

03LG4ZZ Occlusion of Intracranial Artery, Percutaneous Endoscopic Approach

03LH0BZ Occlusion of Right Common Carotid Artery with Bioactive Intraluminal Device, Open Approach

03LH0CZ Occlusion of Right Common Carotid Artery with Extraluminal Device, Open Approach

03LH0DZ Occlusion of Right Common Carotid Artery with Intraluminal Device, Open Approach

03LH0ZZ Occlusion of Right Common Carotid Artery, Open Approach

03LH3BZ Occlusion of Right Common Carotid Artery with Bioactive Intraluminal Device, Percutaneous Approach

03LH3CZ Occlusion of Right Common Carotid Artery with Extraluminal Device, Percutaneous Approach

03LH3DZ Occlusion of Right Common Carotid Artery with Intraluminal Device, Percutaneous Approach

03LH3ZZ Occlusion of Right Common Carotid Artery, Percutaneous Approach

03LH4BZ Occlusion of Right Common Carotid Artery with Bioactive Intraluminal Device, Percutaneous Endoscopic Approach

03LH4CZ Occlusion of Right Common Carotid Artery with Extraluminal Device, Percutaneous Endoscopic Approach

03LH4DZ Occlusion of Right Common Carotid Artery with Intraluminal Device, Percutaneous Endoscopic Approach

03LH4ZZ Occlusion of Right Common Carotid Artery, Percutaneous Endoscopic Approach

03LJ0BZ Occlusion of Left Common Carotid Artery with Bioactive Intraluminal Device, Open Approach

03LJ0CZ Occlusion of Left Common Carotid Artery with Extraluminal Device, Open Approach

03LJ0DZ Occlusion of Left Common Carotid Artery with Intraluminal Device, Open Approach

03LJ0ZZ Occlusion of Left Common Carotid Artery, Open Approach

03LJ3BZ Occlusion of Left Common Carotid Artery with Bioactive Intraluminal Device, Percutaneous Approach

03LJ3CZ Occlusion of Left Common Carotid Artery with Extraluminal Device, Percutaneous Approach

03LJ3DZ Occlusion of Left Common Carotid Artery with Intraluminal Device, Percutaneous Approach

03LJ3ZZ Occlusion of Left Common Carotid Artery, Percutaneous Approach

03LJ4BZ Occlusion of Left Common Carotid Artery with Bioactive Intraluminal Device, Percutaneous Endoscopic Approach

03LJ4CZ Occlusion of Left Common Carotid Artery with Extraluminal Device, Percutaneous Endoscopic Approach

03LJ4DZ Occlusion of Left Common Carotid Artery with Intraluminal Device, Percutaneous Endoscopic Approach

03LJ4ZZ Occlusion of Left Common Carotid Artery, Percutaneous Endoscopic Approach

03LK0BZ Occlusion of Right Internal Carotid Artery with Bioactive Intraluminal Device, Open Approach

03LK0CZ Occlusion of Right Internal Carotid Artery with Extraluminal Device, Open Approach

03LK0DZ Occlusion of Right Internal Carotid Artery with Intraluminal Device, Open Approach

03LK0ZZ Occlusion of Right Internal Carotid Artery, Open Approach

03LK3BZ Occlusion of Right Internal Carotid Artery with Bioactive Intraluminal Device, Percutaneous Approach

03LK3CZ Occlusion of Right Internal Carotid Artery with Extraluminal Device, Percutaneous Approach

03LK3DZ Occlusion of Right Internal Carotid Artery with Intraluminal Device, Percutaneous Approach

03LK3ZZ Occlusion of Right Internal Carotid Artery, Percutaneous Approach

03LK4BZ Occlusion of Right Internal Carotid Artery with Bioactive Intraluminal Device, Percutaneous Endoscopic Approach

03LK4CZ Occlusion of Right Internal Carotid Artery with Extraluminal Device, Percutaneous Endoscopic Approach

03LK4DZ Occlusion of Right Internal Carotid Artery with Intraluminal Device, Percutaneous Endoscopic Approach

03LK4ZZ Occlusion of Right Internal Carotid Artery, Percutaneous Endoscopic Approach

03LL0BZ Occlusion of Left Internal Carotid Artery with Bioactive Intraluminal Device, Open Approach

03LL0CZ Occlusion of Left Internal Carotid Artery with Extraluminal Device, Open Approach

03LL0DZ Occlusion of Left Internal Carotid Artery with Intraluminal Device, Open Approach

03LL0ZZ Occlusion of Left Internal Carotid Artery, Open Approach

03LL3BZ Occlusion of Left Internal Carotid Artery with Bioactive Intraluminal Device, Percutaneous Approach

03LL3CZ Occlusion of Left Internal Carotid Artery with Extraluminal Device, Percutaneous Approach

03LL3DZ Occlusion of Left Internal Carotid Artery with Intraluminal Device, Percutaneous Approach

03LL3ZZ Occlusion of Left Internal Carotid Artery, Percutaneous Approach

03LL4BZ Occlusion of Left Internal Carotid Artery with Bioactive Intraluminal Device, Percutaneous Endoscopic Approach

03LL4CZ Occlusion of Left Internal Carotid Artery with Extraluminal Device, Percutaneous Endoscopic Approach

03LL4DZ Occlusion of Left Internal Carotid Artery with Intraluminal Device, Percutaneous Endoscopic Approach

03LL4ZZ Occlusion of Left Internal Carotid Artery, Percutaneous Endoscopic Approach

03LM0BZ Occlusion of Right External Carotid Artery with Bioactive Intraluminal Device, Open Approach

03LM0CZ Occlusion of Right External Carotid Artery with Extraluminal Device, Open Approach

03LM0DZ Occlusion of Right External Carotid Artery with Intraluminal Device, Open Approach

03LM0ZZ Occlusion of Right External Carotid Artery, Open Approach

03LM3BZ Occlusion of Right External Carotid Artery with Bioactive Intraluminal Device, Percutaneous Approach

03LM3CZ Occlusion of Right External Carotid Artery with Extraluminal Device, Percutaneous Approach

03LM3DZ Occlusion of Right External Carotid Artery with Intraluminal Device, Percutaneous Approach

03LM3ZZ Occlusion of Right External Carotid Artery, Percutaneous Approach

03LM4BZ Occlusion of Right External Carotid Artery with Bioactive Intraluminal Device, Percutaneous Endoscopic Approach

03LM4CZ Occlusion of Right External Carotid Artery with Extraluminal Device, Percutaneous Endoscopic Approach

03LM4DZ Occlusion of Right External Carotid Artery with Intraluminal Device, Percutaneous Endoscopic Approach

03LM4ZZ Occlusion of Right External Carotid Artery, Percutaneous Endoscopic Approach

03LN0BZ Occlusion of Left External Carotid Artery with Bioactive Intraluminal Device, Open Approach

03LN0CZ Occlusion of Left External Carotid Artery with Extraluminal Device, Open Approach

03LN0DZ Occlusion of Left External Carotid Artery with Intraluminal Device, Open Approach

03LN0ZZ Occlusion of Left External Carotid Artery, Open Approach

03LN3BZ Occlusion of Left External Carotid Artery with Bioactive Intraluminal Device, Percutaneous Approach

03LN3CZ Occlusion of Left External Carotid Artery with Extraluminal Device, Percutaneous Approach

03LN3DZ Occlusion of Left External Carotid Artery with Intraluminal Device, Percutaneous Approach

03LN3ZZ Occlusion of Left External Carotid Artery, Percutaneous Approach

03LN4BZ Occlusion of Left External Carotid Artery with Bioactive Intraluminal Device, Percutaneous Endoscopic Approach

03LN4CZ Occlusion of Left External Carotid Artery with Extraluminal Device, Percutaneous Endoscopic Approach

03LN4DZ Occlusion of Left External Carotid Artery with Intraluminal Device, Percutaneous Endoscopic Approach

03LN4ZZ Occlusion of Left External Carotid Artery, Percutaneous Endoscopic Approach

03LP0BZ Occlusion of Right Vertebral Artery with Bioactive Intraluminal Device, Open Approach

03LP0CZ Occlusion of Right Vertebral Artery with Extraluminal Device, Open Approach

03LP0DZ Occlusion of Right Vertebral Artery with Intraluminal Device, Open Approach

03LP0ZZ Occlusion of Right Vertebral Artery, Open Approach

03LP3BZ Occlusion of Right Vertebral Artery with Bioactive Intraluminal Device, Percutaneous Approach

03LP3CZ Occlusion of Right Vertebral Artery with Extraluminal Device, Percutaneous Approach

03LP3DZ Occlusion of Right Vertebral Artery with Intraluminal Device, Percutaneous Approach

03LP3ZZ Occlusion of Right Vertebral Artery, Percutaneous Approach

03LP4BZ Occlusion of Right Vertebral Artery with Bioactive Intraluminal Device, Percutaneous Endoscopic Approach

03LP4CZ Occlusion of Right Vertebral Artery with Extraluminal Device, Percutaneous Endoscopic Approach

03LP4DZ Occlusion of Right Vertebral Artery with Intraluminal Device, Percutaneous Endoscopic Approach

03LP4ZZ Occlusion of Right Vertebral Artery, Percutaneous Endoscopic Approach

03LQ0BZ Occlusion of Left Vertebral Artery with Bioactive Intraluminal Device, Open Approach

03LQ0CZ Occlusion of Left Vertebral Artery with Extraluminal Device, Open Approach

03LQ0DZ Occlusion of Left Vertebral Artery with Intraluminal Device, Open Approach

03LQ0ZZ Occlusion of Left Vertebral Artery, Open Approach

03LQ3BZ Occlusion of Left Vertebral Artery with Bioactive Intraluminal Device, Percutaneous Approach

03LQ3CZ Occlusion of Left Vertebral Artery with Extraluminal Device, Percutaneous Approach

03LQ3DZ Occlusion of Left Vertebral Artery with Intraluminal Device, Percutaneous Approach

03LQ3ZZ Occlusion of Left Vertebral Artery, Percutaneous Approach

03LQ4BZ Occlusion of Left Vertebral Artery with Bioactive Intraluminal Device, Percutaneous Endoscopic Approach

03LQ4CZ Occlusion of Left Vertebral Artery with Extraluminal Device, Percutaneous Endoscopic Approach

03LQ4DZ Occlusion of Left Vertebral Artery with Intraluminal Device, Percutaneous Endoscopic Approach

03LQ4ZZ Occlusion of Left Vertebral Artery, Percutaneous Endoscopic Approach

03LR0CZ Occlusion of Face Artery with Extraluminal Device, Open Approach

03LR0DZ Occlusion of Face Artery with Intraluminal Device, Open Approach

03LR0ZZ Occlusion of Face Artery, Open Approach

03LR3CZ Occlusion of Face Artery with Extraluminal Device, Percutaneous Approach

03LR3DZ Occlusion of Face Artery with Intraluminal Device, Percutaneous Approach

03LR3ZZ Occlusion of Face Artery, Percutaneous Approach

03LR4CZ Occlusion of Face Artery with Extraluminal Device, Percutaneous Endoscopic Approach

03LR4DZ Occlusion of Face Artery with Intraluminal Device, Percutaneous Endoscopic Approach

03LR4ZZ Occlusion of Face Artery, Percutaneous Endoscopic Approach

03LS0CZ Occlusion of Right Temporal Artery with Extraluminal Device, Open Approach

03LS0DZ Occlusion of Right Temporal Artery with Intraluminal Device, Open Approach

03LS0ZZ Occlusion of Right Temporal Artery, Open Approach

03LS3CZ Occlusion of Right Temporal Artery with Extraluminal Device, Percutaneous Approach

03LS3DZ Occlusion of Right Temporal Artery with Intraluminal Device, Percutaneous Approach

03LS3ZZ Occlusion of Right Temporal Artery, Percutaneous Approach

03LS4CZ Occlusion of Right Temporal Artery with Extraluminal Device, Percutaneous Endoscopic Approach

03LS4DZ Occlusion of Right Temporal Artery with Intraluminal Device, Percutaneous Endoscopic Approach

03LS4ZZ Occlusion of Right Temporal Artery, Percutaneous Endoscopic Approach

03LT0CZ Occlusion of Left Temporal Artery with Extraluminal Device, Open Approach

03LT0DZ Occlusion of Left Temporal Artery with Intraluminal Device, Open Approach

03LT0ZZ Occlusion of Left Temporal Artery, Open Approach

03LT3CZ Occlusion of Left Temporal Artery with Extraluminal Device, Percutaneous Approach

03LT3DZ Occlusion of Left Temporal Artery with Intraluminal Device, Percutaneous Approach

03LT3ZZ Occlusion of Left Temporal Artery, Percutaneous Approach

03LT4CZ Occlusion of Left Temporal Artery with Extraluminal Device, Percutaneous Endoscopic Approach

03LT4DZ Occlusion of Left Temporal Artery with Intraluminal Device, Percutaneous Endoscopic Approach

03LT4ZZ Occlusion of Left Temporal Artery, Percutaneous Endoscopic Approach

03LU0CZ Occlusion of Right Thyroid Artery with Extraluminal Device, Open Approach

03LU0DZ Occlusion of Right Thyroid Artery with Intraluminal Device, Open Approach

03LU0ZZ Occlusion of Right Thyroid Artery, Open Approach

03LU3CZ Occlusion of Right Thyroid Artery with Extraluminal Device, Percutaneous Approach

03LU3DZ Occlusion of Right Thyroid Artery with Intraluminal Device, Percutaneous Approach

03LU3ZZ Occlusion of Right Thyroid Artery, Percutaneous Approach

03LU4CZ Occlusion of Right Thyroid Artery with Extraluminal Device, Percutaneous Endoscopic Approach

03LU4DZ Occlusion of Right Thyroid Artery with Intraluminal Device, Percutaneous Endoscopic Approach

03LU4ZZ Occlusion of Right Thyroid Artery, Percutaneous Endoscopic Approach

03LV0CZ Occlusion of Left Thyroid Artery with Extraluminal Device, Open Approach

03LV0DZ Occlusion of Left Thyroid Artery with Intraluminal Device, Open Approach

03LV0ZZ Occlusion of Left Thyroid Artery, Open Approach

03LV3CZ Occlusion of Left Thyroid Artery with Extraluminal Device, Percutaneous Approach

03LV3DZ Occlusion of Left Thyroid Artery with Intraluminal Device, Percutaneous Approach

03LV3ZZ Occlusion of Left Thyroid Artery, Percutaneous Approach

03LV4CZ Occlusion of Left Thyroid Artery with Extraluminal Device, Percutaneous Endoscopic Approach

03LV4DZ Occlusion of Left Thyroid Artery with Intraluminal Device, Percutaneous Endoscopic Approach

03LV4ZZ Occlusion of Left Thyroid Artery, Percutaneous Endoscopic Approach

03LY0CZ Occlusion of Upper Artery with Extraluminal Device, Open Approach

03LY0DZ Occlusion of Upper Artery with Intraluminal Device, Open Approach

03LY0ZZ Occlusion of Upper Artery, Open Approach

03LY3CZ Occlusion of Upper Artery with Extraluminal Device, Percutaneous Approach

03LY3DZ Occlusion of Upper Artery with Intraluminal Device, Percutaneous Approach

03LY3ZZ Occlusion of Upper Artery, Percutaneous Approach

03LY4CZ Occlusion of Upper Artery with Extraluminal Device, Percutaneous Endoscopic Approach

03LY4DZ Occlusion of Upper Artery with Intraluminal Device, Percutaneous Endoscopic Approach

03LY4ZZ Occlusion of Upper Artery, Percutaneous Endoscopic Approach

03N – Upper Arteries, Release

Review Coding Guidelines B3.13 and B3.14

03N00ZZ Release Right Internal Mammary Artery, Open Approach

03N03ZZ Release Right Internal Mammary Artery, Percutaneous Approach

03N04ZZ Release Right Internal Mammary Artery, Percutaneous Endoscopic Approach

03N10ZZ Release Left Internal Mammary Artery, Open Approach

03N13ZZ Release Left Internal Mammary Artery, Percutaneous Approach

03N14ZZ Release Left Internal Mammary Artery, Percutaneous Endoscopic Approach

03N20ZZ Release Innominate Artery, Open Approach

♀ Female-only   ♂ Male-only   ● Limited Coverage   ● Non-OR   ▨ HAC-associated procedure   ● Non-covered procedures   ✚ Combination

03N23ZZ   Release Innominate Artery, Percutaneous Approach
03N24ZZ   Release Innominate Artery, Percutaneous Endoscopic Approach
03N30ZZ   Release Right Subclavian Artery, Open Approach
03N33ZZ   Release Right Subclavian Artery, Percutaneous Approach
03N34ZZ   Release Right Subclavian Artery, Percutaneous Endoscopic Approach
03N40ZZ   Release Left Subclavian Artery, Open Approach
03N43ZZ   Release Left Subclavian Artery, Percutaneous Approach
03N44ZZ   Release Left Subclavian Artery, Percutaneous Endoscopic Approach
03N50ZZ   Release Right Axillary Artery, Open Approach
03N53ZZ   Release Right Axillary Artery, Percutaneous Approach
03N54ZZ   Release Right Axillary Artery, Percutaneous Endoscopic Approach
03N60ZZ   Release Left Axillary Artery, Open Approach
03N63ZZ   Release Left Axillary Artery, Percutaneous Approach
03N64ZZ   Release Left Axillary Artery, Percutaneous Endoscopic Approach
03N70ZZ   Release Right Brachial Artery, Open Approach
03N73ZZ   Release Right Brachial Artery, Percutaneous Approach
03N74ZZ   Release Right Brachial Artery, Percutaneous Endoscopic Approach
03N80ZZ   Release Left Brachial Artery, Open Approach
03N83ZZ   Release Left Brachial Artery, Percutaneous Approach
03N84ZZ   Release Left Brachial Artery, Percutaneous Endoscopic Approach
03N90ZZ   Release Right Ulnar Artery, Open Approach
03N93ZZ   Release Right Ulnar Artery, Percutaneous Approach
03N94ZZ   Release Right Ulnar Artery, Percutaneous Endoscopic Approach
03NA0ZZ   Release Left Ulnar Artery, Open Approach
03NA3ZZ   Release Left Ulnar Artery, Percutaneous Approach
03NA4ZZ   Release Left Ulnar Artery, Percutaneous Endoscopic Approach
03NB0ZZ   Release Right Radial Artery, Open Approach
03NB3ZZ   Release Right Radial Artery, Percutaneous Approach
03NB4ZZ   Release Right Radial Artery, Percutaneous Endoscopic Approach
03NC0ZZ   Release Left Radial Artery, Open Approach
03NC3ZZ   Release Left Radial Artery, Percutaneous Approach
03NC4ZZ   Release Left Radial Artery, Percutaneous Endoscopic Approach
03ND0ZZ   Release Right Hand Artery, Open Approach
03ND3ZZ   Release Right Hand Artery, Percutaneous Approach
03ND4ZZ   Release Right Hand Artery, Percutaneous Endoscopic Approach
03NF0ZZ   Release Left Hand Artery, Open Approach
03NF3ZZ   Release Left Hand Artery, Percutaneous Approach
03NF4ZZ   Release Left Hand Artery, Percutaneous Endoscopic Approach
03NG0ZZ   Release Intracranial Artery, Open Approach
03NG3ZZ   Release Intracranial Artery, Percutaneous Approach
03NG4ZZ   Release Intracranial Artery, Percutaneous Endoscopic Approach
03NH0ZZ   Release Right Common Carotid Artery, Open Approach
03NH3ZZ   Release Right Common Carotid Artery, Percutaneous Approach
03NH4ZZ   Release Right Common Carotid Artery, Percutaneous Endoscopic Approach
03NJ0ZZ   Release Left Common Carotid Artery, Open Approach

03NJ3ZZ   Release Left Common Carotid Artery, Percutaneous Approach
03NJ4ZZ   Release Left Common Carotid Artery, Percutaneous Endoscopic Approach
03NK0ZZ   Release Right Internal Carotid Artery, Open Approach
03NK3ZZ   Release Right Internal Carotid Artery, Percutaneous Approach
03NK4ZZ   Release Right Internal Carotid Artery, Percutaneous Endoscopic Approach
03NL0ZZ   Release Left Internal Carotid Artery, Open Approach
03NL3ZZ   Release Left Internal Carotid Artery, Percutaneous Approach
03NL4ZZ   Release Left Internal Carotid Artery, Percutaneous Endoscopic Approach
03NM0ZZ   Release Right External Carotid Artery, Open Approach
03NM3ZZ   Release Right External Carotid Artery, Percutaneous Approach
03NM4ZZ   Release Right External Carotid Artery, Percutaneous Endoscopic Approach
03NN0ZZ   Release Left External Carotid Artery, Open Approach
03NN3ZZ   Release Left External Carotid Artery, Percutaneous Approach
03NN4ZZ   Release Left External Carotid Artery, Percutaneous Endoscopic Approach
03NP0ZZ   Release Right Vertebral Artery, Open Approach
03NP3ZZ   Release Right Vertebral Artery, Percutaneous Approach
03NP4ZZ   Release Right Vertebral Artery, Percutaneous Endoscopic Approach
03NQ0ZZ   Release Left Vertebral Artery, Open Approach
03NQ3ZZ   Release Left Vertebral Artery, Percutaneous Approach
03NQ4ZZ   Release Left Vertebral Artery, Percutaneous Endoscopic Approach
03NR0ZZ   Release Face Artery, Open Approach
03NR3ZZ   Release Face Artery, Percutaneous Approach
03NR4ZZ   Release Face Artery, Percutaneous Endoscopic Approach
03NS0ZZ   Release Right Temporal Artery, Open Approach
03NS3ZZ   Release Right Temporal Artery, Percutaneous Approach
03NS4ZZ   Release Right Temporal Artery, Percutaneous Endoscopic Approach
03NT0ZZ   Release Left Temporal Artery, Open Approach
03NT3ZZ   Release Left Temporal Artery, Percutaneous Approach
03NT4ZZ   Release Left Temporal Artery, Percutaneous Endoscopic Approach
03NU0ZZ   Release Right Thyroid Artery, Open Approach
03NU3ZZ   Release Right Thyroid Artery, Percutaneous Approach
03NU4ZZ   Release Right Thyroid Artery, Percutaneous Endoscopic Approach
03NV0ZZ   Release Left Thyroid Artery, Open Approach
03NV3ZZ   Release Left Thyroid Artery, Percutaneous Approach
03NV4ZZ   Release Left Thyroid Artery, Percutaneous Endoscopic Approach
03NY0ZZ   Release Upper Artery, Open Approach
03NY3ZZ   Release Upper Artery, Percutaneous Approach
03NY4ZZ   Release Upper Artery, Percutaneous Endoscopic Approach

03P – Upper Arteries, Removal

Review Coding Guideline B6.1c

03PY00Z   Removal of Drainage Device from Upper Artery, Open Approach
03PY02Z   Removal of Monitoring Device from Upper Artery, Open Approach
03PY03Z   Removal of Infusion Device from Upper Artery, Open Approach
03PY07Z   Removal of Autologous Tissue Substitute from Upper Artery, Open Approach
03PY0CZ   Removal of Extraluminal Device from Upper Artery, Open Approach
03PY0DZ   Removal of Intraluminal Device from Upper Artery, Open Approach
03PY0JZ   Removal of Synthetic Substitute from Upper Artery, Open Approach
03PY0KZ   Removal of Nonautologous Tissue Substitute from Upper Artery, Open Approach
03PY0MZ   Removal of Stimulator Lead from Upper Artery, Open Approach
03PY30Z   Removal of Drainage Device from Upper Artery, Percutaneous Approach
03PY32Z   Removal of Monitoring Device from Upper Artery, Percutaneous Approach
03PY33Z   Removal of Infusion Device from Upper Artery, Percutaneous Approach
03PY37Z   Removal of Autologous Tissue Substitute from Upper Artery, Percutaneous Approach
03PY3CZ   Removal of Extraluminal Device from Upper Artery, Percutaneous Approach

03PY3DZ   Removal of Intraluminal Device from Upper Artery, Percutaneous Approach
03PY3JZ   Removal of Synthetic Substitute from Upper Artery, Percutaneous Approach
03PY3KZ   Removal of Nonautologous Tissue Substitute from Upper Artery, Percutaneous Approach
03PY3MZ   Removal of Stimulator Lead from Upper Artery, Percutaneous Approach
03PY40Z   Removal of Drainage Device from Upper Artery, Percutaneous Endoscopic Approach
03PY42Z   Removal of Monitoring Device from Upper Artery, Percutaneous Endoscopic Approach
03PY43Z   Removal of Infusion Device from Upper Artery, Percutaneous Endoscopic Approach
03PY47Z   Removal of Autologous Tissue Substitute from Upper Artery, Percutaneous Endoscopic Approach
03PY4CZ   Removal of Extraluminal Device from Upper Artery, Percutaneous Endoscopic Approach
03PY4DZ   Removal of Intraluminal Device from Upper Artery, Percutaneous Endoscopic Approach
03PY4JZ   Removal of Synthetic Substitute from Upper Artery, Percutaneous Endoscopic Approach

---

♀ Female-only   ♂ Male-only   ● Limited Coverage   ● Non-OR   🅷🅰🅲 HAC-associated procedure   ● Non-covered procedures   ➕ Combination

03PY4KZ Removal of Nonautologous Tissue Substitute from Upper Artery, Percutaneous Endoscopic Approach
03PY4MZ Removal of Stimulator Lead from Upper Artery, Percutaneous Endoscopic Approach
03PYX0Z Removal of Drainage Device from Upper Artery, External Approach

03PYX2Z Removal of Monitoring Device from Upper Artery, External Approach
03PYX3Z Removal of Infusion Device from Upper Artery, External Approach
03PYXDZ Removal of Intraluminal Device from Upper Artery, External Approach
03PYXMZ Removal of Stimulator Lead from Upper Artery, External Approach

03Q – Upper Arteries, Repair

03Q00ZZ Repair Right Internal Mammary Artery, Open Approach
03Q03ZZ Repair Right Internal Mammary Artery, Percutaneous Approach
03Q04ZZ Repair Right Internal Mammary Artery, Percutaneous Endoscopic Approach
03Q10ZZ Repair Left Internal Mammary Artery, Open Approach
03Q13ZZ Repair Left Internal Mammary Artery, Percutaneous Approach
03Q14ZZ Repair Left Internal Mammary Artery, Percutaneous Endoscopic Approach
03Q20ZZ Repair Innominate Artery, Open Approach
03Q23ZZ Repair Innominate Artery, Percutaneous Approach
03Q24ZZ Repair Innominate Artery, Percutaneous Endoscopic Approach
03Q30ZZ Repair Right Subclavian Artery, Open Approach
03Q33ZZ Repair Right Subclavian Artery, Percutaneous Approach
03Q34ZZ Repair Right Subclavian Artery, Percutaneous Endoscopic Approach
03Q40ZZ Repair Left Subclavian Artery, Open Approach
03Q43ZZ Repair Left Subclavian Artery, Percutaneous Approach
03Q44ZZ Repair Left Subclavian Artery, Percutaneous Endoscopic Approach
03Q50ZZ Repair Right Axillary Artery, Open Approach
03Q53ZZ Repair Right Axillary Artery, Percutaneous Approach
03Q54ZZ Repair Right Axillary Artery, Percutaneous Endoscopic Approach
03Q60ZZ Repair Left Axillary Artery, Open Approach
03Q63ZZ Repair Left Axillary Artery, Percutaneous Approach
03Q64ZZ Repair Left Axillary Artery, Percutaneous Endoscopic Approach
03Q70ZZ Repair Right Brachial Artery, Open Approach
03Q73ZZ Repair Right Brachial Artery, Percutaneous Approach
03Q74ZZ Repair Right Brachial Artery, Percutaneous Endoscopic Approach
03Q80ZZ Repair Left Brachial Artery, Open Approach
03Q83ZZ Repair Left Brachial Artery, Percutaneous Approach
03Q84ZZ Repair Left Brachial Artery, Percutaneous Endoscopic Approach
03Q90ZZ Repair Right Ulnar Artery, Open Approach
03Q93ZZ Repair Right Ulnar Artery, Percutaneous Approach
03Q94ZZ Repair Right Ulnar Artery, Percutaneous Endoscopic Approach
03QA0ZZ Repair Left Ulnar Artery, Open Approach
03QA3ZZ Repair Left Ulnar Artery, Percutaneous Approach
03QA4ZZ Repair Left Ulnar Artery, Percutaneous Endoscopic Approach
03QB0ZZ Repair Right Radial Artery, Open Approach
03QB3ZZ Repair Right Radial Artery, Percutaneous Approach
03QB4ZZ Repair Right Radial Artery, Percutaneous Endoscopic Approach
03QC0ZZ Repair Left Radial Artery, Open Approach
03QC3ZZ Repair Left Radial Artery, Percutaneous Approach
03QC4ZZ Repair Left Radial Artery, Percutaneous Endoscopic Approach
03QD0ZZ Repair Right Hand Artery, Open Approach
03QD3ZZ Repair Right Hand Artery, Percutaneous Approach
03QD4ZZ Repair Right Hand Artery, Percutaneous Endoscopic Approach
03QF0ZZ Repair Left Hand Artery, Open Approach
03QF3ZZ Repair Left Hand Artery, Percutaneous Approach
03QF4ZZ Repair Left Hand Artery, Percutaneous Endoscopic Approach
03QG0ZZ Repair Intracranial Artery, Open Approach
03QG3ZZ Repair Intracranial Artery, Percutaneous Approach
03QG4ZZ Repair Intracranial Artery, Percutaneous Endoscopic Approach

03QH0ZZ Repair Right Common Carotid Artery, Open Approach
03QH3ZZ Repair Right Common Carotid Artery, Percutaneous Approach
03QH4ZZ Repair Right Common Carotid Artery, Percutaneous Endoscopic Approach
03QJ0ZZ Repair Left Common Carotid Artery, Open Approach
03QJ3ZZ Repair Left Common Carotid Artery, Percutaneous Approach
03QJ4ZZ Repair Left Common Carotid Artery, Percutaneous Endoscopic Approach
03QK0ZZ Repair Right Internal Carotid Artery, Open Approach
03QK3ZZ Repair Right Internal Carotid Artery, Percutaneous Approach
03QK4ZZ Repair Right Internal Carotid Artery, Percutaneous Endoscopic Approach
03QL0ZZ Repair Left Internal Carotid Artery, Open Approach
03QL3ZZ Repair Left Internal Carotid Artery, Percutaneous Approach
03QL4ZZ Repair Left Internal Carotid Artery, Percutaneous Endoscopic Approach
03QM0ZZ Repair Right External Carotid Artery, Open Approach
03QM3ZZ Repair Right External Carotid Artery, Percutaneous Approach
03QM4ZZ Repair Right External Carotid Artery, Percutaneous Endoscopic Approach
03QN0ZZ Repair Left External Carotid Artery, Open Approach
03QN3ZZ Repair Left External Carotid Artery, Percutaneous Approach
03QN4ZZ Repair Left External Carotid Artery, Percutaneous Endoscopic Approach
03QP0ZZ Repair Right Vertebral Artery, Open Approach
03QP3ZZ Repair Right Vertebral Artery, Percutaneous Approach
03QP4ZZ Repair Right Vertebral Artery, Percutaneous Endoscopic Approach
03QQ0ZZ Repair Left Vertebral Artery, Open Approach
03QQ3ZZ Repair Left Vertebral Artery, Percutaneous Approach
03QQ4ZZ Repair Left Vertebral Artery, Percutaneous Endoscopic Approach
03QR0ZZ Repair Face Artery, Open Approach
03QR3ZZ Repair Face Artery, Percutaneous Approach
03QR4ZZ Repair Face Artery, Percutaneous Endoscopic Approach
03QS0ZZ Repair Right Temporal Artery, Open Approach
03QS3ZZ Repair Right Temporal Artery, Percutaneous Approach
03QS4ZZ Repair Right Temporal Artery, Percutaneous Endoscopic Approach
03QT0ZZ Repair Left Temporal Artery, Open Approach
03QT3ZZ Repair Left Temporal Artery, Percutaneous Approach
03QT4ZZ Repair Left Temporal Artery, Percutaneous Endoscopic Approach
03QU0ZZ Repair Right Thyroid Artery, Open Approach
03QU3ZZ Repair Right Thyroid Artery, Percutaneous Approach
03QU4ZZ Repair Right Thyroid Artery, Percutaneous Endoscopic Approach
03QV0ZZ Repair Left Thyroid Artery, Open Approach
03QV3ZZ Repair Left Thyroid Artery, Percutaneous Approach
03QV4ZZ Repair Left Thyroid Artery, Percutaneous Endoscopic Approach
03QY0ZZ Repair Upper Artery, Open Approach
03QY3ZZ Repair Upper Artery, Percutaneous Approach
03QY4ZZ Repair Upper Artery, Percutaneous Endoscopic Approach

03R – Upper Arteries, Replacement

03R007Z Replacement of Right Internal Mammary Artery with Autologous Tissue Substitute, Open Approach
03R00JZ Replacement of Right Internal Mammary Artery with Synthetic Substitute, Open Approach
03R00KZ Replacement of Right Internal Mammary Artery with Nonautologous Tissue Substitute, Open Approach
03R047Z Replacement of Right Internal Mammary Artery with Autologous Tissue Substitute, Percutaneous Endoscopic Approach
03R04JZ Replacement of Right Internal Mammary Artery with Synthetic Substitute, Percutaneous Endoscopic Approach

03R04KZ Replacement of Right Internal Mammary Artery with Nonautologous Tissue Substitute, Percutaneous Endoscopic Approach
03R107Z Replacement of Left Internal Mammary Artery with Autologous Tissue Substitute, Open Approach
03R10JZ Replacement of Left Internal Mammary Artery with Synthetic Substitute, Open Approach
03R10KZ Replacement of Left Internal Mammary Artery with Nonautologous Tissue Substitute, Open Approach
03R147Z Replacement of Left Internal Mammary Artery with Autologous Tissue Substitute, Percutaneous Endoscopic Approach

03R14JZ Replacement of Left Internal Mammary Artery with Synthetic Substitute, Percutaneous Endoscopic Approach

03R14KZ Replacement of Left Internal Mammary Artery with Nonautologous Tissue Substitute, Percutaneous Endoscopic Approach

03R207Z Replacement of Innominate Artery with Autologous Tissue Substitute, Open Approach

03R20JZ Replacement of Innominate Artery with Synthetic Substitute, Open Approach

03R20KZ Replacement of Innominate Artery with Nonautologous Tissue Substitute, Open Approach

03R247Z Replacement of Innominate Artery with Autologous Tissue Substitute, Percutaneous Endoscopic Approach

03R24JZ Replacement of Innominate Artery with Synthetic Substitute, Percutaneous Endoscopic Approach

03R24KZ Replacement of Innominate Artery with Nonautologous Tissue Substitute, Percutaneous Endoscopic Approach

03R307Z Replacement of Right Subclavian Artery with Autologous Tissue Substitute, Open Approach

03R30JZ Replacement of Right Subclavian Artery with Synthetic Substitute, Open Approach

03R30KZ Replacement of Right Subclavian Artery with Nonautologous Tissue Substitute, Open Approach

03R347Z Replacement of Right Subclavian Artery with Autologous Tissue Substitute, Percutaneous Endoscopic Approach

03R34JZ Replacement of Right Subclavian Artery with Synthetic Substitute, Percutaneous Endoscopic Approach

03R34KZ Replacement of Right Subclavian Artery with Nonautologous Tissue Substitute, Percutaneous Endoscopic Approach

03R407Z Replacement of Left Subclavian Artery with Autologous Tissue Substitute, Open Approach

03R40JZ Replacement of Left Subclavian Artery with Synthetic Substitute, Open Approach

03R40KZ Replacement of Left Subclavian Artery with Nonautologous Tissue Substitute, Open Approach

03R447Z Replacement of Left Subclavian Artery with Autologous Tissue Substitute, Percutaneous Endoscopic Approach

03R44JZ Replacement of Left Subclavian Artery with Synthetic Substitute, Percutaneous Endoscopic Approach

03R44KZ Replacement of Left Subclavian Artery with Nonautologous Tissue Substitute, Percutaneous Endoscopic Approach

03R507Z Replacement of Right Axillary Artery with Autologous Tissue Substitute, Open Approach

03R50JZ Replacement of Right Axillary Artery with Synthetic Substitute, Open Approach

03R50KZ Replacement of Right Axillary Artery with Nonautologous Tissue Substitute, Open Approach

03R547Z Replacement of Right Axillary Artery with Autologous Tissue Substitute, Percutaneous Endoscopic Approach

03R54JZ Replacement of Right Axillary Artery with Synthetic Substitute, Percutaneous Endoscopic Approach

03R54KZ Replacement of Right Axillary Artery with Nonautologous Tissue Substitute, Percutaneous Endoscopic Approach

03R607Z Replacement of Left Axillary Artery with Autologous Tissue Substitute, Open Approach

03R60JZ Replacement of Left Axillary Artery with Synthetic Substitute, Open Approach

03R60KZ Replacement of Left Axillary Artery with Nonautologous Tissue Substitute, Open Approach

03R647Z Replacement of Left Axillary Artery with Autologous Tissue Substitute, Percutaneous Endoscopic Approach

03R64JZ Replacement of Left Axillary Artery with Synthetic Substitute, Percutaneous Endoscopic Approach

03R64KZ Replacement of Left Axillary Artery with Nonautologous Tissue Substitute, Percutaneous Endoscopic Approach

03R707Z Replacement of Right Brachial Artery with Autologous Tissue Substitute, Open Approach

03R70JZ Replacement of Right Brachial Artery with Synthetic Substitute, Open Approach

03R70KZ Replacement of Right Brachial Artery with Nonautologous Tissue Substitute, Open Approach

03R747Z Replacement of Right Brachial Artery with Autologous Tissue Substitute, Percutaneous Endoscopic Approach

03R74JZ Replacement of Right Brachial Artery with Synthetic Substitute, Percutaneous Endoscopic Approach

03R74KZ Replacement of Right Brachial Artery with Nonautologous Tissue Substitute, Percutaneous Endoscopic Approach

03R807Z Replacement of Left Brachial Artery with Autologous Tissue Substitute, Open Approach

03R80JZ Replacement of Left Brachial Artery with Synthetic Substitute, Open Approach

03R80KZ Replacement of Left Brachial Artery with Nonautologous Tissue Substitute, Open Approach

03R847Z Replacement of Left Brachial Artery with Autologous Tissue Substitute, Percutaneous Endoscopic Approach

03R84JZ Replacement of Left Brachial Artery with Synthetic Substitute, Percutaneous Endoscopic Approach

03R84KZ Replacement of Left Brachial Artery with Nonautologous Tissue Substitute, Percutaneous Endoscopic Approach

03R907Z Replacement of Right Ulnar Artery with Autologous Tissue Substitute, Open Approach

03R90JZ Replacement of Right Ulnar Artery with Synthetic Substitute, Open Approach

03R90KZ Replacement of Right Ulnar Artery with Nonautologous Tissue Substitute, Open Approach

03R947Z Replacement of Right Ulnar Artery with Autologous Tissue Substitute, Percutaneous Endoscopic Approach

03R94JZ Replacement of Right Ulnar Artery with Synthetic Substitute, Percutaneous Endoscopic Approach

03R94KZ Replacement of Right Ulnar Artery with Nonautologous Tissue Substitute, Percutaneous Endoscopic Approach

03RA07Z Replacement of Left Ulnar Artery with Autologous Tissue Substitute, Open Approach

03RA0JZ Replacement of Left Ulnar Artery with Synthetic Substitute, Open Approach

03RA0KZ Replacement of Left Ulnar Artery with Nonautologous Tissue Substitute, Open Approach

03RA47Z Replacement of Left Ulnar Artery with Autologous Tissue Substitute, Percutaneous Endoscopic Approach

03RA4JZ Replacement of Left Ulnar Artery with Synthetic Substitute, Percutaneous Endoscopic Approach

03RA4KZ Replacement of Left Ulnar Artery with Nonautologous Tissue Substitute, Percutaneous Endoscopic Approach

03RB07Z Replacement of Right Radial Artery with Autologous Tissue Substitute, Open Approach

03RB0JZ Replacement of Right Radial Artery with Synthetic Substitute, Open Approach

03RB0KZ Replacement of Right Radial Artery with Nonautologous Tissue Substitute, Open Approach

03RB47Z Replacement of Right Radial Artery with Autologous Tissue Substitute, Percutaneous Endoscopic Approach

03RB4JZ Replacement of Right Radial Artery with Synthetic Substitute, Percutaneous Endoscopic Approach

03RB4KZ Replacement of Right Radial Artery with Nonautologous Tissue Substitute, Percutaneous Endoscopic Approach

03RC07Z Replacement of Left Radial Artery with Autologous Tissue Substitute, Open Approach

03RC0JZ Replacement of Left Radial Artery with Synthetic Substitute, Open Approach

03RC0KZ Replacement of Left Radial Artery with Nonautologous Tissue Substitute, Open Approach

03RC47Z Replacement of Left Radial Artery with Autologous Tissue Substitute, Percutaneous Endoscopic Approach

03RC4JZ Replacement of Left Radial Artery with Synthetic Substitute, Percutaneous Endoscopic Approach

03RC4KZ Replacement of Left Radial Artery with Nonautologous Tissue Substitute, Percutaneous Endoscopic Approach

03RD07Z Replacement of Right Hand Artery with Autologous Tissue Substitute, Open Approach

03RD0JZ Replacement of Right Hand Artery with Synthetic Substitute, Open Approach

03RD0KZ Replacement of Right Hand Artery with Nonautologous Tissue Substitute, Open Approach

03RD47Z Replacement of Right Hand Artery with Autologous Tissue Substitute, Percutaneous Endoscopic Approach

03RD4JZ Replacement of Right Hand Artery with Synthetic Substitute, Percutaneous Endoscopic Approach

03RD4KZ Replacement of Right Hand Artery with Nonautologous Tissue Substitute, Percutaneous Endoscopic Approach

03RF07Z   Replacement of Left Hand Artery with Autologous Tissue Substitute, Open Approach

03RF0JZ   Replacement of Left Hand Artery with Synthetic Substitute, Open Approach

03RF0KZ   Replacement of Left Hand Artery with Nonautologous Tissue Substitute, Open Approach

03RF47Z   Replacement of Left Hand Artery with Autologous Tissue Substitute, Percutaneous Endoscopic Approach

03RF4JZ   Replacement of Left Hand Artery with Synthetic Substitute, Percutaneous Endoscopic Approach

03RF4KZ   Replacement of Left Hand Artery with Nonautologous Tissue Substitute, Percutaneous Endoscopic Approach

03RG07Z   Replacement of Intracranial Artery with Autologous Tissue Substitute, Open Approach

03RG0JZ   Replacement of Intracranial Artery with Synthetic Substitute, Open Approach

03RG0KZ   Replacement of Intracranial Artery with Nonautologous Tissue Substitute, Open Approach

03RG47Z   Replacement of Intracranial Artery with Autologous Tissue Substitute, Percutaneous Endoscopic Approach

03RG4JZ   Replacement of Intracranial Artery with Synthetic Substitute, Percutaneous Endoscopic Approach

03RG4KZ   Replacement of Intracranial Artery with Nonautologous Tissue Substitute, Percutaneous Endoscopic Approach

03RH07Z   Replacement of Right Common Carotid Artery with Autologous Tissue Substitute, Open Approach

03RH0JZ   Replacement of Right Common Carotid Artery with Synthetic Substitute, Open Approach

03RH0KZ   Replacement of Right Common Carotid Artery with Nonautologous Tissue Substitute, Open Approach

03RH47Z   Replacement of Right Common Carotid Artery with Autologous Tissue Substitute, Percutaneous Endoscopic Approach

03RH4JZ   Replacement of Right Common Carotid Artery with Synthetic Substitute, Percutaneous Endoscopic Approach

03RH4KZ   Replacement of Right Common Carotid Artery with Nonautologous Tissue Substitute, Percutaneous Endoscopic Approach

03RJ07Z   Replacement of Left Common Carotid Artery with Autologous Tissue Substitute, Open Approach

03RJ0JZ   Replacement of Left Common Carotid Artery with Synthetic Substitute, Open Approach

03RJ0KZ   Replacement of Left Common Carotid Artery with Nonautologous Tissue Substitute, Open Approach

03RJ47Z   Replacement of Left Common Carotid Artery with Autologous Tissue Substitute, Percutaneous Endoscopic Approach

03RJ4JZ   Replacement of Left Common Carotid Artery with Synthetic Substitute, Percutaneous Endoscopic Approach

03RJ4KZ   Replacement of Left Common Carotid Artery with Nonautologous Tissue Substitute, Percutaneous Endoscopic Approach

03RK07Z   Replacement of Right Internal Carotid Artery with Autologous Tissue Substitute, Open Approach

03RK0JZ   Replacement of Right Internal Carotid Artery with Synthetic Substitute, Open Approach

03RK0KZ   Replacement of Right Internal Carotid Artery with Nonautologous Tissue Substitute, Open Approach

03RK47Z   Replacement of Right Internal Carotid Artery with Autologous Tissue Substitute, Percutaneous Endoscopic Approach

03RK4JZ   Replacement of Right Internal Carotid Artery with Synthetic Substitute, Percutaneous Endoscopic Approach

03RK4KZ   Replacement of Right Internal Carotid Artery with Nonautologous Tissue Substitute, Percutaneous Endoscopic Approach

03RL07Z   Replacement of Left Internal Carotid Artery with Autologous Tissue Substitute, Open Approach

03RL0JZ   Replacement of Left Internal Carotid Artery with Synthetic Substitute, Open Approach

03RL0KZ   Replacement of Left Internal Carotid Artery with Nonautologous Tissue Substitute, Open Approach

03RL47Z   Replacement of Left Internal Carotid Artery with Autologous Tissue Substitute, Percutaneous Endoscopic Approach

03RL4JZ   Replacement of Left Internal Carotid Artery with Synthetic Substitute, Percutaneous Endoscopic Approach

03RL4KZ   Replacement of Left Internal Carotid Artery with Nonautologous Tissue Substitute, Percutaneous Endoscopic Approach

03RM07Z   Replacement of Right External Carotid Artery with Autologous Tissue Substitute, Open Approach

03RM0JZ   Replacement of Right External Carotid Artery with Synthetic Substitute, Open Approach

03RM0KZ   Replacement of Right External Carotid Artery with Nonautologous Tissue Substitute, Open Approach

03RM47Z   Replacement of Right External Carotid Artery with Autologous Tissue Substitute, Percutaneous Endoscopic Approach

03RM4JZ   Replacement of Right External Carotid Artery with Synthetic Substitute, Percutaneous Endoscopic Approach

03RM4KZ   Replacement of Right External Carotid Artery with Nonautologous Tissue Substitute, Percutaneous Endoscopic Approach

03RN07Z   Replacement of Left External Carotid Artery with Autologous Tissue Substitute, Open Approach

03RN0JZ   Replacement of Left External Carotid Artery with Synthetic Substitute, Open Approach

03RN0KZ   Replacement of Left External Carotid Artery with Nonautologous Tissue Substitute, Open Approach

03RN47Z   Replacement of Left External Carotid Artery with Autologous Tissue Substitute, Percutaneous Endoscopic Approach

03RN4JZ   Replacement of Left External Carotid Artery with Synthetic Substitute, Percutaneous Endoscopic Approach

03RN4KZ   Replacement of Left External Carotid Artery with Nonautologous Tissue Substitute, Percutaneous Endoscopic Approach

03RP07Z   Replacement of Right Vertebral Artery with Autologous Tissue Substitute, Open Approach

03RP0JZ   Replacement of Right Vertebral Artery with Synthetic Substitute, Open Approach

03RP0KZ   Replacement of Right Vertebral Artery with Nonautologous Tissue Substitute, Open Approach

03RP47Z   Replacement of Right Vertebral Artery with Autologous Tissue Substitute, Percutaneous Endoscopic Approach

03RP4JZ   Replacement of Right Vertebral Artery with Synthetic Substitute, Percutaneous Endoscopic Approach

03RP4KZ   Replacement of Right Vertebral Artery with Nonautologous Tissue Substitute, Percutaneous Endoscopic Approach

03RQ07Z   Replacement of Left Vertebral Artery with Autologous Tissue Substitute, Open Approach

03RQ0JZ   Replacement of Left Vertebral Artery with Synthetic Substitute, Open Approach

03RQ0KZ   Replacement of Left Vertebral Artery with Nonautologous Tissue Substitute, Open Approach

03RQ47Z   Replacement of Left Vertebral Artery with Autologous Tissue Substitute, Percutaneous Endoscopic Approach

03RQ4JZ   Replacement of Left Vertebral Artery with Synthetic Substitute, Percutaneous Endoscopic Approach

03RQ4KZ   Replacement of Left Vertebral Artery with Nonautologous Tissue Substitute, Percutaneous Endoscopic Approach

03RR07Z   Replacement of Face Artery with Autologous Tissue Substitute, Open Approach

03RR0JZ   Replacement of Face Artery with Synthetic Substitute, Open Approach

03RR0KZ   Replacement of Face Artery with Nonautologous Tissue Substitute, Open Approach

03RR47Z   Replacement of Face Artery with Autologous Tissue Substitute, Percutaneous Endoscopic Approach

03RR4JZ   Replacement of Face Artery with Synthetic Substitute, Percutaneous Endoscopic Approach

03RR4KZ   Replacement of Face Artery with Nonautologous Tissue Substitute, Percutaneous Endoscopic Approach

03RS07Z   Replacement of Right Temporal Artery with Autologous Tissue Substitute, Open Approach

03RS0JZ   Replacement of Right Temporal Artery with Synthetic Substitute, Open Approach

03RS0KZ   Replacement of Right Temporal Artery with Nonautologous Tissue Substitute, Open Approach

03RS47Z   Replacement of Right Temporal Artery with Autologous Tissue Substitute, Percutaneous Endoscopic Approach

03RS4JZ   Replacement of Right Temporal Artery with Synthetic Substitute, Percutaneous Endoscopic Approach

03RS4KZ   Replacement of Right Temporal Artery with Nonautologous Tissue Substitute, Percutaneous Endoscopic Approach

03RT07Z   Replacement of Left Temporal Artery with Autologous Tissue Substitute, Open Approach

03RT0JZ   Replacement of Left Temporal Artery with Synthetic Substitute, Open Approach

---

♀ Female-only   ♂ Male-only   ● Limited Coverage   ● Non-OR   [HAC] HAC-associated procedure   ● Non-covered procedures   ✚ Combination

03RT0KZ   Replacement of Left Temporal Artery with Nonautologous Tissue Substitute, Open Approach

03RT47Z   Replacement of Left Temporal Artery with Autologous Tissue Substitute, Percutaneous Endoscopic Approach

03RT4JZ   Replacement of Left Temporal Artery with Synthetic Substitute, Percutaneous Endoscopic Approach

03RT4KZ   Replacement of Left Temporal Artery with Nonautologous Tissue Substitute, Percutaneous Endoscopic Approach

03RU07Z   Replacement of Right Thyroid Artery with Autologous Tissue Substitute, Open Approach

03RU0JZ   Replacement of Right Thyroid Artery with Synthetic Substitute, Open Approach

03RU0KZ   Replacement of Right Thyroid Artery with Nonautologous Tissue Substitute, Open Approach

03RU47Z   Replacement of Right Thyroid Artery with Autologous Tissue Substitute, Percutaneous Endoscopic Approach

03RU4JZ   Replacement of Right Thyroid Artery with Synthetic Substitute, Percutaneous Endoscopic Approach

03RU4KZ   Replacement of Right Thyroid Artery with Nonautologous Tissue Substitute, Percutaneous Endoscopic Approach

03RV07Z   Replacement of Left Thyroid Artery with Autologous Tissue Substitute, Open Approach

03RV0JZ   Replacement of Left Thyroid Artery with Synthetic Substitute, Open Approach

03RV0KZ   Replacement of Left Thyroid Artery with Nonautologous Tissue Substitute, Open Approach

03RV47Z   Replacement of Left Thyroid Artery with Autologous Tissue Substitute, Percutaneous Endoscopic Approach

03RV4JZ   Replacement of Left Thyroid Artery with Synthetic Substitute, Percutaneous Endoscopic Approach

03RV4KZ   Replacement of Left Thyroid Artery with Nonautologous Tissue Substitute, Percutaneous Endoscopic Approach

03RY07Z   Replacement of Upper Artery with Autologous Tissue Substitute, Open Approach

03RY0JZ   Replacement of Upper Artery with Synthetic Substitute, Open Approach

03RY0KZ   Replacement of Upper Artery with Nonautologous Tissue Substitute, Open Approach

03RY47Z   Replacement of Upper Artery with Autologous Tissue Substitute, Percutaneous Endoscopic Approach

03RY4JZ   Replacement of Upper Artery with Synthetic Substitute, Percutaneous Endoscopic Approach

03RY4KZ   Replacement of Upper Artery with Nonautologous Tissue Substitute, Percutaneous Endoscopic Approach

03S – Upper Arteries, Reposition

03S00ZZ   Reposition Right Internal Mammary Artery, Open Approach

03S03ZZ   Reposition Right Internal Mammary Artery, Percutaneous Approach

03S04ZZ   Reposition Right Internal Mammary Artery, Percutaneous Endoscopic Approach

03S10ZZ   Reposition Left Internal Mammary Artery, Open Approach

03S13ZZ   Reposition Left Internal Mammary Artery, Percutaneous Approach

03S14ZZ   Reposition Left Internal Mammary Artery, Percutaneous Endoscopic Approach

03S20ZZ   Reposition Innominate Artery, Open Approach

03S23ZZ   Reposition Innominate Artery, Percutaneous Approach

03S24ZZ   Reposition Innominate Artery, Percutaneous Endoscopic Approach

03S30ZZ   Reposition Right Subclavian Artery, Open Approach

03S33ZZ   Reposition Right Subclavian Artery, Percutaneous Approach

03S34ZZ   Reposition Right Subclavian Artery, Percutaneous Endoscopic Approach

03S40ZZ   Reposition Left Subclavian Artery, Open Approach

03S43ZZ   Reposition Left Subclavian Artery, Percutaneous Approach

03S44ZZ   Reposition Left Subclavian Artery, Percutaneous Endoscopic Approach

03S50ZZ   Reposition Right Axillary Artery, Open Approach

03S53ZZ   Reposition Right Axillary Artery, Percutaneous Approach

03S54ZZ   Reposition Right Axillary Artery, Percutaneous Endoscopic Approach

03S60ZZ   Reposition Left Axillary Artery, Open Approach

03S63ZZ   Reposition Left Axillary Artery, Percutaneous Approach

03S64ZZ   Reposition Left Axillary Artery, Percutaneous Endoscopic Approach

03S70ZZ   Reposition Right Brachial Artery, Open Approach

03S73ZZ   Reposition Right Brachial Artery, Percutaneous Approach

03S74ZZ   Reposition Right Brachial Artery, Percutaneous Endoscopic Approach

03S80ZZ   Reposition Left Brachial Artery, Open Approach

03S83ZZ   Reposition Left Brachial Artery, Percutaneous Approach

03S84ZZ   Reposition Left Brachial Artery, Percutaneous Endoscopic Approach

03S90ZZ   Reposition Right Ulnar Artery, Open Approach

03S93ZZ   Reposition Right Ulnar Artery, Percutaneous Approach

03S94ZZ   Reposition Right Ulnar Artery, Percutaneous Endoscopic Approach

03SA0ZZ   Reposition Left Ulnar Artery, Open Approach

03SA3ZZ   Reposition Left Ulnar Artery, Percutaneous Approach

03SA4ZZ   Reposition Left Ulnar Artery, Percutaneous Endoscopic Approach

03SB0ZZ   Reposition Right Radial Artery, Open Approach

03SB3ZZ   Reposition Right Radial Artery, Percutaneous Approach

03SB4ZZ   Reposition Right Radial Artery, Percutaneous Endoscopic Approach

03SC0ZZ   Reposition Left Radial Artery, Open Approach

03SC3ZZ   Reposition Left Radial Artery, Percutaneous Approach

03SC4ZZ   Reposition Left Radial Artery, Percutaneous Endoscopic Approach

03SD0ZZ   Reposition Right Hand Artery, Open Approach

03SD3ZZ   Reposition Right Hand Artery, Percutaneous Approach

03SD4ZZ   Reposition Right Hand Artery, Percutaneous Endoscopic Approach

03SF0ZZ   Reposition Left Hand Artery, Open Approach

03SF3ZZ   Reposition Left Hand Artery, Percutaneous Approach

03SF4ZZ   Reposition Left Hand Artery, Percutaneous Endoscopic Approach

03SG0ZZ   Reposition Intracranial Artery, Open Approach

03SG3ZZ   Reposition Intracranial Artery, Percutaneous Approach

03SG4ZZ   Reposition Intracranial Artery, Percutaneous Endoscopic Approach

03SH0ZZ   Reposition Right Common Carotid Artery, Open Approach

03SH3ZZ   Reposition Right Common Carotid Artery, Percutaneous Approach

03SH4ZZ   Reposition Right Common Carotid Artery, Percutaneous Endoscopic Approach

03SJ0ZZ   Reposition Left Common Carotid Artery, Open Approach

03SJ3ZZ   Reposition Left Common Carotid Artery, Percutaneous Approach

03SJ4ZZ   Reposition Left Common Carotid Artery, Percutaneous Endoscopic Approach

03SK0ZZ   Reposition Right Internal Carotid Artery, Open Approach

03SK3ZZ   Reposition Right Internal Carotid Artery, Percutaneous Approach

03SK4ZZ   Reposition Right Internal Carotid Artery, Percutaneous Endoscopic Approach

03SL0ZZ   Reposition Left Internal Carotid Artery, Open Approach

03SL3ZZ   Reposition Left Internal Carotid Artery, Percutaneous Approach

03SL4ZZ   Reposition Left Internal Carotid Artery, Percutaneous Endoscopic Approach

03SM0ZZ   Reposition Right External Carotid Artery, Open Approach

03SM3ZZ   Reposition Right External Carotid Artery, Percutaneous Approach

03SM4ZZ   Reposition Right External Carotid Artery, Percutaneous Endoscopic Approach

03SN0ZZ   Reposition Left External Carotid Artery, Open Approach

03SN3ZZ   Reposition Left External Carotid Artery, Percutaneous Approach

03SN4ZZ   Reposition Left External Carotid Artery, Percutaneous Endoscopic Approach

03SP0ZZ   Reposition Right Vertebral Artery, Open Approach

03SP3ZZ   Reposition Right Vertebral Artery, Percutaneous Approach

03SP4ZZ   Reposition Right Vertebral Artery, Percutaneous Endoscopic Approach

03SQ0ZZ   Reposition Left Vertebral Artery, Open Approach

03SQ3ZZ   Reposition Left Vertebral Artery, Percutaneous Approach

03SQ4ZZ   Reposition Left Vertebral Artery, Percutaneous Endoscopic Approach

03SR0ZZ   Reposition Face Artery, Open Approach

03SR3ZZ   Reposition Face Artery, Percutaneous Approach

03SR4ZZ   Reposition Face Artery, Percutaneous Endoscopic Approach

03SS0ZZ   Reposition Right Temporal Artery, Open Approach

03SS3ZZ   Reposition Right Temporal Artery, Percutaneous Approach

03SS4ZZ   Reposition Right Temporal Artery, Percutaneous Endoscopic Approach

03ST0ZZ   Reposition Left Temporal Artery, Open Approach

03ST3ZZ   Reposition Left Temporal Artery, Percutaneous Approach

03ST4ZZ   Reposition Left Temporal Artery, Percutaneous Endoscopic Approach

03SU0ZZ   Reposition Right Thyroid Artery, Open Approach

03SU3ZZ   Reposition Right Thyroid Artery, Percutaneous Approach

03SU4ZZ   Reposition Right Thyroid Artery, Percutaneous Endoscopic Approach

03SV0ZZ Reposition Left Thyroid Artery, Open Approach
03SV3ZZ Reposition Left Thyroid Artery, Percutaneous Approach
03SV4ZZ Reposition Left Thyroid Artery, Percutaneous Endoscopic Approach

03SY0ZZ Reposition Upper Artery, Open Approach
03SY3ZZ Reposition Upper Artery, Percutaneous Approach
03SY4ZZ Reposition Upper Artery, Percutaneous Endoscopic Approach

03U – Upper Arteries, Supplement

03U007Z Supplement Right Internal Mammary Artery with Autologous Tissue Substitute, Open Approach
03U00JZ Supplement Right Internal Mammary Artery with Synthetic Substitute, Open Approach
03U00KZ Supplement Right Internal Mammary Artery with Nonautologous Tissue Substitute, Open Approach
03U037Z Supplement Right Internal Mammary Artery with Autologous Tissue Substitute, Percutaneous Approach
03U03JZ Supplement Right Internal Mammary Artery with Synthetic Substitute, Percutaneous Approach
03U03KZ Supplement Right Internal Mammary Artery with Nonautologous Tissue Substitute, Percutaneous Approach
03U047Z Supplement Right Internal Mammary Artery with Autologous Tissue Substitute, Percutaneous Endoscopic Approach
03U04JZ Supplement Right Internal Mammary Artery with Synthetic Substitute, Percutaneous Endoscopic Approach
03U04KZ Supplement Right Internal Mammary Artery with Nonautologous Tissue Substitute, Percutaneous Endoscopic Approach
03U107Z Supplement Left Internal Mammary Artery with Autologous Tissue Substitute, Open Approach
03U10JZ Supplement Left Internal Mammary Artery with Synthetic Substitute, Open Approach
03U10KZ Supplement Left Internal Mammary Artery with Nonautologous Tissue Substitute, Open Approach
03U137Z Supplement Left Internal Mammary Artery with Autologous Tissue Substitute, Percutaneous Approach
03U13JZ Supplement Left Internal Mammary Artery with Synthetic Substitute, Percutaneous Approach
03U13KZ Supplement Left Internal Mammary Artery with Nonautologous Tissue Substitute, Percutaneous Approach
03U147Z Supplement Left Internal Mammary Artery with Autologous Tissue Substitute, Percutaneous Endoscopic Approach
03U14JZ Supplement Left Internal Mammary Artery with Synthetic Substitute, Percutaneous Endoscopic Approach
03U14KZ Supplement Left Internal Mammary Artery with Nonautologous Tissue Substitute, Percutaneous Endoscopic Approach
03U207Z Supplement Innominate Artery with Autologous Tissue Substitute, Open Approach
03U20JZ Supplement Innominate Artery with Synthetic Substitute, Open Approach
03U20KZ Supplement Innominate Artery with Nonautologous Tissue Substitute, Open Approach
03U237Z Supplement Innominate Artery with Autologous Tissue Substitute, Percutaneous Approach
03U23JZ Supplement Innominate Artery with Synthetic Substitute, Percutaneous Approach
03U23KZ Supplement Innominate Artery with Nonautologous Tissue Substitute, Percutaneous Approach
03U247Z Supplement Innominate Artery with Autologous Tissue Substitute, Percutaneous Endoscopic Approach
03U24JZ Supplement Innominate Artery with Synthetic Substitute, Percutaneous Endoscopic Approach
03U24KZ Supplement Innominate Artery with Nonautologous Tissue Substitute, Percutaneous Endoscopic Approach
03U307Z Supplement Right Subclavian Artery with Autologous Tissue Substitute, Open Approach
03U30JZ Supplement Right Subclavian Artery with Synthetic Substitute, Open Approach
03U30KZ Supplement Right Subclavian Artery with Nonautologous Tissue Substitute, Open Approach
03U337Z Supplement Right Subclavian Artery with Autologous Tissue Substitute, Percutaneous Approach
03U33JZ Supplement Right Subclavian Artery with Synthetic Substitute, Percutaneous Approach
03U33KZ Supplement Right Subclavian Artery with Nonautologous Tissue Substitute, Percutaneous Approach

03U347Z Supplement Right Subclavian Artery with Autologous Tissue Substitute, Percutaneous Endoscopic Approach
03U34JZ Supplement Right Subclavian Artery with Synthetic Substitute, Percutaneous Endoscopic Approach
03U34KZ Supplement Right Subclavian Artery with Nonautologous Tissue Substitute, Percutaneous Endoscopic Approach
03U407Z Supplement Left Subclavian Artery with Autologous Tissue Substitute, Open Approach
03U40JZ Supplement Left Subclavian Artery with Synthetic Substitute, Open Approach
03U40KZ Supplement Left Subclavian Artery with Nonautologous Tissue Substitute, Open Approach
03U437Z Supplement Left Subclavian Artery with Autologous Tissue Substitute, Percutaneous Approach
03U43JZ Supplement Left Subclavian Artery with Synthetic Substitute, Percutaneous Approach
03U43KZ Supplement Left Subclavian Artery with Nonautologous Tissue Substitute, Percutaneous Approach
03U447Z Supplement Left Subclavian Artery with Autologous Tissue Substitute, Percutaneous Endoscopic Approach
03U44JZ Supplement Left Subclavian Artery with Synthetic Substitute, Percutaneous Endoscopic Approach
03U44KZ Supplement Left Subclavian Artery with Nonautologous Tissue Substitute, Percutaneous Endoscopic Approach
03U507Z Supplement Right Axillary Artery with Autologous Tissue Substitute, Open Approach
03U50JZ Supplement Right Axillary Artery with Synthetic Substitute, Open Approach
03U50KZ Supplement Right Axillary Artery with Nonautologous Tissue Substitute, Open Approach
03U537Z Supplement Right Axillary Artery with Autologous Tissue Substitute, Percutaneous Approach
03U53JZ Supplement Right Axillary Artery with Synthetic Substitute, Percutaneous Approach
03U53KZ Supplement Right Axillary Artery with Nonautologous Tissue Substitute, Percutaneous Approach
03U547Z Supplement Right Axillary Artery with Autologous Tissue Substitute, Percutaneous Endoscopic Approach
03U54JZ Supplement Right Axillary Artery with Synthetic Substitute, Percutaneous Endoscopic Approach
03U54KZ Supplement Right Axillary Artery with Nonautologous Tissue Substitute, Percutaneous Endoscopic Approach
03U607Z Supplement Left Axillary Artery with Autologous Tissue Substitute, Open Approach
03U60JZ Supplement Left Axillary Artery with Synthetic Substitute, Open Approach
03U60KZ Supplement Left Axillary Artery with Nonautologous Tissue Substitute, Open Approach
03U637Z Supplement Left Axillary Artery with Autologous Tissue Substitute, Percutaneous Approach
03U63JZ Supplement Left Axillary Artery with Synthetic Substitute, Percutaneous Approach
03U63KZ Supplement Left Axillary Artery with Nonautologous Tissue Substitute, Percutaneous Approach
03U647Z Supplement Left Axillary Artery with Autologous Tissue Substitute, Percutaneous Endoscopic Approach
03U64JZ Supplement Left Axillary Artery with Synthetic Substitute, Percutaneous Endoscopic Approach
03U64KZ Supplement Left Axillary Artery with Nonautologous Tissue Substitute, Percutaneous Endoscopic Approach
03U707Z Supplement Right Brachial Artery with Autologous Tissue Substitute, Open Approach
03U70JZ Supplement Right Brachial Artery with Synthetic Substitute, Open Approach
03U70KZ Supplement Right Brachial Artery with Nonautologous Tissue Substitute, Open Approach

---

03U737Z Supplement Right Brachial Artery with Autologous Tissue Substitute, Percutaneous Approach

03U73JZ Supplement Right Brachial Artery with Synthetic Substitute, Percutaneous Approach

03U73KZ Supplement Right Brachial Artery with Nonautologous Tissue Substitute, Percutaneous Approach

03U747Z Supplement Right Brachial Artery with Autologous Tissue Substitute, Percutaneous Endoscopic Approach

03U74JZ Supplement Right Brachial Artery with Synthetic Substitute, Percutaneous Endoscopic Approach

03U74KZ Supplement Right Brachial Artery with Nonautologous Tissue Substitute, Percutaneous Endoscopic Approach

03U807Z Supplement Left Brachial Artery with Autologous Tissue Substitute, Open Approach

03U80JZ Supplement Left Brachial Artery with Synthetic Substitute, Open Approach

03U80KZ Supplement Left Brachial Artery with Nonautologous Tissue Substitute, Open Approach

03U837Z Supplement Left Brachial Artery with Autologous Tissue Substitute, Percutaneous Approach

03U83JZ Supplement Left Brachial Artery with Synthetic Substitute, Percutaneous Approach

03U83KZ Supplement Left Brachial Artery with Nonautologous Tissue Substitute, Percutaneous Approach

03U847Z Supplement Left Brachial Artery with Autologous Tissue Substitute, Percutaneous Endoscopic Approach

03U84JZ Supplement Left Brachial Artery with Synthetic Substitute, Percutaneous Endoscopic Approach

03U84KZ Supplement Left Brachial Artery with Nonautologous Tissue Substitute, Percutaneous Endoscopic Approach

03U907Z Supplement Right Ulnar Artery with Autologous Tissue Substitute, Open Approach

03U90JZ Supplement Right Ulnar Artery with Synthetic Substitute, Open Approach

03U90KZ Supplement Right Ulnar Artery with Nonautologous Tissue Substitute, Open Approach

03U937Z Supplement Right Ulnar Artery with Autologous Tissue Substitute, Percutaneous Approach

03U93JZ Supplement Right Ulnar Artery with Synthetic Substitute, Percutaneous Approach

03U93KZ Supplement Right Ulnar Artery with Nonautologous Tissue Substitute, Percutaneous Approach

03U947Z Supplement Right Ulnar Artery with Autologous Tissue Substitute, Percutaneous Endoscopic Approach

03U94JZ Supplement Right Ulnar Artery with Synthetic Substitute, Percutaneous Endoscopic Approach

03U94KZ Supplement Right Ulnar Artery with Nonautologous Tissue Substitute, Percutaneous Endoscopic Approach

03UA07Z Supplement Left Ulnar Artery with Autologous Tissue Substitute, Open Approach

03UA0JZ Supplement Left Ulnar Artery with Synthetic Substitute, Open Approach

03UA0KZ Supplement Left Ulnar Artery with Nonautologous Tissue Substitute, Open Approach

03UA37Z Supplement Left Ulnar Artery with Autologous Tissue Substitute, Percutaneous Approach

03UA3JZ Supplement Left Ulnar Artery with Synthetic Substitute, Percutaneous Approach

03UA3KZ Supplement Left Ulnar Artery with Nonautologous Tissue Substitute, Percutaneous Approach

03UA47Z Supplement Left Ulnar Artery with Autologous Tissue Substitute, Percutaneous Endoscopic Approach

03UA4JZ Supplement Left Ulnar Artery with Synthetic Substitute, Percutaneous Endoscopic Approach

03UA4KZ Supplement Left Ulnar Artery with Nonautologous Tissue Substitute, Percutaneous Endoscopic Approach

03UB07Z Supplement Right Radial Artery with Autologous Tissue Substitute, Open Approach

03UB0JZ Supplement Right Radial Artery with Synthetic Substitute, Open Approach

03UB0KZ Supplement Right Radial Artery with Nonautologous Tissue Substitute, Open Approach

03UB37Z Supplement Right Radial Artery with Autologous Tissue Substitute, Percutaneous Approach

03UB3JZ Supplement Right Radial Artery with Synthetic Substitute, Percutaneous Approach

03UB3KZ Supplement Right Radial Artery with Nonautologous Tissue Substitute, Percutaneous Approach

03UB47Z Supplement Right Radial Artery with Autologous Tissue Substitute, Percutaneous Endoscopic Approach

03UB4JZ Supplement Right Radial Artery with Synthetic Substitute, Percutaneous Endoscopic Approach

03UB4KZ Supplement Right Radial Artery with Nonautologous Tissue Substitute, Percutaneous Endoscopic Approach

03UC07Z Supplement Left Radial Artery with Autologous Tissue Substitute, Open Approach

03UC0JZ Supplement Left Radial Artery with Synthetic Substitute, Open Approach

03UC0KZ Supplement Left Radial Artery with Nonautologous Tissue Substitute, Open Approach

03UC37Z Supplement Left Radial Artery with Autologous Tissue Substitute, Percutaneous Approach

03UC3JZ Supplement Left Radial Artery with Synthetic Substitute, Percutaneous Approach

03UC3KZ Supplement Left Radial Artery with Nonautologous Tissue Substitute, Percutaneous Approach

03UC47Z Supplement Left Radial Artery with Autologous Tissue Substitute, Percutaneous Endoscopic Approach

03UC4JZ Supplement Left Radial Artery with Synthetic Substitute, Percutaneous Endoscopic Approach

03UC4KZ Supplement Left Radial Artery with Nonautologous Tissue Substitute, Percutaneous Endoscopic Approach

03UD07Z Supplement Right Hand Artery with Autologous Tissue Substitute, Open Approach

03UD0JZ Supplement Right Hand Artery with Synthetic Substitute, Open Approach

03UD0KZ Supplement Right Hand Artery with Nonautologous Tissue Substitute, Open Approach

03UD37Z Supplement Right Hand Artery with Autologous Tissue Substitute, Percutaneous Approach

03UD3JZ Supplement Right Hand Artery with Synthetic Substitute, Percutaneous Approach

03UD3KZ Supplement Right Hand Artery with Nonautologous Tissue Substitute, Percutaneous Approach

03UD47Z Supplement Right Hand Artery with Autologous Tissue Substitute, Percutaneous Endoscopic Approach

03UD4JZ Supplement Right Hand Artery with Synthetic Substitute, Percutaneous Endoscopic Approach

03UD4KZ Supplement Right Hand Artery with Nonautologous Tissue Substitute, Percutaneous Endoscopic Approach

03UF07Z Supplement Left Hand Artery with Autologous Tissue Substitute, Open Approach

03UF0JZ Supplement Left Hand Artery with Synthetic Substitute, Open Approach

03UF0KZ Supplement Left Hand Artery with Nonautologous Tissue Substitute, Open Approach

03UF37Z Supplement Left Hand Artery with Autologous Tissue Substitute, Percutaneous Approach

03UF3JZ Supplement Left Hand Artery with Synthetic Substitute, Percutaneous Approach

03UF3KZ Supplement Left Hand Artery with Nonautologous Tissue Substitute, Percutaneous Approach

03UF47Z Supplement Left Hand Artery with Autologous Tissue Substitute, Percutaneous Endoscopic Approach

03UF4JZ Supplement Left Hand Artery with Synthetic Substitute, Percutaneous Endoscopic Approach

03UF4KZ Supplement Left Hand Artery with Nonautologous Tissue Substitute, Percutaneous Endoscopic Approach

03UG07Z Supplement Intracranial Artery with Autologous Tissue Substitute, Open Approach

03UG0JZ Supplement Intracranial Artery with Synthetic Substitute, Open Approach

03UG0KZ Supplement Intracranial Artery with Nonautologous Tissue Substitute, Open Approach

03UG37Z Supplement Intracranial Artery with Autologous Tissue Substitute, Percutaneous Approach

03UG3JZ Supplement Intracranial Artery with Synthetic Substitute, Percutaneous Approach

♀ Female-only   ♂ Male-only   ● Limited Coverage   ● Non-OR   HAC HAC-associated procedure   ● Non-covered procedures   ✚ Combination

03UG3KZ Supplement Intracranial Artery with Nonautologous Tissue Substitute, Percutaneous Approach

03UG47Z Supplement Intracranial Artery with Autologous Tissue Substitute, Percutaneous Endoscopic Approach

03UG4JZ Supplement Intracranial Artery with Synthetic Substitute, Percutaneous Endoscopic Approach

03UG4KZ Supplement Intracranial Artery with Nonautologous Tissue Substitute, Percutaneous Endoscopic Approach

03UH07Z Supplement Right Common Carotid Artery with Autologous Tissue Substitute, Open Approach

03UH0JZ Supplement Right Common Carotid Artery with Synthetic Substitute, Open Approach

03UH0KZ Supplement Right Common Carotid Artery with Nonautologous Tissue Substitute, Open Approach

03UH37Z Supplement Right Common Carotid Artery with Autologous Tissue Substitute, Percutaneous Approach

03UH3JZ Supplement Right Common Carotid Artery with Synthetic Substitute, Percutaneous Approach

03UH3KZ Supplement Right Common Carotid Artery with Nonautologous Tissue Substitute, Percutaneous Approach

03UH47Z Supplement Right Common Carotid Artery with Autologous Tissue Substitute, Percutaneous Endoscopic Approach

03UH4JZ Supplement Right Common Carotid Artery with Synthetic Substitute, Percutaneous Endoscopic Approach

03UH4KZ Supplement Right Common Carotid Artery with Nonautologous Tissue Substitute, Percutaneous Endoscopic Approach

03UJ07Z Supplement Left Common Carotid Artery with Autologous Tissue Substitute, Open Approach

03UJ0JZ Supplement Left Common Carotid Artery with Synthetic Substitute, Open Approach

03UJ0KZ Supplement Left Common Carotid Artery with Nonautologous Tissue Substitute, Open Approach

03UJ37Z Supplement Left Common Carotid Artery with Autologous Tissue Substitute, Percutaneous Approach

03UJ3JZ Supplement Left Common Carotid Artery with Synthetic Substitute, Percutaneous Approach

03UJ3KZ Supplement Left Common Carotid Artery with Nonautologous Tissue Substitute, Percutaneous Approach

03UJ47Z Supplement Left Common Carotid Artery with Autologous Tissue Substitute, Percutaneous Endoscopic Approach

03UJ4JZ Supplement Left Common Carotid Artery with Synthetic Substitute, Percutaneous Endoscopic Approach

03UJ4KZ Supplement Left Common Carotid Artery with Nonautologous Tissue Substitute, Percutaneous Endoscopic Approach

03UK07Z Supplement Right Internal Carotid Artery with Autologous Tissue Substitute, Open Approach

03UK0JZ Supplement Right Internal Carotid Artery with Synthetic Substitute, Open Approach

03UK0KZ Supplement Right Internal Carotid Artery with Nonautologous Tissue Substitute, Open Approach

03UK37Z Supplement Right Internal Carotid Artery with Autologous Tissue Substitute, Percutaneous Approach

03UK3JZ Supplement Right Internal Carotid Artery with Synthetic Substitute, Percutaneous Approach

03UK3KZ Supplement Right Internal Carotid Artery with Nonautologous Tissue Substitute, Percutaneous Approach

03UK47Z Supplement Right Internal Carotid Artery with Autologous Tissue Substitute, Percutaneous Endoscopic Approach

03UK4JZ Supplement Right Internal Carotid Artery with Synthetic Substitute, Percutaneous Endoscopic Approach

03UK4KZ Supplement Right Internal Carotid Artery with Nonautologous Tissue Substitute, Percutaneous Endoscopic Approach

03UL07Z Supplement Left Internal Carotid Artery with Autologous Tissue Substitute, Open Approach

03UL0JZ Supplement Left Internal Carotid Artery with Synthetic Substitute, Open Approach

03UL0KZ Supplement Left Internal Carotid Artery with Nonautologous Tissue Substitute, Open Approach

03UL37Z Supplement Left Internal Carotid Artery with Autologous Tissue Substitute, Percutaneous Approach

03UL3JZ Supplement Left Internal Carotid Artery with Synthetic Substitute, Percutaneous Approach

03UL3KZ Supplement Left Internal Carotid Artery with Nonautologous Tissue Substitute, Percutaneous Approach

03UL47Z Supplement Left Internal Carotid Artery with Autologous Tissue Substitute, Percutaneous Endoscopic Approach

03UL4JZ Supplement Left Internal Carotid Artery with Synthetic Substitute, Percutaneous Endoscopic Approach

03UL4KZ Supplement Left Internal Carotid Artery with Nonautologous Tissue Substitute, Percutaneous Endoscopic Approach

03UM07Z Supplement Right External Carotid Artery with Autologous Tissue Substitute, Open Approach

03UM0JZ Supplement Right External Carotid Artery with Synthetic Substitute, Open Approach

03UM0KZ Supplement Right External Carotid Artery with Nonautologous Tissue Substitute, Open Approach

03UM37Z Supplement Right External Carotid Artery with Autologous Tissue Substitute, Percutaneous Approach

03UM3JZ Supplement Right External Carotid Artery with Synthetic Substitute, Percutaneous Approach

03UM3KZ Supplement Right External Carotid Artery with Nonautologous Tissue Substitute, Percutaneous Approach

03UM47Z Supplement Right External Carotid Artery with Autologous Tissue Substitute, Percutaneous Endoscopic Approach

03UM4JZ Supplement Right External Carotid Artery with Synthetic Substitute, Percutaneous Endoscopic Approach

03UM4KZ Supplement Right External Carotid Artery with Nonautologous Tissue Substitute, Percutaneous Endoscopic Approach

03UN07Z Supplement Left External Carotid Artery with Autologous Tissue Substitute, Open Approach

03UN0JZ Supplement Left External Carotid Artery with Synthetic Substitute, Open Approach

03UN0KZ Supplement Left External Carotid Artery with Nonautologous Tissue Substitute, Open Approach

03UN37Z Supplement Left External Carotid Artery with Autologous Tissue Substitute, Percutaneous Approach

03UN3JZ Supplement Left External Carotid Artery with Synthetic Substitute, Percutaneous Approach

03UN3KZ Supplement Left External Carotid Artery with Nonautologous Tissue Substitute, Percutaneous Approach

03UN47Z Supplement Left External Carotid Artery with Autologous Tissue Substitute, Percutaneous Endoscopic Approach

03UN4JZ Supplement Left External Carotid Artery with Synthetic Substitute, Percutaneous Endoscopic Approach

03UN4KZ Supplement Left External Carotid Artery with Nonautologous Tissue Substitute, Percutaneous Endoscopic Approach

03UP07Z Supplement Right Vertebral Artery with Autologous Tissue Substitute, Open Approach

03UP0JZ Supplement Right Vertebral Artery with Synthetic Substitute, Open Approach

03UP0KZ Supplement Right Vertebral Artery with Nonautologous Tissue Substitute, Open Approach

03UP37Z Supplement Right Vertebral Artery with Autologous Tissue Substitute, Percutaneous Approach

03UP3JZ Supplement Right Vertebral Artery with Synthetic Substitute, Percutaneous Approach

03UP3KZ Supplement Right Vertebral Artery with Nonautologous Tissue Substitute, Percutaneous Approach

03UP47Z Supplement Right Vertebral Artery with Autologous Tissue Substitute, Percutaneous Endoscopic Approach

03UP4JZ Supplement Right Vertebral Artery with Synthetic Substitute, Percutaneous Endoscopic Approach

03UP4KZ Supplement Right Vertebral Artery with Nonautologous Tissue Substitute, Percutaneous Endoscopic Approach

03UQ07Z Supplement Left Vertebral Artery with Autologous Tissue Substitute, Open Approach

03UQ0JZ Supplement Left Vertebral Artery with Synthetic Substitute, Open Approach

03UQ0KZ Supplement Left Vertebral Artery with Nonautologous Tissue Substitute, Open Approach

03UQ37Z Supplement Left Vertebral Artery with Autologous Tissue Substitute, Percutaneous Approach

03UQ3JZ Supplement Left Vertebral Artery with Synthetic Substitute, Percutaneous Approach

03UQ3KZ Supplement Left Vertebral Artery with Nonautologous Tissue Substitute, Percutaneous Approach

03UQ47Z Supplement Left Vertebral Artery with Autologous Tissue Substitute, Percutaneous Endoscopic Approach

03UQ4JZ Supplement Left Vertebral Artery with Synthetic Substitute, Percutaneous Endoscopic Approach

03UQ4KZ Supplement Left Vertebral Artery with Nonautologous Tissue Substitute, Percutaneous Endoscopic Approach

03UR07Z Supplement Face Artery with Autologous Tissue Substitute, Open Approach

03UR0JZ Supplement Face Artery with Synthetic Substitute, Open Approach

03UR0KZ Supplement Face Artery with Nonautologous Tissue Substitute, Open Approach

03UR37Z Supplement Face Artery with Autologous Tissue Substitute, Percutaneous Approach

03UR3JZ Supplement Face Artery with Synthetic Substitute, Percutaneous Approach

03UR3KZ Supplement Face Artery with Nonautologous Tissue Substitute, Percutaneous Approach

03UR47Z Supplement Face Artery with Autologous Tissue Substitute, Percutaneous Endoscopic Approach

03UR4JZ Supplement Face Artery with Synthetic Substitute, Percutaneous Endoscopic Approach

03UR4KZ Supplement Face Artery with Nonautologous Tissue Substitute, Percutaneous Endoscopic Approach

03US07Z Supplement Right Temporal Artery with Autologous Tissue Substitute, Open Approach

03US0JZ Supplement Right Temporal Artery with Synthetic Substitute, Open Approach

03US0KZ Supplement Right Temporal Artery with Nonautologous Tissue Substitute, Open Approach

03US37Z Supplement Right Temporal Artery with Autologous Tissue Substitute, Percutaneous Approach

03US3JZ Supplement Right Temporal Artery with Synthetic Substitute, Percutaneous Approach

03US3KZ Supplement Right Temporal Artery with Nonautologous Tissue Substitute, Percutaneous Approach

03US47Z Supplement Right Temporal Artery with Autologous Tissue Substitute, Percutaneous Endoscopic Approach

03US4JZ Supplement Right Temporal Artery with Synthetic Substitute, Percutaneous Endoscopic Approach

03US4KZ Supplement Right Temporal Artery with Nonautologous Tissue Substitute, Percutaneous Endoscopic Approach

03UT07Z Supplement Left Temporal Artery with Autologous Tissue Substitute, Open Approach

03UT0JZ Supplement Left Temporal Artery with Synthetic Substitute, Open Approach

03UT0KZ Supplement Left Temporal Artery with Nonautologous Tissue Substitute, Open Approach

03UT37Z Supplement Left Temporal Artery with Autologous Tissue Substitute, Percutaneous Approach

03UT3JZ Supplement Left Temporal Artery with Synthetic Substitute, Percutaneous Approach

03UT3KZ Supplement Left Temporal Artery with Nonautologous Tissue Substitute, Percutaneous Approach

03UT47Z Supplement Left Temporal Artery with Autologous Tissue Substitute, Percutaneous Endoscopic Approach

03UT4JZ Supplement Left Temporal Artery with Synthetic Substitute, Percutaneous Endoscopic Approach

03UT4KZ Supplement Left Temporal Artery with Nonautologous Tissue Substitute, Percutaneous Endoscopic Approach

03UU07Z Supplement Right Thyroid Artery with Autologous Tissue Substitute, Open Approach

03UU0JZ Supplement Right Thyroid Artery with Synthetic Substitute, Open Approach

03UU0KZ Supplement Right Thyroid Artery with Nonautologous Tissue Substitute, Open Approach

03UU37Z Supplement Right Thyroid Artery with Autologous Tissue Substitute, Percutaneous Approach

03UU3JZ Supplement Right Thyroid Artery with Synthetic Substitute, Percutaneous Approach

03UU3KZ Supplement Right Thyroid Artery with Nonautologous Tissue Substitute, Percutaneous Approach

03UU47Z Supplement Right Thyroid Artery with Autologous Tissue Substitute, Percutaneous Endoscopic Approach

03UU4JZ Supplement Right Thyroid Artery with Synthetic Substitute, Percutaneous Endoscopic Approach

03UU4KZ Supplement Right Thyroid Artery with Nonautologous Tissue Substitute, Percutaneous Endoscopic Approach

03UV07Z Supplement Left Thyroid Artery with Autologous Tissue Substitute, Open Approach

03UV0JZ Supplement Left Thyroid Artery with Synthetic Substitute, Open Approach

03UV0KZ Supplement Left Thyroid Artery with Nonautologous Tissue Substitute, Open Approach

03UV37Z Supplement Left Thyroid Artery with Autologous Tissue Substitute, Percutaneous Approach

03UV3JZ Supplement Left Thyroid Artery with Synthetic Substitute, Percutaneous Approach

03UV3KZ Supplement Left Thyroid Artery with Nonautologous Tissue Substitute, Percutaneous Approach

03UV47Z Supplement Left Thyroid Artery with Autologous Tissue Substitute, Percutaneous Endoscopic Approach

03UV4JZ Supplement Left Thyroid Artery with Synthetic Substitute, Percutaneous Endoscopic Approach

03UV4KZ Supplement Left Thyroid Artery with Nonautologous Tissue Substitute, Percutaneous Endoscopic Approach

03UY07Z Supplement Upper Artery with Autologous Tissue Substitute, Open Approach

03UY0JZ Supplement Upper Artery with Synthetic Substitute, Open Approach

03UY0KZ Supplement Upper Artery with Nonautologous Tissue Substitute, Open Approach

03UY37Z Supplement Upper Artery with Autologous Tissue Substitute, Percutaneous Approach

03UY3JZ Supplement Upper Artery with Synthetic Substitute, Percutaneous Approach

03UY3KZ Supplement Upper Artery with Nonautologous Tissue Substitute, Percutaneous Approach

03UY47Z Supplement Upper Artery with Autologous Tissue Substitute, Percutaneous Endoscopic Approach

03UY4JZ Supplement Upper Artery with Synthetic Substitute, Percutaneous Endoscopic Approach

03UY4KZ Supplement Upper Artery with Nonautologous Tissue Substitute, Percutaneous Endoscopic Approach

03V – Upper Arteries, Restriction

Review Coding Guideline B3.12

03V00CZ Restriction of Right Internal Mammary Artery with Extraluminal Device, Open Approach

03V00DZ Restriction of Right Internal Mammary Artery with Intraluminal Device, Open Approach

03V00ZZ Restriction of Right Internal Mammary Artery, Open Approach

03V03CZ Restriction of Right Internal Mammary Artery with Extraluminal Device, Percutaneous Approach

03V03DZ Restriction of Right Internal Mammary Artery with Intraluminal Device, Percutaneous Approach

03V03ZZ Restriction of Right Internal Mammary Artery, Percutaneous Approach

03V04CZ Restriction of Right Internal Mammary Artery with Extraluminal Device, Percutaneous Endoscopic Approach

03V04DZ Restriction of Right Internal Mammary Artery with Intraluminal Device, Percutaneous Endoscopic Approach

03V04ZZ Restriction of Right Internal Mammary Artery, Percutaneous Endoscopic Approach

03V10CZ Restriction of Left Internal Mammary Artery with Extraluminal Device, Open Approach

03V10DZ Restriction of Left Internal Mammary Artery with Intraluminal Device, Open Approach

03V10ZZ Restriction of Left Internal Mammary Artery, Open Approach

03V13CZ Restriction of Left Internal Mammary Artery with Extraluminal Device, Percutaneous Approach

03V13DZ Restriction of Left Internal Mammary Artery with Intraluminal Device, Percutaneous Approach

03V13ZZ Restriction of Left Internal Mammary Artery, Percutaneous Approach

03V14CZ Restriction of Left Internal Mammary Artery with Extraluminal Device, Percutaneous Endoscopic Approach

03V14DZ Restriction of Left Internal Mammary Artery with Intraluminal Device, Percutaneous Endoscopic Approach

03V14ZZ Restriction of Left Internal Mammary Artery, Percutaneous Endoscopic Approach

03V20CZ Restriction of Innominate Artery with Extraluminal Device, Open Approach

03V20DZ Restriction of Innominate Artery with Intraluminal Device, Open Approach

03V20ZZ Restriction of Innominate Artery, Open Approach

03V23CZ Restriction of Innominate Artery with Extraluminal Device, Percutaneous Approach

03V23DZ Restriction of Innominate Artery with Intraluminal Device, Percutaneous Approach

03V23ZZ Restriction of Innominate Artery, Percutaneous Approach

03V24CZ Restriction of Innominate Artery with Extraluminal Device, Percutaneous Endoscopic Approach

03V24DZ Restriction of Innominate Artery with Intraluminal Device, Percutaneous Endoscopic Approach

03V24ZZ Restriction of Innominate Artery, Percutaneous Endoscopic Approach

03V30CZ Restriction of Right Subclavian Artery with Extraluminal Device, Open Approach

03V30DZ Restriction of Right Subclavian Artery with Intraluminal Device, Open Approach

03V30ZZ Restriction of Right Subclavian Artery, Open Approach

03V33CZ Restriction of Right Subclavian Artery with Extraluminal Device, Percutaneous Approach

03V33DZ Restriction of Right Subclavian Artery with Intraluminal Device, Percutaneous Approach

03V33ZZ Restriction of Right Subclavian Artery, Percutaneous Approach

03V34CZ Restriction of Right Subclavian Artery with Extraluminal Device, Percutaneous Endoscopic Approach

03V34DZ Restriction of Right Subclavian Artery with Intraluminal Device, Percutaneous Endoscopic Approach

03V34ZZ Restriction of Right Subclavian Artery, Percutaneous Endoscopic Approach

03V40CZ Restriction of Left Subclavian Artery with Extraluminal Device, Open Approach

03V40DZ Restriction of Left Subclavian Artery with Intraluminal Device, Open Approach

03V40ZZ Restriction of Left Subclavian Artery, Open Approach

03V43CZ Restriction of Left Subclavian Artery with Extraluminal Device, Percutaneous Approach

03V43DZ Restriction of Left Subclavian Artery with Intraluminal Device, Percutaneous Approach

03V43ZZ Restriction of Left Subclavian Artery, Percutaneous Approach

03V44CZ Restriction of Left Subclavian Artery with Extraluminal Device, Percutaneous Endoscopic Approach

03V44DZ Restriction of Left Subclavian Artery with Intraluminal Device, Percutaneous Endoscopic Approach

03V44ZZ Restriction of Left Subclavian Artery, Percutaneous Endoscopic Approach

03V50CZ Restriction of Right Axillary Artery with Extraluminal Device, Open Approach

03V50DZ Restriction of Right Axillary Artery with Intraluminal Device, Open Approach

03V50ZZ Restriction of Right Axillary Artery, Open Approach

03V53CZ Restriction of Right Axillary Artery with Extraluminal Device, Percutaneous Approach

03V53DZ Restriction of Right Axillary Artery with Intraluminal Device, Percutaneous Approach

03V53ZZ Restriction of Right Axillary Artery, Percutaneous Approach

03V54CZ Restriction of Right Axillary Artery with Extraluminal Device, Percutaneous Endoscopic Approach

03V54DZ Restriction of Right Axillary Artery with Intraluminal Device, Percutaneous Endoscopic Approach

03V54ZZ Restriction of Right Axillary Artery, Percutaneous Endoscopic Approach

03V60CZ Restriction of Left Axillary Artery with Extraluminal Device, Open Approach

03V60DZ Restriction of Left Axillary Artery with Intraluminal Device, Open Approach

03V60ZZ Restriction of Left Axillary Artery, Open Approach

03V63CZ Restriction of Left Axillary Artery with Extraluminal Device, Percutaneous Approach

03V63DZ Restriction of Left Axillary Artery with Intraluminal Device, Percutaneous Approach

03V63ZZ Restriction of Left Axillary Artery, Percutaneous Approach

03V64CZ Restriction of Left Axillary Artery with Extraluminal Device, Percutaneous Endoscopic Approach

03V64DZ Restriction of Left Axillary Artery with Intraluminal Device, Percutaneous Endoscopic Approach

03V64ZZ Restriction of Left Axillary Artery, Percutaneous Endoscopic Approach

03V70CZ Restriction of Right Brachial Artery with Extraluminal Device, Open Approach

03V70DZ Restriction of Right Brachial Artery with Intraluminal Device, Open Approach

03V70ZZ Restriction of Right Brachial Artery, Open Approach

03V73CZ Restriction of Right Brachial Artery with Extraluminal Device, Percutaneous Approach

03V73DZ Restriction of Right Brachial Artery with Intraluminal Device, Percutaneous Approach

03V73ZZ Restriction of Right Brachial Artery, Percutaneous Approach

03V74CZ Restriction of Right Brachial Artery with Extraluminal Device, Percutaneous Endoscopic Approach

03V74DZ Restriction of Right Brachial Artery with Intraluminal Device, Percutaneous Endoscopic Approach

03V74ZZ Restriction of Right Brachial Artery, Percutaneous Endoscopic Approach

03V80CZ Restriction of Left Brachial Artery with Extraluminal Device, Open Approach

03V80DZ Restriction of Left Brachial Artery with Intraluminal Device, Open Approach

03V80ZZ Restriction of Left Brachial Artery, Open Approach

03V83CZ Restriction of Left Brachial Artery with Extraluminal Device, Percutaneous Approach

03V83DZ Restriction of Left Brachial Artery with Intraluminal Device, Percutaneous Approach

03V83ZZ Restriction of Left Brachial Artery, Percutaneous Approach

03V84CZ Restriction of Left Brachial Artery with Extraluminal Device, Percutaneous Endoscopic Approach

03V84DZ Restriction of Left Brachial Artery with Intraluminal Device, Percutaneous Endoscopic Approach

03V84ZZ Restriction of Left Brachial Artery, Percutaneous Endoscopic Approach

03V90CZ Restriction of Right Ulnar Artery with Extraluminal Device, Open Approach

03V90DZ Restriction of Right Ulnar Artery with Intraluminal Device, Open Approach

03V90ZZ Restriction of Right Ulnar Artery, Open Approach

03V93CZ Restriction of Right Ulnar Artery with Extraluminal Device, Percutaneous Approach

03V93DZ Restriction of Right Ulnar Artery with Intraluminal Device, Percutaneous Approach

03V93ZZ Restriction of Right Ulnar Artery, Percutaneous Approach

03V94CZ Restriction of Right Ulnar Artery with Extraluminal Device, Percutaneous Endoscopic Approach

03V94DZ Restriction of Right Ulnar Artery with Intraluminal Device, Percutaneous Endoscopic Approach

03V94ZZ Restriction of Right Ulnar Artery, Percutaneous Endoscopic Approach

03VA0CZ Restriction of Left Ulnar Artery with Extraluminal Device, Open Approach

03VA0DZ Restriction of Left Ulnar Artery with Intraluminal Device, Open Approach

03VA0ZZ Restriction of Left Ulnar Artery, Open Approach

03VA3CZ Restriction of Left Ulnar Artery with Extraluminal Device, Percutaneous Approach

03VA3DZ Restriction of Left Ulnar Artery with Intraluminal Device, Percutaneous Approach

03VA3ZZ Restriction of Left Ulnar Artery, Percutaneous Approach

03VA4CZ Restriction of Left Ulnar Artery with Extraluminal Device, Percutaneous Endoscopic Approach

03VA4DZ   Restriction of Left Ulnar Artery with Intraluminal Device, Percutaneous Endoscopic Approach

03VA4ZZ   Restriction of Left Ulnar Artery, Percutaneous Endoscopic Approach

03VB0CZ   Restriction of Right Radial Artery with Extraluminal Device, Open Approach

03VB0DZ   Restriction of Right Radial Artery with Intraluminal Device, Open Approach

03VB0ZZ   Restriction of Right Radial Artery, Open Approach

03VB3CZ   Restriction of Right Radial Artery with Extraluminal Device, Percutaneous Approach

03VB3DZ   Restriction of Right Radial Artery with Intraluminal Device, Percutaneous Approach

03VB3ZZ   Restriction of Right Radial Artery, Percutaneous Approach

03VB4CZ   Restriction of Right Radial Artery with Extraluminal Device, Percutaneous Endoscopic Approach

03VB4DZ   Restriction of Right Radial Artery with Intraluminal Device, Percutaneous Endoscopic Approach

03VB4ZZ   Restriction of Right Radial Artery, Percutaneous Endoscopic Approach

03VC0CZ   Restriction of Left Radial Artery with Extraluminal Device, Open Approach

03VC0DZ   Restriction of Left Radial Artery with Intraluminal Device, Open Approach

03VC0ZZ   Restriction of Left Radial Artery, Open Approach

03VC3CZ   Restriction of Left Radial Artery with Extraluminal Device, Percutaneous Approach

03VC3DZ   Restriction of Left Radial Artery with Intraluminal Device, Percutaneous Approach

03VC3ZZ   Restriction of Left Radial Artery, Percutaneous Approach

03VC4CZ   Restriction of Left Radial Artery with Extraluminal Device, Percutaneous Endoscopic Approach

03VC4DZ   Restriction of Left Radial Artery with Intraluminal Device, Percutaneous Endoscopic Approach

03VC4ZZ   Restriction of Left Radial Artery, Percutaneous Endoscopic Approach

03VD0CZ   Restriction of Right Hand Artery with Extraluminal Device, Open Approach

03VD0DZ   Restriction of Right Hand Artery with Intraluminal Device, Open Approach

03VD0ZZ   Restriction of Right Hand Artery, Open Approach

03VD3CZ   Restriction of Right Hand Artery with Extraluminal Device, Percutaneous Approach

03VD3DZ   Restriction of Right Hand Artery with Intraluminal Device, Percutaneous Approach

03VD3ZZ   Restriction of Right Hand Artery, Percutaneous Approach

03VD4CZ   Restriction of Right Hand Artery with Extraluminal Device, Percutaneous Endoscopic Approach

03VD4DZ   Restriction of Right Hand Artery with Intraluminal Device, Percutaneous Endoscopic Approach

03VD4ZZ   Restriction of Right Hand Artery, Percutaneous Endoscopic Approach

03VF0CZ   Restriction of Left Hand Artery with Extraluminal Device, Open Approach

03VF0DZ   Restriction of Left Hand Artery with Intraluminal Device, Open Approach

03VF0ZZ   Restriction of Left Hand Artery, Open Approach

03VF3CZ   Restriction of Left Hand Artery with Extraluminal Device, Percutaneous Approach

03VF3DZ   Restriction of Left Hand Artery with Intraluminal Device, Percutaneous Approach

03VF3ZZ   Restriction of Left Hand Artery, Percutaneous Approach

03VF4CZ   Restriction of Left Hand Artery with Extraluminal Device, Percutaneous Endoscopic Approach

03VF4DZ   Restriction of Left Hand Artery with Intraluminal Device, Percutaneous Endoscopic Approach

03VF4ZZ   Restriction of Left Hand Artery, Percutaneous Endoscopic Approach

03VG0BZ   Restriction of Intracranial Artery with Bioactive Intraluminal Device, Open Approach

03VG0CZ   Restriction of Intracranial Artery with Extraluminal Device, Open Approach

03VG0DZ   Restriction of Intracranial Artery with Intraluminal Device, Open Approach

03VG0ZZ   Restriction of Intracranial Artery, Open Approach

03VG3BZ   Restriction of Intracranial Artery with Bioactive Intraluminal Device, Percutaneous Approach

03VG3CZ   Restriction of Intracranial Artery with Extraluminal Device, Percutaneous Approach

03VG3DZ   Restriction of Intracranial Artery with Intraluminal Device, Percutaneous Approach

03VG3ZZ   Restriction of Intracranial Artery, Percutaneous Approach

03VG4BZ   Restriction of Intracranial Artery with Bioactive Intraluminal Device, Percutaneous Endoscopic Approach

03VG4CZ   Restriction of Intracranial Artery with Extraluminal Device, Percutaneous Endoscopic Approach

03VG4DZ   Restriction of Intracranial Artery with Intraluminal Device, Percutaneous Endoscopic Approach

03VG4ZZ   Restriction of Intracranial Artery, Percutaneous Endoscopic Approach

03VH0BZ   Restriction of Right Common Carotid Artery with Bioactive Intraluminal Device, Open Approach

03VH0CZ   Restriction of Right Common Carotid Artery with Extraluminal Device, Open Approach

03VH0DZ   Restriction of Right Common Carotid Artery with Intraluminal Device, Open Approach

03VH0ZZ   Restriction of Right Common Carotid Artery, Open Approach

03VH3BZ   Restriction of Right Common Carotid Artery with Bioactive Intraluminal Device, Percutaneous Approach

03VH3CZ   Restriction of Right Common Carotid Artery with Extraluminal Device, Percutaneous Approach

03VH3DZ   Restriction of Right Common Carotid Artery with Intraluminal Device, Percutaneous Approach

03VH3ZZ   Restriction of Right Common Carotid Artery, Percutaneous Approach

03VH4BZ   Restriction of Right Common Carotid Artery with Bioactive Intraluminal Device, Percutaneous Endoscopic Approach

03VH4CZ   Restriction of Right Common Carotid Artery with Extraluminal Device, Percutaneous Endoscopic Approach

03VH4DZ   Restriction of Right Common Carotid Artery with Intraluminal Device, Percutaneous Endoscopic Approach

03VH4ZZ   Restriction of Right Common Carotid Artery, Percutaneous Endoscopic Approach

03VJ0BZ   Restriction of Left Common Carotid Artery with Bioactive Intraluminal Device, Open Approach

03VJ0CZ   Restriction of Left Common Carotid Artery with Extraluminal Device, Open Approach

03VJ0DZ   Restriction of Left Common Carotid Artery with Intraluminal Device, Open Approach

03VJ0ZZ   Restriction of Left Common Carotid Artery, Open Approach

03VJ3BZ   Restriction of Left Common Carotid Artery with Bioactive Intraluminal Device, Percutaneous Approach

03VJ3CZ   Restriction of Left Common Carotid Artery with Extraluminal Device, Percutaneous Approach

03VJ3DZ   Restriction of Left Common Carotid Artery with Intraluminal Device, Percutaneous Approach

03VJ3ZZ   Restriction of Left Common Carotid Artery, Percutaneous Approach

03VJ4BZ   Restriction of Left Common Carotid Artery with Bioactive Intraluminal Device, Percutaneous Endoscopic Approach

03VJ4CZ   Restriction of Left Common Carotid Artery with Extraluminal Device, Percutaneous Endoscopic Approach

03VJ4DZ   Restriction of Left Common Carotid Artery with Intraluminal Device, Percutaneous Endoscopic Approach

03VJ4ZZ   Restriction of Left Common Carotid Artery, Percutaneous Endoscopic Approach

03VK0BZ   Restriction of Right Internal Carotid Artery with Bioactive Intraluminal Device, Open Approach

03VK0CZ   Restriction of Right Internal Carotid Artery with Extraluminal Device, Open Approach

03VK0DZ   Restriction of Right Internal Carotid Artery with Intraluminal Device, Open Approach

03VK0ZZ   Restriction of Right Internal Carotid Artery, Open Approach

03VK3BZ   Restriction of Right Internal Carotid Artery with Bioactive Intraluminal Device, Percutaneous Approach

03VK3CZ   Restriction of Right Internal Carotid Artery with Extraluminal Device, Percutaneous Approach

03VK3DZ   Restriction of Right Internal Carotid Artery with Intraluminal Device, Percutaneous Approach

03VK3ZZ   Restriction of Right Internal Carotid Artery, Percutaneous Approach

03VK4BZ   Restriction of Right Internal Carotid Artery with Bioactive Intraluminal Device, Percutaneous Endoscopic Approach

03VK4CZ   Restriction of Right Internal Carotid Artery with Extraluminal Device, Percutaneous Endoscopic Approach

03VK4DZ   Restriction of Right Internal Carotid Artery with Intraluminal Device, Percutaneous Endoscopic Approach

03VK4ZZ   Restriction of Right Internal Carotid Artery, Percutaneous Endoscopic Approach

03VL0BZ   Restriction of Left Internal Carotid Artery with Bioactive Intraluminal Device, Open Approach

03VL0CZ   Restriction of Left Internal Carotid Artery with Extraluminal Device, Open Approach

03VL0DZ   Restriction of Left Internal Carotid Artery with Intraluminal Device, Open Approach

03VL0ZZ   Restriction of Left Internal Carotid Artery, Open Approach

03VL3BZ   Restriction of Left Internal Carotid Artery with Bioactive Intraluminal Device, Percutaneous Approach

03VL3CZ   Restriction of Left Internal Carotid Artery with Extraluminal Device, Percutaneous Approach

03VL3DZ   Restriction of Left Internal Carotid Artery with Intraluminal Device, Percutaneous Approach

03VL3ZZ   Restriction of Left Internal Carotid Artery, Percutaneous Approach

03VL4BZ   Restriction of Left Internal Carotid Artery with Bioactive Intraluminal Device, Percutaneous Endoscopic Approach

03VL4CZ   Restriction of Left Internal Carotid Artery with Extraluminal Device, Percutaneous Endoscopic Approach

03VL4DZ   Restriction of Left Internal Carotid Artery with Intraluminal Device, Percutaneous Endoscopic Approach

03VL4ZZ   Restriction of Left Internal Carotid Artery, Percutaneous Endoscopic Approach

03VM0BZ   Restriction of Right External Carotid Artery with Bioactive Intraluminal Device, Open Approach

03VM0CZ   Restriction of Right External Carotid Artery with Extraluminal Device, Open Approach

03VM0DZ   Restriction of Right External Carotid Artery with Intraluminal Device, Open Approach

03VM0ZZ   Restriction of Right External Carotid Artery, Open Approach

03VM3BZ   Restriction of Right External Carotid Artery with Bioactive Intraluminal Device, Percutaneous Approach

03VM3CZ   Restriction of Right External Carotid Artery with Extraluminal Device, Percutaneous Approach

03VM3DZ   Restriction of Right External Carotid Artery with Intraluminal Device, Percutaneous Approach

03VM3ZZ   Restriction of Right External Carotid Artery, Percutaneous Approach

03VM4BZ   Restriction of Right External Carotid Artery with Bioactive Intraluminal Device, Percutaneous Endoscopic Approach

03VM4CZ   Restriction of Right External Carotid Artery with Extraluminal Device, Percutaneous Endoscopic Approach

03VM4DZ   Restriction of Right External Carotid Artery with Intraluminal Device, Percutaneous Endoscopic Approach

03VM4ZZ   Restriction of Right External Carotid Artery, Percutaneous Endoscopic Approach

03VN0BZ   Restriction of Left External Carotid Artery with Bioactive Intraluminal Device, Open Approach

03VN0CZ   Restriction of Left External Carotid Artery with Extraluminal Device, Open Approach

03VN0DZ   Restriction of Left External Carotid Artery with Intraluminal Device, Open Approach

03VN0ZZ   Restriction of Left External Carotid Artery, Open Approach

03VN3BZ   Restriction of Left External Carotid Artery with Bioactive Intraluminal Device, Percutaneous Approach

03VN3CZ   Restriction of Left External Carotid Artery with Extraluminal Device, Percutaneous Approach

03VN3DZ   Restriction of Left External Carotid Artery with Intraluminal Device, Percutaneous Approach

03VN3ZZ   Restriction of Left External Carotid Artery, Percutaneous Approach

03VN4BZ   Restriction of Left External Carotid Artery with Bioactive Intraluminal Device, Percutaneous Endoscopic Approach

03VN4CZ   Restriction of Left External Carotid Artery with Extraluminal Device, Percutaneous Endoscopic Approach

03VN4DZ   Restriction of Left External Carotid Artery with Intraluminal Device, Percutaneous Endoscopic Approach

03VN4ZZ   Restriction of Left External Carotid Artery, Percutaneous Endoscopic Approach

03VP0BZ   Restriction of Right Vertebral Artery with Bioactive Intraluminal Device, Open Approach

03VP0CZ   Restriction of Right Vertebral Artery with Extraluminal Device, Open Approach

03VP0DZ   Restriction of Right Vertebral Artery with Intraluminal Device, Open Approach

03VP0ZZ   Restriction of Right Vertebral Artery, Open Approach

03VP3BZ   Restriction of Right Vertebral Artery with Bioactive Intraluminal Device, Percutaneous Approach

03VP3CZ   Restriction of Right Vertebral Artery with Extraluminal Device, Percutaneous Approach

03VP3DZ   Restriction of Right Vertebral Artery with Intraluminal Device, Percutaneous Approach

03VP3ZZ   Restriction of Right Vertebral Artery, Percutaneous Approach

03VP4BZ   Restriction of Right Vertebral Artery with Bioactive Intraluminal Device, Percutaneous Endoscopic Approach

03VP4CZ   Restriction of Right Vertebral Artery with Extraluminal Device, Percutaneous Endoscopic Approach

03VP4DZ   Restriction of Right Vertebral Artery with Intraluminal Device, Percutaneous Endoscopic Approach

03VP4ZZ   Restriction of Right Vertebral Artery, Percutaneous Endoscopic Approach

03VQ0BZ   Restriction of Left Vertebral Artery with Bioactive Intraluminal Device, Open Approach

03VQ0CZ   Restriction of Left Vertebral Artery with Extraluminal Device, Open Approach

03VQ0DZ   Restriction of Left Vertebral Artery with Intraluminal Device, Open Approach

03VQ0ZZ   Restriction of Left Vertebral Artery, Open Approach

03VQ3BZ   Restriction of Left Vertebral Artery with Bioactive Intraluminal Device, Percutaneous Approach

03VQ3CZ   Restriction of Left Vertebral Artery with Extraluminal Device, Percutaneous Approach

03VQ3DZ   Restriction of Left Vertebral Artery with Intraluminal Device, Percutaneous Approach

03VQ3ZZ   Restriction of Left Vertebral Artery, Percutaneous Approach

03VQ4BZ   Restriction of Left Vertebral Artery with Bioactive Intraluminal Device, Percutaneous Endoscopic Approach

03VQ4CZ   Restriction of Left Vertebral Artery with Extraluminal Device, Percutaneous Endoscopic Approach

03VQ4DZ   Restriction of Left Vertebral Artery with Intraluminal Device, Percutaneous Endoscopic Approach

03VQ4ZZ   Restriction of Left Vertebral Artery, Percutaneous Endoscopic Approach

03VR0CZ   Restriction of Face Artery with Extraluminal Device, Open Approach

03VR0DZ   Restriction of Face Artery with Intraluminal Device, Open Approach

03VR0ZZ   Restriction of Face Artery, Open Approach

03VR3CZ   Restriction of Face Artery with Extraluminal Device, Percutaneous Approach

03VR3DZ   Restriction of Face Artery with Intraluminal Device, Percutaneous Approach

03VR3ZZ   Restriction of Face Artery, Percutaneous Approach

03VR4CZ   Restriction of Face Artery with Extraluminal Device, Percutaneous Endoscopic Approach

03VR4DZ   Restriction of Face Artery with Intraluminal Device, Percutaneous Endoscopic Approach

03VR4ZZ   Restriction of Face Artery, Percutaneous Endoscopic Approach

03VS0CZ   Restriction of Right Temporal Artery with Extraluminal Device, Open Approach

03VS0DZ   Restriction of Right Temporal Artery with Intraluminal Device, Open Approach

03VS0ZZ   Restriction of Right Temporal Artery, Open Approach

03VS3CZ   Restriction of Right Temporal Artery with Extraluminal Device, Percutaneous Approach

03VS3DZ   Restriction of Right Temporal Artery with Intraluminal Device, Percutaneous Approach

03VS3ZZ   Restriction of Right Temporal Artery, Percutaneous Approach

03VS4CZ Restriction of Right Temporal Artery with Extraluminal Device, Percutaneous Endoscopic Approach
03VS4DZ Restriction of Right Temporal Artery with Intraluminal Device, Percutaneous Endoscopic Approach
03VS4ZZ Restriction of Right Temporal Artery, Percutaneous Endoscopic Approach
03VT0CZ Restriction of Left Temporal Artery with Extraluminal Device, Open Approach
03VT0DZ Restriction of Left Temporal Artery with Intraluminal Device, Open Approach
03VT0ZZ Restriction of Left Temporal Artery, Open Approach
03VT3CZ Restriction of Left Temporal Artery with Extraluminal Device, Percutaneous Approach
03VT3DZ Restriction of Left Temporal Artery with Intraluminal Device, Percutaneous Approach
03VT3ZZ Restriction of Left Temporal Artery, Percutaneous Approach
03VT4CZ Restriction of Left Temporal Artery with Extraluminal Device, Percutaneous Endoscopic Approach
03VT4DZ Restriction of Left Temporal Artery with Intraluminal Device, Percutaneous Endoscopic Approach
03VT4ZZ Restriction of Left Temporal Artery, Percutaneous Endoscopic Approach
03VU0CZ Restriction of Right Thyroid Artery with Extraluminal Device, Open Approach
03VU0DZ Restriction of Right Thyroid Artery with Intraluminal Device, Open Approach
03VU0ZZ Restriction of Right Thyroid Artery, Open Approach
03VU3CZ Restriction of Right Thyroid Artery with Extraluminal Device, Percutaneous Approach
03VU3DZ Restriction of Right Thyroid Artery with Intraluminal Device, Percutaneous Approach
03VU3ZZ Restriction of Right Thyroid Artery, Percutaneous Approach
03VU4CZ Restriction of Right Thyroid Artery with Extraluminal Device, Percutaneous Endoscopic Approach

03VU4DZ Restriction of Right Thyroid Artery with Intraluminal Device, Percutaneous Endoscopic Approach
03VU4ZZ Restriction of Right Thyroid Artery, Percutaneous Endoscopic Approach
03VV0CZ Restriction of Left Thyroid Artery with Extraluminal Device, Open Approach
03VV0DZ Restriction of Left Thyroid Artery with Intraluminal Device, Open Approach
03VV0ZZ Restriction of Left Thyroid Artery, Open Approach
03VV3CZ Restriction of Left Thyroid Artery with Extraluminal Device, Percutaneous Approach
03VV3DZ Restriction of Left Thyroid Artery with Intraluminal Device, Percutaneous Approach
03VV3ZZ Restriction of Left Thyroid Artery, Percutaneous Approach
03VV4CZ Restriction of Left Thyroid Artery with Extraluminal Device, Percutaneous Endoscopic Approach
03VV4DZ Restriction of Left Thyroid Artery with Intraluminal Device, Percutaneous Endoscopic Approach
03VV4ZZ Restriction of Left Thyroid Artery, Percutaneous Endoscopic Approach
03VY0CZ Restriction of Upper Artery with Extraluminal Device, Open Approach
03VY0DZ Restriction of Upper Artery with Intraluminal Device, Open Approach
03VY0ZZ Restriction of Upper Artery, Open Approach
03VY3CZ Restriction of Upper Artery with Extraluminal Device, Percutaneous Approach
03VY3DZ Restriction of Upper Artery with Intraluminal Device, Percutaneous Approach
03VY3ZZ Restriction of Upper Artery, Percutaneous Approach
03VY4CZ Restriction of Upper Artery with Extraluminal Device, Percutaneous Endoscopic Approach
03VY4DZ Restriction of Upper Artery with Intraluminal Device, Percutaneous Endoscopic Approach
03VY4ZZ Restriction of Upper Artery, Percutaneous Endoscopic Approach

03W – Upper Arteries, Revision

Review Coding Guideline B6.1c

03WY00Z Revision of Drainage Device in Upper Artery, Open Approach
03WY02Z Revision of Monitoring Device in Upper Artery, Open Approach
03WY03Z Revision of Infusion Device in Upper Artery, Open Approach
03WY07Z Revision of Autologous Tissue Substitute in Upper Artery, Open Approach
03WY0CZ Revision of Extraluminal Device in Upper Artery, Open Approach
03WY0DZ Revision of Intraluminal Device in Upper Artery, Open Approach
03WY0JZ Revision of Synthetic Substitute in Upper Artery, Open Approach
03WY0KZ Revision of Nonautologous Tissue Substitute in Upper Artery, Open Approach
03WY0MZ Revision of Stimulator Lead in Upper Artery, Open Approach
03WY30Z Revision of Drainage Device in Upper Artery, Percutaneous Approach
03WY32Z Revision of Monitoring Device in Upper Artery, Percutaneous Approach
03WY33Z Revision of Infusion Device in Upper Artery, Percutaneous Approach
03WY37Z Revision of Autologous Tissue Substitute in Upper Artery, Percutaneous Approach
03WY3CZ Revision of Extraluminal Device in Upper Artery, Percutaneous Approach
03WY3DZ Revision of Intraluminal Device in Upper Artery, Percutaneous Approach
03WY3JZ Revision of Synthetic Substitute in Upper Artery, Percutaneous Approach
03WY3KZ Revision of Nonautologous Tissue Substitute in Upper Artery, Percutaneous Approach
03WY3MZ Revision of Stimulator Lead in Upper Artery, Percutaneous Approach
03WY40Z Revision of Drainage Device in Upper Artery, Percutaneous Endoscopic Approach
03WY42Z Revision of Monitoring Device in Upper Artery, Percutaneous Endoscopic Approach

03WY43Z Revision of Infusion Device in Upper Artery, Percutaneous Endoscopic Approach
03WY47Z Revision of Autologous Tissue Substitute in Upper Artery, Percutaneous Endoscopic Approach
03WY4CZ Revision of Extraluminal Device in Upper Artery, Percutaneous Endoscopic Approach
03WY4DZ Revision of Intraluminal Device in Upper Artery, Percutaneous Endoscopic Approach
03WY4JZ Revision of Synthetic Substitute in Upper Artery, Percutaneous Endoscopic Approach
03WY4KZ Revision of Nonautologous Tissue Substitute in Upper Artery, Percutaneous Endoscopic Approach
03WY4MZ Revision of Stimulator Lead in Upper Artery, Percutaneous Endoscopic Approach
03WYX0Z Revision of Drainage Device in Upper Artery, External Approach
03WYX2Z Revision of Monitoring Device in Upper Artery, External Approach
03WYX3Z Revision of Infusion Device in Upper Artery, External Approach
03WYX7Z Revision of Autologous Tissue Substitute in Upper Artery, External Approach
03WYXCZ Revision of Extraluminal Device in Upper Artery, External Approach
03WYXDZ Revision of Intraluminal Device in Upper Artery, External Approach
03WYXJZ Revision of Synthetic Substitute in Upper Artery, External Approach
03WYXKZ Revision of Nonautologous Tissue Substitute in Upper Artery, External Approach
03WYXMZ Revision of Stimulator Lead in Upper Artery, External Approach

---

♀ Female-only   ♂ Male-only   ● Limited Coverage   ● Non-OR   🅗🅐🅒 HAC-associated procedure   ● Non-covered procedures   ➕ Combination

Lower Arteries

Arteries

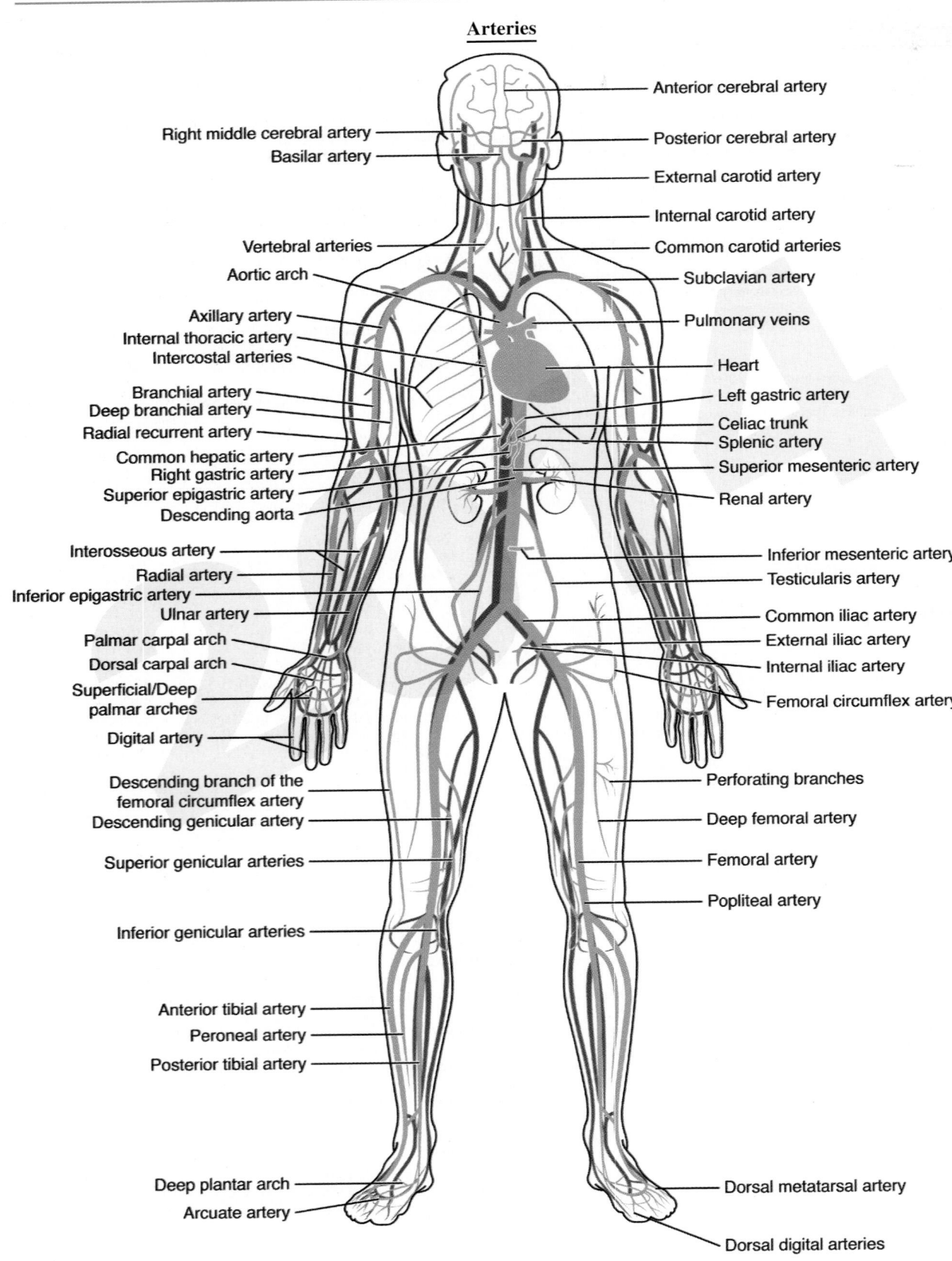

Lower Arteries Tables 041–04W

Section	0	**Medical and Surgical**
Body System	4	**Lower Arteries**
Operation	1	**Bypass:** Altering the route of passage of the contents of a tubular body part

Body Part (4th)	Approach (5th)	Device (6th)	Qualifier (7th)
0 Abdominal Aorta C Common Iliac Artery, Right D Common Iliac Artery, Left	0 Open 4 Percutaneous Endoscopic	9 Autologous Venous Tissue A Autologous Arterial Tissue J Synthetic Substitute K Nonautologous Tissue Substitute Z No Device	0 Abdominal Aorta 1 Celiac Artery 2 Mesenteric Artery 3 Renal Artery, Right 4 Renal Artery, Left 5 Renal Artery, Bilateral 6 Common Iliac Artery, Right 7 Common Iliac Artery, Left 8 Common Iliac Arteries, Bilateral 9 Internal Iliac Artery, Right B Internal Iliac Artery, Left C Internal Iliac Arteries, Bilateral D External Iliac Artery, Right F External Iliac Artery, Left G External Iliac Arteries, Bilateral H Femoral Artery, Right J Femoral Artery, Left K Femoral Arteries, Bilateral Q Lower Extremity Artery R Lower Artery
4 Splenic Artery	0 Open 4 Percutaneous Endoscopic	9 Autologous Venous Tissue A Autologous Arterial Tissue J Synthetic Substitute K Nonautologous Tissue Substitute Z No Device	3 Renal Artery, Right 4 Renal Artery, Left 5 Renal Artery, Bilateral
E Internal Iliac Artery, Right F Internal Iliac Artery, Left H External Iliac Artery, Right J External Iliac Artery, Left	0 Open 4 Percutaneous Endoscopic	9 Autologous Venous Tissue A Autologous Arterial Tissue J Synthetic Substitute K Nonautologous Tissue Substitute Z No Device	9 Internal Iliac Artery, Right B Internal Iliac Artery, Left C Internal Iliac Arteries, Bilateral D External Iliac Artery, Right F External Iliac Artery, Left G External Iliac Arteries, Bilateral H Femoral Artery, Right J Femoral Artery, Left K Femoral Arteries, Bilateral P Foot Artery Q Lower Extremity Artery
K Femoral Artery, Right L Femoral Artery, Left	0 Open 4 Percutaneous Endoscopic	9 Autologous Venous Tissue A Autologous Arterial Tissue J Synthetic Substitute K Nonautologous Tissue Substitute Z No Device	H Femoral Artery, Right J Femoral Artery, Left K Femoral Arteries, Bilateral L Popliteal Artery M Peroneal Artery N Posterior Tibial Artery P Foot Artery Q Lower Extremity Artery S Lower Extremity Vein
M Popliteal Artery, Right N Popliteal Artery, Left	0 Open 4 Percutaneous Endoscopic	9 Autologous Venous Tissue A Autologous Arterial Tissue J Synthetic Substitute K Nonautologous Tissue Substitute Z No Device	L Popliteal Artery M Peroneal Artery P Foot Artery Q Lower Extremity Artery S Lower Extremity Vein

Section	0	Medical and Surgical
Body System	4	Lower Arteries
Operation	5	**Destruction:** Physical eradication of all or a portion of a body part by the direct use of energy, force, or a destructive agent

Body Part (4ᵗʰ)	Approach (5ᵗʰ)	Device (6ᵗʰ)	Qualifier (7ᵗʰ)
0 Abdominal Aorta 1 Celiac Artery 2 Gastric Artery 3 Hepatic Artery 4 Splenic Artery 5 Superior Mesenteric Artery 6 Colic Artery, Right 7 Colic Artery, Left 8 Colic Artery, Middle 9 Renal Artery, Right A Renal Artery, Left B Inferior Mesenteric Artery C Common Iliac Artery, Right D Common Iliac Artery, Left E Internal Iliac Artery, Right F Internal Iliac Artery, Left H External Iliac Artery, Right J External Iliac Artery, Left K Femoral Artery, Right L Femoral Artery, Left M Popliteal Artery, Right N Popliteal Artery, Left P Anterior Tibial Artery, Right Q Anterior Tibial Artery, Left R Posterior Tibial Artery, Right S Posterior Tibial Artery, Left T Peroneal Artery, Right U Peroneal Artery, Left V Foot Artery, Right W Foot Artery, Left Y Lower Artery	0 Open 3 Percutaneous 4 Percutaneous Endoscopic	Z No Device	Z No Qualifier

Section	0	Medical and Surgical
Body System	4	Lower Arteries
Operation	7	Dilation: Expanding an orifice or the lumen of a tubular body part

Body Part (4th)	Approach (5th)	Device (6th)	Qualifier (7th)
0 Abdominal Aorta 1 Celiac Artery 2 Gastric Artery 3 Hepatic Artery 4 Splenic Artery 5 Superior Mesenteric Artery 6 Colic Artery, Right 7 Colic Artery, Left 8 Colic Artery, Middle 9 Renal Artery, Right A Renal Artery, Left B Inferior Mesenteric Artery C Common Iliac Artery, Right D Common Iliac Artery, Left E Internal Iliac Artery, Right F Internal Iliac Artery, Left H External Iliac Artery, Right J External Iliac Artery, Left K Femoral Artery, Right L Femoral Artery, Left M Popliteal Artery, Right N Popliteal Artery, Left P Anterior Tibial Artery, Right Q Anterior Tibial Artery, Left R Posterior Tibial Artery, Right S Posterior Tibial Artery, Left T Peroneal Artery, Right U Peroneal Artery, Left V Foot Artery, Right W Foot Artery, Left Y Lower Artery	0 Open 3 Percutaneous 4 Percutaneous Endoscopic	4 Intraluminal Device, Drug-eluting D Intraluminal Device Z No Device	Z No Qualifier

Section	0	Medical and Surgical
Body System	4	Lower Arteries
Operation	9	**Drainage:** Taking or letting out fluids and/or gases from a body part

Body Part (4th)	Approach (5th)	Device (6th)	Qualifier (7th)
0 Abdominal Aorta 1 Celiac Artery 2 Gastric Artery 3 Hepatic Artery 4 Splenic Artery 5 Superior Mesenteric Artery 6 Colic Artery, Right 7 Colic Artery, Left 8 Colic Artery, Middle 9 Renal Artery, Right A Renal Artery, Left B Inferior Mesenteric Artery C Common Iliac Artery, Right D Common Iliac Artery, Left E Internal Iliac Artery, Right F Internal Iliac Artery, Left H External Iliac Artery, Right J External Iliac Artery, Left K Femoral Artery, Right L Femoral Artery, Left M Popliteal Artery, Right N Popliteal Artery, Left P Anterior Tibial Artery, Right Q Anterior Tibial Artery, Left R Posterior Tibial Artery, Right S Posterior Tibial Artery, Left T Peroneal Artery, Right U Peroneal Artery, Left V Foot Artery, Right W Foot Artery, Left Y Lower Artery	0 Open 3 Percutaneous 4 Percutaneous Endoscopic	0 Drainage Device	Z No Qualifier
0 Abdominal Aorta 1 Celiac Artery 2 Gastric Artery 3 Hepatic Artery 4 Splenic Artery 5 Superior Mesenteric Artery 6 Colic Artery, Right 7 Colic Artery, Left 8 Colic Artery, Middle 9 Renal Artery, Right A Renal Artery, Left B Inferior Mesenteric Artery C Common Iliac Artery, Right D Common Iliac Artery, Left E Internal Iliac Artery, Right F Internal Iliac Artery, Left H External Iliac Artery, Right J External Iliac Artery, Left K Femoral Artery, Right L Femoral Artery, Left M Popliteal Artery, Right N Popliteal Artery, Left P Anterior Tibial Artery, Right Q Anterior Tibial Artery, Left R Posterior Tibial Artery, Right S Posterior Tibial Artery, Left T Peroneal Artery, Right U Peroneal Artery, Left V Foot Artery, Right W Foot Artery, Left Y Lower Artery	0 Open 3 Percutaneous 4 Percutaneous Endoscopic	Z No Device	X Diagnostic Z No Qualifier

Section	0	Medical and Surgical
Body System	4	Lower Arteries
Operation	B	Excision: Cutting out or off, without replacement, a portion of a body part

Body Part (4th)	Approach (5th)	Device (6th)	Qualifier (7th)
0 Abdominal Aorta	0 Open	Z No Device	X Diagnostic
1 Celiac Artery	3 Percutaneous		Z No Qualifier
2 Gastric Artery	4 Percutaneous		
3 Hepatic Artery	Endoscopic		
4 Splenic Artery			
5 Superior Mesenteric Artery			
6 Colic Artery, Right			
7 Colic Artery, Left			
8 Colic Artery, Middle			
9 Renal Artery, Right			
A Renal Artery, Left			
B Inferior Mesenteric Artery			
C Common Iliac Artery, Right			
D Common Iliac Artery, Left			
E Internal Iliac Artery, Right			
F Internal Iliac Artery, Left			
H External Iliac Artery, Right			
J External Iliac Artery, Left			
K Femoral Artery, Right			
L Femoral Artery, Left			
M Popliteal Artery, Right			
N Popliteal Artery, Left			
P Anterior Tibial Artery, Right			
Q Anterior Tibial Artery, Left			
R Posterior Tibial Artery, Right			
S Posterior Tibial Artery, Left			
T Peroneal Artery, Right			
U Peroneal Artery, Left			
V Foot Artery, Right			
W Foot Artery, Left			
Y Lower Artery			

Section	0	**Medical and Surgical**
Body System	**4**	**Lower Arteries**
Operation	**C**	**Extirpation:** Taking or cutting out solid matter from a body part

Body Part (4th)	Approach (5th)	Device (6th)	Qualifier (7th)
0 Abdominal Aorta 1 Celiac Artery 2 Gastric Artery 3 Hepatic Artery 4 Splenic Artery 5 Superior Mesenteric Artery 6 Colic Artery, Right 7 Colic Artery, Left 8 Colic Artery, Middle 9 Renal Artery, Right A Renal Artery, Left B Inferior Mesenteric Artery C Common Iliac Artery, Right D Common Iliac Artery, Left E Internal Iliac Artery, Right F Internal Iliac Artery, Left H External Iliac Artery, Right J External Iliac Artery, Left K Femoral Artery, Right L Femoral Artery, Left M Popliteal Artery, Right N Popliteal Artery, Left P Anterior Tibial Artery, Right Q Anterior Tibial Artery, Left R Posterior Tibial Artery, Right S Posterior Tibial Artery, Left T Peroneal Artery, Right U Peroneal Artery, Left V Foot Artery, Right W Foot Artery, Left Y Lower Artery	0 Open 3 Percutaneous 4 Percutaneous Endoscopic	Z No Device	Z No Qualifier

Section	0	**Medical and Surgical**
Body System	**4**	**Lower Arteries**
Operation	**H**	**Insertion:** Putting in a nonbiological appliance that monitors, assists, performs, or prevents a physiological function but does not physically take the place of a body part

Body Part (4th)	Approach (5th)	Device (6th)	Qualifier (7th)
0 Abdominal Aorta Y Lower Artery	0 Open 3 Percutaneous 4 Percutaneous Endoscopic	2 Monitoring Device 3 Infusion Device D Intraluminal Device	Z No Qualifier

Continued

04H Continued

Section	0	Medical and Surgical
Body System	4	Lower Arteries
Operation	H	**Insertion:** Putting in a nonbiological appliance that monitors, assists, performs, or prevents a physiological function but does not physically take the place of a body part

Body Part (4th)	Approach (5th)	Device (6th)	Qualifier (7th)
1 Celiac Artery 2 Gastric Artery 3 Hepatic Artery 4 Splenic Artery 5 Superior Mesenteric Artery 6 Colic Artery, Right 7 Colic Artery, Left 8 Colic Artery, Middle 9 Renal Artery, Right A Renal Artery, Left B Inferior Mesenteric Artery C Common Iliac Artery, Right D Common Iliac Artery, Left E Internal Iliac Artery, Right F Internal Iliac Artery, Left H External Iliac Artery, Right J External Iliac Artery, Left K Femoral Artery, Right L Femoral Artery, Left M Popliteal Artery, Right N Popliteal Artery, Left P Anterior Tibial Artery, Right Q Anterior Tibial Artery, Left R Posterior Tibial Artery, Right S Posterior Tibial Artery, Left T Peroneal Artery, Right U Peroneal Artery, Left V Foot Artery, Right W Foot Artery, Left	0 Open 3 Percutaneous 4 Percutaneous Endoscopic	3 Infusion Device D Intraluminal Device	Z No Qualifier

Section	0	Medical and Surgical
Body System	4	Lower Arteries
Operation	J	**Inspection:** Visually and/or manually exploring a body part

Body Part (4th)	Approach (5th)	Device (6th)	Qualifier (7th)
Y Lower Artery	0 Open 3 Percutaneous 4 Percutaneous Endoscopic X External	Z No Device	Z No Qualifier

Section	0	Medical and Surgical
Body System	4	Lower Arteries
Operation	L	Occlusion: Completely closing an orifice or the lumen of a tubular body part

Body Part (4th)	Approach (5th)	Device (6th)	Qualifier (7th)
0 Abdominal Aorta 1 Celiac Artery 2 Gastric Artery 3 Hepatic Artery 4 Splenic Artery 5 Superior Mesenteric Artery 6 Colic Artery, Right 7 Colic Artery, Left 8 Colic Artery, Middle 9 Renal Artery, Right A Renal Artery, Left B Inferior Mesenteric Artery C Common Iliac Artery, Right D Common Iliac Artery, Left H External Iliac Artery, Right J External Iliac Artery, Left K Femoral Artery, Right L Femoral Artery, Left M Popliteal Artery, Right N Popliteal Artery, Left P Anterior Tibial Artery, Right Q Anterior Tibial Artery, Left R Posterior Tibial Artery, Right S Posterior Tibial Artery, Left T Peroneal Artery, Right U Peroneal Artery, Left V Foot Artery, Right W Foot Artery, Left Y Lower Artery	0 Open 3 Percutaneous 4 Percutaneous Endoscopic	C Extraluminal Device D Intraluminal Device Z No Device	Z No Qualifier
E Internal Iliac Artery, Right	0 Open 3 Percutaneous 4 Percutaneous Endoscopic	C Extraluminal Device D Intraluminal Device Z No Device	T Uterine Artery, Right Z No Qualifier
F Internal Iliac Artery, Left	0 Open 3 Percutaneous 4 Percutaneous Endoscopic	C Extraluminal Device D Intraluminal Device Z No Device	U Uterine Artery, Left Z No Qualifier

Section	0	**Medical and Surgical**
Body System	4	**Lower Arteries**
Operation	N	**Release:** Freeing a body part from an abnormal physical constraint by cutting or by the use of force

Body Part (4th)	Approach (5th)	Device (6th)	Qualifier (7th)
0 Abdominal Aorta 1 Celiac Artery 2 Gastric Artery 3 Hepatic Artery 4 Splenic Artery 5 Superior Mesenteric Artery 6 Colic Artery, Right 7 Colic Artery, Left 8 Colic Artery, Middle 9 Renal Artery, Right A Renal Artery, Left B Inferior Mesenteric Artery C Common Iliac Artery, Right D Common Iliac Artery, Left E Internal Iliac Artery, Right F Internal Iliac Artery, Left H External Iliac Artery, Right J External Iliac Artery, Left K Femoral Artery, Right L Femoral Artery, Left M Popliteal Artery, Right N Popliteal Artery, Left P Anterior Tibial Artery, Right Q Anterior Tibial Artery, Left R Posterior Tibial Artery, Right S Posterior Tibial Artery, Left T Peroneal Artery, Right U Peroneal Artery, Left V Foot Artery, Right W Foot Artery, Left Y Lower Artery	0 Open 3 Percutaneous 4 Percutaneous Endoscopic	Z No Device	Z No Qualifier

Section	0	**Medical and Surgical**
Body System	4	**Lower Arteries**
Operation	P	**Removal:** Taking out or off a device from a body part

Body Part (4th)	Approach (5th)	Device (6th)	Qualifier (7th)
Y Lower Artery	0 Open 3 Percutaneous 4 Percutaneous Endoscopic	0 Drainage Device 2 Monitoring Device 3 Infusion Device 7 Autologous Tissue Substitute C Extraluminal Device D Intraluminal Device J Synthetic Substitute K Nonautologous Tissue Substitute	Z No Qualifier
Y Lower Artery	X External	0 Drainage Device 1 Radioactive Element 2 Monitoring Device 3 Infusion Device D Intraluminal Device	Z No Qualifier

Section	0	**Medical and Surgical**
Body System	4	**Lower Arteries**
Operation	Q	**Repair:** Restoring, to the extent possible, a body part to its normal anatomic structure and function

Body Part (4th)	Approach (5th)	Device (6th)	Qualifier (7th)
0 Abdominal Aorta 1 Celiac Artery 2 Gastric Artery 3 Hepatic Artery 4 Splenic Artery 5 Superior Mesenteric Artery 6 Colic Artery, Right 7 Colic Artery, Left 8 Colic Artery, Middle 9 Renal Artery, Right A Renal Artery, Left B Inferior Mesenteric Artery C Common Iliac Artery, Right D Common Iliac Artery, Left E Internal Iliac Artery, Right F Internal Iliac Artery, Left H External Iliac Artery, Right J External Iliac Artery, Left K Femoral Artery, Right L Femoral Artery, Left M Popliteal Artery, Right N Popliteal Artery, Left P Anterior Tibial Artery, Right Q Anterior Tibial Artery, Left R Posterior Tibial Artery, Right S Posterior Tibial Artery, Left T Peroneal Artery, Right U Peroneal Artery, Left V Foot Artery, Right W Foot Artery, Left Y Lower Artery	0 Open 3 Percutaneous 4 Percutaneous Endoscopic	Z No Device	Z No Qualifier

Section	0	**Medical and Surgical**
Body System	4	**Lower Arteries**
Operation	R	**Replacement:** Putting in or on biological or synthetic material that physically takes the place and/or function of all or a portion of a body part

Body Part (4th)	Approach (5th)	Device (6th)	Qualifier (7th)
0 Abdominal Aorta 1 Celiac Artery 2 Gastric Artery 3 Hepatic Artery 4 Splenic Artery 5 Superior Mesenteric Artery 6 Colic Artery, Right 7 Colic Artery, Left 8 Colic Artery, Middle 9 Renal Artery, Right A Renal Artery, Left B Inferior Mesenteric Artery C Common Iliac Artery, Right D Common Iliac Artery, Left E Internal Iliac Artery, Right F Internal Iliac Artery, Left H External Iliac Artery, Right J External Iliac Artery, Left K Femoral Artery, Right L Femoral Artery, Left M Popliteal Artery, Right N Popliteal Artery, Left P Anterior Tibial Artery, Right Q Anterior Tibial Artery, Left R Posterior Tibial Artery, Right S Posterior Tibial Artery, Left T Peroneal Artery, Right U Peroneal Artery, Left V Foot Artery, Right W Foot Artery, Left Y Lower Artery	0 Open 4 Percutaneous Endoscopic	7 Autologous Tissue Substitute J Synthetic Substitute K Nonautologous Tissue Substitute	Z No Qualifier

Section	0	Medical and Surgical
Body System	4	Lower Arteries
Operation	S	**Reposition:** Moving to its normal location, or other suitable location, all or a portion of a body part

Body Part (4ᵗʰ)	Approach (5ᵗʰ)	Device (6ᵗʰ)	Qualifier (7ᵗʰ)
0 Abdominal Aorta	0 Open	Z No Device	Z No Qualifier
1 Celiac Artery	3 Percutaneous		
2 Gastric Artery	4 Percutaneous Endoscopic		
3 Hepatic Artery			
4 Splenic Artery			
5 Superior Mesenteric Artery			
6 Colic Artery, Right			
7 Colic Artery, Left			
8 Colic Artery, Middle			
9 Renal Artery, Right			
A Renal Artery, Left			
B Inferior Mesenteric Artery			
C Common Iliac Artery, Right			
D Common Iliac Artery, Left			
E Internal Iliac Artery, Right			
F Internal Iliac Artery, Left			
H External Iliac Artery, Right			
J External Iliac Artery, Left			
K Femoral Artery, Right			
L Femoral Artery, Left			
M Popliteal Artery, Right			
N Popliteal Artery, Left			
P Anterior Tibial Artery, Right			
Q Anterior Tibial Artery, Left			
R Posterior Tibial Artery, Right			
S Posterior Tibial Artery, Left			
T Peroneal Artery, Right			
U Peroneal Artery, Left			
V Foot Artery, Right			
W Foot Artery, Left			
Y Lower Artery			

Section	0	Medical and Surgical
Body System	4	Lower Arteries
Operation	U	Supplement: Putting in or on biological or synthetic material that physically reinforces and/or augments the function of a portion of a body part

Body Part (4th)	Approach (5th)	Device (6th)	Qualifier (7th)
0 Abdominal Aorta 1 Celiac Artery 2 Gastric Artery 3 Hepatic Artery 4 Splenic Artery 5 Superior Mesenteric Artery 6 Colic Artery, Right 7 Colic Artery, Left 8 Colic Artery, Middle 9 Renal Artery, Right A Renal Artery, Left B Inferior Mesenteric Artery C Common Iliac Artery, Right D Common Iliac Artery, Left E Internal Iliac Artery, Right F Internal Iliac Artery, Left H External Iliac Artery, Right J External Iliac Artery, Left K Femoral Artery, Right L Femoral Artery, Left M Popliteal Artery, Right N Popliteal Artery, Left P Anterior Tibial Artery, Right Q Anterior Tibial Artery, Left R Posterior Tibial Artery, Right S Posterior Tibial Artery, Left T Peroneal Artery, Right U Peroneal Artery, Left V Foot Artery, Right W Foot Artery, Left Y Lower Artery	0 Open 3 Percutaneous 4 Percutaneous Endoscopic	7 Autologous Tissue Substitute J Synthetic Substitute K Nonautologous Tissue Substitute	Z No Qualifier

Section	0	Medical and Surgical
Body System	4	Lower Arteries
Operation	V	Restriction: Partially closing an orifice or the lumen of a tubular body part

Body Part (4th)	Approach (5th)	Device (6th)	Qualifier (7th)
0 Abdominal Aorta	0 Open 3 Percutaneous 4 Percutaneous Endoscopic	C Extraluminal Device Z No Device	Z No Qualifier
0 Abdominal Aorta	0 Open 3 Percutaneous 4 Percutaneous Endoscopic	D Intraluminal Device	J Temporary Z No Qualifier

Continued

Section	0	Medical and Surgical
Body System	4	Lower Arteries
Operation	V	**Restriction:** Partially closing an orifice or the lumen of a tubular body part

Body Part (4th)	Approach (5th)	Device (6th)	Qualifier (7th)
1 Celiac Artery 2 Gastric Artery 3 Hepatic Artery 4 Splenic Artery 5 Superior Mesenteric Artery 6 Colic Artery, Right 7 Colic Artery, Left 8 Colic Artery, Middle 9 Renal Artery, Right A Renal Artery, Left B Inferior Mesenteric Artery C Common Iliac Artery, Right D Common Iliac Artery, Left E Internal Iliac Artery, Right F Internal Iliac Artery, Left H External Iliac Artery, Right J External Iliac Artery, Left K Femoral Artery, Right L Femoral Artery, Left M Popliteal Artery, Right N Popliteal Artery, Left P Anterior Tibial Artery, Right Q Anterior Tibial Artery, Left R Posterior Tibial Artery, Right S Posterior Tibial Artery, Left T Peroneal Artery, Right U Peroneal Artery, Left V Foot Artery, Right W Foot Artery, Left Y Lower Artery	0 Open 3 Percutaneous 4 Percutaneous Endoscopic	C Extraluminal Device D Intraluminal Device Z No Device	Z No Qualifier

Section	0	Medical and Surgical
Body System	4	Lower Arteries
Operation	W	**Revision:** Correcting, to the extent possible, a portion of a malfunctioning device or the position of a displaced device

Body Part (4th)	Approach (5th)	Device (6th)	Qualifier (7th)
Y Lower Artery	0 Open 3 Percutaneous 4 Percutaneous Endoscopic X External	0 Drainage Device 2 Monitoring Device 3 Infusion Device 7 Autologous Tissue Substitute C Extraluminal Device D Intraluminal Device J Synthetic Substitute K Nonautologous Tissue Substitute	Z No Qualifier

Lower Arteries Code Listing 041–04W

041 – Lower Arteries, Bypass

Review Coding Guideline B3.6a

0410090 Bypass Abdominal Aorta to Abdominal Aorta with Autologous Venous Tissue, Open Approach

0410091 Bypass Abdominal Aorta to Celiac Artery with Autologous Venous Tissue, Open Approach

0410092 Bypass Abdominal Aorta to Mesenteric Artery with Autologous Venous Tissue, Open Approach

0410093 Bypass Abdominal Aorta to Right Renal Artery with Autologous Venous Tissue, Open Approach

0410094 Bypass Abdominal Aorta to Left Renal Artery with Autologous Venous Tissue, Open Approach

0410095 Bypass Abdominal Aorta to Bilateral Renal Artery with Autologous Venous Tissue, Open Approach

0410096 Bypass Abdominal Aorta to Right Common Iliac Artery with Autologous Venous Tissue, Open Approach

0410097 Bypass Abdominal Aorta to Left Common Iliac Artery with Autologous Venous Tissue, Open Approach

0410098 Bypass Abdominal Aorta to Bilateral Common Iliac Arteries with Autologous Venous Tissue, Open Approach

0410099 Bypass Abdominal Aorta to Right Internal Iliac Artery with Autologous Venous Tissue, Open Approach

041009B Bypass Abdominal Aorta to Left Internal Iliac Artery with Autologous Venous Tissue, Open Approach

041009C Bypass Abdominal Aorta to Bilateral Internal Iliac Arteries with Autologous Venous Tissue, Open Approach

041009D Bypass Abdominal Aorta to Right External Iliac Artery with Autologous Venous Tissue, Open Approach

041009F Bypass Abdominal Aorta to Left External Iliac Artery with Autologous Venous Tissue, Open Approach

041009G Bypass Abdominal Aorta to Bilateral External Iliac Arteries with Autologous Venous Tissue, Open Approach

041009H Bypass Abdominal Aorta to Right Femoral Artery with Autologous Venous Tissue, Open Approach

041009J Bypass Abdominal Aorta to Left Femoral Artery with Autologous Venous Tissue, Open Approach

041009K Bypass Abdominal Aorta to Bilateral Femoral Arteries with Autologous Venous Tissue, Open Approach

041009Q Bypass Abdominal Aorta to Lower Extremity Artery with Autologous Venous Tissue, Open Approach

041009R Bypass Abdominal Aorta to Lower Artery with Autologous Venous Tissue, Open Approach

04100A0 Bypass Abdominal Aorta to Abdominal Aorta with Autologous Arterial Tissue, Open Approach

04100A1 Bypass Abdominal Aorta to Celiac Artery with Autologous Arterial Tissue, Open Approach

04100A2 Bypass Abdominal Aorta to Mesenteric Artery with Autologous Arterial Tissue, Open Approach

04100A3 Bypass Abdominal Aorta to Right Renal Artery with Autologous Arterial Tissue, Open Approach

04100A4 Bypass Abdominal Aorta to Left Renal Artery with Autologous Arterial Tissue, Open Approach

04100A5 Bypass Abdominal Aorta to Bilateral Renal Artery with Autologous Arterial Tissue, Open Approach

04100A6 Bypass Abdominal Aorta to Right Common Iliac Artery with Autologous Arterial Tissue, Open Approach

04100A7 Bypass Abdominal Aorta to Left Common Iliac Artery with Autologous Arterial Tissue, Open Approach

04100A8 Bypass Abdominal Aorta to Bilateral Common Iliac Arteries with Autologous Arterial Tissue, Open Approach

04100A9 Bypass Abdominal Aorta to Right Internal Iliac Artery with Autologous Arterial Tissue, Open Approach

04100AB Bypass Abdominal Aorta to Left Internal Iliac Artery with Autologous Arterial Tissue, Open Approach

04100AC Bypass Abdominal Aorta to Bilateral Internal Iliac Arteries with Autologous Arterial Tissue, Open Approach

04100AD Bypass Abdominal Aorta to Right External Iliac Artery with Autologous Arterial Tissue, Open Approach

04100AF Bypass Abdominal Aorta to Left External Iliac Artery with Autologous Arterial Tissue, Open Approach

04100AG Bypass Abdominal Aorta to Bilateral External Iliac Arteries with Autologous Arterial Tissue, Open Approach

04100AH Bypass Abdominal Aorta to Right Femoral Artery with Autologous Arterial Tissue, Open Approach

04100AJ Bypass Abdominal Aorta to Left Femoral Artery with Autologous Arterial Tissue, Open Approach

04100AK Bypass Abdominal Aorta to Bilateral Femoral Arteries with Autologous Arterial Tissue, Open Approach

04100AQ Bypass Abdominal Aorta to Lower Extremity Artery with Autologous Arterial Tissue, Open Approach

04100AR Bypass Abdominal Aorta to Lower Artery with Autologous Arterial Tissue, Open Approach

04100J0 Bypass Abdominal Aorta to Abdominal Aorta with Synthetic Substitute, Open Approach

04100J1 Bypass Abdominal Aorta to Celiac Artery with Synthetic Substitute, Open Approach

04100J2 Bypass Abdominal Aorta to Mesenteric Artery with Synthetic Substitute, Open Approach

04100J3 Bypass Abdominal Aorta to Right Renal Artery with Synthetic Substitute, Open Approach

04100J4 Bypass Abdominal Aorta to Left Renal Artery with Synthetic Substitute, Open Approach

04100J5 Bypass Abdominal Aorta to Bilateral Renal Artery with Synthetic Substitute, Open Approach

04100J6 Bypass Abdominal Aorta to Right Common Iliac Artery with Synthetic Substitute, Open Approach

04100J7 Bypass Abdominal Aorta to Left Common Iliac Artery with Synthetic Substitute, Open Approach

04100J8 Bypass Abdominal Aorta to Bilateral Common Iliac Arteries with Synthetic Substitute, Open Approach

04100J9 Bypass Abdominal Aorta to Right Internal Iliac Artery with Synthetic Substitute, Open Approach

04100JB Bypass Abdominal Aorta to Left Internal Iliac Artery with Synthetic Substitute, Open Approach

04100JC Bypass Abdominal Aorta to Bilateral Internal Iliac Arteries with Synthetic Substitute, Open Approach

04100JD Bypass Abdominal Aorta to Right External Iliac Artery with Synthetic Substitute, Open Approach

04100JF Bypass Abdominal Aorta to Left External Iliac Artery with Synthetic Substitute, Open Approach

04100JG Bypass Abdominal Aorta to Bilateral External Iliac Arteries with Synthetic Substitute, Open Approach

04100JH Bypass Abdominal Aorta to Right Femoral Artery with Synthetic Substitute, Open Approach

04100JJ Bypass Abdominal Aorta to Left Femoral Artery with Synthetic Substitute, Open Approach

04100JK Bypass Abdominal Aorta to Bilateral Femoral Arteries with Synthetic Substitute, Open Approach

04100JQ Bypass Abdominal Aorta to Lower Extremity Artery with Synthetic Substitute, Open Approach

04100JR Bypass Abdominal Aorta to Lower Artery with Synthetic Substitute, Open Approach

04100K0 Bypass Abdominal Aorta to Abdominal Aorta with Nonautologous Tissue Substitute, Open Approach

04100K1 Bypass Abdominal Aorta to Celiac Artery with Nonautologous Tissue Substitute, Open Approach

04100K2 Bypass Abdominal Aorta to Mesenteric Artery with Nonautologous Tissue Substitute, Open Approach

04100K3 Bypass Abdominal Aorta to Right Renal Artery with Nonautologous Tissue Substitute, Open Approach

04100K4 Bypass Abdominal Aorta to Left Renal Artery with Nonautologous Tissue Substitute, Open Approach

04100K5 Bypass Abdominal Aorta to Bilateral Renal Artery with Nonautologous Tissue Substitute, Open Approach

04100K6 Bypass Abdominal Aorta to Right Common Iliac Artery with Nonautologous Tissue Substitute, Open Approach

04100K7 Bypass Abdominal Aorta to Left Common Iliac Artery with Nonautologous Tissue Substitute, Open Approach

04100K8 Bypass Abdominal Aorta to Bilateral Common Iliac Arteries with Nonautologous Tissue Substitute, Open Approach

04100K9 Bypass Abdominal Aorta to Right Internal Iliac Artery with Nonautologous Tissue Substitute, Open Approach

04100KB Bypass Abdominal Aorta to Left Internal Iliac Artery with Nonautologous Tissue Substitute, Open Approach

04100KC Bypass Abdominal Aorta to Bilateral Internal Iliac Arteries with Nonautologous Tissue Substitute, Open Approach

04100KD Bypass Abdominal Aorta to Right External Iliac Artery with Nonautologous Tissue Substitute, Open Approach

04100KF Bypass Abdominal Aorta to Left External Iliac Artery with Nonautologous Tissue Substitute, Open Approach

04100KG Bypass Abdominal Aorta to Bilateral External Iliac Arteries with Nonautologous Tissue Substitute, Open Approach

04100KH Bypass Abdominal Aorta to Right Femoral Artery with Nonautologous Tissue Substitute, Open Approach

04100KJ Bypass Abdominal Aorta to Left Femoral Artery with Nonautologous Tissue Substitute, Open Approach

04100KK Bypass Abdominal Aorta to Bilateral Femoral Arteries with Nonautologous Tissue Substitute, Open Approach

04100KQ Bypass Abdominal Aorta to Lower Extremity Artery with Nonautologous Tissue Substitute, Open Approach

04100KR Bypass Abdominal Aorta to Lower Artery with Nonautologous Tissue Substitute, Open Approach

04100Z0 Bypass Abdominal Aorta to Abdominal Aorta, Open Approach

04100Z1 Bypass Abdominal Aorta to Celiac Artery, Open Approach

04100Z2 Bypass Abdominal Aorta to Mesenteric Artery, Open Approach

04100Z3 Bypass Abdominal Aorta to Right Renal Artery, Open Approach

04100Z4 Bypass Abdominal Aorta to Left Renal Artery, Open Approach

04100Z5 Bypass Abdominal Aorta to Bilateral Renal Artery, Open Approach

04100Z6 Bypass Abdominal Aorta to Right Common Iliac Artery, Open Approach

04100Z7 Bypass Abdominal Aorta to Left Common Iliac Artery, Open Approach

04100Z8 Bypass Abdominal Aorta to Bilateral Common Iliac Arteries, Open Approach

04100Z9 Bypass Abdominal Aorta to Right Internal Iliac Artery, Open Approach

04100ZB Bypass Abdominal Aorta to Left Internal Iliac Artery, Open Approach

04100ZC Bypass Abdominal Aorta to Bilateral Internal Iliac Arteries, Open Approach

04100ZD Bypass Abdominal Aorta to Right External Iliac Artery, Open Approach

04100ZF Bypass Abdominal Aorta to Left External Iliac Artery, Open Approach

04100ZG Bypass Abdominal Aorta to Bilateral External Iliac Arteries, Open Approach

04100ZH Bypass Abdominal Aorta to Right Femoral Artery, Open Approach

04100ZJ Bypass Abdominal Aorta to Left Femoral Artery, Open Approach

04100ZK Bypass Abdominal Aorta to Bilateral Femoral Arteries, Open Approach

04100ZQ Bypass Abdominal Aorta to Lower Extremity Artery, Open Approach

04100ZR Bypass Abdominal Aorta to Lower Artery, Open Approach

0410490 Bypass Abdominal Aorta to Abdominal Aorta with Autologous Venous Tissue, Percutaneous Endoscopic Approach

0410491 Bypass Abdominal Aorta to Celiac Artery with Autologous Venous Tissue, Percutaneous Endoscopic Approach

0410492 Bypass Abdominal Aorta to Mesenteric Artery with Autologous Venous Tissue, Percutaneous Endoscopic Approach

0410493 Bypass Abdominal Aorta to Right Renal Artery with Autologous Venous Tissue, Percutaneous Endoscopic Approach

0410494 Bypass Abdominal Aorta to Left Renal Artery with Autologous Venous Tissue, Percutaneous Endoscopic Approach

0410495 Bypass Abdominal Aorta to Bilateral Renal Artery with Autologous Venous Tissue, Percutaneous Endoscopic Approach

0410496 Bypass Abdominal Aorta to Right Common Iliac Artery with Autologous Venous Tissue, Percutaneous Endoscopic Approach

0410497 Bypass Abdominal Aorta to Left Common Iliac Artery with Autologous Venous Tissue, Percutaneous Endoscopic Approach

0410498 Bypass Abdominal Aorta to Bilateral Common Iliac Arteries with Autologous Venous Tissue, Percutaneous Endoscopic Approach

0410499 Bypass Abdominal Aorta to Right Internal Iliac Artery with Autologous Venous Tissue, Percutaneous Endoscopic Approach

041049B Bypass Abdominal Aorta to Left Internal Iliac Artery with Autologous Venous Tissue, Percutaneous Endoscopic Approach

041049C Bypass Abdominal Aorta to Bilateral Internal Iliac Arteries with Autologous Venous Tissue, Percutaneous Endoscopic Approach

041049D Bypass Abdominal Aorta to Right External Iliac Artery with Autologous Venous Tissue, Percutaneous Endoscopic Approach

041049F Bypass Abdominal Aorta to Left External Iliac Artery with Autologous Venous Tissue, Percutaneous Endoscopic Approach

041049G Bypass Abdominal Aorta to Bilateral External Iliac Arteries with Autologous Venous Tissue, Percutaneous Endoscopic Approach

041049H Bypass Abdominal Aorta to Right Femoral Artery with Autologous Venous Tissue, Percutaneous Endoscopic Approach

041049J Bypass Abdominal Aorta to Left Femoral Artery with Autologous Venous Tissue, Percutaneous Endoscopic Approach

041049K Bypass Abdominal Aorta to Bilateral Femoral Arteries with Autologous Venous Tissue, Percutaneous Endoscopic Approach

041049Q Bypass Abdominal Aorta to Lower Extremity Artery with Autologous Venous Tissue, Percutaneous Endoscopic Approach

041049R Bypass Abdominal Aorta to Lower Artery with Autologous Venous Tissue, Percutaneous Endoscopic Approach

04104A0 Bypass Abdominal Aorta to Abdominal Aorta with Autologous Arterial Tissue, Percutaneous Endoscopic Approach

04104A1 Bypass Abdominal Aorta to Celiac Artery with Autologous Arterial Tissue, Percutaneous Endoscopic Approach

04104A2 Bypass Abdominal Aorta to Mesenteric Artery with Autologous Arterial Tissue, Percutaneous Endoscopic Approach

04104A3 Bypass Abdominal Aorta to Right Renal Artery with Autologous Arterial Tissue, Percutaneous Endoscopic Approach

04104A4 Bypass Abdominal Aorta to Left Renal Artery with Autologous Arterial Tissue, Percutaneous Endoscopic Approach

04104A5 Bypass Abdominal Aorta to Bilateral Renal Artery with Autologous Arterial Tissue, Percutaneous Endoscopic Approach

04104A6 Bypass Abdominal Aorta to Right Common Iliac Artery with Autologous Arterial Tissue, Percutaneous Endoscopic Approach

04104A7 Bypass Abdominal Aorta to Left Common Iliac Artery with Autologous Arterial Tissue, Percutaneous Endoscopic Approach

04104A8 Bypass Abdominal Aorta to Bilateral Common Iliac Arteries with Autologous Arterial Tissue, Percutaneous Endoscopic Approach

04104A9 Bypass Abdominal Aorta to Right Internal Iliac Artery with Autologous Arterial Tissue, Percutaneous Endoscopic Approach

04104AB Bypass Abdominal Aorta to Left Internal Iliac Artery with Autologous Arterial Tissue, Percutaneous Endoscopic Approach

04104AC Bypass Abdominal Aorta to Bilateral Internal Iliac Arteries with Autologous Arterial Tissue, Percutaneous Endoscopic Approach

04104AD Bypass Abdominal Aorta to Right External Iliac Artery with Autologous Arterial Tissue, Percutaneous Endoscopic Approach

04104AF Bypass Abdominal Aorta to Left External Iliac Artery with Autologous Arterial Tissue, Percutaneous Endoscopic Approach

04104AG Bypass Abdominal Aorta to Bilateral External Iliac Arteries with Autologous Arterial Tissue, Percutaneous Endoscopic Approach

04104AH Bypass Abdominal Aorta to Right Femoral Artery with Autologous Arterial Tissue, Percutaneous Endoscopic Approach

04104AJ Bypass Abdominal Aorta to Left Femoral Artery with Autologous Arterial Tissue, Percutaneous Endoscopic Approach

04104AK Bypass Abdominal Aorta to Bilateral Femoral Arteries with Autologous Arterial Tissue, Percutaneous Endoscopic Approach

04104AQ Bypass Abdominal Aorta to Lower Extremity Artery with Autologous Arterial Tissue, Percutaneous Endoscopic Approach

04104AR Bypass Abdominal Aorta to Lower Artery with Autologous Arterial Tissue, Percutaneous Endoscopic Approach

04104J0 Bypass Abdominal Aorta to Abdominal Aorta with Synthetic Substitute, Percutaneous Endoscopic Approach

04104J1 Bypass Abdominal Aorta to Celiac Artery with Synthetic Substitute, Percutaneous Endoscopic Approach

04104J2 Bypass Abdominal Aorta to Mesenteric Artery with Synthetic Substitute, Percutaneous Endoscopic Approach

04104J3 Bypass Abdominal Aorta to Right Renal Artery with Synthetic Substitute, Percutaneous Endoscopic Approach

04104J4 Bypass Abdominal Aorta to Left Renal Artery with Synthetic Substitute, Percutaneous Endoscopic Approach

04104J5   Bypass Abdominal Aorta to Bilateral Renal Artery with Synthetic Substitute, Percutaneous Endoscopic Approach

04104J6   Bypass Abdominal Aorta to Right Common Iliac Artery with Synthetic Substitute, Percutaneous Endoscopic Approach

04104J7   Bypass Abdominal Aorta to Left Common Iliac Artery with Synthetic Substitute, Percutaneous Endoscopic Approach

04104J8   Bypass Abdominal Aorta to Bilateral Common Iliac Arteries with Synthetic Substitute, Percutaneous Endoscopic Approach

04104J9   Bypass Abdominal Aorta to Right Internal Iliac Artery with Synthetic Substitute, Percutaneous Endoscopic Approach

04104JB   Bypass Abdominal Aorta to Left Internal Iliac Artery with Synthetic Substitute, Percutaneous Endoscopic Approach

04104JC   Bypass Abdominal Aorta to Bilateral Internal Iliac Arteries with Synthetic Substitute, Percutaneous Endoscopic Approach

04104JD   Bypass Abdominal Aorta to Right External Iliac Artery with Synthetic Substitute, Percutaneous Endoscopic Approach

04104JF   Bypass Abdominal Aorta to Left External Iliac Artery with Synthetic Substitute, Percutaneous Endoscopic Approach

04104JG   Bypass Abdominal Aorta to Bilateral External Iliac Arteries with Synthetic Substitute, Percutaneous Endoscopic Approach

04104JH   Bypass Abdominal Aorta to Right Femoral Artery with Synthetic Substitute, Percutaneous Endoscopic Approach

04104JJ   Bypass Abdominal Aorta to Left Femoral Artery with Synthetic Substitute, Percutaneous Endoscopic Approach

04104JK   Bypass Abdominal Aorta to Bilateral Femoral Arteries with Synthetic Substitute, Percutaneous Endoscopic Approach

04104JQ   Bypass Abdominal Aorta to Lower Extremity Artery with Synthetic Substitute, Percutaneous Endoscopic Approach

04104JR   Bypass Abdominal Aorta to Lower Artery with Synthetic Substitute, Percutaneous Endoscopic Approach

04104K0   Bypass Abdominal Aorta to Abdominal Aorta with Nonautologous Tissue Substitute, Percutaneous Endoscopic Approach

04104K1   Bypass Abdominal Aorta to Celiac Artery with Nonautologous Tissue Substitute, Percutaneous Endoscopic Approach

04104K2   Bypass Abdominal Aorta to Mesenteric Artery with Nonautologous Tissue Substitute, Percutaneous Endoscopic Approach

04104K3   Bypass Abdominal Aorta to Right Renal Artery with Nonautologous Tissue Substitute, Percutaneous Endoscopic Approach

04104K4   Bypass Abdominal Aorta to Left Renal Artery with Nonautologous Tissue Substitute, Percutaneous Endoscopic Approach

04104K5   Bypass Abdominal Aorta to Bilateral Renal Artery with Nonautologous Tissue Substitute, Percutaneous Endoscopic Approach

04104K6   Bypass Abdominal Aorta to Right Common Iliac Artery with Nonautologous Tissue Substitute, Percutaneous Endoscopic Approach

04104K7   Bypass Abdominal Aorta to Left Common Iliac Artery with Nonautologous Tissue Substitute, Percutaneous Endoscopic Approach

04104K8   Bypass Abdominal Aorta to Bilateral Common Iliac Arteries with Nonautologous Tissue Substitute, Percutaneous Endoscopic Approach

04104K9   Bypass Abdominal Aorta to Right Internal Iliac Artery with Nonautologous Tissue Substitute, Percutaneous Endoscopic Approach

04104KB   Bypass Abdominal Aorta to Left Internal Iliac Artery with Nonautologous Tissue Substitute, Percutaneous Endoscopic Approach

04104KC   Bypass Abdominal Aorta to Bilateral Internal Iliac Arteries with Nonautologous Tissue Substitute, Percutaneous Endoscopic Approach

04104KD   Bypass Abdominal Aorta to Right External Iliac Artery with Nonautologous Tissue Substitute, Percutaneous Endoscopic Approach

04104KF   Bypass Abdominal Aorta to Left External Iliac Artery with Nonautologous Tissue Substitute, Percutaneous Endoscopic Approach

04104KG   Bypass Abdominal Aorta to Bilateral External Iliac Arteries with Nonautologous Tissue Substitute, Percutaneous Endoscopic Approach

04104KH   Bypass Abdominal Aorta to Right Femoral Artery with Nonautologous Tissue Substitute, Percutaneous Endoscopic Approach

04104KJ   Bypass Abdominal Aorta to Left Femoral Artery with Nonautologous Tissue Substitute, Percutaneous Endoscopic Approach

04104KK   Bypass Abdominal Aorta to Bilateral Femoral Arteries with Nonautologous Tissue Substitute, Percutaneous Endoscopic Approach

04104KQ   Bypass Abdominal Aorta to Lower Extremity Artery with Nonautologous Tissue Substitute, Percutaneous Endoscopic Approach

04104KR   Bypass Abdominal Aorta to Lower Artery with Nonautologous Tissue Substitute, Percutaneous Endoscopic Approach

04104Z0   Bypass Abdominal Aorta to Abdominal Aorta, Percutaneous Endoscopic Approach

04104Z1   Bypass Abdominal Aorta to Celiac Artery, Percutaneous Endoscopic Approach

04104Z2   Bypass Abdominal Aorta to Mesenteric Artery, Percutaneous Endoscopic Approach

04104Z3   Bypass Abdominal Aorta to Right Renal Artery, Percutaneous Endoscopic Approach

04104Z4   Bypass Abdominal Aorta to Left Renal Artery, Percutaneous Endoscopic Approach

04104Z5   Bypass Abdominal Aorta to Bilateral Renal Artery, Percutaneous Endoscopic Approach

04104Z6   Bypass Abdominal Aorta to Right Common Iliac Artery, Percutaneous Endoscopic Approach

04104Z7   Bypass Abdominal Aorta to Left Common Iliac Artery, Percutaneous Endoscopic Approach

04104Z8   Bypass Abdominal Aorta to Bilateral Common Iliac Arteries, Percutaneous Endoscopic Approach

04104Z9   Bypass Abdominal Aorta to Right Internal Iliac Artery, Percutaneous Endoscopic Approach

04104ZB   Bypass Abdominal Aorta to Left Internal Iliac Artery, Percutaneous Endoscopic Approach

04104ZC   Bypass Abdominal Aorta to Bilateral Internal Iliac Arteries, Percutaneous Endoscopic Approach

04104ZD   Bypass Abdominal Aorta to Right External Iliac Artery, Percutaneous Endoscopic Approach

04104ZF   Bypass Abdominal Aorta to Left External Iliac Artery, Percutaneous Endoscopic Approach

04104ZG   Bypass Abdominal Aorta to Bilateral External Iliac Arteries, Percutaneous Endoscopic Approach

04104ZH   Bypass Abdominal Aorta to Right Femoral Artery, Percutaneous Endoscopic Approach

04104ZJ   Bypass Abdominal Aorta to Left Femoral Artery, Percutaneous Endoscopic Approach

04104ZK   Bypass Abdominal Aorta to Bilateral Femoral Arteries, Percutaneous Endoscopic Approach

04104ZQ   Bypass Abdominal Aorta to Lower Extremity Artery, Percutaneous Endoscopic Approach

04104ZR   Bypass Abdominal Aorta to Lower Artery, Percutaneous Endoscopic Approach

0414093   Bypass Splenic Artery to Right Renal Artery with Autologous Venous Tissue, Open Approach

0414094   Bypass Splenic Artery to Left Renal Artery with Autologous Venous Tissue, Open Approach

0414095   Bypass Splenic Artery to Bilateral Renal Artery with Autologous Venous Tissue, Open Approach

04140A3   Bypass Splenic Artery to Right Renal Artery with Autologous Arterial Tissue, Open Approach

04140A4   Bypass Splenic Artery to Left Renal Artery with Autologous Arterial Tissue, Open Approach

04140A5   Bypass Splenic Artery to Bilateral Renal Artery with Autologous Arterial Tissue, Open Approach

04140J3   Bypass Splenic Artery to Right Renal Artery with Synthetic Substitute, Open Approach

04140J4   Bypass Splenic Artery to Left Renal Artery with Synthetic Substitute, Open Approach

04140J5   Bypass Splenic Artery to Bilateral Renal Artery with Synthetic Substitute, Open Approach

04140K3   Bypass Splenic Artery to Right Renal Artery with Nonautologous Tissue Substitute, Open Approach

04140K4   Bypass Splenic Artery to Left Renal Artery with Nonautologous Tissue Substitute, Open Approach

04140K5   Bypass Splenic Artery to Bilateral Renal Artery with Nonautologous Tissue Substitute, Open Approach

04140Z3   Bypass Splenic Artery to Right Renal Artery, Open Approach

04140Z4   Bypass Splenic Artery to Left Renal Artery, Open Approach

04140Z5   Bypass Splenic Artery to Bilateral Renal Artery, Open Approach

414493   Bypass Splenic Artery to Right Renal Artery with Autologous Venous Tissue, Percutaneous Endoscopic Approach

0414494   Bypass Splenic Artery to Left Renal Artery with Autologous Venous Tissue, Percutaneous Endoscopic Approach

0414495   Bypass Splenic Artery to Bilateral Renal Artery with Autologous Venous Tissue, Percutaneous Endoscopic Approach

04144A3   Bypass Splenic Artery to Right Renal Artery with Autologous Arterial Tissue, Percutaneous Endoscopic Approach

04144A4   Bypass Splenic Artery to Left Renal Artery with Autologous Arterial Tissue, Percutaneous Endoscopic Approach

04144A5   Bypass Splenic Artery to Bilateral Renal Artery with Autologous Arterial Tissue, Percutaneous Endoscopic Approach

04144J3   Bypass Splenic Artery to Right Renal Artery with Synthetic Substitute, Percutaneous Endoscopic Approach

04144J4   Bypass Splenic Artery to Left Renal Artery with Synthetic Substitute, Percutaneous Endoscopic Approach

04144J5   Bypass Splenic Artery to Bilateral Renal Artery with Synthetic Substitute, Percutaneous Endoscopic Approach

04144K3   Bypass Splenic Artery to Right Renal Artery with Nonautologous Tissue Substitute, Percutaneous Endoscopic Approach

04144K4   Bypass Splenic Artery to Left Renal Artery with Nonautologous Tissue Substitute, Percutaneous Endoscopic Approach

04144K5   Bypass Splenic Artery to Bilateral Renal Artery with Nonautologous Tissue Substitute, Percutaneous Endoscopic Approach

04144Z3   Bypass Splenic Artery to Right Renal Artery, Percutaneous Endoscopic Approach

04144Z4   Bypass Splenic Artery to Left Renal Artery, Percutaneous Endoscopic Approach

04144Z5   Bypass Splenic Artery to Bilateral Renal Artery, Percutaneous Endoscopic Approach

041C090   Bypass Right Common Iliac Artery to Abdominal Aorta with Autologous Venous Tissue, Open Approach

041C091   Bypass Right Common Iliac Artery to Celiac Artery with Autologous Venous Tissue, Open Approach

041C092   Bypass Right Common Iliac Artery to Mesenteric Artery with Autologous Venous Tissue, Open Approach

041C093   Bypass Right Common Iliac Artery to Right Renal Artery with Autologous Venous Tissue, Open Approach

041C094   Bypass Right Common Iliac Artery to Left Renal Artery with Autologous Venous Tissue, Open Approach

041C095   Bypass Right Common Iliac Artery to Bilateral Renal Artery with Autologous Venous Tissue, Open Approach

041C096   Bypass Right Common Iliac Artery to Right Common Iliac Artery with Autologous Venous Tissue, Open Approach

041C097   Bypass Right Common Iliac Artery to Left Common Iliac Artery with Autologous Venous Tissue, Open Approach

041C098   Bypass Right Common Iliac Artery to Bilateral Common Iliac Arteries with Autologous Venous Tissue, Open Approach

041C099   Bypass Right Common Iliac Artery to Right Internal Iliac Artery with Autologous Venous Tissue, Open Approach

041C09B   Bypass Right Common Iliac Artery to Left Internal Iliac Artery with Autologous Venous Tissue, Open Approach

041C09C   Bypass Right Common Iliac Artery to Bilateral Internal Iliac Arteries with Autologous Venous Tissue, Open Approach

041C09D   Bypass Right Common Iliac Artery to Right External Iliac Artery with Autologous Venous Tissue, Open Approach

041C09F   Bypass Right Common Iliac Artery to Left External Iliac Artery with Autologous Venous Tissue, Open Approach

041C09G   Bypass Right Common Iliac Artery to Bilateral External Iliac Arteries with Autologous Venous Tissue, Open Approach

041C09H   Bypass Right Common Iliac Artery to Right Femoral Artery with Autologous Venous Tissue, Open Approach

041C09J   Bypass Right Common Iliac Artery to Left Femoral Artery with Autologous Venous Tissue, Open Approach

041C09K   Bypass Right Common Iliac Artery to Bilateral Femoral Arteries with Autologous Venous Tissue, Open Approach

041C09Q   Bypass Right Common Iliac Artery to Lower Extremity Artery with Autologous Venous Tissue, Open Approach

041C09R   Bypass Right Common Iliac Artery to Lower Artery with Autologous Venous Tissue, Open Approach

041C0A0   Bypass Right Common Iliac Artery to Abdominal Aorta with Autologous Arterial Tissue, Open Approach

041C0A1   Bypass Right Common Iliac Artery to Celiac Artery with Autologous Arterial Tissue, Open Approach

041C0A2   Bypass Right Common Iliac Artery to Mesenteric Artery with Autologous Arterial Tissue, Open Approach

041C0A3   Bypass Right Common Iliac Artery to Right Renal Artery with Autologous Arterial Tissue, Open Approach

041C0A4   Bypass Right Common Iliac Artery to Left Renal Artery with Autologous Arterial Tissue, Open Approach

041C0A5   Bypass Right Common Iliac Artery to Bilateral Renal Artery with Autologous Arterial Tissue, Open Approach

041C0A6   Bypass Right Common Iliac Artery to Right Common Iliac Artery with Autologous Arterial Tissue, Open Approach

041C0A7   Bypass Right Common Iliac Artery to Left Common Iliac Artery with Autologous Arterial Tissue, Open Approach

041C0A8   Bypass Right Common Iliac Artery to Bilateral Common Iliac Arteries with Autologous Arterial Tissue, Open Approach

041C0A9   Bypass Right Common Iliac Artery to Right Internal Iliac Artery with Autologous Arterial Tissue, Open Approach

041C0AB   Bypass Right Common Iliac Artery to Left Internal Iliac Artery with Autologous Arterial Tissue, Open Approach

041C0AC   Bypass Right Common Iliac Artery to Bilateral Internal Iliac Arteries with Autologous Arterial Tissue, Open Approach

041C0AD   Bypass Right Common Iliac Artery to Right External Iliac Artery with Autologous Arterial Tissue, Open Approach

041C0AF   Bypass Right Common Iliac Artery to Left External Iliac Artery with Autologous Arterial Tissue, Open Approach

041C0AG   Bypass Right Common Iliac Artery to Bilateral External Iliac Arteries with Autologous Arterial Tissue, Open Approach

041C0AH   Bypass Right Common Iliac Artery to Right Femoral Artery with Autologous Arterial Tissue, Open Approach

041C0AJ   Bypass Right Common Iliac Artery to Left Femoral Artery with Autologous Arterial Tissue, Open Approach

041C0AK   Bypass Right Common Iliac Artery to Bilateral Femoral Arteries with Autologous Arterial Tissue, Open Approach

041C0AQ   Bypass Right Common Iliac Artery to Lower Extremity Artery with Autologous Arterial Tissue, Open Approach

041C0AR   Bypass Right Common Iliac Artery to Lower Artery with Autologous Arterial Tissue, Open Approach

041C0J0   Bypass Right Common Iliac Artery to Abdominal Aorta with Synthetic Substitute, Open Approach

041C0J1   Bypass Right Common Iliac Artery to Celiac Artery with Synthetic Substitute, Open Approach

041C0J2   Bypass Right Common Iliac Artery to Mesenteric Artery with Synthetic Substitute, Open Approach

041C0J3   Bypass Right Common Iliac Artery to Right Renal Artery with Synthetic Substitute, Open Approach

041C0J4   Bypass Right Common Iliac Artery to Left Renal Artery with Synthetic Substitute, Open Approach

041C0J5   Bypass Right Common Iliac Artery to Bilateral Renal Artery with Synthetic Substitute, Open Approach

041C0J6   Bypass Right Common Iliac Artery to Right Common Iliac Artery with Synthetic Substitute, Open Approach

041C0J7   Bypass Right Common Iliac Artery to Left Common Iliac Artery with Synthetic Substitute, Open Approach

041C0J8   Bypass Right Common Iliac Artery to Bilateral Common Iliac Arteries with Synthetic Substitute, Open Approach

041C0J9   Bypass Right Common Iliac Artery to Right Internal Iliac Artery with Synthetic Substitute, Open Approach

041C0JB   Bypass Right Common Iliac Artery to Left Internal Iliac Artery with Synthetic Substitute, Open Approach

041C0JC   Bypass Right Common Iliac Artery to Bilateral Internal Iliac Arteries with Synthetic Substitute, Open Approach

041C0JD   Bypass Right Common Iliac Artery to Right External Iliac Artery with Synthetic Substitute, Open Approach

041C0JF   Bypass Right Common Iliac Artery to Left External Iliac Artery with Synthetic Substitute, Open Approach

041C0JG   Bypass Right Common Iliac Artery to Bilateral External Iliac Arteries with Synthetic Substitute, Open Approach

041C0JH Bypass Right Common Iliac Artery to Right Femoral Artery with Synthetic Substitute, Open Approach

041C0JJ Bypass Right Common Iliac Artery to Left Femoral Artery with Synthetic Substitute, Open Approach

041C0JK Bypass Right Common Iliac Artery to Bilateral Femoral Arteries with Synthetic Substitute, Open Approach

041C0JQ Bypass Right Common Iliac Artery to Lower Extremity Artery with Synthetic Substitute, Open Approach

041C0JR Bypass Right Common Iliac Artery to Lower Artery with Synthetic Substitute, Open Approach

041C0K0 Bypass Right Common Iliac Artery to Abdominal Aorta with Nonautologous Tissue Substitute, Open Approach

041C0K1 Bypass Right Common Iliac Artery to Celiac Artery with Nonautologous Tissue Substitute, Open Approach

041C0K2 Bypass Right Common Iliac Artery to Mesenteric Artery with Nonautologous Tissue Substitute, Open Approach

041C0K3 Bypass Right Common Iliac Artery to Right Renal Artery with Nonautologous Tissue Substitute, Open Approach

041C0K4 Bypass Right Common Iliac Artery to Left Renal Artery with Nonautologous Tissue Substitute, Open Approach

041C0K5 Bypass Right Common Iliac Artery to Bilateral Renal Artery with Nonautologous Tissue Substitute, Open Approach

041C0K6 Bypass Right Common Iliac Artery to Right Common Iliac Artery with Nonautologous Tissue Substitute, Open Approach

041C0K7 Bypass Right Common Iliac Artery to Left Common Iliac Artery with Nonautologous Tissue Substitute, Open Approach

041C0K8 Bypass Right Common Iliac Artery to Bilateral Common Iliac Arteries with Nonautologous Tissue Substitute, Open Approach

041C0K9 Bypass Right Common Iliac Artery to Right Internal Iliac Artery with Nonautologous Tissue Substitute, Open Approach

041C0KB Bypass Right Common Iliac Artery to Left Internal Iliac Artery with Nonautologous Tissue Substitute, Open Approach

041C0KC Bypass Right Common Iliac Artery to Bilateral Internal Iliac Arteries with Nonautologous Tissue Substitute, Open Approach

041C0KD Bypass Right Common Iliac Artery to Right External Iliac Artery with Nonautologous Tissue Substitute, Open Approach

041C0KF Bypass Right Common Iliac Artery to Left External Iliac Artery with Nonautologous Tissue Substitute, Open Approach

041C0KG Bypass Right Common Iliac Artery to Bilateral External Iliac Arteries with Nonautologous Tissue Substitute, Open Approach

041C0KH Bypass Right Common Iliac Artery to Right Femoral Artery with Nonautologous Tissue Substitute, Open Approach

041C0KJ Bypass Right Common Iliac Artery to Left Femoral Artery with Nonautologous Tissue Substitute, Open Approach

041C0KK Bypass Right Common Iliac Artery to Bilateral Femoral Arteries with Nonautologous Tissue Substitute, Open Approach

041C0KQ Bypass Right Common Iliac Artery to Lower Extremity Artery with Nonautologous Tissue Substitute, Open Approach

041C0KR Bypass Right Common Iliac Artery to Lower Artery with Nonautologous Tissue Substitute, Open Approach

041C0Z0 Bypass Right Common Iliac Artery to Abdominal Aorta, Open Approach

041C0Z1 Bypass Right Common Iliac Artery to Celiac Artery, Open Approach

041C0Z2 Bypass Right Common Iliac Artery to Mesenteric Artery, Open Approach

041C0Z3 Bypass Right Common Iliac Artery to Right Renal Artery, Open Approach

041C0Z4 Bypass Right Common Iliac Artery to Left Renal Artery, Open Approach

041C0Z5 Bypass Right Common Iliac Artery to Bilateral Renal Artery, Open Approach

041C0Z6 Bypass Right Common Iliac Artery to Right Common Iliac Artery, Open Approach

041C0Z7 Bypass Right Common Iliac Artery to Left Common Iliac Artery, Open Approach

041C0Z8 Bypass Right Common Iliac Artery to Bilateral Common Iliac Arteries, Open Approach

041C0Z9 Bypass Right Common Iliac Artery to Right Internal Iliac Artery, Open Approach

041C0ZB Bypass Right Common Iliac Artery to Left Internal Iliac Artery, Open Approach

041C0ZC Bypass Right Common Iliac Artery to Bilateral Internal Iliac Arteries, Open Approach

041C0ZD Bypass Right Common Iliac Artery to Right External Iliac Artery, Open Approach

041C0ZF Bypass Right Common Iliac Artery to Left External Iliac Artery, Open Approach

041C0ZG Bypass Right Common Iliac Artery to Bilateral External Iliac Arteries, Open Approach

041C0ZH Bypass Right Common Iliac Artery to Right Femoral Artery, Open Approach

041C0ZJ Bypass Right Common Iliac Artery to Left Femoral Artery, Open Approach

041C0ZK Bypass Right Common Iliac Artery to Bilateral Femoral Arteries, Open Approach

041C0ZQ Bypass Right Common Iliac Artery to Lower Extremity Artery, Open Approach

041C0ZR Bypass Right Common Iliac Artery to Lower Artery, Open Approach

041C490 Bypass Right Common Iliac Artery to Abdominal Aorta with Autologous Venous Tissue, Percutaneous Endoscopic Approach

041C491 Bypass Right Common Iliac Artery to Celiac Artery with Autologous Venous Tissue, Percutaneous Endoscopic Approach

041C492 Bypass Right Common Iliac Artery to Mesenteric Artery with Autologous Venous Tissue, Percutaneous Endoscopic Approach

041C493 Bypass Right Common Iliac Artery to Right Renal Artery with Autologous Venous Tissue, Percutaneous Endoscopic Approach

041C494 Bypass Right Common Iliac Artery to Left Renal Artery with Autologous Venous Tissue, Percutaneous Endoscopic Approach

041C495 Bypass Right Common Iliac Artery to Bilateral Renal Artery with Autologous Venous Tissue, Percutaneous Endoscopic Approach

041C496 Bypass Right Common Iliac Artery to Right Common Iliac Artery with Autologous Venous Tissue, Percutaneous Endoscopic Approach

041C497 Bypass Right Common Iliac Artery to Left Common Iliac Artery with Autologous Venous Tissue, Percutaneous Endoscopic Approach

041C498 Bypass Right Common Iliac Artery to Bilateral Common Iliac Arteries with Autologous Venous Tissue, Percutaneous Endoscopic Approach

041C499 Bypass Right Common Iliac Artery to Right Internal Iliac Artery with Autologous Venous Tissue, Percutaneous Endoscopic Approach

041C49B Bypass Right Common Iliac Artery to Left Internal Iliac Artery with Autologous Venous Tissue, Percutaneous Endoscopic Approach

041C49C Bypass Right Common Iliac Artery to Bilateral Internal Iliac Arteries with Autologous Venous Tissue, Percutaneous Endoscopic Approach

041C49D Bypass Right Common Iliac Artery to Right External Iliac Artery with Autologous Venous Tissue, Percutaneous Endoscopic Approach

041C49F Bypass Right Common Iliac Artery to Left External Iliac Artery with Autologous Venous Tissue, Percutaneous Endoscopic Approach

041C49G Bypass Right Common Iliac Artery to Bilateral External Iliac Arteries with Autologous Venous Tissue, Percutaneous Endoscopic Approach

041C49H Bypass Right Common Iliac Artery to Right Femoral Artery with Autologous Venous Tissue, Percutaneous Endoscopic Approach

041C49J Bypass Right Common Iliac Artery to Left Femoral Artery with Autologous Venous Tissue, Percutaneous Endoscopic Approach

041C49K Bypass Right Common Iliac Artery to Bilateral Femoral Arteries with Autologous Venous Tissue, Percutaneous Endoscopic Approach

041C49Q Bypass Right Common Iliac Artery to Lower Extremity Artery with Autologous Venous Tissue, Percutaneous Endoscopic Approach

041C49R Bypass Right Common Iliac Artery to Lower Artery with Autologous Venous Tissue, Percutaneous Endoscopic Approach

041C4A0 Bypass Right Common Iliac Artery to Abdominal Aorta with Autologous Arterial Tissue, Percutaneous Endoscopic Approach

041C4A1 Bypass Right Common Iliac Artery to Celiac Artery with Autologous Arterial Tissue, Percutaneous Endoscopic Approach

041C4A2 Bypass Right Common Iliac Artery to Mesenteric Artery with Autologous Arterial Tissue, Percutaneous Endoscopic Approach

041C4A3   Bypass Right Common Iliac Artery to Right Renal Artery with Autologous Arterial Tissue, Percutaneous Endoscopic Approach

041C4A4   Bypass Right Common Iliac Artery to Left Renal Artery with Autologous Arterial Tissue, Percutaneous Endoscopic Approach

041C4A5   Bypass Right Common Iliac Artery to Bilateral Renal Artery with Autologous Arterial Tissue, Percutaneous Endoscopic Approach

041C4A6   Bypass Right Common Iliac Artery to Right Common Iliac Artery with Autologous Arterial Tissue, Percutaneous Endoscopic Approach

041C4A7   Bypass Right Common Iliac Artery to Left Common Iliac Artery with Autologous Arterial Tissue, Percutaneous Endoscopic Approach

041C4A8   Bypass Right Common Iliac Artery to Bilateral Common Iliac Arteries with Autologous Arterial Tissue, Percutaneous Endoscopic Approach

041C4A9   Bypass Right Common Iliac Artery to Right Internal Iliac Artery with Autologous Arterial Tissue, Percutaneous Endoscopic Approach

041C4AB   Bypass Right Common Iliac Artery to Left Internal Iliac Artery with Autologous Arterial Tissue, Percutaneous Endoscopic Approach

041C4AC   Bypass Right Common Iliac Artery to Bilateral Internal Iliac Arteries with Autologous Arterial Tissue, Percutaneous Endoscopic Approach

041C4AD   Bypass Right Common Iliac Artery to Right External Iliac Artery with Autologous Arterial Tissue, Percutaneous Endoscopic Approach

041C4AF   Bypass Right Common Iliac Artery to Left External Iliac Artery with Autologous Arterial Tissue, Percutaneous Endoscopic Approach

041C4AG   Bypass Right Common Iliac Artery to Bilateral External Iliac Arteries with Autologous Arterial Tissue, Percutaneous Endoscopic Approach

041C4AH   Bypass Right Common Iliac Artery to Right Femoral Artery with Autologous Arterial Tissue, Percutaneous Endoscopic Approach

041C4AJ   Bypass Right Common Iliac Artery to Left Femoral Artery with Autologous Arterial Tissue, Percutaneous Endoscopic Approach

041C4AK   Bypass Right Common Iliac Artery to Bilateral Femoral Arteries with Autologous Arterial Tissue, Percutaneous Endoscopic Approach

041C4AQ   Bypass Right Common Iliac Artery to Lower Extremity Artery with Autologous Arterial Tissue, Percutaneous Endoscopic Approach

041C4AR   Bypass Right Common Iliac Artery to Lower Artery with Autologous Arterial Tissue, Percutaneous Endoscopic Approach

041C4J0   Bypass Right Common Iliac Artery to Abdominal Aorta with Synthetic Substitute, Percutaneous Endoscopic Approach

041C4J1   Bypass Right Common Iliac Artery to Celiac Artery with Synthetic Substitute, Percutaneous Endoscopic Approach

041C4J2   Bypass Right Common Iliac Artery to Mesenteric Artery with Synthetic Substitute, Percutaneous Endoscopic Approach

041C4J3   Bypass Right Common Iliac Artery to Right Renal Artery with Synthetic Substitute, Percutaneous Endoscopic Approach

041C4J4   Bypass Right Common Iliac Artery to Left Renal Artery with Synthetic Substitute, Percutaneous Endoscopic Approach

041C4J5   Bypass Right Common Iliac Artery to Bilateral Renal Artery with Synthetic Substitute, Percutaneous Endoscopic Approach

041C4J6   Bypass Right Common Iliac Artery to Right Common Iliac Artery with Synthetic Substitute, Percutaneous Endoscopic Approach

041C4J7   Bypass Right Common Iliac Artery to Left Common Iliac Artery with Synthetic Substitute, Percutaneous Endoscopic Approach

041C4J8   Bypass Right Common Iliac Artery to Bilateral Common Iliac Arteries with Synthetic Substitute, Percutaneous Endoscopic Approach

041C4J9   Bypass Right Common Iliac Artery to Right Internal Iliac Artery with Synthetic Substitute, Percutaneous Endoscopic Approach

041C4JB   Bypass Right Common Iliac Artery to Left Internal Iliac Artery with Synthetic Substitute, Percutaneous Endoscopic Approach

041C4JC   Bypass Right Common Iliac Artery to Bilateral Internal Iliac Arteries with Synthetic Substitute, Percutaneous Endoscopic Approach

041C4JD   Bypass Right Common Iliac Artery to Right External Iliac Artery with Synthetic Substitute, Percutaneous Endoscopic Approach

041C4JF   Bypass Right Common Iliac Artery to Left External Iliac Artery with Synthetic Substitute, Percutaneous Endoscopic Approach

041C4JG   Bypass Right Common Iliac Artery to Bilateral External Iliac Arteries with Synthetic Substitute, Percutaneous Endoscopic Approach

041C4JH   Bypass Right Common Iliac Artery to Right Femoral Artery with Synthetic Substitute, Percutaneous Endoscopic Approach

041C4JJ   Bypass Right Common Iliac Artery to Left Femoral Artery with Synthetic Substitute, Percutaneous Endoscopic Approach

041C4JK   Bypass Right Common Iliac Artery to Bilateral Femoral Arteries with Synthetic Substitute, Percutaneous Endoscopic Approach

041C4JQ   Bypass Right Common Iliac Artery to Lower Extremity Artery with Synthetic Substitute, Percutaneous Endoscopic Approach

041C4JR   Bypass Right Common Iliac Artery to Lower Artery with Synthetic Substitute, Percutaneous Endoscopic Approach

041C4K0   Bypass Right Common Iliac Artery to Abdominal Aorta with Nonautologous Tissue Substitute, Percutaneous Endoscopic Approach

041C4K1   Bypass Right Common Iliac Artery to Celiac Artery with Nonautologous Tissue Substitute, Percutaneous Endoscopic Approach

041C4K2   Bypass Right Common Iliac Artery to Mesenteric Artery with Nonautologous Tissue Substitute, Percutaneous Endoscopic Approach

041C4K3   Bypass Right Common Iliac Artery to Right Renal Artery with Nonautologous Tissue Substitute, Percutaneous Endoscopic Approach

041C4K4   Bypass Right Common Iliac Artery to Left Renal Artery with Nonautologous Tissue Substitute, Percutaneous Endoscopic Approach

041C4K5   Bypass Right Common Iliac Artery to Bilateral Renal Artery with Nonautologous Tissue Substitute, Percutaneous Endoscopic Approach

041C4K6   Bypass Right Common Iliac Artery to Right Common Iliac Artery with Nonautologous Tissue Substitute, Percutaneous Endoscopic Approach

041C4K7   Bypass Right Common Iliac Artery to Left Common Iliac Artery with Nonautologous Tissue Substitute, Percutaneous Endoscopic Approach

041C4K8   Bypass Right Common Iliac Artery to Bilateral Common Iliac Arteries with Nonautologous Tissue Substitute, Percutaneous Endoscopic Approach

041C4K9   Bypass Right Common Iliac Artery to Right Internal Iliac Artery with Nonautologous Tissue Substitute, Percutaneous Endoscopic Approach

041C4KB   Bypass Right Common Iliac Artery to Left Internal Iliac Artery with Nonautologous Tissue Substitute, Percutaneous Endoscopic Approach

041C4KC   Bypass Right Common Iliac Artery to Bilateral Internal Iliac Arteries with Nonautologous Tissue Substitute, Percutaneous Endoscopic Approach

041C4KD   Bypass Right Common Iliac Artery to Right External Iliac Artery with Nonautologous Tissue Substitute, Percutaneous Endoscopic Approach

041C4KF   Bypass Right Common Iliac Artery to Left External Iliac Artery with Nonautologous Tissue Substitute, Percutaneous Endoscopic Approach

041C4KG   Bypass Right Common Iliac Artery to Bilateral External Iliac Arteries with Nonautologous Tissue Substitute, Percutaneous Endoscopic Approach

041C4KH   Bypass Right Common Iliac Artery to Right Femoral Artery with Nonautologous Tissue Substitute, Percutaneous Endoscopic Approach

041C4KJ   Bypass Right Common Iliac Artery to Left Femoral Artery with Nonautologous Tissue Substitute, Percutaneous Endoscopic Approach

041C4KK   Bypass Right Common Iliac Artery to Bilateral Femoral Arteries with Nonautologous Tissue Substitute, Percutaneous Endoscopic Approach

041C4KQ   Bypass Right Common Iliac Artery to Lower Extremity Artery with Nonautologous Tissue Substitute, Percutaneous Endoscopic Approach

041C4KR   Bypass Right Common Iliac Artery to Lower Artery with Nonautologous Tissue Substitute, Percutaneous Endoscopic Approach

041C4Z0 Bypass Right Common Iliac Artery to Abdominal Aorta, Percutaneous Endoscopic Approach
041C4Z1 Bypass Right Common Iliac Artery to Celiac Artery, Percutaneous Endoscopic Approach
041C4Z2 Bypass Right Common Iliac Artery to Mesenteric Artery, Percutaneous Endoscopic Approach
041C4Z3 Bypass Right Common Iliac Artery to Right Renal Artery, Percutaneous Endoscopic Approach
041C4Z4 Bypass Right Common Iliac Artery to Left Renal Artery, Percutaneous Endoscopic Approach
041C4Z5 Bypass Right Common Iliac Artery to Bilateral Renal Artery, Percutaneous Endoscopic Approach
041C4Z6 Bypass Right Common Iliac Artery to Right Common Iliac Artery, Percutaneous Endoscopic Approach
041C4Z7 Bypass Right Common Iliac Artery to Left Common Iliac Artery, Percutaneous Endoscopic Approach
041C4Z8 Bypass Right Common Iliac Artery to Bilateral Common Iliac Arteries, Percutaneous Endoscopic Approach
041C4Z9 Bypass Right Common Iliac Artery to Right Internal Iliac Artery, Percutaneous Endoscopic Approach
041C4ZB Bypass Right Common Iliac Artery to Left Internal Iliac Artery, Percutaneous Endoscopic Approach
041C4ZC Bypass Right Common Iliac Artery to Bilateral Internal Iliac Arteries, Percutaneous Endoscopic Approach
041C4ZD Bypass Right Common Iliac Artery to Right External Iliac Artery, Percutaneous Endoscopic Approach
041C4ZF Bypass Right Common Iliac Artery to Left External Iliac Artery, Percutaneous Endoscopic Approach
041C4ZG Bypass Right Common Iliac Artery to Bilateral External Iliac Arteries, Percutaneous Endoscopic Approach
041C4ZH Bypass Right Common Iliac Artery to Right Femoral Artery, Percutaneous Endoscopic Approach
041C4ZJ Bypass Right Common Iliac Artery to Left Femoral Artery, Percutaneous Endoscopic Approach
041C4ZK Bypass Right Common Iliac Artery to Bilateral Femoral Arteries, Percutaneous Endoscopic Approach
041C4ZQ Bypass Right Common Iliac Artery to Lower Extremity Artery, Percutaneous Endoscopic Approach
041C4ZR Bypass Right Common Iliac Artery to Lower Artery, Percutaneous Endoscopic Approach
041D090 Bypass Left Common Iliac Artery to Abdominal Aorta with Autologous Venous Tissue, Open Approach
041D091 Bypass Left Common Iliac Artery to Celiac Artery with Autologous Venous Tissue, Open Approach
041D092 Bypass Left Common Iliac Artery to Mesenteric Artery with Autologous Venous Tissue, Open Approach
041D093 Bypass Left Common Iliac Artery to Right Renal Artery with Autologous Venous Tissue, Open Approach
041D094 Bypass Left Common Iliac Artery to Left Renal Artery with Autologous Venous Tissue, Open Approach
041D095 Bypass Left Common Iliac Artery to Bilateral Renal Artery with Autologous Venous Tissue, Open Approach
041D096 Bypass Left Common Iliac Artery to Right Common Iliac Artery with Autologous Venous Tissue, Open Approach
041D097 Bypass Left Common Iliac Artery to Left Common Iliac Artery with Autologous Venous Tissue, Open Approach
041D098 Bypass Left Common Iliac Artery to Bilateral Common Iliac Arteries with Autologous Venous Tissue, Open Approach
041D099 Bypass Left Common Iliac Artery to Right Internal Iliac Artery with Autologous Venous Tissue, Open Approach
041D09B Bypass Left Common Iliac Artery to Left Internal Iliac Artery with Autologous Venous Tissue, Open Approach
041D09C Bypass Left Common Iliac Artery to Bilateral Internal Iliac Arteries with Autologous Venous Tissue, Open Approach
041D09D Bypass Left Common Iliac Artery to Right External Iliac Artery with Autologous Venous Tissue, Open Approach
041D09F Bypass Left Common Iliac Artery to Left External Iliac Artery with Autologous Venous Tissue, Open Approach
041D09G Bypass Left Common Iliac Artery to Bilateral External Iliac Arteries with Autologous Venous Tissue, Open Approach
041D09H Bypass Left Common Iliac Artery to Right Femoral Artery with Autologous Venous Tissue, Open Approach

041D09J Bypass Left Common Iliac Artery to Left Femoral Artery with Autologous Venous Tissue, Open Approach
041D09K Bypass Left Common Iliac Artery to Bilateral Femoral Arteries with Autologous Venous Tissue, Open Approach
041D09Q Bypass Left Common Iliac Artery to Lower Extremity Artery with Autologous Venous Tissue, Open Approach
041D09R Bypass Left Common Iliac Artery to Lower Artery with Autologous Venous Tissue, Open Approach
041D0A0 Bypass Left Common Iliac Artery to Abdominal Aorta with Autologous Arterial Tissue, Open Approach
041D0A1 Bypass Left Common Iliac Artery to Celiac Artery with Autologous Arterial Tissue, Open Approach
041D0A2 Bypass Left Common Iliac Artery to Mesenteric Artery with Autologous Arterial Tissue, Open Approach
041D0A3 Bypass Left Common Iliac Artery to Right Renal Artery with Autologous Arterial Tissue, Open Approach
041D0A4 Bypass Left Common Iliac Artery to Left Renal Artery with Autologous Arterial Tissue, Open Approach
041D0A5 Bypass Left Common Iliac Artery to Bilateral Renal Artery with Autologous Arterial Tissue, Open Approach
041D0A6 Bypass Left Common Iliac Artery to Right Common Iliac Artery with Autologous Arterial Tissue, Open Approach
041D0A7 Bypass Left Common Iliac Artery to Left Common Iliac Artery with Autologous Arterial Tissue, Open Approach
041D0A8 Bypass Left Common Iliac Artery to Bilateral Common Iliac Arteries with Autologous Arterial Tissue, Open Approach
041D0A9 Bypass Left Common Iliac Artery to Right Internal Iliac Artery with Autologous Arterial Tissue, Open Approach
041D0AB Bypass Left Common Iliac Artery to Left Internal Iliac Artery with Autologous Arterial Tissue, Open Approach
041D0AC Bypass Left Common Iliac Artery to Bilateral Internal Iliac Arteries with Autologous Arterial Tissue, Open Approach
041D0AD Bypass Left Common Iliac Artery to Right External Iliac Artery with Autologous Arterial Tissue, Open Approach
041D0AF Bypass Left Common Iliac Artery to Left External Iliac Artery with Autologous Arterial Tissue, Open Approach
041D0AG Bypass Left Common Iliac Artery to Bilateral External Iliac Arteries with Autologous Arterial Tissue, Open Approach
041D0AH Bypass Left Common Iliac Artery to Right Femoral Artery with Autologous Arterial Tissue, Open Approach
041D0AJ Bypass Left Common Iliac Artery to Left Femoral Artery with Autologous Arterial Tissue, Open Approach
041D0AK Bypass Left Common Iliac Artery to Bilateral Femoral Arteries with Autologous Arterial Tissue, Open Approach
041D0AQ Bypass Left Common Iliac Artery to Lower Extremity Artery with Autologous Arterial Tissue, Open Approach
041D0AR Bypass Left Common Iliac Artery to Lower Artery with Autologous Arterial Tissue, Open Approach
041D0J0 Bypass Left Common Iliac Artery to Abdominal Aorta with Synthetic Substitute, Open Approach
041D0J1 Bypass Left Common Iliac Artery to Celiac Artery with Synthetic Substitute, Open Approach
041D0J2 Bypass Left Common Iliac Artery to Mesenteric Artery with Synthetic Substitute, Open Approach
041D0J3 Bypass Left Common Iliac Artery to Right Renal Artery with Synthetic Substitute, Open Approach
041D0J4 Bypass Left Common Iliac Artery to Left Renal Artery with Synthetic Substitute, Open Approach
041D0J5 Bypass Left Common Iliac Artery to Bilateral Renal Artery with Synthetic Substitute, Open Approach
041D0J6 Bypass Left Common Iliac Artery to Right Common Iliac Artery with Synthetic Substitute, Open Approach
041D0J7 Bypass Left Common Iliac Artery to Left Common Iliac Artery with Synthetic Substitute, Open Approach
041D0J8 Bypass Left Common Iliac Artery to Bilateral Common Iliac Arteries with Synthetic Substitute, Open Approach
041D0J9 Bypass Left Common Iliac Artery to Right Internal Iliac Artery with Synthetic Substitute, Open Approach
041D0JB Bypass Left Common Iliac Artery to Left Internal Iliac Artery with Synthetic Substitute, Open Approach
041D0JC Bypass Left Common Iliac Artery to Bilateral Internal Iliac Arteries with Synthetic Substitute, Open Approach

041D0JD Bypass Left Common Iliac Artery to Right External Iliac Artery with Synthetic Substitute, Open Approach

041D0JF Bypass Left Common Iliac Artery to Left External Iliac Artery with Synthetic Substitute, Open Approach

041D0JG Bypass Left Common Iliac Artery to Bilateral External Iliac Arteries with Synthetic Substitute, Open Approach

041D0JH Bypass Left Common Iliac Artery to Right Femoral Artery with Synthetic Substitute, Open Approach

041D0JJ Bypass Left Common Iliac Artery to Left Femoral Artery with Synthetic Substitute, Open Approach

041D0JK Bypass Left Common Iliac Artery to Bilateral Femoral Arteries with Synthetic Substitute, Open Approach

041D0JQ Bypass Left Common Iliac Artery to Lower Extremity Artery with Synthetic Substitute, Open Approach

041D0JR Bypass Left Common Iliac Artery to Lower Artery with Synthetic Substitute, Open Approach

041D0K0 Bypass Left Common Iliac Artery to Abdominal Aorta with Nonautologous Tissue Substitute, Open Approach

041D0K1 Bypass Left Common Iliac Artery to Celiac Artery with Nonautologous Tissue Substitute, Open Approach

041D0K2 Bypass Left Common Iliac Artery to Mesenteric Artery with Nonautologous Tissue Substitute, Open Approach

041D0K3 Bypass Left Common Iliac Artery to Right Renal Artery with Nonautologous Tissue Substitute, Open Approach

041D0K4 Bypass Left Common Iliac Artery to Left Renal Artery with Nonautologous Tissue Substitute, Open Approach

041D0K5 Bypass Left Common Iliac Artery to Bilateral Renal Artery with Nonautologous Tissue Substitute, Open Approach

041D0K6 Bypass Left Common Iliac Artery to Right Common Iliac Artery with Nonautologous Tissue Substitute, Open Approach

041D0K7 Bypass Left Common Iliac Artery to Left Common Iliac Artery with Nonautologous Tissue Substitute, Open Approach

041D0K8 Bypass Left Common Iliac Artery to Bilateral Common Iliac Arteries with Nonautologous Tissue Substitute, Open Approach

041D0K9 Bypass Left Common Iliac Artery to Right Internal Iliac Artery with Nonautologous Tissue Substitute, Open Approach

041D0KB Bypass Left Common Iliac Artery to Left Internal Iliac Artery with Nonautologous Tissue Substitute, Open Approach

041D0KC Bypass Left Common Iliac Artery to Bilateral Internal Iliac Arteries with Nonautologous Tissue Substitute, Open Approach

041D0KD Bypass Left Common Iliac Artery to Right External Iliac Artery with Nonautologous Tissue Substitute, Open Approach

041D0KF Bypass Left Common Iliac Artery to Left External Iliac Artery with Nonautologous Tissue Substitute, Open Approach

041D0KG Bypass Left Common Iliac Artery to Bilateral External Iliac Arteries with Nonautologous Tissue Substitute, Open Approach

041D0KH Bypass Left Common Iliac Artery to Right Femoral Artery with Nonautologous Tissue Substitute, Open Approach

041D0KJ Bypass Left Common Iliac Artery to Left Femoral Artery with Nonautologous Tissue Substitute, Open Approach

041D0KK Bypass Left Common Iliac Artery to Bilateral Femoral Arteries with Nonautologous Tissue Substitute, Open Approach

041D0KQ Bypass Left Common Iliac Artery to Lower Extremity Artery with Nonautologous Tissue Substitute, Open Approach

041D0KR Bypass Left Common Iliac Artery to Lower Artery with Nonautologous Tissue Substitute, Open Approach

041D0Z0 Bypass Left Common Iliac Artery to Abdominal Aorta, Open Approach

041D0Z1 Bypass Left Common Iliac Artery to Celiac Artery, Open Approach

041D0Z2 Bypass Left Common Iliac Artery to Mesenteric Artery, Open Approach

041D0Z3 Bypass Left Common Iliac Artery to Right Renal Artery, Open Approach

041D0Z4 Bypass Left Common Iliac Artery to Left Renal Artery, Open Approach

041D0Z5 Bypass Left Common Iliac Artery to Bilateral Renal Artery, Open Approach

041D0Z6 Bypass Left Common Iliac Artery to Right Common Iliac Artery, Open Approach

041D0Z7 Bypass Left Common Iliac Artery to Left Common Iliac Artery, Open Approach

041D0Z8 Bypass Left Common Iliac Artery to Bilateral Common Iliac Arteries, Open Approach

041D0Z9 Bypass Left Common Iliac Artery to Right Internal Iliac Artery, Open Approach

041D0ZB Bypass Left Common Iliac Artery to Left Internal Iliac Artery, Open Approach

041D0ZC Bypass Left Common Iliac Artery to Bilateral Internal Iliac Arteries, Open Approach

041D0ZD Bypass Left Common Iliac Artery to Right External Iliac Artery, Open Approach

041D0ZF Bypass Left Common Iliac Artery to Left External Iliac Artery, Open Approach

041D0ZG Bypass Left Common Iliac Artery to Bilateral External Iliac Arteries, Open Approach

041D0ZH Bypass Left Common Iliac Artery to Right Femoral Artery, Open Approach

041D0ZJ Bypass Left Common Iliac Artery to Left Femoral Artery, Open Approach

041D0ZK Bypass Left Common Iliac Artery to Bilateral Femoral Arteries, Open Approach

041D0ZQ Bypass Left Common Iliac Artery to Lower Extremity Artery, Open Approach

041D0ZR Bypass Left Common Iliac Artery to Lower Artery, Open Approach

041D490 Bypass Left Common Iliac Artery to Abdominal Aorta with Autologous Venous Tissue, Percutaneous Endoscopic Approach

041D491 Bypass Left Common Iliac Artery to Celiac Artery with Autologous Venous Tissue, Percutaneous Endoscopic Approach

041D492 Bypass Left Common Iliac Artery to Mesenteric Artery with Autologous Venous Tissue, Percutaneous Endoscopic Approach

041D493 Bypass Left Common Iliac Artery to Right Renal Artery with Autologous Venous Tissue, Percutaneous Endoscopic Approach

041D494 Bypass Left Common Iliac Artery to Left Renal Artery with Autologous Venous Tissue, Percutaneous Endoscopic Approach

041D495 Bypass Left Common Iliac Artery to Bilateral Renal Artery with Autologous Venous Tissue, Percutaneous Endoscopic Approach

041D496 Bypass Left Common Iliac Artery to Right Common Iliac Artery with Autologous Venous Tissue, Percutaneous Endoscopic Approach

041D497 Bypass Left Common Iliac Artery to Left Common Iliac Artery with Autologous Venous Tissue, Percutaneous Endoscopic Approach

041D498 Bypass Left Common Iliac Artery to Bilateral Common Iliac Arteries with Autologous Venous Tissue, Percutaneous Endoscopic Approach

041D499 Bypass Left Common Iliac Artery to Right Internal Iliac Artery with Autologous Venous Tissue, Percutaneous Endoscopic Approach

041D49B Bypass Left Common Iliac Artery to Left Internal Iliac Artery with Autologous Venous Tissue, Percutaneous Endoscopic Approach

041D49C Bypass Left Common Iliac Artery to Bilateral Internal Iliac Arteries with Autologous Venous Tissue, Percutaneous Endoscopic Approach

041D49D Bypass Left Common Iliac Artery to Right External Iliac Artery with Autologous Venous Tissue, Percutaneous Endoscopic Approach

041D49F Bypass Left Common Iliac Artery to Left External Iliac Artery with Autologous Venous Tissue, Percutaneous Endoscopic Approach

041D49G Bypass Left Common Iliac Artery to Bilateral External Iliac Arteries with Autologous Venous Tissue, Percutaneous Endoscopic Approach

041D49H Bypass Left Common Iliac Artery to Right Femoral Artery with Autologous Venous Tissue, Percutaneous Endoscopic Approach

041D49J Bypass Left Common Iliac Artery to Left Femoral Artery with Autologous Venous Tissue, Percutaneous Endoscopic Approach

041D49K Bypass Left Common Iliac Artery to Bilateral Femoral Arteries with Autologous Venous Tissue, Percutaneous Endoscopic Approach

041D49Q Bypass Left Common Iliac Artery to Lower Extremity Artery with Autologous Venous Tissue, Percutaneous Endoscopic Approach

041D49R Bypass Left Common Iliac Artery to Lower Artery with Autologous Venous Tissue, Percutaneous Endoscopic Approach

041D4A0 Bypass Left Common Iliac Artery to Abdominal Aorta with Autologous Arterial Tissue, Percutaneous Endoscopic Approach

041D4A1 Bypass Left Common Iliac Artery to Celiac Artery with Autologous Arterial Tissue, Percutaneous Endoscopic Approach

041D4A2 Bypass Left Common Iliac Artery to Mesenteric Artery with Autologous Arterial Tissue, Percutaneous Endoscopic Approach

041D4A3 Bypass Left Common Iliac Artery to Right Renal Artery with Autologous Arterial Tissue, Percutaneous Endoscopic Approach

041D4A4 Bypass Left Common Iliac Artery to Left Renal Artery with Autologous Arterial Tissue, Percutaneous Endoscopic Approach

041D4A5 Bypass Left Common Iliac Artery to Bilateral Renal Artery with Autologous Arterial Tissue, Percutaneous Endoscopic Approach

041D4A6 Bypass Left Common Iliac Artery to Right Common Iliac Artery with Autologous Arterial Tissue, Percutaneous Endoscopic Approach

041D4A7 Bypass Left Common Iliac Artery to Left Common Iliac Artery with Autologous Arterial Tissue, Percutaneous Endoscopic Approach

041D4A8 Bypass Left Common Iliac Artery to Bilateral Common Iliac Arteries with Autologous Arterial Tissue, Percutaneous Endoscopic Approach

041D4A9 Bypass Left Common Iliac Artery to Right Internal Iliac Artery with Autologous Arterial Tissue, Percutaneous Endoscopic Approach

041D4AB Bypass Left Common Iliac Artery to Left Internal Iliac Artery with Autologous Arterial Tissue, Percutaneous Endoscopic Approach

041D4AC Bypass Left Common Iliac Artery to Bilateral Internal Iliac Arteries with Autologous Arterial Tissue, Percutaneous Endoscopic Approach

041D4AD Bypass Left Common Iliac Artery to Right External Iliac Artery with Autologous Arterial Tissue, Percutaneous Endoscopic Approach

041D4AF Bypass Left Common Iliac Artery to Left External Iliac Artery with Autologous Arterial Tissue, Percutaneous Endoscopic Approach

041D4AG Bypass Left Common Iliac Artery to Bilateral External Iliac Arteries with Autologous Arterial Tissue, Percutaneous Endoscopic Approach

041D4AH Bypass Left Common Iliac Artery to Right Femoral Artery with Autologous Arterial Tissue, Percutaneous Endoscopic Approach

041D4AJ Bypass Left Common Iliac Artery to Left Femoral Artery with Autologous Arterial Tissue, Percutaneous Endoscopic Approach

041D4AK Bypass Left Common Iliac Artery to Bilateral Femoral Arteries with Autologous Arterial Tissue, Percutaneous Endoscopic Approach

041D4AQ Bypass Left Common Iliac Artery to Lower Extremity Artery with Autologous Arterial Tissue, Percutaneous Endoscopic Approach

041D4AR Bypass Left Common Iliac Artery to Lower Artery with Autologous Arterial Tissue, Percutaneous Endoscopic Approach

041D4J0 Bypass Left Common Iliac Artery to Abdominal Aorta with Synthetic Substitute, Percutaneous Endoscopic Approach

041D4J1 Bypass Left Common Iliac Artery to Celiac Artery with Synthetic Substitute, Percutaneous Endoscopic Approach

041D4J2 Bypass Left Common Iliac Artery to Mesenteric Artery with Synthetic Substitute, Percutaneous Endoscopic Approach

041D4J3 Bypass Left Common Iliac Artery to Right Renal Artery with Synthetic Substitute, Percutaneous Endoscopic Approach

041D4J4 Bypass Left Common Iliac Artery to Left Renal Artery with Synthetic Substitute, Percutaneous Endoscopic Approach

041D4J5 Bypass Left Common Iliac Artery to Bilateral Renal Artery with Synthetic Substitute, Percutaneous Endoscopic Approach

041D4J6 Bypass Left Common Iliac Artery to Right Common Iliac Artery with Synthetic Substitute, Percutaneous Endoscopic Approach

041D4J7 Bypass Left Common Iliac Artery to Left Common Iliac Artery with Synthetic Substitute, Percutaneous Endoscopic Approach

041D4J8 Bypass Left Common Iliac Artery to Bilateral Common Iliac Arteries with Synthetic Substitute, Percutaneous Endoscopic Approach

041D4J9 Bypass Left Common Iliac Artery to Right Internal Iliac Artery with Synthetic Substitute, Percutaneous Endoscopic Approach

041D4JB Bypass Left Common Iliac Artery to Left Internal Iliac Artery with Synthetic Substitute, Percutaneous Endoscopic Approach

041D4JC Bypass Left Common Iliac Artery to Bilateral Internal Iliac Arteries with Synthetic Substitute, Percutaneous Endoscopic Approach

041D4JD Bypass Left Common Iliac Artery to Right External Iliac Artery with Synthetic Substitute, Percutaneous Endoscopic Approach

041D4JF Bypass Left Common Iliac Artery to Left External Iliac Artery with Synthetic Substitute, Percutaneous Endoscopic Approach

041D4JG Bypass Left Common Iliac Artery to Bilateral External Iliac Arteries with Synthetic Substitute, Percutaneous Endoscopic Approach

041D4JH Bypass Left Common Iliac Artery to Right Femoral Artery with Synthetic Substitute, Percutaneous Endoscopic Approach

041D4JJ Bypass Left Common Iliac Artery to Left Femoral Artery with Synthetic Substitute, Percutaneous Endoscopic Approach

041D4JK Bypass Left Common Iliac Artery to Bilateral Femoral Arteries with Synthetic Substitute, Percutaneous Endoscopic Approach

041D4JQ Bypass Left Common Iliac Artery to Lower Extremity Artery with Synthetic Substitute, Percutaneous Endoscopic Approach

041D4JR Bypass Left Common Iliac Artery to Lower Artery with Synthetic Substitute, Percutaneous Endoscopic Approach

041D4K0 Bypass Left Common Iliac Artery to Abdominal Aorta with Nonautologous Tissue Substitute, Percutaneous Endoscopic Approach

041D4K1 Bypass Left Common Iliac Artery to Celiac Artery with Nonautologous Tissue Substitute, Percutaneous Endoscopic Approach

041D4K2 Bypass Left Common Iliac Artery to Mesenteric Artery with Nonautologous Tissue Substitute, Percutaneous Endoscopic Approach

041D4K3 Bypass Left Common Iliac Artery to Right Renal Artery with Nonautologous Tissue Substitute, Percutaneous Endoscopic Approach

041D4K4 Bypass Left Common Iliac Artery to Left Renal Artery with Nonautologous Tissue Substitute, Percutaneous Endoscopic Approach

041D4K5 Bypass Left Common Iliac Artery to Bilateral Renal Artery with Nonautologous Tissue Substitute, Percutaneous Endoscopic Approach

041D4K6 Bypass Left Common Iliac Artery to Right Common Iliac Artery with Nonautologous Tissue Substitute, Percutaneous Endoscopic Approach

041D4K7 Bypass Left Common Iliac Artery to Left Common Iliac Artery with Nonautologous Tissue Substitute, Percutaneous Endoscopic Approach

041D4K8 Bypass Left Common Iliac Artery to Bilateral Common Iliac Arteries with Nonautologous Tissue Substitute, Percutaneous Endoscopic Approach

041D4K9 Bypass Left Common Iliac Artery to Right Internal Iliac Artery with Nonautologous Tissue Substitute, Percutaneous Endoscopic Approach

041D4KB Bypass Left Common Iliac Artery to Left Internal Iliac Artery with Nonautologous Tissue Substitute, Percutaneous Endoscopic Approach

041D4KC Bypass Left Common Iliac Artery to Bilateral Internal Iliac Arteries with Nonautologous Tissue Substitute, Percutaneous Endoscopic Approach

041D4KD Bypass Left Common Iliac Artery to Right External Iliac Artery with Nonautologous Tissue Substitute, Percutaneous Endoscopic Approach

041D4KF Bypass Left Common Iliac Artery to Left External Iliac Artery with Nonautologous Tissue Substitute, Percutaneous Endoscopic Approach

041D4KG Bypass Left Common Iliac Artery to Bilateral External Iliac Arteries with Nonautologous Tissue Substitute, Percutaneous Endoscopic Approach

041D4KH Bypass Left Common Iliac Artery to Right Femoral Artery with Nonautologous Tissue Substitute, Percutaneous Endoscopic Approach

041D4KJ Bypass Left Common Iliac Artery to Left Femoral Artery with Nonautologous Tissue Substitute, Percutaneous Endoscopic Approach

041D4KK Bypass Left Common Iliac Artery to Bilateral Femoral Arteries with Nonautologous Tissue Substitute, Percutaneous Endoscopic Approach

041D4KQ Bypass Left Common Iliac Artery to Lower Extremity Artery with Nonautologous Tissue Substitute, Percutaneous Endoscopic Approach

041D4KR Bypass Left Common Iliac Artery to Lower Artery with Nonautologous Tissue Substitute, Percutaneous Endoscopic Approach

041D4Z0 Bypass Left Common Iliac Artery to Abdominal Aorta, Percutaneous Endoscopic Approach

041D4Z1 Bypass Left Common Iliac Artery to Celiac Artery, Percutaneous Endoscopic Approach

041D4Z2 Bypass Left Common Iliac Artery to Mesenteric Artery, Percutaneous Endoscopic Approach

041D4Z3 Bypass Left Common Iliac Artery to Right Renal Artery, Percutaneous Endoscopic Approach

041D4Z4 Bypass Left Common Iliac Artery to Left Renal Artery, Percutaneous Endoscopic Approach

041D4Z5 Bypass Left Common Iliac Artery to Bilateral Renal Artery, Percutaneous Endoscopic Approach

041D4Z6 Bypass Left Common Iliac Artery to Right Common Iliac Artery, Percutaneous Endoscopic Approach

041D4Z7 Bypass Left Common Iliac Artery to Left Common Iliac Artery, Percutaneous Endoscopic Approach

041D4Z8 Bypass Left Common Iliac Artery to Bilateral Common Iliac Arteries, Percutaneous Endoscopic Approach

041D4Z9 Bypass Left Common Iliac Artery to Right Internal Iliac Artery, Percutaneous Endoscopic Approach

041D4ZB Bypass Left Common Iliac Artery to Left Internal Iliac Artery, Percutaneous Endoscopic Approach

041D4ZC Bypass Left Common Iliac Artery to Bilateral Internal Iliac Arteries, Percutaneous Endoscopic Approach

041D4ZD Bypass Left Common Iliac Artery to Right External Iliac Artery, Percutaneous Endoscopic Approach

041D4ZF Bypass Left Common Iliac Artery to Left External Iliac Artery, Percutaneous Endoscopic Approach

041D4ZG Bypass Left Common Iliac Artery to Bilateral External Iliac Arteries, Percutaneous Endoscopic Approach

041D4ZH Bypass Left Common Iliac Artery to Right Femoral Artery, Percutaneous Endoscopic Approach

041D4ZJ Bypass Left Common Iliac Artery to Left Femoral Artery, Percutaneous Endoscopic Approach

041D4ZK Bypass Left Common Iliac Artery to Bilateral Femoral Arteries, Percutaneous Endoscopic Approach

041D4ZQ Bypass Left Common Iliac Artery to Lower Extremity Artery, Percutaneous Endoscopic Approach

041D4ZR Bypass Left Common Iliac Artery to Lower Artery, Percutaneous Endoscopic Approach

041E099 Bypass Right Internal Iliac Artery to Right Internal Iliac Artery with Autologous Venous Tissue, Open Approach

041E09B Bypass Right Internal Iliac Artery to Left Internal Iliac Artery with Autologous Venous Tissue, Open Approach

041E09C Bypass Right Internal Iliac Artery to Bilateral Internal Iliac Arteries with Autologous Venous Tissue, Open Approach

041E09D Bypass Right Internal Iliac Artery to Right External Iliac Artery with Autologous Venous Tissue, Open Approach

041E09F Bypass Right Internal Iliac Artery to Left External Iliac Artery with Autologous Venous Tissue, Open Approach

041E09G Bypass Right Internal Iliac Artery to Bilateral External Iliac Arteries with Autologous Venous Tissue, Open Approach

041E09H Bypass Right Internal Iliac Artery to Right Femoral Artery with Autologous Venous Tissue, Open Approach

041E09J Bypass Right Internal Iliac Artery to Left Femoral Artery with Autologous Venous Tissue, Open Approach

041E09K Bypass Right Internal Iliac Artery to Bilateral Femoral Arteries with Autologous Venous Tissue, Open Approach

041E09P Bypass Right Internal Iliac Artery to Foot Artery with Autologous Venous Tissue, Open Approach

041E09Q Bypass Right Internal Iliac Artery to Lower Extremity Artery with Autologous Venous Tissue, Open Approach

041E0A9 Bypass Right Internal Iliac Artery to Right Internal Iliac Artery with Autologous Arterial Tissue, Open Approach

041E0AB Bypass Right Internal Iliac Artery to Left Internal Iliac Artery with Autologous Arterial Tissue, Open Approach

041E0AC Bypass Right Internal Iliac Artery to Bilateral Internal Iliac Arteries with Autologous Arterial Tissue, Open Approach

041E0AD Bypass Right Internal Iliac Artery to Right External Iliac Artery with Autologous Arterial Tissue, Open Approach

041E0AF Bypass Right Internal Iliac Artery to Left External Iliac Artery with Autologous Arterial Tissue, Open Approach

041E0AG Bypass Right Internal Iliac Artery to Bilateral External Iliac Arteries with Autologous Arterial Tissue, Open Approach

041E0AH Bypass Right Internal Iliac Artery to Right Femoral Artery with Autologous Arterial Tissue, Open Approach

041E0AJ Bypass Right Internal Iliac Artery to Left Femoral Artery with Autologous Arterial Tissue, Open Approach

041E0AK Bypass Right Internal Iliac Artery to Bilateral Femoral Arteries with Autologous Arterial Tissue, Open Approach

041E0AP Bypass Right Internal Iliac Artery to Foot Artery with Autologous Arterial Tissue, Open Approach

041E0AQ Bypass Right Internal Iliac Artery to Lower Extremity Artery with Autologous Arterial Tissue, Open Approach

041E0J9 Bypass Right Internal Iliac Artery to Right Internal Iliac Artery with Synthetic Substitute, Open Approach

041E0JB Bypass Right Internal Iliac Artery to Left Internal Iliac Artery with Synthetic Substitute, Open Approach

041E0JC Bypass Right Internal Iliac Artery to Bilateral Internal Iliac Arteries with Synthetic Substitute, Open Approach

041E0JD Bypass Right Internal Iliac Artery to Right External Iliac Artery with Synthetic Substitute, Open Approach

041E0JF Bypass Right Internal Iliac Artery to Left External Iliac Artery with Synthetic Substitute, Open Approach

041E0JG Bypass Right Internal Iliac Artery to Bilateral External Iliac Arteries with Synthetic Substitute, Open Approach

041E0JH Bypass Right Internal Iliac Artery to Right Femoral Artery with Synthetic Substitute, Open Approach

041E0JJ Bypass Right Internal Iliac Artery to Left Femoral Artery with Synthetic Substitute, Open Approach

041E0JK Bypass Right Internal Iliac Artery to Bilateral Femoral Arteries with Synthetic Substitute, Open Approach

041E0JP Bypass Right Internal Iliac Artery to Foot Artery with Synthetic Substitute, Open Approach

041E0JQ Bypass Right Internal Iliac Artery to Lower Extremity Artery with Synthetic Substitute, Open Approach

041E0K9 Bypass Right Internal Iliac Artery to Right Internal Iliac Artery with Nonautologous Tissue Substitute, Open Approach

041E0KB Bypass Right Internal Iliac Artery to Left Internal Iliac Artery with Nonautologous Tissue Substitute, Open Approach

041E0KC Bypass Right Internal Iliac Artery to Bilateral Internal Iliac Arteries with Nonautologous Tissue Substitute, Open Approach

041E0KD Bypass Right Internal Iliac Artery to Right External Iliac Artery with Nonautologous Tissue Substitute, Open Approach

041E0KF Bypass Right Internal Iliac Artery to Left External Iliac Artery with Nonautologous Tissue Substitute, Open Approach

041E0KG Bypass Right Internal Iliac Artery to Bilateral External Iliac Arteries with Nonautologous Tissue Substitute, Open Approach

041E0KH Bypass Right Internal Iliac Artery to Right Femoral Artery with Nonautologous Tissue Substitute, Open Approach

041E0KJ Bypass Right Internal Iliac Artery to Left Femoral Artery with Nonautologous Tissue Substitute, Open Approach

041E0KK Bypass Right Internal Iliac Artery to Bilateral Femoral Arteries with Nonautologous Tissue Substitute, Open Approach

041E0KP Bypass Right Internal Iliac Artery to Foot Artery with Nonautologous Tissue Substitute, Open Approach

041E0KQ Bypass Right Internal Iliac Artery to Lower Extremity Artery with Nonautologous Tissue Substitute, Open Approach

041E0Z9 Bypass Right Internal Iliac Artery to Right Internal Iliac Artery, Open Approach

041E0ZB Bypass Right Internal Iliac Artery to Left Internal Iliac Artery, Open Approach

041E0ZC Bypass Right Internal Iliac Artery to Bilateral Internal Iliac Arteries, Open Approach

041E0ZD Bypass Right Internal Iliac Artery to Right External Iliac Artery, Open Approach

041E0ZF Bypass Right Internal Iliac Artery to Left External Iliac Artery, Open Approach

041E0ZG Bypass Right Internal Iliac Artery to Bilateral External Iliac Arteries, Open Approach

041E0ZH Bypass Right Internal Iliac Artery to Right Femoral Artery, Open Approach

041E0ZJ Bypass Right Internal Iliac Artery to Left Femoral Artery, Open Approach

041E0ZK Bypass Right Internal Iliac Artery to Bilateral Femoral Arteries, Open Approach

041E0ZP Bypass Right Internal Iliac Artery to Foot Artery, Open Approach

041E0ZQ Bypass Right Internal Iliac Artery to Lower Extremity Artery, Open Approach

041E499 Bypass Right Internal Iliac Artery to Right Internal Iliac Artery with Autologous Venous Tissue, Percutaneous Endoscopic Approach

041E49B Bypass Right Internal Iliac Artery to Left Internal Iliac Artery with Autologous Venous Tissue, Percutaneous Endoscopic Approach

041E49C Bypass Right Internal Iliac Artery to Bilateral Internal Iliac Arteries with Autologous Venous Tissue, Percutaneous Endoscopic Approach

041E49D Bypass Right Internal Iliac Artery to Right External Iliac Artery with Autologous Venous Tissue, Percutaneous Endoscopic Approach

041E49F Bypass Right Internal Iliac Artery to Left External Iliac Artery with Autologous Venous Tissue, Percutaneous Endoscopic Approach

041E49G Bypass Right Internal Iliac Artery to Bilateral External Iliac Arteries with Autologous Venous Tissue, Percutaneous Endoscopic Approach

041E49H Bypass Right Internal Iliac Artery to Right Femoral Artery with Autologous Venous Tissue, Percutaneous Endoscopic Approach

041E49J Bypass Right Internal Iliac Artery to Left Femoral Artery with Autologous Venous Tissue, Percutaneous Endoscopic Approach

041E49K Bypass Right Internal Iliac Artery to Bilateral Femoral Arteries with Autologous Venous Tissue, Percutaneous Endoscopic Approach

041E49P Bypass Right Internal Iliac Artery to Foot Artery with Autologous Venous Tissue, Percutaneous Endoscopic Approach

041E49Q Bypass Right Internal Iliac Artery to Lower Extremity Artery with Autologous Venous Tissue, Percutaneous Endoscopic Approach

041E4A9 Bypass Right Internal Iliac Artery to Right Internal Iliac Artery with Autologous Arterial Tissue, Percutaneous Endoscopic Approach

041E4AB Bypass Right Internal Iliac Artery to Left Internal Iliac Artery with Autologous Arterial Tissue, Percutaneous Endoscopic Approach

041E4AC Bypass Right Internal Iliac Artery to Bilateral Internal Iliac Arteries with Autologous Arterial Tissue, Percutaneous Endoscopic Approach

041E4AD Bypass Right Internal Iliac Artery to Right External Iliac Artery with Autologous Arterial Tissue, Percutaneous Endoscopic Approach

041E4AF Bypass Right Internal Iliac Artery to Left External Iliac Artery with Autologous Arterial Tissue, Percutaneous Endoscopic Approach

041E4AG Bypass Right Internal Iliac Artery to Bilateral External Iliac Arteries with Autologous Arterial Tissue, Percutaneous Endoscopic Approach

041E4AH Bypass Right Internal Iliac Artery to Right Femoral Artery with Autologous Arterial Tissue, Percutaneous Endoscopic Approach

041E4AJ Bypass Right Internal Iliac Artery to Left Femoral Artery with Autologous Arterial Tissue, Percutaneous Endoscopic Approach

041E4AK Bypass Right Internal Iliac Artery to Bilateral Femoral Arteries with Autologous Arterial Tissue, Percutaneous Endoscopic Approach

041E4AP Bypass Right Internal Iliac Artery to Foot Artery with Autologous Arterial Tissue, Percutaneous Endoscopic Approach

041E4AQ Bypass Right Internal Iliac Artery to Lower Extremity Artery with Autologous Arterial Tissue, Percutaneous Endoscopic Approach

041E4J9 Bypass Right Internal Iliac Artery to Right Internal Iliac Artery with Synthetic Substitute, Percutaneous Endoscopic Approach

041E4JB Bypass Right Internal Iliac Artery to Left Internal Iliac Artery with Synthetic Substitute, Percutaneous Endoscopic Approach

041E4JC Bypass Right Internal Iliac Artery to Bilateral Internal Iliac Arteries with Synthetic Substitute, Percutaneous Endoscopic Approach

041E4JD Bypass Right Internal Iliac Artery to Right External Iliac Artery with Synthetic Substitute, Percutaneous Endoscopic Approach

041E4JF Bypass Right Internal Iliac Artery to Left External Iliac Artery with Synthetic Substitute, Percutaneous Endoscopic Approach

041E4JG Bypass Right Internal Iliac Artery to Bilateral External Iliac Arteries with Synthetic Substitute, Percutaneous Endoscopic Approach

041E4JH Bypass Right Internal Iliac Artery to Right Femoral Artery with Synthetic Substitute, Percutaneous Endoscopic Approach

041E4JJ Bypass Right Internal Iliac Artery to Left Femoral Artery with Synthetic Substitute, Percutaneous Endoscopic Approach

041E4JK Bypass Right Internal Iliac Artery to Bilateral Femoral Arteries with Synthetic Substitute, Percutaneous Endoscopic Approach

041E4JP Bypass Right Internal Iliac Artery to Foot Artery with Synthetic Substitute, Percutaneous Endoscopic Approach

041E4JQ Bypass Right Internal Iliac Artery to Lower Extremity Artery with Synthetic Substitute, Percutaneous Endoscopic Approach

041E4K9 Bypass Right Internal Iliac Artery to Right Internal Iliac Artery with Nonautologous Tissue Substitute, Percutaneous Endoscopic Approach

041E4KB Bypass Right Internal Iliac Artery to Left Internal Iliac Artery with Nonautologous Tissue Substitute, Percutaneous Endoscopic Approach

041E4KC Bypass Right Internal Iliac Artery to Bilateral Internal Iliac Arteries with Nonautologous Tissue Substitute, Percutaneous Endoscopic Approach

041E4KD Bypass Right Internal Iliac Artery to Right External Iliac Artery with Nonautologous Tissue Substitute, Percutaneous Endoscopic Approach

041E4KF Bypass Right Internal Iliac Artery to Left External Iliac Artery with Nonautologous Tissue Substitute, Percutaneous Endoscopic Approach

041E4KG Bypass Right Internal Iliac Artery to Bilateral External Iliac Arteries with Nonautologous Tissue Substitute, Percutaneous Endoscopic Approach

041E4KH Bypass Right Internal Iliac Artery to Right Femoral Artery with Nonautologous Tissue Substitute, Percutaneous Endoscopic Approach

041E4KJ Bypass Right Internal Iliac Artery to Left Femoral Artery with Nonautologous Tissue Substitute, Percutaneous Endoscopic Approach

041E4KK Bypass Right Internal Iliac Artery to Bilateral Femoral Arteries with Nonautologous Tissue Substitute, Percutaneous Endoscopic Approach

041E4KP Bypass Right Internal Iliac Artery to Foot Artery with Nonautologous Tissue Substitute, Percutaneous Endoscopic Approach

041E4KQ Bypass Right Internal Iliac Artery to Lower Extremity Artery with Nonautologous Tissue Substitute, Percutaneous Endoscopic Approach

041E4Z9 Bypass Right Internal Iliac Artery to Right Internal Iliac Artery, Percutaneous Endoscopic Approach

041E4ZB Bypass Right Internal Iliac Artery to Left Internal Iliac Artery, Percutaneous Endoscopic Approach

041E4ZC Bypass Right Internal Iliac Artery to Bilateral Internal Iliac Arteries, Percutaneous Endoscopic Approach

041E4ZD Bypass Right Internal Iliac Artery to Right External Iliac Artery, Percutaneous Endoscopic Approach

041E4ZF Bypass Right Internal Iliac Artery to Left External Iliac Artery, Percutaneous Endoscopic Approach

041E4ZG Bypass Right Internal Iliac Artery to Bilateral External Iliac Arteries, Percutaneous Endoscopic Approach

041E4ZH Bypass Right Internal Iliac Artery to Right Femoral Artery, Percutaneous Endoscopic Approach

041E4ZJ Bypass Right Internal Iliac Artery to Left Femoral Artery, Percutaneous Endoscopic Approach

041E4ZK Bypass Right Internal Iliac Artery to Bilateral Femoral Arteries, Percutaneous Endoscopic Approach

041E4ZP Bypass Right Internal Iliac Artery to Foot Artery, Percutaneous Endoscopic Approach

041E4ZQ Bypass Right Internal Iliac Artery to Lower Extremity Artery, Percutaneous Endoscopic Approach

041F099 Bypass Left Internal Iliac Artery to Right Internal Iliac Artery with Autologous Venous Tissue, Open Approach

041F09B Bypass Left Internal Iliac Artery to Left Internal Iliac Artery with Autologous Venous Tissue, Open Approach

041F09C Bypass Left Internal Iliac Artery to Bilateral Internal Iliac Arteries with Autologous Venous Tissue, Open Approach

041F09D Bypass Left Internal Iliac Artery to Right External Iliac Artery with Autologous Venous Tissue, Open Approach

041F09F Bypass Left Internal Iliac Artery to Left External Iliac Artery with Autologous Venous Tissue, Open Approach

041F09G Bypass Left Internal Iliac Artery to Bilateral External Iliac Arteries with Autologous Venous Tissue, Open Approach

041F09H Bypass Left Internal Iliac Artery to Right Femoral Artery with Autologous Venous Tissue, Open Approach

041F09J Bypass Left Internal Iliac Artery to Left Femoral Artery with Autologous Venous Tissue, Open Approach

041F09K Bypass Left Internal Iliac Artery to Bilateral Femoral Arteries with Autologous Venous Tissue, Open Approach

041F09P Bypass Left Internal Iliac Artery to Foot Artery with Autologous Venous Tissue, Open Approach

041F09Q Bypass Left Internal Iliac Artery to Lower Extremity Artery with Autologous Venous Tissue, Open Approach

041F0A9 Bypass Left Internal Iliac Artery to Right Internal Iliac Artery with Autologous Arterial Tissue, Open Approach

041F0AB Bypass Left Internal Iliac Artery to Left Internal Iliac Artery with Autologous Arterial Tissue, Open Approach

041F0AC Bypass Left Internal Iliac Artery to Bilateral Internal Iliac Arteries with Autologous Arterial Tissue, Open Approach

041F0AD Bypass Left Internal Iliac Artery to Right External Iliac Artery with Autologous Arterial Tissue, Open Approach

041F0AF Bypass Left Internal Iliac Artery to Left External Iliac Artery with Autologous Arterial Tissue, Open Approach

041F0AG Bypass Left Internal Iliac Artery to Bilateral External Iliac Arteries with Autologous Arterial Tissue, Open Approach

041F0AH Bypass Left Internal Iliac Artery to Right Femoral Artery with Autologous Arterial Tissue, Open Approach

041F0AJ Bypass Left Internal Iliac Artery to Left Femoral Artery with Autologous Arterial Tissue, Open Approach

041F0AK Bypass Left Internal Iliac Artery to Bilateral Femoral Arteries with Autologous Arterial Tissue, Open Approach

041F0AP Bypass Left Internal Iliac Artery to Foot Artery with Autologous Arterial Tissue, Open Approach

041F0AQ Bypass Left Internal Iliac Artery to Lower Extremity Artery with Autologous Arterial Tissue, Open Approach

041F0J9 Bypass Left Internal Iliac Artery to Right Internal Iliac Artery with Synthetic Substitute, Open Approach

041F0JB Bypass Left Internal Iliac Artery to Left Internal Iliac Artery with Synthetic Substitute, Open Approach

041F0JC Bypass Left Internal Iliac Artery to Bilateral Internal Iliac Arteries with Synthetic Substitute, Open Approach

041F0JD Bypass Left Internal Iliac Artery to Right External Iliac Artery with Synthetic Substitute, Open Approach

041F0JF Bypass Left Internal Iliac Artery to Left External Iliac Artery with Synthetic Substitute, Open Approach

041F0JG Bypass Left Internal Iliac Artery to Bilateral External Iliac Arteries with Synthetic Substitute, Open Approach

041F0JH Bypass Left Internal Iliac Artery to Right Femoral Artery with Synthetic Substitute, Open Approach

041F0JJ Bypass Left Internal Iliac Artery to Left Femoral Artery with Synthetic Substitute, Open Approach

041F0JK Bypass Left Internal Iliac Artery to Bilateral Femoral Arteries with Synthetic Substitute, Open Approach

041F0JP Bypass Left Internal Iliac Artery to Foot Artery with Synthetic Substitute, Open Approach

041F0JQ Bypass Left Internal Iliac Artery to Lower Extremity Artery with Synthetic Substitute, Open Approach

041F0K9 Bypass Left Internal Iliac Artery to Right Internal Iliac Artery with Nonautologous Tissue Substitute, Open Approach

041F0KB Bypass Left Internal Iliac Artery to Left Internal Iliac Artery with Nonautologous Tissue Substitute, Open Approach

041F0KC Bypass Left Internal Iliac Artery to Bilateral Internal Iliac Arteries with Nonautologous Tissue Substitute, Open Approach

041F0KD Bypass Left Internal Iliac Artery to Right External Iliac Artery with Nonautologous Tissue Substitute, Open Approach

041F0KF Bypass Left Internal Iliac Artery to Left External Iliac Artery with Nonautologous Tissue Substitute, Open Approach

041F0KG Bypass Left Internal Iliac Artery to Bilateral External Iliac Arteries with Nonautologous Tissue Substitute, Open Approach

041F0KH Bypass Left Internal Iliac Artery to Right Femoral Artery with Nonautologous Tissue Substitute, Open Approach

041F0KJ Bypass Left Internal Iliac Artery to Left Femoral Artery with Nonautologous Tissue Substitute, Open Approach

041F0KK Bypass Left Internal Iliac Artery to Bilateral Femoral Arteries with Nonautologous Tissue Substitute, Open Approach

041F0KP Bypass Left Internal Iliac Artery to Foot Artery with Nonautologous Tissue Substitute, Open Approach

041F0KQ Bypass Left Internal Iliac Artery to Lower Extremity Artery with Nonautologous Tissue Substitute, Open Approach

041F0Z9 Bypass Left Internal Iliac Artery to Right Internal Iliac Artery, Open Approach

041F0ZB Bypass Left Internal Iliac Artery to Left Internal Iliac Artery, Open Approach

041F0ZC Bypass Left Internal Iliac Artery to Bilateral Internal Iliac Arteries, Open Approach

041F0ZD Bypass Left Internal Iliac Artery to Right External Iliac Artery, Open Approach

041F0ZF Bypass Left Internal Iliac Artery to Left External Iliac Artery, Open Approach

041F0ZG Bypass Left Internal Iliac Artery to Bilateral External Iliac Arteries, Open Approach

041F0ZH Bypass Left Internal Iliac Artery to Right Femoral Artery, Open Approach

041F0ZJ Bypass Left Internal Iliac Artery to Left Femoral Artery, Open Approach

041F0ZK Bypass Left Internal Iliac Artery to Bilateral Femoral Arteries, Open Approach

041F0ZP Bypass Left Internal Iliac Artery to Foot Artery, Open Approach

041F0ZQ Bypass Left Internal Iliac Artery to Lower Extremity Artery, Open Approach

041F499 Bypass Left Internal Iliac Artery to Right Internal Iliac Artery with Autologous Venous Tissue, Percutaneous Endoscopic Approach

041F49B Bypass Left Internal Iliac Artery to Left Internal Iliac Artery with Autologous Venous Tissue, Percutaneous Endoscopic Approach

041F49C Bypass Left Internal Iliac Artery to Bilateral Internal Iliac Arteries with Autologous Venous Tissue, Percutaneous Endoscopic Approach

041F49D Bypass Left Internal Iliac Artery to Right External Iliac Artery with Autologous Venous Tissue, Percutaneous Endoscopic Approach

041F49F Bypass Left Internal Iliac Artery to Left External Iliac Artery with Autologous Venous Tissue, Percutaneous Endoscopic Approach

041F49G Bypass Left Internal Iliac Artery to Bilateral External Iliac Arteries with Autologous Venous Tissue, Percutaneous Endoscopic Approach

041F49H Bypass Left Internal Iliac Artery to Right Femoral Artery with Autologous Venous Tissue, Percutaneous Endoscopic Approach

041F49J Bypass Left Internal Iliac Artery to Left Femoral Artery with Autologous Venous Tissue, Percutaneous Endoscopic Approach

041F49K Bypass Left Internal Iliac Artery to Bilateral Femoral Arteries with Autologous Venous Tissue, Percutaneous Endoscopic Approach

041F49P Bypass Left Internal Iliac Artery to Foot Artery with Autologous Venous Tissue, Percutaneous Endoscopic Approach

041F49Q Bypass Left Internal Iliac Artery to Lower Extremity Artery with Autologous Venous Tissue, Percutaneous Endoscopic Approach

041F4A9 Bypass Left Internal Iliac Artery to Right Internal Iliac Artery with Autologous Arterial Tissue, Percutaneous Endoscopic Approach

041F4AB Bypass Left Internal Iliac Artery to Left Internal Iliac Artery with Autologous Arterial Tissue, Percutaneous Endoscopic Approach

041F4AC Bypass Left Internal Iliac Artery to Bilateral Internal Iliac Arteries with Autologous Arterial Tissue, Percutaneous Endoscopic Approach

041F4AD Bypass Left Internal Iliac Artery to Right External Iliac Artery with Autologous Arterial Tissue, Percutaneous Endoscopic Approach

041F4AF Bypass Left Internal Iliac Artery to Left External Iliac Artery with Autologous Arterial Tissue, Percutaneous Endoscopic Approach

041F4AG Bypass Left Internal Iliac Artery to Bilateral External Iliac Arteries with Autologous Arterial Tissue, Percutaneous Endoscopic Approach

041F4AH Bypass Left Internal Iliac Artery to Right Femoral Artery with Autologous Arterial Tissue, Percutaneous Endoscopic Approach

041F4AJ Bypass Left Internal Iliac Artery to Left Femoral Artery with Autologous Arterial Tissue, Percutaneous Endoscopic Approach

041F4AK Bypass Left Internal Iliac Artery to Bilateral Femoral Arteries with Autologous Arterial Tissue, Percutaneous Endoscopic Approach

041F4AP Bypass Left Internal Iliac Artery to Foot Artery with Autologous Arterial Tissue, Percutaneous Endoscopic Approach

041F4AQ Bypass Left Internal Iliac Artery to Lower Extremity Artery with Autologous Arterial Tissue, Percutaneous Endoscopic Approach

041F4J9 Bypass Left Internal Iliac Artery to Right Internal Iliac Artery with Synthetic Substitute, Percutaneous Endoscopic Approach

041F4JB Bypass Left Internal Iliac Artery to Left Internal Iliac Artery with Synthetic Substitute, Percutaneous Endoscopic Approach

041F4JC Bypass Left Internal Iliac Artery to Bilateral Internal Iliac Arteries with Synthetic Substitute, Percutaneous Endoscopic Approach

041F4JD Bypass Left Internal Iliac Artery to Right External Iliac Artery with Synthetic Substitute, Percutaneous Endoscopic Approach

041F4JF Bypass Left Internal Iliac Artery to Left External Iliac Artery with Synthetic Substitute, Percutaneous Endoscopic Approach

041F4JG Bypass Left Internal Iliac Artery to Bilateral External Iliac Arteries with Synthetic Substitute, Percutaneous Endoscopic Approach

041F4JH Bypass Left Internal Iliac Artery to Right Femoral Artery with Synthetic Substitute, Percutaneous Endoscopic Approach

041F4JJ Bypass Left Internal Iliac Artery to Left Femoral Artery with Synthetic Substitute, Percutaneous Endoscopic Approach

041F4JK Bypass Left Internal Iliac Artery to Bilateral Femoral Arteries with Synthetic Substitute, Percutaneous Endoscopic Approach

041F4JP Bypass Left Internal Iliac Artery to Foot Artery with Synthetic Substitute, Percutaneous Endoscopic Approach

041F4JQ Bypass Left Internal Iliac Artery to Lower Extremity Artery with Synthetic Substitute, Percutaneous Endoscopic Approach

041F4K9 Bypass Left Internal Iliac Artery to Right Internal Iliac Artery with Nonautologous Tissue Substitute, Percutaneous Endoscopic Approach

041F4KB Bypass Left Internal Iliac Artery to Left Internal Iliac Artery with Nonautologous Tissue Substitute, Percutaneous Endoscopic Approach

041F4KC Bypass Left Internal Iliac Artery to Bilateral Internal Iliac Arteries with Nonautologous Tissue Substitute, Percutaneous Endoscopic Approach

041F4KD Bypass Left Internal Iliac Artery to Right External Iliac Artery with Nonautologous Tissue Substitute, Percutaneous Endoscopic Approach

041F4KF Bypass Left Internal Iliac Artery to Left External Iliac Artery with Nonautologous Tissue Substitute, Percutaneous Endoscopic Approach

041F4KG Bypass Left Internal Iliac Artery to Bilateral External Iliac Arteries with Nonautologous Tissue Substitute, Percutaneous Endoscopic Approach

041F4KH Bypass Left Internal Iliac Artery to Right Femoral Artery with Nonautologous Tissue Substitute, Percutaneous Endoscopic Approach

041F4KJ Bypass Left Internal Iliac Artery to Left Femoral Artery with Nonautologous Tissue Substitute, Percutaneous Endoscopic Approach

041F4KK Bypass Left Internal Iliac Artery to Bilateral Femoral Arteries with Nonautologous Tissue Substitute, Percutaneous Endoscopic Approach

041F4KP Bypass Left Internal Iliac Artery to Foot Artery with Nonautologous Tissue Substitute, Percutaneous Endoscopic Approach

041F4KQ Bypass Left Internal Iliac Artery to Lower Extremity Artery with Nonautologous Tissue Substitute, Percutaneous Endoscopic Approach

041F4Z9 Bypass Left Internal Iliac Artery to Right Internal Iliac Artery, Percutaneous Endoscopic Approach

041F4ZB Bypass Left Internal Iliac Artery to Left Internal Iliac Artery, Percutaneous Endoscopic Approach

041F4ZC Bypass Left Internal Iliac Artery to Bilateral Internal Iliac Arteries, Percutaneous Endoscopic Approach

041F4ZD Bypass Left Internal Iliac Artery to Right External Iliac Artery, Percutaneous Endoscopic Approach

041F4ZF Bypass Left Internal Iliac Artery to Left External Iliac Artery, Percutaneous Endoscopic Approach

041F4ZG Bypass Left Internal Iliac Artery to Bilateral External Iliac Arteries, Percutaneous Endoscopic Approach

041F4ZH Bypass Left Internal Iliac Artery to Right Femoral Artery, Percutaneous Endoscopic Approach

041F4ZJ Bypass Left Internal Iliac Artery to Left Femoral Artery, Percutaneous Endoscopic Approach

041F4ZK Bypass Left Internal Iliac Artery to Bilateral Femoral Arteries, Percutaneous Endoscopic Approach

041F4ZP Bypass Left Internal Iliac Artery to Foot Artery, Percutaneous Endoscopic Approach

041F4ZQ Bypass Left Internal Iliac Artery to Lower Extremity Artery, Percutaneous Endoscopic Approach

041H099 Bypass Right External Iliac Artery to Right Internal Iliac Artery with Autologous Venous Tissue, Open Approach

041H09B Bypass Right External Iliac Artery to Left Internal Iliac Artery with Autologous Venous Tissue, Open Approach

041H09C Bypass Right External Iliac Artery to Bilateral Internal Iliac Arteries with Autologous Venous Tissue, Open Approach

041H09D Bypass Right External Iliac Artery to Right External Iliac Artery with Autologous Venous Tissue, Open Approach

041H09F Bypass Right External Iliac Artery to Left External Iliac Artery with Autologous Venous Tissue, Open Approach

041H09G Bypass Right External Iliac Artery to Bilateral External Iliac Arteries with Autologous Venous Tissue, Open Approach

041H09H Bypass Right External Iliac Artery to Right Femoral Artery with Autologous Venous Tissue, Open Approach

041H09J Bypass Right External Iliac Artery to Left Femoral Artery with Autologous Venous Tissue, Open Approach

041H09K Bypass Right External Iliac Artery to Bilateral Femoral Arteries with Autologous Venous Tissue, Open Approach

041H09P Bypass Right External Iliac Artery to Foot Artery with Autologous Venous Tissue, Open Approach

041H09Q Bypass Right External Iliac Artery to Lower Extremity Artery with Autologous Venous Tissue, Open Approach

041H0A9 Bypass Right External Iliac Artery to Right Internal Iliac Artery with Autologous Arterial Tissue, Open Approach

041H0AB Bypass Right External Iliac Artery to Left Internal Iliac Artery with Autologous Arterial Tissue, Open Approach

041H0AC Bypass Right External Iliac Artery to Bilateral Internal Iliac Arteries with Autologous Arterial Tissue, Open Approach

041H0AD Bypass Right External Iliac Artery to Right External Iliac Artery with Autologous Arterial Tissue, Open Approach

041H0AF Bypass Right External Iliac Artery to Left External Iliac Artery with Autologous Arterial Tissue, Open Approach

041H0AG Bypass Right External Iliac Artery to Bilateral External Iliac Arteries with Autologous Arterial Tissue, Open Approach

041H0AH Bypass Right External Iliac Artery to Right Femoral Artery with Autologous Arterial Tissue, Open Approach

041H0AJ Bypass Right External Iliac Artery to Left Femoral Artery with Autologous Arterial Tissue, Open Approach

041H0AK Bypass Right External Iliac Artery to Bilateral Femoral Arteries with Autologous Arterial Tissue, Open Approach

041H0AP Bypass Right External Iliac Artery to Foot Artery with Autologous Arterial Tissue, Open Approach

041H0AQ Bypass Right External Iliac Artery to Lower Extremity Artery with Autologous Arterial Tissue, Open Approach

041H0J9 Bypass Right External Iliac Artery to Right Internal Iliac Artery with Synthetic Substitute, Open Approach

041H0JB Bypass Right External Iliac Artery to Left Internal Iliac Artery with Synthetic Substitute, Open Approach

041H0JC Bypass Right External Iliac Artery to Bilateral Internal Iliac Arteries with Synthetic Substitute, Open Approach

041H0JD Bypass Right External Iliac Artery to Right External Iliac Artery with Synthetic Substitute, Open Approach

041H0JF Bypass Right External Iliac Artery to Left External Iliac Artery with Synthetic Substitute, Open Approach

041H0JG Bypass Right External Iliac Artery to Bilateral External Iliac Arteries with Synthetic Substitute, Open Approach

041H0JH Bypass Right External Iliac Artery to Right Femoral Artery with Synthetic Substitute, Open Approach

041H0JJ Bypass Right External Iliac Artery to Left Femoral Artery with Synthetic Substitute, Open Approach

041H0JK Bypass Right External Iliac Artery to Bilateral Femoral Arteries with Synthetic Substitute, Open Approach

041H0JP Bypass Right External Iliac Artery to Foot Artery with Synthetic Substitute, Open Approach

041H0JQ Bypass Right External Iliac Artery to Lower Extremity Artery with Synthetic Substitute, Open Approach

041H0K9 Bypass Right External Iliac Artery to Right Internal Iliac Artery with Nonautologous Tissue Substitute, Open Approach

041H0KB Bypass Right External Iliac Artery to Left Internal Iliac Artery with Nonautologous Tissue Substitute, Open Approach

041H0KC Bypass Right External Iliac Artery to Bilateral Internal Iliac Arteries with Nonautologous Tissue Substitute, Open Approach

041H0KD Bypass Right External Iliac Artery to Right External Iliac Artery with Nonautologous Tissue Substitute, Open Approach

041H0KF Bypass Right External Iliac Artery to Left External Iliac Artery with Nonautologous Tissue Substitute, Open Approach

041H0KG   Bypass Right External Iliac Artery to Bilateral External Iliac Arteries with Nonautologous Tissue Substitute, Open Approach

041H0KH   Bypass Right External Iliac Artery to Right Femoral Artery with Nonautologous Tissue Substitute, Open Approach

041H0KJ   Bypass Right External Iliac Artery to Left Femoral Artery with Nonautologous Tissue Substitute, Open Approach

041H0KK   Bypass Right External Iliac Artery to Bilateral Femoral Arteries with Nonautologous Tissue Substitute, Open Approach

041H0KP   Bypass Right External Iliac Artery to Foot Artery with Nonautologous Tissue Substitute, Open Approach

041H0KQ   Bypass Right External Iliac Artery to Lower Extremity Artery with Nonautologous Tissue Substitute, Open Approach

041H0Z9   Bypass Right External Iliac Artery to Right Internal Iliac Artery, Open Approach

041H0ZB   Bypass Right External Iliac Artery to Left Internal Iliac Artery, Open Approach

041H0ZC   Bypass Right External Iliac Artery to Bilateral Internal Iliac Arteries, Open Approach

041H0ZD   Bypass Right External Iliac Artery to Right External Iliac Artery, Open Approach

041H0ZF   Bypass Right External Iliac Artery to Left External Iliac Artery, Open Approach

041H0ZG   Bypass Right External Iliac Artery to Bilateral External Iliac Arteries, Open Approach

041H0ZH   Bypass Right External Iliac Artery to Right Femoral Artery, Open Approach

041H0ZJ   Bypass Right External Iliac Artery to Left Femoral Artery, Open Approach

041H0ZK   Bypass Right External Iliac Artery to Bilateral Femoral Arteries, Open Approach

041H0ZP   Bypass Right External Iliac Artery to Foot Artery, Open Approach

041H0ZQ   Bypass Right External Iliac Artery to Lower Extremity Artery, Open Approach

041H499   Bypass Right External Iliac Artery to Right Internal Iliac Artery with Autologous Venous Tissue, Percutaneous Endoscopic Approach

041H49B   Bypass Right External Iliac Artery to Left Internal Iliac Artery with Autologous Venous Tissue, Percutaneous Endoscopic Approach

041H49C   Bypass Right External Iliac Artery to Bilateral Internal Iliac Arteries with Autologous Venous Tissue, Percutaneous Endoscopic Approach

041H49D   Bypass Right External Iliac Artery to Right External Iliac Artery with Autologous Venous Tissue, Percutaneous Endoscopic Approach

041H49F   Bypass Right External Iliac Artery to Left External Iliac Artery with Autologous Venous Tissue, Percutaneous Endoscopic Approach

041H49G   Bypass Right External Iliac Artery to Bilateral External Iliac Arteries with Autologous Venous Tissue, Percutaneous Endoscopic Approach

041H49H   Bypass Right External Iliac Artery to Right Femoral Artery with Autologous Venous Tissue, Percutaneous Endoscopic Approach

041H49J   Bypass Right External Iliac Artery to Left Femoral Artery with Autologous Venous Tissue, Percutaneous Endoscopic Approach

041H49K   Bypass Right External Iliac Artery to Bilateral Femoral Arteries with Autologous Venous Tissue, Percutaneous Endoscopic Approach

041H49P   Bypass Right External Iliac Artery to Foot Artery with Autologous Venous Tissue, Percutaneous Endoscopic Approach

041H49Q   Bypass Right External Iliac Artery to Lower Extremity Artery with Autologous Venous Tissue, Percutaneous Endoscopic Approach

041H4A9   Bypass Right External Iliac Artery to Right Internal Iliac Artery with Autologous Arterial Tissue, Percutaneous Endoscopic Approach

041H4AB   Bypass Right External Iliac Artery to Left Internal Iliac Artery with Autologous Arterial Tissue, Percutaneous Endoscopic Approach

041H4AC   Bypass Right External Iliac Artery to Bilateral Internal Iliac Arteries with Autologous Arterial Tissue, Percutaneous Endoscopic Approach

041H4AD   Bypass Right External Iliac Artery to Right External Iliac Artery with Autologous Arterial Tissue, Percutaneous Endoscopic Approach

041H4AF   Bypass Right External Iliac Artery to Left External Iliac Artery with Autologous Arterial Tissue, Percutaneous Endoscopic Approach

041H4AG   Bypass Right External Iliac Artery to Bilateral External Iliac Arteries with Autologous Arterial Tissue, Percutaneous Endoscopic Approach

041H4AH   Bypass Right External Iliac Artery to Right Femoral Artery with Autologous Arterial Tissue, Percutaneous Endoscopic Approach

041H4AJ   Bypass Right External Iliac Artery to Left Femoral Artery with Autologous Arterial Tissue, Percutaneous Endoscopic Approach

041H4AK   Bypass Right External Iliac Artery to Bilateral Femoral Arteries with Autologous Arterial Tissue, Percutaneous Endoscopic Approach

041H4AP   Bypass Right External Iliac Artery to Foot Artery with Autologous Arterial Tissue, Percutaneous Endoscopic Approach

041H4AQ   Bypass Right External Iliac Artery to Lower Extremity Artery with Autologous Arterial Tissue, Percutaneous Endoscopic Approach

041H4J9   Bypass Right External Iliac Artery to Right Internal Iliac Artery with Synthetic Substitute, Percutaneous Endoscopic Approach

041H4JB   Bypass Right External Iliac Artery to Left Internal Iliac Artery with Synthetic Substitute, Percutaneous Endoscopic Approach

041H4JC   Bypass Right External Iliac Artery to Bilateral Internal Iliac Arteries with Synthetic Substitute, Percutaneous Endoscopic Approach

041H4JD   Bypass Right External Iliac Artery to Right External Iliac Artery with Synthetic Substitute, Percutaneous Endoscopic Approach

041H4JF   Bypass Right External Iliac Artery to Left External Iliac Artery with Synthetic Substitute, Percutaneous Endoscopic Approach

041H4JG   Bypass Right External Iliac Artery to Bilateral External Iliac Arteries with Synthetic Substitute, Percutaneous Endoscopic Approach

041H4JH   Bypass Right External Iliac Artery to Right Femoral Artery with Synthetic Substitute, Percutaneous Endoscopic Approach

041H4JJ   Bypass Right External Iliac Artery to Left Femoral Artery with Synthetic Substitute, Percutaneous Endoscopic Approach

041H4JK   Bypass Right External Iliac Artery to Bilateral Femoral Arteries with Synthetic Substitute, Percutaneous Endoscopic Approach

041H4JP   Bypass Right External Iliac Artery to Foot Artery with Synthetic Substitute, Percutaneous Endoscopic Approach

041H4JQ   Bypass Right External Iliac Artery to Lower Extremity Artery with Synthetic Substitute, Percutaneous Endoscopic Approach

041H4K9   Bypass Right External Iliac Artery to Right Internal Iliac Artery with Nonautologous Tissue Substitute, Percutaneous Endoscopic Approach

041H4KB   Bypass Right External Iliac Artery to Left Internal Iliac Artery with Nonautologous Tissue Substitute, Percutaneous Endoscopic Approach

041H4KC   Bypass Right External Iliac Artery to Bilateral Internal Iliac Arteries with Nonautologous Tissue Substitute, Percutaneous Endoscopic Approach

041H4KD   Bypass Right External Iliac Artery to Right External Iliac Artery with Nonautologous Tissue Substitute, Percutaneous Endoscopic Approach

041H4KF   Bypass Right External Iliac Artery to Left External Iliac Artery with Nonautologous Tissue Substitute, Percutaneous Endoscopic Approach

041H4KG   Bypass Right External Iliac Artery to Bilateral External Iliac Arteries with Nonautologous Tissue Substitute, Percutaneous Endoscopic Approach

041H4KH   Bypass Right External Iliac Artery to Right Femoral Artery with Nonautologous Tissue Substitute, Percutaneous Endoscopic Approach

041H4KJ   Bypass Right External Iliac Artery to Left Femoral Artery with Nonautologous Tissue Substitute, Percutaneous Endoscopic Approach

041H4KK   Bypass Right External Iliac Artery to Bilateral Femoral Arteries with Nonautologous Tissue Substitute, Percutaneous Endoscopic Approach

041H4KP   Bypass Right External Iliac Artery to Foot Artery with Nonautologous Tissue Substitute, Percutaneous Endoscopic Approach

041H4KQ   Bypass Right External Iliac Artery to Lower Extremity Artery with Nonautologous Tissue Substitute, Percutaneous Endoscopic Approach

041H4Z9   Bypass Right External Iliac Artery to Right Internal Iliac Artery, Percutaneous Endoscopic Approach

041H4ZB   Bypass Right External Iliac Artery to Left Internal Iliac Artery, Percutaneous Endoscopic Approach

041H4ZC   Bypass Right External Iliac Artery to Bilateral Internal Iliac Arteries, Percutaneous Endoscopic Approach

041H4ZD   Bypass Right External Iliac Artery to Right External Iliac Artery, Percutaneous Endoscopic Approach

041H4ZF   Bypass Right External Iliac Artery to Left External Iliac Artery, Percutaneous Endoscopic Approach

041H4ZG   Bypass Right External Iliac Artery to Bilateral External Iliac Arteries, Percutaneous Endoscopic Approach

041H4ZH   Bypass Right External Iliac Artery to Right Femoral Artery, Percutaneous Endoscopic Approach

041H4ZJ   Bypass Right External Iliac Artery to Left Femoral Artery, Percutaneous Endoscopic Approach

041H4ZK   Bypass Right External Iliac Artery to Bilateral Femoral Arteries, Percutaneous Endoscopic Approach

041H4ZP   Bypass Right External Iliac Artery to Foot Artery, Percutaneous Endoscopic Approach

041H4ZQ   Bypass Right External Iliac Artery to Lower Extremity Artery, Percutaneous Endoscopic Approach

041J099   Bypass Left External Iliac Artery to Right Internal Iliac Artery with Autologous Venous Tissue, Open Approach

041J09B   Bypass Left External Iliac Artery to Left Internal Iliac Artery with Autologous Venous Tissue, Open Approach

041J09C   Bypass Left External Iliac Artery to Bilateral Internal Iliac Arteries with Autologous Venous Tissue, Open Approach

041J09D   Bypass Left External Iliac Artery to Right External Iliac Artery with Autologous Venous Tissue, Open Approach

041J09F   Bypass Left External Iliac Artery to Left External Iliac Artery with Autologous Venous Tissue, Open Approach

041J09G   Bypass Left External Iliac Artery to Bilateral External Iliac Arteries with Autologous Venous Tissue, Open Approach

041J09H   Bypass Left External Iliac Artery to Right Femoral Artery with Autologous Venous Tissue, Open Approach

041J09J   Bypass Left External Iliac Artery to Left Femoral Artery with Autologous Venous Tissue, Open Approach

041J09K   Bypass Left External Iliac Artery to Bilateral Femoral Arteries with Autologous Venous Tissue, Open Approach

041J09P   Bypass Left External Iliac Artery to Foot Artery with Autologous Venous Tissue, Open Approach

041J09Q   Bypass Left External Iliac Artery to Lower Extremity Artery with Autologous Venous Tissue, Open Approach

041J0A9   Bypass Left External Iliac Artery to Right Internal Iliac Artery with Autologous Arterial Tissue, Open Approach

041J0AB   Bypass Left External Iliac Artery to Left Internal Iliac Artery with Autologous Arterial Tissue, Open Approach

041J0AC   Bypass Left External Iliac Artery to Bilateral Internal Iliac Arteries with Autologous Arterial Tissue, Open Approach

041J0AD   Bypass Left External Iliac Artery to Right External Iliac Artery with Autologous Arterial Tissue, Open Approach

041J0AF   Bypass Left External Iliac Artery to Left External Iliac Artery with Autologous Arterial Tissue, Open Approach

041J0AG   Bypass Left External Iliac Artery to Bilateral External Iliac Arteries with Autologous Arterial Tissue, Open Approach

041J0AH   Bypass Left External Iliac Artery to Right Femoral Artery with Autologous Arterial Tissue, Open Approach

041J0AJ   Bypass Left External Iliac Artery to Left Femoral Artery with Autologous Arterial Tissue, Open Approach

041J0AK   Bypass Left External Iliac Artery to Bilateral Femoral Arteries with Autologous Arterial Tissue, Open Approach

041J0AP   Bypass Left External Iliac Artery to Foot Artery with Autologous Arterial Tissue, Open Approach

041J0AQ   Bypass Left External Iliac Artery to Lower Extremity Artery with Autologous Arterial Tissue, Open Approach

041J0J9   Bypass Left External Iliac Artery to Right Internal Iliac Artery with Synthetic Substitute, Open Approach

041J0JB   Bypass Left External Iliac Artery to Left Internal Iliac Artery with Synthetic Substitute, Open Approach

041J0JC   Bypass Left External Iliac Artery to Bilateral Internal Iliac Arteries with Synthetic Substitute, Open Approach

041J0JD   Bypass Left External Iliac Artery to Right External Iliac Artery with Synthetic Substitute, Open Approach

041J0JF   Bypass Left External Iliac Artery to Left External Iliac Artery with Synthetic Substitute, Open Approach

041J0JG   Bypass Left External Iliac Artery to Bilateral External Iliac Arteries with Synthetic Substitute, Open Approach

041J0JH   Bypass Left External Iliac Artery to Right Femoral Artery with Synthetic Substitute, Open Approach

041J0JJ   Bypass Left External Iliac Artery to Left Femoral Artery with Synthetic Substitute, Open Approach

041J0JK   Bypass Left External Iliac Artery to Bilateral Femoral Arteries with Synthetic Substitute, Open Approach

041J0JP   Bypass Left External Iliac Artery to Foot Artery with Synthetic Substitute, Open Approach

041J0JQ   Bypass Left External Iliac Artery to Lower Extremity Artery with Synthetic Substitute, Open Approach

041J0K9   Bypass Left External Iliac Artery to Right Internal Iliac Artery with Nonautologous Tissue Substitute, Open Approach

041J0KB   Bypass Left External Iliac Artery to Left Internal Iliac Artery with Nonautologous Tissue Substitute, Open Approach

041J0KC   Bypass Left External Iliac Artery to Bilateral Internal Iliac Arteries with Nonautologous Tissue Substitute, Open Approach

041J0KD   Bypass Left External Iliac Artery to Right External Iliac Artery with Nonautologous Tissue Substitute, Open Approach

041J0KF   Bypass Left External Iliac Artery to Left External Iliac Artery with Nonautologous Tissue Substitute, Open Approach

041J0KG   Bypass Left External Iliac Artery to Bilateral External Iliac Arteries with Nonautologous Tissue Substitute, Open Approach

041J0KH   Bypass Left External Iliac Artery to Right Femoral Artery with Nonautologous Tissue Substitute, Open Approach

041J0KJ   Bypass Left External Iliac Artery to Left Femoral Artery with Nonautologous Tissue Substitute, Open Approach

041J0KK   Bypass Left External Iliac Artery to Bilateral Femoral Arteries with Nonautologous Tissue Substitute, Open Approach

041J0KP   Bypass Left External Iliac Artery to Foot Artery with Nonautologous Tissue Substitute, Open Approach

041J0KQ   Bypass Left External Iliac Artery to Lower Extremity Artery with Nonautologous Tissue Substitute, Open Approach

041J0Z9   Bypass Left External Iliac Artery to Right Internal Iliac Artery, Open Approach

041J0ZB   Bypass Left External Iliac Artery to Left Internal Iliac Artery, Open Approach

041J0ZC   Bypass Left External Iliac Artery to Bilateral Internal Iliac Arteries, Open Approach

041J0ZD   Bypass Left External Iliac Artery to Right External Iliac Artery, Open Approach

041J0ZF   Bypass Left External Iliac Artery to Left External Iliac Artery, Open Approach

041J0ZG   Bypass Left External Iliac Artery to Bilateral External Iliac Arteries, Open Approach

041J0ZH   Bypass Left External Iliac Artery to Right Femoral Artery, Open Approach

041J0ZJ   Bypass Left External Iliac Artery to Left Femoral Artery, Open Approach

041J0ZK   Bypass Left External Iliac Artery to Bilateral Femoral Arteries, Open Approach

041J0ZP   Bypass Left External Iliac Artery to Foot Artery, Open Approach

041J0ZQ   Bypass Left External Iliac Artery to Lower Extremity Artery, Open Approach

041J499   Bypass Left External Iliac Artery to Right Internal Iliac Artery with Autologous Venous Tissue, Percutaneous Endoscopic Approach

041J49B   Bypass Left External Iliac Artery to Left Internal Iliac Artery with Autologous Venous Tissue, Percutaneous Endoscopic Approach

041J49C   Bypass Left External Iliac Artery to Bilateral Internal Iliac Arteries with Autologous Venous Tissue, Percutaneous Endoscopic Approach

041J49D   Bypass Left External Iliac Artery to Right External Iliac Artery with Autologous Venous Tissue, Percutaneous Endoscopic Approach

041J49F   Bypass Left External Iliac Artery to Left External Iliac Artery with Autologous Venous Tissue, Percutaneous Endoscopic Approach

041J49G   Bypass Left External Iliac Artery to Bilateral External Iliac Arteries with Autologous Venous Tissue, Percutaneous Endoscopic Approach

041J49H   Bypass Left External Iliac Artery to Right Femoral Artery with Autologous Venous Tissue, Percutaneous Endoscopic Approach

041J49J   Bypass Left External Iliac Artery to Left Femoral Artery with Autologous Venous Tissue, Percutaneous Endoscopic Approach

041J49K   Bypass Left External Iliac Artery to Bilateral Femoral Arteries with Autologous Venous Tissue, Percutaneous Endoscopic Approach

041J49P   Bypass Left External Iliac Artery to Foot Artery with Autologous Venous Tissue, Percutaneous Endoscopic Approach

041J49Q   Bypass Left External Iliac Artery to Lower Extremity Artery with Autologous Venous Tissue, Percutaneous Endoscopic Approach

041J4A9   Bypass Left External Iliac Artery to Right Internal Iliac Artery with Autologous Arterial Tissue, Percutaneous Endoscopic Approach

041J4AB   Bypass Left External Iliac Artery to Left Internal Iliac Artery with Autologous Arterial Tissue, Percutaneous Endoscopic Approach

041J4AC   Bypass Left External Iliac Artery to Bilateral Internal Iliac Arteries with Autologous Arterial Tissue, Percutaneous Endoscopic Approach

041J4AD   Bypass Left External Iliac Artery to Right External Iliac Artery with Autologous Arterial Tissue, Percutaneous Endoscopic Approach

041J4AF   Bypass Left External Iliac Artery to Left External Iliac Artery with Autologous Arterial Tissue, Percutaneous Endoscopic Approach

041J4AG   Bypass Left External Iliac Artery to Bilateral External Iliac Arteries with Autologous Arterial Tissue, Percutaneous Endoscopic Approach

041J4AH   Bypass Left External Iliac Artery to Right Femoral Artery with Autologous Arterial Tissue, Percutaneous Endoscopic Approach

041J4AJ   Bypass Left External Iliac Artery to Left Femoral Artery with Autologous Arterial Tissue, Percutaneous Endoscopic Approach

041J4AK   Bypass Left External Iliac Artery to Bilateral Femoral Arteries with Autologous Arterial Tissue, Percutaneous Endoscopic Approach

041J4AP   Bypass Left External Iliac Artery to Foot Artery with Autologous Arterial Tissue, Percutaneous Endoscopic Approach

041J4AQ   Bypass Left External Iliac Artery to Lower Extremity Artery with Autologous Arterial Tissue, Percutaneous Endoscopic Approach

041J4J9   Bypass Left External Iliac Artery to Right Internal Iliac Artery with Synthetic Substitute, Percutaneous Endoscopic Approach

041J4JB   Bypass Left External Iliac Artery to Left Internal Iliac Artery with Synthetic Substitute, Percutaneous Endoscopic Approach

041J4JC   Bypass Left External Iliac Artery to Bilateral Internal Iliac Arteries with Synthetic Substitute, Percutaneous Endoscopic Approach

041J4JD   Bypass Left External Iliac Artery to Right External Iliac Artery with Synthetic Substitute, Percutaneous Endoscopic Approach

041J4JF   Bypass Left External Iliac Artery to Left External Iliac Artery with Synthetic Substitute, Percutaneous Endoscopic Approach

041J4JG   Bypass Left External Iliac Artery to Bilateral External Iliac Arteries with Synthetic Substitute, Percutaneous Endoscopic Approach

041J4JH   Bypass Left External Iliac Artery to Right Femoral Artery with Synthetic Substitute, Percutaneous Endoscopic Approach

041J4JJ   Bypass Left External Iliac Artery to Left Femoral Artery with Synthetic Substitute, Percutaneous Endoscopic Approach

041J4JK   Bypass Left External Iliac Artery to Bilateral Femoral Arteries with Synthetic Substitute, Percutaneous Endoscopic Approach

041J4JP   Bypass Left External Iliac Artery to Foot Artery with Synthetic Substitute, Percutaneous Endoscopic Approach

041J4JQ   Bypass Left External Iliac Artery to Lower Extremity Artery with Synthetic Substitute, Percutaneous Endoscopic Approach

041J4K9   Bypass Left External Iliac Artery to Right Internal Iliac Artery with Nonautologous Tissue Substitute, Percutaneous Endoscopic Approach

041J4KB   Bypass Left External Iliac Artery to Left Internal Iliac Artery with Nonautologous Tissue Substitute, Percutaneous Endoscopic Approach

041J4KC   Bypass Left External Iliac Artery to Bilateral Internal Iliac Arteries with Nonautologous Tissue Substitute, Percutaneous Endoscopic Approach

041J4KD   Bypass Left External Iliac Artery to Right External Iliac Artery with Nonautologous Tissue Substitute, Percutaneous Endoscopic Approach

041J4KF   Bypass Left External Iliac Artery to Left External Iliac Artery with Nonautologous Tissue Substitute, Percutaneous Endoscopic Approach

041J4KG   Bypass Left External Iliac Artery to Bilateral External Iliac Arteries with Nonautologous Tissue Substitute, Percutaneous Endoscopic Approach

041J4KH   Bypass Left External Iliac Artery to Right Femoral Artery with Nonautologous Tissue Substitute, Percutaneous Endoscopic Approach

041J4KJ   Bypass Left External Iliac Artery to Left Femoral Artery with Nonautologous Tissue Substitute, Percutaneous Endoscopic Approach

041J4KK   Bypass Left External Iliac Artery to Bilateral Femoral Arteries with Nonautologous Tissue Substitute, Percutaneous Endoscopic Approach

041J4KP   Bypass Left External Iliac Artery to Foot Artery with Nonautologous Tissue Substitute, Percutaneous Endoscopic Approach

041J4KQ   Bypass Left External Iliac Artery to Lower Extremity Artery with Nonautologous Tissue Substitute, Percutaneous Endoscopic Approach

041J4Z9   Bypass Left External Iliac Artery to Right Internal Iliac Artery, Percutaneous Endoscopic Approach

041J4ZB   Bypass Left External Iliac Artery to Left Internal Iliac Artery, Percutaneous Endoscopic Approach

041J4ZC   Bypass Left External Iliac Artery to Bilateral Internal Iliac Arteries, Percutaneous Endoscopic Approach

041J4ZD   Bypass Left External Iliac Artery to Right External Iliac Artery, Percutaneous Endoscopic Approach

041J4ZF   Bypass Left External Iliac Artery to Left External Iliac Artery, Percutaneous Endoscopic Approach

041J4ZG   Bypass Left External Iliac Artery to Bilateral External Iliac Arteries, Percutaneous Endoscopic Approach

041J4ZH   Bypass Left External Iliac Artery to Right Femoral Artery, Percutaneous Endoscopic Approach

041J4ZJ   Bypass Left External Iliac Artery to Left Femoral Artery, Percutaneous Endoscopic Approach

041J4ZK   Bypass Left External Iliac Artery to Bilateral Femoral Arteries, Percutaneous Endoscopic Approach

041J4ZP   Bypass Left External Iliac Artery to Foot Artery, Percutaneous Endoscopic Approach

041J4ZQ   Bypass Left External Iliac Artery to Lower Extremity Artery, Percutaneous Endoscopic Approach

041K09H   Bypass Right Femoral Artery to Right Femoral Artery with Autologous Venous Tissue, Open Approach

041K09J   Bypass Right Femoral Artery to Left Femoral Artery with Autologous Venous Tissue, Open Approach

041K09K   Bypass Right Femoral Artery to Bilateral Femoral Arteries with Autologous Venous Tissue, Open Approach

041K09L   Bypass Right Femoral Artery to Popliteal Artery with Autologous Venous Tissue, Open Approach

041K09M   Bypass Right Femoral Artery to Peroneal Artery with Autologous Venous Tissue, Open Approach

041K09N   Bypass Right Femoral Artery to Posterior Tibial Artery with Autologous Venous Tissue, Open Approach

041K09P   Bypass Right Femoral Artery to Foot Artery with Autologous Venous Tissue, Open Approach

041K09Q   Bypass Right Femoral Artery to Lower Extremity Artery with Autologous Venous Tissue, Open Approach

041K09S   Bypass Right Femoral Artery to Lower Extremity Vein with Autologous Venous Tissue, Open Approach

041K0AH   Bypass Right Femoral Artery to Right Femoral Artery with Autologous Arterial Tissue, Open Approach

041K0AJ   Bypass Right Femoral Artery to Left Femoral Artery with Autologous Arterial Tissue, Open Approach

041K0AK   Bypass Right Femoral Artery to Bilateral Femoral Arteries with Autologous Arterial Tissue, Open Approach

041K0AL   Bypass Right Femoral Artery to Popliteal Artery with Autologous Arterial Tissue, Open Approach

041K0AM   Bypass Right Femoral Artery to Peroneal Artery with Autologous Arterial Tissue, Open Approach

041K0AN   Bypass Right Femoral Artery to Posterior Tibial Artery with Autologous Arterial Tissue, Open Approach

041K0AP   Bypass Right Femoral Artery to Foot Artery with Autologous Arterial Tissue, Open Approach

041K0AQ   Bypass Right Femoral Artery to Lower Extremity Artery with Autologous Arterial Tissue, Open Approach

041K0AS   Bypass Right Femoral Artery to Lower Extremity Vein with Autologous Arterial Tissue, Open Approach

041K0JH   Bypass Right Femoral Artery to Right Femoral Artery with Synthetic Substitute, Open Approach

041K0JJ   Bypass Right Femoral Artery to Left Femoral Artery with Synthetic Substitute, Open Approach

041K0JK   Bypass Right Femoral Artery to Bilateral Femoral Arteries with Synthetic Substitute, Open Approach

041K0JL   Bypass Right Femoral Artery to Popliteal Artery with Synthetic Substitute, Open Approach

041K0JM   Bypass Right Femoral Artery to Peroneal Artery with Synthetic Substitute, Open Approach

041K0JN   Bypass Right Femoral Artery to Posterior Tibial Artery with Synthetic Substitute, Open Approach

041K0JP   Bypass Right Femoral Artery to Foot Artery with Synthetic Substitute, Open Approach

041K0JQ   Bypass Right Femoral Artery to Lower Extremity Artery with Synthetic Substitute, Open Approach

041K0JS   Bypass Right Femoral Artery to Lower Extremity Vein with Synthetic Substitute, Open Approach

041K0KH   Bypass Right Femoral Artery to Right Femoral Artery with Nonautologous Tissue Substitute, Open Approach

041K0KJ   Bypass Right Femoral Artery to Left Femoral Artery with Nonautologous Tissue Substitute, Open Approach

041K0KK   Bypass Right Femoral Artery to Bilateral Femoral Arteries with Nonautologous Tissue Substitute, Open Approach

041K0KL   Bypass Right Femoral Artery to Popliteal Artery with Nonautologous Tissue Substitute, Open Approach

041K0KM   Bypass Right Femoral Artery to Peroneal Artery with Nonautologous Tissue Substitute, Open Approach

041K0KN   Bypass Right Femoral Artery to Posterior Tibial Artery with Nonautologous Tissue Substitute, Open Approach

041K0KP   Bypass Right Femoral Artery to Foot Artery with Nonautologous Tissue Substitute, Open Approach

041K0KQ   Bypass Right Femoral Artery to Lower Extremity Artery with Nonautologous Tissue Substitute, Open Approach

041K0KS   Bypass Right Femoral Artery to Lower Extremity Vein with Nonautologous Tissue Substitute, Open Approach

041K0ZH   Bypass Right Femoral Artery to Right Femoral Artery, Open Approach

041K0ZJ   Bypass Right Femoral Artery to Left Femoral Artery, Open Approach

041K0ZK   Bypass Right Femoral Artery to Bilateral Femoral Arteries, Open Approach

041K0ZL   Bypass Right Femoral Artery to Popliteal Artery, Open Approach

041K0ZM   Bypass Right Femoral Artery to Peroneal Artery, Open Approach

041K0ZN   Bypass Right Femoral Artery to Posterior Tibial Artery, Open Approach

041K0ZP   Bypass Right Femoral Artery to Foot Artery, Open Approach

041K0ZQ   Bypass Right Femoral Artery to Lower Extremity Artery, Open Approach

041K0ZS   Bypass Right Femoral Artery to Lower Extremity Vein, Open Approach

041K49H   Bypass Right Femoral Artery to Right Femoral Artery with Autologous Venous Tissue, Percutaneous Endoscopic Approach

041K49J   Bypass Right Femoral Artery to Left Femoral Artery with Autologous Venous Tissue, Percutaneous Endoscopic Approach

041K49K   Bypass Right Femoral Artery to Bilateral Femoral Arteries with Autologous Venous Tissue, Percutaneous Endoscopic Approach

041K49L   Bypass Right Femoral Artery to Popliteal Artery with Autologous Venous Tissue, Percutaneous Endoscopic Approach

041K49M   Bypass Right Femoral Artery to Peroneal Artery with Autologous Venous Tissue, Percutaneous Endoscopic Approach

041K49N   Bypass Right Femoral Artery to Posterior Tibial Artery with Autologous Venous Tissue, Percutaneous Endoscopic Approach

041K49P   Bypass Right Femoral Artery to Foot Artery with Autologous Venous Tissue, Percutaneous Endoscopic Approach

041K49Q   Bypass Right Femoral Artery to Lower Extremity Artery with Autologous Venous Tissue, Percutaneous Endoscopic Approach

041K49S   Bypass Right Femoral Artery to Lower Extremity Vein with Autologous Venous Tissue, Percutaneous Endoscopic Approach

041K4AH   Bypass Right Femoral Artery to Right Femoral Artery with Autologous Arterial Tissue, Percutaneous Endoscopic Approach

041K4AJ   Bypass Right Femoral Artery to Left Femoral Artery with Autologous Arterial Tissue, Percutaneous Endoscopic Approach

041K4AK   Bypass Right Femoral Artery to Bilateral Femoral Arteries with Autologous Arterial Tissue, Percutaneous Endoscopic Approach

041K4AL   Bypass Right Femoral Artery to Popliteal Artery with Autologous Arterial Tissue, Percutaneous Endoscopic Approach

041K4AM   Bypass Right Femoral Artery to Peroneal Artery with Autologous Arterial Tissue, Percutaneous Endoscopic Approach

041K4AN   Bypass Right Femoral Artery to Posterior Tibial Artery with Autologous Arterial Tissue, Percutaneous Endoscopic Approach

041K4AP   Bypass Right Femoral Artery to Foot Artery with Autologous Arterial Tissue, Percutaneous Endoscopic Approach

041K4AQ   Bypass Right Femoral Artery to Lower Extremity Artery with Autologous Arterial Tissue, Percutaneous Endoscopic Approach

041K4AS   Bypass Right Femoral Artery to Lower Extremity Vein with Autologous Arterial Tissue, Percutaneous Endoscopic Approach

041K4JH   Bypass Right Femoral Artery to Right Femoral Artery with Synthetic Substitute, Percutaneous Endoscopic Approach

041K4JJ   Bypass Right Femoral Artery to Left Femoral Artery with Synthetic Substitute, Percutaneous Endoscopic Approach

041K4JK   Bypass Right Femoral Artery to Bilateral Femoral Arteries with Synthetic Substitute, Percutaneous Endoscopic Approach

041K4JL   Bypass Right Femoral Artery to Popliteal Artery with Synthetic Substitute, Percutaneous Endoscopic Approach

041K4JM   Bypass Right Femoral Artery to Peroneal Artery with Synthetic Substitute, Percutaneous Endoscopic Approach

041K4JN   Bypass Right Femoral Artery to Posterior Tibial Artery with Synthetic Substitute, Percutaneous Endoscopic Approach

041K4JP   Bypass Right Femoral Artery to Foot Artery with Synthetic Substitute, Percutaneous Endoscopic Approach

041K4JQ   Bypass Right Femoral Artery to Lower Extremity Artery with Synthetic Substitute, Percutaneous Endoscopic Approach

041K4JS   Bypass Right Femoral Artery to Lower Extremity Vein with Synthetic Substitute, Percutaneous Endoscopic Approach

041K4KH   Bypass Right Femoral Artery to Right Femoral Artery with Nonautologous Tissue Substitute, Percutaneous Endoscopic Approach

041K4KJ   Bypass Right Femoral Artery to Left Femoral Artery with Nonautologous Tissue Substitute, Percutaneous Endoscopic Approach

041K4KK   Bypass Right Femoral Artery to Bilateral Femoral Arteries with Nonautologous Tissue Substitute, Percutaneous Endoscopic Approach

041K4KL   Bypass Right Femoral Artery to Popliteal Artery with Nonautologous Tissue Substitute, Percutaneous Endoscopic Approach

041K4KM   Bypass Right Femoral Artery to Peroneal Artery with Nonautologous Tissue Substitute, Percutaneous Endoscopic Approach

041K4KN   Bypass Right Femoral Artery to Posterior Tibial Artery with Nonautologous Tissue Substitute, Percutaneous Endoscopic Approach

041K4KP   Bypass Right Femoral Artery to Foot Artery with Nonautologous Tissue Substitute, Percutaneous Endoscopic Approach

041K4KQ   Bypass Right Femoral Artery to Lower Extremity Artery with Nonautologous Tissue Substitute, Percutaneous Endoscopic Approach

041K4KS   Bypass Right Femoral Artery to Lower Extremity Vein with Nonautologous Tissue Substitute, Percutaneous Endoscopic Approach

041K4ZH   Bypass Right Femoral Artery to Right Femoral Artery, Percutaneous Endoscopic Approach

041K4ZJ   Bypass Right Femoral Artery to Left Femoral Artery, Percutaneous Endoscopic Approach

041K4ZK   Bypass Right Femoral Artery to Bilateral Femoral Arteries, Percutaneous Endoscopic Approach

041K4ZL   Bypass Right Femoral Artery to Popliteal Artery, Percutaneous Endoscopic Approach

041K4ZM   Bypass Right Femoral Artery to Peroneal Artery, Percutaneous Endoscopic Approach

041K4ZN   Bypass Right Femoral Artery to Posterior Tibial Artery, Percutaneous Endoscopic Approach

041K4ZP   Bypass Right Femoral Artery to Foot Artery, Percutaneous Endoscopic Approach

041K4ZQ   Bypass Right Femoral Artery to Lower Extremity Artery, Percutaneous Endoscopic Approach

♀ Female-only   ♂ Male-only   ◯ Limited Coverage   ● Non-OR   HAC HAC-associated procedure   ⬤ Non-covered procedures   ✚ Combination

041K4ZS Bypass Right Femoral Artery to Lower Extremity Vein, Percutaneous Endoscopic Approach

041L09H Bypass Left Femoral Artery to Right Femoral Artery with Autologous Venous Tissue, Open Approach

041L09J Bypass Left Femoral Artery to Left Femoral Artery with Autologous Venous Tissue, Open Approach

041L09K Bypass Left Femoral Artery to Bilateral Femoral Arteries with Autologous Venous Tissue, Open Approach

041L09L Bypass Left Femoral Artery to Popliteal Artery with Autologous Venous Tissue, Open Approach

041L09M Bypass Left Femoral Artery to Peroneal Artery with Autologous Venous Tissue, Open Approach

041L09N Bypass Left Femoral Artery to Posterior Tibial Artery with Autologous Venous Tissue, Open Approach

041L09P Bypass Left Femoral Artery to Foot Artery with Autologous Venous Tissue, Open Approach

041L09Q Bypass Left Femoral Artery to Lower Extremity Artery with Autologous Venous Tissue, Open Approach

041L09S Bypass Left Femoral Artery to Lower Extremity Vein with Autologous Venous Tissue, Open Approach

041L0AH Bypass Left Femoral Artery to Right Femoral Artery with Autologous Arterial Tissue, Open Approach

041L0AJ Bypass Left Femoral Artery to Left Femoral Artery with Autologous Arterial Tissue, Open Approach

041L0AK Bypass Left Femoral Artery to Bilateral Femoral Arteries with Autologous Arterial Tissue, Open Approach

041L0AL Bypass Left Femoral Artery to Popliteal Artery with Autologous Arterial Tissue, Open Approach

041L0AM Bypass Left Femoral Artery to Peroneal Artery with Autologous Arterial Tissue, Open Approach

041L0AN Bypass Left Femoral Artery to Posterior Tibial Artery with Autologous Arterial Tissue, Open Approach

041L0AP Bypass Left Femoral Artery to Foot Artery with Autologous Arterial Tissue, Open Approach

041L0AQ Bypass Left Femoral Artery to Lower Extremity Artery with Autologous Arterial Tissue, Open Approach

041L0AS Bypass Left Femoral Artery to Lower Extremity Vein with Autologous Arterial Tissue, Open Approach

041L0JH Bypass Left Femoral Artery to Right Femoral Artery with Synthetic Substitute, Open Approach

041L0JJ Bypass Left Femoral Artery to Left Femoral Artery with Synthetic Substitute, Open Approach

041L0JK Bypass Left Femoral Artery to Bilateral Femoral Arteries with Synthetic Substitute, Open Approach

041L0JL Bypass Left Femoral Artery to Popliteal Artery with Synthetic Substitute, Open Approach

041L0JM Bypass Left Femoral Artery to Peroneal Artery with Synthetic Substitute, Open Approach

041L0JN Bypass Left Femoral Artery to Posterior Tibial Artery with Synthetic Substitute, Open Approach

041L0JP Bypass Left Femoral Artery to Foot Artery with Synthetic Substitute, Open Approach

041L0JQ Bypass Left Femoral Artery to Lower Extremity Artery with Synthetic Substitute, Open Approach

041L0JS Bypass Left Femoral Artery to Lower Extremity Vein with Synthetic Substitute, Open Approach

041L0KH Bypass Left Femoral Artery to Right Femoral Artery with Nonautologous Tissue Substitute, Open Approach

041L0KJ Bypass Left Femoral Artery to Left Femoral Artery with Nonautologous Tissue Substitute, Open Approach

041L0KK Bypass Left Femoral Artery to Bilateral Femoral Arteries with Nonautologous Tissue Substitute, Open Approach

041L0KL Bypass Left Femoral Artery to Popliteal Artery with Nonautologous Tissue Substitute, Open Approach

041L0KM Bypass Left Femoral Artery to Peroneal Artery with Nonautologous Tissue Substitute, Open Approach

041L0KN Bypass Left Femoral Artery to Posterior Tibial Artery with Nonautologous Tissue Substitute, Open Approach

041L0KP Bypass Left Femoral Artery to Foot Artery with Nonautologous Tissue Substitute, Open Approach

041L0KQ Bypass Left Femoral Artery to Lower Extremity Artery with Nonautologous Tissue Substitute, Open Approach

041L0KS Bypass Left Femoral Artery to Lower Extremity Vein with Nonautologous Tissue Substitute, Open Approach

041L0ZH Bypass Left Femoral Artery to Right Femoral Artery, Open Approach

041L0ZJ Bypass Left Femoral Artery to Left Femoral Artery, Open Approach

041L0ZK Bypass Left Femoral Artery to Bilateral Femoral Arteries, Open Approach

041L0ZL Bypass Left Femoral Artery to Popliteal Artery, Open Approach

041L0ZM Bypass Left Femoral Artery to Peroneal Artery, Open Approach

041L0ZN Bypass Left Femoral Artery to Posterior Tibial Artery, Open Approach

041L0ZP Bypass Left Femoral Artery to Foot Artery, Open Approach

041L0ZQ Bypass Left Femoral Artery to Lower Extremity Artery, Open Approach

041L0ZS Bypass Left Femoral Artery to Lower Extremity Vein, Open Approach

041L49H Bypass Left Femoral Artery to Right Femoral Artery with Autologous Venous Tissue, Percutaneous Endoscopic Approach

041L49J Bypass Left Femoral Artery to Left Femoral Artery with Autologous Venous Tissue, Percutaneous Endoscopic Approach

041L49K Bypass Left Femoral Artery to Bilateral Femoral Arteries with Autologous Venous Tissue, Percutaneous Endoscopic Approach

041L49L Bypass Left Femoral Artery to Popliteal Artery with Autologous Venous Tissue, Percutaneous Endoscopic Approach

041L49M Bypass Left Femoral Artery to Peroneal Artery with Autologous Venous Tissue, Percutaneous Endoscopic Approach

041L49N Bypass Left Femoral Artery to Posterior Tibial Artery with Autologous Venous Tissue, Percutaneous Endoscopic Approach

041L49P Bypass Left Femoral Artery to Foot Artery with Autologous Venous Tissue, Percutaneous Endoscopic Approach

041L49Q Bypass Left Femoral Artery to Lower Extremity Artery with Autologous Venous Tissue, Percutaneous Endoscopic Approach

041L49S Bypass Left Femoral Artery to Lower Extremity Vein with Autologous Venous Tissue, Percutaneous Endoscopic Approach

041L4AH Bypass Left Femoral Artery to Right Femoral Artery with Autologous Arterial Tissue, Percutaneous Endoscopic Approach

041L4AJ Bypass Left Femoral Artery to Left Femoral Artery with Autologous Arterial Tissue, Percutaneous Endoscopic Approach

041L4AK Bypass Left Femoral Artery to Bilateral Femoral Arteries with Autologous Arterial Tissue, Percutaneous Endoscopic Approach

041L4AL Bypass Left Femoral Artery to Popliteal Artery with Autologous Arterial Tissue, Percutaneous Endoscopic Approach

041L4AM Bypass Left Femoral Artery to Peroneal Artery with Autologous Arterial Tissue, Percutaneous Endoscopic Approach

041L4AN Bypass Left Femoral Artery to Posterior Tibial Artery with Autologous Arterial Tissue, Percutaneous Endoscopic Approach

041L4AP Bypass Left Femoral Artery to Foot Artery with Autologous Arterial Tissue, Percutaneous Endoscopic Approach

041L4AQ Bypass Left Femoral Artery to Lower Extremity Artery with Autologous Arterial Tissue, Percutaneous Endoscopic Approach

041L4AS Bypass Left Femoral Artery to Lower Extremity Vein with Autologous Arterial Tissue, Percutaneous Endoscopic Approach

041L4JH Bypass Left Femoral Artery to Right Femoral Artery with Synthetic Substitute, Percutaneous Endoscopic Approach

041L4JJ Bypass Left Femoral Artery to Left Femoral Artery with Synthetic Substitute, Percutaneous Endoscopic Approach

041L4JK Bypass Left Femoral Artery to Bilateral Femoral Arteries with Synthetic Substitute, Percutaneous Endoscopic Approach

041L4JL Bypass Left Femoral Artery to Popliteal Artery with Synthetic Substitute, Percutaneous Endoscopic Approach

041L4JM Bypass Left Femoral Artery to Peroneal Artery with Synthetic Substitute, Percutaneous Endoscopic Approach

041L4JN Bypass Left Femoral Artery to Posterior Tibial Artery with Synthetic Substitute, Percutaneous Endoscopic Approach

041L4JP Bypass Left Femoral Artery to Foot Artery with Synthetic Substitute, Percutaneous Endoscopic Approach

041L4JQ Bypass Left Femoral Artery to Lower Extremity Artery with Synthetic Substitute, Percutaneous Endoscopic Approach

041L4JS Bypass Left Femoral Artery to Lower Extremity Vein with Synthetic Substitute, Percutaneous Endoscopic Approach

041L4KH Bypass Left Femoral Artery to Right Femoral Artery with Nonautologous Tissue Substitute, Percutaneous Endoscopic Approach

041L4KJ Bypass Left Femoral Artery to Left Femoral Artery with Nonautologous Tissue Substitute, Percutaneous Endoscopic Approach

041L4KK Bypass Left Femoral Artery to Bilateral Femoral Arteries with Nonautologous Tissue Substitute, Percutaneous Endoscopic Approach

041L4KL Bypass Left Femoral Artery to Popliteal Artery with Nonautologous Tissue Substitute, Percutaneous Endoscopic Approach

041L4KM Bypass Left Femoral Artery to Peroneal Artery with Nonautologous Tissue Substitute, Percutaneous Endoscopic Approach

041L4KN Bypass Left Femoral Artery to Posterior Tibial Artery with Nonautologous Tissue Substitute, Percutaneous Endoscopic Approach

041L4KP Bypass Left Femoral Artery to Foot Artery with Nonautologous Tissue Substitute, Percutaneous Endoscopic Approach

041L4KQ Bypass Left Femoral Artery to Lower Extremity Artery with Nonautologous Tissue Substitute, Percutaneous Endoscopic Approach

041L4KS Bypass Left Femoral Artery to Lower Extremity Vein with Nonautologous Tissue Substitute, Percutaneous Endoscopic Approach

041L4ZH Bypass Left Femoral Artery to Right Femoral Artery, Percutaneous Endoscopic Approach

041L4ZJ Bypass Left Femoral Artery to Left Femoral Artery, Percutaneous Endoscopic Approach

041L4ZK Bypass Left Femoral Artery to Bilateral Femoral Arteries, Percutaneous Endoscopic Approach

041L4ZL Bypass Left Femoral Artery to Popliteal Artery, Percutaneous Endoscopic Approach

041L4ZM Bypass Left Femoral Artery to Peroneal Artery, Percutaneous Endoscopic Approach

041L4ZN Bypass Left Femoral Artery to Posterior Tibial Artery, Percutaneous Endoscopic Approach

041L4ZP Bypass Left Femoral Artery to Foot Artery, Percutaneous Endoscopic Approach

041L4ZQ Bypass Left Femoral Artery to Lower Extremity Artery, Percutaneous Endoscopic Approach

041L4ZS Bypass Left Femoral Artery to Lower Extremity Vein, Percutaneous Endoscopic Approach

041M09L Bypass Right Popliteal Artery to Popliteal Artery with Autologous Venous Tissue, Open Approach

041M09M Bypass Right Popliteal Artery to Peroneal Artery with Autologous Venous Tissue, Open Approach

041M09P Bypass Right Popliteal Artery to Foot Artery with Autologous Venous Tissue, Open Approach

041M09Q Bypass Right Popliteal Artery to Lower Extremity Artery with Autologous Venous Tissue, Open Approach

041M09S Bypass Right Popliteal Artery to Lower Extremity Vein with Autologous Venous Tissue, Open Approach

041M0AL Bypass Right Popliteal Artery to Popliteal Artery with Autologous Arterial Tissue, Open Approach

041M0AM Bypass Right Popliteal Artery to Peroneal Artery with Autologous Arterial Tissue, Open Approach

041M0AP Bypass Right Popliteal Artery to Foot Artery with Autologous Arterial Tissue, Open Approach

041M0AQ Bypass Right Popliteal Artery to Lower Extremity Artery with Autologous Arterial Tissue, Open Approach

041M0AS Bypass Right Popliteal Artery to Lower Extremity Vein with Autologous Arterial Tissue, Open Approach

041M0JL Bypass Right Popliteal Artery to Popliteal Artery with Synthetic Substitute, Open Approach

041M0JM Bypass Right Popliteal Artery to Peroneal Artery with Synthetic Substitute, Open Approach

041M0JP Bypass Right Popliteal Artery to Foot Artery with Synthetic Substitute, Open Approach

041M0JQ Bypass Right Popliteal Artery to Lower Extremity Artery with Synthetic Substitute, Open Approach

041M0JS Bypass Right Popliteal Artery to Lower Extremity Vein with Synthetic Substitute, Open Approach

041M0KL Bypass Right Popliteal Artery to Popliteal Artery with Nonautologous Tissue Substitute, Open Approach

041M0KM Bypass Right Popliteal Artery to Peroneal Artery with Nonautologous Tissue Substitute, Open Approach

041M0KP Bypass Right Popliteal Artery to Foot Artery with Nonautologous Tissue Substitute, Open Approach

041M0KQ Bypass Right Popliteal Artery to Lower Extremity Artery with Nonautologous Tissue Substitute, Open Approach

041M0KS Bypass Right Popliteal Artery to Lower Extremity Vein with Nonautologous Tissue Substitute, Open Approach

041M0ZL Bypass Right Popliteal Artery to Popliteal Artery, Open Approach

041M0ZM Bypass Right Popliteal Artery to Peroneal Artery, Open Approach

041M0ZP Bypass Right Popliteal Artery to Foot Artery, Open Approach

041M0ZQ Bypass Right Popliteal Artery to Lower Extremity Artery, Open Approach

041M0ZS Bypass Right Popliteal Artery to Lower Extremity Vein, Open Approach

041M49L Bypass Right Popliteal Artery to Popliteal Artery with Autologous Venous Tissue, Percutaneous Endoscopic Approach

041M49M Bypass Right Popliteal Artery to Peroneal Artery with Autologous Venous Tissue, Percutaneous Endoscopic Approach

041M49P Bypass Right Popliteal Artery to Foot Artery with Autologous Venous Tissue, Percutaneous Endoscopic Approach

041M49Q Bypass Right Popliteal Artery to Lower Extremity Artery with Autologous Venous Tissue, Percutaneous Endoscopic Approach

041M49S Bypass Right Popliteal Artery to Lower Extremity Vein with Autologous Venous Tissue, Percutaneous Endoscopic Approach

041M4AL Bypass Right Popliteal Artery to Popliteal Artery with Autologous Arterial Tissue, Percutaneous Endoscopic Approach

041M4AM Bypass Right Popliteal Artery to Peroneal Artery with Autologous Arterial Tissue, Percutaneous Endoscopic Approach

041M4AP Bypass Right Popliteal Artery to Foot Artery with Autologous Arterial Tissue, Percutaneous Endoscopic Approach

041M4AQ Bypass Right Popliteal Artery to Lower Extremity Artery with Autologous Arterial Tissue, Percutaneous Endoscopic Approach

041M4AS Bypass Right Popliteal Artery to Lower Extremity Vein with Autologous Arterial Tissue, Percutaneous Endoscopic Approach

041M4JL Bypass Right Popliteal Artery to Popliteal Artery with Synthetic Substitute, Percutaneous Endoscopic Approach

041M4JM Bypass Right Popliteal Artery to Peroneal Artery with Synthetic Substitute, Percutaneous Endoscopic Approach

041M4JP Bypass Right Popliteal Artery to Foot Artery with Synthetic Substitute, Percutaneous Endoscopic Approach

041M4JQ Bypass Right Popliteal Artery to Lower Extremity Artery with Synthetic Substitute, Percutaneous Endoscopic Approach

041M4JS Bypass Right Popliteal Artery to Lower Extremity Vein with Synthetic Substitute, Percutaneous Endoscopic Approach

041M4KL Bypass Right Popliteal Artery to Popliteal Artery with Nonautologous Tissue Substitute, Percutaneous Endoscopic Approach

041M4KM Bypass Right Popliteal Artery to Peroneal Artery with Nonautologous Tissue Substitute, Percutaneous Endoscopic Approach

041M4KP Bypass Right Popliteal Artery to Foot Artery with Nonautologous Tissue Substitute, Percutaneous Endoscopic Approach

041M4KQ Bypass Right Popliteal Artery to Lower Extremity Artery with Nonautologous Tissue Substitute, Percutaneous Endoscopic Approach

041M4KS Bypass Right Popliteal Artery to Lower Extremity Vein with Nonautologous Tissue Substitute, Percutaneous Endoscopic Approach

041M4ZL Bypass Right Popliteal Artery to Popliteal Artery, Percutaneous Endoscopic Approach

041M4ZM Bypass Right Popliteal Artery to Peroneal Artery, Percutaneous Endoscopic Approach

041M4ZP Bypass Right Popliteal Artery to Foot Artery, Percutaneous Endoscopic Approach

041M4ZQ Bypass Right Popliteal Artery to Lower Extremity Artery, Percutaneous Endoscopic Approach

041M4ZS Bypass Right Popliteal Artery to Lower Extremity Vein, Percutaneous Endoscopic Approach

041N09L Bypass Left Popliteal Artery to Popliteal Artery with Autologous Venous Tissue, Open Approach

041N09M Bypass Left Popliteal Artery to Peroneal Artery with Autologous Venous Tissue, Open Approach

041N09P Bypass Left Popliteal Artery to Foot Artery with Autologous Venous Tissue, Open Approach

041N09Q Bypass Left Popliteal Artery to Lower Extremity Artery with Autologous Venous Tissue, Open Approach

041N09S Bypass Left Popliteal Artery to Lower Extremity Vein with Autologous Venous Tissue, Open Approach

041N0AL	Bypass Left Popliteal Artery to Popliteal Artery with Autologous Arterial Tissue, Open Approach
041N0AM	Bypass Left Popliteal Artery to Peroneal Artery with Autologous Arterial Tissue, Open Approach
041N0AP	Bypass Left Popliteal Artery to Foot Artery with Autologous Arterial Tissue, Open Approach
041N0AQ	Bypass Left Popliteal Artery to Lower Extremity Artery with Autologous Arterial Tissue, Open Approach
041N0AS	Bypass Left Popliteal Artery to Lower Extremity Vein with Autologous Arterial Tissue, Open Approach
041N0JL	Bypass Left Popliteal Artery to Popliteal Artery with Synthetic Substitute, Open Approach
041N0JM	Bypass Left Popliteal Artery to Peroneal Artery with Synthetic Substitute, Open Approach
041N0JP	Bypass Left Popliteal Artery to Foot Artery with Synthetic Substitute, Open Approach
041N0JQ	Bypass Left Popliteal Artery to Lower Extremity Artery with Synthetic Substitute, Open Approach
041N0JS	Bypass Left Popliteal Artery to Lower Extremity Vein with Synthetic Substitute, Open Approach
041N0KL	Bypass Left Popliteal Artery to Popliteal Artery with Nonautologous Tissue Substitute, Open Approach
041N0KM	Bypass Left Popliteal Artery to Peroneal Artery with Nonautologous Tissue Substitute, Open Approach
041N0KP	Bypass Left Popliteal Artery to Foot Artery with Nonautologous Tissue Substitute, Open Approach
041N0KQ	Bypass Left Popliteal Artery to Lower Extremity Artery with Nonautologous Tissue Substitute, Open Approach
041N0KS	Bypass Left Popliteal Artery to Lower Extremity Vein with Nonautologous Tissue Substitute, Open Approach
041N0ZL	Bypass Left Popliteal Artery to Popliteal Artery, Open Approach
041N0ZM	Bypass Left Popliteal Artery to Peroneal Artery, Open Approach
041N0ZP	Bypass Left Popliteal Artery to Foot Artery, Open Approach
041N0ZQ	Bypass Left Popliteal Artery to Lower Extremity Artery, Open Approach
041N0ZS	Bypass Left Popliteal Artery to Lower Extremity Vein, Open Approach
041N49L	Bypass Left Popliteal Artery to Popliteal Artery with Autologous Venous Tissue, Percutaneous Endoscopic Approach
041N49M	Bypass Left Popliteal Artery to Peroneal Artery with Autologous Venous Tissue, Percutaneous Endoscopic Approach
041N49P	Bypass Left Popliteal Artery to Foot Artery with Autologous Venous Tissue, Percutaneous Endoscopic Approach
041N49Q	Bypass Left Popliteal Artery to Lower Extremity Artery with Autologous Venous Tissue, Percutaneous Endoscopic Approach

041N49S	Bypass Left Popliteal Artery to Lower Extremity Vein with Autologous Venous Tissue, Percutaneous Endoscopic Approach
041N4AL	Bypass Left Popliteal Artery to Popliteal Artery with Autologous Arterial Tissue, Percutaneous Endoscopic Approach
041N4AM	Bypass Left Popliteal Artery to Peroneal Artery with Autologous Arterial Tissue, Percutaneous Endoscopic Approach
041N4AP	Bypass Left Popliteal Artery to Foot Artery with Autologous Arterial Tissue, Percutaneous Endoscopic Approach
041N4AQ	Bypass Left Popliteal Artery to Lower Extremity Artery with Autologous Arterial Tissue, Percutaneous Endoscopic Approach
041N4AS	Bypass Left Popliteal Artery to Lower Extremity Vein with Autologous Arterial Tissue, Percutaneous Endoscopic Approach
041N4JL	Bypass Left Popliteal Artery to Popliteal Artery with Synthetic Substitute, Percutaneous Endoscopic Approach
041N4JM	Bypass Left Popliteal Artery to Peroneal Artery with Synthetic Substitute, Percutaneous Endoscopic Approach
041N4JP	Bypass Left Popliteal Artery to Foot Artery with Synthetic Substitute, Percutaneous Endoscopic Approach
041N4JQ	Bypass Left Popliteal Artery to Lower Extremity Artery with Synthetic Substitute, Percutaneous Endoscopic Approach
041N4JS	Bypass Left Popliteal Artery to Lower Extremity Vein with Synthetic Substitute, Percutaneous Endoscopic Approach
041N4KL	Bypass Left Popliteal Artery to Popliteal Artery with Nonautologous Tissue Substitute, Percutaneous Endoscopic Approach
041N4KM	Bypass Left Popliteal Artery to Peroneal Artery with Nonautologous Tissue Substitute, Percutaneous Endoscopic Approach
041N4KP	Bypass Left Popliteal Artery to Foot Artery with Nonautologous Tissue Substitute, Percutaneous Endoscopic Approach
041N4KQ	Bypass Left Popliteal Artery to Lower Extremity Artery with Nonautologous Tissue Substitute, Percutaneous Endoscopic Approach
041N4KS	Bypass Left Popliteal Artery to Lower Extremity Vein with Nonautologous Tissue Substitute, Percutaneous Endoscopic Approach
041N4ZL	Bypass Left Popliteal Artery to Popliteal Artery, Percutaneous Endoscopic Approach
041N4ZM	Bypass Left Popliteal Artery to Peroneal Artery, Percutaneous Endoscopic Approach
041N4ZP	Bypass Left Popliteal Artery to Foot Artery, Percutaneous Endoscopic Approach
041N4ZQ	Bypass Left Popliteal Artery to Lower Extremity Artery, Percutaneous Endoscopic Approach
041N4ZS	Bypass Left Popliteal Artery to Lower Extremity Vein, Percutaneous Endoscopic Approach

045 – Lower Arteries, Destruction

04500ZZ	Destruction of Abdominal Aorta, Open Approach
04503ZZ	Destruction of Abdominal Aorta, Percutaneous Approach
04504ZZ	Destruction of Abdominal Aorta, Percutaneous Endoscopic Approach
04510ZZ	Destruction of Celiac Artery, Open Approach
04513ZZ	Destruction of Celiac Artery, Percutaneous Approach
04514ZZ	Destruction of Celiac Artery, Percutaneous Endoscopic Approach
04520ZZ	Destruction of Gastric Artery, Open Approach
04523ZZ	Destruction of Gastric Artery, Percutaneous Approach
04524ZZ	Destruction of Gastric Artery, Percutaneous Endoscopic Approach
04530ZZ	Destruction of Hepatic Artery, Open Approach
04533ZZ	Destruction of Hepatic Artery, Percutaneous Approach
04534ZZ	Destruction of Hepatic Artery, Percutaneous Endoscopic Approach
04540ZZ	Destruction of Splenic Artery, Open Approach
04543ZZ	Destruction of Splenic Artery, Percutaneous Approach
04544ZZ	Destruction of Splenic Artery, Percutaneous Endoscopic Approach
04550ZZ	Destruction of Superior Mesenteric Artery, Open Approach
04553ZZ	Destruction of Superior Mesenteric Artery, Percutaneous Approach
04554ZZ	Destruction of Superior Mesenteric Artery, Percutaneous Endoscopic Approach
04560ZZ	Destruction of Right Colic Artery, Open Approach
04563ZZ	Destruction of Right Colic Artery, Percutaneous Approach
04564ZZ	Destruction of Right Colic Artery, Percutaneous Endoscopic Approach
04570ZZ	Destruction of Left Colic Artery, Open Approach

04573ZZ	Destruction of Left Colic Artery, Percutaneous Approach
04574ZZ	Destruction of Left Colic Artery, Percutaneous Endoscopic Approach
04580ZZ	Destruction of Middle Colic Artery, Open Approach
04583ZZ	Destruction of Middle Colic Artery, Percutaneous Approach
04584ZZ	Destruction of Middle Colic Artery, Percutaneous Endoscopic Approach
04590ZZ	Destruction of Right Renal Artery, Open Approach
04593ZZ	Destruction of Right Renal Artery, Percutaneous Approach
04594ZZ	Destruction of Right Renal Artery, Percutaneous Endoscopic Approach
045A0ZZ	Destruction of Left Renal Artery, Open Approach
045A3ZZ	Destruction of Left Renal Artery, Percutaneous Approach
045A4ZZ	Destruction of Left Renal Artery, Percutaneous Endoscopic Approach
045B0ZZ	Destruction of Inferior Mesenteric Artery, Open Approach
045B3ZZ	Destruction of Inferior Mesenteric Artery, Percutaneous Approach
045B4ZZ	Destruction of Inferior Mesenteric Artery, Percutaneous Endoscopic Approach
045C0ZZ	Destruction of Right Common Iliac Artery, Open Approach
045C3ZZ	Destruction of Right Common Iliac Artery, Percutaneous Approach
045C4ZZ	Destruction of Right Common Iliac Artery, Percutaneous Endoscopic Approach
045D0ZZ	Destruction of Left Common Iliac Artery, Open Approach
045D3ZZ	Destruction of Left Common Iliac Artery, Percutaneous Approach

045D4ZZ	Destruction of Left Common Iliac Artery, Percutaneous Endoscopic Approach
045E0ZZ	Destruction of Right Internal Iliac Artery, Open Approach
045E3ZZ	Destruction of Right Internal Iliac Artery, Percutaneous Approach
045E4ZZ	Destruction of Right Internal Iliac Artery, Percutaneous Endoscopic Approach
045F0ZZ	Destruction of Left Internal Iliac Artery, Open Approach
045F3ZZ	Destruction of Left Internal Iliac Artery, Percutaneous Approach
045F4ZZ	Destruction of Left Internal Iliac Artery, Percutaneous Endoscopic Approach
045H0ZZ	Destruction of Right External Iliac Artery, Open Approach
045H3ZZ	Destruction of Right External Iliac Artery, Percutaneous Approach
045H4ZZ	Destruction of Right External Iliac Artery, Percutaneous Endoscopic Approach
045J0ZZ	Destruction of Left External Iliac Artery, Open Approach
045J3ZZ	Destruction of Left External Iliac Artery, Percutaneous Approach
045J4ZZ	Destruction of Left External Iliac Artery, Percutaneous Endoscopic Approach
045K0ZZ	Destruction of Right Femoral Artery, Open Approach
045K3ZZ	Destruction of Right Femoral Artery, Percutaneous Approach
045K4ZZ	Destruction of Right Femoral Artery, Percutaneous Endoscopic Approach
045L0ZZ	Destruction of Left Femoral Artery, Open Approach
045L3ZZ	Destruction of Left Femoral Artery, Percutaneous Approach
045L4ZZ	Destruction of Left Femoral Artery, Percutaneous Endoscopic Approach
045M0ZZ	Destruction of Right Popliteal Artery, Open Approach
045M3ZZ	Destruction of Right Popliteal Artery, Percutaneous Approach
045M4ZZ	Destruction of Right Popliteal Artery, Percutaneous Endoscopic Approach
045N0ZZ	Destruction of Left Popliteal Artery, Open Approach
045N3ZZ	Destruction of Left Popliteal Artery, Percutaneous Approach
045N4ZZ	Destruction of Left Popliteal Artery, Percutaneous Endoscopic Approach

045P0ZZ	Destruction of Right Anterior Tibial Artery, Open Approach
045P3ZZ	Destruction of Right Anterior Tibial Artery, Percutaneous Approach
045P4ZZ	Destruction of Right Anterior Tibial Artery, Percutaneous Endoscopic Approach
045Q0ZZ	Destruction of Left Anterior Tibial Artery, Open Approach
045Q3ZZ	Destruction of Left Anterior Tibial Artery, Percutaneous Approach
045Q4ZZ	Destruction of Left Anterior Tibial Artery, Percutaneous Endoscopic Approach
045R0ZZ	Destruction of Right Posterior Tibial Artery, Open Approach
045R3ZZ	Destruction of Right Posterior Tibial Artery, Percutaneous Approach
045R4ZZ	Destruction of Right Posterior Tibial Artery, Percutaneous Endoscopic Approach
045S0ZZ	Destruction of Left Posterior Tibial Artery, Open Approach
045S3ZZ	Destruction of Left Posterior Tibial Artery, Percutaneous Approach
045S4ZZ	Destruction of Left Posterior Tibial Artery, Percutaneous Endoscopic Approach
045T0ZZ	Destruction of Right Peroneal Artery, Open Approach
045T3ZZ	Destruction of Right Peroneal Artery, Percutaneous Approach
045T4ZZ	Destruction of Right Peroneal Artery, Percutaneous Endoscopic Approach
045U0ZZ	Destruction of Left Peroneal Artery, Open Approach
045U3ZZ	Destruction of Left Peroneal Artery, Percutaneous Approach
045U4ZZ	Destruction of Left Peroneal Artery, Percutaneous Endoscopic Approach
045V0ZZ	Destruction of Right Foot Artery, Open Approach
045V3ZZ	Destruction of Right Foot Artery, Percutaneous Approach
045V4ZZ	Destruction of Right Foot Artery, Percutaneous Endoscopic Approach
045W0ZZ	Destruction of Left Foot Artery, Open Approach
045W3ZZ	Destruction of Left Foot Artery, Percutaneous Approach
045W4ZZ	Destruction of Left Foot Artery, Percutaneous Endoscopic Approach
045Y0ZZ	Destruction of Lower Artery, Open Approach
045Y3ZZ	Destruction of Lower Artery, Percutaneous Approach
045Y4ZZ	Destruction of Lower Artery, Percutaneous Endoscopic Approach

047 – Lower Arteries, Dilation

047004Z	Dilation of Abdominal Aorta with Drug-eluting Intraluminal Device, Open Approach
04700DZ	Dilation of Abdominal Aorta with Intraluminal Device, Open Approach
04700ZZ	Dilation of Abdominal Aorta, Open Approach
047034Z	Dilation of Abdominal Aorta with Drug-eluting Intraluminal Device, Percutaneous Approach
04703DZ	Dilation of Abdominal Aorta with Intraluminal Device, Percutaneous Approach
04703ZZ	Dilation of Abdominal Aorta, Percutaneous Approach
047044Z	Dilation of Abdominal Aorta with Drug-eluting Intraluminal Device, Percutaneous Endoscopic Approach
04704DZ	Dilation of Abdominal Aorta with Intraluminal Device, Percutaneous Endoscopic Approach
04704ZZ	Dilation of Abdominal Aorta, Percutaneous Endoscopic Approach
047104Z	Dilation of Celiac Artery with Drug-eluting Intraluminal Device, Open Approach
04710DZ	Dilation of Celiac Artery with Intraluminal Device, Open Approach
04710ZZ	Dilation of Celiac Artery, Open Approach
047134Z	Dilation of Celiac Artery with Drug-eluting Intraluminal Device, Percutaneous Approach
04713DZ	Dilation of Celiac Artery with Intraluminal Device, Percutaneous Approach
04713ZZ	Dilation of Celiac Artery, Percutaneous Approach
047144Z	Dilation of Celiac Artery with Drug-eluting Intraluminal Device, Percutaneous Endoscopic Approach
04714DZ	Dilation of Celiac Artery with Intraluminal Device, Percutaneous Endoscopic Approach
04714ZZ	Dilation of Celiac Artery, Percutaneous Endoscopic Approach
047204Z	Dilation of Gastric Artery with Drug-eluting Intraluminal Device, Open Approach
04720DZ	Dilation of Gastric Artery with Intraluminal Device, Open Approach
04720ZZ	Dilation of Gastric Artery, Open Approach
047234Z	Dilation of Gastric Artery with Drug-eluting Intraluminal Device, Percutaneous Approach

04723DZ	Dilation of Gastric Artery with Intraluminal Device, Percutaneous Approach
04723ZZ	Dilation of Gastric Artery, Percutaneous Approach
047244Z	Dilation of Gastric Artery with Drug-eluting Intraluminal Device, Percutaneous Endoscopic Approach
04724DZ	Dilation of Gastric Artery with Intraluminal Device, Percutaneous Endoscopic Approach
04724ZZ	Dilation of Gastric Artery, Percutaneous Endoscopic Approach
047304Z	Dilation of Hepatic Artery with Drug-eluting Intraluminal Device, Open Approach
04730DZ	Dilation of Hepatic Artery with Intraluminal Device, Open Approach
04730ZZ	Dilation of Hepatic Artery, Open Approach
047334Z	Dilation of Hepatic Artery with Drug-eluting Intraluminal Device, Percutaneous Approach
04733DZ	Dilation of Hepatic Artery with Intraluminal Device, Percutaneous Approach
04733ZZ	Dilation of Hepatic Artery, Percutaneous Approach
047344Z	Dilation of Hepatic Artery with Drug-eluting Intraluminal Device, Percutaneous Endoscopic Approach
04734DZ	Dilation of Hepatic Artery with Intraluminal Device, Percutaneous Endoscopic Approach
04734ZZ	Dilation of Hepatic Artery, Percutaneous Endoscopic Approach
047404Z	Dilation of Splenic Artery with Drug-eluting Intraluminal Device, Open Approach
04740DZ	Dilation of Splenic Artery with Intraluminal Device, Open Approach
04740ZZ	Dilation of Splenic Artery, Open Approach
047434Z	Dilation of Splenic Artery with Drug-eluting Intraluminal Device, Percutaneous Approach
04743DZ	Dilation of Splenic Artery with Intraluminal Device, Percutaneous Approach
04743ZZ	Dilation of Splenic Artery, Percutaneous Approach
047444Z	Dilation of Splenic Artery with Drug-eluting Intraluminal Device, Percutaneous Endoscopic Approach

---

♀ Female-only   ♂ Male-only   ⬤ Limited Coverage   ● Non-OR   ▰▰▰ HAC-associated procedure   ⬤ Non-covered procedures   ➕ Combination

04744DZ Dilation of Splenic Artery with Intraluminal Device, Percutaneous Endoscopic Approach

04744ZZ Dilation of Splenic Artery, Percutaneous Endoscopic Approach

047504Z Dilation of Superior Mesenteric Artery with Drug-eluting Intraluminal Device, Open Approach

04750DZ Dilation of Superior Mesenteric Artery with Intraluminal Device, Open Approach

04750ZZ Dilation of Superior Mesenteric Artery, Open Approach

047534Z Dilation of Superior Mesenteric Artery with Drug-eluting Intraluminal Device, Percutaneous Approach

04753DZ Dilation of Superior Mesenteric Artery with Intraluminal Device, Percutaneous Approach

04753ZZ Dilation of Superior Mesenteric Artery, Percutaneous Approach

047544Z Dilation of Superior Mesenteric Artery with Drug-eluting Intraluminal Device, Percutaneous Endoscopic Approach

04754DZ Dilation of Superior Mesenteric Artery with Intraluminal Device, Percutaneous Endoscopic Approach

04754ZZ Dilation of Superior Mesenteric Artery, Percutaneous Endoscopic Approach

047604Z Dilation of Right Colic Artery with Drug-eluting Intraluminal Device, Open Approach

04760DZ Dilation of Right Colic Artery with Intraluminal Device, Open Approach

04760ZZ Dilation of Right Colic Artery, Open Approach

047634Z Dilation of Right Colic Artery with Drug-eluting Intraluminal Device, Percutaneous Approach

04763DZ Dilation of Right Colic Artery with Intraluminal Device, Percutaneous Approach

04763ZZ Dilation of Right Colic Artery, Percutaneous Approach

047644Z Dilation of Right Colic Artery with Drug-eluting Intraluminal Device, Percutaneous Endoscopic Approach

04764DZ Dilation of Right Colic Artery with Intraluminal Device, Percutaneous Endoscopic Approach

04764ZZ Dilation of Right Colic Artery, Percutaneous Endoscopic Approach

047704Z Dilation of Left Colic Artery with Drug-eluting Intraluminal Device, Open Approach

04770DZ Dilation of Left Colic Artery with Intraluminal Device, Open Approach

04770ZZ Dilation of Left Colic Artery, Open Approach

047734Z Dilation of Left Colic Artery with Drug-eluting Intraluminal Device, Percutaneous Approach

04773DZ Dilation of Left Colic Artery with Intraluminal Device, Percutaneous Approach

04773ZZ Dilation of Left Colic Artery, Percutaneous Approach

047744Z Dilation of Left Colic Artery with Drug-eluting Intraluminal Device, Percutaneous Endoscopic Approach

04774DZ Dilation of Left Colic Artery with Intraluminal Device, Percutaneous Endoscopic Approach

04774ZZ Dilation of Left Colic Artery, Percutaneous Endoscopic Approach

047804Z Dilation of Middle Colic Artery with Drug-eluting Intraluminal Device, Open Approach

04780DZ Dilation of Middle Colic Artery with Intraluminal Device, Open Approach

04780ZZ Dilation of Middle Colic Artery, Open Approach

047834Z Dilation of Middle Colic Artery with Drug-eluting Intraluminal Device, Percutaneous Approach

04783DZ Dilation of Middle Colic Artery with Intraluminal Device, Percutaneous Approach

04783ZZ Dilation of Middle Colic Artery, Percutaneous Approach

047844Z Dilation of Middle Colic Artery with Drug-eluting Intraluminal Device, Percutaneous Endoscopic Approach

04784DZ Dilation of Middle Colic Artery with Intraluminal Device, Percutaneous Endoscopic Approach

04784ZZ Dilation of Middle Colic Artery, Percutaneous Endoscopic Approach

047904Z Dilation of Right Renal Artery with Drug-eluting Intraluminal Device, Open Approach

04790DZ Dilation of Right Renal Artery with Intraluminal Device, Open Approach

04790ZZ Dilation of Right Renal Artery, Open Approach

047934Z Dilation of Right Renal Artery with Drug-eluting Intraluminal Device, Percutaneous Approach

04793DZ Dilation of Right Renal Artery with Intraluminal Device, Percutaneous Approach

04793ZZ Dilation of Right Renal Artery, Percutaneous Approach

047944Z Dilation of Right Renal Artery with Drug-eluting Intraluminal Device, Percutaneous Endoscopic Approach

04794DZ Dilation of Right Renal Artery with Intraluminal Device, Percutaneous Endoscopic Approach

04794ZZ Dilation of Right Renal Artery, Percutaneous Endoscopic Approach

047A04Z Dilation of Left Renal Artery with Drug-eluting Intraluminal Device, Open Approach

047A0DZ Dilation of Left Renal Artery with Intraluminal Device, Open Approach

047A0ZZ Dilation of Left Renal Artery, Open Approach

047A34Z Dilation of Left Renal Artery with Drug-eluting Intraluminal Device, Percutaneous Approach

047A3DZ Dilation of Left Renal Artery with Intraluminal Device, Percutaneous Approach

047A3ZZ Dilation of Left Renal Artery, Percutaneous Approach

047A44Z Dilation of Left Renal Artery with Drug-eluting Intraluminal Device, Percutaneous Endoscopic Approach

047A4DZ Dilation of Left Renal Artery with Intraluminal Device, Percutaneous Endoscopic Approach

047A4ZZ Dilation of Left Renal Artery, Percutaneous Endoscopic Approach

047B04Z Dilation of Inferior Mesenteric Artery with Drug-eluting Intraluminal Device, Open Approach

047B0DZ Dilation of Inferior Mesenteric Artery with Intraluminal Device, Open Approach

047B0ZZ Dilation of Inferior Mesenteric Artery, Open Approach

047B34Z Dilation of Inferior Mesenteric Artery with Drug-eluting Intraluminal Device, Percutaneous Approach

047B3DZ Dilation of Inferior Mesenteric Artery with Intraluminal Device, Percutaneous Approach

047B3ZZ Dilation of Inferior Mesenteric Artery, Percutaneous Approach

047B44Z Dilation of Inferior Mesenteric Artery with Drug-eluting Intraluminal Device, Percutaneous Endoscopic Approach

047B4DZ Dilation of Inferior Mesenteric Artery with Intraluminal Device, Percutaneous Endoscopic Approach

047B4ZZ Dilation of Inferior Mesenteric Artery, Percutaneous Endoscopic Approach

047C04Z Dilation of Right Common Iliac Artery with Drug-eluting Intraluminal Device, Open Approach

047C0DZ Dilation of Right Common Iliac Artery with Intraluminal Device, Open Approach

047C0ZZ Dilation of Right Common Iliac Artery, Open Approach

047C34Z Dilation of Right Common Iliac Artery with Drug-eluting Intraluminal Device, Percutaneous Approach

047C3DZ Dilation of Right Common Iliac Artery with Intraluminal Device, Percutaneous Approach

047C3ZZ Dilation of Right Common Iliac Artery, Percutaneous Approach

047C44Z Dilation of Right Common Iliac Artery with Drug-eluting Intraluminal Device, Percutaneous Endoscopic Approach

047C4DZ Dilation of Right Common Iliac Artery with Intraluminal Device, Percutaneous Endoscopic Approach

047C4ZZ Dilation of Right Common Iliac Artery, Percutaneous Endoscopic Approach

047D04Z Dilation of Left Common Iliac Artery with Drug-eluting Intraluminal Device, Open Approach

047D0DZ Dilation of Left Common Iliac Artery with Intraluminal Device, Open Approach

047D0ZZ Dilation of Left Common Iliac Artery, Open Approach

047D34Z Dilation of Left Common Iliac Artery with Drug-eluting Intraluminal Device, Percutaneous Approach

047D3DZ Dilation of Left Common Iliac Artery with Intraluminal Device, Percutaneous Approach

047D3ZZ Dilation of Left Common Iliac Artery, Percutaneous Approach

047D44Z Dilation of Left Common Iliac Artery with Drug-eluting Intraluminal Device, Percutaneous Endoscopic Approach

047D4DZ Dilation of Left Common Iliac Artery with Intraluminal Device, Percutaneous Endoscopic Approach

047D4ZZ Dilation of Left Common Iliac Artery, Percutaneous Endoscopic Approach

047E04Z Dilation of Right Internal Iliac Artery with Drug-eluting Intraluminal Device, Open Approach

047E0DZ   Dilation of Right Internal Iliac Artery with Intraluminal Device, Open Approach

047E0ZZ   Dilation of Right Internal Iliac Artery, Open Approach

047E34Z   Dilation of Right Internal Iliac Artery with Drug-eluting Intraluminal Device, Percutaneous Approach

047E3DZ   Dilation of Right Internal Iliac Artery with Intraluminal Device, Percutaneous Approach

047E3ZZ   Dilation of Right Internal Iliac Artery, Percutaneous Approach

047E44Z   Dilation of Right Internal Iliac Artery with Drug-eluting Intraluminal Device, Percutaneous Endoscopic Approach

047E4DZ   Dilation of Right Internal Iliac Artery with Intraluminal Device, Percutaneous Endoscopic Approach

047E4ZZ   Dilation of Right Internal Iliac Artery, Percutaneous Endoscopic Approach

047F04Z   Dilation of Left Internal Iliac Artery with Drug-eluting Intraluminal Device, Open Approach

047F0DZ   Dilation of Left Internal Iliac Artery with Intraluminal Device, Open Approach

047F0ZZ   Dilation of Left Internal Iliac Artery, Open Approach

047F34Z   Dilation of Left Internal Iliac Artery with Drug-eluting Intraluminal Device, Percutaneous Approach

047F3DZ   Dilation of Left Internal Iliac Artery with Intraluminal Device, Percutaneous Approach

047F3ZZ   Dilation of Left Internal Iliac Artery, Percutaneous Approach

047F44Z   Dilation of Left Internal Iliac Artery with Drug-eluting Intraluminal Device, Percutaneous Endoscopic Approach

047F4DZ   Dilation of Left Internal Iliac Artery with Intraluminal Device, Percutaneous Endoscopic Approach

047F4ZZ   Dilation of Left Internal Iliac Artery, Percutaneous Endoscopic Approach

047H04Z   Dilation of Right External Iliac Artery with Drug-eluting Intraluminal Device, Open Approach

047H0DZ   Dilation of Right External Iliac Artery with Intraluminal Device, Open Approach

047H0ZZ   Dilation of Right External Iliac Artery, Open Approach

047H34Z   Dilation of Right External Iliac Artery with Drug-eluting Intraluminal Device, Percutaneous Approach

047H3DZ   Dilation of Right External Iliac Artery with Intraluminal Device, Percutaneous Approach

047H3ZZ   Dilation of Right External Iliac Artery, Percutaneous Approach

047H44Z   Dilation of Right External Iliac Artery with Drug-eluting Intraluminal Device, Percutaneous Endoscopic Approach

047H4DZ   Dilation of Right External Iliac Artery with Intraluminal Device, Percutaneous Endoscopic Approach

047H4ZZ   Dilation of Right External Iliac Artery, Percutaneous Endoscopic Approach

047J04Z   Dilation of Left External Iliac Artery with Drug-eluting Intraluminal Device, Open Approach

047J0DZ   Dilation of Left External Iliac Artery with Intraluminal Device, Open Approach

047J0ZZ   Dilation of Left External Iliac Artery, Open Approach

047J34Z   Dilation of Left External Iliac Artery with Drug-eluting Intraluminal Device, Percutaneous Approach

047J3DZ   Dilation of Left External Iliac Artery with Intraluminal Device, Percutaneous Approach

047J3ZZ   Dilation of Left External Iliac Artery, Percutaneous Approach

047J44Z   Dilation of Left External Iliac Artery with Drug-eluting Intraluminal Device, Percutaneous Endoscopic Approach

047J4DZ   Dilation of Left External Iliac Artery with Intraluminal Device, Percutaneous Endoscopic Approach

047J4ZZ   Dilation of Left External Iliac Artery, Percutaneous Endoscopic Approach

047K04Z   Dilation of Right Femoral Artery with Drug-eluting Intraluminal Device, Open Approach

047K0DZ   Dilation of Right Femoral Artery with Intraluminal Device, Open Approach

047K0ZZ   Dilation of Right Femoral Artery, Open Approach

047K34Z   Dilation of Right Femoral Artery with Drug-eluting Intraluminal Device, Percutaneous Approach

047K3DZ   Dilation of Right Femoral Artery with Intraluminal Device, Percutaneous Approach

047K3ZZ   Dilation of Right Femoral Artery, Percutaneous Approach

047K44Z   Dilation of Right Femoral Artery with Drug-eluting Intraluminal Device, Percutaneous Endoscopic Approach

047K4DZ   Dilation of Right Femoral Artery with Intraluminal Device, Percutaneous Endoscopic Approach

047K4ZZ   Dilation of Right Femoral Artery, Percutaneous Endoscopic Approach

047L04Z   Dilation of Left Femoral Artery with Drug-eluting Intraluminal Device, Open Approach

047L0DZ   Dilation of Left Femoral Artery with Intraluminal Device, Open Approach

047L0ZZ   Dilation of Left Femoral Artery, Open Approach

047L34Z   Dilation of Left Femoral Artery with Drug-eluting Intraluminal Device, Percutaneous Approach

047L3DZ   Dilation of Left Femoral Artery with Intraluminal Device, Percutaneous Approach

047L3ZZ   Dilation of Left Femoral Artery, Percutaneous Approach

047L44Z   Dilation of Left Femoral Artery with Drug-eluting Intraluminal Device, Percutaneous Endoscopic Approach

047L4DZ   Dilation of Left Femoral Artery with Intraluminal Device, Percutaneous Endoscopic Approach

047L4ZZ   Dilation of Left Femoral Artery, Percutaneous Endoscopic Approach

047M04Z   Dilation of Right Popliteal Artery with Drug-eluting Intraluminal Device, Open Approach

047M0DZ   Dilation of Right Popliteal Artery with Intraluminal Device, Open Approach

047M0ZZ   Dilation of Right Popliteal Artery, Open Approach

047M34Z   Dilation of Right Popliteal Artery with Drug-eluting Intraluminal Device, Percutaneous Approach

047M3DZ   Dilation of Right Popliteal Artery with Intraluminal Device, Percutaneous Approach

047M3ZZ   Dilation of Right Popliteal Artery, Percutaneous Approach

047M44Z   Dilation of Right Popliteal Artery with Drug-eluting Intraluminal Device, Percutaneous Endoscopic Approach

047M4DZ   Dilation of Right Popliteal Artery with Intraluminal Device, Percutaneous Endoscopic Approach

047M4ZZ   Dilation of Right Popliteal Artery, Percutaneous Endoscopic Approach

047N04Z   Dilation of Left Popliteal Artery with Drug-eluting Intraluminal Device, Open Approach

047N0DZ   Dilation of Left Popliteal Artery with Intraluminal Device, Open Approach

047N0ZZ   Dilation of Left Popliteal Artery, Open Approach

047N34Z   Dilation of Left Popliteal Artery with Drug-eluting Intraluminal Device, Percutaneous Approach

047N3DZ   Dilation of Left Popliteal Artery with Intraluminal Device, Percutaneous Approach

047N3ZZ   Dilation of Left Popliteal Artery, Percutaneous Approach

047N44Z   Dilation of Left Popliteal Artery with Drug-eluting Intraluminal Device, Percutaneous Endoscopic Approach

047N4DZ   Dilation of Left Popliteal Artery with Intraluminal Device, Percutaneous Endoscopic Approach

047N4ZZ   Dilation of Left Popliteal Artery, Percutaneous Endoscopic Approach

047P04Z   Dilation of Right Anterior Tibial Artery with Drug-eluting Intraluminal Device, Open Approach

047P0DZ   Dilation of Right Anterior Tibial Artery with Intraluminal Device, Open Approach

047P0ZZ   Dilation of Right Anterior Tibial Artery, Open Approach

047P34Z   Dilation of Right Anterior Tibial Artery with Drug-eluting Intraluminal Device, Percutaneous Approach

047P3DZ   Dilation of Right Anterior Tibial Artery with Intraluminal Device, Percutaneous Approach

047P3ZZ   Dilation of Right Anterior Tibial Artery, Percutaneous Approach

047P44Z   Dilation of Right Anterior Tibial Artery with Drug-eluting Intraluminal Device, Percutaneous Endoscopic Approach

047P4DZ   Dilation of Right Anterior Tibial Artery with Intraluminal Device, Percutaneous Endoscopic Approach

047P4ZZ   Dilation of Right Anterior Tibial Artery, Percutaneous Endoscopic Approach

047Q04Z   Dilation of Left Anterior Tibial Artery with Drug-eluting Intraluminal Device, Open Approach

---

047Q0DZ Dilation of Left Anterior Tibial Artery with Intraluminal Device, Open Approach

047Q0ZZ Dilation of Left Anterior Tibial Artery, Open Approach

047Q34Z Dilation of Left Anterior Tibial Artery with Drug-eluting Intraluminal Device, Percutaneous Approach

047Q3DZ Dilation of Left Anterior Tibial Artery with Intraluminal Device, Percutaneous Approach

047Q3ZZ Dilation of Left Anterior Tibial Artery, Percutaneous Approach

047Q44Z Dilation of Left Anterior Tibial Artery with Drug-eluting Intraluminal Device, Percutaneous Endoscopic Approach

047Q4DZ Dilation of Left Anterior Tibial Artery with Intraluminal Device, Percutaneous Endoscopic Approach

047Q4ZZ Dilation of Left Anterior Tibial Artery, Percutaneous Endoscopic Approach

047R04Z Dilation of Right Posterior Tibial Artery with Drug-eluting Intraluminal Device, Open Approach

047R0DZ Dilation of Right Posterior Tibial Artery with Intraluminal Device, Open Approach

047R0ZZ Dilation of Right Posterior Tibial Artery, Open Approach

047R34Z Dilation of Right Posterior Tibial Artery with Drug-eluting Intraluminal Device, Percutaneous Approach

047R3DZ Dilation of Right Posterior Tibial Artery with Intraluminal Device, Percutaneous Approach

047R3ZZ Dilation of Right Posterior Tibial Artery, Percutaneous Approach

047R44Z Dilation of Right Posterior Tibial Artery with Drug-eluting Intraluminal Device, Percutaneous Endoscopic Approach

047R4DZ Dilation of Right Posterior Tibial Artery with Intraluminal Device, Percutaneous Endoscopic Approach

047R4ZZ Dilation of Right Posterior Tibial Artery, Percutaneous Endoscopic Approach

047S04Z Dilation of Left Posterior Tibial Artery with Drug-eluting Intraluminal Device, Open Approach

047S0DZ Dilation of Left Posterior Tibial Artery with Intraluminal Device, Open Approach

047S0ZZ Dilation of Left Posterior Tibial Artery, Open Approach

047S34Z Dilation of Left Posterior Tibial Artery with Drug-eluting Intraluminal Device, Percutaneous Approach

047S3DZ Dilation of Left Posterior Tibial Artery with Intraluminal Device, Percutaneous Approach

047S3ZZ Dilation of Left Posterior Tibial Artery, Percutaneous Approach

047S44Z Dilation of Left Posterior Tibial Artery with Drug-eluting Intraluminal Device, Percutaneous Endoscopic Approach

047S4DZ Dilation of Left Posterior Tibial Artery with Intraluminal Device, Percutaneous Endoscopic Approach

047S4ZZ Dilation of Left Posterior Tibial Artery, Percutaneous Endoscopic Approach

047T04Z Dilation of Right Peroneal Artery with Drug-eluting Intraluminal Device, Open Approach

047T0DZ Dilation of Right Peroneal Artery with Intraluminal Device, Open Approach

047T0ZZ Dilation of Right Peroneal Artery, Open Approach

047T34Z Dilation of Right Peroneal Artery with Drug-eluting Intraluminal Device, Percutaneous Approach

047T3DZ Dilation of Right Peroneal Artery with Intraluminal Device, Percutaneous Approach

047T3ZZ Dilation of Right Peroneal Artery, Percutaneous Approach

047T44Z Dilation of Right Peroneal Artery with Drug-eluting Intraluminal Device, Percutaneous Endoscopic Approach

047T4DZ Dilation of Right Peroneal Artery with Intraluminal Device, Percutaneous Endoscopic Approach

047T4ZZ Dilation of Right Peroneal Artery, Percutaneous Endoscopic Approach

047U04Z Dilation of Left Peroneal Artery with Drug-eluting Intraluminal Device, Open Approach

047U0DZ Dilation of Left Peroneal Artery with Intraluminal Device, Open Approach

047U0ZZ Dilation of Left Peroneal Artery, Open Approach

047U34Z Dilation of Left Peroneal Artery with Drug-eluting Intraluminal Device, Percutaneous Approach

047U3DZ Dilation of Left Peroneal Artery with Intraluminal Device, Percutaneous Approach

047U3ZZ Dilation of Left Peroneal Artery, Percutaneous Approach

047U44Z Dilation of Left Peroneal Artery with Drug-eluting Intraluminal Device, Percutaneous Endoscopic Approach

047U4DZ Dilation of Left Peroneal Artery with Intraluminal Device, Percutaneous Endoscopic Approach

047U4ZZ Dilation of Left Peroneal Artery, Percutaneous Endoscopic Approach

047V04Z Dilation of Right Foot Artery with Drug-eluting Intraluminal Device, Open Approach

047V0DZ Dilation of Right Foot Artery with Intraluminal Device, Open Approach

047V0ZZ Dilation of Right Foot Artery, Open Approach

047V34Z Dilation of Right Foot Artery with Drug-eluting Intraluminal Device, Percutaneous Approach

047V3DZ Dilation of Right Foot Artery with Intraluminal Device, Percutaneous Approach

047V3ZZ Dilation of Right Foot Artery, Percutaneous Approach

047V44Z Dilation of Right Foot Artery with Drug-eluting Intraluminal Device, Percutaneous Endoscopic Approach

047V4DZ Dilation of Right Foot Artery with Intraluminal Device, Percutaneous Endoscopic Approach

047V4ZZ Dilation of Right Foot Artery, Percutaneous Endoscopic Approach

047W04Z Dilation of Left Foot Artery with Drug-eluting Intraluminal Device, Open Approach

047W0DZ Dilation of Left Foot Artery with Intraluminal Device, Open Approach

047W0ZZ Dilation of Left Foot Artery, Open Approach

047W34Z Dilation of Left Foot Artery with Drug-eluting Intraluminal Device, Percutaneous Approach

047W3DZ Dilation of Left Foot Artery with Intraluminal Device, Percutaneous Approach

047W3ZZ Dilation of Left Foot Artery, Percutaneous Approach

047W44Z Dilation of Left Foot Artery with Drug-eluting Intraluminal Device, Percutaneous Endoscopic Approach

047W4DZ Dilation of Left Foot Artery with Intraluminal Device, Percutaneous Endoscopic Approach

047W4ZZ Dilation of Left Foot Artery, Percutaneous Endoscopic Approach

047Y04Z Dilation of Lower Artery with Drug-eluting Intraluminal Device, Open Approach

047Y0DZ Dilation of Lower Artery with Intraluminal Device, Open Approach

047Y0ZZ Dilation of Lower Artery, Open Approach

047Y34Z Dilation of Lower Artery with Drug-eluting Intraluminal Device, Percutaneous Approach

047Y3DZ Dilation of Lower Artery with Intraluminal Device, Percutaneous Approach

047Y3ZZ Dilation of Lower Artery, Percutaneous Approach

047Y44Z Dilation of Lower Artery with Drug-eluting Intraluminal Device, Percutaneous Endoscopic Approach

047Y4DZ Dilation of Lower Artery with Intraluminal Device, Percutaneous Endoscopic Approach

047Y4ZZ Dilation of Lower Artery, Percutaneous Endoscopic Approach

049 – Lower Arteries, Drainage

Review Coding Guidelines B3.4a and B3.4b

Review Coding Guideline B6.2

049000Z Drainage of Abdominal Aorta with Drainage Device, Open Approach

04900ZX Drainage of Abdominal Aorta, Open Approach, Diagnostic

04900ZZ Drainage of Abdominal Aorta, Open Approach

049030Z Drainage of Abdominal Aorta with Drainage Device, Percutaneous Approach

04903ZX Drainage of Abdominal Aorta, Percutaneous Approach, Diagnostic

04903ZZ Drainage of Abdominal Aorta, Percutaneous Approach

049040Z   Drainage of Abdominal Aorta with Drainage Device, Percutaneous Endoscopic Approach
04904ZX   Drainage of Abdominal Aorta, Percutaneous Endoscopic Approach, Diagnostic
04904ZZ   Drainage of Abdominal Aorta, Percutaneous Endoscopic Approach
049100Z   Drainage of Celiac Artery with Drainage Device, Open Approach
04910ZX   Drainage of Celiac Artery, Open Approach, Diagnostic
04910ZZ   Drainage of Celiac Artery, Open Approach
049130Z   Drainage of Celiac Artery with Drainage Device, Percutaneous Approach
04913ZX   Drainage of Celiac Artery, Percutaneous Approach, Diagnostic
04913ZZ   Drainage of Celiac Artery, Percutaneous Approach
049140Z   Drainage of Celiac Artery with Drainage Device, Percutaneous Endoscopic Approach
04914ZX   Drainage of Celiac Artery, Percutaneous Endoscopic Approach, Diagnostic
04914ZZ   Drainage of Celiac Artery, Percutaneous Endoscopic Approach
049200Z   Drainage of Gastric Artery with Drainage Device, Open Approach
04920ZX   Drainage of Gastric Artery, Open Approach, Diagnostic
04920ZZ   Drainage of Gastric Artery, Open Approach
049230Z   Drainage of Gastric Artery with Drainage Device, Percutaneous Approach
04923ZX   Drainage of Gastric Artery, Percutaneous Approach, Diagnostic
04923ZZ   Drainage of Gastric Artery, Percutaneous Approach
049240Z   Drainage of Gastric Artery with Drainage Device, Percutaneous Endoscopic Approach
04924ZX   Drainage of Gastric Artery, Percutaneous Endoscopic Approach, Diagnostic
04924ZZ   Drainage of Gastric Artery, Percutaneous Endoscopic Approach
049300Z   Drainage of Hepatic Artery with Drainage Device, Open Approach
04930ZX   Drainage of Hepatic Artery, Open Approach, Diagnostic
04930ZZ   Drainage of Hepatic Artery, Open Approach
049330Z   Drainage of Hepatic Artery with Drainage Device, Percutaneous Approach
04933ZX   Drainage of Hepatic Artery, Percutaneous Approach, Diagnostic
04933ZZ   Drainage of Hepatic Artery, Percutaneous Approach
049340Z   Drainage of Hepatic Artery with Drainage Device, Percutaneous Endoscopic Approach
04934ZX   Drainage of Hepatic Artery, Percutaneous Endoscopic Approach, Diagnostic
04934ZZ   Drainage of Hepatic Artery, Percutaneous Endoscopic Approach
049400Z   Drainage of Splenic Artery with Drainage Device, Open Approach
04940ZX   Drainage of Splenic Artery, Open Approach, Diagnostic
04940ZZ   Drainage of Splenic Artery, Open Approach
049430Z   Drainage of Splenic Artery with Drainage Device, Percutaneous Approach
04943ZX   Drainage of Splenic Artery, Percutaneous Approach, Diagnostic
04943ZZ   Drainage of Splenic Artery, Percutaneous Approach
049440Z   Drainage of Splenic Artery with Drainage Device, Percutaneous Endoscopic Approach
04944ZX   Drainage of Splenic Artery, Percutaneous Endoscopic Approach, Diagnostic
04944ZZ   Drainage of Splenic Artery, Percutaneous Endoscopic Approach
049500Z   Drainage of Superior Mesenteric Artery with Drainage Device, Open Approach
04950ZX   Drainage of Superior Mesenteric Artery, Open Approach, Diagnostic
04950ZZ   Drainage of Superior Mesenteric Artery, Open Approach
049530Z   Drainage of Superior Mesenteric Artery with Drainage Device, Percutaneous Approach
04953ZX   Drainage of Superior Mesenteric Artery, Percutaneous Approach, Diagnostic
04953ZZ   Drainage of Superior Mesenteric Artery, Percutaneous Approach
049540Z   Drainage of Superior Mesenteric Artery with Drainage Device, Percutaneous Endoscopic Approach
04954ZX   Drainage of Superior Mesenteric Artery, Percutaneous Endoscopic Approach, Diagnostic
04954ZZ   Drainage of Superior Mesenteric Artery, Percutaneous Endoscopic Approach
049600Z   Drainage of Right Colic Artery with Drainage Device, Open Approach
04960ZX   Drainage of Right Colic Artery, Open Approach, Diagnostic
04960ZZ   Drainage of Right Colic Artery, Open Approach
049630Z   Drainage of Right Colic Artery with Drainage Device, Percutaneous Approach
04963ZX   Drainage of Right Colic Artery, Percutaneous Approach, Diagnostic
04963ZZ   Drainage of Right Colic Artery, Percutaneous Approach
049640Z   Drainage of Right Colic Artery with Drainage Device, Percutaneous Endoscopic Approach
04964ZX   Drainage of Right Colic Artery, Percutaneous Endoscopic Approach, Diagnostic
04964ZZ   Drainage of Right Colic Artery, Percutaneous Endoscopic Approach
049700Z   Drainage of Left Colic Artery with Drainage Device, Open Approach
04970ZX   Drainage of Left Colic Artery, Open Approach, Diagnostic
04970ZZ   Drainage of Left Colic Artery, Open Approach
049730Z   Drainage of Left Colic Artery with Drainage Device, Percutaneous Approach
04973ZX   Drainage of Left Colic Artery, Percutaneous Approach, Diagnostic
04973ZZ   Drainage of Left Colic Artery, Percutaneous Approach
049740Z   Drainage of Left Colic Artery with Drainage Device, Percutaneous Endoscopic Approach
04974ZX   Drainage of Left Colic Artery, Percutaneous Endoscopic Approach, Diagnostic
04974ZZ   Drainage of Left Colic Artery, Percutaneous Endoscopic Approach
049800Z   Drainage of Middle Colic Artery with Drainage Device, Open Approach
04980ZX   Drainage of Middle Colic Artery, Open Approach, Diagnostic
04980ZZ   Drainage of Middle Colic Artery, Open Approach
049830Z   Drainage of Middle Colic Artery with Drainage Device, Percutaneous Approach
04983ZX   Drainage of Middle Colic Artery, Percutaneous Approach, Diagnostic
04983ZZ   Drainage of Middle Colic Artery, Percutaneous Approach
049840Z   Drainage of Middle Colic Artery with Drainage Device, Percutaneous Endoscopic Approach
04984ZX   Drainage of Middle Colic Artery, Percutaneous Endoscopic Approach, Diagnostic
04984ZZ   Drainage of Middle Colic Artery, Percutaneous Endoscopic Approach
049900Z   Drainage of Right Renal Artery with Drainage Device, Open Approach
04990ZX   Drainage of Right Renal Artery, Open Approach, Diagnostic
04990ZZ   Drainage of Right Renal Artery, Open Approach
049930Z   Drainage of Right Renal Artery with Drainage Device, Percutaneous Approach
04993ZX   Drainage of Right Renal Artery, Percutaneous Approach, Diagnostic
04993ZZ   Drainage of Right Renal Artery, Percutaneous Approach
049940Z   Drainage of Right Renal Artery with Drainage Device, Percutaneous Endoscopic Approach
04994ZX   Drainage of Right Renal Artery, Percutaneous Endoscopic Approach, Diagnostic
04994ZZ   Drainage of Right Renal Artery, Percutaneous Endoscopic Approach
049A00Z   Drainage of Left Renal Artery with Drainage Device, Open Approach
049A0ZX   Drainage of Left Renal Artery, Open Approach, Diagnostic
049A0ZZ   Drainage of Left Renal Artery, Open Approach
049A30Z   Drainage of Left Renal Artery with Drainage Device, Percutaneous Approach
049A3ZX   Drainage of Left Renal Artery, Percutaneous Approach, Diagnostic
049A3ZZ   Drainage of Left Renal Artery, Percutaneous Approach
049A40Z   Drainage of Left Renal Artery with Drainage Device, Percutaneous Endoscopic Approach
049A4ZX   Drainage of Left Renal Artery, Percutaneous Endoscopic Approach, Diagnostic
049A4ZZ   Drainage of Left Renal Artery, Percutaneous Endoscopic Approach
049B00Z   Drainage of Inferior Mesenteric Artery with Drainage Device, Open Approach
049B0ZX   Drainage of Inferior Mesenteric Artery, Open Approach, Diagnostic
049B0ZZ   Drainage of Inferior Mesenteric Artery, Open Approach
049B30Z   Drainage of Inferior Mesenteric Artery with Drainage Device, Percutaneous Approach
049B3ZX   Drainage of Inferior Mesenteric Artery, Percutaneous Approach, Diagnostic
049B3ZZ   Drainage of Inferior Mesenteric Artery, Percutaneous Approach

049B40Z Drainage of Inferior Mesenteric Artery with Drainage Device, Percutaneous Endoscopic Approach

049B4ZX Drainage of Inferior Mesenteric Artery, Percutaneous Endoscopic Approach, Diagnostic

049B4ZZ Drainage of Inferior Mesenteric Artery, Percutaneous Endoscopic Approach

049C00Z Drainage of Right Common Iliac Artery with Drainage Device, Open Approach

049C0ZX Drainage of Right Common Iliac Artery, Open Approach, Diagnostic

049C0ZZ Drainage of Right Common Iliac Artery, Open Approach

049C30Z Drainage of Right Common Iliac Artery with Drainage Device, Percutaneous Approach

049C3ZX Drainage of Right Common Iliac Artery, Percutaneous Approach, Diagnostic

049C3ZZ Drainage of Right Common Iliac Artery, Percutaneous Approach

049C40Z Drainage of Right Common Iliac Artery with Drainage Device, Percutaneous Endoscopic Approach

049C4ZX Drainage of Right Common Iliac Artery, Percutaneous Endoscopic Approach, Diagnostic

049C4ZZ Drainage of Right Common Iliac Artery, Percutaneous Endoscopic Approach

049D00Z Drainage of Left Common Iliac Artery with Drainage Device, Open Approach

049D0ZX Drainage of Left Common Iliac Artery, Open Approach, Diagnostic

049D0ZZ Drainage of Left Common Iliac Artery, Open Approach

049D30Z Drainage of Left Common Iliac Artery with Drainage Device, Percutaneous Approach

049D3ZX Drainage of Left Common Iliac Artery, Percutaneous Approach, Diagnostic

049D3ZZ Drainage of Left Common Iliac Artery, Percutaneous Approach

049D40Z Drainage of Left Common Iliac Artery with Drainage Device, Percutaneous Endoscopic Approach

049D4ZX Drainage of Left Common Iliac Artery, Percutaneous Endoscopic Approach, Diagnostic

049D4ZZ Drainage of Left Common Iliac Artery, Percutaneous Endoscopic Approach

049E00Z Drainage of Right Internal Iliac Artery with Drainage Device, Open Approach

049E0ZX Drainage of Right Internal Iliac Artery, Open Approach, Diagnostic

049E0ZZ Drainage of Right Internal Iliac Artery, Open Approach

049E30Z Drainage of Right Internal Iliac Artery with Drainage Device, Percutaneous Approach

049E3ZX Drainage of Right Internal Iliac Artery, Percutaneous Approach, Diagnostic

049E3ZZ Drainage of Right Internal Iliac Artery, Percutaneous Approach

049E40Z Drainage of Right Internal Iliac Artery with Drainage Device, Percutaneous Endoscopic Approach

049E4ZX Drainage of Right Internal Iliac Artery, Percutaneous Endoscopic Approach, Diagnostic

049E4ZZ Drainage of Right Internal Iliac Artery, Percutaneous Endoscopic Approach

049F00Z Drainage of Left Internal Iliac Artery with Drainage Device, Open Approach

049F0ZX Drainage of Left Internal Iliac Artery, Open Approach, Diagnostic

049F0ZZ Drainage of Left Internal Iliac Artery, Open Approach

049F30Z Drainage of Left Internal Iliac Artery with Drainage Device, Percutaneous Approach

049F3ZX Drainage of Left Internal Iliac Artery, Percutaneous Approach, Diagnostic

049F3ZZ Drainage of Left Internal Iliac Artery, Percutaneous Approach

049F40Z Drainage of Left Internal Iliac Artery with Drainage Device, Percutaneous Endoscopic Approach

049F4ZX Drainage of Left Internal Iliac Artery, Percutaneous Endoscopic Approach, Diagnostic

049F4ZZ Drainage of Left Internal Iliac Artery, Percutaneous Endoscopic Approach

049H00Z Drainage of Right External Iliac Artery with Drainage Device, Open Approach

049H0ZX Drainage of Right External Iliac Artery, Open Approach, Diagnostic

049H0ZZ Drainage of Right External Iliac Artery, Open Approach

049H30Z Drainage of Right External Iliac Artery with Drainage Device, Percutaneous Approach

049H3ZX Drainage of Right External Iliac Artery, Percutaneous Approach, Diagnostic

049H3ZZ Drainage of Right External Iliac Artery, Percutaneous Approach

049H40Z Drainage of Right External Iliac Artery with Drainage Device, Percutaneous Endoscopic Approach

049H4ZX Drainage of Right External Iliac Artery, Percutaneous Endoscopic Approach, Diagnostic

049H4ZZ Drainage of Right External Iliac Artery, Percutaneous Endoscopic Approach

049J00Z Drainage of Left External Iliac Artery with Drainage Device, Open Approach

049J0ZX Drainage of Left External Iliac Artery, Open Approach, Diagnostic

049J0ZZ Drainage of Left External Iliac Artery, Open Approach

049J30Z Drainage of Left External Iliac Artery with Drainage Device, Percutaneous Approach

049J3ZX Drainage of Left External Iliac Artery, Percutaneous Approach, Diagnostic

049J3ZZ Drainage of Left External Iliac Artery, Percutaneous Approach

049J40Z Drainage of Left External Iliac Artery with Drainage Device, Percutaneous Endoscopic Approach

049J4ZX Drainage of Left External Iliac Artery, Percutaneous Endoscopic Approach, Diagnostic

049J4ZZ Drainage of Left External Iliac Artery, Percutaneous Endoscopic Approach

049K00Z Drainage of Right Femoral Artery with Drainage Device, Open Approach

049K0ZX Drainage of Right Femoral Artery, Open Approach, Diagnostic

049K0ZZ Drainage of Right Femoral Artery, Open Approach

049K30Z Drainage of Right Femoral Artery with Drainage Device, Percutaneous Approach

049K3ZX Drainage of Right Femoral Artery, Percutaneous Approach, Diagnostic

049K3ZZ Drainage of Right Femoral Artery, Percutaneous Approach

049K40Z Drainage of Right Femoral Artery with Drainage Device, Percutaneous Endoscopic Approach

049K4ZX Drainage of Right Femoral Artery, Percutaneous Endoscopic Approach, Diagnostic

049K4ZZ Drainage of Right Femoral Artery, Percutaneous Endoscopic Approach

049L00Z Drainage of Left Femoral Artery with Drainage Device, Open Approach

049L0ZX Drainage of Left Femoral Artery, Open Approach, Diagnostic

049L0ZZ Drainage of Left Femoral Artery, Open Approach

049L30Z Drainage of Left Femoral Artery with Drainage Device, Percutaneous Approach

049L3ZX Drainage of Left Femoral Artery, Percutaneous Approach, Diagnostic

049L3ZZ Drainage of Left Femoral Artery, Percutaneous Approach

049L40Z Drainage of Left Femoral Artery with Drainage Device, Percutaneous Endoscopic Approach

049L4ZX Drainage of Left Femoral Artery, Percutaneous Endoscopic Approach, Diagnostic

049L4ZZ Drainage of Left Femoral Artery, Percutaneous Endoscopic Approach

049M00Z Drainage of Right Popliteal Artery with Drainage Device, Open Approach

049M0ZX Drainage of Right Popliteal Artery, Open Approach, Diagnostic

049M0ZZ Drainage of Right Popliteal Artery, Open Approach

049M30Z Drainage of Right Popliteal Artery with Drainage Device, Percutaneous Approach

049M3ZX Drainage of Right Popliteal Artery, Percutaneous Approach, Diagnostic

049M3ZZ Drainage of Right Popliteal Artery, Percutaneous Approach

049M40Z Drainage of Right Popliteal Artery with Drainage Device, Percutaneous Endoscopic Approach

049M4ZX Drainage of Right Popliteal Artery, Percutaneous Endoscopic Approach, Diagnostic

049M4ZZ Drainage of Right Popliteal Artery, Percutaneous Endoscopic Approach

049N00Z Drainage of Left Popliteal Artery with Drainage Device, Open Approach

049N0ZX Drainage of Left Popliteal Artery, Open Approach, Diagnostic

049N0ZZ Drainage of Left Popliteal Artery, Open Approach

049N30Z Drainage of Left Popliteal Artery with Drainage Device, Percutaneous Approach

049N3ZX Drainage of Left Popliteal Artery, Percutaneous Approach, Diagnostic

049N3ZZ Drainage of Left Popliteal Artery, Percutaneous Approach

049N40Z Drainage of Left Popliteal Artery with Drainage Device, Percutaneous Endoscopic Approach

049N4ZX Drainage of Left Popliteal Artery, Percutaneous Endoscopic Approach, Diagnostic

049N4ZZ Drainage of Left Popliteal Artery, Percutaneous Endoscopic Approach

049P00Z Drainage of Right Anterior Tibial Artery with Drainage Device, Open Approach

049P0ZX Drainage of Right Anterior Tibial Artery, Open Approach, Diagnostic

049P0ZZ Drainage of Right Anterior Tibial Artery, Open Approach

049P30Z Drainage of Right Anterior Tibial Artery with Drainage Device, Percutaneous Approach

049P3ZX Drainage of Right Anterior Tibial Artery, Percutaneous Approach, Diagnostic

049P3ZZ Drainage of Right Anterior Tibial Artery, Percutaneous Approach

049P40Z Drainage of Right Anterior Tibial Artery with Drainage Device, Percutaneous Endoscopic Approach

049P4ZX Drainage of Right Anterior Tibial Artery, Percutaneous Endoscopic Approach, Diagnostic

049P4ZZ Drainage of Right Anterior Tibial Artery, Percutaneous Endoscopic Approach

049Q00Z Drainage of Left Anterior Tibial Artery with Drainage Device, Open Approach

049Q0ZX Drainage of Left Anterior Tibial Artery, Open Approach, Diagnostic

049Q0ZZ Drainage of Left Anterior Tibial Artery, Open Approach

049Q30Z Drainage of Left Anterior Tibial Artery with Drainage Device, Percutaneous Approach

049Q3ZX Drainage of Left Anterior Tibial Artery, Percutaneous Approach, Diagnostic

049Q3ZZ Drainage of Left Anterior Tibial Artery, Percutaneous Approach

049Q40Z Drainage of Left Anterior Tibial Artery with Drainage Device, Percutaneous Endoscopic Approach

049Q4ZX Drainage of Left Anterior Tibial Artery, Percutaneous Endoscopic Approach, Diagnostic

049Q4ZZ Drainage of Left Anterior Tibial Artery, Percutaneous Endoscopic Approach

049R00Z Drainage of Right Posterior Tibial Artery with Drainage Device, Open Approach

049R0ZX Drainage of Right Posterior Tibial Artery, Open Approach, Diagnostic

049R0ZZ Drainage of Right Posterior Tibial Artery, Open Approach

049R30Z Drainage of Right Posterior Tibial Artery with Drainage Device, Percutaneous Approach

049R3ZX Drainage of Right Posterior Tibial Artery, Percutaneous Approach, Diagnostic

049R3ZZ Drainage of Right Posterior Tibial Artery, Percutaneous Approach

049R40Z Drainage of Right Posterior Tibial Artery with Drainage Device, Percutaneous Endoscopic Approach

049R4ZX Drainage of Right Posterior Tibial Artery, Percutaneous Endoscopic Approach, Diagnostic

049R4ZZ Drainage of Right Posterior Tibial Artery, Percutaneous Endoscopic Approach

049S00Z Drainage of Left Posterior Tibial Artery with Drainage Device, Open Approach

049S0ZX Drainage of Left Posterior Tibial Artery, Open Approach, Diagnostic

049S0ZZ Drainage of Left Posterior Tibial Artery, Open Approach

049S30Z Drainage of Left Posterior Tibial Artery with Drainage Device, Percutaneous Approach

049S3ZX Drainage of Left Posterior Tibial Artery, Percutaneous Approach, Diagnostic

049S3ZZ Drainage of Left Posterior Tibial Artery, Percutaneous Approach

049S40Z Drainage of Left Posterior Tibial Artery with Drainage Device, Percutaneous Endoscopic Approach

049S4ZX Drainage of Left Posterior Tibial Artery, Percutaneous Endoscopic Approach, Diagnostic

049S4ZZ Drainage of Left Posterior Tibial Artery, Percutaneous Endoscopic Approach

049T00Z Drainage of Right Peroneal Artery with Drainage Device, Open Approach

049T0ZX Drainage of Right Peroneal Artery, Open Approach, Diagnostic

049T0ZZ Drainage of Right Peroneal Artery, Open Approach

049T30Z Drainage of Right Peroneal Artery with Drainage Device, Percutaneous Approach

049T3ZX Drainage of Right Peroneal Artery, Percutaneous Approach, Diagnostic

049T3ZZ Drainage of Right Peroneal Artery, Percutaneous Approach

049T40Z Drainage of Right Peroneal Artery with Drainage Device, Percutaneous Endoscopic Approach

049T4ZX Drainage of Right Peroneal Artery, Percutaneous Endoscopic Approach, Diagnostic

049T4ZZ Drainage of Right Peroneal Artery, Percutaneous Endoscopic Approach

049U00Z Drainage of Left Peroneal Artery with Drainage Device, Open Approach

049U0ZX Drainage of Left Peroneal Artery, Open Approach, Diagnostic

049U0ZZ Drainage of Left Peroneal Artery, Open Approach

049U30Z Drainage of Left Peroneal Artery with Drainage Device, Percutaneous Approach

049U3ZX Drainage of Left Peroneal Artery, Percutaneous Approach, Diagnostic

049U3ZZ Drainage of Left Peroneal Artery, Percutaneous Approach

049U40Z Drainage of Left Peroneal Artery with Drainage Device, Percutaneous Endoscopic Approach

049U4ZX Drainage of Left Peroneal Artery, Percutaneous Endoscopic Approach, Diagnostic

049U4ZZ Drainage of Left Peroneal Artery, Percutaneous Endoscopic Approach

049V00Z Drainage of Right Foot Artery with Drainage Device, Open Approach

049V0ZX Drainage of Right Foot Artery, Open Approach, Diagnostic

049V0ZZ Drainage of Right Foot Artery, Open Approach

049V30Z Drainage of Right Foot Artery with Drainage Device, Percutaneous Approach

049V3ZX Drainage of Right Foot Artery, Percutaneous Approach, Diagnostic

049V3ZZ Drainage of Right Foot Artery, Percutaneous Approach

049V40Z Drainage of Right Foot Artery with Drainage Device, Percutaneous Endoscopic Approach

049V4ZX Drainage of Right Foot Artery, Percutaneous Endoscopic Approach, Diagnostic

049V4ZZ Drainage of Right Foot Artery, Percutaneous Endoscopic Approach

049W00Z Drainage of Left Foot Artery with Drainage Device, Open Approach

049W0ZX Drainage of Left Foot Artery, Open Approach, Diagnostic

049W0ZZ Drainage of Left Foot Artery, Open Approach

049W30Z Drainage of Left Foot Artery with Drainage Device, Percutaneous Approach

049W3ZX Drainage of Left Foot Artery, Percutaneous Approach, Diagnostic

049W3ZZ Drainage of Left Foot Artery, Percutaneous Approach

049W40Z Drainage of Left Foot Artery with Drainage Device, Percutaneous Endoscopic Approach

049W4ZX Drainage of Left Foot Artery, Percutaneous Endoscopic Approach, Diagnostic

049W4ZZ Drainage of Left Foot Artery, Percutaneous Endoscopic Approach

049Y00Z Drainage of Lower Artery with Drainage Device, Open Approach

049Y0ZX Drainage of Lower Artery, Open Approach, Diagnostic

049Y0ZZ Drainage of Lower Artery, Open Approach

049Y30Z Drainage of Lower Artery with Drainage Device, Percutaneous Approach

049Y3ZX Drainage of Lower Artery, Percutaneous Approach, Diagnostic

049Y3ZZ Drainage of Lower Artery, Percutaneous Approach

049Y40Z Drainage of Lower Artery with Drainage Device, Percutaneous Endoscopic Approach

049Y4ZX Drainage of Lower Artery, Percutaneous Endoscopic Approach, Diagnostic

049Y4ZZ Drainage of Lower Artery, Percutaneous Endoscopic Approach

04B – Lower Arteries, Excision

Review Coding Guidelines B3.4a and B3.4b

Review Coding Guideline B3.8

04B00ZX	Excision of Abdominal Aorta, Open Approach, Diagnostic
04B00ZZ	Excision of Abdominal Aorta, Open Approach
04B03ZX	Excision of Abdominal Aorta, Percutaneous Approach, Diagnostic
04B03ZZ	Excision of Abdominal Aorta, Percutaneous Approach
04B04ZX	Excision of Abdominal Aorta, Percutaneous Endoscopic Approach, Diagnostic
04B04ZZ	Excision of Abdominal Aorta, Percutaneous Endoscopic Approach
04B10ZX	Excision of Celiac Artery, Open Approach, Diagnostic
04B10ZZ	Excision of Celiac Artery, Open Approach
04B13ZX	Excision of Celiac Artery, Percutaneous Approach, Diagnostic
04B13ZZ	Excision of Celiac Artery, Percutaneous Approach
04B14ZX	Excision of Celiac Artery, Percutaneous Endoscopic Approach, Diagnostic
04B14ZZ	Excision of Celiac Artery, Percutaneous Endoscopic Approach
04B20ZX	Excision of Gastric Artery, Open Approach, Diagnostic
04B20ZZ	Excision of Gastric Artery, Open Approach
04B23ZX	Excision of Gastric Artery, Percutaneous Approach, Diagnostic
04B23ZZ	Excision of Gastric Artery, Percutaneous Approach
04B24ZX	Excision of Gastric Artery, Percutaneous Endoscopic Approach, Diagnostic
04B24ZZ	Excision of Gastric Artery, Percutaneous Endoscopic Approach
04B30ZX	Excision of Hepatic Artery, Open Approach, Diagnostic
04B30ZZ	Excision of Hepatic Artery, Open Approach
04B33ZX	Excision of Hepatic Artery, Percutaneous Approach, Diagnostic
04B33ZZ	Excision of Hepatic Artery, Percutaneous Approach
04B34ZX	Excision of Hepatic Artery, Percutaneous Endoscopic Approach, Diagnostic
04B34ZZ	Excision of Hepatic Artery, Percutaneous Endoscopic Approach
04B40ZX	Excision of Splenic Artery, Open Approach, Diagnostic
04B40ZZ	Excision of Splenic Artery, Open Approach
04B43ZX	Excision of Splenic Artery, Percutaneous Approach, Diagnostic
04B43ZZ	Excision of Splenic Artery, Percutaneous Approach
04B44ZX	Excision of Splenic Artery, Percutaneous Endoscopic Approach, Diagnostic
04B44ZZ	Excision of Splenic Artery, Percutaneous Endoscopic Approach
04B50ZX	Excision of Superior Mesenteric Artery, Open Approach, Diagnostic
04B50ZZ	Excision of Superior Mesenteric Artery, Open Approach
04B53ZX	Excision of Superior Mesenteric Artery, Percutaneous Approach, Diagnostic
04B53ZZ	Excision of Superior Mesenteric Artery, Percutaneous Approach
04B54ZX	Excision of Superior Mesenteric Artery, Percutaneous Endoscopic Approach, Diagnostic
04B54ZZ	Excision of Superior Mesenteric Artery, Percutaneous Endoscopic Approach
04B60ZX	Excision of Right Colic Artery, Open Approach, Diagnostic
04B60ZZ	Excision of Right Colic Artery, Open Approach
04B63ZX	Excision of Right Colic Artery, Percutaneous Approach, Diagnostic
04B63ZZ	Excision of Right Colic Artery, Percutaneous Approach
04B64ZX	Excision of Right Colic Artery, Percutaneous Endoscopic Approach, Diagnostic
04B64ZZ	Excision of Right Colic Artery, Percutaneous Endoscopic Approach
04B70ZX	Excision of Left Colic Artery, Open Approach, Diagnostic
04B70ZZ	Excision of Left Colic Artery, Open Approach
04B73ZX	Excision of Left Colic Artery, Percutaneous Approach, Diagnostic
04B73ZZ	Excision of Left Colic Artery, Percutaneous Approach
04B74ZX	Excision of Left Colic Artery, Percutaneous Endoscopic Approach, Diagnostic
04B74ZZ	Excision of Left Colic Artery, Percutaneous Endoscopic Approach
04B80ZX	Excision of Middle Colic Artery, Open Approach, Diagnostic
04B80ZZ	Excision of Middle Colic Artery, Open Approach
04B83ZX	Excision of Middle Colic Artery, Percutaneous Approach, Diagnostic
04B83ZZ	Excision of Middle Colic Artery, Percutaneous Approach
04B84ZX	Excision of Middle Colic Artery, Percutaneous Endoscopic Approach, Diagnostic
04B84ZZ	Excision of Middle Colic Artery, Percutaneous Endoscopic Approach
04B90ZX	Excision of Right Renal Artery, Open Approach, Diagnostic
04B90ZZ	Excision of Right Renal Artery, Open Approach
04B93ZX	Excision of Right Renal Artery, Percutaneous Approach, Diagnostic
04B93ZZ	Excision of Right Renal Artery, Percutaneous Approach
04B94ZX	Excision of Right Renal Artery, Percutaneous Endoscopic Approach, Diagnostic
04B94ZZ	Excision of Right Renal Artery, Percutaneous Endoscopic Approach
04BA0ZX	Excision of Left Renal Artery, Open Approach, Diagnostic
04BA0ZZ	Excision of Left Renal Artery, Open Approach
04BA3ZX	Excision of Left Renal Artery, Percutaneous Approach, Diagnostic
04BA3ZZ	Excision of Left Renal Artery, Percutaneous Approach
04BA4ZX	Excision of Left Renal Artery, Percutaneous Endoscopic Approach, Diagnostic
04BA4ZZ	Excision of Left Renal Artery, Percutaneous Endoscopic Approach
04BB0ZX	Excision of Inferior Mesenteric Artery, Open Approach, Diagnostic
04BB0ZZ	Excision of Inferior Mesenteric Artery, Open Approach
04BB3ZX	Excision of Inferior Mesenteric Artery, Percutaneous Approach, Diagnostic
04BB3ZZ	Excision of Inferior Mesenteric Artery, Percutaneous Approach
04BB4ZX	Excision of Inferior Mesenteric Artery, Percutaneous Endoscopic Approach, Diagnostic
04BB4ZZ	Excision of Inferior Mesenteric Artery, Percutaneous Endoscopic Approach
04BC0ZX	Excision of Right Common Iliac Artery, Open Approach, Diagnostic
04BC0ZZ	Excision of Right Common Iliac Artery, Open Approach
04BC3ZX	Excision of Right Common Iliac Artery, Percutaneous Approach, Diagnostic
04BC3ZZ	Excision of Right Common Iliac Artery, Percutaneous Approach
04BC4ZX	Excision of Right Common Iliac Artery, Percutaneous Endoscopic Approach, Diagnostic
04BC4ZZ	Excision of Right Common Iliac Artery, Percutaneous Endoscopic Approach
04BD0ZX	Excision of Left Common Iliac Artery, Open Approach, Diagnostic
04BD0ZZ	Excision of Left Common Iliac Artery, Open Approach
04BD3ZX	Excision of Left Common Iliac Artery, Percutaneous Approach, Diagnostic
04BD3ZZ	Excision of Left Common Iliac Artery, Percutaneous Approach
04BD4ZX	Excision of Left Common Iliac Artery, Percutaneous Endoscopic Approach, Diagnostic
04BD4ZZ	Excision of Left Common Iliac Artery, Percutaneous Endoscopic Approach
04BE0ZX	Excision of Right Internal Iliac Artery, Open Approach, Diagnostic
04BE0ZZ	Excision of Right Internal Iliac Artery, Open Approach
04BE3ZX	Excision of Right Internal Iliac Artery, Percutaneous Approach, Diagnostic
04BE3ZZ	Excision of Right Internal Iliac Artery, Percutaneous Approach
04BE4ZX	Excision of Right Internal Iliac Artery, Percutaneous Endoscopic Approach, Diagnostic
04BE4ZZ	Excision of Right Internal Iliac Artery, Percutaneous Endoscopic Approach
04BF0ZX	Excision of Left Internal Iliac Artery, Open Approach, Diagnostic
04BF0ZZ	Excision of Left Internal Iliac Artery, Open Approach
04BF3ZX	Excision of Left Internal Iliac Artery, Percutaneous Approach, Diagnostic
04BF3ZZ	Excision of Left Internal Iliac Artery, Percutaneous Approach
04BF4ZX	Excision of Left Internal Iliac Artery, Percutaneous Endoscopic Approach, Diagnostic
04BF4ZZ	Excision of Left Internal Iliac Artery, Percutaneous Endoscopic Approach
04BH0ZX	Excision of Right External Iliac Artery, Open Approach, Diagnostic
04BH0ZZ	Excision of Right External Iliac Artery, Open Approach
04BH3ZX	Excision of Right External Iliac Artery, Percutaneous Approach, Diagnostic
04BH3ZZ	Excision of Right External Iliac Artery, Percutaneous Approach
04BH4ZX	Excision of Right External Iliac Artery, Percutaneous Endoscopic Approach, Diagnostic

04BH4ZZ	Excision of Right External Iliac Artery, Percutaneous Endoscopic Approach
04BJ0ZX	Excision of Left External Iliac Artery, Open Approach, Diagnostic
04BJ0ZZ	Excision of Left External Iliac Artery, Open Approach
04BJ3ZX	Excision of Left External Iliac Artery, Percutaneous Approach, Diagnostic
04BJ3ZZ	Excision of Left External Iliac Artery, Percutaneous Approach
04BJ4ZX	Excision of Left External Iliac Artery, Percutaneous Endoscopic Approach, Diagnostic
04BJ4ZZ	Excision of Left External Iliac Artery, Percutaneous Endoscopic Approach
04BK0ZX	Excision of Right Femoral Artery, Open Approach, Diagnostic
04BL4ZZ	Excision of Left Femoral Artery, Percutaneous Endoscopic Approach
04BM0ZX	Excision of Right Popliteal Artery, Open Approach, Diagnostic
04BM0ZZ	Excision of Right Popliteal Artery, Open Approach
04BM3ZX	Excision of Right Popliteal Artery, Percutaneous Approach, Diagnostic
04BM3ZZ	Excision of Right Popliteal Artery, Percutaneous Approach
04BM4ZX	Excision of Right Popliteal Artery, Percutaneous Endoscopic Approach, Diagnostic
04BM4ZZ	Excision of Right Popliteal Artery, Percutaneous Endoscopic Approach
04BN0ZX	Excision of Left Popliteal Artery, Open Approach, Diagnostic
04BN0ZZ	Excision of Left Popliteal Artery, Open Approach
04BN3ZX	Excision of Left Popliteal Artery, Percutaneous Approach, Diagnostic
04BN3ZZ	Excision of Left Popliteal Artery, Percutaneous Approach
04BN4ZX	Excision of Left Popliteal Artery, Percutaneous Endoscopic Approach, Diagnostic
04BN4ZZ	Excision of Left Popliteal Artery, Percutaneous Endoscopic Approach
04BP0ZX	Excision of Right Anterior Tibial Artery, Open Approach, Diagnostic
04BP0ZZ	Excision of Right Anterior Tibial Artery, Open Approach
04BP3ZX	Excision of Right Anterior Tibial Artery, Percutaneous Approach, Diagnostic
04BP3ZZ	Excision of Right Anterior Tibial Artery, Percutaneous Approach
04BP4ZX	Excision of Right Anterior Tibial Artery, Percutaneous Endoscopic Approach, Diagnostic
04BP4ZZ	Excision of Right Anterior Tibial Artery, Percutaneous Endoscopic Approach
04BQ0ZX	Excision of Left Anterior Tibial Artery, Open Approach, Diagnostic
04BQ0ZZ	Excision of Left Anterior Tibial Artery, Open Approach
04BQ3ZX	Excision of Left Anterior Tibial Artery, Percutaneous Approach, Diagnostic
04BQ3ZZ	Excision of Left Anterior Tibial Artery, Percutaneous Approach
04BQ4ZX	Excision of Left Anterior Tibial Artery, Percutaneous Endoscopic Approach, Diagnostic
04BQ4ZZ	Excision of Left Anterior Tibial Artery, Percutaneous Endoscopic Approach
04BR0ZX	Excision of Right Posterior Tibial Artery, Open Approach, Diagnostic
04BR0ZZ	Excision of Right Posterior Tibial Artery, Open Approach

04BR3ZX	Excision of Right Posterior Tibial Artery, Percutaneous Approach, Diagnostic
04BR3ZZ	Excision of Right Posterior Tibial Artery, Percutaneous Approach
04BR4ZX	Excision of Right Posterior Tibial Artery, Percutaneous Endoscopic Approach, Diagnostic
04BR4ZZ	Excision of Right Posterior Tibial Artery, Percutaneous Endoscopic Approach
04BS0ZX	Excision of Left Posterior Tibial Artery, Open Approach, Diagnostic
04BS0ZZ	Excision of Left Posterior Tibial Artery, Open Approach
04BS3ZX	Excision of Left Posterior Tibial Artery, Percutaneous Approach, Diagnostic
04BS3ZZ	Excision of Left Posterior Tibial Artery, Percutaneous Approach
04BS4ZX	Excision of Left Posterior Tibial Artery, Percutaneous Endoscopic Approach, Diagnostic
04BS4ZZ	Excision of Left Posterior Tibial Artery, Percutaneous Endoscopic Approach
04BT0ZX	Excision of Right Peroneal Artery, Open Approach, Diagnostic
04BT0ZZ	Excision of Right Peroneal Artery, Open Approach
04BT3ZX	Excision of Right Peroneal Artery, Percutaneous Approach, Diagnostic
04BT3ZZ	Excision of Right Peroneal Artery, Percutaneous Approach
04BT4ZX	Excision of Right Peroneal Artery, Percutaneous Endoscopic Approach, Diagnostic
04BT4ZZ	Excision of Right Peroneal Artery, Percutaneous Endoscopic Approach
04BU0ZX	Excision of Left Peroneal Artery, Open Approach, Diagnostic
04BU0ZZ	Excision of Left Peroneal Artery, Open Approach
04BU3ZX	Excision of Left Peroneal Artery, Percutaneous Approach, Diagnostic
04BU3ZZ	Excision of Left Peroneal Artery, Percutaneous Approach
04BU4ZX	Excision of Left Peroneal Artery, Percutaneous Endoscopic Approach, Diagnostic
04BU4ZZ	Excision of Left Peroneal Artery, Percutaneous Endoscopic Approach
04BV0ZX	Excision of Right Foot Artery, Open Approach, Diagnostic
04BV0ZZ	Excision of Right Foot Artery, Open Approach
04BV3ZX	Excision of Right Foot Artery, Percutaneous Approach, Diagnostic
04BV3ZZ	Excision of Right Foot Artery, Percutaneous Approach
04BV4ZX	Excision of Right Foot Artery, Percutaneous Endoscopic Approach, Diagnostic
04BV4ZZ	Excision of Right Foot Artery, Percutaneous Endoscopic Approach
04BW0ZX	Excision of Left Foot Artery, Open Approach, Diagnostic
04BW0ZZ	Excision of Left Foot Artery, Open Approach
04BW3ZX	Excision of Left Foot Artery, Percutaneous Approach, Diagnostic
04BW3ZZ	Excision of Left Foot Artery, Percutaneous Approach
04BW4ZX	Excision of Left Foot Artery, Percutaneous Endoscopic Approach, Diagnostic
04BW4ZZ	Excision of Left Foot Artery, Percutaneous Endoscopic Approach
04BY0ZX	Excision of Lower Artery, Open Approach, Diagnostic
04BY0ZZ	Excision of Lower Artery, Open Approach
04BY3ZX	Excision of Lower Artery, Percutaneous Approach, Diagnostic
04BY3ZZ	Excision of Lower Artery, Percutaneous Approach
04BY4ZX	Excision of Lower Artery, Percutaneous Endoscopic Approach, Diagnostic
04BY4ZZ	Excision of Lower Artery, Percutaneous Endoscopic Approach

04C – Lower Arteries, Extirpation

04C00ZZ	Extirpation of Matter from Abdominal Aorta, Open Approach
04C03ZZ	Extirpation of Matter from Abdominal Aorta, Percutaneous Approach
04C04ZZ	Extirpation of Matter from Abdominal Aorta, Percutaneous Endoscopic Approach
04C10ZZ	Extirpation of Matter from Celiac Artery, Open Approach
04C13ZZ	Extirpation of Matter from Celiac Artery, Percutaneous Approach
04C14ZZ	Extirpation of Matter from Celiac Artery, Percutaneous Endoscopic Approach
04C20ZZ	Extirpation of Matter from Gastric Artery, Open Approach
04C23ZZ	Extirpation of Matter from Gastric Artery, Percutaneous Approach
04C24ZZ	Extirpation of Matter from Gastric Artery, Percutaneous Endoscopic Approach
04C30ZZ	Extirpation of Matter from Hepatic Artery, Open Approach
04C33ZZ	Extirpation of Matter from Hepatic Artery, Percutaneous Approach

04C34ZZ	Extirpation of Matter from Hepatic Artery, Percutaneous Endoscopic Approach
04C40ZZ	Extirpation of Matter from Splenic Artery, Open Approach
04C43ZZ	Extirpation of Matter from Splenic Artery, Percutaneous Approach
04C44ZZ	Extirpation of Matter from Splenic Artery, Percutaneous Endoscopic Approach
04C50ZZ	Extirpation of Matter from Superior Mesenteric Artery, Open Approach
04C53ZZ	Extirpation of Matter from Superior Mesenteric Artery, Percutaneous Approach
04C54ZZ	Extirpation of Matter from Superior Mesenteric Artery, Percutaneous Endoscopic Approach
04C60ZZ	Extirpation of Matter from Right Colic Artery, Open Approach
04C63ZZ	Extirpation of Matter from Right Colic Artery, Percutaneous Approach

04C64ZZ   Extirpation of Matter from Right Colic Artery, Percutaneous Endoscopic Approach

04C70ZZ   Extirpation of Matter from Left Colic Artery, Open Approach

04C73ZZ   Extirpation of Matter from Left Colic Artery, Percutaneous Approach

04C74ZZ   Extirpation of Matter from Left Colic Artery, Percutaneous Endoscopic Approach

04C80ZZ   Extirpation of Matter from Middle Colic Artery, Open Approach

04C83ZZ   Extirpation of Matter from Middle Colic Artery, Percutaneous Approach

04C84ZZ   Extirpation of Matter from Middle Colic Artery, Percutaneous Endoscopic Approach

04C90ZZ   Extirpation of Matter from Right Renal Artery, Open Approach

04C93ZZ   Extirpation of Matter from Right Renal Artery, Percutaneous Approach

04C94ZZ   Extirpation of Matter from Right Renal Artery, Percutaneous Endoscopic Approach

04CA0ZZ   Extirpation of Matter from Left Renal Artery, Open Approach

04CA3ZZ   Extirpation of Matter from Left Renal Artery, Percutaneous Approach

04CA4ZZ   Extirpation of Matter from Left Renal Artery, Percutaneous Endoscopic Approach

04CB0ZZ   Extirpation of Matter from Inferior Mesenteric Artery, Open Approach

04CB3ZZ   Extirpation of Matter from Inferior Mesenteric Artery, Percutaneous Approach

04CB4ZZ   Extirpation of Matter from Inferior Mesenteric Artery, Percutaneous Endoscopic Approach

04CC0ZZ   Extirpation of Matter from Right Common Iliac Artery, Open Approach

04CC3ZZ   Extirpation of Matter from Right Common Iliac Artery, Percutaneous Approach

04CC4ZZ   Extirpation of Matter from Right Common Iliac Artery, Percutaneous Endoscopic Approach

04CD0ZZ   Extirpation of Matter from Left Common Iliac Artery, Open Approach

04CD3ZZ   Extirpation of Matter from Left Common Iliac Artery, Percutaneous Approach

04CD4ZZ   Extirpation of Matter from Left Common Iliac Artery, Percutaneous Endoscopic Approach

04CE0ZZ   Extirpation of Matter from Right Internal Iliac Artery, Open Approach

04CE3ZZ   Extirpation of Matter from Right Internal Iliac Artery, Percutaneous Approach

04CE4ZZ   Extirpation of Matter from Right Internal Iliac Artery, Percutaneous Endoscopic Approach

04CF0ZZ   Extirpation of Matter from Left Internal Iliac Artery, Open Approach

04CF3ZZ   Extirpation of Matter from Left Internal Iliac Artery, Percutaneous Approach

04CF4ZZ   Extirpation of Matter from Left Internal Iliac Artery, Percutaneous Endoscopic Approach

04CH0ZZ   Extirpation of Matter from Right External Iliac Artery, Open Approach

04CH3ZZ   Extirpation of Matter from Right External Iliac Artery, Percutaneous Approach

04CH4ZZ   Extirpation of Matter from Right External Iliac Artery, Percutaneous Endoscopic Approach

04CJ0ZZ   Extirpation of Matter from Left External Iliac Artery, Open Approach

04CJ3ZZ   Extirpation of Matter from Left External Iliac Artery, Percutaneous Approach

04CJ4ZZ   Extirpation of Matter from Left External Iliac Artery, Percutaneous Endoscopic Approach

04CK0ZZ   Extirpation of Matter from Right Femoral Artery, Open Approach

04CK3ZZ   Extirpation of Matter from Right Femoral Artery, Percutaneous Approach

04CK4ZZ   Extirpation of Matter from Right Femoral Artery, Percutaneous Endoscopic Approach

04CL0ZZ   Extirpation of Matter from Left Femoral Artery, Open Approach

04CL3ZZ   Extirpation of Matter from Left Femoral Artery, Percutaneous Approach

04CL4ZZ   Extirpation of Matter from Left Femoral Artery, Percutaneous Endoscopic Approach

04CM0ZZ   Extirpation of Matter from Right Popliteal Artery, Open Approach

04CM3ZZ   Extirpation of Matter from Right Popliteal Artery, Percutaneous Approach

04CM4ZZ   Extirpation of Matter from Right Popliteal Artery, Percutaneous Endoscopic Approach

04CN0ZZ   Extirpation of Matter from Left Popliteal Artery, Open Approach

04CN3ZZ   Extirpation of Matter from Left Popliteal Artery, Percutaneous Approach

04CN4ZZ   Extirpation of Matter from Left Popliteal Artery, Percutaneous Endoscopic Approach

04CP0ZZ   Extirpation of Matter from Right Anterior Tibial Artery, Open Approach

04CP3ZZ   Extirpation of Matter from Right Anterior Tibial Artery, Percutaneous Approach

04CP4ZZ   Extirpation of Matter from Right Anterior Tibial Artery, Percutaneous Endoscopic Approach

04CQ0ZZ   Extirpation of Matter from Left Anterior Tibial Artery, Open Approach

04CQ3ZZ   Extirpation of Matter from Left Anterior Tibial Artery, Percutaneous Approach

04CQ4ZZ   Extirpation of Matter from Left Anterior Tibial Artery, Percutaneous Endoscopic Approach

04CR0ZZ   Extirpation of Matter from Right Posterior Tibial Artery, Open Approach

04CR3ZZ   Extirpation of Matter from Right Posterior Tibial Artery, Percutaneous Approach

04CR4ZZ   Extirpation of Matter from Right Posterior Tibial Artery, Percutaneous Endoscopic Approach

04CS0ZZ   Extirpation of Matter from Left Posterior Tibial Artery, Open Approach

04CS3ZZ   Extirpation of Matter from Left Posterior Tibial Artery, Percutaneous Approach

04CS4ZZ   Extirpation of Matter from Left Posterior Tibial Artery, Percutaneous Endoscopic Approach

04CT0ZZ   Extirpation of Matter from Right Peroneal Artery, Open Approach

04CT3ZZ   Extirpation of Matter from Right Peroneal Artery, Percutaneous Approach

04CT4ZZ   Extirpation of Matter from Right Peroneal Artery, Percutaneous Endoscopic Approach

04CU0ZZ   Extirpation of Matter from Left Peroneal Artery, Open Approach

04CU3ZZ   Extirpation of Matter from Left Peroneal Artery, Percutaneous Approach

04CU4ZZ   Extirpation of Matter from Left Peroneal Artery, Percutaneous Endoscopic Approach

04CV0ZZ   Extirpation of Matter from Right Foot Artery, Open Approach

04CV3ZZ   Extirpation of Matter from Right Foot Artery, Percutaneous Approach

04CV4ZZ   Extirpation of Matter from Right Foot Artery, Percutaneous Endoscopic Approach

04CW0ZZ   Extirpation of Matter from Left Foot Artery, Open Approach

04CW3ZZ   Extirpation of Matter from Left Foot Artery, Percutaneous Approach

04CW4ZZ   Extirpation of Matter from Left Foot Artery, Percutaneous Endoscopic Approach

04CY0ZZ   Extirpation of Matter from Lower Artery, Open Approach

04CY3ZZ   Extirpation of Matter from Lower Artery, Percutaneous Approach

04CY4ZZ   Extirpation of Matter from Lower Artery, Percutaneous Endoscopic Approach

04H – Lower Arteries, Insertion

04H002Z   Insertion of Monitoring Device into Abdominal Aorta, Open Approach

04H003Z   Insertion of Infusion Device into Abdominal Aorta, Open Approach

04H00DZ   Insertion of Intraluminal Device into Abdominal Aorta, Open Approach

04H032Z   Insertion of Monitoring Device into Abdominal Aorta, Percutaneous Approach

04H033Z Insertion of Infusion Device into Abdominal Aorta, Percutaneous Approach

04H03DZ Insertion of Intraluminal Device into Abdominal Aorta, Percutaneous Approach

04H042Z Insertion of Monitoring Device into Abdominal Aorta, Percutaneous Endoscopic Approach

04H043Z Insertion of Infusion Device into Abdominal Aorta, Percutaneous Endoscopic Approach

04H04DZ Insertion of Intraluminal Device into Abdominal Aorta, Percutaneous Endoscopic Approach

04H103Z Insertion of Infusion Device into Celiac Artery, Open Approach

04H10DZ Insertion of Intraluminal Device into Celiac Artery, Open Approach

04H133Z Insertion of Infusion Device into Celiac Artery, Percutaneous Approach

04H13DZ Insertion of Intraluminal Device into Celiac Artery, Percutaneous Approach

04H143Z Insertion of Infusion Device into Celiac Artery, Percutaneous Endoscopic Approach

04H14DZ Insertion of Intraluminal Device into Celiac Artery, Percutaneous Endoscopic Approach

04H203Z Insertion of Infusion Device into Gastric Artery, Open Approach

04H20DZ Insertion of Intraluminal Device into Gastric Artery, Open Approach

04H233Z Insertion of Infusion Device into Gastric Artery, Percutaneous Approach

04H23DZ Insertion of Intraluminal Device into Gastric Artery, Percutaneous Approach

04H243Z Insertion of Infusion Device into Gastric Artery, Percutaneous Endoscopic Approach

04H24DZ Insertion of Intraluminal Device into Gastric Artery, Percutaneous Endoscopic Approach

04H303Z Insertion of Infusion Device into Hepatic Artery, Open Approach

04H30DZ Insertion of Intraluminal Device into Hepatic Artery, Open Approach

04H333Z Insertion of Infusion Device into Hepatic Artery, Percutaneous Approach

04H33DZ Insertion of Intraluminal Device into Hepatic Artery, Percutaneous Approach

04H343Z Insertion of Infusion Device into Hepatic Artery, Percutaneous Endoscopic Approach

04H34DZ Insertion of Intraluminal Device into Hepatic Artery, Percutaneous Endoscopic Approach

04H403Z Insertion of Infusion Device into Splenic Artery, Open Approach

04H40DZ Insertion of Intraluminal Device into Splenic Artery, Open Approach

04H433Z Insertion of Infusion Device into Splenic Artery, Percutaneous Approach

04H43DZ Insertion of Intraluminal Device into Splenic Artery, Percutaneous Approach

04H443Z Insertion of Infusion Device into Splenic Artery, Percutaneous Endoscopic Approach

04H44DZ Insertion of Intraluminal Device into Splenic Artery, Percutaneous Endoscopic Approach

04H503Z Insertion of Infusion Device into Superior Mesenteric Artery, Open Approach

04H50DZ Insertion of Intraluminal Device into Superior Mesenteric Artery, Open Approach

04H533Z Insertion of Infusion Device into Superior Mesenteric Artery, Percutaneous Approach

04H53DZ Insertion of Intraluminal Device into Superior Mesenteric Artery, Percutaneous Approach

04H543Z Insertion of Infusion Device into Superior Mesenteric Artery, Percutaneous Endoscopic Approach

04H54DZ Insertion of Intraluminal Device into Superior Mesenteric Artery, Percutaneous Endoscopic Approach

04H603Z Insertion of Infusion Device into Right Colic Artery, Open Approach

04H60DZ Insertion of Intraluminal Device into Right Colic Artery, Open Approach

04H633Z Insertion of Infusion Device into Right Colic Artery, Percutaneous Approach

04H63DZ Insertion of Intraluminal Device into Right Colic Artery, Percutaneous Approach

04H643Z Insertion of Infusion Device into Right Colic Artery, Percutaneous Endoscopic Approach

04H64DZ Insertion of Intraluminal Device into Right Colic Artery, Percutaneous Endoscopic Approach

04H703Z Insertion of Infusion Device into Left Colic Artery, Open Approach

04H70DZ Insertion of Intraluminal Device into Left Colic Artery, Open Approach

04H733Z Insertion of Infusion Device into Left Colic Artery, Percutaneous Approach

04H73DZ Insertion of Intraluminal Device into Left Colic Artery, Percutaneous Approach

04H743Z Insertion of Infusion Device into Left Colic Artery, Percutaneous Endoscopic Approach

04H74DZ Insertion of Intraluminal Device into Left Colic Artery, Percutaneous Endoscopic Approach

04H803Z Insertion of Infusion Device into Middle Colic Artery, Open Approach

04H80DZ Insertion of Intraluminal Device into Middle Colic Artery, Open Approach

04H833Z Insertion of Infusion Device into Middle Colic Artery, Percutaneous Approach

04H83DZ Insertion of Intraluminal Device into Middle Colic Artery, Percutaneous Approach

04H843Z Insertion of Infusion Device into Middle Colic Artery, Percutaneous Endoscopic Approach

04H84DZ Insertion of Intraluminal Device into Middle Colic Artery, Percutaneous Endoscopic Approach

04H903Z Insertion of Infusion Device into Right Renal Artery, Open Approach

04H90DZ Insertion of Intraluminal Device into Right Renal Artery, Open Approach

04H933Z Insertion of Infusion Device into Right Renal Artery, Percutaneous Approach

04H93DZ Insertion of Intraluminal Device into Right Renal Artery, Percutaneous Approach

04H943Z Insertion of Infusion Device into Right Renal Artery, Percutaneous Endoscopic Approach

04H94DZ Insertion of Intraluminal Device into Right Renal Artery, Percutaneous Endoscopic Approach

04HA03Z Insertion of Infusion Device into Left Renal Artery, Open Approach

04HA0DZ Insertion of Intraluminal Device into Left Renal Artery, Open Approach

04HA33Z Insertion of Infusion Device into Left Renal Artery, Percutaneous Approach

04HA3DZ Insertion of Intraluminal Device into Left Renal Artery, Percutaneous Approach

04HA43Z Insertion of Infusion Device into Left Renal Artery, Percutaneous Endoscopic Approach

04HA4DZ Insertion of Intraluminal Device into Left Renal Artery, Percutaneous Endoscopic Approach

04HB03Z Insertion of Infusion Device into Inferior Mesenteric Artery, Open Approach

04HB0DZ Insertion of Intraluminal Device into Inferior Mesenteric Artery, Open Approach

04HB33Z Insertion of Infusion Device into Inferior Mesenteric Artery, Percutaneous Approach

04HB3DZ Insertion of Intraluminal Device into Inferior Mesenteric Artery, Percutaneous Approach

04HB43Z Insertion of Infusion Device into Inferior Mesenteric Artery, Percutaneous Endoscopic Approach

04HB4DZ Insertion of Intraluminal Device into Inferior Mesenteric Artery, Percutaneous Endoscopic Approach

04HC03Z Insertion of Infusion Device into Right Common Iliac Artery, Open Approach

04HC0DZ Insertion of Intraluminal Device into Right Common Iliac Artery, Open Approach

04HC33Z Insertion of Infusion Device into Right Common Iliac Artery, Percutaneous Approach

04HC3DZ Insertion of Intraluminal Device into Right Common Iliac Artery, Percutaneous Approach

04HC43Z Insertion of Infusion Device into Right Common Iliac Artery, Percutaneous Endoscopic Approach

---

♀ Female-only   ♂ Male-only   ◯ Limited Coverage   ● Non-OR   ▣ HAC-associated procedure   ⬤ Non-covered procedures   ✚ Combination

04HC4DZ Insertion of Intraluminal Device into Right Common Iliac Artery, Percutaneous Endoscopic Approach

04HD03Z Insertion of Infusion Device into Left Common Iliac Artery, Open Approach

04HD0DZ Insertion of Intraluminal Device into Left Common Iliac Artery, Open Approach

04HD33Z Insertion of Infusion Device into Left Common Iliac Artery, Percutaneous Approach

04HD3DZ Insertion of Intraluminal Device into Left Common Iliac Artery, Percutaneous Approach

04HD43Z Insertion of Infusion Device into Left Common Iliac Artery, Percutaneous Endoscopic Approach

04HD4DZ Insertion of Intraluminal Device into Left Common Iliac Artery, Percutaneous Endoscopic Approach

04HE03Z Insertion of Infusion Device into Right Internal Iliac Artery, Open Approach

04HE0DZ Insertion of Intraluminal Device into Right Internal Iliac Artery, Open Approach

04HE33Z Insertion of Infusion Device into Right Internal Iliac Artery, Percutaneous Approach

04HE3DZ Insertion of Intraluminal Device into Right Internal Iliac Artery, Percutaneous Approach

04HE43Z Insertion of Infusion Device into Right Internal Iliac Artery, Percutaneous Endoscopic Approach

04HE4DZ Insertion of Intraluminal Device into Right Internal Iliac Artery, Percutaneous Endoscopic Approach

04HF03Z Insertion of Infusion Device into Left Internal Iliac Artery, Open Approach

04HF0DZ Insertion of Intraluminal Device into Left Internal Iliac Artery, Open Approach

04HF33Z Insertion of Infusion Device into Left Internal Iliac Artery, Percutaneous Approach

04HF3DZ Insertion of Intraluminal Device into Left Internal Iliac Artery, Percutaneous Approach

04HF43Z Insertion of Infusion Device into Left Internal Iliac Artery, Percutaneous Endoscopic Approach

04HF4DZ Insertion of Intraluminal Device into Left Internal Iliac Artery, Percutaneous Endoscopic Approach

04HH03Z Insertion of Infusion Device into Right External Iliac Artery, Open Approach

04HH0DZ Insertion of Intraluminal Device into Right External Iliac Artery, Open Approach

04HH33Z Insertion of Infusion Device into Right External Iliac Artery, Percutaneous Approach

04HH3DZ Insertion of Intraluminal Device into Right External Iliac Artery, Percutaneous Approach

04HH43Z Insertion of Infusion Device into Right External Iliac Artery, Percutaneous Endoscopic Approach

04HH4DZ Insertion of Intraluminal Device into Right External Iliac Artery, Percutaneous Endoscopic Approach

04HJ03Z Insertion of Infusion Device into Left External Iliac Artery, Open Approach

04HJ0DZ Insertion of Intraluminal Device into Left External Iliac Artery, Open Approach

04HJ33Z Insertion of Infusion Device into Left External Iliac Artery, Percutaneous Approach

04HJ3DZ Insertion of Intraluminal Device into Left External Iliac Artery, Percutaneous Approach

04HJ43Z Insertion of Infusion Device into Left External Iliac Artery, Percutaneous Endoscopic Approach

04HJ4DZ Insertion of Intraluminal Device into Left External Iliac Artery, Percutaneous Endoscopic Approach

04HK03Z Insertion of Infusion Device into Right Femoral Artery, Open Approach

04HK0DZ Insertion of Intraluminal Device into Right Femoral Artery, Open Approach

04HK33Z Insertion of Infusion Device into Right Femoral Artery, Percutaneous Approach

04HK3DZ Insertion of Intraluminal Device into Right Femoral Artery, Percutaneous Approach

04HK43Z Insertion of Infusion Device into Right Femoral Artery, Percutaneous Endoscopic Approach

04HK4DZ Insertion of Intraluminal Device into Right Femoral Artery, Percutaneous Endoscopic Approach

04HL03Z Insertion of Infusion Device into Left Femoral Artery, Open Approach

04HL0DZ Insertion of Intraluminal Device into Left Femoral Artery, Open Approach

04HL33Z Insertion of Infusion Device into Left Femoral Artery, Percutaneous Approach

04HL3DZ Insertion of Intraluminal Device into Left Femoral Artery, Percutaneous Approach

04HL43Z Insertion of Infusion Device into Left Femoral Artery, Percutaneous Endoscopic Approach

04HL4DZ Insertion of Intraluminal Device into Left Femoral Artery, Percutaneous Endoscopic Approach

04HM03Z Insertion of Infusion Device into Right Popliteal Artery, Open Approach

04HM0DZ Insertion of Intraluminal Device into Right Popliteal Artery, Open Approach

04HM33Z Insertion of Infusion Device into Right Popliteal Artery, Percutaneous Approach

04HM3DZ Insertion of Intraluminal Device into Right Popliteal Artery, Percutaneous Approach

04HM43Z Insertion of Infusion Device into Right Popliteal Artery, Percutaneous Endoscopic Approach

04HM4DZ Insertion of Intraluminal Device into Right Popliteal Artery, Percutaneous Endoscopic Approach

04HN03Z Insertion of Infusion Device into Left Popliteal Artery, Open Approach

04HN0DZ Insertion of Intraluminal Device into Left Popliteal Artery, Open Approach

04HN33Z Insertion of Infusion Device into Left Popliteal Artery, Percutaneous Approach

04HN3DZ Insertion of Intraluminal Device into Left Popliteal Artery, Percutaneous Approach

04HN43Z Insertion of Infusion Device into Left Popliteal Artery, Percutaneous Endoscopic Approach

04HN4DZ Insertion of Intraluminal Device into Left Popliteal Artery, Percutaneous Endoscopic Approach

04HP03Z Insertion of Infusion Device into Right Anterior Tibial Artery, Open Approach

04HP0DZ Insertion of Intraluminal Device into Right Anterior Tibial Artery, Open Approach

04HP33Z Insertion of Infusion Device into Right Anterior Tibial Artery, Percutaneous Approach

04HP3DZ Insertion of Intraluminal Device into Right Anterior Tibial Artery, Percutaneous Approach

04HP43Z Insertion of Infusion Device into Right Anterior Tibial Artery, Percutaneous Endoscopic Approach

04HP4DZ Insertion of Intraluminal Device into Right Anterior Tibial Artery, Percutaneous Endoscopic Approach

04HQ03Z Insertion of Infusion Device into Left Anterior Tibial Artery, Open Approach

04HQ0DZ Insertion of Intraluminal Device into Left Anterior Tibial Artery, Open Approach

04HQ33Z Insertion of Infusion Device into Left Anterior Tibial Artery, Percutaneous Approach

04HQ3DZ Insertion of Intraluminal Device into Left Anterior Tibial Artery, Percutaneous Approach

04HQ43Z Insertion of Infusion Device into Left Anterior Tibial Artery, Percutaneous Endoscopic Approach

04HQ4DZ Insertion of Intraluminal Device into Left Anterior Tibial Artery, Percutaneous Endoscopic Approach

04HR03Z Insertion of Infusion Device into Right Posterior Tibial Artery, Open Approach

04HR0DZ Insertion of Intraluminal Device into Right Posterior Tibial Artery, Open Approach

04HR33Z Insertion of Infusion Device into Right Posterior Tibial Artery, Percutaneous Approach

04HR3DZ Insertion of Intraluminal Device into Right Posterior Tibial Artery, Percutaneous Approach

04HR43Z Insertion of Infusion Device into Right Posterior Tibial Artery, Percutaneous Endoscopic Approach

04HR4DZ Insertion of Intraluminal Device into Right Posterior Tibial Artery, Percutaneous Endoscopic Approach

04HS03Z Insertion of Infusion Device into Left Posterior Tibial Artery, Open Approach

04HS0DZ Insertion of Intraluminal Device into Left Posterior Tibial Artery, Open Approach

04HS33Z Insertion of Infusion Device into Left Posterior Tibial Artery, Percutaneous Approach

04HS3DZ Insertion of Intraluminal Device into Left Posterior Tibial Artery, Percutaneous Approach

04HS43Z Insertion of Infusion Device into Left Posterior Tibial Artery, Percutaneous Endoscopic Approach

04HS4DZ Insertion of Intraluminal Device into Left Posterior Tibial Artery, Percutaneous Endoscopic Approach

04HT03Z Insertion of Infusion Device into Right Peroneal Artery, Open Approach

04HT0DZ Insertion of Intraluminal Device into Right Peroneal Artery, Open Approach

04HT33Z Insertion of Infusion Device into Right Peroneal Artery, Percutaneous Approach

04HT3DZ Insertion of Intraluminal Device into Right Peroneal Artery, Percutaneous Approach

04HT43Z Insertion of Infusion Device into Right Peroneal Artery, Percutaneous Endoscopic Approach

04HT4DZ Insertion of Intraluminal Device into Right Peroneal Artery, Percutaneous Endoscopic Approach

04HU03Z Insertion of Infusion Device into Left Peroneal Artery, Open Approach

04HU0DZ Insertion of Intraluminal Device into Left Peroneal Artery, Open Approach

04HU33Z Insertion of Infusion Device into Left Peroneal Artery, Percutaneous Approach

04HU3DZ Insertion of Intraluminal Device into Left Peroneal Artery, Percutaneous Approach

04HU43Z Insertion of Infusion Device into Left Peroneal Artery, Percutaneous Endoscopic Approach

04HU4DZ Insertion of Intraluminal Device into Left Peroneal Artery, Percutaneous Endoscopic Approach

04HV03Z Insertion of Infusion Device into Right Foot Artery, Open Approach

04HV0DZ Insertion of Intraluminal Device into Right Foot Artery, Open Approach

04HV33Z Insertion of Infusion Device into Right Foot Artery, Percutaneous Approach

04HV3DZ Insertion of Intraluminal Device into Right Foot Artery, Percutaneous Approach

04HV43Z Insertion of Infusion Device into Right Foot Artery, Percutaneous Endoscopic Approach

04HV4DZ Insertion of Intraluminal Device into Right Foot Artery, Percutaneous Endoscopic Approach

04HW03Z Insertion of Infusion Device into Left Foot Artery, Open Approach

04HW0DZ Insertion of Intraluminal Device into Left Foot Artery, Open Approach

04HW33Z Insertion of Infusion Device into Left Foot Artery, Percutaneous Approach

04HW3DZ Insertion of Intraluminal Device into Left Foot Artery, Percutaneous Approach

04HW43Z Insertion of Infusion Device into Left Foot Artery, Percutaneous Endoscopic Approach

04HW4DZ Insertion of Intraluminal Device into Left Foot Artery, Percutaneous Endoscopic Approach

04HY02Z Insertion of Monitoring Device into Lower Artery, Open Approach

04HY03Z Insertion of Infusion Device into Lower Artery, Open Approach

04HY0DZ Insertion of Intraluminal Device into Lower Artery, Open Approach

04HY32Z Insertion of Monitoring Device into Lower Artery, Percutaneous Approach

04HY33Z Insertion of Infusion Device into Lower Artery, Percutaneous Approach

04HY3DZ Insertion of Intraluminal Device into Lower Artery, Percutaneous Approach

04HY42Z Insertion of Monitoring Device into Lower Artery, Percutaneous Endoscopic Approach

04HY43Z Insertion of Infusion Device into Lower Artery, Percutaneous Endoscopic Approach

04HY4DZ Insertion of Intraluminal Device into Lower Artery, Percutaneous Endoscopic Approach

04J – Lower Arteries, Inspection

Review Coding Guidelines B3.11a, B3.11b and B3.11c

04JY0ZZ Inspection of Lower Artery, Open Approach
04JY3ZZ Inspection of Lower Artery, Percutaneous Approach

04JY4ZZ Inspection of Lower Artery, Percutaneous Endoscopic Approach
04JYXZZ Inspection of Lower Artery, External Approach

04L – Lower Arteries, Occlusion

Review Coding Guideline B3.12

04L00CZ Occlusion of Abdominal Aorta with Extraluminal Device, Open Approach

04L00DZ Occlusion of Abdominal Aorta with Intraluminal Device, Open Approach

04L00ZZ Occlusion of Abdominal Aorta, Open Approach

04L03CZ Occlusion of Abdominal Aorta with Extraluminal Device, Percutaneous Approach

04L03DZ Occlusion of Abdominal Aorta with Intraluminal Device, Percutaneous Approach

04L03ZZ Occlusion of Abdominal Aorta, Percutaneous Approach

04L04CZ Occlusion of Abdominal Aorta with Extraluminal Device, Percutaneous Endoscopic Approach

04L04DZ Occlusion of Abdominal Aorta with Intraluminal Device, Percutaneous Endoscopic Approach

04L04ZZ Occlusion of Abdominal Aorta, Percutaneous Endoscopic Approach

04L10CZ Occlusion of Celiac Artery with Extraluminal Device, Open Approach

04L10DZ Occlusion of Celiac Artery with Intraluminal Device, Open Approach

04L10ZZ Occlusion of Celiac Artery, Open Approach

04L13CZ Occlusion of Celiac Artery with Extraluminal Device, Percutaneous Approach

04L13DZ Occlusion of Celiac Artery with Intraluminal Device, Percutaneous Approach

04L13ZZ Occlusion of Celiac Artery, Percutaneous Approach

04L14CZ Occlusion of Celiac Artery with Extraluminal Device, Percutaneous Endoscopic Approach

04L14DZ Occlusion of Celiac Artery with Intraluminal Device, Percutaneous Endoscopic Approach

04L14ZZ Occlusion of Celiac Artery, Percutaneous Endoscopic Approach

04L20CZ Occlusion of Gastric Artery with Extraluminal Device, Open Approach

04L20DZ Occlusion of Gastric Artery with Intraluminal Device, Open Approach

04L20ZZ Occlusion of Gastric Artery, Open Approach

04L23CZ Occlusion of Gastric Artery with Extraluminal Device, Percutaneous Approach

04L23DZ Occlusion of Gastric Artery with Intraluminal Device, Percutaneous Approach

04L23ZZ Occlusion of Gastric Artery, Percutaneous Approach

04L24CZ Occlusion of Gastric Artery with Extraluminal Device, Percutaneous Endoscopic Approach

04L24DZ Occlusion of Gastric Artery with Intraluminal Device, Percutaneous Endoscopic Approach

04L24ZZ   Occlusion of Gastric Artery, Percutaneous Endoscopic Approach
04L30CZ   Occlusion of Hepatic Artery with Extraluminal Device, Open Approach
04L30DZ   Occlusion of Hepatic Artery with Intraluminal Device, Open Approach
04L30ZZ   Occlusion of Hepatic Artery, Open Approach
04L33CZ   Occlusion of Hepatic Artery with Extraluminal Device, Percutaneous Approach
04L33DZ   Occlusion of Hepatic Artery with Intraluminal Device, Percutaneous Approach
04L33ZZ   Occlusion of Hepatic Artery, Percutaneous Approach
04L34CZ   Occlusion of Hepatic Artery with Extraluminal Device, Percutaneous Endoscopic Approach
04L34DZ   Occlusion of Hepatic Artery with Intraluminal Device, Percutaneous Endoscopic Approach
04L34ZZ   Occlusion of Hepatic Artery, Percutaneous Endoscopic Approach
04L40CZ   Occlusion of Splenic Artery with Extraluminal Device, Open Approach
04L40DZ   Occlusion of Splenic Artery with Intraluminal Device, Open Approach
04L40ZZ   Occlusion of Splenic Artery, Open Approach
04L43CZ   Occlusion of Splenic Artery with Extraluminal Device, Percutaneous Approach
04L43DZ   Occlusion of Splenic Artery with Intraluminal Device, Percutaneous Approach
04L43ZZ   Occlusion of Splenic Artery, Percutaneous Approach
04L44CZ   Occlusion of Splenic Artery with Extraluminal Device, Percutaneous Endoscopic Approach
04L44DZ   Occlusion of Splenic Artery with Intraluminal Device, Percutaneous Endoscopic Approach
04L44ZZ   Occlusion of Splenic Artery, Percutaneous Endoscopic Approach
04L50CZ   Occlusion of Superior Mesenteric Artery with Extraluminal Device, Open Approach
04L50DZ   Occlusion of Superior Mesenteric Artery with Intraluminal Device, Open Approach
04L50ZZ   Occlusion of Superior Mesenteric Artery, Open Approach
04L53CZ   Occlusion of Superior Mesenteric Artery with Extraluminal Device, Percutaneous Approach
04L53DZ   Occlusion of Superior Mesenteric Artery with Intraluminal Device, Percutaneous Approach
04L53ZZ   Occlusion of Superior Mesenteric Artery, Percutaneous Approach
04L54CZ   Occlusion of Superior Mesenteric Artery with Extraluminal Device, Percutaneous Endoscopic Approach
04L54DZ   Occlusion of Superior Mesenteric Artery with Intraluminal Device, Percutaneous Endoscopic Approach
04L54ZZ   Occlusion of Superior Mesenteric Artery, Percutaneous Endoscopic Approach
04L60CZ   Occlusion of Right Colic Artery with Extraluminal Device, Open Approach
04L60DZ   Occlusion of Right Colic Artery with Intraluminal Device, Open Approach
04L60ZZ   Occlusion of Right Colic Artery, Open Approach
04L63CZ   Occlusion of Right Colic Artery with Extraluminal Device, Percutaneous Approach
04L63DZ   Occlusion of Right Colic Artery with Intraluminal Device, Percutaneous Approach
04L63ZZ   Occlusion of Right Colic Artery, Percutaneous Approach
04L64CZ   Occlusion of Right Colic Artery with Extraluminal Device, Percutaneous Endoscopic Approach
04L64DZ   Occlusion of Right Colic Artery with Intraluminal Device, Percutaneous Endoscopic Approach
04L64ZZ   Occlusion of Right Colic Artery, Percutaneous Endoscopic Approach
04L70CZ   Occlusion of Left Colic Artery with Extraluminal Device, Open Approach
04L70DZ   Occlusion of Left Colic Artery with Intraluminal Device, Open Approach
04L70ZZ   Occlusion of Left Colic Artery, Open Approach
04L73CZ   Occlusion of Left Colic Artery with Extraluminal Device, Percutaneous Approach
04L73DZ   Occlusion of Left Colic Artery with Intraluminal Device, Percutaneous Approach
04L73ZZ   Occlusion of Left Colic Artery, Percutaneous Approach

04L74CZ   Occlusion of Left Colic Artery with Extraluminal Device, Percutaneous Endoscopic Approach
04L74DZ   Occlusion of Left Colic Artery with Intraluminal Device, Percutaneous Endoscopic Approach
04L74ZZ   Occlusion of Left Colic Artery, Percutaneous Endoscopic Approach
04L80CZ   Occlusion of Middle Colic Artery with Extraluminal Device, Open Approach
04L80DZ   Occlusion of Middle Colic Artery with Intraluminal Device, Open Approach
04L80ZZ   Occlusion of Middle Colic Artery, Open Approach
04L83CZ   Occlusion of Middle Colic Artery with Extraluminal Device, Percutaneous Approach
04L83DZ   Occlusion of Middle Colic Artery with Intraluminal Device, Percutaneous Approach
04L83ZZ   Occlusion of Middle Colic Artery, Percutaneous Approach
04L84CZ   Occlusion of Middle Colic Artery with Extraluminal Device, Percutaneous Endoscopic Approach
04L84DZ   Occlusion of Middle Colic Artery with Intraluminal Device, Percutaneous Endoscopic Approach
04L84ZZ   Occlusion of Middle Colic Artery, Percutaneous Endoscopic Approach
04L90CZ   Occlusion of Right Renal Artery with Extraluminal Device, Open Approach
04L90DZ   Occlusion of Right Renal Artery with Intraluminal Device, Open Approach
04L90ZZ   Occlusion of Right Renal Artery, Open Approach
04L93CZ   Occlusion of Right Renal Artery with Extraluminal Device, Percutaneous Approach
04L93DZ   Occlusion of Right Renal Artery with Intraluminal Device, Percutaneous Approach
04L93ZZ   Occlusion of Right Renal Artery, Percutaneous Approach
04L94CZ   Occlusion of Right Renal Artery with Extraluminal Device, Percutaneous Endoscopic Approach
04L94DZ   Occlusion of Right Renal Artery with Intraluminal Device, Percutaneous Endoscopic Approach
04L94ZZ   Occlusion of Right Renal Artery, Percutaneous Endoscopic Approach
04LA0CZ   Occlusion of Left Renal Artery with Extraluminal Device, Open Approach
04LA0DZ   Occlusion of Left Renal Artery with Intraluminal Device, Open Approach
04LA0ZZ   Occlusion of Left Renal Artery, Open Approach
04LA3CZ   Occlusion of Left Renal Artery with Extraluminal Device, Percutaneous Approach
04LA3DZ   Occlusion of Left Renal Artery with Intraluminal Device, Percutaneous Approach
04LA3ZZ   Occlusion of Left Renal Artery, Percutaneous Approach
04LA4CZ   Occlusion of Left Renal Artery with Extraluminal Device, Percutaneous Endoscopic Approach
04LA4DZ   Occlusion of Left Renal Artery with Intraluminal Device, Percutaneous Endoscopic Approach
04LA4ZZ   Occlusion of Left Renal Artery, Percutaneous Endoscopic Approach
04LB0CZ   Occlusion of Inferior Mesenteric Artery with Extraluminal Device, Open Approach
04LB0DZ   Occlusion of Inferior Mesenteric Artery with Intraluminal Device, Open Approach
04LB0ZZ   Occlusion of Inferior Mesenteric Artery, Open Approach
04LB3CZ   Occlusion of Inferior Mesenteric Artery with Extraluminal Device, Percutaneous Approach
04LB3DZ   Occlusion of Inferior Mesenteric Artery with Intraluminal Device, Percutaneous Approach
04LB3ZZ   Occlusion of Inferior Mesenteric Artery, Percutaneous Approach
04LB4CZ   Occlusion of Inferior Mesenteric Artery with Extraluminal Device, Percutaneous Endoscopic Approach
04LB4DZ   Occlusion of Inferior Mesenteric Artery with Intraluminal Device, Percutaneous Endoscopic Approach
04LB4ZZ   Occlusion of Inferior Mesenteric Artery, Percutaneous Endoscopic Approach
04LC0CZ   Occlusion of Right Common Iliac Artery with Extraluminal Device, Open Approach
04LC0DZ   Occlusion of Right Common Iliac Artery with Intraluminal Device, Open Approach
04LC0ZZ   Occlusion of Right Common Iliac Artery, Open Approach

04LC3CZ Occlusion of Right Common Iliac Artery with Extraluminal Device, Percutaneous Approach

04LC3DZ Occlusion of Right Common Iliac Artery with Intraluminal Device, Percutaneous Approach

04LC3ZZ Occlusion of Right Common Iliac Artery, Percutaneous Approach

04LC4CZ Occlusion of Right Common Iliac Artery with Extraluminal Device, Percutaneous Endoscopic Approach

04LC4DZ Occlusion of Right Common Iliac Artery with Intraluminal Device, Percutaneous Endoscopic Approach

04LC4ZZ Occlusion of Right Common Iliac Artery, Percutaneous Endoscopic Approach

04LD0CZ Occlusion of Left Common Iliac Artery with Extraluminal Device, Open Approach

04LD0DZ Occlusion of Left Common Iliac Artery with Intraluminal Device, Open Approach

04LD0ZZ Occlusion of Left Common Iliac Artery, Open Approach

04LD3CZ Occlusion of Left Common Iliac Artery with Extraluminal Device, Percutaneous Approach

04LD3DZ Occlusion of Left Common Iliac Artery with Intraluminal Device, Percutaneous Approach

04LD3ZZ Occlusion of Left Common Iliac Artery, Percutaneous Approach

04LD4CZ Occlusion of Left Common Iliac Artery with Extraluminal Device, Percutaneous Endoscopic Approach

04LD4DZ Occlusion of Left Common Iliac Artery with Intraluminal Device, Percutaneous Endoscopic Approach

04LD4ZZ Occlusion of Left Common Iliac Artery, Percutaneous Endoscopic Approach

♀ **04LE0CT** Occlusion of Right Uterine Artery with Extraluminal Device, Open Approach

04LE0CZ Occlusion of Right Internal Iliac Artery with Extraluminal Device, Open Approach

♀ **04LE0DT** Occlusion of Right Uterine Artery with Intraluminal Device, Open Approach

04LE0DZ Occlusion of Right Internal Iliac Artery with Intraluminal Device, Open Approach

♀ **04LE0ZT** Occlusion of Right Uterine Artery, Open Approach

04LE0ZZ Occlusion of Right Internal Iliac Artery, Open Approach

♀ **04LE3CT** Occlusion of Right Uterine Artery with Extraluminal Device, Percutaneous Approach

04LE3CZ Occlusion of Right Internal Iliac Artery with Extraluminal Device, Percutaneous Approach

♀ **04LE3DT** Occlusion of Right Uterine Artery with Intraluminal Device, Percutaneous Approach

04LE3DZ Occlusion of Right Internal Iliac Artery with Intraluminal Device, Percutaneous Approach

♀ **04LE3ZT** Occlusion of Right Uterine Artery, Percutaneous Approach

04LE3ZZ Occlusion of Right Internal Iliac Artery, Percutaneous Approach

♀ **04LE4CT** Occlusion of Right Uterine Artery with Extraluminal Device, Percutaneous Endoscopic Approach

04LE4CZ Occlusion of Right Internal Iliac Artery with Extraluminal Device, Percutaneous Endoscopic Approach

♀ **04LE4DT** Occlusion of Right Uterine Artery with Intraluminal Device, Percutaneous Endoscopic Approach

04LE4DZ Occlusion of Right Internal Iliac Artery with Intraluminal Device, Percutaneous Endoscopic Approach

♀ **04LE4ZT** Occlusion of Right Uterine Artery, Percutaneous Endoscopic Approach

04LE4ZZ Occlusion of Right Internal Iliac Artery, Percutaneous Endoscopic Approach

♀ **04LF0CU** Occlusion of Left Uterine Artery with Extraluminal Device, Open Approach

04LF0CZ Occlusion of Left Internal Iliac Artery with Extraluminal Device, Open Approach

♀ **04LF0DU** Occlusion of Left Uterine Artery with Intraluminal Device, Open Approach

04LF0DZ Occlusion of Left Internal Iliac Artery with Intraluminal Device, Open Approach

♀ **04LF0ZU** Occlusion of Left Uterine Artery, Open Approach

04LF0ZZ Occlusion of Left Internal Iliac Artery, Open Approach

♀ **04LF3CU** Occlusion of Left Uterine Artery with Extraluminal Device, Percutaneous Approach

04LF3CZ Occlusion of Left Internal Iliac Artery with Extraluminal Device, Percutaneous Approach

♀ **04LF3DU** Occlusion of Left Uterine Artery with Intraluminal Device, Percutaneous Approach

04LF3DZ Occlusion of Left Internal Iliac Artery with Intraluminal Device, Percutaneous Approach

♀ **04LF3ZU** Occlusion of Left Uterine Artery, Percutaneous Approach

04LF3ZZ Occlusion of Left Internal Iliac Artery, Percutaneous Approach

♀ **04LF4CU** Occlusion of Left Uterine Artery with Extraluminal Device, Percutaneous Endoscopic Approach

04LF4CZ Occlusion of Left Internal Iliac Artery with Extraluminal Device, Percutaneous Endoscopic Approach

♀ **04LF4DU** Occlusion of Left Uterine Artery with Intraluminal Device, Percutaneous Endoscopic Approach

04LF4DZ Occlusion of Left Internal Iliac Artery with Intraluminal Device, Percutaneous Endoscopic Approach

♀ **04LF4ZU** Occlusion of Left Uterine Artery, Percutaneous Endoscopic Approach

04LF4ZZ Occlusion of Left Internal Iliac Artery, Percutaneous Endoscopic Approach

04LH0CZ Occlusion of Right External Iliac Artery with Extraluminal Device, Open Approach

04LH0DZ Occlusion of Right External Iliac Artery with Intraluminal Device, Open Approach

04LH0ZZ Occlusion of Right External Iliac Artery, Open Approach

04LH3CZ Occlusion of Right External Iliac Artery with Extraluminal Device, Percutaneous Approach

04LH3DZ Occlusion of Right External Iliac Artery with Intraluminal Device, Percutaneous Approach

04LH3ZZ Occlusion of Right External Iliac Artery, Percutaneous Approach

04LH4CZ Occlusion of Right External Iliac Artery with Extraluminal Device, Percutaneous Endoscopic Approach

04LH4DZ Occlusion of Right External Iliac Artery with Intraluminal Device, Percutaneous Endoscopic Approach

04LH4ZZ Occlusion of Right External Iliac Artery, Percutaneous Endoscopic Approach

04LJ0CZ Occlusion of Left External Iliac Artery with Extraluminal Device, Open Approach

04LJ0DZ Occlusion of Left External Iliac Artery with Intraluminal Device, Open Approach

04LJ0ZZ Occlusion of Left External Iliac Artery, Open Approach

04LJ3CZ Occlusion of Left External Iliac Artery with Extraluminal Device, Percutaneous Approach

04LJ3DZ Occlusion of Left External Iliac Artery with Intraluminal Device, Percutaneous Approach

04LJ3ZZ Occlusion of Left External Iliac Artery, Percutaneous Approach

04LJ4CZ Occlusion of Left External Iliac Artery with Extraluminal Device, Percutaneous Endoscopic Approach

04LJ4DZ Occlusion of Left External Iliac Artery with Intraluminal Device, Percutaneous Endoscopic Approach

04LJ4ZZ Occlusion of Left External Iliac Artery, Percutaneous Endoscopic Approach

04LK0CZ Occlusion of Right Femoral Artery with Extraluminal Device, Open Approach

04LK0DZ Occlusion of Right Femoral Artery with Intraluminal Device, Open Approach

04LK0ZZ Occlusion of Right Femoral Artery, Open Approach

04LK3CZ Occlusion of Right Femoral Artery with Extraluminal Device, Percutaneous Approach

04LK3DZ Occlusion of Right Femoral Artery with Intraluminal Device, Percutaneous Approach

04LK3ZZ Occlusion of Right Femoral Artery, Percutaneous Approach

04LK4CZ Occlusion of Right Femoral Artery with Extraluminal Device, Percutaneous Endoscopic Approach

04LK4DZ Occlusion of Right Femoral Artery with Intraluminal Device, Percutaneous Endoscopic Approach

04LK4ZZ Occlusion of Right Femoral Artery, Percutaneous Endoscopic Approach

04LL0CZ Occlusion of Left Femoral Artery with Extraluminal Device, Open Approach

04LL0DZ Occlusion of Left Femoral Artery with Intraluminal Device, Open Approach

04LL0ZZ Occlusion of Left Femoral Artery, Open Approach

04LL3CZ Occlusion of Left Femoral Artery with Extraluminal Device, Percutaneous Approach

04LL3DZ Occlusion of Left Femoral Artery with Intraluminal Device, Percutaneous Approach

04LL3ZZ Occlusion of Left Femoral Artery, Percutaneous Approach

04LL4CZ Occlusion of Left Femoral Artery with Extraluminal Device, Percutaneous Endoscopic Approach

04LL4DZ Occlusion of Left Femoral Artery with Intraluminal Device, Percutaneous Endoscopic Approach

04LL4ZZ Occlusion of Left Femoral Artery, Percutaneous Endoscopic Approach

04LM0CZ Occlusion of Right Popliteal Artery with Extraluminal Device, Open Approach

04LM0DZ Occlusion of Right Popliteal Artery with Intraluminal Device, Open Approach

04LM0ZZ Occlusion of Right Popliteal Artery, Open Approach

04LM3CZ Occlusion of Right Popliteal Artery with Extraluminal Device, Percutaneous Approach

04LM3DZ Occlusion of Right Popliteal Artery with Intraluminal Device, Percutaneous Approach

04LM3ZZ Occlusion of Right Popliteal Artery, Percutaneous Approach

04LM4CZ Occlusion of Right Popliteal Artery with Extraluminal Device, Percutaneous Endoscopic Approach

04LM4DZ Occlusion of Right Popliteal Artery with Intraluminal Device, Percutaneous Endoscopic Approach

04LM4ZZ Occlusion of Right Popliteal Artery, Percutaneous Endoscopic Approach

04LN0CZ Occlusion of Left Popliteal Artery with Extraluminal Device, Open Approach

04LN0DZ Occlusion of Left Popliteal Artery with Intraluminal Device, Open Approach

04LN0ZZ Occlusion of Left Popliteal Artery, Open Approach

04LN3CZ Occlusion of Left Popliteal Artery with Extraluminal Device, Percutaneous Approach

04LN3DZ Occlusion of Left Popliteal Artery with Intraluminal Device, Percutaneous Approach

04LN3ZZ Occlusion of Left Popliteal Artery, Percutaneous Approach

04LN4CZ Occlusion of Left Popliteal Artery with Extraluminal Device, Percutaneous Endoscopic Approach

04LN4DZ Occlusion of Left Popliteal Artery with Intraluminal Device, Percutaneous Endoscopic Approach

04LN4ZZ Occlusion of Left Popliteal Artery, Percutaneous Endoscopic Approach

04LP0CZ Occlusion of Right Anterior Tibial Artery with Extraluminal Device, Open Approach

04LP0DZ Occlusion of Right Anterior Tibial Artery with Intraluminal Device, Open Approach

04LP0ZZ Occlusion of Right Anterior Tibial Artery, Open Approach

04LP3CZ Occlusion of Right Anterior Tibial Artery with Extraluminal Device, Percutaneous Approach

04LP3DZ Occlusion of Right Anterior Tibial Artery with Intraluminal Device, Percutaneous Approach

04LP3ZZ Occlusion of Right Anterior Tibial Artery, Percutaneous Approach

04LP4CZ Occlusion of Right Anterior Tibial Artery with Extraluminal Device, Percutaneous Endoscopic Approach

04LP4DZ Occlusion of Right Anterior Tibial Artery with Intraluminal Device, Percutaneous Endoscopic Approach

04LP4ZZ Occlusion of Right Anterior Tibial Artery, Percutaneous Endoscopic Approach

04LQ0CZ Occlusion of Left Anterior Tibial Artery with Extraluminal Device, Open Approach

04LQ0DZ Occlusion of Left Anterior Tibial Artery with Intraluminal Device, Open Approach

04LQ0ZZ Occlusion of Left Anterior Tibial Artery, Open Approach

04LQ3CZ Occlusion of Left Anterior Tibial Artery with Extraluminal Device, Percutaneous Approach

04LQ3DZ Occlusion of Left Anterior Tibial Artery with Intraluminal Device, Percutaneous Approach

04LQ3ZZ Occlusion of Left Anterior Tibial Artery, Percutaneous Approach

04LQ4CZ Occlusion of Left Anterior Tibial Artery with Extraluminal Device, Percutaneous Endoscopic Approach

04LQ4DZ Occlusion of Left Anterior Tibial Artery with Intraluminal Device, Percutaneous Endoscopic Approach

04LQ4ZZ Occlusion of Left Anterior Tibial Artery, Percutaneous Endoscopic Approach

04LR0CZ Occlusion of Right Posterior Tibial Artery with Extraluminal Device, Open Approach

04LR0DZ Occlusion of Right Posterior Tibial Artery with Intraluminal Device, Open Approach

04LR0ZZ Occlusion of Right Posterior Tibial Artery, Open Approach

04LR3CZ Occlusion of Right Posterior Tibial Artery with Extraluminal Device, Percutaneous Approach

04LR3DZ Occlusion of Right Posterior Tibial Artery with Intraluminal Device, Percutaneous Approach

04LR3ZZ Occlusion of Right Posterior Tibial Artery, Percutaneous Approach

04LR4CZ Occlusion of Right Posterior Tibial Artery with Extraluminal Device, Percutaneous Endoscopic Approach

04LR4DZ Occlusion of Right Posterior Tibial Artery with Intraluminal Device, Percutaneous Endoscopic Approach

04LR4ZZ Occlusion of Right Posterior Tibial Artery, Percutaneous Endoscopic Approach

04LS0CZ Occlusion of Left Posterior Tibial Artery with Extraluminal Device, Open Approach

04LS0DZ Occlusion of Left Posterior Tibial Artery with Intraluminal Device, Open Approach

04LS0ZZ Occlusion of Left Posterior Tibial Artery, Open Approach

04LS3CZ Occlusion of Left Posterior Tibial Artery with Extraluminal Device, Percutaneous Approach

04LS3DZ Occlusion of Left Posterior Tibial Artery with Intraluminal Device, Percutaneous Approach

04LS3ZZ Occlusion of Left Posterior Tibial Artery, Percutaneous Approach

04LS4CZ Occlusion of Left Posterior Tibial Artery with Extraluminal Device, Percutaneous Endoscopic Approach

04LS4DZ Occlusion of Left Posterior Tibial Artery with Intraluminal Device, Percutaneous Endoscopic Approach

04LS4ZZ Occlusion of Left Posterior Tibial Artery, Percutaneous Endoscopic Approach

04LT0CZ Occlusion of Right Peroneal Artery with Extraluminal Device, Open Approach

04LT0DZ Occlusion of Right Peroneal Artery with Intraluminal Device, Open Approach

04LT0ZZ Occlusion of Right Peroneal Artery, Open Approach

04LT3CZ Occlusion of Right Peroneal Artery with Extraluminal Device, Percutaneous Approach

04LT3DZ Occlusion of Right Peroneal Artery with Intraluminal Device, Percutaneous Approach

04LT3ZZ Occlusion of Right Peroneal Artery, Percutaneous Approach

04LT4CZ Occlusion of Right Peroneal Artery with Extraluminal Device, Percutaneous Endoscopic Approach

04LT4DZ Occlusion of Right Peroneal Artery with Intraluminal Device, Percutaneous Endoscopic Approach

04LT4ZZ Occlusion of Right Peroneal Artery, Percutaneous Endoscopic Approach

04LU0CZ Occlusion of Left Peroneal Artery with Extraluminal Device, Open Approach

04LU0DZ Occlusion of Left Peroneal Artery with Intraluminal Device, Open Approach

04LU0ZZ Occlusion of Left Peroneal Artery, Open Approach

04LU3CZ Occlusion of Left Peroneal Artery with Extraluminal Device, Percutaneous Approach

04LU3DZ Occlusion of Left Peroneal Artery with Intraluminal Device, Percutaneous Approach

04LU3ZZ Occlusion of Left Peroneal Artery, Percutaneous Approach

04LU4CZ Occlusion of Left Peroneal Artery with Extraluminal Device, Percutaneous Endoscopic Approach

04LU4DZ Occlusion of Left Peroneal Artery with Intraluminal Device, Percutaneous Endoscopic Approach

04LU4ZZ Occlusion of Left Peroneal Artery, Percutaneous Endoscopic Approach

04LV0CZ Occlusion of Right Foot Artery with Extraluminal Device, Open Approach

04LV0DZ Occlusion of Right Foot Artery with Intraluminal Device, Open Approach

04LV0ZZ Occlusion of Right Foot Artery, Open Approach

04LV3CZ Occlusion of Right Foot Artery with Extraluminal Device, Percutaneous Approach

04LV3DZ Occlusion of Right Foot Artery with Intraluminal Device, Percutaneous Approach

04LV3ZZ Occlusion of Right Foot Artery, Percutaneous Approach
04LV4CZ Occlusion of Right Foot Artery with Extraluminal Device, Percutaneous Endoscopic Approach
04LV4DZ Occlusion of Right Foot Artery with Intraluminal Device, Percutaneous Endoscopic Approach
04LV4ZZ Occlusion of Right Foot Artery, Percutaneous Endoscopic Approach
04LW0CZ Occlusion of Left Foot Artery with Extraluminal Device, Open Approach
04LW0DZ Occlusion of Left Foot Artery with Intraluminal Device, Open Approach
04LW0ZZ Occlusion of Left Foot Artery, Open Approach
04LW3CZ Occlusion of Left Foot Artery with Extraluminal Device, Percutaneous Approach
04LW3DZ Occlusion of Left Foot Artery with Intraluminal Device, Percutaneous Approach
04LW3ZZ Occlusion of Left Foot Artery, Percutaneous Approach
04LW4CZ Occlusion of Left Foot Artery with Extraluminal Device, Percutaneous Endoscopic Approach

04LW4DZ Occlusion of Left Foot Artery with Intraluminal Device, Percutaneous Endoscopic Approach
04LW4ZZ Occlusion of Left Foot Artery, Percutaneous Endoscopic Approach
04LY0CZ Occlusion of Lower Artery with Extraluminal Device, Open Approach
04LY0DZ Occlusion of Lower Artery with Intraluminal Device, Open Approach
04LY0ZZ Occlusion of Lower Artery, Open Approach
04LY3CZ Occlusion of Lower Artery with Extraluminal Device, Percutaneous Approach
04LY3DZ Occlusion of Lower Artery with Intraluminal Device, Percutaneous Approach
04LY3ZZ Occlusion of Lower Artery, Percutaneous Approach
04LY4CZ Occlusion of Lower Artery with Extraluminal Device, Percutaneous Endoscopic Approach
04LY4DZ Occlusion of Lower Artery with Intraluminal Device, Percutaneous Endoscopic Approach
04LY4ZZ Occlusion of Lower Artery, Percutaneous Endoscopic Approach

04N – Lower Arteries, Release

Review Coding Guidelines B3.13 and B3.14

04N00ZZ Release Abdominal Aorta, Open Approach
04N03ZZ Release Abdominal Aorta, Percutaneous Approach
04N04ZZ Release Abdominal Aorta, Percutaneous Endoscopic Approach
04N10ZZ Release Celiac Artery, Open Approach
04N13ZZ Release Celiac Artery, Percutaneous Approach
04N14ZZ Release Celiac Artery, Percutaneous Endoscopic Approach
04N20ZZ Release Gastric Artery, Open Approach
04N23ZZ Release Gastric Artery, Percutaneous Approach
04N24ZZ Release Gastric Artery, Percutaneous Endoscopic Approach
04N30ZZ Release Hepatic Artery, Open Approach
04N33ZZ Release Hepatic Artery, Percutaneous Approach
04N34ZZ Release Hepatic Artery, Percutaneous Endoscopic Approach
04N40ZZ Release Splenic Artery, Open Approach
04N43ZZ Release Splenic Artery, Percutaneous Approach
04N44ZZ Release Splenic Artery, Percutaneous Endoscopic Approach
04N50ZZ Release Superior Mesenteric Artery, Open Approach
04N53ZZ Release Superior Mesenteric Artery, Percutaneous Approach
04N54ZZ Release Superior Mesenteric Artery, Percutaneous Endoscopic Approach
04N60ZZ Release Right Colic Artery, Open Approach
04N63ZZ Release Right Colic Artery, Percutaneous Approach
04N64ZZ Release Right Colic Artery, Percutaneous Endoscopic Approach
04N70ZZ Release Left Colic Artery, Open Approach
04N73ZZ Release Left Colic Artery, Percutaneous Approach
04N74ZZ Release Left Colic Artery, Percutaneous Endoscopic Approach
04N80ZZ Release Middle Colic Artery, Open Approach
04N83ZZ Release Middle Colic Artery, Percutaneous Approach
04N84ZZ Release Middle Colic Artery, Percutaneous Endoscopic Approach
04N90ZZ Release Right Renal Artery, Open Approach
04N93ZZ Release Right Renal Artery, Percutaneous Approach
04N94ZZ Release Right Renal Artery, Percutaneous Endoscopic Approach
04NA0ZZ Release Left Renal Artery, Open Approach
04NA3ZZ Release Left Renal Artery, Percutaneous Approach
04NA4ZZ Release Left Renal Artery, Percutaneous Endoscopic Approach
04NB0ZZ Release Inferior Mesenteric Artery, Open Approach
04NB3ZZ Release Inferior Mesenteric Artery, Percutaneous Approach
04NB4ZZ Release Inferior Mesenteric Artery, Percutaneous Endoscopic Approach
04NC0ZZ Release Right Common Iliac Artery, Open Approach
04NC3ZZ Release Right Common Iliac Artery, Percutaneous Approach
04NC4ZZ Release Right Common Iliac Artery, Percutaneous Endoscopic Approach
04ND0ZZ Release Left Common Iliac Artery, Open Approach
04ND3ZZ Release Left Common Iliac Artery, Percutaneous Approach
04ND4ZZ Release Left Common Iliac Artery, Percutaneous Endoscopic Approach
04NE0ZZ Release Right Internal Iliac Artery, Open Approach
04NE3ZZ Release Right Internal Iliac Artery, Percutaneous Approach
04NE4ZZ Release Right Internal Iliac Artery, Percutaneous Endoscopic Approach

04NF0ZZ Release Left Internal Iliac Artery, Open Approach
04NF3ZZ Release Left Internal Iliac Artery, Percutaneous Approach
04NF4ZZ Release Left Internal Iliac Artery, Percutaneous Endoscopic Approach
04NH0ZZ Release Right External Iliac Artery, Open Approach
04NH3ZZ Release Right External Iliac Artery, Percutaneous Approach
04NH4ZZ Release Right External Iliac Artery, Percutaneous Endoscopic Approach
04NJ0ZZ Release Left External Iliac Artery, Open Approach
04NJ3ZZ Release Left External Iliac Artery, Percutaneous Approach
04NJ4ZZ Release Left External Iliac Artery, Percutaneous Endoscopic Approach
04NK0ZZ Release Right Femoral Artery, Open Approach
04NK3ZZ Release Right Femoral Artery, Percutaneous Approach
04NK4ZZ Release Right Femoral Artery, Percutaneous Endoscopic Approach
04NL0ZZ Release Left Femoral Artery, Open Approach
04NL3ZZ Release Left Femoral Artery, Percutaneous Approach
04NL4ZZ Release Left Femoral Artery, Percutaneous Endoscopic Approach
04NM0ZZ Release Right Popliteal Artery, Open Approach
04NM3ZZ Release Right Popliteal Artery, Percutaneous Approach
04NM4ZZ Release Right Popliteal Artery, Percutaneous Endoscopic Approach
04NN0ZZ Release Left Popliteal Artery, Open Approach
04NN3ZZ Release Left Popliteal Artery, Percutaneous Approach
04NN4ZZ Release Left Popliteal Artery, Percutaneous Endoscopic Approach
04NP0ZZ Release Right Anterior Tibial Artery, Open Approach
04NP3ZZ Release Right Anterior Tibial Artery, Percutaneous Approach
04NP4ZZ Release Right Anterior Tibial Artery, Percutaneous Endoscopic Approach
04NQ0ZZ Release Left Anterior Tibial Artery, Open Approach
04NQ3ZZ Release Left Anterior Tibial Artery, Percutaneous Approach
04NQ4ZZ Release Left Anterior Tibial Artery, Percutaneous Endoscopic Approach
04NR0ZZ Release Right Posterior Tibial Artery, Open Approach
04NR3ZZ Release Right Posterior Tibial Artery, Percutaneous Approach
04NR4ZZ Release Right Posterior Tibial Artery, Percutaneous Endoscopic Approach
04NS0ZZ Release Left Posterior Tibial Artery, Open Approach
04NS3ZZ Release Left Posterior Tibial Artery, Percutaneous Approach
04NS4ZZ Release Left Posterior Tibial Artery, Percutaneous Endoscopic Approach
04NT0ZZ Release Right Peroneal Artery, Open Approach
04NT3ZZ Release Right Peroneal Artery, Percutaneous Approach
04NT4ZZ Release Right Peroneal Artery, Percutaneous Endoscopic Approach
04NU0ZZ Release Left Peroneal Artery, Open Approach
04NU3ZZ Release Left Peroneal Artery, Percutaneous Approach
04NU4ZZ Release Left Peroneal Artery, Percutaneous Endoscopic Approach
04NV0ZZ Release Right Foot Artery, Open Approach
04NV3ZZ Release Right Foot Artery, Percutaneous Approach
04NV4ZZ Release Right Foot Artery, Percutaneous Endoscopic Approach
04NW0ZZ Release Left Foot Artery, Open Approach

04NW3ZZ Release Left Foot Artery, Percutaneous Approach
04NW4ZZ Release Left Foot Artery, Percutaneous Endoscopic Approach
04NY0ZZ Release Lower Artery, Open Approach

04NY3ZZ Release Lower Artery, Percutaneous Approach
04NY4ZZ Release Lower Artery, Percutaneous Endoscopic Approach

04P – Lower Arteries, Removal

Review Coding Guideline B6.1c

04PY00Z Removal of Drainage Device from Lower Artery, Open Approach
04PY02Z Removal of Monitoring Device from Lower Artery, Open Approach
04PY03Z Removal of Infusion Device from Lower Artery, Open Approach
04PY07Z Removal of Autologous Tissue Substitute from Lower Artery, Open Approach
04PY0CZ Removal of Extraluminal Device from Lower Artery, Open Approach
04PY0DZ Removal of Intraluminal Device from Lower Artery, Open Approach
04PY0JZ Removal of Synthetic Substitute from Lower Artery, Open Approach
04PY0KZ Removal of Nonautologous Tissue Substitute from Lower Artery, Open Approach
04PY30Z Removal of Drainage Device from Lower Artery, Percutaneous Approach
04PY32Z Removal of Monitoring Device from Lower Artery, Percutaneous Approach
04PY33Z Removal of Infusion Device from Lower Artery, Percutaneous Approach
04PY37Z Removal of Autologous Tissue Substitute from Lower Artery, Percutaneous Approach
04PY3CZ Removal of Extraluminal Device from Lower Artery, Percutaneous Approach
04PY3DZ Removal of Intraluminal Device from Lower Artery, Percutaneous Approach
04PY3JZ Removal of Synthetic Substitute from Lower Artery, Percutaneous Approach

04PY3KZ Removal of Nonautologous Tissue Substitute from Lower Artery, Percutaneous Approach
04PY40Z Removal of Drainage Device from Lower Artery, Percutaneous Endoscopic Approach
04PY42Z Removal of Monitoring Device from Lower Artery, Percutaneous Endoscopic Approach
04PY43Z Removal of Infusion Device from Lower Artery, Percutaneous Endoscopic Approach
04PY47Z Removal of Autologous Tissue Substitute from Lower Artery, Percutaneous Endoscopic Approach
04PY4CZ Removal of Extraluminal Device from Lower Artery, Percutaneous Endoscopic Approach
04PY4DZ Removal of Intraluminal Device from Lower Artery, Percutaneous Endoscopic Approach
04PY4JZ Removal of Synthetic Substitute from Lower Artery, Percutaneous Endoscopic Approach
04PY4KZ Removal of Nonautologous Tissue Substitute from Lower Artery, Percutaneous Endoscopic Approach
04PYX0Z Removal of Drainage Device from Lower Artery, External Approach
04PYX1Z Removal of Radioactive Element from Lower Artery, External Approach
04PYX2Z Removal of Monitoring Device from Lower Artery, External Approach
04PYX3Z Removal of Infusion Device from Lower Artery, External Approach
04PYXDZ Removal of Intraluminal Device from Lower Artery, External Approach

04Q – Lower Arteries, Repair

04Q00ZZ Repair Abdominal Aorta, Open Approach
04Q03ZZ Repair Abdominal Aorta, Percutaneous Approach
04Q04ZZ Repair Abdominal Aorta, Percutaneous Endoscopic Approach
04Q10ZZ Repair Celiac Artery, Open Approach
04Q13ZZ Repair Celiac Artery, Percutaneous Approach
04Q14ZZ Repair Celiac Artery, Percutaneous Endoscopic Approach
04Q20ZZ Repair Gastric Artery, Open Approach
04Q23ZZ Repair Gastric Artery, Percutaneous Approach
04Q24ZZ Repair Gastric Artery, Percutaneous Endoscopic Approach
04Q30ZZ Repair Hepatic Artery, Open Approach
04Q33ZZ Repair Hepatic Artery, Percutaneous Approach
04Q34ZZ Repair Hepatic Artery, Percutaneous Endoscopic Approach
04Q40ZZ Repair Splenic Artery, Open Approach
04Q43ZZ Repair Splenic Artery, Percutaneous Approach
04Q44ZZ Repair Splenic Artery, Percutaneous Endoscopic Approach
04Q50ZZ Repair Superior Mesenteric Artery, Open Approach
04Q53ZZ Repair Superior Mesenteric Artery, Percutaneous Approach
04Q54ZZ Repair Superior Mesenteric Artery, Percutaneous Endoscopic Approach
04Q60ZZ Repair Right Colic Artery, Open Approach
04Q63ZZ Repair Right Colic Artery, Percutaneous Approach
04Q64ZZ Repair Right Colic Artery, Percutaneous Endoscopic Approach
04Q70ZZ Repair Left Colic Artery, Open Approach
04Q73ZZ Repair Left Colic Artery, Percutaneous Approach
04Q74ZZ Repair Left Colic Artery, Percutaneous Endoscopic Approach
04Q80ZZ Repair Middle Colic Artery, Open Approach
04Q83ZZ Repair Middle Colic Artery, Percutaneous Approach
04Q84ZZ Repair Middle Colic Artery, Percutaneous Endoscopic Approach
04Q90ZZ Repair Right Renal Artery, Open Approach
04Q93ZZ Repair Right Renal Artery, Percutaneous Approach
04Q94ZZ Repair Right Renal Artery, Percutaneous Endoscopic Approach
04QA0ZZ Repair Left Renal Artery, Open Approach
04QA3ZZ Repair Left Renal Artery, Percutaneous Approach
04QA4ZZ Repair Left Renal Artery, Percutaneous Endoscopic Approach
04QB0ZZ Repair Inferior Mesenteric Artery, Open Approach

04QB3ZZ Repair Inferior Mesenteric Artery, Percutaneous Approach
04QB4ZZ Repair Inferior Mesenteric Artery, Percutaneous Endoscopic Approach
04QC0ZZ Repair Right Common Iliac Artery, Open Approach
04QC3ZZ Repair Right Common Iliac Artery, Percutaneous Approach
04QC4ZZ Repair Right Common Iliac Artery, Percutaneous Endoscopic Approach
04QD0ZZ Repair Left Common Iliac Artery, Open Approach
04QD3ZZ Repair Left Common Iliac Artery, Percutaneous Approach
04QD4ZZ Repair Left Common Iliac Artery, Percutaneous Endoscopic Approach
04QE0ZZ Repair Right Internal Iliac Artery, Open Approach
04QE3ZZ Repair Right Internal Iliac Artery, Percutaneous Approach
04QE4ZZ Repair Right Internal Iliac Artery, Percutaneous Endoscopic Approach
04QF0ZZ Repair Left Internal Iliac Artery, Open Approach
04QF3ZZ Repair Left Internal Iliac Artery, Percutaneous Approach
04QF4ZZ Repair Left Internal Iliac Artery, Percutaneous Endoscopic Approach
04QH0ZZ Repair Right External Iliac Artery, Open Approach
04QH3ZZ Repair Right External Iliac Artery, Percutaneous Approach
04QH4ZZ Repair Right External Iliac Artery, Percutaneous Endoscopic Approach
04QJ0ZZ Repair Left External Iliac Artery, Open Approach
04QJ3ZZ Repair Left External Iliac Artery, Percutaneous Approach
04QJ4ZZ Repair Left External Iliac Artery, Percutaneous Endoscopic Approach
04QK0ZZ Repair Right Femoral Artery, Open Approach
04QK3ZZ Repair Right Femoral Artery, Percutaneous Approach
04QK4ZZ Repair Right Femoral Artery, Percutaneous Endoscopic Approach
04QL0ZZ Repair Left Femoral Artery, Open Approach
04QL3ZZ Repair Left Femoral Artery, Percutaneous Approach
04QL4ZZ Repair Left Femoral Artery, Percutaneous Endoscopic Approach
04QM0ZZ Repair Right Popliteal Artery, Open Approach
04QM3ZZ Repair Right Popliteal Artery, Percutaneous Approach

04QM4ZZ Repair Right Popliteal Artery, Percutaneous Endoscopic Approach
04QN0ZZ Repair Left Popliteal Artery, Open Approach
04QN3ZZ Repair Left Popliteal Artery, Percutaneous Approach
04QN4ZZ Repair Left Popliteal Artery, Percutaneous Endoscopic Approach
04QP0ZZ Repair Right Anterior Tibial Artery, Open Approach
04QP3ZZ Repair Right Anterior Tibial Artery, Percutaneous Approach
04QP4ZZ Repair Right Anterior Tibial Artery, Percutaneous Endoscopic Approach
04QQ0ZZ Repair Left Anterior Tibial Artery, Open Approach
04QQ3ZZ Repair Left Anterior Tibial Artery, Percutaneous Approach
04QQ4ZZ Repair Left Anterior Tibial Artery, Percutaneous Endoscopic Approach
04QR0ZZ Repair Right Posterior Tibial Artery, Open Approach
04QR3ZZ Repair Right Posterior Tibial Artery, Percutaneous Approach
04QR4ZZ Repair Right Posterior Tibial Artery, Percutaneous Endoscopic Approach
04QS0ZZ Repair Left Posterior Tibial Artery, Open Approach
04QS3ZZ Repair Left Posterior Tibial Artery, Percutaneous Approach
04QS4ZZ Repair Left Posterior Tibial Artery, Percutaneous Endoscopic Approach
04QT0ZZ Repair Right Peroneal Artery, Open Approach
04QT3ZZ Repair Right Peroneal Artery, Percutaneous Approach
04QT4ZZ Repair Right Peroneal Artery, Percutaneous Endoscopic Approach
04QU0ZZ Repair Left Peroneal Artery, Open Approach
04QU3ZZ Repair Left Peroneal Artery, Percutaneous Approach
04QU4ZZ Repair Left Peroneal Artery, Percutaneous Endoscopic Approach
04QV0ZZ Repair Right Foot Artery, Open Approach
04QV3ZZ Repair Right Foot Artery, Percutaneous Approach
04QV4ZZ Repair Right Foot Artery, Percutaneous Endoscopic Approach
04QW0ZZ Repair Left Foot Artery, Open Approach
04QW3ZZ Repair Left Foot Artery, Percutaneous Approach
04QW4ZZ Repair Left Foot Artery, Percutaneous Endoscopic Approach
04QY0ZZ Repair Lower Artery, Open Approach
04QY3ZZ Repair Lower Artery, Percutaneous Approach
04QY4ZZ Repair Lower Artery, Percutaneous Endoscopic Approach

04R – Lower Arteries, Replacement

04R007Z Replacement of Abdominal Aorta with Autologous Tissue Substitute, Open Approach
04R00JZ Replacement of Abdominal Aorta with Synthetic Substitute, Open Approach
04R00KZ Replacement of Abdominal Aorta with Nonautologous Tissue Substitute, Open Approach
04R047Z Replacement of Abdominal Aorta with Autologous Tissue Substitute, Percutaneous Endoscopic Approach
04R04JZ Replacement of Abdominal Aorta with Synthetic Substitute, Percutaneous Endoscopic Approach
04R04KZ Replacement of Abdominal Aorta with Nonautologous Tissue Substitute, Percutaneous Endoscopic Approach
04R107Z Replacement of Celiac Artery with Autologous Tissue Substitute, Open Approach
04R10JZ Replacement of Celiac Artery with Synthetic Substitute, Open Approach
04R10KZ Replacement of Celiac Artery with Nonautologous Tissue Substitute, Open Approach
04R147Z Replacement of Celiac Artery with Autologous Tissue Substitute, Percutaneous Endoscopic Approach
04R14JZ Replacement of Celiac Artery with Synthetic Substitute, Percutaneous Endoscopic Approach
04R14KZ Replacement of Celiac Artery with Nonautologous Tissue Substitute, Percutaneous Endoscopic Approach
04R207Z Replacement of Gastric Artery with Autologous Tissue Substitute, Open Approach
04R20JZ Replacement of Gastric Artery with Synthetic Substitute, Open Approach
04R20KZ Replacement of Gastric Artery with Nonautologous Tissue Substitute, Open Approach
04R247Z Replacement of Gastric Artery with Autologous Tissue Substitute, Percutaneous Endoscopic Approach
04R24JZ Replacement of Gastric Artery with Synthetic Substitute, Percutaneous Endoscopic Approach
04R24KZ Replacement of Gastric Artery with Nonautologous Tissue Substitute, Percutaneous Endoscopic Approach
04R307Z Replacement of Hepatic Artery with Autologous Tissue Substitute, Open Approach
04R30JZ Replacement of Hepatic Artery with Synthetic Substitute, Open Approach
04R30KZ Replacement of Hepatic Artery with Nonautologous Tissue Substitute, Open Approach
04R347Z Replacement of Hepatic Artery with Autologous Tissue Substitute, Percutaneous Endoscopic Approach
04R34JZ Replacement of Hepatic Artery with Synthetic Substitute, Percutaneous Endoscopic Approach
04R34KZ Replacement of Hepatic Artery with Nonautologous Tissue Substitute, Percutaneous Endoscopic Approach
04R407Z Replacement of Splenic Artery with Autologous Tissue Substitute, Open Approach
04R40JZ Replacement of Splenic Artery with Synthetic Substitute, Open Approach
04R40KZ Replacement of Splenic Artery with Nonautologous Tissue Substitute, Open Approach
04R447Z Replacement of Splenic Artery with Autologous Tissue Substitute, Percutaneous Endoscopic Approach
04R44JZ Replacement of Splenic Artery with Synthetic Substitute, Percutaneous Endoscopic Approach
04R44KZ Replacement of Splenic Artery with Nonautologous Tissue Substitute, Percutaneous Endoscopic Approach
04R507Z Replacement of Superior Mesenteric Artery with Autologous Tissue Substitute, Open Approach
04R50JZ Replacement of Superior Mesenteric Artery with Synthetic Substitute, Open Approach
04R50KZ Replacement of Superior Mesenteric Artery with Nonautologous Tissue Substitute, Open Approach
04R547Z Replacement of Superior Mesenteric Artery with Autologous Tissue Substitute, Percutaneous Endoscopic Approach
04R54JZ Replacement of Superior Mesenteric Artery with Synthetic Substitute, Percutaneous Endoscopic Approach
04R54KZ Replacement of Superior Mesenteric Artery with Nonautologous Tissue Substitute, Percutaneous Endoscopic Approach
04R607Z Replacement of Right Colic Artery with Autologous Tissue Substitute, Open Approach
04R60JZ Replacement of Right Colic Artery with Synthetic Substitute, Open Approach
04R60KZ Replacement of Right Colic Artery with Nonautologous Tissue Substitute, Open Approach
04R647Z Replacement of Right Colic Artery with Autologous Tissue Substitute, Percutaneous Endoscopic Approach
04R64JZ Replacement of Right Colic Artery with Synthetic Substitute, Percutaneous Endoscopic Approach
04R64KZ Replacement of Right Colic Artery with Nonautologous Tissue Substitute, Percutaneous Endoscopic Approach
04R707Z Replacement of Left Colic Artery with Autologous Tissue Substitute, Open Approach
04R70JZ Replacement of Left Colic Artery with Synthetic Substitute, Open Approach
04R70KZ Replacement of Left Colic Artery with Nonautologous Tissue Substitute, Open Approach
04R747Z Replacement of Left Colic Artery with Autologous Tissue Substitute, Percutaneous Endoscopic Approach
04R74JZ Replacement of Left Colic Artery with Synthetic Substitute, Percutaneous Endoscopic Approach
04R74KZ Replacement of Left Colic Artery with Nonautologous Tissue Substitute, Percutaneous Endoscopic Approach
04R807Z Replacement of Middle Colic Artery with Autologous Tissue Substitute, Open Approach
04R80JZ Replacement of Middle Colic Artery with Synthetic Substitute, Open Approach
04R80KZ Replacement of Middle Colic Artery with Nonautologous Tissue Substitute, Open Approach
04R847Z Replacement of Middle Colic Artery with Autologous Tissue Substitute, Percutaneous Endoscopic Approach

04R84JZ Replacement of Middle Colic Artery with Synthetic Substitute, Percutaneous Endoscopic Approach

04R84KZ Replacement of Middle Colic Artery with Nonautologous Tissue Substitute, Percutaneous Endoscopic Approach

04R907Z Replacement of Right Renal Artery with Autologous Tissue Substitute, Open Approach

04R90JZ Replacement of Right Renal Artery with Synthetic Substitute, Open Approach

04R90KZ Replacement of Right Renal Artery with Nonautologous Tissue Substitute, Open Approach

04R947Z Replacement of Right Renal Artery with Autologous Tissue Substitute, Percutaneous Endoscopic Approach

04R94JZ Replacement of Right Renal Artery with Synthetic Substitute, Percutaneous Endoscopic Approach

04R94KZ Replacement of Right Renal Artery with Nonautologous Tissue Substitute, Percutaneous Endoscopic Approach

04RA07Z Replacement of Left Renal Artery with Autologous Tissue Substitute, Open Approach

04RA0JZ Replacement of Left Renal Artery with Synthetic Substitute, Open Approach

04RA0KZ Replacement of Left Renal Artery with Nonautologous Tissue Substitute, Open Approach

04RA47Z Replacement of Left Renal Artery with Autologous Tissue Substitute, Percutaneous Endoscopic Approach

04RA4JZ Replacement of Left Renal Artery with Synthetic Substitute, Percutaneous Endoscopic Approach

04RA4KZ Replacement of Left Renal Artery with Nonautologous Tissue Substitute, Percutaneous Endoscopic Approach

04RB07Z Replacement of Inferior Mesenteric Artery with Autologous Tissue Substitute, Open Approach

04RB0JZ Replacement of Inferior Mesenteric Artery with Synthetic Substitute, Open Approach

04RB0KZ Replacement of Inferior Mesenteric Artery with Nonautologous Tissue Substitute, Open Approach

04RB47Z Replacement of Inferior Mesenteric Artery with Autologous Tissue Substitute, Percutaneous Endoscopic Approach

04RB4JZ Replacement of Inferior Mesenteric Artery with Synthetic Substitute, Percutaneous Endoscopic Approach

04RB4KZ Replacement of Inferior Mesenteric Artery with Nonautologous Tissue Substitute, Percutaneous Endoscopic Approach

04RC07Z Replacement of Right Common Iliac Artery with Autologous Tissue Substitute, Open Approach

04RC0JZ Replacement of Right Common Iliac Artery with Synthetic Substitute, Open Approach

04RC0KZ Replacement of Right Common Iliac Artery with Nonautologous Tissue Substitute, Open Approach

04RC47Z Replacement of Right Common Iliac Artery with Autologous Tissue Substitute, Percutaneous Endoscopic Approach

04RC4JZ Replacement of Right Common Iliac Artery with Synthetic Substitute, Percutaneous Endoscopic Approach

04RC4KZ Replacement of Right Common Iliac Artery with Nonautologous Tissue Substitute, Percutaneous Endoscopic Approach

04RD07Z Replacement of Left Common Iliac Artery with Autologous Tissue Substitute, Open Approach

04RD0JZ Replacement of Left Common Iliac Artery with Synthetic Substitute, Open Approach

04RD0KZ Replacement of Left Common Iliac Artery with Nonautologous Tissue Substitute, Open Approach

04RD47Z Replacement of Left Common Iliac Artery with Autologous Tissue Substitute, Percutaneous Endoscopic Approach

04RD4JZ Replacement of Left Common Iliac Artery with Synthetic Substitute, Percutaneous Endoscopic Approach

04RD4KZ Replacement of Left Common Iliac Artery with Nonautologous Tissue Substitute, Percutaneous Endoscopic Approach

04RE07Z Replacement of Right Internal Iliac Artery with Autologous Tissue Substitute, Open Approach

04RE0JZ Replacement of Right Internal Iliac Artery with Synthetic Substitute, Open Approach

04RE0KZ Replacement of Right Internal Iliac Artery with Nonautologous Tissue Substitute, Open Approach

04RE47Z Replacement of Right Internal Iliac Artery with Autologous Tissue Substitute, Percutaneous Endoscopic Approach

04RE4JZ Replacement of Right Internal Iliac Artery with Synthetic Substitute, Percutaneous Endoscopic Approach

04RE4KZ Replacement of Right Internal Iliac Artery with Nonautologous Tissue Substitute, Percutaneous Endoscopic Approach

04RF07Z Replacement of Left Internal Iliac Artery with Autologous Tissue Substitute, Open Approach

04RF0JZ Replacement of Left Internal Iliac Artery with Synthetic Substitute, Open Approach

04RF0KZ Replacement of Left Internal Iliac Artery with Nonautologous Tissue Substitute, Open Approach

04RF47Z Replacement of Left Internal Iliac Artery with Autologous Tissue Substitute, Percutaneous Endoscopic Approach

04RF4JZ Replacement of Left Internal Iliac Artery with Synthetic Substitute, Percutaneous Endoscopic Approach

04RF4KZ Replacement of Left Internal Iliac Artery with Nonautologous Tissue Substitute, Percutaneous Endoscopic Approach

04RH07Z Replacement of Right External Iliac Artery with Autologous Tissue Substitute, Open Approach

04RH0JZ Replacement of Right External Iliac Artery with Synthetic Substitute, Open Approach

04RH0KZ Replacement of Right External Iliac Artery with Nonautologous Tissue Substitute, Open Approach

04RH47Z Replacement of Right External Iliac Artery with Autologous Tissue Substitute, Percutaneous Endoscopic Approach

04RH4JZ Replacement of Right External Iliac Artery with Synthetic Substitute, Percutaneous Endoscopic Approach

04RH4KZ Replacement of Right External Iliac Artery with Nonautologous Tissue Substitute, Percutaneous Endoscopic Approach

04RJ07Z Replacement of Left External Iliac Artery with Autologous Tissue Substitute, Open Approach

04RJ0JZ Replacement of Left External Iliac Artery with Synthetic Substitute, Open Approach

04RJ0KZ Replacement of Left External Iliac Artery with Nonautologous Tissue Substitute, Open Approach

04RJ47Z Replacement of Left External Iliac Artery with Autologous Tissue Substitute, Percutaneous Endoscopic Approach

04RJ4JZ Replacement of Left External Iliac Artery with Synthetic Substitute, Percutaneous Endoscopic Approach

04RJ4KZ Replacement of Left External Iliac Artery with Nonautologous Tissue Substitute, Percutaneous Endoscopic Approach

04RK07Z Replacement of Right Femoral Artery with Autologous Tissue Substitute, Open Approach

04RK0JZ Replacement of Right Femoral Artery with Synthetic Substitute, Open Approach

04RK0KZ Replacement of Right Femoral Artery with Nonautologous Tissue Substitute, Open Approach

04RK47Z Replacement of Right Femoral Artery with Autologous Tissue Substitute, Percutaneous Endoscopic Approach

04RK4JZ Replacement of Right Femoral Artery with Synthetic Substitute, Percutaneous Endoscopic Approach

04RK4KZ Replacement of Right Femoral Artery with Nonautologous Tissue Substitute, Percutaneous Endoscopic Approach

04RL07Z Replacement of Left Femoral Artery with Autologous Tissue Substitute, Open Approach

04RL0JZ Replacement of Left Femoral Artery with Synthetic Substitute, Open Approach

04RL0KZ Replacement of Left Femoral Artery with Nonautologous Tissue Substitute, Open Approach

04RL47Z Replacement of Left Femoral Artery with Autologous Tissue Substitute, Percutaneous Endoscopic Approach

04RL4JZ Replacement of Left Femoral Artery with Synthetic Substitute, Percutaneous Endoscopic Approach

04RL4KZ Replacement of Left Femoral Artery with Nonautologous Tissue Substitute, Percutaneous Endoscopic Approach

04RM07Z Replacement of Right Popliteal Artery with Autologous Tissue Substitute, Open Approach

04RM0JZ Replacement of Right Popliteal Artery with Synthetic Substitute, Open Approach

04RM0KZ Replacement of Right Popliteal Artery with Nonautologous Tissue Substitute, Open Approach

04RM47Z Replacement of Right Popliteal Artery with Autologous Tissue Substitute, Percutaneous Endoscopic Approach

04RM4JZ Replacement of Right Popliteal Artery with Synthetic Substitute, Percutaneous Endoscopic Approach

04RM4KZ Replacement of Right Popliteal Artery with Nonautologous Tissue Substitute, Percutaneous Endoscopic Approach

04RN07Z Replacement of Left Popliteal Artery with Autologous Tissue Substitute, Open Approach

04RN0JZ Replacement of Left Popliteal Artery with Synthetic Substitute, Open Approach

04RN0KZ Replacement of Left Popliteal Artery with Nonautologous Tissue Substitute, Open Approach

04RN47Z Replacement of Left Popliteal Artery with Autologous Tissue Substitute, Percutaneous Endoscopic Approach

04RN4JZ Replacement of Left Popliteal Artery with Synthetic Substitute, Percutaneous Endoscopic Approach

04RN4KZ Replacement of Left Popliteal Artery with Nonautologous Tissue Substitute, Percutaneous Endoscopic Approach

04RP07Z Replacement of Right Anterior Tibial Artery with Autologous Tissue Substitute, Open Approach

04RP0JZ Replacement of Right Anterior Tibial Artery with Synthetic Substitute, Open Approach

04RP0KZ Replacement of Right Anterior Tibial Artery with Nonautologous Tissue Substitute, Open Approach

04RP47Z Replacement of Right Anterior Tibial Artery with Autologous Tissue Substitute, Percutaneous Endoscopic Approach

04RP4JZ Replacement of Right Anterior Tibial Artery with Synthetic Substitute, Percutaneous Endoscopic Approach

04RP4KZ Replacement of Right Anterior Tibial Artery with Nonautologous Tissue Substitute, Percutaneous Endoscopic Approach

04RQ07Z Replacement of Left Anterior Tibial Artery with Autologous Tissue Substitute, Open Approach

04RQ0JZ Replacement of Left Anterior Tibial Artery with Synthetic Substitute, Open Approach

04RQ0KZ Replacement of Left Anterior Tibial Artery with Nonautologous Tissue Substitute, Open Approach

04RQ47Z Replacement of Left Anterior Tibial Artery with Autologous Tissue Substitute, Percutaneous Endoscopic Approach

04RQ4JZ Replacement of Left Anterior Tibial Artery with Synthetic Substitute, Percutaneous Endoscopic Approach

04RQ4KZ Replacement of Left Anterior Tibial Artery with Nonautologous Tissue Substitute, Percutaneous Endoscopic Approach

04RR07Z Replacement of Right Posterior Tibial Artery with Autologous Tissue Substitute, Open Approach

04RR0JZ Replacement of Right Posterior Tibial Artery with Synthetic Substitute, Open Approach

04RR0KZ Replacement of Right Posterior Tibial Artery with Nonautologous Tissue Substitute, Open Approach

04RR47Z Replacement of Right Posterior Tibial Artery with Autologous Tissue Substitute, Percutaneous Endoscopic Approach

04RR4JZ Replacement of Right Posterior Tibial Artery with Synthetic Substitute, Percutaneous Endoscopic Approach

04RR4KZ Replacement of Right Posterior Tibial Artery with Nonautologous Tissue Substitute, Percutaneous Endoscopic Approach

04RS07Z Replacement of Left Posterior Tibial Artery with Autologous Tissue Substitute, Open Approach

04RS0JZ Replacement of Left Posterior Tibial Artery with Synthetic Substitute, Open Approach

04RS0KZ Replacement of Left Posterior Tibial Artery with Nonautologous Tissue Substitute, Open Approach

04RS47Z Replacement of Left Posterior Tibial Artery with Autologous Tissue Substitute, Percutaneous Endoscopic Approach

04RS4JZ Replacement of Left Posterior Tibial Artery with Synthetic Substitute, Percutaneous Endoscopic Approach

04RS4KZ Replacement of Left Posterior Tibial Artery with Nonautologous Tissue Substitute, Percutaneous Endoscopic Approach

04RT07Z Replacement of Right Peroneal Artery with Autologous Tissue Substitute, Open Approach

04RT0JZ Replacement of Right Peroneal Artery with Synthetic Substitute, Open Approach

04RT0KZ Replacement of Right Peroneal Artery with Nonautologous Tissue Substitute, Open Approach

04RT47Z Replacement of Right Peroneal Artery with Autologous Tissue Substitute, Percutaneous Endoscopic Approach

04RT4JZ Replacement of Right Peroneal Artery with Synthetic Substitute, Percutaneous Endoscopic Approach

04RT4KZ Replacement of Right Peroneal Artery with Nonautologous Tissue Substitute, Percutaneous Endoscopic Approach

04RU07Z Replacement of Left Peroneal Artery with Autologous Tissue Substitute, Open Approach

04RU0JZ Replacement of Left Peroneal Artery with Synthetic Substitute, Open Approach

04RU0KZ Replacement of Left Peroneal Artery with Nonautologous Tissue Substitute, Open Approach

04RU47Z Replacement of Left Peroneal Artery with Autologous Tissue Substitute, Percutaneous Endoscopic Approach

04RU4JZ Replacement of Left Peroneal Artery with Synthetic Substitute, Percutaneous Endoscopic Approach

04RU4KZ Replacement of Left Peroneal Artery with Nonautologous Tissue Substitute, Percutaneous Endoscopic Approach

04RV07Z Replacement of Right Foot Artery with Autologous Tissue Substitute, Open Approach

04RV0JZ Replacement of Right Foot Artery with Synthetic Substitute, Open Approach

04RV0KZ Replacement of Right Foot Artery with Nonautologous Tissue Substitute, Open Approach

04RV47Z Replacement of Right Foot Artery with Autologous Tissue Substitute, Percutaneous Endoscopic Approach

04RV4JZ Replacement of Right Foot Artery with Synthetic Substitute, Percutaneous Endoscopic Approach

04RV4KZ Replacement of Right Foot Artery with Nonautologous Tissue Substitute, Percutaneous Endoscopic Approach

04RW07Z Replacement of Left Foot Artery with Autologous Tissue Substitute, Open Approach

04RW0JZ Replacement of Left Foot Artery with Synthetic Substitute, Open Approach

04RW0KZ Replacement of Left Foot Artery with Nonautologous Tissue Substitute, Open Approach

04RW47Z Replacement of Left Foot Artery with Autologous Tissue Substitute, Percutaneous Endoscopic Approach

04RW4JZ Replacement of Left Foot Artery with Synthetic Substitute, Percutaneous Endoscopic Approach

04RW4KZ Replacement of Left Foot Artery with Nonautologous Tissue Substitute, Percutaneous Endoscopic Approach

04RY07Z Replacement of Lower Artery with Autologous Tissue Substitute, Open Approach

04RY0JZ Replacement of Lower Artery with Synthetic Substitute, Open Approach

04RY0KZ Replacement of Lower Artery with Nonautologous Tissue Substitute, Open Approach

04RY47Z Replacement of Lower Artery with Autologous Tissue Substitute, Percutaneous Endoscopic Approach

04RY4JZ Replacement of Lower Artery with Synthetic Substitute, Percutaneous Endoscopic Approach

04RY4KZ Replacement of Lower Artery with Nonautologous Tissue Substitute, Percutaneous Endoscopic Approach

04S – Lower Arteries, Reposition

04S00ZZ Reposition Abdominal Aorta, Open Approach
04S03ZZ Reposition Abdominal Aorta, Percutaneous Approach
04S04ZZ Reposition Abdominal Aorta, Percutaneous Endoscopic Approach
04S10ZZ Reposition Celiac Artery, Open Approach
04S13ZZ Reposition Celiac Artery, Percutaneous Approach
04S14ZZ Reposition Celiac Artery, Percutaneous Endoscopic Approach
04S20ZZ Reposition Gastric Artery, Open Approach
04S23ZZ Reposition Gastric Artery, Percutaneous Approach

04S24ZZ Reposition Gastric Artery, Percutaneous Endoscopic Approach
04S30ZZ Reposition Hepatic Artery, Open Approach
04S33ZZ Reposition Hepatic Artery, Percutaneous Approach
04S34ZZ Reposition Hepatic Artery, Percutaneous Endoscopic Approach
04S40ZZ Reposition Splenic Artery, Open Approach
04S43ZZ Reposition Splenic Artery, Percutaneous Approach
04S44ZZ Reposition Splenic Artery, Percutaneous Endoscopic Approach
04S50ZZ Reposition Superior Mesenteric Artery, Open Approach

04S53ZZ	Reposition Superior Mesenteric Artery, Percutaneous Approach
04S54ZZ	Reposition Superior Mesenteric Artery, Percutaneous Endoscopic Approach
04S60ZZ	Reposition Right Colic Artery, Open Approach
04S63ZZ	Reposition Right Colic Artery, Percutaneous Approach
04S64ZZ	Reposition Right Colic Artery, Percutaneous Endoscopic Approach
04S70ZZ	Reposition Left Colic Artery, Open Approach
04S73ZZ	Reposition Left Colic Artery, Percutaneous Approach
04S74ZZ	Reposition Left Colic Artery, Percutaneous Endoscopic Approach
04S80ZZ	Reposition Middle Colic Artery, Open Approach
04S83ZZ	Reposition Middle Colic Artery, Percutaneous Approach
04S84ZZ	Reposition Middle Colic Artery, Percutaneous Endoscopic Approach
04S90ZZ	Reposition Right Renal Artery, Open Approach
04S93ZZ	Reposition Right Renal Artery, Percutaneous Approach
04S94ZZ	Reposition Right Renal Artery, Percutaneous Endoscopic Approach
04SA0ZZ	Reposition Left Renal Artery, Open Approach
04SA3ZZ	Reposition Left Renal Artery, Percutaneous Approach
04SA4ZZ	Reposition Left Renal Artery, Percutaneous Endoscopic Approach
04SB0ZZ	Reposition Inferior Mesenteric Artery, Open Approach
04SB3ZZ	Reposition Inferior Mesenteric Artery, Percutaneous Approach
04SB4ZZ	Reposition Inferior Mesenteric Artery, Percutaneous Endoscopic Approach
04SC0ZZ	Reposition Right Common Iliac Artery, Open Approach
04SC3ZZ	Reposition Right Common Iliac Artery, Percutaneous Approach
04SC4ZZ	Reposition Right Common Iliac Artery, Percutaneous Endoscopic Approach
04SD0ZZ	Reposition Left Common Iliac Artery, Open Approach
04SD3ZZ	Reposition Left Common Iliac Artery, Percutaneous Approach
04SD4ZZ	Reposition Left Common Iliac Artery, Percutaneous Endoscopic Approach
04SE0ZZ	Reposition Right Internal Iliac Artery, Open Approach
04SE3ZZ	Reposition Right Internal Iliac Artery, Percutaneous Approach
04SE4ZZ	Reposition Right Internal Iliac Artery, Percutaneous Endoscopic Approach
04SF0ZZ	Reposition Left Internal Iliac Artery, Open Approach
04SF3ZZ	Reposition Left Internal Iliac Artery, Percutaneous Approach
04SF4ZZ	Reposition Left Internal Iliac Artery, Percutaneous Endoscopic Approach
04SH0ZZ	Reposition Right External Iliac Artery, Open Approach
04SH3ZZ	Reposition Right External Iliac Artery, Percutaneous Approach
04SH4ZZ	Reposition Right External Iliac Artery, Percutaneous Endoscopic Approach
04SJ0ZZ	Reposition Left External Iliac Artery, Open Approach
04SJ3ZZ	Reposition Left External Iliac Artery, Percutaneous Approach
04SJ4ZZ	Reposition Left External Iliac Artery, Percutaneous Endoscopic Approach
04SK0ZZ	Reposition Right Femoral Artery, Open Approach
04SK3ZZ	Reposition Right Femoral Artery, Percutaneous Approach
04SK4ZZ	Reposition Right Femoral Artery, Percutaneous Endoscopic Approach
04SL0ZZ	Reposition Left Femoral Artery, Open Approach
04SL3ZZ	Reposition Left Femoral Artery, Percutaneous Approach
04SL4ZZ	Reposition Left Femoral Artery, Percutaneous Endoscopic Approach
04SM0ZZ	Reposition Right Popliteal Artery, Open Approach
04SM3ZZ	Reposition Right Popliteal Artery, Percutaneous Approach
04SM4ZZ	Reposition Right Popliteal Artery, Percutaneous Endoscopic Approach
04SN0ZZ	Reposition Left Popliteal Artery, Open Approach
04SN3ZZ	Reposition Left Popliteal Artery, Percutaneous Approach
04SN4ZZ	Reposition Left Popliteal Artery, Percutaneous Endoscopic Approach
04SP0ZZ	Reposition Right Anterior Tibial Artery, Open Approach
04SP3ZZ	Reposition Right Anterior Tibial Artery, Percutaneous Approach
04SP4ZZ	Reposition Right Anterior Tibial Artery, Percutaneous Endoscopic Approach
04SQ0ZZ	Reposition Left Anterior Tibial Artery, Open Approach
04SQ3ZZ	Reposition Left Anterior Tibial Artery, Percutaneous Approach
04SQ4ZZ	Reposition Left Anterior Tibial Artery, Percutaneous Endoscopic Approach
04SR0ZZ	Reposition Right Posterior Tibial Artery, Open Approach
04SR3ZZ	Reposition Right Posterior Tibial Artery, Percutaneous Approach
04SR4ZZ	Reposition Right Posterior Tibial Artery, Percutaneous Endoscopic Approach
04SS0ZZ	Reposition Left Posterior Tibial Artery, Open Approach
04SS3ZZ	Reposition Left Posterior Tibial Artery, Percutaneous Approach
04SS4ZZ	Reposition Left Posterior Tibial Artery, Percutaneous Endoscopic Approach
04ST0ZZ	Reposition Right Peroneal Artery, Open Approach
04ST3ZZ	Reposition Right Peroneal Artery, Percutaneous Approach
04ST4ZZ	Reposition Right Peroneal Artery, Percutaneous Endoscopic Approach
04SU0ZZ	Reposition Left Peroneal Artery, Open Approach
04SU3ZZ	Reposition Left Peroneal Artery, Percutaneous Approach
04SU4ZZ	Reposition Left Peroneal Artery, Percutaneous Endoscopic Approach
04SV0ZZ	Reposition Right Foot Artery, Open Approach
04SV3ZZ	Reposition Right Foot Artery, Percutaneous Approach
04SV4ZZ	Reposition Right Foot Artery, Percutaneous Endoscopic Approach
04SW0ZZ	Reposition Left Foot Artery, Open Approach
04SW3ZZ	Reposition Left Foot Artery, Percutaneous Approach
04SW4ZZ	Reposition Left Foot Artery, Percutaneous Endoscopic Approach
04SY0ZZ	Reposition Lower Artery, Open Approach
04SY3ZZ	Reposition Lower Artery, Percutaneous Approach
04SY4ZZ	Reposition Lower Artery, Percutaneous Endoscopic Approach

04U – Lower Arteries, Supplement

04U007Z	Supplement Abdominal Aorta with Autologous Tissue Substitute, Open Approach
04U00JZ	Supplement Abdominal Aorta with Synthetic Substitute, Open Approach
04U00KZ	Supplement Abdominal Aorta with Nonautologous Tissue Substitute, Open Approach
04U037Z	Supplement Abdominal Aorta with Autologous Tissue Substitute, Percutaneous Approach
04U03JZ	Supplement Abdominal Aorta with Synthetic Substitute, Percutaneous Approach
04U03KZ	Supplement Abdominal Aorta with Nonautologous Tissue Substitute, Percutaneous Approach
04U047Z	Supplement Abdominal Aorta with Autologous Tissue Substitute, Percutaneous Endoscopic Approach
04U04JZ	Supplement Abdominal Aorta with Synthetic Substitute, Percutaneous Endoscopic Approach
04U04KZ	Supplement Abdominal Aorta with Nonautologous Tissue Substitute, Percutaneous Endoscopic Approach
04U107Z	Supplement Celiac Artery with Autologous Tissue Substitute, Open Approach
04U10JZ	Supplement Celiac Artery with Synthetic Substitute, Open Approach
04U10KZ	Supplement Celiac Artery with Nonautologous Tissue Substitute, Open Approach
04U137Z	Supplement Celiac Artery with Autologous Tissue Substitute, Percutaneous Approach
04U13JZ	Supplement Celiac Artery with Synthetic Substitute, Percutaneous Approach
04U13KZ	Supplement Celiac Artery with Nonautologous Tissue Substitute, Percutaneous Approach
04U147Z	Supplement Celiac Artery with Autologous Tissue Substitute, Percutaneous Endoscopic Approach
04U14JZ	Supplement Celiac Artery with Synthetic Substitute, Percutaneous Endoscopic Approach
04U14KZ	Supplement Celiac Artery with Nonautologous Tissue Substitute, Percutaneous Endoscopic Approach
04U207Z	Supplement Gastric Artery with Autologous Tissue Substitute, Open Approach
04U20JZ	Supplement Gastric Artery with Synthetic Substitute, Open Approach
04U20KZ	Supplement Gastric Artery with Nonautologous Tissue Substitute, Open Approach
04U237Z	Supplement Gastric Artery with Autologous Tissue Substitute, Percutaneous Approach

04U23JZ Supplement Gastric Artery with Synthetic Substitute, Percutaneous Approach

04U23KZ Supplement Gastric Artery with Nonautologous Tissue Substitute, Percutaneous Approach

04U247Z Supplement Gastric Artery with Autologous Tissue Substitute, Percutaneous Endoscopic Approach

04U24JZ Supplement Gastric Artery with Synthetic Substitute, Percutaneous Endoscopic Approach

04U24KZ Supplement Gastric Artery with Nonautologous Tissue Substitute, Percutaneous Endoscopic Approach

04U307Z Supplement Hepatic Artery with Autologous Tissue Substitute, Open Approach

04U30JZ Supplement Hepatic Artery with Synthetic Substitute, Open Approach

04U30KZ Supplement Hepatic Artery with Nonautologous Tissue Substitute, Open Approach

04U337Z Supplement Hepatic Artery with Autologous Tissue Substitute, Percutaneous Approach

04U33JZ Supplement Hepatic Artery with Synthetic Substitute, Percutaneous Approach

04U33KZ Supplement Hepatic Artery with Nonautologous Tissue Substitute, Percutaneous Approach

04U347Z Supplement Hepatic Artery with Autologous Tissue Substitute, Percutaneous Endoscopic Approach

04U34JZ Supplement Hepatic Artery with Synthetic Substitute, Percutaneous Endoscopic Approach

04U34KZ Supplement Hepatic Artery with Nonautologous Tissue Substitute, Percutaneous Endoscopic Approach

04U407Z Supplement Splenic Artery with Autologous Tissue Substitute, Open Approach

04U40JZ Supplement Splenic Artery with Synthetic Substitute, Open Approach

04U40KZ Supplement Splenic Artery with Nonautologous Tissue Substitute, Open Approach

04U437Z Supplement Splenic Artery with Autologous Tissue Substitute, Percutaneous Approach

04U43JZ Supplement Splenic Artery with Synthetic Substitute, Percutaneous Approach

04U43KZ Supplement Splenic Artery with Nonautologous Tissue Substitute, Percutaneous Approach

04U447Z Supplement Splenic Artery with Autologous Tissue Substitute, Percutaneous Endoscopic Approach

04U44JZ Supplement Splenic Artery with Synthetic Substitute, Percutaneous Endoscopic Approach

04U44KZ Supplement Splenic Artery with Nonautologous Tissue Substitute, Percutaneous Endoscopic Approach

04U507Z Supplement Superior Mesenteric Artery with Autologous Tissue Substitute, Open Approach

04U50JZ Supplement Superior Mesenteric Artery with Synthetic Substitute, Open Approach

04U50KZ Supplement Superior Mesenteric Artery with Nonautologous Tissue Substitute, Open Approach

04U537Z Supplement Superior Mesenteric Artery with Autologous Tissue Substitute, Percutaneous Approach

04U53JZ Supplement Superior Mesenteric Artery with Synthetic Substitute, Percutaneous Approach

04U53KZ Supplement Superior Mesenteric Artery with Nonautologous Tissue Substitute, Percutaneous Approach

04U547Z Supplement Superior Mesenteric Artery with Autologous Tissue Substitute, Percutaneous Endoscopic Approach

04U54JZ Supplement Superior Mesenteric Artery with Synthetic Substitute, Percutaneous Endoscopic Approach

04U54KZ Supplement Superior Mesenteric Artery with Nonautologous Tissue Substitute, Percutaneous Endoscopic Approach

04U607Z Supplement Right Colic Artery with Autologous Tissue Substitute, Open Approach

04U60JZ Supplement Right Colic Artery with Synthetic Substitute, Open Approach

04U60KZ Supplement Right Colic Artery with Nonautologous Tissue Substitute, Open Approach

04U637Z Supplement Right Colic Artery with Autologous Tissue Substitute, Percutaneous Approach

04U63JZ Supplement Right Colic Artery with Synthetic Substitute, Percutaneous Approach

04U63KZ Supplement Right Colic Artery with Nonautologous Tissue Substitute, Percutaneous Approach

04U647Z Supplement Right Colic Artery with Autologous Tissue Substitute, Percutaneous Endoscopic Approach

04U64JZ Supplement Right Colic Artery with Synthetic Substitute, Percutaneous Endoscopic Approach

04U64KZ Supplement Right Colic Artery with Nonautologous Tissue Substitute, Percutaneous Endoscopic Approach

04U707Z Supplement Left Colic Artery with Autologous Tissue Substitute, Open Approach

04U70JZ Supplement Left Colic Artery with Synthetic Substitute, Open Approach

04U70KZ Supplement Left Colic Artery with Nonautologous Tissue Substitute, Open Approach

04U737Z Supplement Left Colic Artery with Autologous Tissue Substitute, Percutaneous Approach

04U73JZ Supplement Left Colic Artery with Synthetic Substitute, Percutaneous Approach

04U73KZ Supplement Left Colic Artery with Nonautologous Tissue Substitute, Percutaneous Approach

04U747Z Supplement Left Colic Artery with Autologous Tissue Substitute, Percutaneous Endoscopic Approach

04U74JZ Supplement Left Colic Artery with Synthetic Substitute, Percutaneous Endoscopic Approach

04U74KZ Supplement Left Colic Artery with Nonautologous Tissue Substitute, Percutaneous Endoscopic Approach

04U807Z Supplement Middle Colic Artery with Autologous Tissue Substitute, Open Approach

04U80JZ Supplement Middle Colic Artery with Synthetic Substitute, Open Approach

04U80KZ Supplement Middle Colic Artery with Nonautologous Tissue Substitute, Open Approach

04U837Z Supplement Middle Colic Artery with Autologous Tissue Substitute, Percutaneous Approach

04U83JZ Supplement Middle Colic Artery with Synthetic Substitute, Percutaneous Approach

04U83KZ Supplement Middle Colic Artery with Nonautologous Tissue Substitute, Percutaneous Approach

04U847Z Supplement Middle Colic Artery with Autologous Tissue Substitute, Percutaneous Endoscopic Approach

04U84JZ Supplement Middle Colic Artery with Synthetic Substitute, Percutaneous Endoscopic Approach

04U84KZ Supplement Middle Colic Artery with Nonautologous Tissue Substitute, Percutaneous Endoscopic Approach

04U907Z Supplement Right Renal Artery with Autologous Tissue Substitute, Open Approach

04U90JZ Supplement Right Renal Artery with Synthetic Substitute, Open Approach

04U90KZ Supplement Right Renal Artery with Nonautologous Tissue Substitute, Open Approach

04U937Z Supplement Right Renal Artery with Autologous Tissue Substitute, Percutaneous Approach

04U93JZ Supplement Right Renal Artery with Synthetic Substitute, Percutaneous Approach

04U93KZ Supplement Right Renal Artery with Nonautologous Tissue Substitute, Percutaneous Approach

04U947Z Supplement Right Renal Artery with Autologous Tissue Substitute, Percutaneous Endoscopic Approach

04U94JZ Supplement Right Renal Artery with Synthetic Substitute, Percutaneous Endoscopic Approach

04U94KZ Supplement Right Renal Artery with Nonautologous Tissue Substitute, Percutaneous Endoscopic Approach

04UA07Z Supplement Left Renal Artery with Autologous Tissue Substitute, Open Approach

04UA0JZ Supplement Left Renal Artery with Synthetic Substitute, Open Approach

04UA0KZ Supplement Left Renal Artery with Nonautologous Tissue Substitute, Open Approach

04UA37Z Supplement Left Renal Artery with Autologous Tissue Substitute, Percutaneous Approach

04UA3JZ Supplement Left Renal Artery with Synthetic Substitute, Percutaneous Approach

04UA3KZ Supplement Left Renal Artery with Nonautologous Tissue Substitute, Percutaneous Approach

04UA47Z Supplement Left Renal Artery with Autologous Tissue Substitute, Percutaneous Endoscopic Approach

04UA4JZ Supplement Left Renal Artery with Synthetic Substitute, Percutaneous Endoscopic Approach

04UA4KZ Supplement Left Renal Artery with Nonautologous Tissue Substitute, Percutaneous Endoscopic Approach

04UB07Z Supplement Inferior Mesenteric Artery with Autologous Tissue Substitute, Open Approach

04UB0JZ Supplement Inferior Mesenteric Artery with Synthetic Substitute, Open Approach

04UB0KZ Supplement Inferior Mesenteric Artery with Nonautologous Tissue Substitute, Open Approach

04UB37Z Supplement Inferior Mesenteric Artery with Autologous Tissue Substitute, Percutaneous Approach

04UB3JZ Supplement Inferior Mesenteric Artery with Synthetic Substitute, Percutaneous Approach

04UB3KZ Supplement Inferior Mesenteric Artery with Nonautologous Tissue Substitute, Percutaneous Approach

04UB47Z Supplement Inferior Mesenteric Artery with Autologous Tissue Substitute, Percutaneous Endoscopic Approach

04UB4JZ Supplement Inferior Mesenteric Artery with Synthetic Substitute, Percutaneous Endoscopic Approach

04UB4KZ Supplement Inferior Mesenteric Artery with Nonautologous Tissue Substitute, Percutaneous Endoscopic Approach

04UC07Z Supplement Right Common Iliac Artery with Autologous Tissue Substitute, Open Approach

04UC0JZ Supplement Right Common Iliac Artery with Synthetic Substitute, Open Approach

04UC0KZ Supplement Right Common Iliac Artery with Nonautologous Tissue Substitute, Open Approach

04UC37Z Supplement Right Common Iliac Artery with Autologous Tissue Substitute, Percutaneous Approach

04UC3JZ Supplement Right Common Iliac Artery with Synthetic Substitute, Percutaneous Approach

04UC3KZ Supplement Right Common Iliac Artery with Nonautologous Tissue Substitute, Percutaneous Approach

04UC47Z Supplement Right Common Iliac Artery with Autologous Tissue Substitute, Percutaneous Endoscopic Approach

04UC4JZ Supplement Right Common Iliac Artery with Synthetic Substitute, Percutaneous Endoscopic Approach

04UC4KZ Supplement Right Common Iliac Artery with Nonautologous Tissue Substitute, Percutaneous Endoscopic Approach

04UD07Z Supplement Left Common Iliac Artery with Autologous Tissue Substitute, Open Approach

04UD0JZ Supplement Left Common Iliac Artery with Synthetic Substitute, Open Approach

04UD0KZ Supplement Left Common Iliac Artery with Nonautologous Tissue Substitute, Open Approach

04UD37Z Supplement Left Common Iliac Artery with Autologous Tissue Substitute, Percutaneous Approach

04UD3JZ Supplement Left Common Iliac Artery with Synthetic Substitute, Percutaneous Approach

04UD3KZ Supplement Left Common Iliac Artery with Nonautologous Tissue Substitute, Percutaneous Approach

04UD47Z Supplement Left Common Iliac Artery with Autologous Tissue Substitute, Percutaneous Endoscopic Approach

04UD4JZ Supplement Left Common Iliac Artery with Synthetic Substitute, Percutaneous Endoscopic Approach

04UD4KZ Supplement Left Common Iliac Artery with Nonautologous Tissue Substitute, Percutaneous Endoscopic Approach

04UE07Z Supplement Right Internal Iliac Artery with Autologous Tissue Substitute, Open Approach

04UE0JZ Supplement Right Internal Iliac Artery with Synthetic Substitute, Open Approach

04UE0KZ Supplement Right Internal Iliac Artery with Nonautologous Tissue Substitute, Open Approach

04UE37Z Supplement Right Internal Iliac Artery with Autologous Tissue Substitute, Percutaneous Approach

04UE3JZ Supplement Right Internal Iliac Artery with Synthetic Substitute, Percutaneous Approach

04UE3KZ Supplement Right Internal Iliac Artery with Nonautologous Tissue Substitute, Percutaneous Approach

04UE47Z Supplement Right Internal Iliac Artery with Autologous Tissue Substitute, Percutaneous Endoscopic Approach

04UE4JZ Supplement Right Internal Iliac Artery with Synthetic Substitute, Percutaneous Endoscopic Approach

04UE4KZ Supplement Right Internal Iliac Artery with Nonautologous Tissue Substitute, Percutaneous Endoscopic Approach

04UF07Z Supplement Left Internal Iliac Artery with Autologous Tissue Substitute, Open Approach

04UF0JZ Supplement Left Internal Iliac Artery with Synthetic Substitute, Open Approach

04UF0KZ Supplement Left Internal Iliac Artery with Nonautologous Tissue Substitute, Open Approach

04UF37Z Supplement Left Internal Iliac Artery with Autologous Tissue Substitute, Percutaneous Approach

04UF3JZ Supplement Left Internal Iliac Artery with Synthetic Substitute, Percutaneous Approach

04UF3KZ Supplement Left Internal Iliac Artery with Nonautologous Tissue Substitute, Percutaneous Approach

04UF47Z Supplement Left Internal Iliac Artery with Autologous Tissue Substitute, Percutaneous Endoscopic Approach

04UF4JZ Supplement Left Internal Iliac Artery with Synthetic Substitute, Percutaneous Endoscopic Approach

04UF4KZ Supplement Left Internal Iliac Artery with Nonautologous Tissue Substitute, Percutaneous Endoscopic Approach

04UH07Z Supplement Right External Iliac Artery with Autologous Tissue Substitute, Open Approach

04UH0JZ Supplement Right External Iliac Artery with Synthetic Substitute, Open Approach

04UH0KZ Supplement Right External Iliac Artery with Nonautologous Tissue Substitute, Open Approach

04UH37Z Supplement Right External Iliac Artery with Autologous Tissue Substitute, Percutaneous Approach

04UH3JZ Supplement Right External Iliac Artery with Synthetic Substitute, Percutaneous Approach

04UH3KZ Supplement Right External Iliac Artery with Nonautologous Tissue Substitute, Percutaneous Approach

04UH47Z Supplement Right External Iliac Artery with Autologous Tissue Substitute, Percutaneous Endoscopic Approach

04UH4JZ Supplement Right External Iliac Artery with Synthetic Substitute, Percutaneous Endoscopic Approach

04UH4KZ Supplement Right External Iliac Artery with Nonautologous Tissue Substitute, Percutaneous Endoscopic Approach

04UJ07Z Supplement Left External Iliac Artery with Autologous Tissue Substitute, Open Approach

04UJ0JZ Supplement Left External Iliac Artery with Synthetic Substitute, Open Approach

04UJ0KZ Supplement Left External Iliac Artery with Nonautologous Tissue Substitute, Open Approach

04UJ37Z Supplement Left External Iliac Artery with Autologous Tissue Substitute, Percutaneous Approach

04UJ3JZ Supplement Left External Iliac Artery with Synthetic Substitute, Percutaneous Approach

04UJ3KZ Supplement Left External Iliac Artery with Nonautologous Tissue Substitute, Percutaneous Approach

04UJ47Z Supplement Left External Iliac Artery with Autologous Tissue Substitute, Percutaneous Endoscopic Approach

04UJ4JZ Supplement Left External Iliac Artery with Synthetic Substitute, Percutaneous Endoscopic Approach

04UJ4KZ Supplement Left External Iliac Artery with Nonautologous Tissue Substitute, Percutaneous Endoscopic Approach

04UK07Z Supplement Right Femoral Artery with Autologous Tissue Substitute, Open Approach

04UK0JZ Supplement Right Femoral Artery with Synthetic Substitute, Open Approach

04UK0KZ Supplement Right Femoral Artery with Nonautologous Tissue Substitute, Open Approach

04UK37Z Supplement Right Femoral Artery with Autologous Tissue Substitute, Percutaneous Approach

04UK3JZ Supplement Right Femoral Artery with Synthetic Substitute, Percutaneous Approach

04UK3KZ Supplement Right Femoral Artery with Nonautologous Tissue Substitute, Percutaneous Approach

04UK47Z Supplement Right Femoral Artery with Autologous Tissue Substitute, Percutaneous Endoscopic Approach

04UK4JZ Supplement Right Femoral Artery with Synthetic Substitute, Percutaneous Endoscopic Approach

04UK4KZ Supplement Right Femoral Artery with Nonautologous Tissue Substitute, Percutaneous Endoscopic Approach

04UL07Z Supplement Left Femoral Artery with Autologous Tissue Substitute, Open Approach

04UL0JZ Supplement Left Femoral Artery with Synthetic Substitute, Open Approach

04UL0KZ Supplement Left Femoral Artery with Nonautologous Tissue Substitute, Open Approach

04UL37Z Supplement Left Femoral Artery with Autologous Tissue Substitute, Percutaneous Approach

04UL3JZ Supplement Left Femoral Artery with Synthetic Substitute, Percutaneous Approach

04UL3KZ Supplement Left Femoral Artery with Nonautologous Tissue Substitute, Percutaneous Approach

04UL47Z Supplement Left Femoral Artery with Autologous Tissue Substitute, Percutaneous Endoscopic Approach

04UL4JZ Supplement Left Femoral Artery with Synthetic Substitute, Percutaneous Endoscopic Approach

04UL4KZ Supplement Left Femoral Artery with Nonautologous Tissue Substitute, Percutaneous Endoscopic Approach

04UM07Z Supplement Right Popliteal Artery with Autologous Tissue Substitute, Open Approach

04UM0JZ Supplement Right Popliteal Artery with Synthetic Substitute, Open Approach

04UM0KZ Supplement Right Popliteal Artery with Nonautologous Tissue Substitute, Open Approach

04UM37Z Supplement Right Popliteal Artery with Autologous Tissue Substitute, Percutaneous Approach

04UM3JZ Supplement Right Popliteal Artery with Synthetic Substitute, Percutaneous Approach

04UM3KZ Supplement Right Popliteal Artery with Nonautologous Tissue Substitute, Percutaneous Approach

04UM47Z Supplement Right Popliteal Artery with Autologous Tissue Substitute, Percutaneous Endoscopic Approach

04UM4JZ Supplement Right Popliteal Artery with Synthetic Substitute, Percutaneous Endoscopic Approach

04UM4KZ Supplement Right Popliteal Artery with Nonautologous Tissue Substitute, Percutaneous Endoscopic Approach

04UN07Z Supplement Left Popliteal Artery with Autologous Tissue Substitute, Open Approach

04UN0JZ Supplement Left Popliteal Artery with Synthetic Substitute, Open Approach

04UN0KZ Supplement Left Popliteal Artery with Nonautologous Tissue Substitute, Open Approach

04UN37Z Supplement Left Popliteal Artery with Autologous Tissue Substitute, Percutaneous Approach

04UN3JZ Supplement Left Popliteal Artery with Synthetic Substitute, Percutaneous Approach

04UN3KZ Supplement Left Popliteal Artery with Nonautologous Tissue Substitute, Percutaneous Approach

04UN47Z Supplement Left Popliteal Artery with Autologous Tissue Substitute, Percutaneous Endoscopic Approach

04UN4JZ Supplement Left Popliteal Artery with Synthetic Substitute, Percutaneous Endoscopic Approach

04UN4KZ Supplement Left Popliteal Artery with Nonautologous Tissue Substitute, Percutaneous Endoscopic Approach

04UP07Z Supplement Right Anterior Tibial Artery with Autologous Tissue Substitute, Open Approach

04UP0JZ Supplement Right Anterior Tibial Artery with Synthetic Substitute, Open Approach

04UP0KZ Supplement Right Anterior Tibial Artery with Nonautologous Tissue Substitute, Open Approach

04UP37Z Supplement Right Anterior Tibial Artery with Autologous Tissue Substitute, Percutaneous Approach

04UP3JZ Supplement Right Anterior Tibial Artery with Synthetic Substitute, Percutaneous Approach

04UP3KZ Supplement Right Anterior Tibial Artery with Nonautologous Tissue Substitute, Percutaneous Approach

04UP47Z Supplement Right Anterior Tibial Artery with Autologous Tissue Substitute, Percutaneous Endoscopic Approach

04UP4JZ Supplement Right Anterior Tibial Artery with Synthetic Substitute, Percutaneous Endoscopic Approach

04UP4KZ Supplement Right Anterior Tibial Artery with Nonautologous Tissue Substitute, Percutaneous Endoscopic Approach

04UQ07Z Supplement Left Anterior Tibial Artery with Autologous Tissue Substitute, Open Approach

04UQ0JZ Supplement Left Anterior Tibial Artery with Synthetic Substitute, Open Approach

04UQ0KZ Supplement Left Anterior Tibial Artery with Nonautologous Tissue Substitute, Open Approach

04UQ37Z Supplement Left Anterior Tibial Artery with Autologous Tissue Substitute, Percutaneous Approach

04UQ3JZ Supplement Left Anterior Tibial Artery with Synthetic Substitute, Percutaneous Approach

04UQ3KZ Supplement Left Anterior Tibial Artery with Nonautologous Tissue Substitute, Percutaneous Approach

04UQ47Z Supplement Left Anterior Tibial Artery with Autologous Tissue Substitute, Percutaneous Endoscopic Approach

04UQ4JZ Supplement Left Anterior Tibial Artery with Synthetic Substitute, Percutaneous Endoscopic Approach

04UQ4KZ Supplement Left Anterior Tibial Artery with Nonautologous Tissue Substitute, Percutaneous Endoscopic Approach

04UR07Z Supplement Right Posterior Tibial Artery with Autologous Tissue Substitute, Open Approach

04UR0JZ Supplement Right Posterior Tibial Artery with Synthetic Substitute, Open Approach

04UR0KZ Supplement Right Posterior Tibial Artery with Nonautologous Tissue Substitute, Open Approach

04UR37Z Supplement Right Posterior Tibial Artery with Autologous Tissue Substitute, Percutaneous Approach

04UR3JZ Supplement Right Posterior Tibial Artery with Synthetic Substitute, Percutaneous Approach

04UR3KZ Supplement Right Posterior Tibial Artery with Nonautologous Tissue Substitute, Percutaneous Approach

04UR47Z Supplement Right Posterior Tibial Artery with Autologous Tissue Substitute, Percutaneous Endoscopic Approach

04UR4JZ Supplement Right Posterior Tibial Artery with Synthetic Substitute, Percutaneous Endoscopic Approach

04UR4KZ Supplement Right Posterior Tibial Artery with Nonautologous Tissue Substitute, Percutaneous Endoscopic Approach

04US07Z Supplement Left Posterior Tibial Artery with Autologous Tissue Substitute, Open Approach

04US0JZ Supplement Left Posterior Tibial Artery with Synthetic Substitute, Open Approach

04US0KZ Supplement Left Posterior Tibial Artery with Nonautologous Tissue Substitute, Open Approach

04US37Z Supplement Left Posterior Tibial Artery with Autologous Tissue Substitute, Percutaneous Approach

04US3JZ Supplement Left Posterior Tibial Artery with Synthetic Substitute, Percutaneous Approach

04US3KZ Supplement Left Posterior Tibial Artery with Nonautologous Tissue Substitute, Percutaneous Approach

04US47Z Supplement Left Posterior Tibial Artery with Autologous Tissue Substitute, Percutaneous Endoscopic Approach

04US4JZ Supplement Left Posterior Tibial Artery with Synthetic Substitute, Percutaneous Endoscopic Approach

04US4KZ Supplement Left Posterior Tibial Artery with Nonautologous Tissue Substitute, Percutaneous Endoscopic Approach

04UT07Z Supplement Right Peroneal Artery with Autologous Tissue Substitute, Open Approach

04UT0JZ Supplement Right Peroneal Artery with Synthetic Substitute, Open Approach

04UT0KZ Supplement Right Peroneal Artery with Nonautologous Tissue Substitute, Open Approach

04UT37Z Supplement Right Peroneal Artery with Autologous Tissue Substitute, Percutaneous Approach

♀ Female-only ♂ Male-only ● Limited Coverage ● Non-OR HAC HAC-associated procedure ● Non-covered procedures ✚ Combination

04UT3JZ   Supplement Right Peroneal Artery with Synthetic Substitute, Percutaneous Approach

04UT3KZ   Supplement Right Peroneal Artery with Nonautologous Tissue Substitute, Percutaneous Approach

04UT47Z   Supplement Right Peroneal Artery with Autologous Tissue Substitute, Percutaneous Endoscopic Approach

04UT4JZ   Supplement Right Peroneal Artery with Synthetic Substitute, Percutaneous Endoscopic Approach

04UT4KZ   Supplement Right Peroneal Artery with Nonautologous Tissue Substitute, Percutaneous Endoscopic Approach

04UU07Z   Supplement Left Peroneal Artery with Autologous Tissue Substitute, Open Approach

04UU0JZ   Supplement Left Peroneal Artery with Synthetic Substitute, Open Approach

04UU0KZ   Supplement Left Peroneal Artery with Nonautologous Tissue Substitute, Open Approach

04UU37Z   Supplement Left Peroneal Artery with Autologous Tissue Substitute, Percutaneous Approach

04UU3JZ   Supplement Left Peroneal Artery with Synthetic Substitute, Percutaneous Approach

04UU3KZ   Supplement Left Peroneal Artery with Nonautologous Tissue Substitute, Percutaneous Approach

04UU47Z   Supplement Left Peroneal Artery with Autologous Tissue Substitute, Percutaneous Endoscopic Approach

04UU4JZ   Supplement Left Peroneal Artery with Synthetic Substitute, Percutaneous Endoscopic Approach

04UU4KZ   Supplement Left Peroneal Artery with Nonautologous Tissue Substitute, Percutaneous Endoscopic Approach

04UV07Z   Supplement Right Foot Artery with Autologous Tissue Substitute, Open Approach

04UV0JZ   Supplement Right Foot Artery with Synthetic Substitute, Open Approach

04UV0KZ   Supplement Right Foot Artery with Nonautologous Tissue Substitute, Open Approach

04UV37Z   Supplement Right Foot Artery with Autologous Tissue Substitute, Percutaneous Approach

04UV3JZ   Supplement Right Foot Artery with Synthetic Substitute, Percutaneous Approach

04UV3KZ   Supplement Right Foot Artery with Nonautologous Tissue Substitute, Percutaneous Approach

04UV47Z   Supplement Right Foot Artery with Autologous Tissue Substitute, Percutaneous Endoscopic Approach

04UV4JZ   Supplement Right Foot Artery with Synthetic Substitute, Percutaneous Endoscopic Approach

04UV4KZ   Supplement Right Foot Artery with Nonautologous Tissue Substitute, Percutaneous Endoscopic Approach

04UW07Z   Supplement Left Foot Artery with Autologous Tissue Substitute, Open Approach

04UW0JZ   Supplement Left Foot Artery with Synthetic Substitute, Open Approach

04UW0KZ   Supplement Left Foot Artery with Nonautologous Tissue Substitute, Open Approach

04UW37Z   Supplement Left Foot Artery with Autologous Tissue Substitute, Percutaneous Approach

04UW3JZ   Supplement Left Foot Artery with Synthetic Substitute, Percutaneous Approach

04UW3KZ   Supplement Left Foot Artery with Nonautologous Tissue Substitute, Percutaneous Approach

04UW47Z   Supplement Left Foot Artery with Autologous Tissue Substitute, Percutaneous Endoscopic Approach

04UW4JZ   Supplement Left Foot Artery with Synthetic Substitute, Percutaneous Endoscopic Approach

04UW4KZ   Supplement Left Foot Artery with Nonautologous Tissue Substitute, Percutaneous Endoscopic Approach

04UY07Z   Supplement Lower Artery with Autologous Tissue Substitute, Open Approach

04UY0JZ   Supplement Lower Artery with Synthetic Substitute, Open Approach

04UY0KZ   Supplement Lower Artery with Nonautologous Tissue Substitute, Open Approach

04UY37Z   Supplement Lower Artery with Autologous Tissue Substitute, Percutaneous Approach

04UY3JZ   Supplement Lower Artery with Synthetic Substitute, Percutaneous Approach

04UY3KZ   Supplement Lower Artery with Nonautologous Tissue Substitute, Percutaneous Approach

04UY47Z   Supplement Lower Artery with Autologous Tissue Substitute, Percutaneous Endoscopic Approach

04UY4JZ   Supplement Lower Artery with Synthetic Substitute, Percutaneous Endoscopic Approach

04UY4KZ   Supplement Lower Artery with Nonautologous Tissue Substitute, Percutaneous Endoscopic Approach

04V – Lower Arteries, Restriction

Review Coding Guideline B3.12

04V00CZ   Restriction of Abdominal Aorta with Extraluminal Device, Open Approach

04V00DJ   Restriction of Abdominal Aorta with Intraluminal Device, Temporary, Open Approach

04V00DZ   Restriction of Abdominal Aorta with Intraluminal Device, Open Approach

04V00ZZ   Restriction of Abdominal Aorta, Open Approach

04V03CZ   Restriction of Abdominal Aorta with Extraluminal Device, Percutaneous Approach

04V03DJ   Restriction of Abdominal Aorta with Intraluminal Device, Temporary, Percutaneous Approach

04V03DZ   Restriction of Abdominal Aorta with Intraluminal Device, Percutaneous Approach

04V03ZZ   Restriction of Abdominal Aorta, Percutaneous Approach

04V04CZ   Restriction of Abdominal Aorta with Extraluminal Device, Percutaneous Endoscopic Approach

04V04DJ   Restriction of Abdominal Aorta with Intraluminal Device, Temporary, Percutaneous Endoscopic Approach

04V04DZ   Restriction of Abdominal Aorta with Intraluminal Device, Percutaneous Endoscopic Approach

04V04ZZ   Restriction of Abdominal Aorta, Percutaneous Endoscopic Approach

04V10CZ   Restriction of Celiac Artery with Extraluminal Device, Open Approach

04V10DZ   Restriction of Celiac Artery with Intraluminal Device, Open Approach

04V10ZZ   Restriction of Celiac Artery, Open Approach

04V13CZ   Restriction of Celiac Artery with Extraluminal Device, Percutaneous Approach

04V13DZ   Restriction of Celiac Artery with Intraluminal Device, Percutaneous Approach

04V13ZZ   Restriction of Celiac Artery, Percutaneous Approach

04V14CZ   Restriction of Celiac Artery with Extraluminal Device, Percutaneous Endoscopic Approach

04V14DZ   Restriction of Celiac Artery with Intraluminal Device, Percutaneous Endoscopic Approach

04V14ZZ   Restriction of Celiac Artery, Percutaneous Endoscopic Approach

04V20CZ   Restriction of Gastric Artery with Extraluminal Device, Open Approach

04V20DZ   Restriction of Gastric Artery with Intraluminal Device, Open Approach

04V20ZZ   Restriction of Gastric Artery, Open Approach

04V23CZ   Restriction of Gastric Artery with Extraluminal Device, Percutaneous Approach

04V23DZ   Restriction of Gastric Artery with Intraluminal Device, Percutaneous Approach

04V23ZZ   Restriction of Gastric Artery, Percutaneous Approach

04V24CZ   Restriction of Gastric Artery with Extraluminal Device, Percutaneous Endoscopic Approach

04V24DZ   Restriction of Gastric Artery with Intraluminal Device, Percutaneous Endoscopic Approach

04V24ZZ   Restriction of Gastric Artery, Percutaneous Endoscopic Approach

---

♀ Female-only   ♂ Male-only   ● Limited Coverage   ● Non-OR   ᴴᴬᶜ HAC-associated procedure   ● Non-covered procedures   ➕ Combination

04V30CZ Restriction of Hepatic Artery with Extraluminal Device, Open Approach

04V30DZ Restriction of Hepatic Artery with Intraluminal Device, Open Approach

04V30ZZ Restriction of Hepatic Artery, Open Approach

04V33CZ Restriction of Hepatic Artery with Extraluminal Device, Percutaneous Approach

04V33DZ Restriction of Hepatic Artery with Intraluminal Device, Percutaneous Approach

04V33ZZ Restriction of Hepatic Artery, Percutaneous Approach

04V34CZ Restriction of Hepatic Artery with Extraluminal Device, Percutaneous Endoscopic Approach

04V34DZ Restriction of Hepatic Artery with Intraluminal Device, Percutaneous Endoscopic Approach

04V34ZZ Restriction of Hepatic Artery, Percutaneous Endoscopic Approach

04V40CZ Restriction of Splenic Artery with Extraluminal Device, Open Approach

04V40DZ Restriction of Splenic Artery with Intraluminal Device, Open Approach

04V40ZZ Restriction of Splenic Artery, Open Approach

04V43CZ Restriction of Splenic Artery with Extraluminal Device, Percutaneous Approach

04V43DZ Restriction of Splenic Artery with Intraluminal Device, Percutaneous Approach

04V43ZZ Restriction of Splenic Artery, Percutaneous Approach

04V44CZ Restriction of Splenic Artery with Extraluminal Device, Percutaneous Endoscopic Approach

04V44DZ Restriction of Splenic Artery with Intraluminal Device, Percutaneous Endoscopic Approach

04V44ZZ Restriction of Splenic Artery, Percutaneous Endoscopic Approach

04V50CZ Restriction of Superior Mesenteric Artery with Extraluminal Device, Open Approach

04V50DZ Restriction of Superior Mesenteric Artery with Intraluminal Device, Open Approach

04V50ZZ Restriction of Superior Mesenteric Artery, Open Approach

04V53CZ Restriction of Superior Mesenteric Artery with Extraluminal Device, Percutaneous Approach

04V53DZ Restriction of Superior Mesenteric Artery with Intraluminal Device, Percutaneous Approach

04V53ZZ Restriction of Superior Mesenteric Artery, Percutaneous Approach

04V54CZ Restriction of Superior Mesenteric Artery with Extraluminal Device, Percutaneous Endoscopic Approach

04V54DZ Restriction of Superior Mesenteric Artery with Intraluminal Device, Percutaneous Endoscopic Approach

04V54ZZ Restriction of Superior Mesenteric Artery, Percutaneous Endoscopic Approach

04V60CZ Restriction of Right Colic Artery with Extraluminal Device, Open Approach

04V60DZ Restriction of Right Colic Artery with Intraluminal Device, Open Approach

04V60ZZ Restriction of Right Colic Artery, Open Approach

04V63CZ Restriction of Right Colic Artery with Extraluminal Device, Percutaneous Approach

04V63DZ Restriction of Right Colic Artery with Intraluminal Device, Percutaneous Approach

04V63ZZ Restriction of Right Colic Artery, Percutaneous Approach

04V64CZ Restriction of Right Colic Artery with Extraluminal Device, Percutaneous Endoscopic Approach

04V64DZ Restriction of Right Colic Artery with Intraluminal Device, Percutaneous Endoscopic Approach

04V64ZZ Restriction of Right Colic Artery, Percutaneous Endoscopic Approach

04V70CZ Restriction of Left Colic Artery with Extraluminal Device, Open Approach

04V70DZ Restriction of Left Colic Artery with Intraluminal Device, Open Approach

04V70ZZ Restriction of Left Colic Artery, Open Approach

04V73CZ Restriction of Left Colic Artery with Extraluminal Device, Percutaneous Approach

04V73DZ Restriction of Left Colic Artery with Intraluminal Device, Percutaneous Approach

04V73ZZ Restriction of Left Colic Artery, Percutaneous Approach

04V74CZ Restriction of Left Colic Artery with Extraluminal Device, Percutaneous Endoscopic Approach

04V74DZ Restriction of Left Colic Artery with Intraluminal Device, Percutaneous Endoscopic Approach

04V74ZZ Restriction of Left Colic Artery, Percutaneous Endoscopic Approach

04V80CZ Restriction of Middle Colic Artery with Extraluminal Device, Open Approach

04V80DZ Restriction of Middle Colic Artery with Intraluminal Device, Open Approach

04V80ZZ Restriction of Middle Colic Artery, Open Approach

04V83CZ Restriction of Middle Colic Artery with Extraluminal Device, Percutaneous Approach

04V83DZ Restriction of Middle Colic Artery with Intraluminal Device, Percutaneous Approach

04V83ZZ Restriction of Middle Colic Artery, Percutaneous Approach

04V84CZ Restriction of Middle Colic Artery with Extraluminal Device, Percutaneous Endoscopic Approach

04V84DZ Restriction of Middle Colic Artery with Intraluminal Device, Percutaneous Endoscopic Approach

04V84ZZ Restriction of Middle Colic Artery, Percutaneous Endoscopic Approach

04V90CZ Restriction of Right Renal Artery with Extraluminal Device, Open Approach

04V90DZ Restriction of Right Renal Artery with Intraluminal Device, Open Approach

04V90ZZ Restriction of Right Renal Artery, Open Approach

04V93CZ Restriction of Right Renal Artery with Extraluminal Device, Percutaneous Approach

04V93DZ Restriction of Right Renal Artery with Intraluminal Device, Percutaneous Approach

04V93ZZ Restriction of Right Renal Artery, Percutaneous Approach

04V94CZ Restriction of Right Renal Artery with Extraluminal Device, Percutaneous Endoscopic Approach

04V94DZ Restriction of Right Renal Artery with Intraluminal Device, Percutaneous Endoscopic Approach

04V94ZZ Restriction of Right Renal Artery, Percutaneous Endoscopic Approach

04VA0CZ Restriction of Left Renal Artery with Extraluminal Device, Open Approach

04VA0DZ Restriction of Left Renal Artery with Intraluminal Device, Open Approach

04VA0ZZ Restriction of Left Renal Artery, Open Approach

04VA3CZ Restriction of Left Renal Artery with Extraluminal Device, Percutaneous Approach

04VA3DZ Restriction of Left Renal Artery with Intraluminal Device, Percutaneous Approach

04VA3ZZ Restriction of Left Renal Artery, Percutaneous Approach

04VA4CZ Restriction of Left Renal Artery with Extraluminal Device, Percutaneous Endoscopic Approach

04VA4DZ Restriction of Left Renal Artery with Intraluminal Device, Percutaneous Endoscopic Approach

04VA4ZZ Restriction of Left Renal Artery, Percutaneous Endoscopic Approach

04VB0CZ Restriction of Inferior Mesenteric Artery with Extraluminal Device, Open Approach

04VB0DZ Restriction of Inferior Mesenteric Artery with Intraluminal Device, Open Approach

04VB0ZZ Restriction of Inferior Mesenteric Artery, Open Approach

04VB3CZ Restriction of Inferior Mesenteric Artery with Extraluminal Device, Percutaneous Approach

04VB3DZ Restriction of Inferior Mesenteric Artery with Intraluminal Device, Percutaneous Approach

04VB3ZZ Restriction of Inferior Mesenteric Artery, Percutaneous Approach

04VB4CZ Restriction of Inferior Mesenteric Artery with Extraluminal Device, Percutaneous Endoscopic Approach

04VB4DZ Restriction of Inferior Mesenteric Artery with Intraluminal Device, Percutaneous Endoscopic Approach

04VB4ZZ Restriction of Inferior Mesenteric Artery, Percutaneous Endoscopic Approach

04VC0CZ Restriction of Right Common Iliac Artery with Extraluminal Device, Open Approach

04VC0DZ Restriction of Right Common Iliac Artery with Intraluminal Device, Open Approach

---

♀ Female-only   ♂ Male-only   ◯ Limited Coverage   ● Non-OR   🅷🅰🅲 HAC-associated procedure   ⬡ Non-covered procedures   ➕ Combination

04VC0ZZ Restriction of Right Common Iliac Artery, Open Approach

04VC3CZ Restriction of Right Common Iliac Artery with Extraluminal Device, Percutaneous Approach

04VC3DZ Restriction of Right Common Iliac Artery with Intraluminal Device, Percutaneous Approach

04VC3ZZ Restriction of Right Common Iliac Artery, Percutaneous Approach

04VC4CZ Restriction of Right Common Iliac Artery with Extraluminal Device, Percutaneous Endoscopic Approach

04VC4DZ Restriction of Right Common Iliac Artery with Intraluminal Device, Percutaneous Endoscopic Approach

04VC4ZZ Restriction of Right Common Iliac Artery, Percutaneous Endoscopic Approach

04VD0CZ Restriction of Left Common Iliac Artery with Extraluminal Device, Open Approach

04VD0DZ Restriction of Left Common Iliac Artery with Intraluminal Device, Open Approach

04VD0ZZ Restriction of Left Common Iliac Artery, Open Approach

04VD3CZ Restriction of Left Common Iliac Artery with Extraluminal Device, Percutaneous Approach

04VD3DZ Restriction of Left Common Iliac Artery with Intraluminal Device, Percutaneous Approach

04VD3ZZ Restriction of Left Common Iliac Artery, Percutaneous Approach

04VD4CZ Restriction of Left Common Iliac Artery with Extraluminal Device, Percutaneous Endoscopic Approach

04VD4DZ Restriction of Left Common Iliac Artery with Intraluminal Device, Percutaneous Endoscopic Approach

04VD4ZZ Restriction of Left Common Iliac Artery, Percutaneous Endoscopic Approach

04VE0CZ Restriction of Right Internal Iliac Artery with Extraluminal Device, Open Approach

04VE0DZ Restriction of Right Internal Iliac Artery with Intraluminal Device, Open Approach

04VE0ZZ Restriction of Right Internal Iliac Artery, Open Approach

04VE3CZ Restriction of Right Internal Iliac Artery with Extraluminal Device, Percutaneous Approach

04VE3DZ Restriction of Right Internal Iliac Artery with Intraluminal Device, Percutaneous Approach

04VE3ZZ Restriction of Right Internal Iliac Artery, Percutaneous Approach

04VE4CZ Restriction of Right Internal Iliac Artery with Extraluminal Device, Percutaneous Endoscopic Approach

04VE4DZ Restriction of Right Internal Iliac Artery with Intraluminal Device, Percutaneous Endoscopic Approach

04VE4ZZ Restriction of Right Internal Iliac Artery, Percutaneous Endoscopic Approach

04VF0CZ Restriction of Left Internal Iliac Artery with Extraluminal Device, Open Approach

04VF0DZ Restriction of Left Internal Iliac Artery with Intraluminal Device, Open Approach

04VF0ZZ Restriction of Left Internal Iliac Artery, Open Approach

04VF3CZ Restriction of Left Internal Iliac Artery with Extraluminal Device, Percutaneous Approach

04VF3DZ Restriction of Left Internal Iliac Artery with Intraluminal Device, Percutaneous Approach

04VF3ZZ Restriction of Left Internal Iliac Artery, Percutaneous Approach

04VF4CZ Restriction of Left Internal Iliac Artery with Extraluminal Device, Percutaneous Endoscopic Approach

04VF4DZ Restriction of Left Internal Iliac Artery with Intraluminal Device, Percutaneous Endoscopic Approach

04VF4ZZ Restriction of Left Internal Iliac Artery, Percutaneous Endoscopic Approach

04VH0CZ Restriction of Right External Iliac Artery with Extraluminal Device, Open Approach

04VH0DZ Restriction of Right External Iliac Artery with Intraluminal Device, Open Approach

04VH0ZZ Restriction of Right External Iliac Artery, Open Approach

04VH3CZ Restriction of Right External Iliac Artery with Extraluminal Device, Percutaneous Approach

04VH3DZ Restriction of Right External Iliac Artery with Intraluminal Device, Percutaneous Approach

04VH3ZZ Restriction of Right External Iliac Artery, Percutaneous Approach

04VH4CZ Restriction of Right External Iliac Artery with Extraluminal Device, Percutaneous Endoscopic Approach

04VH4DZ Restriction of Right External Iliac Artery with Intraluminal Device, Percutaneous Endoscopic Approach

04VH4ZZ Restriction of Right External Iliac Artery, Percutaneous Endoscopic Approach

04VJ0CZ Restriction of Left External Iliac Artery with Extraluminal Device, Open Approach

04VJ0DZ Restriction of Left External Iliac Artery with Intraluminal Device, Open Approach

04VJ0ZZ Restriction of Left External Iliac Artery, Open Approach

04VJ3CZ Restriction of Left External Iliac Artery with Extraluminal Device, Percutaneous Approach

04VJ3DZ Restriction of Left External Iliac Artery with Intraluminal Device, Percutaneous Approach

04VJ3ZZ Restriction of Left External Iliac Artery, Percutaneous Approach

04VJ4CZ Restriction of Left External Iliac Artery with Extraluminal Device, Percutaneous Endoscopic Approach

04VJ4DZ Restriction of Left External Iliac Artery with Intraluminal Device, Percutaneous Endoscopic Approach

04VJ4ZZ Restriction of Left External Iliac Artery, Percutaneous Endoscopic Approach

04VK0CZ Restriction of Right Femoral Artery with Extraluminal Device, Open Approach

04VK0DZ Restriction of Right Femoral Artery with Intraluminal Device, Open Approach

04VK0ZZ Restriction of Right Femoral Artery, Open Approach

04VK3CZ Restriction of Right Femoral Artery with Extraluminal Device, Percutaneous Approach

04VK3DZ Restriction of Right Femoral Artery with Intraluminal Device, Percutaneous Approach

04VK3ZZ Restriction of Right Femoral Artery, Percutaneous Approach

04VK4CZ Restriction of Right Femoral Artery with Extraluminal Device, Percutaneous Endoscopic Approach

04VK4DZ Restriction of Right Femoral Artery with Intraluminal Device, Percutaneous Endoscopic Approach

04VK4ZZ Restriction of Right Femoral Artery, Percutaneous Endoscopic Approach

04VL0CZ Restriction of Left Femoral Artery with Extraluminal Device, Open Approach

04VL0DZ Restriction of Left Femoral Artery with Intraluminal Device, Open Approach

04VL0ZZ Restriction of Left Femoral Artery, Open Approach

04VL3CZ Restriction of Left Femoral Artery with Extraluminal Device, Percutaneous Approach

04VL3DZ Restriction of Left Femoral Artery with Intraluminal Device, Percutaneous Approach

04VL3ZZ Restriction of Left Femoral Artery, Percutaneous Approach

04VL4CZ Restriction of Left Femoral Artery with Extraluminal Device, Percutaneous Endoscopic Approach

04VL4DZ Restriction of Left Femoral Artery with Intraluminal Device, Percutaneous Endoscopic Approach

04VL4ZZ Restriction of Left Femoral Artery, Percutaneous Endoscopic Approach

04VM0CZ Restriction of Right Popliteal Artery with Extraluminal Device, Open Approach

04VM0DZ Restriction of Right Popliteal Artery with Intraluminal Device, Open Approach

04VM0ZZ Restriction of Right Popliteal Artery, Open Approach

04VM3CZ Restriction of Right Popliteal Artery with Extraluminal Device, Percutaneous Approach

04VM3DZ Restriction of Right Popliteal Artery with Intraluminal Device, Percutaneous Approach

04VM3ZZ Restriction of Right Popliteal Artery, Percutaneous Approach

04VM4CZ Restriction of Right Popliteal Artery with Extraluminal Device, Percutaneous Endoscopic Approach

04VM4DZ Restriction of Right Popliteal Artery with Intraluminal Device, Percutaneous Endoscopic Approach

04VM4ZZ Restriction of Right Popliteal Artery, Percutaneous Endoscopic Approach

04VN0CZ Restriction of Left Popliteal Artery with Extraluminal Device, Open Approach

04VN0DZ Restriction of Left Popliteal Artery with Intraluminal Device, Open Approach

04VN0ZZ Restriction of Left Popliteal Artery, Open Approach

04VN3CZ Restriction of Left Popliteal Artery with Extraluminal Device, Percutaneous Approach

04VN3DZ Restriction of Left Popliteal Artery with Intraluminal Device, Percutaneous Approach

04VN3ZZ Restriction of Left Popliteal Artery, Percutaneous Approach

04VN4CZ Restriction of Left Popliteal Artery with Extraluminal Device, Percutaneous Endoscopic Approach

04VN4DZ Restriction of Left Popliteal Artery with Intraluminal Device, Percutaneous Endoscopic Approach

04VN4ZZ Restriction of Left Popliteal Artery, Percutaneous Endoscopic Approach

04VP0CZ Restriction of Right Anterior Tibial Artery with Extraluminal Device, Open Approach

04VP0DZ Restriction of Right Anterior Tibial Artery with Intraluminal Device, Open Approach

04VP0ZZ Restriction of Right Anterior Tibial Artery, Open Approach

04VP3CZ Restriction of Right Anterior Tibial Artery with Extraluminal Device, Percutaneous Approach

04VP3DZ Restriction of Right Anterior Tibial Artery with Intraluminal Device, Percutaneous Approach

04VP3ZZ Restriction of Right Anterior Tibial Artery, Percutaneous Approach

04VP4CZ Restriction of Right Anterior Tibial Artery with Extraluminal Device, Percutaneous Endoscopic Approach

04VP4DZ Restriction of Right Anterior Tibial Artery with Intraluminal Device, Percutaneous Endoscopic Approach

04VP4ZZ Restriction of Right Anterior Tibial Artery, Percutaneous Endoscopic Approach

04VQ0CZ Restriction of Left Anterior Tibial Artery with Extraluminal Device, Open Approach

04VQ0DZ Restriction of Left Anterior Tibial Artery with Intraluminal Device, Open Approach

04VQ0ZZ Restriction of Left Anterior Tibial Artery, Open Approach

04VQ3CZ Restriction of Left Anterior Tibial Artery with Extraluminal Device, Percutaneous Approach

04VQ3DZ Restriction of Left Anterior Tibial Artery with Intraluminal Device, Percutaneous Approach

04VQ3ZZ Restriction of Left Anterior Tibial Artery, Percutaneous Approach

04VQ4CZ Restriction of Left Anterior Tibial Artery with Extraluminal Device, Percutaneous Endoscopic Approach

04VQ4DZ Restriction of Left Anterior Tibial Artery with Intraluminal Device, Percutaneous Endoscopic Approach

04VQ4ZZ Restriction of Left Anterior Tibial Artery, Percutaneous Endoscopic Approach

04VR0CZ Restriction of Right Posterior Tibial Artery with Extraluminal Device, Open Approach

04VR0DZ Restriction of Right Posterior Tibial Artery with Intraluminal Device, Open Approach

04VR0ZZ Restriction of Right Posterior Tibial Artery, Open Approach

04VR3CZ Restriction of Right Posterior Tibial Artery with Extraluminal Device, Percutaneous Approach

04VR3DZ Restriction of Right Posterior Tibial Artery with Intraluminal Device, Percutaneous Approach

04VR3ZZ Restriction of Right Posterior Tibial Artery, Percutaneous Approach

04VR4CZ Restriction of Right Posterior Tibial Artery with Extraluminal Device, Percutaneous Endoscopic Approach

04VR4DZ Restriction of Right Posterior Tibial Artery with Intraluminal Device, Percutaneous Endoscopic Approach

04VR4ZZ Restriction of Right Posterior Tibial Artery, Percutaneous Endoscopic Approach

04VS0CZ Restriction of Left Posterior Tibial Artery with Extraluminal Device, Open Approach

04VS0DZ Restriction of Left Posterior Tibial Artery with Intraluminal Device, Open Approach

04VS0ZZ Restriction of Left Posterior Tibial Artery, Open Approach

04VS3CZ Restriction of Left Posterior Tibial Artery with Extraluminal Device, Percutaneous Approach

04VS3DZ Restriction of Left Posterior Tibial Artery with Intraluminal Device, Percutaneous Approach

04VS3ZZ Restriction of Left Posterior Tibial Artery, Percutaneous Approach

04VS4CZ Restriction of Left Posterior Tibial Artery with Extraluminal Device, Percutaneous Endoscopic Approach

04VS4DZ Restriction of Left Posterior Tibial Artery with Intraluminal Device, Percutaneous Endoscopic Approach

04VS4ZZ Restriction of Left Posterior Tibial Artery, Percutaneous Endoscopic Approach

04VT0CZ Restriction of Right Peroneal Artery with Extraluminal Device, Open Approach

04VT0DZ Restriction of Right Peroneal Artery with Intraluminal Device, Open Approach

04VT0ZZ Restriction of Right Peroneal Artery, Open Approach

04VT3CZ Restriction of Right Peroneal Artery with Extraluminal Device, Percutaneous Approach

04VT3DZ Restriction of Right Peroneal Artery with Intraluminal Device, Percutaneous Approach

04VT3ZZ Restriction of Right Peroneal Artery, Percutaneous Approach

04VT4CZ Restriction of Right Peroneal Artery with Extraluminal Device, Percutaneous Endoscopic Approach

04VT4DZ Restriction of Right Peroneal Artery with Intraluminal Device, Percutaneous Endoscopic Approach

04VT4ZZ Restriction of Right Peroneal Artery, Percutaneous Endoscopic Approach

04VU0CZ Restriction of Left Peroneal Artery with Extraluminal Device, Open Approach

04VU0DZ Restriction of Left Peroneal Artery with Intraluminal Device, Open Approach

04VU0ZZ Restriction of Left Peroneal Artery, Open Approach

04VU3CZ Restriction of Left Peroneal Artery with Extraluminal Device, Percutaneous Approach

04VU3DZ Restriction of Left Peroneal Artery with Intraluminal Device, Percutaneous Approach

04VU3ZZ Restriction of Left Peroneal Artery, Percutaneous Approach

04VU4CZ Restriction of Left Peroneal Artery with Extraluminal Device, Percutaneous Endoscopic Approach

04VU4DZ Restriction of Left Peroneal Artery with Intraluminal Device, Percutaneous Endoscopic Approach

04VU4ZZ Restriction of Left Peroneal Artery, Percutaneous Endoscopic Approach

04VV0CZ Restriction of Right Foot Artery with Extraluminal Device, Open Approach

04VV0DZ Restriction of Right Foot Artery with Intraluminal Device, Open Approach

04VV0ZZ Restriction of Right Foot Artery, Open Approach

04VV3CZ Restriction of Right Foot Artery with Extraluminal Device, Percutaneous Approach

04VV3DZ Restriction of Right Foot Artery with Intraluminal Device, Percutaneous Approach

04VV3ZZ Restriction of Right Foot Artery, Percutaneous Approach

04VV4CZ Restriction of Right Foot Artery with Extraluminal Device, Percutaneous Endoscopic Approach

04VV4DZ Restriction of Right Foot Artery with Intraluminal Device, Percutaneous Endoscopic Approach

04VV4ZZ Restriction of Right Foot Artery, Percutaneous Endoscopic Approach

04VW0CZ Restriction of Left Foot Artery with Extraluminal Device, Open Approach

04VW0DZ Restriction of Left Foot Artery with Intraluminal Device, Open Approach

04VW0ZZ Restriction of Left Foot Artery, Open Approach

04VW3CZ Restriction of Left Foot Artery with Extraluminal Device, Percutaneous Approach

04VW3DZ Restriction of Left Foot Artery with Intraluminal Device, Percutaneous Approach

04VW3ZZ Restriction of Left Foot Artery, Percutaneous Approach

04VW4CZ Restriction of Left Foot Artery with Extraluminal Device, Percutaneous Endoscopic Approach

04VW4DZ Restriction of Left Foot Artery with Intraluminal Device, Percutaneous Endoscopic Approach

04VW4ZZ Restriction of Left Foot Artery, Percutaneous Endoscopic Approach

04VY0CZ Restriction of Lower Artery with Extraluminal Device, Open Approach

04VY0DZ Restriction of Lower Artery with Intraluminal Device, Open Approach

04VY0ZZ Restriction of Lower Artery, Open Approach

04VY3CZ Restriction of Lower Artery with Extraluminal Device, Percutaneous Approach

04VY3DZ   Restriction of Lower Artery with Intraluminal Device, Percutaneous Approach

04VY3ZZ   Restriction of Lower Artery, Percutaneous Approach

04VY4CZ   Restriction of Lower Artery with Extraluminal Device, Percutaneous Endoscopic Approach

04VY4DZ   Restriction of Lower Artery with Intraluminal Device, Percutaneous Endoscopic Approach

04VY4ZZ   Restriction of Lower Artery, Percutaneous Endoscopic Approach

04W – Lower Arteries, Revision

Review Coding Guideline B6.1c

04WY00Z   Revision of Drainage Device in Lower Artery, Open Approach

04WY02Z   Revision of Monitoring Device in Lower Artery, Open Approach

04WY03Z   Revision of Infusion Device in Lower Artery, Open Approach

04WY07Z   Revision of Autologous Tissue Substitute in Lower Artery, Open Approach

04WY0CZ   Revision of Extraluminal Device in Lower Artery, Open Approach

04WY0DZ   Revision of Intraluminal Device in Lower Artery, Open Approach

04WY0JZ   Revision of Synthetic Substitute in Lower Artery, Open Approach

04WY0KZ   Revision of Nonautologous Tissue Substitute in Lower Artery, Open Approach

04WY30Z   Revision of Drainage Device in Lower Artery, Percutaneous Approach

04WY32Z   Revision of Monitoring Device in Lower Artery, Percutaneous Approach

04WY33Z   Revision of Infusion Device in Lower Artery, Percutaneous Approach

04WY37Z   Revision of Autologous Tissue Substitute in Lower Artery, Percutaneous Approach

04WY3CZ   Revision of Extraluminal Device in Lower Artery, Percutaneous Approach

04WY3DZ   Revision of Intraluminal Device in Lower Artery, Percutaneous Approach

04WY3JZ   Revision of Synthetic Substitute in Lower Artery, Percutaneous Approach

04WY3KZ   Revision of Nonautologous Tissue Substitute in Lower Artery, Percutaneous Approach

04WY40Z   Revision of Drainage Device in Lower Artery, Percutaneous Endoscopic Approach

04WY42Z   Revision of Monitoring Device in Lower Artery, Percutaneous Endoscopic Approach

04WY43Z   Revision of Infusion Device in Lower Artery, Percutaneous Endoscopic Approach

04WY47Z   Revision of Autologous Tissue Substitute in Lower Artery, Percutaneous Endoscopic Approach

04WY4CZ   Revision of Extraluminal Device in Lower Artery, Percutaneous Endoscopic Approach

04WY4DZ   Revision of Intraluminal Device in Lower Artery, Percutaneous Endoscopic Approach

04WY4JZ   Revision of Synthetic Substitute in Lower Artery, Percutaneous Endoscopic Approach

04WY4KZ   Revision of Nonautologous Tissue Substitute in Lower Artery, Percutaneous Endoscopic Approach

04WYX0Z   Revision of Drainage Device in Lower Artery, External Approach

04WYX2Z   Revision of Monitoring Device in Lower Artery, External Approach

04WYX3Z   Revision of Infusion Device in Lower Artery, External Approach

04WYX7Z   Revision of Autologous Tissue Substitute in Lower Artery, External Approach

04WYXCZ   Revision of Extraluminal Device in Lower Artery, External Approach

04WYXDZ   Revision of Intraluminal Device in Lower Artery, External Approach

04WYXJZ   Revision of Synthetic Substitute in Lower Artery, External Approach

04WYXKZ   Revision of Nonautologous Tissue Substitute in Lower Artery, External Approach

Upper Veins

Veins

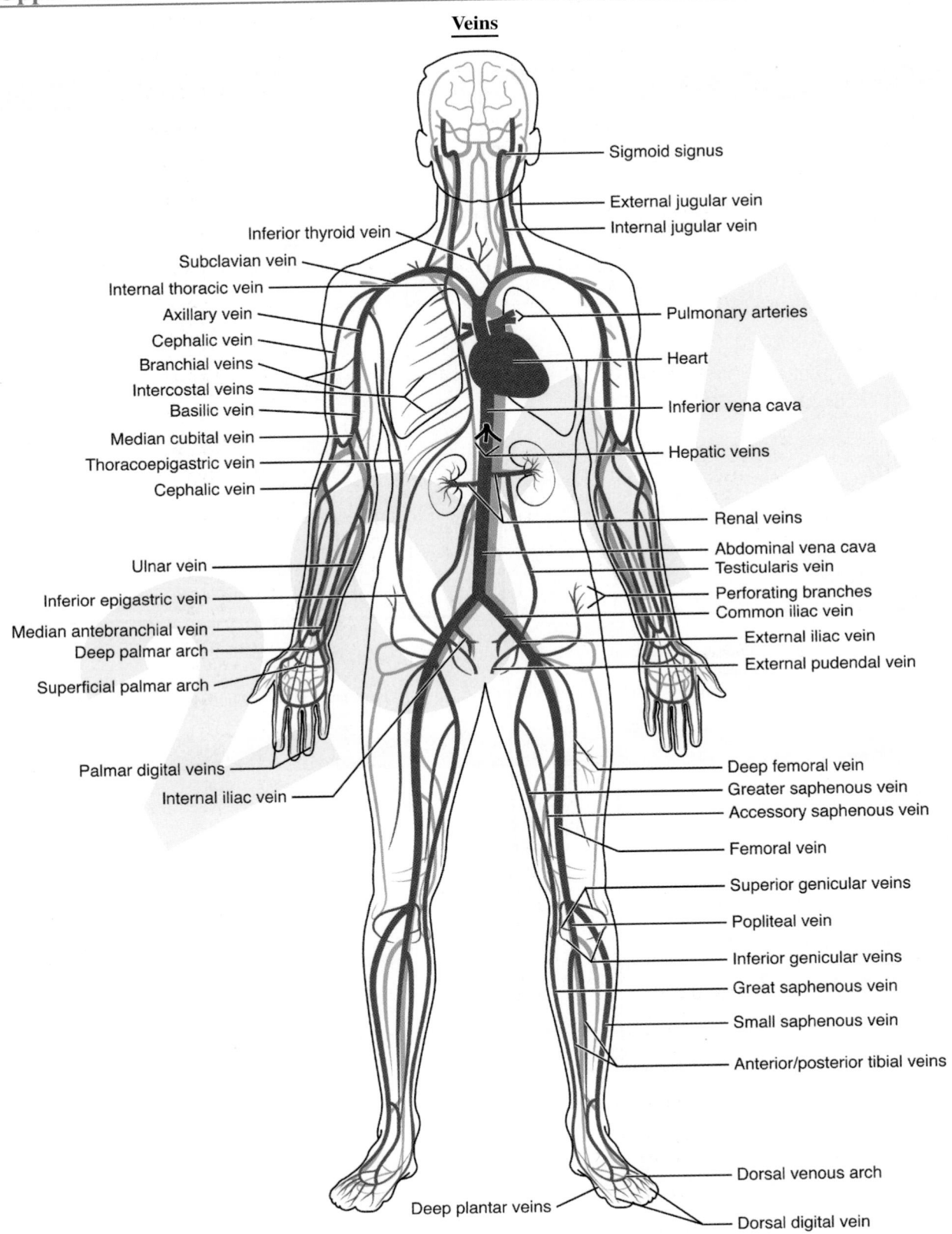

Sigmoid signus

External jugular vein

Internal jugular vein

Inferior thyroid vein

Subclavian vein

Internal thoracic vein

Axillary vein

Cephalic vein

Branchial veins

Intercostal veins

Basilic vein

Median cubital vein

Thoracoepigastric vein

Cephalic vein

Ulnar vein

Inferior epigastric vein

Median antebranchial vein

Deep palmar arch

Superficial palmar arch

Palmar digital veins

Internal iliac vein

Deep plantar veins

Pulmonary arteries

Heart

Inferior vena cava

Hepatic veins

Renal veins

Abdominal vena cava

Testicularis vein

Perforating branches

Common iliac vein

External iliac vein

External pudendal vein

Deep femoral vein

Greater saphenous vein

Accessory saphenous vein

Femoral vein

Superior genicular veins

Popliteal vein

Inferior genicular veins

Great saphenous vein

Small saphenous vein

Anterior/posterior tibial veins

Dorsal venous arch

Dorsal digital vein

Upper Veins Tables 051–05W

Section	0	Medical and Surgical
Body System	5	Upper Veins
Operation	1	Bypass: Altering the route of passage of the contents of a tubular body part

Body Part (4th)	Approach (5th)	Device (6th)	Qualifier (7th)
0 Azygos Vein 1 Hemiazygos Vein 3 Innominate Vein, Right 4 Innominate Vein, Left 5 Subclavian Vein, Right 6 Subclavian Vein, Left 7 Axillary Vein, Right 8 Axillary Vein, Left 9 Brachial Vein, Right A Brachial Vein, Left B Basilic Vein, Right C Basilic Vein, Left D Cephalic Vein, Right F Cephalic Vein, Left G Hand Vein, Right H Hand Vein, Left L Intracranial Vein M Internal Jugular Vein, Right N Internal Jugular Vein, Left P External Jugular Vein, Right Q External Jugular Vein, Left R Vertebral Vein, Right S Vertebral Vein, Left T Face Vein, Right V Face Vein, Left	0 Open 4 Percutaneous Endoscopic	7 Autologous Tissue Substitute 9 Autologous Venous Tissue A Autologous Arterial Tissue J Synthetic Substitute K Nonautologous Tissue Substitute Z No Device	Y Upper Vein

Section	0	Medical and Surgical
Body System	5	Upper Veins
Operation	5	Destruction: Physical eradication of all or a portion of a body part by the direct use of energy, force, or a destructive agent

Body Part (4th)	Approach (5th)	Device (6th)	Qualifier (7th)
0 Azygos Vein 1 Hemiazygos Vein 3 Innominate Vein, Right 4 Innominate Vein, Left 5 Subclavian Vein, Right 6 Subclavian Vein, Left 7 Axillary Vein, Right 8 Axillary Vein, Left 9 Brachial Vein, Right A Brachial Vein, Left B Basilic Vein, Right C Basilic Vein, Left D Cephalic Vein, Right F Cephalic Vein, Left G Hand Vein, Right H Hand Vein, Left L Intracranial Vein M Internal Jugular Vein, Right N Internal Jugular Vein, Left P External Jugular Vein, Right Q External Jugular Vein, Left R Vertebral Vein, Right S Vertebral Vein, Left T Face Vein, Right V Face Vein, Left Y Upper Vein	0 Open 3 Percutaneous 4 Percutaneous Endoscopic	Z No Device	Z No Qualifier

Section	0	**Medical and Surgical**
Body System	5	**Upper Veins**
Operation	7	**Dilation:** Expanding an orifice or the lumen of a tubular body part

Body Part (4th)	Approach (5th)	Device (6th)	Qualifier (7th)
0 Azygos Vein 1 Hemiazygos Vein 3 Innominate Vein, Right 4 Innominate Vein, Left 5 Subclavian Vein, Right 6 Subclavian Vein, Left 7 Axillary Vein, Right 8 Axillary Vein, Left 9 Brachial Vein, Right A Brachial Vein, Left B Basilic Vein, Right C Basilic Vein, Left D Cephalic Vein, Right F Cephalic Vein, Left G Hand Vein, Right H Hand Vein, Left L Intracranial Vein M Internal Jugular Vein, Right N Internal Jugular Vein, Left P External Jugular Vein, Right Q External Jugular Vein, Left R Vertebral Vein, Right S Vertebral Vein, Left T Face Vein, Right V Face Vein, Left Y Upper Vein	0 Open 3 Percutaneous 4 Percutaneous Endoscopic	D Intraluminal Device Z No Device	Z No Qualifier

Section	0	**Medical and Surgical**
Body System	5	**Upper Veins**
Operation	9	**Drainage:** Taking or letting out fluids and/or gases from a body part

Body Part (4th)	Approach (5th)	Device (6th)	Qualifier (7th)
0 Azygos Vein 1 Hemiazygos Vein 3 Innominate Vein, Right 4 Innominate Vein, Left 5 Subclavian Vein, Right 6 Subclavian Vein, Left 7 Axillary Vein, Right 8 Axillary Vein, Left 9 Brachial Vein, Right A Brachial Vein, Left B Basilic Vein, Right C Basilic Vein, Left D Cephalic Vein, Right F Cephalic Vein, Left G Hand Vein, Right H Hand Vein, Left L Intracranial Vein M Internal Jugular Vein, Right N Internal Jugular Vein, Left P External Jugular Vein, Right Q External Jugular Vein, Left R Vertebral Vein, Right S Vertebral Vein, Left T Face Vein, Right V Face Vein, Left Y Upper Vein	0 Open 3 Percutaneous 4 Percutaneous Endoscopic	0 Drainage Device	Z No Qualifier

Continued

059 Continued

Section	0	Medical and Surgical
Body System	5	Upper Veins
Operation	9	Drainage: Taking or letting out fluids and/or gases from a body part

Body Part (4th)	Approach (5th)	Device (6th)	Qualifier (7th)
0 Azygos Vein	0 Open	Z No Device	X Diagnostic
1 Hemiazygos Vein	3 Percutaneous		Z No Qualifier
3 Innominate Vein, Right	4 Percutaneous		
4 Innominate Vein, Left	Endoscopic		
5 Subclavian Vein, Right			
6 Subclavian Vein, Left			
7 Axillary Vein, Right			
8 Axillary Vein, Left			
9 Brachial Vein, Right			
A Brachial Vein, Left			
B Basilic Vein, Right			
C Basilic Vein, Left			
D Cephalic Vein, Right			
F Cephalic Vein, Left			
G Hand Vein, Right			
H Hand Vein, Left			
L Intracranial Vein			
M Internal Jugular Vein, Right			
N Internal Jugular Vein, Left			
P External Jugular Vein, Right			
Q External Jugular Vein, Left			
R Vertebral Vein, Right			
S Vertebral Vein, Left			
T Face Vein, Right			
V Face Vein, Left			
Y Upper Vein			

Section	0	Medical and Surgical
Body System	5	Upper Veins
Operation	B	Excision: Cutting out or off, without replacement, a portion of a body part

Body Part (4th)	Approach (5th)	Device (6th)	Qualifier (7th)
0 Azygos Vein	0 Open	Z No Device	X Diagnostic
1 Hemiazygos Vein	3 Percutaneous		Z No Qualifier
3 Innominate Vein, Right	4 Percutaneous		
4 Innominate Vein, Left	Endoscopic		
5 Subclavian Vein, Right			
6 Subclavian Vein, Left			
7 Axillary Vein, Right			
8 Axillary Vein, Left			
9 Brachial Vein, Right			
A Brachial Vein, Left			
B Basilic Vein, Right			
C Basilic Vein, Left			
D Cephalic Vein, Right			
F Cephalic Vein, Left			
G Hand Vein, Right			
H Hand Vein, Left			
L Intracranial Vein			
M Internal Jugular Vein, Right			
N Internal Jugular Vein, Left			
P External Jugular Vein, Right			
Q External Jugular Vein, Left			
R Vertebral Vein, Right			
S Vertebral Vein, Left			
T Face Vein, Right			
V Face Vein, Left			
Y Upper Vein			

Section	0	Medical and Surgical
Body System	5	Upper Veins
Operation	C	**Extirpation:** Taking or cutting out solid matter from a body part

Body Part (4th)	Approach (5th)	Device (6th)	Qualifier (7th)
0 Azygos Vein	0 Open	Z No Device	Z No Qualifier
1 Hemiazygos Vein	3 Percutaneous		
3 Innominate Vein, Right	4 Percutaneous Endoscopic		
4 Innominate Vein, Left			
5 Subclavian Vein, Right			
6 Subclavian Vein, Left			
7 Axillary Vein, Right			
8 Axillary Vein, Left			
9 Brachial Vein, Right			
A Brachial Vein, Left			
B Basilic Vein, Right			
C Basilic Vein, Left			
D Cephalic Vein, Right			
F Cephalic Vein, Left			
G Hand Vein, Right			
H Hand Vein, Left			
L Intracranial Vein			
M Internal Jugular Vein, Right			
N Internal Jugular Vein, Left			
P External Jugular Vein, Right			
Q External Jugular Vein, Left			
R Vertebral Vein, Right			
S Vertebral Vein, Left			
T Face Vein, Right			
V Face Vein, Left			
Y Upper Vein			

Section	0	Medical and Surgical
Body System	5	Upper Veins
Operation	D	**Extraction:** Pulling or stripping out or off all or a portion of a body part by the use of force

Body Part (4th)	Approach (5th)	Device (6th)	Qualifier (7th)
9 Brachial Vein, Right	0 Open	Z No Device	Z No Qualifier
A Brachial Vein, Left	3 Percutaneous		
B Basilic Vein, Right			
C Basilic Vein, Left			
D Cephalic Vein, Right			
F Cephalic Vein, Left			
G Hand Vein, Right			
H Hand Vein, Left			
Y Upper Vein			

Section	0	Medical and Surgical
Body System	5	Upper Veins
Operation	H	Insertion: Putting in a nonbiological appliance that monitors, assists, performs, or prevents a physiological function but does not physically take the place of a body part

Body Part (4th)	Approach (5th)	Device (6th)	Qualifier (7th)
0 Azygos Vein 1 Hemiazygos Vein 3 Innominate Vein, Right 4 Innominate Vein, Left 5 Subclavian Vein, Right 6 Subclavian Vein, Left 7 Axillary Vein, Right 8 Axillary Vein, Left 9 Brachial Vein, Right A Brachial Vein, Left B Basilic Vein, Right C Basilic Vein, Left D Cephalic Vein, Right F Cephalic Vein, Left G Hand Vein, Right H Hand Vein, Left L Intracranial Vein M Internal Jugular Vein, Right N Internal Jugular Vein, Left P External Jugular Vein, Right Q External Jugular Vein, Left R Vertebral Vein, Right S Vertebral Vein, Left T Face Vein, Right V Face Vein, Left	0 Open 3 Percutaneous 4 Percutaneous Endoscopic	3 Infusion Device D Intraluminal Device	Z No Qualifier
Y Upper Vein	0 Open 3 Percutaneous 4 Percutaneous Endoscopic	2 Monitoring Device 3 Infusion Device D Intraluminal Device	Z No Qualifier

Section	0	Medical and Surgical
Body System	5	Upper Veins
Operation	J	Inspection: Visually and/or manually exploring a body part

Body Part (4th)	Approach (5th)	Device (6th)	Qualifier (7th)
Y Upper Vein	0 Open 3 Percutaneous 4 Percutaneous Endoscopic X External	Z No Device	Z No Qualifier

Section	0	Medical and Surgical
Body System	5	Upper Veins
Operation	L	Occlusion: Completely closing an orifice or the lumen of a tubular body part

Body Part (4th)	Approach (5th)	Device (6th)	Qualifier (7th)
0 Azygos Vein 1 Hemiazygos Vein 3 Innominate Vein, Right 4 Innominate Vein, Left 5 Subclavian Vein, Right 6 Subclavian Vein, Left 7 Axillary Vein, Right 8 Axillary Vein, Left 9 Brachial Vein, Right A Brachial Vein, Left B Basilic Vein, Right C Basilic Vein, Left D Cephalic Vein, Right F Cephalic Vein, Left G Hand Vein, Right H Hand Vein, Left L Intracranial Vein M Internal Jugular Vein, Right N Internal Jugular Vein, Left P External Jugular Vein, Right Q External Jugular Vein, Left R Vertebral Vein, Right S Vertebral Vein, Left T Face Vein, Right V Face Vein, Left Y Upper Vein	0 Open 3 Percutaneous 4 Percutaneous Endoscopic	C Extraluminal Device D Intraluminal Device Z No Device	Z No Qualifier

05L–05N

Section	0	Medical and Surgical
Body System	5	Upper Veins
Operation	N	Release: Freeing a body part from an abnormal physical constraint by cutting or by the use of force

Body Part (4th)	Approach (5th)	Device (6th)	Qualifier (7th)
0 Azygos Vein 1 Hemiazygos Vein 3 Innominate Vein, Right 4 Innominate Vein, Left 5 Subclavian Vein, Right 6 Subclavian Vein, Left 7 Axillary Vein, Right 8 Axillary Vein, Left 9 Brachial Vein, Right A Brachial Vein, Left B Basilic Vein, Right C Basilic Vein, Left D Cephalic Vein, Right F Cephalic Vein, Left G Hand Vein, Right H Hand Vein, Left L Intracranial Vein M Internal Jugular Vein, Right N Internal Jugular Vein, Left P External Jugular Vein, Right Q External Jugular Vein, Left R Vertebral Vein, Right S Vertebral Vein, Left T Face Vein, Right V Face Vein, Left Y Upper Vein	0 Open 3 Percutaneous 4 Percutaneous Endoscopic	Z No Device	Z No Qualifier

Section	0	Medical and Surgical
Body System	5	Upper Veins
Operation	P	Removal: Taking out or off a device from a body part

Body Part (4th)	Approach (5th)	Device (6th)	Qualifier (7th)
Y Upper Vein	0 Open 3 Percutaneous 4 Percutaneous Endoscopic	0 Drainage Device 2 Monitoring Device 3 Infusion Device 7 Autologous Tissue Substitute C Extraluminal Device D Intraluminal Device J Synthetic Substitute K Nonautologous Tissue Substitute	Z No Qualifier
Y Upper Vein	X External	0 Drainage Device 2 Monitoring Device 3 Infusion Device D Intraluminal Device	Z No Qualifier

Section	0	Medical and Surgical
Body System	5	Upper Veins
Operation	Q	Repair: Restoring, to the extent possible, a body part to its normal anatomic structure and function

Body Part (4th)	Approach (5th)	Device (6th)	Qualifier (7th)
0 Azygos Vein 1 Hemiazygos Vein 3 Innominate Vein, Right 4 Innominate Vein, Left 5 Subclavian Vein, Right 6 Subclavian Vein, Left 7 Axillary Vein, Right 8 Axillary Vein, Left 9 Brachial Vein, Right A Brachial Vein, Left B Basilic Vein, Right C Basilic Vein, Left D Cephalic Vein, Right F Cephalic Vein, Left G Hand Vein, Right H Hand Vein, Left L Intracranial Vein M Internal Jugular Vein, Right N Internal Jugular Vein, Left P External Jugular Vein, Right Q External Jugular Vein, Left R Vertebral Vein, Right S Vertebral Vein, Left T Face Vein, Right V Face Vein, Left Y Upper Vein	0 Open 3 Percutaneous 4 Percutaneous Endoscopic	Z No Device	Z No Qualifier

Section	0	Medical and Surgical
Body System	5	Upper Veins
Operation	R	**Replacement:** Putting in or on biological or synthetic material that physically takes the place and/or function of all or a portion of a body part

Body Part (4th)	Approach (5th)	Device (6th)	Qualifier (7th)
0 Azygos Vein 1 Hemiazygos Vein 3 Innominate Vein, Right 4 Innominate Vein, Left 5 Subclavian Vein, Right 6 Subclavian Vein, Left 7 Axillary Vein, Right 8 Axillary Vein, Left 9 Brachial Vein, Right A Brachial Vein, Left B Basilic Vein, Right C Basilic Vein, Left D Cephalic Vein, Right F Cephalic Vein, Left G Hand Vein, Right H Hand Vein, Left L Intracranial Vein M Internal Jugular Vein, Right N Internal Jugular Vein, Left P External Jugular Vein, Right Q External Jugular Vein, Left R Vertebral Vein, Right S Vertebral Vein, Left T Face Vein, Right V Face Vein, Left Y Upper Vein	0 Open 4 Percutaneous Endoscopic	7 Autologous Tissue Substitute J Synthetic Substitute K Nonautologous Tissue Substitute	Z No Qualifier

Section	0	Medical and Surgical
Body System	5	Upper Veins
Operation	S	**Reposition:** Moving to its normal location, or other suitable location, all or a portion of a body part

Body Part (4th)	Approach (5th)	Device (6th)	Qualifier (7th)
0 Azygos Vein 1 Hemiazygos Vein 3 Innominate Vein, Right 4 Innominate Vein, Left 5 Subclavian Vein, Right 6 Subclavian Vein, Left 7 Axillary Vein, Right 8 Axillary Vein, Left 9 Brachial Vein, Right A Brachial Vein, Left B Basilic Vein, Right C Basilic Vein, Left D Cephalic Vein, Right F Cephalic Vein, Left G Hand Vein, Right H Hand Vein, Left L Intracranial Vein M Internal Jugular Vein, Right N Internal Jugular Vein, Left P External Jugular Vein, Right Q External Jugular Vein, Left R Vertebral Vein, Right S Vertebral Vein, Left T Face Vein, Right V Face Vein, Left Y Upper Vein	0 Open 3 Percutaneous 4 Percutaneous Endoscopic	Z No Device	Z No Qualifier

Section	0	Medical and Surgical
Body System	5	Upper Veins
Operation	U	**Supplement:** Putting in or on biological or synthetic material that physically reinforces and/or augments the function of a portion of a body part

Body Part (4th)	Approach (5th)	Device (6th)	Qualifier (7th)
0 Azygos Vein 1 Hemiazygos Vein 3 Innominate Vein, Right 4 Innominate Vein, Left 5 Subclavian Vein, Right 6 Subclavian Vein, Left 7 Axillary Vein, Right 8 Axillary Vein, Left 9 Brachial Vein, Right A Brachial Vein, Left B Basilic Vein, Right C Basilic Vein, Left D Cephalic Vein, Right F Cephalic Vein, Left G Hand Vein, Right H Hand Vein, Left L Intracranial Vein M Internal Jugular Vein, Right N Internal Jugular Vein, Left P External Jugular Vein, Right Q External Jugular Vein, Left R Vertebral Vein, Right S Vertebral Vein, Left T Face Vein, Right V Face Vein, Left Y Upper Vein	0 Open 3 Percutaneous 4 Percutaneous Endoscopic	7 Autologous Tissue Substitute J Synthetic Substitute K Nonautologous Tissue Substitute	Z No Qualifier

Section	0	Medical and Surgical
Body System	5	Upper Veins
Operation	V	**Restriction:** Partially closing an orifice or the lumen of a tubular body part

Body Part (4th)	Approach (5th)	Device (6th)	Qualifier (7th)
0 Azygos Vein 1 Hemiazygos Vein 3 Innominate Vein, Right 4 Innominate Vein, Left 5 Subclavian Vein, Right 6 Subclavian Vein, Left 7 Axillary Vein, Right 8 Axillary Vein, Left 9 Brachial Vein, Right A Brachial Vein, Left B Basilic Vein, Right C Basilic Vein, Left D Cephalic Vein, Right F Cephalic Vein, Left G Hand Vein, Right H Hand Vein, Left L Intracranial Vein M Internal Jugular Vein, Right N Internal Jugular Vein, Left P External Jugular Vein, Right Q External Jugular Vein, Left R Vertebral Vein, Right S Vertebral Vein, Left T Face Vein, Right V Face Vein, Left Y Upper Vein	0 Open 3 Percutaneous 4 Percutaneous Endoscopic	C Extraluminal Device D Intraluminal Device Z No Device	Z No Qualifier

Section	0	**Medical and Surgical**
Body System	5	**Upper Veins**
Operation	W	**Revision:** Correcting, to the extent possible, a portion of a malfunctioning device or the position of a displaced device

Body Part (4ᵗʰ)	Approach (5ᵗʰ)	Device (6ᵗʰ)	Qualifier (7ᵗʰ)
Y Upper Vein	0 Open 3 Percutaneous 4 Percutaneous Endoscopic X External	0 Drainage Device 2 Monitoring Device 3 Infusion Device 7 Autologous Tissue Substitute C Extraluminal Device D Intraluminal Device J Synthetic Substitute K Nonautologous Tissue Substitute	Z No Qualifier

Upper Veins Code Listing 051–05W

051 – Upper Veins, Bypass

Review Coding Guideline B3.6a

051007Y Bypass Azygos Vein to Upper Vein with Autologous Tissue Substitute, Open Approach

051009Y Bypass Azygos Vein to Upper Vein with Autologous Venous Tissue, Open Approach

05100AY Bypass Azygos Vein to Upper Vein with Autologous Arterial Tissue, Open Approach

05100JY Bypass Azygos Vein to Upper Vein with Synthetic Substitute, Open Approach

05100KY Bypass Azygos Vein to Upper Vein with Nonautologous Tissue Substitute, Open Approach

05100ZY Bypass Azygos Vein to Upper Vein, Open Approach

051047Y Bypass Azygos Vein to Upper Vein with Autologous Tissue Substitute, Percutaneous Endoscopic Approach

051049Y Bypass Azygos Vein to Upper Vein with Autologous Venous Tissue, Percutaneous Endoscopic Approach

05104AY Bypass Azygos Vein to Upper Vein with Autologous Arterial Tissue, Percutaneous Endoscopic Approach

05104JY Bypass Azygos Vein to Upper Vein with Synthetic Substitute, Percutaneous Endoscopic Approach

05104KY Bypass Azygos Vein to Upper Vein with Nonautologous Tissue Substitute, Percutaneous Endoscopic Approach

05104ZY Bypass Azygos Vein to Upper Vein, Percutaneous Endoscopic Approach

051107Y Bypass Hemiazygos Vein to Upper Vein with Autologous Tissue Substitute, Open Approach

051109Y Bypass Hemiazygos Vein to Upper Vein with Autologous Venous Tissue, Open Approach

05110AY Bypass Hemiazygos Vein to Upper Vein with Autologous Arterial Tissue, Open Approach

05110JY Bypass Hemiazygos Vein to Upper Vein with Synthetic Substitute, Open Approach

05110KY Bypass Hemiazygos Vein to Upper Vein with Nonautologous Tissue Substitute, Open Approach

05110ZY Bypass Hemiazygos Vein to Upper Vein, Open Approach

051147Y Bypass Hemiazygos Vein to Upper Vein with Autologous Tissue Substitute, Percutaneous Endoscopic Approach

051149Y Bypass Hemiazygos Vein to Upper Vein with Autologous Venous Tissue, Percutaneous Endoscopic Approach

05114AY Bypass Hemiazygos Vein to Upper Vein with Autologous Arterial Tissue, Percutaneous Endoscopic Approach

05114JY Bypass Hemiazygos Vein to Upper Vein with Synthetic Substitute, Percutaneous Endoscopic Approach

05114KY Bypass Hemiazygos Vein to Upper Vein with Nonautologous Tissue Substitute, Percutaneous Endoscopic Approach

05114ZY Bypass Hemiazygos Vein to Upper Vein, Percutaneous Endoscopic Approach

051307Y Bypass Right Innominate Vein to Upper Vein with Autologous Tissue Substitute, Open Approach

051309Y Bypass Right Innominate Vein to Upper Vein with Autologous Venous Tissue, Open Approach

05130AY Bypass Right Innominate Vein to Upper Vein with Autologous Arterial Tissue, Open Approach

05130JY Bypass Right Innominate Vein to Upper Vein with Synthetic Substitute, Open Approach

05130KY Bypass Right Innominate Vein to Upper Vein with Nonautologous Tissue Substitute, Open Approach

05130ZY Bypass Right Innominate Vein to Upper Vein, Open Approach

051347Y Bypass Right Innominate Vein to Upper Vein with Autologous Tissue Substitute, Percutaneous Endoscopic Approach

051349Y Bypass Right Innominate Vein to Upper Vein with Autologous Venous Tissue, Percutaneous Endoscopic Approach

05134AY Bypass Right Innominate Vein to Upper Vein with Autologous Arterial Tissue, Percutaneous Endoscopic Approach

05134JY Bypass Right Innominate Vein to Upper Vein with Synthetic Substitute, Percutaneous Endoscopic Approach

05134KY Bypass Right Innominate Vein to Upper Vein with Nonautologous Tissue Substitute, Percutaneous Endoscopic Approach

05134ZY Bypass Right Innominate Vein to Upper Vein, Percutaneous Endoscopic Approach

051407Y Bypass Left Innominate Vein to Upper Vein with Autologous Tissue Substitute, Open Approach

051409Y Bypass Left Innominate Vein to Upper Vein with Autologous Venous Tissue, Open Approach

05140AY Bypass Left Innominate Vein to Upper Vein with Autologous Arterial Tissue, Open Approach

05140JY Bypass Left Innominate Vein to Upper Vein with Synthetic Substitute, Open Approach

05140KY Bypass Left Innominate Vein to Upper Vein with Nonautologous Tissue Substitute, Open Approach

05140ZY Bypass Left Innominate Vein to Upper Vein, Open Approach

051447Y Bypass Left Innominate Vein to Upper Vein with Autologous Tissue Substitute, Percutaneous Endoscopic Approach

051449Y Bypass Left Innominate Vein to Upper Vein with Autologous Venous Tissue, Percutaneous Endoscopic Approach

05144AY Bypass Left Innominate Vein to Upper Vein with Autologous Arterial Tissue, Percutaneous Endoscopic Approach

05144JY Bypass Left Innominate Vein to Upper Vein with Synthetic Substitute, Percutaneous Endoscopic Approach

05144KY Bypass Left Innominate Vein to Upper Vein with Nonautologous Tissue Substitute, Percutaneous Endoscopic Approach

05144ZY Bypass Left Innominate Vein to Upper Vein, Percutaneous Endoscopic Approach

051507Y Bypass Right Subclavian Vein to Upper Vein with Autologous Tissue Substitute, Open Approach

051509Y Bypass Right Subclavian Vein to Upper Vein with Autologous Venous Tissue, Open Approach

05150AY Bypass Right Subclavian Vein to Upper Vein with Autologous Arterial Tissue, Open Approach

05150JY Bypass Right Subclavian Vein to Upper Vein with Synthetic Substitute, Open Approach

♀ Female-only   ♂ Male-only   ● Limited Coverage   ● Non-OR   🅷🅰🅲 HAC-associated procedure   ● Non-covered procedures   ➕ Combination

05150KY   Bypass Right Subclavian Vein to Upper Vein with Nonautologous Tissue Substitute, Open Approach

05150ZY   Bypass Right Subclavian Vein to Upper Vein, Open Approach

051547Y   Bypass Right Subclavian Vein to Upper Vein with Autologous Tissue Substitute, Percutaneous Endoscopic Approach

051549Y   Bypass Right Subclavian Vein to Upper Vein with Autologous Venous Tissue, Percutaneous Endoscopic Approach

05154AY   Bypass Right Subclavian Vein to Upper Vein with Autologous Arterial Tissue, Percutaneous Endoscopic Approach

05154JY   Bypass Right Subclavian Vein to Upper Vein with Synthetic Substitute, Percutaneous Endoscopic Approach

05154KY   Bypass Right Subclavian Vein to Upper Vein with Nonautologous Tissue Substitute, Percutaneous Endoscopic Approach

05154ZY   Bypass Right Subclavian Vein to Upper Vein, Percutaneous Endoscopic Approach

051607Y   Bypass Left Subclavian Vein to Upper Vein with Autologous Tissue Substitute, Open Approach

051609Y   Bypass Left Subclavian Vein to Upper Vein with Autologous Venous Tissue, Open Approach

05160AY   Bypass Left Subclavian Vein to Upper Vein with Autologous Arterial Tissue, Open Approach

05160JY   Bypass Left Subclavian Vein to Upper Vein with Synthetic Substitute, Open Approach

05160KY   Bypass Left Subclavian Vein to Upper Vein with Nonautologous Tissue Substitute, Open Approach

05160ZY   Bypass Left Subclavian Vein to Upper Vein, Open Approach

051647Y   Bypass Left Subclavian Vein to Upper Vein with Autologous Tissue Substitute, Percutaneous Endoscopic Approach

051649Y   Bypass Left Subclavian Vein to Upper Vein with Autologous Venous Tissue, Percutaneous Endoscopic Approach

05164AY   Bypass Left Subclavian Vein to Upper Vein with Autologous Arterial Tissue, Percutaneous Endoscopic Approach

05164JY   Bypass Left Subclavian Vein to Upper Vein with Synthetic Substitute, Percutaneous Endoscopic Approach

05164KY   Bypass Left Subclavian Vein to Upper Vein with Nonautologous Tissue Substitute, Percutaneous Endoscopic Approach

05164ZY   Bypass Left Subclavian Vein to Upper Vein, Percutaneous Endoscopic Approach

051707Y   Bypass Right Axillary Vein to Upper Vein with Autologous Tissue Substitute, Open Approach

051709Y   Bypass Right Axillary Vein to Upper Vein with Autologous Venous Tissue, Open Approach

05170AY   Bypass Right Axillary Vein to Upper Vein with Autologous Arterial Tissue, Open Approach

05170JY   Bypass Right Axillary Vein to Upper Vein with Synthetic Substitute, Open Approach

05170KY   Bypass Right Axillary Vein to Upper Vein with Nonautologous Tissue Substitute, Open Approach

05170ZY   Bypass Right Axillary Vein to Upper Vein, Open Approach

051747Y   Bypass Right Axillary Vein to Upper Vein with Autologous Tissue Substitute, Percutaneous Endoscopic Approach

051749Y   Bypass Right Axillary Vein to Upper Vein with Autologous Venous Tissue, Percutaneous Endoscopic Approach

05174AY   Bypass Right Axillary Vein to Upper Vein with Autologous Arterial Tissue, Percutaneous Endoscopic Approach

05174JY   Bypass Right Axillary Vein to Upper Vein with Synthetic Substitute, Percutaneous Endoscopic Approach

05174KY   Bypass Right Axillary Vein to Upper Vein with Nonautologous Tissue Substitute, Percutaneous Endoscopic Approach

05174ZY   Bypass Right Axillary Vein to Upper Vein, Percutaneous Endoscopic Approach

051807Y   Bypass Left Axillary Vein to Upper Vein with Autologous Tissue Substitute, Open Approach

051809Y   Bypass Left Axillary Vein to Upper Vein with Autologous Venous Tissue, Open Approach

05180AY   Bypass Left Axillary Vein to Upper Vein with Autologous Arterial Tissue, Open Approach

05180JY   Bypass Left Axillary Vein to Upper Vein with Synthetic Substitute, Open Approach

05180KY   Bypass Left Axillary Vein to Upper Vein with Nonautologous Tissue Substitute, Open Approach

05180ZY   Bypass Left Axillary Vein to Upper Vein, Open Approach

051847Y   Bypass Left Axillary Vein to Upper Vein with Autologous Tissue Substitute, Percutaneous Endoscopic Approach

051849Y   Bypass Left Axillary Vein to Upper Vein with Autologous Venous Tissue, Percutaneous Endoscopic Approach

05184AY   Bypass Left Axillary Vein to Upper Vein with Autologous Arterial Tissue, Percutaneous Endoscopic Approach

05184JY   Bypass Left Axillary Vein to Upper Vein with Synthetic Substitute, Percutaneous Endoscopic Approach

05184KY   Bypass Left Axillary Vein to Upper Vein with Nonautologous Tissue Substitute, Percutaneous Endoscopic Approach

05184ZY   Bypass Left Axillary Vein to Upper Vein, Percutaneous Endoscopic Approach

051907Y   Bypass Right Brachial Vein to Upper Vein with Autologous Tissue Substitute, Open Approach

051909Y   Bypass Right Brachial Vein to Upper Vein with Autologous Venous Tissue, Open Approach

05190AY   Bypass Right Brachial Vein to Upper Vein with Autologous Arterial Tissue, Open Approach

05190JY   Bypass Right Brachial Vein to Upper Vein with Synthetic Substitute, Open Approach

05190KY   Bypass Right Brachial Vein to Upper Vein with Nonautologous Tissue Substitute, Open Approach

05190ZY   Bypass Right Brachial Vein to Upper Vein, Open Approach

051947Y   Bypass Right Brachial Vein to Upper Vein with Autologous Tissue Substitute, Percutaneous Endoscopic Approach

051949Y   Bypass Right Brachial Vein to Upper Vein with Autologous Venous Tissue, Percutaneous Endoscopic Approach

05194AY   Bypass Right Brachial Vein to Upper Vein with Autologous Arterial Tissue, Percutaneous Endoscopic Approach

05194JY   Bypass Right Brachial Vein to Upper Vein with Synthetic Substitute, Percutaneous Endoscopic Approach

05194KY   Bypass Right Brachial Vein to Upper Vein with Nonautologous Tissue Substitute, Percutaneous Endoscopic Approach

05194ZY   Bypass Right Brachial Vein to Upper Vein, Percutaneous Endoscopic Approach

051A07Y   Bypass Left Brachial Vein to Upper Vein with Autologous Tissue Substitute, Open Approach

051A09Y   Bypass Left Brachial Vein to Upper Vein with Autologous Venous Tissue, Open Approach

051A0AY   Bypass Left Brachial Vein to Upper Vein with Autologous Arterial Tissue, Open Approach

051A0JY   Bypass Left Brachial Vein to Upper Vein with Synthetic Substitute, Open Approach

051A0KY   Bypass Left Brachial Vein to Upper Vein with Nonautologous Tissue Substitute, Open Approach

051A0ZY   Bypass Left Brachial Vein to Upper Vein, Open Approach

051A47Y   Bypass Left Brachial Vein to Upper Vein with Autologous Tissue Substitute, Percutaneous Endoscopic Approach

051A49Y   Bypass Left Brachial Vein to Upper Vein with Autologous Venous Tissue, Percutaneous Endoscopic Approach

051A4AY   Bypass Left Brachial Vein to Upper Vein with Autologous Arterial Tissue, Percutaneous Endoscopic Approach

051A4JY   Bypass Left Brachial Vein to Upper Vein with Synthetic Substitute, Percutaneous Endoscopic Approach

051A4KY   Bypass Left Brachial Vein to Upper Vein with Nonautologous Tissue Substitute, Percutaneous Endoscopic Approach

051A4ZY   Bypass Left Brachial Vein to Upper Vein, Percutaneous Endoscopic Approach

051B07Y   Bypass Right Basilic Vein to Upper Vein with Autologous Tissue Substitute, Open Approach

051B09Y   Bypass Right Basilic Vein to Upper Vein with Autologous Venous Tissue, Open Approach

051B0AY   Bypass Right Basilic Vein to Upper Vein with Autologous Arterial Tissue, Open Approach

051B0JY   Bypass Right Basilic Vein to Upper Vein with Synthetic Substitute, Open Approach

051B0KY   Bypass Right Basilic Vein to Upper Vein with Nonautologous Tissue Substitute, Open Approach

051B0ZY   Bypass Right Basilic Vein to Upper Vein, Open Approach

051B47Y   Bypass Right Basilic Vein to Upper Vein with Autologous Tissue Substitute, Percutaneous Endoscopic Approach

051B49Y   Bypass Right Basilic Vein to Upper Vein with Autologous Venous Tissue, Percutaneous Endoscopic Approach

051B4AY   Bypass Right Basilic Vein to Upper Vein with Autologous Arterial Tissue, Percutaneous Endoscopic Approach

---

♀ Female-only   ♂ Male-only   ● Limited Coverage   ● Non-OR   ■ HAC-associated procedure   ⬢ Non-covered procedures   ✚ Combination

051B4JY Bypass Right Basilic Vein to Upper Vein with Synthetic Substitute, Percutaneous Endoscopic Approach

051B4KY Bypass Right Basilic Vein to Upper Vein with Nonautologous Tissue Substitute, Percutaneous Endoscopic Approach

051B4ZY Bypass Right Basilic Vein to Upper Vein, Percutaneous Endoscopic Approach

051C07Y Bypass Left Basilic Vein to Upper Vein with Autologous Tissue Substitute, Open Approach

051C09Y Bypass Left Basilic Vein to Upper Vein with Autologous Venous Tissue, Open Approach

051C0AY Bypass Left Basilic Vein to Upper Vein with Autologous Arterial Tissue, Open Approach

051C0JY Bypass Left Basilic Vein to Upper Vein with Synthetic Substitute, Open Approach

051C0KY Bypass Left Basilic Vein to Upper Vein with Nonautologous Tissue Substitute, Open Approach

051C0ZY Bypass Left Basilic Vein to Upper Vein, Open Approach

051C47Y Bypass Left Basilic Vein to Upper Vein with Autologous Tissue Substitute, Percutaneous Endoscopic Approach

051C49Y Bypass Left Basilic Vein to Upper Vein with Autologous Venous Tissue, Percutaneous Endoscopic Approach

051C4AY Bypass Left Basilic Vein to Upper Vein with Autologous Arterial Tissue, Percutaneous Endoscopic Approach

051C4JY Bypass Left Basilic Vein to Upper Vein with Synthetic Substitute, Percutaneous Endoscopic Approach

051C4KY Bypass Left Basilic Vein to Upper Vein with Nonautologous Tissue Substitute, Percutaneous Endoscopic Approach

051C4ZY Bypass Left Basilic Vein to Upper Vein, Percutaneous Endoscopic Approach

051D07Y Bypass Right Cephalic Vein to Upper Vein with Autologous Tissue Substitute, Open Approach

051D09Y Bypass Right Cephalic Vein to Upper Vein with Autologous Venous Tissue, Open Approach

051D0AY Bypass Right Cephalic Vein to Upper Vein with Autologous Arterial Tissue, Open Approach

051D0JY Bypass Right Cephalic Vein to Upper Vein with Synthetic Substitute, Open Approach

051D0KY Bypass Right Cephalic Vein to Upper Vein with Nonautologous Tissue Substitute, Open Approach

051D0ZY Bypass Right Cephalic Vein to Upper Vein, Open Approach

051D47Y Bypass Right Cephalic Vein to Upper Vein with Autologous Tissue Substitute, Percutaneous Endoscopic Approach

051D49Y Bypass Right Cephalic Vein to Upper Vein with Autologous Venous Tissue, Percutaneous Endoscopic Approach

051D4AY Bypass Right Cephalic Vein to Upper Vein with Autologous Arterial Tissue, Percutaneous Endoscopic Approach

051D4JY Bypass Right Cephalic Vein to Upper Vein with Synthetic Substitute, Percutaneous Endoscopic Approach

051D4KY Bypass Right Cephalic Vein to Upper Vein with Nonautologous Tissue Substitute, Percutaneous Endoscopic Approach

051D4ZY Bypass Right Cephalic Vein to Upper Vein, Percutaneous Endoscopic Approach

051F07Y Bypass Left Cephalic Vein to Upper Vein with Autologous Tissue Substitute, Open Approach

051F09Y Bypass Left Cephalic Vein to Upper Vein with Autologous Venous Tissue, Open Approach

051F0AY Bypass Left Cephalic Vein to Upper Vein with Autologous Arterial Tissue, Open Approach

051F0JY Bypass Left Cephalic Vein to Upper Vein with Synthetic Substitute, Open Approach

051F0KY Bypass Left Cephalic Vein to Upper Vein with Nonautologous Tissue Substitute, Open Approach

051F0ZY Bypass Left Cephalic Vein to Upper Vein, Open Approach

051F47Y Bypass Left Cephalic Vein to Upper Vein with Autologous Tissue Substitute, Percutaneous Endoscopic Approach

051F49Y Bypass Left Cephalic Vein to Upper Vein with Autologous Venous Tissue, Percutaneous Endoscopic Approach

051F4AY Bypass Left Cephalic Vein to Upper Vein with Autologous Arterial Tissue, Percutaneous Endoscopic Approach

051F4JY Bypass Left Cephalic Vein to Upper Vein with Synthetic Substitute, Percutaneous Endoscopic Approach

051F4KY Bypass Left Cephalic Vein to Upper Vein with Nonautologous Tissue Substitute, Percutaneous Endoscopic Approach

051F4ZY Bypass Left Cephalic Vein to Upper Vein, Percutaneous Endoscopic Approach

051G07Y Bypass Right Hand Vein to Upper Vein with Autologous Tissue Substitute, Open Approach

051G09Y Bypass Right Hand Vein to Upper Vein with Autologous Venous Tissue, Open Approach

051G0AY Bypass Right Hand Vein to Upper Vein with Autologous Arterial Tissue, Open Approach

051G0JY Bypass Right Hand Vein to Upper Vein with Synthetic Substitute, Open Approach

051G0KY Bypass Right Hand Vein to Upper Vein with Nonautologous Tissue Substitute, Open Approach

051G0ZY Bypass Right Hand Vein to Upper Vein, Open Approach

051G47Y Bypass Right Hand Vein to Upper Vein with Autologous Tissue Substitute, Percutaneous Endoscopic Approach

051G49Y Bypass Right Hand Vein to Upper Vein with Autologous Venous Tissue, Percutaneous Endoscopic Approach

051G4AY Bypass Right Hand Vein to Upper Vein with Autologous Arterial Tissue, Percutaneous Endoscopic Approach

051G4JY Bypass Right Hand Vein to Upper Vein with Synthetic Substitute, Percutaneous Endoscopic Approach

051G4KY Bypass Right Hand Vein to Upper Vein with Nonautologous Tissue Substitute, Percutaneous Endoscopic Approach

051G4ZY Bypass Right Hand Vein to Upper Vein, Percutaneous Endoscopic Approach

051H07Y Bypass Left Hand Vein to Upper Vein with Autologous Tissue Substitute, Open Approach

051H09Y Bypass Left Hand Vein to Upper Vein with Autologous Venous Tissue, Open Approach

051H0AY Bypass Left Hand Vein to Upper Vein with Autologous Arterial Tissue, Open Approach

051H0JY Bypass Left Hand Vein to Upper Vein with Synthetic Substitute, Open Approach

051H0KY Bypass Left Hand Vein to Upper Vein with Nonautologous Tissue Substitute, Open Approach

051H0ZY Bypass Left Hand Vein to Upper Vein, Open Approach

051H47Y Bypass Left Hand Vein to Upper Vein with Autologous Tissue Substitute, Percutaneous Endoscopic Approach

051H49Y Bypass Left Hand Vein to Upper Vein with Autologous Venous Tissue, Percutaneous Endoscopic Approach

051H4AY Bypass Left Hand Vein to Upper Vein with Autologous Arterial Tissue, Percutaneous Endoscopic Approach

051H4JY Bypass Left Hand Vein to Upper Vein with Synthetic Substitute, Percutaneous Endoscopic Approach

051H4KY Bypass Left Hand Vein to Upper Vein with Nonautologous Tissue Substitute, Percutaneous Endoscopic Approach

051H4ZY Bypass Left Hand Vein to Upper Vein, Percutaneous Endoscopic Approach

051L07Y Bypass Intracranial Vein to Upper Vein with Autologous Tissue Substitute, Open Approach

051L09Y Bypass Intracranial Vein to Upper Vein with Autologous Venous Tissue, Open Approach

051L0AY Bypass Intracranial Vein to Upper Vein with Autologous Arterial Tissue, Open Approach

051L0JY Bypass Intracranial Vein to Upper Vein with Synthetic Substitute, Open Approach

051L0KY Bypass Intracranial Vein to Upper Vein with Nonautologous Tissue Substitute, Open Approach

051L0ZY Bypass Intracranial Vein to Upper Vein, Open Approach

051L47Y Bypass Intracranial Vein to Upper Vein with Autologous Tissue Substitute, Percutaneous Endoscopic Approach

051L49Y Bypass Intracranial Vein to Upper Vein with Autologous Venous Tissue, Percutaneous Endoscopic Approach

051L4AY Bypass Intracranial Vein to Upper Vein with Autologous Arterial Tissue, Percutaneous Endoscopic Approach

051L4JY Bypass Intracranial Vein to Upper Vein with Synthetic Substitute, Percutaneous Endoscopic Approach

051L4KY Bypass Intracranial Vein to Upper Vein with Nonautologous Tissue Substitute, Percutaneous Endoscopic Approach

051L4ZY Bypass Intracranial Vein to Upper Vein, Percutaneous Endoscopic Approach

051M07Y Bypass Right Internal Jugular Vein to Upper Vein with Autologous Tissue Substitute, Open Approach

051M09Y Bypass Right Internal Jugular Vein to Upper Vein with Autologous Venous Tissue, Open Approach

051M0AY Bypass Right Internal Jugular Vein to Upper Vein with Autologous Arterial Tissue, Open Approach

051M0JY Bypass Right Internal Jugular Vein to Upper Vein with Synthetic Substitute, Open Approach

051M0KY Bypass Right Internal Jugular Vein to Upper Vein with Nonautologous Tissue Substitute, Open Approach

051M0ZY Bypass Right Internal Jugular Vein to Upper Vein, Open Approach

051M47Y Bypass Right Internal Jugular Vein to Upper Vein with Autologous Tissue Substitute, Percutaneous Endoscopic Approach

051M49Y Bypass Right Internal Jugular Vein to Upper Vein with Autologous Venous Tissue, Percutaneous Endoscopic Approach

051M4AY Bypass Right Internal Jugular Vein to Upper Vein with Autologous Arterial Tissue, Percutaneous Endoscopic Approach

051M4JY Bypass Right Internal Jugular Vein to Upper Vein with Synthetic Substitute, Percutaneous Endoscopic Approach

051M4KY Bypass Right Internal Jugular Vein to Upper Vein with Nonautologous Tissue Substitute, Percutaneous Endoscopic Approach

051M4ZY Bypass Right Internal Jugular Vein to Upper Vein, Percutaneous Endoscopic Approach

051N07Y Bypass Left Internal Jugular Vein to Upper Vein with Autologous Tissue Substitute, Open Approach

051N09Y Bypass Left Internal Jugular Vein to Upper Vein with Autologous Venous Tissue, Open Approach

051N0AY Bypass Left Internal Jugular Vein to Upper Vein with Autologous Arterial Tissue, Open Approach

051N0JY Bypass Left Internal Jugular Vein to Upper Vein with Synthetic Substitute, Open Approach

051N0KY Bypass Left Internal Jugular Vein to Upper Vein with Nonautologous Tissue Substitute, Open Approach

051N0ZY Bypass Left Internal Jugular Vein to Upper Vein, Open Approach

051N47Y Bypass Left Internal Jugular Vein to Upper Vein with Autologous Tissue Substitute, Percutaneous Endoscopic Approach

051N49Y Bypass Left Internal Jugular Vein to Upper Vein with Autologous Venous Tissue, Percutaneous Endoscopic Approach

051N4AY Bypass Left Internal Jugular Vein to Upper Vein with Autologous Arterial Tissue, Percutaneous Endoscopic Approach

051N4JY Bypass Left Internal Jugular Vein to Upper Vein with Synthetic Substitute, Percutaneous Endoscopic Approach

051N4KY Bypass Left Internal Jugular Vein to Upper Vein with Nonautologous Tissue Substitute, Percutaneous Endoscopic Approach

051N4ZY Bypass Left Internal Jugular Vein to Upper Vein, Percutaneous Endoscopic Approach

051P07Y Bypass Right External Jugular Vein to Upper Vein with Autologous Tissue Substitute, Open Approach

051P09Y Bypass Right External Jugular Vein to Upper Vein with Autologous Venous Tissue, Open Approach

051P0AY Bypass Right External Jugular Vein to Upper Vein with Autologous Arterial Tissue, Open Approach

051P0JY Bypass Right External Jugular Vein to Upper Vein with Synthetic Substitute, Open Approach

051P0KY Bypass Right External Jugular Vein to Upper Vein with Nonautologous Tissue Substitute, Open Approach

051P0ZY Bypass Right External Jugular Vein to Upper Vein, Open Approach

051P47Y Bypass Right External Jugular Vein to Upper Vein with Autologous Tissue Substitute, Percutaneous Endoscopic Approach

051P49Y Bypass Right External Jugular Vein to Upper Vein with Autologous Venous Tissue, Percutaneous Endoscopic Approach

051P4AY Bypass Right External Jugular Vein to Upper Vein with Autologous Arterial Tissue, Percutaneous Endoscopic Approach

051P4JY Bypass Right External Jugular Vein to Upper Vein with Synthetic Substitute, Percutaneous Endoscopic Approach

051P4KY Bypass Right External Jugular Vein to Upper Vein with Nonautologous Tissue Substitute, Percutaneous Endoscopic Approach

051P4ZY Bypass Right External Jugular Vein to Upper Vein, Percutaneous Endoscopic Approach

051Q07Y Bypass Left External Jugular Vein to Upper Vein with Autologous Tissue Substitute, Open Approach

051Q09Y Bypass Left External Jugular Vein to Upper Vein with Autologous Venous Tissue, Open Approach

051Q0AY Bypass Left External Jugular Vein to Upper Vein with Autologous Arterial Tissue, Open Approach

051Q0JY Bypass Left External Jugular Vein to Upper Vein with Synthetic Substitute, Open Approach

051Q0KY Bypass Left External Jugular Vein to Upper Vein with Nonautologous Tissue Substitute, Open Approach

051Q0ZY Bypass Left External Jugular Vein to Upper Vein, Open Approach

051Q47Y Bypass Left External Jugular Vein to Upper Vein with Autologous Tissue Substitute, Percutaneous Endoscopic Approach

051Q49Y Bypass Left External Jugular Vein to Upper Vein with Autologous Venous Tissue, Percutaneous Endoscopic Approach

051Q4AY Bypass Left External Jugular Vein to Upper Vein with Autologous Arterial Tissue, Percutaneous Endoscopic Approach

051Q4JY Bypass Left External Jugular Vein to Upper Vein with Synthetic Substitute, Percutaneous Endoscopic Approach

051Q4KY Bypass Left External Jugular Vein to Upper Vein with Nonautologous Tissue Substitute, Percutaneous Endoscopic Approach

051Q4ZY Bypass Left External Jugular Vein to Upper Vein, Percutaneous Endoscopic Approach

051R07Y Bypass Right Vertebral Vein to Upper Vein with Autologous Tissue Substitute, Open Approach

051R09Y Bypass Right Vertebral Vein to Upper Vein with Autologous Venous Tissue, Open Approach

051R0AY Bypass Right Vertebral Vein to Upper Vein with Autologous Arterial Tissue, Open Approach

051R0JY Bypass Right Vertebral Vein to Upper Vein with Synthetic Substitute, Open Approach

051R0KY Bypass Right Vertebral Vein to Upper Vein with Nonautologous Tissue Substitute, Open Approach

051R0ZY Bypass Right Vertebral Vein to Upper Vein, Open Approach

051R47Y Bypass Right Vertebral Vein to Upper Vein with Autologous Tissue Substitute, Percutaneous Endoscopic Approach

051R49Y Bypass Right Vertebral Vein to Upper Vein with Autologous Venous Tissue, Percutaneous Endoscopic Approach

051R4AY Bypass Right Vertebral Vein to Upper Vein with Autologous Arterial Tissue, Percutaneous Endoscopic Approach

051R4JY Bypass Right Vertebral Vein to Upper Vein with Synthetic Substitute, Percutaneous Endoscopic Approach

051R4KY Bypass Right Vertebral Vein to Upper Vein with Nonautologous Tissue Substitute, Percutaneous Endoscopic Approach

051R4ZY Bypass Right Vertebral Vein to Upper Vein, Percutaneous Endoscopic Approach

051S07Y Bypass Left Vertebral Vein to Upper Vein with Autologous Tissue Substitute, Open Approach

051S09Y Bypass Left Vertebral Vein to Upper Vein with Autologous Venous Tissue, Open Approach

051S0AY Bypass Left Vertebral Vein to Upper Vein with Autologous Arterial Tissue, Open Approach

051S0JY Bypass Left Vertebral Vein to Upper Vein with Synthetic Substitute, Open Approach

051S0KY Bypass Left Vertebral Vein to Upper Vein with Nonautologous Tissue Substitute, Open Approach

051S0ZY Bypass Left Vertebral Vein to Upper Vein, Open Approach

051S47Y Bypass Left Vertebral Vein to Upper Vein with Autologous Tissue Substitute, Percutaneous Endoscopic Approach

051S49Y Bypass Left Vertebral Vein to Upper Vein with Autologous Venous Tissue, Percutaneous Endoscopic Approach

051S4AY Bypass Left Vertebral Vein to Upper Vein with Autologous Arterial Tissue, Percutaneous Endoscopic Approach

051S4JY Bypass Left Vertebral Vein to Upper Vein with Synthetic Substitute, Percutaneous Endoscopic Approach

051S4KY Bypass Left Vertebral Vein to Upper Vein with Nonautologous Tissue Substitute, Percutaneous Endoscopic Approach

051S4ZY Bypass Left Vertebral Vein to Upper Vein, Percutaneous Endoscopic Approach

051T07Y Bypass Right Face Vein to Upper Vein with Autologous Tissue Substitute, Open Approach

051T09Y Bypass Right Face Vein to Upper Vein with Autologous Venous Tissue, Open Approach

051T0AY Bypass Right Face Vein to Upper Vein with Autologous Arterial Tissue, Open Approach

051T0JY Bypass Right Face Vein to Upper Vein with Synthetic Substitute, Open Approach

051T0KY   Bypass Right Face Vein to Upper Vein with Nonautologous Tissue Substitute, Open Approach

051T0ZY   Bypass Right Face Vein to Upper Vein, Open Approach

051T47Y   Bypass Right Face Vein to Upper Vein with Autologous Tissue Substitute, Percutaneous Endoscopic Approach

051T49Y   Bypass Right Face Vein to Upper Vein with Autologous Venous Tissue, Percutaneous Endoscopic Approach

051T4AY   Bypass Right Face Vein to Upper Vein with Autologous Arterial Tissue, Percutaneous Endoscopic Approach

051T4JY   Bypass Right Face Vein to Upper Vein with Synthetic Substitute, Percutaneous Endoscopic Approach

051T4KY   Bypass Right Face Vein to Upper Vein with Nonautologous Tissue Substitute, Percutaneous Endoscopic Approach

051T4ZY   Bypass Right Face Vein to Upper Vein, Percutaneous Endoscopic Approach

051V07Y   Bypass Left Face Vein to Upper Vein with Autologous Tissue Substitute, Open Approach

051V09Y   Bypass Left Face Vein to Upper Vein with Autologous Venous Tissue, Open Approach

051V0AY   Bypass Left Face Vein to Upper Vein with Autologous Arterial Tissue, Open Approach

051V0JY   Bypass Left Face Vein to Upper Vein with Synthetic Substitute, Open Approach

051V0KY   Bypass Left Face Vein to Upper Vein with Nonautologous Tissue Substitute, Open Approach

051V0ZY   Bypass Left Face Vein to Upper Vein, Open Approach

051V47Y   Bypass Left Face Vein to Upper Vein with Autologous Tissue Substitute, Percutaneous Endoscopic Approach

051V49Y   Bypass Left Face Vein to Upper Vein with Autologous Venous Tissue, Percutaneous Endoscopic Approach

051V4AY   Bypass Left Face Vein to Upper Vein with Autologous Arterial Tissue, Percutaneous Endoscopic Approach

051V4JY   Bypass Left Face Vein to Upper Vein with Synthetic Substitute, Percutaneous Endoscopic Approach

051V4KY   Bypass Left Face Vein to Upper Vein with Nonautologous Tissue Substitute, Percutaneous Endoscopic Approach

051V4ZY   Bypass Left Face Vein to Upper Vein, Percutaneous Endoscopic Approach

055 – Upper Veins, Destruction

05500ZZ   Destruction of Azygos Vein, Open Approach

05503ZZ   Destruction of Azygos Vein, Percutaneous Approach

05504ZZ   Destruction of Azygos Vein, Percutaneous Endoscopic Approach

05510ZZ   Destruction of Hemiazygos Vein, Open Approach

05513ZZ   Destruction of Hemiazygos Vein, Percutaneous Approach

05514ZZ   Destruction of Hemiazygos Vein, Percutaneous Endoscopic Approach

05530ZZ   Destruction of Right Innominate Vein, Open Approach

05533ZZ   Destruction of Right Innominate Vein, Percutaneous Approach

05534ZZ   Destruction of Right Innominate Vein, Percutaneous Endoscopic Approach

05540ZZ   Destruction of Left Innominate Vein, Open Approach

05543ZZ   Destruction of Left Innominate Vein, Percutaneous Approach

05544ZZ   Destruction of Left Innominate Vein, Percutaneous Endoscopic Approach

05550ZZ   Destruction of Right Subclavian Vein, Open Approach

05553ZZ   Destruction of Right Subclavian Vein, Percutaneous Approach

05554ZZ   Destruction of Right Subclavian Vein, Percutaneous Endoscopic Approach

05560ZZ   Destruction of Left Subclavian Vein, Open Approach

05563ZZ   Destruction of Left Subclavian Vein, Percutaneous Approach

05564ZZ   Destruction of Left Subclavian Vein, Percutaneous Endoscopic Approach

05570ZZ   Destruction of Right Axillary Vein, Open Approach

05573ZZ   Destruction of Right Axillary Vein, Percutaneous Approach

05574ZZ   Destruction of Right Axillary Vein, Percutaneous Endoscopic Approach

05580ZZ   Destruction of Left Axillary Vein, Open Approach

05583ZZ   Destruction of Left Axillary Vein, Percutaneous Approach

05584ZZ   Destruction of Left Axillary Vein, Percutaneous Endoscopic Approach

05590ZZ   Destruction of Right Brachial Vein, Open Approach

05593ZZ   Destruction of Right Brachial Vein, Percutaneous Approach

05594ZZ   Destruction of Right Brachial Vein, Percutaneous Endoscopic Approach

055A0ZZ   Destruction of Left Brachial Vein, Open Approach

055A3ZZ   Destruction of Left Brachial Vein, Percutaneous Approach

055A4ZZ   Destruction of Left Brachial Vein, Percutaneous Endoscopic Approach

055B0ZZ   Destruction of Right Basilic Vein, Open Approach

055B3ZZ   Destruction of Right Basilic Vein, Percutaneous Approach

055B4ZZ   Destruction of Right Basilic Vein, Percutaneous Endoscopic Approach

055C0ZZ   Destruction of Left Basilic Vein, Open Approach

055C3ZZ   Destruction of Left Basilic Vein, Percutaneous Approach

055C4ZZ   Destruction of Left Basilic Vein, Percutaneous Endoscopic Approach

055D0ZZ   Destruction of Right Cephalic Vein, Open Approach

055D3ZZ   Destruction of Right Cephalic Vein, Percutaneous Approach

055D4ZZ   Destruction of Right Cephalic Vein, Percutaneous Endoscopic Approach

055F0ZZ   Destruction of Left Cephalic Vein, Open Approach

055F3ZZ   Destruction of Left Cephalic Vein, Percutaneous Approach

055F4ZZ   Destruction of Left Cephalic Vein, Percutaneous Endoscopic Approach

055G0ZZ   Destruction of Right Hand Vein, Open Approach

055G3ZZ   Destruction of Right Hand Vein, Percutaneous Approach

055G4ZZ   Destruction of Right Hand Vein, Percutaneous Endoscopic Approach

055H0ZZ   Destruction of Left Hand Vein, Open Approach

055H3ZZ   Destruction of Left Hand Vein, Percutaneous Approach

055H4ZZ   Destruction of Left Hand Vein, Percutaneous Endoscopic Approach

055L0ZZ   Destruction of Intracranial Vein, Open Approach

055L3ZZ   Destruction of Intracranial Vein, Percutaneous Approach

055L4ZZ   Destruction of Intracranial Vein, Percutaneous Endoscopic Approach

055M0ZZ   Destruction of Right Internal Jugular Vein, Open Approach

055M3ZZ   Destruction of Right Internal Jugular Vein, Percutaneous Approach

055M4ZZ   Destruction of Right Internal Jugular Vein, Percutaneous Endoscopic Approach

055N0ZZ   Destruction of Left Internal Jugular Vein, Open Approach

055N3ZZ   Destruction of Left Internal Jugular Vein, Percutaneous Approach

055N4ZZ   Destruction of Left Internal Jugular Vein, Percutaneous Endoscopic Approach

055P0ZZ   Destruction of Right External Jugular Vein, Open Approach

055P3ZZ   Destruction of Right External Jugular Vein, Percutaneous Approach

055P4ZZ   Destruction of Right External Jugular Vein, Percutaneous Endoscopic Approach

055Q0ZZ   Destruction of Left External Jugular Vein, Open Approach

055Q3ZZ   Destruction of Left External Jugular Vein, Percutaneous Approach

055Q4ZZ   Destruction of Left External Jugular Vein, Percutaneous Endoscopic Approach

055R0ZZ   Destruction of Right Vertebral Vein, Open Approach

055R3ZZ   Destruction of Right Vertebral Vein, Percutaneous Approach

055R4ZZ   Destruction of Right Vertebral Vein, Percutaneous Endoscopic Approach

055S0ZZ   Destruction of Left Vertebral Vein, Open Approach

055S3ZZ   Destruction of Left Vertebral Vein, Percutaneous Approach

055S4ZZ   Destruction of Left Vertebral Vein, Percutaneous Endoscopic Approach

055T0ZZ   Destruction of Right Face Vein, Open Approach

055T3ZZ   Destruction of Right Face Vein, Percutaneous Approach

055T4ZZ   Destruction of Right Face Vein, Percutaneous Endoscopic Approach

055V0ZZ   Destruction of Left Face Vein, Open Approach

055V3ZZ   Destruction of Left Face Vein, Percutaneous Approach

055V4ZZ   Destruction of Left Face Vein, Percutaneous Endoscopic Approach

055Y0ZZ   Destruction of Upper Vein, Open Approach

055Y3ZZ   Destruction of Upper Vein, Percutaneous Approach

055Y4ZZ   Destruction of Upper Vein, Percutaneous Endoscopic Approach

---

♀ Female-only   ♂ Male-only   ⬤ Limited Coverage   ⬤ Non-OR   ᴴᴬᶜ HAC-associated procedure   ⬤ Non-covered procedures   ➕ Combination

057 – Upper Veins, Dilation

05700DZ	Dilation of Azygos Vein with Intraluminal Device, Open Approach
05700ZZ	Dilation of Azygos Vein, Open Approach
05703DZ	Dilation of Azygos Vein with Intraluminal Device, Percutaneous Approach
05703ZZ	Dilation of Azygos Vein, Percutaneous Approach
05704DZ	Dilation of Azygos Vein with Intraluminal Device, Percutaneous Endoscopic Approach
05704ZZ	Dilation of Azygos Vein, Percutaneous Endoscopic Approach
05710DZ	Dilation of Hemiazygos Vein with Intraluminal Device, Open Approach
05710ZZ	Dilation of Hemiazygos Vein, Open Approach
05713DZ	Dilation of Hemiazygos Vein with Intraluminal Device, Percutaneous Approach
05713ZZ	Dilation of Hemiazygos Vein, Percutaneous Approach
05714DZ	Dilation of Hemiazygos Vein with Intraluminal Device, Percutaneous Endoscopic Approach
05714ZZ	Dilation of Hemiazygos Vein, Percutaneous Endoscopic Approach
05730DZ	Dilation of Right Innominate Vein with Intraluminal Device, Open Approach
05730ZZ	Dilation of Right Innominate Vein, Open Approach
05733DZ	Dilation of Right Innominate Vein with Intraluminal Device, Percutaneous Approach
05733ZZ	Dilation of Right Innominate Vein, Percutaneous Approach
05734DZ	Dilation of Right Innominate Vein with Intraluminal Device, Percutaneous Endoscopic Approach
05734ZZ	Dilation of Right Innominate Vein, Percutaneous Endoscopic Approach
05740DZ	Dilation of Left Innominate Vein with Intraluminal Device, Open Approach
05740ZZ	Dilation of Left Innominate Vein, Open Approach
05743DZ	Dilation of Left Innominate Vein with Intraluminal Device, Percutaneous Approach
05743ZZ	Dilation of Left Innominate Vein, Percutaneous Approach
05744DZ	Dilation of Left Innominate Vein with Intraluminal Device, Percutaneous Endoscopic Approach
05744ZZ	Dilation of Left Innominate Vein, Percutaneous Endoscopic Approach
05750DZ	Dilation of Right Subclavian Vein with Intraluminal Device, Open Approach
05750ZZ	Dilation of Right Subclavian Vein, Open Approach
05753DZ	Dilation of Right Subclavian Vein with Intraluminal Device, Percutaneous Approach
05753ZZ	Dilation of Right Subclavian Vein, Percutaneous Approach
05754DZ	Dilation of Right Subclavian Vein with Intraluminal Device, Percutaneous Endoscopic Approach
05754ZZ	Dilation of Right Subclavian Vein, Percutaneous Endoscopic Approach
05760DZ	Dilation of Left Subclavian Vein with Intraluminal Device, Open Approach
05760ZZ	Dilation of Left Subclavian Vein, Open Approach
05763DZ	Dilation of Left Subclavian Vein with Intraluminal Device, Percutaneous Approach
05763ZZ	Dilation of Left Subclavian Vein, Percutaneous Approach
05764DZ	Dilation of Left Subclavian Vein with Intraluminal Device, Percutaneous Endoscopic Approach
05764ZZ	Dilation of Left Subclavian Vein, Percutaneous Endoscopic Approach
05770DZ	Dilation of Right Axillary Vein with Intraluminal Device, Open Approach
05770ZZ	Dilation of Right Axillary Vein, Open Approach
05773DZ	Dilation of Right Axillary Vein with Intraluminal Device, Percutaneous Approach
05773ZZ	Dilation of Right Axillary Vein, Percutaneous Approach
05774DZ	Dilation of Right Axillary Vein with Intraluminal Device, Percutaneous Endoscopic Approach
05774ZZ	Dilation of Right Axillary Vein, Percutaneous Endoscopic Approach
05780DZ	Dilation of Left Axillary Vein with Intraluminal Device, Open Approach
05780ZZ	Dilation of Left Axillary Vein, Open Approach
05783DZ	Dilation of Left Axillary Vein with Intraluminal Device, Percutaneous Approach
05783ZZ	Dilation of Left Axillary Vein, Percutaneous Approach
05784DZ	Dilation of Left Axillary Vein with Intraluminal Device, Percutaneous Endoscopic Approach
05784ZZ	Dilation of Left Axillary Vein, Percutaneous Endoscopic Approach
05790DZ	Dilation of Right Brachial Vein with Intraluminal Device, Open Approach
05790ZZ	Dilation of Right Brachial Vein, Open Approach
05793DZ	Dilation of Right Brachial Vein with Intraluminal Device, Percutaneous Approach
05793ZZ	Dilation of Right Brachial Vein, Percutaneous Approach
05794DZ	Dilation of Right Brachial Vein with Intraluminal Device, Percutaneous Endoscopic Approach
05794ZZ	Dilation of Right Brachial Vein, Percutaneous Endoscopic Approach
057A0DZ	Dilation of Left Brachial Vein with Intraluminal Device, Open Approach
057A0ZZ	Dilation of Left Brachial Vein, Open Approach
057A3DZ	Dilation of Left Brachial Vein with Intraluminal Device, Percutaneous Approach
057A3ZZ	Dilation of Left Brachial Vein, Percutaneous Approach
057A4DZ	Dilation of Left Brachial Vein with Intraluminal Device, Percutaneous Endoscopic Approach
057A4ZZ	Dilation of Left Brachial Vein, Percutaneous Endoscopic Approach
057B0DZ	Dilation of Right Basilic Vein with Intraluminal Device, Open Approach
057B0ZZ	Dilation of Right Basilic Vein, Open Approach
057B3DZ	Dilation of Right Basilic Vein with Intraluminal Device, Percutaneous Approach
057B3ZZ	Dilation of Right Basilic Vein, Percutaneous Approach
057B4DZ	Dilation of Right Basilic Vein with Intraluminal Device, Percutaneous Endoscopic Approach
057B4ZZ	Dilation of Right Basilic Vein, Percutaneous Endoscopic Approach
057C0DZ	Dilation of Left Basilic Vein with Intraluminal Device, Open Approach
057C0ZZ	Dilation of Left Basilic Vein, Open Approach
057C3DZ	Dilation of Left Basilic Vein with Intraluminal Device, Percutaneous Approach
057C3ZZ	Dilation of Left Basilic Vein, Percutaneous Approach
057C4DZ	Dilation of Left Basilic Vein with Intraluminal Device, Percutaneous Endoscopic Approach
057C4ZZ	Dilation of Left Basilic Vein, Percutaneous Endoscopic Approach
057D0DZ	Dilation of Right Cephalic Vein with Intraluminal Device, Open Approach
057D0ZZ	Dilation of Right Cephalic Vein, Open Approach
057D3DZ	Dilation of Right Cephalic Vein with Intraluminal Device, Percutaneous Approach
057D3ZZ	Dilation of Right Cephalic Vein, Percutaneous Approach
057D4DZ	Dilation of Right Cephalic Vein with Intraluminal Device, Percutaneous Endoscopic Approach
057D4ZZ	Dilation of Right Cephalic Vein, Percutaneous Endoscopic Approach
057F0DZ	Dilation of Left Cephalic Vein with Intraluminal Device, Open Approach
057F0ZZ	Dilation of Left Cephalic Vein, Open Approach
057F3DZ	Dilation of Left Cephalic Vein with Intraluminal Device, Percutaneous Approach
057F3ZZ	Dilation of Left Cephalic Vein, Percutaneous Approach
057F4DZ	Dilation of Left Cephalic Vein with Intraluminal Device, Percutaneous Endoscopic Approach
057F4ZZ	Dilation of Left Cephalic Vein, Percutaneous Endoscopic Approach
057G0DZ	Dilation of Right Hand Vein with Intraluminal Device, Open Approach
057G0ZZ	Dilation of Right Hand Vein, Open Approach
057G3DZ	Dilation of Right Hand Vein with Intraluminal Device, Percutaneous Approach
057G3ZZ	Dilation of Right Hand Vein, Percutaneous Approach
057G4DZ	Dilation of Right Hand Vein with Intraluminal Device, Percutaneous Endoscopic Approach
057G4ZZ	Dilation of Right Hand Vein, Percutaneous Endoscopic Approach
057H0DZ	Dilation of Left Hand Vein with Intraluminal Device, Open Approach
057H0ZZ	Dilation of Left Hand Vein, Open Approach

057H3DZ Dilation of Left Hand Vein with Intraluminal Device, Percutaneous Approach

057H3ZZ Dilation of Left Hand Vein, Percutaneous Approach

057H4DZ Dilation of Left Hand Vein with Intraluminal Device, Percutaneous Endoscopic Approach

057H4ZZ Dilation of Left Hand Vein, Percutaneous Endoscopic Approach

057L0DZ Dilation of Intracranial Vein with Intraluminal Device, Open Approach

057L0ZZ Dilation of Intracranial Vein, Open Approach

057L3DZ Dilation of Intracranial Vein with Intraluminal Device, Percutaneous Approach

● 057L3ZZ Dilation of Intracranial Vein, Percutaneous Approach

057L4DZ Dilation of Intracranial Vein with Intraluminal Device, Percutaneous Endoscopic Approach

● 057L4ZZ Dilation of Intracranial Vein, Percutaneous Endoscopic Approach

057M0DZ Dilation of Right Internal Jugular Vein with Intraluminal Device, Open Approach

057M0ZZ Dilation of Right Internal Jugular Vein, Open Approach

057M3DZ Dilation of Right Internal Jugular Vein with Intraluminal Device, Percutaneous Approach

057M3ZZ Dilation of Right Internal Jugular Vein, Percutaneous Approach

057M4DZ Dilation of Right Internal Jugular Vein with Intraluminal Device, Percutaneous Endoscopic Approach

057M4ZZ Dilation of Right Internal Jugular Vein, Percutaneous Endoscopic Approach

057N0DZ Dilation of Left Internal Jugular Vein with Intraluminal Device, Open Approach

057N0ZZ Dilation of Left Internal Jugular Vein, Open Approach

057N3DZ Dilation of Left Internal Jugular Vein with Intraluminal Device, Percutaneous Approach

057N3ZZ Dilation of Left Internal Jugular Vein, Percutaneous Approach

057N4DZ Dilation of Left Internal Jugular Vein with Intraluminal Device, Percutaneous Endoscopic Approach

057N4ZZ Dilation of Left Internal Jugular Vein, Percutaneous Endoscopic Approach

057P0DZ Dilation of Right External Jugular Vein with Intraluminal Device, Open Approach

057P0ZZ Dilation of Right External Jugular Vein, Open Approach

057P3DZ Dilation of Right External Jugular Vein with Intraluminal Device, Percutaneous Approach

057P3ZZ Dilation of Right External Jugular Vein, Percutaneous Approach

057P4DZ Dilation of Right External Jugular Vein with Intraluminal Device, Percutaneous Endoscopic Approach

057P4ZZ Dilation of Right External Jugular Vein, Percutaneous Endoscopic Approach

057Q0DZ Dilation of Left External Jugular Vein with Intraluminal Device, Open Approach

057Q0ZZ Dilation of Left External Jugular Vein, Open Approach

057Q3DZ Dilation of Left External Jugular Vein with Intraluminal Device, Percutaneous Approach

057Q3ZZ Dilation of Left External Jugular Vein, Percutaneous Approach

057Q4DZ Dilation of Left External Jugular Vein with Intraluminal Device, Percutaneous Endoscopic Approach

057Q4ZZ Dilation of Left External Jugular Vein, Percutaneous Endoscopic Approach

057R0DZ Dilation of Right Vertebral Vein with Intraluminal Device, Open Approach

057R0ZZ Dilation of Right Vertebral Vein, Open Approach

057R3DZ Dilation of Right Vertebral Vein with Intraluminal Device, Percutaneous Approach

057R3ZZ Dilation of Right Vertebral Vein, Percutaneous Approach

057R4DZ Dilation of Right Vertebral Vein with Intraluminal Device, Percutaneous Endoscopic Approach

057R4ZZ Dilation of Right Vertebral Vein, Percutaneous Endoscopic Approach

057S0DZ Dilation of Left Vertebral Vein with Intraluminal Device, Open Approach

057S0ZZ Dilation of Left Vertebral Vein, Open Approach

057S3DZ Dilation of Left Vertebral Vein with Intraluminal Device, Percutaneous Approach

057S3ZZ Dilation of Left Vertebral Vein, Percutaneous Approach

057S4DZ Dilation of Left Vertebral Vein with Intraluminal Device, Percutaneous Endoscopic Approach

057S4ZZ Dilation of Left Vertebral Vein, Percutaneous Endoscopic Approach

057T0DZ Dilation of Right Face Vein with Intraluminal Device, Open Approach

057T0ZZ Dilation of Right Face Vein, Open Approach

057T3DZ Dilation of Right Face Vein with Intraluminal Device, Percutaneous Approach

057T3ZZ Dilation of Right Face Vein, Percutaneous Approach

057T4DZ Dilation of Right Face Vein with Intraluminal Device, Percutaneous Endoscopic Approach

057T4ZZ Dilation of Right Face Vein, Percutaneous Endoscopic Approach

057V0DZ Dilation of Left Face Vein with Intraluminal Device, Open Approach

057V0ZZ Dilation of Left Face Vein, Open Approach

057V3DZ Dilation of Left Face Vein with Intraluminal Device, Percutaneous Approach

057V3ZZ Dilation of Left Face Vein, Percutaneous Approach

057V4DZ Dilation of Left Face Vein with Intraluminal Device, Percutaneous Endoscopic Approach

057V4ZZ Dilation of Left Face Vein, Percutaneous Endoscopic Approach

057Y0DZ Dilation of Upper Vein with Intraluminal Device, Open Approach

057Y0ZZ Dilation of Upper Vein, Open Approach

057Y3DZ Dilation of Upper Vein with Intraluminal Device, Percutaneous Approach

057Y3ZZ Dilation of Upper Vein, Percutaneous Approach

057Y4DZ Dilation of Upper Vein with Intraluminal Device, Percutaneous Endoscopic Approach

057Y4ZZ Dilation of Upper Vein, Percutaneous Endoscopic Approach

059 – Upper Veins, Drainage

Review Coding Guidelines B3.4a and B3.4b

Review Coding Guideline B6.2

059000Z Drainage of Azygos Vein with Drainage Device, Open Approach

05900ZX Drainage of Azygos Vein, Open Approach, Diagnostic

05900ZZ Drainage of Azygos Vein, Open Approach

059030Z Drainage of Azygos Vein with Drainage Device, Percutaneous Approach

05903ZX Drainage of Azygos Vein, Percutaneous Approach, Diagnostic

05903ZZ Drainage of Azygos Vein, Percutaneous Approach

059040Z Drainage of Azygos Vein with Drainage Device, Percutaneous Endoscopic Approach

05904ZX Drainage of Azygos Vein, Percutaneous Endoscopic Approach, Diagnostic

05904ZZ Drainage of Azygos Vein, Percutaneous Endoscopic Approach

059100Z Drainage of Hemiazygos Vein with Drainage Device, Open Approach

05910ZX Drainage of Hemiazygos Vein, Open Approach, Diagnostic

05910ZZ Drainage of Hemiazygos Vein, Open Approach

059130Z Drainage of Hemiazygos Vein with Drainage Device, Percutaneous Approach

05913ZX Drainage of Hemiazygos Vein, Percutaneous Approach, Diagnostic

05913ZZ Drainage of Hemiazygos Vein, Percutaneous Approach

059140Z Drainage of Hemiazygos Vein with Drainage Device, Percutaneous Endoscopic Approach

05914ZX Drainage of Hemiazygos Vein, Percutaneous Endoscopic Approach, Diagnostic

05914ZZ Drainage of Hemiazygos Vein, Percutaneous Endoscopic Approach

059300Z Drainage of Right Innominate Vein with Drainage Device, Open Approach

05930ZX Drainage of Right Innominate Vein, Open Approach, Diagnostic

05930ZZ Drainage of Right Innominate Vein, Open Approach

059330Z Drainage of Right Innominate Vein with Drainage Device, Percutaneous Approach

05933ZX Drainage of Right Innominate Vein, Percutaneous Approach, Diagnostic

05933ZZ	Drainage of Right Innominate Vein, Percutaneous Approach
059340Z	Drainage of Right Innominate Vein with Drainage Device, Percutaneous Endoscopic Approach
05934ZX	Drainage of Right Innominate Vein, Percutaneous Endoscopic Approach, Diagnostic
05934ZZ	Drainage of Right Innominate Vein, Percutaneous Endoscopic Approach
059400Z	Drainage of Left Innominate Vein with Drainage Device, Open Approach
05940ZX	Drainage of Left Innominate Vein, Open Approach, Diagnostic
05940ZZ	Drainage of Left Innominate Vein, Open Approach
059430Z	Drainage of Left Innominate Vein with Drainage Device, Percutaneous Approach
05943ZX	Drainage of Left Innominate Vein, Percutaneous Approach, Diagnostic
05943ZZ	Drainage of Left Innominate Vein, Percutaneous Approach
059440Z	Drainage of Left Innominate Vein with Drainage Device, Percutaneous Endoscopic Approach
05944ZX	Drainage of Left Innominate Vein, Percutaneous Endoscopic Approach, Diagnostic
05944ZZ	Drainage of Left Innominate Vein, Percutaneous Endoscopic Approach
059500Z	Drainage of Right Subclavian Vein with Drainage Device, Open Approach
05950ZX	Drainage of Right Subclavian Vein, Open Approach, Diagnostic
05950ZZ	Drainage of Right Subclavian Vein, Open Approach
059530Z	Drainage of Right Subclavian Vein with Drainage Device, Percutaneous Approach
05953ZX	Drainage of Right Subclavian Vein, Percutaneous Approach, Diagnostic
05953ZZ	Drainage of Right Subclavian Vein, Percutaneous Approach
059540Z	Drainage of Right Subclavian Vein with Drainage Device, Percutaneous Endoscopic Approach
05954ZX	Drainage of Right Subclavian Vein, Percutaneous Endoscopic Approach, Diagnostic
05954ZZ	Drainage of Right Subclavian Vein, Percutaneous Endoscopic Approach
059600Z	Drainage of Left Subclavian Vein with Drainage Device, Open Approach
05960ZX	Drainage of Left Subclavian Vein, Open Approach, Diagnostic
05960ZZ	Drainage of Left Subclavian Vein, Open Approach
059630Z	Drainage of Left Subclavian Vein with Drainage Device, Percutaneous Approach
05963ZX	Drainage of Left Subclavian Vein, Percutaneous Approach, Diagnostic
05963ZZ	Drainage of Left Subclavian Vein, Percutaneous Approach
059640Z	Drainage of Left Subclavian Vein with Drainage Device, Percutaneous Endoscopic Approach
05964ZX	Drainage of Left Subclavian Vein, Percutaneous Endoscopic Approach, Diagnostic
05964ZZ	Drainage of Left Subclavian Vein, Percutaneous Endoscopic Approach
059700Z	Drainage of Right Axillary Vein with Drainage Device, Open Approach
05970ZX	Drainage of Right Axillary Vein, Open Approach, Diagnostic
05970ZZ	Drainage of Right Axillary Vein, Open Approach
059730Z	Drainage of Right Axillary Vein with Drainage Device, Percutaneous Approach
05973ZX	Drainage of Right Axillary Vein, Percutaneous Approach, Diagnostic
05973ZZ	Drainage of Right Axillary Vein, Percutaneous Approach
059740Z	Drainage of Right Axillary Vein with Drainage Device, Percutaneous Endoscopic Approach
05974ZX	Drainage of Right Axillary Vein, Percutaneous Endoscopic Approach, Diagnostic
05974ZZ	Drainage of Right Axillary Vein, Percutaneous Endoscopic Approach
059800Z	Drainage of Left Axillary Vein with Drainage Device, Open Approach
05980ZX	Drainage of Left Axillary Vein, Open Approach, Diagnostic
05980ZZ	Drainage of Left Axillary Vein, Open Approach
059830Z	Drainage of Left Axillary Vein with Drainage Device, Percutaneous Approach

05983ZX	Drainage of Left Axillary Vein, Percutaneous Approach, Diagnostic
05983ZZ	Drainage of Left Axillary Vein, Percutaneous Approach
059840Z	Drainage of Left Axillary Vein with Drainage Device, Percutaneous Endoscopic Approach
05984ZX	Drainage of Left Axillary Vein, Percutaneous Endoscopic Approach, Diagnostic
05984ZZ	Drainage of Left Axillary Vein, Percutaneous Endoscopic Approach
059900Z	Drainage of Right Brachial Vein with Drainage Device, Open Approach
05990ZX	Drainage of Right Brachial Vein, Open Approach, Diagnostic
05990ZZ	Drainage of Right Brachial Vein, Open Approach
059930Z	Drainage of Right Brachial Vein with Drainage Device, Percutaneous Approach
05993ZX	Drainage of Right Brachial Vein, Percutaneous Approach, Diagnostic
05993ZZ	Drainage of Right Brachial Vein, Percutaneous Approach
059940Z	Drainage of Right Brachial Vein with Drainage Device, Percutaneous Endoscopic Approach
05994ZX	Drainage of Right Brachial Vein, Percutaneous Endoscopic Approach, Diagnostic
05994ZZ	Drainage of Right Brachial Vein, Percutaneous Endoscopic Approach
059A00Z	Drainage of Left Brachial Vein with Drainage Device, Open Approach
059A0ZX	Drainage of Left Brachial Vein, Open Approach, Diagnostic
059A0ZZ	Drainage of Left Brachial Vein, Open Approach
059A30Z	Drainage of Left Brachial Vein with Drainage Device, Percutaneous Approach
059A3ZX	Drainage of Left Brachial Vein, Percutaneous Approach, Diagnostic
059A3ZZ	Drainage of Left Brachial Vein, Percutaneous Approach
059A40Z	Drainage of Left Brachial Vein with Drainage Device, Percutaneous Endoscopic Approach
059A4ZX	Drainage of Left Brachial Vein, Percutaneous Endoscopic Approach, Diagnostic
059A4ZZ	Drainage of Left Brachial Vein, Percutaneous Endoscopic Approach
059B00Z	Drainage of Right Basilic Vein with Drainage Device, Open Approach
059B0ZX	Drainage of Right Basilic Vein, Open Approach, Diagnostic
059B0ZZ	Drainage of Right Basilic Vein, Open Approach
059B30Z	Drainage of Right Basilic Vein with Drainage Device, Percutaneous Approach
059B3ZX	Drainage of Right Basilic Vein, Percutaneous Approach, Diagnostic
059B3ZZ	Drainage of Right Basilic Vein, Percutaneous Approach
059B40Z	Drainage of Right Basilic Vein with Drainage Device, Percutaneous Endoscopic Approach
059B4ZX	Drainage of Right Basilic Vein, Percutaneous Endoscopic Approach, Diagnostic
059B4ZZ	Drainage of Right Basilic Vein, Percutaneous Endoscopic Approach
059C00Z	Drainage of Left Basilic Vein with Drainage Device, Open Approach
059C0ZX	Drainage of Left Basilic Vein, Open Approach, Diagnostic
059C0ZZ	Drainage of Left Basilic Vein, Open Approach
059C30Z	Drainage of Left Basilic Vein with Drainage Device, Percutaneous Approach
059C3ZX	Drainage of Left Basilic Vein, Percutaneous Approach, Diagnostic
059C3ZZ	Drainage of Left Basilic Vein, Percutaneous Approach
059C40Z	Drainage of Left Basilic Vein with Drainage Device, Percutaneous Endoscopic Approach
059C4ZX	Drainage of Left Basilic Vein, Percutaneous Endoscopic Approach, Diagnostic
059C4ZZ	Drainage of Left Basilic Vein, Percutaneous Endoscopic Approach
059D00Z	Drainage of Right Cephalic Vein with Drainage Device, Open Approach
059D0ZX	Drainage of Right Cephalic Vein, Open Approach, Diagnostic
059D0ZZ	Drainage of Right Cephalic Vein, Open Approach
059D30Z	Drainage of Right Cephalic Vein with Drainage Device, Percutaneous Approach
059D3ZX	Drainage of Right Cephalic Vein, Percutaneous Approach, Diagnostic
059D3ZZ	Drainage of Right Cephalic Vein, Percutaneous Approach
059D40Z	Drainage of Right Cephalic Vein with Drainage Device, Percutaneous Endoscopic Approach
059D4ZX	Drainage of Right Cephalic Vein, Percutaneous Endoscopic Approach, Diagnostic

059D4ZZ Drainage of Right Cephalic Vein, Percutaneous Endoscopic Approach

059F00Z Drainage of Left Cephalic Vein with Drainage Device, Open Approach

059F0ZX Drainage of Left Cephalic Vein, Open Approach, Diagnostic

059F0ZZ Drainage of Left Cephalic Vein, Open Approach

059F30Z Drainage of Left Cephalic Vein with Drainage Device, Percutaneous Approach

059F3ZX Drainage of Left Cephalic Vein, Percutaneous Approach, Diagnostic

059F3ZZ Drainage of Left Cephalic Vein, Percutaneous Approach

059F40Z Drainage of Left Cephalic Vein with Drainage Device, Percutaneous Endoscopic Approach

059F4ZX Drainage of Left Cephalic Vein, Percutaneous Endoscopic Approach, Diagnostic

059F4ZZ Drainage of Left Cephalic Vein, Percutaneous Endoscopic Approach

059G00Z Drainage of Right Hand Vein with Drainage Device, Open Approach

059G0ZX Drainage of Right Hand Vein, Open Approach, Diagnostic

059G0ZZ Drainage of Right Hand Vein, Open Approach

059G30Z Drainage of Right Hand Vein with Drainage Device, Percutaneous Approach

059G3ZX Drainage of Right Hand Vein, Percutaneous Approach, Diagnostic

059G3ZZ Drainage of Right Hand Vein, Percutaneous Approach

059G40Z Drainage of Right Hand Vein with Drainage Device, Percutaneous Endoscopic Approach

059G4ZX Drainage of Right Hand Vein, Percutaneous Endoscopic Approach, Diagnostic

059G4ZZ Drainage of Right Hand Vein, Percutaneous Endoscopic Approach

059H00Z Drainage of Left Hand Vein with Drainage Device, Open Approach

059H0ZX Drainage of Left Hand Vein, Open Approach, Diagnostic

059H0ZZ Drainage of Left Hand Vein, Open Approach

059H30Z Drainage of Left Hand Vein with Drainage Device, Percutaneous Approach

059H3ZX Drainage of Left Hand Vein, Percutaneous Approach, Diagnostic

059H3ZZ Drainage of Left Hand Vein, Percutaneous Approach

059H40Z Drainage of Left Hand Vein with Drainage Device, Percutaneous Endoscopic Approach

059H4ZX Drainage of Left Hand Vein, Percutaneous Endoscopic Approach, Diagnostic

059H4ZZ Drainage of Left Hand Vein, Percutaneous Endoscopic Approach

059L00Z Drainage of Intracranial Vein with Drainage Device, Open Approach

059L0ZX Drainage of Intracranial Vein, Open Approach, Diagnostic

059L0ZZ Drainage of Intracranial Vein, Open Approach

059L30Z Drainage of Intracranial Vein with Drainage Device, Percutaneous Approach

059L3ZX Drainage of Intracranial Vein, Percutaneous Approach, Diagnostic

059L3ZZ Drainage of Intracranial Vein, Percutaneous Approach

059L40Z Drainage of Intracranial Vein with Drainage Device, Percutaneous Endoscopic Approach

059L4ZX Drainage of Intracranial Vein, Percutaneous Endoscopic Approach, Diagnostic

059L4ZZ Drainage of Intracranial Vein, Percutaneous Endoscopic Approach

059M00Z Drainage of Right Internal Jugular Vein with Drainage Device, Open Approach

059M0ZX Drainage of Right Internal Jugular Vein, Open Approach, Diagnostic

059M0ZZ Drainage of Right Internal Jugular Vein, Open Approach

059M30Z Drainage of Right Internal Jugular Vein with Drainage Device, Percutaneous Approach

059M3ZX Drainage of Right Internal Jugular Vein, Percutaneous Approach, Diagnostic

059M3ZZ Drainage of Right Internal Jugular Vein, Percutaneous Approach

059M40Z Drainage of Right Internal Jugular Vein with Drainage Device, Percutaneous Endoscopic Approach

059M4ZX Drainage of Right Internal Jugular Vein, Percutaneous Endoscopic Approach, Diagnostic

059M4ZZ Drainage of Right Internal Jugular Vein, Percutaneous Endoscopic Approach

059N00Z Drainage of Left Internal Jugular Vein with Drainage Device, Open Approach

059N0ZX Drainage of Left Internal Jugular Vein, Open Approach, Diagnostic

059N0ZZ Drainage of Left Internal Jugular Vein, Open Approach

059N30Z Drainage of Left Internal Jugular Vein with Drainage Device, Percutaneous Approach

059N3ZX Drainage of Left Internal Jugular Vein, Percutaneous Approach, Diagnostic

059N3ZZ Drainage of Left Internal Jugular Vein, Percutaneous Approach

059N40Z Drainage of Left Internal Jugular Vein with Drainage Device, Percutaneous Endoscopic Approach

059N4ZX Drainage of Left Internal Jugular Vein, Percutaneous Endoscopic Approach, Diagnostic

059N4ZZ Drainage of Left Internal Jugular Vein, Percutaneous Endoscopic Approach

059P00Z Drainage of Right External Jugular Vein with Drainage Device, Open Approach

059P0ZX Drainage of Right External Jugular Vein, Open Approach, Diagnostic

059P0ZZ Drainage of Right External Jugular Vein, Open Approach

059P30Z Drainage of Right External Jugular Vein with Drainage Device, Percutaneous Approach

059P3ZX Drainage of Right External Jugular Vein, Percutaneous Approach, Diagnostic

059P3ZZ Drainage of Right External Jugular Vein, Percutaneous Approach

059P40Z Drainage of Right External Jugular Vein with Drainage Device, Percutaneous Endoscopic Approach

059P4ZX Drainage of Right External Jugular Vein, Percutaneous Endoscopic Approach, Diagnostic

059P4ZZ Drainage of Right External Jugular Vein, Percutaneous Endoscopic Approach

059Q00Z Drainage of Left External Jugular Vein with Drainage Device, Open Approach

059Q0ZX Drainage of Left External Jugular Vein, Open Approach, Diagnostic

059Q0ZZ Drainage of Left External Jugular Vein, Open Approach

059Q30Z Drainage of Left External Jugular Vein with Drainage Device, Percutaneous Approach

059Q3ZX Drainage of Left External Jugular Vein, Percutaneous Approach, Diagnostic

059Q3ZZ Drainage of Left External Jugular Vein, Percutaneous Approach

059Q40Z Drainage of Left External Jugular Vein with Drainage Device, Percutaneous Endoscopic Approach

059Q4ZX Drainage of Left External Jugular Vein, Percutaneous Endoscopic Approach, Diagnostic

059Q4ZZ Drainage of Left External Jugular Vein, Percutaneous Endoscopic Approach

059R00Z Drainage of Right Vertebral Vein with Drainage Device, Open Approach

059R0ZX Drainage of Right Vertebral Vein, Open Approach, Diagnostic

059R0ZZ Drainage of Right Vertebral Vein, Open Approach

059R30Z Drainage of Right Vertebral Vein with Drainage Device, Percutaneous Approach

059R3ZX Drainage of Right Vertebral Vein, Percutaneous Approach, Diagnostic

059R3ZZ Drainage of Right Vertebral Vein, Percutaneous Approach

059R40Z Drainage of Right Vertebral Vein with Drainage Device, Percutaneous Endoscopic Approach

059R4ZX Drainage of Right Vertebral Vein, Percutaneous Endoscopic Approach, Diagnostic

059R4ZZ Drainage of Right Vertebral Vein, Percutaneous Endoscopic Approach

059S00Z Drainage of Left Vertebral Vein with Drainage Device, Open Approach

059S0ZX Drainage of Left Vertebral Vein, Open Approach, Diagnostic

059S0ZZ Drainage of Left Vertebral Vein, Open Approach

059S30Z Drainage of Left Vertebral Vein with Drainage Device, Percutaneous Approach

059S3ZX Drainage of Left Vertebral Vein, Percutaneous Approach, Diagnostic

059S3ZZ Drainage of Left Vertebral Vein, Percutaneous Approach

059S40Z Drainage of Left Vertebral Vein with Drainage Device, Percutaneous Endoscopic Approach

059S4ZX Drainage of Left Vertebral Vein, Percutaneous Endoscopic Approach, Diagnostic

059S4ZZ Drainage of Left Vertebral Vein, Percutaneous Endoscopic Approach

059T00Z Drainage of Right Face Vein with Drainage Device, Open Approach

059T0ZX Drainage of Right Face Vein, Open Approach, Diagnostic

059T0ZZ Drainage of Right Face Vein, Open Approach

♀ Female-only   ♂ Male-only   ◐ Limited Coverage   ● Non-OR   🅷🅰🅲 HAC-associated procedure   ◆ Non-covered procedures   ➕ Combination

059T30Z	Drainage of Right Face Vein with Drainage Device, Percutaneous Approach
059T3ZX	Drainage of Right Face Vein, Percutaneous Approach, Diagnostic
059T3ZZ	Drainage of Right Face Vein, Percutaneous Approach
059T40Z	Drainage of Right Face Vein with Drainage Device, Percutaneous Endoscopic Approach
059T4ZX	Drainage of Right Face Vein, Percutaneous Endoscopic Approach, Diagnostic
059T4ZZ	Drainage of Right Face Vein, Percutaneous Endoscopic Approach
059V00Z	Drainage of Left Face Vein with Drainage Device, Open Approach
059V0ZX	Drainage of Left Face Vein, Open Approach, Diagnostic
059V0ZZ	Drainage of Left Face Vein, Open Approach
059V30Z	Drainage of Left Face Vein with Drainage Device, Percutaneous Approach
059V3ZX	Drainage of Left Face Vein, Percutaneous Approach, Diagnostic
059V3ZZ	Drainage of Left Face Vein, Percutaneous Approach

059V40Z	Drainage of Left Face Vein with Drainage Device, Percutaneous Endoscopic Approach
059V4ZX	Drainage of Left Face Vein, Percutaneous Endoscopic Approach, Diagnostic
059V4ZZ	Drainage of Left Face Vein, Percutaneous Endoscopic Approach
059Y00Z	Drainage of Upper Vein with Drainage Device, Open Approach
059Y0ZX	Drainage of Upper Vein, Open Approach, Diagnostic
059Y0ZZ	Drainage of Upper Vein, Open Approach
059Y30Z	Drainage of Upper Vein with Drainage Device, Percutaneous Approach
059Y3ZX	Drainage of Upper Vein, Percutaneous Approach, Diagnostic
059Y3ZZ	Drainage of Upper Vein, Percutaneous Approach
059Y40Z	Drainage of Upper Vein with Drainage Device, Percutaneous Endoscopic Approach
059Y4ZX	Drainage of Upper Vein, Percutaneous Endoscopic Approach, Diagnostic
059Y4ZZ	Drainage of Upper Vein, Percutaneous Endoscopic Approach

05B – Upper Veins, Excision

Review Coding Guidelines B3.4a and B3.4b

Review Coding Guideline B3.8

05B00ZX	Excision of Azygos Vein, Open Approach, Diagnostic
05B00ZZ	Excision of Azygos Vein, Open Approach
05B03ZX	Excision of Azygos Vein, Percutaneous Approach, Diagnostic
05B03ZZ	Excision of Azygos Vein, Percutaneous Approach
05B04ZX	Excision of Azygos Vein, Percutaneous Endoscopic Approach, Diagnostic
05B04ZZ	Excision of Azygos Vein, Percutaneous Endoscopic Approach
05B10ZX	Excision of Hemiazygos Vein, Open Approach, Diagnostic
05B10ZZ	Excision of Hemiazygos Vein, Open Approach
05B13ZX	Excision of Hemiazygos Vein, Percutaneous Approach, Diagnostic
05B13ZZ	Excision of Hemiazygos Vein, Percutaneous Approach
05B14ZX	Excision of Hemiazygos Vein, Percutaneous Endoscopic Approach, Diagnostic
05B14ZZ	Excision of Hemiazygos Vein, Percutaneous Endoscopic Approach
05B30ZX	Excision of Right Innominate Vein, Open Approach, Diagnostic
05B30ZZ	Excision of Right Innominate Vein, Open Approach
05B33ZX	Excision of Right Innominate Vein, Percutaneous Approach, Diagnostic
05B33ZZ	Excision of Right Innominate Vein, Percutaneous Approach
05B34ZX	Excision of Right Innominate Vein, Percutaneous Endoscopic Approach, Diagnostic
05B34ZZ	Excision of Right Innominate Vein, Percutaneous Endoscopic Approach
05B40ZX	Excision of Left Innominate Vein, Open Approach, Diagnostic
05B40ZZ	Excision of Left Innominate Vein, Open Approach
05B43ZX	Excision of Left Innominate Vein, Percutaneous Approach, Diagnostic
05B43ZZ	Excision of Left Innominate Vein, Percutaneous Approach
05B44ZX	Excision of Left Innominate Vein, Percutaneous Endoscopic Approach, Diagnostic
05B44ZZ	Excision of Left Innominate Vein, Percutaneous Endoscopic Approach
05B50ZX	Excision of Right Subclavian Vein, Open Approach, Diagnostic
05B50ZZ	Excision of Right Subclavian Vein, Open Approach
05B53ZX	Excision of Right Subclavian Vein, Percutaneous Approach, Diagnostic
05B53ZZ	Excision of Right Subclavian Vein, Percutaneous Approach
05B54ZX	Excision of Right Subclavian Vein, Percutaneous Endoscopic Approach, Diagnostic
05B54ZZ	Excision of Right Subclavian Vein, Percutaneous Endoscopic Approach
05B60ZX	Excision of Left Subclavian Vein, Open Approach, Diagnostic
05B60ZZ	Excision of Left Subclavian Vein, Open Approach
05B63ZX	Excision of Left Subclavian Vein, Percutaneous Approach, Diagnostic
05B63ZZ	Excision of Left Subclavian Vein, Percutaneous Approach
05B64ZX	Excision of Left Subclavian Vein, Percutaneous Endoscopic Approach, Diagnostic
05B64ZZ	Excision of Left Subclavian Vein, Percutaneous Endoscopic Approach

05B70ZX	Excision of Right Axillary Vein, Open Approach, Diagnostic
05B70ZZ	Excision of Right Axillary Vein, Open Approach
05B73ZX	Excision of Right Axillary Vein, Percutaneous Approach, Diagnostic
05B73ZZ	Excision of Right Axillary Vein, Percutaneous Approach
05B74ZX	Excision of Right Axillary Vein, Percutaneous Endoscopic Approach, Diagnostic
05B74ZZ	Excision of Right Axillary Vein, Percutaneous Endoscopic Approach
05B80ZX	Excision of Left Axillary Vein, Open Approach, Diagnostic
05B80ZZ	Excision of Left Axillary Vein, Open Approach
05B83ZX	Excision of Left Axillary Vein, Percutaneous Approach, Diagnostic
05B83ZZ	Excision of Left Axillary Vein, Percutaneous Approach
05B84ZX	Excision of Left Axillary Vein, Percutaneous Endoscopic Approach, Diagnostic
05B84ZZ	Excision of Left Axillary Vein, Percutaneous Endoscopic Approach
05B90ZX	Excision of Right Brachial Vein, Open Approach, Diagnostic
05B90ZZ	Excision of Right Brachial Vein, Open Approach
05B93ZX	Excision of Right Brachial Vein, Percutaneous Approach, Diagnostic
05B93ZZ	Excision of Right Brachial Vein, Percutaneous Approach
05B94ZX	Excision of Right Brachial Vein, Percutaneous Endoscopic Approach, Diagnostic
05B94ZZ	Excision of Right Brachial Vein, Percutaneous Endoscopic Approach
05BA0ZX	Excision of Left Brachial Vein, Open Approach, Diagnostic
05BA0ZZ	Excision of Left Brachial Vein, Open Approach
05BA3ZX	Excision of Left Brachial Vein, Percutaneous Approach, Diagnostic
05BA3ZZ	Excision of Left Brachial Vein, Percutaneous Approach
05BA4ZX	Excision of Left Brachial Vein, Percutaneous Endoscopic Approach, Diagnostic
05BA4ZZ	Excision of Left Brachial Vein, Percutaneous Endoscopic Approach
05BB0ZX	Excision of Right Basilic Vein, Open Approach, Diagnostic
05BB0ZZ	Excision of Right Basilic Vein, Open Approach
05BB3ZX	Excision of Right Basilic Vein, Percutaneous Approach, Diagnostic
05BB3ZZ	Excision of Right Basilic Vein, Percutaneous Approach
05BB4ZX	Excision of Right Basilic Vein, Percutaneous Endoscopic Approach, Diagnostic
05BB4ZZ	Excision of Right Basilic Vein, Percutaneous Endoscopic Approach
05BC0ZX	Excision of Left Basilic Vein, Open Approach, Diagnostic
05BC0ZZ	Excision of Left Basilic Vein, Open Approach
05BC3ZX	Excision of Left Basilic Vein, Percutaneous Approach, Diagnostic
05BC3ZZ	Excision of Left Basilic Vein, Percutaneous Approach
05BC4ZX	Excision of Left Basilic Vein, Percutaneous Endoscopic Approach, Diagnostic
05BC4ZZ	Excision of Left Basilic Vein, Percutaneous Endoscopic Approach
05BD0ZX	Excision of Right Cephalic Vein, Open Approach, Diagnostic
05BD0ZZ	Excision of Right Cephalic Vein, Open Approach
05BD3ZX	Excision of Right Cephalic Vein, Percutaneous Approach, Diagnostic
05BD3ZZ	Excision of Right Cephalic Vein, Percutaneous Approach

05BD4ZX   Excision of Right Cephalic Vein, Percutaneous Endoscopic Approach, Diagnostic
05BD4ZZ   Excision of Right Cephalic Vein, Percutaneous Endoscopic Approach
05BF0ZX   Excision of Left Cephalic Vein, Open Approach, Diagnostic
05BF0ZZ   Excision of Left Cephalic Vein, Open Approach
05BF3ZX   Excision of Left Cephalic Vein, Percutaneous Approach, Diagnostic
05BF3ZZ   Excision of Left Cephalic Vein, Percutaneous Approach
05BF4ZX   Excision of Left Cephalic Vein, Percutaneous Endoscopic Approach, Diagnostic
05BF4ZZ   Excision of Left Cephalic Vein, Percutaneous Endoscopic Approach
05BG0ZX   Excision of Right Hand Vein, Open Approach, Diagnostic
05BG0ZZ   Excision of Right Hand Vein, Open Approach
05BG3ZX   Excision of Right Hand Vein, Percutaneous Approach, Diagnostic
05BG3ZZ   Excision of Right Hand Vein, Percutaneous Approach
05BG4ZX   Excision of Right Hand Vein, Percutaneous Endoscopic Approach, Diagnostic
05BG4ZZ   Excision of Right Hand Vein, Percutaneous Endoscopic Approach
05BH0ZX   Excision of Left Hand Vein, Open Approach, Diagnostic
05BH0ZZ   Excision of Left Hand Vein, Open Approach
05BH3ZX   Excision of Left Hand Vein, Percutaneous Approach, Diagnostic
05BH3ZZ   Excision of Left Hand Vein, Percutaneous Approach
05BH4ZX   Excision of Left Hand Vein, Percutaneous Endoscopic Approach, Diagnostic
05BH4ZZ   Excision of Left Hand Vein, Percutaneous Endoscopic Approach
05BL0ZX   Excision of Intracranial Vein, Open Approach, Diagnostic
05BL0ZZ   Excision of Intracranial Vein, Open Approach
05BL3ZX   Excision of Intracranial Vein, Percutaneous Approach, Diagnostic
05BL3ZZ   Excision of Intracranial Vein, Percutaneous Approach
05BL4ZX   Excision of Intracranial Vein, Percutaneous Endoscopic Approach, Diagnostic
05BL4ZZ   Excision of Intracranial Vein, Percutaneous Endoscopic Approach
05BM0ZX   Excision of Right Internal Jugular Vein, Open Approach, Diagnostic
05BM0ZZ   Excision of Right Internal Jugular Vein, Open Approach
05BM3ZX   Excision of Right Internal Jugular Vein, Percutaneous Approach, Diagnostic
05BM3ZZ   Excision of Right Internal Jugular Vein, Percutaneous Approach
05BM4ZX   Excision of Right Internal Jugular Vein, Percutaneous Endoscopic Approach, Diagnostic
05BM4ZZ   Excision of Right Internal Jugular Vein, Percutaneous Endoscopic Approach
05BN0ZX   Excision of Left Internal Jugular Vein, Open Approach, Diagnostic
05BN0ZZ   Excision of Left Internal Jugular Vein, Open Approach
05BN3ZX   Excision of Left Internal Jugular Vein, Percutaneous Approach, Diagnostic
05BN3ZZ   Excision of Left Internal Jugular Vein, Percutaneous Approach
05BN4ZX   Excision of Left Internal Jugular Vein, Percutaneous Endoscopic Approach, Diagnostic
05BN4ZZ   Excision of Left Internal Jugular Vein, Percutaneous Endoscopic Approach
05BP0ZX   Excision of Right External Jugular Vein, Open Approach, Diagnostic
05BP0ZZ   Excision of Right External Jugular Vein, Open Approach
05BP3ZX   Excision of Right External Jugular Vein, Percutaneous Approach, Diagnostic

05BP3ZZ   Excision of Right External Jugular Vein, Percutaneous Approach
05BP4ZX   Excision of Right External Jugular Vein, Percutaneous Endoscopic Approach, Diagnostic
05BP4ZZ   Excision of Right External Jugular Vein, Percutaneous Endoscopic Approach
05BQ0ZX   Excision of Left External Jugular Vein, Open Approach, Diagnostic
05BQ0ZZ   Excision of Left External Jugular Vein, Open Approach
05BQ3ZX   Excision of Left External Jugular Vein, Percutaneous Approach, Diagnostic
05BQ3ZZ   Excision of Left External Jugular Vein, Percutaneous Approach
05BQ4ZX   Excision of Left External Jugular Vein, Percutaneous Endoscopic Approach, Diagnostic
05BQ4ZZ   Excision of Left External Jugular Vein, Percutaneous Endoscopic Approach
05BR0ZX   Excision of Right Vertebral Vein, Open Approach, Diagnostic
05BR0ZZ   Excision of Right Vertebral Vein, Open Approach
05BR3ZX   Excision of Right Vertebral Vein, Percutaneous Approach, Diagnostic
05BR3ZZ   Excision of Right Vertebral Vein, Percutaneous Approach
05BR4ZX   Excision of Right Vertebral Vein, Percutaneous Endoscopic Approach, Diagnostic
05BR4ZZ   Excision of Right Vertebral Vein, Percutaneous Endoscopic Approach
05BS0ZX   Excision of Left Vertebral Vein, Open Approach, Diagnostic
05BS0ZZ   Excision of Left Vertebral Vein, Open Approach
05BS3ZX   Excision of Left Vertebral Vein, Percutaneous Approach, Diagnostic
05BS3ZZ   Excision of Left Vertebral Vein, Percutaneous Approach
05BS4ZX   Excision of Left Vertebral Vein, Percutaneous Endoscopic Approach, Diagnostic
05BS4ZZ   Excision of Left Vertebral Vein, Percutaneous Endoscopic Approach
05BT0ZX   Excision of Right Face Vein, Open Approach, Diagnostic
05BT0ZZ   Excision of Right Face Vein, Open Approach
05BT3ZX   Excision of Right Face Vein, Percutaneous Approach, Diagnostic
05BT3ZZ   Excision of Right Face Vein, Percutaneous Approach
05BT4ZX   Excision of Right Face Vein, Percutaneous Endoscopic Approach, Diagnostic
05BT4ZZ   Excision of Right Face Vein, Percutaneous Endoscopic Approach
05BV0ZX   Excision of Left Face Vein, Open Approach, Diagnostic
05BV0ZZ   Excision of Left Face Vein, Open Approach
05BV3ZX   Excision of Left Face Vein, Percutaneous Approach, Diagnostic
05BV3ZZ   Excision of Left Face Vein, Percutaneous Approach
05BV4ZX   Excision of Left Face Vein, Percutaneous Endoscopic Approach, Diagnostic
05BV4ZZ   Excision of Left Face Vein, Percutaneous Endoscopic Approach
05BY0ZX   Excision of Upper Vein, Open Approach, Diagnostic
05BY0ZZ   Excision of Upper Vein, Open Approach
05BY3ZX   Excision of Upper Vein, Percutaneous Approach, Diagnostic
05BY3ZZ   Excision of Upper Vein, Percutaneous Approach
05BY4ZX   Excision of Upper Vein, Percutaneous Endoscopic Approach, Diagnostic
05BY4ZZ   Excision of Upper Vein, Percutaneous Endoscopic Approach

05C – Upper Veins, Extirpation

05C00ZZ   Extirpation of Matter from Azygos Vein, Open Approach
05C03ZZ   Extirpation of Matter from Azygos Vein, Percutaneous Approach
05C04ZZ   Extirpation of Matter from Azygos Vein, Percutaneous Endoscopic Approach
05C10ZZ   Extirpation of Matter from Hemiazygos Vein, Open Approach
05C13ZZ   Extirpation of Matter from Hemiazygos Vein, Percutaneous Approach
05C14ZZ   Extirpation of Matter from Hemiazygos Vein, Percutaneous Endoscopic Approach
05C30ZZ   Extirpation of Matter from Right Innominate Vein, Open Approach
05C33ZZ   Extirpation of Matter from Right Innominate Vein, Percutaneous Approach
05C34ZZ   Extirpation of Matter from Right Innominate Vein, Percutaneous Endoscopic Approach
05C40ZZ   Extirpation of Matter from Left Innominate Vein, Open Approach

05C43ZZ   Extirpation of Matter from Left Innominate Vein, Percutaneous Approach
05C44ZZ   Extirpation of Matter from Left Innominate Vein, Percutaneous Endoscopic Approach
05C50ZZ   Extirpation of Matter from Right Subclavian Vein, Open Approach
05C53ZZ   Extirpation of Matter from Right Subclavian Vein, Percutaneous Approach
05C54ZZ   Extirpation of Matter from Right Subclavian Vein, Percutaneous Endoscopic Approach
05C60ZZ   Extirpation of Matter from Left Subclavian Vein, Open Approach
05C63ZZ   Extirpation of Matter from Left Subclavian Vein, Percutaneous Approach
05C64ZZ   Extirpation of Matter from Left Subclavian Vein, Percutaneous Endoscopic Approach
05C70ZZ   Extirpation of Matter from Right Axillary Vein, Open Approach

05C73ZZ   Extirpation of Matter from Right Axillary Vein, Percutaneous Approach

05C74ZZ   Extirpation of Matter from Right Axillary Vein, Percutaneous Endoscopic Approach

05C80ZZ   Extirpation of Matter from Left Axillary Vein, Open Approach

05C83ZZ   Extirpation of Matter from Left Axillary Vein, Percutaneous Approach

05C84ZZ   Extirpation of Matter from Left Axillary Vein, Percutaneous Endoscopic Approach

05C90ZZ   Extirpation of Matter from Right Brachial Vein, Open Approach

05C93ZZ   Extirpation of Matter from Right Brachial Vein, Percutaneous Approach

05C94ZZ   Extirpation of Matter from Right Brachial Vein, Percutaneous Endoscopic Approach

05CA0ZZ   Extirpation of Matter from Left Brachial Vein, Open Approach

05CA3ZZ   Extirpation of Matter from Left Brachial Vein, Percutaneous Approach

05CA4ZZ   Extirpation of Matter from Left Brachial Vein, Percutaneous Endoscopic Approach

05CB0ZZ   Extirpation of Matter from Right Basilic Vein, Open Approach

05CB3ZZ   Extirpation of Matter from Right Basilic Vein, Percutaneous Approach

05CB4ZZ   Extirpation of Matter from Right Basilic Vein, Percutaneous Endoscopic Approach

05CC0ZZ   Extirpation of Matter from Left Basilic Vein, Open Approach

05CC3ZZ   Extirpation of Matter from Left Basilic Vein, Percutaneous Approach

05CC4ZZ   Extirpation of Matter from Left Basilic Vein, Percutaneous Endoscopic Approach

05CD0ZZ   Extirpation of Matter from Right Cephalic Vein, Open Approach

05CD3ZZ   Extirpation of Matter from Right Cephalic Vein, Percutaneous Approach

05CD4ZZ   Extirpation of Matter from Right Cephalic Vein, Percutaneous Endoscopic Approach

05CF0ZZ   Extirpation of Matter from Left Cephalic Vein, Open Approach

05CF3ZZ   Extirpation of Matter from Left Cephalic Vein, Percutaneous Approach

05CF4ZZ   Extirpation of Matter from Left Cephalic Vein, Percutaneous Endoscopic Approach

05CG0ZZ   Extirpation of Matter from Right Hand Vein, Open Approach

05CG3ZZ   Extirpation of Matter from Right Hand Vein, Percutaneous Approach

05CG4ZZ   Extirpation of Matter from Right Hand Vein, Percutaneous Endoscopic Approach

05CH0ZZ   Extirpation of Matter from Left Hand Vein, Open Approach

05CH3ZZ   Extirpation of Matter from Left Hand Vein, Percutaneous Approach

05CH4ZZ   Extirpation of Matter from Left Hand Vein, Percutaneous Endoscopic Approach

05CL0ZZ   Extirpation of Matter from Intracranial Vein, Open Approach

⬤ 05CL3ZZ   Extirpation of Matter from Intracranial Vein, Percutaneous Approach

⬤ 05CL4ZZ   Extirpation of Matter from Intracranial Vein, Percutaneous Endoscopic Approach

05CM0ZZ   Extirpation of Matter from Right Internal Jugular Vein, Open Approach

05CM3ZZ   Extirpation of Matter from Right Internal Jugular Vein, Percutaneous Approach

05CM4ZZ   Extirpation of Matter from Right Internal Jugular Vein, Percutaneous Endoscopic Approach

05CN0ZZ   Extirpation of Matter from Left Internal Jugular Vein, Open Approach

05CN3ZZ   Extirpation of Matter from Left Internal Jugular Vein, Percutaneous Approach

05CN4ZZ   Extirpation of Matter from Left Internal Jugular Vein, Percutaneous Endoscopic Approach

05CP0ZZ   Extirpation of Matter from Right External Jugular Vein, Open Approach

05CP3ZZ   Extirpation of Matter from Right External Jugular Vein, Percutaneous Approach

05CP4ZZ   Extirpation of Matter from Right External Jugular Vein, Percutaneous Endoscopic Approach

05CQ0ZZ   Extirpation of Matter from Left External Jugular Vein, Open Approach

05CQ3ZZ   Extirpation of Matter from Left External Jugular Vein, Percutaneous Approach

05CQ4ZZ   Extirpation of Matter from Left External Jugular Vein, Percutaneous Endoscopic Approach

05CR0ZZ   Extirpation of Matter from Right Vertebral Vein, Open Approach

05CR3ZZ   Extirpation of Matter from Right Vertebral Vein, Percutaneous Approach

05CR4ZZ   Extirpation of Matter from Right Vertebral Vein, Percutaneous Endoscopic Approach

05CS0ZZ   Extirpation of Matter from Left Vertebral Vein, Open Approach

05CS3ZZ   Extirpation of Matter from Left Vertebral Vein, Percutaneous Approach

05CS4ZZ   Extirpation of Matter from Left Vertebral Vein, Percutaneous Endoscopic Approach

05CT0ZZ   Extirpation of Matter from Right Face Vein, Open Approach

05CT3ZZ   Extirpation of Matter from Right Face Vein, Percutaneous Approach

05CT4ZZ   Extirpation of Matter from Right Face Vein, Percutaneous Endoscopic Approach

05CV0ZZ   Extirpation of Matter from Left Face Vein, Open Approach

05CV3ZZ   Extirpation of Matter from Left Face Vein, Percutaneous Approach

05CV4ZZ   Extirpation of Matter from Left Face Vein, Percutaneous Endoscopic Approach

05CY0ZZ   Extirpation of Matter from Upper Vein, Open Approach

05CY3ZZ   Extirpation of Matter from Upper Vein, Percutaneous Approach

05CY4ZZ   Extirpation of Matter from Upper Vein, Percutaneous Endoscopic Approach

05D – Upper Veins, Extraction

05D90ZZ   Extraction of Right Brachial Vein, Open Approach

05D93ZZ   Extraction of Right Brachial Vein, Percutaneous Approach

05DA0ZZ   Extraction of Left Brachial Vein, Open Approach

05DA3ZZ   Extraction of Left Brachial Vein, Percutaneous Approach

05DB0ZZ   Extraction of Right Basilic Vein, Open Approach

05DB3ZZ   Extraction of Right Basilic Vein, Percutaneous Approach

05DC0ZZ   Extraction of Left Basilic Vein, Open Approach

05DC3ZZ   Extraction of Left Basilic Vein, Percutaneous Approach

05DD0ZZ   Extraction of Right Cephalic Vein, Open Approach

05DD3ZZ   Extraction of Right Cephalic Vein, Percutaneous Approach

05DF0ZZ   Extraction of Left Cephalic Vein, Open Approach

05DF3ZZ   Extraction of Left Cephalic Vein, Percutaneous Approach

05DG0ZZ   Extraction of Right Hand Vein, Open Approach

05DG3ZZ   Extraction of Right Hand Vein, Percutaneous Approach

05DH0ZZ   Extraction of Left Hand Vein, Open Approach

05DH3ZZ   Extraction of Left Hand Vein, Percutaneous Approach

05DY0ZZ   Extraction of Upper Vein, Open Approach

05DY3ZZ   Extraction of Upper Vein, Percutaneous Approach

05H – Upper Veins, Insertion

05H003Z   Insertion of Infusion Device into Azygos Vein, Open Approach

05H00DZ   Insertion of Intraluminal Device into Azygos Vein, Open Approach

05H033Z   Insertion of Infusion Device into Azygos Vein, Percutaneous Approach

05H03DZ   Insertion of Intraluminal Device into Azygos Vein, Percutaneous Approach

05H043Z   Insertion of Infusion Device into Azygos Vein, Percutaneous Endoscopic Approach

05H04DZ   Insertion of Intraluminal Device into Azygos Vein, Percutaneous Endoscopic Approach

05H103Z   Insertion of Infusion Device into Hemiazygos Vein, Open Approach

05H10DZ   Insertion of Intraluminal Device into Hemiazygos Vein, Open Approach

05H133Z   Insertion of Infusion Device into Hemiazygos Vein, Percutaneous Approach

05H13DZ   Insertion of Intraluminal Device into Hemiazygos Vein, Percutaneous Approach

05H143Z   Insertion of Infusion Device into Hemiazygos Vein, Percutaneous Endoscopic Approach

♀ Female-only   ♂ Male-only   ⬤ Limited Coverage   ⬤ Non-OR   HAC HAC-associated procedure   ⬤ Non-covered procedures   ✚ Combination

05H14DZ   Insertion of Intraluminal Device into Hemiazygos Vein, Percutaneous Endoscopic Approach

05H303Z   Insertion of Infusion Device into Right Innominate Vein, Open Approach

05H30DZ   Insertion of Intraluminal Device into Right Innominate Vein, Open Approach

05H333Z   Insertion of Infusion Device into Right Innominate Vein, Percutaneous Approach

05H33DZ   Insertion of Intraluminal Device into Right Innominate Vein, Percutaneous Approach

05H343Z   Insertion of Infusion Device into Right Innominate Vein, Percutaneous Endoscopic Approach

05H34DZ   Insertion of Intraluminal Device into Right Innominate Vein, Percutaneous Endoscopic Approach

05H403Z   Insertion of Infusion Device into Left Innominate Vein, Open Approach

05H40DZ   Insertion of Intraluminal Device into Left Innominate Vein, Open Approach

05H433Z   Insertion of Infusion Device into Left Innominate Vein, Percutaneous Approach

05H43DZ   Insertion of Intraluminal Device into Left Innominate Vein, Percutaneous Approach

05H443Z   Insertion of Infusion Device into Left Innominate Vein, Percutaneous Endoscopic Approach

05H44DZ   Insertion of Intraluminal Device into Left Innominate Vein, Percutaneous Endoscopic Approach

05H503Z   Insertion of Infusion Device into Right Subclavian Vein, Open Approach

05H50DZ   Insertion of Intraluminal Device into Right Subclavian Vein, Open Approach

05H533Z   Insertion of Infusion Device into Right Subclavian Vein, Percutaneous Approach

05H53DZ   Insertion of Intraluminal Device into Right Subclavian Vein, Percutaneous Approach

05H543Z   Insertion of Infusion Device into Right Subclavian Vein, Percutaneous Endoscopic Approach

05H54DZ   Insertion of Intraluminal Device into Right Subclavian Vein, Percutaneous Endoscopic Approach

05H603Z   Insertion of Infusion Device into Left Subclavian Vein, Open Approach

05H60DZ   Insertion of Intraluminal Device into Left Subclavian Vein, Open Approach

05H633Z   Insertion of Infusion Device into Left Subclavian Vein, Percutaneous Approach

05H63DZ   Insertion of Intraluminal Device into Left Subclavian Vein, Percutaneous Approach

05H643Z   Insertion of Infusion Device into Left Subclavian Vein, Percutaneous Endoscopic Approach

05H64DZ   Insertion of Intraluminal Device into Left Subclavian Vein, Percutaneous Endoscopic Approach

05H703Z   Insertion of Infusion Device into Right Axillary Vein, Open Approach

05H70DZ   Insertion of Intraluminal Device into Right Axillary Vein, Open Approach

05H733Z   Insertion of Infusion Device into Right Axillary Vein, Percutaneous Approach

05H73DZ   Insertion of Intraluminal Device into Right Axillary Vein, Percutaneous Approach

05H743Z   Insertion of Infusion Device into Right Axillary Vein, Percutaneous Endoscopic Approach

05H74DZ   Insertion of Intraluminal Device into Right Axillary Vein, Percutaneous Endoscopic Approach

05H803Z   Insertion of Infusion Device into Left Axillary Vein, Open Approach

05H80DZ   Insertion of Intraluminal Device into Left Axillary Vein, Open Approach

05H833Z   Insertion of Infusion Device into Left Axillary Vein, Percutaneous Approach

05H83DZ   Insertion of Intraluminal Device into Left Axillary Vein, Percutaneous Approach

05H843Z   Insertion of Infusion Device into Left Axillary Vein, Percutaneous Endoscopic Approach

05H84DZ   Insertion of Intraluminal Device into Left Axillary Vein, Percutaneous Endoscopic Approach

05H903Z   Insertion of Infusion Device into Right Brachial Vein, Open Approach

05H90DZ   Insertion of Intraluminal Device into Right Brachial Vein, Open Approach

05H933Z   Insertion of Infusion Device into Right Brachial Vein, Percutaneous Approach

05H93DZ   Insertion of Intraluminal Device into Right Brachial Vein, Percutaneous Approach

05H943Z   Insertion of Infusion Device into Right Brachial Vein, Percutaneous Endoscopic Approach

05H94DZ   Insertion of Intraluminal Device into Right Brachial Vein, Percutaneous Endoscopic Approach

05HA03Z   Insertion of Infusion Device into Left Brachial Vein, Open Approach

05HA0DZ   Insertion of Intraluminal Device into Left Brachial Vein, Open Approach

05HA33Z   Insertion of Infusion Device into Left Brachial Vein, Percutaneous Approach

05HA3DZ   Insertion of Intraluminal Device into Left Brachial Vein, Percutaneous Approach

05HA43Z   Insertion of Infusion Device into Left Brachial Vein, Percutaneous Endoscopic Approach

05HA4DZ   Insertion of Intraluminal Device into Left Brachial Vein, Percutaneous Endoscopic Approach

05HB03Z   Insertion of Infusion Device into Right Basilic Vein, Open Approach

05HB0DZ   Insertion of Intraluminal Device into Right Basilic Vein, Open Approach

05HB33Z   Insertion of Infusion Device into Right Basilic Vein, Percutaneous Approach

05HB3DZ   Insertion of Intraluminal Device into Right Basilic Vein, Percutaneous Approach

05HB43Z   Insertion of Infusion Device into Right Basilic Vein, Percutaneous Endoscopic Approach

05HB4DZ   Insertion of Intraluminal Device into Right Basilic Vein, Percutaneous Endoscopic Approach

05HC03Z   Insertion of Infusion Device into Left Basilic Vein, Open Approach

05HC0DZ   Insertion of Intraluminal Device into Left Basilic Vein, Open Approach

05HC33Z   Insertion of Infusion Device into Left Basilic Vein, Percutaneous Approach

05HC3DZ   Insertion of Intraluminal Device into Left Basilic Vein, Percutaneous Approach

05HC43Z   Insertion of Infusion Device into Left Basilic Vein, Percutaneous Endoscopic Approach

05HC4DZ   Insertion of Intraluminal Device into Left Basilic Vein, Percutaneous Endoscopic Approach

05HD03Z   Insertion of Infusion Device into Right Cephalic Vein, Open Approach

05HD0DZ   Insertion of Intraluminal Device into Right Cephalic Vein, Open Approach

05HD33Z   Insertion of Infusion Device into Right Cephalic Vein, Percutaneous Approach

05HD3DZ   Insertion of Intraluminal Device into Right Cephalic Vein, Percutaneous Approach

05HD43Z   Insertion of Infusion Device into Right Cephalic Vein, Percutaneous Endoscopic Approach

05HD4DZ   Insertion of Intraluminal Device into Right Cephalic Vein, Percutaneous Endoscopic Approach

05HF03Z   Insertion of Infusion Device into Left Cephalic Vein, Open Approach

05HF0DZ   Insertion of Intraluminal Device into Left Cephalic Vein, Open Approach

05HF33Z   Insertion of Infusion Device into Left Cephalic Vein, Percutaneous Approach

05HF3DZ   Insertion of Intraluminal Device into Left Cephalic Vein, Percutaneous Approach

05HF43Z   Insertion of Infusion Device into Left Cephalic Vein, Percutaneous Endoscopic Approach

05HF4DZ   Insertion of Intraluminal Device into Left Cephalic Vein, Percutaneous Endoscopic Approach

05HG03Z   Insertion of Infusion Device into Right Hand Vein, Open Approach

05HG0DZ Insertion of Intraluminal Device into Right Hand Vein, Open Approach

05HG33Z Insertion of Infusion Device into Right Hand Vein, Percutaneous Approach

05HG3DZ Insertion of Intraluminal Device into Right Hand Vein, Percutaneous Approach

05HG43Z Insertion of Infusion Device into Right Hand Vein, Percutaneous Endoscopic Approach

05HG4DZ Insertion of Intraluminal Device into Right Hand Vein, Percutaneous Endoscopic Approach

05HH03Z Insertion of Infusion Device into Left Hand Vein, Open Approach

05HH0DZ Insertion of Intraluminal Device into Left Hand Vein, Open Approach

05HH33Z Insertion of Infusion Device into Left Hand Vein, Percutaneous Approach

05HH3DZ Insertion of Intraluminal Device into Left Hand Vein, Percutaneous Approach

05HH43Z Insertion of Infusion Device into Left Hand Vein, Percutaneous Endoscopic Approach

05HH4DZ Insertion of Intraluminal Device into Left Hand Vein, Percutaneous Endoscopic Approach

05HL03Z Insertion of Infusion Device into Intracranial Vein, Open Approach

05HL0DZ Insertion of Intraluminal Device into Intracranial Vein, Open Approach

05HL33Z Insertion of Infusion Device into Intracranial Vein, Percutaneous Approach

05HL3DZ Insertion of Intraluminal Device into Intracranial Vein, Percutaneous Approach

05HL43Z Insertion of Infusion Device into Intracranial Vein, Percutaneous Endoscopic Approach

05HL4DZ Insertion of Intraluminal Device into Intracranial Vein, Percutaneous Endoscopic Approach

05HM03Z Insertion of Infusion Device into Right Internal Jugular Vein, Open Approach

05HM0DZ Insertion of Intraluminal Device into Right Internal Jugular Vein, Open Approach

05HM33Z Insertion of Infusion Device into Right Internal Jugular Vein, Percutaneous Approach

HAC With secondary diagnosis code J95.811

05HM3DZ Insertion of Intraluminal Device into Right Internal Jugular Vein, Percutaneous Approach

05HM43Z Insertion of Infusion Device into Right Internal Jugular Vein, Percutaneous Endoscopic Approach

05HM4DZ Insertion of Intraluminal Device into Right Internal Jugular Vein, Percutaneous Endoscopic Approach

05HN03Z Insertion of Infusion Device into Left Internal Jugular Vein, Open Approach

05HN0DZ Insertion of Intraluminal Device into Left Internal Jugular Vein, Open Approach

05HN33Z Insertion of Infusion Device into Left Internal Jugular Vein, Percutaneous Approach

HAC With secondary diagnosis code J95.811

05HN3DZ Insertion of Intraluminal Device into Left Internal Jugular Vein, Percutaneous Approach

05HN43Z Insertion of Infusion Device into Left Internal Jugular Vein, Percutaneous Endoscopic Approach

05HN4DZ Insertion of Intraluminal Device into Left Internal Jugular Vein, Percutaneous Endoscopic Approach

05HP03Z Insertion of Infusion Device into Right External Jugular Vein, Open Approach

05HP0DZ Insertion of Intraluminal Device into Right External Jugular Vein, Open Approach

05HP33Z Insertion of Infusion Device into Right External Jugular Vein, Percutaneous Approach

HAC With secondary diagnosis code J95.811

05HP3DZ Insertion of Intraluminal Device into Right External Jugular Vein, Percutaneous Approach

05HP43Z Insertion of Infusion Device into Right External Jugular Vein, Percutaneous Endoscopic Approach

05HP4DZ Insertion of Intraluminal Device into Right External Jugular Vein, Percutaneous Endoscopic Approach

05HQ03Z Insertion of Infusion Device into Left External Jugular Vein, Open Approach

05HQ0DZ Insertion of Intraluminal Device into Left External Jugular Vein, Open Approach

05HQ33Z Insertion of Infusion Device into Left External Jugular Vein, Percutaneous Approach

HAC With secondary diagnosis code J95.811

05HQ3DZ Insertion of Intraluminal Device into Left External Jugular Vein, Percutaneous Approach

05HQ43Z Insertion of Infusion Device into Left External Jugular Vein, Percutaneous Endoscopic Approach

05HQ4DZ Insertion of Intraluminal Device into Left External Jugular Vein, Percutaneous Endoscopic Approach

05HR03Z Insertion of Infusion Device into Right Vertebral Vein, Open Approach

05HR0DZ Insertion of Intraluminal Device into Right Vertebral Vein, Open Approach

05HR33Z Insertion of Infusion Device into Right Vertebral Vein, Percutaneous Approach

05HR3DZ Insertion of Intraluminal Device into Right Vertebral Vein, Percutaneous Approach

05HR43Z Insertion of Infusion Device into Right Vertebral Vein, Percutaneous Endoscopic Approach

05HR4DZ Insertion of Intraluminal Device into Right Vertebral Vein, Percutaneous Endoscopic Approach

05HS03Z Insertion of Infusion Device into Left Vertebral Vein, Open Approach

05HS0DZ Insertion of Intraluminal Device into Left Vertebral Vein, Open Approach

05HS33Z Insertion of Infusion Device into Left Vertebral Vein, Percutaneous Approach

05HS3DZ Insertion of Intraluminal Device into Left Vertebral Vein, Percutaneous Approach

05HS43Z Insertion of Infusion Device into Left Vertebral Vein, Percutaneous Endoscopic Approach

05HS4DZ Insertion of Intraluminal Device into Left Vertebral Vein, Percutaneous Endoscopic Approach

05HT03Z Insertion of Infusion Device into Right Face Vein, Open Approach

05HT0DZ Insertion of Intraluminal Device into Right Face Vein, Open Approach

05HT33Z Insertion of Infusion Device into Right Face Vein, Percutaneous Approach

05HT3DZ Insertion of Intraluminal Device into Right Face Vein, Percutaneous Approach

05HT43Z Insertion of Infusion Device into Right Face Vein, Percutaneous Endoscopic Approach

05HT4DZ Insertion of Intraluminal Device into Right Face Vein, Percutaneous Endoscopic Approach

05HV03Z Insertion of Infusion Device into Left Face Vein, Open Approach

05HV0DZ Insertion of Intraluminal Device into Left Face Vein, Open Approach

05HV33Z Insertion of Infusion Device into Left Face Vein, Percutaneous Approach

05HV3DZ Insertion of Intraluminal Device into Left Face Vein, Percutaneous Approach

05HV43Z Insertion of Infusion Device into Left Face Vein, Percutaneous Endoscopic Approach

05HV4DZ Insertion of Intraluminal Device into Left Face Vein, Percutaneous Endoscopic Approach

05HY02Z Insertion of Monitoring Device into Upper Vein, Open Approach

05HY03Z Insertion of Infusion Device into Upper Vein, Open Approach

05HY0DZ Insertion of Intraluminal Device into Upper Vein, Open Approach

05HY32Z Insertion of Monitoring Device into Upper Vein, Percutaneous Approach

05HY33Z Insertion of Infusion Device into Upper Vein, Percutaneous Approach

05HY3DZ Insertion of Intraluminal Device into Upper Vein, Percutaneous Approach

05HY42Z Insertion of Monitoring Device into Upper Vein, Percutaneous Endoscopic Approach

05HY43Z Insertion of Infusion Device into Upper Vein, Percutaneous Endoscopic Approach

05HY4DZ Insertion of Intraluminal Device into Upper Vein, Percutaneous Endoscopic Approach

---

♀ Female-only   ♂ Male-only   ● Limited Coverage   ● Non-OR   HAC HAC-associated procedure   ● Non-covered procedures   + Combination

05J – Upper Veins, Inspection

Review Coding Guidelines B3.11a, B3.11b and B3.11c

05JY0ZZ Inspection of Upper Vein, Open Approach
05JY3ZZ Inspection of Upper Vein, Percutaneous Approach

05JY4ZZ Inspection of Upper Vein, Percutaneous Endoscopic Approach
05JYXZZ Inspection of Upper Vein, External Approach

05L – Upper Veins, Occlusion

Review Coding Guideline B3.12

05L00CZ Occlusion of Azygos Vein with Extraluminal Device, Open Approach
05L00DZ Occlusion of Azygos Vein with Intraluminal Device, Open Approach
05L00ZZ Occlusion of Azygos Vein, Open Approach
05L03CZ Occlusion of Azygos Vein with Extraluminal Device, Percutaneous Approach
05L03DZ Occlusion of Azygos Vein with Intraluminal Device, Percutaneous Approach
05L03ZZ Occlusion of Azygos Vein, Percutaneous Approach
05L04CZ Occlusion of Azygos Vein with Extraluminal Device, Percutaneous Endoscopic Approach
05L04DZ Occlusion of Azygos Vein with Intraluminal Device, Percutaneous Endoscopic Approach
05L04ZZ Occlusion of Azygos Vein, Percutaneous Endoscopic Approach
05L10CZ Occlusion of Hemiazygos Vein with Extraluminal Device, Open Approach
05L10DZ Occlusion of Hemiazygos Vein with Intraluminal Device, Open Approach
05L10ZZ Occlusion of Hemiazygos Vein, Open Approach
05L13CZ Occlusion of Hemiazygos Vein with Extraluminal Device, Percutaneous Approach
05L13DZ Occlusion of Hemiazygos Vein with Intraluminal Device, Percutaneous Approach
05L13ZZ Occlusion of Hemiazygos Vein, Percutaneous Approach
05L14CZ Occlusion of Hemiazygos Vein with Extraluminal Device, Percutaneous Endoscopic Approach
05L14DZ Occlusion of Hemiazygos Vein with Intraluminal Device, Percutaneous Endoscopic Approach
05L14ZZ Occlusion of Hemiazygos Vein, Percutaneous Endoscopic Approach
05L30CZ Occlusion of Right Innominate Vein with Extraluminal Device, Open Approach
05L30DZ Occlusion of Right Innominate Vein with Intraluminal Device, Open Approach
05L30ZZ Occlusion of Right Innominate Vein, Open Approach
05L33CZ Occlusion of Right Innominate Vein with Extraluminal Device, Percutaneous Approach
05L33DZ Occlusion of Right Innominate Vein with Intraluminal Device, Percutaneous Approach
05L33ZZ Occlusion of Right Innominate Vein, Percutaneous Approach
05L34CZ Occlusion of Right Innominate Vein with Extraluminal Device, Percutaneous Endoscopic Approach
05L34DZ Occlusion of Right Innominate Vein with Intraluminal Device, Percutaneous Endoscopic Approach
05L34ZZ Occlusion of Right Innominate Vein, Percutaneous Endoscopic Approach
05L40CZ Occlusion of Left Innominate Vein with Extraluminal Device, Open Approach
05L40DZ Occlusion of Left Innominate Vein with Intraluminal Device, Open Approach
05L40ZZ Occlusion of Left Innominate Vein, Open Approach
05L43CZ Occlusion of Left Innominate Vein with Extraluminal Device, Percutaneous Approach
05L43DZ Occlusion of Left Innominate Vein with Intraluminal Device, Percutaneous Approach
05L43ZZ Occlusion of Left Innominate Vein, Percutaneous Approach
05L44CZ Occlusion of Left Innominate Vein with Extraluminal Device, Percutaneous Endoscopic Approach
05L44DZ Occlusion of Left Innominate Vein with Intraluminal Device, Percutaneous Endoscopic Approach
05L44ZZ Occlusion of Left Innominate Vein, Percutaneous Endoscopic Approach

05L50CZ Occlusion of Right Subclavian Vein with Extraluminal Device, Open Approach
05L50DZ Occlusion of Right Subclavian Vein with Intraluminal Device, Open Approach
05L50ZZ Occlusion of Right Subclavian Vein, Open Approach
05L53CZ Occlusion of Right Subclavian Vein with Extraluminal Device, Percutaneous Approach
05L53DZ Occlusion of Right Subclavian Vein with Intraluminal Device, Percutaneous Approach
05L53ZZ Occlusion of Right Subclavian Vein, Percutaneous Approach
05L54CZ Occlusion of Right Subclavian Vein with Extraluminal Device, Percutaneous Endoscopic Approach
05L54DZ Occlusion of Right Subclavian Vein with Intraluminal Device, Percutaneous Endoscopic Approach
05L54ZZ Occlusion of Right Subclavian Vein, Percutaneous Endoscopic Approach
05L60CZ Occlusion of Left Subclavian Vein with Extraluminal Device, Open Approach
05L60DZ Occlusion of Left Subclavian Vein with Intraluminal Device, Open Approach
05L60ZZ Occlusion of Left Subclavian Vein, Open Approach
05L63CZ Occlusion of Left Subclavian Vein with Extraluminal Device, Percutaneous Approach
05L63DZ Occlusion of Left Subclavian Vein with Intraluminal Device, Percutaneous Approach
05L63ZZ Occlusion of Left Subclavian Vein, Percutaneous Approach
05L64CZ Occlusion of Left Subclavian Vein with Extraluminal Device, Percutaneous Endoscopic Approach
05L64DZ Occlusion of Left Subclavian Vein with Intraluminal Device, Percutaneous Endoscopic Approach
05L64ZZ Occlusion of Left Subclavian Vein, Percutaneous Endoscopic Approach
05L70CZ Occlusion of Right Axillary Vein with Extraluminal Device, Open Approach
05L70DZ Occlusion of Right Axillary Vein with Intraluminal Device, Open Approach
05L70ZZ Occlusion of Right Axillary Vein, Open Approach
05L73CZ Occlusion of Right Axillary Vein with Extraluminal Device, Percutaneous Approach
05L73DZ Occlusion of Right Axillary Vein with Intraluminal Device, Percutaneous Approach
05L73ZZ Occlusion of Right Axillary Vein, Percutaneous Approach
05L74CZ Occlusion of Right Axillary Vein with Extraluminal Device, Percutaneous Endoscopic Approach
05L74DZ Occlusion of Right Axillary Vein with Intraluminal Device, Percutaneous Endoscopic Approach
05L74ZZ Occlusion of Right Axillary Vein, Percutaneous Endoscopic Approach
05L80CZ Occlusion of Left Axillary Vein with Extraluminal Device, Open Approach
05L80DZ Occlusion of Left Axillary Vein with Intraluminal Device, Open Approach
05L80ZZ Occlusion of Left Axillary Vein, Open Approach
05L83CZ Occlusion of Left Axillary Vein with Extraluminal Device, Percutaneous Approach
05L83DZ Occlusion of Left Axillary Vein with Intraluminal Device, Percutaneous Approach
05L83ZZ Occlusion of Left Axillary Vein, Percutaneous Approach
05L84CZ Occlusion of Left Axillary Vein with Extraluminal Device, Percutaneous Endoscopic Approach
05L84DZ Occlusion of Left Axillary Vein with Intraluminal Device, Percutaneous Endoscopic Approach

05L84ZZ   Occlusion of Left Axillary Vein, Percutaneous Endoscopic Approach

05L90CZ   Occlusion of Right Brachial Vein with Extraluminal Device, Open Approach

05L90DZ   Occlusion of Right Brachial Vein with Intraluminal Device, Open Approach

05L90ZZ   Occlusion of Right Brachial Vein, Open Approach

05L93CZ   Occlusion of Right Brachial Vein with Extraluminal Device, Percutaneous Approach

05L93DZ   Occlusion of Right Brachial Vein with Intraluminal Device, Percutaneous Approach

05L93ZZ   Occlusion of Right Brachial Vein, Percutaneous Approach

05L94CZ   Occlusion of Right Brachial Vein with Extraluminal Device, Percutaneous Endoscopic Approach

05L94DZ   Occlusion of Right Brachial Vein with Intraluminal Device, Percutaneous Endoscopic Approach

05L94ZZ   Occlusion of Right Brachial Vein, Percutaneous Endoscopic Approach

05LA0CZ   Occlusion of Left Brachial Vein with Extraluminal Device, Open Approach

05LA0DZ   Occlusion of Left Brachial Vein with Intraluminal Device, Open Approach

05LA0ZZ   Occlusion of Left Brachial Vein, Open Approach

05LA3CZ   Occlusion of Left Brachial Vein with Extraluminal Device, Percutaneous Approach

05LA3DZ   Occlusion of Left Brachial Vein with Intraluminal Device, Percutaneous Approach

05LA3ZZ   Occlusion of Left Brachial Vein, Percutaneous Approach

05LA4CZ   Occlusion of Left Brachial Vein with Extraluminal Device, Percutaneous Endoscopic Approach

05LA4DZ   Occlusion of Left Brachial Vein with Intraluminal Device, Percutaneous Endoscopic Approach

05LA4ZZ   Occlusion of Left Brachial Vein, Percutaneous Endoscopic Approach

05LB0CZ   Occlusion of Right Basilic Vein with Extraluminal Device, Open Approach

05LB0DZ   Occlusion of Right Basilic Vein with Intraluminal Device, Open Approach

05LB0ZZ   Occlusion of Right Basilic Vein, Open Approach

05LB3CZ   Occlusion of Right Basilic Vein with Extraluminal Device, Percutaneous Approach

05LB3DZ   Occlusion of Right Basilic Vein with Intraluminal Device, Percutaneous Approach

05LB3ZZ   Occlusion of Right Basilic Vein, Percutaneous Approach

05LB4CZ   Occlusion of Right Basilic Vein with Extraluminal Device, Percutaneous Endoscopic Approach

05LB4DZ   Occlusion of Right Basilic Vein with Intraluminal Device, Percutaneous Endoscopic Approach

05LB4ZZ   Occlusion of Right Basilic Vein, Percutaneous Endoscopic Approach

05LC0CZ   Occlusion of Left Basilic Vein with Extraluminal Device, Open Approach

05LC0DZ   Occlusion of Left Basilic Vein with Intraluminal Device, Open Approach

05LC0ZZ   Occlusion of Left Basilic Vein, Open Approach

05LC3CZ   Occlusion of Left Basilic Vein with Extraluminal Device, Percutaneous Approach

05LC3DZ   Occlusion of Left Basilic Vein with Intraluminal Device, Percutaneous Approach

05LC3ZZ   Occlusion of Left Basilic Vein, Percutaneous Approach

05LC4CZ   Occlusion of Left Basilic Vein with Extraluminal Device, Percutaneous Endoscopic Approach

05LC4DZ   Occlusion of Left Basilic Vein with Intraluminal Device, Percutaneous Endoscopic Approach

05LC4ZZ   Occlusion of Left Basilic Vein, Percutaneous Endoscopic Approach

05LD0CZ   Occlusion of Right Cephalic Vein with Extraluminal Device, Open Approach

05LD0DZ   Occlusion of Right Cephalic Vein with Intraluminal Device, Open Approach

05LD0ZZ   Occlusion of Right Cephalic Vein, Open Approach

05LD3CZ   Occlusion of Right Cephalic Vein with Extraluminal Device, Percutaneous Approach

05LD3DZ   Occlusion of Right Cephalic Vein with Intraluminal Device, Percutaneous Approach

05LD3ZZ   Occlusion of Right Cephalic Vein, Percutaneous Approach

05LD4CZ   Occlusion of Right Cephalic Vein with Extraluminal Device, Percutaneous Endoscopic Approach

05LD4DZ   Occlusion of Right Cephalic Vein with Intraluminal Device, Percutaneous Endoscopic Approach

05LD4ZZ   Occlusion of Right Cephalic Vein, Percutaneous Endoscopic Approach

05LF0CZ   Occlusion of Left Cephalic Vein with Extraluminal Device, Open Approach

05LF0DZ   Occlusion of Left Cephalic Vein with Intraluminal Device, Open Approach

05LF0ZZ   Occlusion of Left Cephalic Vein, Open Approach

05LF3CZ   Occlusion of Left Cephalic Vein with Extraluminal Device, Percutaneous Approach

05LF3DZ   Occlusion of Left Cephalic Vein with Intraluminal Device, Percutaneous Approach

05LF3ZZ   Occlusion of Left Cephalic Vein, Percutaneous Approach

05LF4CZ   Occlusion of Left Cephalic Vein with Extraluminal Device, Percutaneous Endoscopic Approach

05LF4DZ   Occlusion of Left Cephalic Vein with Intraluminal Device, Percutaneous Endoscopic Approach

05LF4ZZ   Occlusion of Left Cephalic Vein, Percutaneous Endoscopic Approach

05LG0CZ   Occlusion of Right Hand Vein with Extraluminal Device, Open Approach

05LG0DZ   Occlusion of Right Hand Vein with Intraluminal Device, Open Approach

05LG0ZZ   Occlusion of Right Hand Vein, Open Approach

05LG3CZ   Occlusion of Right Hand Vein with Extraluminal Device, Percutaneous Approach

05LG3DZ   Occlusion of Right Hand Vein with Intraluminal Device, Percutaneous Approach

05LG3ZZ   Occlusion of Right Hand Vein, Percutaneous Approach

05LG4CZ   Occlusion of Right Hand Vein with Extraluminal Device, Percutaneous Endoscopic Approach

05LG4DZ   Occlusion of Right Hand Vein with Intraluminal Device, Percutaneous Endoscopic Approach

05LG4ZZ   Occlusion of Right Hand Vein, Percutaneous Endoscopic Approach

05LH0CZ   Occlusion of Left Hand Vein with Extraluminal Device, Open Approach

05LH0DZ   Occlusion of Left Hand Vein with Intraluminal Device, Open Approach

05LH0ZZ   Occlusion of Left Hand Vein, Open Approach

05LH3CZ   Occlusion of Left Hand Vein with Extraluminal Device, Percutaneous Approach

05LH3DZ   Occlusion of Left Hand Vein with Intraluminal Device, Percutaneous Approach

05LH3ZZ   Occlusion of Left Hand Vein, Percutaneous Approach

05LH4CZ   Occlusion of Left Hand Vein with Extraluminal Device, Percutaneous Endoscopic Approach

05LH4DZ   Occlusion of Left Hand Vein with Intraluminal Device, Percutaneous Endoscopic Approach

05LH4ZZ   Occlusion of Left Hand Vein, Percutaneous Endoscopic Approach

05LL0CZ   Occlusion of Intracranial Vein with Extraluminal Device, Open Approach

05LL0DZ   Occlusion of Intracranial Vein with Intraluminal Device, Open Approach

05LL0ZZ   Occlusion of Intracranial Vein, Open Approach

05LL3CZ   Occlusion of Intracranial Vein with Extraluminal Device, Percutaneous Approach

05LL3DZ   Occlusion of Intracranial Vein with Intraluminal Device, Percutaneous Approach

05LL3ZZ   Occlusion of Intracranial Vein, Percutaneous Approach

05LL4CZ   Occlusion of Intracranial Vein with Extraluminal Device, Percutaneous Endoscopic Approach

05LL4DZ   Occlusion of Intracranial Vein with Intraluminal Device, Percutaneous Endoscopic Approach

05LL4ZZ   Occlusion of Intracranial Vein, Percutaneous Endoscopic Approach

05LM0CZ   Occlusion of Right Internal Jugular Vein with Extraluminal Device, Open Approach

05LM0DZ Occlusion of Right Internal Jugular Vein with Intraluminal Device, Open Approach
05LM0ZZ Occlusion of Right Internal Jugular Vein, Open Approach
05LM3CZ Occlusion of Right Internal Jugular Vein with Extraluminal Device, Percutaneous Approach
05LM3DZ Occlusion of Right Internal Jugular Vein with Intraluminal Device, Percutaneous Approach
05LM3ZZ Occlusion of Right Internal Jugular Vein, Percutaneous Approach
05LM4CZ Occlusion of Right Internal Jugular Vein with Extraluminal Device, Percutaneous Endoscopic Approach
05LM4DZ Occlusion of Right Internal Jugular Vein with Intraluminal Device, Percutaneous Endoscopic Approach
05LM4ZZ Occlusion of Right Internal Jugular Vein, Percutaneous Endoscopic Approach
05LN0CZ Occlusion of Left Internal Jugular Vein with Extraluminal Device, Open Approach
05LN0DZ Occlusion of Left Internal Jugular Vein with Intraluminal Device, Open Approach
05LN0ZZ Occlusion of Left Internal Jugular Vein, Open Approach
05LN3CZ Occlusion of Left Internal Jugular Vein with Extraluminal Device, Percutaneous Approach
05LN3DZ Occlusion of Left Internal Jugular Vein with Intraluminal Device, Percutaneous Approach
05LN3ZZ Occlusion of Left Internal Jugular Vein, Percutaneous Approach
05LN4CZ Occlusion of Left Internal Jugular Vein with Extraluminal Device, Percutaneous Endoscopic Approach
05LN4DZ Occlusion of Left Internal Jugular Vein with Intraluminal Device, Percutaneous Endoscopic Approach
05LN4ZZ Occlusion of Left Internal Jugular Vein, Percutaneous Endoscopic Approach
05LP0CZ Occlusion of Right External Jugular Vein with Extraluminal Device, Open Approach
05LP0DZ Occlusion of Right External Jugular Vein with Intraluminal Device, Open Approach
05LP0ZZ Occlusion of Right External Jugular Vein, Open Approach
05LP3CZ Occlusion of Right External Jugular Vein with Extraluminal Device, Percutaneous Approach
05LP3DZ Occlusion of Right External Jugular Vein with Intraluminal Device, Percutaneous Approach
05LP3ZZ Occlusion of Right External Jugular Vein, Percutaneous Approach
05LP4CZ Occlusion of Right External Jugular Vein with Extraluminal Device, Percutaneous Endoscopic Approach
05LP4DZ Occlusion of Right External Jugular Vein with Intraluminal Device, Percutaneous Endoscopic Approach
05LP4ZZ Occlusion of Right External Jugular Vein, Percutaneous Endoscopic Approach
05LQ0CZ Occlusion of Left External Jugular Vein with Extraluminal Device, Open Approach
05LQ0DZ Occlusion of Left External Jugular Vein with Intraluminal Device, Open Approach
05LQ0ZZ Occlusion of Left External Jugular Vein, Open Approach
05LQ3CZ Occlusion of Left External Jugular Vein with Extraluminal Device, Percutaneous Approach
05LQ3DZ Occlusion of Left External Jugular Vein with Intraluminal Device, Percutaneous Approach
05LQ3ZZ Occlusion of Left External Jugular Vein, Percutaneous Approach
05LQ4CZ Occlusion of Left External Jugular Vein with Extraluminal Device, Percutaneous Endoscopic Approach
05LQ4DZ Occlusion of Left External Jugular Vein with Intraluminal Device, Percutaneous Endoscopic Approach
05LQ4ZZ Occlusion of Left External Jugular Vein, Percutaneous Endoscopic Approach
05LR0CZ Occlusion of Right Vertebral Vein with Extraluminal Device, Open Approach
05LR0DZ Occlusion of Right Vertebral Vein with Intraluminal Device, Open Approach
05LR0ZZ Occlusion of Right Vertebral Vein, Open Approach
05LR3CZ Occlusion of Right Vertebral Vein with Extraluminal Device, Percutaneous Approach
05LR3DZ Occlusion of Right Vertebral Vein with Intraluminal Device, Percutaneous Approach

05LR3ZZ Occlusion of Right Vertebral Vein, Percutaneous Approach
05LR4CZ Occlusion of Right Vertebral Vein with Extraluminal Device, Percutaneous Endoscopic Approach
05LR4DZ Occlusion of Right Vertebral Vein with Intraluminal Device, Percutaneous Endoscopic Approach
05LR4ZZ Occlusion of Right Vertebral Vein, Percutaneous Endoscopic Approach
05LS0CZ Occlusion of Left Vertebral Vein with Extraluminal Device, Open Approach
05LS0DZ Occlusion of Left Vertebral Vein with Intraluminal Device, Open Approach
05LS0ZZ Occlusion of Left Vertebral Vein, Open Approach
05LS3CZ Occlusion of Left Vertebral Vein with Extraluminal Device, Percutaneous Approach
05LS3DZ Occlusion of Left Vertebral Vein with Intraluminal Device, Percutaneous Approach
05LS3ZZ Occlusion of Left Vertebral Vein, Percutaneous Approach
05LS4CZ Occlusion of Left Vertebral Vein with Extraluminal Device, Percutaneous Endoscopic Approach
05LS4DZ Occlusion of Left Vertebral Vein with Intraluminal Device, Percutaneous Endoscopic Approach
05LS4ZZ Occlusion of Left Vertebral Vein, Percutaneous Endoscopic Approach
05LT0CZ Occlusion of Right Face Vein with Extraluminal Device, Open Approach
05LT0DZ Occlusion of Right Face Vein with Intraluminal Device, Open Approach
05LT0ZZ Occlusion of Right Face Vein, Open Approach
05LT3CZ Occlusion of Right Face Vein with Extraluminal Device, Percutaneous Approach
05LT3DZ Occlusion of Right Face Vein with Intraluminal Device, Percutaneous Approach
05LT3ZZ Occlusion of Right Face Vein, Percutaneous Approach
05LT4CZ Occlusion of Right Face Vein with Extraluminal Device, Percutaneous Endoscopic Approach
05LT4DZ Occlusion of Right Face Vein with Intraluminal Device, Percutaneous Endoscopic Approach
05LT4ZZ Occlusion of Right Face Vein, Percutaneous Endoscopic Approach
05LV0CZ Occlusion of Left Face Vein with Extraluminal Device, Open Approach
05LV0DZ Occlusion of Left Face Vein with Intraluminal Device, Open Approach
05LV0ZZ Occlusion of Left Face Vein, Open Approach
05LV3CZ Occlusion of Left Face Vein with Extraluminal Device, Percutaneous Approach
05LV3DZ Occlusion of Left Face Vein with Intraluminal Device, Percutaneous Approach
05LV3ZZ Occlusion of Left Face Vein, Percutaneous Approach
05LV4CZ Occlusion of Left Face Vein with Extraluminal Device, Percutaneous Endoscopic Approach
05LV4DZ Occlusion of Left Face Vein with Intraluminal Device, Percutaneous Endoscopic Approach
05LV4ZZ Occlusion of Left Face Vein, Percutaneous Endoscopic Approach
05LY0CZ Occlusion of Upper Vein with Extraluminal Device, Open Approach
05LY0DZ Occlusion of Upper Vein with Intraluminal Device, Open Approach
05LY0ZZ Occlusion of Upper Vein, Open Approach
05LY3CZ Occlusion of Upper Vein with Extraluminal Device, Percutaneous Approach
05LY3DZ Occlusion of Upper Vein with Intraluminal Device, Percutaneous Approach
05LY3ZZ Occlusion of Upper Vein, Percutaneous Approach
05LY4CZ Occlusion of Upper Vein with Extraluminal Device, Percutaneous Endoscopic Approach
05LY4DZ Occlusion of Upper Vein with Intraluminal Device, Percutaneous Endoscopic Approach
05LY4ZZ Occlusion of Upper Vein, Percutaneous Endoscopic Approach

05N – Upper Veins, Release

Review Coding Guidelines B3.13 and B3.14

05N00ZZ	Release Azygos Vein, Open Approach
05N03ZZ	Release Azygos Vein, Percutaneous Approach
05N04ZZ	Release Azygos Vein, Percutaneous Endoscopic Approach
05N10ZZ	Release Hemiazygos Vein, Open Approach
05N13ZZ	Release Hemiazygos Vein, Percutaneous Approach
05N14ZZ	Release Hemiazygos Vein, Percutaneous Endoscopic Approach
05N30ZZ	Release Right Innominate Vein, Open Approach
05N33ZZ	Release Right Innominate Vein, Percutaneous Approach
05N34ZZ	Release Right Innominate Vein, Percutaneous Endoscopic Approach
05N40ZZ	Release Left Innominate Vein, Open Approach
05N43ZZ	Release Left Innominate Vein, Percutaneous Approach
05N44ZZ	Release Left Innominate Vein, Percutaneous Endoscopic Approach
05N50ZZ	Release Right Subclavian Vein, Open Approach
05N53ZZ	Release Right Subclavian Vein, Percutaneous Approach
05N54ZZ	Release Right Subclavian Vein, Percutaneous Endoscopic Approach
05N60ZZ	Release Left Subclavian Vein, Open Approach
05N63ZZ	Release Left Subclavian Vein, Percutaneous Approach
05N64ZZ	Release Left Subclavian Vein, Percutaneous Endoscopic Approach
05N70ZZ	Release Right Axillary Vein, Open Approach
05N73ZZ	Release Right Axillary Vein, Percutaneous Approach
05N74ZZ	Release Right Axillary Vein, Percutaneous Endoscopic Approach
05N80ZZ	Release Left Axillary Vein, Open Approach
05N83ZZ	Release Left Axillary Vein, Percutaneous Approach
05N84ZZ	Release Left Axillary Vein, Percutaneous Endoscopic Approach
05N90ZZ	Release Right Brachial Vein, Open Approach
05N93ZZ	Release Right Brachial Vein, Percutaneous Approach
05N94ZZ	Release Right Brachial Vein, Percutaneous Endoscopic Approach
05NA0ZZ	Release Left Brachial Vein, Open Approach
05NA3ZZ	Release Left Brachial Vein, Percutaneous Approach
05NA4ZZ	Release Left Brachial Vein, Percutaneous Endoscopic Approach
05NB0ZZ	Release Right Basilic Vein, Open Approach
05NB3ZZ	Release Right Basilic Vein, Percutaneous Approach
05NB4ZZ	Release Right Basilic Vein, Percutaneous Endoscopic Approach
05NC0ZZ	Release Left Basilic Vein, Open Approach
05NC3ZZ	Release Left Basilic Vein, Percutaneous Approach
05NC4ZZ	Release Left Basilic Vein, Percutaneous Endoscopic Approach
05ND0ZZ	Release Right Cephalic Vein, Open Approach
05ND3ZZ	Release Right Cephalic Vein, Percutaneous Approach
05ND4ZZ	Release Right Cephalic Vein, Percutaneous Endoscopic Approach
05NF0ZZ	Release Left Cephalic Vein, Open Approach
05NF3ZZ	Release Left Cephalic Vein, Percutaneous Approach
05NF4ZZ	Release Left Cephalic Vein, Percutaneous Endoscopic Approach
05NG0ZZ	Release Right Hand Vein, Open Approach
05NG3ZZ	Release Right Hand Vein, Percutaneous Approach
05NG4ZZ	Release Right Hand Vein, Percutaneous Endoscopic Approach
05NH0ZZ	Release Left Hand Vein, Open Approach
05NH3ZZ	Release Left Hand Vein, Percutaneous Approach
05NH4ZZ	Release Left Hand Vein, Percutaneous Endoscopic Approach
05NL0ZZ	Release Intracranial Vein, Open Approach
05NL3ZZ	Release Intracranial Vein, Percutaneous Approach
05NL4ZZ	Release Intracranial Vein, Percutaneous Endoscopic Approach
05NM0ZZ	Release Right Internal Jugular Vein, Open Approach
05NM3ZZ	Release Right Internal Jugular Vein, Percutaneous Approach
05NM4ZZ	Release Right Internal Jugular Vein, Percutaneous Endoscopic Approach
05NN0ZZ	Release Left Internal Jugular Vein, Open Approach
05NN3ZZ	Release Left Internal Jugular Vein, Percutaneous Approach
05NN4ZZ	Release Left Internal Jugular Vein, Percutaneous Endoscopic Approach
05NP0ZZ	Release Right External Jugular Vein, Open Approach
05NP3ZZ	Release Right External Jugular Vein, Percutaneous Approach
05NP4ZZ	Release Right External Jugular Vein, Percutaneous Endoscopic Approach
05NQ0ZZ	Release Left External Jugular Vein, Open Approach
05NQ3ZZ	Release Left External Jugular Vein, Percutaneous Approach
05NQ4ZZ	Release Left External Jugular Vein, Percutaneous Endoscopic Approach
05NR0ZZ	Release Right Vertebral Vein, Open Approach
05NR3ZZ	Release Right Vertebral Vein, Percutaneous Approach
05NR4ZZ	Release Right Vertebral Vein, Percutaneous Endoscopic Approach
05NS0ZZ	Release Left Vertebral Vein, Open Approach
05NS3ZZ	Release Left Vertebral Vein, Percutaneous Approach
05NS4ZZ	Release Left Vertebral Vein, Percutaneous Endoscopic Approach
05NT0ZZ	Release Right Face Vein, Open Approach
05NT3ZZ	Release Right Face Vein, Percutaneous Approach
05NT4ZZ	Release Right Face Vein, Percutaneous Endoscopic Approach
05NV0ZZ	Release Left Face Vein, Open Approach
05NV3ZZ	Release Left Face Vein, Percutaneous Approach
05NV4ZZ	Release Left Face Vein, Percutaneous Endoscopic Approach
05NY0ZZ	Release Upper Vein, Open Approach
05NY3ZZ	Release Upper Vein, Percutaneous Approach
05NY4ZZ	Release Upper Vein, Percutaneous Endoscopic Approach

05P – Upper Veins, Removal

Review Coding Guideline B6.1c

05PY00Z	Removal of Drainage Device from Upper Vein, Open Approach
05PY02Z	Removal of Monitoring Device from Upper Vein, Open Approach
05PY03Z	Removal of Infusion Device from Upper Vein, Open Approach
05PY07Z	Removal of Autologous Tissue Substitute from Upper Vein, Open Approach
05PY0CZ	Removal of Extraluminal Device from Upper Vein, Open Approach
05PY0DZ	Removal of Intraluminal Device from Upper Vein, Open Approach
05PY0JZ	Removal of Synthetic Substitute from Upper Vein, Open Approach
05PY0KZ	Removal of Nonautologous Tissue Substitute from Upper Vein, Open Approach
05PY30Z	Removal of Drainage Device from Upper Vein, Percutaneous Approach
05PY32Z	Removal of Monitoring Device from Upper Vein, Percutaneous Approach
05PY33Z	Removal of Infusion Device from Upper Vein, Percutaneous Approach
05PY37Z	Removal of Autologous Tissue Substitute from Upper Vein, Percutaneous Approach
05PY3CZ	Removal of Extraluminal Device from Upper Vein, Percutaneous Approach
05PY3DZ	Removal of Intraluminal Device from Upper Vein, Percutaneous Approach
05PY3JZ	Removal of Synthetic Substitute from Upper Vein, Percutaneous Approach
05PY3KZ	Removal of Nonautologous Tissue Substitute from Upper Vein, Percutaneous Approach
05PY40Z	Removal of Drainage Device from Upper Vein, Percutaneous Endoscopic Approach
05PY42Z	Removal of Monitoring Device from Upper Vein, Percutaneous Endoscopic Approach
05PY43Z	Removal of Infusion Device from Upper Vein, Percutaneous Endoscopic Approach
05PY47Z	Removal of Autologous Tissue Substitute from Upper Vein, Percutaneous Endoscopic Approach
05PY4CZ	Removal of Extraluminal Device from Upper Vein, Percutaneous Endoscopic Approach
05PY4DZ	Removal of Intraluminal Device from Upper Vein, Percutaneous Endoscopic Approach
05PY4JZ	Removal of Synthetic Substitute from Upper Vein, Percutaneous Endoscopic Approach
05PY4KZ	Removal of Nonautologous Tissue Substitute from Upper Vein, Percutaneous Endoscopic Approach
05PYX0Z	Removal of Drainage Device from Upper Vein, External Approach
05PYX2Z	Removal of Monitoring Device from Upper Vein, External Approach
05PYX3Z	Removal of Infusion Device from Upper Vein, External Approach
05PYXDZ	Removal of Intraluminal Device from Upper Vein, External Approach

♀ Female-only   ♂ Male-only   ● Limited Coverage   ● Non-OR   ᴴᴬᶜ HAC-associated procedure   ● Non-covered procedures   ✛ Combination

05Q – Upper Veins, Repair

05Q00ZZ	Repair Azygos Vein, Open Approach
05Q03ZZ	Repair Azygos Vein, Percutaneous Approach
05Q04ZZ	Repair Azygos Vein, Percutaneous Endoscopic Approach
05Q10ZZ	Repair Hemiazygos Vein, Open Approach
05Q13ZZ	Repair Hemiazygos Vein, Percutaneous Approach
05Q14ZZ	Repair Hemiazygos Vein, Percutaneous Endoscopic Approach
05Q30ZZ	Repair Right Innominate Vein, Open Approach
05Q33ZZ	Repair Right Innominate Vein, Percutaneous Approach
05Q34ZZ	Repair Right Innominate Vein, Percutaneous Endoscopic Approach
05Q40ZZ	Repair Left Innominate Vein, Open Approach
05Q43ZZ	Repair Left Innominate Vein, Percutaneous Approach
05Q44ZZ	Repair Left Innominate Vein, Percutaneous Endoscopic Approach
05Q50ZZ	Repair Right Subclavian Vein, Open Approach
05Q53ZZ	Repair Right Subclavian Vein, Percutaneous Approach
05Q54ZZ	Repair Right Subclavian Vein, Percutaneous Endoscopic Approach
05Q60ZZ	Repair Left Subclavian Vein, Open Approach
05Q63ZZ	Repair Left Subclavian Vein, Percutaneous Approach
05Q64ZZ	Repair Left Subclavian Vein, Percutaneous Endoscopic Approach
05Q70ZZ	Repair Right Axillary Vein, Open Approach
05Q73ZZ	Repair Right Axillary Vein, Percutaneous Approach
05Q74ZZ	Repair Right Axillary Vein, Percutaneous Endoscopic Approach
05Q80ZZ	Repair Left Axillary Vein, Open Approach
05Q83ZZ	Repair Left Axillary Vein, Percutaneous Approach
05Q84ZZ	Repair Left Axillary Vein, Percutaneous Endoscopic Approach
05Q90ZZ	Repair Right Brachial Vein, Open Approach
05Q93ZZ	Repair Right Brachial Vein, Percutaneous Approach
05Q94ZZ	Repair Right Brachial Vein, Percutaneous Endoscopic Approach
05QA0ZZ	Repair Left Brachial Vein, Open Approach
05QA3ZZ	Repair Left Brachial Vein, Percutaneous Approach
05QA4ZZ	Repair Left Brachial Vein, Percutaneous Endoscopic Approach
05QB0ZZ	Repair Right Basilic Vein, Open Approach
05QB3ZZ	Repair Right Basilic Vein, Percutaneous Approach
05QB4ZZ	Repair Right Basilic Vein, Percutaneous Endoscopic Approach
05QC0ZZ	Repair Left Basilic Vein, Open Approach
05QC3ZZ	Repair Left Basilic Vein, Percutaneous Approach
05QC4ZZ	Repair Left Basilic Vein, Percutaneous Endoscopic Approach
05QD0ZZ	Repair Right Cephalic Vein, Open Approach
05QD3ZZ	Repair Right Cephalic Vein, Percutaneous Approach
05QD4ZZ	Repair Right Cephalic Vein, Percutaneous Endoscopic Approach
05QF0ZZ	Repair Left Cephalic Vein, Open Approach
05QF3ZZ	Repair Left Cephalic Vein, Percutaneous Approach
05QF4ZZ	Repair Left Cephalic Vein, Percutaneous Endoscopic Approach
05QG0ZZ	Repair Right Hand Vein, Open Approach
05QG3ZZ	Repair Right Hand Vein, Percutaneous Approach
05QG4ZZ	Repair Right Hand Vein, Percutaneous Endoscopic Approach
05QH0ZZ	Repair Left Hand Vein, Open Approach
05QH3ZZ	Repair Left Hand Vein, Percutaneous Approach
05QH4ZZ	Repair Left Hand Vein, Percutaneous Endoscopic Approach
05QL0ZZ	Repair Intracranial Vein, Open Approach
05QL3ZZ	Repair Intracranial Vein, Percutaneous Approach
05QL4ZZ	Repair Intracranial Vein, Percutaneous Endoscopic Approach
05QM0ZZ	Repair Right Internal Jugular Vein, Open Approach
05QM3ZZ	Repair Right Internal Jugular Vein, Percutaneous Approach
05QM4ZZ	Repair Right Internal Jugular Vein, Percutaneous Endoscopic Approach
05QN0ZZ	Repair Left Internal Jugular Vein, Open Approach
05QN3ZZ	Repair Left Internal Jugular Vein, Percutaneous Approach
05QN4ZZ	Repair Left Internal Jugular Vein, Percutaneous Endoscopic Approach
05QP0ZZ	Repair Right External Jugular Vein, Open Approach
05QP3ZZ	Repair Right External Jugular Vein, Percutaneous Approach
05QP4ZZ	Repair Right External Jugular Vein, Percutaneous Endoscopic Approach
05QQ0ZZ	Repair Left External Jugular Vein, Open Approach
05QQ3ZZ	Repair Left External Jugular Vein, Percutaneous Approach
05QQ4ZZ	Repair Left External Jugular Vein, Percutaneous Endoscopic Approach
05QR0ZZ	Repair Right Vertebral Vein, Open Approach
05QR3ZZ	Repair Right Vertebral Vein, Percutaneous Approach
05QR4ZZ	Repair Right Vertebral Vein, Percutaneous Endoscopic Approach
05QS0ZZ	Repair Left Vertebral Vein, Open Approach
05QS3ZZ	Repair Left Vertebral Vein, Percutaneous Approach
05QS4ZZ	Repair Left Vertebral Vein, Percutaneous Endoscopic Approach
05QT0ZZ	Repair Right Face Vein, Open Approach
05QT3ZZ	Repair Right Face Vein, Percutaneous Approach
05QT4ZZ	Repair Right Face Vein, Percutaneous Endoscopic Approach
05QV0ZZ	Repair Left Face Vein, Open Approach
05QV3ZZ	Repair Left Face Vein, Percutaneous Approach
05QV4ZZ	Repair Left Face Vein, Percutaneous Endoscopic Approach
05QY0ZZ	Repair Upper Vein, Open Approach
05QY3ZZ	Repair Upper Vein, Percutaneous Approach
05QY4ZZ	Repair Upper Vein, Percutaneous Endoscopic Approach

05R – Upper Veins, Replacement

05R007Z	Replacement of Azygos Vein with Autologous Tissue Substitute, Open Approach
05R00JZ	Replacement of Azygos Vein with Synthetic Substitute, Open Approach
05R00KZ	Replacement of Azygos Vein with Nonautologous Tissue Substitute, Open Approach
05R047Z	Replacement of Azygos Vein with Autologous Tissue Substitute, Percutaneous Endoscopic Approach
05R04JZ	Replacement of Azygos Vein with Synthetic Substitute, Percutaneous Endoscopic Approach
05R04KZ	Replacement of Azygos Vein with Nonautologous Tissue Substitute, Percutaneous Endoscopic Approach
05R107Z	Replacement of Hemiazygos Vein with Autologous Tissue Substitute, Open Approach
05R10JZ	Replacement of Hemiazygos Vein with Synthetic Substitute, Open Approach
05R10KZ	Replacement of Hemiazygos Vein with Nonautologous Tissue Substitute, Open Approach
05R147Z	Replacement of Hemiazygos Vein with Autologous Tissue Substitute, Percutaneous Endoscopic Approach
05R14JZ	Replacement of Hemiazygos Vein with Synthetic Substitute, Percutaneous Endoscopic Approach
05R14KZ	Replacement of Hemiazygos Vein with Nonautologous Tissue Substitute, Percutaneous Endoscopic Approach
05R307Z	Replacement of Right Innominate Vein with Autologous Tissue Substitute, Open Approach
05R30JZ	Replacement of Right Innominate Vein with Synthetic Substitute, Open Approach
05R30KZ	Replacement of Right Innominate Vein with Nonautologous Tissue Substitute, Open Approach
05R347Z	Replacement of Right Innominate Vein with Autologous Tissue Substitute, Percutaneous Endoscopic Approach
05R34JZ	Replacement of Right Innominate Vein with Synthetic Substitute, Percutaneous Endoscopic Approach
05R34KZ	Replacement of Right Innominate Vein with Nonautologous Tissue Substitute, Percutaneous Endoscopic Approach
05R407Z	Replacement of Left Innominate Vein with Autologous Tissue Substitute, Open Approach
05R40JZ	Replacement of Left Innominate Vein with Synthetic Substitute, Open Approach
05R40KZ	Replacement of Left Innominate Vein with Nonautologous Tissue Substitute, Open Approach
05R447Z	Replacement of Left Innominate Vein with Autologous Tissue Substitute, Percutaneous Endoscopic Approach
05R44JZ	Replacement of Left Innominate Vein with Synthetic Substitute, Percutaneous Endoscopic Approach
05R44KZ	Replacement of Left Innominate Vein with Nonautologous Tissue Substitute, Percutaneous Endoscopic Approach
05R507Z	Replacement of Right Subclavian Vein with Autologous Tissue Substitute, Open Approach
05R50JZ	Replacement of Right Subclavian Vein with Synthetic Substitute, Open Approach
05R50KZ	Replacement of Right Subclavian Vein with Nonautologous Tissue Substitute, Open Approach
05R547Z	Replacement of Right Subclavian Vein with Autologous Tissue Substitute, Percutaneous Endoscopic Approach

05R54JZ   Replacement of Right Subclavian Vein with Synthetic Substitute, Percutaneous Endoscopic Approach

05R54KZ   Replacement of Right Subclavian Vein with Nonautologous Tissue Substitute, Percutaneous Endoscopic Approach

05R607Z   Replacement of Left Subclavian Vein with Autologous Tissue Substitute, Open Approach

05R60JZ   Replacement of Left Subclavian Vein with Synthetic Substitute, Open Approach

05R60KZ   Replacement of Left Subclavian Vein with Nonautologous Tissue Substitute, Open Approach

05R647Z   Replacement of Left Subclavian Vein with Autologous Tissue Substitute, Percutaneous Endoscopic Approach

05R64JZ   Replacement of Left Subclavian Vein with Synthetic Substitute, Percutaneous Endoscopic Approach

05R64KZ   Replacement of Left Subclavian Vein with Nonautologous Tissue Substitute, Percutaneous Endoscopic Approach

05R707Z   Replacement of Right Axillary Vein with Autologous Tissue Substitute, Open Approach

05R70JZ   Replacement of Right Axillary Vein with Synthetic Substitute, Open Approach

05R70KZ   Replacement of Right Axillary Vein with Nonautologous Tissue Substitute, Open Approach

05R747Z   Replacement of Right Axillary Vein with Autologous Tissue Substitute, Percutaneous Endoscopic Approach

05R74JZ   Replacement of Right Axillary Vein with Synthetic Substitute, Percutaneous Endoscopic Approach

05R74KZ   Replacement of Right Axillary Vein with Nonautologous Tissue Substitute, Percutaneous Endoscopic Approach

05R807Z   Replacement of Left Axillary Vein with Autologous Tissue Substitute, Open Approach

05R80JZ   Replacement of Left Axillary Vein with Synthetic Substitute, Open Approach

05R80KZ   Replacement of Left Axillary Vein with Nonautologous Tissue Substitute, Open Approach

05R847Z   Replacement of Left Axillary Vein with Autologous Tissue Substitute, Percutaneous Endoscopic Approach

05R84JZ   Replacement of Left Axillary Vein with Synthetic Substitute, Percutaneous Endoscopic Approach

05R84KZ   Replacement of Left Axillary Vein with Nonautologous Tissue Substitute, Percutaneous Endoscopic Approach

05R907Z   Replacement of Right Brachial Vein with Autologous Tissue Substitute, Open Approach

05R90JZ   Replacement of Right Brachial Vein with Synthetic Substitute, Open Approach

05R90KZ   Replacement of Right Brachial Vein with Nonautologous Tissue Substitute, Open Approach

05R947Z   Replacement of Right Brachial Vein with Autologous Tissue Substitute, Percutaneous Endoscopic Approach

05R94JZ   Replacement of Right Brachial Vein with Synthetic Substitute, Percutaneous Endoscopic Approach

05R94KZ   Replacement of Right Brachial Vein with Nonautologous Tissue Substitute, Percutaneous Endoscopic Approach

05RA07Z   Replacement of Left Brachial Vein with Autologous Tissue Substitute, Open Approach

05RA0JZ   Replacement of Left Brachial Vein with Synthetic Substitute, Open Approach

05RA0KZ   Replacement of Left Brachial Vein with Nonautologous Tissue Substitute, Open Approach

05RA47Z   Replacement of Left Brachial Vein with Autologous Tissue Substitute, Percutaneous Endoscopic Approach

05RA4JZ   Replacement of Left Brachial Vein with Synthetic Substitute, Percutaneous Endoscopic Approach

05RA4KZ   Replacement of Left Brachial Vein with Nonautologous Tissue Substitute, Percutaneous Endoscopic Approach

05RB07Z   Replacement of Right Basilic Vein with Autologous Tissue Substitute, Open Approach

05RB0JZ   Replacement of Right Basilic Vein with Synthetic Substitute, Open Approach

05RB0KZ   Replacement of Right Basilic Vein with Nonautologous Tissue Substitute, Open Approach

05RB47Z   Replacement of Right Basilic Vein with Autologous Tissue Substitute, Percutaneous Endoscopic Approach

05RB4JZ   Replacement of Right Basilic Vein with Synthetic Substitute, Percutaneous Endoscopic Approach

05RB4KZ   Replacement of Right Basilic Vein with Nonautologous Tissue Substitute, Percutaneous Endoscopic Approach

05RC07Z   Replacement of Left Basilic Vein with Autologous Tissue Substitute, Open Approach

05RC0JZ   Replacement of Left Basilic Vein with Synthetic Substitute, Open Approach

05RC0KZ   Replacement of Left Basilic Vein with Nonautologous Tissue Substitute, Open Approach

05RC47Z   Replacement of Left Basilic Vein with Autologous Tissue Substitute, Percutaneous Endoscopic Approach

05RC4JZ   Replacement of Left Basilic Vein with Synthetic Substitute, Percutaneous Endoscopic Approach

05RC4KZ   Replacement of Left Basilic Vein with Nonautologous Tissue Substitute, Percutaneous Endoscopic Approach

05RD07Z   Replacement of Right Cephalic Vein with Autologous Tissue Substitute, Open Approach

05RD0JZ   Replacement of Right Cephalic Vein with Synthetic Substitute, Open Approach

05RD0KZ   Replacement of Right Cephalic Vein with Nonautologous Tissue Substitute, Open Approach

05RD47Z   Replacement of Right Cephalic Vein with Autologous Tissue Substitute, Percutaneous Endoscopic Approach

05RD4JZ   Replacement of Right Cephalic Vein with Synthetic Substitute, Percutaneous Endoscopic Approach

05RD4KZ   Replacement of Right Cephalic Vein with Nonautologous Tissue Substitute, Percutaneous Endoscopic Approach

05RF07Z   Replacement of Left Cephalic Vein with Autologous Tissue Substitute, Open Approach

05RF0JZ   Replacement of Left Cephalic Vein with Synthetic Substitute, Open Approach

05RF0KZ   Replacement of Left Cephalic Vein with Nonautologous Tissue Substitute, Open Approach

05RF47Z   Replacement of Left Cephalic Vein with Autologous Tissue Substitute, Percutaneous Endoscopic Approach

05RF4JZ   Replacement of Left Cephalic Vein with Synthetic Substitute, Percutaneous Endoscopic Approach

05RF4KZ   Replacement of Left Cephalic Vein with Nonautologous Tissue Substitute, Percutaneous Endoscopic Approach

05RG07Z   Replacement of Right Hand Vein with Autologous Tissue Substitute, Open Approach

05RG0JZ   Replacement of Right Hand Vein with Synthetic Substitute, Open Approach

05RG0KZ   Replacement of Right Hand Vein with Nonautologous Tissue Substitute, Open Approach

05RG47Z   Replacement of Right Hand Vein with Autologous Tissue Substitute, Percutaneous Endoscopic Approach

05RG4JZ   Replacement of Right Hand Vein with Synthetic Substitute, Percutaneous Endoscopic Approach

05RG4KZ   Replacement of Right Hand Vein with Nonautologous Tissue Substitute, Percutaneous Endoscopic Approach

05RH07Z   Replacement of Left Hand Vein with Autologous Tissue Substitute, Open Approach

05RH0JZ   Replacement of Left Hand Vein with Synthetic Substitute, Open Approach

05RH0KZ   Replacement of Left Hand Vein with Nonautologous Tissue Substitute, Open Approach

05RH47Z   Replacement of Left Hand Vein with Autologous Tissue Substitute, Percutaneous Endoscopic Approach

05RH4JZ   Replacement of Left Hand Vein with Synthetic Substitute, Percutaneous Endoscopic Approach

05RH4KZ   Replacement of Left Hand Vein with Nonautologous Tissue Substitute, Percutaneous Endoscopic Approach

05RL07Z   Replacement of Intracranial Vein with Autologous Tissue Substitute, Open Approach

05RL0JZ   Replacement of Intracranial Vein with Synthetic Substitute, Open Approach

05RL0KZ   Replacement of Intracranial Vein with Nonautologous Tissue Substitute, Open Approach

05RL47Z   Replacement of Intracranial Vein with Autologous Tissue Substitute, Percutaneous Endoscopic Approach

05RL4JZ   Replacement of Intracranial Vein with Synthetic Substitute, Percutaneous Endoscopic Approach

05RL4KZ   Replacement of Intracranial Vein with Nonautologous Tissue Substitute, Percutaneous Endoscopic Approach

05RM07Z   Replacement of Right Internal Jugular Vein with Autologous Tissue Substitute, Open Approach
05RM0JZ   Replacement of Right Internal Jugular Vein with Synthetic Substitute, Open Approach
05RM0KZ   Replacement of Right Internal Jugular Vein with Nonautologous Tissue Substitute, Open Approach
05RM47Z   Replacement of Right Internal Jugular Vein with Autologous Tissue Substitute, Percutaneous Endoscopic Approach
05RM4JZ   Replacement of Right Internal Jugular Vein with Synthetic Substitute, Percutaneous Endoscopic Approach
05RM4KZ   Replacement of Right Internal Jugular Vein with Nonautologous Tissue Substitute, Percutaneous Endoscopic Approach
05RN07Z   Replacement of Left Internal Jugular Vein with Autologous Tissue Substitute, Open Approach
05RN0JZ   Replacement of Left Internal Jugular Vein with Synthetic Substitute, Open Approach
05RN0KZ   Replacement of Left Internal Jugular Vein with Nonautologous Tissue Substitute, Open Approach
05RN47Z   Replacement of Left Internal Jugular Vein with Autologous Tissue Substitute, Percutaneous Endoscopic Approach
05RN4JZ   Replacement of Left Internal Jugular Vein with Synthetic Substitute, Percutaneous Endoscopic Approach
05RN4KZ   Replacement of Left Internal Jugular Vein with Nonautologous Tissue Substitute, Percutaneous Endoscopic Approach
05RP07Z   Replacement of Right External Jugular Vein with Autologous Tissue Substitute, Open Approach
05RP0JZ   Replacement of Right External Jugular Vein with Synthetic Substitute, Open Approach
05RP0KZ   Replacement of Right External Jugular Vein with Nonautologous Tissue Substitute, Open Approach
05RP47Z   Replacement of Right External Jugular Vein with Autologous Tissue Substitute, Percutaneous Endoscopic Approach
05RP4JZ   Replacement of Right External Jugular Vein with Synthetic Substitute, Percutaneous Endoscopic Approach
05RP4KZ   Replacement of Right External Jugular Vein with Nonautologous Tissue Substitute, Percutaneous Endoscopic Approach
05RQ07Z   Replacement of Left External Jugular Vein with Autologous Tissue Substitute, Open Approach
05RQ0JZ   Replacement of Left External Jugular Vein with Synthetic Substitute, Open Approach
05RQ0KZ   Replacement of Left External Jugular Vein with Nonautologous Tissue Substitute, Open Approach
05RQ47Z   Replacement of Left External Jugular Vein with Autologous Tissue Substitute, Percutaneous Endoscopic Approach
05RQ4JZ   Replacement of Left External Jugular Vein with Synthetic Substitute, Percutaneous Endoscopic Approach
05RQ4KZ   Replacement of Left External Jugular Vein with Nonautologous Tissue Substitute, Percutaneous Endoscopic Approach
05RR07Z   Replacement of Right Vertebral Vein with Autologous Tissue Substitute, Open Approach
05RR0JZ   Replacement of Right Vertebral Vein with Synthetic Substitute, Open Approach
05RR0KZ   Replacement of Right Vertebral Vein with Nonautologous Tissue Substitute, Open Approach

05RR47Z   Replacement of Right Vertebral Vein with Autologous Tissue Substitute, Percutaneous Endoscopic Approach
05RR4JZ   Replacement of Right Vertebral Vein with Synthetic Substitute, Percutaneous Endoscopic Approach
05RR4KZ   Replacement of Right Vertebral Vein with Nonautologous Tissue Substitute, Percutaneous Endoscopic Approach
05RS07Z   Replacement of Left Vertebral Vein with Autologous Tissue Substitute, Open Approach
05RS0JZ   Replacement of Left Vertebral Vein with Synthetic Substitute, Open Approach
05RS0KZ   Replacement of Left Vertebral Vein with Nonautologous Tissue Substitute, Open Approach
05RS47Z   Replacement of Left Vertebral Vein with Autologous Tissue Substitute, Percutaneous Endoscopic Approach
05RS4JZ   Replacement of Left Vertebral Vein with Synthetic Substitute, Percutaneous Endoscopic Approach
05RS4KZ   Replacement of Left Vertebral Vein with Nonautologous Tissue Substitute, Percutaneous Endoscopic Approach
05RT07Z   Replacement of Right Face Vein with Autologous Tissue Substitute, Open Approach
05RT0JZ   Replacement of Right Face Vein with Synthetic Substitute, Open Approach
05RT0KZ   Replacement of Right Face Vein with Nonautologous Tissue Substitute, Open Approach
05RT47Z   Replacement of Right Face Vein with Autologous Tissue Substitute, Percutaneous Endoscopic Approach
05RT4JZ   Replacement of Right Face Vein with Synthetic Substitute, Percutaneous Endoscopic Approach
05RT4KZ   Replacement of Right Face Vein with Nonautologous Tissue Substitute, Percutaneous Endoscopic Approach
05RV07Z   Replacement of Left Face Vein with Autologous Tissue Substitute, Open Approach
05RV0JZ   Replacement of Left Face Vein with Synthetic Substitute, Open Approach
05RV0KZ   Replacement of Left Face Vein with Nonautologous Tissue Substitute, Open Approach
05RV47Z   Replacement of Left Face Vein with Autologous Tissue Substitute, Percutaneous Endoscopic Approach
05RV4JZ   Replacement of Left Face Vein with Synthetic Substitute, Percutaneous Endoscopic Approach
05RV4KZ   Replacement of Left Face Vein with Nonautologous Tissue Substitute, Percutaneous Endoscopic Approach
05RY07Z   Replacement of Upper Vein with Autologous Tissue Substitute, Open Approach
05RY0JZ   Replacement of Upper Vein with Synthetic Substitute, Open Approach
05RY0KZ   Replacement of Upper Vein with Nonautologous Tissue Substitute, Open Approach
05RY47Z   Replacement of Upper Vein with Autologous Tissue Substitute, Percutaneous Endoscopic Approach
05RY4JZ   Replacement of Upper Vein with Synthetic Substitute, Percutaneous Endoscopic Approach
05RY4KZ   Replacement of Upper Vein with Nonautologous Tissue Substitute, Percutaneous Endoscopic Approach

05S – Upper Veins, Reposition

05S00ZZ   Reposition Azygos Vein, Open Approach
05S03ZZ   Reposition Azygos Vein, Percutaneous Approach
05S04ZZ   Reposition Azygos Vein, Percutaneous Endoscopic Approach
05S10ZZ   Reposition Hemiazygos Vein, Open Approach
05S13ZZ   Reposition Hemiazygos Vein, Percutaneous Approach
05S14ZZ   Reposition Hemiazygos Vein, Percutaneous Endoscopic Approach
05S30ZZ   Reposition Right Innominate Vein, Open Approach
05S33ZZ   Reposition Right Innominate Vein, Percutaneous Approach
05S34ZZ   Reposition Right Innominate Vein, Percutaneous Endoscopic Approach
05S40ZZ   Reposition Left Innominate Vein, Open Approach
05S43ZZ   Reposition Left Innominate Vein, Percutaneous Approach
05S44ZZ   Reposition Left Innominate Vein, Percutaneous Endoscopic Approach
05S50ZZ   Reposition Right Subclavian Vein, Open Approach
05S53ZZ   Reposition Right Subclavian Vein, Percutaneous Approach

05S54ZZ   Reposition Right Subclavian Vein, Percutaneous Endoscopic Approach
05S60ZZ   Reposition Left Subclavian Vein, Open Approach
05S63ZZ   Reposition Left Subclavian Vein, Percutaneous Approach
05S64ZZ   Reposition Left Subclavian Vein, Percutaneous Endoscopic Approach
05S70ZZ   Reposition Right Axillary Vein, Open Approach
05S73ZZ   Reposition Right Axillary Vein, Percutaneous Approach
05S74ZZ   Reposition Right Axillary Vein, Percutaneous Endoscopic Approach
05S80ZZ   Reposition Left Axillary Vein, Open Approach
05S83ZZ   Reposition Left Axillary Vein, Percutaneous Approach
05S84ZZ   Reposition Left Axillary Vein, Percutaneous Endoscopic Approach
05S90ZZ   Reposition Right Brachial Vein, Open Approach
05S93ZZ   Reposition Right Brachial Vein, Percutaneous Approach
05S94ZZ   Reposition Right Brachial Vein, Percutaneous Endoscopic Approach
05SA0ZZ   Reposition Left Brachial Vein, Open Approach

05SA3ZZ   Reposition Left Brachial Vein, Percutaneous Approach
05SA4ZZ   Reposition Left Brachial Vein, Percutaneous Endoscopic Approach
05SB0ZZ   Reposition Right Basilic Vein, Open Approach
05SB3ZZ   Reposition Right Basilic Vein, Percutaneous Approach
05SB4ZZ   Reposition Right Basilic Vein, Percutaneous Endoscopic Approach
05SC0ZZ   Reposition Left Basilic Vein, Open Approach
05SC3ZZ   Reposition Left Basilic Vein, Percutaneous Approach
05SC4ZZ   Reposition Left Basilic Vein, Percutaneous Endoscopic Approach
05SD0ZZ   Reposition Right Cephalic Vein, Open Approach
05SD3ZZ   Reposition Right Cephalic Vein, Percutaneous Approach
05SD4ZZ   Reposition Right Cephalic Vein, Percutaneous Endoscopic Approach
05SF0ZZ   Reposition Left Cephalic Vein, Open Approach
05SF3ZZ   Reposition Left Cephalic Vein, Percutaneous Approach
05SF4ZZ   Reposition Left Cephalic Vein, Percutaneous Endoscopic Approach
05SG0ZZ   Reposition Right Hand Vein, Open Approach
05SG3ZZ   Reposition Right Hand Vein, Percutaneous Approach
05SG4ZZ   Reposition Right Hand Vein, Percutaneous Endoscopic Approach
05SH0ZZ   Reposition Left Hand Vein, Open Approach
05SH3ZZ   Reposition Left Hand Vein, Percutaneous Approach
05SH4ZZ   Reposition Left Hand Vein, Percutaneous Endoscopic Approach
05SL0ZZ   Reposition Intracranial Vein, Open Approach
05SL3ZZ   Reposition Intracranial Vein, Percutaneous Approach
05SL4ZZ   Reposition Intracranial Vein, Percutaneous Endoscopic Approach
05SM0ZZ   Reposition Right Internal Jugular Vein, Open Approach
05SM3ZZ   Reposition Right Internal Jugular Vein, Percutaneous Approach
05SM4ZZ   Reposition Right Internal Jugular Vein, Percutaneous Endoscopic Approach

05SN0ZZ   Reposition Left Internal Jugular Vein, Open Approach
05SN3ZZ   Reposition Left Internal Jugular Vein, Percutaneous Approach
05SN4ZZ   Reposition Left Internal Jugular Vein, Percutaneous Endoscopic Approach
05SP0ZZ   Reposition Right External Jugular Vein, Open Approach
05SP3ZZ   Reposition Right External Jugular Vein, Percutaneous Approach
05SP4ZZ   Reposition Right External Jugular Vein, Percutaneous Endoscopic Approach
05SQ0ZZ   Reposition Left External Jugular Vein, Open Approach
05SQ3ZZ   Reposition Left External Jugular Vein, Percutaneous Approach
05SQ4ZZ   Reposition Left External Jugular Vein, Percutaneous Endoscopic Approach
05SR0ZZ   Reposition Right Vertebral Vein, Open Approach
05SR3ZZ   Reposition Right Vertebral Vein, Percutaneous Approach
05SR4ZZ   Reposition Right Vertebral Vein, Percutaneous Endoscopic Approach
05SS0ZZ   Reposition Left Vertebral Vein, Open Approach
05SS3ZZ   Reposition Left Vertebral Vein, Percutaneous Approach
05SS4ZZ   Reposition Left Vertebral Vein, Percutaneous Endoscopic Approach
05ST0ZZ   Reposition Right Face Vein, Open Approach
05ST3ZZ   Reposition Right Face Vein, Percutaneous Approach
05ST4ZZ   Reposition Right Face Vein, Percutaneous Endoscopic Approach
05SV0ZZ   Reposition Left Face Vein, Open Approach
05SV3ZZ   Reposition Left Face Vein, Percutaneous Approach
05SV4ZZ   Reposition Left Face Vein, Percutaneous Endoscopic Approach
05SY0ZZ   Reposition Upper Vein, Open Approach
05SY3ZZ   Reposition Upper Vein, Percutaneous Approach
05SY4ZZ   Reposition Upper Vein, Percutaneous Endoscopic Approach

05U – Upper Veins, Supplement

05U007Z   Supplement Azygos Vein with Autologous Tissue Substitute, Open Approach
05U00JZ   Supplement Azygos Vein with Synthetic Substitute, Open Approach
05U00KZ   Supplement Azygos Vein with Nonautologous Tissue Substitute, Open Approach
05U037Z   Supplement Azygos Vein with Autologous Tissue Substitute, Percutaneous Approach
05U03JZ   Supplement Azygos Vein with Synthetic Substitute, Percutaneous Approach
05U03KZ   Supplement Azygos Vein with Nonautologous Tissue Substitute, Percutaneous Approach
05U047Z   Supplement Azygos Vein with Autologous Tissue Substitute, Percutaneous Endoscopic Approach
05U04JZ   Supplement Azygos Vein with Synthetic Substitute, Percutaneous Endoscopic Approach
05U04KZ   Supplement Azygos Vein with Nonautologous Tissue Substitute, Percutaneous Endoscopic Approach
05U107Z   Supplement Hemiazygos Vein with Autologous Tissue Substitute, Open Approach
05U10JZ   Supplement Hemiazygos Vein with Synthetic Substitute, Open Approach
05U10KZ   Supplement Hemiazygos Vein with Nonautologous Tissue Substitute, Open Approach
05U137Z   Supplement Hemiazygos Vein with Autologous Tissue Substitute, Percutaneous Approach
05U13JZ   Supplement Hemiazygos Vein with Synthetic Substitute, Percutaneous Approach
05U13KZ   Supplement Hemiazygos Vein with Nonautologous Tissue Substitute, Percutaneous Approach
05U147Z   Supplement Hemiazygos Vein with Autologous Tissue Substitute, Percutaneous Endoscopic Approach
05U14JZ   Supplement Hemiazygos Vein with Synthetic Substitute, Percutaneous Endoscopic Approach
05U14KZ   Supplement Hemiazygos Vein with Nonautologous Tissue Substitute, Percutaneous Endoscopic Approach
05U307Z   Supplement Right Innominate Vein with Autologous Tissue Substitute, Open Approach
05U30JZ   Supplement Right Innominate Vein with Synthetic Substitute, Open Approach
05U30KZ   Supplement Right Innominate Vein with Nonautologous Tissue Substitute, Open Approach
05U337Z   Supplement Right Innominate Vein with Autologous Tissue Substitute, Percutaneous Approach

05U33JZ   Supplement Right Innominate Vein with Synthetic Substitute, Percutaneous Approach
05U33KZ   Supplement Right Innominate Vein with Nonautologous Tissue Substitute, Percutaneous Approach
05U347Z   Supplement Right Innominate Vein with Autologous Tissue Substitute, Percutaneous Endoscopic Approach
05U34JZ   Supplement Right Innominate Vein with Synthetic Substitute, Percutaneous Endoscopic Approach
05U34KZ   Supplement Right Innominate Vein with Nonautologous Tissue Substitute, Percutaneous Endoscopic Approach
05U407Z   Supplement Left Innominate Vein with Autologous Tissue Substitute, Open Approach
05U40JZ   Supplement Left Innominate Vein with Synthetic Substitute, Open Approach
05U40KZ   Supplement Left Innominate Vein with Nonautologous Tissue Substitute, Open Approach
05U437Z   Supplement Left Innominate Vein with Autologous Tissue Substitute, Percutaneous Approach
05U43JZ   Supplement Left Innominate Vein with Synthetic Substitute, Percutaneous Approach
05U43KZ   Supplement Left Innominate Vein with Nonautologous Tissue Substitute, Percutaneous Approach
05U447Z   Supplement Left Innominate Vein with Autologous Tissue Substitute, Percutaneous Endoscopic Approach
05U44JZ   Supplement Left Innominate Vein with Synthetic Substitute, Percutaneous Endoscopic Approach
05U44KZ   Supplement Left Innominate Vein with Nonautologous Tissue Substitute, Percutaneous Endoscopic Approach
05U507Z   Supplement Right Subclavian Vein with Autologous Tissue Substitute, Open Approach
05U50JZ   Supplement Right Subclavian Vein with Synthetic Substitute, Open Approach
05U50KZ   Supplement Right Subclavian Vein with Nonautologous Tissue Substitute, Open Approach
05U537Z   Supplement Right Subclavian Vein with Autologous Tissue Substitute, Percutaneous Approach
05U53JZ   Supplement Right Subclavian Vein with Synthetic Substitute, Percutaneous Approach
05U53KZ   Supplement Right Subclavian Vein with Nonautologous Tissue Substitute, Percutaneous Approach
05U547Z   Supplement Right Subclavian Vein with Autologous Tissue Substitute, Percutaneous Endoscopic Approach

05U54JZ Supplement Right Subclavian Vein with Synthetic Substitute, Percutaneous Endoscopic Approach

05U54KZ Supplement Right Subclavian Vein with Nonautologous Tissue Substitute, Percutaneous Endoscopic Approach

05U607Z Supplement Left Subclavian Vein with Autologous Tissue Substitute, Open Approach

05U60JZ Supplement Left Subclavian Vein with Synthetic Substitute, Open Approach

05U60KZ Supplement Left Subclavian Vein with Nonautologous Tissue Substitute, Open Approach

05U637Z Supplement Left Subclavian Vein with Autologous Tissue Substitute, Percutaneous Approach

05U63JZ Supplement Left Subclavian Vein with Synthetic Substitute, Percutaneous Approach

05U63KZ Supplement Left Subclavian Vein with Nonautologous Tissue Substitute, Percutaneous Approach

05U647Z Supplement Left Subclavian Vein with Autologous Tissue Substitute, Percutaneous Endoscopic Approach

05U64JZ Supplement Left Subclavian Vein with Synthetic Substitute, Percutaneous Endoscopic Approach

05U64KZ Supplement Left Subclavian Vein with Nonautologous Tissue Substitute, Percutaneous Endoscopic Approach

05U707Z Supplement Right Axillary Vein with Autologous Tissue Substitute, Open Approach

05U70JZ Supplement Right Axillary Vein with Synthetic Substitute, Open Approach

05U70KZ Supplement Right Axillary Vein with Nonautologous Tissue Substitute, Open Approach

05U737Z Supplement Right Axillary Vein with Autologous Tissue Substitute, Percutaneous Approach

05U73JZ Supplement Right Axillary Vein with Synthetic Substitute, Percutaneous Approach

05U73KZ Supplement Right Axillary Vein with Nonautologous Tissue Substitute, Percutaneous Approach

05U747Z Supplement Right Axillary Vein with Autologous Tissue Substitute, Percutaneous Endoscopic Approach

05U74JZ Supplement Right Axillary Vein with Synthetic Substitute, Percutaneous Endoscopic Approach

05U74KZ Supplement Right Axillary Vein with Nonautologous Tissue Substitute, Percutaneous Endoscopic Approach

05U807Z Supplement Left Axillary Vein with Autologous Tissue Substitute, Open Approach

05U80JZ Supplement Left Axillary Vein with Synthetic Substitute, Open Approach

05U80KZ Supplement Left Axillary Vein with Nonautologous Tissue Substitute, Open Approach

05U837Z Supplement Left Axillary Vein with Autologous Tissue Substitute, Percutaneous Approach

05U83JZ Supplement Left Axillary Vein with Synthetic Substitute, Percutaneous Approach

05U83KZ Supplement Left Axillary Vein with Nonautologous Tissue Substitute, Percutaneous Approach

05U847Z Supplement Left Axillary Vein with Autologous Tissue Substitute, Percutaneous Endoscopic Approach

05U84JZ Supplement Left Axillary Vein with Synthetic Substitute, Percutaneous Endoscopic Approach

05U84KZ Supplement Left Axillary Vein with Nonautologous Tissue Substitute, Percutaneous Endoscopic Approach

05U907Z Supplement Right Brachial Vein with Autologous Tissue Substitute, Open Approach

05U90JZ Supplement Right Brachial Vein with Synthetic Substitute, Open Approach

05U90KZ Supplement Right Brachial Vein with Nonautologous Tissue Substitute, Open Approach

05U937Z Supplement Right Brachial Vein with Autologous Tissue Substitute, Percutaneous Approach

05U93JZ Supplement Right Brachial Vein with Synthetic Substitute, Percutaneous Approach

05U93KZ Supplement Right Brachial Vein with Nonautologous Tissue Substitute, Percutaneous Approach

05U947Z Supplement Right Brachial Vein with Autologous Tissue Substitute, Percutaneous Endoscopic Approach

05U94JZ Supplement Right Brachial Vein with Synthetic Substitute, Percutaneous Endoscopic Approach

05U94KZ Supplement Right Brachial Vein with Nonautologous Tissue Substitute, Percutaneous Endoscopic Approach

05UA07Z Supplement Left Brachial Vein with Autologous Tissue Substitute, Open Approach

05UA0JZ Supplement Left Brachial Vein with Synthetic Substitute, Open Approach

05UA0KZ Supplement Left Brachial Vein with Nonautologous Tissue Substitute, Open Approach

05UA37Z Supplement Left Brachial Vein with Autologous Tissue Substitute, Percutaneous Approach

05UA3JZ Supplement Left Brachial Vein with Synthetic Substitute, Percutaneous Approach

05UA3KZ Supplement Left Brachial Vein with Nonautologous Tissue Substitute, Percutaneous Approach

05UA47Z Supplement Left Brachial Vein with Autologous Tissue Substitute, Percutaneous Endoscopic Approach

05UA4JZ Supplement Left Brachial Vein with Synthetic Substitute, Percutaneous Endoscopic Approach

05UA4KZ Supplement Left Brachial Vein with Nonautologous Tissue Substitute, Percutaneous Endoscopic Approach

05UB07Z Supplement Right Basilic Vein with Autologous Tissue Substitute, Open Approach

05UB0JZ Supplement Right Basilic Vein with Synthetic Substitute, Open Approach

05UB0KZ Supplement Right Basilic Vein with Nonautologous Tissue Substitute, Open Approach

05UB37Z Supplement Right Basilic Vein with Autologous Tissue Substitute, Percutaneous Approach

05UB3JZ Supplement Right Basilic Vein with Synthetic Substitute, Percutaneous Approach

05UB3KZ Supplement Right Basilic Vein with Nonautologous Tissue Substitute, Percutaneous Approach

05UB47Z Supplement Right Basilic Vein with Autologous Tissue Substitute, Percutaneous Endoscopic Approach

05UB4JZ Supplement Right Basilic Vein with Synthetic Substitute, Percutaneous Endoscopic Approach

05UB4KZ Supplement Right Basilic Vein with Nonautologous Tissue Substitute, Percutaneous Endoscopic Approach

05UC07Z Supplement Left Basilic Vein with Autologous Tissue Substitute, Open Approach

05UC0JZ Supplement Left Basilic Vein with Synthetic Substitute, Open Approach

05UC0KZ Supplement Left Basilic Vein with Nonautologous Tissue Substitute, Open Approach

05UC37Z Supplement Left Basilic Vein with Autologous Tissue Substitute, Percutaneous Approach

05UC3JZ Supplement Left Basilic Vein with Synthetic Substitute, Percutaneous Approach

05UC3KZ Supplement Left Basilic Vein with Nonautologous Tissue Substitute, Percutaneous Approach

05UC47Z Supplement Left Basilic Vein with Autologous Tissue Substitute, Percutaneous Endoscopic Approach

05UC4JZ Supplement Left Basilic Vein with Synthetic Substitute, Percutaneous Endoscopic Approach

05UC4KZ Supplement Left Basilic Vein with Nonautologous Tissue Substitute, Percutaneous Endoscopic Approach

05UD07Z Supplement Right Cephalic Vein with Autologous Tissue Substitute, Open Approach

05UD0JZ Supplement Right Cephalic Vein with Synthetic Substitute, Open Approach

05UD0KZ Supplement Right Cephalic Vein with Nonautologous Tissue Substitute, Open Approach

05UD37Z Supplement Right Cephalic Vein with Autologous Tissue Substitute, Percutaneous Approach

05UD3JZ Supplement Right Cephalic Vein with Synthetic Substitute, Percutaneous Approach

05UD3KZ Supplement Right Cephalic Vein with Nonautologous Tissue Substitute, Percutaneous Approach

05UD47Z Supplement Right Cephalic Vein with Autologous Tissue Substitute, Percutaneous Endoscopic Approach

05UD4JZ Supplement Right Cephalic Vein with Synthetic Substitute, Percutaneous Endoscopic Approach

05UD4KZ Supplement Right Cephalic Vein with Nonautologous Tissue Substitute, Percutaneous Endoscopic Approach

---

♀ Female-only   ♂ Male-only   ● Limited Coverage   ● Non-OR   ▨ HAC-associated procedure   ● Non-covered procedures   ✚ Combination

05UF07Z   Supplement Left Cephalic Vein with Autologous Tissue Substitute, Open Approach

05UF0JZ   Supplement Left Cephalic Vein with Synthetic Substitute, Open Approach

05UF0KZ   Supplement Left Cephalic Vein with Nonautologous Tissue Substitute, Open Approach

05UF37Z   Supplement Left Cephalic Vein with Autologous Tissue Substitute, Percutaneous Approach

05UF3JZ   Supplement Left Cephalic Vein with Synthetic Substitute, Percutaneous Approach

05UF3KZ   Supplement Left Cephalic Vein with Nonautologous Tissue Substitute, Percutaneous Approach

05UF47Z   Supplement Left Cephalic Vein with Autologous Tissue Substitute, Percutaneous Endoscopic Approach

05UF4JZ   Supplement Left Cephalic Vein with Synthetic Substitute, Percutaneous Endoscopic Approach

05UF4KZ   Supplement Left Cephalic Vein with Nonautologous Tissue Substitute, Percutaneous Endoscopic Approach

05UG07Z   Supplement Right Hand Vein with Autologous Tissue Substitute, Open Approach

05UG0JZ   Supplement Right Hand Vein with Synthetic Substitute, Open Approach

05UG0KZ   Supplement Right Hand Vein with Nonautologous Tissue Substitute, Open Approach

05UG37Z   Supplement Right Hand Vein with Autologous Tissue Substitute, Percutaneous Approach

05UG3JZ   Supplement Right Hand Vein with Synthetic Substitute, Percutaneous Approach

05UG3KZ   Supplement Right Hand Vein with Nonautologous Tissue Substitute, Percutaneous Approach

05UG47Z   Supplement Right Hand Vein with Autologous Tissue Substitute, Percutaneous Endoscopic Approach

05UG4JZ   Supplement Right Hand Vein with Synthetic Substitute, Percutaneous Endoscopic Approach

05UG4KZ   Supplement Right Hand Vein with Nonautologous Tissue Substitute, Percutaneous Endoscopic Approach

05UH07Z   Supplement Left Hand Vein with Autologous Tissue Substitute, Open Approach

05UH0JZ   Supplement Left Hand Vein with Synthetic Substitute, Open Approach

05UH0KZ   Supplement Left Hand Vein with Nonautologous Tissue Substitute, Open Approach

05UH37Z   Supplement Left Hand Vein with Autologous Tissue Substitute, Percutaneous Approach

05UH3JZ   Supplement Left Hand Vein with Synthetic Substitute, Percutaneous Approach

05UH3KZ   Supplement Left Hand Vein with Nonautologous Tissue Substitute, Percutaneous Approach

05UH47Z   Supplement Left Hand Vein with Autologous Tissue Substitute, Percutaneous Endoscopic Approach

05UH4JZ   Supplement Left Hand Vein with Synthetic Substitute, Percutaneous Endoscopic Approach

05UH4KZ   Supplement Left Hand Vein with Nonautologous Tissue Substitute, Percutaneous Endoscopic Approach

05UL07Z   Supplement Intracranial Vein with Autologous Tissue Substitute, Open Approach

05UL0JZ   Supplement Intracranial Vein with Synthetic Substitute, Open Approach

05UL0KZ   Supplement Intracranial Vein with Nonautologous Tissue Substitute, Open Approach

05UL37Z   Supplement Intracranial Vein with Autologous Tissue Substitute, Percutaneous Approach

05UL3JZ   Supplement Intracranial Vein with Synthetic Substitute, Percutaneous Approach

05UL3KZ   Supplement Intracranial Vein with Nonautologous Tissue Substitute, Percutaneous Approach

05UL47Z   Supplement Intracranial Vein with Autologous Tissue Substitute, Percutaneous Endoscopic Approach

05UL4JZ   Supplement Intracranial Vein with Synthetic Substitute, Percutaneous Endoscopic Approach

05UL4KZ   Supplement Intracranial Vein with Nonautologous Tissue Substitute, Percutaneous Endoscopic Approach

05UM07Z   Supplement Right Internal Jugular Vein with Autologous Tissue Substitute, Open Approach

05UM0JZ   Supplement Right Internal Jugular Vein with Synthetic Substitute, Open Approach

05UM0KZ   Supplement Right Internal Jugular Vein with Nonautologous Tissue Substitute, Open Approach

05UM37Z   Supplement Right Internal Jugular Vein with Autologous Tissue Substitute, Percutaneous Approach

05UM3JZ   Supplement Right Internal Jugular Vein with Synthetic Substitute, Percutaneous Approach

05UM3KZ   Supplement Right Internal Jugular Vein with Nonautologous Tissue Substitute, Percutaneous Approach

05UM47Z   Supplement Right Internal Jugular Vein with Autologous Tissue Substitute, Percutaneous Endoscopic Approach

05UM4JZ   Supplement Right Internal Jugular Vein with Synthetic Substitute, Percutaneous Endoscopic Approach

05UM4KZ   Supplement Right Internal Jugular Vein with Nonautologous Tissue Substitute, Percutaneous Endoscopic Approach

05UN07Z   Supplement Left Internal Jugular Vein with Autologous Tissue Substitute, Open Approach

05UN0JZ   Supplement Left Internal Jugular Vein with Synthetic Substitute, Open Approach

05UN0KZ   Supplement Left Internal Jugular Vein with Nonautologous Tissue Substitute, Open Approach

05UN37Z   Supplement Left Internal Jugular Vein with Autologous Tissue Substitute, Percutaneous Approach

05UN3JZ   Supplement Left Internal Jugular Vein with Synthetic Substitute, Percutaneous Approach

05UN3KZ   Supplement Left Internal Jugular Vein with Nonautologous Tissue Substitute, Percutaneous Approach

05UN47Z   Supplement Left Internal Jugular Vein with Autologous Tissue Substitute, Percutaneous Endoscopic Approach

05UN4JZ   Supplement Left Internal Jugular Vein with Synthetic Substitute, Percutaneous Endoscopic Approach

05UN4KZ   Supplement Left Internal Jugular Vein with Nonautologous Tissue Substitute, Percutaneous Endoscopic Approach

05UP07Z   Supplement Right External Jugular Vein with Autologous Tissue Substitute, Open Approach

05UP0JZ   Supplement Right External Jugular Vein with Synthetic Substitute, Open Approach

05UP0KZ   Supplement Right External Jugular Vein with Nonautologous Tissue Substitute, Open Approach

05UP37Z   Supplement Right External Jugular Vein with Autologous Tissue Substitute, Percutaneous Approach

05UP3JZ   Supplement Right External Jugular Vein with Synthetic Substitute, Percutaneous Approach

05UP3KZ   Supplement Right External Jugular Vein with Nonautologous Tissue Substitute, Percutaneous Approach

05UP47Z   Supplement Right External Jugular Vein with Autologous Tissue Substitute, Percutaneous Endoscopic Approach

05UP4JZ   Supplement Right External Jugular Vein with Synthetic Substitute, Percutaneous Endoscopic Approach

05UP4KZ   Supplement Right External Jugular Vein with Nonautologous Tissue Substitute, Percutaneous Endoscopic Approach

05UQ07Z   Supplement Left External Jugular Vein with Autologous Tissue Substitute, Open Approach

05UQ0JZ   Supplement Left External Jugular Vein with Synthetic Substitute, Open Approach

05UQ0KZ   Supplement Left External Jugular Vein with Nonautologous Tissue Substitute, Open Approach

05UQ37Z   Supplement Left External Jugular Vein with Autologous Tissue Substitute, Percutaneous Approach

05UQ3JZ   Supplement Left External Jugular Vein with Synthetic Substitute, Percutaneous Approach

05UQ3KZ   Supplement Left External Jugular Vein with Nonautologous Tissue Substitute, Percutaneous Approach

05UQ47Z   Supplement Left External Jugular Vein with Autologous Tissue Substitute, Percutaneous Endoscopic Approach

05UQ4JZ   Supplement Left External Jugular Vein with Synthetic Substitute, Percutaneous Endoscopic Approach

05UQ4KZ   Supplement Left External Jugular Vein with Nonautologous Tissue Substitute, Percutaneous Endoscopic Approach

05UR07Z   Supplement Right Vertebral Vein with Autologous Tissue Substitute, Open Approach

05UR0JZ   Supplement Right Vertebral Vein with Synthetic Substitute, Open Approach

---

♀ Female-only   ♂ Male-only   ● Limited Coverage   ● Non-OR   [HAC] HAC-associated procedure   ● Non-covered procedures   + Combination

05UR0KZ Supplement Right Vertebral Vein with Nonautologous Tissue Substitute, Open Approach

05UR37Z Supplement Right Vertebral Vein with Autologous Tissue Substitute, Percutaneous Approach

05UR3JZ Supplement Right Vertebral Vein with Synthetic Substitute, Percutaneous Approach

05UR3KZ Supplement Right Vertebral Vein with Nonautologous Tissue Substitute, Percutaneous Approach

05UR47Z Supplement Right Vertebral Vein with Autologous Tissue Substitute, Percutaneous Endoscopic Approach

05UR4JZ Supplement Right Vertebral Vein with Synthetic Substitute, Percutaneous Endoscopic Approach

05UR4KZ Supplement Right Vertebral Vein with Nonautologous Tissue Substitute, Percutaneous Endoscopic Approach

05US07Z Supplement Left Vertebral Vein with Autologous Tissue Substitute, Open Approach

05US0JZ Supplement Left Vertebral Vein with Synthetic Substitute, Open Approach

05US0KZ Supplement Left Vertebral Vein with Nonautologous Tissue Substitute, Open Approach

05US37Z Supplement Left Vertebral Vein with Autologous Tissue Substitute, Percutaneous Approach

05US3JZ Supplement Left Vertebral Vein with Synthetic Substitute, Percutaneous Approach

05US3KZ Supplement Left Vertebral Vein with Nonautologous Tissue Substitute, Percutaneous Approach

05US47Z Supplement Left Vertebral Vein with Autologous Tissue Substitute, Percutaneous Endoscopic Approach

05US4JZ Supplement Left Vertebral Vein with Synthetic Substitute, Percutaneous Endoscopic Approach

05US4KZ Supplement Left Vertebral Vein with Nonautologous Tissue Substitute, Percutaneous Endoscopic Approach

05UT07Z Supplement Right Face Vein with Autologous Tissue Substitute, Open Approach

05UT0JZ Supplement Right Face Vein with Synthetic Substitute, Open Approach

05UT0KZ Supplement Right Face Vein with Nonautologous Tissue Substitute, Open Approach

05UT37Z Supplement Right Face Vein with Autologous Tissue Substitute, Percutaneous Approach

05UT3JZ Supplement Right Face Vein with Synthetic Substitute, Percutaneous Approach

05UT3KZ Supplement Right Face Vein with Nonautologous Tissue Substitute, Percutaneous Approach

05UT47Z Supplement Right Face Vein with Autologous Tissue Substitute, Percutaneous Endoscopic Approach

05UT4JZ Supplement Right Face Vein with Synthetic Substitute, Percutaneous Endoscopic Approach

05UT4KZ Supplement Right Face Vein with Nonautologous Tissue Substitute, Percutaneous Endoscopic Approach

05UV07Z Supplement Left Face Vein with Autologous Tissue Substitute, Open Approach

05UV0JZ Supplement Left Face Vein with Synthetic Substitute, Open Approach

05UV0KZ Supplement Left Face Vein with Nonautologous Tissue Substitute, Open Approach

05UV37Z Supplement Left Face Vein with Autologous Tissue Substitute, Percutaneous Approach

05UV3JZ Supplement Left Face Vein with Synthetic Substitute, Percutaneous Approach

05UV3KZ Supplement Left Face Vein with Nonautologous Tissue Substitute, Percutaneous Approach

05UV47Z Supplement Left Face Vein with Autologous Tissue Substitute, Percutaneous Endoscopic Approach

05UV4JZ Supplement Left Face Vein with Synthetic Substitute, Percutaneous Endoscopic Approach

05UV4KZ Supplement Left Face Vein with Nonautologous Tissue Substitute, Percutaneous Endoscopic Approach

05UY07Z Supplement Upper Vein with Autologous Tissue Substitute, Open Approach

05UY0JZ Supplement Upper Vein with Synthetic Substitute, Open Approach

05UY0KZ Supplement Upper Vein with Nonautologous Tissue Substitute, Open Approach

05UY37Z Supplement Upper Vein with Autologous Tissue Substitute, Percutaneous Approach

05UY3JZ Supplement Upper Vein with Synthetic Substitute, Percutaneous Approach

05UY3KZ Supplement Upper Vein with Nonautologous Tissue Substitute, Percutaneous Approach

05UY47Z Supplement Upper Vein with Autologous Tissue Substitute, Percutaneous Endoscopic Approach

05UY4JZ Supplement Upper Vein with Synthetic Substitute, Percutaneous Endoscopic Approach

05UY4KZ Supplement Upper Vein with Nonautologous Tissue Substitute, Percutaneous Endoscopic Approach

05V – Upper Veins, Restriction

Review Coding Guideline B3.12

05V00CZ Restriction of Azygos Vein with Extraluminal Device, Open Approach

05V00DZ Restriction of Azygos Vein with Intraluminal Device, Open Approach

05V00ZZ Restriction of Azygos Vein, Open Approach

05V03CZ Restriction of Azygos Vein with Extraluminal Device, Percutaneous Approach

05V03DZ Restriction of Azygos Vein with Intraluminal Device, Percutaneous Approach

05V03ZZ Restriction of Azygos Vein, Percutaneous Approach

05V04CZ Restriction of Azygos Vein with Extraluminal Device, Percutaneous Endoscopic Approach

05V04DZ Restriction of Azygos Vein with Intraluminal Device, Percutaneous Endoscopic Approach

05V04ZZ Restriction of Azygos Vein, Percutaneous Endoscopic Approach

05V10CZ Restriction of Hemiazygos Vein with Extraluminal Device, Open Approach

05V10DZ Restriction of Hemiazygos Vein with Intraluminal Device, Open Approach

05V10ZZ Restriction of Hemiazygos Vein, Open Approach

05V13CZ Restriction of Hemiazygos Vein with Extraluminal Device, Percutaneous Approach

05V13DZ Restriction of Hemiazygos Vein with Intraluminal Device, Percutaneous Approach

05V13ZZ Restriction of Hemiazygos Vein, Percutaneous Approach

05V14CZ Restriction of Hemiazygos Vein with Extraluminal Device, Percutaneous Endoscopic Approach

05V14DZ Restriction of Hemiazygos Vein with Intraluminal Device, Percutaneous Endoscopic Approach

05V14ZZ Restriction of Hemiazygos Vein, Percutaneous Endoscopic Approach

05V30CZ Restriction of Right Innominate Vein with Extraluminal Device, Open Approach

05V30DZ Restriction of Right Innominate Vein with Intraluminal Device, Open Approach

05V30ZZ Restriction of Right Innominate Vein, Open Approach

05V33CZ Restriction of Right Innominate Vein with Extraluminal Device, Percutaneous Approach

05V33DZ Restriction of Right Innominate Vein with Intraluminal Device, Percutaneous Approach

05V33ZZ Restriction of Right Innominate Vein, Percutaneous Approach

05V34CZ Restriction of Right Innominate Vein with Extraluminal Device, Percutaneous Endoscopic Approach

05V34DZ Restriction of Right Innominate Vein with Intraluminal Device, Percutaneous Endoscopic Approach

05V34ZZ Restriction of Right Innominate Vein, Percutaneous Endoscopic Approach

05V40CZ Restriction of Left Innominate Vein with Extraluminal Device, Open Approach

05V40DZ Restriction of Left Innominate Vein with Intraluminal Device, Open Approach

05V40ZZ Restriction of Left Innominate Vein, Open Approach

05V43CZ Restriction of Left Innominate Vein with Extraluminal Device, Percutaneous Approach

05V43DZ Restriction of Left Innominate Vein with Intraluminal Device, Percutaneous Approach

05V43ZZ Restriction of Left Innominate Vein, Percutaneous Approach

05V44CZ Restriction of Left Innominate Vein with Extraluminal Device, Percutaneous Endoscopic Approach

05V44DZ Restriction of Left Innominate Vein with Intraluminal Device, Percutaneous Endoscopic Approach

05V44ZZ Restriction of Left Innominate Vein, Percutaneous Endoscopic Approach

05V50CZ Restriction of Right Subclavian Vein with Extraluminal Device, Open Approach

05V50DZ Restriction of Right Subclavian Vein with Intraluminal Device, Open Approach

05V50ZZ Restriction of Right Subclavian Vein, Open Approach

05V53CZ Restriction of Right Subclavian Vein with Extraluminal Device, Percutaneous Approach

05V53DZ Restriction of Right Subclavian Vein with Intraluminal Device, Percutaneous Approach

05V53ZZ Restriction of Right Subclavian Vein, Percutaneous Approach

05V54CZ Restriction of Right Subclavian Vein with Extraluminal Device, Percutaneous Endoscopic Approach

05V54DZ Restriction of Right Subclavian Vein with Intraluminal Device, Percutaneous Endoscopic Approach

05V54ZZ Restriction of Right Subclavian Vein, Percutaneous Endoscopic Approach

05V60CZ Restriction of Left Subclavian Vein with Extraluminal Device, Open Approach

05V60DZ Restriction of Left Subclavian Vein with Intraluminal Device, Open Approach

05V60ZZ Restriction of Left Subclavian Vein, Open Approach

05V63CZ Restriction of Left Subclavian Vein with Extraluminal Device, Percutaneous Approach

05V63DZ Restriction of Left Subclavian Vein with Intraluminal Device, Percutaneous Approach

05V63ZZ Restriction of Left Subclavian Vein, Percutaneous Approach

05V64CZ Restriction of Left Subclavian Vein with Extraluminal Device, Percutaneous Endoscopic Approach

05V64DZ Restriction of Left Subclavian Vein with Intraluminal Device, Percutaneous Endoscopic Approach

05V64ZZ Restriction of Left Subclavian Vein, Percutaneous Endoscopic Approach

05V70CZ Restriction of Right Axillary Vein with Extraluminal Device, Open Approach

05V70DZ Restriction of Right Axillary Vein with Intraluminal Device, Open Approach

05V70ZZ Restriction of Right Axillary Vein, Open Approach

05V73CZ Restriction of Right Axillary Vein with Extraluminal Device, Percutaneous Approach

05V73DZ Restriction of Right Axillary Vein with Intraluminal Device, Percutaneous Approach

05V73ZZ Restriction of Right Axillary Vein, Percutaneous Approach

05V74CZ Restriction of Right Axillary Vein with Extraluminal Device, Percutaneous Endoscopic Approach

05V74DZ Restriction of Right Axillary Vein with Intraluminal Device, Percutaneous Endoscopic Approach

05V74ZZ Restriction of Right Axillary Vein, Percutaneous Endoscopic Approach

05V80CZ Restriction of Left Axillary Vein with Extraluminal Device, Open Approach

05V80DZ Restriction of Left Axillary Vein with Intraluminal Device, Open Approach

05V80ZZ Restriction of Left Axillary Vein, Open Approach

05V83CZ Restriction of Left Axillary Vein with Extraluminal Device, Percutaneous Approach

05V83DZ Restriction of Left Axillary Vein with Intraluminal Device, Percutaneous Approach

05V83ZZ Restriction of Left Axillary Vein, Percutaneous Approach

05V84CZ Restriction of Left Axillary Vein with Extraluminal Device, Percutaneous Endoscopic Approach

05V84DZ Restriction of Left Axillary Vein with Intraluminal Device, Percutaneous Endoscopic Approach

05V84ZZ Restriction of Left Axillary Vein, Percutaneous Endoscopic Approach

05V90CZ Restriction of Right Brachial Vein with Extraluminal Device, Open Approach

05V90DZ Restriction of Right Brachial Vein with Intraluminal Device, Open Approach

05V90ZZ Restriction of Right Brachial Vein, Open Approach

05V93CZ Restriction of Right Brachial Vein with Extraluminal Device, Percutaneous Approach

05V93DZ Restriction of Right Brachial Vein with Intraluminal Device, Percutaneous Approach

05V93ZZ Restriction of Right Brachial Vein, Percutaneous Approach

05V94CZ Restriction of Right Brachial Vein with Extraluminal Device, Percutaneous Endoscopic Approach

05V94DZ Restriction of Right Brachial Vein with Intraluminal Device, Percutaneous Endoscopic Approach

05V94ZZ Restriction of Right Brachial Vein, Percutaneous Endoscopic Approach

05VA0CZ Restriction of Left Brachial Vein with Extraluminal Device, Open Approach

05VA0DZ Restriction of Left Brachial Vein with Intraluminal Device, Open Approach

05VA0ZZ Restriction of Left Brachial Vein, Open Approach

05VA3CZ Restriction of Left Brachial Vein with Extraluminal Device, Percutaneous Approach

05VA3DZ Restriction of Left Brachial Vein with Intraluminal Device, Percutaneous Approach

05VA3ZZ Restriction of Left Brachial Vein, Percutaneous Approach

05VA4CZ Restriction of Left Brachial Vein with Extraluminal Device, Percutaneous Endoscopic Approach

05VA4DZ Restriction of Left Brachial Vein with Intraluminal Device, Percutaneous Endoscopic Approach

05VA4ZZ Restriction of Left Brachial Vein, Percutaneous Endoscopic Approach

05VB0CZ Restriction of Right Basilic Vein with Extraluminal Device, Open Approach

05VB0DZ Restriction of Right Basilic Vein with Intraluminal Device, Open Approach

05VB0ZZ Restriction of Right Basilic Vein, Open Approach

05VB3CZ Restriction of Right Basilic Vein with Extraluminal Device, Percutaneous Approach

05VB3DZ Restriction of Right Basilic Vein with Intraluminal Device, Percutaneous Approach

05VB3ZZ Restriction of Right Basilic Vein, Percutaneous Approach

05VB4CZ Restriction of Right Basilic Vein with Extraluminal Device, Percutaneous Endoscopic Approach

05VB4DZ Restriction of Right Basilic Vein with Intraluminal Device, Percutaneous Endoscopic Approach

05VB4ZZ Restriction of Right Basilic Vein, Percutaneous Endoscopic Approach

05VC0CZ Restriction of Left Basilic Vein with Extraluminal Device, Open Approach

05VC0DZ Restriction of Left Basilic Vein with Intraluminal Device, Open Approach

05VC0ZZ Restriction of Left Basilic Vein, Open Approach

05VC3CZ Restriction of Left Basilic Vein with Extraluminal Device, Percutaneous Approach

05VC3DZ Restriction of Left Basilic Vein with Intraluminal Device, Percutaneous Approach

05VC3ZZ Restriction of Left Basilic Vein, Percutaneous Approach

05VC4CZ Restriction of Left Basilic Vein with Extraluminal Device, Percutaneous Endoscopic Approach

05VC4DZ Restriction of Left Basilic Vein with Intraluminal Device, Percutaneous Endoscopic Approach

05VC4ZZ Restriction of Left Basilic Vein, Percutaneous Endoscopic Approach

05VD0CZ Restriction of Right Cephalic Vein with Extraluminal Device, Open Approach

05VD0DZ Restriction of Right Cephalic Vein with Intraluminal Device, Open Approach

05VD0ZZ Restriction of Right Cephalic Vein, Open Approach

05VD3CZ Restriction of Right Cephalic Vein with Extraluminal Device, Percutaneous Approach

05VD3DZ Restriction of Right Cephalic Vein with Intraluminal Device, Percutaneous Approach

05VD3ZZ Restriction of Right Cephalic Vein, Percutaneous Approach

05VD4CZ Restriction of Right Cephalic Vein with Extraluminal Device, Percutaneous Endoscopic Approach

05VD4DZ Restriction of Right Cephalic Vein with Intraluminal Device, Percutaneous Endoscopic Approach

05VD4ZZ Restriction of Right Cephalic Vein, Percutaneous Endoscopic Approach

05VF0CZ Restriction of Left Cephalic Vein with Extraluminal Device, Open Approach

05VF0DZ Restriction of Left Cephalic Vein with Intraluminal Device, Open Approach

05VF0ZZ Restriction of Left Cephalic Vein, Open Approach

05VF3CZ Restriction of Left Cephalic Vein with Extraluminal Device, Percutaneous Approach

05VF3DZ Restriction of Left Cephalic Vein with Intraluminal Device, Percutaneous Approach

05VF3ZZ Restriction of Left Cephalic Vein, Percutaneous Approach

05VF4CZ Restriction of Left Cephalic Vein with Extraluminal Device, Percutaneous Endoscopic Approach

05VF4DZ Restriction of Left Cephalic Vein with Intraluminal Device, Percutaneous Endoscopic Approach

05VF4ZZ Restriction of Left Cephalic Vein, Percutaneous Endoscopic Approach

05VG0CZ Restriction of Right Hand Vein with Extraluminal Device, Open Approach

05VG0DZ Restriction of Right Hand Vein with Intraluminal Device, Open Approach

05VG0ZZ Restriction of Right Hand Vein, Open Approach

05VG3CZ Restriction of Right Hand Vein with Extraluminal Device, Percutaneous Approach

05VG3DZ Restriction of Right Hand Vein with Intraluminal Device, Percutaneous Approach

05VG3ZZ Restriction of Right Hand Vein, Percutaneous Approach

05VG4CZ Restriction of Right Hand Vein with Extraluminal Device, Percutaneous Endoscopic Approach

05VG4DZ Restriction of Right Hand Vein with Intraluminal Device, Percutaneous Endoscopic Approach

05VG4ZZ Restriction of Right Hand Vein, Percutaneous Endoscopic Approach

05VH0CZ Restriction of Left Hand Vein with Extraluminal Device, Open Approach

05VH0DZ Restriction of Left Hand Vein with Intraluminal Device, Open Approach

05VH0ZZ Restriction of Left Hand Vein, Open Approach

05VH3CZ Restriction of Left Hand Vein with Extraluminal Device, Percutaneous Approach

05VH3DZ Restriction of Left Hand Vein with Intraluminal Device, Percutaneous Approach

05VH3ZZ Restriction of Left Hand Vein, Percutaneous Approach

05VH4CZ Restriction of Left Hand Vein with Extraluminal Device, Percutaneous Endoscopic Approach

05VH4DZ Restriction of Left Hand Vein with Intraluminal Device, Percutaneous Endoscopic Approach

05VH4ZZ Restriction of Left Hand Vein, Percutaneous Endoscopic Approach

05VL0CZ Restriction of Intracranial Vein with Extraluminal Device, Open Approach

05VL0DZ Restriction of Intracranial Vein with Intraluminal Device, Open Approach

05VL0ZZ Restriction of Intracranial Vein, Open Approach

05VL3CZ Restriction of Intracranial Vein with Extraluminal Device, Percutaneous Approach

05VL3DZ Restriction of Intracranial Vein with Intraluminal Device, Percutaneous Approach

05VL3ZZ Restriction of Intracranial Vein, Percutaneous Approach

05VL4CZ Restriction of Intracranial Vein with Extraluminal Device, Percutaneous Endoscopic Approach

05VL4DZ Restriction of Intracranial Vein with Intraluminal Device, Percutaneous Endoscopic Approach

05VL4ZZ Restriction of Intracranial Vein, Percutaneous Endoscopic Approach

05VM0CZ Restriction of Right Internal Jugular Vein with Extraluminal Device, Open Approach

05VM0DZ Restriction of Right Internal Jugular Vein with Intraluminal Device, Open Approach

05VM0ZZ Restriction of Right Internal Jugular Vein, Open Approach

05VM3CZ Restriction of Right Internal Jugular Vein with Extraluminal Device, Percutaneous Approach

05VM3DZ Restriction of Right Internal Jugular Vein with Intraluminal Device, Percutaneous Approach

05VM3ZZ Restriction of Right Internal Jugular Vein, Percutaneous Approach

05VM4CZ Restriction of Right Internal Jugular Vein with Extraluminal Device, Percutaneous Endoscopic Approach

05VM4DZ Restriction of Right Internal Jugular Vein with Intraluminal Device, Percutaneous Endoscopic Approach

05VM4ZZ Restriction of Right Internal Jugular Vein, Percutaneous Endoscopic Approach

05VN0CZ Restriction of Left Internal Jugular Vein with Extraluminal Device, Open Approach

05VN0DZ Restriction of Left Internal Jugular Vein with Intraluminal Device, Open Approach

05VN0ZZ Restriction of Left Internal Jugular Vein, Open Approach

05VN3CZ Restriction of Left Internal Jugular Vein with Extraluminal Device, Percutaneous Approach

05VN3DZ Restriction of Left Internal Jugular Vein with Intraluminal Device, Percutaneous Approach

05VN3ZZ Restriction of Left Internal Jugular Vein, Percutaneous Approach

05VN4CZ Restriction of Left Internal Jugular Vein with Extraluminal Device, Percutaneous Endoscopic Approach

05VN4DZ Restriction of Left Internal Jugular Vein with Intraluminal Device, Percutaneous Endoscopic Approach

05VN4ZZ Restriction of Left Internal Jugular Vein, Percutaneous Endoscopic Approach

05VP0CZ Restriction of Right External Jugular Vein with Extraluminal Device, Open Approach

05VP0DZ Restriction of Right External Jugular Vein with Intraluminal Device, Open Approach

05VP0ZZ Restriction of Right External Jugular Vein, Open Approach

05VP3CZ Restriction of Right External Jugular Vein with Extraluminal Device, Percutaneous Approach

05VP3DZ Restriction of Right External Jugular Vein with Intraluminal Device, Percutaneous Approach

05VP3ZZ Restriction of Right External Jugular Vein, Percutaneous Approach

05VP4CZ Restriction of Right External Jugular Vein with Extraluminal Device, Percutaneous Endoscopic Approach

05VP4DZ Restriction of Right External Jugular Vein with Intraluminal Device, Percutaneous Endoscopic Approach

05VP4ZZ Restriction of Right External Jugular Vein, Percutaneous Endoscopic Approach

05VQ0CZ Restriction of Left External Jugular Vein with Extraluminal Device, Open Approach

05VQ0DZ Restriction of Left External Jugular Vein with Intraluminal Device, Open Approach

05VQ0ZZ Restriction of Left External Jugular Vein, Open Approach

05VQ3CZ Restriction of Left External Jugular Vein with Extraluminal Device, Percutaneous Approach

05VQ3DZ Restriction of Left External Jugular Vein with Intraluminal Device, Percutaneous Approach

05VQ3ZZ Restriction of Left External Jugular Vein, Percutaneous Approach

05VQ4CZ Restriction of Left External Jugular Vein with Extraluminal Device, Percutaneous Endoscopic Approach

05VQ4DZ Restriction of Left External Jugular Vein with Intraluminal Device, Percutaneous Endoscopic Approach

05VQ4ZZ Restriction of Left External Jugular Vein, Percutaneous Endoscopic Approach

05VR0CZ Restriction of Right Vertebral Vein with Extraluminal Device, Open Approach

05VR0DZ Restriction of Right Vertebral Vein with Intraluminal Device, Open Approach

05VR0ZZ Restriction of Right Vertebral Vein, Open Approach

05VR3CZ Restriction of Right Vertebral Vein with Extraluminal Device, Percutaneous Approach

05VR3DZ Restriction of Right Vertebral Vein with Intraluminal Device, Percutaneous Approach

05VR3ZZ Restriction of Right Vertebral Vein, Percutaneous Approach

05VR4CZ Restriction of Right Vertebral Vein with Extraluminal Device, Percutaneous Endoscopic Approach

05VR4DZ Restriction of Right Vertebral Vein with Intraluminal Device, Percutaneous Endoscopic Approach

05VR4ZZ Restriction of Right Vertebral Vein, Percutaneous Endoscopic Approach

05VS0CZ Restriction of Left Vertebral Vein with Extraluminal Device, Open Approach

05VS0DZ Restriction of Left Vertebral Vein with Intraluminal Device, Open Approach

05VS0ZZ Restriction of Left Vertebral Vein, Open Approach

05VS3CZ Restriction of Left Vertebral Vein with Extraluminal Device, Percutaneous Approach

05VS3DZ Restriction of Left Vertebral Vein with Intraluminal Device, Percutaneous Approach

05VS3ZZ Restriction of Left Vertebral Vein, Percutaneous Approach

05VS4CZ Restriction of Left Vertebral Vein with Extraluminal Device, Percutaneous Endoscopic Approach

05VS4DZ Restriction of Left Vertebral Vein with Intraluminal Device, Percutaneous Endoscopic Approach

05VS4ZZ Restriction of Left Vertebral Vein, Percutaneous Endoscopic Approach

05VT0CZ Restriction of Right Face Vein with Extraluminal Device, Open Approach

05VT0DZ Restriction of Right Face Vein with Intraluminal Device, Open Approach

05VT0ZZ Restriction of Right Face Vein, Open Approach

05VT3CZ Restriction of Right Face Vein with Extraluminal Device, Percutaneous Approach

05VT3DZ Restriction of Right Face Vein with Intraluminal Device, Percutaneous Approach

05VT3ZZ Restriction of Right Face Vein, Percutaneous Approach

05VT4CZ Restriction of Right Face Vein with Extraluminal Device, Percutaneous Endoscopic Approach

05VT4DZ Restriction of Right Face Vein with Intraluminal Device, Percutaneous Endoscopic Approach

05VT4ZZ Restriction of Right Face Vein, Percutaneous Endoscopic Approach

05VV0CZ Restriction of Left Face Vein with Extraluminal Device, Open Approach

05VV0DZ Restriction of Left Face Vein with Intraluminal Device, Open Approach

05VV0ZZ Restriction of Left Face Vein, Open Approach

05VV3CZ Restriction of Left Face Vein with Extraluminal Device, Percutaneous Approach

05VV3DZ Restriction of Left Face Vein with Intraluminal Device, Percutaneous Approach

05VV3ZZ Restriction of Left Face Vein, Percutaneous Approach

05VV4CZ Restriction of Left Face Vein with Extraluminal Device, Percutaneous Endoscopic Approach

05VV4DZ Restriction of Left Face Vein with Intraluminal Device, Percutaneous Endoscopic Approach

05VV4ZZ Restriction of Left Face Vein, Percutaneous Endoscopic Approach

05VY0CZ Restriction of Upper Vein with Extraluminal Device, Open Approach

05VY0DZ Restriction of Upper Vein with Intraluminal Device, Open Approach

05VY0ZZ Restriction of Upper Vein, Open Approach

05VY3CZ Restriction of Upper Vein with Extraluminal Device, Percutaneous Approach

05VY3DZ Restriction of Upper Vein with Intraluminal Device, Percutaneous Approach

05VY3ZZ Restriction of Upper Vein, Percutaneous Approach

05VY4CZ Restriction of Upper Vein with Extraluminal Device, Percutaneous Endoscopic Approach

05VY4DZ Restriction of Upper Vein with Intraluminal Device, Percutaneous Endoscopic Approach

05VY4ZZ Restriction of Upper Vein, Percutaneous Endoscopic Approach

05W – Upper Veins, Revision

Review Coding Guideline B6.1c

05WY00Z Revision of Drainage Device in Upper Vein, Open Approach

05WY02Z Revision of Monitoring Device in Upper Vein, Open Approach

05WY03Z Revision of Infusion Device in Upper Vein, Open Approach

05WY07Z Revision of Autologous Tissue Substitute in Upper Vein, Open Approach

05WY0CZ Revision of Extraluminal Device in Upper Vein, Open Approach

05WY0DZ Revision of Intraluminal Device in Upper Vein, Open Approach

05WY0JZ Revision of Synthetic Substitute in Upper Vein, Open Approach

05WY0KZ Revision of Nonautologous Tissue Substitute in Upper Vein, Open Approach

05WY30Z Revision of Drainage Device in Upper Vein, Percutaneous Approach

05WY32Z Revision of Monitoring Device in Upper Vein, Percutaneous Approach

05WY33Z Revision of Infusion Device in Upper Vein, Percutaneous Approach

05WY37Z Revision of Autologous Tissue Substitute in Upper Vein, Percutaneous Approach

05WY3CZ Revision of Extraluminal Device in Upper Vein, Percutaneous Approach

05WY3DZ Revision of Intraluminal Device in Upper Vein, Percutaneous Approach

05WY3JZ Revision of Synthetic Substitute in Upper Vein, Percutaneous Approach

05WY3KZ Revision of Nonautologous Tissue Substitute in Upper Vein, Percutaneous Approach

05WY40Z Revision of Drainage Device in Upper Vein, Percutaneous Endoscopic Approach

05WY42Z Revision of Monitoring Device in Upper Vein, Percutaneous Endoscopic Approach

05WY43Z Revision of Infusion Device in Upper Vein, Percutaneous Endoscopic Approach

05WY47Z Revision of Autologous Tissue Substitute in Upper Vein, Percutaneous Endoscopic Approach

05WY4CZ Revision of Extraluminal Device in Upper Vein, Percutaneous Endoscopic Approach

05WY4DZ Revision of Intraluminal Device in Upper Vein, Percutaneous Endoscopic Approach

05WY4JZ Revision of Synthetic Substitute in Upper Vein, Percutaneous Endoscopic Approach

05WY4KZ Revision of Nonautologous Tissue Substitute in Upper Vein, Percutaneous Endoscopic Approach

05WYX0Z Revision of Drainage Device in Upper Vein, External Approach

05WYX2Z Revision of Monitoring Device in Upper Vein, External Approach

05WYX3Z Revision of Infusion Device in Upper Vein, External Approach

05WYX7Z Revision of Autologous Tissue Substitute in Upper Vein, External Approach

05WYXCZ Revision of Extraluminal Device in Upper Vein, External Approach

05WYXDZ Revision of Intraluminal Device in Upper Vein, External Approach

05WYXJZ Revision of Synthetic Substitute in Upper Vein, External Approach

05WYXKZ Revision of Nonautologous Tissue Substitute in Upper Vein, External Approach

Lower Veins

Veins

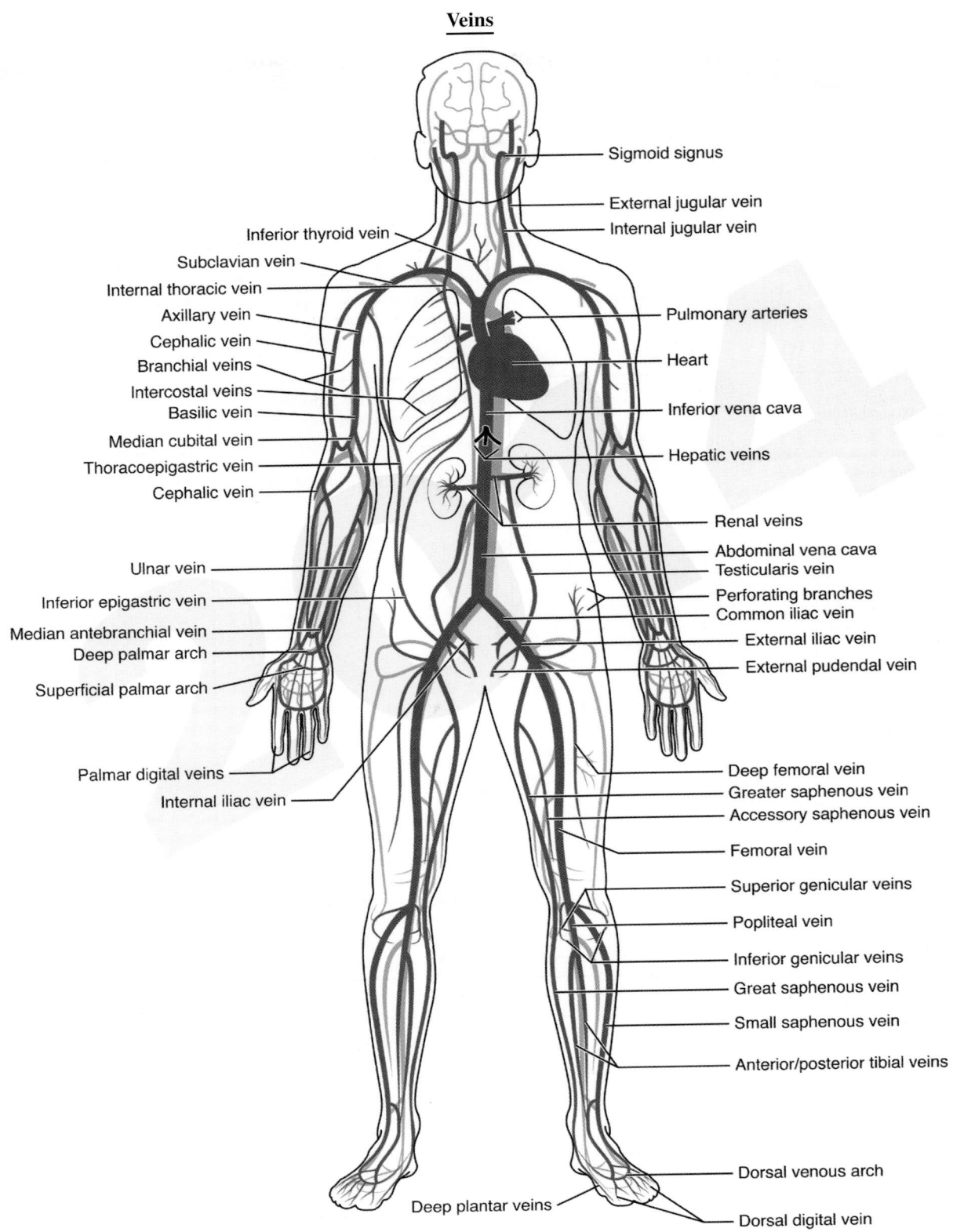

Sigmoid signus

External jugular vein

Internal jugular vein

Inferior thyroid vein

Subclavian vein

Internal thoracic vein

Axillary vein

Cephalic vein

Branchial veins

Intercostal veins

Basilic vein

Median cubital vein

Thoracoepigastric vein

Cephalic vein

Pulmonary arteries

Heart

Inferior vena cava

Hepatic veins

Renal veins

Abdominal vena cava

Testicularis vein

Perforating branches

Common iliac vein

External iliac vein

External pudendal vein

Ulnar vein

Inferior epigastric vein

Median antebranchial vein

Deep palmar arch

Superficial palmar arch

Palmar digital veins

Internal iliac vein

Deep femoral vein

Greater saphenous vein

Accessory saphenous vein

Femoral vein

Superior genicular veins

Popliteal vein

Inferior genicular veins

Great saphenous vein

Small saphenous vein

Anterior/posterior tibial veins

Dorsal venous arch

Deep plantar veins

Dorsal digital vein

Lower Veins Tables 061–06W

Section	0	Medical and Surgical
Body System	6	Lower Veins
Operation	1	Bypass: Altering the route of passage of the contents of a tubular body part

Body Part (4th)	Approach (5th)	Device (6th)	Qualifier (7th)
0 Inferior Vena Cava	0 Open 4 Percutaneous Endoscopic	7 Autologous Tissue Substitute 9 Autologous Venous Tissue A Autologous Arterial Tissue J Synthetic Substitute K Nonautologous Tissue Substitute Z No Device	5 Superior Mesenteric Vein 6 Inferior Mesenteric Vein Y Lower Vein
1 Splenic Vein	0 Open 4 Percutaneous Endoscopic	7 Autologous Tissue Substitute 9 Autologous Venous Tissue A Autologous Arterial Tissue J Synthetic Substitute K Nonautologous Tissue Substitute Z No Device	9 Renal Vein, Right B Renal Vein, Left Y Lower Vein
2 Gastric Vein 3 Esophageal Vein 4 Hepatic Vein 5 Superior Mesenteric Vein 6 Inferior Mesenteric Vein 7 Colic Vein 9 Renal Vein, Right B Renal Vein, Left C Common Iliac Vein, Right D Common Iliac Vein, Left F External Iliac Vein, Right G External Iliac Vein, Left H Hypogastric Vein, Right J Hypogastric Vein, Left M Femoral Vein, Right N Femoral Vein, Left P Greater Saphenous Vein, Right Q Greater Saphenous Vein, Left R Lesser Saphenous Vein, Right S Lesser Saphenous Vein, Left T Foot Vein, Right V Foot Vein, Left	0 Open 4 Percutaneous Endoscopic	7 Autologous Tissue Substitute 9 Autologous Venous Tissue A Autologous Arterial Tissue J Synthetic Substitute K Nonautologous Tissue Substitute Z No Device	Y Lower Vein
8 Portal Vein	0 Open	7 Autologous Tissue Substitute 9 Autologous Venous Tissue A Autologous Arterial Tissue J Synthetic Substitute K Nonautologous Tissue Substitute Z No Device	9 Renal Vein, Right B Renal Vein, Left Y Lower Vein
8 Portal Vein	3 Percutaneous	D Intraluminal Device	Y Lower Vein
8 Portal Vein	4 Percutaneous Endoscopic	7 Autologous Tissue Substitute 9 Autologous Venous Tissue A Autologous Arterial Tissue J Synthetic Substitute K Nonautologous Tissue Substitute Z No Device	9 Renal Vein, Right B Renal Vein, Left Y Lower Vein
8 Portal Vein	4 Percutaneous Endoscopic	D Intraluminal Device	Y Lower Vein

Section	0	**Medical and Surgical**
Body System	6	**Lower Veins**
Operation	5	**Destruction:** Physical eradication of all or a portion of a body part by the direct use of energy, force, or a destructive agent

Body Part (4th)	Approach (5th)	Device (6th)	Qualifier (7th)
0 Inferior Vena Cava 1 Splenic Vein 2 Gastric Vein 3 Esophageal Vein 4 Hepatic Vein 5 Superior Mesenteric Vein 6 Inferior Mesenteric Vein 7 Colic Vein 8 Portal Vein 9 Renal Vein, Right B Renal Vein, Left C Common Iliac Vein, Right D Common Iliac Vein, Left F External Iliac Vein, Right G External Iliac Vein, Left H Hypogastric Vein, Right J Hypogastric Vein, Left M Femoral Vein, Right N Femoral Vein, Left P Greater Saphenous Vein, Right Q Greater Saphenous Vein, Left R Lesser Saphenous Vein, Right S Lesser Saphenous Vein, Left T Foot Vein, Right V Foot Vein, Left	0 Open 3 Percutaneous 4 Percutaneous Endoscopic	Z No Device	Z No Qualifier
Y Lower Vein	0 Open 3 Percutaneous 4 Percutaneous Endoscopic	Z No Device	C Hemorrhoidal Plexus Z No Qualifier

Section	0	**Medical and Surgical**
Body System	6	**Lower Veins**
Operation	7	**Dilation:** Expanding an orifice or the lumen of a tubular body part

Body Part (4th)	Approach (5th)	Device (6th)	Qualifier (7th)
0 Inferior Vena Cava	0 Open	D Intraluminal Device	Z No Qualifier
1 Splenic Vein	3 Percutaneous	Z No Device	
2 Gastric Vein	4 Percutaneous Endoscopic		
3 Esophageal Vein			
4 Hepatic Vein			
5 Superior Mesenteric Vein			
6 Inferior Mesenteric Vein			
7 Colic Vein			
8 Portal Vein			
9 Renal Vein, Right			
B Renal Vein, Left			
C Common Iliac Vein, Right			
D Common Iliac Vein, Left			
F External Iliac Vein, Right			
G External Iliac Vein, Left			
H Hypogastric Vein, Right			
J Hypogastric Vein, Left			
M Femoral Vein, Right			
N Femoral Vein, Left			
P Greater Saphenous Vein, Right			
Q Greater Saphenous Vein, Left			
R Lesser Saphenous Vein, Right			
S Lesser Saphenous Vein, Left			
T Foot Vein, Right			
V Foot Vein, Left			
Y Lower Vein			

Section	0	**Medical and Surgical**
Body System	6	**Lower Veins**
Operation	9	**Drainage:** Taking or letting out fluids and/or gases from a body part

Body Part (4th)	Approach (5th)	Device (6th)	Qualifier (7th)
0 Inferior Vena Cava 1 Splenic Vein 2 Gastric Vein 3 Esophageal Vein 4 Hepatic Vein 5 Superior Mesenteric Vein 6 Inferior Mesenteric Vein 7 Colic Vein 8 Portal Vein 9 Renal Vein, Right B Renal Vein, Left C Common Iliac Vein, Right D Common Iliac Vein, Left F External Iliac Vein, Right G External Iliac Vein, Left H Hypogastric Vein, Right J Hypogastric Vein, Left M Femoral Vein, Right N Femoral Vein, Left P Greater Saphenous Vein, Right Q Greater Saphenous Vein, Left R Lesser Saphenous Vein, Right S Lesser Saphenous Vein, Left T Foot Vein, Right V Foot Vein, Left Y Lower Vein	0 Open 3 Percutaneous 4 Percutaneous Endoscopic	0 Drainage Device	Z No Qualifier
0 Inferior Vena Cava 1 Splenic Vein 2 Gastric Vein 3 Esophageal Vein 4 Hepatic Vein 5 Superior Mesenteric Vein 6 Inferior Mesenteric Vein 7 Colic Vein 8 Portal Vein 9 Renal Vein, Right B Renal Vein, Left C Common Iliac Vein, Right D Common Iliac Vein, Left F External Iliac Vein, Right G External Iliac Vein, Left H Hypogastric Vein, Right J Hypogastric Vein, Left M Femoral Vein, Right N Femoral Vein, Left P Greater Saphenous Vein, Right Q Greater Saphenous Vein, Left R Lesser Saphenous Vein, Right S Lesser Saphenous Vein, Left T Foot Vein, Right V Foot Vein, Left Y Lower Vein	0 Open 3 Percutaneous 4 Percutaneous Endoscopic	Z No Device	X Diagnostic Z No Qualifier

Section	0	Medical and Surgical
Body System	6	Lower Veins
Operation	B	Excision: Cutting out or off, without replacement, a portion of a body part

Body Part (4th)	Approach (5th)	Device (6th)	Qualifier (7th)
0 Inferior Vena Cava 1 Splenic Vein 2 Gastric Vein 3 Esophageal Vein 4 Hepatic Vein 5 Superior Mesenteric Vein 6 Inferior Mesenteric Vein 7 Colic Vein 8 Portal Vein 9 Renal Vein, Right B Renal Vein, Left C Common Iliac Vein, Right D Common Iliac Vein, Left F External Iliac Vein, Right G External Iliac Vein, Left H Hypogastric Vein, Right J Hypogastric Vein, Left M Femoral Vein, Right N Femoral Vein, Left P Greater Saphenous Vein, Right Q Greater Saphenous Vein, Left R Lesser Saphenous Vein, Right S Lesser Saphenous Vein, Left T Foot Vein, Right V Foot Vein, Left	0 Open 3 Percutaneous 4 Percutaneous Endoscopic	Z No Device	X Diagnostic Z No Qualifier
Y Lower Vein	0 Open 3 Percutaneous 4 Percutaneous Endoscopic	Z No Device	C Hemorrhoidal Plexus X Diagnostic Z No Qualifier

Section	0	Medical and Surgical
Body System	6	Lower Veins
Operation	C	Extirpation: Taking or cutting out solid matter from a body part

Body Part (4th)	Approach (5th)	Device (6th)	Qualifier (7th)
0 Inferior Vena Cava 1 Splenic Vein 2 Gastric Vein 3 Esophageal Vein 4 Hepatic Vein 5 Superior Mesenteric Vein 6 Inferior Mesenteric Vein 7 Colic Vein 8 Portal Vein 9 Renal Vein, Right B Renal Vein, Left C Common Iliac Vein, Right D Common Iliac Vein, Left F External Iliac Vein, Right G External Iliac Vein, Left H Hypogastric Vein, Right J Hypogastric Vein, Left M Femoral Vein, Right N Femoral Vein, Left P Greater Saphenous Vein, Right Q Greater Saphenous Vein, Left R Lesser Saphenous Vein, Right S Lesser Saphenous Vein, Left T Foot Vein, Right V Foot Vein, Left Y Lower Vein	0 Open 3 Percutaneous 4 Percutaneous Endoscopic	Z No Device	Z No Qualifier

Section	0	**Medical and Surgical**
Body System	**6**	**Lower Veins**
Operation	**D**	**Extraction:** Pulling or stripping out or off all or a portion of a body part by the use of force

Body Part (4ᵗʰ)	Approach (5ᵗʰ)	Device (6ᵗʰ)	Qualifier (7ᵗʰ)
M Femoral Vein, Right N Femoral Vein, Left P Greater Saphenous Vein, Right Q Greater Saphenous Vein, Left R Lesser Saphenous Vein, Right S Lesser Saphenous Vein, Left T Foot Vein, Right V Foot Vein, Left Y Lower Vein	0 Open 3 Percutaneous 4 Percutaneous Endoscopic	Z No Device	Z No Qualifier

Section	0	**Medical and Surgical**
Body System	**6**	**Lower Veins**
Operation	**H**	**Insertion:** Putting in a nonbiological appliance that monitors, assists, performs, or prevents a physiological function but does not physically take the place of a body part

Body Part (4ᵗʰ)	Approach (5ᵗʰ)	Device (6ᵗʰ)	Qualifier (7ᵗʰ)
0 Inferior Vena Cava	0 Open 3 Percutaneous	3 Infusion Device	T Via Umbilical Vein Z No Qualifier
0 Inferior Vena Cava	0 Open 3 Percutaneous	D Intraluminal Device	Z No Qualifier
0 Inferior Vena Cava	4 Percutaneous Endoscopic	3 Infusion Device D Intraluminal Device	Z No Qualifier
1 Splenic Vein 2 Gastric Vein 3 Esophageal Vein 4 Hepatic Vein 5 Superior Mesenteric Vein 6 Inferior Mesenteric Vein 7 Colic Vein 8 Portal Vein 9 Renal Vein, Right B Renal Vein, Left C Common Iliac Vein, Right D Common Iliac Vein, Left F External Iliac Vein, Right G External Iliac Vein, Left H Hypogastric Vein, Right J Hypogastric Vein, Left M Femoral Vein, Right N Femoral Vein, Left P Greater Saphenous Vein, Right Q Greater Saphenous Vein, Left R Lesser Saphenous Vein, Right S Lesser Saphenous Vein, Left T Foot Vein, Right V Foot Vein, Left	0 Open 3 Percutaneous 4 Percutaneous Endoscopic	3 Infusion Device D Intraluminal Device	Z No Qualifier
Y Lower Vein	0 Open 3 Percutaneous 4 Percutaneous Endoscopic	2 Monitoring Device 3 Infusion Device D Intraluminal Device	Z No Qualifier

Section	0	Medical and Surgical
Body System	6	Lower Veins
Operation	J	Inspection: Visually and/or manually exploring a body part

Body Part (4th)	Approach (5th)	Device (6th)	Qualifier (7th)
Y Lower Vein	0 Open 3 Percutaneous 4 Percutaneous Endoscopic X External	Z No Device	Z No Qualifier

Section	0	Medical and Surgical
Body System	6	Lower Veins
Operation	L	Occlusion: Completely closing an orifice or the lumen of a tubular body part

Body Part (4th)	Approach (5th)	Device (6th)	Qualifier (7th)
0 Inferior Vena Cava 1 Splenic Vein 2 Gastric Vein 3 Esophageal Vein 4 Hepatic Vein 5 Superior Mesenteric Vein 6 Inferior Mesenteric Vein 7 Colic Vein 8 Portal Vein 9 Renal Vein, Right B Renal Vein, Left C Common Iliac Vein, Right D Common Iliac Vein, Left F External Iliac Vein, Right G External Iliac Vein, Left H Hypogastric Vein, Right J Hypogastric Vein, Left M Femoral Vein, Right N Femoral Vein, Left P Greater Saphenous Vein, Right Q Greater Saphenous Vein, Left R Lesser Saphenous Vein, Right S Lesser Saphenous Vein, Left T Foot Vein, Right V Foot Vein, Left	0 Open 3 Percutaneous 4 Percutaneous Endoscopic	C Extraluminal Device D Intraluminal Device Z No Device	Z No Qualifier
Y Lower Vein	0 Open 3 Percutaneous 4 Percutaneous Endoscopic	C Extraluminal Device D Intraluminal Device Z No Device	C Hemorrhoidal Plexus Z No Qualifier

Section	0	Medical and Surgical
Body System	6	Lower Veins
Operation	N	Release: Freeing a body part from an abnormal physical constraint by cutting or by the use of force

Body Part (4th)	Approach (5th)	Device (6th)	Qualifier (7th)
0 Inferior Vena Cava 1 Splenic Vein 2 Gastric Vein 3 Esophageal Vein 4 Hepatic Vein 5 Superior Mesenteric Vein 6 Inferior Mesenteric Vein 7 Colic Vein 8 Portal Vein 9 Renal Vein, Right B Renal Vein, Left C Common Iliac Vein, Right D Common Iliac Vein, Left F External Iliac Vein, Right G External Iliac Vein, Left H Hypogastric Vein, Right J Hypogastric Vein, Left M Femoral Vein, Right N Femoral Vein, Left P Greater Saphenous Vein, Right Q Greater Saphenous Vein, Left R Lesser Saphenous Vein, Right S Lesser Saphenous Vein, Left T Foot Vein, Right V Foot Vein, Left Y Lower Vein	0 Open 3 Percutaneous 4 Percutaneous Endoscopic	Z No Device	Z No Qualifier

Section	0	Medical and Surgical
Body System	6	Lower Veins
Operation	P	Removal: Taking out or off a device from a body part

Body Part (4th)	Approach (5th)	Device (6th)	Qualifier (7th)
Y Lower Vein	0 Open 3 Percutaneous 4 Percutaneous Endoscopic	0 Drainage Device 2 Monitoring Device 3 Infusion Device 7 Autologous Tissue Substitute C Extraluminal Device D Intraluminal Device J Synthetic Substitute K Nonautologous Tissue Substitute	Z No Qualifier
Y Lower Vein	X External	0 Drainage Device 2 Monitoring Device 3 Infusion Device D Intraluminal Device	Z No Qualifier

Section	0	Medical and Surgical
Body System	6	Lower Veins
Operation	Q	Repair: Restoring, to the extent possible, a body part to its normal anatomic structure and function

Body Part (4th)	Approach (5th)	Device (6th)	Qualifier (7th)
0 Inferior Vena Cava 1 Splenic Vein 2 Gastric Vein 3 Esophageal Vein 4 Hepatic Vein 5 Superior Mesenteric Vein 6 Inferior Mesenteric Vein 7 Colic Vein 8 Portal Vein 9 Renal Vein, Right B Renal Vein, Left C Common Iliac Vein, Right D Common Iliac Vein, Left F External Iliac Vein, Right G External Iliac Vein, Left H Hypogastric Vein, Right J Hypogastric Vein, Left M Femoral Vein, Right N Femoral Vein, Left P Greater Saphenous Vein, Right Q Greater Saphenous Vein, Left R Lesser Saphenous Vein, Right S Lesser Saphenous Vein, Left T Foot Vein, Right V Foot Vein, Left Y Lower Vein	0 Open 3 Percutaneous 4 Percutaneous Endoscopic	Z No Device	Z No Qualifier

Section	0	Medical and Surgical
Body System	6	Lower Veins
Operation	R	Replacement: Putting in or on biological or synthetic material that physically takes the place and/or function of all or a portion of a body part

Body Part (4th)	Approach (5th)	Device (6th)	Qualifier (7th)
0 Inferior Vena Cava 1 Splenic Vein 2 Gastric Vein 3 Esophageal Vein 4 Hepatic Vein 5 Superior Mesenteric Vein 6 Inferior Mesenteric Vein 7 Colic Vein 8 Portal Vein 9 Renal Vein, Right B Renal Vein, Left C Common Iliac Vein, Right D Common Iliac Vein, Left F External Iliac Vein, Right G External Iliac Vein, Left H Hypogastric Vein, Right J Hypogastric Vein, Left M Femoral Vein, Right N Femoral Vein, Left P Greater Saphenous Vein, Right Q Greater Saphenous Vein, Left R Lesser Saphenous Vein, Right S Lesser Saphenous Vein, Left T Foot Vein, Right V Foot Vein, Left Y Lower Vein	0 Open 4 Percutaneous Endoscopic	7 Autologous Tissue Substitute J Synthetic Substitute K Nonautologous Tissue Substitute	Z No Qualifier

Section	0	Medical and Surgical
Body System	6	Lower Veins
Operation	S	Reposition: Moving to its normal location, or other suitable location, all or a portion of a body part

Body Part (4th)	Approach (5th)	Device (6th)	Qualifier (7th)
0 Inferior Vena Cava 1 Splenic Vein 2 Gastric Vein 3 Esophageal Vein 4 Hepatic Vein 5 Superior Mesenteric Vein 6 Inferior Mesenteric Vein 7 Colic Vein 8 Portal Vein 9 Renal Vein, Right B Renal Vein, Left C Common Iliac Vein, Right D Common Iliac Vein, Left F External Iliac Vein, Right G External Iliac Vein, Left H Hypogastric Vein, Right J Hypogastric Vein, Left M Femoral Vein, Right N Femoral Vein, Left P Greater Saphenous Vein, Right Q Greater Saphenous Vein, Left R Lesser Saphenous Vein, Right S Lesser Saphenous Vein, Left T Foot Vein, Right V Foot Vein, Left Y Lower Vein	0 Open 3 Percutaneous 4 Percutaneous Endoscopic	Z No Device	Z No Qualifier

Section	0	Medical and Surgical
Body System	6	Lower Veins
Operation	U	Supplement: Putting in or on biological or synthetic material that physically reinforces and/or augments the function of a portion of a body part

Body Part (4th)	Approach (5th)	Device (6th)	Qualifier (7th)
0 Inferior Vena Cava 1 Splenic Vein 2 Gastric Vein 3 Esophageal Vein 4 Hepatic Vein 5 Superior Mesenteric Vein 6 Inferior Mesenteric Vein 7 Colic Vein 8 Portal Vein 9 Renal Vein, Right B Renal Vein, Left C Common Iliac Vein, Right D Common Iliac Vein, Left F External Iliac Vein, Right G External Iliac Vein, Left H Hypogastric Vein, Right J Hypogastric Vein, Left M Femoral Vein, Right N Femoral Vein, Left P Greater Saphenous Vein, Right Q Greater Saphenous Vein, Left R Lesser Saphenous Vein, Right S Lesser Saphenous Vein, Left T Foot Vein, Right V Foot Vein, Left Y Lower Vein	0 Open 3 Percutaneous 4 Percutaneous Endoscopic	7 Autologous Tissue Substitute J Synthetic Substitute K Nonautologous Tissue Substitute	Z No Qualifier

Section	0	Medical and Surgical
Body System	6	Lower Veins
Operation	V	**Restriction:** Partially closing an orifice or the lumen of a tubular body part

Body Part (4th)	Approach (5th)	Device (6th)	Qualifier (7th)
0 Inferior Vena Cava 1 Splenic Vein 2 Gastric Vein 3 Esophageal Vein 4 Hepatic Vein 5 Superior Mesenteric Vein 6 Inferior Mesenteric Vein 7 Colic Vein 8 Portal Vein 9 Renal Vein, Right B Renal Vein, Left C Common Iliac Vein, Right D Common Iliac Vein, Left F External Iliac Vein, Right G External Iliac Vein, Left H Hypogastric Vein, Right J Hypogastric Vein, Left M Femoral Vein, Right N Femoral Vein, Left P Greater Saphenous Vein, Right Q Greater Saphenous Vein, Left R Lesser Saphenous Vein, Right S Lesser Saphenous Vein, Left T Foot Vein, Right V Foot Vein, Left Y Lower Vein	0 Open 3 Percutaneous 4 Percutaneous Endoscopic	C Extraluminal Device D Intraluminal Device Z No Device	Z No Qualifier

Section	0	Medical and Surgical
Body System	6	Lower Veins
Operation	W	**Revision:** Correcting, to the extent possible, a portion of a malfunctioning device or the position of a displaced device

Body Part (4th)	Approach (5th)	Device (6th)	Qualifier (7th)
Y Lower Vein	0 Open 3 Percutaneous 4 Percutaneous Endoscopic X External	0 Drainage Device 2 Monitoring Device 3 Infusion Device 7 Autologous Tissue Substitute C Extraluminal Device D Intraluminal Device J Synthetic Substitute K Nonautologous Tissue Substitute	Z No Qualifier

Lower Veins Code Listing 061–06W

061 – Lower Veins, Bypass

Review Coding Guideline B3.6a

0610075 Bypass Inferior Vena Cava to Superior Mesenteric Vein with Autologous Tissue Substitute, Open Approach

0610076 Bypass Inferior Vena Cava to Inferior Mesenteric Vein with Autologous Tissue Substitute, Open Approach

061007Y Bypass Inferior Vena Cava to Lower Vein with Autologous Tissue Substitute, Open Approach

0610095 Bypass Inferior Vena Cava to Superior Mesenteric Vein with Autologous Venous Tissue, Open Approach

0610096 Bypass Inferior Vena Cava to Inferior Mesenteric Vein with Autologous Venous Tissue, Open Approach

061009Y Bypass Inferior Vena Cava to Lower Vein with Autologous Venous Tissue, Open Approach

06100A5 Bypass Inferior Vena Cava to Superior Mesenteric Vein with Autologous Arterial Tissue, Open Approach

06100A6 Bypass Inferior Vena Cava to Inferior Mesenteric Vein with Autologous Arterial Tissue, Open Approach

06100AY Bypass Inferior Vena Cava to Lower Vein with Autologous Arterial Tissue, Open Approach

06100J5 Bypass Inferior Vena Cava to Superior Mesenteric Vein with Synthetic Substitute, Open Approach

06100J6 Bypass Inferior Vena Cava to Inferior Mesenteric Vein with Synthetic Substitute, Open Approach

06100JY Bypass Inferior Vena Cava to Lower Vein with Synthetic Substitute, Open Approach

♀ Female-only   ♂ Male-only   ● Limited Coverage   ● Non-OR   HAC HAC-associated procedure   ● Non-covered procedures   + Combination

06100K5 Bypass Inferior Vena Cava to Superior Mesenteric Vein with Nonautologous Tissue Substitute, Open Approach

06100K6 Bypass Inferior Vena Cava to Inferior Mesenteric Vein with Nonautologous Tissue Substitute, Open Approach

06100KY Bypass Inferior Vena Cava to Lower Vein with Nonautologous Tissue Substitute, Open Approach

06100Z5 Bypass Inferior Vena Cava to Superior Mesenteric Vein, Open Approach

06100Z6 Bypass Inferior Vena Cava to Inferior Mesenteric Vein, Open Approach

06100ZY Bypass Inferior Vena Cava to Lower Vein, Open Approach

0610475 Bypass Inferior Vena Cava to Superior Mesenteric Vein with Autologous Tissue Substitute, Percutaneous Endoscopic Approach

0610476 Bypass Inferior Vena Cava to Inferior Mesenteric Vein with Autologous Tissue Substitute, Percutaneous Endoscopic Approach

061047Y Bypass Inferior Vena Cava to Lower Vein with Autologous Tissue Substitute, Percutaneous Endoscopic Approach

0610495 Bypass Inferior Vena Cava to Superior Mesenteric Vein with Autologous Venous Tissue, Percutaneous Endoscopic Approach

0610496 Bypass Inferior Vena Cava to Inferior Mesenteric Vein with Autologous Venous Tissue, Percutaneous Endoscopic Approach

061049Y Bypass Inferior Vena Cava to Lower Vein with Autologous Venous Tissue, Percutaneous Endoscopic Approach

06104A5 Bypass Inferior Vena Cava to Superior Mesenteric Vein with Autologous Arterial Tissue, Percutaneous Endoscopic Approach

06104A6 Bypass Inferior Vena Cava to Inferior Mesenteric Vein with Autologous Arterial Tissue, Percutaneous Endoscopic Approach

06104AY Bypass Inferior Vena Cava to Lower Vein with Autologous Arterial Tissue, Percutaneous Endoscopic Approach

06104J5 Bypass Inferior Vena Cava to Superior Mesenteric Vein with Synthetic Substitute, Percutaneous Endoscopic Approach

06104J6 Bypass Inferior Vena Cava to Inferior Mesenteric Vein with Synthetic Substitute, Percutaneous Endoscopic Approach

06104JY Bypass Inferior Vena Cava to Lower Vein with Synthetic Substitute, Percutaneous Endoscopic Approach

06104K5 Bypass Inferior Vena Cava to Superior Mesenteric Vein with Nonautologous Tissue Substitute, Percutaneous Endoscopic Approach

06104K6 Bypass Inferior Vena Cava to Inferior Mesenteric Vein with Nonautologous Tissue Substitute, Percutaneous Endoscopic Approach

06104KY Bypass Inferior Vena Cava to Lower Vein with Nonautologous Tissue Substitute, Percutaneous Endoscopic Approach

06104Z5 Bypass Inferior Vena Cava to Superior Mesenteric Vein, Percutaneous Endoscopic Approach

06104Z6 Bypass Inferior Vena Cava to Inferior Mesenteric Vein, Percutaneous Endoscopic Approach

06104ZY Bypass Inferior Vena Cava to Lower Vein, Percutaneous Endoscopic Approach

0611079 Bypass Splenic Vein to Right Renal Vein with Autologous Tissue Substitute, Open Approach

061107B Bypass Splenic Vein to Left Renal Vein with Autologous Tissue Substitute, Open Approach

061107Y Bypass Splenic Vein to Lower Vein with Autologous Tissue Substitute, Open Approach

0611099 Bypass Splenic Vein to Right Renal Vein with Autologous Venous Tissue, Open Approach

061109B Bypass Splenic Vein to Left Renal Vein with Autologous Venous Tissue, Open Approach

061109Y Bypass Splenic Vein to Lower Vein with Autologous Venous Tissue, Open Approach

06110A9 Bypass Splenic Vein to Right Renal Vein with Autologous Arterial Tissue, Open Approach

06110AB Bypass Splenic Vein to Left Renal Vein with Autologous Arterial Tissue, Open Approach

06110AY Bypass Splenic Vein to Lower Vein with Autologous Arterial Tissue, Open Approach

06110J9 Bypass Splenic Vein to Right Renal Vein with Synthetic Substitute, Open Approach

06110JB Bypass Splenic Vein to Left Renal Vein with Synthetic Substitute, Open Approach

06110JY Bypass Splenic Vein to Lower Vein with Synthetic Substitute, Open Approach

06110K9 Bypass Splenic Vein to Right Renal Vein with Nonautologous Tissue Substitute, Open Approach

06110KB Bypass Splenic Vein to Left Renal Vein with Nonautologous Tissue Substitute, Open Approach

06110KY Bypass Splenic Vein to Lower Vein with Nonautologous Tissue Substitute, Open Approach

06110Z9 Bypass Splenic Vein to Right Renal Vein, Open Approach

06110ZB Bypass Splenic Vein to Left Renal Vein, Open Approach

06110ZY Bypass Splenic Vein to Lower Vein, Open Approach

0611479 Bypass Splenic Vein to Right Renal Vein with Autologous Tissue Substitute, Percutaneous Endoscopic Approach

061147B Bypass Splenic Vein to Left Renal Vein with Autologous Tissue Substitute, Percutaneous Endoscopic Approach

061147Y Bypass Splenic Vein to Lower Vein with Autologous Tissue Substitute, Percutaneous Endoscopic Approach

0611499 Bypass Splenic Vein to Right Renal Vein with Autologous Venous Tissue, Percutaneous Endoscopic Approach

061149B Bypass Splenic Vein to Left Renal Vein with Autologous Venous Tissue, Percutaneous Endoscopic Approach

061149Y Bypass Splenic Vein to Lower Vein with Autologous Venous Tissue, Percutaneous Endoscopic Approach

06114A9 Bypass Splenic Vein to Right Renal Vein with Autologous Arterial Tissue, Percutaneous Endoscopic Approach

06114AB Bypass Splenic Vein to Left Renal Vein with Autologous Arterial Tissue, Percutaneous Endoscopic Approach

06114AY Bypass Splenic Vein to Lower Vein with Autologous Arterial Tissue, Percutaneous Endoscopic Approach

06114J9 Bypass Splenic Vein to Right Renal Vein with Synthetic Substitute, Percutaneous Endoscopic Approach

06114JB Bypass Splenic Vein to Left Renal Vein with Synthetic Substitute, Percutaneous Endoscopic Approach

06114JY Bypass Splenic Vein to Lower Vein with Synthetic Substitute, Percutaneous Endoscopic Approach

06114K9 Bypass Splenic Vein to Right Renal Vein with Nonautologous Tissue Substitute, Percutaneous Endoscopic Approach

06114KB Bypass Splenic Vein to Left Renal Vein with Nonautologous Tissue Substitute, Percutaneous Endoscopic Approach

06114KY Bypass Splenic Vein to Lower Vein with Nonautologous Tissue Substitute, Percutaneous Endoscopic Approach

06114Z9 Bypass Splenic Vein to Right Renal Vein, Percutaneous Endoscopic Approach

06114ZB Bypass Splenic Vein to Left Renal Vein, Percutaneous Endoscopic Approach

06114ZY Bypass Splenic Vein to Lower Vein, Percutaneous Endoscopic Approach

061207Y Bypass Gastric Vein to Lower Vein with Autologous Tissue Substitute, Open Approach

061209Y Bypass Gastric Vein to Lower Vein with Autologous Venous Tissue, Open Approach

06120AY Bypass Gastric Vein to Lower Vein with Autologous Arterial Tissue, Open Approach

06120JY Bypass Gastric Vein to Lower Vein with Synthetic Substitute, Open Approach

06120KY Bypass Gastric Vein to Lower Vein with Nonautologous Tissue Substitute, Open Approach

06120ZY Bypass Gastric Vein to Lower Vein, Open Approach

061247Y Bypass Gastric Vein to Lower Vein with Autologous Tissue Substitute, Percutaneous Endoscopic Approach

061249Y Bypass Gastric Vein to Lower Vein with Autologous Venous Tissue, Percutaneous Endoscopic Approach

06124AY Bypass Gastric Vein to Lower Vein with Autologous Arterial Tissue, Percutaneous Endoscopic Approach

06124JY Bypass Gastric Vein to Lower Vein with Synthetic Substitute, Percutaneous Endoscopic Approach

06124KY Bypass Gastric Vein to Lower Vein with Nonautologous Tissue Substitute, Percutaneous Endoscopic Approach

06124ZY Bypass Gastric Vein to Lower Vein, Percutaneous Endoscopic Approach

061307Y Bypass Esophageal Vein to Lower Vein with Autologous Tissue Substitute, Open Approach

061309Y Bypass Esophageal Vein to Lower Vein with Autologous Venous Tissue, Open Approach

06130AY Bypass Esophageal Vein to Lower Vein with Autologous Arterial Tissue, Open Approach

06130JY Bypass Esophageal Vein to Lower Vein with Synthetic Substitute, Open Approach

06130KY Bypass Esophageal Vein to Lower Vein with Nonautologous Tissue Substitute, Open Approach

06130ZY Bypass Esophageal Vein to Lower Vein, Open Approach

061347Y Bypass Esophageal Vein to Lower Vein with Autologous Tissue Substitute, Percutaneous Endoscopic Approach

061349Y Bypass Esophageal Vein to Lower Vein with Autologous Venous Tissue, Percutaneous Endoscopic Approach

06134AY Bypass Esophageal Vein to Lower Vein with Autologous Arterial Tissue, Percutaneous Endoscopic Approach

06134JY Bypass Esophageal Vein to Lower Vein with Synthetic Substitute, Percutaneous Endoscopic Approach

06134KY Bypass Esophageal Vein to Lower Vein with Nonautologous Tissue Substitute, Percutaneous Endoscopic Approach

06134ZY Bypass Esophageal Vein to Lower Vein, Percutaneous Endoscopic Approach

061407Y Bypass Hepatic Vein to Lower Vein with Autologous Tissue Substitute, Open Approach

061409Y Bypass Hepatic Vein to Lower Vein with Autologous Venous Tissue, Open Approach

06140AY Bypass Hepatic Vein to Lower Vein with Autologous Arterial Tissue, Open Approach

06140JY Bypass Hepatic Vein to Lower Vein with Synthetic Substitute, Open Approach

06140KY Bypass Hepatic Vein to Lower Vein with Nonautologous Tissue Substitute, Open Approach

06140ZY Bypass Hepatic Vein to Lower Vein, Open Approach

061447Y Bypass Hepatic Vein to Lower Vein with Autologous Tissue Substitute, Percutaneous Endoscopic Approach

061449Y Bypass Hepatic Vein to Lower Vein with Autologous Venous Tissue, Percutaneous Endoscopic Approach

06144AY Bypass Hepatic Vein to Lower Vein with Autologous Arterial Tissue, Percutaneous Endoscopic Approach

06144JY Bypass Hepatic Vein to Lower Vein with Synthetic Substitute, Percutaneous Endoscopic Approach

06144KY Bypass Hepatic Vein to Lower Vein with Nonautologous Tissue Substitute, Percutaneous Endoscopic Approach

06144ZY Bypass Hepatic Vein to Lower Vein, Percutaneous Endoscopic Approach

061507Y Bypass Superior Mesenteric Vein to Lower Vein with Autologous Tissue Substitute, Open Approach

061509Y Bypass Superior Mesenteric Vein to Lower Vein with Autologous Venous Tissue, Open Approach

06150AY Bypass Superior Mesenteric Vein to Lower Vein with Autologous Arterial Tissue, Open Approach

06150JY Bypass Superior Mesenteric Vein to Lower Vein with Synthetic Substitute, Open Approach

06150KY Bypass Superior Mesenteric Vein to Lower Vein with Nonautologous Tissue Substitute, Open Approach

06150ZY Bypass Superior Mesenteric Vein to Lower Vein, Open Approach

061547Y Bypass Superior Mesenteric Vein to Lower Vein with Autologous Tissue Substitute, Percutaneous Endoscopic Approach

061549Y Bypass Superior Mesenteric Vein to Lower Vein with Autologous Venous Tissue, Percutaneous Endoscopic Approach

06154AY Bypass Superior Mesenteric Vein to Lower Vein with Autologous Arterial Tissue, Percutaneous Endoscopic Approach

06154JY Bypass Superior Mesenteric Vein to Lower Vein with Synthetic Substitute, Percutaneous Endoscopic Approach

06154KY Bypass Superior Mesenteric Vein to Lower Vein with Nonautologous Tissue Substitute, Percutaneous Endoscopic Approach

06154ZY Bypass Superior Mesenteric Vein to Lower Vein, Percutaneous Endoscopic Approach

061607Y Bypass Inferior Mesenteric Vein to Lower Vein with Autologous Tissue Substitute, Open Approach

061609Y Bypass Inferior Mesenteric Vein to Lower Vein with Autologous Venous Tissue, Open Approach

06160AY Bypass Inferior Mesenteric Vein to Lower Vein with Autologous Arterial Tissue, Open Approach

06160JY Bypass Inferior Mesenteric Vein to Lower Vein with Synthetic Substitute, Open Approach

06160KY Bypass Inferior Mesenteric Vein to Lower Vein with Nonautologous Tissue Substitute, Open Approach

06160ZY Bypass Inferior Mesenteric Vein to Lower Vein, Open Approach

061647Y Bypass Inferior Mesenteric Vein to Lower Vein with Autologous Tissue Substitute, Percutaneous Endoscopic Approach

061649Y Bypass Inferior Mesenteric Vein to Lower Vein with Autologous Venous Tissue, Percutaneous Endoscopic Approach

06164AY Bypass Inferior Mesenteric Vein to Lower Vein with Autologous Arterial Tissue, Percutaneous Endoscopic Approach

06164JY Bypass Inferior Mesenteric Vein to Lower Vein with Synthetic Substitute, Percutaneous Endoscopic Approach

06164KY Bypass Inferior Mesenteric Vein to Lower Vein with Nonautologous Tissue Substitute, Percutaneous Endoscopic Approach

06164ZY Bypass Inferior Mesenteric Vein to Lower Vein, Percutaneous Endoscopic Approach

061707Y Bypass Colic Vein to Lower Vein with Autologous Tissue Substitute, Open Approach

061709Y Bypass Colic Vein to Lower Vein with Autologous Venous Tissue, Open Approach

06170AY Bypass Colic Vein to Lower Vein with Autologous Arterial Tissue, Open Approach

06170JY Bypass Colic Vein to Lower Vein with Synthetic Substitute, Open Approach

06170KY Bypass Colic Vein to Lower Vein with Nonautologous Tissue Substitute, Open Approach

06170ZY Bypass Colic Vein to Lower Vein, Open Approach

061747Y Bypass Colic Vein to Lower Vein with Autologous Tissue Substitute, Percutaneous Endoscopic Approach

061749Y Bypass Colic Vein to Lower Vein with Autologous Venous Tissue, Percutaneous Endoscopic Approach

06174AY Bypass Colic Vein to Lower Vein with Autologous Arterial Tissue, Percutaneous Endoscopic Approach

06174JY Bypass Colic Vein to Lower Vein with Synthetic Substitute, Percutaneous Endoscopic Approach

06174KY Bypass Colic Vein to Lower Vein with Nonautologous Tissue Substitute, Percutaneous Endoscopic Approach

06174ZY Bypass Colic Vein to Lower Vein, Percutaneous Endoscopic Approach

0618079 Bypass Portal Vein to Right Renal Vein with Autologous Tissue Substitute, Open Approach

061807B Bypass Portal Vein to Left Renal Vein with Autologous Tissue Substitute, Open Approach

061807Y Bypass Portal Vein to Lower Vein with Autologous Tissue Substitute, Open Approach

0618099 Bypass Portal Vein to Right Renal Vein with Autologous Venous Tissue, Open Approach

061809B Bypass Portal Vein to Left Renal Vein with Autologous Venous Tissue, Open Approach

061809Y Bypass Portal Vein to Lower Vein with Autologous Venous Tissue, Open Approach

06180A9 Bypass Portal Vein to Right Renal Vein with Autologous Arterial Tissue, Open Approach

06180AB Bypass Portal Vein to Left Renal Vein with Autologous Arterial Tissue, Open Approach

06180AY Bypass Portal Vein to Lower Vein with Autologous Arterial Tissue, Open Approach

06180J9 Bypass Portal Vein to Right Renal Vein with Synthetic Substitute, Open Approach

06180JB Bypass Portal Vein to Left Renal Vein with Synthetic Substitute, Open Approach

06180JY Bypass Portal Vein to Lower Vein with Synthetic Substitute, Open Approach

06180K9 Bypass Portal Vein to Right Renal Vein with Nonautologous Tissue Substitute, Open Approach

06180KB Bypass Portal Vein to Left Renal Vein with Nonautologous Tissue Substitute, Open Approach

06180KY Bypass Portal Vein to Lower Vein with Nonautologous Tissue Substitute, Open Approach

06180Z9 Bypass Portal Vein to Right Renal Vein, Open Approach

06180ZB Bypass Portal Vein to Left Renal Vein, Open Approach

06180ZY Bypass Portal Vein to Lower Vein, Open Approach

06183DY Bypass Portal Vein to Lower Vein with Intraluminal Device, Percutaneous Approach

---

♀ Female-only   ♂ Male-only   ◐ Limited Coverage   ● Non-OR   ▰ HAC-associated procedure   ● Non-covered procedures   ✚ Combination

0618479   Bypass Portal Vein to Right Renal Vein with Autologous Tissue Substitute, Percutaneous Endoscopic Approach

061847B   Bypass Portal Vein to Left Renal Vein with Autologous Tissue Substitute, Percutaneous Endoscopic Approach

061847Y   Bypass Portal Vein to Lower Vein with Autologous Tissue Substitute, Percutaneous Endoscopic Approach

0618499   Bypass Portal Vein to Right Renal Vein with Autologous Venous Tissue, Percutaneous Endoscopic Approach

061849B   Bypass Portal Vein to Left Renal Vein with Autologous Venous Tissue, Percutaneous Endoscopic Approach

061849Y   Bypass Portal Vein to Lower Vein with Autologous Venous Tissue, Percutaneous Endoscopic Approach

06184A9   Bypass Portal Vein to Right Renal Vein with Autologous Arterial Tissue, Percutaneous Endoscopic Approach

06184AB   Bypass Portal Vein to Left Renal Vein with Autologous Arterial Tissue, Percutaneous Endoscopic Approach

06184AY   Bypass Portal Vein to Lower Vein with Autologous Arterial Tissue, Percutaneous Endoscopic Approach

06184DY   Bypass Portal Vein to Lower Vein with Intraluminal Device, Percutaneous Endoscopic Approach

06184J9   Bypass Portal Vein to Right Renal Vein with Synthetic Substitute, Percutaneous Endoscopic Approach

06184JB   Bypass Portal Vein to Left Renal Vein with Synthetic Substitute, Percutaneous Endoscopic Approach

06184JY   Bypass Portal Vein to Lower Vein with Synthetic Substitute, Percutaneous Endoscopic Approach

06184K9   Bypass Portal Vein to Right Renal Vein with Nonautologous Tissue Substitute, Percutaneous Endoscopic Approach

06184KB   Bypass Portal Vein to Left Renal Vein with Nonautologous Tissue Substitute, Percutaneous Endoscopic Approach

06184KY   Bypass Portal Vein to Lower Vein with Nonautologous Tissue Substitute, Percutaneous Endoscopic Approach

06184Z9   Bypass Portal Vein to Right Renal Vein, Percutaneous Endoscopic Approach

06184ZB   Bypass Portal Vein to Left Renal Vein, Percutaneous Endoscopic Approach

06184ZY   Bypass Portal Vein to Lower Vein, Percutaneous Endoscopic Approach

061907Y   Bypass Right Renal Vein to Lower Vein with Autologous Tissue Substitute, Open Approach

061909Y   Bypass Right Renal Vein to Lower Vein with Autologous Venous Tissue, Open Approach

06190AY   Bypass Right Renal Vein to Lower Vein with Autologous Arterial Tissue, Open Approach

06190JY   Bypass Right Renal Vein to Lower Vein with Synthetic Substitute, Open Approach

06190KY   Bypass Right Renal Vein to Lower Vein with Nonautologous Tissue Substitute, Open Approach

06190ZY   Bypass Right Renal Vein to Lower Vein, Open Approach

061947Y   Bypass Right Renal Vein to Lower Vein with Autologous Tissue Substitute, Percutaneous Endoscopic Approach

061949Y   Bypass Right Renal Vein to Lower Vein with Autologous Venous Tissue, Percutaneous Endoscopic Approach

06194AY   Bypass Right Renal Vein to Lower Vein with Autologous Arterial Tissue, Percutaneous Endoscopic Approach

06194JY   Bypass Right Renal Vein to Lower Vein with Synthetic Substitute, Percutaneous Endoscopic Approach

06194KY   Bypass Right Renal Vein to Lower Vein with Nonautologous Tissue Substitute, Percutaneous Endoscopic Approach

06194ZY   Bypass Right Renal Vein to Lower Vein, Percutaneous Endoscopic Approach

061B07Y   Bypass Left Renal Vein to Lower Vein with Autologous Tissue Substitute, Open Approach

061B09Y   Bypass Left Renal Vein to Lower Vein with Autologous Venous Tissue, Open Approach

061B0AY   Bypass Left Renal Vein to Lower Vein with Autologous Arterial Tissue, Open Approach

061B0JY   Bypass Left Renal Vein to Lower Vein with Synthetic Substitute, Open Approach

061B0KY   Bypass Left Renal Vein to Lower Vein with Nonautologous Tissue Substitute, Open Approach

061B0ZY   Bypass Left Renal Vein to Lower Vein, Open Approach

061B47Y   Bypass Left Renal Vein to Lower Vein with Autologous Tissue Substitute, Percutaneous Endoscopic Approach

061B49Y   Bypass Left Renal Vein to Lower Vein with Autologous Venous Tissue, Percutaneous Endoscopic Approach

061B4AY   Bypass Left Renal Vein to Lower Vein with Autologous Arterial Tissue, Percutaneous Endoscopic Approach

061B4JY   Bypass Left Renal Vein to Lower Vein with Synthetic Substitute, Percutaneous Endoscopic Approach

061B4KY   Bypass Left Renal Vein to Lower Vein with Nonautologous Tissue Substitute, Percutaneous Endoscopic Approach

061B4ZY   Bypass Left Renal Vein to Lower Vein, Percutaneous Endoscopic Approach

061C07Y   Bypass Right Common Iliac Vein to Lower Vein with Autologous Tissue Substitute, Open Approach

061C09Y   Bypass Right Common Iliac Vein to Lower Vein with Autologous Venous Tissue, Open Approach

061C0AY   Bypass Right Common Iliac Vein to Lower Vein with Autologous Arterial Tissue, Open Approach

061C0JY   Bypass Right Common Iliac Vein to Lower Vein with Synthetic Substitute, Open Approach

061C0KY   Bypass Right Common Iliac Vein to Lower Vein with Nonautologous Tissue Substitute, Open Approach

061C0ZY   Bypass Right Common Iliac Vein to Lower Vein, Open Approach

061C47Y   Bypass Right Common Iliac Vein to Lower Vein with Autologous Tissue Substitute, Percutaneous Endoscopic Approach

061C49Y   Bypass Right Common Iliac Vein to Lower Vein with Autologous Venous Tissue, Percutaneous Endoscopic Approach

061C4AY   Bypass Right Common Iliac Vein to Lower Vein with Autologous Arterial Tissue, Percutaneous Endoscopic Approach

061C4JY   Bypass Right Common Iliac Vein to Lower Vein with Synthetic Substitute, Percutaneous Endoscopic Approach

061C4KY   Bypass Right Common Iliac Vein to Lower Vein with Nonautologous Tissue Substitute, Percutaneous Endoscopic Approach

061C4ZY   Bypass Right Common Iliac Vein to Lower Vein, Percutaneous Endoscopic Approach

061D07Y   Bypass Left Common Iliac Vein to Lower Vein with Autologous Tissue Substitute, Open Approach

061D09Y   Bypass Left Common Iliac Vein to Lower Vein with Autologous Venous Tissue, Open Approach

061D0AY   Bypass Left Common Iliac Vein to Lower Vein with Autologous Arterial Tissue, Open Approach

061D0JY   Bypass Left Common Iliac Vein to Lower Vein with Synthetic Substitute, Open Approach

061D0KY   Bypass Left Common Iliac Vein to Lower Vein with Nonautologous Tissue Substitute, Open Approach

061D0ZY   Bypass Left Common Iliac Vein to Lower Vein, Open Approach

061D47Y   Bypass Left Common Iliac Vein to Lower Vein with Autologous Tissue Substitute, Percutaneous Endoscopic Approach

061D49Y   Bypass Left Common Iliac Vein to Lower Vein with Autologous Venous Tissue, Percutaneous Endoscopic Approach

061D4AY   Bypass Left Common Iliac Vein to Lower Vein with Autologous Arterial Tissue, Percutaneous Endoscopic Approach

061D4JY   Bypass Left Common Iliac Vein to Lower Vein with Synthetic Substitute, Percutaneous Endoscopic Approach

061D4KY   Bypass Left Common Iliac Vein to Lower Vein with Nonautologous Tissue Substitute, Percutaneous Endoscopic Approach

061D4ZY   Bypass Left Common Iliac Vein to Lower Vein, Percutaneous Endoscopic Approach

061F07Y   Bypass Right External Iliac Vein to Lower Vein with Autologous Tissue Substitute, Open Approach

061F09Y   Bypass Right External Iliac Vein to Lower Vein with Autologous Venous Tissue, Open Approach

061F0AY   Bypass Right External Iliac Vein to Lower Vein with Autologous Arterial Tissue, Open Approach

061F0JY   Bypass Right External Iliac Vein to Lower Vein with Synthetic Substitute, Open Approach

061F0KY   Bypass Right External Iliac Vein to Lower Vein with Nonautologous Tissue Substitute, Open Approach

061F0ZY   Bypass Right External Iliac Vein to Lower Vein, Open Approach

061F47Y   Bypass Right External Iliac Vein to Lower Vein with Autologous Tissue Substitute, Percutaneous Endoscopic Approach

061F49Y Bypass Right External Iliac Vein to Lower Vein with Autologous Venous Tissue, Percutaneous Endoscopic Approach

061F4AY Bypass Right External Iliac Vein to Lower Vein with Autologous Arterial Tissue, Percutaneous Endoscopic Approach

061F4JY Bypass Right External Iliac Vein to Lower Vein with Synthetic Substitute, Percutaneous Endoscopic Approach

061F4KY Bypass Right External Iliac Vein to Lower Vein with Nonautologous Tissue Substitute, Percutaneous Endoscopic Approach

061F4ZY Bypass Right External Iliac Vein to Lower Vein, Percutaneous Endoscopic Approach

061G07Y Bypass Left External Iliac Vein to Lower Vein with Autologous Tissue Substitute, Open Approach

061G09Y Bypass Left External Iliac Vein to Lower Vein with Autologous Venous Tissue, Open Approach

061G0AY Bypass Left External Iliac Vein to Lower Vein with Autologous Arterial Tissue, Open Approach

061G0JY Bypass Left External Iliac Vein to Lower Vein with Synthetic Substitute, Open Approach

061G0KY Bypass Left External Iliac Vein to Lower Vein with Nonautologous Tissue Substitute, Open Approach

061G0ZY Bypass Left External Iliac Vein to Lower Vein, Open Approach

061G47Y Bypass Left External Iliac Vein to Lower Vein with Autologous Tissue Substitute, Percutaneous Endoscopic Approach

061G49Y Bypass Left External Iliac Vein to Lower Vein with Autologous Venous Tissue, Percutaneous Endoscopic Approach

061G4AY Bypass Left External Iliac Vein to Lower Vein with Autologous Arterial Tissue, Percutaneous Endoscopic Approach

061G4JY Bypass Left External Iliac Vein to Lower Vein with Synthetic Substitute, Percutaneous Endoscopic Approach

061G4KY Bypass Left External Iliac Vein to Lower Vein with Nonautologous Tissue Substitute, Percutaneous Endoscopic Approach

061G4ZY Bypass Left External Iliac Vein to Lower Vein, Percutaneous Endoscopic Approach

061H07Y Bypass Right Hypogastric Vein to Lower Vein with Autologous Tissue Substitute, Open Approach

061H09Y Bypass Right Hypogastric Vein to Lower Vein with Autologous Venous Tissue, Open Approach

061H0AY Bypass Right Hypogastric Vein to Lower Vein with Autologous Arterial Tissue, Open Approach

061H0JY Bypass Right Hypogastric Vein to Lower Vein with Synthetic Substitute, Open Approach

061H0KY Bypass Right Hypogastric Vein to Lower Vein with Nonautologous Tissue Substitute, Open Approach

061H0ZY Bypass Right Hypogastric Vein to Lower Vein, Open Approach

061H47Y Bypass Right Hypogastric Vein to Lower Vein with Autologous Tissue Substitute, Percutaneous Endoscopic Approach

061H49Y Bypass Right Hypogastric Vein to Lower Vein with Autologous Venous Tissue, Percutaneous Endoscopic Approach

061H4AY Bypass Right Hypogastric Vein to Lower Vein with Autologous Arterial Tissue, Percutaneous Endoscopic Approach

061H4JY Bypass Right Hypogastric Vein to Lower Vein with Synthetic Substitute, Percutaneous Endoscopic Approach

061H4KY Bypass Right Hypogastric Vein to Lower Vein with Nonautologous Tissue Substitute, Percutaneous Endoscopic Approach

061H4ZY Bypass Right Hypogastric Vein to Lower Vein, Percutaneous Endoscopic Approach

061J07Y Bypass Left Hypogastric Vein to Lower Vein with Autologous Tissue Substitute, Open Approach

061J09Y Bypass Left Hypogastric Vein to Lower Vein with Autologous Venous Tissue, Open Approach

061J0AY Bypass Left Hypogastric Vein to Lower Vein with Autologous Arterial Tissue, Open Approach

061J0JY Bypass Left Hypogastric Vein to Lower Vein with Synthetic Substitute, Open Approach

061J0KY Bypass Left Hypogastric Vein to Lower Vein with Nonautologous Tissue Substitute, Open Approach

061J0ZY Bypass Left Hypogastric Vein to Lower Vein, Open Approach

061J47Y Bypass Left Hypogastric Vein to Lower Vein with Autologous Tissue Substitute, Percutaneous Endoscopic Approach

061J49Y Bypass Left Hypogastric Vein to Lower Vein with Autologous Venous Tissue, Percutaneous Endoscopic Approach

061J4AY Bypass Left Hypogastric Vein to Lower Vein with Autologous Arterial Tissue, Percutaneous Endoscopic Approach

061J4JY Bypass Left Hypogastric Vein to Lower Vein with Synthetic Substitute, Percutaneous Endoscopic Approach

061J4KY Bypass Left Hypogastric Vein to Lower Vein with Nonautologous Tissue Substitute, Percutaneous Endoscopic Approach

061J4ZY Bypass Left Hypogastric Vein to Lower Vein, Percutaneous Endoscopic Approach

061M07Y Bypass Right Femoral Vein to Lower Vein with Autologous Tissue Substitute, Open Approach

061M09Y Bypass Right Femoral Vein to Lower Vein with Autologous Venous Tissue, Open Approach

061M0AY Bypass Right Femoral Vein to Lower Vein with Autologous Arterial Tissue, Open Approach

061M0JY Bypass Right Femoral Vein to Lower Vein with Synthetic Substitute, Open Approach

061M0KY Bypass Right Femoral Vein to Lower Vein with Nonautologous Tissue Substitute, Open Approach

061M0ZY Bypass Right Femoral Vein to Lower Vein, Open Approach

061M47Y Bypass Right Femoral Vein to Lower Vein with Autologous Tissue Substitute, Percutaneous Endoscopic Approach

061M49Y Bypass Right Femoral Vein to Lower Vein with Autologous Venous Tissue, Percutaneous Endoscopic Approach

061M4AY Bypass Right Femoral Vein to Lower Vein with Autologous Arterial Tissue, Percutaneous Endoscopic Approach

061M4JY Bypass Right Femoral Vein to Lower Vein with Synthetic Substitute, Percutaneous Endoscopic Approach

061M4KY Bypass Right Femoral Vein to Lower Vein with Nonautologous Tissue Substitute, Percutaneous Endoscopic Approach

061M4ZY Bypass Right Femoral Vein to Lower Vein, Percutaneous Endoscopic Approach

061N07Y Bypass Left Femoral Vein to Lower Vein with Autologous Tissue Substitute, Open Approach

061N09Y Bypass Left Femoral Vein to Lower Vein with Autologous Venous Tissue, Open Approach

061N0AY Bypass Left Femoral Vein to Lower Vein with Autologous Arterial Tissue, Open Approach

061N0JY Bypass Left Femoral Vein to Lower Vein with Synthetic Substitute, Open Approach

061N0KY Bypass Left Femoral Vein to Lower Vein with Nonautologous Tissue Substitute, Open Approach

061N0ZY Bypass Left Femoral Vein to Lower Vein, Open Approach

061N47Y Bypass Left Femoral Vein to Lower Vein with Autologous Tissue Substitute, Percutaneous Endoscopic Approach

061N49Y Bypass Left Femoral Vein to Lower Vein with Autologous Venous Tissue, Percutaneous Endoscopic Approach

061N4AY Bypass Left Femoral Vein to Lower Vein with Autologous Arterial Tissue, Percutaneous Endoscopic Approach

061N4JY Bypass Left Femoral Vein to Lower Vein with Synthetic Substitute, Percutaneous Endoscopic Approach

061N4KY Bypass Left Femoral Vein to Lower Vein with Nonautologous Tissue Substitute, Percutaneous Endoscopic Approach

061N4ZY Bypass Left Femoral Vein to Lower Vein, Percutaneous Endoscopic Approach

061P07Y Bypass Right Greater Saphenous Vein to Lower Vein with Autologous Tissue Substitute, Open Approach

061P09Y Bypass Right Greater Saphenous Vein to Lower Vein with Autologous Venous Tissue, Open Approach

061P0AY Bypass Right Greater Saphenous Vein to Lower Vein with Autologous Arterial Tissue, Open Approach

061P0JY Bypass Right Greater Saphenous Vein to Lower Vein with Synthetic Substitute, Open Approach

061P0KY Bypass Right Greater Saphenous Vein to Lower Vein with Nonautologous Tissue Substitute, Open Approach

061P0ZY Bypass Right Greater Saphenous Vein to Lower Vein, Open Approach

061P47Y Bypass Right Greater Saphenous Vein to Lower Vein with Autologous Tissue Substitute, Percutaneous Endoscopic Approach

061P49Y Bypass Right Greater Saphenous Vein to Lower Vein with Autologous Venous Tissue, Percutaneous Endoscopic Approach

061P4AY Bypass Right Greater Saphenous Vein to Lower Vein with Autologous Arterial Tissue, Percutaneous Endoscopic Approach

061P4JY Bypass Right Greater Saphenous Vein to Lower Vein with Synthetic Substitute, Percutaneous Endoscopic Approach

061P4KY Bypass Right Greater Saphenous Vein to Lower Vein with Nonautologous Tissue Substitute, Percutaneous Endoscopic Approach

061P4ZY Bypass Right Greater Saphenous Vein to Lower Vein, Percutaneous Endoscopic Approach

061Q07Y Bypass Left Greater Saphenous Vein to Lower Vein with Autologous Tissue Substitute, Open Approach

061Q09Y Bypass Left Greater Saphenous Vein to Lower Vein with Autologous Venous Tissue, Open Approach

061Q0AY Bypass Left Greater Saphenous Vein to Lower Vein with Autologous Arterial Tissue, Open Approach

061Q0JY Bypass Left Greater Saphenous Vein to Lower Vein with Synthetic Substitute, Open Approach

061Q0KY Bypass Left Greater Saphenous Vein to Lower Vein with Nonautologous Tissue Substitute, Open Approach

061Q0ZY Bypass Left Greater Saphenous Vein to Lower Vein, Open Approach

061Q47Y Bypass Left Greater Saphenous Vein to Lower Vein with Autologous Tissue Substitute, Percutaneous Endoscopic Approach

061Q49Y Bypass Left Greater Saphenous Vein to Lower Vein with Autologous Venous Tissue, Percutaneous Endoscopic Approach

061Q4AY Bypass Left Greater Saphenous Vein to Lower Vein with Autologous Arterial Tissue, Percutaneous Endoscopic Approach

061Q4JY Bypass Left Greater Saphenous Vein to Lower Vein with Synthetic Substitute, Percutaneous Endoscopic Approach

061Q4KY Bypass Left Greater Saphenous Vein to Lower Vein with Nonautologous Tissue Substitute, Percutaneous Endoscopic Approach

061Q4ZY Bypass Left Greater Saphenous Vein to Lower Vein, Percutaneous Endoscopic Approach

061R07Y Bypass Right Lesser Saphenous Vein to Lower Vein with Autologous Tissue Substitute, Open Approach

061R09Y Bypass Right Lesser Saphenous Vein to Lower Vein with Autologous Venous Tissue, Open Approach

061R0AY Bypass Right Lesser Saphenous Vein to Lower Vein with Autologous Arterial Tissue, Open Approach

061R0JY Bypass Right Lesser Saphenous Vein to Lower Vein with Synthetic Substitute, Open Approach

061R0KY Bypass Right Lesser Saphenous Vein to Lower Vein with Nonautologous Tissue Substitute, Open Approach

061R0ZY Bypass Right Lesser Saphenous Vein to Lower Vein, Open Approach

061R47Y Bypass Right Lesser Saphenous Vein to Lower Vein with Autologous Tissue Substitute, Percutaneous Endoscopic Approach

061R49Y Bypass Right Lesser Saphenous Vein to Lower Vein with Autologous Venous Tissue, Percutaneous Endoscopic Approach

061R4AY Bypass Right Lesser Saphenous Vein to Lower Vein with Autologous Arterial Tissue, Percutaneous Endoscopic Approach

061R4JY Bypass Right Lesser Saphenous Vein to Lower Vein with Synthetic Substitute, Percutaneous Endoscopic Approach

061R4KY Bypass Right Lesser Saphenous Vein to Lower Vein with Nonautologous Tissue Substitute, Percutaneous Endoscopic Approach

061R4ZY Bypass Right Lesser Saphenous Vein to Lower Vein, Percutaneous Endoscopic Approach

061S07Y Bypass Left Lesser Saphenous Vein to Lower Vein with Autologous Tissue Substitute, Open Approach

061S09Y Bypass Left Lesser Saphenous Vein to Lower Vein with Autologous Venous Tissue, Open Approach

061S0AY Bypass Left Lesser Saphenous Vein to Lower Vein with Autologous Arterial Tissue, Open Approach

061S0JY Bypass Left Lesser Saphenous Vein to Lower Vein with Synthetic Substitute, Open Approach

061S0KY Bypass Left Lesser Saphenous Vein to Lower Vein with Nonautologous Tissue Substitute, Open Approach

061S0ZY Bypass Left Lesser Saphenous Vein to Lower Vein, Open Approach

061S47Y Bypass Left Lesser Saphenous Vein to Lower Vein with Autologous Tissue Substitute, Percutaneous Endoscopic Approach

061S49Y Bypass Left Lesser Saphenous Vein to Lower Vein with Autologous Venous Tissue, Percutaneous Endoscopic Approach

061S4AY Bypass Left Lesser Saphenous Vein to Lower Vein with Autologous Arterial Tissue, Percutaneous Endoscopic Approach

061S4JY Bypass Left Lesser Saphenous Vein to Lower Vein with Synthetic Substitute, Percutaneous Endoscopic Approach

061S4KY Bypass Left Lesser Saphenous Vein to Lower Vein with Nonautologous Tissue Substitute, Percutaneous Endoscopic Approach

061S4ZY Bypass Left Lesser Saphenous Vein to Lower Vein, Percutaneous Endoscopic Approach

061T07Y Bypass Right Foot Vein to Lower Vein with Autologous Tissue Substitute, Open Approach

061T09Y Bypass Right Foot Vein to Lower Vein with Autologous Venous Tissue, Open Approach

061T0AY Bypass Right Foot Vein to Lower Vein with Autologous Arterial Tissue, Open Approach

061T0JY Bypass Right Foot Vein to Lower Vein with Synthetic Substitute, Open Approach

061T0KY Bypass Right Foot Vein to Lower Vein with Nonautologous Tissue Substitute, Open Approach

061T0ZY Bypass Right Foot Vein to Lower Vein, Open Approach

061T47Y Bypass Right Foot Vein to Lower Vein with Autologous Tissue Substitute, Percutaneous Endoscopic Approach

061T49Y Bypass Right Foot Vein to Lower Vein with Autologous Venous Tissue, Percutaneous Endoscopic Approach

061T4AY Bypass Right Foot Vein to Lower Vein with Autologous Arterial Tissue, Percutaneous Endoscopic Approach

061T4JY Bypass Right Foot Vein to Lower Vein with Synthetic Substitute, Percutaneous Endoscopic Approach

061T4KY Bypass Right Foot Vein to Lower Vein with Nonautologous Tissue Substitute, Percutaneous Endoscopic Approach

061T4ZY Bypass Right Foot Vein to Lower Vein, Percutaneous Endoscopic Approach

061V07Y Bypass Left Foot Vein to Lower Vein with Autologous Tissue Substitute, Open Approach

061V09Y Bypass Left Foot Vein to Lower Vein with Autologous Venous Tissue, Open Approach

061V0AY Bypass Left Foot Vein to Lower Vein with Autologous Arterial Tissue, Open Approach

061V0JY Bypass Left Foot Vein to Lower Vein with Synthetic Substitute, Open Approach

061V0KY Bypass Left Foot Vein to Lower Vein with Nonautologous Tissue Substitute, Open Approach

061V0ZY Bypass Left Foot Vein to Lower Vein, Open Approach

061V47Y Bypass Left Foot Vein to Lower Vein with Autologous Tissue Substitute, Percutaneous Endoscopic Approach

061V49Y Bypass Left Foot Vein to Lower Vein with Autologous Venous Tissue, Percutaneous Endoscopic Approach

061V4AY Bypass Left Foot Vein to Lower Vein with Autologous Arterial Tissue, Percutaneous Endoscopic Approach

061V4JY Bypass Left Foot Vein to Lower Vein with Synthetic Substitute, Percutaneous Endoscopic Approach

061V4KY Bypass Left Foot Vein to Lower Vein with Nonautologous Tissue Substitute, Percutaneous Endoscopic Approach

061V4ZY Bypass Left Foot Vein to Lower Vein, Percutaneous Endoscopic Approach

065 – Lower Veins, Destruction

06500ZZ Destruction of Inferior Vena Cava, Open Approach

06503ZZ Destruction of Inferior Vena Cava, Percutaneous Approach

06504ZZ Destruction of Inferior Vena Cava, Percutaneous Endoscopic Approach

06510ZZ Destruction of Splenic Vein, Open Approach

06513ZZ Destruction of Splenic Vein, Percutaneous Approach

06514ZZ Destruction of Splenic Vein, Percutaneous Endoscopic Approach

06520ZZ Destruction of Gastric Vein, Open Approach

06523ZZ Destruction of Gastric Vein, Percutaneous Approach

06524ZZ Destruction of Gastric Vein, Percutaneous Endoscopic Approach

06530ZZ Destruction of Esophageal Vein, Open Approach

06533ZZ Destruction of Esophageal Vein, Percutaneous Approach

06534ZZ Destruction of Esophageal Vein, Percutaneous Endoscopic Approach

06540ZZ Destruction of Hepatic Vein, Open Approach

06543ZZ Destruction of Hepatic Vein, Percutaneous Approach

06544ZZ	Destruction of Hepatic Vein, Percutaneous Endoscopic Approach
06550ZZ	Destruction of Superior Mesenteric Vein, Open Approach
06553ZZ	Destruction of Superior Mesenteric Vein, Percutaneous Approach
06554ZZ	Destruction of Superior Mesenteric Vein, Percutaneous Endoscopic Approach
06560ZZ	Destruction of Inferior Mesenteric Vein, Open Approach
06563ZZ	Destruction of Inferior Mesenteric Vein, Percutaneous Approach
06564ZZ	Destruction of Inferior Mesenteric Vein, Percutaneous Endoscopic Approach
06570ZZ	Destruction of Colic Vein, Open Approach
06573ZZ	Destruction of Colic Vein, Percutaneous Approach
06574ZZ	Destruction of Colic Vein, Percutaneous Endoscopic Approach
06580ZZ	Destruction of Portal Vein, Open Approach
06583ZZ	Destruction of Portal Vein, Percutaneous Approach
06584ZZ	Destruction of Portal Vein, Percutaneous Endoscopic Approach
06590ZZ	Destruction of Right Renal Vein, Open Approach
06593ZZ	Destruction of Right Renal Vein, Percutaneous Approach
06594ZZ	Destruction of Right Renal Vein, Percutaneous Endoscopic Approach
065B0ZZ	Destruction of Left Renal Vein, Open Approach
065B3ZZ	Destruction of Left Renal Vein, Percutaneous Approach
065B4ZZ	Destruction of Left Renal Vein, Percutaneous Endoscopic Approach
065C0ZZ	Destruction of Right Common Iliac Vein, Open Approach
065C3ZZ	Destruction of Right Common Iliac Vein, Percutaneous Approach
065C4ZZ	Destruction of Right Common Iliac Vein, Percutaneous Endoscopic Approach
065D0ZZ	Destruction of Left Common Iliac Vein, Open Approach
065D3ZZ	Destruction of Left Common Iliac Vein, Percutaneous Approach
065D4ZZ	Destruction of Left Common Iliac Vein, Percutaneous Endoscopic Approach
065F0ZZ	Destruction of Right External Iliac Vein, Open Approach
065F3ZZ	Destruction of Right External Iliac Vein, Percutaneous Approach
065F4ZZ	Destruction of Right External Iliac Vein, Percutaneous Endoscopic Approach
065G0ZZ	Destruction of Left External Iliac Vein, Open Approach
065G3ZZ	Destruction of Left External Iliac Vein, Percutaneous Approach
065G4ZZ	Destruction of Left External Iliac Vein, Percutaneous Endoscopic Approach
065H0ZZ	Destruction of Right Hypogastric Vein, Open Approach
065H3ZZ	Destruction of Right Hypogastric Vein, Percutaneous Approach
065H4ZZ	Destruction of Right Hypogastric Vein, Percutaneous Endoscopic Approach
065J0ZZ	Destruction of Left Hypogastric Vein, Open Approach
065J3ZZ	Destruction of Left Hypogastric Vein, Percutaneous Approach
065J4ZZ	Destruction of Left Hypogastric Vein, Percutaneous Endoscopic Approach
065M0ZZ	Destruction of Right Femoral Vein, Open Approach
065M3ZZ	Destruction of Right Femoral Vein, Percutaneous Approach
065M4ZZ	Destruction of Right Femoral Vein, Percutaneous Endoscopic Approach
065N0ZZ	Destruction of Left Femoral Vein, Open Approach
065N3ZZ	Destruction of Left Femoral Vein, Percutaneous Approach
065N4ZZ	Destruction of Left Femoral Vein, Percutaneous Endoscopic Approach
065P0ZZ	Destruction of Right Greater Saphenous Vein, Open Approach
065P3ZZ	Destruction of Right Greater Saphenous Vein, Percutaneous Approach
065P4ZZ	Destruction of Right Greater Saphenous Vein, Percutaneous Endoscopic Approach
065Q0ZZ	Destruction of Left Greater Saphenous Vein, Open Approach
065Q3ZZ	Destruction of Left Greater Saphenous Vein, Percutaneous Approach
065Q4ZZ	Destruction of Left Greater Saphenous Vein, Percutaneous Endoscopic Approach
065R0ZZ	Destruction of Right Lesser Saphenous Vein, Open Approach
065R3ZZ	Destruction of Right Lesser Saphenous Vein, Percutaneous Approach
065R4ZZ	Destruction of Right Lesser Saphenous Vein, Percutaneous Endoscopic Approach
065S0ZZ	Destruction of Left Lesser Saphenous Vein, Open Approach
065S3ZZ	Destruction of Left Lesser Saphenous Vein, Percutaneous Approach
065S4ZZ	Destruction of Left Lesser Saphenous Vein, Percutaneous Endoscopic Approach
065T0ZZ	Destruction of Right Foot Vein, Open Approach
065T3ZZ	Destruction of Right Foot Vein, Percutaneous Approach
065T4ZZ	Destruction of Right Foot Vein, Percutaneous Endoscopic Approach
065V0ZZ	Destruction of Left Foot Vein, Open Approach
065V3ZZ	Destruction of Left Foot Vein, Percutaneous Approach
065V4ZZ	Destruction of Left Foot Vein, Percutaneous Endoscopic Approach
065Y0ZC	Destruction of Hemorrhoidal Plexus, Open Approach
065Y0ZZ	Destruction of Lower Vein, Open Approach
065Y3ZC	Destruction of Hemorrhoidal Plexus, Percutaneous Approach
065Y3ZZ	Destruction of Lower Vein, Percutaneous Approach
065Y4ZC	Destruction of Hemorrhoidal Plexus, Percutaneous Endoscopic Approach
065Y4ZZ	Destruction of Lower Vein, Percutaneous Endoscopic Approach

067 – Lower Veins, Dilation

06700DZ	Dilation of Inferior Vena Cava with Intraluminal Device, Open Approach
06700ZZ	Dilation of Inferior Vena Cava, Open Approach
06703DZ	Dilation of Inferior Vena Cava with Intraluminal Device, Percutaneous Approach
06703ZZ	Dilation of Inferior Vena Cava, Percutaneous Approach
06704DZ	Dilation of Inferior Vena Cava with Intraluminal Device, Percutaneous Endoscopic Approach
06704ZZ	Dilation of Inferior Vena Cava, Percutaneous Endoscopic Approach
06710DZ	Dilation of Splenic Vein with Intraluminal Device, Open Approach
06710ZZ	Dilation of Splenic Vein, Open Approach
06713DZ	Dilation of Splenic Vein with Intraluminal Device, Percutaneous Approach
06713ZZ	Dilation of Splenic Vein, Percutaneous Approach
06714DZ	Dilation of Splenic Vein with Intraluminal Device, Percutaneous Endoscopic Approach
06714ZZ	Dilation of Splenic Vein, Percutaneous Endoscopic Approach
06720DZ	Dilation of Gastric Vein with Intraluminal Device, Open Approach
06720ZZ	Dilation of Gastric Vein, Open Approach
06723DZ	Dilation of Gastric Vein with Intraluminal Device, Percutaneous Approach
06723ZZ	Dilation of Gastric Vein, Percutaneous Approach
06724DZ	Dilation of Gastric Vein with Intraluminal Device, Percutaneous Endoscopic Approach
06724ZZ	Dilation of Gastric Vein, Percutaneous Endoscopic Approach
06730DZ	Dilation of Esophageal Vein with Intraluminal Device, Open Approach
06730ZZ	Dilation of Esophageal Vein, Open Approach
06733DZ	Dilation of Esophageal Vein with Intraluminal Device, Percutaneous Approach
06733ZZ	Dilation of Esophageal Vein, Percutaneous Approach
06734DZ	Dilation of Esophageal Vein with Intraluminal Device, Percutaneous Endoscopic Approach
06734ZZ	Dilation of Esophageal Vein, Percutaneous Endoscopic Approach
06740DZ	Dilation of Hepatic Vein with Intraluminal Device, Open Approach
06740ZZ	Dilation of Hepatic Vein, Open Approach
06743DZ	Dilation of Hepatic Vein with Intraluminal Device, Percutaneous Approach
06743ZZ	Dilation of Hepatic Vein, Percutaneous Approach
06744DZ	Dilation of Hepatic Vein with Intraluminal Device, Percutaneous Endoscopic Approach
06744ZZ	Dilation of Hepatic Vein, Percutaneous Endoscopic Approach
06750DZ	Dilation of Superior Mesenteric Vein with Intraluminal Device, Open Approach
06750ZZ	Dilation of Superior Mesenteric Vein, Open Approach
06753DZ	Dilation of Superior Mesenteric Vein with Intraluminal Device, Percutaneous Approach
06753ZZ	Dilation of Superior Mesenteric Vein, Percutaneous Approach
06754DZ	Dilation of Superior Mesenteric Vein with Intraluminal Device, Percutaneous Endoscopic Approach
06754ZZ	Dilation of Superior Mesenteric Vein, Percutaneous Endoscopic Approach
06760DZ	Dilation of Inferior Mesenteric Vein with Intraluminal Device, Open Approach

06760ZZ   Dilation of Inferior Mesenteric Vein, Open Approach

06763DZ   Dilation of Inferior Mesenteric Vein with Intraluminal Device, Percutaneous Approach

06763ZZ   Dilation of Inferior Mesenteric Vein, Percutaneous Approach

06764DZ   Dilation of Inferior Mesenteric Vein with Intraluminal Device, Percutaneous Endoscopic Approach

06764ZZ   Dilation of Inferior Mesenteric Vein, Percutaneous Endoscopic Approach

06770DZ   Dilation of Colic Vein with Intraluminal Device, Open Approach

06770ZZ   Dilation of Colic Vein, Open Approach

06773DZ   Dilation of Colic Vein with Intraluminal Device, Percutaneous Approach

06773ZZ   Dilation of Colic Vein, Percutaneous Approach

06774DZ   Dilation of Colic Vein with Intraluminal Device, Percutaneous Endoscopic Approach

06774ZZ   Dilation of Colic Vein, Percutaneous Endoscopic Approach

06780DZ   Dilation of Portal Vein with Intraluminal Device, Open Approach

06780ZZ   Dilation of Portal Vein, Open Approach

06783DZ   Dilation of Portal Vein with Intraluminal Device, Percutaneous Approach

06783ZZ   Dilation of Portal Vein, Percutaneous Approach

06784DZ   Dilation of Portal Vein with Intraluminal Device, Percutaneous Endoscopic Approach

06784ZZ   Dilation of Portal Vein, Percutaneous Endoscopic Approach

06790DZ   Dilation of Right Renal Vein with Intraluminal Device, Open Approach

06790ZZ   Dilation of Right Renal Vein, Open Approach

06793DZ   Dilation of Right Renal Vein with Intraluminal Device, Percutaneous Approach

06793ZZ   Dilation of Right Renal Vein, Percutaneous Approach

06794DZ   Dilation of Right Renal Vein with Intraluminal Device, Percutaneous Endoscopic Approach

06794ZZ   Dilation of Right Renal Vein, Percutaneous Endoscopic Approach

067B0DZ   Dilation of Left Renal Vein with Intraluminal Device, Open Approach

067B0ZZ   Dilation of Left Renal Vein, Open Approach

067B3DZ   Dilation of Left Renal Vein with Intraluminal Device, Percutaneous Approach

067B3ZZ   Dilation of Left Renal Vein, Percutaneous Approach

067B4DZ   Dilation of Left Renal Vein with Intraluminal Device, Percutaneous Endoscopic Approach

067B4ZZ   Dilation of Left Renal Vein, Percutaneous Endoscopic Approach

067C0DZ   Dilation of Right Common Iliac Vein with Intraluminal Device, Open Approach

067C0ZZ   Dilation of Right Common Iliac Vein, Open Approach

067C3DZ   Dilation of Right Common Iliac Vein with Intraluminal Device, Percutaneous Approach

067C3ZZ   Dilation of Right Common Iliac Vein, Percutaneous Approach

067C4DZ   Dilation of Right Common Iliac Vein with Intraluminal Device, Percutaneous Endoscopic Approach

067C4ZZ   Dilation of Right Common Iliac Vein, Percutaneous Endoscopic Approach

067D0DZ   Dilation of Left Common Iliac Vein with Intraluminal Device, Open Approach

067D0ZZ   Dilation of Left Common Iliac Vein, Open Approach

067D3DZ   Dilation of Left Common Iliac Vein with Intraluminal Device, Percutaneous Approach

067D3ZZ   Dilation of Left Common Iliac Vein, Percutaneous Approach

067D4DZ   Dilation of Left Common Iliac Vein with Intraluminal Device, Percutaneous Endoscopic Approach

067D4ZZ   Dilation of Left Common Iliac Vein, Percutaneous Endoscopic Approach

067F0DZ   Dilation of Right External Iliac Vein with Intraluminal Device, Open Approach

067F0ZZ   Dilation of Right External Iliac Vein, Open Approach

067F3DZ   Dilation of Right External Iliac Vein with Intraluminal Device, Percutaneous Approach

067F3ZZ   Dilation of Right External Iliac Vein, Percutaneous Approach

067F4DZ   Dilation of Right External Iliac Vein with Intraluminal Device, Percutaneous Endoscopic Approach

067F4ZZ   Dilation of Right External Iliac Vein, Percutaneous Endoscopic Approach

067G0DZ   Dilation of Left External Iliac Vein with Intraluminal Device, Open Approach

067G0ZZ   Dilation of Left External Iliac Vein, Open Approach

067G3DZ   Dilation of Left External Iliac Vein with Intraluminal Device, Percutaneous Approach

067G3ZZ   Dilation of Left External Iliac Vein, Percutaneous Approach

067G4DZ   Dilation of Left External Iliac Vein with Intraluminal Device, Percutaneous Endoscopic Approach

067G4ZZ   Dilation of Left External Iliac Vein, Percutaneous Endoscopic Approach

067H0DZ   Dilation of Right Hypogastric Vein with Intraluminal Device, Open Approach

067H0ZZ   Dilation of Right Hypogastric Vein, Open Approach

067H3DZ   Dilation of Right Hypogastric Vein with Intraluminal Device, Percutaneous Approach

067H3ZZ   Dilation of Right Hypogastric Vein, Percutaneous Approach

067H4DZ   Dilation of Right Hypogastric Vein with Intraluminal Device, Percutaneous Endoscopic Approach

067H4ZZ   Dilation of Right Hypogastric Vein, Percutaneous Endoscopic Approach

067J0DZ   Dilation of Left Hypogastric Vein with Intraluminal Device, Open Approach

067J0ZZ   Dilation of Left Hypogastric Vein, Open Approach

067J3DZ   Dilation of Left Hypogastric Vein with Intraluminal Device, Percutaneous Approach

067J3ZZ   Dilation of Left Hypogastric Vein, Percutaneous Approach

067J4DZ   Dilation of Left Hypogastric Vein with Intraluminal Device, Percutaneous Endoscopic Approach

067J4ZZ   Dilation of Left Hypogastric Vein, Percutaneous Endoscopic Approach

067M0DZ   Dilation of Right Femoral Vein with Intraluminal Device, Open Approach

067M0ZZ   Dilation of Right Femoral Vein, Open Approach

067M3DZ   Dilation of Right Femoral Vein with Intraluminal Device, Percutaneous Approach

067M3ZZ   Dilation of Right Femoral Vein, Percutaneous Approach

067M4DZ   Dilation of Right Femoral Vein with Intraluminal Device, Percutaneous Endoscopic Approach

067M4ZZ   Dilation of Right Femoral Vein, Percutaneous Endoscopic Approach

067N0DZ   Dilation of Left Femoral Vein with Intraluminal Device, Open Approach

067N0ZZ   Dilation of Left Femoral Vein, Open Approach

067N3DZ   Dilation of Left Femoral Vein with Intraluminal Device, Percutaneous Approach

067N3ZZ   Dilation of Left Femoral Vein, Percutaneous Approach

067N4DZ   Dilation of Left Femoral Vein with Intraluminal Device, Percutaneous Endoscopic Approach

067N4ZZ   Dilation of Left Femoral Vein, Percutaneous Endoscopic Approach

067P0DZ   Dilation of Right Greater Saphenous Vein with Intraluminal Device, Open Approach

067P0ZZ   Dilation of Right Greater Saphenous Vein, Open Approach

067P3DZ   Dilation of Right Greater Saphenous Vein with Intraluminal Device, Percutaneous Approach

067P3ZZ   Dilation of Right Greater Saphenous Vein, Percutaneous Approach

067P4DZ   Dilation of Right Greater Saphenous Vein with Intraluminal Device, Percutaneous Endoscopic Approach

067P4ZZ   Dilation of Right Greater Saphenous Vein, Percutaneous Endoscopic Approach

067Q0DZ   Dilation of Left Greater Saphenous Vein with Intraluminal Device, Open Approach

067Q0ZZ   Dilation of Left Greater Saphenous Vein, Open Approach

067Q3DZ   Dilation of Left Greater Saphenous Vein with Intraluminal Device, Percutaneous Approach

067Q3ZZ   Dilation of Left Greater Saphenous Vein, Percutaneous Approach

067Q4DZ   Dilation of Left Greater Saphenous Vein with Intraluminal Device, Percutaneous Endoscopic Approach

067Q4ZZ   Dilation of Left Greater Saphenous Vein, Percutaneous Endoscopic Approach

067R0DZ   Dilation of Right Lesser Saphenous Vein with Intraluminal Device, Open Approach

067R0ZZ   Dilation of Right Lesser Saphenous Vein, Open Approach

067R3DZ   Dilation of Right Lesser Saphenous Vein with Intraluminal Device, Percutaneous Approach

067R3ZZ   Dilation of Right Lesser Saphenous Vein, Percutaneous Approach

067R4DZ   Dilation of Right Lesser Saphenous Vein with Intraluminal Device, Percutaneous Endoscopic Approach

067R4ZZ   Dilation of Right Lesser Saphenous Vein, Percutaneous Endoscopic Approach

067S0DZ   Dilation of Left Lesser Saphenous Vein with Intraluminal Device, Open Approach

067S0ZZ   Dilation of Left Lesser Saphenous Vein, Open Approach

067S3DZ   Dilation of Left Lesser Saphenous Vein with Intraluminal Device, Percutaneous Approach

067S3ZZ   Dilation of Left Lesser Saphenous Vein, Percutaneous Approach

067S4DZ   Dilation of Left Lesser Saphenous Vein with Intraluminal Device, Percutaneous Endoscopic Approach

067S4ZZ   Dilation of Left Lesser Saphenous Vein, Percutaneous Endoscopic Approach

067T0DZ   Dilation of Right Foot Vein with Intraluminal Device, Open Approach

067T0ZZ   Dilation of Right Foot Vein, Open Approach

067T3DZ   Dilation of Right Foot Vein with Intraluminal Device, Percutaneous Approach

067T3ZZ   Dilation of Right Foot Vein, Percutaneous Approach

067T4DZ   Dilation of Right Foot Vein with Intraluminal Device, Percutaneous Endoscopic Approach

067T4ZZ   Dilation of Right Foot Vein, Percutaneous Endoscopic Approach

067V0DZ   Dilation of Left Foot Vein with Intraluminal Device, Open Approach

067V0ZZ   Dilation of Left Foot Vein, Open Approach

067V3DZ   Dilation of Left Foot Vein with Intraluminal Device, Percutaneous Approach

067V3ZZ   Dilation of Left Foot Vein, Percutaneous Approach

067V4DZ   Dilation of Left Foot Vein with Intraluminal Device, Percutaneous Endoscopic Approach

067V4ZZ   Dilation of Left Foot Vein, Percutaneous Endoscopic Approach

067Y0DZ   Dilation of Lower Vein with Intraluminal Device, Open Approach

067Y0ZZ   Dilation of Lower Vein, Open Approach

067Y3DZ   Dilation of Lower Vein with Intraluminal Device, Percutaneous Approach

067Y3ZZ   Dilation of Lower Vein, Percutaneous Approach

067Y4DZ   Dilation of Lower Vein with Intraluminal Device, Percutaneous Endoscopic Approach

067Y4ZZ   Dilation of Lower Vein, Percutaneous Endoscopic Approach

069 – Lower Veins, Drainage

Review Coding Guidelines B3.4a and B3.4b

Review Coding Guideline B6.2

069000Z   Drainage of Inferior Vena Cava with Drainage Device, Open Approach

06900ZX   Drainage of Inferior Vena Cava, Open Approach, Diagnostic

06900ZZ   Drainage of Inferior Vena Cava, Open Approach

069030Z   Drainage of Inferior Vena Cava with Drainage Device, Percutaneous Approach

06903ZX   Drainage of Inferior Vena Cava, Percutaneous Approach, Diagnostic

06903ZZ   Drainage of Inferior Vena Cava, Percutaneous Approach

069040Z   Drainage of Inferior Vena Cava with Drainage Device, Percutaneous Endoscopic Approach

06904ZX   Drainage of Inferior Vena Cava, Percutaneous Endoscopic Approach, Diagnostic

06904ZZ   Drainage of Inferior Vena Cava, Percutaneous Endoscopic Approach

069100Z   Drainage of Splenic Vein with Drainage Device, Open Approach

06910ZX   Drainage of Splenic Vein, Open Approach, Diagnostic

06910ZZ   Drainage of Splenic Vein, Open Approach

069130Z   Drainage of Splenic Vein with Drainage Device, Percutaneous Approach

06913ZX   Drainage of Splenic Vein, Percutaneous Approach, Diagnostic

06913ZZ   Drainage of Splenic Vein, Percutaneous Approach

069140Z   Drainage of Splenic Vein with Drainage Device, Percutaneous Endoscopic Approach

06914ZX   Drainage of Splenic Vein, Percutaneous Endoscopic Approach, Diagnostic

06914ZZ   Drainage of Splenic Vein, Percutaneous Endoscopic Approach

069200Z   Drainage of Gastric Vein with Drainage Device, Open Approach

06920ZX   Drainage of Gastric Vein, Open Approach, Diagnostic

06920ZZ   Drainage of Gastric Vein, Open Approach

069230Z   Drainage of Gastric Vein with Drainage Device, Percutaneous Approach

06923ZX   Drainage of Gastric Vein, Percutaneous Approach, Diagnostic

06923ZZ   Drainage of Gastric Vein, Percutaneous Approach

069240Z   Drainage of Gastric Vein with Drainage Device, Percutaneous Endoscopic Approach

06924ZX   Drainage of Gastric Vein, Percutaneous Endoscopic Approach, Diagnostic

06924ZZ   Drainage of Gastric Vein, Percutaneous Endoscopic Approach

069300Z   Drainage of Esophageal Vein with Drainage Device, Open Approach

06930ZX   Drainage of Esophageal Vein, Open Approach, Diagnostic

06930ZZ   Drainage of Esophageal Vein, Open Approach

069330Z   Drainage of Esophageal Vein with Drainage Device, Percutaneous Approach

06933ZX   Drainage of Esophageal Vein, Percutaneous Approach, Diagnostic

06933ZZ   Drainage of Esophageal Vein, Percutaneous Approach

069340Z   Drainage of Esophageal Vein with Drainage Device, Percutaneous Endoscopic Approach

06934ZX   Drainage of Esophageal Vein, Percutaneous Endoscopic Approach, Diagnostic

06934ZZ   Drainage of Esophageal Vein, Percutaneous Endoscopic Approach

069400Z   Drainage of Hepatic Vein with Drainage Device, Open Approach

06940ZX   Drainage of Hepatic Vein, Open Approach, Diagnostic

06940ZZ   Drainage of Hepatic Vein, Open Approach

069430Z   Drainage of Hepatic Vein with Drainage Device, Percutaneous Approach

06943ZX   Drainage of Hepatic Vein, Percutaneous Approach, Diagnostic

06943ZZ   Drainage of Hepatic Vein, Percutaneous Approach

069440Z   Drainage of Hepatic Vein with Drainage Device, Percutaneous Endoscopic Approach

06944ZX   Drainage of Hepatic Vein, Percutaneous Endoscopic Approach, Diagnostic

06944ZZ   Drainage of Hepatic Vein, Percutaneous Endoscopic Approach

069500Z   Drainage of Superior Mesenteric Vein with Drainage Device, Open Approach

06950ZX   Drainage of Superior Mesenteric Vein, Open Approach, Diagnostic

06950ZZ   Drainage of Superior Mesenteric Vein, Open Approach

069530Z   Drainage of Superior Mesenteric Vein with Drainage Device, Percutaneous Approach

06953ZX   Drainage of Superior Mesenteric Vein, Percutaneous Approach, Diagnostic

06953ZZ   Drainage of Superior Mesenteric Vein, Percutaneous Approach

069540Z   Drainage of Superior Mesenteric Vein with Drainage Device, Percutaneous Endoscopic Approach

06954ZX   Drainage of Superior Mesenteric Vein, Percutaneous Endoscopic Approach, Diagnostic

06954ZZ   Drainage of Superior Mesenteric Vein, Percutaneous Endoscopic Approach

069600Z   Drainage of Inferior Mesenteric Vein with Drainage Device, Open Approach

06960ZX   Drainage of Inferior Mesenteric Vein, Open Approach, Diagnostic

06960ZZ   Drainage of Inferior Mesenteric Vein, Open Approach

069630Z   Drainage of Inferior Mesenteric Vein with Drainage Device, Percutaneous Approach

06963ZX   Drainage of Inferior Mesenteric Vein, Percutaneous Approach, Diagnostic

06963ZZ   Drainage of Inferior Mesenteric Vein, Percutaneous Approach

069640Z   Drainage of Inferior Mesenteric Vein with Drainage Device, Percutaneous Endoscopic Approach

06964ZX   Drainage of Inferior Mesenteric Vein, Percutaneous Endoscopic Approach, Diagnostic

06964ZZ   Drainage of Inferior Mesenteric Vein, Percutaneous Endoscopic Approach

069700Z   Drainage of Colic Vein with Drainage Device, Open Approach

06970ZX	Drainage of Colic Vein, Open Approach, Diagnostic
06970ZZ	Drainage of Colic Vein, Open Approach
069730Z	Drainage of Colic Vein with Drainage Device, Percutaneous Approach
06973ZX	Drainage of Colic Vein, Percutaneous Approach, Diagnostic
06973ZZ	Drainage of Colic Vein, Percutaneous Approach
069740Z	Drainage of Colic Vein with Drainage Device, Percutaneous Endoscopic Approach
06974ZX	Drainage of Colic Vein, Percutaneous Endoscopic Approach, Diagnostic
06974ZZ	Drainage of Colic Vein, Percutaneous Endoscopic Approach
069800Z	Drainage of Portal Vein with Drainage Device, Open Approach
06980ZX	Drainage of Portal Vein, Open Approach, Diagnostic
06980ZZ	Drainage of Portal Vein, Open Approach
069830Z	Drainage of Portal Vein with Drainage Device, Percutaneous Approach
06983ZX	Drainage of Portal Vein, Percutaneous Approach, Diagnostic
06983ZZ	Drainage of Portal Vein, Percutaneous Approach
069840Z	Drainage of Portal Vein with Drainage Device, Percutaneous Endoscopic Approach
06984ZX	Drainage of Portal Vein, Percutaneous Endoscopic Approach, Diagnostic
06984ZZ	Drainage of Portal Vein, Percutaneous Endoscopic Approach
069900Z	Drainage of Right Renal Vein with Drainage Device, Open Approach
06990ZX	Drainage of Right Renal Vein, Open Approach, Diagnostic
06990ZZ	Drainage of Right Renal Vein, Open Approach
069930Z	Drainage of Right Renal Vein with Drainage Device, Percutaneous Approach
06993ZX	Drainage of Right Renal Vein, Percutaneous Approach, Diagnostic
06993ZZ	Drainage of Right Renal Vein, Percutaneous Approach
069940Z	Drainage of Right Renal Vein with Drainage Device, Percutaneous Endoscopic Approach
06994ZX	Drainage of Right Renal Vein, Percutaneous Endoscopic Approach, Diagnostic
06994ZZ	Drainage of Right Renal Vein, Percutaneous Endoscopic Approach
069B00Z	Drainage of Left Renal Vein with Drainage Device, Open Approach
069B0ZX	Drainage of Left Renal Vein, Open Approach, Diagnostic
069B0ZZ	Drainage of Left Renal Vein, Open Approach
069B30Z	Drainage of Left Renal Vein with Drainage Device, Percutaneous Approach
069B3ZX	Drainage of Left Renal Vein, Percutaneous Approach, Diagnostic
069B3ZZ	Drainage of Left Renal Vein, Percutaneous Approach
069B40Z	Drainage of Left Renal Vein with Drainage Device, Percutaneous Endoscopic Approach
069B4ZX	Drainage of Left Renal Vein, Percutaneous Endoscopic Approach, Diagnostic
069B4ZZ	Drainage of Left Renal Vein, Percutaneous Endoscopic Approach
069C00Z	Drainage of Right Common Iliac Vein with Drainage Device, Open Approach
069C0ZX	Drainage of Right Common Iliac Vein, Open Approach, Diagnostic
069C0ZZ	Drainage of Right Common Iliac Vein, Open Approach
069C30Z	Drainage of Right Common Iliac Vein with Drainage Device, Percutaneous Approach
069C3ZX	Drainage of Right Common Iliac Vein, Percutaneous Approach, Diagnostic
069C3ZZ	Drainage of Right Common Iliac Vein, Percutaneous Approach
069C40Z	Drainage of Right Common Iliac Vein with Drainage Device, Percutaneous Endoscopic Approach
069C4ZX	Drainage of Right Common Iliac Vein, Percutaneous Endoscopic Approach, Diagnostic
069C4ZZ	Drainage of Right Common Iliac Vein, Percutaneous Endoscopic Approach
069D00Z	Drainage of Left Common Iliac Vein with Drainage Device, Open Approach
069D0ZX	Drainage of Left Common Iliac Vein, Open Approach, Diagnostic
069D0ZZ	Drainage of Left Common Iliac Vein, Open Approach
069D30Z	Drainage of Left Common Iliac Vein with Drainage Device, Percutaneous Approach
069D3ZX	Drainage of Left Common Iliac Vein, Percutaneous Approach, Diagnostic
069D3ZZ	Drainage of Left Common Iliac Vein, Percutaneous Approach
069D40Z	Drainage of Left Common Iliac Vein with Drainage Device, Percutaneous Endoscopic Approach
069D4ZX	Drainage of Left Common Iliac Vein, Percutaneous Endoscopic Approach, Diagnostic
069D4ZZ	Drainage of Left Common Iliac Vein, Percutaneous Endoscopic Approach
069F00Z	Drainage of Right External Iliac Vein with Drainage Device, Open Approach
069F0ZX	Drainage of Right External Iliac Vein, Open Approach, Diagnostic
069F0ZZ	Drainage of Right External Iliac Vein, Open Approach
069F30Z	Drainage of Right External Iliac Vein with Drainage Device, Percutaneous Approach
069F3ZX	Drainage of Right External Iliac Vein, Percutaneous Approach, Diagnostic
069F3ZZ	Drainage of Right External Iliac Vein, Percutaneous Approach
069F40Z	Drainage of Right External Iliac Vein with Drainage Device, Percutaneous Endoscopic Approach
069F4ZX	Drainage of Right External Iliac Vein, Percutaneous Endoscopic Approach, Diagnostic
069F4ZZ	Drainage of Right External Iliac Vein, Percutaneous Endoscopic Approach
069G00Z	Drainage of Left External Iliac Vein with Drainage Device, Open Approach
069G0ZX	Drainage of Left External Iliac Vein, Open Approach, Diagnostic
069G0ZZ	Drainage of Left External Iliac Vein, Open Approach
069G30Z	Drainage of Left External Iliac Vein with Drainage Device, Percutaneous Approach
069G3ZX	Drainage of Left External Iliac Vein, Percutaneous Approach, Diagnostic
069G3ZZ	Drainage of Left External Iliac Vein, Percutaneous Approach
069G40Z	Drainage of Left External Iliac Vein with Drainage Device, Percutaneous Endoscopic Approach
069G4ZX	Drainage of Left External Iliac Vein, Percutaneous Endoscopic Approach, Diagnostic
069G4ZZ	Drainage of Left External Iliac Vein, Percutaneous Endoscopic Approach
069H00Z	Drainage of Right Hypogastric Vein with Drainage Device, Open Approach
069H0ZX	Drainage of Right Hypogastric Vein, Open Approach, Diagnostic
069H0ZZ	Drainage of Right Hypogastric Vein, Open Approach
069H30Z	Drainage of Right Hypogastric Vein with Drainage Device, Percutaneous Approach
069H3ZX	Drainage of Right Hypogastric Vein, Percutaneous Approach, Diagnostic
069H3ZZ	Drainage of Right Hypogastric Vein, Percutaneous Approach
069H40Z	Drainage of Right Hypogastric Vein with Drainage Device, Percutaneous Endoscopic Approach
069H4ZX	Drainage of Right Hypogastric Vein, Percutaneous Endoscopic Approach, Diagnostic
069H4ZZ	Drainage of Right Hypogastric Vein, Percutaneous Endoscopic Approach
069J00Z	Drainage of Left Hypogastric Vein with Drainage Device, Open Approach
069J0ZX	Drainage of Left Hypogastric Vein, Open Approach, Diagnostic
069J0ZZ	Drainage of Left Hypogastric Vein, Open Approach
069J30Z	Drainage of Left Hypogastric Vein with Drainage Device, Percutaneous Approach
069J3ZX	Drainage of Left Hypogastric Vein, Percutaneous Approach, Diagnostic
069J3ZZ	Drainage of Left Hypogastric Vein, Percutaneous Approach
069J40Z	Drainage of Left Hypogastric Vein with Drainage Device, Percutaneous Endoscopic Approach
069J4ZX	Drainage of Left Hypogastric Vein, Percutaneous Endoscopic Approach, Diagnostic
069J4ZZ	Drainage of Left Hypogastric Vein, Percutaneous Endoscopic Approach
069M00Z	Drainage of Right Femoral Vein with Drainage Device, Open Approach
069M0ZX	Drainage of Right Femoral Vein, Open Approach, Diagnostic
069M0ZZ	Drainage of Right Femoral Vein, Open Approach
069M30Z	Drainage of Right Femoral Vein with Drainage Device, Percutaneous Approach

069M3ZX	Drainage of Right Femoral Vein, Percutaneous Approach, Diagnostic
069M3ZZ	Drainage of Right Femoral Vein, Percutaneous Approach
069M40Z	Drainage of Right Femoral Vein with Drainage Device, Percutaneous Endoscopic Approach
069M4ZX	Drainage of Right Femoral Vein, Percutaneous Endoscopic Approach, Diagnostic
069M4ZZ	Drainage of Right Femoral Vein, Percutaneous Endoscopic Approach
069N00Z	Drainage of Left Femoral Vein with Drainage Device, Open Approach
069N0ZX	Drainage of Left Femoral Vein, Open Approach, Diagnostic
069N0ZZ	Drainage of Left Femoral Vein, Open Approach
069N30Z	Drainage of Left Femoral Vein with Drainage Device, Percutaneous Approach
069N3ZX	Drainage of Left Femoral Vein, Percutaneous Approach, Diagnostic
069N3ZZ	Drainage of Left Femoral Vein, Percutaneous Approach
069N40Z	Drainage of Left Femoral Vein with Drainage Device, Percutaneous Endoscopic Approach
069N4ZX	Drainage of Left Femoral Vein, Percutaneous Endoscopic Approach, Diagnostic
069N4ZZ	Drainage of Left Femoral Vein, Percutaneous Endoscopic Approach
069P00Z	Drainage of Right Greater Saphenous Vein with Drainage Device, Open Approach
069P0ZX	Drainage of Right Greater Saphenous Vein, Open Approach, Diagnostic
069P0ZZ	Drainage of Right Greater Saphenous Vein, Open Approach
069P30Z	Drainage of Right Greater Saphenous Vein with Drainage Device, Percutaneous Approach
069P3ZX	Drainage of Right Greater Saphenous Vein, Percutaneous Approach, Diagnostic
069P3ZZ	Drainage of Right Greater Saphenous Vein, Percutaneous Approach
069P40Z	Drainage of Right Greater Saphenous Vein with Drainage Device, Percutaneous Endoscopic Approach
069P4ZX	Drainage of Right Greater Saphenous Vein, Percutaneous Endoscopic Approach, Diagnostic
069P4ZZ	Drainage of Right Greater Saphenous Vein, Percutaneous Endoscopic Approach
069Q00Z	Drainage of Left Greater Saphenous Vein with Drainage Device, Open Approach
069Q0ZX	Drainage of Left Greater Saphenous Vein, Open Approach, Diagnostic
069Q0ZZ	Drainage of Left Greater Saphenous Vein, Open Approach
069Q30Z	Drainage of Left Greater Saphenous Vein with Drainage Device, Percutaneous Approach
069Q3ZX	Drainage of Left Greater Saphenous Vein, Percutaneous Approach, Diagnostic
069Q3ZZ	Drainage of Left Greater Saphenous Vein, Percutaneous Approach
069Q40Z	Drainage of Left Greater Saphenous Vein with Drainage Device, Percutaneous Endoscopic Approach
069Q4ZX	Drainage of Left Greater Saphenous Vein, Percutaneous Endoscopic Approach, Diagnostic
069Q4ZZ	Drainage of Left Greater Saphenous Vein, Percutaneous Endoscopic Approach
069R00Z	Drainage of Right Lesser Saphenous Vein with Drainage Device, Open Approach
069R0ZX	Drainage of Right Lesser Saphenous Vein, Open Approach, Diagnostic
069R0ZZ	Drainage of Right Lesser Saphenous Vein, Open Approach
069R30Z	Drainage of Right Lesser Saphenous Vein with Drainage Device, Percutaneous Approach
069R3ZX	Drainage of Right Lesser Saphenous Vein, Percutaneous Approach, Diagnostic
069R3ZZ	Drainage of Right Lesser Saphenous Vein, Percutaneous Approach
069R40Z	Drainage of Right Lesser Saphenous Vein with Drainage Device, Percutaneous Endoscopic Approach
069R4ZX	Drainage of Right Lesser Saphenous Vein, Percutaneous Endoscopic Approach, Diagnostic
069R4ZZ	Drainage of Right Lesser Saphenous Vein, Percutaneous Endoscopic Approach
069S00Z	Drainage of Left Lesser Saphenous Vein with Drainage Device, Open Approach
069S0ZX	Drainage of Left Lesser Saphenous Vein, Open Approach, Diagnostic
069S0ZZ	Drainage of Left Lesser Saphenous Vein, Open Approach
069S30Z	Drainage of Left Lesser Saphenous Vein with Drainage Device, Percutaneous Approach
069S3ZX	Drainage of Left Lesser Saphenous Vein, Percutaneous Approach, Diagnostic
069S3ZZ	Drainage of Left Lesser Saphenous Vein, Percutaneous Approach
069S40Z	Drainage of Left Lesser Saphenous Vein with Drainage Device, Percutaneous Endoscopic Approach
069S4ZX	Drainage of Left Lesser Saphenous Vein, Percutaneous Endoscopic Approach, Diagnostic
069S4ZZ	Drainage of Left Lesser Saphenous Vein, Percutaneous Endoscopic Approach
069T00Z	Drainage of Right Foot Vein with Drainage Device, Open Approach
069T0ZX	Drainage of Right Foot Vein, Open Approach, Diagnostic
069T0ZZ	Drainage of Right Foot Vein, Open Approach
069T30Z	Drainage of Right Foot Vein with Drainage Device, Percutaneous Approach
069T3ZX	Drainage of Right Foot Vein, Percutaneous Approach, Diagnostic
069T3ZZ	Drainage of Right Foot Vein, Percutaneous Approach
069T40Z	Drainage of Right Foot Vein with Drainage Device, Percutaneous Endoscopic Approach
069T4ZX	Drainage of Right Foot Vein, Percutaneous Endoscopic Approach, Diagnostic
069T4ZZ	Drainage of Right Foot Vein, Percutaneous Endoscopic Approach
069V00Z	Drainage of Left Foot Vein with Drainage Device, Open Approach
069V0ZX	Drainage of Left Foot Vein, Open Approach, Diagnostic
069V0ZZ	Drainage of Left Foot Vein, Open Approach
069V30Z	Drainage of Left Foot Vein with Drainage Device, Percutaneous Approach
069V3ZX	Drainage of Left Foot Vein, Percutaneous Approach, Diagnostic
069V3ZZ	Drainage of Left Foot Vein, Percutaneous Approach
069V40Z	Drainage of Left Foot Vein with Drainage Device, Percutaneous Endoscopic Approach
069V4ZX	Drainage of Left Foot Vein, Percutaneous Endoscopic Approach, Diagnostic
069V4ZZ	Drainage of Left Foot Vein, Percutaneous Endoscopic Approach
069Y00Z	Drainage of Lower Vein with Drainage Device, Open Approach
069Y0ZX	Drainage of Lower Vein, Open Approach, Diagnostic
069Y0ZZ	Drainage of Lower Vein, Open Approach
069Y30Z	Drainage of Lower Vein with Drainage Device, Percutaneous Approach
069Y3ZX	Drainage of Lower Vein, Percutaneous Approach, Diagnostic
069Y3ZZ	Drainage of Lower Vein, Percutaneous Approach
069Y40Z	Drainage of Lower Vein with Drainage Device, Percutaneous Endoscopic Approach
069Y4ZX	Drainage of Lower Vein, Percutaneous Endoscopic Approach, Diagnostic
069Y4ZZ	Drainage of Lower Vein, Percutaneous Endoscopic Approach

06B – Lower Veins, Excision

Review Coding Guidelines B3.4a and B3.4b

Review Coding Guideline B3.8

06B00ZX	Excision of Inferior Vena Cava, Open Approach, Diagnostic
06B00ZZ	Excision of Inferior Vena Cava, Open Approach
06B03ZX	Excision of Inferior Vena Cava, Percutaneous Approach, Diagnostic
06B03ZZ	Excision of Inferior Vena Cava, Percutaneous Approach
06B04ZX	Excision of Inferior Vena Cava, Percutaneous Endoscopic Approach, Diagnostic
06B04ZZ	Excision of Inferior Vena Cava, Percutaneous Endoscopic Approach
06B10ZX	Excision of Splenic Vein, Open Approach, Diagnostic
06B10ZZ	Excision of Splenic Vein, Open Approach
06B13ZX	Excision of Splenic Vein, Percutaneous Approach, Diagnostic
06B13ZZ	Excision of Splenic Vein, Percutaneous Approach

06B14ZX Excision of Splenic Vein, Percutaneous Endoscopic Approach, Diagnostic

06B14ZZ Excision of Splenic Vein, Percutaneous Endoscopic Approach

06B20ZX Excision of Gastric Vein, Open Approach, Diagnostic

06B20ZZ Excision of Gastric Vein, Open Approach

06B23ZX Excision of Gastric Vein, Percutaneous Approach, Diagnostic

06B23ZZ Excision of Gastric Vein, Percutaneous Approach

06B24ZX Excision of Gastric Vein, Percutaneous Endoscopic Approach, Diagnostic

06B24ZZ Excision of Gastric Vein, Percutaneous Endoscopic Approach

06B30ZX Excision of Esophageal Vein, Open Approach, Diagnostic

06B30ZZ Excision of Esophageal Vein, Open Approach

06B33ZX Excision of Esophageal Vein, Percutaneous Approach, Diagnostic

06B33ZZ Excision of Esophageal Vein, Percutaneous Approach

06B34ZX Excision of Esophageal Vein, Percutaneous Endoscopic Approach, Diagnostic

06B34ZZ Excision of Esophageal Vein, Percutaneous Endoscopic Approach

06B40ZX Excision of Hepatic Vein, Open Approach, Diagnostic

06B40ZZ Excision of Hepatic Vein, Open Approach

06B43ZX Excision of Hepatic Vein, Percutaneous Approach, Diagnostic

06B43ZZ Excision of Hepatic Vein, Percutaneous Approach

06B44ZX Excision of Hepatic Vein, Percutaneous Endoscopic Approach, Diagnostic

06B44ZZ Excision of Hepatic Vein, Percutaneous Endoscopic Approach

06B50ZX Excision of Superior Mesenteric Vein, Open Approach, Diagnostic

06B50ZZ Excision of Superior Mesenteric Vein, Open Approach

06B53ZX Excision of Superior Mesenteric Vein, Percutaneous Approach, Diagnostic

06B53ZZ Excision of Superior Mesenteric Vein, Percutaneous Approach

06B54ZX Excision of Superior Mesenteric Vein, Percutaneous Endoscopic Approach, Diagnostic

06B54ZZ Excision of Superior Mesenteric Vein, Percutaneous Endoscopic Approach

06B60ZX Excision of Inferior Mesenteric Vein, Open Approach, Diagnostic

06B60ZZ Excision of Inferior Mesenteric Vein, Open Approach

06B63ZX Excision of Inferior Mesenteric Vein, Percutaneous Approach, Diagnostic

06B63ZZ Excision of Inferior Mesenteric Vein, Percutaneous Approach

06B64ZX Excision of Inferior Mesenteric Vein, Percutaneous Endoscopic Approach, Diagnostic

06B64ZZ Excision of Inferior Mesenteric Vein, Percutaneous Endoscopic Approach

06B70ZX Excision of Colic Vein, Open Approach, Diagnostic

06B70ZZ Excision of Colic Vein, Open Approach

06B73ZX Excision of Colic Vein, Percutaneous Approach, Diagnostic

06B73ZZ Excision of Colic Vein, Percutaneous Approach

06B74ZX Excision of Colic Vein, Percutaneous Endoscopic Approach, Diagnostic

06B74ZZ Excision of Colic Vein, Percutaneous Endoscopic Approach

06B80ZX Excision of Portal Vein, Open Approach, Diagnostic

06B80ZZ Excision of Portal Vein, Open Approach

06B83ZX Excision of Portal Vein, Percutaneous Approach, Diagnostic

06B83ZZ Excision of Portal Vein, Percutaneous Approach

06B84ZX Excision of Portal Vein, Percutaneous Endoscopic Approach, Diagnostic

06B84ZZ Excision of Portal Vein, Percutaneous Endoscopic Approach

06B90ZX Excision of Right Renal Vein, Open Approach, Diagnostic

06B90ZZ Excision of Right Renal Vein, Open Approach

06B93ZX Excision of Right Renal Vein, Percutaneous Approach, Diagnostic

06B93ZZ Excision of Right Renal Vein, Percutaneous Approach

06B94ZX Excision of Right Renal Vein, Percutaneous Endoscopic Approach, Diagnostic

06B94ZZ Excision of Right Renal Vein, Percutaneous Endoscopic Approach

06BB0ZX Excision of Left Renal Vein, Open Approach, Diagnostic

06BB0ZZ Excision of Left Renal Vein, Open Approach

06BB3ZX Excision of Left Renal Vein, Percutaneous Approach, Diagnostic

06BB3ZZ Excision of Left Renal Vein, Percutaneous Approach

06BB4ZX Excision of Left Renal Vein, Percutaneous Endoscopic Approach, Diagnostic

06BB4ZZ Excision of Left Renal Vein, Percutaneous Endoscopic Approach

06BC0ZX Excision of Right Common Iliac Vein, Open Approach, Diagnostic

06BC0ZZ Excision of Right Common Iliac Vein, Open Approach

06BC3ZX Excision of Right Common Iliac Vein, Percutaneous Approach, Diagnostic

06BC3ZZ Excision of Right Common Iliac Vein, Percutaneous Approach

06BC4ZX Excision of Right Common Iliac Vein, Percutaneous Endoscopic Approach, Diagnostic

06BC4ZZ Excision of Right Common Iliac Vein, Percutaneous Endoscopic Approach

06BD0ZX Excision of Left Common Iliac Vein, Open Approach, Diagnostic

06BD0ZZ Excision of Left Common Iliac Vein, Open Approach

06BD3ZX Excision of Left Common Iliac Vein, Percutaneous Approach, Diagnostic

06BD3ZZ Excision of Left Common Iliac Vein, Percutaneous Approach

06BD4ZX Excision of Left Common Iliac Vein, Percutaneous Endoscopic Approach, Diagnostic

06BD4ZZ Excision of Left Common Iliac Vein, Percutaneous Endoscopic Approach

06BF0ZX Excision of Right External Iliac Vein, Open Approach, Diagnostic

06BF0ZZ Excision of Right External Iliac Vein, Open Approach

06BF3ZX Excision of Right External Iliac Vein, Percutaneous Approach, Diagnostic

06BF3ZZ Excision of Right External Iliac Vein, Percutaneous Approach

06BF4ZX Excision of Right External Iliac Vein, Percutaneous Endoscopic Approach, Diagnostic

06BF4ZZ Excision of Right External Iliac Vein, Percutaneous Endoscopic Approach

06BG0ZX Excision of Left External Iliac Vein, Open Approach, Diagnostic

06BG0ZZ Excision of Left External Iliac Vein, Open Approach

06BG3ZX Excision of Left External Iliac Vein, Percutaneous Approach, Diagnostic

06BG3ZZ Excision of Left External Iliac Vein, Percutaneous Approach

06BG4ZX Excision of Left External Iliac Vein, Percutaneous Endoscopic Approach, Diagnostic

06BG4ZZ Excision of Left External Iliac Vein, Percutaneous Endoscopic Approach

06BH0ZX Excision of Right Hypogastric Vein, Open Approach, Diagnostic

06BH0ZZ Excision of Right Hypogastric Vein, Open Approach

06BH3ZX Excision of Right Hypogastric Vein, Percutaneous Approach, Diagnostic

06BH3ZZ Excision of Right Hypogastric Vein, Percutaneous Approach

06BH4ZX Excision of Right Hypogastric Vein, Percutaneous Endoscopic Approach, Diagnostic

06BH4ZZ Excision of Right Hypogastric Vein, Percutaneous Endoscopic Approach

06BJ0ZX Excision of Left Hypogastric Vein, Open Approach, Diagnostic

06BJ0ZZ Excision of Left Hypogastric Vein, Open Approach

06BJ3ZX Excision of Left Hypogastric Vein, Percutaneous Approach, Diagnostic

06BJ3ZZ Excision of Left Hypogastric Vein, Percutaneous Approach

06BJ4ZX Excision of Left Hypogastric Vein, Percutaneous Endoscopic Approach, Diagnostic

06BJ4ZZ Excision of Left Hypogastric Vein, Percutaneous Endoscopic Approach

06BM0ZX Excision of Right Femoral Vein, Open Approach, Diagnostic

06BM0ZZ Excision of Right Femoral Vein, Open Approach

06BM3ZX Excision of Right Femoral Vein, Percutaneous Approach, Diagnostic

06BM3ZZ Excision of Right Femoral Vein, Percutaneous Approach

06BM4ZX Excision of Right Femoral Vein, Percutaneous Endoscopic Approach, Diagnostic

06BM4ZZ Excision of Right Femoral Vein, Percutaneous Endoscopic Approach

06BN0ZX Excision of Left Femoral Vein, Open Approach, Diagnostic

06BN0ZZ Excision of Left Femoral Vein, Open Approach

06BN3ZX Excision of Left Femoral Vein, Percutaneous Approach, Diagnostic

06BN3ZZ Excision of Left Femoral Vein, Percutaneous Approach

06BN4ZX Excision of Left Femoral Vein, Percutaneous Endoscopic Approach, Diagnostic

06BN4ZZ Excision of Left Femoral Vein, Percutaneous Endoscopic Approach

06BP0ZX Excision of Right Greater Saphenous Vein, Open Approach, Diagnostic

06BP0ZZ Excision of Right Greater Saphenous Vein, Open Approach

06BP3ZX Excision of Right Greater Saphenous Vein, Percutaneous Approach, Diagnostic

♀ Female-only   ♂ Male-only   ● Limited Coverage   ● Non-OR   🅷🅰🅲 HAC-associated procedure   ⬣ Non-covered procedures   ➕ Combination

06BP3ZZ   Excision of Right Greater Saphenous Vein, Percutaneous Approach

06BP4ZX   Excision of Right Greater Saphenous Vein, Percutaneous Endoscopic Approach, Diagnostic

06BP4ZZ   Excision of Right Greater Saphenous Vein, Percutaneous Endoscopic Approach

06BQ0ZX   Excision of Left Greater Saphenous Vein, Open Approach, Diagnostic

06BQ0ZZ   Excision of Left Greater Saphenous Vein, Open Approach

06BQ3ZX   Excision of Left Greater Saphenous Vein, Percutaneous Approach, Diagnostic

06BQ3ZZ   Excision of Left Greater Saphenous Vein, Percutaneous Approach

06BQ4ZX   Excision of Left Greater Saphenous Vein, Percutaneous Endoscopic Approach, Diagnostic

06BQ4ZZ   Excision of Left Greater Saphenous Vein, Percutaneous Endoscopic Approach

06BR0ZX   Excision of Right Lesser Saphenous Vein, Open Approach, Diagnostic

06BR0ZZ   Excision of Right Lesser Saphenous Vein, Open Approach

06BR3ZX   Excision of Right Lesser Saphenous Vein, Percutaneous Approach, Diagnostic

06BR3ZZ   Excision of Right Lesser Saphenous Vein, Percutaneous Approach

06BR4ZX   Excision of Right Lesser Saphenous Vein, Percutaneous Endoscopic Approach, Diagnostic

06BR4ZZ   Excision of Right Lesser Saphenous Vein, Percutaneous Endoscopic Approach

06BS0ZX   Excision of Left Lesser Saphenous Vein, Open Approach, Diagnostic

06BS0ZZ   Excision of Left Lesser Saphenous Vein, Open Approach

06BS3ZX   Excision of Left Lesser Saphenous Vein, Percutaneous Approach, Diagnostic

06BS3ZZ   Excision of Left Lesser Saphenous Vein, Percutaneous Approach

06BS4ZX   Excision of Left Lesser Saphenous Vein, Percutaneous Endoscopic Approach, Diagnostic

06BS4ZZ   Excision of Left Lesser Saphenous Vein, Percutaneous Endoscopic Approach

06BT0ZX   Excision of Right Foot Vein, Open Approach, Diagnostic

06BT0ZZ   Excision of Right Foot Vein, Open Approach

06BT3ZX   Excision of Right Foot Vein, Percutaneous Approach, Diagnostic

06BT3ZZ   Excision of Right Foot Vein, Percutaneous Approach

06BT4ZX   Excision of Right Foot Vein, Percutaneous Endoscopic Approach, Diagnostic

06BT4ZZ   Excision of Right Foot Vein, Percutaneous Endoscopic Approach

06BV0ZX   Excision of Left Foot Vein, Open Approach, Diagnostic

06BV0ZZ   Excision of Left Foot Vein, Open Approach

06BV3ZX   Excision of Left Foot Vein, Percutaneous Approach, Diagnostic

06BV3ZZ   Excision of Left Foot Vein, Percutaneous Approach

06BV4ZX   Excision of Left Foot Vein, Percutaneous Endoscopic Approach, Diagnostic

06BV4ZZ   Excision of Left Foot Vein, Percutaneous Endoscopic Approach

06BY0ZC   Excision of Hemorrhoidal Plexus, Open Approach

06BY0ZX   Excision of Lower Vein, Open Approach, Diagnostic

06BY0ZZ   Excision of Lower Vein, Open Approach

06BY3ZC   Excision of Hemorrhoidal Plexus, Percutaneous Approach

06BY3ZX   Excision of Lower Vein, Percutaneous Approach, Diagnostic

06BY3ZZ   Excision of Lower Vein, Percutaneous Approach

06BY4ZC   Excision of Hemorrhoidal Plexus, Percutaneous Endoscopic Approach

06BY4ZX   Excision of Lower Vein, Percutaneous Endoscopic Approach, Diagnostic

06BY4ZZ   Excision of Lower Vein, Percutaneous Endoscopic Approach

06C – Lower Veins, Extirpation

06C00ZZ   Extirpation of Matter from Inferior Vena Cava, Open Approach

06C03ZZ   Extirpation of Matter from Inferior Vena Cava, Percutaneous Approach

06C04ZZ   Extirpation of Matter from Inferior Vena Cava, Percutaneous Endoscopic Approach

06C10ZZ   Extirpation of Matter from Splenic Vein, Open Approach

06C13ZZ   Extirpation of Matter from Splenic Vein, Percutaneous Approach

06C14ZZ   Extirpation of Matter from Splenic Vein, Percutaneous Endoscopic Approach

06C20ZZ   Extirpation of Matter from Gastric Vein, Open Approach

06C23ZZ   Extirpation of Matter from Gastric Vein, Percutaneous Approach

06C24ZZ   Extirpation of Matter from Gastric Vein, Percutaneous Endoscopic Approach

06C30ZZ   Extirpation of Matter from Esophageal Vein, Open Approach

06C33ZZ   Extirpation of Matter from Esophageal Vein, Percutaneous Approach

06C34ZZ   Extirpation of Matter from Esophageal Vein, Percutaneous Endoscopic Approach

06C40ZZ   Extirpation of Matter from Hepatic Vein, Open Approach

06C43ZZ   Extirpation of Matter from Hepatic Vein, Percutaneous Approach

06C44ZZ   Extirpation of Matter from Hepatic Vein, Percutaneous Endoscopic Approach

06C50ZZ   Extirpation of Matter from Superior Mesenteric Vein, Open Approach

06C53ZZ   Extirpation of Matter from Superior Mesenteric Vein, Percutaneous Approach

06C54ZZ   Extirpation of Matter from Superior Mesenteric Vein, Percutaneous Endoscopic Approach

06C60ZZ   Extirpation of Matter from Inferior Mesenteric Vein, Open Approach

06C63ZZ   Extirpation of Matter from Inferior Mesenteric Vein, Percutaneous Approach

06C64ZZ   Extirpation of Matter from Inferior Mesenteric Vein, Percutaneous Endoscopic Approach

06C70ZZ   Extirpation of Matter from Colic Vein, Open Approach

06C73ZZ   Extirpation of Matter from Colic Vein, Percutaneous Approach

06C74ZZ   Extirpation of Matter from Colic Vein, Percutaneous Endoscopic Approach

06C80ZZ   Extirpation of Matter from Portal Vein, Open Approach

06C83ZZ   Extirpation of Matter from Portal Vein, Percutaneous Approach

06C84ZZ   Extirpation of Matter from Portal Vein, Percutaneous Endoscopic Approach

06C90ZZ   Extirpation of Matter from Right Renal Vein, Open Approach

06C93ZZ   Extirpation of Matter from Right Renal Vein, Percutaneous Approach

06C94ZZ   Extirpation of Matter from Right Renal Vein, Percutaneous Endoscopic Approach

06CB0ZZ   Extirpation of Matter from Left Renal Vein, Open Approach

06CB3ZZ   Extirpation of Matter from Left Renal Vein, Percutaneous Approach

06CB4ZZ   Extirpation of Matter from Left Renal Vein, Percutaneous Endoscopic Approach

06CC0ZZ   Extirpation of Matter from Right Common Iliac Vein, Open Approach

06CC3ZZ   Extirpation of Matter from Right Common Iliac Vein, Percutaneous Approach

06CC4ZZ   Extirpation of Matter from Right Common Iliac Vein, Percutaneous Endoscopic Approach

06CD0ZZ   Extirpation of Matter from Left Common Iliac Vein, Open Approach

06CD3ZZ   Extirpation of Matter from Left Common Iliac Vein, Percutaneous Approach

06CD4ZZ   Extirpation of Matter from Left Common Iliac Vein, Percutaneous Endoscopic Approach

06CF0ZZ   Extirpation of Matter from Right External Iliac Vein, Open Approach

06CF3ZZ   Extirpation of Matter from Right External Iliac Vein, Percutaneous Approach

06CF4ZZ   Extirpation of Matter from Right External Iliac Vein, Percutaneous Endoscopic Approach

06CG0ZZ   Extirpation of Matter from Left External Iliac Vein, Open Approach

06CG3ZZ   Extirpation of Matter from Left External Iliac Vein, Percutaneous Approach

06CG4ZZ   Extirpation of Matter from Left External Iliac Vein, Percutaneous Endoscopic Approach

06CH0ZZ   Extirpation of Matter from Right Hypogastric Vein, Open Approach

06CH3ZZ   Extirpation of Matter from Right Hypogastric Vein, Percutaneous Approach

06CH4ZZ   Extirpation of Matter from Right Hypogastric Vein, Percutaneous Endoscopic Approach

06CJ0ZZ   Extirpation of Matter from Left Hypogastric Vein, Open Approach

06CJ3ZZ	Extirpation of Matter from Left Hypogastric Vein, Percutaneous Approach
06CJ4ZZ	Extirpation of Matter from Left Hypogastric Vein, Percutaneous Endoscopic Approach
06CM0ZZ	Extirpation of Matter from Right Femoral Vein, Open Approach
06CM3ZZ	Extirpation of Matter from Right Femoral Vein, Percutaneous Approach
06CM4ZZ	Extirpation of Matter from Right Femoral Vein, Percutaneous Endoscopic Approach
06CN0ZZ	Extirpation of Matter from Left Femoral Vein, Open Approach
06CN3ZZ	Extirpation of Matter from Left Femoral Vein, Percutaneous Approach
06CN4ZZ	Extirpation of Matter from Left Femoral Vein, Percutaneous Endoscopic Approach
06CP0ZZ	Extirpation of Matter from Right Greater Saphenous Vein, Open Approach
06CP3ZZ	Extirpation of Matter from Right Greater Saphenous Vein, Percutaneous Approach
06CP4ZZ	Extirpation of Matter from Right Greater Saphenous Vein, Percutaneous Endoscopic Approach
06CQ0ZZ	Extirpation of Matter from Left Greater Saphenous Vein, Open Approach
06CQ3ZZ	Extirpation of Matter from Left Greater Saphenous Vein, Percutaneous Approach
06CQ4ZZ	Extirpation of Matter from Left Greater Saphenous Vein, Percutaneous Endoscopic Approach
06CR0ZZ	Extirpation of Matter from Right Lesser Saphenous Vein, Open Approach
06CR3ZZ	Extirpation of Matter from Right Lesser Saphenous Vein, Percutaneous Approach
06CR4ZZ	Extirpation of Matter from Right Lesser Saphenous Vein, Percutaneous Endoscopic Approach
06CS0ZZ	Extirpation of Matter from Left Lesser Saphenous Vein, Open Approach
06CS3ZZ	Extirpation of Matter from Left Lesser Saphenous Vein, Percutaneous Approach
06CS4ZZ	Extirpation of Matter from Left Lesser Saphenous Vein, Percutaneous Endoscopic Approach
06CT0ZZ	Extirpation of Matter from Right Foot Vein, Open Approach
06CT3ZZ	Extirpation of Matter from Right Foot Vein, Percutaneous Approach
06CT4ZZ	Extirpation of Matter from Right Foot Vein, Percutaneous Endoscopic Approach
06CV0ZZ	Extirpation of Matter from Left Foot Vein, Open Approach
06CV3ZZ	Extirpation of Matter from Left Foot Vein, Percutaneous Approach
06CV4ZZ	Extirpation of Matter from Left Foot Vein, Percutaneous Endoscopic Approach
06CY0ZZ	Extirpation of Matter from Lower Vein, Open Approach
06CY3ZZ	Extirpation of Matter from Lower Vein, Percutaneous Approach
06CY4ZZ	Extirpation of Matter from Lower Vein, Percutaneous Endoscopic Approach

06D – Lower Veins, Extraction

06DM0ZZ	Extraction of Right Femoral Vein, Open Approach
06DM3ZZ	Extraction of Right Femoral Vein, Percutaneous Approach
06DM4ZZ	Extraction of Right Femoral Vein, Percutaneous Endoscopic Approach
06DN0ZZ	Extraction of Left Femoral Vein, Open Approach
06DN3ZZ	Extraction of Left Femoral Vein, Percutaneous Approach
06DN4ZZ	Extraction of Left Femoral Vein, Percutaneous Endoscopic Approach
06DP0ZZ	Extraction of Right Greater Saphenous Vein, Open Approach
06DP3ZZ	Extraction of Right Greater Saphenous Vein, Percutaneous Approach
06DP4ZZ	Extraction of Right Greater Saphenous Vein, Percutaneous Endoscopic Approach
06DQ0ZZ	Extraction of Left Greater Saphenous Vein, Open Approach
06DQ3ZZ	Extraction of Left Greater Saphenous Vein, Percutaneous Approach
06DQ4ZZ	Extraction of Left Greater Saphenous Vein, Percutaneous Endoscopic Approach
06DR0ZZ	Extraction of Right Lesser Saphenous Vein, Open Approach
06DR3ZZ	Extraction of Right Lesser Saphenous Vein, Percutaneous Approach
06DR4ZZ	Extraction of Right Lesser Saphenous Vein, Percutaneous Endoscopic Approach
06DS0ZZ	Extraction of Left Lesser Saphenous Vein, Open Approach
06DS3ZZ	Extraction of Left Lesser Saphenous Vein, Percutaneous Approach
06DS4ZZ	Extraction of Left Lesser Saphenous Vein, Percutaneous Endoscopic Approach
06DT0ZZ	Extraction of Right Foot Vein, Open Approach
06DT3ZZ	Extraction of Right Foot Vein, Percutaneous Approach
06DT4ZZ	Extraction of Right Foot Vein, Percutaneous Endoscopic Approach
06DV0ZZ	Extraction of Left Foot Vein, Open Approach
06DV3ZZ	Extraction of Left Foot Vein, Percutaneous Approach
06DV4ZZ	Extraction of Left Foot Vein, Percutaneous Endoscopic Approach
06DY0ZZ	Extraction of Lower Vein, Open Approach
06DY3ZZ	Extraction of Lower Vein, Percutaneous Approach
06DY4ZZ	Extraction of Lower Vein, Percutaneous Endoscopic Approach

06H – Lower Veins, Insertion

06H003T	Insertion of Infusion Device, Via Umbilical Vein, into Inferior Vena Cava, Open Approach
06H003Z	Insertion of Infusion Device into Inferior Vena Cava, Open Approach
06H00DZ	Insertion of Intraluminal Device into Inferior Vena Cava, Open Approach
06H033T	Insertion of Infusion Device, Via Umbilical Vein, into Inferior Vena Cava, Percutaneous Approach
06H033Z	Insertion of Infusion Device into Inferior Vena Cava, Percutaneous Approach
06H03DZ	Insertion of Intraluminal Device into Inferior Vena Cava, Percutaneous Approach
06H043Z	Insertion of Infusion Device into Inferior Vena Cava, Percutaneous Endoscopic Approach
06H04DZ	Insertion of Intraluminal Device into Inferior Vena Cava, Percutaneous Endoscopic Approach
06H103Z	Insertion of Infusion Device into Splenic Vein, Open Approach
06H10DZ	Insertion of Intraluminal Device into Splenic Vein, Open Approach
06H133Z	Insertion of Infusion Device into Splenic Vein, Percutaneous Approach
06H13DZ	Insertion of Intraluminal Device into Splenic Vein, Percutaneous Approach
06H143Z	Insertion of Infusion Device into Splenic Vein, Percutaneous Endoscopic Approach
06H14DZ	Insertion of Intraluminal Device into Splenic Vein, Percutaneous Endoscopic Approach
06H203Z	Insertion of Infusion Device into Gastric Vein, Open Approach
06H20DZ	Insertion of Intraluminal Device into Gastric Vein, Open Approach
06H233Z	Insertion of Infusion Device into Gastric Vein, Percutaneous Approach
06H23DZ	Insertion of Intraluminal Device into Gastric Vein, Percutaneous Approach
06H243Z	Insertion of Infusion Device into Gastric Vein, Percutaneous Endoscopic Approach
06H24DZ	Insertion of Intraluminal Device into Gastric Vein, Percutaneous Endoscopic Approach
06H303Z	Insertion of Infusion Device into Esophageal Vein, Open Approach
06H30DZ	Insertion of Intraluminal Device into Esophageal Vein, Open Approach
06H333Z	Insertion of Infusion Device into Esophageal Vein, Percutaneous Approach
06H33DZ	Insertion of Intraluminal Device into Esophageal Vein, Percutaneous Approach
06H343Z	Insertion of Infusion Device into Esophageal Vein, Percutaneous Endoscopic Approach
06H34DZ	Insertion of Intraluminal Device into Esophageal Vein, Percutaneous Endoscopic Approach

06H403Z   Insertion of Infusion Device into Hepatic Vein, Open Approach

06H40DZ   Insertion of Intraluminal Device into Hepatic Vein, Open Approach

06H433Z   Insertion of Infusion Device into Hepatic Vein, Percutaneous Approach

06H43DZ   Insertion of Intraluminal Device into Hepatic Vein, Percutaneous Approach

06H443Z   Insertion of Infusion Device into Hepatic Vein, Percutaneous Endoscopic Approach

06H44DZ   Insertion of Intraluminal Device into Hepatic Vein, Percutaneous Endoscopic Approach

06H503Z   Insertion of Infusion Device into Superior Mesenteric Vein, Open Approach

06H50DZ   Insertion of Intraluminal Device into Superior Mesenteric Vein, Open Approach

06H533Z   Insertion of Infusion Device into Superior Mesenteric Vein, Percutaneous Approach

06H53DZ   Insertion of Intraluminal Device into Superior Mesenteric Vein, Percutaneous Approach

06H543Z   Insertion of Infusion Device into Superior Mesenteric Vein, Percutaneous Endoscopic Approach

06H54DZ   Insertion of Intraluminal Device into Superior Mesenteric Vein, Percutaneous Endoscopic Approach

06H603Z   Insertion of Infusion Device into Inferior Mesenteric Vein, Open Approach

06H60DZ   Insertion of Intraluminal Device into Inferior Mesenteric Vein, Open Approach

06H633Z   Insertion of Infusion Device into Inferior Mesenteric Vein, Percutaneous Approach

06H63DZ   Insertion of Intraluminal Device into Inferior Mesenteric Vein, Percutaneous Approach

06H643Z   Insertion of Infusion Device into Inferior Mesenteric Vein, Percutaneous Endoscopic Approach

06H64DZ   Insertion of Intraluminal Device into Inferior Mesenteric Vein, Percutaneous Endoscopic Approach

06H703Z   Insertion of Infusion Device into Colic Vein, Open Approach

06H70DZ   Insertion of Intraluminal Device into Colic Vein, Open Approach

06H733Z   Insertion of Infusion Device into Colic Vein, Percutaneous Approach

06H73DZ   Insertion of Intraluminal Device into Colic Vein, Percutaneous Approach

06H743Z   Insertion of Infusion Device into Colic Vein, Percutaneous Endoscopic Approach

06H74DZ   Insertion of Intraluminal Device into Colic Vein, Percutaneous Endoscopic Approach

06H803Z   Insertion of Infusion Device into Portal Vein, Open Approach

06H80DZ   Insertion of Intraluminal Device into Portal Vein, Open Approach

06H833Z   Insertion of Infusion Device into Portal Vein, Percutaneous Approach

06H83DZ   Insertion of Intraluminal Device into Portal Vein, Percutaneous Approach

06H843Z   Insertion of Infusion Device into Portal Vein, Percutaneous Endoscopic Approach

06H84DZ   Insertion of Intraluminal Device into Portal Vein, Percutaneous Endoscopic Approach

06H903Z   Insertion of Infusion Device into Right Renal Vein, Open Approach

06H90DZ   Insertion of Intraluminal Device into Right Renal Vein, Open Approach

06H933Z   Insertion of Infusion Device into Right Renal Vein, Percutaneous Approach

06H93DZ   Insertion of Intraluminal Device into Right Renal Vein, Percutaneous Approach

06H943Z   Insertion of Infusion Device into Right Renal Vein, Percutaneous Endoscopic Approach

06H94DZ   Insertion of Intraluminal Device into Right Renal Vein, Percutaneous Endoscopic Approach

06HB03Z   Insertion of Infusion Device into Left Renal Vein, Open Approach

06HB0DZ   Insertion of Intraluminal Device into Left Renal Vein, Open Approach

06HB33Z   Insertion of Infusion Device into Left Renal Vein, Percutaneous Approach

06HB3DZ   Insertion of Intraluminal Device into Left Renal Vein, Percutaneous Approach

06HB43Z   Insertion of Infusion Device into Left Renal Vein, Percutaneous Endoscopic Approach

06HB4DZ   Insertion of Intraluminal Device into Left Renal Vein, Percutaneous Endoscopic Approach

06HC03Z   Insertion of Infusion Device into Right Common Iliac Vein, Open Approach

06HC0DZ   Insertion of Intraluminal Device into Right Common Iliac Vein, Open Approach

06HC33Z   Insertion of Infusion Device into Right Common Iliac Vein, Percutaneous Approach

06HC3DZ   Insertion of Intraluminal Device into Right Common Iliac Vein, Percutaneous Approach

06HC43Z   Insertion of Infusion Device into Right Common Iliac Vein, Percutaneous Endoscopic Approach

06HC4DZ   Insertion of Intraluminal Device into Right Common Iliac Vein, Percutaneous Endoscopic Approach

06HD03Z   Insertion of Infusion Device into Left Common Iliac Vein, Open Approach

06HD0DZ   Insertion of Intraluminal Device into Left Common Iliac Vein, Open Approach

06HD33Z   Insertion of Infusion Device into Left Common Iliac Vein, Percutaneous Approach

06HD3DZ   Insertion of Intraluminal Device into Left Common Iliac Vein, Percutaneous Approach

06HD43Z   Insertion of Infusion Device into Left Common Iliac Vein, Percutaneous Endoscopic Approach

06HD4DZ   Insertion of Intraluminal Device into Left Common Iliac Vein, Percutaneous Endoscopic Approach

06HF03Z   Insertion of Infusion Device into Right External Iliac Vein, Open Approach

06HF0DZ   Insertion of Intraluminal Device into Right External Iliac Vein, Open Approach

06HF33Z   Insertion of Infusion Device into Right External Iliac Vein, Percutaneous Approach

06HF3DZ   Insertion of Intraluminal Device into Right External Iliac Vein, Percutaneous Approach

06HF43Z   Insertion of Infusion Device into Right External Iliac Vein, Percutaneous Endoscopic Approach

06HF4DZ   Insertion of Intraluminal Device into Right External Iliac Vein, Percutaneous Endoscopic Approach

06HG03Z   Insertion of Infusion Device into Left External Iliac Vein, Open Approach

06HG0DZ   Insertion of Intraluminal Device into Left External Iliac Vein, Open Approach

06HG33Z   Insertion of Infusion Device into Left External Iliac Vein, Percutaneous Approach

06HG3DZ   Insertion of Intraluminal Device into Left External Iliac Vein, Percutaneous Approach

06HG43Z   Insertion of Infusion Device into Left External Iliac Vein, Percutaneous Endoscopic Approach

06HG4DZ   Insertion of Intraluminal Device into Left External Iliac Vein, Percutaneous Endoscopic Approach

06HH03Z   Insertion of Infusion Device into Right Hypogastric Vein, Open Approach

06HH0DZ   Insertion of Intraluminal Device into Right Hypogastric Vein, Open Approach

06HH33Z   Insertion of Infusion Device into Right Hypogastric Vein, Percutaneous Approach

06HH3DZ   Insertion of Intraluminal Device into Right Hypogastric Vein, Percutaneous Approach

06HH43Z   Insertion of Infusion Device into Right Hypogastric Vein, Percutaneous Endoscopic Approach

06HH4DZ   Insertion of Intraluminal Device into Right Hypogastric Vein, Percutaneous Endoscopic Approach

06HJ03Z   Insertion of Infusion Device into Left Hypogastric Vein, Open Approach

06HJ0DZ   Insertion of Intraluminal Device into Left Hypogastric Vein, Open Approach

06HJ33Z   Insertion of Infusion Device into Left Hypogastric Vein, Percutaneous Approach

06HJ3DZ   Insertion of Intraluminal Device into Left Hypogastric Vein, Percutaneous Approach

06HJ43Z   Insertion of Infusion Device into Left Hypogastric Vein, Percutaneous Endoscopic Approach

06HJ4DZ   Insertion of Intraluminal Device into Left Hypogastric Vein, Percutaneous Endoscopic Approach

06HM03Z   Insertion of Infusion Device into Right Femoral Vein, Open Approach

06HM0DZ   Insertion of Intraluminal Device into Right Femoral Vein, Open Approach

06HM33Z   Insertion of Infusion Device into Right Femoral Vein, Percutaneous Approach

06HM3DZ   Insertion of Intraluminal Device into Right Femoral Vein, Percutaneous Approach

06HM43Z   Insertion of Infusion Device into Right Femoral Vein, Percutaneous Endoscopic Approach

06HM4DZ   Insertion of Intraluminal Device into Right Femoral Vein, Percutaneous Endoscopic Approach

06HN03Z   Insertion of Infusion Device into Left Femoral Vein, Open Approach

06HN0DZ   Insertion of Intraluminal Device into Left Femoral Vein, Open Approach

06HN33Z   Insertion of Infusion Device into Left Femoral Vein, Percutaneous Approach

06HN3DZ   Insertion of Intraluminal Device into Left Femoral Vein, Percutaneous Approach

06HN43Z   Insertion of Infusion Device into Left Femoral Vein, Percutaneous Endoscopic Approach

06HN4DZ   Insertion of Intraluminal Device into Left Femoral Vein, Percutaneous Endoscopic Approach

06HP03Z   Insertion of Infusion Device into Right Greater Saphenous Vein, Open Approach

06HP0DZ   Insertion of Intraluminal Device into Right Greater Saphenous Vein, Open Approach

06HP33Z   Insertion of Infusion Device into Right Greater Saphenous Vein, Percutaneous Approach

06HP3DZ   Insertion of Intraluminal Device into Right Greater Saphenous Vein, Percutaneous Approach

06HP43Z   Insertion of Infusion Device into Right Greater Saphenous Vein, Percutaneous Endoscopic Approach

06HP4DZ   Insertion of Intraluminal Device into Right Greater Saphenous Vein, Percutaneous Endoscopic Approach

06HQ03Z   Insertion of Infusion Device into Left Greater Saphenous Vein, Open Approach

06HQ0DZ   Insertion of Intraluminal Device into Left Greater Saphenous Vein, Open Approach

06HQ33Z   Insertion of Infusion Device into Left Greater Saphenous Vein, Percutaneous Approach

06HQ3DZ   Insertion of Intraluminal Device into Left Greater Saphenous Vein, Percutaneous Approach

06HQ43Z   Insertion of Infusion Device into Left Greater Saphenous Vein, Percutaneous Endoscopic Approach

06HQ4DZ   Insertion of Intraluminal Device into Left Greater Saphenous Vein, Percutaneous Endoscopic Approach

06HR03Z   Insertion of Infusion Device into Right Lesser Saphenous Vein, Open Approach

06HR0DZ   Insertion of Intraluminal Device into Right Lesser Saphenous Vein, Open Approach

06HR33Z   Insertion of Infusion Device into Right Lesser Saphenous Vein, Percutaneous Approach

06HR3DZ   Insertion of Intraluminal Device into Right Lesser Saphenous Vein, Percutaneous Approach

06HR43Z   Insertion of Infusion Device into Right Lesser Saphenous Vein, Percutaneous Endoscopic Approach

06HR4DZ   Insertion of Intraluminal Device into Right Lesser Saphenous Vein, Percutaneous Endoscopic Approach

06HS03Z   Insertion of Infusion Device into Left Lesser Saphenous Vein, Open Approach

06HS0DZ   Insertion of Intraluminal Device into Left Lesser Saphenous Vein, Open Approach

06HS33Z   Insertion of Infusion Device into Left Lesser Saphenous Vein, Percutaneous Approach

06HS3DZ   Insertion of Intraluminal Device into Left Lesser Saphenous Vein, Percutaneous Approach

06HS43Z   Insertion of Infusion Device into Left Lesser Saphenous Vein, Percutaneous Endoscopic Approach

06HS4DZ   Insertion of Intraluminal Device into Left Lesser Saphenous Vein, Percutaneous Endoscopic Approach

06HT03Z   Insertion of Infusion Device into Right Foot Vein, Open Approach

06HT0DZ   Insertion of Intraluminal Device into Right Foot Vein, Open Approach

06HT33Z   Insertion of Infusion Device into Right Foot Vein, Percutaneous Approach

06HT3DZ   Insertion of Intraluminal Device into Right Foot Vein, Percutaneous Approach

06HT43Z   Insertion of Infusion Device into Right Foot Vein, Percutaneous Endoscopic Approach

06HT4DZ   Insertion of Intraluminal Device into Right Foot Vein, Percutaneous Endoscopic Approach

06HV03Z   Insertion of Infusion Device into Left Foot Vein, Open Approach

06HV0DZ   Insertion of Intraluminal Device into Left Foot Vein, Open Approach

06HV33Z   Insertion of Infusion Device into Left Foot Vein, Percutaneous Approach

06HV3DZ   Insertion of Intraluminal Device into Left Foot Vein, Percutaneous Approach

06HV43Z   Insertion of Infusion Device into Left Foot Vein, Percutaneous Endoscopic Approach

06HV4DZ   Insertion of Intraluminal Device into Left Foot Vein, Percutaneous Endoscopic Approach

06HY02Z   Insertion of Monitoring Device into Lower Vein, Open Approach

06HY03Z   Insertion of Infusion Device into Lower Vein, Open Approach

06HY0DZ   Insertion of Intraluminal Device into Lower Vein, Open Approach

06HY32Z   Insertion of Monitoring Device into Lower Vein, Percutaneous Approach

06HY33Z   Insertion of Infusion Device into Lower Vein, Percutaneous Approach

06HY3DZ   Insertion of Intraluminal Device into Lower Vein, Percutaneous Approach

06HY42Z   Insertion of Monitoring Device into Lower Vein, Percutaneous Endoscopic Approach

06HY43Z   Insertion of Infusion Device into Lower Vein, Percutaneous Endoscopic Approach

06HY4DZ   Insertion of Intraluminal Device into Lower Vein, Percutaneous Endoscopic Approach

06J – Lower Veins, Inspection

Review Coding Guidelines B3.11a, B3.11b and B3.11c

06JY0ZZ   Inspection of Lower Vein, Open Approach
06JY3ZZ   Inspection of Lower Vein, Percutaneous Approach

06JY4ZZ   Inspection of Lower Vein, Percutaneous Endoscopic Approach
06JYXZZ   Inspection of Lower Vein, External Approach

06L – Lower Veins, Occlusion

Review Coding Guideline B3.12

06L00CZ   Occlusion of Inferior Vena Cava with Extraluminal Device, Open Approach

06L00DZ   Occlusion of Inferior Vena Cava with Intraluminal Device, Open Approach

06L00ZZ   Occlusion of Inferior Vena Cava, Open Approach

06L03CZ   Occlusion of Inferior Vena Cava with Extraluminal Device, Percutaneous Approach

06L03DZ   Occlusion of Inferior Vena Cava with Intraluminal Device, Percutaneous Approach

06L03ZZ   Occlusion of Inferior Vena Cava, Percutaneous Approach

06L04CZ   Occlusion of Inferior Vena Cava with Extraluminal Device, Percutaneous Endoscopic Approach

06L04DZ   Occlusion of Inferior Vena Cava with Intraluminal Device, Percutaneous Endoscopic Approach

06L04ZZ   Occlusion of Inferior Vena Cava, Percutaneous Endoscopic Approach

06L10CZ   Occlusion of Splenic Vein with Extraluminal Device, Open Approach

06L10DZ   Occlusion of Splenic Vein with Intraluminal Device, Open Approach

06L10ZZ   Occlusion of Splenic Vein, Open Approach

06L13CZ   Occlusion of Splenic Vein with Extraluminal Device, Percutaneous Approach

06L13DZ   Occlusion of Splenic Vein with Intraluminal Device, Percutaneous Approach

06L13ZZ   Occlusion of Splenic Vein, Percutaneous Approach

06L14CZ   Occlusion of Splenic Vein with Extraluminal Device, Percutaneous Endoscopic Approach

06L14DZ   Occlusion of Splenic Vein with Intraluminal Device, Percutaneous Endoscopic Approach

06L14ZZ   Occlusion of Splenic Vein, Percutaneous Endoscopic Approach

06L20CZ   Occlusion of Gastric Vein with Extraluminal Device, Open Approach

06L20DZ   Occlusion of Gastric Vein with Intraluminal Device, Open Approach

06L20ZZ   Occlusion of Gastric Vein, Open Approach

06L23CZ   Occlusion of Gastric Vein with Extraluminal Device, Percutaneous Approach

06L23DZ   Occlusion of Gastric Vein with Intraluminal Device, Percutaneous Approach

06L23ZZ   Occlusion of Gastric Vein, Percutaneous Approach

06L24CZ   Occlusion of Gastric Vein with Extraluminal Device, Percutaneous Endoscopic Approach

06L24DZ   Occlusion of Gastric Vein with Intraluminal Device, Percutaneous Endoscopic Approach

06L24ZZ   Occlusion of Gastric Vein, Percutaneous Endoscopic Approach

06L30CZ   Occlusion of Esophageal Vein with Extraluminal Device, Open Approach

06L30DZ   Occlusion of Esophageal Vein with Intraluminal Device, Open Approach

06L30ZZ   Occlusion of Esophageal Vein, Open Approach

06L33CZ   Occlusion of Esophageal Vein with Extraluminal Device, Percutaneous Approach

06L33DZ   Occlusion of Esophageal Vein with Intraluminal Device, Percutaneous Approach

06L33ZZ   Occlusion of Esophageal Vein, Percutaneous Approach

06L34CZ   Occlusion of Esophageal Vein with Extraluminal Device, Percutaneous Endoscopic Approach

06L34DZ   Occlusion of Esophageal Vein with Intraluminal Device, Percutaneous Endoscopic Approach

06L34ZZ   Occlusion of Esophageal Vein, Percutaneous Endoscopic Approach

06L40CZ   Occlusion of Hepatic Vein with Extraluminal Device, Open Approach

06L40DZ   Occlusion of Hepatic Vein with Intraluminal Device, Open Approach

06L40ZZ   Occlusion of Hepatic Vein, Open Approach

06L43CZ   Occlusion of Hepatic Vein with Extraluminal Device, Percutaneous Approach

06L43DZ   Occlusion of Hepatic Vein with Intraluminal Device, Percutaneous Approach

06L43ZZ   Occlusion of Hepatic Vein, Percutaneous Approach

06L44CZ   Occlusion of Hepatic Vein with Extraluminal Device, Percutaneous Endoscopic Approach

06L44DZ   Occlusion of Hepatic Vein with Intraluminal Device, Percutaneous Endoscopic Approach

06L44ZZ   Occlusion of Hepatic Vein, Percutaneous Endoscopic Approach

06L50CZ   Occlusion of Superior Mesenteric Vein with Extraluminal Device, Open Approach

06L50DZ   Occlusion of Superior Mesenteric Vein with Intraluminal Device, Open Approach

06L50ZZ   Occlusion of Superior Mesenteric Vein, Open Approach

06L53CZ   Occlusion of Superior Mesenteric Vein with Extraluminal Device, Percutaneous Approach

06L53DZ   Occlusion of Superior Mesenteric Vein with Intraluminal Device, Percutaneous Approach

06L53ZZ   Occlusion of Superior Mesenteric Vein, Percutaneous Approach

06L54CZ   Occlusion of Superior Mesenteric Vein with Extraluminal Device, Percutaneous Endoscopic Approach

06L54DZ   Occlusion of Superior Mesenteric Vein with Intraluminal Device, Percutaneous Endoscopic Approach

06L54ZZ   Occlusion of Superior Mesenteric Vein, Percutaneous Endoscopic Approach

06L60CZ   Occlusion of Inferior Mesenteric Vein with Extraluminal Device, Open Approach

06L60DZ   Occlusion of Inferior Mesenteric Vein with Intraluminal Device, Open Approach

06L60ZZ   Occlusion of Inferior Mesenteric Vein, Open Approach

06L63CZ   Occlusion of Inferior Mesenteric Vein with Extraluminal Device, Percutaneous Approach

06L63DZ   Occlusion of Inferior Mesenteric Vein with Intraluminal Device, Percutaneous Approach

06L63ZZ   Occlusion of Inferior Mesenteric Vein, Percutaneous Approach

06L64CZ   Occlusion of Inferior Mesenteric Vein with Extraluminal Device, Percutaneous Endoscopic Approach

06L64DZ   Occlusion of Inferior Mesenteric Vein with Intraluminal Device, Percutaneous Endoscopic Approach

06L64ZZ   Occlusion of Inferior Mesenteric Vein, Percutaneous Endoscopic Approach

06L70CZ   Occlusion of Colic Vein with Extraluminal Device, Open Approach

06L70DZ   Occlusion of Colic Vein with Intraluminal Device, Open Approach

06L70ZZ   Occlusion of Colic Vein, Open Approach

06L73CZ   Occlusion of Colic Vein with Extraluminal Device, Percutaneous Approach

06L73DZ   Occlusion of Colic Vein with Intraluminal Device, Percutaneous Approach

06L73ZZ   Occlusion of Colic Vein, Percutaneous Approach

06L74CZ   Occlusion of Colic Vein with Extraluminal Device, Percutaneous Endoscopic Approach

06L74DZ   Occlusion of Colic Vein with Intraluminal Device, Percutaneous Endoscopic Approach

06L74ZZ   Occlusion of Colic Vein, Percutaneous Endoscopic Approach

06L80CZ   Occlusion of Portal Vein with Extraluminal Device, Open Approach

06L80DZ   Occlusion of Portal Vein with Intraluminal Device, Open Approach

06L80ZZ   Occlusion of Portal Vein, Open Approach

06L83CZ   Occlusion of Portal Vein with Extraluminal Device, Percutaneous Approach

06L83DZ   Occlusion of Portal Vein with Intraluminal Device, Percutaneous Approach

06L83ZZ   Occlusion of Portal Vein, Percutaneous Approach

06L84CZ   Occlusion of Portal Vein with Extraluminal Device, Percutaneous Endoscopic Approach

06L84DZ   Occlusion of Portal Vein with Intraluminal Device, Percutaneous Endoscopic Approach

06L84ZZ   Occlusion of Portal Vein, Percutaneous Endoscopic Approach

06L90CZ   Occlusion of Right Renal Vein with Extraluminal Device, Open Approach

06L90DZ   Occlusion of Right Renal Vein with Intraluminal Device, Open Approach

06L90ZZ   Occlusion of Right Renal Vein, Open Approach

06L93CZ   Occlusion of Right Renal Vein with Extraluminal Device, Percutaneous Approach

06L93DZ   Occlusion of Right Renal Vein with Intraluminal Device, Percutaneous Approach

06L93ZZ   Occlusion of Right Renal Vein, Percutaneous Approach

06L94CZ   Occlusion of Right Renal Vein with Extraluminal Device, Percutaneous Endoscopic Approach

06L94DZ   Occlusion of Right Renal Vein with Intraluminal Device, Percutaneous Endoscopic Approach

06L94ZZ   Occlusion of Right Renal Vein, Percutaneous Endoscopic Approach

06LB0CZ   Occlusion of Left Renal Vein with Extraluminal Device, Open Approach

06LB0DZ   Occlusion of Left Renal Vein with Intraluminal Device, Open Approach

06LB0ZZ   Occlusion of Left Renal Vein, Open Approach

06LB3CZ   Occlusion of Left Renal Vein with Extraluminal Device, Percutaneous Approach

06LB3DZ Occlusion of Left Renal Vein with Intraluminal Device, Percutaneous Approach

06LB3ZZ Occlusion of Left Renal Vein, Percutaneous Approach

06LB4CZ Occlusion of Left Renal Vein with Extraluminal Device, Percutaneous Endoscopic Approach

06LB4DZ Occlusion of Left Renal Vein with Intraluminal Device, Percutaneous Endoscopic Approach

06LB4ZZ Occlusion of Left Renal Vein, Percutaneous Endoscopic Approach

06LC0CZ Occlusion of Right Common Iliac Vein with Extraluminal Device, Open Approach

06LC0DZ Occlusion of Right Common Iliac Vein with Intraluminal Device, Open Approach

06LC0ZZ Occlusion of Right Common Iliac Vein, Open Approach

06LC3CZ Occlusion of Right Common Iliac Vein with Extraluminal Device, Percutaneous Approach

06LC3DZ Occlusion of Right Common Iliac Vein with Intraluminal Device, Percutaneous Approach

06LC3ZZ Occlusion of Right Common Iliac Vein, Percutaneous Approach

06LC4CZ Occlusion of Right Common Iliac Vein with Extraluminal Device, Percutaneous Endoscopic Approach

06LC4DZ Occlusion of Right Common Iliac Vein with Intraluminal Device, Percutaneous Endoscopic Approach

06LC4ZZ Occlusion of Right Common Iliac Vein, Percutaneous Endoscopic Approach

06LD0CZ Occlusion of Left Common Iliac Vein with Extraluminal Device, Open Approach

06LD0DZ Occlusion of Left Common Iliac Vein with Intraluminal Device, Open Approach

06LD0ZZ Occlusion of Left Common Iliac Vein, Open Approach

06LD3CZ Occlusion of Left Common Iliac Vein with Extraluminal Device, Percutaneous Approach

06LD3DZ Occlusion of Left Common Iliac Vein with Intraluminal Device, Percutaneous Approach

06LD3ZZ Occlusion of Left Common Iliac Vein, Percutaneous Approach

06LD4CZ Occlusion of Left Common Iliac Vein with Extraluminal Device, Percutaneous Endoscopic Approach

06LD4DZ Occlusion of Left Common Iliac Vein with Intraluminal Device, Percutaneous Endoscopic Approach

06LD4ZZ Occlusion of Left Common Iliac Vein, Percutaneous Endoscopic Approach

06LF0CZ Occlusion of Right External Iliac Vein with Extraluminal Device, Open Approach

06LF0DZ Occlusion of Right External Iliac Vein with Intraluminal Device, Open Approach

06LF0ZZ Occlusion of Right External Iliac Vein, Open Approach

06LF3CZ Occlusion of Right External Iliac Vein with Extraluminal Device, Percutaneous Approach

06LF3DZ Occlusion of Right External Iliac Vein with Intraluminal Device, Percutaneous Approach

06LF3ZZ Occlusion of Right External Iliac Vein, Percutaneous Approach

06LF4CZ Occlusion of Right External Iliac Vein with Extraluminal Device, Percutaneous Endoscopic Approach

06LF4DZ Occlusion of Right External Iliac Vein with Intraluminal Device, Percutaneous Endoscopic Approach

06LF4ZZ Occlusion of Right External Iliac Vein, Percutaneous Endoscopic Approach

06LG0CZ Occlusion of Left External Iliac Vein with Extraluminal Device, Open Approach

06LG0DZ Occlusion of Left External Iliac Vein with Intraluminal Device, Open Approach

06LG0ZZ Occlusion of Left External Iliac Vein, Open Approach

06LG3CZ Occlusion of Left External Iliac Vein with Extraluminal Device, Percutaneous Approach

06LG3DZ Occlusion of Left External Iliac Vein with Intraluminal Device, Percutaneous Approach

06LG3ZZ Occlusion of Left External Iliac Vein, Percutaneous Approach

06LG4CZ Occlusion of Left External Iliac Vein with Extraluminal Device, Percutaneous Endoscopic Approach

06LG4DZ Occlusion of Left External Iliac Vein with Intraluminal Device, Percutaneous Endoscopic Approach

06LG4ZZ Occlusion of Left External Iliac Vein, Percutaneous Endoscopic Approach

06LH0CZ Occlusion of Right Hypogastric Vein with Extraluminal Device, Open Approach

06LH0DZ Occlusion of Right Hypogastric Vein with Intraluminal Device, Open Approach

06LH0ZZ Occlusion of Right Hypogastric Vein, Open Approach

06LH3CZ Occlusion of Right Hypogastric Vein with Extraluminal Device, Percutaneous Approach

06LH3DZ Occlusion of Right Hypogastric Vein with Intraluminal Device, Percutaneous Approach

06LH3ZZ Occlusion of Right Hypogastric Vein, Percutaneous Approach

06LH4CZ Occlusion of Right Hypogastric Vein with Extraluminal Device, Percutaneous Endoscopic Approach

06LH4DZ Occlusion of Right Hypogastric Vein with Intraluminal Device, Percutaneous Endoscopic Approach

06LH4ZZ Occlusion of Right Hypogastric Vein, Percutaneous Endoscopic Approach

06LJ0CZ Occlusion of Left Hypogastric Vein with Extraluminal Device, Open Approach

06LJ0DZ Occlusion of Left Hypogastric Vein with Intraluminal Device, Open Approach

06LJ0ZZ Occlusion of Left Hypogastric Vein, Open Approach

06LJ3CZ Occlusion of Left Hypogastric Vein with Extraluminal Device, Percutaneous Approach

06LJ3DZ Occlusion of Left Hypogastric Vein with Intraluminal Device, Percutaneous Approach

06LJ3ZZ Occlusion of Left Hypogastric Vein, Percutaneous Approach

06LJ4CZ Occlusion of Left Hypogastric Vein with Extraluminal Device, Percutaneous Endoscopic Approach

06LJ4DZ Occlusion of Left Hypogastric Vein with Intraluminal Device, Percutaneous Endoscopic Approach

06LJ4ZZ Occlusion of Left Hypogastric Vein, Percutaneous Endoscopic Approach

06LM0CZ Occlusion of Right Femoral Vein with Extraluminal Device, Open Approach

06LM0DZ Occlusion of Right Femoral Vein with Intraluminal Device, Open Approach

06LM0ZZ Occlusion of Right Femoral Vein, Open Approach

06LM3CZ Occlusion of Right Femoral Vein with Extraluminal Device, Percutaneous Approach

06LM3DZ Occlusion of Right Femoral Vein with Intraluminal Device, Percutaneous Approach

06LM3ZZ Occlusion of Right Femoral Vein, Percutaneous Approach

06LM4CZ Occlusion of Right Femoral Vein with Extraluminal Device, Percutaneous Endoscopic Approach

06LM4DZ Occlusion of Right Femoral Vein with Intraluminal Device, Percutaneous Endoscopic Approach

06LM4ZZ Occlusion of Right Femoral Vein, Percutaneous Endoscopic Approach

06LN0CZ Occlusion of Left Femoral Vein with Extraluminal Device, Open Approach

06LN0DZ Occlusion of Left Femoral Vein with Intraluminal Device, Open Approach

06LN0ZZ Occlusion of Left Femoral Vein, Open Approach

06LN3CZ Occlusion of Left Femoral Vein with Extraluminal Device, Percutaneous Approach

06LN3DZ Occlusion of Left Femoral Vein with Intraluminal Device, Percutaneous Approach

06LN3ZZ Occlusion of Left Femoral Vein, Percutaneous Approach

06LN4CZ Occlusion of Left Femoral Vein with Extraluminal Device, Percutaneous Endoscopic Approach

06LN4DZ Occlusion of Left Femoral Vein with Intraluminal Device, Percutaneous Endoscopic Approach

06LN4ZZ Occlusion of Left Femoral Vein, Percutaneous Endoscopic Approach

06LP0CZ Occlusion of Right Greater Saphenous Vein with Extraluminal Device, Open Approach

06LP0DZ Occlusion of Right Greater Saphenous Vein with Intraluminal Device, Open Approach

06LP0ZZ Occlusion of Right Greater Saphenous Vein, Open Approach

06LP3CZ Occlusion of Right Greater Saphenous Vein with Extraluminal Device, Percutaneous Approach

06LP3DZ Occlusion of Right Greater Saphenous Vein with Intraluminal Device, Percutaneous Approach

06LP3ZZ	Occlusion of Right Greater Saphenous Vein, Percutaneous Approach
06LP4CZ	Occlusion of Right Greater Saphenous Vein with Extraluminal Device, Percutaneous Endoscopic Approach
06LP4DZ	Occlusion of Right Greater Saphenous Vein with Intraluminal Device, Percutaneous Endoscopic Approach
06LP4ZZ	Occlusion of Right Greater Saphenous Vein, Percutaneous Endoscopic Approach
06LQ0CZ	Occlusion of Left Greater Saphenous Vein with Extraluminal Device, Open Approach
06LQ0DZ	Occlusion of Left Greater Saphenous Vein with Intraluminal Device, Open Approach
06LQ0ZZ	Occlusion of Left Greater Saphenous Vein, Open Approach
06LQ3CZ	Occlusion of Left Greater Saphenous Vein with Extraluminal Device, Percutaneous Approach
06LQ3DZ	Occlusion of Left Greater Saphenous Vein with Intraluminal Device, Percutaneous Approach
06LQ3ZZ	Occlusion of Left Greater Saphenous Vein, Percutaneous Approach
06LQ4CZ	Occlusion of Left Greater Saphenous Vein with Extraluminal Device, Percutaneous Endoscopic Approach
06LQ4DZ	Occlusion of Left Greater Saphenous Vein with Intraluminal Device, Percutaneous Endoscopic Approach
06LQ4ZZ	Occlusion of Left Greater Saphenous Vein, Percutaneous Endoscopic Approach
06LR0CZ	Occlusion of Right Lesser Saphenous Vein with Extraluminal Device, Open Approach
06LR0DZ	Occlusion of Right Lesser Saphenous Vein with Intraluminal Device, Open Approach
06LR0ZZ	Occlusion of Right Lesser Saphenous Vein, Open Approach
06LR3CZ	Occlusion of Right Lesser Saphenous Vein with Extraluminal Device, Percutaneous Approach
06LR3DZ	Occlusion of Right Lesser Saphenous Vein with Intraluminal Device, Percutaneous Approach
06LR3ZZ	Occlusion of Right Lesser Saphenous Vein, Percutaneous Approach
06LR4CZ	Occlusion of Right Lesser Saphenous Vein with Extraluminal Device, Percutaneous Endoscopic Approach
06LR4DZ	Occlusion of Right Lesser Saphenous Vein with Intraluminal Device, Percutaneous Endoscopic Approach
06LR4ZZ	Occlusion of Right Lesser Saphenous Vein, Percutaneous Endoscopic Approach
06LS0CZ	Occlusion of Left Lesser Saphenous Vein with Extraluminal Device, Open Approach
06LS0DZ	Occlusion of Left Lesser Saphenous Vein with Intraluminal Device, Open Approach
06LS0ZZ	Occlusion of Left Lesser Saphenous Vein, Open Approach
06LS3CZ	Occlusion of Left Lesser Saphenous Vein with Extraluminal Device, Percutaneous Approach
06LS3DZ	Occlusion of Left Lesser Saphenous Vein with Intraluminal Device, Percutaneous Approach
06LS3ZZ	Occlusion of Left Lesser Saphenous Vein, Percutaneous Approach
06LS4CZ	Occlusion of Left Lesser Saphenous Vein with Extraluminal Device, Percutaneous Endoscopic Approach
06LS4DZ	Occlusion of Left Lesser Saphenous Vein with Intraluminal Device, Percutaneous Endoscopic Approach
06LS4ZZ	Occlusion of Left Lesser Saphenous Vein, Percutaneous Endoscopic Approach
06LT0CZ	Occlusion of Right Foot Vein with Extraluminal Device, Open Approach
06LT0DZ	Occlusion of Right Foot Vein with Intraluminal Device, Open Approach

06LT0ZZ	Occlusion of Right Foot Vein, Open Approach
06LT3CZ	Occlusion of Right Foot Vein with Extraluminal Device, Percutaneous Approach
06LT3DZ	Occlusion of Right Foot Vein with Intraluminal Device, Percutaneous Approach
06LT3ZZ	Occlusion of Right Foot Vein, Percutaneous Approach
06LT4CZ	Occlusion of Right Foot Vein with Extraluminal Device, Percutaneous Endoscopic Approach
06LT4DZ	Occlusion of Right Foot Vein with Intraluminal Device, Percutaneous Endoscopic Approach
06LT4ZZ	Occlusion of Right Foot Vein, Percutaneous Endoscopic Approach
06LV0CZ	Occlusion of Left Foot Vein with Extraluminal Device, Open Approach
06LV0DZ	Occlusion of Left Foot Vein with Intraluminal Device, Open Approach
06LV0ZZ	Occlusion of Left Foot Vein, Open Approach
06LV3CZ	Occlusion of Left Foot Vein with Extraluminal Device, Percutaneous Approach
06LV3DZ	Occlusion of Left Foot Vein with Intraluminal Device, Percutaneous Approach
06LV3ZZ	Occlusion of Left Foot Vein, Percutaneous Approach
06LV4CZ	Occlusion of Left Foot Vein with Extraluminal Device, Percutaneous Endoscopic Approach
06LV4DZ	Occlusion of Left Foot Vein with Intraluminal Device, Percutaneous Endoscopic Approach
06LV4ZZ	Occlusion of Left Foot Vein, Percutaneous Endoscopic Approach
06LY0CC	Occlusion of Hemorrhoidal Plexus with Extraluminal Device, Open Approach
06LY0CZ	Occlusion of Lower Vein with Extraluminal Device, Open Approach
06LY0DC	Occlusion of Hemorrhoidal Plexus with Intraluminal Device, Open Approach
06LY0DZ	Occlusion of Lower Vein with Intraluminal Device, Open Approach
06LY0ZC	Occlusion of Hemorrhoidal Plexus, Open Approach
06LY0ZZ	Occlusion of Lower Vein, Open Approach
06LY3CC	Occlusion of Hemorrhoidal Plexus with Extraluminal Device, Percutaneous Approach
06LY3CZ	Occlusion of Lower Vein with Extraluminal Device, Percutaneous Approach
06LY3DC	Occlusion of Hemorrhoidal Plexus with Intraluminal Device, Percutaneous Approach
06LY3DZ	Occlusion of Lower Vein with Intraluminal Device, Percutaneous Approach
06LY3ZC	Occlusion of Hemorrhoidal Plexus, Percutaneous Approach
06LY3ZZ	Occlusion of Lower Vein, Percutaneous Approach
06LY4CC	Occlusion of Hemorrhoidal Plexus with Extraluminal Device, Percutaneous Endoscopic Approach
06LY4CZ	Occlusion of Lower Vein with Extraluminal Device, Percutaneous Endoscopic Approach
06LY4DC	Occlusion of Hemorrhoidal Plexus with Intraluminal Device, Percutaneous Endoscopic Approach
06LY4DZ	Occlusion of Lower Vein with Intraluminal Device, Percutaneous Endoscopic Approach
06LY4ZC	Occlusion of Hemorrhoidal Plexus, Percutaneous Endoscopic Approach
06LY4ZZ	Occlusion of Lower Vein, Percutaneous Endoscopic Approach

06N – Lower Veins, Release

Review Coding Guidelines B3.13 and B3.14

06N00ZZ	Release Inferior Vena Cava, Open Approach
06N03ZZ	Release Inferior Vena Cava, Percutaneous Approach
06N04ZZ	Release Inferior Vena Cava, Percutaneous Endoscopic Approach
06N10ZZ	Release Splenic Vein, Open Approach
06N13ZZ	Release Splenic Vein, Percutaneous Approach
06N14ZZ	Release Splenic Vein, Percutaneous Endoscopic Approach
06N20ZZ	Release Gastric Vein, Open Approach
06N23ZZ	Release Gastric Vein, Percutaneous Approach
06N24ZZ	Release Gastric Vein, Percutaneous Endoscopic Approach

06N30ZZ	Release Esophageal Vein, Open Approach
06N33ZZ	Release Esophageal Vein, Percutaneous Approach
06N34ZZ	Release Esophageal Vein, Percutaneous Endoscopic Approach
06N40ZZ	Release Hepatic Vein, Open Approach
06N43ZZ	Release Hepatic Vein, Percutaneous Approach
06N44ZZ	Release Hepatic Vein, Percutaneous Endoscopic Approach
06N50ZZ	Release Superior Mesenteric Vein, Open Approach
06N53ZZ	Release Superior Mesenteric Vein, Percutaneous Approach

06N54ZZ Release Superior Mesenteric Vein, Percutaneous Endoscopic Approach
06N60ZZ Release Inferior Mesenteric Vein, Open Approach
06N63ZZ Release Inferior Mesenteric Vein, Percutaneous Approach
06N64ZZ Release Inferior Mesenteric Vein, Percutaneous Endoscopic Approach
06N70ZZ Release Colic Vein, Open Approach
06N73ZZ Release Colic Vein, Percutaneous Approach
06N74ZZ Release Colic Vein, Percutaneous Endoscopic Approach
06N80ZZ Release Portal Vein, Open Approach
06N83ZZ Release Portal Vein, Percutaneous Approach
06N84ZZ Release Portal Vein, Percutaneous Endoscopic Approach
06N90ZZ Release Right Renal Vein, Open Approach
06N93ZZ Release Right Renal Vein, Percutaneous Approach
06N94ZZ Release Right Renal Vein, Percutaneous Endoscopic Approach
06NB0ZZ Release Left Renal Vein, Open Approach
06NB3ZZ Release Left Renal Vein, Percutaneous Approach
06NB4ZZ Release Left Renal Vein, Percutaneous Endoscopic Approach
06NC0ZZ Release Right Common Iliac Vein, Open Approach
06NC3ZZ Release Right Common Iliac Vein, Percutaneous Approach
06NC4ZZ Release Right Common Iliac Vein, Percutaneous Endoscopic Approach
06ND0ZZ Release Left Common Iliac Vein, Open Approach
06ND3ZZ Release Left Common Iliac Vein, Percutaneous Approach
06ND4ZZ Release Left Common Iliac Vein, Percutaneous Endoscopic Approach
06NF0ZZ Release Right External Iliac Vein, Open Approach
06NF3ZZ Release Right External Iliac Vein, Percutaneous Approach
06NF4ZZ Release Right External Iliac Vein, Percutaneous Endoscopic Approach
06NG0ZZ Release Left External Iliac Vein, Open Approach
06NG3ZZ Release Left External Iliac Vein, Percutaneous Approach
06NG4ZZ Release Left External Iliac Vein, Percutaneous Endoscopic Approach
06NH0ZZ Release Right Hypogastric Vein, Open Approach
06NH3ZZ Release Right Hypogastric Vein, Percutaneous Approach

06NH4ZZ Release Right Hypogastric Vein, Percutaneous Endoscopic Approach
06NJ0ZZ Release Left Hypogastric Vein, Open Approach
06NJ3ZZ Release Left Hypogastric Vein, Percutaneous Approach
06NJ4ZZ Release Left Hypogastric Vein, Percutaneous Endoscopic Approach
06NM0ZZ Release Right Femoral Vein, Open Approach
06NM3ZZ Release Right Femoral Vein, Percutaneous Approach
06NM4ZZ Release Right Femoral Vein, Percutaneous Endoscopic Approach
06NN0ZZ Release Left Femoral Vein, Open Approach
06NN3ZZ Release Left Femoral Vein, Percutaneous Approach
06NN4ZZ Release Left Femoral Vein, Percutaneous Endoscopic Approach
06NP0ZZ Release Right Greater Saphenous Vein, Open Approach
06NP3ZZ Release Right Greater Saphenous Vein, Percutaneous Approach
06NP4ZZ Release Right Greater Saphenous Vein, Percutaneous Endoscopic Approach
06NQ0ZZ Release Left Greater Saphenous Vein, Open Approach
06NQ3ZZ Release Left Greater Saphenous Vein, Percutaneous Approach
06NQ4ZZ Release Left Greater Saphenous Vein, Percutaneous Endoscopic Approach
06NR0ZZ Release Right Lesser Saphenous Vein, Open Approach
06NR3ZZ Release Right Lesser Saphenous Vein, Percutaneous Approach
06NR4ZZ Release Right Lesser Saphenous Vein, Percutaneous Endoscopic Approach
06NS0ZZ Release Left Lesser Saphenous Vein, Open Approach
06NS3ZZ Release Left Lesser Saphenous Vein, Percutaneous Approach
06NS4ZZ Release Left Lesser Saphenous Vein, Percutaneous Endoscopic Approach
06NT0ZZ Release Right Foot Vein, Open Approach
06NT3ZZ Release Right Foot Vein, Percutaneous Approach
06NT4ZZ Release Right Foot Vein, Percutaneous Endoscopic Approach
06NV0ZZ Release Left Foot Vein, Open Approach
06NV3ZZ Release Left Foot Vein, Percutaneous Approach
06NV4ZZ Release Left Foot Vein, Percutaneous Endoscopic Approach
06NY0ZZ Release Lower Vein, Open Approach
06NY3ZZ Release Lower Vein, Percutaneous Approach
06NY4ZZ Release Lower Vein, Percutaneous Endoscopic Approach

06P – Lower Veins, Removal

Review Coding Guideline B6.1c

06PY00Z Removal of Drainage Device from Lower Vein, Open Approach
06PY02Z Removal of Monitoring Device from Lower Vein, Open Approach
06PY03Z Removal of Infusion Device from Lower Vein, Open Approach
06PY07Z Removal of Autologous Tissue Substitute from Lower Vein, Open Approach
06PY0CZ Removal of Extraluminal Device from Lower Vein, Open Approach
06PY0DZ Removal of Intraluminal Device from Lower Vein, Open Approach
06PY0JZ Removal of Synthetic Substitute from Lower Vein, Open Approach
06PY0KZ Removal of Nonautologous Tissue Substitute from Lower Vein, Open Approach
06PY30Z Removal of Drainage Device from Lower Vein, Percutaneous Approach
06PY32Z Removal of Monitoring Device from Lower Vein, Percutaneous Approach
06PY33Z Removal of Infusion Device from Lower Vein, Percutaneous Approach
06PY37Z Removal of Autologous Tissue Substitute from Lower Vein, Percutaneous Approach
06PY3CZ Removal of Extraluminal Device from Lower Vein, Percutaneous Approach
06PY3DZ Removal of Intraluminal Device from Lower Vein, Percutaneous Approach
06PY3JZ Removal of Synthetic Substitute from Lower Vein, Percutaneous Approach

06PY3KZ Removal of Nonautologous Tissue Substitute from Lower Vein, Percutaneous Approach
06PY40Z Removal of Drainage Device from Lower Vein, Percutaneous Endoscopic Approach
06PY42Z Removal of Monitoring Device from Lower Vein, Percutaneous Endoscopic Approach
06PY43Z Removal of Infusion Device from Lower Vein, Percutaneous Endoscopic Approach
06PY47Z Removal of Autologous Tissue Substitute from Lower Vein, Percutaneous Endoscopic Approach
06PY4CZ Removal of Extraluminal Device from Lower Vein, Percutaneous Endoscopic Approach
06PY4DZ Removal of Intraluminal Device from Lower Vein, Percutaneous Endoscopic Approach
06PY4JZ Removal of Synthetic Substitute from Lower Vein, Percutaneous Endoscopic Approach
06PY4KZ Removal of Nonautologous Tissue Substitute from Lower Vein, Percutaneous Endoscopic Approach
06PYX0Z Removal of Drainage Device from Lower Vein, External Approach
06PYX2Z Removal of Monitoring Device from Lower Vein, External Approach
06PYX3Z Removal of Infusion Device from Lower Vein, External Approach
06PYXDZ Removal of Intraluminal Device from Lower Vein, External Approach

06Q – Lower Veins, Repair

06Q00ZZ Repair Inferior Vena Cava, Open Approach
06Q03ZZ Repair Inferior Vena Cava, Percutaneous Approach
06Q04ZZ Repair Inferior Vena Cava, Percutaneous Endoscopic Approach
06Q10ZZ Repair Splenic Vein, Open Approach
06Q13ZZ Repair Splenic Vein, Percutaneous Approach

06Q14ZZ Repair Splenic Vein, Percutaneous Endoscopic Approach
06Q20ZZ Repair Gastric Vein, Open Approach
06Q23ZZ Repair Gastric Vein, Percutaneous Approach
06Q24ZZ Repair Gastric Vein, Percutaneous Endoscopic Approach
06Q30ZZ Repair Esophageal Vein, Open Approach

♀ Female-only   ♂ Male-only   ● Limited Coverage   ● Non-OR   **HAC** HAC-associated procedure   ● Non-covered procedures   ✚ Combination

06Q33ZZ	Repair Esophageal Vein, Percutaneous Approach
06Q34ZZ	Repair Esophageal Vein, Percutaneous Endoscopic Approach
06Q40ZZ	Repair Hepatic Vein, Open Approach
06Q43ZZ	Repair Hepatic Vein, Percutaneous Approach
06Q44ZZ	Repair Hepatic Vein, Percutaneous Endoscopic Approach
06Q50ZZ	Repair Superior Mesenteric Vein, Open Approach
06Q53ZZ	Repair Superior Mesenteric Vein, Percutaneous Approach
06Q54ZZ	Repair Superior Mesenteric Vein, Percutaneous Endoscopic Approach
06Q60ZZ	Repair Inferior Mesenteric Vein, Open Approach
06Q63ZZ	Repair Inferior Mesenteric Vein, Percutaneous Approach
06Q64ZZ	Repair Inferior Mesenteric Vein, Percutaneous Endoscopic Approach
06Q70ZZ	Repair Colic Vein, Open Approach
06Q73ZZ	Repair Colic Vein, Percutaneous Approach
06Q74ZZ	Repair Colic Vein, Percutaneous Endoscopic Approach
06Q80ZZ	Repair Portal Vein, Open Approach
06Q83ZZ	Repair Portal Vein, Percutaneous Approach
06Q84ZZ	Repair Portal Vein, Percutaneous Endoscopic Approach
06Q90ZZ	Repair Right Renal Vein, Open Approach
06Q93ZZ	Repair Right Renal Vein, Percutaneous Approach
06Q94ZZ	Repair Right Renal Vein, Percutaneous Endoscopic Approach
06QB0ZZ	Repair Left Renal Vein, Open Approach
06QB3ZZ	Repair Left Renal Vein, Percutaneous Approach
06QB4ZZ	Repair Left Renal Vein, Percutaneous Endoscopic Approach
06QC0ZZ	Repair Right Common Iliac Vein, Open Approach
06QC3ZZ	Repair Right Common Iliac Vein, Percutaneous Approach
06QC4ZZ	Repair Right Common Iliac Vein, Percutaneous Endoscopic Approach
06QD0ZZ	Repair Left Common Iliac Vein, Open Approach
06QD3ZZ	Repair Left Common Iliac Vein, Percutaneous Approach
06QD4ZZ	Repair Left Common Iliac Vein, Percutaneous Endoscopic Approach
06QF0ZZ	Repair Right External Iliac Vein, Open Approach
06QF3ZZ	Repair Right External Iliac Vein, Percutaneous Approach
06QF4ZZ	Repair Right External Iliac Vein, Percutaneous Endoscopic Approach
06QG0ZZ	Repair Left External Iliac Vein, Open Approach
06QG3ZZ	Repair Left External Iliac Vein, Percutaneous Approach
06QG4ZZ	Repair Left External Iliac Vein, Percutaneous Endoscopic Approach
06QH0ZZ	Repair Right Hypogastric Vein, Open Approach
06QH3ZZ	Repair Right Hypogastric Vein, Percutaneous Approach
06QH4ZZ	Repair Right Hypogastric Vein, Percutaneous Endoscopic Approach
06QJ0ZZ	Repair Left Hypogastric Vein, Open Approach
06QJ3ZZ	Repair Left Hypogastric Vein, Percutaneous Approach
06QJ4ZZ	Repair Left Hypogastric Vein, Percutaneous Endoscopic Approach
06QM0ZZ	Repair Right Femoral Vein, Open Approach
06QM3ZZ	Repair Right Femoral Vein, Percutaneous Approach
06QM4ZZ	Repair Right Femoral Vein, Percutaneous Endoscopic Approach
06QN0ZZ	Repair Left Femoral Vein, Open Approach
06QN3ZZ	Repair Left Femoral Vein, Percutaneous Approach
06QN4ZZ	Repair Left Femoral Vein, Percutaneous Endoscopic Approach
06QP0ZZ	Repair Right Greater Saphenous Vein, Open Approach
06QP3ZZ	Repair Right Greater Saphenous Vein, Percutaneous Approach
06QP4ZZ	Repair Right Greater Saphenous Vein, Percutaneous Endoscopic Approach
06QQ0ZZ	Repair Left Greater Saphenous Vein, Open Approach
06QQ3ZZ	Repair Left Greater Saphenous Vein, Percutaneous Approach
06QQ4ZZ	Repair Left Greater Saphenous Vein, Percutaneous Endoscopic Approach
06QR0ZZ	Repair Right Lesser Saphenous Vein, Open Approach
06QR3ZZ	Repair Right Lesser Saphenous Vein, Percutaneous Approach
06QR4ZZ	Repair Right Lesser Saphenous Vein, Percutaneous Endoscopic Approach
06QS0ZZ	Repair Left Lesser Saphenous Vein, Open Approach
06QS3ZZ	Repair Left Lesser Saphenous Vein, Percutaneous Approach
06QS4ZZ	Repair Left Lesser Saphenous Vein, Percutaneous Endoscopic Approach
06QT0ZZ	Repair Right Foot Vein, Open Approach
06QT3ZZ	Repair Right Foot Vein, Percutaneous Approach
06QT4ZZ	Repair Right Foot Vein, Percutaneous Endoscopic Approach
06QV0ZZ	Repair Left Foot Vein, Open Approach
06QV3ZZ	Repair Left Foot Vein, Percutaneous Approach
06QV4ZZ	Repair Left Foot Vein, Percutaneous Endoscopic Approach
06QY0ZZ	Repair Lower Vein, Open Approach
06QY3ZZ	Repair Lower Vein, Percutaneous Approach
06QY4ZZ	Repair Lower Vein, Percutaneous Endoscopic Approach

06R – Lower Veins, Replacement

06R007Z	Replacement of Inferior Vena Cava with Autologous Tissue Substitute, Open Approach
06R00JZ	Replacement of Inferior Vena Cava with Synthetic Substitute, Open Approach
06R00KZ	Replacement of Inferior Vena Cava with Nonautologous Tissue Substitute, Open Approach
06R047Z	Replacement of Inferior Vena Cava with Autologous Tissue Substitute, Percutaneous Endoscopic Approach
06R04JZ	Replacement of Inferior Vena Cava with Synthetic Substitute, Percutaneous Endoscopic Approach
06R04KZ	Replacement of Inferior Vena Cava with Nonautologous Tissue Substitute, Percutaneous Endoscopic Approach
06R107Z	Replacement of Splenic Vein with Autologous Tissue Substitute, Open Approach
06R10JZ	Replacement of Splenic Vein with Synthetic Substitute, Open Approach
06R10KZ	Replacement of Splenic Vein with Nonautologous Tissue Substitute, Open Approach
06R147Z	Replacement of Splenic Vein with Autologous Tissue Substitute, Percutaneous Endoscopic Approach
06R14JZ	Replacement of Splenic Vein with Synthetic Substitute, Percutaneous Endoscopic Approach
06R14KZ	Replacement of Splenic Vein with Nonautologous Tissue Substitute, Percutaneous Endoscopic Approach
06R207Z	Replacement of Gastric Vein with Autologous Tissue Substitute, Open Approach
06R20JZ	Replacement of Gastric Vein with Synthetic Substitute, Open Approach
06R20KZ	Replacement of Gastric Vein with Nonautologous Tissue Substitute, Open Approach
06R247Z	Replacement of Gastric Vein with Autologous Tissue Substitute, Percutaneous Endoscopic Approach
06R24JZ	Replacement of Gastric Vein with Synthetic Substitute, Percutaneous Endoscopic Approach
06R24KZ	Replacement of Gastric Vein with Nonautologous Tissue Substitute, Percutaneous Endoscopic Approach
06R307Z	Replacement of Esophageal Vein with Autologous Tissue Substitute, Open Approach
06R30JZ	Replacement of Esophageal Vein with Synthetic Substitute, Open Approach
06R30KZ	Replacement of Esophageal Vein with Nonautologous Tissue Substitute, Open Approach
06R347Z	Replacement of Esophageal Vein with Autologous Tissue Substitute, Percutaneous Endoscopic Approach
06R34JZ	Replacement of Esophageal Vein with Synthetic Substitute, Percutaneous Endoscopic Approach
06R34KZ	Replacement of Esophageal Vein with Nonautologous Tissue Substitute, Percutaneous Endoscopic Approach
06R407Z	Replacement of Hepatic Vein with Autologous Tissue Substitute, Open Approach
06R40JZ	Replacement of Hepatic Vein with Synthetic Substitute, Open Approach
06R40KZ	Replacement of Hepatic Vein with Nonautologous Tissue Substitute, Open Approach
06R447Z	Replacement of Hepatic Vein with Autologous Tissue Substitute, Percutaneous Endoscopic Approach
06R44JZ	Replacement of Hepatic Vein with Synthetic Substitute, Percutaneous Endoscopic Approach
06R44KZ	Replacement of Hepatic Vein with Nonautologous Tissue Substitute, Percutaneous Endoscopic Approach

♀ Female-only   ♂ Male-only   ● Limited Coverage   ● Non-OR   HAC HAC-associated procedure   ● Non-covered procedures   ＋ Combination

06R507Z Replacement of Superior Mesenteric Vein with Autologous Tissue Substitute, Open Approach

06R50JZ Replacement of Superior Mesenteric Vein with Synthetic Substitute, Open Approach

06R50KZ Replacement of Superior Mesenteric Vein with Nonautologous Tissue Substitute, Open Approach

06R547Z Replacement of Superior Mesenteric Vein with Autologous Tissue Substitute, Percutaneous Endoscopic Approach

06R54JZ Replacement of Superior Mesenteric Vein with Synthetic Substitute, Percutaneous Endoscopic Approach

06R54KZ Replacement of Superior Mesenteric Vein with Nonautologous Tissue Substitute, Percutaneous Endoscopic Approach

06R607Z Replacement of Inferior Mesenteric Vein with Autologous Tissue Substitute, Open Approach

06R60JZ Replacement of Inferior Mesenteric Vein with Synthetic Substitute, Open Approach

06R60KZ Replacement of Inferior Mesenteric Vein with Nonautologous Tissue Substitute, Open Approach

06R647Z Replacement of Inferior Mesenteric Vein with Autologous Tissue Substitute, Percutaneous Endoscopic Approach

06R64JZ Replacement of Inferior Mesenteric Vein with Synthetic Substitute, Percutaneous Endoscopic Approach

06R64KZ Replacement of Inferior Mesenteric Vein with Nonautologous Tissue Substitute, Percutaneous Endoscopic Approach

06R707Z Replacement of Colic Vein with Autologous Tissue Substitute, Open Approach

06R70JZ Replacement of Colic Vein with Synthetic Substitute, Open Approach

06R70KZ Replacement of Colic Vein with Nonautologous Tissue Substitute, Open Approach

06R747Z Replacement of Colic Vein with Autologous Tissue Substitute, Percutaneous Endoscopic Approach

06R74JZ Replacement of Colic Vein with Synthetic Substitute, Percutaneous Endoscopic Approach

06R74KZ Replacement of Colic Vein with Nonautologous Tissue Substitute, Percutaneous Endoscopic Approach

06R807Z Replacement of Portal Vein with Autologous Tissue Substitute, Open Approach

06R80JZ Replacement of Portal Vein with Synthetic Substitute, Open Approach

06R80KZ Replacement of Portal Vein with Nonautologous Tissue Substitute, Open Approach

06R847Z Replacement of Portal Vein with Autologous Tissue Substitute, Percutaneous Endoscopic Approach

06R84JZ Replacement of Portal Vein with Synthetic Substitute, Percutaneous Endoscopic Approach

06R84KZ Replacement of Portal Vein with Nonautologous Tissue Substitute, Percutaneous Endoscopic Approach

06R907Z Replacement of Right Renal Vein with Autologous Tissue Substitute, Open Approach

06R90JZ Replacement of Right Renal Vein with Synthetic Substitute, Open Approach

06R90KZ Replacement of Right Renal Vein with Nonautologous Tissue Substitute, Open Approach

06R947Z Replacement of Right Renal Vein with Autologous Tissue Substitute, Percutaneous Endoscopic Approach

06R94JZ Replacement of Right Renal Vein with Synthetic Substitute, Percutaneous Endoscopic Approach

06R94KZ Replacement of Right Renal Vein with Nonautologous Tissue Substitute, Percutaneous Endoscopic Approach

06RB07Z Replacement of Left Renal Vein with Autologous Tissue Substitute, Open Approach

06RB0JZ Replacement of Left Renal Vein with Synthetic Substitute, Open Approach

06RB0KZ Replacement of Left Renal Vein with Nonautologous Tissue Substitute, Open Approach

06RB47Z Replacement of Left Renal Vein with Autologous Tissue Substitute, Percutaneous Endoscopic Approach

06RB4JZ Replacement of Left Renal Vein with Synthetic Substitute, Percutaneous Endoscopic Approach

06RB4KZ Replacement of Left Renal Vein with Nonautologous Tissue Substitute, Percutaneous Endoscopic Approach

06RC07Z Replacement of Right Common Iliac Vein with Autologous Tissue Substitute, Open Approach

06RC0JZ Replacement of Right Common Iliac Vein with Synthetic Substitute, Open Approach

06RC0KZ Replacement of Right Common Iliac Vein with Nonautologous Tissue Substitute, Open Approach

06RC47Z Replacement of Right Common Iliac Vein with Autologous Tissue Substitute, Percutaneous Endoscopic Approach

06RC4JZ Replacement of Right Common Iliac Vein with Synthetic Substitute, Percutaneous Endoscopic Approach

06RC4KZ Replacement of Right Common Iliac Vein with Nonautologous Tissue Substitute, Percutaneous Endoscopic Approach

06RD07Z Replacement of Left Common Iliac Vein with Autologous Tissue Substitute, Open Approach

06RD0JZ Replacement of Left Common Iliac Vein with Synthetic Substitute, Open Approach

06RD0KZ Replacement of Left Common Iliac Vein with Nonautologous Tissue Substitute, Open Approach

06RD47Z Replacement of Left Common Iliac Vein with Autologous Tissue Substitute, Percutaneous Endoscopic Approach

06RD4JZ Replacement of Left Common Iliac Vein with Synthetic Substitute, Percutaneous Endoscopic Approach

06RD4KZ Replacement of Left Common Iliac Vein with Nonautologous Tissue Substitute, Percutaneous Endoscopic Approach

06RF07Z Replacement of Right External Iliac Vein with Autologous Tissue Substitute, Open Approach

06RF0JZ Replacement of Right External Iliac Vein with Synthetic Substitute, Open Approach

06RF0KZ Replacement of Right External Iliac Vein with Nonautologous Tissue Substitute, Open Approach

06RF47Z Replacement of Right External Iliac Vein with Autologous Tissue Substitute, Percutaneous Endoscopic Approach

06RF4JZ Replacement of Right External Iliac Vein with Synthetic Substitute, Percutaneous Endoscopic Approach

06RF4KZ Replacement of Right External Iliac Vein with Nonautologous Tissue Substitute, Percutaneous Endoscopic Approach

06RG07Z Replacement of Left External Iliac Vein with Autologous Tissue Substitute, Open Approach

06RG0JZ Replacement of Left External Iliac Vein with Synthetic Substitute, Open Approach

06RG0KZ Replacement of Left External Iliac Vein with Nonautologous Tissue Substitute, Open Approach

06RG47Z Replacement of Left External Iliac Vein with Autologous Tissue Substitute, Percutaneous Endoscopic Approach

06RG4JZ Replacement of Left External Iliac Vein with Synthetic Substitute, Percutaneous Endoscopic Approach

06RG4KZ Replacement of Left External Iliac Vein with Nonautologous Tissue Substitute, Percutaneous Endoscopic Approach

06RH07Z Replacement of Right Hypogastric Vein with Autologous Tissue Substitute, Open Approach

06RH0JZ Replacement of Right Hypogastric Vein with Synthetic Substitute, Open Approach

06RH0KZ Replacement of Right Hypogastric Vein with Nonautologous Tissue Substitute, Open Approach

06RH47Z Replacement of Right Hypogastric Vein with Autologous Tissue Substitute, Percutaneous Endoscopic Approach

06RH4JZ Replacement of Right Hypogastric Vein with Synthetic Substitute, Percutaneous Endoscopic Approach

06RH4KZ Replacement of Right Hypogastric Vein with Nonautologous Tissue Substitute, Percutaneous Endoscopic Approach

06RJ07Z Replacement of Left Hypogastric Vein with Autologous Tissue Substitute, Open Approach

06RJ0JZ Replacement of Left Hypogastric Vein with Synthetic Substitute, Open Approach

06RJ0KZ Replacement of Left Hypogastric Vein with Nonautologous Tissue Substitute, Open Approach

06RJ47Z Replacement of Left Hypogastric Vein with Autologous Tissue Substitute, Percutaneous Endoscopic Approach

06RJ4JZ Replacement of Left Hypogastric Vein with Synthetic Substitute, Percutaneous Endoscopic Approach

06RJ4KZ Replacement of Left Hypogastric Vein with Nonautologous Tissue Substitute, Percutaneous Endoscopic Approach

06RM07Z   Replacement of Right Femoral Vein with Autologous Tissue Substitute, Open Approach
06RM0JZ   Replacement of Right Femoral Vein with Synthetic Substitute, Open Approach
06RM0KZ   Replacement of Right Femoral Vein with Nonautologous Tissue Substitute, Open Approach
06RM47Z   Replacement of Right Femoral Vein with Autologous Tissue Substitute, Percutaneous Endoscopic Approach
06RM4JZ   Replacement of Right Femoral Vein with Synthetic Substitute, Percutaneous Endoscopic Approach
06RM4KZ   Replacement of Right Femoral Vein with Nonautologous Tissue Substitute, Percutaneous Endoscopic Approach
06RN07Z   Replacement of Left Femoral Vein with Autologous Tissue Substitute, Open Approach
06RN0JZ   Replacement of Left Femoral Vein with Synthetic Substitute, Open Approach
06RN0KZ   Replacement of Left Femoral Vein with Nonautologous Tissue Substitute, Open Approach
06RN47Z   Replacement of Left Femoral Vein with Autologous Tissue Substitute, Percutaneous Endoscopic Approach
06RN4JZ   Replacement of Left Femoral Vein with Synthetic Substitute, Percutaneous Endoscopic Approach
06RN4KZ   Replacement of Left Femoral Vein with Nonautologous Tissue Substitute, Percutaneous Endoscopic Approach
06RP07Z   Replacement of Right Greater Saphenous Vein with Autologous Tissue Substitute, Open Approach
06RP0JZ   Replacement of Right Greater Saphenous Vein with Synthetic Substitute, Open Approach
06RP0KZ   Replacement of Right Greater Saphenous Vein with Nonautologous Tissue Substitute, Open Approach
06RP47Z   Replacement of Right Greater Saphenous Vein with Autologous Tissue Substitute, Percutaneous Endoscopic Approach
06RP4JZ   Replacement of Right Greater Saphenous Vein with Synthetic Substitute, Percutaneous Endoscopic Approach
06RP4KZ   Replacement of Right Greater Saphenous Vein with Nonautologous Tissue Substitute, Percutaneous Endoscopic Approach
06RQ07Z   Replacement of Left Greater Saphenous Vein with Autologous Tissue Substitute, Open Approach
06RQ0JZ   Replacement of Left Greater Saphenous Vein with Synthetic Substitute, Open Approach
06RQ0KZ   Replacement of Left Greater Saphenous Vein with Nonautologous Tissue Substitute, Open Approach
06RQ47Z   Replacement of Left Greater Saphenous Vein with Autologous Tissue Substitute, Percutaneous Endoscopic Approach
06RQ4JZ   Replacement of Left Greater Saphenous Vein with Synthetic Substitute, Percutaneous Endoscopic Approach
06RQ4KZ   Replacement of Left Greater Saphenous Vein with Nonautologous Tissue Substitute, Percutaneous Endoscopic Approach
06RR07Z   Replacement of Right Lesser Saphenous Vein with Autologous Tissue Substitute, Open Approach
06RR0JZ   Replacement of Right Lesser Saphenous Vein with Synthetic Substitute, Open Approach
06RR0KZ   Replacement of Right Lesser Saphenous Vein with Nonautologous Tissue Substitute, Open Approach

06RR47Z   Replacement of Right Lesser Saphenous Vein with Autologous Tissue Substitute, Percutaneous Endoscopic Approach
06RR4JZ   Replacement of Right Lesser Saphenous Vein with Synthetic Substitute, Percutaneous Endoscopic Approach
06RR4KZ   Replacement of Right Lesser Saphenous Vein with Nonautologous Tissue Substitute, Percutaneous Endoscopic Approach
06RS07Z   Replacement of Left Lesser Saphenous Vein with Autologous Tissue Substitute, Open Approach
06RS0JZ   Replacement of Left Lesser Saphenous Vein with Synthetic Substitute, Open Approach
06RS0KZ   Replacement of Left Lesser Saphenous Vein with Nonautologous Tissue Substitute, Open Approach
06RS47Z   Replacement of Left Lesser Saphenous Vein with Autologous Tissue Substitute, Percutaneous Endoscopic Approach
06RS4JZ   Replacement of Left Lesser Saphenous Vein with Synthetic Substitute, Percutaneous Endoscopic Approach
06RS4KZ   Replacement of Left Lesser Saphenous Vein with Nonautologous Tissue Substitute, Percutaneous Endoscopic Approach
06RT07Z   Replacement of Right Foot Vein with Autologous Tissue Substitute, Open Approach
06RT0JZ   Replacement of Right Foot Vein with Synthetic Substitute, Open Approach
06RT0KZ   Replacement of Right Foot Vein with Nonautologous Tissue Substitute, Open Approach
06RT47Z   Replacement of Right Foot Vein with Autologous Tissue Substitute, Percutaneous Endoscopic Approach
06RT4JZ   Replacement of Right Foot Vein with Synthetic Substitute, Percutaneous Endoscopic Approach
06RT4KZ   Replacement of Right Foot Vein with Nonautologous Tissue Substitute, Percutaneous Endoscopic Approach
06RV07Z   Replacement of Left Foot Vein with Autologous Tissue Substitute, Open Approach
06RV0JZ   Replacement of Left Foot Vein with Synthetic Substitute, Open Approach
06RV0KZ   Replacement of Left Foot Vein with Nonautologous Tissue Substitute, Open Approach
06RV47Z   Replacement of Left Foot Vein with Autologous Tissue Substitute, Percutaneous Endoscopic Approach
06RV4JZ   Replacement of Left Foot Vein with Synthetic Substitute, Percutaneous Endoscopic Approach
06RV4KZ   Replacement of Left Foot Vein with Nonautologous Tissue Substitute, Percutaneous Endoscopic Approach
06RY07Z   Replacement of Lower Vein with Autologous Tissue Substitute, Open Approach
06RY0JZ   Replacement of Lower Vein with Synthetic Substitute, Open Approach
06RY0KZ   Replacement of Lower Vein with Nonautologous Tissue Substitute, Open Approach
06RY47Z   Replacement of Lower Vein with Autologous Tissue Substitute, Percutaneous Endoscopic Approach
06RY4JZ   Replacement of Lower Vein with Synthetic Substitute, Percutaneous Endoscopic Approach
06RY4KZ   Replacement of Lower Vein with Nonautologous Tissue Substitute, Percutaneous Endoscopic Approach

06S – Lower Veins, Reposition

06S00ZZ   Reposition Inferior Vena Cava, Open Approach
06S03ZZ   Reposition Inferior Vena Cava, Percutaneous Approach
06S04ZZ   Reposition Inferior Vena Cava, Percutaneous Endoscopic Approach
06S10ZZ   Reposition Splenic Vein, Open Approach
06S13ZZ   Reposition Splenic Vein, Percutaneous Approach
06S14ZZ   Reposition Splenic Vein, Percutaneous Endoscopic Approach
06S20ZZ   Reposition Gastric Vein, Open Approach
06S23ZZ   Reposition Gastric Vein, Percutaneous Approach
06S24ZZ   Reposition Gastric Vein, Percutaneous Endoscopic Approach
06S30ZZ   Reposition Esophageal Vein, Open Approach
06S33ZZ   Reposition Esophageal Vein, Percutaneous Approach
06S34ZZ   Reposition Esophageal Vein, Percutaneous Endoscopic Approach
06S40ZZ   Reposition Hepatic Vein, Open Approach
06S43ZZ   Reposition Hepatic Vein, Percutaneous Approach
06S44ZZ   Reposition Hepatic Vein, Percutaneous Endoscopic Approach
06S50ZZ   Reposition Superior Mesenteric Vein, Open Approach

06S53ZZ   Reposition Superior Mesenteric Vein, Percutaneous Approach
06S54ZZ   Reposition Superior Mesenteric Vein, Percutaneous Endoscopic Approach
06S60ZZ   Reposition Inferior Mesenteric Vein, Open Approach
06S63ZZ   Reposition Inferior Mesenteric Vein, Percutaneous Approach
06S64ZZ   Reposition Inferior Mesenteric Vein, Percutaneous Endoscopic Approach
06S70ZZ   Reposition Colic Vein, Open Approach
06S73ZZ   Reposition Colic Vein, Percutaneous Approach
06S74ZZ   Reposition Colic Vein, Percutaneous Endoscopic Approach
06S80ZZ   Reposition Portal Vein, Open Approach
06S83ZZ   Reposition Portal Vein, Percutaneous Approach
06S84ZZ   Reposition Portal Vein, Percutaneous Endoscopic Approach
06S90ZZ   Reposition Right Renal Vein, Open Approach
06S93ZZ   Reposition Right Renal Vein, Percutaneous Approach
06S94ZZ   Reposition Right Renal Vein, Percutaneous Endoscopic Approach

06SB0ZZ	Reposition Left Renal Vein, Open Approach
06SB3ZZ	Reposition Left Renal Vein, Percutaneous Approach
06SB4ZZ	Reposition Left Renal Vein, Percutaneous Endoscopic Approach
06SC0ZZ	Reposition Right Common Iliac Vein, Open Approach
06SC3ZZ	Reposition Right Common Iliac Vein, Percutaneous Approach
06SC4ZZ	Reposition Right Common Iliac Vein, Percutaneous Endoscopic Approach
06SD0ZZ	Reposition Left Common Iliac Vein, Open Approach
06SD3ZZ	Reposition Left Common Iliac Vein, Percutaneous Approach
06SD4ZZ	Reposition Left Common Iliac Vein, Percutaneous Endoscopic Approach
06SF0ZZ	Reposition Right External Iliac Vein, Open Approach
06SF3ZZ	Reposition Right External Iliac Vein, Percutaneous Approach
06SF4ZZ	Reposition Right External Iliac Vein, Percutaneous Endoscopic Approach
06SG0ZZ	Reposition Left External Iliac Vein, Open Approach
06SG3ZZ	Reposition Left External Iliac Vein, Percutaneous Approach
06SG4ZZ	Reposition Left External Iliac Vein, Percutaneous Endoscopic Approach
06SH0ZZ	Reposition Right Hypogastric Vein, Open Approach
06SH3ZZ	Reposition Right Hypogastric Vein, Percutaneous Approach
06SH4ZZ	Reposition Right Hypogastric Vein, Percutaneous Endoscopic Approach
06SJ0ZZ	Reposition Left Hypogastric Vein, Open Approach
06SJ3ZZ	Reposition Left Hypogastric Vein, Percutaneous Approach
06SJ4ZZ	Reposition Left Hypogastric Vein, Percutaneous Endoscopic Approach
06SM0ZZ	Reposition Right Femoral Vein, Open Approach
06SM3ZZ	Reposition Right Femoral Vein, Percutaneous Approach
06SM4ZZ	Reposition Right Femoral Vein, Percutaneous Endoscopic Approach
06SN0ZZ	Reposition Left Femoral Vein, Open Approach
06SN3ZZ	Reposition Left Femoral Vein, Percutaneous Approach
06SN4ZZ	Reposition Left Femoral Vein, Percutaneous Endoscopic Approach
06SP0ZZ	Reposition Right Greater Saphenous Vein, Open Approach
06SP3ZZ	Reposition Right Greater Saphenous Vein, Percutaneous Approach
06SP4ZZ	Reposition Right Greater Saphenous Vein, Percutaneous Endoscopic Approach
06SQ0ZZ	Reposition Left Greater Saphenous Vein, Open Approach
06SQ3ZZ	Reposition Left Greater Saphenous Vein, Percutaneous Approach
06SQ4ZZ	Reposition Left Greater Saphenous Vein, Percutaneous Endoscopic Approach
06SR0ZZ	Reposition Right Lesser Saphenous Vein, Open Approach
06SR3ZZ	Reposition Right Lesser Saphenous Vein, Percutaneous Approach
06SR4ZZ	Reposition Right Lesser Saphenous Vein, Percutaneous Endoscopic Approach
06SS0ZZ	Reposition Left Lesser Saphenous Vein, Open Approach
06SS3ZZ	Reposition Left Lesser Saphenous Vein, Percutaneous Approach
06SS4ZZ	Reposition Left Lesser Saphenous Vein, Percutaneous Endoscopic Approach
06ST0ZZ	Reposition Right Foot Vein, Open Approach
06ST3ZZ	Reposition Right Foot Vein, Percutaneous Approach
06ST4ZZ	Reposition Right Foot Vein, Percutaneous Endoscopic Approach
06SV0ZZ	Reposition Left Foot Vein, Open Approach
06SV3ZZ	Reposition Left Foot Vein, Percutaneous Approach
06SV4ZZ	Reposition Left Foot Vein, Percutaneous Endoscopic Approach
06SY0ZZ	Reposition Lower Vein, Open Approach
06SY3ZZ	Reposition Lower Vein, Percutaneous Approach
06SY4ZZ	Reposition Lower Vein, Percutaneous Endoscopic Approach

06U – Lower Veins, Supplement

06U007Z	Supplement Inferior Vena Cava with Autologous Tissue Substitute, Open Approach
06U00JZ	Supplement Inferior Vena Cava with Synthetic Substitute, Open Approach
06U00KZ	Supplement Inferior Vena Cava with Nonautologous Tissue Substitute, Open Approach
06U037Z	Supplement Inferior Vena Cava with Autologous Tissue Substitute, Percutaneous Approach
06U03JZ	Supplement Inferior Vena Cava with Synthetic Substitute, Percutaneous Approach
06U03KZ	Supplement Inferior Vena Cava with Nonautologous Tissue Substitute, Percutaneous Approach
06U047Z	Supplement Inferior Vena Cava with Autologous Tissue Substitute, Percutaneous Endoscopic Approach
06U04JZ	Supplement Inferior Vena Cava with Synthetic Substitute, Percutaneous Endoscopic Approach
06U04KZ	Supplement Inferior Vena Cava with Nonautologous Tissue Substitute, Percutaneous Endoscopic Approach
06U107Z	Supplement Splenic Vein with Autologous Tissue Substitute, Open Approach
06U10JZ	Supplement Splenic Vein with Synthetic Substitute, Open Approach
06U10KZ	Supplement Splenic Vein with Nonautologous Tissue Substitute, Open Approach
06U137Z	Supplement Splenic Vein with Autologous Tissue Substitute, Percutaneous Approach
06U13JZ	Supplement Splenic Vein with Synthetic Substitute, Percutaneous Approach
06U13KZ	Supplement Splenic Vein with Nonautologous Tissue Substitute, Percutaneous Approach
06U147Z	Supplement Splenic Vein with Autologous Tissue Substitute, Percutaneous Endoscopic Approach
06U14JZ	Supplement Splenic Vein with Synthetic Substitute, Percutaneous Endoscopic Approach
06U14KZ	Supplement Splenic Vein with Nonautologous Tissue Substitute, Percutaneous Endoscopic Approach
06U207Z	Supplement Gastric Vein with Autologous Tissue Substitute, Open Approach
06U20JZ	Supplement Gastric Vein with Synthetic Substitute, Open Approach
06U20KZ	Supplement Gastric Vein with Nonautologous Tissue Substitute, Open Approach
06U237Z	Supplement Gastric Vein with Autologous Tissue Substitute, Percutaneous Approach
06U23JZ	Supplement Gastric Vein with Synthetic Substitute, Percutaneous Approach
06U23KZ	Supplement Gastric Vein with Nonautologous Tissue Substitute, Percutaneous Approach
06U247Z	Supplement Gastric Vein with Autologous Tissue Substitute, Percutaneous Endoscopic Approach
06U24JZ	Supplement Gastric Vein with Synthetic Substitute, Percutaneous Endoscopic Approach
06U24KZ	Supplement Gastric Vein with Nonautologous Tissue Substitute, Percutaneous Endoscopic Approach
06U307Z	Supplement Esophageal Vein with Autologous Tissue Substitute, Open Approach
06U30JZ	Supplement Esophageal Vein with Synthetic Substitute, Open Approach
06U30KZ	Supplement Esophageal Vein with Nonautologous Tissue Substitute, Open Approach
06U337Z	Supplement Esophageal Vein with Autologous Tissue Substitute, Percutaneous Approach
06U33JZ	Supplement Esophageal Vein with Synthetic Substitute, Percutaneous Approach
06U33KZ	Supplement Esophageal Vein with Nonautologous Tissue Substitute, Percutaneous Approach
06U347Z	Supplement Esophageal Vein with Autologous Tissue Substitute, Percutaneous Endoscopic Approach
06U34JZ	Supplement Esophageal Vein with Synthetic Substitute, Percutaneous Endoscopic Approach
06U34KZ	Supplement Esophageal Vein with Nonautologous Tissue Substitute, Percutaneous Endoscopic Approach
06U407Z	Supplement Hepatic Vein with Autologous Tissue Substitute, Open Approach
06U40JZ	Supplement Hepatic Vein with Synthetic Substitute, Open Approach
06U40KZ	Supplement Hepatic Vein with Nonautologous Tissue Substitute, Open Approach
06U437Z	Supplement Hepatic Vein with Autologous Tissue Substitute, Percutaneous Approach
06U43JZ	Supplement Hepatic Vein with Synthetic Substitute, Percutaneous Approach
06U43KZ	Supplement Hepatic Vein with Nonautologous Tissue Substitute, Percutaneous Approach

♀ Female-only ♂ Male-only ● Limited Coverage ● Non-OR ▦ HAC-associated procedure ● Non-covered procedures ✚ Combination

06U447Z Supplement Hepatic Vein with Autologous Tissue Substitute, Percutaneous Endoscopic Approach

06U44JZ Supplement Hepatic Vein with Synthetic Substitute, Percutaneous Endoscopic Approach

06U44KZ Supplement Hepatic Vein with Nonautologous Tissue Substitute, Percutaneous Endoscopic Approach

06U507Z Supplement Superior Mesenteric Vein with Autologous Tissue Substitute, Open Approach

06U50JZ Supplement Superior Mesenteric Vein with Synthetic Substitute, Open Approach

06U50KZ Supplement Superior Mesenteric Vein with Nonautologous Tissue Substitute, Open Approach

06U537Z Supplement Superior Mesenteric Vein with Autologous Tissue Substitute, Percutaneous Approach

06U53JZ Supplement Superior Mesenteric Vein with Synthetic Substitute, Percutaneous Approach

06U53KZ Supplement Superior Mesenteric Vein with Nonautologous Tissue Substitute, Percutaneous Approach

06U547Z Supplement Superior Mesenteric Vein with Autologous Tissue Substitute, Percutaneous Endoscopic Approach

06U54JZ Supplement Superior Mesenteric Vein with Synthetic Substitute, Percutaneous Endoscopic Approach

06U54KZ Supplement Superior Mesenteric Vein with Nonautologous Tissue Substitute, Percutaneous Endoscopic Approach

06U607Z Supplement Inferior Mesenteric Vein with Autologous Tissue Substitute, Open Approach

06U60JZ Supplement Inferior Mesenteric Vein with Synthetic Substitute, Open Approach

06U60KZ Supplement Inferior Mesenteric Vein with Nonautologous Tissue Substitute, Open Approach

06U637Z Supplement Inferior Mesenteric Vein with Autologous Tissue Substitute, Percutaneous Approach

06U63JZ Supplement Inferior Mesenteric Vein with Synthetic Substitute, Percutaneous Approach

06U63KZ Supplement Inferior Mesenteric Vein with Nonautologous Tissue Substitute, Percutaneous Approach

06U647Z Supplement Inferior Mesenteric Vein with Autologous Tissue Substitute, Percutaneous Endoscopic Approach

06U64JZ Supplement Inferior Mesenteric Vein with Synthetic Substitute, Percutaneous Endoscopic Approach

06U64KZ Supplement Inferior Mesenteric Vein with Nonautologous Tissue Substitute, Percutaneous Endoscopic Approach

06U707Z Supplement Colic Vein with Autologous Tissue Substitute, Open Approach

06U70JZ Supplement Colic Vein with Synthetic Substitute, Open Approach

06U70KZ Supplement Colic Vein with Nonautologous Tissue Substitute, Open Approach

06U737Z Supplement Colic Vein with Autologous Tissue Substitute, Percutaneous Approach

06U73JZ Supplement Colic Vein with Synthetic Substitute, Percutaneous Approach

06U73KZ Supplement Colic Vein with Nonautologous Tissue Substitute, Percutaneous Approach

06U747Z Supplement Colic Vein with Autologous Tissue Substitute, Percutaneous Endoscopic Approach

06U74JZ Supplement Colic Vein with Synthetic Substitute, Percutaneous Endoscopic Approach

06U74KZ Supplement Colic Vein with Nonautologous Tissue Substitute, Percutaneous Endoscopic Approach

06U807Z Supplement Portal Vein with Autologous Tissue Substitute, Open Approach

06U80JZ Supplement Portal Vein with Synthetic Substitute, Open Approach

06U80KZ Supplement Portal Vein with Nonautologous Tissue Substitute, Open Approach

06U837Z Supplement Portal Vein with Autologous Tissue Substitute, Percutaneous Approach

06U83JZ Supplement Portal Vein with Synthetic Substitute, Percutaneous Approach

06U83KZ Supplement Portal Vein with Nonautologous Tissue Substitute, Percutaneous Approach

06U847Z Supplement Portal Vein with Autologous Tissue Substitute, Percutaneous Endoscopic Approach

06U84JZ Supplement Portal Vein with Synthetic Substitute, Percutaneous Endoscopic Approach

06U84KZ Supplement Portal Vein with Nonautologous Tissue Substitute, Percutaneous Endoscopic Approach

06U907Z Supplement Right Renal Vein with Autologous Tissue Substitute, Open Approach

06U90JZ Supplement Right Renal Vein with Synthetic Substitute, Open Approach

06U90KZ Supplement Right Renal Vein with Nonautologous Tissue Substitute, Open Approach

06U937Z Supplement Right Renal Vein with Autologous Tissue Substitute, Percutaneous Approach

06U93JZ Supplement Right Renal Vein with Synthetic Substitute, Percutaneous Approach

06U93KZ Supplement Right Renal Vein with Nonautologous Tissue Substitute, Percutaneous Approach

06U947Z Supplement Right Renal Vein with Autologous Tissue Substitute, Percutaneous Endoscopic Approach

06U94JZ Supplement Right Renal Vein with Synthetic Substitute, Percutaneous Endoscopic Approach

06U94KZ Supplement Right Renal Vein with Nonautologous Tissue Substitute, Percutaneous Endoscopic Approach

06UB07Z Supplement Left Renal Vein with Autologous Tissue Substitute, Open Approach

06UB0JZ Supplement Left Renal Vein with Synthetic Substitute, Open Approach

06UB0KZ Supplement Left Renal Vein with Nonautologous Tissue Substitute, Open Approach

06UB37Z Supplement Left Renal Vein with Autologous Tissue Substitute, Percutaneous Approach

06UB3JZ Supplement Left Renal Vein with Synthetic Substitute, Percutaneous Approach

06UB3KZ Supplement Left Renal Vein with Nonautologous Tissue Substitute, Percutaneous Approach

06UB47Z Supplement Left Renal Vein with Autologous Tissue Substitute, Percutaneous Endoscopic Approach

06UB4JZ Supplement Left Renal Vein with Synthetic Substitute, Percutaneous Endoscopic Approach

06UB4KZ Supplement Left Renal Vein with Nonautologous Tissue Substitute, Percutaneous Endoscopic Approach

06UC07Z Supplement Right Common Iliac Vein with Autologous Tissue Substitute, Open Approach

06UC0JZ Supplement Right Common Iliac Vein with Synthetic Substitute, Open Approach

06UC0KZ Supplement Right Common Iliac Vein with Nonautologous Tissue Substitute, Open Approach

06UC37Z Supplement Right Common Iliac Vein with Autologous Tissue Substitute, Percutaneous Approach

06UC3JZ Supplement Right Common Iliac Vein with Synthetic Substitute, Percutaneous Approach

06UC3KZ Supplement Right Common Iliac Vein with Nonautologous Tissue Substitute, Percutaneous Approach

06UC47Z Supplement Right Common Iliac Vein with Autologous Tissue Substitute, Percutaneous Endoscopic Approach

06UC4JZ Supplement Right Common Iliac Vein with Synthetic Substitute, Percutaneous Endoscopic Approach

06UC4KZ Supplement Right Common Iliac Vein with Nonautologous Tissue Substitute, Percutaneous Endoscopic Approach

06UD07Z Supplement Left Common Iliac Vein with Autologous Tissue Substitute, Open Approach

06UD0JZ Supplement Left Common Iliac Vein with Synthetic Substitute, Open Approach

06UD0KZ Supplement Left Common Iliac Vein with Nonautologous Tissue Substitute, Open Approach

06UD37Z Supplement Left Common Iliac Vein with Autologous Tissue Substitute, Percutaneous Approach

06UD3JZ Supplement Left Common Iliac Vein with Synthetic Substitute, Percutaneous Approach

06UD3KZ Supplement Left Common Iliac Vein with Nonautologous Tissue Substitute, Percutaneous Approach

06UD47Z Supplement Left Common Iliac Vein with Autologous Tissue Substitute, Percutaneous Endoscopic Approach

06UD4JZ   Supplement Left Common Iliac Vein with Synthetic Substitute, Percutaneous Endoscopic Approach

06UD4KZ   Supplement Left Common Iliac Vein with Nonautologous Tissue Substitute, Percutaneous Endoscopic Approach

06UF07Z   Supplement Right External Iliac Vein with Autologous Tissue Substitute, Open Approach

06UF0JZ   Supplement Right External Iliac Vein with Synthetic Substitute, Open Approach

06UF0KZ   Supplement Right External Iliac Vein with Nonautologous Tissue Substitute, Open Approach

06UF37Z   Supplement Right External Iliac Vein with Autologous Tissue Substitute, Percutaneous Approach

06UF3JZ   Supplement Right External Iliac Vein with Synthetic Substitute, Percutaneous Approach

06UF3KZ   Supplement Right External Iliac Vein with Nonautologous Tissue Substitute, Percutaneous Approach

06UF47Z   Supplement Right External Iliac Vein with Autologous Tissue Substitute, Percutaneous Endoscopic Approach

06UF4JZ   Supplement Right External Iliac Vein with Synthetic Substitute, Percutaneous Endoscopic Approach

06UF4KZ   Supplement Right External Iliac Vein with Nonautologous Tissue Substitute, Percutaneous Endoscopic Approach

06UG07Z   Supplement Left External Iliac Vein with Autologous Tissue Substitute, Open Approach

06UG0JZ   Supplement Left External Iliac Vein with Synthetic Substitute, Open Approach

06UG0KZ   Supplement Left External Iliac Vein with Nonautologous Tissue Substitute, Open Approach

06UG37Z   Supplement Left External Iliac Vein with Autologous Tissue Substitute, Percutaneous Approach

06UG3JZ   Supplement Left External Iliac Vein with Synthetic Substitute, Percutaneous Approach

06UG3KZ   Supplement Left External Iliac Vein with Nonautologous Tissue Substitute, Percutaneous Approach

06UG47Z   Supplement Left External Iliac Vein with Autologous Tissue Substitute, Percutaneous Endoscopic Approach

06UG4JZ   Supplement Left External Iliac Vein with Synthetic Substitute, Percutaneous Endoscopic Approach

06UG4KZ   Supplement Left External Iliac Vein with Nonautologous Tissue Substitute, Percutaneous Endoscopic Approach

06UH07Z   Supplement Right Hypogastric Vein with Autologous Tissue Substitute, Open Approach

06UH0JZ   Supplement Right Hypogastric Vein with Synthetic Substitute, Open Approach

06UH0KZ   Supplement Right Hypogastric Vein with Nonautologous Tissue Substitute, Open Approach

06UH37Z   Supplement Right Hypogastric Vein with Autologous Tissue Substitute, Percutaneous Approach

06UH3JZ   Supplement Right Hypogastric Vein with Synthetic Substitute, Percutaneous Approach

06UH3KZ   Supplement Right Hypogastric Vein with Nonautologous Tissue Substitute, Percutaneous Approach

06UH47Z   Supplement Right Hypogastric Vein with Autologous Tissue Substitute, Percutaneous Endoscopic Approach

06UH4JZ   Supplement Right Hypogastric Vein with Synthetic Substitute, Percutaneous Endoscopic Approach

06UH4KZ   Supplement Right Hypogastric Vein with Nonautologous Tissue Substitute, Percutaneous Endoscopic Approach

06UJ07Z   Supplement Left Hypogastric Vein with Autologous Tissue Substitute, Open Approach

06UJ0JZ   Supplement Left Hypogastric Vein with Synthetic Substitute, Open Approach

06UJ0KZ   Supplement Left Hypogastric Vein with Nonautologous Tissue Substitute, Open Approach

06UJ37Z   Supplement Left Hypogastric Vein with Autologous Tissue Substitute, Percutaneous Approach

06UJ3JZ   Supplement Left Hypogastric Vein with Synthetic Substitute, Percutaneous Approach

06UJ3KZ   Supplement Left Hypogastric Vein with Nonautologous Tissue Substitute, Percutaneous Approach

06UJ47Z   Supplement Left Hypogastric Vein with Autologous Tissue Substitute, Percutaneous Endoscopic Approach

06UJ4JZ   Supplement Left Hypogastric Vein with Synthetic Substitute, Percutaneous Endoscopic Approach

06UJ4KZ   Supplement Left Hypogastric Vein with Nonautologous Tissue Substitute, Percutaneous Endoscopic Approach

06UM07Z   Supplement Right Femoral Vein with Autologous Tissue Substitute, Open Approach

06UM0JZ   Supplement Right Femoral Vein with Synthetic Substitute, Open Approach

06UM0KZ   Supplement Right Femoral Vein with Nonautologous Tissue Substitute, Open Approach

06UM37Z   Supplement Right Femoral Vein with Autologous Tissue Substitute, Percutaneous Approach

06UM3JZ   Supplement Right Femoral Vein with Synthetic Substitute, Percutaneous Approach

06UM3KZ   Supplement Right Femoral Vein with Nonautologous Tissue Substitute, Percutaneous Approach

06UM47Z   Supplement Right Femoral Vein with Autologous Tissue Substitute, Percutaneous Endoscopic Approach

06UM4JZ   Supplement Right Femoral Vein with Synthetic Substitute, Percutaneous Endoscopic Approach

06UM4KZ   Supplement Right Femoral Vein with Nonautologous Tissue Substitute, Percutaneous Endoscopic Approach

06UN07Z   Supplement Left Femoral Vein with Autologous Tissue Substitute, Open Approach

06UN0JZ   Supplement Left Femoral Vein with Synthetic Substitute, Open Approach

06UN0KZ   Supplement Left Femoral Vein with Nonautologous Tissue Substitute, Open Approach

06UN37Z   Supplement Left Femoral Vein with Autologous Tissue Substitute, Percutaneous Approach

06UN3JZ   Supplement Left Femoral Vein with Synthetic Substitute, Percutaneous Approach

06UN3KZ   Supplement Left Femoral Vein with Nonautologous Tissue Substitute, Percutaneous Approach

06UN47Z   Supplement Left Femoral Vein with Autologous Tissue Substitute, Percutaneous Endoscopic Approach

06UN4JZ   Supplement Left Femoral Vein with Synthetic Substitute, Percutaneous Endoscopic Approach

06UN4KZ   Supplement Left Femoral Vein with Nonautologous Tissue Substitute, Percutaneous Endoscopic Approach

06UP07Z   Supplement Right Greater Saphenous Vein with Autologous Tissue Substitute, Open Approach

06UP0JZ   Supplement Right Greater Saphenous Vein with Synthetic Substitute, Open Approach

06UP0KZ   Supplement Right Greater Saphenous Vein with Nonautologous Tissue Substitute, Open Approach

06UP37Z   Supplement Right Greater Saphenous Vein with Autologous Tissue Substitute, Percutaneous Approach

06UP3JZ   Supplement Right Greater Saphenous Vein with Synthetic Substitute, Percutaneous Approach

06UP3KZ   Supplement Right Greater Saphenous Vein with Nonautologous Tissue Substitute, Percutaneous Approach

06UP47Z   Supplement Right Greater Saphenous Vein with Autologous Tissue Substitute, Percutaneous Endoscopic Approach

06UP4JZ   Supplement Right Greater Saphenous Vein with Synthetic Substitute, Percutaneous Endoscopic Approach

06UP4KZ   Supplement Right Greater Saphenous Vein with Nonautologous Tissue Substitute, Percutaneous Endoscopic Approach

06UQ07Z   Supplement Left Greater Saphenous Vein with Autologous Tissue Substitute, Open Approach

06UQ0JZ   Supplement Left Greater Saphenous Vein with Synthetic Substitute, Open Approach

06UQ0KZ   Supplement Left Greater Saphenous Vein with Nonautologous Tissue Substitute, Open Approach

06UQ37Z   Supplement Left Greater Saphenous Vein with Autologous Tissue Substitute, Percutaneous Approach

06UQ3JZ   Supplement Left Greater Saphenous Vein with Synthetic Substitute, Percutaneous Approach

06UQ3KZ   Supplement Left Greater Saphenous Vein with Nonautologous Tissue Substitute, Percutaneous Approach

06UQ47Z   Supplement Left Greater Saphenous Vein with Autologous Tissue Substitute, Percutaneous Endoscopic Approach

06UQ4JZ   Supplement Left Greater Saphenous Vein with Synthetic Substitute, Percutaneous Endoscopic Approach

06UQ4KZ   Supplement Left Greater Saphenous Vein with Nonautologous Tissue Substitute, Percutaneous Endoscopic Approach

06UR07Z   Supplement Right Lesser Saphenous Vein with Autologous Tissue Substitute, Open Approach

06UR0JZ   Supplement Right Lesser Saphenous Vein with Synthetic Substitute, Open Approach

06UR0KZ   Supplement Right Lesser Saphenous Vein with Nonautologous Tissue Substitute, Open Approach

06UR37Z   Supplement Right Lesser Saphenous Vein with Autologous Tissue Substitute, Percutaneous Approach

06UR3JZ   Supplement Right Lesser Saphenous Vein with Synthetic Substitute, Percutaneous Approach

06UR3KZ   Supplement Right Lesser Saphenous Vein with Nonautologous Tissue Substitute, Percutaneous Approach

06UR47Z   Supplement Right Lesser Saphenous Vein with Autologous Tissue Substitute, Percutaneous Endoscopic Approach

06UR4JZ   Supplement Right Lesser Saphenous Vein with Synthetic Substitute, Percutaneous Endoscopic Approach

06UR4KZ   Supplement Right Lesser Saphenous Vein with Nonautologous Tissue Substitute, Percutaneous Endoscopic Approach

06US07Z   Supplement Left Lesser Saphenous Vein with Autologous Tissue Substitute, Open Approach

06US0JZ   Supplement Left Lesser Saphenous Vein with Synthetic Substitute, Open Approach

06US0KZ   Supplement Left Lesser Saphenous Vein with Nonautologous Tissue Substitute, Open Approach

06US37Z   Supplement Left Lesser Saphenous Vein with Autologous Tissue Substitute, Percutaneous Approach

06US3JZ   Supplement Left Lesser Saphenous Vein with Synthetic Substitute, Percutaneous Approach

06US3KZ   Supplement Left Lesser Saphenous Vein with Nonautologous Tissue Substitute, Percutaneous Approach

06US47Z   Supplement Left Lesser Saphenous Vein with Autologous Tissue Substitute, Percutaneous Endoscopic Approach

06US4JZ   Supplement Left Lesser Saphenous Vein with Synthetic Substitute, Percutaneous Endoscopic Approach

06US4KZ   Supplement Left Lesser Saphenous Vein with Nonautologous Tissue Substitute, Percutaneous Endoscopic Approach

06UT07Z   Supplement Right Foot Vein with Autologous Tissue Substitute, Open Approach

06UT0JZ   Supplement Right Foot Vein with Synthetic Substitute, Open Approach

06UT0KZ   Supplement Right Foot Vein with Nonautologous Tissue Substitute, Open Approach

06UT37Z   Supplement Right Foot Vein with Autologous Tissue Substitute, Percutaneous Approach

06UT3JZ   Supplement Right Foot Vein with Synthetic Substitute, Percutaneous Approach

06UT3KZ   Supplement Right Foot Vein with Nonautologous Tissue Substitute, Percutaneous Approach

06UT47Z   Supplement Right Foot Vein with Autologous Tissue Substitute, Percutaneous Endoscopic Approach

06UT4JZ   Supplement Right Foot Vein with Synthetic Substitute, Percutaneous Endoscopic Approach

06UT4KZ   Supplement Right Foot Vein with Nonautologous Tissue Substitute, Percutaneous Endoscopic Approach

06UV07Z   Supplement Left Foot Vein with Autologous Tissue Substitute, Open Approach

06UV0JZ   Supplement Left Foot Vein with Synthetic Substitute, Open Approach

06UV0KZ   Supplement Left Foot Vein with Nonautologous Tissue Substitute, Open Approach

06UV37Z   Supplement Left Foot Vein with Autologous Tissue Substitute, Percutaneous Approach

06UV3JZ   Supplement Left Foot Vein with Synthetic Substitute, Percutaneous Approach

06UV3KZ   Supplement Left Foot Vein with Nonautologous Tissue Substitute, Percutaneous Approach

06UV47Z   Supplement Left Foot Vein with Autologous Tissue Substitute, Percutaneous Endoscopic Approach

06UV4JZ   Supplement Left Foot Vein with Synthetic Substitute, Percutaneous Endoscopic Approach

06UV4KZ   Supplement Left Foot Vein with Nonautologous Tissue Substitute, Percutaneous Endoscopic Approach

06UY07Z   Supplement Lower Vein with Autologous Tissue Substitute, Open Approach

06UY0JZ   Supplement Lower Vein with Synthetic Substitute, Open Approach

06UY0KZ   Supplement Lower Vein with Nonautologous Tissue Substitute, Open Approach

06UY37Z   Supplement Lower Vein with Autologous Tissue Substitute, Percutaneous Approach

06UY3JZ   Supplement Lower Vein with Synthetic Substitute, Percutaneous Approach

06UY3KZ   Supplement Lower Vein with Nonautologous Tissue Substitute, Percutaneous Approach

06UY47Z   Supplement Lower Vein with Autologous Tissue Substitute, Percutaneous Endoscopic Approach

06UY4JZ   Supplement Lower Vein with Synthetic Substitute, Percutaneous Endoscopic Approach

06UY4KZ   Supplement Lower Vein with Nonautologous Tissue Substitute, Percutaneous Endoscopic Approach

06V   Lower Veins, Restriction

Review Coding Guideline B3.12

06V00CZ   Restriction of Inferior Vena Cava with Extraluminal Device, Open Approach

06V00DZ   Restriction of Inferior Vena Cava with Intraluminal Device, Open Approach

06V00ZZ   Restriction of Inferior Vena Cava, Open Approach

06V03CZ   Restriction of Inferior Vena Cava with Extraluminal Device, Percutaneous Approach

06V03DZ   Restriction of Inferior Vena Cava with Intraluminal Device, Percutaneous Approach

06V03ZZ   Restriction of Inferior Vena Cava, Percutaneous Approach

06V04CZ   Restriction of Inferior Vena Cava with Extraluminal Device, Percutaneous Endoscopic Approach

06V04DZ   Restriction of Inferior Vena Cava with Intraluminal Device, Percutaneous Endoscopic Approach

06V04ZZ   Restriction of Inferior Vena Cava, Percutaneous Endoscopic Approach

06V10CZ   Restriction of Splenic Vein with Extraluminal Device, Open Approach

06V10DZ   Restriction of Splenic Vein with Intraluminal Device, Open Approach

06V10ZZ   Restriction of Splenic Vein, Open Approach

06V13CZ   Restriction of Splenic Vein with Extraluminal Device, Percutaneous Approach

06V13DZ   Restriction of Splenic Vein with Intraluminal Device, Percutaneous Approach

06V13ZZ   Restriction of Splenic Vein, Percutaneous Approach

06V14CZ   Restriction of Splenic Vein with Extraluminal Device, Percutaneous Endoscopic Approach

06V14DZ   Restriction of Splenic Vein with Intraluminal Device, Percutaneous Endoscopic Approach

06V14ZZ   Restriction of Splenic Vein, Percutaneous Endoscopic Approach

06V20CZ   Restriction of Gastric Vein with Extraluminal Device, Open Approach

06V20DZ   Restriction of Gastric Vein with Intraluminal Device, Open Approach

06V20ZZ   Restriction of Gastric Vein, Open Approach

06V23CZ   Restriction of Gastric Vein with Extraluminal Device, Percutaneous Approach

06V23DZ   Restriction of Gastric Vein with Intraluminal Device, Percutaneous Approach

06V23ZZ   Restriction of Gastric Vein, Percutaneous Approach

06V24CZ Restriction of Gastric Vein with Extraluminal Device, Percutaneous Endoscopic Approach

06V24DZ Restriction of Gastric Vein with Intraluminal Device, Percutaneous Endoscopic Approach

06V24ZZ Restriction of Gastric Vein, Percutaneous Endoscopic Approach

06V30CZ Restriction of Esophageal Vein with Extraluminal Device, Open Approach

06V30DZ Restriction of Esophageal Vein with Intraluminal Device, Open Approach

06V30ZZ Restriction of Esophageal Vein, Open Approach

06V33CZ Restriction of Esophageal Vein with Extraluminal Device, Percutaneous Approach

06V33DZ Restriction of Esophageal Vein with Intraluminal Device, Percutaneous Approach

06V33ZZ Restriction of Esophageal Vein, Percutaneous Approach

06V34CZ Restriction of Esophageal Vein with Extraluminal Device, Percutaneous Endoscopic Approach

06V34DZ Restriction of Esophageal Vein with Intraluminal Device, Percutaneous Endoscopic Approach

06V34ZZ Restriction of Esophageal Vein, Percutaneous Endoscopic Approach

06V40CZ Restriction of Hepatic Vein with Extraluminal Device, Open Approach

06V40DZ Restriction of Hepatic Vein with Intraluminal Device, Open Approach

06V40ZZ Restriction of Hepatic Vein, Open Approach

06V43CZ Restriction of Hepatic Vein with Extraluminal Device, Percutaneous Approach

06V43DZ Restriction of Hepatic Vein with Intraluminal Device, Percutaneous Approach

06V43ZZ Restriction of Hepatic Vein, Percutaneous Approach

06V44CZ Restriction of Hepatic Vein with Extraluminal Device, Percutaneous Endoscopic Approach

06V44DZ Restriction of Hepatic Vein with Intraluminal Device, Percutaneous Endoscopic Approach

06V44ZZ Restriction of Hepatic Vein, Percutaneous Endoscopic Approach

06V50CZ Restriction of Superior Mesenteric Vein with Extraluminal Device, Open Approach

06V50DZ Restriction of Superior Mesenteric Vein with Intraluminal Device, Open Approach

06V50ZZ Restriction of Superior Mesenteric Vein, Open Approach

06V53CZ Restriction of Superior Mesenteric Vein with Extraluminal Device, Percutaneous Approach

06V53DZ Restriction of Superior Mesenteric Vein with Intraluminal Device, Percutaneous Approach

06V53ZZ Restriction of Superior Mesenteric Vein, Percutaneous Approach

06V54CZ Restriction of Superior Mesenteric Vein with Extraluminal Device, Percutaneous Endoscopic Approach

06V54DZ Restriction of Superior Mesenteric Vein with Intraluminal Device, Percutaneous Endoscopic Approach

06V54ZZ Restriction of Superior Mesenteric Vein, Percutaneous Endoscopic Approach

06V60CZ Restriction of Inferior Mesenteric Vein with Extraluminal Device, Open Approach

06V60DZ Restriction of Inferior Mesenteric Vein with Intraluminal Device, Open Approach

06V60ZZ Restriction of Inferior Mesenteric Vein, Open Approach

06V63CZ Restriction of Inferior Mesenteric Vein with Extraluminal Device, Percutaneous Approach

06V63DZ Restriction of Inferior Mesenteric Vein with Intraluminal Device, Percutaneous Approach

06V63ZZ Restriction of Inferior Mesenteric Vein, Percutaneous Approach

06V64CZ Restriction of Inferior Mesenteric Vein with Extraluminal Device, Percutaneous Endoscopic Approach

06V64DZ Restriction of Inferior Mesenteric Vein with Intraluminal Device, Percutaneous Endoscopic Approach

06V64ZZ Restriction of Inferior Mesenteric Vein, Percutaneous Endoscopic Approach

06V70CZ Restriction of Colic Vein with Extraluminal Device, Open Approach

06V70DZ Restriction of Colic Vein with Intraluminal Device, Open Approach

06V70ZZ Restriction of Colic Vein, Open Approach

06V73CZ Restriction of Colic Vein with Extraluminal Device, Percutaneous Approach

06V73DZ Restriction of Colic Vein with Intraluminal Device, Percutaneous Approach

06V73ZZ Restriction of Colic Vein, Percutaneous Approach

06V74CZ Restriction of Colic Vein with Extraluminal Device, Percutaneous Endoscopic Approach

06V74DZ Restriction of Colic Vein with Intraluminal Device, Percutaneous Endoscopic Approach

06V74ZZ Restriction of Colic Vein, Percutaneous Endoscopic Approach

06V80CZ Restriction of Portal Vein with Extraluminal Device, Open Approach

06V80DZ Restriction of Portal Vein with Intraluminal Device, Open Approach

06V80ZZ Restriction of Portal Vein, Open Approach

06V83CZ Restriction of Portal Vein with Extraluminal Device, Percutaneous Approach

06V83DZ Restriction of Portal Vein with Intraluminal Device, Percutaneous Approach

06V83ZZ Restriction of Portal Vein, Percutaneous Approach

06V84CZ Restriction of Portal Vein with Extraluminal Device, Percutaneous Endoscopic Approach

06V84DZ Restriction of Portal Vein with Intraluminal Device, Percutaneous Endoscopic Approach

06V84ZZ Restriction of Portal Vein, Percutaneous Endoscopic Approach

06V90CZ Restriction of Right Renal Vein with Extraluminal Device, Open Approach

06V90DZ Restriction of Right Renal Vein with Intraluminal Device, Open Approach

06V90ZZ Restriction of Right Renal Vein, Open Approach

06V93CZ Restriction of Right Renal Vein with Extraluminal Device, Percutaneous Approach

06V93DZ Restriction of Right Renal Vein with Intraluminal Device, Percutaneous Approach

06V93ZZ Restriction of Right Renal Vein, Percutaneous Approach

06V94CZ Restriction of Right Renal Vein with Extraluminal Device, Percutaneous Endoscopic Approach

06V94DZ Restriction of Right Renal Vein with Intraluminal Device, Percutaneous Endoscopic Approach

06V94ZZ Restriction of Right Renal Vein, Percutaneous Endoscopic Approach

06VB0CZ Restriction of Left Renal Vein with Extraluminal Device, Open Approach

06VB0DZ Restriction of Left Renal Vein with Intraluminal Device, Open Approach

06VB0ZZ Restriction of Left Renal Vein, Open Approach

06VB3CZ Restriction of Left Renal Vein with Extraluminal Device, Percutaneous Approach

06VB3DZ Restriction of Left Renal Vein with Intraluminal Device, Percutaneous Approach

06VB3ZZ Restriction of Left Renal Vein, Percutaneous Approach

06VB4CZ Restriction of Left Renal Vein with Extraluminal Device, Percutaneous Endoscopic Approach

06VB4DZ Restriction of Left Renal Vein with Intraluminal Device, Percutaneous Endoscopic Approach

06VB4ZZ Restriction of Left Renal Vein, Percutaneous Endoscopic Approach

06VC0CZ Restriction of Right Common Iliac Vein with Extraluminal Device, Open Approach

06VC0DZ Restriction of Right Common Iliac Vein with Intraluminal Device, Open Approach

06VC0ZZ Restriction of Right Common Iliac Vein, Open Approach

06VC3CZ Restriction of Right Common Iliac Vein with Extraluminal Device, Percutaneous Approach

06VC3DZ Restriction of Right Common Iliac Vein with Intraluminal Device, Percutaneous Approach

06VC3ZZ Restriction of Right Common Iliac Vein, Percutaneous Approach

06VC4CZ Restriction of Right Common Iliac Vein with Extraluminal Device, Percutaneous Endoscopic Approach

06VC4DZ Restriction of Right Common Iliac Vein with Intraluminal Device, Percutaneous Endoscopic Approach

06VC4ZZ Restriction of Right Common Iliac Vein, Percutaneous Endoscopic Approach

06VD0CZ Restriction of Left Common Iliac Vein with Extraluminal Device, Open Approach

06VD0DZ Restriction of Left Common Iliac Vein with Intraluminal Device, Open Approach

06VD0ZZ Restriction of Left Common Iliac Vein, Open Approach

06VD3CZ   Restriction of Left Common Iliac Vein with Extraluminal Device, Percutaneous Approach

06VD3DZ   Restriction of Left Common Iliac Vein with Intraluminal Device, Percutaneous Approach

06VD3ZZ   Restriction of Left Common Iliac Vein, Percutaneous Approach

06VD4CZ   Restriction of Left Common Iliac Vein with Extraluminal Device, Percutaneous Endoscopic Approach

06VD4DZ   Restriction of Left Common Iliac Vein with Intraluminal Device, Percutaneous Endoscopic Approach

06VD4ZZ   Restriction of Left Common Iliac Vein, Percutaneous Endoscopic Approach

06VF0CZ   Restriction of Right External Iliac Vein with Extraluminal Device, Open Approach

06VF0DZ   Restriction of Right External Iliac Vein with Intraluminal Device, Open Approach

06VF0ZZ   Restriction of Right External Iliac Vein, Open Approach

06VF3CZ   Restriction of Right External Iliac Vein with Extraluminal Device, Percutaneous Approach

06VF3DZ   Restriction of Right External Iliac Vein with Intraluminal Device, Percutaneous Approach

06VF3ZZ   Restriction of Right External Iliac Vein, Percutaneous Approach

06VF4CZ   Restriction of Right External Iliac Vein with Extraluminal Device, Percutaneous Endoscopic Approach

06VF4DZ   Restriction of Right External Iliac Vein with Intraluminal Device, Percutaneous Endoscopic Approach

06VF4ZZ   Restriction of Right External Iliac Vein, Percutaneous Endoscopic Approach

06VG0CZ   Restriction of Left External Iliac Vein with Extraluminal Device, Open Approach

06VG0DZ   Restriction of Left External Iliac Vein with Intraluminal Device, Open Approach

06VG0ZZ   Restriction of Left External Iliac Vein, Open Approach

06VG3CZ   Restriction of Left External Iliac Vein with Extraluminal Device, Percutaneous Approach

06VG3DZ   Restriction of Left External Iliac Vein with Intraluminal Device, Percutaneous Approach

06VG3ZZ   Restriction of Left External Iliac Vein, Percutaneous Approach

06VG4CZ   Restriction of Left External Iliac Vein with Extraluminal Device, Percutaneous Endoscopic Approach

06VG4DZ   Restriction of Left External Iliac Vein with Intraluminal Device, Percutaneous Endoscopic Approach

06VG4ZZ   Restriction of Left External Iliac Vein, Percutaneous Endoscopic Approach

06VH0CZ   Restriction of Right Hypogastric Vein with Extraluminal Device, Open Approach

06VH0DZ   Restriction of Right Hypogastric Vein with Intraluminal Device, Open Approach

06VH0ZZ   Restriction of Right Hypogastric Vein, Open Approach

06VH3CZ   Restriction of Right Hypogastric Vein with Extraluminal Device, Percutaneous Approach

06VH3DZ   Restriction of Right Hypogastric Vein with Intraluminal Device, Percutaneous Approach

06VH3ZZ   Restriction of Right Hypogastric Vein, Percutaneous Approach

06VH4CZ   Restriction of Right Hypogastric Vein with Extraluminal Device, Percutaneous Endoscopic Approach

06VH4DZ   Restriction of Right Hypogastric Vein with Intraluminal Device, Percutaneous Endoscopic Approach

06VH4ZZ   Restriction of Right Hypogastric Vein, Percutaneous Endoscopic Approach

06VJ0CZ   Restriction of Left Hypogastric Vein with Extraluminal Device, Open Approach

06VJ0DZ   Restriction of Left Hypogastric Vein with Intraluminal Device, Open Approach

06VJ0ZZ   Restriction of Left Hypogastric Vein, Open Approach

06VJ3CZ   Restriction of Left Hypogastric Vein with Extraluminal Device, Percutaneous Approach

06VJ3DZ   Restriction of Left Hypogastric Vein with Intraluminal Device, Percutaneous Approach

06VJ3ZZ   Restriction of Left Hypogastric Vein, Percutaneous Approach

06VJ4CZ   Restriction of Left Hypogastric Vein with Extraluminal Device, Percutaneous Endoscopic Approach

06VJ4DZ   Restriction of Left Hypogastric Vein with Intraluminal Device, Percutaneous Endoscopic Approach

06VJ4ZZ   Restriction of Left Hypogastric Vein, Percutaneous Endoscopic Approach

06VM0CZ   Restriction of Right Femoral Vein with Extraluminal Device, Open Approach

06VM0DZ   Restriction of Right Femoral Vein with Intraluminal Device, Open Approach

06VM0ZZ   Restriction of Right Femoral Vein, Open Approach

06VM3CZ   Restriction of Right Femoral Vein with Extraluminal Device, Percutaneous Approach

06VM3DZ   Restriction of Right Femoral Vein with Intraluminal Device, Percutaneous Approach

06VM3ZZ   Restriction of Right Femoral Vein, Percutaneous Approach

06VM4CZ   Restriction of Right Femoral Vein with Extraluminal Device, Percutaneous Endoscopic Approach

06VM4DZ   Restriction of Right Femoral Vein with Intraluminal Device, Percutaneous Endoscopic Approach

06VM4ZZ   Restriction of Right Femoral Vein, Percutaneous Endoscopic Approach

06VN0CZ   Restriction of Left Femoral Vein with Extraluminal Device, Open Approach

06VN0DZ   Restriction of Left Femoral Vein with Intraluminal Device, Open Approach

06VN0ZZ   Restriction of Left Femoral Vein, Open Approach

06VN3CZ   Restriction of Left Femoral Vein with Extraluminal Device, Percutaneous Approach

06VN3DZ   Restriction of Left Femoral Vein with Intraluminal Device, Percutaneous Approach

06VN3ZZ   Restriction of Left Femoral Vein, Percutaneous Approach

06VN4CZ   Restriction of Left Femoral Vein with Extraluminal Device, Percutaneous Endoscopic Approach

06VN4DZ   Restriction of Left Femoral Vein with Intraluminal Device, Percutaneous Endoscopic Approach

06VN4ZZ   Restriction of Left Femoral Vein, Percutaneous Endoscopic Approach

06VP0CZ   Restriction of Right Greater Saphenous Vein with Extraluminal Device, Open Approach

06VP0DZ   Restriction of Right Greater Saphenous Vein with Intraluminal Device, Open Approach

06VP0ZZ   Restriction of Right Greater Saphenous Vein, Open Approach

06VP3CZ   Restriction of Right Greater Saphenous Vein with Extraluminal Device, Percutaneous Approach

06VP3DZ   Restriction of Right Greater Saphenous Vein with Intraluminal Device, Percutaneous Approach

06VP3ZZ   Restriction of Right Greater Saphenous Vein, Percutaneous Approach

06VP4CZ   Restriction of Right Greater Saphenous Vein with Extraluminal Device, Percutaneous Endoscopic Approach

06VP4DZ   Restriction of Right Greater Saphenous Vein with Intraluminal Device, Percutaneous Endoscopic Approach

06VP4ZZ   Restriction of Right Greater Saphenous Vein, Percutaneous Endoscopic Approach

06VQ0CZ   Restriction of Left Greater Saphenous Vein with Extraluminal Device, Open Approach

06VQ0DZ   Restriction of Left Greater Saphenous Vein with Intraluminal Device, Open Approach

06VQ0ZZ   Restriction of Left Greater Saphenous Vein, Open Approach

06VQ3CZ   Restriction of Left Greater Saphenous Vein with Extraluminal Device, Percutaneous Approach

06VQ3DZ   Restriction of Left Greater Saphenous Vein with Intraluminal Device, Percutaneous Approach

06VQ3ZZ   Restriction of Left Greater Saphenous Vein, Percutaneous Approach

06VQ4CZ   Restriction of Left Greater Saphenous Vein with Extraluminal Device, Percutaneous Endoscopic Approach

06VQ4DZ   Restriction of Left Greater Saphenous Vein with Intraluminal Device, Percutaneous Endoscopic Approach

06VQ4ZZ   Restriction of Left Greater Saphenous Vein, Percutaneous Endoscopic Approach

06VR0CZ   Restriction of Right Lesser Saphenous Vein with Extraluminal Device, Open Approach

06VR0DZ   Restriction of Right Lesser Saphenous Vein with Intraluminal Device, Open Approach

06VR0ZZ   Restriction of Right Lesser Saphenous Vein, Open Approach

06VR3CZ   Restriction of Right Lesser Saphenous Vein with Extraluminal Device, Percutaneous Approach
06VR3DZ   Restriction of Right Lesser Saphenous Vein with Intraluminal Device, Percutaneous Approach
06VR3ZZ   Restriction of Right Lesser Saphenous Vein, Percutaneous Approach
06VR4CZ   Restriction of Right Lesser Saphenous Vein with Extraluminal Device, Percutaneous Endoscopic Approach
06VR4DZ   Restriction of Right Lesser Saphenous Vein with Intraluminal Device, Percutaneous Endoscopic Approach
06VR4ZZ   Restriction of Right Lesser Saphenous Vein, Percutaneous Endoscopic Approach
06VS0CZ   Restriction of Left Lesser Saphenous Vein with Extraluminal Device, Open Approach
06VS0DZ   Restriction of Left Lesser Saphenous Vein with Intraluminal Device, Open Approach
06VS0ZZ   Restriction of Left Lesser Saphenous Vein, Open Approach
06VS3CZ   Restriction of Left Lesser Saphenous Vein with Extraluminal Device, Percutaneous Approach
06VS3DZ   Restriction of Left Lesser Saphenous Vein with Intraluminal Device, Percutaneous Approach
06VS3ZZ   Restriction of Left Lesser Saphenous Vein, Percutaneous Approach
06VS4CZ   Restriction of Left Lesser Saphenous Vein with Extraluminal Device, Percutaneous Endoscopic Approach
06VS4DZ   Restriction of Left Lesser Saphenous Vein with Intraluminal Device, Percutaneous Endoscopic Approach
06VS4ZZ   Restriction of Left Lesser Saphenous Vein, Percutaneous Endoscopic Approach
06VT0CZ   Restriction of Right Foot Vein with Extraluminal Device, Open Approach
06VT0DZ   Restriction of Right Foot Vein with Intraluminal Device, Open Approach
06VT0ZZ   Restriction of Right Foot Vein, Open Approach
06VT3CZ   Restriction of Right Foot Vein with Extraluminal Device, Percutaneous Approach
06VT3DZ   Restriction of Right Foot Vein with Intraluminal Device, Percutaneous Approach

06VT3ZZ   Restriction of Right Foot Vein, Percutaneous Approach
06VT4CZ   Restriction of Right Foot Vein with Extraluminal Device, Percutaneous Endoscopic Approach
06VT4DZ   Restriction of Right Foot Vein with Intraluminal Device, Percutaneous Endoscopic Approach
06VT4ZZ   Restriction of Right Foot Vein, Percutaneous Endoscopic Approach
06VV0CZ   Restriction of Left Foot Vein with Extraluminal Device, Open Approach
06VV0DZ   Restriction of Left Foot Vein with Intraluminal Device, Open Approach
06VV0ZZ   Restriction of Left Foot Vein, Open Approach
06VV3CZ   Restriction of Left Foot Vein with Extraluminal Device, Percutaneous Approach
06VV3DZ   Restriction of Left Foot Vein with Intraluminal Device, Percutaneous Approach
06VV3ZZ   Restriction of Left Foot Vein, Percutaneous Approach
06VV4CZ   Restriction of Left Foot Vein with Extraluminal Device, Percutaneous Endoscopic Approach
06VV4DZ   Restriction of Left Foot Vein with Intraluminal Device, Percutaneous Endoscopic Approach
06VV4ZZ   Restriction of Left Foot Vein, Percutaneous Endoscopic Approach
06VY0CZ   Restriction of Lower Vein with Extraluminal Device, Open Approach
06VY0DZ   Restriction of Lower Vein with Intraluminal Device, Open Approach
06VY0ZZ   Restriction of Lower Vein, Open Approach
06VY3CZ   Restriction of Lower Vein with Extraluminal Device, Percutaneous Approach
06VY3DZ   Restriction of Lower Vein with Intraluminal Device, Percutaneous Approach
06VY3ZZ   Restriction of Lower Vein, Percutaneous Approach
06VY4CZ   Restriction of Lower Vein with Extraluminal Device, Percutaneous Endoscopic Approach
06VY4DZ   Restriction of Lower Vein with Intraluminal Device, Percutaneous Endoscopic Approach
06VY4ZZ   Restriction of Lower Vein, Percutaneous Endoscopic Approach

06W – Lower Veins, Revision

Review Coding Guideline B6.1c

06WY00Z   Revision of Drainage Device in Lower Vein, Open Approach
06WY02Z   Revision of Monitoring Device in Lower Vein, Open Approach
06WY03Z   Revision of Infusion Device in Lower Vein, Open Approach
06WY07Z   Revision of Autologous Tissue Substitute in Lower Vein, Open Approach
06WY0CZ   Revision of Extraluminal Device in Lower Vein, Open Approach
06WY0DZ   Revision of Intraluminal Device in Lower Vein, Open Approach
06WY0JZ   Revision of Synthetic Substitute in Lower Vein, Open Approach
06WY0KZ   Revision of Nonautologous Tissue Substitute in Lower Vein, Open Approach
06WY30Z   Revision of Drainage Device in Lower Vein, Percutaneous Approach
06WY32Z   Revision of Monitoring Device in Lower Vein, Percutaneous Approach
06WY33Z   Revision of Infusion Device in Lower Vein, Percutaneous Approach
06WY37Z   Revision of Autologous Tissue Substitute in Lower Vein, Percutaneous Approach
06WY3CZ   Revision of Extraluminal Device in Lower Vein, Percutaneous Approach
06WY3DZ   Revision of Intraluminal Device in Lower Vein, Percutaneous Approach
06WY3JZ   Revision of Synthetic Substitute in Lower Vein, Percutaneous Approach
06WY3KZ   Revision of Nonautologous Tissue Substitute in Lower Vein, Percutaneous Approach
06WY40Z   Revision of Drainage Device in Lower Vein, Percutaneous Endoscopic Approach

06WY42Z   Revision of Monitoring Device in Lower Vein, Percutaneous Endoscopic Approach
06WY43Z   Revision of Infusion Device in Lower Vein, Percutaneous Endoscopic Approach
06WY47Z   Revision of Autologous Tissue Substitute in Lower Vein, Percutaneous Endoscopic Approach
06WY4CZ   Revision of Extraluminal Device in Lower Vein, Percutaneous Endoscopic Approach
06WY4DZ   Revision of Intraluminal Device in Lower Vein, Percutaneous Endoscopic Approach
06WY4JZ   Revision of Synthetic Substitute in Lower Vein, Percutaneous Endoscopic Approach
06WY4KZ   Revision of Nonautologous Tissue Substitute in Lower Vein, Percutaneous Endoscopic Approach
06WYX0Z   Revision of Drainage Device in Lower Vein, External Approach
06WYX2Z   Revision of Monitoring Device in Lower Vein, External Approach
06WYX3Z   Revision of Infusion Device in Lower Vein, External Approach
06WYX7Z   Revision of Autologous Tissue Substitute in Lower Vein, External Approach
06WYXCZ   Revision of Extraluminal Device in Lower Vein, External Approach
06WYXDZ   Revision of Intraluminal Device in Lower Vein, External Approach
06WYXJZ   Revision of Synthetic Substitute in Lower Vein, External Approach
06WYXKZ   Revision of Nonautologous Tissue Substitute in Lower Vein, External Approach

Lymphatic and Hemic System

Lymphatic System

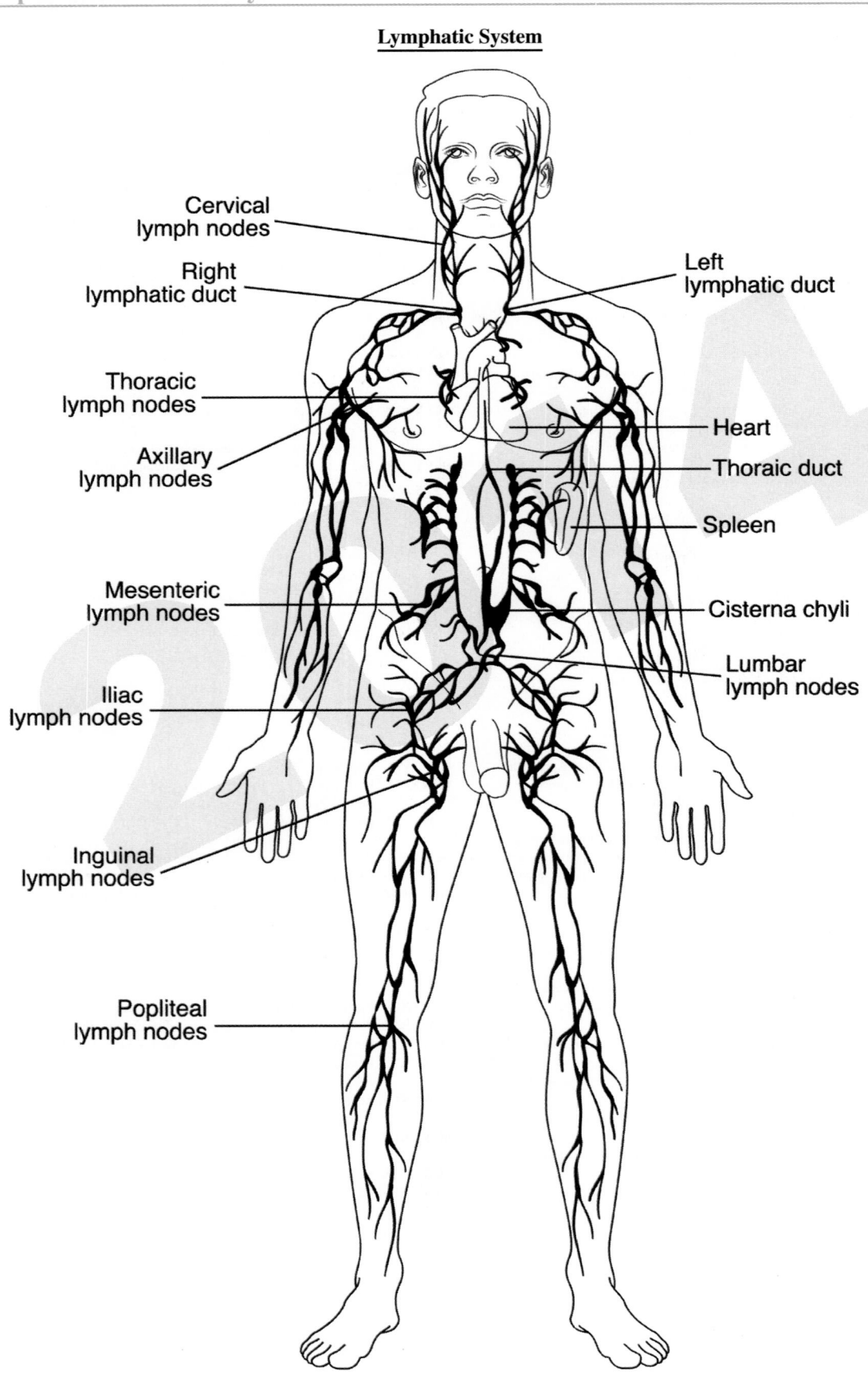

Lymphatic and Hemic Systems Tables 072–07Y

Section	0	Medical and Surgical
Body System	7	Lymphatic and Hemic Systems
Operation	2	**Change:** Taking out or off a device from a body part and putting back an identical or similar device in or on the same body part without cutting or puncturing the skin or a mucous membrane

Body Part (4th)	Approach (5th)	Device (6th)	Qualifier (7th)
K Thoracic Duct L Cisterna Chyli M Thymus N Lymphatic P Spleen T Bone Marrow	X External	0 Drainage Device Y Other Device	Z No Qualifier

Section	0	Medical and Surgical
Body System	7	Lymphatic and Hemic Systems
Operation	5	**Destruction:** Physical eradication of all or a portion of a body part by the direct use of energy, force, or a destructive agent

Body Part (4th)	Approach (5th)	Device (6th)	Qualifier (7th)
0 Lymphatic, Head 1 Lymphatic, Right Neck 2 Lymphatic, Left Neck 3 Lymphatic, Right Upper Extremity 4 Lymphatic, Left Upper Extremity 5 Lymphatic, Right Axillary 6 Lymphatic, Left Axillary 7 Lymphatic, Thorax 8 Lymphatic, Internal Mammary, Right 9 Lymphatic, Internal Mammary, Left B Lymphatic, Mesenteric C Lymphatic, Pelvis D Lymphatic, Aortic F Lymphatic, Right Lower Extremity G Lymphatic, Left Lower Extremity H Lymphatic, Right Inguinal J Lymphatic, Left Inguinal K Thoracic Duct L Cisterna Chyli M Thymus P Spleen	0 Open 3 Percutaneous 4 Percutaneous Endoscopic	Z No Device	Z No Qualifier

Section	**0**	**Medical and Surgical**
Body System	**7**	**Lymphatic and Hemic Systems**
Operation	**9**	**Drainage:** Taking or letting out fluids and/or gases from a body part

Body Part (4th)	Approach (5th)	Device (6th)	Qualifier (7th)
0 Lymphatic, Head **1** Lymphatic, Right Neck **2** Lymphatic, Left Neck **3** Lymphatic, Right Upper Extremity **4** Lymphatic, Left Upper Extremity **5** Lymphatic, Right Axillary **6** Lymphatic, Left Axillary **7** Lymphatic, Thorax **8** Lymphatic, Internal Mammary, Right **9** Lymphatic, Internal Mammary, Left **B** Lymphatic, Mesenteric **C** Lymphatic, Pelvis **D** Lymphatic, Aortic **F** Lymphatic, Right Lower Extremity **G** Lymphatic, Left Lower Extremity **H** Lymphatic, Right Inguinal **J** Lymphatic, Left Inguinal **K** Thoracic Duct **L** Cisterna Chyli **M** Thymus **P** Spleen **T** Bone Marrow	**0** Open **3** Percutaneous **4** Percutaneous Endoscopic	**0** Drainage Device	**Z** No Qualifier
0 Lymphatic, Head **1** Lymphatic, Right Neck **2** Lymphatic, Left Neck **3** Lymphatic, Right Upper Extremity **4** Lymphatic, Left Upper Extremity **5** Lymphatic, Right Axillary **6** Lymphatic, Left Axillary **7** Lymphatic, Thorax **8** Lymphatic, Internal Mammary, Right **9** Lymphatic, Internal Mammary, Left **B** Lymphatic, Mesenteric **C** Lymphatic, Pelvis **D** Lymphatic, Aortic **F** Lymphatic, Right Lower Extremity **G** Lymphatic, Left Lower Extremity **H** Lymphatic, Right Inguinal **J** Lymphatic, Left Inguinal **K** Thoracic Duct **L** Cisterna Chyli **M** Thymus **P** Spleen **T** Bone Marrow	**0** Open **3** Percutaneous **4** Percutaneous Endoscopic	**Z** No Device	**X** Diagnostic **Z** No Qualifier

Section	0	**Medical and Surgical**
Body System	7	**Lymphatic and Hemic Systems**
Operation	B	**Excision:** Cutting out or off, without replacement, a portion of a body part

Body Part (4th)	Approach (5th)	Device (6th)	Qualifier (7th)
0 Lymphatic, Head 1 Lymphatic, Right Neck 2 Lymphatic, Left Neck 3 Lymphatic, Right Upper Extremity 4 Lymphatic, Left Upper Extremity 5 Lymphatic, Right Axillary 6 Lymphatic, Left Axillary 7 Lymphatic, Thorax 8 Lymphatic, Internal Mammary, Right 9 Lymphatic, Internal Mammary, Left B Lymphatic, Mesenteric C Lymphatic, Pelvis D Lymphatic, Aortic F Lymphatic, Right Lower Extremity G Lymphatic, Left Lower Extremity H Lymphatic, Right Inguinal J Lymphatic, Left Inguinal K Thoracic Duct L Cisterna Chyli M Thymus P Spleen	0 Open 3 Percutaneous 4 Percutaneous Endoscopic	Z No Device	X Diagnostic Z No Qualifier

Section	0	**Medical and Surgical**
Body System	7	**Lymphatic and Hemic Systems**
Operation	C	**Extirpation:** Taking or cutting out solid matter from a body part

Body Part (4th)	Approach (5th)	Device (6th)	Qualifier (7th)
0 Lymphatic, Head 1 Lymphatic, Right Neck 2 Lymphatic, Left Neck 3 Lymphatic, Right Upper Extremity 4 Lymphatic, Left Upper Extremity 5 Lymphatic, Right Axillary 6 Lymphatic, Left Axillary 7 Lymphatic, Thorax 8 Lymphatic, Internal Mammary, Right 9 Lymphatic, Internal Mammary, Left B Lymphatic, Mesenteric C Lymphatic, Pelvis D Lymphatic, Aortic F Lymphatic, Right Lower Extremity G Lymphatic, Left Lower Extremity H Lymphatic, Right Inguinal J Lymphatic, Left Inguinal K Thoracic Duct L Cisterna Chyli M Thymus P Spleen	0 Open 3 Percutaneous 4 Percutaneous Endoscopic	Z No Device	Z No Qualifier

Section	0	**Medical and Surgical**
Body System	7	**Lymphatic and Hemic Systems**
Operation	D	**Extraction:** Pulling or stripping out or off all or a portion of a body part by the use of force

Body Part (4th)	Approach (5th)	Device (6th)	Qualifier (7th)
Q Bone Marrow, Sternum R Bone Marrow, Iliac S Bone Marrow, Vertebral	0 Open 3 Percutaneous	Z No Device	X Diagnostic Z No Qualifier

Section	0	Medical and Surgical
Body System	7	Lymphatic and Hemic Systems
Operation	H	Insertion: Putting in a nonbiological appliance that monitors, assists, performs, or prevents a physiological function but does not physically take the place of a body part

Body Part (4th)	Approach (5th)	Device (6th)	Qualifier (7th)
K Thoracic Duct L Cisterna Chyli M Thymus N Lymphatic P Spleen	0 Open 3 Percutaneous 4 Percutaneous Endoscopic	3 Infusion Device	Z No Qualifier

Section	0	Medical and Surgical
Body System	7	Lymphatic and Hemic Systems
Operation	J	Inspection: Visually and/or manually exploring a body part

Body Part (4th)	Approach (5th)	Device (6th)	Qualifier (7th)
K Thoracic Duct L Cisterna Chyli M Thymus T Bone Marrow	0 Open 3 Percutaneous 4 Percutaneous Endoscopic	Z No Device	Z No Qualifier
N Lymphatic P Spleen	0 Open 3 Percutaneous 4 Percutaneous Endoscopic X External	Z No Device	Z No Qualifier

Section	0	Medical and Surgical
Body System	7	Lymphatic and Hemic Systems
Operation	L	Occlusion: Completely closing an orifice or the lumen of a tubular body part

Body Part (4th)	Approach (5th)	Device (6th)	Qualifier (7th)
0 Lymphatic, Head 1 Lymphatic, Right Neck 2 Lymphatic, Left Neck 3 Lymphatic, Right Upper Extremity 4 Lymphatic, Left Upper Extremity 5 Lymphatic, Right Axillary 6 Lymphatic, Left Axillary 7 Lymphatic, Thorax 8 Lymphatic, Internal Mammary, Right 9 Lymphatic, Internal Mammary, Left B Lymphatic, Mesenteric C Lymphatic, Pelvis D Lymphatic, Aortic F Lymphatic, Right Lower Extremity G Lymphatic, Left Lower Extremity H Lymphatic, Right Inguinal J Lymphatic, Left Inguinal K Thoracic Duct L Cisterna Chyli	0 Open 3 Percutaneous 4 Percutaneous Endoscopic	C Extraluminal Device D Intraluminal Device Z No Device	Z No Qualifier

Section	0	Medical and Surgical
Body System	7	Lymphatic and Hemic Systems
Operation	N	Release: Freeing a body part from an abnormal physical constraint by cutting or by the use of force

Body Part (4th)	Approach (5th)	Device (6th)	Qualifier (7th)
0 Lymphatic, Head 1 Lymphatic, Right Neck 2 Lymphatic, Left Neck 3 Lymphatic, Right Upper Extremity 4 Lymphatic, Left Upper Extremity 5 Lymphatic, Right Axillary 6 Lymphatic, Left Axillary 7 Lymphatic, Thorax 8 Lymphatic, Internal Mammary, Right 9 Lymphatic, Internal Mammary, Left B Lymphatic, Mesenteric C Lymphatic, Pelvis D Lymphatic, Aortic F Lymphatic, Right Lower Extremity G Lymphatic, Left Lower Extremity H Lymphatic, Right Inguinal J Lymphatic, Left Inguinal K Thoracic Duct L Cisterna Chyli M Thymus P Spleen	0 Open 3 Percutaneous 4 Percutaneous Endoscopic	Z No Device	Z No Qualifier

Section	0	Medical and Surgical
Body System	7	Lymphatic and Hemic Systems
Operation	P	Removal: Taking out or off a device from a body part

Body Part (4th)	Approach (5th)	Device (6th)	Qualifier (7th)
K Thoracic Duct L Cisterna Chyli N Lymphatic	0 Open 3 Percutaneous 4 Percutaneous Endoscopic	0 Drainage Device 3 Infusion Device 7 Autologous Tissue Substitute C Extraluminal Device D Intraluminal Device J Synthetic Substitute K Nonautologous Tissue Substitute	Z No Qualifier
K Thoracic Duct L Cisterna Chyli N Lymphatic	X External	0 Drainage Device 3 Infusion Device D Intraluminal Device	Z No Qualifier
M Thymus P Spleen	0 Open 3 Percutaneous 4 Percutaneous Endoscopic X External	0 Drainage Device 3 Infusion Device	Z No Qualifier
T Bone Marrow	0 Open 3 Percutaneous 4 Percutaneous Endoscopic X External	0 Drainage Device	Z No Qualifier

Section	0	Medical and Surgical
Body System	7	Lymphatic and Hemic Systems
Operation	Q	Repair: Restoring, to the extent possible, a body part to its normal anatomic structure and function

Body Part (4th)	Approach (5th)	Device (6th)	Qualifier (7th)
0 Lymphatic, Head 1 Lymphatic, Right Neck 2 Lymphatic, Left Neck 3 Lymphatic, Right Upper Extremity 4 Lymphatic, Left Upper Extremity 5 Lymphatic, Right Axillary 6 Lymphatic, Left Axillary 7 Lymphatic, Thorax 8 Lymphatic, Internal Mammary, Right 9 Lymphatic, Internal Mammary, Left B Lymphatic, Mesenteric C Lymphatic, Pelvis D Lymphatic, Aortic F Lymphatic, Right Lower Extremity G Lymphatic, Left Lower Extremity H Lymphatic, Right Inguinal J Lymphatic, Left Inguinal K Thoracic Duct L Cisterna Chyli M Thymus P Spleen	0 Open 3 Percutaneous 4 Percutaneous Endoscopic	Z No Device	Z No Qualifier

Section	0	Medical and Surgical
Body System	7	Lymphatic and Hemic Systems
Operation	S	Reposition: Moving to its normal location, or other suitable location, all or a portion of a body part

Body Part (4th)	Approach (5th)	Device (6th)	Qualifier (7th)
M Thymus P Spleen	0 Open	Z No Device	Z No Qualifier

Section	0	Medical and Surgical
Body System	7	Lymphatic and Hemic Systems
Operation	T	Resection: Cutting out or off, without replacement, all of a body part

Body Part (4th)	Approach (5th)	Device (6th)	Qualifier (7th)
0 Lymphatic, Head 1 Lymphatic, Right Neck 2 Lymphatic, Left Neck 3 Lymphatic, Right Upper Extremity 4 Lymphatic, Left Upper Extremity 5 Lymphatic, Right Axillary 6 Lymphatic, Left Axillary 7 Lymphatic, Thorax 8 Lymphatic, Internal Mammary, Right 9 Lymphatic, Internal Mammary, Left B Lymphatic, Mesenteric C Lymphatic, Pelvis D Lymphatic, Aortic F Lymphatic, Right Lower Extremity G Lymphatic, Left Lower Extremity H Lymphatic, Right Inguinal J Lymphatic, Left Inguinal K Thoracic Duct L Cisterna Chyli M Thymus P Spleen	0 Open 4 Percutaneous Endoscopic	Z No Device	Z No Qualifier

Section	0	Medical and Surgical
Body System	7	Lymphatic and Hemic Systems
Operation	U	Supplement: Putting in or on biological or synthetic material that physically reinforces and/or augments the function of a portion of a body part

Body Part (4th)	Approach (5th)	Device (6th)	Qualifier (7th)
0 Lymphatic, Head 1 Lymphatic, Right Neck 2 Lymphatic, Left Neck 3 Lymphatic, Right Upper Extremity 4 Lymphatic, Left Upper Extremity 5 Lymphatic, Right Axillary 6 Lymphatic, Left Axillary 7 Lymphatic, Thorax 8 Lymphatic, Internal Mammary, Right 9 Lymphatic, Internal Mammary, Left B Lymphatic, Mesenteric C Lymphatic, Pelvis D Lymphatic, Aortic F Lymphatic, Right Lower Extremity G Lymphatic, Left Lower Extremity H Lymphatic, Right Inguinal J Lymphatic, Left Inguinal K Thoracic Duct L Cisterna Chyli	0 Open 4 Percutaneous Endoscopic	7 Autologous Tissue Substitute J Synthetic Substitute K Nonautologous Tissue Substitute	Z No Qualifier

Section	0	Medical and Surgical
Body System	7	Lymphatic and Hemic Systems
Operation	V	Restriction: Partially closing an orifice or the lumen of a tubular body part

Body Part (4th)	Approach (5th)	Device (6th)	Qualifier (7th)
0 Lymphatic, Head 1 Lymphatic, Right Neck 2 Lymphatic, Left Neck 3 Lymphatic, Right Upper Extremity 4 Lymphatic, Left Upper Extremity 5 Lymphatic, Right Axillary 6 Lymphatic, Left Axillary 7 Lymphatic, Thorax 8 Lymphatic, Internal Mammary, Right 9 Lymphatic, Internal Mammary, Left B Lymphatic, Mesenteric C Lymphatic, Pelvis D Lymphatic, Aortic F Lymphatic, Right Lower Extremity G Lymphatic, Left Lower Extremity H Lymphatic, Right Inguinal J Lymphatic, Left Inguinal K Thoracic Duct L Cisterna Chyli	0 Open 3 Percutaneous 4 Percutaneous Endoscopic	C Extraluminal Device D Intraluminal Device Z No Device	Z No Qualifier

Section	0	Medical and Surgical
Body System	7	Lymphatic and Hemic Systems
Operation	W	Revision: Correcting, to the extent possible, a portion of a malfunctioning device or the position of a displaced device

Body Part (4th)	Approach (5th)	Device (6th)	Qualifier (7th)
K Thoracic Duct L Cisterna Chyli N Lymphatic	0 Open 3 Percutaneous 4 Percutaneous Endoscopic X External	0 Drainage Device 3 Infusion Device 7 Autologous Tissue Substitute C Extraluminal Device D Intraluminal Device J Synthetic Substitute K Nonautologous Tissue Substitute	Z No Qualifier

Continued

Section	0	Medical and Surgical
Body System	7	Lymphatic and Hemic Systems
Operation	W	Revision: Correcting, to the extent possible, a portion of a malfunctioning device or the position of a displaced device

07W Continued

Body Part (4th)	Approach (5th)	Device (6th)	Qualifier (7th)
M Thymus P Spleen	0 Open 3 Percutaneous 4 Percutaneous Endoscopic X External	0 Drainage Device 3 Infusion Device	Z No Qualifier
T Bone Marrow	0 Open 3 Percutaneous 4 Percutaneous Endoscopic X External	0 Drainage Device	Z No Qualifier

Section	0	Medical and Surgical
Body System	7	Lymphatic and Hemic Systems
Operation	Y	Transplantation: Putting in or on all or a portion of a living body part taken from another individual or animal to physically take the place and/or function of all or a portion of a similar body part

Body Part (4th)	Approach (5th)	Device (6th)	Qualifier (7th)
M Thymus P Spleen	0 Open	Z No Device	0 Allogeneic 1 Syngeneic 2 Zooplastic

Lymphatic and Hemic Systems Code Listing 072–07Y

072 – Lymphatic and Hemic Systems, Change

Review Coding Guideline B6.1c

072KX0Z   Change Drainage Device in Thoracic Duct, External Approach
072KXYZ   Change Other Device in Thoracic Duct, External Approach
072LX0Z   Change Drainage Device in Cisterna Chyli, External Approach
072LXYZ   Change Other Device in Cisterna Chyli, External Approach
072MX0Z   Change Drainage Device in Thymus, External Approach
072MXYZ   Change Other Device in Thymus, External Approach

072NX0Z   Change Drainage Device in Lymphatic, External Approach
072NXYZ   Change Other Device in Lymphatic, External Approach
072PX0Z   Change Drainage Device in Spleen, External Approach
072PXYZ   Change Other Device in Spleen, External Approach
072TX0Z   Change Drainage Device in Bone Marrow, External Approach
072TXYZ   Change Other Device in Bone Marrow, External Approach

075 – Lymphatic and Hemic Systems, Destruction

07500ZZ   Destruction of Head Lymphatic, Open Approach
07503ZZ   Destruction of Head Lymphatic, Percutaneous Approach
07504ZZ   Destruction of Head Lymphatic, Percutaneous Endoscopic Approach
07510ZZ   Destruction of Right Neck Lymphatic, Open Approach
07513ZZ   Destruction of Right Neck Lymphatic, Percutaneous Approach
07514ZZ   Destruction of Right Neck Lymphatic, Percutaneous Endoscopic Approach
07520ZZ   Destruction of Left Neck Lymphatic, Open Approach
07523ZZ   Destruction of Left Neck Lymphatic, Percutaneous Approach
07524ZZ   Destruction of Left Neck Lymphatic, Percutaneous Endoscopic Approach
07530ZZ   Destruction of Right Upper Extremity Lymphatic, Open Approach
07533ZZ   Destruction of Right Upper Extremity Lymphatic, Percutaneous Approach
07534ZZ   Destruction of Right Upper Extremity Lymphatic, Percutaneous Endoscopic Approach
07540ZZ   Destruction of Left Upper Extremity Lymphatic, Open Approach
07543ZZ   Destruction of Left Upper Extremity Lymphatic, Percutaneous Approach
07544ZZ   Destruction of Left Upper Extremity Lymphatic, Percutaneous Endoscopic Approach
07550ZZ   Destruction of Right Axillary Lymphatic, Open Approach
07553ZZ   Destruction of Right Axillary Lymphatic, Percutaneous Approach

07554ZZ   Destruction of Right Axillary Lymphatic, Percutaneous Endoscopic Approach
07560ZZ   Destruction of Left Axillary Lymphatic, Open Approach
07563ZZ   Destruction of Left Axillary Lymphatic, Percutaneous Approach
07564ZZ   Destruction of Left Axillary Lymphatic, Percutaneous Endoscopic Approach
07570ZZ   Destruction of Thorax Lymphatic, Open Approach
07573ZZ   Destruction of Thorax Lymphatic, Percutaneous Approach
07574ZZ   Destruction of Thorax Lymphatic, Percutaneous Endoscopic Approach
07580ZZ   Destruction of Right Internal Mammary Lymphatic, Open Approach
07583ZZ   Destruction of Right Internal Mammary Lymphatic, Percutaneous Approach
07584ZZ   Destruction of Right Internal Mammary Lymphatic, Percutaneous Endoscopic Approach
07590ZZ   Destruction of Left Internal Mammary Lymphatic, Open Approach
07593ZZ   Destruction of Left Internal Mammary Lymphatic, Percutaneous Approach
07594ZZ   Destruction of Left Internal Mammary Lymphatic, Percutaneous Endoscopic Approach
075B0ZZ   Destruction of Mesenteric Lymphatic, Open Approach
075B3ZZ   Destruction of Mesenteric Lymphatic, Percutaneous Approach
075B4ZZ   Destruction of Mesenteric Lymphatic, Percutaneous Endoscopic Approach

---

♀ Female-only   ♂ Male-only   ◐ Limited Coverage   ● Non-OR   **HAC** HAC-associated procedure   ⬢ Non-covered procedures   ✛ Combination

075C0ZZ	Destruction of Pelvis Lymphatic, Open Approach	075H3ZZ	Destruction of Right Inguinal Lymphatic, Percutaneous Approach
075C3ZZ	Destruction of Pelvis Lymphatic, Percutaneous Approach	075H4ZZ	Destruction of Right Inguinal Lymphatic, Percutaneous Endoscopic Approach
075C4ZZ	Destruction of Pelvis Lymphatic, Percutaneous Endoscopic Approach	075J0ZZ	Destruction of Left Inguinal Lymphatic, Open Approach
075D0ZZ	Destruction of Aortic Lymphatic, Open Approach	075J3ZZ	Destruction of Left Inguinal Lymphatic, Percutaneous Approach
075D3ZZ	Destruction of Aortic Lymphatic, Percutaneous Approach	075J4ZZ	Destruction of Left Inguinal Lymphatic, Percutaneous Endoscopic Approach
075D4ZZ	Destruction of Aortic Lymphatic, Percutaneous Endoscopic Approach	075K0ZZ	Destruction of Thoracic Duct, Open Approach
075F0ZZ	Destruction of Right Lower Extremity Lymphatic, Open Approach	075K3ZZ	Destruction of Thoracic Duct, Percutaneous Approach
075F3ZZ	Destruction of Right Lower Extremity Lymphatic, Percutaneous Approach	075K4ZZ	Destruction of Thoracic Duct, Percutaneous Endoscopic Approach
075F4ZZ	Destruction of Right Lower Extremity Lymphatic, Percutaneous Endoscopic Approach	075L0ZZ	Destruction of Cisterna Chyli, Open Approach
		075L3ZZ	Destruction of Cisterna Chyli, Percutaneous Approach
075G0ZZ	Destruction of Left Lower Extremity Lymphatic, Open Approach	075L4ZZ	Destruction of Cisterna Chyli, Percutaneous Endoscopic Approach
075G3ZZ	Destruction of Left Lower Extremity Lymphatic, Percutaneous Approach	075M0ZZ	Destruction of Thymus, Open Approach
		075M3ZZ	Destruction of Thymus, Percutaneous Approach
075G4ZZ	Destruction of Left Lower Extremity Lymphatic, Percutaneous Endoscopic Approach	075M4ZZ	Destruction of Thymus, Percutaneous Endoscopic Approach
		075P0ZZ	Destruction of Spleen, Open Approach
075H0ZZ	Destruction of Right Inguinal Lymphatic, Open Approach	075P3ZZ	Destruction of Spleen, Percutaneous Approach
		075P4ZZ	Destruction of Spleen, Percutaneous Endoscopic Approach

079 – Lymphatic and Hemic Systems, Drainage

Review Coding Guidelines B3.4a and B3.4b

Review Coding Guideline B6.2

079000Z	Drainage of Head Lymphatic with Drainage Device, Open Approach	079330Z	Drainage of Right Upper Extremity Lymphatic with Drainage Device, Percutaneous Approach
07900ZX	Drainage of Head Lymphatic, Open Approach, Diagnostic	07933ZX	Drainage of Right Upper Extremity Lymphatic, Percutaneous Approach, Diagnostic
07900ZZ	Drainage of Head Lymphatic, Open Approach		
079030Z	Drainage of Head Lymphatic with Drainage Device, Percutaneous Approach	07933ZZ	Drainage of Right Upper Extremity Lymphatic, Percutaneous Approach
07903ZX	Drainage of Head Lymphatic, Percutaneous Approach, Diagnostic	079340Z	Drainage of Right Upper Extremity Lymphatic with Drainage Device, Percutaneous Endoscopic Approach
07903ZZ	Drainage of Head Lymphatic, Percutaneous Approach	07934ZX	Drainage of Right Upper Extremity Lymphatic, Percutaneous Endoscopic Approach, Diagnostic
079040Z	Drainage of Head Lymphatic with Drainage Device, Percutaneous Endoscopic Approach	07934ZZ	Drainage of Right Upper Extremity Lymphatic, Percutaneous Endoscopic Approach
07904ZX	Drainage of Head Lymphatic, Percutaneous Endoscopic Approach, Diagnostic		
07904ZZ	Drainage of Head Lymphatic, Percutaneous Endoscopic Approach	079400Z	Drainage of Left Upper Extremity Lymphatic with Drainage Device, Open Approach
079100Z	Drainage of Right Neck Lymphatic with Drainage Device, Open Approach	07940ZX	Drainage of Left Upper Extremity Lymphatic, Open Approach, Diagnostic
07910ZX	Drainage of Right Neck Lymphatic, Open Approach, Diagnostic	07940ZZ	Drainage of Left Upper Extremity Lymphatic, Open Approach
07910ZZ	Drainage of Right Neck Lymphatic, Open Approach	079430Z	Drainage of Left Upper Extremity Lymphatic with Drainage Device, Percutaneous Approach
079130Z	Drainage of Right Neck Lymphatic with Drainage Device, Percutaneous Approach	07943ZX	Drainage of Left Upper Extremity Lymphatic, Percutaneous Approach, Diagnostic
07913ZX	Drainage of Right Neck Lymphatic, Percutaneous Approach, Diagnostic	07943ZZ	Drainage of Left Upper Extremity Lymphatic, Percutaneous Approach
07913ZZ	Drainage of Right Neck Lymphatic, Percutaneous Approach	079440Z	Drainage of Left Upper Extremity Lymphatic with Drainage Device, Percutaneous Endoscopic Approach
079140Z	Drainage of Right Neck Lymphatic with Drainage Device, Percutaneous Endoscopic Approach	07944ZX	Drainage of Left Upper Extremity Lymphatic, Percutaneous Endoscopic Approach, Diagnostic
07914ZX	Drainage of Right Neck Lymphatic, Percutaneous Endoscopic Approach, Diagnostic	07944ZZ	Drainage of Left Upper Extremity Lymphatic, Percutaneous Endoscopic Approach
07914ZZ	Drainage of Right Neck Lymphatic, Percutaneous Endoscopic Approach	079500Z	Drainage of Right Axillary Lymphatic with Drainage Device, Open Approach
079200Z	Drainage of Left Neck Lymphatic with Drainage Device, Open Approach	07950ZX	Drainage of Right Axillary Lymphatic, Open Approach, Diagnostic
07920ZX	Drainage of Left Neck Lymphatic, Open Approach, Diagnostic	07950ZZ	Drainage of Right Axillary Lymphatic, Open Approach
07920ZZ	Drainage of Left Neck Lymphatic, Open Approach	079530Z	Drainage of Right Axillary Lymphatic with Drainage Device, Percutaneous Approach
079230Z	Drainage of Left Neck Lymphatic with Drainage Device, Percutaneous Approach	07953ZX	Drainage of Right Axillary Lymphatic, Percutaneous Approach, Diagnostic
07923ZX	Drainage of Left Neck Lymphatic, Percutaneous Approach, Diagnostic	07953ZZ	Drainage of Right Axillary Lymphatic, Percutaneous Approach
07923ZZ	Drainage of Left Neck Lymphatic, Percutaneous Approach	079540Z	Drainage of Right Axillary Lymphatic with Drainage Device, Percutaneous Endoscopic Approach
079240Z	Drainage of Left Neck Lymphatic with Drainage Device, Percutaneous Endoscopic Approach	07954ZX	Drainage of Right Axillary Lymphatic, Percutaneous Endoscopic Approach, Diagnostic
07924ZX	Drainage of Left Neck Lymphatic, Percutaneous Endoscopic Approach, Diagnostic		
07924ZZ	Drainage of Left Neck Lymphatic, Percutaneous Endoscopic Approach	07954ZZ	Drainage of Right Axillary Lymphatic, Percutaneous Endoscopic Approach
079300Z	Drainage of Right Upper Extremity Lymphatic with Drainage Device, Open Approach	079600Z	Drainage of Left Axillary Lymphatic with Drainage Device, Open Approach
07930ZX	Drainage of Right Upper Extremity Lymphatic, Open Approach, Diagnostic	07960ZX	Drainage of Left Axillary Lymphatic, Open Approach, Diagnostic
07930ZZ	Drainage of Right Upper Extremity Lymphatic, Open Approach		

♀ Female-only   ♂ Male-only   ⬤ Limited Coverage   ● Non-OR   ▨ HAC-associated procedure   ⬤ Non-covered procedures   ➕ Combination

07960ZZ	Drainage of Left Axillary Lymphatic, Open Approach
079630Z	Drainage of Left Axillary Lymphatic with Drainage Device, Percutaneous Approach
07963ZX	Drainage of Left Axillary Lymphatic, Percutaneous Approach, Diagnostic
07963ZZ	Drainage of Left Axillary Lymphatic, Percutaneous Approach
079640Z	Drainage of Left Axillary Lymphatic with Drainage Device, Percutaneous Endoscopic Approach
07964ZX	Drainage of Left Axillary Lymphatic, Percutaneous Endoscopic Approach, Diagnostic
07964ZZ	Drainage of Left Axillary Lymphatic, Percutaneous Endoscopic Approach
079700Z	Drainage of Thorax Lymphatic with Drainage Device, Open Approach
07970ZX	Drainage of Thorax Lymphatic, Open Approach, Diagnostic
07970ZZ	Drainage of Thorax Lymphatic, Open Approach
079730Z	Drainage of Thorax Lymphatic with Drainage Device, Percutaneous Approach
07973ZX	Drainage of Thorax Lymphatic, Percutaneous Approach, Diagnostic
07973ZZ	Drainage of Thorax Lymphatic, Percutaneous Approach
079740Z	Drainage of Thorax Lymphatic with Drainage Device, Percutaneous Endoscopic Approach
07974ZX	Drainage of Thorax Lymphatic, Percutaneous Endoscopic Approach, Diagnostic
07974ZZ	Drainage of Thorax Lymphatic, Percutaneous Endoscopic Approach
079800Z	Drainage of Right Internal Mammary Lymphatic with Drainage Device, Open Approach
07980ZX	Drainage of Right Internal Mammary Lymphatic, Open Approach, Diagnostic
07980ZZ	Drainage of Right Internal Mammary Lymphatic, Open Approach
079830Z	Drainage of Right Internal Mammary Lymphatic with Drainage Device, Percutaneous Approach
07983ZX	Drainage of Right Internal Mammary Lymphatic, Percutaneous Approach, Diagnostic
07983ZZ	Drainage of Right Internal Mammary Lymphatic, Percutaneous Approach
079840Z	Drainage of Right Internal Mammary Lymphatic with Drainage Device, Percutaneous Endoscopic Approach
07984ZX	Drainage of Right Internal Mammary Lymphatic, Percutaneous Endoscopic Approach, Diagnostic
07984ZZ	Drainage of Right Internal Mammary Lymphatic, Percutaneous Endoscopic Approach
079900Z	Drainage of Left Internal Mammary Lymphatic with Drainage Device, Open Approach
07990ZX	Drainage of Left Internal Mammary Lymphatic, Open Approach, Diagnostic
07990ZZ	Drainage of Left Internal Mammary Lymphatic, Open Approach
079930Z	Drainage of Left Internal Mammary Lymphatic with Drainage Device, Percutaneous Approach
07993ZX	Drainage of Left Internal Mammary Lymphatic, Percutaneous Approach, Diagnostic
07993ZZ	Drainage of Left Internal Mammary Lymphatic, Percutaneous Approach
079940Z	Drainage of Left Internal Mammary Lymphatic with Drainage Device, Percutaneous Endoscopic Approach
07994ZX	Drainage of Left Internal Mammary Lymphatic, Percutaneous Endoscopic Approach, Diagnostic
07994ZZ	Drainage of Left Internal Mammary Lymphatic, Percutaneous Endoscopic Approach
079B00Z	Drainage of Mesenteric Lymphatic with Drainage Device, Open Approach
079B0ZX	Drainage of Mesenteric Lymphatic, Open Approach, Diagnostic
079B0ZZ	Drainage of Mesenteric Lymphatic, Open Approach
079B30Z	Drainage of Mesenteric Lymphatic with Drainage Device, Percutaneous Approach
079B3ZX	Drainage of Mesenteric Lymphatic, Percutaneous Approach, Diagnostic
079B3ZZ	Drainage of Mesenteric Lymphatic, Percutaneous Approach
079B40Z	Drainage of Mesenteric Lymphatic with Drainage Device, Percutaneous Endoscopic Approach
079B4ZX	Drainage of Mesenteric Lymphatic, Percutaneous Endoscopic Approach, Diagnostic
079B4ZZ	Drainage of Mesenteric Lymphatic, Percutaneous Endoscopic Approach
079C00Z	Drainage of Pelvis Lymphatic with Drainage Device, Open Approach
079C0ZX	Drainage of Pelvis Lymphatic, Open Approach, Diagnostic
079C0ZZ	Drainage of Pelvis Lymphatic, Open Approach
079C30Z	Drainage of Pelvis Lymphatic with Drainage Device, Percutaneous Approach
079C3ZX	Drainage of Pelvis Lymphatic, Percutaneous Approach, Diagnostic
079C3ZZ	Drainage of Pelvis Lymphatic, Percutaneous Approach
079C40Z	Drainage of Pelvis Lymphatic with Drainage Device, Percutaneous Endoscopic Approach
079C4ZX	Drainage of Pelvis Lymphatic, Percutaneous Endoscopic Approach, Diagnostic
079C4ZZ	Drainage of Pelvis Lymphatic, Percutaneous Endoscopic Approach
079D00Z	Drainage of Aortic Lymphatic with Drainage Device, Open Approach
079D0ZX	Drainage of Aortic Lymphatic, Open Approach, Diagnostic
079D0ZZ	Drainage of Aortic Lymphatic, Open Approach
079D30Z	Drainage of Aortic Lymphatic with Drainage Device, Percutaneous Approach
079D3ZX	Drainage of Aortic Lymphatic, Percutaneous Approach, Diagnostic
079D3ZZ	Drainage of Aortic Lymphatic, Percutaneous Approach
079D40Z	Drainage of Aortic Lymphatic with Drainage Device, Percutaneous Endoscopic Approach
079D4ZX	Drainage of Aortic Lymphatic, Percutaneous Endoscopic Approach, Diagnostic
079D4ZZ	Drainage of Aortic Lymphatic, Percutaneous Endoscopic Approach
079F00Z	Drainage of Right Lower Extremity Lymphatic with Drainage Device, Open Approach
079F0ZX	Drainage of Right Lower Extremity Lymphatic, Open Approach, Diagnostic
079F0ZZ	Drainage of Right Lower Extremity Lymphatic, Open Approach
079F30Z	Drainage of Right Lower Extremity Lymphatic with Drainage Device, Percutaneous Approach
079F3ZX	Drainage of Right Lower Extremity Lymphatic, Percutaneous Approach, Diagnostic
079F3ZZ	Drainage of Right Lower Extremity Lymphatic, Percutaneous Approach
079F40Z	Drainage of Right Lower Extremity Lymphatic with Drainage Device, Percutaneous Endoscopic Approach
079F4ZX	Drainage of Right Lower Extremity Lymphatic, Percutaneous Endoscopic Approach, Diagnostic
079F4ZZ	Drainage of Right Lower Extremity Lymphatic, Percutaneous Endoscopic Approach
079G00Z	Drainage of Left Lower Extremity Lymphatic with Drainage Device, Open Approach
079G0ZX	Drainage of Left Lower Extremity Lymphatic, Open Approach, Diagnostic
079G0ZZ	Drainage of Left Lower Extremity Lymphatic, Open Approach
079G30Z	Drainage of Left Lower Extremity Lymphatic with Drainage Device, Percutaneous Approach
079G3ZX	Drainage of Left Lower Extremity Lymphatic, Percutaneous Approach, Diagnostic
079G3ZZ	Drainage of Left Lower Extremity Lymphatic, Percutaneous Approach
079G40Z	Drainage of Left Lower Extremity Lymphatic with Drainage Device, Percutaneous Endoscopic Approach
079G4ZX	Drainage of Left Lower Extremity Lymphatic, Percutaneous Endoscopic Approach, Diagnostic
079G4ZZ	Drainage of Left Lower Extremity Lymphatic, Percutaneous Endoscopic Approach
079H00Z	Drainage of Right Inguinal Lymphatic with Drainage Device, Open Approach
079H0ZX	Drainage of Right Inguinal Lymphatic, Open Approach, Diagnostic
079H0ZZ	Drainage of Right Inguinal Lymphatic, Open Approach
079H30Z	Drainage of Right Inguinal Lymphatic with Drainage Device, Percutaneous Approach
079H3ZX	Drainage of Right Inguinal Lymphatic, Percutaneous Approach, Diagnostic
079H3ZZ	Drainage of Right Inguinal Lymphatic, Percutaneous Approach

079H40Z	Drainage of Right Inguinal Lymphatic with Drainage Device, Percutaneous Endoscopic Approach
079H4ZX	Drainage of Right Inguinal Lymphatic, Percutaneous Endoscopic Approach, Diagnostic
079H4ZZ	Drainage of Right Inguinal Lymphatic, Percutaneous Endoscopic Approach
079J00Z	Drainage of Left Inguinal Lymphatic with Drainage Device, Open Approach
079J0ZX	Drainage of Left Inguinal Lymphatic, Open Approach, Diagnostic
079J0ZZ	Drainage of Left Inguinal Lymphatic, Open Approach
079J30Z	Drainage of Left Inguinal Lymphatic with Drainage Device, Percutaneous Approach
079J3ZX	Drainage of Left Inguinal Lymphatic, Percutaneous Approach, Diagnostic
079J3ZZ	Drainage of Left Inguinal Lymphatic, Percutaneous Approach
079J40Z	Drainage of Left Inguinal Lymphatic with Drainage Device, Percutaneous Endoscopic Approach
079J4ZX	Drainage of Left Inguinal Lymphatic, Percutaneous Endoscopic Approach, Diagnostic
079J4ZZ	Drainage of Left Inguinal Lymphatic, Percutaneous Endoscopic Approach
079K00Z	Drainage of Thoracic Duct with Drainage Device, Open Approach
079K0ZX	Drainage of Thoracic Duct, Open Approach, Diagnostic
079K0ZZ	Drainage of Thoracic Duct, Open Approach
079K30Z	Drainage of Thoracic Duct with Drainage Device, Percutaneous Approach
079K3ZX	Drainage of Thoracic Duct, Percutaneous Approach, Diagnostic
079K3ZZ	Drainage of Thoracic Duct, Percutaneous Approach
079K40Z	Drainage of Thoracic Duct with Drainage Device, Percutaneous Endoscopic Approach
079K4ZX	Drainage of Thoracic Duct, Percutaneous Endoscopic Approach, Diagnostic
079K4ZZ	Drainage of Thoracic Duct, Percutaneous Endoscopic Approach
079L00Z	Drainage of Cisterna Chyli with Drainage Device, Open Approach
079L0ZX	Drainage of Cisterna Chyli, Open Approach, Diagnostic
079L0ZZ	Drainage of Cisterna Chyli, Open Approach
079L30Z	Drainage of Cisterna Chyli with Drainage Device, Percutaneous Approach
079L3ZX	Drainage of Cisterna Chyli, Percutaneous Approach, Diagnostic
079L3ZZ	Drainage of Cisterna Chyli, Percutaneous Approach
079L40Z	Drainage of Cisterna Chyli with Drainage Device, Percutaneous Approach
079L4ZX	Drainage of Cisterna Chyli, Percutaneous Endoscopic Approach, Diagnostic
079L4ZZ	Drainage of Cisterna Chyli, Percutaneous Endoscopic Approach
079M00Z	Drainage of Thymus with Drainage Device, Open Approach
079M0ZX	Drainage of Thymus, Open Approach, Diagnostic
079M0ZZ	Drainage of Thymus, Open Approach
079M30Z	Drainage of Thymus with Drainage Device, Percutaneous Approach
079M3ZX	Drainage of Thymus, Percutaneous Approach, Diagnostic
079M3ZZ	Drainage of Thymus, Percutaneous Approach
079M40Z	Drainage of Thymus with Drainage Device, Percutaneous Endoscopic Approach
079M4ZX	Drainage of Thymus, Percutaneous Endoscopic Approach, Diagnostic
079M4ZZ	Drainage of Thymus, Percutaneous Endoscopic Approach
079P00Z	Drainage of Spleen with Drainage Device, Open Approach
079P0ZX	Drainage of Spleen, Open Approach, Diagnostic
079P0ZZ	Drainage of Spleen, Open Approach
079P30Z	Drainage of Spleen with Drainage Device, Percutaneous Approach
079P3ZX	Drainage of Spleen, Percutaneous Approach, Diagnostic
079P3ZZ	Drainage of Spleen, Percutaneous Approach
079P40Z	Drainage of Spleen with Drainage Device, Percutaneous Endoscopic Approach
079P4ZX	Drainage of Spleen, Percutaneous Endoscopic Approach, Diagnostic
079P4ZZ	Drainage of Spleen, Percutaneous Endoscopic Approach
079T00Z	Drainage of Bone Marrow with Drainage Device, Open Approach
079T0ZX	Drainage of Bone Marrow, Open Approach, Diagnostic
079T0ZZ	Drainage of Bone Marrow, Open Approach
079T30Z	Drainage of Bone Marrow with Drainage Device, Percutaneous Approach
079T3ZX	Drainage of Bone Marrow, Percutaneous Approach, Diagnostic
079T3ZZ	Drainage of Bone Marrow, Percutaneous Approach
079T40Z	Drainage of Bone Marrow with Drainage Device, Percutaneous Endoscopic Approach
079T4ZX	Drainage of Bone Marrow, Percutaneous Endoscopic Approach, Diagnostic
079T4ZZ	Drainage of Bone Marrow, Percutaneous Endoscopic Approach

07B – Lymphatic and Hemic Systems, Excision

Review Coding Guidelines B3.4a and B3.4b

Review Coding Guideline B3.8

07B00ZX	Excision of Head Lymphatic, Open Approach, Diagnostic
07B00ZZ	Excision of Head Lymphatic, Open Approach
07B03ZX	Excision of Head Lymphatic, Percutaneous Approach, Diagnostic
07B03ZZ	Excision of Head Lymphatic, Percutaneous Approach
07B04ZX	Excision of Head Lymphatic, Percutaneous Endoscopic Approach, Diagnostic
07B04ZZ	Excision of Head Lymphatic, Percutaneous Endoscopic Approach
07B10ZX	Excision of Right Neck Lymphatic, Open Approach, Diagnostic
07B10ZZ	Excision of Right Neck Lymphatic, Open Approach
07B13ZX	Excision of Right Neck Lymphatic, Percutaneous Approach, Diagnostic
07B13ZZ	Excision of Right Neck Lymphatic, Percutaneous Approach
07B14ZX	Excision of Right Neck Lymphatic, Percutaneous Endoscopic Approach, Diagnostic
07B14ZZ	Excision of Right Neck Lymphatic, Percutaneous Endoscopic Approach
07B20ZX	Excision of Left Neck Lymphatic, Open Approach, Diagnostic
07B20ZZ	Excision of Left Neck Lymphatic, Open Approach
07B23ZX	Excision of Left Neck Lymphatic, Percutaneous Approach, Diagnostic
07B23ZZ	Excision of Left Neck Lymphatic, Percutaneous Approach
07B24ZX	Excision of Left Neck Lymphatic, Percutaneous Endoscopic Approach, Diagnostic
07B24ZZ	Excision of Left Neck Lymphatic, Percutaneous Endoscopic Approach
07B30ZX	Excision of Right Upper Extremity Lymphatic, Open Approach, Diagnostic
07B30ZZ	Excision of Right Upper Extremity Lymphatic, Open Approach
07B33ZX	Excision of Right Upper Extremity Lymphatic, Percutaneous Approach, Diagnostic
07B33ZZ	Excision of Right Upper Extremity Lymphatic, Percutaneous Approach
07B34ZX	Excision of Right Upper Extremity Lymphatic, Percutaneous Endoscopic Approach, Diagnostic
07B34ZZ	Excision of Right Upper Extremity Lymphatic, Percutaneous Endoscopic Approach
07B40ZX	Excision of Left Upper Extremity Lymphatic, Open Approach, Diagnostic
07B40ZZ	Excision of Left Upper Extremity Lymphatic, Open Approach
07B43ZX	Excision of Left Upper Extremity Lymphatic, Percutaneous Approach, Diagnostic
07B43ZZ	Excision of Left Upper Extremity Lymphatic, Percutaneous Approach
07B44ZX	Excision of Left Upper Extremity Lymphatic, Percutaneous Endoscopic Approach, Diagnostic
07B44ZZ	Excision of Left Upper Extremity Lymphatic, Percutaneous Endoscopic Approach
07B50ZX	Excision of Right Axillary Lymphatic, Open Approach, Diagnostic
07B50ZZ	Excision of Right Axillary Lymphatic, Open Approach
07B53ZX	Excision of Right Axillary Lymphatic, Percutaneous Approach, Diagnostic
07B53ZZ	Excision of Right Axillary Lymphatic, Percutaneous Approach
07B54ZX	Excision of Right Axillary Lymphatic, Percutaneous Endoscopic Approach, Diagnostic

07B54ZZ	Excision of Right Axillary Lymphatic, Percutaneous Endoscopic Approach
07B60ZX	Excision of Left Axillary Lymphatic, Open Approach, Diagnostic
07B60ZZ	Excision of Left Axillary Lymphatic, Open Approach
07B63ZX	Excision of Left Axillary Lymphatic, Percutaneous Approach, Diagnostic
07B63ZZ	Excision of Left Axillary Lymphatic, Percutaneous Approach
07B64ZX	Excision of Left Axillary Lymphatic, Percutaneous Endoscopic Approach, Diagnostic
07B64ZZ	Excision of Left Axillary Lymphatic, Percutaneous Endoscopic Approach
07B70ZX	Excision of Thorax Lymphatic, Open Approach, Diagnostic
07B70ZZ	Excision of Thorax Lymphatic, Open Approach
07B73ZX	Excision of Thorax Lymphatic, Percutaneous Approach, Diagnostic
07B73ZZ	Excision of Thorax Lymphatic, Percutaneous Approach
07B74ZX	Excision of Thorax Lymphatic, Percutaneous Endoscopic Approach, Diagnostic
07B74ZZ	Excision of Thorax Lymphatic, Percutaneous Endoscopic Approach
07B80ZX	Excision of Right Internal Mammary Lymphatic, Open Approach, Diagnostic
07B80ZZ	Excision of Right Internal Mammary Lymphatic, Open Approach
07B83ZX	Excision of Right Internal Mammary Lymphatic, Percutaneous Approach, Diagnostic
07B83ZZ	Excision of Right Internal Mammary Lymphatic, Percutaneous Approach
07B84ZX	Excision of Right Internal Mammary Lymphatic, Percutaneous Endoscopic Approach, Diagnostic
07B84ZZ	Excision of Right Internal Mammary Lymphatic, Percutaneous Endoscopic Approach
07B90ZX	Excision of Left Internal Mammary Lymphatic, Open Approach, Diagnostic
07B90ZZ	Excision of Left Internal Mammary Lymphatic, Open Approach
07B93ZX	Excision of Left Internal Mammary Lymphatic, Percutaneous Approach, Diagnostic
07B93ZZ	Excision of Left Internal Mammary Lymphatic, Percutaneous Approach
07B94ZX	Excision of Left Internal Mammary Lymphatic, Percutaneous Endoscopic Approach, Diagnostic
07B94ZZ	Excision of Left Internal Mammary Lymphatic, Percutaneous Endoscopic Approach
07BB0ZX	Excision of Mesenteric Lymphatic, Open Approach, Diagnostic
07BB0ZZ	Excision of Mesenteric Lymphatic, Open Approach
07BB3ZX	Excision of Mesenteric Lymphatic, Percutaneous Approach, Diagnostic
07BB3ZZ	Excision of Mesenteric Lymphatic, Percutaneous Approach
07BB4ZX	Excision of Mesenteric Lymphatic, Percutaneous Endoscopic Approach, Diagnostic
07BB4ZZ	Excision of Mesenteric Lymphatic, Percutaneous Endoscopic Approach
07BC0ZX	Excision of Pelvis Lymphatic, Open Approach, Diagnostic
07BC0ZZ	Excision of Pelvis Lymphatic, Open Approach
07BC3ZX	Excision of Pelvis Lymphatic, Percutaneous Approach, Diagnostic
07BC3ZZ	Excision of Pelvis Lymphatic, Percutaneous Approach
07BC4ZX	Excision of Pelvis Lymphatic, Percutaneous Endoscopic Approach, Diagnostic
07BC4ZZ	Excision of Pelvis Lymphatic, Percutaneous Endoscopic Approach
07BD0ZX	Excision of Aortic Lymphatic, Open Approach, Diagnostic
07BD0ZZ	Excision of Aortic Lymphatic, Open Approach
07BD3ZX	Excision of Aortic Lymphatic, Percutaneous Approach, Diagnostic
07BD3ZZ	Excision of Aortic Lymphatic, Percutaneous Approach
07BD4ZX	Excision of Aortic Lymphatic, Percutaneous Endoscopic Approach, Diagnostic
07BD4ZZ	Excision of Aortic Lymphatic, Percutaneous Endoscopic Approach
07BF0ZX	Excision of Right Lower Extremity Lymphatic, Open Approach, Diagnostic

07BF0ZZ	Excision of Right Lower Extremity Lymphatic, Open Approach
07BF3ZX	Excision of Right Lower Extremity Lymphatic, Percutaneous Approach, Diagnostic
07BF3ZZ	Excision of Right Lower Extremity Lymphatic, Percutaneous Approach
07BF4ZX	Excision of Right Lower Extremity Lymphatic, Percutaneous Endoscopic Approach, Diagnostic
07BF4ZZ	Excision of Right Lower Extremity Lymphatic, Percutaneous Endoscopic Approach
07BG0ZX	Excision of Left Lower Extremity Lymphatic, Open Approach, Diagnostic
07BG0ZZ	Excision of Left Lower Extremity Lymphatic, Open Approach
07BG3ZX	Excision of Left Lower Extremity Lymphatic, Percutaneous Approach, Diagnostic
07BG3ZZ	Excision of Left Lower Extremity Lymphatic, Percutaneous Approach
07BG4ZX	Excision of Left Lower Extremity Lymphatic, Percutaneous Endoscopic Approach, Diagnostic
07BG4ZZ	Excision of Left Lower Extremity Lymphatic, Percutaneous Endoscopic Approach
07BH0ZX	Excision of Right Inguinal Lymphatic, Open Approach, Diagnostic
07BH0ZZ	Excision of Right Inguinal Lymphatic, Open Approach
07BH3ZX	Excision of Right Inguinal Lymphatic, Percutaneous Approach, Diagnostic
07BH3ZZ	Excision of Right Inguinal Lymphatic, Percutaneous Approach
07BH4ZX	Excision of Right Inguinal Lymphatic, Percutaneous Endoscopic Approach, Diagnostic
07BH4ZZ	Excision of Right Inguinal Lymphatic, Percutaneous Endoscopic Approach
07BJ0ZX	Excision of Left Inguinal Lymphatic, Open Approach, Diagnostic
07BJ0ZZ	Excision of Left Inguinal Lymphatic, Open Approach
07BJ3ZX	Excision of Left Inguinal Lymphatic, Percutaneous Approach, Diagnostic
07BJ3ZZ	Excision of Left Inguinal Lymphatic, Percutaneous Approach
07BJ4ZX	Excision of Left Inguinal Lymphatic, Percutaneous Endoscopic Approach, Diagnostic
07BJ4ZZ	Excision of Left Inguinal Lymphatic, Percutaneous Endoscopic Approach
07BK0ZX	Excision of Thoracic Duct, Open Approach, Diagnostic
07BK0ZZ	Excision of Thoracic Duct, Open Approach
07BK3ZX	Excision of Thoracic Duct, Percutaneous Approach, Diagnostic
07BK3ZZ	Excision of Thoracic Duct, Percutaneous Approach
07BK4ZX	Excision of Thoracic Duct, Percutaneous Endoscopic Approach, Diagnostic
07BK4ZZ	Excision of Thoracic Duct, Percutaneous Endoscopic Approach
07BL0ZX	Excision of Cisterna Chyli, Open Approach, Diagnostic
07BL0ZZ	Excision of Cisterna Chyli, Open Approach
07BL3ZX	Excision of Cisterna Chyli, Percutaneous Approach, Diagnostic
07BL3ZZ	Excision of Cisterna Chyli, Percutaneous Approach
07BL4ZX	Excision of Cisterna Chyli, Percutaneous Endoscopic Approach, Diagnostic
07BL4ZZ	Excision of Cisterna Chyli, Percutaneous Endoscopic Approach
07BM0ZX	Excision of Thymus, Open Approach, Diagnostic
07BM0ZZ	Excision of Thymus, Open Approach
07BM3ZX	Excision of Thymus, Percutaneous Approach, Diagnostic
07BM3ZZ	Excision of Thymus, Percutaneous Approach
07BM4ZX	Excision of Thymus, Percutaneous Endoscopic Approach, Diagnostic
07BM4ZZ	Excision of Thymus, Percutaneous Endoscopic Approach
07BP0ZX	Excision of Spleen, Open Approach, Diagnostic
07BP0ZZ	Excision of Spleen, Open Approach
07BP3ZX	Excision of Spleen, Percutaneous Approach, Diagnostic
07BP3ZZ	Excision of Spleen, Percutaneous Approach
07BP4ZX	Excision of Spleen, Percutaneous Endoscopic Approach, Diagnostic
07BP4ZZ	Excision of Spleen, Percutaneous Endoscopic Approach

07C – Lymphatic and Hemic Systems, Extirpation

07C00ZZ	Extirpation of Matter from Head Lymphatic, Open Approach
07C03ZZ	Extirpation of Matter from Head Lymphatic, Percutaneous Approach
07C04ZZ	Extirpation of Matter from Head Lymphatic, Percutaneous Endoscopic Approach
07C10ZZ	Extirpation of Matter from Right Neck Lymphatic, Open Approach
07C13ZZ	Extirpation of Matter from Right Neck Lymphatic, Percutaneous Approach
07C14ZZ	Extirpation of Matter from Right Neck Lymphatic, Percutaneous Endoscopic Approach
07C20ZZ	Extirpation of Matter from Left Neck Lymphatic, Open Approach

07C23ZZ Extirpation of Matter from Left Neck Lymphatic, Percutaneous Approach
07C24ZZ Extirpation of Matter from Left Neck Lymphatic, Percutaneous Endoscopic Approach
07C30ZZ Extirpation of Matter from Right Upper Extremity Lymphatic, Open Approach
07C33ZZ Extirpation of Matter from Right Upper Extremity Lymphatic, Percutaneous Approach
07C34ZZ Extirpation of Matter from Right Upper Extremity Lymphatic, Percutaneous Endoscopic Approach
07C40ZZ Extirpation of Matter from Left Upper Extremity Lymphatic, Open Approach
07C43ZZ Extirpation of Matter from Left Upper Extremity Lymphatic, Percutaneous Approach
07C44ZZ Extirpation of Matter from Left Upper Extremity Lymphatic, Percutaneous Endoscopic Approach
07C50ZZ Extirpation of Matter from Right Axillary Lymphatic, Open Approach
07C53ZZ Extirpation of Matter from Right Axillary Lymphatic, Percutaneous Approach
07C54ZZ Extirpation of Matter from Right Axillary Lymphatic, Percutaneous Endoscopic Approach
07C60ZZ Extirpation of Matter from Left Axillary Lymphatic, Open Approach
07C63ZZ Extirpation of Matter from Left Axillary Lymphatic, Percutaneous Approach
07C64ZZ Extirpation of Matter from Left Axillary Lymphatic, Percutaneous Endoscopic Approach
07C70ZZ Extirpation of Matter from Thorax Lymphatic, Open Approach
07C73ZZ Extirpation of Matter from Thorax Lymphatic, Percutaneous Approach
07C74ZZ Extirpation of Matter from Thorax Lymphatic, Percutaneous Endoscopic Approach
07C80ZZ Extirpation of Matter from Right Internal Mammary Lymphatic, Open Approach
07C83ZZ Extirpation of Matter from Right Internal Mammary Lymphatic, Percutaneous Approach
07C84ZZ Extirpation of Matter from Right Internal Mammary Lymphatic, Percutaneous Endoscopic Approach
07C90ZZ Extirpation of Matter from Left Internal Mammary Lymphatic, Open Approach
07C93ZZ Extirpation of Matter from Left Internal Mammary Lymphatic, Percutaneous Approach
07C94ZZ Extirpation of Matter from Left Internal Mammary Lymphatic, Percutaneous Endoscopic Approach
07CB0ZZ Extirpation of Matter from Mesenteric Lymphatic, Open Approach
07CB3ZZ Extirpation of Matter from Mesenteric Lymphatic, Percutaneous Approach
07CB4ZZ Extirpation of Matter from Mesenteric Lymphatic, Percutaneous Endoscopic Approach

07CC0ZZ Extirpation of Matter from Pelvis Lymphatic, Open Approach
07CC3ZZ Extirpation of Matter from Pelvis Lymphatic, Percutaneous Approach
07CC4ZZ Extirpation of Matter from Pelvis Lymphatic, Percutaneous Endoscopic Approach
07CD0ZZ Extirpation of Matter from Aortic Lymphatic, Open Approach
07CD3ZZ Extirpation of Matter from Aortic Lymphatic, Percutaneous Approach
07CD4ZZ Extirpation of Matter from Aortic Lymphatic, Percutaneous Endoscopic Approach
07CF0ZZ Extirpation of Matter from Right Lower Extremity Lymphatic, Open Approach
07CF3ZZ Extirpation of Matter from Right Lower Extremity Lymphatic, Percutaneous Approach
07CF4ZZ Extirpation of Matter from Right Lower Extremity Lymphatic, Percutaneous Endoscopic Approach
07CG0ZZ Extirpation of Matter from Left Lower Extremity Lymphatic, Open Approach
07CG3ZZ Extirpation of Matter from Left Lower Extremity Lymphatic, Percutaneous Approach
07CG4ZZ Extirpation of Matter from Left Lower Extremity Lymphatic, Percutaneous Endoscopic Approach
07CH0ZZ Extirpation of Matter from Right Inguinal Lymphatic, Open Approach
07CH3ZZ Extirpation of Matter from Right Inguinal Lymphatic, Percutaneous Approach
07CH4ZZ Extirpation of Matter from Right Inguinal Lymphatic, Percutaneous Endoscopic Approach
07CJ0ZZ Extirpation of Matter from Left Inguinal Lymphatic, Open Approach
07CJ3ZZ Extirpation of Matter from Left Inguinal Lymphatic, Percutaneous Approach
07CJ4ZZ Extirpation of Matter from Left Inguinal Lymphatic, Percutaneous Endoscopic Approach
07CK0ZZ Extirpation of Matter from Thoracic Duct, Open Approach
07CK3ZZ Extirpation of Matter from Thoracic Duct, Percutaneous Approach
07CK4ZZ Extirpation of Matter from Thoracic Duct, Percutaneous Endoscopic Approach
07CL0ZZ Extirpation of Matter from Cisterna Chyli, Open Approach
07CL3ZZ Extirpation of Matter from Cisterna Chyli, Percutaneous Approach
07CL4ZZ Extirpation of Matter from Cisterna Chyli, Percutaneous Endoscopic Approach
07CM0ZZ Extirpation of Matter from Thymus, Open Approach
07CM3ZZ Extirpation of Matter from Thymus, Percutaneous Approach
07CM4ZZ Extirpation of Matter from Thymus, Percutaneous Endoscopic Approach
07CP0ZZ Extirpation of Matter from Spleen, Open Approach
07CP3ZZ Extirpation of Matter from Spleen, Percutaneous Approach
07CP4ZZ Extirpation of Matter from Spleen, Percutaneous Endoscopic Approach

07D – Lymphatic and Hemic Systems, Extraction

Review Coding Guidelines B3.4a and B3.4b

07DQ0ZX Extraction of Sternum Bone Marrow, Open Approach, Diagnostic
07DQ0ZZ Extraction of Sternum Bone Marrow, Open Approach
07DQ3ZX Extraction of Sternum Bone Marrow, Percutaneous Approach, Diagnostic
07DQ3ZZ Extraction of Sternum Bone Marrow, Percutaneous Approach
07DR0ZX Extraction of Iliac Bone Marrow, Open Approach, Diagnostic
07DR0ZZ Extraction of Iliac Bone Marrow, Open Approach

07DR3ZX Extraction of Iliac Bone Marrow, Percutaneous Approach, Diagnostic
07DR3ZZ Extraction of Iliac Bone Marrow, Percutaneous Approach
07DS0ZX Extraction of Vertebral Bone Marrow, Open Approach, Diagnostic
07DS0ZZ Extraction of Vertebral Bone Marrow, Open Approach
07DS3ZX Extraction of Vertebral Bone Marrow, Percutaneous Approach, Diagnostic
07DS3ZZ Extraction of Vertebral Bone Marrow, Percutaneous Approach

07H – Lymphatic and Hemic Systems, Insertion

07HK03Z Insertion of Infusion Device into Thoracic Duct, Open Approach
07HK33Z Insertion of Infusion Device into Thoracic Duct, Percutaneous Approach
07HK43Z Insertion of Infusion Device into Thoracic Duct, Percutaneous Endoscopic Approach
07HL03Z Insertion of Infusion Device into Cisterna Chyli, Open Approach
07HL33Z Insertion of Infusion Device into Cisterna Chyli, Percutaneous Approach

07HL43Z Insertion of Infusion Device into Cisterna Chyli, Percutaneous Endoscopic Approach
07HM03Z Insertion of Infusion Device into Thymus, Open Approach
07HM33Z Insertion of Infusion Device into Thymus, Percutaneous Approach
07HM43Z Insertion of Infusion Device into Thymus, Percutaneous Endoscopic Approach
07HN03Z Insertion of Infusion Device into Lymphatic, Open Approach
07HN33Z Insertion of Infusion Device into Lymphatic, Percutaneous Approach

---

♀ Female-only   ♂ Male-only   ● Limited Coverage   ● Non-OR   ᴴᴬᶜ HAC-associated procedure   ● Non-covered procedures   ✚ Combination

07HN43Z	Insertion of Infusion Device into Lymphatic, Percutaneous Endoscopic Approach
07HP03Z	Insertion of Infusion Device into Spleen, Open Approach

07HP33Z	Insertion of Infusion Device into Spleen, Percutaneous Approach
07HP43Z	Insertion of Infusion Device into Spleen, Percutaneous Endoscopic Approach

07J – Lymphatic and Hemic Systems, Inspection

Review Coding Guidelines B3.11a, B3.11b and B3.11c

07JK0ZZ	Inspection of Thoracic Duct, Open Approach
07JK3ZZ	Inspection of Thoracic Duct, Percutaneous Approach
07JK4ZZ	Inspection of Thoracic Duct, Percutaneous Endoscopic Approach
07JL0ZZ	Inspection of Cisterna Chyli, Open Approach
07JL3ZZ	Inspection of Cisterna Chyli, Percutaneous Approach
07JL4ZZ	Inspection of Cisterna Chyli, Percutaneous Endoscopic Approach
07JM0ZZ	Inspection of Thymus, Open Approach
07JM3ZZ	Inspection of Thymus, Percutaneous Approach
07JM4ZZ	Inspection of Thymus, Percutaneous Endoscopic Approach
07JN0ZZ	Inspection of Lymphatic, Open Approach

07JN3ZZ	Inspection of Lymphatic, Percutaneous Approach
07JN4ZZ	Inspection of Lymphatic, Percutaneous Endoscopic Approach
07JNXZZ	Inspection of Lymphatic, External Approach
07JP0ZZ	Inspection of Spleen, Open Approach
07JP3ZZ	Inspection of Spleen, Percutaneous Approach
07JP4ZZ	Inspection of Spleen, Percutaneous Endoscopic Approach
07JPXZZ	Inspection of Spleen, External Approach
07JT0ZZ	Inspection of Bone Marrow, Open Approach
07JT3ZZ	Inspection of Bone Marrow, Percutaneous Approach
07JT4ZZ	Inspection of Bone Marrow, Percutaneous Endoscopic Approach

07L – Lymphatic and Hemic Systems, Occlusion

07L00CZ	Occlusion of Head Lymphatic with Extraluminal Device, Open Approach
07L00DZ	Occlusion of Head Lymphatic with Intraluminal Device, Open Approach
07L00ZZ	Occlusion of Head Lymphatic, Open Approach
07L03CZ	Occlusion of Head Lymphatic with Extraluminal Device, Percutaneous Approach
07L03DZ	Occlusion of Head Lymphatic with Intraluminal Device, Percutaneous Approach
07L03ZZ	Occlusion of Head Lymphatic, Percutaneous Approach
07L04CZ	Occlusion of Head Lymphatic with Extraluminal Device, Percutaneous Endoscopic Approach
07L04DZ	Occlusion of Head Lymphatic with Intraluminal Device, Percutaneous Endoscopic Approach
07L04ZZ	Occlusion of Head Lymphatic, Percutaneous Endoscopic Approach
07L10CZ	Occlusion of Right Neck Lymphatic with Extraluminal Device, Open Approach
07L10DZ	Occlusion of Right Neck Lymphatic with Intraluminal Device, Open Approach
07L10ZZ	Occlusion of Right Neck Lymphatic, Open Approach
07L13CZ	Occlusion of Right Neck Lymphatic with Extraluminal Device, Percutaneous Approach
07L13DZ	Occlusion of Right Neck Lymphatic with Intraluminal Device, Percutaneous Approach
07L13ZZ	Occlusion of Right Neck Lymphatic, Percutaneous Approach
07L14CZ	Occlusion of Right Neck Lymphatic with Extraluminal Device, Percutaneous Endoscopic Approach
07L14DZ	Occlusion of Right Neck Lymphatic with Intraluminal Device, Percutaneous Endoscopic Approach
07L14ZZ	Occlusion of Right Neck Lymphatic, Percutaneous Endoscopic Approach
07L20CZ	Occlusion of Left Neck Lymphatic with Extraluminal Device, Open Approach
07L20DZ	Occlusion of Left Neck Lymphatic with Intraluminal Device, Open Approach
07L20ZZ	Occlusion of Left Neck Lymphatic, Open Approach
07L23CZ	Occlusion of Left Neck Lymphatic with Extraluminal Device, Percutaneous Approach
07L23DZ	Occlusion of Left Neck Lymphatic with Intraluminal Device, Percutaneous Approach
07L23ZZ	Occlusion of Left Neck Lymphatic, Percutaneous Approach
07L24CZ	Occlusion of Left Neck Lymphatic with Extraluminal Device, Percutaneous Endoscopic Approach
07L24DZ	Occlusion of Left Neck Lymphatic with Intraluminal Device, Percutaneous Endoscopic Approach
07L24ZZ	Occlusion of Left Neck Lymphatic, Percutaneous Endoscopic Approach
07L30CZ	Occlusion of Right Upper Extremity Lymphatic with Extraluminal Device, Open Approach
07L30DZ	Occlusion of Right Upper Extremity Lymphatic with Intraluminal Device, Open Approach
07L30ZZ	Occlusion of Right Upper Extremity Lymphatic, Open Approach

07L33CZ	Occlusion of Right Upper Extremity Lymphatic with Extraluminal Device, Percutaneous Approach
07L33DZ	Occlusion of Right Upper Extremity Lymphatic with Intraluminal Device, Percutaneous Approach
07L33ZZ	Occlusion of Right Upper Extremity Lymphatic, Percutaneous Approach
07L34CZ	Occlusion of Right Upper Extremity Lymphatic with Extraluminal Device, Percutaneous Endoscopic Approach
07L34DZ	Occlusion of Right Upper Extremity Lymphatic with Intraluminal Device, Percutaneous Endoscopic Approach
07L34ZZ	Occlusion of Right Upper Extremity Lymphatic, Percutaneous Endoscopic Approach
07L40CZ	Occlusion of Left Upper Extremity Lymphatic with Extraluminal Device, Open Approach
07L40DZ	Occlusion of Left Upper Extremity Lymphatic with Intraluminal Device, Open Approach
07L40ZZ	Occlusion of Left Upper Extremity Lymphatic, Open Approach
07L43CZ	Occlusion of Left Upper Extremity Lymphatic with Extraluminal Device, Percutaneous Approach
07L43DZ	Occlusion of Left Upper Extremity Lymphatic with Intraluminal Device, Percutaneous Approach
07L43ZZ	Occlusion of Left Upper Extremity Lymphatic, Percutaneous Approach
07L44CZ	Occlusion of Left Upper Extremity Lymphatic with Extraluminal Device, Percutaneous Endoscopic Approach
07L44DZ	Occlusion of Left Upper Extremity Lymphatic with Intraluminal Device, Percutaneous Endoscopic Approach
07L44ZZ	Occlusion of Left Upper Extremity Lymphatic, Percutaneous Endoscopic Approach
07L50CZ	Occlusion of Right Axillary Lymphatic with Extraluminal Device, Open Approach
07L50DZ	Occlusion of Right Axillary Lymphatic with Intraluminal Device, Open Approach
07L50ZZ	Occlusion of Right Axillary Lymphatic, Open Approach
07L53CZ	Occlusion of Right Axillary Lymphatic with Extraluminal Device, Percutaneous Approach
07L53DZ	Occlusion of Right Axillary Lymphatic with Intraluminal Device, Percutaneous Approach
07L53ZZ	Occlusion of Right Axillary Lymphatic, Percutaneous Approach
07L54CZ	Occlusion of Right Axillary Lymphatic with Extraluminal Device, Percutaneous Endoscopic Approach
07L54DZ	Occlusion of Right Axillary Lymphatic with Intraluminal Device, Percutaneous Endoscopic Approach
07L54ZZ	Occlusion of Right Axillary Lymphatic, Percutaneous Endoscopic Approach
07L60CZ	Occlusion of Left Axillary Lymphatic with Extraluminal Device, Open Approach
07L60DZ	Occlusion of Left Axillary Lymphatic with Intraluminal Device, Open Approach
07L60ZZ	Occlusion of Left Axillary Lymphatic, Open Approach
07L63CZ	Occlusion of Left Axillary Lymphatic with Extraluminal Device, Percutaneous Approach

07L63DZ Occlusion of Left Axillary Lymphatic with Intraluminal Device, Percutaneous Approach

07L63ZZ Occlusion of Left Axillary Lymphatic, Percutaneous Approach

07L64CZ Occlusion of Left Axillary Lymphatic with Extraluminal Device, Percutaneous Endoscopic Approach

07L64DZ Occlusion of Left Axillary Lymphatic with Intraluminal Device, Percutaneous Endoscopic Approach

07L64ZZ Occlusion of Left Axillary Lymphatic, Percutaneous Endoscopic Approach

07L70CZ Occlusion of Thorax Lymphatic with Extraluminal Device, Open Approach

07L70DZ Occlusion of Thorax Lymphatic with Intraluminal Device, Open Approach

07L70ZZ Occlusion of Thorax Lymphatic, Open Approach

07L73CZ Occlusion of Thorax Lymphatic with Extraluminal Device, Percutaneous Approach

07L73DZ Occlusion of Thorax Lymphatic with Intraluminal Device, Percutaneous Approach

07L73ZZ Occlusion of Thorax Lymphatic, Percutaneous Approach

07L74CZ Occlusion of Thorax Lymphatic with Extraluminal Device, Percutaneous Endoscopic Approach

07L74DZ Occlusion of Thorax Lymphatic with Intraluminal Device, Percutaneous Endoscopic Approach

07L74ZZ Occlusion of Thorax Lymphatic, Percutaneous Endoscopic Approach

07L80CZ Occlusion of Right Internal Mammary Lymphatic with Extraluminal Device, Open Approach

07L80DZ Occlusion of Right Internal Mammary Lymphatic with Intraluminal Device, Open Approach

07L80ZZ Occlusion of Right Internal Mammary Lymphatic, Open Approach

07L83CZ Occlusion of Right Internal Mammary Lymphatic with Extraluminal Device, Percutaneous Approach

07L83DZ Occlusion of Right Internal Mammary Lymphatic with Intraluminal Device, Percutaneous Approach

07L83ZZ Occlusion of Right Internal Mammary Lymphatic, Percutaneous Approach

07L84CZ Occlusion of Right Internal Mammary Lymphatic with Extraluminal Device, Percutaneous Endoscopic Approach

07L84DZ Occlusion of Right Internal Mammary Lymphatic with Intraluminal Device, Percutaneous Endoscopic Approach

07L84ZZ Occlusion of Right Internal Mammary Lymphatic, Percutaneous Endoscopic Approach

07L90CZ Occlusion of Left Internal Mammary Lymphatic with Extraluminal Device, Open Approach

07L90DZ Occlusion of Left Internal Mammary Lymphatic with Intraluminal Device, Open Approach

07L90ZZ Occlusion of Left Internal Mammary Lymphatic, Open Approach

07L93CZ Occlusion of Left Internal Mammary Lymphatic with Extraluminal Device, Percutaneous Approach

07L93DZ Occlusion of Left Internal Mammary Lymphatic with Intraluminal Device, Percutaneous Approach

07L93ZZ Occlusion of Left Internal Mammary Lymphatic, Percutaneous Approach

07L94CZ Occlusion of Left Internal Mammary Lymphatic with Extraluminal Device, Percutaneous Endoscopic Approach

07L94DZ Occlusion of Left Internal Mammary Lymphatic with Intraluminal Device, Percutaneous Endoscopic Approach

07L94ZZ Occlusion of Left Internal Mammary Lymphatic, Percutaneous Endoscopic Approach

07LB0CZ Occlusion of Mesenteric Lymphatic with Extraluminal Device, Open Approach

07LB0DZ Occlusion of Mesenteric Lymphatic with Intraluminal Device, Open Approach

07LB0ZZ Occlusion of Mesenteric Lymphatic, Open Approach

07LB3CZ Occlusion of Mesenteric Lymphatic with Extraluminal Device, Percutaneous Approach

07LB3DZ Occlusion of Mesenteric Lymphatic with Intraluminal Device, Percutaneous Approach

07LB3ZZ Occlusion of Mesenteric Lymphatic, Percutaneous Approach

07LB4CZ Occlusion of Mesenteric Lymphatic with Extraluminal Device, Percutaneous Endoscopic Approach

07LB4DZ Occlusion of Mesenteric Lymphatic with Intraluminal Device, Percutaneous Endoscopic Approach

07LB4ZZ Occlusion of Mesenteric Lymphatic, Percutaneous Endoscopic Approach

07LC0CZ Occlusion of Pelvis Lymphatic with Extraluminal Device, Open Approach

07LC0DZ Occlusion of Pelvis Lymphatic with Intraluminal Device, Open Approach

07LC0ZZ Occlusion of Pelvis Lymphatic, Open Approach

07LC3CZ Occlusion of Pelvis Lymphatic with Extraluminal Device, Percutaneous Approach

07LC3DZ Occlusion of Pelvis Lymphatic with Intraluminal Device, Percutaneous Approach

07LC3ZZ Occlusion of Pelvis Lymphatic, Percutaneous Approach

07LC4CZ Occlusion of Pelvis Lymphatic with Extraluminal Device, Percutaneous Endoscopic Approach

07LC4DZ Occlusion of Pelvis Lymphatic with Intraluminal Device, Percutaneous Endoscopic Approach

07LC4ZZ Occlusion of Pelvis Lymphatic, Percutaneous Endoscopic Approach

07LD0CZ Occlusion of Aortic Lymphatic with Extraluminal Device, Open Approach

07LD0DZ Occlusion of Aortic Lymphatic with Intraluminal Device, Open Approach

07LD0ZZ Occlusion of Aortic Lymphatic, Open Approach

07LD3CZ Occlusion of Aortic Lymphatic with Extraluminal Device, Percutaneous Approach

07LD3DZ Occlusion of Aortic Lymphatic with Intraluminal Device, Percutaneous Approach

07LD3ZZ Occlusion of Aortic Lymphatic, Percutaneous Approach

07LD4CZ Occlusion of Aortic Lymphatic with Extraluminal Device, Percutaneous Endoscopic Approach

07LD4DZ Occlusion of Aortic Lymphatic with Intraluminal Device, Percutaneous Endoscopic Approach

07LD4ZZ Occlusion of Aortic Lymphatic, Percutaneous Endoscopic Approach

07LF0CZ Occlusion of Right Lower Extremity Lymphatic with Extraluminal Device, Open Approach

07LF0DZ Occlusion of Right Lower Extremity Lymphatic with Intraluminal Device, Open Approach

07LF0ZZ Occlusion of Right Lower Extremity Lymphatic, Open Approach

07LF3CZ Occlusion of Right Lower Extremity Lymphatic with Extraluminal Device, Percutaneous Approach

07LF3DZ Occlusion of Right Lower Extremity Lymphatic with Intraluminal Device, Percutaneous Approach

07LF3ZZ Occlusion of Right Lower Extremity Lymphatic, Percutaneous Approach

07LF4CZ Occlusion of Right Lower Extremity Lymphatic with Extraluminal Device, Percutaneous Endoscopic Approach

07LF4DZ Occlusion of Right Lower Extremity Lymphatic with Intraluminal Device, Percutaneous Endoscopic Approach

07LF4ZZ Occlusion of Right Lower Extremity Lymphatic, Percutaneous Endoscopic Approach

07LG0CZ Occlusion of Left Lower Extremity Lymphatic with Extraluminal Device, Open Approach

07LG0DZ Occlusion of Left Lower Extremity Lymphatic with Intraluminal Device, Open Approach

07LG0ZZ Occlusion of Left Lower Extremity Lymphatic, Open Approach

07LG3CZ Occlusion of Left Lower Extremity Lymphatic with Extraluminal Device, Percutaneous Approach

07LG3DZ Occlusion of Left Lower Extremity Lymphatic with Intraluminal Device, Percutaneous Approach

07LG3ZZ Occlusion of Left Lower Extremity Lymphatic, Percutaneous Approach

07LG4CZ Occlusion of Left Lower Extremity Lymphatic with Extraluminal Device, Percutaneous Endoscopic Approach

07LG4DZ Occlusion of Left Lower Extremity Lymphatic with Intraluminal Device, Percutaneous Endoscopic Approach

07LG4ZZ Occlusion of Left Lower Extremity Lymphatic, Percutaneous Endoscopic Approach

07LH0CZ Occlusion of Right Inguinal Lymphatic with Extraluminal Device, Open Approach

07LH0DZ Occlusion of Right Inguinal Lymphatic with Intraluminal Device, Open Approach

07LH0ZZ Occlusion of Right Inguinal Lymphatic, Open Approach

07LH3CZ Occlusion of Right Inguinal Lymphatic with Extraluminal Device, Percutaneous Approach

07LH3DZ   Occlusion of Right Inguinal Lymphatic with Intraluminal Device, Percutaneous Approach

07LH3ZZ   Occlusion of Right Inguinal Lymphatic, Percutaneous Approach

07LH4CZ   Occlusion of Right Inguinal Lymphatic with Extraluminal Device, Percutaneous Endoscopic Approach

07LH4DZ   Occlusion of Right Inguinal Lymphatic with Intraluminal Device, Percutaneous Endoscopic Approach

07LH4ZZ   Occlusion of Right Inguinal Lymphatic, Percutaneous Endoscopic Approach

07LJ0CZ   Occlusion of Left Inguinal Lymphatic with Extraluminal Device, Open Approach

07LJ0DZ   Occlusion of Left Inguinal Lymphatic with Intraluminal Device, Open Approach

07LJ0ZZ   Occlusion of Left Inguinal Lymphatic, Open Approach

07LJ3CZ   Occlusion of Left Inguinal Lymphatic with Extraluminal Device, Percutaneous Approach

07LJ3DZ   Occlusion of Left Inguinal Lymphatic with Intraluminal Device, Percutaneous Approach

07LJ3ZZ   Occlusion of Left Inguinal Lymphatic, Percutaneous Approach

07LJ4CZ   Occlusion of Left Inguinal Lymphatic with Extraluminal Device, Percutaneous Endoscopic Approach

07LJ4DZ   Occlusion of Left Inguinal Lymphatic with Intraluminal Device, Percutaneous Endoscopic Approach

07LJ4ZZ   Occlusion of Left Inguinal Lymphatic, Percutaneous Endoscopic Approach

07LK0CZ   Occlusion of Thoracic Duct with Extraluminal Device, Open Approach

07LK0DZ   Occlusion of Thoracic Duct with Intraluminal Device, Open Approach

07LK0ZZ   Occlusion of Thoracic Duct, Open Approach

07LK3CZ   Occlusion of Thoracic Duct with Extraluminal Device, Percutaneous Approach

07LK3DZ   Occlusion of Thoracic Duct with Intraluminal Device, Percutaneous Approach

07LK3ZZ   Occlusion of Thoracic Duct, Percutaneous Approach

07LK4CZ   Occlusion of Thoracic Duct with Extraluminal Device, Percutaneous Endoscopic Approach

07LK4DZ   Occlusion of Thoracic Duct with Intraluminal Device, Percutaneous Endoscopic Approach

07LK4ZZ   Occlusion of Thoracic Duct, Percutaneous Endoscopic Approach

07LL0CZ   Occlusion of Cisterna Chyli with Extraluminal Device, Open Approach

07LL0DZ   Occlusion of Cisterna Chyli with Intraluminal Device, Open Approach

07LL0ZZ   Occlusion of Cisterna Chyli, Open Approach

07LL3CZ   Occlusion of Cisterna Chyli with Extraluminal Device, Percutaneous Approach

07LL3DZ   Occlusion of Cisterna Chyli with Intraluminal Device, Percutaneous Approach

07LL3ZZ   Occlusion of Cisterna Chyli, Percutaneous Approach

07LL4CZ   Occlusion of Cisterna Chyli with Extraluminal Device, Percutaneous Endoscopic Approach

07LL4DZ   Occlusion of Cisterna Chyli with Intraluminal Device, Percutaneous Endoscopic Approach

07LL4ZZ   Occlusion of Cisterna Chyli, Percutaneous Endoscopic Approach

07N – Lymphatic and Hemic Systems, Release

Review Coding Guidelines B3.13 and B3.14

07N00ZZ   Release Head Lymphatic, Open Approach
07N03ZZ   Release Head Lymphatic, Percutaneous Approach
07N04ZZ   Release Head Lymphatic, Percutaneous Endoscopic Approach
07N10ZZ   Release Right Neck Lymphatic, Open Approach
07N13ZZ   Release Right Neck Lymphatic, Percutaneous Approach
07N14ZZ   Release Right Neck Lymphatic, Percutaneous Endoscopic Approach
07N20ZZ   Release Left Neck Lymphatic, Open Approach
07N23ZZ   Release Left Neck Lymphatic, Percutaneous Approach
07N24ZZ   Release Left Neck Lymphatic, Percutaneous Endoscopic Approach
07N30ZZ   Release Right Upper Extremity Lymphatic, Open Approach
07N33ZZ   Release Right Upper Extremity Lymphatic, Percutaneous Approach
07N34ZZ   Release Right Upper Extremity Lymphatic, Percutaneous Endoscopic Approach
07N40ZZ   Release Left Upper Extremity Lymphatic, Open Approach
07N43ZZ   Release Left Upper Extremity Lymphatic, Percutaneous Approach
07N44ZZ   Release Left Upper Extremity Lymphatic, Percutaneous Endoscopic Approach
07N50ZZ   Release Right Axillary Lymphatic, Open Approach
07N53ZZ   Release Right Axillary Lymphatic, Percutaneous Approach
07N54ZZ   Release Right Axillary Lymphatic, Percutaneous Endoscopic Approach
07N60ZZ   Release Left Axillary Lymphatic, Open Approach
07N63ZZ   Release Left Axillary Lymphatic, Percutaneous Approach
07N64ZZ   Release Left Axillary Lymphatic, Percutaneous Endoscopic Approach
07N70ZZ   Release Thorax Lymphatic, Open Approach
07N73ZZ   Release Thorax Lymphatic, Percutaneous Approach
07N74ZZ   Release Thorax Lymphatic, Percutaneous Endoscopic Approach
07N80ZZ   Release Right Internal Mammary Lymphatic, Open Approach
07N83ZZ   Release Right Internal Mammary Lymphatic, Percutaneous Approach
07N84ZZ   Release Right Internal Mammary Lymphatic, Percutaneous Endoscopic Approach
07N90ZZ   Release Left Internal Mammary Lymphatic, Open Approach
07N93ZZ   Release Left Internal Mammary Lymphatic, Percutaneous Approach
07N94ZZ   Release Left Internal Mammary Lymphatic, Percutaneous Endoscopic Approach

07NB0ZZ   Release Mesenteric Lymphatic, Open Approach
07NB3ZZ   Release Mesenteric Lymphatic, Percutaneous Approach
07NB4ZZ   Release Mesenteric Lymphatic, Percutaneous Endoscopic Approach
07NC0ZZ   Release Pelvis Lymphatic, Open Approach
07NC3ZZ   Release Pelvis Lymphatic, Percutaneous Approach
07NC4ZZ   Release Pelvis Lymphatic, Percutaneous Endoscopic Approach
07ND0ZZ   Release Aortic Lymphatic, Open Approach
07ND3ZZ   Release Aortic Lymphatic, Percutaneous Approach
07ND4ZZ   Release Aortic Lymphatic, Percutaneous Endoscopic Approach
07NF0ZZ   Release Right Lower Extremity Lymphatic, Open Approach
07NF3ZZ   Release Right Lower Extremity Lymphatic, Percutaneous Approach
07NF4ZZ   Release Right Lower Extremity Lymphatic, Percutaneous Endoscopic Approach
07NG0ZZ   Release Left Lower Extremity Lymphatic, Open Approach
07NG3ZZ   Release Left Lower Extremity Lymphatic, Percutaneous Approach
07NG4ZZ   Release Left Lower Extremity Lymphatic, Percutaneous Endoscopic Approach
07NH0ZZ   Release Right Inguinal Lymphatic, Open Approach
07NH3ZZ   Release Right Inguinal Lymphatic, Percutaneous Approach
07NH4ZZ   Release Right Inguinal Lymphatic, Percutaneous Endoscopic Approach
07NJ0ZZ   Release Left Inguinal Lymphatic, Open Approach
07NJ3ZZ   Release Left Inguinal Lymphatic, Percutaneous Approach
07NJ4ZZ   Release Left Inguinal Lymphatic, Percutaneous Endoscopic Approach
07NK0ZZ   Release Thoracic Duct, Open Approach
07NK3ZZ   Release Thoracic Duct, Percutaneous Approach
07NK4ZZ   Release Thoracic Duct, Percutaneous Endoscopic Approach
07NL0ZZ   Release Cisterna Chyli, Open Approach
07NL3ZZ   Release Cisterna Chyli, Percutaneous Approach
07NL4ZZ   Release Cisterna Chyli, Percutaneous Endoscopic Approach
07NM0ZZ   Release Thymus, Open Approach
07NM3ZZ   Release Thymus, Percutaneous Approach
07NM4ZZ   Release Thymus, Percutaneous Endoscopic Approach
07NP0ZZ   Release Spleen, Open Approach
07NP3ZZ   Release Spleen, Percutaneous Approach
07NP4ZZ   Release Spleen, Percutaneous Endoscopic Approach

♀ Female-only   ♂ Male-only   ● Limited Coverage   ● Non-OR   ᴴᴬᶜ HAC-associated procedure   ● Non-covered procedures   ✚ Combination

07P – Lymphatic and Hemic Systems, Removal

Review Coding Guideline B6.1c

07PK00Z Removal of Drainage Device from Thoracic Duct, Open Approach

07PK03Z Removal of Infusion Device from Thoracic Duct, Open Approach

07PK07Z Removal of Autologous Tissue Substitute from Thoracic Duct, Open Approach

07PK0CZ Removal of Extraluminal Device from Thoracic Duct, Open Approach

07PK0DZ Removal of Intraluminal Device from Thoracic Duct, Open Approach

07PK0JZ Removal of Synthetic Substitute from Thoracic Duct, Open Approach

07PK0KZ Removal of Nonautologous Tissue Substitute from Thoracic Duct, Open Approach

07PK30Z Removal of Drainage Device from Thoracic Duct, Percutaneous Approach

07PK33Z Removal of Infusion Device from Thoracic Duct, Percutaneous Approach

07PK37Z Removal of Autologous Tissue Substitute from Thoracic Duct, Percutaneous Approach

07PK3CZ Removal of Extraluminal Device from Thoracic Duct, Percutaneous Approach

07PK3DZ Removal of Intraluminal Device from Thoracic Duct, Percutaneous Approach

07PK3JZ Removal of Synthetic Substitute from Thoracic Duct, Percutaneous Approach

07PK3KZ Removal of Nonautologous Tissue Substitute from Thoracic Duct, Percutaneous Approach

07PK40Z Removal of Drainage Device from Thoracic Duct, Percutaneous Endoscopic Approach

07PK43Z Removal of Infusion Device from Thoracic Duct, Percutaneous Endoscopic Approach

07PK47Z Removal of Autologous Tissue Substitute from Thoracic Duct, Percutaneous Endoscopic Approach

07PK4CZ Removal of Extraluminal Device from Thoracic Duct, Percutaneous Endoscopic Approach

07PK4DZ Removal of Intraluminal Device from Thoracic Duct, Percutaneous Endoscopic Approach

07PK4JZ Removal of Synthetic Substitute from Thoracic Duct, Percutaneous Endoscopic Approach

07PK4KZ Removal of Nonautologous Tissue Substitute from Thoracic Duct, Percutaneous Endoscopic Approach

07PKX0Z Removal of Drainage Device from Thoracic Duct, External Approach

07PKX3Z Removal of Infusion Device from Thoracic Duct, External Approach

07PKXDZ Removal of Intraluminal Device from Thoracic Duct, External Approach

07PL00Z Removal of Drainage Device from Cisterna Chyli, Open Approach

07PL03Z Removal of Infusion Device from Cisterna Chyli, Open Approach

07PL07Z Removal of Autologous Tissue Substitute from Cisterna Chyli, Open Approach

07PL0CZ Removal of Extraluminal Device from Cisterna Chyli, Open Approach

07PL0DZ Removal of Intraluminal Device from Cisterna Chyli, Open Approach

07PL0JZ Removal of Synthetic Substitute from Cisterna Chyli, Open Approach

07PL0KZ Removal of Nonautologous Tissue Substitute from Cisterna Chyli, Open Approach

07PL30Z Removal of Drainage Device from Cisterna Chyli, Percutaneous Approach

07PL33Z Removal of Infusion Device from Cisterna Chyli, Percutaneous Approach

07PL37Z Removal of Autologous Tissue Substitute from Cisterna Chyli, Percutaneous Approach

07PL3CZ Removal of Extraluminal Device from Cisterna Chyli, Percutaneous Approach

07PL3DZ Removal of Intraluminal Device from Cisterna Chyli, Percutaneous Approach

07PL3JZ Removal of Synthetic Substitute from Cisterna Chyli, Percutaneous Approach

07PL3KZ Removal of Nonautologous Tissue Substitute from Cisterna Chyli, Percutaneous Approach

07PL40Z Removal of Drainage Device from Cisterna Chyli, Percutaneous Endoscopic Approach

07PL43Z Removal of Infusion Device from Cisterna Chyli, Percutaneous Endoscopic Approach

07PL47Z Removal of Autologous Tissue Substitute from Cisterna Chyli, Percutaneous Endoscopic Approach

07PL4CZ Removal of Extraluminal Device from Cisterna Chyli, Percutaneous Endoscopic Approach

07PL4DZ Removal of Intraluminal Device from Cisterna Chyli, Percutaneous Endoscopic Approach

07PL4JZ Removal of Synthetic Substitute from Cisterna Chyli, Percutaneous Endoscopic Approach

07PL4KZ Removal of Nonautologous Tissue Substitute from Cisterna Chyli, Percutaneous Endoscopic Approach

07PLX0Z Removal of Drainage Device from Cisterna Chyli, External Approach

07PLX3Z Removal of Infusion Device from Cisterna Chyli, External Approach

07PLXDZ Removal of Intraluminal Device from Cisterna Chyli, External Approach

07PM00Z Removal of Drainage Device from Thymus, Open Approach

07PM03Z Removal of Infusion Device from Thymus, Open Approach

07PM30Z Removal of Drainage Device from Thymus, Percutaneous Approach

07PM33Z Removal of Infusion Device from Thymus, Percutaneous Approach

07PM40Z Removal of Drainage Device from Thymus, Percutaneous Endoscopic Approach

07PM43Z Removal of Infusion Device from Thymus, Percutaneous Endoscopic Approach

07PMX0Z Removal of Drainage Device from Thymus, External Approach

07PMX3Z Removal of Infusion Device from Thymus, External Approach

07PN00Z Removal of Drainage Device from Lymphatic, Open Approach

07PN03Z Removal of Infusion Device from Lymphatic, Open Approach

07PN07Z Removal of Autologous Tissue Substitute from Lymphatic, Open Approach

07PN0CZ Removal of Extraluminal Device from Lymphatic, Open Approach

07PN0DZ Removal of Intraluminal Device from Lymphatic, Open Approach

07PN0JZ Removal of Synthetic Substitute from Lymphatic, Open Approach

07PN0KZ Removal of Nonautologous Tissue Substitute from Lymphatic, Open Approach

07PN30Z Removal of Drainage Device from Lymphatic, Percutaneous Approach

07PN33Z Removal of Infusion Device from Lymphatic, Percutaneous Approach

07PN37Z Removal of Autologous Tissue Substitute from Lymphatic, Percutaneous Approach

07PN3CZ Removal of Extraluminal Device from Lymphatic, Percutaneous Approach

07PN3DZ Removal of Intraluminal Device from Lymphatic, Percutaneous Approach

07PN3JZ Removal of Synthetic Substitute from Lymphatic, Percutaneous Approach

07PN3KZ Removal of Nonautologous Tissue Substitute from Lymphatic, Percutaneous Approach

07PN40Z Removal of Drainage Device from Lymphatic, Percutaneous Endoscopic Approach

07PN43Z Removal of Infusion Device from Lymphatic, Percutaneous Endoscopic Approach

07PN47Z Removal of Autologous Tissue Substitute from Lymphatic, Percutaneous Endoscopic Approach

07PN4CZ Removal of Extraluminal Device from Lymphatic, Percutaneous Endoscopic Approach

07PN4DZ Removal of Intraluminal Device from Lymphatic, Percutaneous Endoscopic Approach

07PN4JZ Removal of Synthetic Substitute from Lymphatic, Percutaneous Endoscopic Approach

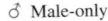 Female-only   ♂ Male-only   ● Limited Coverage   ● Non-OR   🅷🅰🅲 HAC-associated procedure   ● Non-covered procedures   ➕ Combination

07PN4KZ Removal of Nonautologous Tissue Substitute from Lymphatic, Percutaneous Endoscopic Approach
07PNX0Z Removal of Drainage Device from Lymphatic, External Approach
07PNX3Z Removal of Infusion Device from Lymphatic, External Approach
07PNXDZ Removal of Intraluminal Device from Lymphatic, External Approach
07PP00Z Removal of Drainage Device from Spleen, Open Approach
07PP03Z Removal of Infusion Device from Spleen, Open Approach
07PP30Z Removal of Drainage Device from Spleen, Percutaneous Approach
07PP33Z Removal of Infusion Device from Spleen, Percutaneous Approach
07PP40Z Removal of Drainage Device from Spleen, Percutaneous Endoscopic Approach

07PP43Z Removal of Infusion Device from Spleen, Percutaneous Endoscopic Approach
07PPX0Z Removal of Drainage Device from Spleen, External Approach
07PPX3Z Removal of Infusion Device from Spleen, External Approach
07PT00Z Removal of Drainage Device from Bone Marrow, Open Approach
07PT30Z Removal of Drainage Device from Bone Marrow, Percutaneous Approach
07PT40Z Removal of Drainage Device from Bone Marrow, Percutaneous Endoscopic Approach
07PTX0Z Removal of Drainage Device from Bone Marrow, External Approach

07Q – Lymphatic and Hemic Systems, Repair

07Q00ZZ Repair Head Lymphatic, Open Approach
07Q03ZZ Repair Head Lymphatic, Percutaneous Approach
07Q04ZZ Repair Head Lymphatic, Percutaneous Endoscopic Approach
07Q10ZZ Repair Right Neck Lymphatic, Open Approach
07Q13ZZ Repair Right Neck Lymphatic, Percutaneous Approach
07Q14ZZ Repair Right Neck Lymphatic, Percutaneous Endoscopic Approach
07Q20ZZ Repair Left Neck Lymphatic, Open Approach
07Q23ZZ Repair Left Neck Lymphatic, Percutaneous Approach
07Q24ZZ Repair Left Neck Lymphatic, Percutaneous Endoscopic Approach
07Q30ZZ Repair Right Upper Extremity Lymphatic, Open Approach
07Q33ZZ Repair Right Upper Extremity Lymphatic, Percutaneous Approach
07Q34ZZ Repair Right Upper Extremity Lymphatic, Percutaneous Endoscopic Approach
07Q40ZZ Repair Left Upper Extremity Lymphatic, Open Approach
07Q43ZZ Repair Left Upper Extremity Lymphatic, Percutaneous Approach
07Q44ZZ Repair Left Upper Extremity Lymphatic, Percutaneous Endoscopic Approach
07Q50ZZ Repair Right Axillary Lymphatic, Open Approach
07Q53ZZ Repair Right Axillary Lymphatic, Percutaneous Approach
07Q54ZZ Repair Right Axillary Lymphatic, Percutaneous Endoscopic Approach
07Q60ZZ Repair Left Axillary Lymphatic, Open Approach
07Q63ZZ Repair Left Axillary Lymphatic, Percutaneous Approach
07Q64ZZ Repair Left Axillary Lymphatic, Percutaneous Endoscopic Approach
07Q70ZZ Repair Thorax Lymphatic, Open Approach
07Q73ZZ Repair Thorax Lymphatic, Percutaneous Approach
07Q74ZZ Repair Thorax Lymphatic, Percutaneous Endoscopic Approach
07Q80ZZ Repair Right Internal Mammary Lymphatic, Open Approach
07Q83ZZ Repair Right Internal Mammary Lymphatic, Percutaneous Approach
07Q84ZZ Repair Right Internal Mammary Lymphatic, Percutaneous Endoscopic Approach
07Q90ZZ Repair Left Internal Mammary Lymphatic, Open Approach
07Q93ZZ Repair Left Internal Mammary Lymphatic, Percutaneous Approach
07Q94ZZ Repair Left Internal Mammary Lymphatic, Percutaneous Endoscopic Approach
07QB0ZZ Repair Mesenteric Lymphatic, Open Approach

07QB3ZZ Repair Mesenteric Lymphatic, Percutaneous Approach
07QB4ZZ Repair Mesenteric Lymphatic, Percutaneous Endoscopic Approach
07QC0ZZ Repair Pelvis Lymphatic, Open Approach
07QC3ZZ Repair Pelvis Lymphatic, Percutaneous Approach
07QC4ZZ Repair Pelvis Lymphatic, Percutaneous Endoscopic Approach
07QD0ZZ Repair Aortic Lymphatic, Open Approach
07QD3ZZ Repair Aortic Lymphatic, Percutaneous Approach
07QD4ZZ Repair Aortic Lymphatic, Percutaneous Endoscopic Approach
07QF0ZZ Repair Right Lower Extremity Lymphatic, Open Approach
07QF3ZZ Repair Right Lower Extremity Lymphatic, Percutaneous Approach
07QF4ZZ Repair Right Lower Extremity Lymphatic, Percutaneous Endoscopic Approach
07QG0ZZ Repair Left Lower Extremity Lymphatic, Open Approach
07QG3ZZ Repair Left Lower Extremity Lymphatic, Percutaneous Approach
07QG4ZZ Repair Left Lower Extremity Lymphatic, Percutaneous Endoscopic Approach
07QH0ZZ Repair Right Inguinal Lymphatic, Open Approach
07QH3ZZ Repair Right Inguinal Lymphatic, Percutaneous Approach
07QH4ZZ Repair Right Inguinal Lymphatic, Percutaneous Endoscopic Approach
07QJ0ZZ Repair Left Inguinal Lymphatic, Open Approach
07QJ3ZZ Repair Left Inguinal Lymphatic, Percutaneous Approach
07QJ4ZZ Repair Left Inguinal Lymphatic, Percutaneous Endoscopic Approach
07QK0ZZ Repair Thoracic Duct, Open Approach
07QK3ZZ Repair Thoracic Duct, Percutaneous Approach
07QK4ZZ Repair Thoracic Duct, Percutaneous Endoscopic Approach
07QL0ZZ Repair Cisterna Chyli, Open Approach
07QL3ZZ Repair Cisterna Chyli, Percutaneous Approach
07QL4ZZ Repair Cisterna Chyli, Percutaneous Endoscopic Approach
07QM0ZZ Repair Thymus, Open Approach
07QM3ZZ Repair Thymus, Percutaneous Approach
07QM4ZZ Repair Thymus, Percutaneous Endoscopic Approach
07QP0ZZ Repair Spleen, Open Approach
07QP3ZZ Repair Spleen, Percutaneous Approach
07QP4ZZ Repair Spleen, Percutaneous Endoscopic Approach

07S – Lymphatic and Hemic Systems, Reposition

07SM0ZZ Reposition Thymus, Open Approach
07SP0ZZ Reposition Spleen, Open Approach

07T – Lymphatic and Hemic Systems, Resection

Review Coding Guideline B3.8

07T00ZZ Resection of Head Lymphatic, Open Approach
07T04ZZ Resection of Head Lymphatic, Percutaneous Endoscopic Approach
07T10ZZ Resection of Right Neck Lymphatic, Open Approach
07T14ZZ Resection of Right Neck Lymphatic, Percutaneous Endoscopic Approach
07T20ZZ Resection of Left Neck Lymphatic, Open Approach
07T24ZZ Resection of Left Neck Lymphatic, Percutaneous Endoscopic Approach
07T30ZZ Resection of Right Upper Extremity Lymphatic, Open Approach

07T34ZZ Resection of Right Upper Extremity Lymphatic, Percutaneous Endoscopic Approach
07T40ZZ Resection of Left Upper Extremity Lymphatic, Open Approach
07T44ZZ Resection of Left Upper Extremity Lymphatic, Percutaneous Endoscopic Approach
07T50ZZ Resection of Right Axillary Lymphatic, Open Approach
07T54ZZ Resection of Right Axillary Lymphatic, Percutaneous Endoscopic Approach
07T60ZZ Resection of Left Axillary Lymphatic, Open Approach

♀ Female-only   ♂ Male-only   ● Limited Coverage   ● Non-OR   HAC HAC-associated procedure   ⬣ Non-covered procedures   ➕ Combination

07T64ZZ Resection of Left Axillary Lymphatic, Percutaneous Endoscopic Approach

07T70ZZ Resection of Thorax Lymphatic, Open Approach

07T74ZZ Resection of Thorax Lymphatic, Percutaneous Endoscopic Approach

07T80ZZ Resection of Right Internal Mammary Lymphatic, Open Approach

07T84ZZ Resection of Right Internal Mammary Lymphatic, Percutaneous Endoscopic Approach

07T90ZZ Resection of Left Internal Mammary Lymphatic, Open Approach

07T94ZZ Resection of Left Internal Mammary Lymphatic, Percutaneous Endoscopic Approach

07TB0ZZ Resection of Mesenteric Lymphatic, Open Approach

07TB4ZZ Resection of Mesenteric Lymphatic, Percutaneous Endoscopic Approach

07TC0ZZ Resection of Pelvis Lymphatic, Open Approach

07TC4ZZ Resection of Pelvis Lymphatic, Percutaneous Endoscopic Approach

07TD0ZZ Resection of Aortic Lymphatic, Open Approach

07TD4ZZ Resection of Aortic Lymphatic, Percutaneous Endoscopic Approach

07TF0ZZ Resection of Right Lower Extremity Lymphatic, Open Approach

07TF4ZZ Resection of Right Lower Extremity Lymphatic, Percutaneous Endoscopic Approach

07TG0ZZ Resection of Left Lower Extremity Lymphatic, Open Approach

07TG4ZZ Resection of Left Lower Extremity Lymphatic, Percutaneous Endoscopic Approach

07TH0ZZ Resection of Right Inguinal Lymphatic, Open Approach

07TH4ZZ Resection of Right Inguinal Lymphatic, Percutaneous Endoscopic Approach

07TJ0ZZ Resection of Left Inguinal Lymphatic, Open Approach

07TJ4ZZ Resection of Left Inguinal Lymphatic, Percutaneous Endoscopic Approach

07TK0ZZ Resection of Thoracic Duct, Open Approach

07TK4ZZ Resection of Thoracic Duct, Percutaneous Endoscopic Approach

07TL0ZZ Resection of Cisterna Chyli, Open Approach

07TL4ZZ Resection of Cisterna Chyli, Percutaneous Endoscopic Approach

07TM0ZZ Resection of Thymus, Open Approach

07TM4ZZ Resection of Thymus, Percutaneous Endoscopic Approach

07TP0ZZ Resection of Spleen, Open Approach

07TP4ZZ Resection of Spleen, Percutaneous Endoscopic Approach

07U – Lymphatic and Hemic Systems, Supplement

07U007Z Supplement Head Lymphatic with Autologous Tissue Substitute, Open Approach

07U00JZ Supplement Head Lymphatic with Synthetic Substitute, Open Approach

07U00KZ Supplement Head Lymphatic with Nonautologous Tissue Substitute, Open Approach

07U047Z Supplement Head Lymphatic with Autologous Tissue Substitute, Percutaneous Endoscopic Approach

07U04JZ Supplement Head Lymphatic with Synthetic Substitute, Percutaneous Endoscopic Approach

07U04KZ Supplement Head Lymphatic with Nonautologous Tissue Substitute, Percutaneous Endoscopic Approach

07U107Z Supplement Right Neck Lymphatic with Autologous Tissue Substitute, Open Approach

07U10JZ Supplement Right Neck Lymphatic with Synthetic Substitute, Open Approach

07U10KZ Supplement Right Neck Lymphatic with Nonautologous Tissue Substitute, Open Approach

07U147Z Supplement Right Neck Lymphatic with Autologous Tissue Substitute, Percutaneous Endoscopic Approach

07U14JZ Supplement Right Neck Lymphatic with Synthetic Substitute, Percutaneous Endoscopic Approach

07U14KZ Supplement Right Neck Lymphatic with Nonautologous Tissue Substitute, Percutaneous Endoscopic Approach

07U207Z Supplement Left Neck Lymphatic with Autologous Tissue Substitute, Open Approach

07U20JZ Supplement Left Neck Lymphatic with Synthetic Substitute, Open Approach

07U20KZ Supplement Left Neck Lymphatic with Nonautologous Tissue Substitute, Open Approach

07U247Z Supplement Left Neck Lymphatic with Autologous Tissue Substitute, Percutaneous Endoscopic Approach

07U24JZ Supplement Left Neck Lymphatic with Synthetic Substitute, Percutaneous Endoscopic Approach

07U24KZ Supplement Left Neck Lymphatic with Nonautologous Tissue Substitute, Percutaneous Endoscopic Approach

07U307Z Supplement Right Upper Extremity Lymphatic with Autologous Tissue Substitute, Open Approach

07U30JZ Supplement Right Upper Extremity Lymphatic with Synthetic Substitute, Open Approach

07U30KZ Supplement Right Upper Extremity Lymphatic with Nonautologous Tissue Substitute, Open Approach

07U347Z Supplement Right Upper Extremity Lymphatic with Autologous Tissue Substitute, Percutaneous Endoscopic Approach

07U34JZ Supplement Right Upper Extremity Lymphatic with Synthetic Substitute, Percutaneous Endoscopic Approach

07U34KZ Supplement Right Upper Extremity Lymphatic with Nonautologous Tissue Substitute, Percutaneous Endoscopic Approach

07U407Z Supplement Left Upper Extremity Lymphatic with Autologous Tissue Substitute, Open Approach

07U40JZ Supplement Left Upper Extremity Lymphatic with Synthetic Substitute, Open Approach

07U40KZ Supplement Left Upper Extremity Lymphatic with Nonautologous Tissue Substitute, Open Approach

07U447Z Supplement Left Upper Extremity Lymphatic with Autologous Tissue Substitute, Percutaneous Endoscopic Approach

07U44JZ Supplement Left Upper Extremity Lymphatic with Synthetic Substitute, Percutaneous Endoscopic Approach

07U44KZ Supplement Left Upper Extremity Lymphatic with Nonautologous Tissue Substitute, Percutaneous Endoscopic Approach

07U507Z Supplement Right Axillary Lymphatic with Autologous Tissue Substitute, Open Approach

07U50JZ Supplement Right Axillary Lymphatic with Synthetic Substitute, Open Approach

07U50KZ Supplement Right Axillary Lymphatic with Nonautologous Tissue Substitute, Open Approach

07U547Z Supplement Right Axillary Lymphatic with Autologous Tissue Substitute, Percutaneous Endoscopic Approach

07U54JZ Supplement Right Axillary Lymphatic with Synthetic Substitute, Percutaneous Endoscopic Approach

07U54KZ Supplement Right Axillary Lymphatic with Nonautologous Tissue Substitute, Percutaneous Endoscopic Approach

07U607Z Supplement Left Axillary Lymphatic with Autologous Tissue Substitute, Open Approach

07U60JZ Supplement Left Axillary Lymphatic with Synthetic Substitute, Open Approach

07U60KZ Supplement Left Axillary Lymphatic with Nonautologous Tissue Substitute, Open Approach

07U647Z Supplement Left Axillary Lymphatic with Autologous Tissue Substitute, Percutaneous Endoscopic Approach

07U64JZ Supplement Left Axillary Lymphatic with Synthetic Substitute, Percutaneous Endoscopic Approach

07U64KZ Supplement Left Axillary Lymphatic with Nonautologous Tissue Substitute, Percutaneous Endoscopic Approach

07U707Z Supplement Thorax Lymphatic with Autologous Tissue Substitute, Open Approach

07U70JZ Supplement Thorax Lymphatic with Synthetic Substitute, Open Approach

07U70KZ Supplement Thorax Lymphatic with Nonautologous Tissue Substitute, Open Approach

07U747Z Supplement Thorax Lymphatic with Autologous Tissue Substitute, Percutaneous Endoscopic Approach

07U74JZ Supplement Thorax Lymphatic with Synthetic Substitute, Percutaneous Endoscopic Approach

07U74KZ Supplement Thorax Lymphatic with Nonautologous Tissue Substitute, Percutaneous Endoscopic Approach

07U807Z Supplement Right Internal Mammary Lymphatic with Autologous Tissue Substitute, Open Approach

07U80JZ Supplement Right Internal Mammary Lymphatic with Synthetic Substitute, Open Approach

07U80KZ   Supplement Right Internal Mammary Lymphatic with Nonautologous Tissue Substitute, Open Approach

07U847Z   Supplement Right Internal Mammary Lymphatic with Autologous Tissue Substitute, Percutaneous Endoscopic Approach

07U84JZ   Supplement Right Internal Mammary Lymphatic with Synthetic Substitute, Percutaneous Endoscopic Approach

07U84KZ   Supplement Right Internal Mammary Lymphatic with Nonautologous Tissue Substitute, Percutaneous Endoscopic Approach

07U907Z   Supplement Left Internal Mammary Lymphatic with Autologous Tissue Substitute, Open Approach

07U90JZ   Supplement Left Internal Mammary Lymphatic with Synthetic Substitute, Open Approach

07U90KZ   Supplement Left Internal Mammary Lymphatic with Nonautologous Tissue Substitute, Open Approach

07U947Z   Supplement Left Internal Mammary Lymphatic with Autologous Tissue Substitute, Percutaneous Endoscopic Approach

07U94JZ   Supplement Left Internal Mammary Lymphatic with Synthetic Substitute, Percutaneous Endoscopic Approach

07U94KZ   Supplement Left Internal Mammary Lymphatic with Nonautologous Tissue Substitute, Percutaneous Endoscopic Approach

07UB07Z   Supplement Mesenteric Lymphatic with Autologous Tissue Substitute, Open Approach

07UB0JZ   Supplement Mesenteric Lymphatic with Synthetic Substitute, Open Approach

07UB0KZ   Supplement Mesenteric Lymphatic with Nonautologous Tissue Substitute, Open Approach

07UB47Z   Supplement Mesenteric Lymphatic with Autologous Tissue Substitute, Percutaneous Endoscopic Approach

07UB4JZ   Supplement Mesenteric Lymphatic with Synthetic Substitute, Percutaneous Endoscopic Approach

07UB4KZ   Supplement Mesenteric Lymphatic with Nonautologous Tissue Substitute, Percutaneous Endoscopic Approach

07UC07Z   Supplement Pelvis Lymphatic with Autologous Tissue Substitute, Open Approach

07UC0JZ   Supplement Pelvis Lymphatic with Synthetic Substitute, Open Approach

07UC0KZ   Supplement Pelvis Lymphatic with Nonautologous Tissue Substitute, Open Approach

07UC47Z   Supplement Pelvis Lymphatic with Autologous Tissue Substitute, Percutaneous Endoscopic Approach

07UC4JZ   Supplement Pelvis Lymphatic with Synthetic Substitute, Percutaneous Endoscopic Approach

07UC4KZ   Supplement Pelvis Lymphatic with Nonautologous Tissue Substitute, Percutaneous Endoscopic Approach

07UD07Z   Supplement Aortic Lymphatic with Autologous Tissue Substitute, Open Approach

07UD0JZ   Supplement Aortic Lymphatic with Synthetic Substitute, Open Approach

07UD0KZ   Supplement Aortic Lymphatic with Nonautologous Tissue Substitute, Open Approach

07UD47Z   Supplement Aortic Lymphatic with Autologous Tissue Substitute, Percutaneous Endoscopic Approach

07UD4JZ   Supplement Aortic Lymphatic with Synthetic Substitute, Percutaneous Endoscopic Approach

07UD4KZ   Supplement Aortic Lymphatic with Nonautologous Tissue Substitute, Percutaneous Endoscopic Approach

07UF07Z   Supplement Right Lower Extremity Lymphatic with Autologous Tissue Substitute, Open Approach

07UF0JZ   Supplement Right Lower Extremity Lymphatic with Synthetic Substitute, Open Approach

07UF0KZ   Supplement Right Lower Extremity Lymphatic with Nonautologous Tissue Substitute, Open Approach

07UF47Z   Supplement Right Lower Extremity Lymphatic with Autologous Tissue Substitute, Percutaneous Endoscopic Approach

07UF4JZ   Supplement Right Lower Extremity Lymphatic with Synthetic Substitute, Percutaneous Endoscopic Approach

07UF4KZ   Supplement Right Lower Extremity Lymphatic with Nonautologous Tissue Substitute, Percutaneous Endoscopic Approach

07UG07Z   Supplement Left Lower Extremity Lymphatic with Autologous Tissue Substitute, Open Approach

07UG0JZ   Supplement Left Lower Extremity Lymphatic with Synthetic Substitute, Open Approach

07UG0KZ   Supplement Left Lower Extremity Lymphatic with Nonautologous Tissue Substitute, Open Approach

07UG47Z   Supplement Left Lower Extremity Lymphatic with Autologous Tissue Substitute, Percutaneous Endoscopic Approach

07UG4JZ   Supplement Left Lower Extremity Lymphatic with Synthetic Substitute, Percutaneous Endoscopic Approach

07UG4KZ   Supplement Left Lower Extremity Lymphatic with Nonautologous Tissue Substitute, Percutaneous Endoscopic Approach

07UH07Z   Supplement Right Inguinal Lymphatic with Autologous Tissue Substitute, Open Approach

07UH0JZ   Supplement Right Inguinal Lymphatic with Synthetic Substitute, Open Approach

07UH0KZ   Supplement Right Inguinal Lymphatic with Nonautologous Tissue Substitute, Open Approach

07UH47Z   Supplement Right Inguinal Lymphatic with Autologous Tissue Substitute, Percutaneous Endoscopic Approach

07UH4JZ   Supplement Right Inguinal Lymphatic with Synthetic Substitute, Percutaneous Endoscopic Approach

07UH4KZ   Supplement Right Inguinal Lymphatic with Nonautologous Tissue Substitute, Percutaneous Endoscopic Approach

07UJ07Z   Supplement Left Inguinal Lymphatic with Autologous Tissue Substitute, Open Approach

07UJ0JZ   Supplement Left Inguinal Lymphatic with Synthetic Substitute, Open Approach

07UJ0KZ   Supplement Left Inguinal Lymphatic with Nonautologous Tissue Substitute, Open Approach

07UJ47Z   Supplement Left Inguinal Lymphatic with Autologous Tissue Substitute, Percutaneous Endoscopic Approach

07UJ4JZ   Supplement Left Inguinal Lymphatic with Synthetic Substitute, Percutaneous Endoscopic Approach

07UJ4KZ   Supplement Left Inguinal Lymphatic with Nonautologous Tissue Substitute, Percutaneous Endoscopic Approach

07UK07Z   Supplement Thoracic Duct with Autologous Tissue Substitute, Open Approach

07UK0JZ   Supplement Thoracic Duct with Synthetic Substitute, Open Approach

07UK0KZ   Supplement Thoracic Duct with Nonautologous Tissue Substitute, Open Approach

07UK47Z   Supplement Thoracic Duct with Autologous Tissue Substitute, Percutaneous Endoscopic Approach

07UK4JZ   Supplement Thoracic Duct with Synthetic Substitute, Percutaneous Endoscopic Approach

07UK4KZ   Supplement Thoracic Duct with Nonautologous Tissue Substitute, Percutaneous Endoscopic Approach

07UL07Z   Supplement Cisterna Chyli with Autologous Tissue Substitute, Open Approach

07UL0JZ   Supplement Cisterna Chyli with Synthetic Substitute, Open Approach

07UL0KZ   Supplement Cisterna Chyli with Nonautologous Tissue Substitute, Open Approach

07UL47Z   Supplement Cisterna Chyli with Autologous Tissue Substitute, Percutaneous Endoscopic Approach

07UL4JZ   Supplement Cisterna Chyli with Synthetic Substitute, Percutaneous Endoscopic Approach

07UL4KZ   Supplement Cisterna Chyli with Nonautologous Tissue Substitute, Percutaneous Endoscopic Approach

07V – Lymphatic and Hemic Systems, Restriction

07V00CZ   Restriction of Head Lymphatic with Extraluminal Device, Open Approach

07V00DZ   Restriction of Head Lymphatic with Intraluminal Device, Open Approach

07V00ZZ   Restriction of Head Lymphatic, Open Approach

07V03CZ   Restriction of Head Lymphatic with Extraluminal Device, Percutaneous Approach

07V03DZ   Restriction of Head Lymphatic with Intraluminal Device, Percutaneous Approach

07V03ZZ   Restriction of Head Lymphatic, Percutaneous Approach

---

♀ Female-only   ♂ Male-only   ◐ Limited Coverage   ● Non-OR   [HAC] HAC-associated procedure   ● Non-covered procedures   ✚ Combination

07V04CZ   Restriction of Head Lymphatic with Extraluminal Device, Percutaneous Endoscopic Approach

07V04DZ   Restriction of Head Lymphatic with Intraluminal Device, Percutaneous Endoscopic Approach

07V04ZZ   Restriction of Head Lymphatic, Percutaneous Endoscopic Approach

07V10CZ   Restriction of Right Neck Lymphatic with Extraluminal Device, Open Approach

07V10DZ   Restriction of Right Neck Lymphatic with Intraluminal Device, Open Approach

07V10ZZ   Restriction of Right Neck Lymphatic, Open Approach

07V13CZ   Restriction of Right Neck Lymphatic with Extraluminal Device, Percutaneous Approach

07V13DZ   Restriction of Right Neck Lymphatic with Intraluminal Device, Percutaneous Approach

07V13ZZ   Restriction of Right Neck Lymphatic, Percutaneous Approach

07V14CZ   Restriction of Right Neck Lymphatic with Extraluminal Device, Percutaneous Endoscopic Approach

07V14DZ   Restriction of Right Neck Lymphatic with Intraluminal Device, Percutaneous Endoscopic Approach

07V14ZZ   Restriction of Right Neck Lymphatic, Percutaneous Endoscopic Approach

07V20CZ   Restriction of Left Neck Lymphatic with Extraluminal Device, Open Approach

07V20DZ   Restriction of Left Neck Lymphatic with Intraluminal Device, Open Approach

07V20ZZ   Restriction of Left Neck Lymphatic, Open Approach

07V23CZ   Restriction of Left Neck Lymphatic with Extraluminal Device, Percutaneous Approach

07V23DZ   Restriction of Left Neck Lymphatic with Intraluminal Device, Percutaneous Approach

07V23ZZ   Restriction of Left Neck Lymphatic, Percutaneous Approach

07V24CZ   Restriction of Left Neck Lymphatic with Extraluminal Device, Percutaneous Endoscopic Approach

07V24DZ   Restriction of Left Neck Lymphatic with Intraluminal Device, Percutaneous Endoscopic Approach

07V24ZZ   Restriction of Left Neck Lymphatic, Percutaneous Endoscopic Approach

07V30CZ   Restriction of Right Upper Extremity Lymphatic with Extraluminal Device, Open Approach

07V30DZ   Restriction of Right Upper Extremity Lymphatic with Intraluminal Device, Open Approach

07V30ZZ   Restriction of Right Upper Extremity Lymphatic, Open Approach

07V33CZ   Restriction of Right Upper Extremity Lymphatic with Extraluminal Device, Percutaneous Approach

07V33DZ   Restriction of Right Upper Extremity Lymphatic with Intraluminal Device, Percutaneous Approach

07V33ZZ   Restriction of Right Upper Extremity Lymphatic, Percutaneous Approach

07V34CZ   Restriction of Right Upper Extremity Lymphatic with Extraluminal Device, Percutaneous Endoscopic Approach

07V34DZ   Restriction of Right Upper Extremity Lymphatic with Intraluminal Device, Percutaneous Endoscopic Approach

07V34ZZ   Restriction of Right Upper Extremity Lymphatic, Percutaneous Endoscopic Approach

07V40CZ   Restriction of Left Upper Extremity Lymphatic with Extraluminal Device, Open Approach

07V40DZ   Restriction of Left Upper Extremity Lymphatic with Intraluminal Device, Open Approach

07V40ZZ   Restriction of Left Upper Extremity Lymphatic, Open Approach

07V43CZ   Restriction of Left Upper Extremity Lymphatic with Extraluminal Device, Percutaneous Approach

07V43DZ   Restriction of Left Upper Extremity Lymphatic with Intraluminal Device, Percutaneous Approach

07V43ZZ   Restriction of Left Upper Extremity Lymphatic, Percutaneous Approach

07V44CZ   Restriction of Left Upper Extremity Lymphatic with Extraluminal Device, Percutaneous Endoscopic Approach

07V44DZ   Restriction of Left Upper Extremity Lymphatic with Intraluminal Device, Percutaneous Endoscopic Approach

07V44ZZ   Restriction of Left Upper Extremity Lymphatic, Percutaneous Endoscopic Approach

07V50CZ   Restriction of Right Axillary Lymphatic with Extraluminal Device, Open Approach

07V50DZ   Restriction of Right Axillary Lymphatic with Intraluminal Device, Open Approach

07V50ZZ   Restriction of Right Axillary Lymphatic, Open Approach

07V53CZ   Restriction of Right Axillary Lymphatic with Extraluminal Device, Percutaneous Approach

07V53DZ   Restriction of Right Axillary Lymphatic with Intraluminal Device, Percutaneous Approach

07V53ZZ   Restriction of Right Axillary Lymphatic, Percutaneous Approach

07V54CZ   Restriction of Right Axillary Lymphatic with Extraluminal Device, Percutaneous Endoscopic Approach

07V54DZ   Restriction of Right Axillary Lymphatic with Intraluminal Device, Percutaneous Endoscopic Approach

07V54ZZ   Restriction of Right Axillary Lymphatic, Percutaneous Endoscopic Approach

07V60CZ   Restriction of Left Axillary Lymphatic with Extraluminal Device, Open Approach

07V60DZ   Restriction of Left Axillary Lymphatic with Intraluminal Device, Open Approach

07V60ZZ   Restriction of Left Axillary Lymphatic, Open Approach

07V63CZ   Restriction of Left Axillary Lymphatic with Extraluminal Device, Percutaneous Approach

07V63DZ   Restriction of Left Axillary Lymphatic with Intraluminal Device, Percutaneous Approach

07V63ZZ   Restriction of Left Axillary Lymphatic, Percutaneous Approach

07V64CZ   Restriction of Left Axillary Lymphatic with Extraluminal Device, Percutaneous Endoscopic Approach

07V64DZ   Restriction of Left Axillary Lymphatic with Intraluminal Device, Percutaneous Endoscopic Approach

07V64ZZ   Restriction of Left Axillary Lymphatic, Percutaneous Endoscopic Approach

07V70CZ   Restriction of Thorax Lymphatic with Extraluminal Device, Open Approach

07V70DZ   Restriction of Thorax Lymphatic with Intraluminal Device, Open Approach

07V70ZZ   Restriction of Thorax Lymphatic, Open Approach

07V73CZ   Restriction of Thorax Lymphatic with Extraluminal Device, Percutaneous Approach

07V73DZ   Restriction of Thorax Lymphatic with Intraluminal Device, Percutaneous Approach

07V73ZZ   Restriction of Thorax Lymphatic, Percutaneous Approach

07V74CZ   Restriction of Thorax Lymphatic with Extraluminal Device, Percutaneous Endoscopic Approach

07V74DZ   Restriction of Thorax Lymphatic with Intraluminal Device, Percutaneous Endoscopic Approach

07V74ZZ   Restriction of Thorax Lymphatic, Percutaneous Endoscopic Approach

07V80CZ   Restriction of Right Internal Mammary Lymphatic with Extraluminal Device, Open Approach

07V80DZ   Restriction of Right Internal Mammary Lymphatic with Intraluminal Device, Open Approach

07V80ZZ   Restriction of Right Internal Mammary Lymphatic, Open Approach

07V83CZ   Restriction of Right Internal Mammary Lymphatic with Extraluminal Device, Percutaneous Approach

07V83DZ   Restriction of Right Internal Mammary Lymphatic with Intraluminal Device, Percutaneous Approach

07V83ZZ   Restriction of Right Internal Mammary Lymphatic, Percutaneous Approach

07V84CZ   Restriction of Right Internal Mammary Lymphatic with Extraluminal Device, Percutaneous Endoscopic Approach

07V84DZ   Restriction of Right Internal Mammary Lymphatic with Intraluminal Device, Percutaneous Endoscopic Approach

07V84ZZ   Restriction of Right Internal Mammary Lymphatic, Percutaneous Endoscopic Approach

07V90CZ   Restriction of Left Internal Mammary Lymphatic with Extraluminal Device, Open Approach

07V90DZ   Restriction of Left Internal Mammary Lymphatic with Intraluminal Device, Open Approach

07V90ZZ   Restriction of Left Internal Mammary Lymphatic, Open Approach

07V93CZ   Restriction of Left Internal Mammary Lymphatic with Extraluminal Device, Percutaneous Approach

07V93DZ   Restriction of Left Internal Mammary Lymphatic with Intraluminal Device, Percutaneous Approach

07V93ZZ Restriction of Left Internal Mammary Lymphatic, Percutaneous Approach

07V94CZ Restriction of Left Internal Mammary Lymphatic with Extraluminal Device, Percutaneous Endoscopic Approach

07V94DZ Restriction of Left Internal Mammary Lymphatic with Intraluminal Device, Percutaneous Endoscopic Approach

07V94ZZ Restriction of Left Internal Mammary Lymphatic, Percutaneous Endoscopic Approach

07VB0CZ Restriction of Mesenteric Lymphatic with Extraluminal Device, Open Approach

07VB0DZ Restriction of Mesenteric Lymphatic with Intraluminal Device, Open Approach

07VB0ZZ Restriction of Mesenteric Lymphatic, Open Approach

07VB3CZ Restriction of Mesenteric Lymphatic with Extraluminal Device, Percutaneous Approach

07VB3DZ Restriction of Mesenteric Lymphatic with Intraluminal Device, Percutaneous Approach

07VB3ZZ Restriction of Mesenteric Lymphatic, Percutaneous Approach

07VB4CZ Restriction of Mesenteric Lymphatic with Extraluminal Device, Percutaneous Endoscopic Approach

07VB4DZ Restriction of Mesenteric Lymphatic with Intraluminal Device, Percutaneous Endoscopic Approach

07VB4ZZ Restriction of Mesenteric Lymphatic, Percutaneous Endoscopic Approach

07VC0CZ Restriction of Pelvis Lymphatic with Extraluminal Device, Open Approach

07VC0DZ Restriction of Pelvis Lymphatic with Intraluminal Device, Open Approach

07VC0ZZ Restriction of Pelvis Lymphatic, Open Approach

07VC3CZ Restriction of Pelvis Lymphatic with Extraluminal Device, Percutaneous Approach

07VC3DZ Restriction of Pelvis Lymphatic with Intraluminal Device, Percutaneous Approach

07VC3ZZ Restriction of Pelvis Lymphatic, Percutaneous Approach

07VC4CZ Restriction of Pelvis Lymphatic with Extraluminal Device, Percutaneous Endoscopic Approach

07VC4DZ Restriction of Pelvis Lymphatic with Intraluminal Device, Percutaneous Endoscopic Approach

07VC4ZZ Restriction of Pelvis Lymphatic, Percutaneous Endoscopic Approach

07VD0CZ Restriction of Aortic Lymphatic with Extraluminal Device, Open Approach

07VD0DZ Restriction of Aortic Lymphatic with Intraluminal Device, Open Approach

07VD0ZZ Restriction of Aortic Lymphatic, Open Approach

07VD3CZ Restriction of Aortic Lymphatic with Extraluminal Device, Percutaneous Approach

07VD3DZ Restriction of Aortic Lymphatic with Intraluminal Device, Percutaneous Approach

07VD3ZZ Restriction of Aortic Lymphatic, Percutaneous Approach

07VD4CZ Restriction of Aortic Lymphatic with Extraluminal Device, Percutaneous Endoscopic Approach

07VD4DZ Restriction of Aortic Lymphatic with Intraluminal Device, Percutaneous Endoscopic Approach

07VD4ZZ Restriction of Aortic Lymphatic, Percutaneous Endoscopic Approach

07VF0CZ Restriction of Right Lower Extremity Lymphatic with Extraluminal Device, Open Approach

07VF0DZ Restriction of Right Lower Extremity Lymphatic with Intraluminal Device, Open Approach

07VF0ZZ Restriction of Right Lower Extremity Lymphatic, Open Approach

07VF3CZ Restriction of Right Lower Extremity Lymphatic with Extraluminal Device, Percutaneous Approach

07VF3DZ Restriction of Right Lower Extremity Lymphatic with Intraluminal Device, Percutaneous Approach

07VF3ZZ Restriction of Right Lower Extremity Lymphatic, Percutaneous Approach

07VF4CZ Restriction of Right Lower Extremity Lymphatic with Extraluminal Device, Percutaneous Endoscopic Approach

07VF4DZ Restriction of Right Lower Extremity Lymphatic with Intraluminal Device, Percutaneous Endoscopic Approach

07VF4ZZ Restriction of Right Lower Extremity Lymphatic, Percutaneous Endoscopic Approach

07VG0CZ Restriction of Left Lower Extremity Lymphatic with Extraluminal Device, Open Approach

07VG0DZ Restriction of Left Lower Extremity Lymphatic with Intraluminal Device, Open Approach

07VG0ZZ Restriction of Left Lower Extremity Lymphatic, Open Approach

07VG3CZ Restriction of Left Lower Extremity Lymphatic with Extraluminal Device, Percutaneous Approach

07VG3DZ Restriction of Left Lower Extremity Lymphatic with Intraluminal Device, Percutaneous Approach

07VG3ZZ Restriction of Left Lower Extremity Lymphatic, Percutaneous Approach

07VG4CZ Restriction of Left Lower Extremity Lymphatic with Extraluminal Device, Percutaneous Endoscopic Approach

07VG4DZ Restriction of Left Lower Extremity Lymphatic with Intraluminal Device, Percutaneous Endoscopic Approach

07VG4ZZ Restriction of Left Lower Extremity Lymphatic, Percutaneous Endoscopic Approach

07VH0CZ Restriction of Right Inguinal Lymphatic with Extraluminal Device, Open Approach

07VH0DZ Restriction of Right Inguinal Lymphatic with Intraluminal Device, Open Approach

07VH0ZZ Restriction of Right Inguinal Lymphatic, Open Approach

07VH3CZ Restriction of Right Inguinal Lymphatic with Extraluminal Device, Percutaneous Approach

07VH3DZ Restriction of Right Inguinal Lymphatic with Intraluminal Device, Percutaneous Approach

07VH3ZZ Restriction of Right Inguinal Lymphatic, Percutaneous Approach

07VH4CZ Restriction of Right Inguinal Lymphatic with Extraluminal Device, Percutaneous Endoscopic Approach

07VH4DZ Restriction of Right Inguinal Lymphatic with Intraluminal Device, Percutaneous Endoscopic Approach

07VH4ZZ Restriction of Right Inguinal Lymphatic, Percutaneous Endoscopic Approach

07VJ0CZ Restriction of Left Inguinal Lymphatic with Extraluminal Device, Open Approach

07VJ0DZ Restriction of Left Inguinal Lymphatic with Intraluminal Device, Open Approach

07VJ0ZZ Restriction of Left Inguinal Lymphatic, Open Approach

07VJ3CZ Restriction of Left Inguinal Lymphatic with Extraluminal Device, Percutaneous Approach

07VJ3DZ Restriction of Left Inguinal Lymphatic with Intraluminal Device, Percutaneous Approach

07VJ3ZZ Restriction of Left Inguinal Lymphatic, Percutaneous Approach

07VJ4CZ Restriction of Left Inguinal Lymphatic with Extraluminal Device, Percutaneous Endoscopic Approach

07VJ4DZ Restriction of Left Inguinal Lymphatic with Intraluminal Device, Percutaneous Endoscopic Approach

07VJ4ZZ Restriction of Left Inguinal Lymphatic, Percutaneous Endoscopic Approach

07VK0CZ Restriction of Thoracic Duct with Extraluminal Device, Open Approach

07VK0DZ Restriction of Thoracic Duct with Intraluminal Device, Open Approach

07VK0ZZ Restriction of Thoracic Duct, Open Approach

07VK3CZ Restriction of Thoracic Duct with Extraluminal Device, Percutaneous Approach

07VK3DZ Restriction of Thoracic Duct with Intraluminal Device, Percutaneous Approach

07VK3ZZ Restriction of Thoracic Duct, Percutaneous Approach

07VK4CZ Restriction of Thoracic Duct with Extraluminal Device, Percutaneous Endoscopic Approach

07VK4DZ Restriction of Thoracic Duct with Intraluminal Device, Percutaneous Endoscopic Approach

07VK4ZZ Restriction of Thoracic Duct, Percutaneous Endoscopic Approach

07VL0CZ Restriction of Cisterna Chyli with Extraluminal Device, Open Approach

07VL0DZ Restriction of Cisterna Chyli with Intraluminal Device, Open Approach

07VL0ZZ Restriction of Cisterna Chyli, Open Approach

07VL3CZ Restriction of Cisterna Chyli with Extraluminal Device, Percutaneous Approach

07VL3DZ Restriction of Cisterna Chyli with Intraluminal Device, Percutaneous Approach

07VL3ZZ Restriction of Cisterna Chyli, Percutaneous Approach
07VL4CZ Restriction of Cisterna Chyli with Extraluminal Device, Percutaneous Endoscopic Approach

07VL4DZ Restriction of Cisterna Chyli with Intraluminal Device, Percutaneous Endoscopic Approach
07VL4ZZ Restriction of Cisterna Chyli, Percutaneous Endoscopic Approach

07W – Lymphatic and Hemic Systems, Revision

Review Coding Guideline B6.1c

07WK00Z Revision of Drainage Device in Thoracic Duct, Open Approach
07WK03Z Revision of Infusion Device in Thoracic Duct, Open Approach
07WK07Z Revision of Autologous Tissue Substitute in Thoracic Duct, Open Approach
07WK0CZ Revision of Extraluminal Device in Thoracic Duct, Open Approach
07WK0DZ Revision of Intraluminal Device in Thoracic Duct, Open Approach
07WK0JZ Revision of Synthetic Substitute in Thoracic Duct, Open Approach
07WK0KZ Revision of Nonautologous Tissue Substitute in Thoracic Duct, Open Approach
07WK30Z Revision of Drainage Device in Thoracic Duct, Percutaneous Approach
07WK33Z Revision of Infusion Device in Thoracic Duct, Percutaneous Approach
07WK37Z Revision of Autologous Tissue Substitute in Thoracic Duct, Percutaneous Approach
07WK3CZ Revision of Extraluminal Device in Thoracic Duct, Percutaneous Approach
07WK3DZ Revision of Intraluminal Device in Thoracic Duct, Percutaneous Approach
07WK3JZ Revision of Synthetic Substitute in Thoracic Duct, Percutaneous Approach
07WK3KZ Revision of Nonautologous Tissue Substitute in Thoracic Duct, Percutaneous Approach
07WK40Z Revision of Drainage Device in Thoracic Duct, Percutaneous Endoscopic Approach
07WK43Z Revision of Infusion Device in Thoracic Duct, Percutaneous Endoscopic Approach
07WK47Z Revision of Autologous Tissue Substitute in Thoracic Duct, Percutaneous Endoscopic Approach
07WK4CZ Revision of Extraluminal Device in Thoracic Duct, Percutaneous Endoscopic Approach
07WK4DZ Revision of Intraluminal Device in Thoracic Duct, Percutaneous Endoscopic Approach
07WK4JZ Revision of Synthetic Substitute in Thoracic Duct, Percutaneous Endoscopic Approach
07WK4KZ Revision of Nonautologous Tissue Substitute in Thoracic Duct, Percutaneous Endoscopic Approach
07WKX0Z Revision of Drainage Device in Thoracic Duct, External Approach
07WKX3Z Revision of Infusion Device in Thoracic Duct, External Approach
07WKX7Z Revision of Autologous Tissue Substitute in Thoracic Duct, External Approach
07WKXCZ Revision of Extraluminal Device in Thoracic Duct, External Approach
07WKXDZ Revision of Intraluminal Device in Thoracic Duct, External Approach
07WKXJZ Revision of Synthetic Substitute in Thoracic Duct, External Approach
07WKXKZ Revision of Nonautologous Tissue Substitute in Thoracic Duct, External Approach
07WL00Z Revision of Drainage Device in Cisterna Chyli, Open Approach
07WL03Z Revision of Infusion Device in Cisterna Chyli, Open Approach
07WL07Z Revision of Autologous Tissue Substitute in Cisterna Chyli, Open Approach
07WL0CZ Revision of Extraluminal Device in Cisterna Chyli, Open Approach
07WL0DZ Revision of Intraluminal Device in Cisterna Chyli, Open Approach
07WL0JZ Revision of Synthetic Substitute in Cisterna Chyli, Open Approach
07WL0KZ Revision of Nonautologous Tissue Substitute in Cisterna Chyli, Open Approach
07WL30Z Revision of Drainage Device in Cisterna Chyli, Percutaneous Approach
07WL33Z Revision of Infusion Device in Cisterna Chyli, Percutaneous Approach
07WL37Z Revision of Autologous Tissue Substitute in Cisterna Chyli, Percutaneous Approach

07WL3CZ Revision of Extraluminal Device in Cisterna Chyli, Percutaneous Approach
07WL3DZ Revision of Intraluminal Device in Cisterna Chyli, Percutaneous Approach
07WL3JZ Revision of Synthetic Substitute in Cisterna Chyli, Percutaneous Approach
07WL3KZ Revision of Nonautologous Tissue Substitute in Cisterna Chyli, Percutaneous Approach
07WL40Z Revision of Drainage Device in Cisterna Chyli, Percutaneous Endoscopic Approach
07WL43Z Revision of Infusion Device in Cisterna Chyli, Percutaneous Endoscopic Approach
07WL47Z Revision of Autologous Tissue Substitute in Cisterna Chyli, Percutaneous Endoscopic Approach
07WL4CZ Revision of Extraluminal Device in Cisterna Chyli, Percutaneous Endoscopic Approach
07WL4DZ Revision of Intraluminal Device in Cisterna Chyli, Percutaneous Endoscopic Approach
07WL4JZ Revision of Synthetic Substitute in Cisterna Chyli, Percutaneous Endoscopic Approach
07WL4KZ Revision of Nonautologous Tissue Substitute in Cisterna Chyli, Percutaneous Endoscopic Approach
07WLX0Z Revision of Drainage Device in Cisterna Chyli, External Approach
07WLX3Z Revision of Infusion Device in Cisterna Chyli, External Approach
07WLX7Z Revision of Autologous Tissue Substitute in Cisterna Chyli, External Approach
07WLXCZ Revision of Extraluminal Device in Cisterna Chyli, External Approach
07WLXDZ Revision of Intraluminal Device in Cisterna Chyli, External Approach
07WLXJZ Revision of Synthetic Substitute in Cisterna Chyli, External Approach
07WLXKZ Revision of Nonautologous Tissue Substitute in Cisterna Chyli, External Approach
07WM00Z Revision of Drainage Device in Thymus, Open Approach
07WM03Z Revision of Infusion Device in Thymus, Open Approach
07WM30Z Revision of Drainage Device in Thymus, Percutaneous Approach
07WM33Z Revision of Infusion Device in Thymus, Percutaneous Approach
07WM40Z Revision of Drainage Device in Thymus, Percutaneous Endoscopic Approach
07WM43Z Revision of Infusion Device in Thymus, Percutaneous Endoscopic Approach
07WMX0Z Revision of Drainage Device in Thymus, External Approach
07WMX3Z Revision of Infusion Device in Thymus, External Approach
07WN00Z Revision of Drainage Device in Lymphatic, Open Approach
07WN03Z Revision of Infusion Device in Lymphatic, Open Approach
07WN07Z Revision of Autologous Tissue Substitute in Lymphatic, Open Approach
07WN0CZ Revision of Extraluminal Device in Lymphatic, Open Approach
07WN0DZ Revision of Intraluminal Device in Lymphatic, Open Approach
07WN0JZ Revision of Synthetic Substitute in Lymphatic, Open Approach
07WN0KZ Revision of Nonautologous Tissue Substitute in Lymphatic, Open Approach
07WN30Z Revision of Drainage Device in Lymphatic, Percutaneous Approach
07WN33Z Revision of Infusion Device in Lymphatic, Percutaneous Approach
07WN37Z Revision of Autologous Tissue Substitute in Lymphatic, Percutaneous Approach
07WN3CZ Revision of Extraluminal Device in Lymphatic, Percutaneous Approach
07WN3DZ Revision of Intraluminal Device in Lymphatic, Percutaneous Approach
07WN3JZ Revision of Synthetic Substitute in Lymphatic, Percutaneous Approach
07WN3KZ Revision of Nonautologous Tissue Substitute in Lymphatic, Percutaneous Approach

07WN40Z   Revision of Drainage Device in Lymphatic, Percutaneous Endoscopic Approach
07WN43Z   Revision of Infusion Device in Lymphatic, Percutaneous Endoscopic Approach
07WN47Z   Revision of Autologous Tissue Substitute in Lymphatic, Percutaneous Endoscopic Approach
07WN4CZ   Revision of Extraluminal Device in Lymphatic, Percutaneous Endoscopic Approach
07WN4DZ   Revision of Intraluminal Device in Lymphatic, Percutaneous Endoscopic Approach
07WN4JZ   Revision of Synthetic Substitute in Lymphatic, Percutaneous Endoscopic Approach
07WN4KZ   Revision of Nonautologous Tissue Substitute in Lymphatic, Percutaneous Endoscopic Approach
07WNX0Z   Revision of Drainage Device in Lymphatic, External Approach
07WNX3Z   Revision of Infusion Device in Lymphatic, External Approach
07WNX7Z   Revision of Autologous Tissue Substitute in Lymphatic, External Approach
07WNXCZ   Revision of Extraluminal Device in Lymphatic, External Approach
07WNXDZ   Revision of Intraluminal Device in Lymphatic, External Approach

07WNXJZ   Revision of Synthetic Substitute in Lymphatic, External Approach
07WNXKZ   Revision of Nonautologous Tissue Substitute in Lymphatic, External Approach
07WP00Z   Revision of Drainage Device in Spleen, Open Approach
07WP03Z   Revision of Infusion Device in Spleen, Open Approach
07WP30Z   Revision of Drainage Device in Spleen, Percutaneous Approach
07WP33Z   Revision of Infusion Device in Spleen, Percutaneous Approach
07WP40Z   Revision of Drainage Device in Spleen, Percutaneous Endoscopic Approach
07WP43Z   Revision of Infusion Device in Spleen, Percutaneous Endoscopic Approach
07WPX0Z   Revision of Drainage Device in Spleen, External Approach
07WPX3Z   Revision of Infusion Device in Spleen, External Approach
07WT00Z   Revision of Drainage Device in Bone Marrow, Open Approach
07WT30Z   Revision of Drainage Device in Bone Marrow, Percutaneous Approach
07WT40Z   Revision of Drainage Device in Bone Marrow, Percutaneous Endoscopic Approach
07WTX0Z   Revision of Drainage Device in Bone Marrow, External Approach

07Y – Lymphatic and Hemic Systems, Transplantation

Review Coding Guideline B3.16

07YM0Z0   Transplantation of Thymus, Allogeneic, Open Approach
07YM0Z1   Transplantation of Thymus, Syngeneic, Open Approach
07YM0Z2   Transplantation of Thymus, Zooplastic, Open Approach

07YP0Z0   Transplantation of Spleen, Allogeneic, Open Approach
07YP0Z1   Transplantation of Spleen, Syngeneic, Open Approach
07YP0Z2   Transplantation of Spleen, Zooplastic, Open Approach

---

♀ Female-only   ♂ Male-only   ○ Limited Coverage   ● Non-OR   ▨ HAC-associated procedure   ● Non-covered procedures   ➕ Combination

Eye

<u>Eye</u>

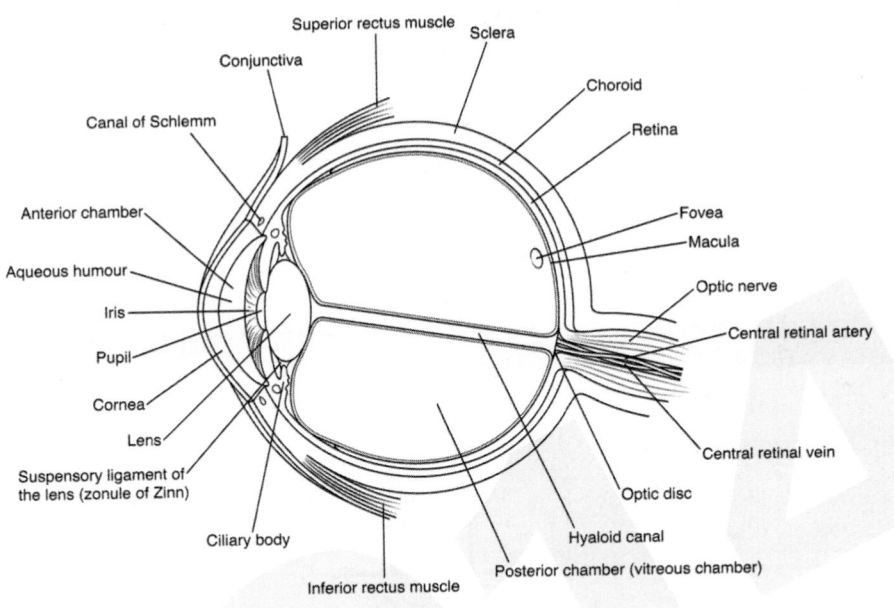

Superior rectus muscle   Sclera
Conjunctiva   Choroid
Canal of Schlemm   Retina
Anterior chamber   Fovea
Aqueous humour   Macula
Iris   Optic nerve
Pupil   Central retinal artery
Cornea
Lens   Central retinal vein
Suspensory ligament of
the lens (zonule of Zinn)
Ciliary body   Optic disc
Inferior rectus muscle   Hyaloid canal
                          Posterior chamber (vitreous chamber)

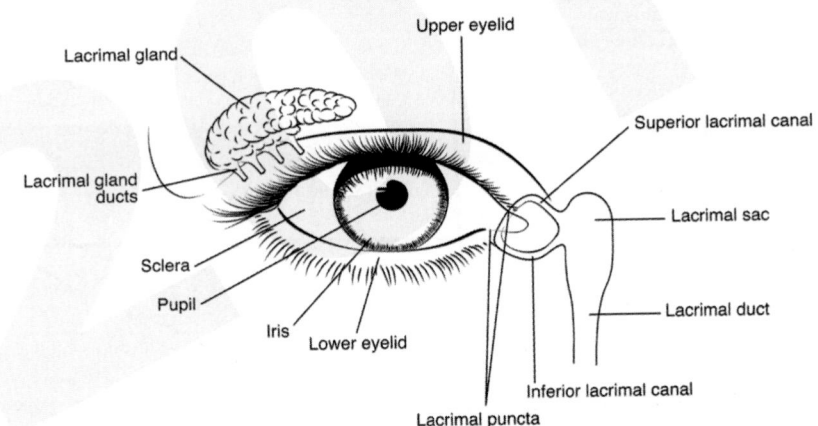

Lacrimal gland   Upper eyelid
Lacrimal gland   Superior lacrimal canal
ducts
                          Lacrimal sac
Sclera
Pupil   Lacrimal duct
Iris   Lower eyelid
                          Inferior lacrimal canal
Lacrimal puncta

Eye Muscles

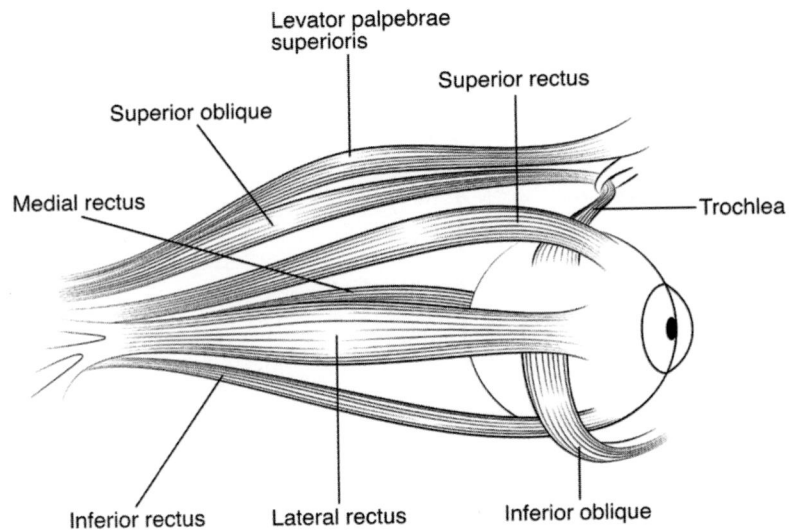

Levator palpebrae
superioris
Superior oblique   Superior rectus
Medial rectus   Trochlea
Inferior rectus   Lateral rectus   Inferior oblique

Section	0	Medical and Surgical
Body System	8	Eye
Operation	0	**Alteration:** Modifying the anatomic structure of a body part without affecting the function of the body part

Body Part (4ᵗʰ)	Approach (5ᵗʰ)	Device (6ᵗʰ)	Qualifier (7ᵗʰ)
N Upper Eyelid, Right **P** Upper Eyelid, Left **Q** Lower Eyelid, Right **R** Lower Eyelid, Left	**0** Open **3** Percutaneous **X** External	**7** Autologous Tissue Substitute **J** Synthetic Substitute **K** Nonautologous Tissue Substitute **Z** No Device	**Z** No Qualifier

Section	0	Medical and Surgical
Body System	8	Eye
Operation	1	**Bypass:** Altering the route of passage of the contents of a tubular body part

Body Part (4ᵗʰ)	Approach (5ᵗʰ)	Device (6ᵗʰ)	Qualifier (7ᵗʰ)
2 Anterior Chamber, Right **3** Anterior Chamber, Left	**3** Percutaneous	**J** Synthetic Substitute **K** Nonautologous Tissue Substitute **Z** No Device	**4** Sclera
X Lacrimal Duct, Right **Y** Lacrimal Duct, Left	**0** Open **3** Percutaneous	**J** Synthetic Substitute **K** Nonautologous Tissue Substitute **Z** No Device	**3** Nasal Cavity

Section	0	Medical and Surgical
Body System	8	Eye
Operation	2	**Change:** Taking out or off a device from a body part and putting back an identical or similar device in or on the same body part without cutting or puncturing the skin or a mucous membrane

Body Part (4ᵗʰ)	Approach (5ᵗʰ)	Device (6ᵗʰ)	Qualifier (7ᵗʰ)
0 Eye, Right **1** Eye, Left	**X** External	**0** Drainage Device **Y** Other Device	**Z** No Qualifier

Section	0	Medical and Surgical
Body System	8	Eye
Operation	5	**Destruction:** Physical eradication of all or a portion of a body part by the direct use of energy, force, or a destructive agent

Body Part (4ᵗʰ)	Approach (5ᵗʰ)	Device (6ᵗʰ)	Qualifier (7ᵗʰ)
0 Eye, Right **1** Eye, Left **6** Sclera, Right **7** Sclera, Left **8** Cornea, Right **9** Cornea, Left **S** Conjunctiva, Right **T** Conjunctiva, Left	**X** External	**Z** No Device	**Z** No Qualifier
2 Anterior Chamber, Right **3** Anterior Chamber, Left **4** Vitreous, Right **5** Vitreous, Left **C** Iris, Right **D** Iris, Left **E** Retina, Right **F** Retina, Left **G** Retinal Vessel, Right **H** Retinal Vessel, Left **J** Lens, Right **K** Lens, Left	**3** Percutaneous	**Z** No Device	**Z** No Qualifier

Continued

085 Continued

Section	0	**Medical and Surgical**
Body System	8	Eye
Operation	5	**Destruction:** Physical eradication of all or a portion of a body part by the direct use of energy, force, or a destructive agent

Body Part (4th)	Approach (5th)	Device (6th)	Qualifier (7th)
A Choroid, Right B Choroid, Left L Extraocular Muscle, Right M Extraocular Muscle, Left V Lacrimal Gland, Right W Lacrimal Gland, Left	0 Open 3 Percutaneous	Z No Device	Z No Qualifier
N Upper Eyelid, Right P Upper Eyelid, Left Q Lower Eyelid, Right R Lower Eyelid, Left	0 Open 3 Percutaneous X External	Z No Device	Z No Qualifier
X Lacrimal Duct, Right Y Lacrimal Duct, Left	0 Open 3 Percutaneous 7 Via Natural or Artificial Opening 8 Via Natural or Artificial Opening Endoscopic	Z No Device	Z No Qualifier

Section	0	**Medical and Surgical**
Body System	8	Eye
Operation	7	**Dilation:** Expanding an orifice or the lumen of a tubular body part

Body Part (4th)	Approach (5th)	Device (6th)	Qualifier (7th)
X Lacrimal Duct, Right Y Lacrimal Duct, Left	0 Open 3 Percutaneous 7 Via Natural or Artificial Opening 8 Via Natural or Artificial Opening Endoscopic	D Intraluminal Device Z No Device	Z No Qualifier

Section	0	**Medical and Surgical**
Body System	8	Eye
Operation	9	**Drainage:** Taking or letting out fluids and/or gases from a body part

Body Part (4th)	Approach (5th)	Device (6th)	Qualifier (7th)
0 Eye, Right 1 Eye, Left 6 Sclera, Right 7 Sclera, Left 8 Cornea, Right 9 Cornea, Left S Conjunctiva, Right T Conjunctiva, Left	X External	0 Drainage Device	Z No Qualifier
0 Eye, Right 1 Eye, Left 6 Sclera, Right 7 Sclera, Left 8 Cornea, Right 9 Cornea, Left S Conjunctiva, Right T Conjunctiva, Left	X External	Z No Device	X Diagnostic Z No Qualifier

Continued

Medical and Surgical Section (0)

089

Section	0	Medical and Surgical
Body System	8	Eye
Operation	9	**Drainage:** Taking or letting out fluids and/or gases from a body part

Body Part (4th)	Approach (5th)	Device (6th)	Qualifier (7th)
2 Anterior Chamber, Right 3 Anterior Chamber, Left 4 Vitreous, Right 5 Vitreous, Left C Iris, Right D Iris, Left E Retina, Right F Retina, Left G Retinal Vessel, Right H Retinal Vessel, Left J Lens, Right K Lens, Left	3 Percutaneous	0 Drainage Device	Z No Qualifier
2 Anterior Chamber, Right 3 Anterior Chamber, Left 4 Vitreous, Right 5 Vitreous, Left C Iris, Right D Iris, Left E Retina, Right F Retina, Left G Retinal Vessel, Right H Retinal Vessel, Left J Lens, Right K Lens, Left	3 Percutaneous	Z No Device	X Diagnostic Z No Qualifier
A Choroid, Right B Choroid, Left L Extraocular Muscle, Right M Extraocular Muscle, Left V Lacrimal Gland, Right W Lacrimal Gland, Left	0 Open 3 Percutaneous	0 Drainage Device	Z No Qualifier
A Choroid, Right B Choroid, Left L Extraocular Muscle, Right M Extraocular Muscle, Left V Lacrimal Gland, Right W Lacrimal Gland, Left	0 Open 3 Percutaneous	Z No Device	X Diagnostic Z No Qualifier
N Upper Eyelid, Right P Upper Eyelid, Left Q Lower Eyelid, Right R Lower Eyelid, Left	0 Open 3 Percutaneous X External	0 Drainage Device	Z No Qualifier
N Upper Eyelid, Right P Upper Eyelid, Left Q Lower Eyelid, Right R Lower Eyelid, Left	0 Open 3 Percutaneous X External	Z No Device	X Diagnostic Z No Qualifier
X Lacrimal Duct, Right Y Lacrimal Duct, Left	0 Open 3 Percutaneous 7 Via Natural or Artificial Opening 8 Via Natural or Artificial Opening Endoscopic	0 Drainage Device	Z No Qualifier
X Lacrimal Duct, Right Y Lacrimal Duct, Left	0 Open 3 Percutaneous 7 Via Natural or Artificial Opening 8 Via Natural or Artificial Opening Endoscopic	Z No Device	X Diagnostic Z No Qualifier

Section	0	**Medical and Surgical**
Body System	8	**Eye**
Operation	B	**Excision:** Cutting out or off, without replacement, a portion of a body part

Body Part (4ᵗʰ)	Approach (5ᵗʰ)	Device (6ᵗʰ)	Qualifier (7ᵗʰ)
0 Eye, Right 1 Eye, Left N Upper Eyelid, Right P Upper Eyelid, Left Q Lower Eyelid, Right R Lower Eyelid, Left	0 Open 3 Percutaneous X External	Z No Device	X Diagnostic Z No Qualifier
4 Vitreous, Right 5 Vitreous, Left C Iris, Right D Iris, Left E Retina, Right F Retina, Left J Lens, Right K Lens, Left	3 Percutaneous	Z No Device	X Diagnostic Z No Qualifier
6 Sclera, Right 7 Sclera, Left 8 Cornea, Right 9 Cornea, Left S Conjunctiva, Right T Conjunctiva, Left	X External	Z No Device	X Diagnostic Z No Qualifier
A Choroid, Right B Choroid, Left L Extraocular Muscle, Right M Extraocular Muscle, Left V Lacrimal Gland, Right W Lacrimal Gland, Left	0 Open 3 Percutaneous	Z No Device	X Diagnostic Z No Qualifier
X Lacrimal Duct, Right Y Lacrimal Duct, Left	0 Open 3 Percutaneous 7 Via Natural or Artificial Opening 8 Via Natural or Artificial Opening Endoscopic	Z No Device	X Diagnostic Z No Qualifier

Section	0	Medical and Surgical
Body System	8	Eye
Operation	C	**Extirpation:** Taking or cutting out solid matter from a body part

Body Part (4th)	Approach (5th)	Device (6th)	Qualifier (7th)
0 Eye, Right 1 Eye, Left 6 Sclera, Right 7 Sclera, Left 8 Cornea, Right 9 Cornea, Left S Conjunctiva, Right T Conjunctiva, Left	X External	Z No Device	Z No Qualifier
2 Anterior Chamber, Right 3 Anterior Chamber, Left 4 Vitreous, Right 5 Vitreous, Left C Iris, Right D Iris, Left E Retina, Right F Retina, Left G Retinal Vessel, Right H Retinal Vessel, Left J Lens, Right K Lens, Left	3 Percutaneous X External	Z No Device	Z No Qualifier
A Choroid, Right B Choroid, Left L Extraocular Muscle, Right M Extraocular Muscle, Left N Upper Eyelid, Right P Upper Eyelid, Left Q Lower Eyelid, Right R Lower Eyelid, Left V Lacrimal Gland, Right W Lacrimal Gland, Left	0 Open 3 Percutaneous X External	Z No Device	Z No Qualifier
X Lacrimal Duct, Right Y Lacrimal Duct, Left	0 Open 3 Percutaneous 7 Via Natural or Artificial Opening 8 Via Natural or Artificial Opening Endoscopic	Z No Device	Z No Qualifier

Section	0	Medical and Surgical
Body System	8	Eye
Operation	D	**Extraction:** Pulling or stripping out or off all or a portion of a body part by the use of force

Body Part (4th)	Approach (5th)	Device (6th)	Qualifier (7th)
8 Cornea, Right 9 Cornea, Left	X External	Z No Device	X Diagnostic Z No Qualifier
J Lens, Right K Lens, Left	3 Percutaneous	Z No Device	Z No Qualifier

Section	0	Medical and Surgical
Body System	8	Eye
Operation	F	**Fragmentation:** Breaking solid matter in a body part into pieces

Body Part (4th)	Approach (5th)	Device (6th)	Qualifier (7th)
4 Vitreous, Right 5 Vitreous, Left	3 Percutaneous X External	Z No Device	Z No Qualifier

Section	0	Medical and Surgical
Body System	8	Eye
Operation	H	**Insertion:** Putting in a nonbiological appliance that monitors, assists, performs, or prevents a physiological function but does not physically take the place of a body part

Body Part (4th)	Approach (5th)	Device (6th)	Qualifier (7th)
0 Eye, Right 1 Eye, Left	0 Open	5 Epiretinal Visual Prosthesis	Z No Qualifier
0 Eye, Right 1 Eye, Left	3 Percutaneous X External	1 Radioactive Element 3 Infusion Device	Z No Qualifier

Section	0	Medical and Surgical
Body System	8	Eye
Operation	J	**Inspection:** Visually and/or manually exploring a body part

Body Part (4th)	Approach (5th)	Device (6th)	Qualifier (7th)
0 Eye, Right 1 Eye, Left J Lens, Right K Lens, Left	X External	Z No Device	Z No Qualifier
L Extraocular Muscle, Right M Extraocular Muscle, Left	0 Open X External	Z No Device	Z No Qualifier

Section	0	Medical and Surgical
Body System	8	Eye
Operation	L	**Occlusion:** Completely closing an orifice or the lumen of a tubular body part

Body Part (4th)	Approach (5th)	Device (6th)	Qualifier (7th)
X Lacrimal Duct, Right Y Lacrimal Duct, Left	0 Open 3 Percutaneous	C Extraluminal Device D Intraluminal Device Z No Device	Z No Qualifier
X Lacrimal Duct, Right Y Lacrimal Duct, Left	7 Via Natural or Artificial Opening 8 Via Natural or Artificial Opening Endoscopic	D Intraluminal Device Z No Device	Z No Qualifier

Section	0	Medical and Surgical
Body System	8	Eye
Operation	M	**Reattachment:** Putting back in or on all or a portion of a separated body part to its normal location or other suitable location

Body Part (4th)	Approach (5th)	Device (6th)	Qualifier (7th)
N Upper Eyelid, Right P Upper Eyelid, Left Q Lower Eyelid, Right R Lower Eyelid, Left	X External	Z No Device	Z No Qualifier

Section	0	Medical and Surgical
Body System	8	Eye
Operation	N	Release: Freeing a body part from an abnormal physical constraint by cutting or by the use of force

Body Part (4th)	Approach (5th)	Device (6th)	Qualifier (7th)
0 Eye, Right 1 Eye, Left 6 Sclera, Right 7 Sclera, Left 8 Cornea, Right 9 Cornea, Left S Conjunctiva, Right T Conjunctiva, Left	X External	Z No Device	Z No Qualifier
2 Anterior Chamber, Right 3 Anterior Chamber, Left 4 Vitreous, Right 5 Vitreous, Left C Iris, Right D Iris, Left E Retina, Right F Retina, Left G Retinal Vessel, Right H Retinal Vessel, Left J Lens, Right K Lens, Left	3 Percutaneous	Z No Device	Z No Qualifier
A Choroid, Right B Choroid, Left L Extraocular Muscle, Right M Extraocular Muscle, Left V Lacrimal Gland, Right W Lacrimal Gland, Left	0 Open 3 Percutaneous	Z No Device	Z No Qualifier
N Upper Eyelid, Right P Upper Eyelid, Left Q Lower Eyelid, Right R Lower Eyelid, Left	0 Open 3 Percutaneous X External	Z No Device	Z No Qualifier
X Lacrimal Duct, Right Y Lacrimal Duct, Left	0 Open 3 Percutaneous 7 Via Natural or Artificial Opening 8 Via Natural or Artificial Opening Endoscopic	Z No Device	Z No Qualifier

Section	0	Medical and Surgical
Body System	8	Eye
Operation	P	Removal: Taking out or off a device from a body part

Body Part (4th)	Approach (5th)	Device (6th)	Qualifier (7th)
0 Eye, Right 1 Eye, Left	0 Open 3 Percutaneous 7 Via Natural or Artificial Opening 8 Via Natural or Artificial Opening Endoscopic X External	0 Drainage Device 1 Radioactive Element 3 Infusion Device 7 Autologous Tissue Substitute C Extraluminal Device D Intraluminal Device J Synthetic Substitute K Nonautologous Tissue Substitute	Z No Qualifier
J Lens, Right K Lens, Left	3 Percutaneous	J Synthetic Substitute	Z No Qualifier
L Extraocular Muscle, Right M Extraocular Muscle, Left	0 Open 3 Percutaneous	0 Drainage Device 7 Autologous Tissue Substitute J Synthetic Substitute K Nonautologous Tissue Substitute	Z No Qualifier

Section	0	Medical and Surgical
Body System	8	Eye
Operation	Q	**Repair:** Restoring, to the extent possible, a body part to its normal anatomic structure and function

Body Part (4th)	Approach (5th)	Device (6th)	Qualifier (7th)
0 Eye, Right 1 Eye, Left 6 Sclera, Right 7 Sclera, Left 8 Cornea, Right 9 Cornea, Left S Conjunctiva, Right T Conjunctiva, Left	X External	Z No Device	Z No Qualifier
2 Anterior Chamber, Right 3 Anterior Chamber, Left 4 Vitreous, Right 5 Vitreous, Left C Iris, Right D Iris, Left E Retina, Right F Retina, Left G Retinal Vessel, Right H Retinal Vessel, Left J Lens, Right K Lens, Left	3 Percutaneous	Z No Device	Z No Qualifier
A Choroid, Right B Choroid, Left L Extraocular Muscle, Right M Extraocular Muscle, Left V Lacrimal Gland, Right W Lacrimal Gland, Left	0 Open 3 Percutaneous	Z No Device	Z No Qualifier
N Upper Eyelid, Right P Upper Eyelid, Left Q Lower Eyelid, Right R Lower Eyelid, Left	0 Open 3 Percutaneous X External	Z No Device	Z No Qualifier
X Lacrimal Duct, Right Y Lacrimal Duct, Left	0 Open 3 Percutaneous 7 Via Natural or Artificial Opening 8 Via Natural or Artificial Opening Endoscopic	Z No Device	Z No Qualifier

Section	0	Medical and Surgical
Body System	8	Eye
Operation	R	**Replacement:** Putting in or on biological or synthetic material that physically takes the place and/or function of all or a portion of a body part

Body Part (4th)	Approach (5th)	Device (6th)	Qualifier (7th)
0 Eye, Right 1 Eye, Left A Choroid, Right B Choroid, Left	0 Open 3 Percutaneous	7 Autologous Tissue Substitute J Synthetic Substitute K Nonautologous Tissue Substitute	Z No Qualifier
4 Vitreous, Right 5 Vitreous, Left C Iris, Right D Iris, Left G Retinal Vessel, Right H Retinal Vessel, Left	3 Percutaneous	7 Autologous Tissue Substitute J Synthetic Substitute K Nonautologous Tissue Substitute	Z No Qualifier

Continued

08R *Continued*

Section	0	Medical and Surgical
Body System	8	Eye
Operation	R	**Replacement:** Putting in or on biological or synthetic material that physically takes the place and/or function of all or a portion of a body part

Body Part (4th)	Approach (5th)	Device (6th)	Qualifier (7th)
6 Sclera, Right 7 Sclera, Left S Conjunctiva, Right T Conjunctiva, Left	X External	7 Autologous Tissue Substitute J Synthetic Substitute K Nonautologous Tissue Substitute	Z No Qualifier
8 Cornea, Right 9 Cornea, Left	3 Percutaneous X External	7 Autologous Tissue Substitute J Synthetic Substitute K Nonautologous Tissue Substitute	Z No Qualifier
J Lens, Right K Lens, Left	3 Percutaneous	0 Synthetic Substitute, Intraocular Telescope 7 Autologous Tissue Substitute J Synthetic Substitute K Nonautologous Tissue Substitute	Z No Qualifier
N Upper Eyelid, Right P Upper Eyelid, Left Q Lower Eyelid, Right R Lower Eyelid, Left	0 Open 3 Percutaneous X External	7 Autologous Tissue Substitute J Synthetic Substitute K Nonautologous Tissue Substitute	Z No Qualifier
X Lacrimal Duct, Right Y Lacrimal Duct, Left	0 Open 3 Percutaneous 7 Via Natural or Artificial Opening 8 Via Natural or Artificial Opening Endoscopic	7 Autologous Tissue Substitute J Synthetic Substitute K Nonautologous Tissue Substitute	Z No Qualifier

Section	0	Medical and Surgical
Body System	8	Eye
Operation	S	**Reposition:** Moving to its normal location, or other suitable location, all or a portion of a body part

Body Part (4th)	Approach (5th)	Device (6th)	Qualifier (7th)
C Iris, Right D Iris, Left G Retinal Vessel, Right H Retinal Vessel, Left J Lens, Right K Lens, Left	3 Percutaneous	Z No Device	Z No Qualifier
L Extraocular Muscle, Right M Extraocular Muscle, Left V Lacrimal Gland, Right W Lacrimal Gland, Left	0 Open 3 Percutaneous	Z No Device	Z No Qualifier
N Upper Eyelid, Right P Upper Eyelid, Left Q Lower Eyelid, Right R Lower Eyelid, Left	0 Open 3 Percutaneous X External	Z No Device	Z No Qualifier
X Lacrimal Duct, Right Y Lacrimal Duct, Left	0 Open 3 Percutaneous 7 Via Natural or Artificial Opening 8 Via Natural or Artificial Opening Endoscopic	Z No Device	Z No Qualifier

Section	0	**Medical and Surgical**
Body System	8	**Eye**
Operation	T	**Resection:** Cutting out or off, without replacement, all of a body part

Body Part (4th)	Approach (5th)	Device (6th)	Qualifier (7th)
0 Eye, Right **1** Eye, Left **8** Cornea, Right **9** Cornea, Left	**X** External	**Z** No Device	**Z** No Qualifier
4 Vitreous, Right **5** Vitreous, Left **C** Iris, Right **D** Iris, Left **J** Lens, Right **K** Lens, Left	**3** Percutaneous	**Z** No Device	**Z** No Qualifier
L Extraocular Muscle, Right **M** Extraocular Muscle, Left **V** Lacrimal Gland, Right **W** Lacrimal Gland, Left	**0** Open **3** Percutaneous	**Z** No Device	**Z** No Qualifier
N Upper Eyelid, Right **P** Upper Eyelid, Left **Q** Lower Eyelid, Right **R** Lower Eyelid, Left	**0** Open **X** External	**Z** No Device	**Z** No Qualifier
X Lacrimal Duct, Right **Y** Lacrimal Duct, Left	**0** Open **3** Percutaneous **7** Via Natural or Artificial Opening **8** Via Natural or Artificial Opening Endoscopic	**Z** No Device	**Z** No Qualifier

Section	0	**Medical and Surgical**
Body System	8	**Eye**
Operation	U	**Supplement:** Putting in or on biological or synthetic material that physically reinforces and/or augments the function of a portion of a body part

Body Part (4th)	Approach (5th)	Device (6th)	Qualifier (7th)
0 Eye, Right **1** Eye, Left **C** Iris, Right **D** Iris, Left **E** Retina, Right **F** Retina, Left **G** Retinal Vessel, Right **H** Retinal Vessel, Left **L** Extraocular Muscle, Right **M** Extraocular Muscle, Left	**0** Open **3** Percutaneous	**7** Autologous Tissue Substitute **J** Synthetic Substitute **K** Nonautologous Tissue Substitute	**Z** No Qualifier
8 Cornea, Right **9** Cornea, Left **N** Upper Eyelid, Right **P** Upper Eyelid, Left **Q** Lower Eyelid, Right **R** Lower Eyelid, Left	**0** Open **3** Percutaneous **X** External	**7** Autologous Tissue Substitute **J** Synthetic Substitute **K** Nonautologous Tissue Substitute	**Z** No Qualifier
X Lacrimal Duct, Right **Y** Lacrimal Duct, Left	**0** Open **3** Percutaneous **7** Via Natural or Artificial Opening **8** Via Natural or Artificial Opening Endoscopic	**7** Autologous Tissue Substitute **J** Synthetic Substitute **K** Nonautologous Tissue Substitute	**Z** No Qualifier

Section	0	Medical and Surgical
Body System	8	Eye
Operation	V	**Restriction:** Partially closing an orifice or the lumen of a tubular body part

Body Part (4th)	Approach (5th)	Device (6th)	Qualifier (7th)
X Lacrimal Duct, Right Y Lacrimal Duct, Left	0 Open 3 Percutaneous	C Extraluminal Device D Intraluminal Device Z No Device	Z No Qualifier
X Lacrimal Duct, Right Y Lacrimal Duct, Left	7 Via Natural or Artificial Opening 8 Via Natural or Artificial Opening Endoscopic	D Intraluminal Device Z No Device	Z No Qualifier

Section	0	Medical and Surgical
Body System	8	Eye
Operation	W	**Revision:** Correcting, to the extent possible, a portion of a malfunctioning device or the position of a displaced device

Body Part (4th)	Approach (5th)	Device (6th)	Qualifier (7th)
0 Eye, Right 1 Eye, Left	0 Open 3 Percutaneous 7 Via Natural or Artificial Opening 8 Via Natural or Artificial Opening Endoscopic X External	0 Drainage Device 3 Infusion Device 7 Autologous Tissue Substitute C Extraluminal Device D Intraluminal Device J Synthetic Substitute K Nonautologous Tissue Substitute	Z No Qualifier
J Lens, Right K Lens, Left	3 Percutaneous X External	J Synthetic Substitute	Z No Qualifier
L Extraocular Muscle, Right M Extraocular Muscle, Left	0 Open 3 Percutaneous	0 Drainage Device 7 Autologous Tissue Substitute J Synthetic Substitute K Nonautologous Tissue Substitute	Z No Qualifier

Section	0	Medical and Surgical
Body System	8	Eye
Operation	X	**Transfer:** Moving, without taking out, all or a portion of a body part to another location to take over the function of all or a portion of a body part

Body Part (4th)	Approach (5th)	Device (6th)	Qualifier (7th)
L Extraocular Muscle, Right M Extraocular Muscle, Left	0 Open 3 Percutaneous	Z No Device	Z No Qualifier

Eye Code Listing 080–08X

080 – Eye, Alteration

080N07Z Alteration of Right Upper Eyelid with Autologous Tissue Substitute, Open Approach

080N0JZ Alteration of Right Upper Eyelid with Synthetic Substitute, Open Approach

080N0KZ Alteration of Right Upper Eyelid with Nonautologous Tissue Substitute, Open Approach

080N0ZZ Alteration of Right Upper Eyelid, Open Approach

080N37Z Alteration of Right Upper Eyelid with Autologous Tissue Substitute, Percutaneous Approach

080N3JZ Alteration of Right Upper Eyelid with Synthetic Substitute, Percutaneous Approach

080N3KZ Alteration of Right Upper Eyelid with Nonautologous Tissue Substitute, Percutaneous Approach

080N3ZZ Alteration of Right Upper Eyelid, Percutaneous Approach

080NX7Z Alteration of Right Upper Eyelid with Autologous Tissue Substitute, External Approach

080NXJZ Alteration of Right Upper Eyelid with Synthetic Substitute, External Approach

080NXKZ Alteration of Right Upper Eyelid with Nonautologous Tissue Substitute, External Approach

080NXZZ Alteration of Right Upper Eyelid, External Approach

080P07Z Alteration of Left Upper Eyelid with Autologous Tissue Substitute, Open Approach

080P0JZ Alteration of Left Upper Eyelid with Synthetic Substitute, Open Approach

080P0KZ Alteration of Left Upper Eyelid with Nonautologous Tissue Substitute, Open Approach

080P0ZZ Alteration of Left Upper Eyelid, Open Approach

080P37Z	Alteration of Left Upper Eyelid with Autologous Tissue Substitute, Percutaneous Approach
080P3JZ	Alteration of Left Upper Eyelid with Synthetic Substitute, Percutaneous Approach
080P3KZ	Alteration of Left Upper Eyelid with Nonautologous Tissue Substitute, Percutaneous Approach
080P3ZZ	Alteration of Left Upper Eyelid, Percutaneous Approach
080PX7Z	Alteration of Left Upper Eyelid with Autologous Tissue Substitute, External Approach
080PXJZ	Alteration of Left Upper Eyelid with Synthetic Substitute, External Approach
080PXKZ	Alteration of Left Upper Eyelid with Nonautologous Tissue Substitute, External Approach
080PXZZ	Alteration of Left Upper Eyelid, External Approach
080Q07Z	Alteration of Right Lower Eyelid with Autologous Tissue Substitute, Open Approach
080Q0JZ	Alteration of Right Lower Eyelid with Synthetic Substitute, Open Approach
080Q0KZ	Alteration of Right Lower Eyelid with Nonautologous Tissue Substitute, Open Approach
080Q0ZZ	Alteration of Right Lower Eyelid, Open Approach
080Q37Z	Alteration of Right Lower Eyelid with Autologous Tissue Substitute, Percutaneous Approach
080Q3JZ	Alteration of Right Lower Eyelid with Synthetic Substitute, Percutaneous Approach
080Q3KZ	Alteration of Right Lower Eyelid with Nonautologous Tissue Substitute, Percutaneous Approach
080Q3ZZ	Alteration of Right Lower Eyelid, Percutaneous Approach

080QX7Z	Alteration of Right Lower Eyelid with Autologous Tissue Substitute, External Approach
080QXJZ	Alteration of Right Lower Eyelid with Synthetic Substitute, External Approach
080QXKZ	Alteration of Right Lower Eyelid with Nonautologous Tissue Substitute, External Approach
080QXZZ	Alteration of Right Lower Eyelid, External Approach
080R07Z	Alteration of Left Lower Eyelid with Autologous Tissue Substitute, Open Approach
080R0JZ	Alteration of Left Lower Eyelid with Synthetic Substitute, Open Approach
080R0KZ	Alteration of Left Lower Eyelid with Nonautologous Tissue Substitute, Open Approach
080R0ZZ	Alteration of Left Lower Eyelid, Open Approach
080R37Z	Alteration of Left Lower Eyelid with Autologous Tissue Substitute, Percutaneous Approach
080R3JZ	Alteration of Left Lower Eyelid with Synthetic Substitute, Percutaneous Approach
080R3KZ	Alteration of Left Lower Eyelid with Nonautologous Tissue Substitute, Percutaneous Approach
080R3ZZ	Alteration of Left Lower Eyelid, Percutaneous Approach
080RX7Z	Alteration of Left Lower Eyelid with Autologous Tissue Substitute, External Approach
080RXJZ	Alteration of Left Lower Eyelid with Synthetic Substitute, External Approach
080RXKZ	Alteration of Left Lower Eyelid with Nonautologous Tissue Substitute, External Approach
080RXZZ	Alteration of Left Lower Eyelid, External Approach

081 – Eye, Bypass

Review Coding Guideline B3.6a

08123J4	Bypass Right Anterior Chamber to Sclera with Synthetic Substitute, Percutaneous Approach
08123K4	Bypass Right Anterior Chamber to Sclera with Nonautologous Tissue Substitute, Percutaneous Approach
08123Z4	Bypass Right Anterior Chamber to Sclera, Percutaneous Approach
08133J4	Bypass Left Anterior Chamber to Sclera with Synthetic Substitute, Percutaneous Approach
08133K4	Bypass Left Anterior Chamber to Sclera with Nonautologous Tissue Substitute, Percutaneous Approach
08133Z4	Bypass Left Anterior Chamber to Sclera, Percutaneous Approach
081X0J3	Bypass Right Lacrimal Duct to Nasal Cavity with Synthetic Substitute, Open Approach
081X0K3	Bypass Right Lacrimal Duct to Nasal Cavity with Nonautologous Tissue Substitute, Open Approach
081X0Z3	Bypass Right Lacrimal Duct to Nasal Cavity, Open Approach

081X3J3	Bypass Right Lacrimal Duct to Nasal Cavity with Synthetic Substitute, Percutaneous Approach
081X3K3	Bypass Right Lacrimal Duct to Nasal Cavity with Nonautologous Tissue Substitute, Percutaneous Approach
081X3Z3	Bypass Right Lacrimal Duct to Nasal Cavity, Percutaneous Approach
081Y0J3	Bypass Left Lacrimal Duct to Nasal Cavity with Synthetic Substitute, Open Approach
081Y0K3	Bypass Left Lacrimal Duct to Nasal Cavity with Nonautologous Tissue Substitute, Open Approach
081Y0Z3	Bypass Left Lacrimal Duct to Nasal Cavity, Open Approach
081Y3J3	Bypass Left Lacrimal Duct to Nasal Cavity with Synthetic Substitute, Percutaneous Approach
081Y3K3	Bypass Left Lacrimal Duct to Nasal Cavity with Nonautologous Tissue Substitute, Percutaneous Approach
081Y3Z3	Bypass Left Lacrimal Duct to Nasal Cavity, Percutaneous Approach

082 – Eye, Change

Review Coding Guideline B6.1c

0820X0Z	Change Drainage Device in Right Eye, External Approach
0820XYZ	Change Other Device in Right Eye, External Approach

0821X0Z	Change Drainage Device in Left Eye, External Approach
0821XYZ	Change Other Device in Left Eye, External Approach

085 – Eye, Destruction

0850XZZ	Destruction of Right Eye, External Approach
0851XZZ	Destruction of Left Eye, External Approach
08523ZZ	Destruction of Right Anterior Chamber, Percutaneous Approach
08533ZZ	Destruction of Left Anterior Chamber, Percutaneous Approach
08543ZZ	Destruction of Right Vitreous, Percutaneous Approach
08553ZZ	Destruction of Left Vitreous, Percutaneous Approach
0856XZZ	Destruction of Right Sclera, External Approach
0857XZZ	Destruction of Left Sclera, External Approach
0858XZZ	Destruction of Right Cornea, External Approach
0859XZZ	Destruction of Left Cornea, External Approach
085A0ZZ	Destruction of Right Choroid, Open Approach
085A3ZZ	Destruction of Right Choroid, Percutaneous Approach
085B0ZZ	Destruction of Left Choroid, Open Approach

085B3ZZ	Destruction of Left Choroid, Percutaneous Approach
085C3ZZ	Destruction of Right Iris, Percutaneous Approach
085D3ZZ	Destruction of Left Iris, Percutaneous Approach
085E3ZZ	Destruction of Right Retina, Percutaneous Approach
085F3ZZ	Destruction of Left Retina, Percutaneous Approach
085G3ZZ	Destruction of Right Retinal Vessel, Percutaneous Approach
085H3ZZ	Destruction of Left Retinal Vessel, Percutaneous Approach
085J3ZZ	Destruction of Right Lens, Percutaneous Approach
085K3ZZ	Destruction of Left Lens, Percutaneous Approach
085L0ZZ	Destruction of Right Extraocular Muscle, Open Approach
085L3ZZ	Destruction of Right Extraocular Muscle, Percutaneous Approach
085M0ZZ	Destruction of Left Extraocular Muscle, Open Approach
085M3ZZ	Destruction of Left Extraocular Muscle, Percutaneous Approach

085N0ZZ	Destruction of Right Upper Eyelid, Open Approach
085N3ZZ	Destruction of Right Upper Eyelid, Percutaneous Approach
085NXZZ	Destruction of Right Upper Eyelid, External Approach
085P0ZZ	Destruction of Left Upper Eyelid, Open Approach
085P3ZZ	Destruction of Left Upper Eyelid, Percutaneous Approach
085PXZZ	Destruction of Left Upper Eyelid, External Approach
085Q0ZZ	Destruction of Right Lower Eyelid, Open Approach
085Q3ZZ	Destruction of Right Lower Eyelid, Percutaneous Approach
085QXZZ	Destruction of Right Lower Eyelid, External Approach
085R0ZZ	Destruction of Left Lower Eyelid, Open Approach
085R3ZZ	Destruction of Left Lower Eyelid, Percutaneous Approach
085RXZZ	Destruction of Left Lower Eyelid, External Approach
085SXZZ	Destruction of Right Conjunctiva, External Approach
085TXZZ	Destruction of Left Conjunctiva, External Approach
085V0ZZ	Destruction of Right Lacrimal Gland, Open Approach
085V3ZZ	Destruction of Right Lacrimal Gland, Percutaneous Approach
085W0ZZ	Destruction of Left Lacrimal Gland, Open Approach
085W3ZZ	Destruction of Left Lacrimal Gland, Percutaneous Approach
085X0ZZ	Destruction of Right Lacrimal Duct, Open Approach
085X3ZZ	Destruction of Right Lacrimal Duct, Percutaneous Approach
085X7ZZ	Destruction of Right Lacrimal Duct, Via Natural or Artificial Opening
085X8ZZ	Destruction of Right Lacrimal Duct, Via Natural or Artificial Opening Endoscopic
085Y0ZZ	Destruction of Left Lacrimal Duct, Open Approach
085Y3ZZ	Destruction of Left Lacrimal Duct, Percutaneous Approach
085Y7ZZ	Destruction of Left Lacrimal Duct, Via Natural or Artificial Opening
085Y8ZZ	Destruction of Left Lacrimal Duct, Via Natural or Artificial Opening Endoscopic

087 – Eye, Dilation

087X0DZ	Dilation of Right Lacrimal Duct with Intraluminal Device, Open Approach
087X0ZZ	Dilation of Right Lacrimal Duct, Open Approach
087X3DZ	Dilation of Right Lacrimal Duct with Intraluminal Device, Percutaneous Approach
087X3ZZ	Dilation of Right Lacrimal Duct, Percutaneous Approach
087X7DZ	Dilation of Right Lacrimal Duct with Intraluminal Device, Via Natural or Artificial Opening
087X7ZZ	Dilation of Right Lacrimal Duct, Via Natural or Artificial Opening
087X8DZ	Dilation of Right Lacrimal Duct with Intraluminal Device, Via Natural or Artificial Opening Endoscopic
087X8ZZ	Dilation of Right Lacrimal Duct, Via Natural or Artificial Opening Endoscopic
087Y0DZ	Dilation of Left Lacrimal Duct with Intraluminal Device, Open Approach
087Y0ZZ	Dilation of Left Lacrimal Duct, Open Approach
087Y3DZ	Dilation of Left Lacrimal Duct with Intraluminal Device, Percutaneous Approach
087Y3ZZ	Dilation of Left Lacrimal Duct, Percutaneous Approach
087Y7DZ	Dilation of Left Lacrimal Duct with Intraluminal Device, Via Natural or Artificial Opening
087Y7ZZ	Dilation of Left Lacrimal Duct, Via Natural or Artificial Opening
087Y8DZ	Dilation of Left Lacrimal Duct with Intraluminal Device, Via Natural or Artificial Opening Endoscopic
087Y8ZZ	Dilation of Left Lacrimal Duct, Via Natural or Artificial Opening Endoscopic

089 – Eye, Drainage

Review Coding Guidelines B3.4a and B3.4b

Review Coding Guideline B6.2

0890X0Z	Drainage of Right Eye with Drainage Device, External Approach
0890XZX	Drainage of Right Eye, External Approach, Diagnostic
0890XZZ	Drainage of Right Eye, External Approach
0891X0Z	Drainage of Left Eye with Drainage Device, External Approach
0891XZX	Drainage of Left Eye, External Approach, Diagnostic
0891XZZ	Drainage of Left Eye, External Approach
089230Z	Drainage of Right Anterior Chamber with Drainage Device, Percutaneous Approach
08923ZX	Drainage of Right Anterior Chamber, Percutaneous Approach, Diagnostic
08923ZZ	Drainage of Right Anterior Chamber, Percutaneous Approach
089330Z	Drainage of Left Anterior Chamber with Drainage Device, Percutaneous Approach
08933ZX	Drainage of Left Anterior Chamber, Percutaneous Approach, Diagnostic
08933ZZ	Drainage of Left Anterior Chamber, Percutaneous Approach
089430Z	Drainage of Right Vitreous with Drainage Device, Percutaneous Approach
08943ZX	Drainage of Right Vitreous, Percutaneous Approach, Diagnostic
08943ZZ	Drainage of Right Vitreous, Percutaneous Approach
089530Z	Drainage of Left Vitreous with Drainage Device, Percutaneous Approach
08953ZX	Drainage of Left Vitreous, Percutaneous Approach, Diagnostic
08953ZZ	Drainage of Left Vitreous, Percutaneous Approach
0896X0Z	Drainage of Right Sclera with Drainage Device, External Approach
0896XZX	Drainage of Right Sclera, External Approach, Diagnostic
0896XZZ	Drainage of Right Sclera, External Approach
0897X0Z	Drainage of Left Sclera with Drainage Device, External Approach
0897XZX	Drainage of Left Sclera, External Approach, Diagnostic
0897XZZ	Drainage of Left Sclera, External Approach
0898X0Z	Drainage of Right Cornea with Drainage Device, External Approach
0898XZX	Drainage of Right Cornea, External Approach, Diagnostic
0898XZZ	Drainage of Right Cornea, External Approach
0899X0Z	Drainage of Left Cornea with Drainage Device, External Approach
0899XZX	Drainage of Left Cornea, External Approach, Diagnostic
0899XZZ	Drainage of Left Cornea, External Approach
089A00Z	Drainage of Right Choroid with Drainage Device, Open Approach
089A0ZX	Drainage of Right Choroid, Open Approach, Diagnostic
089A0ZZ	Drainage of Right Choroid, Open Approach
089A30Z	Drainage of Right Choroid with Drainage Device, Percutaneous Approach
089A3ZX	Drainage of Right Choroid, Percutaneous Approach, Diagnostic
089A3ZZ	Drainage of Right Choroid, Percutaneous Approach
089B00Z	Drainage of Left Choroid with Drainage Device, Open Approach
089B0ZX	Drainage of Left Choroid, Open Approach, Diagnostic
089B0ZZ	Drainage of Left Choroid, Open Approach
089B30Z	Drainage of Left Choroid with Drainage Device, Percutaneous Approach
089B3ZX	Drainage of Left Choroid, Percutaneous Approach, Diagnostic
089B3ZZ	Drainage of Left Choroid, Percutaneous Approach
089C30Z	Drainage of Right Iris with Drainage Device, Percutaneous Approach
089C3ZX	Drainage of Right Iris, Percutaneous Approach, Diagnostic
089C3ZZ	Drainage of Right Iris, Percutaneous Approach
089D30Z	Drainage of Left Iris with Drainage Device, Percutaneous Approach
089D3ZX	Drainage of Left Iris, Percutaneous Approach, Diagnostic
089D3ZZ	Drainage of Left Iris, Percutaneous Approach
089E30Z	Drainage of Right Retina with Drainage Device, Percutaneous Approach
089E3ZX	Drainage of Right Retina, Percutaneous Approach, Diagnostic
089E3ZZ	Drainage of Right Retina, Percutaneous Approach
089F30Z	Drainage of Left Retina with Drainage Device, Percutaneous Approach
089F3ZX	Drainage of Left Retina, Percutaneous Approach, Diagnostic
089F3ZZ	Drainage of Left Retina, Percutaneous Approach
089G30Z	Drainage of Right Retinal Vessel with Drainage Device, Percutaneous Approach
089G3ZX	Drainage of Right Retinal Vessel, Percutaneous Approach, Diagnostic
089G3ZZ	Drainage of Right Retinal Vessel, Percutaneous Approach

089H30Z	Drainage of Left Retinal Vessel with Drainage Device, Percutaneous Approach
089H3ZX	Drainage of Left Retinal Vessel, Percutaneous Approach, Diagnostic
089H3ZZ	Drainage of Left Retinal Vessel, Percutaneous Approach
089J30Z	Drainage of Right Lens with Drainage Device, Percutaneous Approach
089J3ZX	Drainage of Right Lens, Percutaneous Approach, Diagnostic
089J3ZZ	Drainage of Right Lens, Percutaneous Approach
089K30Z	Drainage of Left Lens with Drainage Device, Percutaneous Approach
089K3ZX	Drainage of Left Lens, Percutaneous Approach, Diagnostic
089K3ZZ	Drainage of Left Lens, Percutaneous Approach
089L00Z	Drainage of Right Extraocular Muscle with Drainage Device, Open Approach
089L0ZX	Drainage of Right Extraocular Muscle, Open Approach, Diagnostic
089L0ZZ	Drainage of Right Extraocular Muscle, Open Approach
089L30Z	Drainage of Right Extraocular Muscle with Drainage Device, Percutaneous Approach
089L3ZX	Drainage of Right Extraocular Muscle, Percutaneous Approach, Diagnostic
089L3ZZ	Drainage of Right Extraocular Muscle, Percutaneous Approach
089M00Z	Drainage of Left Extraocular Muscle with Drainage Device, Open Approach
089M0ZX	Drainage of Left Extraocular Muscle, Open Approach, Diagnostic
089M0ZZ	Drainage of Left Extraocular Muscle, Open Approach
089M30Z	Drainage of Left Extraocular Muscle with Drainage Device, Percutaneous Approach
089M3ZX	Drainage of Left Extraocular Muscle, Percutaneous Approach, Diagnostic
089M3ZZ	Drainage of Left Extraocular Muscle, Percutaneous Approach
089N00Z	Drainage of Right Upper Eyelid with Drainage Device, Open Approach
089N0ZX	Drainage of Right Upper Eyelid, Open Approach, Diagnostic
089N0ZZ	Drainage of Right Upper Eyelid, Open Approach
089N30Z	Drainage of Right Upper Eyelid with Drainage Device, Percutaneous Approach
089N3ZX	Drainage of Right Upper Eyelid, Percutaneous Approach, Diagnostic
089N3ZZ	Drainage of Right Upper Eyelid, Percutaneous Approach
089NX0Z	Drainage of Right Upper Eyelid with Drainage Device, External Approach
089NXZX	Drainage of Right Upper Eyelid, External Approach, Diagnostic
089NXZZ	Drainage of Right Upper Eyelid, External Approach
089P00Z	Drainage of Left Upper Eyelid with Drainage Device, Open Approach
089P0ZX	Drainage of Left Upper Eyelid, Open Approach, Diagnostic
089P0ZZ	Drainage of Left Upper Eyelid, Open Approach
089P30Z	Drainage of Left Upper Eyelid with Drainage Device, Percutaneous Approach
089P3ZX	Drainage of Left Upper Eyelid, Percutaneous Approach, Diagnostic
089P3ZZ	Drainage of Left Upper Eyelid, Percutaneous Approach
089PX0Z	Drainage of Left Upper Eyelid with Drainage Device, External Approach
089PXZX	Drainage of Left Upper Eyelid, External Approach, Diagnostic
089PXZZ	Drainage of Left Upper Eyelid, External Approach
089Q00Z	Drainage of Right Lower Eyelid with Drainage Device, Open Approach
089Q0ZX	Drainage of Right Lower Eyelid, Open Approach, Diagnostic
089Q0ZZ	Drainage of Right Lower Eyelid, Open Approach
089Q30Z	Drainage of Right Lower Eyelid with Drainage Device, Percutaneous Approach
089Q3ZX	Drainage of Right Lower Eyelid, Percutaneous Approach, Diagnostic
089Q3ZZ	Drainage of Right Lower Eyelid, Percutaneous Approach
089QX0Z	Drainage of Right Lower Eyelid with Drainage Device, External Approach
089QXZX	Drainage of Right Lower Eyelid, External Approach, Diagnostic
089QXZZ	Drainage of Right Lower Eyelid, External Approach
089R00Z	Drainage of Left Lower Eyelid with Drainage Device, Open Approach
089R0ZX	Drainage of Left Lower Eyelid, Open Approach, Diagnostic
089R0ZZ	Drainage of Left Lower Eyelid, Open Approach
089R30Z	Drainage of Left Lower Eyelid with Drainage Device, Percutaneous Approach
089R3ZX	Drainage of Left Lower Eyelid, Percutaneous Approach, Diagnostic
089R3ZZ	Drainage of Left Lower Eyelid, Percutaneous Approach
089RX0Z	Drainage of Left Lower Eyelid with Drainage Device, External Approach
089RXZX	Drainage of Left Lower Eyelid, External Approach, Diagnostic
089RXZZ	Drainage of Left Lower Eyelid, External Approach
089SX0Z	Drainage of Right Conjunctiva with Drainage Device, External Approach
089SXZX	Drainage of Right Conjunctiva, External Approach, Diagnostic
089SXZZ	Drainage of Right Conjunctiva, External Approach
089TX0Z	Drainage of Left Conjunctiva with Drainage Device, External Approach
089TXZX	Drainage of Left Conjunctiva, External Approach, Diagnostic
089TXZZ	Drainage of Left Conjunctiva, External Approach
089V00Z	Drainage of Right Lacrimal Gland with Drainage Device, Open Approach
089V0ZX	Drainage of Right Lacrimal Gland, Open Approach, Diagnostic
089V0ZZ	Drainage of Right Lacrimal Gland, Open Approach
089V30Z	Drainage of Right Lacrimal Gland with Drainage Device, Percutaneous Approach
089V3ZX	Drainage of Right Lacrimal Gland, Percutaneous Approach, Diagnostic
089V3ZZ	Drainage of Right Lacrimal Gland, Percutaneous Approach
089W00Z	Drainage of Left Lacrimal Gland with Drainage Device, Open Approach
089W0ZX	Drainage of Left Lacrimal Gland, Open Approach, Diagnostic
089W0ZZ	Drainage of Left Lacrimal Gland, Open Approach
089W30Z	Drainage of Left Lacrimal Gland with Drainage Device, Percutaneous Approach
089W3ZX	Drainage of Left Lacrimal Gland, Percutaneous Approach, Diagnostic
089W3ZZ	Drainage of Left Lacrimal Gland, Percutaneous Approach
089X00Z	Drainage of Right Lacrimal Duct with Drainage Device, Open Approach
089X0ZX	Drainage of Right Lacrimal Duct, Open Approach, Diagnostic
089X0ZZ	Drainage of Right Lacrimal Duct, Open Approach
089X30Z	Drainage of Right Lacrimal Duct with Drainage Device, Percutaneous Approach
089X3ZX	Drainage of Right Lacrimal Duct, Percutaneous Approach, Diagnostic
089X3ZZ	Drainage of Right Lacrimal Duct, Percutaneous Approach
089X70Z	Drainage of Right Lacrimal Duct with Drainage Device, Via Natural or Artificial Opening
089X7ZX	Drainage of Right Lacrimal Duct, Via Natural or Artificial Opening, Diagnostic
089X7ZZ	Drainage of Right Lacrimal Duct, Via Natural or Artificial Opening
089X80Z	Drainage of Right Lacrimal Duct with Drainage Device, Via Natural or Artificial Opening Endoscopic
089X8ZX	Drainage of Right Lacrimal Duct, Via Natural or Artificial Opening Endoscopic, Diagnostic
089X8ZZ	Drainage of Right Lacrimal Duct, Via Natural or Artificial Opening Endoscopic
089Y00Z	Drainage of Left Lacrimal Duct with Drainage Device, Open Approach
089Y0ZX	Drainage of Left Lacrimal Duct, Open Approach, Diagnostic
089Y0ZZ	Drainage of Left Lacrimal Duct, Open Approach
089Y30Z	Drainage of Left Lacrimal Duct with Drainage Device, Percutaneous Approach
089Y3ZX	Drainage of Left Lacrimal Duct, Percutaneous Approach, Diagnostic
089Y3ZZ	Drainage of Left Lacrimal Duct, Percutaneous Approach
089Y70Z	Drainage of Left Lacrimal Duct with Drainage Device, Via Natural or Artificial Opening
089Y7ZX	Drainage of Left Lacrimal Duct, Via Natural or Artificial Opening, Diagnostic
089Y7ZZ	Drainage of Left Lacrimal Duct, Via Natural or Artificial Opening
089Y80Z	Drainage of Left Lacrimal Duct with Drainage Device, Via Natural or Artificial Opening Endoscopic
089Y8ZX	Drainage of Left Lacrimal Duct, Via Natural or Artificial Opening Endoscopic, Diagnostic
089Y8ZZ	Drainage of Left Lacrimal Duct, Via Natural or Artificial Opening Endoscopic

08B – Eye, Excision

Review Coding Guidelines B3.4a and B3.4b

Review Coding Guideline B3.8

08B00ZX	Excision of Right Eye, Open Approach, Diagnostic
08B00ZZ	Excision of Right Eye, Open Approach
08B03ZX	Excision of Right Eye, Percutaneous Approach, Diagnostic
08B03ZZ	Excision of Right Eye, Percutaneous Approach
08B0XZX	Excision of Right Eye, External Approach, Diagnostic
08B0XZZ	Excision of Right Eye, External Approach
08B10ZX	Excision of Left Eye, Open Approach, Diagnostic
08B10ZZ	Excision of Left Eye, Open Approach
08B13ZX	Excision of Left Eye, Percutaneous Approach, Diagnostic
08B13ZZ	Excision of Left Eye, Percutaneous Approach
08B1XZX	Excision of Left Eye, External Approach, Diagnostic
08B1XZZ	Excision of Left Eye, External Approach
08B43ZX	Excision of Right Vitreous, Percutaneous Approach, Diagnostic
08B43ZZ	Excision of Right Vitreous, Percutaneous Approach
08B53ZX	Excision of Left Vitreous, Percutaneous Approach, Diagnostic
08B53ZZ	Excision of Left Vitreous, Percutaneous Approach
08B6XZX	Excision of Right Sclera, External Approach, Diagnostic
08B6XZZ	Excision of Right Sclera, External Approach
08B7XZX	Excision of Left Sclera, External Approach, Diagnostic
08B7XZZ	Excision of Left Sclera, External Approach
08B8XZX	Excision of Right Cornea, External Approach, Diagnostic
08B8XZZ	Excision of Right Cornea, External Approach
08B9XZX	Excision of Left Cornea, External Approach, Diagnostic
08B9XZZ	Excision of Left Cornea, External Approach
08BA0ZX	Excision of Right Choroid, Open Approach, Diagnostic
08BA0ZZ	Excision of Right Choroid, Open Approach
08BA3ZX	Excision of Right Choroid, Percutaneous Approach, Diagnostic
08BA3ZZ	Excision of Right Choroid, Percutaneous Approach
08BB0ZX	Excision of Left Choroid, Open Approach, Diagnostic
08BB0ZZ	Excision of Left Choroid, Open Approach
08BB3ZX	Excision of Left Choroid, Percutaneous Approach, Diagnostic
08BB3ZZ	Excision of Left Choroid, Percutaneous Approach
08BC3ZX	Excision of Right Iris, Percutaneous Approach, Diagnostic
08BC3ZZ	Excision of Right Iris, Percutaneous Approach
08BD3ZX	Excision of Left Iris, Percutaneous Approach, Diagnostic
08BD3ZZ	Excision of Left Iris, Percutaneous Approach
08BE3ZX	Excision of Right Retina, Percutaneous Approach, Diagnostic
08BE3ZZ	Excision of Right Retina, Percutaneous Approach
08BF3ZX	Excision of Left Retina, Percutaneous Approach, Diagnostic
08BF3ZZ	Excision of Left Retina, Percutaneous Approach
08BJ3ZX	Excision of Right Lens, Percutaneous Approach, Diagnostic
08BJ3ZZ	Excision of Right Lens, Percutaneous Approach
08BK3ZX	Excision of Left Lens, Percutaneous Approach, Diagnostic
08BK3ZZ	Excision of Left Lens, Percutaneous Approach
08BL0ZX	Excision of Right Extraocular Muscle, Open Approach, Diagnostic
08BL0ZZ	Excision of Right Extraocular Muscle, Open Approach
08BL3ZX	Excision of Right Extraocular Muscle, Percutaneous Approach, Diagnostic
08BL3ZZ	Excision of Right Extraocular Muscle, Percutaneous Approach
08BM0ZX	Excision of Left Extraocular Muscle, Open Approach, Diagnostic
08BM0ZZ	Excision of Left Extraocular Muscle, Open Approach
08BM3ZX	Excision of Left Extraocular Muscle, Percutaneous Approach, Diagnostic
08BM3ZZ	Excision of Left Extraocular Muscle, Percutaneous Approach
08BN0ZX	Excision of Right Upper Eyelid, Open Approach, Diagnostic
08BN0ZZ	Excision of Right Upper Eyelid, Open Approach
08BN3ZX	Excision of Right Upper Eyelid, Percutaneous Approach, Diagnostic
08BN3ZZ	Excision of Right Upper Eyelid, Percutaneous Approach
08BNXZX	Excision of Right Upper Eyelid, External Approach, Diagnostic
08BNXZZ	Excision of Right Upper Eyelid, External Approach
08BP0ZX	Excision of Left Upper Eyelid, Open Approach, Diagnostic
08BP0ZZ	Excision of Left Upper Eyelid, Open Approach
08BP3ZX	Excision of Left Upper Eyelid, Percutaneous Approach, Diagnostic
08BP3ZZ	Excision of Left Upper Eyelid, Percutaneous Approach
08BPXZX	Excision of Left Upper Eyelid, External Approach, Diagnostic
08BPXZZ	Excision of Left Upper Eyelid, External Approach
08BQ0ZX	Excision of Right Lower Eyelid, Open Approach, Diagnostic
08BQ0ZZ	Excision of Right Lower Eyelid, Open Approach
08BQ3ZX	Excision of Right Lower Eyelid, Percutaneous Approach, Diagnostic
08BQ3ZZ	Excision of Right Lower Eyelid, Percutaneous Approach
08BQXZX	Excision of Right Lower Eyelid, External Approach, Diagnostic
08BQXZZ	Excision of Right Lower Eyelid, External Approach
08BR0ZX	Excision of Left Lower Eyelid, Open Approach, Diagnostic
08BR0ZZ	Excision of Left Lower Eyelid, Open Approach
08BR3ZX	Excision of Left Lower Eyelid, Percutaneous Approach, Diagnostic
08BR3ZZ	Excision of Left Lower Eyelid, Percutaneous Approach
08BRXZX	Excision of Left Lower Eyelid, External Approach, Diagnostic
08BRXZZ	Excision of Left Lower Eyelid, External Approach
08BSXZX	Excision of Right Conjunctiva, External Approach, Diagnostic
08BSXZZ	Excision of Right Conjunctiva, External Approach
08BTXZX	Excision of Left Conjunctiva, External Approach, Diagnostic
08BTXZZ	Excision of Left Conjunctiva, External Approach
08BV0ZX	Excision of Right Lacrimal Gland, Open Approach, Diagnostic
08BV0ZZ	Excision of Right Lacrimal Gland, Open Approach
08BV3ZX	Excision of Right Lacrimal Gland, Percutaneous Approach, Diagnostic
08BV3ZZ	Excision of Right Lacrimal Gland, Percutaneous Approach
08BW0ZX	Excision of Left Lacrimal Gland, Open Approach, Diagnostic
08BW0ZZ	Excision of Left Lacrimal Gland, Open Approach
08BW3ZX	Excision of Left Lacrimal Gland, Percutaneous Approach, Diagnostic
08BW3ZZ	Excision of Left Lacrimal Gland, Percutaneous Approach
08BX0ZX	Excision of Right Lacrimal Duct, Open Approach, Diagnostic
08BX0ZZ	Excision of Right Lacrimal Duct, Open Approach
08BX3ZX	Excision of Right Lacrimal Duct, Percutaneous Approach, Diagnostic
08BX3ZZ	Excision of Right Lacrimal Duct, Percutaneous Approach
08BX7ZX	Excision of Right Lacrimal Duct, Via Natural or Artificial Opening, Diagnostic
08BX7ZZ	Excision of Right Lacrimal Duct, Via Natural or Artificial Opening
08BX8ZX	Excision of Right Lacrimal Duct, Via Natural or Artificial Opening Endoscopic, Diagnostic
08BX8ZZ	Excision of Right Lacrimal Duct, Via Natural or Artificial Opening Endoscopic
08BY0ZX	Excision of Left Lacrimal Duct, Open Approach, Diagnostic
08BY0ZZ	Excision of Left Lacrimal Duct, Open Approach
08BY3ZX	Excision of Left Lacrimal Duct, Percutaneous Approach, Diagnostic
08BY3ZZ	Excision of Left Lacrimal Duct, Percutaneous Approach
08BY7ZX	Excision of Left Lacrimal Duct, Via Natural or Artificial Opening, Diagnostic
08BY7ZZ	Excision of Left Lacrimal Duct, Via Natural or Artificial Opening
08BY8ZX	Excision of Left Lacrimal Duct, Via Natural or Artificial Opening Endoscopic, Diagnostic
08BY8ZZ	Excision of Left Lacrimal Duct, Via Natural or Artificial Opening Endoscopic

08C – Eye, Extirpation

08C0XZZ	Extirpation of Matter from Right Eye, External Approach
08C1XZZ	Extirpation of Matter from Left Eye, External Approach
08C23ZZ	Extirpation of Matter from Right Anterior Chamber, Percutaneous Approach
08C2XZZ	Extirpation of Matter from Right Anterior Chamber, External Approach
08C33ZZ	Extirpation of Matter from Left Anterior Chamber, Percutaneous Approach
08C3XZZ	Extirpation of Matter from Left Anterior Chamber, External Approach
08C43ZZ	Extirpation of Matter from Right Vitreous, Percutaneous Approach
08C4XZZ	Extirpation of Matter from Right Vitreous, External Approach

08C53ZZ	Extirpation of Matter from Left Vitreous, Percutaneous Approach	**08CN0ZZ**	Extirpation of Matter from Right Upper Eyelid, Open Approach
08C5XZZ	Extirpation of Matter from Left Vitreous, External Approach	**08CN3ZZ**	Extirpation of Matter from Right Upper Eyelid, Percutaneous Approach
08C6XZZ	Extirpation of Matter from Right Sclera, External Approach	**08CNXZZ**	Extirpation of Matter from Right Upper Eyelid, External Approach
08C7XZZ	Extirpation of Matter from Left Sclera, External Approach	**08CP0ZZ**	Extirpation of Matter from Left Upper Eyelid, Open Approach
08C8XZZ	Extirpation of Matter from Right Cornea, External Approach	**08CP3ZZ**	Extirpation of Matter from Left Upper Eyelid, Percutaneous Approach
08C9XZZ	Extirpation of Matter from Left Cornea, External Approach	**08CPXZZ**	Extirpation of Matter from Left Upper Eyelid, External Approach
08CA0ZZ	Extirpation of Matter from Right Choroid, Open Approach	**08CQ0ZZ**	Extirpation of Matter from Right Lower Eyelid, Open Approach
08CA3ZZ	Extirpation of Matter from Right Choroid, Percutaneous Approach	**08CQ3ZZ**	Extirpation of Matter from Right Lower Eyelid, Percutaneous Approach
08CAXZZ	Extirpation of Matter from Right Choroid, External Approach	**08CQXZZ**	Extirpation of Matter from Right Lower Eyelid, External Approach
08CB0ZZ	Extirpation of Matter from Left Choroid, Open Approach	**08CR0ZZ**	Extirpation of Matter from Left Lower Eyelid, Open Approach
08CB3ZZ	Extirpation of Matter from Left Choroid, Percutaneous Approach	**08CR3ZZ**	Extirpation of Matter from Left Lower Eyelid, Percutaneous Approach
08CBXZZ	Extirpation of Matter from Left Choroid, External Approach	**08CRXZZ**	Extirpation of Matter from Left Lower Eyelid, External Approach
08CC3ZZ	Extirpation of Matter from Right Iris, Percutaneous Approach	**08CSXZZ**	Extirpation of Matter from Right Conjunctiva, External Approach
08CCXZZ	Extirpation of Matter from Right Iris, External Approach	**08CTXZZ**	Extirpation of Matter from Left Conjunctiva, External Approach
08CD3ZZ	Extirpation of Matter from Left Iris, Percutaneous Approach	**08CV0ZZ**	Extirpation of Matter from Right Lacrimal Gland, Open Approach
08CDXZZ	Extirpation of Matter from Left Iris, External Approach	**08CV3ZZ**	Extirpation of Matter from Right Lacrimal Gland, Percutaneous Approach
08CE3ZZ	Extirpation of Matter from Right Retina, Percutaneous Approach	**08CVXZZ**	Extirpation of Matter from Right Lacrimal Gland, External Approach
08CEXZZ	Extirpation of Matter from Right Retina, External Approach	**08CW0ZZ**	Extirpation of Matter from Left Lacrimal Gland, Open Approach
08CF3ZZ	Extirpation of Matter from Left Retina, Percutaneous Approach	**08CW3ZZ**	Extirpation of Matter from Left Lacrimal Gland, Percutaneous Approach
08CFXZZ	Extirpation of Matter from Left Retina, External Approach	**08CWXZZ**	Extirpation of Matter from Left Lacrimal Gland, External Approach
08CG3ZZ	Extirpation of Matter from Right Retinal Vessel, Percutaneous Approach	**08CX0ZZ**	Extirpation of Matter from Right Lacrimal Duct, Open Approach
08CGXZZ	Extirpation of Matter from Right Retinal Vessel, External Approach	**08CX3ZZ**	Extirpation of Matter from Right Lacrimal Duct, Percutaneous Approach
08CH3ZZ	Extirpation of Matter from Left Retinal Vessel, Percutaneous Approach	**08CX7ZZ**	Extirpation of Matter from Right Lacrimal Duct, Via Natural or Artificial Opening
08CHXZZ	Extirpation of Matter from Left Retinal Vessel, External Approach	**08CX8ZZ**	Extirpation of Matter from Right Lacrimal Duct, Via Natural or Artificial Opening Endoscopic
08CJ3ZZ	Extirpation of Matter from Right Lens, Percutaneous Approach	**08CY0ZZ**	Extirpation of Matter from Left Lacrimal Duct, Open Approach
08CJXZZ	Extirpation of Matter from Right Lens, External Approach	**08CY3ZZ**	Extirpation of Matter from Left Lacrimal Duct, Percutaneous Approach
08CK3ZZ	Extirpation of Matter from Left Lens, Percutaneous Approach	**08CY7ZZ**	Extirpation of Matter from Left Lacrimal Duct, Via Natural or Artificial Opening
08CKXZZ	Extirpation of Matter from Left Lens, External Approach	**08CY8ZZ**	Extirpation of Matter from Left Lacrimal Duct, Via Natural or Artificial Opening Endoscopic
08CL0ZZ	Extirpation of Matter from Right Extraocular Muscle, Open Approach		
08CL3ZZ	Extirpation of Matter from Right Extraocular Muscle, Percutaneous Approach		
08CLXZZ	Extirpation of Matter from Right Extraocular Muscle, External Approach		
08CM0ZZ	Extirpation of Matter from Left Extraocular Muscle, Open Approach		
08CM3ZZ	Extirpation of Matter from Left Extraocular Muscle, Percutaneous Approach		
08CMXZZ	Extirpation of Matter from Left Extraocular Muscle, External Approach		

08D – Eye, Extraction

Review Coding Guidelines B3.4a and B3.4b

08D8XZX	Extraction of Right Cornea, External Approach, Diagnostic	**08D9XZZ**	Extraction of Left Cornea, External Approach
08D8XZZ	Extraction of Right Cornea, External Approach	**08DJ3ZZ**	Extraction of Right Lens, Percutaneous Approach
08D9XZX	Extraction of Left Cornea, External Approach, Diagnostic	**08DK3ZZ**	Extraction of Left Lens, Percutaneous Approach

08F – Eye, Fragmentation

08F43ZZ	Fragmentation in Right Vitreous, Percutaneous Approach	**08F53ZZ**	Fragmentation in Left Vitreous, Percutaneous Approach
● **08F4XZZ**	Fragmentation in Right Vitreous, External Approach	● **08F5XZZ**	Fragmentation in Left Vitreous, External Approach

08H – Eye, Insertion

08H005Z	Insertion of Epiretinal Visual Prosthesis into Right Eye, Open Approach	**08H105Z**	Insertion of Epiretinal Visual Prosthesis into Left Eye, Open Approach
08H031Z	Insertion of Radioactive Element into Right Eye, Percutaneous Approach	**08H131Z**	Insertion of Radioactive Element into Left Eye, Percutaneous Approach
08H033Z	Insertion of Infusion Device into Right Eye, Percutaneous Approach	**08H133Z**	Insertion of Infusion Device into Left Eye, Percutaneous Approach
08H0X1Z	Insertion of Radioactive Element into Right Eye, External Approach	**08H1X1Z**	Insertion of Radioactive Element into Left Eye, External Approach
08H0X3Z	Insertion of Infusion Device into Right Eye, External Approach	**08H1X3Z**	Insertion of Infusion Device into Left Eye, External Approach

08J – Eye, Inspection

Review Coding Guidelines B3.11a, B3.11b and B3.11c

08J0XZZ	Inspection of Right Eye, External Approach	**08JJXZZ**	Inspection of Right Lens, External Approach
08J1XZZ	Inspection of Left Eye, External Approach	**08JKXZZ**	Inspection of Left Lens, External Approach

---

♀ Female-only   ♂ Male-only   ● Limited Coverage   ● Non-OR   **HAC** HAC-associated procedure   ● Non-covered procedures   ✛ Combination

08JL0ZZ Inspection of Right Extraocular Muscle, Open Approach
08JLXZZ Inspection of Right Extraocular Muscle, External Approach

08JM0ZZ Inspection of Left Extraocular Muscle, Open Approach
08JMXZZ Inspection of Left Extraocular Muscle, External Approach

08L – Eye, Occlusion

08LX0CZ Occlusion of Right Lacrimal Duct with Extraluminal Device, Open Approach
08LX0DZ Occlusion of Right Lacrimal Duct with Intraluminal Device, Open Approach
08LX0ZZ Occlusion of Right Lacrimal Duct, Open Approach
08LX3CZ Occlusion of Right Lacrimal Duct with Extraluminal Device, Percutaneous Approach
08LX3DZ Occlusion of Right Lacrimal Duct with Intraluminal Device, Percutaneous Approach
08LX3ZZ Occlusion of Right Lacrimal Duct, Percutaneous Approach
08LX7DZ Occlusion of Right Lacrimal Duct with Intraluminal Device, Via Natural or Artificial Opening
08LX7ZZ Occlusion of Right Lacrimal Duct, Via Natural or Artificial Opening
08LX8DZ Occlusion of Right Lacrimal Duct with Intraluminal Device, Via Natural or Artificial Opening Endoscopic
08LX8ZZ Occlusion of Right Lacrimal Duct, Via Natural or Artificial Opening Endoscopic

08LY0CZ Occlusion of Left Lacrimal Duct with Extraluminal Device, Open Approach
08LY0DZ Occlusion of Left Lacrimal Duct with Intraluminal Device, Open Approach
08LY0ZZ Occlusion of Left Lacrimal Duct, Open Approach
08LY3CZ Occlusion of Left Lacrimal Duct with Extraluminal Device, Percutaneous Approach
08LY3DZ Occlusion of Left Lacrimal Duct with Intraluminal Device, Percutaneous Approach
08LY3ZZ Occlusion of Left Lacrimal Duct, Percutaneous Approach
08LY7DZ Occlusion of Left Lacrimal Duct with Intraluminal Device, Via Natural or Artificial Opening
08LY7ZZ Occlusion of Left Lacrimal Duct, Via Natural or Artificial Opening
08LY8DZ Occlusion of Left Lacrimal Duct with Intraluminal Device, Via Natural or Artificial Opening Endoscopic
08LY8ZZ Occlusion of Left Lacrimal Duct, Via Natural or Artificial Opening Endoscopic

08M – Eye, Reattachment

08MNXZZ Reattachment of Right Upper Eyelid, External Approach
08MPXZZ Reattachment of Left Upper Eyelid, External Approach

08MQXZZ Reattachment of Right Lower Eyelid, External Approach
08MRXZZ Reattachment of Left Lower Eyelid, External Approach

08N – Eye, Release

Review Coding Guidelines B3.13 and B3.14

08N0XZZ Release Right Eye, External Approach
08N1XZZ Release Left Eye, External Approach
08N23ZZ Release Right Anterior Chamber, Percutaneous Approach
08N33ZZ Release Left Anterior Chamber, Percutaneous Approach
08N43ZZ Release Right Vitreous, Percutaneous Approach
08N53ZZ Release Left Vitreous, Percutaneous Approach
08N6XZZ Release Right Sclera, External Approach
08N7XZZ Release Left Sclera, External Approach
08N8XZZ Release Right Cornea, External Approach
08N9XZZ Release Left Cornea, External Approach
08NA0ZZ Release Right Choroid, Open Approach
08NA3ZZ Release Right Choroid, Percutaneous Approach
08NB0ZZ Release Left Choroid, Open Approach
08NB3ZZ Release Left Choroid, Percutaneous Approach
08NC3ZZ Release Right Iris, Percutaneous Approach
08ND3ZZ Release Left Iris, Percutaneous Approach
08NE3ZZ Release Right Retina, Percutaneous Approach
08NF3ZZ Release Left Retina, Percutaneous Approach
08NG3ZZ Release Right Retinal Vessel, Percutaneous Approach
08NH3ZZ Release Left Retinal Vessel, Percutaneous Approach
08NJ3ZZ Release Right Lens, Percutaneous Approach
08NK3ZZ Release Left Lens, Percutaneous Approach
08NL0ZZ Release Right Extraocular Muscle, Open Approach
08NL3ZZ Release Right Extraocular Muscle, Percutaneous Approach
08NM0ZZ Release Left Extraocular Muscle, Open Approach
08NM3ZZ Release Left Extraocular Muscle, Percutaneous Approach
08NN0ZZ Release Right Upper Eyelid, Open Approach

08NN3ZZ Release Right Upper Eyelid, Percutaneous Approach
08NNXZZ Release Right Upper Eyelid, External Approach
08NP0ZZ Release Left Upper Eyelid, Open Approach
08NP3ZZ Release Left Upper Eyelid, Percutaneous Approach
08NPXZZ Release Left Upper Eyelid, External Approach
08NQ0ZZ Release Right Lower Eyelid, Open Approach
08NQ3ZZ Release Right Lower Eyelid, Percutaneous Approach
08NQXZZ Release Right Lower Eyelid, External Approach
08NR0ZZ Release Left Lower Eyelid, Open Approach
08NR3ZZ Release Left Lower Eyelid, Percutaneous Approach
08NRXZZ Release Left Lower Eyelid, External Approach
08NSXZZ Release Right Conjunctiva, External Approach
08NTXZZ Release Left Conjunctiva, External Approach
08NV0ZZ Release Right Lacrimal Gland, Open Approach
08NV3ZZ Release Right Lacrimal Gland, Percutaneous Approach
08NW0ZZ Release Left Lacrimal Gland, Open Approach
08NW3ZZ Release Left Lacrimal Gland, Percutaneous Approach
08NX0ZZ Release Right Lacrimal Duct, Open Approach
08NX3ZZ Release Right Lacrimal Duct, Percutaneous Approach
08NX7ZZ Release Right Lacrimal Duct, Via Natural or Artificial Opening
08NX8ZZ Release Right Lacrimal Duct, Via Natural or Artificial Opening Endoscopic
08NY0ZZ Release Left Lacrimal Duct, Open Approach
08NY3ZZ Release Left Lacrimal Duct, Percutaneous Approach
08NY7ZZ Release Left Lacrimal Duct, Via Natural or Artificial Opening
08NY8ZZ Release Left Lacrimal Duct, Via Natural or Artificial Opening Endoscopic

08P – Eye, Removal

Review Coding Guideline B6.1c

08P000Z Removal of Drainage Device from Right Eye, Open Approach
08P001Z Removal of Radioactive Element from Right Eye, Open Approach
08P003Z Removal of Infusion Device from Right Eye, Open Approach
08P007Z Removal of Autologous Tissue Substitute from Right Eye, Open Approach
08P00CZ Removal of Extraluminal Device from Right Eye, Open Approach
08P00DZ Removal of Intraluminal Device from Right Eye, Open Approach

08P00JZ Removal of Synthetic Substitute from Right Eye, Open Approach
08P00KZ Removal of Nonautologous Tissue Substitute from Right Eye, Open Approach
08P030Z Removal of Drainage Device from Right Eye, Percutaneous Approach
08P031Z Removal of Radioactive Element from Right Eye, Percutaneous Approach

08P033Z   Removal of Infusion Device from Right Eye, Percutaneous Approach

08P037Z   Removal of Autologous Tissue Substitute from Right Eye, Percutaneous Approach

08P03CZ   Removal of Extraluminal Device from Right Eye, Percutaneous Approach

08P03DZ   Removal of Intraluminal Device from Right Eye, Percutaneous Approach

08P03JZ   Removal of Synthetic Substitute from Right Eye, Percutaneous Approach

08P03KZ   Removal of Nonautologous Tissue Substitute from Right Eye, Percutaneous Approach

08P070Z   Removal of Drainage Device from Right Eye, Via Natural or Artificial Opening

08P071Z   Removal of Radioactive Element from Right Eye, Via Natural or Artificial Opening

08P073Z   Removal of Infusion Device from Right Eye, Via Natural or Artificial Opening

08P077Z   Removal of Autologous Tissue Substitute from Right Eye, Via Natural or Artificial Opening

08P07CZ   Removal of Extraluminal Device from Right Eye, Via Natural or Artificial Opening

08P07DZ   Removal of Intraluminal Device from Right Eye, Via Natural or Artificial Opening

08P07JZ   Removal of Synthetic Substitute from Right Eye, Via Natural or Artificial Opening

08P07KZ   Removal of Nonautologous Tissue Substitute from Right Eye, Via Natural or Artificial Opening

08P080Z   Removal of Drainage Device from Right Eye, Via Natural or Artificial Opening Endoscopic

08P081Z   Removal of Radioactive Element from Right Eye, Via Natural or Artificial Opening Endoscopic

08P083Z   Removal of Infusion Device from Right Eye, Via Natural or Artificial Opening Endoscopic

08P087Z   Removal of Autologous Tissue Substitute from Right Eye, Via Natural or Artificial Opening Endoscopic

08P08CZ   Removal of Extraluminal Device from Right Eye, Via Natural or Artificial Opening Endoscopic

08P08DZ   Removal of Intraluminal Device from Right Eye, Via Natural or Artificial Opening Endoscopic

08P08JZ   Removal of Synthetic Substitute from Right Eye, Via Natural or Artificial Opening Endoscopic

08P08KZ   Removal of Nonautologous Tissue Substitute from Right Eye, Via Natural or Artificial Opening Endoscopic

08P0X0Z   Removal of Drainage Device from Right Eye, External Approach

08P0X1Z   Removal of Radioactive Element from Right Eye, External Approach

08P0X3Z   Removal of Infusion Device from Right Eye, External Approach

08P0X7Z   Removal of Autologous Tissue Substitute from Right Eye, External Approach

08P0XCZ   Removal of Extraluminal Device from Right Eye, External Approach

08P0XDZ   Removal of Intraluminal Device from Right Eye, External Approach

08P0XJZ   Removal of Synthetic Substitute from Right Eye, External Approach

08P0XKZ   Removal of Nonautologous Tissue Substitute from Right Eye, External Approach

08P100Z   Removal of Drainage Device from Left Eye, Open Approach

08P101Z   Removal of Radioactive Element from Left Eye, Open Approach

08P103Z   Removal of Infusion Device from Left Eye, Open Approach

08P107Z   Removal of Autologous Tissue Substitute from Left Eye, Open Approach

08P10CZ   Removal of Extraluminal Device from Left Eye, Open Approach

08P10DZ   Removal of Intraluminal Device from Left Eye, Open Approach

08P10JZ   Removal of Synthetic Substitute from Left Eye, Open Approach

08P10KZ   Removal of Nonautologous Tissue Substitute from Left Eye, Open Approach

08P130Z   Removal of Drainage Device from Left Eye, Percutaneous Approach

08P131Z   Removal of Radioactive Element from Left Eye, Percutaneous Approach

08P133Z   Removal of Infusion Device from Left Eye, Percutaneous Approach

08P137Z   Removal of Autologous Tissue Substitute from Left Eye, Percutaneous Approach

08P13CZ   Removal of Extraluminal Device from Left Eye, Percutaneous Approach

08P13DZ   Removal of Intraluminal Device from Left Eye, Percutaneous Approach

08P13JZ   Removal of Synthetic Substitute from Left Eye, Percutaneous Approach

08P13KZ   Removal of Nonautologous Tissue Substitute from Left Eye, Percutaneous Approach

08P170Z   Removal of Drainage Device from Left Eye, Via Natural or Artificial Opening

08P171Z   Removal of Radioactive Element from Left Eye, Via Natural or Artificial Opening

08P173Z   Removal of Infusion Device from Left Eye, Via Natural or Artificial Opening

08P177Z   Removal of Autologous Tissue Substitute from Left Eye, Via Natural or Artificial Opening

08P17CZ   Removal of Extraluminal Device from Left Eye, Via Natural or Artificial Opening

08P17DZ   Removal of Intraluminal Device from Left Eye, Via Natural or Artificial Opening

08P17JZ   Removal of Synthetic Substitute from Left Eye, Via Natural or Artificial Opening

08P17KZ   Removal of Nonautologous Tissue Substitute from Left Eye, Via Natural or Artificial Opening

08P180Z   Removal of Drainage Device from Left Eye, Via Natural or Artificial Opening Endoscopic

08P181Z   Removal of Radioactive Element from Left Eye, Via Natural or Artificial Opening Endoscopic

08P183Z   Removal of Infusion Device from Left Eye, Via Natural or Artificial Opening Endoscopic

08P187Z   Removal of Autologous Tissue Substitute from Left Eye, Via Natural or Artificial Opening Endoscopic

08P18CZ   Removal of Extraluminal Device from Left Eye, Via Natural or Artificial Opening Endoscopic

08P18DZ   Removal of Intraluminal Device from Left Eye, Via Natural or Artificial Opening Endoscopic

08P18JZ   Removal of Synthetic Substitute from Left Eye, Via Natural or Artificial Opening Endoscopic

08P18KZ   Removal of Nonautologous Tissue Substitute from Left Eye, Via Natural or Artificial Opening Endoscopic

08P1X0Z   Removal of Drainage Device from Left Eye, External Approach

08P1X1Z   Removal of Radioactive Element from Left Eye, External Approach

08P1X3Z   Removal of Infusion Device from Left Eye, External Approach

08P1X7Z   Removal of Autologous Tissue Substitute from Left Eye, External Approach

08P1XCZ   Removal of Extraluminal Device from Left Eye, External Approach

08P1XDZ   Removal of Intraluminal Device from Left Eye, External Approach

08P1XJZ   Removal of Synthetic Substitute from Left Eye, External Approach

08P1XKZ   Removal of Nonautologous Tissue Substitute from Left Eye, External Approach

08PJ3JZ   Removal of Synthetic Substitute from Right Lens, Percutaneous Approach

08PK3JZ   Removal of Synthetic Substitute from Left Lens, Percutaneous Approach

08PL00Z   Removal of Drainage Device from Right Extraocular Muscle, Open Approach

08PL07Z   Removal of Autologous Tissue Substitute from Right Extraocular Muscle, Open Approach

08PL0JZ   Removal of Synthetic Substitute from Right Extraocular Muscle, Open Approach

08PL0KZ   Removal of Nonautologous Tissue Substitute from Right Extraocular Muscle, Open Approach

08PL30Z   Removal of Drainage Device from Right Extraocular Muscle, Percutaneous Approach

08PL37Z   Removal of Autologous Tissue Substitute from Right Extraocular Muscle, Percutaneous Approach

08PL3JZ   Removal of Synthetic Substitute from Right Extraocular Muscle, Percutaneous Approach

08PL3KZ   Removal of Nonautologous Tissue Substitute from Right Extraocular Muscle, Percutaneous Approach

08PM00Z   Removal of Drainage Device from Left Extraocular Muscle, Open Approach

08PM07Z Removal of Autologous Tissue Substitute from Left Extraocular Muscle, Open Approach

08PM0JZ Removal of Synthetic Substitute from Left Extraocular Muscle, Open Approach

08PM0KZ Removal of Nonautologous Tissue Substitute from Left Extraocular Muscle, Open Approach

08PM30Z Removal of Drainage Device from Left Extraocular Muscle, Percutaneous Approach

08PM37Z Removal of Autologous Tissue Substitute from Left Extraocular Muscle, Percutaneous Approach

08PM3JZ Removal of Synthetic Substitute from Left Extraocular Muscle, Percutaneous Approach

08PM3KZ Removal of Nonautologous Tissue Substitute from Left Extraocular Muscle, Percutaneous Approach

08Q – Eye, Repair

08Q0XZZ Repair Right Eye, External Approach
08Q1XZZ Repair Left Eye, External Approach
08Q23ZZ Repair Right Anterior Chamber, Percutaneous Approach
08Q33ZZ Repair Left Anterior Chamber, Percutaneous Approach
08Q43ZZ Repair Right Vitreous, Percutaneous Approach
08Q53ZZ Repair Left Vitreous, Percutaneous Approach
08Q6XZZ Repair Right Sclera, External Approach
08Q7XZZ Repair Left Sclera, External Approach
⬤ **08Q8XZZ** Repair Right Cornea, External Approach
⬤ **08Q9XZZ** Repair Left Cornea, External Approach
08QA0ZZ Repair Right Choroid, Open Approach
08QA3ZZ Repair Right Choroid, Percutaneous Approach
08QB0ZZ Repair Left Choroid, Open Approach
08QB3ZZ Repair Left Choroid, Percutaneous Approach
08QC3ZZ Repair Right Iris, Percutaneous Approach
08QD3ZZ Repair Left Iris, Percutaneous Approach
08QE3ZZ Repair Right Retina, Percutaneous Approach
08QF3ZZ Repair Left Retina, Percutaneous Approach
08QG3ZZ Repair Right Retinal Vessel, Percutaneous Approach
08QH3ZZ Repair Left Retinal Vessel, Percutaneous Approach
08QJ3ZZ Repair Right Lens, Percutaneous Approach
08QK3ZZ Repair Left Lens, Percutaneous Approach
08QL0ZZ Repair Right Extraocular Muscle, Open Approach
08QL3ZZ Repair Right Extraocular Muscle, Percutaneous Approach
08QM0ZZ Repair Left Extraocular Muscle, Open Approach
08QM3ZZ Repair Left Extraocular Muscle, Percutaneous Approach
08QN0ZZ Repair Right Upper Eyelid, Open Approach

08QN3ZZ Repair Right Upper Eyelid, Percutaneous Approach
08QNXZZ Repair Right Upper Eyelid, External Approach
08QP0ZZ Repair Left Upper Eyelid, Open Approach
08QP3ZZ Repair Left Upper Eyelid, Percutaneous Approach
08QPXZZ Repair Left Upper Eyelid, External Approach
08QQ0ZZ Repair Right Lower Eyelid, Open Approach
08QQ3ZZ Repair Right Lower Eyelid, Percutaneous Approach
08QQXZZ Repair Right Lower Eyelid, External Approach
08QR0ZZ Repair Left Lower Eyelid, Open Approach
08QR3ZZ Repair Left Lower Eyelid, Percutaneous Approach
08QRXZZ Repair Left Lower Eyelid, External Approach
08QSXZZ Repair Right Conjunctiva, External Approach
08QTXZZ Repair Left Conjunctiva, External Approach
08QV0ZZ Repair Right Lacrimal Gland, Open Approach
08QV3ZZ Repair Right Lacrimal Gland, Percutaneous Approach
08QW0ZZ Repair Left Lacrimal Gland, Open Approach
08QW3ZZ Repair Left Lacrimal Gland, Percutaneous Approach
08QX0ZZ Repair Right Lacrimal Duct, Open Approach
08QX3ZZ Repair Right Lacrimal Duct, Percutaneous Approach
08QX7ZZ Repair Right Lacrimal Duct, Via Natural or Artificial Opening
08QX8ZZ Repair Right Lacrimal Duct, Via Natural or Artificial Opening Endoscopic
08QY0ZZ Repair Left Lacrimal Duct, Open Approach
08QY3ZZ Repair Left Lacrimal Duct, Percutaneous Approach
08QY7ZZ Repair Left Lacrimal Duct, Via Natural or Artificial Opening
08QY8ZZ Repair Left Lacrimal Duct, Via Natural or Artificial Opening Endoscopic

08R – Eye, Replacement

08R007Z Replacement of Right Eye with Autologous Tissue Substitute, Open Approach

08R00JZ Replacement of Right Eye with Synthetic Substitute, Open Approach

08R00KZ Replacement of Right Eye with Nonautologous Tissue Substitute, Open Approach

08R037Z Replacement of Right Eye with Autologous Tissue Substitute, Percutaneous Approach

08R03JZ Replacement of Right Eye with Synthetic Substitute, Percutaneous Approach

08R03KZ Replacement of Right Eye with Nonautologous Tissue Substitute, Percutaneous Approach

08R107Z Replacement of Left Eye with Autologous Tissue Substitute, Open Approach

08R10JZ Replacement of Left Eye with Synthetic Substitute, Open Approach

08R10KZ Replacement of Left Eye with Nonautologous Tissue Substitute, Open Approach

08R137Z Replacement of Left Eye with Autologous Tissue Substitute, Percutaneous Approach

08R13JZ Replacement of Left Eye with Synthetic Substitute, Percutaneous Approach

08R13KZ Replacement of Left Eye with Nonautologous Tissue Substitute, Percutaneous Approach

08R437Z Replacement of Right Vitreous with Autologous Tissue Substitute, Percutaneous Approach

08R43JZ Replacement of Right Vitreous with Synthetic Substitute, Percutaneous Approach

08R43KZ Replacement of Right Vitreous with Nonautologous Tissue Substitute, Percutaneous Approach

08R537Z Replacement of Left Vitreous with Autologous Tissue Substitute, Percutaneous Approach

08R53JZ Replacement of Left Vitreous with Synthetic Substitute, Percutaneous Approach

08R53KZ Replacement of Left Vitreous with Nonautologous Tissue Substitute, Percutaneous Approach

08R6X7Z Replacement of Right Sclera with Autologous Tissue Substitute, External Approach

08R6XJZ Replacement of Right Sclera with Synthetic Substitute, External Approach

08R6XKZ Replacement of Right Sclera with Nonautologous Tissue Substitute, External Approach

08R7X7Z Replacement of Left Sclera with Autologous Tissue Substitute, External Approach

08R7XJZ Replacement of Left Sclera with Synthetic Substitute, External Approach

08R7XKZ Replacement of Left Sclera with Nonautologous Tissue Substitute, External Approach

08R837Z Replacement of Right Cornea with Autologous Tissue Substitute, Percutaneous Approach

08R83JZ Replacement of Right Cornea with Synthetic Substitute, Percutaneous Approach

08R83KZ Replacement of Right Cornea with Nonautologous Tissue Substitute, Percutaneous Approach

08R8X7Z Replacement of Right Cornea with Autologous Tissue Substitute, External Approach

08R8XJZ Replacement of Right Cornea with Synthetic Substitute, External Approach

08R8XKZ Replacement of Right Cornea with Nonautologous Tissue Substitute, External Approach

08R937Z Replacement of Left Cornea with Autologous Tissue Substitute, Percutaneous Approach

08R93JZ Replacement of Left Cornea with Synthetic Substitute, Percutaneous Approach

♀ Female-only   ♂ Male-only   ⬤ Limited Coverage   ⬤ Non-OR   [HAC] HAC-associated procedure   ⬤ Non-covered procedures   ✚ Combination

08R93KZ Replacement of Left Cornea with Nonautologous Tissue Substitute, Percutaneous Approach

08R9X7Z Replacement of Left Cornea with Autologous Tissue Substitute, External Approach

08R9XJZ Replacement of Left Cornea with Synthetic Substitute, External Approach

08R9XKZ Replacement of Left Cornea with Nonautologous Tissue Substitute, External Approach

08RA07Z Replacement of Right Choroid with Autologous Tissue Substitute, Open Approach

08RA0JZ Replacement of Right Choroid with Synthetic Substitute, Open Approach

08RA0KZ Replacement of Right Choroid with Nonautologous Tissue Substitute, Open Approach

08RA37Z Replacement of Right Choroid with Autologous Tissue Substitute, Percutaneous Approach

08RA3JZ Replacement of Right Choroid with Synthetic Substitute, Percutaneous Approach

08RA3KZ Replacement of Right Choroid with Nonautologous Tissue Substitute, Percutaneous Approach

08RB07Z Replacement of Left Choroid with Autologous Tissue Substitute, Open Approach

08RB0JZ Replacement of Left Choroid with Synthetic Substitute, Open Approach

08RB0KZ Replacement of Left Choroid with Nonautologous Tissue Substitute, Open Approach

08RB37Z Replacement of Left Choroid with Autologous Tissue Substitute, Percutaneous Approach

08RB3JZ Replacement of Left Choroid with Synthetic Substitute, Percutaneous Approach

08RB3KZ Replacement of Left Choroid with Nonautologous Tissue Substitute, Percutaneous Approach

08RC37Z Replacement of Right Iris with Autologous Tissue Substitute, Percutaneous Approach

08RC3JZ Replacement of Right Iris with Synthetic Substitute, Percutaneous Approach

08RC3KZ Replacement of Right Iris with Nonautologous Tissue Substitute, Percutaneous Approach

08RD37Z Replacement of Left Iris with Autologous Tissue Substitute, Percutaneous Approach

08RD3JZ Replacement of Left Iris with Synthetic Substitute, Percutaneous Approach

08RD3KZ Replacement of Left Iris with Nonautologous Tissue Substitute, Percutaneous Approach

08RG37Z Replacement of Right Retinal Vessel with Autologous Tissue Substitute, Percutaneous Approach

08RG3JZ Replacement of Right Retinal Vessel with Synthetic Substitute, Percutaneous Approach

08RG3KZ Replacement of Right Retinal Vessel with Nonautologous Tissue Substitute, Percutaneous Approach

08RH37Z Replacement of Left Retinal Vessel with Autologous Tissue Substitute, Percutaneous Approach

08RH3JZ Replacement of Left Retinal Vessel with Synthetic Substitute, Percutaneous Approach

08RH3KZ Replacement of Left Retinal Vessel with Nonautologous Tissue Substitute, Percutaneous Approach

08RJ30Z Replacement of Right Lens with Intraocular Telescope, Percutaneous Approach

08RJ37Z Replacement of Right Lens with Autologous Tissue Substitute, Percutaneous Approach

08RJ3JZ Replacement of Right Lens with Synthetic Substitute, Percutaneous Approach

08RJ3KZ Replacement of Right Lens with Nonautologous Tissue Substitute, Percutaneous Approach

08RK30Z Replacement of Left Lens with Intraocular Telescope, Percutaneous Approach

08RK37Z Replacement of Left Lens with Autologous Tissue Substitute, Percutaneous Approach

08RK3JZ Replacement of Left Lens with Synthetic Substitute, Percutaneous Approach

08RK3KZ Replacement of Left Lens with Nonautologous Tissue Substitute, Percutaneous Approach

08RN07Z Replacement of Right Upper Eyelid with Autologous Tissue Substitute, Open Approach

08RN0JZ Replacement of Right Upper Eyelid with Synthetic Substitute, Open Approach

08RN0KZ Replacement of Right Upper Eyelid with Nonautologous Tissue Substitute, Open Approach

08RN37Z Replacement of Right Upper Eyelid with Autologous Tissue Substitute, Percutaneous Approach

08RN3JZ Replacement of Right Upper Eyelid with Synthetic Substitute, Percutaneous Approach

08RN3KZ Replacement of Right Upper Eyelid with Nonautologous Tissue Substitute, Percutaneous Approach

08RNX7Z Replacement of Right Upper Eyelid with Autologous Tissue Substitute, External Approach

08RNXJZ Replacement of Right Upper Eyelid with Synthetic Substitute, External Approach

08RNXKZ Replacement of Right Upper Eyelid with Nonautologous Tissue Substitute, External Approach

08RP07Z Replacement of Left Upper Eyelid with Autologous Tissue Substitute, Open Approach

08RP0JZ Replacement of Left Upper Eyelid with Synthetic Substitute, Open Approach

08RP0KZ Replacement of Left Upper Eyelid with Nonautologous Tissue Substitute, Open Approach

08RP37Z Replacement of Left Upper Eyelid with Autologous Tissue Substitute, Percutaneous Approach

08RP3JZ Replacement of Left Upper Eyelid with Synthetic Substitute, Percutaneous Approach

08RP3KZ Replacement of Left Upper Eyelid with Nonautologous Tissue Substitute, Percutaneous Approach

08RPX7Z Replacement of Left Upper Eyelid with Autologous Tissue Substitute, External Approach

08RPXJZ Replacement of Left Upper Eyelid with Synthetic Substitute, External Approach

08RPXKZ Replacement of Left Upper Eyelid with Nonautologous Tissue Substitute, External Approach

08RQ07Z Replacement of Right Lower Eyelid with Autologous Tissue Substitute, Open Approach

08RQ0JZ Replacement of Right Lower Eyelid with Synthetic Substitute, Open Approach

08RQ0KZ Replacement of Right Lower Eyelid with Nonautologous Tissue Substitute, Open Approach

08RQ37Z Replacement of Right Lower Eyelid with Autologous Tissue Substitute, Percutaneous Approach

08RQ3JZ Replacement of Right Lower Eyelid with Synthetic Substitute, Percutaneous Approach

08RQ3KZ Replacement of Right Lower Eyelid with Nonautologous Tissue Substitute, Percutaneous Approach

08RQX7Z Replacement of Right Lower Eyelid with Autologous Tissue Substitute, External Approach

08RQXJZ Replacement of Right Lower Eyelid with Synthetic Substitute, External Approach

08RQXKZ Replacement of Right Lower Eyelid with Nonautologous Tissue Substitute, External Approach

08RR07Z Replacement of Left Lower Eyelid with Autologous Tissue Substitute, Open Approach

08RR0JZ Replacement of Left Lower Eyelid with Synthetic Substitute, Open Approach

08RR0KZ Replacement of Left Lower Eyelid with Nonautologous Tissue Substitute, Open Approach

08RR37Z Replacement of Left Lower Eyelid with Autologous Tissue Substitute, Percutaneous Approach

08RR3JZ Replacement of Left Lower Eyelid with Synthetic Substitute, Percutaneous Approach

08RR3KZ Replacement of Left Lower Eyelid with Nonautologous Tissue Substitute, Percutaneous Approach

08RRX7Z Replacement of Left Lower Eyelid with Autologous Tissue Substitute, External Approach

08RRXJZ Replacement of Left Lower Eyelid with Synthetic Substitute, External Approach

08RRXKZ Replacement of Left Lower Eyelid with Nonautologous Tissue Substitute, External Approach

08RSX7Z Replacement of Right Conjunctiva with Autologous Tissue Substitute, External Approach

08RSXJZ Replacement of Right Conjunctiva with Synthetic Substitute, External Approach

08RSXKZ Replacement of Right Conjunctiva with Nonautologous Tissue Substitute, External Approach

08RTX7Z Replacement of Left Conjunctiva with Autologous Tissue Substitute, External Approach

08RTXJZ Replacement of Left Conjunctiva with Synthetic Substitute, External Approach

08RTXKZ Replacement of Left Conjunctiva with Nonautologous Tissue Substitute, External Approach

08RX07Z Replacement of Right Lacrimal Duct with Autologous Tissue Substitute, Open Approach

08RX0JZ Replacement of Right Lacrimal Duct with Synthetic Substitute, Open Approach

08RX0KZ Replacement of Right Lacrimal Duct with Nonautologous Tissue Substitute, Open Approach

08RX37Z Replacement of Right Lacrimal Duct with Autologous Tissue Substitute, Percutaneous Approach

08RX3JZ Replacement of Right Lacrimal Duct with Synthetic Substitute, Percutaneous Approach

08RX3KZ Replacement of Right Lacrimal Duct with Nonautologous Tissue Substitute, Percutaneous Approach

08RX77Z Replacement of Right Lacrimal Duct with Autologous Tissue Substitute, Via Natural or Artificial Opening

08RX7JZ Replacement of Right Lacrimal Duct with Synthetic Substitute, Via Natural or Artificial Opening

08RX7KZ Replacement of Right Lacrimal Duct with Nonautologous Tissue Substitute, Via Natural or Artificial Opening

08RX87Z Replacement of Right Lacrimal Duct with Autologous Tissue Substitute, Via Natural or Artificial Opening Endoscopic

08RX8JZ Replacement of Right Lacrimal Duct with Synthetic Substitute, Via Natural or Artificial Opening Endoscopic

08RX8KZ Replacement of Right Lacrimal Duct with Nonautologous Tissue Substitute, Via Natural or Artificial Opening Endoscopic

08RY07Z Replacement of Left Lacrimal Duct with Autologous Tissue Substitute, Open Approach

08RY0JZ Replacement of Left Lacrimal Duct with Synthetic Substitute, Open Approach

08RY0KZ Replacement of Left Lacrimal Duct with Nonautologous Tissue Substitute, Open Approach

08RY37Z Replacement of Left Lacrimal Duct with Autologous Tissue Substitute, Percutaneous Approach

08RY3JZ Replacement of Left Lacrimal Duct with Synthetic Substitute, Percutaneous Approach

08RY3KZ Replacement of Left Lacrimal Duct with Nonautologous Tissue Substitute, Percutaneous Approach

08RY77Z Replacement of Left Lacrimal Duct with Autologous Tissue Substitute, Via Natural or Artificial Opening

08RY7JZ Replacement of Left Lacrimal Duct with Synthetic Substitute, Via Natural or Artificial Opening

08RY7KZ Replacement of Left Lacrimal Duct with Nonautologous Tissue Substitute, Via Natural or Artificial Opening

08RY87Z Replacement of Left Lacrimal Duct with Autologous Tissue Substitute, Via Natural or Artificial Opening Endoscopic

08RY8JZ Replacement of Left Lacrimal Duct with Synthetic Substitute, Via Natural or Artificial Opening Endoscopic

08RY8KZ Replacement of Left Lacrimal Duct with Nonautologous Tissue Substitute, Via Natural or Artificial Opening Endoscopic

08S – Eye, Reposition

08SC3ZZ Reposition Right Iris, Percutaneous Approach

08SD3ZZ Reposition Left Iris, Percutaneous Approach

08SG3ZZ Reposition Right Retinal Vessel, Percutaneous Approach

08SH3ZZ Reposition Left Retinal Vessel, Percutaneous Approach

08SJ3ZZ Reposition Right Lens, Percutaneous Approach

08SK3ZZ Reposition Left Lens, Percutaneous Approach

08SL0ZZ Reposition Right Extraocular Muscle, Open Approach

08SL3ZZ Reposition Right Extraocular Muscle, Percutaneous Approach

08SM0ZZ Reposition Left Extraocular Muscle, Open Approach

08SM3ZZ Reposition Left Extraocular Muscle, Percutaneous Approach

08SN0ZZ Reposition Right Upper Eyelid, Open Approach

08SN3ZZ Reposition Right Upper Eyelid, Percutaneous Approach

08SNXZZ Reposition Right Upper Eyelid, External Approach

08SP0ZZ Reposition Left Upper Eyelid, Open Approach

08SP3ZZ Reposition Left Upper Eyelid, Percutaneous Approach

08SPXZZ Reposition Left Upper Eyelid, External Approach

08SQ0ZZ Reposition Right Lower Eyelid, Open Approach

08SQ3ZZ Reposition Right Lower Eyelid, Percutaneous Approach

08SQXZZ Reposition Right Lower Eyelid, External Approach

08SR0ZZ Reposition Left Lower Eyelid, Open Approach

08SR3ZZ Reposition Left Lower Eyelid, Percutaneous Approach

08SRXZZ Reposition Left Lower Eyelid, External Approach

08SV0ZZ Reposition Right Lacrimal Gland, Open Approach

08SV3ZZ Reposition Right Lacrimal Gland, Percutaneous Approach

08SW0ZZ Reposition Left Lacrimal Gland, Open Approach

08SW3ZZ Reposition Left Lacrimal Gland, Percutaneous Approach

08SX0ZZ Reposition Right Lacrimal Duct, Open Approach

08SX3ZZ Reposition Right Lacrimal Duct, Percutaneous Approach

08SX7ZZ Reposition Right Lacrimal Duct, Via Natural or Artificial Opening

08SX8ZZ Reposition Right Lacrimal Duct, Via Natural or Artificial Opening Endoscopic

08SY0ZZ Reposition Left Lacrimal Duct, Open Approach

08SY3ZZ Reposition Left Lacrimal Duct, Percutaneous Approach

08SY7ZZ Reposition Left Lacrimal Duct, Via Natural or Artificial Opening

08SY8ZZ Reposition Left Lacrimal Duct, Via Natural or Artificial Opening Endoscopic

08T – Eye, Resection

Review Coding Guideline B3.8

08T0XZZ Resection of Right Eye, External Approach

08T1XZZ Resection of Left Eye, External Approach

08T43ZZ Resection of Right Vitreous, Percutaneous Approach

08T53ZZ Resection of Left Vitreous, Percutaneous Approach

08T8XZZ Resection of Right Cornea, External Approach

08T9XZZ Resection of Left Cornea, External Approach

08TC3ZZ Resection of Right Iris, Percutaneous Approach

08TD3ZZ Resection of Left Iris, Percutaneous Approach

08TJ3ZZ Resection of Right Lens, Percutaneous Approach

08TK3ZZ Resection of Left Lens, Percutaneous Approach

08TL0ZZ Resection of Right Extraocular Muscle, Open Approach

08TL3ZZ Resection of Right Extraocular Muscle, Percutaneous Approach

08TM0ZZ Resection of Left Extraocular Muscle, Open Approach

08TM3ZZ Resection of Left Extraocular Muscle, Percutaneous Approach

08TN0ZZ Resection of Right Upper Eyelid, Open Approach

08TNXZZ Resection of Right Upper Eyelid, External Approach

08TP0ZZ Resection of Left Upper Eyelid, Open Approach

08TPXZZ Resection of Left Upper Eyelid, External Approach

08TQ0ZZ Resection of Right Lower Eyelid, Open Approach

08TQXZZ Resection of Right Lower Eyelid, External Approach

08TR0ZZ Resection of Left Lower Eyelid, Open Approach

08TRXZZ Resection of Left Lower Eyelid, External Approach

08TV0ZZ Resection of Right Lacrimal Gland, Open Approach

08TV3ZZ Resection of Right Lacrimal Gland, Percutaneous Approach

08TW0ZZ Resection of Left Lacrimal Gland, Open Approach

08TW3ZZ Resection of Left Lacrimal Gland, Percutaneous Approach

08TX0ZZ Resection of Right Lacrimal Duct, Open Approach

08TX3ZZ Resection of Right Lacrimal Duct, Percutaneous Approach

08TX7ZZ Resection of Right Lacrimal Duct, Via Natural or Artificial Opening

08TX8ZZ Resection of Right Lacrimal Duct, Via Natural or Artificial Opening Endoscopic

08TY0ZZ Resection of Left Lacrimal Duct, Open Approach

08TY3ZZ   Resection of Left Lacrimal Duct, Percutaneous Approach

08TY7ZZ   Resection of Left Lacrimal Duct, Via Natural or Artificial Opening

08TY8ZZ   Resection of Left Lacrimal Duct, Via Natural or Artificial Opening Endoscopic

08U – Eye, Supplement

08U007Z   Supplement of Right Eye with Autologous Tissue Substitute, Open Approach

08U00JZ   Supplement of Right Eye with Synthetic Substitute, Open Approach

08U00KZ   Supplement of Right Eye with Nonautologous Tissue Substitute, Open Approach

08U037Z   Supplement of Right Eye with Autologous Tissue Substitute, Percutaneous Approach

08U03JZ   Supplement of Right Eye with Synthetic Substitute, Percutaneous Approach

08U03KZ   Supplement of Right Eye with Nonautologous Tissue Substitute, Percutaneous Approach

08U107Z   Supplement of Left Eye with Autologous Tissue Substitute, Open Approach

08U10JZ   Supplement of Left Eye with Synthetic Substitute, Open Approach

08U10KZ   Supplement of Left Eye with Nonautologous Tissue Substitute, Open Approach

08U137Z   Supplement of Left Eye with Autologous Tissue Substitute, Percutaneous Approach

08U13JZ   Supplement of Left Eye with Synthetic Substitute, Percutaneous Approach

08U13KZ   Supplement of Left Eye with Nonautologous Tissue Substitute, Percutaneous Approach

08U807Z   Supplement Right Cornea with Autologous Tissue Substitute, Open Approach

08U80JZ   Supplement Right Cornea with Synthetic Substitute, Open Approach

● 08U80KZ   Supplement Right Cornea with Nonautologous Tissue Substitute, Open Approach

08U837Z   Supplement Right Cornea with Autologous Tissue Substitute, Percutaneous Approach

08U83JZ   Supplement Right Cornea with Synthetic Substitute, Percutaneous Approach

● 08U83KZ   Supplement Right Cornea with Nonautologous Tissue Substitute, Percutaneous Approach

08U8X7Z   Supplement Right Cornea with Autologous Tissue Substitute, External Approach

08U8XJZ   Supplement Right Cornea with Synthetic Substitute, External Approach

● 08U8XKZ   Supplement Right Cornea with Nonautologous Tissue Substitute, External Approach

08U907Z   Supplement Left Cornea with Autologous Tissue Substitute, Open Approach

08U90JZ   Supplement Left Cornea with Synthetic Substitute, Open Approach

● 08U90KZ   Supplement Left Cornea with Nonautologous Tissue Substitute, Open Approach

08U937Z   Supplement Left Cornea with Autologous Tissue Substitute, Percutaneous Approach

08U93JZ   Supplement Left Cornea with Synthetic Substitute, Percutaneous Approach

● 08U93KZ   Supplement Left Cornea with Nonautologous Tissue Substitute, Percutaneous Approach

08U9X7Z   Supplement Left Cornea with Autologous Tissue Substitute, External Approach

08U9XJZ   Supplement Left Cornea with Synthetic Substitute, External Approach

● 08U9XKZ   Supplement Left Cornea with Nonautologous Tissue Substitute, External Approach

08UC07Z   Supplement Right Iris with Autologous Tissue Substitute, Open Approach

08UC0JZ   Supplement Right Iris with Synthetic Substitute, Open Approach

08UC0KZ   Supplement Right Iris with Nonautologous Tissue Substitute, Open Approach

08UC37Z   Supplement Right Iris with Autologous Tissue Substitute, Percutaneous Approach

08UC3JZ   Supplement Right Iris with Synthetic Substitute, Percutaneous Approach

08UC3KZ   Supplement Right Iris with Nonautologous Tissue Substitute, Percutaneous Approach

08UD07Z   Supplement Left Iris with Autologous Tissue Substitute, Open Approach

08UD0JZ   Supplement Left Iris with Synthetic Substitute, Open Approach

08UD0KZ   Supplement Left Iris with Nonautologous Tissue Substitute, Open Approach

08UD37Z   Supplement Left Iris with Autologous Tissue Substitute, Percutaneous Approach

08UD3JZ   Supplement Left Iris with Synthetic Substitute, Percutaneous Approach

08UD3KZ   Supplement Left Iris with Nonautologous Tissue Substitute, Percutaneous Approach

08UE07Z   Supplement Right Retina with Autologous Tissue Substitute, Open Approach

08UE0JZ   Supplement Right Retina with Synthetic Substitute, Open Approach

08UE0KZ   Supplement Right Retina with Nonautologous Tissue Substitute, Open Approach

08UE37Z   Supplement Right Retina with Autologous Tissue Substitute, Percutaneous Approach

08UE3JZ   Supplement Right Retina with Synthetic Substitute, Percutaneous Approach

08UE3KZ   Supplement Right Retina with Nonautologous Tissue Substitute, Percutaneous Approach

08UF07Z   Supplement Left Retina with Autologous Tissue Substitute, Open Approach

08UF0JZ   Supplement Left Retina with Synthetic Substitute, Open Approach

08UF0KZ   Supplement Left Retina with Nonautologous Tissue Substitute, Open Approach

08UF37Z   Supplement Left Retina with Autologous Tissue Substitute, Percutaneous Approach

08UF3JZ   Supplement Left Retina with Synthetic Substitute, Percutaneous Approach

08UF3KZ   Supplement Left Retina with Nonautologous Tissue Substitute, Percutaneous Approach

08UG07Z   Supplement Right Retinal Vessel with Autologous Tissue Substitute, Open Approach

08UG0JZ   Supplement Right Retinal Vessel with Synthetic Substitute, Open Approach

08UG0KZ   Supplement Right Retinal Vessel with Nonautologous Tissue Substitute, Open Approach

08UG37Z   Supplement Right Retinal Vessel with Autologous Tissue Substitute, Percutaneous Approach

08UG3JZ   Supplement Right Retinal Vessel with Synthetic Substitute, Percutaneous Approach

08UG3KZ   Supplement Right Retinal Vessel with Nonautologous Tissue Substitute, Percutaneous Approach

08UH07Z   Supplement Left Retinal Vessel with Autologous Tissue Substitute, Open Approach

08UH0JZ   Supplement Left Retinal Vessel with Synthetic Substitute, Open Approach

08UH0KZ   Supplement Left Retinal Vessel with Nonautologous Tissue Substitute, Open Approach

08UH37Z   Supplement Left Retinal Vessel with Autologous Tissue Substitute, Percutaneous Approach

08UH3JZ   Supplement Left Retinal Vessel with Synthetic Substitute, Percutaneous Approach

08UH3KZ   Supplement Left Retinal Vessel with Nonautologous Tissue Substitute, Percutaneous Approach

08UL07Z   Supplement Right Extraocular Muscle with Autologous Tissue Substitute, Open Approach

08UL0JZ   Supplement Right Extraocular Muscle with Synthetic Substitute, Open Approach

08UL0KZ   Supplement Right Extraocular Muscle with Nonautologous Tissue Substitute, Open Approach

08UL37Z   Supplement Right Extraocular Muscle with Autologous Tissue Substitute, Percutaneous Approach

08UL3JZ   Supplement Right Extraocular Muscle with Synthetic Substitute, Percutaneous Approach

08UL3KZ Supplement Right Extraocular Muscle with Nonautologous Tissue Substitute, Percutaneous Approach

08UM07Z Supplement Left Extraocular Muscle with Autologous Tissue Substitute, Open Approach

08UM0JZ Supplement Left Extraocular Muscle with Synthetic Substitute, Open Approach

08UM0KZ Supplement Left Extraocular Muscle with Nonautologous Tissue Substitute, Open Approach

08UM37Z Supplement Left Extraocular Muscle with Autologous Tissue Substitute, Percutaneous Approach

08UM3JZ Supplement Left Extraocular Muscle with Synthetic Substitute, Percutaneous Approach

08UM3KZ Supplement Left Extraocular Muscle with Nonautologous Tissue Substitute, Percutaneous Approach

08UN07Z Supplement Right Upper Eyelid with Autologous Tissue Substitute, Open Approach

08UN0JZ Supplement Right Upper Eyelid with Synthetic Substitute, Open Approach

08UN0KZ Supplement Right Upper Eyelid with Nonautologous Tissue Substitute, Open Approach

08UN37Z Supplement Right Upper Eyelid with Autologous Tissue Substitute, Percutaneous Approach

08UN3JZ Supplement Right Upper Eyelid with Synthetic Substitute, Percutaneous Approach

08UN3KZ Supplement Right Upper Eyelid with Nonautologous Tissue Substitute, Percutaneous Approach

08UNX7Z Supplement Right Upper Eyelid with Autologous Tissue Substitute, External Approach

08UNXJZ Supplement Right Upper Eyelid with Synthetic Substitute, External Approach

08UNXKZ Supplement Right Upper Eyelid with Nonautologous Tissue Substitute, External Approach

08UP07Z Supplement Left Upper Eyelid with Autologous Tissue Substitute, Open Approach

08UP0JZ Supplement Left Upper Eyelid with Synthetic Substitute, Open Approach

08UP0KZ Supplement Left Upper Eyelid with Nonautologous Tissue Substitute, Open Approach

08UP37Z Supplement Left Upper Eyelid with Autologous Tissue Substitute, Percutaneous Approach

08UP3JZ Supplement Left Upper Eyelid with Synthetic Substitute, Percutaneous Approach

08UP3KZ Supplement Left Upper Eyelid with Nonautologous Tissue Substitute, Percutaneous Approach

08UPX7Z Supplement Left Upper Eyelid with Autologous Tissue Substitute, External Approach

08UPXJZ Supplement Left Upper Eyelid with Synthetic Substitute, External Approach

08UPXKZ Supplement Left Upper Eyelid with Nonautologous Tissue Substitute, External Approach

08UQ07Z Supplement Right Lower Eyelid with Autologous Tissue Substitute, Open Approach

08UQ0JZ Supplement Right Lower Eyelid with Synthetic Substitute, Open Approach

08UQ0KZ Supplement Right Lower Eyelid with Nonautologous Tissue Substitute, Open Approach

08UQ37Z Supplement Right Lower Eyelid with Autologous Tissue Substitute, Percutaneous Approach

08UQ3JZ Supplement Right Lower Eyelid with Synthetic Substitute, Percutaneous Approach

08UQ3KZ Supplement Right Lower Eyelid with Nonautologous Tissue Substitute, Percutaneous Approach

08UQX7Z Supplement Right Lower Eyelid with Autologous Tissue Substitute, External Approach

08UQXJZ Supplement Right Lower Eyelid with Synthetic Substitute, External Approach

08UQXKZ Supplement Right Lower Eyelid with Nonautologous Tissue Substitute, External Approach

08UR07Z Supplement Left Lower Eyelid with Autologous Tissue Substitute, Open Approach

08UR0JZ Supplement Left Lower Eyelid with Synthetic Substitute, Open Approach

08UR0KZ Supplement Left Lower Eyelid with Nonautologous Tissue Substitute, Open Approach

08UR37Z Supplement Left Lower Eyelid with Autologous Tissue Substitute, Percutaneous Approach

08UR3JZ Supplement Left Lower Eyelid with Synthetic Substitute, Percutaneous Approach

08UR3KZ Supplement Left Lower Eyelid with Nonautologous Tissue Substitute, Percutaneous Approach

08URX7Z Supplement Left Lower Eyelid with Autologous Tissue Substitute, External Approach

08URXJZ Supplement Left Lower Eyelid with Synthetic Substitute, External Approach

08URXKZ Supplement Left Lower Eyelid with Nonautologous Tissue Substitute, External Approach

08UX07Z Supplement Right Lacrimal Duct with Autologous Tissue Substitute, Open Approach

08UX0JZ Supplement Right Lacrimal Duct with Synthetic Substitute, Open Approach

08UX0KZ Supplement Right Lacrimal Duct with Nonautologous Tissue Substitute, Open Approach

08UX37Z Supplement Right Lacrimal Duct with Autologous Tissue Substitute, Percutaneous Approach

08UX3JZ Supplement Right Lacrimal Duct with Synthetic Substitute, Percutaneous Approach

08UX3KZ Supplement Right Lacrimal Duct with Nonautologous Tissue Substitute, Percutaneous Approach

08UX77Z Supplement Right Lacrimal Duct with Autologous Tissue Substitute, Via Natural or Artificial Opening

08UX7JZ Supplement Right Lacrimal Duct with Synthetic Substitute, Via Natural or Artificial Opening

08UX7KZ Supplement Right Lacrimal Duct with Nonautologous Tissue Substitute, Via Natural or Artificial Opening

08UX87Z Supplement Right Lacrimal Duct with Autologous Tissue Substitute, Via Natural or Artificial Opening Endoscopic

08UX8JZ Supplement Right Lacrimal Duct with Synthetic Substitute, Via Natural or Artificial Opening Endoscopic

08UX8KZ Supplement Right Lacrimal Duct with Nonautologous Tissue Substitute, Via Natural or Artificial Opening Endoscopic

08UY07Z Supplement Left Lacrimal Duct with Autologous Tissue Substitute, Open Approach

08UY0JZ Supplement Left Lacrimal Duct with Synthetic Substitute, Open Approach

08UY0KZ Supplement Left Lacrimal Duct with Nonautologous Tissue Substitute, Open Approach

08UY37Z Supplement Left Lacrimal Duct with Autologous Tissue Substitute, Percutaneous Approach

08UY3JZ Supplement Left Lacrimal Duct with Synthetic Substitute, Percutaneous Approach

08UY3KZ Supplement Left Lacrimal Duct with Nonautologous Tissue Substitute, Percutaneous Approach

08UY77Z Supplement Left Lacrimal Duct with Autologous Tissue Substitute, Via Natural or Artificial Opening

08UY7JZ Supplement Left Lacrimal Duct with Synthetic Substitute, Via Natural or Artificial Opening

08UY7KZ Supplement Left Lacrimal Duct with Nonautologous Tissue Substitute, Via Natural or Artificial Opening

08UY87Z Supplement Left Lacrimal Duct with Autologous Tissue Substitute, Via Natural or Artificial Opening Endoscopic

08UY8JZ Supplement Left Lacrimal Duct with Synthetic Substitute, Via Natural or Artificial Opening Endoscopic

08UY8KZ Supplement Left Lacrimal Duct with Nonautologous Tissue Substitute, Via Natural or Artificial Opening Endoscopic

08V – Eye, Restriction

08VX0CZ Restriction of Right Lacrimal Duct with Extraluminal Device, Open Approach

08VX0DZ Restriction of Right Lacrimal Duct with Intraluminal Device, Open Approach

08VX0ZZ   Restriction of Right Lacrimal Duct, Open Approach
08VX3CZ   Restriction of Right Lacrimal Duct with Extraluminal Device, Percutaneous Approach
08VX3DZ   Restriction of Right Lacrimal Duct with Intraluminal Device, Percutaneous Approach
08VX3ZZ   Restriction of Right Lacrimal Duct, Percutaneous Approach
08VX7DZ   Restriction of Right Lacrimal Duct with Intraluminal Device, Via Natural or Artificial Opening
08VX7ZZ   Restriction of Right Lacrimal Duct, Via Natural or Artificial Opening
08VX8DZ   Restriction of Right Lacrimal Duct with Intraluminal Device, Via Natural or Artificial Opening Endoscopic
08VX8ZZ   Restriction of Right Lacrimal Duct, Via Natural or Artificial Opening Endoscopic
08VY0CZ   Restriction of Left Lacrimal Duct with Extraluminal Device, Open Approach

08VY0DZ   Restriction of Left Lacrimal Duct with Intraluminal Device, Open Approach
08VY0ZZ   Restriction of Left Lacrimal Duct, Open Approach
08VY3CZ   Restriction of Left Lacrimal Duct with Extraluminal Device, Percutaneous Approach
08VY3DZ   Restriction of Left Lacrimal Duct with Intraluminal Device, Percutaneous Approach
08VY3ZZ   Restriction of Left Lacrimal Duct, Percutaneous Approach
08VY7DZ   Restriction of Left Lacrimal Duct with Intraluminal Device, Via Natural or Artificial Opening
08VY7ZZ   Restriction of Left Lacrimal Duct, Via Natural or Artificial Opening
08VY8DZ   Restriction of Left Lacrimal Duct with Intraluminal Device, Via Natural or Artificial Opening Endoscopic
08VY8ZZ   Restriction of Left Lacrimal Duct, Via Natural or Artificial Opening Endoscopic

08W – Eye, Revision

Review Coding Guideline B6.1c

08W000Z   Revision of Drainage Device in Right Eye, Open Approach
08W003Z   Revision of Infusion Device in Right Eye, Open Approach
08W007Z   Revision of Autologous Tissue Substitute in Right Eye, Open Approach
08W00CZ   Revision of Extraluminal Device in Right Eye, Open Approach
08W00DZ   Revision of Intraluminal Device in Right Eye, Open Approach
08W00JZ   Revision of Synthetic Substitute in Right Eye, Open Approach
08W00KZ   Revision of Nonautologous Tissue Substitute in Right Eye, Open Approach
08W030Z   Revision of Drainage Device in Right Eye, Percutaneous Approach
08W033Z   Revision of Infusion Device in Right Eye, Percutaneous Approach
08W037Z   Revision of Autologous Tissue Substitute in Right Eye, Percutaneous Approach
08W03CZ   Revision of Extraluminal Device in Right Eye, Percutaneous Approach
08W03DZ   Revision of Intraluminal Device in Right Eye, Percutaneous Approach
08W03JZ   Revision of Synthetic Substitute in Right Eye, Percutaneous Approach
08W03KZ   Revision of Nonautologous Tissue Substitute in Right Eye, Percutaneous Approach
08W070Z   Revision of Drainage Device in Right Eye, Via Natural or Artificial Opening
08W073Z   Revision of Infusion Device in Right Eye, Via Natural or Artificial Opening
08W077Z   Revision of Autologous Tissue Substitute in Right Eye, Via Natural or Artificial Opening
08W07CZ   Revision of Extraluminal Device in Right Eye, Via Natural or Artificial Opening
08W07DZ   Revision of Intraluminal Device in Right Eye, Via Natural or Artificial Opening
08W07JZ   Revision of Synthetic Substitute in Right Eye, Via Natural or Artificial Opening
08W07KZ   Revision of Nonautologous Tissue Substitute in Right Eye, Via Natural or Artificial Opening
08W080Z   Revision of Drainage Device in Right Eye, Via Natural or Artificial Opening Endoscopic
08W083Z   Revision of Infusion Device in Right Eye, Via Natural or Artificial Opening Endoscopic
08W087Z   Revision of Autologous Tissue Substitute in Right Eye, Via Natural or Artificial Opening Endoscopic
08W08CZ   Revision of Extraluminal Device in Right Eye, Via Natural or Artificial Opening Endoscopic
08W08DZ   Revision of Intraluminal Device in Right Eye, Via Natural or Artificial Opening Endoscopic
08W08JZ   Revision of Synthetic Substitute in Right Eye, Via Natural or Artificial Opening Endoscopic
08W08KZ   Revision of Nonautologous Tissue Substitute in Right Eye, Via Natural or Artificial Opening Endoscopic
08W0X0Z   Revision of Drainage Device in Right Eye, External Approach
08W0X3Z   Revision of Infusion Device in Right Eye, External Approach
08W0X7Z   Revision of Autologous Tissue Substitute in Right Eye, External Approach

08W0XCZ   Revision of Extraluminal Device in Right Eye, External Approach
08W0XDZ   Revision of Intraluminal Device in Right Eye, External Approach
08W0XJZ   Revision of Synthetic Substitute in Right Eye, External Approach
08W0XKZ   Revision of Nonautologous Tissue Substitute in Right Eye, External Approach
08W100Z   Revision of Drainage Device in Left Eye, Open Approach
08W103Z   Revision of Infusion Device in Left Eye, Open Approach
08W107Z   Revision of Autologous Tissue Substitute in Left Eye, Open Approach
08W10CZ   Revision of Extraluminal Device in Left Eye, Open Approach
08W10DZ   Revision of Intraluminal Device in Left Eye, Open Approach
08W10JZ   Revision of Synthetic Substitute in Left Eye, Open Approach
08W10KZ   Revision of Nonautologous Tissue Substitute in Left Eye, Open Approach
08W130Z   Revision of Drainage Device in Left Eye, Percutaneous Approach
08W133Z   Revision of Infusion Device in Left Eye, Percutaneous Approach
08W137Z   Revision of Autologous Tissue Substitute in Left Eye, Percutaneous Approach
08W13CZ   Revision of Extraluminal Device in Left Eye, Percutaneous Approach
08W13DZ   Revision of Intraluminal Device in Left Eye, Percutaneous Approach
08W13JZ   Revision of Synthetic Substitute in Left Eye, Percutaneous Approach
08W13KZ   Revision of Nonautologous Tissue Substitute in Left Eye, Percutaneous Approach
08W170Z   Revision of Drainage Device in Left Eye, Via Natural or Artificial Opening
08W173Z   Revision of Infusion Device in Left Eye, Via Natural or Artificial Opening
08W177Z   Revision of Autologous Tissue Substitute in Left Eye, Via Natural or Artificial Opening
08W17CZ   Revision of Extraluminal Device in Left Eye, Via Natural or Artificial Opening
08W17DZ   Revision of Intraluminal Device in Left Eye, Via Natural or Artificial Opening
08W17JZ   Revision of Synthetic Substitute in Left Eye, Via Natural or Artificial Opening
08W17KZ   Revision of Nonautologous Tissue Substitute in Left Eye, Via Natural or Artificial Opening
08W180Z   Revision of Drainage Device in Left Eye, Via Natural or Artificial Opening Endoscopic
08W183Z   Revision of Infusion Device in Left Eye, Via Natural or Artificial Opening Endoscopic
08W187Z   Revision of Autologous Tissue Substitute in Left Eye, Via Natural or Artificial Opening Endoscopic
08W18CZ   Revision of Extraluminal Device in Left Eye, Via Natural or Artificial Opening Endoscopic
08W18DZ   Revision of Intraluminal Device in Left Eye, Via Natural or Artificial Opening Endoscopic
08W18JZ   Revision of Synthetic Substitute in Left Eye, Via Natural or Artificial Opening Endoscopic

08W18KZ Revision of Nonautologous Tissue Substitute in Left Eye, Via Natural or Artificial Opening Endoscopic

08W1X0Z Revision of Drainage Device in Left Eye, External Approach

08W1X3Z Revision of Infusion Device in Left Eye, External Approach

08W1X7Z Revision of Autologous Tissue Substitute in Left Eye, External Approach

08W1XCZ Revision of Extraluminal Device in Left Eye, External Approach

08W1XDZ Revision of Intraluminal Device in Left Eye, External Approach

08W1XJZ Revision of Synthetic Substitute in Left Eye, External Approach

08W1XKZ Revision of Nonautologous Tissue Substitute in Left Eye, External Approach

08WJ3JZ Revision of Synthetic Substitute in Right Lens, Percutaneous Approach

08WJXJZ Revision of Synthetic Substitute in Right Lens, External Approach

08WK3JZ Revision of Synthetic Substitute in Left Lens, Percutaneous Approach

08WKXJZ Revision of Synthetic Substitute in Left Lens, External Approach

08WL00Z Revision of Drainage Device in Right Extraocular Muscle, Open Approach

08WL07Z Revision of Autologous Tissue Substitute in Right Extraocular Muscle, Open Approach

08WL0JZ Revision of Synthetic Substitute in Right Extraocular Muscle, Open Approach

08WL0KZ Revision of Nonautologous Tissue Substitute in Right Extraocular Muscle, Open Approach

08WL30Z Revision of Drainage Device in Right Extraocular Muscle, Percutaneous Approach

08WL37Z Revision of Autologous Tissue Substitute in Right Extraocular Muscle, Percutaneous Approach

08WL3JZ Revision of Synthetic Substitute in Right Extraocular Muscle, Percutaneous Approach

08WL3KZ Revision of Nonautologous Tissue Substitute in Right Extraocular Muscle, Percutaneous Approach

08WM00Z Revision of Drainage Device in Left Extraocular Muscle, Open Approach

08WM07Z Revision of Autologous Tissue Substitute in Left Extraocular Muscle, Open Approach

08WM0JZ Revision of Synthetic Substitute in Left Extraocular Muscle, Open Approach

08WM0KZ Revision of Nonautologous Tissue Substitute in Left Extraocular Muscle, Open Approach

08WM30Z Revision of Drainage Device in Left Extraocular Muscle, Percutaneous Approach

08WM37Z Revision of Autologous Tissue Substitute in Left Extraocular Muscle, Percutaneous Approach

08WM3JZ Revision of Synthetic Substitute in Left Extraocular Muscle, Percutaneous Approach

08WM3KZ Revision of Nonautologous Tissue Substitute in Left Extraocular Muscle, Percutaneous Approach

08X – Eye, Transfer

08XL0ZZ Transfer Right Extraocular Muscle, Open Approach

08XL3ZZ Transfer Right Extraocular Muscle, Percutaneous Approach

08XM0ZZ Transfer Left Extraocular Muscle, Open Approach

08XM3ZZ Transfer Left Extraocular Muscle, Percutaneous Approach

---

♀ Female-only   ♂ Male-only   ● Limited Coverage   ● Non-OR   ᴴᴬᶜ HAC-associated procedure   ● Non-covered procedures   ✚ Combination

Nose and Sinus

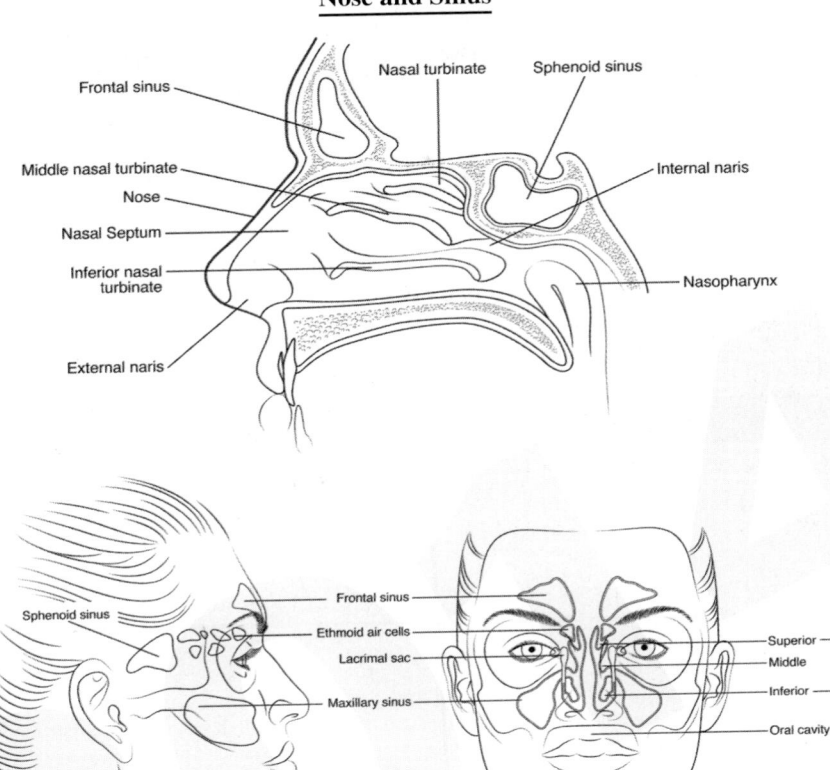

Ear

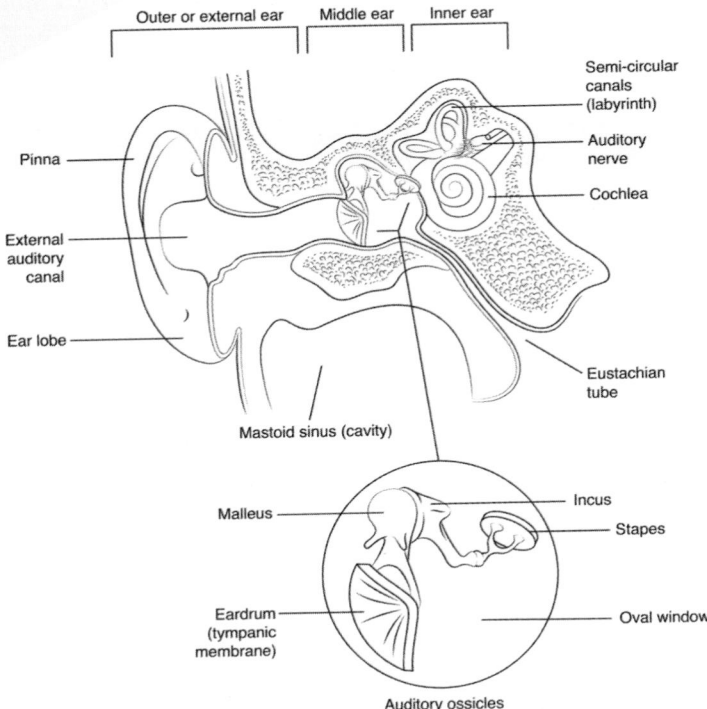

Medical and Surgical Section (0)

090–095

Section	0	Medical and Surgical
Body System	9	Ear, Nose, Sinus
Operation	0	**Alteration:** Modifying the anatomic structure of a body part without affecting the function of the body part

Body Part (4th)	Approach (5th)	Device (6th)	Qualifier (7th)
0 External Ear, Right 1 External Ear, Left 2 External Ear, Bilateral K Nose	0 Open 3 Percutaneous 4 Percutaneous Endoscopic X External	7 Autologous Tissue Substitute J Synthetic Substitute K Nonautologous Tissue Substitute Z No Device	Z No Qualifier

Section	0	Medical and Surgical
Body System	9	Ear, Nose, Sinus
Operation	1	**Bypass:** Altering the route of passage of the contents of a tubular body part

Body Part (4th)	Approach (5th)	Device (6th)	Qualifier (7th)
D Inner Ear, Right E Inner Ear, Left	0 Open	7 Autologous Tissue Substitute J Synthetic Substitute K Nonautologous Tissue Substitute Z No Device	0 Endolymphatic

Section	0	Medical and Surgical
Body System	9	Ear, Nose, Sinus
Operation	2	**Change:** Taking out or off a device from a body part and putting back an identical or similar device in or on the same body part without cutting or puncturing the skin or a mucous membrane

Body Part (4th)	Approach (5th)	Device (6th)	Qualifier (7th)
H Ear, Right J Ear, Left K Nose Y Sinus	X External	0 Drainage Device Y Other Device	Z No Qualifier

Section	0	Medical and Surgical
Body System	9	Ear, Nose, Sinus
Operation	5	**Destruction:** Physical eradication of all or a portion of a body part by the direct use of energy, force, or a destructive agent

Body Part (4th)	Approach (5th)	Device (6th)	Qualifier (7th)
0 External Ear, Right 1 External Ear, Left K Nose	0 Open 3 Percutaneous 4 Percutaneous Endoscopic X External	Z No Device	Z No Qualifier
3 External Auditory Canal, Right 4 External Auditory Canal, Left	0 Open 3 Percutaneous 4 Percutaneous Endoscopic 7 Via Natural or Artificial Opening 8 Via Natural or Artificial Opening Endoscopic X External	Z No Device	Z No Qualifier
5 Middle Ear, Right 6 Middle Ear, Left 9 Auditory Ossicle, Right A Auditory Ossicle, Left D Inner Ear, Right E Inner Ear, Left	0 Open	Z No Device	Z No Qualifier

Continued

Section	0	Medical and Surgical	095 *Continued*
Body System	9	Ear, Nose, Sinus	
Operation	5	Destruction: Physical eradication of all or a portion of a body part by the direct use of energy, force, or a destructive agent	

Body Part (4th)	Approach (5th)	Device (6th)	Qualifier (7th)
7 Tympanic Membrane, Right 8 Tympanic Membrane, Left F Eustachian Tube, Right G Eustachian Tube, Left L Nasal Turbinate N Nasopharynx	0 Open 3 Percutaneous 4 Percutaneous Endoscopic 7 Via Natural or Artificial Opening 8 Via Natural or Artificial Opening Endoscopic	Z No Device	Z No Qualifier
B Mastoid Sinus, Right C Mastoid Sinus, Left M Nasal Septum P Accessory Sinus Q Maxillary Sinus, Right R Maxillary Sinus, Left S Frontal Sinus, Right T Frontal Sinus, Left U Ethmoid Sinus, Right V Ethmoid Sinus, Left W Sphenoid Sinus, Right X Sphenoid Sinus, Left	0 Open 3 Percutaneous 4 Percutaneous Endoscopic	Z No Device	Z No Qualifier

Section	0	Medical and Surgical
Body System	9	Ear, Nose, Sinus
Operation	7	Dilation: Expanding an orifice or the lumen of a tubular body part

Body Part (4th)	Approach (5th)	Device (6th)	Qualifier (7th)
F Eustachian Tube, Right G Eustachian Tube, Left	0 Open 7 Via Natural or Artificial Opening 8 Via Natural or Artificial Opening Endoscopic	D Intraluminal Device Z No Device	Z No Qualifier
F Eustachian Tube, Right G Eustachian Tube, Left	3 Percutaneous 4 Percutaneous Endoscopic	Z No Device	Z No Qualifier

Section	0	Medical and Surgical
Body System	9	Ear, Nose, Sinus
Operation	8	Division: Cutting into a body part, without draining fluids and/or gases from the body part, in order to separate or transect a body part

Body Part (4th)	Approach (5th)	Device (6th)	Qualifier (7th)
L Nasal Turbinate	0 Open 3 Percutaneous 4 Percutaneous Endoscopic 7 Via Natural or Artificial Opening 8 Via Natural or Artificial Opening Endoscopic	Z No Device	Z No Qualifier

Section	0	Medical and Surgical
Body System	9	Ear, Nose, Sinus
Operation	9	Drainage: Taking or letting out fluids and/or gases from a body part

Body Part (4th)	Approach (5th)	Device (6th)	Qualifier (7th)
0 External Ear, Right 1 External Ear, Left K Nose	0 Open 3 Percutaneous 4 Percutaneous Endoscopic X External	0 Drainage Device	Z No Qualifier

Continued

Section	0	Medical and Surgical
Body System	9	Ear, Nose, Sinus
Operation	9	Drainage: Taking or letting out fluids and/or gases from a body part

Body Part (4th)	Approach (5th)	Device (6th)	Qualifier (7th)
0 External Ear, Right **1** External Ear, Left **K** Nose	**0** Open **3** Percutaneous **4** Percutaneous Endoscopic **X** External	**Z** No Device	**X** Diagnostic **Z** No Qualifier
3 External Auditory Canal, Right **4** External Auditory Canal, Left	**0** Open **3** Percutaneous **4** Percutaneous Endoscopic **7** Via Natural or Artificial Opening **8** Via Natural or Artificial Opening Endoscopic **X** External	**0** Drainage Device	**Z** No Qualifier
3 External Auditory Canal, Right **4** External Auditory Canal, Left	**0** Open **3** Percutaneous **4** Percutaneous Endoscopic **7** Via Natural or Artificial Opening **8** Via Natural or Artificial Opening Endoscopic **X** External	**Z** No Device	**X** Diagnostic **Z** No Qualifier
5 Middle Ear, Right **6** Middle Ear, Left **9** Auditory Ossicle, Right **A** Auditory Ossicle, Left **D** Inner Ear, Right **E** Inner Ear, Left	**0** Open	**0** Drainage Device	**Z** No Qualifier
5 Middle Ear, Right **6** Middle Ear, Left **9** Auditory Ossicle, Right **A** Auditory Ossicle, Left **D** Inner Ear, Right **E** Inner Ear, Left	**0** Open	**Z** No Device	**X** Diagnostic **Z** No Qualifier
7 Tympanic Membrane, Right **8** Tympanic Membrane, Left **F** Eustachian Tube, Right **G** Eustachian Tube, Left **L** Nasal Turbinate **N** Nasopharynx	**0** Open **3** Percutaneous **4** Percutaneous Endoscopic **7** Via Natural or Artificial Opening **8** Via Natural or Artificial Opening Endoscopic	**0** Drainage Device	**Z** No Qualifier
7 Tympanic Membrane, Right **8** Tympanic Membrane, Left **F** Eustachian Tube, Right **G** Eustachian Tube, Left **L** Nasal Turbinate **N** Nasopharynx	**0** Open **3** Percutaneous **4** Percutaneous Endoscopic **7** Via Natural or Artificial Opening **8** Via Natural or Artificial Opening Endoscopic	**Z** No Device	**X** Diagnostic **Z** No Qualifier
B Mastoid Sinus, Right **C** Mastoid Sinus, Left **M** Nasal Septum **P** Accessory Sinus **Q** Maxillary Sinus, Right **R** Maxillary Sinus, Left **S** Frontal Sinus, Right **T** Frontal Sinus, Left **U** Ethmoid Sinus, Right **V** Ethmoid Sinus, Left **W** Sphenoid Sinus, Right **X** Sphenoid Sinus, Left	**0** Open **3** Percutaneous **4** Percutaneous Endoscopic	**0** Drainage Device	**Z** No Qualifier

Continued

Section	0	**Medical and Surgical**
Body System	9	**Ear, Nose, Sinus**
Operation	9	**Drainage:** Taking or letting out fluids and/or gases from a body part

Body Part (4th)	Approach (5th)	Device (6th)	Qualifier (7th)
B Mastoid Sinus, Right **C** Mastoid Sinus, Left **M** Nasal Septum **P** Accessory Sinus **Q** Maxillary Sinus, Right **R** Maxillary Sinus, Left **S** Frontal Sinus, Right **T** Frontal Sinus, Left **U** Ethmoid Sinus, Right **V** Ethmoid Sinus, Left **W** Sphenoid Sinus, Right **X** Sphenoid Sinus, Left	**0** Open **3** Percutaneous **4** Percutaneous Endoscopic	**Z** No Device	**X** Diagnostic **Z** No Qualifier

Section	0	**Medical and Surgical**
Body System	9	**Ear, Nose, Sinus**
Operation	B	**Excision:** Cutting out or off, without replacement, a portion of a body part

Body Part (4th)	Approach (5th)	Device (6th)	Qualifier (7th)
0 External Ear, Right **1** External Ear, Left **K** Nose	**0** Open **3** Percutaneous **4** Percutaneous Endoscopic **X** External	**Z** No Device	**X** Diagnostic **Z** No Qualifier
3 External Auditory Canal, Right **4** External Auditory Canal, Left	**0** Open **3** Percutaneous **4** Percutaneous Endoscopic **7** Via Natural or Artificial Opening **8** Via Natural or Artificial Opening Endoscopic **X** External	**Z** No Device	**X** Diagnostic **Z** No Qualifier
5 Middle Ear, Right **6** Middle Ear, Left **9** Auditory Ossicle, Right **A** Auditory Ossicle, Left **D** Inner Ear, Right **E** Inner Ear, Left	**0** Open	**Z** No Device	**X** Diagnostic **Z** No Qualifier
7 Tympanic Membrane, Right **8** Tympanic Membrane, Left **F** Eustachian Tube, Right **G** Eustachian Tube, Left **L** Nasal Turbinate **N** Nasopharynx	**0** Open **3** Percutaneous **4** Percutaneous Endoscopic **7** Via Natural or Artificial Opening **8** Via Natural or Artificial Opening Endoscopic	**Z** No Device	**X** Diagnostic **Z** No Qualifier
B Mastoid Sinus, Right **C** Mastoid Sinus, Left **M** Nasal Septum **P** Accessory Sinus **Q** Maxillary Sinus, Right **R** Maxillary Sinus, Left **S** Frontal Sinus, Right **T** Frontal Sinus, Left **U** Ethmoid Sinus, Right **V** Ethmoid Sinus, Left **W** Sphenoid Sinus, Right **X** Sphenoid Sinus, Left	**0** Open **3** Percutaneous **4** Percutaneous Endoscopic	**Z** No Device	**X** Diagnostic **Z** No Qualifier

Section	0	Medical and Surgical
Body System	9	Ear, Nose, Sinus
Operation	C	**Extirpation:** Taking or cutting out solid matter from a body part

Body Part (4th)	Approach (5th)	Device (6th)	Qualifier (7th)
0 External Ear, Right **1** External Ear, Left **K** Nose	**0** Open **3** Percutaneous **4** Percutaneous Endoscopic **X** External	**Z** No Device	**Z** No Qualifier
3 External Auditory Canal, Right **4** External Auditory Canal, Left	**0** Open **3** Percutaneous **4** Percutaneous Endoscopic **7** Via Natural or Artificial Opening **8** Via Natural or Artificial Opening Endoscopic **X** External	**Z** No Device	**Z** No Qualifier
5 Middle Ear, Right **6** Middle Ear, Left **9** Auditory Ossicle, Right **A** Auditory Ossicle, Left **D** Inner Ear, Right **E** Inner Ear, Left	**0** Open	**Z** No Device	**Z** No Qualifier
7 Tympanic Membrane, Right **8** Tympanic Membrane, Left **F** Eustachian Tube, Right **G** Eustachian Tube, Left **L** Nasal Turbinate **N** Nasopharynx	**0** Open **3** Percutaneous **4** Percutaneous Endoscopic **7** Via Natural or Artificial Opening **8** Via Natural or Artificial Opening Endoscopic	**Z** No Device	**Z** No Qualifier
B Mastoid Sinus, Right **C** Mastoid Sinus, Left **M** Nasal Septum **P** Accessory Sinus **Q** Maxillary Sinus, Right **R** Maxillary Sinus, Left **S** Frontal Sinus, Right **T** Frontal Sinus, Left **U** Ethmoid Sinus, Right **V** Ethmoid Sinus, Left **W** Sphenoid Sinus, Right **X** Sphenoid Sinus, Left	**0** Open **3** Percutaneous **4** Percutaneous Endoscopic	**Z** No Device	**Z** No Qualifier

Section	0	Medical and Surgical
Body System	9	Ear, Nose, Sinus
Operation	D	**Extraction:** Pulling or stripping out or off all or a portion of a body part by the use of force

Body Part (4th)	Approach (5th)	Device (6th)	Qualifier (7th)
7 Tympanic Membrane, Right **8** Tympanic Membrane, Left **L** Nasal Turbinate	**0** Open **3** Percutaneous **4** Percutaneous Endoscopic **7** Via Natural or Artificial Opening **8** Via Natural or Artificial Opening Endoscopic	**Z** No Device	**Z** No Qualifier
9 Auditory Ossicle, Right **A** Auditory Ossicle, Left	**0** Open	**Z** No Device	**Z** No Qualifier

Continued

Section	0	Medical and Surgical
Body System	9	Ear, Nose, Sinus
Operation	D	Extraction: Pulling or stripping out or off all or a portion of a body part by the use of force

Body Part (4th)	Approach (5th)	Device (6th)	Qualifier (7th)
B Mastoid Sinus, Right C Mastoid Sinus, Left M Nasal Septum P Accessory Sinus Q Maxillary Sinus, Right R Maxillary Sinus, Left S Frontal Sinus, Right T Frontal Sinus, Left U Ethmoid Sinus, Right V Ethmoid Sinus, Left W Sphenoid Sinus, Right X Sphenoid Sinus, Left	0 Open 3 Percutaneous 4 Percutaneous Endoscopic	Z No Device	Z No Qualifier

Section	0	Medical and Surgical
Body System	9	Ear, Nose, Sinus
Operation	H	Insertion: Putting in a nonbiological appliance that monitors, assists, performs, or prevents a physiological function but does not physically take the place of a body part

Body Part (4th)	Approach (5th)	Device (6th)	Qualifier (7th)
D Inner Ear, Right E Inner Ear, Left	0 Open 3 Percutaneous 4 Percutaneous Endoscopic	4 Hearing Device, Bone Conduction 5 Hearing Device, Single Channel Cochlear Prosthesis 6 Hearing Device, Multiple Channel Cochlear Prosthesis S Hearing Device	Z No Qualifier
N Nasopharynx	7 Via Natural or Artificial Opening 8 Via Natural or Artificial Opening Endoscopic	B Intraluminal Device, Airway	Z No Qualifier

Section	0	Medical and Surgical
Body System	9	Ear, Nose, Sinus
Operation	J	Inspection: Visually and/or manually exploring a body part

Body Part (4th)	Approach (5th)	Device (6th)	Qualifier (7th)
7 Tympanic Membrane, Right 8 Tympanic Membrane, Left H Ear, Right J Ear, Left	0 Open 3 Percutaneous 4 Percutaneous Endoscopic 7 Via Natural or Artificial Opening 8 Via Natural or Artificial Opening Endoscopic X External	Z No Device	Z No Qualifier
D Inner Ear, Right E Inner Ear, Left K Nose Y Sinus	0 Open 3 Percutaneous 4 Percutaneous Endoscopic X External	Z No Device	Z No Qualifier

Section	0	Medical and Surgical
Body System	9	Ear, Nose, Sinus
Operation	M	Reattachment: Putting back in or on all or a portion of a separated body part to its normal location or other suitable location

Body Part (4th)	Approach (5th)	Device (6th)	Qualifier (7th)
0 External Ear, Right 1 External Ear, Left K Nose	X External	Z No Device	Z No Qualifier

Section	0	Medical and Surgical
Body System	9	Ear, Nose, Sinus
Operation	N	Release: Freeing a body part from an abnormal physical constraint by cutting or by the use of force

Body Part (4th)	Approach (5th)	Device (6th)	Qualifier (7th)
0 External Ear, Right 1 External Ear, Left K Nose	0 Open 3 Percutaneous 4 Percutaneous Endoscopic X External	Z No Device	Z No Qualifier
3 External Auditory Canal, Right 4 External Auditory Canal, Left	0 Open 3 Percutaneous 4 Percutaneous Endoscopic 7 Via Natural or Artificial Opening 8 Via Natural or Artificial Opening Endoscopic X External	Z No Device	Z No Qualifier
5 Middle Ear, Right 6 Middle Ear, Left 9 Auditory Ossicle, Right A Auditory Ossicle, Left D Inner Ear, Right E Inner Ear, Left	0 Open	Z No Device	Z No Qualifier
7 Tympanic Membrane, Right 8 Tympanic Membrane, Left F Eustachian Tube, Right G Eustachian Tube, Left L Nasal Turbinate N Nasopharynx	0 Open 3 Percutaneous 4 Percutaneous Endoscopic 7 Via Natural or Artificial Opening 8 Via Natural or Artificial Opening Endoscopic	Z No Device	Z No Qualifier
B Mastoid Sinus, Right C Mastoid Sinus, Left M Nasal Septum P Accessory Sinus Q Maxillary Sinus, Right R Maxillary Sinus, Left S Frontal Sinus, Right T Frontal Sinus, Left U Ethmoid Sinus, Right V Ethmoid Sinus, Left W Sphenoid Sinus, Right X Sphenoid Sinus, Left	0 Open 3 Percutaneous 4 Percutaneous Endoscopic	Z No Device	Z No Qualifier

Section	0	Medical and Surgical
Body System	9	Ear, Nose, Sinus
Operation	P	Removal: Taking out or off a device from a body part

Body Part (4th)	Approach (5th)	Device (6th)	Qualifier (7th)
7 Tympanic Membrane, Right 8 Tympanic Membrane, Left	0 Open 7 Via Natural or Artificial Opening 8 Via Natural or Artificial Opening Endoscopic X External	0 Drainage Device	Z No Qualifier
D Inner Ear, Right E Inner Ear, Left	0 Open 7 Via Natural or Artificial Opening 8 Via Natural or Artificial Opening Endoscopic	S Hearing Device	Z No Qualifier

Continued

Section	0	Medical and Surgical
Body System	9	Ear, Nose, Sinus
Operation	P	**Removal:** Taking out or off a device from a body part

Body Part (4th)	Approach (5th)	Device (6th)	Qualifier (7th)
H Ear, Right J Ear, Left K Nose	0 Open 3 Percutaneous 4 Percutaneous Endoscopic 7 Via Natural or Artificial Opening 8 Via Natural or Artificial Opening Endoscopic X External	0 Drainage Device 7 Autologous Tissue Substitute D Intraluminal Device J Synthetic Substitute K Nonautologous Tissue Substitute	Z No Qualifier
Y Sinus	0 Open 3 Percutaneous 4 Percutaneous Endoscopic X External	0 Drainage Device	Z No Qualifier

Section	0	Medical and Surgical
Body System	9	Ear, Nose, Sinus
Operation	Q	**Repair:** Restoring, to the extent possible, a body part to its normal anatomic structure and function

Body Part (4th)	Approach (5th)	Device (6th)	Qualifier (7th)
0 External Ear, Right 1 External Ear, Left 2 External Ear, Bilateral K Nose	0 Open 3 Percutaneous 4 Percutaneous Endoscopic X External	Z No Device	Z No Qualifier
3 External Auditory Canal, Right 4 External Auditory Canal, Left F Eustachian Tube, Right G Eustachian Tube, Left	0 Open 3 Percutaneous 4 Percutaneous Endoscopic 7 Via Natural or Artificial Opening 8 Via Natural or Artificial Opening Endoscopic X External	Z No Device	Z No Qualifier
5 Middle Ear, Right 6 Middle Ear, Left 9 Auditory Ossicle, Right A Auditory Ossicle, Left D Inner Ear, Right E Inner Ear, Left	0 Open	Z No Device	Z No Qualifier
7 Tympanic Membrane, Right 8 Tympanic Membrane, Left L Nasal Turbinate N Nasopharynx	0 Open 3 Percutaneous 4 Percutaneous Endoscopic 7 Via Natural or Artificial Opening 8 Via Natural or Artificial Opening Endoscopic	Z No Device	Z No Qualifier
B Mastoid Sinus, Right C Mastoid Sinus, Left M Nasal Septum P Accessory Sinus Q Maxillary Sinus, Right R Maxillary Sinus, Left S Frontal Sinus, Right T Frontal Sinus, Left U Ethmoid Sinus, Right V Ethmoid Sinus, Left W Sphenoid Sinus, Right X Sphenoid Sinus, Left	0 Open 3 Percutaneous 4 Percutaneous Endoscopic	Z No Device	Z No Qualifier

Section	0	Medical and Surgical
Body System	9	Ear, Nose, Sinus
Operation	R	**Replacement:** Putting in or on biological or synthetic material that physically takes the place and/or function of all or a portion of a body part

Body Part (4th)	Approach (5th)	Device (6th)	Qualifier (7th)
0 External Ear, Right 1 External Ear, Left 2 External Ear, Bilateral K Nose	0 Open X External	7 Autologous Tissue Substitute J Synthetic Substitute K Nonautologous Tissue Substitute	Z No Qualifier
5 Middle Ear, Right 6 Middle Ear, Left 9 Auditory Ossicle, Right A Auditory Ossicle, Left D Inner Ear, Right E Inner Ear, Left	0 Open	7 Autologous Tissue Substitute J Synthetic Substitute K Nonautologous Tissue Substitute	Z No Qualifier
7 Tympanic Membrane, Right 8 Tympanic Membrane, Left N Nasopharynx	0 Open 7 Via Natural or Artificial Opening 8 Via Natural or Artificial Opening Endoscopic	7 Autologous Tissue Substitute J Synthetic Substitute K Nonautologous Tissue Substitute	Z No Qualifier
L Nasal Turbinate	0 Open 3 Percutaneous 4 Percutaneous Endoscopic 7 Via Natural or Artificial Opening 8 Via Natural or Artificial Opening Endoscopic	7 Autologous Tissue Substitute J Synthetic Substitute K Nonautologous Tissue Substitute	Z No Qualifier
M Nasal Septum	0 Open 3 Percutaneous 4 Percutaneous Endoscopic	7 Autologous Tissue Substitute J Synthetic Substitute K Nonautologous Tissue Substitute	Z No Qualifier

Section	0	Medical and Surgical
Body System	9	Ear, Nose, Sinus
Operation	S	**Reposition:** Moving to its normal location, or other suitable location, all or a portion of a body part

Body Part (4th)	Approach (5th)	Device (6th)	Qualifier (7th)
0 External Ear, Right 1 External Ear, Left 2 External Ear, Bilateral K Nose	0 Open 4 Percutaneous Endoscopic X External	Z No Device	Z No Qualifier
7 Tympanic Membrane, Right 8 Tympanic Membrane, Left F Eustachian Tube, Right G Eustachian Tube, Left L Nasal Turbinate	0 Open 4 Percutaneous Endoscopic 7 Via Natural or Artificial Opening 8 Via Natural or Artificial Opening Endoscopic	Z No Device	Z No Qualifier
9 Auditory Ossicle, Right A Auditory Ossicle, Left M Nasal Septum	0 Open 4 Percutaneous Endoscopic	Z No Device	Z No Qualifier

Section	0	Medical and Surgical
Body System	9	Ear, Nose, Sinus
Operation	T	Resection: Cutting out or off, without replacement, all of a body part

Body Part (4th)	Approach (5th)	Device (6th)	Qualifier (7th)
0 External Ear, Right 1 External Ear, Left K Nose	0 Open 4 Percutaneous Endoscopic X External	Z No Device	Z No Qualifier
5 Middle Ear, Right 6 Middle Ear, Left 9 Auditory Ossicle, Right A Auditory Ossicle, Left D Inner Ear, Right E Inner Ear, Left	0 Open	Z No Device	Z No Qualifier
7 Tympanic Membrane, Right 8 Tympanic Membrane, Left F Eustachian Tube, Right G Eustachian Tube, Left L Nasal Turbinate N Nasopharynx	0 Open 4 Percutaneous Endoscopic 7 Via Natural or Artificial Opening 8 Via Natural or Artificial Opening Endoscopic	Z No Device	Z No Qualifier
B Mastoid Sinus, Right C Mastoid Sinus, Left M Nasal Septum P Accessory Sinus Q Maxillary Sinus, Right R Maxillary Sinus, Left S Frontal Sinus, Right T Frontal Sinus, Left U Ethmoid Sinus, Right V Ethmoid Sinus, Left W Sphenoid Sinus, Right X Sphenoid Sinus, Left	0 Open 4 Percutaneous Endoscopic	Z No Device	Z No Qualifier

Section	0	Medical and Surgical
Body System	9	Ear, Nose, Sinus
Operation	U	Supplement: Putting in or on biological or synthetic material that physically reinforces and/or augments the function of a portion of a body part

Body Part (4th)	Approach (5th)	Device (6th)	Qualifier (7th)
0 External Ear, Right 1 External Ear, Left 2 External Ear, Bilateral K Nose	0 Open X External	7 Autologous Tissue Substitute J Synthetic Substitute K Nonautologous Tissue Substitute	Z No Qualifier
5 Middle Ear, Right 6 Middle Ear, Left 9 Auditory Ossicle, Right A Auditory Ossicle, Left D Inner Ear, Right E Inner Ear, Left	0 Open	7 Autologous Tissue Substitute J Synthetic Substitute K Nonautologous Tissue Substitute	Z No Qualifier
7 Tympanic Membrane, Right 8 Tympanic Membrane, Left N Nasopharynx	0 Open 7 Via Natural or Artificial Opening 8 Via Natural or Artificial Opening Endoscopic	7 Autologous Tissue Substitute J Synthetic Substitute K Nonautologous Tissue Substitute	Z No Qualifier

Continued

Section	0	Medical and Surgical	*09U Continued*
Body System	9	Ear, Nose, Sinus	
Operation	U	**Supplement:** Putting in or on biological or synthetic material that physically reinforces and/or augments the function of a portion of a body part	

Body Part (4ᵗʰ)	Approach (5ᵗʰ)	Device (6ᵗʰ)	Qualifier (7ᵗʰ)
L Nasal Turbinate	0 Open 3 Percutaneous 4 Percutaneous Endoscopic 7 Via Natural or Artificial Opening 8 Via Natural or Artificial Opening Endoscopic	7 Autologous Tissue Substitute J Synthetic Substitute K Nonautologous Tissue Substitute	Z No Qualifier
M Nasal Septum	0 Open 3 Percutaneous 4 Percutaneous Endoscopic	7 Autologous Tissue Substitute J Synthetic Substitute K Nonautologous Tissue Substitute	Z No Qualifier

Section	0	Medical and Surgical
Body System	9	Ear, Nose, Sinus
Operation	W	**Revision:** Correcting, to the extent possible, a portion of a malfunctioning device or the position of a displaced device

Body Part (4ᵗʰ)	Approach (5ᵗʰ)	Device (6ᵗʰ)	Qualifier (7ᵗʰ)
7 Tympanic Membrane, Right 8 Tympanic Membrane, Left 9 Auditory Ossicle, Right A Auditory Ossicle, Left	0 Open 7 Via Natural or Artificial Opening 8 Via Natural or Artificial Opening Endoscopic	7 Autologous Tissue Substitute J Synthetic Substitute K Nonautologous Tissue Substitute	Z No Qualifier
D Inner Ear, Right E Inner Ear, Left	0 Open 7 Via Natural or Artificial Opening 8 Via Natural or Artificial Opening Endoscopic	S Hearing Device	Z No Qualifier
H Ear, Right J Ear, Left K Nose	0 Open 3 Percutaneous 4 Percutaneous Endoscopic 7 Via Natural or Artificial Opening 8 Via Natural or Artificial Opening Endoscopic X External	0 Drainage Device 7 Autologous Tissue Substitute D Intraluminal Device J Synthetic Substitute K Nonautologous Tissue Substitute	Z No Qualifier
Y Sinus	0 Open 3 Percutaneous 4 Percutaneous Endoscopic X External	0 Drainage Device	Z No Qualifier

Ear, Nose, Sinus Coding Listing 090–09W

090 – Ear, Nose, Sinus, Alteration

090007Z Alteration of Right External Ear with Autologous Tissue Substitute, Open Approach

09000JZ Alteration of Right External Ear with Synthetic Substitute, Open Approach

09000KZ Alteration of Right External Ear with Nonautologous Tissue Substitute, Open Approach

09000ZZ Alteration of Right External Ear, Open Approach

090037Z Alteration of Right External Ear with Autologous Tissue Substitute, Percutaneous Approach

09003JZ Alteration of Right External Ear with Synthetic Substitute, Percutaneous Approach

09003KZ Alteration of Right External Ear with Nonautologous Tissue Substitute, Percutaneous Approach

09003ZZ Alteration of Right External Ear, Percutaneous Approach

090047Z Alteration of Right External Ear with Autologous Tissue Substitute, Percutaneous Endoscopic Approach

09004JZ Alteration of Right External Ear with Synthetic Substitute, Percutaneous Endoscopic Approach

09004KZ Alteration of Right External Ear with Nonautologous Tissue Substitute, Percutaneous Endoscopic Approach

09004ZZ Alteration of Right External Ear, Percutaneous Endoscopic Approach

0900X7Z Alteration of Right External Ear with Autologous Tissue Substitute, External Approach

0900XJZ Alteration of Right External Ear with Synthetic Substitute, External Approach

0900XKZ Alteration of Right External Ear with Nonautologous Tissue Substitute, External Approach

---

♀ Female-only   ♂ Male-only   ● Limited Coverage   ● Non-OR   ▥ HAC-associated procedure   ● Non-covered procedures   ✚ Combination

0900XZZ	Alteration of Right External Ear, External Approach
090107Z	Alteration of Left External Ear with Autologous Tissue Substitute, Open Approach
09010JZ	Alteration of Left External Ear with Synthetic Substitute, Open Approach
09010KZ	Alteration of Left External Ear with Nonautologous Tissue Substitute, Open Approach
09010ZZ	Alteration of Left External Ear, Open Approach
090137Z	Alteration of Left External Ear with Autologous Tissue Substitute, Percutaneous Approach
09013JZ	Alteration of Left External Ear with Synthetic Substitute, Percutaneous Approach
09013KZ	Alteration of Left External Ear with Nonautologous Tissue Substitute, Percutaneous Approach
09013ZZ	Alteration of Left External Ear, Percutaneous Approach
090147Z	Alteration of Left External Ear with Autologous Tissue Substitute, Percutaneous Endoscopic Approach
09014JZ	Alteration of Left External Ear with Synthetic Substitute, Percutaneous Endoscopic Approach
09014KZ	Alteration of Left External Ear with Nonautologous Tissue Substitute, Percutaneous Endoscopic Approach
09014ZZ	Alteration of Left External Ear, Percutaneous Endoscopic Approach
0901X7Z	Alteration of Left External Ear with Autologous Tissue Substitute, External Approach
0901XJZ	Alteration of Left External Ear with Synthetic Substitute, External Approach
0901XKZ	Alteration of Left External Ear with Nonautologous Tissue Substitute, External Approach
0901XZZ	Alteration of Left External Ear, External Approach
090207Z	Alteration of Bilateral External Ear with Autologous Tissue Substitute, Open Approach
09020JZ	Alteration of Bilateral External Ear with Synthetic Substitute, Open Approach
09020KZ	Alteration of Bilateral External Ear with Nonautologous Tissue Substitute, Open Approach
09020ZZ	Alteration of Bilateral External Ear, Open Approach
090237Z	Alteration of Bilateral External Ear with Autologous Tissue Substitute, Percutaneous Approach
09023JZ	Alteration of Bilateral External Ear with Synthetic Substitute, Percutaneous Approach
09023KZ	Alteration of Bilateral External Ear with Nonautologous Tissue Substitute, Percutaneous Approach
09023ZZ	Alteration of Bilateral External Ear, Percutaneous Approach
090247Z	Alteration of Bilateral External Ear with Autologous Tissue Substitute, Percutaneous Endoscopic Approach
09024JZ	Alteration of Bilateral External Ear with Synthetic Substitute, Percutaneous Endoscopic Approach
09024KZ	Alteration of Bilateral External Ear with Nonautologous Tissue Substitute, Percutaneous Endoscopic Approach
09024ZZ	Alteration of Bilateral External Ear, Percutaneous Endoscopic Approach
0902X7Z	Alteration of Bilateral External Ear with Autologous Tissue Substitute, External Approach
0902XJZ	Alteration of Bilateral External Ear with Synthetic Substitute, External Approach
0902XKZ	Alteration of Bilateral External Ear with Nonautologous Tissue Substitute, External Approach
0902XZZ	Alteration of Bilateral External Ear, External Approach
090K07Z	Alteration of Nose with Autologous Tissue Substitute, Open Approach
090K0JZ	Alteration of Nose with Synthetic Substitute, Open Approach
090K0KZ	Alteration of Nose with Nonautologous Tissue Substitute, Open Approach
090K0ZZ	Alteration of Nose, Open Approach
090K37Z	Alteration of Nose with Autologous Tissue Substitute, Percutaneous Approach
090K3JZ	Alteration of Nose with Synthetic Substitute, Percutaneous Approach
090K3KZ	Alteration of Nose with Nonautologous Tissue Substitute, Percutaneous Approach
090K3ZZ	Alteration of Nose, Percutaneous Approach
090K47Z	Alteration of Nose with Autologous Tissue Substitute, Percutaneous Endoscopic Approach
090K4JZ	Alteration of Nose with Synthetic Substitute, Percutaneous Endoscopic Approach
090K4KZ	Alteration of Nose with Nonautologous Tissue Substitute, Percutaneous Endoscopic Approach
090K4ZZ	Alteration of Nose, Percutaneous Endoscopic Approach
090KX7Z	Alteration of Nose with Autologous Tissue Substitute, External Approach
090KXJZ	Alteration of Nose with Synthetic Substitute, External Approach
090KXKZ	Alteration of Nose with Nonautologous Tissue Substitute, External Approach
090KXZZ	Alteration of Nose, External Approach

091 – Ear, Nose, Sinus, Bypass

Review Coding Guideline B3.6a

091D070	Bypass Right Inner Ear to Endolymphatic with Autologous Tissue Substitute, Open Approach
091D0J0	Bypass Right Inner Ear to Endolymphatic with Synthetic Substitute, Open Approach
091D0K0	Bypass Right Inner Ear to Endolymphatic with Nonautologous Tissue Substitute, Open Approach
091D0Z0	Bypass Right Inner Ear to Endolymphatic, Open Approach
091E070	Bypass Left Inner Ear to Endolymphatic with Autologous Tissue Substitute, Open Approach
091E0J0	Bypass Left Inner Ear to Endolymphatic with Synthetic Substitute, Open Approach
091E0K0	Bypass Left Inner Ear to Endolymphatic with Nonautologous Tissue Substitute, Open Approach
091E0Z0	Bypass Left Inner Ear to Endolymphatic, Open Approach

092 – Ear, Nose, Sinus, Change

Review Coding Guideline B6.1c

092HX0Z	Change Drainage Device in Right Ear, External Approach
092HXYZ	Change Other Device in Right Ear, External Approach
092JX0Z	Change Drainage Device in Left Ear, External Approach
092JXYZ	Change Other Device in Left Ear, External Approach
092KX0Z	Change Drainage Device in Nose, External Approach
092KXYZ	Change Other Device in Nose, External Approach
092YX0Z	Change Drainage Device in Sinus, External Approach
092YXYZ	Change Other Device in Sinus, External Approach

095 – Ear, Nose, Sinus, Destruction

09500ZZ	Destruction of Right External Ear, Open Approach
09503ZZ	Destruction of Right External Ear, Percutaneous Approach
09504ZZ	Destruction of Right External Ear, Percutaneous Endoscopic Approach
0950XZZ	Destruction of Right External Ear, External Approach
09510ZZ	Destruction of Left External Ear, Open Approach
09513ZZ	Destruction of Left External Ear, Percutaneous Approach
09514ZZ	Destruction of Left External Ear, Percutaneous Endoscopic Approach
0951XZZ	Destruction of Left External Ear, External Approach
09530ZZ	Destruction of Right External Auditory Canal, Open Approach
09533ZZ	Destruction of Right External Auditory Canal, Percutaneous Approach

♀ Female-only   ♂ Male-only   ● Limited Coverage   ● Non-OR   ▥ HAC-associated procedure   ● Non-covered procedures   ✛ Combination

09534ZZ	Destruction of Right External Auditory Canal, Percutaneous Endoscopic Approach
09537ZZ	Destruction of Right External Auditory Canal, Via Natural or Artificial Opening
09538ZZ	Destruction of Right External Auditory Canal, Via Natural or Artificial Opening Endoscopic
0953XZZ	Destruction of Right External Auditory Canal, External Approach
09540ZZ	Destruction of Left External Auditory Canal, Open Approach
09543ZZ	Destruction of Left External Auditory Canal, Percutaneous Approach
09544ZZ	Destruction of Left External Auditory Canal, Percutaneous Endoscopic Approach
09547ZZ	Destruction of Left External Auditory Canal, Via Natural or Artificial Opening
09548ZZ	Destruction of Left External Auditory Canal, Via Natural or Artificial Opening Endoscopic
0954XZZ	Destruction of Left External Auditory Canal, External Approach
09550ZZ	Destruction of Right Middle Ear, Open Approach
09560ZZ	Destruction of Left Middle Ear, Open Approach
09570ZZ	Destruction of Right Tympanic Membrane, Open Approach
09573ZZ	Destruction of Right Tympanic Membrane, Percutaneous Approach
09574ZZ	Destruction of Right Tympanic Membrane, Percutaneous Endoscopic Approach
09577ZZ	Destruction of Right Tympanic Membrane, Via Natural or Artificial Opening
09578ZZ	Destruction of Right Tympanic Membrane, Via Natural or Artificial Opening Endoscopic
09580ZZ	Destruction of Left Tympanic Membrane, Open Approach
09583ZZ	Destruction of Left Tympanic Membrane, Percutaneous Approach
09584ZZ	Destruction of Left Tympanic Membrane, Percutaneous Endoscopic Approach
09587ZZ	Destruction of Left Tympanic Membrane, Via Natural or Artificial Opening
09588ZZ	Destruction of Left Tympanic Membrane, Via Natural or Artificial Opening Endoscopic
09590ZZ	Destruction of Right Auditory Ossicle, Open Approach
095A0ZZ	Destruction of Left Auditory Ossicle, Open Approach
095B0ZZ	Destruction of Right Mastoid Sinus, Open Approach
095B3ZZ	Destruction of Right Mastoid Sinus, Percutaneous Approach
095B4ZZ	Destruction of Right Mastoid Sinus, Percutaneous Endoscopic Approach
095C0ZZ	Destruction of Left Mastoid Sinus, Open Approach
095C3ZZ	Destruction of Left Mastoid Sinus, Percutaneous Approach
095C4ZZ	Destruction of Left Mastoid Sinus, Percutaneous Endoscopic Approach
095D0ZZ	Destruction of Right Inner Ear, Open Approach
095E0ZZ	Destruction of Left Inner Ear, Open Approach
095F0ZZ	Destruction of Right Eustachian Tube, Open Approach
095F3ZZ	Destruction of Right Eustachian Tube, Percutaneous Approach
095F4ZZ	Destruction of Right Eustachian Tube, Percutaneous Endoscopic Approach
095F7ZZ	Destruction of Right Eustachian Tube, Via Natural or Artificial Opening
095F8ZZ	Destruction of Right Eustachian Tube, Via Natural or Artificial Opening Endoscopic
095G0ZZ	Destruction of Left Eustachian Tube, Open Approach
095G3ZZ	Destruction of Left Eustachian Tube, Percutaneous Approach
095G4ZZ	Destruction of Left Eustachian Tube, Percutaneous Endoscopic Approach
095G7ZZ	Destruction of Left Eustachian Tube, Via Natural or Artificial Opening
095G8ZZ	Destruction of Left Eustachian Tube, Via Natural or Artificial Opening Endoscopic
095K0ZZ	Destruction of Nose, Open Approach
095K3ZZ	Destruction of Nose, Percutaneous Approach
095K4ZZ	Destruction of Nose, Percutaneous Endoscopic Approach
095KXZZ	Destruction of Nose, External Approach
095L0ZZ	Destruction of Nasal Turbinate, Open Approach
095L3ZZ	Destruction of Nasal Turbinate, Percutaneous Approach
095L4ZZ	Destruction of Nasal Turbinate, Percutaneous Endoscopic Approach
095L7ZZ	Destruction of Nasal Turbinate, Via Natural or Artificial Opening
095L8ZZ	Destruction of Nasal Turbinate, Via Natural or Artificial Opening Endoscopic
095M0ZZ	Destruction of Nasal Septum, Open Approach
095M3ZZ	Destruction of Nasal Septum, Percutaneous Approach
095M4ZZ	Destruction of Nasal Septum, Percutaneous Endoscopic Approach
095N0ZZ	Destruction of Nasopharynx, Open Approach
095N3ZZ	Destruction of Nasopharynx, Percutaneous Approach
095N4ZZ	Destruction of Nasopharynx, Percutaneous Endoscopic Approach
095N7ZZ	Destruction of Nasopharynx, Via Natural or Artificial Opening
095N8ZZ	Destruction of Nasopharynx, Via Natural or Artificial Opening Endoscopic
095P0ZZ	Destruction of Accessory Sinus, Open Approach
095P3ZZ	Destruction of Accessory Sinus, Percutaneous Approach
095P4ZZ	Destruction of Accessory Sinus, Percutaneous Endoscopic Approach
095Q0ZZ	Destruction of Right Maxillary Sinus, Open Approach
095Q3ZZ	Destruction of Right Maxillary Sinus, Percutaneous Approach
095Q4ZZ	Destruction of Right Maxillary Sinus, Percutaneous Endoscopic Approach
095R0ZZ	Destruction of Left Maxillary Sinus, Open Approach
095R3ZZ	Destruction of Left Maxillary Sinus, Percutaneous Approach
095R4ZZ	Destruction of Left Maxillary Sinus, Percutaneous Endoscopic Approach
095S0ZZ	Destruction of Right Frontal Sinus, Open Approach
095S3ZZ	Destruction of Right Frontal Sinus, Percutaneous Approach
095S4ZZ	Destruction of Right Frontal Sinus, Percutaneous Endoscopic Approach
095T0ZZ	Destruction of Left Frontal Sinus, Open Approach
095T3ZZ	Destruction of Left Frontal Sinus, Percutaneous Approach
095T4ZZ	Destruction of Left Frontal Sinus, Percutaneous Endoscopic Approach
095U0ZZ	Destruction of Right Ethmoid Sinus, Open Approach
095U3ZZ	Destruction of Right Ethmoid Sinus, Percutaneous Approach
095U4ZZ	Destruction of Right Ethmoid Sinus, Percutaneous Endoscopic Approach
095V0ZZ	Destruction of Left Ethmoid Sinus, Open Approach
095V3ZZ	Destruction of Left Ethmoid Sinus, Percutaneous Approach
095V4ZZ	Destruction of Left Ethmoid Sinus, Percutaneous Endoscopic Approach
095W0ZZ	Destruction of Right Sphenoid Sinus, Open Approach
095W3ZZ	Destruction of Right Sphenoid Sinus, Percutaneous Approach
095W4ZZ	Destruction of Right Sphenoid Sinus, Percutaneous Endoscopic Approach
095X0ZZ	Destruction of Left Sphenoid Sinus, Open Approach
095X3ZZ	Destruction of Left Sphenoid Sinus, Percutaneous Approach
095X4ZZ	Destruction of Left Sphenoid Sinus, Percutaneous Endoscopic Approach

097 – Ear, Nose, Sinus, Dilation

097F0DZ	Dilation of Right Eustachian Tube with Intraluminal Device, Open Approach
097F0ZZ	Dilation of Right Eustachian Tube, Open Approach
097F3ZZ	Dilation of Right Eustachian Tube, Percutaneous Approach
097F4ZZ	Dilation of Right Eustachian Tube, Percutaneous Endoscopic Approach
097F7DZ	Dilation of Right Eustachian Tube with Intraluminal Device, Via Natural or Artificial Opening
097F7ZZ	Dilation of Right Eustachian Tube, Via Natural or Artificial Opening
097F8DZ	Dilation of Right Eustachian Tube with Intraluminal Device, Via Natural or Artificial Opening Endoscopic
097F8ZZ	Dilation of Right Eustachian Tube, Via Natural or Artificial Opening Endoscopic
097G0DZ	Dilation of Left Eustachian Tube with Intraluminal Device, Open Approach
097G0ZZ	Dilation of Left Eustachian Tube, Open Approach
097G3ZZ	Dilation of Left Eustachian Tube, Percutaneous Approach

097G4ZZ   Dilation of Left Eustachian Tube, Percutaneous Endoscopic Approach

097G7DZ   Dilation of Left Eustachian Tube with Intraluminal Device, Via Natural or Artificial Opening

097G7ZZ   Dilation of Left Eustachian Tube, Via Natural or Artificial Opening

097G8DZ   Dilation of Left Eustachian Tube with Intraluminal Device, Via Natural or Artificial Opening Endoscopic

097G8ZZ   Dilation of Left Eustachian Tube, Via Natural or Artificial Opening Endoscopic

098 – Ear, Nose, Sinus, Division

098L0ZZ   Division of Nasal Turbinate, Open Approach
098L3ZZ   Division of Nasal Turbinate, Percutaneous Approach
098L4ZZ   Division of Nasal Turbinate, Percutaneous Endoscopic Approach

098L7ZZ   Division of Nasal Turbinate, Via Natural or Artificial Opening
098L8ZZ   Division of Nasal Turbinate, Via Natural or Artificial Opening Endoscopic

099 – Ear, Nose, Sinus, Drainage

Review Coding Guidelines B3.4a and B3.4b

Review Coding Guideline B6.2

099000Z   Drainage of Right External Ear with Drainage Device, Open Approach
09900ZX   Drainage of Right External Ear, Open Approach, Diagnostic
09900ZZ   Drainage of Right External Ear, Open Approach
099030Z   Drainage of Right External Ear with Drainage Device, Percutaneous Approach
09903ZX   Drainage of Right External Ear, Percutaneous Approach, Diagnostic
09903ZZ   Drainage of Right External Ear, Percutaneous Approach
099040Z   Drainage of Right External Ear with Drainage Device, Percutaneous Endoscopic Approach
09904ZX   Drainage of Right External Ear, Percutaneous Endoscopic Approach, Diagnostic
09904ZZ   Drainage of Right External Ear, Percutaneous Endoscopic Approach
0990X0Z   Drainage of Right External Ear with Drainage Device, External Approach
0990XZX   Drainage of Right External Ear, External Approach, Diagnostic
0990XZZ   Drainage of Right External Ear, External Approach
099100Z   Drainage of Left External Ear with Drainage Device, Open Approach
09910ZX   Drainage of Left External Ear, Open Approach, Diagnostic
09910ZZ   Drainage of Left External Ear, Open Approach
099130Z   Drainage of Left External Ear with Drainage Device, Percutaneous Approach
09913ZX   Drainage of Left External Ear, Percutaneous Approach, Diagnostic
09913ZZ   Drainage of Left External Ear, Percutaneous Approach
099140Z   Drainage of Left External Ear with Drainage Device, Percutaneous Endoscopic Approach
09914ZX   Drainage of Left External Ear, Percutaneous Endoscopic Approach, Diagnostic
09914ZZ   Drainage of Left External Ear, Percutaneous Endoscopic Approach
0991X0Z   Drainage of Left External Ear with Drainage Device, External Approach
0991XZX   Drainage of Left External Ear, External Approach, Diagnostic
0991XZZ   Drainage of Left External Ear, External Approach
099300Z   Drainage of Right External Auditory Canal with Drainage Device, Open Approach
09930ZX   Drainage of Right External Auditory Canal, Open Approach, Diagnostic
09930ZZ   Drainage of Right External Auditory Canal, Open Approach
099330Z   Drainage of Right External Auditory Canal with Drainage Device, Percutaneous Approach
09933ZX   Drainage of Right External Auditory Canal, Percutaneous Approach, Diagnostic
09933ZZ   Drainage of Right External Auditory Canal, Percutaneous Approach
099340Z   Drainage of Right External Auditory Canal with Drainage Device, Percutaneous Endoscopic Approach
09934ZX   Drainage of Right External Auditory Canal, Percutaneous Endoscopic Approach, Diagnostic
09934ZZ   Drainage of Right External Auditory Canal, Percutaneous Endoscopic Approach
099370Z   Drainage of Right External Auditory Canal with Drainage Device, Via Natural or Artificial Opening
09937ZX   Drainage of Right External Auditory Canal, Via Natural or Artificial Opening, Diagnostic

09937ZZ   Drainage of Right External Auditory Canal, Via Natural or Artificial Opening
099380Z   Drainage of Right External Auditory Canal with Drainage Device, Via Natural or Artificial Opening Endoscopic
09938ZX   Drainage of Right External Auditory Canal, Via Natural or Artificial Opening Endoscopic, Diagnostic
09938ZZ   Drainage of Right External Auditory Canal, Via Natural or Artificial Opening Endoscopic
0993X0Z   Drainage of Right External Auditory Canal with Drainage Device, External Approach
0993XZX   Drainage of Right External Auditory Canal, External Approach, Diagnostic
0993XZZ   Drainage of Right External Auditory Canal, External Approach
099400Z   Drainage of Left External Auditory Canal with Drainage Device, Open Approach
09940ZX   Drainage of Left External Auditory Canal, Open Approach, Diagnostic
09940ZZ   Drainage of Left External Auditory Canal, Open Approach
099430Z   Drainage of Left External Auditory Canal with Drainage Device, Percutaneous Approach
09943ZX   Drainage of Left External Auditory Canal, Percutaneous Approach, Diagnostic
09943ZZ   Drainage of Left External Auditory Canal, Percutaneous Approach
099440Z   Drainage of Left External Auditory Canal with Drainage Device, Percutaneous Endoscopic Approach
09944ZX   Drainage of Left External Auditory Canal, Percutaneous Endoscopic Approach, Diagnostic
09944ZZ   Drainage of Left External Auditory Canal, Percutaneous Endoscopic Approach
099470Z   Drainage of Left External Auditory Canal with Drainage Device, Via Natural or Artificial Opening
09947ZX   Drainage of Left External Auditory Canal, Via Natural or Artificial Opening, Diagnostic
09947ZZ   Drainage of Left External Auditory Canal, Via Natural or Artificial Opening
099480Z   Drainage of Left External Auditory Canal with Drainage Device, Via Natural or Artificial Opening Endoscopic
09948ZX   Drainage of Left External Auditory Canal, Via Natural or Artificial Opening Endoscopic, Diagnostic
09948ZZ   Drainage of Left External Auditory Canal, Via Natural or Artificial Opening Endoscopic
0994X0Z   Drainage of Left External Auditory Canal with Drainage Device, External Approach
0994XZX   Drainage of Left External Auditory Canal, External Approach, Diagnostic
0994XZZ   Drainage of Left External Auditory Canal, External Approach
099500Z   Drainage of Right Middle Ear with Drainage Device, Open Approach
09950ZX   Drainage of Right Middle Ear, Open Approach, Diagnostic
09950ZZ   Drainage of Right Middle Ear, Open Approach
099600Z   Drainage of Left Middle Ear with Drainage Device, Open Approach
09960ZX   Drainage of Left Middle Ear, Open Approach, Diagnostic
09960ZZ   Drainage of Left Middle Ear, Open Approach
099700Z   Drainage of Right Tympanic Membrane with Drainage Device, Open Approach

09970ZX Drainage of Right Tympanic Membrane, Open Approach, Diagnostic

09970ZZ Drainage of Right Tympanic Membrane, Open Approach

099730Z Drainage of Right Tympanic Membrane with Drainage Device, Percutaneous Approach

09973ZX Drainage of Right Tympanic Membrane, Percutaneous Approach, Diagnostic

09973ZZ Drainage of Right Tympanic Membrane, Percutaneous Approach

099740Z Drainage of Right Tympanic Membrane with Drainage Device, Percutaneous Endoscopic Approach

09974ZX Drainage of Right Tympanic Membrane, Percutaneous Endoscopic Approach, Diagnostic

09974ZZ Drainage of Right Tympanic Membrane, Percutaneous Endoscopic Approach

099770Z Drainage of Right Tympanic Membrane with Drainage Device, Via Natural or Artificial Opening

09977ZX Drainage of Right Tympanic Membrane, Via Natural or Artificial Opening, Diagnostic

09977ZZ Drainage of Right Tympanic Membrane, Via Natural or Artificial Opening

099780Z Drainage of Right Tympanic Membrane with Drainage Device, Via Natural or Artificial Opening Endoscopic

09978ZX Drainage of Right Tympanic Membrane, Via Natural or Artificial Opening Endoscopic, Diagnostic

09978ZZ Drainage of Right Tympanic Membrane, Via Natural or Artificial Opening Endoscopic

099800Z Drainage of Left Tympanic Membrane with Drainage Device, Open Approach

09980ZX Drainage of Left Tympanic Membrane, Open Approach, Diagnostic

09980ZZ Drainage of Left Tympanic Membrane, Open Approach

099830Z Drainage of Left Tympanic Membrane with Drainage Device, Percutaneous Approach

09983ZX Drainage of Left Tympanic Membrane, Percutaneous Approach, Diagnostic

09983ZZ Drainage of Left Tympanic Membrane, Percutaneous Approach

099840Z Drainage of Left Tympanic Membrane with Drainage Device, Percutaneous Endoscopic Approach

09984ZX Drainage of Left Tympanic Membrane, Percutaneous Endoscopic Approach, Diagnostic

09984ZZ Drainage of Left Tympanic Membrane, Percutaneous Endoscopic Approach

099870Z Drainage of Left Tympanic Membrane with Drainage Device, Via Natural or Artificial Opening

09987ZX Drainage of Left Tympanic Membrane, Via Natural or Artificial Opening, Diagnostic

09987ZZ Drainage of Left Tympanic Membrane, Via Natural or Artificial Opening

099880Z Drainage of Left Tympanic Membrane with Drainage Device, Via Natural or Artificial Opening Endoscopic

09988ZX Drainage of Left Tympanic Membrane, Via Natural or Artificial Opening Endoscopic, Diagnostic

09988ZZ Drainage of Left Tympanic Membrane, Via Natural or Artificial Opening Endoscopic

099900Z Drainage of Right Auditory Ossicle with Drainage Device, Open Approach

09990ZX Drainage of Right Auditory Ossicle, Open Approach, Diagnostic

09990ZZ Drainage of Right Auditory Ossicle, Open Approach

099A00Z Drainage of Left Auditory Ossicle with Drainage Device, Open Approach

099A0ZX Drainage of Left Auditory Ossicle, Open Approach, Diagnostic

099A0ZZ Drainage of Left Auditory Ossicle, Open Approach

099B00Z Drainage of Right Mastoid Sinus with Drainage Device, Open Approach

099B0ZX Drainage of Right Mastoid Sinus, Open Approach, Diagnostic

099B0ZZ Drainage of Right Mastoid Sinus, Open Approach

099B30Z Drainage of Right Mastoid Sinus with Drainage Device, Percutaneous Approach

099B3ZX Drainage of Right Mastoid Sinus, Percutaneous Approach, Diagnostic

099B3ZZ Drainage of Right Mastoid Sinus, Percutaneous Approach

099B40Z Drainage of Right Mastoid Sinus with Drainage Device, Percutaneous Endoscopic Approach

099B4ZX Drainage of Right Mastoid Sinus, Percutaneous Endoscopic Approach, Diagnostic

099B4ZZ Drainage of Right Mastoid Sinus, Percutaneous Endoscopic Approach

099C00Z Drainage of Left Mastoid Sinus with Drainage Device, Open Approach

099C0ZX Drainage of Left Mastoid Sinus, Open Approach, Diagnostic

099C0ZZ Drainage of Left Mastoid Sinus, Open Approach

099C30Z Drainage of Left Mastoid Sinus with Drainage Device, Percutaneous Approach

099C3ZX Drainage of Left Mastoid Sinus, Percutaneous Approach, Diagnostic

099C3ZZ Drainage of Left Mastoid Sinus, Percutaneous Approach

099C40Z Drainage of Left Mastoid Sinus with Drainage Device, Percutaneous Endoscopic Approach

099C4ZX Drainage of Left Mastoid Sinus, Percutaneous Endoscopic Approach, Diagnostic

099C4ZZ Drainage of Left Mastoid Sinus, Percutaneous Endoscopic Approach

099D00Z Drainage of Right Inner Ear with Drainage Device, Open Approach

099D0ZX Drainage of Right Inner Ear, Open Approach, Diagnostic

099D0ZZ Drainage of Right Inner Ear, Open Approach

099E00Z Drainage of Left Inner Ear with Drainage Device, Open Approach

099E0ZX Drainage of Left Inner Ear, Open Approach, Diagnostic

099E0ZZ Drainage of Left Inner Ear, Open Approach

099F00Z Drainage of Right Eustachian Tube with Drainage Device, Open Approach

099F0ZX Drainage of Right Eustachian Tube, Open Approach, Diagnostic

099F0ZZ Drainage of Right Eustachian Tube, Open Approach

099F30Z Drainage of Right Eustachian Tube with Drainage Device, Percutaneous Approach

099F3ZX Drainage of Right Eustachian Tube, Percutaneous Approach, Diagnostic

099F3ZZ Drainage of Right Eustachian Tube, Percutaneous Approach

099F40Z Drainage of Right Eustachian Tube with Drainage Device, Percutaneous Endoscopic Approach

099F4ZX Drainage of Right Eustachian Tube, Percutaneous Endoscopic Approach, Diagnostic

099F4ZZ Drainage of Right Eustachian Tube, Percutaneous Endoscopic Approach

099F70Z Drainage of Right Eustachian Tube with Drainage Device, Via Natural or Artificial Opening

099F7ZX Drainage of Right Eustachian Tube, Via Natural or Artificial Opening, Diagnostic

099F7ZZ Drainage of Right Eustachian Tube, Via Natural or Artificial Opening

099F80Z Drainage of Right Eustachian Tube with Drainage Device, Via Natural or Artificial Opening Endoscopic

099F8ZX Drainage of Right Eustachian Tube, Via Natural or Artificial Opening Endoscopic, Diagnostic

099F8ZZ Drainage of Right Eustachian Tube, Via Natural or Artificial Opening Endoscopic

099G00Z Drainage of Left Eustachian Tube with Drainage Device, Open Approach

099G0ZX Drainage of Left Eustachian Tube, Open Approach, Diagnostic

099G0ZZ Drainage of Left Eustachian Tube, Open Approach

099G30Z Drainage of Left Eustachian Tube with Drainage Device, Percutaneous Approach

099G3ZX Drainage of Left Eustachian Tube, Percutaneous Approach, Diagnostic

099G3ZZ Drainage of Left Eustachian Tube, Percutaneous Approach

099G40Z Drainage of Left Eustachian Tube with Drainage Device, Percutaneous Endoscopic Approach

099G4ZX Drainage of Left Eustachian Tube, Percutaneous Endoscopic Approach, Diagnostic

099G4ZZ Drainage of Left Eustachian Tube, Percutaneous Endoscopic Approach

099G70Z Drainage of Left Eustachian Tube with Drainage Device, Via Natural or Artificial Opening

099G7ZX Drainage of Left Eustachian Tube, Via Natural or Artificial Opening, Diagnostic

099G7ZZ Drainage of Left Eustachian Tube, Via Natural or Artificial Opening

099G80Z Drainage of Left Eustachian Tube with Drainage Device, Via Natural or Artificial Opening Endoscopic

099G8ZX Drainage of Left Eustachian Tube, Via Natural or Artificial Opening Endoscopic, Diagnostic

099G8ZZ Drainage of Left Eustachian Tube, Via Natural or Artificial Opening Endoscopic

099K00Z Drainage of Nose with Drainage Device, Open Approach

099K0ZX Drainage of Nose, Open Approach, Diagnostic

099K0ZZ Drainage of Nose, Open Approach

099K30Z Drainage of Nose with Drainage Device, Percutaneous Approach

099K3ZX Drainage of Nose, Percutaneous Approach, Diagnostic

099K3ZZ Drainage of Nose, Percutaneous Approach

099K40Z Drainage of Nose with Drainage Device, Percutaneous Endoscopic Approach

099K4ZX Drainage of Nose, Percutaneous Endoscopic Approach, Diagnostic

099K4ZZ Drainage of Nose, Percutaneous Endoscopic Approach

099KX0Z Drainage of Nose with Drainage Device, External Approach

099KXZX Drainage of Nose, External Approach, Diagnostic

099KXZZ Drainage of Nose, External Approach

099L00Z Drainage of Nasal Turbinate with Drainage Device, Open Approach

099L0ZX Drainage of Nasal Turbinate, Open Approach, Diagnostic

099L0ZZ Drainage of Nasal Turbinate, Open Approach

099L30Z Drainage of Nasal Turbinate with Drainage Device, Percutaneous Approach

099L3ZX Drainage of Nasal Turbinate, Percutaneous Approach, Diagnostic

099L3ZZ Drainage of Nasal Turbinate, Percutaneous Approach

099L40Z Drainage of Nasal Turbinate with Drainage Device, Percutaneous Endoscopic Approach

099L4ZX Drainage of Nasal Turbinate, Percutaneous Endoscopic Approach, Diagnostic

099L4ZZ Drainage of Nasal Turbinate, Percutaneous Endoscopic Approach

099L70Z Drainage of Nasal Turbinate with Drainage Device, Via Natural or Artificial Opening

099L7ZX Drainage of Nasal Turbinate, Via Natural or Artificial Opening, Diagnostic

099L7ZZ Drainage of Nasal Turbinate, Via Natural or Artificial Opening

099L80Z Drainage of Nasal Turbinate with Drainage Device, Via Natural or Artificial Opening Endoscopic

099L8ZX Drainage of Nasal Turbinate, Via Natural or Artificial Opening Endoscopic, Diagnostic

099L8ZZ Drainage of Nasal Turbinate, Via Natural or Artificial Opening Endoscopic

099M00Z Drainage of Nasal Septum with Drainage Device, Open Approach

099M0ZX Drainage of Nasal Septum, Open Approach, Diagnostic

099M0ZZ Drainage of Nasal Septum, Open Approach

099M30Z Drainage of Nasal Septum with Drainage Device, Percutaneous Approach

099M3ZX Drainage of Nasal Septum, Percutaneous Approach, Diagnostic

099M3ZZ Drainage of Nasal Septum, Percutaneous Approach

099M40Z Drainage of Nasal Septum with Drainage Device, Percutaneous Endoscopic Approach

099M4ZX Drainage of Nasal Septum, Percutaneous Endoscopic Approach, Diagnostic

099M4ZZ Drainage of Nasal Septum, Percutaneous Endoscopic Approach

099N00Z Drainage of Nasopharynx with Drainage Device, Open Approach

099N0ZX Drainage of Nasopharynx, Open Approach, Diagnostic

099N0ZZ Drainage of Nasopharynx, Open Approach

099N30Z Drainage of Nasopharynx with Drainage Device, Percutaneous Approach

099N3ZX Drainage of Nasopharynx, Percutaneous Approach, Diagnostic

099N3ZZ Drainage of Nasopharynx, Percutaneous Approach

099N40Z Drainage of Nasopharynx with Drainage Device, Percutaneous Endoscopic Approach

099N4ZX Drainage of Nasopharynx, Percutaneous Endoscopic Approach, Diagnostic

099N4ZZ Drainage of Nasopharynx, Percutaneous Endoscopic Approach

099N70Z Drainage of Nasopharynx with Drainage Device, Via Natural or Artificial Opening

099N7ZX Drainage of Nasopharynx, Via Natural or Artificial Opening, Diagnostic

099N7ZZ Drainage of Nasopharynx, Via Natural or Artificial Opening

099N80Z Drainage of Nasopharynx with Drainage Device, Via Natural or Artificial Opening Endoscopic

099N8ZX Drainage of Nasopharynx, Via Natural or Artificial Opening Endoscopic, Diagnostic

099N8ZZ Drainage of Nasopharynx, Via Natural or Artificial Opening Endoscopic

099P00Z Drainage of Accessory Sinus with Drainage Device, Open Approach

099P0ZX Drainage of Accessory Sinus, Open Approach, Diagnostic

099P0ZZ Drainage of Accessory Sinus, Open Approach

099P30Z Drainage of Accessory Sinus with Drainage Device, Percutaneous Approach

099P3ZX Drainage of Accessory Sinus, Percutaneous Approach, Diagnostic

099P3ZZ Drainage of Accessory Sinus, Percutaneous Approach

099P40Z Drainage of Accessory Sinus with Drainage Device, Percutaneous Endoscopic Approach

099P4ZX Drainage of Accessory Sinus, Percutaneous Endoscopic Approach, Diagnostic

099P4ZZ Drainage of Accessory Sinus, Percutaneous Endoscopic Approach

099Q00Z Drainage of Right Maxillary Sinus with Drainage Device, Open Approach

099Q0ZX Drainage of Right Maxillary Sinus, Open Approach, Diagnostic

099Q0ZZ Drainage of Right Maxillary Sinus, Open Approach

099Q30Z Drainage of Right Maxillary Sinus with Drainage Device, Percutaneous Approach

099Q3ZX Drainage of Right Maxillary Sinus, Percutaneous Approach, Diagnostic

099Q3ZZ Drainage of Right Maxillary Sinus, Percutaneous Approach

099Q40Z Drainage of Right Maxillary Sinus with Drainage Device, Percutaneous Endoscopic Approach

099Q4ZX Drainage of Right Maxillary Sinus, Percutaneous Endoscopic Approach, Diagnostic

099Q4ZZ Drainage of Right Maxillary Sinus, Percutaneous Endoscopic Approach

099R00Z Drainage of Left Maxillary Sinus with Drainage Device, Open Approach

099R0ZX Drainage of Left Maxillary Sinus, Open Approach, Diagnostic

099R0ZZ Drainage of Left Maxillary Sinus, Open Approach

099R30Z Drainage of Left Maxillary Sinus with Drainage Device, Percutaneous Approach

099R3ZX Drainage of Left Maxillary Sinus, Percutaneous Approach, Diagnostic

099R3ZZ Drainage of Left Maxillary Sinus, Percutaneous Approach

099R40Z Drainage of Left Maxillary Sinus with Drainage Device, Percutaneous Endoscopic Approach

099R4ZX Drainage of Left Maxillary Sinus, Percutaneous Endoscopic Approach, Diagnostic

099R4ZZ Drainage of Left Maxillary Sinus, Percutaneous Endoscopic Approach

099S00Z Drainage of Right Frontal Sinus with Drainage Device, Open Approach

099S0ZX Drainage of Right Frontal Sinus, Open Approach, Diagnostic

099S0ZZ Drainage of Right Frontal Sinus, Open Approach

099S30Z Drainage of Right Frontal Sinus with Drainage Device, Percutaneous Approach

099S3ZX Drainage of Right Frontal Sinus, Percutaneous Approach, Diagnostic

099S3ZZ Drainage of Right Frontal Sinus, Percutaneous Approach

099S40Z Drainage of Right Frontal Sinus with Drainage Device, Percutaneous Endoscopic Approach

099S4ZX Drainage of Right Frontal Sinus, Percutaneous Endoscopic Approach, Diagnostic

099S4ZZ Drainage of Right Frontal Sinus, Percutaneous Endoscopic Approach

099T00Z Drainage of Left Frontal Sinus with Drainage Device, Open Approach

099T0ZX Drainage of Left Frontal Sinus, Open Approach, Diagnostic

099T0ZZ Drainage of Left Frontal Sinus, Open Approach

099T30Z Drainage of Left Frontal Sinus with Drainage Device, Percutaneous Approach

099T3ZX Drainage of Left Frontal Sinus, Percutaneous Approach, Diagnostic

099T3ZZ Drainage of Left Frontal Sinus, Percutaneous Approach

099T40Z Drainage of Left Frontal Sinus with Drainage Device, Percutaneous Endoscopic Approach

099T4ZX Drainage of Left Frontal Sinus, Percutaneous Endoscopic Approach, Diagnostic

099T4ZZ Drainage of Left Frontal Sinus, Percutaneous Endoscopic Approach

099U00Z Drainage of Right Ethmoid Sinus with Drainage Device, Open Approach

---

♀ Female-only   ♂ Male-only   ● Limited Coverage   ● Non-OR   🄷🄰🄲 HAC-associated procedure   ● Non-covered procedures   ✚ Combination

099U0ZX	Drainage of Right Ethmoid Sinus, Open Approach, Diagnostic
099U0ZZ	Drainage of Right Ethmoid Sinus, Open Approach
099U30Z	Drainage of Right Ethmoid Sinus with Drainage Device, Percutaneous Approach
099U3ZX	Drainage of Right Ethmoid Sinus, Percutaneous Approach, Diagnostic
099U3ZZ	Drainage of Right Ethmoid Sinus, Percutaneous Approach
099U40Z	Drainage of Right Ethmoid Sinus with Drainage Device, Percutaneous Endoscopic Approach
099U4ZX	Drainage of Right Ethmoid Sinus, Percutaneous Endoscopic Approach, Diagnostic
099U4ZZ	Drainage of Right Ethmoid Sinus, Percutaneous Endoscopic Approach
099V00Z	Drainage of Left Ethmoid Sinus with Drainage Device, Open Approach
099V0ZX	Drainage of Left Ethmoid Sinus, Open Approach, Diagnostic
099V0ZZ	Drainage of Left Ethmoid Sinus, Open Approach
099V30Z	Drainage of Left Ethmoid Sinus with Drainage Device, Percutaneous Approach
099V3ZX	Drainage of Left Ethmoid Sinus, Percutaneous Approach, Diagnostic
099V3ZZ	Drainage of Left Ethmoid Sinus, Percutaneous Approach
099V40Z	Drainage of Left Ethmoid Sinus with Drainage Device, Percutaneous Endoscopic Approach
099V4ZX	Drainage of Left Ethmoid Sinus, Percutaneous Endoscopic Approach, Diagnostic
099V4ZZ	Drainage of Left Ethmoid Sinus, Percutaneous Endoscopic Approach
099W00Z	Drainage of Right Sphenoid Sinus with Drainage Device, Open Approach
099W0ZX	Drainage of Right Sphenoid Sinus, Open Approach, Diagnostic
099W0ZZ	Drainage of Right Sphenoid Sinus, Open Approach
099W30Z	Drainage of Right Sphenoid Sinus with Drainage Device, Percutaneous Approach
099W3ZX	Drainage of Right Sphenoid Sinus, Percutaneous Approach, Diagnostic
099W3ZZ	Drainage of Right Sphenoid Sinus, Percutaneous Approach
099W40Z	Drainage of Right Sphenoid Sinus with Drainage Device, Percutaneous Endoscopic Approach
099W4ZX	Drainage of Right Sphenoid Sinus, Percutaneous Endoscopic Approach, Diagnostic
099W4ZZ	Drainage of Right Sphenoid Sinus, Percutaneous Endoscopic Approach
099X00Z	Drainage of Left Sphenoid Sinus with Drainage Device, Open Approach
099X0ZX	Drainage of Left Sphenoid Sinus, Open Approach, Diagnostic
099X0ZZ	Drainage of Left Sphenoid Sinus, Open Approach
099X30Z	Drainage of Left Sphenoid Sinus with Drainage Device, Percutaneous Approach
099X3ZX	Drainage of Left Sphenoid Sinus, Percutaneous Approach, Diagnostic
099X3ZZ	Drainage of Left Sphenoid Sinus, Percutaneous Approach
099X40Z	Drainage of Left Sphenoid Sinus with Drainage Device, Percutaneous Endoscopic Approach
099X4ZX	Drainage of Left Sphenoid Sinus, Percutaneous Endoscopic Approach, Diagnostic
099X4ZZ	Drainage of Left Sphenoid Sinus, Percutaneous Endoscopic Approach

09B – Ear, Nose, Sinus, Excision

Review Coding Guidelines B3.4a and B3.4b

Review Coding Guideline B3.8

09B00ZX	Excision of Right External Ear, Open Approach, Diagnostic
09B00ZZ	Excision of Right External Ear, Open Approach
09B03ZX	Excision of Right External Ear, Percutaneous Approach, Diagnostic
09B03ZZ	Excision of Right External Ear, Percutaneous Approach
09B04ZX	Excision of Right External Ear, Percutaneous Endoscopic Approach, Diagnostic
09B04ZZ	Excision of Right External Ear, Percutaneous Endoscopic Approach
09B0XZX	Excision of Right External Ear, External Approach, Diagnostic
09B0XZZ	Excision of Right External Ear, External Approach
09B10ZX	Excision of Left External Ear, Open Approach, Diagnostic
09B10ZZ	Excision of Left External Ear, Open Approach
09B13ZX	Excision of Left External Ear, Percutaneous Approach, Diagnostic
09B13ZZ	Excision of Left External Ear, Percutaneous Approach
09B14ZX	Excision of Left External Ear, Percutaneous Endoscopic Approach, Diagnostic
09B14ZZ	Excision of Left External Ear, Percutaneous Endoscopic Approach
09B1XZX	Excision of Left External Ear, External Approach, Diagnostic
09B1XZZ	Excision of Left External Ear, External Approach
09B30ZX	Excision of Right External Auditory Canal, Open Approach, Diagnostic
09B30ZZ	Excision of Right External Auditory Canal, Open Approach
09B33ZX	Excision of Right External Auditory Canal, Percutaneous Approach, Diagnostic
09B33ZZ	Excision of Right External Auditory Canal, Percutaneous Approach
09B34ZX	Excision of Right External Auditory Canal, Percutaneous Endoscopic Approach, Diagnostic
09B34ZZ	Excision of Right External Auditory Canal, Percutaneous Endoscopic Approach
09B37ZX	Excision of Right External Auditory Canal, Via Natural or Artificial Opening, Diagnostic
09B37ZZ	Excision of Right External Auditory Canal, Via Natural or Artificial Opening
09B38ZX	Excision of Right External Auditory Canal, Via Natural or Artificial Opening Endoscopic, Diagnostic
09B38ZZ	Excision of Right External Auditory Canal, Via Natural or Artificial Opening Endoscopic
09B3XZX	Excision of Right External Auditory Canal, External Approach, Diagnostic
09B3XZZ	Excision of Right External Auditory Canal, External Approach
09B40ZX	Excision of Left External Auditory Canal, Open Approach, Diagnostic
09B40ZZ	Excision of Left External Auditory Canal, Open Approach
09B43ZX	Excision of Left External Auditory Canal, Percutaneous Approach, Diagnostic
09B43ZZ	Excision of Left External Auditory Canal, Percutaneous Approach
09B44ZX	Excision of Left External Auditory Canal, Percutaneous Endoscopic Approach, Diagnostic
09B44ZZ	Excision of Left External Auditory Canal, Percutaneous Endoscopic Approach
09B47ZX	Excision of Left External Auditory Canal, Via Natural or Artificial Opening, Diagnostic
09B47ZZ	Excision of Left External Auditory Canal, Via Natural or Artificial Opening
09B48ZX	Excision of Left External Auditory Canal, Via Natural or Artificial Opening Endoscopic, Diagnostic
09B48ZZ	Excision of Left External Auditory Canal, Via Natural or Artificial Opening Endoscopic
09B4XZX	Excision of Left External Auditory Canal, External Approach, Diagnostic
09B4XZZ	Excision of Left External Auditory Canal, External Approach
09B50ZX	Excision of Right Middle Ear, Open Approach, Diagnostic
09B50ZZ	Excision of Right Middle Ear, Open Approach
09B60ZX	Excision of Left Middle Ear, Open Approach, Diagnostic
09B60ZZ	Excision of Left Middle Ear, Open Approach
09B70ZX	Excision of Right Tympanic Membrane, Open Approach, Diagnostic
09B70ZZ	Excision of Right Tympanic Membrane, Open Approach
09B73ZX	Excision of Right Tympanic Membrane, Percutaneous Approach, Diagnostic
09B73ZZ	Excision of Right Tympanic Membrane, Percutaneous Approach
09B74ZX	Excision of Right Tympanic Membrane, Percutaneous Endoscopic Approach, Diagnostic

09B74ZZ   Excision of Right Tympanic Membrane, Percutaneous Endoscopic Approach

09B77ZX   Excision of Right Tympanic Membrane, Via Natural or Artificial Opening, Diagnostic

09B77ZZ   Excision of Right Tympanic Membrane, Via Natural or Artificial Opening

09B78ZX   Excision of Right Tympanic Membrane, Via Natural or Artificial Opening Endoscopic, Diagnostic

09B78ZZ   Excision of Right Tympanic Membrane, Via Natural or Artificial Opening Endoscopic

09B80ZX   Excision of Left Tympanic Membrane, Open Approach, Diagnostic

09B80ZZ   Excision of Left Tympanic Membrane, Open Approach

09B83ZX   Excision of Left Tympanic Membrane, Percutaneous Approach, Diagnostic

09B83ZZ   Excision of Left Tympanic Membrane, Percutaneous Approach

09B84ZX   Excision of Left Tympanic Membrane, Percutaneous Endoscopic Approach, Diagnostic

09B84ZZ   Excision of Left Tympanic Membrane, Percutaneous Endoscopic Approach

09B87ZX   Excision of Left Tympanic Membrane, Via Natural or Artificial Opening, Diagnostic

09B87ZZ   Excision of Left Tympanic Membrane, Via Natural or Artificial Opening

09B88ZX   Excision of Left Tympanic Membrane, Via Natural or Artificial Opening Endoscopic, Diagnostic

09B88ZZ   Excision of Left Tympanic Membrane, Via Natural or Artificial Opening Endoscopic

09B90ZX   Excision of Right Auditory Ossicle, Open Approach, Diagnostic

09B90ZZ   Excision of Right Auditory Ossicle, Open Approach

09BA0ZX   Excision of Left Auditory Ossicle, Open Approach, Diagnostic

09BA0ZZ   Excision of Left Auditory Ossicle, Open Approach

09BB0ZX   Excision of Right Mastoid Sinus, Open Approach, Diagnostic

09BB0ZZ   Excision of Right Mastoid Sinus, Open Approach

09BB3ZX   Excision of Right Mastoid Sinus, Percutaneous Approach, Diagnostic

09BB3ZZ   Excision of Right Mastoid Sinus, Percutaneous Approach

09BB4ZX   Excision of Right Mastoid Sinus, Percutaneous Endoscopic Approach, Diagnostic

09BB4ZZ   Excision of Right Mastoid Sinus, Percutaneous Endoscopic Approach

09BC0ZX   Excision of Left Mastoid Sinus, Open Approach, Diagnostic

09BC0ZZ   Excision of Left Mastoid Sinus, Open Approach

09BC3ZX   Excision of Left Mastoid Sinus, Percutaneous Approach, Diagnostic

09BC3ZZ   Excision of Left Mastoid Sinus, Percutaneous Approach

09BC4ZX   Excision of Left Mastoid Sinus, Percutaneous Endoscopic Approach, Diagnostic

09BC4ZZ   Excision of Left Mastoid Sinus, Percutaneous Endoscopic Approach

09BD0ZX   Excision of Right Inner Ear, Open Approach, Diagnostic

09BD0ZZ   Excision of Right Inner Ear, Open Approach

09BE0ZX   Excision of Left Inner Ear, Open Approach, Diagnostic

09BE0ZZ   Excision of Left Inner Ear, Open Approach

09BF0ZX   Excision of Right Eustachian Tube, Open Approach, Diagnostic

09BF0ZZ   Excision of Right Eustachian Tube, Open Approach

09BF3ZX   Excision of Right Eustachian Tube, Percutaneous Approach, Diagnostic

09BF3ZZ   Excision of Right Eustachian Tube, Percutaneous Approach

09BF4ZX   Excision of Right Eustachian Tube, Percutaneous Endoscopic Approach, Diagnostic

09BF4ZZ   Excision of Right Eustachian Tube, Percutaneous Endoscopic Approach

09BF7ZX   Excision of Right Eustachian Tube, Via Natural or Artificial Opening, Diagnostic

09BF7ZZ   Excision of Right Eustachian Tube, Via Natural or Artificial Opening

09BF8ZX   Excision of Right Eustachian Tube, Via Natural or Artificial Opening Endoscopic, Diagnostic

09BF8ZZ   Excision of Right Eustachian Tube, Via Natural or Artificial Opening Endoscopic

09BG0ZX   Excision of Left Eustachian Tube, Open Approach, Diagnostic

09BG0ZZ   Excision of Left Eustachian Tube, Open Approach

09BG3ZX   Excision of Left Eustachian Tube, Percutaneous Approach, Diagnostic

09BG3ZZ   Excision of Left Eustachian Tube, Percutaneous Approach

09BG4ZX   Excision of Left Eustachian Tube, Percutaneous Endoscopic Approach, Diagnostic

09BG4ZZ   Excision of Left Eustachian Tube, Percutaneous Endoscopic Approach

09BG7ZX   Excision of Left Eustachian Tube, Via Natural or Artificial Opening, Diagnostic

09BG7ZZ   Excision of Left Eustachian Tube, Via Natural or Artificial Opening

09BG8ZX   Excision of Left Eustachian Tube, Via Natural or Artificial Opening Endoscopic, Diagnostic

09BG8ZZ   Excision of Left Eustachian Tube, Via Natural or Artificial Opening Endoscopic

09BK0ZX   Excision of Nose, Open Approach, Diagnostic

09BK0ZZ   Excision of Nose, Open Approach

09BK3ZX   Excision of Nose, Percutaneous Approach, Diagnostic

09BK3ZZ   Excision of Nose, Percutaneous Approach

09BK4ZX   Excision of Nose, Percutaneous Endoscopic Approach, Diagnostic

09BK4ZZ   Excision of Nose, Percutaneous Endoscopic Approach

09BKXZX   Excision of Nose, External Approach, Diagnostic

09BKXZZ   Excision of Nose, External Approach

09BL0ZX   Excision of Nasal Turbinate, Open Approach, Diagnostic

09BL0ZZ   Excision of Nasal Turbinate, Open Approach

09BL3ZX   Excision of Nasal Turbinate, Percutaneous Approach, Diagnostic

09BL3ZZ   Excision of Nasal Turbinate, Percutaneous Approach

09BL4ZX   Excision of Nasal Turbinate, Percutaneous Endoscopic Approach, Diagnostic

09BL4ZZ   Excision of Nasal Turbinate, Percutaneous Endoscopic Approach

09BL7ZX   Excision of Nasal Turbinate, Via Natural or Artificial Opening, Diagnostic

09BL7ZZ   Excision of Nasal Turbinate, Via Natural or Artificial Opening

09BL8ZX   Excision of Nasal Turbinate, Via Natural or Artificial Opening Endoscopic, Diagnostic

09BL8ZZ   Excision of Nasal Turbinate, Via Natural or Artificial Opening Endoscopic

09BM0ZX   Excision of Nasal Septum, Open Approach, Diagnostic

09BM0ZZ   Excision of Nasal Septum, Open Approach

09BM3ZX   Excision of Nasal Septum, Percutaneous Approach, Diagnostic

09BM3ZZ   Excision of Nasal Septum, Percutaneous Approach

09BM4ZX   Excision of Nasal Septum, Percutaneous Endoscopic Approach, Diagnostic

09BM4ZZ   Excision of Nasal Septum, Percutaneous Endoscopic Approach

09BN0ZX   Excision of Nasopharynx, Open Approach, Diagnostic

09BN0ZZ   Excision of Nasopharynx, Open Approach

09BN3ZX   Excision of Nasopharynx, Percutaneous Approach, Diagnostic

09BN3ZZ   Excision of Nasopharynx, Percutaneous Approach

09BN4ZX   Excision of Nasopharynx, Percutaneous Endoscopic Approach, Diagnostic

09BN4ZZ   Excision of Nasopharynx, Percutaneous Endoscopic Approach

09BN7ZX   Excision of Nasopharynx, Via Natural or Artificial Opening, Diagnostic

09BN7ZZ   Excision of Nasopharynx, Via Natural or Artificial Opening

09BN8ZX   Excision of Nasopharynx, Via Natural or Artificial Opening Endoscopic, Diagnostic

09BN8ZZ   Excision of Nasopharynx, Via Natural or Artificial Opening Endoscopic

09BP0ZX   Excision of Accessory Sinus, Open Approach, Diagnostic

09BP0ZZ   Excision of Accessory Sinus, Open Approach

09BP3ZX   Excision of Accessory Sinus, Percutaneous Approach, Diagnostic

09BP3ZZ   Excision of Accessory Sinus, Percutaneous Approach

09BP4ZX   Excision of Accessory Sinus, Percutaneous Endoscopic Approach, Diagnostic

09BP4ZZ   Excision of Accessory Sinus, Percutaneous Endoscopic Approach

09BQ0ZX   Excision of Right Maxillary Sinus, Open Approach, Diagnostic

09BQ0ZZ   Excision of Right Maxillary Sinus, Open Approach

09BQ3ZX   Excision of Right Maxillary Sinus, Percutaneous Approach, Diagnostic

09BQ3ZZ   Excision of Right Maxillary Sinus, Percutaneous Approach

09BQ4ZX   Excision of Right Maxillary Sinus, Percutaneous Endoscopic Approach, Diagnostic

09BQ4ZZ   Excision of Right Maxillary Sinus, Percutaneous Endoscopic Approach

09BR0ZX   Excision of Left Maxillary Sinus, Open Approach, Diagnostic

09BR0ZZ   Excision of Left Maxillary Sinus, Open Approach

09BR3ZX Excision of Left Maxillary Sinus, Percutaneous Approach, Diagnostic
09BR3ZZ Excision of Left Maxillary Sinus, Percutaneous Approach
09BR4ZX Excision of Left Maxillary Sinus, Percutaneous Endoscopic Approach, Diagnostic
09BR4ZZ Excision of Left Maxillary Sinus, Percutaneous Endoscopic Approach
09BS0ZX Excision of Right Frontal Sinus, Open Approach, Diagnostic
09BS0ZZ Excision of Right Frontal Sinus, Open Approach
09BS3ZX Excision of Right Frontal Sinus, Percutaneous Approach, Diagnostic
09BS3ZZ Excision of Right Frontal Sinus, Percutaneous Approach
09BS4ZX Excision of Right Frontal Sinus, Percutaneous Endoscopic Approach, Diagnostic
09BS4ZZ Excision of Right Frontal Sinus, Percutaneous Endoscopic Approach
09BT0ZX Excision of Left Frontal Sinus, Open Approach, Diagnostic
09BT0ZZ Excision of Left Frontal Sinus, Open Approach
09BT3ZX Excision of Left Frontal Sinus, Percutaneous Approach, Diagnostic
09BT3ZZ Excision of Left Frontal Sinus, Percutaneous Approach
09BT4ZX Excision of Left Frontal Sinus, Percutaneous Endoscopic Approach, Diagnostic
09BT4ZZ Excision of Left Frontal Sinus, Percutaneous Endoscopic Approach
09BU0ZX Excision of Right Ethmoid Sinus, Open Approach, Diagnostic
09BU0ZZ Excision of Right Ethmoid Sinus, Open Approach
09BU3ZX Excision of Right Ethmoid Sinus, Percutaneous Approach, Diagnostic
09BU3ZZ Excision of Right Ethmoid Sinus, Percutaneous Approach
09BU4ZX Excision of Right Ethmoid Sinus, Percutaneous Endoscopic Approach, Diagnostic

09BU4ZZ Excision of Right Ethmoid Sinus, Percutaneous Endoscopic Approach
09BV0ZX Excision of Left Ethmoid Sinus, Open Approach, Diagnostic
09BV0ZZ Excision of Left Ethmoid Sinus, Open Approach
09BV3ZX Excision of Left Ethmoid Sinus, Percutaneous Approach, Diagnostic
09BV3ZZ Excision of Left Ethmoid Sinus, Percutaneous Approach
09BV4ZX Excision of Left Ethmoid Sinus, Percutaneous Endoscopic Approach, Diagnostic
09BV4ZZ Excision of Left Ethmoid Sinus, Percutaneous Endoscopic Approach
09BW0ZX Excision of Right Sphenoid Sinus, Open Approach, Diagnostic
09BW0ZZ Excision of Right Sphenoid Sinus, Open Approach
09BW3ZX Excision of Right Sphenoid Sinus, Percutaneous Approach, Diagnostic
09BW3ZZ Excision of Right Sphenoid Sinus, Percutaneous Approach
09BW4ZX Excision of Right Sphenoid Sinus, Percutaneous Endoscopic Approach, Diagnostic
09BW4ZZ Excision of Right Sphenoid Sinus, Percutaneous Endoscopic Approach
09BX0ZX Excision of Left Sphenoid Sinus, Open Approach, Diagnostic
09BX0ZZ Excision of Left Sphenoid Sinus, Open Approach
09BX3ZX Excision of Left Sphenoid Sinus, Percutaneous Approach, Diagnostic
09BX3ZZ Excision of Left Sphenoid Sinus, Percutaneous Approach
09BX4ZX Excision of Left Sphenoid Sinus, Percutaneous Endoscopic Approach, Diagnostic
09BX4ZZ Excision of Left Sphenoid Sinus, Percutaneous Endoscopic Approach

09C – Ear, Nose, Sinus, Extirpation

09C00ZZ Extirpation of Matter from Right External Ear, Open Approach
09C03ZZ Extirpation of Matter from Right External Ear, Percutaneous Approach
09C04ZZ Extirpation of Matter from Right External Ear, Percutaneous Endoscopic Approach
09C0XZZ Extirpation of Matter from Right External Ear, External Approach
09C10ZZ Extirpation of Matter from Left External Ear, Open Approach
09C13ZZ Extirpation of Matter from Left External Ear, Percutaneous Approach
09C14ZZ Extirpation of Matter from Left External Ear, Percutaneous Endoscopic Approach
09C1XZZ Extirpation of Matter from Left External Ear, External Approach
09C30ZZ Extirpation of Matter from Right External Auditory Canal, Open Approach
09C33ZZ Extirpation of Matter from Right External Auditory Canal, Percutaneous Approach
09C34ZZ Extirpation of Matter from Right External Auditory Canal, Percutaneous Endoscopic Approach
09C37ZZ Extirpation of Matter from Right External Auditory Canal, Via Natural or Artificial Opening
09C38ZZ Extirpation of Matter from Right External Auditory Canal, Via Natural or Artificial Opening Endoscopic
09C3XZZ Extirpation of Matter from Right External Auditory Canal, External Approach
09C40ZZ Extirpation of Matter from Left External Auditory Canal, Open Approach
09C43ZZ Extirpation of Matter from Left External Auditory Canal, Percutaneous Approach
09C44ZZ Extirpation of Matter from Left External Auditory Canal, Percutaneous Endoscopic Approach
09C47ZZ Extirpation of Matter from Left External Auditory Canal, Via Natural or Artificial Opening
09C48ZZ Extirpation of Matter from Left External Auditory Canal, Via Natural or Artificial Opening Endoscopic
09C4XZZ Extirpation of Matter from Left External Auditory Canal, External Approach
09C50ZZ Extirpation of Matter from Right Middle Ear, Open Approach
09C60ZZ Extirpation of Matter from Left Middle Ear, Open Approach
09C70ZZ Extirpation of Matter from Right Tympanic Membrane, Open Approach

09C73ZZ Extirpation of Matter from Right Tympanic Membrane, Percutaneous Approach
09C74ZZ Extirpation of Matter from Right Tympanic Membrane, Percutaneous Endoscopic Approach
09C77ZZ Extirpation of Matter from Right Tympanic Membrane, Via Natural or Artificial Opening
09C78ZZ Extirpation of Matter from Right Tympanic Membrane, Via Natural or Artificial Opening Endoscopic
09C80ZZ Extirpation of Matter from Left Tympanic Membrane, Open Approach
09C83ZZ Extirpation of Matter from Left Tympanic Membrane, Percutaneous Approach
09C84ZZ Extirpation of Matter from Left Tympanic Membrane, Percutaneous Endoscopic Approach
09C87ZZ Extirpation of Matter from Left Tympanic Membrane, Via Natural or Artificial Opening
09C88ZZ Extirpation of Matter from Left Tympanic Membrane, Via Natural or Artificial Opening Endoscopic
09C90ZZ Extirpation of Matter from Right Auditory Ossicle, Open Approach
09CA0ZZ Extirpation of Matter from Left Auditory Ossicle, Open Approach
09CB0ZZ Extirpation of Matter from Right Mastoid Sinus, Open Approach
09CB3ZZ Extirpation of Matter from Right Mastoid Sinus, Percutaneous Approach
09CB4ZZ Extirpation of Matter from Right Mastoid Sinus, Percutaneous Endoscopic Approach
09CC0ZZ Extirpation of Matter from Left Mastoid Sinus, Open Approach
09CC3ZZ Extirpation of Matter from Left Mastoid Sinus, Percutaneous Approach
09CC4ZZ Extirpation of Matter from Left Mastoid Sinus, Percutaneous Endoscopic Approach
09CD0ZZ Extirpation of Matter from Right Inner Ear, Open Approach
09CE0ZZ Extirpation of Matter from Left Inner Ear, Open Approach
09CF0ZZ Extirpation of Matter from Right Eustachian Tube, Open Approach
09CF3ZZ Extirpation of Matter from Right Eustachian Tube, Percutaneous Approach
09CF4ZZ Extirpation of Matter from Right Eustachian Tube, Percutaneous Endoscopic Approach
09CF7ZZ Extirpation of Matter from Right Eustachian Tube, Via Natural or Artificial Opening
09CF8ZZ Extirpation of Matter from Right Eustachian Tube, Via Natural or Artificial Opening Endoscopic

---

09CG0ZZ Extirpation of Matter from Left Eustachian Tube, Open Approach

09CG3ZZ Extirpation of Matter from Left Eustachian Tube, Percutaneous Approach

09CG4ZZ Extirpation of Matter from Left Eustachian Tube, Percutaneous Endoscopic Approach

09CG7ZZ Extirpation of Matter from Left Eustachian Tube, Via Natural or Artificial Opening

09CG8ZZ Extirpation of Matter from Left Eustachian Tube, Via Natural or Artificial Opening Endoscopic

09CK0ZZ Extirpation of Matter from Nose, Open Approach

09CK3ZZ Extirpation of Matter from Nose, Percutaneous Approach

09CK4ZZ Extirpation of Matter from Nose, Percutaneous Endoscopic Approach

09CKXZZ Extirpation of Matter from Nose, External Approach

09CL0ZZ Extirpation of Matter from Nasal Turbinate, Open Approach

09CL3ZZ Extirpation of Matter from Nasal Turbinate, Percutaneous Approach

09CL4ZZ Extirpation of Matter from Nasal Turbinate, Percutaneous Endoscopic Approach

09CL7ZZ Extirpation of Matter from Nasal Turbinate, Via Natural or Artificial Opening

09CL8ZZ Extirpation of Matter from Nasal Turbinate, Via Natural or Artificial Opening Endoscopic

09CM0ZZ Extirpation of Matter from Nasal Septum, Open Approach

09CM3ZZ Extirpation of Matter from Nasal Septum, Percutaneous Approach

09CM4ZZ Extirpation of Matter from Nasal Septum, Percutaneous Endoscopic Approach

09CN0ZZ Extirpation of Matter from Nasopharynx, Open Approach

09CN3ZZ Extirpation of Matter from Nasopharynx, Percutaneous Approach

09CN4ZZ Extirpation of Matter from Nasopharynx, Percutaneous Endoscopic Approach

09CN7ZZ Extirpation of Matter from Nasopharynx, Via Natural or Artificial Opening

09CN8ZZ Extirpation of Matter from Nasopharynx, Via Natural or Artificial Opening Endoscopic

09CP0ZZ Extirpation of Matter from Accessory Sinus, Open Approach

09CP3ZZ Extirpation of Matter from Accessory Sinus, Percutaneous Approach

09CP4ZZ Extirpation of Matter from Accessory Sinus, Percutaneous Endoscopic Approach

09CQ0ZZ Extirpation of Matter from Right Maxillary Sinus, Open Approach

09CQ3ZZ Extirpation of Matter from Right Maxillary Sinus, Percutaneous Approach

09CQ4ZZ Extirpation of Matter from Right Maxillary Sinus, Percutaneous Endoscopic Approach

09CR0ZZ Extirpation of Matter from Left Maxillary Sinus, Open Approach

09CR3ZZ Extirpation of Matter from Left Maxillary Sinus, Percutaneous Approach

09CR4ZZ Extirpation of Matter from Left Maxillary Sinus, Percutaneous Endoscopic Approach

09CS0ZZ Extirpation of Matter from Right Frontal Sinus, Open Approach

09CS3ZZ Extirpation of Matter from Right Frontal Sinus, Percutaneous Approach

09CS4ZZ Extirpation of Matter from Right Frontal Sinus, Percutaneous Endoscopic Approach

09CT0ZZ Extirpation of Matter from Left Frontal Sinus, Open Approach

09CT3ZZ Extirpation of Matter from Left Frontal Sinus, Percutaneous Approach

09CT4ZZ Extirpation of Matter from Left Frontal Sinus, Percutaneous Endoscopic Approach

09CU0ZZ Extirpation of Matter from Right Ethmoid Sinus, Open Approach

09CU3ZZ Extirpation of Matter from Right Ethmoid Sinus, Percutaneous Approach

09CU4ZZ Extirpation of Matter from Right Ethmoid Sinus, Percutaneous Endoscopic Approach

09CV0ZZ Extirpation of Matter from Left Ethmoid Sinus, Open Approach

09CV3ZZ Extirpation of Matter from Left Ethmoid Sinus, Percutaneous Approach

09CV4ZZ Extirpation of Matter from Left Ethmoid Sinus, Percutaneous Endoscopic Approach

09CW0ZZ Extirpation of Matter from Right Sphenoid Sinus, Open Approach

09CW3ZZ Extirpation of Matter from Right Sphenoid Sinus, Percutaneous Approach

09CW4ZZ Extirpation of Matter from Right Sphenoid Sinus, Percutaneous Endoscopic Approach

09CX0ZZ Extirpation of Matter from Left Sphenoid Sinus, Open Approach

09CX3ZZ Extirpation of Matter from Left Sphenoid Sinus, Percutaneous Approach

09CX4ZZ Extirpation of Matter from Left Sphenoid Sinus, Percutaneous Endoscopic Approach

09D – Ear, Nose, Sinus, Extraction

09D70ZZ Extraction of Right Tympanic Membrane, Open Approach

09D73ZZ Extraction of Right Tympanic Membrane, Percutaneous Approach

09D74ZZ Extraction of Right Tympanic Membrane, Percutaneous Endoscopic Approach

09D77ZZ Extraction of Right Tympanic Membrane, Via Natural or Artificial Opening

09D78ZZ Extraction of Right Tympanic Membrane, Via Natural or Artificial Opening Endoscopic

09D80ZZ Extraction of Left Tympanic Membrane, Open Approach

09D83ZZ Extraction of Left Tympanic Membrane, Percutaneous Approach

09D84ZZ Extraction of Left Tympanic Membrane, Percutaneous Endoscopic Approach

09D87ZZ Extraction of Left Tympanic Membrane, Via Natural or Artificial Opening

09D88ZZ Extraction of Left Tympanic Membrane, Via Natural or Artificial Opening Endoscopic

09D90ZZ Extraction of Right Auditory Ossicle, Open Approach

09DA0ZZ Extraction of Left Auditory Ossicle, Open Approach

09DB0ZZ Extraction of Right Mastoid Sinus, Open Approach

09DB3ZZ Extraction of Right Mastoid Sinus, Percutaneous Approach

09DB4ZZ Extraction of Right Mastoid Sinus, Percutaneous Endoscopic Approach

09DC0ZZ Extraction of Left Mastoid Sinus, Open Approach

09DC3ZZ Extraction of Left Mastoid Sinus, Percutaneous Approach

09DC4ZZ Extraction of Left Mastoid Sinus, Percutaneous Endoscopic Approach

09DL0ZZ Extraction of Nasal Turbinate, Open Approach

09DL3ZZ Extraction of Nasal Turbinate, Percutaneous Approach

09DL4ZZ Extraction of Nasal Turbinate, Percutaneous Endoscopic Approach

09DL7ZZ Extraction of Nasal Turbinate, Via Natural or Artificial Opening

09DL8ZZ Extraction of Nasal Turbinate, Via Natural or Artificial Opening Endoscopic

09DM0ZZ Extraction of Nasal Septum, Open Approach

09DM3ZZ Extraction of Nasal Septum, Percutaneous Approach

09DM4ZZ Extraction of Nasal Septum, Percutaneous Endoscopic Approach

09DP0ZZ Extraction of Accessory Sinus, Open Approach

09DP3ZZ Extraction of Accessory Sinus, Percutaneous Approach

09DP4ZZ Extraction of Accessory Sinus, Percutaneous Endoscopic Approach

09DQ0ZZ Extraction of Right Maxillary Sinus, Open Approach

09DQ3ZZ Extraction of Right Maxillary Sinus, Percutaneous Approach

09DQ4ZZ Extraction of Right Maxillary Sinus, Percutaneous Endoscopic Approach

09DR0ZZ Extraction of Left Maxillary Sinus, Open Approach

09DR3ZZ Extraction of Left Maxillary Sinus, Percutaneous Approach

09DR4ZZ Extraction of Left Maxillary Sinus, Percutaneous Endoscopic Approach

09DS0ZZ Extraction of Right Frontal Sinus, Open Approach

09DS3ZZ Extraction of Right Frontal Sinus, Percutaneous Approach

09DS4ZZ Extraction of Right Frontal Sinus, Percutaneous Endoscopic Approach

09DT0ZZ Extraction of Left Frontal Sinus, Open Approach

09DT3ZZ Extraction of Left Frontal Sinus, Percutaneous Approach

09DT4ZZ Extraction of Left Frontal Sinus, Percutaneous Endoscopic Approach

09DU0ZZ Extraction of Right Ethmoid Sinus, Open Approach

09DU3ZZ Extraction of Right Ethmoid Sinus, Percutaneous Approach

09DU4ZZ Extraction of Right Ethmoid Sinus, Percutaneous Endoscopic Approach

09DV0ZZ	Extraction of Left Ethmoid Sinus, Open Approach
09DV3ZZ	Extraction of Left Ethmoid Sinus, Percutaneous Approach
09DV4ZZ	Extraction of Left Ethmoid Sinus, Percutaneous Endoscopic Approach
09DW0ZZ	Extraction of Right Sphenoid Sinus, Open Approach
09DW3ZZ	Extraction of Right Sphenoid Sinus, Percutaneous Approach
09DW4ZZ	Extraction of Right Sphenoid Sinus, Percutaneous Endoscopic Approach

09DX0ZZ	Extraction of Left Sphenoid Sinus, Open Approach
09DX3ZZ	Extraction of Left Sphenoid Sinus, Percutaneous Approach
09DX4ZZ	Extraction of Left Sphenoid Sinus, Percutaneous Endoscopic Approach

09H – Ear, Nose, Sinus, Insertion

09HD04Z	Insertion of Bone Conduction Hearing Device into Right Inner Ear, Open Approach
09HD05Z	Insertion of Single Channel Cochlear Prosthesis into Right Inner Ear, Open Approach
09HD06Z	Insertion of Multiple Channel Cochlear Prosthesis into Right Inner Ear, Open Approach
09HD0SZ	Insertion of Hearing Device into Right Inner Ear, Open Approach
09HD34Z	Insertion of Bone Conduction Hearing Device into Right Inner Ear, Percutaneous Approach
09HD35Z	Insertion of Single Channel Cochlear Prosthesis into Right Inner Ear, Percutaneous Approach
09HD36Z	Insertion of Multiple Channel Cochlear Prosthesis into Right Inner Ear, Percutaneous Approach
09HD3SZ	Insertion of Hearing Device into Right Inner Ear, Percutaneous Approach
09HD44Z	Insertion of Bone Conduction Hearing Device into Right Inner Ear, Percutaneous Endoscopic Approach
09HD45Z	Insertion of Single Channel Cochlear Prosthesis into Right Inner Ear, Percutaneous Endoscopic Approach
09HD46Z	Insertion of Multiple Channel Cochlear Prosthesis into Right Inner Ear, Percutaneous Endoscopic Approach
09HD4SZ	Insertion of Hearing Device into Right Inner Ear, Percutaneous Endoscopic Approach
09HE04Z	Insertion of Bone Conduction Hearing Device into Left Inner Ear, Open Approach

09HE05Z	Insertion of Single Channel Cochlear Prosthesis into Left Inner Ear, Open Approach
09HE06Z	Insertion of Multiple Channel Cochlear Prosthesis into Left Inner Ear, Open Approach
09HE0SZ	Insertion of Hearing Device into Left Inner Ear, Open Approach
09HE34Z	Insertion of Bone Conduction Hearing Device into Left Inner Ear, Percutaneous Approach
09HE35Z	Insertion of Single Channel Cochlear Prosthesis into Left Inner Ear, Percutaneous Approach
09HE36Z	Insertion of Multiple Channel Cochlear Prosthesis into Left Inner Ear, Percutaneous Approach
09HE3SZ	Insertion of Hearing Device into Left Inner Ear, Percutaneous Approach
09HE44Z	Insertion of Bone Conduction Hearing Device into Left Inner Ear, Percutaneous Endoscopic Approach
09HE45Z	Insertion of Single Channel Cochlear Prosthesis into Left Inner Ear, Percutaneous Endoscopic Approach
09HE46Z	Insertion of Multiple Channel Cochlear Prosthesis into Left Inner Ear, Percutaneous Endoscopic Approach
09HE4SZ	Insertion of Hearing Device into Left Inner Ear, Percutaneous Endoscopic Approach
09HN7BZ	Insertion of Airway into Nasopharynx, Via Natural or Artificial Opening
09HN8BZ	Insertion of Airway into Nasopharynx, Via Natural or Artificial Opening Endoscopic

09J – Ear, Nose, Sinus, Inspection

Review Coding Guidelines B3.11a, B3.11b and B3.11c

09J70ZZ	Inspection of Right Tympanic Membrane, Open Approach
09J73ZZ	Inspection of Right Tympanic Membrane, Percutaneous Approach
09J74ZZ	Inspection of Right Tympanic Membrane, Percutaneous Endoscopic Approach
09J77ZZ	Inspection of Right Tympanic Membrane, Via Natural or Artificial Opening
09J78ZZ	Inspection of Right Tympanic Membrane, Via Natural or Artificial Opening Endoscopic
09J7XZZ	Inspection of Right Tympanic Membrane, External Approach
09J80ZZ	Inspection of Left Tympanic Membrane, Open Approach
09J83ZZ	Inspection of Left Tympanic Membrane, Percutaneous Approach
09J84ZZ	Inspection of Left Tympanic Membrane, Percutaneous Endoscopic Approach
09J87ZZ	Inspection of Left Tympanic Membrane, Via Natural or Artificial Opening
09J88ZZ	Inspection of Left Tympanic Membrane, Via Natural or Artificial Opening Endoscopic
09J8XZZ	Inspection of Left Tympanic Membrane, External Approach
09JD0ZZ	Inspection of Right Inner Ear, Open Approach
09JD3ZZ	Inspection of Right Inner Ear, Percutaneous Approach
09JD4ZZ	Inspection of Right Inner Ear, Percutaneous Endoscopic Approach
09JDXZZ	Inspection of Right Inner Ear, External Approach
09JE0ZZ	Inspection of Left Inner Ear, Open Approach
09JE3ZZ	Inspection of Left Inner Ear, Percutaneous Approach

09JE4ZZ	Inspection of Left Inner Ear, Percutaneous Endoscopic Approach
09JEXZZ	Inspection of Left Inner Ear, External Approach
09JH0ZZ	Inspection of Right Ear, Open Approach
09JH3ZZ	Inspection of Right Ear, Percutaneous Approach
09JH4ZZ	Inspection of Right Ear, Percutaneous Endoscopic Approach
09JH7ZZ	Inspection of Right Ear, Via Natural or Artificial Opening
09JH8ZZ	Inspection of Right Ear, Via Natural or Artificial Opening Endoscopic
09JHXZZ	Inspection of Right Ear, External Approach
09JJ0ZZ	Inspection of Left Ear, Open Approach
09JJ3ZZ	Inspection of Left Ear, Percutaneous Approach
09JJ4ZZ	Inspection of Left Ear, Percutaneous Endoscopic Approach
09JJ7ZZ	Inspection of Left Ear, Via Natural or Artificial Opening
09JJ8ZZ	Inspection of Left Ear, Via Natural or Artificial Opening Endoscopic
09JJXZZ	Inspection of Left Ear, External Approach
09JK0ZZ	Inspection of Nose, Open Approach
09JK3ZZ	Inspection of Nose, Percutaneous Approach
09JK4ZZ	Inspection of Nose, Percutaneous Endoscopic Approach
09JKXZZ	Inspection of Nose, External Approach
09JY0ZZ	Inspection of Sinus, Open Approach
09JY3ZZ	Inspection of Sinus, Percutaneous Approach
09JY4ZZ	Inspection of Sinus, Percutaneous Endoscopic Approach
09JYXZZ	Inspection of Sinus, External Approach

09M – Ear, Nose, Sinus, Reattachment

09M0XZZ	Reattachment of Right External Ear, External Approach
09M1XZZ	Reattachment of Left External Ear, External Approach

09MKXZZ	Reattachment of Nose, External Approach

09N – Ear, Nose, Sinus, Release

Review Coding Guidelines B3.13 and B3.14

09N00ZZ	Release Right External Ear, Open Approach
09N03ZZ	Release Right External Ear, Percutaneous Approach
09N04ZZ	Release Right External Ear, Percutaneous Endoscopic Approach
09N0XZZ	Release Right External Ear, External Approach
09N10ZZ	Release Left External Ear, Open Approach
09N13ZZ	Release Left External Ear, Percutaneous Approach
09N14ZZ	Release Left External Ear, Percutaneous Endoscopic Approach
09N1XZZ	Release Left External Ear, External Approach
09N30ZZ	Release Right External Auditory Canal, Open Approach
09N33ZZ	Release Right External Auditory Canal, Percutaneous Approach
09N34ZZ	Release Right External Auditory Canal, Percutaneous Endoscopic Approach
09N37ZZ	Release Right External Auditory Canal, Via Natural or Artificial Opening
09N38ZZ	Release Right External Auditory Canal, Via Natural or Artificial Opening Endoscopic
09N3XZZ	Release Right External Auditory Canal, External Approach
09N40ZZ	Release Left External Auditory Canal, Open Approach
09N43ZZ	Release Left External Auditory Canal, Percutaneous Approach
09N44ZZ	Release Left External Auditory Canal, Percutaneous Endoscopic Approach
09N47ZZ	Release Left External Auditory Canal, Via Natural or Artificial Opening
09N48ZZ	Release Left External Auditory Canal, Via Natural or Artificial Opening Endoscopic
09N4XZZ	Release Left External Auditory Canal, External Approach
09N50ZZ	Release Right Middle Ear, Open Approach
09N60ZZ	Release Left Middle Ear, Open Approach
09N70ZZ	Release Right Tympanic Membrane, Open Approach
09N73ZZ	Release Right Tympanic Membrane, Percutaneous Approach
09N74ZZ	Release Right Tympanic Membrane, Percutaneous Endoscopic Approach
09N77ZZ	Release Right Tympanic Membrane, Via Natural or Artificial Opening
09N78ZZ	Release Right Tympanic Membrane, Via Natural or Artificial Opening Endoscopic
09N80ZZ	Release Left Tympanic Membrane, Open Approach
09N83ZZ	Release Left Tympanic Membrane, Percutaneous Approach
09N84ZZ	Release Left Tympanic Membrane, Percutaneous Endoscopic Approach
09N87ZZ	Release Left Tympanic Membrane, Via Natural or Artificial Opening
09N88ZZ	Release Left Tympanic Membrane, Via Natural or Artificial Opening Endoscopic
09N90ZZ	Release Right Auditory Ossicle, Open Approach
09NA0ZZ	Release Left Auditory Ossicle, Open Approach
09NB0ZZ	Release Right Mastoid Sinus, Open Approach
09NB3ZZ	Release Right Mastoid Sinus, Percutaneous Approach
09NB4ZZ	Release Right Mastoid Sinus, Percutaneous Endoscopic Approach
09NC0ZZ	Release Left Mastoid Sinus, Open Approach
09NC3ZZ	Release Left Mastoid Sinus, Percutaneous Approach
09NC4ZZ	Release Left Mastoid Sinus, Percutaneous Endoscopic Approach
09ND0ZZ	Release Right Inner Ear, Open Approach
09NE0ZZ	Release Left Inner Ear, Open Approach
09NF0ZZ	Release Right Eustachian Tube, Open Approach
09NF3ZZ	Release Right Eustachian Tube, Percutaneous Approach
09NF4ZZ	Release Right Eustachian Tube, Percutaneous Endoscopic Approach
09NF7ZZ	Release Right Eustachian Tube, Via Natural or Artificial Opening
09NF8ZZ	Release Right Eustachian Tube, Via Natural or Artificial Opening Endoscopic
09NG0ZZ	Release Left Eustachian Tube, Open Approach
09NG3ZZ	Release Left Eustachian Tube, Percutaneous Approach
09NG4ZZ	Release Left Eustachian Tube, Percutaneous Endoscopic Approach
09NG7ZZ	Release Left Eustachian Tube, Via Natural or Artificial Opening
09NG8ZZ	Release Left Eustachian Tube, Via Natural or Artificial Opening Endoscopic
09NK0ZZ	Release Nose, Open Approach
09NK3ZZ	Release Nose, Percutaneous Approach
09NK4ZZ	Release Nose, Percutaneous Endoscopic Approach
09NKXZZ	Release Nose, External Approach
09NL0ZZ	Release Nasal Turbinate, Open Approach
09NL3ZZ	Release Nasal Turbinate, Percutaneous Approach
09NL4ZZ	Release Nasal Turbinate, Percutaneous Endoscopic Approach
09NL7ZZ	Release Nasal Turbinate, Via Natural or Artificial Opening
09NL8ZZ	Release Nasal Turbinate, Via Natural or Artificial Opening Endoscopic
09NM0ZZ	Release Nasal Septum, Open Approach
09NM3ZZ	Release Nasal Septum, Percutaneous Approach
09NM4ZZ	Release Nasal Septum, Percutaneous Endoscopic Approach
09NN0ZZ	Release Nasopharynx, Open Approach
09NN3ZZ	Release Nasopharynx, Percutaneous Approach
09NN4ZZ	Release Nasopharynx, Percutaneous Endoscopic Approach
09NN7ZZ	Release Nasopharynx, Via Natural or Artificial Opening
09NN8ZZ	Release Nasopharynx, Via Natural or Artificial Opening Endoscopic
09NP0ZZ	Release Accessory Sinus, Open Approach
09NP3ZZ	Release Accessory Sinus, Percutaneous Approach
09NP4ZZ	Release Accessory Sinus, Percutaneous Endoscopic Approach
09NQ0ZZ	Release Right Maxillary Sinus, Open Approach
09NQ3ZZ	Release Right Maxillary Sinus, Percutaneous Approach
09NQ4ZZ	Release Right Maxillary Sinus, Percutaneous Endoscopic Approach
09NR0ZZ	Release Left Maxillary Sinus, Open Approach
09NR3ZZ	Release Left Maxillary Sinus, Percutaneous Approach
09NR4ZZ	Release Left Maxillary Sinus, Percutaneous Endoscopic Approach
09NS0ZZ	Release Right Frontal Sinus, Open Approach
09NS3ZZ	Release Right Frontal Sinus, Percutaneous Approach
09NS4ZZ	Release Right Frontal Sinus, Percutaneous Endoscopic Approach
09NT0ZZ	Release Left Frontal Sinus, Open Approach
09NT3ZZ	Release Left Frontal Sinus, Percutaneous Approach
09NT4ZZ	Release Left Frontal Sinus, Percutaneous Endoscopic Approach
09NU0ZZ	Release Right Ethmoid Sinus, Open Approach
09NU3ZZ	Release Right Ethmoid Sinus, Percutaneous Approach
09NU4ZZ	Release Right Ethmoid Sinus, Percutaneous Endoscopic Approach
09NV0ZZ	Release Left Ethmoid Sinus, Open Approach
09NV3ZZ	Release Left Ethmoid Sinus, Percutaneous Approach
09NV4ZZ	Release Left Ethmoid Sinus, Percutaneous Endoscopic Approach
09NW0ZZ	Release Right Sphenoid Sinus, Open Approach
09NW3ZZ	Release Right Sphenoid Sinus, Percutaneous Approach
09NW4ZZ	Release Right Sphenoid Sinus, Percutaneous Endoscopic Approach
09NX0ZZ	Release Left Sphenoid Sinus, Open Approach
09NX3ZZ	Release Left Sphenoid Sinus, Percutaneous Approach
09NX4ZZ	Release Left Sphenoid Sinus, Percutaneous Endoscopic Approach

09P – Ear, Nose, Sinus, Removal

Review Coding Guideline B6.1c

09P700Z	Removal of Drainage Device from Right Tympanic Membrane, Open Approach
09P770Z	Removal of Drainage Device from Right Tympanic Membrane, Via Natural or Artificial Opening
09P780Z	Removal of Drainage Device from Right Tympanic Membrane, Via Natural or Artificial Opening Endoscopic
09P7X0Z	Removal of Drainage Device from Right Tympanic Membrane, External Approach
09P800Z	Removal of Drainage Device from Left Tympanic Membrane, Open Approach
09P870Z	Removal of Drainage Device from Left Tympanic Membrane, Via Natural or Artificial Opening
09P880Z	Removal of Drainage Device from Left Tympanic Membrane, Via Natural or Artificial Opening Endoscopic
09P8X0Z	Removal of Drainage Device from Left Tympanic Membrane, External Approach

♀ Female-only   ♂ Male-only   ● Limited Coverage   ● Non-OR   ▨ HAC-associated procedure   ● Non-covered procedures   ✚ Combination

09PD0SZ   Removal of Hearing Device from Right Inner Ear, Open Approach

09PD7SZ   Removal of Hearing Device from Right Inner Ear, Via Natural or Artificial Opening

09PD8SZ   Removal of Hearing Device from Right Inner Ear, Via Natural or Artificial Opening Endoscopic

09PE0SZ   Removal of Hearing Device from Left Inner Ear, Open Approach

09PE7SZ   Removal of Hearing Device from Left Inner Ear, Via Natural or Artificial Opening

09PE8SZ   Removal of Hearing Device from Left Inner Ear, Via Natural or Artificial Opening Endoscopic

09PH00Z   Removal of Drainage Device from Right Ear, Open Approach

09PH07Z   Removal of Autologous Tissue Substitute from Right Ear, Open Approach

09PH0DZ   Removal of Intraluminal Device from Right Ear, Open Approach

09PH0JZ   Removal of Synthetic Substitute from Right Ear, Open Approach

09PH0KZ   Removal of Nonautologous Tissue Substitute from Right Ear, Open Approach

09PH30Z   Removal of Drainage Device from Right Ear, Percutaneous Approach

09PH37Z   Removal of Autologous Tissue Substitute from Right Ear, Percutaneous Approach

09PH3DZ   Removal of Intraluminal Device from Right Ear, Percutaneous Approach

09PH3JZ   Removal of Synthetic Substitute from Right Ear, Percutaneous Approach

09PH3KZ   Removal of Nonautologous Tissue Substitute from Right Ear, Percutaneous Approach

09PH40Z   Removal of Drainage Device from Right Ear, Percutaneous Endoscopic Approach

09PH47Z   Removal of Autologous Tissue Substitute from Right Ear, Percutaneous Endoscopic Approach

09PH4DZ   Removal of Intraluminal Device from Right Ear, Percutaneous Endoscopic Approach

09PH4JZ   Removal of Synthetic Substitute from Right Ear, Percutaneous Endoscopic Approach

09PH4KZ   Removal of Nonautologous Tissue Substitute from Right Ear, Percutaneous Endoscopic Approach

09PH70Z   Removal of Drainage Device from Right Ear, Via Natural or Artificial Opening

09PH77Z   Removal of Autologous Tissue Substitute from Right Ear, Via Natural or Artificial Opening

09PH7DZ   Removal of Intraluminal Device from Right Ear, Via Natural or Artificial Opening

09PH7JZ   Removal of Synthetic Substitute from Right Ear, Via Natural or Artificial Opening

09PH7KZ   Removal of Nonautologous Tissue Substitute from Right Ear, Via Natural or Artificial Opening

09PH80Z   Removal of Drainage Device from Right Ear, Via Natural or Artificial Opening Endoscopic

09PH87Z   Removal of Autologous Tissue Substitute from Right Ear, Via Natural or Artificial Opening Endoscopic

09PH8DZ   Removal of Intraluminal Device from Right Ear, Via Natural or Artificial Opening Endoscopic

09PH8JZ   Removal of Synthetic Substitute from Right Ear, Via Natural or Artificial Opening Endoscopic

09PH8KZ   Removal of Nonautologous Tissue Substitute from Right Ear, Via Natural or Artificial Opening Endoscopic

09PHX0Z   Removal of Drainage Device from Right Ear, External Approach

09PHX7Z   Removal of Autologous Tissue Substitute from Right Ear, External Approach

09PHXDZ   Removal of Intraluminal Device from Right Ear, External Approach

09PHXJZ   Removal of Synthetic Substitute from Right Ear, External Approach

09PHXKZ   Removal of Nonautologous Tissue Substitute from Right Ear, External Approach

09PJ00Z   Removal of Drainage Device from Left Ear, Open Approach

09PJ07Z   Removal of Autologous Tissue Substitute from Left Ear, Open Approach

09PJ0DZ   Removal of Intraluminal Device from Left Ear, Open Approach

09PJ0JZ   Removal of Synthetic Substitute from Left Ear, Open Approach

09PJ0KZ   Removal of Nonautologous Tissue Substitute from Left Ear, Open Approach

09PJ30Z   Removal of Drainage Device from Left Ear, Percutaneous Approach

09PJ37Z   Removal of Autologous Tissue Substitute from Left Ear, Percutaneous Approach

09PJ3DZ   Removal of Intraluminal Device from Left Ear, Percutaneous Approach

09PJ3JZ   Removal of Synthetic Substitute from Left Ear, Percutaneous Approach

09PJ3KZ   Removal of Nonautologous Tissue Substitute from Left Ear, Percutaneous Approach

09PJ40Z   Removal of Drainage Device from Left Ear, Percutaneous Endoscopic Approach

09PJ47Z   Removal of Autologous Tissue Substitute from Left Ear, Percutaneous Endoscopic Approach

09PJ4DZ   Removal of Intraluminal Device from Left Ear, Percutaneous Endoscopic Approach

09PJ4JZ   Removal of Synthetic Substitute from Left Ear, Percutaneous Endoscopic Approach

09PJ4KZ   Removal of Nonautologous Tissue Substitute from Left Ear, Percutaneous Endoscopic Approach

09PJ70Z   Removal of Drainage Device from Left Ear, Via Natural or Artificial Opening

09PJ77Z   Removal of Autologous Tissue Substitute from Left Ear, Via Natural or Artificial Opening

09PJ7DZ   Removal of Intraluminal Device from Left Ear, Via Natural or Artificial Opening

09PJ7JZ   Removal of Synthetic Substitute from Left Ear, Via Natural or Artificial Opening

09PJ7KZ   Removal of Nonautologous Tissue Substitute from Left Ear, Via Natural or Artificial Opening

09PJ80Z   Removal of Drainage Device from Left Ear, Via Natural or Artificial Opening Endoscopic

09PJ87Z   Removal of Autologous Tissue Substitute from Left Ear, Via Natural or Artificial Opening Endoscopic

09PJ8DZ   Removal of Intraluminal Device from Left Ear, Via Natural or Artificial Opening Endoscopic

09PJ8JZ   Removal of Synthetic Substitute from Left Ear, Via Natural or Artificial Opening Endoscopic

09PJ8KZ   Removal of Nonautologous Tissue Substitute from Left Ear, Via Natural or Artificial Opening Endoscopic

09PJX0Z   Removal of Drainage Device from Left Ear, External Approach

09PJX7Z   Removal of Autologous Tissue Substitute from Left Ear, External Approach

09PJXDZ   Removal of Intraluminal Device from Left Ear, External Approach

09PJXJZ   Removal of Synthetic Substitute from Left Ear, External Approach

09PJXKZ   Removal of Nonautologous Tissue Substitute from Left Ear, External Approach

09PK00Z   Removal of Drainage Device from Nose, Open Approach

09PK07Z   Removal of Autologous Tissue Substitute from Nose, Open Approach

09PK0DZ   Removal of Intraluminal Device from Nose, Open Approach

09PK0JZ   Removal of Synthetic Substitute from Nose, Open Approach

09PK0KZ   Removal of Nonautologous Tissue Substitute from Nose, Open Approach

09PK30Z   Removal of Drainage Device from Nose, Percutaneous Approach

09PK37Z   Removal of Autologous Tissue Substitute from Nose, Percutaneous Approach

09PK3DZ   Removal of Intraluminal Device from Nose, Percutaneous Approach

09PK3JZ   Removal of Synthetic Substitute from Nose, Percutaneous Approach

09PK3KZ   Removal of Nonautologous Tissue Substitute from Nose, Percutaneous Approach

09PK40Z   Removal of Drainage Device from Nose, Percutaneous Endoscopic Approach

09PK47Z   Removal of Autologous Tissue Substitute from Nose, Percutaneous Endoscopic Approach

09PK4DZ   Removal of Intraluminal Device from Nose, Percutaneous Endoscopic Approach

09PK4JZ   Removal of Synthetic Substitute from Nose, Percutaneous Endoscopic Approach

09PK4KZ   Removal of Nonautologous Tissue Substitute from Nose, Percutaneous Endoscopic Approach

09PK70Z   Removal of Drainage Device from Nose, Via Natural or Artificial Opening

09PK77Z   Removal of Autologous Tissue Substitute from Nose, Via Natural or Artificial Opening

09PK7DZ Removal of Intraluminal Device from Nose, Via Natural or Artificial Opening

09PK7JZ Removal of Synthetic Substitute from Nose, Via Natural or Artificial Opening

09PK7KZ Removal of Nonautologous Tissue Substitute from Nose, Via Natural or Artificial Opening

09PK80Z Removal of Drainage Device from Nose, Via Natural or Artificial Opening Endoscopic

09PK87Z Removal of Autologous Tissue Substitute from Nose, Via Natural or Artificial Opening Endoscopic

09PK8DZ Removal of Intraluminal Device from Nose, Via Natural or Artificial Opening Endoscopic

09PK8JZ Removal of Synthetic Substitute from Nose, Via Natural or Artificial Opening Endoscopic

09PK8KZ Removal of Nonautologous Tissue Substitute from Nose, Via Natural or Artificial Opening Endoscopic

09PKX0Z Removal of Drainage Device from Nose, External Approach

09PKX7Z Removal of Autologous Tissue Substitute from Nose, External Approach

09PKXDZ Removal of Intraluminal Device from Nose, External Approach

09PKXJZ Removal of Synthetic Substitute from Nose, External Approach

09PKXKZ Removal of Nonautologous Tissue Substitute from Nose, External Approach

09PY00Z Removal of Drainage Device from Sinus, Open Approach

09PY30Z Removal of Drainage Device from Sinus, Percutaneous Approach

09PY40Z Removal of Drainage Device from Sinus, Percutaneous Endoscopic Approach

09PYX0Z Removal of Drainage Device from Sinus, External Approach

09Q – Ear, Nose, Sinus, Repair

09Q00ZZ Repair Right External Ear, Open Approach
09Q03ZZ Repair Right External Ear, Percutaneous Approach
09Q04ZZ Repair Right External Ear, Percutaneous Endoscopic Approach
09Q0XZZ Repair Right External Ear, External Approach
09Q10ZZ Repair Left External Ear, Open Approach
09Q13ZZ Repair Left External Ear, Percutaneous Approach
09Q14ZZ Repair Left External Ear, Percutaneous Endoscopic Approach
09Q1XZZ Repair Left External Ear, External Approach
09Q20ZZ Repair Bilateral External Ear, Open Approach
09Q23ZZ Repair Bilateral External Ear, Percutaneous Approach
09Q24ZZ Repair Bilateral External Ear, Percutaneous Endoscopic Approach
09Q2XZZ Repair Bilateral External Ear, External Approach
09Q30ZZ Repair Right External Auditory Canal, Open Approach
09Q33ZZ Repair Right External Auditory Canal, Percutaneous Approach
09Q34ZZ Repair Right External Auditory Canal, Percutaneous Endoscopic Approach
09Q37ZZ Repair Right External Auditory Canal, Via Natural or Artificial Opening
09Q38ZZ Repair Right External Auditory Canal, Via Natural or Artificial Opening Endoscopic
09Q3XZZ Repair Right External Auditory Canal, External Approach
09Q40ZZ Repair Left External Auditory Canal, Open Approach
09Q43ZZ Repair Left External Auditory Canal, Percutaneous Approach
09Q44ZZ Repair Left External Auditory Canal, Percutaneous Endoscopic Approach
09Q47ZZ Repair Left External Auditory Canal, Via Natural or Artificial Opening
09Q48ZZ Repair Left External Auditory Canal, Via Natural or Artificial Opening Endoscopic
09Q4XZZ Repair Left External Auditory Canal, External Approach
09Q50ZZ Repair Right Middle Ear, Open Approach
09Q60ZZ Repair Left Middle Ear, Open Approach
09Q70ZZ Repair Right Tympanic Membrane, Open Approach
09Q73ZZ Repair Right Tympanic Membrane, Percutaneous Approach
09Q74ZZ Repair Right Tympanic Membrane, Percutaneous Endoscopic Approach
09Q77ZZ Repair Right Tympanic Membrane, Via Natural or Artificial Opening
09Q78ZZ Repair Right Tympanic Membrane, Via Natural or Artificial Opening Endoscopic
09Q80ZZ Repair Left Tympanic Membrane, Open Approach
09Q83ZZ Repair Left Tympanic Membrane, Percutaneous Approach
09Q84ZZ Repair Left Tympanic Membrane, Percutaneous Endoscopic Approach
09Q87ZZ Repair Left Tympanic Membrane, Via Natural or Artificial Opening
09Q88ZZ Repair Left Tympanic Membrane, Via Natural or Artificial Opening Endoscopic
09Q90ZZ Repair Right Auditory Ossicle, Open Approach
09QA0ZZ Repair Left Auditory Ossicle, Open Approach
09QB0ZZ Repair Right Mastoid Sinus, Open Approach
09QB3ZZ Repair Right Mastoid Sinus, Percutaneous Approach
09QB4ZZ Repair Right Mastoid Sinus, Percutaneous Endoscopic Approach
09QC0ZZ Repair Left Mastoid Sinus, Open Approach
09QC3ZZ Repair Left Mastoid Sinus, Percutaneous Approach
09QC4ZZ Repair Left Mastoid Sinus, Percutaneous Endoscopic Approach
09QD0ZZ Repair Right Inner Ear, Open Approach

09QE0ZZ Repair Left Inner Ear, Open Approach
09QF0ZZ Repair Right Eustachian Tube, Open Approach
09QF3ZZ Repair Right Eustachian Tube, Percutaneous Approach
09QF4ZZ Repair Right Eustachian Tube, Percutaneous Endoscopic Approach
09QF7ZZ Repair Right Eustachian Tube, Via Natural or Artificial Opening
09QF8ZZ Repair Right Eustachian Tube, Via Natural or Artificial Opening Endoscopic
09QFXZZ Repair Right Eustachian Tube, External Approach
09QG0ZZ Repair Left Eustachian Tube, Open Approach
09QG3ZZ Repair Left Eustachian Tube, Percutaneous Approach
09QG4ZZ Repair Left Eustachian Tube, Percutaneous Endoscopic Approach
09QG7ZZ Repair Left Eustachian Tube, Via Natural or Artificial Opening
09QG8ZZ Repair Left Eustachian Tube, Via Natural or Artificial Opening Endoscopic
09QGXZZ Repair Left Eustachian Tube, External Approach
09QK0ZZ Repair Nose, Open Approach
09QK3ZZ Repair Nose, Percutaneous Approach
09QK4ZZ Repair Nose, Percutaneous Endoscopic Approach
09QKXZZ Repair Nose, External Approach
09QL0ZZ Repair Nasal Turbinate, Open Approach
09QL3ZZ Repair Nasal Turbinate, Percutaneous Approach
09QL4ZZ Repair Nasal Turbinate, Percutaneous Endoscopic Approach
09QL7ZZ Repair Nasal Turbinate, Via Natural or Artificial Opening
09QL8ZZ Repair Nasal Turbinate, Via Natural or Artificial Opening Endoscopic
09QM0ZZ Repair Nasal Septum, Open Approach
09QM3ZZ Repair Nasal Septum, Percutaneous Approach
09QM4ZZ Repair Nasal Septum, Percutaneous Endoscopic Approach
09QN0ZZ Repair Nasopharynx, Open Approach
09QN3ZZ Repair Nasopharynx, Percutaneous Approach
09QN4ZZ Repair Nasopharynx, Percutaneous Endoscopic Approach
09QN7ZZ Repair Nasopharynx, Via Natural or Artificial Opening
09QN8ZZ Repair Nasopharynx, Via Natural or Artificial Opening Endoscopic
09QP0ZZ Repair Accessory Sinus, Open Approach
09QP3ZZ Repair Accessory Sinus, Percutaneous Approach
09QP4ZZ Repair Accessory Sinus, Percutaneous Endoscopic Approach
09QQ0ZZ Repair Right Maxillary Sinus, Open Approach
09QQ3ZZ Repair Right Maxillary Sinus, Percutaneous Approach
09QQ4ZZ Repair Right Maxillary Sinus, Percutaneous Endoscopic Approach
09QR0ZZ Repair Left Maxillary Sinus, Open Approach
09QR3ZZ Repair Left Maxillary Sinus, Percutaneous Approach
09QR4ZZ Repair Left Maxillary Sinus, Percutaneous Endoscopic Approach
09QS0ZZ Repair Right Frontal Sinus, Open Approach
09QS3ZZ Repair Right Frontal Sinus, Percutaneous Approach
09QS4ZZ Repair Right Frontal Sinus, Percutaneous Endoscopic Approach
09QT0ZZ Repair Left Frontal Sinus, Open Approach
09QT3ZZ Repair Left Frontal Sinus, Percutaneous Approach
09QT4ZZ Repair Left Frontal Sinus, Percutaneous Endoscopic Approach
09QU0ZZ Repair Right Ethmoid Sinus, Open Approach
09QU3ZZ Repair Right Ethmoid Sinus, Percutaneous Approach
09QU4ZZ Repair Right Ethmoid Sinus, Percutaneous Endoscopic Approach
09QV0ZZ Repair Left Ethmoid Sinus, Open Approach
09QV3ZZ Repair Left Ethmoid Sinus, Percutaneous Approach
09QV4ZZ Repair Left Ethmoid Sinus, Percutaneous Endoscopic Approach
09QW0ZZ Repair Right Sphenoid Sinus, Open Approach
09QW3ZZ Repair Right Sphenoid Sinus, Percutaneous Approach

09QW4ZZ Repair Right Sphenoid Sinus, Percutaneous Endoscopic Approach

09QX0ZZ Repair Left Sphenoid Sinus, Open Approach

09QX3ZZ Repair Left Sphenoid Sinus, Percutaneous Approach

09QX4ZZ Repair Left Sphenoid Sinus, Percutaneous Endoscopic Approach

09R – Ear, Nose, Sinus, Replacement

09R007Z Replacement of Right External Ear with Autologous Tissue Substitute, Open Approach

09R00JZ Replacement of Right External Ear with Synthetic Substitute, Open Approach

09R00KZ Replacement of Right External Ear with Nonautologous Tissue Substitute, Open Approach

09R0X7Z Replacement of Right External Ear with Autologous Tissue Substitute, External Approach

09R0XJZ Replacement of Right External Ear with Synthetic Substitute, External Approach

09R0XKZ Replacement of Right External Ear with Nonautologous Tissue Substitute, External Approach

09R107Z Replacement of Left External Ear with Autologous Tissue Substitute, Open Approach

09R10JZ Replacement of Left External Ear with Synthetic Substitute, Open Approach

09R10KZ Replacement of Left External Ear with Nonautologous Tissue Substitute, Open Approach

09R1X7Z Replacement of Left External Ear with Autologous Tissue Substitute, External Approach

09R1XJZ Replacement of Left External Ear with Synthetic Substitute, External Approach

09R1XKZ Replacement of Left External Ear with Nonautologous Tissue Substitute, External Approach

09R207Z Replacement of Bilateral External Ear with Autologous Tissue Substitute, Open Approach

09R20JZ Replacement of Bilateral External Ear with Synthetic Substitute, Open Approach

09R20KZ Replacement of Bilateral External Ear with Nonautologous Tissue Substitute, Open Approach

09R2X7Z Replacement of Bilateral External Ear with Autologous Tissue Substitute, External Approach

09R2XJZ Replacement of Bilateral External Ear with Synthetic Substitute, External Approach

09R2XKZ Replacement of Bilateral External Ear with Nonautologous Tissue Substitute, External Approach

09R507Z Replacement of Right Middle Ear with Autologous Tissue Substitute, Open Approach

09R50JZ Replacement of Right Middle Ear with Synthetic Substitute, Open Approach

09R50KZ Replacement of Right Middle Ear with Nonautologous Tissue Substitute, Open Approach

09R607Z Replacement of Left Middle Ear with Autologous Tissue Substitute, Open Approach

09R60JZ Replacement of Left Middle Ear with Synthetic Substitute, Open Approach

09R60KZ Replacement of Left Middle Ear with Nonautologous Tissue Substitute, Open Approach

09R707Z Replacement of Right Tympanic Membrane with Autologous Tissue Substitute, Open Approach

09R70JZ Replacement of Right Tympanic Membrane with Synthetic Substitute, Open Approach

09R70KZ Replacement of Right Tympanic Membrane with Nonautologous Tissue Substitute, Open Approach

09R777Z Replacement of Right Tympanic Membrane with Autologous Tissue Substitute, Via Natural or Artificial Opening

09R77JZ Replacement of Right Tympanic Membrane with Synthetic Substitute, Via Natural or Artificial Opening

09R77KZ Replacement of Right Tympanic Membrane with Nonautologous Tissue Substitute, Via Natural or Artificial Opening

09R787Z Replacement of Right Tympanic Membrane with Autologous Tissue Substitute, Via Natural or Artificial Opening Endoscopic

09R78JZ Replacement of Right Tympanic Membrane with Synthetic Substitute, Via Natural or Artificial Opening Endoscopic

09R78KZ Replacement of Right Tympanic Membrane with Nonautologous Tissue Substitute, Via Natural or Artificial Opening Endoscopic

09R807Z Replacement of Left Tympanic Membrane with Autologous Tissue Substitute, Open Approach

09R80JZ Replacement of Left Tympanic Membrane with Synthetic Substitute, Open Approach

09R80KZ Replacement of Left Tympanic Membrane with Nonautologous Tissue Substitute, Open Approach

09R877Z Replacement of Left Tympanic Membrane with Autologous Tissue Substitute, Via Natural or Artificial Opening

09R87JZ Replacement of Left Tympanic Membrane with Synthetic Substitute, Via Natural or Artificial Opening

09R87KZ Replacement of Left Tympanic Membrane with Nonautologous Tissue Substitute, Via Natural or Artificial Opening

09R887Z Replacement of Left Tympanic Membrane with Autologous Tissue Substitute, Via Natural or Artificial Opening Endoscopic

09R88JZ Replacement of Left Tympanic Membrane with Synthetic Substitute, Via Natural or Artificial Opening Endoscopic

09R88KZ Replacement of Left Tympanic Membrane with Nonautologous Tissue Substitute, Via Natural or Artificial Opening Endoscopic

09R907Z Replacement of Right Auditory Ossicle with Autologous Tissue Substitute, Open Approach

09R90JZ Replacement of Right Auditory Ossicle with Synthetic Substitute, Open Approach

09R90KZ Replacement of Right Auditory Ossicle with Nonautologous Tissue Substitute, Open Approach

09RA07Z Replacement of Left Auditory Ossicle with Autologous Tissue Substitute, Open Approach

09RA0JZ Replacement of Left Auditory Ossicle with Synthetic Substitute, Open Approach

09RA0KZ Replacement of Left Auditory Ossicle with Nonautologous Tissue Substitute, Open Approach

09RD07Z Replacement of Right Inner Ear with Autologous Tissue Substitute, Open Approach

09RD0JZ Replacement of Right Inner Ear with Synthetic Substitute, Open Approach

09RD0KZ Replacement of Right Inner Ear with Nonautologous Tissue Substitute, Open Approach

09RE07Z Replacement of Left Inner Ear with Autologous Tissue Substitute, Open Approach

09RE0JZ Replacement of Left Inner Ear with Synthetic Substitute, Open Approach

09RE0KZ Replacement of Left Inner Ear with Nonautologous Tissue Substitute, Open Approach

09RK07Z Replacement of Nose with Autologous Tissue Substitute, Open Approach

09RK0JZ Replacement of Nose with Synthetic Substitute, Open Approach

09RK0KZ Replacement of Nose with Nonautologous Tissue Substitute, Open Approach

09RKX7Z Replacement of Nose with Autologous Tissue Substitute, External Approach

09RKXJZ Replacement of Nose with Synthetic Substitute, External Approach

09RKXKZ Replacement of Nose with Nonautologous Tissue Substitute, External Approach

09RL07Z Replacement of Nasal Turbinate with Autologous Tissue Substitute, Open Approach

09RL0JZ Replacement of Nasal Turbinate with Synthetic Substitute, Open Approach

09RL0KZ Replacement of Nasal Turbinate with Nonautologous Tissue Substitute, Open Approach

09RL37Z Replacement of Nasal Turbinate with Autologous Tissue Substitute, Percutaneous Approach

09RL3JZ Replacement of Nasal Turbinate with Synthetic Substitute, Percutaneous Approach

09RL3KZ Replacement of Nasal Turbinate with Nonautologous Tissue Substitute, Percutaneous Approach

09RL47Z Replacement of Nasal Turbinate with Autologous Tissue Substitute, Percutaneous Endoscopic Approach

09RL4JZ Replacement of Nasal Turbinate with Synthetic Substitute, Percutaneous Endoscopic Approach

09RL4KZ Replacement of Nasal Turbinate with Nonautologous Tissue Substitute, Percutaneous Endoscopic Approach

---

09RL77Z   Replacement of Nasal Turbinate with Autologous Tissue Substitute, Via Natural or Artificial Opening

09RL7JZ   Replacement of Nasal Turbinate with Synthetic Substitute, Via Natural or Artificial Opening

09RL7KZ   Replacement of Nasal Turbinate with Nonautologous Tissue Substitute, Via Natural or Artificial Opening

09RL87Z   Replacement of Nasal Turbinate with Autologous Tissue Substitute, Via Natural or Artificial Opening Endoscopic

09RL8JZ   Replacement of Nasal Turbinate with Synthetic Substitute, Via Natural or Artificial Opening Endoscopic

09RL8KZ   Replacement of Nasal Turbinate with Nonautologous Tissue Substitute, Via Natural or Artificial Opening Endoscopic

09RM07Z   Replacement of Nasal Septum with Autologous Tissue Substitute, Open Approach

09RM0JZ   Replacement of Nasal Septum with Synthetic Substitute, Open Approach

09RM0KZ   Replacement of Nasal Septum with Nonautologous Tissue Substitute, Open Approach

09RM37Z   Replacement of Nasal Septum with Autologous Tissue Substitute, Percutaneous Approach

09RM3JZ   Replacement of Nasal Septum with Synthetic Substitute, Percutaneous Approach

09RM3KZ   Replacement of Nasal Septum with Nonautologous Tissue Substitute, Percutaneous Approach

09RM47Z   Replacement of Nasal Septum with Autologous Tissue Substitute, Percutaneous Endoscopic Approach

09RM4JZ   Replacement of Nasal Septum with Synthetic Substitute, Percutaneous Endoscopic Approach

09RM4KZ   Replacement of Nasal Septum with Nonautologous Tissue Substitute, Percutaneous Endoscopic Approach

09RN07Z   Replacement of Nasopharynx with Autologous Tissue Substitute, Open Approach

09RN0JZ   Replacement of Nasopharynx with Synthetic Substitute, Open Approach

09RN0KZ   Replacement of Nasopharynx with Nonautologous Tissue Substitute, Open Approach

09RN77Z   Replacement of Nasopharynx with Autologous Tissue Substitute, Via Natural or Artificial Opening

09RN7JZ   Replacement of Nasopharynx with Synthetic Substitute, Via Natural or Artificial Opening

09RN7KZ   Replacement of Nasopharynx with Nonautologous Tissue Substitute, Via Natural or Artificial Opening

09RN87Z   Replacement of Nasopharynx with Autologous Tissue Substitute, Via Natural or Artificial Opening Endoscopic

09RN8JZ   Replacement of Nasopharynx with Synthetic Substitute, Via Natural or Artificial Opening Endoscopic

09RN8KZ   Replacement of Nasopharynx with Nonautologous Tissue Substitute, Via Natural or Artificial Opening Endoscopic

09S – Ear, Nose, Sinus, Reposition

09S00ZZ   Reposition Right External Ear, Open Approach
09S04ZZ   Reposition Right External Ear, Percutaneous Endoscopic Approach
09S0XZZ   Reposition Right External Ear, External Approach
09S10ZZ   Reposition Left External Ear, Open Approach
09S14ZZ   Reposition Left External Ear, Percutaneous Endoscopic Approach
09S1XZZ   Reposition Left External Ear, External Approach
09S20ZZ   Reposition Bilateral External Ear, Open Approach
09S24ZZ   Reposition Bilateral External Ear, Percutaneous Endoscopic Approach
09S2XZZ   Reposition Bilateral External Ear, External Approach
09S70ZZ   Reposition Right Tympanic Membrane, Open Approach
09S74ZZ   Reposition Right Tympanic Membrane, Percutaneous Endoscopic Approach
09S77ZZ   Reposition Right Tympanic Membrane, Via Natural or Artificial Opening
09S78ZZ   Reposition Right Tympanic Membrane, Via Natural or Artificial Opening Endoscopic
09S80ZZ   Reposition Left Tympanic Membrane, Open Approach
09S84ZZ   Reposition Left Tympanic Membrane, Percutaneous Endoscopic Approach
09S87ZZ   Reposition Left Tympanic Membrane, Via Natural or Artificial Opening
09S88ZZ   Reposition Left Tympanic Membrane, Via Natural or Artificial Opening Endoscopic
09S90ZZ   Reposition Right Auditory Ossicle, Open Approach
09S94ZZ   Reposition Right Auditory Ossicle, Percutaneous Endoscopic Approach

09SA0ZZ   Reposition Left Auditory Ossicle, Open Approach
09SA4ZZ   Reposition Left Auditory Ossicle, Percutaneous Endoscopic Approach
09SF0ZZ   Reposition Right Eustachian Tube, Open Approach
09SF4ZZ   Reposition Right Eustachian Tube, Percutaneous Endoscopic Approach
09SF7ZZ   Reposition Right Eustachian Tube, Via Natural or Artificial Opening
09SF8ZZ   Reposition Right Eustachian Tube, Via Natural or Artificial Opening Endoscopic
09SG0ZZ   Reposition Left Eustachian Tube, Open Approach
09SG4ZZ   Reposition Left Eustachian Tube, Percutaneous Endoscopic Approach
09SG7ZZ   Reposition Left Eustachian Tube, Via Natural or Artificial Opening
09SG8ZZ   Reposition Left Eustachian Tube, Via Natural or Artificial Opening Endoscopic
09SK0ZZ   Reposition Nose, Open Approach
09SK4ZZ   Reposition Nose, Percutaneous Endoscopic Approach
09SKXZZ   Reposition Nose, External Approach
09SL0ZZ   Reposition Nasal Turbinate, Open Approach
09SL4ZZ   Reposition Nasal Turbinate, Percutaneous Endoscopic Approach
09SL7ZZ   Reposition Nasal Turbinate, Via Natural or Artificial Opening
09SL8ZZ   Reposition Nasal Turbinate, Via Natural or Artificial Opening Endoscopic
09SM0ZZ   Reposition Nasal Septum, Open Approach
09SM4ZZ   Reposition Nasal Septum, Percutaneous Endoscopic Approach

09T – Ear, Nose, Sinus, Resection

Review Coding Guideline B3.8

09T00ZZ   Resection of Right External Ear, Open Approach
09T04ZZ   Resection of Right External Ear, Percutaneous Endoscopic Approach
09T0XZZ   Resection of Right External Ear, External Approach
09T10ZZ   Resection of Left External Ear, Open Approach
09T14ZZ   Resection of Left External Ear, Percutaneous Endoscopic Approach
09T1XZZ   Resection of Left External Ear, External Approach
09T50ZZ   Resection of Right Middle Ear, Open Approach
09T60ZZ   Resection of Left Middle Ear, Open Approach
09T70ZZ   Resection of Right Tympanic Membrane, Open Approach
09T74ZZ   Resection of Right Tympanic Membrane, Percutaneous Endoscopic Approach
09T77ZZ   Resection of Right Tympanic Membrane, Via Natural or Artificial Opening

09T78ZZ   Resection of Right Tympanic Membrane, Via Natural or Artificial Opening Endoscopic
09T80ZZ   Resection of Left Tympanic Membrane, Open Approach
09T84ZZ   Resection of Left Tympanic Membrane, Percutaneous Endoscopic Approach
09T87ZZ   Resection of Left Tympanic Membrane, Via Natural or Artificial Opening
09T88ZZ   Resection of Left Tympanic Membrane, Via Natural or Artificial Opening Endoscopic
09T90ZZ   Resection of Right Auditory Ossicle, Open Approach
09TA0ZZ   Resection of Left Auditory Ossicle, Open Approach
09TB0ZZ   Resection of Right Mastoid Sinus, Open Approach
09TB4ZZ   Resection of Right Mastoid Sinus, Percutaneous Endoscopic Approach

09TC0ZZ	Resection of Left Mastoid Sinus, Open Approach
09TC4ZZ	Resection of Left Mastoid Sinus, Percutaneous Endoscopic Approach
09TD0ZZ	Resection of Right Inner Ear, Open Approach
09TE0ZZ	Resection of Left Inner Ear, Open Approach
09TF0ZZ	Resection of Right Eustachian Tube, Open Approach
09TF4ZZ	Resection of Right Eustachian Tube, Percutaneous Endoscopic Approach
09TF7ZZ	Resection of Right Eustachian Tube, Via Natural or Artificial Opening
09TF8ZZ	Resection of Right Eustachian Tube, Via Natural or Artificial Opening Endoscopic
09TG0ZZ	Resection of Left Eustachian Tube, Open Approach
09TG4ZZ	Resection of Left Eustachian Tube, Percutaneous Endoscopic Approach
09TG7ZZ	Resection of Left Eustachian Tube, Via Natural or Artificial Opening
09TG8ZZ	Resection of Left Eustachian Tube, Via Natural or Artificial Opening Endoscopic
09TK0ZZ	Resection of Nose, Open Approach
09TK4ZZ	Resection of Nose, Percutaneous Endoscopic Approach
09TKXZZ	Resection of Nose, External Approach
09TL0ZZ	Resection of Nasal Turbinate, Open Approach
09TL4ZZ	Resection of Nasal Turbinate, Percutaneous Endoscopic Approach
09TL7ZZ	Resection of Nasal Turbinate, Via Natural or Artificial Opening
09TL8ZZ	Resection of Nasal Turbinate, Via Natural or Artificial Opening Endoscopic
09TM0ZZ	Resection of Nasal Septum, Open Approach
09TM4ZZ	Resection of Nasal Septum, Percutaneous Endoscopic Approach
09TN0ZZ	Resection of Nasopharynx, Open Approach
09TN4ZZ	Resection of Nasopharynx, Percutaneous Endoscopic Approach
09TN7ZZ	Resection of Nasopharynx, Via Natural or Artificial Opening
09TN8ZZ	Resection of Nasopharynx, Via Natural or Artificial Opening Endoscopic
09TP0ZZ	Resection of Accessory Sinus, Open Approach
09TP4ZZ	Resection of Accessory Sinus, Percutaneous Endoscopic Approach
09TQ0ZZ	Resection of Right Maxillary Sinus, Open Approach
09TQ4ZZ	Resection of Right Maxillary Sinus, Percutaneous Endoscopic Approach
09TR0ZZ	Resection of Left Maxillary Sinus, Open Approach
09TR4ZZ	Resection of Left Maxillary Sinus, Percutaneous Endoscopic Approach
09TS0ZZ	Resection of Right Frontal Sinus, Open Approach
09TS4ZZ	Resection of Right Frontal Sinus, Percutaneous Endoscopic Approach
09TT0ZZ	Resection of Left Frontal Sinus, Open Approach
09TT4ZZ	Resection of Left Frontal Sinus, Percutaneous Endoscopic Approach
09TU0ZZ	Resection of Right Ethmoid Sinus, Open Approach
09TU4ZZ	Resection of Right Ethmoid Sinus, Percutaneous Endoscopic Approach
09TV0ZZ	Resection of Left Ethmoid Sinus, Open Approach
09TV4ZZ	Resection of Left Ethmoid Sinus, Percutaneous Endoscopic Approach
09TW0ZZ	Resection of Right Sphenoid Sinus, Open Approach
09TW4ZZ	Resection of Right Sphenoid Sinus, Percutaneous Endoscopic Approach
09TX0ZZ	Resection of Left Sphenoid Sinus, Open Approach
09TX4ZZ	Resection of Left Sphenoid Sinus, Percutaneous Endoscopic Approach

09U – Ear, Nose, Sinus, Supplement

09U007Z	Supplement Right External Ear with Autologous Tissue Substitute, Open Approach
09U00JZ	Supplement Right External Ear with Synthetic Substitute, Open Approach
09U00KZ	Supplement Right External Ear with Nonautologous Tissue Substitute, Open Approach
09U0X7Z	Supplement Right External Ear with Autologous Tissue Substitute, External Approach
09U0XJZ	Supplement Right External Ear with Synthetic Substitute, External Approach
09U0XKZ	Supplement Right External Ear with Nonautologous Tissue Substitute, External Approach
09U107Z	Supplement Left External Ear with Autologous Tissue Substitute, Open Approach
09U10JZ	Supplement Left External Ear with Synthetic Substitute, Open Approach
09U10KZ	Supplement Left External Ear with Nonautologous Tissue Substitute, Open Approach
09U1X7Z	Supplement Left External Ear with Autologous Tissue Substitute, External Approach
09U1XJZ	Supplement Left External Ear with Synthetic Substitute, External Approach
09U1XKZ	Supplement Left External Ear with Nonautologous Tissue Substitute, External Approach
09U207Z	Supplement Bilateral External Ear with Autologous Tissue Substitute, Open Approach
09U20JZ	Supplement Bilateral External Ear with Synthetic Substitute, Open Approach
09U20KZ	Supplement Bilateral External Ear with Nonautologous Tissue Substitute, Open Approach
09U2X7Z	Supplement Bilateral External Ear with Autologous Tissue Substitute, External Approach
09U2XJZ	Supplement Bilateral External Ear with Synthetic Substitute, External Approach
09U2XKZ	Supplement Bilateral External Ear with Nonautologous Tissue Substitute, External Approach
09U507Z	Supplement Right Middle Ear with Autologous Tissue Substitute, Open Approach
09U50JZ	Supplement Right Middle Ear with Synthetic Substitute, Open Approach
09U50KZ	Supplement Right Middle Ear with Nonautologous Tissue Substitute, Open Approach
09U607Z	Supplement Left Middle Ear with Autologous Tissue Substitute, Open Approach
09U60JZ	Supplement Left Middle Ear with Synthetic Substitute, Open Approach
09U60KZ	Supplement Left Middle Ear with Nonautologous Tissue Substitute, Open Approach
09U707Z	Supplement Right Tympanic Membrane with Autologous Tissue Substitute, Open Approach
09U70JZ	Supplement Right Tympanic Membrane with Synthetic Substitute, Open Approach
09U70KZ	Supplement Right Tympanic Membrane with Nonautologous Tissue Substitute, Open Approach
09U777Z	Supplement Right Tympanic Membrane with Autologous Tissue Substitute, Via Natural or Artificial Opening
09U77JZ	Supplement Right Tympanic Membrane with Synthetic Substitute, Via Natural or Artificial Opening
09U77KZ	Supplement Right Tympanic Membrane with Nonautologous Tissue Substitute, Via Natural or Artificial Opening
09U787Z	Supplement Right Tympanic Membrane with Autologous Tissue Substitute, Via Natural or Artificial Opening Endoscopic
09U78JZ	Supplement Right Tympanic Membrane with Synthetic Substitute, Via Natural or Artificial Opening Endoscopic
09U78KZ	Supplement Right Tympanic Membrane with Nonautologous Tissue Substitute, Via Natural or Artificial Opening Endoscopic
09U807Z	Supplement Left Tympanic Membrane with Autologous Tissue Substitute, Open Approach
09U80JZ	Supplement Left Tympanic Membrane with Synthetic Substitute, Open Approach
09U80KZ	Supplement Left Tympanic Membrane with Nonautologous Tissue Substitute, Open Approach
09U877Z	Supplement Left Tympanic Membrane with Autologous Tissue Substitute, Via Natural or Artificial Opening
09U87JZ	Supplement Left Tympanic Membrane with Synthetic Substitute, Via Natural or Artificial Opening
09U87KZ	Supplement Left Tympanic Membrane with Nonautologous Tissue Substitute, Via Natural or Artificial Opening
09U887Z	Supplement Left Tympanic Membrane with Autologous Tissue Substitute, Via Natural or Artificial Opening Endoscopic

09U88JZ	Supplement Left Tympanic Membrane with Synthetic Substitute, Via Natural or Artificial Opening Endoscopic
09U88KZ	Supplement Left Tympanic Membrane with Nonautologous Tissue Substitute, Via Natural or Artificial Opening Endoscopic
09U907Z	Supplement Right Auditory Ossicle with Autologous Tissue Substitute, Open Approach
09U90JZ	Supplement Right Auditory Ossicle with Synthetic Substitute, Open Approach
09U90KZ	Supplement Right Auditory Ossicle with Nonautologous Tissue Substitute, Open Approach
09UA07Z	Supplement Left Auditory Ossicle with Autologous Tissue Substitute, Open Approach
09UA0JZ	Supplement Left Auditory Ossicle with Synthetic Substitute, Open Approach
09UA0KZ	Supplement Left Auditory Ossicle with Nonautologous Tissue Substitute, Open Approach
09UD07Z	Supplement Right Inner Ear with Autologous Tissue Substitute, Open Approach
09UD0JZ	Supplement Right Inner Ear with Synthetic Substitute, Open Approach
09UD0KZ	Supplement Right Inner Ear with Nonautologous Tissue Substitute, Open Approach
09UE07Z	Supplement Left Inner Ear with Autologous Tissue Substitute, Open Approach
09UE0JZ	Supplement Left Inner Ear with Synthetic Substitute, Open Approach
09UE0KZ	Supplement Left Inner Ear with Nonautologous Tissue Substitute, Open Approach
09UK07Z	Supplement Nose with Autologous Tissue Substitute, Open Approach
09UK0JZ	Supplement Nose with Synthetic Substitute, Open Approach
09UK0KZ	Supplement Nose with Nonautologous Tissue Substitute, Open Approach
09UKX7Z	Supplement Nose with Autologous Tissue Substitute, External Approach
09UKXJZ	Supplement Nose with Synthetic Substitute, External Approach
09UKXKZ	Supplement Nose with Nonautologous Tissue Substitute, External Approach
09UL07Z	Supplement Nasal Turbinate with Autologous Tissue Substitute, Open Approach
09UL0JZ	Supplement Nasal Turbinate with Synthetic Substitute, Open Approach
09UL0KZ	Supplement Nasal Turbinate with Nonautologous Tissue Substitute, Open Approach
09UL37Z	Supplement Nasal Turbinate with Autologous Tissue Substitute, Percutaneous Approach
09UL3JZ	Supplement Nasal Turbinate with Synthetic Substitute, Percutaneous Approach
09UL3KZ	Supplement Nasal Turbinate with Nonautologous Tissue Substitute, Percutaneous Approach
09UL47Z	Supplement Nasal Turbinate with Autologous Tissue Substitute, Percutaneous Endoscopic Approach
09UL4JZ	Supplement Nasal Turbinate with Synthetic Substitute, Percutaneous Endoscopic Approach
09UL4KZ	Supplement Nasal Turbinate with Nonautologous Tissue Substitute, Percutaneous Endoscopic Approach
09UL77Z	Supplement Nasal Turbinate with Autologous Tissue Substitute, Via Natural or Artificial Opening
09UL7JZ	Supplement Nasal Turbinate with Synthetic Substitute, Via Natural or Artificial Opening
09UL7KZ	Supplement Nasal Turbinate with Nonautologous Tissue Substitute, Via Natural or Artificial Opening
09UL87Z	Supplement Nasal Turbinate with Autologous Tissue Substitute, Via Natural or Artificial Opening Endoscopic
09UL8JZ	Supplement Nasal Turbinate with Synthetic Substitute, Via Natural or Artificial Opening Endoscopic
09UL8KZ	Supplement Nasal Turbinate with Nonautologous Tissue Substitute, Via Natural or Artificial Opening Endoscopic
09UM07Z	Supplement Nasal Septum with Autologous Tissue Substitute, Open Approach
09UM0JZ	Supplement Nasal Septum with Synthetic Substitute, Open Approach
09UM0KZ	Supplement Nasal Septum with Nonautologous Tissue Substitute, Open Approach
09UM37Z	Supplement Nasal Septum with Autologous Tissue Substitute, Percutaneous Approach
09UM3JZ	Supplement Nasal Septum with Synthetic Substitute, Percutaneous Approach
09UM3KZ	Supplement Nasal Septum with Nonautologous Tissue Substitute, Percutaneous Approach
09UM47Z	Supplement Nasal Septum with Autologous Tissue Substitute, Percutaneous Endoscopic Approach
09UM4JZ	Supplement Nasal Septum with Synthetic Substitute, Percutaneous Endoscopic Approach
09UM4KZ	Supplement Nasal Septum with Nonautologous Tissue Substitute, Percutaneous Endoscopic Approach
09UN07Z	Supplement Nasopharynx with Autologous Tissue Substitute, Open Approach
09UN0JZ	Supplement Nasopharynx with Synthetic Substitute, Open Approach
09UN0KZ	Supplement Nasopharynx with Nonautologous Tissue Substitute, Open Approach
09UN77Z	Supplement Nasopharynx with Autologous Tissue Substitute, Via Natural or Artificial Opening
09UN7JZ	Supplement Nasopharynx with Synthetic Substitute, Via Natural or Artificial Opening
09UN7KZ	Supplement Nasopharynx with Nonautologous Tissue Substitute, Via Natural or Artificial Opening
09UN87Z	Supplement Nasopharynx with Autologous Tissue Substitute, Via Natural or Artificial Opening Endoscopic
09UN8JZ	Supplement Nasopharynx with Synthetic Substitute, Via Natural or Artificial Opening Endoscopic
09UN8KZ	Supplement Nasopharynx with Nonautologous Tissue Substitute, Via Natural or Artificial Opening Endoscopic

09W – Ear, Nose, Sinus, Revision

Review Coding Guideline B6.1c

09W707Z	Revision of Autologous Tissue Substitute in Right Tympanic Membrane, Open Approach
09W70JZ	Revision of Synthetic Substitute in Right Tympanic Membrane, Open Approach
09W70KZ	Revision of Nonautologous Tissue Substitute in Right Tympanic Membrane, Open Approach
09W777Z	Revision of Autologous Tissue Substitute in Right Tympanic Membrane, Via Natural or Artificial Opening
09W77JZ	Revision of Synthetic Substitute in Right Tympanic Membrane, Via Natural or Artificial Opening
09W77KZ	Revision of Nonautologous Tissue Substitute in Right Tympanic Membrane, Via Natural or Artificial Opening
09W787Z	Revision of Autologous Tissue Substitute in Right Tympanic Membrane, Via Natural or Artificial Opening Endoscopic
09W78JZ	Revision of Synthetic Substitute in Right Tympanic Membrane, Via Natural or Artificial Opening Endoscopic
09W78KZ	Revision of Nonautologous Tissue Substitute in Right Tympanic Membrane, Via Natural or Artificial Opening Endoscopic
09W807Z	Revision of Autologous Tissue Substitute in Left Tympanic Membrane, Open Approach
09W80JZ	Revision of Synthetic Substitute in Left Tympanic Membrane, Open Approach
09W80KZ	Revision of Nonautologous Tissue Substitute in Left Tympanic Membrane, Open Approach
09W877Z	Revision of Autologous Tissue Substitute in Left Tympanic Membrane, Via Natural or Artificial Opening
09W87JZ	Revision of Synthetic Substitute in Left Tympanic Membrane, Via Natural or Artificial Opening
09W87KZ	Revision of Nonautologous Tissue Substitute in Left Tympanic Membrane, Via Natural or Artificial Opening
09W887Z	Revision of Autologous Tissue Substitute in Left Tympanic Membrane, Via Natural or Artificial Opening Endoscopic

09W88JZ Revision of Synthetic Substitute in Left Tympanic Membrane, Via Natural or Artificial Opening Endoscopic

09W88KZ Revision of Nonautologous Tissue Substitute in Left Tympanic Membrane, Via Natural or Artificial Opening Endoscopic

09W907Z Revision of Autologous Tissue Substitute in Right Auditory Ossicle, Open Approach

09W90JZ Revision of Synthetic Substitute in Right Auditory Ossicle, Open Approach

09W90KZ Revision of Nonautologous Tissue Substitute in Right Auditory Ossicle, Open Approach

09W977Z Revision of Autologous Tissue Substitute in Right Auditory Ossicle, Via Natural or Artificial Opening

09W97JZ Revision of Synthetic Substitute in Right Auditory Ossicle, Via Natural or Artificial Opening

09W97KZ Revision of Nonautologous Tissue Substitute in Right Auditory Ossicle, Via Natural or Artificial Opening

09W987Z Revision of Autologous Tissue Substitute in Right Auditory Ossicle, Via Natural or Artificial Opening Endoscopic

09W98JZ Revision of Synthetic Substitute in Right Auditory Ossicle, Via Natural or Artificial Opening Endoscopic

09W98KZ Revision of Nonautologous Tissue Substitute in Right Auditory Ossicle, Via Natural or Artificial Opening Endoscopic

09WA07Z Revision of Autologous Tissue Substitute in Left Auditory Ossicle, Open Approach

09WA0JZ Revision of Synthetic Substitute in Left Auditory Ossicle, Open Approach

09WA0KZ Revision of Nonautologous Tissue Substitute in Left Auditory Ossicle, Open Approach

09WA77Z Revision of Autologous Tissue Substitute in Left Auditory Ossicle, Via Natural or Artificial Opening

09WA7JZ Revision of Synthetic Substitute in Left Auditory Ossicle, Via Natural or Artificial Opening

09WA7KZ Revision of Nonautologous Tissue Substitute in Left Auditory Ossicle, Via Natural or Artificial Opening

09WA87Z Revision of Autologous Tissue Substitute in Left Auditory Ossicle, Via Natural or Artificial Opening Endoscopic

09WA8JZ Revision of Synthetic Substitute in Left Auditory Ossicle, Via Natural or Artificial Opening Endoscopic

09WA8KZ Revision of Nonautologous Tissue Substitute in Left Auditory Ossicle, Via Natural or Artificial Opening Endoscopic

09WD0SZ Revision of Hearing Device in Right Inner Ear, Open Approach

09WD7SZ Revision of Hearing Device in Right Inner Ear, Via Natural or Artificial Opening

09WD8SZ Revision of Hearing Device in Right Inner Ear, Via Natural or Artificial Opening Endoscopic

09WE0SZ Revision of Hearing Device in Left Inner Ear, Open Approach

09WE7SZ Revision of Hearing Device in Left Inner Ear, Via Natural or Artificial Opening

09WE8SZ Revision of Hearing Device in Left Inner Ear, Via Natural or Artificial Opening Endoscopic

09WH00Z Revision of Drainage Device in Right Ear, Open Approach

09WH07Z Revision of Autologous Tissue Substitute in Right Ear, Open Approach

09WH0DZ Revision of Intraluminal Device in Right Ear, Open Approach

09WH0JZ Revision of Synthetic Substitute in Right Ear, Open Approach

09WH0KZ Revision of Nonautologous Tissue Substitute in Right Ear, Open Approach

09WH30Z Revision of Drainage Device in Right Ear, Percutaneous Approach

09WH37Z Revision of Autologous Tissue Substitute in Right Ear, Percutaneous Approach

09WH3DZ Revision of Intraluminal Device in Right Ear, Percutaneous Approach

09WH3JZ Revision of Synthetic Substitute in Right Ear, Percutaneous Approach

09WH3KZ Revision of Nonautologous Tissue Substitute in Right Ear, Percutaneous Approach

09WH40Z Revision of Drainage Device in Right Ear, Percutaneous Endoscopic Approach

09WH47Z Revision of Autologous Tissue Substitute in Right Ear, Percutaneous Endoscopic Approach

09WH4DZ Revision of Intraluminal Device in Right Ear, Percutaneous Endoscopic Approach

09WH4JZ Revision of Synthetic Substitute in Right Ear, Percutaneous Endoscopic Approach

09WH4KZ Revision of Nonautologous Tissue Substitute in Right Ear, Percutaneous Endoscopic Approach

09WH70Z Revision of Drainage Device in Right Ear, Via Natural or Artificial Opening

09WH77Z Revision of Autologous Tissue Substitute in Right Ear, Via Natural or Artificial Opening

09WH7DZ Revision of Intraluminal Device in Right Ear, Via Natural or Artificial Opening

09WH7JZ Revision of Synthetic Substitute in Right Ear, Via Natural or Artificial Opening

09WH7KZ Revision of Nonautologous Tissue Substitute in Right Ear, Via Natural or Artificial Opening

09WH80Z Revision of Drainage Device in Right Ear, Via Natural or Artificial Opening Endoscopic

09WH87Z Revision of Autologous Tissue Substitute in Right Ear, Via Natural or Artificial Opening Endoscopic

09WH8DZ Revision of Intraluminal Device in Right Ear, Via Natural or Artificial Opening Endoscopic

09WH8JZ Revision of Synthetic Substitute in Right Ear, Via Natural or Artificial Opening Endoscopic

09WH8KZ Revision of Nonautologous Tissue Substitute in Right Ear, Via Natural or Artificial Opening Endoscopic

09WHX0Z Revision of Drainage Device in Right Ear, External Approach

09WHX7Z Revision of Autologous Tissue Substitute in Right Ear, External Approach

09WHXDZ Revision of Intraluminal Device in Right Ear, External Approach

09WHXJZ Revision of Synthetic Substitute in Right Ear, External Approach

09WHXKZ Revision of Nonautologous Tissue Substitute in Right Ear, External Approach

09WJ00Z Revision of Drainage Device in Left Ear, Open Approach

09WJ07Z Revision of Autologous Tissue Substitute in Left Ear, Open Approach

09WJ0DZ Revision of Intraluminal Device in Left Ear, Open Approach

09WJ0JZ Revision of Synthetic Substitute in Left Ear, Open Approach

09WJ0KZ Revision of Nonautologous Tissue Substitute in Left Ear, Open Approach

09WJ30Z Revision of Drainage Device in Left Ear, Percutaneous Approach

09WJ37Z Revision of Autologous Tissue Substitute in Left Ear, Percutaneous Approach

09WJ3DZ Revision of Intraluminal Device in Left Ear, Percutaneous Approach

09WJ3JZ Revision of Synthetic Substitute in Left Ear, Percutaneous Approach

09WJ3KZ Revision of Nonautologous Tissue Substitute in Left Ear, Percutaneous Approach

09WJ40Z Revision of Drainage Device in Left Ear, Percutaneous Endoscopic Approach

09WJ47Z Revision of Autologous Tissue Substitute in Left Ear, Percutaneous Endoscopic Approach

09WJ4DZ Revision of Intraluminal Device in Left Ear, Percutaneous Endoscopic Approach

09WJ4JZ Revision of Synthetic Substitute in Left Ear, Percutaneous Endoscopic Approach

09WJ4KZ Revision of Nonautologous Tissue Substitute in Left Ear, Percutaneous Endoscopic Approach

09WJ70Z Revision of Drainage Device in Left Ear, Via Natural or Artificial Opening

09WJ77Z Revision of Autologous Tissue Substitute in Left Ear, Via Natural or Artificial Opening

09WJ7DZ Revision of Intraluminal Device in Left Ear, Via Natural or Artificial Opening

09WJ7JZ Revision of Synthetic Substitute in Left Ear, Via Natural or Artificial Opening

09WJ7KZ Revision of Nonautologous Tissue Substitute in Left Ear, Via Natural or Artificial Opening

09WJ80Z Revision of Drainage Device in Left Ear, Via Natural or Artificial Opening Endoscopic

09WJ87Z Revision of Autologous Tissue Substitute in Left Ear, Via Natural or Artificial Opening Endoscopic

09WJ8DZ Revision of Intraluminal Device in Left Ear, Via Natural or Artificial Opening Endoscopic

09WJ8JZ Revision of Synthetic Substitute in Left Ear, Via Natural or Artificial Opening Endoscopic

09WJ8KZ Revision of Nonautologous Tissue Substitute in Left Ear, Via Natural or Artificial Opening Endoscopic

09WJX0Z Revision of Drainage Device in Left Ear, External Approach

09WJX7Z Revision of Autologous Tissue Substitute in Left Ear, External Approach

09WJXDZ Revision of Intraluminal Device in Left Ear, External Approach

09WJXJZ Revision of Synthetic Substitute in Left Ear, External Approach

09WJXKZ Revision of Nonautologous Tissue Substitute in Left Ear, External Approach

09WK00Z Revision of Drainage Device in Nose, Open Approach

09WK07Z Revision of Autologous Tissue Substitute in Nose, Open Approach

09WK0DZ Revision of Intraluminal Device in Nose, Open Approach

09WK0JZ Revision of Synthetic Substitute in Nose, Open Approach

09WK0KZ Revision of Nonautologous Tissue Substitute in Nose, Open Approach

09WK30Z Revision of Drainage Device in Nose, Percutaneous Approach

09WK37Z Revision of Autologous Tissue Substitute in Nose, Percutaneous Approach

09WK3DZ Revision of Intraluminal Device in Nose, Percutaneous Approach

09WK3JZ Revision of Synthetic Substitute in Nose, Percutaneous Approach

09WK3KZ Revision of Nonautologous Tissue Substitute in Nose, Percutaneous Approach

09WK40Z Revision of Drainage Device in Nose, Percutaneous Endoscopic Approach

09WK47Z Revision of Autologous Tissue Substitute in Nose, Percutaneous Endoscopic Approach

09WK4DZ Revision of Intraluminal Device in Nose, Percutaneous Endoscopic Approach

09WK4JZ Revision of Synthetic Substitute in Nose, Percutaneous Endoscopic Approach

09WK4KZ Revision of Nonautologous Tissue Substitute in Nose, Percutaneous Endoscopic Approach

09WK70Z Revision of Drainage Device in Nose, Via Natural or Artificial Opening

09WK77Z Revision of Autologous Tissue Substitute in Nose, Via Natural or Artificial Opening

09WK7DZ Revision of Intraluminal Device in Nose, Via Natural or Artificial Opening

09WK7JZ Revision of Synthetic Substitute in Nose, Via Natural or Artificial Opening

09WK7KZ Revision of Nonautologous Tissue Substitute in Nose, Via Natural or Artificial Opening

09WK80Z Revision of Drainage Device in Nose, Via Natural or Artificial Opening Endoscopic

09WK87Z Revision of Autologous Tissue Substitute in Nose, Via Natural or Artificial Opening Endoscopic

09WK8DZ Revision of Intraluminal Device in Nose, Via Natural or Artificial Opening Endoscopic

09WK8JZ Revision of Synthetic Substitute in Nose, Via Natural or Artificial Opening Endoscopic

09WK8KZ Revision of Nonautologous Tissue Substitute in Nose, Via Natural or Artificial Opening Endoscopic

09WKX0Z Revision of Drainage Device in Nose, External Approach

09WKX7Z Revision of Autologous Tissue Substitute in Nose, External Approach

09WKXDZ Revision of Intraluminal Device in Nose, External Approach

09WKXJZ Revision of Synthetic Substitute in Nose, External Approach

09WKXKZ Revision of Nonautologous Tissue Substitute in Nose, External Approach

09WY00Z Revision of Drainage Device in Sinus, Open Approach

09WY30Z Revision of Drainage Device in Sinus, Percutaneous Approach

09WY40Z Revision of Drainage Device in Sinus, Percutaneous Endoscopic Approach

09WYX0Z Revision of Drainage Device in Sinus, External Approach

Respiratory System

Lungs

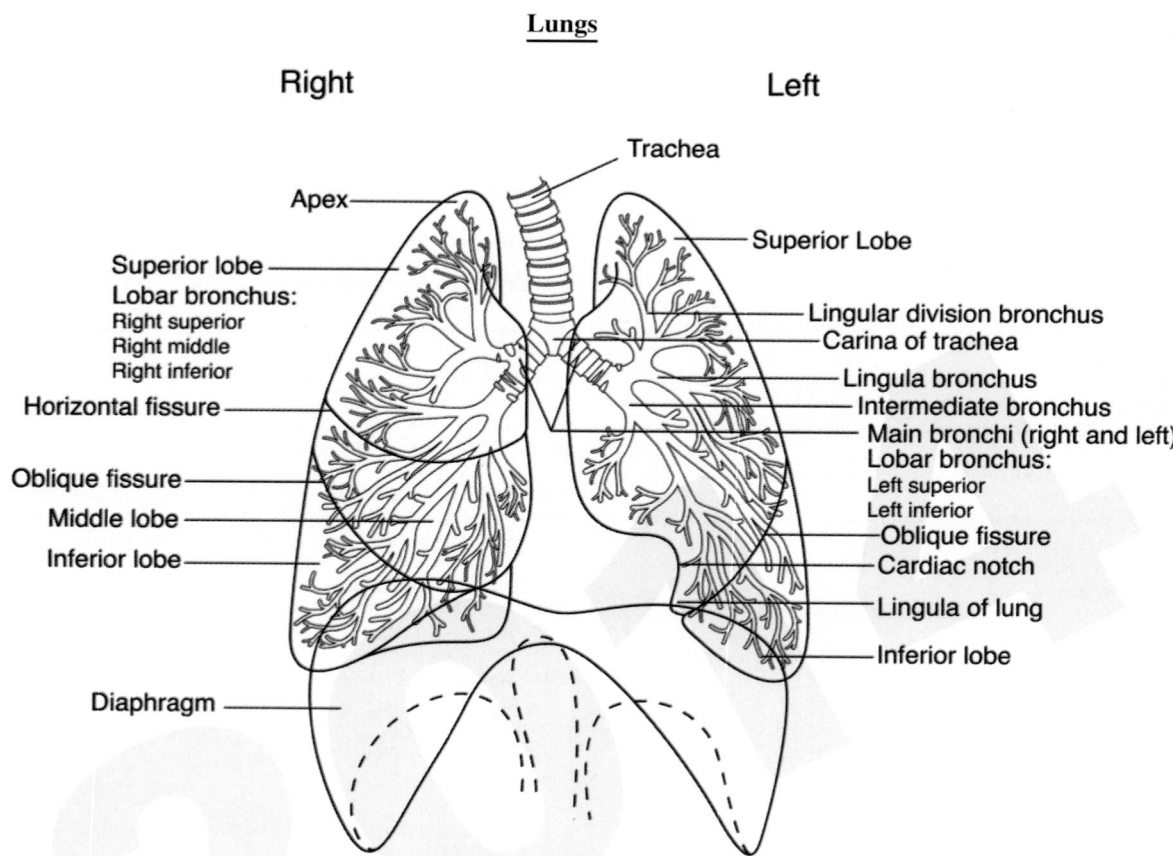

Respiratory System Tables 0B1–0BY

Section	0	Medical and Surgical
Body System	B	Respiratory System
Operation	1	**Bypass:** Altering the route of passage of the contents of a tubular body part

Body Part (4th)	Approach (5th)	Device (6th)	Qualifier (7th)
1 Trachea	0 Open	D Intraluminal Device	6 Esophagus
1 Trachea	0 Open	F Tracheostomy Device Z No Device	4 Cutaneous
1 Trachea	3 Percutaneous 4 Percutaneous Endoscopic	F Tracheostomy Device Z No Device	4 Cutaneous

Section	0	Medical and Surgical
Body System	B	Respiratory System
Operation	2	**Change:** Taking out or off a device from a body part and putting back an identical or similar device in or on the same body part without cutting or puncturing the skin or a mucous membrane

Body Part (4th)	Approach (5th)	Device (6th)	Qualifier (7th)
0 Tracheobronchial Tree K Lung, Right L Lung, Left Q Pleura T Diaphragm	X External	0 Drainage Device Y Other Device	Z No Qualifier
1 Trachea	X External	0 Drainage Device E Intraluminal Device, Endotracheal Airway F Tracheostomy Device Y Other Device	Z No Qualifier

Section	0	Medical and Surgical
Body System	B	Respiratory System
Operation	5	**Destruction:** Physical eradication of all or a portion of a body part by the direct use of energy, force, or a destructive agent

Body Part (4th)	Approach (5th)	Device (6th)	Qualifier (7th)
1 Trachea 2 Carina 3 Main Bronchus, Right 4 Upper Lobe Bronchus, Right 5 Middle Lobe Bronchus, Right 6 Lower Lobe Bronchus, Right 7 Main Bronchus, Left 8 Upper Lobe Bronchus, Left 9 Lingula Bronchus B Lower Lobe Bronchus, Left C Upper Lung Lobe, Right D Middle Lung Lobe, Right F Lower Lung Lobe, Right G Upper Lung Lobe, Left H Lung Lingula J Lower Lung Lobe, Left K Lung, Right L Lung, Left M Lungs, Bilateral	0 Open 3 Percutaneous 4 Percutaneous Endoscopic 7 Via Natural or Artificial Opening 8 Via Natural or Artificial Opening Endoscopic	Z No Device	Z No Qualifier
N Pleura, Right P Pleura, Left R Diaphragm, Right S Diaphragm, Left	0 Open 3 Percutaneous 4 Percutaneous Endoscopic	Z No Device	Z No Qualifier

Section	0	Medical and Surgical
Body System	B	Respiratory System
Operation	7	**Dilation:** Expanding an orifice or the lumen of a tubular body part

Body Part (4ᵗʰ)	Approach (5ᵗʰ)	Device (6ᵗʰ)	Qualifier (7ᵗʰ)
1 Trachea 2 Carina 3 Main Bronchus, Right 4 Upper Lobe Bronchus, Right 5 Middle Lobe Bronchus, Right 6 Lower Lobe Bronchus, Right 7 Main Bronchus, Left 8 Upper Lobe Bronchus, Left 9 Lingula Bronchus B Lower Lobe Bronchus, Left	0 Open 3 Percutaneous 4 Percutaneous Endoscopic 7 Via Natural or Artificial Opening 8 Via Natural or Artificial Opening Endoscopic	D Intraluminal Device Z No Device	Z No Qualifier

Section	0	Medical and Surgical
Body System	B	Respiratory System
Operation	9	**Drainage:** Taking or letting out fluids and/or gases from a body part

Body Part (4ᵗʰ)	Approach (5ᵗʰ)	Device (6ᵗʰ)	Qualifier (7ᵗʰ)
1 Trachea 2 Carina 3 Main Bronchus, Right 4 Upper Lobe Bronchus, Right 5 Middle Lobe Bronchus, Right 6 Lower Lobe Bronchus, Right 7 Main Bronchus, Left 8 Upper Lobe Bronchus, Left 9 Lingula Bronchus B Lower Lobe Bronchus, Left C Upper Lung Lobe, Right D Middle Lung Lobe, Right F Lower Lung Lobe, Right G Upper Lung Lobe, Left H Lung Lingula J Lower Lung Lobe, Left K Lung, Right L Lung, Left M Lungs, Bilateral	0 Open 3 Percutaneous 4 Percutaneous Endoscopic 7 Via Natural or Artificial Opening 8 Via Natural or Artificial Opening Endoscopic	0 Drainage Device	Z No Qualifier
1 Trachea 2 Carina 3 Main Bronchus, Right 4 Upper Lobe Bronchus, Right 5 Middle Lobe Bronchus, Right 6 Lower Lobe Bronchus, Right 7 Main Bronchus, Left 8 Upper Lobe Bronchus, Left 9 Lingula Bronchus B Lower Lobe Bronchus, Left C Upper Lung Lobe, Right D Middle Lung Lobe, Right F Lower Lung Lobe, Right G Upper Lung Lobe, Left H Lung Lingula J Lower Lung Lobe, Left K Lung, Right L Lung, Left M Lungs, Bilateral	0 Open 3 Percutaneous 4 Percutaneous Endoscopic 7 Via Natural or Artificial Opening 8 Via Natural or Artificial Opening Endoscopic	Z No Device	X Diagnostic Z No Qualifier

Continued

Section	0	Medical and Surgical
Body System	B	Respiratory System
Operation	9	Drainage: Taking or letting out fluids and/or gases from a body part

Body Part (4th)	Approach (5th)	Device (6th)	Qualifier (7th)
N Pleura, Right P Pleura, Left R Diaphragm, Right S Diaphragm, Left	0 Open 3 Percutaneous 4 Percutaneous Endoscopic	0 Drainage Device	Z No Qualifier
N Pleura, Right P Pleura, Left R Diaphragm, Right S Diaphragm, Left	0 Open 3 Percutaneous 4 Percutaneous Endoscopic	Z No Device	X Diagnostic Z No Qualifier

Section	0	Medical and Surgical
Body System	B	Respiratory System
Operation	B	Excision: Cutting out or off, without replacement, a portion of a body part

Body Part (4th)	Approach (5th)	Device (6th)	Qualifier (7th)
1 Trachea 2 Carina 3 Main Bronchus, Right 4 Upper Lobe Bronchus, Right 5 Middle Lobe Bronchus, Right 6 Lower Lobe Bronchus, Right 7 Main Bronchus, Left 8 Upper Lobe Bronchus, Left 9 Lingula Bronchus B Lower Lobe Bronchus, Left C Upper Lung Lobe, Right D Middle Lung Lobe, Right F Lower Lung Lobe, Right G Upper Lung Lobe, Left H Lung Lingula J Lower Lung Lobe, Left K Lung, Right L Lung, Left M Lungs, Bilateral	0 Open 3 Percutaneous 4 Percutaneous Endoscopic 7 Via Natural or Artificial Opening 8 Via Natural or Artificial Opening Endoscopic	Z No Device	X Diagnostic Z No Qualifier
N Pleura, Right P Pleura, Left R Diaphragm, Right S Diaphragm, Left	0 Open 3 Percutaneous 4 Percutaneous Endoscopic	Z No Device	X Diagnostic Z No Qualifier

Section	0	Medical and Surgical
Body System	B	Respiratory System
Operation	C	**Extirpation:** Taking or cutting out solid matter from a body part

Body Part (4th)	Approach (5th)	Device (6th)	Qualifier (7th)
1 Trachea 2 Carina 3 Main Bronchus, Right 4 Upper Lobe Bronchus, Right 5 Middle Lobe Bronchus, Right 6 Lower Lobe Bronchus, Right 7 Main Bronchus, Left 8 Upper Lobe Bronchus, Left 9 Lingula Bronchus B Lower Lobe Bronchus, Left C Upper Lung Lobe, Right D Middle Lung Lobe, Right F Lower Lung Lobe, Right G Upper Lung Lobe, Left H Lung Lingula J Lower Lung Lobe, Left K Lung, Right L Lung, Left M Lungs, Bilateral	0 Open 3 Percutaneous 4 Percutaneous Endoscopic 7 Via Natural or Artificial Opening 8 Via Natural or Artificial Opening Endoscopic	Z No Device	Z No Qualifier
N Pleura, Right P Pleura, Left R Diaphragm, Right S Diaphragm, Left	0 Open 3 Percutaneous 4 Percutaneous Endoscopic	Z No Device	Z No Qualifier

Section	0	Medical and Surgical
Body System	B	Respiratory System
Operation	D	**Extraction:** Pulling or stripping out or off all or a portion of a body part by the use of force

Body Part (4th)	Approach (5th)	Device (6th)	Qualifier (7th)
N Pleura, Right P Pleura, Left	0 Open 3 Percutaneous 4 Percutaneous Endoscopic	Z No Device	X Diagnostic Z No Qualifier

Section	0	Medical and Surgical
Body System	B	Respiratory System
Operation	F	**Fragmentation:** Breaking solid matter in a body part into pieces

Body Part (4th)	Approach (5th)	Device (6th)	Qualifier (7th)
1 Trachea 2 Carina 3 Main Bronchus, Right 4 Upper Lobe Bronchus, Right 5 Middle Lobe Bronchus, Right 6 Lower Lobe Bronchus, Right 7 Main Bronchus, Left 8 Upper Lobe Bronchus, Left 9 Lingula Bronchus B Lower Lobe Bronchus, Left	0 Open 3 Percutaneous 4 Percutaneous Endoscopic 7 Via Natural or Artificial Opening 8 Via Natural or Artificial Opening Endoscopic X External	Z No Device	Z No Qualifier

Section   0   **Medical and Surgical**
Body System   B   **Respiratory System**
Operation   H   **Insertion:** Putting in a nonbiological appliance that monitors, assists, performs, or prevents a physiological function but does not physically take the place of a body part

Body Part (4th)	Approach (5th)	Device (6th)	Qualifier (7th)
0 Tracheobronchial Tree	0 Open 3 Percutaneous 4 Percutaneous Endoscopic 7 Via Natural or Artificial Opening 8 Via Natural or Artificial Opening Endoscopic	1 Radioactive Element 2 Monitoring Device 3 Infusion Device D Intraluminal Device	Z No Qualifier
1 Trachea	0 Open	2 Monitoring Device D Intraluminal Device	Z No Qualifier
1 Trachea	3 Percutaneous	D Intraluminal Device E Intraluminal Device, Endotracheal Airway	Z No Qualifier
1 Trachea	4 Percutaneous Endoscopic	D Intraluminal Device	Z No Qualifier
1 Trachea	7 Via Natural or Artificial Opening 8 Via Natural or Artificial Opening Endoscopic	2 Monitoring Device D Intraluminal Device E Intraluminal Device, Endotracheal Airway	Z No Qualifier
3 Main Bronchus, Right 4 Upper Lobe Bronchus, Right 5 Middle Lobe Bronchus, Right 6 Lower Lobe Bronchus, Right 7 Main Bronchus, Left 8 Upper Lobe Bronchus, Left 9 Lingula Bronchus B Lower Lobe Bronchus, Left	0 Open 3 Percutaneous 4 Percutaneous Endoscopic 7 Via Natural or Artificial Opening 8 Via Natural or Artificial Opening Endoscopic	G Intraluminal Device, Endobronchial Valve	Z No Qualifier
K Lung, Right L Lung, Left	0 Open 3 Percutaneous 4 Percutaneous Endoscopic 7 Via Natural or Artificial Opening 8 Via Natural or Artificial Opening Endoscopic	1 Radioactive Element 2 Monitoring Device 3 Infusion Device	Z No Qualifier
R Diaphragm, Right S Diaphragm, Left	0 Open 3 Percutaneous 4 Percutaneous Endoscopic	2 Monitoring Device M Diaphragmatic Pacemaker Lead	Z No Qualifier

Section   0   **Medical and Surgical**
Body System   B   **Respiratory System**
Operation   J   **Inspection:** Visually and/or manually exploring a body part

Body Part (4th)	Approach (5th)	Device (6th)	Qualifier (7th)
0 Tracheobronchial Tree 1 Trachea K Lung, Right L Lung, Left Q Pleura T Diaphragm	0 Open 3 Percutaneous 4 Percutaneous Endoscopic 7 Via Natural or Artificial Opening 8 Via Natural or Artificial Opening Endoscopic X External	Z No Device	Z No Qualifier

Section	0	Medical and Surgical
Body System	B	Respiratory System
Operation	L	Occlusion: Completely closing an orifice or the lumen of a tubular body part

Body Part (4th)	Approach (5th)	Device (6th)	Qualifier (7th)
1 Trachea 2 Carina 3 Main Bronchus, Right 4 Upper Lobe Bronchus, Right 5 Middle Lobe Bronchus, Right 6 Lower Lobe Bronchus, Right 7 Main Bronchus, Left 8 Upper Lobe Bronchus, Left 9 Lingula Bronchus B Lower Lobe Bronchus, Left	0 Open 3 Percutaneous 4 Percutaneous Endoscopic	C Extraluminal Device D Intraluminal Device Z No Device	Z No Qualifier
1 Trachea 2 Carina 3 Main Bronchus, Right 4 Upper Lobe Bronchus, Right 5 Middle Lobe Bronchus, Right 6 Lower Lobe Bronchus, Right 7 Main Bronchus, Left 8 Upper Lobe Bronchus, Left 9 Lingula Bronchus B Lower Lobe Bronchus, Left	7 Via Natural or Artificial Opening 8 Via Natural or Artificial Opening Endoscopic	D Intraluminal Device Z No Device	Z No Qualifier

Section	0	Medical and Surgical
Body System	B	Respiratory System
Operation	M	Reattachment: Putting back in or on all or a portion of a separated body part to its normal location or other suitable location

Body Part (4th)	Approach (5th)	Device (6th)	Qualifier (7th)
1 Trachea 2 Carina 3 Main Bronchus, Right 4 Upper Lobe Bronchus, Right 5 Middle Lobe Bronchus, Right 6 Lower Lobe Bronchus, Right 7 Main Bronchus, Left 8 Upper Lobe Bronchus, Left 9 Lingula Bronchus B Lower Lobe Bronchus, Left C Upper Lung Lobe, Right D Middle Lung Lobe, Right F Lower Lung Lobe, Right G Upper Lung Lobe, Left H Lung Lingula J Lower Lung Lobe, Left K Lung, Right L Lung, Left R Diaphragm, Right S Diaphragm, Left	0 Open	Z No Device	Z No Qualifier

Section   0   **Medical and Surgical**
Body System   B   **Respiratory System**
Operation   N   **Release:** Freeing a body part from an abnormal physical constraint by cutting or by the use of force

Body Part (4ᵗʰ)	Approach (5ᵗʰ)	Device (6ᵗʰ)	Qualifier (7ᵗʰ)
1 Trachea 2 Carina 3 Main Bronchus, Right 4 Upper Lobe Bronchus, Right 5 Middle Lobe Bronchus, Right 6 Lower Lobe Bronchus, Right 7 Main Bronchus, Left 8 Upper Lobe Bronchus, Left 9 Lingula Bronchus B Lower Lobe Bronchus, Left C Upper Lung Lobe, Right D Middle Lung Lobe, Right F Lower Lung Lobe, Right G Upper Lung Lobe, Left H Lung Lingula J Lower Lung Lobe, Left K Lung, Right L Lung, Left M Lungs, Bilateral	0 Open 3 Percutaneous 4 Percutaneous Endoscopic 7 Via Natural or Artificial Opening 8 Via Natural or Artificial Opening Endoscopic	Z No Device	Z No Qualifier
N Pleura, Right P Pleura, Left R Diaphragm, Right S Diaphragm, Left	0 Open 3 Percutaneous 4 Percutaneous Endoscopic	Z No Device	Z No Qualifier

Section   0   **Medical and Surgical**
Body System   B   **Respiratory System**
Operation   P   **Removal:** Taking out or off a device from a body part

Body Part (4ᵗʰ)	Approach (5ᵗʰ)	Device (6ᵗʰ)	Qualifier (7ᵗʰ)
0 Tracheobronchial Tree	0 Open 3 Percutaneous 4 Percutaneous Endoscopic 7 Via Natural or Artificial Opening 8 Via Natural or Artificial Opening Endoscopic	0 Drainage Device 1 Radioactive Element 2 Monitoring Device 3 Infusion Device 7 Autologous Tissue Substitute C Extraluminal Device D Intraluminal Device J Synthetic Substitute K Nonautologous Tissue Substitute	Z No Qualifier
0 Tracheobronchial Tree	X External	0 Drainage Device 1 Radioactive Element 2 Monitoring Device 3 Infusion Device D Intraluminal Device	Z No Qualifier
1 Trachea	0 Open 3 Percutaneous 4 Percutaneous Endoscopic 7 Via Natural or Artificial Opening 8 Via Natural or Artificial Opening Endoscopic	0 Drainage Device 2 Monitoring Device 7 Autologous Tissue Substitute C Extraluminal Device D Intraluminal Device F Tracheostomy Device J Synthetic Substitute K Nonautologous Tissue Substitute	Z No Qualifier

Continued

Section	0	Medical and Surgical
Body System	B	Respiratory System
Operation	P	Removal: Taking out or off a device from a body part

0BP Continued

Body Part (4th)	Approach (5th)	Device (6th)	Qualifier (7th)
1 Trachea	X External	0 Drainage Device 2 Monitoring Device D Intraluminal Device F Tracheostomy Device	Z No Qualifier
K Lung, Right L Lung, Left	0 Open 3 Percutaneous 4 Percutaneous Endoscopic 7 Via Natural or Artificial Opening 8 Via Natural or Artificial Opening Endoscopic X External	0 Drainage Device 1 Radioactive Element 2 Monitoring Device 3 Infusion Device	Z No Qualifier
Q Pleura	0 Open 3 Percutaneous 4 Percutaneous Endoscopic 7 Via Natural or Artificial Opening 8 Via Natural or Artificial Opening Endoscopic X External	0 Drainage Device 1 Radioactive Element 2 Monitoring Device	Z No Qualifier
T Diaphragm	0 Open 3 Percutaneous 4 Percutaneous Endoscopic 7 Via Natural or Artificial Opening 8 Via Natural or Artificial Opening Endoscopic	0 Drainage Device 2 Monitoring Device 7 Autologous Tissue Substitute J Synthetic Substitute K Nonautologous Tissue Substitute M Diaphragmatic Pacemaker Lead	Z No Qualifier
T Diaphragm	X External	0 Drainage Device 2 Monitoring Device M Diaphragmatic Pacemaker Lead	Z No Qualifier

Section	0	Medical and Surgical
Body System	B	Respiratory System
Operation	Q	Repair: Restoring, to the extent possible, a body part to its normal anatomic structure and function

Body Part (4th)	Approach (5th)	Device (6th)	Qualifier (7th)
1 Trachea 2 Carina 3 Main Bronchus, Right 4 Upper Lobe Bronchus, Right 5 Middle Lobe Bronchus, Right 6 Lower Lobe Bronchus, Right 7 Main Bronchus, Left 8 Upper Lobe Bronchus, Left 9 Lingula Bronchus B Lower Lobe Bronchus, Left C Upper Lung Lobe, Right D Middle Lung Lobe, Right F Lower Lung Lobe, Right G Upper Lung Lobe, Left H Lung Lingula J Lower Lung Lobe, Left K Lung, Right L Lung, Left M Lungs, Bilateral	0 Open 3 Percutaneous 4 Percutaneous Endoscopic 7 Via Natural or Artificial Opening 8 Via Natural or Artificial Opening Endoscopic	Z No Device	Z No Qualifier
N Pleura, Right P Pleura, Left R Diaphragm, Right S Diaphragm, Left	0 Open 3 Percutaneous 4 Percutaneous Endoscopic	Z No Device	Z No Qualifier

Section	0	Medical and Surgical
Body System	B	Respiratory System
Operation	S	**Reposition:** Moving to its normal location, or other suitable location, all or a portion of a body part

Body Part (4th)	Approach (5th)	Device (6th)	Qualifier (7th)
1 Trachea 2 Carina 3 Main Bronchus, Right 4 Upper Lobe Bronchus, Right 5 Middle Lobe Bronchus, Right 6 Lower Lobe Bronchus, Right 7 Main Bronchus, Left 8 Upper Lobe Bronchus, Left 9 Lingula Bronchus B Lower Lobe Bronchus, Left C Upper Lung Lobe, Right D Middle Lung Lobe, Right F Lower Lung Lobe, Right G Upper Lung Lobe, Left H Lung Lingula J Lower Lung Lobe, Left K Lung, Right L Lung, Left R Diaphragm, Right S Diaphragm, Left	0 Open	Z No Device	Z No Qualifier

Section	0	Medical and Surgical
Body System	B	Respiratory System
Operation	T	**Resection:** Cutting out or off, without replacement, all of a body part

Body Part (4th)	Approach (5th)	Device (6th)	Qualifier (7th)
1 Trachea 2 Carina 3 Main Bronchus, Right 4 Upper Lobe Bronchus, Right 5 Middle Lobe Bronchus, Right 6 Lower Lobe Bronchus, Right 7 Main Bronchus, Left 8 Upper Lobe Bronchus, Left 9 Lingula Bronchus B Lower Lobe Bronchus, Left C Upper Lung Lobe, Right D Middle Lung Lobe, Right F Lower Lung Lobe, Right G Upper Lung Lobe, Left H Lung Lingula J Lower Lung Lobe, Left K Lung, Right L Lung, Left M Lungs, Bilateral R Diaphragm, Right S Diaphragm, Left	0 Open 4 Percutaneous Endoscopic	Z No Device	Z No Qualifier

Section	0	Medical and Surgical
Body System	B	Respiratory System
Operation	U	**Supplement:** Putting in or on biological or synthetic material that physically reinforces and/or augments the function of a portion of a body part

Body Part (4th)	Approach (5th)	Device (6th)	Qualifier (7th)
1 Trachea 2 Carina 3 Main Bronchus, Right 4 Upper Lobe Bronchus, Right 5 Middle Lobe Bronchus, Right 6 Lower Lobe Bronchus, Right 7 Main Bronchus, Left 8 Upper Lobe Bronchus, Left 9 Lingula Bronchus B Lower Lobe Bronchus, Left R Diaphragm, Right S Diaphragm, Left	0 Open 4 Percutaneous Endoscopic	7 Autologous Tissue Substitute J Synthetic Substitute K Nonautologous Tissue Substitute	Z No Qualifier

Section	0	Medical and Surgical
Body System	B	Respiratory System
Operation	V	**Restriction:** Partially closing an orifice or the lumen of a tubular body part

Body Part (4th)	Approach (5th)	Device (6th)	Qualifier (7th)
1 Trachea 2 Carina 3 Main Bronchus, Right 4 Upper Lobe Bronchus, Right 5 Middle Lobe Bronchus, Right 6 Lower Lobe Bronchus, Right 7 Main Bronchus, Left 8 Upper Lobe Bronchus, Left 9 Lingula Bronchus B Lower Lobe Bronchus, Left	0 Open 3 Percutaneous 4 Percutaneous Endoscopic	C Extraluminal Device D Intraluminal Device Z No Device	Z No Qualifier
1 Trachea 2 Carina 3 Main Bronchus, Right 4 Upper Lobe Bronchus, Right 5 Middle Lobe Bronchus, Right 6 Lower Lobe Bronchus, Right 7 Main Bronchus, Left 8 Upper Lobe Bronchus, Left 9 Lingula Bronchus B Lower Lobe Bronchus, Left	7 Via Natural or Artificial Opening 8 Via Natural or Artificial Opening Endoscopic	D Intraluminal Device Z No Device	Z No Qualifier

Section	0	Medical and Surgical
Body System	B	Respiratory System
Operation	W	**Revision:** Correcting, to the extent possible, a portion of a malfunctioning device or the position of a displaced device

Body Part (4th)	Approach (5th)	Device (6th)	Qualifier (7th)
0 Tracheobronchial Tree	0 Open 3 Percutaneous 4 Percutaneous Endoscopic 7 Via Natural or Artificial Opening 8 Via Natural or Artificial Opening Endoscopic X External	0 Drainage Device 2 Monitoring Device 3 Infusion Device 7 Autologous Tissue Substitute C Extraluminal Device D Intraluminal Device J Synthetic Substitute K Nonautologous Tissue Substitute	Z No Qualifier

Continued

Section   0   **Medical and Surgical**
Body System   B   **Respiratory System**
Operation   W   **Revision:** Correcting, to the extent possible, a portion of a malfunctioning device or the position of a displaced device

Body Part (4th)	Approach (5th)	Device (6th)	Qualifier (7th)
1 Trachea	0 Open 3 Percutaneous 4 Percutaneous Endoscopic 7 Via Natural or Artificial Opening 8 Via Natural or Artificial Opening Endoscopic X External	0 Drainage Device 2 Monitoring Device 7 Autologous Tissue Substitute C Extraluminal Device D Intraluminal Device F Tracheostomy Device J Synthetic Substitute K Nonautologous Tissue Substitute	Z No Qualifier
K Lung, Right L Lung, Left	0 Open 3 Percutaneous 4 Percutaneous Endoscopic 7 Via Natural or Artificial Opening 8 Via Natural or Artificial Opening Endoscopic X External	0 Drainage Device 2 Monitoring Device 3 Infusion Device	Z No Qualifier
Q Pleura	0 Open 3 Percutaneous 4 Percutaneous Endoscopic 7 Via Natural or Artificial Opening 8 Via Natural or Artificial Opening Endoscopic X External	0 Drainage Device 2 Monitoring Device	Z No Qualifier
T Diaphragm	0 Open 3 Percutaneous 4 Percutaneous Endoscopic 7 Via Natural or Artificial Opening 8 Via Natural or Artificial Opening Endoscopic X External	0 Drainage Device 2 Monitoring Device 7 Autologous Tissue Substitute J Synthetic Substitute K Nonautologous Tissue Substitute M Diaphragmatic Pacemaker Lead	Z No Qualifier

Section   0   **Medical and Surgical**
Body System   B   **Respiratory System**
Operation   Y   **Transplantation:** Putting in or on all or a portion of a living body part taken from another individual or animal to physically take the place and/or function of all or a portion of a similar body part

Body Part (4th)	Approach (5th)	Device (6th)	Qualifier (7th)
C Upper Lung Lobe, Right D Middle Lung Lobe, Right F Lower Lung Lobe, Right G Upper Lung Lobe, Left H Lung Lingula J Lower Lung Lobe, Left K Lung, Right L Lung, Left M Lungs, Bilateral	0 Open	Z No Device	0 Allogeneic 1 Syngeneic 2 Zooplastic

Respiratory System Code Listing 0B1–0BY

0B1 – Respiratory System, Bypass

Review Coding Guideline B3.6a

0B110D6 Bypass Trachea to Esophagus with Intraluminal Device, Open Approach

0B110F4 Bypass Trachea to Cutaneous with Tracheostomy Device, Open Approach

0B110Z4 Bypass Trachea to Cutaneous, Open Approach

● **0B113F4** Bypass Trachea to Cutaneous with Tracheostomy Device, Percutaneous Approach

● **0B113Z4** Bypass Trachea to Cutaneous, Percutaneous Approach

0B114F4 Bypass Trachea to Cutaneous with Tracheostomy Device, Percutaneous Endoscopic Approach

0B114Z4 Bypass Trachea to Cutaneous, Percutaneous Endoscopic Approach

0B2 – Respiratory System, Change

Review Coding Guideline B6.1c

0B20X0Z Change Drainage Device in Tracheobronchial Tree, External Approach

0B20XYZ Change Other Device in Tracheobronchial Tree, External Approach

0B21X0Z Change Drainage Device in Trachea, External Approach

0B21XEZ Change Endotracheal Airway in Trachea, External Approach

0B21XFZ Change Tracheostomy Device in Trachea, External Approach

0B21XYZ Change Other Device in Trachea, External Approach

0B2KX0Z Change Drainage Device in Right Lung, External Approach

0B2KXYZ Change Other Device in Right Lung, External Approach

0B2LX0Z Change Drainage Device in Left Lung, External Approach

0B2LXYZ Change Other Device in Left Lung, External Approach

0B2QX0Z Change Drainage Device in Pleura, External Approach

0B2QXYZ Change Other Device in Pleura, External Approach

0B2TX0Z Change Drainage Device in Diaphragm, External Approach

0B2TXYZ Change Other Device in Diaphragm, External Approach

0B5 – Respiratory System, Destruction

0B510ZZ Destruction of Trachea, Open Approach

0B513ZZ Destruction of Trachea, Percutaneous Approach

0B514ZZ Destruction of Trachea, Percutaneous Endoscopic Approach

0B517ZZ Destruction of Trachea, Via Natural or Artificial Opening

0B518ZZ Destruction of Trachea, Via Natural or Artificial Opening Endoscopic

0B520ZZ Destruction of Carina, Open Approach

0B523ZZ Destruction of Carina, Percutaneous Approach

0B524ZZ Destruction of Carina, Percutaneous Endoscopic Approach

0B527ZZ Destruction of Carina, Via Natural or Artificial Opening

0B528ZZ Destruction of Carina, Via Natural or Artificial Opening Endoscopic

0B530ZZ Destruction of Right Main Bronchus, Open Approach

0B533ZZ Destruction of Right Main Bronchus, Percutaneous Approach

0B534ZZ Destruction of Right Main Bronchus, Percutaneous Endoscopic Approach

0B537ZZ Destruction of Right Main Bronchus, Via Natural or Artificial Opening

0B538ZZ Destruction of Right Main Bronchus, Via Natural or Artificial Opening Endoscopic

0B540ZZ Destruction of Right Upper Lobe Bronchus, Open Approach

0B543ZZ Destruction of Right Upper Lobe Bronchus, Percutaneous Approach

0B544ZZ Destruction of Right Upper Lobe Bronchus, Percutaneous Endoscopic Approach

0B547ZZ Destruction of Right Upper Lobe Bronchus, Via Natural or Artificial Opening

0B548ZZ Destruction of Right Upper Lobe Bronchus, Via Natural or Artificial Opening Endoscopic

0B550ZZ Destruction of Right Middle Lobe Bronchus, Open Approach

0B553ZZ Destruction of Right Middle Lobe Bronchus, Percutaneous Approach

0B554ZZ Destruction of Right Middle Lobe Bronchus, Percutaneous Endoscopic Approach

0B557ZZ Destruction of Right Middle Lobe Bronchus, Via Natural or Artificial Opening

0B558ZZ Destruction of Right Middle Lobe Bronchus, Via Natural or Artificial Opening Endoscopic

0B560ZZ Destruction of Right Lower Lobe Bronchus, Open Approach

0B563ZZ Destruction of Right Lower Lobe Bronchus, Percutaneous Approach

0B564ZZ Destruction of Right Lower Lobe Bronchus, Percutaneous Endoscopic Approach

0B567ZZ Destruction of Right Lower Lobe Bronchus, Via Natural or Artificial Opening

0B568ZZ Destruction of Right Lower Lobe Bronchus, Via Natural or Artificial Opening Endoscopic

0B570ZZ Destruction of Left Main Bronchus, Open Approach

0B573ZZ Destruction of Left Main Bronchus, Percutaneous Approach

0B574ZZ Destruction of Left Main Bronchus, Percutaneous Endoscopic Approach

0B577ZZ Destruction of Left Main Bronchus, Via Natural or Artificial Opening

0B578ZZ Destruction of Left Main Bronchus, Via Natural or Artificial Opening Endoscopic

0B580ZZ Destruction of Left Upper Lobe Bronchus, Open Approach

0B583ZZ Destruction of Left Upper Lobe Bronchus, Percutaneous Approach

0B584ZZ Destruction of Left Upper Lobe Bronchus, Percutaneous Endoscopic Approach

0B587ZZ Destruction of Left Upper Lobe Bronchus, Via Natural or Artificial Opening

0B588ZZ Destruction of Left Upper Lobe Bronchus, Via Natural or Artificial Opening Endoscopic

0B590ZZ Destruction of Lingula Bronchus, Open Approach

0B593ZZ Destruction of Lingula Bronchus, Percutaneous Approach

0B594ZZ Destruction of Lingula Bronchus, Percutaneous Endoscopic Approach

0B597ZZ Destruction of Lingula Bronchus, Via Natural or Artificial Opening

0B598ZZ Destruction of Lingula Bronchus, Via Natural or Artificial Opening Endoscopic

0B5B0ZZ Destruction of Left Lower Lobe Bronchus, Open Approach

0B5B3ZZ Destruction of Left Lower Lobe Bronchus, Percutaneous Approach

0B5B4ZZ Destruction of Left Lower Lobe Bronchus, Percutaneous Endoscopic Approach

0B5B7ZZ Destruction of Left Lower Lobe Bronchus, Via Natural or Artificial Opening

0B5B8ZZ Destruction of Left Lower Lobe Bronchus, Via Natural or Artificial Opening Endoscopic

0B5C0ZZ Destruction of Right Upper Lung Lobe, Open Approach

0B5C3ZZ Destruction of Right Upper Lung Lobe, Percutaneous Approach

0B5C4ZZ Destruction of Right Upper Lung Lobe, Percutaneous Endoscopic Approach

0B5C7ZZ Destruction of Right Upper Lung Lobe, Via Natural or Artificial Opening

0B5C8ZZ Destruction of Right Upper Lung Lobe, Via Natural or Artificial Opening Endoscopic

0B5D0ZZ Destruction of Right Middle Lung Lobe, Open Approach

0B5D3ZZ Destruction of Right Middle Lung Lobe, Percutaneous Approach

0B5D4ZZ Destruction of Right Middle Lung Lobe, Percutaneous Endoscopic Approach

0B5D7ZZ Destruction of Right Middle Lung Lobe, Via Natural or Artificial Opening

0B5D8ZZ Destruction of Right Middle Lung Lobe, Via Natural or Artificial Opening Endoscopic

0B5F0ZZ Destruction of Right Lower Lung Lobe, Open Approach

0B5F3ZZ	Destruction of Right Lower Lung Lobe, Percutaneous Approach
0B5F4ZZ	Destruction of Right Lower Lung Lobe, Percutaneous Endoscopic Approach
0B5F7ZZ	Destruction of Right Lower Lung Lobe, Via Natural or Artificial Opening
0B5F8ZZ	Destruction of Right Lower Lung Lobe, Via Natural or Artificial Opening Endoscopic
0B5G0ZZ	Destruction of Left Upper Lung Lobe, Open Approach
0B5G3ZZ	Destruction of Left Upper Lung Lobe, Percutaneous Approach
0B5G4ZZ	Destruction of Left Upper Lung Lobe, Percutaneous Endoscopic Approach
0B5G7ZZ	Destruction of Left Upper Lung Lobe, Via Natural or Artificial Opening
0B5G8ZZ	Destruction of Left Upper Lung Lobe, Via Natural or Artificial Opening Endoscopic
0B5H0ZZ	Destruction of Lung Lingula, Open Approach
0B5H3ZZ	Destruction of Lung Lingula, Percutaneous Approach
0B5H4ZZ	Destruction of Lung Lingula, Percutaneous Endoscopic Approach
0B5H7ZZ	Destruction of Lung Lingula, Via Natural or Artificial Opening
0B5H8ZZ	Destruction of Lung Lingula, Via Natural or Artificial Opening Endoscopic
0B5J0ZZ	Destruction of Left Lower Lung Lobe, Open Approach
0B5J3ZZ	Destruction of Left Lower Lung Lobe, Percutaneous Approach
0B5J4ZZ	Destruction of Left Lower Lung Lobe, Percutaneous Endoscopic Approach
0B5J7ZZ	Destruction of Left Lower Lung Lobe, Via Natural or Artificial Opening
0B5J8ZZ	Destruction of Left Lower Lung Lobe, Via Natural or Artificial Opening Endoscopic
0B5K0ZZ	Destruction of Right Lung, Open Approach
0B5K3ZZ	Destruction of Right Lung, Percutaneous Approach
0B5K4ZZ	Destruction of Right Lung, Percutaneous Endoscopic Approach
0B5K7ZZ	Destruction of Right Lung, Via Natural or Artificial Opening
0B5K8ZZ	Destruction of Right Lung, Via Natural or Artificial Opening Endoscopic
0B5L0ZZ	Destruction of Left Lung, Open Approach
0B5L3ZZ	Destruction of Left Lung, Percutaneous Approach
0B5L4ZZ	Destruction of Left Lung, Percutaneous Endoscopic Approach
0B5L7ZZ	Destruction of Left Lung, Via Natural or Artificial Opening
0B5L8ZZ	Destruction of Left Lung, Via Natural or Artificial Opening Endoscopic
0B5M0ZZ	Destruction of Bilateral Lungs, Open Approach
0B5M3ZZ	Destruction of Bilateral Lungs, Percutaneous Approach
0B5M4ZZ	Destruction of Bilateral Lungs, Percutaneous Endoscopic Approach
0B5M7ZZ	Destruction of Bilateral Lungs, Via Natural or Artificial Opening
0B5M8ZZ	Destruction of Bilateral Lungs, Via Natural or Artificial Opening Endoscopic
0B5N0ZZ	Destruction of Right Pleura, Open Approach
0B5N3ZZ	Destruction of Right Pleura, Percutaneous Approach
0B5N4ZZ	Destruction of Right Pleura, Percutaneous Endoscopic Approach
0B5P0ZZ	Destruction of Left Pleura, Open Approach
0B5P3ZZ	Destruction of Left Pleura, Percutaneous Approach
0B5P4ZZ	Destruction of Left Pleura, Percutaneous Endoscopic Approach
0B5R0ZZ	Destruction of Right Diaphragm, Open Approach
0B5R3ZZ	Destruction of Right Diaphragm, Percutaneous Approach
0B5R4ZZ	Destruction of Right Diaphragm, Percutaneous Endoscopic Approach
0B5S0ZZ	Destruction of Left Diaphragm, Open Approach
0B5S3ZZ	Destruction of Left Diaphragm, Percutaneous Approach
0B5S4ZZ	Destruction of Left Diaphragm, Percutaneous Endoscopic Approach

0B7 – Respiratory System, Dilation

0B710DZ	Dilation of Trachea with Intraluminal Device, Open Approach
0B710ZZ	Dilation of Trachea, Open Approach
0B713DZ	Dilation of Trachea with Intraluminal Device, Percutaneous Approach
0B713ZZ	Dilation of Trachea, Percutaneous Approach
0B714DZ	Dilation of Trachea with Intraluminal Device, Percutaneous Endoscopic Approach
0B714ZZ	Dilation of Trachea, Percutaneous Endoscopic Approach
0B717DZ	Dilation of Trachea with Intraluminal Device, Via Natural or Artificial Opening
0B717ZZ	Dilation of Trachea, Via Natural or Artificial Opening
0B718DZ	Dilation of Trachea with Intraluminal Device, Via Natural or Artificial Opening Endoscopic
0B718ZZ	Dilation of Trachea, Via Natural or Artificial Opening Endoscopic
0B720DZ	Dilation of Carina with Intraluminal Device, Open Approach
0B720ZZ	Dilation of Carina, Open Approach
0B723DZ	Dilation of Carina with Intraluminal Device, Percutaneous Approach
0B723ZZ	Dilation of Carina, Percutaneous Approach
0B724DZ	Dilation of Carina with Intraluminal Device, Percutaneous Endoscopic Approach
0B724ZZ	Dilation of Carina, Percutaneous Endoscopic Approach
0B727DZ	Dilation of Carina with Intraluminal Device, Via Natural or Artificial Opening
0B727ZZ	Dilation of Carina, Via Natural or Artificial Opening
0B728DZ	Dilation of Carina with Intraluminal Device, Via Natural or Artificial Opening Endoscopic
0B728ZZ	Dilation of Carina, Via Natural or Artificial Opening Endoscopic
0B730DZ	Dilation of Right Main Bronchus with Intraluminal Device, Open Approach
0B730ZZ	Dilation of Right Main Bronchus, Open Approach
0B733DZ	Dilation of Right Main Bronchus with Intraluminal Device, Percutaneous Approach
0B733ZZ	Dilation of Right Main Bronchus, Percutaneous Approach
0B734DZ	Dilation of Right Main Bronchus with Intraluminal Device, Percutaneous Endoscopic Approach
0B734ZZ	Dilation of Right Main Bronchus, Percutaneous Endoscopic Approach
0B737DZ	Dilation of Right Main Bronchus with Intraluminal Device, Via Natural or Artificial Opening
0B737ZZ	Dilation of Right Main Bronchus, Via Natural or Artificial Opening
0B738DZ	Dilation of Right Main Bronchus with Intraluminal Device, Via Natural or Artificial Opening Endoscopic
0B738ZZ	Dilation of Right Main Bronchus, Via Natural or Artificial Opening Endoscopic
0B740DZ	Dilation of Right Upper Lobe Bronchus with Intraluminal Device, Open Approach
0B740ZZ	Dilation of Right Upper Lobe Bronchus, Open Approach
0B743DZ	Dilation of Right Upper Lobe Bronchus with Intraluminal Device, Percutaneous Approach
0B743ZZ	Dilation of Right Upper Lobe Bronchus, Percutaneous Approach
0B744DZ	Dilation of Right Upper Lobe Bronchus with Intraluminal Device, Percutaneous Endoscopic Approach
0B744ZZ	Dilation of Right Upper Lobe Bronchus, Percutaneous Endoscopic Approach
0B747DZ	Dilation of Right Upper Lobe Bronchus with Intraluminal Device, Via Natural or Artificial Opening
0B747ZZ	Dilation of Right Upper Lobe Bronchus, Via Natural or Artificial Opening
0B748DZ	Dilation of Right Upper Lobe Bronchus with Intraluminal Device, Via Natural or Artificial Opening Endoscopic
0B748ZZ	Dilation of Right Upper Lobe Bronchus, Via Natural or Artificial Opening Endoscopic
0B750DZ	Dilation of Right Middle Lobe Bronchus with Intraluminal Device, Open Approach
0B750ZZ	Dilation of Right Middle Lobe Bronchus, Open Approach
0B753DZ	Dilation of Right Middle Lobe Bronchus with Intraluminal Device, Percutaneous Approach
0B753ZZ	Dilation of Right Middle Lobe Bronchus, Percutaneous Approach
0B754DZ	Dilation of Right Middle Lobe Bronchus with Intraluminal Device, Percutaneous Endoscopic Approach
0B754ZZ	Dilation of Right Middle Lobe Bronchus, Percutaneous Endoscopic Approach
0B757DZ	Dilation of Right Middle Lobe Bronchus with Intraluminal Device, Via Natural or Artificial Opening
0B757ZZ	Dilation of Right Middle Lobe Bronchus, Via Natural or Artificial Opening
0B758DZ	Dilation of Right Middle Lobe Bronchus with Intraluminal Device, Via Natural or Artificial Opening Endoscopic

0B758ZZ Dilation of Right Middle Lobe Bronchus, Via Natural or Artificial Opening Endoscopic

0B760DZ Dilation of Right Lower Lobe Bronchus with Intraluminal Device, Open Approach

0B760ZZ Dilation of Right Lower Lobe Bronchus, Open Approach

0B763DZ Dilation of Right Lower Lobe Bronchus with Intraluminal Device, Percutaneous Approach

0B763ZZ Dilation of Right Lower Lobe Bronchus, Percutaneous Approach

0B764DZ Dilation of Right Lower Lobe Bronchus with Intraluminal Device, Percutaneous Endoscopic Approach

0B764ZZ Dilation of Right Lower Lobe Bronchus, Percutaneous Endoscopic Approach

0B767DZ Dilation of Right Lower Lobe Bronchus with Intraluminal Device, Via Natural or Artificial Opening

0B767ZZ Dilation of Right Lower Lobe Bronchus, Via Natural or Artificial Opening

0B768DZ Dilation of Right Lower Lobe Bronchus with Intraluminal Device, Via Natural or Artificial Opening Endoscopic

0B768ZZ Dilation of Right Lower Lobe Bronchus, Via Natural or Artificial Opening Endoscopic

0B770DZ Dilation of Left Main Bronchus with Intraluminal Device, Open Approach

0B770ZZ Dilation of Left Main Bronchus, Open Approach

0B773DZ Dilation of Left Main Bronchus with Intraluminal Device, Percutaneous Approach

0B773ZZ Dilation of Left Main Bronchus, Percutaneous Approach

0B774DZ Dilation of Left Main Bronchus with Intraluminal Device, Percutaneous Endoscopic Approach

0B774ZZ Dilation of Left Main Bronchus, Percutaneous Endoscopic Approach

0B777DZ Dilation of Left Main Bronchus with Intraluminal Device, Via Natural or Artificial Opening

0B777ZZ Dilation of Left Main Bronchus, Via Natural or Artificial Opening

0B778DZ Dilation of Left Main Bronchus with Intraluminal Device, Via Natural or Artificial Opening Endoscopic

0B778ZZ Dilation of Left Main Bronchus, Via Natural or Artificial Opening Endoscopic

0B780DZ Dilation of Left Upper Lobe Bronchus with Intraluminal Device, Open Approach

0B780ZZ Dilation of Left Upper Lobe Bronchus, Open Approach

0B783DZ Dilation of Left Upper Lobe Bronchus with Intraluminal Device, Percutaneous Approach

0B783ZZ Dilation of Left Upper Lobe Bronchus, Percutaneous Approach

0B784DZ Dilation of Left Upper Lobe Bronchus with Intraluminal Device, Percutaneous Endoscopic Approach

0B784ZZ Dilation of Left Upper Lobe Bronchus, Percutaneous Endoscopic Approach

0B787DZ Dilation of Left Upper Lobe Bronchus with Intraluminal Device, Via Natural or Artificial Opening

0B787ZZ Dilation of Left Upper Lobe Bronchus, Via Natural or Artificial Opening

0B788DZ Dilation of Left Upper Lobe Bronchus with Intraluminal Device, Via Natural or Artificial Opening Endoscopic

0B788ZZ Dilation of Left Upper Lobe Bronchus, Via Natural or Artificial Opening Endoscopic

0B790DZ Dilation of Lingula Bronchus with Intraluminal Device, Open Approach

0B790ZZ Dilation of Lingula Bronchus, Open Approach

0B793DZ Dilation of Lingula Bronchus with Intraluminal Device, Percutaneous Approach

0B793ZZ Dilation of Lingula Bronchus, Percutaneous Approach

0B794DZ Dilation of Lingula Bronchus with Intraluminal Device, Percutaneous Endoscopic Approach

0B794ZZ Dilation of Lingula Bronchus, Percutaneous Endoscopic Approach

0B797DZ Dilation of Lingula Bronchus with Intraluminal Device, Via Natural or Artificial Opening

0B797ZZ Dilation of Lingula Bronchus, Via Natural or Artificial Opening

0B798DZ Dilation of Lingula Bronchus with Intraluminal Device, Via Natural or Artificial Opening Endoscopic

0B798ZZ Dilation of Lingula Bronchus, Via Natural or Artificial Opening Endoscopic

0B7B0DZ Dilation of Left Lower Lobe Bronchus with Intraluminal Device, Open Approach

0B7B0ZZ Dilation of Left Lower Lobe Bronchus, Open Approach

0B7B3DZ Dilation of Left Lower Lobe Bronchus with Intraluminal Device, Percutaneous Approach

0B7B3ZZ Dilation of Left Lower Lobe Bronchus, Percutaneous Approach

0B7B4DZ Dilation of Left Lower Lobe Bronchus with Intraluminal Device, Percutaneous Endoscopic Approach

0B7B4ZZ Dilation of Left Lower Lobe Bronchus, Percutaneous Endoscopic Approach

0B7B7DZ Dilation of Left Lower Lobe Bronchus with Intraluminal Device, Via Natural or Artificial Opening

0B7B7ZZ Dilation of Left Lower Lobe Bronchus, Via Natural or Artificial Opening

0B7B8DZ Dilation of Left Lower Lobe Bronchus with Intraluminal Device, Via Natural or Artificial Opening Endoscopic

0B7B8ZZ Dilation of Left Lower Lobe Bronchus, Via Natural or Artificial Opening Endoscopic

0B9 – Respiratory System, Drainage

Review Coding Guidelines B3.4a and B3.4b

Review Coding Guideline B6.2

0B9100Z Drainage of Trachea with Drainage Device, Open Approach

0B910ZX Drainage of Trachea, Open Approach, Diagnostic

0B910ZZ Drainage of Trachea, Open Approach

0B9130Z Drainage of Trachea with Drainage Device, Percutaneous Approach

0B913ZX Drainage of Trachea, Percutaneous Approach, Diagnostic

0B913ZZ Drainage of Trachea, Percutaneous Approach

0B9140Z Drainage of Trachea with Drainage Device, Percutaneous Endoscopic Approach

0B914ZX Drainage of Trachea, Percutaneous Endoscopic Approach, Diagnostic

0B914ZZ Drainage of Trachea, Percutaneous Endoscopic Approach

0B9170Z Drainage of Trachea with Drainage Device, Via Natural or Artificial Opening

0B917ZX Drainage of Trachea, Via Natural or Artificial Opening, Diagnostic

0B917ZZ Drainage of Trachea, Via Natural or Artificial Opening

0B9180Z Drainage of Trachea with Drainage Device, Via Natural or Artificial Opening Endoscopic

0B918ZX Drainage of Trachea, Via Natural or Artificial Opening Endoscopic, Diagnostic

0B918ZZ Drainage of Trachea, Via Natural or Artificial Opening Endoscopic

0B9200Z Drainage of Carina with Drainage Device, Open Approach

0B920ZX Drainage of Carina, Open Approach, Diagnostic

0B920ZZ Drainage of Carina, Open Approach

0B9230Z Drainage of Carina with Drainage Device, Percutaneous Approach

0B923ZX Drainage of Carina, Percutaneous Approach, Diagnostic

0B923ZZ Drainage of Carina, Percutaneous Approach

0B9240Z Drainage of Carina with Drainage Device, Percutaneous Endoscopic Approach

0B924ZX Drainage of Carina, Percutaneous Endoscopic Approach, Diagnostic

0B924ZZ Drainage of Carina, Percutaneous Endoscopic Approach

0B9270Z Drainage of Carina with Drainage Device, Via Natural or Artificial Opening

0B927ZX Drainage of Carina, Via Natural or Artificial Opening, Diagnostic

0B927ZZ Drainage of Carina, Via Natural or Artificial Opening

0B9280Z Drainage of Carina with Drainage Device, Via Natural or Artificial Opening Endoscopic

0B928ZX Drainage of Carina, Via Natural or Artificial Opening Endoscopic, Diagnostic

0B928ZZ Drainage of Carina, Via Natural or Artificial Opening Endoscopic

0B9300Z Drainage of Right Main Bronchus with Drainage Device, Open Approach

0B930ZX Drainage of Right Main Bronchus, Open Approach, Diagnostic

0B930ZZ Drainage of Right Main Bronchus, Open Approach
0B9330Z Drainage of Right Main Bronchus with Drainage Device, Percutaneous Approach
0B933ZX Drainage of Right Main Bronchus, Percutaneous Approach, Diagnostic
0B933ZZ Drainage of Right Main Bronchus, Percutaneous Approach
0B9340Z Drainage of Right Main Bronchus with Drainage Device, Percutaneous Endoscopic Approach
0B934ZX Drainage of Right Main Bronchus, Percutaneous Endoscopic Approach, Diagnostic
0B934ZZ Drainage of Right Main Bronchus, Percutaneous Endoscopic Approach
0B9370Z Drainage of Right Main Bronchus with Drainage Device, Via Natural or Artificial Opening
0B937ZX Drainage of Right Main Bronchus, Via Natural or Artificial Opening, Diagnostic
0B937ZZ Drainage of Right Main Bronchus, Via Natural or Artificial Opening
0B9380Z Drainage of Right Main Bronchus with Drainage Device, Via Natural or Artificial Opening Endoscopic
0B938ZX Drainage of Right Main Bronchus, Via Natural or Artificial Opening Endoscopic, Diagnostic
0B938ZZ Drainage of Right Main Bronchus, Via Natural or Artificial Opening Endoscopic
0B9400Z Drainage of Right Upper Lobe Bronchus with Drainage Device, Open Approach
0B940ZX Drainage of Right Upper Lobe Bronchus, Open Approach, Diagnostic
0B940ZZ Drainage of Right Upper Lobe Bronchus, Open Approach
0B9430Z Drainage of Right Upper Lobe Bronchus with Drainage Device, Percutaneous Approach
0B943ZX Drainage of Right Upper Lobe Bronchus, Percutaneous Approach, Diagnostic
0B943ZZ Drainage of Right Upper Lobe Bronchus, Percutaneous Approach
0B9440Z Drainage of Right Upper Lobe Bronchus with Drainage Device, Percutaneous Endoscopic Approach
0B944ZX Drainage of Right Upper Lobe Bronchus, Percutaneous Endoscopic Approach, Diagnostic
0B944ZZ Drainage of Right Upper Lobe Bronchus, Percutaneous Endoscopic Approach
0B9470Z Drainage of Right Upper Lobe Bronchus with Drainage Device, Via Natural or Artificial Opening
0B947ZX Drainage of Right Upper Lobe Bronchus, Via Natural or Artificial Opening, Diagnostic
0B947ZZ Drainage of Right Upper Lobe Bronchus, Via Natural or Artificial Opening
0B9480Z Drainage of Right Upper Lobe Bronchus with Drainage Device, Via Natural or Artificial Opening Endoscopic
0B948ZX Drainage of Right Upper Lobe Bronchus, Via Natural or Artificial Opening Endoscopic, Diagnostic
0B948ZZ Drainage of Right Upper Lobe Bronchus, Via Natural or Artificial Opening Endoscopic
0B9500Z Drainage of Right Middle Lobe Bronchus with Drainage Device, Open Approach
0B950ZX Drainage of Right Middle Lobe Bronchus, Open Approach, Diagnostic
0B950ZZ Drainage of Right Middle Lobe Bronchus, Open Approach
0B9530Z Drainage of Right Middle Lobe Bronchus with Drainage Device, Percutaneous Approach
0B953ZX Drainage of Right Middle Lobe Bronchus, Percutaneous Approach, Diagnostic
0B953ZZ Drainage of Right Middle Lobe Bronchus, Percutaneous Approach
0B9540Z Drainage of Right Middle Lobe Bronchus with Drainage Device, Percutaneous Endoscopic Approach
0B954ZX Drainage of Right Middle Lobe Bronchus, Percutaneous Endoscopic Approach, Diagnostic
0B954ZZ Drainage of Right Middle Lobe Bronchus, Percutaneous Endoscopic Approach
0B9570Z Drainage of Right Middle Lobe Bronchus with Drainage Device, Via Natural or Artificial Opening
0B957ZX Drainage of Right Middle Lobe Bronchus, Via Natural or Artificial Opening, Diagnostic
0B957ZZ Drainage of Right Middle Lobe Bronchus, Via Natural or Artificial Opening

0B9580Z Drainage of Right Middle Lobe Bronchus with Drainage Device, Via Natural or Artificial Opening Endoscopic
0B958ZX Drainage of Right Middle Lobe Bronchus, Via Natural or Artificial Opening Endoscopic, Diagnostic
0B958ZZ Drainage of Right Middle Lobe Bronchus, Via Natural or Artificial Opening Endoscopic
0B9600Z Drainage of Right Lower Lobe Bronchus with Drainage Device, Open Approach
0B960ZX Drainage of Right Lower Lobe Bronchus, Open Approach, Diagnostic
0B960ZZ Drainage of Right Lower Lobe Bronchus, Open Approach
0B9630Z Drainage of Right Lower Lobe Bronchus with Drainage Device, Percutaneous Approach
0B963ZX Drainage of Right Lower Lobe Bronchus, Percutaneous Approach, Diagnostic
0B963ZZ Drainage of Right Lower Lobe Bronchus, Percutaneous Approach
0B9640Z Drainage of Right Lower Lobe Bronchus with Drainage Device, Percutaneous Endoscopic Approach
0B964ZX Drainage of Right Lower Lobe Bronchus, Percutaneous Endoscopic Approach, Diagnostic
0B964ZZ Drainage of Right Lower Lobe Bronchus, Percutaneous Endoscopic Approach
0B9670Z Drainage of Right Lower Lobe Bronchus with Drainage Device, Via Natural or Artificial Opening
0B967ZX Drainage of Right Lower Lobe Bronchus, Via Natural or Artificial Opening, Diagnostic
0B967ZZ Drainage of Right Lower Lobe Bronchus, Via Natural or Artificial Opening
0B9680Z Drainage of Right Lower Lobe Bronchus with Drainage Device, Via Natural or Artificial Opening Endoscopic
0B968ZX Drainage of Right Lower Lobe Bronchus, Via Natural or Artificial Opening Endoscopic, Diagnostic
0B968ZZ Drainage of Right Lower Lobe Bronchus, Via Natural or Artificial Opening Endoscopic
0B9700Z Drainage of Left Main Bronchus with Drainage Device, Open Approach
0B970ZX Drainage of Left Main Bronchus, Open Approach, Diagnostic
0B970ZZ Drainage of Left Main Bronchus, Open Approach
0B9730Z Drainage of Left Main Bronchus with Drainage Device, Percutaneous Approach
0B973ZX Drainage of Left Main Bronchus, Percutaneous Approach, Diagnostic
0B973ZZ Drainage of Left Main Bronchus, Percutaneous Approach
0B9740Z Drainage of Left Main Bronchus with Drainage Device, Percutaneous Endoscopic Approach
0B974ZX Drainage of Left Main Bronchus, Percutaneous Endoscopic Approach, Diagnostic
0B974ZZ Drainage of Left Main Bronchus, Percutaneous Endoscopic Approach
0B9770Z Drainage of Left Main Bronchus with Drainage Device, Via Natural or Artificial Opening
0B977ZX Drainage of Left Main Bronchus, Via Natural or Artificial Opening, Diagnostic
0B977ZZ Drainage of Left Main Bronchus, Via Natural or Artificial Opening
0B9780Z Drainage of Left Main Bronchus with Drainage Device, Via Natural or Artificial Opening Endoscopic
0B978ZX Drainage of Left Main Bronchus, Via Natural or Artificial Opening Endoscopic, Diagnostic
0B978ZZ Drainage of Left Main Bronchus, Via Natural or Artificial Opening Endoscopic
0B9800Z Drainage of Left Upper Lobe Bronchus with Drainage Device, Open Approach
0B980ZX Drainage of Left Upper Lobe Bronchus, Open Approach, Diagnostic
0B980ZZ Drainage of Left Upper Lobe Bronchus, Open Approach
0B9830Z Drainage of Left Upper Lobe Bronchus with Drainage Device, Percutaneous Approach
0B983ZX Drainage of Left Upper Lobe Bronchus, Percutaneous Approach, Diagnostic
0B983ZZ Drainage of Left Upper Lobe Bronchus, Percutaneous Approach
0B9840Z Drainage of Left Upper Lobe Bronchus with Drainage Device, Percutaneous Endoscopic Approach
0B984ZX Drainage of Left Upper Lobe Bronchus, Percutaneous Endoscopic Approach, Diagnostic

---

♀ Female-only   ♂ Male-only   ● Limited Coverage   ● Non-OR   🅷🅰🅲 HAC-associated procedure   ⬣ Non-covered procedures   ➕ Combination

0B984ZZ	Drainage of Left Upper Lobe Bronchus, Percutaneous Endoscopic Approach
0B9870Z	Drainage of Left Upper Lobe Bronchus with Drainage Device, Via Natural or Artificial Opening
0B987ZX	Drainage of Left Upper Lobe Bronchus, Via Natural or Artificial Opening, Diagnostic
0B987ZZ	Drainage of Left Upper Lobe Bronchus, Via Natural or Artificial Opening
0B9880Z	Drainage of Left Upper Lobe Bronchus with Drainage Device, Via Natural or Artificial Opening Endoscopic
0B988ZX	Drainage of Left Upper Lobe Bronchus, Via Natural or Artificial Opening Endoscopic, Diagnostic
0B988ZZ	Drainage of Left Upper Lobe Bronchus, Via Natural or Artificial Opening Endoscopic
0B9900Z	Drainage of Lingula Bronchus with Drainage Device, Open Approach
0B990ZX	Drainage of Lingula Bronchus, Open Approach, Diagnostic
0B990ZZ	Drainage of Lingula Bronchus, Open Approach
0B9930Z	Drainage of Lingula Bronchus with Drainage Device, Percutaneous Approach
0B993ZX	Drainage of Lingula Bronchus, Percutaneous Approach, Diagnostic
0B993ZZ	Drainage of Lingula Bronchus, Percutaneous Approach
0B9940Z	Drainage of Lingula Bronchus with Drainage Device, Percutaneous Endoscopic Approach
0B994ZX	Drainage of Lingula Bronchus, Percutaneous Endoscopic Approach, Diagnostic
0B994ZZ	Drainage of Lingula Bronchus, Percutaneous Endoscopic Approach
0B9970Z	Drainage of Lingula Bronchus with Drainage Device, Via Natural or Artificial Opening
0B997ZX	Drainage of Lingula Bronchus, Via Natural or Artificial Opening, Diagnostic
0B997ZZ	Drainage of Lingula Bronchus, Via Natural or Artificial Opening
0B9980Z	Drainage of Lingula Bronchus with Drainage Device, Via Natural or Artificial Opening Endoscopic
0B998ZX	Drainage of Lingula Bronchus, Via Natural or Artificial Opening Endoscopic, Diagnostic
0B998ZZ	Drainage of Lingula Bronchus, Via Natural or Artificial Opening Endoscopic
0B9B00Z	Drainage of Left Lower Lobe Bronchus with Drainage Device, Open Approach
0B9B0ZX	Drainage of Left Lower Lobe Bronchus, Open Approach, Diagnostic
0B9B0ZZ	Drainage of Left Lower Lobe Bronchus, Open Approach
0B9B30Z	Drainage of Left Lower Lobe Bronchus with Drainage Device, Percutaneous Approach
0B9B3ZX	Drainage of Left Lower Lobe Bronchus, Percutaneous Approach, Diagnostic
0B9B3ZZ	Drainage of Left Lower Lobe Bronchus, Percutaneous Approach
0B9B40Z	Drainage of Left Lower Lobe Bronchus with Drainage Device, Percutaneous Endoscopic Approach
0B9B4ZX	Drainage of Left Lower Lobe Bronchus, Percutaneous Endoscopic Approach, Diagnostic
0B9B4ZZ	Drainage of Left Lower Lobe Bronchus, Percutaneous Endoscopic Approach
0B9B70Z	Drainage of Left Lower Lobe Bronchus with Drainage Device, Via Natural or Artificial Opening
0B9B7ZX	Drainage of Left Lower Lobe Bronchus, Via Natural or Artificial Opening, Diagnostic
0B9B7ZZ	Drainage of Left Lower Lobe Bronchus, Via Natural or Artificial Opening
0B9B80Z	Drainage of Left Lower Lobe Bronchus with Drainage Device, Via Natural or Artificial Opening Endoscopic
0B9B8ZX	Drainage of Left Lower Lobe Bronchus, Via Natural or Artificial Opening Endoscopic, Diagnostic
0B9B8ZZ	Drainage of Left Lower Lobe Bronchus, Via Natural or Artificial Opening Endoscopic
0B9C00Z	Drainage of Right Upper Lung Lobe with Drainage Device, Open Approach
0B9C0ZX	Drainage of Right Upper Lung Lobe, Open Approach, Diagnostic
0B9C0ZZ	Drainage of Right Upper Lung Lobe, Open Approach
0B9C30Z	Drainage of Right Upper Lung Lobe with Drainage Device, Percutaneous Approach

0B9C3ZX	Drainage of Right Upper Lung Lobe, Percutaneous Approach, Diagnostic
0B9C3ZZ	Drainage of Right Upper Lung Lobe, Percutaneous Approach
0B9C40Z	Drainage of Right Upper Lung Lobe with Drainage Device, Percutaneous Endoscopic Approach
0B9C4ZX	Drainage of Right Upper Lung Lobe, Percutaneous Endoscopic Approach, Diagnostic
0B9C4ZZ	Drainage of Right Upper Lung Lobe, Percutaneous Endoscopic Approach
0B9C70Z	Drainage of Right Upper Lung Lobe with Drainage Device, Via Natural or Artificial Opening
0B9C7ZX	Drainage of Right Upper Lung Lobe, Via Natural or Artificial Opening, Diagnostic
0B9C7ZZ	Drainage of Right Upper Lung Lobe, Via Natural or Artificial Opening
0B9C80Z	Drainage of Right Upper Lung Lobe with Drainage Device, Via Natural or Artificial Opening Endoscopic
0B9C8ZX	Drainage of Right Upper Lung Lobe, Via Natural or Artificial Opening Endoscopic, Diagnostic
0B9C8ZZ	Drainage of Right Upper Lung Lobe, Via Natural or Artificial Opening Endoscopic
0B9D00Z	Drainage of Right Middle Lung Lobe with Drainage Device, Open Approach
0B9D0ZX	Drainage of Right Middle Lung Lobe, Open Approach, Diagnostic
0B9D0ZZ	Drainage of Right Middle Lung Lobe, Open Approach
0B9D30Z	Drainage of Right Middle Lung Lobe with Drainage Device, Percutaneous Approach
0B9D3ZX	Drainage of Right Middle Lung Lobe, Percutaneous Approach, Diagnostic
0B9D3ZZ	Drainage of Right Middle Lung Lobe, Percutaneous Approach
0B9D40Z	Drainage of Right Middle Lung Lobe with Drainage Device, Percutaneous Endoscopic Approach
0B9D4ZX	Drainage of Right Middle Lung Lobe, Percutaneous Endoscopic Approach, Diagnostic
0B9D4ZZ	Drainage of Right Middle Lung Lobe, Percutaneous Endoscopic Approach
0B9D70Z	Drainage of Right Middle Lung Lobe with Drainage Device, Via Natural or Artificial Opening
0B9D7ZX	Drainage of Right Middle Lung Lobe, Via Natural or Artificial Opening, Diagnostic
0B9D7ZZ	Drainage of Right Middle Lung Lobe, Via Natural or Artificial Opening
0B9D80Z	Drainage of Right Middle Lung Lobe with Drainage Device, Via Natural or Artificial Opening Endoscopic
0B9D8ZX	Drainage of Right Middle Lung Lobe, Via Natural or Artificial Opening Endoscopic, Diagnostic
0B9D8ZZ	Drainage of Right Middle Lung Lobe, Via Natural or Artificial Opening Endoscopic
0B9F00Z	Drainage of Right Lower Lung Lobe with Drainage Device, Open Approach
0B9F0ZX	Drainage of Right Lower Lung Lobe, Open Approach, Diagnostic
0B9F0ZZ	Drainage of Right Lower Lung Lobe, Open Approach
0B9F30Z	Drainage of Right Lower Lung Lobe with Drainage Device, Percutaneous Approach
0B9F3ZX	Drainage of Right Lower Lung Lobe, Percutaneous Approach, Diagnostic
0B9F3ZZ	Drainage of Right Lower Lung Lobe, Percutaneous Approach
0B9F40Z	Drainage of Right Lower Lung Lobe with Drainage Device, Percutaneous Endoscopic Approach
0B9F4ZX	Drainage of Right Lower Lung Lobe, Percutaneous Endoscopic Approach, Diagnostic
0B9F4ZZ	Drainage of Right Lower Lung Lobe, Percutaneous Endoscopic Approach
0B9F70Z	Drainage of Right Lower Lung Lobe with Drainage Device, Via Natural or Artificial Opening
0B9F7ZX	Drainage of Right Lower Lung Lobe, Via Natural or Artificial Opening, Diagnostic
0B9F7ZZ	Drainage of Right Lower Lung Lobe, Via Natural or Artificial Opening
0B9F80Z	Drainage of Right Lower Lung Lobe with Drainage Device, Via Natural or Artificial Opening Endoscopic
0B9F8ZX	Drainage of Right Lower Lung Lobe, Via Natural or Artificial Opening Endoscopic, Diagnostic

0B9F8ZZ Drainage of Right Lower Lung Lobe, Via Natural or Artificial Opening Endoscopic

0B9G00Z Drainage of Left Upper Lung Lobe with Drainage Device, Open Approach

0B9G0ZX Drainage of Left Upper Lung Lobe, Open Approach, Diagnostic

0B9G0ZZ Drainage of Left Upper Lung Lobe, Open Approach

0B9G30Z Drainage of Left Upper Lung Lobe with Drainage Device, Percutaneous Approach

0B9G3ZX Drainage of Left Upper Lung Lobe, Percutaneous Approach, Diagnostic

0B9G3ZZ Drainage of Left Upper Lung Lobe, Percutaneous Approach

0B9G40Z Drainage of Left Upper Lung Lobe with Drainage Device, Percutaneous Endoscopic Approach

0B9G4ZX Drainage of Left Upper Lung Lobe, Percutaneous Endoscopic Approach, Diagnostic

0B9G4ZZ Drainage of Left Upper Lung Lobe, Percutaneous Endoscopic Approach

0B9G70Z Drainage of Left Upper Lung Lobe with Drainage Device, Via Natural or Artificial Opening

0B9G7ZX Drainage of Left Upper Lung Lobe, Via Natural or Artificial Opening, Diagnostic

0B9G7ZZ Drainage of Left Upper Lung Lobe, Via Natural or Artificial Opening

0B9G80Z Drainage of Left Upper Lung Lobe with Drainage Device, Via Natural or Artificial Opening Endoscopic

0B9G8ZX Drainage of Left Upper Lung Lobe, Via Natural or Artificial Opening Endoscopic, Diagnostic

0B9G8ZZ Drainage of Left Upper Lung Lobe, Via Natural or Artificial Opening Endoscopic

0B9H00Z Drainage of Lung Lingula with Drainage Device, Open Approach

0B9H0ZX Drainage of Lung Lingula, Open Approach, Diagnostic

0B9H0ZZ Drainage of Lung Lingula, Open Approach

0B9H30Z Drainage of Lung Lingula with Drainage Device, Percutaneous Approach

0B9H3ZX Drainage of Lung Lingula, Percutaneous Approach, Diagnostic

0B9H3ZZ Drainage of Lung Lingula, Percutaneous Approach

0B9H40Z Drainage of Lung Lingula with Drainage Device, Percutaneous Endoscopic Approach

0B9H4ZX Drainage of Lung Lingula, Percutaneous Endoscopic Approach, Diagnostic

0B9H4ZZ Drainage of Lung Lingula, Percutaneous Endoscopic Approach

0B9H70Z Drainage of Lung Lingula with Drainage Device, Via Natural or Artificial Opening

0B9H7ZX Drainage of Lung Lingula, Via Natural or Artificial Opening, Diagnostic

0B9H7ZZ Drainage of Lung Lingula, Via Natural or Artificial Opening

0B9H80Z Drainage of Lung Lingula with Drainage Device, Via Natural or Artificial Opening Endoscopic

0B9H8ZX Drainage of Lung Lingula, Via Natural or Artificial Opening Endoscopic, Diagnostic

0B9H8ZZ Drainage of Lung Lingula, Via Natural or Artificial Opening Endoscopic

0B9J00Z Drainage of Left Lower Lung Lobe with Drainage Device, Open Approach

0B9J0ZX Drainage of Left Lower Lung Lobe, Open Approach, Diagnostic

0B9J0ZZ Drainage of Left Lower Lung Lobe, Open Approach

0B9J30Z Drainage of Left Lower Lung Lobe with Drainage Device, Percutaneous Approach

0B9J3ZX Drainage of Left Lower Lung Lobe, Percutaneous Approach, Diagnostic

0B9J3ZZ Drainage of Left Lower Lung Lobe, Percutaneous Approach

0B9J40Z Drainage of Left Lower Lung Lobe with Drainage Device, Percutaneous Endoscopic Approach

0B9J4ZX Drainage of Left Lower Lung Lobe, Percutaneous Endoscopic Approach, Diagnostic

0B9J4ZZ Drainage of Left Lower Lung Lobe, Percutaneous Endoscopic Approach

0B9J70Z Drainage of Left Lower Lung Lobe with Drainage Device, Via Natural or Artificial Opening

0B9J7ZX Drainage of Left Lower Lung Lobe, Via Natural or Artificial Opening, Diagnostic

0B9J7ZZ Drainage of Left Lower Lung Lobe, Via Natural or Artificial Opening

0B9J80Z Drainage of Left Lower Lung Lobe with Drainage Device, Via Natural or Artificial Opening Endoscopic

0B9J8ZX Drainage of Left Lower Lung Lobe, Via Natural or Artificial Opening Endoscopic, Diagnostic

0B9J8ZZ Drainage of Left Lower Lung Lobe, Via Natural or Artificial Opening Endoscopic

0B9K00Z Drainage of Right Lung with Drainage Device, Open Approach

0B9K0ZX Drainage of Right Lung, Open Approach, Diagnostic

0B9K0ZZ Drainage of Right Lung, Open Approach

0B9K30Z Drainage of Right Lung with Drainage Device, Percutaneous Approach

0B9K3ZX Drainage of Right Lung, Percutaneous Approach, Diagnostic

0B9K3ZZ Drainage of Right Lung, Percutaneous Approach

0B9K40Z Drainage of Right Lung with Drainage Device, Percutaneous Endoscopic Approach

0B9K4ZX Drainage of Right Lung, Percutaneous Endoscopic Approach, Diagnostic

0B9K4ZZ Drainage of Right Lung, Percutaneous Endoscopic Approach

0B9K70Z Drainage of Right Lung with Drainage Device, Via Natural or Artificial Opening

0B9K7ZX Drainage of Right Lung, Via Natural or Artificial Opening, Diagnostic

0B9K7ZZ Drainage of Right Lung, Via Natural or Artificial Opening

0B9K80Z Drainage of Right Lung with Drainage Device, Via Natural or Artificial Opening Endoscopic

0B9K8ZX Drainage of Right Lung, Via Natural or Artificial Opening Endoscopic, Diagnostic

0B9K8ZZ Drainage of Right Lung, Via Natural or Artificial Opening Endoscopic

0B9L00Z Drainage of Left Lung with Drainage Device, Open Approach

0B9L0ZX Drainage of Left Lung, Open Approach, Diagnostic

0B9L0ZZ Drainage of Left Lung, Open Approach

0B9L30Z Drainage of Left Lung with Drainage Device, Percutaneous Approach

0B9L3ZX Drainage of Left Lung, Percutaneous Approach, Diagnostic

0B9L3ZZ Drainage of Left Lung, Percutaneous Approach

0B9L40Z Drainage of Left Lung with Drainage Device, Percutaneous Endoscopic Approach

0B9L4ZX Drainage of Left Lung, Percutaneous Endoscopic Approach, Diagnostic

0B9L4ZZ Drainage of Left Lung, Percutaneous Endoscopic Approach

0B9L70Z Drainage of Left Lung with Drainage Device, Via Natural or Artificial Opening

0B9L7ZX Drainage of Left Lung, Via Natural or Artificial Opening, Diagnostic

0B9L7ZZ Drainage of Left Lung, Via Natural or Artificial Opening

0B9L80Z Drainage of Left Lung with Drainage Device, Via Natural or Artificial Opening Endoscopic

0B9L8ZX Drainage of Left Lung, Via Natural or Artificial Opening Endoscopic, Diagnostic

0B9L8ZZ Drainage of Left Lung, Via Natural or Artificial Opening Endoscopic

0B9M00Z Drainage of Bilateral Lungs with Drainage Device, Open Approach

0B9M0ZX Drainage of Bilateral Lungs, Open Approach, Diagnostic

0B9M0ZZ Drainage of Bilateral Lungs, Open Approach

0B9M30Z Drainage of Bilateral Lungs with Drainage Device, Percutaneous Approach

0B9M3ZX Drainage of Bilateral Lungs, Percutaneous Approach, Diagnostic

0B9M3ZZ Drainage of Bilateral Lungs, Percutaneous Approach

0B9M40Z Drainage of Bilateral Lungs with Drainage Device, Percutaneous Endoscopic Approach

0B9M4ZX Drainage of Bilateral Lungs, Percutaneous Endoscopic Approach, Diagnostic

0B9M4ZZ Drainage of Bilateral Lungs, Percutaneous Endoscopic Approach

0B9M70Z Drainage of Bilateral Lungs with Drainage Device, Via Natural or Artificial Opening

0B9M7ZX Drainage of Bilateral Lungs, Via Natural or Artificial Opening, Diagnostic

0B9M7ZZ Drainage of Bilateral Lungs, Via Natural or Artificial Opening

0B9M80Z Drainage of Bilateral Lungs with Drainage Device, Via Natural or Artificial Opening Endoscopic

0B9M8ZX Drainage of Bilateral Lungs, Via Natural or Artificial Opening Endoscopic, Diagnostic

0B9M8ZZ	Drainage of Bilateral Lungs, Via Natural or Artificial Opening Endoscopic
0B9N00Z	Drainage of Right Pleura with Drainage Device, Open Approach
0B9N0ZX	Drainage of Right Pleura, Open Approach, Diagnostic
0B9N0ZZ	Drainage of Right Pleura, Open Approach
0B9N30Z	Drainage of Right Pleura with Drainage Device, Percutaneous Approach
0B9N3ZX	Drainage of Right Pleura, Percutaneous Approach, Diagnostic
0B9N3ZZ	Drainage of Right Pleura, Percutaneous Approach
0B9N40Z	Drainage of Right Pleura with Drainage Device, Percutaneous Endoscopic Approach
0B9N4ZX	Drainage of Right Pleura, Percutaneous Endoscopic Approach, Diagnostic
0B9N4ZZ	Drainage of Right Pleura, Percutaneous Endoscopic Approach
0B9P00Z	Drainage of Left Pleura with Drainage Device, Open Approach
0B9P0ZX	Drainage of Left Pleura, Open Approach, Diagnostic
0B9P0ZZ	Drainage of Left Pleura, Open Approach
0B9P30Z	Drainage of Left Pleura with Drainage Device, Percutaneous Approach
0B9P3ZX	Drainage of Left Pleura, Percutaneous Approach, Diagnostic
0B9P3ZZ	Drainage of Left Pleura, Percutaneous Approach
0B9P40Z	Drainage of Left Pleura with Drainage Device, Percutaneous Endoscopic Approach
0B9P4ZX	Drainage of Left Pleura, Percutaneous Endoscopic Approach, Diagnostic
0B9P4ZZ	Drainage of Left Pleura, Percutaneous Endoscopic Approach

0B9R00Z	Drainage of Right Diaphragm with Drainage Device, Open Approach
0B9R0ZX	Drainage of Right Diaphragm, Open Approach, Diagnostic
0B9R0ZZ	Drainage of Right Diaphragm, Open Approach
0B9R30Z	Drainage of Right Diaphragm with Drainage Device, Percutaneous Approach
0B9R3ZX	Drainage of Right Diaphragm, Percutaneous Approach, Diagnostic
0B9R3ZZ	Drainage of Right Diaphragm, Percutaneous Approach
0B9R40Z	Drainage of Right Diaphragm with Drainage Device, Percutaneous Endoscopic Approach
0B9R4ZX	Drainage of Right Diaphragm, Percutaneous Endoscopic Approach, Diagnostic
0B9R4ZZ	Drainage of Right Diaphragm, Percutaneous Endoscopic Approach
0B9S00Z	Drainage of Left Diaphragm with Drainage Device, Open Approach
0B9S0ZX	Drainage of Left Diaphragm, Open Approach, Diagnostic
0B9S0ZZ	Drainage of Left Diaphragm, Open Approach
0B9S30Z	Drainage of Left Diaphragm with Drainage Device, Percutaneous Approach
0B9S3ZX	Drainage of Left Diaphragm, Percutaneous Approach, Diagnostic
0B9S3ZZ	Drainage of Left Diaphragm, Percutaneous Approach
0B9S40Z	Drainage of Left Diaphragm with Drainage Device, Percutaneous Endoscopic Approach
0B9S4ZX	Drainage of Left Diaphragm, Percutaneous Endoscopic Approach, Diagnostic
0B9S4ZZ	Drainage of Left Diaphragm, Percutaneous Endoscopic Approach

0BB – Respiratory System, Excision

Review Coding Guidelines B3.4a and B3.4b

Review Coding Guideline B3.8

0BB10ZX	Excision of Trachea, Open Approach, Diagnostic
0BB10ZZ	Excision of Trachea, Open Approach
0BB13ZX	Excision of Trachea, Percutaneous Approach, Diagnostic
0BB13ZZ	Excision of Trachea, Percutaneous Approach
0BB14ZX	Excision of Trachea, Percutaneous Endoscopic Approach, Diagnostic
0BB14ZZ	Excision of Trachea, Percutaneous Endoscopic Approach
0BB17ZX	Excision of Trachea, Via Natural or Artificial Opening, Diagnostic
0BB17ZZ	Excision of Trachea, Via Natural or Artificial Opening
0BB18ZX	Excision of Trachea, Via Natural or Artificial Opening Endoscopic, Diagnostic
0BB18ZZ	Excision of Trachea, Via Natural or Artificial Opening Endoscopic
0BB20ZX	Excision of Carina, Open Approach, Diagnostic
0BB20ZZ	Excision of Carina, Open Approach
0BB23ZX	Excision of Carina, Percutaneous Approach, Diagnostic
0BB23ZZ	Excision of Carina, Percutaneous Approach
0BB24ZX	Excision of Carina, Percutaneous Endoscopic Approach, Diagnostic
0BB24ZZ	Excision of Carina, Percutaneous Endoscopic Approach
0BB27ZX	Excision of Carina, Via Natural or Artificial Opening, Diagnostic
0BB27ZZ	Excision of Carina, Via Natural or Artificial Opening
0BB28ZX	Excision of Carina, Via Natural or Artificial Opening Endoscopic, Diagnostic
0BB28ZZ	Excision of Carina, Via Natural or Artificial Opening Endoscopic
0BB30ZX	Excision of Right Main Bronchus, Open Approach, Diagnostic
0BB30ZZ	Excision of Right Main Bronchus, Open Approach
0BB33ZX	Excision of Right Main Bronchus, Percutaneous Approach, Diagnostic
0BB33ZZ	Excision of Right Main Bronchus, Percutaneous Approach
0BB34ZX	Excision of Right Main Bronchus, Percutaneous Endoscopic Approach, Diagnostic
0BB34ZZ	Excision of Right Main Bronchus, Percutaneous Endoscopic Approach
0BB37ZX	Excision of Right Main Bronchus, Via Natural or Artificial Opening, Diagnostic
0BB37ZZ	Excision of Right Main Bronchus, Via Natural or Artificial Opening
0BB38ZX	Excision of Right Main Bronchus, Via Natural or Artificial Opening Endoscopic, Diagnostic
0BB38ZZ	Excision of Right Main Bronchus, Via Natural or Artificial Opening Endoscopic
0BB40ZX	Excision of Right Upper Lobe Bronchus, Open Approach, Diagnostic

0BB40ZZ	Excision of Right Upper Lobe Bronchus, Open Approach
0BB43ZX	Excision of Right Upper Lobe Bronchus, Percutaneous Approach, Diagnostic
0BB43ZZ	Excision of Right Upper Lobe Bronchus, Percutaneous Approach
0BB44ZX	Excision of Right Upper Lobe Bronchus, Percutaneous Endoscopic Approach, Diagnostic
0BB44ZZ	Excision of Right Upper Lobe Bronchus, Percutaneous Endoscopic Approach
0BB47ZX	Excision of Right Upper Lobe Bronchus, Via Natural or Artificial Opening, Diagnostic
0BB47ZZ	Excision of Right Upper Lobe Bronchus, Via Natural or Artificial Opening
0BB48ZX	Excision of Right Upper Lobe Bronchus, Via Natural or Artificial Opening Endoscopic, Diagnostic
0BB48ZZ	Excision of Right Upper Lobe Bronchus, Via Natural or Artificial Opening Endoscopic
0BB50ZX	Excision of Right Middle Lobe Bronchus, Open Approach, Diagnostic
0BB50ZZ	Excision of Right Middle Lobe Bronchus, Open Approach
0BB53ZX	Excision of Right Middle Lobe Bronchus, Percutaneous Approach, Diagnostic
0BB53ZZ	Excision of Right Middle Lobe Bronchus, Percutaneous Approach
0BB54ZX	Excision of Right Middle Lobe Bronchus, Percutaneous Endoscopic Approach, Diagnostic
0BB54ZZ	Excision of Right Middle Lobe Bronchus, Percutaneous Endoscopic Approach
0BB57ZX	Excision of Right Middle Lobe Bronchus, Via Natural or Artificial Opening, Diagnostic
0BB57ZZ	Excision of Right Middle Lobe Bronchus, Via Natural or Artificial Opening
0BB58ZX	Excision of Right Middle Lobe Bronchus, Via Natural or Artificial Opening Endoscopic, Diagnostic
0BB58ZZ	Excision of Right Middle Lobe Bronchus, Via Natural or Artificial Opening Endoscopic
0BB60ZX	Excision of Right Lower Lobe Bronchus, Open Approach, Diagnostic
0BB60ZZ	Excision of Right Lower Lobe Bronchus, Open Approach
0BB63ZX	Excision of Right Lower Lobe Bronchus, Percutaneous Approach, Diagnostic
0BB63ZZ	Excision of Right Lower Lobe Bronchus, Percutaneous Approach

0BB64ZX   Excision of Right Lower Lobe Bronchus, Percutaneous Endoscopic Approach, Diagnostic

0BB64ZZ   Excision of Right Lower Lobe Bronchus, Percutaneous Endoscopic Approach

0BB67ZX   Excision of Right Lower Lobe Bronchus, Via Natural or Artificial Opening, Diagnostic

0BB67ZZ   Excision of Right Lower Lobe Bronchus, Via Natural or Artificial Opening

0BB68ZX   Excision of Right Lower Lobe Bronchus, Via Natural or Artificial Opening Endoscopic, Diagnostic

0BB68ZZ   Excision of Right Lower Lobe Bronchus, Via Natural or Artificial Opening Endoscopic

0BB70ZX   Excision of Left Main Bronchus, Open Approach, Diagnostic

0BB70ZZ   Excision of Left Main Bronchus, Open Approach

0BB73ZX   Excision of Left Main Bronchus, Percutaneous Approach, Diagnostic

0BB73ZZ   Excision of Left Main Bronchus, Percutaneous Approach

0BB74ZX   Excision of Left Main Bronchus, Percutaneous Endoscopic Approach, Diagnostic

0BB74ZZ   Excision of Left Main Bronchus, Percutaneous Endoscopic Approach

0BB77ZX   Excision of Left Main Bronchus, Via Natural or Artificial Opening, Diagnostic

0BB77ZZ   Excision of Left Main Bronchus, Via Natural or Artificial Opening

0BB78ZX   Excision of Left Main Bronchus, Via Natural or Artificial Opening Endoscopic, Diagnostic

0BB78ZZ   Excision of Left Main Bronchus, Via Natural or Artificial Opening Endoscopic

0BB80ZX   Excision of Left Upper Lobe Bronchus, Open Approach, Diagnostic

0BB80ZZ   Excision of Left Upper Lobe Bronchus, Open Approach

0BB83ZX   Excision of Left Upper Lobe Bronchus, Percutaneous Approach, Diagnostic

0BB83ZZ   Excision of Left Upper Lobe Bronchus, Percutaneous Approach

0BB84ZX   Excision of Left Upper Lobe Bronchus, Percutaneous Endoscopic Approach, Diagnostic

0BB84ZZ   Excision of Left Upper Lobe Bronchus, Percutaneous Endoscopic Approach

0BB87ZX   Excision of Left Upper Lobe Bronchus, Via Natural or Artificial Opening, Diagnostic

0BB87ZZ   Excision of Left Upper Lobe Bronchus, Via Natural or Artificial Opening

0BB88ZX   Excision of Left Upper Lobe Bronchus, Via Natural or Artificial Opening Endoscopic, Diagnostic

0BB88ZZ   Excision of Left Upper Lobe Bronchus, Via Natural or Artificial Opening Endoscopic

0BB90ZX   Excision of Lingula Bronchus, Open Approach, Diagnostic

0BB90ZZ   Excision of Lingula Bronchus, Open Approach

0BB93ZX   Excision of Lingula Bronchus, Percutaneous Approach, Diagnostic

0BB93ZZ   Excision of Lingula Bronchus, Percutaneous Approach

0BB94ZX   Excision of Lingula Bronchus, Percutaneous Endoscopic Approach, Diagnostic

0BB94ZZ   Excision of Lingula Bronchus, Percutaneous Endoscopic Approach

0BB97ZX   Excision of Lingula Bronchus, Via Natural or Artificial Opening, Diagnostic

0BB97ZZ   Excision of Lingula Bronchus, Via Natural or Artificial Opening

0BB98ZX   Excision of Lingula Bronchus, Via Natural or Artificial Opening Endoscopic, Diagnostic

0BB98ZZ   Excision of Lingula Bronchus, Via Natural or Artificial Opening Endoscopic

0BBB0ZX   Excision of Left Lower Lobe Bronchus, Open Approach, Diagnostic

0BBB0ZZ   Excision of Left Lower Lobe Bronchus, Open Approach

0BBB3ZX   Excision of Left Lower Lobe Bronchus, Percutaneous Approach, Diagnostic

0BBB3ZZ   Excision of Left Lower Lobe Bronchus, Percutaneous Approach

0BBB4ZX   Excision of Left Lower Lobe Bronchus, Percutaneous Endoscopic Approach, Diagnostic

0BBB4ZZ   Excision of Left Lower Lobe Bronchus, Percutaneous Endoscopic Approach

0BBB7ZX   Excision of Left Lower Lobe Bronchus, Via Natural or Artificial Opening, Diagnostic

0BBB7ZZ   Excision of Left Lower Lobe Bronchus, Via Natural or Artificial Opening

0BBB8ZX   Excision of Left Lower Lobe Bronchus, Via Natural or Artificial Opening Endoscopic, Diagnostic

0BBB8ZZ   Excision of Left Lower Lobe Bronchus, Via Natural or Artificial Opening Endoscopic

0BBC0ZX   Excision of Right Upper Lung Lobe, Open Approach, Diagnostic

0BBC0ZZ   Excision of Right Upper Lung Lobe, Open Approach

0BBC3ZX   Excision of Right Upper Lung Lobe, Percutaneous Approach, Diagnostic

0BBC3ZZ   Excision of Right Upper Lung Lobe, Percutaneous Approach

0BBC4ZX   Excision of Right Upper Lung Lobe, Percutaneous Endoscopic Approach, Diagnostic

0BBC4ZZ   Excision of Right Upper Lung Lobe, Percutaneous Endoscopic Approach

0BBC7ZX   Excision of Right Upper Lung Lobe, Via Natural or Artificial Opening, Diagnostic

0BBC7ZZ   Excision of Right Upper Lung Lobe, Via Natural or Artificial Opening

0BBC8ZX   Excision of Right Upper Lung Lobe, Via Natural or Artificial Opening Endoscopic, Diagnostic

0BBC8ZZ   Excision of Right Upper Lung Lobe, Via Natural or Artificial Opening Endoscopic

0BBD0ZX   Excision of Right Middle Lung Lobe, Open Approach, Diagnostic

0BBD0ZZ   Excision of Right Middle Lung Lobe, Open Approach

0BBD3ZX   Excision of Right Middle Lung Lobe, Percutaneous Approach, Diagnostic

0BBD3ZZ   Excision of Right Middle Lung Lobe, Percutaneous Approach

0BBD4ZX   Excision of Right Middle Lung Lobe, Percutaneous Endoscopic Approach, Diagnostic

0BBD4ZZ   Excision of Right Middle Lung Lobe, Percutaneous Endoscopic Approach

0BBD7ZX   Excision of Right Middle Lung Lobe, Via Natural or Artificial Opening, Diagnostic

0BBD7ZZ   Excision of Right Middle Lung Lobe, Via Natural or Artificial Opening

0BBD8ZX   Excision of Right Middle Lung Lobe, Via Natural or Artificial Opening Endoscopic, Diagnostic

0BBD8ZZ   Excision of Right Middle Lung Lobe, Via Natural or Artificial Opening Endoscopic

0BBF0ZX   Excision of Right Lower Lung Lobe, Open Approach, Diagnostic

0BBF0ZZ   Excision of Right Lower Lung Lobe, Open Approach

0BBF3ZX   Excision of Right Lower Lung Lobe, Percutaneous Approach, Diagnostic

0BBF3ZZ   Excision of Right Lower Lung Lobe, Percutaneous Approach

0BBF4ZX   Excision of Right Lower Lung Lobe, Percutaneous Endoscopic Approach, Diagnostic

0BBF4ZZ   Excision of Right Lower Lung Lobe, Percutaneous Endoscopic Approach

0BBF7ZX   Excision of Right Lower Lung Lobe, Via Natural or Artificial Opening, Diagnostic

0BBF7ZZ   Excision of Right Lower Lung Lobe, Via Natural or Artificial Opening

0BBF8ZX   Excision of Right Lower Lung Lobe, Via Natural or Artificial Opening Endoscopic, Diagnostic

0BBF8ZZ   Excision of Right Lower Lung Lobe, Via Natural or Artificial Opening Endoscopic

0BBG0ZX   Excision of Left Upper Lung Lobe, Open Approach, Diagnostic

0BBG0ZZ   Excision of Left Upper Lung Lobe, Open Approach

0BBG3ZX   Excision of Left Upper Lung Lobe, Percutaneous Approach, Diagnostic

0BBG3ZZ   Excision of Left Upper Lung Lobe, Percutaneous Approach

0BBG4ZX   Excision of Left Upper Lung Lobe, Percutaneous Endoscopic Approach, Diagnostic

0BBG4ZZ   Excision of Left Upper Lung Lobe, Percutaneous Endoscopic Approach

0BBG7ZX   Excision of Left Upper Lung Lobe, Via Natural or Artificial Opening, Diagnostic

0BBG7ZZ   Excision of Left Upper Lung Lobe, Via Natural or Artificial Opening

0BBG8ZX   Excision of Left Upper Lung Lobe, Via Natural or Artificial Opening Endoscopic, Diagnostic

0BBG8ZZ   Excision of Left Upper Lung Lobe, Via Natural or Artificial Opening Endoscopic

0BBH0ZX   Excision of Lung Lingula, Open Approach, Diagnostic

0BBH0ZZ   Excision of Lung Lingula, Open Approach

0BBH3ZX   Excision of Lung Lingula, Percutaneous Approach, Diagnostic

0BBH3ZZ	Excision of Lung Lingula, Percutaneous Approach
0BBH4ZX	Excision of Lung Lingula, Percutaneous Endoscopic Approach, Diagnostic
0BBH4ZZ	Excision of Lung Lingula, Percutaneous Endoscopic Approach
0BBH7ZX	Excision of Lung Lingula, Via Natural or Artificial Opening, Diagnostic
0BBH7ZZ	Excision of Lung Lingula, Via Natural or Artificial Opening
0BBH8ZX	Excision of Lung Lingula, Via Natural or Artificial Opening Endoscopic, Diagnostic
0BBH8ZZ	Excision of Lung Lingula, Via Natural or Artificial Opening Endoscopic
0BBJ0ZX	Excision of Left Lower Lung Lobe, Open Approach, Diagnostic
0BBJ0ZZ	Excision of Left Lower Lung Lobe, Open Approach
0BBJ3ZX	Excision of Left Lower Lung Lobe, Percutaneous Approach, Diagnostic
0BBJ3ZZ	Excision of Left Lower Lung Lobe, Percutaneous Approach
0BBJ4ZX	Excision of Left Lower Lung Lobe, Percutaneous Endoscopic Approach, Diagnostic
0BBJ4ZZ	Excision of Left Lower Lung Lobe, Percutaneous Endoscopic Approach
0BBJ7ZX	Excision of Left Lower Lung Lobe, Via Natural or Artificial Opening, Diagnostic
0BBJ7ZZ	Excision of Left Lower Lung Lobe, Via Natural or Artificial Opening
0BBJ8ZX	Excision of Left Lower Lung Lobe, Via Natural or Artificial Opening Endoscopic, Diagnostic
0BBJ8ZZ	Excision of Left Lower Lung Lobe, Via Natural or Artificial Opening Endoscopic
0BBK0ZX	Excision of Right Lung, Open Approach, Diagnostic
0BBK0ZZ	Excision of Right Lung, Open Approach
0BBK3ZX	Excision of Right Lung, Percutaneous Approach, Diagnostic
0BBK3ZZ	Excision of Right Lung, Percutaneous Approach
0BBK4ZX	Excision of Right Lung, Percutaneous Endoscopic Approach, Diagnostic
0BBK4ZZ	Excision of Right Lung, Percutaneous Endoscopic Approach
0BBK7ZX	Excision of Right Lung, Via Natural or Artificial Opening, Diagnostic
0BBK7ZZ	Excision of Right Lung, Via Natural or Artificial Opening
0BBK8ZX	Excision of Right Lung, Via Natural or Artificial Opening Endoscopic, Diagnostic
0BBK8ZZ	Excision of Right Lung, Via Natural or Artificial Opening Endoscopic
0BBL0ZX	Excision of Left Lung, Open Approach, Diagnostic
0BBL0ZZ	Excision of Left Lung, Open Approach
0BBL3ZX	Excision of Left Lung, Percutaneous Approach, Diagnostic
0BBL3ZZ	Excision of Left Lung, Percutaneous Approach
0BBL4ZX	Excision of Left Lung, Percutaneous Endoscopic Approach, Diagnostic
0BBL4ZZ	Excision of Left Lung, Percutaneous Endoscopic Approach
0BBL7ZX	Excision of Left Lung, Via Natural or Artificial Opening, Diagnostic
0BBL7ZZ	Excision of Left Lung, Via Natural or Artificial Opening
0BBL8ZX	Excision of Left Lung, Via Natural or Artificial Opening Endoscopic, Diagnostic
0BBL8ZZ	Excision of Left Lung, Via Natural or Artificial Opening Endoscopic
0BBM0ZX	Excision of Bilateral Lungs, Open Approach, Diagnostic
0BBM0ZZ	Excision of Bilateral Lungs, Open Approach
0BBM3ZX	Excision of Bilateral Lungs, Percutaneous Approach, Diagnostic
0BBM3ZZ	Excision of Bilateral Lungs, Percutaneous Approach
0BBM4ZX	Excision of Bilateral Lungs, Percutaneous Endoscopic Approach, Diagnostic
0BBM4ZZ	Excision of Bilateral Lungs, Percutaneous Endoscopic Approach
0BBM7ZX	Excision of Bilateral Lungs, Via Natural or Artificial Opening, Diagnostic
0BBM7ZZ	Excision of Bilateral Lungs, Via Natural or Artificial Opening
0BBM8ZX	Excision of Bilateral Lungs, Via Natural or Artificial Opening Endoscopic, Diagnostic
0BBM8ZZ	Excision of Bilateral Lungs, Via Natural or Artificial Opening Endoscopic
0BBN0ZX	Excision of Right Pleura, Open Approach, Diagnostic
0BBN0ZZ	Excision of Right Pleura, Open Approach
0BBN3ZX	Excision of Right Pleura, Percutaneous Approach, Diagnostic
0BBN3ZZ	Excision of Right Pleura, Percutaneous Approach
0BBN4ZX	Excision of Right Pleura, Percutaneous Endoscopic Approach, Diagnostic
0BBN4ZZ	Excision of Right Pleura, Percutaneous Endoscopic Approach
0BBP0ZX	Excision of Left Pleura, Open Approach, Diagnostic
0BBP0ZZ	Excision of Left Pleura, Open Approach
0BBP3ZX	Excision of Left Pleura, Percutaneous Approach, Diagnostic
0BBP3ZZ	Excision of Left Pleura, Percutaneous Approach
0BBP4ZX	Excision of Left Pleura, Percutaneous Endoscopic Approach, Diagnostic
0BBP4ZZ	Excision of Left Pleura, Percutaneous Endoscopic Approach
0BBR0ZX	Excision of Right Diaphragm, Open Approach, Diagnostic
0BBR0ZZ	Excision of Right Diaphragm, Open Approach
0BBR3ZX	Excision of Right Diaphragm, Percutaneous Approach, Diagnostic
0BBR3ZZ	Excision of Right Diaphragm, Percutaneous Approach
0BBR4ZX	Excision of Right Diaphragm, Percutaneous Endoscopic Approach, Diagnostic
0BBR4ZZ	Excision of Right Diaphragm, Percutaneous Endoscopic Approach
0BBS0ZX	Excision of Left Diaphragm, Open Approach, Diagnostic
0BBS0ZZ	Excision of Left Diaphragm, Open Approach
0BBS3ZX	Excision of Left Diaphragm, Percutaneous Approach, Diagnostic
0BBS3ZZ	Excision of Left Diaphragm, Percutaneous Approach
0BBS4ZX	Excision of Left Diaphragm, Percutaneous Endoscopic Approach, Diagnostic
0BBS4ZZ	Excision of Left Diaphragm, Percutaneous Endoscopic Approach

0BC – Respiratory System, Extirpation

0BC10ZZ	Extirpation of Matter from Trachea, Open Approach
0BC13ZZ	Extirpation of Matter from Trachea, Percutaneous Approach
0BC14ZZ	Extirpation of Matter from Trachea, Percutaneous Endoscopic Approach
0BC17ZZ	Extirpation of Matter from Trachea, Via Natural or Artificial Opening
0BC18ZZ	Extirpation of Matter from Trachea, Via Natural or Artificial Opening Endoscopic
0BC20ZZ	Extirpation of Matter from Carina, Open Approach
0BC23ZZ	Extirpation of Matter from Carina, Percutaneous Approach
0BC24ZZ	Extirpation of Matter from Carina, Percutaneous Endoscopic Approach
0BC27ZZ	Extirpation of Matter from Carina, Via Natural or Artificial Opening
0BC28ZZ	Extirpation of Matter from Carina, Via Natural or Artificial Opening Endoscopic
0BC30ZZ	Extirpation of Matter from Right Main Bronchus, Open Approach
0BC33ZZ	Extirpation of Matter from Right Main Bronchus, Percutaneous Approach
0BC34ZZ	Extirpation of Matter from Right Main Bronchus, Percutaneous Endoscopic Approach
0BC37ZZ	Extirpation of Matter from Right Main Bronchus, Via Natural or Artificial Opening
0BC38ZZ	Extirpation of Matter from Right Main Bronchus, Via Natural or Artificial Opening Endoscopic
0BC40ZZ	Extirpation of Matter from Right Upper Lobe Bronchus, Open Approach
0BC43ZZ	Extirpation of Matter from Right Upper Lobe Bronchus, Percutaneous Approach
0BC44ZZ	Extirpation of Matter from Right Upper Lobe Bronchus, Percutaneous Endoscopic Approach
0BC47ZZ	Extirpation of Matter from Right Upper Lobe Bronchus, Via Natural or Artificial Opening
0BC48ZZ	Extirpation of Matter from Right Upper Lobe Bronchus, Via Natural or Artificial Opening Endoscopic
0BC50ZZ	Extirpation of Matter from Right Middle Lobe Bronchus, Open Approach
0BC53ZZ	Extirpation of Matter from Right Middle Lobe Bronchus, Percutaneous Approach
0BC54ZZ	Extirpation of Matter from Right Middle Lobe Bronchus, Percutaneous Endoscopic Approach
0BC57ZZ	Extirpation of Matter from Right Middle Lobe Bronchus, Via Natural or Artificial Opening
0BC58ZZ	Extirpation of Matter from Right Middle Lobe Bronchus, Via Natural or Artificial Opening Endoscopic

0BC60ZZ   Extirpation of Matter from Right Lower Lobe Bronchus, Open Approach

0BC63ZZ   Extirpation of Matter from Right Lower Lobe Bronchus, Percutaneous Approach

0BC64ZZ   Extirpation of Matter from Right Lower Lobe Bronchus, Percutaneous Endoscopic Approach

0BC67ZZ   Extirpation of Matter from Right Lower Lobe Bronchus, Via Natural or Artificial Opening

0BC68ZZ   Extirpation of Matter from Right Lower Lobe Bronchus, Via Natural or Artificial Opening Endoscopic

0BC70ZZ   Extirpation of Matter from Left Main Bronchus, Open Approach

0BC73ZZ   Extirpation of Matter from Left Main Bronchus, Percutaneous Approach

0BC74ZZ   Extirpation of Matter from Left Main Bronchus, Percutaneous Endoscopic Approach

0BC77ZZ   Extirpation of Matter from Left Main Bronchus, Via Natural or Artificial Opening

0BC78ZZ   Extirpation of Matter from Left Main Bronchus, Via Natural or Artificial Opening Endoscopic

0BC80ZZ   Extirpation of Matter from Left Upper Lobe Bronchus, Open Approach

0BC83ZZ   Extirpation of Matter from Left Upper Lobe Bronchus, Percutaneous Approach

0BC84ZZ   Extirpation of Matter from Left Upper Lobe Bronchus, Percutaneous Endoscopic Approach

0BC87ZZ   Extirpation of Matter from Left Upper Lobe Bronchus, Via Natural or Artificial Opening

0BC88ZZ   Extirpation of Matter from Left Upper Lobe Bronchus, Via Natural or Artificial Opening Endoscopic

0BC90ZZ   Extirpation of Matter from Lingula Bronchus, Open Approach

0BC93ZZ   Extirpation of Matter from Lingula Bronchus, Percutaneous Approach

0BC94ZZ   Extirpation of Matter from Lingula Bronchus, Percutaneous Endoscopic Approach

0BC97ZZ   Extirpation of Matter from Lingula Bronchus, Via Natural or Artificial Opening

0BC98ZZ   Extirpation of Matter from Lingula Bronchus, Via Natural or Artificial Opening Endoscopic

0BCB0ZZ   Extirpation of Matter from Left Lower Lobe Bronchus, Open Approach

0BCB3ZZ   Extirpation of Matter from Left Lower Lobe Bronchus, Percutaneous Approach

0BCB4ZZ   Extirpation of Matter from Left Lower Lobe Bronchus, Percutaneous Endoscopic Approach

0BCB7ZZ   Extirpation of Matter from Left Lower Lobe Bronchus, Via Natural or Artificial Opening

0BCB8ZZ   Extirpation of Matter from Left Lower Lobe Bronchus, Via Natural or Artificial Opening Endoscopic

0BCC0ZZ   Extirpation of Matter from Right Upper Lung Lobe, Open Approach

0BCC3ZZ   Extirpation of Matter from Right Upper Lung Lobe, Percutaneous Approach

0BCC4ZZ   Extirpation of Matter from Right Upper Lung Lobe, Percutaneous Endoscopic Approach

0BCC7ZZ   Extirpation of Matter from Right Upper Lung Lobe, Via Natural or Artificial Opening

0BCC8ZZ   Extirpation of Matter from Right Upper Lung Lobe, Via Natural or Artificial Opening Endoscopic

0BCD0ZZ   Extirpation of Matter from Right Middle Lung Lobe, Open Approach

0BCD3ZZ   Extirpation of Matter from Right Middle Lung Lobe, Percutaneous Approach

0BCD4ZZ   Extirpation of Matter from Right Middle Lung Lobe, Percutaneous Endoscopic Approach

0BCD7ZZ   Extirpation of Matter from Right Middle Lung Lobe, Via Natural or Artificial Opening

0BCD8ZZ   Extirpation of Matter from Right Middle Lung Lobe, Via Natural or Artificial Opening Endoscopic

0BCF0ZZ   Extirpation of Matter from Right Lower Lung Lobe, Open Approach

0BCF3ZZ   Extirpation of Matter from Right Lower Lung Lobe, Percutaneous Approach

0BCF4ZZ   Extirpation of Matter from Right Lower Lung Lobe, Percutaneous Endoscopic Approach

0BCF7ZZ   Extirpation of Matter from Right Lower Lung Lobe, Via Natural or Artificial Opening

0BCF8ZZ   Extirpation of Matter from Right Lower Lung Lobe, Via Natural or Artificial Opening Endoscopic

0BCG0ZZ   Extirpation of Matter from Left Upper Lung Lobe, Open Approach

0BCG3ZZ   Extirpation of Matter from Left Upper Lung Lobe, Percutaneous Approach

0BCG4ZZ   Extirpation of Matter from Left Upper Lung Lobe, Percutaneous Endoscopic Approach

0BCG7ZZ   Extirpation of Matter from Left Upper Lung Lobe, Via Natural or Artificial Opening

0BCG8ZZ   Extirpation of Matter from Left Upper Lung Lobe, Via Natural or Artificial Opening Endoscopic

0BCH0ZZ   Extirpation of Matter from Lung Lingula, Open Approach

0BCH3ZZ   Extirpation of Matter from Lung Lingula, Percutaneous Approach

0BCH4ZZ   Extirpation of Matter from Lung Lingula, Percutaneous Endoscopic Approach

0BCH7ZZ   Extirpation of Matter from Lung Lingula, Via Natural or Artificial Opening

0BCH8ZZ   Extirpation of Matter from Lung Lingula, Via Natural or Artificial Opening Endoscopic

0BCJ0ZZ   Extirpation of Matter from Left Lower Lung Lobe, Open Approach

0BCJ3ZZ   Extirpation of Matter from Left Lower Lung Lobe, Percutaneous Approach

0BCJ4ZZ   Extirpation of Matter from Left Lower Lung Lobe, Percutaneous Endoscopic Approach

0BCJ7ZZ   Extirpation of Matter from Left Lower Lung Lobe, Via Natural or Artificial Opening

0BCJ8ZZ   Extirpation of Matter from Left Lower Lung Lobe, Via Natural or Artificial Opening Endoscopic

0BCK0ZZ   Extirpation of Matter from Right Lung, Open Approach

0BCK3ZZ   Extirpation of Matter from Right Lung, Percutaneous Approach

0BCK4ZZ   Extirpation of Matter from Right Lung, Percutaneous Endoscopic Approach

0BCK7ZZ   Extirpation of Matter from Right Lung, Via Natural or Artificial Opening

0BCK8ZZ   Extirpation of Matter from Right Lung, Via Natural or Artificial Opening Endoscopic

0BCL0ZZ   Extirpation of Matter from Left Lung, Open Approach

0BCL3ZZ   Extirpation of Matter from Left Lung, Percutaneous Approach

0BCL4ZZ   Extirpation of Matter from Left Lung, Percutaneous Endoscopic Approach

0BCL7ZZ   Extirpation of Matter from Left Lung, Via Natural or Artificial Opening

0BCL8ZZ   Extirpation of Matter from Left Lung, Via Natural or Artificial Opening Endoscopic

0BCM0ZZ   Extirpation of Matter from Bilateral Lungs, Open Approach

0BCM3ZZ   Extirpation of Matter from Bilateral Lungs, Percutaneous Approach

0BCM4ZZ   Extirpation of Matter from Bilateral Lungs, Percutaneous Endoscopic Approach

0BCM7ZZ   Extirpation of Matter from Bilateral Lungs, Via Natural or Artificial Opening

0BCM8ZZ   Extirpation of Matter from Bilateral Lungs, Via Natural or Artificial Opening Endoscopic

0BCN0ZZ   Extirpation of Matter from Right Pleura, Open Approach

0BCN3ZZ   Extirpation of Matter from Right Pleura, Percutaneous Approach

0BCN4ZZ   Extirpation of Matter from Right Pleura, Percutaneous Endoscopic Approach

0BCP0ZZ   Extirpation of Matter from Left Pleura, Open Approach

0BCP3ZZ   Extirpation of Matter from Left Pleura, Percutaneous Approach

0BCP4ZZ   Extirpation of Matter from Left Pleura, Percutaneous Endoscopic Approach

0BCR0ZZ   Extirpation of Matter from Right Diaphragm, Open Approach

0BCR3ZZ   Extirpation of Matter from Right Diaphragm, Percutaneous Approach

0BCR4ZZ   Extirpation of Matter from Right Diaphragm, Percutaneous Endoscopic Approach

0BCS0ZZ   Extirpation of Matter from Left Diaphragm, Open Approach

0BCS3ZZ   Extirpation of Matter from Left Diaphragm, Percutaneous Approach

0BCS4ZZ   Extirpation of Matter from Left Diaphragm, Percutaneous Endoscopic Approach

0BD – Respiratory System, Extraction

Review Coding Guidelines B3.4a and B3.4b

0BDN0ZX Extraction of Right Pleura, Open Approach, Diagnostic
0BDN0ZZ Extraction of Right Pleura, Open Approach
0BDN3ZX Extraction of Right Pleura, Percutaneous Approach, Diagnostic
0BDN3ZZ Extraction of Right Pleura, Percutaneous Approach
0BDN4ZX Extraction of Right Pleura, Percutaneous Endoscopic Approach, Diagnostic
0BDN4ZZ Extraction of Right Pleura, Percutaneous Endoscopic Approach

0BDP0ZX Extraction of Left Pleura, Open Approach, Diagnostic
0BDP0ZZ Extraction of Left Pleura, Open Approach
0BDP3ZX Extraction of Left Pleura, Percutaneous Approach, Diagnostic
0BDP3ZZ Extraction of Left Pleura, Percutaneous Approach
0BDP4ZX Extraction of Left Pleura, Percutaneous Endoscopic Approach, Diagnostic
0BDP4ZZ Extraction of Left Pleura, Percutaneous Endoscopic Approach

0BF – Respiratory System, Fragmentation

0BF10ZZ Fragmentation in Trachea, Open Approach
0BF13ZZ Fragmentation in Trachea, Percutaneous Approach
0BF14ZZ Fragmentation in Trachea, Percutaneous Endoscopic Approach
0BF17ZZ Fragmentation in Trachea, Via Natural or Artificial Opening
0BF18ZZ Fragmentation in Trachea, Via Natural or Artificial Opening Endoscopic
● **0BF1XZZ** Fragmentation in Trachea, External Approach
0BF20ZZ Fragmentation in Carina, Open Approach
0BF23ZZ Fragmentation in Carina, Percutaneous Approach
0BF24ZZ Fragmentation in Carina, Percutaneous Endoscopic Approach
0BF27ZZ Fragmentation in Carina, Via Natural or Artificial Opening
0BF28ZZ Fragmentation in Carina, Via Natural or Artificial Opening Endoscopic
● **0BF2XZZ** Fragmentation in Carina, External Approach
0BF30ZZ Fragmentation in Right Main Bronchus, Open Approach
0BF33ZZ Fragmentation in Right Main Bronchus, Percutaneous Approach
0BF34ZZ Fragmentation in Right Main Bronchus, Percutaneous Endoscopic Approach
0BF37ZZ Fragmentation in Right Main Bronchus, Via Natural or Artificial Opening
0BF38ZZ Fragmentation in Right Main Bronchus, Via Natural or Artificial Opening Endoscopic
● **0BF3XZZ** Fragmentation in Right Main Bronchus, External Approach
0BF40ZZ Fragmentation in Right Upper Lobe Bronchus, Open Approach
0BF43ZZ Fragmentation in Right Upper Lobe Bronchus, Percutaneous Approach
0BF44ZZ Fragmentation in Right Upper Lobe Bronchus, Percutaneous Endoscopic Approach
0BF47ZZ Fragmentation in Right Upper Lobe Bronchus, Via Natural or Artificial Opening
0BF48ZZ Fragmentation in Right Upper Lobe Bronchus, Via Natural or Artificial Opening Endoscopic
● **0BF4XZZ** Fragmentation in Right Upper Lobe Bronchus, External Approach
0BF50ZZ Fragmentation in Right Middle Lobe Bronchus, Open Approach
0BF53ZZ Fragmentation in Right Middle Lobe Bronchus, Percutaneous Approach
0BF54ZZ Fragmentation in Right Middle Lobe Bronchus, Percutaneous Endoscopic Approach
0BF57ZZ Fragmentation in Right Middle Lobe Bronchus, Via Natural or Artificial Opening
0BF58ZZ Fragmentation in Right Middle Lobe Bronchus, Via Natural or Artificial Opening Endoscopic
● **0BF5XZZ** Fragmentation in Right Middle Lobe Bronchus, External Approach
0BF60ZZ Fragmentation in Right Lower Lobe Bronchus, Open Approach
0BF63ZZ Fragmentation in Right Lower Lobe Bronchus, Percutaneous Approach

0BF64ZZ Fragmentation in Right Lower Lobe Bronchus, Percutaneous Endoscopic Approach
0BF67ZZ Fragmentation in Right Lower Lobe Bronchus, Via Natural or Artificial Opening
0BF68ZZ Fragmentation in Right Lower Lobe Bronchus, Via Natural or Artificial Opening Endoscopic
● **0BF6XZZ** Fragmentation in Right Lower Lobe Bronchus, External Approach
0BF70ZZ Fragmentation in Left Main Bronchus, Open Approach
0BF73ZZ Fragmentation in Left Main Bronchus, Percutaneous Approach
0BF74ZZ Fragmentation in Left Main Bronchus, Percutaneous Endoscopic Approach
0BF77ZZ Fragmentation in Left Main Bronchus, Via Natural or Artificial Opening
0BF78ZZ Fragmentation in Left Main Bronchus, Via Natural or Artificial Opening Endoscopic
● **0BF7XZZ** Fragmentation in Left Main Bronchus, External Approach
0BF80ZZ Fragmentation in Left Upper Lobe Bronchus, Open Approach
0BF83ZZ Fragmentation in Left Upper Lobe Bronchus, Percutaneous Approach
0BF84ZZ Fragmentation in Left Upper Lobe Bronchus, Percutaneous Endoscopic Approach
0BF87ZZ Fragmentation in Left Upper Lobe Bronchus, Via Natural or Artificial Opening
0BF88ZZ Fragmentation in Left Upper Lobe Bronchus, Via Natural or Artificial Opening Endoscopic
● **0BF8XZZ** Fragmentation in Left Upper Lobe Bronchus, External Approach
0BF90ZZ Fragmentation in Lingula Bronchus, Open Approach
0BF93ZZ Fragmentation in Lingula Bronchus, Percutaneous Approach
0BF94ZZ Fragmentation in Lingula Bronchus, Percutaneous Endoscopic Approach
0BF97ZZ Fragmentation in Lingula Bronchus, Via Natural or Artificial Opening
0BF98ZZ Fragmentation in Lingula Bronchus, Via Natural or Artificial Opening Endoscopic
● **0BF9XZZ** Fragmentation in Lingula Bronchus, External Approach
0BFB0ZZ Fragmentation in Left Lower Lobe Bronchus, Open Approach
0BFB3ZZ Fragmentation in Left Lower Lobe Bronchus, Percutaneous Approach
0BFB4ZZ Fragmentation in Left Lower Lobe Bronchus, Percutaneous Endoscopic Approach
0BFB7ZZ Fragmentation in Left Lower Lobe Bronchus, Via Natural or Artificial Opening
0BFB8ZZ Fragmentation in Left Lower Lobe Bronchus, Via Natural or Artificial Opening Endoscopic
● **0BFBXZZ** Fragmentation in Left Lower Lobe Bronchus, External Approach

0BH – Respiratory System, Insertion

0BH001Z Insertion of Radioactive Element into Tracheobronchial Tree, Open Approach
0BH002Z Insertion of Monitoring Device into Tracheobronchial Tree, Open Approach
0BH003Z Insertion of Infusion Device into Tracheobronchial Tree, Open Approach
0BH00DZ Insertion of Intraluminal Device into Tracheobronchial Tree, Open Approach
0BH031Z Insertion of Radioactive Element into Tracheobronchial Tree, Percutaneous Approach
0BH032Z Insertion of Monitoring Device into Tracheobronchial Tree, Percutaneous Approach

0BH033Z Insertion of Infusion Device into Tracheobronchial Tree, Percutaneous Approach
0BH03DZ Insertion of Intraluminal Device into Tracheobronchial Tree, Percutaneous Approach
0BH041Z Insertion of Radioactive Element into Tracheobronchial Tree, Percutaneous Endoscopic Approach
0BH042Z Insertion of Monitoring Device into Tracheobronchial Tree, Percutaneous Endoscopic Approach
0BH043Z Insertion of Infusion Device into Tracheobronchial Tree, Percutaneous Endoscopic Approach
0BH04DZ Insertion of Intraluminal Device into Tracheobronchial Tree, Percutaneous Endoscopic Approach

 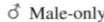

0BH071Z Insertion of Radioactive Element into Tracheobronchial Tree, Via Natural or Artificial Opening

0BH072Z Insertion of Monitoring Device into Tracheobronchial Tree, Via Natural or Artificial Opening

0BH073Z Insertion of Infusion Device into Tracheobronchial Tree, Via Natural or Artificial Opening

0BH07DZ Insertion of Intraluminal Device into Tracheobronchial Tree, Via Natural or Artificial Opening

0BH081Z Insertion of Radioactive Element into Tracheobronchial Tree, Via Natural or Artificial Opening Endoscopic

0BH082Z Insertion of Monitoring Device into Tracheobronchial Tree, Via Natural or Artificial Opening Endoscopic

0BH083Z Insertion of Infusion Device into Tracheobronchial Tree, Via Natural or Artificial Opening Endoscopic

0BH08DZ Insertion of Intraluminal Device into Tracheobronchial Tree, Via Natural or Artificial Opening Endoscopic

0BH102Z Insertion of Monitoring Device into Trachea, Open Approach

0BH10DZ Insertion of Intraluminal Device into Trachea, Open Approach

0BH13DZ Insertion of Intraluminal Device into Trachea, Percutaneous Approach

0BH13EZ Insertion of Endotracheal Airway into Trachea, Percutaneous Approach

0BH14DZ Insertion of Intraluminal Device into Trachea, Percutaneous Endoscopic Approach

0BH172Z Insertion of Monitoring Device into Trachea, Via Natural or Artificial Opening

0BH17DZ Insertion of Intraluminal Device into Trachea, Via Natural or Artificial Opening

0BH17EZ Insertion of Endotracheal Airway into Trachea, Via Natural or Artificial Opening

0BH182Z Insertion of Monitoring Device into Trachea, Via Natural or Artificial Opening Endoscopic

0BH18DZ Insertion of Intraluminal Device into Trachea, Via Natural or Artificial Opening Endoscopic

0BH18EZ Insertion of Endotracheal Airway into Trachea, Via Natural or Artificial Opening Endoscopic

0BH30GZ Insertion of Endobronchial Valve into Right Main Bronchus, Open Approach

0BH33GZ Insertion of Endobronchial Valve into Right Main Bronchus, Percutaneous Approach

0BH34GZ Insertion of Endobronchial Valve into Right Main Bronchus, Percutaneous Endoscopic Approach

0BH37GZ Insertion of Endobronchial Valve into Right Main Bronchus, Via Natural or Artificial Opening

0BH38GZ Insertion of Endobronchial Valve into Right Main Bronchus, Via Natural or Artificial Opening Endoscopic

0BH40GZ Insertion of Endobronchial Valve into Right Upper Lobe Bronchus, Open Approach

0BH43GZ Insertion of Endobronchial Valve into Right Upper Lobe Bronchus, Percutaneous Approach

0BH44GZ Insertion of Endobronchial Valve into Right Upper Lobe Bronchus, Percutaneous Endoscopic Approach

0BH47GZ Insertion of Endobronchial Valve into Right Upper Lobe Bronchus, Via Natural or Artificial Opening

0BH48GZ Insertion of Endobronchial Valve into Right Upper Lobe Bronchus, Via Natural or Artificial Opening Endoscopic

0BH50GZ Insertion of Endobronchial Valve into Right Middle Lobe Bronchus, Open Approach

0BH53GZ Insertion of Endobronchial Valve into Right Middle Lobe Bronchus, Percutaneous Approach

0BH54GZ Insertion of Endobronchial Valve into Right Middle Lobe Bronchus, Percutaneous Endoscopic Approach

0BH57GZ Insertion of Endobronchial Valve into Right Middle Lobe Bronchus, Via Natural or Artificial Opening

0BH58GZ Insertion of Endobronchial Valve into Right Middle Lobe Bronchus, Via Natural or Artificial Opening Endoscopic

0BH60GZ Insertion of Endobronchial Valve into Right Lower Lobe Bronchus, Open Approach

0BH63GZ Insertion of Endobronchial Valve into Right Lower Lobe Bronchus, Percutaneous Approach

0BH64GZ Insertion of Endobronchial Valve into Right Lower Lobe Bronchus, Percutaneous Endoscopic Approach

0BH67GZ Insertion of Endobronchial Valve into Right Lower Lobe Bronchus, Via Natural or Artificial Opening

0BH68GZ Insertion of Endobronchial Valve into Right Lower Lobe Bronchus, Via Natural or Artificial Opening Endoscopic

0BH70GZ Insertion of Endobronchial Valve into Left Main Bronchus, Open Approach

0BH73GZ Insertion of Endobronchial Valve into Left Main Bronchus, Percutaneous Approach

0BH74GZ Insertion of Endobronchial Valve into Left Main Bronchus, Percutaneous Endoscopic Approach

0BH77GZ Insertion of Endobronchial Valve into Left Main Bronchus, Via Natural or Artificial Opening

0BH78GZ Insertion of Endobronchial Valve into Left Main Bronchus, Via Natural or Artificial Opening Endoscopic

0BH80GZ Insertion of Endobronchial Valve into Left Upper Lobe Bronchus, Open Approach

0BH83GZ Insertion of Endobronchial Valve into Left Upper Lobe Bronchus, Percutaneous Approach

0BH84GZ Insertion of Endobronchial Valve into Left Upper Lobe Bronchus, Percutaneous Endoscopic Approach

0BH87GZ Insertion of Endobronchial Valve into Left Upper Lobe Bronchus, Via Natural or Artificial Opening

0BH88GZ Insertion of Endobronchial Valve into Left Upper Lobe Bronchus, Via Natural or Artificial Opening Endoscopic

0BH90GZ Insertion of Endobronchial Valve into Lingula Bronchus, Open Approach

0BH93GZ Insertion of Endobronchial Valve into Lingula Bronchus, Percutaneous Approach

0BH94GZ Insertion of Endobronchial Valve into Lingula Bronchus, Percutaneous Endoscopic Approach

0BH97GZ Insertion of Endobronchial Valve into Lingula Bronchus, Via Natural or Artificial Opening

0BH98GZ Insertion of Endobronchial Valve into Lingula Bronchus, Via Natural or Artificial Opening Endoscopic

0BHB0GZ Insertion of Endobronchial Valve into Left Lower Lobe Bronchus, Open Approach

0BHB3GZ Insertion of Endobronchial Valve into Left Lower Lobe Bronchus, Percutaneous Approach

0BHB4GZ Insertion of Endobronchial Valve into Left Lower Lobe Bronchus, Percutaneous Endoscopic Approach

0BHB7GZ Insertion of Endobronchial Valve into Left Lower Lobe Bronchus, Via Natural or Artificial Opening

0BHB8GZ Insertion of Endobronchial Valve into Left Lower Lobe Bronchus, Via Natural or Artificial Opening Endoscopic

0BHK01Z Insertion of Radioactive Element into Right Lung, Open Approach

0BHK02Z Insertion of Monitoring Device into Right Lung, Open Approach

0BHK03Z Insertion of Infusion Device into Right Lung, Open Approach

0BHK31Z Insertion of Radioactive Element into Right Lung, Percutaneous Approach

0BHK32Z Insertion of Monitoring Device into Right Lung, Percutaneous Approach

0BHK33Z Insertion of Infusion Device into Right Lung, Percutaneous Approach

0BHK41Z Insertion of Radioactive Element into Right Lung, Percutaneous Endoscopic Approach

0BHK42Z Insertion of Monitoring Device into Right Lung, Percutaneous Endoscopic Approach

0BHK43Z Insertion of Infusion Device into Right Lung, Percutaneous Endoscopic Approach

0BHK71Z Insertion of Radioactive Element into Right Lung, Via Natural or Artificial Opening

0BHK72Z Insertion of Monitoring Device into Right Lung, Via Natural or Artificial Opening

0BHK73Z Insertion of Infusion Device into Right Lung, Via Natural or Artificial Opening

0BHK81Z Insertion of Radioactive Element into Right Lung, Via Natural or Artificial Opening Endoscopic

0BHK82Z Insertion of Monitoring Device into Right Lung, Via Natural or Artificial Opening Endoscopic

0BHK83Z Insertion of Infusion Device into Right Lung, Via Natural or Artificial Opening Endoscopic

0BHL01Z Insertion of Radioactive Element into Left Lung, Open Approach

0BHL02Z Insertion of Monitoring Device into Left Lung, Open Approach

0BHL03Z Insertion of Infusion Device into Left Lung, Open Approach

0BHL31Z Insertion of Radioactive Element into Left Lung, Percutaneous Approach

0BHL32Z Insertion of Monitoring Device into Left Lung, Percutaneous Approach

---

♀ Female-only   ♂ Male-only   ● Limited Coverage   ● Non-OR   **HAC** HAC-associated procedure   ● Non-covered procedures   ✚ Combination

0BHL33Z Insertion of Infusion Device into Left Lung, Percutaneous Approach

0BHL41Z Insertion of Radioactive Element into Left Lung, Percutaneous Endoscopic Approach

0BHL42Z Insertion of Monitoring Device into Left Lung, Percutaneous Endoscopic Approach

0BHL43Z Insertion of Infusion Device into Left Lung, Percutaneous Endoscopic Approach

0BHL71Z Insertion of Radioactive Element into Left Lung, Via Natural or Artificial Opening

0BHL72Z Insertion of Monitoring Device into Left Lung, Via Natural or Artificial Opening

0BHL73Z Insertion of Infusion Device into Left Lung, Via Natural or Artificial Opening

0BHL81Z Insertion of Radioactive Element into Left Lung, Via Natural or Artificial Opening Endoscopic

0BHL82Z Insertion of Monitoring Device into Left Lung, Via Natural or Artificial Opening Endoscopic

0BHL83Z Insertion of Infusion Device into Left Lung, Via Natural or Artificial Opening Endoscopic

0BHR02Z Insertion of Monitoring Device into Right Diaphragm, Open Approach

0BHR0MZ Insertion of Diaphragmatic Pacemaker Lead into Right Diaphragm, Open Approach

0BHR32Z Insertion of Monitoring Device into Right Diaphragm, Percutaneous Approach

0BHR3MZ Insertion of Diaphragmatic Pacemaker Lead into Right Diaphragm, Percutaneous Approach

0BHR42Z Insertion of Monitoring Device into Right Diaphragm, Percutaneous Endoscopic Approach

0BHR4MZ Insertion of Diaphragmatic Pacemaker Lead into Right Diaphragm, Percutaneous Endoscopic Approach

0BHS02Z Insertion of Monitoring Device into Left Diaphragm, Open Approach

0BHS0MZ Insertion of Diaphragmatic Pacemaker Lead into Left Diaphragm, Open Approach

0BHS32Z Insertion of Monitoring Device into Left Diaphragm, Percutaneous Approach

0BHS3MZ Insertion of Diaphragmatic Pacemaker Lead into Left Diaphragm, Percutaneous Approach

0BHS42Z Insertion of Monitoring Device into Left Diaphragm, Percutaneous Endoscopic Approach

0BHS4MZ Insertion of Diaphragmatic Pacemaker Lead into Left Diaphragm, Percutaneous Endoscopic Approach

0BJ – Respiratory System, Inspection

Review Coding Guidelines B3.11a, B3.11b and B3.11c

0BJ00ZZ Inspection of Tracheobronchial Tree, Open Approach

0BJ03ZZ Inspection of Tracheobronchial Tree, Percutaneous Approach

0BJ04ZZ Inspection of Tracheobronchial Tree, Percutaneous Endoscopic Approach

0BJ07ZZ Inspection of Tracheobronchial Tree, Via Natural or Artificial Opening

0BJ08ZZ Inspection of Tracheobronchial Tree, Via Natural or Artificial Opening Endoscopic

0BJ0XZZ Inspection of Tracheobronchial Tree, External Approach

0BJ10ZZ Inspection of Trachea, Open Approach

0BJ13ZZ Inspection of Trachea, Percutaneous Approach

0BJ14ZZ Inspection of Trachea, Percutaneous Endoscopic Approach

0BJ17ZZ Inspection of Trachea, Via Natural or Artificial Opening

0BJ18ZZ Inspection of Trachea, Via Natural or Artificial Opening Endoscopic

0BJ1XZZ Inspection of Trachea, External Approach

0BJK0ZZ Inspection of Right Lung, Open Approach

0BJK3ZZ Inspection of Right Lung, Percutaneous Approach

0BJK4ZZ Inspection of Right Lung, Percutaneous Endoscopic Approach

0BJK7ZZ Inspection of Right Lung, Via Natural or Artificial Opening

0BJK8ZZ Inspection of Right Lung, Via Natural or Artificial Opening Endoscopic

0BJKXZZ Inspection of Right Lung, External Approach

0BJL0ZZ Inspection of Left Lung, Open Approach

0BJL3ZZ Inspection of Left Lung, Percutaneous Approach

0BJL4ZZ Inspection of Left Lung, Percutaneous Endoscopic Approach

0BJL7ZZ Inspection of Left Lung, Via Natural or Artificial Opening

0BJL8ZZ Inspection of Left Lung, Via Natural or Artificial Opening Endoscopic

0BJLXZZ Inspection of Left Lung, External Approach

0BJQ0ZZ Inspection of Pleura, Open Approach

0BJQ3ZZ Inspection of Pleura, Percutaneous Approach

0BJQ4ZZ Inspection of Pleura, Percutaneous Endoscopic Approach

0BJQ7ZZ Inspection of Pleura, Via Natural or Artificial Opening

0BJQ8ZZ Inspection of Pleura, Via Natural or Artificial Opening Endoscopic

0BJQXZZ Inspection of Pleura, External Approach

0BJT0ZZ Inspection of Diaphragm, Open Approach

0BJT3ZZ Inspection of Diaphragm, Percutaneous Approach

0BJT4ZZ Inspection of Diaphragm, Percutaneous Endoscopic Approach

0BJT7ZZ Inspection of Diaphragm, Via Natural or Artificial Opening

0BJT8ZZ Inspection of Diaphragm, Via Natural or Artificial Opening Endoscopic

0BJTXZZ Inspection of Diaphragm, External Approach

0BL – Respiratory System, Occlusion

0BL10CZ Occlusion of Trachea with Extraluminal Device, Open Approach

0BL10DZ Occlusion of Trachea with Intraluminal Device, Open Approach

0BL10ZZ Occlusion of Trachea, Open Approach

0BL13CZ Occlusion of Trachea with Extraluminal Device, Percutaneous Approach

0BL13DZ Occlusion of Trachea with Intraluminal Device, Percutaneous Approach

0BL13ZZ Occlusion of Trachea, Percutaneous Approach

0BL14CZ Occlusion of Trachea with Extraluminal Device, Percutaneous Endoscopic Approach

0BL14DZ Occlusion of Trachea with Intraluminal Device, Percutaneous Endoscopic Approach

0BL14ZZ Occlusion of Trachea, Percutaneous Endoscopic Approach

0BL17DZ Occlusion of Trachea with Intraluminal Device, Via Natural or Artificial Opening

0BL17ZZ Occlusion of Trachea, Via Natural or Artificial Opening

0BL18DZ Occlusion of Trachea with Intraluminal Device, Via Natural or Artificial Opening Endoscopic

0BL18ZZ Occlusion of Trachea, Via Natural or Artificial Opening Endoscopic

0BL20CZ Occlusion of Carina with Extraluminal Device, Open Approach

0BL20DZ Occlusion of Carina with Intraluminal Device, Open Approach

0BL20ZZ Occlusion of Carina, Open Approach

0BL23CZ Occlusion of Carina with Extraluminal Device, Percutaneous Approach

0BL23DZ Occlusion of Carina with Intraluminal Device, Percutaneous Approach

0BL23ZZ Occlusion of Carina, Percutaneous Approach

0BL24CZ Occlusion of Carina with Extraluminal Device, Percutaneous Endoscopic Approach

0BL24DZ Occlusion of Carina with Intraluminal Device, Percutaneous Endoscopic Approach

0BL24ZZ Occlusion of Carina, Percutaneous Endoscopic Approach

0BL27DZ Occlusion of Carina with Intraluminal Device, Via Natural or Artificial Opening

0BL27ZZ Occlusion of Carina, Via Natural or Artificial Opening

0BL28DZ Occlusion of Carina with Intraluminal Device, Via Natural or Artificial Opening Endoscopic

0BL28ZZ Occlusion of Carina, Via Natural or Artificial Opening Endoscopic

0BL30CZ Occlusion of Right Main Bronchus with Extraluminal Device, Open Approach

0BL30DZ Occlusion of Right Main Bronchus with Intraluminal Device, Open Approach

0BL30ZZ Occlusion of Right Main Bronchus, Open Approach

0BL33CZ Occlusion of Right Main Bronchus with Extraluminal Device, Percutaneous Approach

0BL33DZ Occlusion of Right Main Bronchus with Intraluminal Device, Percutaneous Approach

0BL33ZZ Occlusion of Right Main Bronchus, Percutaneous Approach

0BL34CZ Occlusion of Right Main Bronchus with Extraluminal Device, Percutaneous Endoscopic Approach

0BL34DZ Occlusion of Right Main Bronchus with Intraluminal Device, Percutaneous Endoscopic Approach

0BL34ZZ Occlusion of Right Main Bronchus, Percutaneous Endoscopic Approach

0BL37DZ Occlusion of Right Main Bronchus with Intraluminal Device, Via Natural or Artificial Opening

0BL37ZZ Occlusion of Right Main Bronchus, Via Natural or Artificial Opening

0BL38DZ Occlusion of Right Main Bronchus with Intraluminal Device, Via Natural or Artificial Opening Endoscopic

0BL38ZZ Occlusion of Right Main Bronchus, Via Natural or Artificial Opening Endoscopic

0BL40CZ Occlusion of Right Upper Lobe Bronchus with Extraluminal Device, Open Approach

0BL40DZ Occlusion of Right Upper Lobe Bronchus with Intraluminal Device, Open Approach

0BL40ZZ Occlusion of Right Upper Lobe Bronchus, Open Approach

0BL43CZ Occlusion of Right Upper Lobe Bronchus with Extraluminal Device, Percutaneous Approach

0BL43DZ Occlusion of Right Upper Lobe Bronchus with Intraluminal Device, Percutaneous Approach

0BL43ZZ Occlusion of Right Upper Lobe Bronchus, Percutaneous Approach

0BL44CZ Occlusion of Right Upper Lobe Bronchus with Extraluminal Device, Percutaneous Endoscopic Approach

0BL44DZ Occlusion of Right Upper Lobe Bronchus with Intraluminal Device, Percutaneous Endoscopic Approach

0BL44ZZ Occlusion of Right Upper Lobe Bronchus, Percutaneous Endoscopic Approach

0BL47DZ Occlusion of Right Upper Lobe Bronchus with Intraluminal Device, Via Natural or Artificial Opening

0BL47ZZ Occlusion of Right Upper Lobe Bronchus, Via Natural or Artificial Opening

0BL48DZ Occlusion of Right Upper Lobe Bronchus with Intraluminal Device, Via Natural or Artificial Opening Endoscopic

0BL48ZZ Occlusion of Right Upper Lobe Bronchus, Via Natural or Artificial Opening Endoscopic

0BL50CZ Occlusion of Right Middle Lobe Bronchus with Extraluminal Device, Open Approach

0BL50DZ Occlusion of Right Middle Lobe Bronchus with Intraluminal Device, Open Approach

0BL50ZZ Occlusion of Right Middle Lobe Bronchus, Open Approach

0BL53CZ Occlusion of Right Middle Lobe Bronchus with Extraluminal Device, Percutaneous Approach

0BL53DZ Occlusion of Right Middle Lobe Bronchus with Intraluminal Device, Percutaneous Approach

0BL53ZZ Occlusion of Right Middle Lobe Bronchus, Percutaneous Approach

0BL54CZ Occlusion of Right Middle Lobe Bronchus with Extraluminal Device, Percutaneous Endoscopic Approach

0BL54DZ Occlusion of Right Middle Lobe Bronchus with Intraluminal Device, Percutaneous Endoscopic Approach

0BL54ZZ Occlusion of Right Middle Lobe Bronchus, Percutaneous Endoscopic Approach

0BL57DZ Occlusion of Right Middle Lobe Bronchus with Intraluminal Device, Via Natural or Artificial Opening

0BL57ZZ Occlusion of Right Middle Lobe Bronchus, Via Natural or Artificial Opening

0BL58DZ Occlusion of Right Middle Lobe Bronchus with Intraluminal Device, Via Natural or Artificial Opening Endoscopic

0BL58ZZ Occlusion of Right Middle Lobe Bronchus, Via Natural or Artificial Opening Endoscopic

0BL60CZ Occlusion of Right Lower Lobe Bronchus with Extraluminal Device, Open Approach

0BL60DZ Occlusion of Right Lower Lobe Bronchus with Intraluminal Device, Open Approach

0BL60ZZ Occlusion of Right Lower Lobe Bronchus, Open Approach

0BL63CZ Occlusion of Right Lower Lobe Bronchus with Extraluminal Device, Percutaneous Approach

0BL63DZ Occlusion of Right Lower Lobe Bronchus with Intraluminal Device, Percutaneous Approach

0BL63ZZ Occlusion of Right Lower Lobe Bronchus, Percutaneous Approach

0BL64CZ Occlusion of Right Lower Lobe Bronchus with Extraluminal Device, Percutaneous Endoscopic Approach

0BL64DZ Occlusion of Right Lower Lobe Bronchus with Intraluminal Device, Percutaneous Endoscopic Approach

0BL64ZZ Occlusion of Right Lower Lobe Bronchus, Percutaneous Endoscopic Approach

0BL67DZ Occlusion of Right Lower Lobe Bronchus with Intraluminal Device, Via Natural or Artificial Opening

0BL67ZZ Occlusion of Right Lower Lobe Bronchus, Via Natural or Artificial Opening

0BL68DZ Occlusion of Right Lower Lobe Bronchus with Intraluminal Device, Via Natural or Artificial Opening Endoscopic

0BL68ZZ Occlusion of Right Lower Lobe Bronchus, Via Natural or Artificial Opening Endoscopic

0BL70CZ Occlusion of Left Main Bronchus with Extraluminal Device, Open Approach

0BL70DZ Occlusion of Left Main Bronchus with Intraluminal Device, Open Approach

0BL70ZZ Occlusion of Left Main Bronchus, Open Approach

0BL73CZ Occlusion of Left Main Bronchus with Extraluminal Device, Percutaneous Approach

0BL73DZ Occlusion of Left Main Bronchus with Intraluminal Device, Percutaneous Approach

0BL73ZZ Occlusion of Left Main Bronchus, Percutaneous Approach

0BL74CZ Occlusion of Left Main Bronchus with Extraluminal Device, Percutaneous Endoscopic Approach

0BL74DZ Occlusion of Left Main Bronchus with Intraluminal Device, Percutaneous Endoscopic Approach

0BL74ZZ Occlusion of Left Main Bronchus, Percutaneous Endoscopic Approach

0BL77DZ Occlusion of Left Main Bronchus with Intraluminal Device, Via Natural or Artificial Opening

0BL77ZZ Occlusion of Left Main Bronchus, Via Natural or Artificial Opening

0BL78DZ Occlusion of Left Main Bronchus with Intraluminal Device, Via Natural or Artificial Opening Endoscopic

0BL78ZZ Occlusion of Left Main Bronchus, Via Natural or Artificial Opening Endoscopic

0BL80CZ Occlusion of Left Upper Lobe Bronchus with Extraluminal Device, Open Approach

0BL80DZ Occlusion of Left Upper Lobe Bronchus with Intraluminal Device, Open Approach

0BL80ZZ Occlusion of Left Upper Lobe Bronchus, Open Approach

0BL83CZ Occlusion of Left Upper Lobe Bronchus with Extraluminal Device, Percutaneous Approach

0BL83DZ Occlusion of Left Upper Lobe Bronchus with Intraluminal Device, Percutaneous Approach

0BL83ZZ Occlusion of Left Upper Lobe Bronchus, Percutaneous Approach

0BL84CZ Occlusion of Left Upper Lobe Bronchus with Extraluminal Device, Percutaneous Endoscopic Approach

0BL84DZ Occlusion of Left Upper Lobe Bronchus with Intraluminal Device, Percutaneous Endoscopic Approach

0BL84ZZ Occlusion of Left Upper Lobe Bronchus, Percutaneous Endoscopic Approach

0BL87DZ Occlusion of Left Upper Lobe Bronchus with Intraluminal Device, Via Natural or Artificial Opening

0BL87ZZ Occlusion of Left Upper Lobe Bronchus, Via Natural or Artificial Opening

0BL88DZ Occlusion of Left Upper Lobe Bronchus with Intraluminal Device, Via Natural or Artificial Opening Endoscopic

0BL88ZZ Occlusion of Left Upper Lobe Bronchus, Via Natural or Artificial Opening Endoscopic

0BL90CZ Occlusion of Lingula Bronchus with Extraluminal Device, Open Approach

0BL90DZ Occlusion of Lingula Bronchus with Intraluminal Device, Open Approach

0BL90ZZ Occlusion of Lingula Bronchus, Open Approach

0BL93CZ Occlusion of Lingula Bronchus with Extraluminal Device, Percutaneous Approach

---

♀ Female-only   ♂ Male-only   ● Limited Coverage   ● Non-OR   ▉HAC HAC-associated procedure   ⬢ Non-covered procedures   ✚ Combination

0BL93DZ   Occlusion of Lingula Bronchus with Intraluminal Device, Percutaneous Approach
0BL93ZZ   Occlusion of Lingula Bronchus, Percutaneous Approach
0BL94CZ   Occlusion of Lingula Bronchus with Extraluminal Device, Percutaneous Endoscopic Approach
0BL94DZ   Occlusion of Lingula Bronchus with Intraluminal Device, Percutaneous Endoscopic Approach
0BL94ZZ   Occlusion of Lingula Bronchus, Percutaneous Endoscopic Approach
0BL97DZ   Occlusion of Lingula Bronchus with Intraluminal Device, Via Natural or Artificial Opening
0BL97ZZ   Occlusion of Lingula Bronchus, Via Natural or Artificial Opening
0BL98DZ   Occlusion of Lingula Bronchus with Intraluminal Device, Via Natural or Artificial Opening Endoscopic
0BL98ZZ   Occlusion of Lingula Bronchus, Via Natural or Artificial Opening Endoscopic
0BLB0CZ   Occlusion of Left Lower Lobe Bronchus with Extraluminal Device, Open Approach
0BLB0DZ   Occlusion of Left Lower Lobe Bronchus with Intraluminal Device, Open Approach
0BLB0ZZ   Occlusion of Left Lower Lobe Bronchus, Open Approach

0BLB3CZ   Occlusion of Left Lower Lobe Bronchus with Extraluminal Device, Percutaneous Approach
0BLB3DZ   Occlusion of Left Lower Lobe Bronchus with Intraluminal Device, Percutaneous Approach
0BLB3ZZ   Occlusion of Left Lower Lobe Bronchus, Percutaneous Approach
0BLB4CZ   Occlusion of Left Lower Lobe Bronchus with Extraluminal Device, Percutaneous Endoscopic Approach
0BLB4DZ   Occlusion of Left Lower Lobe Bronchus with Intraluminal Device, Percutaneous Endoscopic Approach
0BLB4ZZ   Occlusion of Left Lower Lobe Bronchus, Percutaneous Endoscopic Approach
0BLB7DZ   Occlusion of Left Lower Lobe Bronchus with Intraluminal Device, Via Natural or Artificial Opening
0BLB7ZZ   Occlusion of Left Lower Lobe Bronchus, Via Natural or Artificial Opening
0BLB8DZ   Occlusion of Left Lower Lobe Bronchus with Intraluminal Device, Via Natural or Artificial Opening Endoscopic
0BLB8ZZ   Occlusion of Left Lower Lobe Bronchus, Via Natural or Artificial Opening Endoscopic

0BM – Respiratory System, Reattachment

0BM10ZZ   Reattachment of Trachea, Open Approach
0BM20ZZ   Reattachment of Carina, Open Approach
0BM30ZZ   Reattachment of Right Main Bronchus, Open Approach
0BM40ZZ   Reattachment of Right Upper Lobe Bronchus, Open Approach
0BM50ZZ   Reattachment of Right Middle Lobe Bronchus, Open Approach
0BM60ZZ   Reattachment of Right Lower Lobe Bronchus, Open Approach
0BM70ZZ   Reattachment of Left Main Bronchus, Open Approach
0BM80ZZ   Reattachment of Left Upper Lobe Bronchus, Open Approach
0BM90ZZ   Reattachment of Lingula Bronchus, Open Approach
0BMB0ZZ   Reattachment of Left Lower Lobe Bronchus, Open Approach

0BMC0ZZ   Reattachment of Right Upper Lung Lobe, Open Approach
0BMD0ZZ   Reattachment of Right Middle Lung Lobe, Open Approach
0BMF0ZZ   Reattachment of Right Lower Lung Lobe, Open Approach
0BMG0ZZ   Reattachment of Left Upper Lung Lobe, Open Approach
0BMH0ZZ   Reattachment of Lung Lingula, Open Approach
0BMJ0ZZ   Reattachment of Left Lower Lung Lobe, Open Approach
0BMK0ZZ   Reattachment of Right Lung, Open Approach
0BML0ZZ   Reattachment of Left Lung, Open Approach
0BMR0ZZ   Reattachment of Right Diaphragm, Open Approach
0BMS0ZZ   Reattachment of Left Diaphragm, Open Approach

0BN – Respiratory System, Release

Review Coding Guidelines B3.13 and B3.14

0BN10ZZ   Release Trachea, Open Approach
0BN13ZZ   Release Trachea, Percutaneous Approach
0BN14ZZ   Release Trachea, Percutaneous Endoscopic Approach
0BN17ZZ   Release Trachea, Via Natural or Artificial Opening
0BN18ZZ   Release Trachea, Via Natural or Artificial Opening Endoscopic
0BN20ZZ   Release Carina, Open Approach
0BN23ZZ   Release Carina, Percutaneous Approach
0BN24ZZ   Release Carina, Percutaneous Endoscopic Approach
0BN27ZZ   Release Carina, Via Natural or Artificial Opening
0BN28ZZ   Release Carina, Via Natural or Artificial Opening Endoscopic
0BN30ZZ   Release Right Main Bronchus, Open Approach
0BN33ZZ   Release Right Main Bronchus, Percutaneous Approach
0BN34ZZ   Release Right Main Bronchus, Percutaneous Endoscopic Approach
0BN37ZZ   Release Right Main Bronchus, Via Natural or Artificial Opening
0BN38ZZ   Release Right Main Bronchus, Via Natural or Artificial Opening Endoscopic
0BN40ZZ   Release Right Upper Lobe Bronchus, Open Approach
0BN43ZZ   Release Right Upper Lobe Bronchus, Percutaneous Approach
0BN44ZZ   Release Right Upper Lobe Bronchus, Percutaneous Endoscopic Approach
0BN47ZZ   Release Right Upper Lobe Bronchus, Via Natural or Artificial Opening
0BN48ZZ   Release Right Upper Lobe Bronchus, Via Natural or Artificial Opening Endoscopic
0BN50ZZ   Release Right Middle Lobe Bronchus, Open Approach
0BN53ZZ   Release Right Middle Lobe Bronchus, Percutaneous Approach
0BN54ZZ   Release Right Middle Lobe Bronchus, Percutaneous Endoscopic Approach
0BN57ZZ   Release Right Middle Lobe Bronchus, Via Natural or Artificial Opening
0BN58ZZ   Release Right Middle Lobe Bronchus, Via Natural or Artificial Opening Endoscopic
0BN60ZZ   Release Right Lower Lobe Bronchus, Open Approach
0BN63ZZ   Release Right Lower Lobe Bronchus, Percutaneous Approach

0BN64ZZ   Release Right Lower Lobe Bronchus, Percutaneous Endoscopic Approach
0BN67ZZ   Release Right Lower Lobe Bronchus, Via Natural or Artificial Opening
0BN68ZZ   Release Right Lower Lobe Bronchus, Via Natural or Artificial Opening Endoscopic
0BN70ZZ   Release Left Main Bronchus, Open Approach
0BN73ZZ   Release Left Main Bronchus, Percutaneous Approach
0BN74ZZ   Release Left Main Bronchus, Percutaneous Endoscopic Approach
0BN77ZZ   Release Left Main Bronchus, Via Natural or Artificial Opening
0BN78ZZ   Release Left Main Bronchus, Via Natural or Artificial Opening Endoscopic
0BN80ZZ   Release Left Upper Lobe Bronchus, Open Approach
0BN83ZZ   Release Left Upper Lobe Bronchus, Percutaneous Approach
0BN84ZZ   Release Left Upper Lobe Bronchus, Percutaneous Endoscopic Approach
0BN87ZZ   Release Left Upper Lobe Bronchus, Via Natural or Artificial Opening
0BN88ZZ   Release Left Upper Lobe Bronchus, Via Natural or Artificial Opening Endoscopic
0BN90ZZ   Release Lingula Bronchus, Open Approach
0BN93ZZ   Release Lingula Bronchus, Percutaneous Approach
0BN94ZZ   Release Lingula Bronchus, Percutaneous Endoscopic Approach
0BN97ZZ   Release Lingula Bronchus, Via Natural or Artificial Opening
0BN98ZZ   Release Lingula Bronchus, Via Natural or Artificial Opening Endoscopic
0BNB0ZZ   Release Left Lower Lobe Bronchus, Open Approach
0BNB3ZZ   Release Left Lower Lobe Bronchus, Percutaneous Approach
0BNB4ZZ   Release Left Lower Lobe Bronchus, Percutaneous Endoscopic Approach
0BNB7ZZ   Release Left Lower Lobe Bronchus, Via Natural or Artificial Opening
0BNB8ZZ   Release Left Lower Lobe Bronchus, Via Natural or Artificial Opening Endoscopic
0BNC0ZZ   Release Right Upper Lung Lobe, Open Approach

0BNC3ZZ Release Right Upper Lung Lobe, Percutaneous Approach
0BNC4ZZ Release Right Upper Lung Lobe, Percutaneous Endoscopic Approach
0BNC7ZZ Release Right Upper Lung Lobe, Via Natural or Artificial Opening
0BNC8ZZ Release Right Upper Lung Lobe, Via Natural or Artificial Opening Endoscopic
0BND0ZZ Release Right Middle Lung Lobe, Open Approach
0BND3ZZ Release Right Middle Lung Lobe, Percutaneous Approach
0BND4ZZ Release Right Middle Lung Lobe, Percutaneous Endoscopic Approach
0BND7ZZ Release Right Middle Lung Lobe, Via Natural or Artificial Opening
0BND8ZZ Release Right Middle Lung Lobe, Via Natural or Artificial Opening Endoscopic
0BNF0ZZ Release Right Lower Lung Lobe, Open Approach
0BNF3ZZ Release Right Lower Lung Lobe, Percutaneous Approach
0BNF4ZZ Release Right Lower Lung Lobe, Percutaneous Endoscopic Approach
0BNF7ZZ Release Right Lower Lung Lobe, Via Natural or Artificial Opening
0BNF8ZZ Release Right Lower Lung Lobe, Via Natural or Artificial Opening Endoscopic
0BNG0ZZ Release Left Upper Lung Lobe, Open Approach
0BNG3ZZ Release Left Upper Lung Lobe, Percutaneous Approach
0BNG4ZZ Release Left Upper Lung Lobe, Percutaneous Endoscopic Approach
0BNG7ZZ Release Left Upper Lung Lobe, Via Natural or Artificial Opening
0BNG8ZZ Release Left Upper Lung Lobe, Via Natural or Artificial Opening Endoscopic
0BNH0ZZ Release Lung Lingula, Open Approach
0BNH3ZZ Release Lung Lingula, Percutaneous Approach
0BNH4ZZ Release Lung Lingula, Percutaneous Endoscopic Approach
0BNH7ZZ Release Lung Lingula, Via Natural or Artificial Opening
0BNH8ZZ Release Lung Lingula, Via Natural or Artificial Opening Endoscopic
0BNJ0ZZ Release Left Lower Lung Lobe, Open Approach
0BNJ3ZZ Release Left Lower Lung Lobe, Percutaneous Approach

0BNJ4ZZ Release Left Lower Lung Lobe, Percutaneous Endoscopic Approach
0BNJ7ZZ Release Left Lower Lung Lobe, Via Natural or Artificial Opening
0BNJ8ZZ Release Left Lower Lung Lobe, Via Natural or Artificial Opening Endoscopic
0BNK0ZZ Release Right Lung, Open Approach
0BNK3ZZ Release Right Lung, Percutaneous Approach
0BNK4ZZ Release Right Lung, Percutaneous Endoscopic Approach
0BNK7ZZ Release Right Lung, Via Natural or Artificial Opening
0BNK8ZZ Release Right Lung, Via Natural or Artificial Opening Endoscopic
0BNL0ZZ Release Left Lung, Open Approach
0BNL3ZZ Release Left Lung, Percutaneous Approach
0BNL4ZZ Release Left Lung, Percutaneous Endoscopic Approach
0BNL7ZZ Release Left Lung, Via Natural or Artificial Opening
0BNL8ZZ Release Left Lung, Via Natural or Artificial Opening Endoscopic
0BNM0ZZ Release Bilateral Lungs, Open Approach
0BNM3ZZ Release Bilateral Lungs, Percutaneous Approach
0BNM4ZZ Release Bilateral Lungs, Percutaneous Endoscopic Approach
0BNM7ZZ Release Bilateral Lungs, Via Natural or Artificial Opening
0BNM8ZZ Release Bilateral Lungs, Via Natural or Artificial Opening Endoscopic
0BNN0ZZ Release Right Pleura, Open Approach
0BNN3ZZ Release Right Pleura, Percutaneous Approach
0BNN4ZZ Release Right Pleura, Percutaneous Endoscopic Approach
0BNP0ZZ Release Left Pleura, Open Approach
0BNP3ZZ Release Left Pleura, Percutaneous Approach
0BNP4ZZ Release Left Pleura, Percutaneous Endoscopic Approach
0BNR0ZZ Release Right Diaphragm, Open Approach
0BNR3ZZ Release Right Diaphragm, Percutaneous Approach
0BNR4ZZ Release Right Diaphragm, Percutaneous Endoscopic Approach
0BNS0ZZ Release Left Diaphragm, Open Approach
0BNS3ZZ Release Left Diaphragm, Percutaneous Approach
0BNS4ZZ Release Left Diaphragm, Percutaneous Endoscopic Approach

0BP – Respiratory System, Removal

Review Coding Guideline B6.1c

0BP000Z Removal of Drainage Device from Tracheobronchial Tree, Open Approach
0BP001Z Removal of Radioactive Element from Tracheobronchial Tree, Open Approach
0BP002Z Removal of Monitoring Device from Tracheobronchial Tree, Open Approach
0BP003Z Removal of Infusion Device from Tracheobronchial Tree, Open Approach
0BP007Z Removal of Autologous Tissue Substitute from Tracheobronchial Tree, Open Approach
0BP00CZ Removal of Extraluminal Device from Tracheobronchial Tree, Open Approach
0BP00DZ Removal of Intraluminal Device from Tracheobronchial Tree, Open Approach
0BP00JZ Removal of Synthetic Substitute from Tracheobronchial Tree, Open Approach
0BP00KZ Removal of Nonautologous Tissue Substitute from Tracheobronchial Tree, Open Approach
0BP030Z Removal of Drainage Device from Tracheobronchial Tree, Percutaneous Approach
0BP031Z Removal of Radioactive Element from Tracheobronchial Tree, Percutaneous Approach
0BP032Z Removal of Monitoring Device from Tracheobronchial Tree, Percutaneous Approach
0BP033Z Removal of Infusion Device from Tracheobronchial Tree, Percutaneous Approach
0BP037Z Removal of Autologous Tissue Substitute from Tracheobronchial Tree, Percutaneous Approach
0BP03CZ Removal of Extraluminal Device from Tracheobronchial Tree, Percutaneous Approach
0BP03DZ Removal of Intraluminal Device from Tracheobronchial Tree, Percutaneous Approach
0BP03JZ Removal of Synthetic Substitute from Tracheobronchial Tree, Percutaneous Approach
0BP03KZ Removal of Nonautologous Tissue Substitute from Tracheobronchial Tree, Percutaneous Approach

0BP040Z Removal of Drainage Device from Tracheobronchial Tree, Percutaneous Endoscopic Approach
0BP041Z Removal of Radioactive Element from Tracheobronchial Tree, Percutaneous Endoscopic Approach
0BP042Z Removal of Monitoring Device from Tracheobronchial Tree, Percutaneous Endoscopic Approach
0BP043Z Removal of Infusion Device from Tracheobronchial Tree, Percutaneous Endoscopic Approach
0BP047Z Removal of Autologous Tissue Substitute from Tracheobronchial Tree, Percutaneous Endoscopic Approach
0BP04CZ Removal of Extraluminal Device from Tracheobronchial Tree, Percutaneous Endoscopic Approach
0BP04DZ Removal of Intraluminal Device from Tracheobronchial Tree, Percutaneous Endoscopic Approach
0BP04JZ Removal of Synthetic Substitute from Tracheobronchial Tree, Percutaneous Endoscopic Approach
0BP04KZ Removal of Nonautologous Tissue Substitute from Tracheobronchial Tree, Percutaneous Endoscopic Approach
0BP070Z Removal of Drainage Device from Tracheobronchial Tree, Via Natural or Artificial Opening
0BP071Z Removal of Radioactive Element from Tracheobronchial Tree, Via Natural or Artificial Opening
0BP072Z Removal of Monitoring Device from Tracheobronchial Tree, Via Natural or Artificial Opening
0BP073Z Removal of Infusion Device from Tracheobronchial Tree, Via Natural or Artificial Opening
0BP077Z Removal of Autologous Tissue Substitute from Tracheobronchial Tree, Via Natural or Artificial Opening
0BP07CZ Removal of Extraluminal Device from Tracheobronchial Tree, Via Natural or Artificial Opening
0BP07DZ Removal of Intraluminal Device from Tracheobronchial Tree, Via Natural or Artificial Opening
0BP07JZ Removal of Synthetic Substitute from Tracheobronchial Tree, Via Natural or Artificial Opening
0BP07KZ Removal of Nonautologous Tissue Substitute from Tracheobronchial Tree, Via Natural or Artificial Opening

0BP080Z   Removal of Drainage Device from Tracheobronchial Tree, Via Natural or Artificial Opening Endoscopic

0BP081Z   Removal of Radioactive Element from Tracheobronchial Tree, Via Natural or Artificial Opening Endoscopic

0BP082Z   Removal of Monitoring Device from Tracheobronchial Tree, Via Natural or Artificial Opening Endoscopic

0BP083Z   Removal of Infusion Device from Tracheobronchial Tree, Via Natural or Artificial Opening Endoscopic

0BP087Z   Removal of Autologous Tissue Substitute from Tracheobronchial Tree, Via Natural or Artificial Opening Endoscopic

0BP08CZ   Removal of Extraluminal Device from Tracheobronchial Tree, Via Natural or Artificial Opening Endoscopic

0BP08DZ   Removal of Intraluminal Device from Tracheobronchial Tree, Via Natural or Artificial Opening Endoscopic

0BP08JZ   Removal of Synthetic Substitute from Tracheobronchial Tree, Via Natural or Artificial Opening Endoscopic

0BP08KZ   Removal of Nonautologous Tissue Substitute from Tracheobronchial Tree, Via Natural or Artificial Opening Endoscopic

0BP0X0Z   Removal of Drainage Device from Tracheobronchial Tree, External Approach

0BP0X1Z   Removal of Radioactive Element from Tracheobronchial Tree, External Approach

0BP0X2Z   Removal of Monitoring Device from Tracheobronchial Tree, External Approach

0BP0X3Z   Removal of Infusion Device from Tracheobronchial Tree, External Approach

0BP0XDZ   Removal of Intraluminal Device from Tracheobronchial Tree, External Approach

0BP100Z   Removal of Drainage Device from Trachea, Open Approach

0BP102Z   Removal of Monitoring Device from Trachea, Open Approach

0BP107Z   Removal of Autologous Tissue Substitute from Trachea, Open Approach

0BP10CZ   Removal of Extraluminal Device from Trachea, Open Approach

0BP10DZ   Removal of Intraluminal Device from Trachea, Open Approach

0BP10FZ   Removal of Tracheostomy Device from Trachea, Open Approach

0BP10JZ   Removal of Synthetic Substitute from Trachea, Open Approach

0BP10KZ   Removal of Nonautologous Tissue Substitute from Trachea, Open Approach

0BP130Z   Removal of Drainage Device from Trachea, Percutaneous Approach

0BP132Z   Removal of Monitoring Device from Trachea, Percutaneous Approach

0BP137Z   Removal of Autologous Tissue Substitute from Trachea, Percutaneous Approach

0BP13CZ   Removal of Extraluminal Device from Trachea, Percutaneous Approach

0BP13DZ   Removal of Intraluminal Device from Trachea, Percutaneous Approach

0BP13FZ   Removal of Tracheostomy Device from Trachea, Percutaneous Approach

0BP13JZ   Removal of Synthetic Substitute from Trachea, Percutaneous Approach

0BP13KZ   Removal of Nonautologous Tissue Substitute from Trachea, Percutaneous Approach

0BP140Z   Removal of Drainage Device from Trachea, Percutaneous Endoscopic Approach

0BP142Z   Removal of Monitoring Device from Trachea, Percutaneous Endoscopic Approach

0BP147Z   Removal of Autologous Tissue Substitute from Trachea, Percutaneous Endoscopic Approach

0BP14CZ   Removal of Extraluminal Device from Trachea, Percutaneous Endoscopic Approach

0BP14DZ   Removal of Intraluminal Device from Trachea, Percutaneous Endoscopic Approach

0BP14FZ   Removal of Tracheostomy Device from Trachea, Percutaneous Endoscopic Approach

0BP14JZ   Removal of Synthetic Substitute from Trachea, Percutaneous Endoscopic Approach

0BP14KZ   Removal of Nonautologous Tissue Substitute from Trachea, Percutaneous Endoscopic Approach

0BP170Z   Removal of Drainage Device from Trachea, Via Natural or Artificial Opening

0BP172Z   Removal of Monitoring Device from Trachea, Via Natural or Artificial Opening

0BP177Z   Removal of Autologous Tissue Substitute from Trachea, Via Natural or Artificial Opening

0BP17CZ   Removal of Extraluminal Device from Trachea, Via Natural or Artificial Opening

0BP17DZ   Removal of Intraluminal Device from Trachea, Via Natural or Artificial Opening

0BP17FZ   Removal of Tracheostomy Device from Trachea, Via Natural or Artificial Opening

0BP17JZ   Removal of Synthetic Substitute from Trachea, Via Natural or Artificial Opening

0BP17KZ   Removal of Nonautologous Tissue Substitute from Trachea, Via Natural or Artificial Opening

0BP180Z   Removal of Drainage Device from Trachea, Via Natural or Artificial Opening Endoscopic

0BP182Z   Removal of Monitoring Device from Trachea, Via Natural or Artificial Opening Endoscopic

0BP187Z   Removal of Autologous Tissue Substitute from Trachea, Via Natural or Artificial Opening Endoscopic

0BP18CZ   Removal of Extraluminal Device from Trachea, Via Natural or Artificial Opening Endoscopic

0BP18DZ   Removal of Intraluminal Device from Trachea, Via Natural or Artificial Opening Endoscopic

0BP18FZ   Removal of Tracheostomy Device from Trachea, Via Natural or Artificial Opening Endoscopic

0BP18JZ   Removal of Synthetic Substitute from Trachea, Via Natural or Artificial Opening Endoscopic

0BP18KZ   Removal of Nonautologous Tissue Substitute from Trachea, Via Natural or Artificial Opening Endoscopic

0BP1X0Z   Removal of Drainage Device from Trachea, External Approach

0BP1X2Z   Removal of Monitoring Device from Trachea, External Approach

0BP1XDZ   Removal of Intraluminal Device from Trachea, External Approach

0BP1XFZ   Removal of Tracheostomy Device from Trachea, External Approach

0BPK00Z   Removal of Drainage Device from Right Lung, Open Approach

0BPK01Z   Removal of Radioactive Element from Right Lung, Open Approach

0BPK02Z   Removal of Monitoring Device from Right Lung, Open Approach

0BPK03Z   Removal of Infusion Device from Right Lung, Open Approach

0BPK30Z   Removal of Drainage Device from Right Lung, Percutaneous Approach

0BPK31Z   Removal of Radioactive Element from Right Lung, Percutaneous Approach

0BPK32Z   Removal of Monitoring Device from Right Lung, Percutaneous Approach

0BPK33Z   Removal of Infusion Device from Right Lung, Percutaneous Approach

0BPK40Z   Removal of Drainage Device from Right Lung, Percutaneous Endoscopic Approach

0BPK41Z   Removal of Radioactive Element from Right Lung, Percutaneous Endoscopic Approach

0BPK42Z   Removal of Monitoring Device from Right Lung, Percutaneous Endoscopic Approach

0BPK43Z   Removal of Infusion Device from Right Lung, Percutaneous Endoscopic Approach

0BPK70Z   Removal of Drainage Device from Right Lung, Via Natural or Artificial Opening

0BPK71Z   Removal of Radioactive Element from Right Lung, Via Natural or Artificial Opening

0BPK72Z   Removal of Monitoring Device from Right Lung, Via Natural or Artificial Opening

0BPK73Z   Removal of Infusion Device from Right Lung, Via Natural or Artificial Opening

0BPK80Z   Removal of Drainage Device from Right Lung, Via Natural or Artificial Opening Endoscopic

0BPK81Z   Removal of Radioactive Element from Right Lung, Via Natural or Artificial Opening Endoscopic

0BPK82Z   Removal of Monitoring Device from Right Lung, Via Natural or Artificial Opening Endoscopic

0BPK83Z   Removal of Infusion Device from Right Lung, Via Natural or Artificial Opening Endoscopic

0BPKX0Z   Removal of Drainage Device from Right Lung, External Approach

0BPKX1Z   Removal of Radioactive Element from Right Lung, External Approach

0BPKX2Z   Removal of Monitoring Device from Right Lung, External Approach

0BPKX3Z   Removal of Infusion Device from Right Lung, External Approach

---

♀ Female-only   ♂ Male-only   ● Limited Coverage   ● Non-OR   HAC HAC-associated procedure   ● Non-covered procedures   ✚ Combination

0BPL00Z Removal of Drainage Device from Left Lung, Open Approach
0BPL01Z Removal of Radioactive Element from Left Lung, Open Approach
0BPL02Z Removal of Monitoring Device from Left Lung, Open Approach
0BPL03Z Removal of Infusion Device from Left Lung, Open Approach
0BPL30Z Removal of Drainage Device from Left Lung, Percutaneous Approach
0BPL31Z Removal of Radioactive Element from Left Lung, Percutaneous Approach
0BPL32Z Removal of Monitoring Device from Left Lung, Percutaneous Approach
0BPL33Z Removal of Infusion Device from Left Lung, Percutaneous Approach
0BPL40Z Removal of Drainage Device from Left Lung, Percutaneous Endoscopic Approach
0BPL41Z Removal of Radioactive Element from Left Lung, Percutaneous Endoscopic Approach
0BPL42Z Removal of Monitoring Device from Left Lung, Percutaneous Endoscopic Approach
0BPL43Z Removal of Infusion Device from Left Lung, Percutaneous Endoscopic Approach
0BPL70Z Removal of Drainage Device from Left Lung, Via Natural or Artificial Opening
0BPL71Z Removal of Radioactive Element from Left Lung, Via Natural or Artificial Opening
0BPL72Z Removal of Monitoring Device from Left Lung, Via Natural or Artificial Opening
0BPL73Z Removal of Infusion Device from Left Lung, Via Natural or Artificial Opening
0BPL80Z Removal of Drainage Device from Left Lung, Via Natural or Artificial Opening Endoscopic
0BPL81Z Removal of Radioactive Element from Left Lung, Via Natural or Artificial Opening Endoscopic
0BPL82Z Removal of Monitoring Device from Left Lung, Via Natural or Artificial Opening Endoscopic
0BPL83Z Removal of Infusion Device from Left Lung, Via Natural or Artificial Opening Endoscopic
0BPLX0Z Removal of Drainage Device from Left Lung, External Approach
0BPLX1Z Removal of Radioactive Element from Left Lung, External Approach
0BPLX2Z Removal of Monitoring Device from Left Lung, External Approach
0BPLX3Z Removal of Infusion Device from Left Lung, External Approach
0BPQ00Z Removal of Drainage Device from Pleura, Open Approach
0BPQ01Z Removal of Radioactive Element from Pleura, Open Approach
0BPQ02Z Removal of Monitoring Device from Pleura, Open Approach
0BPQ30Z Removal of Drainage Device from Pleura, Percutaneous Approach
0BPQ31Z Removal of Radioactive Element from Pleura, Percutaneous Approach
0BPQ32Z Removal of Monitoring Device from Pleura, Percutaneous Approach
0BPQ40Z Removal of Drainage Device from Pleura, Percutaneous Endoscopic Approach
0BPQ41Z Removal of Radioactive Element from Pleura, Percutaneous Endoscopic Approach
0BPQ42Z Removal of Monitoring Device from Pleura, Percutaneous Endoscopic Approach
0BPQ70Z Removal of Drainage Device from Pleura, Via Natural or Artificial Opening
0BPQ71Z Removal of Radioactive Element from Pleura, Via Natural or Artificial Opening
0BPQ72Z Removal of Monitoring Device from Pleura, Via Natural or Artificial Opening
0BPQ80Z Removal of Drainage Device from Pleura, Via Natural or Artificial Opening Endoscopic
0BPQ81Z Removal of Radioactive Element from Pleura, Via Natural or Artificial Opening Endoscopic
0BPQ82Z Removal of Monitoring Device from Pleura, Via Natural or Artificial Opening Endoscopic

0BPQX0Z Removal of Drainage Device from Pleura, External Approach
0BPQX1Z Removal of Radioactive Element from Pleura, External Approach
0BPQX2Z Removal of Monitoring Device from Pleura, External Approach
0BPT00Z Removal of Drainage Device from Diaphragm, Open Approach
0BPT02Z Removal of Monitoring Device from Diaphragm, Open Approach
0BPT07Z Removal of Autologous Tissue Substitute from Diaphragm, Open Approach
0BPT0JZ Removal of Synthetic Substitute from Diaphragm, Open Approach
0BPT0KZ Removal of Nonautologous Tissue Substitute from Diaphragm, Open Approach
0BPT0MZ Removal of Diaphragmatic Pacemaker Lead from Diaphragm, Open Approach
0BPT30Z Removal of Drainage Device from Diaphragm, Percutaneous Approach
0BPT32Z Removal of Monitoring Device from Diaphragm, Percutaneous Approach
0BPT37Z Removal of Autologous Tissue Substitute from Diaphragm, Percutaneous Approach
0BPT3JZ Removal of Synthetic Substitute from Diaphragm, Percutaneous Approach
0BPT3KZ Removal of Nonautologous Tissue Substitute from Diaphragm, Percutaneous Approach
0BPT3MZ Removal of Diaphragmatic Pacemaker Lead from Diaphragm, Percutaneous Approach
0BPT40Z Removal of Drainage Device from Diaphragm, Percutaneous Endoscopic Approach
0BPT42Z Removal of Monitoring Device from Diaphragm, Percutaneous Endoscopic Approach
0BPT47Z Removal of Autologous Tissue Substitute from Diaphragm, Percutaneous Endoscopic Approach
0BPT4JZ Removal of Synthetic Substitute from Diaphragm, Percutaneous Endoscopic Approach
0BPT4KZ Removal of Nonautologous Tissue Substitute from Diaphragm, Percutaneous Endoscopic Approach
0BPT4MZ Removal of Diaphragmatic Pacemaker Lead from Diaphragm, Percutaneous Endoscopic Approach
0BPT70Z Removal of Drainage Device from Diaphragm, Via Natural or Artificial Opening
0BPT72Z Removal of Monitoring Device from Diaphragm, Via Natural or Artificial Opening
0BPT77Z Removal of Autologous Tissue Substitute from Diaphragm, Via Natural or Artificial Opening
0BPT7JZ Removal of Synthetic Substitute from Diaphragm, Via Natural or Artificial Opening
0BPT7KZ Removal of Nonautologous Tissue Substitute from Diaphragm, Via Natural or Artificial Opening
0BPT7MZ Removal of Diaphragmatic Pacemaker Lead from Diaphragm, Via Natural or Artificial Opening
0BPT80Z Removal of Drainage Device from Diaphragm, Via Natural or Artificial Opening Endoscopic
0BPT82Z Removal of Monitoring Device from Diaphragm, Via Natural or Artificial Opening Endoscopic
0BPT87Z Removal of Autologous Tissue Substitute from Diaphragm, Via Natural or Artificial Opening Endoscopic
0BPT8JZ Removal of Synthetic Substitute from Diaphragm, Via Natural or Artificial Opening Endoscopic
0BPT8KZ Removal of Nonautologous Tissue Substitute from Diaphragm, Via Natural or Artificial Opening Endoscopic
0BPT8MZ Removal of Diaphragmatic Pacemaker Lead from Diaphragm, Via Natural or Artificial Opening Endoscopic
0BPTX0Z Removal of Drainage Device from Diaphragm, External Approach
0BPTX2Z Removal of Monitoring Device from Diaphragm, External Approach
0BPTXMZ Removal of Diaphragmatic Pacemaker Lead from Diaphragm, External Approach

0BQ – Respiratory System, Repair

0BQ10ZZ Repair Trachea, Open Approach
0BQ13ZZ Repair Trachea, Percutaneous Approach
0BQ14ZZ Repair Trachea, Percutaneous Endoscopic Approach

0BQ17ZZ Repair Trachea, Via Natural or Artificial Opening
0BQ18ZZ Repair Trachea, Via Natural or Artificial Opening Endoscopic
0BQ20ZZ Repair Carina, Open Approach

♀ Female-only   ♂ Male-only   ⬤ Limited Coverage   ● Non-OR   🄷🄰🄲 HAC-associated procedure   ⬤ Non-covered procedures   ➕ Combination

0BQ23ZZ	Repair Carina, Percutaneous Approach
0BQ24ZZ	Repair Carina, Percutaneous Endoscopic Approach
0BQ27ZZ	Repair Carina, Via Natural or Artificial Opening
0BQ28ZZ	Repair Carina, Via Natural or Artificial Opening Endoscopic
0BQ30ZZ	Repair Right Main Bronchus, Open Approach
0BQ33ZZ	Repair Right Main Bronchus, Percutaneous Approach
0BQ34ZZ	Repair Right Main Bronchus, Percutaneous Endoscopic Approach
0BQ37ZZ	Repair Right Main Bronchus, Via Natural or Artificial Opening
0BQ38ZZ	Repair Right Main Bronchus, Via Natural or Artificial Opening Endoscopic
0BQ40ZZ	Repair Right Upper Lobe Bronchus, Open Approach
0BQ43ZZ	Repair Right Upper Lobe Bronchus, Percutaneous Approach
0BQ44ZZ	Repair Right Upper Lobe Bronchus, Percutaneous Endoscopic Approach
0BQ47ZZ	Repair Right Upper Lobe Bronchus, Via Natural or Artificial Opening
0BQ48ZZ	Repair Right Upper Lobe Bronchus, Via Natural or Artificial Opening Endoscopic
0BQ50ZZ	Repair Right Middle Lobe Bronchus, Open Approach
0BQ53ZZ	Repair Right Middle Lobe Bronchus, Percutaneous Approach
0BQ54ZZ	Repair Right Middle Lobe Bronchus, Percutaneous Endoscopic Approach
0BQ57ZZ	Repair Right Middle Lobe Bronchus, Via Natural or Artificial Opening
0BQ58ZZ	Repair Right Middle Lobe Bronchus, Via Natural or Artificial Opening Endoscopic
0BQ60ZZ	Repair Right Lower Lobe Bronchus, Open Approach
0BQ63ZZ	Repair Right Lower Lobe Bronchus, Percutaneous Approach
0BQ64ZZ	Repair Right Lower Lobe Bronchus, Percutaneous Endoscopic Approach
0BQ67ZZ	Repair Right Lower Lobe Bronchus, Via Natural or Artificial Opening
0BQ68ZZ	Repair Right Lower Lobe Bronchus, Via Natural or Artificial Opening Endoscopic
0BQ70ZZ	Repair Left Main Bronchus, Open Approach
0BQ73ZZ	Repair Left Main Bronchus, Percutaneous Approach
0BQ74ZZ	Repair Left Main Bronchus, Percutaneous Endoscopic Approach
0BQ77ZZ	Repair Left Main Bronchus, Via Natural or Artificial Opening
0BQ78ZZ	Repair Left Main Bronchus, Via Natural or Artificial Opening Endoscopic
0BQ80ZZ	Repair Left Upper Lobe Bronchus, Open Approach
0BQ83ZZ	Repair Left Upper Lobe Bronchus, Percutaneous Approach
0BQ84ZZ	Repair Left Upper Lobe Bronchus, Percutaneous Endoscopic Approach
0BQ87ZZ	Repair Left Upper Lobe Bronchus, Via Natural or Artificial Opening
0BQ88ZZ	Repair Left Upper Lobe Bronchus, Via Natural or Artificial Opening Endoscopic
0BQ90ZZ	Repair Lingula Bronchus, Open Approach
0BQ93ZZ	Repair Lingula Bronchus, Percutaneous Approach
0BQ94ZZ	Repair Lingula Bronchus, Percutaneous Endoscopic Approach
0BQ97ZZ	Repair Lingula Bronchus, Via Natural or Artificial Opening
0BQ98ZZ	Repair Lingula Bronchus, Via Natural or Artificial Opening Endoscopic
0BQB0ZZ	Repair Left Lower Lobe Bronchus, Open Approach
0BQB3ZZ	Repair Left Lower Lobe Bronchus, Percutaneous Approach
0BQB4ZZ	Repair Left Lower Lobe Bronchus, Percutaneous Endoscopic Approach
0BQB7ZZ	Repair Left Lower Lobe Bronchus, Via Natural or Artificial Opening
0BQB8ZZ	Repair Left Lower Lobe Bronchus, Via Natural or Artificial Opening Endoscopic
0BQC0ZZ	Repair Right Upper Lung Lobe, Open Approach
0BQC3ZZ	Repair Right Upper Lung Lobe, Percutaneous Approach
0BQC4ZZ	Repair Right Upper Lung Lobe, Percutaneous Endoscopic Approach
0BQC7ZZ	Repair Right Upper Lung Lobe, Via Natural or Artificial Opening
0BQC8ZZ	Repair Right Upper Lung Lobe, Via Natural or Artificial Opening Endoscopic
0BQD0ZZ	Repair Right Middle Lung Lobe, Open Approach
0BQD3ZZ	Repair Right Middle Lung Lobe, Percutaneous Approach
0BQD4ZZ	Repair Right Middle Lung Lobe, Percutaneous Endoscopic Approach
0BQD7ZZ	Repair Right Middle Lung Lobe, Via Natural or Artificial Opening
0BQD8ZZ	Repair Right Middle Lung Lobe, Via Natural or Artificial Opening Endoscopic
0BQF0ZZ	Repair Right Lower Lung Lobe, Open Approach
0BQF3ZZ	Repair Right Lower Lung Lobe, Percutaneous Approach
0BQF4ZZ	Repair Right Lower Lung Lobe, Percutaneous Endoscopic Approach
0BQF7ZZ	Repair Right Lower Lung Lobe, Via Natural or Artificial Opening
0BQF8ZZ	Repair Right Lower Lung Lobe, Via Natural or Artificial Opening Endoscopic
0BQG0ZZ	Repair Left Upper Lung Lobe, Open Approach
0BQG3ZZ	Repair Left Upper Lung Lobe, Percutaneous Approach
0BQG4ZZ	Repair Left Upper Lung Lobe, Percutaneous Endoscopic Approach
0BQG7ZZ	Repair Left Upper Lung Lobe, Via Natural or Artificial Opening
0BQG8ZZ	Repair Left Upper Lung Lobe, Via Natural or Artificial Opening Endoscopic
0BQH0ZZ	Repair Lung Lingula, Open Approach
0BQH3ZZ	Repair Lung Lingula, Percutaneous Approach
0BQH4ZZ	Repair Lung Lingula, Percutaneous Endoscopic Approach
0BQH7ZZ	Repair Lung Lingula, Via Natural or Artificial Opening
0BQH8ZZ	Repair Lung Lingula, Via Natural or Artificial Opening Endoscopic
0BQJ0ZZ	Repair Left Lower Lung Lobe, Open Approach
0BQJ3ZZ	Repair Left Lower Lung Lobe, Percutaneous Approach
0BQJ4ZZ	Repair Left Lower Lung Lobe, Percutaneous Endoscopic Approach
0BQJ7ZZ	Repair Left Lower Lung Lobe, Via Natural or Artificial Opening
0BQJ8ZZ	Repair Left Lower Lung Lobe, Via Natural or Artificial Opening Endoscopic
0BQK0ZZ	Repair Right Lung, Open Approach
0BQK3ZZ	Repair Right Lung, Percutaneous Approach
0BQK4ZZ	Repair Right Lung, Percutaneous Endoscopic Approach
0BQK7ZZ	Repair Right Lung, Via Natural or Artificial Opening
0BQK8ZZ	Repair Right Lung, Via Natural or Artificial Opening Endoscopic
0BQL0ZZ	Repair Left Lung, Open Approach
0BQL3ZZ	Repair Left Lung, Percutaneous Approach
0BQL4ZZ	Repair Left Lung, Percutaneous Endoscopic Approach
0BQL7ZZ	Repair Left Lung, Via Natural or Artificial Opening
0BQL8ZZ	Repair Left Lung, Via Natural or Artificial Opening Endoscopic
0BQM0ZZ	Repair Bilateral Lungs, Open Approach
0BQM3ZZ	Repair Bilateral Lungs, Percutaneous Approach
0BQM4ZZ	Repair Bilateral Lungs, Percutaneous Endoscopic Approach
0BQM7ZZ	Repair Bilateral Lungs, Via Natural or Artificial Opening
0BQM8ZZ	Repair Bilateral Lungs, Via Natural or Artificial Opening Endoscopic
0BQN0ZZ	Repair Right Pleura, Open Approach
0BQN3ZZ	Repair Right Pleura, Percutaneous Approach
0BQN4ZZ	Repair Right Pleura, Percutaneous Endoscopic Approach
0BQP0ZZ	Repair Left Pleura, Open Approach
0BQP3ZZ	Repair Left Pleura, Percutaneous Approach
0BQP4ZZ	Repair Left Pleura, Percutaneous Endoscopic Approach
0BQR0ZZ	Repair Right Diaphragm, Open Approach
0BQR3ZZ	Repair Right Diaphragm, Percutaneous Approach
0BQR4ZZ	Repair Right Diaphragm, Percutaneous Endoscopic Approach
0BQS0ZZ	Repair Left Diaphragm, Open Approach
0BQS3ZZ	Repair Left Diaphragm, Percutaneous Approach
0BQS4ZZ	Repair Left Diaphragm, Percutaneous Endoscopic Approach

0BS – Respiratory System, Reposition

0BS10ZZ	Reposition Trachea, Open Approach
0BS20ZZ	Reposition Carina, Open Approach
0BS30ZZ	Reposition Right Main Bronchus, Open Approach
0BS40ZZ	Reposition Right Upper Lobe Bronchus, Open Approach
0BS50ZZ	Reposition Right Middle Lobe Bronchus, Open Approach
0BS60ZZ	Reposition Right Lower Lobe Bronchus, Open Approach
0BS70ZZ	Reposition Left Main Bronchus, Open Approach
0BS80ZZ	Reposition Left Upper Lobe Bronchus, Open Approach
0BS90ZZ	Reposition Lingula Bronchus, Open Approach
0BSB0ZZ	Reposition Left Lower Lobe Bronchus, Open Approach
0BSC0ZZ	Reposition Right Upper Lung Lobe, Open Approach
0BSD0ZZ	Reposition Right Middle Lung Lobe, Open Approach
0BSF0ZZ	Reposition Right Lower Lung Lobe, Open Approach
0BSG0ZZ	Reposition Left Upper Lung Lobe, Open Approach

0BSH0ZZ	Reposition Lung Lingula, Open Approach
0BSJ0ZZ	Reposition Left Lower Lung Lobe, Open Approach
0BSK0ZZ	Reposition Right Lung, Open Approach
0BSL0ZZ	Reposition Left Lung, Open Approach
0BSR0ZZ	Reposition Right Diaphragm, Open Approach
0BSS0ZZ	Reposition Left Diaphragm, Open Approach

0BT – Respiratory System, Resection

Review Coding Guideline B3.8

0BT10ZZ	Resection of Trachea, Open Approach
0BT14ZZ	Resection of Trachea, Percutaneous Endoscopic Approach
0BT20ZZ	Resection of Carina, Open Approach
0BT24ZZ	Resection of Carina, Percutaneous Endoscopic Approach
0BT30ZZ	Resection of Right Main Bronchus, Open Approach
0BT34ZZ	Resection of Right Main Bronchus, Percutaneous Endoscopic Approach
0BT40ZZ	Resection of Right Upper Lobe Bronchus, Open Approach
0BT44ZZ	Resection of Right Upper Lobe Bronchus, Percutaneous Endoscopic Approach
0BT50ZZ	Resection of Right Middle Lobe Bronchus, Open Approach
0BT54ZZ	Resection of Right Middle Lobe Bronchus, Percutaneous Endoscopic Approach
0BT60ZZ	Resection of Right Lower Lobe Bronchus, Open Approach
0BT64ZZ	Resection of Right Lower Lobe Bronchus, Percutaneous Endoscopic Approach
0BT70ZZ	Resection of Left Main Bronchus, Open Approach
0BT74ZZ	Resection of Left Main Bronchus, Percutaneous Endoscopic Approach
0BT80ZZ	Resection of Left Upper Lobe Bronchus, Open Approach
0BT84ZZ	Resection of Left Upper Lobe Bronchus, Percutaneous Endoscopic Approach
0BT90ZZ	Resection of Lingula Bronchus, Open Approach
0BT94ZZ	Resection of Lingula Bronchus, Percutaneous Endoscopic Approach
0BTB0ZZ	Resection of Left Lower Lobe Bronchus, Open Approach
0BTB4ZZ	Resection of Left Lower Lobe Bronchus, Percutaneous Endoscopic Approach
0BTC0ZZ	Resection of Right Upper Lung Lobe, Open Approach
0BTC4ZZ	Resection of Right Upper Lung Lobe, Percutaneous Endoscopic Approach
0BTD0ZZ	Resection of Right Middle Lung Lobe, Open Approach
0BTD4ZZ	Resection of Right Middle Lung Lobe, Percutaneous Endoscopic Approach
0BTF0ZZ	Resection of Right Lower Lung Lobe, Open Approach
0BTF4ZZ	Resection of Right Lower Lung Lobe, Percutaneous Endoscopic Approach
0BTG0ZZ	Resection of Left Upper Lung Lobe, Open Approach
0BTG4ZZ	Resection of Left Upper Lung Lobe, Percutaneous Endoscopic Approach
0BTH0ZZ	Resection of Lung Lingula, Open Approach
0BTH4ZZ	Resection of Lung Lingula, Percutaneous Endoscopic Approach
0BTJ0ZZ	Resection of Left Lower Lung Lobe, Open Approach
0BTJ4ZZ	Resection of Left Lower Lung Lobe, Percutaneous Endoscopic Approach
0BTK0ZZ	Resection of Right Lung, Open Approach
0BTK4ZZ	Resection of Right Lung, Percutaneous Endoscopic Approach
0BTL0ZZ	Resection of Left Lung, Open Approach
0BTL4ZZ	Resection of Left Lung, Percutaneous Endoscopic Approach
0BTM0ZZ	Resection of Bilateral Lungs, Open Approach
0BTM4ZZ	Resection of Bilateral Lungs, Percutaneous Endoscopic Approach
0BTR0ZZ	Resection of Right Diaphragm, Open Approach
0BTR4ZZ	Resection of Right Diaphragm, Percutaneous Endoscopic Approach
0BTS0ZZ	Resection of Left Diaphragm, Open Approach
0BTS4ZZ	Resection of Left Diaphragm, Percutaneous Endoscopic Approach

0BU – Respiratory System, Supplement

0BU107Z	Supplement Trachea with Autologous Tissue Substitute, Open Approach
0BU10JZ	Supplement Trachea with Synthetic Substitute, Open Approach
0BU10KZ	Supplement Trachea with Nonautologous Tissue Substitute, Open Approach
0BU147Z	Supplement Trachea with Autologous Tissue Substitute, Percutaneous Endoscopic Approach
0BU14JZ	Supplement Trachea with Synthetic Substitute, Percutaneous Endoscopic Approach
0BU14KZ	Supplement Trachea with Nonautologous Tissue Substitute, Percutaneous Endoscopic Approach
0BU207Z	Supplement Carina with Autologous Tissue Substitute, Open Approach
0BU20JZ	Supplement Carina with Synthetic Substitute, Open Approach
0BU20KZ	Supplement Carina with Nonautologous Tissue Substitute, Open Approach
0BU247Z	Supplement Carina with Autologous Tissue Substitute, Percutaneous Endoscopic Approach
0BU24JZ	Supplement Carina with Synthetic Substitute, Percutaneous Endoscopic Approach
0BU24KZ	Supplement Carina with Nonautologous Tissue Substitute, Percutaneous Endoscopic Approach
0BU307Z	Supplement Right Main Bronchus with Autologous Tissue Substitute, Open Approach
0BU30JZ	Supplement Right Main Bronchus with Synthetic Substitute, Open Approach
0BU30KZ	Supplement Right Main Bronchus with Nonautologous Tissue Substitute, Open Approach
0BU347Z	Supplement Right Main Bronchus with Autologous Tissue Substitute, Percutaneous Endoscopic Approach
0BU34JZ	Supplement Right Main Bronchus with Synthetic Substitute, Percutaneous Endoscopic Approach
0BU34KZ	Supplement Right Main Bronchus with Nonautologous Tissue Substitute, Percutaneous Endoscopic Approach
0BU407Z	Supplement Right Upper Lobe Bronchus with Autologous Tissue Substitute, Open Approach
0BU40JZ	Supplement Right Upper Lobe Bronchus with Synthetic Substitute, Open Approach
0BU40KZ	Supplement Right Upper Lobe Bronchus with Nonautologous Tissue Substitute, Open Approach
0BU447Z	Supplement Right Upper Lobe Bronchus with Autologous Tissue Substitute, Percutaneous Endoscopic Approach
0BU44JZ	Supplement Right Upper Lobe Bronchus with Synthetic Substitute, Percutaneous Endoscopic Approach
0BU44KZ	Supplement Right Upper Lobe Bronchus with Nonautologous Tissue Substitute, Percutaneous Endoscopic Approach
0BU507Z	Supplement Right Middle Lobe Bronchus with Autologous Tissue Substitute, Open Approach
0BU50JZ	Supplement Right Middle Lobe Bronchus with Synthetic Substitute, Open Approach
0BU50KZ	Supplement Right Middle Lobe Bronchus with Nonautologous Tissue Substitute, Open Approach
0BU547Z	Supplement Right Middle Lobe Bronchus with Autologous Tissue Substitute, Percutaneous Endoscopic Approach
0BU54JZ	Supplement Right Middle Lobe Bronchus with Synthetic Substitute, Percutaneous Endoscopic Approach
0BU54KZ	Supplement Right Middle Lobe Bronchus with Nonautologous Tissue Substitute, Percutaneous Endoscopic Approach
0BU607Z	Supplement Right Lower Lobe Bronchus with Autologous Tissue Substitute, Open Approach
0BU60JZ	Supplement Right Lower Lobe Bronchus with Synthetic Substitute, Open Approach
0BU60KZ	Supplement Right Lower Lobe Bronchus with Nonautologous Tissue Substitute, Open Approach
0BU647Z	Supplement Right Lower Lobe Bronchus with Autologous Tissue Substitute, Percutaneous Endoscopic Approach
0BU64JZ	Supplement Right Lower Lobe Bronchus with Synthetic Substitute, Percutaneous Endoscopic Approach
0BU64KZ	Supplement Right Lower Lobe Bronchus with Nonautologous Tissue Substitute, Percutaneous Endoscopic Approach
0BU707Z	Supplement Left Main Bronchus with Autologous Tissue Substitute, Open Approach

0BU70JZ   Supplement Left Main Bronchus with Synthetic Substitute, Open Approach

0BU70KZ   Supplement Left Main Bronchus with Nonautologous Tissue Substitute, Open Approach

0BU747Z   Supplement Left Main Bronchus with Autologous Tissue Substitute, Percutaneous Endoscopic Approach

0BU74JZ   Supplement Left Main Bronchus with Synthetic Substitute, Percutaneous Endoscopic Approach

0BU74KZ   Supplement Left Main Bronchus with Nonautologous Tissue Substitute, Percutaneous Endoscopic Approach

0BU807Z   Supplement Left Upper Lobe Bronchus with Autologous Tissue Substitute, Open Approach

0BU80JZ   Supplement Left Upper Lobe Bronchus with Synthetic Substitute, Open Approach

0BU80KZ   Supplement Left Upper Lobe Bronchus with Nonautologous Tissue Substitute, Open Approach

0BU847Z   Supplement Left Upper Lobe Bronchus with Autologous Tissue Substitute, Percutaneous Endoscopic Approach

0BU84JZ   Supplement Left Upper Lobe Bronchus with Synthetic Substitute, Percutaneous Endoscopic Approach

0BU84KZ   Supplement Left Upper Lobe Bronchus with Nonautologous Tissue Substitute, Percutaneous Endoscopic Approach

0BU907Z   Supplement Lingula Bronchus with Autologous Tissue Substitute, Open Approach

0BU90JZ   Supplement Lingula Bronchus with Synthetic Substitute, Open Approach

0BU90KZ   Supplement Lingula Bronchus with Nonautologous Tissue Substitute, Open Approach

0BU947Z   Supplement Lingula Bronchus with Autologous Tissue Substitute, Percutaneous Endoscopic Approach

0BU94JZ   Supplement Lingula Bronchus with Synthetic Substitute, Percutaneous Endoscopic Approach

0BU94KZ   Supplement Lingula Bronchus with Nonautologous Tissue Substitute, Percutaneous Endoscopic Approach

0BUB07Z   Supplement Left Lower Lobe Bronchus with Autologous Tissue Substitute, Open Approach

0BUB0JZ   Supplement Left Lower Lobe Bronchus with Synthetic Substitute, Open Approach

0BUB0KZ   Supplement Left Lower Lobe Bronchus with Nonautologous Tissue Substitute, Open Approach

0BUB47Z   Supplement Left Lower Lobe Bronchus with Autologous Tissue Substitute, Percutaneous Endoscopic Approach

0BUB4JZ   Supplement Left Lower Lobe Bronchus with Synthetic Substitute, Percutaneous Endoscopic Approach

0BUB4KZ   Supplement Left Lower Lobe Bronchus with Nonautologous Tissue Substitute, Percutaneous Endoscopic Approach

0BUR07Z   Supplement Right Diaphragm with Autologous Tissue Substitute, Open Approach

0BUR0JZ   Supplement Right Diaphragm with Synthetic Substitute, Open Approach

0BUR0KZ   Supplement Right Diaphragm with Nonautologous Tissue Substitute, Open Approach

0BUR47Z   Supplement Right Diaphragm with Autologous Tissue Substitute, Percutaneous Endoscopic Approach

0BUR4JZ   Supplement Right Diaphragm with Synthetic Substitute, Percutaneous Endoscopic Approach

0BUR4KZ   Supplement Right Diaphragm with Nonautologous Tissue Substitute, Percutaneous Endoscopic Approach

0BUS07Z   Supplement Left Diaphragm with Autologous Tissue Substitute, Open Approach

0BUS0JZ   Supplement Left Diaphragm with Synthetic Substitute, Open Approach

0BUS0KZ   Supplement Left Diaphragm with Nonautologous Tissue Substitute, Open Approach

0BUS47Z   Supplement Left Diaphragm with Autologous Tissue Substitute, Percutaneous Endoscopic Approach

0BUS4JZ   Supplement Left Diaphragm with Synthetic Substitute, Percutaneous Endoscopic Approach

0BUS4KZ   Supplement Left Diaphragm with Nonautologous Tissue Substitute, Percutaneous Endoscopic Approach

0BV – Respiratory System, Restriction

0BV10CZ   Restriction of Trachea with Extraluminal Device, Open Approach

0BV10DZ   Restriction of Trachea with Intraluminal Device, Open Approach

0BV10ZZ   Restriction of Trachea, Open Approach

0BV13CZ   Restriction of Trachea with Extraluminal Device, Percutaneous Approach

0BV13DZ   Restriction of Trachea with Intraluminal Device, Percutaneous Approach

0BV13ZZ   Restriction of Trachea, Percutaneous Approach

0BV14CZ   Restriction of Trachea with Extraluminal Device, Percutaneous Endoscopic Approach

0BV14DZ   Restriction of Trachea with Intraluminal Device, Percutaneous Endoscopic Approach

0BV14ZZ   Restriction of Trachea, Percutaneous Endoscopic Approach

0BV17DZ   Restriction of Trachea with Intraluminal Device, Via Natural or Artificial Opening

0BV17ZZ   Restriction of Trachea, Via Natural or Artificial Opening

0BV18DZ   Restriction of Trachea with Intraluminal Device, Via Natural or Artificial Opening Endoscopic

0BV18ZZ   Restriction of Trachea, Via Natural or Artificial Opening Endoscopic

0BV20CZ   Restriction of Carina with Extraluminal Device, Open Approach

0BV20DZ   Restriction of Carina with Intraluminal Device, Open Approach

0BV20ZZ   Restriction of Carina, Open Approach

0BV23CZ   Restriction of Carina with Extraluminal Device, Percutaneous Approach

0BV23DZ   Restriction of Carina with Intraluminal Device, Percutaneous Approach

0BV23ZZ   Restriction of Carina, Percutaneous Approach

0BV24CZ   Restriction of Carina with Extraluminal Device, Percutaneous Endoscopic Approach

0BV24DZ   Restriction of Carina with Intraluminal Device, Percutaneous Endoscopic Approach

0BV24ZZ   Restriction of Carina, Percutaneous Endoscopic Approach

0BV27DZ   Restriction of Carina with Intraluminal Device, Via Natural or Artificial Opening

0BV27ZZ   Restriction of Carina, Via Natural or Artificial Opening

0BV28DZ   Restriction of Carina with Intraluminal Device, Via Natural or Artificial Opening Endoscopic

0BV28ZZ   Restriction of Carina, Via Natural or Artificial Opening Endoscopic

0BV30CZ   Restriction of Right Main Bronchus with Extraluminal Device, Open Approach

0BV30DZ   Restriction of Right Main Bronchus with Intraluminal Device, Open Approach

0BV30ZZ   Restriction of Right Main Bronchus, Open Approach

0BV33CZ   Restriction of Right Main Bronchus with Extraluminal Device, Percutaneous Approach

0BV33DZ   Restriction of Right Main Bronchus with Intraluminal Device, Percutaneous Approach

0BV33ZZ   Restriction of Right Main Bronchus, Percutaneous Approach

0BV34CZ   Restriction of Right Main Bronchus with Extraluminal Device, Percutaneous Endoscopic Approach

0BV34DZ   Restriction of Right Main Bronchus with Intraluminal Device, Percutaneous Endoscopic Approach

0BV34ZZ   Restriction of Right Main Bronchus, Percutaneous Endoscopic Approach

0BV37DZ   Restriction of Right Main Bronchus with Intraluminal Device, Via Natural or Artificial Opening

0BV37ZZ   Restriction of Right Main Bronchus, Via Natural or Artificial Opening

0BV38DZ   Restriction of Right Main Bronchus with Intraluminal Device, Via Natural or Artificial Opening Endoscopic

0BV38ZZ   Restriction of Right Main Bronchus, Via Natural or Artificial Opening Endoscopic

0BV40CZ   Restriction of Right Upper Lobe Bronchus with Extraluminal Device, Open Approach

0BV40DZ   Restriction of Right Upper Lobe Bronchus with Intraluminal Device, Open Approach

0BV40ZZ   Restriction of Right Upper Lobe Bronchus, Open Approach

0BV43CZ   Restriction of Right Upper Lobe Bronchus with Extraluminal Device, Percutaneous Approach

0BV43DZ Restriction of Right Upper Lobe Bronchus with Intraluminal Device, Percutaneous Approach

0BV43ZZ Restriction of Right Upper Lobe Bronchus, Percutaneous Approach

0BV44CZ Restriction of Right Upper Lobe Bronchus with Extraluminal Device, Percutaneous Endoscopic Approach

0BV44DZ Restriction of Right Upper Lobe Bronchus with Intraluminal Device, Percutaneous Endoscopic Approach

0BV44ZZ Restriction of Right Upper Lobe Bronchus, Percutaneous Endoscopic Approach

0BV47DZ Restriction of Right Upper Lobe Bronchus with Intraluminal Device, Via Natural or Artificial Opening

0BV47ZZ Restriction of Right Upper Lobe Bronchus, Via Natural or Artificial Opening

0BV48DZ Restriction of Right Upper Lobe Bronchus with Intraluminal Device, Via Natural or Artificial Opening Endoscopic

0BV48ZZ Restriction of Right Upper Lobe Bronchus, Via Natural or Artificial Opening Endoscopic

0BV50CZ Restriction of Right Middle Lobe Bronchus with Extraluminal Device, Open Approach

0BV50DZ Restriction of Right Middle Lobe Bronchus with Intraluminal Device, Open Approach

0BV50ZZ Restriction of Right Middle Lobe Bronchus, Open Approach

0BV53CZ Restriction of Right Middle Lobe Bronchus with Extraluminal Device, Percutaneous Approach

0BV53DZ Restriction of Right Middle Lobe Bronchus with Intraluminal Device, Percutaneous Approach

0BV53ZZ Restriction of Right Middle Lobe Bronchus, Percutaneous Approach

0BV54CZ Restriction of Right Middle Lobe Bronchus with Extraluminal Device, Percutaneous Endoscopic Approach

0BV54DZ Restriction of Right Middle Lobe Bronchus with Intraluminal Device, Percutaneous Endoscopic Approach

0BV54ZZ Restriction of Right Middle Lobe Bronchus, Percutaneous Endoscopic Approach

0BV57DZ Restriction of Right Middle Lobe Bronchus with Intraluminal Device, Via Natural or Artificial Opening

0BV57ZZ Restriction of Right Middle Lobe Bronchus, Via Natural or Artificial Opening

0BV58DZ Restriction of Right Middle Lobe Bronchus with Intraluminal Device, Via Natural or Artificial Opening Endoscopic

0BV58ZZ Restriction of Right Middle Lobe Bronchus, Via Natural or Artificial Opening Endoscopic

0BV60CZ Restriction of Right Lower Lobe Bronchus with Extraluminal Device, Open Approach

0BV60DZ Restriction of Right Lower Lobe Bronchus with Intraluminal Device, Open Approach

0BV60ZZ Restriction of Right Lower Lobe Bronchus, Open Approach

0BV63CZ Restriction of Right Lower Lobe Bronchus with Extraluminal Device, Percutaneous Approach

0BV63DZ Restriction of Right Lower Lobe Bronchus with Intraluminal Device, Percutaneous Approach

0BV63ZZ Restriction of Right Lower Lobe Bronchus, Percutaneous Approach

0BV64CZ Restriction of Right Lower Lobe Bronchus with Extraluminal Device, Percutaneous Endoscopic Approach

0BV64DZ Restriction of Right Lower Lobe Bronchus with Intraluminal Device, Percutaneous Endoscopic Approach

0BV64ZZ Restriction of Right Lower Lobe Bronchus, Percutaneous Endoscopic Approach

0BV67DZ Restriction of Right Lower Lobe Bronchus with Intraluminal Device, Via Natural or Artificial Opening

0BV67ZZ Restriction of Right Lower Lobe Bronchus, Via Natural or Artificial Opening

0BV68DZ Restriction of Right Lower Lobe Bronchus with Intraluminal Device, Via Natural or Artificial Opening Endoscopic

0BV68ZZ Restriction of Right Lower Lobe Bronchus, Via Natural or Artificial Opening Endoscopic

0BV70CZ Restriction of Left Main Bronchus with Extraluminal Device, Open Approach

0BV70DZ Restriction of Left Main Bronchus with Intraluminal Device, Open Approach

0BV70ZZ Restriction of Left Main Bronchus, Open Approach

0BV73CZ Restriction of Left Main Bronchus with Extraluminal Device, Percutaneous Approach

0BV73DZ Restriction of Left Main Bronchus with Intraluminal Device, Percutaneous Approach

0BV73ZZ Restriction of Left Main Bronchus, Percutaneous Approach

0BV74CZ Restriction of Left Main Bronchus with Extraluminal Device, Percutaneous Endoscopic Approach

0BV74DZ Restriction of Left Main Bronchus with Intraluminal Device, Percutaneous Endoscopic Approach

0BV74ZZ Restriction of Left Main Bronchus, Percutaneous Endoscopic Approach

0BV77DZ Restriction of Left Main Bronchus with Intraluminal Device, Via Natural or Artificial Opening

0BV77ZZ Restriction of Left Main Bronchus, Via Natural or Artificial Opening

0BV78DZ Restriction of Left Main Bronchus with Intraluminal Device, Via Natural or Artificial Opening Endoscopic

0BV78ZZ Restriction of Left Main Bronchus, Via Natural or Artificial Opening Endoscopic

0BV80CZ Restriction of Left Upper Lobe Bronchus with Extraluminal Device, Open Approach

0BV80DZ Restriction of Left Upper Lobe Bronchus with Intraluminal Device, Open Approach

0BV80ZZ Restriction of Left Upper Lobe Bronchus, Open Approach

0BV83CZ Restriction of Left Upper Lobe Bronchus with Extraluminal Device, Percutaneous Approach

0BV83DZ Restriction of Left Upper Lobe Bronchus with Intraluminal Device, Percutaneous Approach

0BV83ZZ Restriction of Left Upper Lobe Bronchus, Percutaneous Approach

0BV84CZ Restriction of Left Upper Lobe Bronchus with Extraluminal Device, Percutaneous Endoscopic Approach

0BV84DZ Restriction of Left Upper Lobe Bronchus with Intraluminal Device, Percutaneous Endoscopic Approach

0BV84ZZ Restriction of Left Upper Lobe Bronchus, Percutaneous Endoscopic Approach

0BV87DZ Restriction of Left Upper Lobe Bronchus with Intraluminal Device, Via Natural or Artificial Opening

0BV87ZZ Restriction of Left Upper Lobe Bronchus, Via Natural or Artificial Opening

0BV88DZ Restriction of Left Upper Lobe Bronchus with Intraluminal Device, Via Natural or Artificial Opening Endoscopic

0BV88ZZ Restriction of Left Upper Lobe Bronchus, Via Natural or Artificial Opening Endoscopic

0BV90CZ Restriction of Lingula Bronchus with Extraluminal Device, Open Approach

0BV90DZ Restriction of Lingula Bronchus with Intraluminal Device, Open Approach

0BV90ZZ Restriction of Lingula Bronchus, Open Approach

0BV93CZ Restriction of Lingula Bronchus with Extraluminal Device, Percutaneous Approach

0BV93DZ Restriction of Lingula Bronchus with Intraluminal Device, Percutaneous Approach

0BV93ZZ Restriction of Lingula Bronchus, Percutaneous Approach

0BV94CZ Restriction of Lingula Bronchus with Extraluminal Device, Percutaneous Endoscopic Approach

0BV94DZ Restriction of Lingula Bronchus with Intraluminal Device, Percutaneous Endoscopic Approach

0BV94ZZ Restriction of Lingula Bronchus, Percutaneous Endoscopic Approach

0BV97DZ Restriction of Lingula Bronchus with Intraluminal Device, Via Natural or Artificial Opening

0BV97ZZ Restriction of Lingula Bronchus, Via Natural or Artificial Opening

0BV98DZ Restriction of Lingula Bronchus with Intraluminal Device, Via Natural or Artificial Opening Endoscopic

0BV98ZZ Restriction of Lingula Bronchus, Via Natural or Artificial Opening Endoscopic

0BVB0CZ Restriction of Left Lower Lobe Bronchus with Extraluminal Device, Open Approach

0BVB0DZ Restriction of Left Lower Lobe Bronchus with Intraluminal Device, Open Approach

0BVB0ZZ Restriction of Left Lower Lobe Bronchus, Open Approach

0BVB3CZ Restriction of Left Lower Lobe Bronchus with Extraluminal Device, Percutaneous Approach

0BVB3DZ Restriction of Left Lower Lobe Bronchus with Intraluminal Device, Percutaneous Approach

0BVB3ZZ Restriction of Left Lower Lobe Bronchus, Percutaneous Approach

0BVB4CZ Restriction of Left Lower Lobe Bronchus with Extraluminal Device, Percutaneous Endoscopic Approach

0BVB4DZ Restriction of Left Lower Lobe Bronchus with Intraluminal Device, Percutaneous Endoscopic Approach

0BVB4ZZ Restriction of Left Lower Lobe Bronchus, Percutaneous Endoscopic Approach

0BVB7DZ Restriction of Left Lower Lobe Bronchus with Intraluminal Device, Via Natural or Artificial Opening

0BVB7ZZ Restriction of Left Lower Lobe Bronchus, Via Natural or Artificial Opening

0BVB8DZ Restriction of Left Lower Lobe Bronchus with Intraluminal Device, Via Natural or Artificial Opening Endoscopic

0BVB8ZZ Restriction of Left Lower Lobe Bronchus, Via Natural or Artificial Opening Endoscopic

0BW – Respiratory System, Revision

Review Coding Guideline B6.1c

0BW000Z Revision of Drainage Device in Tracheobronchial Tree, Open Approach

0BW002Z Revision of Monitoring Device in Tracheobronchial Tree, Open Approach

0BW003Z Revision of Infusion Device in Tracheobronchial Tree, Open Approach

0BW007Z Revision of Autologous Tissue Substitute in Tracheobronchial Tree, Open Approach

0BW00CZ Revision of Extraluminal Device in Tracheobronchial Tree, Open Approach

0BW00DZ Revision of Intraluminal Device in Tracheobronchial Tree, Open Approach

0BW00JZ Revision of Synthetic Substitute in Tracheobronchial Tree, Open Approach

0BW00KZ Revision of Nonautologous Tissue Substitute in Tracheobronchial Tree, Open Approach

0BW030Z Revision of Drainage Device in Tracheobronchial Tree, Percutaneous Approach

0BW032Z Revision of Monitoring Device in Tracheobronchial Tree, Percutaneous Approach

0BW033Z Revision of Infusion Device in Tracheobronchial Tree, Percutaneous Approach

0BW037Z Revision of Autologous Tissue Substitute in Tracheobronchial Tree, Percutaneous Approach

0BW03CZ Revision of Extraluminal Device in Tracheobronchial Tree, Percutaneous Approach

0BW03DZ Revision of Intraluminal Device in Tracheobronchial Tree, Percutaneous Approach

0BW03JZ Revision of Synthetic Substitute in Tracheobronchial Tree, Percutaneous Approach

0BW03KZ Revision of Nonautologous Tissue Substitute in Tracheobronchial Tree, Percutaneous Approach

0BW040Z Revision of Drainage Device in Tracheobronchial Tree, Percutaneous Endoscopic Approach

0BW042Z Revision of Monitoring Device in Tracheobronchial Tree, Percutaneous Endoscopic Approach

0BW043Z Revision of Infusion Device in Tracheobronchial Tree, Percutaneous Endoscopic Approach

0BW047Z Revision of Autologous Tissue Substitute in Tracheobronchial Tree, Percutaneous Endoscopic Approach

0BW04CZ Revision of Extraluminal Device in Tracheobronchial Tree, Percutaneous Endoscopic Approach

0BW04DZ Revision of Intraluminal Device in Tracheobronchial Tree, Percutaneous Endoscopic Approach

0BW04JZ Revision of Synthetic Substitute in Tracheobronchial Tree, Percutaneous Endoscopic Approach

0BW04KZ Revision of Nonautologous Tissue Substitute in Tracheobronchial Tree, Percutaneous Endoscopic Approach

0BW070Z Revision of Drainage Device in Tracheobronchial Tree, Via Natural or Artificial Opening

0BW072Z Revision of Monitoring Device in Tracheobronchial Tree, Via Natural or Artificial Opening

0BW073Z Revision of Infusion Device in Tracheobronchial Tree, Via Natural or Artificial Opening

0BW077Z Revision of Autologous Tissue Substitute in Tracheobronchial Tree, Via Natural or Artificial Opening

0BW07CZ Revision of Extraluminal Device in Tracheobronchial Tree, Via Natural or Artificial Opening

0BW07DZ Revision of Intraluminal Device in Tracheobronchial Tree, Via Natural or Artificial Opening

0BW07JZ Revision of Synthetic Substitute in Tracheobronchial Tree, Via Natural or Artificial Opening

0BW07KZ Revision of Nonautologous Tissue Substitute in Tracheobronchial Tree, Via Natural or Artificial Opening

0BW080Z Revision of Drainage Device in Tracheobronchial Tree, Via Natural or Artificial Opening Endoscopic

0BW082Z Revision of Monitoring Device in Tracheobronchial Tree, Via Natural or Artificial Opening Endoscopic

0BW083Z Revision of Infusion Device in Tracheobronchial Tree, Via Natural or Artificial Opening Endoscopic

0BW087Z Revision of Autologous Tissue Substitute in Tracheobronchial Tree, Via Natural or Artificial Opening Endoscopic

0BW08CZ Revision of Extraluminal Device in Tracheobronchial Tree, Via Natural or Artificial Opening Endoscopic

0BW08DZ Revision of Intraluminal Device in Tracheobronchial Tree, Via Natural or Artificial Opening Endoscopic

0BW08JZ Revision of Synthetic Substitute in Tracheobronchial Tree, Via Natural or Artificial Opening Endoscopic

0BW08KZ Revision of Nonautologous Tissue Substitute in Tracheobronchial Tree, Via Natural or Artificial Opening Endoscopic

0BW0X0Z Revision of Drainage Device in Tracheobronchial Tree, External Approach

0BW0X2Z Revision of Monitoring Device in Tracheobronchial Tree, External Approach

0BW0X3Z Revision of Infusion Device in Tracheobronchial Tree, External Approach

0BW0X7Z Revision of Autologous Tissue Substitute in Tracheobronchial Tree, External Approach

0BW0XCZ Revision of Extraluminal Device in Tracheobronchial Tree, External Approach

0BW0XDZ Revision of Intraluminal Device in Tracheobronchial Tree, External Approach

0BW0XJZ Revision of Synthetic Substitute in Tracheobronchial Tree, External Approach

0BW0XKZ Revision of Nonautologous Tissue Substitute in Tracheobronchial Tree, External Approach

0BW100Z Revision of Drainage Device in Trachea, Open Approach

0BW102Z Revision of Monitoring Device in Trachea, Open Approach

0BW107Z Revision of Autologous Tissue Substitute in Trachea, Open Approach

0BW10CZ Revision of Extraluminal Device in Trachea, Open Approach

0BW10DZ Revision of Intraluminal Device in Trachea, Open Approach

0BW10FZ Revision of Tracheostomy Device in Trachea, Open Approach

0BW10JZ Revision of Synthetic Substitute in Trachea, Open Approach

0BW10KZ Revision of Nonautologous Tissue Substitute in Trachea, Open Approach

0BW130Z Revision of Drainage Device in Trachea, Percutaneous Approach

0BW132Z Revision of Monitoring Device in Trachea, Percutaneous Approach

0BW137Z Revision of Autologous Tissue Substitute in Trachea, Percutaneous Approach

0BW13CZ Revision of Extraluminal Device in Trachea, Percutaneous Approach

0BW13DZ Revision of Intraluminal Device in Trachea, Percutaneous Approach

0BW13FZ Revision of Tracheostomy Device in Trachea, Percutaneous Approach

0BW13JZ Revision of Synthetic Substitute in Trachea, Percutaneous Approach

0BW13KZ Revision of Nonautologous Tissue Substitute in Trachea, Percutaneous Approach

0BW140Z Revision of Drainage Device in Trachea, Percutaneous Endoscopic Approach

0BW142Z Revision of Monitoring Device in Trachea, Percutaneous Endoscopic Approach

0BW147Z Revision of Autologous Tissue Substitute in Trachea, Percutaneous Endoscopic Approach

0BW14CZ Revision of Extraluminal Device in Trachea, Percutaneous Endoscopic Approach

0BW14DZ Revision of Intraluminal Device in Trachea, Percutaneous Endoscopic Approach

0BW14FZ Revision of Tracheostomy Device in Trachea, Percutaneous Endoscopic Approach

0BW14JZ Revision of Synthetic Substitute in Trachea, Percutaneous Endoscopic Approach

0BW14KZ Revision of Nonautologous Tissue Substitute in Trachea, Percutaneous Endoscopic Approach

0BW170Z Revision of Drainage Device in Trachea, Via Natural or Artificial Opening

0BW172Z Revision of Monitoring Device in Trachea, Via Natural or Artificial Opening

0BW177Z Revision of Autologous Tissue Substitute in Trachea, Via Natural or Artificial Opening

0BW17CZ Revision of Extraluminal Device in Trachea, Via Natural or Artificial Opening

0BW17DZ Revision of Intraluminal Device in Trachea, Via Natural or Artificial Opening

0BW17FZ Revision of Tracheostomy Device in Trachea, Via Natural or Artificial Opening

0BW17JZ Revision of Synthetic Substitute in Trachea, Via Natural or Artificial Opening

0BW17KZ Revision of Nonautologous Tissue Substitute in Trachea, Via Natural or Artificial Opening

0BW180Z Revision of Drainage Device in Trachea, Via Natural or Artificial Opening Endoscopic

0BW182Z Revision of Monitoring Device in Trachea, Via Natural or Artificial Opening Endoscopic

0BW187Z Revision of Autologous Tissue Substitute in Trachea, Via Natural or Artificial Opening Endoscopic

0BW18CZ Revision of Extraluminal Device in Trachea, Via Natural or Artificial Opening Endoscopic

0BW18DZ Revision of Intraluminal Device in Trachea, Via Natural or Artificial Opening Endoscopic

0BW18FZ Revision of Tracheostomy Device in Trachea, Via Natural or Artificial Opening Endoscopic

0BW18JZ Revision of Synthetic Substitute in Trachea, Via Natural or Artificial Opening Endoscopic

0BW18KZ Revision of Nonautologous Tissue Substitute in Trachea, Via Natural or Artificial Opening Endoscopic

0BW1X0Z Revision of Drainage Device in Trachea, External Approach

0BW1X2Z Revision of Monitoring Device in Trachea, External Approach

0BW1X7Z Revision of Autologous Tissue Substitute in Trachea, External Approach

0BW1XCZ Revision of Extraluminal Device in Trachea, External Approach

0BW1XDZ Revision of Intraluminal Device in Trachea, External Approach

0BW1XFZ Revision of Tracheostomy Device in Trachea, External Approach

0BW1XJZ Revision of Synthetic Substitute in Trachea, External Approach

0BW1XKZ Revision of Nonautologous Tissue Substitute in Trachea, External Approach

0BWK00Z Revision of Drainage Device in Right Lung, Open Approach

0BWK02Z Revision of Monitoring Device in Right Lung, Open Approach

0BWK03Z Revision of Infusion Device in Right Lung, Open Approach

0BWK30Z Revision of Drainage Device in Right Lung, Percutaneous Approach

0BWK32Z Revision of Monitoring Device in Right Lung, Percutaneous Approach

0BWK33Z Revision of Infusion Device in Right Lung, Percutaneous Approach

0BWK40Z Revision of Drainage Device in Right Lung, Percutaneous Endoscopic Approach

0BWK42Z Revision of Monitoring Device in Right Lung, Percutaneous Endoscopic Approach

0BWK43Z Revision of Infusion Device in Right Lung, Percutaneous Endoscopic Approach

0BWK70Z Revision of Drainage Device in Right Lung, Via Natural or Artificial Opening

0BWK72Z Revision of Monitoring Device in Right Lung, Via Natural or Artificial Opening

0BWK73Z Revision of Infusion Device in Right Lung, Via Natural or Artificial Opening

0BWK80Z Revision of Drainage Device in Right Lung, Via Natural or Artificial Opening Endoscopic

0BWK82Z Revision of Monitoring Device in Right Lung, Via Natural or Artificial Opening Endoscopic

0BWK83Z Revision of Infusion Device in Right Lung, Via Natural or Artificial Opening Endoscopic

0BWKX0Z Revision of Drainage Device in Right Lung, External Approach

0BWKX2Z Revision of Monitoring Device in Right Lung, External Approach

0BWKX3Z Revision of Infusion Device in Right Lung, External Approach

0BWL00Z Revision of Drainage Device in Left Lung, Open Approach

0BWL02Z Revision of Monitoring Device in Left Lung, Open Approach

0BWL03Z Revision of Infusion Device in Left Lung, Open Approach

0BWL30Z Revision of Drainage Device in Left Lung, Percutaneous Approach

0BWL32Z Revision of Monitoring Device in Left Lung, Percutaneous Approach

0BWL33Z Revision of Infusion Device in Left Lung, Percutaneous Approach

0BWL40Z Revision of Drainage Device in Left Lung, Percutaneous Endoscopic Approach

0BWL42Z Revision of Monitoring Device in Left Lung, Percutaneous Endoscopic Approach

0BWL43Z Revision of Infusion Device in Left Lung, Percutaneous Endoscopic Approach

0BWL70Z Revision of Drainage Device in Left Lung, Via Natural or Artificial Opening

0BWL72Z Revision of Monitoring Device in Left Lung, Via Natural or Artificial Opening

0BWL73Z Revision of Infusion Device in Left Lung, Via Natural or Artificial Opening

0BWL80Z Revision of Drainage Device in Left Lung, Via Natural or Artificial Opening Endoscopic

0BWL82Z Revision of Monitoring Device in Left Lung, Via Natural or Artificial Opening Endoscopic

0BWL83Z Revision of Infusion Device in Left Lung, Via Natural or Artificial Opening Endoscopic

0BWLX0Z Revision of Drainage Device in Left Lung, External Approach

0BWLX2Z Revision of Monitoring Device in Left Lung, External Approach

0BWLX3Z Revision of Infusion Device in Left Lung, External Approach

0BWQ00Z Revision of Drainage Device in Pleura, Open Approach

0BWQ02Z Revision of Monitoring Device in Pleura, Open Approach

0BWQ30Z Revision of Drainage Device in Pleura, Percutaneous Approach

0BWQ32Z Revision of Monitoring Device in Pleura, Percutaneous Approach

0BWQ40Z Revision of Drainage Device in Pleura, Percutaneous Endoscopic Approach

0BWQ42Z Revision of Monitoring Device in Pleura, Percutaneous Endoscopic Approach

0BWQ70Z Revision of Drainage Device in Pleura, Via Natural or Artificial Opening

0BWQ72Z Revision of Monitoring Device in Pleura, Via Natural or Artificial Opening

0BWQ80Z Revision of Drainage Device in Pleura, Via Natural or Artificial Opening Endoscopic

0BWQ82Z Revision of Monitoring Device in Pleura, Via Natural or Artificial Opening Endoscopic

0BWQX0Z Revision of Drainage Device in Pleura, External Approach

0BWQX2Z Revision of Monitoring Device in Pleura, External Approach

0BWT00Z Revision of Drainage Device in Diaphragm, Open Approach

0BWT02Z Revision of Monitoring Device in Diaphragm, Open Approach

0BWT07Z Revision of Autologous Tissue Substitute in Diaphragm, Open Approach

0BWT0JZ Revision of Synthetic Substitute in Diaphragm, Open Approach

0BWT0KZ Revision of Nonautologous Tissue Substitute in Diaphragm, Open Approach

0BWT0MZ Revision of Diaphragmatic Pacemaker Lead in Diaphragm, Open Approach

0BWT30Z Revision of Drainage Device in Diaphragm, Percutaneous Approach

0BWT32Z Revision of Monitoring Device in Diaphragm, Percutaneous Approach

0BWT37Z Revision of Autologous Tissue Substitute in Diaphragm, Percutaneous Approach

0BWT3JZ Revision of Synthetic Substitute in Diaphragm, Percutaneous Approach

0BWT3KZ Revision of Nonautologous Tissue Substitute in Diaphragm, Percutaneous Approach

0BWT3MZ Revision of Diaphragmatic Pacemaker Lead in Diaphragm, Percutaneous Approach

0BWT40Z Revision of Drainage Device in Diaphragm, Percutaneous Endoscopic Approach

0BWT42Z Revision of Monitoring Device in Diaphragm, Percutaneous Endoscopic Approach

0BWT47Z Revision of Autologous Tissue Substitute in Diaphragm, Percutaneous Endoscopic Approach

0BWT4JZ Revision of Synthetic Substitute in Diaphragm, Percutaneous Endoscopic Approach

0BWT4KZ Revision of Nonautologous Tissue Substitute in Diaphragm, Percutaneous Endoscopic Approach

0BWT4MZ Revision of Diaphragmatic Pacemaker Lead in Diaphragm, Percutaneous Endoscopic Approach

0BWT70Z Revision of Drainage Device in Diaphragm, Via Natural or Artificial Opening

0BWT72Z Revision of Monitoring Device in Diaphragm, Via Natural or Artificial Opening

0BWT77Z Revision of Autologous Tissue Substitute in Diaphragm, Via Natural or Artificial Opening

0BWT7JZ Revision of Synthetic Substitute in Diaphragm, Via Natural or Artificial Opening

0BWT7KZ Revision of Nonautologous Tissue Substitute in Diaphragm, Via Natural or Artificial Opening

0BWT7MZ Revision of Diaphragmatic Pacemaker Lead in Diaphragm, Via Natural or Artificial Opening

0BWT80Z Revision of Drainage Device in Diaphragm, Via Natural or Artificial Opening Endoscopic

0BWT82Z Revision of Monitoring Device in Diaphragm, Via Natural or Artificial Opening Endoscopic

0BWT87Z Revision of Autologous Tissue Substitute in Diaphragm, Via Natural or Artificial Opening Endoscopic

0BWT8JZ Revision of Synthetic Substitute in Diaphragm, Via Natural or Artificial Opening Endoscopic

0BWT8KZ Revision of Nonautologous Tissue Substitute in Diaphragm, Via Natural or Artificial Opening Endoscopic

0BWT8MZ Revision of Diaphragmatic Pacemaker Lead in Diaphragm, Via Natural or Artificial Opening Endoscopic

0BWTX0Z Revision of Drainage Device in Diaphragm, External Approach

0BWTX2Z Revision of Monitoring Device in Diaphragm, External Approach

0BWTX7Z Revision of Autologous Tissue Substitute in Diaphragm, External Approach

0BWTXJZ Revision of Synthetic Substitute in Diaphragm, External Approach

0BWTXKZ Revision of Nonautologous Tissue Substitute in Diaphragm, External Approach

0BWTXMZ Revision of Diaphragmatic Pacemaker Lead in Diaphragm, External Approach

0BY – Respiratory System, Transplantation

Review Coding Guideline B3.16

0BYC0Z0 Transplantation of Right Upper Lung Lobe, Allogeneic, Open Approach

0BYC0Z1 Transplantation of Right Upper Lung Lobe, Syngeneic, Open Approach

0BYC0Z2 Transplantation of Right Upper Lung Lobe, Zooplastic, Open Approach

0BYD0Z0 Transplantation of Right Middle Lung Lobe, Allogeneic, Open Approach

0BYD0Z1 Transplantation of Right Middle Lung Lobe, Syngeneic, Open Approach

0BYD0Z2 Transplantation of Right Middle Lung Lobe, Zooplastic, Open Approach

0BYF0Z0 Transplantation of Right Lower Lung Lobe, Allogeneic, Open Approach

0BYF0Z1 Transplantation of Right Lower Lung Lobe, Syngeneic, Open Approach

0BYF0Z2 Transplantation of Right Lower Lung Lobe, Zooplastic, Open Approach

0BYG0Z0 Transplantation of Left Upper Lung Lobe, Allogeneic, Open Approach

0BYG0Z1 Transplantation of Left Upper Lung Lobe, Syngeneic, Open Approach

0BYG0Z2 Transplantation of Left Upper Lung Lobe, Zooplastic, Open Approach

0BYH0Z0 Transplantation of Lung Lingula, Allogeneic, Open Approach

0BYH0Z1 Transplantation of Lung Lingula, Syngeneic, Open Approach

0BYH0Z2 Transplantation of Lung Lingula, Zooplastic, Open Approach

0BYJ0Z0 Transplantation of Left Lower Lung Lobe, Allogeneic, Open Approach

0BYJ0Z1 Transplantation of Left Lower Lung Lobe, Syngeneic, Open Approach

0BYJ0Z2 Transplantation of Left Lower Lung Lobe, Zooplastic, Open Approach

0BYK0Z0 Transplantation of Right Lung, Allogeneic, Open Approach

0BYK0Z1 Transplantation of Right Lung, Syngeneic, Open Approach

0BYK0Z2 Transplantation of Right Lung, Zooplastic, Open Approach

0BYL0Z0 Transplantation of Left Lung, Allogeneic, Open Approach

0BYL0Z1 Transplantation of Left Lung, Syngeneic, Open Approach

0BYL0Z2 Transplantation of Left Lung, Zooplastic, Open Approach

0BYM0Z0 Transplantation of Bilateral Lungs, Allogeneic, Open Approach

0BYM0Z1 Transplantation of Bilateral Lungs, Syngeneic, Open Approach

0BYM0Z2 Transplantation of Bilateral Lungs, Zooplastic, Open Approach

Mouth and Throat

Oral Cavity

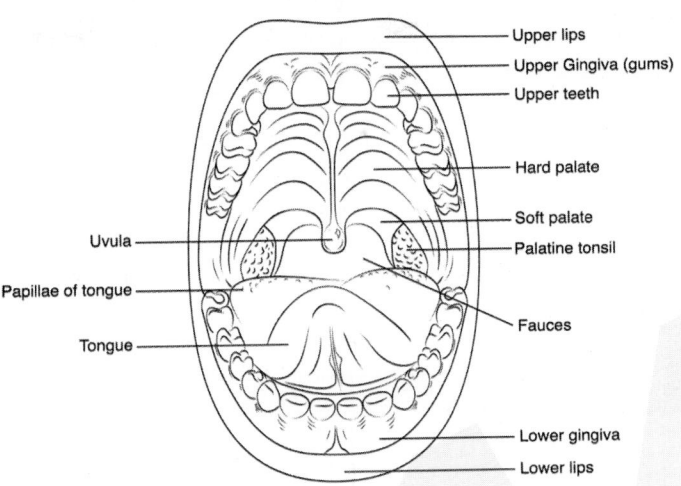

Upper lips
Upper Gingiva (gums)
Upper teeth

Hard palate

Soft palate
Palatine tonsil

Uvula
Papillae of tongue
Tongue

Fauces

Lower gingiva
Lower lips

Glands of the Oral Cavity

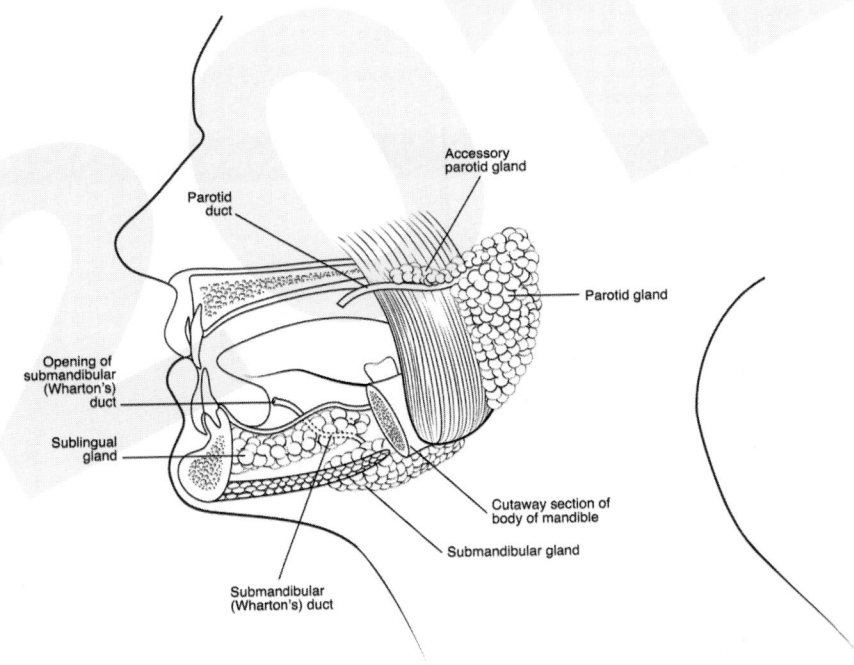

Accessory
parotid gland

Parotid
duct

Parotid gland

Opening of
submandibular
(Wharton's)
duct

Sublingual
gland

Cutaway section of
body of mandible

Submandibular gland

Submandibular
(Wharton's) duct

Throat

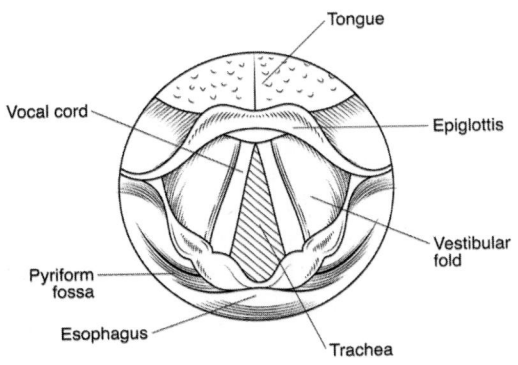

Tongue

Vocal cord

Epiglottis

Vestibular
fold

Pyriform
fossa

Esophagus

Trachea

Mouth and Throat Tables 0C0–0CX

Section	**0**	**Medical and Surgical**
Body System	**C**	**Mouth and Throat**
Operation	**0**	**Alteration:** Modifying the anatomic structure of a body part without affecting the function of the body part

Body Part (4ᵗʰ)	Approach (5ᵗʰ)	Device (6ᵗʰ)	Qualifier (7ᵗʰ)
0 Upper Lip **1** Lower Lip	**X** External	**7** Autologous Tissue Substitute **J** Synthetic Substitute **K** Nonautologous Tissue Substitute **Z** No Device	**Z** No Qualifier

Section	**0**	**Medical and Surgical**
Body System	**C**	**Mouth and Throat**
Operation	**2**	**Change:** Taking out or off a device from a body part and putting back an identical or similar device in or on the same body part without cutting or puncturing the skin or a mucous membrane

Body Part (4ᵗʰ)	Approach (5ᵗʰ)	Device (6ᵗʰ)	Qualifier (7ᵗʰ)
A Salivary Gland **S** Larynx **Y** Mouth and Throat	**X** External	**0** Drainage Device **Y** Other Device	**Z** No Qualifier

Section	**0**	**Medical and Surgical**
Body System	**C**	**Mouth and Throat**
Operation	**5**	**Destruction:** Physical eradication of all or a portion of a body part by the direct use of energy, force, or a destructive agent

Body Part (4ᵗʰ)	Approach (5ᵗʰ)	Device (6ᵗʰ)	Qualifier (7ᵗʰ)
0 Upper Lip **1** Lower Lip **2** Hard Palate **3** Soft Palate **4** Buccal Mucosa **5** Upper Gingiva **6** Lower Gingiva **7** Tongue **N** Uvula **P** Tonsils **Q** Adenoids	**0** Open **3** Percutaneous **X** External	**Z** No Device	**Z** No Qualifier
8 Parotid Gland, Right **9** Parotid Gland, Left **B** Parotid Duct, Right **C** Parotid Duct, Left **D** Sublingual Gland, Right **F** Sublingual Gland, Left **G** Submaxillary Gland, Right **H** Submaxillary Gland, Left **J** Minor Salivary Gland	**0** Open **3** Percutaneous	**Z** No Device	**Z** No Qualifier
M Pharynx **R** Epiglottis **S** Larynx **T** Vocal Cord, Right **V** Vocal Cord, Left	**0** Open **3** Percutaneous **4** Percutaneous Endoscopic **7** Via Natural or Artificial Opening **8** Via Natural or Artificial Opening Endoscopic	**Z** No Device	**Z** No Qualifier
W Upper Tooth **X** Lower Tooth	**0** Open **X** External	**Z** No Device	**0** Single **1** Multiple **2** All

Section	0	**Medical and Surgical**
Body System	C	**Mouth and Throat**
Operation	7	**Dilation:** Expanding an orifice or the lumen of a tubular body part

Body Part (4th)	Approach (5th)	Device (6th)	Qualifier (7th)
B Parotid Duct, Right **C** Parotid Duct, Left	**0** Open **3** Percutaneous **7** Via Natural or Artificial Opening	**D** Intraluminal Device **Z** No Device	**Z** No Qualifier
M Pharynx	**7** Via Natural or Artificial Opening **8** Via Natural or Artificial Opening Endoscopic	**D** Intraluminal Device **Z** No Device	**Z** No Qualifier
S Larynx	**0** Open **3** Percutaneous **4** Percutaneous Endoscopic **7** Via Natural or Artificial Opening **8** Via Natural or Artificial Opening Endoscopic	**D** Intraluminal Device **Z** No Device	**Z** No Qualifier

Section	0	**Medical and Surgical**
Body System	C	**Mouth and Throat**
Operation	9	**Drainage:** Taking or letting out fluids and/or gases from a body part

Body Part (4th)	Approach (5th)	Device (6th)	Qualifier (7th)
0 Upper Lip **1** Lower Lip **2** Hard Palate **3** Soft Palate **4** Buccal Mucosa **5** Upper Gingiva **6** Lower Gingiva **7** Tongue **N** Uvula **P** Tonsils **Q** Adenoids	**0** Open **3** Percutaneous **X** External	**0** Drainage Device	**Z** No Qualifier
0 Upper Lip **1** Lower Lip **2** Hard Palate **3** Soft Palate **4** Buccal Mucosa **5** Upper Gingiva **6** Lower Gingiva **7** Tongue **N** Uvula **P** Tonsils **Q** Adenoids	**0** Open **3** Percutaneous **X** External	**Z** No Device	**X** Diagnostic **Z** No Qualifier
8 Parotid Gland, Right **9** Parotid Gland, Left **B** Parotid Duct, Right **C** Parotid Duct, Left **D** Sublingual Gland, Right **F** Sublingual Gland, Left **G** Submaxillary Gland, Right **H** Submaxillary Gland, Left **J** Minor Salivary Gland	**0** Open **3** Percutaneous	**0** Drainage Device	**Z** No Qualifier

Continued

Section	0	Medical and Surgical	
Body System	C	Mouth and Throat	
Operation	9	Drainage: Taking or letting out fluids and/or gases from a body part	0C9 *Continued*

Body Part (4th)	Approach (5th)	Device (6th)	Qualifier (7th)
8 Parotid Gland, Right 9 Parotid Gland, Left B Parotid Duct, Right C Parotid Duct, Left D Sublingual Gland, Right F Sublingual Gland, Left G Submaxillary Gland, Right H Submaxillary Gland, Left J Minor Salivary Gland	0 Open 3 Percutaneous	Z No Device	X Diagnostic Z No Qualifier
M Pharynx R Epiglottis S Larynx T Vocal Cord, Right V Vocal Cord, Left	0 Open 3 Percutaneous 4 Percutaneous Endoscopic 7 Via Natural or Artificial Opening 8 Via Natural or Artificial Opening Endoscopic	0 Drainage Device	Z No Qualifier
M Pharynx R Epiglottis S Larynx T Vocal Cord, Right V Vocal Cord, Left	0 Open 3 Percutaneous 4 Percutaneous Endoscopic 7 Via Natural or Artificial Opening 8 Via Natural or Artificial Opening Endoscopic	Z No Device	X Diagnostic Z No Qualifier
W Upper Tooth X Lower Tooth	0 Open X External	0 Drainage Device Z No Device	0 Single 1 Multiple 2 All

Section	0	Medical and Surgical	
Body System	C	Mouth and Throat	
Operation	B	Excision: Cutting out or off, without replacement, a portion of a body part	

Body Part (4th)	Approach (5th)	Device (6th)	Qualifier (7th)
0 Upper Lip 1 Lower Lip 2 Hard Palate 3 Soft Palate 4 Buccal Mucosa 5 Upper Gingiva 6 Lower Gingiva 7 Tongue N Uvula P Tonsils Q Adenoids	0 Open 3 Percutaneous X External	Z No Device	X Diagnostic Z No Qualifier
8 Parotid Gland, Right 9 Parotid Gland, Left B Parotid Duct, Right C Parotid Duct, Left D Sublingual Gland, Right F Sublingual Gland, Left G Submaxillary Gland, Right H Submaxillary Gland, Left J Minor Salivary Gland	0 Open 3 Percutaneous	Z No Device	X Diagnostic Z No Qualifier

Continued

Section	0	Medical and Surgical	0CB *Continued*
Body System	C	Mouth and Throat	
Operation	B	Excision: Cutting out or off, without replacement, a portion of a body part	

Body Part (4th)	Approach (5th)	Device (6th)	Qualifier (7th)
M Pharynx R Epiglottis S Larynx T Vocal Cord, Right V Vocal Cord, Left	0 Open 3 Percutaneous 4 Percutaneous Endoscopic 7 Via Natural or Artificial Opening 8 Via Natural or Artificial Opening Endoscopic	Z No Device	X Diagnostic Z No Qualifier
W Upper Tooth X Lower Tooth	0 Open X External	Z No Device	0 Single 1 Multiple 2 All

Section	0	Medical and Surgical
Body System	C	Mouth and Throat
Operation	C	Extirpation: Taking or cutting out solid matter from a body part

Body Part (4th)	Approach (5th)	Device (6th)	Qualifier (7th)
0 Upper Lip 1 Lower Lip 2 Hard Palate 3 Soft Palate 4 Buccal Mucosa 5 Upper Gingiva 6 Lower Gingiva 7 Tongue N Uvula P Tonsils Q Adenoids	0 Open 3 Percutaneous X External	Z No Device	Z No Qualifier
8 Parotid Gland, Right 9 Parotid Gland, Left B Parotid Duct, Right C Parotid Duct, Left D Sublingual Gland, Right F Sublingual Gland, Left G Submaxillary Gland, Right H Submaxillary Gland, Left J Minor Salivary Gland	0 Open 3 Percutaneous	Z No Device	Z No Qualifier
M Pharynx R Epiglottis S Larynx T Vocal Cord, Right V Vocal Cord, Left	0 Open 3 Percutaneous 4 Percutaneous Endoscopic 7 Via Natural or Artificial Opening 8 Via Natural or Artificial Opening Endoscopic	Z No Device	Z No Qualifier
W Upper Tooth X Lower Tooth	0 Open X External	Z No Device	0 Single 1 Multiple 2 All

Section	0	Medical and Surgical
Body System	C	Mouth and Throat
Operation	D	Extraction: Pulling or stripping out or off all or a portion of a body part by the use of force

Body Part (4th)	Approach (5th)	Device (6th)	Qualifier (7th)
T Vocal Cord, Right V Vocal Cord, Left	0 Open 3 Percutaneous 4 Percutaneous Endoscopic 7 Via Natural or Artificial Opening 8 Via Natural or Artificial Opening Endoscopic	Z No Device	Z No Qualifier
W Upper Tooth X Lower Tooth	X External	Z No Device	0 Single 1 Multiple 2 All

Section	0	Medical and Surgical
Body System	C	Mouth and Throat
Operation	F	Fragmentation: Breaking solid matter in a body part into pieces

Body Part (4th)	Approach (5th)	Device (6th)	Qualifier (7th)
B Parotid Duct, Right C Parotid Duct, Left	0 Open 3 Percutaneous 7 Via Natural or Artificial Opening X External	Z No Device	Z No Qualifier

Section	0	Medical and Surgical
Body System	C	Mouth and Throat
Operation	H	Insertion: Putting in a nonbiological appliance that monitors, assists, performs, or prevents a physiological function but does not physically take the place of a body part

Body Part (4th)	Approach (5th)	Device (6th)	Qualifier (7th)
7 Tongue	0 Open 3 Percutaneous X External	1 Radioactive Element	Z No Qualifier
Y Mouth and Throat	7 Via Natural or Artificial Opening 8 Via Natural or Artificial Opening Endoscopic	B Intraluminal Device, Airway	Z No Qualifier

Section	0	Medical and Surgical
Body System	C	Mouth and Throat
Operation	J	Inspection: Visually and/or manually exploring a body part

Body Part (4th)	Approach (5th)	Device (6th)	Qualifier (7th)
A SalivaryGland	0 Open 3 Percutaneous X External	Z No Device	Z No Qualifier
S Larynx Y Mouth and Throat	0 Open 3 Percutaneous 4 Percutaneous Endoscopic 7 Via Natural or Artificial Opening 8 Via Natural or Artificial Opening Endoscopic X External	Z No Device	Z No Qualifier

Section	0	Medical and Surgical
Body System	C	Mouth and Throat
Operation	L	**Occlusion:** Completely closing an orifice or the lumen of a tubular body part

Body Part (4th)	Approach (5th)	Device (6th)	Qualifier (7th)
B Parotid Duct, Right C Parotid Duct, Left	0 Open 3 Percutaneous 4 Percutaneous Endoscopic	C Extraluminal Device D Intraluminal Device Z No Device	Z No Qualifier
B Parotid Duct, Right C Parotid Duct, Left	7 Via Natural or Artificial Opening 8 Via Natural or Artificial Opening Endoscopic	D Intraluminal Device Z No Device	Z No Qualifier

Section	0	Medical and Surgical
Body System	C	Mouth and Throat
Operation	M	**Reattachment:** Putting back in or on all or a portion of a separated body part to its normal location or other suitable location

Body Part (4th)	Approach (5th)	Device (6th)	Qualifier (7th)
0 Upper Lip 1 Lower Lip 3 Soft Palate 7 Tongue N Uvula	0 Open	Z No Device	Z No Qualifier
W Upper Tooth X Lower Tooth	0 Open X External	Z No Device	0 Single 1 Multiple 2 All

Section	0	Medical and Surgical
Body System	C	Mouth and Throat
Operation	N	**Release:** Freeing a body part from an abnormal physical constraint by cutting or by the use of force

Body Part (4th)	Approach (5th)	Device (6th)	Qualifier (7th)
0 Upper Lip 1 Lower Lip 2 Hard Palate 3 Soft Palate 4 Buccal Mucosa 5 Upper Gingiva 6 Lower Gingiva 7 Tongue N Uvula P Tonsils Q Adenoids	0 Open 3 Percutaneous X External	Z No Device	Z No Qualifier
8 Parotid Gland, Right 9 Parotid Gland, Left B Parotid Duct, Right C Parotid Duct, Left D Sublingual Gland, Right F Sublingual Gland, Left G Submaxillary Gland, Right H Submaxillary Gland, Left J Minor Salivary Gland	0 Open 3 Percutaneous	Z No Device	Z No Qualifier

Continued

Section	0	Medical and Surgical
Body System	C	Mouth and Throat
Operation	N	**Release:** Freeing a body part from an abnormal physical constraint by cutting or by the use of force

Body Part (4th)	Approach (5th)	Device (6th)	Qualifier (7th)
M Pharynx R Epiglottis S Larynx T Vocal Cord, Right V Vocal Cord, Left	0 Open 3 Percutaneous 4 Percutaneous Endoscopic 7 Via Natural or Artificial Opening 8 Via Natural or Artificial Opening Endoscopic	Z No Device	Z No Qualifier
W Upper Tooth X Lower Tooth	0 Open X External	Z No Device	0 Single 1 Multiple 2 All

Section	0	Medical and Surgical
Body System	C	Mouth and Throat
Operation	P	**Removal:** Taking out or off a device from a body part

Body Part (4th)	Approach (5th)	Device (6th)	Qualifier (7th)
A Salivary Gland	0 Open 3 Percutaneous	0 Drainage Device C Extraluminal Device	Z No Qualifier
S Larynx	0 Open 3 Percutaneous 7 Via Natural or Artificial Opening 8 Via Natural or Artificial Opening Endoscopic X External	0 Drainage Device 7 Autologous Tissue Substitute D Intraluminal Device J Synthetic Substitute K Nonautologous Tissue Substitute	Z No Qualifier
Y Mouth and Throat	0 Open 3 Percutaneous 7 Via Natural or Artificial Opening 8 Via Natural or Artificial Opening Endoscopic X External	0 Drainage Device 1 Radioactive Element 7 Autologous Tissue Substitute D Intraluminal Device J Synthetic Substitute K Nonautologous Tissue Substitute	Z No Qualifier

Section	0	Medical and Surgical
Body System	C	Mouth and Throat
Operation	Q	**Repair:** Restoring, to the extent possible, a body part to its normal anatomic structure and function

Body Part (4th)	Approach (5th)	Device (6th)	Qualifier (7th)
0 Upper Lip 1 Lower Lip 2 Hard Palate 3 Soft Palate 4 Buccal Mucosa 5 Upper Gingiva 6 Lower Gingiva 7 Tongue N Uvula P Tonsils Q Adenoids	0 Open 3 Percutaneous X External	Z No Device	Z No Qualifier

Continued

0CQ *Continued*

Section	0	Medical and Surgical
Body System	C	Mouth and Throat
Operation	Q	**Repair:** Restoring, to the extent possible, a body part to its normal anatomic structure and function

Body Part (4th)	Approach (5th)	Device (6th)	Qualifier (7th)
8 Parotid Gland, Right 9 Parotid Gland, Left B Parotid Duct, Right C Parotid Duct, Left D Sublingual Gland, Right F Sublingual Gland, Left G Submaxillary Gland, Right H Submaxillary Gland, Left J Minor Salivary Gland	0 Open 3 Percutaneous	Z No Device	Z No Qualifier
M Pharynx R Epiglottis S Larynx T Vocal Cord, Right V Vocal Cord, Left	0 Open 3 Percutaneous 4 Percutaneous Endoscopic 7 Via Natural or Artificial Opening 8 Via Natural or Artificial Opening Endoscopic	Z No Device	Z No Qualifier
W Upper Tooth X Lower Tooth	0 Open X External	Z No Device	0 Single 1 Multiple 2 All

Section	0	Medical and Surgical
Body System	C	Mouth and Throat
Operation	R	**Replacement:** Putting in or on biological or synthetic material that physically takes the place and/or function of all or a portion of a body part

Body Part (4th)	Approach (5th)	Device (6th)	Qualifier (7th)
0 Upper Lip 1 Lower Lip 2 Hard Palate 3 Soft Palate 4 Buccal Mucosa 5 Upper Gingiva 6 Lower Gingiva 7 Tongue N Uvula	0 Open 3 Percutaneous X External	7 Autologous Tissue Substitute J Synthetic Substitute K Nonautologous Tissue Substitute	Z No Qualifier
B Parotid Duct, Right C Parotid Duct, Left	0 Open 3 Percutaneous	7 Autologous Tissue Substitute J Synthetic Substitute K Nonautologous Tissue Substitute	Z No Qualifier
M Pharynx R Epiglottis S Larynx T Vocal Cord, Right V Vocal Cord, Left	0 Open 7 Via Natural or Artificial Opening 8 Via Natural or Artificial Opening Endoscopic	7 Autologous Tissue Substitute J Synthetic Substitute K Nonautologous Tissue Substitute	Z No Qualifier
W Upper Tooth X Lower Tooth	0 Open X External	7 Autologous Tissue Substitute J Synthetic Substitute K Nonautologous Tissue Substitute	0 Single 1 Multiple 2 All

Section   0   **Medical and Surgical**
Body System   C   **Mouth and Throat**
Operation   S   **Reposition:** Moving to its normal location, or other suitable location, all or a portion of a body part

Body Part (4th)	Approach (5th)	Device (6th)	Qualifier (7th)
0 Upper Lip 1 Lower Lip 2 Hard Palate 3 Soft Palate 7 Tongue N Uvula	0 Open X External	Z No Device	Z No Qualifier
B Parotid Duct, Right C Parotid Duct, Left	0 Open 3 Percutaneous	Z No Device	Z No Qualifier
R Epiglottis T Vocal Cord, Right V Vocal Cord, Left	0 Open 7 Via Natural or Artificial Opening 8 Via Natural or Artificial Opening Endoscopic	Z No Device	Z No Qualifier
W Upper Tooth X Lower Tooth	0 Open X External	5 External Fixation Device Z No Device	0 Single 1 Multiple 2 All

Section   0   **Medical and Surgical**
Body System   C   **Mouth and Throat**
Operation   T   **Resection:** Cutting out or off, without replacement, all of a body part

Body Part (4th)	Approach (5th)	Device (6th)	Qualifier (7th)
0 Upper Lip 1 Lower Lip 2 Hard Palate 3 Soft Palate 7 Tongue N Uvula P Tonsils Q Adenoids	0 Open X External	Z No Device	Z No Qualifier
8 Parotid Gland, Right 9 Parotid Gland, Left B Parotid Duct, Right C Parotid Duct, Left D Sublingual Gland, Right F Sublingual Gland, Left G Submaxillary Gland, Right H Submaxillary Gland, Left J Minor Salivary Gland	0 Open	Z No Device	Z No Qualifier
M Pharynx R Epiglottis S Larynx T Vocal Cord, Right V Vocal Cord, Left	0 Open 4 Percutaneous Endoscopic 7 Via Natural or Artificial Opening 8 Via Natural or Artificial Opening Endoscopic	Z No Device	Z No Qualifier
W Upper Tooth X Lower Tooth	0 Open	Z No Device	0 Single 1 Multiple 2 All

Section	0	Medical and Surgical
Body System	C	Mouth and Throat
Operation	U	**Supplement:** Putting in or on biological or synthetic material that physically reinforces and/or augments the function of a portion of a body part

Body Part (4th)	Approach (5th)	Device (6th)	Qualifier (7th)
0 Upper Lip 1 Lower Lip 2 Hard Palate 3 Soft Palate 4 Buccal Mucosa 5 Upper Gingiva 6 Lower Gingiva 7 Tongue N Uvula	0 Open 3 Percutaneous X External	7 Autologous Tissue Substitute J Synthetic Substitute K Nonautologous Tissue Substitute	Z No Qualifier
M Pharynx R Epiglottis S Larynx T Vocal Cord, Right V Vocal Cord, Left	0 Open 7 Via Natural or Artificial Opening 8 Via Natural or Artificial Opening Endoscopic	7 Autologous Tissue Substitute J Synthetic Substitute K Nonautologous Tissue Substitute	Z No Qualifier

Section	0	Medical and Surgical
Body System	C	Mouth and Throat
Operation	V	**Restriction:** Partially closing an orifice or the lumen of a tubular body part

Body Part (4th)	Approach (5th)	Device (6th)	Qualifier (7th)
B Parotid Duct, Right C Parotid Duct, Left	0 Open 3 Percutaneous	C Extraluminal Device D Intraluminal Device Z No Device	Z No Qualifier
B Parotid Duct, Right C Parotid Duct, Left	7 Via Natural or Artificial Opening 8 Via Natural or Artificial Opening Endoscopic	D Intraluminal Device Z No Device	Z No Qualifier

Section	0	Medical and Surgical
Body System	C	Mouth and Throat
Operation	W	**Revision:** Correcting, to the extent possible, a portion of a malfunctioning device or the position of a displaced device

Body Part (4th)	Approach (5th)	Device (6th)	Qualifier (7th)
A Salivary Gland	0 Open 3 Percutaneous X External	0 Drainage Device C Extraluminal Device	Z No Qualifier
S Larynx	0 Open 3 Percutaneous 7 Via Natural or Artificial Opening 8 Via Natural or Artificial Opening Endoscopic X External	0 Drainage Device 7 Autologous Tissue Substitute D Intraluminal Device J Synthetic Substitute K Nonautologous Tissue Substitute	Z No Qualifier
Y Mouth and Throat	0 Open 3 Percutaneous 7 Via Natural or Artificial Opening 8 Via Natural or Artificial Opening Endoscopic X External	0 Drainage Device 1 Radioactive Element 7 Autologous Tissue Substitute D Intraluminal Device J Synthetic Substitute K Nonautologous Tissue Substitute	Z No Qualifier

Section	0	Medical and Surgical
Body System	C	Mouth and Throat
Operation	X	**Transfer:** Moving, without taking out, all or a portion of a body part to another location to take over the function of all or a portion of a body part

Body Part (4th)	Approach (5th)	Device (6th)	Qualifier (7th)
0 Upper Lip 1 Lower Lip 3 Soft Palate 4 Buccal Mucosa 5 Upper Gingiva 6 Lower Gingiva 7 Tongue	0 Open X External	Z No Device	Z No Qualifier

Mouth and Throat Code Listing 0C0–0CX

0C0 – Mouth and Throat, Alteration

0C00X7Z Alteration of Upper Lip with Autologous Tissue Substitute, External Approach

0C00XJZ Alteration of Upper Lip with Synthetic Substitute, External Approach

0C00XKZ Alteration of Upper Lip with Nonautologous Tissue Substitute, External Approach

0C00XZZ Alteration of Upper Lip, External Approach

0C01X7Z Alteration of Lower Lip with Autologous Tissue Substitute, External Approach

0C01XJZ Alteration of Lower Lip with Synthetic Substitute, External Approach

0C01XKZ Alteration of Lower Lip with Nonautologous Tissue Substitute, External Approach

0C01XZZ Alteration of Lower Lip, External Approach

0C2 – Mouth and Throat, Change

Review Coding Guideline B6.1c

0C2AX0Z Change Drainage Device in Salivary Gland, External Approach

0C2AXYZ Change Other Device in Salivary Gland, External Approach

0C2SX0Z Change Drainage Device in Larynx, External Approach

0C2SXYZ Change Other Device in Larynx, External Approach

0C2YX0Z Change Drainage Device in Mouth and Throat, External Approach

0C2YXYZ Change Other Device in Mouth and Throat, External Approach

0C5 – Mouth and Throat, Destruction

0C500ZZ Destruction of Upper Lip, Open Approach

0C503ZZ Destruction of Upper Lip, Percutaneous Approach

0C50XZZ Destruction of Upper Lip, External Approach

0C510ZZ Destruction of Lower Lip, Open Approach

0C513ZZ Destruction of Lower Lip, Percutaneous Approach

0C51XZZ Destruction of Lower Lip, External Approach

0C520ZZ Destruction of Hard Palate, Open Approach

0C523ZZ Destruction of Hard Palate, Percutaneous Approach

0C52XZZ Destruction of Hard Palate, External Approach

0C530ZZ Destruction of Soft Palate, Open Approach

0C533ZZ Destruction of Soft Palate, Percutaneous Approach

0C53XZZ Destruction of Soft Palate, External Approach

0C540ZZ Destruction of Buccal Mucosa, Open Approach

0C543ZZ Destruction of Buccal Mucosa, Percutaneous Approach

0C54XZZ Destruction of Buccal Mucosa, External Approach

0C550ZZ Destruction of Upper Gingiva, Open Approach

0C553ZZ Destruction of Upper Gingiva, Percutaneous Approach

0C55XZZ Destruction of Upper Gingiva, External Approach

0C560ZZ Destruction of Lower Gingiva, Open Approach

0C563ZZ Destruction of Lower Gingiva, Percutaneous Approach

0C56XZZ Destruction of Lower Gingiva, External Approach

0C570ZZ Destruction of Tongue, Open Approach

0C573ZZ Destruction of Tongue, Percutaneous Approach

0C57XZZ Destruction of Tongue, External Approach

0C580ZZ Destruction of Right Parotid Gland, Open Approach

0C583ZZ Destruction of Right Parotid Gland, Percutaneous Approach

0C590ZZ Destruction of Left Parotid Gland, Open Approach

0C593ZZ Destruction of Left Parotid Gland, Percutaneous Approach

0C5B0ZZ Destruction of Right Parotid Duct, Open Approach

0C5B3ZZ Destruction of Right Parotid Duct, Percutaneous Approach

0C5C0ZZ Destruction of Left Parotid Duct, Open Approach

0C5C3ZZ Destruction of Left Parotid Duct, Percutaneous Approach

0C5D0ZZ Destruction of Right Sublingual Gland, Open Approach

0C5D3ZZ Destruction of Right Sublingual Gland, Percutaneous Approach

0C5F0ZZ Destruction of Left Sublingual Gland, Open Approach

0C5F3ZZ Destruction of Left Sublingual Gland, Percutaneous Approach

0C5G0ZZ Destruction of Right Submaxillary Gland, Open Approach

0C5G3ZZ Destruction of Right Submaxillary Gland, Percutaneous Approach

0C5H0ZZ Destruction of Left Submaxillary Gland, Open Approach

0C5H3ZZ Destruction of Left Submaxillary Gland, Percutaneous Approach

0C5J0ZZ Destruction of Minor Salivary Gland, Open Approach

0C5J3ZZ Destruction of Minor Salivary Gland, Percutaneous Approach

0C5M0ZZ Destruction of Pharynx, Open Approach

0C5M3ZZ Destruction of Pharynx, Percutaneous Approach

0C5M4ZZ Destruction of Pharynx, Percutaneous Endoscopic Approach

0C5M7ZZ Destruction of Pharynx, Via Natural or Artificial Opening

0C5M8ZZ Destruction of Pharynx, Via Natural or Artificial Opening Endoscopic

0C5N0ZZ Destruction of Uvula, Open Approach

0C5N3ZZ Destruction of Uvula, Percutaneous Approach

0C5NXZZ Destruction of Uvula, External Approach

0C5P0ZZ Destruction of Tonsils, Open Approach

0C5P3ZZ Destruction of Tonsils, Percutaneous Approach

0C5PXZZ Destruction of Tonsils, External Approach

0C5Q0ZZ Destruction of Adenoids, Open Approach

0C5Q3ZZ Destruction of Adenoids, Percutaneous Approach

0C5QXZZ Destruction of Adenoids, External Approach

0C5R0ZZ Destruction of Epiglottis, Open Approach

0C5R3ZZ Destruction of Epiglottis, Percutaneous Approach

0C5R4ZZ Destruction of Epiglottis, Percutaneous Endoscopic Approach

0C5R7ZZ Destruction of Epiglottis, Via Natural or Artificial Opening

0C5R8ZZ Destruction of Epiglottis, Via Natural or Artificial Opening Endoscopic

0C5S0ZZ Destruction of Larynx, Open Approach

♀ Female-only   ♂ Male-only   ● Limited Coverage   ● Non-OR   ▨ HAC-associated procedure   ● Non-covered procedures   ✚ Combination

0C5S3ZZ   Destruction of Larynx, Percutaneous Approach
0C5S4ZZ   Destruction of Larynx, Percutaneous Endoscopic Approach
0C5S7ZZ   Destruction of Larynx, Via Natural or Artificial Opening
0C5S8ZZ   Destruction of Larynx, Via Natural or Artificial Opening Endoscopic
0C5T0ZZ   Destruction of Right Vocal Cord, Open Approach
0C5T3ZZ   Destruction of Right Vocal Cord, Percutaneous Approach
0C5T4ZZ   Destruction of Right Vocal Cord, Percutaneous Endoscopic Approach
0C5T7ZZ   Destruction of Right Vocal Cord, Via Natural or Artificial Opening
0C5T8ZZ   Destruction of Right Vocal Cord, Via Natural or Artificial Opening Endoscopic
0C5V0ZZ   Destruction of Left Vocal Cord, Open Approach
0C5V3ZZ   Destruction of Left Vocal Cord, Percutaneous Approach
0C5V4ZZ   Destruction of Left Vocal Cord, Percutaneous Endoscopic Approach
0C5V7ZZ   Destruction of Left Vocal Cord, Via Natural or Artificial Opening

0C5V8ZZ   Destruction of Left Vocal Cord, Via Natural or Artificial Opening Endoscopic
0C5W0Z0   Destruction of Upper Tooth, Single, Open Approach
0C5W0Z1   Destruction of Upper Tooth, Multiple, Open Approach
0C5W0Z2   Destruction of Upper Tooth, All, Open Approach
0C5WXZ0   Destruction of Upper Tooth, Single, External Approach
0C5WXZ1   Destruction of Upper Tooth, Multiple, External Approach
0C5WXZ2   Destruction of Upper Tooth, All, External Approach
0C5X0Z0   Destruction of Lower Tooth, Single, Open Approach
0C5X0Z1   Destruction of Lower Tooth, Multiple, Open Approach
0C5X0Z2   Destruction of Lower Tooth, All, Open Approach
0C5XXZ0   Destruction of Lower Tooth, Single, External Approach
0C5XXZ1   Destruction of Lower Tooth, Multiple, External Approach
0C5XXZ2   Destruction of Lower Tooth, All, External Approach

0C7 – Mouth and Throat, Dilation

0C7B0DZ   Dilation of Right Parotid Duct with Intraluminal Device, Open Approach
0C7B0ZZ   Dilation of Right Parotid Duct, Open Approach
0C7B3DZ   Dilation of Right Parotid Duct with Intraluminal Device, Percutaneous Approach
0C7B3ZZ   Dilation of Right Parotid Duct, Percutaneous Approach
0C7B7DZ   Dilation of Right Parotid Duct with Intraluminal Device, Via Natural or Artificial Opening
0C7B7ZZ   Dilation of Right Parotid Duct, Via Natural or Artificial Opening
0C7C0DZ   Dilation of Left Parotid Duct with Intraluminal Device, Open Approach
0C7C0ZZ   Dilation of Left Parotid Duct, Open Approach
0C7C3DZ   Dilation of Left Parotid Duct with Intraluminal Device, Percutaneous Approach
0C7C3ZZ   Dilation of Left Parotid Duct, Percutaneous Approach
0C7C7DZ   Dilation of Left Parotid Duct with Intraluminal Device, Via Natural or Artificial Opening
0C7C7ZZ   Dilation of Left Parotid Duct, Via Natural or Artificial Opening
0C7M7DZ   Dilation of Pharynx with Intraluminal Device, Via Natural or Artificial Opening

0C7M7ZZ   Dilation of Pharynx, Via Natural or Artificial Opening
0C7M8DZ   Dilation of Pharynx with Intraluminal Device, Via Natural or Artificial Opening Endoscopic
0C7M8ZZ   Dilation of Pharynx, Via Natural or Artificial Opening Endoscopic
0C7S0DZ   Dilation of Larynx with Intraluminal Device, Open Approach
0C7S0ZZ   Dilation of Larynx, Open Approach
0C7S3DZ   Dilation of Larynx with Intraluminal Device, Percutaneous Approach
0C7S3ZZ   Dilation of Larynx, Percutaneous Approach
0C7S4DZ   Dilation of Larynx with Intraluminal Device, Percutaneous Endoscopic Approach
0C7S4ZZ   Dilation of Larynx, Percutaneous Endoscopic Approach
0C7S7DZ   Dilation of Larynx with Intraluminal Device, Via Natural or Artificial Opening
0C7S7ZZ   Dilation of Larynx, Via Natural or Artificial Opening
0C7S8DZ   Dilation of Larynx with Intraluminal Device, Via Natural or Artificial Opening Endoscopic
0C7S8ZZ   Dilation of Larynx, Via Natural or Artificial Opening Endoscopic

0C9 – Mouth and Throat, Drainage

Review Coding Guidelines B3.4a and B3.4b

Review Coding Guideline B6.2

0C9000Z   Drainage of Upper Lip with Drainage Device, Open Approach
0C900ZX   Drainage of Upper Lip, Open Approach, Diagnostic
0C900ZZ   Drainage of Upper Lip, Open Approach
0C9030Z   Drainage of Upper Lip with Drainage Device, Percutaneous Approach
0C903ZX   Drainage of Upper Lip, Percutaneous Approach, Diagnostic
0C903ZZ   Drainage of Upper Lip, Percutaneous Approach
0C90X0Z   Drainage of Upper Lip with Drainage Device, External Approach
0C90XZX   Drainage of Upper Lip, External Approach, Diagnostic
0C90XZZ   Drainage of Upper Lip, External Approach
0C9100Z   Drainage of Lower Lip with Drainage Device, Open Approach
0C910ZX   Drainage of Lower Lip, Open Approach, Diagnostic
0C910ZZ   Drainage of Lower Lip, Open Approach
0C9130Z   Drainage of Lower Lip with Drainage Device, Percutaneous Approach
0C913ZX   Drainage of Lower Lip, Percutaneous Approach, Diagnostic
0C913ZZ   Drainage of Lower Lip, Percutaneous Approach
0C91X0Z   Drainage of Lower Lip with Drainage Device, External Approach
0C91XZX   Drainage of Lower Lip, External Approach, Diagnostic
0C91XZZ   Drainage of Lower Lip, External Approach
0C9200Z   Drainage of Hard Palate with Drainage Device, Open Approach
0C920ZX   Drainage of Hard Palate, Open Approach, Diagnostic
0C920ZZ   Drainage of Hard Palate, Open Approach
0C9230Z   Drainage of Hard Palate with Drainage Device, Percutaneous Approach
0C923ZX   Drainage of Hard Palate, Percutaneous Approach, Diagnostic
0C923ZZ   Drainage of Hard Palate, Percutaneous Approach
0C92X0Z   Drainage of Hard Palate with Drainage Device, External Approach
0C92XZX   Drainage of Hard Palate, External Approach, Diagnostic

0C92XZZ   Drainage of Hard Palate, External Approach
0C9300Z   Drainage of Soft Palate with Drainage Device, Open Approach
0C930ZX   Drainage of Soft Palate, Open Approach, Diagnostic
0C930ZZ   Drainage of Soft Palate, Open Approach
0C9330Z   Drainage of Soft Palate with Drainage Device, Percutaneous Approach
0C933ZX   Drainage of Soft Palate, Percutaneous Approach, Diagnostic
0C933ZZ   Drainage of Soft Palate, Percutaneous Approach
0C93X0Z   Drainage of Soft Palate with Drainage Device, External Approach
0C93XZX   Drainage of Soft Palate, External Approach, Diagnostic
0C93XZZ   Drainage of Soft Palate, External Approach
0C9400Z   Drainage of Buccal Mucosa with Drainage Device, Open Approach
0C940ZX   Drainage of Buccal Mucosa, Open Approach, Diagnostic
0C940ZZ   Drainage of Buccal Mucosa, Open Approach
0C9430Z   Drainage of Buccal Mucosa with Drainage Device, Percutaneous Approach
0C943ZX   Drainage of Buccal Mucosa, Percutaneous Approach, Diagnostic
0C943ZZ   Drainage of Buccal Mucosa, Percutaneous Approach
0C94X0Z   Drainage of Buccal Mucosa with Drainage Device, External Approach
0C94XZX   Drainage of Buccal Mucosa, External Approach, Diagnostic
0C94XZZ   Drainage of Buccal Mucosa, External Approach
0C9500Z   Drainage of Upper Gingiva with Drainage Device, Open Approach
0C950ZX   Drainage of Upper Gingiva, Open Approach, Diagnostic
0C950ZZ   Drainage of Upper Gingiva, Open Approach
0C9530Z   Drainage of Upper Gingiva with Drainage Device, Percutaneous Approach
0C953ZX   Drainage of Upper Gingiva, Percutaneous Approach, Diagnostic
0C953ZZ   Drainage of Upper Gingiva, Percutaneous Approach

♀ Female-only   ♂ Male-only   ● Limited Coverage   ● Non-OR   HAC HAC-associated procedure   ● Non-covered procedures   ✚ Combination

0C95X0Z	Drainage of Upper Gingiva with Drainage Device, External Approach
0C95XZX	Drainage of Upper Gingiva, External Approach, Diagnostic
0C95XZZ	Drainage of Upper Gingiva, External Approach
0C9600Z	Drainage of Lower Gingiva with Drainage Device, Open Approach
0C960ZX	Drainage of Lower Gingiva, Open Approach, Diagnostic
0C960ZZ	Drainage of Lower Gingiva, Open Approach
0C9630Z	Drainage of Lower Gingiva with Drainage Device, Percutaneous Approach
0C963ZX	Drainage of Lower Gingiva, Percutaneous Approach, Diagnostic
0C963ZZ	Drainage of Lower Gingiva, Percutaneous Approach
0C96X0Z	Drainage of Lower Gingiva with Drainage Device, External Approach
0C96XZX	Drainage of Lower Gingiva, External Approach, Diagnostic
0C96XZZ	Drainage of Lower Gingiva, External Approach
0C9700Z	Drainage of Tongue with Drainage Device, Open Approach
0C970ZX	Drainage of Tongue, Open Approach, Diagnostic
0C970ZZ	Drainage of Tongue, Open Approach
0C9730Z	Drainage of Tongue with Drainage Device, Percutaneous Approach
0C973ZX	Drainage of Tongue, Percutaneous Approach, Diagnostic
0C973ZZ	Drainage of Tongue, Percutaneous Approach
0C97X0Z	Drainage of Tongue with Drainage Device, External Approach
0C97XZX	Drainage of Tongue, External Approach, Diagnostic
0C97XZZ	Drainage of Tongue, External Approach
0C9800Z	Drainage of Right Parotid Gland with Drainage Device, Open Approach
0C980ZX	Drainage of Right Parotid Gland, Open Approach, Diagnostic
0C980ZZ	Drainage of Right Parotid Gland, Open Approach
0C9830Z	Drainage of Right Parotid Gland with Drainage Device, Percutaneous Approach
0C983ZX	Drainage of Right Parotid Gland, Percutaneous Approach, Diagnostic
0C983ZZ	Drainage of Right Parotid Gland, Percutaneous Approach
0C9900Z	Drainage of Left Parotid Gland with Drainage Device, Open Approach
0C990ZX	Drainage of Left Parotid Gland, Open Approach, Diagnostic
0C990ZZ	Drainage of Left Parotid Gland, Open Approach
0C9930Z	Drainage of Left Parotid Gland with Drainage Device, Percutaneous Approach
0C993ZX	Drainage of Left Parotid Gland, Percutaneous Approach, Diagnostic
0C993ZZ	Drainage of Left Parotid Gland, Percutaneous Approach
0C9B00Z	Drainage of Right Parotid Duct with Drainage Device, Open Approach
0C9B0ZX	Drainage of Right Parotid Duct, Open Approach, Diagnostic
0C9B0ZZ	Drainage of Right Parotid Duct, Open Approach
0C9B30Z	Drainage of Right Parotid Duct with Drainage Device, Percutaneous Approach
0C9B3ZX	Drainage of Right Parotid Duct, Percutaneous Approach, Diagnostic
0C9B3ZZ	Drainage of Right Parotid Duct, Percutaneous Approach
0C9C00Z	Drainage of Left Parotid Duct with Drainage Device, Open Approach
0C9C0ZX	Drainage of Left Parotid Duct, Open Approach, Diagnostic
0C9C0ZZ	Drainage of Left Parotid Duct, Open Approach
0C9C30Z	Drainage of Left Parotid Duct with Drainage Device, Percutaneous Approach
0C9C3ZX	Drainage of Left Parotid Duct, Percutaneous Approach, Diagnostic
0C9C3ZZ	Drainage of Left Parotid Duct, Percutaneous Approach
0C9D00Z	Drainage of Right Sublingual Gland with Drainage Device, Open Approach
0C9D0ZX	Drainage of Right Sublingual Gland, Open Approach, Diagnostic
0C9D0ZZ	Drainage of Right Sublingual Gland, Open Approach
0C9D30Z	Drainage of Right Sublingual Gland with Drainage Device, Percutaneous Approach
0C9D3ZX	Drainage of Right Sublingual Gland, Percutaneous Approach, Diagnostic
0C9D3ZZ	Drainage of Right Sublingual Gland, Percutaneous Approach
0C9F00Z	Drainage of Left Sublingual Gland with Drainage Device, Open Approach
0C9F0ZX	Drainage of Left Sublingual Gland, Open Approach, Diagnostic
0C9F0ZZ	Drainage of Left Sublingual Gland, Open Approach
0C9F30Z	Drainage of Left Sublingual Gland with Drainage Device, Percutaneous Approach
0C9F3ZX	Drainage of Left Sublingual Gland, Percutaneous Approach, Diagnostic
0C9F3ZZ	Drainage of Left Sublingual Gland, Percutaneous Approach
0C9G00Z	Drainage of Right Submaxillary Gland with Drainage Device, Open Approach
0C9G0ZX	Drainage of Right Submaxillary Gland, Open Approach, Diagnostic
0C9G0ZZ	Drainage of Right Submaxillary Gland, Open Approach
0C9G30Z	Drainage of Right Submaxillary Gland with Drainage Device, Percutaneous Approach
0C9G3ZX	Drainage of Right Submaxillary Gland, Percutaneous Approach, Diagnostic
0C9G3ZZ	Drainage of Right Submaxillary Gland, Percutaneous Approach
0C9H00Z	Drainage of Left Submaxillary Gland with Drainage Device, Open Approach
0C9H0ZX	Drainage of Left Submaxillary Gland, Open Approach, Diagnostic
0C9H0ZZ	Drainage of Left Submaxillary Gland, Open Approach
0C9H30Z	Drainage of Left Submaxillary Gland with Drainage Device, Percutaneous Approach
0C9H3ZX	Drainage of Left Submaxillary Gland, Percutaneous Approach, Diagnostic
0C9H3ZZ	Drainage of Left Submaxillary Gland, Percutaneous Approach
0C9J00Z	Drainage of Minor Salivary Gland with Drainage Device, Open Approach
0C9J0ZX	Drainage of Minor Salivary Gland, Open Approach, Diagnostic
0C9J0ZZ	Drainage of Minor Salivary Gland, Open Approach
0C9J30Z	Drainage of Minor Salivary Gland with Drainage Device, Percutaneous Approach
0C9J3ZX	Drainage of Minor Salivary Gland, Percutaneous Approach, Diagnostic
0C9J3ZZ	Drainage of Minor Salivary Gland, Percutaneous Approach
0C9M00Z	Drainage of Pharynx with Drainage Device, Open Approach
0C9M0ZX	Drainage of Pharynx, Open Approach, Diagnostic
0C9M0ZZ	Drainage of Pharynx, Open Approach
0C9M30Z	Drainage of Pharynx with Drainage Device, Percutaneous Approach
0C9M3ZX	Drainage of Pharynx, Percutaneous Approach, Diagnostic
0C9M3ZZ	Drainage of Pharynx, Percutaneous Approach
0C9M40Z	Drainage of Pharynx with Drainage Device, Percutaneous Endoscopic Approach
0C9M4ZX	Drainage of Pharynx, Percutaneous Endoscopic Approach, Diagnostic
0C9M4ZZ	Drainage of Pharynx, Percutaneous Endoscopic Approach
0C9M70Z	Drainage of Pharynx with Drainage Device, Via Natural or Artificial Opening
0C9M7ZX	Drainage of Pharynx, Via Natural or Artificial Opening, Diagnostic
0C9M7ZZ	Drainage of Pharynx, Via Natural or Artificial Opening
0C9M80Z	Drainage of Pharynx with Drainage Device, Via Natural or Artificial Opening Endoscopic
0C9M8ZX	Drainage of Pharynx, Via Natural or Artificial Opening Endoscopic, Diagnostic
0C9M8ZZ	Drainage of Pharynx, Via Natural or Artificial Opening Endoscopic
0C9N00Z	Drainage of Uvula with Drainage Device, Open Approach
0C9N0ZX	Drainage of Uvula, Open Approach, Diagnostic
0C9N0ZZ	Drainage of Uvula, Open Approach
0C9N30Z	Drainage of Uvula with Drainage Device, Percutaneous Approach
0C9N3ZX	Drainage of Uvula, Percutaneous Approach, Diagnostic
0C9N3ZZ	Drainage of Uvula, Percutaneous Approach
0C9NX0Z	Drainage of Uvula with Drainage Device, External Approach
0C9NXZX	Drainage of Uvula, External Approach, Diagnostic
0C9NXZZ	Drainage of Uvula, External Approach
0C9P00Z	Drainage of Tonsils with Drainage Device, Open Approach
0C9P0ZX	Drainage of Tonsils, Open Approach, Diagnostic
0C9P0ZZ	Drainage of Tonsils, Open Approach
0C9P30Z	Drainage of Tonsils with Drainage Device, Percutaneous Approach
0C9P3ZX	Drainage of Tonsils, Percutaneous Approach, Diagnostic
0C9P3ZZ	Drainage of Tonsils, Percutaneous Approach
0C9PX0Z	Drainage of Tonsils with Drainage Device, External Approach
0C9PXZX	Drainage of Tonsils, External Approach, Diagnostic
0C9PXZZ	Drainage of Tonsils, External Approach
0C9Q00Z	Drainage of Adenoids with Drainage Device, Open Approach
0C9Q0ZX	Drainage of Adenoids, Open Approach, Diagnostic
0C9Q0ZZ	Drainage of Adenoids, Open Approach

0C9Q30Z	Drainage of Adenoids with Drainage Device, Percutaneous Approach
0C9Q3ZX	Drainage of Adenoids, Percutaneous Approach, Diagnostic
0C9Q3ZZ	Drainage of Adenoids, Percutaneous Approach
0C9QX0Z	Drainage of Adenoids with Drainage Device, External Approach
0C9QXZX	Drainage of Adenoids, External Approach, Diagnostic
0C9QXZZ	Drainage of Adenoids, External Approach
0C9R00Z	Drainage of Epiglottis with Drainage Device, Open Approach
0C9R0ZX	Drainage of Epiglottis, Open Approach, Diagnostic
0C9R0ZZ	Drainage of Epiglottis, Open Approach
0C9R30Z	Drainage of Epiglottis with Drainage Device, Percutaneous Approach
0C9R3ZX	Drainage of Epiglottis, Percutaneous Approach, Diagnostic
0C9R3ZZ	Drainage of Epiglottis, Percutaneous Approach
0C9R40Z	Drainage of Epiglottis with Drainage Device, Percutaneous Endoscopic Approach
0C9R4ZX	Drainage of Epiglottis, Percutaneous Endoscopic Approach, Diagnostic
0C9R4ZZ	Drainage of Epiglottis, Percutaneous Endoscopic Approach
0C9R70Z	Drainage of Epiglottis with Drainage Device, Via Natural or Artificial Opening
0C9R7ZX	Drainage of Epiglottis, Via Natural or Artificial Opening, Diagnostic
0C9R7ZZ	Drainage of Epiglottis, Via Natural or Artificial Opening
0C9R80Z	Drainage of Epiglottis with Drainage Device, Via Natural or Artificial Opening Endoscopic
0C9R8ZX	Drainage of Epiglottis, Via Natural or Artificial Opening Endoscopic, Diagnostic
0C9R8ZZ	Drainage of Epiglottis, Via Natural or Artificial Opening Endoscopic
0C9S00Z	Drainage of Larynx with Drainage Device, Open Approach
0C9S0ZX	Drainage of Larynx, Open Approach, Diagnostic
0C9S0ZZ	Drainage of Larynx, Open Approach
0C9S30Z	Drainage of Larynx with Drainage Device, Percutaneous Approach
0C9S3ZX	Drainage of Larynx, Percutaneous Approach, Diagnostic
0C9S3ZZ	Drainage of Larynx, Percutaneous Approach
0C9S40Z	Drainage of Larynx with Drainage Device, Percutaneous Endoscopic Approach
0C9S4ZX	Drainage of Larynx, Percutaneous Endoscopic Approach, Diagnostic
0C9S4ZZ	Drainage of Larynx, Percutaneous Endoscopic Approach
0C9S70Z	Drainage of Larynx with Drainage Device, Via Natural or Artificial Opening
0C9S7ZX	Drainage of Larynx, Via Natural or Artificial Opening, Diagnostic
0C9S7ZZ	Drainage of Larynx, Via Natural or Artificial Opening
0C9S80Z	Drainage of Larynx with Drainage Device, Via Natural or Artificial Opening Endoscopic
0C9S8ZX	Drainage of Larynx, Via Natural or Artificial Opening Endoscopic, Diagnostic
0C9S8ZZ	Drainage of Larynx, Via Natural or Artificial Opening Endoscopic
0C9T00Z	Drainage of Right Vocal Cord with Drainage Device, Open Approach
0C9T0ZX	Drainage of Right Vocal Cord, Open Approach, Diagnostic
0C9T0ZZ	Drainage of Right Vocal Cord, Open Approach
0C9T30Z	Drainage of Right Vocal Cord with Drainage Device, Percutaneous Approach
0C9T3ZX	Drainage of Right Vocal Cord, Percutaneous Approach, Diagnostic
0C9T3ZZ	Drainage of Right Vocal Cord, Percutaneous Approach
0C9T40Z	Drainage of Right Vocal Cord with Drainage Device, Percutaneous Endoscopic Approach
0C9T4ZX	Drainage of Right Vocal Cord, Percutaneous Endoscopic Approach, Diagnostic
0C9T4ZZ	Drainage of Right Vocal Cord, Percutaneous Endoscopic Approach
0C9T70Z	Drainage of Right Vocal Cord with Drainage Device, Via Natural or Artificial Opening
0C9T7ZX	Drainage of Right Vocal Cord, Via Natural or Artificial Opening, Diagnostic

0C9T7ZZ	Drainage of Right Vocal Cord, Via Natural or Artificial Opening
0C9T80Z	Drainage of Right Vocal Cord with Drainage Device, Via Natural or Artificial Opening Endoscopic
0C9T8ZX	Drainage of Right Vocal Cord, Via Natural or Artificial Opening Endoscopic, Diagnostic
0C9T8ZZ	Drainage of Right Vocal Cord, Via Natural or Artificial Opening Endoscopic
0C9V00Z	Drainage of Left Vocal Cord with Drainage Device, Open Approach
0C9V0ZX	Drainage of Left Vocal Cord, Open Approach, Diagnostic
0C9V0ZZ	Drainage of Left Vocal Cord, Open Approach
0C9V30Z	Drainage of Left Vocal Cord with Drainage Device, Percutaneous Approach
0C9V3ZX	Drainage of Left Vocal Cord, Percutaneous Approach, Diagnostic
0C9V3ZZ	Drainage of Left Vocal Cord, Percutaneous Approach
0C9V40Z	Drainage of Left Vocal Cord with Drainage Device, Percutaneous Endoscopic Approach
0C9V4ZX	Drainage of Left Vocal Cord, Percutaneous Endoscopic Approach, Diagnostic
0C9V4ZZ	Drainage of Left Vocal Cord, Percutaneous Endoscopic Approach
0C9V70Z	Drainage of Left Vocal Cord with Drainage Device, Via Natural or Artificial Opening
0C9V7ZX	Drainage of Left Vocal Cord, Via Natural or Artificial Opening, Diagnostic
0C9V7ZZ	Drainage of Left Vocal Cord, Via Natural or Artificial Opening
0C9V80Z	Drainage of Left Vocal Cord with Drainage Device, Via Natural or Artificial Opening Endoscopic
0C9V8ZX	Drainage of Left Vocal Cord, Via Natural or Artificial Opening Endoscopic, Diagnostic
0C9V8ZZ	Drainage of Left Vocal Cord, Via Natural or Artificial Opening Endoscopic
0C9W000	Drainage of Upper Tooth with Drainage Device, Open Approach, Single
0C9W001	Drainage of Upper Tooth with Drainage Device, Open Approach, Multiple
0C9W002	Drainage of Upper Tooth with Drainage Device, Open Approach, All
0C9W0Z0	Drainage of Upper Tooth, Open Approach, Single
0C9W0Z1	Drainage of Upper Tooth, Open Approach, Multiple
0C9W0Z2	Drainage of Upper Tooth, Open Approach, All
0C9WX00	Drainage of Upper Tooth with Drainage Device, External Approach, Single
0C9WX01	Drainage of Upper Tooth with Drainage Device, External Approach, Multiple
0C9WX02	Drainage of Upper Tooth with Drainage Device, External Approach, All
0C9WXZ0	Drainage of Upper Tooth, External Approach, Single
0C9WXZ1	Drainage of Upper Tooth, External Approach, Multiple
0C9WXZ2	Drainage of Upper Tooth, External Approach, All
0C9X000	Drainage of Lower Tooth with Drainage Device, Open Approach, Single
0C9X001	Drainage of Lower Tooth with Drainage Device, Open Approach, Multiple
0C9X002	Drainage of Lower Tooth with Drainage Device, Open Approach, All
0C9X0Z0	Drainage of Lower Tooth, Open Approach, Single
0C9X0Z1	Drainage of Lower Tooth, Open Approach, Multiple
0C9X0Z2	Drainage of Lower Tooth, Open Approach, All
0C9XX00	Drainage of Lower Tooth with Drainage Device, External Approach, Single
0C9XX01	Drainage of Lower Tooth with Drainage Device, External Approach, Multiple
0C9XX02	Drainage of Lower Tooth with Drainage Device, External Approach, All
0C9XXZ0	Drainage of Lower Tooth, External Approach, Single
0C9XXZ1	Drainage of Lower Tooth, External Approach, Multiple
0C9XXZ2	Drainage of Lower Tooth, External Approach, All

0CB – Mouth and Throat, Excision

Review Coding Guidelines B3.4a and B3.4b

Review Coding Guideline B3.8

0CB00ZX	Excision of Upper Lip, Open Approach, Diagnostic
0CB00ZZ	Excision of Upper Lip, Open Approach
0CB03ZX	Excision of Upper Lip, Percutaneous Approach, Diagnostic
0CB03ZZ	Excision of Upper Lip, Percutaneous Approach
0CB0XZX	Excision of Upper Lip, External Approach, Diagnostic
0CB0XZZ	Excision of Upper Lip, External Approach
0CB10ZX	Excision of Lower Lip, Open Approach, Diagnostic
0CB10ZZ	Excision of Lower Lip, Open Approach
0CB13ZX	Excision of Lower Lip, Percutaneous Approach, Diagnostic
0CB13ZZ	Excision of Lower Lip, Percutaneous Approach
0CB1XZX	Excision of Lower Lip, External Approach, Diagnostic
0CB1XZZ	Excision of Lower Lip, External Approach
0CB20ZX	Excision of Hard Palate, Open Approach, Diagnostic
0CB20ZZ	Excision of Hard Palate, Open Approach
0CB23ZX	Excision of Hard Palate, Percutaneous Approach, Diagnostic
0CB23ZZ	Excision of Hard Palate, Percutaneous Approach
0CB2XZX	Excision of Hard Palate, External Approach, Diagnostic
0CB2XZZ	Excision of Hard Palate, External Approach
0CB30ZX	Excision of Soft Palate, Open Approach, Diagnostic
0CB30ZZ	Excision of Soft Palate, Open Approach
0CB33ZX	Excision of Soft Palate, Percutaneous Approach, Diagnostic
0CB33ZZ	Excision of Soft Palate, Percutaneous Approach
0CB3XZX	Excision of Soft Palate, External Approach, Diagnostic
0CB3XZZ	Excision of Soft Palate, External Approach
0CB40ZX	Excision of Buccal Mucosa, Open Approach, Diagnostic
0CB40ZZ	Excision of Buccal Mucosa, Open Approach
0CB43ZX	Excision of Buccal Mucosa, Percutaneous Approach, Diagnostic
0CB43ZZ	Excision of Buccal Mucosa, Percutaneous Approach
0CB4XZX	Excision of Buccal Mucosa, External Approach, Diagnostic
0CB4XZZ	Excision of Buccal Mucosa, External Approach
0CB50ZX	Excision of Upper Gingiva, Open Approach, Diagnostic
0CB50ZZ	Excision of Upper Gingiva, Open Approach
0CB53ZX	Excision of Upper Gingiva, Percutaneous Approach, Diagnostic
0CB53ZZ	Excision of Upper Gingiva, Percutaneous Approach
0CB5XZX	Excision of Upper Gingiva, External Approach, Diagnostic
0CB5XZZ	Excision of Upper Gingiva, External Approach
0CB60ZX	Excision of Lower Gingiva, Open Approach, Diagnostic
0CB60ZZ	Excision of Lower Gingiva, Open Approach
0CB63ZX	Excision of Lower Gingiva, Percutaneous Approach, Diagnostic
0CB63ZZ	Excision of Lower Gingiva, Percutaneous Approach
0CB6XZX	Excision of Lower Gingiva, External Approach, Diagnostic
0CB6XZZ	Excision of Lower Gingiva, External Approach
0CB70ZX	Excision of Tongue, Open Approach, Diagnostic
0CB70ZZ	Excision of Tongue, Open Approach
0CB73ZX	Excision of Tongue, Percutaneous Approach, Diagnostic
0CB73ZZ	Excision of Tongue, Percutaneous Approach
0CB7XZX	Excision of Tongue, External Approach, Diagnostic
0CB7XZZ	Excision of Tongue, External Approach
0CB80ZX	Excision of Right Parotid Gland, Open Approach, Diagnostic
0CB80ZZ	Excision of Right Parotid Gland, Open Approach
0CB83ZX	Excision of Right Parotid Gland, Percutaneous Approach, Diagnostic
0CB83ZZ	Excision of Right Parotid Gland, Percutaneous Approach
0CB90ZX	Excision of Left Parotid Gland, Open Approach, Diagnostic
0CB90ZZ	Excision of Left Parotid Gland, Open Approach
0CB93ZX	Excision of Left Parotid Gland, Percutaneous Approach, Diagnostic
0CB93ZZ	Excision of Left Parotid Gland, Percutaneous Approach
0CBB0ZX	Excision of Right Parotid Duct, Open Approach, Diagnostic
0CBB0ZZ	Excision of Right Parotid Duct, Open Approach
0CBB3ZX	Excision of Right Parotid Duct, Percutaneous Approach, Diagnostic
0CBB3ZZ	Excision of Right Parotid Duct, Percutaneous Approach
0CBC0ZX	Excision of Left Parotid Duct, Open Approach, Diagnostic
0CBC0ZZ	Excision of Left Parotid Duct, Open Approach
0CBC3ZX	Excision of Left Parotid Duct, Percutaneous Approach, Diagnostic
0CBC3ZZ	Excision of Left Parotid Duct, Percutaneous Approach
0CBD0ZX	Excision of Right Sublingual Gland, Open Approach, Diagnostic
0CBD0ZZ	Excision of Right Sublingual Gland, Open Approach
0CBD3ZX	Excision of Right Sublingual Gland, Percutaneous Approach, Diagnostic
0CBD3ZZ	Excision of Right Sublingual Gland, Percutaneous Approach
0CBF0ZX	Excision of Left Sublingual Gland, Open Approach, Diagnostic
0CBF0ZZ	Excision of Left Sublingual Gland, Open Approach
0CBF3ZX	Excision of Left Sublingual Gland, Percutaneous Approach, Diagnostic
0CBF3ZZ	Excision of Left Sublingual Gland, Percutaneous Approach
0CBG0ZX	Excision of Right Submaxillary Gland, Open Approach, Diagnostic
0CBG0ZZ	Excision of Right Submaxillary Gland, Open Approach
0CBG3ZX	Excision of Right Submaxillary Gland, Percutaneous Approach, Diagnostic
0CBG3ZZ	Excision of Right Submaxillary Gland, Percutaneous Approach
0CBH0ZX	Excision of Left Submaxillary Gland, Open Approach, Diagnostic
0CBH0ZZ	Excision of Left Submaxillary Gland, Open Approach
0CBH3ZX	Excision of Left Submaxillary Gland, Percutaneous Approach, Diagnostic
0CBH3ZZ	Excision of Left Submaxillary Gland, Percutaneous Approach
0CBJ0ZX	Excision of Minor Salivary Gland, Open Approach, Diagnostic
0CBJ0ZZ	Excision of Minor Salivary Gland, Open Approach
0CBJ3ZX	Excision of Minor Salivary Gland, Percutaneous Approach, Diagnostic
0CBJ3ZZ	Excision of Minor Salivary Gland, Percutaneous Approach
0CBM0ZX	Excision of Pharynx, Open Approach, Diagnostic
0CBM0ZZ	Excision of Pharynx, Open Approach
0CBM3ZX	Excision of Pharynx, Percutaneous Approach, Diagnostic
0CBM3ZZ	Excision of Pharynx, Percutaneous Approach
0CBM4ZX	Excision of Pharynx, Percutaneous Endoscopic Approach, Diagnostic
0CBM4ZZ	Excision of Pharynx, Percutaneous Endoscopic Approach
0CBM7ZX	Excision of Pharynx, Via Natural or Artificial Opening, Diagnostic
0CBM7ZZ	Excision of Pharynx, Via Natural or Artificial Opening
0CBM8ZX	Excision of Pharynx, Via Natural or Artificial Opening Endoscopic, Diagnostic
0CBM8ZZ	Excision of Pharynx, Via Natural or Artificial Opening Endoscopic
0CBN0ZX	Excision of Uvula, Open Approach, Diagnostic
0CBN0ZZ	Excision of Uvula, Open Approach
0CBN3ZX	Excision of Uvula, Percutaneous Approach, Diagnostic
0CBN3ZZ	Excision of Uvula, Percutaneous Approach
0CBNXZX	Excision of Uvula, External Approach, Diagnostic
0CBNXZZ	Excision of Uvula, External Approach
0CBP0ZX	Excision of Tonsils, Open Approach, Diagnostic
0CBP0ZZ	Excision of Tonsils, Open Approach
0CBP3ZX	Excision of Tonsils, Percutaneous Approach, Diagnostic
0CBP3ZZ	Excision of Tonsils, Percutaneous Approach
0CBPXZX	Excision of Tonsils, External Approach, Diagnostic
0CBPXZZ	Excision of Tonsils, External Approach
0CBQ0ZX	Excision of Adenoids, Open Approach, Diagnostic
0CBQ0ZZ	Excision of Adenoids, Open Approach
0CBQ3ZX	Excision of Adenoids, Percutaneous Approach, Diagnostic
0CBQ3ZZ	Excision of Adenoids, Percutaneous Approach
0CBQXZX	Excision of Adenoids, External Approach, Diagnostic
0CBQXZZ	Excision of Adenoids, External Approach
0CBR0ZX	Excision of Epiglottis, Open Approach, Diagnostic
0CBR0ZZ	Excision of Epiglottis, Open Approach
0CBR3ZX	Excision of Epiglottis, Percutaneous Approach, Diagnostic
0CBR3ZZ	Excision of Epiglottis, Percutaneous Approach
0CBR4ZX	Excision of Epiglottis, Percutaneous Endoscopic Approach, Diagnostic
0CBR4ZZ	Excision of Epiglottis, Percutaneous Endoscopic Approach
0CBR7ZX	Excision of Epiglottis, Via Natural or Artificial Opening, Diagnostic
0CBR7ZZ	Excision of Epiglottis, Via Natural or Artificial Opening
0CBR8ZX	Excision of Epiglottis, Via Natural or Artificial Opening Endoscopic, Diagnostic
0CBR8ZZ	Excision of Epiglottis, Via Natural or Artificial Opening Endoscopic

0CBS0ZX   Excision of Larynx, Open Approach, Diagnostic
0CBS0ZZ   Excision of Larynx, Open Approach
0CBS3ZX   Excision of Larynx, Percutaneous Approach, Diagnostic
0CBS3ZZ   Excision of Larynx, Percutaneous Approach
0CBS4ZX   Excision of Larynx, Percutaneous Endoscopic Approach, Diagnostic
0CBS4ZZ   Excision of Larynx, Percutaneous Endoscopic Approach
0CBS7ZX   Excision of Larynx, Via Natural or Artificial Opening, Diagnostic
0CBS7ZZ   Excision of Larynx, Via Natural or Artificial Opening
0CBS8ZX   Excision of Larynx, Via Natural or Artificial Opening Endoscopic, Diagnostic
0CBS8ZZ   Excision of Larynx, Via Natural or Artificial Opening Endoscopic
0CBT0ZX   Excision of Right Vocal Cord, Open Approach, Diagnostic
0CBT0ZZ   Excision of Right Vocal Cord, Open Approach
0CBT3ZX   Excision of Right Vocal Cord, Percutaneous Approach, Diagnostic
0CBT3ZZ   Excision of Right Vocal Cord, Percutaneous Approach
0CBT4ZX   Excision of Right Vocal Cord, Percutaneous Endoscopic Approach, Diagnostic
0CBT4ZZ   Excision of Right Vocal Cord, Percutaneous Endoscopic Approach
0CBT7ZX   Excision of Right Vocal Cord, Via Natural or Artificial Opening, Diagnostic
0CBT7ZZ   Excision of Right Vocal Cord, Via Natural or Artificial Opening
0CBT8ZX   Excision of Right Vocal Cord, Via Natural or Artificial Opening Endoscopic, Diagnostic
0CBT8ZZ   Excision of Right Vocal Cord, Via Natural or Artificial Opening Endoscopic
0CBV0ZX   Excision of Left Vocal Cord, Open Approach, Diagnostic
0CBV0ZZ   Excision of Left Vocal Cord, Open Approach
0CBV3ZX   Excision of Left Vocal Cord, Percutaneous Approach, Diagnostic
0CBV3ZZ   Excision of Left Vocal Cord, Percutaneous Approach
0CBV4ZX   Excision of Left Vocal Cord, Percutaneous Endoscopic Approach, Diagnostic
0CBV4ZZ   Excision of Left Vocal Cord, Percutaneous Endoscopic Approach
0CBV7ZX   Excision of Left Vocal Cord, Via Natural or Artificial Opening, Diagnostic
0CBV7ZZ   Excision of Left Vocal Cord, Via Natural or Artificial Opening
0CBV8ZX   Excision of Left Vocal Cord, Via Natural or Artificial Opening Endoscopic, Diagnostic
0CBV8ZZ   Excision of Left Vocal Cord, Via Natural or Artificial Opening Endoscopic
0CBW0Z0   Excision of Upper Tooth, Open Approach, Single
0CBW0Z1   Excision of Upper Tooth, Open Approach, Multiple
0CBW0Z2   Excision of Upper Tooth, Open Approach, All
0CBWXZ0   Excision of Upper Tooth, External Approach, Single
0CBWXZ1   Excision of Upper Tooth, External Approach, Multiple
0CBWXZ2   Excision of Upper Tooth, External Approach, All
0CBX0Z0   Excision of Lower Tooth, Open Approach, Single
0CBX0Z1   Excision of Lower Tooth, Open Approach, Multiple
0CBX0Z2   Excision of Lower Tooth, Open Approach, All
0CBXXZ0   Excision of Lower Tooth, External Approach, Single
0CBXXZ1   Excision of Lower Tooth, External Approach, Multiple
0CBXXZ2   Excision of Lower Tooth, External Approach, All

0CC – Mouth and Throat, Extirpation

0CC00ZZ   Extirpation of Matter from Upper Lip, Open Approach
0CC03ZZ   Extirpation of Matter from Upper Lip, Percutaneous Approach
0CC0XZZ   Extirpation of Matter from Upper Lip, External Approach
0CC10ZZ   Extirpation of Matter from Lower Lip, Open Approach
0CC13ZZ   Extirpation of Matter from Lower Lip, Percutaneous Approach
0CC1XZZ   Extirpation of Matter from Lower Lip, External Approach
0CC20ZZ   Extirpation of Matter from Hard Palate, Open Approach
0CC23ZZ   Extirpation of Matter from Hard Palate, Percutaneous Approach
0CC2XZZ   Extirpation of Matter from Hard Palate, External Approach
0CC30ZZ   Extirpation of Matter from Soft Palate, Open Approach
0CC33ZZ   Extirpation of Matter from Soft Palate, Percutaneous Approach
0CC3XZZ   Extirpation of Matter from Soft Palate, External Approach
0CC40ZZ   Extirpation of Matter from Buccal Mucosa, Open Approach
0CC43ZZ   Extirpation of Matter from Buccal Mucosa, Percutaneous Approach
0CC4XZZ   Extirpation of Matter from Buccal Mucosa, External Approach
0CC50ZZ   Extirpation of Matter from Upper Gingiva, Open Approach
0CC53ZZ   Extirpation of Matter from Upper Gingiva, Percutaneous Approach
0CC5XZZ   Extirpation of Matter from Upper Gingiva, External Approach
0CC60ZZ   Extirpation of Matter from Lower Gingiva, Open Approach
0CC63ZZ   Extirpation of Matter from Lower Gingiva, Percutaneous Approach
0CC6XZZ   Extirpation of Matter from Lower Gingiva, External Approach
0CC70ZZ   Extirpation of Matter from Tongue, Open Approach
0CC73ZZ   Extirpation of Matter from Tongue, Percutaneous Approach
0CC7XZZ   Extirpation of Matter from Tongue, External Approach
0CC80ZZ   Extirpation of Matter from Right Parotid Gland, Open Approach
0CC83ZZ   Extirpation of Matter from Right Parotid Gland, Percutaneous Approach
0CC90ZZ   Extirpation of Matter from Left Parotid Gland, Open Approach
0CC93ZZ   Extirpation of Matter from Left Parotid Gland, Percutaneous Approach
0CCB0ZZ   Extirpation of Matter from Right Parotid Duct, Open Approach
0CCB3ZZ   Extirpation of Matter from Right Parotid Duct, Percutaneous Approach
0CCC0ZZ   Extirpation of Matter from Left Parotid Duct, Open Approach
0CCC3ZZ   Extirpation of Matter from Left Parotid Duct, Percutaneous Approach
0CCD0ZZ   Extirpation of Matter from Right Sublingual Gland, Open Approach
0CCD3ZZ   Extirpation of Matter from Right Sublingual Gland, Percutaneous Approach
0CCF0ZZ   Extirpation of Matter from Left Sublingual Gland, Open Approach
0CCF3ZZ   Extirpation of Matter from Left Sublingual Gland, Percutaneous Approach

0CCG0ZZ   Extirpation of Matter from Right Submaxillary Gland, Open Approach
0CCG3ZZ   Extirpation of Matter from Right Submaxillary Gland, Percutaneous Approach
0CCH0ZZ   Extirpation of Matter from Left Submaxillary Gland, Open Approach
0CCH3ZZ   Extirpation of Matter from Left Submaxillary Gland, Percutaneous Approach
0CCJ0ZZ   Extirpation of Matter from Minor Salivary Gland, Open Approach
0CCJ3ZZ   Extirpation of Matter from Minor Salivary Gland, Percutaneous Approach
0CCM0ZZ   Extirpation of Matter from Pharynx, Open Approach
0CCM3ZZ   Extirpation of Matter from Pharynx, Percutaneous Approach
0CCM4ZZ   Extirpation of Matter from Pharynx, Percutaneous Endoscopic Approach
0CCM7ZZ   Extirpation of Matter from Pharynx, Via Natural or Artificial Opening
0CCM8ZZ   Extirpation of Matter from Pharynx, Via Natural or Artificial Opening Endoscopic
0CCN0ZZ   Extirpation of Matter from Uvula, Open Approach
0CCN3ZZ   Extirpation of Matter from Uvula, Percutaneous Approach
0CCNXZZ   Extirpation of Matter from Uvula, External Approach
0CCP0ZZ   Extirpation of Matter from Tonsils, Open Approach
0CCP3ZZ   Extirpation of Matter from Tonsils, Percutaneous Approach
0CCPXZZ   Extirpation of Matter from Tonsils, External Approach
0CCQ0ZZ   Extirpation of Matter from Adenoids, Open Approach
0CCQ3ZZ   Extirpation of Matter from Adenoids, Percutaneous Approach
0CCQXZZ   Extirpation of Matter from Adenoids, External Approach
0CCR0ZZ   Extirpation of Matter from Epiglottis, Open Approach
0CCR3ZZ   Extirpation of Matter from Epiglottis, Percutaneous Approach
0CCR4ZZ   Extirpation of Matter from Epiglottis, Percutaneous Endoscopic Approach
0CCR7ZZ   Extirpation of Matter from Epiglottis, Via Natural or Artificial Opening
0CCR8ZZ   Extirpation of Matter from Epiglottis, Via Natural or Artificial Opening Endoscopic
0CCS0ZZ   Extirpation of Matter from Larynx, Open Approach
0CCS3ZZ   Extirpation of Matter from Larynx, Percutaneous Approach
0CCS4ZZ   Extirpation of Matter from Larynx, Percutaneous Endoscopic Approach
0CCS7ZZ   Extirpation of Matter from Larynx, Via Natural or Artificial Opening
0CCS8ZZ   Extirpation of Matter from Larynx, Via Natural or Artificial Opening Endoscopic
0CCT0ZZ   Extirpation of Matter from Right Vocal Cord, Open Approach

0CCT3ZZ	Extirpation of Matter from Right Vocal Cord, Percutaneous Approach
0CCT4ZZ	Extirpation of Matter from Right Vocal Cord, Percutaneous Endoscopic Approach
0CCT7ZZ	Extirpation of Matter from Right Vocal Cord, Via Natural or Artificial Opening
0CCT8ZZ	Extirpation of Matter from Right Vocal Cord, Via Natural or Artificial Opening Endoscopic
0CCV0ZZ	Extirpation of Matter from Left Vocal Cord, Open Approach
0CCV3ZZ	Extirpation of Matter from Left Vocal Cord, Percutaneous Approach
0CCV4ZZ	Extirpation of Matter from Left Vocal Cord, Percutaneous Endoscopic Approach
0CCV7ZZ	Extirpation of Matter from Left Vocal Cord, Via Natural or Artificial Opening
0CCV8ZZ	Extirpation of Matter from Left Vocal Cord, Via Natural or Artificial Opening Endoscopic

0CCW0Z0	Extirpation of Matter from Upper Tooth, Single, Open Approach
0CCW0Z1	Extirpation of Matter from Upper Tooth, Multiple, Open Approach
0CCW0Z2	Extirpation of Matter from Upper Tooth, All, Open Approach
0CCWXZ0	Extirpation of Matter from Upper Tooth, Single, External Approach
0CCWXZ1	Extirpation of Matter from Upper Tooth, Multiple, External Approach
0CCWXZ2	Extirpation of Matter from Upper Tooth, All, External Approach
0CCX0Z0	Extirpation of Matter from Lower Tooth, Single, Open Approach
0CCX0Z1	Extirpation of Matter from Lower Tooth, Multiple, Open Approach
0CCX0Z2	Extirpation of Matter from Lower Tooth, All, Open Approach
0CCXXZ0	Extirpation of Matter from Lower Tooth, Single, External Approach
0CCXXZ1	Extirpation of Matter from Lower Tooth, Multiple, External Approach
0CCXXZ2	Extirpation of Matter from Lower Tooth, All, External Approach

0CD – Mouth and Throat, Extraction

0CDT0ZZ	Extraction of Right Vocal Cord, Open Approach
0CDT3ZZ	Extraction of Right Vocal Cord, Percutaneous Approach
0CDT4ZZ	Extraction of Right Vocal Cord, Percutaneous Endoscopic Approach
0CDT7ZZ	Extraction of Right Vocal Cord, Via Natural or Artificial Opening
0CDT8ZZ	Extraction of Right Vocal Cord, Via Natural or Artificial Opening Endoscopic
0CDV0ZZ	Extraction of Left Vocal Cord, Open Approach
0CDV3ZZ	Extraction of Left Vocal Cord, Percutaneous Approach
0CDV4ZZ	Extraction of Left Vocal Cord, Percutaneous Endoscopic Approach

0CDV7ZZ	Extraction of Left Vocal Cord, Via Natural or Artificial Opening
0CDV8ZZ	Extraction of Left Vocal Cord, Via Natural or Artificial Opening Endoscopic
0CDWXZ0	Extraction of Upper Tooth, Single, External Approach
0CDWXZ1	Extraction of Upper Tooth, Multiple, External Approach
0CDWXZ2	Extraction of Upper Tooth, All, External Approach
0CDXXZ0	Extraction of Lower Tooth, Single, External Approach
0CDXXZ1	Extraction of Lower Tooth, Multiple, External Approach
0CDXXZ2	Extraction of Lower Tooth, All, External Approach

0CF – Mouth and Throat, Fragmentation

0CFB0ZZ	Fragmentation in Right Parotid Duct, Open Approach
0CFB3ZZ	Fragmentation in Right Parotid Duct, Percutaneous Approach
0CFB7ZZ	Fragmentation in Right Parotid Duct, Via Natural or Artificial Opening
⬗ 0CFBXZZ	Fragmentation in Right Parotid Duct, External Approach

0CFC0ZZ	Fragmentation in Left Parotid Duct, Open Approach
0CFC3ZZ	Fragmentation in Left Parotid Duct, Percutaneous Approach
0CFC7ZZ	Fragmentation in Left Parotid Duct, Via Natural or Artificial Opening
⬗ 0CFCXZZ	Fragmentation in Left Parotid Duct, External Approach

0CH – Mouth and Throat, Insertion

0CH701Z	Insertion of Radioactive Element into Tongue, Open Approach
0CH731Z	Insertion of Radioactive Element into Tongue, Percutaneous Approach
0CH7X1Z	Insertion of Radioactive Element into Tongue, External Approach

0CHY7BZ	Insertion of Airway into Mouth and Throat, Via Natural or Artificial Opening
0CHY8BZ	Insertion of Airway into Mouth and Throat, Via Natural or Artificial Opening Endoscopic

0CJ – Mouth and Throat, Inspection

Review Coding Guidelines B3.11a, B3.11b and B3.11c

0CJA0ZZ	Inspection of Salivary Gland, Open Approach
0CJA3ZZ	Inspection of Salivary Gland, Percutaneous Approach
0CJAXZZ	Inspection of Salivary Gland, External Approach
0CJS0ZZ	Inspection of Larynx, Open Approach
0CJS3ZZ	Inspection of Larynx, Percutaneous Approach
0CJS4ZZ	Inspection of Larynx, Percutaneous Endoscopic Approach
0CJS7ZZ	Inspection of Larynx, Via Natural or Artificial Opening
0CJS8ZZ	Inspection of Larynx, Via Natural or Artificial Opening Endoscopic

0CJSXZZ	Inspection of Larynx, External Approach
0CJY0ZZ	Inspection of Mouth and Throat, Open Approach
0CJY3ZZ	Inspection of Mouth and Throat, Percutaneous Approach
0CJY4ZZ	Inspection of Mouth and Throat, Percutaneous Endoscopic Approach
0CJY7ZZ	Inspection of Mouth and Throat, Via Natural or Artificial Opening
0CJY8ZZ	Inspection of Mouth and Throat, Via Natural or Artificial Opening Endoscopic
0CJYXZZ	Inspection of Mouth and Throat, External Approach

0CL – Mouth and Throat, Occlusion

0CLB0CZ	Occlusion of Right Parotid Duct with Extraluminal Device, Open Approach
0CLB0DZ	Occlusion of Right Parotid Duct with Intraluminal Device, Open Approach
0CLB0ZZ	Occlusion of Right Parotid Duct, Open Approach
0CLB3CZ	Occlusion of Right Parotid Duct with Extraluminal Device, Percutaneous Approach
0CLB3DZ	Occlusion of Right Parotid Duct with Intraluminal Device, Percutaneous Approach
0CLB3ZZ	Occlusion of Right Parotid Duct, Percutaneous Approach

0CLB4CZ	Occlusion of Right Parotid Duct with Extraluminal Device, Percutaneous Endoscopic Approach
0CLB4DZ	Occlusion of Right Parotid Duct with Intraluminal Device, Percutaneous Endoscopic Approach
0CLB4ZZ	Occlusion of Right Parotid Duct, Percutaneous Endoscopic Approach
0CLB7DZ	Occlusion of Right Parotid Duct with Intraluminal Device, Via Natural or Artificial Opening
0CLB7ZZ	Occlusion of Right Parotid Duct, Via Natural or Artificial Opening
0CLB8DZ	Occlusion of Right Parotid Duct with Intraluminal Device, Via Natural or Artificial Opening Endoscopic

0CLB8ZZ   Occlusion of Right Parotid Duct, Via Natural or Artificial Opening Endoscopic

0CLC0CZ   Occlusion of Left Parotid Duct with Extraluminal Device, Open Approach

0CLC0DZ   Occlusion of Left Parotid Duct with Intraluminal Device, Open Approach

0CLC0ZZ   Occlusion of Left Parotid Duct, Open Approach

0CLC3CZ   Occlusion of Left Parotid Duct with Extraluminal Device, Percutaneous Approach

0CLC3DZ   Occlusion of Left Parotid Duct with Intraluminal Device, Percutaneous Approach

0CLC3ZZ   Occlusion of Left Parotid Duct, Percutaneous Approach

0CLC4CZ   Occlusion of Left Parotid Duct with Extraluminal Device, Percutaneous Endoscopic Approach

0CLC4DZ   Occlusion of Left Parotid Duct with Intraluminal Device, Percutaneous Endoscopic Approach

0CLC4ZZ   Occlusion of Left Parotid Duct, Percutaneous Endoscopic Approach

0CLC7DZ   Occlusion of Left Parotid Duct with Intraluminal Device, Via Natural or Artificial Opening

0CLC7ZZ   Occlusion of Left Parotid Duct, Via Natural or Artificial Opening

0CLC8DZ   Occlusion of Left Parotid Duct with Intraluminal Device, Via Natural or Artificial Opening Endoscopic

0CLC8ZZ   Occlusion of Left Parotid Duct, Via Natural or Artificial Opening Endoscopic

0CM – Mouth and Throat, Reattachment

0CM00ZZ   Reattachment of Upper Lip, Open Approach
0CM10ZZ   Reattachment of Lower Lip, Open Approach
0CM30ZZ   Reattachment of Soft Palate, Open Approach
0CM70ZZ   Reattachment of Tongue, Open Approach
0CMN0ZZ   Reattachment of Uvula, Open Approach
0CMW0Z0   Reattachment of Upper Tooth, Single, Open Approach
0CMW0Z1   Reattachment of Upper Tooth, Multiple, Open Approach
0CMW0Z2   Reattachment of Upper Tooth, All, Open Approach
0CMWXZ0   Reattachment of Upper Tooth, Single, External Approach

0CMWXZ1   Reattachment of Upper Tooth, Multiple, External Approach
0CMWXZ2   Reattachment of Upper Tooth, All, External Approach
0CMX0Z0   Reattachment of Lower Tooth, Single, Open Approach
0CMX0Z1   Reattachment of Lower Tooth, Multiple, Open Approach
0CMX0Z2   Reattachment of Lower Tooth, All, Open Approach
0CMXXZ0   Reattachment of Lower Tooth, Single, External Approach
0CMXXZ1   Reattachment of Lower Tooth, Multiple, External Approach
0CMXXZ2   Reattachment of Lower Tooth, All, External Approach

0CN – Mouth and Throat, Release

Review Coding Guidelines B3.13 and B3.14

0CN00ZZ   Release Upper Lip, Open Approach
0CN03ZZ   Release Upper Lip, Percutaneous Approach
0CN0XZZ   Release Upper Lip, External Approach
0CN10ZZ   Release Lower Lip, Open Approach
0CN13ZZ   Release Lower Lip, Percutaneous Approach
0CN1XZZ   Release Lower Lip, External Approach
0CN20ZZ   Release Hard Palate, Open Approach
0CN23ZZ   Release Hard Palate, Percutaneous Approach
0CN2XZZ   Release Hard Palate, External Approach
0CN30ZZ   Release Soft Palate, Open Approach
0CN33ZZ   Release Soft Palate, Percutaneous Approach
0CN3XZZ   Release Soft Palate, External Approach
0CN40ZZ   Release Buccal Mucosa, Open Approach
0CN43ZZ   Release Buccal Mucosa, Percutaneous Approach
0CN4XZZ   Release Buccal Mucosa, External Approach
0CN50ZZ   Release Upper Gingiva, Open Approach
0CN53ZZ   Release Upper Gingiva, Percutaneous Approach
0CN5XZZ   Release Upper Gingiva, External Approach
0CN60ZZ   Release Lower Gingiva, Open Approach
0CN63ZZ   Release Lower Gingiva, Percutaneous Approach
0CN6XZZ   Release Lower Gingiva, External Approach
0CN70ZZ   Release Tongue, Open Approach
0CN73ZZ   Release Tongue, Percutaneous Approach
0CN7XZZ   Release Tongue, External Approach
0CN80ZZ   Release Right Parotid Gland, Open Approach
0CN83ZZ   Release Right Parotid Gland, Percutaneous Approach
0CN90ZZ   Release Left Parotid Gland, Open Approach
0CN93ZZ   Release Left Parotid Gland, Percutaneous Approach
0CNB0ZZ   Release Right Parotid Duct, Open Approach
0CNB3ZZ   Release Right Parotid Duct, Percutaneous Approach
0CNC0ZZ   Release Left Parotid Duct, Open Approach
0CNC3ZZ   Release Left Parotid Duct, Percutaneous Approach
0CND0ZZ   Release Right Sublingual Gland, Open Approach
0CND3ZZ   Release Right Sublingual Gland, Percutaneous Approach
0CNF0ZZ   Release Left Sublingual Gland, Open Approach
0CNF3ZZ   Release Left Sublingual Gland, Percutaneous Approach
0CNG0ZZ   Release Right Submaxillary Gland, Open Approach
0CNG3ZZ   Release Right Submaxillary Gland, Percutaneous Approach
0CNH0ZZ   Release Left Submaxillary Gland, Open Approach
0CNH3ZZ   Release Left Submaxillary Gland, Percutaneous Approach
0CNJ0ZZ   Release Minor Salivary Gland, Open Approach
0CNJ3ZZ   Release Minor Salivary Gland, Percutaneous Approach
0CNM0ZZ   Release Pharynx, Open Approach

0CNM3ZZ   Release Pharynx, Percutaneous Approach
0CNM4ZZ   Release Pharynx, Percutaneous Endoscopic Approach
0CNM7ZZ   Release Pharynx, Via Natural or Artificial Opening
0CNM8ZZ   Release Pharynx, Via Natural or Artificial Opening Endoscopic
0CNN0ZZ   Release Uvula, Open Approach
0CNN3ZZ   Release Uvula, Percutaneous Approach
0CNNXZZ   Release Uvula, External Approach
0CNP0ZZ   Release Tonsils, Open Approach
0CNP3ZZ   Release Tonsils, Percutaneous Approach
0CNPXZZ   Release Tonsils, External Approach
0CNQ0ZZ   Release Adenoids, Open Approach
0CNQ3ZZ   Release Adenoids, Percutaneous Approach
0CNQXZZ   Release Adenoids, External Approach
0CNR0ZZ   Release Epiglottis, Open Approach
0CNR3ZZ   Release Epiglottis, Percutaneous Approach
0CNR4ZZ   Release Epiglottis, Percutaneous Endoscopic Approach
0CNR7ZZ   Release Epiglottis, Via Natural or Artificial Opening
0CNR8ZZ   Release Epiglottis, Via Natural or Artificial Opening Endoscopic
0CNS0ZZ   Release Larynx, Open Approach
0CNS3ZZ   Release Larynx, Percutaneous Approach
0CNS4ZZ   Release Larynx, Percutaneous Endoscopic Approach
0CNS7ZZ   Release Larynx, Via Natural or Artificial Opening
0CNS8ZZ   Release Larynx, Via Natural or Artificial Opening Endoscopic
0CNT0ZZ   Release Right Vocal Cord, Open Approach
0CNT3ZZ   Release Right Vocal Cord, Percutaneous Approach
0CNT4ZZ   Release Right Vocal Cord, Percutaneous Endoscopic Approach
0CNT7ZZ   Release Right Vocal Cord, Via Natural or Artificial Opening
0CNT8ZZ   Release Right Vocal Cord, Via Natural or Artificial Opening Endoscopic
0CNV0ZZ   Release Left Vocal Cord, Open Approach
0CNV3ZZ   Release Left Vocal Cord, Percutaneous Approach
0CNV4ZZ   Release Left Vocal Cord, Percutaneous Endoscopic Approach
0CNV7ZZ   Release Left Vocal Cord, Via Natural or Artificial Opening
0CNV8ZZ   Release Left Vocal Cord, Via Natural or Artificial Opening Endoscopic
0CNW0Z0   Release Upper Tooth, Single, Open Approach
0CNW0Z1   Release Upper Tooth, Multiple, Open Approach
0CNW0Z2   Release Upper Tooth, All, Open Approach
0CNWXZ0   Release Upper Tooth, Single, External Approach
0CNWXZ1   Release Upper Tooth, Multiple, External Approach

0CNWXZ2   Release Upper Tooth, All, External Approach
0CNX0Z0   Release Lower Tooth, Single, Open Approach
0CNX0Z1   Release Lower Tooth, Multiple, Open Approach
0CNX0Z2   Release Lower Tooth, All, Open Approach

0CNXXZ0   Release Lower Tooth, Single, External Approach
0CNXXZ1   Release Lower Tooth, Multiple, External Approach
0CNXXZ2   Release Lower Tooth, All, External Approach

0CP – Mouth and Throat, Removal

Review Coding Guideline B6.1c

0CPA00Z   Removal of Drainage Device from Salivary Gland, Open Approach
0CPA0CZ   Removal of Extraluminal Device from Salivary Gland, Open Approach
0CPA30Z   Removal of Drainage Device from Salivary Gland, Percutaneous Approach
0CPA3CZ   Removal of Extraluminal Device from Salivary Gland, Percutaneous Approach
0CPS00Z   Removal of Drainage Device from Larynx, Open Approach
0CPS07Z   Removal of Autologous Tissue Substitute from Larynx, Open Approach
0CPS0DZ   Removal of Intraluminal Device from Larynx, Open Approach
0CPS0JZ   Removal of Synthetic Substitute from Larynx, Open Approach
0CPS0KZ   Removal of Nonautologous Tissue Substitute from Larynx, Open Approach
0CPS30Z   Removal of Drainage Device from Larynx, Percutaneous Approach
0CPS37Z   Removal of Autologous Tissue Substitute from Larynx, Percutaneous Approach
0CPS3DZ   Removal of Intraluminal Device from Larynx, Percutaneous Approach
0CPS3JZ   Removal of Synthetic Substitute from Larynx, Percutaneous Approach
0CPS3KZ   Removal of Nonautologous Tissue Substitute from Larynx, Percutaneous Approach
0CPS70Z   Removal of Drainage Device from Larynx, Via Natural or Artificial Opening
0CPS77Z   Removal of Autologous Tissue Substitute from Larynx, Via Natural or Artificial Opening
0CPS7DZ   Removal of Intraluminal Device from Larynx, Via Natural or Artificial Opening
0CPS7JZ   Removal of Synthetic Substitute from Larynx, Via Natural or Artificial Opening
0CPS7KZ   Removal of Nonautologous Tissue Substitute from Larynx, Via Natural or Artificial Opening
0CPS80Z   Removal of Drainage Device from Larynx, Via Natural or Artificial Opening Endoscopic
0CPS87Z   Removal of Autologous Tissue Substitute from Larynx, Via Natural or Artificial Opening Endoscopic
0CPS8DZ   Removal of Intraluminal Device from Larynx, Via Natural or Artificial Opening Endoscopic
0CPS8JZ   Removal of Synthetic Substitute from Larynx, Via Natural or Artificial Opening Endoscopic
0CPS8KZ   Removal of Nonautologous Tissue Substitute from Larynx, Via Natural or Artificial Opening Endoscopic
0CPSX0Z   Removal of Drainage Device from Larynx, External Approach
0CPSX7Z   Removal of Autologous Tissue Substitute from Larynx, External Approach
0CPSXDZ   Removal of Intraluminal Device from Larynx, External Approach
0CPSXJZ   Removal of Synthetic Substitute from Larynx, External Approach
0CPSXKZ   Removal of Nonautologous Tissue Substitute from Larynx, External Approach
0CPY00Z   Removal of Drainage Device from Mouth and Throat, Open Approach

0CPY01Z   Removal of Radioactive Element from Mouth and Throat, Open Approach
0CPY07Z   Removal of Autologous Tissue Substitute from Mouth and Throat, Open Approach
0CPY0DZ   Removal of Intraluminal Device from Mouth and Throat, Open Approach
0CPY0JZ   Removal of Synthetic Substitute from Mouth and Throat, Open Approach
0CPY0KZ   Removal of Nonautologous Tissue Substitute from Mouth and Throat, Open Approach
0CPY30Z   Removal of Drainage Device from Mouth and Throat, Percutaneous Approach
0CPY31Z   Removal of Radioactive Element from Mouth and Throat, Percutaneous Approach
0CPY37Z   Removal of Autologous Tissue Substitute from Mouth and Throat, Percutaneous Approach
0CPY3DZ   Removal of Intraluminal Device from Mouth and Throat, Percutaneous Approach
0CPY3JZ   Removal of Synthetic Substitute from Mouth and Throat, Percutaneous Approach
0CPY3KZ   Removal of Nonautologous Tissue Substitute from Mouth and Throat, Percutaneous Approach
0CPY70Z   Removal of Drainage Device from Mouth and Throat, Via Natural or Artificial Opening
0CPY71Z   Removal of Radioactive Element from Mouth and Throat, Via Natural or Artificial Opening
0CPY77Z   Removal of Autologous Tissue Substitute from Mouth and Throat, Via Natural or Artificial Opening
0CPY7DZ   Removal of Intraluminal Device from Mouth and Throat, Via Natural or Artificial Opening
0CPY7JZ   Removal of Synthetic Substitute from Mouth and Throat, Via Natural or Artificial Opening
0CPY7KZ   Removal of Nonautologous Tissue Substitute from Mouth and Throat, Via Natural or Artificial Opening
0CPY80Z   Removal of Drainage Device from Mouth and Throat, Via Natural or Artificial Opening Endoscopic
0CPY81Z   Removal of Radioactive Element from Mouth and Throat, Via Natural or Artificial Opening Endoscopic
0CPY87Z   Removal of Autologous Tissue Substitute from Mouth and Throat, Via Natural or Artificial Opening Endoscopic
0CPY8DZ   Removal of Intraluminal Device from Mouth and Throat, Via Natural or Artificial Opening Endoscopic
0CPY8JZ   Removal of Synthetic Substitute from Mouth and Throat, Via Natural or Artificial Opening Endoscopic
0CPY8KZ   Removal of Nonautologous Tissue Substitute from Mouth and Throat, Via Natural or Artificial Opening Endoscopic
0CPYX0Z   Removal of Drainage Device from Mouth and Throat, External Approach
0CPYX1Z   Removal of Radioactive Element from Mouth and Throat, External Approach
0CPYX7Z   Removal of Autologous Tissue Substitute from Mouth and Throat, External Approach
0CPYXDZ   Removal of Intraluminal Device from Mouth and Throat, External Approach
0CPYXJZ   Removal of Synthetic Substitute from Mouth and Throat, External Approach
0CPYXKZ   Removal of Nonautologous Tissue Substitute from Mouth and Throat, External Approach

0CQ – Mouth and Throat, Repair

0CQ00ZZ   Repair Upper Lip, Open Approach
0CQ03ZZ   Repair Upper Lip, Percutaneous Approach

0CQ0XZZ   Repair Upper Lip, External Approach
0CQ10ZZ   Repair Lower Lip, Open Approach

0CQ13ZZ	Repair Lower Lip, Percutaneous Approach
0CQ1XZZ	Repair Lower Lip, External Approach
0CQ20ZZ	Repair Hard Palate, Open Approach
0CQ23ZZ	Repair Hard Palate, Percutaneous Approach
0CQ2XZZ	Repair Hard Palate, External Approach
0CQ30ZZ	Repair Soft Palate, Open Approach
0CQ33ZZ	Repair Soft Palate, Percutaneous Approach
0CQ3XZZ	Repair Soft Palate, External Approach
0CQ40ZZ	Repair Buccal Mucosa, Open Approach
0CQ43ZZ	Repair Buccal Mucosa, Percutaneous Approach
0CQ4XZZ	Repair Buccal Mucosa, External Approach
0CQ50ZZ	Repair Upper Gingiva, Open Approach
0CQ53ZZ	Repair Upper Gingiva, Percutaneous Approach
0CQ5XZZ	Repair Upper Gingiva, External Approach
0CQ60ZZ	Repair Lower Gingiva, Open Approach
0CQ63ZZ	Repair Lower Gingiva, Percutaneous Approach
0CQ6XZZ	Repair Lower Gingiva, External Approach
0CQ70ZZ	Repair Tongue, Open Approach
0CQ73ZZ	Repair Tongue, Percutaneous Approach
0CQ7XZZ	Repair Tongue, External Approach
0CQ80ZZ	Repair Right Parotid Gland, Open Approach
0CQ83ZZ	Repair Right Parotid Gland, Percutaneous Approach
0CQ90ZZ	Repair Left Parotid Gland, Open Approach
0CQ93ZZ	Repair Left Parotid Gland, Percutaneous Approach
0CQB0ZZ	Repair Right Parotid Duct, Open Approach
0CQB3ZZ	Repair Right Parotid Duct, Percutaneous Approach
0CQC0ZZ	Repair Left Parotid Duct, Open Approach
0CQC3ZZ	Repair Left Parotid Duct, Percutaneous Approach
0CQD0ZZ	Repair Right Sublingual Gland, Open Approach
0CQD3ZZ	Repair Right Sublingual Gland, Percutaneous Approach
0CQF0ZZ	Repair Left Sublingual Gland, Open Approach
0CQF3ZZ	Repair Left Sublingual Gland, Percutaneous Approach
0CQG0ZZ	Repair Right Submaxillary Gland, Open Approach
0CQG3ZZ	Repair Right Submaxillary Gland, Percutaneous Approach
0CQH0ZZ	Repair Left Submaxillary Gland, Open Approach
0CQH3ZZ	Repair Left Submaxillary Gland, Percutaneous Approach
0CQJ0ZZ	Repair Minor Salivary Gland, Open Approach
0CQJ3ZZ	Repair Minor Salivary Gland, Percutaneous Approach
0CQM0ZZ	Repair Pharynx, Open Approach
0CQM3ZZ	Repair Pharynx, Percutaneous Approach
0CQM4ZZ	Repair Pharynx, Percutaneous Endoscopic Approach
0CQM7ZZ	Repair Pharynx, Via Natural or Artificial Opening
0CQM8ZZ	Repair Pharynx, Via Natural or Artificial Opening Endoscopic
0CQN0ZZ	Repair Uvula, Open Approach
0CQN3ZZ	Repair Uvula, Percutaneous Approach
0CQNXZZ	Repair Uvula, External Approach
0CQP0ZZ	Repair Tonsils, Open Approach
0CQP3ZZ	Repair Tonsils, Percutaneous Approach
0CQPXZZ	Repair Tonsils, External Approach
0CQQ0ZZ	Repair Adenoids, Open Approach
0CQQ3ZZ	Repair Adenoids, Percutaneous Approach
0CQQXZZ	Repair Adenoids, External Approach
0CQR0ZZ	Repair Epiglottis, Open Approach
0CQR3ZZ	Repair Epiglottis, Percutaneous Approach
0CQR4ZZ	Repair Epiglottis, Percutaneous Endoscopic Approach
0CQR7ZZ	Repair Epiglottis, Via Natural or Artificial Opening
0CQR8ZZ	Repair Epiglottis, Via Natural or Artificial Opening Endoscopic
0CQS0ZZ	Repair Larynx, Open Approach
0CQS3ZZ	Repair Larynx, Percutaneous Approach
0CQS4ZZ	Repair Larynx, Percutaneous Endoscopic Approach
0CQS7ZZ	Repair Larynx, Via Natural or Artificial Opening
0CQS8ZZ	Repair Larynx, Via Natural or Artificial Opening Endoscopic
0CQT0ZZ	Repair Right Vocal Cord, Open Approach
0CQT3ZZ	Repair Right Vocal Cord, Percutaneous Approach
0CQT4ZZ	Repair Right Vocal Cord, Percutaneous Endoscopic Approach
0CQT7ZZ	Repair Right Vocal Cord, Via Natural or Artificial Opening
0CQT8ZZ	Repair Right Vocal Cord, Via Natural or Artificial Opening Endoscopic
0CQV0ZZ	Repair Left Vocal Cord, Open Approach
0CQV3ZZ	Repair Left Vocal Cord, Percutaneous Approach
0CQV4ZZ	Repair Left Vocal Cord, Percutaneous Endoscopic Approach
0CQV7ZZ	Repair Left Vocal Cord, Via Natural or Artificial Opening
0CQV8ZZ	Repair Left Vocal Cord, Via Natural or Artificial Opening Endoscopic
0CQW0Z0	Repair of Upper Tooth, Single, Open Approach
0CQW0Z1	Repair of Upper Tooth, Multiple, Open Approach
0CQW0Z2	Repair of Upper Tooth, All, Open Approach
0CQWXZ0	Repair of Upper Tooth, Single, External Approach
0CQWXZ1	Repair of Upper Tooth, Multiple, External Approach
0CQWXZ2	Repair of Upper Tooth, All, External Approach
0CQX0Z0	Repair of Lower Tooth, Single, Open Approach
0CQX0Z1	Repair of Lower Tooth, Multiple, Open Approach
0CQX0Z2	Repair of Lower Tooth, All, Open Approach
0CQXXZ0	Repair of Lower Tooth, Single, External Approach
0CQXXZ1	Repair of Lower Tooth, Multiple, External Approach
0CQXXZ2	Repair of Lower Tooth, All, External Approach

0CR – Mouth and Throat, Replacement

0CR007Z	Replacement of Upper Lip with Autologous Tissue Substitute, Open Approach
0CR00JZ	Replacement of Upper Lip with Synthetic Substitute, Open Approach
0CR00KZ	Replacement of Upper Lip with Nonautologous Tissue Substitute, Open Approach
0CR037Z	Replacement of Upper Lip with Autologous Tissue Substitute, Percutaneous Approach
0CR03JZ	Replacement of Upper Lip with Synthetic Substitute, Percutaneous Approach
0CR03KZ	Replacement of Upper Lip with Nonautologous Tissue Substitute, Percutaneous Approach
0CR0X7Z	Replacement of Upper Lip with Autologous Tissue Substitute, External Approach
0CR0XJZ	Replacement of Upper Lip with Synthetic Substitute, External Approach
0CR0XKZ	Replacement of Upper Lip with Nonautologous Tissue Substitute, External Approach
0CR107Z	Replacement of Lower Lip with Autologous Tissue Substitute, Open Approach
0CR10JZ	Replacement of Lower Lip with Synthetic Substitute, Open Approach
0CR10KZ	Replacement of Lower Lip with Nonautologous Tissue Substitute, Open Approach
0CR137Z	Replacement of Lower Lip with Autologous Tissue Substitute, Percutaneous Approach
0CR13JZ	Replacement of Lower Lip with Synthetic Substitute, Percutaneous Approach
0CR13KZ	Replacement of Lower Lip with Nonautologous Tissue Substitute, Percutaneous Approach
0CR1X7Z	Replacement of Lower Lip with Autologous Tissue Substitute, External Approach
0CR1XJZ	Replacement of Lower Lip with Synthetic Substitute, External Approach
0CR1XKZ	Replacement of Lower Lip with Nonautologous Tissue Substitute, External Approach
0CR207Z	Replacement of Hard Palate with Autologous Tissue Substitute, Open Approach
0CR20JZ	Replacement of Hard Palate with Synthetic Substitute, Open Approach
0CR20KZ	Replacement of Hard Palate with Nonautologous Tissue Substitute, Open Approach
0CR237Z	Replacement of Hard Palate with Autologous Tissue Substitute, Percutaneous Approach
0CR23JZ	Replacement of Hard Palate with Synthetic Substitute, Percutaneous Approach
0CR23KZ	Replacement of Hard Palate with Nonautologous Tissue Substitute, Percutaneous Approach

0CR2X7Z	Replacement of Hard Palate with Autologous Tissue Substitute, External Approach
0CR2XJZ	Replacement of Hard Palate with Synthetic Substitute, External Approach
0CR2XKZ	Replacement of Hard Palate with Nonautologous Tissue Substitute, External Approach
0CR307Z	Replacement of Soft Palate with Autologous Tissue Substitute, Open Approach
0CR30JZ	Replacement of Soft Palate with Synthetic Substitute, Open Approach
0CR30KZ	Replacement of Soft Palate with Nonautologous Tissue Substitute, Open Approach
0CR337Z	Replacement of Soft Palate with Autologous Tissue Substitute, Percutaneous Approach
0CR33JZ	Replacement of Soft Palate with Synthetic Substitute, Percutaneous Approach
0CR33KZ	Replacement of Soft Palate with Nonautologous Tissue Substitute, Percutaneous Approach
0CR3X7Z	Replacement of Soft Palate with Autologous Tissue Substitute, External Approach
0CR3XJZ	Replacement of Soft Palate with Synthetic Substitute, External Approach
0CR3XKZ	Replacement of Soft Palate with Nonautologous Tissue Substitute, External Approach
0CR407Z	Replacement of Buccal Mucosa with Autologous Tissue Substitute, Open Approach
0CR40JZ	Replacement of Buccal Mucosa with Synthetic Substitute, Open Approach
0CR40KZ	Replacement of Buccal Mucosa with Nonautologous Tissue Substitute, Open Approach
0CR437Z	Replacement of Buccal Mucosa with Autologous Tissue Substitute, Percutaneous Approach
0CR43JZ	Replacement of Buccal Mucosa with Synthetic Substitute, Percutaneous Approach
0CR43KZ	Replacement of Buccal Mucosa with Nonautologous Tissue Substitute, Percutaneous Approach
0CR4X7Z	Replacement of Buccal Mucosa with Autologous Tissue Substitute, External Approach
0CR4XJZ	Replacement of Buccal Mucosa with Synthetic Substitute, External Approach
0CR4XKZ	Replacement of Buccal Mucosa with Nonautologous Tissue Substitute, External Approach
0CR507Z	Replacement of Upper Gingiva with Autologous Tissue Substitute, Open Approach
0CR50JZ	Replacement of Upper Gingiva with Synthetic Substitute, Open Approach
0CR50KZ	Replacement of Upper Gingiva with Nonautologous Tissue Substitute, Open Approach
0CR537Z	Replacement of Upper Gingiva with Autologous Tissue Substitute, Percutaneous Approach
0CR53JZ	Replacement of Upper Gingiva with Synthetic Substitute, Percutaneous Approach
0CR53KZ	Replacement of Upper Gingiva with Nonautologous Tissue Substitute, Percutaneous Approach
0CR5X7Z	Replacement of Upper Gingiva with Autologous Tissue Substitute, External Approach
0CR5XJZ	Replacement of Upper Gingiva with Synthetic Substitute, External Approach
0CR5XKZ	Replacement of Upper Gingiva with Nonautologous Tissue Substitute, External Approach
0CR607Z	Replacement of Lower Gingiva with Autologous Tissue Substitute, Open Approach
0CR60JZ	Replacement of Lower Gingiva with Synthetic Substitute, Open Approach
0CR60KZ	Replacement of Lower Gingiva with Nonautologous Tissue Substitute, Open Approach
0CR637Z	Replacement of Lower Gingiva with Autologous Tissue Substitute, Percutaneous Approach
0CR63JZ	Replacement of Lower Gingiva with Synthetic Substitute, Percutaneous Approach
0CR63KZ	Replacement of Lower Gingiva with Nonautologous Tissue Substitute, Percutaneous Approach
0CR6X7Z	Replacement of Lower Gingiva with Autologous Tissue Substitute, External Approach
0CR6XJZ	Replacement of Lower Gingiva with Synthetic Substitute, External Approach
0CR6XKZ	Replacement of Lower Gingiva with Nonautologous Tissue Substitute, External Approach
0CR707Z	Replacement of Tongue with Autologous Tissue Substitute, Open Approach
0CR70JZ	Replacement of Tongue with Synthetic Substitute, Open Approach
0CR70KZ	Replacement of Tongue with Nonautologous Tissue Substitute, Open Approach
0CR737Z	Replacement of Tongue with Autologous Tissue Substitute, Percutaneous Approach
0CR73JZ	Replacement of Tongue with Synthetic Substitute, Percutaneous Approach
0CR73KZ	Replacement of Tongue with Nonautologous Tissue Substitute, Percutaneous Approach
0CR7X7Z	Replacement of Tongue with Autologous Tissue Substitute, External Approach
0CR7XJZ	Replacement of Tongue with Synthetic Substitute, External Approach
0CR7XKZ	Replacement of Tongue with Nonautologous Tissue Substitute, External Approach
0CRB07Z	Replacement of Right Parotid Duct with Autologous Tissue Substitute, Open Approach
0CRB0JZ	Replacement of Right Parotid Duct with Synthetic Substitute, Open Approach
0CRB0KZ	Replacement of Right Parotid Duct with Nonautologous Tissue Substitute, Open Approach
0CRB37Z	Replacement of Right Parotid Duct with Autologous Tissue Substitute, Percutaneous Approach
0CRB3JZ	Replacement of Right Parotid Duct with Synthetic Substitute, Percutaneous Approach
0CRB3KZ	Replacement of Right Parotid Duct with Nonautologous Tissue Substitute, Percutaneous Approach
0CRC07Z	Replacement of Left Parotid Duct with Autologous Tissue Substitute, Open Approach
0CRC0JZ	Replacement of Left Parotid Duct with Synthetic Substitute, Open Approach
0CRC0KZ	Replacement of Left Parotid Duct with Nonautologous Tissue Substitute, Open Approach
0CRC37Z	Replacement of Left Parotid Duct with Autologous Tissue Substitute, Percutaneous Approach
0CRC3JZ	Replacement of Left Parotid Duct with Synthetic Substitute, Percutaneous Approach
0CRC3KZ	Replacement of Left Parotid Duct with Nonautologous Tissue Substitute, Percutaneous Approach
0CRM07Z	Replacement of Pharynx with Autologous Tissue Substitute, Open Approach
0CRM0JZ	Replacement of Pharynx with Synthetic Substitute, Open Approach
0CRM0KZ	Replacement of Pharynx with Nonautologous Tissue Substitute, Open Approach
0CRM77Z	Replacement of Pharynx with Autologous Tissue Substitute, Via Natural or Artificial Opening
0CRM7JZ	Replacement of Pharynx with Synthetic Substitute, Via Natural or Artificial Opening
0CRM7KZ	Replacement of Pharynx with Nonautologous Tissue Substitute, Via Natural or Artificial Opening
0CRM87Z	Replacement of Pharynx with Autologous Tissue Substitute, Via Natural or Artificial Opening Endoscopic
0CRM8JZ	Replacement of Pharynx with Synthetic Substitute, Via Natural or Artificial Opening Endoscopic
0CRM8KZ	Replacement of Pharynx with Nonautologous Tissue Substitute, Via Natural or Artificial Opening Endoscopic
0CRN07Z	Replacement of Uvula with Autologous Tissue Substitute, Open Approach
0CRN0JZ	Replacement of Uvula with Synthetic Substitute, Open Approach
0CRN0KZ	Replacement of Uvula with Nonautologous Tissue Substitute, Open Approach

0CRN37Z	Replacement of Uvula with Autologous Tissue Substitute, Percutaneous Approach
0CRN3JZ	Replacement of Uvula with Synthetic Substitute, Percutaneous Approach
0CRN3KZ	Replacement of Uvula with Nonautologous Tissue Substitute, Percutaneous Approach
0CRNX7Z	Replacement of Uvula with Autologous Tissue Substitute, External Approach
0CRNXJZ	Replacement of Uvula with Synthetic Substitute, External Approach
0CRNXKZ	Replacement of Uvula with Nonautologous Tissue Substitute, External Approach
0CRR07Z	Replacement of Epiglottis with Autologous Tissue Substitute, Open Approach
0CRR0JZ	Replacement of Epiglottis with Synthetic Substitute, Open Approach
0CRR0KZ	Replacement of Epiglottis with Nonautologous Tissue Substitute, Open Approach
0CRR77Z	Replacement of Epiglottis with Autologous Tissue Substitute, Via Natural or Artificial Opening
0CRR7JZ	Replacement of Epiglottis with Synthetic Substitute, Via Natural or Artificial Opening
0CRR7KZ	Replacement of Epiglottis with Nonautologous Tissue Substitute, Via Natural or Artificial Opening
0CRR87Z	Replacement of Epiglottis with Autologous Tissue Substitute, Via Natural or Artificial Opening Endoscopic
0CRR8JZ	Replacement of Epiglottis with Synthetic Substitute, Via Natural or Artificial Opening Endoscopic
0CRR8KZ	Replacement of Epiglottis with Nonautologous Tissue Substitute, Via Natural or Artificial Opening Endoscopic
0CRS07Z	Replacement of Larynx with Autologous Tissue Substitute, Open Approach
0CRS0JZ	Replacement of Larynx with Synthetic Substitute, Open Approach
0CRS0KZ	Replacement of Larynx with Nonautologous Tissue Substitute, Open Approach
0CRS77Z	Replacement of Larynx with Autologous Tissue Substitute, Via Natural or Artificial Opening
0CRS7JZ	Replacement of Larynx with Synthetic Substitute, Via Natural or Artificial Opening
0CRS7KZ	Replacement of Larynx with Nonautologous Tissue Substitute, Via Natural or Artificial Opening
0CRS87Z	Replacement of Larynx with Autologous Tissue Substitute, Via Natural or Artificial Opening Endoscopic
0CRS8JZ	Replacement of Larynx with Synthetic Substitute, Via Natural or Artificial Opening Endoscopic
0CRS8KZ	Replacement of Larynx with Nonautologous Tissue Substitute, Via Natural or Artificial Opening Endoscopic
0CRT07Z	Replacement of Right Vocal Cord with Autologous Tissue Substitute, Open Approach
0CRT0JZ	Replacement of Right Vocal Cord with Synthetic Substitute, Open Approach
0CRT0KZ	Replacement of Right Vocal Cord with Nonautologous Tissue Substitute, Open Approach
0CRT77Z	Replacement of Right Vocal Cord with Autologous Tissue Substitute, Via Natural or Artificial Opening
0CRT7JZ	Replacement of Right Vocal Cord with Synthetic Substitute, Via Natural or Artificial Opening
0CRT7KZ	Replacement of Right Vocal Cord with Nonautologous Tissue Substitute, Via Natural or Artificial Opening
0CRT87Z	Replacement of Right Vocal Cord with Autologous Tissue Substitute, Via Natural or Artificial Opening Endoscopic
0CRT8JZ	Replacement of Right Vocal Cord with Synthetic Substitute, Via Natural or Artificial Opening Endoscopic
0CRT8KZ	Replacement of Right Vocal Cord with Nonautologous Tissue Substitute, Via Natural or Artificial Opening Endoscopic
0CRV07Z	Replacement of Left Vocal Cord with Autologous Tissue Substitute, Open Approach
0CRV0JZ	Replacement of Left Vocal Cord with Synthetic Substitute, Open Approach
0CRV0KZ	Replacement of Left Vocal Cord with Nonautologous Tissue Substitute, Open Approach
0CRV77Z	Replacement of Left Vocal Cord with Autologous Tissue Substitute, Via Natural or Artificial Opening
0CRV7JZ	Replacement of Left Vocal Cord with Synthetic Substitute, Via Natural or Artificial Opening
0CRV7KZ	Replacement of Left Vocal Cord with Nonautologous Tissue Substitute, Via Natural or Artificial Opening
0CRV87Z	Replacement of Left Vocal Cord with Autologous Tissue Substitute, Via Natural or Artificial Opening Endoscopic
0CRV8JZ	Replacement of Left Vocal Cord with Synthetic Substitute, Via Natural or Artificial Opening Endoscopic
0CRV8KZ	Replacement of Left Vocal Cord with Nonautologous Tissue Substitute, Via Natural or Artificial Opening Endoscopic
0CRW070	Replacement of Upper Tooth, Single, with Autologous Tissue Substitute, Open Approach
0CRW071	Replacement of Upper Tooth, Multiple, with Autologous Tissue Substitute, Open Approach
0CRW072	Replacement of Upper Tooth, All, with Autologous Tissue Substitute, Open Approach
0CRW0J0	Replacement of Upper Tooth, Single, with Synthetic Substitute, Open Approach
0CRW0J1	Replacement of Upper Tooth, Multiple, with Synthetic Substitute, Open Approach
0CRW0J2	Replacement of Upper Tooth, All, with Synthetic Substitute, Open Approach
0CRW0K0	Replacement of Upper Tooth, Single, with Nonautologous Tissue Substitute, Open Approach
0CRW0K1	Replacement of Upper Tooth, Multiple, with Nonautologous Tissue Substitute, Open Approach
0CRW0K2	Replacement of Upper Tooth, All, with Nonautologous Tissue Substitute, Open Approach
0CRWX70	Replacement of Upper Tooth, Single, with Autologous Tissue Substitute, External Approach
0CRWX71	Replacement of Upper Tooth, Multiple, with Autologous Tissue Substitute, External Approach
0CRWX72	Replacement of Upper Tooth, All, with Autologous Tissue Substitute, External Approach
0CRWXJ0	Replacement of Upper Tooth, Single, with Synthetic Substitute, External Approach
0CRWXJ1	Replacement of Upper Tooth, Multiple, with Synthetic Substitute, External Approach
0CRWXJ2	Replacement of Upper Tooth, All, with Synthetic Substitute, External Approach
0CRWXK0	Replacement of Upper Tooth, Single, with Nonautologous Tissue Substitute, External Approach
0CRWXK1	Replacement of Upper Tooth, Multiple, with Nonautologous Tissue Substitute, External Approach
0CRWXK2	Replacement of Upper Tooth, All, with Nonautologous Tissue Substitute, External Approach
0CRX070	Replacement of Lower Tooth, Single, with Autologous Tissue Substitute, Open Approach
0CRX071	Replacement of Lower Tooth, Multiple, with Autologous Tissue Substitute, Open Approach
0CRX072	Replacement of Lower Tooth, All, with Autologous Tissue Substitute, Open Approach
0CRX0J0	Replacement of Lower Tooth, Single, with Synthetic Substitute, Open Approach
0CRX0J1	Replacement of Lower Tooth, Multiple, with Synthetic Substitute, Open Approach
0CRX0J2	Replacement of Lower Tooth, All, with Synthetic Substitute, Open Approach
0CRX0K0	Replacement of Lower Tooth, Single, with Nonautologous Tissue Substitute, Open Approach
0CRX0K1	Replacement of Lower Tooth, Multiple, with Nonautologous Tissue Substitute, Open Approach
0CRX0K2	Replacement of Lower Tooth, All, with Nonautologous Tissue Substitute, Open Approach
0CRXX70	Replacement of Lower Tooth, Single, with Autologous Tissue Substitute, External Approach

0CRXX71	Replacement of Lower Tooth, Multiple, with Autologous Tissue Substitute, External Approach
0CRXX72	Replacement of Lower Tooth, All, with Autologous Tissue Substitute, External Approach
0CRXXJ0	Replacement of Lower Tooth, Single, with Synthetic Substitute, External Approach
0CRXXJ1	Replacement of Lower Tooth, Multiple, with Synthetic Substitute, External Approach
0CRXXJ2	Replacement of Lower Tooth, All, with Synthetic Substitute, External Approach
0CRXXK0	Replacement of Lower Tooth, Single, with Nonautologous Tissue Substitute, External Approach
0CRXXK1	Replacement of Lower Tooth, Multiple, with Nonautologous Tissue Substitute, External Approach
0CRXXK2	Replacement of Lower Tooth, All, with Nonautologous Tissue Substitute, External Approach

0CS – Mouth and Throat, Reposition

0CS00ZZ	Reposition Upper Lip, Open Approach
0CS0XZZ	Reposition Upper Lip, External Approach
0CS10ZZ	Reposition Lower Lip, Open Approach
0CS1XZZ	Reposition Lower Lip, External Approach
0CS20ZZ	Reposition Hard Palate, Open Approach
0CS2XZZ	Reposition Hard Palate, External Approach
0CS30ZZ	Reposition Soft Palate, Open Approach
0CS3XZZ	Reposition Soft Palate, External Approach
0CS70ZZ	Reposition Tongue, Open Approach
0CS7XZZ	Reposition Tongue, External Approach
0CSB0ZZ	Reposition Right Parotid Duct, Open Approach
0CSB3ZZ	Reposition Right Parotid Duct, Percutaneous Approach
0CSC0ZZ	Reposition Left Parotid Duct, Open Approach
0CSC3ZZ	Reposition Left Parotid Duct, Percutaneous Approach
0CSN0ZZ	Reposition Uvula, Open Approach
0CSNXZZ	Reposition Uvula, External Approach
0CSR0ZZ	Reposition Epiglottis, Open Approach
0CSR7ZZ	Reposition Epiglottis, Via Natural or Artificial Opening
0CSR8ZZ	Reposition Epiglottis, Via Natural or Artificial Opening Endoscopic
0CST0ZZ	Reposition Right Vocal Cord, Open Approach
0CST7ZZ	Reposition Right Vocal Cord, Via Natural or Artificial Opening
0CST8ZZ	Reposition Right Vocal Cord, Via Natural or Artificial Opening Endoscopic
0CSV0ZZ	Reposition Left Vocal Cord, Open Approach
0CSV7ZZ	Reposition Left Vocal Cord, Via Natural or Artificial Opening
0CSV8ZZ	Reposition Left Vocal Cord, Via Natural or Artificial Opening Endoscopic
0CSW050	Reposition Upper Tooth with External Fixation Device, Single, Open Approach
0CSW051	Reposition Upper Tooth with External Fixation Device, Multiple, Open Approach
0CSW052	Reposition Upper Tooth with External Fixation Device, All, Open Approach
0CSW0Z0	Reposition Upper Tooth, Single, Open Approach
0CSW0Z1	Reposition Upper Tooth, Multiple, Open Approach
0CSW0Z2	Reposition Upper Tooth, All, Open Approach
0CSWX50	Reposition Upper Tooth, Single, with External Fixation Device, External Approach
0CSWX51	Reposition Upper Tooth, Multiple, with External Fixation Device, External Approach
0CSWX52	Reposition Upper Tooth, All, with External Fixation Device, External Approach
0CSWXZ0	Reposition Upper Tooth, Single, External Approach
0CSWXZ1	Reposition Upper Tooth, Multiple, External Approach
0CSWXZ2	Reposition Upper Tooth, All, External Approach
0CSX050	Reposition Lower Tooth with External Fixation Device, Single, Open Approach
0CSX051	Reposition Lower Tooth with External Fixation Device, Multiple, Open Approach
0CSX052	Reposition Lower Tooth with External Fixation Device, All, Open Approach
0CSX0Z0	Reposition Lower Tooth, Single, Open Approach
0CSX0Z1	Reposition Lower Tooth, Multiple, Open Approach
0CSX0Z2	Reposition Lower Tooth, All, Open Approach
0CSXX50	Reposition Lower Tooth, Single, with External Fixation Device, External Approach
0CSXX51	Reposition Lower Tooth, Multiple, with External Fixation Device, External Approach
0CSXX52	Reposition Lower Tooth, All, with External Fixation Device, External Approach
0CSXXZ0	Reposition Lower Tooth, Single, External Approach
0CSXXZ1	Reposition Lower Tooth, Multiple, External Approach
0CSXXZ2	Reposition Lower Tooth, All, External Approach

0CT – Mouth and Throat, Resection

Review Coding Guideline B3.8

0CT00ZZ	Resection of Upper Lip, Open Approach
0CT0XZZ	Resection of Upper Lip, External Approach
0CT10ZZ	Resection of Lower Lip, Open Approach
0CT1XZZ	Resection of Lower Lip, External Approach
0CT20ZZ	Resection of Hard Palate, Open Approach
0CT2XZZ	Resection of Hard Palate, External Approach
0CT30ZZ	Resection of Soft Palate, Open Approach
0CT3XZZ	Resection of Soft Palate, External Approach
0CT70ZZ	Resection of Tongue, Open Approach
0CT7XZZ	Resection of Tongue, External Approach
0CT80ZZ	Resection of Right Parotid Gland, Open Approach
0CT90ZZ	Resection of Left Parotid Gland, Open Approach
0CTB0ZZ	Resection of Right Parotid Duct, Open Approach
0CTC0ZZ	Resection of Left Parotid Duct, Open Approach
0CTD0ZZ	Resection of Right Sublingual Gland, Open Approach
0CTF0ZZ	Resection of Left Sublingual Gland, Open Approach
0CTG0ZZ	Resection of Right Submaxillary Gland, Open Approach
0CTH0ZZ	Resection of Left Submaxillary Gland, Open Approach
0CTJ0ZZ	Resection of Minor Salivary Gland, Open Approach
0CTM0ZZ	Resection of Pharynx, Open Approach
0CTM4ZZ	Resection of Pharynx, Percutaneous Endoscopic Approach
0CTM7ZZ	Resection of Pharynx, Via Natural or Artificial Opening
0CTM8ZZ	Resection of Pharynx, Via Natural or Artificial Opening Endoscopic
0CTN0ZZ	Resection of Uvula, Open Approach
0CTNXZZ	Resection of Uvula, External Approach
0CTP0ZZ	Resection of Tonsils, Open Approach
0CTPXZZ	Resection of Tonsils, External Approach
0CTQ0ZZ	Resection of Adenoids, Open Approach
0CTQXZZ	Resection of Adenoids, External Approach
0CTR0ZZ	Resection of Epiglottis, Open Approach
0CTR4ZZ	Resection of Epiglottis, Percutaneous Endoscopic Approach
0CTR7ZZ	Resection of Epiglottis, Via Natural or Artificial Opening
0CTR8ZZ	Resection of Epiglottis, Via Natural or Artificial Opening Endoscopic
0CTS0ZZ	Resection of Larynx, Open Approach
0CTS4ZZ	Resection of Larynx, Percutaneous Endoscopic Approach
0CTS7ZZ	Resection of Larynx, Via Natural or Artificial Opening
0CTS8ZZ	Resection of Larynx, Via Natural or Artificial Opening Endoscopic
0CTT0ZZ	Resection of Right Vocal Cord, Open Approach
0CTT4ZZ	Resection of Right Vocal Cord, Percutaneous Endoscopic Approach
0CTT7ZZ	Resection of Right Vocal Cord, Via Natural or Artificial Opening
0CTT8ZZ	Resection of Right Vocal Cord, Via Natural or Artificial Opening Endoscopic
0CTV0ZZ	Resection of Left Vocal Cord, Open Approach

0CTV4ZZ	Resection of Left Vocal Cord, Percutaneous Endoscopic Approach	0CTW0Z1	Resection of Upper Tooth, Multiple, Open Approach
0CTV7ZZ	Resection of Left Vocal Cord, Via Natural or Artificial Opening	0CTW0Z2	Resection of Upper Tooth, All, Open Approach
0CTV8ZZ	Resection of Left Vocal Cord, Via Natural or Artificial Opening Endoscopic	0CTX0Z0	Resection of Lower Tooth, Single, Open Approach
		0CTX0Z1	Resection of Lower Tooth, Multiple, Open Approach
0CTW0Z0	Resection of Upper Tooth, Single, Open Approach	0CTX0Z2	Resection of Lower Tooth, All, Open Approach

0CU – Mouth and Throat, Supplement

0CU007Z	Supplement Upper Lip with Autologous Tissue Substitute, Open Approach	0CU3XJZ	Supplement Soft Palate with Synthetic Substitute, External Approach
0CU00JZ	Supplement Upper Lip with Synthetic Substitute, Open Approach	0CU3XKZ	Supplement Soft Palate with Nonautologous Tissue Substitute, External Approach
0CU00KZ	Supplement Upper Lip with Nonautologous Tissue Substitute, Open Approach	0CU407Z	Supplement Buccal Mucosa with Autologous Tissue Substitute, Open Approach
0CU037Z	Supplement Upper Lip with Autologous Tissue Substitute, Percutaneous Approach	0CU40JZ	Supplement Buccal Mucosa with Synthetic Substitute, Open Approach
0CU03JZ	Supplement Upper Lip with Synthetic Substitute, Percutaneous Approach	0CU40KZ	Supplement Buccal Mucosa with Nonautologous Tissue Substitute, Open Approach
0CU03KZ	Supplement Upper Lip with Nonautologous Tissue Substitute, Percutaneous Approach	0CU437Z	Supplement Buccal Mucosa with Autologous Tissue Substitute, Percutaneous Approach
0CU0X7Z	Supplement Upper Lip with Autologous Tissue Substitute, External Approach	0CU43JZ	Supplement Buccal Mucosa with Synthetic Substitute, Percutaneous Approach
0CU0XJZ	Supplement Upper Lip with Synthetic Substitute, External Approach	0CU43KZ	Supplement Buccal Mucosa with Nonautologous Tissue Substitute, Percutaneous Approach
0CU0XKZ	Supplement Upper Lip with Nonautologous Tissue Substitute, External Approach	0CU4X7Z	Supplement Buccal Mucosa with Autologous Tissue Substitute, External Approach
0CU107Z	Supplement Lower Lip with Autologous Tissue Substitute, Open Approach	0CU4XJZ	Supplement Buccal Mucosa with Synthetic Substitute, External Approach
0CU10JZ	Supplement Lower Lip with Synthetic Substitute, Open Approach	0CU4XKZ	Supplement Buccal Mucosa with Nonautologous Tissue Substitute, External Approach
0CU10KZ	Supplement Lower Lip with Nonautologous Tissue Substitute, Open Approach	0CU507Z	Supplement Upper Gingiva with Autologous Tissue Substitute, Open Approach
0CU137Z	Supplement Lower Lip with Autologous Tissue Substitute, Percutaneous Approach	0CU50JZ	Supplement Upper Gingiva with Synthetic Substitute, Open Approach
0CU13JZ	Supplement Lower Lip with Synthetic Substitute, Percutaneous Approach	0CU50KZ	Supplement Upper Gingiva with Nonautologous Tissue Substitute, Open Approach
0CU13KZ	Supplement Lower Lip with Nonautologous Tissue Substitute, Percutaneous Approach	0CU537Z	Supplement Upper Gingiva with Autologous Tissue Substitute, Percutaneous Approach
0CU1X7Z	Supplement Lower Lip with Autologous Tissue Substitute, External Approach	0CU53JZ	Supplement Upper Gingiva with Synthetic Substitute, Percutaneous Approach
0CU1XJZ	Supplement Lower Lip with Synthetic Substitute, External Approach	0CU53KZ	Supplement Upper Gingiva with Nonautologous Tissue Substitute, Percutaneous Approach
0CU1XKZ	Supplement Lower Lip with Nonautologous Tissue Substitute, External Approach	0CU5X7Z	Supplement Upper Gingiva with Autologous Tissue Substitute, External Approach
0CU207Z	Supplement Hard Palate with Autologous Tissue Substitute, Open Approach	0CU5XJZ	Supplement Upper Gingiva with Synthetic Substitute, External Approach
0CU20JZ	Supplement Hard Palate with Synthetic Substitute, Open Approach	0CU5XKZ	Supplement Upper Gingiva with Nonautologous Tissue Substitute, External Approach
0CU20KZ	Supplement Hard Palate with Nonautologous Tissue Substitute, Open Approach	0CU607Z	Supplement Lower Gingiva with Autologous Tissue Substitute, Open Approach
0CU237Z	Supplement Hard Palate with Autologous Tissue Substitute, Percutaneous Approach	0CU60JZ	Supplement Lower Gingiva with Synthetic Substitute, Open Approach
0CU23JZ	Supplement Hard Palate with Synthetic Substitute, Percutaneous Approach	0CU60KZ	Supplement Lower Gingiva with Nonautologous Tissue Substitute, Open Approach
0CU23KZ	Supplement Hard Palate with Nonautologous Tissue Substitute, Percutaneous Approach	0CU637Z	Supplement Lower Gingiva with Autologous Tissue Substitute, Percutaneous Approach
0CU2X7Z	Supplement Hard Palate with Autologous Tissue Substitute, External Approach	0CU63JZ	Supplement Lower Gingiva with Synthetic Substitute, Percutaneous Approach
0CU2XJZ	Supplement Hard Palate with Synthetic Substitute, External Approach	0CU63KZ	Supplement Lower Gingiva with Nonautologous Tissue Substitute, Percutaneous Approach
0CU2XKZ	Supplement Hard Palate with Nonautologous Tissue Substitute, External Approach	0CU6X7Z	Supplement Lower Gingiva with Autologous Tissue Substitute, External Approach
0CU307Z	Supplement Soft Palate with Autologous Tissue Substitute, Open Approach	0CU6XJZ	Supplement Lower Gingiva with Synthetic Substitute, External Approach
0CU30JZ	Supplement Soft Palate with Synthetic Substitute, Open Approach	0CU6XKZ	Supplement Lower Gingiva with Nonautologous Tissue Substitute, External Approach
0CU30KZ	Supplement Soft Palate with Nonautologous Tissue Substitute, Open Approach	0CU707Z	Supplement Tongue with Autologous Tissue Substitute, Open Approach
0CU337Z	Supplement Soft Palate with Autologous Tissue Substitute, Percutaneous Approach	0CU70JZ	Supplement Tongue with Synthetic Substitute, Open Approach
0CU33JZ	Supplement Soft Palate with Synthetic Substitute, Percutaneous Approach	0CU70KZ	Supplement Tongue with Nonautologous Tissue Substitute, Open Approach
0CU33KZ	Supplement Soft Palate with Nonautologous Tissue Substitute, Percutaneous Approach	0CU737Z	Supplement Tongue with Autologous Tissue Substitute, Percutaneous Approach
0CU3X7Z	Supplement Soft Palate with Autologous Tissue Substitute, External Approach		

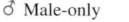

♀ Female-only   ♂ Male-only   ● Limited Coverage   ● Non-OR   HAC HAC-associated procedure   ● Non-covered procedures   ✚ Combination

0CU73JZ	Supplement Tongue with Synthetic Substitute, Percutaneous Approach
0CU73KZ	Supplement Tongue with Nonautologous Tissue Substitute, Percutaneous Approach
0CU7X7Z	Supplement Tongue with Autologous Tissue Substitute, External Approach
0CU7XJZ	Supplement Tongue with Synthetic Substitute, External Approach
0CU7XKZ	Supplement Tongue with Nonautologous Tissue Substitute, External Approach
0CUM07Z	Supplement Pharynx with Autologous Tissue Substitute, Open Approach
0CUM0JZ	Supplement Pharynx with Synthetic Substitute, Open Approach
0CUM0KZ	Supplement Pharynx with Nonautologous Tissue Substitute, Open Approach
0CUM77Z	Supplement Pharynx with Autologous Tissue Substitute, Via Natural or Artificial Opening
0CUM7JZ	Supplement Pharynx with Synthetic Substitute, Via Natural or Artificial Opening
0CUM7KZ	Supplement Pharynx with Nonautologous Tissue Substitute, Via Natural or Artificial Opening
0CUM87Z	Supplement Pharynx with Autologous Tissue Substitute, Via Natural or Artificial Opening Endoscopic
0CUM8JZ	Supplement Pharynx with Synthetic Substitute, Via Natural or Artificial Opening Endoscopic
0CUM8KZ	Supplement Pharynx with Nonautologous Tissue Substitute, Via Natural or Artificial Opening Endoscopic
0CUN07Z	Supplement Uvula with Autologous Tissue Substitute, Open Approach
0CUN0JZ	Supplement Uvula with Synthetic Substitute, Open Approach
0CUN0KZ	Supplement Uvula with Nonautologous Tissue Substitute, Open Approach
0CUN37Z	Supplement Uvula with Autologous Tissue Substitute, Percutaneous Approach
0CUN3JZ	Supplement Uvula with Synthetic Substitute, Percutaneous Approach
0CUN3KZ	Supplement Uvula with Nonautologous Tissue Substitute, Percutaneous Approach
0CUNX7Z	Supplement Uvula with Autologous Tissue Substitute, External Approach
0CUNXJZ	Supplement Uvula with Synthetic Substitute, External Approach
0CUNXKZ	Supplement Uvula with Nonautologous Tissue Substitute, External Approach
0CUR07Z	Supplement Epiglottis with Autologous Tissue Substitute, Open Approach
0CUR0JZ	Supplement Epiglottis with Synthetic Substitute, Open Approach
0CUR0KZ	Supplement Epiglottis with Nonautologous Tissue Substitute, Open Approach
0CUR77Z	Supplement Epiglottis with Autologous Tissue Substitute, Via Natural or Artificial Opening
0CUR7JZ	Supplement Epiglottis with Synthetic Substitute, Via Natural or Artificial Opening
0CUR7KZ	Supplement Epiglottis with Nonautologous Tissue Substitute, Via Natural or Artificial Opening
0CUR87Z	Supplement Epiglottis with Autologous Tissue Substitute, Via Natural or Artificial Opening Endoscopic
0CUR8JZ	Supplement Epiglottis with Synthetic Substitute, Via Natural or Artificial Opening Endoscopic
0CUR8KZ	Supplement Epiglottis with Nonautologous Tissue Substitute, Via Natural or Artificial Opening Endoscopic
0CUS07Z	Supplement Larynx with Autologous Tissue Substitute, Open Approach
0CUS0JZ	Supplement Larynx with Synthetic Substitute, Open Approach
0CUS0KZ	Supplement Larynx with Nonautologous Tissue Substitute, Open Approach
0CUS77Z	Supplement Larynx with Autologous Tissue Substitute, Via Natural or Artificial Opening
0CUS7JZ	Supplement Larynx with Synthetic Substitute, Via Natural or Artificial Opening
0CUS7KZ	Supplement Larynx with Nonautologous Tissue Substitute, Via Natural or Artificial Opening
0CUS87Z	Supplement Larynx with Autologous Tissue Substitute, Via Natural or Artificial Opening Endoscopic
0CUS8JZ	Supplement Larynx with Synthetic Substitute, Via Natural or Artificial Opening Endoscopic
0CUS8KZ	Supplement Larynx with Nonautologous Tissue Substitute, Via Natural or Artificial Opening Endoscopic
0CUT07Z	Supplement Right Vocal Cord with Autologous Tissue Substitute, Open Approach
0CUT0JZ	Supplement Right Vocal Cord with Synthetic Substitute, Open Approach
0CUT0KZ	Supplement Right Vocal Cord with Nonautologous Tissue Substitute, Open Approach
0CUT77Z	Supplement Right Vocal Cord with Autologous Tissue Substitute, Via Natural or Artificial Opening
0CUT7JZ	Supplement Right Vocal Cord with Synthetic Substitute, Via Natural or Artificial Opening
0CUT7KZ	Supplement Right Vocal Cord with Nonautologous Tissue Substitute, Via Natural or Artificial Opening
0CUT87Z	Supplement Right Vocal Cord with Autologous Tissue Substitute, Via Natural or Artificial Opening Endoscopic
0CUT8JZ	Supplement Right Vocal Cord with Synthetic Substitute, Via Natural or Artificial Opening Endoscopic
0CUT8KZ	Supplement Right Vocal Cord with Nonautologous Tissue Substitute, Via Natural or Artificial Opening Endoscopic
0CUV07Z	Supplement Left Vocal Cord with Autologous Tissue Substitute, Open Approach
0CUV0JZ	Supplement Left Vocal Cord with Synthetic Substitute, Open Approach
0CUV0KZ	Supplement Left Vocal Cord with Nonautologous Tissue Substitute, Open Approach
0CUV77Z	Supplement Left Vocal Cord with Autologous Tissue Substitute, Via Natural or Artificial Opening
0CUV7JZ	Supplement Left Vocal Cord with Synthetic Substitute, Via Natural or Artificial Opening
0CUV7KZ	Supplement Left Vocal Cord with Nonautologous Tissue Substitute, Via Natural or Artificial Opening
0CUV87Z	Supplement Left Vocal Cord with Autologous Tissue Substitute, Via Natural or Artificial Opening Endoscopic
0CUV8JZ	Supplement Left Vocal Cord with Synthetic Substitute, Via Natural or Artificial Opening Endoscopic
0CUV8KZ	Supplement Left Vocal Cord with Nonautologous Tissue Substitute, Via Natural or Artificial Opening Endoscopic

0CV – Mouth and Throat, Restriction

0CVB0CZ	Restriction of Right Parotid Duct with Extraluminal Device, Open Approach
0CVB0DZ	Restriction of Right Parotid Duct with Intraluminal Device, Open Approach
0CVB0ZZ	Restriction of Right Parotid Duct, Open Approach
0CVB3CZ	Restriction of Right Parotid Duct with Extraluminal Device, Percutaneous Approach
0CVB3DZ	Restriction of Right Parotid Duct with Intraluminal Device, Percutaneous Approach
0CVB3ZZ	Restriction of Right Parotid Duct, Percutaneous Approach
0CVB7DZ	Restriction of Right Parotid Duct with Intraluminal Device, Via Natural or Artificial Opening
0CVB7ZZ	Restriction of Right Parotid Duct, Via Natural or Artificial Opening
0CVB8DZ	Restriction of Right Parotid Duct with Intraluminal Device, Via Natural or Artificial Opening Endoscopic
0CVB8ZZ	Restriction of Right Parotid Duct, Via Natural or Artificial Opening Endoscopic
0CVC0CZ	Restriction of Left Parotid Duct with Extraluminal Device, Open Approach

0CVC0DZ   Restriction of Left Parotid Duct with Intraluminal Device, Open Approach

0CVC0ZZ   Restriction of Left Parotid Duct, Open Approach

0CVC3CZ   Restriction of Left Parotid Duct with Extraluminal Device, Percutaneous Approach

0CVC3DZ   Restriction of Left Parotid Duct with Intraluminal Device, Percutaneous Approach

0CVC3ZZ   Restriction of Left Parotid Duct, Percutaneous Approach

0CVC7DZ   Restriction of Left Parotid Duct with Intraluminal Device, Via Natural or Artificial Opening

0CVC7ZZ   Restriction of Left Parotid Duct, Via Natural or Artificial Opening

0CVC8DZ   Restriction of Left Parotid Duct with Intraluminal Device, Via Natural or Artificial Opening Endoscopic

0CVC8ZZ   Restriction of Left Parotid Duct, Via Natural or Artificial Opening Endoscopic

0CW – Mouth and Throat, Revision

Review Coding Guideline B6.1c

0CWA00Z   Revision of Drainage Device in Salivary Gland, Open Approach

0CWA0CZ   Revision of Extraluminal Device in Salivary Gland, Open Approach

0CWA30Z   Revision of Drainage Device in Salivary Gland, Percutaneous Approach

0CWA3CZ   Revision of Extraluminal Device in Salivary Gland, Percutaneous Approach

0CWAX0Z   Revision of Drainage Device in Salivary Gland, External Approach

0CWAXCZ   Revision of Extraluminal Device in Salivary Gland, External Approach

0CWS00Z   Revision of Drainage Device in Larynx, Open Approach

0CWS07Z   Revision of Autologous Tissue Substitute in Larynx, Open Approach

0CWS0DZ   Revision of Intraluminal Device in Larynx, Open Approach

0CWS0JZ   Revision of Synthetic Substitute in Larynx, Open Approach

0CWS0KZ   Revision of Nonautologous Tissue Substitute in Larynx, Open Approach

0CWS30Z   Revision of Drainage Device in Larynx, Percutaneous Approach

0CWS37Z   Revision of Autologous Tissue Substitute in Larynx, Percutaneous Approach

0CWS3DZ   Revision of Intraluminal Device in Larynx, Percutaneous Approach

0CWS3JZ   Revision of Synthetic Substitute in Larynx, Percutaneous Approach

0CWS3KZ   Revision of Nonautologous Tissue Substitute in Larynx, Percutaneous Approach

0CWS70Z   Revision of Drainage Device in Larynx, Via Natural or Artificial Opening

0CWS77Z   Revision of Autologous Tissue Substitute in Larynx, Via Natural or Artificial Opening

0CWS7DZ   Revision of Intraluminal Device in Larynx, Via Natural or Artificial Opening

0CWS7JZ   Revision of Synthetic Substitute in Larynx, Via Natural or Artificial Opening

0CWS7KZ   Revision of Nonautologous Tissue Substitute in Larynx, Via Natural or Artificial Opening

0CWS80Z   Revision of Drainage Device in Larynx, Via Natural or Artificial Opening Endoscopic

0CWS87Z   Revision of Autologous Tissue Substitute in Larynx, Via Natural or Artificial Opening Endoscopic

0CWS8DZ   Revision of Intraluminal Device in Larynx, Via Natural or Artificial Opening Endoscopic

0CWS8JZ   Revision of Synthetic Substitute in Larynx, Via Natural or Artificial Opening Endoscopic

0CWS8KZ   Revision of Nonautologous Tissue Substitute in Larynx, Via Natural or Artificial Opening Endoscopic

0CWSX0Z   Revision of Drainage Device in Larynx, External Approach

0CWSX7Z   Revision of Autologous Tissue Substitute in Larynx, External Approach

0CWSXDZ   Revision of Intraluminal Device in Larynx, External Approach

0CWSXJZ   Revision of Synthetic Substitute in Larynx, External Approach

0CWSXKZ   Revision of Nonautologous Tissue Substitute in Larynx, External Approach

0CWY00Z   Revision of Drainage Device in Mouth and Throat, Open Approach

0CWY01Z   Revision of Radioactive Element in Mouth and Throat, Open Approach

0CWY07Z   Revision of Autologous Tissue Substitute in Mouth and Throat, Open Approach

0CWY0DZ   Revision of Intraluminal Device in Mouth and Throat, Open Approach

0CWY0JZ   Revision of Synthetic Substitute in Mouth and Throat, Open Approach

0CWY0KZ   Revision of Nonautologous Tissue Substitute in Mouth and Throat, Open Approach

0CWY30Z   Revision of Drainage Device in Mouth and Throat, Percutaneous Approach

0CWY31Z   Revision of Radioactive Element in Mouth and Throat, Percutaneous Approach

0CWY37Z   Revision of Autologous Tissue Substitute in Mouth and Throat, Percutaneous Approach

0CWY3DZ   Revision of Intraluminal Device in Mouth and Throat, Percutaneous Approach

0CWY3JZ   Revision of Synthetic Substitute in Mouth and Throat, Percutaneous Approach

0CWY3KZ   Revision of Nonautologous Tissue Substitute in Mouth and Throat, Percutaneous Approach

0CWY70Z   Revision of Drainage Device in Mouth and Throat, Via Natural or Artificial Opening

0CWY71Z   Revision of Radioactive Element in Mouth and Throat, Via Natural or Artificial Opening

0CWY77Z   Revision of Autologous Tissue Substitute in Mouth and Throat, Via Natural or Artificial Opening

0CWY7DZ   Revision of Intraluminal Device in Mouth and Throat, Via Natural or Artificial Opening

0CWY7JZ   Revision of Synthetic Substitute in Mouth and Throat, Via Natural or Artificial Opening

0CWY7KZ   Revision of Nonautologous Tissue Substitute in Mouth and Throat, Via Natural or Artificial Opening

0CWY80Z   Revision of Drainage Device in Mouth and Throat, Via Natural or Artificial Opening Endoscopic

0CWY81Z   Revision of Radioactive Element in Mouth and Throat, Via Natural or Artificial Opening Endoscopic

0CWY87Z   Revision of Autologous Tissue Substitute in Mouth and Throat, Via Natural or Artificial Opening Endoscopic

0CWY8DZ   Revision of Intraluminal Device in Mouth and Throat, Via Natural or Artificial Opening Endoscopic

0CWY8JZ   Revision of Synthetic Substitute in Mouth and Throat, Via Natural or Artificial Opening Endoscopic

0CWY8KZ   Revision of Nonautologous Tissue Substitute in Mouth and Throat, Via Natural or Artificial Opening Endoscopic

0CWYX0Z   Revision of Drainage Device in Mouth and Throat, External Approach

0CWYX1Z   Revision of Radioactive Element in Mouth and Throat, External Approach

0CWYX7Z   Revision of Autologous Tissue Substitute in Mouth and Throat, External Approach

0CWYXDZ   Revision of Intraluminal Device in Mouth and Throat, External Approach

0CWYXJZ   Revision of Synthetic Substitute in Mouth and Throat, External Approach

0CWYXKZ   Revision of Nonautologous Tissue Substitute in Mouth and Throat, External Approach

0CX – Mouth and Throat, Transfer

0CX00ZZ   Transfer Upper Lip, Open Approach

0CX0XZZ   Transfer Upper Lip, External Approach

0CX10ZZ   Transfer Lower Lip, Open Approach

0CX1XZZ   Transfer Lower Lip, External Approach

♀ Female-only   ♂ Male-only   ● Limited Coverage   ● Non-OR   🅗🅐🅒 HAC-associated procedure   ⬟ Non-covered procedures   ➕ Combination

0CX30ZZ	Transfer Soft Palate, Open Approach
0CX3XZZ	Transfer Soft Palate, External Approach
0CX40ZZ	Transfer Buccal Mucosa, Open Approach
0CX4XZZ	Transfer Buccal Mucosa, External Approach
0CX50ZZ	Transfer Upper Gingiva, Open Approach

0CX5XZZ	Transfer Upper Gingiva, External Approach
0CX60ZZ	Transfer Lower Gingiva, Open Approach
0CX6XZZ	Transfer Lower Gingiva, External Approach
0CX70ZZ	Transfer Tongue, Open Approach
0CX7XZZ	Transfer Tongue, External Approach

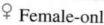 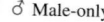

Gastrointestinal System

Upper Gastrointestinal System

Gastrointestinal System

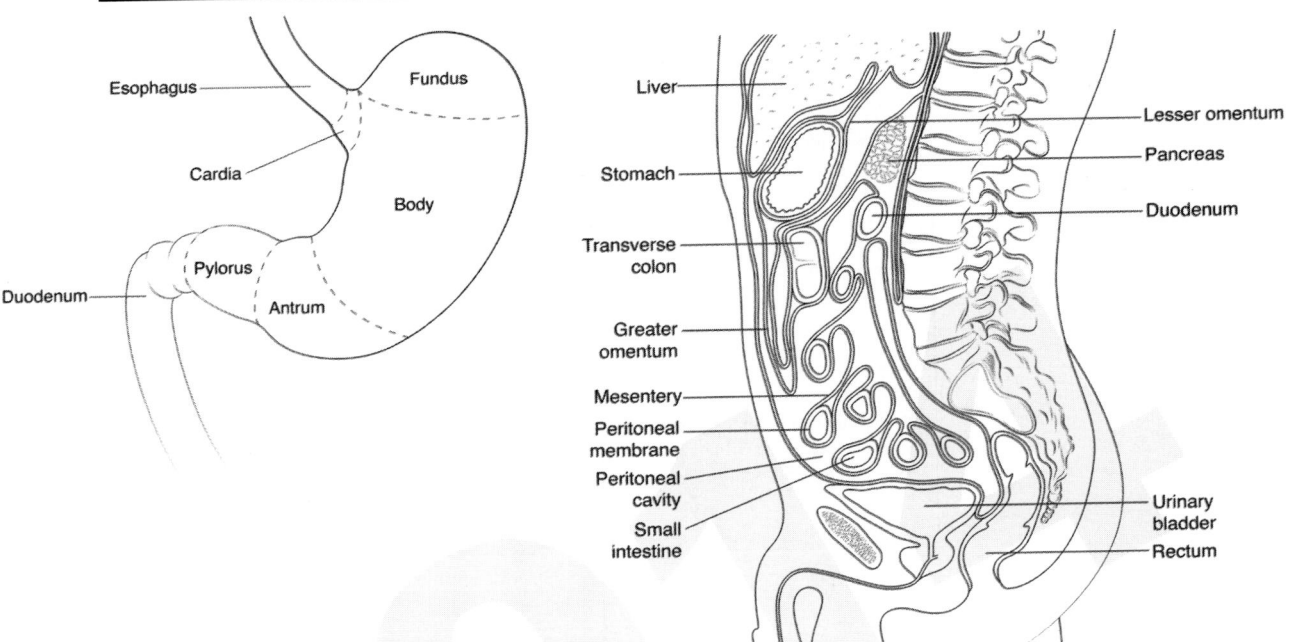

Gastrointestinal System

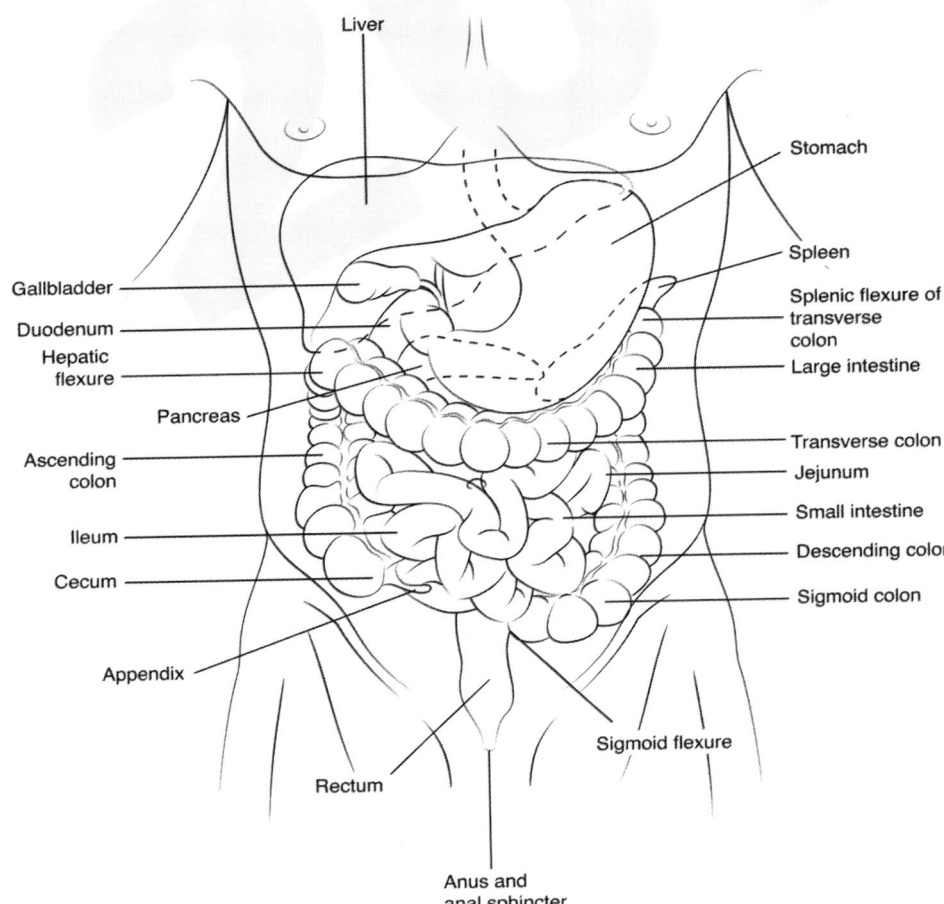

Gastrointestinal System Tables 0D1–0DY

Section	0	Medical and Surgical
Body System	D	Gastrointestinal System
Operation	1	Bypass: Altering the route of passage of the contents of a tubular body part

Body Part (4th)	Approach (4th)	Device (4th)	Qualifier (4th)
1 Esophagus, Upper 2 Esophagus, Middle 3 Esophagus, Lower 5 Esophagus	0 Open 4 Percutaneous Endoscopic 8 Via Natural or Artificial Opening Endoscopic	7 Autologous Tissue Substitute J Synthetic Substitute K Nonautologous Tissue Substitute Z No Device	4 Cutaneous 6 Stomach 9 Duodenum A Jejunum B Ileum
1 Esophagus, Upper 2 Esophagus, Middle 3 Esophagus, Lower 5 Esophagus	3 Percutaneous	J Synthetic Substitute	4 Cutaneous
6 Stomach 9 Duodenum	0 Open 4 Percutaneous Endoscopic 8 Via Natural or Artificial Opening Endoscopic	7 Autologous Tissue Substitute J Synthetic Substitute K Nonautologous Tissue Substitute Z No Device	4 Cutaneous 9 Duodenum A Jejunum B Ileum L Transverse Colon
6 Stomach 9 Duodenum	3 Percutaneous	J Synthetic Substitute	4 Cutaneous
A Jejunum	0 Open 4 Percutaneous Endoscopic 8 Via Natural or Artificial Opening Endoscopic	7 Autologous Tissue Substitute J Synthetic Substitute K Nonautologous Tissue Substitute Z No Device	4 Cutaneous A Jejunum B Ileum H Cecum K Ascending Colon L Transverse Colon M Descending Colon N Sigmoid Colon P Rectum Q Anus
A Jejunum	3 Percutaneous	J Synthetic Substitute	4 Cutaneous
B Ileum	0 Open 4 Percutaneous Endoscopic 8 Via Natural or Artificial Opening Endoscopic	7 Autologous Tissue Substitute J Synthetic Substitute K Nonautologous Tissue Substitute Z No Device	4 Cutaneous B Ileum H Cecum K Ascending Colon L Transverse Colon M Descending Colon N Sigmoid Colon P Rectum Q Anus
B Ileum	3 Percutaneous	J Synthetic Substitute	4 Cutaneous
H Cecum	0 Open 4 Percutaneous Endoscopic 8 Via Natural or Artificial Opening Endoscopic	7 Autologous Tissue Substitute J Synthetic Substitute K Nonautologous Tissue Substitute Z No Device	4 Cutaneous H Cecum K Ascending Colon L Transverse Colon M Descending Colon N Sigmoid Colon P Rectum
H Cecum	3 Percutaneous	J Synthetic Substitute	4 Cutaneous

Continued

0D1 Continued

Section	0	**Medical and Surgical**
Body System	D	**Gastrointestinal System**
Operation	1	**Bypass:** Altering the route of passage of the contents of a tubular body part

Body Part (4th)	Approach (4th)	Device (4th)	Qualifier (4th)
K Ascending Colon	0 Open 4 Percutaneous Endoscopic 8 Via Natural or Artificial Opening Endoscopic	7 Autologous Tissue Substitute J Synthetic Substitute K Nonautologous Tissue Substitute Z No Device	4 Cutaneous K Ascending Colon L Transverse Colon M Descending Colon N Sigmoid Colon P Rectum
K Ascending Colon	3 Percutaneous	J Synthetic Substitute	4 Cutaneous
L Transverse Colon	0 Open 4 Percutaneous Endoscopic 8 Via Natural or Artificial Opening Endoscopic	7 Autologous Tissue Substitute J Synthetic Substitute K Nonautologous Tissue Substitute Z No Device	4 Cutaneous L Transverse Colon M escending Colon N Sigmoid Colon P Rectum
L Transverse Colon	3 Percutaneous	J Synthetic Substitute	4 Cutaneous
M Descending Colon	0 Open 4 Percutaneous Endoscopic 8 Via Natural or Artificial Opening Endoscopic	7 Autologous Tissue Substitute J Synthetic Substitute K Nonautologous Tissue Substitute Z No Device	4 Cutaneous M Descending Colon N Sigmoid Colon P Rectum
M Descending Colon	3 Percutaneous	J Synthetic Substitute	4 Cutaneous
N Sigmoid Colon	0 Open 4 Percutaneous Endoscopic 8 Via Natural or Artificial Opening Endoscopic	7 Autologous Tissue Substitute J Synthetic Substitute K Nonautologous Tissue Substitute Z No Device	4 Cutaneous N Sigmoid Colon P Rectum
N Sigmoid Colon	3 Percutaneous	J Synthetic Substitute	4 Cutaneous

Section	0	**Medical and Surgical**
Body System	D	**Gastrointestinal System**
Operation	2	**Change:** Taking out or off a device from a body part and putting back an identical or similar device in or on the same body part without cutting or puncturing the skin or a mucous membrane

Body Part (4th)	Approach (4th)	Device (4th)	Qualifier (4th)
0 Upper Intestinal Tract D Lower Intestinal Tract	X External	0 Drainage Device U Feeding Device Y Other Device	Z No Qualifier
U Omentum V Mesentery W Peritoneum	X External	0 Drainage Device Y Other Device	Z No Qualifier

Section	0	Medical and Surgical
Body System	D	Gastrointestinal System
Operation	5	**Destruction:** Physical eradication of all or a portion of a body part by the direct use of energy, force, or a destructive agent

Body Part (4ᵗʰ)	Approach (4ᵗʰ)	Device (4ᵗʰ)	Qualifier (4ᵗʰ)
1 Esophagus, Upper 2 Esophagus, Middle 3 Esophagus, Lower 4 Esophagogastric Junction 5 Esophagus 6 Stomach 7 Stomach, Pylorus 8 Small Intestine 9 Duodenum A Jejunum B Ileum C Ileocecal Valve E Large Intestine F Large Intestine, Right G Large Intestine, Left H Cecum J Appendix K Ascending Colon L Transverse Colon M Descending Colon N Sigmoid Colon P Rectum	0 Open 3 Percutaneous 4 Percutaneous Endoscopic 7 Via Natural or Artificial Opening 8 Via Natural or Artificial Opening Endoscopic	Z No Device	Z No Qualifier
Q Anus	0 Open 3 Percutaneous 4 Percutaneous Endoscopic 7 Via Natural or Artificial Opening 8 Via Natural or Artificial Opening Endoscopic X External	Z No Device	Z No Qualifier
R Anal Sphincter S Greater Omentum T Lesser Omentum V Mesentery W Peritoneum	0 Open 3 Percutaneous 4 Percutaneous Endoscopic	Z No Device	Z No Qualifier

Section	0	Medical and Surgical
Body System	D	Gastrointestinal System
Operation	7	Dilation: Expanding an orifice or the lumen of a tubular body part

Body Part (4th)	Approach (4th)	Device (4th)	Qualifier (4th)
1 Esophagus, Upper 2 Esophagus, Middle 3 Esophagus, Lower 4 Esophagogastric Junction 5 Esophagus 6 Stomach 7 Stomach, Pylorus 8 Small Intestine 9 Duodenum A Jejunum B Ileum C Ileocecal Valve E Large Intestine F Large Intestine, Right G Large Intestine, Left H Cecum K Ascending Colon L Transverse Colon M Descending Colon N Sigmoid Colon P Rectum Q Anus	0 Open 3 Percutaneous 4 Percutaneous Endoscopic 7 Via Natural or Artificial Opening 8 Via Natural or Artificial Opening Endoscopic	D Intraluminal Device Z No Device	Z No Qualifier

Section	0	Medical and Surgical
Body System	D	Gastrointestinal System
Operation	8	Division: Cutting into a body part, without draining fluids and/or gases from the body part, in order to separate or transect a body part

Body Part (4th)	Approach (4th)	Device (4th)	Qualifier (4th)
4 Esophagogastric Junction 7 Stomach, Pylorus	0 Open 3 Percutaneous 4 Percutaneous Endoscopic 7 Via Natural or Artificial Opening 8 Via Natural or Artificial Opening Endoscopic	Z No Device	Z No Qualifier
R Anal Sphincter	0 Open 3 Percutaneous	Z No Device	Z No Qualifier

Section	0	Medical and Surgical
Body System	D	Gastrointestinal System
Operation	9	**Drainage:** Taking or letting out fluids and/or gases from a body part

Body Part (4th)	Approach (4th)	Device (4th)	Qualifier (4th)
1 Esophagus, Upper 2 Esophagus, Middle 3 Esophagus, Lower 4 Esophagogastric Junction 5 Esophagus 6 Stomach 7 Stomach, Pylorus 8 Small Intestine 9 Duodenum A Jejunum B Ileum C Ileocecal Valve E Large Intestine F Large Intestine, Right G Large Intestine, Left H Cecum J Appendix K Ascending Colon L Transverse Colon M Descending Colon N Sigmoid Colon P Rectum	0 Open 3 Percutaneous 4 Percutaneous Endoscopic 7 Via Natural or Artificial Opening 8 Via Natural or Artificial Opening Endoscopic	0 Drainage Device	Z No Qualifier
1 Esophagus, Upper 2 Esophagus, Middle 3 Esophagus, Lower 4 Esophagogastric Junction 5 Esophagus 6 Stomach 7 Stomach, Pylorus 8 Small Intestine 9 Duodenum A Jejunum B Ileum C Ileocecal Valve E Large Intestine F Large Intestine, Right G Large Intestine, Left H Cecum J Appendix K Ascending Colon L Transverse Colon M Descending Colon N Sigmoid Colon P Rectum	0 Open 3 Percutaneous 4 Percutaneous Endoscopic 7 Via Natural or Artificial Opening 8 Via Natural or Artificial Opening Endoscopic	Z No Device	X Diagnostic Z No Qualifier
Q Anus	0 Open 3 Percutaneous 4 Percutaneous Endoscopic 7 Via Natural or Artificial Opening 8 Via Natural or Artificial Opening Endoscopic X External	0 Drainage Device	Z No Qualifier

Continued

0D9 Continued

Section	0	**Medical and Surgical**
Body System	D	**Gastrointestinal System**
Operation	9	**Drainage:** Taking or letting out fluids and/or gases from a body part

Body Part (4th)	Approach (4th)	Device (4th)	Qualifier (4th)
Q Anus	**0** Open **3** Percutaneous **4** Percutaneous Endoscopic **7** Via Natural or Artificial Opening **8** Via Natural or Artificial Opening Endoscopic **X** External	**Z** No Device	**X** Diagnostic **Z** No Qualifier
R Anal Sphincter **S** Greater Omentum **T** Lesser Omentum **V** Mesentery **W** Peritoneum	**0** Open **3** Percutaneous **4** Percutaneous Endoscopic	**0** Drainage Device	**Z** No Qualifier
R Anal Sphincter **S** Greater Omentum **T** Lesser Omentum **V** Mesentery **W** Peritoneum	**0** Open **3** Percutaneous **4** Percutaneous Endoscopic	**Z** No Device	**X** Diagnostic **Z** No Qualifier

Section	0	**Medical and Surgical**
Body System	D	**Gastrointestinal System**
Operation	B	**Excision:** Cutting out or off, without replacement, a portion of a body part

Body Part (4th)	Approach (4th)	Device (4th)	Qualifier (4th)
1 Esophagus, Upper **2** Esophagus, Middle **3** Esophagus, Lower **4** Esophagogastric Junction **5** Esophagus **7** Stomach, Pylorus **8** Small Intestine **9** Duodenum **A** Jejunum **B** Ileum **C** Ileocecal Valve **E** Large Intestine **F** Large Intestine, Right **G** Large Intestine, Left **H** Cecum **J** Appendix **K** Ascending Colon **L** Transverse Colon **M** Descending Colon **N** Sigmoid Colon **P** Rectum	**0** Open **3** Percutaneous **4** Percutaneous Endoscopic **7** Via Natural or Artificial Opening **8** Via Natural or Artificial Opening Endoscopic	**Z** No Device	**X** Diagnostic **Z** No Qualifier
6 Stomach	**0** Open **3** Percutaneous **4** Percutaneous Endoscopic **7** Via Natural or Artificial Opening **8** Via Natural or Artificial Opening Endoscopic	**Z** No Device	**3** Vertical **X** Diagnostic **Z** No Qualifier

Continued

0DB Continued

Section	0	Medical and Surgical
Body System	D	Gastrointestinal System
Operation	B	Excision: Cutting out or off, without replacement, a portion of a body part

Body Part (4th)	Approach (4th)	Device (4th)	Qualifier (4th)
Q Anus	0 Open 3 Percutaneous 4 Percutaneous Endoscopic 7 Via Natural or Artificial Opening 8 Via Natural or Artificial Opening Endoscopic X External	Z No Device	X Diagnostic Z No Qualifier
R Anal Sphincter S Greater Omentum T Lesser Omentum V Mesentery W Peritoneum	0 Open 3 Percutaneous 4 Percutaneous Endoscopic	Z No Device	X Diagnostic Z No Qualifier

Section	0	Medical and Surgical
Body System	D	Gastrointestinal System
Operation	C	Extirpation: Taking or cutting out solid matter from a body part

Body Part (4th)	Approach (4th)	Device (4th)	Qualifier (4th)
1 Esophagus, Upper 2 Esophagus, Middle 3 Esophagus, Lower 4 Esophagogastric Junction 5 Esophagus 6 Stomach 7 Stomach, Pylorus 8 Small Intestine 9 Duodenum A Jejunum B Ileum C Ileocecal Valve E Large Intestine F Large Intestine, Right G Large Intestine, Left H Cecum J Appendix K Ascending Colon L Transverse Colon M Descending Colon N Sigmoid Colon P Rectum	0 Open 3 Percutaneous 4 Percutaneous Endoscopic 7 Via Natural or Artificial Opening 8 Via Natural or Artificial Opening Endoscopic	Z No Device	Z No Qualifier
Q Anus	0 Open 3 Percutaneous 4 Percutaneous Endoscopic 7 Via Natural or Artificial Opening 8 Via Natural or Artificial Opening Endoscopic X External	Z No Device	Z No Qualifier
R Anal Sphincter S Greater Omentum T Lesser Omentum V Mesentery W Peritoneum	0 Open 3 Percutaneous 4 Percutaneous Endoscopic	Z No Device	Z No Qualifier

Section	0	**Medical and Surgical**
Body System	D	**Gastrointestinal System**
Operation	F	**Fragmentation:** Breaking solid matter in a body part into pieces

Body Part (4th)	Approach (4th)	Device (4th)	Qualifier (4th)
5 Esophagus 6 Stomach 8 Small Intestine 9 Duodenum A Jejunum B Ileum E Large Intestine F Large Intestine, Right G Large Intestine, Left H Cecum J Appendix K Ascending Colon L Transverse Colon M Descending Colon N Sigmoid Colon P Rectum Q Anus	0 Open 3 Percutaneous 4 Percutaneous Endoscopic 7 Via Natural or Artificial Opening 8 Via Natural or Artificial Opening Endoscopic X External	Z No Device	Z No Qualifier

Section	0	**Medical and Surgical**
Body System	D	**Gastrointestinal System**
Operation	H	**Insertion:** Putting in a nonbiological appliance that monitors, assists, performs, or prevents a physiological function but does not physically take the place of a body part

Body Part (4th)	Approach (4th)	Device (4th)	Qualifier (4th)
5 Esophagus	0 Open 3 Percutaneous 4 Percutaneous Endoscopic	1 Radioactive Element 2 Monitoring Device 3 Infusion Device D Intraluminal Device U Feeding Device	Z No Qualifier
5 Esophagus	7 Via Natural or Artificial Opening 8 Via Natural or Artificial Opening Endoscopic	1 Radioactive Element 2 Monitoring Device 3 Infusion Device B Intraluminal Device, Airway D Intraluminal Device U Feeding Device	Z No Qualifier
6 Stomach	0 Open 3 Percutaneous 4 Percutaneous Endoscopic	2 Monitoring Device 3 Infusion Device D Intraluminal Device M Stimulator Lead U Feeding Device	Z No Qualifier
6 Stomach	7 Via Natural or Artificial Opening 8 Via Natural or Artificial Opening Endoscopic	2 Monitoring Device 3 Infusion Device D Intraluminal Device U Feeding Device	Z No Qualifier
8 Small Intestine 9 Duodenum A Jejunum B Ileum	0 Open 3 Percutaneous 4 Percutaneous Endoscopic 7 Via Natural or Artificial Opening 8 Via Natural or Artificial Opening Endoscopic	2 Monitoring Device 3 Infusion Device D Intraluminal Device U Feeding Device	Z No Qualifier

Continued

Section	0	Medical and Surgical
Body System	D	Gastrointestinal System
Operation	H	Insertion: Putting in a nonbiological appliance that monitors, assists, performs, or prevents a physiological function but does not physically take the place of a body part

0DH *Continued*

Body Part (4th)	Approach (4th)	Device (4th)	Qualifier (4th)
E Large Intestine	0 Open 3 Percutaneous 4 Percutaneous Endoscopic 7 Via Natural or Artificial Opening 8 Via Natural or Artificial Opening Endoscopic	D Intraluminal Device	Z No Qualifier
P Rectum	0 Open 3 Percutaneous 4 Percutaneous Endoscopic 7 Via Natural or Artificial Opening 8 Via Natural or Artificial Opening Endoscopic	1 Radioactive Element D Intraluminal Device	Z No Qualifier
Q Anus	0 Open 3 Percutaneous 4 Percutaneous Endoscopic	D Intraluminal Device L Artificial Sphincter	Z No Qualifier
Q Anus	7 Via Natural or Artificial Opening 8 Via Natural or Artificial Opening Endoscopic	D Intraluminal Device	Z No Qualifier
R Anal Sphincter	0 Open 3 Percutaneous 4 Percutaneous Endoscopic	M Stimulator Lead	Z No Qualifier

Section	0	Medical and Surgical
Body System	D	Gastrointestinal System
Operation	J	Inspection: Visually and/or manually exploring a body part

Body Part (4th)	Approach (4th)	Device (4th)	Qualifier (4th)
0 Upper Intestinal Tract 6 Stomach D Lower Intestinal Tract	0 Open 3 Percutaneous 4 Percutaneous Endoscopic 7 Via Natural or Artificial Opening 8 Via Natural or Artificial Opening Endoscopic X External	Z No Device	Z No Qualifier
U Omentum V Mesentery W Peritoneum	0 Open 3 Percutaneous 4 Percutaneous Endoscopic X External	Z No Device	Z No Qualifier

Section	0	**Medical and Surgical**
Body System	D	**Gastrointestinal System**
Operation	L	**Occlusion:** Completely closing an orifice or the lumen of a tubular body part

Body Part (4ᵗʰ)	Approach (4ᵗʰ)	Device (4ᵗʰ)	Qualifier (4ᵗʰ)
1 Esophagus, Upper **2** Esophagus, Middle **3** Esophagus, Lower **4** Esophagogastric Junction **5** Esophagus **6** Stomach **7** Stomach, Pylorus **8** Small Intestine **9** Duodenum **A** Jejunum **B** Ileum **C** Ileocecal Valve **E** Large Intestine **F** Large Intestine, Right **G** Large Intestine, Left **H** Cecum **K** Ascending Colon **L** Transverse Colon **M** Descending Colon **N** Sigmoid Colon **P** Rectum	**0** Open **3** Percutaneous **4** Percutaneous Endoscopic	**C** Extraluminal Device **D** Intraluminal Device **Z** No Device	**Z** No Qualifier
1 Esophagus, Upper **2** Esophagus, Middle **3** Esophagus, Lower **4** Esophagogastric Junction **5** Esophagus **6** Stomach **7** Stomach, Pylorus **8** Small Intestine **9** Duodenum **A** Jejunum **B** Ileum **C** Ileocecal Valve **E** Large Intestine **F** Large Intestine, Right **G** Large Intestine, Left **H** Cecum **K** Ascending Colon **L** Transverse Colon **M** Descending Colon **N** Sigmoid Colon **P** Rectum	**7** Via Natural or Artificial Opening **8** Via Natural or Artificial Opening Endoscopic	**D** Intraluminal Device **Z** No Device	**Z** No Qualifier
Q Anus	**0** Open **3** Percutaneous **4** Percutaneous Endoscopic **X** External	**C** Extraluminal Device **D** Intraluminal Device **Z** No Device	**Z** No Qualifier
Q Anus	**7** Via Natural or Artificial Opening **8** Via Natural or Artificial Opening Endoscopic	**D** Intraluminal Device **Z** No Device	**Z** No Qualifier

Section	0	Medical and Surgical
Body System	D	Gastrointestinal System
Operation	M	**Reattachment:** Putting back in or on all or a portion of a separated body part to its normal location or other suitable location

Body Part (4ᵗʰ)	Approach (4ᵗʰ)	Device (4ᵗʰ)	Qualifier (4ᵗʰ)
5 Esophagus 6 Stomach 8 Small Intestine 9 Duodenum A Jejunum B Ileum E Large Intestine F Large Intestine, Right G Large Intestine, Left H Cecum K Ascending Colon L Transverse Colon M Descending Colon N Sigmoid Colon P Rectum	0 Open 4 Percutaneous Endoscopic	Z No Device	Z No Qualifier

Section	0	Medical and Surgical
Body System	D	Gastrointestinal System
Operation	N	**Release:** Freeing a body part from an abnormal physical constraint by cutting or by the use of force

Body Part (4ᵗʰ)	Approach (4ᵗʰ)	Device (4ᵗʰ)	Qualifier (4ᵗʰ)
1 Esophagus, Upper 2 Esophagus, Middle 3 Esophagus, Lower 4 Esophagogastric Junction 5 Esophagus 6 Stomach 7 Stomach, Pylorus 8 Small Intestine 9 Duodenum A Jejunum B Ileum C Ileocecal Valve E Large Intestine F Large Intestine, Right G Large Intestine, Left H Cecum J Appendix K Ascending Colon L Transverse Colon M Descending Colon N Sigmoid Colon P Rectum	0 Open 3 Percutaneous 4 Percutaneous Endoscopic 7 Via Natural or Artificial Opening 8 Via Natural or Artificial Opening Endoscopic	Z No Device	Z No Qualifier

Continued

Section	0	Medical and Surgical
Body System	D	Gastrointestinal System
Operation	N	Release: Freeing a body part from an abnormal physical constraint by cutting or by the use of force

Body Part (4th)	Approach (4th)	Device (4th)	Qualifier (4th)
Q Anus	0 Open 3 Percutaneous 4 Percutaneous Endoscopic 7 Via Natural or Artificial Opening 8 Via Natural or Artificial Opening Endoscopic X External	Z No Device	Z No Qualifier
R Anal Sphincter S Greater Omentum T Lesser Omentum V Mesentery W Peritoneum	0 Open 3 Percutaneous 4 Percutaneous Endoscopic	Z No Device	Z No Qualifier

Section	0	Medical and Surgical
Body System	D	Gastrointestinal System
Operation	P	Removal: Taking out or off a device from a body part

Body Part (4th)	Approach (4th)	Device (4th)	Qualifier (4th)
0 Upper Intestinal Tract D Lower Intestinal Tract	0 Open 3 Percutaneous 4 Percutaneous Endoscopic 7 Via Natural or Artificial Opening 8 Via Natural or Artificial Opening Endoscopic	0 Drainage Device 2 Monitoring Device 3 Infusion Device 7 Autologous Tissue Substitute C Extraluminal Device D Intraluminal Device J Synthetic Substitute K Nonautologous Tissue Substitute U Feeding Device	Z No Qualifier
0 Upper Intestinal Tract D Lower Intestinal Tract	X External	0 Drainage Device 2 Monitoring Device 3 Infusion Device D Intraluminal Device U Feeding Device	Z No Qualifier
5 Esophagus	0 Open 3 Percutaneous 4 Percutaneous Endoscopic	1 Radioactive Element 2 Monitoring Device 3 Infusion Device U Feeding Device	Z No Qualifier
5 Esophagus	7 Via Natural or Artificial Opening 8 Via Natural or Artificial Opening Endoscopic	1 Radioactive Element D Intraluminal Device	Z No Qualifier
5 Esophagus	X External	1 Radioactive Element 2 Monitoring Device 3 Infusion Device D Intraluminal Device U Feeding Device	Z No Qualifier

Continued

Section	0	Medical and Surgical
Body System	D	Gastrointestinal System
Operation	P	Removal: Taking out or off a device from a body part

Body Part (4th)	Approach (4th)	Device (4th)	Qualifier (4th)
6 Stomach	0 Open 3 Percutaneous 4 Percutaneous Endoscopic	0 Drainage Device 2 Monitoring Device 3 Infusion Device 7 Autologous Tissue Substitute C Extraluminal Device D Intraluminal Device J Synthetic Substitute K Nonautologous Tissue Substitute M Stimulator Lead U Feeding Device	Z No Qualifier
6 Stomach	7 Via Natural or Artificial Opening 8 Via Natural or Artificial Opening Endoscopic	0 Drainage Device 2 Monitoring Device 3 Infusion Device 7 Autologous Tissue Substitute C Extraluminal Device D Intraluminal Device J Synthetic Substitute K Nonautologous Tissue Substitute U Feeding Device	Z No Qualifier
6 Stomach	X External	0 Drainage Device 2 Monitoring Device 3 Infusion Device D Intraluminal Device U Feeding Device	Z No Qualifier
P Rectum	0 Open 3 Percutaneous 4 Percutaneous Endoscopic 7 Via Natural or Artificial Opening 8 Via Natural or Artificial Opening Endoscopic X External	1 Radioactive Element	Z No Qualifier
Q Anus	0 Open 3 Percutaneous 4 Percutaneous Endoscopic 7 Via Natural or Artificial Opening 8 Via Natural or Artificial Opening Endoscopic	L Artificial Sphincter	Z No Qualifier
R Anal Sphincter	0 Open 3 Percutaneous 4 Percutaneous Endoscopic	M Stimulator Lead	Z No Qualifier
U Omentum V Mesentery W Peritoneum	0 Open 3 Percutaneous 4 Percutaneous Endoscopic	0 Drainage Device 1 Radioactive Element 7 Autologous Tissue Substitute J Synthetic Substitute K Nonautologous Tissue Substitute	Z No Qualifier

Section	0	Medical and Surgical
Body System	D	Gastrointestinal System
Operation	Q	**Repair:** Restoring, to the extent possible, a body part to its normal anatomic structure and function

Body Part (4th)	Approach (4th)	Device (4th)	Qualifier (4th)
1 Esophagus, Upper 2 Esophagus, Middle 3 Esophagus, Lower 4 Esophagogastric Junction 5 Esophagus 6 Stomach 7 Stomach, Pylorus 8 Small Intestine 9 Duodenum A Jejunum B Ileum C Ileocecal Valve E Large Intestine F Large Intestine, Right G Large Intestine, Left H Cecum J Appendix K Ascending Colon L Transverse Colon M Descending Colon N Sigmoid Colon P Rectum	0 Open 3 Percutaneous 4 Percutaneous Endoscopic 7 Via Natural or Artificial Opening 8 Via Natural or Artificial Opening Endoscopic	Z No Device	Z No Qualifier
Q Anus	0 Open 3 Percutaneous 4 Percutaneous Endoscopic 7 Via Natural or Artificial Opening 8 Via Natural or Artificial Opening Endoscopic X External	Z No Device	Z No Qualifier
R Anal Sphincter S Greater Omentum T Lesser Omentum V Mesentery W Peritoneum	0 Open 3 Percutaneous 4 Percutaneous Endoscopic	Z No Device	Z No Qualifier

Section	0	Medical and Surgical
Body System	D	Gastrointestinal System
Operation	R	**Replacement:** Putting in or on biological or synthetic material that physically takes the place and/or function of all or a portion of a body part

Body Part (4th)	Approach (4th)	Device (4th)	Qualifier (4th)
5 Esophagus	0 Open 4 Percutaneous Endoscopic 7 Via Natural or Artificial Opening 8 Via Natural or Artificial Opening Endoscopic	7 Autologous Tissue Substitute J Synthetic Substitute K Nonautologous Tissue Substitute	Z No Qualifier
R Anal Sphincter S Greater Omentum T Lesser Omentum V Mesentery W Peritoneum	0 Open 4 Percutaneous Endoscopic	7 Autologous Tissue Substitute J Synthetic Substitute K Nonautologous Tissue Substitute	Z No Qualifier

Section	0	Medical and Surgical
Body System	D	Gastrointestinal System
Operation	S	**Reposition:** Moving to its normal location, or other suitable location, all or a portion of a body part

Body Part (4ᵗʰ)	Approach (4ᵗʰ)	Device (4ᵗʰ)	Qualifier (4ᵗʰ)
5 Esophagus 6 Stomach 9 Duodenum A Jejunum B Ileum H Cecum K Ascending Colon L Transverse Colon M Descending Colon N Sigmoid Colon P Rectum Q Anus	0 Open 4 Percutaneous Endoscopic 7 Via Natural or Artificial Opening 8 Via Natural or Artificial Opening Endoscopic X External	Z No Device	Z No Qualifier

Section	0	Medical and Surgical
Body System	D	Gastrointestinal System
Operation	T	**Resection:** Cutting out or off, without replacement, all of a body part

Body Part (4ᵗʰ)	Approach (4ᵗʰ)	Device (4ᵗʰ)	Qualifier (4ᵗʰ)
1 Esophagus, Upper 2 Esophagus, Middle 3 Esophagus, Lower 4 Esophagogastric Junction 5 Esophagus 6 Stomach 7 Stomach, Pylorus 8 Small Intestine 9 Duodenum A Jejunum B Ileum C Ileocecal Valve E Large Intestine F Large Intestine, Right G Large Intestine, Left H Cecum J Appendix K Ascending Colon L Transverse Colon M Descending Colon N Sigmoid Colon P Rectum Q Anus	0 Open 4 Percutaneous Endoscopic 7 Via Natural or Artificial Opening 8 Via Natural or Artificial Opening Endoscopic	Z No Device	Z No Qualifier
R Anal Sphincter S Greater Omentum T Lesser Omentum	0 Open 4 Percutaneous Endoscopic	Z No Device	Z No Qualifier

Section	0	**Medical and Surgical**
Body System	D	**Gastrointestinal System**
Operation	U	**Supplement:** Putting in or on biological or synthetic material that physically reinforces and/or augments the function of a portion of a body part

Body Part (4ᵗʰ)	Approach (4ᵗʰ)	Device (4ᵗʰ)	Qualifier (4ᵗʰ)
1 Esophagus, Upper 2 Esophagus, Middle 3 Esophagus, Lower 4 Esophagogastric Junction 5 Esophagus 6 Stomach 7 Stomach, Pylorus 8 Small Intestine 9 Duodenum A Jejunum B Ileum C Ileocecal Valve E Large Intestine F Large Intestine, Right G Large Intestine, Left H Cecum K Ascending Colon L Transverse Colon M Descending Colon N Sigmoid Colon P Rectum	0 Open 4 Percutaneous Endoscopic 7 Via Natural or Artificial Opening 8 Via Natural or Artificial Opening Endoscopic	7 Autologous Tissue Substitute J Synthetic Substitute K Nonautologous Tissue Substitute	Z No Qualifier
Q Anus	0 Open 4 Percutaneous Endoscopic 7 Via Natural or Artificial Opening 8 Via Natural or Artificial Opening Endoscopic X External	7 Autologous Tissue Substitute J Synthetic Substitute K Nonautologous Tissue Substitute	Z No Qualifier
R Anal Sphincter S Greater Omentum T Lesser Omentum V Mesentery W Peritoneum	0 Open 4 Percutaneous Endoscopic	7 Autologous Tissue Substitute J Synthetic Substitute K Nonautologous Tissue Substitute	Z No Qualifier

Section	0	**Medical and Surgical**
Body System	D	**Gastrointestinal System**
Operation	V	**Restriction:** Partially closing an orifice or the lumen of a tubular body part

Body Part (4th)	Approach (4th)	Device (4th)	Qualifier (4th)
1 Esophagus, Upper 2 Esophagus, Middle 3 Esophagus, Lower 4 Esophagogastric Junction 5 Esophagus 6 Stomach 7 Stomach, Pylorus 8 Small Intestine 9 Duodenum A Jejunum B Ileum C Ileocecal Valve E Large Intestine F Large Intestine, Right G Large Intestine, Left H Cecum K Ascending Colon L Transverse Colon M Descending Colon N Sigmoid Colon P Rectum	0 Open 3 Percutaneous 4 Percutaneous Endoscopic	C Extraluminal Device D Intraluminal Device Z No Device	Z No Qualifier
1 Esophagus, Upper 2 Esophagus, Middle 3 Esophagus, Lower 4 Esophagogastric Junction 5 Esophagus 6 Stomach 7 Stomach, Pylorus 8 Small Intestine 9 Duodenum A Jejunum B Ileum C Ileocecal Valve E Large Intestine F Large Intestine, Right G Large Intestine, Left H Cecum K Ascending Colon L Transverse Colon M Descending Colon N Sigmoid Colon P Rectum	7 Via Natural or Artificial Opening 8 Via Natural or Artificial Opening Endoscopic	D Intraluminal Device Z No Device	Z No Qualifier
Q Anus	0 Open 3 Percutaneous 4 Percutaneous Endoscopic X External	C Extraluminal Device D Intraluminal Device Z No Device	Z No Qualifier
Q Anus	7 Via Natural or Artificial Opening 8 Via Natural or Artificial Opening Endoscopic	D Intraluminal Device Z No Device	Z No Qualifier

Section	0	Medical and Surgical
Body System	D	Gastrointestinal System
Operation	W	Revision: Correcting, to the extent possible, a portion of a malfunctioning device or the position of a displaced device

Body Part (4th)	Approach (4th)	Device (4th)	Qualifier (4th)
0 Upper Intestinal Tract D Lower Intestinal Tract	0 Open 3 Percutaneous 4 Percutaneous Endoscopic 7 Via Natural or Artificial Opening 8 Via Natural or Artificial Opening Endoscopic X External	0 Drainage Device 2 Monitoring Device 3 Infusion Device 7 Autologous Tissue Substitute C Extraluminal Device D Intraluminal Device J Synthetic Substitute K Nonautologous Tissue Substitute U Feeding Device	Z No Qualifier
5 Esophagus	7 Via Natural or Artificial Opening 8 Via Natural or Artificial Opening Endoscopic X External	D Intraluminal Device	Z No Qualifier
6 Stomach	0 Open 3 Percutaneous 4 Percutaneous Endoscopic	0 Drainage Device 2 Monitoring Device 3 Infusion Device 7 Autologous Tissue Substitute C Extraluminal Device D Intraluminal Device J Synthetic Substitute K Nonautologous Tissue Substitute M Stimulator Lead U Feeding Device	Z No Qualifier
6 Stomach	7 Via Natural or Artificial Opening 8 Via Natural or Artificial Opening Endoscopic X External	0 Drainage Device 2 Monitoring Device 3 Infusion Device 7 Autologous Tissue Substitute C Extraluminal Device D Intraluminal Device J Synthetic Substitute K Nonautologous Tissue Substitute U Feeding Device	Z No Qualifier
8 Small Intestine E Large Intestine	0 Open 4 Percutaneous Endoscopic 7 Via Natural or Artificial Opening 8 Via Natural or Artificial Opening Endoscopic	7 Autologous Tissue Substitute J Synthetic Substitute K Nonautologous Tissue Substitute	Z No Qualifier

Continued

Section	0	Medical and Surgical
Body System	D	Gastrointestinal System
Operation	W	**Revision:** Correcting, to the extent possible, a portion of a malfunctioning device or the position of a displaced device

Body Part (4ᵗʰ)	Approach (4ᵗʰ)	Device (4ᵗʰ)	Qualifier (4ᵗʰ)
Q Anus	0 Open 3 Percutaneous 4 Percutaneous Endoscopic 7 Via Natural or Artificial Opening 8 Via Natural or Artificial Opening Endoscopic	L Artificial Sphincter	Z No Qualifier
R Anal Sphincter	0 Open 3 Percutaneous 4 Percutaneous Endoscopic	M Stimulator Lead	Z No Qualifier
U Omentum V Mesentery W Peritoneum	0 Open 3 Percutaneous 4 Percutaneous Endoscopic	0 Drainage Device 7 Autologous Tissue Substitute J Synthetic Substitute K Nonautologous Tissue Substitute	Z No Qualifier

Section	0	Medical and Surgical
Body System	D	Gastrointestinal System
Operation	X	**Transfer:** Moving, without taking out, all or a portion of a body part to another location to take over the function of all or a portion of a body part

Body Part (4ᵗʰ)	Approach (4ᵗʰ)	Device (4ᵗʰ)	Qualifier (4ᵗʰ)
6 Stomach 8 Small Intestine E Large Intestine	0 Open 4 Percutaneous Endoscopic	Z No Device	5 Esophagus

Section	0	Medical and Surgical
Body System	D	Gastrointestinal System
Operation	Y	**Transplantation:** Putting in or on all or a portion of a living body part taken from another individual or animal to physically take the place and/or function of all or a portion of a similar body part

Body Part (4ᵗʰ)	Approach (4ᵗʰ)	Device (4ᵗʰ)	Qualifier (4ᵗʰ)
5 Esophagus 6 Stomach 8 Small Intestine E Large Intestine	0 Open	Z No Device	0 Allogeneic 1 Syngeneic 2 Zooplastic

Gastrointestinal System Code Listing 0D1–0DY

Review Coding Guideline B4.8

0D1 – Gastrointestinal System, Bypass

Review Coding Guideline B3.6a

0D11074	Bypass Upper Esophagus to Cutaneous with Autologous Tissue Substitute, Open Approach	**0D1107A**	Bypass Upper Esophagus to Jejunum with Autologous Tissue Substitute, Open Approach
0D11076	Bypass Upper Esophagus to Stomach with Autologous Tissue Substitute, Open Approach	**0D1107B**	Bypass Upper Esophagus to Ileum with Autologous Tissue Substitute, Open Approach
0D11079	Bypass Upper Esophagus to Duodenum with Autologous Tissue Substitute, Open Approach	**0D110J4**	Bypass Upper Esophagus to Cutaneous with Synthetic Substitute, Open Approach

♀ Female-only ♂ Male-only ● Limited Coverage ● Non-OR ▨ HAC-associated procedure ● Non-covered procedures ✚ Combination

0D110J6   Bypass Upper Esophagus to Stomach with Synthetic Substitute, Open Approach

0D110J9   Bypass Upper Esophagus to Duodenum with Synthetic Substitute, Open Approach

0D110JA   Bypass Upper Esophagus to Jejunum with Synthetic Substitute, Open Approach

0D110JB   Bypass Upper Esophagus to Ileum with Synthetic Substitute, Open Approach

0D110K4   Bypass Upper Esophagus to Cutaneous with Nonautologous Tissue Substitute, Open Approach

0D110K6   Bypass Upper Esophagus to Stomach with Nonautologous Tissue Substitute, Open Approach

0D110K9   Bypass Upper Esophagus to Duodenum with Nonautologous Tissue Substitute, Open Approach

0D110KA   Bypass Upper Esophagus to Jejunum with Nonautologous Tissue Substitute, Open Approach

0D110KB   Bypass Upper Esophagus to Ileum with Nonautologous Tissue Substitute, Open Approach

0D110Z4   Bypass Upper Esophagus to Cutaneous, Open Approach

0D110Z6   Bypass Upper Esophagus to Stomach, Open Approach

0D110Z9   Bypass Upper Esophagus to Duodenum, Open Approach

0D110ZA   Bypass Upper Esophagus to Jejunum, Open Approach

0D110ZB   Bypass Upper Esophagus to Ileum, Open Approach

0D113J4   Bypass Upper Esophagus to Cutaneous with Synthetic Substitute, Percutaneous Approach

0D11474   Bypass Upper Esophagus to Cutaneous with Autologous Tissue Substitute, Percutaneous Endoscopic Approach

0D11476   Bypass Upper Esophagus to Stomach with Autologous Tissue Substitute, Percutaneous Endoscopic Approach

0D11479   Bypass Upper Esophagus to Duodenum with Autologous Tissue Substitute, Percutaneous Endoscopic Approach

0D1147A   Bypass Upper Esophagus to Jejunum with Autologous Tissue Substitute, Percutaneous Endoscopic Approach

0D1147B   Bypass Upper Esophagus to Ileum with Autologous Tissue Substitute, Percutaneous Endoscopic Approach

0D114J4   Bypass Upper Esophagus to Cutaneous with Synthetic Substitute, Percutaneous Endoscopic Approach

0D114J6   Bypass Upper Esophagus to Stomach with Synthetic Substitute, Percutaneous Endoscopic Approach

0D114J9   Bypass Upper Esophagus to Duodenum with Synthetic Substitute, Percutaneous Endoscopic Approach

0D114JA   Bypass Upper Esophagus to Jejunum with Synthetic Substitute, Percutaneous Endoscopic Approach

0D114JB   Bypass Upper Esophagus to Ileum with Synthetic Substitute, Percutaneous Endoscopic Approach

0D114K4   Bypass Upper Esophagus to Cutaneous with Nonautologous Tissue Substitute, Percutaneous Endoscopic Approach

0D114K6   Bypass Upper Esophagus to Stomach with Nonautologous Tissue Substitute, Percutaneous Endoscopic Approach

0D114K9   Bypass Upper Esophagus to Duodenum with Nonautologous Tissue Substitute, Percutaneous Endoscopic Approach

0D114KA   Bypass Upper Esophagus to Jejunum with Nonautologous Tissue Substitute, Percutaneous Endoscopic Approach

0D114KB   Bypass Upper Esophagus to Ileum with Nonautologous Tissue Substitute, Percutaneous Endoscopic Approach

0D114Z4   Bypass Upper Esophagus to Cutaneous, Percutaneous Endoscopic Approach

0D114Z6   Bypass Upper Esophagus to Stomach, Percutaneous Endoscopic Approach

0D114Z9   Bypass Upper Esophagus to Duodenum, Percutaneous Endoscopic Approach

0D114ZA   Bypass Upper Esophagus to Jejunum, Percutaneous Endoscopic Approach

0D114ZB   Bypass Upper Esophagus to Ileum, Percutaneous Endoscopic Approach

0D11874   Bypass Upper Esophagus to Cutaneous with Autologous Tissue Substitute, Via Natural or Artificial Opening Endoscopic

0D11876   Bypass Upper Esophagus to Stomach with Autologous Tissue Substitute, Via Natural or Artificial Opening Endoscopic

0D11879   Bypass Upper Esophagus to Duodenum with Autologous Tissue Substitute, Via Natural or Artificial Opening Endoscopic

0D1187A   Bypass Upper Esophagus to Jejunum with Autologous Tissue Substitute, Via Natural or Artificial Opening Endoscopic

0D1187B   Bypass Upper Esophagus to Ileum with Autologous Tissue Substitute, Via Natural or Artificial Opening Endoscopic

0D118J4   Bypass Upper Esophagus to Cutaneous with Synthetic Substitute, Via Natural or Artificial Opening Endoscopic

0D118J6   Bypass Upper Esophagus to Stomach with Synthetic Substitute, Via Natural or Artificial Opening Endoscopic

0D118J9   Bypass Upper Esophagus to Duodenum with Synthetic Substitute, Via Natural or Artificial Opening Endoscopic

0D118JA   Bypass Upper Esophagus to Jejunum with Synthetic Substitute, Via Natural or Artificial Opening Endoscopic

0D118JB   Bypass Upper Esophagus to Ileum with Synthetic Substitute, Via Natural or Artificial Opening Endoscopic

0D118K4   Bypass Upper Esophagus to Cutaneous with Nonautologous Tissue Substitute, Via Natural or Artificial Opening Endoscopic

0D118K6   Bypass Upper Esophagus to Stomach with Nonautologous Tissue Substitute, Via Natural or Artificial Opening Endoscopic

0D118K9   Bypass Upper Esophagus to Duodenum with Nonautologous Tissue Substitute, Via Natural or Artificial Opening Endoscopic

0D118KA   Bypass Upper Esophagus to Jejunum with Nonautologous Tissue Substitute, Via Natural or Artificial Opening Endoscopic

0D118KB   Bypass Upper Esophagus to Ileum with Nonautologous Tissue Substitute, Via Natural or Artificial Opening Endoscopic

0D118Z4   Bypass Upper Esophagus to Cutaneous, Via Natural or Artificial Opening Endoscopic

0D118Z6   Bypass Upper Esophagus to Stomach, Via Natural or Artificial Opening Endoscopic

0D118Z9   Bypass Upper Esophagus to Duodenum, Via Natural or Artificial Opening Endoscopic

0D118ZA   Bypass Upper Esophagus to Jejunum, Via Natural or Artificial Opening Endoscopic

0D118ZB   Bypass Upper Esophagus to Ileum, Via Natural or Artificial Opening Endoscopic

0D12074   Bypass Middle Esophagus to Cutaneous with Autologous Tissue Substitute, Open Approach

0D12076   Bypass Middle Esophagus to Stomach with Autologous Tissue Substitute, Open Approach

0D12079   Bypass Middle Esophagus to Duodenum with Autologous Tissue Substitute, Open Approach

0D1207A   Bypass Middle Esophagus to Jejunum with Autologous Tissue Substitute, Open Approach

0D1207B   Bypass Middle Esophagus to Ileum with Autologous Tissue Substitute, Open Approach

0D120J4   Bypass Middle Esophagus to Cutaneous with Synthetic Substitute, Open Approach

0D120J6   Bypass Middle Esophagus to Stomach with Synthetic Substitute, Open Approach

0D120J9   Bypass Middle Esophagus to Duodenum with Synthetic Substitute, Open Approach

0D120JA   Bypass Middle Esophagus to Jejunum with Synthetic Substitute, Open Approach

0D120JB   Bypass Middle Esophagus to Ileum with Synthetic Substitute, Open Approach

0D120K4   Bypass Middle Esophagus to Cutaneous with Nonautologous Tissue Substitute, Open Approach

0D120K6   Bypass Middle Esophagus to Stomach with Nonautologous Tissue Substitute, Open Approach

0D120K9   Bypass Middle Esophagus to Duodenum with Nonautologous Tissue Substitute, Open Approach

0D120KA   Bypass Middle Esophagus to Jejunum with Nonautologous Tissue Substitute, Open Approach

0D120KB   Bypass Middle Esophagus to Ileum with Nonautologous Tissue Substitute, Open Approach

0D120Z4   Bypass Middle Esophagus to Cutaneous, Open Approach

0D120Z6   Bypass Middle Esophagus to Stomach, Open Approach

0D120Z9   Bypass Middle Esophagus to Duodenum, Open Approach

0D120ZA   Bypass Middle Esophagus to Jejunum, Open Approach

0D120ZB   Bypass Middle Esophagus to Ileum, Open Approach

0D123J4   Bypass Middle Esophagus to Cutaneous with Synthetic Substitute, Percutaneous Approach

0D12474   Bypass Middle Esophagus to Cutaneous with Autologous Tissue Substitute, Percutaneous Endoscopic Approach

0D12476   Bypass Middle Esophagus to Stomach with Autologous Tissue Substitute, Percutaneous Endoscopic Approach

0D12479   Bypass Middle Esophagus to Duodenum with Autologous Tissue Substitute, Percutaneous Endoscopic Approach

0D1247A   Bypass Middle Esophagus to Jejunum with Autologous Tissue Substitute, Percutaneous Endoscopic Approach

0D1247B   Bypass Middle Esophagus to Ileum with Autologous Tissue Substitute, Percutaneous Endoscopic Approach

0D124J4   Bypass Middle Esophagus to Cutaneous with Synthetic Substitute, Percutaneous Endoscopic Approach

0D124J6   Bypass Middle Esophagus to Stomach with Synthetic Substitute, Percutaneous Endoscopic Approach

0D124J9   Bypass Middle Esophagus to Duodenum with Synthetic Substitute, Percutaneous Endoscopic Approach

0D124JA   Bypass Middle Esophagus to Jejunum with Synthetic Substitute, Percutaneous Endoscopic Approach

0D124JB   Bypass Middle Esophagus to Ileum with Synthetic Substitute, Percutaneous Endoscopic Approach

0D124K4   Bypass Middle Esophagus to Cutaneous with Nonautologous Tissue Substitute, Percutaneous Endoscopic Approach

0D124K6   Bypass Middle Esophagus to Stomach with Nonautologous Tissue Substitute, Percutaneous Endoscopic Approach

0D124K9   Bypass Middle Esophagus to Duodenum with Nonautologous Tissue Substitute, Percutaneous Endoscopic Approach

0D124KA   Bypass Middle Esophagus to Jejunum with Nonautologous Tissue Substitute, Percutaneous Endoscopic Approach

0D124KB   Bypass Middle Esophagus to Ileum with Nonautologous Tissue Substitute, Percutaneous Endoscopic Approach

0D124Z4   Bypass Middle Esophagus to Cutaneous, Percutaneous Endoscopic Approach

0D124Z6   Bypass Middle Esophagus to Stomach, Percutaneous Endoscopic Approach

0D124Z9   Bypass Middle Esophagus to Duodenum, Percutaneous Endoscopic Approach

0D124ZA   Bypass Middle Esophagus to Jejunum, Percutaneous Endoscopic Approach

0D124ZB   Bypass Middle Esophagus to Ileum, Percutaneous Endoscopic Approach

0D12874   Bypass Middle Esophagus to Cutaneous with Autologous Tissue Substitute, Via Natural or Artificial Opening Endoscopic

0D12876   Bypass Middle Esophagus to Stomach with Autologous Tissue Substitute, Via Natural or Artificial Opening Endoscopic

0D12879   Bypass Middle Esophagus to Duodenum with Autologous Tissue Substitute, Via Natural or Artificial Opening Endoscopic

0D1287A   Bypass Middle Esophagus to Jejunum with Autologous Tissue Substitute, Via Natural or Artificial Opening Endoscopic

0D1287B   Bypass Middle Esophagus to Ileum with Autologous Tissue Substitute, Via Natural or Artificial Opening Endoscopic

0D128J4   Bypass Middle Esophagus to Cutaneous with Synthetic Substitute, Via Natural or Artificial Opening Endoscopic

0D128J6   Bypass Middle Esophagus to Stomach with Synthetic Substitute, Via Natural or Artificial Opening Endoscopic

0D128J9   Bypass Middle Esophagus to Duodenum with Synthetic Substitute, Via Natural or Artificial Opening Endoscopic

0D128JA   Bypass Middle Esophagus to Jejunum with Synthetic Substitute, Via Natural or Artificial Opening Endoscopic

0D128JB   Bypass Middle Esophagus to Ileum with Synthetic Substitute, Via Natural or Artificial Opening Endoscopic

0D128K4   Bypass Middle Esophagus to Cutaneous with Nonautologous Tissue Substitute, Via Natural or Artificial Opening Endoscopic

0D128K6   Bypass Middle Esophagus to Stomach with Nonautologous Tissue Substitute, Via Natural or Artificial Opening Endoscopic

0D128K9   Bypass Middle Esophagus to Duodenum with Nonautologous Tissue Substitute, Via Natural or Artificial Opening Endoscopic

0D128KA   Bypass Middle Esophagus to Jejunum with Nonautologous Tissue Substitute, Via Natural or Artificial Opening Endoscopic

0D128KB   Bypass Middle Esophagus to Ileum with Nonautologous Tissue Substitute, Via Natural or Artificial Opening Endoscopic

0D128Z4   Bypass Middle Esophagus to Cutaneous, Via Natural or Artificial Opening Endoscopic

0D128Z6   Bypass Middle Esophagus to Stomach, Via Natural or Artificial Opening Endoscopic

0D128Z9   Bypass Middle Esophagus to Duodenum, Via Natural or Artificial Opening Endoscopic

0D128ZA   Bypass Middle Esophagus to Jejunum, Via Natural or Artificial Opening Endoscopic

0D128ZB   Bypass Middle Esophagus to Ileum, Via Natural or Artificial Opening Endoscopic

0D13074   Bypass Lower Esophagus to Cutaneous with Autologous Tissue Substitute, Open Approach

0D13076   Bypass Lower Esophagus to Stomach with Autologous Tissue Substitute, Open Approach

0D13079   Bypass Lower Esophagus to Duodenum with Autologous Tissue Substitute, Open Approach

0D1307A   Bypass Lower Esophagus to Jejunum with Autologous Tissue Substitute, Open Approach

0D1307B   Bypass Lower Esophagus to Ileum with Autologous Tissue Substitute, Open Approach

0D130J4   Bypass Lower Esophagus to Cutaneous with Synthetic Substitute, Open Approach

0D130J6   Bypass Lower Esophagus to Stomach with Synthetic Substitute, Open Approach

0D130J9   Bypass Lower Esophagus to Duodenum with Synthetic Substitute, Open Approach

0D130JA   Bypass Lower Esophagus to Jejunum with Synthetic Substitute, Open Approach

0D130JB   Bypass Lower Esophagus to Ileum with Synthetic Substitute, Open Approach

0D130K4   Bypass Lower Esophagus to Cutaneous with Nonautologous Tissue Substitute, Open Approach

0D130K6   Bypass Lower Esophagus to Stomach with Nonautologous Tissue Substitute, Open Approach

0D130K9   Bypass Lower Esophagus to Duodenum with Nonautologous Tissue Substitute, Open Approach

0D130KA   Bypass Lower Esophagus to Jejunum with Nonautologous Tissue Substitute, Open Approach

0D130KB   Bypass Lower Esophagus to Ileum with Nonautologous Tissue Substitute, Open Approach

0D130Z4   Bypass Lower Esophagus to Cutaneous, Open Approach

0D130Z6   Bypass Lower Esophagus to Stomach, Open Approach

0D130Z9   Bypass Lower Esophagus to Duodenum, Open Approach

0D130ZA   Bypass Lower Esophagus to Jejunum, Open Approach

0D130ZB   Bypass Lower Esophagus to Ileum, Open Approach

0D133J4   Bypass Lower Esophagus to Cutaneous with Synthetic Substitute, Percutaneous Approach

0D13474   Bypass Lower Esophagus to Cutaneous with Autologous Tissue Substitute, Percutaneous Endoscopic Approach

0D13476   Bypass Lower Esophagus to Stomach with Autologous Tissue Substitute, Percutaneous Endoscopic Approach

0D13479   Bypass Lower Esophagus to Duodenum with Autologous Tissue Substitute, Percutaneous Endoscopic Approach

0D1347A   Bypass Lower Esophagus to Jejunum with Autologous Tissue Substitute, Percutaneous Endoscopic Approach

0D1347B   Bypass Lower Esophagus to Ileum with Autologous Tissue Substitute, Percutaneous Endoscopic Approach

0D134J4   Bypass Lower Esophagus to Cutaneous with Synthetic Substitute, Percutaneous Endoscopic Approach

0D134J6   Bypass Lower Esophagus to Stomach with Synthetic Substitute, Percutaneous Endoscopic Approach

0D134J9   Bypass Lower Esophagus to Duodenum with Synthetic Substitute, Percutaneous Endoscopic Approach

0D134JA   Bypass Lower Esophagus to Jejunum with Synthetic Substitute, Percutaneous Endoscopic Approach

0D134JB   Bypass Lower Esophagus to Ileum with Synthetic Substitute, Percutaneous Endoscopic Approach

0D134K4   Bypass Lower Esophagus to Cutaneous with Nonautologous Tissue Substitute, Percutaneous Endoscopic Approach

0D134K6   Bypass Lower Esophagus to Stomach with Nonautologous Tissue Substitute, Percutaneous Endoscopic Approach

0D134K9   Bypass Lower Esophagus to Duodenum with Nonautologous Tissue Substitute, Percutaneous Endoscopic Approach

0D134KA   Bypass Lower Esophagus to Jejunum with Nonautologous Tissue Substitute, Percutaneous Endoscopic Approach

0D134KB Bypass Lower Esophagus to Ileum with Nonautologous Tissue Substitute, Percutaneous Endoscopic Approach

0D134Z4 Bypass Lower Esophagus to Cutaneous, Percutaneous Endoscopic Approach

0D134Z6 Bypass Lower Esophagus to Stomach, Percutaneous Endoscopic Approach

0D134Z9 Bypass Lower Esophagus to Duodenum, Percutaneous Endoscopic Approach

0D134ZA Bypass Lower Esophagus to Jejunum, Percutaneous Endoscopic Approach

0D134ZB Bypass Lower Esophagus to Ileum, Percutaneous Endoscopic Approach

0D13874 Bypass Lower Esophagus to Cutaneous with Autologous Tissue Substitute, Via Natural or Artificial Opening Endoscopic

0D13876 Bypass Lower Esophagus to Stomach with Autologous Tissue Substitute, Via Natural or Artificial Opening Endoscopic

0D13879 Bypass Lower Esophagus to Duodenum with Autologous Tissue Substitute, Via Natural or Artificial Opening Endoscopic

0D1387A Bypass Lower Esophagus to Jejunum with Autologous Tissue Substitute, Via Natural or Artificial Opening Endoscopic

0D1387B Bypass Lower Esophagus to Ileum with Autologous Tissue Substitute, Via Natural or Artificial Opening Endoscopic

0D138J4 Bypass Lower Esophagus to Cutaneous with Synthetic Substitute, Via Natural or Artificial Opening Endoscopic

0D138J6 Bypass Lower Esophagus to Stomach with Synthetic Substitute, Via Natural or Artificial Opening Endoscopic

0D138J9 Bypass Lower Esophagus to Duodenum with Synthetic Substitute, Via Natural or Artificial Opening Endoscopic

0D138JA Bypass Lower Esophagus to Jejunum with Synthetic Substitute, Via Natural or Artificial Opening Endoscopic

0D138JB Bypass Lower Esophagus to Ileum with Synthetic Substitute, Via Natural or Artificial Opening Endoscopic

0D138K4 Bypass Lower Esophagus to Cutaneous with Nonautologous Tissue Substitute, Via Natural or Artificial Opening Endoscopic

0D138K6 Bypass Lower Esophagus to Stomach with Nonautologous Tissue Substitute, Via Natural or Artificial Opening Endoscopic

0D138K9 Bypass Lower Esophagus to Duodenum with Nonautologous Tissue Substitute, Via Natural or Artificial Opening Endoscopic

0D138KA Bypass Lower Esophagus to Jejunum with Nonautologous Tissue Substitute, Via Natural or Artificial Opening Endoscopic

0D138KB Bypass Lower Esophagus to Ileum with Nonautologous Tissue Substitute, Via Natural or Artificial Opening Endoscopic

0D138Z4 Bypass Lower Esophagus to Cutaneous, Via Natural or Artificial Opening Endoscopic

0D138Z6 Bypass Lower Esophagus to Stomach, Via Natural or Artificial Opening Endoscopic

0D138Z9 Bypass Lower Esophagus to Duodenum, Via Natural or Artificial Opening Endoscopic

0D138ZA Bypass Lower Esophagus to Jejunum, Via Natural or Artificial Opening Endoscopic

0D138ZB Bypass Lower Esophagus to Ileum, Via Natural or Artificial Opening Endoscopic

0D15074 Bypass Esophagus to Cutaneous with Autologous Tissue Substitute, Open Approach

0D15076 Bypass Esophagus to Stomach with Autologous Tissue Substitute, Open Approach

0D15079 Bypass Esophagus to Duodenum with Autologous Tissue Substitute, Open Approach

0D1507A Bypass Esophagus to Jejunum with Autologous Tissue Substitute, Open Approach

0D1507B Bypass Esophagus to Ileum with Autologous Tissue Substitute, Open Approach

0D150J4 Bypass Esophagus to Cutaneous with Synthetic Substitute, Open Approach

0D150J6 Bypass Esophagus to Stomach with Synthetic Substitute, Open Approach

0D150J9 Bypass Esophagus to Duodenum with Synthetic Substitute, Open Approach

0D150JA Bypass Esophagus to Jejunum with Synthetic Substitute, Open Approach

0D150JB Bypass Esophagus to Ileum with Synthetic Substitute, Open Approach

0D150K4 Bypass Esophagus to Cutaneous with Nonautologous Tissue Substitute, Open Approach

0D150K6 Bypass Esophagus to Stomach with Nonautologous Tissue Substitute, Open Approach

0D150K9 Bypass Esophagus to Duodenum with Nonautologous Tissue Substitute, Open Approach

0D150KA Bypass Esophagus to Jejunum with Nonautologous Tissue Substitute, Open Approach

0D150KB Bypass Esophagus to Ileum with Nonautologous Tissue Substitute, Open Approach

0D150Z4 Bypass Esophagus to Cutaneous, Open Approach

0D150Z6 Bypass Esophagus to Stomach, Open Approach

0D150Z9 Bypass Esophagus to Duodenum, Open Approach

0D150ZA Bypass Esophagus to Jejunum, Open Approach

0D150ZB Bypass Esophagus to Ileum, Open Approach

0D153J4 Bypass Esophagus to Cutaneous with Synthetic Substitute, Percutaneous Approach

0D15474 Bypass Esophagus to Cutaneous with Autologous Tissue Substitute, Percutaneous Endoscopic Approach

0D15476 Bypass Esophagus to Stomach with Autologous Tissue Substitute, Percutaneous Endoscopic Approach

0D15479 Bypass Esophagus to Duodenum with Autologous Tissue Substitute, Percutaneous Endoscopic Approach

0D1547A Bypass Esophagus to Jejunum with Autologous Tissue Substitute, Percutaneous Endoscopic Approach

0D1547B Bypass Esophagus to Ileum with Autologous Tissue Substitute, Percutaneous Endoscopic Approach

0D154J4 Bypass Esophagus to Cutaneous with Synthetic Substitute, Percutaneous Endoscopic Approach

0D154J6 Bypass Esophagus to Stomach with Synthetic Substitute, Percutaneous Endoscopic Approach

0D154J9 Bypass Esophagus to Duodenum with Synthetic Substitute, Percutaneous Endoscopic Approach

0D154JA Bypass Esophagus to Jejunum with Synthetic Substitute, Percutaneous Endoscopic Approach

0D154JB Bypass Esophagus to Ileum with Synthetic Substitute, Percutaneous Endoscopic Approach

0D154K4 Bypass Esophagus to Cutaneous with Nonautologous Tissue Substitute, Percutaneous Endoscopic Approach

0D154K6 Bypass Esophagus to Stomach with Nonautologous Tissue Substitute, Percutaneous Endoscopic Approach

0D154K9 Bypass Esophagus to Duodenum with Nonautologous Tissue Substitute, Percutaneous Endoscopic Approach

0D154KA Bypass Esophagus to Jejunum with Nonautologous Tissue Substitute, Percutaneous Endoscopic Approach

0D154KB Bypass Esophagus to Ileum with Nonautologous Tissue Substitute, Percutaneous Endoscopic Approach

0D154Z4 Bypass Esophagus to Cutaneous, Percutaneous Endoscopic Approach

0D154Z6 Bypass Esophagus to Stomach, Percutaneous Endoscopic Approach

0D154Z9 Bypass Esophagus to Duodenum, Percutaneous Endoscopic Approach

0D154ZA Bypass Esophagus to Jejunum, Percutaneous Endoscopic Approach

0D154ZB Bypass Esophagus to Ileum, Percutaneous Endoscopic Approach

0D15874 Bypass Esophagus to Cutaneous with Autologous Tissue Substitute, Via Natural or Artificial Opening Endoscopic

0D15876 Bypass Esophagus to Stomach with Autologous Tissue Substitute, Via Natural or Artificial Opening Endoscopic

0D15879 Bypass Esophagus to Duodenum with Autologous Tissue Substitute, Via Natural or Artificial Opening Endoscopic

0D1587A Bypass Esophagus to Jejunum with Autologous Tissue Substitute, Via Natural or Artificial Opening Endoscopic

0D1587B Bypass Esophagus to Ileum with Autologous Tissue Substitute, Via Natural or Artificial Opening Endoscopic

0D158J4 Bypass Esophagus to Cutaneous with Synthetic Substitute, Via Natural or Artificial Opening Endoscopic

0D158J6 Bypass Esophagus to Stomach with Synthetic Substitute, Via Natural or Artificial Opening Endoscopic

0D158J9 Bypass Esophagus to Duodenum with Synthetic Substitute, Via Natural or Artificial Opening Endoscopic

0D158JA   Bypass Esophagus to Jejunum with Synthetic Substitute, Via Natural or Artificial Opening Endoscopic

0D158JB   Bypass Esophagus to Ileum with Synthetic Substitute, Via Natural or Artificial Opening Endoscopic

0D158K4   Bypass Esophagus to Cutaneous with Nonautologous Tissue Substitute, Via Natural or Artificial Opening Endoscopic

0D158K6   Bypass Esophagus to Stomach with Nonautologous Tissue Substitute, Via Natural or Artificial Opening Endoscopic

0D158K9   Bypass Esophagus to Duodenum with Nonautologous Tissue Substitute, Via Natural or Artificial Opening Endoscopic

0D158KA   Bypass Esophagus to Jejunum with Nonautologous Tissue Substitute, Via Natural or Artificial Opening Endoscopic

0D158KB   Bypass Esophagus to Ileum with Nonautologous Tissue Substitute, Via Natural or Artificial Opening Endoscopic

0D158Z4   Bypass Esophagus to Cutaneous, Via Natural or Artificial Opening Endoscopic

0D158Z6   Bypass Esophagus to Stomach, Via Natural or Artificial Opening Endoscopic

0D158Z9   Bypass Esophagus to Duodenum, Via Natural or Artificial Opening Endoscopic

0D158ZA   Bypass Esophagus to Jejunum, Via Natural or Artificial Opening Endoscopic

0D158ZB   Bypass Esophagus to Ileum, Via Natural or Artificial Opening Endoscopic

0D16074   Bypass Stomach to Cutaneous with Autologous Tissue Substitute, Open Approach

0D16079   Bypass Stomach to Duodenum with Autologous Tissue Substitute, Open Approach

HAC   When reported with principal diagnosis code K66.01 and secondary diagnosis code K68.11, K95.01, K95.81 or T81.4XXA

0D1607A   Bypass Stomach to Jejunum with Autologous Tissue Substitute, Open Approach

0D1607B   Bypass Stomach to Ileum with Autologous Tissue Substitute, Open Approach

HAC   When reported with principal diagnosis code K66.01 and secondary diagnosis code K68.11, K95.01, K95.81 or T81.4XXA

0D1607L   Bypass Stomach to Transverse Colon with Autologous Tissue Substitute, Open Approach

HAC   When reported with principal diagnosis code K66.01 and secondary diagnosis code K68.11, K95.01, K95.81 or T81.4XXA

0D160J4   Bypass Stomach to Cutaneous with Synthetic Substitute, Open Approach

0D160J9   Bypass Stomach to Duodenum with Synthetic Substitute, Open Approach

HAC   When reported with principal diagnosis code K66.01 and secondary diagnosis code K68.11, K95.01, K95.81 or T81.4XXA

0D160JA   Bypass Stomach to Jejunum with Synthetic Substitute, Open Approach

HAC   When reported with principal diagnosis code K66.01 and secondary diagnosis code K68.11, K95.01, K95.81 or T81.4XXA

0D160JB   Bypass Stomach to Ileum with Synthetic Substitute, Open Approach

HAC   When reported with principal diagnosis code K66.01 and secondary diagnosis code K68.11, K95.01, K95.81 or T81.4XXA

0D160JL   Bypass Stomach to Transverse Colon with Synthetic Substitute, Open Approach

HAC   When reported with principal diagnosis code K66.01 and secondary diagnosis code K68.11, K95.01, K95.81 or T81.4XXA

0D160K4   Bypass Stomach to Cutaneous with Nonautologous Tissue Substitute, Open Approach

0D160K9   Bypass Stomach to Duodenum with Nonautologous Tissue Substitute, Open Approach

HAC   When reported with principal diagnosis code K66.01 and secondary diagnosis code K68.11, K95.01, K95.81 or T81.4XXA

0D160KA   Bypass Stomach to Jejunum with Nonautologous Tissue Substitute, Open Approach

HAC   When reported with principal diagnosis code K66.01 and secondary diagnosis code K68.11, K95.01, K95.81 or T81.4XXA

0D160KB   Bypass Stomach to Ileum with Nonautologous Tissue Substitute, Open Approach

HAC   When reported with principal diagnosis code K66.01 and secondary diagnosis code K68.11, K95.01, K95.81 or T81.4XXA

0D160KL   Bypass Stomach to Transverse Colon with Nonautologous Tissue Substitute, Open Approach

HAC   When reported with principal diagnosis code K66.01 and secondary diagnosis code K68.11, K95.01, K95.81 or T81.4XXA

0D160Z4   Bypass Stomach to Cutaneous, Open Approach

0D160Z9   Bypass Stomach to Duodenum, Open Approach

HAC   When reported with principal diagnosis code K66.01 and secondary diagnosis code K68.11, K95.01, K95.81 or T81.4XXA

0D160ZA   Bypass Stomach to Jejunum, Open Approach

HAC   When reported with principal diagnosis code K66.01 and secondary diagnosis code K68.11, K95.01, K95.81 or T81.4XXA

0D160ZB   Bypass Stomach to Ileum, Open Approach

HAC   When reported with principal diagnosis code K66.01 and secondary diagnosis code K68.11, K95.01, K95.81 or T81.4XXA

0D160ZL   Bypass Stomach to Transverse Colon, Open Approach

HAC   When reported with principal diagnosis code K66.01 and secondary diagnosis code K68.11, K95.01, K95.81 or T81.4XXA

0D163J4   Bypass Stomach to Cutaneous with Synthetic Substitute, Percutaneous Approach

0D16474   Bypass Stomach to Cutaneous with Autologous Tissue Substitute, Percutaneous Endoscopic Approach

0D16479   Bypass Stomach to Duodenum with Autologous Tissue Substitute, Percutaneous Endoscopic Approach

HAC   When reported with principal diagnosis code K66.01 and secondary diagnosis code K68.11, K95.01, K95.81 or T81.4XXA

0D1647A   Bypass Stomach to Jejunum with Autologous Tissue Substitute, Percutaneous Endoscopic Approach

HAC   When reported with principal diagnosis code K66.01 and secondary diagnosis code K68.11, K95.01, K95.81 or T81.4XXA

0D1647B   Bypass Stomach to Ileum with Autologous Tissue Substitute, Percutaneous Endoscopic Approach

HAC   When reported with principal diagnosis code K66.01 and secondary diagnosis code K68.11, K95.01, K95.81 or T81.4XXA

0D1647L   Bypass Stomach to Transverse Colon with Autologous Tissue Substitute, Percutaneous Endoscopic Approach

HAC   When reported with principal diagnosis code K66.01 and secondary diagnosis code K68.11, K95.01, K95.81 or T81.4XXA

0D164J4   Bypass Stomach to Cutaneous with Synthetic Substitute, Percutaneous Endoscopic Approach

0D164J9   Bypass Stomach to Duodenum with Synthetic Substitute, Percutaneous Endoscopic Approach

HAC   When reported with principal diagnosis code K66.01 and secondary diagnosis code K68.11, K95.01, K95.81 or T81.4XXA

0D164JA   Bypass Stomach to Jejunum with Synthetic Substitute, Percutaneous Endoscopic Approach

HAC   When reported with principal diagnosis code K66.01 and secondary diagnosis code K68.11, K95.01, K95.81 or T81.4XXA

0D164JB   Bypass Stomach to Ileum with Synthetic Substitute, Percutaneous Endoscopic Approach

HAC   When reported with principal diagnosis code K66.01 and secondary diagnosis code K68.11, K95.01, K95.81 or T81.4XXA

0D164JL   Bypass Stomach to Transverse Colon with Synthetic Substitute, Percutaneous Endoscopic Approach

HAC   When reported with principal diagnosis code K66.01 and secondary diagnosis code K68.11, K95.01, K95.81 or T81.4XXA

0D164K4   Bypass Stomach to Cutaneous with Nonautologous Tissue Substitute, Percutaneous Endoscopic Approach

0D164K9   Bypass Stomach to Duodenum with Nonautologous Tissue Substitute, Percutaneous Endoscopic Approach

HAC   When reported with principal diagnosis code K66.01 and secondary diagnosis code K68.11, K95.01, K95.81 or T81.4XXA

0D164KA   Bypass Stomach to Jejunum with Nonautologous Tissue Substitute, Percutaneous Endoscopic Approach

HAC   When reported with principal diagnosis code K66.01 and secondary diagnosis code K68.11, K95.01, K95.81 or T81.4XXA

0D164KB   Bypass Stomach to Ileum with Nonautologous Tissue Substitute, Percutaneous Endoscopic Approach

HAC   When reported with principal diagnosis code K66.01 and secondary diagnosis code K68.11, K95.01, K95.81 or T81.4XXA

0D164KL   Bypass Stomach to Transverse Colon with Nonautologous Tissue Substitute, Percutaneous Endoscopic Approach

HAC   When reported with principal diagnosis code K66.01 and secondary diagnosis code K68.11, K95.01, K95.81 or T81.4XXA

0D164Z4   Bypass Stomach to Cutaneous, Percutaneous Endoscopic Approach

0D164Z9   Bypass Stomach to Duodenum, Percutaneous Endoscopic Approach

HAC   When reported with principal diagnosis code K66.01 and secondary diagnosis code K68.11, K95.01, K95.81 or T81.4XXA

0D164ZA   Bypass Stomach to Jejunum, Percutaneous Endoscopic Approach

HAC   When reported with principal diagnosis code K66.01 and secondary diagnosis code K68.11, K95.01, K95.81 or T81.4XXA

0D164ZB   Bypass Stomach to Ileum, Percutaneous Endoscopic Approach

HAC   When reported with principal diagnosis code K66.01 and secondary diagnosis code K68.11, K95.01, K95.81 or T81.4XXA

0D164ZL   Bypass Stomach to Transverse Colon, Percutaneous Endoscopic Approach

0D16874   Bypass Stomach to Cutaneous with Autologous Tissue Substitute, Via Natural or Artificial Opening Endoscopic

0D16879   Bypass Stomach to Duodenum with Autologous Tissue Substitute, Via Natural or Artificial Opening Endoscopic

HAC   When reported with principal diagnosis code K66.01 and secondary diagnosis code K68.11, K95.01, K95.81 or T81.4XXA

0D1687A   Bypass Stomach to Jejunum with Autologous Tissue Substitute, Via Natural or Artificial Opening Endoscopic

HAC   When reported with principal diagnosis code K66.01 and secondary diagnosis code K68.11, K95.01, K95.81 or T81.4XXA

0D1687B   Bypass Stomach to Ileum with Autologous Tissue Substitute, Via Natural or Artificial Opening Endoscopic

HAC   When reported with principal diagnosis code K66.01 and secondary diagnosis code K68.11, K95.01, K95.81 or T81.4XXA

0D1687L   Bypass Stomach to Transverse Colon with Autologous Tissue Substitute, Via Natural or Artificial Opening Endoscopic

HAC   When reported with principal diagnosis code K66.01 and secondary diagnosis code K68.11, K95.01, K95.81 or T81.4XXA

0D168J4   Bypass Stomach to Cutaneous with Synthetic Substitute, Via Natural or Artificial Opening Endoscopic

0D168J9   Bypass Stomach to Duodenum with Synthetic Substitute, Via Natural or Artificial Opening Endoscopic

HAC   When reported with principal diagnosis code K66.01 and secondary diagnosis code K68.11, K95.01, K95.81 or T81.4XXA

0D168JA   Bypass Stomach to Jejunum with Synthetic Substitute, Via Natural or Artificial Opening Endoscopic

HAC   When reported with principal diagnosis code K66.01 and secondary diagnosis code K68.11, K95.01, K95.81 or T81.4XXA

0D168JB   Bypass Stomach to Ileum with Synthetic Substitute, Via Natural or Artificial Opening Endoscopic

HAC   When reported with principal diagnosis code K66.01 and secondary diagnosis code K68.11, K95.01, K95.81 or T81.4XXA

0D168JL   Bypass Stomach to Transverse Colon with Synthetic Substitute, Via Natural or Artificial Opening Endoscopic

HAC   When reported with principal diagnosis code K66.01 and secondary diagnosis code K68.11, K95.01, K95.81 or T81.4XXA

0D168K4   Bypass Stomach to Cutaneous with Nonautologous Tissue Substitute, Via Natural or Artificial Opening Endoscopic

0D168K9   Bypass Stomach to Duodenum with Nonautologous Tissue Substitute, Via Natural or Artificial Opening Endoscopic

HAC   When reported with principal diagnosis code K66.01 and secondary diagnosis code K68.11, K95.01, K95.81 or T81.4XXA

0D168KA   Bypass Stomach to Jejunum with Nonautologous Tissue Substitute, Via Natural or Artificial Opening Endoscopic

HAC   When reported with principal diagnosis code K66.01 and secondary diagnosis code K68.11, K95.01, K95.81 or T81.4XXA

0D168KB   Bypass Stomach to Ileum with Nonautologous Tissue Substitute, Via Natural or Artificial Opening Endoscopic

0D168KL   Bypass Stomach to Transverse Colon with Nonautologous Tissue Substitute, Via Natural or Artificial Opening Endoscopic

HAC   When reported with principal diagnosis code K66.01 and secondary diagnosis code K68.11, K95.01, K95.81 or T81.4XXA

0D168Z4   Bypass Stomach to Cutaneous, Via Natural or Artificial Opening Endoscopic

0D168Z9   Bypass Stomach to Duodenum, Via Natural or Artificial Opening Endoscopic

HAC   When reported with principal diagnosis code K66.01 and secondary diagnosis code K68.11, K95.01, K95.81 or T81.4XXA

0D168ZA   Bypass Stomach to Jejunum, Via Natural or Artificial Opening Endoscopic

HAC   When reported with principal diagnosis code K66.01 and secondary diagnosis code K68.11, K95.01, K95.81 or T81.4XXA

0D168ZB   Bypass Stomach to Ileum, Via Natural or Artificial Opening Endoscopic

HAC   When reported with principal diagnosis code K66.01 and secondary diagnosis code K68.11, K95.01, K95.81 or T81.4XXA

0D168ZL   Bypass Stomach to Transverse Colon, Via Natural or Artificial Opening Endoscopic

HAC   When reported with principal diagnosis code K66.01 and secondary diagnosis code K68.11, K95.01, K95.81 or T81.4XXA

0D19074   Bypass Duodenum to Cutaneous with Autologous Tissue Substitute, Open Approach

0D19079   Bypass Duodenum to Duodenum with Autologous Tissue Substitute, Open Approach

0D1907A   Bypass Duodenum to Jejunum with Autologous Tissue Substitute, Open Approach

0D1907B   Bypass Duodenum to Ileum with Autologous Tissue Substitute, Open Approach

0D1907L   Bypass Duodenum to Transverse Colon with Autologous Tissue Substitute, Open Approach

0D190J4   Bypass Duodenum to Cutaneous with Synthetic Substitute, Open Approach

0D190J9   Bypass Duodenum to Duodenum with Synthetic Substitute, Open Approach

0D190JA   Bypass Duodenum to Jejunum with Synthetic Substitute, Open Approach

0D190JB   Bypass Duodenum to Ileum with Synthetic Substitute, Open Approach

0D190JL   Bypass Duodenum to Transverse Colon with Synthetic Substitute, Open Approach

0D190K4   Bypass Duodenum to Cutaneous with Nonautologous Tissue Substitute, Open Approach

0D190K9   Bypass Duodenum to Duodenum with Nonautologous Tissue Substitute, Open Approach

0D190KA   Bypass Duodenum to Jejunum with Nonautologous Tissue Substitute, Open Approach

0D190KB   Bypass Duodenum to Ileum with Nonautologous Tissue Substitute, Open Approach

0D190KL   Bypass Duodenum to Transverse Colon with Nonautologous Tissue Substitute, Open Approach

0D190Z4   Bypass Duodenum to Cutaneous, Open Approach

0D190Z9   Bypass Duodenum to Duodenum, Open Approach

0D190ZA   Bypass Duodenum to Jejunum, Open Approach

0D190ZB   Bypass Duodenum to Ileum, Open Approach

0D190ZL   Bypass Duodenum to Transverse Colon, Open Approach

0D193J4   Bypass Duodenum to Cutaneous with Synthetic Substitute, Percutaneous Approach

0D19474   Bypass Duodenum to Cutaneous with Autologous Tissue Substitute, Percutaneous Endoscopic Approach

0D19479   Bypass Duodenum to Duodenum with Autologous Tissue Substitute, Percutaneous Endoscopic Approach

0D1947A   Bypass Duodenum to Jejunum with Autologous Tissue Substitute, Percutaneous Endoscopic Approach

0D1947B   Bypass Duodenum to Ileum with Autologous Tissue Substitute, Percutaneous Endoscopic Approach

0D1947L   Bypass Duodenum to Transverse Colon with Autologous Tissue Substitute, Percutaneous Endoscopic Approach

0D194J4   Bypass Duodenum to Cutaneous with Synthetic Substitute, Percutaneous Endoscopic Approach

0D194J9   Bypass Duodenum to Duodenum with Synthetic Substitute, Percutaneous Endoscopic Approach

0D194JA   Bypass Duodenum to Jejunum with Synthetic Substitute, Percutaneous Endoscopic Approach

0D194JB   Bypass Duodenum to Ileum with Synthetic Substitute, Percutaneous Endoscopic Approach

0D194JL   Bypass Duodenum to Transverse Colon with Synthetic Substitute, Percutaneous Endoscopic Approach

0D194K4   Bypass Duodenum to Cutaneous with Nonautologous Tissue Substitute, Percutaneous Endoscopic Approach

0D194K9   Bypass Duodenum to Duodenum with Nonautologous Tissue Substitute, Percutaneous Endoscopic Approach

0D194KA Bypass Duodenum to Jejunum with Nonautologous Tissue Substitute, Percutaneous Endoscopic Approach

0D194KB Bypass Duodenum to Ileum with Nonautologous Tissue Substitute, Percutaneous Endoscopic Approach

0D194KL Bypass Duodenum to Transverse Colon with Nonautologous Tissue Substitute, Percutaneous Endoscopic Approach

0D194Z4 Bypass Duodenum to Cutaneous, Percutaneous Endoscopic Approach

0D194Z9 Bypass Duodenum to Duodenum, Percutaneous Endoscopic Approach

0D194ZA Bypass Duodenum to Jejunum, Percutaneous Endoscopic Approach

0D194ZB Bypass Duodenum to Ileum, Percutaneous Endoscopic Approach

0D194ZL Bypass Duodenum to Transverse Colon, Percutaneous Endoscopic Approach

0D19874 Bypass Duodenum to Cutaneous with Autologous Tissue Substitute, Via Natural or Artificial Opening Endoscopic

0D19879 Bypass Duodenum to Duodenum with Autologous Tissue Substitute, Via Natural or Artificial Opening Endoscopic

0D1987A Bypass Duodenum to Jejunum with Autologous Tissue Substitute, Via Natural or Artificial Opening Endoscopic

0D1987B Bypass Duodenum to Ileum with Autologous Tissue Substitute, Via Natural or Artificial Opening Endoscopic

0D1987L Bypass Duodenum to Transverse Colon with Autologous Tissue Substitute, Via Natural or Artificial Opening Endoscopic

0D198J4 Bypass Duodenum to Cutaneous with Synthetic Substitute, Via Natural or Artificial Opening Endoscopic

0D198J9 Bypass Duodenum to Duodenum with Synthetic Substitute, Via Natural or Artificial Opening Endoscopic

0D198JA Bypass Duodenum to Jejunum with Synthetic Substitute, Via Natural or Artificial Opening Endoscopic

0D198JB Bypass Duodenum to Ileum with Synthetic Substitute, Via Natural or Artificial Opening Endoscopic

0D198JL Bypass Duodenum to Transverse Colon with Synthetic Substitute, Via Natural or Artificial Opening Endoscopic

0D198K4 Bypass Duodenum to Cutaneous with Nonautologous Tissue Substitute, Via Natural or Artificial Opening Endoscopic

0D198K9 Bypass Duodenum to Duodenum with Nonautologous Tissue Substitute, Via Natural or Artificial Opening Endoscopic

0D198KA Bypass Duodenum to Jejunum with Nonautologous Tissue Substitute, Via Natural or Artificial Opening Endoscopic

0D198KB Bypass Duodenum to Ileum with Nonautologous Tissue Substitute, Via Natural or Artificial Opening Endoscopic

0D198KL Bypass Duodenum to Transverse Colon with Nonautologous Tissue Substitute, Via Natural or Artificial Opening Endoscopic

0D198Z4 Bypass Duodenum to Cutaneous, Via Natural or Artificial Opening Endoscopic

0D198Z9 Bypass Duodenum to Duodenum, Via Natural or Artificial Opening Endoscopic

0D198ZA Bypass Duodenum to Jejunum, Via Natural or Artificial Opening Endoscopic

0D198ZB Bypass Duodenum to Ileum, Via Natural or Artificial Opening Endoscopic

0D198ZL Bypass Duodenum to Transverse Colon, Via Natural or Artificial Opening Endoscopic

0D1A074 Bypass Jejunum to Cutaneous with Autologous Tissue Substitute, Open Approach

0D1A07A Bypass Jejunum to Jejunum with Autologous Tissue Substitute, Open Approach

0D1A07B Bypass Jejunum to Ileum with Autologous Tissue Substitute, Open Approach

0D1A07H Bypass Jejunum to Cecum with Autologous Tissue Substitute, Open Approach

0D1A07K Bypass Jejunum to Ascending Colon with Autologous Tissue Substitute, Open Approach

0D1A07L Bypass Jejunum to Transverse Colon with Autologous Tissue Substitute, Open Approach

0D1A07M Bypass Jejunum to Descending Colon with Autologous Tissue Substitute, Open Approach

0D1A07N Bypass Jejunum to Sigmoid Colon with Autologous Tissue Substitute, Open Approach

0D1A07P Bypass Jejunum to Rectum with Autologous Tissue Substitute, Open Approach

0D1A07Q Bypass Jejunum to Anus with Autologous Tissue Substitute, Open Approach

0D1A0J4 Bypass Jejunum to Cutaneous with Synthetic Substitute, Open Approach

0D1A0JA Bypass Jejunum to Jejunum with Synthetic Substitute, Open Approach

0D1A0JB Bypass Jejunum to Ileum with Synthetic Substitute, Open Approach

0D1A0JH Bypass Jejunum to Cecum with Synthetic Substitute, Open Approach

0D1A0JK Bypass Jejunum to Ascending Colon with Synthetic Substitute, Open Approach

0D1A0JL Bypass Jejunum to Transverse Colon with Synthetic Substitute, Open Approach

0D1A0JM Bypass Jejunum to Descending Colon with Synthetic Substitute, Open Approach

0D1A0JN Bypass Jejunum to Sigmoid Colon with Synthetic Substitute, Open Approach

0D1A0JP Bypass Jejunum to Rectum with Synthetic Substitute, Open Approach

0D1A0JQ Bypass Jejunum to Anus with Synthetic Substitute, Open Approach

0D1A0K4 Bypass Jejunum to Cutaneous with Nonautologous Tissue Substitute, Open Approach

0D1A0KA Bypass Jejunum to Jejunum with Nonautologous Tissue Substitute, Open Approach

0D1A0KB Bypass Jejunum to Ileum with Nonautologous Tissue Substitute, Open Approach

0D1A0KH Bypass Jejunum to Cecum with Nonautologous Tissue Substitute, Open Approach

0D1A0KK Bypass Jejunum to Ascending Colon with Nonautologous Tissue Substitute, Open Approach

0D1A0KL Bypass Jejunum to Transverse Colon with Nonautologous Tissue Substitute, Open Approach

0D1A0KM Bypass Jejunum to Descending Colon with Nonautologous Tissue Substitute, Open Approach

0D1A0KN Bypass Jejunum to Sigmoid Colon with Nonautologous Tissue Substitute, Open Approach

0D1A0KP Bypass Jejunum to Rectum with Nonautologous Tissue Substitute, Open Approach

0D1A0KQ Bypass Jejunum to Anus with Nonautologous Tissue Substitute, Open Approach

0D1A0Z4 Bypass Jejunum to Cutaneous, Open Approach

0D1A0ZA Bypass Jejunum to Jejunum, Open Approach

0D1A0ZB Bypass Jejunum to Ileum, Open Approach

0D1A0ZH Bypass Jejunum to Cecum, Open Approach

0D1A0ZK Bypass Jejunum to Ascending Colon, Open Approach

0D1A0ZL Bypass Jejunum to Transverse Colon, Open Approach

0D1A0ZM Bypass Jejunum to Descending Colon, Open Approach

0D1A0ZN Bypass Jejunum to Sigmoid Colon, Open Approach

0D1A0ZP Bypass Jejunum to Rectum, Open Approach

0D1A0ZQ Bypass Jejunum to Anus, Open Approach

0D1A3J4 Bypass Jejunum to Cutaneous with Synthetic Substitute, Percutaneous Approach

0D1A474 Bypass Jejunum to Cutaneous with Autologous Tissue Substitute, Percutaneous Endoscopic Approach

0D1A47A Bypass Jejunum to Jejunum with Autologous Tissue Substitute, Percutaneous Endoscopic Approach

0D1A47B Bypass Jejunum to Ileum with Autologous Tissue Substitute, Percutaneous Endoscopic Approach

0D1A47H Bypass Jejunum to Cecum with Autologous Tissue Substitute, Percutaneous Endoscopic Approach

0D1A47K Bypass Jejunum to Ascending Colon with Autologous Tissue Substitute, Percutaneous Endoscopic Approach

0D1A47L Bypass Jejunum to Transverse Colon with Autologous Tissue Substitute, Percutaneous Endoscopic Approach

0D1A47M Bypass Jejunum to Descending Colon with Autologous Tissue Substitute, Percutaneous Endoscopic Approach

0D1A47N Bypass Jejunum to Sigmoid Colon with Autologous Tissue Substitute, Percutaneous Endoscopic Approach

0D1A47P Bypass Jejunum to Rectum with Autologous Tissue Substitute, Percutaneous Endoscopic Approach

0D1A47Q Bypass Jejunum to Anus with Autologous Tissue Substitute, Percutaneous Endoscopic Approach

0D1A4J4 Bypass Jejunum to Cutaneous with Synthetic Substitute, Percutaneous Endoscopic Approach

0D1A4JA Bypass Jejunum to Jejunum with Synthetic Substitute, Percutaneous Endoscopic Approach

0D1A4JB Bypass Jejunum to Ileum with Synthetic Substitute, Percutaneous Endoscopic Approach

0D1A4JH Bypass Jejunum to Cecum with Synthetic Substitute, Percutaneous Endoscopic Approach

0D1A4JK Bypass Jejunum to Ascending Colon with Synthetic Substitute, Percutaneous Endoscopic Approach

0D1A4JL Bypass Jejunum to Transverse Colon with Synthetic Substitute, Percutaneous Endoscopic Approach

0D1A4JM Bypass Jejunum to Descending Colon with Synthetic Substitute, Percutaneous Endoscopic Approach

0D1A4JN Bypass Jejunum to Sigmoid Colon with Synthetic Substitute, Percutaneous Endoscopic Approach

0D1A4JP Bypass Jejunum to Rectum with Synthetic Substitute, Percutaneous Endoscopic Approach

0D1A4JQ Bypass Jejunum to Anus with Synthetic Substitute, Percutaneous Endoscopic Approach

0D1A4K4 Bypass Jejunum to Cutaneous with Nonautologous Tissue Substitute, Percutaneous Endoscopic Approach

0D1A4KA Bypass Jejunum to Jejunum with Nonautologous Tissue Substitute, Percutaneous Endoscopic Approach

0D1A4KB Bypass Jejunum to Ileum with Nonautologous Tissue Substitute, Percutaneous Endoscopic Approach

0D1A4KH Bypass Jejunum to Cecum with Nonautologous Tissue Substitute, Percutaneous Endoscopic Approach

0D1A4KK Bypass Jejunum to Ascending Colon with Nonautologous Tissue Substitute, Percutaneous Endoscopic Approach

0D1A4KL Bypass Jejunum to Transverse Colon with Nonautologous Tissue Substitute, Percutaneous Endoscopic Approach

0D1A4KM Bypass Jejunum to Descending Colon with Nonautologous Tissue Substitute, Percutaneous Endoscopic Approach

0D1A4KN Bypass Jejunum to Sigmoid Colon with Nonautologous Tissue Substitute, Percutaneous Endoscopic Approach

0D1A4KP Bypass Jejunum to Rectum with Nonautologous Tissue Substitute, Percutaneous Endoscopic Approach

0D1A4KQ Bypass Jejunum to Anus with Nonautologous Tissue Substitute, Percutaneous Endoscopic Approach

0D1A4Z4 Bypass Jejunum to Cutaneous, Percutaneous Endoscopic Approach

0D1A4ZA Bypass Jejunum to Jejunum, Percutaneous Endoscopic Approach

0D1A4ZB Bypass Jejunum to Ileum, Percutaneous Endoscopic Approach

0D1A4ZH Bypass Jejunum to Cecum, Percutaneous Endoscopic Approach

0D1A4ZK Bypass Jejunum to Ascending Colon, Percutaneous Endoscopic Approach

0D1A4ZL Bypass Jejunum to Transverse Colon, Percutaneous Endoscopic Approach

0D1A4ZM Bypass Jejunum to Descending Colon, Percutaneous Endoscopic Approach

0D1A4ZN Bypass Jejunum to Sigmoid Colon, Percutaneous Endoscopic Approach

0D1A4ZP Bypass Jejunum to Rectum, Percutaneous Endoscopic Approach

0D1A4ZQ Bypass Jejunum to Anus, Percutaneous Endoscopic Approach

0D1A874 Bypass Jejunum to Cutaneous with Autologous Tissue Substitute, Via Natural or Artificial Opening Endoscopic

0D1A87A Bypass Jejunum to Jejunum with Autologous Tissue Substitute, Via Natural or Artificial Opening Endoscopic

0D1A87B Bypass Jejunum to Ileum with Autologous Tissue Substitute, Via Natural or Artificial Opening Endoscopic

0D1A87H Bypass Jejunum to Cecum with Autologous Tissue Substitute, Via Natural or Artificial Opening Endoscopic

0D1A87K Bypass Jejunum to Ascending Colon with Autologous Tissue Substitute, Via Natural or Artificial Opening Endoscopic

0D1A87L Bypass Jejunum to Transverse Colon with Autologous Tissue Substitute, Via Natural or Artificial Opening Endoscopic

0D1A87M Bypass Jejunum to Descending Colon with Autologous Tissue Substitute, Via Natural or Artificial Opening Endoscopic

0D1A87N Bypass Jejunum to Sigmoid Colon with Autologous Tissue Substitute, Via Natural or Artificial Opening Endoscopic

0D1A87P Bypass Jejunum to Rectum with Autologous Tissue Substitute, Via Natural or Artificial Opening Endoscopic

0D1A87Q Bypass Jejunum to Anus with Autologous Tissue Substitute, Via Natural or Artificial Opening Endoscopic

0D1A8J4 Bypass Jejunum to Cutaneous with Synthetic Substitute, Via Natural or Artificial Opening Endoscopic

0D1A8JA Bypass Jejunum to Jejunum with Synthetic Substitute, Via Natural or Artificial Opening Endoscopic

0D1A8JB Bypass Jejunum to Ileum with Synthetic Substitute, Via Natural or Artificial Opening Endoscopic

0D1A8JH Bypass Jejunum to Cecum with Synthetic Substitute, Via Natural or Artificial Opening Endoscopic

0D1A8JK Bypass Jejunum to Ascending Colon with Synthetic Substitute, Via Natural or Artificial Opening Endoscopic

0D1A8JL Bypass Jejunum to Transverse Colon with Synthetic Substitute, Via Natural or Artificial Opening Endoscopic

0D1A8JM Bypass Jejunum to Descending Colon with Synthetic Substitute, Via Natural or Artificial Opening Endoscopic

0D1A8JN Bypass Jejunum to Sigmoid Colon with Synthetic Substitute, Via Natural or Artificial Opening Endoscopic

0D1A8JP Bypass Jejunum to Rectum with Synthetic Substitute, Via Natural or Artificial Opening Endoscopic

0D1A8JQ Bypass Jejunum to Anus with Synthetic Substitute, Via Natural or Artificial Opening Endoscopic

0D1A8K4 Bypass Jejunum to Cutaneous with Nonautologous Tissue Substitute, Via Natural or Artificial Opening Endoscopic

0D1A8KA Bypass Jejunum to Jejunum with Nonautologous Tissue Substitute, Via Natural or Artificial Opening Endoscopic

0D1A8KB Bypass Jejunum to Ileum with Nonautologous Tissue Substitute, Via Natural or Artificial Opening Endoscopic

0D1A8KH Bypass Jejunum to Cecum with Nonautologous Tissue Substitute, Via Natural or Artificial Opening Endoscopic

0D1A8KK Bypass Jejunum to Ascending Colon with Nonautologous Tissue Substitute, Via Natural or Artificial Opening Endoscopic

0D1A8KL Bypass Jejunum to Transverse Colon with Nonautologous Tissue Substitute, Via Natural or Artificial Opening Endoscopic

0D1A8KM Bypass Jejunum to Descending Colon with Nonautologous Tissue Substitute, Via Natural or Artificial Opening Endoscopic

0D1A8KN Bypass Jejunum to Sigmoid Colon with Nonautologous Tissue Substitute, Via Natural or Artificial Opening Endoscopic

0D1A8KP Bypass Jejunum to Rectum with Nonautologous Tissue Substitute, Via Natural or Artificial Opening Endoscopic

0D1A8KQ Bypass Jejunum to Anus with Nonautologous Tissue Substitute, Via Natural or Artificial Opening Endoscopic

0D1A8Z4 Bypass Jejunum to Cutaneous, Via Natural or Artificial Opening Endoscopic

0D1A8ZA Bypass Jejunum to Jejunum, Via Natural or Artificial Opening Endoscopic

0D1A8ZB Bypass Jejunum to Ileum, Via Natural or Artificial Opening Endoscopic

0D1A8ZH Bypass Jejunum to Cecum, Via Natural or Artificial Opening Endoscopic

0D1A8ZK Bypass Jejunum to Ascending Colon, Via Natural or Artificial Opening Endoscopic

0D1A8ZL Bypass Jejunum to Transverse Colon, Via Natural or Artificial Opening Endoscopic

0D1A8ZM Bypass Jejunum to Descending Colon, Via Natural or Artificial Opening Endoscopic

0D1A8ZN Bypass Jejunum to Sigmoid Colon, Via Natural or Artificial Opening Endoscopic

0D1A8ZP Bypass Jejunum to Rectum, Via Natural or Artificial Opening Endoscopic

0D1A8ZQ Bypass Jejunum to Anus, Via Natural or Artificial Opening Endoscopic

0D1B074 Bypass Ileum to Cutaneous with Autologous Tissue Substitute, Open Approach

0D1B07B Bypass Ileum to Ileum with Autologous Tissue Substitute, Open Approach

0D1B07H Bypass Ileum to Cecum with Autologous Tissue Substitute, Open Approach

0D1B07K Bypass Ileum to Ascending Colon with Autologous Tissue Substitute, Open Approach

0D1B07L Bypass Ileum to Transverse Colon with Autologous Tissue Substitute, Open Approach

0D1B07M Bypass Ileum to Descending Colon with Autologous Tissue Substitute, Open Approach

0D1B07N Bypass Ileum to Sigmoid Colon with Autologous Tissue Substitute, Open Approach

0D1B07P Bypass Ileum to Rectum with Autologous Tissue Substitute, Open Approach

0D1B07Q Bypass Ileum to Anus with Autologous Tissue Substitute, Open Approach

0D1B0J4 Bypass Ileum to Cutaneous with Synthetic Substitute, Open Approach

0D1B0JB Bypass Ileum to Ileum with Synthetic Substitute, Open Approach

0D1B0JH Bypass Ileum to Cecum with Synthetic Substitute, Open Approach

0D1B0JK Bypass Ileum to Ascending Colon with Synthetic Substitute, Open Approach

0D1B0JL Bypass Ileum to Transverse Colon with Synthetic Substitute, Open Approach

0D1B0JM Bypass Ileum to Descending Colon with Synthetic Substitute, Open Approach

0D1B0JN Bypass Ileum to Sigmoid Colon with Synthetic Substitute, Open Approach

0D1B0JP Bypass Ileum to Rectum with Synthetic Substitute, Open Approach

0D1B0JQ Bypass Ileum to Anus with Synthetic Substitute, Open Approach

0D1B0K4 Bypass Ileum to Cutaneous with Nonautologous Tissue Substitute, Open Approach

0D1B0KB Bypass Ileum to Ileum with Nonautologous Tissue Substitute, Open Approach

0D1B0KH Bypass Ileum to Cecum with Nonautologous Tissue Substitute, Open Approach

0D1B0KK Bypass Ileum to Ascending Colon with Nonautologous Tissue Substitute, Open Approach

0D1B0KL Bypass Ileum to Transverse Colon with Nonautologous Tissue Substitute, Open Approach

0D1B0KM Bypass Ileum to Descending Colon with Nonautologous Tissue Substitute, Open Approach

0D1B0KN Bypass Ileum to Sigmoid Colon with Nonautologous Tissue Substitute, Open Approach

0D1B0KP Bypass Ileum to Rectum with Nonautologous Tissue Substitute, Open Approach

0D1B0KQ Bypass Ileum to Anus with Nonautologous Tissue Substitute, Open Approach

0D1B0Z4 Bypass Ileum to Cutaneous, Open Approach

0D1B0ZB Bypass Ileum to Ileum, Open Approach

0D1B0ZH Bypass Ileum to Cecum, Open Approach

0D1B0ZK Bypass Ileum to Ascending Colon, Open Approach

0D1B0ZL Bypass Ileum to Transverse Colon, Open Approach

0D1B0ZM Bypass Ileum to Descending Colon, Open Approach

0D1B0ZN Bypass Ileum to Sigmoid Colon, Open Approach

0D1B0ZP Bypass Ileum to Rectum, Open Approach

0D1B0ZQ Bypass Ileum to Anus, Open Approach

0D1B3J4 Bypass Ileum to Cutaneous with Synthetic Substitute, Percutaneous Approach

0D1B474 Bypass Ileum to Cutaneous with Autologous Tissue Substitute, Percutaneous Endoscopic Approach

0D1B47B Bypass Ileum to Ileum with Autologous Tissue Substitute, Percutaneous Endoscopic Approach

0D1B47H Bypass Ileum to Cecum with Autologous Tissue Substitute, Percutaneous Endoscopic Approach

0D1B47K Bypass Ileum to Ascending Colon with Autologous Tissue Substitute, Percutaneous Endoscopic Approach

0D1B47L Bypass Ileum to Transverse Colon with Autologous Tissue Substitute, Percutaneous Endoscopic Approach

0D1B47M Bypass Ileum to Descending Colon with Autologous Tissue Substitute, Percutaneous Endoscopic Approach

0D1B47N Bypass Ileum to Sigmoid Colon with Autologous Tissue Substitute, Percutaneous Endoscopic Approach

0D1B47P Bypass Ileum to Rectum with Autologous Tissue Substitute, Percutaneous Endoscopic Approach

0D1B47Q Bypass Ileum to Anus with Autologous Tissue Substitute, Percutaneous Endoscopic Approach

0D1B4J4 Bypass Ileum to Cutaneous with Synthetic Substitute, Percutaneous Endoscopic Approach

0D1B4JB Bypass Ileum to Ileum with Synthetic Substitute, Percutaneous Endoscopic Approach

0D1B4JH Bypass Ileum to Cecum with Synthetic Substitute, Percutaneous Endoscopic Approach

0D1B4JK Bypass Ileum to Ascending Colon with Synthetic Substitute, Percutaneous Endoscopic Approach

0D1B4JL Bypass Ileum to Transverse Colon with Synthetic Substitute, Percutaneous Endoscopic Approach

0D1B4JM Bypass Ileum to Descending Colon with Synthetic Substitute, Percutaneous Endoscopic Approach

0D1B4JN Bypass Ileum to Sigmoid Colon with Synthetic Substitute, Percutaneous Endoscopic Approach

0D1B4JP Bypass Ileum to Rectum with Synthetic Substitute, Percutaneous Endoscopic Approach

0D1B4JQ Bypass Ileum to Anus with Synthetic Substitute, Percutaneous Endoscopic Approach

0D1B4K4 Bypass Ileum to Cutaneous with Nonautologous Tissue Substitute, Percutaneous Endoscopic Approach

0D1B4KB Bypass Ileum to Ileum with Nonautologous Tissue Substitute, Percutaneous Endoscopic Approach

0D1B4KH Bypass Ileum to Cecum with Nonautologous Tissue Substitute, Percutaneous Endoscopic Approach

0D1B4KK Bypass Ileum to Ascending Colon with Nonautologous Tissue Substitute, Percutaneous Endoscopic Approach

0D1B4KL Bypass Ileum to Transverse Colon with Nonautologous Tissue Substitute, Percutaneous Endoscopic Approach

0D1B4KM Bypass Ileum to Descending Colon with Nonautologous Tissue Substitute, Percutaneous Endoscopic Approach

0D1B4KN Bypass Ileum to Sigmoid Colon with Nonautologous Tissue Substitute, Percutaneous Endoscopic Approach

0D1B4KP Bypass Ileum to Rectum with Nonautologous Tissue Substitute, Percutaneous Endoscopic Approach

0D1B4KQ Bypass Ileum to Anus with Nonautologous Tissue Substitute, Percutaneous Endoscopic Approach

0D1B4Z4 Bypass Ileum to Cutaneous, Percutaneous Endoscopic Approach

0D1B4ZB Bypass Ileum to Ileum, Percutaneous Endoscopic Approach

0D1B4ZH Bypass Ileum to Cecum, Percutaneous Endoscopic Approach

0D1B4ZK Bypass Ileum to Ascending Colon, Percutaneous Endoscopic Approach

0D1B4ZL Bypass Ileum to Transverse Colon, Percutaneous Endoscopic Approach

0D1B4ZM Bypass Ileum to Descending Colon, Percutaneous Endoscopic Approach

0D1B4ZN Bypass Ileum to Sigmoid Colon, Percutaneous Endoscopic Approach

0D1B4ZP Bypass Ileum to Rectum, Percutaneous Endoscopic Approach

0D1B4ZQ Bypass Ileum to Anus, Percutaneous Endoscopic Approach

0D1B874 Bypass Ileum to Cutaneous with Autologous Tissue Substitute, Via Natural or Artificial Opening Endoscopic

0D1B87B Bypass Ileum to Ileum with Autologous Tissue Substitute, Via Natural or Artificial Opening Endoscopic

0D1B87H Bypass Ileum to Cecum with Autologous Tissue Substitute, Via Natural or Artificial Opening Endoscopic

0D1B87K Bypass Ileum to Ascending Colon with Autologous Tissue Substitute, Via Natural or Artificial Opening Endoscopic

0D1B87L Bypass Ileum to Transverse Colon with Autologous Tissue Substitute, Via Natural or Artificial Opening Endoscopic

0D1B87M Bypass Ileum to Descending Colon with Autologous Tissue Substitute, Via Natural or Artificial Opening Endoscopic

0D1B87N Bypass Ileum to Sigmoid Colon with Autologous Tissue Substitute, Via Natural or Artificial Opening Endoscopic

0D1B87P Bypass Ileum to Rectum with Autologous Tissue Substitute, Via Natural or Artificial Opening Endoscopic

0D1B87Q Bypass Ileum to Anus with Autologous Tissue Substitute, Via Natural or Artificial Opening Endoscopic

0D1B8J4 Bypass Ileum to Cutaneous with Synthetic Substitute, Via Natural or Artificial Opening Endoscopic

0D1B8JB Bypass Ileum to Ileum with Synthetic Substitute, Via Natural or Artificial Opening Endoscopic

0D1B8JH Bypass Ileum to Cecum with Synthetic Substitute, Via Natural or Artificial Opening Endoscopic

0D1B8JK Bypass Ileum to Ascending Colon with Synthetic Substitute, Via Natural or Artificial Opening Endoscopic

0D1B8JL Bypass Ileum to Transverse Colon with Synthetic Substitute, Via Natural or Artificial Opening Endoscopic

0D1B8JM Bypass Ileum to Descending Colon with Synthetic Substitute, Via Natural or Artificial Opening Endoscopic

0D1B8JN Bypass Ileum to Sigmoid Colon with Synthetic Substitute, Via Natural or Artificial Opening Endoscopic

0D1B8JP Bypass Ileum to Rectum with Synthetic Substitute, Via Natural or Artificial Opening Endoscopic

0D1B8JQ Bypass Ileum to Anus with Synthetic Substitute, Via Natural or Artificial Opening Endoscopic

0D1B8K4 Bypass Ileum to Cutaneous with Nonautologous Tissue Substitute, Via Natural or Artificial Opening Endoscopic

0D1B8KB Bypass Ileum to Ileum with Nonautologous Tissue Substitute, Via Natural or Artificial Opening Endoscopic

0D1B8KH Bypass Ileum to Cecum with Nonautologous Tissue Substitute, Via Natural or Artificial Opening Endoscopic

0D1B8KK Bypass Ileum to Ascending Colon with Nonautologous Tissue Substitute, Via Natural or Artificial Opening Endoscopic

0D1B8KL Bypass Ileum to Transverse Colon with Nonautologous Tissue Substitute, Via Natural or Artificial Opening Endoscopic

0D1B8KM Bypass Ileum to Descending Colon with Nonautologous Tissue Substitute, Via Natural or Artificial Opening Endoscopic

0D1B8KN Bypass Ileum to Sigmoid Colon with Nonautologous Tissue Substitute, Via Natural or Artificial Opening Endoscopic

0D1B8KP Bypass Ileum to Rectum with Nonautologous Tissue Substitute, Via Natural or Artificial Opening Endoscopic

0D1B8KQ Bypass Ileum to Anus with Nonautologous Tissue Substitute, Via Natural or Artificial Opening Endoscopic

0D1B8Z4 Bypass Ileum to Cutaneous, Via Natural or Artificial Opening Endoscopic

0D1B8ZB Bypass Ileum to Ileum, Via Natural or Artificial Opening Endoscopic

0D1B8ZH Bypass Ileum to Cecum, Via Natural or Artificial Opening Endoscopic

0D1B8ZK Bypass Ileum to Ascending Colon, Via Natural or Artificial Opening Endoscopic

0D1B8ZL Bypass Ileum to Transverse Colon, Via Natural or Artificial Opening Endoscopic

0D1B8ZM Bypass Ileum to Descending Colon, Via Natural or Artificial Opening Endoscopic

0D1B8ZN Bypass Ileum to Sigmoid Colon, Via Natural or Artificial Opening Endoscopic

0D1B8ZP Bypass Ileum to Rectum, Via Natural or Artificial Opening Endoscopic

0D1B8ZQ Bypass Ileum to Anus, Via Natural or Artificial Opening Endoscopic

0D1H074 Bypass Cecum to Cutaneous with Autologous Tissue Substitute, Open Approach

0D1H07H Bypass Cecum to Cecum with Autologous Tissue Substitute, Open Approach

0D1H07K Bypass Cecum to Ascending Colon with Autologous Tissue Substitute, Open Approach

0D1H07L Bypass Cecum to Transverse Colon with Autologous Tissue Substitute, Open Approach

0D1H07M Bypass Cecum to Descending Colon with Autologous Tissue Substitute, Open Approach

0D1H07N Bypass Cecum to Sigmoid Colon with Autologous Tissue Substitute, Open Approach

0D1H07P Bypass Cecum to Rectum with Autologous Tissue Substitute, Open Approach

0D1H0J4 Bypass Cecum to Cutaneous with Synthetic Substitute, Open Approach

0D1H0JH Bypass Cecum to Cecum with Synthetic Substitute, Open Approach

0D1H0JK Bypass Cecum to Ascending Colon with Synthetic Substitute, Open Approach

0D1H0JL Bypass Cecum to Transverse Colon with Synthetic Substitute, Open Approach

0D1H0JM Bypass Cecum to Descending Colon with Synthetic Substitute, Open Approach

0D1H0JN Bypass Cecum to Sigmoid Colon with Synthetic Substitute, Open Approach

0D1H0JP Bypass Cecum to Rectum with Synthetic Substitute, Open Approach

0D1H0K4 Bypass Cecum to Cutaneous with Nonautologous Tissue Substitute, Open Approach

0D1H0KH Bypass Cecum to Cecum with Nonautologous Tissue Substitute, Open Approach

0D1H0KK Bypass Cecum to Ascending Colon with Nonautologous Tissue Substitute, Open Approach

0D1H0KL Bypass Cecum to Transverse Colon with Nonautologous Tissue Substitute, Open Approach

0D1H0KM Bypass Cecum to Descending Colon with Nonautologous Tissue Substitute, Open Approach

0D1H0KN Bypass Cecum to Sigmoid Colon with Nonautologous Tissue Substitute, Open Approach

0D1H0KP Bypass Cecum to Rectum with Nonautologous Tissue Substitute, Open Approach

0D1H0Z4 Bypass Cecum to Cutaneous, Open Approach

0D1H0ZH Bypass Cecum to Cecum, Open Approach

0D1H0ZK Bypass Cecum to Ascending Colon, Open Approach

0D1H0ZL Bypass Cecum to Transverse Colon, Open Approach

0D1H0ZM Bypass Cecum to Descending Colon, Open Approach

0D1H0ZN Bypass Cecum to Sigmoid Colon, Open Approach

0D1H0ZP Bypass Cecum to Rectum, Open Approach

0D1H3J4 Bypass Cecum to Cutaneous with Synthetic Substitute, Percutaneous Approach

0D1H474 Bypass Cecum to Cutaneous with Autologous Tissue Substitute, Percutaneous Endoscopic Approach

0D1H47H Bypass Cecum to Cecum with Autologous Tissue Substitute, Percutaneous Endoscopic Approach

0D1H47K Bypass Cecum to Ascending Colon with Autologous Tissue Substitute, Percutaneous Endoscopic Approach

0D1H47L Bypass Cecum to Transverse Colon with Autologous Tissue Substitute, Percutaneous Endoscopic Approach

0D1H47M Bypass Cecum to Descending Colon with Autologous Tissue Substitute, Percutaneous Endoscopic Approach

0D1H47N Bypass Cecum to Sigmoid Colon with Autologous Tissue Substitute, Percutaneous Endoscopic Approach

0D1H47P Bypass Cecum to Rectum with Autologous Tissue Substitute, Percutaneous Endoscopic Approach

0D1H4J4 Bypass Cecum to Cutaneous with Synthetic Substitute, Percutaneous Endoscopic Approach

0D1H4JH Bypass Cecum to Cecum with Synthetic Substitute, Percutaneous Endoscopic Approach

0D1H4JK Bypass Cecum to Ascending Colon with Synthetic Substitute, Percutaneous Endoscopic Approach

0D1H4JL Bypass Cecum to Transverse Colon with Synthetic Substitute, Percutaneous Endoscopic Approach

0D1H4JM Bypass Cecum to Descending Colon with Synthetic Substitute, Percutaneous Endoscopic Approach

0D1H4JN Bypass Cecum to Sigmoid Colon with Synthetic Substitute, Percutaneous Endoscopic Approach

0D1H4JP Bypass Cecum to Rectum with Synthetic Substitute, Percutaneous Endoscopic Approach

0D1H4K4 Bypass Cecum to Cutaneous with Nonautologous Tissue Substitute, Percutaneous Endoscopic Approach

0D1H4KH Bypass Cecum to Cecum with Nonautologous Tissue Substitute, Percutaneous Endoscopic Approach

0D1H4KK Bypass Cecum to Ascending Colon with Nonautologous Tissue Substitute, Percutaneous Endoscopic Approach

0D1H4KL Bypass Cecum to Transverse Colon with Nonautologous Tissue Substitute, Percutaneous Endoscopic Approach

0D1H4KM Bypass Cecum to Descending Colon with Nonautologous Tissue Substitute, Percutaneous Endoscopic Approach

0D1H4KN Bypass Cecum to Sigmoid Colon with Nonautologous Tissue Substitute, Percutaneous Endoscopic Approach

0D1H4KP Bypass Cecum to Rectum with Nonautologous Tissue Substitute, Percutaneous Endoscopic Approach

0D1H4Z4 Bypass Cecum to Cutaneous, Percutaneous Endoscopic Approach

0D1H4ZH Bypass Cecum to Cecum, Percutaneous Endoscopic Approach

0D1H4ZK Bypass Cecum to Ascending Colon, Percutaneous Endoscopic Approach

0D1H4ZL Bypass Cecum to Transverse Colon, Percutaneous Endoscopic Approach

0D1H4ZM Bypass Cecum to Descending Colon, Percutaneous Endoscopic Approach

0D1H4ZN Bypass Cecum to Sigmoid Colon, Percutaneous Endoscopic Approach

0D1H4ZP Bypass Cecum to Rectum, Percutaneous Endoscopic Approach

0D1H874 Bypass Cecum to Cutaneous with Autologous Tissue Substitute, Via Natural or Artificial Opening Endoscopic

0D1H87H Bypass Cecum to Cecum with Autologous Tissue Substitute, Via Natural or Artificial Opening Endoscopic

0D1H87K Bypass Cecum to Ascending Colon with Autologous Tissue Substitute, Via Natural or Artificial Opening Endoscopic

0D1H87L Bypass Cecum to Transverse Colon with Autologous Tissue Substitute, Via Natural or Artificial Opening Endoscopic

0D1H87M Bypass Cecum to Descending Colon with Autologous Tissue Substitute, Via Natural or Artificial Opening Endoscopic

0D1H87N Bypass Cecum to Sigmoid Colon with Autologous Tissue Substitute, Via Natural or Artificial Opening Endoscopic

0D1H87P Bypass Cecum to Rectum with Autologous Tissue Substitute, Via Natural or Artificial Opening Endoscopic

0D1H8J4 Bypass Cecum to Cutaneous with Synthetic Substitute, Via Natural or Artificial Opening Endoscopic

0D1H8JH Bypass Cecum to Cecum with Synthetic Substitute, Via Natural or Artificial Opening Endoscopic

0D1H8JK Bypass Cecum to Ascending Colon with Synthetic Substitute, Via Natural or Artificial Opening Endoscopic

0D1H8JL Bypass Cecum to Transverse Colon with Synthetic Substitute, Via Natural or Artificial Opening Endoscopic

0D1H8JM Bypass Cecum to Descending Colon with Synthetic Substitute, Via Natural or Artificial Opening Endoscopic

0D1H8JN Bypass Cecum to Sigmoid Colon with Synthetic Substitute, Via Natural or Artificial Opening Endoscopic

0D1H8JP Bypass Cecum to Rectum with Synthetic Substitute, Via Natural or Artificial Opening Endoscopic

0D1H8K4 Bypass Cecum to Cutaneous with Nonautologous Tissue Substitute, Via Natural or Artificial Opening Endoscopic

0D1H8KH Bypass Cecum to Cecum with Nonautologous Tissue Substitute, Via Natural or Artificial Opening Endoscopic

0D1H8KK Bypass Cecum to Ascending Colon with Nonautologous Tissue Substitute, Via Natural or Artificial Opening Endoscopic

0D1H8KL Bypass Cecum to Transverse Colon with Nonautologous Tissue Substitute, Via Natural or Artificial Opening Endoscopic

0D1H8KM Bypass Cecum to Descending Colon with Nonautologous Tissue Substitute, Via Natural or Artificial Opening Endoscopic

0D1H8KN Bypass Cecum to Sigmoid Colon with Nonautologous Tissue Substitute, Via Natural or Artificial Opening Endoscopic

0D1H8KP Bypass Cecum to Rectum with Nonautologous Tissue Substitute, Via Natural or Artificial Opening Endoscopic

0D1H8Z4 Bypass Cecum to Cutaneous, Via Natural or Artificial Opening Endoscopic

0D1H8ZH Bypass Cecum to Cecum, Via Natural or Artificial Opening Endoscopic

0D1H8ZK Bypass Cecum to Ascending Colon, Via Natural or Artificial Opening Endoscopic

0D1H8ZL Bypass Cecum to Transverse Colon, Via Natural or Artificial Opening Endoscopic

0D1H8ZM Bypass Cecum to Descending Colon, Via Natural or Artificial Opening Endoscopic

0D1H8ZN Bypass Cecum to Sigmoid Colon, Via Natural or Artificial Opening Endoscopic

0D1H8ZP Bypass Cecum to Rectum, Via Natural or Artificial Opening Endoscopic

0D1K074 Bypass Ascending Colon to Cutaneous with Autologous Tissue Substitute, Open Approach

0D1K07K Bypass Ascending Colon to Ascending Colon with Autologous Tissue Substitute, Open Approach

0D1K07L Bypass Ascending Colon to Transverse Colon with Autologous Tissue Substitute, Open Approach

0D1K07M Bypass Ascending Colon to Descending Colon with Autologous Tissue Substitute, Open Approach

0D1K07N Bypass Ascending Colon to Sigmoid Colon with Autologous Tissue Substitute, Open Approach

0D1K07P Bypass Ascending Colon to Rectum with Autologous Tissue Substitute, Open Approach

0D1K0J4 Bypass Ascending Colon to Cutaneous with Synthetic Substitute, Open Approach

0D1K0JK Bypass Ascending Colon to Ascending Colon with Synthetic Substitute, Open Approach

0D1K0JL Bypass Ascending Colon to Transverse Colon with Synthetic Substitute, Open Approach

0D1K0JM Bypass Ascending Colon to Descending Colon with Synthetic Substitute, Open Approach

0D1K0JN Bypass Ascending Colon to Sigmoid Colon with Synthetic Substitute, Open Approach

0D1K0JP Bypass Ascending Colon to Rectum with Synthetic Substitute, Open Approach

0D1K0K4 Bypass Ascending Colon to Cutaneous with Nonautologous Tissue Substitute, Open Approach

0D1K0KK Bypass Ascending Colon to Ascending Colon with Nonautologous Tissue Substitute, Open Approach

0D1K0KL Bypass Ascending Colon to Transverse Colon with Nonautologous Tissue Substitute, Open Approach

0D1K0KM Bypass Ascending Colon to Descending Colon with Nonautologous Tissue Substitute, Open Approach

0D1K0KN Bypass Ascending Colon to Sigmoid Colon with Nonautologous Tissue Substitute, Open Approach

0D1K0KP Bypass Ascending Colon to Rectum with Nonautologous Tissue Substitute, Open Approach

0D1K0Z4 Bypass Ascending Colon to Cutaneous, Open Approach

0D1K0ZK Bypass Ascending Colon to Ascending Colon, Open Approach

0D1K0ZL Bypass Ascending Colon to Transverse Colon, Open Approach

0D1K0ZM Bypass Ascending Colon to Descending Colon, Open Approach

0D1K0ZN Bypass Ascending Colon to Sigmoid Colon, Open Approach

0D1K0ZP Bypass Ascending Colon to Rectum, Open Approach

0D1K3J4 Bypass Ascending Colon to Cutaneous with Synthetic Substitute, Percutaneous Approach

0D1K474 Bypass Ascending Colon to Cutaneous with Autologous Tissue Substitute, Percutaneous Endoscopic Approach

0D1K47K Bypass Ascending Colon to Ascending Colon with Autologous Tissue Substitute, Percutaneous Endoscopic Approach

0D1K47L Bypass Ascending Colon to Transverse Colon with Autologous Tissue Substitute, Percutaneous Endoscopic Approach

0D1K47M Bypass Ascending Colon to Descending Colon with Autologous Tissue Substitute, Percutaneous Endoscopic Approach

0D1K47N Bypass Ascending Colon to Sigmoid Colon with Autologous Tissue Substitute, Percutaneous Endoscopic Approach

0D1K47P Bypass Ascending Colon to Rectum with Autologous Tissue Substitute, Percutaneous Endoscopic Approach

0D1K4J4 Bypass Ascending Colon to Cutaneous with Synthetic Substitute, Percutaneous Endoscopic Approach

0D1K4JK Bypass Ascending Colon to Ascending Colon with Synthetic Substitute, Percutaneous Endoscopic Approach

0D1K4JL Bypass Ascending Colon to Transverse Colon with Synthetic Substitute, Percutaneous Endoscopic Approach

0D1K4JM Bypass Ascending Colon to Descending Colon with Synthetic Substitute, Percutaneous Endoscopic Approach

0D1K4JN Bypass Ascending Colon to Sigmoid Colon with Synthetic Substitute, Percutaneous Endoscopic Approach

0D1K4JP Bypass Ascending Colon to Rectum with Synthetic Substitute, Percutaneous Endoscopic Approach

0D1K4K4 Bypass Ascending Colon to Cutaneous with Nonautologous Tissue Substitute, Percutaneous Endoscopic Approach

0D1K4KK Bypass Ascending Colon to Ascending Colon with Nonautologous Tissue Substitute, Percutaneous Endoscopic Approach

0D1K4KL Bypass Ascending Colon to Transverse Colon with Nonautologous Tissue Substitute, Percutaneous Endoscopic Approach

0D1K4KM Bypass Ascending Colon to Descending Colon with Nonautologous Tissue Substitute, Percutaneous Endoscopic Approach

0D1K4KN Bypass Ascending Colon to Sigmoid Colon with Nonautologous Tissue Substitute, Percutaneous Endoscopic Approach

0D1K4KP Bypass Ascending Colon to Rectum with Nonautologous Tissue Substitute, Percutaneous Endoscopic Approach

0D1K4Z4 Bypass Ascending Colon to Cutaneous, Percutaneous Endoscopic Approach

0D1K4ZK Bypass Ascending Colon to Ascending Colon, Percutaneous Endoscopic Approach

0D1K4ZL Bypass Ascending Colon to Transverse Colon, Percutaneous Endoscopic Approach

0D1K4ZM Bypass Ascending Colon to Descending Colon, Percutaneous Endoscopic Approach

0D1K4ZN Bypass Ascending Colon to Sigmoid Colon, Percutaneous Endoscopic Approach

0D1K4ZP   Bypass Ascending Colon to Rectum, Percutaneous Endoscopic Approach

0D1K874   Bypass Ascending Colon to Cutaneous with Autologous Tissue Substitute, Via Natural or Artificial Opening Endoscopic

0D1K87K   Bypass Ascending Colon to Ascending Colon with Autologous Tissue Substitute, Via Natural or Artificial Opening Endoscopic

0D1K87L   Bypass Ascending Colon to Transverse Colon with Autologous Tissue Substitute, Via Natural or Artificial Opening Endoscopic

0D1K87M   Bypass Ascending Colon to Descending Colon with Autologous Tissue Substitute, Via Natural or Artificial Opening Endoscopic

0D1K87N   Bypass Ascending Colon to Sigmoid Colon with Autologous Tissue Substitute, Via Natural or Artificial Opening Endoscopic

0D1K87P   Bypass Ascending Colon to Rectum with Autologous Tissue Substitute, Via Natural or Artificial Opening Endoscopic

0D1K8J4   Bypass Ascending Colon to Cutaneous with Synthetic Substitute, Via Natural or Artificial Opening Endoscopic

0D1K8JK   Bypass Ascending Colon to Ascending Colon with Synthetic Substitute, Via Natural or Artificial Opening Endoscopic

0D1K8JL   Bypass Ascending Colon to Transverse Colon with Synthetic Substitute, Via Natural or Artificial Opening Endoscopic

0D1K8JM   Bypass Ascending Colon to Descending Colon with Synthetic Substitute, Via Natural or Artificial Opening Endoscopic

0D1K8JN   Bypass Ascending Colon to Sigmoid Colon with Synthetic Substitute, Via Natural or Artificial Opening Endoscopic

0D1K8JP   Bypass Ascending Colon to Rectum with Synthetic Substitute, Via Natural or Artificial Opening Endoscopic

0D1K8K4   Bypass Ascending Colon to Cutaneous with Nonautologous Tissue Substitute, Via Natural or Artificial Opening Endoscopic

0D1K8KK   Bypass Ascending Colon to Ascending Colon with Nonautologous Tissue Substitute, Via Natural or Artificial Opening Endoscopic

0D1K8KL   Bypass Ascending Colon to Transverse Colon with Nonautologous Tissue Substitute, Via Natural or Artificial Opening Endoscopic

0D1K8KM   Bypass Ascending Colon to Descending Colon with Nonautologous Tissue Substitute, Via Natural or Artificial Opening Endoscopic

0D1K8KN   Bypass Ascending Colon to Sigmoid Colon with Nonautologous Tissue Substitute, Via Natural or Artificial Opening Endoscopic

0D1K8KP   Bypass Ascending Colon to Rectum with Nonautologous Tissue Substitute, Via Natural or Artificial Opening Endoscopic

0D1K8Z4   Bypass Ascending Colon to Cutaneous, Via Natural or Artificial Opening Endoscopic

0D1K8ZK   Bypass Ascending Colon to Ascending Colon, Via Natural or Artificial Opening Endoscopic

0D1K8ZL   Bypass Ascending Colon to Transverse Colon, Via Natural or Artificial Opening Endoscopic

0D1K8ZM   Bypass Ascending Colon to Descending Colon, Via Natural or Artificial Opening Endoscopic

0D1K8ZN   Bypass Ascending Colon to Sigmoid Colon, Via Natural or Artificial Opening Endoscopic

0D1K8ZP   Bypass Ascending Colon to Rectum, Via Natural or Artificial Opening Endoscopic

0D1L074   Bypass Transverse Colon to Cutaneous with Autologous Tissue Substitute, Open Approach

0D1L07L   Bypass Transverse Colon to Transverse Colon with Autologous Tissue Substitute, Open Approach

0D1L07M   Bypass Transverse Colon to Descending Colon with Autologous Tissue Substitute, Open Approach

0D1L07N   Bypass Transverse Colon to Sigmoid Colon with Autologous Tissue Substitute, Open Approach

0D1L07P   Bypass Transverse Colon to Rectum with Autologous Tissue Substitute, Open Approach

0D1L0J4   Bypass Transverse Colon to Cutaneous with Synthetic Substitute, Open Approach

0D1L0JL   Bypass Transverse Colon to Transverse Colon with Synthetic Substitute, Open Approach

0D1L0JM   Bypass Transverse Colon to Descending Colon with Synthetic Substitute, Open Approach

0D1L0JN   Bypass Transverse Colon to Sigmoid Colon with Synthetic Substitute, Open Approach

0D1L0JP   Bypass Transverse Colon to Rectum with Synthetic Substitute, Open Approach

0D1L0K4   Bypass Transverse Colon to Cutaneous with Nonautologous Tissue Substitute, Open Approach

0D1L0KL   Bypass Transverse Colon to Transverse Colon with Nonautologous Tissue Substitute, Open Approach

0D1L0KM   Bypass Transverse Colon to Descending Colon with Nonautologous Tissue Substitute, Open Approach

0D1L0KN   Bypass Transverse Colon to Sigmoid Colon with Nonautologous Tissue Substitute, Open Approach

0D1L0KP   Bypass Transverse Colon to Rectum with Nonautologous Tissue Substitute, Open Approach

0D1L0Z4   Bypass Transverse Colon to Cutaneous, Open Approach

0D1L0ZL   Bypass Transverse Colon to Transverse Colon, Open Approach

0D1L0ZM   Bypass Transverse Colon to Descending Colon, Open Approach

0D1L0ZN   Bypass Transverse Colon to Sigmoid Colon, Open Approach

0D1L0ZP   Bypass Transverse Colon to Rectum, Open Approach

0D1L3J4   Bypass Transverse Colon to Cutaneous with Synthetic Substitute, Percutaneous Approach

0D1L474   Bypass Transverse Colon to Cutaneous with Autologous Tissue Substitute, Percutaneous Endoscopic Approach

0D1L47L   Bypass Transverse Colon to Transverse Colon with Autologous Tissue Substitute, Percutaneous Endoscopic Approach

0D1L47M   Bypass Transverse Colon to Descending Colon with Autologous Tissue Substitute, Percutaneous Endoscopic Approach

0D1L47N   Bypass Transverse Colon to Sigmoid Colon with Autologous Tissue Substitute, Percutaneous Endoscopic Approach

0D1L47P   Bypass Transverse Colon to Rectum with Autologous Tissue Substitute, Percutaneous Endoscopic Approach

0D1L4J4   Bypass Transverse Colon to Cutaneous with Synthetic Substitute, Percutaneous Endoscopic Approach

0D1L4JL   Bypass Transverse Colon to Transverse Colon with Synthetic Substitute, Percutaneous Endoscopic Approach

0D1L4JM   Bypass Transverse Colon to Descending Colon with Synthetic Substitute, Percutaneous Endoscopic Approach

0D1L4JN   Bypass Transverse Colon to Sigmoid Colon with Synthetic Substitute, Percutaneous Endoscopic Approach

0D1L4JP   Bypass Transverse Colon to Rectum with Synthetic Substitute, Percutaneous Endoscopic Approach

0D1L4K4   Bypass Transverse Colon to Cutaneous with Nonautologous Tissue Substitute, Percutaneous Endoscopic Approach

0D1L4KL   Bypass Transverse Colon to Transverse Colon with Nonautologous Tissue Substitute, Percutaneous Endoscopic Approach

0D1L4KM   Bypass Transverse Colon to Descending Colon with Nonautologous Tissue Substitute, Percutaneous Endoscopic Approach

0D1L4KN   Bypass Transverse Colon to Sigmoid Colon with Nonautologous Tissue Substitute, Percutaneous Endoscopic Approach

0D1L4KP   Bypass Transverse Colon to Rectum with Nonautologous Tissue Substitute, Percutaneous Endoscopic Approach

0D1L4Z4   Bypass Transverse Colon to Cutaneous, Percutaneous Endoscopic Approach

0D1L4ZL   Bypass Transverse Colon to Transverse Colon, Percutaneous Endoscopic Approach

0D1L4ZM   Bypass Transverse Colon to Descending Colon, Percutaneous Endoscopic Approach

0D1L4ZN   Bypass Transverse Colon to Sigmoid Colon, Percutaneous Endoscopic Approach

0D1L4ZP   Bypass Transverse Colon to Rectum, Percutaneous Endoscopic Approach

0D1L874   Bypass Transverse Colon to Cutaneous with Autologous Tissue Substitute, Via Natural or Artificial Opening Endoscopic

0D1L87L   Bypass Transverse Colon to Transverse Colon with Autologous Tissue Substitute, Via Natural or Artificial Opening Endoscopic

0D1L87M   Bypass Transverse Colon to Descending Colon with Autologous Tissue Substitute, Via Natural or Artificial Opening Endoscopic

0D1L87N   Bypass Transverse Colon to Sigmoid Colon with Autologous Tissue Substitute, Via Natural or Artificial Opening Endoscopic

0D1L87P   Bypass Transverse Colon to Rectum with Autologous Tissue Substitute, Via Natural or Artificial Opening Endoscopic

0D1L8J4   Bypass Transverse Colon to Cutaneous with Synthetic Substitute, Via Natural or Artificial Opening Endoscopic

0D1L8JL   Bypass Transverse Colon to Transverse Colon with Synthetic Substitute, Via Natural or Artificial Opening Endoscopic

0D1L8JM   Bypass Transverse Colon to Descending Colon with Synthetic Substitute, Via Natural or Artificial Opening Endoscopic

0D1L8JN Bypass Transverse Colon to Sigmoid Colon with Synthetic Substitute, Via Natural or Artificial Opening Endoscopic

0D1L8JP Bypass Transverse Colon to Rectum with Synthetic Substitute, Via Natural or Artificial Opening Endoscopic

0D1L8K4 Bypass Transverse Colon to Cutaneous with Nonautologous Tissue Substitute, Via Natural or Artificial Opening Endoscopic

0D1L8KL Bypass Transverse Colon to Transverse Colon with Nonautologous Tissue Substitute, Via Natural or Artificial Opening Endoscopic

0D1L8KM Bypass Transverse Colon to Descending Colon with Nonautologous Tissue Substitute, Via Natural or Artificial Opening Endoscopic

0D1L8KN Bypass Transverse Colon to Sigmoid Colon with Nonautologous Tissue Substitute, Via Natural or Artificial Opening Endoscopic

0D1L8KP Bypass Transverse Colon to Rectum with Nonautologous Tissue Substitute, Via Natural or Artificial Opening Endoscopic

0D1L8Z4 Bypass Transverse Colon to Cutaneous, Via Natural or Artificial Opening Endoscopic

0D1L8ZL Bypass Transverse Colon to Transverse Colon, Via Natural or Artificial Opening Endoscopic

0D1L8ZM Bypass Transverse Colon to Descending Colon, Via Natural or Artificial Opening Endoscopic

0D1L8ZN Bypass Transverse Colon to Sigmoid Colon, Via Natural or Artificial Opening Endoscopic

0D1L8ZP Bypass Transverse Colon to Rectum, Via Natural or Artificial Opening Endoscopic

0D1M074 Bypass Descending Colon to Cutaneous with Autologous Tissue Substitute, Open Approach

0D1M07M Bypass Descending Colon to Descending Colon with Autologous Tissue Substitute, Open Approach

0D1M07N Bypass Descending Colon to Sigmoid Colon with Autologous Tissue Substitute, Open Approach

0D1M07P Bypass Descending Colon to Rectum with Autologous Tissue Substitute, Open Approach

0D1M0J4 Bypass Descending Colon to Cutaneous with Synthetic Substitute, Open Approach

0D1M0JM Bypass Descending Colon to Descending Colon with Synthetic Substitute, Open Approach

0D1M0JN Bypass Descending Colon to Sigmoid Colon with Synthetic Substitute, Open Approach

0D1M0JP Bypass Descending Colon to Rectum with Synthetic Substitute, Open Approach

0D1M0K4 Bypass Descending Colon to Cutaneous with Nonautologous Tissue Substitute, Open Approach

0D1M0KM Bypass Descending Colon to Descending Colon with Nonautologous Tissue Substitute, Open Approach

0D1M0KN Bypass Descending Colon to Sigmoid Colon with Nonautologous Tissue Substitute, Open Approach

0D1M0KP Bypass Descending Colon to Rectum with Nonautologous Tissue Substitute, Open Approach

0D1M0Z4 Bypass Descending Colon to Cutaneous, Open Approach

0D1M0ZM Bypass Descending Colon to Descending Colon, Open Approach

0D1M0ZN Bypass Descending Colon to Sigmoid Colon, Open Approach

0D1M0ZP Bypass Descending Colon to Rectum, Open Approach

0D1M3J4 Bypass Descending Colon to Cutaneous with Synthetic Substitute, Percutaneous Approach

0D1M474 Bypass Descending Colon to Cutaneous with Autologous Tissue Substitute, Percutaneous Endoscopic Approach

0D1M47M Bypass Descending Colon to Descending Colon with Autologous Tissue Substitute, Percutaneous Endoscopic Approach

0D1M47N Bypass Descending Colon to Sigmoid Colon with Autologous Tissue Substitute, Percutaneous Endoscopic Approach

0D1M47P Bypass Descending Colon to Rectum with Autologous Tissue Substitute, Percutaneous Endoscopic Approach

0D1M4J4 Bypass Descending Colon to Cutaneous with Synthetic Substitute, Percutaneous Endoscopic Approach

0D1M4JM Bypass Descending Colon to Descending Colon with Synthetic Substitute, Percutaneous Endoscopic Approach

0D1M4JN Bypass Descending Colon to Sigmoid Colon with Synthetic Substitute, Percutaneous Endoscopic Approach

0D1M4JP Bypass Descending Colon to Rectum with Synthetic Substitute, Percutaneous Endoscopic Approach

0D1M4K4 Bypass Descending Colon to Cutaneous with Nonautologous Tissue Substitute, Percutaneous Endoscopic Approach

0D1M4KM Bypass Descending Colon to Descending Colon with Nonautologous Tissue Substitute, Percutaneous Endoscopic Approach

0D1M4KN Bypass Descending Colon to Sigmoid Colon with Nonautologous Tissue Substitute, Percutaneous Endoscopic Approach

0D1M4KP Bypass Descending Colon to Rectum with Nonautologous Tissue Substitute, Percutaneous Endoscopic Approach

0D1M4Z4 Bypass Descending Colon to Cutaneous, Percutaneous Endoscopic Approach

0D1M4ZM Bypass Descending Colon to Descending Colon, Percutaneous Endoscopic Approach

0D1M4ZN Bypass Descending Colon to Sigmoid Colon, Percutaneous Endoscopic Approach

0D1M4ZP Bypass Descending Colon to Rectum, Percutaneous Endoscopic Approach

0D1M874 Bypass Descending Colon to Cutaneous with Autologous Tissue Substitute, Via Natural or Artificial Opening Endoscopic

0D1M87M Bypass Descending Colon to Descending Colon with Autologous Tissue Substitute, Via Natural or Artificial Opening Endoscopic

0D1M87N Bypass Descending Colon to Sigmoid Colon with Autologous Tissue Substitute, Via Natural or Artificial Opening Endoscopic

0D1M87P Bypass Descending Colon to Rectum with Autologous Tissue Substitute, Via Natural or Artificial Opening Endoscopic

0D1M8J4 Bypass Descending Colon to Cutaneous with Synthetic Substitute, Via Natural or Artificial Opening Endoscopic

0D1M8JM Bypass Descending Colon to Descending Colon with Synthetic Substitute, Via Natural or Artificial Opening Endoscopic

0D1M8JN Bypass Descending Colon to Sigmoid Colon with Synthetic Substitute, Via Natural or Artificial Opening Endoscopic

0D1M8JP Bypass Descending Colon to Rectum with Synthetic Substitute, Via Natural or Artificial Opening Endoscopic

0D1M8K4 Bypass Descending Colon to Cutaneous with Nonautologous Tissue Substitute, Via Natural or Artificial Opening Endoscopic

0D1M8KM Bypass Descending Colon to Descending Colon with Nonautologous Tissue Substitute, Via Natural or Artificial Opening Endoscopic

0D1M8KN Bypass Descending Colon to Sigmoid Colon with Nonautologous Tissue Substitute, Via Natural or Artificial Opening Endoscopic

0D1M8KP Bypass Descending Colon to Rectum with Nonautologous Tissue Substitute, Via Natural or Artificial Opening Endoscopic

0D1M8Z4 Bypass Descending Colon to Cutaneous, Via Natural or Artificial Opening Endoscopic

0D1M8ZM Bypass Descending Colon to Descending Colon, Via Natural or Artificial Opening Endoscopic

0D1M8ZN Bypass Descending Colon to Sigmoid Colon, Via Natural or Artificial Opening Endoscopic

0D1M8ZP Bypass Descending Colon to Rectum, Via Natural or Artificial Opening Endoscopic

0D1N074 Bypass Sigmoid Colon to Cutaneous with Autologous Tissue Substitute, Open Approach

0D1N07N Bypass Sigmoid Colon to Sigmoid Colon with Autologous Tissue Substitute, Open Approach

0D1N07P Bypass Sigmoid Colon to Rectum with Autologous Tissue Substitute, Open Approach

0D1N0J4 Bypass Sigmoid Colon to Cutaneous with Synthetic Substitute, Open Approach

0D1N0JN Bypass Sigmoid Colon to Sigmoid Colon with Synthetic Substitute, Open Approach

0D1N0JP Bypass Sigmoid Colon to Rectum with Synthetic Substitute, Open Approach

0D1N0K4 Bypass Sigmoid Colon to Cutaneous with Nonautologous Tissue Substitute, Open Approach

0D1N0KN Bypass Sigmoid Colon to Sigmoid Colon with Nonautologous Tissue Substitute, Open Approach

0D1N0KP Bypass Sigmoid Colon to Rectum with Nonautologous Tissue Substitute, Open Approach

0D1N0Z4 Bypass Sigmoid Colon to Cutaneous, Open Approach

0D1N0ZN Bypass Sigmoid Colon to Sigmoid Colon, Open Approach

0D1N0ZP Bypass Sigmoid Colon to Rectum, Open Approach

0D1N3J4 Bypass Sigmoid Colon to Cutaneous with Synthetic Substitute, Percutaneous Approach

0D1N474	Bypass Sigmoid Colon to Cutaneous with Autologous Tissue Substitute, Percutaneous Endoscopic Approach
0D1N47N	Bypass Sigmoid Colon to Sigmoid Colon with Autologous Tissue Substitute, Percutaneous Endoscopic Approach
0D1N47P	Bypass Sigmoid Colon to Rectum with Autologous Tissue Substitute, Percutaneous Endoscopic Approach
0D1N4J4	Bypass Sigmoid Colon to Cutaneous with Synthetic Substitute, Percutaneous Endoscopic Approach
0D1N4JN	Bypass Sigmoid Colon to Sigmoid Colon with Synthetic Substitute, Percutaneous Endoscopic Approach
0D1N4JP	Bypass Sigmoid Colon to Rectum with Synthetic Substitute, Percutaneous Endoscopic Approach
0D1N4K4	Bypass Sigmoid Colon to Cutaneous with Nonautologous Tissue Substitute, Percutaneous Endoscopic Approach
0D1N4KN	Bypass Sigmoid Colon to Sigmoid Colon with Nonautologous Tissue Substitute, Percutaneous Endoscopic Approach
0D1N4KP	Bypass Sigmoid Colon to Rectum with Nonautologous Tissue Substitute, Percutaneous Endoscopic Approach
0D1N4Z4	Bypass Sigmoid Colon to Cutaneous, Percutaneous Endoscopic Approach
0D1N4ZN	Bypass Sigmoid Colon to Sigmoid Colon, Percutaneous Endoscopic Approach
0D1N4ZP	Bypass Sigmoid Colon to Rectum, Percutaneous Endoscopic Approach
0D1N874	Bypass Sigmoid Colon to Cutaneous with Autologous Tissue Substitute, Via Natural or Artificial Opening Endoscopic
0D1N87N	Bypass Sigmoid Colon to Sigmoid Colon with Autologous Tissue Substitute, Via Natural or Artificial Opening Endoscopic
0D1N87P	Bypass Sigmoid Colon to Rectum with Autologous Tissue Substitute, Via Natural or Artificial Opening Endoscopic
0D1N8J4	Bypass Sigmoid Colon to Cutaneous with Synthetic Substitute, Via Natural or Artificial Opening Endoscopic
0D1N8JN	Bypass Sigmoid Colon to Sigmoid Colon with Synthetic Substitute, Via Natural or Artificial Opening Endoscopic
0D1N8JP	Bypass Sigmoid Colon to Rectum with Synthetic Substitute, Via Natural or Artificial Opening Endoscopic
0D1N8K4	Bypass Sigmoid Colon to Cutaneous with Nonautologous Tissue Substitute, Via Natural or Artificial Opening Endoscopic
0D1N8KN	Bypass Sigmoid Colon to Sigmoid Colon with Nonautologous Tissue Substitute, Via Natural or Artificial Opening Endoscopic
0D1N8KP	Bypass Sigmoid Colon to Rectum with Nonautologous Tissue Substitute, Via Natural or Artificial Opening Endoscopic
0D1N8Z4	Bypass Sigmoid Colon to Cutaneous, Via Natural or Artificial Opening Endoscopic
0D1N8ZN	Bypass Sigmoid Colon to Sigmoid Colon, Via Natural or Artificial Opening Endoscopic
0D1N8ZP	Bypass Sigmoid Colon to Rectum, Via Natural or Artificial Opening Endoscopic

0D2 – Gastrointestinal System, Change

Review Coding Guideline B6.1c

0D20X0Z	Change Drainage Device in Upper Intestinal Tract, External Approach
0D20XUZ	Change Feeding Device in Upper Intestinal Tract, External Approach
0D20XYZ	Change Other Device in Upper Intestinal Tract, External Approach
0D2DX0Z	Change Drainage Device in Lower Intestinal Tract, External Approach
0D2DXUZ	Change Feeding Device in Lower Intestinal Tract, External Approach
0D2DXYZ	Change Other Device in Lower Intestinal Tract, External Approach
0D2UX0Z	Change Drainage Device in Omentum, External Approach
0D2UXYZ	Change Other Device in Omentum, External Approach
0D2VX0Z	Change Drainage Device in Mesentery, External Approach
0D2VXYZ	Change Other Device in Mesentery, External Approach
0D2WX0Z	Change Drainage Device in Peritoneum, External Approach
0D2WXYZ	Change Other Device in Peritoneum, External Approach

0D5 – Gastrointestinal System, Destruction

0D510ZZ	Destruction of Upper Esophagus, Open Approach
0D513ZZ	Destruction of Upper Esophagus, Percutaneous Approach
0D514ZZ	Destruction of Upper Esophagus, Percutaneous Endoscopic Approach
0D517ZZ	Destruction of Upper Esophagus, Via Natural or Artificial Opening
0D518ZZ	Destruction of Upper Esophagus, Via Natural or Artificial Opening Endoscopic
0D520ZZ	Destruction of Middle Esophagus, Open Approach
0D523ZZ	Destruction of Middle Esophagus, Percutaneous Approach
0D524ZZ	Destruction of Middle Esophagus, Percutaneous Endoscopic Approach
0D527ZZ	Destruction of Middle Esophagus, Via Natural or Artificial Opening
0D528ZZ	Destruction of Middle Esophagus, Via Natural or Artificial Opening Endoscopic
0D530ZZ	Destruction of Lower Esophagus, Open Approach
0D533ZZ	Destruction of Lower Esophagus, Percutaneous Approach
0D534ZZ	Destruction of Lower Esophagus, Percutaneous Endoscopic Approach
0D537ZZ	Destruction of Lower Esophagus, Via Natural or Artificial Opening
0D538ZZ	Destruction of Lower Esophagus, Via Natural or Artificial Opening Endoscopic
0D540ZZ	Destruction of Esophagogastric Junction, Open Approach
0D543ZZ	Destruction of Esophagogastric Junction, Percutaneous Approach
0D544ZZ	Destruction of Esophagogastric Junction, Percutaneous Endoscopic Approach
0D547ZZ	Destruction of Esophagogastric Junction, Via Natural or Artificial Opening
0D548ZZ	Destruction of Esophagogastric Junction, Via Natural or Artificial Opening Endoscopic
0D550ZZ	Destruction of Esophagus, Open Approach
0D553ZZ	Destruction of Esophagus, Percutaneous Approach
0D554ZZ	Destruction of Esophagus, Percutaneous Endoscopic Approach
0D557ZZ	Destruction of Esophagus, Via Natural or Artificial Opening
0D558ZZ	Destruction of Esophagus, Via Natural or Artificial Opening Endoscopic
0D560ZZ	Destruction of Stomach, Open Approach
0D563ZZ	Destruction of Stomach, Percutaneous Approach
0D564ZZ	Destruction of Stomach, Percutaneous Endoscopic Approach
0D567ZZ	Destruction of Stomach, Via Natural or Artificial Opening
0D568ZZ	Destruction of Stomach, Via Natural or Artificial Opening Endoscopic
0D570ZZ	Destruction of Stomach, Pylorus, Open Approach
0D573ZZ	Destruction of Stomach, Pylorus, Percutaneous Approach
0D574ZZ	Destruction of Stomach, Pylorus, Percutaneous Endoscopic Approach
0D577ZZ	Destruction of Stomach, Pylorus, Via Natural or Artificial Opening
0D578ZZ	Destruction of Stomach, Pylorus, Via Natural or Artificial Opening Endoscopic
0D580ZZ	Destruction of Small Intestine, Open Approach
0D583ZZ	Destruction of Small Intestine, Percutaneous Approach
0D584ZZ	Destruction of Small Intestine, Percutaneous Endoscopic Approach
0D587ZZ	Destruction of Small Intestine, Via Natural or Artificial Opening
0D588ZZ	Destruction of Small Intestine, Via Natural or Artificial Opening Endoscopic
0D590ZZ	Destruction of Duodenum, Open Approach
0D593ZZ	Destruction of Duodenum, Percutaneous Approach
0D594ZZ	Destruction of Duodenum, Percutaneous Endoscopic Approach
0D597ZZ	Destruction of Duodenum, Via Natural or Artificial Opening
0D598ZZ	Destruction of Duodenum, Via Natural or Artificial Opening Endoscopic
0D5A0ZZ	Destruction of Jejunum, Open Approach

0D5A3ZZ	Destruction of Jejunum, Percutaneous Approach
0D5A4ZZ	Destruction of Jejunum, Percutaneous Endoscopic Approach
0D5A7ZZ	Destruction of Jejunum, Via Natural or Artificial Opening
0D5A8ZZ	Destruction of Jejunum, Via Natural or Artificial Opening Endoscopic
0D5B0ZZ	Destruction of Ileum, Open Approach
0D5B3ZZ	Destruction of Ileum, Percutaneous Approach
0D5B4ZZ	Destruction of Ileum, Percutaneous Endoscopic Approach
0D5B7ZZ	Destruction of Ileum, Via Natural or Artificial Opening
0D5B8ZZ	Destruction of Ileum, Via Natural or Artificial Opening Endoscopic
0D5C0ZZ	Destruction of Ileocecal Valve, Open Approach
0D5C3ZZ	Destruction of Ileocecal Valve, Percutaneous Approach
0D5C4ZZ	Destruction of Ileocecal Valve, Percutaneous Endoscopic Approach
0D5C7ZZ	Destruction of Ileocecal Valve, Via Natural or Artificial Opening
0D5C8ZZ	Destruction of Ileocecal Valve, Via Natural or Artificial Opening Endoscopic
0D5E0ZZ	Destruction of Large Intestine, Open Approach
0D5E3ZZ	Destruction of Large Intestine, Percutaneous Approach
0D5E4ZZ	Destruction of Large Intestine, Percutaneous Endoscopic Approach
0D5E7ZZ	Destruction of Large Intestine, Via Natural or Artificial Opening
0D5E8ZZ	Destruction of Large Intestine, Via Natural or Artificial Opening Endoscopic
0D5F0ZZ	Destruction of Right Large Intestine, Open Approach
0D5F3ZZ	Destruction of Right Large Intestine, Percutaneous Approach
0D5F4ZZ	Destruction of Right Large Intestine, Percutaneous Endoscopic Approach
0D5F7ZZ	Destruction of Right Large Intestine, Via Natural or Artificial Opening
0D5F8ZZ	Destruction of Right Large Intestine, Via Natural or Artificial Opening Endoscopic
0D5G0ZZ	Destruction of Left Large Intestine, Open Approach
0D5G3ZZ	Destruction of Left Large Intestine, Percutaneous Approach
0D5G4ZZ	Destruction of Left Large Intestine, Percutaneous Endoscopic Approach
0D5G7ZZ	Destruction of Left Large Intestine, Via Natural or Artificial Opening
0D5G8ZZ	Destruction of Left Large Intestine, Via Natural or Artificial Opening Endoscopic
0D5H0ZZ	Destruction of Cecum, Open Approach
0D5H3ZZ	Destruction of Cecum, Percutaneous Approach
0D5H4ZZ	Destruction of Cecum, Percutaneous Endoscopic Approach
0D5H7ZZ	Destruction of Cecum, Via Natural or Artificial Opening
0D5H8ZZ	Destruction of Cecum, Via Natural or Artificial Opening Endoscopic
0D5J0ZZ	Destruction of Appendix, Open Approach
0D5J3ZZ	Destruction of Appendix, Percutaneous Approach
0D5J4ZZ	Destruction of Appendix, Percutaneous Endoscopic Approach
0D5J7ZZ	Destruction of Appendix, Via Natural or Artificial Opening
0D5J8ZZ	Destruction of Appendix, Via Natural or Artificial Opening Endoscopic
0D5K0ZZ	Destruction of Ascending Colon, Open Approach
0D5K3ZZ	Destruction of Ascending Colon, Percutaneous Approach
0D5K4ZZ	Destruction of Ascending Colon, Percutaneous Endoscopic Approach

0D5K7ZZ	Destruction of Ascending Colon, Via Natural or Artificial Opening
0D5K8ZZ	Destruction of Ascending Colon, Via Natural or Artificial Opening Endoscopic
0D5L0ZZ	Destruction of Transverse Colon, Open Approach
0D5L3ZZ	Destruction of Transverse Colon, Percutaneous Approach
0D5L4ZZ	Destruction of Transverse Colon, Percutaneous Endoscopic Approach
0D5L7ZZ	Destruction of Transverse Colon, Via Natural or Artificial Opening
0D5L8ZZ	Destruction of Transverse Colon, Via Natural or Artificial Opening Endoscopic
0D5M0ZZ	Destruction of Descending Colon, Open Approach
0D5M3ZZ	Destruction of Descending Colon, Percutaneous Approach
0D5M4ZZ	Destruction of Descending Colon, Percutaneous Endoscopic Approach
0D5M7ZZ	Destruction of Descending Colon, Via Natural or Artificial Opening
0D5M8ZZ	Destruction of Descending Colon, Via Natural or Artificial Opening Endoscopic
0D5N0ZZ	Destruction of Sigmoid Colon, Open Approach
0D5N3ZZ	Destruction of Sigmoid Colon, Percutaneous Approach
0D5N4ZZ	Destruction of Sigmoid Colon, Percutaneous Endoscopic Approach
0D5N7ZZ	Destruction of Sigmoid Colon, Via Natural or Artificial Opening
0D5N8ZZ	Destruction of Sigmoid Colon, Via Natural or Artificial Opening Endoscopic
0D5P0ZZ	Destruction of Rectum, Open Approach
0D5P3ZZ	Destruction of Rectum, Percutaneous Approach
0D5P4ZZ	Destruction of Rectum, Percutaneous Endoscopic Approach
0D5P7ZZ	Destruction of Rectum, Via Natural or Artificial Opening
0D5P8ZZ	Destruction of Rectum, Via Natural or Artificial Opening Endoscopic
0D5Q0ZZ	Destruction of Anus, Open Approach
0D5Q3ZZ	Destruction of Anus, Percutaneous Approach
0D5Q4ZZ	Destruction of Anus, Percutaneous Endoscopic Approach
0D5Q7ZZ	Destruction of Anus, Via Natural or Artificial Opening
0D5Q8ZZ	Destruction of Anus, Via Natural or Artificial Opening Endoscopic
0D5QXZZ	Destruction of Anus, External Approach
0D5R0ZZ	Destruction of Anal Sphincter, Open Approach
0D5R3ZZ	Destruction of Anal Sphincter, Percutaneous Approach
0D5R4ZZ	Destruction of Anal Sphincter, Percutaneous Endoscopic Approach
0D5S0ZZ	Destruction of Greater Omentum, Open Approach
0D5S3ZZ	Destruction of Greater Omentum, Percutaneous Approach
0D5S4ZZ	Destruction of Greater Omentum, Percutaneous Endoscopic Approach
0D5T0ZZ	Destruction of Lesser Omentum, Open Approach
0D5T3ZZ	Destruction of Lesser Omentum, Percutaneous Approach
0D5T4ZZ	Destruction of Lesser Omentum, Percutaneous Endoscopic Approach
0D5V0ZZ	Destruction of Mesentery, Open Approach
0D5V3ZZ	Destruction of Mesentery, Percutaneous Approach
0D5V4ZZ	Destruction of Mesentery, Percutaneous Endoscopic Approach
0D5W0ZZ	Destruction of Peritoneum, Open Approach
0D5W3ZZ	Destruction of Peritoneum, Percutaneous Approach
0D5W4ZZ	Destruction of Peritoneum, Percutaneous Endoscopic Approach

0D7 – Gastrointestinal System, Dilation

0D710DZ	Dilation of Upper Esophagus with Intraluminal Device, Open Approach
0D710ZZ	Dilation of Upper Esophagus, Open Approach
0D713DZ	Dilation of Upper Esophagus with Intraluminal Device, Percutaneous Approach
0D713ZZ	Dilation of Upper Esophagus, Percutaneous Approach
0D714DZ	Dilation of Upper Esophagus with Intraluminal Device, Percutaneous Endoscopic Approach
0D714ZZ	Dilation of Upper Esophagus, Percutaneous Endoscopic Approach
0D717DZ	Dilation of Upper Esophagus with Intraluminal Device, Via Natural or Artificial Opening
0D717ZZ	Dilation of Upper Esophagus, Via Natural or Artificial Opening
0D718DZ	Dilation of Upper Esophagus with Intraluminal Device, Via Natural or Artificial Opening Endoscopic
0D718ZZ	Dilation of Upper Esophagus, Via Natural or Artificial Opening Endoscopic

0D720DZ	Dilation of Middle Esophagus with Intraluminal Device, Open Approach
0D720ZZ	Dilation of Middle Esophagus, Open Approach
0D723DZ	Dilation of Middle Esophagus with Intraluminal Device, Percutaneous Approach
0D723ZZ	Dilation of Middle Esophagus, Percutaneous Approach
0D724DZ	Dilation of Middle Esophagus with Intraluminal Device, Percutaneous Endoscopic Approach
0D724ZZ	Dilation of Middle Esophagus, Percutaneous Endoscopic Approach
0D727DZ	Dilation of Middle Esophagus with Intraluminal Device, Via Natural or Artificial Opening
0D727ZZ	Dilation of Middle Esophagus, Via Natural or Artificial Opening
0D728DZ	Dilation of Middle Esophagus with Intraluminal Device, Via Natural or Artificial Opening Endoscopic
0D728ZZ	Dilation of Middle Esophagus, Via Natural or Artificial Opening Endoscopic

♀ Female-only   ♂ Male-only   ● Limited Coverage   ● Non-OR   HAC HAC-associated procedure   ● Non-covered procedures   ✚ Combination

0D730DZ Dilation of Lower Esophagus with Intraluminal Device, Open Approach

0D730ZZ Dilation of Lower Esophagus, Open Approach

0D733DZ Dilation of Lower Esophagus with Intraluminal Device, Percutaneous Approach

0D733ZZ Dilation of Lower Esophagus, Percutaneous Approach

0D734DZ Dilation of Lower Esophagus with Intraluminal Device, Percutaneous Endoscopic Approach

0D734ZZ Dilation of Lower Esophagus, Percutaneous Endoscopic Approach

0D737DZ Dilation of Lower Esophagus with Intraluminal Device, Via Natural or Artificial Opening

0D737ZZ Dilation of Lower Esophagus, Via Natural or Artificial Opening

0D738DZ Dilation of Lower Esophagus with Intraluminal Device, Via Natural or Artificial Opening Endoscopic

0D738ZZ Dilation of Lower Esophagus, Via Natural or Artificial Opening Endoscopic

0D740DZ Dilation of Esophagogastric Junction with Intraluminal Device, Open Approach

0D740ZZ Dilation of Esophagogastric Junction, Open Approach

0D743DZ Dilation of Esophagogastric Junction with Intraluminal Device, Percutaneous Approach

0D743ZZ Dilation of Esophagogastric Junction, Percutaneous Approach

0D744DZ Dilation of Esophagogastric Junction with Intraluminal Device, Percutaneous Endoscopic Approach

0D744ZZ Dilation of Esophagogastric Junction, Percutaneous Endoscopic Approach

0D747DZ Dilation of Esophagogastric Junction with Intraluminal Device, Via Natural or Artificial Opening

0D747ZZ Dilation of Esophagogastric Junction, Via Natural or Artificial Opening

0D748DZ Dilation of Esophagogastric Junction with Intraluminal Device, Via Natural or Artificial Opening Endoscopic

0D748ZZ Dilation of Esophagogastric Junction, Via Natural or Artificial Opening Endoscopic

0D750DZ Dilation of Esophagus with Intraluminal Device, Open Approach

0D750ZZ Dilation of Esophagus, Open Approach

0D753DZ Dilation of Esophagus with Intraluminal Device, Percutaneous Approach

0D753ZZ Dilation of Esophagus, Percutaneous Approach

0D754DZ Dilation of Esophagus with Intraluminal Device, Percutaneous Endoscopic Approach

0D754ZZ Dilation of Esophagus, Percutaneous Endoscopic Approach

0D757DZ Dilation of Esophagus with Intraluminal Device, Via Natural or Artificial Opening

0D757ZZ Dilation of Esophagus, Via Natural or Artificial Opening

0D758DZ Dilation of Esophagus with Intraluminal Device, Via Natural or Artificial Opening Endoscopic

0D758ZZ Dilation of Esophagus, Via Natural or Artificial Opening Endoscopic

0D760DZ Dilation of Stomach with Intraluminal Device, Open Approach

0D760ZZ Dilation of Stomach, Open Approach

0D763DZ Dilation of Stomach with Intraluminal Device, Percutaneous Approach

0D763ZZ Dilation of Stomach, Percutaneous Approach

0D764DZ Dilation of Stomach with Intraluminal Device, Percutaneous Endoscopic Approach

0D764ZZ Dilation of Stomach, Percutaneous Endoscopic Approach

0D767DZ Dilation of Stomach with Intraluminal Device, Via Natural or Artificial Opening

0D767ZZ Dilation of Stomach, Via Natural or Artificial Opening

0D768DZ Dilation of Stomach with Intraluminal Device, Via Natural or Artificial Opening Endoscopic

0D768ZZ Dilation of Stomach, Via Natural or Artificial Opening Endoscopic

0D770DZ Dilation of Stomach, Pylorus with Intraluminal Device, Open Approach

0D770ZZ Dilation of Stomach, Pylorus, Open Approach

0D773DZ Dilation of Stomach, Pylorus with Intraluminal Device, Percutaneous Approach

0D773ZZ Dilation of Stomach, Pylorus, Percutaneous Approach

0D774DZ Dilation of Stomach, Pylorus with Intraluminal Device, Percutaneous Endoscopic Approach

0D774ZZ Dilation of Stomach, Pylorus, Percutaneous Endoscopic Approach

0D777DZ Dilation of Stomach, Pylorus with Intraluminal Device, Via Natural or Artificial Opening

0D777ZZ Dilation of Stomach, Pylorus, Via Natural or Artificial Opening

0D778DZ Dilation of Stomach, Pylorus with Intraluminal Device, Via Natural or Artificial Opening Endoscopic

0D778ZZ Dilation of Stomach, Pylorus, Via Natural or Artificial Opening Endoscopic

0D780DZ Dilation of Small Intestine with Intraluminal Device, Open Approach

0D780ZZ Dilation of Small Intestine, Open Approach

0D783DZ Dilation of Small Intestine with Intraluminal Device, Percutaneous Approach

0D783ZZ Dilation of Small Intestine, Percutaneous Approach

0D784DZ Dilation of Small Intestine with Intraluminal Device, Percutaneous Endoscopic Approach

0D784ZZ Dilation of Small Intestine, Percutaneous Endoscopic Approach

0D787DZ Dilation of Small Intestine with Intraluminal Device, Via Natural or Artificial Opening

0D787ZZ Dilation of Small Intestine, Via Natural or Artificial Opening

0D788DZ Dilation of Small Intestine with Intraluminal Device, Via Natural or Artificial Opening Endoscopic

0D788ZZ Dilation of Small Intestine, Via Natural or Artificial Opening Endoscopic

0D790DZ Dilation of Duodenum with Intraluminal Device, Open Approach

0D790ZZ Dilation of Duodenum, Open Approach

0D793DZ Dilation of Duodenum with Intraluminal Device, Percutaneous Approach

0D793ZZ Dilation of Duodenum, Percutaneous Approach

0D794DZ Dilation of Duodenum with Intraluminal Device, Percutaneous Endoscopic Approach

0D794ZZ Dilation of Duodenum, Percutaneous Endoscopic Approach

0D797DZ Dilation of Duodenum with Intraluminal Device, Via Natural or Artificial Opening

0D797ZZ Dilation of Duodenum, Via Natural or Artificial Opening

0D798DZ Dilation of Duodenum with Intraluminal Device, Via Natural or Artificial Opening Endoscopic

0D798ZZ Dilation of Duodenum, Via Natural or Artificial Opening Endoscopic

0D7A0DZ Dilation of Jejunum with Intraluminal Device, Open Approach

0D7A0ZZ Dilation of Jejunum, Open Approach

0D7A3DZ Dilation of Jejunum with Intraluminal Device, Percutaneous Approach

0D7A3ZZ Dilation of Jejunum, Percutaneous Approach

0D7A4DZ Dilation of Jejunum with Intraluminal Device, Percutaneous Endoscopic Approach

0D7A4ZZ Dilation of Jejunum, Percutaneous Endoscopic Approach

0D7A7DZ Dilation of Jejunum with Intraluminal Device, Via Natural or Artificial Opening

0D7A7ZZ Dilation of Jejunum, Via Natural or Artificial Opening

0D7A8DZ Dilation of Jejunum with Intraluminal Device, Via Natural or Artificial Opening Endoscopic

0D7A8ZZ Dilation of Jejunum, Via Natural or Artificial Opening Endoscopic

0D7B0DZ Dilation of Ileum with Intraluminal Device, Open Approach

0D7B0ZZ Dilation of Ileum, Open Approach

0D7B3DZ Dilation of Ileum with Intraluminal Device, Percutaneous Approach

0D7B3ZZ Dilation of Ileum, Percutaneous Approach

0D7B4DZ Dilation of Ileum with Intraluminal Device, Percutaneous Endoscopic Approach

0D7B4ZZ Dilation of Ileum, Percutaneous Endoscopic Approach

0D7B7DZ Dilation of Ileum with Intraluminal Device, Via Natural or Artificial Opening

0D7B7ZZ Dilation of Ileum, Via Natural or Artificial Opening

0D7B8DZ Dilation of Ileum with Intraluminal Device, Via Natural or Artificial Opening Endoscopic

0D7B8ZZ Dilation of Ileum, Via Natural or Artificial Opening Endoscopic

0D7C0DZ Dilation of Ileocecal Valve with Intraluminal Device, Open Approach

0D7C0ZZ Dilation of Ileocecal Valve, Open Approach

0D7C3DZ Dilation of Ileocecal Valve with Intraluminal Device, Percutaneous Approach

0D7C3ZZ Dilation of Ileocecal Valve, Percutaneous Approach

0D7C4DZ Dilation of Ileocecal Valve with Intraluminal Device, Percutaneous Endoscopic Approach

0D7C4ZZ Dilation of Ileocecal Valve, Percutaneous Endoscopic Approach

0D7C7DZ Dilation of Ileocecal Valve with Intraluminal Device, Via Natural or Artificial Opening

0D7C7ZZ Dilation of Ileocecal Valve, Via Natural or Artificial Opening

0D7C8DZ Dilation of Ileocecal Valve with Intraluminal Device, Via Natural or Artificial Opening Endoscopic

0D7C8ZZ Dilation of Ileocecal Valve, Via Natural or Artificial Opening Endoscopic

0D7E0DZ Dilation of Large Intestine with Intraluminal Device, Open Approach

0D7E0ZZ Dilation of Large Intestine, Open Approach

0D7E3DZ Dilation of Large Intestine with Intraluminal Device, Percutaneous Approach

0D7E3ZZ Dilation of Large Intestine, Percutaneous Approach

0D7E4DZ Dilation of Large Intestine with Intraluminal Device, Percutaneous Endoscopic Approach

0D7E4ZZ Dilation of Large Intestine, Percutaneous Endoscopic Approach

0D7E7DZ Dilation of Large Intestine with Intraluminal Device, Via Natural or Artificial Opening

0D7E7ZZ Dilation of Large Intestine, Via Natural or Artificial Opening

0D7E8DZ Dilation of Large Intestine with Intraluminal Device, Via Natural or Artificial Opening Endoscopic

0D7E8ZZ Dilation of Large Intestine, Via Natural or Artificial Opening Endoscopic

0D7F0DZ Dilation of Right Large Intestine with Intraluminal Device, Open Approach

0D7F0ZZ Dilation of Right Large Intestine, Open Approach

0D7F3DZ Dilation of Right Large Intestine with Intraluminal Device, Percutaneous Approach

0D7F3ZZ Dilation of Right Large Intestine, Percutaneous Approach

0D7F4DZ Dilation of Right Large Intestine with Intraluminal Device, Percutaneous Endoscopic Approach

0D7F4ZZ Dilation of Right Large Intestine, Percutaneous Endoscopic Approach

0D7F7DZ Dilation of Right Large Intestine with Intraluminal Device, Via Natural or Artificial Opening

0D7F7ZZ Dilation of Right Large Intestine, Via Natural or Artificial Opening

0D7F8DZ Dilation of Right Large Intestine with Intraluminal Device, Via Natural or Artificial Opening Endoscopic

0D7F8ZZ Dilation of Right Large Intestine, Via Natural or Artificial Opening Endoscopic

0D7G0DZ Dilation of Left Large Intestine with Intraluminal Device, Open Approach

0D7G0ZZ Dilation of Left Large Intestine, Open Approach

0D7G3DZ Dilation of Left Large Intestine with Intraluminal Device, Percutaneous Approach

0D7G3ZZ Dilation of Left Large Intestine, Percutaneous Approach

0D7G4DZ Dilation of Left Large Intestine with Intraluminal Device, Percutaneous Endoscopic Approach

0D7G4ZZ Dilation of Left Large Intestine, Percutaneous Endoscopic Approach

0D7G7DZ Dilation of Left Large Intestine with Intraluminal Device, Via Natural or Artificial Opening

0D7G7ZZ Dilation of Left Large Intestine, Via Natural or Artificial Opening

0D7G8DZ Dilation of Left Large Intestine with Intraluminal Device, Via Natural or Artificial Opening Endoscopic

0D7G8ZZ Dilation of Left Large Intestine, Via Natural or Artificial Opening Endoscopic

0D7H0DZ Dilation of Cecum with Intraluminal Device, Open Approach

0D7H0ZZ Dilation of Cecum, Open Approach

0D7H3DZ Dilation of Cecum with Intraluminal Device, Percutaneous Approach

0D7H3ZZ Dilation of Cecum, Percutaneous Approach

0D7H4DZ Dilation of Cecum with Intraluminal Device, Percutaneous Endoscopic Approach

0D7H4ZZ Dilation of Cecum, Percutaneous Endoscopic Approach

0D7H7DZ Dilation of Cecum with Intraluminal Device, Via Natural or Artificial Opening

0D7H7ZZ Dilation of Cecum, Via Natural or Artificial Opening

0D7H8DZ Dilation of Cecum with Intraluminal Device, Via Natural or Artificial Opening Endoscopic

0D7H8ZZ Dilation of Cecum, Via Natural or Artificial Opening Endoscopic

0D7K0DZ Dilation of Ascending Colon with Intraluminal Device, Open Approach

0D7K0ZZ Dilation of Ascending Colon, Open Approach

0D7K3DZ Dilation of Ascending Colon with Intraluminal Device, Percutaneous Approach

0D7K3ZZ Dilation of Ascending Colon, Percutaneous Approach

0D7K4DZ Dilation of Ascending Colon with Intraluminal Device, Percutaneous Endoscopic Approach

0D7K4ZZ Dilation of Ascending Colon, Percutaneous Endoscopic Approach

0D7K7DZ Dilation of Ascending Colon with Intraluminal Device, Via Natural or Artificial Opening

0D7K7ZZ Dilation of Ascending Colon, Via Natural or Artificial Opening

0D7K8DZ Dilation of Ascending Colon with Intraluminal Device, Via Natural or Artificial Opening Endoscopic

0D7K8ZZ Dilation of Ascending Colon, Via Natural or Artificial Opening Endoscopic

0D7L0DZ Dilation of Transverse Colon with Intraluminal Device, Open Approach

0D7L0ZZ Dilation of Transverse Colon, Open Approach

0D7L3DZ Dilation of Transverse Colon with Intraluminal Device, Percutaneous Approach

0D7L3ZZ Dilation of Transverse Colon, Percutaneous Approach

0D7L4DZ Dilation of Transverse Colon with Intraluminal Device, Percutaneous Endoscopic Approach

0D7L4ZZ Dilation of Transverse Colon, Percutaneous Endoscopic Approach

0D7L7DZ Dilation of Transverse Colon with Intraluminal Device, Via Natural or Artificial Opening

0D7L7ZZ Dilation of Transverse Colon, Via Natural or Artificial Opening

0D7L8DZ Dilation of Transverse Colon with Intraluminal Device, Via Natural or Artificial Opening Endoscopic

0D7L8ZZ Dilation of Transverse Colon, Via Natural or Artificial Opening Endoscopic

0D7M0DZ Dilation of Descending Colon with Intraluminal Device, Open Approach

0D7M0ZZ Dilation of Descending Colon, Open Approach

0D7M3DZ Dilation of Descending Colon with Intraluminal Device, Percutaneous Approach

0D7M3ZZ Dilation of Descending Colon, Percutaneous Approach

0D7M4DZ Dilation of Descending Colon with Intraluminal Device, Percutaneous Endoscopic Approach

0D7M4ZZ Dilation of Descending Colon, Percutaneous Endoscopic Approach

0D7M7DZ Dilation of Descending Colon with Intraluminal Device, Via Natural or Artificial Opening

0D7M7ZZ Dilation of Descending Colon, Via Natural or Artificial Opening

0D7M8DZ Dilation of Descending Colon with Intraluminal Device, Via Natural or Artificial Opening Endoscopic

0D7M8ZZ Dilation of Descending Colon, Via Natural or Artificial Opening Endoscopic

0D7N0DZ Dilation of Sigmoid Colon with Intraluminal Device, Open Approach

0D7N0ZZ Dilation of Sigmoid Colon, Open Approach

0D7N3DZ Dilation of Sigmoid Colon with Intraluminal Device, Percutaneous Approach

0D7N3ZZ Dilation of Sigmoid Colon, Percutaneous Approach

0D7N4DZ Dilation of Sigmoid Colon with Intraluminal Device, Percutaneous Endoscopic Approach

0D7N4ZZ Dilation of Sigmoid Colon, Percutaneous Endoscopic Approach

0D7N7DZ Dilation of Sigmoid Colon with Intraluminal Device, Via Natural or Artificial Opening

0D7N7ZZ Dilation of Sigmoid Colon, Via Natural or Artificial Opening

0D7N8DZ Dilation of Sigmoid Colon with Intraluminal Device, Via Natural or Artificial Opening Endoscopic

0D7N8ZZ Dilation of Sigmoid Colon, Via Natural or Artificial Opening Endoscopic

0D7P0DZ Dilation of Rectum with Intraluminal Device, Open Approach

0D7P0ZZ Dilation of Rectum, Open Approach

0D7P3DZ Dilation of Rectum with Intraluminal Device, Percutaneous Approach

0D7P3ZZ Dilation of Rectum, Percutaneous Approach

0D7P4DZ Dilation of Rectum with Intraluminal Device, Percutaneous Endoscopic Approach

0D7P4ZZ   Dilation of Rectum, Percutaneous Endoscopic Approach
0D7P7DZ   Dilation of Rectum with Intraluminal Device, Via Natural or Artificial Opening
0D7P7ZZ   Dilation of Rectum, Via Natural or Artificial Opening
0D7P8DZ   Dilation of Rectum with Intraluminal Device, Via Natural or Artificial Opening Endoscopic
0D7P8ZZ   Dilation of Rectum, Via Natural or Artificial Opening Endoscopic
0D7Q0DZ   Dilation of Anus with Intraluminal Device, Open Approach
0D7Q0ZZ   Dilation of Anus, Open Approach
0D7Q3DZ   Dilation of Anus with Intraluminal Device, Percutaneous Approach

0D7Q3ZZ   Dilation of Anus, Percutaneous Approach
0D7Q4DZ   Dilation of Anus with Intraluminal Device, Percutaneous Endoscopic Approach
0D7Q4ZZ   Dilation of Anus, Percutaneous Endoscopic Approach
0D7Q7DZ   Dilation of Anus with Intraluminal Device, Via Natural or Artificial Opening
0D7Q7ZZ   Dilation of Anus, Via Natural or Artificial Opening
0D7Q8DZ   Dilation of Anus with Intraluminal Device, Via Natural or Artificial Opening Endoscopic
0D7Q8ZZ   Dilation of Anus, Via Natural or Artificial Opening Endoscopic

0D8 – Gastrointestinal System, Division

Review Coding Guideline B3.14

0D840ZZ   Division of Esophagogastric Junction, Open Approach
0D843ZZ   Division of Esophagogastric Junction, Percutaneous Approach
0D844ZZ   Division of Esophagogastric Junction, Percutaneous Endoscopic Approach
0D847ZZ   Division of Esophagogastric Junction, Via Natural or Artificial Opening
0D848ZZ   Division of Esophagogastric Junction, Via Natural or Artificial Opening Endoscopic

0D870ZZ   Division of Stomach, Pylorus, Open Approach
0D873ZZ   Division of Stomach, Pylorus, Percutaneous Approach
0D874ZZ   Division of Stomach, Pylorus, Percutaneous Endoscopic Approach
0D877ZZ   Division of Stomach, Pylorus, Via Natural or Artificial Opening
0D878ZZ   Division of Stomach, Pylorus, Via Natural or Artificial Opening Endoscopic
0D8R0ZZ   Division of Anal Sphincter, Open Approach
0D8R3ZZ   Division of Anal Sphincter, Percutaneous Approach

0D9 – Gastrointestinal System, Drainage

Review Coding Guidelines B3.4a and B3.4b

Review Coding Guideline B6.2

0D9100Z   Drainage of Upper Esophagus with Drainage Device, Open Approach
0D910ZX   Drainage of Upper Esophagus, Open Approach, Diagnostic
0D910ZZ   Drainage of Upper Esophagus, Open Approach
0D9130Z   Drainage of Upper Esophagus with Drainage Device, Percutaneous Approach
0D913ZX   Drainage of Upper Esophagus, Percutaneous Approach, Diagnostic
0D913ZZ   Drainage of Upper Esophagus, Percutaneous Approach
0D9140Z   Drainage of Upper Esophagus with Drainage Device, Percutaneous Endoscopic Approach
0D914ZX   Drainage of Upper Esophagus, Percutaneous Endoscopic Approach, Diagnostic
0D914ZZ   Drainage of Upper Esophagus, Percutaneous Endoscopic Approach
0D9170Z   Drainage of Upper Esophagus with Drainage Device, Via Natural or Artificial Opening
0D917ZX   Drainage of Upper Esophagus, Via Natural or Artificial Opening, Diagnostic
0D917ZZ   Drainage of Upper Esophagus, Via Natural or Artificial Opening
0D9180Z   Drainage of Upper Esophagus with Drainage Device, Via Natural or Artificial Opening Endoscopic
0D918ZX   Drainage of Upper Esophagus, Via Natural or Artificial Opening Endoscopic, Diagnostic
0D918ZZ   Drainage of Upper Esophagus, Via Natural or Artificial Opening Endoscopic
0D9200Z   Drainage of Middle Esophagus with Drainage Device, Open Approach
0D920ZX   Drainage of Middle Esophagus, Open Approach, Diagnostic
0D920ZZ   Drainage of Middle Esophagus, Open Approach
0D9230Z   Drainage of Middle Esophagus with Drainage Device, Percutaneous Approach
0D923ZX   Drainage of Middle Esophagus, Percutaneous Approach, Diagnostic
0D923ZZ   Drainage of Middle Esophagus, Percutaneous Approach
0D9240Z   Drainage of Middle Esophagus with Drainage Device, Percutaneous Endoscopic Approach
0D924ZX   Drainage of Middle Esophagus, Percutaneous Endoscopic Approach, Diagnostic
0D924ZZ   Drainage of Middle Esophagus, Percutaneous Endoscopic Approach
0D9270Z   Drainage of Middle Esophagus with Drainage Device, Via Natural or Artificial Opening
0D927ZX   Drainage of Middle Esophagus, Via Natural or Artificial Opening, Diagnostic

0D927ZZ   Drainage of Middle Esophagus, Via Natural or Artificial Opening
0D9280Z   Drainage of Middle Esophagus with Drainage Device, Via Natural or Artificial Opening Endoscopic
0D928ZX   Drainage of Middle Esophagus, Via Natural or Artificial Opening Endoscopic, Diagnostic
0D928ZZ   Drainage of Middle Esophagus, Via Natural or Artificial Opening Endoscopic
0D9300Z   Drainage of Lower Esophagus with Drainage Device, Open Approach
0D930ZX   Drainage of Lower Esophagus, Open Approach, Diagnostic
0D930ZZ   Drainage of Lower Esophagus, Open Approach
0D9330Z   Drainage of Lower Esophagus with Drainage Device, Percutaneous Approach
0D933ZX   Drainage of Lower Esophagus, Percutaneous Approach, Diagnostic
0D933ZZ   Drainage of Lower Esophagus, Percutaneous Approach
0D9340Z   Drainage of Lower Esophagus with Drainage Device, Percutaneous Endoscopic Approach
0D934ZX   Drainage of Lower Esophagus, Percutaneous Endoscopic Approach, Diagnostic
0D934ZZ   Drainage of Lower Esophagus, Percutaneous Endoscopic Approach
0D9370Z   Drainage of Lower Esophagus with Drainage Device, Via Natural or Artificial Opening
0D937ZX   Drainage of Lower Esophagus, Via Natural or Artificial Opening, Diagnostic
0D937ZZ   Drainage of Lower Esophagus, Via Natural or Artificial Opening
0D9380Z   Drainage of Lower Esophagus with Drainage Device, Via Natural or Artificial Opening Endoscopic
0D938ZX   Drainage of Lower Esophagus, Via Natural or Artificial Opening Endoscopic, Diagnostic
0D938ZZ   Drainage of Lower Esophagus, Via Natural or Artificial Opening Endoscopic
0D9400Z   Drainage of Esophagogastric Junction with Drainage Device, Open Approach
0D940ZX   Drainage of Esophagogastric Junction, Open Approach, Diagnostic
0D940ZZ   Drainage of Esophagogastric Junction, Open Approach
0D9430Z   Drainage of Esophagogastric Junction with Drainage Device, Percutaneous Approach
0D943ZX   Drainage of Esophagogastric Junction, Percutaneous Approach, Diagnostic
0D943ZZ   Drainage of Esophagogastric Junction, Percutaneous Approach
0D9440Z   Drainage of Esophagogastric Junction with Drainage Device, Percutaneous Endoscopic Approach

0D944ZX   Drainage of Esophagogastric Junction, Percutaneous Endoscopic Approach, Diagnostic

0D944ZZ   Drainage of Esophagogastric Junction, Percutaneous Endoscopic Approach

0D9470Z   Drainage of Esophagogastric Junction with Drainage Device, Via Natural or Artificial Opening

0D947ZX   Drainage of Esophagogastric Junction, Via Natural or Artificial Opening, Diagnostic

0D947ZZ   Drainage of Esophagogastric Junction, Via Natural or Artificial Opening

0D9480Z   Drainage of Esophagogastric Junction with Drainage Device, Via Natural or Artificial Opening Endoscopic

0D948ZX   Drainage of Esophagogastric Junction, Via Natural or Artificial Opening Endoscopic, Diagnostic

0D948ZZ   Drainage of Esophagogastric Junction, Via Natural or Artificial Opening Endoscopic

0D9500Z   Drainage of Esophagus with Drainage Device, Open Approach

0D950ZX   Drainage of Esophagus, Open Approach, Diagnostic

0D950ZZ   Drainage of Esophagus, Open Approach

0D9530Z   Drainage of Esophagus with Drainage Device, Percutaneous Approach

0D953ZX   Drainage of Esophagus, Percutaneous Approach, Diagnostic

0D953ZZ   Drainage of Esophagus, Percutaneous Approach

0D9540Z   Drainage of Esophagus with Drainage Device, Percutaneous Endoscopic Approach

0D954ZX   Drainage of Esophagus, Percutaneous Endoscopic Approach, Diagnostic

0D954ZZ   Drainage of Esophagus, Percutaneous Endoscopic Approach

0D9570Z   Drainage of Esophagus with Drainage Device, Via Natural or Artificial Opening

0D957ZX   Drainage of Esophagus, Via Natural or Artificial Opening, Diagnostic

0D957ZZ   Drainage of Esophagus, Via Natural or Artificial Opening

0D9580Z   Drainage of Esophagus with Drainage Device, Via Natural or Artificial Opening Endoscopic

0D958ZX   Drainage of Esophagus, Via Natural or Artificial Opening Endoscopic, Diagnostic

0D958ZZ   Drainage of Esophagus, Via Natural or Artificial Opening Endoscopic

0D9600Z   Drainage of Stomach with Drainage Device, Open Approach

0D960ZX   Drainage of Stomach, Open Approach, Diagnostic

0D960ZZ   Drainage of Stomach, Open Approach

0D9630Z   Drainage of Stomach with Drainage Device, Percutaneous Approach

0D963ZX   Drainage of Stomach, Percutaneous Approach, Diagnostic

0D963ZZ   Drainage of Stomach, Percutaneous Approach

0D9640Z   Drainage of Stomach with Drainage Device, Percutaneous Endoscopic Approach

0D964ZX   Drainage of Stomach, Percutaneous Endoscopic Approach, Diagnostic

0D964ZZ   Drainage of Stomach, Percutaneous Endoscopic Approach

0D9670Z   Drainage of Stomach with Drainage Device, Via Natural or Artificial Opening

0D967ZX   Drainage of Stomach, Via Natural or Artificial Opening, Diagnostic

0D967ZZ   Drainage of Stomach, Via Natural or Artificial Opening

0D9680Z   Drainage of Stomach with Drainage Device, Via Natural or Artificial Opening Endoscopic

0D968ZX   Drainage of Stomach, Via Natural or Artificial Opening Endoscopic, Diagnostic

0D968ZZ   Drainage of Stomach, Via Natural or Artificial Opening Endoscopic

0D9700Z   Drainage of Stomach, Pylorus with Drainage Device, Open Approach

0D970ZX   Drainage of Stomach, Pylorus, Open Approach, Diagnostic

0D970ZZ   Drainage of Stomach, Pylorus, Open Approach

0D9730Z   Drainage of Stomach, Pylorus with Drainage Device, Percutaneous Approach

0D973ZX   Drainage of Stomach, Pylorus, Percutaneous Approach, Diagnostic

0D973ZZ   Drainage of Stomach, Pylorus, Percutaneous Approach

0D9740Z   Drainage of Stomach, Pylorus with Drainage Device, Percutaneous Endoscopic Approach

0D974ZX   Drainage of Stomach, Pylorus, Percutaneous Endoscopic Approach, Diagnostic

0D974ZZ   Drainage of Stomach, Pylorus, Percutaneous Endoscopic Approach

0D9770Z   Drainage of Stomach, Pylorus with Drainage Device, Via Natural or Artificial Opening

0D977ZX   Drainage of Stomach, Pylorus, Via Natural or Artificial Opening, Diagnostic

0D977ZZ   Drainage of Stomach, Pylorus, Via Natural or Artificial Opening

0D9780Z   Drainage of Stomach, Pylorus with Drainage Device, Via Natural or Artificial Opening Endoscopic

0D978ZX   Drainage of Stomach, Pylorus, Via Natural or Artificial Opening Endoscopic, Diagnostic

0D978ZZ   Drainage of Stomach, Pylorus, Via Natural or Artificial Opening Endoscopic

0D9800Z   Drainage of Small Intestine with Drainage Device, Open Approach

0D980ZX   Drainage of Small Intestine, Open Approach, Diagnostic

0D980ZZ   Drainage of Small Intestine, Open Approach

0D9830Z   Drainage of Small Intestine with Drainage Device, Percutaneous Approach

0D983ZX   Drainage of Small Intestine, Percutaneous Approach, Diagnostic

0D983ZZ   Drainage of Small Intestine, Percutaneous Approach

0D9840Z   Drainage of Small Intestine with Drainage Device, Percutaneous Endoscopic Approach

0D984ZX   Drainage of Small Intestine, Percutaneous Endoscopic Approach, Diagnostic

0D984ZZ   Drainage of Small Intestine, Percutaneous Endoscopic Approach

0D9870Z   Drainage of Small Intestine with Drainage Device, Via Natural or Artificial Opening

0D987ZX   Drainage of Small Intestine, Via Natural or Artificial Opening, Diagnostic

0D987ZZ   Drainage of Small Intestine, Via Natural or Artificial Opening

0D9880Z   Drainage of Small Intestine with Drainage Device, Via Natural or Artificial Opening Endoscopic

0D988ZX   Drainage of Small Intestine, Via Natural or Artificial Opening Endoscopic, Diagnostic

0D988ZZ   Drainage of Small Intestine, Via Natural or Artificial Opening Endoscopic

0D9900Z   Drainage of Duodenum with Drainage Device, Open Approach

0D990ZX   Drainage of Duodenum, Open Approach, Diagnostic

0D990ZZ   Drainage of Duodenum, Open Approach

0D9930Z   Drainage of Duodenum with Drainage Device, Percutaneous Approach

0D993ZX   Drainage of Duodenum, Percutaneous Approach, Diagnostic

0D993ZZ   Drainage of Duodenum, Percutaneous Approach

0D9940Z   Drainage of Duodenum with Drainage Device, Percutaneous Endoscopic Approach

0D994ZX   Drainage of Duodenum, Percutaneous Endoscopic Approach, Diagnostic

0D994ZZ   Drainage of Duodenum, Percutaneous Endoscopic Approach

0D9970Z   Drainage of Duodenum with Drainage Device, Via Natural or Artificial Opening

0D997ZX   Drainage of Duodenum, Via Natural or Artificial Opening, Diagnostic

0D997ZZ   Drainage of Duodenum, Via Natural or Artificial Opening

0D9980Z   Drainage of Duodenum with Drainage Device, Via Natural or Artificial Opening Endoscopic

0D998ZX   Drainage of Duodenum, Via Natural or Artificial Opening Endoscopic, Diagnostic

0D998ZZ   Drainage of Duodenum, Via Natural or Artificial Opening Endoscopic

0D9A00Z   Drainage of Jejunum with Drainage Device, Open Approach

0D9A0ZX   Drainage of Jejunum, Open Approach, Diagnostic

0D9A0ZZ   Drainage of Jejunum, Open Approach

0D9A30Z   Drainage of Jejunum with Drainage Device, Percutaneous Approach

0D9A3ZX   Drainage of Jejunum, Percutaneous Approach, Diagnostic

0D9A3ZZ   Drainage of Jejunum, Percutaneous Approach

0D9A40Z   Drainage of Jejunum with Drainage Device, Percutaneous Endoscopic Approach

0D9A4ZX   Drainage of Jejunum, Percutaneous Endoscopic Approach, Diagnostic

0D9A4ZZ   Drainage of Jejunum, Percutaneous Endoscopic Approach

0D9A70Z   Drainage of Jejunum with Drainage Device, Via Natural or Artificial Opening

0D9A7ZX   Drainage of Jejunum, Via Natural or Artificial Opening, Diagnostic

0D9A7ZZ   Drainage of Jejunum, Via Natural or Artificial Opening

0D9A80Z   Drainage of Jejunum with Drainage Device, Via Natural or Artificial Opening Endoscopic

0D9A8ZX   Drainage of Jejunum, Via Natural or Artificial Opening Endoscopic, Diagnostic

0D9A8ZZ	Drainage of Jejunum, Via Natural or Artificial Opening Endoscopic
0D9B00Z	Drainage of Ileum with Drainage Device, Open Approach
0D9B0ZX	Drainage of Ileum, Open Approach, Diagnostic
0D9B0ZZ	Drainage of Ileum, Open Approach
0D9B30Z	Drainage of Ileum with Drainage Device, Percutaneous Approach
0D9B3ZX	Drainage of Ileum, Percutaneous Approach, Diagnostic
0D9B3ZZ	Drainage of Ileum, Percutaneous Approach
0D9B40Z	Drainage of Ileum with Drainage Device, Percutaneous Endoscopic Approach
0D9B4ZX	Drainage of Ileum, Percutaneous Endoscopic Approach, Diagnostic
0D9B4ZZ	Drainage of Ileum, Percutaneous Endoscopic Approach
0D9B70Z	Drainage of Ileum with Drainage Device, Via Natural or Artificial Opening
0D9B7ZX	Drainage of Ileum, Via Natural or Artificial Opening, Diagnostic
0D9B7ZZ	Drainage of Ileum, Via Natural or Artificial Opening
0D9B80Z	Drainage of Ileum with Drainage Device, Via Natural or Artificial Opening Endoscopic
0D9B8ZX	Drainage of Ileum, Via Natural or Artificial Opening Endoscopic, Diagnostic
0D9B8ZZ	Drainage of Ileum, Via Natural or Artificial Opening Endoscopic
0D9C00Z	Drainage of Ileocecal Valve with Drainage Device, Open Approach
0D9C0ZX	Drainage of Ileocecal Valve, Open Approach, Diagnostic
0D9C0ZZ	Drainage of Ileocecal Valve, Open Approach
0D9C30Z	Drainage of Ileocecal Valve with Drainage Device, Percutaneous Approach
0D9C3ZX	Drainage of Ileocecal Valve, Percutaneous Approach, Diagnostic
0D9C3ZZ	Drainage of Ileocecal Valve, Percutaneous Approach
0D9C40Z	Drainage of Ileocecal Valve with Drainage Device, Percutaneous Endoscopic Approach
0D9C4ZX	Drainage of Ileocecal Valve, Percutaneous Endoscopic Approach, Diagnostic
0D9C4ZZ	Drainage of Ileocecal Valve, Percutaneous Endoscopic Approach
0D9C70Z	Drainage of Ileocecal Valve with Drainage Device, Via Natural or Artificial Opening
0D9C7ZX	Drainage of Ileocecal Valve, Via Natural or Artificial Opening, Diagnostic
0D9C7ZZ	Drainage of Ileocecal Valve, Via Natural or Artificial Opening
0D9C80Z	Drainage of Ileocecal Valve with Drainage Device, Via Natural or Artificial Opening Endoscopic
0D9C8ZX	Drainage of Ileocecal Valve, Via Natural or Artificial Opening Endoscopic, Diagnostic
0D9C8ZZ	Drainage of Ileocecal Valve, Via Natural or Artificial Opening Endoscopic
0D9E00Z	Drainage of Large Intestine with Drainage Device, Open Approach
0D9E0ZX	Drainage of Large Intestine, Open Approach, Diagnostic
0D9E0ZZ	Drainage of Large Intestine, Open Approach
0D9E30Z	Drainage of Large Intestine with Drainage Device, Percutaneous Approach
0D9E3ZX	Drainage of Large Intestine, Percutaneous Approach, Diagnostic
0D9E3ZZ	Drainage of Large Intestine, Percutaneous Approach
0D9E40Z	Drainage of Large Intestine with Drainage Device, Percutaneous Endoscopic Approach
0D9E4ZX	Drainage of Large Intestine, Percutaneous Endoscopic Approach, Diagnostic
0D9E4ZZ	Drainage of Large Intestine, Percutaneous Endoscopic Approach
0D9E70Z	Drainage of Large Intestine with Drainage Device, Via Natural or Artificial Opening
0D9E7ZX	Drainage of Large Intestine, Via Natural or Artificial Opening, Diagnostic
0D9E7ZZ	Drainage of Large Intestine, Via Natural or Artificial Opening
0D9E80Z	Drainage of Large Intestine with Drainage Device, Via Natural or Artificial Opening Endoscopic
0D9E8ZX	Drainage of Large Intestine, Via Natural or Artificial Opening Endoscopic, Diagnostic
0D9E8ZZ	Drainage of Large Intestine, Via Natural or Artificial Opening Endoscopic
0D9F00Z	Drainage of Right Large Intestine with Drainage Device, Open Approach
0D9F0ZX	Drainage of Right Large Intestine, Open Approach, Diagnostic
0D9F0ZZ	Drainage of Right Large Intestine, Open Approach
0D9F30Z	Drainage of Right Large Intestine with Drainage Device, Percutaneous Approach
0D9F3ZX	Drainage of Right Large Intestine, Percutaneous Approach, Diagnostic
0D9F3ZZ	Drainage of Right Large Intestine, Percutaneous Approach
0D9F40Z	Drainage of Right Large Intestine with Drainage Device, Percutaneous Endoscopic Approach
0D9F4ZX	Drainage of Right Large Intestine, Percutaneous Endoscopic Approach, Diagnostic
0D9F4ZZ	Drainage of Right Large Intestine, Percutaneous Endoscopic Approach
0D9F70Z	Drainage of Right Large Intestine with Drainage Device, Via Natural or Artificial Opening
0D9F7ZX	Drainage of Right Large Intestine, Via Natural or Artificial Opening, Diagnostic
0D9F7ZZ	Drainage of Right Large Intestine, Via Natural or Artificial Opening
0D9F80Z	Drainage of Right Large Intestine with Drainage Device, Via Natural or Artificial Opening Endoscopic
0D9F8ZX	Drainage of Right Large Intestine, Via Natural or Artificial Opening Endoscopic, Diagnostic
0D9F8ZZ	Drainage of Right Large Intestine, Via Natural or Artificial Opening Endoscopic
0D9G00Z	Drainage of Left Large Intestine with Drainage Device, Open Approach
0D9G0ZX	Drainage of Left Large Intestine, Open Approach, Diagnostic
0D9G0ZZ	Drainage of Left Large Intestine, Open Approach
0D9G30Z	Drainage of Left Large Intestine with Drainage Device, Percutaneous Approach
0D9G3ZX	Drainage of Left Large Intestine, Percutaneous Approach, Diagnostic
0D9G3ZZ	Drainage of Left Large Intestine, Percutaneous Approach
0D9G40Z	Drainage of Left Large Intestine with Drainage Device, Percutaneous Endoscopic Approach
0D9G4ZX	Drainage of Left Large Intestine, Percutaneous Endoscopic Approach, Diagnostic
0D9G4ZZ	Drainage of Left Large Intestine, Percutaneous Endoscopic Approach
0D9G70Z	Drainage of Left Large Intestine with Drainage Device, Via Natural or Artificial Opening
0D9G7ZX	Drainage of Left Large Intestine, Via Natural or Artificial Opening, Diagnostic
0D9G7ZZ	Drainage of Left Large Intestine, Via Natural or Artificial Opening
0D9G80Z	Drainage of Left Large Intestine with Drainage Device, Via Natural or Artificial Opening Endoscopic
0D9G8ZX	Drainage of Left Large Intestine, Via Natural or Artificial Opening Endoscopic, Diagnostic
0D9G8ZZ	Drainage of Left Large Intestine, Via Natural or Artificial Opening Endoscopic
0D9H00Z	Drainage of Cecum with Drainage Device, Open Approach
0D9H0ZX	Drainage of Cecum, Open Approach, Diagnostic
0D9H0ZZ	Drainage of Cecum, Open Approach
0D9H30Z	Drainage of Cecum with Drainage Device, Percutaneous Approach
0D9H3ZX	Drainage of Cecum, Percutaneous Approach, Diagnostic
0D9H3ZZ	Drainage of Cecum, Percutaneous Approach
0D9H40Z	Drainage of Cecum with Drainage Device, Percutaneous Endoscopic Approach
0D9H4ZX	Drainage of Cecum, Percutaneous Endoscopic Approach, Diagnostic
0D9H4ZZ	Drainage of Cecum, Percutaneous Endoscopic Approach
0D9H70Z	Drainage of Cecum with Drainage Device, Via Natural or Artificial Opening
0D9H7ZX	Drainage of Cecum, Via Natural or Artificial Opening, Diagnostic
0D9H7ZZ	Drainage of Cecum, Via Natural or Artificial Opening
0D9H80Z	Drainage of Cecum with Drainage Device, Via Natural or Artificial Opening Endoscopic
0D9H8ZX	Drainage of Cecum, Via Natural or Artificial Opening Endoscopic, Diagnostic
0D9H8ZZ	Drainage of Cecum, Via Natural or Artificial Opening Endoscopic
0D9J00Z	Drainage of Appendix with Drainage Device, Open Approach
0D9J0ZX	Drainage of Appendix, Open Approach, Diagnostic
0D9J0ZZ	Drainage of Appendix, Open Approach
0D9J30Z	Drainage of Appendix with Drainage Device, Percutaneous Approach
0D9J3ZX	Drainage of Appendix, Percutaneous Approach, Diagnostic
0D9J3ZZ	Drainage of Appendix, Percutaneous Approach

0D9J40Z Drainage of Appendix with Drainage Device, Percutaneous Endoscopic Approach

0D9J4ZX Drainage of Appendix, Percutaneous Endoscopic Approach, Diagnostic

0D9J4ZZ Drainage of Appendix, Percutaneous Endoscopic Approach

0D9J70Z Drainage of Appendix with Drainage Device, Via Natural or Artificial Opening

0D9J7ZX Drainage of Appendix, Via Natural or Artificial Opening, Diagnostic

0D9J7ZZ Drainage of Appendix, Via Natural or Artificial Opening

0D9J80Z Drainage of Appendix with Drainage Device, Via Natural or Artificial Opening Endoscopic

0D9J8ZX Drainage of Appendix, Via Natural or Artificial Opening Endoscopic, Diagnostic

0D9J8ZZ Drainage of Appendix, Via Natural or Artificial Opening Endoscopic

0D9K00Z Drainage of Ascending Colon with Drainage Device, Open Approach

0D9K0ZX Drainage of Ascending Colon, Open Approach, Diagnostic

0D9K0ZZ Drainage of Ascending Colon, Open Approach

0D9K30Z Drainage of Ascending Colon with Drainage Device, Percutaneous Approach

0D9K3ZX Drainage of Ascending Colon, Percutaneous Approach, Diagnostic

0D9K3ZZ Drainage of Ascending Colon, Percutaneous Approach

0D9K40Z Drainage of Ascending Colon with Drainage Device, Percutaneous Endoscopic Approach

0D9K4ZX Drainage of Ascending Colon, Percutaneous Endoscopic Approach, Diagnostic

0D9K4ZZ Drainage of Ascending Colon, Percutaneous Endoscopic Approach

0D9K70Z Drainage of Ascending Colon with Drainage Device, Via Natural or Artificial Opening

0D9K7ZX Drainage of Ascending Colon, Via Natural or Artificial Opening, Diagnostic

0D9K7ZZ Drainage of Ascending Colon, Via Natural or Artificial Opening

0D9K80Z Drainage of Ascending Colon with Drainage Device, Via Natural or Artificial Opening Endoscopic

0D9K8ZX Drainage of Ascending Colon, Via Natural or Artificial Opening Endoscopic, Diagnostic

0D9K8ZZ Drainage of Ascending Colon, Via Natural or Artificial Opening Endoscopic

0D9L00Z Drainage of Transverse Colon with Drainage Device, Open Approach

0D9L0ZX Drainage of Transverse Colon, Open Approach, Diagnostic

0D9L0ZZ Drainage of Transverse Colon, Open Approach

0D9L30Z Drainage of Transverse Colon with Drainage Device, Percutaneous Approach

0D9L3ZX Drainage of Transverse Colon, Percutaneous Approach, Diagnostic

0D9L3ZZ Drainage of Transverse Colon, Percutaneous Approach

0D9L40Z Drainage of Transverse Colon with Drainage Device, Percutaneous Endoscopic Approach

0D9L4ZX Drainage of Transverse Colon, Percutaneous Endoscopic Approach, Diagnostic

0D9L4ZZ Drainage of Transverse Colon, Percutaneous Endoscopic Approach

0D9L70Z Drainage of Transverse Colon with Drainage Device, Via Natural or Artificial Opening

0D9L7ZX Drainage of Transverse Colon, Via Natural or Artificial Opening, Diagnostic

0D9L7ZZ Drainage of Transverse Colon, Via Natural or Artificial Opening

0D9L80Z Drainage of Transverse Colon with Drainage Device, Via Natural or Artificial Opening Endoscopic

0D9L8ZX Drainage of Transverse Colon, Via Natural or Artificial Opening Endoscopic, Diagnostic

0D9L8ZZ Drainage of Transverse Colon, Via Natural or Artificial Opening Endoscopic

0D9M00Z Drainage of Descending Colon with Drainage Device, Open Approach

0D9M0ZX Drainage of Descending Colon, Open Approach, Diagnostic

0D9M0ZZ Drainage of Descending Colon, Open Approach

0D9M30Z Drainage of Descending Colon with Drainage Device, Percutaneous Approach

0D9M3ZX Drainage of Descending Colon, Percutaneous Approach, Diagnostic

0D9M3ZZ Drainage of Descending Colon, Percutaneous Approach

0D9M40Z Drainage of Descending Colon with Drainage Device, Percutaneous Endoscopic Approach

0D9M4ZX Drainage of Descending Colon, Percutaneous Endoscopic Approach, Diagnostic

0D9M4ZZ Drainage of Descending Colon, Percutaneous Endoscopic Approach

0D9M70Z Drainage of Descending Colon with Drainage Device, Via Natural or Artificial Opening

0D9M7ZX Drainage of Descending Colon, Via Natural or Artificial Opening, Diagnostic

0D9M7ZZ Drainage of Descending Colon, Via Natural or Artificial Opening

0D9M80Z Drainage of Descending Colon with Drainage Device, Via Natural or Artificial Opening Endoscopic

0D9M8ZX Drainage of Descending Colon, Via Natural or Artificial Opening Endoscopic, Diagnostic

0D9M8ZZ Drainage of Descending Colon, Via Natural or Artificial Opening Endoscopic

0D9N00Z Drainage of Sigmoid Colon with Drainage Device, Open Approach

0D9N0ZX Drainage of Sigmoid Colon, Open Approach, Diagnostic

0D9N0ZZ Drainage of Sigmoid Colon, Open Approach

0D9N30Z Drainage of Sigmoid Colon with Drainage Device, Percutaneous Approach

0D9N3ZX Drainage of Sigmoid Colon, Percutaneous Approach, Diagnostic

0D9N3ZZ Drainage of Sigmoid Colon, Percutaneous Approach

0D9N40Z Drainage of Sigmoid Colon with Drainage Device, Percutaneous Endoscopic Approach

0D9N4ZX Drainage of Sigmoid Colon, Percutaneous Endoscopic Approach, Diagnostic

0D9N4ZZ Drainage of Sigmoid Colon, Percutaneous Endoscopic Approach

0D9N70Z Drainage of Sigmoid Colon with Drainage Device, Via Natural or Artificial Opening

0D9N7ZX Drainage of Sigmoid Colon, Via Natural or Artificial Opening, Diagnostic

0D9N7ZZ Drainage of Sigmoid Colon, Via Natural or Artificial Opening

0D9N80Z Drainage of Sigmoid Colon with Drainage Device, Via Natural or Artificial Opening Endoscopic

0D9N8ZX Drainage of Sigmoid Colon, Via Natural or Artificial Opening Endoscopic, Diagnostic

0D9N8ZZ Drainage of Sigmoid Colon, Via Natural or Artificial Opening Endoscopic

0D9P00Z Drainage of Rectum with Drainage Device, Open Approach

0D9P0ZX Drainage of Rectum, Open Approach, Diagnostic

0D9P0ZZ Drainage of Rectum, Open Approach

0D9P30Z Drainage of Rectum with Drainage Device, Percutaneous Approach

0D9P3ZX Drainage of Rectum, Percutaneous Approach, Diagnostic

0D9P3ZZ Drainage of Rectum, Percutaneous Approach

0D9P40Z Drainage of Rectum with Drainage Device, Percutaneous Endoscopic Approach

0D9P4ZX Drainage of Rectum, Percutaneous Endoscopic Approach, Diagnostic

0D9P4ZZ Drainage of Rectum, Percutaneous Endoscopic Approach

0D9P70Z Drainage of Rectum with Drainage Device, Via Natural or Artificial Opening

0D9P7ZX Drainage of Rectum, Via Natural or Artificial Opening, Diagnostic

0D9P7ZZ Drainage of Rectum, Via Natural or Artificial Opening

0D9P80Z Drainage of Rectum with Drainage Device, Via Natural or Artificial Opening Endoscopic

0D9P8ZX Drainage of Rectum, Via Natural or Artificial Opening Endoscopic, Diagnostic

0D9P8ZZ Drainage of Rectum, Via Natural or Artificial Opening Endoscopic

0D9Q00Z Drainage of Anus with Drainage Device, Open Approach

0D9Q0ZX Drainage of Anus, Open Approach, Diagnostic

0D9Q0ZZ Drainage of Anus, Open Approach

0D9Q30Z Drainage of Anus with Drainage Device, Percutaneous Approach

0D9Q3ZX Drainage of Anus, Percutaneous Approach, Diagnostic

0D9Q3ZZ Drainage of Anus, Percutaneous Approach

0D9Q40Z Drainage of Anus with Drainage Device, Percutaneous Endoscopic Approach

0D9Q4ZX Drainage of Anus, Percutaneous Endoscopic Approach, Diagnostic

0D9Q4ZZ Drainage of Anus, Percutaneous Endoscopic Approach

0D9Q70Z Drainage of Anus with Drainage Device, Via Natural or Artificial Opening

0D9Q7ZX	Drainage of Anus, Via Natural or Artificial Opening, Diagnostic
0D9Q7ZZ	Drainage of Anus, Via Natural or Artificial Opening
0D9Q80Z	Drainage of Anus with Drainage Device, Via Natural or Artificial Opening Endoscopic
0D9Q8ZX	Drainage of Anus, Via Natural or Artificial Opening Endoscopic, Diagnostic
0D9Q8ZZ	Drainage of Anus, Via Natural or Artificial Opening Endoscopic
0D9QX0Z	Drainage of Anus with Drainage Device, External Approach
0D9QXZX	Drainage of Anus, External Approach, Diagnostic
0D9QXZZ	Drainage of Anus, External Approach
0D9R00Z	Drainage of Anal Sphincter with Drainage Device, Open Approach
0D9R0ZX	Drainage of Anal Sphincter, Open Approach, Diagnostic
0D9R0ZZ	Drainage of Anal Sphincter, Open Approach
0D9R30Z	Drainage of Anal Sphincter with Drainage Device, Percutaneous Approach
0D9R3ZX	Drainage of Anal Sphincter, Percutaneous Approach, Diagnostic
0D9R3ZZ	Drainage of Anal Sphincter, Percutaneous Approach
0D9R40Z	Drainage of Anal Sphincter with Drainage Device, Percutaneous Endoscopic Approach
0D9R4ZX	Drainage of Anal Sphincter, Percutaneous Endoscopic Approach, Diagnostic
0D9R4ZZ	Drainage of Anal Sphincter, Percutaneous Endoscopic Approach
0D9S00Z	Drainage of Greater Omentum with Drainage Device, Open Approach
0D9S0ZX	Drainage of Greater Omentum, Open Approach, Diagnostic
0D9S0ZZ	Drainage of Greater Omentum, Open Approach
0D9S30Z	Drainage of Greater Omentum with Drainage Device, Percutaneous Approach
0D9S3ZX	Drainage of Greater Omentum, Percutaneous Approach, Diagnostic
0D9S3ZZ	Drainage of Greater Omentum, Percutaneous Approach
0D9S40Z	Drainage of Greater Omentum with Drainage Device, Percutaneous Endoscopic Approach
0D9S4ZX	Drainage of Greater Omentum, Percutaneous Endoscopic Approach, Diagnostic
0D9S4ZZ	Drainage of Greater Omentum, Percutaneous Endoscopic Approach
0D9T00Z	Drainage of Lesser Omentum with Drainage Device, Open Approach
0D9T0ZX	Drainage of Lesser Omentum, Open Approach, Diagnostic
0D9T0ZZ	Drainage of Lesser Omentum, Open Approach
0D9T30Z	Drainage of Lesser Omentum with Drainage Device, Percutaneous Approach
0D9T3ZX	Drainage of Lesser Omentum, Percutaneous Approach, Diagnostic
0D9T3ZZ	Drainage of Lesser Omentum, Percutaneous Approach
0D9T40Z	Drainage of Lesser Omentum with Drainage Device, Percutaneous Endoscopic Approach
0D9T4ZX	Drainage of Lesser Omentum, Percutaneous Endoscopic Approach, Diagnostic
0D9T4ZZ	Drainage of Lesser Omentum, Percutaneous Endoscopic Approach
0D9V00Z	Drainage of Mesentery with Drainage Device, Open Approach
0D9V0ZX	Drainage of Mesentery, Open Approach, Diagnostic
0D9V0ZZ	Drainage of Mesentery, Open Approach
0D9V30Z	Drainage of Mesentery with Drainage Device, Percutaneous Approach
0D9V3ZX	Drainage of Mesentery, Percutaneous Approach, Diagnostic
0D9V3ZZ	Drainage of Mesentery, Percutaneous Approach
0D9V40Z	Drainage of Mesentery with Drainage Device, Percutaneous Endoscopic Approach
0D9V4ZX	Drainage of Mesentery, Percutaneous Endoscopic Approach, Diagnostic
0D9V4ZZ	Drainage of Mesentery, Percutaneous Endoscopic Approach
0D9W00Z	Drainage of Peritoneum with Drainage Device, Open Approach
0D9W0ZX	Drainage of Peritoneum, Open Approach, Diagnostic
0D9W0ZZ	Drainage of Peritoneum, Open Approach
0D9W30Z	Drainage of Peritoneum with Drainage Device, Percutaneous Approach
0D9W3ZX	Drainage of Peritoneum, Percutaneous Approach, Diagnostic
0D9W3ZZ	Drainage of Peritoneum, Percutaneous Approach
0D9W40Z	Drainage of Peritoneum with Drainage Device, Percutaneous Endoscopic Approach
0D9W4ZX	Drainage of Peritoneum, Percutaneous Endoscopic Approach, Diagnostic
0D9W4ZZ	Drainage of Peritoneum, Percutaneous Endoscopic Approach

0DB – Gastrointestinal System, Excision

Review Coding Guidelines B3.4a and B3.4b

Review Coding Guideline B3.8

0DB10ZX	Excision of Upper Esophagus, Open Approach, Diagnostic
0DB10ZZ	Excision of Upper Esophagus, Open Approach
0DB13ZX	Excision of Upper Esophagus, Percutaneous Approach, Diagnostic
0DB13ZZ	Excision of Upper Esophagus, Percutaneous Approach
0DB14ZX	Excision of Upper Esophagus, Percutaneous Endoscopic Approach, Diagnostic
0DB14ZZ	Excision of Upper Esophagus, Percutaneous Endoscopic Approach
0DB17ZX	Excision of Upper Esophagus, Via Natural or Artificial Opening, Diagnostic
0DB17ZZ	Excision of Upper Esophagus, Via Natural or Artificial Opening
0DB18ZX	Excision of Upper Esophagus, Via Natural or Artificial Opening Endoscopic, Diagnostic
0DB18ZZ	Excision of Upper Esophagus, Via Natural or Artificial Opening Endoscopic
0DB20ZX	Excision of Middle Esophagus, Open Approach, Diagnostic
0DB20ZZ	Excision of Middle Esophagus, Open Approach
0DB23ZX	Excision of Middle Esophagus, Percutaneous Approach, Diagnostic
0DB23ZZ	Excision of Middle Esophagus, Percutaneous Approach
0DB24ZX	Excision of Middle Esophagus, Percutaneous Endoscopic Approach, Diagnostic
0DB24ZZ	Excision of Middle Esophagus, Percutaneous Endoscopic Approach
0DB27ZX	Excision of Middle Esophagus, Via Natural or Artificial Opening, Diagnostic
0DB27ZZ	Excision of Middle Esophagus, Via Natural or Artificial Opening
0DB28ZX	Excision of Middle Esophagus, Via Natural or Artificial Opening Endoscopic, Diagnostic
0DB28ZZ	Excision of Middle Esophagus, Via Natural or Artificial Opening Endoscopic
0DB30ZX	Excision of Lower Esophagus, Open Approach, Diagnostic
0DB30ZZ	Excision of Lower Esophagus, Open Approach
0DB33ZX	Excision of Lower Esophagus, Percutaneous Approach, Diagnostic
0DB33ZZ	Excision of Lower Esophagus, Percutaneous Approach
0DB34ZX	Excision of Lower Esophagus, Percutaneous Endoscopic Approach, Diagnostic
0DB34ZZ	Excision of Lower Esophagus, Percutaneous Endoscopic Approach
0DB37ZX	Excision of Lower Esophagus, Via Natural or Artificial Opening, Diagnostic
0DB37ZZ	Excision of Lower Esophagus, Via Natural or Artificial Opening
0DB38ZX	Excision of Lower Esophagus, Via Natural or Artificial Opening Endoscopic, Diagnostic
0DB38ZZ	Excision of Lower Esophagus, Via Natural or Artificial Opening Endoscopic
0DB40ZX	Excision of Esophagogastric Junction, Open Approach, Diagnostic
0DB40ZZ	Excision of Esophagogastric Junction, Open Approach
0DB43ZX	Excision of Esophagogastric Junction, Percutaneous Approach, Diagnostic
0DB43ZZ	Excision of Esophagogastric Junction, Percutaneous Approach
0DB44ZX	Excision of Esophagogastric Junction, Percutaneous Endoscopic Approach, Diagnostic
0DB44ZZ	Excision of Esophagogastric Junction, Percutaneous Endoscopic Approach

0DB47ZX Excision of Esophagogastric Junction, Via Natural or Artificial Opening, Diagnostic

0DB47ZZ Excision of Esophagogastric Junction, Via Natural or Artificial Opening

0DB48ZX Excision of Esophagogastric Junction, Via Natural or Artificial Opening Endoscopic, Diagnostic

0DB48ZZ Excision of Esophagogastric Junction, Via Natural or Artificial Opening Endoscopic

0DB50ZX Excision of Esophagus, Open Approach, Diagnostic

0DB50ZZ Excision of Esophagus, Open Approach

0DB53ZX Excision of Esophagus, Percutaneous Approach, Diagnostic

0DB53ZZ Excision of Esophagus, Percutaneous Approach

0DB54ZX Excision of Esophagus, Percutaneous Endoscopic Approach, Diagnostic

0DB54ZZ Excision of Esophagus, Percutaneous Endoscopic Approach

0DB57ZX Excision of Esophagus, Via Natural or Artificial Opening, Diagnostic

0DB57ZZ Excision of Esophagus, Via Natural or Artificial Opening

0DB58ZX Excision of Esophagus, Via Natural or Artificial Opening Endoscopic, Diagnostic

0DB58ZZ Excision of Esophagus, Via Natural or Artificial Opening Endoscopic

0DB60Z3 Excision of Stomach, Open Approach, Vertical

0DB60ZX Excision of Stomach, Open Approach, Diagnostic

0DB60ZZ Excision of Stomach, Open Approach

0DB63Z3 Excision of Stomach, Percutaneous Approach, Vertical

0DB63ZX Excision of Stomach, Percutaneous Approach, Diagnostic

0DB63ZZ Excision of Stomach, Percutaneous Approach

0DB64Z3 Excision of Stomach, Percutaneous Endoscopic Approach, Vertical

0DB64ZX Excision of Stomach, Percutaneous Endoscopic Approach, Diagnostic

0DB64ZZ Excision of Stomach, Percutaneous Endoscopic Approach

0DB67Z3 Excision of Stomach, Via Natural or Artificial Opening, Vertical

0DB67ZX Excision of Stomach, Via Natural or Artificial Opening, Diagnostic

0DB67ZZ Excision of Stomach, Via Natural or Artificial Opening

0DB68Z3 Excision of Stomach, Via Natural or Artificial Opening Endoscopic, Vertical

0DB68ZX Excision of Stomach, Via Natural or Artificial Opening Endoscopic, Diagnostic

0DB68ZZ Excision of Stomach, Via Natural or Artificial Opening Endoscopic

0DB70ZX Excision of Stomach, Pylorus, Open Approach, Diagnostic

0DB70ZZ Excision of Stomach, Pylorus, Open Approach

0DB73ZX Excision of Stomach, Pylorus, Percutaneous Approach, Diagnostic

0DB73ZZ Excision of Stomach, Pylorus, Percutaneous Approach

0DB74ZX Excision of Stomach, Pylorus, Percutaneous Endoscopic Approach, Diagnostic

0DB74ZZ Excision of Stomach, Pylorus, Percutaneous Endoscopic Approach

0DB77ZX Excision of Stomach, Pylorus, Via Natural or Artificial Opening, Diagnostic

0DB77ZZ Excision of Stomach, Pylorus, Via Natural or Artificial Opening

0DB78ZX Excision of Stomach, Pylorus, Via Natural or Artificial Opening Endoscopic, Diagnostic

0DB78ZZ Excision of Stomach, Pylorus, Via Natural or Artificial Opening Endoscopic

0DB80ZX Excision of Small Intestine, Open Approach, Diagnostic

0DB80ZZ Excision of Small Intestine, Open Approach

0DB83ZX Excision of Small Intestine, Percutaneous Approach, Diagnostic

0DB83ZZ Excision of Small Intestine, Percutaneous Approach

0DB84ZX Excision of Small Intestine, Percutaneous Endoscopic Approach, Diagnostic

0DB84ZZ Excision of Small Intestine, Percutaneous Endoscopic Approach

0DB87ZX Excision of Small Intestine, Via Natural or Artificial Opening, Diagnostic

0DB87ZZ Excision of Small Intestine, Via Natural or Artificial Opening

0DB88ZX Excision of Small Intestine, Via Natural or Artificial Opening Endoscopic, Diagnostic

0DB88ZZ Excision of Small Intestine, Via Natural or Artificial Opening Endoscopic

0DB90ZX Excision of Duodenum, Open Approach, Diagnostic

0DB90ZZ Excision of Duodenum, Open Approach

0DB93ZX Excision of Duodenum, Percutaneous Approach, Diagnostic

0DB93ZZ Excision of Duodenum, Percutaneous Approach

0DB94ZX Excision of Duodenum, Percutaneous Endoscopic Approach, Diagnostic

0DB94ZZ Excision of Duodenum, Percutaneous Endoscopic Approach

0DB97ZX Excision of Duodenum, Via Natural or Artificial Opening, Diagnostic

0DB97ZZ Excision of Duodenum, Via Natural or Artificial Opening

0DB98ZX Excision of Duodenum, Via Natural or Artificial Opening Endoscopic, Diagnostic

0DB98ZZ Excision of Duodenum, Via Natural or Artificial Opening Endoscopic

0DBA0ZX Excision of Jejunum, Open Approach, Diagnostic

0DBA0ZZ Excision of Jejunum, Open Approach

0DBA3ZX Excision of Jejunum, Percutaneous Approach, Diagnostic

0DBA3ZZ Excision of Jejunum, Percutaneous Approach

0DBA4ZX Excision of Jejunum, Percutaneous Endoscopic Approach, Diagnostic

0DBA4ZZ Excision of Jejunum, Percutaneous Endoscopic Approach

0DBA7ZX Excision of Jejunum, Via Natural or Artificial Opening, Diagnostic

0DBA7ZZ Excision of Jejunum, Via Natural or Artificial Opening

0DBA8ZX Excision of Jejunum, Via Natural or Artificial Opening Endoscopic, Diagnostic

0DBA8ZZ Excision of Jejunum, Via Natural or Artificial Opening Endoscopic

0DBB0ZX Excision of Ileum, Open Approach, Diagnostic

0DBB0ZZ Excision of Ileum, Open Approach

0DBB3ZX Excision of Ileum, Percutaneous Approach, Diagnostic

0DBB3ZZ Excision of Ileum, Percutaneous Approach

0DBB4ZX Excision of Ileum, Percutaneous Endoscopic Approach, Diagnostic

0DBB4ZZ Excision of Ileum, Percutaneous Endoscopic Approach

0DBB7ZX Excision of Ileum, Via Natural or Artificial Opening, Diagnostic

0DBB7ZZ Excision of Ileum, Via Natural or Artificial Opening

0DBB8ZX Excision of Ileum, Via Natural or Artificial Opening Endoscopic, Diagnostic

0DBB8ZZ Excision of Ileum, Via Natural or Artificial Opening Endoscopic

0DBC0ZX Excision of Ileocecal Valve, Open Approach, Diagnostic

0DBC0ZZ Excision of Ileocecal Valve, Open Approach

0DBC3ZX Excision of Ileocecal Valve, Percutaneous Approach, Diagnostic

0DBC3ZZ Excision of Ileocecal Valve, Percutaneous Approach

0DBC4ZX Excision of Ileocecal Valve, Percutaneous Endoscopic Approach, Diagnostic

0DBC4ZZ Excision of Ileocecal Valve, Percutaneous Endoscopic Approach

0DBC7ZX Excision of Ileocecal Valve, Via Natural or Artificial Opening, Diagnostic

0DBC7ZZ Excision of Ileocecal Valve, Via Natural or Artificial Opening

0DBC8ZX Excision of Ileocecal Valve, Via Natural or Artificial Opening Endoscopic, Diagnostic

0DBC8ZZ Excision of Ileocecal Valve, Via Natural or Artificial Opening Endoscopic

0DBE0ZX Excision of Large Intestine, Open Approach, Diagnostic

0DBE0ZZ Excision of Large Intestine, Open Approach

0DBE3ZX Excision of Large Intestine, Percutaneous Approach, Diagnostic

0DBE3ZZ Excision of Large Intestine, Percutaneous Approach

0DBE4ZX Excision of Large Intestine, Percutaneous Endoscopic Approach, Diagnostic

0DBE4ZZ Excision of Large Intestine, Percutaneous Endoscopic Approach

0DBE7ZX Excision of Large Intestine, Via Natural or Artificial Opening, Diagnostic

0DBE7ZZ Excision of Large Intestine, Via Natural or Artificial Opening

0DBE8ZX Excision of Large Intestine, Via Natural or Artificial Opening Endoscopic, Diagnostic

0DBE8ZZ Excision of Large Intestine, Via Natural or Artificial Opening Endoscopic

0DBF0ZX Excision of Right Large Intestine, Open Approach, Diagnostic

0DBF0ZZ Excision of Right Large Intestine, Open Approach

0DBF3ZX Excision of Right Large Intestine, Percutaneous Approach, Diagnostic

0DBF3ZZ Excision of Right Large Intestine, Percutaneous Approach

0DBF4ZX Excision of Right Large Intestine, Percutaneous Endoscopic Approach, Diagnostic

0DBF4ZZ Excision of Right Large Intestine, Percutaneous Endoscopic Approach

0DBF7ZX Excision of Right Large Intestine, Via Natural or Artificial Opening, Diagnostic

0DBF7ZZ Excision of Right Large Intestine, Via Natural or Artificial Opening

0DBF8ZX Excision of Right Large Intestine, Via Natural or Artificial Opening Endoscopic, Diagnostic

0DBF8ZZ Excision of Right Large Intestine, Via Natural or Artificial Opening Endoscopic

0DBG0ZX Excision of Left Large Intestine, Open Approach, Diagnostic

0DBG0ZZ Excision of Left Large Intestine, Open Approach

0DBG3ZX Excision of Left Large Intestine, Percutaneous Approach, Diagnostic

0DBG3ZZ Excision of Left Large Intestine, Percutaneous Approach

0DBG4ZX Excision of Left Large Intestine, Percutaneous Endoscopic Approach, Diagnostic

0DBG4ZZ Excision of Left Large Intestine, Percutaneous Endoscopic Approach

0DBG7ZX Excision of Left Large Intestine, Via Natural or Artificial Opening, Diagnostic

0DBG7ZZ Excision of Left Large Intestine, Via Natural or Artificial Opening

0DBG8ZX Excision of Left Large Intestine, Via Natural or Artificial Opening Endoscopic, Diagnostic

0DBG8ZZ Excision of Left Large Intestine, Via Natural or Artificial Opening Endoscopic

0DBH0ZX Excision of Cecum, Open Approach, Diagnostic

0DBH0ZZ Excision of Cecum, Open Approach

0DBH3ZX Excision of Cecum, Percutaneous Approach, Diagnostic

0DBH3ZZ Excision of Cecum, Percutaneous Approach

0DBH4ZX Excision of Cecum, Percutaneous Endoscopic Approach, Diagnostic

0DBH4ZZ Excision of Cecum, Percutaneous Endoscopic Approach

0DBH7ZX Excision of Cecum, Via Natural or Artificial Opening, Diagnostic

0DBH7ZZ Excision of Cecum, Via Natural or Artificial Opening

0DBH8ZX Excision of Cecum, Via Natural or Artificial Opening Endoscopic, Diagnostic

0DBH8ZZ Excision of Cecum, Via Natural or Artificial Opening Endoscopic

0DBJ0ZX Excision of Appendix, Open Approach, Diagnostic

0DBJ0ZZ Excision of Appendix, Open Approach

0DBJ3ZX Excision of Appendix, Percutaneous Approach, Diagnostic

0DBJ3ZZ Excision of Appendix, Percutaneous Approach

0DBJ4ZX Excision of Appendix, Percutaneous Endoscopic Approach, Diagnostic

0DBJ4ZZ Excision of Appendix, Percutaneous Endoscopic Approach

0DBJ7ZX Excision of Appendix, Via Natural or Artificial Opening, Diagnostic

0DBJ7ZZ Excision of Appendix, Via Natural or Artificial Opening

0DBJ8ZX Excision of Appendix, Via Natural or Artificial Opening Endoscopic, Diagnostic

0DBJ8ZZ Excision of Appendix, Via Natural or Artificial Opening Endoscopic

0DBK0ZX Excision of Ascending Colon, Open Approach, Diagnostic

0DBK0ZZ Excision of Ascending Colon, Open Approach

0DBK3ZX Excision of Ascending Colon, Percutaneous Approach, Diagnostic

0DBK3ZZ Excision of Ascending Colon, Percutaneous Approach

0DBK4ZX Excision of Ascending Colon, Percutaneous Endoscopic Approach, Diagnostic

0DBK4ZZ Excision of Ascending Colon, Percutaneous Endoscopic Approach

0DBK7ZX Excision of Ascending Colon, Via Natural or Artificial Opening, Diagnostic

0DBK7ZZ Excision of Ascending Colon, Via Natural or Artificial Opening

0DBK8ZX Excision of Ascending Colon, Via Natural or Artificial Opening Endoscopic, Diagnostic

0DBK8ZZ Excision of Ascending Colon, Via Natural or Artificial Opening Endoscopic

0DBL0ZX Excision of Transverse Colon, Open Approach, Diagnostic

0DBL0ZZ Excision of Transverse Colon, Open Approach

0DBL3ZX Excision of Transverse Colon, Percutaneous Approach, Diagnostic

0DBL3ZZ Excision of Transverse Colon, Percutaneous Approach

0DBL4ZX Excision of Transverse Colon, Percutaneous Endoscopic Approach, Diagnostic

0DBL4ZZ Excision of Transverse Colon, Percutaneous Endoscopic Approach

0DBL7ZX Excision of Transverse Colon, Via Natural or Artificial Opening, Diagnostic

0DBL7ZZ Excision of Transverse Colon, Via Natural or Artificial Opening

0DBL8ZX Excision of Transverse Colon, Via Natural or Artificial Opening Endoscopic, Diagnostic

0DBL8ZZ Excision of Transverse Colon, Via Natural or Artificial Opening Endoscopic

0DBM0ZX Excision of Descending Colon, Open Approach, Diagnostic

0DBM0ZZ Excision of Descending Colon, Open Approach

0DBM3ZX Excision of Descending Colon, Percutaneous Approach, Diagnostic

0DBM3ZZ Excision of Descending Colon, Percutaneous Approach

0DBM4ZX Excision of Descending Colon, Percutaneous Endoscopic Approach, Diagnostic

0DBM4ZZ Excision of Descending Colon, Percutaneous Endoscopic Approach

0DBM7ZX Excision of Descending Colon, Via Natural or Artificial Opening, Diagnostic

0DBM7ZZ Excision of Descending Colon, Via Natural or Artificial Opening

0DBM8ZX Excision of Descending Colon, Via Natural or Artificial Opening Endoscopic, Diagnostic

0DBM8ZZ Excision of Descending Colon, Via Natural or Artificial Opening Endoscopic

0DBN0ZX Excision of Sigmoid Colon, Open Approach, Diagnostic

0DBN0ZZ Excision of Sigmoid Colon, Open Approach

0DBN3ZX Excision of Sigmoid Colon, Percutaneous Approach, Diagnostic

0DBN3ZZ Excision of Sigmoid Colon, Percutaneous Approach

0DBN4ZX Excision of Sigmoid Colon, Percutaneous Endoscopic Approach, Diagnostic

0DBN4ZZ Excision of Sigmoid Colon, Percutaneous Endoscopic Approach

0DBN7ZX Excision of Sigmoid Colon, Via Natural or Artificial Opening, Diagnostic

0DBN7ZZ Excision of Sigmoid Colon, Via Natural or Artificial Opening

0DBN8ZX Excision of Sigmoid Colon, Via Natural or Artificial Opening Endoscopic, Diagnostic

0DBN8ZZ Excision of Sigmoid Colon, Via Natural or Artificial Opening Endoscopic

0DBP0ZX Excision of Rectum, Open Approach, Diagnostic

0DBP0ZZ Excision of Rectum, Open Approach

0DBP3ZX Excision of Rectum, Percutaneous Approach, Diagnostic

0DBP3ZZ Excision of Rectum, Percutaneous Approach

0DBP4ZX Excision of Rectum, Percutaneous Endoscopic Approach, Diagnostic

0DBP4ZZ Excision of Rectum, Percutaneous Endoscopic Approach

0DBP7ZX Excision of Rectum, Via Natural or Artificial Opening, Diagnostic

0DBP7ZZ Excision of Rectum, Via Natural or Artificial Opening

0DBP8ZX Excision of Rectum, Via Natural or Artificial Opening Endoscopic, Diagnostic

0DBP8ZZ Excision of Rectum, Via Natural or Artificial Opening Endoscopic

0DBQ0ZX Excision of Anus, Open Approach, Diagnostic

0DBQ0ZZ Excision of Anus, Open Approach

0DBQ3ZX Excision of Anus, Percutaneous Approach, Diagnostic

0DBQ3ZZ Excision of Anus, Percutaneous Approach

0DBQ4ZX Excision of Anus, Percutaneous Endoscopic Approach, Diagnostic

0DBQ4ZZ Excision of Anus, Percutaneous Endoscopic Approach

0DBQ7ZX Excision of Anus, Via Natural or Artificial Opening, Diagnostic

0DBQ7ZZ Excision of Anus, Via Natural or Artificial Opening

0DBQ8ZX Excision of Anus, Via Natural or Artificial Opening Endoscopic, Diagnostic

0DBQ8ZZ Excision of Anus, Via Natural or Artificial Opening Endoscopic

0DBQXZX Excision of Anus, External Approach, Diagnostic

0DBQXZZ Excision of Anus, External Approach

0DBR0ZX Excision of Anal Sphincter, Open Approach, Diagnostic

0DBR0ZZ Excision of Anal Sphincter, Open Approach

0DBR3ZX Excision of Anal Sphincter, Percutaneous Approach, Diagnostic

0DBR3ZZ Excision of Anal Sphincter, Percutaneous Approach

0DBR4ZX Excision of Anal Sphincter, Percutaneous Endoscopic Approach, Diagnostic

0DBR4ZZ Excision of Anal Sphincter, Percutaneous Endoscopic Approach

0DBS0ZX Excision of Greater Omentum, Open Approach, Diagnostic

0DBS0ZZ Excision of Greater Omentum, Open Approach

0DBS3ZX Excision of Greater Omentum, Percutaneous Approach, Diagnostic

0DBS3ZZ Excision of Greater Omentum, Percutaneous Approach

0DBS4ZX Excision of Greater Omentum, Percutaneous Endoscopic Approach, Diagnostic

0DBS4ZZ Excision of Greater Omentum, Percutaneous Endoscopic Approach

0DBT0ZX Excision of Lesser Omentum, Open Approach, Diagnostic

0DBT0ZZ Excision of Lesser Omentum, Open Approach

0DBT3ZX Excision of Lesser Omentum, Percutaneous Approach, Diagnostic

0DBT3ZZ Excision of Lesser Omentum, Percutaneous Approach

♀ Female-only   ♂ Male-only   ◯ Limited Coverage   ● Non-OR   🅷🅰🅲 HAC-associated procedure   ⬢ Non-covered procedures   ✚ Combination

0DBT4ZX Excision of Lesser Omentum, Percutaneous Endoscopic Approach, Diagnostic
0DBT4ZZ Excision of Lesser Omentum, Percutaneous Endoscopic Approach
0DBV0ZX Excision of Mesentery, Open Approach, Diagnostic
0DBV0ZZ Excision of Mesentery, Open Approach
0DBV3ZX Excision of Mesentery, Percutaneous Approach, Diagnostic
0DBV3ZZ Excision of Mesentery, Percutaneous Approach
0DBV4ZX Excision of Mesentery, Percutaneous Endoscopic Approach, Diagnostic

0DBV4ZZ Excision of Mesentery, Percutaneous Endoscopic Approach
0DBW0ZX Excision of Peritoneum, Open Approach, Diagnostic
0DBW0ZZ Excision of Peritoneum, Open Approach
0DBW3ZX Excision of Peritoneum, Percutaneous Approach, Diagnostic
0DBW3ZZ Excision of Peritoneum, Percutaneous Approach
0DBW4ZX Excision of Peritoneum, Percutaneous Endoscopic Approach, Diagnostic
0DBW4ZZ Excision of Peritoneum, Percutaneous Endoscopic Approach

0DC – Gastrointestinal System, Extirpation

0DC10ZZ Extirpation of Matter from Upper Esophagus, Open Approach
0DC13ZZ Extirpation of Matter from Upper Esophagus, Percutaneous Approach
0DC14ZZ Extirpation of Matter from Upper Esophagus, Percutaneous Endoscopic Approach
0DC17ZZ Extirpation of Matter from Upper Esophagus, Via Natural or Artificial Opening
0DC18ZZ Extirpation of Matter from Upper Esophagus, Via Natural or Artificial Opening Endoscopic
0DC20ZZ Extirpation of Matter from Middle Esophagus, Open Approach
0DC23ZZ Extirpation of Matter from Middle Esophagus, Percutaneous Approach
0DC24ZZ Extirpation of Matter from Middle Esophagus, Percutaneous Endoscopic Approach
0DC27ZZ Extirpation of Matter from Middle Esophagus, Via Natural or Artificial Opening
0DC28ZZ Extirpation of Matter from Middle Esophagus, Via Natural or Artificial Opening Endoscopic
0DC30ZZ Extirpation of Matter from Lower Esophagus, Open Approach
0DC33ZZ Extirpation of Matter from Lower Esophagus, Percutaneous Approach
0DC34ZZ Extirpation of Matter from Lower Esophagus, Percutaneous Endoscopic Approach
0DC37ZZ Extirpation of Matter from Lower Esophagus, Via Natural or Artificial Opening
0DC38ZZ Extirpation of Matter from Lower Esophagus, Via Natural or Artificial Opening Endoscopic
0DC40ZZ Extirpation of Matter from Esophagogastric Junction, Open Approach
0DC43ZZ Extirpation of Matter from Esophagogastric Junction, Percutaneous Approach
0DC44ZZ Extirpation of Matter from Esophagogastric Junction, Percutaneous Endoscopic Approach
0DC47ZZ Extirpation of Matter from Esophagogastric Junction, Via Natural or Artificial Opening
0DC48ZZ Extirpation of Matter from Esophagogastric Junction, Via Natural or Artificial Opening Endoscopic
0DC50ZZ Extirpation of Matter from Esophagus, Open Approach
0DC53ZZ Extirpation of Matter from Esophagus, Percutaneous Approach
0DC54ZZ Extirpation of Matter from Esophagus, Percutaneous Endoscopic Approach
0DC57ZZ Extirpation of Matter from Esophagus, Via Natural or Artificial Opening
0DC58ZZ Extirpation of Matter from Esophagus, Via Natural or Artificial Opening Endoscopic
0DC60ZZ Extirpation of Matter from Stomach, Open Approach
0DC63ZZ Extirpation of Matter from Stomach, Percutaneous Approach
0DC64ZZ Extirpation of Matter from Stomach, Percutaneous Endoscopic Approach
0DC67ZZ Extirpation of Matter from Stomach, Via Natural or Artificial Opening
0DC68ZZ Extirpation of Matter from Stomach, Via Natural or Artificial Opening Endoscopic
0DC70ZZ Extirpation of Matter from Stomach, Pylorus, Open Approach
0DC73ZZ Extirpation of Matter from Stomach, Pylorus, Percutaneous Approach
0DC74ZZ Extirpation of Matter from Stomach, Pylorus, Percutaneous Endoscopic Approach
0DC77ZZ Extirpation of Matter from Stomach, Pylorus, Via Natural or Artificial Opening

0DC78ZZ Extirpation of Matter from Stomach, Pylorus, Via Natural or Artificial Opening Endoscopic
0DC80ZZ Extirpation of Matter from Small Intestine, Open Approach
0DC83ZZ Extirpation of Matter from Small Intestine, Percutaneous Approach
0DC84ZZ Extirpation of Matter from Small Intestine, Percutaneous Endoscopic Approach
0DC87ZZ Extirpation of Matter from Small Intestine, Via Natural or Artificial Opening
0DC88ZZ Extirpation of Matter from Small Intestine, Via Natural or Artificial Opening Endoscopic
0DC90ZZ Extirpation of Matter from Duodenum, Open Approach
0DC93ZZ Extirpation of Matter from Duodenum, Percutaneous Approach
0DC94ZZ Extirpation of Matter from Duodenum, Percutaneous Endoscopic Approach
0DC97ZZ Extirpation of Matter from Duodenum, Via Natural or Artificial Opening
0DC98ZZ Extirpation of Matter from Duodenum, Via Natural or Artificial Opening Endoscopic
0DCA0ZZ Extirpation of Matter from Jejunum, Open Approach
0DCA3ZZ Extirpation of Matter from Jejunum, Percutaneous Approach
0DCA4ZZ Extirpation of Matter from Jejunum, Percutaneous Endoscopic Approach
0DCA7ZZ Extirpation of Matter from Jejunum, Via Natural or Artificial Opening
0DCA8ZZ Extirpation of Matter from Jejunum, Via Natural or Artificial Opening Endoscopic
0DCB0ZZ Extirpation of Matter from Ileum, Open Approach
0DCB3ZZ Extirpation of Matter from Ileum, Percutaneous Approach
0DCB4ZZ Extirpation of Matter from Ileum, Percutaneous Endoscopic Approach
0DCB7ZZ Extirpation of Matter from Ileum, Via Natural or Artificial Opening
0DCB8ZZ Extirpation of Matter from Ileum, Via Natural or Artificial Opening Endoscopic
0DCC0ZZ Extirpation of Matter from Ileocecal Valve, Open Approach
0DCC3ZZ Extirpation of Matter from Ileocecal Valve, Percutaneous Approach
0DCC4ZZ Extirpation of Matter from Ileocecal Valve, Percutaneous Endoscopic Approach
0DCC7ZZ Extirpation of Matter from Ileocecal Valve, Via Natural or Artificial Opening
0DCC8ZZ Extirpation of Matter from Ileocecal Valve, Via Natural or Artificial Opening Endoscopic
0DCE0ZZ Extirpation of Matter from Large Intestine, Open Approach
0DCE3ZZ Extirpation of Matter from Large Intestine, Percutaneous Approach
0DCE4ZZ Extirpation of Matter from Large Intestine, Percutaneous Endoscopic Approach
0DCE7ZZ Extirpation of Matter from Large Intestine, Via Natural or Artificial Opening
0DCE8ZZ Extirpation of Matter from Large Intestine, Via Natural or Artificial Opening Endoscopic
0DCF0ZZ Extirpation of Matter from Right Large Intestine, Open Approach
0DCF3ZZ Extirpation of Matter from Right Large Intestine, Percutaneous Approach
0DCF4ZZ Extirpation of Matter from Right Large Intestine, Percutaneous Endoscopic Approach
0DCF7ZZ Extirpation of Matter from Right Large Intestine, Via Natural or Artificial Opening
0DCF8ZZ Extirpation of Matter from Right Large Intestine, Via Natural or Artificial Opening Endoscopic
0DCG0ZZ Extirpation of Matter from Left Large Intestine, Open Approach

0DCG3ZZ Extirpation of Matter from Left Large Intestine, Percutaneous Approach

0DCG4ZZ Extirpation of Matter from Left Large Intestine, Percutaneous Endoscopic Approach

0DCG7ZZ Extirpation of Matter from Left Large Intestine, Via Natural or Artificial Opening

0DCG8ZZ Extirpation of Matter from Left Large Intestine, Via Natural or Artificial Opening Endoscopic

0DCH0ZZ Extirpation of Matter from Cecum, Open Approach

0DCH3ZZ Extirpation of Matter from Cecum, Percutaneous Approach

0DCH4ZZ Extirpation of Matter from Cecum, Percutaneous Endoscopic Approach

0DCH7ZZ Extirpation of Matter from Cecum, Via Natural or Artificial Opening

0DCH8ZZ Extirpation of Matter from Cecum, Via Natural or Artificial Opening Endoscopic

0DCJ0ZZ Extirpation of Matter from Appendix, Open Approach

0DCJ3ZZ Extirpation of Matter from Appendix, Percutaneous Approach

0DCJ4ZZ Extirpation of Matter from Appendix, Percutaneous Endoscopic Approach

0DCJ7ZZ Extirpation of Matter from Appendix, Via Natural or Artificial Opening

0DCJ8ZZ Extirpation of Matter from Appendix, Via Natural or Artificial Opening Endoscopic

0DCK0ZZ Extirpation of Matter from Ascending Colon, Open Approach

0DCK3ZZ Extirpation of Matter from Ascending Colon, Percutaneous Approach

0DCK4ZZ Extirpation of Matter from Ascending Colon, Percutaneous Endoscopic Approach

0DCK7ZZ Extirpation of Matter from Ascending Colon, Via Natural or Artificial Opening

0DCK8ZZ Extirpation of Matter from Ascending Colon, Via Natural or Artificial Opening Endoscopic

0DCL0ZZ Extirpation of Matter from Transverse Colon, Open Approach

0DCL3ZZ Extirpation of Matter from Transverse Colon, Percutaneous Approach

0DCL4ZZ Extirpation of Matter from Transverse Colon, Percutaneous Endoscopic Approach

0DCL7ZZ Extirpation of Matter from Transverse Colon, Via Natural or Artificial Opening

0DCL8ZZ Extirpation of Matter from Transverse Colon, Via Natural or Artificial Opening Endoscopic

0DCM0ZZ Extirpation of Matter from Descending Colon, Open Approach

0DCM3ZZ Extirpation of Matter from Descending Colon, Percutaneous Approach

0DCM4ZZ Extirpation of Matter from Descending Colon, Percutaneous Endoscopic Approach

0DCM7ZZ Extirpation of Matter from Descending Colon, Via Natural or Artificial Opening

0DCM8ZZ Extirpation of Matter from Descending Colon, Via Natural or Artificial Opening Endoscopic

0DCN0ZZ Extirpation of Matter from Sigmoid Colon, Open Approach

0DCN3ZZ Extirpation of Matter from Sigmoid Colon, Percutaneous Approach

0DCN4ZZ Extirpation of Matter from Sigmoid Colon, Percutaneous Endoscopic Approach

0DCN7ZZ Extirpation of Matter from Sigmoid Colon, Via Natural or Artificial Opening

0DCN8ZZ Extirpation of Matter from Sigmoid Colon, Via Natural or Artificial Opening Endoscopic

0DCP0ZZ Extirpation of Matter from Rectum, Open Approach

0DCP3ZZ Extirpation of Matter from Rectum, Percutaneous Approach

0DCP4ZZ Extirpation of Matter from Rectum, Percutaneous Endoscopic Approach

0DCP7ZZ Extirpation of Matter from Rectum, Via Natural or Artificial Opening

0DCP8ZZ Extirpation of Matter from Rectum, Via Natural or Artificial Opening Endoscopic

0DCQ0ZZ Extirpation of Matter from Anus, Open Approach

0DCQ3ZZ Extirpation of Matter from Anus, Percutaneous Approach

0DCQ4ZZ Extirpation of Matter from Anus, Percutaneous Endoscopic Approach

0DCQ7ZZ Extirpation of Matter from Anus, Via Natural or Artificial Opening

0DCQ8ZZ Extirpation of Matter from Anus, Via Natural or Artificial Opening Endoscopic

0DCQXZZ Extirpation of Matter from Anus, External Approach

0DCR0ZZ Extirpation of Matter from Anal Sphincter, Open Approach

0DCR3ZZ Extirpation of Matter from Anal Sphincter, Percutaneous Approach

0DCR4ZZ Extirpation of Matter from Anal Sphincter, Percutaneous Endoscopic Approach

0DCS0ZZ Extirpation of Matter from Greater Omentum, Open Approach

0DCS3ZZ Extirpation of Matter from Greater Omentum, Percutaneous Approach

0DCS4ZZ Extirpation of Matter from Greater Omentum, Percutaneous Endoscopic Approach

0DCT0ZZ Extirpation of Matter from Lesser Omentum, Open Approach

0DCT3ZZ Extirpation of Matter from Lesser Omentum, Percutaneous Approach

0DCT4ZZ Extirpation of Matter from Lesser Omentum, Percutaneous Endoscopic Approach

0DCV0ZZ Extirpation of Matter from Mesentery, Open Approach

0DCV3ZZ Extirpation of Matter from Mesentery, Percutaneous Approach

0DCV4ZZ Extirpation of Matter from Mesentery, Percutaneous Endoscopic Approach

0DCW0ZZ Extirpation of Matter from Peritoneum, Open Approach

0DCW3ZZ Extirpation of Matter from Peritoneum, Percutaneous Approach

0DCW4ZZ Extirpation of Matter from Peritoneum, Percutaneous Endoscopic Approach

0DF – Gastrointestinal System, Fragmentation

0DF50ZZ Fragmentation in Esophagus, Open Approach

0DF53ZZ Fragmentation in Esophagus, Percutaneous Approach

0DF54ZZ Fragmentation in Esophagus, Percutaneous Endoscopic Approach

0DF57ZZ Fragmentation in Esophagus, Via Natural or Artificial Opening

0DF58ZZ Fragmentation in Esophagus, Via Natural or Artificial Opening Endoscopic

● **0DF5XZZ** Fragmentation in Esophagus, External Approach

0DF60ZZ Fragmentation in Stomach, Open Approach

0DF63ZZ Fragmentation in Stomach, Percutaneous Approach

0DF64ZZ Fragmentation in Stomach, Percutaneous Endoscopic Approach

0DF67ZZ Fragmentation in Stomach, Via Natural or Artificial Opening

0DF68ZZ Fragmentation in Stomach, Via Natural or Artificial Opening Endoscopic

● **0DF6XZZ** Fragmentation in Stomach, External Approach

0DF80ZZ Fragmentation in Small Intestine, Open Approach

0DF83ZZ Fragmentation in Small Intestine, Percutaneous Approach

0DF84ZZ Fragmentation in Small Intestine, Percutaneous Endoscopic Approach

0DF87ZZ Fragmentation in Small Intestine, Via Natural or Artificial Opening

0DF88ZZ Fragmentation in Small Intestine, Via Natural or Artificial Opening Endoscopic

● **0DF8XZZ** Fragmentation in Small Intestine, External Approach

0DF90ZZ Fragmentation in Duodenum, Open Approach

0DF93ZZ Fragmentation in Duodenum, Percutaneous Approach

0DF94ZZ Fragmentation in Duodenum, Percutaneous Endoscopic Approach

0DF97ZZ Fragmentation in Duodenum, Via Natural or Artificial Opening

0DF98ZZ Fragmentation in Duodenum, Via Natural or Artificial Opening Endoscopic

● **0DF9XZZ** Fragmentation in Duodenum, External Approach

0DFA0ZZ Fragmentation in Jejunum, Open Approach

0DFA3ZZ Fragmentation in Jejunum, Percutaneous Approach

0DFA4ZZ Fragmentation in Jejunum, Percutaneous Endoscopic Approach

0DFA7ZZ Fragmentation in Jejunum, Via Natural or Artificial Opening

0DFA8ZZ Fragmentation in Jejunum, Via Natural or Artificial Opening Endoscopic

● **0DFAXZZ** Fragmentation in Jejunum, External Approach

0DFB0ZZ Fragmentation in Ileum, Open Approach

0DFB3ZZ Fragmentation in Ileum, Percutaneous Approach

0DFB4ZZ Fragmentation in Ileum, Percutaneous Endoscopic Approach

0DFB7ZZ Fragmentation in Ileum, Via Natural or Artificial Opening

0DFB8ZZ Fragmentation in Ileum, Via Natural or Artificial Opening Endoscopic

◉ 0DFBXZZ Fragmentation in Ileum, External Approach
0DFE0ZZ Fragmentation in Large Intestine, Open Approach
0DFE3ZZ Fragmentation in Large Intestine, Percutaneous Approach
0DFE4ZZ Fragmentation in Large Intestine, Percutaneous Endoscopic Approach
0DFE7ZZ Fragmentation in Large Intestine, Via Natural or Artificial Opening
0DFE8ZZ Fragmentation in Large Intestine, Via Natural or Artificial Opening Endoscopic
◉ 0DFEXZZ Fragmentation in Large Intestine, External Approach
0DFF0ZZ Fragmentation in Right Large Intestine, Open Approach
0DFF3ZZ Fragmentation in Right Large Intestine, Percutaneous Approach
0DFF4ZZ Fragmentation in Right Large Intestine, Percutaneous Endoscopic Approach
0DFF7ZZ Fragmentation in Right Large Intestine, Via Natural or Artificial Opening
0DFF8ZZ Fragmentation in Right Large Intestine, Via Natural or Artificial Opening Endoscopic
◉ 0DFFXZZ Fragmentation in Right Large Intestine, External Approach
0DFG0ZZ Fragmentation in Left Large Intestine, Open Approach
0DFG3ZZ Fragmentation in Left Large Intestine, Percutaneous Approach
0DFG4ZZ Fragmentation in Left Large Intestine, Percutaneous Endoscopic Approach
0DFG7ZZ Fragmentation in Left Large Intestine, Via Natural or Artificial Opening
0DFG8ZZ Fragmentation in Left Large Intestine, Via Natural or Artificial Opening Endoscopic
◉ 0DFGXZZ Fragmentation in Left Large Intestine, External Approach
0DFH0ZZ Fragmentation in Cecum, Open Approach
0DFH3ZZ Fragmentation in Cecum, Percutaneous Approach
0DFH4ZZ Fragmentation in Cecum, Percutaneous Endoscopic Approach
0DFH7ZZ Fragmentation in Cecum, Via Natural or Artificial Opening
0DFH8ZZ Fragmentation in Cecum, Via Natural or Artificial Opening Endoscopic
◉ 0DFHXZZ Fragmentation in Cecum, External Approach
0DFJ0ZZ Fragmentation in Appendix, Open Approach
0DFJ3ZZ Fragmentation in Appendix, Percutaneous Approach
0DFJ4ZZ Fragmentation in Appendix, Percutaneous Endoscopic Approach
0DFJ7ZZ Fragmentation in Appendix, Via Natural or Artificial Opening
0DFJ8ZZ Fragmentation in Appendix, Via Natural or Artificial Opening Endoscopic
◉ 0DFJXZZ Fragmentation in Appendix, External Approach
0DFK0ZZ Fragmentation in Ascending Colon, Open Approach
0DFK3ZZ Fragmentation in Ascending Colon, Percutaneous Approach
0DFK4ZZ Fragmentation in Ascending Colon, Percutaneous Endoscopic Approach

0DFK7ZZ Fragmentation in Ascending Colon, Via Natural or Artificial Opening
0DFK8ZZ Fragmentation in Ascending Colon, Via Natural or Artificial Opening Endoscopic
◉ 0DFKXZZ Fragmentation in Ascending Colon, External Approach
0DFL0ZZ Fragmentation in Transverse Colon, Open Approach
0DFL3ZZ Fragmentation in Transverse Colon, Percutaneous Approach
0DFL4ZZ Fragmentation in Transverse Colon, Percutaneous Endoscopic Approach
0DFL7ZZ Fragmentation in Transverse Colon, Via Natural or Artificial Opening
0DFL8ZZ Fragmentation in Transverse Colon, Via Natural or Artificial Opening Endoscopic
◉ 0DFLXZZ Fragmentation in Transverse Colon, External Approach
0DFM0ZZ Fragmentation in Descending Colon, Open Approach
0DFM3ZZ Fragmentation in Descending Colon, Percutaneous Approach
0DFM4ZZ Fragmentation in Descending Colon, Percutaneous Endoscopic Approach
0DFM7ZZ Fragmentation in Descending Colon, Via Natural or Artificial Opening
0DFM8ZZ Fragmentation in Descending Colon, Via Natural or Artificial Opening Endoscopic
◉ 0DFMXZZ Fragmentation in Descending Colon, External Approach
0DFN0ZZ Fragmentation in Sigmoid Colon, Open Approach
0DFN3ZZ Fragmentation in Sigmoid Colon, Percutaneous Approach
0DFN4ZZ Fragmentation in Sigmoid Colon, Percutaneous Endoscopic Approach
0DFN7ZZ Fragmentation in Sigmoid Colon, Via Natural or Artificial Opening
0DFN8ZZ Fragmentation in Sigmoid Colon, Via Natural or Artificial Opening Endoscopic
◉ 0DFNXZZ Fragmentation in Sigmoid Colon, External Approach
0DFP0ZZ Fragmentation in Rectum, Open Approach
0DFP3ZZ Fragmentation in Rectum, Percutaneous Approach
0DFP4ZZ Fragmentation in Rectum, Percutaneous Endoscopic Approach
0DFP7ZZ Fragmentation in Rectum, Via Natural or Artificial Opening
0DFP8ZZ Fragmentation in Rectum, Via Natural or Artificial Opening Endoscopic
◉ 0DFPXZZ Fragmentation in Rectum, External Approach
0DFQ0ZZ Fragmentation in Anus, Open Approach
0DFQ3ZZ Fragmentation in Anus, Percutaneous Approach
0DFQ4ZZ Fragmentation in Anus, Percutaneous Endoscopic Approach
0DFQ7ZZ Fragmentation in Anus, Via Natural or Artificial Opening
0DFQ8ZZ Fragmentation in Anus, Via Natural or Artificial Opening Endoscopic
◉ 0DFQXZZ Fragmentation in Anus, External Approach

0DH – Gastrointestinal System, Insertion

0DH501Z Insertion of Radioactive Element into Esophagus, Open Approach
0DH502Z Insertion of Monitoring Device into Esophagus, Open Approach
0DH503Z Insertion of Infusion Device into Esophagus, Open Approach
0DH50DZ Insertion of Intraluminal Device into Esophagus, Open Approach
0DH50UZ Insertion of Feeding Device into Esophagus, Open Approach
0DH531Z Insertion of Radioactive Element into Esophagus, Percutaneous Approach
0DH532Z Insertion of Monitoring Device into Esophagus, Percutaneous Approach
0DH533Z Insertion of Infusion Device into Esophagus, Percutaneous Approach
0DH53DZ Insertion of Intraluminal Device into Esophagus, Percutaneous Approach
0DH53UZ Insertion of Feeding Device into Esophagus, Percutaneous Approach
0DH541Z Insertion of Radioactive Element into Esophagus, Percutaneous Endoscopic Approach
0DH542Z Insertion of Monitoring Device into Esophagus, Percutaneous Endoscopic Approach
0DH543Z Insertion of Infusion Device into Esophagus, Percutaneous Endoscopic Approach
0DH54DZ Insertion of Intraluminal Device into Esophagus, Percutaneous Endoscopic Approach
0DH54UZ Insertion of Feeding Device into Esophagus, Percutaneous Endoscopic Approach

0DH571Z Insertion of Radioactive Element into Esophagus, Via Natural or Artificial Opening
0DH572Z Insertion of Monitoring Device into Esophagus, Via Natural or Artificial Opening
0DH573Z Insertion of Infusion Device into Esophagus, Via Natural or Artificial Opening
0DH57BZ Insertion of Airway into Esophagus, Via Natural or Artificial Opening
0DH57DZ Insertion of Intraluminal Device into Esophagus, Via Natural or Artificial Opening
0DH57UZ Insertion of Feeding Device into Esophagus, Via Natural or Artificial Opening
0DH581Z Insertion of Radioactive Element into Esophagus, Via Natural or Artificial Opening Endoscopic
0DH582Z Insertion of Monitoring Device into Esophagus, Via Natural or Artificial Opening Endoscopic
0DH583Z Insertion of Infusion Device into Esophagus, Via Natural or Artificial Opening Endoscopic
0DH58BZ Insertion of Airway into Esophagus, Via Natural or Artificial Opening Endoscopic
0DH58DZ Insertion of Intraluminal Device into Esophagus, Via Natural or Artificial Opening Endoscopic
0DH58UZ Insertion of Feeding Device into Esophagus, Via Natural or Artificial Opening Endoscopic
0DH602Z Insertion of Monitoring Device into Stomach, Open Approach

0DH603Z Insertion of Infusion Device into Stomach, Open Approach
0DH60DZ Insertion of Intraluminal Device into Stomach, Open Approach
0DH60MZ Insertion of Stimulator Lead into Stomach, Open Approach
0DH60UZ Insertion of Feeding Device into Stomach, Open Approach
0DH632Z Insertion of Monitoring Device into Stomach, Percutaneous Approach
0DH633Z Insertion of Infusion Device into Stomach, Percutaneous Approach
0DH63DZ Insertion of Intraluminal Device into Stomach, Percutaneous Approach
0DH63MZ Insertion of Stimulator Lead into Stomach, Percutaneous Approach
0DH63UZ Insertion of Feeding Device into Stomach, Percutaneous Approach
0DH642Z Insertion of Monitoring Device into Stomach, Percutaneous Endoscopic Approach
0DH643Z Insertion of Infusion Device into Stomach, Percutaneous Endoscopic Approach
0DH64DZ Insertion of Intraluminal Device into Stomach, Percutaneous Endoscopic Approach
0DH64MZ Insertion of Stimulator Lead into Stomach, Percutaneous Endoscopic Approach
0DH64UZ Insertion of Feeding Device into Stomach, Percutaneous Endoscopic Approach
0DH672Z Insertion of Monitoring Device into Stomach, Via Natural or Artificial Opening
0DH673Z Insertion of Infusion Device into Stomach, Via Natural or Artificial Opening
0DH67DZ Insertion of Intraluminal Device into Stomach, Via Natural or Artificial Opening
0DH67UZ Insertion of Feeding Device into Stomach, Via Natural or Artificial Opening
0DH682Z Insertion of Monitoring Device into Stomach, Via Natural or Artificial Opening Endoscopic
0DH683Z Insertion of Infusion Device into Stomach, Via Natural or Artificial Opening Endoscopic
0DH68DZ Insertion of Intraluminal Device into Stomach, Via Natural or Artificial Opening Endoscopic
0DH68UZ Insertion of Feeding Device into Stomach, Via Natural or Artificial Opening Endoscopic
0DH802Z Insertion of Monitoring Device into Small Intestine, Open Approach
0DH803Z Insertion of Infusion Device into Small Intestine, Open Approach
0DH80DZ Insertion of Intraluminal Device into Small Intestine, Open Approach
0DH80UZ Insertion of Feeding Device into Small Intestine, Open Approach
0DH832Z Insertion of Monitoring Device into Small Intestine, Percutaneous Approach
0DH833Z Insertion of Infusion Device into Small Intestine, Percutaneous Approach
0DH83DZ Insertion of Intraluminal Device into Small Intestine, Percutaneous Approach
0DH83UZ Insertion of Feeding Device into Small Intestine, Percutaneous Approach
0DH842Z Insertion of Monitoring Device into Small Intestine, Percutaneous Endoscopic Approach
0DH843Z Insertion of Infusion Device into Small Intestine, Percutaneous Endoscopic Approach
0DH84DZ Insertion of Intraluminal Device into Small Intestine, Percutaneous Endoscopic Approach
0DH84UZ Insertion of Feeding Device into Small Intestine, Percutaneous Endoscopic Approach
0DH872Z Insertion of Monitoring Device into Small Intestine, Via Natural or Artificial Opening
0DH873Z Insertion of Infusion Device into Small Intestine, Via Natural or Artificial Opening
0DH87DZ Insertion of Intraluminal Device into Small Intestine, Via Natural or Artificial Opening
0DH87UZ Insertion of Feeding Device into Small Intestine, Via Natural or Artificial Opening
0DH882Z Insertion of Monitoring Device into Small Intestine, Via Natural or Artificial Opening Endoscopic
0DH883Z Insertion of Infusion Device into Small Intestine, Via Natural or Artificial Opening Endoscopic
0DH88DZ Insertion of Intraluminal Device into Small Intestine, Via Natural or Artificial Opening Endoscopic

0DH88UZ Insertion of Feeding Device into Small Intestine, Via Natural or Artificial Opening Endoscopic
0DH902Z Insertion of Monitoring Device into Duodenum, Open Approach
0DH903Z Insertion of Infusion Device into Duodenum, Open Approach
0DH90DZ Insertion of Intraluminal Device into Duodenum, Open Approach
0DH90UZ Insertion of Feeding Device into Duodenum, Open Approach
0DH932Z Insertion of Monitoring Device into Duodenum, Percutaneous Approach
0DH933Z Insertion of Infusion Device into Duodenum, Percutaneous Approach
0DH93DZ Insertion of Intraluminal Device into Duodenum, Percutaneous Approach
0DH93UZ Insertion of Feeding Device into Duodenum, Percutaneous Approach
0DH942Z Insertion of Monitoring Device into Duodenum, Percutaneous Endoscopic Approach
0DH943Z Insertion of Infusion Device into Duodenum, Percutaneous Endoscopic Approach
0DH94DZ Insertion of Intraluminal Device into Duodenum, Percutaneous Endoscopic Approach
0DH94UZ Insertion of Feeding Device into Duodenum, Percutaneous Endoscopic Approach
0DH972Z Insertion of Monitoring Device into Duodenum, Via Natural or Artificial Opening
0DH973Z Insertion of Infusion Device into Duodenum, Via Natural or Artificial Opening
0DH97DZ Insertion of Intraluminal Device into Duodenum, Via Natural or Artificial Opening
0DH97UZ Insertion of Feeding Device into Duodenum, Via Natural or Artificial Opening
0DH982Z Insertion of Monitoring Device into Duodenum, Via Natural or Artificial Opening Endoscopic
0DH983Z Insertion of Infusion Device into Duodenum, Via Natural or Artificial Opening Endoscopic
0DH98DZ Insertion of Intraluminal Device into Duodenum, Via Natural or Artificial Opening Endoscopic
0DH98UZ Insertion of Feeding Device into Duodenum, Via Natural or Artificial Opening Endoscopic
0DHA02Z Insertion of Monitoring Device into Jejunum, Open Approach
0DHA03Z Insertion of Infusion Device into Jejunum, Open Approach
0DHA0DZ Insertion of Intraluminal Device into Jejunum, Open Approach
0DHA0UZ Insertion of Feeding Device into Jejunum, Open Approach
0DHA32Z Insertion of Monitoring Device into Jejunum, Percutaneous Approach
0DHA33Z Insertion of Infusion Device into Jejunum, Percutaneous Approach
0DHA3DZ Insertion of Intraluminal Device into Jejunum, Percutaneous Approach
0DHA3UZ Insertion of Feeding Device into Jejunum, Percutaneous Approach
0DHA42Z Insertion of Monitoring Device into Jejunum, Percutaneous Endoscopic Approach
0DHA43Z Insertion of Infusion Device into Jejunum, Percutaneous Endoscopic Approach
0DHA4DZ Insertion of Intraluminal Device into Jejunum, Percutaneous Endoscopic Approach
0DHA4UZ Insertion of Feeding Device into Jejunum, Percutaneous Endoscopic Approach
0DHA72Z Insertion of Monitoring Device into Jejunum, Via Natural or Artificial Opening
0DHA73Z Insertion of Infusion Device into Jejunum, Via Natural or Artificial Opening
0DHA7DZ Insertion of Intraluminal Device into Jejunum, Via Natural or Artificial Opening
0DHA7UZ Insertion of Feeding Device into Jejunum, Via Natural or Artificial Opening
0DHA82Z Insertion of Monitoring Device into Jejunum, Via Natural or Artificial Opening Endoscopic
0DHA83Z Insertion of Infusion Device into Jejunum, Via Natural or Artificial Opening Endoscopic
0DHA8DZ Insertion of Intraluminal Device into Jejunum, Via Natural or Artificial Opening Endoscopic
0DHA8UZ Insertion of Feeding Device into Jejunum, Via Natural or Artificial Opening Endoscopic
0DHB02Z Insertion of Monitoring Device into Ileum, Open Approach

0DHB03Z	Insertion of Infusion Device into Ileum, Open Approach
0DHB0DZ	Insertion of Intraluminal Device into Ileum, Open Approach
0DHB0UZ	Insertion of Feeding Device into Ileum, Open Approach
0DHB32Z	Insertion of Monitoring Device into Ileum, Percutaneous Approach
0DHB33Z	Insertion of Infusion Device into Ileum, Percutaneous Approach
0DHB3DZ	Insertion of Intraluminal Device into Ileum, Percutaneous Approach
0DHB3UZ	Insertion of Feeding Device into Ileum, Percutaneous Approach
0DHB42Z	Insertion of Monitoring Device into Ileum, Percutaneous Endoscopic Approach
0DHB43Z	Insertion of Infusion Device into Ileum, Percutaneous Endoscopic Approach
0DHB4DZ	Insertion of Intraluminal Device into Ileum, Percutaneous Endoscopic Approach
0DHB4UZ	Insertion of Feeding Device into Ileum, Percutaneous Endoscopic Approach
0DHB72Z	Insertion of Monitoring Device into Ileum, Via Natural or Artificial Opening
0DHB73Z	Insertion of Infusion Device into Ileum, Via Natural or Artificial Opening
0DHB7DZ	Insertion of Intraluminal Device into Ileum, Via Natural or Artificial Opening
0DHB7UZ	Insertion of Feeding Device into Ileum, Via Natural or Artificial Opening
0DHB82Z	Insertion of Monitoring Device into Ileum, Via Natural or Artificial Opening Endoscopic
0DHB83Z	Insertion of Infusion Device into Ileum, Via Natural or Artificial Opening Endoscopic
0DHB8DZ	Insertion of Intraluminal Device into Ileum, Via Natural or Artificial Opening Endoscopic
0DHB8UZ	Insertion of Feeding Device into Ileum, Via Natural or Artificial Opening Endoscopic
0DHE0DZ	Insertion of Intraluminal Device into Large Intestine, Open Approach
0DHE3DZ	Insertion of Intraluminal Device into Large Intestine, Percutaneous Approach
0DHE4DZ	Insertion of Intraluminal Device into Large Intestine, Percutaneous Endoscopic Approach
0DHE7DZ	Insertion of Intraluminal Device into Large Intestine, Via Natural or Artificial Opening
0DHE8DZ	Insertion of Intraluminal Device into Large Intestine, Via Natural or Artificial Opening Endoscopic
0DHP01Z	Insertion of Radioactive Element into Rectum, Open Approach
0DHP0DZ	Insertion of Intraluminal Device into Rectum, Open Approach
0DHP31Z	Insertion of Radioactive Element into Rectum, Percutaneous Approach
0DHP3DZ	Insertion of Intraluminal Device into Rectum, Percutaneous Approach
0DHP41Z	Insertion of Radioactive Element into Rectum, Percutaneous Endoscopic Approach
0DHP4DZ	Insertion of Intraluminal Device into Rectum, Percutaneous Endoscopic Approach
0DHP71Z	Insertion of Radioactive Element into Rectum, Via Natural or Artificial Opening
0DHP7DZ	Insertion of Intraluminal Device into Rectum, Via Natural or Artificial Opening
0DHP81Z	Insertion of Radioactive Element into Rectum, Via Natural or Artificial Opening Endoscopic
0DHP8DZ	Insertion of Intraluminal Device into Rectum, Via Natural or Artificial Opening Endoscopic
0DHQ0DZ	Insertion of Intraluminal Device into Anus, Open Approach
0DHQ0LZ	Insertion of Artificial Sphincter into Anus, Open Approach
0DHQ3DZ	Insertion of Intraluminal Device into Anus, Percutaneous Approach
0DHQ3LZ	Insertion of Artificial Sphincter into Anus, Percutaneous Approach
0DHQ4DZ	Insertion of Intraluminal Device into Anus, Percutaneous Endoscopic Approach
0DHQ4LZ	Insertion of Artificial Sphincter into Anus, Percutaneous Endoscopic Approach
0DHQ7DZ	Insertion of Intraluminal Device into Anus, Via Natural or Artificial Opening
0DHQ8DZ	Insertion of Intraluminal Device into Anus, Via Natural or Artificial Opening Endoscopic
0DHR0MZ	Insertion of Stimulator Lead into Anal Sphincter, Open Approach
0DHR3MZ	Insertion of Stimulator Lead into Anal Sphincter, Percutaneous Approach
0DHR4MZ	Insertion of Stimulator Lead into Anal Sphincter, Percutaneous Endoscopic Approach

0DJ – Gastrointestinal System, Inspection

Review Coding Guidelines B3.11a, B3.11b and B3.11c

0DJ00ZZ	Inspection of Upper Intestinal Tract, Open Approach
0DJ03ZZ	Inspection of Upper Intestinal Tract, Percutaneous Approach
0DJ04ZZ	Inspection of Upper Intestinal Tract, Percutaneous Endoscopic Approach
0DJ07ZZ	Inspection of Upper Intestinal Tract, Via Natural or Artificial Opening
0DJ08ZZ	Inspection of Upper Intestinal Tract, Via Natural or Artificial Opening Endoscopic
0DJ0XZZ	Inspection of Upper Intestinal Tract, External Approach
0DJ60ZZ	Inspection of Stomach, Open Approach
0DJ63ZZ	Inspection of Stomach, Percutaneous Approach
0DJ64ZZ	Inspection of Stomach, Percutaneous Endoscopic Approach
0DJ67ZZ	Inspection of Stomach, Via Natural or Artificial Opening
0DJ68ZZ	Inspection of Stomach, Via Natural or Artificial Opening Endoscopic
0DJ6XZZ	Inspection of Stomach, External Approach
0DJD0ZZ	Inspection of Lower Intestinal Tract, Open Approach
0DJD3ZZ	Inspection of Lower Intestinal Tract, Percutaneous Approach
0DJD4ZZ	Inspection of Lower Intestinal Tract, Percutaneous Endoscopic Approach
0DJD7ZZ	Inspection of Lower Intestinal Tract, Via Natural or Artificial Opening
0DJD8ZZ	Inspection of Lower Intestinal Tract, Via Natural or Artificial Opening Endoscopic
0DJDXZZ	Inspection of Lower Intestinal Tract, External Approach
0DJU0ZZ	Inspection of Omentum, Open Approach
0DJU3ZZ	Inspection of Omentum, Percutaneous Approach
0DJU4ZZ	Inspection of Omentum, Percutaneous Endoscopic Approach
0DJUXZZ	Inspection of Omentum, External Approach
0DJV0ZZ	Inspection of Mesentery, Open Approach
0DJV3ZZ	Inspection of Mesentery, Percutaneous Approach
0DJV4ZZ	Inspection of Mesentery, Percutaneous Endoscopic Approach
0DJVXZZ	Inspection of Mesentery, External Approach
0DJW0ZZ	Inspection of Peritoneum, Open Approach
0DJW3ZZ	Inspection of Peritoneum, Percutaneous Approach
0DJW4ZZ	Inspection of Peritoneum, Percutaneous Endoscopic Approach
0DJWXZZ	Inspection of Peritoneum, External Approach

0DL – Gastrointestinal System, Occlusion

0DL10CZ	Occlusion of Upper Esophagus with Extraluminal Device, Open Approach
0DL10DZ	Occlusion of Upper Esophagus with Intraluminal Device, Open Approach
0DL10ZZ	Occlusion of Upper Esophagus, Open Approach
0DL13CZ	Occlusion of Upper Esophagus with Extraluminal Device, Percutaneous Approach
0DL13DZ	Occlusion of Upper Esophagus with Intraluminal Device, Percutaneous Approach
0DL13ZZ	Occlusion of Upper Esophagus, Percutaneous Approach
0DL14CZ	Occlusion of Upper Esophagus with Extraluminal Device, Percutaneous Endoscopic Approach
0DL14DZ	Occlusion of Upper Esophagus with Intraluminal Device, Percutaneous Endoscopic Approach

0DL14ZZ Occlusion of Upper Esophagus, Percutaneous Endoscopic Approach

0DL17DZ Occlusion of Upper Esophagus with Intraluminal Device, Via Natural or Artificial Opening

0DL17ZZ Occlusion of Upper Esophagus, Via Natural or Artificial Opening

0DL18DZ Occlusion of Upper Esophagus with Intraluminal Device, Via Natural or Artificial Opening Endoscopic

0DL18ZZ Occlusion of Upper Esophagus, Via Natural or Artificial Opening Endoscopic

0DL20CZ Occlusion of Middle Esophagus with Extraluminal Device, Open Approach

0DL20DZ Occlusion of Middle Esophagus with Intraluminal Device, Open Approach

0DL20ZZ Occlusion of Middle Esophagus, Open Approach

0DL23CZ Occlusion of Middle Esophagus with Extraluminal Device, Percutaneous Approach

0DL23DZ Occlusion of Middle Esophagus with Intraluminal Device, Percutaneous Approach

0DL23ZZ Occlusion of Middle Esophagus, Percutaneous Approach

0DL24CZ Occlusion of Middle Esophagus with Extraluminal Device, Percutaneous Endoscopic Approach

0DL24DZ Occlusion of Middle Esophagus with Intraluminal Device, Percutaneous Endoscopic Approach

0DL24ZZ Occlusion of Middle Esophagus, Percutaneous Endoscopic Approach

0DL27DZ Occlusion of Middle Esophagus with Intraluminal Device, Via Natural or Artificial Opening

0DL27ZZ Occlusion of Middle Esophagus, Via Natural or Artificial Opening

0DL28DZ Occlusion of Middle Esophagus with Intraluminal Device, Via Natural or Artificial Opening Endoscopic

0DL28ZZ Occlusion of Middle Esophagus, Via Natural or Artificial Opening Endoscopic

0DL30CZ Occlusion of Lower Esophagus with Extraluminal Device, Open Approach

0DL30DZ Occlusion of Lower Esophagus with Intraluminal Device, Open Approach

0DL30ZZ Occlusion of Lower Esophagus, Open Approach

0DL33CZ Occlusion of Lower Esophagus with Extraluminal Device, Percutaneous Approach

0DL33DZ Occlusion of Lower Esophagus with Intraluminal Device, Percutaneous Approach

0DL33ZZ Occlusion of Lower Esophagus, Percutaneous Approach

0DL34CZ Occlusion of Lower Esophagus with Extraluminal Device, Percutaneous Endoscopic Approach

0DL34DZ Occlusion of Lower Esophagus with Intraluminal Device, Percutaneous Endoscopic Approach

0DL34ZZ Occlusion of Lower Esophagus, Percutaneous Endoscopic Approach

0DL37DZ Occlusion of Lower Esophagus with Intraluminal Device, Via Natural or Artificial Opening

0DL37ZZ Occlusion of Lower Esophagus, Via Natural or Artificial Opening

0DL38DZ Occlusion of Lower Esophagus with Intraluminal Device, Via Natural or Artificial Opening Endoscopic

0DL38ZZ Occlusion of Lower Esophagus, Via Natural or Artificial Opening Endoscopic

0DL40CZ Occlusion of Esophagogastric Junction with Extraluminal Device, Open Approach

0DL40DZ Occlusion of Esophagogastric Junction with Intraluminal Device, Open Approach

0DL40ZZ Occlusion of Esophagogastric Junction, Open Approach

0DL43CZ Occlusion of Esophagogastric Junction with Extraluminal Device, Percutaneous Approach

0DL43DZ Occlusion of Esophagogastric Junction with Intraluminal Device, Percutaneous Approach

0DL43ZZ Occlusion of Esophagogastric Junction, Percutaneous Approach

0DL44CZ Occlusion of Esophagogastric Junction with Extraluminal Device, Percutaneous Endoscopic Approach

0DL44DZ Occlusion of Esophagogastric Junction with Intraluminal Device, Percutaneous Endoscopic Approach

0DL44ZZ Occlusion of Esophagogastric Junction, Percutaneous Endoscopic Approach

0DL47DZ Occlusion of Esophagogastric Junction with Intraluminal Device, Via Natural or Artificial Opening

0DL47ZZ Occlusion of Esophagogastric Junction, Via Natural or Artificial Opening

0DL48DZ Occlusion of Esophagogastric Junction with Intraluminal Device, Via Natural or Artificial Opening Endoscopic

0DL48ZZ Occlusion of Esophagogastric Junction, Via Natural or Artificial Opening Endoscopic

0DL50CZ Occlusion of Esophagus with Extraluminal Device, Open Approach

0DL50DZ Occlusion of Esophagus with Intraluminal Device, Open Approach

0DL50ZZ Occlusion of Esophagus, Open Approach

0DL53CZ Occlusion of Esophagus with Extraluminal Device, Percutaneous Approach

0DL53DZ Occlusion of Esophagus with Intraluminal Device, Percutaneous Approach

0DL53ZZ Occlusion of Esophagus, Percutaneous Approach

0DL54CZ Occlusion of Esophagus with Extraluminal Device, Percutaneous Endoscopic Approach

0DL54DZ Occlusion of Esophagus with Intraluminal Device, Percutaneous Endoscopic Approach

0DL54ZZ Occlusion of Esophagus, Percutaneous Endoscopic Approach

0DL57DZ Occlusion of Esophagus with Intraluminal Device, Via Natural or Artificial Opening

0DL57ZZ Occlusion of Esophagus, Via Natural or Artificial Opening

0DL58DZ Occlusion of Esophagus with Intraluminal Device, Via Natural or Artificial Opening Endoscopic

0DL58ZZ Occlusion of Esophagus, Via Natural or Artificial Opening Endoscopic

0DL60CZ Occlusion of Stomach with Extraluminal Device, Open Approach

0DL60DZ Occlusion of Stomach with Intraluminal Device, Open Approach

0DL60ZZ Occlusion of Stomach, Open Approach

0DL63CZ Occlusion of Stomach with Extraluminal Device, Percutaneous Approach

0DL63DZ Occlusion of Stomach with Intraluminal Device, Percutaneous Approach

0DL63ZZ Occlusion of Stomach, Percutaneous Approach

0DL64CZ Occlusion of Stomach with Extraluminal Device, Percutaneous Endoscopic Approach

0DL64DZ Occlusion of Stomach with Intraluminal Device, Percutaneous Endoscopic Approach

0DL64ZZ Occlusion of Stomach, Percutaneous Endoscopic Approach

0DL67DZ Occlusion of Stomach with Intraluminal Device, Via Natural or Artificial Opening

0DL67ZZ Occlusion of Stomach, Via Natural or Artificial Opening

0DL68DZ Occlusion of Stomach with Intraluminal Device, Via Natural or Artificial Opening Endoscopic

0DL68ZZ Occlusion of Stomach, Via Natural or Artificial Opening Endoscopic

0DL70CZ Occlusion of Stomach, Pylorus with Extraluminal Device, Open Approach

0DL70DZ Occlusion of Stomach, Pylorus with Intraluminal Device, Open Approach

0DL70ZZ Occlusion of Stomach, Pylorus, Open Approach

0DL73CZ Occlusion of Stomach, Pylorus with Extraluminal Device, Percutaneous Approach

0DL73DZ Occlusion of Stomach, Pylorus with Intraluminal Device, Percutaneous Approach

0DL73ZZ Occlusion of Stomach, Pylorus, Percutaneous Approach

0DL74CZ Occlusion of Stomach, Pylorus with Extraluminal Device, Percutaneous Endoscopic Approach

0DL74DZ Occlusion of Stomach, Pylorus with Intraluminal Device, Percutaneous Endoscopic Approach

0DL74ZZ Occlusion of Stomach, Pylorus, Percutaneous Endoscopic Approach

0DL77DZ Occlusion of Stomach, Pylorus with Intraluminal Device, Via Natural or Artificial Opening

0DL77ZZ Occlusion of Stomach, Pylorus, Via Natural or Artificial Opening

0DL78DZ Occlusion of Stomach, Pylorus with Intraluminal Device, Via Natural or Artificial Opening Endoscopic

0DL78ZZ Occlusion of Stomach, Pylorus, Via Natural or Artificial Opening Endoscopic

0DL80CZ Occlusion of Small Intestine with Extraluminal Device, Open Approach

0DL80DZ Occlusion of Small Intestine with Intraluminal Device, Open Approach

0DL80ZZ Occlusion of Small Intestine, Open Approach
0DL83CZ Occlusion of Small Intestine with Extraluminal Device, Percutaneous Approach
0DL83DZ Occlusion of Small Intestine with Intraluminal Device, Percutaneous Approach
0DL83ZZ Occlusion of Small Intestine, Percutaneous Approach
0DL84CZ Occlusion of Small Intestine with Extraluminal Device, Percutaneous Endoscopic Approach
0DL84DZ Occlusion of Small Intestine with Intraluminal Device, Percutaneous Endoscopic Approach
0DL84ZZ Occlusion of Small Intestine, Percutaneous Endoscopic Approach
0DL87DZ Occlusion of Small Intestine with Intraluminal Device, Via Natural or Artificial Opening
0DL87ZZ Occlusion of Small Intestine, Via Natural or Artificial Opening
0DL88DZ Occlusion of Small Intestine with Intraluminal Device, Via Natural or Artificial Opening Endoscopic
0DL88ZZ Occlusion of Small Intestine, Via Natural or Artificial Opening Endoscopic
0DL90CZ Occlusion of Duodenum with Extraluminal Device, Open Approach
0DL90DZ Occlusion of Duodenum with Intraluminal Device, Open Approach
0DL90ZZ Occlusion of Duodenum, Open Approach
0DL93CZ Occlusion of Duodenum with Extraluminal Device, Percutaneous Approach
0DL93DZ Occlusion of Duodenum with Intraluminal Device, Percutaneous Approach
0DL93ZZ Occlusion of Duodenum, Percutaneous Approach
0DL94CZ Occlusion of Duodenum with Extraluminal Device, Percutaneous Endoscopic Approach
0DL94DZ Occlusion of Duodenum with Intraluminal Device, Percutaneous Endoscopic Approach
0DL94ZZ Occlusion of Duodenum, Percutaneous Endoscopic Approach
0DL97DZ Occlusion of Duodenum with Intraluminal Device, Via Natural or Artificial Opening
0DL97ZZ Occlusion of Duodenum, Via Natural or Artificial Opening
0DL98DZ Occlusion of Duodenum with Intraluminal Device, Via Natural or Artificial Opening Endoscopic
0DL98ZZ Occlusion of Duodenum, Via Natural or Artificial Opening Endoscopic
0DLA0CZ Occlusion of Jejunum with Extraluminal Device, Open Approach
0DLA0DZ Occlusion of Jejunum with Intraluminal Device, Open Approach
0DLA0ZZ Occlusion of Jejunum, Open Approach
0DLA3CZ Occlusion of Jejunum with Extraluminal Device, Percutaneous Approach
0DLA3DZ Occlusion of Jejunum with Intraluminal Device, Percutaneous Approach
0DLA3ZZ Occlusion of Jejunum, Percutaneous Approach
0DLA4CZ Occlusion of Jejunum with Extraluminal Device, Percutaneous Endoscopic Approach
0DLA4DZ Occlusion of Jejunum with Intraluminal Device, Percutaneous Endoscopic Approach
0DLA4ZZ Occlusion of Jejunum, Percutaneous Endoscopic Approach
0DLA7DZ Occlusion of Jejunum with Intraluminal Device, Via Natural or Artificial Opening
0DLA7ZZ Occlusion of Jejunum, Via Natural or Artificial Opening
0DLA8DZ Occlusion of Jejunum with Intraluminal Device, Via Natural or Artificial Opening Endoscopic
0DLA8ZZ Occlusion of Jejunum, Via Natural or Artificial Opening Endoscopic
0DLB0CZ Occlusion of Ileum with Extraluminal Device, Open Approach
0DLB0DZ Occlusion of Ileum with Intraluminal Device, Open Approach
0DLB0ZZ Occlusion of Ileum, Open Approach
0DLB3CZ Occlusion of Ileum with Extraluminal Device, Percutaneous Approach
0DLB3DZ Occlusion of Ileum with Intraluminal Device, Percutaneous Approach
0DLB3ZZ Occlusion of Ileum, Percutaneous Approach
0DLB4CZ Occlusion of Ileum with Extraluminal Device, Percutaneous Endoscopic Approach
0DLB4DZ Occlusion of Ileum with Intraluminal Device, Percutaneous Endoscopic Approach
0DLB4ZZ Occlusion of Ileum, Percutaneous Endoscopic Approach

0DLB7DZ Occlusion of Ileum with Intraluminal Device, Via Natural or Artificial Opening
0DLB7ZZ Occlusion of Ileum, Via Natural or Artificial Opening
0DLB8DZ Occlusion of Ileum with Intraluminal Device, Via Natural or Artificial Opening Endoscopic
0DLB8ZZ Occlusion of Ileum, Via Natural or Artificial Opening Endoscopic
0DLC0CZ Occlusion of Ileocecal Valve with Extraluminal Device, Open Approach
0DLC0DZ Occlusion of Ileocecal Valve with Intraluminal Device, Open Approach
0DLC0ZZ Occlusion of Ileocecal Valve, Open Approach
0DLC3CZ Occlusion of Ileocecal Valve with Extraluminal Device, Percutaneous Approach
0DLC3DZ Occlusion of Ileocecal Valve with Intraluminal Device, Percutaneous Approach
0DLC3ZZ Occlusion of Ileocecal Valve, Percutaneous Approach
0DLC4CZ Occlusion of Ileocecal Valve with Extraluminal Device, Percutaneous Endoscopic Approach
0DLC4DZ Occlusion of Ileocecal Valve with Intraluminal Device, Percutaneous Endoscopic Approach
0DLC4ZZ Occlusion of Ileocecal Valve, Percutaneous Endoscopic Approach
0DLC7DZ Occlusion of Ileocecal Valve with Intraluminal Device, Via Natural or Artificial Opening
0DLC7ZZ Occlusion of Ileocecal Valve, Via Natural or Artificial Opening
0DLC8DZ Occlusion of Ileocecal Valve with Intraluminal Device, Via Natural or Artificial Opening Endoscopic
0DLC8ZZ Occlusion of Ileocecal Valve, Via Natural or Artificial Opening Endoscopic
0DLE0CZ Occlusion of Large Intestine with Extraluminal Device, Open Approach
0DLE0DZ Occlusion of Large Intestine with Intraluminal Device, Open Approach
0DLE0ZZ Occlusion of Large Intestine, Open Approach
0DLE3CZ Occlusion of Large Intestine with Extraluminal Device, Percutaneous Approach
0DLE3DZ Occlusion of Large Intestine with Intraluminal Device, Percutaneous Approach
0DLE3ZZ Occlusion of Large Intestine, Percutaneous Approach
0DLE4CZ Occlusion of Large Intestine with Extraluminal Device, Percutaneous Endoscopic Approach
0DLE4DZ Occlusion of Large Intestine with Intraluminal Device, Percutaneous Endoscopic Approach
0DLE4ZZ Occlusion of Large Intestine, Percutaneous Endoscopic Approach
0DLE7DZ Occlusion of Large Intestine with Intraluminal Device, Via Natural or Artificial Opening
0DLE7ZZ Occlusion of Large Intestine, Via Natural or Artificial Opening
0DLE8DZ Occlusion of Large Intestine with Intraluminal Device, Via Natural or Artificial Opening Endoscopic
0DLE8ZZ Occlusion of Large Intestine, Via Natural or Artificial Opening Endoscopic
0DLF0CZ Occlusion of Right Large Intestine with Extraluminal Device, Open Approach
0DLF0DZ Occlusion of Right Large Intestine with Intraluminal Device, Open Approach
0DLF0ZZ Occlusion of Right Large Intestine, Open Approach
0DLF3CZ Occlusion of Right Large Intestine with Extraluminal Device, Percutaneous Approach
0DLF3DZ Occlusion of Right Large Intestine with Intraluminal Device, Percutaneous Approach
0DLF3ZZ Occlusion of Right Large Intestine, Percutaneous Approach
0DLF4CZ Occlusion of Right Large Intestine with Extraluminal Device, Percutaneous Endoscopic Approach
0DLF4DZ Occlusion of Right Large Intestine with Intraluminal Device, Percutaneous Endoscopic Approach
0DLF4ZZ Occlusion of Right Large Intestine, Percutaneous Endoscopic Approach
0DLF7DZ Occlusion of Right Large Intestine with Intraluminal Device, Via Natural or Artificial Opening
0DLF7ZZ Occlusion of Right Large Intestine, Via Natural or Artificial Opening
0DLF8DZ Occlusion of Right Large Intestine with Intraluminal Device, Via Natural or Artificial Opening Endoscopic

♀ Female-only   ♂ Male-only   ● Limited Coverage   ● Non-OR   [HAC] HAC-associated procedure   ● Non-covered procedures   ✚ Combination

0DLF8ZZ Occlusion of Right Large Intestine, Via Natural or Artificial Opening Endoscopic

0DLG0CZ Occlusion of Left Large Intestine with Extraluminal Device, Open Approach

0DLG0DZ Occlusion of Left Large Intestine with Intraluminal Device, Open Approach

0DLG0ZZ Occlusion of Left Large Intestine, Open Approach

0DLG3CZ Occlusion of Left Large Intestine with Extraluminal Device, Percutaneous Approach

0DLG3DZ Occlusion of Left Large Intestine with Intraluminal Device, Percutaneous Approach

0DLG3ZZ Occlusion of Left Large Intestine, Percutaneous Approach

0DLG4CZ Occlusion of Left Large Intestine with Extraluminal Device, Percutaneous Endoscopic Approach

0DLG4DZ Occlusion of Left Large Intestine with Intraluminal Device, Percutaneous Endoscopic Approach

0DLG4ZZ Occlusion of Left Large Intestine, Percutaneous Endoscopic Approach

0DLG7DZ Occlusion of Left Large Intestine with Intraluminal Device, Via Natural or Artificial Opening

0DLG7ZZ Occlusion of Left Large Intestine, Via Natural or Artificial Opening

0DLG8DZ Occlusion of Left Large Intestine with Intraluminal Device, Via Natural or Artificial Opening Endoscopic

0DLG8ZZ Occlusion of Left Large Intestine, Via Natural or Artificial Opening Endoscopic

0DLH0CZ Occlusion of Cecum with Extraluminal Device, Open Approach

0DLH0DZ Occlusion of Cecum with Intraluminal Device, Open Approach

0DLH0ZZ Occlusion of Cecum, Open Approach

0DLH3CZ Occlusion of Cecum with Extraluminal Device, Percutaneous Approach

0DLH3DZ Occlusion of Cecum with Intraluminal Device, Percutaneous Approach

0DLH3ZZ Occlusion of Cecum, Percutaneous Approach

0DLH4CZ Occlusion of Cecum with Extraluminal Device, Percutaneous Endoscopic Approach

0DLH4DZ Occlusion of Cecum with Intraluminal Device, Percutaneous Endoscopic Approach

0DLH4ZZ Occlusion of Cecum, Percutaneous Endoscopic Approach

0DLH7DZ Occlusion of Cecum with Intraluminal Device, Via Natural or Artificial Opening

0DLH7ZZ Occlusion of Cecum, Via Natural or Artificial Opening

0DLH8DZ Occlusion of Cecum with Intraluminal Device, Via Natural or Artificial Opening Endoscopic

0DLH8ZZ Occlusion of Cecum, Via Natural or Artificial Opening Endoscopic

0DLK0CZ Occlusion of Ascending Colon with Extraluminal Device, Open Approach

0DLK0DZ Occlusion of Ascending Colon with Intraluminal Device, Open Approach

0DLK0ZZ Occlusion of Ascending Colon, Open Approach

0DLK3CZ Occlusion of Ascending Colon with Extraluminal Device, Percutaneous Approach

0DLK3DZ Occlusion of Ascending Colon with Intraluminal Device, Percutaneous Approach

0DLK3ZZ Occlusion of Ascending Colon, Percutaneous Approach

0DLK4CZ Occlusion of Ascending Colon with Extraluminal Device, Percutaneous Endoscopic Approach

0DLK4DZ Occlusion of Ascending Colon with Intraluminal Device, Percutaneous Endoscopic Approach

0DLK4ZZ Occlusion of Ascending Colon, Percutaneous Endoscopic Approach

0DLK7DZ Occlusion of Ascending Colon with Intraluminal Device, Via Natural or Artificial Opening

0DLK7ZZ Occlusion of Ascending Colon, Via Natural or Artificial Opening

0DLK8DZ Occlusion of Ascending Colon with Intraluminal Device, Via Natural or Artificial Opening Endoscopic

0DLK8ZZ Occlusion of Ascending Colon, Via Natural or Artificial Opening Endoscopic

0DLL0CZ Occlusion of Transverse Colon with Extraluminal Device, Open Approach

0DLL0DZ Occlusion of Transverse Colon with Intraluminal Device, Open Approach

0DLL0ZZ Occlusion of Transverse Colon, Open Approach

0DLL3CZ Occlusion of Transverse Colon with Extraluminal Device, Percutaneous Approach

0DLL3DZ Occlusion of Transverse Colon with Intraluminal Device, Percutaneous Approach

0DLL3ZZ Occlusion of Transverse Colon, Percutaneous Approach

0DLL4CZ Occlusion of Transverse Colon with Extraluminal Device, Percutaneous Endoscopic Approach

0DLL4DZ Occlusion of Transverse Colon with Intraluminal Device, Percutaneous Endoscopic Approach

0DLL4ZZ Occlusion of Transverse Colon, Percutaneous Endoscopic Approach

0DLL7DZ Occlusion of Transverse Colon with Intraluminal Device, Via Natural or Artificial Opening

0DLL7ZZ Occlusion of Transverse Colon, Via Natural or Artificial Opening

0DLL8DZ Occlusion of Transverse Colon with Intraluminal Device, Via Natural or Artificial Opening Endoscopic

0DLL8ZZ Occlusion of Transverse Colon, Via Natural or Artificial Opening Endoscopic

0DLM0CZ Occlusion of Descending Colon with Extraluminal Device, Open Approach

0DLM0DZ Occlusion of Descending Colon with Intraluminal Device, Open Approach

0DLM0ZZ Occlusion of Descending Colon, Open Approach

0DLM3CZ Occlusion of Descending Colon with Extraluminal Device, Percutaneous Approach

0DLM3DZ Occlusion of Descending Colon with Intraluminal Device, Percutaneous Approach

0DLM3ZZ Occlusion of Descending Colon, Percutaneous Approach

0DLM4CZ Occlusion of Descending Colon with Extraluminal Device, Percutaneous Endoscopic Approach

0DLM4DZ Occlusion of Descending Colon with Intraluminal Device, Percutaneous Endoscopic Approach

0DLM4ZZ Occlusion of Descending Colon, Percutaneous Endoscopic Approach

0DLM7DZ Occlusion of Descending Colon with Intraluminal Device, Via Natural or Artificial Opening

0DLM7ZZ Occlusion of Descending Colon, Via Natural or Artificial Opening

0DLM8DZ Occlusion of Descending Colon with Intraluminal Device, Via Natural or Artificial Opening Endoscopic

0DLM8ZZ Occlusion of Descending Colon, Via Natural or Artificial Opening Endoscopic

0DLN0CZ Occlusion of Sigmoid Colon with Extraluminal Device, Open Approach

0DLN0DZ Occlusion of Sigmoid Colon with Intraluminal Device, Open Approach

0DLN0ZZ Occlusion of Sigmoid Colon, Open Approach

0DLN3CZ Occlusion of Sigmoid Colon with Extraluminal Device, Percutaneous Approach

0DLN3DZ Occlusion of Sigmoid Colon with Intraluminal Device, Percutaneous Approach

0DLN3ZZ Occlusion of Sigmoid Colon, Percutaneous Approach

0DLN4CZ Occlusion of Sigmoid Colon with Extraluminal Device, Percutaneous Endoscopic Approach

0DLN4DZ Occlusion of Sigmoid Colon with Intraluminal Device, Percutaneous Endoscopic Approach

0DLN4ZZ Occlusion of Sigmoid Colon, Percutaneous Endoscopic Approach

0DLN7DZ Occlusion of Sigmoid Colon with Intraluminal Device, Via Natural or Artificial Opening

0DLN7ZZ Occlusion of Sigmoid Colon, Via Natural or Artificial Opening

0DLN8DZ Occlusion of Sigmoid Colon with Intraluminal Device, Via Natural or Artificial Opening Endoscopic

0DLN8ZZ Occlusion of Sigmoid Colon, Via Natural or Artificial Opening Endoscopic

0DLP0CZ Occlusion of Rectum with Extraluminal Device, Open Approach

0DLP0DZ Occlusion of Rectum with Intraluminal Device, Open Approach

0DLP0ZZ Occlusion of Rectum, Open Approach

0DLP3CZ Occlusion of Rectum with Extraluminal Device, Percutaneous Approach

0DLP3DZ Occlusion of Rectum with Intraluminal Device, Percutaneous Approach

0DLP3ZZ Occlusion of Rectum, Percutaneous Approach

0DLP4CZ Occlusion of Rectum with Extraluminal Device, Percutaneous Endoscopic Approach

0DLP4DZ Occlusion of Rectum with Intraluminal Device, Percutaneous Endoscopic Approach

0DLP4ZZ Occlusion of Rectum, Percutaneous Endoscopic Approach

0DLP7DZ Occlusion of Rectum with Intraluminal Device, Via Natural or Artificial Opening

0DLP7ZZ Occlusion of Rectum, Via Natural or Artificial Opening

0DLP8DZ Occlusion of Rectum with Intraluminal Device, Via Natural or Artificial Opening Endoscopic

0DLP8ZZ Occlusion of Rectum, Via Natural or Artificial Opening Endoscopic

0DLQ0CZ Occlusion of Anus with Extraluminal Device, Open Approach

0DLQ0DZ Occlusion of Anus with Intraluminal Device, Open Approach
0DLQ0ZZ Occlusion of Anus, Open Approach
0DLQ3CZ Occlusion of Anus with Extraluminal Device, Percutaneous Approach
0DLQ3DZ Occlusion of Anus with Intraluminal Device, Percutaneous Approach
0DLQ3ZZ Occlusion of Anus, Percutaneous Approach
0DLQ4CZ Occlusion of Anus with Extraluminal Device, Percutaneous Endoscopic Approach
0DLQ4DZ Occlusion of Anus with Intraluminal Device, Percutaneous Endoscopic Approach
0DLQ4ZZ Occlusion of Anus, Percutaneous Endoscopic Approach

0DLQ7DZ Occlusion of Anus with Intraluminal Device, Via Natural or Artificial Opening
0DLQ7ZZ Occlusion of Anus, Via Natural or Artificial Opening
0DLQ8DZ Occlusion of Anus with Intraluminal Device, Via Natural or Artificial Opening Endoscopic
0DLQ8ZZ Occlusion of Anus, Via Natural or Artificial Opening Endoscopic
0DLQXCZ Occlusion of Anus with Extraluminal Device, External Approach
0DLQXDZ Occlusion of Anus with Intraluminal Device, External Approach
0DLQXZZ Occlusion of Anus, External Approach

0DM – Gastrointestinal System, Reattachment

0DM50ZZ Reattachment of Esophagus, Open Approach
0DM54ZZ Reattachment of Esophagus, Percutaneous Endoscopic Approach
0DM60ZZ Reattachment of Stomach, Open Approach
0DM64ZZ Reattachment of Stomach, Percutaneous Endoscopic Approach
0DM80ZZ Reattachment of Small Intestine, Open Approach
0DM84ZZ Reattachment of Small Intestine, Percutaneous Endoscopic Approach
0DM90ZZ Reattachment of Duodenum, Open Approach
0DM94ZZ Reattachment of Duodenum, Percutaneous Endoscopic Approach
0DMA0ZZ Reattachment of Jejunum, Open Approach
0DMA4ZZ Reattachment of Jejunum, Percutaneous Endoscopic Approach
0DMB0ZZ Reattachment of Ileum, Open Approach
0DMB4ZZ Reattachment of Ileum, Percutaneous Endoscopic Approach
0DME0ZZ Reattachment of Large Intestine, Open Approach
0DME4ZZ Reattachment of Large Intestine, Percutaneous Endoscopic Approach
0DMF0ZZ Reattachment of Right Large Intestine, Open Approach
0DMF4ZZ Reattachment of Right Large Intestine, Percutaneous Endoscopic Approach
0DMG0ZZ Reattachment of Left Large Intestine, Open Approach

0DMG4ZZ Reattachment of Left Large Intestine, Percutaneous Endoscopic Approach
0DMH0ZZ Reattachment of Cecum, Open Approach
0DMH4ZZ Reattachment of Cecum, Percutaneous Endoscopic Approach
0DMK0ZZ Reattachment of Ascending Colon, Open Approach
0DMK4ZZ Reattachment of Ascending Colon, Percutaneous Endoscopic Approach
0DML0ZZ Reattachment of Transverse Colon, Open Approach
0DML4ZZ Reattachment of Transverse Colon, Percutaneous Endoscopic Approach
0DMM0ZZ Reattachment of Descending Colon, Open Approach
0DMM4ZZ Reattachment of Descending Colon, Percutaneous Endoscopic Approach
0DMN0ZZ Reattachment of Sigmoid Colon, Open Approach
0DMN4ZZ Reattachment of Sigmoid Colon, Percutaneous Endoscopic Approach
0DMP0ZZ Reattachment of Rectum, Open Approach
0DMP4ZZ Reattachment of Rectum, Percutaneous Endoscopic Approach

0DN – Gastrointestinal System, Release

Review Coding Guideline B3.13

Review Coding Guideline B3.14

0DN10ZZ Release Upper Esophagus, Open Approach
0DN13ZZ Release Upper Esophagus, Percutaneous Approach
0DN14ZZ Release Upper Esophagus, Percutaneous Endoscopic Approach
0DN17ZZ Release Upper Esophagus, Via Natural or Artificial Opening
0DN18ZZ Release Upper Esophagus, Via Natural or Artificial Opening Endoscopic
0DN20ZZ Release Middle Esophagus, Open Approach
0DN23ZZ Release Middle Esophagus, Percutaneous Approach
0DN24ZZ Release Middle Esophagus, Percutaneous Endoscopic Approach
0DN27ZZ Release Middle Esophagus, Via Natural or Artificial Opening
0DN28ZZ Release Middle Esophagus, Via Natural or Artificial Opening Endoscopic
0DN30ZZ Release Lower Esophagus, Open Approach
0DN33ZZ Release Lower Esophagus, Percutaneous Approach
0DN34ZZ Release Lower Esophagus, Percutaneous Endoscopic Approach
0DN37ZZ Release Lower Esophagus, Via Natural or Artificial Opening
0DN38ZZ Release Lower Esophagus, Via Natural or Artificial Opening Endoscopic
0DN40ZZ Release Esophagogastric Junction, Open Approach
0DN43ZZ Release Esophagogastric Junction, Percutaneous Approach
0DN44ZZ Release Esophagogastric Junction, Percutaneous Endoscopic Approach
0DN47ZZ Release Esophagogastric Junction, Via Natural or Artificial Opening
0DN48ZZ Release Esophagogastric Junction, Via Natural or Artificial Opening Endoscopic
0DN50ZZ Release Esophagus, Open Approach
0DN53ZZ Release Esophagus, Percutaneous Approach
0DN54ZZ Release Esophagus, Percutaneous Endoscopic Approach
0DN57ZZ Release Esophagus, Via Natural or Artificial Opening
0DN58ZZ Release Esophagus, Via Natural or Artificial Opening Endoscopic
0DN60ZZ Release Stomach, Open Approach
0DN63ZZ Release Stomach, Percutaneous Approach
0DN64ZZ Release Stomach, Percutaneous Endoscopic Approach
0DN67ZZ Release Stomach, Via Natural or Artificial Opening
0DN68ZZ Release Stomach, Via Natural or Artificial Opening Endoscopic

0DN70ZZ Release Stomach, Pylorus, Open Approach
0DN73ZZ Release Stomach, Pylorus, Percutaneous Approach
0DN74ZZ Release Stomach, Pylorus, Percutaneous Endoscopic Approach
0DN77ZZ Release Stomach, Pylorus, Via Natural or Artificial Opening
0DN78ZZ Release Stomach, Pylorus, Via Natural or Artificial Opening Endoscopic
0DN80ZZ Release Small Intestine, Open Approach
0DN83ZZ Release Small Intestine, Percutaneous Approach
0DN84ZZ Release Small Intestine, Percutaneous Endoscopic Approach
0DN87ZZ Release Small Intestine, Via Natural or Artificial Opening
0DN88ZZ Release Small Intestine, Via Natural or Artificial Opening Endoscopic
0DN90ZZ Release Duodenum, Open Approach
0DN93ZZ Release Duodenum, Percutaneous Approach
0DN94ZZ Release Duodenum, Percutaneous Endoscopic Approach
0DN97ZZ Release Duodenum, Via Natural or Artificial Opening
0DN98ZZ Release Duodenum, Via Natural or Artificial Opening Endoscopic
0DNA0ZZ Release Jejunum, Open Approach
0DNA3ZZ Release Jejunum, Percutaneous Approach
0DNA4ZZ Release Jejunum, Percutaneous Endoscopic Approach
0DNA7ZZ Release Jejunum, Via Natural or Artificial Opening
0DNA8ZZ Release Jejunum, Via Natural or Artificial Opening Endoscopic
0DNB0ZZ Release Ileum, Open Approach
0DNB3ZZ Release Ileum, Percutaneous Approach
0DNB4ZZ Release Ileum, Percutaneous Endoscopic Approach
0DNB7ZZ Release Ileum, Via Natural or Artificial Opening
0DNB8ZZ Release Ileum, Via Natural or Artificial Opening Endoscopic
0DNC0ZZ Release Ileocecal Valve, Open Approach
0DNC3ZZ Release Ileocecal Valve, Percutaneous Approach
0DNC4ZZ Release Ileocecal Valve, Percutaneous Endoscopic Approach
0DNC7ZZ Release Ileocecal Valve, Via Natural or Artificial Opening
0DNC8ZZ Release Ileocecal Valve, Via Natural or Artificial Opening Endoscopic
0DNE0ZZ Release Large Intestine, Open Approach
0DNE3ZZ Release Large Intestine, Percutaneous Approach
0DNE4ZZ Release Large Intestine, Percutaneous Endoscopic Approach
0DNE7ZZ Release Large Intestine, Via Natural or Artificial Opening
0DNE8ZZ Release Large Intestine, Via Natural or Artificial Opening Endoscopic

0DNF0ZZ Release Right Large Intestine, Open Approach
0DNF3ZZ Release Right Large Intestine, Percutaneous Approach
0DNF4ZZ Release Right Large Intestine, Percutaneous Endoscopic Approach
0DNF7ZZ Release Right Large Intestine, Via Natural or Artificial Opening
0DNF8ZZ Release Right Large Intestine, Via Natural or Artificial Opening Endoscopic
0DNG0ZZ Release Left Large Intestine, Open Approach
0DNG3ZZ Release Left Large Intestine, Percutaneous Approach
0DNG4ZZ Release Left Large Intestine, Percutaneous Endoscopic Approach
0DNG7ZZ Release Left Large Intestine, Via Natural or Artificial Opening
0DNG8ZZ Release Left Large Intestine, Via Natural or Artificial Opening Endoscopic
0DNH0ZZ Release Cecum, Open Approach
0DNH3ZZ Release Cecum, Percutaneous Approach
0DNH4ZZ Release Cecum, Percutaneous Endoscopic Approach
0DNH7ZZ Release Cecum, Via Natural or Artificial Opening
0DNH8ZZ Release Cecum, Via Natural or Artificial Opening Endoscopic
0DNJ0ZZ Release Appendix, Open Approach
0DNJ3ZZ Release Appendix, Percutaneous Approach
0DNJ4ZZ Release Appendix, Percutaneous Endoscopic Approach
0DNJ7ZZ Release Appendix, Via Natural or Artificial Opening
0DNJ8ZZ Release Appendix, Via Natural or Artificial Opening Endoscopic
0DNK0ZZ Release Ascending Colon, Open Approach
0DNK3ZZ Release Ascending Colon, Percutaneous Approach
0DNK4ZZ Release Ascending Colon, Percutaneous Endoscopic Approach
0DNK7ZZ Release Ascending Colon, Via Natural or Artificial Opening
0DNK8ZZ Release Ascending Colon, Via Natural or Artificial Opening Endoscopic
0DNL0ZZ Release Transverse Colon, Open Approach
0DNL3ZZ Release Transverse Colon, Percutaneous Approach
0DNL4ZZ Release Transverse Colon, Percutaneous Endoscopic Approach
0DNL7ZZ Release Transverse Colon, Via Natural or Artificial Opening
0DNL8ZZ Release Transverse Colon, Via Natural or Artificial Opening Endoscopic
0DNM0ZZ Release Descending Colon, Open Approach
0DNM3ZZ Release Descending Colon, Percutaneous Approach

0DNM4ZZ Release Descending Colon, Percutaneous Endoscopic Approach
0DNM7ZZ Release Descending Colon, Via Natural or Artificial Opening
0DNM8ZZ Release Descending Colon, Via Natural or Artificial Opening Endoscopic
0DNN0ZZ Release Sigmoid Colon, Open Approach
0DNN3ZZ Release Sigmoid Colon, Percutaneous Approach
0DNN4ZZ Release Sigmoid Colon, Percutaneous Endoscopic Approach
0DNN7ZZ Release Sigmoid Colon, Via Natural or Artificial Opening
0DNN8ZZ Release Sigmoid Colon, Via Natural or Artificial Opening Endoscopic
0DNP0ZZ Release Rectum, Open Approach
0DNP3ZZ Release Rectum, Percutaneous Approach
0DNP4ZZ Release Rectum, Percutaneous Endoscopic Approach
0DNP7ZZ Release Rectum, Via Natural or Artificial Opening
0DNP8ZZ Release Rectum, Via Natural or Artificial Opening Endoscopic
0DNQ0ZZ Release Anus, Open Approach
0DNQ3ZZ Release Anus, Percutaneous Approach
0DNQ4ZZ Release Anus, Percutaneous Endoscopic Approach
0DNQ7ZZ Release Anus, Via Natural or Artificial Opening
0DNQ8ZZ Release Anus, Via Natural or Artificial Opening Endoscopic
0DNQXZZ Release Anus, External Approach
0DNR0ZZ Release Anal Sphincter, Open Approach
0DNR3ZZ Release Anal Sphincter, Percutaneous Approach
0DNR4ZZ Release Anal Sphincter, Percutaneous Endoscopic Approach
0DNS0ZZ Release Greater Omentum, Open Approach
0DNS3ZZ Release Greater Omentum, Percutaneous Approach
0DNS4ZZ Release Greater Omentum, Percutaneous Endoscopic Approach
0DNT0ZZ Release Lesser Omentum, Open Approach
0DNT3ZZ Release Lesser Omentum, Percutaneous Approach
0DNT4ZZ Release Lesser Omentum, Percutaneous Endoscopic Approach
0DNV0ZZ Release Mesentery, Open Approach
0DNV3ZZ Release Mesentery, Percutaneous Approach
0DNV4ZZ Release Mesentery, Percutaneous Endoscopic Approach
0DNW0ZZ Release Peritoneum, Open Approach
0DNW3ZZ Release Peritoneum, Percutaneous Approach
0DNW4ZZ Release Peritoneum, Percutaneous Endoscopic Approach

0DP – Gastrointestinal System, Removal

Review Coding Guideline B6.1c

0DP000Z Removal of Drainage Device from Upper Intestinal Tract, Open Approach
0DP002Z Removal of Monitoring Device from Upper Intestinal Tract, Open Approach
0DP003Z Removal of Infusion Device from Upper Intestinal Tract, Open Approach
0DP007Z Removal of Autologous Tissue Substitute from Upper Intestinal Tract, Open Approach
0DP00CZ Removal of Extraluminal Device from Upper Intestinal Tract, Open Approach
0DP00DZ Removal of Intraluminal Device from Upper Intestinal Tract, Open Approach
0DP00JZ Removal of Synthetic Substitute from Upper Intestinal Tract, Open Approach
0DP00KZ Removal of Nonautologous Tissue Substitute from Upper Intestinal Tract, Open Approach
0DP00UZ Removal of Feeding Device from Upper Intestinal Tract, Open Approach
0DP030Z Removal of Drainage Device from Upper Intestinal Tract, Percutaneous Approach
0DP032Z Removal of Monitoring Device from Upper Intestinal Tract, Percutaneous Approach
0DP033Z Removal of Infusion Device from Upper Intestinal Tract, Percutaneous Approach
0DP037Z Removal of Autologous Tissue Substitute from Upper Intestinal Tract, Percutaneous Approach
0DP03CZ Removal of Extraluminal Device from Upper Intestinal Tract, Percutaneous Approach
0DP03DZ Removal of Intraluminal Device from Upper Intestinal Tract, Percutaneous Approach
0DP03JZ Removal of Synthetic Substitute from Upper Intestinal Tract, Percutaneous Approach

0DP03KZ Removal of Nonautologous Tissue Substitute from Upper Intestinal Tract, Percutaneous Approach
0DP03UZ Removal of Feeding Device from Upper Intestinal Tract, Percutaneous Approach
0DP040Z Removal of Drainage Device from Upper Intestinal Tract, Percutaneous Endoscopic Approach
0DP042Z Removal of Monitoring Device from Upper Intestinal Tract, Percutaneous Endoscopic Approach
0DP043Z Removal of Infusion Device from Upper Intestinal Tract, Percutaneous Endoscopic Approach
0DP047Z Removal of Autologous Tissue Substitute from Upper Intestinal Tract, Percutaneous Endoscopic Approach
0DP04CZ Removal of Extraluminal Device from Upper Intestinal Tract, Percutaneous Endoscopic Approach
0DP04DZ Removal of Intraluminal Device from Upper Intestinal Tract, Percutaneous Endoscopic Approach
0DP04JZ Removal of Synthetic Substitute from Upper Intestinal Tract, Percutaneous Endoscopic Approach
0DP04KZ Removal of Nonautologous Tissue Substitute from Upper Intestinal Tract, Percutaneous Endoscopic Approach
0DP04UZ Removal of Feeding Device from Upper Intestinal Tract, Percutaneous Endoscopic Approach
0DP070Z Removal of Drainage Device from Upper Intestinal Tract, Via Natural or Artificial Opening
0DP072Z Removal of Monitoring Device from Upper Intestinal Tract, Via Natural or Artificial Opening
0DP073Z Removal of Infusion Device from Upper Intestinal Tract, Via Natural or Artificial Opening
0DP077Z Removal of Autologous Tissue Substitute from Upper Intestinal Tract, Via Natural or Artificial Opening
0DP07CZ Removal of Extraluminal Device from Upper Intestinal Tract, Via Natural or Artificial Opening

0DP07DZ Removal of Intraluminal Device from Upper Intestinal Tract, Via Natural or Artificial Opening

0DP07JZ Removal of Synthetic Substitute from Upper Intestinal Tract, Via Natural or Artificial Opening

0DP07KZ Removal of Nonautologous Tissue Substitute from Upper Intestinal Tract, Via Natural or Artificial Opening

0DP07UZ Removal of Feeding Device from Upper Intestinal Tract, Via Natural or Artificial Opening

0DP080Z Removal of Drainage Device from Upper Intestinal Tract, Via Natural or Artificial Opening Endoscopic

0DP082Z Removal of Monitoring Device from Upper Intestinal Tract, Via Natural or Artificial Opening Endoscopic

0DP083Z Removal of Infusion Device from Upper Intestinal Tract, Via Natural or Artificial Opening Endoscopic

0DP087Z Removal of Autologous Tissue Substitute from Upper Intestinal Tract, Via Natural or Artificial Opening Endoscopic

0DP08CZ Removal of Extraluminal Device from Upper Intestinal Tract, Via Natural or Artificial Opening Endoscopic

0DP08DZ Removal of Intraluminal Device from Upper Intestinal Tract, Via Natural or Artificial Opening Endoscopic

0DP08JZ Removal of Synthetic Substitute from Upper Intestinal Tract, Via Natural or Artificial Opening Endoscopic

0DP08KZ Removal of Nonautologous Tissue Substitute from Upper Intestinal Tract, Via Natural or Artificial Opening Endoscopic

0DP08UZ Removal of Feeding Device from Upper Intestinal Tract, Via Natural or Artificial Opening Endoscopic

0DP0X0Z Removal of Drainage Device from Upper Intestinal Tract, External Approach

0DP0X2Z Removal of Monitoring Device from Upper Intestinal Tract, External Approach

0DP0X3Z Removal of Infusion Device from Upper Intestinal Tract, External Approach

0DP0XDZ Removal of Intraluminal Device from Upper Intestinal Tract, External Approach

0DP0XUZ Removal of Feeding Device from Upper Intestinal Tract, External Approach

0DP501Z Removal of Radioactive Element from Esophagus, Open Approach

0DP502Z Removal of Monitoring Device from Esophagus, Open Approach

0DP503Z Removal of Infusion Device from Esophagus, Open Approach

0DP50UZ Removal of Feeding Device from Esophagus, Open Approach

0DP531Z Removal of Radioactive Element from Esophagus, Percutaneous Approach

0DP532Z Removal of Monitoring Device from Esophagus, Percutaneous Approach

0DP533Z Removal of Infusion Device from Esophagus, Percutaneous Approach

0DP53UZ Removal of Feeding Device from Esophagus, Percutaneous Approach

0DP541Z Removal of Radioactive Element from Esophagus, Percutaneous Endoscopic Approach

0DP542Z Removal of Monitoring Device from Esophagus, Percutaneous Endoscopic Approach

0DP543Z Removal of Infusion Device from Esophagus, Percutaneous Endoscopic Approach

0DP54UZ Removal of Feeding Device from Esophagus, Percutaneous Endoscopic Approach

0DP571Z Removal of Radioactive Element from Esophagus, Via Natural or Artificial Opening

0DP57DZ Removal of Intraluminal Device from Esophagus, Via Natural or Artificial Opening

0DP581Z Removal of Radioactive Element from Esophagus, Via Natural or Artificial Opening Endoscopic

0DP58DZ Removal of Intraluminal Device from Esophagus, Via Natural or Artificial Opening Endoscopic

0DP5X1Z Removal of Radioactive Element from Esophagus, External Approach

0DP5X2Z Removal of Monitoring Device from Esophagus, External Approach

0DP5X3Z Removal of Infusion Device from Esophagus, External Approach

0DP5XDZ Removal of Intraluminal Device from Esophagus, External Approach

0DP5XUZ Removal of Feeding Device from Esophagus, External Approach

0DP600Z Removal of Drainage Device from Stomach, Open Approach

0DP602Z Removal of Monitoring Device from Stomach, Open Approach

0DP603Z Removal of Infusion Device from Stomach, Open Approach

0DP607Z Removal of Autologous Tissue Substitute from Stomach, Open Approach

0DP60CZ Removal of Extraluminal Device from Stomach, Open Approach

0DP60DZ Removal of Intraluminal Device from Stomach, Open Approach

0DP60JZ Removal of Synthetic Substitute from Stomach, Open Approach

0DP60KZ Removal of Nonautologous Tissue Substitute from Stomach, Open Approach

0DP60MZ Removal of Stimulator Lead from Stomach, Open Approach

0DP60UZ Removal of Feeding Device from Stomach, Open Approach

0DP630Z Removal of Drainage Device from Stomach, Percutaneous Approach

0DP632Z Removal of Monitoring Device from Stomach, Percutaneous Approach

0DP633Z Removal of Infusion Device from Stomach, Percutaneous Approach

0DP637Z Removal of Autologous Tissue Substitute from Stomach, Percutaneous Approach

0DP63CZ Removal of Extraluminal Device from Stomach, Percutaneous Approach

0DP63DZ Removal of Intraluminal Device from Stomach, Percutaneous Approach

0DP63JZ Removal of Synthetic Substitute from Stomach, Percutaneous Approach

0DP63KZ Removal of Nonautologous Tissue Substitute from Stomach, Percutaneous Approach

0DP63MZ Removal of Stimulator Lead from Stomach, Percutaneous Approach

0DP63UZ Removal of Feeding Device from Stomach, Percutaneous Approach

0DP640Z Removal of Drainage Device from Stomach, Percutaneous Endoscopic Approach

0DP642Z Removal of Monitoring Device from Stomach, Percutaneous Endoscopic Approach

0DP643Z Removal of Infusion Device from Stomach, Percutaneous Endoscopic Approach

0DP647Z Removal of Autologous Tissue Substitute from Stomach, Percutaneous Endoscopic Approach

0DP64CZ Removal of Extraluminal Device from Stomach, Percutaneous Endoscopic Approach

0DP64DZ Removal of Intraluminal Device from Stomach, Percutaneous Endoscopic Approach

0DP64JZ Removal of Synthetic Substitute from Stomach, Percutaneous Endoscopic Approach

0DP64KZ Removal of Nonautologous Tissue Substitute from Stomach, Percutaneous Endoscopic Approach

0DP64MZ Removal of Stimulator Lead from Stomach, Percutaneous Endoscopic Approach

0DP64UZ Removal of Feeding Device from Stomach, Percutaneous Endoscopic Approach

0DP670Z Removal of Drainage Device from Stomach, Via Natural or Artificial Opening

0DP672Z Removal of Monitoring Device from Stomach, Via Natural or Artificial Opening

0DP673Z Removal of Infusion Device from Stomach, Via Natural or Artificial Opening

0DP677Z Removal of Autologous Tissue Substitute from Stomach, Via Natural or Artificial Opening

0DP67CZ Removal of Extraluminal Device from Stomach, Via Natural or Artificial Opening

0DP67DZ Removal of Intraluminal Device from Stomach, Via Natural or Artificial Opening

0DP67JZ Removal of Synthetic Substitute from Stomach, Via Natural or Artificial Opening

0DP67KZ Removal of Nonautologous Tissue Substitute from Stomach, Via Natural or Artificial Opening

0DP67UZ Removal of Feeding Device from Stomach, Via Natural or Artificial Opening

0DP680Z Removal of Drainage Device from Stomach, Via Natural or Artificial Opening Endoscopic

0DP682Z Removal of Monitoring Device from Stomach, Via Natural or Artificial Opening Endoscopic

0DP683Z Removal of Infusion Device from Stomach, Via Natural or Artificial Opening Endoscopic

0DP687Z Removal of Autologous Tissue Substitute from Stomach, Via Natural or Artificial Opening Endoscopic

0DP68CZ Removal of Extraluminal Device from Stomach, Via Natural or Artificial Opening Endoscopic

0DP68DZ Removal of Intraluminal Device from Stomach, Via Natural or Artificial Opening Endoscopic

0DP68JZ Removal of Synthetic Substitute from Stomach, Via Natural or Artificial Opening Endoscopic

0DP68KZ Removal of Nonautologous Tissue Substitute from Stomach, Via Natural or Artificial Opening Endoscopic

0DP68UZ Removal of Feeding Device from Stomach, Via Natural or Artificial Opening Endoscopic

0DP6X0Z Removal of Drainage Device from Stomach, External Approach

0DP6X2Z Removal of Monitoring Device from Stomach, External Approach

0DP6X3Z Removal of Infusion Device from Stomach, External Approach

0DP6XDZ Removal of Intraluminal Device from Stomach, External Approach

0DP6XUZ Removal of Feeding Device from Stomach, External Approach

0DPD00Z Removal of Drainage Device from Lower Intestinal Tract, Open Approach

0DPD02Z Removal of Monitoring Device from Lower Intestinal Tract, Open Approach

0DPD03Z Removal of Infusion Device from Lower Intestinal Tract, Open Approach

0DPD07Z Removal of Autologous Tissue Substitute from Lower Intestinal Tract, Open Approach

0DPD0CZ Removal of Extraluminal Device from Lower Intestinal Tract, Open Approach

0DPD0DZ Removal of Intraluminal Device from Lower Intestinal Tract, Open Approach

0DPD0JZ Removal of Synthetic Substitute from Lower Intestinal Tract, Open Approach

0DPD0KZ Removal of Nonautologous Tissue Substitute from Lower Intestinal Tract, Open Approach

0DPD0UZ Removal of Feeding Device from Lower Intestinal Tract, Open Approach

0DPD30Z Removal of Drainage Device from Lower Intestinal Tract, Percutaneous Approach

0DPD32Z Removal of Monitoring Device from Lower Intestinal Tract, Percutaneous Approach

0DPD33Z Removal of Infusion Device from Lower Intestinal Tract, Percutaneous Approach

0DPD37Z Removal of Autologous Tissue Substitute from Lower Intestinal Tract, Percutaneous Approach

0DPD3CZ Removal of Extraluminal Device from Lower Intestinal Tract, Percutaneous Approach

0DPD3DZ Removal of Intraluminal Device from Lower Intestinal Tract, Percutaneous Approach

0DPD3JZ Removal of Synthetic Substitute from Lower Intestinal Tract, Percutaneous Approach

0DPD3KZ Removal of Nonautologous Tissue Substitute from Lower Intestinal Tract, Percutaneous Approach

0DPD3UZ Removal of Feeding Device from Lower Intestinal Tract, Percutaneous Approach

0DPD40Z Removal of Drainage Device from Lower Intestinal Tract, Percutaneous Endoscopic Approach

0DPD42Z Removal of Monitoring Device from Lower Intestinal Tract, Percutaneous Endoscopic Approach

0DPD43Z Removal of Infusion Device from Lower Intestinal Tract, Percutaneous Endoscopic Approach

0DPD47Z Removal of Autologous Tissue Substitute from Lower Intestinal Tract, Percutaneous Endoscopic Approach

0DPD4CZ Removal of Extraluminal Device from Lower Intestinal Tract, Percutaneous Endoscopic Approach

0DPD4DZ Removal of Intraluminal Device from Lower Intestinal Tract, Percutaneous Endoscopic Approach

0DPD4JZ Removal of Synthetic Substitute from Lower Intestinal Tract, Percutaneous Endoscopic Approach

0DPD4KZ Removal of Nonautologous Tissue Substitute from Lower Intestinal Tract, Percutaneous Endoscopic Approach

0DPD4UZ Removal of Feeding Device from Lower Intestinal Tract, Percutaneous Endoscopic Approach

0DPD70Z Removal of Drainage Device from Lower Intestinal Tract, Via Natural or Artificial Opening

0DPD72Z Removal of Monitoring Device from Lower Intestinal Tract, Via Natural or Artificial Opening

0DPD73Z Removal of Infusion Device from Lower Intestinal Tract, Via Natural or Artificial Opening

0DPD77Z Removal of Autologous Tissue Substitute from Lower Intestinal Tract, Via Natural or Artificial Opening

0DPD7CZ Removal of Extraluminal Device from Lower Intestinal Tract, Via Natural or Artificial Opening

0DPD7DZ Removal of Intraluminal Device from Lower Intestinal Tract, Via Natural or Artificial Opening

0DPD7JZ Removal of Synthetic Substitute from Lower Intestinal Tract, Via Natural or Artificial Opening

0DPD7KZ Removal of Nonautologous Tissue Substitute from Lower Intestinal Tract, Via Natural or Artificial Opening

0DPD7UZ Removal of Feeding Device from Lower Intestinal Tract, Via Natural or Artificial Opening

0DPD80Z Removal of Drainage Device from Lower Intestinal Tract, Via Natural or Artificial Opening Endoscopic

0DPD82Z Removal of Monitoring Device from Lower Intestinal Tract, Via Natural or Artificial Opening Endoscopic

0DPD83Z Removal of Infusion Device from Lower Intestinal Tract, Via Natural or Artificial Opening Endoscopic

0DPD87Z Removal of Autologous Tissue Substitute from Lower Intestinal Tract, Via Natural or Artificial Opening Endoscopic

0DPD8CZ Removal of Extraluminal Device from Lower Intestinal Tract, Via Natural or Artificial Opening Endoscopic

0DPD8DZ Removal of Intraluminal Device from Lower Intestinal Tract, Via Natural or Artificial Opening Endoscopic

0DPD8JZ Removal of Synthetic Substitute from Lower Intestinal Tract, Via Natural or Artificial Opening Endoscopic

0DPD8KZ Removal of Nonautologous Tissue Substitute from Lower Intestinal Tract, Via Natural or Artificial Opening Endoscopic

0DPD8UZ Removal of Feeding Device from Lower Intestinal Tract, Via Natural or Artificial Opening Endoscopic

0DPDX0Z Removal of Drainage Device from Lower Intestinal Tract, External Approach

0DPDX2Z Removal of Monitoring Device from Lower Intestinal Tract, External Approach

0DPDX3Z Removal of Infusion Device from Lower Intestinal Tract, External Approach

0DPDXDZ Removal of Intraluminal Device from Lower Intestinal Tract, External Approach

0DPDXUZ Removal of Feeding Device from Lower Intestinal Tract, External Approach

0DPP01Z Removal of Radioactive Element from Rectum, Open Approach

0DPP31Z Removal of Radioactive Element from Rectum, Percutaneous Approach

0DPP41Z Removal of Radioactive Element from Rectum, Percutaneous Endoscopic Approach

0DPP71Z Removal of Radioactive Element from Rectum, Via Natural or Artificial Opening

0DPP81Z Removal of Radioactive Element from Rectum, Via Natural or Artificial Opening Endoscopic

0DPPX1Z Removal of Radioactive Element from Rectum, External Approach

0DPQ0LZ Removal of Artificial Sphincter from Anus, Open Approach

0DPQ3LZ Removal of Artificial Sphincter from Anus, Percutaneous Approach

0DPQ4LZ Removal of Artificial Sphincter from Anus, Percutaneous Endoscopic Approach

0DPQ7LZ Removal of Artificial Sphincter from Anus, Via Natural or Artificial Opening

0DPQ8LZ Removal of Artificial Sphincter from Anus, Via Natural or Artificial Opening Endoscopic

0DPR0MZ Removal of Stimulator Lead from Anal Sphincter, Open Approach

0DPR3MZ Removal of Stimulator Lead from Anal Sphincter, Percutaneous Approach

0DPR4MZ Removal of Stimulator Lead from Anal Sphincter, Percutaneous Endoscopic Approach

0DPU00Z Removal of Drainage Device from Omentum, Open Approach

0DPU01Z Removal of Radioactive Element from Omentum, Open Approach

0DPU07Z Removal of Autologous Tissue Substitute from Omentum, Open Approach

0DPU0JZ Removal of Synthetic Substitute from Omentum, Open Approach

0DPU0KZ Removal of Nonautologous Tissue Substitute from Omentum, Open Approach

0DPU30Z Removal of Drainage Device from Omentum, Percutaneous Approach

---

♀ Female-only   ♂ Male-only   ⬤ Limited Coverage   ⬤ Non-OR   🆑 HAC-associated procedure   ⬤ Non-covered procedures   ➕ Combination

0DPU31Z Removal of Radioactive Element from Omentum, Percutaneous Approach

0DPU37Z Removal of Autologous Tissue Substitute from Omentum, Percutaneous Approach

0DPU3JZ Removal of Synthetic Substitute from Omentum, Percutaneous Approach

0DPU3KZ Removal of Nonautologous Tissue Substitute from Omentum, Percutaneous Approach

0DPU40Z Removal of Drainage Device from Omentum, Percutaneous Endoscopic Approach

0DPU41Z Removal of Radioactive Element from Omentum, Percutaneous Endoscopic Approach

0DPU47Z Removal of Autologous Tissue Substitute from Omentum, Percutaneous Endoscopic Approach

0DPU4JZ Removal of Synthetic Substitute from Omentum, Percutaneous Endoscopic Approach

0DPU4KZ Removal of Nonautologous Tissue Substitute from Omentum, Percutaneous Endoscopic Approach

0DPV00Z Removal of Drainage Device from Mesentery, Open Approach

0DPV01Z Removal of Radioactive Element from Mesentery, Open Approach

0DPV07Z Removal of Autologous Tissue Substitute from Mesentery, Open Approach

0DPV0JZ Removal of Synthetic Substitute from Mesentery, Open Approach

0DPV0KZ Removal of Nonautologous Tissue Substitute from Mesentery, Open Approach

0DPV30Z Removal of Drainage Device from Mesentery, Percutaneous Approach

0DPV31Z Removal of Radioactive Element from Mesentery, Percutaneous Approach

0DPV37Z Removal of Autologous Tissue Substitute from Mesentery, Percutaneous Approach

0DPV3JZ Removal of Synthetic Substitute from Mesentery, Percutaneous Approach

0DPV3KZ Removal of Nonautologous Tissue Substitute from Mesentery, Percutaneous Approach

0DPV40Z Removal of Drainage Device from Mesentery, Percutaneous Endoscopic Approach

0DPV41Z Removal of Radioactive Element from Mesentery, Percutaneous Endoscopic Approach

0DPV47Z Removal of Autologous Tissue Substitute from Mesentery, Percutaneous Endoscopic Approach

0DPV4JZ Removal of Synthetic Substitute from Mesentery, Percutaneous Endoscopic Approach

0DPV4KZ Removal of Nonautologous Tissue Substitute from Mesentery, Percutaneous Endoscopic Approach

0DPW00Z Removal of Drainage Device from Peritoneum, Open Approach

0DPW01Z Removal of Radioactive Element from Peritoneum, Open Approach

0DPW07Z Removal of Autologous Tissue Substitute from Peritoneum, Open Approach

0DPW0JZ Removal of Synthetic Substitute from Peritoneum, Open Approach

0DPW0KZ Removal of Nonautologous Tissue Substitute from Peritoneum, Open Approach

0DPW30Z Removal of Drainage Device from Peritoneum, Percutaneous Approach

0DPW31Z Removal of Radioactive Element from Peritoneum, Percutaneous Approach

0DPW37Z Removal of Autologous Tissue Substitute from Peritoneum, Percutaneous Approach

0DPW3JZ Removal of Synthetic Substitute from Peritoneum, Percutaneous Approach

0DPW3KZ Removal of Nonautologous Tissue Substitute from Peritoneum, Percutaneous Approach

0DPW40Z Removal of Drainage Device from Peritoneum, Percutaneous Endoscopic Approach

0DPW41Z Removal of Radioactive Element from Peritoneum, Percutaneous Endoscopic Approach

0DPW47Z Removal of Autologous Tissue Substitute from Peritoneum, Percutaneous Endoscopic Approach

0DPW4JZ Removal of Synthetic Substitute from Peritoneum, Percutaneous Endoscopic Approach

0DPW4KZ Removal of Nonautologous Tissue Substitute from Peritoneum, Percutaneous Endoscopic Approach

0DQ – Gastrointestinal System, Repair

0DQ10ZZ Repair Upper Esophagus, Open Approach

0DQ13ZZ Repair Upper Esophagus, Percutaneous Approach

0DQ14ZZ Repair Upper Esophagus, Percutaneous Endoscopic Approach

0DQ17ZZ Repair Upper Esophagus, Via Natural or Artificial Opening

0DQ18ZZ Repair Upper Esophagus, Via Natural or Artificial Opening Endoscopic

0DQ20ZZ Repair Middle Esophagus, Open Approach

0DQ23ZZ Repair Middle Esophagus, Percutaneous Approach

0DQ24ZZ Repair Middle Esophagus, Percutaneous Endoscopic Approach

0DQ27ZZ Repair Middle Esophagus, Via Natural or Artificial Opening

0DQ28ZZ Repair Middle Esophagus, Via Natural or Artificial Opening Endoscopic

0DQ30ZZ Repair Lower Esophagus, Open Approach

0DQ33ZZ Repair Lower Esophagus, Percutaneous Approach

0DQ34ZZ Repair Lower Esophagus, Percutaneous Endoscopic Approach

0DQ37ZZ Repair Lower Esophagus, Via Natural or Artificial Opening

0DQ38ZZ Repair Lower Esophagus, Via Natural or Artificial Opening Endoscopic

0DQ40ZZ Repair Esophagogastric Junction, Open Approach

0DQ43ZZ Repair Esophagogastric Junction, Percutaneous Approach

0DQ44ZZ Repair Esophagogastric Junction, Percutaneous Endoscopic Approach

0DQ47ZZ Repair Esophagogastric Junction, Via Natural or Artificial Opening

0DQ48ZZ Repair Esophagogastric Junction, Via Natural or Artificial Opening Endoscopic

0DQ50ZZ Repair Esophagus, Open Approach

0DQ53ZZ Repair Esophagus, Percutaneous Approach

0DQ54ZZ Repair Esophagus, Percutaneous Endoscopic Approach

0DQ57ZZ Repair Esophagus, Via Natural or Artificial Opening

0DQ58ZZ Repair Esophagus, Via Natural or Artificial Opening Endoscopic

0DQ60ZZ Repair Stomach, Open Approach

0DQ63ZZ Repair Stomach, Percutaneous Approach

0DQ64ZZ Repair Stomach, Percutaneous Endoscopic Approach

0DQ67ZZ Repair Stomach, Via Natural or Artificial Opening

0DQ68ZZ Repair Stomach, Via Natural or Artificial Opening Endoscopic

0DQ70ZZ Repair Stomach, Pylorus, Open Approach

0DQ73ZZ Repair Stomach, Pylorus, Percutaneous Approach

0DQ74ZZ Repair Stomach, Pylorus, Percutaneous Endoscopic Approach

0DQ77ZZ Repair Stomach, Pylorus, Via Natural or Artificial Opening

0DQ78ZZ Repair Stomach, Pylorus, Via Natural or Artificial Opening Endoscopic

0DQ80ZZ Repair Small Intestine, Open Approach

0DQ83ZZ Repair Small Intestine, Percutaneous Approach

0DQ84ZZ Repair Small Intestine, Percutaneous Endoscopic Approach

0DQ87ZZ Repair Small Intestine, Via Natural or Artificial Opening

0DQ88ZZ Repair Small Intestine, Via Natural or Artificial Opening Endoscopic

0DQ90ZZ Repair Duodenum, Open Approach

0DQ93ZZ Repair Duodenum, Percutaneous Approach

0DQ94ZZ Repair Duodenum, Percutaneous Endoscopic Approach

0DQ97ZZ Repair Duodenum, Via Natural or Artificial Opening

0DQ98ZZ Repair Duodenum, Via Natural or Artificial Opening Endoscopic

0DQA0ZZ Repair Jejunum, Open Approach

0DQA3ZZ Repair Jejunum, Percutaneous Approach

0DQA4ZZ Repair Jejunum, Percutaneous Endoscopic Approach

0DQA7ZZ Repair Jejunum, Via Natural or Artificial Opening

0DQA8ZZ Repair Jejunum, Via Natural or Artificial Opening Endoscopic

0DQB0ZZ Repair Ileum, Open Approach

0DQB3ZZ Repair Ileum, Percutaneous Approach

0DQB4ZZ Repair Ileum, Percutaneous Endoscopic Approach

0DQB7ZZ Repair Ileum, Via Natural or Artificial Opening

0DQB8ZZ Repair Ileum, Via Natural or Artificial Opening Endoscopic

0DQC0ZZ Repair Ileocecal Valve, Open Approach

0DQC3ZZ Repair Ileocecal Valve, Percutaneous Approach

0DQC4ZZ Repair Ileocecal Valve, Percutaneous Endoscopic Approach

0DQC7ZZ Repair Ileocecal Valve, Via Natural or Artificial Opening

0DQC8ZZ Repair Ileocecal Valve, Via Natural or Artificial Opening Endoscopic
0DQE0ZZ Repair Large Intestine, Open Approach
0DQE3ZZ Repair Large Intestine, Percutaneous Approach
0DQE4ZZ Repair Large Intestine, Percutaneous Endoscopic Approach
0DQE7ZZ Repair Large Intestine, Via Natural or Artificial Opening
0DQE8ZZ Repair Large Intestine, Via Natural or Artificial Opening Endoscopic
0DQF0ZZ Repair Right Large Intestine, Open Approach
0DQF3ZZ Repair Right Large Intestine, Percutaneous Approach
0DQF4ZZ Repair Right Large Intestine, Percutaneous Endoscopic Approach
0DQF7ZZ Repair Right Large Intestine, Via Natural or Artificial Opening
0DQF8ZZ Repair Right Large Intestine, Via Natural or Artificial Opening Endoscopic
0DQG0ZZ Repair Left Large Intestine, Open Approach
0DQG3ZZ Repair Left Large Intestine, Percutaneous Approach
0DQG4ZZ Repair Left Large Intestine, Percutaneous Endoscopic Approach
0DQG7ZZ Repair Left Large Intestine, Via Natural or Artificial Opening
0DQG8ZZ Repair Left Large Intestine, Via Natural or Artificial Opening Endoscopic
0DQH0ZZ Repair Cecum, Open Approach
0DQH3ZZ Repair Cecum, Percutaneous Approach
0DQH4ZZ Repair Cecum, Percutaneous Endoscopic Approach
0DQH7ZZ Repair Cecum, Via Natural or Artificial Opening
0DQH8ZZ Repair Cecum, Via Natural or Artificial Opening Endoscopic
0DQJ0ZZ Repair Appendix, Open Approach
0DQJ3ZZ Repair Appendix, Percutaneous Approach
0DQJ4ZZ Repair Appendix, Percutaneous Endoscopic Approach
0DQJ7ZZ Repair Appendix, Via Natural or Artificial Opening
0DQJ8ZZ Repair Appendix, Via Natural or Artificial Opening Endoscopic
0DQK0ZZ Repair Ascending Colon, Open Approach
0DQK3ZZ Repair Ascending Colon, Percutaneous Approach
0DQK4ZZ Repair Ascending Colon, Percutaneous Endoscopic Approach
0DQK7ZZ Repair Ascending Colon, Via Natural or Artificial Opening
0DQK8ZZ Repair Ascending Colon, Via Natural or Artificial Opening Endoscopic
0DQL0ZZ Repair Transverse Colon, Open Approach
0DQL3ZZ Repair Transverse Colon, Percutaneous Approach
0DQL4ZZ Repair Transverse Colon, Percutaneous Endoscopic Approach
0DQL7ZZ Repair Transverse Colon, Via Natural or Artificial Opening

0DQL8ZZ Repair Transverse Colon, Via Natural or Artificial Opening Endoscopic
0DQM0ZZ Repair Descending Colon, Open Approach
0DQM3ZZ Repair Descending Colon, Percutaneous Approach
0DQM4ZZ Repair Descending Colon, Percutaneous Endoscopic Approach
0DQM7ZZ Repair Descending Colon, Via Natural or Artificial Opening
0DQM8ZZ Repair Descending Colon, Via Natural or Artificial Opening Endoscopic
0DQN0ZZ Repair Sigmoid Colon, Open Approach
0DQN3ZZ Repair Sigmoid Colon, Percutaneous Approach
0DQN4ZZ Repair Sigmoid Colon, Percutaneous Endoscopic Approach
0DQN7ZZ Repair Sigmoid Colon, Via Natural or Artificial Opening
0DQN8ZZ Repair Sigmoid Colon, Via Natural or Artificial Opening Endoscopic
0DQP0ZZ Repair Rectum, Open Approach
0DQP3ZZ Repair Rectum, Percutaneous Approach
0DQP4ZZ Repair Rectum, Percutaneous Endoscopic Approach
0DQP7ZZ Repair Rectum, Via Natural or Artificial Opening
0DQP8ZZ Repair Rectum, Via Natural or Artificial Opening Endoscopic
0DQQ0ZZ Repair Anus, Open Approach
0DQQ3ZZ Repair Anus, Percutaneous Approach
0DQQ4ZZ Repair Anus, Percutaneous Endoscopic Approach
0DQQ7ZZ Repair Anus, Via Natural or Artificial Opening
0DQQ8ZZ Repair Anus, Via Natural or Artificial Opening Endoscopic
0DQQXZZ Repair Anus, External Approach
0DQR0ZZ Repair Anal Sphincter, Open Approach
0DQR3ZZ Repair Anal Sphincter, Percutaneous Approach
0DQR4ZZ Repair Anal Sphincter, Percutaneous Endoscopic Approach
0DQS0ZZ Repair Greater Omentum, Open Approach
0DQS3ZZ Repair Greater Omentum, Percutaneous Approach
0DQS4ZZ Repair Greater Omentum, Percutaneous Endoscopic Approach
0DQT0ZZ Repair Lesser Omentum, Open Approach
0DQT3ZZ Repair Lesser Omentum, Percutaneous Approach
0DQT4ZZ Repair Lesser Omentum, Percutaneous Endoscopic Approach
0DQV0ZZ Repair Mesentery, Open Approach
0DQV3ZZ Repair Mesentery, Percutaneous Approach
0DQV4ZZ Repair Mesentery, Percutaneous Endoscopic Approach
0DQW0ZZ Repair Peritoneum, Open Approach
0DQW3ZZ Repair Peritoneum, Percutaneous Approach
0DQW4ZZ Repair Peritoneum, Percutaneous Endoscopic Approach

0DR – Gastrointestinal System, Replacement

0DR507Z Replacement of Esophagus with Autologous Tissue Substitute, Open Approach
0DR50JZ Replacement of Esophagus with Synthetic Substitute, Open Approach
0DR50KZ Replacement of Esophagus with Nonautologous Tissue Substitute, Open Approach
0DR547Z Replacement of Esophagus with Autologous Tissue Substitute, Percutaneous Endoscopic Approach
0DR54JZ Replacement of Esophagus with Synthetic Substitute, Percutaneous Endoscopic Approach
0DR54KZ Replacement of Esophagus with Nonautologous Tissue Substitute, Percutaneous Endoscopic Approach
0DR577Z Replacement of Esophagus with Autologous Tissue Substitute, Via Natural or Artificial Opening
0DR57JZ Replacement of Esophagus with Synthetic Substitute, Via Natural or Artificial Opening
0DR57KZ Replacement of Esophagus with Nonautologous Tissue Substitute, Via Natural or Artificial Opening
0DR587Z Replacement of Esophagus with Autologous Tissue Substitute, Via Natural or Artificial Opening Endoscopic
0DR58JZ Replacement of Esophagus with Synthetic Substitute, Via Natural or Artificial Opening Endoscopic
0DR58KZ Replacement of Esophagus with Nonautologous Tissue Substitute, Via Natural or Artificial Opening Endoscopic
0DRR07Z Replacement of Anal Sphincter with Autologous Tissue Substitute, Open Approach
0DRR0JZ Replacement of Anal Sphincter with Synthetic Substitute, Open Approach
0DRR0KZ Replacement of Anal Sphincter with Nonautologous Tissue Substitute, Open Approach

0DRR47Z Replacement of Anal Sphincter with Autologous Tissue Substitute, Percutaneous Endoscopic Approach
0DRR4JZ Replacement of Anal Sphincter with Synthetic Substitute, Percutaneous Endoscopic Approach
0DRR4KZ Replacement of Anal Sphincter with Nonautologous Tissue Substitute, Percutaneous Endoscopic Approach
0DRS07Z Replacement of Greater Omentum with Autologous Tissue Substitute, Open Approach
0DRS0JZ Replacement of Greater Omentum with Synthetic Substitute, Open Approach
0DRS0KZ Replacement of Greater Omentum with Nonautologous Tissue Substitute, Open Approach
0DRS47Z Replacement of Greater Omentum with Autologous Tissue Substitute, Percutaneous Endoscopic Approach
0DRS4JZ Replacement of Greater Omentum with Synthetic Substitute, Percutaneous Endoscopic Approach
0DRS4KZ Replacement of Greater Omentum with Nonautologous Tissue Substitute, Percutaneous Endoscopic Approach
0DRT07Z Replacement of Lesser Omentum with Autologous Tissue Substitute, Open Approach
0DRT0JZ Replacement of Lesser Omentum with Synthetic Substitute, Open Approach
0DRT0KZ Replacement of Lesser Omentum with Nonautologous Tissue Substitute, Open Approach
0DRT47Z Replacement of Lesser Omentum with Autologous Tissue Substitute, Percutaneous Endoscopic Approach
0DRT4JZ Replacement of Lesser Omentum with Synthetic Substitute, Percutaneous Endoscopic Approach
0DRT4KZ Replacement of Lesser Omentum with Nonautologous Tissue Substitute, Percutaneous Endoscopic Approach

0DRV07Z Replacement of Mesentery with Autologous Tissue Substitute, Open Approach

0DRV0JZ Replacement of Mesentery with Synthetic Substitute, Open Approach

0DRV0KZ Replacement of Mesentery with Nonautologous Tissue Substitute, Open Approach

0DRV47Z Replacement of Mesentery with Autologous Tissue Substitute, Percutaneous Endoscopic Approach

0DRV4JZ Replacement of Mesentery with Synthetic Substitute, Percutaneous Endoscopic Approach

0DRV4KZ Replacement of Mesentery with Nonautologous Tissue Substitute, Percutaneous Endoscopic Approach

0DRW07Z Replacement of Peritoneum with Autologous Tissue Substitute, Open Approach

0DRW0JZ Replacement of Peritoneum with Synthetic Substitute, Open Approach

0DRW0KZ Replacement of Peritoneum with Nonautologous Tissue Substitute, Open Approach

0DRW47Z Replacement of Peritoneum with Autologous Tissue Substitute, Percutaneous Endoscopic Approach

0DRW4JZ Replacement of Peritoneum with Synthetic Substitute, Percutaneous Endoscopic Approach

0DRW4KZ Replacement of Peritoneum with Nonautologous Tissue Substitute, Percutaneous Endoscopic Approach

0DS – Gastrointestinal System, Reposition

0DS50ZZ Reposition Esophagus, Open Approach
0DS54ZZ Reposition Esophagus, Percutaneous Endoscopic Approach
0DS57ZZ Reposition Esophagus, Via Natural or Artificial Opening
0DS58ZZ Reposition Esophagus, Via Natural or Artificial Opening Endoscopic
0DS5XZZ Reposition Esophagus, External Approach
0DS60ZZ Reposition Stomach, Open Approach
0DS64ZZ Reposition Stomach, Percutaneous Endoscopic Approach
0DS67ZZ Reposition Stomach, Via Natural or Artificial Opening
0DS68ZZ Reposition Stomach, Via Natural or Artificial Opening Endoscopic
0DS6XZZ Reposition Stomach, External Approach
0DS90ZZ Reposition Duodenum, Open Approach
0DS94ZZ Reposition Duodenum, Percutaneous Endoscopic Approach
0DS97ZZ Reposition Duodenum, Via Natural or Artificial Opening
0DS98ZZ Reposition Duodenum, Via Natural or Artificial Opening Endoscopic
0DS9XZZ Reposition Duodenum, External Approach
0DSA0ZZ Reposition Jejunum, Open Approach
0DSA4ZZ Reposition Jejunum, Percutaneous Endoscopic Approach
0DSA7ZZ Reposition Jejunum, Via Natural or Artificial Opening
0DSA8ZZ Reposition Jejunum, Via Natural or Artificial Opening Endoscopic
0DSAXZZ Reposition Jejunum, External Approach
0DSB0ZZ Reposition Ileum, Open Approach
0DSB4ZZ Reposition Ileum, Percutaneous Endoscopic Approach
0DSB7ZZ Reposition Ileum, Via Natural or Artificial Opening
0DSB8ZZ Reposition Ileum, Via Natural or Artificial Opening Endoscopic
0DSBXZZ Reposition Ileum, External Approach
0DSH0ZZ Reposition Cecum, Open Approach
0DSH4ZZ Reposition Cecum, Percutaneous Endoscopic Approach
0DSH7ZZ Reposition Cecum, Via Natural or Artificial Opening
0DSH8ZZ Reposition Cecum, Via Natural or Artificial Opening Endoscopic
0DSHXZZ Reposition Cecum, External Approach
0DSK0ZZ Reposition Ascending Colon, Open Approach

0DSK4ZZ Reposition Ascending Colon, Percutaneous Endoscopic Approach
0DSK7ZZ Reposition Ascending Colon, Via Natural or Artificial Opening
0DSK8ZZ Reposition Ascending Colon, Via Natural or Artificial Opening Endoscopic
0DSKXZZ Reposition Ascending Colon, External Approach
0DSL0ZZ Reposition Transverse Colon, Open Approach
0DSL4ZZ Reposition Transverse Colon, Percutaneous Endoscopic Approach
0DSL7ZZ Reposition Transverse Colon, Via Natural or Artificial Opening
0DSL8ZZ Reposition Transverse Colon, Via Natural or Artificial Opening Endoscopic
0DSLXZZ Reposition Transverse Colon, External Approach
0DSM0ZZ Reposition Descending Colon, Open Approach
0DSM4ZZ Reposition Descending Colon, Percutaneous Endoscopic Approach
0DSM7ZZ Reposition Descending Colon, Via Natural or Artificial Opening
0DSM8ZZ Reposition Descending Colon, Via Natural or Artificial Opening Endoscopic
0DSMXZZ Reposition Descending Colon, External Approach
0DSN0ZZ Reposition Sigmoid Colon, Open Approach
0DSN4ZZ Reposition Sigmoid Colon, Percutaneous Endoscopic Approach
0DSN7ZZ Reposition Sigmoid Colon, Via Natural or Artificial Opening
0DSN8ZZ Reposition Sigmoid Colon, Via Natural or Artificial Opening Endoscopic
0DSNXZZ Reposition Sigmoid Colon, External Approach
0DSP0ZZ Reposition Rectum, Open Approach
0DSP4ZZ Reposition Rectum, Percutaneous Endoscopic Approach
0DSP7ZZ Reposition Rectum, Via Natural or Artificial Opening
0DSP8ZZ Reposition Rectum, Via Natural or Artificial Opening Endoscopic
0DSPXZZ Reposition Rectum, External Approach
0DSQ0ZZ Reposition Anus, Open Approach
0DSQ4ZZ Reposition Anus, Percutaneous Endoscopic Approach
0DSQ7ZZ Reposition Anus, Via Natural or Artificial Opening
0DSQ8ZZ Reposition Anus, Via Natural or Artificial Opening Endoscopic
0DSQXZZ Reposition Anus, External Approach

0DT – Gastrointestinal System, Resection

Review Coding Guideline B3.8

0DT10ZZ Resection of Upper Esophagus, Open Approach
0DT14ZZ Resection of Upper Esophagus, Percutaneous Endoscopic Approach
0DT17ZZ Resection of Upper Esophagus, Via Natural or Artificial Opening
0DT18ZZ Resection of Upper Esophagus, Via Natural or Artificial Opening Endoscopic
0DT20ZZ Resection of Middle Esophagus, Open Approach
0DT24ZZ Resection of Middle Esophagus, Percutaneous Endoscopic Approach
0DT27ZZ Resection of Middle Esophagus, Via Natural or Artificial Opening
0DT28ZZ Resection of Middle Esophagus, Via Natural or Artificial Opening Endoscopic
0DT30ZZ Resection of Lower Esophagus, Open Approach
0DT34ZZ Resection of Lower Esophagus, Percutaneous Endoscopic Approach
0DT37ZZ Resection of Lower Esophagus, Via Natural or Artificial Opening
0DT38ZZ Resection of Lower Esophagus, Via Natural or Artificial Opening Endoscopic
0DT40ZZ Resection of Esophagogastric Junction, Open Approach
0DT44ZZ Resection of Esophagogastric Junction, Percutaneous Endoscopic Approach
0DT47ZZ Resection of Esophagogastric Junction, Via Natural or Artificial Opening

0DT48ZZ Resection of Esophagogastric Junction, Via Natural or Artificial Opening Endoscopic
0DT50ZZ Resection of Esophagus, Open Approach
0DT54ZZ Resection of Esophagus, Percutaneous Endoscopic Approach
0DT57ZZ Resection of Esophagus, Via Natural or Artificial Opening
0DT58ZZ Resection of Esophagus, Via Natural or Artificial Opening Endoscopic
0DT60ZZ Resection of Stomach, Open Approach
0DT64ZZ Resection of Stomach, Percutaneous Endoscopic Approach
0DT67ZZ Resection of Stomach, Via Natural or Artificial Opening
0DT68ZZ Resection of Stomach, Via Natural or Artificial Opening Endoscopic
0DT70ZZ Resection of Stomach, Pylorus, Open Approach
0DT74ZZ Resection of Stomach, Pylorus, Percutaneous Endoscopic Approach
0DT77ZZ Resection of Stomach, Pylorus, Via Natural or Artificial Opening
0DT78ZZ Resection of Stomach, Pylorus, Via Natural or Artificial Opening Endoscopic
0DT80ZZ Resection of Small Intestine, Open Approach
0DT84ZZ Resection of Small Intestine, Percutaneous Endoscopic Approach
0DT87ZZ Resection of Small Intestine, Via Natural or Artificial Opening

0DT88ZZ Resection of Small Intestine, Via Natural or Artificial Opening Endoscopic
0DT90ZZ Resection of Duodenum, Open Approach
0DT94ZZ Resection of Duodenum, Percutaneous Endoscopic Approach
0DT97ZZ Resection of Duodenum, Via Natural or Artificial Opening
0DT98ZZ Resection of Duodenum, Via Natural or Artificial Opening Endoscopic
0DTA0ZZ Resection of Jejunum, Open Approach
0DTA4ZZ Resection of Jejunum, Percutaneous Endoscopic Approach
0DTA7ZZ Resection of Jejunum, Via Natural or Artificial Opening
0DTA8ZZ Resection of Jejunum, Via Natural or Artificial Opening Endoscopic
0DTB0ZZ Resection of Ileum, Open Approach
0DTB4ZZ Resection of Ileum, Percutaneous Endoscopic Approach
0DTB7ZZ Resection of Ileum, Via Natural or Artificial Opening
0DTB8ZZ Resection of Ileum, Via Natural or Artificial Opening Endoscopic
0DTC0ZZ Resection of Ileocecal Valve, Open Approach
0DTC4ZZ Resection of Ileocecal Valve, Percutaneous Endoscopic Approach
0DTC7ZZ Resection of Ileocecal Valve, Via Natural or Artificial Opening
0DTC8ZZ Resection of Ileocecal Valve, Via Natural or Artificial Opening Endoscopic
0DTE0ZZ Resection of Large Intestine, Open Approach
0DTE4ZZ Resection of Large Intestine, Percutaneous Endoscopic Approach
0DTE7ZZ Resection of Large Intestine, Via Natural or Artificial Opening
0DTE8ZZ Resection of Large Intestine, Via Natural or Artificial Opening Endoscopic
0DTF0ZZ Resection of Right Large Intestine, Open Approach
0DTF4ZZ Resection of Right Large Intestine, Percutaneous Endoscopic Approach
0DTF7ZZ Resection of Right Large Intestine, Via Natural or Artificial Opening
0DTF8ZZ Resection of Right Large Intestine, Via Natural or Artificial Opening Endoscopic
0DTG0ZZ Resection of Left Large Intestine, Open Approach
0DTG4ZZ Resection of Left Large Intestine, Percutaneous Endoscopic Approach
0DTG7ZZ Resection of Left Large Intestine, Via Natural or Artificial Opening
0DTG8ZZ Resection of Left Large Intestine, Via Natural or Artificial Opening Endoscopic
0DTH0ZZ Resection of Cecum, Open Approach
0DTH4ZZ Resection of Cecum, Percutaneous Endoscopic Approach
0DTH7ZZ Resection of Cecum, Via Natural or Artificial Opening
0DTH8ZZ Resection of Cecum, Via Natural or Artificial Opening Endoscopic

0DTJ0ZZ Resection of Appendix, Open Approach
0DTJ4ZZ Resection of Appendix, Percutaneous Endoscopic Approach
0DTJ7ZZ Resection of Appendix, Via Natural or Artificial Opening
0DTJ8ZZ Resection of Appendix, Via Natural or Artificial Opening Endoscopic
0DTK0ZZ Resection of Ascending Colon, Open Approach
0DTK4ZZ Resection of Ascending Colon, Percutaneous Endoscopic Approach
0DTK7ZZ Resection of Ascending Colon, Via Natural or Artificial Opening
0DTK8ZZ Resection of Ascending Colon, Via Natural or Artificial Opening Endoscopic
0DTL0ZZ Resection of Transverse Colon, Open Approach
0DTL4ZZ Resection of Transverse Colon, Percutaneous Endoscopic Approach
0DTL7ZZ Resection of Transverse Colon, Via Natural or Artificial Opening
0DTL8ZZ Resection of Transverse Colon, Via Natural or Artificial Opening Endoscopic
0DTM0ZZ Resection of Descending Colon, Open Approach
0DTM4ZZ Resection of Descending Colon, Percutaneous Endoscopic Approach
0DTM7ZZ Resection of Descending Colon, Via Natural or Artificial Opening
0DTM8ZZ Resection of Descending Colon, Via Natural or Artificial Opening Endoscopic
0DTN0ZZ Resection of Sigmoid Colon, Open Approach
0DTN4ZZ Resection of Sigmoid Colon, Percutaneous Endoscopic Approach
0DTN7ZZ Resection of Sigmoid Colon, Via Natural or Artificial Opening
0DTN8ZZ Resection of Sigmoid Colon, Via Natural or Artificial Opening Endoscopic
0DTP0ZZ Resection of Rectum, Open Approach
0DTP4ZZ Resection of Rectum, Percutaneous Endoscopic Approach
0DTP7ZZ Resection of Rectum, Via Natural or Artificial Opening
0DTP8ZZ Resection of Rectum, Via Natural or Artificial Opening Endoscopic
0DTQ0ZZ Resection of Anus, Open Approach
0DTQ4ZZ Resection of Anus, Percutaneous Endoscopic Approach
0DTQ7ZZ Resection of Anus, Via Natural or Artificial Opening
0DTQ8ZZ Resection of Anus, Via Natural or Artificial Opening Endoscopic
0DTR0ZZ Resection of Anal Sphincter, Open Approach
0DTR4ZZ Resection of Anal Sphincter, Percutaneous Endoscopic Approach
0DTS0ZZ Resection of Greater Omentum, Open Approach
0DTS4ZZ Resection of Greater Omentum, Percutaneous Endoscopic Approach
0DTT0ZZ Resection of Lesser Omentum, Open Approach
0DTT4ZZ Resection of Lesser Omentum, Percutaneous Endoscopic Approach

0DU – Gastrointestinal System, Supplement

0DU107Z Supplement Upper Esophagus with Autologous Tissue Substitute, Open Approach
0DU10JZ Supplement Upper Esophagus with Synthetic Substitute, Open Approach
0DU10KZ Supplement Upper Esophagus with Nonautologous Tissue Substitute, Open Approach
0DU147Z Supplement Upper Esophagus with Autologous Tissue Substitute, Percutaneous Endoscopic Approach
0DU14JZ Supplement Upper Esophagus with Synthetic Substitute, Percutaneous Endoscopic Approach
0DU14KZ Supplement Upper Esophagus with Nonautologous Tissue Substitute, Percutaneous Endoscopic Approach
0DU177Z Supplement Upper Esophagus with Autologous Tissue Substitute, Via Natural or Artificial Opening
0DU17JZ Supplement Upper Esophagus with Synthetic Substitute, Via Natural or Artificial Opening
0DU17KZ Supplement Upper Esophagus with Nonautologous Tissue Substitute, Via Natural or Artificial Opening
0DU187Z Supplement Upper Esophagus with Autologous Tissue Substitute, Via Natural or Artificial Opening Endoscopic
0DU18JZ Supplement Upper Esophagus with Synthetic Substitute, Via Natural or Artificial Opening Endoscopic
0DU18KZ Supplement Upper Esophagus with Nonautologous Tissue Substitute, Via Natural or Artificial Opening Endoscopic
0DU207Z Supplement Middle Esophagus with Autologous Tissue Substitute, Open Approach
0DU20JZ Supplement Middle Esophagus with Synthetic Substitute, Open Approach
0DU20KZ Supplement Middle Esophagus with Nonautologous Tissue Substitute, Open Approach

0DU247Z Supplement Middle Esophagus with Autologous Tissue Substitute, Percutaneous Endoscopic Approach
0DU24JZ Supplement Middle Esophagus with Synthetic Substitute, Percutaneous Endoscopic Approach
0DU24KZ Supplement Middle Esophagus with Nonautologous Tissue Substitute, Percutaneous Endoscopic Approach
0DU277Z Supplement Middle Esophagus with Autologous Tissue Substitute, Via Natural or Artificial Opening
0DU27JZ Supplement Middle Esophagus with Synthetic Substitute, Via Natural or Artificial Opening
0DU27KZ Supplement Middle Esophagus with Nonautologous Tissue Substitute, Via Natural or Artificial Opening
0DU287Z Supplement Middle Esophagus with Autologous Tissue Substitute, Via Natural or Artificial Opening Endoscopic
0DU28JZ Supplement Middle Esophagus with Synthetic Substitute, Via Natural or Artificial Opening Endoscopic
0DU28KZ Supplement Middle Esophagus with Nonautologous Tissue Substitute, Via Natural or Artificial Opening Endoscopic
0DU307Z Supplement Lower Esophagus with Autologous Tissue Substitute, Open Approach
0DU30JZ Supplement Lower Esophagus with Synthetic Substitute, Open Approach
0DU30KZ Supplement Lower Esophagus with Nonautologous Tissue Substitute, Open Approach
0DU347Z Supplement Lower Esophagus with Autologous Tissue Substitute, Percutaneous Endoscopic Approach
0DU34JZ Supplement Lower Esophagus with Synthetic Substitute, Percutaneous Endoscopic Approach
0DU34KZ Supplement Lower Esophagus with Nonautologous Tissue Substitute, Percutaneous Endoscopic Approach

0DU377Z   Supplement Lower Esophagus with Autologous Tissue Substitute, Via Natural or Artificial Opening

0DU37JZ   Supplement Lower Esophagus with Synthetic Substitute, Via Natural or Artificial Opening

0DU37KZ   Supplement Lower Esophagus with Nonautologous Tissue Substitute, Via Natural or Artificial Opening

0DU387Z   Supplement Lower Esophagus with Autologous Tissue Substitute, Via Natural or Artificial Opening Endoscopic

0DU38JZ   Supplement Lower Esophagus with Synthetic Substitute, Via Natural or Artificial Opening Endoscopic

0DU38KZ   Supplement Lower Esophagus with Nonautologous Tissue Substitute, Via Natural or Artificial Opening Endoscopic

0DU407Z   Supplement Esophagogastric Junction with Autologous Tissue Substitute, Open Approach

0DU40JZ   Supplement Esophagogastric Junction with Synthetic Substitute, Open Approach

0DU40KZ   Supplement Esophagogastric Junction with Nonautologous Tissue Substitute, Open Approach

0DU447Z   Supplement Esophagogastric Junction with Autologous Tissue Substitute, Percutaneous Endoscopic Approach

0DU44JZ   Supplement Esophagogastric Junction with Synthetic Substitute, Percutaneous Endoscopic Approach

0DU44KZ   Supplement Esophagogastric Junction with Nonautologous Tissue Substitute, Percutaneous Endoscopic Approach

0DU477Z   Supplement Esophagogastric Junction with Autologous Tissue Substitute, Via Natural or Artificial Opening

0DU47JZ   Supplement Esophagogastric Junction with Synthetic Substitute, Via Natural or Artificial Opening

0DU47KZ   Supplement Esophagogastric Junction with Nonautologous Tissue Substitute, Via Natural or Artificial Opening

0DU487Z   Supplement Esophagogastric Junction with Autologous Tissue Substitute, Via Natural or Artificial Opening Endoscopic

0DU48JZ   Supplement Esophagogastric Junction with Synthetic Substitute, Via Natural or Artificial Opening Endoscopic

0DU48KZ   Supplement Esophagogastric Junction with Nonautologous Tissue Substitute, Via Natural or Artificial Opening Endoscopic

0DU507Z   Supplement Esophagus with Autologous Tissue Substitute, Open Approach

0DU50JZ   Supplement Esophagus with Synthetic Substitute, Open Approach

0DU50KZ   Supplement Esophagus with Nonautologous Tissue Substitute, Open Approach

0DU547Z   Supplement Esophagus with Autologous Tissue Substitute, Percutaneous Endoscopic Approach

0DU54JZ   Supplement Esophagus with Synthetic Substitute, Percutaneous Endoscopic Approach

0DU54KZ   Supplement Esophagus with Nonautologous Tissue Substitute, Percutaneous Endoscopic Approach

0DU577Z   Supplement Esophagus with Autologous Tissue Substitute, Via Natural or Artificial Opening

0DU57JZ   Supplement Esophagus with Synthetic Substitute, Via Natural or Artificial Opening

0DU57KZ   Supplement Esophagus with Nonautologous Tissue Substitute, Via Natural or Artificial Opening

0DU587Z   Supplement Esophagus with Autologous Tissue Substitute, Via Natural or Artificial Opening Endoscopic

0DU58JZ   Supplement Esophagus with Synthetic Substitute, Via Natural or Artificial Opening Endoscopic

0DU58KZ   Supplement Esophagus with Nonautologous Tissue Substitute, Via Natural or Artificial Opening Endoscopic

0DU607Z   Supplement Stomach with Autologous Tissue Substitute, Open Approach

0DU60JZ   Supplement Stomach with Synthetic Substitute, Open Approach

0DU60KZ   Supplement Stomach with Nonautologous Tissue Substitute, Open Approach

0DU647Z   Supplement Stomach with Autologous Tissue Substitute, Percutaneous Endoscopic Approach

0DU64JZ   Supplement Stomach with Synthetic Substitute, Percutaneous Endoscopic Approach

0DU64KZ   Supplement Stomach with Nonautologous Tissue Substitute, Percutaneous Endoscopic Approach

0DU677Z   Supplement Stomach with Autologous Tissue Substitute, Via Natural or Artificial Opening

0DU67JZ   Supplement Stomach with Synthetic Substitute, Via Natural or Artificial Opening

0DU67KZ   Supplement Stomach with Nonautologous Tissue Substitute, Via Natural or Artificial Opening

0DU687Z   Supplement Stomach with Autologous Tissue Substitute, Via Natural or Artificial Opening Endoscopic

0DU68JZ   Supplement Stomach with Synthetic Substitute, Via Natural or Artificial Opening Endoscopic

0DU68KZ   Supplement Stomach with Nonautologous Tissue Substitute, Via Natural or Artificial Opening Endoscopic

0DU707Z   Supplement Stomach, Pylorus with Autologous Tissue Substitute, Open Approach

0DU70JZ   Supplement Stomach, Pylorus with Synthetic Substitute, Open Approach

0DU70KZ   Supplement Stomach, Pylorus with Nonautologous Tissue Substitute, Open Approach

0DU747Z   Supplement Stomach, Pylorus with Autologous Tissue Substitute, Percutaneous Endoscopic Approach

0DU74JZ   Supplement Stomach, Pylorus with Synthetic Substitute, Percutaneous Endoscopic Approach

0DU74KZ   Supplement Stomach, Pylorus with Nonautologous Tissue Substitute, Percutaneous Endoscopic Approach

0DU777Z   Supplement Stomach, Pylorus with Autologous Tissue Substitute, Via Natural or Artificial Opening

0DU77JZ   Supplement Stomach, Pylorus with Synthetic Substitute, Via Natural or Artificial Opening

0DU77KZ   Supplement Stomach, Pylorus with Nonautologous Tissue Substitute, Via Natural or Artificial Opening

0DU787Z   Supplement Stomach, Pylorus with Autologous Tissue Substitute, Via Natural or Artificial Opening Endoscopic

0DU78JZ   Supplement Stomach, Pylorus with Synthetic Substitute, Via Natural or Artificial Opening Endoscopic

0DU78KZ   Supplement Stomach, Pylorus with Nonautologous Tissue Substitute, Via Natural or Artificial Opening Endoscopic

0DU807Z   Supplement Small Intestine with Autologous Tissue Substitute, Open Approach

0DU80JZ   Supplement Small Intestine with Synthetic Substitute, Open Approach

0DU80KZ   Supplement Small Intestine with Nonautologous Tissue Substitute, Open Approach

0DU847Z   Supplement Small Intestine with Autologous Tissue Substitute, Percutaneous Endoscopic Approach

0DU84JZ   Supplement Small Intestine with Synthetic Substitute, Percutaneous Endoscopic Approach

0DU84KZ   Supplement Small Intestine with Nonautologous Tissue Substitute, Percutaneous Endoscopic Approach

0DU877Z   Supplement Small Intestine with Autologous Tissue Substitute, Via Natural or Artificial Opening

0DU87JZ   Supplement Small Intestine with Synthetic Substitute, Via Natural or Artificial Opening

0DU87KZ   Supplement Small Intestine with Nonautologous Tissue Substitute, Via Natural or Artificial Opening

0DU887Z   Supplement Small Intestine with Autologous Tissue Substitute, Via Natural or Artificial Opening Endoscopic

0DU88JZ   Supplement Small Intestine with Synthetic Substitute, Via Natural or Artificial Opening Endoscopic

0DU88KZ   Supplement Small Intestine with Nonautologous Tissue Substitute, Via Natural or Artificial Opening Endoscopic

0DU907Z   Supplement Duodenum with Autologous Tissue Substitute, Open Approach

0DU90JZ   Supplement Duodenum with Synthetic Substitute, Open Approach

0DU90KZ   Supplement Duodenum with Nonautologous Tissue Substitute, Open Approach

0DU947Z   Supplement Duodenum with Autologous Tissue Substitute, Percutaneous Endoscopic Approach

0DU94JZ   Supplement Duodenum with Synthetic Substitute, Percutaneous Endoscopic Approach

0DU94KZ   Supplement Duodenum with Nonautologous Tissue Substitute, Percutaneous Endoscopic Approach

0DU977Z   Supplement Duodenum with Autologous Tissue Substitute, Via Natural or Artificial Opening

0DU97JZ   Supplement Duodenum with Synthetic Substitute, Via Natural or Artificial Opening

0DU97KZ   Supplement Duodenum with Nonautologous Tissue Substitute, Via Natural or Artificial Opening

0DU987Z   Supplement Duodenum with Autologous Tissue Substitute, Via Natural or Artificial Opening Endoscopic

0DU98JZ   Supplement Duodenum with Synthetic Substitute, Via Natural or Artificial Opening Endoscopic

0DU98KZ   Supplement Duodenum with Nonautologous Tissue Substitute, Via Natural or Artificial Opening Endoscopic

0DUA07Z   Supplement Jejunum with Autologous Tissue Substitute, Open Approach

0DUA0JZ   Supplement Jejunum with Synthetic Substitute, Open Approach

0DUA0KZ   Supplement Jejunum with Nonautologous Tissue Substitute, Open Approach

0DUA47Z   Supplement Jejunum with Autologous Tissue Substitute, Percutaneous Endoscopic Approach

0DUA4JZ   Supplement Jejunum with Synthetic Substitute, Percutaneous Endoscopic Approach

0DUA4KZ   Supplement Jejunum with Nonautologous Tissue Substitute, Percutaneous Endoscopic Approach

0DUA77Z   Supplement Jejunum with Autologous Tissue Substitute, Via Natural or Artificial Opening

0DUA7JZ   Supplement Jejunum with Synthetic Substitute, Via Natural or Artificial Opening

0DUA7KZ   Supplement Jejunum with Nonautologous Tissue Substitute, Via Natural or Artificial Opening

0DUA87Z   Supplement Jejunum with Autologous Tissue Substitute, Via Natural or Artificial Opening Endoscopic

0DUA8JZ   Supplement Jejunum with Synthetic Substitute, Via Natural or Artificial Opening Endoscopic

0DUA8KZ   Supplement Jejunum with Nonautologous Tissue Substitute, Via Natural or Artificial Opening Endoscopic

0DUB07Z   Supplement Ileum with Autologous Tissue Substitute, Open Approach

0DUB0JZ   Supplement Ileum with Synthetic Substitute, Open Approach

0DUB0KZ   Supplement Ileum with Nonautologous Tissue Substitute, Open Approach

0DUB47Z   Supplement Ileum with Autologous Tissue Substitute, Percutaneous Endoscopic Approach

0DUB4JZ   Supplement Ileum with Synthetic Substitute, Percutaneous Endoscopic Approach

0DUB4KZ   Supplement Ileum with Nonautologous Tissue Substitute, Percutaneous Endoscopic Approach

0DUB77Z   Supplement Ileum with Autologous Tissue Substitute, Via Natural or Artificial Opening

0DUB7JZ   Supplement Ileum with Synthetic Substitute, Via Natural or Artificial Opening

0DUB7KZ   Supplement Ileum with Nonautologous Tissue Substitute, Via Natural or Artificial Opening

0DUB87Z   Supplement Ileum with Autologous Tissue Substitute, Via Natural or Artificial Opening Endoscopic

0DUB8JZ   Supplement Ileum with Synthetic Substitute, Via Natural or Artificial Opening Endoscopic

0DUB8KZ   Supplement Ileum with Nonautologous Tissue Substitute, Via Natural or Artificial Opening Endoscopic

0DUC07Z   Supplement Ileocecal Valve with Autologous Tissue Substitute, Open Approach

0DUC0JZ   Supplement Ileocecal Valve with Synthetic Substitute, Open Approach

0DUC0KZ   Supplement Ileocecal Valve with Nonautologous Tissue Substitute, Open Approach

0DUC47Z   Supplement Ileocecal Valve with Autologous Tissue Substitute, Percutaneous Endoscopic Approach

0DUC4JZ   Supplement Ileocecal Valve with Synthetic Substitute, Percutaneous Endoscopic Approach

0DUC4KZ   Supplement Ileocecal Valve with Nonautologous Tissue Substitute, Percutaneous Endoscopic Approach

0DUC77Z   Supplement Ileocecal Valve with Autologous Tissue Substitute, Via Natural or Artificial Opening

0DUC7JZ   Supplement Ileocecal Valve with Synthetic Substitute, Via Natural or Artificial Opening

0DUC7KZ   Supplement Ileocecal Valve with Nonautologous Tissue Substitute, Via Natural or Artificial Opening

0DUC87Z   Supplement Ileocecal Valve with Autologous Tissue Substitute, Via Natural or Artificial Opening Endoscopic

0DUC8JZ   Supplement Ileocecal Valve with Synthetic Substitute, Via Natural or Artificial Opening Endoscopic

0DUC8KZ   Supplement Ileocecal Valve with Nonautologous Tissue Substitute, Via Natural or Artificial Opening Endoscopic

0DUE07Z   Supplement Large Intestine with Autologous Tissue Substitute, Open Approach

0DUE0JZ   Supplement Large Intestine with Synthetic Substitute, Open Approach

0DUE0KZ   Supplement Large Intestine with Nonautologous Tissue Substitute, Open Approach

0DUE47Z   Supplement Large Intestine with Autologous Tissue Substitute, Percutaneous Endoscopic Approach

0DUE4JZ   Supplement Large Intestine with Synthetic Substitute, Percutaneous Endoscopic Approach

0DUE4KZ   Supplement Large Intestine with Nonautologous Tissue Substitute, Percutaneous Endoscopic Approach

0DUE77Z   Supplement Large Intestine with Autologous Tissue Substitute, Via Natural or Artificial Opening

0DUE7JZ   Supplement Large Intestine with Synthetic Substitute, Via Natural or Artificial Opening

0DUE7KZ   Supplement Large Intestine with Nonautologous Tissue Substitute, Via Natural or Artificial Opening

0DUE87Z   Supplement Large Intestine with Autologous Tissue Substitute, Via Natural or Artificial Opening Endoscopic

0DUE8JZ   Supplement Large Intestine with Synthetic Substitute, Via Natural or Artificial Opening Endoscopic

0DUE8KZ   Supplement Large Intestine with Nonautologous Tissue Substitute, Via Natural or Artificial Opening Endoscopic

0DUF07Z   Supplement Right Large Intestine with Autologous Tissue Substitute, Open Approach

0DUF0JZ   Supplement Right Large Intestine with Synthetic Substitute, Open Approach

0DUF0KZ   Supplement Right Large Intestine with Nonautologous Tissue Substitute, Open Approach

0DUF47Z   Supplement Right Large Intestine with Autologous Tissue Substitute, Percutaneous Endoscopic Approach

0DUF4JZ   Supplement Right Large Intestine with Synthetic Substitute, Percutaneous Endoscopic Approach

0DUF4KZ   Supplement Right Large Intestine with Nonautologous Tissue Substitute, Percutaneous Endoscopic Approach

0DUF77Z   Supplement Right Large Intestine with Autologous Tissue Substitute, Via Natural or Artificial Opening

0DUF7JZ   Supplement Right Large Intestine with Synthetic Substitute, Via Natural or Artificial Opening

0DUF7KZ   Supplement Right Large Intestine with Nonautologous Tissue Substitute, Via Natural or Artificial Opening

0DUF87Z   Supplement Right Large Intestine with Autologous Tissue Substitute, Via Natural or Artificial Opening Endoscopic

0DUF8JZ   Supplement Right Large Intestine with Synthetic Substitute, Via Natural or Artificial Opening Endoscopic

0DUF8KZ   Supplement Right Large Intestine with Nonautologous Tissue Substitute, Via Natural or Artificial Opening Endoscopic

0DUG07Z   Supplement Left Large Intestine with Autologous Tissue Substitute, Open Approach

0DUG0JZ   Supplement Left Large Intestine with Synthetic Substitute, Open Approach

0DUG0KZ   Supplement Left Large Intestine with Nonautologous Tissue Substitute, Open Approach

0DUG47Z   Supplement Left Large Intestine with Autologous Tissue Substitute, Percutaneous Endoscopic Approach

0DUG4JZ   Supplement Left Large Intestine with Synthetic Substitute, Percutaneous Endoscopic Approach

0DUG4KZ   Supplement Left Large Intestine with Nonautologous Tissue Substitute, Percutaneous Endoscopic Approach

0DUG77Z   Supplement Left Large Intestine with Autologous Tissue Substitute, Via Natural or Artificial Opening

0DUG7JZ   Supplement Left Large Intestine with Synthetic Substitute, Via Natural or Artificial Opening

0DUG7KZ   Supplement Left Large Intestine with Nonautologous Tissue Substitute, Via Natural or Artificial Opening

0DUG87Z   Supplement Left Large Intestine with Autologous Tissue Substitute, Via Natural or Artificial Opening Endoscopic

0DUG8JZ   Supplement Left Large Intestine with Synthetic Substitute, Via Natural or Artificial Opening Endoscopic

0DUG8KZ   Supplement Left Large Intestine with Nonautologous Tissue Substitute, Via Natural or Artificial Opening Endoscopic

0DUH07Z   Supplement Cecum with Autologous Tissue Substitute, Open Approach

0DUH0JZ   Supplement Cecum with Synthetic Substitute, Open Approach

0DUH0KZ   Supplement Cecum with Nonautologous Tissue Substitute, Open Approach

0DUH47Z   Supplement Cecum with Autologous Tissue Substitute, Percutaneous Endoscopic Approach

0DUH4JZ   Supplement Cecum with Synthetic Substitute, Percutaneous Endoscopic Approach

0DUH4KZ   Supplement Cecum with Nonautologous Tissue Substitute, Percutaneous Endoscopic Approach

0DUH77Z   Supplement Cecum with Autologous Tissue Substitute, Via Natural or Artificial Opening

0DUH7JZ   Supplement Cecum with Synthetic Substitute, Via Natural or Artificial Opening

0DUH7KZ   Supplement Cecum with Nonautologous Tissue Substitute, Via Natural or Artificial Opening

0DUH87Z   Supplement Cecum with Autologous Tissue Substitute, Via Natural or Artificial Opening Endoscopic

0DUH8JZ   Supplement Cecum with Synthetic Substitute, Via Natural or Artificial Opening Endoscopic

0DUH8KZ   Supplement Cecum with Nonautologous Tissue Substitute, Via Natural or Artificial Opening Endoscopic

0DUK07Z   Supplement Ascending Colon with Autologous Tissue Substitute, Open Approach

0DUK0JZ   Supplement Ascending Colon with Synthetic Substitute, Open Approach

0DUK0KZ   Supplement Ascending Colon with Nonautologous Tissue Substitute, Open Approach

0DUK47Z   Supplement Ascending Colon with Autologous Tissue Substitute, Percutaneous Endoscopic Approach

0DUK4JZ   Supplement Ascending Colon with Synthetic Substitute, Percutaneous Endoscopic Approach

0DUK4KZ   Supplement Ascending Colon with Nonautologous Tissue Substitute, Percutaneous Endoscopic Approach

0DUK77Z   Supplement Ascending Colon with Autologous Tissue Substitute, Via Natural or Artificial Opening

0DUK7JZ   Supplement Ascending Colon with Synthetic Substitute, Via Natural or Artificial Opening

0DUK7KZ   Supplement Ascending Colon with Nonautologous Tissue Substitute, Via Natural or Artificial Opening

0DUK87Z   Supplement Ascending Colon with Autologous Tissue Substitute, Via Natural or Artificial Opening Endoscopic

0DUK8JZ   Supplement Ascending Colon with Synthetic Substitute, Via Natural or Artificial Opening Endoscopic

0DUK8KZ   Supplement Ascending Colon with Nonautologous Tissue Substitute, Via Natural or Artificial Opening Endoscopic

0DUL07Z   Supplement Transverse Colon with Autologous Tissue Substitute, Open Approach

0DUL0JZ   Supplement Transverse Colon with Synthetic Substitute, Open Approach

0DUL0KZ   Supplement Transverse Colon with Nonautologous Tissue Substitute, Open Approach

0DUL47Z   Supplement Transverse Colon with Autologous Tissue Substitute, Percutaneous Endoscopic Approach

0DUL4JZ   Supplement Transverse Colon with Synthetic Substitute, Percutaneous Endoscopic Approach

0DUL4KZ   Supplement Transverse Colon with Nonautologous Tissue Substitute, Percutaneous Endoscopic Approach

0DUL77Z   Supplement Transverse Colon with Autologous Tissue Substitute, Via Natural or Artificial Opening

0DUL7JZ   Supplement Transverse Colon with Synthetic Substitute, Via Natural or Artificial Opening

0DUL7KZ   Supplement Transverse Colon with Nonautologous Tissue Substitute, Via Natural or Artificial Opening

0DUL87Z   Supplement Transverse Colon with Autologous Tissue Substitute, Via Natural or Artificial Opening Endoscopic

0DUL8JZ   Supplement Transverse Colon with Synthetic Substitute, Via Natural or Artificial Opening Endoscopic

0DUL8KZ   Supplement Transverse Colon with Nonautologous Tissue Substitute, Via Natural or Artificial Opening Endoscopic

0DUM07Z   Supplement Descending Colon with Autologous Tissue Substitute, Open Approach

0DUM0JZ   Supplement Descending Colon with Synthetic Substitute, Open Approach

0DUM0KZ   Supplement Descending Colon with Nonautologous Tissue Substitute, Open Approach

0DUM47Z   Supplement Descending Colon with Autologous Tissue Substitute, Percutaneous Endoscopic Approach

0DUM4JZ   Supplement Descending Colon with Synthetic Substitute, Percutaneous Endoscopic Approach

0DUM4KZ   Supplement Descending Colon with Nonautologous Tissue Substitute, Percutaneous Endoscopic Approach

0DUM77Z   Supplement Descending Colon with Autologous Tissue Substitute, Via Natural or Artificial Opening

0DUM7JZ   Supplement Descending Colon with Synthetic Substitute, Via Natural or Artificial Opening

0DUM7KZ   Supplement Descending Colon with Nonautologous Tissue Substitute, Via Natural or Artificial Opening

0DUM87Z   Supplement Descending Colon with Autologous Tissue Substitute, Via Natural or Artificial Opening Endoscopic

0DUM8JZ   Supplement Descending Colon with Synthetic Substitute, Via Natural or Artificial Opening Endoscopic

0DUM8KZ   Supplement Descending Colon with Nonautologous Tissue Substitute, Via Natural or Artificial Opening Endoscopic

0DUN07Z   Supplement Sigmoid Colon with Autologous Tissue Substitute, Open Approach

0DUN0JZ   Supplement Sigmoid Colon with Synthetic Substitute, Open Approach

0DUN0KZ   Supplement Sigmoid Colon with Nonautologous Tissue Substitute, Open Approach

0DUN47Z   Supplement Sigmoid Colon with Autologous Tissue Substitute, Percutaneous Endoscopic Approach

0DUN4JZ   Supplement Sigmoid Colon with Synthetic Substitute, Percutaneous Endoscopic Approach

0DUN4KZ   Supplement Sigmoid Colon with Nonautologous Tissue Substitute, Percutaneous Endoscopic Approach

0DUN77Z   Supplement Sigmoid Colon with Autologous Tissue Substitute, Via Natural or Artificial Opening

0DUN7JZ   Supplement Sigmoid Colon with Synthetic Substitute, Via Natural or Artificial Opening

0DUN7KZ   Supplement Sigmoid Colon with Nonautologous Tissue Substitute, Via Natural or Artificial Opening

0DUN87Z   Supplement Sigmoid Colon with Autologous Tissue Substitute, Via Natural or Artificial Opening Endoscopic

0DUN8JZ   Supplement Sigmoid Colon with Synthetic Substitute, Via Natural or Artificial Opening Endoscopic

0DUN8KZ   Supplement Sigmoid Colon with Nonautologous Tissue Substitute, Via Natural or Artificial Opening Endoscopic

0DUP07Z   Supplement Rectum with Autologous Tissue Substitute, Open Approach

0DUP0JZ   Supplement Rectum with Synthetic Substitute, Open Approach

0DUP0KZ   Supplement Rectum with Nonautologous Tissue Substitute, Open Approach

0DUP47Z   Supplement Rectum with Autologous Tissue Substitute, Percutaneous Endoscopic Approach

0DUP4JZ   Supplement Rectum with Synthetic Substitute, Percutaneous Endoscopic Approach

0DUP4KZ   Supplement Rectum with Nonautologous Tissue Substitute, Percutaneous Endoscopic Approach

0DUP77Z   Supplement Rectum with Autologous Tissue Substitute, Via Natural or Artificial Opening

0DUP7JZ   Supplement Rectum with Synthetic Substitute, Via Natural or Artificial Opening

0DUP7KZ   Supplement Rectum with Nonautologous Tissue Substitute, Via Natural or Artificial Opening

0DUP87Z   Supplement Rectum with Autologous Tissue Substitute, Via Natural or Artificial Opening Endoscopic

0DUP8JZ   Supplement Rectum with Synthetic Substitute, Via Natural or Artificial Opening Endoscopic

0DUP8KZ Supplement Rectum with Nonautologous Tissue Substitute, Via Natural or Artificial Opening Endoscopic

0DUQ07Z Supplement Anus with Autologous Tissue Substitute, Open Approach

0DUQ0JZ Supplement Anus with Synthetic Substitute, Open Approach

0DUQ0KZ Supplement Anus with Nonautologous Tissue Substitute, Open Approach

0DUQ47Z Supplement Anus with Autologous Tissue Substitute, Percutaneous Endoscopic Approach

0DUQ4JZ Supplement Anus with Synthetic Substitute, Percutaneous Endoscopic Approach

0DUQ4KZ Supplement Anus with Nonautologous Tissue Substitute, Percutaneous Endoscopic Approach

0DUQ77Z Supplement Anus with Autologous Tissue Substitute, Via Natural or Artificial Opening

0DUQ7JZ Supplement Anus with Synthetic Substitute, Via Natural or Artificial Opening

0DUQ7KZ Supplement Anus with Nonautologous Tissue Substitute, Via Natural or Artificial Opening

0DUQ87Z Supplement Anus with Autologous Tissue Substitute, Via Natural or Artificial Opening Endoscopic

0DUQ8JZ Supplement Anus with Synthetic Substitute, Via Natural or Artificial Opening Endoscopic

0DUQ8KZ Supplement Anus with Nonautologous Tissue Substitute, Via Natural or Artificial Opening Endoscopic

0DUQX7Z Supplement Anus with Autologous Tissue Substitute, External Approach

0DUQXJZ Supplement Anus with Synthetic Substitute, External Approach

0DUQXKZ Supplement Anus with Nonautologous Tissue Substitute, External Approach

0DUR07Z Supplement Anal Sphincter with Autologous Tissue Substitute, Open Approach

0DUR0JZ Supplement Anal Sphincter with Synthetic Substitute, Open Approach

0DUR0KZ Supplement Anal Sphincter with Nonautologous Tissue Substitute, Open Approach

0DUR47Z Supplement Anal Sphincter with Autologous Tissue Substitute, Percutaneous Endoscopic Approach

0DUR4JZ Supplement Anal Sphincter with Synthetic Substitute, Percutaneous Endoscopic Approach

0DUR4KZ Supplement Anal Sphincter with Nonautologous Tissue Substitute, Percutaneous Endoscopic Approach

0DUS07Z Supplement Greater Omentum with Autologous Tissue Substitute, Open Approach

0DUS0JZ Supplement Greater Omentum with Synthetic Substitute, Open Approach

0DUS0KZ Supplement Greater Omentum with Nonautologous Tissue Substitute, Open Approach

0DUS47Z Supplement Greater Omentum with Autologous Tissue Substitute, Percutaneous Endoscopic Approach

0DUS4JZ Supplement Greater Omentum with Synthetic Substitute, Percutaneous Endoscopic Approach

0DUS4KZ Supplement Greater Omentum with Nonautologous Tissue Substitute, Percutaneous Endoscopic Approach

0DUT07Z Supplement Lesser Omentum with Autologous Tissue Substitute, Open Approach

0DUT0JZ Supplement Lesser Omentum with Synthetic Substitute, Open Approach

0DUT0KZ Supplement Lesser Omentum with Nonautologous Tissue Substitute, Open Approach

0DUT47Z Supplement Lesser Omentum with Autologous Tissue Substitute, Percutaneous Endoscopic Approach

0DUT4JZ Supplement Lesser Omentum with Synthetic Substitute, Percutaneous Endoscopic Approach

0DUT4KZ Supplement Lesser Omentum with Nonautologous Tissue Substitute, Percutaneous Endoscopic Approach

0DUV07Z Supplement Mesentery with Autologous Tissue Substitute, Open Approach

0DUV0JZ Supplement Mesentery with Synthetic Substitute, Open Approach

0DUV0KZ Supplement Mesentery with Nonautologous Tissue Substitute, Open Approach

0DUV47Z Supplement Mesentery with Autologous Tissue Substitute, Percutaneous Endoscopic Approach

0DUV4JZ Supplement Mesentery with Synthetic Substitute, Percutaneous Endoscopic Approach

0DUV4KZ Supplement Mesentery with Nonautologous Tissue Substitute, Percutaneous Endoscopic Approach

0DUW07Z Supplement Peritoneum with Autologous Tissue Substitute, Open Approach

0DUW0JZ Supplement Peritoneum with Synthetic Substitute, Open Approach

0DUW0KZ Supplement Peritoneum with Nonautologous Tissue Substitute, Open Approach

0DUW47Z Supplement Peritoneum with Autologous Tissue Substitute, Percutaneous Endoscopic Approach

0DUW4JZ Supplement Peritoneum with Synthetic Substitute, Percutaneous Endoscopic Approach

0DUW4KZ Supplement Peritoneum with Nonautologous Tissue Substitute, Percutaneous Endoscopic Approach

0DV – Gastrointestinal System, Restriction

0DV10CZ Restriction of Upper Esophagus with Extraluminal Device, Open Approach

0DV10DZ Restriction of Upper Esophagus with Intraluminal Device, Open Approach

0DV10ZZ Restriction of Upper Esophagus, Open Approach

0DV13CZ Restriction of Upper Esophagus with Extraluminal Device, Percutaneous Approach

0DV13DZ Restriction of Upper Esophagus with Intraluminal Device, Percutaneous Approach

0DV13ZZ Restriction of Upper Esophagus, Percutaneous Approach

0DV14CZ Restriction of Upper Esophagus with Extraluminal Device, Percutaneous Endoscopic Approach

0DV14DZ Restriction of Upper Esophagus with Intraluminal Device, Percutaneous Endoscopic Approach

0DV14ZZ Restriction of Upper Esophagus, Percutaneous Endoscopic Approach

0DV17DZ Restriction of Upper Esophagus with Intraluminal Device, Via Natural or Artificial Opening

0DV17ZZ Restriction of Upper Esophagus, Via Natural or Artificial Opening

0DV18DZ Restriction of Upper Esophagus with Intraluminal Device, Via Natural or Artificial Opening Endoscopic

0DV18ZZ Restriction of Upper Esophagus, Via Natural or Artificial Opening Endoscopic

0DV20CZ Restriction of Middle Esophagus with Extraluminal Device, Open Approach

0DV20DZ Restriction of Middle Esophagus with Intraluminal Device, Open Approach

0DV20ZZ Restriction of Middle Esophagus, Open Approach

0DV23CZ Restriction of Middle Esophagus with Extraluminal Device, Percutaneous Approach

0DV23DZ Restriction of Middle Esophagus with Intraluminal Device, Percutaneous Approach

0DV23ZZ Restriction of Middle Esophagus, Percutaneous Approach

0DV24CZ Restriction of Middle Esophagus with Extraluminal Device, Percutaneous Endoscopic Approach

0DV24DZ Restriction of Middle Esophagus with Intraluminal Device, Percutaneous Endoscopic Approach

0DV24ZZ Restriction of Middle Esophagus, Percutaneous Endoscopic Approach

0DV27DZ Restriction of Middle Esophagus with Intraluminal Device, Via Natural or Artificial Opening

0DV27ZZ Restriction of Middle Esophagus, Via Natural or Artificial Opening

0DV28DZ Restriction of Middle Esophagus with Intraluminal Device, Via Natural or Artificial Opening Endoscopic

0DV28ZZ Restriction of Middle Esophagus, Via Natural or Artificial Opening Endoscopic

0DV30CZ Restriction of Lower Esophagus with Extraluminal Device, Open Approach

0DV30DZ Restriction of Lower Esophagus with Intraluminal Device, Open Approach

0DV30ZZ Restriction of Lower Esophagus, Open Approach

0DV33CZ Restriction of Lower Esophagus with Extraluminal Device, Percutaneous Approach

0DV33DZ Restriction of Lower Esophagus with Intraluminal Device, Percutaneous Approach

0DV33ZZ Restriction of Lower Esophagus, Percutaneous Approach

0DV34CZ Restriction of Lower Esophagus with Extraluminal Device, Percutaneous Endoscopic Approach

0DV34DZ Restriction of Lower Esophagus with Intraluminal Device, Percutaneous Endoscopic Approach

0DV34ZZ Restriction of Lower Esophagus, Percutaneous Endoscopic Approach

0DV37DZ Restriction of Lower Esophagus with Intraluminal Device, Via Natural or Artificial Opening

0DV37ZZ Restriction of Lower Esophagus, Via Natural or Artificial Opening

0DV38DZ Restriction of Lower Esophagus with Intraluminal Device, Via Natural or Artificial Opening Endoscopic

0DV38ZZ Restriction of Lower Esophagus, Via Natural or Artificial Opening Endoscopic

0DV40CZ Restriction of Esophagogastric Junction with Extraluminal Device, Open Approach

0DV40DZ Restriction of Esophagogastric Junction with Intraluminal Device, Open Approach

0DV40ZZ Restriction of Esophagogastric Junction, Open Approach

0DV43CZ Restriction of Esophagogastric Junction with Extraluminal Device, Percutaneous Approach

0DV43DZ Restriction of Esophagogastric Junction with Intraluminal Device, Percutaneous Approach

0DV43ZZ Restriction of Esophagogastric Junction, Percutaneous Approach

0DV44CZ Restriction of Esophagogastric Junction with Extraluminal Device, Percutaneous Endoscopic Approach

0DV44DZ Restriction of Esophagogastric Junction with Intraluminal Device, Percutaneous Endoscopic Approach

0DV44ZZ Restriction of Esophagogastric Junction, Percutaneous Endoscopic Approach

0DV47DZ Restriction of Esophagogastric Junction with Intraluminal Device, Via Natural or Artificial Opening

0DV47ZZ Restriction of Esophagogastric Junction, Via Natural or Artificial Opening

0DV48DZ Restriction of Esophagogastric Junction with Intraluminal Device, Via Natural or Artificial Opening Endoscopic

0DV48ZZ Restriction of Esophagogastric Junction, Via Natural or Artificial Opening Endoscopic

0DV50CZ Restriction of Esophagus with Extraluminal Device, Open Approach

0DV50DZ Restriction of Esophagus with Intraluminal Device, Open Approach

0DV50ZZ Restriction of Esophagus, Open Approach

0DV53CZ Restriction of Esophagus with Extraluminal Device, Percutaneous Approach

0DV53DZ Restriction of Esophagus with Intraluminal Device, Percutaneous Approach

0DV53ZZ Restriction of Esophagus, Percutaneous Approach

0DV54CZ Restriction of Esophagus with Extraluminal Device, Percutaneous Endoscopic Approach

0DV54DZ Restriction of Esophagus with Intraluminal Device, Percutaneous Endoscopic Approach

0DV54ZZ Restriction of Esophagus, Percutaneous Endoscopic Approach

0DV57DZ Restriction of Esophagus with Intraluminal Device, Via Natural or Artificial Opening

0DV57ZZ Restriction of Esophagus, Via Natural or Artificial Opening

0DV58DZ Restriction of Esophagus with Intraluminal Device, Via Natural or Artificial Opening Endoscopic

0DV58ZZ Restriction of Esophagus, Via Natural or Artificial Opening Endoscopic

0DV60CZ Restriction of Stomach with Extraluminal Device, Open Approach

0DV60DZ Restriction of Stomach with Intraluminal Device, Open Approach

0DV60ZZ Restriction of Stomach, Open Approach

0DV63CZ Restriction of Stomach with Extraluminal Device, Percutaneous Approach

0DV63DZ Restriction of Stomach with Intraluminal Device, Percutaneous Approach

0DV63ZZ Restriction of Stomach, Percutaneous Approach

0DV64CZ Restriction of Stomach with Extraluminal Device, Percutaneous Endoscopic Approach

  ℍᴬᶜ *When reported with principal diagnosis code K66.01 and secondary diagnosis code K68.11, K95.01, K95.81 or T81.4XXA*

0DV64DZ Restriction of Stomach with Intraluminal Device, Percutaneous Endoscopic Approach

0DV64ZZ Restriction of Stomach, Percutaneous Endoscopic Approach

● **0DV67DZ** Restriction of Stomach with Intraluminal Device, Via Natural or Artificial Opening

0DV67ZZ Restriction of Stomach, Via Natural or Artificial Opening

● **0DV68DZ** Restriction of Stomach with Intraluminal Device, Via Natural or Artificial Opening Endoscopic

0DV68ZZ Restriction of Stomach, Via Natural or Artificial Opening Endoscopic

0DV70CZ Restriction of Stomach, Pylorus with Extraluminal Device, Open Approach

0DV70DZ Restriction of Stomach, Pylorus with Intraluminal Device, Open Approach

0DV70ZZ Restriction of Stomach, Pylorus, Open Approach

0DV73CZ Restriction of Stomach, Pylorus with Extraluminal Device, Percutaneous Approach

0DV73DZ Restriction of Stomach, Pylorus with Intraluminal Device, Percutaneous Approach

0DV73ZZ Restriction of Stomach, Pylorus, Percutaneous Approach

0DV74CZ Restriction of Stomach, Pylorus with Extraluminal Device, Percutaneous Endoscopic Approach

0DV74DZ Restriction of Stomach, Pylorus with Intraluminal Device, Percutaneous Endoscopic Approach

0DV74ZZ Restriction of Stomach, Pylorus, Percutaneous Endoscopic Approach

0DV77DZ Restriction of Stomach, Pylorus with Intraluminal Device, Via Natural or Artificial Opening

0DV77ZZ Restriction of Stomach, Pylorus, Via Natural or Artificial Opening

0DV78DZ Restriction of Stomach, Pylorus with Intraluminal Device, Via Natural or Artificial Opening Endoscopic

0DV78ZZ Restriction of Stomach, Pylorus, Via Natural or Artificial Opening Endoscopic

0DV80CZ Restriction of Small Intestine with Extraluminal Device, Open Approach

0DV80DZ Restriction of Small Intestine with Intraluminal Device, Open Approach

0DV80ZZ Restriction of Small Intestine, Open Approach

0DV83CZ Restriction of Small Intestine with Extraluminal Device, Percutaneous Approach

0DV83DZ Restriction of Small Intestine with Intraluminal Device, Percutaneous Approach

0DV83ZZ Restriction of Small Intestine, Percutaneous Approach

0DV84CZ Restriction of Small Intestine with Extraluminal Device, Percutaneous Endoscopic Approach

0DV84DZ Restriction of Small Intestine with Intraluminal Device, Percutaneous Endoscopic Approach

0DV84ZZ Restriction of Small Intestine, Percutaneous Endoscopic Approach

0DV87DZ Restriction of Small Intestine with Intraluminal Device, Via Natural or Artificial Opening

0DV87ZZ Restriction of Small Intestine, Via Natural or Artificial Opening

0DV88DZ Restriction of Small Intestine with Intraluminal Device, Via Natural or Artificial Opening Endoscopic

0DV88ZZ Restriction of Small Intestine, Via Natural or Artificial Opening Endoscopic

0DV90CZ Restriction of Duodenum with Extraluminal Device, Open Approach

0DV90DZ Restriction of Duodenum with Intraluminal Device, Open Approach

0DV90ZZ Restriction of Duodenum, Open Approach

0DV93CZ Restriction of Duodenum with Extraluminal Device, Percutaneous Approach

0DV93DZ Restriction of Duodenum with Intraluminal Device, Percutaneous Approach

0DV93ZZ Restriction of Duodenum, Percutaneous Approach

0DV94CZ Restriction of Duodenum with Extraluminal Device, Percutaneous Endoscopic Approach

0DV94DZ Restriction of Duodenum with Intraluminal Device, Percutaneous Endoscopic Approach

0DV94ZZ Restriction of Duodenum, Percutaneous Endoscopic Approach

0DV97DZ Restriction of Duodenum with Intraluminal Device, Via Natural or Artificial Opening

0DV97ZZ Restriction of Duodenum, Via Natural or Artificial Opening

0DV98DZ Restriction of Duodenum with Intraluminal Device, Via Natural or Artificial Opening Endoscopic

0DV98ZZ Restriction of Duodenum, Via Natural or Artificial Opening Endoscopic

0DVA0CZ Restriction of Jejunum with Extraluminal Device, Open Approach

0DVA0DZ Restriction of Jejunum with Intraluminal Device, Open Approach

0DVA0ZZ Restriction of Jejunum, Open Approach

0DVA3CZ Restriction of Jejunum with Extraluminal Device, Percutaneous Approach

0DVA3DZ Restriction of Jejunum with Intraluminal Device, Percutaneous Approach

0DVA3ZZ Restriction of Jejunum, Percutaneous Approach

0DVA4CZ Restriction of Jejunum with Extraluminal Device, Percutaneous Endoscopic Approach

0DVA4DZ Restriction of Jejunum with Intraluminal Device, Percutaneous Endoscopic Approach

0DVA4ZZ Restriction of Jejunum, Percutaneous Endoscopic Approach

0DVA7DZ Restriction of Jejunum with Intraluminal Device, Via Natural or Artificial Opening

0DVA7ZZ Restriction of Jejunum, Via Natural or Artificial Opening

0DVA8DZ Restriction of Jejunum with Intraluminal Device, Via Natural or Artificial Opening Endoscopic

0DVA8ZZ Restriction of Jejunum, Via Natural or Artificial Opening Endoscopic

0DVB0CZ Restriction of Ileum with Extraluminal Device, Open Approach

0DVB0DZ Restriction of Ileum with Intraluminal Device, Open Approach

0DVB0ZZ Restriction of Ileum, Open Approach

0DVB3CZ Restriction of Ileum with Extraluminal Device, Percutaneous Approach

0DVB3DZ Restriction of Ileum with Intraluminal Device, Percutaneous Approach

0DVB3ZZ Restriction of Ileum, Percutaneous Approach

0DVB4CZ Restriction of Ileum with Extraluminal Device, Percutaneous Endoscopic Approach

0DVB4DZ Restriction of Ileum with Intraluminal Device, Percutaneous Endoscopic Approach

0DVB4ZZ Restriction of Ileum, Percutaneous Endoscopic Approach

0DVB7DZ Restriction of Ileum with Intraluminal Device, Via Natural or Artificial Opening

0DVB7ZZ Restriction of Ileum, Via Natural or Artificial Opening

0DVB8DZ Restriction of Ileum with Intraluminal Device, Via Natural or Artificial Opening Endoscopic

0DVB8ZZ Restriction of Ileum, Via Natural or Artificial Opening Endoscopic

0DVC0CZ Restriction of Ileocecal Valve with Extraluminal Device, Open Approach

0DVC0DZ Restriction of Ileocecal Valve with Intraluminal Device, Open Approach

0DVC0ZZ Restriction of Ileocecal Valve, Open Approach

0DVC3CZ Restriction of Ileocecal Valve with Extraluminal Device, Percutaneous Approach

0DVC3DZ Restriction of Ileocecal Valve with Intraluminal Device, Percutaneous Approach

0DVC3ZZ Restriction of Ileocecal Valve, Percutaneous Approach

0DVC4CZ Restriction of Ileocecal Valve with Extraluminal Device, Percutaneous Endoscopic Approach

0DVC4DZ Restriction of Ileocecal Valve with Intraluminal Device, Percutaneous Endoscopic Approach

0DVC4ZZ Restriction of Ileocecal Valve, Percutaneous Endoscopic Approach

0DVC7DZ Restriction of Ileocecal Valve with Intraluminal Device, Via Natural or Artificial Opening

0DVC7ZZ Restriction of Ileocecal Valve, Via Natural or Artificial Opening

0DVC8DZ Restriction of Ileocecal Valve with Intraluminal Device, Via Natural or Artificial Opening Endoscopic

0DVC8ZZ Restriction of Ileocecal Valve, Via Natural or Artificial Opening Endoscopic

0DVE0CZ Restriction of Large Intestine with Extraluminal Device, Open Approach

0DVE0DZ Restriction of Large Intestine with Intraluminal Device, Open Approach

0DVE0ZZ Restriction of Large Intestine, Open Approach

0DVE3CZ Restriction of Large Intestine with Extraluminal Device, Percutaneous Approach

0DVE3DZ Restriction of Large Intestine with Intraluminal Device, Percutaneous Approach

0DVE3ZZ Restriction of Large Intestine, Percutaneous Approach

0DVE4CZ Restriction of Large Intestine with Extraluminal Device, Percutaneous Endoscopic Approach

0DVE4DZ Restriction of Large Intestine with Intraluminal Device, Percutaneous Endoscopic Approach

0DVE4ZZ Restriction of Large Intestine, Percutaneous Endoscopic Approach

0DVE7DZ Restriction of Large Intestine with Intraluminal Device, Via Natural or Artificial Opening

0DVE7ZZ Restriction of Large Intestine, Via Natural or Artificial Opening

0DVE8DZ Restriction of Large Intestine with Intraluminal Device, Via Natural or Artificial Opening Endoscopic

0DVE8ZZ Restriction of Large Intestine, Via Natural or Artificial Opening Endoscopic

0DVF0CZ Restriction of Right Large Intestine with Extraluminal Device, Open Approach

0DVF0DZ Restriction of Right Large Intestine with Intraluminal Device, Open Approach

0DVF0ZZ Restriction of Right Large Intestine, Open Approach

0DVF3CZ Restriction of Right Large Intestine with Extraluminal Device, Percutaneous Approach

0DVF3DZ Restriction of Right Large Intestine with Intraluminal Device, Percutaneous Approach

0DVF3ZZ Restriction of Right Large Intestine, Percutaneous Approach

0DVF4CZ Restriction of Right Large Intestine with Extraluminal Device, Percutaneous Endoscopic Approach

0DVF4DZ Restriction of Right Large Intestine with Intraluminal Device, Percutaneous Endoscopic Approach

0DVF4ZZ Restriction of Right Large Intestine, Percutaneous Endoscopic Approach

0DVF7DZ Restriction of Right Large Intestine with Intraluminal Device, Via Natural or Artificial Opening

0DVF7ZZ Restriction of Right Large Intestine, Via Natural or Artificial Opening

0DVF8DZ Restriction of Right Large Intestine with Intraluminal Device, Via Natural or Artificial Opening Endoscopic

0DVF8ZZ Restriction of Right Large Intestine, Via Natural or Artificial Opening Endoscopic

0DVG0CZ Restriction of Left Large Intestine with Extraluminal Device, Open Approach

0DVG0DZ Restriction of Left Large Intestine with Intraluminal Device, Open Approach

0DVG0ZZ Restriction of Left Large Intestine, Open Approach

0DVG3CZ Restriction of Left Large Intestine with Extraluminal Device, Percutaneous Approach

0DVG3DZ Restriction of Left Large Intestine with Intraluminal Device, Percutaneous Approach

0DVG3ZZ Restriction of Left Large Intestine, Percutaneous Approach

0DVG4CZ Restriction of Left Large Intestine with Extraluminal Device, Percutaneous Endoscopic Approach

0DVG4DZ Restriction of Left Large Intestine with Intraluminal Device, Percutaneous Endoscopic Approach

0DVG4ZZ Restriction of Left Large Intestine, Percutaneous Endoscopic Approach

0DVG7DZ Restriction of Left Large Intestine with Intraluminal Device, Via Natural or Artificial Opening

0DVG7ZZ Restriction of Left Large Intestine, Via Natural or Artificial Opening

0DVG8DZ Restriction of Left Large Intestine with Intraluminal Device, Via Natural or Artificial Opening Endoscopic

0DVG8ZZ Restriction of Left Large Intestine, Via Natural or Artificial Opening Endoscopic

0DVH0CZ Restriction of Cecum with Extraluminal Device, Open Approach

0DVH0DZ Restriction of Cecum with Intraluminal Device, Open Approach

0DVH0ZZ Restriction of Cecum, Open Approach

0DVH3CZ Restriction of Cecum with Extraluminal Device, Percutaneous Approach

0DVH3DZ Restriction of Cecum with Intraluminal Device, Percutaneous Approach

0DVH3ZZ Restriction of Cecum, Percutaneous Approach

0DVH4CZ Restriction of Cecum with Extraluminal Device, Percutaneous Endoscopic Approach

0DVH4DZ Restriction of Cecum with Intraluminal Device, Percutaneous Endoscopic Approach

0DVH4ZZ Restriction of Cecum, Percutaneous Endoscopic Approach

0DVH7DZ Restriction of Cecum with Intraluminal Device, Via Natural or Artificial Opening

0DVH7ZZ Restriction of Cecum, Via Natural or Artificial Opening

0DVH8DZ Restriction of Cecum with Intraluminal Device, Via Natural or Artificial Opening Endoscopic

0DVH8ZZ Restriction of Cecum, Via Natural or Artificial Opening Endoscopic

0DVK0CZ Restriction of Ascending Colon with Extraluminal Device, Open Approach

0DVK0DZ Restriction of Ascending Colon with Intraluminal Device, Open Approach

0DVK0ZZ Restriction of Ascending Colon, Open Approach

0DVK3CZ Restriction of Ascending Colon with Extraluminal Device, Percutaneous Approach

0DVK3DZ Restriction of Ascending Colon with Intraluminal Device, Percutaneous Approach

0DVK3ZZ Restriction of Ascending Colon, Percutaneous Approach

0DVK4CZ Restriction of Ascending Colon with Extraluminal Device, Percutaneous Endoscopic Approach

0DVK4DZ Restriction of Ascending Colon with Intraluminal Device, Percutaneous Endoscopic Approach

0DVK4ZZ Restriction of Ascending Colon, Percutaneous Endoscopic Approach

0DVK7DZ Restriction of Ascending Colon with Intraluminal Device, Via Natural or Artificial Opening

0DVK7ZZ Restriction of Ascending Colon, Via Natural or Artificial Opening

0DVK8DZ Restriction of Ascending Colon with Intraluminal Device, Via Natural or Artificial Opening Endoscopic

0DVK8ZZ Restriction of Ascending Colon, Via Natural or Artificial Opening Endoscopic

0DVL0CZ Restriction of Transverse Colon with Extraluminal Device, Open Approach

0DVL0DZ Restriction of Transverse Colon with Intraluminal Device, Open Approach

0DVL0ZZ Restriction of Transverse Colon, Open Approach

0DVL3CZ Restriction of Transverse Colon with Extraluminal Device, Percutaneous Approach

0DVL3DZ Restriction of Transverse Colon with Intraluminal Device, Percutaneous Approach

0DVL3ZZ Restriction of Transverse Colon, Percutaneous Approach

0DVL4CZ Restriction of Transverse Colon with Extraluminal Device, Percutaneous Endoscopic Approach

0DVL4DZ Restriction of Transverse Colon with Intraluminal Device, Percutaneous Endoscopic Approach

0DVL4ZZ Restriction of Transverse Colon, Percutaneous Endoscopic Approach

0DVL7DZ Restriction of Transverse Colon with Intraluminal Device, Via Natural or Artificial Opening

0DVL7ZZ Restriction of Transverse Colon, Via Natural or Artificial Opening

0DVL8DZ Restriction of Transverse Colon with Intraluminal Device, Via Natural or Artificial Opening Endoscopic

0DVL8ZZ Restriction of Transverse Colon, Via Natural or Artificial Opening Endoscopic

0DVM0CZ Restriction of Descending Colon with Extraluminal Device, Open Approach

0DVM0DZ Restriction of Descending Colon with Intraluminal Device, Open Approach

0DVM0ZZ Restriction of Descending Colon, Open Approach

0DVM3CZ Restriction of Descending Colon with Extraluminal Device, Percutaneous Approach

0DVM3DZ Restriction of Descending Colon with Intraluminal Device, Percutaneous Approach

0DVM3ZZ Restriction of Descending Colon, Percutaneous Approach

0DVM4CZ Restriction of Descending Colon with Extraluminal Device, Percutaneous Endoscopic Approach

0DVM4DZ Restriction of Descending Colon with Intraluminal Device, Percutaneous Endoscopic Approach

0DVM4ZZ Restriction of Descending Colon, Percutaneous Endoscopic Approach

0DVM7DZ Restriction of Descending Colon with Intraluminal Device, Via Natural or Artificial Opening

0DVM7ZZ Restriction of Descending Colon, Via Natural or Artificial Opening

0DVM8DZ Restriction of Descending Colon with Intraluminal Device, Via Natural or Artificial Opening Endoscopic

0DVM8ZZ Restriction of Descending Colon, Via Natural or Artificial Opening Endoscopic

0DVN0CZ Restriction of Sigmoid Colon with Extraluminal Device, Open Approach

0DVN0DZ Restriction of Sigmoid Colon with Intraluminal Device, Open Approach

0DVN0ZZ Restriction of Sigmoid Colon, Open Approach

0DVN3CZ Restriction of Sigmoid Colon with Extraluminal Device, Percutaneous Approach

0DVN3DZ Restriction of Sigmoid Colon with Intraluminal Device, Percutaneous Approach

0DVN3ZZ Restriction of Sigmoid Colon, Percutaneous Approach

0DVN4CZ Restriction of Sigmoid Colon with Extraluminal Device, Percutaneous Endoscopic Approach

0DVN4DZ Restriction of Sigmoid Colon with Intraluminal Device, Percutaneous Endoscopic Approach

0DVN4ZZ Restriction of Sigmoid Colon, Percutaneous Endoscopic Approach

0DVN7DZ Restriction of Sigmoid Colon with Intraluminal Device, Via Natural or Artificial Opening

0DVN7ZZ Restriction of Sigmoid Colon, Via Natural or Artificial Opening

0DVN8DZ Restriction of Sigmoid Colon with Intraluminal Device, Via Natural or Artificial Opening Endoscopic

0DVN8ZZ Restriction of Sigmoid Colon, Via Natural or Artificial Opening Endoscopic

0DVP0CZ Restriction of Rectum with Extraluminal Device, Open Approach

0DVP0DZ Restriction of Rectum with Intraluminal Device, Open Approach

0DVP0ZZ Restriction of Rectum, Open Approach

0DVP3CZ Restriction of Rectum with Extraluminal Device, Percutaneous Approach

0DVP3DZ Restriction of Rectum with Intraluminal Device, Percutaneous Approach

0DVP3ZZ Restriction of Rectum, Percutaneous Approach

0DVP4CZ Restriction of Rectum with Extraluminal Device, Percutaneous Endoscopic Approach

0DVP4DZ Restriction of Rectum with Intraluminal Device, Percutaneous Endoscopic Approach

0DVP4ZZ Restriction of Rectum, Percutaneous Endoscopic Approach

0DVP7DZ Restriction of Rectum with Intraluminal Device, Via Natural or Artificial Opening

0DVP7ZZ Restriction of Rectum, Via Natural or Artificial Opening

0DVP8DZ Restriction of Rectum with Intraluminal Device, Via Natural or Artificial Opening Endoscopic

0DVP8ZZ Restriction of Rectum, Via Natural or Artificial Opening Endoscopic

0DVQ0CZ Restriction of Anus with Extraluminal Device, Open Approach

0DVQ0DZ Restriction of Anus with Intraluminal Device, Open Approach

0DVQ0ZZ Restriction of Anus, Open Approach

0DVQ3CZ Restriction of Anus with Extraluminal Device, Percutaneous Approach

0DVQ3DZ Restriction of Anus with Intraluminal Device, Percutaneous Approach

0DVQ3ZZ Restriction of Anus, Percutaneous Approach

0DVQ4CZ Restriction of Anus with Extraluminal Device, Percutaneous Endoscopic Approach

0DVQ4DZ Restriction of Anus with Intraluminal Device, Percutaneous Endoscopic Approach

0DVQ4ZZ Restriction of Anus, Percutaneous Endoscopic Approach

0DVQ7DZ Restriction of Anus with Intraluminal Device, Via Natural or Artificial Opening

0DVQ7ZZ Restriction of Anus, Via Natural or Artificial Opening

0DVQ8DZ Restriction of Anus with Intraluminal Device, Via Natural or Artificial Opening Endoscopic

0DVQ8ZZ Restriction of Anus, Via Natural or Artificial Opening Endoscopic

0DVQXCZ Restriction of Anus with Extraluminal Device, External Approach

0DVQXDZ Restriction of Anus with Intraluminal Device, External Approach

0DVQXZZ Restriction of Anus, External Approach

0DW – Gastrointestinal System, Revision

Review Coding Guideline B6.1c

0DW000Z Revision of Drainage Device in Upper Intestinal Tract, Open Approach

0DW002Z Revision of Monitoring Device in Upper Intestinal Tract, Open Approach

0DW003Z Revision of Infusion Device in Upper Intestinal Tract, Open Approach

0DW007Z Revision of Autologous Tissue Substitute in Upper Intestinal Tract, Open Approach

0DW00CZ Revision of Extraluminal Device in Upper Intestinal Tract, Open Approach

0DW00DZ Revision of Intraluminal Device in Upper Intestinal Tract, Open Approach

0DW00JZ Revision of Synthetic Substitute in Upper Intestinal Tract, Open Approach

0DW00KZ Revision of Nonautologous Tissue Substitute in Upper Intestinal Tract, Open Approach

0DW00UZ Revision of Feeding Device in Upper Intestinal Tract, Open Approach

0DW030Z Revision of Drainage Device in Upper Intestinal Tract, Percutaneous Approach

0DW032Z Revision of Monitoring Device in Upper Intestinal Tract, Percutaneous Approach

0DW033Z Revision of Infusion Device in Upper Intestinal Tract, Percutaneous Approach

0DW037Z Revision of Autologous Tissue Substitute in Upper Intestinal Tract, Percutaneous Approach

0DW03CZ Revision of Extraluminal Device in Upper Intestinal Tract, Percutaneous Approach

0DW03DZ Revision of Intraluminal Device in Upper Intestinal Tract, Percutaneous Approach

0DW03JZ Revision of Synthetic Substitute in Upper Intestinal Tract, Percutaneous Approach

0DW03KZ Revision of Nonautologous Tissue Substitute in Upper Intestinal Tract, Percutaneous Approach

0DW03UZ Revision of Feeding Device in Upper Intestinal Tract, Percutaneous Approach

0DW040Z Revision of Drainage Device in Upper Intestinal Tract, Percutaneous Endoscopic Approach

0DW042Z Revision of Monitoring Device in Upper Intestinal Tract, Percutaneous Endoscopic Approach

0DW043Z Revision of Infusion Device in Upper Intestinal Tract, Percutaneous Endoscopic Approach

0DW047Z Revision of Autologous Tissue Substitute in Upper Intestinal Tract, Percutaneous Endoscopic Approach

0DW04CZ Revision of Extraluminal Device in Upper Intestinal Tract, Percutaneous Endoscopic Approach

0DW04DZ Revision of Intraluminal Device in Upper Intestinal Tract, Percutaneous Endoscopic Approach

0DW04JZ Revision of Synthetic Substitute in Upper Intestinal Tract, Percutaneous Endoscopic Approach

0DW04KZ Revision of Nonautologous Tissue Substitute in Upper Intestinal Tract, Percutaneous Endoscopic Approach

0DW04UZ Revision of Feeding Device in Upper Intestinal Tract, Percutaneous Endoscopic Approach

0DW070Z Revision of Drainage Device in Upper Intestinal Tract, Via Natural or Artificial Opening

0DW072Z Revision of Monitoring Device in Upper Intestinal Tract, Via Natural or Artificial Opening

0DW073Z Revision of Infusion Device in Upper Intestinal Tract, Via Natural or Artificial Opening

0DW077Z Revision of Autologous Tissue Substitute in Upper Intestinal Tract, Via Natural or Artificial Opening

0DW07CZ Revision of Extraluminal Device in Upper Intestinal Tract, Via Natural or Artificial Opening

0DW07DZ Revision of Intraluminal Device in Upper Intestinal Tract, Via Natural or Artificial Opening

0DW07JZ Revision of Synthetic Substitute in Upper Intestinal Tract, Via Natural or Artificial Opening

0DW07KZ Revision of Nonautologous Tissue Substitute in Upper Intestinal Tract, Via Natural or Artificial Opening

0DW07UZ Revision of Feeding Device in Upper Intestinal Tract, Via Natural or Artificial Opening

0DW080Z Revision of Drainage Device in Upper Intestinal Tract, Via Natural or Artificial Opening Endoscopic

0DW082Z Revision of Monitoring Device in Upper Intestinal Tract, Via Natural or Artificial Opening Endoscopic

0DW083Z Revision of Infusion Device in Upper Intestinal Tract, Via Natural or Artificial Opening Endoscopic

0DW087Z Revision of Autologous Tissue Substitute in Upper Intestinal Tract, Via Natural or Artificial Opening Endoscopic

0DW08CZ Revision of Extraluminal Device in Upper Intestinal Tract, Via Natural or Artificial Opening Endoscopic

0DW08DZ Revision of Intraluminal Device in Upper Intestinal Tract, Via Natural or Artificial Opening Endoscopic

0DW08JZ Revision of Synthetic Substitute in Upper Intestinal Tract, Via Natural or Artificial Opening Endoscopic

0DW08KZ Revision of Nonautologous Tissue Substitute in Upper Intestinal Tract, Via Natural or Artificial Opening Endoscopic

0DW08UZ Revision of Feeding Device in Upper Intestinal Tract, Via Natural or Artificial Opening Endoscopic

0DW0X0Z Revision of Drainage Device in Upper Intestinal Tract, External Approach

0DW0X2Z Revision of Monitoring Device in Upper Intestinal Tract, External Approach

0DW0X3Z Revision of Infusion Device in Upper Intestinal Tract, External Approach

0DW0X7Z Revision of Autologous Tissue Substitute in Upper Intestinal Tract, External Approach

0DW0XCZ Revision of Extraluminal Device in Upper Intestinal Tract, External Approach

0DW0XDZ Revision of Intraluminal Device in Upper Intestinal Tract, External Approach

0DW0XJZ Revision of Synthetic Substitute in Upper Intestinal Tract, External Approach

0DW0XKZ Revision of Nonautologous Tissue Substitute in Upper Intestinal Tract, External Approach

0DW0XUZ Revision of Feeding Device in Upper Intestinal Tract, External Approach

0DW57DZ Revision of Intraluminal Device in Esophagus, Via Natural or Artificial Opening

0DW58DZ Revision of Intraluminal Device in Esophagus, Via Natural or Artificial Opening Endoscopic

0DW5XDZ Revision of Intraluminal Device in Esophagus, External Approach

0DW600Z Revision of Drainage Device in Stomach, Open Approach

0DW602Z Revision of Monitoring Device in Stomach, Open Approach

0DW603Z Revision of Infusion Device in Stomach, Open Approach

0DW607Z Revision of Autologous Tissue Substitute in Stomach, Open Approach

0DW60CZ Revision of Extraluminal Device in Stomach, Open Approach

0DW60DZ Revision of Intraluminal Device in Stomach, Open Approach

0DW60JZ Revision of Synthetic Substitute in Stomach, Open Approach

0DW60KZ Revision of Nonautologous Tissue Substitute in Stomach, Open Approach

0DW60MZ Revision of Stimulator Lead in Stomach, Open Approach

0DW60UZ Revision of Feeding Device in Stomach, Open Approach

0DW630Z Revision of Drainage Device in Stomach, Percutaneous Approach

0DW632Z Revision of Monitoring Device in Stomach, Percutaneous Approach

0DW633Z Revision of Infusion Device in Stomach, Percutaneous Approach

0DW637Z Revision of Autologous Tissue Substitute in Stomach, Percutaneous Approach

0DW63CZ Revision of Extraluminal Device in Stomach, Percutaneous Approach

0DW63DZ Revision of Intraluminal Device in Stomach, Percutaneous Approach

0DW63JZ Revision of Synthetic Substitute in Stomach, Percutaneous Approach

0DW63KZ Revision of Nonautologous Tissue Substitute in Stomach, Percutaneous Approach

0DW63MZ Revision of Stimulator Lead in Stomach, Percutaneous Approach

0DW63UZ Revision of Feeding Device in Stomach, Percutaneous Approach

---

♀ Female-only   ♂ Male-only   ⬤ Limited Coverage   ● Non-OR   🅷🅰🅲 HAC-associated procedure   ⬤ Non-covered procedures   ➕ Combination

0DW640Z Revision of Drainage Device in Stomach, Percutaneous Endoscopic Approach

0DW642Z Revision of Monitoring Device in Stomach, Percutaneous Endoscopic Approach

0DW643Z Revision of Infusion Device in Stomach, Percutaneous Endoscopic Approach

0DW647Z Revision of Autologous Tissue Substitute in Stomach, Percutaneous Endoscopic Approach

0DW64CZ Revision of Extraluminal Device in Stomach, Percutaneous Endoscopic Approach

0DW64DZ Revision of Intraluminal Device in Stomach, Percutaneous Endoscopic Approach

0DW64JZ Revision of Synthetic Substitute in Stomach, Percutaneous Endoscopic Approach

0DW64KZ Revision of Nonautologous Tissue Substitute in Stomach, Percutaneous Endoscopic Approach

0DW64MZ Revision of Stimulator Lead in Stomach, Percutaneous Endoscopic Approach

0DW64UZ Revision of Feeding Device in Stomach, Percutaneous Endoscopic Approach

0DW670Z Revision of Drainage Device in Stomach, Via Natural or Artificial Opening

0DW672Z Revision of Monitoring Device in Stomach, Via Natural or Artificial Opening

0DW673Z Revision of Infusion Device in Stomach, Via Natural or Artificial Opening

0DW677Z Revision of Autologous Tissue Substitute in Stomach, Via Natural or Artificial Opening

0DW67CZ Revision of Extraluminal Device in Stomach, Via Natural or Artificial Opening

0DW67DZ Revision of Intraluminal Device in Stomach, Via Natural or Artificial Opening

0DW67JZ Revision of Synthetic Substitute in Stomach, Via Natural or Artificial Opening

0DW67KZ Revision of Nonautologous Tissue Substitute in Stomach, Via Natural or Artificial Opening

0DW67UZ Revision of Feeding Device in Stomach, Via Natural or Artificial Opening

0DW680Z Revision of Drainage Device in Stomach, Via Natural or Artificial Opening Endoscopic

0DW682Z Revision of Monitoring Device in Stomach, Via Natural or Artificial Opening Endoscopic

0DW683Z Revision of Infusion Device in Stomach, Via Natural or Artificial Opening Endoscopic

0DW687Z Revision of Autologous Tissue Substitute in Stomach, Via Natural or Artificial Opening Endoscopic

0DW68CZ Revision of Extraluminal Device in Stomach, Via Natural or Artificial Opening Endoscopic

0DW68DZ Revision of Intraluminal Device in Stomach, Via Natural or Artificial Opening Endoscopic

0DW68JZ Revision of Synthetic Substitute in Stomach, Via Natural or Artificial Opening Endoscopic

0DW68KZ Revision of Nonautologous Tissue Substitute in Stomach, Via Natural or Artificial Opening Endoscopic

0DW68UZ Revision of Feeding Device in Stomach, Via Natural or Artificial Opening Endoscopic

0DW6X0Z Revision of Drainage Device in Stomach, External Approach

0DW6X2Z Revision of Monitoring Device in Stomach, External Approach

0DW6X3Z Revision of Infusion Device in Stomach, External Approach

0DW6X7Z Revision of Autologous Tissue Substitute in Stomach, External Approach

0DW6XCZ Revision of Extraluminal Device in Stomach, External Approach

0DW6XDZ Revision of Intraluminal Device in Stomach, External Approach

0DW6XJZ Revision of Synthetic Substitute in Stomach, External Approach

0DW6XKZ Revision of Nonautologous Tissue Substitute in Stomach, External Approach

0DW6XUZ Revision of Feeding Device in Stomach, External Approach

0DW807Z Revision of Autologous Tissue Substitute in Small Intestine, Open Approach

0DW80JZ Revision of Synthetic Substitute in Small Intestine, Open Approach

0DW80KZ Revision of Nonautologous Tissue Substitute in Small Intestine, Open Approach

0DW847Z Revision of Autologous Tissue Substitute in Small Intestine, Percutaneous Endoscopic Approach

0DW84JZ Revision of Synthetic Substitute in Small Intestine, Percutaneous Endoscopic Approach

0DW84KZ Revision of Nonautologous Tissue Substitute in Small Intestine, Percutaneous Endoscopic Approach

0DW877Z Revision of Autologous Tissue Substitute in Small Intestine, Via Natural or Artificial Opening

0DW87JZ Revision of Synthetic Substitute in Small Intestine, Via Natural or Artificial Opening

0DW87KZ Revision of Nonautologous Tissue Substitute in Small Intestine, Via Natural or Artificial Opening

0DW887Z Revision of Autologous Tissue Substitute in Small Intestine, Via Natural or Artificial Opening Endoscopic

0DW88JZ Revision of Synthetic Substitute in Small Intestine, Via Natural or Artificial Opening Endoscopic

0DW88KZ Revision of Nonautologous Tissue Substitute in Small Intestine, Via Natural or Artificial Opening Endoscopic

0DWD00Z Revision of Drainage Device in Lower Intestinal Tract, Open Approach

0DWD02Z Revision of Monitoring Device in Lower Intestinal Tract, Open Approach

0DWD03Z Revision of Infusion Device in Lower Intestinal Tract, Open Approach

0DWD07Z Revision of Autologous Tissue Substitute in Lower Intestinal Tract, Open Approach

0DWD0CZ Revision of Extraluminal Device in Lower Intestinal Tract, Open Approach

0DWD0DZ Revision of Intraluminal Device in Lower Intestinal Tract, Open Approach

0DWD0JZ Revision of Synthetic Substitute in Lower Intestinal Tract, Open Approach

0DWD0KZ Revision of Nonautologous Tissue Substitute in Lower Intestinal Tract, Open Approach

0DWD0UZ Revision of Feeding Device in Lower Intestinal Tract, Open Approach

0DWD30Z Revision of Drainage Device in Lower Intestinal Tract, Percutaneous Approach

0DWD32Z Revision of Monitoring Device in Lower Intestinal Tract, Percutaneous Approach

0DWD33Z Revision of Infusion Device in Lower Intestinal Tract, Percutaneous Approach

0DWD37Z Revision of Autologous Tissue Substitute in Lower Intestinal Tract, Percutaneous Approach

0DWD3CZ Revision of Extraluminal Device in Lower Intestinal Tract, Percutaneous Approach

0DWD3DZ Revision of Intraluminal Device in Lower Intestinal Tract, Percutaneous Approach

0DWD3JZ Revision of Synthetic Substitute in Lower Intestinal Tract, Percutaneous Approach

0DWD3KZ Revision of Nonautologous Tissue Substitute in Lower Intestinal Tract, Percutaneous Approach

0DWD3UZ Revision of Feeding Device in Lower Intestinal Tract, Percutaneous Approach

0DWD40Z Revision of Drainage Device in Lower Intestinal Tract, Percutaneous Endoscopic Approach

0DWD42Z Revision of Monitoring Device in Lower Intestinal Tract, Percutaneous Endoscopic Approach

0DWD43Z Revision of Infusion Device in Lower Intestinal Tract, Percutaneous Endoscopic Approach

0DWD47Z Revision of Autologous Tissue Substitute in Lower Intestinal Tract, Percutaneous Endoscopic Approach

0DWD4CZ Revision of Extraluminal Device in Lower Intestinal Tract, Percutaneous Endoscopic Approach

0DWD4DZ Revision of Intraluminal Device in Lower Intestinal Tract, Percutaneous Endoscopic Approach

0DWD4JZ Revision of Synthetic Substitute in Lower Intestinal Tract, Percutaneous Endoscopic Approach

0DWD4KZ Revision of Nonautologous Tissue Substitute in Lower Intestinal Tract, Percutaneous Endoscopic Approach

0DWD4UZ Revision of Feeding Device in Lower Intestinal Tract, Percutaneous Endoscopic Approach

0DWD70Z Revision of Drainage Device in Lower Intestinal Tract, Via Natural or Artificial Opening

0DWD72Z Revision of Monitoring Device in Lower Intestinal Tract, Via Natural or Artificial Opening

0DWD73Z   Revision of Infusion Device in Lower Intestinal Tract, Via Natural or Artificial Opening

0DWD77Z   Revision of Autologous Tissue Substitute in Lower Intestinal Tract, Via Natural or Artificial Opening

0DWD7CZ   Revision of Extraluminal Device in Lower Intestinal Tract, Via Natural or Artificial Opening

0DWD7DZ   Revision of Intraluminal Device in Lower Intestinal Tract, Via Natural or Artificial Opening

0DWD7JZ   Revision of Synthetic Substitute in Lower Intestinal Tract, Via Natural or Artificial Opening

0DWD7KZ   Revision of Nonautologous Tissue Substitute in Lower Intestinal Tract, Via Natural or Artificial Opening

0DWD7UZ   Revision of Feeding Device in Lower Intestinal Tract, Via Natural or Artificial Opening

0DWD80Z   Revision of Drainage Device in Lower Intestinal Tract, Via Natural or Artificial Opening Endoscopic

0DWD82Z   Revision of Monitoring Device in Lower Intestinal Tract, Via Natural or Artificial Opening Endoscopic

0DWD83Z   Revision of Infusion Device in Lower Intestinal Tract, Via Natural or Artificial Opening Endoscopic

0DWD87Z   Revision of Autologous Tissue Substitute in Lower Intestinal Tract, Via Natural or Artificial Opening Endoscopic

0DWD8CZ   Revision of Extraluminal Device in Lower Intestinal Tract, Via Natural or Artificial Opening Endoscopic

0DWD8DZ   Revision of Intraluminal Device in Lower Intestinal Tract, Via Natural or Artificial Opening Endoscopic

0DWD8JZ   Revision of Synthetic Substitute in Lower Intestinal Tract, Via Natural or Artificial Opening Endoscopic

0DWD8KZ   Revision of Nonautologous Tissue Substitute in Lower Intestinal Tract, Via Natural or Artificial Opening Endoscopic

0DWD8UZ   Revision of Feeding Device in Lower Intestinal Tract, Via Natural or Artificial Opening Endoscopic

0DWDX0Z   Revision of Drainage Device in Lower Intestinal Tract, External Approach

0DWDX2Z   Revision of Monitoring Device in Lower Intestinal Tract, External Approach

0DWDX3Z   Revision of Infusion Device in Lower Intestinal Tract, External Approach

0DWDX7Z   Revision of Autologous Tissue Substitute in Lower Intestinal Tract, External Approach

0DWDXCZ   Revision of Extraluminal Device in Lower Intestinal Tract, External Approach

0DWDXDZ   Revision of Intraluminal Device in Lower Intestinal Tract, External Approach

0DWDXJZ   Revision of Synthetic Substitute in Lower Intestinal Tract, External Approach

0DWDXKZ   Revision of Nonautologous Tissue Substitute in Lower Intestinal Tract, External Approach

0DWDXUZ   Revision of Feeding Device in Lower Intestinal Tract, External Approach

0DWE07Z   Revision of Autologous Tissue Substitute in Large Intestine, Open Approach

0DWE0JZ   Revision of Synthetic Substitute in Large Intestine, Open Approach

0DWE0KZ   Revision of Nonautologous Tissue Substitute in Large Intestine, Open Approach

0DWE47Z   Revision of Autologous Tissue Substitute in Large Intestine, Percutaneous Endoscopic Approach

0DWE4JZ   Revision of Synthetic Substitute in Large Intestine, Percutaneous Endoscopic Approach

0DWE4KZ   Revision of Nonautologous Tissue Substitute in Large Intestine, Percutaneous Endoscopic Approach

0DWE77Z   Revision of Autologous Tissue Substitute in Large Intestine, Via Natural or Artificial Opening

0DWE7JZ   Revision of Synthetic Substitute in Large Intestine, Via Natural or Artificial Opening

0DWE7KZ   Revision of Nonautologous Tissue Substitute in Large Intestine, Via Natural or Artificial Opening

0DWE87Z   Revision of Autologous Tissue Substitute in Large Intestine, Via Natural or Artificial Opening Endoscopic

0DWE8JZ   Revision of Synthetic Substitute in Large Intestine, Via Natural or Artificial Opening Endoscopic

0DWE8KZ   Revision of Nonautologous Tissue Substitute in Large Intestine, Via Natural or Artificial Opening Endoscopic

0DWQ0LZ   Revision of Artificial Sphincter in Anus, Open Approach

0DWQ3LZ   Revision of Artificial Sphincter in Anus, Percutaneous Approach

0DWQ4LZ   Revision of Artificial Sphincter in Anus, Percutaneous Endoscopic Approach

0DWQ7LZ   Revision of Artificial Sphincter in Anus, Via Natural or Artificial Opening

0DWQ8LZ   Revision of Artificial Sphincter in Anus, Via Natural or Artificial Opening Endoscopic

0DWR0MZ   Revision of Stimulator Lead in Anal Sphincter, Open Approach

0DWR3MZ   Revision of Stimulator Lead in Anal Sphincter, Percutaneous Approach

0DWR4MZ   Revision of Stimulator Lead in Anal Sphincter, Percutaneous Endoscopic Approach

0DWU00Z   Revision of Drainage Device in Omentum, Open Approach

0DWU07Z   Revision of Autologous Tissue Substitute in Omentum, Open Approach

0DWU0JZ   Revision of Synthetic Substitute in Omentum, Open Approach

0DWU0KZ   Revision of Nonautologous Tissue Substitute in Omentum, Open Approach

0DWU30Z   Revision of Drainage Device in Omentum, Percutaneous Approach

0DWU37Z   Revision of Autologous Tissue Substitute in Omentum, Percutaneous Approach

0DWU3JZ   Revision of Synthetic Substitute in Omentum, Percutaneous Approach

0DWU3KZ   Revision of Nonautologous Tissue Substitute in Omentum, Percutaneous Approach

0DWU40Z   Revision of Drainage Device in Omentum, Percutaneous Endoscopic Approach

0DWU47Z   Revision of Autologous Tissue Substitute in Omentum, Percutaneous Endoscopic Approach

0DWU4JZ   Revision of Synthetic Substitute in Omentum, Percutaneous Endoscopic Approach

0DWU4KZ   Revision of Nonautologous Tissue Substitute in Omentum, Percutaneous Endoscopic Approach

0DWV00Z   Revision of Drainage Device in Mesentery, Open Approach

0DWV07Z   Revision of Autologous Tissue Substitute in Mesentery, Open Approach

0DWV0JZ   Revision of Synthetic Substitute in Mesentery, Open Approach

0DWV0KZ   Revision of Nonautologous Tissue Substitute in Mesentery, Open Approach

0DWV30Z   Revision of Drainage Device in Mesentery, Percutaneous Approach

0DWV37Z   Revision of Autologous Tissue Substitute in Mesentery, Percutaneous Approach

0DWV3JZ   Revision of Synthetic Substitute in Mesentery, Percutaneous Approach

0DWV3KZ   Revision of Nonautologous Tissue Substitute in Mesentery, Percutaneous Approach

0DWV40Z   Revision of Drainage Device in Mesentery, Percutaneous Endoscopic Approach

0DWV47Z   Revision of Autologous Tissue Substitute in Mesentery, Percutaneous Endoscopic Approach

0DWV4JZ   Revision of Synthetic Substitute in Mesentery, Percutaneous Endoscopic Approach

0DWV4KZ   Revision of Nonautologous Tissue Substitute in Mesentery, Percutaneous Endoscopic Approach

0DWW00Z   Revision of Drainage Device in Peritoneum, Open Approach

0DWW07Z   Revision of Autologous Tissue Substitute in Peritoneum, Open Approach

0DWW0JZ   Revision of Synthetic Substitute in Peritoneum, Open Approach

0DWW0KZ   Revision of Nonautologous Tissue Substitute in Peritoneum, Open Approach

0DWW30Z   Revision of Drainage Device in Peritoneum, Percutaneous Approach

0DWW37Z   Revision of Autologous Tissue Substitute in Peritoneum, Percutaneous Approach

0DWW3JZ   Revision of Synthetic Substitute in Peritoneum, Percutaneous Approach

0DWW3KZ   Revision of Nonautologous Tissue Substitute in Peritoneum, Percutaneous Approach

♀ Female-only   ♂ Male-only   ◖ Limited Coverage   ● Non-OR   ▨ HAC-associated procedure   ⬢ Non-covered procedures   ✚ Combination

| 0DWW40Z | Revision of Drainage Device in Peritoneum, Percutaneous Endoscopic Approach |
| 0DWW47Z | Revision of Autologous Tissue Substitute in Peritoneum, Percutaneous Endoscopic Approach |

| 0DWW4JZ | Revision of Synthetic Substitute in Peritoneum, Percutaneous Endoscopic Approach |
| 0DWW4KZ | Revision of Nonautologous Tissue Substitute in Peritoneum, Percutaneous Endoscopic Approach |

0DX – Gastrointestinal System, Transfer

0DX60Z5	Transfer Stomach to Esophagus, Open Approach
0DX64Z5	Transfer Stomach to Esophagus, Percutaneous Endoscopic Approach
0DX80Z5	Transfer Small Intestine to Esophagus, Open Approach

0DX84Z5	Transfer Small Intestine to Esophagus, Percutaneous Endoscopic Approach
0DXE0Z5	Transfer Large Intestine to Esophagus, Open Approach
0DXE4Z5	Transfer Large Intestine to Esophagus, Percutaneous Endoscopic Approach

0DY – Gastrointestinal System, Transplantation

Review Coding Guideline B3.16

0DY50Z0	Transplantation of Esophagus, Allogeneic, Open Approach
0DY50Z1	Transplantation of Esophagus, Syngeneic, Open Approach
0DY50Z2	Transplantation of Esophagus, Zooplastic, Open Approach
0DY60Z0	Transplantation of Stomach, Allogeneic, Open Approach
0DY60Z1	Transplantation of Stomach, Syngeneic, Open Approach
0DY60Z2	Transplantation of Stomach, Zooplastic, Open Approach

0DY80Z0	Transplantation of Small Intestine, Allogeneic, Open Approach
0DY80Z1	Transplantation of Small Intestine, Syngeneic, Open Approach
0DY80Z2	Transplantation of Small Intestine, Zooplastic, Open Approach
0DYE0Z0	Transplantation of Large Intestine, Allogeneic, Open Approach
0DYE0Z1	Transplantation of Large Intestine, Syngeneic, Open Approach`
0DYE0Z2	Transplantation of Large Intestine, Zooplastic, Open Approach

 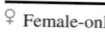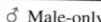

Hepatobiliary System and Pancreas

Hepatobiliary System and Pancreas

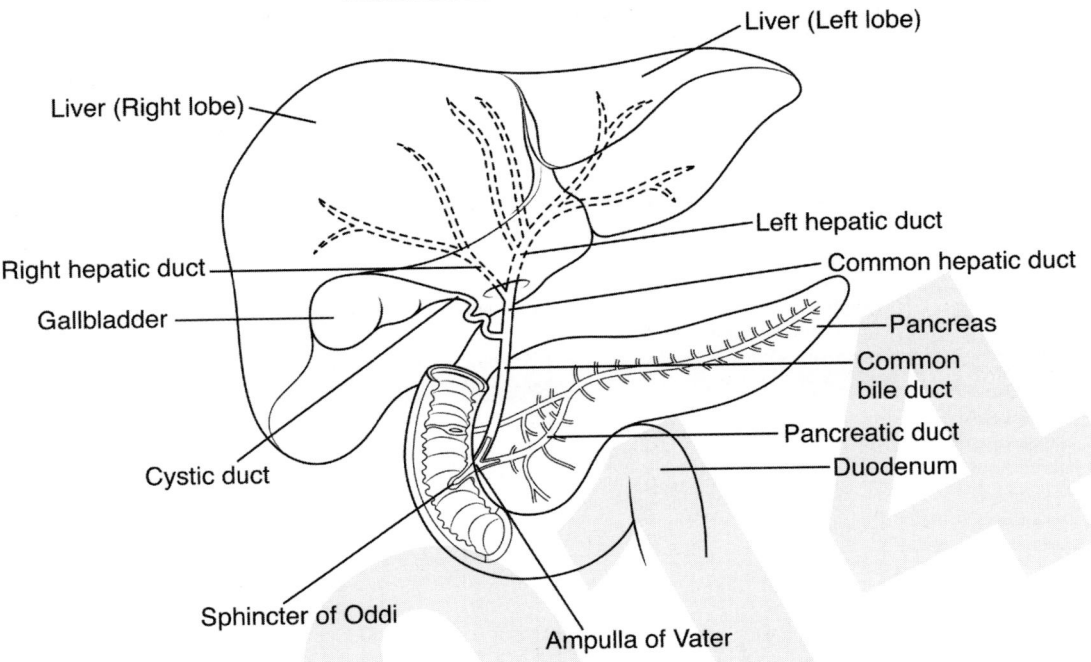

Hepatobiliary System and Pancreas Tables 0F1–0FY

Section	0	Medical and Surgical
Body System	F	Hepatobiliary System and Pancreas
Operation	1	**Bypass:** Altering the route of passage of the contents of a tubular body part

Body Part (4th)	Approach (5th)	Device (6th)	Qualifier (7th)
4 Gallbladder 5 Hepatic Duct, Right 6 Hepatic Duct, Left 8 Cystic Duct 9 Common Bile Duct	0 Open 4 Percutaneous Endoscopic	D Intraluminal Device Z No Device	3 Duodenum 4 Stomach 5 Hepatic Duct, Right 6 Hepatic Duct, Left 7 Hepatic Duct, Caudate 8 Cystic Duct 9 Common Bile Duct B Small Intestine
D Pancreatic Duct F Pancreatic Duct, Accessory G Pancreas	0 Open 4 Percutaneous Endoscopic	D Intraluminal Device Z No Device	3 Duodenum B Small Intestine C Large Intestine

Section	0	Medical and Surgical
Body System	F	Hepatobiliary System and Pancreas
Operation	2	**Change:** Taking out or off a device from a body part and putting back an identical or similar device in or on the same body part without cutting or puncturing the skin or a mucous membrane

Body Part (4th)	Approach (5th)	Device (6th)	Qualifier (7th)
0 Liver 4 Gallbladder B Hepatobiliary Duct D Pancreatic Duct G Pancreas	X External	0 Drainage Device Y Other Device	Z No Qualifier

Section	0	Medical and Surgical
Body System	F	Hepatobiliary System and Pancreas
Operation	5	**Destruction:** Physical eradication of all or a portion of a body part by the direct use of energy, force, or a destructive agent

Body Part (4th)	Approach (5th)	Device (6th)	Qualifier (7th)
0 Liver 1 Liver, Right Lobe 2 Liver, Left Lobe 4 Gallbladder G Pancreas	0 Open 3 Percutaneous 4 Percutaneous Endoscopic	Z No Device	Z No Qualifier
5 Hepatic Duct, Right 6 Hepatic Duct, Left 8 Cystic Duct 9 Common Bile Duct C Ampulla of Vater D Pancreatic Duct F Pancreatic Duct, Accessory	0 Open 3 Percutaneous 4 Percutaneous Endoscopic 7 Via Natural or Artificial Opening 8 Via Natural or Artificial Opening Endoscopic	Z No Device	Z No Qualifier

Section	0	Medical and Surgical
Body System	F	Hepatobiliary System and Pancreas
Operation	7	**Dilation:** Expanding an orifice or the lumen of a tubular body part

Body Part (4th)	Approach (5th)	Device (6th)	Qualifier (7th)
5 Hepatic Duct, Right 6 Hepatic Duct, Left 8 Cystic Duct 9 Common Bile Duct C Ampulla of Vater D Pancreatic Duct F Pancreatic Duct, Accessory	0 Open 3 Percutaneous 4 Percutaneous Endoscopic 7 Via Natural or Artificial Opening 8 Via Natural or Artificial Opening Endoscopic	D Intraluminal Device Z No Device	Z No Qualifier

Section	0	Medical and Surgical
Body System	F	Hepatobiliary System and Pancreas
Operation	8	**Division:** Cutting into a body part, without draining fluids and/or gases from the body part, in order to separate or transect a body part

Body Part (4th)	Approach (5th)	Device (6th)	Qualifier (7th)
G Pancreas	0 Open 3 Percutaneous 4 Percutaneous Endoscopic	Z No Device	Z No Qualifier

Section	0	**Medical and Surgical**
Body System	F	**Hepatobiliary System and Pancreas**
Operation	9	**Drainage:** Taking or letting out fluids and/or gases from a body part

Body Part (4th)	Approach (5th)	Device (6th)	Qualifier (7th)
0 Liver 1 Liver, Right Lobe 2 Liver, Left Lobe 4 Gallbladder G Pancreas	0 Open 3 Percutaneous 4 Percutaneous Endoscopic	0 Drainage Device	Z No Qualifier
0 Liver 1 Liver, Right Lobe 2 Liver, Left Lobe 4 Gallbladder G Pancreas	0 Open 3 Percutaneous 4 Percutaneous Endoscopic	Z No Device	X Diagnostic Z No Qualifier
5 Hepatic Duct, Right 6 Hepatic Duct, Left 8 Cystic Duct 9 Common Bile Duct C Ampulla of Vater D Pancreatic Duct F Pancreatic Duct, Accessory	0 Open 3 Percutaneous 4 Percutaneous Endoscopic 7 Via Natural or Artificial Opening 8 Via Natural or Artificial Opening Endoscopic	0 Drainage Device	Z No Qualifier
5 Hepatic Duct, Right 6 Hepatic Duct, Left 8 Cystic Duct 9 Common Bile Duct C Ampulla of Vater D Pancreatic Duct F Pancreatic Duct, Accessory	0 Open 3 Percutaneous 4 Percutaneous Endoscopic 7 Via Natural or Artificial Opening 8 Via Natural or Artificial Opening Endoscopic	Z No Device	X Diagnostic Z No Qualifier

Section	0	**Medical and Surgical**
Body System	F	**Hepatobiliary System and Pancreas**
Operation	B	**Excision:** Cutting out or off, without replacement, a portion of a body part

Body Part (4th)	Approach (5th)	Device (6th)	Qualifier (7th)
0 Liver 1 Liver, Right Lobe 2 Liver, Left Lobe 4 Gallbladder G Pancreas	0 Open 3 Percutaneous 4 Percutaneous Endoscopic	Z No Device	X Diagnostic Z No Qualifier
5 Hepatic Duct, Right 6 Hepatic Duct, Left 8 Cystic Duct 9 Common Bile Duct C Ampulla of Vater D Pancreatic Duct F Pancreatic Duct, Accessory	0 Open 3 Percutaneous 4 Percutaneous Endoscopic 7 Via Natural or Artificial Opening 8 Via Natural or Artificial Opening Endoscopic	Z No Device	X Diagnostic Z No Qualifier

Section	0	Medical and Surgical
Body System	F	Hepatobiliary System and Pancreas
Operation	C	Extirpation: Taking or cutting out solid matter from a body part

Body Part (4th)	Approach (5th)	Device (6th)	Qualifier (7th)
0 Liver 1 Liver, Right Lobe 2 Liver, Left Lobe 4 Gallbladder G Pancreas	0 Open 3 Percutaneous 4 Percutaneous Endoscopic	Z No Device	Z No Qualifier
5 Hepatic Duct, Right 6 Hepatic Duct, Left 8 Cystic Duct 9 Common Bile Duct C Ampulla of Vater D Pancreatic Duct F Pancreatic Duct, Accessory	0 Open 3 Percutaneous 4 Percutaneous Endoscopic 7 Via Natural or Artificial Opening 8 Via Natural or Artificial Opening Endoscopic	Z No Device	Z No Qualifier

Section	0	Medical and Surgical
Body System	F	Hepatobiliary System and Pancreas
Operation	F	Fragmentation: Breaking solid matter in a body part into pieces

Body Part (4th)	Approach (5th)	Device (6th)	Qualifier (7th)
4 Gallbladder 5 Hepatic Duct, Right 6 Hepatic Duct, Left 8 Cystic Duct 9 Common Bile Duct C Ampulla of Vater D Pancreatic Duct F Pancreatic Duct, Accessory	0 Open 3 Percutaneous 4 Percutaneous Endoscopic 7 Via Natural or Artificial Opening 8 Via Natural or Artificial Opening Endoscopic X External	Z No Device	Z No Qualifier

Section	0	Medical and Surgical
Body System	F	Hepatobiliary System and Pancreas
Operation	H	Insertion: Putting in a nonbiological appliance that monitors, assists, performs, or prevents a physiological function but does not physically take the place of a body part

Body Part (4th)	Approach (5th)	Device (6th)	Qualifier (7th)
0 Liver 1 Liver, Right Lobe 2 Liver, Left Lobe 4 Gallbladder G Pancreas	0 Open 3 Percutaneous 4 Percutaneous Endoscopic	2 Monitoring Device 3 Infusion Device	Z No Qualifier
B Hepatobiliary Duct D Pancreatic Duct	0 Open 3 Percutaneous 4 Percutaneous Endoscopic 7 Via Natural or Artificial Opening 8 Via Natural or Artificial Opening Endoscopic	1 Radioactive Element 2 Monitoring Device 3 Infusion Device D Intraluminal Device	Z No Qualifier

Section	0	Medical and Surgical
Body System	F	Hepatobiliary System and Pancreas
Operation	J	Inspection: Visually and/or manually exploring a body part

Body Part (4th)	Approach (5th)	Device (6th)	Qualifier (7th)
0 Liver 4 Gallbladder G Pancreas	0 Open 3 Percutaneous 4 Percutaneous Endoscopic X External	Z No Device	Z No Qualifier
B Hepatobiliary Duct D Pancreatic Duct	0 Open 3 Percutaneous 4 Percutaneous Endoscopic 7 Via Natural or Artificial Opening 8 Via Natural or Artificial Opening Endoscopic	Z No Device	Z No Qualifier

Section	0	Medical and Surgical
Body System	F	Hepatobiliary System and Pancreas
Operation	L	Occlusion: Completely closing an orifice or the lumen of a tubular body part

Body Part (4th)	Approach (5th)	Device (6th)	Qualifier (7th)
5 Hepatic Duct, Right 6 Hepatic Duct, Left 8 Cystic Duct 9 Common Bile Duct C Ampulla of Vater D Pancreatic Duct F Pancreatic Duct, Accessory	0 Open 3 Percutaneous 4 Percutaneous Endoscopic	C Extraluminal Device D Intraluminal Device Z No Device	Z No Qualifier
5 Hepatic Duct, Right 6 Hepatic Duct, Left 8 Cystic Duct 9 Common Bile Duct C Ampulla of Vater D Pancreatic Duct F Pancreatic Duct, Accessory	7 Via Natural or Artificial Opening 8 Via Natural or Artificial Opening Endoscopic	D Intraluminal Device Z No Device	Z No Qualifier

Section	0	Medical and Surgical
Body System	F	Hepatobiliary System and Pancreas
Operation	M	Reattachment: Putting back in or on all or a portion of a separated body part to its normal location or other suitable location

Body Part (4th)	Approach (5th)	Device (6th)	Qualifier (7th)
0 Liver 1 Liver, Right Lobe 2 Liver, Left Lobe 4 Gallbladder 5 Hepatic Duct, Right 6 Hepatic Duct, Left 8 Cystic Duct 9 Common Bile Duct C Ampulla of Vater D Pancreatic Duct F Pancreatic Duct, Accessory G Pancreas	0 Open 4 Percutaneous Endoscopic	Z No Device	Z No Qualifier

Section	0	Medical and Surgical
Body System	F	Hepatobiliary System and Pancreas
Operation	N	Release: Freeing a body part from an abnormal physical constraint by cutting or by the use of force

Body Part (4th)	Approach (5th)	Device (6th)	Qualifier (7th)
0 Liver 1 Liver, Right Lobe 2 Liver, Left Lobe 4 Gallbladder G Pancreas	0 Open 3 Percutaneous 4 Percutaneous Endoscopic	Z No Device	Z No Qualifier
5 Hepatic Duct, Right 6 Hepatic Duct, Left 8 Cystic Duct 9 Common Bile Duct C Ampulla of Vater D Pancreatic Duct F Pancreatic Duct, Accessory	0 Open 3 Percutaneous 4 Percutaneous Endoscopic 7 Via Natural or Artificial Opening 8 Via Natural or Artificial Opening Endoscopic	Z No Device	Z No Qualifier

Section	0	Medical and Surgical
Body System	F	Hepatobiliary System and Pancreas
Operation	P	Removal: Taking out or off a device from a body part

Body Part (4th)	Approach (5th)	Device (6th)	Qualifier (7th)
0 Liver	0 Open 3 Percutaneous 4 Percutaneous Endoscopic X External	0 Drainage Device 2 Monitoring Device 3 Infusion Device	Z No Qualifier
4 Gallbladder G Pancreas	0 Open 3 Percutaneous 4 Percutaneous Endoscopic X External	0 Drainage Device 2 Monitoring Device 3 Infusion Device D Intraluminal Device	Z No Qualifier
B Hepatobiliary Duct D Pancreatic Duct	0 Open 3 Percutaneous 4 Percutaneous Endoscopic 7 Via Natural or Artificial Opening 8 Via Natural or Artificial Opening Endoscopic	0 Drainage Device 1 Radioactive Element 2 Monitoring Device 3 Infusion Device 7 Autologous Tissue Substitute C Extraluminal Device D Intraluminal Device J Synthetic Substitute K Nonautologous Tissue Substitute	Z No Qualifier
B Hepatobiliary Duct D Pancreatic Duct	X External	0 Drainage Device 1 Radioactive Element 2 Monitoring Device 3 Infusion Device D Intraluminal Device	Z No Qualifier

Section	0	Medical and Surgical
Body System	F	Hepatobiliary System and Pancreas
Operation	Q	Repair: Restoring, to the extent possible, a body part to its normal anatomic structure and function

Body Part (4th)	Approach (5th)	Device (6th)	Qualifier (7th)
0 Liver 1 Liver, Right Lobe 2 Liver, Left Lobe 4 Gallbladder G Pancreas	0 Open 3 Percutaneous 4 Percutaneous Endoscopic	Z No Device	Z No Qualifier

Continued

Section	0	Medical and Surgical
Body System	F	Hepatobiliary System and Pancreas
Operation	Q	**Repair:** Restoring, to the extent possible, a body part to its normal anatomic structure and function

Body Part (4th)	Approach (5th)	Device (6th)	Qualifier (7th)
5 Hepatic Duct, Right 6 Hepatic Duct, Left 8 Cystic Duct 9 Common Bile Duct C Ampulla of Vater D Pancreatic Duct F Pancreatic Duct, Accessory	0 Open 3 Percutaneous 4 Percutaneous Endoscopic 7 Via Natural or Artificial Opening 8 Via Natural or Artificial Opening Endoscopic	Z No Device	Z No Qualifier

Section	0	Medical and Surgical
Body System	F	Hepatobiliary System and Pancreas
Operation	R	**Replacement:** Putting in or on biological or synthetic material that physically takes the place and/or function of all or a portion of a body part

Body Part (4th)	Approach (5th)	Device (6th)	Qualifier (7th)
5 Hepatic Duct, Right 6 Hepatic Duct, Left 8 Cystic Duct 9 Common Bile Duct C Ampulla of Vater D Pancreatic Duct F Pancreatic Duct, Accessory	0 Open 4 Percutaneous Endoscopic	7 Autologous Tissue Substitute J Synthetic Substitute K Nonautologous Tissue Substitute	Z No Qualifier

Section	0	Medical and Surgical
Body System	F	Hepatobiliary System and Pancreas
Operation	S	**Reposition:** Moving to its normal location, or other suitable location, all or a portion of a body part

Body Part (4th)	Approach (5th)	Device (6th)	Qualifier (7th)
0 Liver 4 Gallbladder 5 Hepatic Duct, Right 6 Hepatic Duct, Left 8 Cystic Duct 9 Common Bile Duct C Ampulla of Vater D Pancreatic Duct F Pancreatic Duct, Accessory G Pancreas	0 Open 4 Percutaneous Endoscopic	Z No Device	Z No Qualifier

Section	0	Medical and Surgical
Body System	F	Hepatobiliary System and Pancreas
Operation	T	**Resection:** Cutting out or off, without replacement, all of a body part

Body Part (4th)	Approach (5th)	Device (6th)	Qualifier (7th)
0 Liver 1 Liver, Right Lobe 2 Liver, Left Lobe 4 Gallbladder G Pancreas	0 Open 4 Percutaneous Endoscopic	Z No Device	Z No Qualifier
5 Hepatic Duct, Right 6 Hepatic Duct, Left 8 Cystic Duct 9 Common Bile Duct C Ampulla of Vater D Pancreatic Duct F Pancreatic Duct, Accessory	0 Open 4 Percutaneous Endoscopic 7 Via Natural or Artificial Opening 8 Via Natural or Artificial Opening Endoscopic	Z No Device	Z No Qualifier

Section	0	Medical and Surgical
Body System	F	Hepatobiliary System and Pancreas
Operation	U	Supplement: Putting in or on biological or synthetic material that physically reinforces and/or augments the function of a portion of a body part

Body Part (4th)	Approach (5th)	Device (6th)	Qualifier (7th)
5 Hepatic Duct, Right 6 Hepatic Duct, Left 8 Cystic Duct 9 Common Bile Duct C Ampulla of Vater D Pancreatic Duct F Pancreatic Duct, Accessory	0 Open 3 Percutaneous 4 Percutaneous Endoscopic	7 Autologous Tissue Substitute J Synthetic Substitute K Nonautologous Tissue Substitute	Z No Qualifier

Section	0	Medical and Surgical
Body System	F	Hepatobiliary System and Pancreas
Operation	V	Restriction: Partially closing an orifice or the lumen of a tubular body part

Body Part (4th)	Approach (5th)	Device (6th)	Qualifier (7th)
5 Hepatic Duct, Right 6 Hepatic Duct, Left 8 Cystic Duct 9 Common Bile Duct C Ampulla of Vater D Pancreatic Duct F Pancreatic Duct, Accessory	0 Open 3 Percutaneous 4 Percutaneous Endoscopic	C Extraluminal Device D Intraluminal Device Z No Device	Z No Qualifier
5 Hepatic Duct, Right 6 Hepatic Duct, Left 8 Cystic Duct 9 Common Bile Duct C Ampulla of Vater D Pancreatic Duct F Pancreatic Duct, Accessory	7 Via Natural or Artificial Opening 8 Via Natural or Artificial Opening Endoscopic	D Intraluminal Device Z No Device	Z No Qualifier

Section	0	Medical and Surgical
Body System	F	Hepatobiliary System and Pancreas
Operation	W	Revision: Correcting, to the extent possible, a portion of a malfunctioning device or the position of a displaced device

Body Part (4th)	Approach (5th)	Device (6th)	Qualifier (7th)
0 Liver	0 Open 3 Percutaneous 4 Percutaneous Endoscopic X External	0 Drainage Device 2 Monitoring Device 3 Infusion Device	Z No Qualifier
4 Gallbladder G Pancreas	0 Open 3 Percutaneous 4 Percutaneous Endoscopic X External	0 Drainage Device 2 Monitoring Device 3 Infusion Device D Intraluminal Device	Z No Qualifier
B Hepatobiliary Duct D Pancreatic Duct	0 Open 3 Percutaneous 4 Percutaneous Endoscopic 7 Via Natural or Artificial Opening 8 Via Natural or Artificial Opening Endoscopic X External	0 Drainage Device 2 Monitoring Device 3 Infusion Device 7 Autologous Tissue Substitute C Extraluminal Device D Intraluminal Device J Synthetic Substitute K Nonautologous Tissue Substitute	Z No Qualifier

Section	0	Medical and Surgical
Body System	F	Hepatobiliary System and Pancreas
Operation	Y	**Transplantation:** Putting in or on all or a portion of a living body part taken from another individual or animal to physically take the place and/or function of all or a portion of a similar body part

Body Part (4ᵗʰ)	Approach (5ᵗʰ)	Device (6ᵗʰ)	Qualifier (7ᵗʰ)
0 Liver G Pancreas	0 Open	Z No Device	0 Allogeneic 1 Syngeneic 2 Zooplastic

Hepatobiliary System and Pancreas Code Listing 0F1–0FY

0F1 – Hepatobiliary System and Pancreas, Bypass

Review Coding Guideline B3.6a

0F140D3	Bypass Gallbladder to Duodenum with Intraluminal Device, Open Approach
0F140D4	Bypass Gallbladder to Stomach with Intraluminal Device, Open Approach
0F140D5	Bypass Gallbladder to Right Hepatic Duct with Intraluminal Device, Open Approach
0F140D6	Bypass Gallbladder to Left Hepatic Duct with Intraluminal Device, Open Approach
0F140D7	Bypass Gallbladder to Caudate Hepatic Duct with Intraluminal Device, Open Approach
0F140D8	Bypass Gallbladder to Cystic Duct with Intraluminal Device, Open Approach
0F140D9	Bypass Gallbladder to Common Bile Duct with Intraluminal Device, Open Approach
0F140DB	Bypass Gallbladder to Small Intestine with Intraluminal Device, Open Approach
0F140Z3	Bypass Gallbladder to Duodenum, Open Approach
0F140Z4	Bypass Gallbladder to Stomach, Open Approach
0F140Z5	Bypass Gallbladder to Right Hepatic Duct, Open Approach
0F140Z6	Bypass Gallbladder to Left Hepatic Duct, Open Approach
0F140Z7	Bypass Gallbladder to Caudate Hepatic Duct, Open Approach
0F140Z8	Bypass Gallbladder to Cystic Duct, Open Approach
0F140Z9	Bypass Gallbladder to Common Bile Duct, Open Approach
0F140ZB	Bypass Gallbladder to Small Intestine, Open Approach
0F144D3	Bypass Gallbladder to Duodenum with Intraluminal Device, Percutaneous Endoscopic Approach
0F144D4	Bypass Gallbladder to Stomach with Intraluminal Device, Percutaneous Endoscopic Approach
0F144D5	Bypass Gallbladder to Right Hepatic Duct with Intraluminal Device, Percutaneous Endoscopic Approach
0F144D6	Bypass Gallbladder to Left Hepatic Duct with Intraluminal Device, Percutaneous Endoscopic Approach
0F144D7	Bypass Gallbladder to Caudate Hepatic Duct with Intraluminal Device, Percutaneous Endoscopic Approach
0F144D8	Bypass Gallbladder to Cystic Duct with Intraluminal Device, Percutaneous Endoscopic Approach
0F144D9	Bypass Gallbladder to Common Bile Duct with Intraluminal Device, Percutaneous Endoscopic Approach
0F144DB	Bypass Gallbladder to Small Intestine with Intraluminal Device, Percutaneous Endoscopic Approach
0F144Z3	Bypass Gallbladder to Duodenum, Percutaneous Endoscopic Approach
0F144Z4	Bypass Gallbladder to Stomach, Percutaneous Endoscopic Approach
0F144Z5	Bypass Gallbladder to Right Hepatic Duct, Percutaneous Endoscopic Approach
0F144Z6	Bypass Gallbladder to Left Hepatic Duct, Percutaneous Endoscopic Approach
0F144Z7	Bypass Gallbladder to Caudate Hepatic Duct, Percutaneous Endoscopic Approach
0F144Z8	Bypass Gallbladder to Cystic Duct, Percutaneous Endoscopic Approach
0F144Z9	Bypass Gallbladder to Common Bile Duct, Percutaneous Endoscopic Approach
0F144ZB	Bypass Gallbladder to Small Intestine, Percutaneous Endoscopic Approach
0F150D3	Bypass Right Hepatic Duct to Duodenum with Intraluminal Device, Open Approach
0F150D4	Bypass Right Hepatic Duct to Stomach with Intraluminal Device, Open Approach
0F150D5	Bypass Right Hepatic Duct to Right Hepatic Duct with Intraluminal Device, Open Approach
0F150D6	Bypass Right Hepatic Duct to Left Hepatic Duct with Intraluminal Device, Open Approach
0F150D7	Bypass Right Hepatic Duct to Caudate Hepatic Duct with Intraluminal Device, Open Approach
0F150D8	Bypass Right Hepatic Duct to Cystic Duct with Intraluminal Device, Open Approach
0F150D9	Bypass Right Hepatic Duct to Common Bile Duct with Intraluminal Device, Open Approach
0F150DB	Bypass Right Hepatic Duct to Small Intestine with Intraluminal Device, Open Approach
0F150Z3	Bypass Right Hepatic Duct to Duodenum, Open Approach
0F150Z4	Bypass Right Hepatic Duct to Stomach, Open Approach
0F150Z5	Bypass Right Hepatic Duct to Right Hepatic Duct, Open Approach
0F150Z6	Bypass Right Hepatic Duct to Left Hepatic Duct, Open Approach
0F150Z7	Bypass Right Hepatic Duct to Caudate Hepatic Duct, Open Approach
0F150Z8	Bypass Right Hepatic Duct to Cystic Duct, Open Approach
0F150Z9	Bypass Right Hepatic Duct to Common Bile Duct, Open Approach
0F150ZB	Bypass Right Hepatic Duct to Small Intestine, Open Approach
0F154D3	Bypass Right Hepatic Duct to Duodenum with Intraluminal Device, Percutaneous Endoscopic Approach
0F154D4	Bypass Right Hepatic Duct to Stomach with Intraluminal Device, Percutaneous Endoscopic Approach
0F154D5	Bypass Right Hepatic Duct to Right Hepatic Duct with Intraluminal Device, Percutaneous Endoscopic Approach
0F154D6	Bypass Right Hepatic Duct to Left Hepatic Duct with Intraluminal Device, Percutaneous Endoscopic Approach
0F154D7	Bypass Right Hepatic Duct to Caudate Hepatic Duct with Intraluminal Device, Percutaneous Endoscopic Approach
0F154D8	Bypass Right Hepatic Duct to Cystic Duct with Intraluminal Device, Percutaneous Endoscopic Approach
0F154D9	Bypass Right Hepatic Duct to Common Bile Duct with Intraluminal Device, Percutaneous Endoscopic Approach
0F154DB	Bypass Right Hepatic Duct to Small Intestine with Intraluminal Device, Percutaneous Endoscopic Approach
0F154Z3	Bypass Right Hepatic Duct to Duodenum, Percutaneous Endoscopic Approach
0F154Z4	Bypass Right Hepatic Duct to Stomach, Percutaneous Endoscopic Approach
0F154Z5	Bypass Right Hepatic Duct to Right Hepatic Duct, Percutaneous Endoscopic Approach
0F154Z6	Bypass Right Hepatic Duct to Left Hepatic Duct, Percutaneous Endoscopic Approach
0F154Z7	Bypass Right Hepatic Duct to Caudate Hepatic Duct, Percutaneous Endoscopic Approach

0F154Z8 Bypass Right Hepatic Duct to Cystic Duct, Percutaneous Endoscopic Approach

0F154Z9 Bypass Right Hepatic Duct to Common Bile Duct, Percutaneous Endoscopic Approach

0F154ZB Bypass Right Hepatic Duct to Small Intestine, Percutaneous Endoscopic Approach

0F160D3 Bypass Left Hepatic Duct to Duodenum with Intraluminal Device, Open Approach

0F160D4 Bypass Left Hepatic Duct to Stomach with Intraluminal Device, Open Approach

0F160D5 Bypass Left Hepatic Duct to Right Hepatic Duct with Intraluminal Device, Open Approach

0F160D6 Bypass Left Hepatic Duct to Left Hepatic Duct with Intraluminal Device, Open Approach

0F160D7 Bypass Left Hepatic Duct to Caudate Hepatic Duct with Intraluminal Device, Open Approach

0F160D8 Bypass Left Hepatic Duct to Cystic Duct with Intraluminal Device, Open Approach

0F160D9 Bypass Left Hepatic Duct to Common Bile Duct with Intraluminal Device, Open Approach

0F160DB Bypass Left Hepatic Duct to Small Intestine with Intraluminal Device, Open Approach

0F160Z3 Bypass Left Hepatic Duct to Duodenum, Open Approach

0F160Z4 Bypass Left Hepatic Duct to Stomach, Open Approach

0F160Z5 Bypass Left Hepatic Duct to Right Hepatic Duct, Open Approach

0F160Z6 Bypass Left Hepatic Duct to Left Hepatic Duct, Open Approach

0F160Z7 Bypass Left Hepatic Duct to Caudate Hepatic Duct, Open Approach

0F160Z8 Bypass Left Hepatic Duct to Cystic Duct, Open Approach

0F160Z9 Bypass Left Hepatic Duct to Common Bile Duct, Open Approach

0F160ZB Bypass Left Hepatic Duct to Small Intestine, Open Approach

0F164D3 Bypass Left Hepatic Duct to Duodenum with Intraluminal Device, Percutaneous Endoscopic Approach

0F164D4 Bypass Left Hepatic Duct to Stomach with Intraluminal Device, Percutaneous Endoscopic Approach

0F164D5 Bypass Left Hepatic Duct to Right Hepatic Duct with Intraluminal Device, Percutaneous Endoscopic Approach

0F164D6 Bypass Left Hepatic Duct to Left Hepatic Duct with Intraluminal Device, Percutaneous Endoscopic Approach

0F164D7 Bypass Left Hepatic Duct to Caudate Hepatic Duct with Intraluminal Device, Percutaneous Endoscopic Approach

0F164D8 Bypass Left Hepatic Duct to Cystic Duct with Intraluminal Device, Percutaneous Endoscopic Approach

0F164D9 Bypass Left Hepatic Duct to Common Bile Duct with Intraluminal Device, Percutaneous Endoscopic Approach

0F164DB Bypass Left Hepatic Duct to Small Intestine with Intraluminal Device, Percutaneous Endoscopic Approach

0F164Z3 Bypass Left Hepatic Duct to Duodenum, Percutaneous Endoscopic Approach

0F164Z4 Bypass Left Hepatic Duct to Stomach, Percutaneous Endoscopic Approach

0F164Z5 Bypass Left Hepatic Duct to Right Hepatic Duct, Percutaneous Endoscopic Approach

0F164Z6 Bypass Left Hepatic Duct to Left Hepatic Duct, Percutaneous Endoscopic Approach

0F164Z7 Bypass Left Hepatic Duct to Caudate Hepatic Duct, Percutaneous Endoscopic Approach

0F164Z8 Bypass Left Hepatic Duct to Cystic Duct, Percutaneous Endoscopic Approach

0F164Z9 Bypass Left Hepatic Duct to Common Bile Duct, Percutaneous Endoscopic Approach

0F164ZB Bypass Left Hepatic Duct to Small Intestine, Percutaneous Endoscopic Approach

0F180D3 Bypass Cystic Duct to Duodenum with Intraluminal Device, Open Approach

0F180D4 Bypass Cystic Duct to Stomach with Intraluminal Device, Open Approach

0F180D5 Bypass Cystic Duct to Right Hepatic Duct with Intraluminal Device, Open Approach

0F180D6 Bypass Cystic Duct to Left Hepatic Duct with Intraluminal Device, Open Approach

0F180D7 Bypass Cystic Duct to Caudate Hepatic Duct with Intraluminal Device, Open Approach

0F180D8 Bypass Cystic Duct to Cystic Duct with Intraluminal Device, Open Approach

0F180D9 Bypass Cystic Duct to Common Bile Duct with Intraluminal Device, Open Approach

0F180DB Bypass Cystic Duct to Small Intestine with Intraluminal Device, Open Approach

0F180Z3 Bypass Cystic Duct to Duodenum, Open Approach

0F180Z4 Bypass Cystic Duct to Stomach, Open Approach

0F180Z5 Bypass Cystic Duct to Right Hepatic Duct, Open Approach

0F180Z6 Bypass Cystic Duct to Left Hepatic Duct, Open Approach

0F180Z7 Bypass Cystic Duct to Caudate Hepatic Duct, Open Approach

0F180Z8 Bypass Cystic Duct to Cystic Duct, Open Approach

0F180Z9 Bypass Cystic Duct to Common Bile Duct, Open Approach

0F180ZB Bypass Cystic Duct to Small Intestine, Open Approach

0F184D3 Bypass Cystic Duct to Duodenum with Intraluminal Device, Percutaneous Endoscopic Approach

0F184D4 Bypass Cystic Duct to Stomach with Intraluminal Device, Percutaneous Endoscopic Approach

0F184D5 Bypass Cystic Duct to Right Hepatic Duct with Intraluminal Device, Percutaneous Endoscopic Approach

0F184D6 Bypass Cystic Duct to Left Hepatic Duct with Intraluminal Device, Percutaneous Endoscopic Approach

0F184D7 Bypass Cystic Duct to Caudate Hepatic Duct with Intraluminal Device, Percutaneous Endoscopic Approach

0F184D8 Bypass Cystic Duct to Cystic Duct with Intraluminal Device, Percutaneous Endoscopic Approach

0F184D9 Bypass Cystic Duct to Common Bile Duct with Intraluminal Device, Percutaneous Endoscopic Approach

0F184DB Bypass Cystic Duct to Small Intestine with Intraluminal Device, Percutaneous Endoscopic Approach

0F184Z3 Bypass Cystic Duct to Duodenum, Percutaneous Endoscopic Approach

0F184Z4 Bypass Cystic Duct to Stomach, Percutaneous Endoscopic Approach

0F184Z5 Bypass Cystic Duct to Right Hepatic Duct, Percutaneous Endoscopic Approach

0F184Z6 Bypass Cystic Duct to Left Hepatic Duct, Percutaneous Endoscopic Approach

0F184Z7 Bypass Cystic Duct to Caudate Hepatic Duct, Percutaneous Endoscopic Approach

0F184Z8 Bypass Cystic Duct to Cystic Duct, Percutaneous Endoscopic Approach

0F184Z9 Bypass Cystic Duct to Common Bile Duct, Percutaneous Endoscopic Approach

0F184ZB Bypass Cystic Duct to Small Intestine, Percutaneous Endoscopic Approach

0F190D3 Bypass Common Bile Duct to Duodenum with Intraluminal Device, Open Approach

0F190D4 Bypass Common Bile Duct to Stomach with Intraluminal Device, Open Approach

0F190D5 Bypass Common Bile Duct to Right Hepatic Duct with Intraluminal Device, Open Approach

0F190D6 Bypass Common Bile Duct to Left Hepatic Duct with Intraluminal Device, Open Approach

0F190D7 Bypass Common Bile Duct to Caudate Hepatic Duct with Intraluminal Device, Open Approach

0F190D8 Bypass Common Bile Duct to Cystic Duct with Intraluminal Device, Open Approach

0F190D9 Bypass Common Bile Duct to Common Bile Duct with Intraluminal Device, Open Approach

0F190DB Bypass Common Bile Duct to Small Intestine with Intraluminal Device, Open Approach

0F190Z3 Bypass Common Bile Duct to Duodenum, Open Approach

0F190Z4 Bypass Common Bile Duct to Stomach, Open Approach

0F190Z5 Bypass Common Bile Duct to Right Hepatic Duct, Open Approach

0F190Z6 Bypass Common Bile Duct to Left Hepatic Duct, Open Approach

0F190Z7 Bypass Common Bile Duct to Caudate Hepatic Duct, Open Approach

0F190Z8 Bypass Common Bile Duct to Cystic Duct, Open Approach

0F190Z9 Bypass Common Bile Duct to Common Bile Duct, Open Approach

0F190ZB Bypass Common Bile Duct to Small Intestine, Open Approach

0F194D3 Bypass Common Bile Duct to Duodenum with Intraluminal Device, Percutaneous Endoscopic Approach

0F194D4 Bypass Common Bile Duct to Stomach with Intraluminal Device, Percutaneous Endoscopic Approach

0F194D5 Bypass Common Bile Duct to Right Hepatic Duct with Intraluminal Device, Percutaneous Endoscopic Approach

0F194D6 Bypass Common Bile Duct to Left Hepatic Duct with Intraluminal Device, Percutaneous Endoscopic Approach

0F194D7 Bypass Common Bile Duct to Caudate Hepatic Duct with Intraluminal Device, Percutaneous Endoscopic Approach

0F194D8 Bypass Common Bile Duct to Cystic Duct with Intraluminal Device, Percutaneous Endoscopic Approach

0F194D9 Bypass Common Bile Duct to Common Bile Duct with Intraluminal Device, Percutaneous Endoscopic Approach

0F194DB Bypass Common Bile Duct to Small Intestine with Intraluminal Device, Percutaneous Endoscopic Approach

0F194Z3 Bypass Common Bile Duct to Duodenum, Percutaneous Endoscopic Approach

0F194Z4 Bypass Common Bile Duct to Stomach, Percutaneous Endoscopic Approach

0F194Z5 Bypass Common Bile Duct to Right Hepatic Duct, Percutaneous Endoscopic Approach

0F194Z6 Bypass Common Bile Duct to Left Hepatic Duct, Percutaneous Endoscopic Approach

0F194Z7 Bypass Common Bile Duct to Caudate Hepatic Duct, Percutaneous Endoscopic Approach

0F194Z8 Bypass Common Bile Duct to Cystic Duct, Percutaneous Endoscopic Approach

0F194Z9 Bypass Common Bile Duct to Common Bile Duct, Percutaneous Endoscopic Approach

0F194ZB Bypass Common Bile Duct to Small Intestine, Percutaneous Endoscopic Approach

0F1D0D3 Bypass Pancreatic Duct to Duodenum with Intraluminal Device, Open Approach

0F1D0DB Bypass Pancreatic Duct to Small Intestine with Intraluminal Device, Open Approach

0F1D0DC Bypass Pancreatic Duct to Large Intestine with Intraluminal Device, Open Approach

0F1D0Z3 Bypass Pancreatic Duct to Duodenum, Open Approach

0F1D0ZB Bypass Pancreatic Duct to Small Intestine, Open Approach

0F1D0ZC Bypass Pancreatic Duct to Large Intestine, Open Approach

0F1D4D3 Bypass Pancreatic Duct to Duodenum with Intraluminal Device, Percutaneous Endoscopic Approach

0F1D4DB Bypass Pancreatic Duct to Small Intestine with Intraluminal Device, Percutaneous Endoscopic Approach

0F1D4DC Bypass Pancreatic Duct to Large Intestine with Intraluminal Device, Percutaneous Endoscopic Approach

0F1D4Z3 Bypass Pancreatic Duct to Duodenum, Percutaneous Endoscopic Approach

0F1D4ZB Bypass Pancreatic Duct to Small Intestine, Percutaneous Endoscopic Approach

0F1D4ZC Bypass Pancreatic Duct to Large Intestine, Percutaneous Endoscopic Approach

0F1F0D3 Bypass Accessory Pancreatic Duct to Duodenum with Intraluminal Device, Open Approach

0F1F0DB Bypass Accessory Pancreatic Duct to Small Intestine with Intraluminal Device, Open Approach

0F1F0DC Bypass Accessory Pancreatic Duct to Large Intestine with Intraluminal Device, Open Approach

0F1F0Z3 Bypass Accessory Pancreatic Duct to Duodenum, Open Approach

0F1F0ZB Bypass Accessory Pancreatic Duct to Small Intestine, Open Approach

0F1F0ZC Bypass Accessory Pancreatic Duct to Large Intestine, Open Approach

0F1F4D3 Bypass Accessory Pancreatic Duct to Duodenum with Intraluminal Device, Percutaneous Endoscopic Approach

0F1F4DB Bypass Accessory Pancreatic Duct to Small Intestine with Intraluminal Device, Percutaneous Endoscopic Approach

0F1F4DC Bypass Accessory Pancreatic Duct to Large Intestine with Intraluminal Device, Percutaneous Endoscopic Approach

0F1F4Z3 Bypass Accessory Pancreatic Duct to Duodenum, Percutaneous Endoscopic Approach

0F1F4ZB Bypass Accessory Pancreatic Duct to Small Intestine, Percutaneous Endoscopic Approach

0F1F4ZC Bypass Accessory Pancreatic Duct to Large Intestine, Percutaneous Endoscopic Approach

0F1G0D3 Bypass Pancreas to Duodenum with Intraluminal Device, Open Approach

0F1G0DB Bypass Pancreas to Small Intestine with Intraluminal Device, Open Approach

0F1G0DC Bypass Pancreas to Large Intestine with Intraluminal Device, Open Approach

0F1G0Z3 Bypass Pancreas to Duodenum, Open Approach

0F1G0ZB Bypass Pancreas to Small Intestine, Open Approach

0F1G0ZC Bypass Pancreas to Large Intestine, Open Approach

0F1G4D3 Bypass Pancreas to Duodenum with Intraluminal Device, Percutaneous Endoscopic Approach

0F1G4DB Bypass Pancreas to Small Intestine with Intraluminal Device, Percutaneous Endoscopic Approach

0F1G4DC Bypass Pancreas to Large Intestine with Intraluminal Device, Percutaneous Endoscopic Approach

0F1G4Z3 Bypass Pancreas to Duodenum, Percutaneous Endoscopic Approach

0F1G4ZB Bypass Pancreas to Small Intestine, Percutaneous Endoscopic Approach

0F1G4ZC Bypass Pancreas to Large Intestine, Percutaneous Endoscopic Approach

0F2 – Hepatobiliary System and Pancreas, Change

Review Coding Guideline B6.1c

0F20X0Z Change Drainage Device in Liver, External Approach

0F20XYZ Change Other Device in Liver, External Approach

0F24X0Z Change Drainage Device in Gallbladder, External Approach

0F24XYZ Change Other Device in Gallbladder, External Approach

0F2BX0Z Change Drainage Device in Hepatobiliary Duct, External Approach

0F2BXYZ Change Other Device in Hepatobiliary Duct, External Approach

0F2DX0Z Change Drainage Device in Pancreatic Duct, External Approach

0F2DXYZ Change Other Device in Pancreatic Duct, External Approach

0F2GX0Z Change Drainage Device in Pancreas, External Approach

0F2GXYZ Change Other Device in Pancreas, External Approach

0F5 – Hepatobiliary System and Pancreas, Destruction

0F500ZZ Destruction of Liver, Open Approach

0F503ZZ Destruction of Liver, Percutaneous Approach

0F504ZZ Destruction of Liver, Percutaneous Endoscopic Approach

0F510ZZ Destruction of Right Lobe Liver, Open Approach

0F513ZZ Destruction of Right Lobe Liver, Percutaneous Approach

0F514ZZ Destruction of Right Lobe Liver, Percutaneous Endoscopic Approach

0F520ZZ Destruction of Left Lobe Liver, Open Approach

0F523ZZ Destruction of Left Lobe Liver, Percutaneous Approach

0F524ZZ Destruction of Left Lobe Liver, Percutaneous Endoscopic Approach

0F540ZZ Destruction of Gallbladder, Open Approach

0F543ZZ Destruction of Gallbladder, Percutaneous Approach

0F544ZZ Destruction of Gallbladder, Percutaneous Endoscopic Approach

0F550ZZ Destruction of Right Hepatic Duct, Open Approach

0F553ZZ Destruction of Right Hepatic Duct, Percutaneous Approach

0F554ZZ Destruction of Right Hepatic Duct, Percutaneous Endoscopic Approach

0F557ZZ Destruction of Right Hepatic Duct, Via Natural or Artificial Opening

0F558ZZ Destruction of Right Hepatic Duct, Via Natural or Artificial Opening Endoscopic

0F560ZZ	Destruction of Left Hepatic Duct, Open Approach
0F563ZZ	Destruction of Left Hepatic Duct, Percutaneous Approach
0F564ZZ	Destruction of Left Hepatic Duct, Percutaneous Endoscopic Approach
0F567ZZ	Destruction of Left Hepatic Duct, Via Natural or Artificial Opening
0F568ZZ	Destruction of Left Hepatic Duct, Via Natural or Artificial Opening Endoscopic
0F580ZZ	Destruction of Cystic Duct, Open Approach
0F583ZZ	Destruction of Cystic Duct, Percutaneous Approach
0F584ZZ	Destruction of Cystic Duct, Percutaneous Endoscopic Approach
0F587ZZ	Destruction of Cystic Duct, Via Natural or Artificial Opening
0F588ZZ	Destruction of Cystic Duct, Via Natural or Artificial Opening Endoscopic
0F590ZZ	Destruction of Common Bile Duct, Open Approach
0F593ZZ	Destruction of Common Bile Duct, Percutaneous Approach
0F594ZZ	Destruction of Common Bile Duct, Percutaneous Endoscopic Approach
0F597ZZ	Destruction of Common Bile Duct, Via Natural or Artificial Opening
0F598ZZ	Destruction of Common Bile Duct, Via Natural or Artificial Opening Endoscopic
0F5C0ZZ	Destruction of Ampulla of Vater, Open Approach
0F5C3ZZ	Destruction of Ampulla of Vater, Percutaneous Approach

0F5C4ZZ	Destruction of Ampulla of Vater, Percutaneous Endoscopic Approach
0F5C7ZZ	Destruction of Ampulla of Vater, Via Natural or Artificial Opening
0F5C8ZZ	Destruction of Ampulla of Vater, Via Natural or Artificial Opening Endoscopic
0F5D0ZZ	Destruction of Pancreatic Duct, Open Approach
0F5D3ZZ	Destruction of Pancreatic Duct, Percutaneous Approach
0F5D4ZZ	Destruction of Pancreatic Duct, Percutaneous Endoscopic Approach
0F5D7ZZ	Destruction of Pancreatic Duct, Via Natural or Artificial Opening
0F5D8ZZ	Destruction of Pancreatic Duct, Via Natural or Artificial Opening Endoscopic
0F5F0ZZ	Destruction of Accessory Pancreatic Duct, Open Approach
0F5F3ZZ	Destruction of Accessory Pancreatic Duct, Percutaneous Approach
0F5F4ZZ	Destruction of Accessory Pancreatic Duct, Percutaneous Endoscopic Approach
0F5F7ZZ	Destruction of Accessory Pancreatic Duct, Via Natural or Artificial Opening
0F5F8ZZ	Destruction of Accessory Pancreatic Duct, Via Natural or Artificial Opening Endoscopic
0F5G0ZZ	Destruction of Pancreas, Open Approach
0F5G3ZZ	Destruction of Pancreas, Percutaneous Approach
0F5G4ZZ	Destruction of Pancreas, Percutaneous Endoscopic Approach

0F7 – Hepatobiliary System and Pancreas, Dilation

0F750DZ	Dilation of Right Hepatic Duct with Intraluminal Device, Open Approach
0F750ZZ	Dilation of Right Hepatic Duct, Open Approach
0F753DZ	Dilation of Right Hepatic Duct with Intraluminal Device, Percutaneous Approach
0F753ZZ	Dilation of Right Hepatic Duct, Percutaneous Approach
0F754DZ	Dilation of Right Hepatic Duct with Intraluminal Device, Percutaneous Endoscopic Approach
0F754ZZ	Dilation of Right Hepatic Duct, Percutaneous Endoscopic Approach
0F757DZ	Dilation of Right Hepatic Duct with Intraluminal Device, Via Natural or Artificial Opening
0F757ZZ	Dilation of Right Hepatic Duct, Via Natural or Artificial Opening
0F758DZ	Dilation of Right Hepatic Duct with Intraluminal Device, Via Natural or Artificial Opening Endoscopic
0F758ZZ	Dilation of Right Hepatic Duct, Via Natural or Artificial Opening Endoscopic
0F760DZ	Dilation of Left Hepatic Duct with Intraluminal Device, Open Approach
0F760ZZ	Dilation of Left Hepatic Duct, Open Approach
0F763DZ	Dilation of Left Hepatic Duct with Intraluminal Device, Percutaneous Approach
0F763ZZ	Dilation of Left Hepatic Duct, Percutaneous Approach
0F764DZ	Dilation of Left Hepatic Duct with Intraluminal Device, Percutaneous Endoscopic Approach
0F764ZZ	Dilation of Left Hepatic Duct, Percutaneous Endoscopic Approach
0F767DZ	Dilation of Left Hepatic Duct with Intraluminal Device, Via Natural or Artificial Opening
0F767ZZ	Dilation of Left Hepatic Duct, Via Natural or Artificial Opening
0F768DZ	Dilation of Left Hepatic Duct with Intraluminal Device, Via Natural or Artificial Opening Endoscopic
0F768ZZ	Dilation of Left Hepatic Duct, Via Natural or Artificial Opening Endoscopic
0F780DZ	Dilation of Cystic Duct with Intraluminal Device, Open Approach
0F780ZZ	Dilation of Cystic Duct, Open Approach
0F783DZ	Dilation of Cystic Duct with Intraluminal Device, Percutaneous Approach
0F783ZZ	Dilation of Cystic Duct, Percutaneous Approach
0F784DZ	Dilation of Cystic Duct with Intraluminal Device, Percutaneous Endoscopic Approach
0F784ZZ	Dilation of Cystic Duct, Percutaneous Endoscopic Approach
0F787DZ	Dilation of Cystic Duct with Intraluminal Device, Via Natural or Artificial Opening
0F787ZZ	Dilation of Cystic Duct, Via Natural or Artificial Opening
0F788DZ	Dilation of Cystic Duct with Intraluminal Device, Via Natural or Artificial Opening Endoscopic
0F788ZZ	Dilation of Cystic Duct, Via Natural or Artificial Opening Endoscopic

0F790DZ	Dilation of Common Bile Duct with Intraluminal Device, Open Approach
0F790ZZ	Dilation of Common Bile Duct, Open Approach
0F793DZ	Dilation of Common Bile Duct with Intraluminal Device, Percutaneous Approach
0F793ZZ	Dilation of Common Bile Duct, Percutaneous Approach
0F794DZ	Dilation of Common Bile Duct with Intraluminal Device, Percutaneous Endoscopic Approach
0F794ZZ	Dilation of Common Bile Duct, Percutaneous Endoscopic Approach
0F797DZ	Dilation of Common Bile Duct with Intraluminal Device, Via Natural or Artificial Opening
0F797ZZ	Dilation of Common Bile Duct, Via Natural or Artificial Opening
0F798DZ	Dilation of Common Bile Duct with Intraluminal Device, Via Natural or Artificial Opening Endoscopic
0F798ZZ	Dilation of Common Bile Duct, Via Natural or Artificial Opening Endoscopic
0F7C0DZ	Dilation of Ampulla of Vater with Intraluminal Device, Open Approach
0F7C0ZZ	Dilation of Ampulla of Vater, Open Approach
0F7C3DZ	Dilation of Ampulla of Vater with Intraluminal Device, Percutaneous Approach
0F7C3ZZ	Dilation of Ampulla of Vater, Percutaneous Approach
0F7C4DZ	Dilation of Ampulla of Vater with Intraluminal Device, Percutaneous Endoscopic Approach
0F7C4ZZ	Dilation of Ampulla of Vater, Percutaneous Endoscopic Approach
0F7C7DZ	Dilation of Ampulla of Vater with Intraluminal Device, Via Natural or Artificial Opening
0F7C7ZZ	Dilation of Ampulla of Vater, Via Natural or Artificial Opening
0F7C8DZ	Dilation of Ampulla of Vater with Intraluminal Device, Via Natural or Artificial Opening Endoscopic
0F7C8ZZ	Dilation of Ampulla of Vater, Via Natural or Artificial Opening Endoscopic
0F7D0DZ	Dilation of Pancreatic Duct with Intraluminal Device, Open Approach
0F7D0ZZ	Dilation of Pancreatic Duct, Open Approach
0F7D3DZ	Dilation of Pancreatic Duct with Intraluminal Device, Percutaneous Approach
0F7D3ZZ	Dilation of Pancreatic Duct, Percutaneous Approach
0F7D4DZ	Dilation of Pancreatic Duct with Intraluminal Device, Percutaneous Endoscopic Approach
0F7D4ZZ	Dilation of Pancreatic Duct, Percutaneous Endoscopic Approach
● **0F7D7DZ**	Dilation of Pancreatic Duct with Intraluminal Device, Via Natural or Artificial Opening
0F7D7ZZ	Dilation of Pancreatic Duct, Via Natural or Artificial Opening
0F7D8DZ	Dilation of Pancreatic Duct with Intraluminal Device, Via Natural or Artificial Opening Endoscopic

---

♀ Female-only   ♂ Male-only   ◐ Limited Coverage   ● Non-OR   **HAC** HAC-associated procedure   ● Non-covered procedures   ✚ Combination

0F7D8ZZ	Dilation of Pancreatic Duct, Via Natural or Artificial Opening Endoscopic
0F7F0DZ	Dilation of Accessory Pancreatic Duct with Intraluminal Device, Open Approach
0F7F0ZZ	Dilation of Accessory Pancreatic Duct, Open Approach
0F7F3DZ	Dilation of Accessory Pancreatic Duct with Intraluminal Device, Percutaneous Approach
0F7F3ZZ	Dilation of Accessory Pancreatic Duct, Percutaneous Approach
0F7F4DZ	Dilation of Accessory Pancreatic Duct with Intraluminal Device, Percutaneous Endoscopic Approach
0F7F4ZZ	Dilation of Accessory Pancreatic Duct, Percutaneous Endoscopic Approach
0F7F7DZ	Dilation of Accessory Pancreatic Duct with Intraluminal Device, Via Natural or Artificial Opening
0F7F7ZZ	Dilation of Accessory Pancreatic Duct, Via Natural or Artificial Opening
0F7F8DZ	Dilation of Accessory Pancreatic Duct with Intraluminal Device, Via Natural or Artificial Opening Endoscopic
0F7F8ZZ	Dilation of Accessory Pancreatic Duct, Via Natural or Artificial Opening Endoscopic

0F8 – Hepatobiliary System and Pancreas, Division

Review Coding Guideline B3.14

0F8G0ZZ	Division of Pancreas, Open Approach
0F8G3ZZ	Division of Pancreas, Percutaneous Approach
0F8G4ZZ	Division of Pancreas, Percutaneous Endoscopic Approach

0F9 – Hepatobiliary System and Pancreas, Drainage

Review Coding Guidelines B3.4a and B3.4b

Review Coding Guideline B6.2

0F9000Z	Drainage of Liver with Drainage Device, Open Approach
0F900ZX	Drainage of Liver, Open Approach, Diagnostic
0F900ZZ	Drainage of Liver, Open Approach
0F9030Z	Drainage of Liver with Drainage Device, Percutaneous Approach
0F903ZX	Drainage of Liver, Percutaneous Approach, Diagnostic
0F903ZZ	Drainage of Liver, Percutaneous Approach
0F9040Z	Drainage of Liver with Drainage Device, Percutaneous Endoscopic Approach
0F904ZX	Drainage of Liver, Percutaneous Endoscopic Approach, Diagnostic
0F904ZZ	Drainage of Liver, Percutaneous Endoscopic Approach
0F9100Z	Drainage of Right Lobe Liver with Drainage Device, Open Approach
0F910ZX	Drainage of Right Lobe Liver, Open Approach, Diagnostic
0F910ZZ	Drainage of Right Lobe Liver, Open Approach
0F9130Z	Drainage of Right Lobe Liver with Drainage Device, Percutaneous Approach
0F913ZX	Drainage of Right Lobe Liver, Percutaneous Approach, Diagnostic
0F913ZZ	Drainage of Right Lobe Liver, Percutaneous Approach
0F9140Z	Drainage of Right Lobe Liver with Drainage Device, Percutaneous Endoscopic Approach
0F914ZX	Drainage of Right Lobe Liver, Percutaneous Endoscopic Approach, Diagnostic
0F914ZZ	Drainage of Right Lobe Liver, Percutaneous Endoscopic Approach
0F9200Z	Drainage of Left Lobe Liver with Drainage Device, Open Approach
0F920ZX	Drainage of Left Lobe Liver, Open Approach, Diagnostic
0F920ZZ	Drainage of Left Lobe Liver, Open Approach
0F9230Z	Drainage of Left Lobe Liver with Drainage Device, Percutaneous Approach
0F923ZX	Drainage of Left Lobe Liver, Percutaneous Approach, Diagnostic
0F923ZZ	Drainage of Left Lobe Liver, Percutaneous Approach
0F9240Z	Drainage of Left Lobe Liver with Drainage Device, Percutaneous Endoscopic Approach
0F924ZX	Drainage of Left Lobe Liver, Percutaneous Endoscopic Approach, Diagnostic
0F924ZZ	Drainage of Left Lobe Liver, Percutaneous Endoscopic Approach
0F9400Z	Drainage of Gallbladder with Drainage Device, Open Approach
0F940ZX	Drainage of Gallbladder, Open Approach, Diagnostic
0F940ZZ	Drainage of Gallbladder, Open Approach
0F9430Z	Drainage of Gallbladder with Drainage Device, Percutaneous Approach
0F943ZX	Drainage of Gallbladder, Percutaneous Approach, Diagnostic
0F943ZZ	Drainage of Gallbladder, Percutaneous Approach
0F9440Z	Drainage of Gallbladder with Drainage Device, Percutaneous Endoscopic Approach
0F944ZX	Drainage of Gallbladder, Percutaneous Endoscopic Approach, Diagnostic
0F944ZZ	Drainage of Gallbladder, Percutaneous Endoscopic Approach
0F9500Z	Drainage of Right Hepatic Duct with Drainage Device, Open Approach
0F950ZX	Drainage of Right Hepatic Duct, Open Approach, Diagnostic
0F950ZZ	Drainage of Right Hepatic Duct, Open Approach
0F9530Z	Drainage of Right Hepatic Duct with Drainage Device, Percutaneous Approach
0F953ZX	Drainage of Right Hepatic Duct, Percutaneous Approach, Diagnostic
0F953ZZ	Drainage of Right Hepatic Duct, Percutaneous Approach
0F9540Z	Drainage of Right Hepatic Duct with Drainage Device, Percutaneous Endoscopic Approach
0F954ZX	Drainage of Right Hepatic Duct, Percutaneous Endoscopic Approach, Diagnostic
0F954ZZ	Drainage of Right Hepatic Duct, Percutaneous Endoscopic Approach
0F9570Z	Drainage of Right Hepatic Duct with Drainage Device, Via Natural or Artificial Opening
0F957ZX	Drainage of Right Hepatic Duct, Via Natural or Artificial Opening, Diagnostic
0F957ZZ	Drainage of Right Hepatic Duct, Via Natural or Artificial Opening
0F9580Z	Drainage of Right Hepatic Duct with Drainage Device, Via Natural or Artificial Opening Endoscopic
0F958ZX	Drainage of Right Hepatic Duct, Via Natural or Artificial Opening Endoscopic, Diagnostic
0F958ZZ	Drainage of Right Hepatic Duct, Via Natural or Artificial Opening Endoscopic
0F9600Z	Drainage of Left Hepatic Duct with Drainage Device, Open Approach
0F960ZX	Drainage of Left Hepatic Duct, Open Approach, Diagnostic
0F960ZZ	Drainage of Left Hepatic Duct, Open Approach
0F9630Z	Drainage of Left Hepatic Duct with Drainage Device, Percutaneous Approach
0F963ZX	Drainage of Left Hepatic Duct, Percutaneous Approach, Diagnostic
0F963ZZ	Drainage of Left Hepatic Duct, Percutaneous Approach
0F9640Z	Drainage of Left Hepatic Duct with Drainage Device, Percutaneous Endoscopic Approach
0F964ZX	Drainage of Left Hepatic Duct, Percutaneous Endoscopic Approach, Diagnostic
0F964ZZ	Drainage of Left Hepatic Duct, Percutaneous Endoscopic Approach
0F9670Z	Drainage of Left Hepatic Duct with Drainage Device, Via Natural or Artificial Opening
0F967ZX	Drainage of Left Hepatic Duct, Via Natural or Artificial Opening, Diagnostic
0F967ZZ	Drainage of Left Hepatic Duct, Via Natural or Artificial Opening
0F9680Z	Drainage of Left Hepatic Duct with Drainage Device, Via Natural or Artificial Opening Endoscopic

0F968ZX Drainage of Left Hepatic Duct, Via Natural or Artificial Opening Endoscopic, Diagnostic

0F968ZZ Drainage of Left Hepatic Duct, Via Natural or Artificial Opening Endoscopic

0F9800Z Drainage of Cystic Duct with Drainage Device, Open Approach

0F980ZX Drainage of Cystic Duct, Open Approach, Diagnostic

0F980ZZ Drainage of Cystic Duct, Open Approach

0F9830Z Drainage of Cystic Duct with Drainage Device, Percutaneous Approach

0F983ZX Drainage of Cystic Duct, Percutaneous Approach, Diagnostic

0F983ZZ Drainage of Cystic Duct, Percutaneous Approach

0F9840Z Drainage of Cystic Duct with Drainage Device, Percutaneous Endoscopic Approach

0F984ZX Drainage of Cystic Duct, Percutaneous Endoscopic Approach, Diagnostic

0F984ZZ Drainage of Cystic Duct, Percutaneous Endoscopic Approach

0F9870Z Drainage of Cystic Duct with Drainage Device, Via Natural or Artificial Opening

0F987ZX Drainage of Cystic Duct, Via Natural or Artificial Opening, Diagnostic

0F987ZZ Drainage of Cystic Duct, Via Natural or Artificial Opening

0F9880Z Drainage of Cystic Duct with Drainage Device, Via Natural or Artificial Opening Endoscopic

0F988ZX Drainage of Cystic Duct, Via Natural or Artificial Opening Endoscopic, Diagnostic

0F988ZZ Drainage of Cystic Duct, Via Natural or Artificial Opening Endoscopic

0F9900Z Drainage of Common Bile Duct with Drainage Device, Open Approach

0F990ZX Drainage of Common Bile Duct, Open Approach, Diagnostic

0F990ZZ Drainage of Common Bile Duct, Open Approach

0F9930Z Drainage of Common Bile Duct with Drainage Device, Percutaneous Approach

0F993ZX Drainage of Common Bile Duct, Percutaneous Approach, Diagnostic

0F993ZZ Drainage of Common Bile Duct, Percutaneous Approach

0F9940Z Drainage of Common Bile Duct with Drainage Device, Percutaneous Endoscopic Approach

0F994ZX Drainage of Common Bile Duct, Percutaneous Endoscopic Approach, Diagnostic

0F994ZZ Drainage of Common Bile Duct, Percutaneous Endoscopic Approach

0F9970Z Drainage of Common Bile Duct with Drainage Device, Via Natural or Artificial Opening

0F997ZX Drainage of Common Bile Duct, Via Natural or Artificial Opening, Diagnostic

0F997ZZ Drainage of Common Bile Duct, Via Natural or Artificial Opening

0F9980Z Drainage of Common Bile Duct with Drainage Device, Via Natural or Artificial Opening Endoscopic

0F998ZX Drainage of Common Bile Duct, Via Natural or Artificial Opening Endoscopic, Diagnostic

0F998ZZ Drainage of Common Bile Duct, Via Natural or Artificial Opening Endoscopic

0F9C00Z Drainage of Ampulla of Vater with Drainage Device, Open Approach

0F9C0ZX Drainage of Ampulla of Vater, Open Approach, Diagnostic

0F9C0ZZ Drainage of Ampulla of Vater, Open Approach

0F9C30Z Drainage of Ampulla of Vater with Drainage Device, Percutaneous Approach

0F9C3ZX Drainage of Ampulla of Vater, Percutaneous Approach, Diagnostic

0F9C3ZZ Drainage of Ampulla of Vater, Percutaneous Approach

0F9C40Z Drainage of Ampulla of Vater with Drainage Device, Percutaneous Endoscopic Approach

0F9C4ZX Drainage of Ampulla of Vater, Percutaneous Endoscopic Approach, Diagnostic

0F9C4ZZ Drainage of Ampulla of Vater, Percutaneous Endoscopic Approach

0F9C70Z Drainage of Ampulla of Vater with Drainage Device, Via Natural or Artificial Opening

0F9C7ZX Drainage of Ampulla of Vater, Via Natural or Artificial Opening, Diagnostic

0F9C7ZZ Drainage of Ampulla of Vater, Via Natural or Artificial Opening

0F9C80Z Drainage of Ampulla of Vater with Drainage Device, Via Natural or Artificial Opening Endoscopic

0F9C8ZX Drainage of Ampulla of Vater, Via Natural or Artificial Opening Endoscopic, Diagnostic

0F9C8ZZ Drainage of Ampulla of Vater, Via Natural or Artificial Opening Endoscopic

0F9D00Z Drainage of Pancreatic Duct with Drainage Device, Open Approach

0F9D0ZX Drainage of Pancreatic Duct, Open Approach, Diagnostic

0F9D0ZZ Drainage of Pancreatic Duct, Open Approach

0F9D30Z Drainage of Pancreatic Duct with Drainage Device, Percutaneous Approach

0F9D3ZX Drainage of Pancreatic Duct, Percutaneous Approach, Diagnostic

0F9D3ZZ Drainage of Pancreatic Duct, Percutaneous Approach

0F9D40Z Drainage of Pancreatic Duct with Drainage Device, Percutaneous Endoscopic Approach

0F9D4ZX Drainage of Pancreatic Duct, Percutaneous Endoscopic Approach, Diagnostic

0F9D4ZZ Drainage of Pancreatic Duct, Percutaneous Endoscopic Approach

0F9D70Z Drainage of Pancreatic Duct with Drainage Device, Via Natural or Artificial Opening

0F9D7ZX Drainage of Pancreatic Duct, Via Natural or Artificial Opening, Diagnostic

0F9D7ZZ Drainage of Pancreatic Duct, Via Natural or Artificial Opening

0F9D80Z Drainage of Pancreatic Duct with Drainage Device, Via Natural or Artificial Opening Endoscopic

0F9D8ZX Drainage of Pancreatic Duct, Via Natural or Artificial Opening Endoscopic, Diagnostic

0F9D8ZZ Drainage of Pancreatic Duct, Via Natural or Artificial Opening Endoscopic

0F9F00Z Drainage of Accessory Pancreatic Duct with Drainage Device, Open Approach

0F9F0ZX Drainage of Accessory Pancreatic Duct, Open Approach, Diagnostic

0F9F0ZZ Drainage of Accessory Pancreatic Duct, Open Approach

0F9F30Z Drainage of Accessory Pancreatic Duct with Drainage Device, Percutaneous Approach

0F9F3ZX Drainage of Accessory Pancreatic Duct, Percutaneous Approach, Diagnostic

0F9F3ZZ Drainage of Accessory Pancreatic Duct, Percutaneous Approach

0F9F40Z Drainage of Accessory Pancreatic Duct with Drainage Device, Percutaneous Endoscopic Approach

0F9F4ZX Drainage of Accessory Pancreatic Duct, Percutaneous Endoscopic Approach, Diagnostic

0F9F4ZZ Drainage of Accessory Pancreatic Duct, Percutaneous Endoscopic Approach

0F9F70Z Drainage of Accessory Pancreatic Duct with Drainage Device, Via Natural or Artificial Opening

0F9F7ZX Drainage of Accessory Pancreatic Duct, Via Natural or Artificial Opening, Diagnostic

0F9F7ZZ Drainage of Accessory Pancreatic Duct, Via Natural or Artificial Opening

0F9F80Z Drainage of Accessory Pancreatic Duct with Drainage Device, Via Natural or Artificial Opening Endoscopic

0F9F8ZX Drainage of Accessory Pancreatic Duct, Via Natural or Artificial Opening Endoscopic, Diagnostic

0F9F8ZZ Drainage of Accessory Pancreatic Duct, Via Natural or Artificial Opening Endoscopic

0F9G00Z Drainage of Pancreas with Drainage Device, Open Approach

0F9G0ZX Drainage of Pancreas, Open Approach, Diagnostic

0F9G0ZZ Drainage of Pancreas, Open Approach

0F9G30Z Drainage of Pancreas with Drainage Device, Percutaneous Approach

0F9G3ZX Drainage of Pancreas, Percutaneous Approach, Diagnostic

0F9G3ZZ Drainage of Pancreas, Percutaneous Approach

0F9G40Z Drainage of Pancreas with Drainage Device, Percutaneous Endoscopic Approach

0F9G4ZX Drainage of Pancreas, Percutaneous Endoscopic Approach, Diagnostic

0F9G4ZZ Drainage of Pancreas, Percutaneous Endoscopic Approach

0FB – Hepatobiliary System and Pancreas, Excision

Review Coding Guidelines B3.4a and B3.4b

Review Coding Guideline B3.8

0FB00ZX	Excision of Liver, Open Approach, Diagnostic
0FB00ZZ	Excision of Liver, Open Approach
0FB03ZX	Excision of Liver, Percutaneous Approach, Diagnostic
0FB03ZZ	Excision of Liver, Percutaneous Approach
0FB04ZX	Excision of Liver, Percutaneous Endoscopic Approach, Diagnostic
0FB04ZZ	Excision of Liver, Percutaneous Endoscopic Approach
0FB10ZX	Excision of Right Lobe Liver, Open Approach, Diagnostic
0FB10ZZ	Excision of Right Lobe Liver, Open Approach
0FB13ZX	Excision of Right Lobe Liver, Percutaneous Approach, Diagnostic
0FB13ZZ	Excision of Right Lobe Liver, Percutaneous Approach
0FB14ZX	Excision of Right Lobe Liver, Percutaneous Endoscopic Approach, Diagnostic
0FB14ZZ	Excision of Right Lobe Liver, Percutaneous Endoscopic Approach
0FB20ZX	Excision of Left Lobe Liver, Open Approach, Diagnostic
0FB20ZZ	Excision of Left Lobe Liver, Open Approach
0FB23ZX	Excision of Left Lobe Liver, Percutaneous Approach, Diagnostic
0FB23ZZ	Excision of Left Lobe Liver, Percutaneous Approach
0FB24ZX	Excision of Left Lobe Liver, Percutaneous Endoscopic Approach, Diagnostic
0FB24ZZ	Excision of Left Lobe Liver, Percutaneous Endoscopic Approach
0FB40ZX	Excision of Gallbladder, Open Approach, Diagnostic
0FB40ZZ	Excision of Gallbladder, Open Approach
0FB43ZX	Excision of Gallbladder, Percutaneous Approach, Diagnostic
0FB43ZZ	Excision of Gallbladder, Percutaneous Approach
0FB44ZX	Excision of Gallbladder, Percutaneous Endoscopic Approach, Diagnostic
0FB44ZZ	Excision of Gallbladder, Percutaneous Endoscopic Approach
0FB50ZX	Excision of Right Hepatic Duct, Open Approach, Diagnostic
0FB50ZZ	Excision of Right Hepatic Duct, Open Approach
0FB53ZX	Excision of Right Hepatic Duct, Percutaneous Approach, Diagnostic
0FB53ZZ	Excision of Right Hepatic Duct, Percutaneous Approach
0FB54ZX	Excision of Right Hepatic Duct, Percutaneous Endoscopic Approach, Diagnostic
0FB54ZZ	Excision of Right Hepatic Duct, Percutaneous Endoscopic Approach
0FB57ZX	Excision of Right Hepatic Duct, Via Natural or Artificial Opening, Diagnostic
0FB57ZZ	Excision of Right Hepatic Duct, Via Natural or Artificial Opening
0FB58ZX	Excision of Right Hepatic Duct, Via Natural or Artificial Opening Endoscopic, Diagnostic
0FB58ZZ	Excision of Right Hepatic Duct, Via Natural or Artificial Opening Endoscopic
0FB60ZX	Excision of Left Hepatic Duct, Open Approach, Diagnostic
0FB60ZZ	Excision of Left Hepatic Duct, Open Approach
0FB63ZX	Excision of Left Hepatic Duct, Percutaneous Approach, Diagnostic
0FB63ZZ	Excision of Left Hepatic Duct, Percutaneous Approach
0FB64ZX	Excision of Left Hepatic Duct, Percutaneous Endoscopic Approach, Diagnostic
0FB64ZZ	Excision of Left Hepatic Duct, Percutaneous Endoscopic Approach
0FB67ZX	Excision of Left Hepatic Duct, Via Natural or Artificial Opening, Diagnostic
0FB67ZZ	Excision of Left Hepatic Duct, Via Natural or Artificial Opening
0FB68ZX	Excision of Left Hepatic Duct, Via Natural or Artificial Opening Endoscopic, Diagnostic
0FB68ZZ	Excision of Left Hepatic Duct, Via Natural or Artificial Opening Endoscopic
0FB80ZX	Excision of Cystic Duct, Open Approach, Diagnostic
0FB80ZZ	Excision of Cystic Duct, Open Approach
0FB83ZX	Excision of Cystic Duct, Percutaneous Approach, Diagnostic
0FB83ZZ	Excision of Cystic Duct, Percutaneous Approach
0FB84ZX	Excision of Cystic Duct, Percutaneous Endoscopic Approach, Diagnostic
0FB84ZZ	Excision of Cystic Duct, Percutaneous Endoscopic Approach
0FB87ZX	Excision of Cystic Duct, Via Natural or Artificial Opening, Diagnostic
0FB87ZZ	Excision of Cystic Duct, Via Natural or Artificial Opening
0FB88ZX	Excision of Cystic Duct, Via Natural or Artificial Opening Endoscopic, Diagnostic
0FB88ZZ	Excision of Cystic Duct, Via Natural or Artificial Opening Endoscopic
0FB90ZX	Excision of Common Bile Duct, Open Approach, Diagnostic
0FB90ZZ	Excision of Common Bile Duct, Open Approach
0FB93ZX	Excision of Common Bile Duct, Percutaneous Approach, Diagnostic
0FB93ZZ	Excision of Common Bile Duct, Percutaneous Approach
0FB94ZX	Excision of Common Bile Duct, Percutaneous Endoscopic Approach, Diagnostic
0FB94ZZ	Excision of Common Bile Duct, Percutaneous Endoscopic Approach
0FB97ZX	Excision of Common Bile Duct, Via Natural or Artificial Opening, Diagnostic
0FB97ZZ	Excision of Common Bile Duct, Via Natural or Artificial Opening
0FB98ZX	Excision of Common Bile Duct, Via Natural or Artificial Opening Endoscopic, Diagnostic
0FB98ZZ	Excision of Common Bile Duct, Via Natural or Artificial Opening Endoscopic
0FBC0ZX	Excision of Ampulla of Vater, Open Approach, Diagnostic
0FBC0ZZ	Excision of Ampulla of Vater, Open Approach
0FBC3ZX	Excision of Ampulla of Vater, Percutaneous Approach, Diagnostic
0FBC3ZZ	Excision of Ampulla of Vater, Percutaneous Approach
0FBC4ZX	Excision of Ampulla of Vater, Percutaneous Endoscopic Approach, Diagnostic
0FBC4ZZ	Excision of Ampulla of Vater, Percutaneous Endoscopic Approach
0FBC7ZX	Excision of Ampulla of Vater, Via Natural or Artificial Opening, Diagnostic
0FBC7ZZ	Excision of Ampulla of Vater, Via Natural or Artificial Opening
0FBC8ZX	Excision of Ampulla of Vater, Via Natural or Artificial Opening Endoscopic, Diagnostic
0FBC8ZZ	Excision of Ampulla of Vater, Via Natural or Artificial Opening Endoscopic
0FBD0ZX	Excision of Pancreatic Duct, Open Approach, Diagnostic
0FBD0ZZ	Excision of Pancreatic Duct, Open Approach
0FBD3ZX	Excision of Pancreatic Duct, Percutaneous Approach, Diagnostic
0FBD3ZZ	Excision of Pancreatic Duct, Percutaneous Approach
0FBD4ZX	Excision of Pancreatic Duct, Percutaneous Endoscopic Approach, Diagnostic
0FBD4ZZ	Excision of Pancreatic Duct, Percutaneous Endoscopic Approach
0FBD7ZX	Excision of Pancreatic Duct, Via Natural or Artificial Opening, Diagnostic
0FBD7ZZ	Excision of Pancreatic Duct, Via Natural or Artificial Opening
0FBD8ZX	Excision of Pancreatic Duct, Via Natural or Artificial Opening Endoscopic, Diagnostic
0FBD8ZZ	Excision of Pancreatic Duct, Via Natural or Artificial Opening Endoscopic
0FBF0ZX	Excision of Accessory Pancreatic Duct, Open Approach, Diagnostic
0FBF0ZZ	Excision of Accessory Pancreatic Duct, Open Approach
0FBF3ZX	Excision of Accessory Pancreatic Duct, Percutaneous Approach, Diagnostic
0FBF3ZZ	Excision of Accessory Pancreatic Duct, Percutaneous Approach
0FBF4ZX	Excision of Accessory Pancreatic Duct, Percutaneous Endoscopic Approach, Diagnostic
0FBF4ZZ	Excision of Accessory Pancreatic Duct, Percutaneous Endoscopic Approach
0FBF7ZX	Excision of Accessory Pancreatic Duct, Via Natural or Artificial Opening, Diagnostic
0FBF7ZZ	Excision of Accessory Pancreatic Duct, Via Natural or Artificial Opening
0FBF8ZX	Excision of Accessory Pancreatic Duct, Via Natural or Artificial Opening Endoscopic, Diagnostic
0FBF8ZZ	Excision of Accessory Pancreatic Duct, Via Natural or Artificial Opening Endoscopic
0FBG0ZX	Excision of Pancreas, Open Approach, Diagnostic
0FBG0ZZ	Excision of Pancreas, Open Approach
0FBG3ZX	Excision of Pancreas, Percutaneous Approach, Diagnostic
0FBG3ZZ	Excision of Pancreas, Percutaneous Approach
0FBG4ZX	Excision of Pancreas, Percutaneous Endoscopic Approach, Diagnostic
0FBG4ZZ	Excision of Pancreas, Percutaneous Endoscopic Approach

♀ Female-only   ♂ Male-only   ● Limited Coverage   ● Non-OR   ᴴᴬᶜ HAC-associated procedure   ● Non-covered procedures   ✚ Combination

0FC – Hepatobiliary System and Pancreas, Extirpation

0FC00ZZ	Extirpation of Matter from Liver, Open Approach
0FC03ZZ	Extirpation of Matter from Liver, Percutaneous Approach
0FC04ZZ	Extirpation of Matter from Liver, Percutaneous Endoscopic Approach
0FC10ZZ	Extirpation of Matter from Right Lobe Liver, Open Approach
0FC13ZZ	Extirpation of Matter from Right Lobe Liver, Percutaneous Approach
0FC14ZZ	Extirpation of Matter from Right Lobe Liver, Percutaneous Endoscopic Approach
0FC20ZZ	Extirpation of Matter from Left Lobe Liver, Open Approach
0FC23ZZ	Extirpation of Matter from Left Lobe Liver, Percutaneous Approach
0FC24ZZ	Extirpation of Matter from Left Lobe Liver, Percutaneous Endoscopic Approach
0FC40ZZ	Extirpation of Matter from Gallbladder, Open Approach
0FC43ZZ	Extirpation of Matter from Gallbladder, Percutaneous Approach
0FC44ZZ	Extirpation of Matter from Gallbladder, Percutaneous Endoscopic Approach
0FC50ZZ	Extirpation of Matter from Right Hepatic Duct, Open Approach
0FC53ZZ	Extirpation of Matter from Right Hepatic Duct, Percutaneous Approach
0FC54ZZ	Extirpation of Matter from Right Hepatic Duct, Percutaneous Endoscopic Approach
0FC57ZZ	Extirpation of Matter from Right Hepatic Duct, Via Natural or Artificial Opening
0FC58ZZ	Extirpation of Matter from Right Hepatic Duct, Via Natural or Artificial Opening Endoscopic
0FC60ZZ	Extirpation of Matter from Left Hepatic Duct, Open Approach
0FC63ZZ	Extirpation of Matter from Left Hepatic Duct, Percutaneous Approach
0FC64ZZ	Extirpation of Matter from Left Hepatic Duct, Percutaneous Endoscopic Approach
0FC67ZZ	Extirpation of Matter from Left Hepatic Duct, Via Natural or Artificial Opening
0FC68ZZ	Extirpation of Matter from Left Hepatic Duct, Via Natural or Artificial Opening Endoscopic
0FC80ZZ	Extirpation of Matter from Cystic Duct, Open Approach
0FC83ZZ	Extirpation of Matter from Cystic Duct, Percutaneous Approach
0FC84ZZ	Extirpation of Matter from Cystic Duct, Percutaneous Endoscopic Approach
0FC87ZZ	Extirpation of Matter from Cystic Duct, Via Natural or Artificial Opening
0FC88ZZ	Extirpation of Matter from Cystic Duct, Via Natural or Artificial Opening Endoscopic
0FC90ZZ	Extirpation of Matter from Common Bile Duct, Open Approach
0FC93ZZ	Extirpation of Matter from Common Bile Duct, Percutaneous Approach
0FC94ZZ	Extirpation of Matter from Common Bile Duct, Percutaneous Endoscopic Approach
0FC97ZZ	Extirpation of Matter from Common Bile Duct, Via Natural or Artificial Opening
0FC98ZZ	Extirpation of Matter from Common Bile Duct, Via Natural or Artificial Opening Endoscopic
0FCC0ZZ	Extirpation of Matter from Ampulla of Vater, Open Approach
0FCC3ZZ	Extirpation of Matter from Ampulla of Vater, Percutaneous Approach
0FCC4ZZ	Extirpation of Matter from Ampulla of Vater, Percutaneous Endoscopic Approach
0FCC7ZZ	Extirpation of Matter from Ampulla of Vater, Via Natural or Artificial Opening
0FCC8ZZ	Extirpation of Matter from Ampulla of Vater, Via Natural or Artificial Opening Endoscopic
0FCD0ZZ	Extirpation of Matter from Pancreatic Duct, Open Approach
0FCD3ZZ	Extirpation of Matter from Pancreatic Duct, Percutaneous Approach
0FCD4ZZ	Extirpation of Matter from Pancreatic Duct, Percutaneous Endoscopic Approach
0FCD7ZZ	Extirpation of Matter from Pancreatic Duct, Via Natural or Artificial Opening
0FCD8ZZ	Extirpation of Matter from Pancreatic Duct, Via Natural or Artificial Opening Endoscopic
0FCF0ZZ	Extirpation of Matter from Accessory Pancreatic Duct, Open Approach
0FCF3ZZ	Extirpation of Matter from Accessory Pancreatic Duct, Percutaneous Approach
0FCF4ZZ	Extirpation of Matter from Accessory Pancreatic Duct, Percutaneous Endoscopic Approach
0FCF7ZZ	Extirpation of Matter from Accessory Pancreatic Duct, Via Natural or Artificial Opening
0FCF8ZZ	Extirpation of Matter from Accessory Pancreatic Duct, Via Natural or Artificial Opening Endoscopic
0FCG0ZZ	Extirpation of Matter from Pancreas, Open Approach
0FCG3ZZ	Extirpation of Matter from Pancreas, Percutaneous Approach
0FCG4ZZ	Extirpation of Matter from Pancreas, Percutaneous Endoscopic Approach

0FF – Hepatobiliary System and Pancreas, Fragmentation

0FF40ZZ	Fragmentation in Gallbladder, Open Approach
0FF43ZZ	Fragmentation in Gallbladder, Percutaneous Approach
0FF44ZZ	Fragmentation in Gallbladder, Percutaneous Endoscopic Approach
0FF47ZZ	Fragmentation in Gallbladder, Via Natural or Artificial Opening
0FF48ZZ	Fragmentation in Gallbladder, Via Natural or Artificial Opening Endoscopic
● 0FF4XZZ	Fragmentation in Gallbladder, External Approach
0FF50ZZ	Fragmentation in Right Hepatic Duct, Open Approach
0FF53ZZ	Fragmentation in Right Hepatic Duct, Percutaneous Approach
0FF54ZZ	Fragmentation in Right Hepatic Duct, Percutaneous Endoscopic Approach
0FF57ZZ	Fragmentation in Right Hepatic Duct, Via Natural or Artificial Opening
0FF58ZZ	Fragmentation in Right Hepatic Duct, Via Natural or Artificial Opening Endoscopic
● 0FF5XZZ	Fragmentation in Right Hepatic Duct, External Approach
0FF60ZZ	Fragmentation in Left Hepatic Duct, Open Approach
0FF63ZZ	Fragmentation in Left Hepatic Duct, Percutaneous Approach
0FF64ZZ	Fragmentation in Left Hepatic Duct, Percutaneous Endoscopic Approach
0FF67ZZ	Fragmentation in Left Hepatic Duct, Via Natural or Artificial Opening
0FF68ZZ	Fragmentation in Left Hepatic Duct, Via Natural or Artificial Opening Endoscopic
● 0FF6XZZ	Fragmentation in Left Hepatic Duct, External Approach
0FF80ZZ	Fragmentation in Cystic Duct, Open Approach
0FF83ZZ	Fragmentation in Cystic Duct, Percutaneous Approach
0FF84ZZ	Fragmentation in Cystic Duct, Percutaneous Endoscopic Approach
0FF87ZZ	Fragmentation in Cystic Duct, Via Natural or Artificial Opening
0FF88ZZ	Fragmentation in Cystic Duct, Via Natural or Artificial Opening Endoscopic
● 0FF8XZZ	Fragmentation in Cystic Duct, External Approach
0FF90ZZ	Fragmentation in Common Bile Duct, Open Approach
0FF93ZZ	Fragmentation in Common Bile Duct, Percutaneous Approach
0FF94ZZ	Fragmentation in Common Bile Duct, Percutaneous Endoscopic Approach
0FF97ZZ	Fragmentation in Common Bile Duct, Via Natural or Artificial Opening
0FF98ZZ	Fragmentation in Common Bile Duct, Via Natural or Artificial Opening Endoscopic
● 0FF9XZZ	Fragmentation in Common Bile Duct, External Approach
0FFC0ZZ	Fragmentation in Ampulla of Vater, Open Approach
0FFC3ZZ	Fragmentation in Ampulla of Vater, Percutaneous Approach
0FFC4ZZ	Fragmentation in Ampulla of Vater, Percutaneous Endoscopic Approach
0FFC7ZZ	Fragmentation in Ampulla of Vater, Via Natural or Artificial Opening

0FFC8ZZ Fragmentation in Ampulla of Vater, Via Natural or Artificial Opening Endoscopic

⬤ 0FFCXZZ Fragmentation in Ampulla of Vater, External Approach

0FFD0ZZ Fragmentation in Pancreatic Duct, Open Approach

0FFD3ZZ Fragmentation in Pancreatic Duct, Percutaneous Approach

0FFD4ZZ Fragmentation in Pancreatic Duct, Percutaneous Endoscopic Approach

0FFD7ZZ Fragmentation in Pancreatic Duct, Via Natural or Artificial Opening

0FFD8ZZ Fragmentation in Pancreatic Duct, Via Natural or Artificial Opening Endoscopic

⬤ 0FFDXZZ Fragmentation in Pancreatic Duct, External Approach

0FFF0ZZ Fragmentation in Accessory Pancreatic Duct, Open Approach

0FFF3ZZ Fragmentation in Accessory Pancreatic Duct, Percutaneous Approach

0FFF4ZZ Fragmentation in Accessory Pancreatic Duct, Percutaneous Endoscopic Approach

0FFF7ZZ Fragmentation in Accessory Pancreatic Duct, Via Natural or Artificial Opening

0FFF8ZZ Fragmentation in Accessory Pancreatic Duct, Via Natural or Artificial Opening Endoscopic

⬣ 0FFFXZZ Fragmentation in Accessory Pancreatic Duct, External Approach

0FH *Hepatobiliary System and Pancreas, Insertion*

0FH002Z Insertion of Monitoring Device into Liver, Open Approach

0FH003Z Insertion of Infusion Device into Liver, Open Approach

0FH032Z Insertion of Monitoring Device into Liver, Percutaneous Approach

0FH033Z Insertion of Infusion Device into Liver, Percutaneous Approach

0FH042Z Insertion of Monitoring Device into Liver, Percutaneous Endoscopic Approach

0FH043Z Insertion of Infusion Device into Liver, Percutaneous Endoscopic Approach

0FH102Z Insertion of Monitoring Device into Right Lobe Liver, Open Approach

0FH103Z Insertion of Infusion Device into Right Lobe Liver, Open Approach

0FH132Z Insertion of Monitoring Device into Right Lobe Liver, Percutaneous Approach

0FH133Z Insertion of Infusion Device into Right Lobe Liver, Percutaneous Approach

0FH142Z Insertion of Monitoring Device into Right Lobe Liver, Percutaneous Endoscopic Approach

0FH143Z Insertion of Infusion Device into Right Lobe Liver, Percutaneous Endoscopic Approach

0FH202Z Insertion of Monitoring Device into Left Lobe Liver, Open Approach

0FH203Z Insertion of Infusion Device into Left Lobe Liver, Open Approach

0FH232Z Insertion of Monitoring Device into Left Lobe Liver, Percutaneous Approach

0FH233Z Insertion of Infusion Device into Left Lobe Liver, Percutaneous Approach

0FH242Z Insertion of Monitoring Device into Left Lobe Liver, Percutaneous Endoscopic Approach

0FH243Z Insertion of Infusion Device into Left Lobe Liver, Percutaneous Endoscopic Approach

0FH402Z Insertion of Monitoring Device into Gallbladder, Open Approach

0FH403Z Insertion of Infusion Device into Gallbladder, Open Approach

0FH432Z Insertion of Monitoring Device into Gallbladder, Percutaneous Approach

0FH433Z Insertion of Infusion Device into Gallbladder, Percutaneous Approach

0FH442Z Insertion of Monitoring Device into Gallbladder, Percutaneous Endoscopic Approach

0FH443Z Insertion of Infusion Device into Gallbladder, Percutaneous Endoscopic Approach

0FHB01Z Insertion of Radioactive Element into Hepatobiliary Duct, Open Approach

0FHB02Z Insertion of Monitoring Device into Hepatobiliary Duct, Open Approach

0FHB03Z Insertion of Infusion Device into Hepatobiliary Duct, Open Approach

0FHB0DZ Insertion of Intraluminal Device into Hepatobiliary Duct, Open Approach

0FHB31Z Insertion of Radioactive Element into Hepatobiliary Duct, Percutaneous Approach

0FHB32Z Insertion of Monitoring Device into Hepatobiliary Duct, Percutaneous Approach

0FHB33Z Insertion of Infusion Device into Hepatobiliary Duct, Percutaneous Approach

0FHB3DZ Insertion of Intraluminal Device into Hepatobiliary Duct, Percutaneous Approach

0FHB41Z Insertion of Radioactive Element into Hepatobiliary Duct, Percutaneous Endoscopic Approach

0FHB42Z Insertion of Monitoring Device into Hepatobiliary Duct, Percutaneous Endoscopic Approach

0FHB43Z Insertion of Infusion Device into Hepatobiliary Duct, Percutaneous Endoscopic Approach

0FHB4DZ Insertion of Intraluminal Device into Hepatobiliary Duct, Percutaneous Endoscopic Approach

0FHB71Z Insertion of Radioactive Element into Hepatobiliary Duct, Via Natural or Artificial Opening

0FHB72Z Insertion of Monitoring Device into Hepatobiliary Duct, Via Natural or Artificial Opening

0FHB73Z Insertion of Infusion Device into Hepatobiliary Duct, Via Natural or Artificial Opening

0FHB7DZ Insertion of Intraluminal Device into Hepatobiliary Duct, Via Natural or Artificial Opening

0FHB81Z Insertion of Radioactive Element into Hepatobiliary Duct, Via Natural or Artificial Opening Endoscopic

0FHB82Z Insertion of Monitoring Device into Hepatobiliary Duct, Via Natural or Artificial Opening Endoscopic

0FHB83Z Insertion of Infusion Device into Hepatobiliary Duct, Via Natural or Artificial Opening Endoscopic

0FHB8DZ Insertion of Intraluminal Device into Hepatobiliary Duct, Via Natural or Artificial Opening Endoscopic

0FHD01Z Insertion of Radioactive Element into Pancreatic Duct, Open Approach

0FHD02Z Insertion of Monitoring Device into Pancreatic Duct, Open Approach

0FHD03Z Insertion of Infusion Device into Pancreatic Duct, Open Approach

0FHD0DZ Insertion of Intraluminal Device into Pancreatic Duct, Open Approach

0FHD31Z Insertion of Radioactive Element into Pancreatic Duct, Percutaneous Approach

0FHD32Z Insertion of Monitoring Device into Pancreatic Duct, Percutaneous Approach

0FHD33Z Insertion of Infusion Device into Pancreatic Duct, Percutaneous Approach

0FHD3DZ Insertion of Intraluminal Device into Pancreatic Duct, Percutaneous Approach

0FHD41Z Insertion of Radioactive Element into Pancreatic Duct, Percutaneous Endoscopic Approach

0FHD42Z Insertion of Monitoring Device into Pancreatic Duct, Percutaneous Endoscopic Approach

0FHD43Z Insertion of Infusion Device into Pancreatic Duct, Percutaneous Endoscopic Approach

0FHD4DZ Insertion of Intraluminal Device into Pancreatic Duct, Percutaneous Endoscopic Approach

0FHD71Z Insertion of Radioactive Element into Pancreatic Duct, Via Natural or Artificial Opening

0FHD72Z Insertion of Monitoring Device into Pancreatic Duct, Via Natural or Artificial Opening

0FHD73Z Insertion of Infusion Device into Pancreatic Duct, Via Natural or Artificial Opening

0FHD7DZ Insertion of Intraluminal Device into Pancreatic Duct, Via Natural or Artificial Opening

0FHD81Z Insertion of Radioactive Element into Pancreatic Duct, Via Natural or Artificial Opening Endoscopic

0FHD82Z Insertion of Monitoring Device into Pancreatic Duct, Via Natural or Artificial Opening Endoscopic

0FHD83Z   Insertion of Infusion Device into Pancreatic Duct, Via Natural or Artificial Opening Endoscopic

0FHD8DZ   Insertion of Intraluminal Device into Pancreatic Duct, Via Natural or Artificial Opening Endoscopic

0FHG02Z   Insertion of Monitoring Device into Pancreas, Open Approach

0FHG03Z   Insertion of Infusion Device into Pancreas, Open Approach

0FHG32Z   Insertion of Monitoring Device into Pancreas, Percutaneous Approach

0FHG33Z   Insertion of Infusion Device into Pancreas, Percutaneous Approach

0FHG42Z   Insertion of Monitoring Device into Pancreas, Percutaneous Endoscopic Approach

0FHG43Z   Insertion of Infusion Device into Pancreas, Percutaneous Endoscopic Approach

0FJ – Hepatobiliary System and Pancreas, Inspection

Review Coding Guidelines B3.11a, B3.11b and B3.11c

0FJ00ZZ   Inspection of Liver, Open Approach

0FJ03ZZ   Inspection of Liver, Percutaneous Approach

0FJ04ZZ   Inspection of Liver, Percutaneous Endoscopic Approach

0FJ0XZZ   Inspection of Liver, External Approach

0FJ40ZZ   Inspection of Gallbladder, Open Approach

0FJ43ZZ   Inspection of Gallbladder, Percutaneous Approach

0FJ44ZZ   Inspection of Gallbladder, Percutaneous Endoscopic Approach

0FJ4XZZ   Inspection of Gallbladder, External Approach

0FJB0ZZ   Inspection of Hepatobiliary Duct, Open Approach

0FJB3ZZ   Inspection of Hepatobiliary Duct, Percutaneous Approach

0FJB4ZZ   Inspection of Hepatobiliary Duct, Percutaneous Endoscopic Approach

0FJB7ZZ   Inspection of Hepatobiliary Duct, Via Natural or Artificial Opening

0FJB8ZZ   Inspection of Hepatobiliary Duct, Via Natural or Artificial Opening Endoscopic

0FJD0ZZ   Inspection of Pancreatic Duct, Open Approach

0FJD3ZZ   Inspection of Pancreatic Duct, Percutaneous Approach

0FJD4ZZ   Inspection of Pancreatic Duct, Percutaneous Endoscopic Approach

0FJD7ZZ   Inspection of Pancreatic Duct, Via Natural or Artificial Opening

0FJD8ZZ   Inspection of Pancreatic Duct, Via Natural or Artificial Opening Endoscopic

0FJG0ZZ   Inspection of Pancreas, Open Approach

0FJG3ZZ   Inspection of Pancreas, Percutaneous Approach

0FJG4ZZ   Inspection of Pancreas, Percutaneous Endoscopic Approach

0FJGXZZ   Inspection of Pancreas, External Approach

0FL – Hepatobiliary System and Pancreas, Occlusion

0FL50CZ   Occlusion of Right Hepatic Duct with Extraluminal Device, Open Approach

0FL50DZ   Occlusion of Right Hepatic Duct with Intraluminal Device, Open Approach

0FL50ZZ   Occlusion of Right Hepatic Duct, Open Approach

0FL53CZ   Occlusion of Right Hepatic Duct with Extraluminal Device, Percutaneous Approach

0FL53DZ   Occlusion of Right Hepatic Duct with Intraluminal Device, Percutaneous Approach

0FL53ZZ   Occlusion of Right Hepatic Duct, Percutaneous Approach

0FL54CZ   Occlusion of Right Hepatic Duct with Extraluminal Device, Percutaneous Endoscopic Approach

0FL54DZ   Occlusion of Right Hepatic Duct with Intraluminal Device, Percutaneous Endoscopic Approach

0FL54ZZ   Occlusion of Right Hepatic Duct, Percutaneous Endoscopic Approach

0FL57DZ   Occlusion of Right Hepatic Duct with Intraluminal Device, Via Natural or Artificial Opening

0FL57ZZ   Occlusion of Right Hepatic Duct, Via Natural or Artificial Opening

0FL58DZ   Occlusion of Right Hepatic Duct with Intraluminal Device, Via Natural or Artificial Opening Endoscopic

0FL58ZZ   Occlusion of Right Hepatic Duct, Via Natural or Artificial Opening Endoscopic

0FL60CZ   Occlusion of Left Hepatic Duct with Extraluminal Device, Open Approach

0FL60DZ   Occlusion of Left Hepatic Duct with Intraluminal Device, Open Approach

0FL60ZZ   Occlusion of Left Hepatic Duct, Open Approach

0FL63CZ   Occlusion of Left Hepatic Duct with Extraluminal Device, Percutaneous Approach

0FL63DZ   Occlusion of Left Hepatic Duct with Intraluminal Device, Percutaneous Approach

0FL63ZZ   Occlusion of Left Hepatic Duct, Percutaneous Approach

0FL64CZ   Occlusion of Left Hepatic Duct with Extraluminal Device, Percutaneous Endoscopic Approach

0FL64DZ   Occlusion of Left Hepatic Duct with Intraluminal Device, Percutaneous Endoscopic Approach

0FL64ZZ   Occlusion of Left Hepatic Duct, Percutaneous Endoscopic Approach

0FL67DZ   Occlusion of Left Hepatic Duct with Intraluminal Device, Via Natural or Artificial Opening

0FL67ZZ   Occlusion of Left Hepatic Duct, Via Natural or Artificial Opening

0FL68DZ   Occlusion of Left Hepatic Duct with Intraluminal Device, Via Natural or Artificial Opening Endoscopic

0FL68ZZ   Occlusion of Left Hepatic Duct, Via Natural or Artificial Opening Endoscopic

0FL80CZ   Occlusion of Cystic Duct with Extraluminal Device, Open Approach

0FL80DZ   Occlusion of Cystic Duct with Intraluminal Device, Open Approach

0FL80ZZ   Occlusion of Cystic Duct, Open Approach

0FL83CZ   Occlusion of Cystic Duct with Extraluminal Device, Percutaneous Approach

0FL83DZ   Occlusion of Cystic Duct with Intraluminal Device, Percutaneous Approach

0FL83ZZ   Occlusion of Cystic Duct, Percutaneous Approach

0FL84CZ   Occlusion of Cystic Duct with Extraluminal Device, Percutaneous Endoscopic Approach

0FL84DZ   Occlusion of Cystic Duct with Intraluminal Device, Percutaneous Endoscopic Approach

0FL84ZZ   Occlusion of Cystic Duct, Percutaneous Endoscopic Approach

0FL87DZ   Occlusion of Cystic Duct with Intraluminal Device, Via Natural or Artificial Opening

0FL87ZZ   Occlusion of Cystic Duct, Via Natural or Artificial Opening

0FL88DZ   Occlusion of Cystic Duct with Intraluminal Device, Via Natural or Artificial Opening Endoscopic

0FL88ZZ   Occlusion of Cystic Duct, Via Natural or Artificial Opening Endoscopic

0FL90CZ   Occlusion of Common Bile Duct with Extraluminal Device, Open Approach

0FL90DZ   Occlusion of Common Bile Duct with Intraluminal Device, Open Approach

0FL90ZZ   Occlusion of Common Bile Duct, Open Approach

0FL93CZ   Occlusion of Common Bile Duct with Extraluminal Device, Percutaneous Approach

0FL93DZ   Occlusion of Common Bile Duct with Intraluminal Device, Percutaneous Approach

0FL93ZZ   Occlusion of Common Bile Duct, Percutaneous Approach

0FL94CZ   Occlusion of Common Bile Duct with Extraluminal Device, Percutaneous Endoscopic Approach

0FL94DZ   Occlusion of Common Bile Duct with Intraluminal Device, Percutaneous Endoscopic Approach

0FL94ZZ   Occlusion of Common Bile Duct, Percutaneous Endoscopic Approach

0FL97DZ   Occlusion of Common Bile Duct with Intraluminal Device, Via Natural or Artificial Opening

0FL97ZZ   Occlusion of Common Bile Duct, Via Natural or Artificial Opening

0FL98DZ   Occlusion of Common Bile Duct with Intraluminal Device, Via Natural or Artificial Opening Endoscopic

0FL98ZZ Occlusion of Common Bile Duct, Via Natural or Artificial Opening Endoscopic

0FLC0CZ Occlusion of Ampulla of Vater with Extraluminal Device, Open Approach

0FLC0DZ Occlusion of Ampulla of Vater with Intraluminal Device, Open Approach

0FLC0ZZ Occlusion of Ampulla of Vater, Open Approach

0FLC3CZ Occlusion of Ampulla of Vater with Extraluminal Device, Percutaneous Approach

0FLC3DZ Occlusion of Ampulla of Vater with Intraluminal Device, Percutaneous Approach

0FLC3ZZ Occlusion of Ampulla of Vater, Percutaneous Approach

0FLC4CZ Occlusion of Ampulla of Vater with Extraluminal Device, Percutaneous Endoscopic Approach

0FLC4DZ Occlusion of Ampulla of Vater with Intraluminal Device, Percutaneous Endoscopic Approach

0FLC4ZZ Occlusion of Ampulla of Vater, Percutaneous Endoscopic Approach

0FLC7DZ Occlusion of Ampulla of Vater with Intraluminal Device, Via Natural or Artificial Opening

0FLC7ZZ Occlusion of Ampulla of Vater, Via Natural or Artificial Opening

0FLC8DZ Occlusion of Ampulla of Vater with Intraluminal Device, Via Natural or Artificial Opening Endoscopic

0FLC8ZZ Occlusion of Ampulla of Vater, Via Natural or Artificial Opening Endoscopic

0FLD0CZ Occlusion of Pancreatic Duct with Extraluminal Device, Open Approach

0FLD0DZ Occlusion of Pancreatic Duct with Intraluminal Device, Open Approach

0FLD0ZZ Occlusion of Pancreatic Duct, Open Approach

0FLD3CZ Occlusion of Pancreatic Duct with Extraluminal Device, Percutaneous Approach

0FLD3DZ Occlusion of Pancreatic Duct with Intraluminal Device, Percutaneous Approach

0FLD3ZZ Occlusion of Pancreatic Duct, Percutaneous Approach

0FLD4CZ Occlusion of Pancreatic Duct with Extraluminal Device, Percutaneous Endoscopic Approach

0FLD4DZ Occlusion of Pancreatic Duct with Intraluminal Device, Percutaneous Endoscopic Approach

0FLD4ZZ Occlusion of Pancreatic Duct, Percutaneous Endoscopic Approach

0FLD7DZ Occlusion of Pancreatic Duct with Intraluminal Device, Via Natural or Artificial Opening

0FLD7ZZ Occlusion of Pancreatic Duct, Via Natural or Artificial Opening

0FLD8DZ Occlusion of Pancreatic Duct with Intraluminal Device, Via Natural or Artificial Opening Endoscopic

0FLD8ZZ Occlusion of Pancreatic Duct, Via Natural or Artificial Opening Endoscopic

0FLF0CZ Occlusion of Accessory Pancreatic Duct with Extraluminal Device, Open Approach

0FLF0DZ Occlusion of Accessory Pancreatic Duct with Intraluminal Device, Open Approach

0FLF0ZZ Occlusion of Accessory Pancreatic Duct, Open Approach

0FLF3CZ Occlusion of Accessory Pancreatic Duct with Extraluminal Device, Percutaneous Approach

0FLF3DZ Occlusion of Accessory Pancreatic Duct with Intraluminal Device, Percutaneous Approach

0FLF3ZZ Occlusion of Accessory Pancreatic Duct, Percutaneous Approach

0FLF4CZ Occlusion of Accessory Pancreatic Duct with Extraluminal Device, Percutaneous Endoscopic Approach

0FLF4DZ Occlusion of Accessory Pancreatic Duct with Intraluminal Device, Percutaneous Endoscopic Approach

0FLF4ZZ Occlusion of Accessory Pancreatic Duct, Percutaneous Endoscopic Approach

0FLF7DZ Occlusion of Accessory Pancreatic Duct with Intraluminal Device, Via Natural or Artificial Opening

0FLF7ZZ Occlusion of Accessory Pancreatic Duct, Via Natural or Artificial Opening

0FLF8DZ Occlusion of Accessory Pancreatic Duct with Intraluminal Device, Via Natural or Artificial Opening Endoscopic

0FLF8ZZ Occlusion of Accessory Pancreatic Duct, Via Natural or Artificial Opening Endoscopic

0FM – Hepatobiliary System and Pancreas, Reattachment

0FM00ZZ Reattachment of Liver, Open Approach

0FM04ZZ Reattachment of Liver, Percutaneous Endoscopic Approach

0FM10ZZ Reattachment of Right Lobe Liver, Open Approach

0FM14ZZ Reattachment of Right Lobe Liver, Percutaneous Endoscopic Approach

0FM20ZZ Reattachment of Left Lobe Liver, Open Approach

0FM24ZZ Reattachment of Left Lobe Liver, Percutaneous Endoscopic Approach

0FM40ZZ Reattachment of Gallbladder, Open Approach

0FM44ZZ Reattachment of Gallbladder, Percutaneous Endoscopic Approach

0FM50ZZ Reattachment of Right Hepatic Duct, Open Approach

0FM54ZZ Reattachment of Right Hepatic Duct, Percutaneous Endoscopic Approach

0FM60ZZ Reattachment of Left Hepatic Duct, Open Approach

0FM64ZZ Reattachment of Left Hepatic Duct, Percutaneous Endoscopic Approach

0FM80ZZ Reattachment of Cystic Duct, Open Approach

0FM84ZZ Reattachment of Cystic Duct, Percutaneous Endoscopic Approach

0FM90ZZ Reattachment of Common Bile Duct, Open Approach

0FM94ZZ Reattachment of Common Bile Duct, Percutaneous Endoscopic Approach

0FMC0ZZ Reattachment of Ampulla of Vater, Open Approach

0FMC4ZZ Reattachment of Ampulla of Vater, Percutaneous Endoscopic Approach

0FMD0ZZ Reattachment of Pancreatic Duct, Open Approach

0FMD4ZZ Reattachment of Pancreatic Duct, Percutaneous Endoscopic Approach

0FMF0ZZ Reattachment of Accessory Pancreatic Duct, Open Approach

0FMF4ZZ Reattachment of Accessory Pancreatic Duct, Percutaneous Endoscopic Approach

0FMG0ZZ Reattachment of Pancreas, Open Approach

0FMG4ZZ Reattachment of Pancreas, Percutaneous Endoscopic Approach

0FN – Hepatobiliary System and Pancreas, Release

Review Coding Guideline B3.13

Review Coding Guideline B3.14

0FN00ZZ Release Liver, Open Approach

0FN03ZZ Release Liver, Percutaneous Approach

0FN04ZZ Release Liver, Percutaneous Endoscopic Approach

0FN10ZZ Release Right Lobe Liver, Open Approach

0FN13ZZ Release Right Lobe Liver, Percutaneous Approach

0FN14ZZ Release Right Lobe Liver, Percutaneous Endoscopic Approach

0FN20ZZ Release Left Lobe Liver, Open Approach

0FN23ZZ Release Left Lobe Liver, Percutaneous Approach

0FN24ZZ Release Left Lobe Liver, Percutaneous Endoscopic Approach

0FN40ZZ Release Gallbladder, Open Approach

0FN43ZZ Release Gallbladder, Percutaneous Approach

0FN44ZZ Release Gallbladder, Percutaneous Endoscopic Approach

0FN50ZZ Release Right Hepatic Duct, Open Approach

0FN53ZZ Release Right Hepatic Duct, Percutaneous Approach

0FN54ZZ Release Right Hepatic Duct, Percutaneous Endoscopic Approach

0FN57ZZ Release Right Hepatic Duct, Via Natural or Artificial Opening

0FN58ZZ Release Right Hepatic Duct, Via Natural or Artificial Opening Endoscopic

0FN60ZZ Release Left Hepatic Duct, Open Approach

0FN63ZZ Release Left Hepatic Duct, Percutaneous Approach

0FN64ZZ Release Left Hepatic Duct, Percutaneous Endoscopic Approach

0FN67ZZ Release Left Hepatic Duct, Via Natural or Artificial Opening

0FN68ZZ	Release Left Hepatic Duct, Via Natural or Artificial Opening Endoscopic
0FN80ZZ	Release Cystic Duct, Open Approach
0FN83ZZ	Release Cystic Duct, Percutaneous Approach
0FN84ZZ	Release Cystic Duct, Percutaneous Endoscopic Approach
0FN87ZZ	Release Cystic Duct, Via Natural or Artificial Opening
0FN88ZZ	Release Cystic Duct, Via Natural or Artificial Opening Endoscopic
0FN90ZZ	Release Common Bile Duct, Open Approach
0FN93ZZ	Release Common Bile Duct, Percutaneous Approach
0FN94ZZ	Release Common Bile Duct, Percutaneous Endoscopic Approach
0FN97ZZ	Release Common Bile Duct, Via Natural or Artificial Opening
0FN98ZZ	Release Common Bile Duct, Via Natural or Artificial Opening Endoscopic
0FNC0ZZ	Release Ampulla of Vater, Open Approach
0FNC3ZZ	Release Ampulla of Vater, Percutaneous Approach
0FNC4ZZ	Release Ampulla of Vater, Percutaneous Endoscopic Approach
0FNC7ZZ	Release Ampulla of Vater, Via Natural or Artificial Opening
0FNC8ZZ	Release Ampulla of Vater, Via Natural or Artificial Opening Endoscopic

0FND0ZZ	Release Pancreatic Duct, Open Approach
0FND3ZZ	Release Pancreatic Duct, Percutaneous Approach
0FND4ZZ	Release Pancreatic Duct, Percutaneous Endoscopic Approach
0FND7ZZ	Release Pancreatic Duct, Via Natural or Artificial Opening
0FND8ZZ	Release Pancreatic Duct, Via Natural or Artificial Opening Endoscopic
0FNF0ZZ	Release Accessory Pancreatic Duct, Open Approach
0FNF3ZZ	Release Accessory Pancreatic Duct, Percutaneous Approach
0FNF4ZZ	Release Accessory Pancreatic Duct, Percutaneous Endoscopic Approach
0FNF7ZZ	Release Accessory Pancreatic Duct, Via Natural or Artificial Opening
0FNF8ZZ	Release Accessory Pancreatic Duct, Via Natural or Artificial Opening Endoscopic
0FNG0ZZ	Release Pancreas, Open Approach
0FNG3ZZ	Release Pancreas, Percutaneous Approach
0FNG4ZZ	Release Pancreas, Percutaneous Endoscopic Approach

0FP – Hepatobiliary System and Pancreas, Removal

Review Coding Guideline B6.1c

0FP000Z	Removal of Drainage Device from Liver, Open Approach
0FP002Z	Removal of Monitoring Device from Liver, Open Approach
0FP003Z	Removal of Infusion Device from Liver, Open Approach
0FP030Z	Removal of Drainage Device from Liver, Percutaneous Approach
0FP032Z	Removal of Monitoring Device from Liver, Percutaneous Approach
0FP033Z	Removal of Infusion Device from Liver, Percutaneous Approach
0FP040Z	Removal of Drainage Device from Liver, Percutaneous Endoscopic Approach
0FP042Z	Removal of Monitoring Device from Liver, Percutaneous Endoscopic Approach
0FP043Z	Removal of Infusion Device from Liver, Percutaneous Endoscopic Approach
0FP0X0Z	Removal of Drainage Device from Liver, External Approach
0FP0X2Z	Removal of Monitoring Device from Liver, External Approach
0FP0X3Z	Removal of Infusion Device from Liver, External Approach
0FP400Z	Removal of Drainage Device from Gallbladder, Open Approach
0FP402Z	Removal of Monitoring Device from Gallbladder, Open Approach
0FP403Z	Removal of Infusion Device from Gallbladder, Open Approach
0FP40DZ	Removal of Intraluminal Device from Gallbladder, Open Approach
0FP430Z	Removal of Drainage Device from Gallbladder, Percutaneous Approach
0FP432Z	Removal of Monitoring Device from Gallbladder, Percutaneous Approach
0FP433Z	Removal of Infusion Device from Gallbladder, Percutaneous Approach
0FP43DZ	Removal of Intraluminal Device from Gallbladder, Percutaneous Approach
0FP440Z	Removal of Drainage Device from Gallbladder, Percutaneous Endoscopic Approach
0FP442Z	Removal of Monitoring Device from Gallbladder, Percutaneous Endoscopic Approach
0FP443Z	Removal of Infusion Device from Gallbladder, Percutaneous Endoscopic Approach
0FP44DZ	Removal of Intraluminal Device from Gallbladder, Percutaneous Endoscopic Approach
0FP4X0Z	Removal of Drainage Device from Gallbladder, External Approach
0FP4X2Z	Removal of Monitoring Device from Gallbladder, External Approach
0FP4X3Z	Removal of Infusion Device from Gallbladder, External Approach
0FP4XDZ	Removal of Intraluminal Device from Gallbladder, External Approach
0FPB00Z	Removal of Drainage Device from Hepatobiliary Duct, Open Approach
0FPB01Z	Removal of Radioactive Element from Hepatobiliary Duct, Open Approach
0FPB02Z	Removal of Monitoring Device from Hepatobiliary Duct, Open Approach
0FPB03Z	Removal of Infusion Device from Hepatobiliary Duct, Open Approach

0FPB07Z	Removal of Autologous Tissue Substitute from Hepatobiliary Duct, Open Approach
0FPB0CZ	Removal of Extraluminal Device from Hepatobiliary Duct, Open Approach
0FPB0DZ	Removal of Intraluminal Device from Hepatobiliary Duct, Open Approach
0FPB0JZ	Removal of Synthetic Substitute from Hepatobiliary Duct, Open Approach
0FPB0KZ	Removal of Nonautologous Tissue Substitute from Hepatobiliary Duct, Open Approach
0FPB30Z	Removal of Drainage Device from Hepatobiliary Duct, Percutaneous Approach
0FPB31Z	Removal of Radioactive Element from Hepatobiliary Duct, Percutaneous Approach
0FPB32Z	Removal of Monitoring Device from Hepatobiliary Duct, Percutaneous Approach
0FPB33Z	Removal of Infusion Device from Hepatobiliary Duct, Percutaneous Approach
0FPB37Z	Removal of Autologous Tissue Substitute from Hepatobiliary Duct, Percutaneous Approach
0FPB3CZ	Removal of Extraluminal Device from Hepatobiliary Duct, Percutaneous Approach
0FPB3DZ	Removal of Intraluminal Device from Hepatobiliary Duct, Percutaneous Approach
0FPB3JZ	Removal of Synthetic Substitute from Hepatobiliary Duct, Percutaneous Approach
0FPB3KZ	Removal of Nonautologous Tissue Substitute from Hepatobiliary Duct, Percutaneous Approach
0FPB40Z	Removal of Drainage Device from Hepatobiliary Duct, Percutaneous Endoscopic Approach
0FPB41Z	Removal of Radioactive Element from Hepatobiliary Duct, Percutaneous Endoscopic Approach
0FPB42Z	Removal of Monitoring Device from Hepatobiliary Duct, Percutaneous Endoscopic Approach
0FPB43Z	Removal of Infusion Device from Hepatobiliary Duct, Percutaneous Endoscopic Approach
0FPB47Z	Removal of Autologous Tissue Substitute from Hepatobiliary Duct, Percutaneous Endoscopic Approach
0FPB4CZ	Removal of Extraluminal Device from Hepatobiliary Duct, Percutaneous Endoscopic Approach
0FPB4DZ	Removal of Intraluminal Device from Hepatobiliary Duct, Percutaneous Endoscopic Approach
0FPB4JZ	Removal of Synthetic Substitute from Hepatobiliary Duct, Percutaneous Endoscopic Approach
0FPB4KZ	Removal of Nonautologous Tissue Substitute from Hepatobiliary Duct, Percutaneous Endoscopic Approach
0FPB70Z	Removal of Drainage Device from Hepatobiliary Duct, Via Natural or Artificial Opening
0FPB71Z	Removal of Radioactive Element from Hepatobiliary Duct, Via Natural or Artificial Opening

 Female-only   ♂ Male-only   ◐ Limited Coverage   ● Non-OR   ▥ HAC-associated procedure   ● Non-covered procedures   ✚ Combination

0FPB72Z Removal of Monitoring Device from Hepatobiliary Duct, Via Natural or Artificial Opening

0FPB73Z Removal of Infusion Device from Hepatobiliary Duct, Via Natural or Artificial Opening

0FPB77Z Removal of Autologous Tissue Substitute from Hepatobiliary Duct, Via Natural or Artificial Opening

0FPB7CZ Removal of Extraluminal Device from Hepatobiliary Duct, Via Natural or Artificial Opening

0FPB7DZ Removal of Intraluminal Device from Hepatobiliary Duct, Via Natural or Artificial Opening

0FPB7JZ Removal of Synthetic Substitute from Hepatobiliary Duct, Via Natural or Artificial Opening

0FPB7KZ Removal of Nonautologous Tissue Substitute from Hepatobiliary Duct, Via Natural or Artificial Opening

0FPB80Z Removal of Drainage Device from Hepatobiliary Duct, Via Natural or Artificial Opening Endoscopic

0FPB81Z Removal of Radioactive Element from Hepatobiliary Duct, Via Natural or Artificial Opening Endoscopic

0FPB82Z Removal of Monitoring Device from Hepatobiliary Duct, Via Natural or Artificial Opening Endoscopic

0FPB83Z Removal of Infusion Device from Hepatobiliary Duct, Via Natural or Artificial Opening Endoscopic

0FPB87Z Removal of Autologous Tissue Substitute from Hepatobiliary Duct, Via Natural or Artificial Opening Endoscopic

0FPB8CZ Removal of Extraluminal Device from Hepatobiliary Duct, Via Natural or Artificial Opening Endoscopic

0FPB8DZ Removal of Intraluminal Device from Hepatobiliary Duct, Via Natural or Artificial Opening Endoscopic

0FPB8JZ Removal of Synthetic Substitute from Hepatobiliary Duct, Via Natural or Artificial Opening Endoscopic

0FPB8KZ Removal of Nonautologous Tissue Substitute from Hepatobiliary Duct, Via Natural or Artificial Opening Endoscopic

0FPBX0Z Removal of Drainage Device from Hepatobiliary Duct, External Approach

0FPBX1Z Removal of Radioactive Element from Hepatobiliary Duct, External Approach

0FPBX2Z Removal of Monitoring Device from Hepatobiliary Duct, External Approach

0FPBX3Z Removal of Infusion Device from Hepatobiliary Duct, External Approach

0FPBXDZ Removal of Intraluminal Device from Hepatobiliary Duct, External Approach

0FPD00Z Removal of Drainage Device from Pancreatic Duct, Open Approach

0FPD01Z Removal of Radioactive Element from Pancreatic Duct, Open Approach

0FPD02Z Removal of Monitoring Device from Pancreatic Duct, Open Approach

0FPD03Z Removal of Infusion Device from Pancreatic Duct, Open Approach

0FPD07Z Removal of Autologous Tissue Substitute from Pancreatic Duct, Open Approach

0FPD0CZ Removal of Extraluminal Device from Pancreatic Duct, Open Approach

0FPD0DZ Removal of Intraluminal Device from Pancreatic Duct, Open Approach

0FPD0JZ Removal of Synthetic Substitute from Pancreatic Duct, Open Approach

0FPD0KZ Removal of Nonautologous Tissue Substitute from Pancreatic Duct, Open Approach

0FPD30Z Removal of Drainage Device from Pancreatic Duct, Percutaneous Approach

0FPD31Z Removal of Radioactive Element from Pancreatic Duct, Percutaneous Approach

0FPD32Z Removal of Monitoring Device from Pancreatic Duct, Percutaneous Approach

0FPD33Z Removal of Infusion Device from Pancreatic Duct, Percutaneous Approach

0FPD37Z Removal of Autologous Tissue Substitute from Pancreatic Duct, Percutaneous Approach

0FPD3CZ Removal of Extraluminal Device from Pancreatic Duct, Percutaneous Approach

0FPD3DZ Removal of Intraluminal Device from Pancreatic Duct, Percutaneous Approach

0FPD3JZ Removal of Synthetic Substitute from Pancreatic Duct, Percutaneous Approach

0FPD3KZ Removal of Nonautologous Tissue Substitute from Pancreatic Duct, Percutaneous Approach

0FPD40Z Removal of Drainage Device from Pancreatic Duct, Percutaneous Endoscopic Approach

0FPD41Z Removal of Radioactive Element from Pancreatic Duct, Percutaneous Endoscopic Approach

0FPD42Z Removal of Monitoring Device from Pancreatic Duct, Percutaneous Endoscopic Approach

0FPD43Z Removal of Infusion Device from Pancreatic Duct, Percutaneous Endoscopic Approach

0FPD47Z Removal of Autologous Tissue Substitute from Pancreatic Duct, Percutaneous Endoscopic Approach

0FPD4CZ Removal of Extraluminal Device from Pancreatic Duct, Percutaneous Endoscopic Approach

0FPD4DZ Removal of Intraluminal Device from Pancreatic Duct, Percutaneous Endoscopic Approach

0FPD4JZ Removal of Synthetic Substitute from Pancreatic Duct, Percutaneous Endoscopic Approach

0FPD4KZ Removal of Nonautologous Tissue Substitute from Pancreatic Duct, Percutaneous Endoscopic Approach

0FPD70Z Removal of Drainage Device from Pancreatic Duct, Via Natural or Artificial Opening

0FPD71Z Removal of Radioactive Element from Pancreatic Duct, Via Natural or Artificial Opening

0FPD72Z Removal of Monitoring Device from Pancreatic Duct, Via Natural or Artificial Opening

0FPD73Z Removal of Infusion Device from Pancreatic Duct, Via Natural or Artificial Opening

0FPD77Z Removal of Autologous Tissue Substitute from Pancreatic Duct, Via Natural or Artificial Opening

0FPD7CZ Removal of Extraluminal Device from Pancreatic Duct, Via Natural or Artificial Opening

0FPD7DZ Removal of Intraluminal Device from Pancreatic Duct, Via Natural or Artificial Opening

0FPD7JZ Removal of Synthetic Substitute from Pancreatic Duct, Via Natural or Artificial Opening

0FPD7KZ Removal of Nonautologous Tissue Substitute from Pancreatic Duct, Via Natural or Artificial Opening

0FPD80Z Removal of Drainage Device from Pancreatic Duct, Via Natural or Artificial Opening Endoscopic

0FPD81Z Removal of Radioactive Element from Pancreatic Duct, Via Natural or Artificial Opening Endoscopic

0FPD82Z Removal of Monitoring Device from Pancreatic Duct, Via Natural or Artificial Opening Endoscopic

0FPD83Z Removal of Infusion Device from Pancreatic Duct, Via Natural or Artificial Opening Endoscopic

0FPD87Z Removal of Autologous Tissue Substitute from Pancreatic Duct, Via Natural or Artificial Opening Endoscopic

0FPD8CZ Removal of Extraluminal Device from Pancreatic Duct, Via Natural or Artificial Opening Endoscopic

0FPD8DZ Removal of Intraluminal Device from Pancreatic Duct, Via Natural or Artificial Opening Endoscopic

0FPD8JZ Removal of Synthetic Substitute from Pancreatic Duct, Via Natural or Artificial Opening Endoscopic

0FPD8KZ Removal of Nonautologous Tissue Substitute from Pancreatic Duct, Via Natural or Artificial Opening Endoscopic

0FPDX0Z Removal of Drainage Device from Pancreatic Duct, External Approach

0FPDX1Z Removal of Radioactive Element from Pancreatic Duct, External Approach

0FPDX2Z Removal of Monitoring Device from Pancreatic Duct, External Approach

0FPDX3Z Removal of Infusion Device from Pancreatic Duct, External Approach

0FPDXDZ Removal of Intraluminal Device from Pancreatic Duct, External Approach

0FPG00Z Removal of Drainage Device from Pancreas, Open Approach

0FPG02Z Removal of Monitoring Device from Pancreas, Open Approach

0FPG03Z Removal of Infusion Device from Pancreas, Open Approach

0FPG0DZ Removal of Intraluminal Device from Pancreas, Open Approach

0FPG30Z Removal of Drainage Device from Pancreas, Percutaneous Approach

0FPG32Z Removal of Monitoring Device from Pancreas, Percutaneous Approach

---

♀ Female-only   ♂ Male-only   ◯ Limited Coverage   ● Non-OR   🅷🅰🅲 HAC-associated procedure   ⬡ Non-covered procedures   ✚ Combination

0FPG33Z Removal of Infusion Device from Pancreas, Percutaneous Approach
0FPG3DZ Removal of Intraluminal Device from Pancreas, Percutaneous Approach
0FPG40Z Removal of Drainage Device from Pancreas, Percutaneous Endoscopic Approach
0FPG42Z Removal of Monitoring Device from Pancreas, Percutaneous Endoscopic Approach

0FPG43Z Removal of Infusion Device from Pancreas, Percutaneous Endoscopic Approach
0FPG4DZ Removal of Intraluminal Device from Pancreas, Percutaneous Endoscopic Approach
0FPGX0Z Removal of Drainage Device from Pancreas, External Approach
0FPGX2Z Removal of Monitoring Device from Pancreas, External Approach
0FPGX3Z Removal of Infusion Device from Pancreas, External Approach
0FPGXDZ Removal of Intraluminal Device from Pancreas, External Approach

0FQ – Hepatobiliary System and Pancreas, Repair

0FQ00ZZ Repair Liver, Open Approach
0FQ03ZZ Repair Liver, Percutaneous Approach
0FQ04ZZ Repair Liver, Percutaneous Endoscopic Approach
0FQ10ZZ Repair Right Lobe Liver, Open Approach
0FQ13ZZ Repair Right Lobe Liver, Percutaneous Approach
0FQ14ZZ Repair Right Lobe Liver, Percutaneous Endoscopic Approach
0FQ20ZZ Repair Left Lobe Liver, Open Approach
0FQ23ZZ Repair Left Lobe Liver, Percutaneous Approach
0FQ24ZZ Repair Left Lobe Liver, Percutaneous Endoscopic Approach
0FQ40ZZ Repair Gallbladder, Open Approach
0FQ43ZZ Repair Gallbladder, Percutaneous Approach
0FQ44ZZ Repair Gallbladder, Percutaneous Endoscopic Approach
0FQ50ZZ Repair Right Hepatic Duct, Open Approach
0FQ53ZZ Repair Right Hepatic Duct, Percutaneous Approach
0FQ54ZZ Repair Right Hepatic Duct, Percutaneous Endoscopic Approach
0FQ57ZZ Repair Right Hepatic Duct, Via Natural or Artificial Opening
0FQ58ZZ Repair Right Hepatic Duct, Via Natural or Artificial Opening Endoscopic
0FQ60ZZ Repair Left Hepatic Duct, Open Approach
0FQ63ZZ Repair Left Hepatic Duct, Percutaneous Approach
0FQ64ZZ Repair Left Hepatic Duct, Percutaneous Endoscopic Approach
0FQ67ZZ Repair Left Hepatic Duct, Via Natural or Artificial Opening
0FQ68ZZ Repair Left Hepatic Duct, Via Natural or Artificial Opening Endoscopic
0FQ80ZZ Repair Cystic Duct, Open Approach
0FQ83ZZ Repair Cystic Duct, Percutaneous Approach
0FQ84ZZ Repair Cystic Duct, Percutaneous Endoscopic Approach
0FQ87ZZ Repair Cystic Duct, Via Natural or Artificial Opening
0FQ88ZZ Repair Cystic Duct, Via Natural or Artificial Opening Endoscopic

0FQ90ZZ Repair Common Bile Duct, Open Approach
0FQ93ZZ Repair Common Bile Duct, Percutaneous Approach
0FQ94ZZ Repair Common Bile Duct, Percutaneous Endoscopic Approach
0FQ97ZZ Repair Common Bile Duct, Via Natural or Artificial Opening
0FQ98ZZ Repair Common Bile Duct, Via Natural or Artificial Opening Endoscopic
0FQC0ZZ Repair Ampulla of Vater, Open Approach
0FQC3ZZ Repair Ampulla of Vater, Percutaneous Approach
0FQC4ZZ Repair Ampulla of Vater, Percutaneous Endoscopic Approach
0FQC7ZZ Repair Ampulla of Vater, Via Natural or Artificial Opening
0FQC8ZZ Repair Ampulla of Vater, Via Natural or Artificial Opening Endoscopic
0FQD0ZZ Repair Pancreatic Duct, Open Approach
0FQD3ZZ Repair Pancreatic Duct, Percutaneous Approach
0FQD4ZZ Repair Pancreatic Duct, Percutaneous Endoscopic Approach
0FQD7ZZ Repair Pancreatic Duct, Via Natural or Artificial Opening
0FQD8ZZ Repair Pancreatic Duct, Via Natural or Artificial Opening Endoscopic
0FQF0ZZ Repair Accessory Pancreatic Duct, Open Approach
0FQF3ZZ Repair Accessory Pancreatic Duct, Percutaneous Approach
0FQF4ZZ Repair Accessory Pancreatic Duct, Percutaneous Endoscopic Approach
0FQF7ZZ Repair Accessory Pancreatic Duct, Via Natural or Artificial Opening
0FQF8ZZ Repair Accessory Pancreatic Duct, Via Natural or Artificial Opening Endoscopic
0FQG0ZZ Repair Pancreas, Open Approach
0FQG3ZZ Repair Pancreas, Percutaneous Approach
0FQG4ZZ Repair Pancreas, Percutaneous Endoscopic Approach

0FR – Hepatobiliary System and Pancreas, Replacement

0FR507Z Replacement of Right Hepatic Duct with Autologous Tissue Substitute, Open Approach
0FR50JZ Replacement of Right Hepatic Duct with Synthetic Substitute, Open Approach
0FR50KZ Replacement of Right Hepatic Duct with Nonautologous Tissue Substitute, Open Approach
0FR547Z Replacement of Right Hepatic Duct with Autologous Tissue Substitute, Percutaneous Endoscopic Approach
0FR54JZ Replacement of Right Hepatic Duct with Synthetic Substitute, Percutaneous Endoscopic Approach
0FR54KZ Replacement of Right Hepatic Duct with Nonautologous Tissue Substitute, Percutaneous Endoscopic Approach
0FR607Z Replacement of Left Hepatic Duct with Autologous Tissue Substitute, Open Approach
0FR60JZ Replacement of Left Hepatic Duct with Synthetic Substitute, Open Approach
0FR60KZ Replacement of Left Hepatic Duct with Nonautologous Tissue Substitute, Open Approach
0FR647Z Replacement of Left Hepatic Duct with Autologous Tissue Substitute, Percutaneous Endoscopic Approach
0FR64JZ Replacement of Left Hepatic Duct with Synthetic Substitute, Percutaneous Endoscopic Approach
0FR64KZ Replacement of Left Hepatic Duct with Nonautologous Tissue Substitute, Percutaneous Endoscopic Approach
0FR807Z Replacement of Cystic Duct with Autologous Tissue Substitute, Open Approach
0FR80JZ Replacement of Cystic Duct with Synthetic Substitute, Open Approach
0FR80KZ Replacement of Cystic Duct with Nonautologous Tissue Substitute, Open Approach

0FR847Z Replacement of Cystic Duct with Autologous Tissue Substitute, Percutaneous Endoscopic Approach
0FR84JZ Replacement of Cystic Duct with Synthetic Substitute, Percutaneous Endoscopic Approach
0FR84KZ Replacement of Cystic Duct with Nonautologous Tissue Substitute, Percutaneous Endoscopic Approach
0FR907Z Replacement of Common Bile Duct with Autologous Tissue Substitute, Open Approach
0FR90JZ Replacement of Common Bile Duct with Synthetic Substitute, Open Approach
0FR90KZ Replacement of Common Bile Duct with Nonautologous Tissue Substitute, Open Approach
0FR947Z Replacement of Common Bile Duct with Autologous Tissue Substitute, Percutaneous Endoscopic Approach
0FR94JZ Replacement of Common Bile Duct with Synthetic Substitute, Percutaneous Endoscopic Approach
0FR94KZ Replacement of Common Bile Duct with Nonautologous Tissue Substitute, Percutaneous Endoscopic Approach
0FRC07Z Replacement of Ampulla of Vater with Autologous Tissue Substitute, Open Approach
0FRC0JZ Replacement of Ampulla of Vater with Synthetic Substitute, Open Approach
0FRC0KZ Replacement of Ampulla of Vater with Nonautologous Tissue Substitute, Open Approach
0FRC47Z Replacement of Ampulla of Vater with Autologous Tissue Substitute, Percutaneous Endoscopic Approach
0FRC4JZ Replacement of Ampulla of Vater with Synthetic Substitute, Percutaneous Endoscopic Approach
0FRC4KZ Replacement of Ampulla of Vater with Nonautologous Tissue Substitute, Percutaneous Endoscopic Approach

0FRD07Z Replacement of Pancreatic Duct with Autologous Tissue Substitute, Open Approach

0FRD0JZ Replacement of Pancreatic Duct with Synthetic Substitute, Open Approach

0FRD0KZ Replacement of Pancreatic Duct with Nonautologous Tissue Substitute, Open Approach

0FRD47Z Replacement of Pancreatic Duct with Autologous Tissue Substitute, Percutaneous Endoscopic Approach

0FRD4JZ Replacement of Pancreatic Duct with Synthetic Substitute, Percutaneous Endoscopic Approach

0FRD4KZ Replacement of Pancreatic Duct with Nonautologous Tissue Substitute, Percutaneous Endoscopic Approach

0FRF07Z Replacement of Accessory Pancreatic Duct with Autologous Tissue Substitute, Open Approach

0FRF0JZ Replacement of Accessory Pancreatic Duct with Synthetic Substitute, Open Approach

0FRF0KZ Replacement of Accessory Pancreatic Duct with Nonautologous Tissue Substitute, Open Approach

0FRF47Z Replacement of Accessory Pancreatic Duct with Autologous Tissue Substitute, Percutaneous Endoscopic Approach

0FRF4JZ Replacement of Accessory Pancreatic Duct with Synthetic Substitute, Percutaneous Endoscopic Approach

0FRF4KZ Replacement of Accessory Pancreatic Duct with Nonautologous Tissue Substitute, Percutaneous Endoscopic Approach

0FS – Hepatobiliary System and Pancreas, Reposition

0FS00ZZ Reposition Liver, Open Approach

0FS04ZZ Reposition Liver, Percutaneous Endoscopic Approach

0FS40ZZ Reposition Gallbladder, Open Approach

0FS44ZZ Reposition Gallbladder, Percutaneous Endoscopic Approach

0FS50ZZ Reposition Right Hepatic Duct, Open Approach

0FS54ZZ Reposition Right Hepatic Duct, Percutaneous Endoscopic Approach

0FS60ZZ Reposition Left Hepatic Duct, Open Approach

0FS64ZZ Reposition Left Hepatic Duct, Percutaneous Endoscopic Approach

0FS80ZZ Reposition Cystic Duct, Open Approach

0FS84ZZ Reposition Cystic Duct, Percutaneous Endoscopic Approach

0FS90ZZ Reposition Common Bile Duct, Open Approach

0FS94ZZ Reposition Common Bile Duct, Percutaneous Endoscopic Approach

0FSC0ZZ Reposition Ampulla of Vater, Open Approach

0FSC4ZZ Reposition Ampulla of Vater, Percutaneous Endoscopic Approach

0FSD0ZZ Reposition Pancreatic Duct, Open Approach

0FSD4ZZ Reposition Pancreatic Duct, Percutaneous Endoscopic Approach

0FSF0ZZ Reposition Accessory Pancreatic Duct, Open Approach

0FSF4ZZ Reposition Accessory Pancreatic Duct, Percutaneous Endoscopic Approach

0FSG0ZZ Reposition Pancreas, Open Approach

0FSG4ZZ Reposition Pancreas, Percutaneous Endoscopic Approach

0FT – Hepatobiliary System and Pancreas, Resection

Review Coding Guideline B3.8

0FT00ZZ Resection of Liver, Open Approach

0FT04ZZ Resection of Liver, Percutaneous Endoscopic Approach

0FT10ZZ Resection of Right Lobe Liver, Open Approach

0FT14ZZ Resection of Right Lobe Liver, Percutaneous Endoscopic Approach

0FT20ZZ Resection of Left Lobe Liver, Open Approach

0FT24ZZ Resection of Left Lobe Liver, Percutaneous Endoscopic Approach

0FT40ZZ Resection of Gallbladder, Open Approach

0FT44ZZ Resection of Gallbladder, Percutaneous Endoscopic Approach

0FT50ZZ Resection of Right Hepatic Duct, Open Approach

0FT54ZZ Resection of Right Hepatic Duct, Percutaneous Endoscopic Approach

0FT57ZZ Resection of Right Hepatic Duct, Via Natural or Artificial Opening

0FT58ZZ Resection of Right Hepatic Duct, Via Natural or Artificial Opening Endoscopic

0FT60ZZ Resection of Left Hepatic Duct, Open Approach

0FT64ZZ Resection of Left Hepatic Duct, Percutaneous Endoscopic Approach

0FT67ZZ Resection of Left Hepatic Duct, Via Natural or Artificial Opening

0FT68ZZ Resection of Left Hepatic Duct, Via Natural or Artificial Opening Endoscopic

0FT80ZZ Resection of Cystic Duct, Open Approach

0FT84ZZ Resection of Cystic Duct, Percutaneous Endoscopic Approach

0FT87ZZ Resection of Cystic Duct, Via Natural or Artificial Opening

0FT88ZZ Resection of Cystic Duct, Via Natural or Artificial Opening Endoscopic

0FT90ZZ Resection of Common Bile Duct, Open Approach

0FT94ZZ Resection of Common Bile Duct, Percutaneous Endoscopic Approach

0FT97ZZ Resection of Common Bile Duct, Via Natural or Artificial Opening

0FT98ZZ Resection of Common Bile Duct, Via Natural or Artificial Opening Endoscopic

0FTC0ZZ Resection of Ampulla of Vater, Open Approach

0FTC4ZZ Resection of Ampulla of Vater, Percutaneous Endoscopic Approach

0FTC7ZZ Resection of Ampulla of Vater, Via Natural or Artificial Opening

0FTC8ZZ Resection of Ampulla of Vater, Via Natural or Artificial Opening Endoscopic

0FTD0ZZ Resection of Pancreatic Duct, Open Approach

0FTD4ZZ Resection of Pancreatic Duct, Percutaneous Endoscopic Approach

0FTD7ZZ Resection of Pancreatic Duct, Via Natural or Artificial Opening

0FTD8ZZ Resection of Pancreatic Duct, Via Natural or Artificial Opening Endoscopic

0FTF0ZZ Resection of Accessory Pancreatic Duct, Open Approach

0FTF4ZZ Resection of Accessory Pancreatic Duct, Percutaneous Endoscopic Approach

0FTF7ZZ Resection of Accessory Pancreatic Duct, Via Natural or Artificial Opening

0FTF8ZZ Resection of Accessory Pancreatic Duct, Via Natural or Artificial Opening Endoscopic

0FTG0ZZ Resection of Pancreas, Open Approach

0FTG4ZZ Resection of Pancreas, Percutaneous Endoscopic Approach

0FU – Hepatobiliary System and Pancreas, Supplement

0FU507Z Supplement Right Hepatic Duct with Autologous Tissue Substitute, Open Approach

0FU50JZ Supplement Right Hepatic Duct with Synthetic Substitute, Open Approach

0FU50KZ Supplement Right Hepatic Duct with Nonautologous Tissue Substitute, Open Approach

0FU537Z Supplement Right Hepatic Duct with Autologous Tissue Substitute, Percutaneous Approach

0FU53JZ Supplement Right Hepatic Duct with Synthetic Substitute, Percutaneous Approach

0FU53KZ Supplement Right Hepatic Duct with Nonautologous Tissue Substitute, Percutaneous Approach

0FU547Z Supplement Right Hepatic Duct with Autologous Tissue Substitute, Percutaneous Endoscopic Approach

0FU54JZ Supplement Right Hepatic Duct with Synthetic Substitute, Percutaneous Endoscopic Approach

0FU54KZ Supplement Right Hepatic Duct with Nonautologous Tissue Substitute, Percutaneous Endoscopic Approach

0FU607Z Supplement Left Hepatic Duct with Autologous Tissue Substitute, Open Approach

0FU60JZ Supplement Left Hepatic Duct with Synthetic Substitute, Open Approach

0FU60KZ Supplement Left Hepatic Duct with Nonautologous Tissue Substitute, Open Approach

0FU637Z Supplement Left Hepatic Duct with Autologous Tissue Substitute, Percutaneous Approach

0FU63JZ Supplement Left Hepatic Duct with Synthetic Substitute, Percutaneous Approach

0FU63KZ   Supplement Left Hepatic Duct with Nonautologous Tissue Substitute, Percutaneous Approach

0FU647Z   Supplement Left Hepatic Duct with Autologous Tissue Substitute, Percutaneous Endoscopic Approach

0FU64JZ   Supplement Left Hepatic Duct with Synthetic Substitute, Percutaneous Endoscopic Approach

0FU64KZ   Supplement Left Hepatic Duct with Nonautologous Tissue Substitute, Percutaneous Endoscopic Approach

0FU807Z   Supplement Cystic Duct with Autologous Tissue Substitute, Open Approach

0FU80JZ   Supplement Cystic Duct with Synthetic Substitute, Open Approach

0FU80KZ   Supplement Cystic Duct with Nonautologous Tissue Substitute, Open Approach

0FU837Z   Supplement Cystic Duct with Autologous Tissue Substitute, Percutaneous Approach

0FU83JZ   Supplement Cystic Duct with Synthetic Substitute, Percutaneous Approach

0FU83KZ   Supplement Cystic Duct with Nonautologous Tissue Substitute, Percutaneous Approach

0FU847Z   Supplement Cystic Duct with Autologous Tissue Substitute, Percutaneous Endoscopic Approach

0FU84JZ   Supplement Cystic Duct with Synthetic Substitute, Percutaneous Endoscopic Approach

0FU84KZ   Supplement Cystic Duct with Nonautologous Tissue Substitute, Percutaneous Endoscopic Approach

0FU907Z   Supplement Common Bile Duct with Autologous Tissue Substitute, Open Approach

0FU90JZ   Supplement Common Bile Duct with Synthetic Substitute, Open Approach

0FU90KZ   Supplement Common Bile Duct with Nonautologous Tissue Substitute, Open Approach

0FU937Z   Supplement Common Bile Duct with Autologous Tissue Substitute, Percutaneous Approach

0FU93JZ   Supplement Common Bile Duct with Synthetic Substitute, Percutaneous Approach

0FU93KZ   Supplement Common Bile Duct with Nonautologous Tissue Substitute, Percutaneous Approach

0FU947Z   Supplement Common Bile Duct with Autologous Tissue Substitute, Percutaneous Endoscopic Approach

0FU94JZ   Supplement Common Bile Duct with Synthetic Substitute, Percutaneous Endoscopic Approach

0FU94KZ   Supplement Common Bile Duct with Nonautologous Tissue Substitute, Percutaneous Endoscopic Approach

0FUC07Z   Supplement Ampulla of Vater with Autologous Tissue Substitute, Open Approach

0FUC0JZ   Supplement Ampulla of Vater with Synthetic Substitute, Open Approach

0FUC0KZ   Supplement Ampulla of Vater with Nonautologous Tissue Substitute, Open Approach

0FUC37Z   Supplement Ampulla of Vater with Autologous Tissue Substitute, Percutaneous Approach

0FUC3JZ   Supplement Ampulla of Vater with Synthetic Substitute, Percutaneous Approach

0FUC3KZ   Supplement Ampulla of Vater with Nonautologous Tissue Substitute, Percutaneous Approach

0FUC47Z   Supplement Ampulla of Vater with Autologous Tissue Substitute, Percutaneous Endoscopic Approach

0FUC4JZ   Supplement Ampulla of Vater with Synthetic Substitute, Percutaneous Endoscopic Approach

0FUC4KZ   Supplement Ampulla of Vater with Nonautologous Tissue Substitute, Percutaneous Endoscopic Approach

0FUD07Z   Supplement Pancreatic Duct with Autologous Tissue Substitute, Open Approach

0FUD0JZ   Supplement Pancreatic Duct with Synthetic Substitute, Open Approach

0FUD0KZ   Supplement Pancreatic Duct with Nonautologous Tissue Substitute, Open Approach

0FUD37Z   Supplement Pancreatic Duct with Autologous Tissue Substitute, Percutaneous Approach

0FUD3JZ   Supplement Pancreatic Duct with Synthetic Substitute, Percutaneous Approach

0FUD3KZ   Supplement Pancreatic Duct with Nonautologous Tissue Substitute, Percutaneous Approach

0FUD47Z   Supplement Pancreatic Duct with Autologous Tissue Substitute, Percutaneous Endoscopic Approach

0FUD4JZ   Supplement Pancreatic Duct with Synthetic Substitute, Percutaneous Endoscopic Approach

0FUD4KZ   Supplement Pancreatic Duct with Nonautologous Tissue Substitute, Percutaneous Endoscopic Approach

0FUF07Z   Supplement Accessory Pancreatic Duct with Autologous Tissue Substitute, Open Approach

0FUF0JZ   Supplement Accessory Pancreatic Duct with Synthetic Substitute, Open Approach

0FUF0KZ   Supplement Accessory Pancreatic Duct with Nonautologous Tissue Substitute, Open Approach

0FUF37Z   Supplement Accessory Pancreatic Duct with Autologous Tissue Substitute, Percutaneous Approach

0FUF3JZ   Supplement Accessory Pancreatic Duct with Synthetic Substitute, Percutaneous Approach

0FUF3KZ   Supplement Accessory Pancreatic Duct with Nonautologous Tissue Substitute, Percutaneous Approach

0FUF47Z   Supplement Accessory Pancreatic Duct with Autologous Tissue Substitute, Percutaneous Endoscopic Approach

0FUF4JZ   Supplement Accessory Pancreatic Duct with Synthetic Substitute, Percutaneous Endoscopic Approach

0FUF4KZ   Supplement Accessory Pancreatic Duct with Nonautologous Tissue Substitute, Percutaneous Endoscopic Approach

0FV – Hepatobiliary System and Pancreas, Restriction

0FV50CZ   Restriction of Right Hepatic Duct with Extraluminal Device, Open Approach

0FV50DZ   Restriction of Right Hepatic Duct with Intraluminal Device, Open Approach

0FV50ZZ   Restriction of Right Hepatic Duct, Open Approach

0FV53CZ   Restriction of Right Hepatic Duct with Extraluminal Device, Percutaneous Approach

0FV53DZ   Restriction of Right Hepatic Duct with Intraluminal Device, Percutaneous Approach

0FV53ZZ   Restriction of Right Hepatic Duct, Percutaneous Approach

0FV54CZ   Restriction of Right Hepatic Duct with Extraluminal Device, Percutaneous Endoscopic Approach

0FV54DZ   Restriction of Right Hepatic Duct with Intraluminal Device, Percutaneous Endoscopic Approach

0FV54ZZ   Restriction of Right Hepatic Duct, Percutaneous Endoscopic Approach

0FV57DZ   Restriction of Right Hepatic Duct with Intraluminal Device, Via Natural or Artificial Opening

0FV57ZZ   Restriction of Right Hepatic Duct, Via Natural or Artificial Opening

0FV58DZ   Restriction of Right Hepatic Duct with Intraluminal Device, Via Natural or Artificial Opening Endoscopic

0FV58ZZ   Restriction of Right Hepatic Duct, Via Natural or Artificial Opening Endoscopic

0FV60CZ   Restriction of Left Hepatic Duct with Extraluminal Device, Open Approach

0FV60DZ   Restriction of Left Hepatic Duct with Intraluminal Device, Open Approach

0FV60ZZ   Restriction of Left Hepatic Duct, Open Approach

0FV63CZ   Restriction of Left Hepatic Duct with Extraluminal Device, Percutaneous Approach

0FV63DZ   Restriction of Left Hepatic Duct with Intraluminal Device, Percutaneous Approach

0FV63ZZ   Restriction of Left Hepatic Duct, Percutaneous Approach

0FV64CZ   Restriction of Left Hepatic Duct with Extraluminal Device, Percutaneous Endoscopic Approach

0FV64DZ   Restriction of Left Hepatic Duct with Intraluminal Device, Percutaneous Endoscopic Approach

0FV64ZZ   Restriction of Left Hepatic Duct, Percutaneous Endoscopic Approach

0FV67DZ   Restriction of Left Hepatic Duct with Intraluminal Device, Via Natural or Artificial Opening

0GN80ZZ Release Bilateral Carotid Bodies, Open Approach
0GN83ZZ Release Bilateral Carotid Bodies, Percutaneous Approach
0GN84ZZ Release Bilateral Carotid Bodies, Percutaneous Endoscopic Approach
0GN90ZZ Release Para-aortic Body, Open Approach
0GN93ZZ Release Para-aortic Body, Percutaneous Approach
0GN94ZZ Release Para-aortic Body, Percutaneous Endoscopic Approach
0GNB0ZZ Release Coccygeal Glomus, Open Approach
0GNB3ZZ Release Coccygeal Glomus, Percutaneous Approach
0GNB4ZZ Release Coccygeal Glomus, Percutaneous Endoscopic Approach
0GNC0ZZ Release Glomus Jugulare, Open Approach
0GNC3ZZ Release Glomus Jugulare, Percutaneous Approach
0GNC4ZZ Release Glomus Jugulare, Percutaneous Endoscopic Approach
0GND0ZZ Release Aortic Body, Open Approach
0GND3ZZ Release Aortic Body, Percutaneous Approach
0GND4ZZ Release Aortic Body, Percutaneous Endoscopic Approach
0GNF0ZZ Release Paraganglion Extremity, Open Approach
0GNF3ZZ Release Paraganglion Extremity, Percutaneous Approach
0GNF4ZZ Release Paraganglion Extremity, Percutaneous Endoscopic Approach
0GNG0ZZ Release Left Thyroid Gland Lobe, Open Approach
0GNG3ZZ Release Left Thyroid Gland Lobe, Percutaneous Approach
0GNG4ZZ Release Left Thyroid Gland Lobe, Percutaneous Endoscopic Approach
0GNH0ZZ Release Right Thyroid Gland Lobe, Open Approach
0GNH3ZZ Release Right Thyroid Gland Lobe, Percutaneous Approach
0GNH4ZZ Release Right Thyroid Gland Lobe, Percutaneous Endoscopic Approach

0GNK0ZZ Release Thyroid Gland, Open Approach
0GNK3ZZ Release Thyroid Gland, Percutaneous Approach
0GNK4ZZ Release Thyroid Gland, Percutaneous Endoscopic Approach
0GNL0ZZ Release Right Superior Parathyroid Gland, Open Approach
0GNL3ZZ Release Right Superior Parathyroid Gland, Percutaneous Approach
0GNL4ZZ Release Right Superior Parathyroid Gland, Percutaneous Endoscopic Approach
0GNM0ZZ Release Left Superior Parathyroid Gland, Open Approach
0GNM3ZZ Release Left Superior Parathyroid Gland, Percutaneous Approach
0GNM4ZZ Release Left Superior Parathyroid Gland, Percutaneous Endoscopic Approach
0GNN0ZZ Release Right Inferior Parathyroid Gland, Open Approach
0GNN3ZZ Release Right Inferior Parathyroid Gland, Percutaneous Approach
0GNN4ZZ Release Right Inferior Parathyroid Gland, Percutaneous Endoscopic Approach
0GNP0ZZ Release Left Inferior Parathyroid Gland, Open Approach
0GNP3ZZ Release Left Inferior Parathyroid Gland, Percutaneous Approach
0GNP4ZZ Release Left Inferior Parathyroid Gland, Percutaneous Endoscopic Approach
0GNQ0ZZ Release Multiple Parathyroid Glands, Open Approach
0GNQ3ZZ Release Multiple Parathyroid Glands, Percutaneous Approach
0GNQ4ZZ Release Multiple Parathyroid Glands, Percutaneous Endoscopic Approach
0GNR0ZZ Release Parathyroid Gland, Open Approach
0GNR3ZZ Release Parathyroid Gland, Percutaneous Approach
0GNR4ZZ Release Parathyroid Gland, Percutaneous Endoscopic Approach

0GP – Endocrine System, Removal

Review Coding Guideline B6.1c

0GP000Z Removal of Drainage Device from Pituitary Gland, Open Approach
0GP030Z Removal of Drainage Device from Pituitary Gland, Percutaneous Approach
0GP040Z Removal of Drainage Device from Pituitary Gland, Percutaneous Endoscopic Approach
0GP0X0Z Removal of Drainage Device from Pituitary Gland, External Approach
0GP100Z Removal of Drainage Device from Pineal Body, Open Approach
0GP130Z Removal of Drainage Device from Pineal Body, Percutaneous Approach
0GP140Z Removal of Drainage Device from Pineal Body, Percutaneous Endoscopic Approach
0GP1X0Z Removal of Drainage Device from Pineal Body, External Approach
0GP500Z Removal of Drainage Device from Adrenal Gland, Open Approach
0GP530Z Removal of Drainage Device from Adrenal Gland, Percutaneous Approach
0GP540Z Removal of Drainage Device from Adrenal Gland, Percutaneous Endoscopic Approach
0GP5X0Z Removal of Drainage Device from Adrenal Gland, External Approach
0GPK00Z Removal of Drainage Device from Thyroid Gland, Open Approach
0GPK30Z Removal of Drainage Device from Thyroid Gland, Percutaneous Approach
0GPK40Z Removal of Drainage Device from Thyroid Gland, Percutaneous Endoscopic Approach
0GPKX0Z Removal of Drainage Device from Thyroid Gland, External Approach
0GPR00Z Removal of Drainage Device from Parathyroid Gland, Open Approach

0GPR30Z Removal of Drainage Device from Parathyroid Gland, Percutaneous Approach
0GPR40Z Removal of Drainage Device from Parathyroid Gland, Percutaneous Endoscopic Approach
0GPRX0Z Removal of Drainage Device from Parathyroid Gland, External Approach
0GPS00Z Removal of Drainage Device from Endocrine Gland, Open Approach
0GPS02Z Removal of Monitoring Device from Endocrine Gland, Open Approach
0GPS03Z Removal of Infusion Device from Endocrine Gland, Open Approach
0GPS30Z Removal of Drainage Device from Endocrine Gland, Percutaneous Approach
0GPS32Z Removal of Monitoring Device from Endocrine Gland, Percutaneous Approach
0GPS33Z Removal of Infusion Device from Endocrine Gland, Percutaneous Approach
0GPS40Z Removal of Drainage Device from Endocrine Gland, Percutaneous Endoscopic Approach
0GPS42Z Removal of Monitoring Device from Endocrine Gland, Percutaneous Endoscopic Approach
0GPS43Z Removal of Infusion Device from Endocrine Gland, Percutaneous Endoscopic Approach
0GPSX0Z Removal of Drainage Device from Endocrine Gland, External Approach
0GPSX2Z Removal of Monitoring Device from Endocrine Gland, External Approach
0GPSX3Z Removal of Infusion Device from Endocrine Gland, External Approach

0GQ – Endocrine System, Repair

0GQ00ZZ Repair Pituitary Gland, Open Approach
0GQ03ZZ Repair Pituitary Gland, Percutaneous Approach
0GQ04ZZ Repair Pituitary Gland, Percutaneous Endoscopic Approach
0GQ10ZZ Repair Pineal Body, Open Approach
0GQ13ZZ Repair Pineal Body, Percutaneous Approach
0GQ14ZZ Repair Pineal Body, Percutaneous Endoscopic Approach
0GQ20ZZ Repair Left Adrenal Gland, Open Approach
0GQ23ZZ Repair Left Adrenal Gland, Percutaneous Approach

0GQ24ZZ Repair Left Adrenal Gland, Percutaneous Endoscopic Approach
0GQ30ZZ Repair Right Adrenal Gland, Open Approach
0GQ33ZZ Repair Right Adrenal Gland, Percutaneous Approach
0GQ34ZZ Repair Right Adrenal Gland, Percutaneous Endoscopic Approach
0GQ40ZZ Repair Bilateral Adrenal Glands, Open Approach
0GQ43ZZ Repair Bilateral Adrenal Glands, Percutaneous Approach
0GQ44ZZ Repair Bilateral Adrenal Glands, Percutaneous Endoscopic Approach

---

♀ Female-only   ♂ Male-only   ● Limited Coverage   ● Non-OR   🅷🅰🅲 HAC-associated procedure   ● Non-covered procedures   ➕ Combination

0GQ60ZZ   Repair Left Carotid Body, Open Approach
0GQ63ZZ   Repair Left Carotid Body, Percutaneous Approach
0GQ64ZZ   Repair Left Carotid Body, Percutaneous Endoscopic Approach
0GQ70ZZ   Repair Right Carotid Body, Open Approach
0GQ73ZZ   Repair Right Carotid Body, Percutaneous Approach
0GQ74ZZ   Repair Right Carotid Body, Percutaneous Endoscopic Approach
0GQ80ZZ   Repair Bilateral Carotid Bodies, Open Approach
0GQ83ZZ   Repair Bilateral Carotid Bodies, Percutaneous Approach
0GQ84ZZ   Repair Bilateral Carotid Bodies, Percutaneous Endoscopic Approach
0GQ90ZZ   Repair Para-aortic Body, Open Approach
0GQ93ZZ   Repair Para-aortic Body, Percutaneous Approach
0GQ94ZZ   Repair Para-aortic Body, Percutaneous Endoscopic Approach
0GQB0ZZ   Repair Coccygeal Glomus, Open Approach
0GQB3ZZ   Repair Coccygeal Glomus, Percutaneous Approach
0GQB4ZZ   Repair Coccygeal Glomus, Percutaneous Endoscopic Approach
0GQC0ZZ   Repair Glomus Jugulare, Open Approach
0GQC3ZZ   Repair Glomus Jugulare, Percutaneous Approach
0GQC4ZZ   Repair Glomus Jugulare, Percutaneous Endoscopic Approach
0GQD0ZZ   Repair Aortic Body, Open Approach
0GQD3ZZ   Repair Aortic Body, Percutaneous Approach
0GQD4ZZ   Repair Aortic Body, Percutaneous Endoscopic Approach
0GQF0ZZ   Repair Paraganglion Extremity, Open Approach
0GQF3ZZ   Repair Paraganglion Extremity, Percutaneous Approach
0GQF4ZZ   Repair Paraganglion Extremity, Percutaneous Endoscopic Approach
0GQG0ZZ   Repair Left Thyroid Gland Lobe, Open Approach
0GQG3ZZ   Repair Left Thyroid Gland Lobe, Percutaneous Approach
0GQG4ZZ   Repair Left Thyroid Gland Lobe, Percutaneous Endoscopic Approach
0GQH0ZZ   Repair Right Thyroid Gland Lobe, Open Approach
0GQH3ZZ   Repair Right Thyroid Gland Lobe, Percutaneous Approach

0GQH4ZZ   Repair Right Thyroid Gland Lobe, Percutaneous Endoscopic Approach
0GQJ0ZZ   Repair Thyroid Gland Isthmus, Open Approach
0GQJ3ZZ   Repair Thyroid Gland Isthmus, Percutaneous Approach
0GQJ4ZZ   Repair Thyroid Gland Isthmus, Percutaneous Endoscopic Approach
0GQK0ZZ   Repair Thyroid Gland, Open Approach
0GQK3ZZ   Repair Thyroid Gland, Percutaneous Approach
0GQK4ZZ   Repair Thyroid Gland, Percutaneous Endoscopic Approach
0GQL0ZZ   Repair Right Superior Parathyroid Gland, Open Approach
0GQL3ZZ   Repair Right Superior Parathyroid Gland, Percutaneous Approach
0GQL4ZZ   Repair Right Superior Parathyroid Gland, Percutaneous Endoscopic Approach
0GQM0ZZ   Repair Left Superior Parathyroid Gland, Open Approach
0GQM3ZZ   Repair Left Superior Parathyroid Gland, Percutaneous Approach
0GQM4ZZ   Repair Left Superior Parathyroid Gland, Percutaneous Endoscopic Approach
0GQN0ZZ   Repair Right Inferior Parathyroid Gland, Open Approach
0GQN3ZZ   Repair Right Inferior Parathyroid Gland, Percutaneous Approach
0GQN4ZZ   Repair Right Inferior Parathyroid Gland, Percutaneous Endoscopic Approach
0GQP0ZZ   Repair Left Inferior Parathyroid Gland, Open Approach
0GQP3ZZ   Repair Left Inferior Parathyroid Gland, Percutaneous Approach
0GQP4ZZ   Repair Left Inferior Parathyroid Gland, Percutaneous Endoscopic Approach
0GQQ0ZZ   Repair Multiple Parathyroid Glands, Open Approach
0GQQ3ZZ   Repair Multiple Parathyroid Glands, Percutaneous Approach
0GQQ4ZZ   Repair Multiple Parathyroid Glands, Percutaneous Endoscopic Approach
0GQR0ZZ   Repair Parathyroid Gland, Open Approach
0GQR3ZZ   Repair Parathyroid Gland, Percutaneous Approach
0GQR4ZZ   Repair Parathyroid Gland, Percutaneous Endoscopic Approach

0GS – Endocrine System, Reposition

0GS20ZZ   Reposition Left Adrenal Gland, Open Approach
0GS24ZZ   Reposition Left Adrenal Gland, Percutaneous Endoscopic Approach
0GS30ZZ   Reposition Right Adrenal Gland, Open Approach
0GS34ZZ   Reposition Right Adrenal Gland, Percutaneous Endoscopic Approach
0GSG0ZZ   Reposition Left Thyroid Gland Lobe, Open Approach
0GSG4ZZ   Reposition Left Thyroid Gland Lobe, Percutaneous Endoscopic Approach
0GSH0ZZ   Reposition Right Thyroid Gland Lobe, Open Approach
0GSH4ZZ   Reposition Right Thyroid Gland Lobe, Percutaneous Endoscopic Approach
0GSL0ZZ   Reposition Right Superior Parathyroid Gland, Open Approach
0GSL4ZZ   Reposition Right Superior Parathyroid Gland, Percutaneous Endoscopic Approach

0GSM0ZZ   Reposition Left Superior Parathyroid Gland, Open Approach
0GSM4ZZ   Reposition Left Superior Parathyroid Gland, Percutaneous Endoscopic Approach
0GSN0ZZ   Reposition Right Inferior Parathyroid Gland, Open Approach
0GSN4ZZ   Reposition Right Inferior Parathyroid Gland, Percutaneous Endoscopic Approach
0GSP0ZZ   Reposition Left Inferior Parathyroid Gland, Open Approach
0GSP4ZZ   Reposition Left Inferior Parathyroid Gland, Percutaneous Endoscopic Approach
0GSQ0ZZ   Reposition Multiple Parathyroid Glands, Open Approach
0GSQ4ZZ   Reposition Multiple Parathyroid Glands, Percutaneous Endoscopic Approach
0GSR0ZZ   Reposition Parathyroid Gland, Open Approach
0GSR4ZZ   Reposition Parathyroid Gland, Percutaneous Endoscopic Approach

0GT – Endocrine System, Resection

Review Coding Guideline B3.8

0GT00ZZ   Resection of Pituitary Gland, Open Approach
0GT04ZZ   Resection of Pituitary Gland, Percutaneous Endoscopic Approach
0GT10ZZ   Resection of Pineal Body, Open Approach
0GT14ZZ   Resection of Pineal Body, Percutaneous Endoscopic Approach
0GT20ZZ   Resection of Left Adrenal Gland, Open Approach
0GT24ZZ   Resection of Left Adrenal Gland, Percutaneous Endoscopic Approach
0GT30ZZ   Resection of Right Adrenal Gland, Open Approach
0GT34ZZ   Resection of Right Adrenal Gland, Percutaneous Endoscopic Approach
0GT40ZZ   Resection of Bilateral Adrenal Glands, Open Approach
0GT44ZZ   Resection of Bilateral Adrenal Glands, Percutaneous Endoscopic Approach
0GT60ZZ   Resection of Left Carotid Body, Open Approach
0GT64ZZ   Resection of Left Carotid Body, Percutaneous Endoscopic Approach
0GT70ZZ   Resection of Right Carotid Body, Open Approach
0GT74ZZ   Resection of Right Carotid Body, Percutaneous Endoscopic Approach
0GT80ZZ   Resection of Bilateral Carotid Bodies, Open Approach

0GT84ZZ   Resection of Bilateral Carotid Bodies, Percutaneous Endoscopic Approach
0GT90ZZ   Resection of Para-aortic Body, Open Approach
0GT94ZZ   Resection of Para-aortic Body, Percutaneous Endoscopic Approach
0GTB0ZZ   Resection of Coccygeal Glomus, Open Approach
0GTB4ZZ   Resection of Coccygeal Glomus, Percutaneous Endoscopic Approach
0GTC0ZZ   Resection of Glomus Jugulare, Open Approach
0GTC4ZZ   Resection of Glomus Jugulare, Percutaneous Endoscopic Approach
0GTD0ZZ   Resection of Aortic Body, Open Approach
0GTD4ZZ   Resection of Aortic Body, Percutaneous Endoscopic Approach
0GTF0ZZ   Resection of Paraganglion Extremity, Open Approach
0GTF4ZZ   Resection of Paraganglion Extremity, Percutaneous Endoscopic Approach
0GTG0ZZ   Resection of Left Thyroid Gland Lobe, Open Approach
0GTG4ZZ   Resection of Left Thyroid Gland Lobe, Percutaneous Endoscopic Approach
0GTH0ZZ   Resection of Right Thyroid Gland Lobe, Open Approach
0GTH4ZZ   Resection of Right Thyroid Gland Lobe, Percutaneous Endoscopic Approach

0GTK0ZZ Resection of Thyroid Gland, Open Approach
0GTK4ZZ Resection of Thyroid Gland, Percutaneous Endoscopic Approach
0GTL0ZZ Resection of Right Superior Parathyroid Gland, Open Approach
0GTL4ZZ Resection of Right Superior Parathyroid Gland, Percutaneous Endoscopic Approach
0GTM0ZZ Resection of Left Superior Parathyroid Gland, Open Approach
0GTM4ZZ Resection of Left Superior Parathyroid Gland, Percutaneous Endoscopic Approach
0GTN0ZZ Resection of Right Inferior Parathyroid Gland, Open Approach
0GTN4ZZ Resection of Right Inferior Parathyroid Gland, Percutaneous Endoscopic Approach

0GTP0ZZ Resection of Left Inferior Parathyroid Gland, Open Approach
0GTP4ZZ Resection of Left Inferior Parathyroid Gland, Percutaneous Endoscopic Approach
0GTQ0ZZ Resection of Multiple Parathyroid Glands, Open Approach
0GTQ4ZZ Resection of Multiple Parathyroid Glands, Percutaneous Endoscopic Approach
0GTR0ZZ Resection of Parathyroid Gland, Open Approach
0GTR4ZZ Resection of Parathyroid Gland, Percutaneous Endoscopic Approach

0GW – Endocrine System, Revision

Review Coding Guideline B6.1c

0GW000Z Revision of Drainage Device in Pituitary Gland, Open Approach
0GW030Z Revision of Drainage Device in Pituitary Gland, Percutaneous Approach
0GW040Z Revision of Drainage Device in Pituitary Gland, Percutaneous Endoscopic Approach
0GW0X0Z Revision of Drainage Device in Pituitary Gland, External Approach
0GW100Z Revision of Drainage Device in Pineal Body, Open Approach
0GW130Z Revision of Drainage Device in Pineal Body, Percutaneous Approach
0GW140Z Revision of Drainage Device in Pineal Body, Percutaneous Endoscopic Approach
0GW1X0Z Revision of Drainage Device in Pineal Body, External Approach
0GW500Z Revision of Drainage Device in Adrenal Gland, Open Approach
0GW530Z Revision of Drainage Device in Adrenal Gland, Percutaneous Approach
0GW540Z Revision of Drainage Device in Adrenal Gland, Percutaneous Endoscopic Approach
0GW5X0Z Revision of Drainage Device in Adrenal Gland, External Approach
0GWK00Z Revision of Drainage Device in Thyroid Gland, Open Approach
0GWK30Z Revision of Drainage Device in Thyroid Gland, Percutaneous Approach
0GWK40Z Revision of Drainage Device in Thyroid Gland, Percutaneous Endoscopic Approach
0GWKX0Z Revision of Drainage Device in Thyroid Gland, External Approach
0GWR00Z Revision of Drainage Device in Parathyroid Gland, Open Approach

0GWR30Z Revision of Drainage Device in Parathyroid Gland, Percutaneous Approach
0GWR40Z Revision of Drainage Device in Parathyroid Gland, Percutaneous Endoscopic Approach
0GWRX0Z Revision of Drainage Device in Parathyroid Gland, External Approach
0GWS00Z Revision of Drainage Device in Endocrine Gland, Open Approach
0GWS02Z Revision of Monitoring Device in Endocrine Gland, Open Approach
0GWS03Z Revision of Infusion Device in Endocrine Gland, Open Approach
0GWS30Z Revision of Drainage Device in Endocrine Gland, Percutaneous Approach
0GWS32Z Revision of Monitoring Device in Endocrine Gland, Percutaneous Approach
0GWS33Z Revision of Infusion Device in Endocrine Gland, Percutaneous Approach
0GWS40Z Revision of Drainage Device in Endocrine Gland, Percutaneous Endoscopic Approach
0GWS42Z Revision of Monitoring Device in Endocrine Gland, Percutaneous Endoscopic Approach
0GWS43Z Revision of Infusion Device in Endocrine Gland, Percutaneous Endoscopic Approach
0GWSX0Z Revision of Drainage Device in Endocrine Gland, External Approach
0GWSX2Z Revision of Monitoring Device in Endocrine Gland, External Approach
0GWSX3Z Revision of Infusion Device in Endocrine Gland, External Approach

Medical and Surgical Section (0)

Skin and Breast

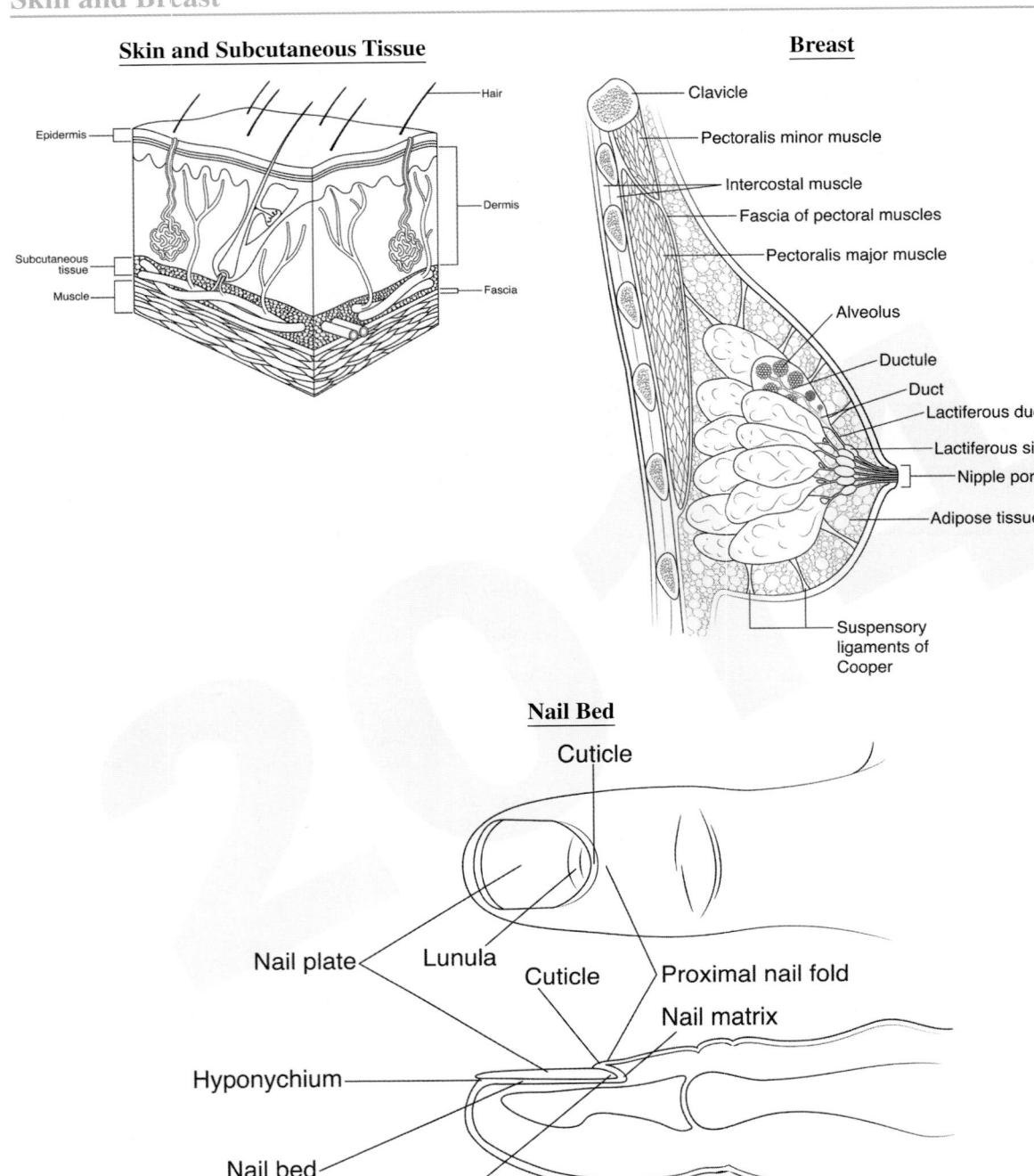

Skin and Subcutaneous Tissue

Hair

Epidermis

Dermis

Subcutaneous tissue

Muscle

Fascia

Breast

Clavicle

Pectoralis minor muscle

Intercostal muscle

Fascia of pectoral muscles

Pectoralis major muscle

Alveolus

Ductule

Duct

Lactiferous duct

Lactiferous sinus

Nipple pores

Adipose tissue

Suspensory ligaments of Cooper

Nail Bed

Cuticle

Nail plate

Lunula

Cuticle

Proximal nail fold

Nail matrix

Hyponychium

Nail bed

Nail root

Skin and Breast Tables 0H0–0HX

Section	0	**Medical and Surgical**
Body System	H	**Skin and Breast**
Operation	0	**Alteration:** Modifying the anatomic structure of a body part without affecting the function of the body part

Body Part (4th)	Approach (5th)	Device (6th)	Qualifier (7th)
T Breast, Right U Breast, Left V Breast, Bilateral	0 Open 3 Percutaneous X External	7 Autologous Tissue Substitute J Synthetic Substitute K Nonautologous Tissue Substitute Z No Device	Z No Qualifier

Section	0	**Medical and Surgical**
Body System	H	**Skin and Breast**
Operation	2	**Change:** Taking out or off a device from a body part and putting back an identical or similar device in or on the same body part without cutting or puncturing the skin or a mucous membrane

Body Part (4th)	Approach (5th)	Device (6th)	Qualifier (7th)
P Skin T Breast, Right U Breast, Left	X External	0 Drainage Device Y Other Device	Z No Qualifier

Section	0	**Medical and Surgical**
Body System	H	**Skin and Breast**
Operation	5	**Destruction:** Physical eradication of all or a portion of a body part by the direct use of energy, force, or a destructive agent

Body Part (4th)	Approach (5th)	Device (6th)	Qualifier (7th)
0 Skin, Scalp 1 Skin, Face 2 Skin, Right Ear 3 Skin, Left Ear 4 Skin, Neck 5 Skin, Chest 6 Skin, Back 7 Skin, Abdomen 8 Skin, Buttock 9 Skin, Perineum A Skin, Genitalia B Skin, Right Upper Arm C Skin, Left Upper Arm D Skin, Right Lower Arm E Skin, Left Lower Arm F Skin, Right Hand G Skin, Left Hand H Skin, Right Upper Leg J Skin, Left Upper Leg K Skin, Right Lower Leg L Skin, Left Lower Leg M Skin, Right Foot N Skin, Left Foot	X External	Z No Device	D Multiple Z No Qualifier
Q Finger Nail R Toe Nail	X External	Z No Device	Z No Qualifier
T Breast, Right U Breast, Left V Breast, Bilateral W Nipple, Right X Nipple, Left	0 Open 3 Percutaneous 7 Via Natural or Artificial Opening 8 Via Natural or Artificial Opening Endoscopic X External	Z No Device	Z No Qualifier

Section	0	Medical and Surgical
Body System	H	Skin and Breast
Operation	8	**Division:** Cutting into a body part, without draining fluids and/or gases from the body part, in order to separate or transect a body part

Body Part (4th)	Approach (5th)	Device (6th)	Qualifier (7th)
0 Skin, Scalp 1 Skin, Face 2 Skin, Right Ear 3 Skin, Left Ear 4 Skin, Neck 5 Skin, Chest 6 Skin, Back 7 Skin, Abdomen 8 Skin, Buttock 9 Skin, Perineum A Skin, Genitalia B Skin, Right Upper Arm C Skin, Left Upper Arm D Skin, Right Lower Arm E Skin, Left Lower Arm F Skin, Right Hand G Skin, Left Hand H Skin, Right Upper Leg J Skin, Left Upper Leg K Skin, Right Lower Leg L Skin, Left Lower Leg M Skin, Right Foot N Skin, Left Foot	X External	Z No Device	Z No Qualifier

Section	0	Medical and Surgical
Body System	H	Skin and Breast
Operation	9	**Drainage:** Taking or letting out fluids and/or gases from a body part

Body Part (4th)	Approach (5th)	Device (6th)	Qualifier (7th)
0 Skin, Scalp 1 Skin, Face 2 Skin, Right Ear 3 Skin, Left Ear 4 Skin, Neck 5 Skin, Chest 6 Skin, Back 7 Skin, Abdomen 8 Skin, Buttock 9 Skin, Perineum A Skin, Genitalia B Skin, Right Upper Arm C Skin, Left Upper Arm D Skin, Right Lower Arm E Skin, Left Lower Arm F Skin, Right Hand G Skin, Left Hand H Skin, Right Upper Leg J Skin, Left Upper Leg K Skin, Right Lower Leg L Skin, Left Lower Leg M Skin, Right Foot N Skin, Left Foot Q Finger Nail R Toe Nail	X External	0 Drainage Device	Z No Qualifier

Continued

Section	0	**Medical and Surgical**
Body System	H	**Skin and Breast**
Operation	9	**Drainage:** Taking or letting out fluids and/or gases from a body part

Body Part (4th)	Approach (5th)	Device (6th)	Qualifier (7th)
0 Skin, Scalp 1 Skin, Face 2 Skin, Right Ear 3 Skin, Left Ear 4 Skin, Neck 5 Skin, Chest 6 Skin, Back 7 Skin, Abdomen 8 Skin, Buttock 9 Skin, Perineum A Skin, Genitalia B Skin, Right Upper Arm C Skin, Left Upper Arm D Skin, Right Lower Arm E Skin, Left Lower Arm F Skin, Right Hand G Skin, Left Hand H Skin, Right Upper Leg J Skin, Left Upper Leg K Skin, Right Lower Leg L Skin, Left Lower Leg M Skin, Right Foot N Skin, Left Foot Q Finger Nail R Toe Nail	X External	Z No Device	X Diagnostic Z No Qualifier
T Breast, Right U Breast, Left V Breast, Bilateral W Nipple, Right X Nipple, Left	0 Open 3 Percutaneous 7 Via Natural or Artificial Opening 8 Via Natural or Artificial Opening Endoscopic X External	0 Drainage Device	Z No Qualifier
T Breast, Right U Breast, Left V Breast, Bilateral W Nipple, Right X Nipple, Left	0 Open 3 Percutaneous 7 Via Natural or Artificial Opening 8 Via Natural or Artificial Opening Endoscopic X External	Z No Device	X Diagnostic Z No Qualifier

Section	0	**Medical and Surgical**
Body System	H	**Skin and Breast**
Operation	B	**Excision:** Cutting out or off, without replacement, a portion of a body part

Body Part (4th)	Approach (5th)	Device (6th)	Qualifier (7th)
0 Skin, Scalp 1 Skin, Face 2 Skin, Right Ear 3 Skin, Left Ear 4 Skin, Neck 5 Skin, Chest 6 Skin, Back 7 Skin, Abdomen 8 Skin, Buttock 9 Skin, Perineum A Skin, Genitalia B Skin, Right Upper Arm C Skin, Left Upper Arm D Skin, Right Lower Arm E Skin, Left Lower Arm F Skin, Right Hand G Skin, Left Hand H Skin, Right Upper Leg J Skin, Left Upper Leg K Skin, Right Lower Leg L Skin, Left Lower Leg M Skin, Right Foot N Skin, Left Foot Q Finger Nail R Toe Nail	X External	Z No Device	X Diagnostic Z No Qualifier
T Breast, Right U Breast, Left V Breast, Bilateral W Nipple, Right X Nipple, Left Y Supernumerary Breast	0 Open 3 Percutaneous 7 Via Natural or Artificial Opening 8 Via Natural or Artificial Opening Endoscopic X External	Z No Device	X Diagnostic Z No Qualifier

Section	0	Medical and Surgical
Body System	H	Skin and Breast
Operation	C	Extirpation: Taking or cutting out solid matter from a body part

Body Part (4th)	Approach (5th)	Device (6th)	Qualifier (7th)
0 Skin, Scalp 1 Skin, Face 2 Skin, Right Ear 3 Skin, Left Ear 4 Skin, Neck 5 Skin, Chest 6 Skin, Back 7 Skin, Abdomen 8 Skin, Buttock 9 Skin, Perineum A Skin, Genitalia B Skin, Right Upper Arm C Skin, Left Upper Arm D Skin, Right Lower Arm E Skin, Left Lower Arm F Skin, Right Hand G Skin, Left Hand H Skin, Right Upper Leg J Skin, Left Upper Leg K Skin, Right Lower Leg L Skin, Left Lower Leg M Skin, Right Foot N Skin, Left Foot Q Finger Nail R Toe Nail	X External	Z No Device	Z No Qualifier
T Breast, Right U Breast, Left V Breast, Bilateral W Nipple, Right X Nipple, Left	0 Open 3 Percutaneous 7 Via Natural or Artificial Opening 8 Via Natural or Artificial Opening Endoscopic X External	Z No Device	Z No Qualifier

Section	0	Medical and Surgical
Body System	H	Skin and Breast
Operation	D	**Extraction:** Pulling or stripping out or off all or a portion of a body part by the use of force

Body Part (4th)	Approach (5th)	Device (6th)	Qualifier (7th)
0 Skin, Scalp 1 Skin, Face 2 Skin, Right Ear 3 Skin, Left Ear 4 Skin, Neck 5 Skin, Chest 6 Skin, Back 7 Skin, Abdomen 8 Skin, Buttock 9 Skin, Perineum A Skin, Genitalia B Skin, Right Upper Arm C Skin, Left Upper Arm D Skin, Right Lower Arm E Skin, Left Lower Arm F Skin, Right Hand G Skin, Left Hand H Skin, Right Upper Leg J Skin, Left Upper Leg K Skin, Right Lower Leg L Skin, Left Lower Leg M Skin, Right Foot N Skin, Left Foot Q Finger Nail R Toe Nail S Hair	X External	Z No Device	Z No Qualifier

Section	0	Medical and Surgical
Body System	H	Skin and Breast
Operation	H	**Insertion:** Putting in a nonbiological appliance that monitors, assists, performs, or prevents a physiological function but does not physically take the place of a body part

Body Part (4th)	Approach (5th)	Device (6th)	Qualifier (7th)
T Breast, Right U Breast, Left V Breast, Bilateral W Nipple, Right X Nipple, Left	0 Open 3 Percutaneous 7 Via Natural or Artificial Opening 8 Via Natural or Artificial Opening Endoscopic	1 Radioactive Element N Tissue Expander	Z No Qualifier
T Breast, Right U Breast, Left V Breast, Bilateral W Nipple, Right X Nipple, Left	X External	1 Radioactive Element	Z No Qualifier

Section	0	Medical and Surgical	
Body System	H	Skin and Breast	
Operation	J	**Inspection:** Visually and/or manually exploring a body part	

Body Part (4th)	Approach (5th)	Device (6th)	Qualifier (7th)
P Skin **Q** Finger Nail **R** Toe Nail	**X** External	**Z** No Device	**Z** No Qualifier
T Breast, Right **U** Breast, Left	**0** Open **3** Percutaneous **7** Via Natural or Artificial Opening **8** Via Natural or Artificial Opening Endoscopic **X** External	**Z** No Device	**Z** No Qualifier

Section	0	Medical and Surgical	
Body System	H	Skin and Breast	
Operation	M	**Reattachment:** Putting back in or on all or a portion of a separated body part to its normal location or other suitable location	

Body Part (4th)	Approach (5th)	Device (6th)	Qualifier (7th)
0 Skin, Scalp **1** Skin, Face **2** Skin, Right Ear **3** Skin, Left Ear **4** Skin, Neck **5** Skin, Chest **6** Skin, Back **7** Skin, Abdomen **8** Skin, Buttock **9** Skin, Perineum **A** Skin, Genitalia **B** Skin, Right Upper Arm **C** Skin, Left Upper Arm **D** Skin, Right Lower Arm **E** Skin, Left Lower Arm **F** Skin, Right Hand **G** Skin, Left Hand **H** Skin, Right Upper Leg **J** Skin, Left Upper Leg **K** Skin, Right Lower Leg **L** Skin, Left Lower Leg **M** Skin, Right Foot **N** Skin, Left Foot **T** Breast, Right **U** Breast, Left **V** Breast, Bilateral **W** Nipple, Right **X** Nipple, Left	**X** External	**Z** No Device	**Z** No Qualifier

Section	0	Medical and Surgical
Body System	H	Skin and Breast
Operation	N	Release: Freeing a body part from an abnormal physical constraint by cutting or by the use of force

Body Part (4th)	Approach (5th)	Device (6th)	Qualifier (7th)
0 Skin, Scalp 1 Skin, Face 2 Skin, Right Ear 3 Skin, Left Ear 4 Skin, Neck 5 Skin, Chest 6 Skin, Back 7 Skin, Abdomen 8 Skin, Buttock 9 Skin, Perineum A Skin, Genitalia B Skin, Right Upper Arm C Skin, Left Upper Arm D Skin, Right Lower Arm E Skin, Left Lower Arm F Skin, Right Hand G Skin, Left Hand H Skin, Right Upper Leg J Skin, Left Upper Leg	X External	Z No Device	Z No Qualifier
K Skin, Right Lower Leg L Skin, Left Lower Leg M Skin, Right Foot N Skin, Left Foot Q Finger Nail R Toe Nail T Breast, Right U Breast, Left V Breast, Bilateral W Nipple, Right X Nipple, Left	0 Open 3 Percutaneous 7 Via Natural or Artificial Opening 8 Via Natural or Artificial Opening Endoscopic X External	Z No Device	Z No Qualifier

Section	0	Medical and Surgical
Body System	H	Skin and Breast
Operation	P	Removal: Taking out or off a device from a body part

Body Part (4th)	Approach (5th)	Device (6th)	Qualifier (7th)
P Skin Q Finger Nail R Toe Nail	X External	0 Drainage Device 7 Autologous Tissue Substitute J Synthetic Substitute K Nonautologous Tissue Substitute	Z No Qualifier
S Hair	X External	7 Autologous Tissue Substitute J Synthetic Substitute K Nonautologous Tissue Substitute	Z No Qualifier
T Breast, Right U Breast, Left	0 Open 3 Percutaneous 7 Via Natural or Artificial Opening 8 Via Natural or Artificial Opening Endoscopic	0 Drainage Device 1 Radioactive Element 7 Autologous Tissue Substitute J Synthetic Substitute K Nonautologous Tissue Substitute N Tissue Expander	Z No Qualifier
T Breast, Right U Breast, Left	X External	0 Drainage Device 1 Radioactive Element 7 Autologous Tissue Substitute J Synthetic Substitute K Nonautologous Tissue Substitute	Z No Qualifier

Section	0	Medical and Surgical
Body System	H	Skin and Breast
Operation	Q	**Repair:** Restoring, to the extent possible, a body part to its normal anatomic structure and function

Body Part (4th)	Approach (5th)	Device (6th)	Qualifier (7th)
0 Skin, Scalp 1 Skin, Face 2 Skin, Right Ear 3 Skin, Left Ear 4 Skin, Neck 5 Skin, Chest 6 Skin, Back 7 Skin, Abdomen 8 Skin, Buttock 9 Skin, Perineum A Skin, Genitalia B Skin, Right Upper Arm C Skin, Left Upper Arm D Skin, Right Lower Arm E Skin, Left Lower Arm F Skin, Right Hand G Skin, Left Hand H Skin, Right Upper Leg J Skin, Left Upper Leg K Skin, Right Lower Leg L Skin, Left Lower Leg M Skin, Right Foot N Skin, Left Foot Q Finger Nail R Toe Nail	X External	Z No Device	Z No Qualifier
T Breast, Right U Breast, Left V Breast, Bilateral W Nipple, Right X Nipple, Left Y Supernumerary Breast	0 Open 3 Percutaneous 7 Via Natural or Artificial Opening 8 Via Natural or Artificial Opening Endoscopic X External	Z No Device	Z No Qualifier

Section	0	Medical and Surgical
Body System	H	Skin and Breast
Operation	R	Replacement: Putting in or on biological or synthetic material that physically takes the place and/or function of all or a portion of a body part

Body Part (4th)	Approach (5th)	Device (6th)	Qualifier (7th)
0 Skin, Scalp 1 Skin, Face 2 Skin, Right Ear 3 Skin, Left Ear 4 Skin, Neck 5 Skin, Chest 6 Skin, Back 7 Skin, Abdomen 8 Skin, Buttock 9 Skin, Perineum A Skin, Genitalia B Skin, Right Upper Arm C Skin, Left Upper Arm D Skin, Right Lower Arm E Skin, Left Lower Arm F Skin, Right Hand G Skin, Left Hand H Skin, Right Upper Leg J Skin, Left Upper Leg K Skin, Right Lower Leg L Skin, Left Lower Leg M Skin, Right Foot N Skin, Left Foot	X External	7 Autologous Tissue Substitute K Nonautologous Tissue Substitute	3 Full Thickness 4 Partial Thickness
0 Skin, Scalp 1 Skin, Face 2 Skin, Right Ear 3 Skin, Left Ear 4 Skin, Neck 5 Skin, Chest 6 Skin, Back 7 Skin, Abdomen 8 Skin, Buttock 9 Skin, Perineum A Skin, Genitalia B Skin, Right Upper Arm C Skin, Left Upper Arm D Skin, Right Lower Arm E Skin, Left Lower Arm F Skin, Right Hand G Skin, Left Hand H Skin, Right Upper Leg J Skin, Left Upper Leg K Skin, Right Lower Leg L Skin, Left Lower Leg M Skin, Right Foot N Skin, Left Foot	X External	J Synthetic Substitute	3 Full Thickness 4 Partial Thickness Z No Qualifier
Q Finger Nail R Toe Nail S Hair	X External	7 Autologous Tissue Substitute J Synthetic Substitute K Nonautologous Tissue Substitute	Z No Qualifier
T Breast, Right U Breast, Left V Breast, Bilateral	0 Open	7 Autologous Tissue Substitute	5 Latissimus Dorsi Myocutaneous Flap 6 Transverse Rectus Abdominis Myocutaneous Flap 7 Deep Inferior Epigastric Artery Perforator Flap 8 Superficial Inferior Epigastric Artery Flap 9 Gluteal Artery Perforator Flap Z No Qualifier

Continued

Section	0	Medical and Surgical
Body System	H	Skin and Breast
Operation	R	Replacement: Putting in or on biological or synthetic material that physically takes the place and/or function of all or a portion of a body part

Body Part (4th)	Approach (5th)	Device (6th)	Qualifier (7th)
T Breast, Right U Breast, Left V Breast, Bilateral	0 Open	J Synthetic Substitute K Nonautologous Tissue Substitute	Z No Qualifier
T Breast, Right U Breast, Left V Breast, Bilateral	3 Percutaneous X External	7 Autologous Tissue Substitute J Synthetic Substitute K Nonautologous Tissue Substitute	Z No Qualifier
W Nipple, Right X Nipple, Left	0 Open 3 Percutaneous X External	7 Autologous Tissue Substitute J Synthetic Substitute K Nonautologous Tissue Substitute	Z No Qualifier

Section	0	Medical and Surgical
Body System	H	Skin and Breast
Operation	S	Reposition: Moving to its normal location, or other suitable location, all or a portion of a body part

Body Part (4th)	Approach (5th)	Device (6th)	Qualifier (7th)
S Hair W Nipple, Right X Nipple, Left	X External	Z No Device	Z No Qualifier
T Breast, Right U Breast, Left V Breast, Bilateral	0 Open	Z No Device	Z No Qualifier

Section	0	Medical and Surgical
Body System	H	Skin and Breast
Operation	T	Resection: Cutting out or off, without replacement, all of a body part

Body Part (4th)	Approach (5th)	Device (6th)	Qualifier (7th)
Q Finger Nail R Toe Nail W Nipple, Right X Nipple, Left	X External	Z No Device	Z No Qualifier
T Breast, Right U Breast, Left V Breast, Bilateral Y Supernumerary Breast	0 Open	Z No Device	Z No Qualifier

Section	0	Medical and Surgical
Body System	H	Skin and Breast
Operation	U	Supplement: Putting in or on biological or synthetic material that physically reinforces and/or augments the function of a portion of a body part

Body Part (4th)	Approach (5th)	Device (6th)	Qualifier (7th)
T Breast, Right U Breast, Left V Breast, Bilateral W Nipple, Right X Nipple, Left	0 Open 3 Percutaneous 7 Via Natural or Artificial Opening 8 Via Natural or Artificial Opening Endoscopic X External	7 Autologous Tissue Substitute J Synthetic Substitute K Nonautologous Tissue Substitute	Z No Qualifier

Section	0	Medical and Surgical
Body System	H	Skin and Breast
Operation	W	**Revision:** Correcting, to the extent possible, a portion of a malfunctioning device or the position of a displaced device

Body Part (4th)	Approach (5th)	Device (6th)	Qualifier (7th)
P Skin Q Finger Nail R Toe Nail	X External	0 Drainage Device 7 Autologous Tissue Substitute J Synthetic Substitute K Nonautologous Tissue Substitute	Z No Qualifier
S Hair	X External	7 Autologous Tissue Substitute J Synthetic Substitute K Nonautologous Tissue Substitute	Z No Qualifier
T Breast, Right U Breast, Left	0 Open 3 Percutaneous 7 Via Natural or Artificial Opening 8 Via Natural or Artificial Opening Endoscopic	0 Drainage Device 7 Autologous Tissue Substitute J Synthetic Substitute K Nonautologous Tissue Substitute N Tissue Expander	Z No Qualifier
T Breast, Right U Breast, Left	X External	0 Drainage Device 7 Autologous Tissue Substitute J Synthetic Substitute K Nonautologous Tissue Substitute	Z No Qualifier

Section	0	Medical and Surgical
Body System	H	Skin and Breast
Operation	X	**Transfer:** Moving, without taking out, all or a portion of a body part to another location to take over the function of all or a portion of a body part

Body Part (4th)	Approach (5th)	Device (6th)	Qualifier (7th)
0 Skin, Scalp 1 Skin, Face 2 Skin, Right Ear 3 Skin, Left Ear 4 Skin, Neck 5 Skin, Chest 6 Skin, Back 7 Skin, Abdomen 8 Skin, Buttock 9 Skin, Perineum A Skin, Genitalia B Skin, Right Upper Arm C Skin, Left Upper Arm D Skin, Right Lower Arm E Skin, Left Lower Arm F Skin, Right Hand G Skin, Left Hand H Skin, Right Upper Leg J Skin, Left Upper Leg K Skin, Right Lower Leg L Skin, Left Lower Leg M Skin, Right Foot N Skin, Left Foot	X External	Z No Device	Z No Qualifier

0GN80ZZ   Release Bilateral Carotid Bodies, Open Approach
0GN83ZZ   Release Bilateral Carotid Bodies, Percutaneous Approach
0GN84ZZ   Release Bilateral Carotid Bodies, Percutaneous Endoscopic Approach
0GN90ZZ   Release Para-aortic Body, Open Approach
0GN93ZZ   Release Para-aortic Body, Percutaneous Approach
0GN94ZZ   Release Para-aortic Body, Percutaneous Endoscopic Approach
0GNB0ZZ   Release Coccygeal Glomus, Open Approach
0GNB3ZZ   Release Coccygeal Glomus, Percutaneous Approach
0GNB4ZZ   Release Coccygeal Glomus, Percutaneous Endoscopic Approach
0GNC0ZZ   Release Glomus Jugulare, Open Approach
0GNC3ZZ   Release Glomus Jugulare, Percutaneous Approach
0GNC4ZZ   Release Glomus Jugulare, Percutaneous Endoscopic Approach
0GND0ZZ   Release Aortic Body, Open Approach
0GND3ZZ   Release Aortic Body, Percutaneous Approach
0GND4ZZ   Release Aortic Body, Percutaneous Endoscopic Approach
0GNF0ZZ   Release Paraganglion Extremity, Open Approach
0GNF3ZZ   Release Paraganglion Extremity, Percutaneous Approach
0GNF4ZZ   Release Paraganglion Extremity, Percutaneous Endoscopic Approach
0GNG0ZZ   Release Left Thyroid Gland Lobe, Open Approach
0GNG3ZZ   Release Left Thyroid Gland Lobe, Percutaneous Approach
0GNG4ZZ   Release Left Thyroid Gland Lobe, Percutaneous Endoscopic Approach
0GNH0ZZ   Release Right Thyroid Gland Lobe, Open Approach
0GNH3ZZ   Release Right Thyroid Gland Lobe, Percutaneous Approach
0GNH4ZZ   Release Right Thyroid Gland Lobe, Percutaneous Endoscopic Approach

0GNK0ZZ   Release Thyroid Gland, Open Approach
0GNK3ZZ   Release Thyroid Gland, Percutaneous Approach
0GNK4ZZ   Release Thyroid Gland, Percutaneous Endoscopic Approach
0GNL0ZZ   Release Right Superior Parathyroid Gland, Open Approach
0GNL3ZZ   Release Right Superior Parathyroid Gland, Percutaneous Approach
0GNL4ZZ   Release Right Superior Parathyroid Gland, Percutaneous Endoscopic Approach
0GNM0ZZ   Release Left Superior Parathyroid Gland, Open Approach
0GNM3ZZ   Release Left Superior Parathyroid Gland, Percutaneous Approach
0GNM4ZZ   Release Left Superior Parathyroid Gland, Percutaneous Endoscopic Approach
0GNN0ZZ   Release Right Inferior Parathyroid Gland, Open Approach
0GNN3ZZ   Release Right Inferior Parathyroid Gland, Percutaneous Approach
0GNN4ZZ   Release Right Inferior Parathyroid Gland, Percutaneous Endoscopic Approach
0GNP0ZZ   Release Left Inferior Parathyroid Gland, Open Approach
0GNP3ZZ   Release Left Inferior Parathyroid Gland, Percutaneous Approach
0GNP4ZZ   Release Left Inferior Parathyroid Gland, Percutaneous Endoscopic Approach
0GNQ0ZZ   Release Multiple Parathyroid Glands, Open Approach
0GNQ3ZZ   Release Multiple Parathyroid Glands, Percutaneous Approach
0GNQ4ZZ   Release Multiple Parathyroid Glands, Percutaneous Endoscopic Approach
0GNR0ZZ   Release Parathyroid Gland, Open Approach
0GNR3ZZ   Release Parathyroid Gland, Percutaneous Approach
0GNR4ZZ   Release Parathyroid Gland, Percutaneous Endoscopic Approach

0GP – Endocrine System, Removal

Review Coding Guideline B6.1c

0GP000Z   Removal of Drainage Device from Pituitary Gland, Open Approach
0GP030Z   Removal of Drainage Device from Pituitary Gland, Percutaneous Approach
0GP040Z   Removal of Drainage Device from Pituitary Gland, Percutaneous Endoscopic Approach
0GP0X0Z   Removal of Drainage Device from Pituitary Gland, External Approach
0GP100Z   Removal of Drainage Device from Pineal Body, Open Approach
0GP130Z   Removal of Drainage Device from Pineal Body, Percutaneous Approach
0GP140Z   Removal of Drainage Device from Pineal Body, Percutaneous Endoscopic Approach
0GP1X0Z   Removal of Drainage Device from Pineal Body, External Approach
0GP500Z   Removal of Drainage Device from Adrenal Gland, Open Approach
0GP530Z   Removal of Drainage Device from Adrenal Gland, Percutaneous Approach
0GP540Z   Removal of Drainage Device from Adrenal Gland, Percutaneous Endoscopic Approach
0GP5X0Z   Removal of Drainage Device from Adrenal Gland, External Approach
0GPK00Z   Removal of Drainage Device from Thyroid Gland, Open Approach
0GPK30Z   Removal of Drainage Device from Thyroid Gland, Percutaneous Approach
0GPK40Z   Removal of Drainage Device from Thyroid Gland, Percutaneous Endoscopic Approach
0GPKX0Z   Removal of Drainage Device from Thyroid Gland, External Approach
0GPR00Z   Removal of Drainage Device from Parathyroid Gland, Open Approach

0GPR30Z   Removal of Drainage Device from Parathyroid Gland, Percutaneous Approach
0GPR40Z   Removal of Drainage Device from Parathyroid Gland, Percutaneous Endoscopic Approach
0GPRX0Z   Removal of Drainage Device from Parathyroid Gland, External Approach
0GPS00Z   Removal of Drainage Device from Endocrine Gland, Open Approach
0GPS02Z   Removal of Monitoring Device from Endocrine Gland, Open Approach
0GPS03Z   Removal of Infusion Device from Endocrine Gland, Open Approach
0GPS30Z   Removal of Drainage Device from Endocrine Gland, Percutaneous Approach
0GPS32Z   Removal of Monitoring Device from Endocrine Gland, Percutaneous Approach
0GPS33Z   Removal of Infusion Device from Endocrine Gland, Percutaneous Approach
0GPS40Z   Removal of Drainage Device from Endocrine Gland, Percutaneous Endoscopic Approach
0GPS42Z   Removal of Monitoring Device from Endocrine Gland, Percutaneous Endoscopic Approach
0GPS43Z   Removal of Infusion Device from Endocrine Gland, Percutaneous Endoscopic Approach
0GPSX0Z   Removal of Drainage Device from Endocrine Gland, External Approach
0GPSX2Z   Removal of Monitoring Device from Endocrine Gland, External Approach
0GPSX3Z   Removal of Infusion Device from Endocrine Gland, External Approach

0GQ – Endocrine System, Repair

0GQ00ZZ   Repair Pituitary Gland, Open Approach
0GQ03ZZ   Repair Pituitary Gland, Percutaneous Approach
0GQ04ZZ   Repair Pituitary Gland, Percutaneous Endoscopic Approach
0GQ10ZZ   Repair Pineal Body, Open Approach
0GQ13ZZ   Repair Pineal Body, Percutaneous Approach
0GQ14ZZ   Repair Pineal Body, Percutaneous Endoscopic Approach
0GQ20ZZ   Repair Left Adrenal Gland, Open Approach
0GQ23ZZ   Repair Left Adrenal Gland, Percutaneous Approach

0GQ24ZZ   Repair Left Adrenal Gland, Percutaneous Endoscopic Approach
0GQ30ZZ   Repair Right Adrenal Gland, Open Approach
0GQ33ZZ   Repair Right Adrenal Gland, Percutaneous Approach
0GQ34ZZ   Repair Right Adrenal Gland, Percutaneous Endoscopic Approach
0GQ40ZZ   Repair Bilateral Adrenal Glands, Open Approach
0GQ43ZZ   Repair Bilateral Adrenal Glands, Percutaneous Approach
0GQ44ZZ   Repair Bilateral Adrenal Glands, Percutaneous Endoscopic Approach

♀ Female-only   ♂ Male-only   ● Limited Coverage   ● Non-OR   HAC HAC-associated procedure   ● Non-covered procedures   + Combination

0GQ60ZZ Repair Left Carotid Body, Open Approach
0GQ63ZZ Repair Left Carotid Body, Percutaneous Approach
0GQ64ZZ Repair Left Carotid Body, Percutaneous Endoscopic Approach
0GQ70ZZ Repair Right Carotid Body, Open Approach
0GQ73ZZ Repair Right Carotid Body, Percutaneous Approach
0GQ74ZZ Repair Right Carotid Body, Percutaneous Endoscopic Approach
0GQ80ZZ Repair Bilateral Carotid Bodies, Open Approach
0GQ83ZZ Repair Bilateral Carotid Bodies, Percutaneous Approach
0GQ84ZZ Repair Bilateral Carotid Bodies, Percutaneous Endoscopic Approach
0GQ90ZZ Repair Para-aortic Body, Open Approach
0GQ93ZZ Repair Para-aortic Body, Percutaneous Approach
0GQ94ZZ Repair Para-aortic Body, Percutaneous Endoscopic Approach
0GQB0ZZ Repair Coccygeal Glomus, Open Approach
0GQB3ZZ Repair Coccygeal Glomus, Percutaneous Approach
0GQB4ZZ Repair Coccygeal Glomus, Percutaneous Endoscopic Approach
0GQC0ZZ Repair Glomus Jugulare, Open Approach
0GQC3ZZ Repair Glomus Jugulare, Percutaneous Approach
0GQC4ZZ Repair Glomus Jugulare, Percutaneous Endoscopic Approach
0GQD0ZZ Repair Aortic Body, Open Approach
0GQD3ZZ Repair Aortic Body, Percutaneous Approach
0GQD4ZZ Repair Aortic Body, Percutaneous Endoscopic Approach
0GQF0ZZ Repair Paraganglion Extremity, Open Approach
0GQF3ZZ Repair Paraganglion Extremity, Percutaneous Approach
0GQF4ZZ Repair Paraganglion Extremity, Percutaneous Endoscopic Approach
0GQG0ZZ Repair Left Thyroid Gland Lobe, Open Approach
0GQG3ZZ Repair Left Thyroid Gland Lobe, Percutaneous Approach
0GQG4ZZ Repair Left Thyroid Gland Lobe, Percutaneous Endoscopic Approach
0GQH0ZZ Repair Right Thyroid Gland Lobe, Open Approach
0GQH3ZZ Repair Right Thyroid Gland Lobe, Percutaneous Approach

0GQH4ZZ Repair Right Thyroid Gland Lobe, Percutaneous Endoscopic Approach
0GQJ0ZZ Repair Thyroid Gland Isthmus, Open Approach
0GQJ3ZZ Repair Thyroid Gland Isthmus, Percutaneous Approach
0GQJ4ZZ Repair Thyroid Gland Isthmus, Percutaneous Endoscopic Approach
0GQK0ZZ Repair Thyroid Gland, Open Approach
0GQK3ZZ Repair Thyroid Gland, Percutaneous Approach
0GQK4ZZ Repair Thyroid Gland, Percutaneous Endoscopic Approach
0GQL0ZZ Repair Right Superior Parathyroid Gland, Open Approach
0GQL3ZZ Repair Right Superior Parathyroid Gland, Percutaneous Approach
0GQL4ZZ Repair Right Superior Parathyroid Gland, Percutaneous Endoscopic Approach
0GQM0ZZ Repair Left Superior Parathyroid Gland, Open Approach
0GQM3ZZ Repair Left Superior Parathyroid Gland, Percutaneous Approach
0GQM4ZZ Repair Left Superior Parathyroid Gland, Percutaneous Endoscopic Approach
0GQN0ZZ Repair Right Inferior Parathyroid Gland, Open Approach
0GQN3ZZ Repair Right Inferior Parathyroid Gland, Percutaneous Approach
0GQN4ZZ Repair Right Inferior Parathyroid Gland, Percutaneous Endoscopic Approach
0GQP0ZZ Repair Left Inferior Parathyroid Gland, Open Approach
0GQP3ZZ Repair Left Inferior Parathyroid Gland, Percutaneous Approach
0GQP4ZZ Repair Left Inferior Parathyroid Gland, Percutaneous Endoscopic Approach
0GQQ0ZZ Repair Multiple Parathyroid Glands, Open Approach
0GQQ3ZZ Repair Multiple Parathyroid Glands, Percutaneous Approach
0GQQ4ZZ Repair Multiple Parathyroid Glands, Percutaneous Endoscopic Approach
0GQR0ZZ Repair Parathyroid Gland, Open Approach
0GQR3ZZ Repair Parathyroid Gland, Percutaneous Approach
0GQR4ZZ Repair Parathyroid Gland, Percutaneous Endoscopic Approach

0GS – Endocrine System, Reposition

0GS20ZZ Reposition Left Adrenal Gland, Open Approach
0GS24ZZ Reposition Left Adrenal Gland, Percutaneous Endoscopic Approach
0GS30ZZ Reposition Right Adrenal Gland, Open Approach
0GS34ZZ Reposition Right Adrenal Gland, Percutaneous Endoscopic Approach
0GSG0ZZ Reposition Left Thyroid Gland Lobe, Open Approach
0GSG4ZZ Reposition Left Thyroid Gland Lobe, Percutaneous Endoscopic Approach
0GSH0ZZ Reposition Right Thyroid Gland Lobe, Open Approach
0GSH4ZZ Reposition Right Thyroid Gland Lobe, Percutaneous Endoscopic Approach
0GSL0ZZ Reposition Right Superior Parathyroid Gland, Open Approach
0GSL4ZZ Reposition Right Superior Parathyroid Gland, Percutaneous Endoscopic Approach

0GSM0ZZ Reposition Left Superior Parathyroid Gland, Open Approach
0GSM4ZZ Reposition Left Superior Parathyroid Gland, Percutaneous Endoscopic Approach
0GSN0ZZ Reposition Right Inferior Parathyroid Gland, Open Approach
0GSN4ZZ Reposition Right Inferior Parathyroid Gland, Percutaneous Endoscopic Approach
0GSP0ZZ Reposition Left Inferior Parathyroid Gland, Open Approach
0GSP4ZZ Reposition Left Inferior Parathyroid Gland, Percutaneous Endoscopic Approach
0GSQ0ZZ Reposition Multiple Parathyroid Glands, Open Approach
0GSQ4ZZ Reposition Multiple Parathyroid Glands, Percutaneous Endoscopic Approach
0GSR0ZZ Reposition Parathyroid Gland, Open Approach
0GSR4ZZ Reposition Parathyroid Gland, Percutaneous Endoscopic Approach

0GT – Endocrine System, Resection

Review Coding Guideline B3.8

0GT00ZZ Resection of Pituitary Gland, Open Approach
0GT04ZZ Resection of Pituitary Gland, Percutaneous Endoscopic Approach
0GT10ZZ Resection of Pineal Body, Open Approach
0GT14ZZ Resection of Pineal Body, Percutaneous Endoscopic Approach
0GT20ZZ Resection of Left Adrenal Gland, Open Approach
0GT24ZZ Resection of Left Adrenal Gland, Percutaneous Endoscopic Approach
0GT30ZZ Resection of Right Adrenal Gland, Open Approach
0GT34ZZ Resection of Right Adrenal Gland, Percutaneous Endoscopic Approach
0GT40ZZ Resection of Bilateral Adrenal Glands, Open Approach
0GT44ZZ Resection of Bilateral Adrenal Glands, Percutaneous Endoscopic Approach
0GT60ZZ Resection of Left Carotid Body, Open Approach
0GT64ZZ Resection of Left Carotid Body, Percutaneous Endoscopic Approach
0GT70ZZ Resection of Right Carotid Body, Open Approach
0GT74ZZ Resection of Right Carotid Body, Percutaneous Endoscopic Approach
0GT80ZZ Resection of Bilateral Carotid Bodies, Open Approach

0GT84ZZ Resection of Bilateral Carotid Bodies, Percutaneous Endoscopic Approach
0GT90ZZ Resection of Para-aortic Body, Open Approach
0GT94ZZ Resection of Para-aortic Body, Percutaneous Endoscopic Approach
0GTB0ZZ Resection of Coccygeal Glomus, Open Approach
0GTB4ZZ Resection of Coccygeal Glomus, Percutaneous Endoscopic Approach
0GTC0ZZ Resection of Glomus Jugulare, Open Approach
0GTC4ZZ Resection of Glomus Jugulare, Percutaneous Endoscopic Approach
0GTD0ZZ Resection of Aortic Body, Open Approach
0GTD4ZZ Resection of Aortic Body, Percutaneous Endoscopic Approach
0GTF0ZZ Resection of Paraganglion Extremity, Open Approach
0GTF4ZZ Resection of Paraganglion Extremity, Percutaneous Endoscopic Approach
0GTG0ZZ Resection of Left Thyroid Gland Lobe, Open Approach
0GTG4ZZ Resection of Left Thyroid Gland Lobe, Percutaneous Endoscopic Approach
0GTH0ZZ Resection of Right Thyroid Gland Lobe, Open Approach
0GTH4ZZ Resection of Right Thyroid Gland Lobe, Percutaneous Endoscopic Approach

0GTK0ZZ Resection of Thyroid Gland, Open Approach
0GTK4ZZ Resection of Thyroid Gland, Percutaneous Endoscopic Approach
0GTL0ZZ Resection of Right Superior Parathyroid Gland, Open Approach
0GTL4ZZ Resection of Right Superior Parathyroid Gland, Percutaneous Endoscopic Approach
0GTM0ZZ Resection of Left Superior Parathyroid Gland, Open Approach
0GTM4ZZ Resection of Left Superior Parathyroid Gland, Percutaneous Endoscopic Approach
0GTN0ZZ Resection of Right Inferior Parathyroid Gland, Open Approach
0GTN4ZZ Resection of Right Inferior Parathyroid Gland, Percutaneous Endoscopic Approach

0GTP0ZZ Resection of Left Inferior Parathyroid Gland, Open Approach
0GTP4ZZ Resection of Left Inferior Parathyroid Gland, Percutaneous Endoscopic Approach
0GTQ0ZZ Resection of Multiple Parathyroid Glands, Open Approach
0GTQ4ZZ Resection of Multiple Parathyroid Glands, Percutaneous Endoscopic Approach
0GTR0ZZ Resection of Parathyroid Gland, Open Approach
0GTR4ZZ Resection of Parathyroid Gland, Percutaneous Endoscopic Approach

0GW – Endocrine System, Revision

Review Coding Guideline B6.1c

0GW000Z Revision of Drainage Device in Pituitary Gland, Open Approach
0GW030Z Revision of Drainage Device in Pituitary Gland, Percutaneous Approach
0GW040Z Revision of Drainage Device in Pituitary Gland, Percutaneous Endoscopic Approach
0GW0X0Z Revision of Drainage Device in Pituitary Gland, External Approach
0GW100Z Revision of Drainage Device in Pineal Body, Open Approach
0GW130Z Revision of Drainage Device in Pineal Body, Percutaneous Approach
0GW140Z Revision of Drainage Device in Pineal Body, Percutaneous Endoscopic Approach
0GW1X0Z Revision of Drainage Device in Pineal Body, External Approach
0GW500Z Revision of Drainage Device in Adrenal Gland, Open Approach
0GW530Z Revision of Drainage Device in Adrenal Gland, Percutaneous Approach
0GW540Z Revision of Drainage Device in Adrenal Gland, Percutaneous Endoscopic Approach
0GW5X0Z Revision of Drainage Device in Adrenal Gland, External Approach
0GWK00Z Revision of Drainage Device in Thyroid Gland, Open Approach
0GWK30Z Revision of Drainage Device in Thyroid Gland, Percutaneous Approach
0GWK40Z Revision of Drainage Device in Thyroid Gland, Percutaneous Endoscopic Approach
0GWKX0Z Revision of Drainage Device in Thyroid Gland, External Approach
0GWR00Z Revision of Drainage Device in Parathyroid Gland, Open Approach

0GWR30Z Revision of Drainage Device in Parathyroid Gland, Percutaneous Approach
0GWR40Z Revision of Drainage Device in Parathyroid Gland, Percutaneous Endoscopic Approach
0GWRX0Z Revision of Drainage Device in Parathyroid Gland, External Approach
0GWS00Z Revision of Drainage Device in Endocrine Gland, Open Approach
0GWS02Z Revision of Monitoring Device in Endocrine Gland, Open Approach
0GWS03Z Revision of Infusion Device in Endocrine Gland, Open Approach
0GWS30Z Revision of Drainage Device in Endocrine Gland, Percutaneous Approach
0GWS32Z Revision of Monitoring Device in Endocrine Gland, Percutaneous Approach
0GWS33Z Revision of Infusion Device in Endocrine Gland, Percutaneous Approach
0GWS40Z Revision of Drainage Device in Endocrine Gland, Percutaneous Endoscopic Approach
0GWS42Z Revision of Monitoring Device in Endocrine Gland, Percutaneous Endoscopic Approach
0GWS43Z Revision of Infusion Device in Endocrine Gland, Percutaneous Endoscopic Approach
0GWSX0Z Revision of Drainage Device in Endocrine Gland, External Approach
0GWSX2Z Revision of Monitoring Device in Endocrine Gland, External Approach
0GWSX3Z Revision of Infusion Device in Endocrine Gland, External Approach

♀ Female-only   ♂ Male-only   ◐ Limited Coverage   ● Non-OR   ▨ HAC-associated procedure   ⬤ Non-covered procedures   ✚ Combination

Skin and Breast

Skin and Subcutaneous Tissue

Hair

Epidermis

Dermis

Subcutaneous tissue

Muscle

Fascia

Breast

Clavicle

Pectoralis minor muscle

Intercostal muscle

Fascia of pectoral muscles

Pectoralis major muscle

Alveolus

Ductule

Duct

Lactiferous duct

Lactiferous sinus

Nipple pores

Adipose tissue

Suspensory ligaments of Cooper

Nail Bed

Cuticle

Nail plate

Lunula

Cuticle

Proximal nail fold

Nail matrix

Hyponychium

Nail bed

Nail root

Skin and Breast Tables 0H0–0HX

Section	0	Medical and Surgical
Body System	H	Skin and Breast
Operation	0	**Alteration:** Modifying the anatomic structure of a body part without affecting the function of the body part

Body Part (4th)	Approach (5th)	Device (6th)	Qualifier (7th)
T Breast, Right U Breast, Left V Breast, Bilateral	0 Open 3 Percutaneous X External	7 Autologous Tissue Substitute J Synthetic Substitute K Nonautologous Tissue Substitute Z No Device	Z No Qualifier

Section	0	Medical and Surgical
Body System	H	Skin and Breast
Operation	2	**Change:** Taking out or off a device from a body part and putting back an identical or similar device in or on the same body part without cutting or puncturing the skin or a mucous membrane

Body Part (4th)	Approach (5th)	Device (6th)	Qualifier (7th)
P Skin T Breast, Right U Breast, Left	X External	0 Drainage Device Y Other Device	Z No Qualifier

Section	0	Medical and Surgical
Body System	H	Skin and Breast
Operation	5	**Destruction:** Physical eradication of all or a portion of a body part by the direct use of energy, force, or a destructive agent

Body Part (4th)	Approach (5th)	Device (6th)	Qualifier (7th)
0 Skin, Scalp 1 Skin, Face 2 Skin, Right Ear 3 Skin, Left Ear 4 Skin, Neck 5 Skin, Chest 6 Skin, Back 7 Skin, Abdomen 8 Skin, Buttock 9 Skin, Perineum A Skin, Genitalia B Skin, Right Upper Arm C Skin, Left Upper Arm D Skin, Right Lower Arm E Skin, Left Lower Arm F Skin, Right Hand G Skin, Left Hand H Skin, Right Upper Leg J Skin, Left Upper Leg K Skin, Right Lower Leg L Skin, Left Lower Leg M Skin, Right Foot N Skin, Left Foot	X External	Z No Device	D Multiple Z No Qualifier
Q Finger Nail R Toe Nail	X External	Z No Device	Z No Qualifier
T Breast, Right U Breast, Left V Breast, Bilateral W Nipple, Right X Nipple, Left	0 Open 3 Percutaneous 7 Via Natural or Artificial Opening 8 Via Natural or Artificial Opening Endoscopic X External	Z No Device	Z No Qualifier

Section	0	Medical and Surgical
Body System	H	Skin and Breast
Operation	8	**Division:** Cutting into a body part, without draining fluids and/or gases from the body part, in order to separate or transect a body part

Body Part (4th)	Approach (5th)	Device (6th)	Qualifier (7th)
0 Skin, Scalp	X External	Z No Device	Z No Qualifier
1 Skin, Face			
2 Skin, Right Ear			
3 Skin, Left Ear			
4 Skin, Neck			
5 Skin, Chest			
6 Skin, Back			
7 Skin, Abdomen			
8 Skin, Buttock			
9 Skin, Perineum			
A Skin, Genitalia			
B Skin, Right Upper Arm			
C Skin, Left Upper Arm			
D Skin, Right Lower Arm			
E Skin, Left Lower Arm			
F Skin, Right Hand			
G Skin, Left Hand			
H Skin, Right Upper Leg			
J Skin, Left Upper Leg			
K Skin, Right Lower Leg			
L Skin, Left Lower Leg			
M Skin, Right Foot			
N Skin, Left Foot			

Section	0	Medical and Surgical
Body System	H	Skin and Breast
Operation	9	**Drainage:** Taking or letting out fluids and/or gases from a body part

Body Part (4th)	Approach (5th)	Device (6th)	Qualifier (7th)
0 Skin, Scalp	X External	0 Drainage Device	Z No Qualifier
1 Skin, Face			
2 Skin, Right Ear			
3 Skin, Left Ear			
4 Skin, Neck			
5 Skin, Chest			
6 Skin, Back			
7 Skin, Abdomen			
8 Skin, Buttock			
9 Skin, Perineum			
A Skin, Genitalia			
B Skin, Right Upper Arm			
C Skin, Left Upper Arm			
D Skin, Right Lower Arm			
E Skin, Left Lower Arm			
F Skin, Right Hand			
G Skin, Left Hand			
H Skin, Right Upper Leg			
J Skin, Left Upper Leg			
K Skin, Right Lower Leg			
L Skin, Left Lower Leg			
M Skin, Right Foot			
N Skin, Left Foot			
Q Finger Nail			
R Toe Nail			

Continued

Section	0	Medical and Surgical
Body System	H	Skin and Breast
Operation	9	**Drainage:** Taking or letting out fluids and/or gases from a body part

0H9 *Continued*

Body Part (4ᵗʰ)	Approach (5ᵗʰ)	Device (6ᵗʰ)	Qualifier (7ᵗʰ)
0 Skin, Scalp 1 Skin, Face 2 Skin, Right Ear 3 Skin, Left Ear 4 Skin, Neck 5 Skin, Chest 6 Skin, Back 7 Skin, Abdomen 8 Skin, Buttock 9 Skin, Perineum A Skin, Genitalia B Skin, Right Upper Arm C Skin, Left Upper Arm D Skin, Right Lower Arm E Skin, Left Lower Arm F Skin, Right Hand G Skin, Left Hand H Skin, Right Upper Leg J Skin, Left Upper Leg K Skin, Right Lower Leg L Skin, Left Lower Leg M Skin, Right Foot N Skin, Left Foot Q Finger Nail R Toe Nail	X External	Z No Device	X Diagnostic Z No Qualifier
T Breast, Right U Breast, Left V Breast, Bilateral W Nipple, Right X Nipple, Left	0 Open 3 Percutaneous 7 Via Natural or Artificial Opening 8 Via Natural or Artificial Opening Endoscopic X External	0 Drainage Device	Z No Qualifier
T Breast, Right U Breast, Left V Breast, Bilateral W Nipple, Right X Nipple, Left	0 Open 3 Percutaneous 7 Via Natural or Artificial Opening 8 Via Natural or Artificial Opening Endoscopic X External	Z No Device	X Diagnostic Z No Qualifier

Section	0	Medical and Surgical
Body System	H	Skin and Breast
Operation	B	Excision: Cutting out or off, without replacement, a portion of a body part

Body Part (4th)	Approach (5th)	Device (6th)	Qualifier (7th)
0 Skin, Scalp 1 Skin, Face 2 Skin, Right Ear 3 Skin, Left Ear 4 Skin, Neck 5 Skin, Chest 6 Skin, Back 7 Skin, Abdomen 8 Skin, Buttock 9 Skin, Perineum A Skin, Genitalia B Skin, Right Upper Arm C Skin, Left Upper Arm D Skin, Right Lower Arm E Skin, Left Lower Arm F Skin, Right Hand G Skin, Left Hand H Skin, Right Upper Leg J Skin, Left Upper Leg K Skin, Right Lower Leg L Skin, Left Lower Leg M Skin, Right Foot N Skin, Left Foot Q Finger Nail R Toe Nail	X External	Z No Device	X Diagnostic Z No Qualifier
T Breast, Right U Breast, Left V Breast, Bilateral W Nipple, Right X Nipple, Left Y Supernumerary Breast	0 Open 3 Percutaneous 7 Via Natural or Artificial Opening 8 Via Natural or Artificial Opening Endoscopic X External	Z No Device	X Diagnostic Z No Qualifier

Section	0	**Medical and Surgical**
Body System	H	**Skin and Breast**
Operation	C	**Extirpation:** Taking or cutting out solid matter from a body part

Body Part (4th)	Approach (5th)	Device (6th)	Qualifier (7th)
0 Skin, Scalp 1 Skin, Face 2 Skin, Right Ear 3 Skin, Left Ear 4 Skin, Neck 5 Skin, Chest 6 Skin, Back 7 Skin, Abdomen 8 Skin, Buttock 9 Skin, Perineum A Skin, Genitalia B Skin, Right Upper Arm C Skin, Left Upper Arm D Skin, Right Lower Arm E Skin, Left Lower Arm F Skin, Right Hand G Skin, Left Hand H Skin, Right Upper Leg J Skin, Left Upper Leg K Skin, Right Lower Leg L Skin, Left Lower Leg M Skin, Right Foot N Skin, Left Foot Q Finger Nail R Toe Nail	X External	Z No Device	Z No Qualifier
T Breast, Right U Breast, Left V Breast, Bilateral W Nipple, Right X Nipple, Left	0 Open 3 Percutaneous 7 Via Natural or Artificial Opening 8 Via Natural or Artificial Opening Endoscopic X External	Z No Device	Z No Qualifier

Section	0	Medical and Surgical
Body System	H	Skin and Breast
Operation	D	**Extraction:** Pulling or stripping out or off all or a portion of a body part by the use of force

Body Part (4th)	Approach (5th)	Device (6th)	Qualifier (7th)
0 Skin, Scalp	X External	Z No Device	Z No Qualifier
1 Skin, Face			
2 Skin, Right Ear			
3 Skin, Left Ear			
4 Skin, Neck			
5 Skin, Chest			
6 Skin, Back			
7 Skin, Abdomen			
8 Skin, Buttock			
9 Skin, Perineum			
A Skin, Genitalia			
B Skin, Right Upper Arm			
C Skin, Left Upper Arm			
D Skin, Right Lower Arm			
E Skin, Left Lower Arm			
F Skin, Right Hand			
G Skin, Left Hand			
H Skin, Right Upper Leg			
J Skin, Left Upper Leg			
K Skin, Right Lower Leg			
L Skin, Left Lower Leg			
M Skin, Right Foot			
N Skin, Left Foot			
Q Finger Nail			
R Toe Nail			
S Hair			

Section	0	Medical and Surgical
Body System	H	Skin and Breast
Operation	H	**Insertion:** Putting in a nonbiological appliance that monitors, assists, performs, or prevents a physiological function but does not physically take the place of a body part

Body Part (4th)	Approach (5th)	Device (6th)	Qualifier (7th)
T Breast, Right	0 Open	1 Radioactive Element	Z No Qualifier
U Breast, Left	3 Percutaneous	N Tissue Expander	
V Breast, Bilateral	7 Via Natural or Artificial Opening		
W Nipple, Right	8 Via Natural or Artificial Opening Endoscopic		
X Nipple, Left			
T Breast, Right	X External	1 Radioactive Element	Z No Qualifier
U Breast, Left			
V Breast, Bilateral			
W Nipple, Right			
X Nipple, Left			

Section   **0**   **Medical and Surgical**
Body System   **H**   **Skin and Breast**
Operation   **J**   **Inspection:** Visually and/or manually exploring a body part

Body Part (4ᵗʰ)	Approach (5ᵗʰ)	Device (6ᵗʰ)	Qualifier (7ᵗʰ)
P Skin Q Finger Nail R Toe Nail	X External	Z No Device	Z No Qualifier
T Breast, Right U Breast, Left	0 Open 3 Percutaneous 7 Via Natural or Artificial Opening 8 Via Natural or Artificial Opening Endoscopic X External	Z No Device	Z No Qualifier

Section   **0**   **Medical and Surgical**
Body System   **H**   **Skin and Breast**
Operation   **M**   **Reattachment:** Putting back in or on all or a portion of a separated body part to its normal location or other suitable location

Body Part (4ᵗʰ)	Approach (5ᵗʰ)	Device (6ᵗʰ)	Qualifier (7ᵗʰ)
0 Skin, Scalp 1 Skin, Face 2 Skin, Right Ear 3 Skin, Left Ear 4 Skin, Neck 5 Skin, Chest 6 Skin, Back 7 Skin, Abdomen 8 Skin, Buttock 9 Skin, Perineum A Skin, Genitalia B Skin, Right Upper Arm C Skin, Left Upper Arm D Skin, Right Lower Arm E Skin, Left Lower Arm F Skin, Right Hand G Skin, Left Hand H Skin, Right Upper Leg J Skin, Left Upper Leg K Skin, Right Lower Leg L Skin, Left Lower Leg M Skin, Right Foot N Skin, Left Foot T Breast, Right U Breast, Left V Breast, Bilateral W Nipple, Right X Nipple, Left	X External	Z No Device	Z No Qualifier

Section	0	Medical and Surgical
Body System	H	Skin and Breast
Operation	N	Release: Freeing a body part from an abnormal physical constraint by cutting or by the use of force

Body Part (4th)	Approach (5th)	Device (6th)	Qualifier (7th)
0 Skin, Scalp 1 Skin, Face 2 Skin, Right Ear 3 Skin, Left Ear 4 Skin, Neck 5 Skin, Chest 6 Skin, Back 7 Skin, Abdomen 8 Skin, Buttock 9 Skin, Perineum A Skin, Genitalia B Skin, Right Upper Arm C Skin, Left Upper Arm D Skin, Right Lower Arm E Skin, Left Lower Arm F Skin, Right Hand G Skin, Left Hand H Skin, Right Upper Leg J Skin, Left Upper Leg	X External	Z No Device	Z No Qualifier
K Skin, Right Lower Leg L Skin, Left Lower Leg M Skin, Right Foot N Skin, Left Foot Q Finger Nail R Toe Nail T Breast, Right U Breast, Left V Breast, Bilateral W Nipple, Right X Nipple, Left	0 Open 3 Percutaneous 7 Via Natural or Artificial Opening 8 Via Natural or Artificial Opening Endoscopic X External	Z No Device	Z No Qualifier

Section	0	Medical and Surgical
Body System	H	Skin and Breast
Operation	P	Removal: Taking out or off a device from a body part

Body Part (4th)	Approach (5th)	Device (6th)	Qualifier (7th)
P Skin Q Finger Nail R Toe Nail	X External	0 Drainage Device 7 Autologous Tissue Substitute J Synthetic Substitute K Nonautologous Tissue Substitute	Z No Qualifier
S Hair	X External	7 Autologous Tissue Substitute J Synthetic Substitute K Nonautologous Tissue Substitute	Z No Qualifier
T Breast, Right U Breast, Left	0 Open 3 Percutaneous 7 Via Natural or Artificial Opening 8 Via Natural or Artificial Opening Endoscopic	0 Drainage Device 1 Radioactive Element 7 Autologous Tissue Substitute J Synthetic Substitute K Nonautologous Tissue Substitute N Tissue Expander	Z No Qualifier
T Breast, Right U Breast, Left	X External	0 Drainage Device 1 Radioactive Element 7 Autologous Tissue Substitute J Synthetic Substitute K Nonautologous Tissue Substitute	Z No Qualifier

Section	0	**Medical and Surgical**
Body System	H	**Skin and Breast**
Operation	Q	**Repair:** Restoring, to the extent possible, a body part to its normal anatomic structure and function

Body Part (4ᵗʰ)	Approach (5ᵗʰ)	Device (6ᵗʰ)	Qualifier (7ᵗʰ)
0 Skin, Scalp 1 Skin, Face 2 Skin, Right Ear 3 Skin, Left Ear 4 Skin, Neck 5 Skin, Chest 6 Skin, Back 7 Skin, Abdomen 8 Skin, Buttock 9 Skin, Perineum A Skin, Genitalia B Skin, Right Upper Arm C Skin, Left Upper Arm D Skin, Right Lower Arm E Skin, Left Lower Arm F Skin, Right Hand G Skin, Left Hand H Skin, Right Upper Leg J Skin, Left Upper Leg K Skin, Right Lower Leg L Skin, Left Lower Leg M Skin, Right Foot N Skin, Left Foot Q Finger Nail R Toe Nail	X External	Z No Device	Z No Qualifier
T Breast, Right U Breast, Left V Breast, Bilateral W Nipple, Right X Nipple, Left Y Supernumerary Breast	0 Open 3 Percutaneous 7 Via Natural or Artificial Opening 8 Via Natural or Artificial Opening Endoscopic X External	Z No Device	Z No Qualifier

Section	0	**Medical and Surgical**
Body System	H	**Skin and Breast**
Operation	R	**Replacement:** Putting in or on biological or synthetic material that physically takes the place and/or function of all or a portion of a body part

Body Part (4th)	Approach (5th)	Device (6th)	Qualifier (7th)
0 Skin, Scalp 1 Skin, Face 2 Skin, Right Ear 3 Skin, Left Ear 4 Skin, Neck 5 Skin, Chest 6 Skin, Back 7 Skin, Abdomen 8 Skin, Buttock 9 Skin, Perineum A Skin, Genitalia B Skin, Right Upper Arm C Skin, Left Upper Arm D Skin, Right Lower Arm E Skin, Left Lower Arm F Skin, Right Hand G Skin, Left Hand H Skin, Right Upper Leg J Skin, Left Upper Leg K Skin, Right Lower Leg L Skin, Left Lower Leg M Skin, Right Foot N Skin, Left Foot	X External	7 Autologous Tissue Substitute K Nonautologous Tissue Substitute	3 Full Thickness 4 Partial Thickness
0 Skin, Scalp 1 Skin, Face 2 Skin, Right Ear 3 Skin, Left Ear 4 Skin, Neck 5 Skin, Chest 6 Skin, Back 7 Skin, Abdomen 8 Skin, Buttock 9 Skin, Perineum A Skin, Genitalia B Skin, Right Upper Arm C Skin, Left Upper Arm D Skin, Right Lower Arm E Skin, Left Lower Arm F Skin, Right Hand G Skin, Left Hand H Skin, Right Upper Leg J Skin, Left Upper Leg K Skin, Right Lower Leg L Skin, Left Lower Leg M Skin, Right Foot N Skin, Left Foot	X External	J Synthetic Substitute	3 Full Thickness 4 Partial Thickness Z No Qualifier
Q Finger Nail R Toe Nail S Hair	X External	7 Autologous Tissue Substitute J Synthetic Substitute K Nonautologous Tissue Substitute	Z No Qualifier
T Breast, Right U Breast, Left V Breast, Bilateral	0 Open	7 Autologous Tissue Substitute	5 Latissimus Dorsi Myocutaneous Flap 6 Transverse Rectus Abdominis Myocutaneous Flap 7 Deep Inferior Epigastric Artery Perforator Flap 8 Superficial Inferior Epigastric Artery Flap 9 Gluteal Artery Perforator Flap Z No Qualifier

Continued

Section	0	Medical and Surgical
Body System	H	Skin and Breast
Operation	R	Replacement: Putting in or on biological or synthetic material that physically takes the place and/or function of all or a portion of a body part

Body Part (4th)	Approach (5th)	Device (6th)	Qualifier (7th)
T Breast, Right U Breast, Left V Breast, Bilateral	0 Open	J Synthetic Substitute K Nonautologous Tissue Substitute	Z No Qualifier
T Breast, Right U Breast, Left V Breast, Bilateral	3 Percutaneous X External	7 Autologous Tissue Substitute J Synthetic Substitute K Nonautologous Tissue Substitute	Z No Qualifier
W Nipple, Right X Nipple, Left	0 Open 3 Percutaneous X External	7 Autologous Tissue Substitute J Synthetic Substitute K Nonautologous Tissue Substitute	Z No Qualifier

Section	0	Medical and Surgical
Body System	H	Skin and Breast
Operation	S	Reposition: Moving to its normal location, or other suitable location, all or a portion of a body part

Body Part (4th)	Approach (5th)	Device (6th)	Qualifier (7th)
S Hair W Nipple, Right X Nipple, Left	X External	Z No Device	Z No Qualifier
T Breast, Right U Breast, Left V Breast, Bilateral	0 Open	Z No Device	Z No Qualifier

Section	0	Medical and Surgical
Body System	H	Skin and Breast
Operation	T	Resection: Cutting out or off, without replacement, all of a body part

Body Part (4th)	Approach (5th)	Device (6th)	Qualifier (7th)
Q Finger Nail R Toe Nail W Nipple, Right X Nipple, Left	X External	Z No Device	Z No Qualifier
T Breast, Right U Breast, Left V Breast, Bilateral Y Supernumerary Breast	0 Open	Z No Device	Z No Qualifier

Section	0	Medical and Surgical
Body System	H	Skin and Breast
Operation	U	Supplement: Putting in or on biological or synthetic material that physically reinforces and/or augments the function of a portion of a body part

Body Part (4th)	Approach (5th)	Device (6th)	Qualifier (7th)
T Breast, Right U Breast, Left V Breast, Bilateral W Nipple, Right X Nipple, Left	0 Open 3 Percutaneous 7 Via Natural or Artificial Opening 8 Via Natural or Artificial Opening Endoscopic X External	7 Autologous Tissue Substitute J Synthetic Substitute K Nonautologous Tissue Substitute	Z No Qualifier

Section	0	Medical and Surgical
Body System	H	Skin and Breast
Operation	W	**Revision:** Correcting, to the extent possible, a portion of a malfunctioning device or the position of a displaced device

Body Part (4th)	Approach (5th)	Device (6th)	Qualifier (7th)
P Skin **Q** Finger Nail **R** Toe Nail	**X** External	**0** Drainage Device **7** Autologous Tissue Substitute **J** Synthetic Substitute **K** Nonautologous Tissue Substitute	**Z** No Qualifier
S Hair	**X** External	**7** Autologous Tissue Substitute **J** Synthetic Substitute **K** Nonautologous Tissue Substitute	**Z** No Qualifier
T Breast, Right **U** Breast, Left	**0** Open **3** Percutaneous **7** Via Natural or Artificial Opening **8** Via Natural or Artificial Opening Endoscopic	**0** Drainage Device **7** Autologous Tissue Substitute **J** Synthetic Substitute **K** Nonautologous Tissue Substitute **N** Tissue Expander	**Z** No Qualifier
T Breast, Right **U** Breast, Left	**X** External	**0** Drainage Device **7** Autologous Tissue Substitute **J** Synthetic Substitute **K** Nonautologous Tissue Substitute	**Z** No Qualifier

Section	0	Medical and Surgical
Body System	H	Skin and Breast
Operation	X	**Transfer:** Moving, without taking out, all or a portion of a body part to another location to take over the function of all or a portion of a body part

Body Part (4th)	Approach (5th)	Device (6th)	Qualifier (7th)
0 Skin, Scalp **1** Skin, Face **2** Skin, Right Ear **3** Skin, Left Ear **4** Skin, Neck **5** Skin, Chest **6** Skin, Back **7** Skin, Abdomen **8** Skin, Buttock **9** Skin, Perineum **A** Skin, Genitalia **B** Skin, Right Upper Arm **C** Skin, Left Upper Arm **D** Skin, Right Lower Arm **E** Skin, Left Lower Arm **F** Skin, Right Hand **G** Skin, Left Hand **H** Skin, Right Upper Leg **J** Skin, Left Upper Leg **K** Skin, Right Lower Leg **L** Skin, Left Lower Leg **M** Skin, Right Foot **N** Skin, Left Foot	**X** External	**Z** No Device	**Z** No Qualifier

Skin and Breast Code Listing 0H0-0HX

H0 – Skin and Breast, Alteration

0H0T07Z Alteration of Right Breast with Autologous Tissue Substitute, Open Approach

0H0T0JZ Alteration of Right Breast with Synthetic Substitute, Open Approach

0H0T0KZ Alteration of Right Breast with Nonautologous Tissue Substitute, Open Approach

0H0T0ZZ Alteration of Right Breast, Open Approach

0H0T37Z Alteration of Right Breast with Autologous Tissue Substitute, Percutaneous Approach

0H0T3JZ Alteration of Right Breast with Synthetic Substitute, Percutaneous Approach

0H0T3KZ Alteration of Right Breast with Nonautologous Tissue Substitute, Percutaneous Approach

0H0T3ZZ Alteration of Right Breast, Percutaneous Approach

0H0TX7Z Alteration of Right Breast with Autologous Tissue Substitute, External Approach

0H0TXJZ Alteration of Right Breast with Synthetic Substitute, External Approach

0H0TXKZ Alteration of Right Breast with Nonautologous Tissue Substitute, External Approach

0H0TXZZ Alteration of Right Breast, External Approach

0H0U07Z Alteration of Left Breast with Autologous Tissue Substitute, Open Approach

0H0U0JZ Alteration of Left Breast with Synthetic Substitute, Open Approach

0H0U0KZ Alteration of Left Breast with Nonautologous Tissue Substitute, Open Approach

0H0U0ZZ Alteration of Left Breast, Open Approach

0H0U37Z Alteration of Left Breast with Autologous Tissue Substitute, Percutaneous Approach

0H0U3JZ Alteration of Left Breast with Synthetic Substitute, Percutaneous Approach

0H0U3KZ Alteration of Left Breast with Nonautologous Tissue Substitute, Percutaneous Approach

0H0U3ZZ Alteration of Left Breast, Percutaneous Approach

0H0UX7Z Alteration of Left Breast with Autologous Tissue Substitute, External Approach

0H0UXJZ Alteration of Left Breast with Synthetic Substitute, External Approach

0H0UXKZ Alteration of Left Breast with Nonautologous Tissue Substitute, External Approach

0H0UXZZ Alteration of Left Breast, External Approach

0H0V07Z Alteration of Bilateral Breast with Autologous Tissue Substitute, Open Approach

0H0V0JZ Alteration of Bilateral Breast with Synthetic Substitute, Open Approach

0H0V0KZ Alteration of Bilateral Breast with Nonautologous Tissue Substitute, Open Approach

0H0V0ZZ Alteration of Bilateral Breast, Open Approach

0H0V37Z Alteration of Bilateral Breast with Autologous Tissue Substitute, Percutaneous Approach

0H0V3JZ Alteration of Bilateral Breast with Synthetic Substitute, Percutaneous Approach

0H0V3KZ Alteration of Bilateral Breast with Nonautologous Tissue Substitute, Percutaneous Approach

0H0V3ZZ Alteration of Bilateral Breast, Percutaneous Approach

0H0VX7Z Alteration of Bilateral Breast with Autologous Tissue Substitute, External Approach

0H0VXJZ Alteration of Bilateral Breast with Synthetic Substitute, External Approach

0H0VXKZ Alteration of Bilateral Breast with Nonautologous Tissue Substitute, External Approach

0H0VXZZ Alteration of Bilateral Breast, External Approach

0H2 – Skin and Breast, Change

Review Coding Guideline B6.1c

0H2PX0Z Change Drainage Device in Skin, External Approach

0H2PXYZ Change Other Device in Skin, External Approach

0H2TX0Z Change Drainage Device in Right Breast, External Approach

0H2TXYZ Change Other Device in Right Breast, External Approach

0H2UX0Z Change Drainage Device in Left Breast, External Approach

0H2UXYZ Change Other Device in Left Breast, External Approach

0H5 – Skin and Breast, Destruction

- **0H50XZD** Destruction of Scalp Skin, Multiple, External Approach
- **0H50XZZ** Destruction of Scalp Skin, External Approach
- **0H51XZD** Destruction of Face Skin, Multiple, External Approach
- **0H51XZZ** Destruction of Face Skin, External Approach
  0H52XZD Destruction of Right Ear Skin, Multiple, External Approach
  0H52XZZ Destruction of Right Ear Skin, External Approach
  0H53XZD Destruction of Left Ear Skin, Multiple, External Approach
  0H53XZZ Destruction of Left Ear Skin, External Approach
- **0H54XZD** Destruction of Neck Skin, Multiple, External Approach
- **0H54XZZ** Destruction of Neck Skin, External Approach
- **0H55XZD** Destruction of Chest Skin, Multiple, External Approach
- **0H55XZZ** Destruction of Chest Skin, External Approach
- **0H56XZD** Destruction of Back Skin, Multiple, External Approach
- **0H56XZZ** Destruction of Back Skin, External Approach
- **0H57XZD** Destruction of Abdomen Skin, Multiple, External Approach
- **0H57XZZ** Destruction of Abdomen Skin, External Approach
- **0H58XZD** Destruction of Buttock Skin, Multiple, External Approach
- **0H58XZZ** Destruction of Buttock Skin, External Approach
- **0H59XZD** Destruction of Perineum Skin, Multiple, External Approach
- **0H59XZZ** Destruction of Perineum Skin, External Approach
- **0H5AXZD** Destruction of Genitalia Skin, Multiple, External Approach
- **0H5AXZZ** Destruction of Genitalia Skin, External Approach
- **0H5BXZD** Destruction of Right Upper Arm Skin, Multiple, External Approach
- **0H5BXZZ** Destruction of Right Upper Arm Skin, External Approach
- **0H5CXZD** Destruction of Left Upper Arm Skin, Multiple, External Approach
- **0H5CXZZ** Destruction of Left Upper Arm Skin, External Approach
- **0H5DXZD** Destruction of Right Lower Arm Skin, Multiple, External Approach
- **0H5DXZZ** Destruction of Right Lower Arm Skin, External Approach
- **0H5EXZD** Destruction of Left Lower Arm Skin, Multiple, External Approach
- **0H5EXZZ** Destruction of Left Lower Arm Skin, External Approach
- **0H5FXZD** Destruction of Right Hand Skin, Multiple, External Approach
- **0H5FXZZ** Destruction of Right Hand Skin, External Approach
- **0H5GXZD** Destruction of Left Hand Skin, Multiple, External Approach
- **0H5GXZZ** Destruction of Left Hand Skin, External Approach
- **0H5HXZD** Destruction of Right Upper Leg Skin, Multiple, External Approach
- **0H5HXZZ** Destruction of Right Upper Leg Skin, External Approach
- **0H5JXZD** Destruction of Left Upper Leg Skin, Multiple, External Approach
- **0H5JXZZ** Destruction of Left Upper Leg Skin, External Approach
- **0H5KXZD** Destruction of Right Lower Leg Skin, Multiple, External Approach
- **0H5KXZZ** Destruction of Right Lower Leg Skin, External Approach
- **0H5LXZD** Destruction of Left Lower Leg Skin, Multiple, External Approach
- **0H5LXZZ** Destruction of Left Lower Leg Skin, External Approach
- **0H5MXZD** Destruction of Right Foot Skin, Multiple, External Approach
- **0H5MXZZ** Destruction of Right Foot Skin, External Approach
- **0H5NXZD** Destruction of Left Foot Skin, Multiple, External Approach
- **0H5NXZZ** Destruction of Left Foot Skin, External Approach
- **0H5QXZZ** Destruction of Finger Nail, External Approach
- **0H5RXZZ** Destruction of Toe Nail, External Approach
  0H5T0ZZ Destruction of Right Breast, Open Approach
  0H5T3ZZ Destruction of Right Breast, Percutaneous Approach
  0H5T7ZZ Destruction of Right Breast, Via Natural or Artificial Opening
  0H5T8ZZ Destruction of Right Breast, Via Natural or Artificial Opening Endoscopic
  0H5TXZZ Destruction of Right Breast, External Approach

♀ Female-only   ♂ Male-only   ◯ Limited Coverage   ● Non-OR   �▪ HAC-associated procedure   ⬤ Non-covered procedures   ⊞ Combination

0H5U0ZZ	Destruction of Left Breast, Open Approach
0H5U3ZZ	Destruction of Left Breast, Percutaneous Approach
0H5U7ZZ	Destruction of Left Breast, Via Natural or Artificial Opening
0H5U8ZZ	Destruction of Left Breast, Via Natural or Artificial Opening Endoscopic
0H5UXZZ	Destruction of Left Breast, External Approach
0H5V0ZZ	Destruction of Bilateral Breast, Open Approach
0H5V3ZZ	Destruction of Bilateral Breast, Percutaneous Approach
0H5V7ZZ	Destruction of Bilateral Breast, Via Natural or Artificial Opening
0H5V8ZZ	Destruction of Bilateral Breast, Via Natural or Artificial Opening Endoscopic
0H5VXZZ	Destruction of Bilateral Breast, External Approach

0H5W0ZZ	Destruction of Right Nipple, Open Approach
0H5W3ZZ	Destruction of Right Nipple, Percutaneous Approach
0H5W7ZZ	Destruction of Right Nipple, Via Natural or Artificial Opening
0H5W8ZZ	Destruction of Right Nipple, Via Natural or Artificial Opening Endoscopic
0H5WXZZ	Destruction of Right Nipple, External Approach
0H5X0ZZ	Destruction of Left Nipple, Open Approach
0H5X3ZZ	Destruction of Left Nipple, Percutaneous Approach
0H5X7ZZ	Destruction of Left Nipple, Via Natural or Artificial Opening
0H5X8ZZ	Destruction of Left Nipple, Via Natural or Artificial Opening Endoscopic
0H5XXZZ	Destruction of Left Nipple, External Approach

0H8 – Skin and Breast, Division

Review Coding Guideline B3.14

0H80XZZ	Division of Scalp Skin, External Approach
0H81XZZ	Division of Face Skin, External Approach
0H82XZZ	Division of Right Ear Skin, External Approach
0H83XZZ	Division of Left Ear Skin, External Approach
0H84XZZ	Division of Neck Skin, External Approach
0H85XZZ	Division of Chest Skin, External Approach
0H86XZZ	Division of Back Skin, External Approach
0H87XZZ	Division of Abdomen Skin, External Approach
0H88XZZ	Division of Buttock Skin, External Approach
0H89XZZ	Division of Perineum Skin, External Approach
0H8AXZZ	Division of Genitalia Skin, External Approach
0H8BXZZ	Division of Right Upper Arm Skin, External Approach

0H8CXZZ	Division of Left Upper Arm Skin, External Approach
0H8DXZZ	Division of Right Lower Arm Skin, External Approach
0H8EXZZ	Division of Left Lower Arm Skin, External Approach
0H8FXZZ	Division of Right Hand Skin, External Approach
0H8GXZZ	Division of Left Hand Skin, External Approach
0H8HXZZ	Division of Right Upper Leg Skin, External Approach
0H8JXZZ	Division of Left Upper Leg Skin, External Approach
0H8KXZZ	Division of Right Lower Leg Skin, External Approach
0H8LXZZ	Division of Left Lower Leg Skin, External Approach
0H8MXZZ	Division of Right Foot Skin, External Approach
0H8NXZZ	Division of Left Foot Skin, External Approach

0H9 – Skin and Breast, Drainage

Review Coding Guidelines B3.4a and B3.4b

Review Coding Guideline B6.2

0H90X0Z	Drainage of Scalp Skin with Drainage Device, External Approach
0H90XZX	Drainage of Scalp Skin, External Approach, Diagnostic
0H90XZZ	Drainage of Scalp Skin, External Approach
0H91X0Z	Drainage of Face Skin with Drainage Device, External Approach
0H91XZX	Drainage of Face Skin, External Approach, Diagnostic
0H91XZZ	Drainage of Face Skin, External Approach
0H92X0Z	Drainage of Right Ear Skin with Drainage Device, External Approach
0H92XZX	Drainage of Right Ear Skin, External Approach, Diagnostic
0H92XZZ	Drainage of Right Ear Skin, External Approach
0H93X0Z	Drainage of Left Ear Skin with Drainage Device, External Approach
0H93XZX	Drainage of Left Ear Skin, External Approach, Diagnostic
0H93XZZ	Drainage of Left Ear Skin, External Approach
0H94X0Z	Drainage of Neck Skin with Drainage Device, External Approach
0H94XZX	Drainage of Neck Skin, External Approach, Diagnostic
0H94XZZ	Drainage of Neck Skin, External Approach
0H95X0Z	Drainage of Chest Skin with Drainage Device, External Approach
0H95XZX	Drainage of Chest Skin, External Approach, Diagnostic
0H95XZZ	Drainage of Chest Skin, External Approach
0H96X0Z	Drainage of Back Skin with Drainage Device, External Approach
0H96XZX	Drainage of Back Skin, External Approach, Diagnostic
0H96XZZ	Drainage of Back Skin, External Approach
0H97X0Z	Drainage of Abdomen Skin with Drainage Device, External Approach
0H97XZX	Drainage of Abdomen Skin, External Approach, Diagnostic
0H97XZZ	Drainage of Abdomen Skin, External Approach
0H98X0Z	Drainage of Buttock Skin with Drainage Device, External Approach
0H98XZX	Drainage of Buttock Skin, External Approach, Diagnostic
0H98XZZ	Drainage of Buttock Skin, External Approach
0H99X0Z	Drainage of Perineum Skin with Drainage Device, External Approach
0H99XZX	Drainage of Perineum Skin, External Approach, Diagnostic
0H99XZZ	Drainage of Perineum Skin, External Approach
0H9AX0Z	Drainage of Genitalia Skin with Drainage Device, External Approach
0H9AXZX	Drainage of Genitalia Skin, External Approach, Diagnostic
0H9AXZZ	Drainage of Genitalia Skin, External Approach
0H9BX0Z	Drainage of Right Upper Arm Skin with Drainage Device, External Approach

0H9BXZX	Drainage of Right Upper Arm Skin, External Approach, Diagnostic
0H9BXZZ	Drainage of Right Upper Arm Skin, External Approach
0H9CX0Z	Drainage of Left Upper Arm Skin with Drainage Device, External Approach
0H9CXZX	Drainage of Left Upper Arm Skin, External Approach, Diagnostic
0H9CXZZ	Drainage of Left Upper Arm Skin, External Approach
0H9DX0Z	Drainage of Right Lower Arm Skin with Drainage Device, External Approach
0H9DXZX	Drainage of Right Lower Arm Skin, External Approach, Diagnostic
0H9DXZZ	Drainage of Right Lower Arm Skin, External Approach
0H9EX0Z	Drainage of Left Lower Arm Skin with Drainage Device, External Approach
0H9EXZX	Drainage of Left Lower Arm Skin, External Approach, Diagnostic
0H9EXZZ	Drainage of Left Lower Arm Skin, External Approach
0H9FX0Z	Drainage of Right Hand Skin with Drainage Device, External Approach
0H9FXZX	Drainage of Right Hand Skin, External Approach, Diagnostic
0H9FXZZ	Drainage of Right Hand Skin, External Approach
0H9GX0Z	Drainage of Left Hand Skin with Drainage Device, External Approach
0H9GXZX	Drainage of Left Hand Skin, External Approach, Diagnostic
0H9GXZZ	Drainage of Left Hand Skin, External Approach
0H9HX0Z	Drainage of Right Upper Leg Skin with Drainage Device, External Approach
0H9HXZX	Drainage of Right Upper Leg Skin, External Approach, Diagnostic
0H9HXZZ	Drainage of Right Upper Leg Skin, External Approach
0H9JX0Z	Drainage of Left Upper Leg Skin with Drainage Device, External Approach
0H9JXZX	Drainage of Left Upper Leg Skin, External Approach, Diagnostic
0H9JXZZ	Drainage of Left Upper Leg Skin, External Approach
0H9KX0Z	Drainage of Right Lower Leg Skin with Drainage Device, External Approach
0H9KXZX	Drainage of Right Lower Leg Skin, External Approach, Diagnostic
0H9KXZZ	Drainage of Right Lower Leg Skin, External Approach
0H9LX0Z	Drainage of Left Lower Leg Skin with Drainage Device, External Approach
0H9LXZX	Drainage of Left Lower Leg Skin, External Approach, Diagnostic
0H9LXZZ	Drainage of Left Lower Leg Skin, External Approach

♀ Female-only   ♂ Male-only   ⬤ Limited Coverage   ● Non-OR   ▦ HAC-associated procedure   ● Non-covered procedures   ✚ Combination

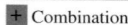

0H9MX0Z Drainage of Right Foot Skin with Drainage Device, External Approach
0H9MXZX Drainage of Right Foot Skin, External Approach, Diagnostic
0H9MXZZ Drainage of Right Foot Skin, External Approach
0H9NX0Z Drainage of Left Foot Skin with Drainage Device, External Approach
0H9NXZX Drainage of Left Foot Skin, External Approach, Diagnostic
0H9NXZZ Drainage of Left Foot Skin, External Approach
0H9QX0Z Drainage of Finger Nail with Drainage Device, External Approach
0H9QXZX Drainage of Finger Nail, External Approach, Diagnostic
0H9QXZZ Drainage of Finger Nail, External Approach
0H9RX0Z Drainage of Toe Nail with Drainage Device, External Approach
0H9RXZX Drainage of Toe Nail, External Approach, Diagnostic
0H9RXZZ Drainage of Toe Nail, External Approach
0H9T00Z Drainage of Right Breast with Drainage Device, Open Approach
0H9T0ZX Drainage of Right Breast, Open Approach, Diagnostic
0H9T0ZZ Drainage of Right Breast, Open Approach
0H9T30Z Drainage of Right Breast with Drainage Device, Percutaneous Approach
0H9T3ZX Drainage of Right Breast, Percutaneous Approach, Diagnostic
0H9T3ZZ Drainage of Right Breast, Percutaneous Approach
0H9T70Z Drainage of Right Breast with Drainage Device, Via Natural or Artificial Opening
0H9T7ZX Drainage of Right Breast, Via Natural or Artificial Opening, Diagnostic
0H9T7ZZ Drainage of Right Breast, Via Natural or Artificial Opening
0H9T80Z Drainage of Right Breast with Drainage Device, Via Natural or Artificial Opening Endoscopic
0H9T8ZX Drainage of Right Breast, Via Natural or Artificial Opening Endoscopic, Diagnostic
0H9T8ZZ Drainage of Right Breast, Via Natural or Artificial Opening Endoscopic
0H9TX0Z Drainage of Right Breast with Drainage Device, External Approach
0H9TXZX Drainage of Right Breast, External Approach, Diagnostic
0H9TXZZ Drainage of Right Breast, External Approach
0H9U00Z Drainage of Left Breast with Drainage Device, Open Approach
0H9U0ZX Drainage of Left Breast, Open Approach, Diagnostic
0H9U0ZZ Drainage of Left Breast, Open Approach
0H9U30Z Drainage of Left Breast with Drainage Device, Percutaneous Approach
0H9U3ZX Drainage of Left Breast, Percutaneous Approach, Diagnostic
0H9U3ZZ Drainage of Left Breast, Percutaneous Approach
0H9U70Z Drainage of Left Breast with Drainage Device, Via Natural or Artificial Opening
0H9U7ZX Drainage of Left Breast, Via Natural or Artificial Opening, Diagnostic
0H9U7ZZ Drainage of Left Breast, Via Natural or Artificial Opening
0H9U80Z Drainage of Left Breast with Drainage Device, Via Natural or Artificial Opening Endoscopic
0H9U8ZX Drainage of Left Breast, Via Natural or Artificial Opening Endoscopic, Diagnostic
0H9U8ZZ Drainage of Left Breast, Via Natural or Artificial Opening Endoscopic
0H9UX0Z Drainage of Left Breast with Drainage Device, External Approach
0H9UXZX Drainage of Left Breast, External Approach, Diagnostic
0H9UXZZ Drainage of Left Breast, External Approach
0H9V00Z Drainage of Bilateral Breast with Drainage Device, Open Approach
0H9V0ZX Drainage of Bilateral Breast, Open Approach, Diagnostic
0H9V0ZZ Drainage of Bilateral Breast, Open Approach
0H9V30Z Drainage of Bilateral Breast with Drainage Device, Percutaneous Approach
0H9V3ZX Drainage of Bilateral Breast, Percutaneous Approach, Diagnostic

0H9V3ZZ Drainage of Bilateral Breast, Percutaneous Approach
0H9V70Z Drainage of Bilateral Breast with Drainage Device, Via Natural or Artificial Opening
0H9V7ZX Drainage of Bilateral Breast, Via Natural or Artificial Opening, Diagnostic
0H9V7ZZ Drainage of Bilateral Breast, Via Natural or Artificial Opening
0H9V80Z Drainage of Bilateral Breast with Drainage Device, Via Natural or Artificial Opening Endoscopic
0H9V8ZX Drainage of Bilateral Breast, Via Natural or Artificial Opening Endoscopic, Diagnostic
0H9V8ZZ Drainage of Bilateral Breast, Via Natural or Artificial Opening Endoscopic
0H9VX0Z Drainage of Bilateral Breast with Drainage Device, External Approach
0H9VXZX Drainage of Bilateral Breast, External Approach, Diagnostic
0H9VXZZ Drainage of Bilateral Breast, External Approach
0H9W00Z Drainage of Right Nipple with Drainage Device, Open Approach
0H9W0ZX Drainage of Right Nipple, Open Approach, Diagnostic
0H9W0ZZ Drainage of Right Nipple, Open Approach
0H9W30Z Drainage of Right Nipple with Drainage Device, Percutaneous Approach
0H9W3ZX Drainage of Right Nipple, Percutaneous Approach, Diagnostic
0H9W3ZZ Drainage of Right Nipple, Percutaneous Approach
0H9W70Z Drainage of Right Nipple with Drainage Device, Via Natural or Artificial Opening
0H9W7ZX Drainage of Right Nipple, Via Natural or Artificial Opening, Diagnostic
0H9W7ZZ Drainage of Right Nipple, Via Natural or Artificial Opening
0H9W80Z Drainage of Right Nipple with Drainage Device, Via Natural or Artificial Opening Endoscopic
0H9W8ZX Drainage of Right Nipple, Via Natural or Artificial Opening Endoscopic, Diagnostic
0H9W8ZZ Drainage of Right Nipple, Via Natural or Artificial Opening Endoscopic
0H9WX0Z Drainage of Right Nipple with Drainage Device, External Approach
0H9WXZX Drainage of Right Nipple, External Approach, Diagnostic
0H9WXZZ Drainage of Right Nipple, External Approach
0H9X00Z Drainage of Left Nipple with Drainage Device, Open Approach
0H9X0ZX Drainage of Left Nipple, Open Approach, Diagnostic
0H9X0ZZ Drainage of Left Nipple, Open Approach
0H9X30Z Drainage of Left Nipple with Drainage Device, Percutaneous Approach
0H9X3ZX Drainage of Left Nipple, Percutaneous Approach, Diagnostic
0H9X3ZZ Drainage of Left Nipple, Percutaneous Approach
0H9X70Z Drainage of Left Nipple with Drainage Device, Via Natural or Artificial Opening
0H9X7ZX Drainage of Left Nipple, Via Natural or Artificial Opening, Diagnostic
0H9X7ZZ Drainage of Left Nipple, Via Natural or Artificial Opening
0H9X80Z Drainage of Left Nipple with Drainage Device, Via Natural or Artificial Opening Endoscopic
0H9X8ZX Drainage of Left Nipple, Via Natural or Artificial Opening Endoscopic, Diagnostic
0H9X8ZZ Drainage of Left Nipple, Via Natural or Artificial Opening Endoscopic
0H9XX0Z Drainage of Left Nipple with Drainage Device, External Approach
0H9XXZX Drainage of Left Nipple, External Approach, Diagnostic
0H9XXZZ Drainage of Left Nipple, External Approach

0HB – Skin and Breast, Excision

Review Coding Guidelines 3B.4a and 3B.4b

Review Coding Guideline B3.5

Review Coding Guideline B3.8

0HB0XZX Excision of Scalp Skin, External Approach, Diagnostic
0HB0XZZ Excision of Scalp Skin, External Approach
0HB1XZX Excision of Face Skin, External Approach, Diagnostic
0HB1XZZ Excision of Face Skin, External Approach
0HB2XZX Excision of Right Ear Skin, External Approach, Diagnostic
0HB2XZZ Excision of Right Ear Skin, External Approach

0HB3XZX Excision of Left Ear Skin, External Approach, Diagnostic
0HB3XZZ Excision of Left Ear Skin, External Approach
0HB4XZX Excision of Neck Skin, External Approach, Diagnostic
0HB4XZZ Excision of Neck Skin, External Approach
0HB5XZX Excision of Chest Skin, External Approach, Diagnostic
0HB5XZZ Excision of Chest Skin, External Approach

♀ Female-only   ♂ Male-only   ◯ Limited Coverage   ● Non-OR   ▨ HAC-associated procedure   ⬣ Non-covered procedures   ✚ Combination

0HB6XZX Excision of Back Skin, External Approach, Diagnostic
0HB6XZZ Excision of Back Skin, External Approach
0HB7XZX Excision of Abdomen Skin, External Approach, Diagnostic
0HB7XZZ Excision of Abdomen Skin, External Approach
0HB8XZX Excision of Buttock Skin, External Approach, Diagnostic
0HB8XZZ Excision of Buttock Skin, External Approach
0HB9XZX Excision of Perineum Skin, External Approach, Diagnostic
● **0HB9XZZ** Excision of Perineum Skin, External Approach
0HBAXZX Excision of Genitalia Skin, External Approach, Diagnostic
0HBAXZZ Excision of Genitalia Skin, External Approach
0HBBXZX Excision of Right Upper Arm Skin, External Approach, Diagnostic
0HBBXZZ Excision of Right Upper Arm Skin, External Approach
0HBCXZX Excision of Left Upper Arm Skin, External Approach, Diagnostic
0HBCXZZ Excision of Left Upper Arm Skin, External Approach
0HBDXZX Excision of Right Lower Arm Skin, External Approach, Diagnostic
0HBDXZZ Excision of Right Lower Arm Skin, External Approach
0HBEXZX Excision of Left Lower Arm Skin, External Approach, Diagnostic
0HBEXZZ Excision of Left Lower Arm Skin, External Approach
0HBFXZX Excision of Right Hand Skin, External Approach, Diagnostic
0HBFXZZ Excision of Right Hand Skin, External Approach
0HBGXZX Excision of Left Hand Skin, External Approach, Diagnostic
0HBGXZZ Excision of Left Hand Skin, External Approach
0HBHXZX Excision of Right Upper Leg Skin, External Approach, Diagnostic
0HBHXZZ Excision of Right Upper Leg Skin, External Approach
0HBJXZX Excision of Left Upper Leg Skin, External Approach, Diagnostic
0HBJXZZ Excision of Left Upper Leg Skin, External Approach
0HBKXZX Excision of Right Lower Leg Skin, External Approach, Diagnostic
0HBKXZZ Excision of Right Lower Leg Skin, External Approach
0HBLXZX Excision of Left Lower Leg Skin, External Approach, Diagnostic
0HBLXZZ Excision of Left Lower Leg Skin, External Approach
0HBMXZX Excision of Right Foot Skin, External Approach, Diagnostic
0HBMXZZ Excision of Right Foot Skin, External Approach
0HBNXZX Excision of Left Foot Skin, External Approach, Diagnostic
0HBNXZZ Excision of Left Foot Skin, External Approach
0HBQXZX Excision of Finger Nail, External Approach, Diagnostic
0HBQXZZ Excision of Finger Nail, External Approach
0HBRXZX Excision of Toe Nail, External Approach, Diagnostic
0HBRXZZ Excision of Toe Nail, External Approach
0HBT0ZX Excision of Right Breast, Open Approach, Diagnostic
0HBT0ZZ Excision of Right Breast, Open Approach
0HBT3ZX Excision of Right Breast, Percutaneous Approach, Diagnostic
0HBT3ZZ Excision of Right Breast, Percutaneous Approach
0HBT7ZX Excision of Right Breast, Via Natural or Artificial Opening, Diagnostic
0HBT7ZZ Excision of Right Breast, Via Natural or Artificial Opening
0HBT8ZX Excision of Right Breast, Via Natural or Artificial Opening Endoscopic, Diagnostic
0HBT8ZZ Excision of Right Breast, Via Natural or Artificial Opening Endoscopic
0HBTXZX Excision of Right Breast, External Approach, Diagnostic
0HBTXZZ Excision of Right Breast, External Approach
0HBU0ZX Excision of Left Breast, Open Approach, Diagnostic
0HBU0ZZ Excision of Left Breast, Open Approach
0HBU3ZX Excision of Left Breast, Percutaneous Approach, Diagnostic
0HBU3ZZ Excision of Left Breast, Percutaneous Approach
0HBU7ZX Excision of Left Breast, Via Natural or Artificial Opening, Diagnostic
0HBU7ZZ Excision of Left Breast, Via Natural or Artificial Opening
0HBU8ZX Excision of Left Breast, Via Natural or Artificial Opening Endoscopic, Diagnostic

0HBU8ZZ Excision of Left Breast, Via Natural or Artificial Opening Endoscopic
0HBUXZX Excision of Left Breast, External Approach, Diagnostic
0HBUXZZ Excision of Left Breast, External Approach
0HBV0ZX Excision of Bilateral Breast, Open Approach, Diagnostic
0HBV0ZZ Excision of Bilateral Breast, Open Approach
0HBV3ZX Excision of Bilateral Breast, Percutaneous Approach, Diagnostic
0HBV3ZZ Excision of Bilateral Breast, Percutaneous Approach
0HBV7ZX Excision of Bilateral Breast, Via Natural or Artificial Opening, Diagnostic
0HBV7ZZ Excision of Bilateral Breast, Via Natural or Artificial Opening
0HBV8ZX Excision of Bilateral Breast, Via Natural or Artificial Opening Endoscopic, Diagnostic
0HBV8ZZ Excision of Bilateral Breast, Via Natural or Artificial Opening Endoscopic
0HBVXZX Excision of Bilateral Breast, External Approach, Diagnostic
0HBVXZZ Excision of Bilateral Breast, External Approach
0HBW0ZX Excision of Right Nipple, Open Approach, Diagnostic
0HBW0ZZ Excision of Right Nipple, Open Approach
0HBW3ZX Excision of Right Nipple, Percutaneous Approach, Diagnostic
0HBW3ZZ Excision of Right Nipple, Percutaneous Approach
0HBW7ZX Excision of Right Nipple, Via Natural or Artificial Opening, Diagnostic
0HBW7ZZ Excision of Right Nipple, Via Natural or Artificial Opening
0HBW8ZX Excision of Right Nipple, Via Natural or Artificial Opening Endoscopic, Diagnostic
0HBW8ZZ Excision of Right Nipple, Via Natural or Artificial Opening Endoscopic
0HBWXZX Excision of Right Nipple, External Approach, Diagnostic
0HBWXZZ Excision of Right Nipple, External Approach
0HBX0ZX Excision of Left Nipple, Open Approach, Diagnostic
0HBX0ZZ Excision of Left Nipple, Open Approach
0HBX3ZX Excision of Left Nipple, Percutaneous Approach, Diagnostic
0HBX3ZZ Excision of Left Nipple, Percutaneous Approach
0HBX7ZX Excision of Left Nipple, Via Natural or Artificial Opening, Diagnostic
0HBX7ZZ Excision of Left Nipple, Via Natural or Artificial Opening
0HBX8ZX Excision of Left Nipple, Via Natural or Artificial Opening Endoscopic, Diagnostic
0HBX8ZZ Excision of Left Nipple, Via Natural or Artificial Opening Endoscopic
0HBXXZX Excision of Left Nipple, External Approach, Diagnostic
0HBXXZZ Excision of Left Nipple, External Approach
0HBY0ZX Excision of Supernumerary Breast, Open Approach, Diagnostic
0HBY0ZZ Excision of Supernumerary Breast, Open Approach
0HBY3ZX Excision of Supernumerary Breast, Percutaneous Approach, Diagnostic
0HBY3ZZ Excision of Supernumerary Breast, Percutaneous Approach
0HBY7ZX Excision of Supernumerary Breast, Via Natural or Artificial Opening, Diagnostic
0HBY7ZZ Excision of Supernumerary Breast, Via Natural or Artificial Opening
0HBY8ZX Excision of Supernumerary Breast, Via Natural or Artificial Opening Endoscopic, Diagnostic
0HBY8ZZ Excision of Supernumerary Breast, Via Natural or Artificial Opening Endoscopic
0HBYXZX Excision of Supernumerary Breast, External Approach, Diagnostic
0HBYXZZ Excision of Supernumerary Breast, External Approach

0HC – Skin and Breast, Extirpation

0HC0XZZ Extirpation of Matter from Scalp Skin, External Approach
0HC1XZZ Extirpation of Matter from Face Skin, External Approach
0HC2XZZ Extirpation of Matter from Right Ear Skin, External Approach
0HC3XZZ Extirpation of Matter from Left Ear Skin, External Approach
0HC4XZZ Extirpation of Matter from Neck Skin, External Approach
0HC5XZZ Extirpation of Matter from Chest Skin, External Approach
0HC6XZZ Extirpation of Matter from Back Skin, External Approach
0HC7XZZ Extirpation of Matter from Abdomen Skin, External Approach
0HC8XZZ Extirpation of Matter from Buttock Skin, External Approach
0HC9XZZ Extirpation of Matter from Perineum Skin, External Approach
0HCAXZZ Extirpation of Matter from Genitalia Skin, External Approach

0HCBXZZ Extirpation of Matter from Right Upper Arm Skin, External Approach
0HCCXZZ Extirpation of Matter from Left Upper Arm Skin, External Approach
0HCDXZZ Extirpation of Matter from Right Lower Arm Skin, External Approach
0HCEXZZ Extirpation of Matter from Left Lower Arm Skin, External Approach
0HCFXZZ Extirpation of Matter from Right Hand Skin, External Approach
0HCGXZZ Extirpation of Matter from Left Hand Skin, External Approach

0HCHXZZ Extirpation of Matter from Right Upper Leg Skin, External Approach

0HCJXZZ Extirpation of Matter from Left Upper Leg Skin, External Approach

0HCKXZZ Extirpation of Matter from Right Lower Leg Skin, External Approach

0HCLXZZ Extirpation of Matter from Left Lower Leg Skin, External Approach

0HCMXZZ Extirpation of Matter from Right Foot Skin, External Approach

0HCNXZZ Extirpation of Matter from Left Foot Skin, External Approach

0HCQXZZ Extirpation of Matter from Finger Nail, External Approach

0HCRXZZ Extirpation of Matter from Toe Nail, External Approach

0HCT0ZZ Extirpation of Matter from Right Breast, Open Approach

0HCT3ZZ Extirpation of Matter from Right Breast, Percutaneous Approach

0HCT7ZZ Extirpation of Matter from Right Breast, Via Natural or Artificial Opening

0HCT8ZZ Extirpation of Matter from Right Breast, Via Natural or Artificial Opening Endoscopic

0HCTXZZ Extirpation of Matter from Right Breast, External Approach

0HCU0ZZ Extirpation of Matter from Left Breast, Open Approach

0HCU3ZZ Extirpation of Matter from Left Breast, Percutaneous Approach

0HCU7ZZ Extirpation of Matter from Left Breast, Via Natural or Artificial Opening

0HCU8ZZ Extirpation of Matter from Left Breast, Via Natural or Artificial Opening Endoscopic

0HCUXZZ Extirpation of Matter from Left Breast, External Approach

0HCV0ZZ Extirpation of Matter from Bilateral Breast, Open Approach

0HCV3ZZ Extirpation of Matter from Bilateral Breast, Percutaneous Approach

0HCV7ZZ Extirpation of Matter from Bilateral Breast, Via Natural or Artificial Opening

0HCV8ZZ Extirpation of Matter from Bilateral Breast, Via Natural or Artificial Opening Endoscopic

0HCVXZZ Extirpation of Matter from Bilateral Breast, External Approach

0HCW0ZZ Extirpation of Matter from Right Nipple, Open Approach

0HCW3ZZ Extirpation of Matter from Right Nipple, Percutaneous Approach

0HCW7ZZ Extirpation of Matter from Right Nipple, Via Natural or Artificial Opening

0HCW8ZZ Extirpation of Matter from Right Nipple, Via Natural or Artificial Opening Endoscopic

0HCWXZZ Extirpation of Matter from Right Nipple, External Approach

0HCX0ZZ Extirpation of Matter from Left Nipple, Open Approach

0HCX3ZZ Extirpation of Matter from Left Nipple, Percutaneous Approach

0HCX7ZZ Extirpation of Matter from Left Nipple, Via Natural or Artificial Opening

0HCX8ZZ Extirpation of Matter from Left Nipple, Via Natural or Artificial Opening Endoscopic

0HCXXZZ Extirpation of Matter from Left Nipple, External Approach

0HD – Skin and Breast, Extraction

0HD0XZZ Extraction of Scalp Skin, External Approach

0HD1XZZ Extraction of Face Skin, External Approach

0HD2XZZ Extraction of Right Ear Skin, External Approach

0HD3XZZ Extraction of Left Ear Skin, External Approach

0HD4XZZ Extraction of Neck Skin, External Approach

0HD5XZZ Extraction of Chest Skin, External Approach

0HD6XZZ Extraction of Back Skin, External Approach

0HD7XZZ Extraction of Abdomen Skin, External Approach

0HD8XZZ Extraction of Buttock Skin, External Approach

0HD9XZZ Extraction of Perineum Skin, External Approach

0HDAXZZ Extraction of Genitalia Skin, External Approach

0HDBXZZ Extraction of Right Upper Arm Skin, External Approach

0HDCXZZ Extraction of Left Upper Arm Skin, External Approach

0HDDXZZ Extraction of Right Lower Arm Skin, External Approach

0HDEXZZ Extraction of Left Lower Arm Skin, External Approach

0HDFXZZ Extraction of Right Hand Skin, External Approach

0HDGXZZ Extraction of Left Hand Skin, External Approach

0HDHXZZ Extraction of Right Upper Leg Skin, External Approach

0HDJXZZ Extraction of Left Upper Leg Skin, External Approach

0HDKXZZ Extraction of Right Lower Leg Skin, External Approach

0HDLXZZ Extraction of Left Lower Leg Skin, External Approach

0HDMXZZ Extraction of Right Foot Skin, External Approach

0HDNXZZ Extraction of Left Foot Skin, External Approach

0HDQXZZ Extraction of Finger Nail, External Approach

0HDRXZZ Extraction of Toe Nail, External Approach

0HDSXZZ Extraction of Hair, External Approach

0HH – Skin and Breast, Insertion

0HHT01Z Insertion of Radioactive Element into Right Breast, Open Approach

0HHT0NZ Insertion of Tissue Expander into Right Breast, Open Approach

0HHT31Z Insertion of Radioactive Element into Right Breast, Percutaneous Approach

0HHT3NZ Insertion of Tissue Expander into Right Breast, Percutaneous Approach

0HHT71Z Insertion of Radioactive Element into Right Breast, Via Natural or Artificial Opening

0HHT7NZ Insertion of Tissue Expander into Right Breast, Via Natural or Artificial Opening

0HHT81Z Insertion of Radioactive Element into Right Breast, Via Natural or Artificial Opening Endoscopic

0HHT8NZ Insertion of Tissue Expander into Right Breast, Via Natural or Artificial Opening Endoscopic

0HHTX1Z Insertion of Radioactive Element into Right Breast, External Approach

0HHU01Z Insertion of Radioactive Element into Left Breast, Open Approach

0HHU0NZ Insertion of Tissue Expander into Left Breast, Open Approach

0HHU31Z Insertion of Radioactive Element into Left Breast, Percutaneous Approach

0HHU3NZ Insertion of Tissue Expander into Left Breast, Percutaneous Approach

0HHU71Z Insertion of Radioactive Element into Left Breast, Via Natural or Artificial Opening

0HHU7NZ Insertion of Tissue Expander into Left Breast, Via Natural or Artificial Opening

0HHU81Z Insertion of Radioactive Element into Left Breast, Via Natural or Artificial Opening Endoscopic

0HHU8NZ Insertion of Tissue Expander into Left Breast, Via Natural or Artificial Opening Endoscopic

0HHUX1Z Insertion of Radioactive Element into Left Breast, External Approach

0HHV01Z Insertion of Radioactive Element into Bilateral Breast, Open Approach

0HHV0NZ Insertion of Tissue Expander into Bilateral Breast, Open Approach

0HHV31Z Insertion of Radioactive Element into Bilateral Breast, Percutaneous Approach

0HHV3NZ Insertion of Tissue Expander into Bilateral Breast, Percutaneous Approach

0HHV71Z Insertion of Radioactive Element into Bilateral Breast, Via Natural or Artificial Opening

0HHV7NZ Insertion of Tissue Expander into Bilateral Breast, Via Natural or Artificial Opening

0HHV81Z Insertion of Radioactive Element into Bilateral Breast, Via Natural or Artificial Opening Endoscopic

0HHV8NZ Insertion of Tissue Expander into Bilateral Breast, Via Natural or Artificial Opening Endoscopic

0HHVX1Z Insertion of Radioactive Element into Bilateral Breast, External Approach

0HHW01Z Insertion of Radioactive Element into Right Nipple, Open Approach

0HHW0NZ Insertion of Tissue Expander into Right Nipple, Open Approach

0HHW31Z Insertion of Radioactive Element into Right Nipple, Percutaneous Approach

0HHW3NZ Insertion of Tissue Expander into Right Nipple, Percutaneous Approach

0HHW71Z Insertion of Radioactive Element into Right Nipple, Via Natural or Artificial Opening

0HHW7NZ Insertion of Tissue Expander into Right Nipple, Via Natural or Artificial Opening

0HHW81Z Insertion of Radioactive Element into Right Nipple, Via Natural or Artificial Opening Endoscopic

0HHW8NZ Insertion of Tissue Expander into Right Nipple, Via Natural or Artificial Opening Endoscopic

0HHWX1Z Insertion of Radioactive Element into Right Nipple, External Approach

0HHX01Z Insertion of Radioactive Element into Left Nipple, Open Approach

0HHX0NZ Insertion of Tissue Expander into Left Nipple, Open Approach

0HHX31Z Insertion of Radioactive Element into Left Nipple, Percutaneous Approach
0HHX3NZ Insertion of Tissue Expander into Left Nipple, Percutaneous Approach
0HHX71Z Insertion of Radioactive Element into Left Nipple, Via Natural or Artificial Opening
0HHX7NZ Insertion of Tissue Expander into Left Nipple, Via Natural or Artificial Opening

0HHX81Z Insertion of Radioactive Element into Left Nipple, Via Natural or Artificial Opening Endoscopic
0HHX8NZ Insertion of Tissue Expander into Left Nipple, Via Natural or Artificial Opening Endoscopic
0HHXX1Z Insertion of Radioactive Element into Left Nipple, External Approach

0HJ – Skin and Breast, Inspection

Review Coding Guideline B3.5

Review Coding Guidelines B3.11a, B3.11b and B3.11c

0HJPXZZ Inspection of Skin, External Approach
0HJQXZZ Inspection of Finger Nail, External Approach
0HJRXZZ Inspection of Toe Nail, External Approach
0HJT0ZZ Inspection of Right Breast, Open Approach
0HJT3ZZ Inspection of Right Breast, Percutaneous Approach
0HJT7ZZ Inspection of Right Breast, Via Natural or Artificial Opening
0HJT8ZZ Inspection of Right Breast, Via Natural or Artificial Opening Endoscopic

0HJTXZZ Inspection of Right Breast, External Approach
0HJU0ZZ Inspection of Left Breast, Open Approach
0HJU3ZZ Inspection of Left Breast, Percutaneous Approach
0HJU7ZZ Inspection of Left Breast, Via Natural or Artificial Opening
0HJU8ZZ Inspection of Left Breast, Via Natural or Artificial Opening Endoscopic
0HJUXZZ Inspection of Left Breast, External Approach

0HM – Skin and Breast, Reattachment

0HM0XZZ Reattachment of Scalp Skin, External Approach
0HM1XZZ Reattachment of Face Skin, External Approach
0HM2XZZ Reattachment of Right Ear Skin, External Approach
0HM3XZZ Reattachment of Left Ear Skin, External Approach
0HM4XZZ Reattachment of Neck Skin, External Approach
0HM5XZZ Reattachment of Chest Skin, External Approach
0HM6XZZ Reattachment of Back Skin, External Approach
0HM7XZZ Reattachment of Abdomen Skin, External Approach
0HM8XZZ Reattachment of Buttock Skin, External Approach
0HM9XZZ Reattachment of Perineum Skin, External Approach
0HMAXZZ Reattachment of Genitalia Skin, External Approach
0HMBXZZ Reattachment of Right Upper Arm Skin, External Approach
0HMCXZZ Reattachment of Left Upper Arm Skin, External Approach
0HMDXZZ Reattachment of Right Lower Arm Skin, External Approach

0HMEXZZ Reattachment of Left Lower Arm Skin, External Approach
0HMFXZZ Reattachment of Right Hand Skin, External Approach
0HMGXZZ Reattachment of Left Hand Skin, External Approach
0HMHXZZ Reattachment of Right Upper Leg Skin, External Approach
0HMJXZZ Reattachment of Left Upper Leg Skin, External Approach
0HMKXZZ Reattachment of Right Lower Leg Skin, External Approach
0HMLXZZ Reattachment of Left Lower Leg Skin, External Approach
0HMMXZZ Reattachment of Right Foot Skin, External Approach
0HMNXZZ Reattachment of Left Foot Skin, External Approach
0HMTXZZ Reattachment of Right Breast, External Approach
0HMUXZZ Reattachment of Left Breast, External Approach
0HMVXZZ Reattachment of Bilateral Breast, External Approach
0HMWXZZ Reattachment of Right Nipple, External Approach
0HMXXZZ Reattachment of Left Nipple, External Approach

0HN – Skin and Breast, Release

Review Coding Guideline B3.13

Review Coding Guideline B3.14

0HN0XZZ Release Scalp Skin, External Approach
0HN1XZZ Release Face Skin, External Approach
0HN2XZZ Release Right Ear Skin, External Approach
0HN3XZZ Release Left Ear Skin, External Approach
0HN4XZZ Release Neck Skin, External Approach
0HN5XZZ Release Chest Skin, External Approach
0HN6XZZ Release Back Skin, External Approach
0HN7XZZ Release Abdomen Skin, External Approach
0HN8XZZ Release Buttock Skin, External Approach
0HN9XZZ Release Perineum Skin, External Approach
0HNAXZZ Release Genitalia Skin, External Approach
0HNBXZZ Release Right Upper Arm Skin, External Approach
0HNCXZZ Release Left Upper Arm Skin, External Approach
0HNDXZZ Release Right Lower Arm Skin, External Approach
0HNEXZZ Release Left Lower Arm Skin, External Approach
0HNFXZZ Release Right Hand Skin, External Approach
0HNGXZZ Release Left Hand Skin, External Approach
0HNHXZZ Release Right Upper Leg Skin, External Approach
0HNJXZZ Release Left Upper Leg Skin, External Approach
0HNKXZZ Release Right Lower Leg Skin, External Approach
0HNLXZZ Release Left Lower Leg Skin, External Approach
0HNMXZZ Release Right Foot Skin, External Approach
0HNNXZZ Release Left Foot Skin, External Approach
0HNQXZZ Release Finger Nail, External Approach
0HNRXZZ Release Toe Nail, External Approach

0HNT0ZZ Release Right Breast, Open Approach
0HNT3ZZ Release Right Breast, Percutaneous Approach
0HNT7ZZ Release Right Breast, Via Natural or Artificial Opening
0HNT8ZZ Release Right Breast, Via Natural or Artificial Opening Endoscopic
0HNTXZZ Release Right Breast, External Approach
0HNU0ZZ Release Left Breast, Open Approach
0HNU3ZZ Release Left Breast, Percutaneous Approach
0HNU7ZZ Release Left Breast, Via Natural or Artificial Opening
0HNU8ZZ Release Left Breast, Via Natural or Artificial Opening Endoscopic
0HNUXZZ Release Left Breast, External Approach
0HNV0ZZ Release Bilateral Breast, Open Approach
0HNV3ZZ Release Bilateral Breast, Percutaneous Approach
0HNV7ZZ Release Bilateral Breast, Via Natural or Artificial Opening
0HNV8ZZ Release Bilateral Breast, Via Natural or Artificial Opening Endoscopic
0HNVXZZ Release Bilateral Breast, External Approach
0HNW0ZZ Release Right Nipple, Open Approach
0HNW3ZZ Release Right Nipple, Percutaneous Approach
0HNW7ZZ Release Right Nipple, Via Natural or Artificial Opening
0HNW8ZZ Release Right Nipple, Via Natural or Artificial Opening Endoscopic
0HNWXZZ Release Right Nipple, External Approach
0HNX0ZZ Release Left Nipple, Open Approach
0HNX3ZZ Release Left Nipple, Percutaneous Approach
0HNX7ZZ Release Left Nipple, Via Natural or Artificial Opening
0HNX8ZZ Release Left Nipple, Via Natural or Artificial Opening Endoscopic
0HNXXZZ Release Left Nipple, External Approach

0HP – Skin and Breast, Removal

Review Coding Guideline B6.1c

0HPPX0Z Removal of Drainage Device from Skin, External Approach
0HPPX7Z Removal of Autologous Tissue Substitute from Skin, External Approach
0HPPXJZ Removal of Synthetic Substitute from Skin, External Approach
0HPPXKZ Removal of Nonautologous Tissue Substitute from Skin, External Approach
0HPQX0Z Removal of Drainage Device from Finger Nail, External Approach
0HPQX7Z Removal of Autologous Tissue Substitute from Finger Nail, External Approach
0HPQXJZ Removal of Synthetic Substitute from Finger Nail, External Approach
0HPQXKZ Removal of Nonautologous Tissue Substitute from Finger Nail, External Approach
0HPRX0Z Removal of Drainage Device from Toe Nail, External Approach
0HPRX7Z Removal of Autologous Tissue Substitute from Toe Nail, External Approach
0HPRXJZ Removal of Synthetic Substitute from Toe Nail, External Approach
0HPRXKZ Removal of Nonautologous Tissue Substitute from Toe Nail, External Approach
0HPSX7Z Removal of Autologous Tissue Substitute from Hair, External Approach
0HPSXJZ Removal of Synthetic Substitute from Hair, External Approach
0HPSXKZ Removal of Nonautologous Tissue Substitute from Hair, External Approach
0HPT00Z Removal of Drainage Device from Right Breast, Open Approach
0HPT01Z Removal of Radioactive Element from Right Breast, Open Approach
0HPT07Z Removal of Autologous Tissue Substitute from Right Breast, Open Approach
0HPT0JZ Removal of Synthetic Substitute from Right Breast, Open Approach
0HPT0KZ Removal of Nonautologous Tissue Substitute from Right Breast, Open Approach
0HPT0NZ Removal of Tissue Expander from Right Breast, Open Approach
0HPT30Z Removal of Drainage Device from Right Breast, Percutaneous Approach
0HPT31Z Removal of Radioactive Element from Right Breast, Percutaneous Approach
0HPT37Z Removal of Autologous Tissue Substitute from Right Breast, Percutaneous Approach
0HPT3JZ Removal of Synthetic Substitute from Right Breast, Percutaneous Approach
0HPT3KZ Removal of Nonautologous Tissue Substitute from Right Breast, Percutaneous Approach
0HPT3NZ Removal of Tissue Expander from Right Breast, Percutaneous Approach
0HPT70Z Removal of Drainage Device from Right Breast, Via Natural or Artificial Opening
0HPT71Z Removal of Radioactive Element from Right Breast, Via Natural or Artificial Opening
0HPT77Z Removal of Autologous Tissue Substitute from Right Breast, Via Natural or Artificial Opening
0HPT7JZ Removal of Synthetic Substitute from Right Breast, Via Natural or Artificial Opening
0HPT7KZ Removal of Nonautologous Tissue Substitute from Right Breast, Via Natural or Artificial Opening
0HPT7NZ Removal of Tissue Expander from Right Breast, Via Natural or Artificial Opening
0HPT80Z Removal of Drainage Device from Right Breast, Via Natural or Artificial Opening Endoscopic
0HPT81Z Removal of Radioactive Element from Right Breast, Via Natural or Artificial Opening Endoscopic
0HPT87Z Removal of Autologous Tissue Substitute from Right Breast, Via Natural or Artificial Opening Endoscopic
0HPT8JZ Removal of Synthetic Substitute from Right Breast, Via Natural or Artificial Opening Endoscopic

0HPT8KZ Removal of Nonautologous Tissue Substitute from Right Breast, Via Natural or Artificial Opening Endoscopic
0HPT8NZ Removal of Tissue Expander from Right Breast, Via Natural or Artificial Opening Endoscopic
0HPTX0Z Removal of Drainage Device from Right Breast, External Approach
0HPTX1Z Removal of Radioactive Element from Right Breast, External Approach
0HPTX7Z Removal of Autologous Tissue Substitute from Right Breast, External Approach
0HPTXJZ Removal of Synthetic Substitute from Right Breast, External Approach
0HPTXKZ Removal of Nonautologous Tissue Substitute from Right Breast, External Approach
0HPU00Z Removal of Drainage Device from Left Breast, Open Approach
0HPU01Z Removal of Radioactive Element from Left Breast, Open Approach
0HPU07Z Removal of Autologous Tissue Substitute from Left Breast, Open Approach
0HPU0JZ Removal of Synthetic Substitute from Left Breast, Open Approach
0HPU0KZ Removal of Nonautologous Tissue Substitute from Left Breast, Open Approach
0HPU0NZ Removal of Tissue Expander from Left Breast, Open Approach
0HPU30Z Removal of Drainage Device from Left Breast, Percutaneous Approach
0HPU31Z Removal of Radioactive Element from Left Breast, Percutaneous Approach
0HPU37Z Removal of Autologous Tissue Substitute from Left Breast, Percutaneous Approach
0HPU3JZ Removal of Synthetic Substitute from Left Breast, Percutaneous Approach
0HPU3KZ Removal of Nonautologous Tissue Substitute from Left Breast, Percutaneous Approach
0HPU3NZ Removal of Tissue Expander from Left Breast, Percutaneous Approach
0HPU70Z Removal of Drainage Device from Left Breast, Via Natural or Artificial Opening
0HPU71Z Removal of Radioactive Element from Left Breast, Via Natural or Artificial Opening
0HPU77Z Removal of Autologous Tissue Substitute from Left Breast, Via Natural or Artificial Opening
0HPU7JZ Removal of Synthetic Substitute from Left Breast, Via Natural or Artificial Opening
0HPU7KZ Removal of Nonautologous Tissue Substitute from Left Breast, Via Natural or Artificial Opening
0HPU7NZ Removal of Tissue Expander from Left Breast, Via Natural or Artificial Opening
0HPU80Z Removal of Drainage Device from Left Breast, Via Natural or Artificial Opening Endoscopic
0HPU81Z Removal of Radioactive Element from Left Breast, Via Natural or Artificial Opening Endoscopic
0HPU87Z Removal of Autologous Tissue Substitute from Left Breast, Via Natural or Artificial Opening Endoscopic
0HPU8JZ Removal of Synthetic Substitute from Left Breast, Via Natural or Artificial Opening Endoscopic
0HPU8KZ Removal of Nonautologous Tissue Substitute from Left Breast, Via Natural or Artificial Opening Endoscopic
0HPU8NZ Removal of Tissue Expander from Left Breast, Via Natural or Artificial Opening Endoscopic
0HPUX0Z Removal of Drainage Device from Left Breast, External Approach
0HPUX1Z Removal of Radioactive Element from Left Breast, External Approach
0HPUX7Z Removal of Autologous Tissue Substitute from Left Breast, External Approach
0HPUXJZ Removal of Synthetic Substitute from Left Breast, External Approach
0HPUXKZ Removal of Nonautologous Tissue Substitute from Left Breast, External Approach

0HQ – Skin and Breast, Repair

Review Coding Guideline B3.5

0HQ0XZZ Repair Scalp Skin, External Approach
0HQ1XZZ Repair Face Skin, External Approach
0HQ2XZZ Repair Right Ear Skin, External Approach
0HQ3XZZ Repair Left Ear Skin, External Approach

0HQ4XZZ	Repair Neck Skin, External Approach
0HQ5XZZ	Repair Chest Skin, External Approach
0HQ6XZZ	Repair Back Skin, External Approach
0HQ7XZZ	Repair Abdomen Skin, External Approach
0HQ8XZZ	Repair Buttock Skin, External Approach
● 0HQ9XZZ	Repair Perineum Skin, External Approach
0HQAXZZ	Repair Genitalia Skin, External Approach
0HQBXZZ	Repair Right Upper Arm Skin, External Approach
0HQCXZZ	Repair Left Upper Arm Skin, External Approach
0HQDXZZ	Repair Right Lower Arm Skin, External Approach
0HQEXZZ	Repair Left Lower Arm Skin, External Approach
0HQFXZZ	Repair Right Hand Skin, External Approach
0HQGXZZ	Repair Left Hand Skin, External Approach
0HQHXZZ	Repair Right Upper Leg Skin, External Approach
0HQJXZZ	Repair Left Upper Leg Skin, External Approach
0HQKXZZ	Repair Right Lower Leg Skin, External Approach
0HQLXZZ	Repair Left Lower Leg Skin, External Approach
0HQMXZZ	Repair Right Foot Skin, External Approach
0HQNXZZ	Repair Left Foot Skin, External Approach
0HQQXZZ	Repair Finger Nail, External Approach
0HQRXZZ	Repair Toe Nail, External Approach
0HQT0ZZ	Repair Right Breast, Open Approach
0HQT3ZZ	Repair Right Breast, Percutaneous Approach
0HQT7ZZ	Repair Right Breast, Via Natural or Artificial Opening
0HQT8ZZ	Repair Right Breast, Via Natural or Artificial Opening Endoscopic
0HQTXZZ	Repair Right Breast, External Approach
0HQU0ZZ	Repair Left Breast, Open Approach
0HQU3ZZ	Repair Left Breast, Percutaneous Approach
0HQU7ZZ	Repair Left Breast, Via Natural or Artificial Opening
0HQU8ZZ	Repair Left Breast, Via Natural or Artificial Opening Endoscopic
0HQUXZZ	Repair Left Breast, External Approach
0HQV0ZZ	Repair Bilateral Breast, Open Approach
0HQV3ZZ	Repair Bilateral Breast, Percutaneous Approach
0HQV7ZZ	Repair Bilateral Breast, Via Natural or Artificial Opening
0HQV8ZZ	Repair Bilateral Breast, Via Natural or Artificial Opening Endoscopic
0HQVXZZ	Repair Bilateral Breast, External Approach
0HQW0ZZ	Repair Right Nipple, Open Approach
0HQW3ZZ	Repair Right Nipple, Percutaneous Approach
0HQW7ZZ	Repair Right Nipple, Via Natural or Artificial Opening
0HQW8ZZ	Repair Right Nipple, Via Natural or Artificial Opening Endoscopic
0HQWXZZ	Repair Right Nipple, External Approach
0HQX0ZZ	Repair Left Nipple, Open Approach
0HQX3ZZ	Repair Left Nipple, Percutaneous Approach
0HQX7ZZ	Repair Left Nipple, Via Natural or Artificial Opening
0HQX8ZZ	Repair Left Nipple, Via Natural or Artificial Opening Endoscopic
0HQXXZZ	Repair Left Nipple, External Approach
0HQY0ZZ	Repair Supernumerary Breast, Open Approach
0HQY3ZZ	Repair Supernumerary Breast, Percutaneous Approach
0HQY7ZZ	Repair Supernumerary Breast, Via Natural or Artificial Opening
0HQY8ZZ	Repair Supernumerary Breast, Via Natural or Artificial Opening Endoscopic
0HQYXZZ	Repair Supernumerary Breast, External Approach

0HR – Skin and Breast, Replacement

0HR0X73	Replacement of Scalp Skin with Autologous Tissue Substitute, Full Thickness, External Approach
0HR0X74	Replacement of Scalp Skin with Autologous Tissue Substitute, Partial Thickness, External Approach
0HR0XJ3	Replacement of Scalp Skin with Synthetic Substitute, Full Thickness, External Approach
0HR0XJ4	Replacement of Scalp Skin with Synthetic Substitute, Partial Thickness, External Approach
0HR0XJZ	Replacement of Scalp Skin with Synthetic Substitute, External Approach
0HR0XK3	Replacement of Scalp Skin with Nonautologous Tissue Substitute, Full Thickness, External Approach
0HR0XK4	Replacement of Scalp Skin with Nonautologous Tissue Substitute, Partial Thickness, External Approach
0HR1X73	Replacement of Face Skin with Autologous Tissue Substitute, Full Thickness, External Approach
0HR1X74	Replacement of Face Skin with Autologous Tissue Substitute, Partial Thickness, External Approach
0HR1XJ3	Replacement of Face Skin with Synthetic Substitute, Full Thickness, External Approach
0HR1XJ4	Replacement of Face Skin with Synthetic Substitute, Partial Thickness, External Approach
0HR1XJZ	Replacement of Face Skin with Synthetic Substitute, External Approach
0HR1XK3	Replacement of Face Skin with Nonautologous Tissue Substitute, Full Thickness, External Approach
0HR1XK4	Replacement of Face Skin with Nonautologous Tissue Substitute, Partial Thickness, External Approach
0HR2X73	Replacement of Right Ear Skin with Autologous Tissue Substitute, Full Thickness, External Approach
0HR2X74	Replacement of Right Ear Skin with Autologous Tissue Substitute, Partial Thickness, External Approach
0HR2XJ3	Replacement of Right Ear Skin with Synthetic Substitute, Full Thickness, External Approach
0HR2XJ4	Replacement of Right Ear Skin with Synthetic Substitute, Partial Thickness, External Approach
0HR2XJZ	Replacement of Right Ear Skin with Synthetic Substitute, External Approach
0HR2XK3	Replacement of Right Ear Skin with Nonautologous Tissue Substitute, Full Thickness, External Approach
0HR2XK4	Replacement of Right Ear Skin with Nonautologous Tissue Substitute, Partial Thickness, External Approach
0HR3X73	Replacement of Left Ear Skin with Autologous Tissue Substitute, Full Thickness, External Approach
0HR3X74	Replacement of Left Ear Skin with Autologous Tissue Substitute, Partial Thickness, External Approach
0HR3XJ3	Replacement of Left Ear Skin with Synthetic Substitute, Full Thickness, External Approach
0HR3XJ4	Replacement of Left Ear Skin with Synthetic Substitute, Partial Thickness, External Approach
0HR3XJZ	Replacement of Left Ear Skin with Synthetic Substitute, External Approach
0HR3XK3	Replacement of Left Ear Skin with Nonautologous Tissue Substitute, Full Thickness, External Approach
0HR3XK4	Replacement of Left Ear Skin with Nonautologous Tissue Substitute, Partial Thickness, External Approach
0HR4X73	Replacement of Neck Skin with Autologous Tissue Substitute, Full Thickness, External Approach
0HR4X74	Replacement of Neck Skin with Autologous Tissue Substitute, Partial Thickness, External Approach
0HR4XJ3	Replacement of Neck Skin with Synthetic Substitute, Full Thickness, External Approach
0HR4XJ4	Replacement of Neck Skin with Synthetic Substitute, Partial Thickness, External Approach
0HR4XJZ	Replacement of Neck Skin with Synthetic Substitute, External Approach
0HR4XK3	Replacement of Neck Skin with Nonautologous Tissue Substitute, Full Thickness, External Approach
0HR4XK4	Replacement of Neck Skin with Nonautologous Tissue Substitute, Partial Thickness, External Approach
0HR5X73	Replacement of Chest Skin with Autologous Tissue Substitute, Full Thickness, External Approach
0HR5X74	Replacement of Chest Skin with Autologous Tissue Substitute, Partial Thickness, External Approach
0HR5XJ3	Replacement of Chest Skin with Synthetic Substitute, Full Thickness, External Approach
0HR5XJ4	Replacement of Chest Skin with Synthetic Substitute, Partial Thickness, External Approach
0HR5XJZ	Replacement of Chest Skin with Synthetic Substitute, External Approach
0HR5XK3	Replacement of Chest Skin with Nonautologous Tissue Substitute, Full Thickness, External Approach
0HR5XK4	Replacement of Chest Skin with Nonautologous Tissue Substitute, Partial Thickness, External Approach
0HR6X73	Replacement of Back Skin with Autologous Tissue Substitute, Full Thickness, External Approach
0HR6X74	Replacement of Back Skin with Autologous Tissue Substitute, Partial Thickness, External Approach

0HR6XJ3 Replacement of Back Skin with Synthetic Substitute, Full Thickness, External Approach

0HR6XJ4 Replacement of Back Skin with Synthetic Substitute, Partial Thickness, External Approach

0HR6XJZ Replacement of Back Skin with Synthetic Substitute, External Approach

0HR6XK3 Replacement of Back Skin with Nonautologous Tissue Substitute, Full Thickness, External Approach

0HR6XK4 Replacement of Back Skin with Nonautologous Tissue Substitute, Partial Thickness, External Approach

0HR7X73 Replacement of Abdomen Skin with Autologous Tissue Substitute, Full Thickness, External Approach

0HR7X74 Replacement of Abdomen Skin with Autologous Tissue Substitute, Partial Thickness, External Approach

0HR7XJ3 Replacement of Abdomen Skin with Synthetic Substitute, Full Thickness, External Approach

0HR7XJ4 Replacement of Abdomen Skin with Synthetic Substitute, Partial Thickness, External Approach

0HR7XJZ Replacement of Abdomen Skin with Synthetic Substitute, External Approach

0HR7XK3 Replacement of Abdomen Skin with Nonautologous Tissue Substitute, Full Thickness, External Approach

0HR7XK4 Replacement of Abdomen Skin with Nonautologous Tissue Substitute, Partial Thickness, External Approach

0HR8X73 Replacement of Buttock Skin with Autologous Tissue Substitute, Full Thickness, External Approach

0HR8X74 Replacement of Buttock Skin with Autologous Tissue Substitute, Partial Thickness, External Approach

0HR8XJ3 Replacement of Buttock Skin with Synthetic Substitute, Full Thickness, External Approach

0HR8XJ4 Replacement of Buttock Skin with Synthetic Substitute, Partial Thickness, External Approach

0HR8XJZ Replacement of Buttock Skin with Synthetic Substitute, External Approach

0HR8XK3 Replacement of Buttock Skin with Nonautologous Tissue Substitute, Full Thickness, External Approach

0HR8XK4 Replacement of Buttock Skin with Nonautologous Tissue Substitute, Partial Thickness, External Approach

0HR9X73 Replacement of Perineum Skin with Autologous Tissue Substitute, Full Thickness, External Approach

0HR9X74 Replacement of Perineum Skin with Autologous Tissue Substitute, Partial Thickness, External Approach

0HR9XJ3 Replacement of Perineum Skin with Synthetic Substitute, Full Thickness, External Approach

0HR9XJ4 Replacement of Perineum Skin with Synthetic Substitute, Partial Thickness, External Approach

0HR9XJZ Replacement of Perineum Skin with Synthetic Substitute, External Approach

0HR9XK3 Replacement of Perineum Skin with Nonautologous Tissue Substitute, Full Thickness, External Approach

0HR9XK4 Replacement of Perineum Skin with Nonautologous Tissue Substitute, Partial Thickness, External Approach

0HRAX73 Replacement of Genitalia Skin with Autologous Tissue Substitute, Full Thickness, External Approach

0HRAX74 Replacement of Genitalia Skin with Autologous Tissue Substitute, Partial Thickness, External Approach

0HRAXJ3 Replacement of Genitalia Skin with Synthetic Substitute, Full Thickness, External Approach

0HRAXJ4 Replacement of Genitalia Skin with Synthetic Substitute, Partial Thickness, External Approach

0HRAXJZ Replacement of Genitalia Skin with Synthetic Substitute, External Approach

0HRAXK3 Replacement of Genitalia Skin with Nonautologous Tissue Substitute, Full Thickness, External Approach

0HRAXK4 Replacement of Genitalia Skin with Nonautologous Tissue Substitute, Partial Thickness, External Approach

0HRBX73 Replacement of Right Upper Arm Skin with Autologous Tissue Substitute, Full Thickness, External Approach

0HRBX74 Replacement of Right Upper Arm Skin with Autologous Tissue Substitute, Partial Thickness, External Approach

0HRBXJ3 Replacement of Right Upper Arm Skin with Synthetic Substitute, Full Thickness, External Approach

0HRBXJ4 Replacement of Right Upper Arm Skin with Synthetic Substitute, Partial Thickness, External Approach

0HRBXJZ Replacement of Right Upper Arm Skin with Synthetic Substitute, External Approach

0HRBXK3 Replacement of Right Upper Arm Skin with Nonautologous Tissue Substitute, Full Thickness, External Approach

0HRBXK4 Replacement of Right Upper Arm Skin with Nonautologous Tissue Substitute, Partial Thickness, External Approach

0HRCX73 Replacement of Left Upper Arm Skin with Autologous Tissue Substitute, Full Thickness, External Approach

0HRCX74 Replacement of Left Upper Arm Skin with Autologous Tissue Substitute, Partial Thickness, External Approach

0HRCXJ3 Replacement of Left Upper Arm Skin with Synthetic Substitute, Full Thickness, External Approach

0HRCXJ4 Replacement of Left Upper Arm Skin with Synthetic Substitute, Partial Thickness, External Approach

0HRCXJZ Replacement of Left Upper Arm Skin with Synthetic Substitute, External Approach

0HRCXK3 Replacement of Left Upper Arm Skin with Nonautologous Tissue Substitute, Full Thickness, External Approach

0HRCXK4 Replacement of Left Upper Arm Skin with Nonautologous Tissue Substitute, Partial Thickness, External Approach

0HRDX73 Replacement of Right Lower Arm Skin with Autologous Tissue Substitute, Full Thickness, External Approach

0HRDX74 Replacement of Right Lower Arm Skin with Autologous Tissue Substitute, Partial Thickness, External Approach

0HRDXJ3 Replacement of Right Lower Arm Skin with Synthetic Substitute, Full Thickness, External Approach

0HRDXJ4 Replacement of Right Lower Arm Skin with Synthetic Substitute, Partial Thickness, External Approach

0HRDXJZ Replacement of Right Lower Arm Skin with Synthetic Substitute, External Approach

0HRDXK3 Replacement of Right Lower Arm Skin with Nonautologous Tissue Substitute, Full Thickness, External Approach

0HRDXK4 Replacement of Right Lower Arm Skin with Nonautologous Tissue Substitute, Partial Thickness, External Approach

0HREX73 Replacement of Left Lower Arm Skin with Autologous Tissue Substitute, Full Thickness, External Approach

0HREX74 Replacement of Left Lower Arm Skin with Autologous Tissue Substitute, Partial Thickness, External Approach

0HREXJ3 Replacement of Left Lower Arm Skin with Synthetic Substitute, Full Thickness, External Approach

0HREXJ4 Replacement of Left Lower Arm Skin with Synthetic Substitute, Partial Thickness, External Approach

0HREXJZ Replacement of Left Lower Arm Skin with Synthetic Substitute, External Approach

0HREXK3 Replacement of Left Lower Arm Skin with Nonautologous Tissue Substitute, Full Thickness, External Approach

0HREXK4 Replacement of Left Lower Arm Skin with Nonautologous Tissue Substitute, Partial Thickness, External Approach

0HRFX73 Replacement of Right Hand Skin with Autologous Tissue Substitute, Full Thickness, External Approach

0HRFX74 Replacement of Right Hand Skin with Autologous Tissue Substitute, Partial Thickness, External Approach

0HRFXJ3 Replacement of Right Hand Skin with Synthetic Substitute, Full Thickness, External Approach

0HRFXJ4 Replacement of Right Hand Skin with Synthetic Substitute, Partial Thickness, External Approach

0HRFXJZ Replacement of Right Hand Skin with Synthetic Substitute, External Approach

0HRFXK3 Replacement of Right Hand Skin with Nonautologous Tissue Substitute, Full Thickness, External Approach

0HRFXK4 Replacement of Right Hand Skin with Nonautologous Tissue Substitute, Partial Thickness, External Approach

0HRGX73 Replacement of Left Hand Skin with Autologous Tissue Substitute, Full Thickness, External Approach

0HRGX74 Replacement of Left Hand Skin with Autologous Tissue Substitute, Partial Thickness, External Approach

0HRGXJ3 Replacement of Left Hand Skin with Synthetic Substitute, Full Thickness, External Approach

0HRGXJ4 Replacement of Left Hand Skin with Synthetic Substitute, Partial Thickness, External Approach

0HRGXJZ Replacement of Left Hand Skin with Synthetic Substitute, External Approach

0HRGXK3 Replacement of Left Hand Skin with Nonautologous Tissue Substitute, Full Thickness, External Approach

---

0HRGXK4 Replacement of Left Hand Skin with Nonautologous Tissue Substitute, Partial Thickness, External Approach

0HRHX73 Replacement of Right Upper Leg Skin with Autologous Tissue Substitute, Full Thickness, External Approach

0HRHX74 Replacement of Right Upper Leg Skin with Autologous Tissue Substitute, Partial Thickness, External Approach

0HRHXJ3 Replacement of Right Upper Leg Skin with Synthetic Substitute, Full Thickness, External Approach

0HRHXJ4 Replacement of Right Upper Leg Skin with Synthetic Substitute, Partial Thickness, External Approach

0HRHXJZ Replacement of Right Upper Leg Skin with Synthetic Substitute, External Approach

0HRHXK3 Replacement of Right Upper Leg Skin with Nonautologous Tissue Substitute, Full Thickness, External Approach

0HRHXK4 Replacement of Right Upper Leg Skin with Nonautologous Tissue Substitute, Partial Thickness, External Approach

0HRJX73 Replacement of Left Upper Leg Skin with Autologous Tissue Substitute, Full Thickness, External Approach

0HRJX74 Replacement of Left Upper Leg Skin with Autologous Tissue Substitute, Partial Thickness, External Approach

0HRJXJ3 Replacement of Left Upper Leg Skin with Synthetic Substitute, Full Thickness, External Approach

0HRJXJ4 Replacement of Left Upper Leg Skin with Synthetic Substitute, Partial Thickness, External Approach

0HRJXJZ Replacement of Left Upper Leg Skin with Synthetic Substitute, External Approach

0HRJXK3 Replacement of Left Upper Leg Skin with Nonautologous Tissue Substitute, Full Thickness, External Approach

0HRJXK4 Replacement of Left Upper Leg Skin with Nonautologous Tissue Substitute, Partial Thickness, External Approach

0HRKX73 Replacement of Right Lower Leg Skin with Autologous Tissue Substitute, Full Thickness, External Approach

0HRKX74 Replacement of Right Lower Leg Skin with Autologous Tissue Substitute, Partial Thickness, External Approach

0HRKXJ3 Replacement of Right Lower Leg Skin with Synthetic Substitute, Full Thickness, External Approach

0HRKXJ4 Replacement of Right Lower Leg Skin with Synthetic Substitute, Partial Thickness, External Approach

0HRKXJZ Replacement of Right Lower Leg Skin with Synthetic Substitute, External Approach

0HRKXK3 Replacement of Right Lower Leg Skin with Nonautologous Tissue Substitute, Full Thickness, External Approach

0HRKXK4 Replacement of Right Lower Leg Skin with Nonautologous Tissue Substitute, Partial Thickness, External Approach

0HRLX73 Replacement of Left Lower Leg Skin with Autologous Tissue Substitute, Full Thickness, External Approach

0HRLX74 Replacement of Left Lower Leg Skin with Autologous Tissue Substitute, Partial Thickness, External Approach

0HRLXJ3 Replacement of Left Lower Leg Skin with Synthetic Substitute, Full Thickness, External Approach

0HRLXJ4 Replacement of Left Lower Leg Skin with Synthetic Substitute, Partial Thickness, External Approach

0HRLXJZ Replacement of Left Lower Leg Skin with Synthetic Substitute, External Approach

0HRLXK3 Replacement of Left Lower Leg Skin with Nonautologous Tissue Substitute, Full Thickness, External Approach

0HRLXK4 Replacement of Left Lower Leg Skin with Nonautologous Tissue Substitute, Partial Thickness, External Approach

0HRMX73 Replacement of Right Foot Skin with Autologous Tissue Substitute, Full Thickness, External Approach

0HRMX74 Replacement of Right Foot Skin with Autologous Tissue Substitute, Partial Thickness, External Approach

0HRMXJ3 Replacement of Right Foot Skin with Synthetic Substitute, Full Thickness, External Approach

0HRMXJ4 Replacement of Right Foot Skin with Synthetic Substitute, Partial Thickness, External Approach

0HRMXJZ Replacement of Right Foot Skin with Synthetic Substitute, External Approach

0HRMXK3 Replacement of Right Foot Skin with Nonautologous Tissue Substitute, Full Thickness, External Approach

0HRMXK4 Replacement of Right Foot Skin with Nonautologous Tissue Substitute, Partial Thickness, External Approach

0HRNX73 Replacement of Left Foot Skin with Autologous Tissue Substitute, Full Thickness, External Approach

0HRNX74 Replacement of Left Foot Skin with Autologous Tissue Substitute, Partial Thickness, External Approach

0HRNXJ3 Replacement of Left Foot Skin with Synthetic Substitute, Full Thickness, External Approach

0HRNXJ4 Replacement of Left Foot Skin with Synthetic Substitute, Partial Thickness, External Approach

0HRNXJZ Replacement of Left Foot Skin with Synthetic Substitute, External Approach

0HRNXK3 Replacement of Left Foot Skin with Nonautologous Tissue Substitute, Full Thickness, External Approach

0HRNXK4 Replacement of Left Foot Skin with Nonautologous Tissue Substitute, Partial Thickness, External Approach

0HRQX7Z Replacement of Finger Nail with Autologous Tissue Substitute, External Approach

0HRQXJZ Replacement of Finger Nail with Synthetic Substitute, External Approach

0HRQXKZ Replacement of Finger Nail with Nonautologous Tissue Substitute, External Approach

0HRRX7Z Replacement of Toe Nail with Autologous Tissue Substitute, External Approach

0HRRXJZ Replacement of Toe Nail with Synthetic Substitute, External Approach

0HRRXKZ Replacement of Toe Nail with Nonautologous Tissue Substitute, External Approach

0HRSX7Z Replacement of Hair with Autologous Tissue Substitute, External Approach

0HRSXJZ Replacement of Hair with Synthetic Substitute, External Approach

0HRSXKZ Replacement of Hair with Nonautologous Tissue Substitute, External Approach

0HRT075 Replacement of Right Breast using Latissimus Dorsi Myocutaneous Flap, Open Approach

0HRT076 Replacement of Right Breast using Transverse Rectus Abdominis Myocutaneous Flap, Open Approach

0HRT077 Replacement of Right Breast using Deep Inferior Epigastric Artery Perforator Flap, Open Approach

0HRT078 Replacement of Right Breast using Superficial Inferior Epigastric Artery Flap, Open Approach

0HRT079 Replacement of Right Breast using Gluteal Artery Perforator Flap, Open Approach

0HRT07Z Replacement of Right Breast with Autologous Tissue Substitute, Open Approach

0HRT0JZ Replacement of Right Breast with Synthetic Substitute, Open Approach

0HRT0KZ Replacement of Right Breast with Nonautologous Tissue Substitute, Open Approach

0HRT37Z Replacement of Right Breast with Autologous Tissue Substitute, Percutaneous Approach

0HRT3JZ Replacement of Right Breast with Synthetic Substitute, Percutaneous Approach

0HRT3KZ Replacement of Right Breast with Nonautologous Tissue Substitute, Percutaneous Approach

0HRTX7Z Replacement of Right Breast with Autologous Tissue Substitute, External Approach

0HRTXJZ Replacement of Right Breast with Synthetic Substitute, External Approach

0HRTXKZ Replacement of Right Breast with Nonautologous Tissue Substitute, External Approach

0HRU075 Replacement of Left Breast using Latissimus Dorsi Myocutaneous Flap, Open Approach

0HRU076 Replacement of Left Breast using Transverse Rectus Abdominis Myocutaneous Flap, Open Approach

0HRU077 Replacement of Left Breast using Deep Inferior Epigastric Artery Perforator Flap, Open Approach

0HRU078 Replacement of Left Breast using Superficial Inferior Epigastric Artery Flap, Open Approach

0HRU079 Replacement of Left Breast using Gluteal Artery Perforator Flap, Open Approach

0HRU07Z Replacement of Left Breast with Autologous Tissue Substitute, Open Approach

0HRU0JZ Replacement of Left Breast with Synthetic Substitute, Open Approach

0HRU0KZ Replacement of Left Breast with Nonautologous Tissue Substitute, Open Approach

---

0HRU37Z	Replacement of Left Breast with Autologous Tissue Substitute, Percutaneous Approach
0HRU3JZ	Replacement of Left Breast with Synthetic Substitute, Percutaneous Approach
0HRU3KZ	Replacement of Left Breast with Nonautologous Tissue Substitute, Percutaneous Approach
0HRUX7Z	Replacement of Left Breast with Autologous Tissue Substitute, External Approach
0HRUXJZ	Replacement of Left Breast with Synthetic Substitute, External Approach
0HRUXKZ	Replacement of Left Breast with Nonautologous Tissue Substitute, External Approach
0HRV075	Replacement of Bilateral Breast using Latissimus Dorsi Myocutaneous Flap, Open Approach
0HRV076	Replacement of Bilateral Breast using Transverse Rectus Abdominis Myocutaneous Flap, Open Approach
0HRV077	Replacement of Bilateral Breast using Deep Inferior Epigastric Artery Perforator Flap, Open Approach
0HRV078	Replacement of Bilateral Breast using Superficial Inferior Epigastric Artery Flap, Open Approach
0HRV079	Replacement of Bilateral Breast using Gluteal Artery Perforator Flap, Open Approach
0HRV07Z	Replacement of Bilateral Breast with Autologous Tissue Substitute, Open Approach
0HRV0JZ	Replacement of Bilateral Breast with Synthetic Substitute, Open Approach
0HRV0KZ	Replacement of Bilateral Breast with Nonautologous Tissue Substitute, Open Approach
0HRV37Z	Replacement of Bilateral Breast with Autologous Tissue Substitute, Percutaneous Approach
0HRV3JZ	Replacement of Bilateral Breast with Synthetic Substitute, Percutaneous Approach
0HRV3KZ	Replacement of Bilateral Breast with Nonautologous Tissue Substitute, Percutaneous Approach
0HRVX7Z	Replacement of Bilateral Breast with Autologous Tissue Substitute, External Approach
0HRVXJZ	Replacement of Bilateral Breast with Synthetic Substitute, External Approach

0HRVXKZ	Replacement of Bilateral Breast with Nonautologous Tissue Substitute, External Approach
0HRW07Z	Replacement of Right Nipple with Autologous Tissue Substitute, Open Approach
0HRW0JZ	Replacement of Right Nipple with Synthetic Substitute, Open Approach
0HRW0KZ	Replacement of Right Nipple with Nonautologous Tissue Substitute, Open Approach
0HRW37Z	Replacement of Right Nipple with Autologous Tissue Substitute, Percutaneous Approach
0HRW3JZ	Replacement of Right Nipple with Synthetic Substitute, Percutaneous Approach
0HRW3KZ	Replacement of Right Nipple with Nonautologous Tissue Substitute, Percutaneous Approach
0HRWX7Z	Replacement of Right Nipple with Autologous Tissue Substitute, External Approach
0HRWXJZ	Replacement of Right Nipple with Synthetic Substitute, External Approach
0HRWXKZ	Replacement of Right Nipple with Nonautologous Tissue Substitute, External Approach
0HRX07Z	Replacement of Left Nipple with Autologous Tissue Substitute, Open Approach
0HRX0JZ	Replacement of Left Nipple with Synthetic Substitute, Open Approach
0HRX0KZ	Replacement of Left Nipple with Nonautologous Tissue Substitute, Open Approach
0HRX37Z	Replacement of Left Nipple with Autologous Tissue Substitute, Percutaneous Approach
0HRX3JZ	Replacement of Left Nipple with Synthetic Substitute, Percutaneous Approach
0HRX3KZ	Replacement of Left Nipple with Nonautologous Tissue Substitute, Percutaneous Approach
0HRXX7Z	Replacement of Left Nipple with Autologous Tissue Substitute, External Approach
0HRXXJZ	Replacement of Left Nipple with Synthetic Substitute, External Approach
0HRXXKZ	Replacement of Left Nipple with Nonautologous Tissue Substitute, External Approach

0HS – Skin and Breast, Reposition

0HSSXZZ	Reposition Hair, External Approach
0HST0ZZ	Reposition Right Breast, Open Approach
0HSU0ZZ	Reposition Left Breast, Open Approach

0HSV0ZZ	Reposition Bilateral Breast, Open Approach
0HSWXZZ	Reposition Right Nipple, External Approach
0HSXXZZ	Reposition Left Nipple, External Approach

0HT – Skin and Breast, Resection

Review Coding Guideline B3.8

0HTQXZZ	Resection of Finger Nail, External Approach
0HTRXZZ	Resection of Toe Nail, External Approach
0HTT0ZZ	Resection of Right Breast, Open Approach
0HTU0ZZ	Resection of Left Breast, Open Approach

0HTV0ZZ	Resection of Bilateral Breast, Open Approach
0HTWXZZ	Resection of Right Nipple, External Approach
0HTXXZZ	Resection of Left Nipple, External Approach
0HTY0ZZ	Resection of Supernumerary Breast, Open Approach

0HU – Skin and Breast, Supplement

0HUT07Z	Supplement Right Breast with Autologous Tissue Substitute, Open Approach
0HUT0JZ	Supplement Right Breast with Synthetic Substitute, Open Approach
0HUT0KZ	Supplement Right Breast with Nonautologous Tissue Substitute, Open Approach
0HUT37Z	Supplement Right Breast with Autologous Tissue Substitute, Percutaneous Approach
0HUT3JZ	Supplement Right Breast with Synthetic Substitute, Percutaneous Approach
0HUT3KZ	Supplement Right Breast with Nonautologous Tissue Substitute, Percutaneous Approach
0HUT77Z	Supplement Right Breast with Autologous Tissue Substitute, Via Natural or Artificial Opening
0HUT7JZ	Supplement Right Breast with Synthetic Substitute, Via Natural or Artificial Opening

0HUT7KZ	Supplement Right Breast with Nonautologous Tissue Substitute, Via Natural or Artificial Opening
0HUT87Z	Supplement Right Breast with Autologous Tissue Substitute, Via Natural or Artificial Opening Endoscopic
0HUT8JZ	Supplement Right Breast with Synthetic Substitute, Via Natural or Artificial Opening Endoscopic
0HUT8KZ	Supplement Right Breast with Nonautologous Tissue Substitute, Via Natural or Artificial Opening Endoscopic
0HUTX7Z	Supplement Right Breast with Autologous Tissue Substitute, External Approach
0HUTXJZ	Supplement Right Breast with Synthetic Substitute, External Approach
0HUTXKZ	Supplement Right Breast with Nonautologous Tissue Substitute, External Approach
0HUU07Z	Supplement Left Breast with Autologous Tissue Substitute, Open Approach
0HUU0JZ	Supplement Left Breast with Synthetic Substitute, Open Approach

0HUU0KZ Supplement Left Breast with Nonautologous Tissue Substitute, Open Approach

0HUU37Z Supplement Left Breast with Autologous Tissue Substitute, Percutaneous Approach

0HUU3JZ Supplement Left Breast with Synthetic Substitute, Percutaneous Approach

0HUU3KZ Supplement Left Breast with Nonautologous Tissue Substitute, Percutaneous Approach

0HUU77Z Supplement Left Breast with Autologous Tissue Substitute, Via Natural or Artificial Opening

0HUU7JZ Supplement Left Breast with Synthetic Substitute, Via Natural or Artificial Opening

0HUU7KZ Supplement Left Breast with Nonautologous Tissue Substitute, Via Natural or Artificial Opening

0HUU87Z Supplement Left Breast with Autologous Tissue Substitute, Via Natural or Artificial Opening Endoscopic

0HUU8JZ Supplement Left Breast with Synthetic Substitute, Via Natural or Artificial Opening Endoscopic

0HUU8KZ Supplement Left Breast with Nonautologous Tissue Substitute, Via Natural or Artificial Opening Endoscopic

0HUUX7Z Supplement Left Breast with Autologous Tissue Substitute, External Approach

0HUUXJZ Supplement Left Breast with Synthetic Substitute, External Approach

0HUUXKZ Supplement Left Breast with Nonautologous Tissue Substitute, External Approach

0HUV07Z Supplement Bilateral Breast with Autologous Tissue Substitute, Open Approach

0HUV0JZ Supplement Bilateral Breast with Synthetic Substitute, Open Approach

0HUV0KZ Supplement Bilateral Breast with Nonautologous Tissue Substitute, Open Approach

0HUV37Z Supplement Bilateral Breast with Autologous Tissue Substitute, Percutaneous Approach

0HUV3JZ Supplement Bilateral Breast with Synthetic Substitute, Percutaneous Approach

0HUV3KZ Supplement Bilateral Breast with Nonautologous Tissue Substitute, Percutaneous Approach

0HUV77Z Supplement Bilateral Breast with Autologous Tissue Substitute, Via Natural or Artificial Opening

0HUV7JZ Supplement Bilateral Breast with Synthetic Substitute, Via Natural or Artificial Opening

0HUV7KZ Supplement Bilateral Breast with Nonautologous Tissue Substitute, Via Natural or Artificial Opening

0HUV87Z Supplement Bilateral Breast with Autologous Tissue Substitute, Via Natural or Artificial Opening Endoscopic

0HUV8JZ Supplement Bilateral Breast with Synthetic Substitute, Via Natural or Artificial Opening Endoscopic

0HUV8KZ Supplement Bilateral Breast with Nonautologous Tissue Substitute, Via Natural or Artificial Opening Endoscopic

0HUVX7Z Supplement Bilateral Breast with Autologous Tissue Substitute, External Approach

0HUVXJZ Supplement Bilateral Breast with Synthetic Substitute, External Approach

0HUVXKZ Supplement Bilateral Breast with Nonautologous Tissue Substitute, External Approach

0HUW07Z Supplement Right Nipple with Autologous Tissue Substitute, Open Approach

0HUW0JZ Supplement Right Nipple with Synthetic Substitute, Open Approach

0HUW0KZ Supplement Right Nipple with Nonautologous Tissue Substitute, Open Approach

0HUW37Z Supplement Right Nipple with Autologous Tissue Substitute, Percutaneous Approach

0HUW3JZ Supplement Right Nipple with Synthetic Substitute, Percutaneous Approach

0HUW3KZ Supplement Right Nipple with Nonautologous Tissue Substitute, Percutaneous Approach

0HUW77Z Supplement Right Nipple with Autologous Tissue Substitute, Via Natural or Artificial Opening

0HUW7JZ Supplement Right Nipple with Synthetic Substitute, Via Natural or Artificial Opening

0HUW7KZ Supplement Right Nipple with Nonautologous Tissue Substitute, Via Natural or Artificial Opening

0HUW87Z Supplement Right Nipple with Autologous Tissue Substitute, Via Natural or Artificial Opening Endoscopic

0HUW8JZ Supplement Right Nipple with Synthetic Substitute, Via Natural or Artificial Opening Endoscopic

0HUW8KZ Supplement Right Nipple with Nonautologous Tissue Substitute, Via Natural or Artificial Opening Endoscopic

0HUWX7Z Supplement Right Nipple with Autologous Tissue Substitute, External Approach

0HUWXJZ Supplement Right Nipple with Synthetic Substitute, External Approach

0HUWXKZ Supplement Right Nipple with Nonautologous Tissue Substitute, External Approach

0HUX07Z Supplement Left Nipple with Autologous Tissue Substitute, Open Approach

0HUX0JZ Supplement Left Nipple with Synthetic Substitute, Open Approach

0HUX0KZ Supplement Left Nipple with Nonautologous Tissue Substitute, Open Approach

0HUX37Z Supplement Left Nipple with Autologous Tissue Substitute, Percutaneous Approach

0HUX3JZ Supplement Left Nipple with Synthetic Substitute, Percutaneous Approach

0HUX3KZ Supplement Left Nipple with Nonautologous Tissue Substitute, Percutaneous Approach

0HUX77Z Supplement Left Nipple with Autologous Tissue Substitute, Via Natural or Artificial Opening

0HUX7JZ Supplement Left Nipple with Synthetic Substitute, Via Natural or Artificial Opening

0HUX7KZ Supplement Left Nipple with Nonautologous Tissue Substitute, Via Natural or Artificial Opening

0HUX87Z Supplement Left Nipple with Autologous Tissue Substitute, Via Natural or Artificial Opening Endoscopic

0HUX8JZ Supplement Left Nipple with Synthetic Substitute, Via Natural or Artificial Opening Endoscopic

0HUX8KZ Supplement Left Nipple with Nonautologous Tissue Substitute, Via Natural or Artificial Opening Endoscopic

0HUXX7Z Supplement Left Nipple with Autologous Tissue Substitute, External Approach

0HUXXJZ Supplement Left Nipple with Synthetic Substitute, External Approach

0HUXXKZ Supplement Left Nipple with Nonautologous Tissue Substitute, External Approach

0HW – Skin and Breast, Revision

Review Coding Guideline B6.1c

0HWPX0Z Revision of Drainage Device in Skin, External Approach

0HWPX7Z Revision of Autologous Tissue Substitute in Skin, External Approach

0HWPXJZ Revision of Synthetic Substitute in Skin, External Approach

0HWPXKZ Revision of Nonautologous Tissue Substitute in Skin, External Approach

0HWQX0Z Revision of Drainage Device in Finger Nail, External Approach

0HWQX7Z Revision of Autologous Tissue Substitute in Finger Nail, External Approach

0HWQXJZ Revision of Synthetic Substitute in Finger Nail, External Approach

0HWQXKZ Revision of Nonautologous Tissue Substitute in Finger Nail, External Approach

0HWRX0Z Revision of Drainage Device in Toe Nail, External Approach

0HWRX7Z Revision of Autologous Tissue Substitute in Toe Nail, External Approach

0HWRXJZ Revision of Synthetic Substitute in Toe Nail, External Approach

0HWRXKZ Revision of Nonautologous Tissue Substitute in Toe Nail, External Approach

0HWSX7Z Revision of Autologous Tissue Substitute in Hair, External Approach

0HWSXJZ   Revision of Synthetic Substitute in Hair, External Approach

0HWSXKZ   Revision of Nonautologous Tissue Substitute in Hair, External Approach

0HWT00Z   Revision of Drainage Device in Right Breast, Open Approach

0HWT07Z   Revision of Autologous Tissue Substitute in Right Breast, Open Approach

0HWT0JZ   Revision of Synthetic Substitute in Right Breast, Open Approach

0HWT0KZ   Revision of Nonautologous Tissue Substitute in Right Breast, Open Approach

0HWT0NZ   Revision of Tissue Expander in Right Breast, Open Approach

0HWT30Z   Revision of Drainage Device in Right Breast, Percutaneous Approach

0HWT37Z   Revision of Autologous Tissue Substitute in Right Breast, Percutaneous Approach

0HWT3JZ   Revision of Synthetic Substitute in Right Breast, Percutaneous Approach

0HWT3KZ   Revision of Nonautologous Tissue Substitute in Right Breast, Percutaneous Approach

0HWT3NZ   Revision of Tissue Expander in Right Breast, Percutaneous Approach

0HWT70Z   Revision of Drainage Device in Right Breast, Via Natural or Artificial Opening

0HWT77Z   Revision of Autologous Tissue Substitute in Right Breast, Via Natural or Artificial Opening

0HWT7JZ   Revision of Synthetic Substitute in Right Breast, Via Natural or Artificial Opening

0HWT7KZ   Revision of Nonautologous Tissue Substitute in Right Breast, Via Natural or Artificial Opening

0HWT7NZ   Revision of Tissue Expander in Right Breast, Via Natural or Artificial Opening

0HWT80Z   Revision of Drainage Device in Right Breast, Via Natural or Artificial Opening Endoscopic

0HWT87Z   Revision of Autologous Tissue Substitute in Right Breast, Via Natural or Artificial Opening Endoscopic

0HWT8JZ   Revision of Synthetic Substitute in Right Breast, Via Natural or Artificial Opening Endoscopic

0HWT8KZ   Revision of Nonautologous Tissue Substitute in Right Breast, Via Natural or Artificial Opening Endoscopic

0HWT8NZ   Revision of Tissue Expander in Right Breast, Via Natural or Artificial Opening Endoscopic

0HWTX0Z   Revision of Drainage Device in Right Breast, External Approach

0HWTX7Z   Revision of Autologous Tissue Substitute in Right Breast, External Approach

0HWTXJZ   Revision of Synthetic Substitute in Right Breast, External Approach

0HWTXKZ   Revision of Nonautologous Tissue Substitute in Right Breast, External Approach

0HWU00Z   Revision of Drainage Device in Left Breast, Open Approach

0HWU07Z   Revision of Autologous Tissue Substitute in Left Breast, Open Approach

0HWU0JZ   Revision of Synthetic Substitute in Left Breast, Open Approach

0HWU0KZ   Revision of Nonautologous Tissue Substitute in Left Breast, Open Approach

0HWU0NZ   Revision of Tissue Expander in Left Breast, Open Approach

0HWU30Z   Revision of Drainage Device in Left Breast, Percutaneous Approach

0HWU37Z   Revision of Autologous Tissue Substitute in Left Breast, Percutaneous Approach

0HWU3JZ   Revision of Synthetic Substitute in Left Breast, Percutaneous Approach

0HWU3KZ   Revision of Nonautologous Tissue Substitute in Left Breast, Percutaneous Approach

0HWU3NZ   Revision of Tissue Expander in Left Breast, Percutaneous Approach

0HWU70Z   Revision of Drainage Device in Left Breast, Via Natural or Artificial Opening

0HWU77Z   Revision of Autologous Tissue Substitute in Left Breast, Via Natural or Artificial Opening

0HWU7JZ   Revision of Synthetic Substitute in Left Breast, Via Natural or Artificial Opening

0HWU7KZ   Revision of Nonautologous Tissue Substitute in Left Breast, Via Natural or Artificial Opening

0HWU7NZ   Revision of Tissue Expander in Left Breast, Via Natural or Artificial Opening

0HWU80Z   Revision of Drainage Device in Left Breast, Via Natural or Artificial Opening Endoscopic

0HWU87Z   Revision of Autologous Tissue Substitute in Left Breast, Via Natural or Artificial Opening Endoscopic

0HWU8JZ   Revision of Synthetic Substitute in Left Breast, Via Natural or Artificial Opening Endoscopic

0HWU8KZ   Revision of Nonautologous Tissue Substitute in Left Breast, Via Natural or Artificial Opening Endoscopic

0HWU8NZ   Revision of Tissue Expander in Left Breast, Via Natural or Artificial Opening Endoscopic

0HWUX0Z   Revision of Drainage Device in Left Breast, External Approach

0HWUX7Z   Revision of Autologous Tissue Substitute in Left Breast, External Approach

0HWUXJZ   Revision of Synthetic Substitute in Left Breast, External Approach

0HWUXKZ   Revision of Nonautologous Tissue Substitute in Left Breast, External Approach

0HX – Skin and Breast, Transfer

0HX0XZZ   Transfer Scalp Skin, External Approach

0HX1XZZ   Transfer Face Skin, External Approach

0HX2XZZ   Transfer Right Ear Skin, External Approach

0HX3XZZ   Transfer Left Ear Skin, External Approach

0HX4XZZ   Transfer Neck Skin, External Approach

0HX5XZZ   Transfer Chest Skin, External Approach

0HX6XZZ   Transfer Back Skin, External Approach

0HX7XZZ   Transfer Abdomen Skin, External Approach

0HX8XZZ   Transfer Buttock Skin, External Approach

0HX9XZZ   Transfer Perineum Skin, External Approach

0HXAXZZ   Transfer Genitalia Skin, External Approach

0HXBXZZ   Transfer Right Upper Arm Skin, External Approach

0HXCXZZ   Transfer Left Upper Arm Skin, External Approach

0HXDXZZ   Transfer Right Lower Arm Skin, External Approach

0HXEXZZ   Transfer Left Lower Arm Skin, External Approach

0HXFXZZ   Transfer Right Hand Skin, External Approach

0HXGXZZ   Transfer Left Hand Skin, External Approach

0HXHXZZ   Transfer Right Upper Leg Skin, External Approach

0HXJXZZ   Transfer Left Upper Leg Skin, External Approach

0HXKXZZ   Transfer Right Lower Leg Skin, External Approach

0HXLXZZ   Transfer Left Lower Leg Skin, External Approach

0HXMXZZ   Transfer Right Foot Skin, External Approach

0HXNXZZ   Transfer Left Foot Skin, External Approach

♀ Female-only   ♂ Male-only   ● Limited Coverage   ● Non-OR   HAC HAC-associated procedure   ● Non-covered procedures   ✚ Combination

Subcutaneous Tissue and Fascia

Subcutaneous Tissue and Fascia

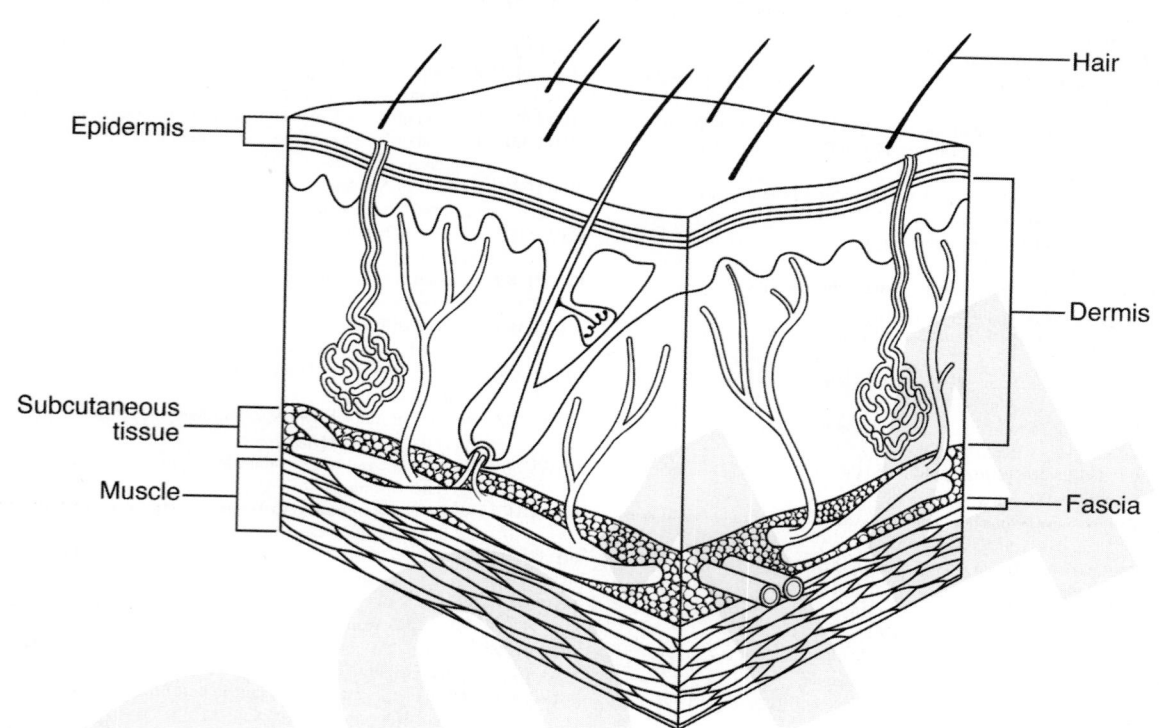

Subcutaneous Tissue and Fascia Tables 0J0–0JX

Section	0	Medical and Surgical
Body System	J	Subcutaneous Tissue and Fascia
Operation	0	Alteration: Modifying the anatomic structure of a body part without affecting the function of the body part

Body Part (4th)	Approach (5th)	Device (6th)	Qualifier (7th)
1 Subcutaneous Tissue and Fascia, Face 4 Subcutaneous Tissue and Fascia, Anterior Neck 5 Subcutaneous Tissue and Fascia, Posterior Neck 6 Subcutaneous Tissue and Fascia, Chest 7 Subcutaneous Tissue and Fascia, Back 8 Subcutaneous Tissue and Fascia, Abdomen 9 Subcutaneous Tissue and Fascia, Buttock D Subcutaneous Tissue and Fascia, Right Upper Arm F Subcutaneous Tissue and Fascia, Left Upper Arm G Subcutaneous Tissue and Fascia, Right Lower Arm H Subcutaneous Tissue and Fascia, Left Lower Arm L Subcutaneous Tissue and Fascia, Right Upper Leg M Subcutaneous Tissue and Fascia, Left Upper Leg N Subcutaneous Tissue and Fascia, Right Lower Leg P Subcutaneous Tissue and Fascia, Left Lower Leg	0 Open 3 Percutaneous	Z No Device	Z No Qualifier

Section	0	Medical and Surgical
Body System	J	Subcutaneous Tissue and Fascia
Operation	2	Change: Taking out or off a device from a body part and putting back an identical or similar device in or on the same body part without cutting or puncturing the skin or a mucous membrane

Body Part (4th)	Approach (5th)	Device (6th)	Qualifier (7th)
S Subcutaneous Tissue and Fascia, Head and Neck T Subcutaneous Tissue and Fascia, Trunk V Subcutaneous Tissue and Fascia, Upper Extremity W Subcutaneous Tissue and Fascia, Lower Extremity	X External	0 Drainage Device Y Other Device	Z No Qualifier

Section	0	Medical and Surgical
Body System	J	Subcutaneous Tissue and Fascia
Operation	5	Destruction: Physical eradication of all or a portion of a body part by the direct use of energy, force, or a destructive agent

Body Part (4th)	Approach (5th)	Device (6th)	Qualifier (7th)
0 Subcutaneous Tissue and Fascia, Scalp 1 Subcutaneous Tissue and Fascia, Face 4 Subcutaneous Tissue and Fascia, Anterior Neck 5 Subcutaneous Tissue and Fascia, Posterior Neck 6 Subcutaneous Tissue and Fascia, Chest 7 Subcutaneous Tissue and Fascia, Back 8 Subcutaneous Tissue and Fascia, Abdomen 9 Subcutaneous Tissue and Fascia, Buttock B Subcutaneous Tissue and Fascia, Perineum C Subcutaneous Tissue and Fascia, Pelvic Region D Subcutaneous Tissue and Fascia, Right Upper Arm F Subcutaneous Tissue and Fascia, Left Upper Arm G Subcutaneous Tissue and Fascia, Right Lower Arm H Subcutaneous Tissue and Fascia, Left Lower Arm J Subcutaneous Tissue and Fascia, Right Hand K Subcutaneous Tissue and Fascia, Left Hand L Subcutaneous Tissue and Fascia, Right Upper Leg M Subcutaneous Tissue and Fascia, Left Upper Leg N Subcutaneous Tissue and Fascia, Right Lower Leg P Subcutaneous Tissue and Fascia, Left Lower Leg Q Subcutaneous Tissue and Fascia, Right Foot R Subcutaneous Tissue and Fascia, Left Foot	0 Open 3 Percutaneous	Z No Device	Z No Qualifier

Section	0	Medical and Surgical
Body System	J	Subcutaneous Tissue and Fascia
Operation	8	Division: Cutting into a body part, without draining fluids and/or gases from the body part, in order to separate or transect a body part

Body Part (4th)	Approach (5th)	Device (6th)	Qualifier (7th)
0 Subcutaneous Tissue and Fascia, Scalp	0 Open	Z No Device	Z No Qualifier
1 Subcutaneous Tissue and Fascia, Face	3 Percutaneous		
4 Subcutaneous Tissue and Fascia, Anterior Neck			
5 Subcutaneous Tissue and Fascia, Posterior Neck			
6 Subcutaneous Tissue and Fascia, Chest			
7 Subcutaneous Tissue and Fascia, Back			
8 Subcutaneous Tissue and Fascia, Abdomen			
9 Subcutaneous Tissue and Fascia, Buttock			
B Subcutaneous Tissue and Fascia, Perineum			
C Subcutaneous Tissue and Fascia, Pelvic Region			
D Subcutaneous Tissue and Fascia, Right Upper Arm			
F Subcutaneous Tissue and Fascia, Left Upper Arm			
G Subcutaneous Tissue and Fascia, Right Lower Arm			
H Subcutaneous Tissue and Fascia, Left Lower Arm			
J Subcutaneous Tissue and Fascia, Right Hand			
K Subcutaneous Tissue and Fascia, Left Hand			
L Subcutaneous Tissue and Fascia, Right Upper Leg			
M Subcutaneous Tissue and Fascia, Left Upper Leg			
N Subcutaneous Tissue and Fascia, Right Lower Leg			
P Subcutaneous Tissue and Fascia, Left Lower Leg			
Q Subcutaneous Tissue and Fascia, Right Foot			
R Subcutaneous Tissue and Fascia, Left Foot			
S Subcutaneous Tissue and Fascia, Head and Neck			
T Subcutaneous Tissue and Fascia, Trunk			
V Subcutaneous Tissue and Fascia, Upper Extremity			
W Subcutaneous Tissue and Fascia, Lower Extremity			

Section	0	Medical and Surgical
Body System	J	Subcutaneous Tissue and Fascia
Operation	9	Drainage: Taking or letting out fluids and/or gases from a body part

Body Part (4th)	Approach (5th)	Device (6th)	Qualifier (7th)
0 Subcutaneous Tissue and Fascia, Scalp	0 Open	0 Drainage Device	Z No Qualifier
1 Subcutaneous Tissue and Fascia, Face	3 Percutaneous		
4 Subcutaneous Tissue and Fascia, Anterior Neck			
5 Subcutaneous Tissue and Fascia, Posterior Neck			
6 Subcutaneous Tissue and Fascia, Chest			
7 Subcutaneous Tissue and Fascia, Back			
8 Subcutaneous Tissue and Fascia, Abdomen			
9 Subcutaneous Tissue and Fascia, Buttock			
B Subcutaneous Tissue and Fascia, Perineum			
C Subcutaneous Tissue and Fascia, Pelvic Region			
D Subcutaneous Tissue and Fascia, Right Upper Arm			
F Subcutaneous Tissue and Fascia, Left Upper Arm			
G Subcutaneous Tissue and Fascia, Right Lower Arm			
H Subcutaneous Tissue and Fascia, Left Lower Arm			
J Subcutaneous Tissue and Fascia, Right Hand			
K Subcutaneous Tissue and Fascia, Left Hand			
L Subcutaneous Tissue and Fascia, Right Upper Leg			
M Subcutaneous Tissue and Fascia, Left Upper Leg			
N Subcutaneous Tissue and Fascia, Right Lower Leg			
P Subcutaneous Tissue and Fascia, Left Lower Leg			
Q Subcutaneous Tissue and Fascia, Right Foot			
R Subcutaneous Tissue and Fascia, Left Foot			

Continued

Skin and Breast Code Listing 0H0–0HX

H0 – Skin and Breast, Alteration

0H0T07Z Alteration of Right Breast with Autologous Tissue Substitute, Open Approach

0H0T0JZ Alteration of Right Breast with Synthetic Substitute, Open Approach

0H0T0KZ Alteration of Right Breast with Nonautologous Tissue Substitute, Open Approach

0H0T0ZZ Alteration of Right Breast, Open Approach

0H0T37Z Alteration of Right Breast with Autologous Tissue Substitute, Percutaneous Approach

0H0T3JZ Alteration of Right Breast with Synthetic Substitute, Percutaneous Approach

0H0T3KZ Alteration of Right Breast with Nonautologous Tissue Substitute, Percutaneous Approach

0H0T3ZZ Alteration of Right Breast, Percutaneous Approach

0H0TX7Z Alteration of Right Breast with Autologous Tissue Substitute, External Approach

0H0TXJZ Alteration of Right Breast with Synthetic Substitute, External Approach

0H0TXKZ Alteration of Right Breast with Nonautologous Tissue Substitute, External Approach

0H0TXZZ Alteration of Right Breast, External Approach

0H0U07Z Alteration of Left Breast with Autologous Tissue Substitute, Open Approach

0H0U0JZ Alteration of Left Breast with Synthetic Substitute, Open Approach

0H0U0KZ Alteration of Left Breast with Nonautologous Tissue Substitute, Open Approach

0H0U0ZZ Alteration of Left Breast, Open Approach

0H0U37Z Alteration of Left Breast with Autologous Tissue Substitute, Percutaneous Approach

0H0U3JZ Alteration of Left Breast with Synthetic Substitute, Percutaneous Approach

0H0U3KZ Alteration of Left Breast with Nonautologous Tissue Substitute, Percutaneous Approach

0H0U3ZZ Alteration of Left Breast, Percutaneous Approach

0H0UX7Z Alteration of Left Breast with Autologous Tissue Substitute, External Approach

0H0UXJZ Alteration of Left Breast with Synthetic Substitute, External Approach

0H0UXKZ Alteration of Left Breast with Nonautologous Tissue Substitute, External Approach

0H0UXZZ Alteration of Left Breast, External Approach

0H0V07Z Alteration of Bilateral Breast with Autologous Tissue Substitute, Open Approach

0H0V0JZ Alteration of Bilateral Breast with Synthetic Substitute, Open Approach

0H0V0KZ Alteration of Bilateral Breast with Nonautologous Tissue Substitute, Open Approach

0H0V0ZZ Alteration of Bilateral Breast, Open Approach

0H0V37Z Alteration of Bilateral Breast with Autologous Tissue Substitute, Percutaneous Approach

0H0V3JZ Alteration of Bilateral Breast with Synthetic Substitute, Percutaneous Approach

0H0V3KZ Alteration of Bilateral Breast with Nonautologous Tissue Substitute, Percutaneous Approach

0H0V3ZZ Alteration of Bilateral Breast, Percutaneous Approach

0H0VX7Z Alteration of Bilateral Breast with Autologous Tissue Substitute, External Approach

0H0VXJZ Alteration of Bilateral Breast with Synthetic Substitute, External Approach

0H0VXKZ Alteration of Bilateral Breast with Nonautologous Tissue Substitute, External Approach

0H0VXZZ Alteration of Bilateral Breast, External Approach

0H2 – Skin and Breast, Change

Review Coding Guideline B6.1c

0H2PX0Z Change Drainage Device in Skin, External Approach

0H2PXYZ Change Other Device in Skin, External Approach

0H2TX0Z Change Drainage Device in Right Breast, External Approach

0H2TXYZ Change Other Device in Right Breast, External Approach

0H2UX0Z Change Drainage Device in Left Breast, External Approach

0H2UXYZ Change Other Device in Left Breast, External Approach

0H5 – Skin and Breast, Destruction

● **0H50XZD** Destruction of Scalp Skin, Multiple, External Approach

● **0H50XZZ** Destruction of Scalp Skin, External Approach

● **0H51XZD** Destruction of Face Skin, Multiple, External Approach

● **0H51XZZ** Destruction of Face Skin, External Approach

0H52XZD Destruction of Right Ear Skin, Multiple, External Approach

0H52XZZ Destruction of Right Ear Skin, External Approach

0H53XZD Destruction of Left Ear Skin, Multiple, External Approach

0H53XZZ Destruction of Left Ear Skin, External Approach

● **0H54XZD** Destruction of Neck Skin, Multiple, External Approach

● **0H54XZZ** Destruction of Neck Skin, External Approach

● **0H55XZD** Destruction of Chest Skin, Multiple, External Approach

● **0H55XZZ** Destruction of Chest Skin, External Approach

● **0H56XZD** Destruction of Back Skin, Multiple, External Approach

● **0H56XZZ** Destruction of Back Skin, External Approach

● **0H57XZD** Destruction of Abdomen Skin, Multiple, External Approach

● **0H57XZZ** Destruction of Abdomen Skin, External Approach

● **0H58XZD** Destruction of Buttock Skin, Multiple, External Approach

● **0H58XZZ** Destruction of Buttock Skin, External Approach

● **0H59XZD** Destruction of Perineum Skin, Multiple, External Approach

● **0H59XZZ** Destruction of Perineum Skin, External Approach

● **0H5AXZD** Destruction of Genitalia Skin, Multiple, External Approach

● **0H5AXZZ** Destruction of Genitalia Skin, External Approach

● **0H5BXZD** Destruction of Right Upper Arm Skin, Multiple, External Approach

● **0H5BXZZ** Destruction of Right Upper Arm Skin, External Approach

● **0H5CXZD** Destruction of Left Upper Arm Skin, Multiple, External Approach

● **0H5CXZZ** Destruction of Left Upper Arm Skin, External Approach

● **0H5DXZD** Destruction of Right Lower Arm Skin, Multiple, External Approach

● **0H5DXZZ** Destruction of Right Lower Arm Skin, External Approach

● **0H5EXZD** Destruction of Left Lower Arm Skin, Multiple, External Approach

● **0H5EXZZ** Destruction of Left Lower Arm Skin, External Approach

● **0H5FXZD** Destruction of Right Hand Skin, Multiple, External Approach

● **0H5FXZZ** Destruction of Right Hand Skin, External Approach

● **0H5GXZD** Destruction of Left Hand Skin, Multiple, External Approach

● **0H5GXZZ** Destruction of Left Hand Skin, External Approach

● **0H5HXZD** Destruction of Right Upper Leg Skin, Multiple, External Approach

● **0H5HXZZ** Destruction of Right Upper Leg Skin, External Approach

● **0H5JXZD** Destruction of Left Upper Leg Skin, Multiple, External Approach

● **0H5JXZZ** Destruction of Left Upper Leg Skin, External Approach

● **0H5KXZD** Destruction of Right Lower Leg Skin, Multiple, External Approach

● **0H5KXZZ** Destruction of Right Lower Leg Skin, External Approach

● **0H5LXZD** Destruction of Left Lower Leg Skin, Multiple, External Approach

● **0H5LXZZ** Destruction of Left Lower Leg Skin, External Approach

● **0H5MXZD** Destruction of Right Foot Skin, Multiple, External Approach

● **0H5MXZZ** Destruction of Right Foot Skin, External Approach

● **0H5NXZD** Destruction of Left Foot Skin, Multiple, External Approach

● **0H5NXZZ** Destruction of Left Foot Skin, External Approach

● **0H5QXZZ** Destruction of Finger Nail, External Approach

● **0H5RXZZ** Destruction of Toe Nail, External Approach

0H5T0ZZ Destruction of Right Breast, Open Approach

0H5T3ZZ Destruction of Right Breast, Percutaneous Approach

0H5T7ZZ Destruction of Right Breast, Via Natural or Artificial Opening

0H5T8ZZ Destruction of Right Breast, Via Natural or Artificial Opening Endoscopic

0H5TXZZ Destruction of Right Breast, External Approach

0H5U0ZZ   Destruction of Left Breast, Open Approach
0H5U3ZZ   Destruction of Left Breast, Percutaneous Approach
0H5U7ZZ   Destruction of Left Breast, Via Natural or Artificial Opening
0H5U8ZZ   Destruction of Left Breast, Via Natural or Artificial Opening Endoscopic
0H5UXZZ   Destruction of Left Breast, External Approach
0H5V0ZZ   Destruction of Bilateral Breast, Open Approach
0H5V3ZZ   Destruction of Bilateral Breast, Percutaneous Approach
0H5V7ZZ   Destruction of Bilateral Breast, Via Natural or Artificial Opening
0H5V8ZZ   Destruction of Bilateral Breast, Via Natural or Artificial Opening Endoscopic
0H5VXZZ   Destruction of Bilateral Breast, External Approach

0H5W0ZZ   Destruction of Right Nipple, Open Approach
0H5W3ZZ   Destruction of Right Nipple, Percutaneous Approach
0H5W7ZZ   Destruction of Right Nipple, Via Natural or Artificial Opening
0H5W8ZZ   Destruction of Right Nipple, Via Natural or Artificial Opening Endoscopic
0H5WXZZ   Destruction of Right Nipple, External Approach
0H5X0ZZ   Destruction of Left Nipple, Open Approach
0H5X3ZZ   Destruction of Left Nipple, Percutaneous Approach
0H5X7ZZ   Destruction of Left Nipple, Via Natural or Artificial Opening
0H5X8ZZ   Destruction of Left Nipple, Via Natural or Artificial Opening Endoscopic
0H5XXZZ   Destruction of Left Nipple, External Approach

0H8 – Skin and Breast, Division

Review Coding Guideline B3.14

0H80XZZ   Division of Scalp Skin, External Approach
0H81XZZ   Division of Face Skin, External Approach
0H82XZZ   Division of Right Ear Skin, External Approach
0H83XZZ   Division of Left Ear Skin, External Approach
0H84XZZ   Division of Neck Skin, External Approach
0H85XZZ   Division of Chest Skin, External Approach
0H86XZZ   Division of Back Skin, External Approach
0H87XZZ   Division of Abdomen Skin, External Approach
0H88XZZ   Division of Buttock Skin, External Approach
0H89XZZ   Division of Perineum Skin, External Approach
0H8AXZZ   Division of Genitalia Skin, External Approach
0H8BXZZ   Division of Right Upper Arm Skin, External Approach

0H8CXZZ   Division of Left Upper Arm Skin, External Approach
0H8DXZZ   Division of Right Lower Arm Skin, External Approach
0H8EXZZ   Division of Left Lower Arm Skin, External Approach
0H8FXZZ   Division of Right Hand Skin, External Approach
0H8GXZZ   Division of Left Hand Skin, External Approach
0H8HXZZ   Division of Right Upper Leg Skin, External Approach
0H8JXZZ   Division of Left Upper Leg Skin, External Approach
0H8KXZZ   Division of Right Lower Leg Skin, External Approach
0H8LXZZ   Division of Left Lower Leg Skin, External Approach
0H8MXZZ   Division of Right Foot Skin, External Approach
0H8NXZZ   Division of Left Foot Skin, External Approach

0H9 – Skin and Breast, Drainage

Review Coding Guidelines B3.4a and B3.4b

Review Coding Guideline B6.2

0H90X0Z   Drainage of Scalp Skin with Drainage Device, External Approach
0H90XZX   Drainage of Scalp Skin, External Approach, Diagnostic
0H90XZZ   Drainage of Scalp Skin, External Approach
0H91X0Z   Drainage of Face Skin with Drainage Device, External Approach
0H91XZX   Drainage of Face Skin, External Approach, Diagnostic
0H91XZZ   Drainage of Face Skin, External Approach
0H92X0Z   Drainage of Right Ear Skin with Drainage Device, External Approach
0H92XZX   Drainage of Right Ear Skin, External Approach, Diagnostic
0H92XZZ   Drainage of Right Ear Skin, External Approach
0H93X0Z   Drainage of Left Ear Skin with Drainage Device, External Approach
0H93XZX   Drainage of Left Ear Skin, External Approach, Diagnostic
0H93XZZ   Drainage of Left Ear Skin, External Approach
0H94X0Z   Drainage of Neck Skin with Drainage Device, External Approach
0H94XZX   Drainage of Neck Skin, External Approach, Diagnostic
0H94XZZ   Drainage of Neck Skin, External Approach
0H95X0Z   Drainage of Chest Skin with Drainage Device, External Approach
0H95XZX   Drainage of Chest Skin, External Approach, Diagnostic
0H95XZZ   Drainage of Chest Skin, External Approach
0H96X0Z   Drainage of Back Skin with Drainage Device, External Approach
0H96XZX   Drainage of Back Skin, External Approach, Diagnostic
0H96XZZ   Drainage of Back Skin, External Approach
0H97X0Z   Drainage of Abdomen Skin with Drainage Device, External Approach
0H97XZX   Drainage of Abdomen Skin, External Approach, Diagnostic
0H97XZZ   Drainage of Abdomen Skin, External Approach
0H98X0Z   Drainage of Buttock Skin with Drainage Device, External Approach
0H98XZX   Drainage of Buttock Skin, External Approach, Diagnostic
0H98XZZ   Drainage of Buttock Skin, External Approach
0H99X0Z   Drainage of Perineum Skin with Drainage Device, External Approach
0H99XZX   Drainage of Perineum Skin, External Approach, Diagnostic
0H99XZZ   Drainage of Perineum Skin, External Approach
0H9AX0Z   Drainage of Genitalia Skin with Drainage Device, External Approach
0H9AXZX   Drainage of Genitalia Skin, External Approach, Diagnostic
0H9AXZZ   Drainage of Genitalia Skin, External Approach
0H9BX0Z   Drainage of Right Upper Arm Skin with Drainage Device, External Approach

0H9BXZX   Drainage of Right Upper Arm Skin, External Approach, Diagnostic
0H9BXZZ   Drainage of Right Upper Arm Skin, External Approach
0H9CX0Z   Drainage of Left Upper Arm Skin with Drainage Device, External Approach
0H9CXZX   Drainage of Left Upper Arm Skin, External Approach, Diagnostic
0H9CXZZ   Drainage of Left Upper Arm Skin, External Approach
0H9DX0Z   Drainage of Right Lower Arm Skin with Drainage Device, External Approach
0H9DXZX   Drainage of Right Lower Arm Skin, External Approach, Diagnostic
0H9DXZZ   Drainage of Right Lower Arm Skin, External Approach
0H9EX0Z   Drainage of Left Lower Arm Skin with Drainage Device, External Approach
0H9EXZX   Drainage of Left Lower Arm Skin, External Approach, Diagnostic
0H9EXZZ   Drainage of Left Lower Arm Skin, External Approach
0H9FX0Z   Drainage of Right Hand Skin with Drainage Device, External Approach
0H9FXZX   Drainage of Right Hand Skin, External Approach, Diagnostic
0H9FXZZ   Drainage of Right Hand Skin, External Approach
0H9GX0Z   Drainage of Left Hand Skin with Drainage Device, External Approach
0H9GXZX   Drainage of Left Hand Skin, External Approach, Diagnostic
0H9GXZZ   Drainage of Left Hand Skin, External Approach
0H9HX0Z   Drainage of Right Upper Leg Skin with Drainage Device, External Approach
0H9HXZX   Drainage of Right Upper Leg Skin, External Approach, Diagnostic
0H9HXZZ   Drainage of Right Upper Leg Skin, External Approach
0H9JX0Z   Drainage of Left Upper Leg Skin with Drainage Device, External Approach
0H9JXZX   Drainage of Left Upper Leg Skin, External Approach, Diagnostic
0H9JXZZ   Drainage of Left Upper Leg Skin, External Approach
0H9KX0Z   Drainage of Right Lower Leg Skin with Drainage Device, External Approach
0H9KXZX   Drainage of Right Lower Leg Skin, External Approach, Diagnostic
0H9KXZZ   Drainage of Right Lower Leg Skin, External Approach
0H9LX0Z   Drainage of Left Lower Leg Skin with Drainage Device, External Approach
0H9LXZX   Drainage of Left Lower Leg Skin, External Approach, Diagnostic
0H9LXZZ   Drainage of Left Lower Leg Skin, External Approach

0H9MX0Z Drainage of Right Foot Skin with Drainage Device, External Approach
0H9MXZX Drainage of Right Foot Skin, External Approach, Diagnostic
0H9MXZZ Drainage of Right Foot Skin, External Approach
0H9NX0Z Drainage of Left Foot Skin with Drainage Device, External Approach
0H9NXZX Drainage of Left Foot Skin, External Approach, Diagnostic
0H9NXZZ Drainage of Left Foot Skin, External Approach
0H9QX0Z Drainage of Finger Nail with Drainage Device, External Approach
0H9QXZX Drainage of Finger Nail, External Approach, Diagnostic
0H9QXZZ Drainage of Finger Nail, External Approach
0H9RX0Z Drainage of Toe Nail with Drainage Device, External Approach
0H9RXZX Drainage of Toe Nail, External Approach, Diagnostic
0H9RXZZ Drainage of Toe Nail, External Approach
0H9T00Z Drainage of Right Breast with Drainage Device, Open Approach
0H9T0ZX Drainage of Right Breast, Open Approach, Diagnostic
0H9T0ZZ Drainage of Right Breast, Open Approach
0H9T30Z Drainage of Right Breast with Drainage Device, Percutaneous Approach
0H9T3ZX Drainage of Right Breast, Percutaneous Approach, Diagnostic
0H9T3ZZ Drainage of Right Breast, Percutaneous Approach
0H9T70Z Drainage of Right Breast with Drainage Device, Via Natural or Artificial Opening
0H9T7ZX Drainage of Right Breast, Via Natural or Artificial Opening, Diagnostic
0H9T7ZZ Drainage of Right Breast, Via Natural or Artificial Opening
0H9T80Z Drainage of Right Breast with Drainage Device, Via Natural or Artificial Opening Endoscopic
0H9T8ZX Drainage of Right Breast, Via Natural or Artificial Opening Endoscopic, Diagnostic
0H9T8ZZ Drainage of Right Breast, Via Natural or Artificial Opening Endoscopic
0H9TX0Z Drainage of Right Breast with Drainage Device, External Approach
0H9TXZX Drainage of Right Breast, External Approach, Diagnostic
0H9TXZZ Drainage of Right Breast, External Approach
0H9U00Z Drainage of Left Breast with Drainage Device, Open Approach
0H9U0ZX Drainage of Left Breast, Open Approach, Diagnostic
0H9U0ZZ Drainage of Left Breast, Open Approach
0H9U30Z Drainage of Left Breast with Drainage Device, Percutaneous Approach
0H9U3ZX Drainage of Left Breast, Percutaneous Approach, Diagnostic
0H9U3ZZ Drainage of Left Breast, Percutaneous Approach
0H9U70Z Drainage of Left Breast with Drainage Device, Via Natural or Artificial Opening
0H9U7ZX Drainage of Left Breast, Via Natural or Artificial Opening, Diagnostic
0H9U7ZZ Drainage of Left Breast, Via Natural or Artificial Opening
0H9U80Z Drainage of Left Breast with Drainage Device, Via Natural or Artificial Opening Endoscopic
0H9U8ZX Drainage of Left Breast, Via Natural or Artificial Opening Endoscopic, Diagnostic
0H9U8ZZ Drainage of Left Breast, Via Natural or Artificial Opening Endoscopic
0H9UX0Z Drainage of Left Breast with Drainage Device, External Approach
0H9UXZX Drainage of Left Breast, External Approach, Diagnostic
0H9UXZZ Drainage of Left Breast, External Approach
0H9V00Z Drainage of Bilateral Breast with Drainage Device, Open Approach
0H9V0ZX Drainage of Bilateral Breast, Open Approach, Diagnostic
0H9V0ZZ Drainage of Bilateral Breast, Open Approach
0H9V30Z Drainage of Bilateral Breast with Drainage Device, Percutaneous Approach
0H9V3ZX Drainage of Bilateral Breast, Percutaneous Approach, Diagnostic

0H9V3ZZ Drainage of Bilateral Breast, Percutaneous Approach
0H9V70Z Drainage of Bilateral Breast with Drainage Device, Via Natural or Artificial Opening
0H9V7ZX Drainage of Bilateral Breast, Via Natural or Artificial Opening, Diagnostic
0H9V7ZZ Drainage of Bilateral Breast, Via Natural or Artificial Opening
0H9V80Z Drainage of Bilateral Breast with Drainage Device, Via Natural or Artificial Opening Endoscopic
0H9V8ZX Drainage of Bilateral Breast, Via Natural or Artificial Opening Endoscopic, Diagnostic
0H9V8ZZ Drainage of Bilateral Breast, Via Natural or Artificial Opening Endoscopic
0H9VX0Z Drainage of Bilateral Breast with Drainage Device, External Approach
0H9VXZX Drainage of Bilateral Breast, External Approach, Diagnostic
0H9VXZZ Drainage of Bilateral Breast, External Approach
0H9W00Z Drainage of Right Nipple with Drainage Device, Open Approach
0H9W0ZX Drainage of Right Nipple, Open Approach, Diagnostic
0H9W0ZZ Drainage of Right Nipple, Open Approach
0H9W30Z Drainage of Right Nipple with Drainage Device, Percutaneous Approach
0H9W3ZX Drainage of Right Nipple, Percutaneous Approach, Diagnostic
0H9W3ZZ Drainage of Right Nipple, Percutaneous Approach
0H9W70Z Drainage of Right Nipple with Drainage Device, Via Natural or Artificial Opening
0H9W7ZX Drainage of Right Nipple, Via Natural or Artificial Opening, Diagnostic
0H9W7ZZ Drainage of Right Nipple, Via Natural or Artificial Opening
0H9W80Z Drainage of Right Nipple with Drainage Device, Via Natural or Artificial Opening Endoscopic
0H9W8ZX Drainage of Right Nipple, Via Natural or Artificial Opening Endoscopic, Diagnostic
0H9W8ZZ Drainage of Right Nipple, Via Natural or Artificial Opening Endoscopic
0H9WX0Z Drainage of Right Nipple with Drainage Device, External Approach
0H9WXZX Drainage of Right Nipple, External Approach, Diagnostic
0H9WXZZ Drainage of Right Nipple, External Approach
0H9X00Z Drainage of Left Nipple with Drainage Device, Open Approach
0H9X0ZX Drainage of Left Nipple, Open Approach, Diagnostic
0H9X0ZZ Drainage of Left Nipple, Open Approach
0H9X30Z Drainage of Left Nipple with Drainage Device, Percutaneous Approach
0H9X3ZX Drainage of Left Nipple, Percutaneous Approach, Diagnostic
0H9X3ZZ Drainage of Left Nipple, Percutaneous Approach
0H9X70Z Drainage of Left Nipple with Drainage Device, Via Natural or Artificial Opening
0H9X7ZX Drainage of Left Nipple, Via Natural or Artificial Opening, Diagnostic
0H9X7ZZ Drainage of Left Nipple, Via Natural or Artificial Opening
0H9X80Z Drainage of Left Nipple with Drainage Device, Via Natural or Artificial Opening Endoscopic
0H9X8ZX Drainage of Left Nipple, Via Natural or Artificial Opening Endoscopic, Diagnostic
0H9X8ZZ Drainage of Left Nipple, Via Natural or Artificial Opening Endoscopic
0H9XX0Z Drainage of Left Nipple with Drainage Device, External Approach
0H9XXZX Drainage of Left Nipple, External Approach, Diagnostic
0H9XXZZ Drainage of Left Nipple, External Approach

0HB – Skin and Breast, Excision

Review Coding Guidelines 3B.4a and 3B.4b

Review Coding Guideline B3.5

Review Coding Guideline B3.8

0HB0XZX Excision of Scalp Skin, External Approach, Diagnostic
0HB0XZZ Excision of Scalp Skin, External Approach
0HB1XZX Excision of Face Skin, External Approach, Diagnostic
0HB1XZZ Excision of Face Skin, External Approach
0HB2XZX Excision of Right Ear Skin, External Approach, Diagnostic
0HB2XZZ Excision of Right Ear Skin, External Approach

0HB3XZX Excision of Left Ear Skin, External Approach, Diagnostic
0HB3XZZ Excision of Left Ear Skin, External Approach
0HB4XZX Excision of Neck Skin, External Approach, Diagnostic
0HB4XZZ Excision of Neck Skin, External Approach
0HB5XZX Excision of Chest Skin, External Approach, Diagnostic
0HB5XZZ Excision of Chest Skin, External Approach

♀ Female-only   ♂ Male-only   ◐ Limited Coverage   ● Non-OR   🅷🅰🅲 HAC-associated procedure   ⬤ Non-covered procedures   ➕ Combination

0HB6XZX Excision of Back Skin, External Approach, Diagnostic
0HB6XZZ Excision of Back Skin, External Approach
0HB7XZX Excision of Abdomen Skin, External Approach, Diagnostic
0HB7XZZ Excision of Abdomen Skin, External Approach
0HB8XZX Excision of Buttock Skin, External Approach, Diagnostic
0HB8XZZ Excision of Buttock Skin, External Approach
0HB9XZX Excision of Perineum Skin, External Approach, Diagnostic
● 0HB9XZZ Excision of Perineum Skin, External Approach
0HBAXZX Excision of Genitalia Skin, External Approach, Diagnostic
0HBAXZZ Excision of Genitalia Skin, External Approach
0HBBXZX Excision of Right Upper Arm Skin, External Approach, Diagnostic
0HBBXZZ Excision of Right Upper Arm Skin, External Approach
0HBCXZX Excision of Left Upper Arm Skin, External Approach, Diagnostic
0HBCXZZ Excision of Left Upper Arm Skin, External Approach
0HBDXZX Excision of Right Lower Arm Skin, External Approach, Diagnostic
0HBDXZZ Excision of Right Lower Arm Skin, External Approach
0HBEXZX Excision of Left Lower Arm Skin, External Approach, Diagnostic
0HBEXZZ Excision of Left Lower Arm Skin, External Approach
0HBFXZX Excision of Right Hand Skin, External Approach, Diagnostic
0HBFXZZ Excision of Right Hand Skin, External Approach
0HBGXZX Excision of Left Hand Skin, External Approach, Diagnostic
0HBGXZZ Excision of Left Hand Skin, External Approach
0HBHXZX Excision of Right Upper Leg Skin, External Approach, Diagnostic
0HBHXZZ Excision of Right Upper Leg Skin, External Approach
0HBJXZX Excision of Left Upper Leg Skin, External Approach, Diagnostic
0HBJXZZ Excision of Left Upper Leg Skin, External Approach
0HBKXZX Excision of Right Lower Leg Skin, External Approach, Diagnostic
0HBKXZZ Excision of Right Lower Leg Skin, External Approach
0HBLXZX Excision of Left Lower Leg Skin, External Approach, Diagnostic
0HBLXZZ Excision of Left Lower Leg Skin, External Approach
0HBMXZX Excision of Right Foot Skin, External Approach, Diagnostic
0HBMXZZ Excision of Right Foot Skin, External Approach
0HBNXZX Excision of Left Foot Skin, External Approach, Diagnostic
0HBNXZZ Excision of Left Foot Skin, External Approach
0HBQXZX Excision of Finger Nail, External Approach, Diagnostic
0HBQXZZ Excision of Finger Nail, External Approach
0HBRXZX Excision of Toe Nail, External Approach, Diagnostic
0HBRXZZ Excision of Toe Nail, External Approach
0HBT0ZX Excision of Right Breast, Open Approach, Diagnostic
0HBT0ZZ Excision of Right Breast, Open Approach
0HBT3ZX Excision of Right Breast, Percutaneous Approach, Diagnostic
0HBT3ZZ Excision of Right Breast, Percutaneous Approach
0HBT7ZX Excision of Right Breast, Via Natural or Artificial Opening, Diagnostic
0HBT7ZZ Excision of Right Breast, Via Natural or Artificial Opening
0HBT8ZX Excision of Right Breast, Via Natural or Artificial Opening Endoscopic, Diagnostic
0HBT8ZZ Excision of Right Breast, Via Natural or Artificial Opening Endoscopic
0HBTXZX Excision of Right Breast, External Approach, Diagnostic
0HBTXZZ Excision of Right Breast, External Approach
0HBU0ZX Excision of Left Breast, Open Approach, Diagnostic
0HBU0ZZ Excision of Left Breast, Open Approach
0HBU3ZX Excision of Left Breast, Percutaneous Approach, Diagnostic
0HBU3ZZ Excision of Left Breast, Percutaneous Approach
0HBU7ZX Excision of Left Breast, Via Natural or Artificial Opening, Diagnostic
0HBU7ZZ Excision of Left Breast, Via Natural or Artificial Opening
0HBU8ZX Excision of Left Breast, Via Natural or Artificial Opening Endoscopic, Diagnostic

0HBU8ZZ Excision of Left Breast, Via Natural or Artificial Opening Endoscopic
0HBUXZX Excision of Left Breast, External Approach, Diagnostic
0HBUXZZ Excision of Left Breast, External Approach
0HBV0ZX Excision of Bilateral Breast, Open Approach, Diagnostic
0HBV0ZZ Excision of Bilateral Breast, Open Approach
0HBV3ZX Excision of Bilateral Breast, Percutaneous Approach, Diagnostic
0HBV3ZZ Excision of Bilateral Breast, Percutaneous Approach
0HBV7ZX Excision of Bilateral Breast, Via Natural or Artificial Opening, Diagnostic
0HBV7ZZ Excision of Bilateral Breast, Via Natural or Artificial Opening
0HBV8ZX Excision of Bilateral Breast, Via Natural or Artificial Opening Endoscopic, Diagnostic
0HBV8ZZ Excision of Bilateral Breast, Via Natural or Artificial Opening Endoscopic
0HBVXZX Excision of Bilateral Breast, External Approach, Diagnostic
0HBVXZZ Excision of Bilateral Breast, External Approach
0HBW0ZX Excision of Right Nipple, Open Approach, Diagnostic
0HBW0ZZ Excision of Right Nipple, Open Approach
0HBW3ZX Excision of Right Nipple, Percutaneous Approach, Diagnostic
0HBW3ZZ Excision of Right Nipple, Percutaneous Approach
0HBW7ZX Excision of Right Nipple, Via Natural or Artificial Opening, Diagnostic
0HBW7ZZ Excision of Right Nipple, Via Natural or Artificial Opening
0HBW8ZX Excision of Right Nipple, Via Natural or Artificial Opening Endoscopic, Diagnostic
0HBW8ZZ Excision of Right Nipple, Via Natural or Artificial Opening Endoscopic
0HBWXZX Excision of Right Nipple, External Approach, Diagnostic
0HBWXZZ Excision of Right Nipple, External Approach
0HBX0ZX Excision of Left Nipple, Open Approach, Diagnostic
0HBX0ZZ Excision of Left Nipple, Open Approach
0HBX3ZX Excision of Left Nipple, Percutaneous Approach, Diagnostic
0HBX3ZZ Excision of Left Nipple, Percutaneous Approach
0HBX7ZX Excision of Left Nipple, Via Natural or Artificial Opening, Diagnostic
0HBX7ZZ Excision of Left Nipple, Via Natural or Artificial Opening
0HBX8ZX Excision of Left Nipple, Via Natural or Artificial Opening Endoscopic, Diagnostic
0HBX8ZZ Excision of Left Nipple, Via Natural or Artificial Opening Endoscopic
0HBXXZX Excision of Left Nipple, External Approach, Diagnostic
0HBXXZZ Excision of Left Nipple, External Approach
0HBY0ZX Excision of Supernumerary Breast, Open Approach, Diagnostic
0HBY0ZZ Excision of Supernumerary Breast, Open Approach
0HBY3ZX Excision of Supernumerary Breast, Percutaneous Approach, Diagnostic
0HBY3ZZ Excision of Supernumerary Breast, Percutaneous Approach
0HBY7ZX Excision of Supernumerary Breast, Via Natural or Artificial Opening, Diagnostic
0HBY7ZZ Excision of Supernumerary Breast, Via Natural or Artificial Opening
0HBY8ZX Excision of Supernumerary Breast, Via Natural or Artificial Opening Endoscopic, Diagnostic
0HBY8ZZ Excision of Supernumerary Breast, Via Natural or Artificial Opening Endoscopic
0HBYXZX Excision of Supernumerary Breast, External Approach, Diagnostic
0HBYXZZ Excision of Supernumerary Breast, External Approach

0HC – Skin and Breast, Extirpation

0HC0XZZ Extirpation of Matter from Scalp Skin, External Approach
0HC1XZZ Extirpation of Matter from Face Skin, External Approach
0HC2XZZ Extirpation of Matter from Right Ear Skin, External Approach
0HC3XZZ Extirpation of Matter from Left Ear Skin, External Approach
0HC4XZZ Extirpation of Matter from Neck Skin, External Approach
0HC5XZZ Extirpation of Matter from Chest Skin, External Approach
0HC6XZZ Extirpation of Matter from Back Skin, External Approach
0HC7XZZ Extirpation of Matter from Abdomen Skin, External Approach
0HC8XZZ Extirpation of Matter from Buttock Skin, External Approach
0HC9XZZ Extirpation of Matter from Perineum Skin, External Approach
0HCAXZZ Extirpation of Matter from Genitalia Skin, External Approach

0HCBXZZ Extirpation of Matter from Right Upper Arm Skin, External Approach
0HCCXZZ Extirpation of Matter from Left Upper Arm Skin, External Approach
0HCDXZZ Extirpation of Matter from Right Lower Arm Skin, External Approach
0HCEXZZ Extirpation of Matter from Left Lower Arm Skin, External Approach
0HCFXZZ Extirpation of Matter from Right Hand Skin, External Approach
0HCGXZZ Extirpation of Matter from Left Hand Skin, External Approach

0HCHXZZ Extirpation of Matter from Right Upper Leg Skin, External Approach

0HCJXZZ Extirpation of Matter from Left Upper Leg Skin, External Approach

0HCKXZZ Extirpation of Matter from Right Lower Leg Skin, External Approach

0HCLXZZ Extirpation of Matter from Left Lower Leg Skin, External Approach

0HCMXZZ Extirpation of Matter from Right Foot Skin, External Approach

0HCNXZZ Extirpation of Matter from Left Foot Skin, External Approach

0HCQXZZ Extirpation of Matter from Finger Nail, External Approach

0HCRXZZ Extirpation of Matter from Toe Nail, External Approach

0HCT0ZZ Extirpation of Matter from Right Breast, Open Approach

0HCT3ZZ Extirpation of Matter from Right Breast, Percutaneous Approach

0HCT7ZZ Extirpation of Matter from Right Breast, Via Natural or Artificial Opening

0HCT8ZZ Extirpation of Matter from Right Breast, Via Natural or Artificial Opening Endoscopic

0HCTXZZ Extirpation of Matter from Right Breast, External Approach

0HCU0ZZ Extirpation of Matter from Left Breast, Open Approach

0HCU3ZZ Extirpation of Matter from Left Breast, Percutaneous Approach

0HCU7ZZ Extirpation of Matter from Left Breast, Via Natural or Artificial Opening

0HCU8ZZ Extirpation of Matter from Left Breast, Via Natural or Artificial Opening Endoscopic

0HCUXZZ Extirpation of Matter from Left Breast, External Approach

0HCV0ZZ Extirpation of Matter from Bilateral Breast, Open Approach

0HCV3ZZ Extirpation of Matter from Bilateral Breast, Percutaneous Approach

0HCV7ZZ Extirpation of Matter from Bilateral Breast, Via Natural or Artificial Opening

0HCV8ZZ Extirpation of Matter from Bilateral Breast, Via Natural or Artificial Opening Endoscopic

0HCVXZZ Extirpation of Matter from Bilateral Breast, External Approach

0HCW0ZZ Extirpation of Matter from Right Nipple, Open Approach

0HCW3ZZ Extirpation of Matter from Right Nipple, Percutaneous Approach

0HCW7ZZ Extirpation of Matter from Right Nipple, Via Natural or Artificial Opening

0HCW8ZZ Extirpation of Matter from Right Nipple, Via Natural or Artificial Opening Endoscopic

0HCWXZZ Extirpation of Matter from Right Nipple, External Approach

0HCX0ZZ Extirpation of Matter from Left Nipple, Open Approach

0HCX3ZZ Extirpation of Matter from Left Nipple, Percutaneous Approach

0HCX7ZZ Extirpation of Matter from Left Nipple, Via Natural or Artificial Opening

0HCX8ZZ Extirpation of Matter from Left Nipple, Via Natural or Artificial Opening Endoscopic

0HCXXZZ Extirpation of Matter from Left Nipple, External Approach

0HD – Skin and Breast, Extraction

0HD0XZZ Extraction of Scalp Skin, External Approach

0HD1XZZ Extraction of Face Skin, External Approach

0HD2XZZ Extraction of Right Ear Skin, External Approach

0HD3XZZ Extraction of Left Ear Skin, External Approach

0HD4XZZ Extraction of Neck Skin, External Approach

0HD5XZZ Extraction of Chest Skin, External Approach

0HD6XZZ Extraction of Back Skin, External Approach

0HD7XZZ Extraction of Abdomen Skin, External Approach

0HD8XZZ Extraction of Buttock Skin, External Approach

0HD9XZZ Extraction of Perineum Skin, External Approach

0HDAXZZ Extraction of Genitalia Skin, External Approach

0HDBXZZ Extraction of Right Upper Arm Skin, External Approach

0HDCXZZ Extraction of Left Upper Arm Skin, External Approach

0HDDXZZ Extraction of Right Lower Arm Skin, External Approach

0HDEXZZ Extraction of Left Lower Arm Skin, External Approach

0HDFXZZ Extraction of Right Hand Skin, External Approach

0HDGXZZ Extraction of Left Hand Skin, External Approach

0HDHXZZ Extraction of Right Upper Leg Skin, External Approach

0HDJXZZ Extraction of Left Upper Leg Skin, External Approach

0HDKXZZ Extraction of Right Lower Leg Skin, External Approach

0HDLXZZ Extraction of Left Lower Leg Skin, External Approach

0HDMXZZ Extraction of Right Foot Skin, External Approach

0HDNXZZ Extraction of Left Foot Skin, External Approach

0HDQXZZ Extraction of Finger Nail, External Approach

0HDRXZZ Extraction of Toe Nail, External Approach

0HDSXZZ Extraction of Hair, External Approach

0HH – Skin and Breast, Insertion

0HHT01Z Insertion of Radioactive Element into Right Breast, Open Approach

0HHT0NZ Insertion of Tissue Expander into Right Breast, Open Approach

0HHT31Z Insertion of Radioactive Element into Right Breast, Percutaneous Approach

0HHT3NZ Insertion of Tissue Expander into Right Breast, Percutaneous Approach

0HHT71Z Insertion of Radioactive Element into Right Breast, Via Natural or Artificial Opening

0HHT7NZ Insertion of Tissue Expander into Right Breast, Via Natural or Artificial Opening

0HHT81Z Insertion of Radioactive Element into Right Breast, Via Natural or Artificial Opening Endoscopic

0HHT8NZ Insertion of Tissue Expander into Right Breast, Via Natural or Artificial Opening Endoscopic

0HHTX1Z Insertion of Radioactive Element into Right Breast, External Approach

0HHU01Z Insertion of Radioactive Element into Left Breast, Open Approach

0HHU0NZ Insertion of Tissue Expander into Left Breast, Open Approach

0HHU31Z Insertion of Radioactive Element into Left Breast, Percutaneous Approach

0HHU3NZ Insertion of Tissue Expander into Left Breast, Percutaneous Approach

0HHU71Z Insertion of Radioactive Element into Left Breast, Via Natural or Artificial Opening

0HHU7NZ Insertion of Tissue Expander into Left Breast, Via Natural or Artificial Opening

0HHU81Z Insertion of Radioactive Element into Left Breast, Via Natural or Artificial Opening Endoscopic

0HHU8NZ Insertion of Tissue Expander into Left Breast, Via Natural or Artificial Opening Endoscopic

0HHUX1Z Insertion of Radioactive Element into Left Breast, External Approach

0HHV01Z Insertion of Radioactive Element into Bilateral Breast, Open Approach

0HHV0NZ Insertion of Tissue Expander into Bilateral Breast, Open Approach

0HHV31Z Insertion of Radioactive Element into Bilateral Breast, Percutaneous Approach

0HHV3NZ Insertion of Tissue Expander into Bilateral Breast, Percutaneous Approach

0HHV71Z Insertion of Radioactive Element into Bilateral Breast, Via Natural or Artificial Opening

0HHV7NZ Insertion of Tissue Expander into Bilateral Breast, Via Natural or Artificial Opening

0HHV81Z Insertion of Radioactive Element into Bilateral Breast, Via Natural or Artificial Opening Endoscopic

0HHV8NZ Insertion of Tissue Expander into Bilateral Breast, Via Natural or Artificial Opening Endoscopic

0HHVX1Z Insertion of Radioactive Element into Bilateral Breast, External Approach

0HHW01Z Insertion of Radioactive Element into Right Nipple, Open Approach

0HHW0NZ Insertion of Tissue Expander into Right Nipple, Open Approach

0HHW31Z Insertion of Radioactive Element into Right Nipple, Percutaneous Approach

0HHW3NZ Insertion of Tissue Expander into Right Nipple, Percutaneous Approach

0HHW71Z Insertion of Radioactive Element into Right Nipple, Via Natural or Artificial Opening

0HHW7NZ Insertion of Tissue Expander into Right Nipple, Via Natural or Artificial Opening

0HHW81Z Insertion of Radioactive Element into Right Nipple, Via Natural or Artificial Opening Endoscopic

0HHW8NZ Insertion of Tissue Expander into Right Nipple, Via Natural or Artificial Opening Endoscopic

0HHWX1Z Insertion of Radioactive Element into Right Nipple, External Approach

0HHX01Z Insertion of Radioactive Element into Left Nipple, Open Approach

0HHX0NZ Insertion of Tissue Expander into Left Nipple, Open Approach

0HHX31Z Insertion of Radioactive Element into Left Nipple, Percutaneous Approach
0HHX3NZ Insertion of Tissue Expander into Left Nipple, Percutaneous Approach
0HHX71Z Insertion of Radioactive Element into Left Nipple, Via Natural or Artificial Opening
0HHX7NZ Insertion of Tissue Expander into Left Nipple, Via Natural or Artificial Opening

0HHX81Z Insertion of Radioactive Element into Left Nipple, Via Natural or Artificial Opening Endoscopic
0HHX8NZ Insertion of Tissue Expander into Left Nipple, Via Natural or Artificial Opening Endoscopic
0HHXX1Z Insertion of Radioactive Element into Left Nipple, External Approach

0HJ – Skin and Breast, Inspection

Review Coding Guideline B3.5

Review Coding Guidelines B3.11a, B3.11b and B3.11c

0HJPXZZ Inspection of Skin, External Approach
0HJQXZZ Inspection of Finger Nail, External Approach
0HJRXZZ Inspection of Toe Nail, External Approach
0HJT0ZZ Inspection of Right Breast, Open Approach
0HJT3ZZ Inspection of Right Breast, Percutaneous Approach
0HJT7ZZ Inspection of Right Breast, Via Natural or Artificial Opening
0HJT8ZZ Inspection of Right Breast, Via Natural or Artificial Opening Endoscopic

0HJTXZZ Inspection of Right Breast, External Approach
0HJU0ZZ Inspection of Left Breast, Open Approach
0HJU3ZZ Inspection of Left Breast, Percutaneous Approach
0HJU7ZZ Inspection of Left Breast, Via Natural or Artificial Opening
0HJU8ZZ Inspection of Left Breast, Via Natural or Artificial Opening Endoscopic
0HJUXZZ Inspection of Left Breast, External Approach

0HM – Skin and Breast, Reattachment

0HM0XZZ Reattachment of Scalp Skin, External Approach
0HM1XZZ Reattachment of Face Skin, External Approach
0HM2XZZ Reattachment of Right Ear Skin, External Approach
0HM3XZZ Reattachment of Left Ear Skin, External Approach
0HM4XZZ Reattachment of Neck Skin, External Approach
0HM5XZZ Reattachment of Chest Skin, External Approach
0HM6XZZ Reattachment of Back Skin, External Approach
0HM7XZZ Reattachment of Abdomen Skin, External Approach
0HM8XZZ Reattachment of Buttock Skin, External Approach
0HM9XZZ Reattachment of Perineum Skin, External Approach
0HMAXZZ Reattachment of Genitalia Skin, External Approach
0HMBXZZ Reattachment of Right Upper Arm Skin, External Approach
0HMCXZZ Reattachment of Left Upper Arm Skin, External Approach
0HMDXZZ Reattachment of Right Lower Arm Skin, External Approach

0HMEXZZ Reattachment of Left Lower Arm Skin, External Approach
0HMFXZZ Reattachment of Right Hand Skin, External Approach
0HMGXZZ Reattachment of Left Hand Skin, External Approach
0HMHXZZ Reattachment of Right Upper Leg Skin, External Approach
0HMJXZZ Reattachment of Left Upper Leg Skin, External Approach
0HMKXZZ Reattachment of Right Lower Leg Skin, External Approach
0HMLXZZ Reattachment of Left Lower Leg Skin, External Approach
0HMMXZZ Reattachment of Right Foot Skin, External Approach
0HMNXZZ Reattachment of Left Foot Skin, External Approach
0HMTXZZ Reattachment of Right Breast, External Approach
0HMUXZZ Reattachment of Left Breast, External Approach
0HMVXZZ Reattachment of Bilateral Breast, External Approach
0HMWXZZ Reattachment of Right Nipple, External Approach
0HMXXZZ Reattachment of Left Nipple, External Approach

0HN – Skin and Breast, Release

Review Coding Guideline B3.13

Review Coding Guideline B3.14

0HN0XZZ Release Scalp Skin, External Approach
0HN1XZZ Release Face Skin, External Approach
0HN2XZZ Release Right Ear Skin, External Approach
0HN3XZZ Release Left Ear Skin, External Approach
0HN4XZZ Release Neck Skin, External Approach
0HN5XZZ Release Chest Skin, External Approach
0HN6XZZ Release Back Skin, External Approach
0HN7XZZ Release Abdomen Skin, External Approach
0HN8XZZ Release Buttock Skin, External Approach
0HN9XZZ Release Perineum Skin, External Approach
0HNAXZZ Release Genitalia Skin, External Approach
0HNBXZZ Release Right Upper Arm Skin, External Approach
0HNCXZZ Release Left Upper Arm Skin, External Approach
0HNDXZZ Release Right Lower Arm Skin, External Approach
0HNEXZZ Release Left Lower Arm Skin, External Approach
0HNFXZZ Release Right Hand Skin, External Approach
0HNGXZZ Release Left Hand Skin, External Approach
0HNHXZZ Release Right Upper Leg Skin, External Approach
0HNJXZZ Release Left Upper Leg Skin, External Approach
0HNKXZZ Release Right Lower Leg Skin, External Approach
0HNLXZZ Release Left Lower Leg Skin, External Approach
0HNMXZZ Release Right Foot Skin, External Approach
0HNNXZZ Release Left Foot Skin, External Approach
0HNQXZZ Release Finger Nail, External Approach
0HNRXZZ Release Toe Nail, External Approach

0HNT0ZZ Release Right Breast, Open Approach
0HNT3ZZ Release Right Breast, Percutaneous Approach
0HNT7ZZ Release Right Breast, Via Natural or Artificial Opening
0HNT8ZZ Release Right Breast, Via Natural or Artificial Opening Endoscopic
0HNTXZZ Release Right Breast, External Approach
0HNU0ZZ Release Left Breast, Open Approach
0HNU3ZZ Release Left Breast, Percutaneous Approach
0HNU7ZZ Release Left Breast, Via Natural or Artificial Opening
0HNU8ZZ Release Left Breast, Via Natural or Artificial Opening Endoscopic
0HNUXZZ Release Left Breast, External Approach
0HNV0ZZ Release Bilateral Breast, Open Approach
0HNV3ZZ Release Bilateral Breast, Percutaneous Approach
0HNV7ZZ Release Bilateral Breast, Via Natural or Artificial Opening
0HNV8ZZ Release Bilateral Breast, Via Natural or Artificial Opening Endoscopic
0HNVXZZ Release Bilateral Breast, External Approach
0HNW0ZZ Release Right Nipple, Open Approach
0HNW3ZZ Release Right Nipple, Percutaneous Approach
0HNW7ZZ Release Right Nipple, Via Natural or Artificial Opening
0HNW8ZZ Release Right Nipple, Via Natural or Artificial Opening Endoscopic
0HNWXZZ Release Right Nipple, External Approach
0HNX0ZZ Release Left Nipple, Open Approach
0HNX3ZZ Release Left Nipple, Percutaneous Approach
0HNX7ZZ Release Left Nipple, Via Natural or Artificial Opening
0HNX8ZZ Release Left Nipple, Via Natural or Artificial Opening Endoscopic
0HNXXZZ Release Left Nipple, External Approach

0HP – Skin and Breast, Removal

Review Coding Guideline B6.1c

0HPPX0Z Removal of Drainage Device from Skin, External Approach
0HPPX7Z Removal of Autologous Tissue Substitute from Skin, External Approach
0HPPXJZ Removal of Synthetic Substitute from Skin, External Approach
0HPPXKZ Removal of Nonautologous Tissue Substitute from Skin, External Approach
0HPQX0Z Removal of Drainage Device from Finger Nail, External Approach
0HPQX7Z Removal of Autologous Tissue Substitute from Finger Nail, External Approach
0HPQXJZ Removal of Synthetic Substitute from Finger Nail, External Approach
0HPQXKZ Removal of Nonautologous Tissue Substitute from Finger Nail, External Approach
0HPRX0Z Removal of Drainage Device from Toe Nail, External Approach
0HPRX7Z Removal of Autologous Tissue Substitute from Toe Nail, External Approach
0HPRXJZ Removal of Synthetic Substitute from Toe Nail, External Approach
0HPRXKZ Removal of Nonautologous Tissue Substitute from Toe Nail, External Approach
0HPSX7Z Removal of Autologous Tissue Substitute from Hair, External Approach
0HPSXJZ Removal of Synthetic Substitute from Hair, External Approach
0HPSXKZ Removal of Nonautologous Tissue Substitute from Hair, External Approach
0HPT00Z Removal of Drainage Device from Right Breast, Open Approach
0HPT01Z Removal of Radioactive Element from Right Breast, Open Approach
0HPT07Z Removal of Autologous Tissue Substitute from Right Breast, Open Approach
0HPT0JZ Removal of Synthetic Substitute from Right Breast, Open Approach
0HPT0KZ Removal of Nonautologous Tissue Substitute from Right Breast, Open Approach
0HPT0NZ Removal of Tissue Expander from Right Breast, Open Approach
0HPT30Z Removal of Drainage Device from Right Breast, Percutaneous Approach
0HPT31Z Removal of Radioactive Element from Right Breast, Percutaneous Approach
0HPT37Z Removal of Autologous Tissue Substitute from Right Breast, Percutaneous Approach
0HPT3JZ Removal of Synthetic Substitute from Right Breast, Percutaneous Approach
0HPT3KZ Removal of Nonautologous Tissue Substitute from Right Breast, Percutaneous Approach
0HPT3NZ Removal of Tissue Expander from Right Breast, Percutaneous Approach
0HPT70Z Removal of Drainage Device from Right Breast, Via Natural or Artificial Opening
0HPT71Z Removal of Radioactive Element from Right Breast, Via Natural or Artificial Opening
0HPT77Z Removal of Autologous Tissue Substitute from Right Breast, Via Natural or Artificial Opening
0HPT7JZ Removal of Synthetic Substitute from Right Breast, Via Natural or Artificial Opening
0HPT7KZ Removal of Nonautologous Tissue Substitute from Right Breast, Via Natural or Artificial Opening
0HPT7NZ Removal of Tissue Expander from Right Breast, Via Natural or Artificial Opening
0HPT80Z Removal of Drainage Device from Right Breast, Via Natural or Artificial Opening Endoscopic
0HPT81Z Removal of Radioactive Element from Right Breast, Via Natural or Artificial Opening Endoscopic
0HPT87Z Removal of Autologous Tissue Substitute from Right Breast, Via Natural or Artificial Opening Endoscopic
0HPT8JZ Removal of Synthetic Substitute from Right Breast, Via Natural or Artificial Opening Endoscopic

0HPT8KZ Removal of Nonautologous Tissue Substitute from Right Breast, Via Natural or Artificial Opening Endoscopic
0HPT8NZ Removal of Tissue Expander from Right Breast, Via Natural or Artificial Opening Endoscopic
0HPTX0Z Removal of Drainage Device from Right Breast, External Approach
0HPTX1Z Removal of Radioactive Element from Right Breast, External Approach
0HPTX7Z Removal of Autologous Tissue Substitute from Right Breast, External Approach
0HPTXJZ Removal of Synthetic Substitute from Right Breast, External Approach
0HPTXKZ Removal of Nonautologous Tissue Substitute from Right Breast, External Approach
0HPU00Z Removal of Drainage Device from Left Breast, Open Approach
0HPU01Z Removal of Radioactive Element from Left Breast, Open Approach
0HPU07Z Removal of Autologous Tissue Substitute from Left Breast, Open Approach
0HPU0JZ Removal of Synthetic Substitute from Left Breast, Open Approach
0HPU0KZ Removal of Nonautologous Tissue Substitute from Left Breast, Open Approach
0HPU0NZ Removal of Tissue Expander from Left Breast, Open Approach
0HPU30Z Removal of Drainage Device from Left Breast, Percutaneous Approach
0HPU31Z Removal of Radioactive Element from Left Breast, Percutaneous Approach
0HPU37Z Removal of Autologous Tissue Substitute from Left Breast, Percutaneous Approach
0HPU3JZ Removal of Synthetic Substitute from Left Breast, Percutaneous Approach
0HPU3KZ Removal of Nonautologous Tissue Substitute from Left Breast, Percutaneous Approach
0HPU3NZ Removal of Tissue Expander from Left Breast, Percutaneous Approach
0HPU70Z Removal of Drainage Device from Left Breast, Via Natural or Artificial Opening
0HPU71Z Removal of Radioactive Element from Left Breast, Via Natural or Artificial Opening
0HPU77Z Removal of Autologous Tissue Substitute from Left Breast, Via Natural or Artificial Opening
0HPU7JZ Removal of Synthetic Substitute from Left Breast, Via Natural or Artificial Opening
0HPU7KZ Removal of Nonautologous Tissue Substitute from Left Breast, Via Natural or Artificial Opening
0HPU7NZ Removal of Tissue Expander from Left Breast, Via Natural or Artificial Opening
0HPU80Z Removal of Drainage Device from Left Breast, Via Natural or Artificial Opening Endoscopic
0HPU81Z Removal of Radioactive Element from Left Breast, Via Natural or Artificial Opening Endoscopic
0HPU87Z Removal of Autologous Tissue Substitute from Left Breast, Via Natural or Artificial Opening Endoscopic
0HPU8JZ Removal of Synthetic Substitute from Left Breast, Via Natural or Artificial Opening Endoscopic
0HPU8KZ Removal of Nonautologous Tissue Substitute from Left Breast, Via Natural or Artificial Opening Endoscopic
0HPU8NZ Removal of Tissue Expander from Left Breast, Via Natural or Artificial Opening Endoscopic
0HPUX0Z Removal of Drainage Device from Left Breast, External Approach
0HPUX1Z Removal of Radioactive Element from Left Breast, External Approach
0HPUX7Z Removal of Autologous Tissue Substitute from Left Breast, External Approach
0HPUXJZ Removal of Synthetic Substitute from Left Breast, External Approach
0HPUXKZ Removal of Nonautologous Tissue Substitute from Left Breast, External Approach

0HQ – Skin and Breast, Repair

Review Coding Guideline B3.5

0HQ0XZZ Repair Scalp Skin, External Approach
0HQ1XZZ Repair Face Skin, External Approach
0HQ2XZZ Repair Right Ear Skin, External Approach
0HQ3XZZ Repair Left Ear Skin, External Approach

♀ Female-only   ♂ Male-only   ● Limited Coverage   ● Non-OR   HAC HAC-associated procedure   ⬡ Non-covered procedures   ➕ Combination

0HQ4XZZ	Repair Neck Skin, External Approach
0HQ5XZZ	Repair Chest Skin, External Approach
0HQ6XZZ	Repair Back Skin, External Approach
0HQ7XZZ	Repair Abdomen Skin, External Approach
0HQ8XZZ	Repair Buttock Skin, External Approach
● 0HQ9XZZ	Repair Perineum Skin, External Approach
0HQAXZZ	Repair Genitalia Skin, External Approach
0HQBXZZ	Repair Right Upper Arm Skin, External Approach
0HQCXZZ	Repair Left Upper Arm Skin, External Approach
0HQDXZZ	Repair Right Lower Arm Skin, External Approach
0HQEXZZ	Repair Left Lower Arm Skin, External Approach
0HQFXZZ	Repair Right Hand Skin, External Approach
0HQGXZZ	Repair Left Hand Skin, External Approach
0HQHXZZ	Repair Right Upper Leg Skin, External Approach
0HQJXZZ	Repair Left Upper Leg Skin, External Approach
0HQKXZZ	Repair Right Lower Leg Skin, External Approach
0HQLXZZ	Repair Left Lower Leg Skin, External Approach
0HQMXZZ	Repair Right Foot Skin, External Approach
0HQNXZZ	Repair Left Foot Skin, External Approach
0HQQXZZ	Repair Finger Nail, External Approach
0HQRXZZ	Repair Toe Nail, External Approach
0HQT0ZZ	Repair Right Breast, Open Approach
0HQT3ZZ	Repair Right Breast, Percutaneous Approach
0HQT7ZZ	Repair Right Breast, Via Natural or Artificial Opening
0HQT8ZZ	Repair Right Breast, Via Natural or Artificial Opening Endoscopic
0HQTXZZ	Repair Right Breast, External Approach
0HQU0ZZ	Repair Left Breast, Open Approach
0HQU3ZZ	Repair Left Breast, Percutaneous Approach
0HQU7ZZ	Repair Left Breast, Via Natural or Artificial Opening
0HQU8ZZ	Repair Left Breast, Via Natural or Artificial Opening Endoscopic
0HQUXZZ	Repair Left Breast, External Approach
0HQV0ZZ	Repair Bilateral Breast, Open Approach
0HQV3ZZ	Repair Bilateral Breast, Percutaneous Approach
0HQV7ZZ	Repair Bilateral Breast, Via Natural or Artificial Opening
0HQV8ZZ	Repair Bilateral Breast, Via Natural or Artificial Opening Endoscopic
0HQVXZZ	Repair Bilateral Breast, External Approach
0HQW0ZZ	Repair Right Nipple, Open Approach
0HQW3ZZ	Repair Right Nipple, Percutaneous Approach
0HQW7ZZ	Repair Right Nipple, Via Natural or Artificial Opening
0HQW8ZZ	Repair Right Nipple, Via Natural or Artificial Opening Endoscopic
0HQWXZZ	Repair Right Nipple, External Approach
0HQX0ZZ	Repair Left Nipple, Open Approach
0HQX3ZZ	Repair Left Nipple, Percutaneous Approach
0HQX7ZZ	Repair Left Nipple, Via Natural or Artificial Opening
0HQX8ZZ	Repair Left Nipple, Via Natural or Artificial Opening Endoscopic
0HQXXZZ	Repair Left Nipple, External Approach
0HQY0ZZ	Repair Supernumerary Breast, Open Approach
0HQY3ZZ	Repair Supernumerary Breast, Percutaneous Approach
0HQY7ZZ	Repair Supernumerary Breast, Via Natural or Artificial Opening
0HQY8ZZ	Repair Supernumerary Breast, Via Natural or Artificial Opening Endoscopic
0HQYXZZ	Repair Supernumerary Breast, External Approach

0HR – Skin and Breast, Replacement

0HR0X73	Replacement of Scalp Skin with Autologous Tissue Substitute, Full Thickness, External Approach
0HR0X74	Replacement of Scalp Skin with Autologous Tissue Substitute, Partial Thickness, External Approach
0HR0XJ3	Replacement of Scalp Skin with Synthetic Substitute, Full Thickness, External Approach
0HR0XJ4	Replacement of Scalp Skin with Synthetic Substitute, Partial Thickness, External Approach
0HR0XJZ	Replacement of Scalp Skin with Synthetic Substitute, External Approach
0HR0XK3	Replacement of Scalp Skin with Nonautologous Tissue Substitute, Full Thickness, External Approach
0HR0XK4	Replacement of Scalp Skin with Nonautologous Tissue Substitute, Partial Thickness, External Approach
0HR1X73	Replacement of Face Skin with Autologous Tissue Substitute, Full Thickness, External Approach
0HR1X74	Replacement of Face Skin with Autologous Tissue Substitute, Partial Thickness, External Approach
0HR1XJ3	Replacement of Face Skin with Synthetic Substitute, Full Thickness, External Approach
0HR1XJ4	Replacement of Face Skin with Synthetic Substitute, Partial Thickness, External Approach
0HR1XJZ	Replacement of Face Skin with Synthetic Substitute, External Approach
0HR1XK3	Replacement of Face Skin with Nonautologous Tissue Substitute, Full Thickness, External Approach
0HR1XK4	Replacement of Face Skin with Nonautologous Tissue Substitute, Partial Thickness, External Approach
0HR2X73	Replacement of Right Ear Skin with Autologous Tissue Substitute, Full Thickness, External Approach
0HR2X74	Replacement of Right Ear Skin with Autologous Tissue Substitute, Partial Thickness, External Approach
0HR2XJ3	Replacement of Right Ear Skin with Synthetic Substitute, Full Thickness, External Approach
0HR2XJ4	Replacement of Right Ear Skin with Synthetic Substitute, Partial Thickness, External Approach
0HR2XJZ	Replacement of Right Ear Skin with Synthetic Substitute, External Approach
0HR2XK3	Replacement of Right Ear Skin with Nonautologous Tissue Substitute, Full Thickness, External Approach
0HR2XK4	Replacement of Right Ear Skin with Nonautologous Tissue Substitute, Partial Thickness, External Approach
0HR3X73	Replacement of Left Ear Skin with Autologous Tissue Substitute, Full Thickness, External Approach
0HR3X74	Replacement of Left Ear Skin with Autologous Tissue Substitute, Partial Thickness, External Approach
0HR3XJ3	Replacement of Left Ear Skin with Synthetic Substitute, Full Thickness, External Approach
0HR3XJ4	Replacement of Left Ear Skin with Synthetic Substitute, Partial Thickness, External Approach
0HR3XJZ	Replacement of Left Ear Skin with Synthetic Substitute, External Approach
0HR3XK3	Replacement of Left Ear Skin with Nonautologous Tissue Substitute, Full Thickness, External Approach
0HR3XK4	Replacement of Left Ear Skin with Nonautologous Tissue Substitute, Partial Thickness, External Approach
0HR4X73	Replacement of Neck Skin with Autologous Tissue Substitute, Full Thickness, External Approach
0HR4X74	Replacement of Neck Skin with Autologous Tissue Substitute, Partial Thickness, External Approach
0HR4XJ3	Replacement of Neck Skin with Synthetic Substitute, Full Thickness, External Approach
0HR4XJ4	Replacement of Neck Skin with Synthetic Substitute, Partial Thickness, External Approach
0HR4XJZ	Replacement of Neck Skin with Synthetic Substitute, External Approach
0HR4XK3	Replacement of Neck Skin with Nonautologous Tissue Substitute, Full Thickness, External Approach
0HR4XK4	Replacement of Neck Skin with Nonautologous Tissue Substitute, Partial Thickness, External Approach
0HR5X73	Replacement of Chest Skin with Autologous Tissue Substitute, Full Thickness, External Approach
0HR5X74	Replacement of Chest Skin with Autologous Tissue Substitute, Partial Thickness, External Approach
0HR5XJ3	Replacement of Chest Skin with Synthetic Substitute, Full Thickness, External Approach
0HR5XJ4	Replacement of Chest Skin with Synthetic Substitute, Partial Thickness, External Approach
0HR5XJZ	Replacement of Chest Skin with Synthetic Substitute, External Approach
0HR5XK3	Replacement of Chest Skin with Nonautologous Tissue Substitute, Full Thickness, External Approach
0HR5XK4	Replacement of Chest Skin with Nonautologous Tissue Substitute, Partial Thickness, External Approach
0HR6X73	Replacement of Back Skin with Autologous Tissue Substitute, Full Thickness, External Approach
0HR6X74	Replacement of Back Skin with Autologous Tissue Substitute, Partial Thickness, External Approach

0HR6XJ3 Replacement of Back Skin with Synthetic Substitute, Full Thickness, External Approach

0HR6XJ4 Replacement of Back Skin with Synthetic Substitute, Partial Thickness, External Approach

0HR6XJZ Replacement of Back Skin with Synthetic Substitute, External Approach

0HR6XK3 Replacement of Back Skin with Nonautologous Tissue Substitute, Full Thickness, External Approach

0HR6XK4 Replacement of Back Skin with Nonautologous Tissue Substitute, Partial Thickness, External Approach

0HR7X73 Replacement of Abdomen Skin with Autologous Tissue Substitute, Full Thickness, External Approach

0HR7X74 Replacement of Abdomen Skin with Autologous Tissue Substitute, Partial Thickness, External Approach

0HR7XJ3 Replacement of Abdomen Skin with Synthetic Substitute, Full Thickness, External Approach

0HR7XJ4 Replacement of Abdomen Skin with Synthetic Substitute, Partial Thickness, External Approach

0HR7XJZ Replacement of Abdomen Skin with Synthetic Substitute, External Approach

0HR7XK3 Replacement of Abdomen Skin with Nonautologous Tissue Substitute, Full Thickness, External Approach

0HR7XK4 Replacement of Abdomen Skin with Nonautologous Tissue Substitute, Partial Thickness, External Approach

0HR8X73 Replacement of Buttock Skin with Autologous Tissue Substitute, Full Thickness, External Approach

0HR8X74 Replacement of Buttock Skin with Autologous Tissue Substitute, Partial Thickness, External Approach

0HR8XJ3 Replacement of Buttock Skin with Synthetic Substitute, Full Thickness, External Approach

0HR8XJ4 Replacement of Buttock Skin with Synthetic Substitute, Partial Thickness, External Approach

0HR8XJZ Replacement of Buttock Skin with Synthetic Substitute, External Approach

0HR8XK3 Replacement of Buttock Skin with Nonautologous Tissue Substitute, Full Thickness, External Approach

0HR8XK4 Replacement of Buttock Skin with Nonautologous Tissue Substitute, Partial Thickness, External Approach

0HR9X73 Replacement of Perineum Skin with Autologous Tissue Substitute, Full Thickness, External Approach

0HR9X74 Replacement of Perineum Skin with Autologous Tissue Substitute, Partial Thickness, External Approach

0HR9XJ3 Replacement of Perineum Skin with Synthetic Substitute, Full Thickness, External Approach

0HR9XJ4 Replacement of Perineum Skin with Synthetic Substitute, Partial Thickness, External Approach

0HR9XJZ Replacement of Perineum Skin with Synthetic Substitute, External Approach

0HR9XK3 Replacement of Perineum Skin with Nonautologous Tissue Substitute, Full Thickness, External Approach

0HR9XK4 Replacement of Perineum Skin with Nonautologous Tissue Substitute, Partial Thickness, External Approach

0HRAX73 Replacement of Genitalia Skin with Autologous Tissue Substitute, Full Thickness, External Approach

0HRAX74 Replacement of Genitalia Skin with Autologous Tissue Substitute, Partial Thickness, External Approach

0HRAXJ3 Replacement of Genitalia Skin with Synthetic Substitute, Full Thickness, External Approach

0HRAXJ4 Replacement of Genitalia Skin with Synthetic Substitute, Partial Thickness, External Approach

0HRAXJZ Replacement of Genitalia Skin with Synthetic Substitute, External Approach

0HRAXK3 Replacement of Genitalia Skin with Nonautologous Tissue Substitute, Full Thickness, External Approach

0HRAXK4 Replacement of Genitalia Skin with Nonautologous Tissue Substitute, Partial Thickness, External Approach

0HRBX73 Replacement of Right Upper Arm Skin with Autologous Tissue Substitute, Full Thickness, External Approach

0HRBX74 Replacement of Right Upper Arm Skin with Autologous Tissue Substitute, Partial Thickness, External Approach

0HRBXJ3 Replacement of Right Upper Arm Skin with Synthetic Substitute, Full Thickness, External Approach

0HRBXJ4 Replacement of Right Upper Arm Skin with Synthetic Substitute, Partial Thickness, External Approach

0HRBXJZ Replacement of Right Upper Arm Skin with Synthetic Substitute, External Approach

0HRBXK3 Replacement of Right Upper Arm Skin with Nonautologous Tissue Substitute, Full Thickness, External Approach

0HRBXK4 Replacement of Right Upper Arm Skin with Nonautologous Tissue Substitute, Partial Thickness, External Approach

0HRCX73 Replacement of Left Upper Arm Skin with Autologous Tissue Substitute, Full Thickness, External Approach

0HRCX74 Replacement of Left Upper Arm Skin with Autologous Tissue Substitute, Partial Thickness, External Approach

0HRCXJ3 Replacement of Left Upper Arm Skin with Synthetic Substitute, Full Thickness, External Approach

0HRCXJ4 Replacement of Left Upper Arm Skin with Synthetic Substitute, Partial Thickness, External Approach

0HRCXJZ Replacement of Left Upper Arm Skin with Synthetic Substitute, External Approach

0HRCXK3 Replacement of Left Upper Arm Skin with Nonautologous Tissue Substitute, Full Thickness, External Approach

0HRCXK4 Replacement of Left Upper Arm Skin with Nonautologous Tissue Substitute, Partial Thickness, External Approach

0HRDX73 Replacement of Right Lower Arm Skin with Autologous Tissue Substitute, Full Thickness, External Approach

0HRDX74 Replacement of Right Lower Arm Skin with Autologous Tissue Substitute, Partial Thickness, External Approach

0HRDXJ3 Replacement of Right Lower Arm Skin with Synthetic Substitute, Full Thickness, External Approach

0HRDXJ4 Replacement of Right Lower Arm Skin with Synthetic Substitute, Partial Thickness, External Approach

0HRDXJZ Replacement of Right Lower Arm Skin with Synthetic Substitute, External Approach

0HRDXK3 Replacement of Right Lower Arm Skin with Nonautologous Tissue Substitute, Full Thickness, External Approach

0HRDXK4 Replacement of Right Lower Arm Skin with Nonautologous Tissue Substitute, Partial Thickness, External Approach

0HREX73 Replacement of Left Lower Arm Skin with Autologous Tissue Substitute, Full Thickness, External Approach

0HREX74 Replacement of Left Lower Arm Skin with Autologous Tissue Substitute, Partial Thickness, External Approach

0HREXJ3 Replacement of Left Lower Arm Skin with Synthetic Substitute, Full Thickness, External Approach

0HREXJ4 Replacement of Left Lower Arm Skin with Synthetic Substitute, Partial Thickness, External Approach

0HREXJZ Replacement of Left Lower Arm Skin with Synthetic Substitute, External Approach

0HREXK3 Replacement of Left Lower Arm Skin with Nonautologous Tissue Substitute, Full Thickness, External Approach

0HREXK4 Replacement of Left Lower Arm Skin with Nonautologous Tissue Substitute, Partial Thickness, External Approach

0HRFX73 Replacement of Right Hand Skin with Autologous Tissue Substitute, Full Thickness, External Approach

0HRFX74 Replacement of Right Hand Skin with Autologous Tissue Substitute, Partial Thickness, External Approach

0HRFXJ3 Replacement of Right Hand Skin with Synthetic Substitute, Full Thickness, External Approach

0HRFXJ4 Replacement of Right Hand Skin with Synthetic Substitute, Partial Thickness, External Approach

0HRFXJZ Replacement of Right Hand Skin with Synthetic Substitute, External Approach

0HRFXK3 Replacement of Right Hand Skin with Nonautologous Tissue Substitute, Full Thickness, External Approach

0HRFXK4 Replacement of Right Hand Skin with Nonautologous Tissue Substitute, Partial Thickness, External Approach

0HRGX73 Replacement of Left Hand Skin with Autologous Tissue Substitute, Full Thickness, External Approach

0HRGX74 Replacement of Left Hand Skin with Autologous Tissue Substitute, Partial Thickness, External Approach

0HRGXJ3 Replacement of Left Hand Skin with Synthetic Substitute, Full Thickness, External Approach

0HRGXJ4 Replacement of Left Hand Skin with Synthetic Substitute, Partial Thickness, External Approach

0HRGXJZ Replacement of Left Hand Skin with Synthetic Substitute, External Approach

0HRGXK3 Replacement of Left Hand Skin with Nonautologous Tissue Substitute, Full Thickness, External Approach

0HRGXK4 Replacement of Left Hand Skin with Nonautologous Tissue Substitute, Partial Thickness, External Approach

0HRHX73 Replacement of Right Upper Leg Skin with Autologous Tissue Substitute, Full Thickness, External Approach

0HRHX74 Replacement of Right Upper Leg Skin with Autologous Tissue Substitute, Partial Thickness, External Approach

0HRHXJ3 Replacement of Right Upper Leg Skin with Synthetic Substitute, Full Thickness, External Approach

0HRHXJ4 Replacement of Right Upper Leg Skin with Synthetic Substitute, Partial Thickness, External Approach

0HRHXJZ Replacement of Right Upper Leg Skin with Synthetic Substitute, External Approach

0HRHXK3 Replacement of Right Upper Leg Skin with Nonautologous Tissue Substitute, Full Thickness, External Approach

0HRHXK4 Replacement of Right Upper Leg Skin with Nonautologous Tissue Substitute, Partial Thickness, External Approach

0HRJX73 Replacement of Left Upper Leg Skin with Autologous Tissue Substitute, Full Thickness, External Approach

0HRJX74 Replacement of Left Upper Leg Skin with Autologous Tissue Substitute, Partial Thickness, External Approach

0HRJXJ3 Replacement of Left Upper Leg Skin with Synthetic Substitute, Full Thickness, External Approach

0HRJXJ4 Replacement of Left Upper Leg Skin with Synthetic Substitute, Partial Thickness, External Approach

0HRJXJZ Replacement of Left Upper Leg Skin with Synthetic Substitute, External Approach

0HRJXK3 Replacement of Left Upper Leg Skin with Nonautologous Tissue Substitute, Full Thickness, External Approach

0HRJXK4 Replacement of Left Upper Leg Skin with Nonautologous Tissue Substitute, Partial Thickness, External Approach

0HRKX73 Replacement of Right Lower Leg Skin with Autologous Tissue Substitute, Full Thickness, External Approach

0HRKX74 Replacement of Right Lower Leg Skin with Autologous Tissue Substitute, Partial Thickness, External Approach

0HRKXJ3 Replacement of Right Lower Leg Skin with Synthetic Substitute, Full Thickness, External Approach

0HRKXJ4 Replacement of Right Lower Leg Skin with Synthetic Substitute, Partial Thickness, External Approach

0HRKXJZ Replacement of Right Lower Leg Skin with Synthetic Substitute, External Approach

0HRKXK3 Replacement of Right Lower Leg Skin with Nonautologous Tissue Substitute, Full Thickness, External Approach

0HRKXK4 Replacement of Right Lower Leg Skin with Nonautologous Tissue Substitute, Partial Thickness, External Approach

0HRLX73 Replacement of Left Lower Leg Skin with Autologous Tissue Substitute, Full Thickness, External Approach

0HRLX74 Replacement of Left Lower Leg Skin with Autologous Tissue Substitute, Partial Thickness, External Approach

0HRLXJ3 Replacement of Left Lower Leg Skin with Synthetic Substitute, Full Thickness, External Approach

0HRLXJ4 Replacement of Left Lower Leg Skin with Synthetic Substitute, Partial Thickness, External Approach

0HRLXJZ Replacement of Left Lower Leg Skin with Synthetic Substitute, External Approach

0HRLXK3 Replacement of Left Lower Leg Skin with Nonautologous Tissue Substitute, Full Thickness, External Approach

0HRLXK4 Replacement of Left Lower Leg Skin with Nonautologous Tissue Substitute, Partial Thickness, External Approach

0HRMX73 Replacement of Right Foot Skin with Autologous Tissue Substitute, Full Thickness, External Approach

0HRMX74 Replacement of Right Foot Skin with Autologous Tissue Substitute, Partial Thickness, External Approach

0HRMXJ3 Replacement of Right Foot Skin with Synthetic Substitute, Full Thickness, External Approach

0HRMXJ4 Replacement of Right Foot Skin with Synthetic Substitute, Partial Thickness, External Approach

0HRMXJZ Replacement of Right Foot Skin with Synthetic Substitute, External Approach

0HRMXK3 Replacement of Right Foot Skin with Nonautologous Tissue Substitute, Full Thickness, External Approach

0HRMXK4 Replacement of Right Foot Skin with Nonautologous Tissue Substitute, Partial Thickness, External Approach

0HRNX73 Replacement of Left Foot Skin with Autologous Tissue Substitute, Full Thickness, External Approach

0HRNX74 Replacement of Left Foot Skin with Autologous Tissue Substitute, Partial Thickness, External Approach

0HRNXJ3 Replacement of Left Foot Skin with Synthetic Substitute, Full Thickness, External Approach

0HRNXJ4 Replacement of Left Foot Skin with Synthetic Substitute, Partial Thickness, External Approach

0HRNXJZ Replacement of Left Foot Skin with Synthetic Substitute, External Approach

0HRNXK3 Replacement of Left Foot Skin with Nonautologous Tissue Substitute, Full Thickness, External Approach

0HRNXK4 Replacement of Left Foot Skin with Nonautologous Tissue Substitute, Partial Thickness, External Approach

0HRQX7Z Replacement of Finger Nail with Autologous Tissue Substitute, External Approach

0HRQXJZ Replacement of Finger Nail with Synthetic Substitute, External Approach

0HRQXKZ Replacement of Finger Nail with Nonautologous Tissue Substitute, External Approach

0HRRX7Z Replacement of Toe Nail with Autologous Tissue Substitute, External Approach

0HRRXJZ Replacement of Toe Nail with Synthetic Substitute, External Approach

0HRRXKZ Replacement of Toe Nail with Nonautologous Tissue Substitute, External Approach

0HRSX7Z Replacement of Hair with Autologous Tissue Substitute, External Approach

0HRSXJZ Replacement of Hair with Synthetic Substitute, External Approach

0HRSXKZ Replacement of Hair with Nonautologous Tissue Substitute, External Approach

0HRT075 Replacement of Right Breast using Latissimus Dorsi Myocutaneous Flap, Open Approach

0HRT076 Replacement of Right Breast using Transverse Rectus Abdominis Myocutaneous Flap, Open Approach

0HRT077 Replacement of Right Breast using Deep Inferior Epigastric Artery Perforator Flap, Open Approach

0HRT078 Replacement of Right Breast using Superficial Inferior Epigastric Artery Flap, Open Approach

0HRT079 Replacement of Right Breast using Gluteal Artery Perforator Flap, Open Approach

0HRT07Z Replacement of Right Breast with Autologous Tissue Substitute, Open Approach

0HRT0JZ Replacement of Right Breast with Synthetic Substitute, Open Approach

0HRT0KZ Replacement of Right Breast with Nonautologous Tissue Substitute, Open Approach

0HRT37Z Replacement of Right Breast with Autologous Tissue Substitute, Percutaneous Approach

0HRT3JZ Replacement of Right Breast with Synthetic Substitute, Percutaneous Approach

0HRT3KZ Replacement of Right Breast with Nonautologous Tissue Substitute, Percutaneous Approach

0HRTX7Z Replacement of Right Breast with Autologous Tissue Substitute, External Approach

0HRTXJZ Replacement of Right Breast with Synthetic Substitute, External Approach

0HRTXKZ Replacement of Right Breast with Nonautologous Tissue Substitute, External Approach

0HRU075 Replacement of Left Breast using Latissimus Dorsi Myocutaneous Flap, Open Approach

0HRU076 Replacement of Left Breast using Transverse Rectus Abdominis Myocutaneous Flap, Open Approach

0HRU077 Replacement of Left Breast using Deep Inferior Epigastric Artery Perforator Flap, Open Approach

0HRU078 Replacement of Left Breast using Superficial Inferior Epigastric Artery Flap, Open Approach

0HRU079 Replacement of Left Breast using Gluteal Artery Perforator Flap, Open Approach

0HRU07Z Replacement of Left Breast with Autologous Tissue Substitute, Open Approach

0HRU0JZ Replacement of Left Breast with Synthetic Substitute, Open Approach

0HRU0KZ Replacement of Left Breast with Nonautologous Tissue Substitute, Open Approach

0HRU37Z   Replacement of Left Breast with Autologous Tissue Substitute, Percutaneous Approach

0HRU3JZ   Replacement of Left Breast with Synthetic Substitute, Percutaneous Approach

0HRU3KZ   Replacement of Left Breast with Nonautologous Tissue Substitute, Percutaneous Approach

0HRUX7Z   Replacement of Left Breast with Autologous Tissue Substitute, External Approach

0HRUXJZ   Replacement of Left Breast with Synthetic Substitute, External Approach

0HRUXKZ   Replacement of Left Breast with Nonautologous Tissue Substitute, External Approach

0HRV075   Replacement of Bilateral Breast using Latissimus Dorsi Myocutaneous Flap, Open Approach

0HRV076   Replacement of Bilateral Breast using Transverse Rectus Abdominis Myocutaneous Flap, Open Approach

0HRV077   Replacement of Bilateral Breast using Deep Inferior Epigastric Artery Perforator Flap, Open Approach

0HRV078   Replacement of Bilateral Breast using Superficial Inferior Epigastric Artery Flap, Open Approach

0HRV079   Replacement of Bilateral Breast using Gluteal Artery Perforator Flap, Open Approach

0HRV07Z   Replacement of Bilateral Breast with Autologous Tissue Substitute, Open Approach

0HRV0JZ   Replacement of Bilateral Breast with Synthetic Substitute, Open Approach

0HRV0KZ   Replacement of Bilateral Breast with Nonautologous Tissue Substitute, Open Approach

0HRV37Z   Replacement of Bilateral Breast with Autologous Tissue Substitute, Percutaneous Approach

0HRV3JZ   Replacement of Bilateral Breast with Synthetic Substitute, Percutaneous Approach

0HRV3KZ   Replacement of Bilateral Breast with Nonautologous Tissue Substitute, Percutaneous Approach

0HRVX7Z   Replacement of Bilateral Breast with Autologous Tissue Substitute, External Approach

0HRVXJZ   Replacement of Bilateral Breast with Synthetic Substitute, External Approach

0HRVXKZ   Replacement of Bilateral Breast with Nonautologous Tissue Substitute, External Approach

0HRW07Z   Replacement of Right Nipple with Autologous Tissue Substitute, Open Approach

0HRW0JZ   Replacement of Right Nipple with Synthetic Substitute, Open Approach

0HRW0KZ   Replacement of Right Nipple with Nonautologous Tissue Substitute, Open Approach

0HRW37Z   Replacement of Right Nipple with Autologous Tissue Substitute, Percutaneous Approach

0HRW3JZ   Replacement of Right Nipple with Synthetic Substitute, Percutaneous Approach

0HRW3KZ   Replacement of Right Nipple with Nonautologous Tissue Substitute, Percutaneous Approach

0HRWX7Z   Replacement of Right Nipple with Autologous Tissue Substitute, External Approach

0HRWXJZ   Replacement of Right Nipple with Synthetic Substitute, External Approach

0HRWXKZ   Replacement of Right Nipple with Nonautologous Tissue Substitute, External Approach

0HRX07Z   Replacement of Left Nipple with Autologous Tissue Substitute, Open Approach

0HRX0JZ   Replacement of Left Nipple with Synthetic Substitute, Open Approach

0HRX0KZ   Replacement of Left Nipple with Nonautologous Tissue Substitute, Open Approach

0HRX37Z   Replacement of Left Nipple with Autologous Tissue Substitute, Percutaneous Approach

0HRX3JZ   Replacement of Left Nipple with Synthetic Substitute, Percutaneous Approach

0HRX3KZ   Replacement of Left Nipple with Nonautologous Tissue Substitute, Percutaneous Approach

0HRXX7Z   Replacement of Left Nipple with Autologous Tissue Substitute, External Approach

0HRXXJZ   Replacement of Left Nipple with Synthetic Substitute, External Approach

0HRXXKZ   Replacement of Left Nipple with Nonautologous Tissue Substitute, External Approach

0HS – Skin and Breast, Reposition

0HSSXZZ   Reposition Hair, External Approach
0HST0ZZ   Reposition Right Breast, Open Approach
0HSU0ZZ   Reposition Left Breast, Open Approach

0HSV0ZZ   Reposition Bilateral Breast, Open Approach
0HSWXZZ   Reposition Right Nipple, External Approach
0HSXXZZ   Reposition Left Nipple, External Approach

0HT – Skin and Breast, Resection

Review Coding Guideline B3.8

0HTQXZZ   Resection of Finger Nail, External Approach
0HTRXZZ   Resection of Toe Nail, External Approach
0HTT0ZZ   Resection of Right Breast, Open Approach
0HTU0ZZ   Resection of Left Breast, Open Approach

0HTV0ZZ   Resection of Bilateral Breast, Open Approach
0HTWXZZ   Resection of Right Nipple, External Approach
0HTXXZZ   Resection of Left Nipple, External Approach
0HTY0ZZ   Resection of Supernumerary Breast, Open Approach

0HU – Skin and Breast, Supplement

0HUT07Z   Supplement Right Breast with Autologous Tissue Substitute, Open Approach

0HUT0JZ   Supplement Right Breast with Synthetic Substitute, Open Approach

0HUT0KZ   Supplement Right Breast with Nonautologous Tissue Substitute, Open Approach

0HUT37Z   Supplement Right Breast with Autologous Tissue Substitute, Percutaneous Approach

0HUT3JZ   Supplement Right Breast with Synthetic Substitute, Percutaneous Approach

0HUT3KZ   Supplement Right Breast with Nonautologous Tissue Substitute, Percutaneous Approach

0HUT77Z   Supplement Right Breast with Autologous Tissue Substitute, Via Natural or Artificial Opening

0HUT7JZ   Supplement Right Breast with Synthetic Substitute, Via Natural or Artificial Opening

0HUT7KZ   Supplement Right Breast with Nonautologous Tissue Substitute, Via Natural or Artificial Opening

0HUT87Z   Supplement Right Breast with Autologous Tissue Substitute, Via Natural or Artificial Opening Endoscopic

0HUT8JZ   Supplement Right Breast with Synthetic Substitute, Via Natural or Artificial Opening Endoscopic

0HUT8KZ   Supplement Right Breast with Nonautologous Tissue Substitute, Via Natural or Artificial Opening Endoscopic

0HUTX7Z   Supplement Right Breast with Autologous Tissue Substitute, External Approach

0HUTXJZ   Supplement Right Breast with Synthetic Substitute, External Approach

0HUTXKZ   Supplement Right Breast with Nonautologous Tissue Substitute, External Approach

0HUU07Z   Supplement Left Breast with Autologous Tissue Substitute, Open Approach

0HUU0JZ   Supplement Left Breast with Synthetic Substitute, Open Approach

---

♀ Female-only   ♂ Male-only   ● Limited Coverage   ● Non-OR   ▨ HAC-associated procedure   ⬣ Non-covered procedures   ✚ Combination

0HUU0KZ Supplement Left Breast with Nonautologous Tissue Substitute, Open Approach

0HUU37Z Supplement Left Breast with Autologous Tissue Substitute, Percutaneous Approach

0HUU3JZ Supplement Left Breast with Synthetic Substitute, Percutaneous Approach

0HUU3KZ Supplement Left Breast with Nonautologous Tissue Substitute, Percutaneous Approach

0HUU77Z Supplement Left Breast with Autologous Tissue Substitute, Via Natural or Artificial Opening

0HUU7JZ Supplement Left Breast with Synthetic Substitute, Via Natural or Artificial Opening

0HUU7KZ Supplement Left Breast with Nonautologous Tissue Substitute, Via Natural or Artificial Opening

0HUU87Z Supplement Left Breast with Autologous Tissue Substitute, Via Natural or Artificial Opening Endoscopic

0HUU8JZ Supplement Left Breast with Synthetic Substitute, Via Natural or Artificial Opening Endoscopic

0HUU8KZ Supplement Left Breast with Nonautologous Tissue Substitute, Via Natural or Artificial Opening Endoscopic

0HUUX7Z Supplement Left Breast with Autologous Tissue Substitute, External Approach

0HUUXJZ Supplement Left Breast with Synthetic Substitute, External Approach

0HUUXKZ Supplement Left Breast with Nonautologous Tissue Substitute, External Approach

0HUV07Z Supplement Bilateral Breast with Autologous Tissue Substitute, Open Approach

0HUV0JZ Supplement Bilateral Breast with Synthetic Substitute, Open Approach

0HUV0KZ Supplement Bilateral Breast with Nonautologous Tissue Substitute, Open Approach

0HUV37Z Supplement Bilateral Breast with Autologous Tissue Substitute, Percutaneous Approach

0HUV3JZ Supplement Bilateral Breast with Synthetic Substitute, Percutaneous Approach

0HUV3KZ Supplement Bilateral Breast with Nonautologous Tissue Substitute, Percutaneous Approach

0HUV77Z Supplement Bilateral Breast with Autologous Tissue Substitute, Via Natural or Artificial Opening

0HUV7JZ Supplement Bilateral Breast with Synthetic Substitute, Via Natural or Artificial Opening

0HUV7KZ Supplement Bilateral Breast with Nonautologous Tissue Substitute, Via Natural or Artificial Opening

0HUV87Z Supplement Bilateral Breast with Autologous Tissue Substitute, Via Natural or Artificial Opening Endoscopic

0HUV8JZ Supplement Bilateral Breast with Synthetic Substitute, Via Natural or Artificial Opening Endoscopic

0HUV8KZ Supplement Bilateral Breast with Nonautologous Tissue Substitute, Via Natural or Artificial Opening Endoscopic

0HUVX7Z Supplement Bilateral Breast with Autologous Tissue Substitute, External Approach

0HUVXJZ Supplement Bilateral Breast with Synthetic Substitute, External Approach

0HUVXKZ Supplement Bilateral Breast with Nonautologous Tissue Substitute, External Approach

0HUW07Z Supplement Right Nipple with Autologous Tissue Substitute, Open Approach

0HUW0JZ Supplement Right Nipple with Synthetic Substitute, Open Approach

0HUW0KZ Supplement Right Nipple with Nonautologous Tissue Substitute, Open Approach

0HUW37Z Supplement Right Nipple with Autologous Tissue Substitute, Percutaneous Approach

0HUW3JZ Supplement Right Nipple with Synthetic Substitute, Percutaneous Approach

0HUW3KZ Supplement Right Nipple with Nonautologous Tissue Substitute, Percutaneous Approach

0HUW77Z Supplement Right Nipple with Autologous Tissue Substitute, Via Natural or Artificial Opening

0HUW7JZ Supplement Right Nipple with Synthetic Substitute, Via Natural or Artificial Opening

0HUW7KZ Supplement Right Nipple with Nonautologous Tissue Substitute, Via Natural or Artificial Opening

0HUW87Z Supplement Right Nipple with Autologous Tissue Substitute, Via Natural or Artificial Opening Endoscopic

0HUW8JZ Supplement Right Nipple with Synthetic Substitute, Via Natural or Artificial Opening Endoscopic

0HUW8KZ Supplement Right Nipple with Nonautologous Tissue Substitute, Via Natural or Artificial Opening Endoscopic

0HUWX7Z Supplement Right Nipple with Autologous Tissue Substitute, External Approach

0HUWXJZ Supplement Right Nipple with Synthetic Substitute, External Approach

0HUWXKZ Supplement Right Nipple with Nonautologous Tissue Substitute, External Approach

0HUX07Z Supplement Left Nipple with Autologous Tissue Substitute, Open Approach

0HUX0JZ Supplement Left Nipple with Synthetic Substitute, Open Approach

0HUX0KZ Supplement Left Nipple with Nonautologous Tissue Substitute, Open Approach

0HUX37Z Supplement Left Nipple with Autologous Tissue Substitute, Percutaneous Approach

0HUX3JZ Supplement Left Nipple with Synthetic Substitute, Percutaneous Approach

0HUX3KZ Supplement Left Nipple with Nonautologous Tissue Substitute, Percutaneous Approach

0HUX77Z Supplement Left Nipple with Autologous Tissue Substitute, Via Natural or Artificial Opening

0HUX7JZ Supplement Left Nipple with Synthetic Substitute, Via Natural or Artificial Opening

0HUX7KZ Supplement Left Nipple with Nonautologous Tissue Substitute, Via Natural or Artificial Opening

0HUX87Z Supplement Left Nipple with Autologous Tissue Substitute, Via Natural or Artificial Opening Endoscopic

0HUX8JZ Supplement Left Nipple with Synthetic Substitute, Via Natural or Artificial Opening Endoscopic

0HUX8KZ Supplement Left Nipple with Nonautologous Tissue Substitute, Via Natural or Artificial Opening Endoscopic

0HUXX7Z Supplement Left Nipple with Autologous Tissue Substitute, External Approach

0HUXXJZ Supplement Left Nipple with Synthetic Substitute, External Approach

0HUXXKZ Supplement Left Nipple with Nonautologous Tissue Substitute, External Approach

0HW – Skin and Breast, Revision

Review Coding Guideline B6.1c

0HWPX0Z Revision of Drainage Device in Skin, External Approach

0HWPX7Z Revision of Autologous Tissue Substitute in Skin, External Approach

0HWPXJZ Revision of Synthetic Substitute in Skin, External Approach

0HWPXKZ Revision of Nonautologous Tissue Substitute in Skin, External Approach

0HWQX0Z Revision of Drainage Device in Finger Nail, External Approach

0HWQX7Z Revision of Autologous Tissue Substitute in Finger Nail, External Approach

0HWQXJZ Revision of Synthetic Substitute in Finger Nail, External Approach

0HWQXKZ Revision of Nonautologous Tissue Substitute in Finger Nail, External Approach

0HWRX0Z Revision of Drainage Device in Toe Nail, External Approach

0HWRX7Z Revision of Autologous Tissue Substitute in Toe Nail, External Approach

0HWRXJZ Revision of Synthetic Substitute in Toe Nail, External Approach

0HWRXKZ Revision of Nonautologous Tissue Substitute in Toe Nail, External Approach

0HWSX7Z Revision of Autologous Tissue Substitute in Hair, External Approach

---

0HWSXJZ	Revision of Synthetic Substitute in Hair, External Approach
0HWSXKZ	Revision of Nonautologous Tissue Substitute in Hair, External Approach
0HWT00Z	Revision of Drainage Device in Right Breast, Open Approach
0HWT07Z	Revision of Autologous Tissue Substitute in Right Breast, Open Approach
0HWT0JZ	Revision of Synthetic Substitute in Right Breast, Open Approach
0HWT0KZ	Revision of Nonautologous Tissue Substitute in Right Breast, Open Approach
0HWT0NZ	Revision of Tissue Expander in Right Breast, Open Approach
0HWT30Z	Revision of Drainage Device in Right Breast, Percutaneous Approach
0HWT37Z	Revision of Autologous Tissue Substitute in Right Breast, Percutaneous Approach
0HWT3JZ	Revision of Synthetic Substitute in Right Breast, Percutaneous Approach
0HWT3KZ	Revision of Nonautologous Tissue Substitute in Right Breast, Percutaneous Approach
0HWT3NZ	Revision of Tissue Expander in Right Breast, Percutaneous Approach
0HWT70Z	Revision of Drainage Device in Right Breast, Via Natural or Artificial Opening
0HWT77Z	Revision of Autologous Tissue Substitute in Right Breast, Via Natural or Artificial Opening
0HWT7JZ	Revision of Synthetic Substitute in Right Breast, Via Natural or Artificial Opening
0HWT7KZ	Revision of Nonautologous Tissue Substitute in Right Breast, Via Natural or Artificial Opening
0HWT7NZ	Revision of Tissue Expander in Right Breast, Via Natural or Artificial Opening
0HWT80Z	Revision of Drainage Device in Right Breast, Via Natural or Artificial Opening Endoscopic
0HWT87Z	Revision of Autologous Tissue Substitute in Right Breast, Via Natural or Artificial Opening Endoscopic
0HWT8JZ	Revision of Synthetic Substitute in Right Breast, Via Natural or Artificial Opening Endoscopic
0HWT8KZ	Revision of Nonautologous Tissue Substitute in Right Breast, Via Natural or Artificial Opening Endoscopic
0HWT8NZ	Revision of Tissue Expander in Right Breast, Via Natural or Artificial Opening Endoscopic
0HWTX0Z	Revision of Drainage Device in Right Breast, External Approach
0HWTX7Z	Revision of Autologous Tissue Substitute in Right Breast, External Approach
0HWTXJZ	Revision of Synthetic Substitute in Right Breast, External Approach
0HWTXKZ	Revision of Nonautologous Tissue Substitute in Right Breast, External Approach
0HWU00Z	Revision of Drainage Device in Left Breast, Open Approach
0HWU07Z	Revision of Autologous Tissue Substitute in Left Breast, Open Approach
0HWU0JZ	Revision of Synthetic Substitute in Left Breast, Open Approach
0HWU0KZ	Revision of Nonautologous Tissue Substitute in Left Breast, Open Approach
0HWU0NZ	Revision of Tissue Expander in Left Breast, Open Approach
0HWU30Z	Revision of Drainage Device in Left Breast, Percutaneous Approach
0HWU37Z	Revision of Autologous Tissue Substitute in Left Breast, Percutaneous Approach
0HWU3JZ	Revision of Synthetic Substitute in Left Breast, Percutaneous Approach
0HWU3KZ	Revision of Nonautologous Tissue Substitute in Left Breast, Percutaneous Approach
0HWU3NZ	Revision of Tissue Expander in Left Breast, Percutaneous Approach
0HWU70Z	Revision of Drainage Device in Left Breast, Via Natural or Artificial Opening
0HWU77Z	Revision of Autologous Tissue Substitute in Left Breast, Via Natural or Artificial Opening
0HWU7JZ	Revision of Synthetic Substitute in Left Breast, Via Natural or Artificial Opening
0HWU7KZ	Revision of Nonautologous Tissue Substitute in Left Breast, Via Natural or Artificial Opening
0HWU7NZ	Revision of Tissue Expander in Left Breast, Via Natural or Artificial Opening
0HWU80Z	Revision of Drainage Device in Left Breast, Via Natural or Artificial Opening Endoscopic
0HWU87Z	Revision of Autologous Tissue Substitute in Left Breast, Via Natural or Artificial Opening Endoscopic
0HWU8JZ	Revision of Synthetic Substitute in Left Breast, Via Natural or Artificial Opening Endoscopic
0HWU8KZ	Revision of Nonautologous Tissue Substitute in Left Breast, Via Natural or Artificial Opening Endoscopic
0HWU8NZ	Revision of Tissue Expander in Left Breast, Via Natural or Artificial Opening Endoscopic
0HWUX0Z	Revision of Drainage Device in Left Breast, External Approach
0HWUX7Z	Revision of Autologous Tissue Substitute in Left Breast, External Approach
0HWUXJZ	Revision of Synthetic Substitute in Left Breast, External Approach
0HWUXKZ	Revision of Nonautologous Tissue Substitute in Left Breast, External Approach

0HX – Skin and Breast, Transfer

0HX0XZZ	Transfer Scalp Skin, External Approach
0HX1XZZ	Transfer Face Skin, External Approach
0HX2XZZ	Transfer Right Ear Skin, External Approach
0HX3XZZ	Transfer Left Ear Skin, External Approach
0HX4XZZ	Transfer Neck Skin, External Approach
0HX5XZZ	Transfer Chest Skin, External Approach
0HX6XZZ	Transfer Back Skin, External Approach
0HX7XZZ	Transfer Abdomen Skin, External Approach
0HX8XZZ	Transfer Buttock Skin, External Approach
0HX9XZZ	Transfer Perineum Skin, External Approach
0HXAXZZ	Transfer Genitalia Skin, External Approach
0HXBXZZ	Transfer Right Upper Arm Skin, External Approach
0HXCXZZ	Transfer Left Upper Arm Skin, External Approach
0HXDXZZ	Transfer Right Lower Arm Skin, External Approach
0HXEXZZ	Transfer Left Lower Arm Skin, External Approach
0HXFXZZ	Transfer Right Hand Skin, External Approach
0HXGXZZ	Transfer Left Hand Skin, External Approach
0HXHXZZ	Transfer Right Upper Leg Skin, External Approach
0HXJXZZ	Transfer Left Upper Leg Skin, External Approach
0HXKXZZ	Transfer Right Lower Leg Skin, External Approach
0HXLXZZ	Transfer Left Lower Leg Skin, External Approach
0HXMXZZ	Transfer Right Foot Skin, External Approach
0HXNXZZ	Transfer Left Foot Skin, External Approach

Subcutaneous Tissue and Fascia

Subcutaneous Tissue and Fascia

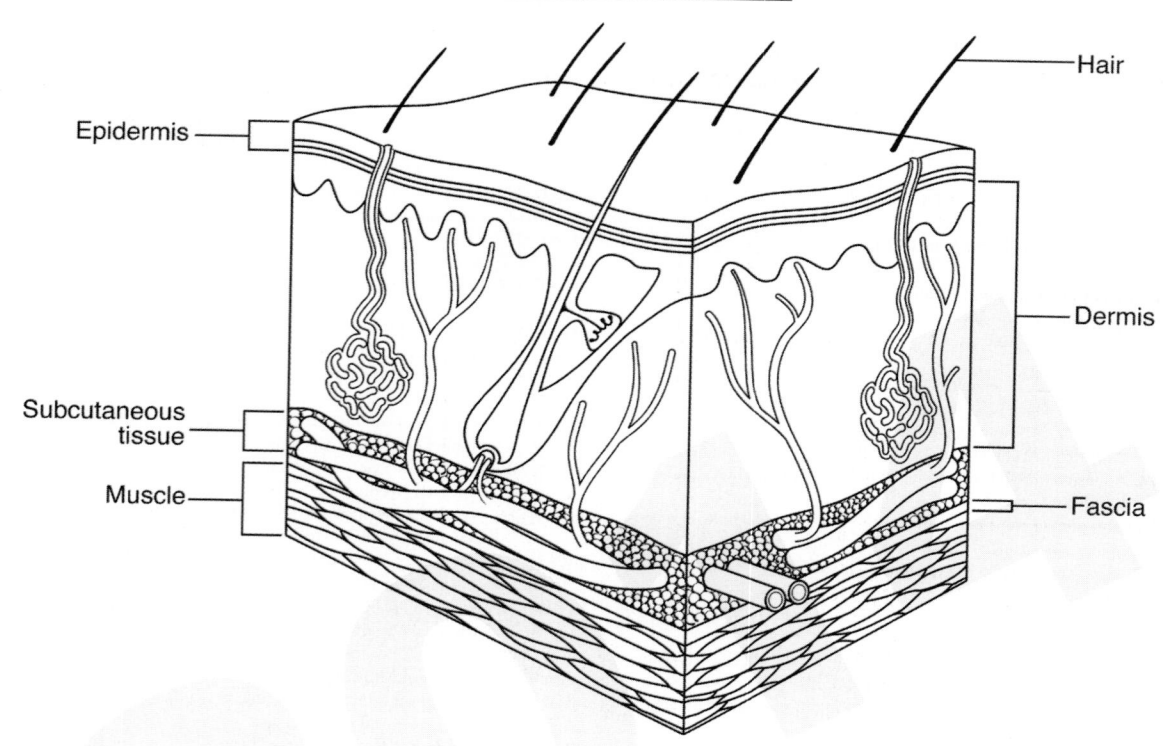

Subcutaneous Tissue and Fascia Tables 0J0–0JX

Section	0	Medical and Surgical
Body System	J	Subcutaneous Tissue and Fascia
Operation	0	Alteration: Modifying the anatomic structure of a body part without affecting the function of the body part

Body Part (4th)	Approach (5th)	Device (6th)	Qualifier (7th)
1 Subcutaneous Tissue and Fascia, Face 4 Subcutaneous Tissue and Fascia, Anterior Neck 5 Subcutaneous Tissue and Fascia, Posterior Neck 6 Subcutaneous Tissue and Fascia, Chest 7 Subcutaneous Tissue and Fascia, Back 8 Subcutaneous Tissue and Fascia, Abdomen 9 Subcutaneous Tissue and Fascia, Buttock D Subcutaneous Tissue and Fascia, Right Upper Arm F Subcutaneous Tissue and Fascia, Left Upper Arm G Subcutaneous Tissue and Fascia, Right Lower Arm H Subcutaneous Tissue and Fascia, Left Lower Arm L Subcutaneous Tissue and Fascia, Right Upper Leg M Subcutaneous Tissue and Fascia, Left Upper Leg N Subcutaneous Tissue and Fascia, Right Lower Leg P Subcutaneous Tissue and Fascia, Left Lower Leg	0 Open 3 Percutaneous	Z No Device	Z No Qualifier

Section	0	Medical and Surgical
Body System	J	Subcutaneous Tissue and Fascia
Operation	2	Change: Taking out or off a device from a body part and putting back an identical or similar device in or on the same body part without cutting or puncturing the skin or a mucous membrane

Body Part (4th)	Approach (5th)	Device (6th)	Qualifier (7th)
S Subcutaneous Tissue and Fascia, Head and Neck T Subcutaneous Tissue and Fascia, Trunk V Subcutaneous Tissue and Fascia, Upper Extremity W Subcutaneous Tissue and Fascia, Lower Extremity	X External	0 Drainage Device Y Other Device	Z No Qualifier

Section	0	Medical and Surgical
Body System	J	Subcutaneous Tissue and Fascia
Operation	5	Destruction: Physical eradication of all or a portion of a body part by the direct use of energy, force, or a destructive agent

Body Part (4th)	Approach (5th)	Device (6th)	Qualifier (7th)
0 Subcutaneous Tissue and Fascia, Scalp 1 Subcutaneous Tissue and Fascia, Face 4 Subcutaneous Tissue and Fascia, Anterior Neck 5 Subcutaneous Tissue and Fascia, Posterior Neck 6 Subcutaneous Tissue and Fascia, Chest 7 Subcutaneous Tissue and Fascia, Back 8 Subcutaneous Tissue and Fascia, Abdomen 9 Subcutaneous Tissue and Fascia, Buttock B Subcutaneous Tissue and Fascia, Perineum C Subcutaneous Tissue and Fascia, Pelvic Region D Subcutaneous Tissue and Fascia, Right Upper Arm F Subcutaneous Tissue and Fascia, Left Upper Arm G Subcutaneous Tissue and Fascia, Right Lower Arm H Subcutaneous Tissue and Fascia, Left Lower Arm J Subcutaneous Tissue and Fascia, Right Hand K Subcutaneous Tissue and Fascia, Left Hand L Subcutaneous Tissue and Fascia, Right Upper Leg M Subcutaneous Tissue and Fascia, Left Upper Leg N Subcutaneous Tissue and Fascia, Right Lower Leg P Subcutaneous Tissue and Fascia, Left Lower Leg Q Subcutaneous Tissue and Fascia, Right Foot R Subcutaneous Tissue and Fascia, Left Foot	0 Open 3 Percutaneous	Z No Device	Z No Qualifier

Section	0	Medical and Surgical
Body System	J	Subcutaneous Tissue and Fascia
Operation	8	Division: Cutting into a body part, without draining fluids and/or gases from the body part, in order to separate or transect a body part

Body Part (4th)	Approach (5th)	Device (6th)	Qualifier (7th)
0 Subcutaneous Tissue and Fascia, Scalp 1 Subcutaneous Tissue and Fascia, Face 4 Subcutaneous Tissue and Fascia, Anterior Neck 5 Subcutaneous Tissue and Fascia, Posterior Neck 6 Subcutaneous Tissue and Fascia, Chest 7 Subcutaneous Tissue and Fascia, Back 8 Subcutaneous Tissue and Fascia, Abdomen 9 Subcutaneous Tissue and Fascia, Buttock B Subcutaneous Tissue and Fascia, Perineum C Subcutaneous Tissue and Fascia, Pelvic Region D Subcutaneous Tissue and Fascia, Right Upper Arm F Subcutaneous Tissue and Fascia, Left Upper Arm G Subcutaneous Tissue and Fascia, Right Lower Arm H Subcutaneous Tissue and Fascia, Left Lower Arm J Subcutaneous Tissue and Fascia, Right Hand K Subcutaneous Tissue and Fascia, Left Hand L Subcutaneous Tissue and Fascia, Right Upper Leg M Subcutaneous Tissue and Fascia, Left Upper Leg N Subcutaneous Tissue and Fascia, Right Lower Leg P Subcutaneous Tissue and Fascia, Left Lower Leg Q Subcutaneous Tissue and Fascia, Right Foot R Subcutaneous Tissue and Fascia, Left Foot S Subcutaneous Tissue and Fascia, Head and Neck T Subcutaneous Tissue and Fascia, Trunk V Subcutaneous Tissue and Fascia, Upper Extremity W Subcutaneous Tissue and Fascia, Lower Extremity	0 Open 3 Percutaneous	Z No Device	Z No Qualifier

Section	0	Medical and Surgical
Body System	J	Subcutaneous Tissue and Fascia
Operation	9	Drainage: Taking or letting out fluids and/or gases from a body part

Body Part (4th)	Approach (5th)	Device (6th)	Qualifier (7th)
0 Subcutaneous Tissue and Fascia, Scalp 1 Subcutaneous Tissue and Fascia, Face 4 Subcutaneous Tissue and Fascia, Anterior Neck 5 Subcutaneous Tissue and Fascia, Posterior Neck 6 Subcutaneous Tissue and Fascia, Chest 7 Subcutaneous Tissue and Fascia, Back 8 Subcutaneous Tissue and Fascia, Abdomen 9 Subcutaneous Tissue and Fascia, Buttock B Subcutaneous Tissue and Fascia, Perineum C Subcutaneous Tissue and Fascia, Pelvic Region D Subcutaneous Tissue and Fascia, Right Upper Arm F Subcutaneous Tissue and Fascia, Left Upper Arm G Subcutaneous Tissue and Fascia, Right Lower Arm H Subcutaneous Tissue and Fascia, Left Lower Arm J Subcutaneous Tissue and Fascia, Right Hand K Subcutaneous Tissue and Fascia, Left Hand L Subcutaneous Tissue and Fascia, Right Upper Leg M Subcutaneous Tissue and Fascia, Left Upper Leg N Subcutaneous Tissue and Fascia, Right Lower Leg P Subcutaneous Tissue and Fascia, Left Lower Leg Q Subcutaneous Tissue and Fascia, Right Foot R Subcutaneous Tissue and Fascia, Left Foot	0 Open 3 Percutaneous	0 Drainage Device	Z No Qualifier

Continued

0JH63NZ   Insertion of Tissue Expander into Chest Subcutaneous Tissue and Fascia, Percutaneous Approach

0JH63PZ   Insertion of Cardiac Rhythm Related Device into Chest Subcutaneous Tissue and Fascia, Percutaneous Approach

HAC   With a secondary diagnosis code of K68.11, T81.4XXA, T82.6XXA, T82.7XXA

+   Pacemaker device when reported with an Insertion of a cardiac lead (6th character J or M) into the coronary vein, atrium, ventricle or pericardium (4th characters 4, 6, 7, K, L and N). *See table 02H to construct the Insertion code.* When a cardiac lead is replaced, also report the Removal of the cardiac lead (6th character M) from the heart. *See table 02P to construct the Removal code.*

0JH63VZ   Insertion of Infusion Pump into Chest Subcutaneous Tissue and Fascia, Percutaneous Approach

● **0JH63WZ**   Insertion of Reservoir into Chest Subcutaneous Tissue and Fascia, Percutaneous Approach

● **0JH63XZ**   Insertion of Vascular Access Device into Chest Subcutaneous Tissue and Fascia, Percutaneous Approach

HAC   With secondary diagnosis code J95.811

0JH70BZ   Insertion of Single Array Stimulator Generator into Back Subcutaneous Tissue and Fascia, Open Approach

+   Neurotransmitter/Neurostimulator when reported with an Insertion of a neurostimulator lead (6th character M) into the cranial nerve, spinal canal or spinal cord. *See table 00H to construct the Insertion code.* Also applicable when reported with Insertion of neurostimulator lead (6th character M) into the peripheral nerve. *See table 01H to construct the Insertion code.* Also applicable when reported with Insertion of a stimulator lead (6th character M) into the stomach. *See table 0DH to construct the Insertion code.*

0JH70CZ   Insertion of Single Array Rechargeable Stimulator Generator into Back Subcutaneous Tissue and Fascia, Open Approach

+   Neurotransmitter/Neurostimulator when reported with an Insertion of a neurostimulator lead (6th character M) into the cranial nerve, spinal canal or spinal cord. *See table 00H to construct the Insertion code.* Also applicable when reported with Insertion of neurostimulator lead (6th character M) into the peripheral nerve. *See table 01H to construct the Insertion code.* Also applicable when reported with Insertion of a stimulator lead (6th character M) into the stomach. *See table 0DH to construct the Insertion code.*

0JH70DZ   Insertion of Multiple Array Stimulator Generator into Back Subcutaneous Tissue and Fascia, Open Approach

+   Major brain device implant when reported with an Insertion of a neurostimulator lead (6th character M) into the brain or cerebral ventricle. *See table 00H to construct the Insertion code.*

+   Neurotransmitter/Neurostimulator when reported with an Insertion of a neurostimulator lead (6th character M) into the cranial nerve, spinal canal or spinal cord. *See table 00H to construct the Insertion code.* Also applicable when reported with Insertion of neurostimulator lead (6th character M) into the peripheral nerve. *See table 01H to construct the Insertion code.* Also applicable when reported with Insertion of a stimulator lead (6th character M) into the stomach. *See table 0DH to construct the Insertion code.*

0JH70EZ   Insertion of Multiple Array Rechargeable Stimulator Generator into Back Subcutaneous Tissue and Fascia, Open Approach

+   Major brain device implant when reported with an Insertion of a neurostimulator lead (6th character M) into the brain or cerebral ventricle. *See table 00H to construct the Insertion code.*

+   Neurotransmitter/Neurostimulator when reported with an Insertion of a neurostimulator lead (6th character M) into the cranial nerve, spinal canal or spinal cord. *See table 00H to construct the Insertion code.* Also applicable when reported with Insertion of neurostimulator lead (6th character M) into the peripheral nerve. *See table 01H to construct the Insertion code.* Also applicable when reported with Insertion of a stimulator lead (6th character M) into the stomach. *See table 0DH to construct the Insertion code.*

● **0JH70MZ**   Insertion of Stimulator Generator into Back Subcutaneous Tissue and Fascia, Open Approach

0JH70NZ   Insertion of Tissue Expander into Back Subcutaneous Tissue and Fascia, Open Approach

0JH70VZ   Insertion of Infusion Pump into Back Subcutaneous Tissue and Fascia, Open Approach

0JH73BZ   Insertion of Single Array Stimulator Generator into Back Subcutaneous Tissue and Fascia, Percutaneous Approach

+   Neurotransmitter/Neurostimulator when reported with an Insertion of a neurostimulator lead (6th character M) into the cranial nerve, spinal canal or spinal cord. *See table 00H to construct the Insertion code.* Also applicable when reported with Insertion of neurostimulator lead (6th character M) into the peripheral nerve. *See table 01H to construct the Insertion code.* Also applicable when reported with Insertion of a stimulator lead (6th character M) into the stomach. *See table 0DH to construct the Insertion code.*

0JH73CZ   Insertion of Single Array Rechargeable Stimulator Generator into Back Subcutaneous Tissue and Fascia, Percutaneous Approach

+   Neurotransmitter/Neurostimulator when reported with an Insertion of a neurostimulator lead (6th character M) into the cranial nerve, spinal canal or spinal cord. *See table 00H to construct the Insertion code.* Also applicable when reported with Insertion of neurostimulator lead (6th character M) into the peripheral nerve. *See table 01H to construct the Insertion code.* Also applicable when reported with Insertion of a stimulator lead (6th character M) into the stomach. *See table 0DH to construct the Insertion code.*

0JH73DZ   Insertion of Multiple Array Stimulator Generator into Back Subcutaneous Tissue and Fascia, Percutaneous Approach

+   Major brain device implant when reported with an Insertion of a neurostimulator lead (6th character M) into the brain or cerebral ventricle. *See table 00H to construct the Insertion code.*

+   Neurotransmitter/Neurostimulator when reported with an Insertion of a neurostimulator lead (6th character M) into the cranial nerve, spinal canal or spinal cord. *See table 00H to construct the Insertion code.* Also applicable when reported with Insertion of neurostimulator lead (6th character M) into the peripheral nerve. *See table 01H to construct the Insertion code.* Also applicable when reported with Insertion of a stimulator lead (6th character M) into the stomach. *See table 0DH to construct the Insertion code.*

0JH73EZ   Insertion of Multiple Array Rechargeable Stimulator Generator into Back Subcutaneous Tissue and Fascia, Percutaneous Approach

+   Major brain device implant when reported with an Insertion of a neurostimulator lead (6th character M) into the brain or cerebral ventricle. *See table 00H to construct the Insertion code.*

+   Neurotransmitter/Neurostimulator when reported with an Insertion of a neurostimulator lead (6th character M) into the cranial nerve, spinal canal or spinal cord. *See table 00H to construct the Insertion code.* Also applicable when reported with Insertion of neurostimulator lead (6th character M) into the peripheral nerve. *See table 01H to construct the Insertion code.* Also applicable when reported with Insertion of a stimulator lead (6th character M) into the stomach. *See table 0DH to construct the Insertion code.*

● **0JH73MZ**   Insertion of Stimulator Generator into Back Subcutaneous Tissue and Fascia, Percutaneous Approach

0JH73NZ   Insertion of Tissue Expander into Back Subcutaneous Tissue and Fascia, Percutaneous Approach

0JH73VZ   Insertion of Infusion Pump into Back Subcutaneous Tissue and Fascia, Percutaneous Approach

0JH800Z   Insertion of Hemodynamic Monitoring Device into Abdomen Subcutaneous Tissue and Fascia, Open Approach

● **0JH802Z**   Insertion of Monitoring Device into Abdomen Subcutaneous Tissue and Fascia, Open Approach

0JH804Z   Insertion of Pacemaker, Single Chamber into Abdomen Subcutaneous Tissue and Fascia, Open Approach

HAC   With a secondary diagnosis code of K68.11, T81.4XXA, T82.6XXA, T82.7XXA

+   Pacemaker device when reported with an Insertion of a cardiac lead (6th character J or M) into the coronary vein, atrium, ventricle or pericardium (4th characters 4, 6, 7, K, L and N). *See table 02H to construct the Insertion code.* When a device is replaced, also report the Removal of the cardiac rhythm device (6th character P) from the trunk subcutaneous tissue and fascia. *See table 0JP to construct the Removal code.* When a cardiac lead is replaced, also report the Removal of the cardiac lead (6th character M) from the heart. *See table 02P to construct the Removal code.*

0JH805Z   Insertion of Pacemaker, Single Chamber Rate Responsive into Abdomen Subcutaneous Tissue and Fascia, Open Approach

HAC   With a secondary diagnosis code of K68.11, T81.4XXA, T82.6XXA, T82.7XXA

+   Pacemaker device when reported with an Insertion of a cardiac lead (6th character J or M) into the coronary vein, atrium, ventricle or pericardium (4th characters 4, 6, 7, K, L and N). *See table 02H to construct the Insertion code.* When a device is replaced, also report the Removal of the cardiac rhythm device (6th character P) from the trunk subcutaneous tissue and fascia. *See table 0JP to construct the Removal code.* When a cardiac lead is replaced, also report the Removal of the cardiac lead (6th character M) from the heart. *See table 02P to construct the Removal code.*

0JH806Z   Insertion of Pacemaker, Dual Chamber into Abdomen Subcutaneous Tissue and Fascia, Open Approach

HAC   With a secondary diagnosis code of K68.11, T81.4XXA, T82.6XXA, T82.7XXA

+   Pacemaker device when reported with an Insertion of a cardiac lead (6th character J or M) into the coronary vein, atrium, ventricle or pericardium (4th characters 4, 6, 7, K, L and N). *See table 02H to construct the Insertion code.* When a device is replaced, also report the Removal of the cardiac rhythm device (6th character P) from the trunk subcutaneous tissue and fascia. *See table 0JP to construct the Removal code.* When a cardiac lead is replaced, also report the Removal of the cardiac lead (6th character M) from the heart. *See table 02P to construct the Removal code.*

0JH807Z   Insertion of Cardiac Resynchronization Pacemaker Pulse Generator into Abdomen Subcutaneous Tissue and Fascia, Open Approach

HAC   With a secondary diagnosis code of K68.11, T81.4XXA, T82.6XXA, T82.7XXA

+   Pacemaker device when reported with an Insertion of a cardiac lead (6th character J or M) into the coronary vein, atrium, ventricle or pericardium (4th characters 4, 6, 7, K, L and N). *See table 02H to construct the Insertion code.* When a cardiac lead is replaced, also report the Removal of the cardiac lead (6th character M) from the heart. See table 02P to construct the Removal code.

0JH808Z   Insertion of Defibrillator Generator into Abdomen Subcutaneous Tissue and Fascia, Open Approach

HAC   With a secondary diagnosis code of K68.11, T81.4XXA, T82.6XXA, T82.7XXA

+   Cardioverter-Defibrillator lead(s)/generator when reported with Insertion of a defibrillator cardiac lead (6th character K) into the coronary vein, atrium, or ventricle. Also applicable with Insertion of pacemaker cardiac lead, defibrillator cardiac lead or cardiac lead (6th characters J, K, M) into the pericardium. *See table 02H to construct the Insertion code.*

0JH809Z   Insertion of Cardiac Resynchronization Defibrillator Pulse Generator into Abdomen Subcutaneous Tissue and Fascia, Open Approach

HAC   With a secondary diagnosis code of K68.11, T81.4XXA, T82.6XXA, T82.7XXA

+   Cardioverter-Defibrillator lead(s)/generator when reported with Insertion of a defibrillator cardiac lead (6th character K) into the atrium, or ventricle. Also applicable with Insertion of pacemaker cardiac lead, defibrillator cardiac lead or cardiac lead (6th characters J, K, M) into the coronary vein or pericardium. *See table 02H to construct the Insertion code.*

0JH80AZ   Insertion of Contractility Modulation Device into Abdomen Subcutaneous Tissue and Fascia, Open Approach

+   Cardioverter-Defibrillator lead(s)/generator when reported with Insertion of a cardiac lead (6th character M) into the left ventricle. *See table 02H to construct the Insertion code.*

0JH80BZ   Insertion of Single Array Stimulator Generator into Abdomen Subcutaneous Tissue and Fascia, Open Approach

+   Neurotransmitter/Neurostimulator when reported with an Insertion of a neurostimulator lead (6th character M) into the cranial nerve, spinal canal or spinal cord. *See table 00H to construct the Insertion code.* Also applicable when reported with Insertion of neurostimulator lead (6th character M) into the peripheral nerve. *See table 01H to construct the Insertion code.* Also applicable when reported with Insertion of a stimulator lead (6th character M) into the stomach. *See table 0DH to construct the Insertion code.*

0JH80CZ   Insertion of Single Array Rechargeable Stimulator Generator into Abdomen Subcutaneous Tissue and Fascia, Open Approach

+   Neurotransmitter/Neurostimulator when reported with an Insertion of a neurostimulator lead (6th character M) into the cranial nerve, spinal canal or spinal cord. *See table 00H to construct the Insertion code.* Also applicable when reported with Insertion of neurostimulator lead (6th character M) into the peripheral nerve. *See table 01H to construct the Insertion code.* Also applicable when reported with Insertion of a stimulator lead (6th character M) into the stomach. *See table 0DH to construct the Insertion code.*

0JH80DZ   Insertion of Multiple Array Stimulator Generator into Abdomen Subcutaneous Tissue and Fascia, Open Approach

+   Major brain device implant when reported with an Insertion of a neurostimulator lead (6th character M) into the brain or cerebral ventricle. *See table 00H to construct the Insertion code.*

+   Neurotransmitter/Neurostimulator when reported with an Insertion of a neurostimulator lead (6th character M) into the cranial nerve, spinal canal or spinal cord. *See table 00H to construct the Insertion code.* Also applicable when reported with Insertion of neurostimulator lead (6th character M) into the peripheral nerve. *See table 01H to construct the Insertion code.* Also applicable when reported with Insertion of a stimulator lead (6th character M) into the stomach. *See table 0DH to construct the Insertion code.*

0JH80EZ   Insertion of Multiple Array Rechargeable Stimulator Generator into Abdomen Subcutaneous Tissue and Fascia, Open Approach

+   Major brain device implant when reported with an Insertion of a neurostimulator lead (6th character M) into the brain or cerebral ventricle. *See table 00H to construct the Insertion code.*

+   Neurotransmitter/Neurostimulator when reported with an Insertion of a neurostimulator lead (6th character M) into the cranial nerve, spinal canal or spinal cord. *See table 00H to construct the Insertion code.* Also applicable when reported with Insertion of neurostimulator lead (6th character M) into the peripheral nerve. *See table 01H to construct the Insertion code.* Also applicable when reported with Insertion of a stimulator lead (6th character M) into the stomach. *See table 0DH to construct the Insertion code.*

● **0JH80HZ**   Insertion of Contraceptive Device into Abdomen Subcutaneous Tissue and Fascia, Open Approach

● **0JH80MZ**   Insertion of Stimulator Generator into Abdomen Subcutaneous Tissue and Fascia, Open Approach

0JH80NZ   Insertion of Tissue Expander into Abdomen Subcutaneous Tissue and Fascia, Open Approach

0JH80PZ   Insertion of Cardiac Rhythm Related Device into Abdomen Subcutaneous Tissue and Fascia, Open Approach

HAC   With a secondary diagnosis code of K68.11, T81.4XXA, T82.6XXA, T82.7XXA

+   Pacemaker device when reported with an Insertion of a cardiac lead (6th character J or M) into the coronary vein, atrium, ventricle or pericardium (4th characters 4, 6, 7, K, L and N). *See table 02H to construct the Insertion code.* When a cardiac lead is replaced, also report the Removal of the cardiac lead (6th character M) from the heart. *See table 02P to construct the Removal code.*

0JH80VZ   Insertion of Infusion Pump into Abdomen Subcutaneous Tissue and Fascia, Open Approach

● **0JH80WZ**   Insertion of Reservoir into Abdomen Subcutaneous Tissue and Fascia, Open Approach

● **0JH80XZ**   Insertion of Vascular Access Device into Abdomen Subcutaneous Tissue and Fascia, Open Approach

0JH830Z   Insertion of Hemodynamic Monitoring Device into Abdomen Subcutaneous Tissue and Fascia, Percutaneous Approach

● **0JH832Z**   Insertion of Monitoring Device into Abdomen Subcutaneous Tissue and Fascia, Percutaneous Approach

0JH834Z   Insertion of Pacemaker, Single Chamber into Abdomen Subcutaneous Tissue and Fascia, Percutaneous Approach

HAC   With a secondary diagnosis code of K68.11, T81.4XXA, T82.6XXA, T82.7XXA

+   Pacemaker device when reported with an Insertion of a cardiac lead (6th character J or M) into the coronary vein, atrium, ventricle or pericardium (4th characters 4, 6, 7, K, L and N). *See table 02H to construct the Insertion code.* When a device is replaced, also report the Removal of the cardiac rhythm device (6th character P) from the trunk subcutaneous tissue and fascia. *See table 0JP to construct the Removal code.* When a cardiac lead is replaced, also report the Removal of the cardiac lead (6th character M) from the heart. *See table 02P to construct the Removal code.*

♀ Female-only   ♂ Male-only   ◒ Limited Coverage   ● Non-OR   HAC HAC-associated procedure   ⬢ Non-covered procedures   + Combination

0JH835Z Insertion of Pacemaker, Single Chamber Rate Responsive into Abdomen Subcutaneous Tissue and Fascia, Percutaneous Approach

HAC With a secondary diagnosis code of K68.11, T81.4XXA, T82.6XXA, T82.7XXA

+ Pacemaker device when reported with an Insertion of a cardiac lead (6th character J or M) into the coronary vein, atrium, ventricle or pericardium (4th characters 4, 6, 7, K, L and N). *See table 02H to construct the Insertion code. When a device is replaced, also report the Removal of the cardiac rhythm device (6th character P) from the trunk subcutaneous tissue and fascia. See table 0JP to construct the Removal code. When a cardiac lead is replaced, also report the Removal of the cardiac lead (6th character M) from the heart. See table 02P to construct the Removal code.*

0JH836Z Insertion of Pacemaker, Dual Chamber into Abdomen Subcutaneous Tissue and Fascia, Percutaneous Approach

HAC With a secondary diagnosis code of K68.11, T81.4XXA, T82.6XXA, T82.7XXA

+ Pacemaker device when reported with an Insertion of a cardiac lead (6th character J or M) into the coronary vein, atrium, ventricle or pericardium (4th characters 4, 6, 7, K, L and N). *See table 02H to construct the Insertion code. When a device is replaced, also report the Removal of the cardiac rhythm device (6th character P) from the trunk subcutaneous tissue and fascia. See table 0JP to construct the Removal code. When a cardiac lead is replaced, also report the Removal of the cardiac lead (6th character M) from the heart. See table 02P to construct the Removal code.*

0JH837Z Insertion of Cardiac Resynchronization Pacemaker Pulse Generator into Abdomen Subcutaneous Tissue and Fascia, Percutaneous Approach

HAC With a secondary diagnosis code of K68.11, T81.4XXA, T82.6XXA, T82.7XXA

+ Pacemaker device when reported with an Insertion of a cardiac lead (6th character J or M) into the coronary vein, atrium, ventricle or pericardium (4th characters 4, 6, 7, K, L and N). *See table 02H to construct the Insertion code. When a cardiac lead is replaced, also report the Removal of the cardiac lead (6th character M) from the heart. See table 02P to construct the Removal code.*

0JH838Z Insertion of Defibrillator Generator into Abdomen Subcutaneous Tissue and Fascia, Percutaneous Approach

HAC With a secondary diagnosis code of K68.11, T81.4XXA, T82.6XXA, T82.7XXA

+ Cardioverter-Defibrillator lead(s)/generator when reported with Insertion of a defibrillator cardiac lead (6th character K) into the coronary vein, atrium, or ventricle. Also applicable with Insertion of pacemaker cardiac lead, defibrillator cardiac lead or cardiac lead (6th characters J, K, M) into the pericardium. *See table 02H to construct the Insertion code.*

0JH839Z Insertion of Cardiac Resynchronization Defibrillator Pulse Generator into Abdomen Subcutaneous Tissue and Fascia, Percutaneous Approach

HAC With a secondary diagnosis code of K68.11, T81.4XXA, T82.6XXA, T82.7XXA

+ Cardioverter-Defibrillator lead(s)/generator when reported with Insertion of a defibrillator cardiac lead (6th character K) into the atrium, or ventricle. Also applicable with Insertion of pacemaker cardiac lead, defibrillator cardiac lead or cardiac lead (6th characters J, K, M) into the coronary vein or pericardium. *See table 02H to construct the Insertion code.*

0JH83AZ Insertion of Contractility Modulation Device into Abdomen Subcutaneous Tissue and Fascia, Percutaneous Approach

+ Cardioverter-Defibrillator lead(s)/generator when reported with Insertion of a cardiac lead (6th character M) into the left ventricle. *See table 02H to construct the Insertion code.*

0JH83BZ Insertion of Single Array Stimulator Generator into Abdomen Subcutaneous Tissue and Fascia, Percutaneous Approach

+ Neurotransmitter/Neurostimulator when reported with an Insertion of a neurostimulator lead (6th character M) into the cranial nerve, spinal canal or spinal cord. *See table 00H to construct the Insertion code. Also applicable when reported with Insertion of neurostimulator lead (6th character M) into the peripheral nerve. See table 01H to construct the Insertion code. Also applicable when reported with Insertion of a stimulator lead (6th character M) into the stomach. See table 0DH to construct the Insertion code.*

0JH83CZ Insertion of Single Array Rechargeable Stimulator Generator into Abdomen Subcutaneous Tissue and Fascia, Percutaneous Approach

+ Neurotransmitter/Neurostimulator when reported with an Insertion of a neurostimulator lead (6th character M) into the cranial nerve, spinal canal or spinal cord. *See table 00H to construct the Insertion code. Also applicable when reported with Insertion of neurostimulator lead (6th character M) into the peripheral nerve. See table 01H to construct the Insertion code. Also applicable when reported with Insertion of a stimulator lead (6th character M) into the stomach. See table 0DH to construct the Insertion code.*

0JH83DZ Insertion of Multiple Array Stimulator Generator into Abdomen Subcutaneous Tissue and Fascia, Percutaneous Approach

+ Major brain device implant when reported with an Insertion of a neurostimulator lead (6th character M) into the brain or cerebral ventricle. *See table 00H to construct the Insertion code.*

+ Neurotransmitter/Neurostimulator when reported with an Insertion of a neurostimulator lead (6th character M) into the cranial nerve, spinal canal or spinal cord. *See table 00H to construct the Insertion code. Also applicable when reported with Insertion of neurostimulator lead (6th character M) into the peripheral nerve. See table 01H to construct the Insertion code. Also applicable when reported with Insertion of a stimulator lead (6th character M) into the stomach. See table 0DH to construct the Insertion code.*

0JH83EZ Insertion of Multiple Array Rechargeable Stimulator Generator into Abdomen Subcutaneous Tissue and Fascia, Percutaneous Approach

+ Major brain device implant when reported with an Insertion of a neurostimulator lead (6th character M) into the brain or cerebral ventricle. *See table 00H to construct the Insertion code.*

+ Neurotransmitter/Neurostimulator when reported with an Insertion of a neurostimulator lead (6th character M) into the cranial nerve, spinal canal or spinal cord. *See table 00H to construct the Insertion code. Also applicable when reported with Insertion of neurostimulator lead (6th character M) into the peripheral nerve. See table 01H to construct the Insertion code. Also applicable when reported with Insertion of a stimulator lead (6th character M) into the stomach. See table 0DH to construct the Insertion code.*

● **0JH83HZ** Insertion of Contraceptive Device into Abdomen Subcutaneous Tissue and Fascia, Percutaneous Approach

● **0JH83MZ** Insertion of Stimulator Generator into Abdomen Subcutaneous Tissue and Fascia, Percutaneous Approach

0JH83NZ Insertion of Tissue Expander into Abdomen Subcutaneous Tissue and Fascia, Percutaneous Approach

0JH83PZ Insertion of Cardiac Rhythm Related Device into Abdomen Subcutaneous Tissue and Fascia, Percutaneous Approach

HAC With a secondary diagnosis code of K68.11, T81.4XXA, T82.6XXA, T82.7XXA

+ Pacemaker device when reported with an Insertion of a cardiac lead (6th character J or M) into the coronary vein, atrium, ventricle or pericardium (4th characters 4, 6, 7, K, L and N). *See table 02H to construct the Insertion code. When a cardiac lead is replaced, also report the Removal of the cardiac lead (6th character M) from the heart. See table 02P to construct the Removal code.*

0JH83VZ Insertion of Infusion Pump into Abdomen Subcutaneous Tissue and Fascia, Percutaneous Approach

● **0JH83WZ** Insertion of Reservoir into Abdomen Subcutaneous Tissue and Fascia, Percutaneous Approach

● **0JH83XZ** Insertion of Vascular Access Device into Abdomen Subcutaneous Tissue and Fascia, Percutaneous Approach

0JH90NZ Insertion of Tissue Expander into Buttock Subcutaneous Tissue and Fascia, Open Approach

0JH93NZ Insertion of Tissue Expander into Buttock Subcutaneous Tissue and Fascia, Percutaneous Approach

0JHB0NZ Insertion of Tissue Expander into Perineum Subcutaneous Tissue and Fascia, Open Approach

0JHB3NZ Insertion of Tissue Expander into Perineum Subcutaneous Tissue and Fascia, Percutaneous Approach

0JHC0NZ Insertion of Tissue Expander into Pelvic Region Subcutaneous Tissue and Fascia, Open Approach

0JHC3NZ Insertion of Tissue Expander into Pelvic Region Subcutaneous Tissue and Fascia, Percutaneous Approach

0JHD0HZ Insertion of Contraceptive Device into Right Upper Arm Subcutaneous Tissue and Fascia, Open Approach

0JHD0NZ Insertion of Tissue Expander into Right Upper Arm Subcutaneous Tissue and Fascia, Open Approach

0JHD0VZ Insertion of Infusion Pump into Right Upper Arm Subcutaneous Tissue and Fascia, Open Approach

● **0JHD0WZ** Insertion of Reservoir into Right Upper Arm Subcutaneous Tissue and Fascia, Open Approach

● **0JHD0XZ** Insertion of Vascular Access Device into Right Upper Arm Subcutaneous Tissue and Fascia, Open Approach

0JHD3HZ Insertion of Contraceptive Device into Right Upper Arm Subcutaneous Tissue and Fascia, Percutaneous Approach

0JHD3NZ Insertion of Tissue Expander into Right Upper Arm Subcutaneous Tissue and Fascia, Percutaneous Approach

0JHD3VZ Insertion of Infusion Pump into Right Upper Arm Subcutaneous Tissue and Fascia, Percutaneous Approach

● **0JHD3WZ** Insertion of Reservoir into Right Upper Arm Subcutaneous Tissue and Fascia, Percutaneous Approach

● **0JHD3XZ** Insertion of Vascular Access Device into Right Upper Arm Subcutaneous Tissue and Fascia, Percutaneous Approach

0JHF0HZ Insertion of Contraceptive Device into Left Upper Arm Subcutaneous Tissue and Fascia, Open Approach

0JHF0NZ Insertion of Tissue Expander into Left Upper Arm Subcutaneous Tissue and Fascia, Open Approach

0JHF0VZ Insertion of Infusion Pump into Left Upper Arm Subcutaneous Tissue and Fascia, Open Approach

● **0JHF0WZ** Insertion of Reservoir into Left Upper Arm Subcutaneous Tissue and Fascia, Open Approach

● **0JHF0XZ** Insertion of Vascular Access Device into Left Upper Arm Subcutaneous Tissue and Fascia, Open Approach

0JHF3HZ Insertion of Contraceptive Device into Left Upper Arm Subcutaneous Tissue and Fascia, Percutaneous Approach

0JHF3NZ Insertion of Tissue Expander into Left Upper Arm Subcutaneous Tissue and Fascia, Percutaneous Approach

0JHF3VZ Insertion of Infusion Pump into Left Upper Arm Subcutaneous Tissue and Fascia, Percutaneous Approach

● **0JHF3WZ** Insertion of Reservoir into Left Upper Arm Subcutaneous Tissue and Fascia, Percutaneous Approach

● **0JHF3XZ** Insertion of Vascular Access Device into Left Upper Arm Subcutaneous Tissue and Fascia, Percutaneous Approach

0JHG0HZ Insertion of Contraceptive Device into Right Lower Arm Subcutaneous Tissue and Fascia, Open Approach

0JHG0NZ Insertion of Tissue Expander into Right Lower Arm Subcutaneous Tissue and Fascia, Open Approach

0JHG0VZ Insertion of Infusion Pump into Right Lower Arm Subcutaneous Tissue and Fascia, Open Approach

● **0JHG0WZ** Insertion of Reservoir into Right Lower Arm Subcutaneous Tissue and Fascia, Open Approach

● **0JHG0XZ** Insertion of Vascular Access Device into Right Lower Arm Subcutaneous Tissue and Fascia, Open Approach

0JHG3HZ Insertion of Contraceptive Device into Right Lower Arm Subcutaneous Tissue and Fascia, Percutaneous Approach

0JHG3NZ Insertion of Tissue Expander into Right Lower Arm Subcutaneous Tissue and Fascia, Percutaneous Approach

0JHG3VZ Insertion of Infusion Pump into Right Lower Arm Subcutaneous Tissue and Fascia, Percutaneous Approach

● **0JHG3WZ** Insertion of Reservoir into Right Lower Arm Subcutaneous Tissue and Fascia, Percutaneous Approach

● **0JHG3XZ** Insertion of Vascular Access Device into Right Lower Arm Subcutaneous Tissue and Fascia, Percutaneous Approach

0JHH0HZ Insertion of Contraceptive Device into Left Lower Arm Subcutaneous Tissue and Fascia, Open Approach

0JHH0NZ Insertion of Tissue Expander into Left Lower Arm Subcutaneous Tissue and Fascia, Open Approach

0JHH0VZ Insertion of Infusion Pump into Left Lower Arm Subcutaneous Tissue and Fascia, Open Approach

● **0JHH0WZ** Insertion of Reservoir into Left Lower Arm Subcutaneous Tissue and Fascia, Open Approach

● **0JHH0XZ** Insertion of Vascular Access Device into Left Lower Arm Subcutaneous Tissue and Fascia, Open Approach

0JHH3HZ Insertion of Contraceptive Device into Left Lower Arm Subcutaneous Tissue and Fascia, Percutaneous Approach

0JHH3NZ Insertion of Tissue Expander into Left Lower Arm Subcutaneous Tissue and Fascia, Percutaneous Approach

0JHH3VZ Insertion of Infusion Pump into Left Lower Arm Subcutaneous Tissue and Fascia, Percutaneous Approach

● **0JHH3WZ** Insertion of Reservoir into Left Lower Arm Subcutaneous Tissue and Fascia, Percutaneous Approach

● **0JHH3XZ** Insertion of Vascular Access Device into Left Lower Arm Subcutaneous Tissue and Fascia, Percutaneous Approach

0JHJ0NZ Insertion of Tissue Expander into Right Hand Subcutaneous Tissue and Fascia, Open Approach

0JHJ3NZ Insertion of Tissue Expander into Right Hand Subcutaneous Tissue and Fascia, Percutaneous Approach

0JHK0NZ Insertion of Tissue Expander into Left Hand Subcutaneous Tissue and Fascia, Open Approach

0JHK3NZ Insertion of Tissue Expander into Left Hand Subcutaneous Tissue and Fascia, Percutaneous Approach

0JHL0HZ Insertion of Contraceptive Device into Right Upper Leg Subcutaneous Tissue and Fascia, Open Approach

0JHL0NZ Insertion of Tissue Expander into Right Upper Leg Subcutaneous Tissue and Fascia, Open Approach

0JHL0VZ Insertion of Infusion Pump into Right Upper Leg Subcutaneous Tissue and Fascia, Open Approach

● **0JHL0WZ** Insertion of Reservoir into Right Upper Leg Subcutaneous Tissue and Fascia, Open Approach

● **0JHL0XZ** Insertion of Vascular Access Device into Right Upper Leg Subcutaneous Tissue and Fascia, Open Approach

0JHL3HZ Insertion of Contraceptive Device into Right Upper Leg Subcutaneous Tissue and Fascia, Percutaneous Approach

0JHL3NZ Insertion of Tissue Expander into Right Upper Leg Subcutaneous Tissue and Fascia, Percutaneous Approach

0JHL3VZ Insertion of Infusion Pump into Right Upper Leg Subcutaneous Tissue and Fascia, Percutaneous Approach

● **0JHL3WZ** Insertion of Reservoir into Right Upper Leg Subcutaneous Tissue and Fascia, Percutaneous Approach

● **0JHL3XZ** Insertion of Vascular Access Device into Right Upper Leg Subcutaneous Tissue and Fascia, Percutaneous Approach

0JHM0HZ Insertion of Contraceptive Device into Left Upper Leg Subcutaneous Tissue and Fascia, Open Approach

0JHM0NZ Insertion of Tissue Expander into Left Upper Leg Subcutaneous Tissue and Fascia, Open Approach

0JHM0VZ Insertion of Infusion Pump into Left Upper Leg Subcutaneous Tissue and Fascia, Open Approach

● **0JHM0WZ** Insertion of Reservoir into Left Upper Leg Subcutaneous Tissue and Fascia, Open Approach

● **0JHM0XZ** Insertion of Vascular Access Device into Left Upper Leg Subcutaneous Tissue and Fascia, Open Approach

0JHM3HZ Insertion of Contraceptive Device into Left Upper Leg Subcutaneous Tissue and Fascia, Percutaneous Approach

0JHM3NZ Insertion of Tissue Expander into Left Upper Leg Subcutaneous Tissue and Fascia, Percutaneous Approach

0JHM3VZ Insertion of Infusion Pump into Left Upper Leg Subcutaneous Tissue and Fascia, Percutaneous Approach

● **0JHM3WZ** Insertion of Reservoir into Left Upper Leg Subcutaneous Tissue and Fascia, Percutaneous Approach

● **0JHM3XZ** Insertion of Vascular Access Device into Left Upper Leg Subcutaneous Tissue and Fascia, Percutaneous Approach

0JHN0HZ Insertion of Contraceptive Device into Right Lower Leg Subcutaneous Tissue and Fascia, Open Approach

0JHN0NZ Insertion of Tissue Expander into Right Lower Leg Subcutaneous Tissue and Fascia, Open Approach

0JHN0VZ Insertion of Infusion Pump into Right Lower Leg Subcutaneous Tissue and Fascia, Open Approach

● **0JHN0WZ** Insertion of Reservoir into Right Lower Leg Subcutaneous Tissue and Fascia, Open Approach

● **0JHN0XZ** Insertion of Vascular Access Device into Right Lower Leg Subcutaneous Tissue and Fascia, Open Approach

● **0JHN3HZ** Insertion of Contraceptive Device into Right Lower Leg Subcutaneous Tissue and Fascia, Percutaneous Approach

0JHN3NZ Insertion of Tissue Expander into Right Lower Leg Subcutaneous Tissue and Fascia, Percutaneous Approach

0JHN3VZ Insertion of Infusion Pump into Right Lower Leg Subcutaneous Tissue and Fascia, Percutaneous Approach

● **0JHN3WZ** Insertion of Reservoir into Right Lower Leg Subcutaneous Tissue and Fascia, Percutaneous Approach

● **0JHN3XZ** Insertion of Vascular Access Device into Right Lower Leg Subcutaneous Tissue and Fascia, Percutaneous Approach

● **0JHP0HZ** Insertion of Contraceptive Device into Left Lower Leg Subcutaneous Tissue and Fascia, Open Approach

0JHP0NZ   Insertion of Tissue Expander into Left Lower Leg Subcutaneous Tissue and Fascia, Open Approach

0JHP0VZ   Insertion of Infusion Pump into Left Lower Leg Subcutaneous Tissue and Fascia, Open Approach

● 0JHP0WZ   Insertion of Reservoir into Left Lower Leg Subcutaneous Tissue and Fascia, Open Approach

● 0JHP0XZ   Insertion of Vascular Access Device into Left Lower Leg Subcutaneous Tissue and Fascia, Open Approach

● 0JHP3HZ   Insertion of Contraceptive Device into Left Lower Leg Subcutaneous Tissue and Fascia, Percutaneous Approach

0JHP3NZ   Insertion of Tissue Expander into Left Lower Leg Subcutaneous Tissue and Fascia, Percutaneous Approach

0JHP3VZ   Insertion of Infusion Pump into Left Lower Leg Subcutaneous Tissue and Fascia, Percutaneous Approach

● 0JHP3WZ   Insertion of Reservoir into Left Lower Leg Subcutaneous Tissue and Fascia, Percutaneous Approach

● 0JHP3XZ   Insertion of Vascular Access Device into Left Lower Leg Subcutaneous Tissue and Fascia, Percutaneous Approach

0JHQ0NZ   Insertion of Tissue Expander into Right Foot Subcutaneous Tissue and Fascia, Open Approach

0JHQ3NZ   Insertion of Tissue Expander into Right Foot Subcutaneous Tissue and Fascia, Percutaneous Approach

0JHR0NZ   Insertion of Tissue Expander into Left Foot Subcutaneous Tissue and Fascia, Open Approach

0JHR3NZ   Insertion of Tissue Expander into Left Foot Subcutaneous Tissue and Fascia, Percutaneous Approach

0JHS01Z   Insertion of Radioactive Element into Head and Neck Subcutaneous Tissue and Fascia, Open Approach

0JHS03Z   Insertion of Infusion Device into Head and Neck Subcutaneous Tissue and Fascia, Open Approach

0JHS31Z   Insertion of Radioactive Element into Head and Neck Subcutaneous Tissue and Fascia, Percutaneous Approach

0JHS33Z   Insertion of Infusion Device into Head and Neck Subcutaneous Tissue and Fascia, Percutaneous Approach

0JHT01Z   Insertion of Radioactive Element into Trunk Subcutaneous Tissue and Fascia, Open Approach

0JHT03Z   Insertion of Infusion Device into Trunk Subcutaneous Tissue and Fascia, Open Approach

0JHT0VZ   Insertion of Infusion Pump into Trunk Subcutaneous Tissue and Fascia, Open Approach

0JHT31Z   Insertion of Radioactive Element into Trunk Subcutaneous Tissue and Fascia, Percutaneous Approach

0JHT33Z   Insertion of Infusion Device into Trunk Subcutaneous Tissue and Fascia, Percutaneous Approach

0JHT3VZ   Insertion of Infusion Pump into Trunk Subcutaneous Tissue and Fascia, Percutaneous Approach

0JHV01Z   Insertion of Radioactive Element into Upper Extremity Subcutaneous Tissue and Fascia, Open Approach

0JHV03Z   Insertion of Infusion Device into Upper Extremity Subcutaneous Tissue and Fascia, Open Approach

0JHV31Z   Insertion of Radioactive Element into Upper Extremity Subcutaneous Tissue and Fascia, Percutaneous Approach

0JHV33Z   Insertion of Infusion Device into Upper Extremity Subcutaneous Tissue and Fascia, Percutaneous Approach

0JHW01Z   Insertion of Radioactive Element into Lower Extremity Subcutaneous Tissue and Fascia, Open Approach

0JHW03Z   Insertion of Infusion Device into Lower Extremity Subcutaneous Tissue and Fascia, Open Approach

0JHW31Z   Insertion of Radioactive Element into Lower Extremity Subcutaneous Tissue and Fascia, Percutaneous Approach

0JHW33Z   Insertion of Infusion Device into Lower Extremity Subcutaneous Tissue and Fascia, Percutaneous Approach

0JJ – Subcutaneous Tissue and Fascia, Inspection

Review Coding Guideline B3.5

Review Coding Guidelines B3.11a, B3.11b and B3.11c

0JJS0ZZ   Inspection of Head and Neck Subcutaneous Tissue and Fascia, Open Approach

0JJS3ZZ   Inspection of Head and Neck Subcutaneous Tissue and Fascia, Percutaneous Approach

0JJSXZZ   Inspection of Head and Neck Subcutaneous Tissue and Fascia, External Approach

0JJT0ZZ   Inspection of Trunk Subcutaneous Tissue and Fascia, Open Approach

0JJT3ZZ   Inspection of Trunk Subcutaneous Tissue and Fascia, Percutaneous Approach

0JJTXZZ   Inspection of Trunk Subcutaneous Tissue and Fascia, External Approach

0JJV0ZZ   Inspection of Upper Extremity Subcutaneous Tissue and Fascia, Open Approach

0JJV3ZZ   Inspection of Upper Extremity Subcutaneous Tissue and Fascia, Percutaneous Approach

0JJVXZZ   Inspection of Upper Extremity Subcutaneous Tissue and Fascia, External Approach

0JJW0ZZ   Inspection of Lower Extremity Subcutaneous Tissue and Fascia, Open Approach

0JJW3ZZ   Inspection of Lower Extremity Subcutaneous Tissue and Fascia, Percutaneous Approach

0JJWXZZ   Inspection of Lower Extremity Subcutaneous Tissue and Fascia, External Approach

0JN – Subcutaneous Tissue and Fascia, Release

Review Coding Guideline B3.13

Review Coding Guideline B3.14

0JN00ZZ   Release Scalp Subcutaneous Tissue and Fascia, Open Approach

0JN03ZZ   Release Scalp Subcutaneous Tissue and Fascia, Percutaneous Approach

0JN0XZZ   Release Scalp Subcutaneous Tissue and Fascia, External Approach

0JN10ZZ   Release Face Subcutaneous Tissue and Fascia, Open Approach

0JN13ZZ   Release Face Subcutaneous Tissue and Fascia, Percutaneous Approach

0JN1XZZ   Release Face Subcutaneous Tissue and Fascia, External Approach

0JN40ZZ   Release Anterior Neck Subcutaneous Tissue and Fascia, Open Approach

0JN43ZZ   Release Anterior Neck Subcutaneous Tissue and Fascia, Percutaneous Approach

0JN4XZZ   Release Anterior Neck Subcutaneous Tissue and Fascia, External Approach

0JN50ZZ   Release Posterior Neck Subcutaneous Tissue and Fascia, Open Approach

0JN53ZZ   Release Posterior Neck Subcutaneous Tissue and Fascia, Percutaneous Approach

0JN5XZZ   Release Posterior Neck Subcutaneous Tissue and Fascia, External Approach

0JN60ZZ   Release Chest Subcutaneous Tissue and Fascia, Open Approach

0JN63ZZ   Release Chest Subcutaneous Tissue and Fascia, Percutaneous Approach

0JN6XZZ   Release Chest Subcutaneous Tissue and Fascia, External Approach

0JN70ZZ   Release Back Subcutaneous Tissue and Fascia, Open Approach

0JN73ZZ   Release Back Subcutaneous Tissue and Fascia, Percutaneous Approach

0JN7XZZ   Release Back Subcutaneous Tissue and Fascia, External Approach

0JN80ZZ   Release Abdomen Subcutaneous Tissue and Fascia, Open Approach

0JN83ZZ   Release Abdomen Subcutaneous Tissue and Fascia, Percutaneous Approach

0JN8XZZ   Release Abdomen Subcutaneous Tissue and Fascia, External Approach

0JN90ZZ Release Buttock Subcutaneous Tissue and Fascia, Open Approach
0JN93ZZ Release Buttock Subcutaneous Tissue and Fascia, Percutaneous Approach
0JN9XZZ Release Buttock Subcutaneous Tissue and Fascia, External Approach
0JNB0ZZ Release Perineum Subcutaneous Tissue and Fascia, Open Approach
0JNB3ZZ Release Perineum Subcutaneous Tissue and Fascia, Percutaneous Approach
0JNBXZZ Release Perineum Subcutaneous Tissue and Fascia, External Approach
0JNC0ZZ Release Pelvic Region Subcutaneous Tissue and Fascia, Open Approach
0JNC3ZZ Release Pelvic Region Subcutaneous Tissue and Fascia, Percutaneous Approach
0JNCXZZ Release Pelvic Region Subcutaneous Tissue and Fascia, External Approach
0JND0ZZ Release Right Upper Arm Subcutaneous Tissue and Fascia, Open Approach
0JND3ZZ Release Right Upper Arm Subcutaneous Tissue and Fascia, Percutaneous Approach
0JNDXZZ Release Right Upper Arm Subcutaneous Tissue and Fascia, External Approach
0JNF0ZZ Release Left Upper Arm Subcutaneous Tissue and Fascia, Open Approach
0JNF3ZZ Release Left Upper Arm Subcutaneous Tissue and Fascia, Percutaneous Approach
0JNFXZZ Release Left Upper Arm Subcutaneous Tissue and Fascia, External Approach
0JNG0ZZ Release Right Lower Arm Subcutaneous Tissue and Fascia, Open Approach
0JNG3ZZ Release Right Lower Arm Subcutaneous Tissue and Fascia, Percutaneous Approach
0JNGXZZ Release Right Lower Arm Subcutaneous Tissue and Fascia, External Approach
0JNH0ZZ Release Left Lower Arm Subcutaneous Tissue and Fascia, Open Approach
0JNH3ZZ Release Left Lower Arm Subcutaneous Tissue and Fascia, Percutaneous Approach
0JNHXZZ Release Left Lower Arm Subcutaneous Tissue and Fascia, External Approach
0JNJ0ZZ Release Right Hand Subcutaneous Tissue and Fascia, Open Approach
0JNJ3ZZ Release Right Hand Subcutaneous Tissue and Fascia, Percutaneous Approach

0JNJXZZ Release Right Hand Subcutaneous Tissue and Fascia, External Approach
0JNK0ZZ Release Left Hand Subcutaneous Tissue and Fascia, Open Approach
0JNK3ZZ Release Left Hand Subcutaneous Tissue and Fascia, Percutaneous Approach
0JNKXZZ Release Left Hand Subcutaneous Tissue and Fascia, External Approach
0JNL0ZZ Release Right Upper Leg Subcutaneous Tissue and Fascia, Open Approach
0JNL3ZZ Release Right Upper Leg Subcutaneous Tissue and Fascia, Percutaneous Approach
0JNLXZZ Release Right Upper Leg Subcutaneous Tissue and Fascia, External Approach
0JNM0ZZ Release Left Upper Leg Subcutaneous Tissue and Fascia, Open Approach
0JNM3ZZ Release Left Upper Leg Subcutaneous Tissue and Fascia, Percutaneous Approach
0JNMXZZ Release Left Upper Leg Subcutaneous Tissue and Fascia, External Approach
0JNN0ZZ Release Right Lower Leg Subcutaneous Tissue and Fascia, Open Approach
0JNN3ZZ Release Right Lower Leg Subcutaneous Tissue and Fascia, Percutaneous Approach
0JNNXZZ Release Right Lower Leg Subcutaneous Tissue and Fascia, External Approach
0JNP0ZZ Release Left Lower Leg Subcutaneous Tissue and Fascia, Open Approach
0JNP3ZZ Release Left Lower Leg Subcutaneous Tissue and Fascia, Percutaneous Approach
0JNPXZZ Release Left Lower Leg Subcutaneous Tissue and Fascia, External Approach
0JNQ0ZZ Release Right Foot Subcutaneous Tissue and Fascia, Open Approach
0JNQ3ZZ Release Right Foot Subcutaneous Tissue and Fascia, Percutaneous Approach
0JNQXZZ Release Right Foot Subcutaneous Tissue and Fascia, External Approach
0JNR0ZZ Release Left Foot Subcutaneous Tissue and Fascia, Open Approach
0JNR3ZZ Release Left Foot Subcutaneous Tissue and Fascia, Percutaneous Approach
0JNRXZZ Release Left Foot Subcutaneous Tissue and Fascia, External Approach

0JP – Subcutaneous Tissue and Fascia, Removal

Review Coding Guideline B6.1c

0JPS00Z Removal of Drainage Device from Head and Neck Subcutaneous Tissue and Fascia, Open Approach
0JPS01Z Removal of Radioactive Element from Head and Neck Subcutaneous Tissue and Fascia, Open Approach
0JPS03Z Removal of Infusion Device from Head and Neck Subcutaneous Tissue and Fascia, Open Approach
0JPS07Z Removal of Autologous Tissue Substitute from Head and Neck Subcutaneous Tissue and Fascia, Open Approach
0JPS0JZ Removal of Synthetic Substitute from Head and Neck Subcutaneous Tissue and Fascia, Open Approach
0JPS0KZ Removal of Nonautologous Tissue Substitute from Head and Neck Subcutaneous Tissue and Fascia, Open Approach
0JPS0NZ Removal of Tissue Expander from Head and Neck Subcutaneous Tissue and Fascia, Open Approach
0JPS30Z Removal of Drainage Device from Head and Neck Subcutaneous Tissue and Fascia, Percutaneous Approach
0JPS31Z Removal of Radioactive Element from Head and Neck Subcutaneous Tissue and Fascia, Percutaneous Approach
0JPS33Z Removal of Infusion Device from Head and Neck Subcutaneous Tissue and Fascia, Percutaneous Approach
0JPS37Z Removal of Autologous Tissue Substitute from Head and Neck Subcutaneous Tissue and Fascia, Percutaneous Approach
0JPS3JZ Removal of Synthetic Substitute from Head and Neck Subcutaneous Tissue and Fascia, Percutaneous Approach
0JPS3KZ Removal of Nonautologous Tissue Substitute from Head and Neck Subcutaneous Tissue and Fascia, Percutaneous Approach

0JPS3NZ Removal of Tissue Expander from Head and Neck Subcutaneous Tissue and Fascia, Percutaneous Approach
0JPSX0Z Removal of Drainage Device from Head and Neck Subcutaneous Tissue and Fascia, External Approach
0JPSX1Z Removal of Radioactive Element from Head and Neck Subcutaneous Tissue and Fascia, External Approach
0JPSX3Z Removal of Infusion Device from Head and Neck Subcutaneous Tissue and Fascia, External Approach
0JPT00Z Removal of Drainage Device from Trunk Subcutaneous Tissue and Fascia, Open Approach
0JPT01Z Removal of Radioactive Element from Trunk Subcutaneous Tissue and Fascia, Open Approach
0JPT02Z Removal of Monitoring Device from Trunk Subcutaneous Tissue and Fascia, Open Approach
0JPT03Z Removal of Infusion Device from Trunk Subcutaneous Tissue and Fascia, Open Approach
0JPT07Z Removal of Autologous Tissue Substitute from Trunk Subcutaneous Tissue and Fascia, Open Approach
0JPT0HZ Removal of Contraceptive Device from Trunk Subcutaneous Tissue and Fascia, Open Approach
0JPT0JZ Removal of Synthetic Substitute from Trunk Subcutaneous Tissue and Fascia, Open Approach
0JPT0KZ Removal of Nonautologous Tissue Substitute from Trunk Subcutaneous Tissue and Fascia, Open Approach
0JPT0MZ Removal of Stimulator Generator from Trunk Subcutaneous Tissue and Fascia, Open Approach

0JPT0NZ   Removal of Tissue Expander from Trunk Subcutaneous Tissue and Fascia, Open Approach

0JPT0PZ   Removal of Cardiac Rhythm Related Device from Trunk Subcutaneous Tissue and Fascia, Open Approach

HAC   With a secondary diagnosis code of K68.11, T81.4XXA, T82.6XXA, T82.7XXA

0JPT0VZ   Removal of Infusion Pump from Trunk Subcutaneous Tissue and Fascia, Open Approach

0JPT0WZ   Removal of Reservoir from Trunk Subcutaneous Tissue and Fascia, Open Approach

0JPT0XZ   Removal of Vascular Access Device from Trunk Subcutaneous Tissue and Fascia, Open Approach

0JPT30Z   Removal of Drainage Device from Trunk Subcutaneous Tissue and Fascia, Percutaneous Approach

0JPT31Z   Removal of Radioactive Element from Trunk Subcutaneous Tissue and Fascia, Percutaneous Approach

0JPT32Z   Removal of Monitoring Device from Trunk Subcutaneous Tissue and Fascia, Percutaneous Approach

0JPT33Z   Removal of Infusion Device from Trunk Subcutaneous Tissue and Fascia, Percutaneous Approach

0JPT37Z   Removal of Autologous Tissue Substitute from Trunk Subcutaneous Tissue and Fascia, Percutaneous Approach

0JPT3HZ   Removal of Contraceptive Device from Trunk Subcutaneous Tissue and Fascia, Percutaneous Approach

0JPT3JZ   Removal of Synthetic Substitute from Trunk Subcutaneous Tissue and Fascia, Percutaneous Approach

0JPT3KZ   Removal of Nonautologous Tissue Substitute from Trunk Subcutaneous Tissue and Fascia, Percutaneous Approach

0JPT3MZ   Removal of Stimulator Generator from Trunk Subcutaneous Tissue and Fascia, Percutaneous Approach

0JPT3NZ   Removal of Tissue Expander from Trunk Subcutaneous Tissue and Fascia, Percutaneous Approach

0JPT3PZ   Removal of Cardiac Rhythm Related Device from Trunk Subcutaneous Tissue and Fascia, Percutaneous Approach

HAC   With a secondary diagnosis code of K68.11, T81.4XXA, T82.6XXA, T82.7XXA

0JPT3VZ   Removal of Infusion Pump from Trunk Subcutaneous Tissue and Fascia, Percutaneous Approach

0JPT3WZ   Removal of Reservoir from Trunk Subcutaneous Tissue and Fascia, Percutaneous Approach

0JPT3XZ   Removal of Vascular Access Device from Trunk Subcutaneous Tissue and Fascia, Percutaneous Approach

0JPTX0Z   Removal of Drainage Device from Trunk Subcutaneous Tissue and Fascia, External Approach

0JPTX1Z   Removal of Radioactive Element from Trunk Subcutaneous Tissue and Fascia, External Approach

0JPTX2Z   Removal of Monitoring Device from Trunk Subcutaneous Tissue and Fascia, External Approach

0JPTX3Z   Removal of Infusion Device from Trunk Subcutaneous Tissue and Fascia, External Approach

0JPTXHZ   Removal of Contraceptive Device from Trunk Subcutaneous Tissue and Fascia, External Approach

0JPTXVZ   Removal of Infusion Pump from Trunk Subcutaneous Tissue and Fascia, External Approach

0JPTXXZ   Removal of Vascular Access Device from Trunk Subcutaneous Tissue and Fascia, External Approach

0JPV00Z   Removal of Drainage Device from Upper Extremity Subcutaneous Tissue and Fascia, Open Approach

0JPV01Z   Removal of Radioactive Element from Upper Extremity Subcutaneous Tissue and Fascia, Open Approach

0JPV03Z   Removal of Infusion Device from Upper Extremity Subcutaneous Tissue and Fascia, Open Approach

0JPV07Z   Removal of Autologous Tissue Substitute from Upper Extremity Subcutaneous Tissue and Fascia, Open Approach

0JPV0HZ   Removal of Contraceptive Device from Upper Extremity Subcutaneous Tissue and Fascia, Open Approach

0JPV0JZ   Removal of Synthetic Substitute from Upper Extremity Subcutaneous Tissue and Fascia, Open Approach

0JPV0KZ   Removal of Nonautologous Tissue Substitute from Upper Extremity Subcutaneous Tissue and Fascia, Open Approach

0JPV0NZ   Removal of Tissue Expander from Upper Extremity Subcutaneous Tissue and Fascia, Open Approach

0JPV0VZ   Removal of Infusion Pump from Upper Extremity Subcutaneous Tissue and Fascia, Open Approach

0JPV0WZ   Removal of Reservoir from Upper Extremity Subcutaneous Tissue and Fascia, Open Approach

0JPV0XZ   Removal of Vascular Access Device from Upper Extremity Subcutaneous Tissue and Fascia, Open Approach

0JPV30Z   Removal of Drainage Device from Upper Extremity Subcutaneous Tissue and Fascia, Percutaneous Approach

0JPV31Z   Removal of Radioactive Element from Upper Extremity Subcutaneous Tissue and Fascia, Percutaneous Approach

0JPV33Z   Removal of Infusion Device from Upper Extremity Subcutaneous Tissue and Fascia, Percutaneous Approach

0JPV37Z   Removal of Autologous Tissue Substitute from Upper Extremity Subcutaneous Tissue and Fascia, Percutaneous Approach

0JPV3HZ   Removal of Contraceptive Device from Upper Extremity Subcutaneous Tissue and Fascia, Percutaneous Approach

0JPV3JZ   Removal of Synthetic Substitute from Upper Extremity Subcutaneous Tissue and Fascia, Percutaneous Approach

0JPV3KZ   Removal of Nonautologous Tissue Substitute from Upper Extremity Subcutaneous Tissue and Fascia, Percutaneous Approach

0JPV3NZ   Removal of Tissue Expander from Upper Extremity Subcutaneous Tissue and Fascia, Percutaneous Approach

0JPV3VZ   Removal of Infusion Pump from Upper Extremity Subcutaneous Tissue and Fascia, Percutaneous Approach

0JPV3WZ   Removal of Reservoir from Upper Extremity Subcutaneous Tissue and Fascia, Percutaneous Approach

0JPV3XZ   Removal of Vascular Access Device from Upper Extremity Subcutaneous Tissue and Fascia, Percutaneous Approach

0JPVX0Z   Removal of Drainage Device from Upper Extremity Subcutaneous Tissue and Fascia, External Approach

0JPVX1Z   Removal of Radioactive Element from Upper Extremity Subcutaneous Tissue and Fascia, External Approach

0JPVX3Z   Removal of Infusion Device from Upper Extremity Subcutaneous Tissue and Fascia, External Approach

0JPVXHZ   Removal of Contraceptive Device from Upper Extremity Subcutaneous Tissue and Fascia, External Approach

0JPVXVZ   Removal of Infusion Pump from Upper Extremity Subcutaneous Tissue and Fascia, External Approach

0JPVXXZ   Removal of Vascular Access Device from Upper Extremity Subcutaneous Tissue and Fascia, External Approach

0JPW00Z   Removal of Drainage Device from Lower Extremity Subcutaneous Tissue and Fascia, Open Approach

0JPW01Z   Removal of Radioactive Element from Lower Extremity Subcutaneous Tissue and Fascia, Open Approach

0JPW03Z   Removal of Infusion Device from Lower Extremity Subcutaneous Tissue and Fascia, Open Approach

0JPW07Z   Removal of Autologous Tissue Substitute from Lower Extremity Subcutaneous Tissue and Fascia, Open Approach

0JPW0HZ   Removal of Contraceptive Device from Lower Extremity Subcutaneous Tissue and Fascia, Open Approach

0JPW0JZ   Removal of Synthetic Substitute from Lower Extremity Subcutaneous Tissue and Fascia, Open Approach

0JPW0KZ   Removal of Nonautologous Tissue Substitute from Lower Extremity Subcutaneous Tissue and Fascia, Open Approach

0JPW0NZ   Removal of Tissue Expander from Lower Extremity Subcutaneous Tissue and Fascia, Open Approach

0JPW0VZ   Removal of Infusion Pump from Lower Extremity Subcutaneous Tissue and Fascia, Open Approach

0JPW0WZ   Removal of Reservoir from Lower Extremity Subcutaneous Tissue and Fascia, Open Approach

0JPW0XZ   Removal of Vascular Access Device from Lower Extremity Subcutaneous Tissue and Fascia, Open Approach

0JPW30Z   Removal of Drainage Device from Lower Extremity Subcutaneous Tissue and Fascia, Percutaneous Approach

0JPW31Z   Removal of Radioactive Element from Lower Extremity Subcutaneous Tissue and Fascia, Percutaneous Approach

0JPW33Z   Removal of Infusion Device from Lower Extremity Subcutaneous Tissue and Fascia, Percutaneous Approach

0JPW37Z   Removal of Autologous Tissue Substitute from Lower Extremity Subcutaneous Tissue and Fascia, Percutaneous Approach

0JPW3HZ   Removal of Contraceptive Device from Lower Extremity Subcutaneous Tissue and Fascia, Percutaneous Approach

0JPW3JZ Removal of Synthetic Substitute from Lower Extremity Subcutaneous Tissue and Fascia, Percutaneous Approach

0JPW3KZ Removal of Nonautologous Tissue Substitute from Lower Extremity Subcutaneous Tissue and Fascia, Percutaneous Approach

0JPW3NZ Removal of Tissue Expander from Lower Extremity Subcutaneous Tissue and Fascia, Percutaneous Approach

0JPW3VZ Removal of Infusion Pump from Lower Extremity Subcutaneous Tissue and Fascia, Percutaneous Approach

0JPW3WZ Removal of Reservoir from Lower Extremity Subcutaneous Tissue and Fascia, Percutaneous Approach

0JPW3XZ Removal of Vascular Access Device from Lower Extremity Subcutaneous Tissue and Fascia, Percutaneous Approach

0JPWX0Z Removal of Drainage Device from Lower Extremity Subcutaneous Tissue and Fascia, External Approach

0JPWX1Z Removal of Radioactive Element from Lower Extremity Subcutaneous Tissue and Fascia, External Approach

0JPWX3Z Removal of Infusion Device from Lower Extremity Subcutaneous Tissue and Fascia, External Approach

0JPWXHZ Removal of Contraceptive Device from Lower Extremity Subcutaneous Tissue and Fascia, External Approach

0JPWXVZ Removal of Infusion Pump from Lower Extremity Subcutaneous Tissue and Fascia, External Approach

0JPWXXZ Removal of Vascular Access Device from Lower Extremity Subcutaneous Tissue and Fascia, External Approach

0JQ – Subcutaneous Tissue and Fascia, Repair

Review Coding Guideline B3.5

0JQ00ZZ Repair Scalp Subcutaneous Tissue and Fascia, Open Approach

0JQ03ZZ Repair Scalp Subcutaneous Tissue and Fascia, Percutaneous Approach

0JQ10ZZ Repair Face Subcutaneous Tissue and Fascia, Open Approach

0JQ13ZZ Repair Face Subcutaneous Tissue and Fascia, Percutaneous Approach

0JQ40ZZ Repair Anterior Neck Subcutaneous Tissue and Fascia, Open Approach

0JQ43ZZ Repair Anterior Neck Subcutaneous Tissue and Fascia, Percutaneous Approach

0JQ50ZZ Repair Posterior Neck Subcutaneous Tissue and Fascia, Open Approach

0JQ53ZZ Repair Posterior Neck Subcutaneous Tissue and Fascia, Percutaneous Approach

0JQ60ZZ Repair Chest Subcutaneous Tissue and Fascia, Open Approach

0JQ63ZZ Repair Chest Subcutaneous Tissue and Fascia, Percutaneous Approach

0JQ70ZZ Repair Back Subcutaneous Tissue and Fascia, Open Approach

0JQ73ZZ Repair Back Subcutaneous Tissue and Fascia, Percutaneous Approach

0JQ80ZZ Repair Abdomen Subcutaneous Tissue and Fascia, Open Approach

0JQ83ZZ Repair Abdomen Subcutaneous Tissue and Fascia, Percutaneous Approach

0JQ90ZZ Repair Buttock Subcutaneous Tissue and Fascia, Open Approach

0JQ93ZZ Repair Buttock Subcutaneous Tissue and Fascia, Percutaneous Approach

0JQB0ZZ Repair Perineum Subcutaneous Tissue and Fascia, Open Approach

0JQB3ZZ Repair Perineum Subcutaneous Tissue and Fascia, Percutaneous Approach

0JQC0ZZ Repair Pelvic Region Subcutaneous Tissue and Fascia, Open Approach

0JQC3ZZ Repair Pelvic Region Subcutaneous Tissue and Fascia, Percutaneous Approach

0JQD0ZZ Repair Right Upper Arm Subcutaneous Tissue and Fascia, Open Approach

0JQD3ZZ Repair Right Upper Arm Subcutaneous Tissue and Fascia, Percutaneous Approach

0JQF0ZZ Repair Left Upper Arm Subcutaneous Tissue and Fascia, Open Approach

0JQF3ZZ Repair Left Upper Arm Subcutaneous Tissue and Fascia, Percutaneous Approach

0JQG0ZZ Repair Right Lower Arm Subcutaneous Tissue and Fascia, Open Approach

0JQG3ZZ Repair Right Lower Arm Subcutaneous Tissue and Fascia, Percutaneous Approach

0JQH0ZZ Repair Left Lower Arm Subcutaneous Tissue and Fascia, Open Approach

0JQH3ZZ Repair Left Lower Arm Subcutaneous Tissue and Fascia, Percutaneous Approach

0JQJ0ZZ Repair Right Hand Subcutaneous Tissue and Fascia, Open Approach

0JQJ3ZZ Repair Right Hand Subcutaneous Tissue and Fascia, Percutaneous Approach

0JQK0ZZ Repair Left Hand Subcutaneous Tissue and Fascia, Open Approach

0JQK3ZZ Repair Left Hand Subcutaneous Tissue and Fascia, Percutaneous Approach

0JQL0ZZ Repair Right Upper Leg Subcutaneous Tissue and Fascia, Open Approach

0JQL3ZZ Repair Right Upper Leg Subcutaneous Tissue and Fascia, Percutaneous Approach

0JQM0ZZ Repair Left Upper Leg Subcutaneous Tissue and Fascia, Open Approach

0JQM3ZZ Repair Left Upper Leg Subcutaneous Tissue and Fascia, Percutaneous Approach

0JQN0ZZ Repair Right Lower Leg Subcutaneous Tissue and Fascia, Open Approach

0JQN3ZZ Repair Right Lower Leg Subcutaneous Tissue and Fascia, Percutaneous Approach

0JQP0ZZ Repair Left Lower Leg Subcutaneous Tissue and Fascia, Open Approach

0JQP3ZZ Repair Left Lower Leg Subcutaneous Tissue and Fascia, Percutaneous Approach

0JQQ0ZZ Repair Right Foot Subcutaneous Tissue and Fascia, Open Approach

0JQQ3ZZ Repair Right Foot Subcutaneous Tissue and Fascia, Percutaneous Approach

0JQR0ZZ Repair Left Foot Subcutaneous Tissue and Fascia, Open Approach

0JQR3ZZ Repair Left Foot Subcutaneous Tissue and Fascia, Percutaneous Approach

0JR – Subcutaneous Tissue and Fascia, Replacement

0JR007Z Replacement of Scalp Subcutaneous Tissue and Fascia with Autologous Tissue Substitute, Open Approach

0JR00JZ Replacement of Scalp Subcutaneous Tissue and Fascia with Synthetic Substitute, Open Approach

0JR00KZ Replacement of Scalp Subcutaneous Tissue and Fascia with Nonautologous Tissue Substitute, Open Approach

0JR037Z Replacement of Scalp Subcutaneous Tissue and Fascia with Autologous Tissue Substitute, Percutaneous Approach

0JR03JZ Replacement of Scalp Subcutaneous Tissue and Fascia with Synthetic Substitute, Percutaneous Approach

0JR03KZ Replacement of Scalp Subcutaneous Tissue and Fascia with Nonautologous Tissue Substitute, Percutaneous Approach

0JR107Z Replacement of Face Subcutaneous Tissue and Fascia with Autologous Tissue Substitute, Open Approach

0JR10JZ Replacement of Face Subcutaneous Tissue and Fascia with Synthetic Substitute, Open Approach

0JR10KZ Replacement of Face Subcutaneous Tissue and Fascia with Nonautologous Tissue Substitute, Open Approach

0JR137Z Replacement of Face Subcutaneous Tissue and Fascia with Autologous Tissue Substitute, Percutaneous Approach

0JR13JZ Replacement of Face Subcutaneous Tissue and Fascia with Synthetic Substitute, Percutaneous Approach

0JR13KZ Replacement of Face Subcutaneous Tissue and Fascia with Nonautologous Tissue Substitute, Percutaneous Approach

0JR407Z Replacement of Anterior Neck Subcutaneous Tissue and Fascia with Autologous Tissue Substitute, Open Approach

0JR40JZ Replacement of Anterior Neck Subcutaneous Tissue and Fascia with Synthetic Substitute, Open Approach

0JR40KZ Replacement of Anterior Neck Subcutaneous Tissue and Fascia with Nonautologous Tissue Substitute, Open Approach

0JR437Z Replacement of Anterior Neck Subcutaneous Tissue and Fascia with Autologous Tissue Substitute, Percutaneous Approach

0JR43JZ Replacement of Anterior Neck Subcutaneous Tissue and Fascia with Synthetic Substitute, Percutaneous Approach

0JR43KZ Replacement of Anterior Neck Subcutaneous Tissue and Fascia with Nonautologous Tissue Substitute, Percutaneous Approach

0JR507Z Replacement of Posterior Neck Subcutaneous Tissue and Fascia with Autologous Tissue Substitute, Open Approach

0JR50JZ Replacement of Posterior Neck Subcutaneous Tissue and Fascia with Synthetic Substitute, Open Approach

0JR50KZ Replacement of Posterior Neck Subcutaneous Tissue and Fascia with Nonautologous Tissue Substitute, Open Approach

0JR537Z Replacement of Posterior Neck Subcutaneous Tissue and Fascia with Autologous Tissue Substitute, Percutaneous Approach

0JR53JZ Replacement of Posterior Neck Subcutaneous Tissue and Fascia with Synthetic Substitute, Percutaneous Approach

0JR53KZ Replacement of Posterior Neck Subcutaneous Tissue and Fascia with Nonautologous Tissue Substitute, Percutaneous Approach

0JR607Z Replacement of Chest Subcutaneous Tissue and Fascia with Autologous Tissue Substitute, Open Approach

0JR60JZ Replacement of Chest Subcutaneous Tissue and Fascia with Synthetic Substitute, Open Approach

0JR60KZ Replacement of Chest Subcutaneous Tissue and Fascia with Nonautologous Tissue Substitute, Open Approach

0JR637Z Replacement of Chest Subcutaneous Tissue and Fascia with Autologous Tissue Substitute, Percutaneous Approach

0JR63JZ Replacement of Chest Subcutaneous Tissue and Fascia with Synthetic Substitute, Percutaneous Approach

0JR63KZ Replacement of Chest Subcutaneous Tissue and Fascia with Nonautologous Tissue Substitute, Percutaneous Approach

0JR707Z Replacement of Back Subcutaneous Tissue and Fascia with Autologous Tissue Substitute, Open Approach

0JR70JZ Replacement of Back Subcutaneous Tissue and Fascia with Synthetic Substitute, Open Approach

0JR70KZ Replacement of Back Subcutaneous Tissue and Fascia with Nonautologous Tissue Substitute, Open Approach

0JR737Z Replacement of Back Subcutaneous Tissue and Fascia with Autologous Tissue Substitute, Percutaneous Approach

0JR73JZ Replacement of Back Subcutaneous Tissue and Fascia with Synthetic Substitute, Percutaneous Approach

0JR73KZ Replacement of Back Subcutaneous Tissue and Fascia with Nonautologous Tissue Substitute, Percutaneous Approach

0JR807Z Replacement of Abdomen Subcutaneous Tissue and Fascia with Autologous Tissue Substitute, Open Approach

0JR80JZ Replacement of Abdomen Subcutaneous Tissue and Fascia with Synthetic Substitute, Open Approach

0JR80KZ Replacement of Abdomen Subcutaneous Tissue and Fascia with Nonautologous Tissue Substitute, Open Approach

0JR837Z Replacement of Abdomen Subcutaneous Tissue and Fascia with Autologous Tissue Substitute, Percutaneous Approach

0JR83JZ Replacement of Abdomen Subcutaneous Tissue and Fascia with Synthetic Substitute, Percutaneous Approach

0JR83KZ Replacement of Abdomen Subcutaneous Tissue and Fascia with Nonautologous Tissue Substitute, Percutaneous Approach

0JR907Z Replacement of Buttock Subcutaneous Tissue and Fascia with Autologous Tissue Substitute, Open Approach

0JR90JZ Replacement of Buttock Subcutaneous Tissue and Fascia with Synthetic Substitute, Open Approach

0JR90KZ Replacement of Buttock Subcutaneous Tissue and Fascia with Nonautologous Tissue Substitute, Open Approach

0JR937Z Replacement of Buttock Subcutaneous Tissue and Fascia with Autologous Tissue Substitute, Percutaneous Approach

0JR93JZ Replacement of Buttock Subcutaneous Tissue and Fascia with Synthetic Substitute, Percutaneous Approach

0JR93KZ Replacement of Buttock Subcutaneous Tissue and Fascia with Nonautologous Tissue Substitute, Percutaneous Approach

0JRB07Z Replacement of Perineum Subcutaneous Tissue and Fascia with Autologous Tissue Substitute, Open Approach

0JRB0JZ Replacement of Perineum Subcutaneous Tissue and Fascia with Synthetic Substitute, Open Approach

0JRB0KZ Replacement of Perineum Subcutaneous Tissue and Fascia with Nonautologous Tissue Substitute, Open Approach

0JRB37Z Replacement of Perineum Subcutaneous Tissue and Fascia with Autologous Tissue Substitute, Percutaneous Approach

0JRB3JZ Replacement of Perineum Subcutaneous Tissue and Fascia with Synthetic Substitute, Percutaneous Approach

0JRB3KZ Replacement of Perineum Subcutaneous Tissue and Fascia with Nonautologous Tissue Substitute, Percutaneous Approach

0JRC07Z Replacement of Pelvic Region Subcutaneous Tissue and Fascia with Autologous Tissue Substitute, Open Approach

0JRC0JZ Replacement of Pelvic Region Subcutaneous Tissue and Fascia with Synthetic Substitute, Open Approach

0JRC0KZ Replacement of Pelvic Region Subcutaneous Tissue and Fascia with Nonautologous Tissue Substitute, Open Approach

0JRC37Z Replacement of Pelvic Region Subcutaneous Tissue and Fascia with Autologous Tissue Substitute, Percutaneous Approach

0JRC3JZ Replacement of Pelvic Region Subcutaneous Tissue and Fascia with Synthetic Substitute, Percutaneous Approach

0JRC3KZ Replacement of Pelvic Region Subcutaneous Tissue and Fascia with Nonautologous Tissue Substitute, Percutaneous Approach

0JRD07Z Replacement of Right Upper Arm Subcutaneous Tissue and Fascia with Autologous Tissue Substitute, Open Approach

0JRD0JZ Replacement of Right Upper Arm Subcutaneous Tissue and Fascia with Synthetic Substitute, Open Approach

0JRD0KZ Replacement of Right Upper Arm Subcutaneous Tissue and Fascia with Nonautologous Tissue Substitute, Open Approach

0JRD37Z Replacement of Right Upper Arm Subcutaneous Tissue and Fascia with Autologous Tissue Substitute, Percutaneous Approach

0JRD3JZ Replacement of Right Upper Arm Subcutaneous Tissue and Fascia with Synthetic Substitute, Percutaneous Approach

0JRD3KZ Replacement of Right Upper Arm Subcutaneous Tissue and Fascia with Nonautologous Tissue Substitute, Percutaneous Approach

0JRF07Z Replacement of Left Upper Arm Subcutaneous Tissue and Fascia with Autologous Tissue Substitute, Open Approach

0JRF0JZ Replacement of Left Upper Arm Subcutaneous Tissue and Fascia with Synthetic Substitute, Open Approach

0JRF0KZ Replacement of Left Upper Arm Subcutaneous Tissue and Fascia with Nonautologous Tissue Substitute, Open Approach

0JRF37Z Replacement of Left Upper Arm Subcutaneous Tissue and Fascia with Autologous Tissue Substitute, Percutaneous Approach

0JRF3JZ Replacement of Left Upper Arm Subcutaneous Tissue and Fascia with Synthetic Substitute, Percutaneous Approach

0JRF3KZ Replacement of Left Upper Arm Subcutaneous Tissue and Fascia with Nonautologous Tissue Substitute, Percutaneous Approach

0JRG07Z Replacement of Right Lower Arm Subcutaneous Tissue and Fascia with Autologous Tissue Substitute, Open Approach

0JRG0JZ Replacement of Right Lower Arm Subcutaneous Tissue and Fascia with Synthetic Substitute, Open Approach

0JRG0KZ Replacement of Right Lower Arm Subcutaneous Tissue and Fascia with Nonautologous Tissue Substitute, Open Approach

0JRG37Z Replacement of Right Lower Arm Subcutaneous Tissue and Fascia with Autologous Tissue Substitute, Percutaneous Approach

0JRG3JZ Replacement of Right Lower Arm Subcutaneous Tissue and Fascia with Synthetic Substitute, Percutaneous Approach

0JRG3KZ Replacement of Right Lower Arm Subcutaneous Tissue and Fascia with Nonautologous Tissue Substitute, Percutaneous Approach

0JRH07Z Replacement of Left Lower Arm Subcutaneous Tissue and Fascia with Autologous Tissue Substitute, Open Approach

0JRH0JZ Replacement of Left Lower Arm Subcutaneous Tissue and Fascia with Synthetic Substitute, Open Approach

0JRH0KZ Replacement of Left Lower Arm Subcutaneous Tissue and Fascia with Nonautologous Tissue Substitute, Open Approach

0JRH37Z Replacement of Left Lower Arm Subcutaneous Tissue and Fascia with Autologous Tissue Substitute, Percutaneous Approach

0JRH3JZ Replacement of Left Lower Arm Subcutaneous Tissue and Fascia with Synthetic Substitute, Percutaneous Approach

0JRH3KZ Replacement of Left Lower Arm Subcutaneous Tissue and Fascia with Nonautologous Tissue Substitute, Percutaneous Approach

0JRJ07Z Replacement of Right Hand Subcutaneous Tissue and Fascia with Autologous Tissue Substitute, Open Approach

0JRJ0JZ Replacement of Right Hand Subcutaneous Tissue and Fascia with Synthetic Substitute, Open Approach

0JRJ0KZ	Replacement of Right Hand Subcutaneous Tissue and Fascia with Nonautologous Tissue Substitute, Open Approach
0JRJ37Z	Replacement of Right Hand Subcutaneous Tissue and Fascia with Autologous Tissue Substitute, Percutaneous Approach
0JRJ3JZ	Replacement of Right Hand Subcutaneous Tissue and Fascia with Synthetic Substitute, Percutaneous Approach
0JRJ3KZ	Replacement of Right Hand Subcutaneous Tissue and Fascia with Nonautologous Tissue Substitute, Percutaneous Approach
0JRK07Z	Replacement of Left Hand Subcutaneous Tissue and Fascia with Autologous Tissue Substitute, Open Approach
0JRK0JZ	Replacement of Left Hand Subcutaneous Tissue and Fascia with Synthetic Substitute, Open Approach
0JRK0KZ	Replacement of Left Hand Subcutaneous Tissue and Fascia with Nonautologous Tissue Substitute, Open Approach
0JRK37Z	Replacement of Left Hand Subcutaneous Tissue and Fascia with Autologous Tissue Substitute, Percutaneous Approach
0JRK3JZ	Replacement of Left Hand Subcutaneous Tissue and Fascia with Synthetic Substitute, Percutaneous Approach
0JRK3KZ	Replacement of Left Hand Subcutaneous Tissue and Fascia with Nonautologous Tissue Substitute, Percutaneous Approach
0JRL07Z	Replacement of Right Upper Leg Subcutaneous Tissue and Fascia with Autologous Tissue Substitute, Open Approach
0JRL0JZ	Replacement of Right Upper Leg Subcutaneous Tissue and Fascia with Synthetic Substitute, Open Approach
0JRL0KZ	Replacement of Right Upper Leg Subcutaneous Tissue and Fascia with Nonautologous Tissue Substitute, Open Approach
0JRL37Z	Replacement of Right Upper Leg Subcutaneous Tissue and Fascia with Autologous Tissue Substitute, Percutaneous Approach
0JRL3JZ	Replacement of Right Upper Leg Subcutaneous Tissue and Fascia with Synthetic Substitute, Percutaneous Approach
0JRL3KZ	Replacement of Right Upper Leg Subcutaneous Tissue and Fascia with Nonautologous Tissue Substitute, Percutaneous Approach
0JRM07Z	Replacement of Left Upper Leg Subcutaneous Tissue and Fascia with Autologous Tissue Substitute, Open Approach
0JRM0JZ	Replacement of Left Upper Leg Subcutaneous Tissue and Fascia with Synthetic Substitute, Open Approach
0JRM0KZ	Replacement of Left Upper Leg Subcutaneous Tissue and Fascia with Nonautologous Tissue Substitute, Open Approach
0JRM37Z	Replacement of Left Upper Leg Subcutaneous Tissue and Fascia with Autologous Tissue Substitute, Percutaneous Approach
0JRM3JZ	Replacement of Left Upper Leg Subcutaneous Tissue and Fascia with Synthetic Substitute, Percutaneous Approach
0JRM3KZ	Replacement of Left Upper Leg Subcutaneous Tissue and Fascia with Nonautologous Tissue Substitute, Percutaneous Approach
0JRN07Z	Replacement of Right Lower Leg Subcutaneous Tissue and Fascia with Autologous Tissue Substitute, Open Approach
0JRN0JZ	Replacement of Right Lower Leg Subcutaneous Tissue and Fascia with Synthetic Substitute, Open Approach
0JRN0KZ	Replacement of Right Lower Leg Subcutaneous Tissue and Fascia with Nonautologous Tissue Substitute, Open Approach
0JRN37Z	Replacement of Right Lower Leg Subcutaneous Tissue and Fascia with Autologous Tissue Substitute, Percutaneous Approach
0JRN3JZ	Replacement of Right Lower Leg Subcutaneous Tissue and Fascia with Synthetic Substitute, Percutaneous Approach
0JRN3KZ	Replacement of Right Lower Leg Subcutaneous Tissue and Fascia with Nonautologous Tissue Substitute, Percutaneous Approach
0JRP07Z	Replacement of Left Lower Leg Subcutaneous Tissue and Fascia with Autologous Tissue Substitute, Open Approach
0JRP0JZ	Replacement of Left Lower Leg Subcutaneous Tissue and Fascia with Synthetic Substitute, Open Approach
0JRP0KZ	Replacement of Left Lower Leg Subcutaneous Tissue and Fascia with Nonautologous Tissue Substitute, Open Approach
0JRP37Z	Replacement of Left Lower Leg Subcutaneous Tissue and Fascia with Autologous Tissue Substitute, Percutaneous Approach
0JRP3JZ	Replacement of Left Lower Leg Subcutaneous Tissue and Fascia with Synthetic Substitute, Percutaneous Approach
0JRP3KZ	Replacement of Left Lower Leg Subcutaneous Tissue and Fascia with Nonautologous Tissue Substitute, Percutaneous Approach
0JRQ07Z	Replacement of Right Foot Subcutaneous Tissue and Fascia with Autologous Tissue Substitute, Open Approach
0JRQ0JZ	Replacement of Right Foot Subcutaneous Tissue and Fascia with Synthetic Substitute, Open Approach
0JRQ0KZ	Replacement of Right Foot Subcutaneous Tissue and Fascia with Nonautologous Tissue Substitute, Open Approach
0JRQ37Z	Replacement of Right Foot Subcutaneous Tissue and Fascia with Autologous Tissue Substitute, Percutaneous Approach
0JRQ3JZ	Replacement of Right Foot Subcutaneous Tissue and Fascia with Synthetic Substitute, Percutaneous Approach
0JRQ3KZ	Replacement of Right Foot Subcutaneous Tissue and Fascia with Nonautologous Tissue Substitute, Percutaneous Approach
0JRR07Z	Replacement of Left Foot Subcutaneous Tissue and Fascia with Autologous Tissue Substitute, Open Approach
0JRR0JZ	Replacement of Left Foot Subcutaneous Tissue and Fascia with Synthetic Substitute, Open Approach
0JRR0KZ	Replacement of Left Foot Subcutaneous Tissue and Fascia with Nonautologous Tissue Substitute, Open Approach
0JRR37Z	Replacement of Left Foot Subcutaneous Tissue and Fascia with Autologous Tissue Substitute, Percutaneous Approach
0JRR3JZ	Replacement of Left Foot Subcutaneous Tissue and Fascia with Synthetic Substitute, Percutaneous Approach
0JRR3KZ	Replacement of Left Foot Subcutaneous Tissue and Fascia with Nonautologous Tissue Substitute, Percutaneous Approach

0JU – Subcutaneous Tissue and Fascia, Supplement

0JU007Z	Supplement of Scalp Subcutaneous Tissue and Fascia with Autologous Tissue Substitute, Open Approach
0JU00JZ	Supplement of Scalp Subcutaneous Tissue and Fascia with Synthetic Substitute, Open Approach
0JU00KZ	Supplement of Scalp Subcutaneous Tissue and Fascia with Nonautologous Tissue Substitute, Open Approach
0JU037Z	Supplement of Scalp Subcutaneous Tissue and Fascia with Autologous Tissue Substitute, Percutaneous Approach
0JU03JZ	Supplement of Scalp Subcutaneous Tissue and Fascia with Synthetic Substitute, Percutaneous Approach
0JU03KZ	Supplement of Scalp Subcutaneous Tissue and Fascia with Nonautologous Tissue Substitute, Percutaneous Approach
0JU107Z	Supplement of Face Subcutaneous Tissue and Fascia with Autologous Tissue Substitute, Open Approach
0JU10JZ	Supplement of Face Subcutaneous Tissue and Fascia with Synthetic Substitute, Open Approach
0JU10KZ	Supplement of Face Subcutaneous Tissue and Fascia with Nonautologous Tissue Substitute, Open Approach
0JU137Z	Supplement of Face Subcutaneous Tissue and Fascia with Autologous Tissue Substitute, Percutaneous Approach
0JU13JZ	Supplement of Face Subcutaneous Tissue and Fascia with Synthetic Substitute, Percutaneous Approach
0JU13KZ	Supplement of Face Subcutaneous Tissue and Fascia with Nonautologous Tissue Substitute, Percutaneous Approach
0JU407Z	Supplement of Anterior Neck Subcutaneous Tissue and Fascia with Autologous Tissue Substitute, Open Approach
0JU40JZ	Supplement of Anterior Neck Subcutaneous Tissue and Fascia with Synthetic Substitute, Open Approach
0JU40KZ	Supplement of Anterior Neck Subcutaneous Tissue and Fascia with Nonautologous Tissue Substitute, Open Approach
0JU437Z	Supplement of Anterior Neck Subcutaneous Tissue and Fascia with Autologous Tissue Substitute, Percutaneous Approach
0JU43JZ	Supplement of Anterior Neck Subcutaneous Tissue and Fascia with Synthetic Substitute, Percutaneous Approach
0JU43KZ	Supplement of Anterior Neck Subcutaneous Tissue and Fascia with Nonautologous Tissue Substitute, Percutaneous Approach
0JU507Z	Supplement of Posterior Neck Subcutaneous Tissue and Fascia with Autologous Tissue Substitute, Open Approach
0JU50JZ	Supplement of Posterior Neck Subcutaneous Tissue and Fascia with Synthetic Substitute, Open Approach
0JU50KZ	Supplement of Posterior Neck Subcutaneous Tissue and Fascia with Nonautologous Tissue Substitute, Open Approach
0JU537Z	Supplement of Posterior Neck Subcutaneous Tissue and Fascia with Autologous Tissue Substitute, Percutaneous Approach
0JU53JZ	Supplement of Posterior Neck Subcutaneous Tissue and Fascia with Synthetic Substitute, Percutaneous Approach
0JU53KZ	Supplement of Posterior Neck Subcutaneous Tissue and Fascia with Nonautologous Tissue Substitute, Percutaneous Approach

0JU607Z Supplement of Chest Subcutaneous Tissue and Fascia with Autologous Tissue Substitute, Open Approach

0JU60JZ Supplement of Chest Subcutaneous Tissue and Fascia with Synthetic Substitute, Open Approach

0JU60KZ Supplement of Chest Subcutaneous Tissue and Fascia with Nonautologous Tissue Substitute, Open Approach

0JU637Z Supplement of Chest Subcutaneous Tissue and Fascia with Autologous Tissue Substitute, Percutaneous Approach

0JU63JZ Supplement of Chest Subcutaneous Tissue and Fascia with Synthetic Substitute, Percutaneous Approach

0JU63KZ Supplen.ent of Chest Subcutaneous Tissue and Fascia with Nonautologous Tissue Substitute, Percutaneous Approach

0JU707Z Supplement of Back Subcutaneous Tissue and Fascia with Autologous Tissue Substitute, Open Approach

0JU70JZ Supplement of Back Subcutaneous Tissue and Fascia with Synthetic Substitute, Open Approach

0JU70KZ Supplement of Back Subcutaneous Tissue and Fascia with Nonautologous Tissue Substitute, Open Approach

0JU737Z Supplement of Back Subcutaneous Tissue and Fascia with Autologous Tissue Substitute, Percutaneous Approach

0JU73JZ Supplement of Back Subcutaneous Tissue and Fascia with Synthetic Substitute, Percutaneous Approach

0JU73KZ Supplement of Back Subcutaneous Tissue and Fascia with Nonautologous Tissue Substitute, Percutaneous Approach

0JU807Z Supplement of Abdomen Subcutaneous Tissue and Fascia with Autologous Tissue Substitute, Open Approach

0JU80JZ Supplement of Abdomen Subcutaneous Tissue and Fascia with Synthetic Substitute, Open Approach

0JU80KZ Supplement of Abdomen Subcutaneous Tissue and Fascia with Nonautologous Tissue Substitute, Open Approach

0JU837Z Supplement of Abdomen Subcutaneous Tissue and Fascia with Autologous Tissue Substitute, Percutaneous Approach

0JU83JZ Supplement of Abdomen Subcutaneous Tissue and Fascia with Synthetic Substitute, Percutaneous Approach

0JU83KZ Supplement of Abdomen Subcutaneous Tissue and Fascia with Nonautologous Tissue Substitute, Percutaneous Approach

0JU907Z Supplement of Buttock Subcutaneous Tissue and Fascia with Autologous Tissue Substitute, Open Approach

0JU90JZ Supplement of Buttock Subcutaneous Tissue and Fascia with Synthetic Substitute, Open Approach

0JU90KZ Supplement of Buttock Subcutaneous Tissue and Fascia with Nonautologous Tissue Substitute, Open Approach

0JU937Z Supplement of Buttock Subcutaneous Tissue and Fascia with Autologous Tissue Substitute, Percutaneous Approach

0JU93JZ Supplement of Buttock Subcutaneous Tissue and Fascia with Synthetic Substitute, Percutaneous Approach

0JU93KZ Supplement of Buttock Subcutaneous Tissue and Fascia with Nonautologous Tissue Substitute, Percutaneous Approach

0JUB07Z Supplement of Perineum Subcutaneous Tissue and Fascia with Autologous Tissue Substitute, Open Approach

0JUB0JZ Supplement of Perineum Subcutaneous Tissue and Fascia with Synthetic Substitute, Open Approach

0JUB0KZ Supplement of Perineum Subcutaneous Tissue and Fascia with Nonautologous Tissue Substitute, Open Approach

0JUB37Z Supplement of Perineum Subcutaneous Tissue and Fascia with Autologous Tissue Substitute, Percutaneous Approach

0JUB3JZ Supplement of Perineum Subcutaneous Tissue and Fascia with Synthetic Substitute, Percutaneous Approach

0JUB3KZ Supplement of Perineum Subcutaneous Tissue and Fascia with Nonautologous Tissue Substitute, Percutaneous Approach

0JUC07Z Supplement of Pelvic Region Subcutaneous Tissue and Fascia with Autologous Tissue Substitute, Open Approach

0JUC0JZ Supplement of Pelvic Region Subcutaneous Tissue and Fascia with Synthetic Substitute, Open Approach

0JUC0KZ Supplement of Pelvic Region Subcutaneous Tissue and Fascia with Nonautologous Tissue Substitute, Open Approach

0JUC37Z Supplement of Pelvic Region Subcutaneous Tissue and Fascia with Autologous Tissue Substitute, Percutaneous Approach

0JUC3JZ Supplement of Pelvic Region Subcutaneous Tissue and Fascia with Synthetic Substitute, Percutaneous Approach

0JUC3KZ Supplement of Pelvic Region Subcutaneous Tissue and Fascia with Nonautologous Tissue Substitute, Percutaneous Approach

0JUD07Z Supplement of Right Upper Arm Subcutaneous Tissue and Fascia with Autologous Tissue Substitute, Open Approach

0JUD0JZ Supplement of Right Upper Arm Subcutaneous Tissue and Fascia with Synthetic Substitute, Open Approach

0JUD0KZ Supplement of Right Upper Arm Subcutaneous Tissue and Fascia with Nonautologous Tissue Substitute, Open Approach

0JUD37Z Supplement of Right Upper Arm Subcutaneous Tissue and Fascia with Autologous Tissue Substitute, Percutaneous Approach

0JUD3JZ Supplement of Right Upper Arm Subcutaneous Tissue and Fascia with Synthetic Substitute, Percutaneous Approach

0JUD3KZ Supplement of Right Upper Arm Subcutaneous Tissue and Fascia with Nonautologous Tissue Substitute, Percutaneous Approach

0JUF07Z Supplement of Left Upper Arm Subcutaneous Tissue and Fascia with Autologous Tissue Substitute, Open Approach

0JUF0JZ Supplement of Left Upper Arm Subcutaneous Tissue and Fascia with Synthetic Substitute, Open Approach

0JUF0KZ Supplement of Left Upper Arm Subcutaneous Tissue and Fascia with Nonautologous Tissue Substitute, Open Approach

0JUF37Z Supplement of Left Upper Arm Subcutaneous Tissue and Fascia with Autologous Tissue Substitute, Percutaneous Approach

0JUF3JZ Supplement of Left Upper Arm Subcutaneous Tissue and Fascia with Synthetic Substitute, Percutaneous Approach

0JUF3KZ Supplement of Left Upper Arm Subcutaneous Tissue and Fascia with Nonautologous Tissue Substitute, Percutaneous Approach

0JUG07Z Supplement of Right Lower Arm Subcutaneous Tissue and Fascia with Autologous Tissue Substitute, Open Approach

0JUG0JZ Supplement of Right Lower Arm Subcutaneous Tissue and Fascia with Synthetic Substitute, Open Approach

0JUG0KZ Supplement of Right Lower Arm Subcutaneous Tissue and Fascia with Nonautologous Tissue Substitute, Open Approach

0JUG37Z Supplement of Right Lower Arm Subcutaneous Tissue and Fascia with Autologous Tissue Substitute, Percutaneous Approach

0JUG3JZ Supplement of Right Lower Arm Subcutaneous Tissue and Fascia with Synthetic Substitute, Percutaneous Approach

0JUG3KZ Supplement of Right Lower Arm Subcutaneous Tissue and Fascia with Nonautologous Tissue Substitute, Percutaneous Approach

0JUH07Z Supplement of Left Lower Arm Subcutaneous Tissue and Fascia with Autologous Tissue Substitute, Open Approach

0JUH0JZ Supplement of Left Lower Arm Subcutaneous Tissue and Fascia with Synthetic Substitute, Open Approach

0JUH0KZ Supplement of Left Lower Arm Subcutaneous Tissue and Fascia with Nonautologous Tissue Substitute, Open Approach

0JUH37Z Supplement of Left Lower Arm Subcutaneous Tissue and Fascia with Autologous Tissue Substitute, Percutaneous Approach

0JUH3JZ Supplement of Left Lower Arm Subcutaneous Tissue and Fascia with Synthetic Substitute, Percutaneous Approach

0JUH3KZ Supplement of Left Lower Arm Subcutaneous Tissue and Fascia with Nonautologous Tissue Substitute, Percutaneous Approach

0JUJ07Z Supplement of Right Hand Subcutaneous Tissue and Fascia with Autologous Tissue Substitute, Open Approach

0JUJ0JZ Supplement of Right Hand Subcutaneous Tissue and Fascia with Synthetic Substitute, Open Approach

0JUJ0KZ Supplement of Right Hand Subcutaneous Tissue and Fascia with Nonautologous Tissue Substitute, Open Approach

0JUJ37Z Supplement of Right Hand Subcutaneous Tissue and Fascia with Autologous Tissue Substitute, Percutaneous Approach

0JUJ3JZ Supplement of Right Hand Subcutaneous Tissue and Fascia with Synthetic Substitute, Percutaneous Approach

0JUJ3KZ Supplement of Right Hand Subcutaneous Tissue and Fascia with Nonautologous Tissue Substitute, Percutaneous Approach

0JUK07Z Supplement of Left Hand Subcutaneous Tissue and Fascia with Autologous Tissue Substitute, Open Approach

0JUK0JZ Supplement of Left Hand Subcutaneous Tissue and Fascia with Synthetic Substitute, Open Approach

0JUK0KZ Supplement of Left Hand Subcutaneous Tissue and Fascia with Nonautologous Tissue Substitute, Open Approach

0JUK37Z Supplement of Left Hand Subcutaneous Tissue and Fascia with Autologous Tissue Substitute, Percutaneous Approach

0JUK3JZ Supplement of Left Hand Subcutaneous Tissue and Fascia with Synthetic Substitute, Percutaneous Approach

0JUK3KZ Supplement of Left Hand Subcutaneous Tissue and Fascia with Nonautologous Tissue Substitute, Percutaneous Approach

0JUL07Z	Supplement of Right Upper Leg Subcutaneous Tissue and Fascia with Autologous Tissue Substitute, Open Approach
0JUL0JZ	Supplement of Right Upper Leg Subcutaneous Tissue and Fascia with Synthetic Substitute, Open Approach
0JUL0KZ	Supplement of Right Upper Leg Subcutaneous Tissue and Fascia with Nonautologous Tissue Substitute, Open Approach
0JUL37Z	Supplement of Right Upper Leg Subcutaneous Tissue and Fascia with Autologous Tissue Substitute, Percutaneous Approach
0JUL3JZ	Supplement of Right Upper Leg Subcutaneous Tissue and Fascia with Synthetic Substitute, Percutaneous Approach
0JUL3KZ	Supplement of Right Upper Leg Subcutaneous Tissue and Fascia with Nonautologous Tissue Substitute, Percutaneous Approach
0JUM07Z	Supplement of Left Upper Leg Subcutaneous Tissue and Fascia with Autologous Tissue Substitute, Open Approach
0JUM0JZ	Supplement of Left Upper Leg Subcutaneous Tissue and Fascia with Synthetic Substitute, Open Approach
0JUM0KZ	Supplement of Left Upper Leg Subcutaneous Tissue and Fascia with Nonautologous Tissue Substitute, Open Approach
0JUM37Z	Supplement of Left Upper Leg Subcutaneous Tissue and Fascia with Autologous Tissue Substitute, Percutaneous Approach
0JUM3JZ	Supplement of Left Upper Leg Subcutaneous Tissue and Fascia with Synthetic Substitute, Percutaneous Approach
0JUM3KZ	Supplement of Left Upper Leg Subcutaneous Tissue and Fascia with Nonautologous Tissue Substitute, Percutaneous Approach
0JUN07Z	Supplement of Right Lower Leg Subcutaneous Tissue and Fascia with Autologous Tissue Substitute, Open Approach
0JUN0JZ	Supplement of Right Lower Leg Subcutaneous Tissue and Fascia with Synthetic Substitute, Open Approach
0JUN0KZ	Supplement of Right Lower Leg Subcutaneous Tissue and Fascia with Nonautologous Tissue Substitute, Open Approach
0JUN37Z	Supplement of Right Lower Leg Subcutaneous Tissue and Fascia with Autologous Tissue Substitute, Percutaneous Approach
0JUN3JZ	Supplement of Right Lower Leg Subcutaneous Tissue and Fascia with Synthetic Substitute, Percutaneous Approach
0JUN3KZ	Supplement of Right Lower Leg Subcutaneous Tissue and Fascia with Nonautologous Tissue Substitute, Percutaneous Approach

0JUP07Z	Supplement of Left Lower Leg Subcutaneous Tissue and Fascia with Autologous Tissue Substitute, Open Approach
0JUP0JZ	Supplement of Left Lower Leg Subcutaneous Tissue and Fascia with Synthetic Substitute, Open Approach
0JUP0KZ	Supplement of Left Lower Leg Subcutaneous Tissue and Fascia with Nonautologous Tissue Substitute, Open Approach
0JUP37Z	Supplement of Left Lower Leg Subcutaneous Tissue and Fascia with Autologous Tissue Substitute, Percutaneous Approach
0JUP3JZ	Supplement of Left Lower Leg Subcutaneous Tissue and Fascia with Synthetic Substitute, Percutaneous Approach
0JUP3KZ	Supplement of Left Lower Leg Subcutaneous Tissue and Fascia with Nonautologous Tissue Substitute, Percutaneous Approach
0JUQ07Z	Supplement of Right Foot Subcutaneous Tissue and Fascia with Autologous Tissue Substitute, Open Approach
0JUQ0JZ	Supplement of Right Foot Subcutaneous Tissue and Fascia with Synthetic Substitute, Open Approach
0JUQ0KZ	Supplement of Right Foot Subcutaneous Tissue and Fascia with Nonautologous Tissue Substitute, Open Approach
0JUQ37Z	Supplement of Right Foot Subcutaneous Tissue and Fascia with Autologous Tissue Substitute, Percutaneous Approach
0JUQ3JZ	Supplement of Right Foot Subcutaneous Tissue and Fascia with Synthetic Substitute, Percutaneous Approach
0JUQ3KZ	Supplement of Right Foot Subcutaneous Tissue and Fascia with Nonautologous Tissue Substitute, Percutaneous Approach
0JUR07Z	Supplement of Left Foot Subcutaneous Tissue and Fascia with Autologous Tissue Substitute, Open Approach
0JUR0JZ	Supplement of Left Foot Subcutaneous Tissue and Fascia with Synthetic Substitute, Open Approach
0JUR0KZ	Supplement of Left Foot Subcutaneous Tissue and Fascia with Nonautologous Tissue Substitute, Open Approach
0JUR37Z	Supplement of Left Foot Subcutaneous Tissue and Fascia with Autologous Tissue Substitute, Percutaneous Approach
0JUR3JZ	Supplement of Left Foot Subcutaneous Tissue and Fascia with Synthetic Substitute, Percutaneous Approach
0JUR3KZ	Supplement of Left Foot Subcutaneous Tissue and Fascia with Nonautologous Tissue Substitute, Percutaneous Approach

0JW – Subcutaneous Tissue and Fascia, Revision

Review Coding Guideline B6.1c

● 0JWS00Z	Revision of Drainage Device in Head and Neck Subcutaneous Tissue and Fascia, Open Approach
● 0JWS03Z	Revision of Infusion Device in Head and Neck Subcutaneous Tissue and Fascia, Open Approach
● 0JWS07Z	Revision of Autologous Tissue Substitute in Head and Neck Subcutaneous Tissue and Fascia, Open Approach
● 0JWS0JZ	Revision of Synthetic Substitute in Head and Neck Subcutaneous Tissue and Fascia, Open Approach
● 0JWS0KZ	Revision of Nonautologous Tissue Substitute in Head and Neck Subcutaneous Tissue and Fascia, Open Approach
● 0JWS0NZ	Revision of Tissue Expander in Head and Neck Subcutaneous Tissue and Fascia, Open Approach
● 0JWS30Z	Revision of Drainage Device in Head and Neck Subcutaneous Tissue and Fascia, Percutaneous Approach
● 0JWS33Z	Revision of Infusion Device in Head and Neck Subcutaneous Tissue and Fascia, Percutaneous Approach
● 0JWS37Z	Revision of Autologous Tissue Substitute in Head and Neck Subcutaneous Tissue and Fascia, Percutaneous Approach
● 0JWS3JZ	Revision of Synthetic Substitute in Head and Neck Subcutaneous Tissue and Fascia, Percutaneous Approach
● 0JWS3KZ	Revision of Nonautologous Tissue Substitute in Head and Neck Subcutaneous Tissue and Fascia, Percutaneous Approach
● 0JWS3NZ	Revision of Tissue Expander in Head and Neck Subcutaneous Tissue and Fascia, Percutaneous Approach
0JWSX0Z	Revision of Drainage Device in Head and Neck Subcutaneous Tissue and Fascia, External Approach
0JWSX3Z	Revision of Infusion Device in Head and Neck Subcutaneous Tissue and Fascia, External Approach
0JWSX7Z	Revision of Autologous Tissue Substitute in Head and Neck Subcutaneous Tissue and Fascia, External Approach
0JWSXJZ	Revision of Synthetic Substitute in Head and Neck Subcutaneous Tissue and Fascia, External Approach

0JWSXKZ	Revision of Nonautologous Tissue Substitute in Head and Neck Subcutaneous Tissue and Fascia, External Approach
0JWSXNZ	Revision of Tissue Expander in Head and Neck Subcutaneous Tissue and Fascia, External Approach
● 0JWT00Z	Revision of Drainage Device in Trunk Subcutaneous Tissue and Fascia, Open Approach
● 0JWT02Z	Revision of Monitoring Device in Trunk Subcutaneous Tissue and Fascia, Open Approach
● 0JWT03Z	Revision of Infusion Device in Trunk Subcutaneous Tissue and Fascia, Open Approach
● 0JWT07Z	Revision of Autologous Tissue Substitute in Trunk Subcutaneous Tissue and Fascia, Open Approach
● 0JWT0HZ	Revision of Contraceptive Device in Trunk Subcutaneous Tissue and Fascia, Open Approach
● 0JWT0JZ	Revision of Synthetic Substitute in Trunk Subcutaneous Tissue and Fascia, Open Approach
● 0JWT0KZ	Revision of Nonautologous Tissue Substitute in Trunk Subcutaneous Tissue and Fascia, Open Approach
0JWT0MZ	Revision of Stimulator Generator in Trunk Subcutaneous Tissue and Fascia, Open Approach
● 0JWT0NZ	Revision of Tissue Expander in Trunk Subcutaneous Tissue and Fascia, Open Approach
0JWT0PZ	Revision of Cardiac Rhythm Related Device in Trunk Subcutaneous Tissue and Fascia, Open Approach
HAC	With a secondary diagnosis code of K68.11, T81.4XXA, T82.6XXA, T82.7XXA
● 0JWT0VZ	Revision of Infusion Pump in Trunk Subcutaneous Tissue and Fascia, Open Approach
● 0JWT0WZ	Revision of Reservoir in Trunk Subcutaneous Tissue and Fascia, Open Approach
● 0JWT0XZ	Revision of Vascular Access Device in Trunk Subcutaneous Tissue and Fascia, Open Approach

● **0JWT30Z** Revision of Drainage Device in Trunk Subcutaneous Tissue and Fascia, Percutaneous Approach

● **0JWT32Z** Revision of Monitoring Device in Trunk Subcutaneous Tissue and Fascia, Percutaneous Approach

● **0JWT33Z** Revision of Infusion Device in Trunk Subcutaneous Tissue and Fascia, Percutaneous Approach

● **0JWT37Z** Revision of Autologous Tissue Substitute in Trunk Subcutaneous Tissue and Fascia, Percutaneous Approach

● **0JWT3HZ** Revision of Contraceptive Device in Trunk Subcutaneous Tissue and Fascia, Percutaneous Approach

● **0JWT3JZ** Revision of Synthetic Substitute in Trunk Subcutaneous Tissue and Fascia, Percutaneous Approach

● **0JWT3KZ** Revision of Nonautologous Tissue Substitute in Trunk Subcutaneous Tissue and Fascia, Percutaneous Approach

0JWT3MZ Revision of Stimulator Generator in Trunk Subcutaneous Tissue and Fascia, Percutaneous Approach

● **0JWT3NZ** Revision of Tissue Expander in Trunk Subcutaneous Tissue and Fascia, Percutaneous Approach

0JWT3PZ Revision of Cardiac Rhythm Related Device in Trunk Subcutaneous Tissue and Fascia, Percutaneous Approach

HAC With a secondary diagnosis code of K68.11, T81.4XXA, T82.6XXA, T82.7XXA

● **0JWT3VZ** Revision of Infusion Pump in Trunk Subcutaneous Tissue and Fascia, Percutaneous Approach

● **0JWT3WZ** Revision of Reservoir in Trunk Subcutaneous Tissue and Fascia, Percutaneous Approach

● **0JWT3XZ** Revision of Vascular Access Device in Trunk Subcutaneous Tissue and Fascia, Percutaneous Approach

0JWTX0Z Revision of Drainage Device in Trunk Subcutaneous Tissue and Fascia, External Approach

0JWTX2Z Revision of Monitoring Device in Trunk Subcutaneous Tissue and Fascia, External Approach

0JWTX3Z Revision of Infusion Device in Trunk Subcutaneous Tissue and Fascia, External Approach

0JWTX7Z Revision of Autologous Tissue Substitute in Trunk Subcutaneous Tissue and Fascia, External Approach

0JWTXHZ Revision of Contraceptive Device in Trunk Subcutaneous Tissue and Fascia, External Approach

0JWTXJZ Revision of Synthetic Substitute in Trunk Subcutaneous Tissue and Fascia, External Approach

0JWTXKZ Revision of Nonautologous Tissue Substitute in Trunk Subcutaneous Tissue and Fascia, External Approach

0JWTXMZ Revision of Stimulator Generator in Trunk Subcutaneous Tissue and Fascia, External Approach

0JWTXNZ Revision of Tissue Expander in Trunk Subcutaneous Tissue and Fascia, External Approach

0JWTXPZ Revision of Cardiac Rhythm Related Device in Trunk Subcutaneous Tissue and Fascia, External Approach

0JWTXVZ Revision of Infusion Pump in Trunk Subcutaneous Tissue and Fascia, External Approach

0JWTXWZ Revision of Reservoir in Trunk Subcutaneous Tissue and Fascia, External Approach

0JWTXXZ Revision of Vascular Access Device in Trunk Subcutaneous Tissue and Fascia, External Approach

● **0JWV00Z** Revision of Drainage Device in Upper Extremity Subcutaneous Tissue and Fascia, Open Approach

● **0JWV03Z** Revision of Infusion Device in Upper Extremity Subcutaneous Tissue and Fascia, Open Approach

● **0JWV07Z** Revision of Autologous Tissue Substitute in Upper Extremity Subcutaneous Tissue and Fascia, Open Approach

● **0JWV0HZ** Revision of Contraceptive Device in Upper Extremity Subcutaneous Tissue and Fascia, Open Approach

● **0JWV0JZ** Revision of Synthetic Substitute in Upper Extremity Subcutaneous Tissue and Fascia, Open Approach

● **0JWV0KZ** Revision of Nonautologous Tissue Substitute in Upper Extremity Subcutaneous Tissue and Fascia, Open Approach

● **0JWV0NZ** Revision of Tissue Expander in Upper Extremity Subcutaneous Tissue and Fascia, Open Approach

● **0JWV0VZ** Revision of Infusion Pump in Upper Extremity Subcutaneous Tissue and Fascia, Open Approach

● **0JWV0WZ** Revision of Reservoir in Upper Extremity Subcutaneous Tissue and Fascia, Open Approach

● **0JWV0XZ** Revision of Vascular Access Device in Upper Extremity Subcutaneous Tissue and Fascia, Open Approach

● **0JWV30Z** Revision of Drainage Device in Upper Extremity Subcutaneous Tissue and Fascia, Percutaneous Approach

● **0JWV33Z** Revision of Infusion Device in Upper Extremity Subcutaneous Tissue and Fascia, Percutaneous Approach

● **0JWV37Z** Revision of Autologous Tissue Substitute in Upper Extremity Subcutaneous Tissue and Fascia, Percutaneous Approach

● **0JWV3HZ** Revision of Contraceptive Device in Upper Extremity Subcutaneous Tissue and Fascia, Percutaneous Approach

● **0JWV3JZ** Revision of Synthetic Substitute in Upper Extremity Subcutaneous Tissue and Fascia, Percutaneous Approach

● **0JWV3KZ** Revision of Nonautologous Tissue Substitute in Upper Extremity Subcutaneous Tissue and Fascia, Percutaneous Approach

● **0JWV3NZ** Revision of Tissue Expander in Upper Extremity Subcutaneous Tissue and Fascia, Percutaneous Approach

● **0JWV3VZ** Revision of Infusion Pump in Upper Extremity Subcutaneous Tissue and Fascia, Percutaneous Approach

● **0JWV3WZ** Revision of Reservoir in Upper Extremity Subcutaneous Tissue and Fascia, Percutaneous Approach

● **0JWV3XZ** Revision of Vascular Access Device in Upper Extremity Subcutaneous Tissue and Fascia, Percutaneous Approach

0JWVX0Z Revision of Drainage Device in Upper Extremity Subcutaneous Tissue and Fascia, External Approach

0JWVX3Z Revision of Infusion Device in Upper Extremity Subcutaneous Tissue and Fascia, External Approach

0JWVX7Z Revision of Autologous Tissue Substitute in Upper Extremity Subcutaneous Tissue and Fascia, External Approach

0JWVXHZ Revision of Contraceptive Device in Upper Extremity Subcutaneous Tissue and Fascia, External Approach

0JWVXJZ Revision of Synthetic Substitute in Upper Extremity Subcutaneous Tissue and Fascia, External Approach

0JWVXKZ Revision of Nonautologous Tissue Substitute in Upper Extremity Subcutaneous Tissue and Fascia, External Approach

0JWVXNZ Revision of Tissue Expander in Upper Extremity Subcutaneous Tissue and Fascia, External Approach

0JWVXVZ Revision of Infusion Pump in Upper Extremity Subcutaneous Tissue and Fascia, External Approach

0JWVXWZ Revision of Reservoir in Upper Extremity Subcutaneous Tissue and Fascia, External Approach

0JWVXXZ Revision of Vascular Access Device in Upper Extremity Subcutaneous Tissue and Fascia, External Approach

● **0JWW00Z** Revision of Drainage Device in Lower Extremity Subcutaneous Tissue and Fascia, Open Approach

● **0JWW03Z** Revision of Infusion Device in Lower Extremity Subcutaneous Tissue and Fascia, Open Approach

● **0JWW07Z** Revision of Autologous Tissue Substitute in Lower Extremity Subcutaneous Tissue and Fascia, Open Approach

● **0JWW0HZ** Revision of Contraceptive Device in Lower Extremity Subcutaneous Tissue and Fascia, Open Approach

● **0JWW0JZ** Revision of Synthetic Substitute in Lower Extremity Subcutaneous Tissue and Fascia, Open Approach

● **0JWW0KZ** Revision of Nonautologous Tissue Substitute in Lower Extremity Subcutaneous Tissue and Fascia, Open Approach

● **0JWW0NZ** Revision of Tissue Expander in Lower Extremity Subcutaneous Tissue and Fascia, Open Approach

● **0JWW0VZ** Revision of Infusion Pump in Lower Extremity Subcutaneous Tissue and Fascia, Open Approach

● **0JWW0WZ** Revision of Reservoir in Lower Extremity Subcutaneous Tissue and Fascia, Open Approach

● **0JWW0XZ** Revision of Vascular Access Device in Lower Extremity Subcutaneous Tissue and Fascia, Open Approach

● **0JWW30Z** Revision of Drainage Device in Lower Extremity Subcutaneous Tissue and Fascia, Percutaneous Approach

● **0JWW33Z** Revision of Infusion Device in Lower Extremity Subcutaneous Tissue and Fascia, Percutaneous Approach

● **0JWW37Z** Revision of Autologous Tissue Substitute in Lower Extremity Subcutaneous Tissue and Fascia, Percutaneous Approach

● **0JWW3HZ** Revision of Contraceptive Device in Lower Extremity Subcutaneous Tissue and Fascia, Percutaneous Approach

● **0JWW3JZ** Revision of Synthetic Substitute in Lower Extremity Subcutaneous Tissue and Fascia, Percutaneous Approach

● **0JWW3KZ**   Revision of Nonautologous Tissue Substitute in Lower Extremity Subcutaneous Tissue and Fascia, Percutaneous Approach

● **0JWW3NZ**   Revision of Tissue Expander in Lower Extremity Subcutaneous Tissue and Fascia, Percutaneous Approach

● **0JWW3VZ**   Revision of Infusion Pump in Lower Extremity Subcutaneous Tissue and Fascia, Percutaneous Approach

● **0JWW3WZ**   Revision of Reservoir in Lower Extremity Subcutaneous Tissue and Fascia, Percutaneous Approach

● **0JWW3XZ**   Revision of Vascular Access Device in Lower Extremity Subcutaneous Tissue and Fascia, Percutaneous Approach

0JWWX0Z   Revision of Drainage Device in Lower Extremity Subcutaneous Tissue and Fascia, External Approach

0JWWX3Z   Revision of Infusion Device in Lower Extremity Subcutaneous Tissue and Fascia, External Approach

0JWWX7Z   Revision of Autologous Tissue Substitute in Lower Extremity Subcutaneous Tissue and Fascia, External Approach

0JWWXHZ   Revision of Contraceptive Device in Lower Extremity Subcutaneous Tissue and Fascia, External Approach

0JWWXJZ   Revision of Synthetic Substitute in Lower Extremity Subcutaneous Tissue and Fascia, External Approach

0JWWXKZ   Revision of Nonautologous Tissue Substitute in Lower Extremity Subcutaneous Tissue and Fascia, External Approach

0JWWXNZ   Revision of Tissue Expander in Lower Extremity Subcutaneous Tissue and Fascia, External Approach

0JWWXVZ   Revision of Infusion Pump in Lower Extremity Subcutaneous Tissue and Fascia, External Approach

0JWWXWZ   Revision of Reservoir in Lower Extremity Subcutaneous Tissue and Fascia, External Approach

0JWWXXZ   Revision of Vascular Access Device in Lower Extremity Subcutaneous Tissue and Fascia, External Approach

0JX – Subcutaneous Tissue and Fascia, Transfer

0JX00ZB   Transfer Scalp Subcutaneous Tissue and Fascia with Skin and Subcutaneous Tissue, Open Approach

0JX00ZC   Transfer Scalp Subcutaneous Tissue and Fascia with Skin, Subcutaneous Tissue and Fascia, Open Approach

0JX00ZZ   Transfer Scalp Subcutaneous Tissue and Fascia, Open Approach

0JX03ZB   Transfer Scalp Subcutaneous Tissue and Fascia with Skin and Subcutaneous Tissue, Percutaneous Approach

0JX03ZC   Transfer Scalp Subcutaneous Tissue and Fascia with Skin, Subcutaneous Tissue and Fascia, Percutaneous Approach

0JX03ZZ   Transfer Scalp Subcutaneous Tissue and Fascia, Percutaneous Approach

0JX10ZB   Transfer Face Subcutaneous Tissue and Fascia with Skin and Subcutaneous Tissue, Open Approach

0JX10ZC   Transfer Face Subcutaneous Tissue and Fascia with Skin, Subcutaneous Tissue and Fascia, Open Approach

0JX10ZZ   Transfer Face Subcutaneous Tissue and Fascia, Open Approach

0JX13ZB   Transfer Face Subcutaneous Tissue and Fascia with Skin and Subcutaneous Tissue, Percutaneous Approach

0JX13ZC   Transfer Face Subcutaneous Tissue and Fascia with Skin, Subcutaneous Tissue and Fascia, Percutaneous Approach

0JX13ZZ   Transfer Face Subcutaneous Tissue and Fascia, Percutaneous Approach

0JX40ZB   Transfer Anterior Neck Subcutaneous Tissue and Fascia with Skin and Subcutaneous Tissue, Open Approach

0JX40ZC   Transfer Anterior Neck Subcutaneous Tissue and Fascia with Skin, Subcutaneous Tissue and Fascia, Open Approach

0JX40ZZ   Transfer Anterior Neck Subcutaneous Tissue and Fascia, Open Approach

0JX43ZB   Transfer Anterior Neck Subcutaneous Tissue and Fascia with Skin and Subcutaneous Tissue, Percutaneous Approach

0JX43ZC   Transfer Anterior Neck Subcutaneous Tissue and Fascia with Skin, Subcutaneous Tissue and Fascia, Percutaneous Approach

0JX43ZZ   Transfer Anterior Neck Subcutaneous Tissue and Fascia, Percutaneous Approach

0JX50ZB   Transfer Posterior Neck Subcutaneous Tissue and Fascia with Skin and Subcutaneous Tissue, Open Approach

0JX50ZC   Transfer Posterior Neck Subcutaneous Tissue and Fascia with Skin, Subcutaneous Tissue and Fascia, Open Approach

0JX50ZZ   Transfer Posterior Neck Subcutaneous Tissue and Fascia, Open Approach

0JX53ZB   Transfer Posterior Neck Subcutaneous Tissue and Fascia with Skin and Subcutaneous Tissue, Percutaneous Approach

0JX53ZC   Transfer Posterior Neck Subcutaneous Tissue and Fascia with Skin, Subcutaneous Tissue and Fascia, Percutaneous Approach

0JX53ZZ   Transfer Posterior Neck Subcutaneous Tissue and Fascia, Percutaneous Approach

0JX60ZB   Transfer Chest Subcutaneous Tissue and Fascia with Skin and Subcutaneous Tissue, Open Approach

0JX60ZC   Transfer Chest Subcutaneous Tissue and Fascia with Skin, Subcutaneous Tissue and Fascia, Open Approach

0JX60ZZ   Transfer Chest Subcutaneous Tissue and Fascia, Open Approach

0JX63ZB   Transfer Chest Subcutaneous Tissue and Fascia with Skin and Subcutaneous Tissue, Percutaneous Approach

0JX63ZC   Transfer Chest Subcutaneous Tissue and Fascia with Skin, Subcutaneous Tissue and Fascia, Percutaneous Approach

0JX63ZZ   Transfer Chest Subcutaneous Tissue and Fascia, Percutaneous Approach

0JX70ZB   Transfer Back Subcutaneous Tissue and Fascia with Skin and Subcutaneous Tissue, Open Approach

0JX70ZC   Transfer Back Subcutaneous Tissue and Fascia with Skin, Subcutaneous Tissue and Fascia, Open Approach

0JX70ZZ   Transfer Back Subcutaneous Tissue and Fascia, Open Approach

0JX73ZB   Transfer Back Subcutaneous Tissue and Fascia with Skin and Subcutaneous Tissue, Percutaneous Approach

0JX73ZC   Transfer Back Subcutaneous Tissue and Fascia with Skin, Subcutaneous Tissue and Fascia, Percutaneous Approach

0JX73ZZ   Transfer Back Subcutaneous Tissue and Fascia, Percutaneous Approach

0JX80ZB   Transfer Abdomen Subcutaneous Tissue and Fascia with Skin and Subcutaneous Tissue, Open Approach

0JX80ZC   Transfer Abdomen Subcutaneous Tissue and Fascia with Skin, Subcutaneous Tissue and Fascia, Open Approach

0JX80ZZ   Transfer Abdomen Subcutaneous Tissue and Fascia, Open Approach

0JX83ZB   Transfer Abdomen Subcutaneous Tissue and Fascia with Skin and Subcutaneous Tissue, Percutaneous Approach

0JX83ZC   Transfer Abdomen Subcutaneous Tissue and Fascia with Skin, Subcutaneous Tissue and Fascia, Percutaneous Approach

0JX83ZZ   Transfer Abdomen Subcutaneous Tissue and Fascia, Percutaneous Approach

0JX90ZB   Transfer Buttock Subcutaneous Tissue and Fascia with Skin and Subcutaneous Tissue, Open Approach

0JX90ZC   Transfer Buttock Subcutaneous Tissue and Fascia with Skin, Subcutaneous Tissue and Fascia, Open Approach

0JX90ZZ   Transfer Buttock Subcutaneous Tissue and Fascia, Open Approach

0JX93ZB   Transfer Buttock Subcutaneous Tissue and Fascia with Skin and Subcutaneous Tissue, Percutaneous Approach

0JX93ZC   Transfer Buttock Subcutaneous Tissue and Fascia with Skin, Subcutaneous Tissue and Fascia, Percutaneous Approach

0JX93ZZ   Transfer Buttock Subcutaneous Tissue and Fascia, Percutaneous Approach

0JXB0ZB   Transfer Perineum Subcutaneous Tissue and Fascia with Skin and Subcutaneous Tissue, Open Approach

0JXB0ZC   Transfer Perineum Subcutaneous Tissue and Fascia with Skin, Subcutaneous Tissue and Fascia, Open Approach

0JXB0ZZ   Transfer Perineum Subcutaneous Tissue and Fascia, Open Approach

0JXB3ZB   Transfer Perineum Subcutaneous Tissue and Fascia with Skin and Subcutaneous Tissue, Percutaneous Approach

0JXB3ZC   Transfer Perineum Subcutaneous Tissue and Fascia with Skin, Subcutaneous Tissue and Fascia, Percutaneous Approach

0JXB3ZZ Transfer Perineum Subcutaneous Tissue and Fascia, Percutaneous Approach

0JXC0ZB Transfer Pelvic Region Subcutaneous Tissue and Fascia with Skin and Subcutaneous Tissue, Open Approach

0JXC0ZC Transfer Pelvic Region Subcutaneous Tissue and Fascia with Skin, Subcutaneous Tissue and Fascia, Open Approach

0JXC0ZZ Transfer Pelvic Region Subcutaneous Tissue and Fascia, Open Approach

0JXC3ZB Transfer Pelvic Region Subcutaneous Tissue and Fascia with Skin and Subcutaneous Tissue, Percutaneous Approach

0JXC3ZC Transfer Pelvic Region Subcutaneous Tissue and Fascia with Skin, Subcutaneous Tissue and Fascia, Percutaneous Approach

0JXC3ZZ Transfer Pelvic Region Subcutaneous Tissue and Fascia, Percutaneous Approach

0JXD0ZB Transfer Right Upper Arm Subcutaneous Tissue and Fascia with Skin and Subcutaneous Tissue, Open Approach

0JXD0ZC Transfer Right Upper Arm Subcutaneous Tissue and Fascia with Skin, Subcutaneous Tissue and Fascia, Open Approach

0JXD0ZZ Transfer Right Upper Arm Subcutaneous Tissue and Fascia, Open Approach

0JXD3ZB Transfer Right Upper Arm Subcutaneous Tissue and Fascia with Skin and Subcutaneous Tissue, Percutaneous Approach

0JXD3ZC Transfer Right Upper Arm Subcutaneous Tissue and Fascia with Skin, Subcutaneous Tissue and Fascia, Percutaneous Approach

0JXD3ZZ Transfer Right Upper Arm Subcutaneous Tissue and Fascia, Percutaneous Approach

0JXF0ZB Transfer Left Upper Arm Subcutaneous Tissue and Fascia with Skin and Subcutaneous Tissue, Open Approach

0JXF0ZC Transfer Left Upper Arm Subcutaneous Tissue and Fascia with Skin, Subcutaneous Tissue and Fascia, Open Approach

0JXF0ZZ Transfer Left Upper Arm Subcutaneous Tissue and Fascia, Open Approach

0JXF3ZB Transfer Left Upper Arm Subcutaneous Tissue and Fascia with Skin and Subcutaneous Tissue, Percutaneous Approach

0JXF3ZC Transfer Left Upper Arm Subcutaneous Tissue and Fascia with Skin, Subcutaneous Tissue and Fascia, Percutaneous Approach

0JXF3ZZ Transfer Left Upper Arm Subcutaneous Tissue and Fascia, Percutaneous Approach

0JXG0ZB Transfer Right Lower Arm Subcutaneous Tissue and Fascia with Skin and Subcutaneous Tissue, Open Approach

0JXG0ZC Transfer Right Lower Arm Subcutaneous Tissue and Fascia with Skin, Subcutaneous Tissue and Fascia, Open Approach

0JXG0ZZ Transfer Right Lower Arm Subcutaneous Tissue and Fascia, Open Approach

0JXG3ZB Transfer Right Lower Arm Subcutaneous Tissue and Fascia with Skin and Subcutaneous Tissue, Percutaneous Approach

0JXG3ZC Transfer Right Lower Arm Subcutaneous Tissue and Fascia with Skin, Subcutaneous Tissue and Fascia, Percutaneous Approach

0JXG3ZZ Transfer Right Lower Arm Subcutaneous Tissue and Fascia, Percutaneous Approach

0JXH0ZB Transfer Left Lower Arm Subcutaneous Tissue and Fascia with Skin and Subcutaneous Tissue, Open Approach

0JXH0ZC Transfer Left Lower Arm Subcutaneous Tissue and Fascia with Skin, Subcutaneous Tissue and Fascia, Open Approach

0JXH0ZZ Transfer Left Lower Arm Subcutaneous Tissue and Fascia, Open Approach

0JXH3ZB Transfer Left Lower Arm Subcutaneous Tissue and Fascia with Skin and Subcutaneous Tissue, Percutaneous Approach

0JXH3ZC Transfer Left Lower Arm Subcutaneous Tissue and Fascia with Skin, Subcutaneous Tissue and Fascia, Percutaneous Approach

0JXH3ZZ Transfer Left Lower Arm Subcutaneous Tissue and Fascia, Percutaneous Approach

0JXJ0ZB Transfer Right Hand Subcutaneous Tissue and Fascia with Skin and Subcutaneous Tissue, Open Approach

0JXJ0ZC Transfer Right Hand Subcutaneous Tissue and Fascia with Skin, Subcutaneous Tissue and Fascia, Open Approach

0JXJ0ZZ Transfer Right Hand Subcutaneous Tissue and Fascia, Open Approach

0JXJ3ZB Transfer Right Hand Subcutaneous Tissue and Fascia with Skin and Subcutaneous Tissue, Percutaneous Approach

0JXJ3ZC Transfer Right Hand Subcutaneous Tissue and Fascia with Skin, Subcutaneous Tissue and Fascia, Percutaneous Approach

0JXJ3ZZ Transfer Right Hand Subcutaneous Tissue and Fascia, Percutaneous Approach

0JXK0ZB Transfer Left Hand Subcutaneous Tissue and Fascia with Skin and Subcutaneous Tissue, Open Approach

0JXK0ZC Transfer Left Hand Subcutaneous Tissue and Fascia with Skin, Subcutaneous Tissue and Fascia, Open Approach

0JXK0ZZ Transfer Left Hand Subcutaneous Tissue and Fascia, Open Approach

0JXK3ZB Transfer Left Hand Subcutaneous Tissue and Fascia with Skin and Subcutaneous Tissue, Percutaneous Approach

0JXK3ZC Transfer Left Hand Subcutaneous Tissue and Fascia with Skin, Subcutaneous Tissue and Fascia, Percutaneous Approach

0JXK3ZZ Transfer Left Hand Subcutaneous Tissue and Fascia, Percutaneous Approach

0JXL0ZB Transfer Right Upper Leg Subcutaneous Tissue and Fascia with Skin and Subcutaneous Tissue, Open Approach

0JXL0ZC Transfer Right Upper Leg Subcutaneous Tissue and Fascia with Skin, Subcutaneous Tissue and Fascia, Open Approach

0JXL0ZZ Transfer Right Upper Leg Subcutaneous Tissue and Fascia, Open Approach

0JXL3ZB Transfer Right Upper Leg Subcutaneous Tissue and Fascia with Skin and Subcutaneous Tissue, Percutaneous Approach

0JXL3ZC Transfer Right Upper Leg Subcutaneous Tissue and Fascia with Skin, Subcutaneous Tissue and Fascia, Percutaneous Approach

0JXL3ZZ Transfer Right Upper Leg Subcutaneous Tissue and Fascia, Percutaneous Approach

0JXM0ZB Transfer Left Upper Leg Subcutaneous Tissue and Fascia with Skin and Subcutaneous Tissue, Open Approach

0JXM0ZC Transfer Left Upper Leg Subcutaneous Tissue and Fascia with Skin, Subcutaneous Tissue and Fascia, Open Approach

0JXM0ZZ Transfer Left Upper Leg Subcutaneous Tissue and Fascia, Open Approach

0JXM3ZB Transfer Left Upper Leg Subcutaneous Tissue and Fascia with Skin and Subcutaneous Tissue, Percutaneous Approach

0JXM3ZC Transfer Left Upper Leg Subcutaneous Tissue and Fascia with Skin, Subcutaneous Tissue and Fascia, Percutaneous Approach

0JXM3ZZ Transfer Left Upper Leg Subcutaneous Tissue and Fascia, Percutaneous Approach

0JXN0ZB Transfer Right Lower Leg Subcutaneous Tissue and Fascia with Skin and Subcutaneous Tissue, Open Approach

0JXN0ZC Transfer Right Lower Leg Subcutaneous Tissue and Fascia with Skin, Subcutaneous Tissue and Fascia, Open Approach

0JXN0ZZ Transfer Right Lower Leg Subcutaneous Tissue and Fascia, Open Approach

0JXN3ZB Transfer Right Lower Leg Subcutaneous Tissue and Fascia with Skin and Subcutaneous Tissue, Percutaneous Approach

0JXN3ZC Transfer Right Lower Leg Subcutaneous Tissue and Fascia with Skin, Subcutaneous Tissue and Fascia, Percutaneous Approach

0JXN3ZZ Transfer Right Lower Leg Subcutaneous Tissue and Fascia, Percutaneous Approach

0JXP0ZB Transfer Left Lower Leg Subcutaneous Tissue and Fascia with Skin and Subcutaneous Tissue, Open Approach

0JXP0ZC Transfer Left Lower Leg Subcutaneous Tissue and Fascia with Skin, Subcutaneous Tissue and Fascia, Open Approach

0JXP0ZZ Transfer Left Lower Leg Subcutaneous Tissue and Fascia, Open Approach

0JXP3ZB Transfer Left Lower Leg Subcutaneous Tissue and Fascia with Skin and Subcutaneous Tissue, Percutaneous Approach

0JXP3ZC Transfer Left Lower Leg Subcutaneous Tissue and Fascia with Skin, Subcutaneous Tissue and Fascia, Percutaneous Approach

0JXP3ZZ Transfer Left Lower Leg Subcutaneous Tissue and Fascia, Percutaneous Approach

0JXQ0ZB Transfer Right Foot Subcutaneous Tissue and Fascia with Skin and Subcutaneous Tissue, Open Approach

0JXQ0ZC Transfer Right Foot Subcutaneous Tissue and Fascia with Skin, Subcutaneous Tissue and Fascia, Open Approach

0JXQ0ZZ Transfer Right Foot Subcutaneous Tissue and Fascia, Open Approach

0JXQ3ZB Transfer Right Foot Subcutaneous Tissue and Fascia with Skin and Subcutaneous Tissue, Percutaneous Approach

0JXQ3ZC Transfer Right Foot Subcutaneous Tissue and Fascia with Skin, Subcutaneous Tissue and Fascia, Percutaneous Approach

0JXQ3ZZ Transfer Right Foot Subcutaneous Tissue and Fascia, Percutaneous Approach

0JXR0ZB Transfer Left Foot Subcutaneous Tissue and Fascia with Skin and Subcutaneous Tissue, Open Approach

0JXR0ZC Transfer Left Foot Subcutaneous Tissue and Fascia with Skin, Subcutaneous Tissue and Fascia, Open Approach

0JXR0ZZ Transfer Left Foot Subcutaneous Tissue and Fascia, Open Approach

0JXR3ZB Transfer Left Foot Subcutaneous Tissue and Fascia with Skin and Subcutaneous Tissue, Percutaneous Approach

0JXR3ZC Transfer Left Foot Subcutaneous Tissue and Fascia with Skin, Subcutaneous Tissue and Fascia, Percutaneous Approach

0JXR3ZZ Transfer Left Foot Subcutaneous Tissue and Fascia, Percutaneous Approach

Muscles

Muscles

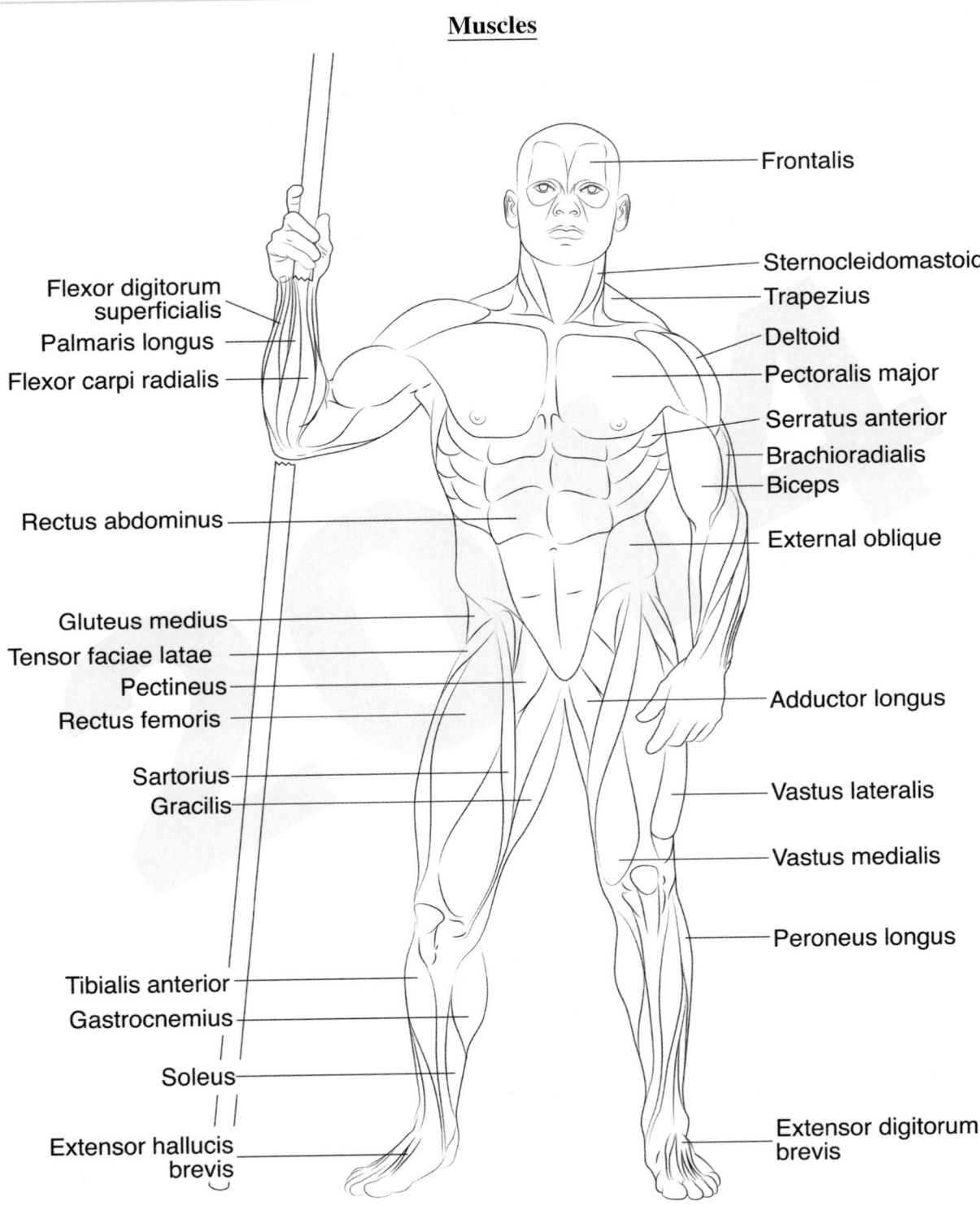

Flexor digitorum superficialis

Palmaris longus

Flexor carpi radialis

Frontalis

Sternocleidomastoid

Trapezius

Deltoid

Pectoralis major

Serratus anterior

Brachioradialis

Biceps

Rectus abdominus

External oblique

Gluteus medius

Tensor faciae latae

Pectineus

Rectus femoris

Adductor longus

Sartorius

Gracilis

Vastus lateralis

Vastus medialis

Peroneus longus

Tibialis anterior

Gastrocnemius

Soleus

Extensor hallucis brevis

Extensor digitorum brevis

Muscles of the Hand

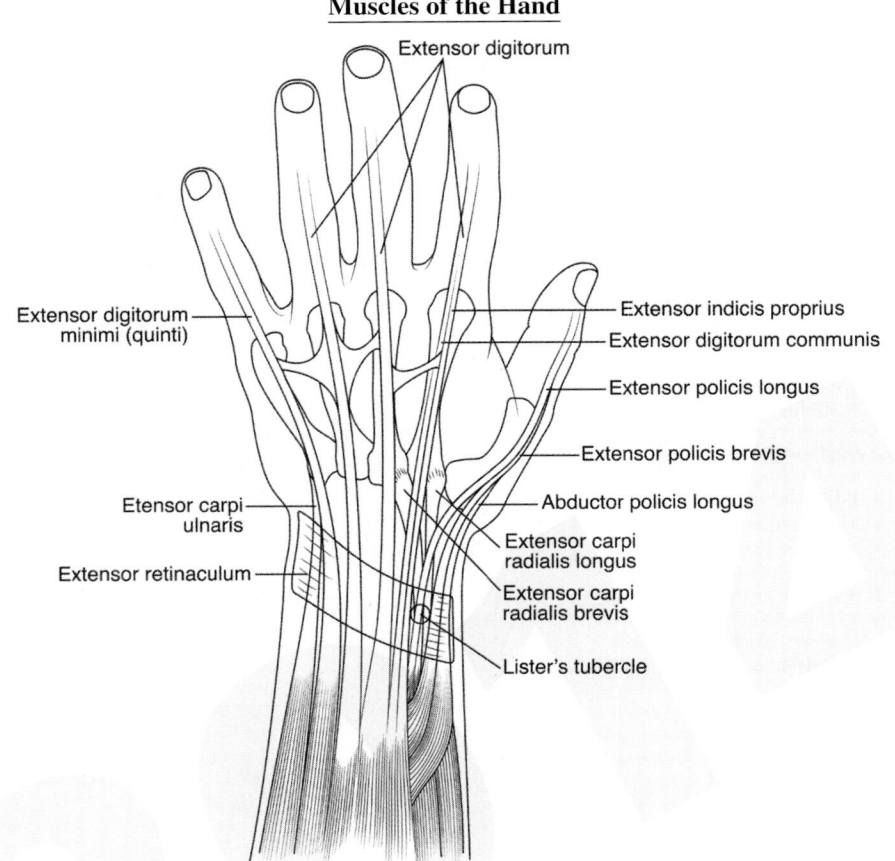

Muscles of the Foot

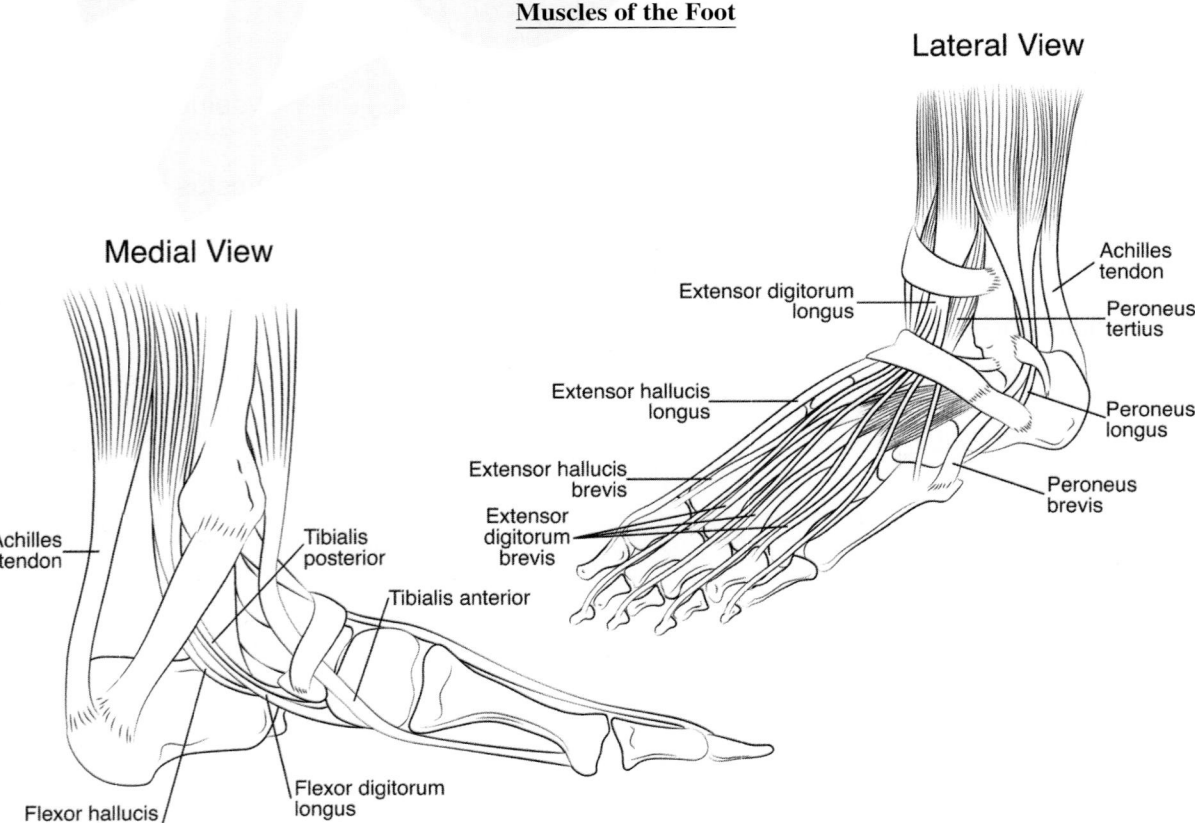

Muscles Tables 0K2–0KX

Section	0	Medical and Surgical
Body System	K	Muscles
Operation	2	**Change:** Taking out or off a device from a body part and putting back an identical or similar device in or on the same body part without cutting or puncturing the skin or a mucous membrane

Body Part (4th)	Approach (5th)	Device (6th)	Qualifier (7th)
X Upper Muscle Y Lower Muscle	X External	0 Drainage Device Y Other Device	Z No Qualifier

Section	0	Medical and Surgical
Body System	K	Muscles
Operation	5	**Destruction:** Physical eradication of all or a portion of a body part by the direct use of energy, force, or a destructive agent

Body Part (4th)	Approach (5th)	Device (6th)	Qualifier (7th)
0 Head Muscle 1 Facial Muscle 2 Neck Muscle, Right 3 Neck Muscle, Left 4 Tongue, Palate, Pharynx Muscle 5 Shoulder Muscle, Right 6 Shoulder Muscle, Left 7 Upper Arm Muscle, Right 8 Upper Arm Muscle, Left 9 Lower Arm and Wrist Muscle, Right B Lower Arm and Wrist Muscle, Left C Hand Muscle, Right D Hand Muscle, Left F Trunk Muscle, Right G Trunk Muscle, Left H Thorax Muscle, Right J Thorax Muscle, Left K Abdomen Muscle, Right L Abdomen Muscle, Left M Perineum Muscle N Hip Muscle, Right P Hip Muscle, Left Q Upper Leg Muscle, Right R Upper Leg Muscle, Left S Lower Leg Muscle, Right T Lower Leg Muscle, Left V Foot Muscle, Right W Foot Muscle, Left	0 Open 3 Percutaneous 4 Percutaneous Endoscopic	Z No Device	Z No Qualifier

Section	0	Medical and Surgical
Body System	K	Muscles
Operation	8	**Division:** Cutting into a body part, without draining fluids and/or gases from the body part, in order to separate or transect a body part

Body Part (4th)	Approach (5th)	Device (6th)	Qualifier (7th)
0 Head Muscle 1 Facial Muscle 2 Neck Muscle, Right 3 Neck Muscle, Left 4 Tongue, Palate, Pharynx Muscle 5 Shoulder Muscle, Right 6 Shoulder Muscle, Left 7 Upper Arm Muscle, Right 8 Upper Arm Muscle, Left 9 Lower Arm and Wrist Muscle, Right B Lower Arm and Wrist Muscle, Left C Hand Muscle, Right D Hand Muscle, Left F Trunk Muscle, Right G Trunk Muscle, Left H Thorax Muscle, Right J Thorax Muscle, Left K Abdomen Muscle, Right L Abdomen Muscle, Left M Perineum Muscle N Hip Muscle, Right P Hip Muscle, Left Q Upper Leg Muscle, Right R Upper Leg Muscle, Left S Lower Leg Muscle, Right T Lower Leg Muscle, Left V Foot Muscle, Right W Foot Muscle, Left	0 Open 3 Percutaneous 4 Percutaneous Endoscopic	Z No Device	Z No Qualifier

Section	0	**Medical and Surgical**
Body System	K	**Muscles**
Operation	9	**Drainage:** Taking or letting out fluids and/or gases from a body part

Body Part (4th)	Approach (5th)	Device (6th)	Qualifier (7th)
0 Head Muscle 1 Facial Muscle 2 Neck Muscle, Right 3 Neck Muscle, Left 4 Tongue, Palate, Pharynx Muscle 5 Shoulder Muscle, Right 6 Shoulder Muscle, Left 7 Upper Arm Muscle, Right 8 Upper Arm Muscle, Left 9 Lower Arm and Wrist Muscle, Right B Lower Arm and Wrist Muscle, Left C Hand Muscle, Right D Hand Muscle, Left F Trunk Muscle, Right G Trunk Muscle, Left H Thorax Muscle, Right J Thorax Muscle, Left K Abdomen Muscle, Right L Abdomen Muscle, Left M Perineum Muscle N Hip Muscle, Right P Hip Muscle, Left Q Upper Leg Muscle, Right R Upper Leg Muscle, Left S Lower Leg Muscle, Right T Lower Leg Muscle, Left V Foot Muscle, Right W Foot Muscle, Left	0 Open 3 Percutaneous 4 Percutaneous Endoscopic	0 Drainage Device	Z No Qualifier
0 Head Muscle 1 Facial Muscle 2 Neck Muscle, Right 3 Neck Muscle, Left 4 Tongue, Palate, Pharynx Muscle 5 Shoulder Muscle, Right 6 Shoulder Muscle, Left 7 Upper Arm Muscle, Right 8 Upper Arm Muscle, Left 9 Lower Arm and Wrist Muscle, Right B Lower Arm and Wrist Muscle, Left C Hand Muscle, Right D Hand Muscle, Left F Trunk Muscle, Right G Trunk Muscle, Left H Thorax Muscle, Right J Thorax Muscle, Left K Abdomen Muscle, Right L Abdomen Muscle, Left M Perineum Muscle N Hip Muscle, Right P Hip Muscle, Left Q Upper Leg Muscle, Right R Upper Leg Muscle, Left S Lower Leg Muscle, Right T Lower Leg Muscle, Left V Foot Muscle, Right W Foot Muscle, Left	0 Open 3 Percutaneous 4 Percutaneous Endoscopic	Z No Device	X Diagnostic Z No Qualifier

Section	0	Medical and Surgical
Body System	K	Muscles
Operation	B	**Excision:** Cutting out or off, without replacement, a portion of a body part

Body Part (4th)	Approach (5th)	Device (6th)	Qualifier (7th)
0 Head Muscle	0 Open	Z No Device	X Diagnostic
1 Facial Muscle	3 Percutaneous		Z No Qualifier
2 Neck Muscle, Right	4 Percutaneous Endoscopic		
3 Neck Muscle, Left			
4 Tongue, Palate, Pharynx Muscle			
5 Shoulder Muscle, Right			
6 Shoulder Muscle, Left			
7 Upper Arm Muscle, Right			
8 Upper Arm Muscle, Left			
9 Lower Arm and Wrist Muscle, Right			
B Lower Arm and Wrist Muscle, Left			
C Hand Muscle, Right			
D Hand Muscle, Left			
F Trunk Muscle, Right			
G Trunk Muscle, Left			
H Thorax Muscle, Right			
J Thorax Muscle, Left			
K Abdomen Muscle, Right			
L Abdomen Muscle, Left			
M Perineum Muscle			
N Hip Muscle, Right			
P Hip Muscle, Left			
Q Upper Leg Muscle, Right			
R Upper Leg Muscle, Left			
S Lower Leg Muscle, Right			
T Lower Leg Muscle, Left			
V Foot Muscle, Right			
W Foot Muscle, Left			

Section	0	Medical and Surgical
Body System	K	Muscles
Operation	C	**Extirpation:** Taking or cutting out solid matter from a body part

Body Part (4th)	Approach (5th)	Device (6th)	Qualifier (7th)
0 Head Muscle	0 Open	Z No Device	Z No Qualifier
1 Facial Muscle	3 Percutaneous		
2 Neck Muscle, Right	4 Percutaneous Endoscopic		
3 Neck Muscle, Left			
4 Tongue, Palate, Pharynx Muscle			
5 Shoulder Muscle, Right			
6 Shoulder Muscle, Left			
7 Upper Arm Muscle, Right			
8 Upper Arm Muscle, Left			
9 Lower Arm and Wrist Muscle, Right			
B Lower Arm and Wrist Muscle, Left			
C Hand Muscle, Right			
D Hand Muscle, Left			
F Trunk Muscle, Right			
G Trunk Muscle, Left			
H Thorax Muscle, Right			
J Thorax Muscle, Left			
K Abdomen Muscle, Right			
L Abdomen Muscle, Left			
M Perineum Muscle			
N Hip Muscle, Right			
P Hip Muscle, Left			
Q Upper Leg Muscle, Right			
R Upper Leg Muscle, Left			
S Lower Leg Muscle, Right			
T Lower Leg Muscle, Left			
V Foot Muscle, Right			
W Foot Muscle, Left			

Section	0	Medical and Surgical
Body System	K	Muscles
Operation	H	**Insertion:** Putting in a nonbiological appliance that monitors, assists, performs, or prevents a physiological function but does not physically take the place of a body part

Body Part (4th)	Approach (5th)	Device (6th)	Qualifier (7th)
X Upper Muscle Y Lower Muscle	0 Open 3 Percutaneous 4 Percutaneous Endoscopic	M Stimulator Lead	Z No Qualifier

Section	0	Medical and Surgical
Body System	K	Muscles
Operation	J	**Inspection:** Visually and/or manually exploring a body part

Body Part (4th)	Approach (5th)	Device (6th)	Qualifier (7th)
X Upper Muscle Y Lower Muscle	0 Open 3 Percutaneous 4 Percutaneous Endoscopic X External	Z No Device	Z No Qualifier

Section	0	Medical and Surgical
Body System	K	Muscles
Operation	M	**Reattachment:** Putting back in or on all or a portion of a separated body part to its normal location or other suitable location

Body Part (4th)	Approach (5th)	Device (6th)	Qualifier (7th)
0 Head Muscle 1 Facial Muscle 2 Neck Muscle, Right 3 Neck Muscle, Left 4 Tongue, Palate, Pharynx Muscle 5 Shoulder Muscle, Right 6 Shoulder Muscle, Left 7 Upper Arm Muscle, Right 8 Upper Arm Muscle, Left 9 Lower Arm and Wrist Muscle, Right B Lower Arm and Wrist Muscle, Left C Hand Muscle, Right D Hand Muscle, Left F Trunk Muscle, Right G Trunk Muscle, Left H Thorax Muscle, Right J Thorax Muscle, Left K Abdomen Muscle, Right L Abdomen Muscle, Left M Perineum Muscle N Hip Muscle, Right P Hip Muscle, Left Q Upper Leg Muscle, Right R Upper Leg Muscle, Left S Lower Leg Muscle, Right T Lower Leg Muscle, Left V Foot Muscle, Right W Foot Muscle, Left	0 Open 4 Percutaneous Endoscopic	Z No Device	Z No Qualifier

Section	0	Medical and Surgical
Body System	K	Muscles
Operation	N	**Release:** Freeing a body part from an abnormal physical constraint by cutting or by the use of force

Body Part (4th)	Approach (5th)	Device (6th)	Qualifier (7th)
0 Head Muscle 1 Facial Muscle 2 Neck Muscle, Right 3 Neck Muscle, Left 4 Tongue, Palate, Pharynx Muscle 5 Shoulder Muscle, Right 6 Shoulder Muscle, Left 7 Upper Arm Muscle, Right 8 Upper Arm Muscle, Left 9 Lower Arm and Wrist Muscle, Right B Lower Arm and Wrist Muscle, Left C Hand Muscle, Right D Hand Muscle, Left F Trunk Muscle, Right G Trunk Muscle, Left H Thorax Muscle, Right J Thorax Muscle, Left K Abdomen Muscle, Right L Abdomen Muscle, Left M Perineum Muscle N Hip Muscle, Right P Hip Muscle, Left Q Upper Leg Muscle, Right R Upper Leg Muscle, Left S Lower Leg Muscle, Right T Lower Leg Muscle, Left V Foot Muscle, Right W Foot Muscle, Left	0 Open 3 Percutaneous 4 Percutaneous Endoscopic X External	Z No Device	Z No Qualifier

Section	0	Medical and Surgical
Body System	K	Muscles
Operation	P	**Removal:** Taking out or off a device from a body part

Body Part (4th)	Approach (5th)	Device (6th)	Qualifier (7th)
X Upper Muscle Y Lower Muscle	0 Open 3 Percutaneous 4 Percutaneous Endoscopic	0 Drainage Device 7 Autologous Tissue Substitute J Synthetic Substitute K Nonautologous Tissue Substitute M Stimulator Lead	Z No Qualifier
X Upper Muscle Y Lower Muscle	X External	0 Drainage Device M Stimulator Lead	Z No Qualifier

Section	0	**Medical and Surgical**
Body System	K	**Muscles**
Operation	Q	**Repair:** Restoring, to the extent possible, a body part to its normal anatomic structure and function

Body Part (4th)	Approach (5th)	Device (6th)	Qualifier (7th)
0 Head Muscle	0 Open	Z No Device	Z No Qualifier
1 Facial Muscle	3 Percutaneous		
2 Neck Muscle, Right	4 Percutaneous Endoscopic		
3 Neck Muscle, Left			
4 Tongue, Palate, Pharynx Muscle			
5 Shoulder Muscle, Right			
6 Shoulder Muscle, Left			
7 Upper Arm Muscle, Right			
8 Upper Arm Muscle, Left			
9 Lower Arm and Wrist Muscle, Right			
B Lower Arm and Wrist Muscle, Left			
C Hand Muscle, Right			
D Hand Muscle, Left			
F Trunk Muscle, Right			
G Trunk Muscle, Left			
H Thorax Muscle, Right			
J Thorax Muscle, Left			
K Abdomen Muscle, Right			
L Abdomen Muscle, Left			
M Perineum Muscle			
N Hip Muscle, Right			
P Hip Muscle, Left			
Q Upper Leg Muscle, Right			
R Upper Leg Muscle, Left			
S Lower Leg Muscle, Right			
T Lower Leg Muscle, Left			
V Foot Muscle, Right			
W Foot Muscle, Left			

0KQ

Section	0	Medical and Surgical
Body System	K	Muscles
Operation	S	Reposition: Moving to its normal location, or other suitable location, all or a portion of a body part

Body Part (4th)	Approach (5th)	Device (6th)	Qualifier (7th)
0 Head Muscle 1 Facial Muscle 2 Neck Muscle, Right 3 Neck Muscle, Left 4 Tongue, Palate, Pharynx Muscle 5 Shoulder Muscle, Right 6 Shoulder Muscle, Left 7 Upper Arm Muscle, Right 8 Upper Arm Muscle, Left 9 Lower Arm and Wrist Muscle, Right B Lower Arm and Wrist Muscle, Left C Hand Muscle, Right D Hand Muscle, Left F Trunk Muscle, Right G Trunk Muscle, Left H Thorax Muscle, Right J Thorax Muscle, Left K Abdomen Muscle, Right L Abdomen Muscle, Left M Perineum Muscle N Hip Muscle, Right P Hip Muscle, Left Q Upper Leg Muscle, Right R Upper Leg Muscle, Left S Lower Leg Muscle, Right T Lower Leg Muscle, Left V Foot Muscle, Right W Foot Muscle, Left	0 Open 4 Percutaneous Endoscopic	Z No Device	Z No Qualifier

Section	0	Medical and Surgical
Body System	K	Muscles
Operation	T	Resection: Cutting out or off, without replacement, all of a body part

Body Part (4th)	Approach (5th)	Device (6th)	Qualifier (7th)
0 Head Muscle 1 Facial Muscle 2 Neck Muscle, Right 3 Neck Muscle, Left 4 Tongue, Palate, Pharynx Muscle 5 Shoulder Muscle, Right 6 Shoulder Muscle, Left 7 Upper Arm Muscle, Right 8 Upper Arm Muscle, Left 9 Lower Arm and Wrist Muscle, Right B Lower Arm and Wrist Muscle, Left C Hand Muscle, Right D Hand Muscle, Left F Trunk Muscle, Right G Trunk Muscle, Left H Thorax Muscle, Right J Thorax Muscle, Left K Abdomen Muscle, Right L Abdomen Muscle, Left M Perineum Muscle N Hip Muscle, Right P Hip Muscle, Left Q Upper Leg Muscle, Right R Upper Leg Muscle, Left S Lower Leg Muscle, Right T Lower Leg Muscle, Left V Foot Muscle, Right W Foot Muscle, Left	0 Open 4 Percutaneous Endoscopic	Z No Device	Z No Qualifier

Section	0	Medical and Surgical
Body System	K	Muscles
Operation	U	**Supplement:** Putting in or on biological or synthetic material that physically reinforces and/or augments the function of a portion of a body part

Body Part (4th)	Approach (5th)	Device (6th)	Qualifier (7th)
0 Head Muscle 1 Facial Muscle 2 Neck Muscle, Right 3 Neck Muscle, Left 4 Tongue, Palate, Pharynx Muscle 5 Shoulder Muscle, Right 6 Shoulder Muscle, Left 7 Upper Arm Muscle, Right 8 Upper Arm Muscle, Left 9 Lower Arm and Wrist Muscle, Right B Lower Arm and Wrist Muscle, Left C Hand Muscle, Right D Hand Muscle, Left F Trunk Muscle, Right G Trunk Muscle, Left H Thorax Muscle, Right J Thorax Muscle, Left K Abdomen Muscle, Right L Abdomen Muscle, Left M Perineum Muscle N Hip Muscle, Right P Hip Muscle, Left Q Upper Leg Muscle, Right R Upper Leg Muscle, Left S Lower Leg Muscle, Right T Lower Leg Muscle, Left V Foot Muscle, Right W Foot Muscle, Left	0 Open 4 Percutaneous Endoscopic	7 Autologous Tissue Substitute J Synthetic Substitute K Nonautologous Tissue Substitute	Z No Qualifier

Section	0	Medical and Surgical
Body System	K	Muscles
Operation	W	**Revision:** Correcting, to the extent possible, a portion of a malfunctioning device or the position of a displaced device

Body Part (4th)	Approach (5th)	Device (6th)	Qualifier (7th)
X Upper Muscle Y Lower Muscle	0 Open 3 Percutaneous 4 Percutaneous Endoscopic X External	0 Drainage Device 7 Autologous Tissue Substitute J Synthetic Substitute K Nonautologous Tissue Substitute M Stimulator Lead	Z No Qualifier

Section	0	**Medical and Surgical**
Body System	K	**Muscles**
Operation	X	**Transfer:** Moving, without taking out, all or a portion of a body part to another location to take over the function of all or a portion of a body part

Body Part (4th)	Approach (5th)	Device (6th)	Qualifier (7th)
0 Head Muscle 1 Facial Muscle 2 Neck Muscle, Right 3 Neck Muscle, Left 4 Tongue, Palate, Pharynx Muscle 5 Shoulder Muscle, Right 6 Shoulder Muscle, Left 7 Upper Arm Muscle, Right 8 Upper Arm Muscle, Left 9 Lower Arm and Wrist Muscle, Right B Lower Arm and Wrist Muscle, Left C Hand Muscle, Right D Hand Muscle, Left F Trunk Muscle, Right G Trunk Muscle, Left H Thorax Muscle, Right J Thorax Muscle, Left M Perineum Muscle N Hip Muscle, Right P Hip Muscle, Left Q Upper Leg Muscle, Right R Upper Leg Muscle, Left S Lower Leg Muscle, Right T Lower Leg Muscle, Left V Foot Muscle, Right W Foot Muscle, Left	0 Open 4 Percutaneous Endoscopic	Z No Device	0 Skin 1 Subcutaneous Tissue 2 Skin and Subcutaneous Tissue Z No Qualifier
K Abdomen Muscle, Right L Abdomen Muscle, Left	0 Open 4 Percutaneous Endoscopic	Z No Device	0 Skin 1 Subcutaneous Tissue 2 Skin and Subcutaneous Tissue 6 Transverse Rectus Abdominis Myocutaneous Flap Z No Qualifier

Muscles Code Listing 0K2–0KX

0K2 – Muscles, Change

Review Coding Guideline B6.1c

0K2XX0Z Change Drainage Device in Upper Muscle, External Approach
0K2XXYZ Change Other Device in Upper Muscle, External Approach

0K2YX0Z Change Drainage Device in Lower Muscle, External Approach
0K2YXYZ Change Other Device in Lower Muscle, External Approach

0K5 – Muscles, Destruction

0K500ZZ Destruction of Head Muscle, Open Approach
0K503ZZ Destruction of Head Muscle, Percutaneous Approach
0K504ZZ Destruction of Head Muscle, Percutaneous Endoscopic Approach
0K510ZZ Destruction of Facial Muscle, Open Approach
0K513ZZ Destruction of Facial Muscle, Percutaneous Approach
0K514ZZ Destruction of Facial Muscle, Percutaneous Endoscopic Approach
0K520ZZ Destruction of Right Neck Muscle, Open Approach
0K523ZZ Destruction of Right Neck Muscle, Percutaneous Approach
0K524ZZ Destruction of Right Neck Muscle, Percutaneous Endoscopic Approach
0K530ZZ Destruction of Left Neck Muscle, Open Approach
0K533ZZ Destruction of Left Neck Muscle, Percutaneous Approach
0K534ZZ Destruction of Left Neck Muscle, Percutaneous Endoscopic Approach

0K540ZZ Destruction of Tongue, Palate, Pharynx Muscle, Open Approach
0K543ZZ Destruction of Tongue, Palate, Pharynx Muscle, Percutaneous Approach
0K544ZZ Destruction of Tongue, Palate, Pharynx Muscle, Percutaneous Endoscopic Approach
0K550ZZ Destruction of Right Shoulder Muscle, Open Approach
0K553ZZ Destruction of Right Shoulder Muscle, Percutaneous Approach
0K554ZZ Destruction of Right Shoulder Muscle, Percutaneous Endoscopic Approach
0K560ZZ Destruction of Left Shoulder Muscle, Open Approach
0K563ZZ Destruction of Left Shoulder Muscle, Percutaneous Approach
0K564ZZ Destruction of Left Shoulder Muscle, Percutaneous Endoscopic Approach
0K570ZZ Destruction of Right Upper Arm Muscle, Open Approach

0K573ZZ	Destruction of Right Upper Arm Muscle, Percutaneous Approach
0K574ZZ	Destruction of Right Upper Arm Muscle, Percutaneous Endoscopic Approach
0K580ZZ	Destruction of Left Upper Arm Muscle, Open Approach
0K583ZZ	Destruction of Left Upper Arm Muscle, Percutaneous Approach
0K584ZZ	Destruction of Left Upper Arm Muscle, Percutaneous Endoscopic Approach
0K590ZZ	Destruction of Right Lower Arm and Wrist Muscle, Open Approach
0K593ZZ	Destruction of Right Lower Arm and Wrist Muscle, Percutaneous Approach
0K594ZZ	Destruction of Right Lower Arm and Wrist Muscle, Percutaneous Endoscopic Approach
0K5B0ZZ	Destruction of Left Lower Arm and Wrist Muscle, Open Approach
0K5B3ZZ	Destruction of Left Lower Arm and Wrist Muscle, Percutaneous Approach
0K5B4ZZ	Destruction of Left Lower Arm and Wrist Muscle, Percutaneous Endoscopic Approach
0K5C0ZZ	Destruction of Right Hand Muscle, Open Approach
0K5C3ZZ	Destruction of Right Hand Muscle, Percutaneous Approach
0K5C4ZZ	Destruction of Right Hand Muscle, Percutaneous Endoscopic Approach
0K5D0ZZ	Destruction of Left Hand Muscle, Open Approach
0K5D3ZZ	Destruction of Left Hand Muscle, Percutaneous Approach
0K5D4ZZ	Destruction of Left Hand Muscle, Percutaneous Endoscopic Approach
0K5F0ZZ	Destruction of Right Trunk Muscle, Open Approach
0K5F3ZZ	Destruction of Right Trunk Muscle, Percutaneous Approach
0K5F4ZZ	Destruction of Right Trunk Muscle, Percutaneous Endoscopic Approach
0K5G0ZZ	Destruction of Left Trunk Muscle, Open Approach
0K5G3ZZ	Destruction of Left Trunk Muscle, Percutaneous Approach
0K5G4ZZ	Destruction of Left Trunk Muscle, Percutaneous Endoscopic Approach
0K5H0ZZ	Destruction of Right Thorax Muscle, Open Approach
0K5H3ZZ	Destruction of Right Thorax Muscle, Percutaneous Approach
0K5H4ZZ	Destruction of Right Thorax Muscle, Percutaneous Endoscopic Approach
0K5J0ZZ	Destruction of Left Thorax Muscle, Open Approach
0K5J3ZZ	Destruction of Left Thorax Muscle, Percutaneous Approach
0K5J4ZZ	Destruction of Left Thorax Muscle, Percutaneous Endoscopic Approach
0K5K0ZZ	Destruction of Right Abdomen Muscle, Open Approach
0K5K3ZZ	Destruction of Right Abdomen Muscle, Percutaneous Approach
0K5K4ZZ	Destruction of Right Abdomen Muscle, Percutaneous Endoscopic Approach
0K5L0ZZ	Destruction of Left Abdomen Muscle, Open Approach
0K5L3ZZ	Destruction of Left Abdomen Muscle, Percutaneous Approach
0K5L4ZZ	Destruction of Left Abdomen Muscle, Percutaneous Endoscopic Approach
0K5M0ZZ	Destruction of Perineum Muscle, Open Approach
0K5M3ZZ	Destruction of Perineum Muscle, Percutaneous Approach
0K5M4ZZ	Destruction of Perineum Muscle, Percutaneous Endoscopic Approach
0K5N0ZZ	Destruction of Right Hip Muscle, Open Approach
0K5N3ZZ	Destruction of Right Hip Muscle, Percutaneous Approach
0K5N4ZZ	Destruction of Right Hip Muscle, Percutaneous Endoscopic Approach
0K5P0ZZ	Destruction of Left Hip Muscle, Open Approach
0K5P3ZZ	Destruction of Left Hip Muscle, Percutaneous Approach
0K5P4ZZ	Destruction of Left Hip Muscle, Percutaneous Endoscopic Approach
0K5Q0ZZ	Destruction of Right Upper Leg Muscle, Open Approach
0K5Q3ZZ	Destruction of Right Upper Leg Muscle, Percutaneous Approach
0K5Q4ZZ	Destruction of Right Upper Leg Muscle, Percutaneous Endoscopic Approach
0K5R0ZZ	Destruction of Left Upper Leg Muscle, Open Approach
0K5R3ZZ	Destruction of Left Upper Leg Muscle, Percutaneous Approach
0K5R4ZZ	Destruction of Left Upper Leg Muscle, Percutaneous Endoscopic Approach
0K5S0ZZ	Destruction of Right Lower Leg Muscle, Open Approach
0K5S3ZZ	Destruction of Right Lower Leg Muscle, Percutaneous Approach
0K5S4ZZ	Destruction of Right Lower Leg Muscle, Percutaneous Endoscopic Approach
0K5T0ZZ	Destruction of Left Lower Leg Muscle, Open Approach
0K5T3ZZ	Destruction of Left Lower Leg Muscle, Percutaneous Approach
0K5T4ZZ	Destruction of Left Lower Leg Muscle, Percutaneous Endoscopic Approach
0K5V0ZZ	Destruction of Right Foot Muscle, Open Approach
0K5V3ZZ	Destruction of Right Foot Muscle, Percutaneous Approach
0K5V4ZZ	Destruction of Right Foot Muscle, Percutaneous Endoscopic Approach
0K5W0ZZ	Destruction of Left Foot Muscle, Open Approach
0K5W3ZZ	Destruction of Left Foot Muscle, Percutaneous Approach
0K5W4ZZ	Destruction of Left Foot Muscle, Percutaneous Endoscopic Approach

0K8 – Muscles, Division

Review Coding Guideline B3.14

0K800ZZ	Division of Head Muscle, Open Approach
0K803ZZ	Division of Head Muscle, Percutaneous Approach
0K804ZZ	Division of Head Muscle, Percutaneous Endoscopic Approach
0K810ZZ	Division of Facial Muscle, Open Approach
0K813ZZ	Division of Facial Muscle, Percutaneous Approach
0K814ZZ	Division of Facial Muscle, Percutaneous Endoscopic Approach
0K820ZZ	Division of Right Neck Muscle, Open Approach
0K823ZZ	Division of Right Neck Muscle, Percutaneous Approach
0K824ZZ	Division of Right Neck Muscle, Percutaneous Endoscopic Approach
0K830ZZ	Division of Left Neck Muscle, Open Approach
0K833ZZ	Division of Left Neck Muscle, Percutaneous Approach
0K834ZZ	Division of Left Neck Muscle, Percutaneous Endoscopic Approach
0K840ZZ	Division of Tongue, Palate, Pharynx Muscle, Open Approach
0K843ZZ	Division of Tongue, Palate, Pharynx Muscle, Percutaneous Approach
0K844ZZ	Division of Tongue, Palate, Pharynx Muscle, Percutaneous Endoscopic Approach
0K850ZZ	Division of Right Shoulder Muscle, Open Approach
0K853ZZ	Division of Right Shoulder Muscle, Percutaneous Approach
0K854ZZ	Division of Right Shoulder Muscle, Percutaneous Endoscopic Approach
0K860ZZ	Division of Left Shoulder Muscle, Open Approach
0K863ZZ	Division of Left Shoulder Muscle, Percutaneous Approach
0K864ZZ	Division of Left Shoulder Muscle, Percutaneous Endoscopic Approach
0K870ZZ	Division of Right Upper Arm Muscle, Open Approach
0K873ZZ	Division of Right Upper Arm Muscle, Percutaneous Approach
0K874ZZ	Division of Right Upper Arm Muscle, Percutaneous Endoscopic Approach
0K880ZZ	Division of Left Upper Arm Muscle, Open Approach
0K883ZZ	Division of Left Upper Arm Muscle, Percutaneous Approach
0K884ZZ	Division of Left Upper Arm Muscle, Percutaneous Endoscopic Approach
0K890ZZ	Division of Right Lower Arm and Wrist Muscle, Open Approach
0K893ZZ	Division of Right Lower Arm and Wrist Muscle, Percutaneous Approach
0K894ZZ	Division of Right Lower Arm and Wrist Muscle, Percutaneous Endoscopic Approach
0K8B0ZZ	Division of Left Lower Arm and Wrist Muscle, Open Approach
0K8B3ZZ	Division of Left Lower Arm and Wrist Muscle, Percutaneous Approach
0K8B4ZZ	Division of Left Lower Arm and Wrist Muscle, Percutaneous Endoscopic Approach
0K8C0ZZ	Division of Right Hand Muscle, Open Approach
0K8C3ZZ	Division of Right Hand Muscle, Percutaneous Approach
0K8C4ZZ	Division of Right Hand Muscle, Percutaneous Endoscopic Approach
0K8D0ZZ	Division of Left Hand Muscle, Open Approach
0K8D3ZZ	Division of Left Hand Muscle, Percutaneous Approach
0K8D4ZZ	Division of Left Hand Muscle, Percutaneous Endoscopic Approach

0K8F0ZZ	Division of Right Trunk Muscle, Open Approach
0K8F3ZZ	Division of Right Trunk Muscle, Percutaneous Approach
0K8F4ZZ	Division of Right Trunk Muscle, Percutaneous Endoscopic Approach
0K8G0ZZ	Division of Left Trunk Muscle, Open Approach
0K8G3ZZ	Division of Left Trunk Muscle, Percutaneous Approach
0K8G4ZZ	Division of Left Trunk Muscle, Percutaneous Endoscopic Approach
0K8H0ZZ	Division of Right Thorax Muscle, Open Approach
0K8H3ZZ	Division of Right Thorax Muscle, Percutaneous Approach
0K8H4ZZ	Division of Right Thorax Muscle, Percutaneous Endoscopic Approach
0K8J0ZZ	Division of Left Thorax Muscle, Open Approach
0K8J3ZZ	Division of Left Thorax Muscle, Percutaneous Approach
0K8J4ZZ	Division of Left Thorax Muscle, Percutaneous Endoscopic Approach
0K8K0ZZ	Division of Right Abdomen Muscle, Open Approach
0K8K3ZZ	Division of Right Abdomen Muscle, Percutaneous Approach
0K8K4ZZ	Division of Right Abdomen Muscle, Percutaneous Endoscopic Approach
0K8L0ZZ	Division of Left Abdomen Muscle, Open Approach
0K8L3ZZ	Division of Left Abdomen Muscle, Percutaneous Approach
0K8L4ZZ	Division of Left Abdomen Muscle, Percutaneous Endoscopic Approach
0K8M0ZZ	Division of Perineum Muscle, Open Approach
0K8M3ZZ	Division of Perineum Muscle, Percutaneous Approach
0K8M4ZZ	Division of Perineum Muscle, Percutaneous Endoscopic Approach
0K8N0ZZ	Division of Right Hip Muscle, Open Approach
0K8N3ZZ	Division of Right Hip Muscle, Percutaneous Approach
0K8N4ZZ	Division of Right Hip Muscle, Percutaneous Endoscopic Approach
0K8P0ZZ	Division of Left Hip Muscle, Open Approach
0K8P3ZZ	Division of Left Hip Muscle, Percutaneous Approach
0K8P4ZZ	Division of Left Hip Muscle, Percutaneous Endoscopic Approach
0K8Q0ZZ	Division of Right Upper Leg Muscle, Open Approach
0K8Q3ZZ	Division of Right Upper Leg Muscle, Percutaneous Approach
0K8Q4ZZ	Division of Right Upper Leg Muscle, Percutaneous Endoscopic Approach
0K8R0ZZ	Division of Left Upper Leg Muscle, Open Approach
0K8R3ZZ	Division of Left Upper Leg Muscle, Percutaneous Approach
0K8R4ZZ	Division of Left Upper Leg Muscle, Percutaneous Endoscopic Approach
0K8S0ZZ	Division of Right Lower Leg Muscle, Open Approach
0K8S3ZZ	Division of Right Lower Leg Muscle, Percutaneous Approach
0K8S4ZZ	Division of Right Lower Leg Muscle, Percutaneous Endoscopic Approach
0K8T0ZZ	Division of Left Lower Leg Muscle, Open Approach
0K8T3ZZ	Division of Left Lower Leg Muscle, Percutaneous Approach
0K8T4ZZ	Division of Left Lower Leg Muscle, Percutaneous Endoscopic Approach
0K8V0ZZ	Division of Right Foot Muscle, Open Approach
0K8V3ZZ	Division of Right Foot Muscle, Percutaneous Approach
0K8V4ZZ	Division of Right Foot Muscle, Percutaneous Endoscopic Approach
0K8W0ZZ	Division of Left Foot Muscle, Open Approach
0K8W3ZZ	Division of Left Foot Muscle, Percutaneous Approach
0K8W4ZZ	Division of Left Foot Muscle, Percutaneous Endoscopic Approach

0K9 – Muscles, Drainage

Review Coding Guidelines B3.4a and B3.4b

Review Coding Guideline B6.2

0K9000Z	Drainage of Head Muscle with Drainage Device, Open Approach
0K900ZX	Drainage of Head Muscle, Open Approach, Diagnostic
0K900ZZ	Drainage of Head Muscle, Open Approach
0K9030Z	Drainage of Head Muscle with Drainage Device, Percutaneous Approach
0K903ZX	Drainage of Head Muscle, Percutaneous Approach, Diagnostic
0K903ZZ	Drainage of Head Muscle, Percutaneous Approach
0K9040Z	Drainage of Head Muscle with Drainage Device, Percutaneous Endoscopic Approach
0K904ZX	Drainage of Head Muscle, Percutaneous Endoscopic Approach, Diagnostic
0K904ZZ	Drainage of Head Muscle, Percutaneous Endoscopic Approach
0K9100Z	Drainage of Facial Muscle with Drainage Device, Open Approach
0K910ZX	Drainage of Facial Muscle, Open Approach, Diagnostic
0K910ZZ	Drainage of Facial Muscle, Open Approach
0K9130Z	Drainage of Facial Muscle with Drainage Device, Percutaneous Approach
0K913ZX	Drainage of Facial Muscle, Percutaneous Approach, Diagnostic
0K913ZZ	Drainage of Facial Muscle, Percutaneous Approach
0K9140Z	Drainage of Facial Muscle with Drainage Device, Percutaneous Endoscopic Approach
0K914ZX	Drainage of Facial Muscle, Percutaneous Endoscopic Approach, Diagnostic
0K914ZZ	Drainage of Facial Muscle, Percutaneous Endoscopic Approach
0K9200Z	Drainage of Right Neck Muscle with Drainage Device, Open Approach
0K920ZX	Drainage of Right Neck Muscle, Open Approach, Diagnostic
0K920ZZ	Drainage of Right Neck Muscle, Open Approach
0K9230Z	Drainage of Right Neck Muscle with Drainage Device, Percutaneous Approach
0K923ZX	Drainage of Right Neck Muscle, Percutaneous Approach, Diagnostic
0K923ZZ	Drainage of Right Neck Muscle, Percutaneous Approach
0K9240Z	Drainage of Right Neck Muscle with Drainage Device, Percutaneous Endoscopic Approach
0K924ZX	Drainage of Right Neck Muscle, Percutaneous Endoscopic Approach, Diagnostic
0K924ZZ	Drainage of Right Neck Muscle, Percutaneous Endoscopic Approach
0K9300Z	Drainage of Left Neck Muscle with Drainage Device, Open Approach
0K930ZX	Drainage of Left Neck Muscle, Open Approach, Diagnostic
0K930ZZ	Drainage of Left Neck Muscle, Open Approach
0K9330Z	Drainage of Left Neck Muscle with Drainage Device, Percutaneous Approach
0K933ZX	Drainage of Left Neck Muscle, Percutaneous Approach, Diagnostic
0K933ZZ	Drainage of Left Neck Muscle, Percutaneous Approach
0K9340Z	Drainage of Left Neck Muscle with Drainage Device, Percutaneous Endoscopic Approach
0K934ZX	Drainage of Left Neck Muscle, Percutaneous Endoscopic Approach, Diagnostic
0K934ZZ	Drainage of Left Neck Muscle, Percutaneous Endoscopic Approach
0K9400Z	Drainage of Tongue, Palate, Pharynx Muscle with Drainage Device, Open Approach
0K940ZX	Drainage of Tongue, Palate, Pharynx Muscle, Open Approach, Diagnostic
0K940ZZ	Drainage of Tongue, Palate, Pharynx Muscle, Open Approach
0K9430Z	Drainage of Tongue, Palate, Pharynx Muscle with Drainage Device, Percutaneous Approach
0K943ZX	Drainage of Tongue, Palate, Pharynx Muscle, Percutaneous Approach, Diagnostic
0K943ZZ	Drainage of Tongue, Palate, Pharynx Muscle, Percutaneous Approach
0K9440Z	Drainage of Tongue, Palate, Pharynx Muscle with Drainage Device, Percutaneous Endoscopic Approach
0K944ZX	Drainage of Tongue, Palate, Pharynx Muscle, Percutaneous Endoscopic Approach, Diagnostic
0K944ZZ	Drainage of Tongue, Palate, Pharynx Muscle, Percutaneous Endoscopic Approach
0K9500Z	Drainage of Right Shoulder Muscle with Drainage Device, Open Approach
0K950ZX	Drainage of Right Shoulder Muscle, Open Approach, Diagnostic
0K950ZZ	Drainage of Right Shoulder Muscle, Open Approach
0K9530Z	Drainage of Right Shoulder Muscle with Drainage Device, Percutaneous Approach
0K953ZX	Drainage of Right Shoulder Muscle, Percutaneous Approach, Diagnostic

0K953ZZ   Drainage of Right Shoulder Muscle, Percutaneous Approach

0K9540Z   Drainage of Right Shoulder Muscle with Drainage Device, Percutaneous Endoscopic Approach

0K954ZX   Drainage of Right Shoulder Muscle, Percutaneous Endoscopic Approach, Diagnostic

0K954ZZ   Drainage of Right Shoulder Muscle, Percutaneous Endoscopic Approach

0K9600Z   Drainage of Left Shoulder Muscle with Drainage Device, Open Approach

0K960ZX   Drainage of Left Shoulder Muscle, Open Approach, Diagnostic

0K960ZZ   Drainage of Left Shoulder Muscle, Open Approach

0K9630Z   Drainage of Left Shoulder Muscle with Drainage Device, Percutaneous Approach

0K963ZX   Drainage of Left Shoulder Muscle, Percutaneous Approach, Diagnostic

0K963ZZ   Drainage of Left Shoulder Muscle, Percutaneous Approach

0K9640Z   Drainage of Left Shoulder Muscle with Drainage Device, Percutaneous Endoscopic Approach

0K964ZX   Drainage of Left Shoulder Muscle, Percutaneous Endoscopic Approach, Diagnostic

0K964ZZ   Drainage of Left Shoulder Muscle, Percutaneous Endoscopic Approach

0K9700Z   Drainage of Right Upper Arm Muscle with Drainage Device, Open Approach

0K970ZX   Drainage of Right Upper Arm Muscle, Open Approach, Diagnostic

0K970ZZ   Drainage of Right Upper Arm Muscle, Open Approach

0K9730Z   Drainage of Right Upper Arm Muscle with Drainage Device, Percutaneous Approach

0K973ZX   Drainage of Right Upper Arm Muscle, Percutaneous Approach, Diagnostic

0K973ZZ   Drainage of Right Upper Arm Muscle, Percutaneous Approach

0K9740Z   Drainage of Right Upper Arm Muscle with Drainage Device, Percutaneous Endoscopic Approach

0K974ZX   Drainage of Right Upper Arm Muscle, Percutaneous Endoscopic Approach, Diagnostic

0K974ZZ   Drainage of Right Upper Arm Muscle, Percutaneous Endoscopic Approach

0K9800Z   Drainage of Left Upper Arm Muscle with Drainage Device, Open Approach

0K980ZX   Drainage of Left Upper Arm Muscle, Open Approach, Diagnostic

0K980ZZ   Drainage of Left Upper Arm Muscle, Open Approach

0K9830Z   Drainage of Left Upper Arm Muscle with Drainage Device, Percutaneous Approach

0K983ZX   Drainage of Left Upper Arm Muscle, Percutaneous Approach, Diagnostic

0K983ZZ   Drainage of Left Upper Arm Muscle, Percutaneous Approach

0K9840Z   Drainage of Left Upper Arm Muscle with Drainage Device, Percutaneous Endoscopic Approach

0K984ZX   Drainage of Left Upper Arm Muscle, Percutaneous Endoscopic Approach, Diagnostic

0K984ZZ   Drainage of Left Upper Arm Muscle, Percutaneous Endoscopic Approach

0K9900Z   Drainage of Right Lower Arm and Wrist Muscle with Drainage Device, Open Approach

0K990ZX   Drainage of Right Lower Arm and Wrist Muscle, Open Approach, Diagnostic

0K990ZZ   Drainage of Right Lower Arm and Wrist Muscle, Open Approach

0K9930Z   Drainage of Right Lower Arm and Wrist Muscle with Drainage Device, Percutaneous Approach

0K993ZX   Drainage of Right Lower Arm and Wrist Muscle, Percutaneous Approach, Diagnostic

0K993ZZ   Drainage of Right Lower Arm and Wrist Muscle, Percutaneous Approach

0K9940Z   Drainage of Right Lower Arm and Wrist Muscle with Drainage Device, Percutaneous Endoscopic Approach

0K994ZX   Drainage of Right Lower Arm and Wrist Muscle, Percutaneous Endoscopic Approach, Diagnostic

0K994ZZ   Drainage of Right Lower Arm and Wrist Muscle, Percutaneous Endoscopic Approach

0K9B00Z   Drainage of Left Lower Arm and Wrist Muscle with Drainage Device, Open Approach

0K9B0ZX   Drainage of Left Lower Arm and Wrist Muscle, Open Approach, Diagnostic

0K9B0ZZ   Drainage of Left Lower Arm and Wrist Muscle, Open Approach

0K9B30Z   Drainage of Left Lower Arm and Wrist Muscle with Drainage Device, Percutaneous Approach

0K9B3ZX   Drainage of Left Lower Arm and Wrist Muscle, Percutaneous Approach, Diagnostic

0K9B3ZZ   Drainage of Left Lower Arm and Wrist Muscle, Percutaneous Approach

0K9B40Z   Drainage of Left Lower Arm and Wrist Muscle with Drainage Device, Percutaneous Endoscopic Approach

0K9B4ZX   Drainage of Left Lower Arm and Wrist Muscle, Percutaneous Endoscopic Approach, Diagnostic

0K9B4ZZ   Drainage of Left Lower Arm and Wrist Muscle, Percutaneous Endoscopic Approach

0K9C00Z   Drainage of Right Hand Muscle with Drainage Device, Open Approach

0K9C0ZX   Drainage of Right Hand Muscle, Open Approach, Diagnostic

0K9C0ZZ   Drainage of Right Hand Muscle, Open Approach

0K9C30Z   Drainage of Right Hand Muscle with Drainage Device, Percutaneous Approach

0K9C3ZX   Drainage of Right Hand Muscle, Percutaneous Approach, Diagnostic

0K9C3ZZ   Drainage of Right Hand Muscle, Percutaneous Approach

0K9C40Z   Drainage of Right Hand Muscle with Drainage Device, Percutaneous Endoscopic Approach

0K9C4ZX   Drainage of Right Hand Muscle, Percutaneous Endoscopic Approach, Diagnostic

0K9C4ZZ   Drainage of Right Hand Muscle, Percutaneous Endoscopic Approach

0K9D00Z   Drainage of Left Hand Muscle with Drainage Device, Open Approach

0K9D0ZX   Drainage of Left Hand Muscle, Open Approach, Diagnostic

0K9D0ZZ   Drainage of Left Hand Muscle, Open Approach

0K9D30Z   Drainage of Left Hand Muscle with Drainage Device, Percutaneous Approach

0K9D3ZX   Drainage of Left Hand Muscle, Percutaneous Approach, Diagnostic

0K9D3ZZ   Drainage of Left Hand Muscle, Percutaneous Approach

0K9D40Z   Drainage of Left Hand Muscle with Drainage Device, Percutaneous Endoscopic Approach

0K9D4ZX   Drainage of Left Hand Muscle, Percutaneous Endoscopic Approach, Diagnostic

0K9D4ZZ   Drainage of Left Hand Muscle, Percutaneous Endoscopic Approach

0K9F00Z   Drainage of Right Trunk Muscle with Drainage Device, Open Approach

0K9F0ZX   Drainage of Right Trunk Muscle, Open Approach, Diagnostic

0K9F0ZZ   Drainage of Right Trunk Muscle, Open Approach

0K9F30Z   Drainage of Right Trunk Muscle with Drainage Device, Percutaneous Approach

0K9F3ZX   Drainage of Right Trunk Muscle, Percutaneous Approach, Diagnostic

0K9F3ZZ   Drainage of Right Trunk Muscle, Percutaneous Approach

0K9F40Z   Drainage of Right Trunk Muscle with Drainage Device, Percutaneous Endoscopic Approach

0K9F4ZX   Drainage of Right Trunk Muscle, Percutaneous Endoscopic Approach, Diagnostic

0K9F4ZZ   Drainage of Right Trunk Muscle, Percutaneous Endoscopic Approach

0K9G00Z   Drainage of Left Trunk Muscle with Drainage Device, Open Approach

0K9G0ZX   Drainage of Left Trunk Muscle, Open Approach, Diagnostic

0K9G0ZZ   Drainage of Left Trunk Muscle, Open Approach

0K9G30Z   Drainage of Left Trunk Muscle with Drainage Device, Percutaneous Approach

0K9G3ZX   Drainage of Left Trunk Muscle, Percutaneous Approach, Diagnostic

0K9G3ZZ   Drainage of Left Trunk Muscle, Percutaneous Approach

0K9G40Z   Drainage of Left Trunk Muscle with Drainage Device, Percutaneous Endoscopic Approach

0K9G4ZX   Drainage of Left Trunk Muscle, Percutaneous Endoscopic Approach, Diagnostic

0K9G4ZZ   Drainage of Left Trunk Muscle, Percutaneous Endoscopic Approach

0K9H00Z   Drainage of Right Thorax Muscle with Drainage Device, Open Approach

0K9H0ZX   Drainage of Right Thorax Muscle, Open Approach, Diagnostic

0K9H0ZZ   Drainage of Right Thorax Muscle, Open Approach

0K9H30Z   Drainage of Right Thorax Muscle with Drainage Device, Percutaneous Approach

0K9H3ZX   Drainage of Right Thorax Muscle, Percutaneous Approach, Diagnostic

0K9H3ZZ   Drainage of Right Thorax Muscle, Percutaneous Approach

0K9H40Z   Drainage of Right Thorax Muscle with Drainage Device, Percutaneous Endoscopic Approach

0K9H4ZX   Drainage of Right Thorax Muscle, Percutaneous Endoscopic Approach, Diagnostic

0K9H4ZZ   Drainage of Right Thorax Muscle, Percutaneous Endoscopic Approach

0K9J00Z   Drainage of Left Thorax Muscle with Drainage Device, Open Approach

0K9J0ZX   Drainage of Left Thorax Muscle, Open Approach, Diagnostic

0K9J0ZZ   Drainage of Left Thorax Muscle, Open Approach

0K9J30Z   Drainage of Left Thorax Muscle with Drainage Device, Percutaneous Approach

0K9J3ZX   Drainage of Left Thorax Muscle, Percutaneous Approach, Diagnostic

0K9J3ZZ   Drainage of Left Thorax Muscle, Percutaneous Approach

0K9J40Z   Drainage of Left Thorax Muscle with Drainage Device, Percutaneous Endoscopic Approach

0K9J4ZX   Drainage of Left Thorax Muscle, Percutaneous Endoscopic Approach, Diagnostic

0K9J4ZZ   Drainage of Left Thorax Muscle, Percutaneous Endoscopic Approach

0K9K00Z   Drainage of Right Abdomen Muscle with Drainage Device, Open Approach

0K9K0ZX   Drainage of Right Abdomen Muscle, Open Approach, Diagnostic

0K9K0ZZ   Drainage of Right Abdomen Muscle, Open Approach

0K9K30Z   Drainage of Right Abdomen Muscle with Drainage Device, Percutaneous Approach

0K9K3ZX   Drainage of Right Abdomen Muscle, Percutaneous Approach, Diagnostic

0K9K3ZZ   Drainage of Right Abdomen Muscle, Percutaneous Approach

0K9K40Z   Drainage of Right Abdomen Muscle with Drainage Device, Percutaneous Endoscopic Approach

0K9K4ZX   Drainage of Right Abdomen Muscle, Percutaneous Endoscopic Approach, Diagnostic

0K9K4ZZ   Drainage of Right Abdomen Muscle, Percutaneous Endoscopic Approach

0K9L00Z   Drainage of Left Abdomen Muscle with Drainage Device, Open Approach

0K9L0ZX   Drainage of Left Abdomen Muscle, Open Approach, Diagnostic

0K9L0ZZ   Drainage of Left Abdomen Muscle, Open Approach

0K9L30Z   Drainage of Left Abdomen Muscle with Drainage Device, Percutaneous Approach

0K9L3ZX   Drainage of Left Abdomen Muscle, Percutaneous Approach, Diagnostic

0K9L3ZZ   Drainage of Left Abdomen Muscle, Percutaneous Approach

0K9L40Z   Drainage of Left Abdomen Muscle with Drainage Device, Percutaneous Endoscopic Approach

0K9L4ZX   Drainage of Left Abdomen Muscle, Percutaneous Endoscopic Approach, Diagnostic

0K9L4ZZ   Drainage of Left Abdomen Muscle, Percutaneous Endoscopic Approach

0K9M00Z   Drainage of Perineum Muscle with Drainage Device, Open Approach

0K9M0ZX   Drainage of Perineum Muscle, Open Approach, Diagnostic

0K9M0ZZ   Drainage of Perineum Muscle, Open Approach

0K9M30Z   Drainage of Perineum Muscle with Drainage Device, Percutaneous Approach

0K9M3ZX   Drainage of Perineum Muscle, Percutaneous Approach, Diagnostic

0K9M3ZZ   Drainage of Perineum Muscle, Percutaneous Approach

0K9M40Z   Drainage of Perineum Muscle with Drainage Device, Percutaneous Endoscopic Approach

0K9M4ZX   Drainage of Perineum Muscle, Percutaneous Endoscopic Approach, Diagnostic

0K9M4ZZ   Drainage of Perineum Muscle, Percutaneous Endoscopic Approach

0K9N00Z   Drainage of Right Hip Muscle with Drainage Device, Open Approach

0K9N0ZX   Drainage of Right Hip Muscle, Open Approach, Diagnostic

0K9N0ZZ   Drainage of Right Hip Muscle, Open Approach

0K9N30Z   Drainage of Right Hip Muscle with Drainage Device, Percutaneous Approach

0K9N3ZX   Drainage of Right Hip Muscle, Percutaneous Approach, Diagnostic

0K9N3ZZ   Drainage of Right Hip Muscle, Percutaneous Approach

0K9N40Z   Drainage of Right Hip Muscle with Drainage Device, Percutaneous Endoscopic Approach

0K9N4ZX   Drainage of Right Hip Muscle, Percutaneous Endoscopic Approach, Diagnostic

0K9N4ZZ   Drainage of Right Hip Muscle, Percutaneous Endoscopic Approach

0K9P00Z   Drainage of Left Hip Muscle with Drainage Device, Open Approach

0K9P0ZX   Drainage of Left Hip Muscle, Open Approach, Diagnostic

0K9P0ZZ   Drainage of Left Hip Muscle, Open Approach

0K9P30Z   Drainage of Left Hip Muscle with Drainage Device, Percutaneous Approach

0K9P3ZX   Drainage of Left Hip Muscle, Percutaneous Approach, Diagnostic

0K9P3ZZ   Drainage of Left Hip Muscle, Percutaneous Approach

0K9P40Z   Drainage of Left Hip Muscle with Drainage Device, Percutaneous Endoscopic Approach

0K9P4ZX   Drainage of Left Hip Muscle, Percutaneous Endoscopic Approach, Diagnostic

0K9P4ZZ   Drainage of Left Hip Muscle, Percutaneous Endoscopic Approach

0K9Q00Z   Drainage of Right Upper Leg Muscle with Drainage Device, Open Approach

0K9Q0ZX   Drainage of Right Upper Leg Muscle, Open Approach, Diagnostic

0K9Q0ZZ   Drainage of Right Upper Leg Muscle, Open Approach

0K9Q30Z   Drainage of Right Upper Leg Muscle with Drainage Device, Percutaneous Approach

0K9Q3ZX   Drainage of Right Upper Leg Muscle, Percutaneous Approach, Diagnostic

0K9Q3ZZ   Drainage of Right Upper Leg Muscle, Percutaneous Approach

0K9Q40Z   Drainage of Right Upper Leg Muscle with Drainage Device, Percutaneous Endoscopic Approach

0K9Q4ZX   Drainage of Right Upper Leg Muscle, Percutaneous Endoscopic Approach, Diagnostic

0K9Q4ZZ   Drainage of Right Upper Leg Muscle, Percutaneous Endoscopic Approach

0K9R00Z   Drainage of Left Upper Leg Muscle with Drainage Device, Open Approach

0K9R0ZX   Drainage of Left Upper Leg Muscle, Open Approach, Diagnostic

0K9R0ZZ   Drainage of Left Upper Leg Muscle, Open Approach

0K9R30Z   Drainage of Left Upper Leg Muscle with Drainage Device, Percutaneous Approach

0K9R3ZX   Drainage of Left Upper Leg Muscle, Percutaneous Approach, Diagnostic

0K9R3ZZ   Drainage of Left Upper Leg Muscle, Percutaneous Approach

0K9R40Z   Drainage of Left Upper Leg Muscle with Drainage Device, Percutaneous Endoscopic Approach

0K9R4ZX   Drainage of Left Upper Leg Muscle, Percutaneous Endoscopic Approach, Diagnostic

0K9R4ZZ   Drainage of Left Upper Leg Muscle, Percutaneous Endoscopic Approach

0K9S00Z   Drainage of Right Lower Leg Muscle with Drainage Device, Open Approach

0K9S0ZX   Drainage of Right Lower Leg Muscle, Open Approach, Diagnostic

0K9S0ZZ   Drainage of Right Lower Leg Muscle, Open Approach

0K9S30Z   Drainage of Right Lower Leg Muscle with Drainage Device, Percutaneous Approach

0K9S3ZX   Drainage of Right Lower Leg Muscle, Percutaneous Approach, Diagnostic

0K9S3ZZ   Drainage of Right Lower Leg Muscle, Percutaneous Approach

0K9S40Z   Drainage of Right Lower Leg Muscle with Drainage Device, Percutaneous Endoscopic Approach

0K9S4ZX   Drainage of Right Lower Leg Muscle, Percutaneous Endoscopic Approach, Diagnostic

0K9S4ZZ   Drainage of Right Lower Leg Muscle, Percutaneous Endoscopic Approach

0K9T00Z   Drainage of Left Lower Leg Muscle with Drainage Device, Open Approach

0K9T0ZX   Drainage of Left Lower Leg Muscle, Open Approach, Diagnostic

0K9T0ZZ   Drainage of Left Lower Leg Muscle, Open Approach

0K9T30Z   Drainage of Left Lower Leg Muscle with Drainage Device, Percutaneous Approach

0K9T3ZX Drainage of Left Lower Leg Muscle, Percutaneous Approach, Diagnostic
0K9T3ZZ Drainage of Left Lower Leg Muscle, Percutaneous Approach
0K9T40Z Drainage of Left Lower Leg Muscle with Drainage Device, Percutaneous Endoscopic Approach
0K9T4ZX Drainage of Left Lower Leg Muscle, Percutaneous Endoscopic Approach, Diagnostic
0K9T4ZZ Drainage of Left Lower Leg Muscle, Percutaneous Endoscopic Approach
0K9V00Z Drainage of Right Foot Muscle with Drainage Device, Open Approach
0K9V0ZX Drainage of Right Foot Muscle, Open Approach, Diagnostic
0K9V0ZZ Drainage of Right Foot Muscle, Open Approach
0K9V30Z Drainage of Right Foot Muscle with Drainage Device, Percutaneous Approach
0K9V3ZX Drainage of Right Foot Muscle, Percutaneous Approach, Diagnostic
0K9V3ZZ Drainage of Right Foot Muscle, Percutaneous Approach
0K9V40Z Drainage of Right Foot Muscle with Drainage Device, Percutaneous Endoscopic Approach

0K9V4ZX Drainage of Right Foot Muscle, Percutaneous Endoscopic Approach, Diagnostic
0K9V4ZZ Drainage of Right Foot Muscle, Percutaneous Endoscopic Approach
0K9W00Z Drainage of Left Foot Muscle with Drainage Device, Open Approach
0K9W0ZX Drainage of Left Foot Muscle, Open Approach, Diagnostic
0K9W0ZZ Drainage of Left Foot Muscle, Open Approach
0K9W30Z Drainage of Left Foot Muscle with Drainage Device, Percutaneous Approach
0K9W3ZX Drainage of Left Foot Muscle, Percutaneous Approach, Diagnostic
0K9W3ZZ Drainage of Left Foot Muscle, Percutaneous Approach
0K9W40Z Drainage of Left Foot Muscle with Drainage Device, Percutaneous Endoscopic Approach
0K9W4ZX Drainage of Left Foot Muscle, Percutaneous Endoscopic Approach, Diagnostic
0K9W4ZZ Drainage of Left Foot Muscle, Percutaneous Endoscopic Approach

0KB – Muscles, Excision

Review Coding Guidelines B3.4a and B3.4b

Review Coding Guideline B3.5

Review Coding Guideline B3.8

0KB00ZX Excision of Head Muscle, Open Approach, Diagnostic
0KB00ZZ Excision of Head Muscle, Open Approach
0KB03ZX Excision of Head Muscle, Percutaneous Approach, Diagnostic
0KB03ZZ Excision of Head Muscle, Percutaneous Approach
0KB04ZX Excision of Head Muscle, Percutaneous Endoscopic Approach, Diagnostic
0KB04ZZ Excision of Head Muscle, Percutaneous Endoscopic Approach
0KB10ZX Excision of Facial Muscle, Open Approach, Diagnostic
0KB10ZZ Excision of Facial Muscle, Open Approach
0KB13ZX Excision of Facial Muscle, Percutaneous Approach, Diagnostic
0KB13ZZ Excision of Facial Muscle, Percutaneous Approach
0KB14ZX Excision of Facial Muscle, Percutaneous Endoscopic Approach, Diagnostic
0KB14ZZ Excision of Facial Muscle, Percutaneous Endoscopic Approach
0KB20ZX Excision of Right Neck Muscle, Open Approach, Diagnostic
0KB20ZZ Excision of Right Neck Muscle, Open Approach
0KB23ZX Excision of Right Neck Muscle, Percutaneous Approach, Diagnostic
0KB23ZZ Excision of Right Neck Muscle, Percutaneous Approach
0KB24ZX Excision of Right Neck Muscle, Percutaneous Endoscopic Approach, Diagnostic
0KB24ZZ Excision of Right Neck Muscle, Percutaneous Endoscopic Approach
0KB30ZX Excision of Left Neck Muscle, Open Approach, Diagnostic
0KB30ZZ Excision of Left Neck Muscle, Open Approach
0KB33ZX Excision of Left Neck Muscle, Percutaneous Approach, Diagnostic
0KB33ZZ Excision of Left Neck Muscle, Percutaneous Approach
0KB34ZX Excision of Left Neck Muscle, Percutaneous Endoscopic Approach, Diagnostic
0KB34ZZ Excision of Left Neck Muscle, Percutaneous Endoscopic Approach
0KB40ZX Excision of Tongue, Palate, Pharynx Muscle, Open Approach, Diagnostic
0KB40ZZ Excision of Tongue, Palate, Pharynx Muscle, Open Approach
0KB43ZX Excision of Tongue, Palate, Pharynx Muscle, Percutaneous Approach, Diagnostic
0KB43ZZ Excision of Tongue, Palate, Pharynx Muscle, Percutaneous Approach
0KB44ZX Excision of Tongue, Palate, Pharynx Muscle, Percutaneous Endoscopic Approach, Diagnostic
0KB44ZZ Excision of Tongue, Palate, Pharynx Muscle, Percutaneous Endoscopic Approach
0KB50ZX Excision of Right Shoulder Muscle, Open Approach, Diagnostic
0KB50ZZ Excision of Right Shoulder Muscle, Open Approach
0KB53ZX Excision of Right Shoulder Muscle, Percutaneous Approach, Diagnostic
0KB53ZZ Excision of Right Shoulder Muscle, Percutaneous Approach

0KB54ZX Excision of Right Shoulder Muscle, Percutaneous Endoscopic Approach, Diagnostic
0KB54ZZ Excision of Right Shoulder Muscle, Percutaneous Endoscopic Approach
0KB60ZX Excision of Left Shoulder Muscle, Open Approach, Diagnostic
0KB60ZZ Excision of Left Shoulder Muscle, Open Approach
0KB63ZX Excision of Left Shoulder Muscle, Percutaneous Approach, Diagnostic
0KB63ZZ Excision of Left Shoulder Muscle, Percutaneous Approach
0KB64ZX Excision of Left Shoulder Muscle, Percutaneous Endoscopic Approach, Diagnostic
0KB64ZZ Excision of Left Shoulder Muscle, Percutaneous Endoscopic Approach
0KB70ZX Excision of Right Upper Arm Muscle, Open Approach, Diagnostic
0KB70ZZ Excision of Right Upper Arm Muscle, Open Approach
0KB73ZX Excision of Right Upper Arm Muscle, Percutaneous Approach, Diagnostic
0KB73ZZ Excision of Right Upper Arm Muscle, Percutaneous Approach
0KB74ZX Excision of Right Upper Arm Muscle, Percutaneous Endoscopic Approach, Diagnostic
0KB74ZZ Excision of Right Upper Arm Muscle, Percutaneous Endoscopic Approach
0KB80ZX Excision of Left Upper Arm Muscle, Open Approach, Diagnostic
0KB80ZZ Excision of Left Upper Arm Muscle, Open Approach
0KB83ZX Excision of Left Upper Arm Muscle, Percutaneous Approach, Diagnostic
0KB83ZZ Excision of Left Upper Arm Muscle, Percutaneous Approach
0KB84ZX Excision of Left Upper Arm Muscle, Percutaneous Endoscopic Approach, Diagnostic
0KB84ZZ Excision of Left Upper Arm Muscle, Percutaneous Endoscopic Approach
0KB90ZX Excision of Right Lower Arm and Wrist Muscle, Open Approach, Diagnostic
0KB90ZZ Excision of Right Lower Arm and Wrist Muscle, Open Approach
0KB93ZX Excision of Right Lower Arm and Wrist Muscle, Percutaneous Approach, Diagnostic
0KB93ZZ Excision of Right Lower Arm and Wrist Muscle, Percutaneous Approach
0KB94ZX Excision of Right Lower Arm and Wrist Muscle, Percutaneous Endoscopic Approach, Diagnostic
0KB94ZZ Excision of Right Lower Arm and Wrist Muscle, Percutaneous Endoscopic Approach
0KBB0ZX Excision of Left Lower Arm and Wrist Muscle, Open Approach, Diagnostic
0KBB0ZZ Excision of Left Lower Arm and Wrist Muscle, Open Approach

0KBB3ZX Excision of Left Lower Arm and Wrist Muscle, Percutaneous Approach, Diagnostic

0KBB3ZZ Excision of Left Lower Arm and Wrist Muscle, Percutaneous Approach

0KBB4ZX Excision of Left Lower Arm and Wrist Muscle, Percutaneous Endoscopic Approach, Diagnostic

0KBB4ZZ Excision of Left Lower Arm and Wrist Muscle, Percutaneous Endoscopic Approach

0KBC0ZX Excision of Right Hand Muscle, Open Approach, Diagnostic

0KBC0ZZ Excision of Right Hand Muscle, Open Approach

0KBC3ZX Excision of Right Hand Muscle, Percutaneous Approach, Diagnostic

0KBC3ZZ Excision of Right Hand Muscle, Percutaneous Approach

0KBC4ZX Excision of Right Hand Muscle, Percutaneous Endoscopic Approach, Diagnostic

0KBC4ZZ Excision of Right Hand Muscle, Percutaneous Endoscopic Approach

0KBD0ZX Excision of Left Hand Muscle, Open Approach, Diagnostic

0KBD0ZZ Excision of Left Hand Muscle, Open Approach

0KBD3ZX Excision of Left Hand Muscle, Percutaneous Approach, Diagnostic

0KBD3ZZ Excision of Left Hand Muscle, Percutaneous Approach

0KBD4ZX Excision of Left Hand Muscle, Percutaneous Endoscopic Approach, Diagnostic

0KBD4ZZ Excision of Left Hand Muscle, Percutaneous Endoscopic Approach

0KBF0ZX Excision of Right Trunk Muscle, Open Approach, Diagnostic

0KBF0ZZ Excision of Right Trunk Muscle, Open Approach

0KBF3ZX Excision of Right Trunk Muscle, Percutaneous Approach, Diagnostic

0KBF3ZZ Excision of Right Trunk Muscle, Percutaneous Approach

0KBF4ZX Excision of Right Trunk Muscle, Percutaneous Endoscopic Approach, Diagnostic

0KBF4ZZ Excision of Right Trunk Muscle, Percutaneous Endoscopic Approach

0KBG0ZX Excision of Left Trunk Muscle, Open Approach, Diagnostic

0KBG0ZZ Excision of Left Trunk Muscle, Open Approach

0KBG3ZX Excision of Left Trunk Muscle, Percutaneous Approach, Diagnostic

0KBG3ZZ Excision of Left Trunk Muscle, Percutaneous Approach

0KBG4ZX Excision of Left Trunk Muscle, Percutaneous Endoscopic Approach, Diagnostic

0KBG4ZZ Excision of Left Trunk Muscle, Percutaneous Endoscopic Approach

0KBH0ZX Excision of Right Thorax Muscle, Open Approach, Diagnostic

0KBH0ZZ Excision of Right Thorax Muscle, Open Approach

0KBH3ZX Excision of Right Thorax Muscle, Percutaneous Approach, Diagnostic

0KBH3ZZ Excision of Right Thorax Muscle, Percutaneous Approach

0KBH4ZX Excision of Right Thorax Muscle, Percutaneous Endoscopic Approach, Diagnostic

0KBH4ZZ Excision of Right Thorax Muscle, Percutaneous Endoscopic Approach

0KBJ0ZX Excision of Left Thorax Muscle, Open Approach, Diagnostic

0KBJ0ZZ Excision of Left Thorax Muscle, Open Approach

0KBJ3ZX Excision of Left Thorax Muscle, Percutaneous Approach, Diagnostic

0KBJ3ZZ Excision of Left Thorax Muscle, Percutaneous Approach

0KBJ4ZX Excision of Left Thorax Muscle, Percutaneous Endoscopic Approach, Diagnostic

0KBJ4ZZ Excision of Left Thorax Muscle, Percutaneous Endoscopic Approach

0KBK0ZX Excision of Right Abdomen Muscle, Open Approach, Diagnostic

0KBK0ZZ Excision of Right Abdomen Muscle, Open Approach

0KBK3ZX Excision of Right Abdomen Muscle, Percutaneous Approach, Diagnostic

0KBK3ZZ Excision of Right Abdomen Muscle, Percutaneous Approach

0KBK4ZX Excision of Right Abdomen Muscle, Percutaneous Endoscopic Approach, Diagnostic

0KBK4ZZ Excision of Right Abdomen Muscle, Percutaneous Endoscopic Approach

0KBL0ZX Excision of Left Abdomen Muscle, Open Approach, Diagnostic

0KBL0ZZ Excision of Left Abdomen Muscle, Open Approach

0KBL3ZX Excision of Left Abdomen Muscle, Percutaneous Approach, Diagnostic

0KBL3ZZ Excision of Left Abdomen Muscle, Percutaneous Approach

0KBL4ZX Excision of Left Abdomen Muscle, Percutaneous Endoscopic Approach, Diagnostic

0KBL4ZZ Excision of Left Abdomen Muscle, Percutaneous Endoscopic Approach

0KBM0ZX Excision of Perineum Muscle, Open Approach, Diagnostic

0KBM0ZZ Excision of Perineum Muscle, Open Approach

0KBM3ZX Excision of Perineum Muscle, Percutaneous Approach, Diagnostic

0KBM3ZZ Excision of Perineum Muscle, Percutaneous Approach

0KBM4ZX Excision of Perineum Muscle, Percutaneous Endoscopic Approach, Diagnostic

0KBM4ZZ Excision of Perineum Muscle, Percutaneous Endoscopic Approach

0KBN0ZX Excision of Right Hip Muscle, Open Approach, Diagnostic

0KBN0ZZ Excision of Right Hip Muscle, Open Approach

0KBN3ZX Excision of Right Hip Muscle, Percutaneous Approach, Diagnostic

0KBN3ZZ Excision of Right Hip Muscle, Percutaneous Approach

0KBN4ZX Excision of Right Hip Muscle, Percutaneous Endoscopic Approach, Diagnostic

0KBN4ZZ Excision of Right Hip Muscle, Percutaneous Endoscopic Approach

0KBP0ZX Excision of Left Hip Muscle, Open Approach, Diagnostic

0KBP0ZZ Excision of Left Hip Muscle, Open Approach

0KBP3ZX Excision of Left Hip Muscle, Percutaneous Approach, Diagnostic

0KBP3ZZ Excision of Left Hip Muscle, Percutaneous Approach

0KBP4ZX Excision of Left Hip Muscle, Percutaneous Endoscopic Approach, Diagnostic

0KBP4ZZ Excision of Left Hip Muscle, Percutaneous Endoscopic Approach

0KBQ0ZX Excision of Right Upper Leg Muscle, Open Approach, Diagnostic

0KBQ0ZZ Excision of Right Upper Leg Muscle, Open Approach

0KBQ3ZX Excision of Right Upper Leg Muscle, Percutaneous Approach, Diagnostic

0KBQ3ZZ Excision of Right Upper Leg Muscle, Percutaneous Approach

0KBQ4ZX Excision of Right Upper Leg Muscle, Percutaneous Endoscopic Approach, Diagnostic

0KBQ4ZZ Excision of Right Upper Leg Muscle, Percutaneous Endoscopic Approach

0KBR0ZX Excision of Left Upper Leg Muscle, Open Approach, Diagnostic

0KBR0ZZ Excision of Left Upper Leg Muscle, Open Approach

0KBR3ZX Excision of Left Upper Leg Muscle, Percutaneous Approach, Diagnostic

0KBR3ZZ Excision of Left Upper Leg Muscle, Percutaneous Approach

0KBR4ZX Excision of Left Upper Leg Muscle, Percutaneous Endoscopic Approach, Diagnostic

0KBR4ZZ Excision of Left Upper Leg Muscle, Percutaneous Endoscopic Approach

0KBS0ZX Excision of Right Lower Leg Muscle, Open Approach, Diagnostic

0KBS0ZZ Excision of Right Lower Leg Muscle, Open Approach

0KBS3ZX Excision of Right Lower Leg Muscle, Percutaneous Approach, Diagnostic

0KBS3ZZ Excision of Right Lower Leg Muscle, Percutaneous Approach

0KBS4ZX Excision of Right Lower Leg Muscle, Percutaneous Endoscopic Approach, Diagnostic

0KBS4ZZ Excision of Right Lower Leg Muscle, Percutaneous Endoscopic Approach

0KBT0ZX Excision of Left Lower Leg Muscle, Open Approach, Diagnostic

0KBT0ZZ Excision of Left Lower Leg Muscle, Open Approach

0KBT3ZX Excision of Left Lower Leg Muscle, Percutaneous Approach, Diagnostic

0KBT3ZZ Excision of Left Lower Leg Muscle, Percutaneous Approach

0KBT4ZX Excision of Left Lower Leg Muscle, Percutaneous Endoscopic Approach, Diagnostic

0KBT4ZZ Excision of Left Lower Leg Muscle, Percutaneous Endoscopic Approach

0KBV0ZX Excision of Right Foot Muscle, Open Approach, Diagnostic

0KBV0ZZ Excision of Right Foot Muscle, Open Approach

0KBV3ZX Excision of Right Foot Muscle, Percutaneous Approach, Diagnostic

0KBV3ZZ Excision of Right Foot Muscle, Percutaneous Approach

0KBV4ZX Excision of Right Foot Muscle, Percutaneous Endoscopic Approach, Diagnostic

0KBV4ZZ Excision of Right Foot Muscle, Percutaneous Endoscopic Approach

0KBW0ZX Excision of Left Foot Muscle, Open Approach, Diagnostic

0KBW0ZZ Excision of Left Foot Muscle, Open Approach

0KBW3ZX Excision of Left Foot Muscle, Percutaneous Approach, Diagnostic

0KBW3ZZ Excision of Left Foot Muscle, Percutaneous Approach

0KBW4ZX Excision of Left Foot Muscle, Percutaneous Endoscopic Approach, Diagnostic

0KBW4ZZ Excision of Left Foot Muscle, Percutaneous Endoscopic Approach

0KC – Muscles, Extirpation

0KC00ZZ	Extirpation of Matter from Head Muscle, Open Approach	**0KCG0ZZ**	Extirpation of Matter from Left Trunk Muscle, Open Approach
0KC03ZZ	Extirpation of Matter from Head Muscle, Percutaneous Approach	**0KCG3ZZ**	Extirpation of Matter from Left Trunk Muscle, Percutaneous Approach
0KC04ZZ	Extirpation of Matter from Head Muscle, Percutaneous Endoscopic Approach	**0KCG4ZZ**	Extirpation of Matter from Left Trunk Muscle, Percutaneous Endoscopic Approach
0KC10ZZ	Extirpation of Matter from Facial Muscle, Open Approach	**0KCH0ZZ**	Extirpation of Matter from Right Thorax Muscle, Open Approach
0KC13ZZ	Extirpation of Matter from Facial Muscle, Percutaneous Approach	**0KCH3ZZ**	Extirpation of Matter from Right Thorax Muscle, Percutaneous Approach
0KC14ZZ	Extirpation of Matter from Facial Muscle, Percutaneous Endoscopic Approach	**0KCH4ZZ**	Extirpation of Matter from Right Thorax Muscle, Percutaneous Endoscopic Approach
0KC20ZZ	Extirpation of Matter from Right Neck Muscle, Open Approach	**0KCJ0ZZ**	Extirpation of Matter from Left Thorax Muscle, Open Approach
0KC23ZZ	Extirpation of Matter from Right Neck Muscle, Percutaneous Approach	**0KCJ3ZZ**	Extirpation of Matter from Left Thorax Muscle, Percutaneous Approach
0KC24ZZ	Extirpation of Matter from Right Neck Muscle, Percutaneous Endoscopic Approach	**0KCJ4ZZ**	Extirpation of Matter from Left Thorax Muscle, Percutaneous Endoscopic Approach
0KC30ZZ	Extirpation of Matter from Left Neck Muscle, Open Approach	**0KCK0ZZ**	Extirpation of Matter from Right Abdomen Muscle, Open Approach
0KC33ZZ	Extirpation of Matter from Left Neck Muscle, Percutaneous Approach	**0KCK3ZZ**	Extirpation of Matter from Right Abdomen Muscle, Percutaneous Approach
0KC34ZZ	Extirpation of Matter from Left Neck Muscle, Percutaneous Endoscopic Approach	**0KCK4ZZ**	Extirpation of Matter from Right Abdomen Muscle, Percutaneous Endoscopic Approach
0KC40ZZ	Extirpation of Matter from Tongue, Palate, Pharynx Muscle, Open Approach	**0KCL0ZZ**	Extirpation of Matter from Left Abdomen Muscle, Open Approach
0KC43ZZ	Extirpation of Matter from Tongue, Palate, Pharynx Muscle, Percutaneous Approach	**0KCL3ZZ**	Extirpation of Matter from Left Abdomen Muscle, Percutaneous Approach
0KC44ZZ	Extirpation of Matter from Tongue, Palate, Pharynx Muscle, Percutaneous Endoscopic Approach	**0KCL4ZZ**	Extirpation of Matter from Left Abdomen Muscle, Percutaneous Endoscopic Approach
0KC50ZZ	Extirpation of Matter from Right Shoulder Muscle, Open Approach	**0KCM0ZZ**	Extirpation of Matter from Perineum Muscle, Open Approach
0KC53ZZ	Extirpation of Matter from Right Shoulder Muscle, Percutaneous Approach	**0KCM3ZZ**	Extirpation of Matter from Perineum Muscle, Percutaneous Approach
0KC54ZZ	Extirpation of Matter from Right Shoulder Muscle, Percutaneous Endoscopic Approach	**0KCM4ZZ**	Extirpation of Matter from Perineum Muscle, Percutaneous Endoscopic Approach
0KC60ZZ	Extirpation of Matter from Left Shoulder Muscle, Open Approach	**0KCN0ZZ**	Extirpation of Matter from Right Hip Muscle, Open Approach
0KC63ZZ	Extirpation of Matter from Left Shoulder Muscle, Percutaneous Approach	**0KCN3ZZ**	Extirpation of Matter from Right Hip Muscle, Percutaneous Approach
0KC64ZZ	Extirpation of Matter from Left Shoulder Muscle, Percutaneous Endoscopic Approach	**0KCN4ZZ**	Extirpation of Matter from Right Hip Muscle, Percutaneous Endoscopic Approach
0KC70ZZ	Extirpation of Matter from Right Upper Arm Muscle, Open Approach	**0KCP0ZZ**	Extirpation of Matter from Left Hip Muscle, Open Approach
0KC73ZZ	Extirpation of Matter from Right Upper Arm Muscle, Percutaneous Approach	**0KCP3ZZ**	Extirpation of Matter from Left Hip Muscle, Percutaneous Approach
0KC74ZZ	Extirpation of Matter from Right Upper Arm Muscle, Percutaneous Endoscopic Approach	**0KCP4ZZ**	Extirpation of Matter from Left Hip Muscle, Percutaneous Endoscopic Approach
0KC80ZZ	Extirpation of Matter from Left Upper Arm Muscle, Open Approach	**0KCQ0ZZ**	Extirpation of Matter from Right Upper Leg Muscle, Open Approach
0KC83ZZ	Extirpation of Matter from Left Upper Arm Muscle, Percutaneous Approach	**0KCQ3ZZ**	Extirpation of Matter from Right Upper Leg Muscle, Percutaneous Approach
0KC84ZZ	Extirpation of Matter from Left Upper Arm Muscle, Percutaneous Endoscopic Approach	**0KCQ4ZZ**	Extirpation of Matter from Right Upper Leg Muscle, Percutaneous Endoscopic Approach
0KC90ZZ	Extirpation of Matter from Right Lower Arm and Wrist Muscle, Open Approach	**0KCR0ZZ**	Extirpation of Matter from Left Upper Leg Muscle, Open Approach
0KC93ZZ	Extirpation of Matter from Right Lower Arm and Wrist Muscle, Percutaneous Approach	**0KCR3ZZ**	Extirpation of Matter from Left Upper Leg Muscle, Percutaneous Approach
0KC94ZZ	Extirpation of Matter from Right Lower Arm and Wrist Muscle, Percutaneous Endoscopic Approach	**0KCR4ZZ**	Extirpation of Matter from Left Upper Leg Muscle, Percutaneous Endoscopic Approach
0KCB0ZZ	Extirpation of Matter from Left Lower Arm and Wrist Muscle, Open Approach	**0KCS0ZZ**	Extirpation of Matter from Right Lower Leg Muscle, Open Approach
0KCB3ZZ	Extirpation of Matter from Left Lower Arm and Wrist Muscle, Percutaneous Approach	**0KCS3ZZ**	Extirpation of Matter from Right Lower Leg Muscle, Percutaneous Approach
0KCB4ZZ	Extirpation of Matter from Left Lower Arm and Wrist Muscle, Percutaneous Endoscopic Approach	**0KCS4ZZ**	Extirpation of Matter from Right Lower Leg Muscle, Percutaneous Endoscopic Approach
0KCC0ZZ	Extirpation of Matter from Right Hand Muscle, Open Approach	**0KCT0ZZ**	Extirpation of Matter from Left Lower Leg Muscle, Open Approach
0KCC3ZZ	Extirpation of Matter from Right Hand Muscle, Percutaneous Approach	**0KCT3ZZ**	Extirpation of Matter from Left Lower Leg Muscle, Percutaneous Approach
0KCC4ZZ	Extirpation of Matter from Right Hand Muscle, Percutaneous Endoscopic Approach	**0KCT4ZZ**	Extirpation of Matter from Left Lower Leg Muscle, Percutaneous Endoscopic Approach
0KCD0ZZ	Extirpation of Matter from Left Hand Muscle, Open Approach	**0KCV0ZZ**	Extirpation of Matter from Right Foot Muscle, Open Approach
0KCD3ZZ	Extirpation of Matter from Left Hand Muscle, Percutaneous Approach	**0KCV3ZZ**	Extirpation of Matter from Right Foot Muscle, Percutaneous Approach
0KCD4ZZ	Extirpation of Matter from Left Hand Muscle, Percutaneous Endoscopic Approach	**0KCV4ZZ**	Extirpation of Matter from Right Foot Muscle, Percutaneous Endoscopic Approach
0KCF0ZZ	Extirpation of Matter from Right Trunk Muscle, Open Approach	**0KCW0ZZ**	Extirpation of Matter from Left Foot Muscle, Open Approach
0KCF3ZZ	Extirpation of Matter from Right Trunk Muscle, Percutaneous Approach	**0KCW3ZZ**	Extirpation of Matter from Left Foot Muscle, Percutaneous Approach
0KCF4ZZ	Extirpation of Matter from Right Trunk Muscle, Percutaneous Endoscopic Approach	**0KCW4ZZ**	Extirpation of Matter from Left Foot Muscle, Percutaneous Endoscopic Approach

---

♀ Female-only   ♂ Male-only   ○ Limited Coverage   ● Non-OR   **HAC** HAC-associated procedure   ◆ Non-covered procedures   ✚ Combination

0KH – Muscles, Insertion

0KHX0MZ Insertion of Stimulator Lead into Upper Muscle, Open Approach
0KHX3MZ Insertion of Stimulator Lead into Upper Muscle, Percutaneous Approach
0KHX4MZ Insertion of Stimulator Lead into Upper Muscle, Percutaneous Endoscopic Approach

0KHY0MZ Insertion of Stimulator Lead into Lower Muscle, Open Approach
0KHY3MZ Insertion of Stimulator Lead into Lower Muscle, Percutaneous Approach
0KHY4MZ Insertion of Stimulator Lead into Lower Muscle, Percutaneous Endoscopic Approach

0KJ – Muscles, Inspection

Review Coding Guideline B3.5

Review Coding Guidelines B3.11a, B3.11b and B3.11c

0KJX0ZZ Inspection of Upper Muscle, Open Approach
0KJX3ZZ Inspection of Upper Muscle, Percutaneous Approach
0KJX4ZZ Inspection of Upper Muscle, Percutaneous Endoscopic Approach
0KJXXZZ Inspection of Upper Muscle, External Approach

0KJY0ZZ Inspection of Lower Muscle, Open Approach
0KJY3ZZ Inspection of Lower Muscle, Percutaneous Approach
0KJY4ZZ Inspection of Lower Muscle, Percutaneous Endoscopic Approach
0KJYXZZ Inspection of Lower Muscle, External Approach

0KM – Muscles, Reattachment

0KM00ZZ Reattachment of Head Muscle, Open Approach
0KM04ZZ Reattachment of Head Muscle, Percutaneous Endoscopic Approach
0KM10ZZ Reattachment of Facial Muscle, Open Approach
0KM14ZZ Reattachment of Facial Muscle, Percutaneous Endoscopic Approach
0KM20ZZ Reattachment of Right Neck Muscle, Open Approach
0KM24ZZ Reattachment of Right Neck Muscle, Percutaneous Endoscopic Approach
0KM30ZZ Reattachment of Left Neck Muscle, Open Approach
0KM34ZZ Reattachment of Left Neck Muscle, Percutaneous Endoscopic Approach
0KM40ZZ Reattachment of Tongue, Palate, Pharynx Muscle, Open Approach
0KM44ZZ Reattachment of Tongue, Palate, Pharynx Muscle, Percutaneous Endoscopic Approach
0KM50ZZ Reattachment of Right Shoulder Muscle, Open Approach
0KM54ZZ Reattachment of Right Shoulder Muscle, Percutaneous Endoscopic Approach
0KM60ZZ Reattachment of Left Shoulder Muscle, Open Approach
0KM64ZZ Reattachment of Left Shoulder Muscle, Percutaneous Endoscopic Approach
0KM70ZZ Reattachment of Right Upper Arm Muscle, Open Approach
0KM74ZZ Reattachment of Right Upper Arm Muscle, Percutaneous Endoscopic Approach
0KM80ZZ Reattachment of Left Upper Arm Muscle, Open Approach
0KM84ZZ Reattachment of Left Upper Arm Muscle, Percutaneous Endoscopic Approach
0KM90ZZ Reattachment of Right Lower Arm and Wrist Muscle, Open Approach
0KM94ZZ Reattachment of Right Lower Arm and Wrist Muscle, Percutaneous Endoscopic Approach
0KMB0ZZ Reattachment of Left Lower Arm and Wrist Muscle, Open Approach
0KMB4ZZ Reattachment of Left Lower Arm and Wrist Muscle, Percutaneous Endoscopic Approach
0KMC0ZZ Reattachment of Right Hand Muscle, Open Approach
0KMC4ZZ Reattachment of Right Hand Muscle, Percutaneous Endoscopic Approach
0KMD0ZZ Reattachment of Left Hand Muscle, Open Approach
0KMD4ZZ Reattachment of Left Hand Muscle, Percutaneous Endoscopic Approach
0KMF0ZZ Reattachment of Right Trunk Muscle, Open Approach
0KMF4ZZ Reattachment of Right Trunk Muscle, Percutaneous Endoscopic Approach

0KMG0ZZ Reattachment of Left Trunk Muscle, Open Approach
0KMG4ZZ Reattachment of Left Trunk Muscle, Percutaneous Endoscopic Approach
0KMH0ZZ Reattachment of Right Thorax Muscle, Open Approach
0KMH4ZZ Reattachment of Right Thorax Muscle, Percutaneous Endoscopic Approach
0KMJ0ZZ Reattachment of Left Thorax Muscle, Open Approach
0KMJ4ZZ Reattachment of Left Thorax Muscle, Percutaneous Endoscopic Approach
0KMK0ZZ Reattachment of Right Abdomen Muscle, Open Approach
0KMK4ZZ Reattachment of Right Abdomen Muscle, Percutaneous Endoscopic Approach
0KML0ZZ Reattachment of Left Abdomen Muscle, Open Approach
0KML4ZZ Reattachment of Left Abdomen Muscle, Percutaneous Endoscopic Approach
0KMM0ZZ Reattachment of Perineum Muscle, Open Approach
0KMM4ZZ Reattachment of Perineum Muscle, Percutaneous Endoscopic Approach
0KMN0ZZ Reattachment of Right Hip Muscle, Open Approach
0KMN4ZZ Reattachment of Right Hip Muscle, Percutaneous Endoscopic Approach
0KMP0ZZ Reattachment of Left Hip Muscle, Open Approach
0KMP4ZZ Reattachment of Left Hip Muscle, Percutaneous Endoscopic Approach
0KMQ0ZZ Reattachment of Right Upper Leg Muscle, Open Approach
0KMQ4ZZ Reattachment of Right Upper Leg Muscle, Percutaneous Endoscopic Approach
0KMR0ZZ Reattachment of Left Upper Leg Muscle, Open Approach
0KMR4ZZ Reattachment of Left Upper Leg Muscle, Percutaneous Endoscopic Approach
0KMS0ZZ Reattachment of Right Lower Leg Muscle, Open Approach
0KMS4ZZ Reattachment of Right Lower Leg Muscle, Percutaneous Endoscopic Approach
0KMT0ZZ Reattachment of Left Lower Leg Muscle, Open Approach
0KMT4ZZ Reattachment of Left Lower Leg Muscle, Percutaneous Endoscopic Approach
0KMV0ZZ Reattachment of Right Foot Muscle, Open Approach
0KMV4ZZ Reattachment of Right Foot Muscle, Percutaneous Endoscopic Approach
0KMW0ZZ Reattachment of Left Foot Muscle, Open Approach
0KMW4ZZ Reattachment of Left Foot Muscle, Percutaneous Endoscopic Approach

0KN – Muscles, Release

Review Coding Guideline B3.13

Review Coding Guideline B3.14

0KN00ZZ Release Head Muscle, Open Approach
0KN03ZZ Release Head Muscle, Percutaneous Approach
0KN04ZZ Release Head Muscle, Percutaneous Endoscopic Approach

0KN0XZZ Release Head Muscle, External Approach
0KN10ZZ Release Facial Muscle, Open Approach
0KN13ZZ Release Facial Muscle, Percutaneous Approach

0KN14ZZ	Release Facial Muscle, Percutaneous Endoscopic Approach
0KN1XZZ	Release Facial Muscle, External Approach
0KN20ZZ	Release Right Neck Muscle, Open Approach
0KN23ZZ	Release Right Neck Muscle, Percutaneous Approach
0KN24ZZ	Release Right Neck Muscle, Percutaneous Endoscopic Approach
0KN2XZZ	Release Right Neck Muscle, External Approach
0KN30ZZ	Release Left Neck Muscle, Open Approach
0KN33ZZ	Release Left Neck Muscle, Percutaneous Approach
0KN34ZZ	Release Left Neck Muscle, Percutaneous Endoscopic Approach
0KN3XZZ	Release Left Neck Muscle, External Approach
0KN40ZZ	Release Tongue, Palate, Pharynx Muscle, Open Approach
0KN43ZZ	Release Tongue, Palate, Pharynx Muscle, Percutaneous Approach
0KN44ZZ	Release Tongue, Palate, Pharynx Muscle, Percutaneous Endoscopic Approach
0KN4XZZ	Release Tongue, Palate, Pharynx Muscle, External Approach
0KN50ZZ	Release Right Shoulder Muscle, Open Approach
0KN53ZZ	Release Right Shoulder Muscle, Percutaneous Approach
0KN54ZZ	Release Right Shoulder Muscle, Percutaneous Endoscopic Approach
0KN5XZZ	Release Right Shoulder Muscle, External Approach
0KN60ZZ	Release Left Shoulder Muscle, Open Approach
0KN63ZZ	Release Left Shoulder Muscle, Percutaneous Approach
0KN64ZZ	Release Left Shoulder Muscle, Percutaneous Endoscopic Approach
0KN6XZZ	Release Left Shoulder Muscle, External Approach
0KN70ZZ	Release Right Upper Arm Muscle, Open Approach
0KN73ZZ	Release Right Upper Arm Muscle, Percutaneous Approach
0KN74ZZ	Release Right Upper Arm Muscle, Percutaneous Endoscopic Approach
0KN7XZZ	Release Right Upper Arm Muscle, External Approach
0KN80ZZ	Release Left Upper Arm Muscle, Open Approach
0KN83ZZ	Release Left Upper Arm Muscle, Percutaneous Approach
0KN84ZZ	Release Left Upper Arm Muscle, Percutaneous Endoscopic Approach
0KN8XZZ	Release Left Upper Arm Muscle, External Approach
0KN90ZZ	Release Right Lower Arm and Wrist Muscle, Open Approach
0KN93ZZ	Release Right Lower Arm and Wrist Muscle, Percutaneous Approach
0KN94ZZ	Release Right Lower Arm and Wrist Muscle, Percutaneous Endoscopic Approach
0KN9XZZ	Release Right Lower Arm and Wrist Muscle, External Approach
0KNB0ZZ	Release Left Lower Arm and Wrist Muscle, Open Approach
0KNB3ZZ	Release Left Lower Arm and Wrist Muscle, Percutaneous Approach
0KNB4ZZ	Release Left Lower Arm and Wrist Muscle, Percutaneous Endoscopic Approach
0KNBXZZ	Release Left Lower Arm and Wrist Muscle, External Approach
0KNC0ZZ	Release Right Hand Muscle, Open Approach
0KNC3ZZ	Release Right Hand Muscle, Percutaneous Approach
0KNC4ZZ	Release Right Hand Muscle, Percutaneous Endoscopic Approach
0KNCXZZ	Release Right Hand Muscle, External Approach
0KND0ZZ	Release Left Hand Muscle, Open Approach
0KND3ZZ	Release Left Hand Muscle, Percutaneous Approach
0KND4ZZ	Release Left Hand Muscle, Percutaneous Endoscopic Approach
0KNDXZZ	Release Left Hand Muscle, External Approach
0KNF0ZZ	Release Right Trunk Muscle, Open Approach
0KNF3ZZ	Release Right Trunk Muscle, Percutaneous Approach
0KNF4ZZ	Release Right Trunk Muscle, Percutaneous Endoscopic Approach
0KNFXZZ	Release Right Trunk Muscle, External Approach
0KNG0ZZ	Release Left Trunk Muscle, Open Approach
0KNG3ZZ	Release Left Trunk Muscle, Percutaneous Approach
0KNG4ZZ	Release Left Trunk Muscle, Percutaneous Endoscopic Approach
0KNGXZZ	Release Left Trunk Muscle, External Approach
0KNH0ZZ	Release Right Thorax Muscle, Open Approach
0KNH3ZZ	Release Right Thorax Muscle, Percutaneous Approach
0KNH4ZZ	Release Right Thorax Muscle, Percutaneous Endoscopic Approach
0KNHXZZ	Release Right Thorax Muscle, External Approach
0KNJ0ZZ	Release Left Thorax Muscle, Open Approach
0KNJ3ZZ	Release Left Thorax Muscle, Percutaneous Approach
0KNJ4ZZ	Release Left Thorax Muscle, Percutaneous Endoscopic Approach
0KNJXZZ	Release Left Thorax Muscle, External Approach
0KNK0ZZ	Release Right Abdomen Muscle, Open Approach
0KNK3ZZ	Release Right Abdomen Muscle, Percutaneous Approach
0KNK4ZZ	Release Right Abdomen Muscle, Percutaneous Endoscopic Approach
0KNKXZZ	Release Right Abdomen Muscle, External Approach
0KNL0ZZ	Release Left Abdomen Muscle, Open Approach
0KNL3ZZ	Release Left Abdomen Muscle, Percutaneous Approach
0KNL4ZZ	Release Left Abdomen Muscle, Percutaneous Endoscopic Approach
0KNLXZZ	Release Left Abdomen Muscle, External Approach
0KNM0ZZ	Release Perineum Muscle, Open Approach
0KNM3ZZ	Release Perineum Muscle, Percutaneous Approach
0KNM4ZZ	Release Perineum Muscle, Percutaneous Endoscopic Approach
0KNMXZZ	Release Perineum Muscle, External Approach
0KNN0ZZ	Release Right Hip Muscle, Open Approach
0KNN3ZZ	Release Right Hip Muscle, Percutaneous Approach
0KNN4ZZ	Release Right Hip Muscle, Percutaneous Endoscopic Approach
0KNNXZZ	Release Right Hip Muscle, External Approach
0KNP0ZZ	Release Left Hip Muscle, Open Approach
0KNP3ZZ	Release Left Hip Muscle, Percutaneous Approach
0KNP4ZZ	Release Left Hip Muscle, Percutaneous Endoscopic Approach
0KNPXZZ	Release Left Hip Muscle, External Approach
0KNQ0ZZ	Release Right Upper Leg Muscle, Open Approach
0KNQ3ZZ	Release Right Upper Leg Muscle, Percutaneous Approach
0KNQ4ZZ	Release Right Upper Leg Muscle, Percutaneous Endoscopic Approach
0KNQXZZ	Release Right Upper Leg Muscle, External Approach
0KNR0ZZ	Release Left Upper Leg Muscle, Open Approach
0KNR3ZZ	Release Left Upper Leg Muscle, Percutaneous Approach
0KNR4ZZ	Release Left Upper Leg Muscle, Percutaneous Endoscopic Approach
0KNRXZZ	Release Left Upper Leg Muscle, External Approach
0KNS0ZZ	Release Right Lower Leg Muscle, Open Approach
0KNS3ZZ	Release Right Lower Leg Muscle, Percutaneous Approach
0KNS4ZZ	Release Right Lower Leg Muscle, Percutaneous Endoscopic Approach
0KNSXZZ	Release Right Lower Leg Muscle, External Approach
0KNT0ZZ	Release Left Lower Leg Muscle, Open Approach
0KNT3ZZ	Release Left Lower Leg Muscle, Percutaneous Approach
0KNT4ZZ	Release Left Lower Leg Muscle, Percutaneous Endoscopic Approach
0KNTXZZ	Release Left Lower Leg Muscle, External Approach
0KNV0ZZ	Release Right Foot Muscle, Open Approach
0KNV3ZZ	Release Right Foot Muscle, Percutaneous Approach
0KNV4ZZ	Release Right Foot Muscle, Percutaneous Endoscopic Approach
0KNVXZZ	Release Right Foot Muscle, External Approach
0KNW0ZZ	Release Left Foot Muscle, Open Approach
0KNW3ZZ	Release Left Foot Muscle, Percutaneous Approach
0KNW4ZZ	Release Left Foot Muscle, Percutaneous Endoscopic Approach
0KNWXZZ	Release Left Foot Muscle, External Approach

0KP – Muscles, Removal

Review Coding Guideline B6.1c

0KPX00Z	Removal of Drainage Device from Upper Muscle, Open Approach
0KPX07Z	Removal of Autologous Tissue Substitute from Upper Muscle, Open Approach
0KPX0JZ	Removal of Synthetic Substitute from Upper Muscle, Open Approach
0KPX0KZ	Removal of Nonautologous Tissue Substitute from Upper Muscle, Open Approach
0KPX0MZ	Removal of Stimulator Lead from Upper Muscle, Open Approach
0KPX30Z	Removal of Drainage Device from Upper Muscle, Percutaneous Approach
0KPX37Z	Removal of Autologous Tissue Substitute from Upper Muscle, Percutaneous Approach
0KPX3JZ	Removal of Synthetic Substitute from Upper Muscle, Percutaneous Approach
0KPX3KZ	Removal of Nonautologous Tissue Substitute from Upper Muscle, Percutaneous Approach

0KPX3MZ	Removal of Stimulator Lead from Upper Muscle, Percutaneous Approach
0KPX40Z	Removal of Drainage Device from Upper Muscle, Percutaneous Endoscopic Approach
0KPX47Z	Removal of Autologous Tissue Substitute from Upper Muscle, Percutaneous Endoscopic Approach
0KPX4JZ	Removal of Synthetic Substitute from Upper Muscle, Percutaneous Endoscopic Approach
0KPX4KZ	Removal of Nonautologous Tissue Substitute from Upper Muscle, Percutaneous Endoscopic Approach
0KPX4MZ	Removal of Stimulator Lead from Upper Muscle, Percutaneous Endoscopic Approach
0KPXX0Z	Removal of Drainage Device from Upper Muscle, External Approach
0KPXXMZ	Removal of Stimulator Lead from Upper Muscle, External Approach
0KPY00Z	Removal of Drainage Device from Lower Muscle, Open Approach
0KPY07Z	Removal of Autologous Tissue Substitute from Lower Muscle, Open Approach
0KPY0JZ	Removal of Synthetic Substitute from Lower Muscle, Open Approach
0KPY0KZ	Removal of Nonautologous Tissue Substitute from Lower Muscle, Open Approach
0KPY0MZ	Removal of Stimulator Lead from Lower Muscle, Open Approach
0KPY30Z	Removal of Drainage Device from Lower Muscle, Percutaneous Approach
0KPY37Z	Removal of Autologous Tissue Substitute from Lower Muscle, Percutaneous Approach
0KPY3JZ	Removal of Synthetic Substitute from Lower Muscle, Percutaneous Approach
0KPY3KZ	Removal of Nonautologous Tissue Substitute from Lower Muscle, Percutaneous Approach
0KPY3MZ	Removal of Stimulator Lead from Lower Muscle, Percutaneous Approach
0KPY40Z	Removal of Drainage Device from Lower Muscle, Percutaneous Endoscopic Approach
0KPY47Z	Removal of Autologous Tissue Substitute from Lower Muscle, Percutaneous Endoscopic Approach
0KPY4JZ	Removal of Synthetic Substitute from Lower Muscle, Percutaneous Endoscopic Approach
0KPY4KZ	Removal of Nonautologous Tissue Substitute from Lower Muscle, Percutaneous Endoscopic Approach
0KPY4MZ	Removal of Stimulator Lead from Lower Muscle, Percutaneous Endoscopic Approach
0KPYX0Z	Removal of Drainage Device from Lower Muscle, External Approach
0KPYXMZ	Removal of Stimulator Lead from Lower Muscle, External Approach

0KQ – Muscles, Repair

Review Coding Guideline B3.5

0KQ00ZZ	Repair Head Muscle, Open Approach
0KQ03ZZ	Repair Head Muscle, Percutaneous Approach
0KQ04ZZ	Repair Head Muscle, Percutaneous Endoscopic Approach
0KQ10ZZ	Repair Facial Muscle, Open Approach
0KQ13ZZ	Repair Facial Muscle, Percutaneous Approach
0KQ14ZZ	Repair Facial Muscle, Percutaneous Endoscopic Approach
0KQ20ZZ	Repair Right Neck Muscle, Open Approach
0KQ23ZZ	Repair Right Neck Muscle, Percutaneous Approach
0KQ24ZZ	Repair Right Neck Muscle, Percutaneous Endoscopic Approach
0KQ30ZZ	Repair Left Neck Muscle, Open Approach
0KQ33ZZ	Repair Left Neck Muscle, Percutaneous Approach
0KQ34ZZ	Repair Left Neck Muscle, Percutaneous Endoscopic Approach
0KQ40ZZ	Repair Tongue, Palate, Pharynx Muscle, Open Approach
0KQ43ZZ	Repair Tongue, Palate, Pharynx Muscle, Percutaneous Approach
0KQ44ZZ	Repair Tongue, Palate, Pharynx Muscle, Percutaneous Endoscopic Approach
0KQ50ZZ	Repair Right Shoulder Muscle, Open Approach
0KQ53ZZ	Repair Right Shoulder Muscle, Percutaneous Approach
0KQ54ZZ	Repair Right Shoulder Muscle, Percutaneous Endoscopic Approach
0KQ60ZZ	Repair Left Shoulder Muscle, Open Approach
0KQ63ZZ	Repair Left Shoulder Muscle, Percutaneous Approach
0KQ64ZZ	Repair Left Shoulder Muscle, Percutaneous Endoscopic Approach
0KQ70ZZ	Repair Right Upper Arm Muscle, Open Approach
0KQ73ZZ	Repair Right Upper Arm Muscle, Percutaneous Approach
0KQ74ZZ	Repair Right Upper Arm Muscle, Percutaneous Endoscopic Approach
0KQ80ZZ	Repair Left Upper Arm Muscle, Open Approach
0KQ83ZZ	Repair Left Upper Arm Muscle, Percutaneous Approach
0KQ84ZZ	Repair Left Upper Arm Muscle, Percutaneous Endoscopic Approach
0KQ90ZZ	Repair Right Lower Arm and Wrist Muscle, Open Approach
0KQ93ZZ	Repair Right Lower Arm and Wrist Muscle, Percutaneous Approach
0KQ94ZZ	Repair Right Lower Arm and Wrist Muscle, Percutaneous Endoscopic Approach
0KQB0ZZ	Repair Left Lower Arm and Wrist Muscle, Open Approach
0KQB3ZZ	Repair Left Lower Arm and Wrist Muscle, Percutaneous Approach
0KQB4ZZ	Repair Left Lower Arm and Wrist Muscle, Percutaneous Endoscopic Approach
0KQC0ZZ	Repair Right Hand Muscle, Open Approach
0KQC3ZZ	Repair Right Hand Muscle, Percutaneous Approach
0KQC4ZZ	Repair Right Hand Muscle, Percutaneous Endoscopic Approach
0KQD0ZZ	Repair Left Hand Muscle, Open Approach
0KQD3ZZ	Repair Left Hand Muscle, Percutaneous Approach
0KQD4ZZ	Repair Left Hand Muscle, Percutaneous Endoscopic Approach
0KQF0ZZ	Repair Right Trunk Muscle, Open Approach
0KQF3ZZ	Repair Right Trunk Muscle, Percutaneous Approach
0KQF4ZZ	Repair Right Trunk Muscle, Percutaneous Endoscopic Approach
0KQG0ZZ	Repair Left Trunk Muscle, Open Approach
0KQG3ZZ	Repair Left Trunk Muscle, Percutaneous Approach
0KQG4ZZ	Repair Left Trunk Muscle, Percutaneous Endoscopic Approach
0KQH0ZZ	Repair Right Thorax Muscle, Open Approach
0KQH3ZZ	Repair Right Thorax Muscle, Percutaneous Approach
0KQH4ZZ	Repair Right Thorax Muscle, Percutaneous Endoscopic Approach
0KQJ0ZZ	Repair Left Thorax Muscle, Open Approach
0KQJ3ZZ	Repair Left Thorax Muscle, Percutaneous Approach
0KQJ4ZZ	Repair Left Thorax Muscle, Percutaneous Endoscopic Approach
0KQK0ZZ	Repair Right Abdomen Muscle, Open Approach
0KQK3ZZ	Repair Right Abdomen Muscle, Percutaneous Approach
0KQK4ZZ	Repair Right Abdomen Muscle, Percutaneous Endoscopic Approach
0KQL0ZZ	Repair Left Abdomen Muscle, Open Approach
0KQL3ZZ	Repair Left Abdomen Muscle, Percutaneous Approach
0KQL4ZZ	Repair Left Abdomen Muscle, Percutaneous Endoscopic Approach
0KQM0ZZ	Repair Perineum Muscle, Open Approach
0KQM3ZZ	Repair Perineum Muscle, Percutaneous Approach
0KQM4ZZ	Repair Perineum Muscle, Percutaneous Endoscopic Approach
0KQN0ZZ	Repair Right Hip Muscle, Open Approach
0KQN3ZZ	Repair Right Hip Muscle, Percutaneous Approach
0KQN4ZZ	Repair Right Hip Muscle, Percutaneous Endoscopic Approach
0KQP0ZZ	Repair Left Hip Muscle, Open Approach
0KQP3ZZ	Repair Left Hip Muscle, Percutaneous Approach
0KQP4ZZ	Repair Left Hip Muscle, Percutaneous Endoscopic Approach
0KQQ0ZZ	Repair Right Upper Leg Muscle, Open Approach
0KQQ3ZZ	Repair Right Upper Leg Muscle, Percutaneous Approach
0KQQ4ZZ	Repair Right Upper Leg Muscle, Percutaneous Endoscopic Approach
0KQR0ZZ	Repair Left Upper Leg Muscle, Open Approach
0KQR3ZZ	Repair Left Upper Leg Muscle, Percutaneous Approach
0KQR4ZZ	Repair Left Upper Leg Muscle, Percutaneous Endoscopic Approach
0KQS0ZZ	Repair Right Lower Leg Muscle, Open Approach
0KQS3ZZ	Repair Right Lower Leg Muscle, Percutaneous Approach
0KQS4ZZ	Repair Right Lower Leg Muscle, Percutaneous Endoscopic Approach
0KQT0ZZ	Repair Left Lower Leg Muscle, Open Approach
0KQT3ZZ	Repair Left Lower Leg Muscle, Percutaneous Approach

0KQT4ZZ	Repair Left Lower Leg Muscle, Percutaneous Endoscopic Approach
0KQV0ZZ	Repair Right Foot Muscle, Open Approach
0KQV3ZZ	Repair Right Foot Muscle, Percutaneous Approach

0KQV4ZZ	Repair Right Foot Muscle, Percutaneous Endoscopic Approach
0KQW0ZZ	Repair Left Foot Muscle, Open Approach
0KQW3ZZ	Repair Left Foot Muscle, Percutaneous Approach
0KQW4ZZ	Repair Left Foot Muscle, Percutaneous Endoscopic Approach

0KS – Muscles, Reposition

0KS00ZZ	Reposition Head Muscle, Open Approach	0KSG0ZZ	Reposition Left Trunk Muscle, Open Approach
0KS04ZZ	Reposition Head Muscle, Percutaneous Endoscopic Approach	0KSG4ZZ	Reposition Left Trunk Muscle, Percutaneous Endoscopic Approach
0KS10ZZ	Reposition Facial Muscle, Open Approach	0KSH0ZZ	Reposition Right Thorax Muscle, Open Approach
0KS14ZZ	Reposition Facial Muscle, Percutaneous Endoscopic Approach	0KSH4ZZ	Reposition Right Thorax Muscle, Percutaneous Endoscopic Approach
0KS20ZZ	Reposition Right Neck Muscle, Open Approach	0KSJ0ZZ	Reposition Left Thorax Muscle, Open Approach
0KS24ZZ	Reposition Right Neck Muscle, Percutaneous Endoscopic Approach	0KSJ4ZZ	Reposition Left Thorax Muscle, Percutaneous Endoscopic Approach
0KS30ZZ	Reposition Left Neck Muscle, Open Approach	0KSK0ZZ	Reposition Right Abdomen Muscle, Open Approach
0KS34ZZ	Reposition Left Neck Muscle, Percutaneous Endoscopic Approach	0KSK4ZZ	Reposition Right Abdomen Muscle, Percutaneous Endoscopic Approach
0KS40ZZ	Reposition Tongue, Palate, Pharynx Muscle, Open Approach	0KSL0ZZ	Reposition Left Abdomen Muscle, Open Approach
0KS44ZZ	Reposition Tongue, Palate, Pharynx Muscle, Percutaneous Endoscopic Approach	0KSL4ZZ	Reposition Left Abdomen Muscle, Percutaneous Endoscopic Approach
0KS50ZZ	Reposition Right Shoulder Muscle, Open Approach	0KSM0ZZ	Reposition Perineum Muscle, Open Approach
0KS54ZZ	Reposition Right Shoulder Muscle, Percutaneous Endoscopic Approach	0KSM4ZZ	Reposition Perineum Muscle, Percutaneous Endoscopic Approach
0KS60ZZ	Reposition Left Shoulder Muscle, Open Approach	0KSN0ZZ	Reposition Right Hip Muscle, Open Approach
0KS64ZZ	Reposition Left Shoulder Muscle, Percutaneous Endoscopic Approach	0KSN4ZZ	Reposition Right Hip Muscle, Percutaneous Endoscopic Approach
0KS70ZZ	Reposition Right Upper Arm Muscle, Open Approach	0KSP0ZZ	Reposition Left Hip Muscle, Open Approach
0KS74ZZ	Reposition Right Upper Arm Muscle, Percutaneous Endoscopic Approach	0KSP4ZZ	Reposition Left Hip Muscle, Percutaneous Endoscopic Approach
0KS80ZZ	Reposition Left Upper Arm Muscle, Open Approach	0KSQ0ZZ	Reposition Right Upper Leg Muscle, Open Approach
0KS84ZZ	Reposition Left Upper Arm Muscle, Percutaneous Endoscopic Approach	0KSQ4ZZ	Reposition Right Upper Leg Muscle, Percutaneous Endoscopic Approach
0KS90ZZ	Reposition Right Lower Arm and Wrist Muscle, Open Approach	0KSR0ZZ	Reposition Left Upper Leg Muscle, Open Approach
0KS94ZZ	Reposition Right Lower Arm and Wrist Muscle, Percutaneous Endoscopic Approach	0KSR4ZZ	Reposition Left Upper Leg Muscle, Percutaneous Endoscopic Approach
0KSB0ZZ	Reposition Left Lower Arm and Wrist Muscle, Open Approach	0KSS0ZZ	Reposition Right Lower Leg Muscle, Open Approach
0KSB4ZZ	Reposition Left Lower Arm and Wrist Muscle, Percutaneous Endoscopic Approach	0KSS4ZZ	Reposition Right Lower Leg Muscle, Percutaneous Endoscopic Approach
0KSC0ZZ	Reposition Right Hand Muscle, Open Approach	0KST0ZZ	Reposition Left Lower Leg Muscle, Open Approach
0KSC4ZZ	Reposition Right Hand Muscle, Percutaneous Endoscopic Approach	0KST4ZZ	Reposition Left Lower Leg Muscle, Percutaneous Endoscopic Approach
0KSD0ZZ	Reposition Left Hand Muscle, Open Approach	0KSV0ZZ	Reposition Right Foot Muscle, Open Approach
0KSD4ZZ	Reposition Left Hand Muscle, Percutaneous Endoscopic Approach	0KSV4ZZ	Reposition Right Foot Muscle, Percutaneous Endoscopic Approach
0KSF0ZZ	Reposition Right Trunk Muscle, Open Approach	0KSW0ZZ	Reposition Left Foot Muscle, Open Approach
0KSF4ZZ	Reposition Right Trunk Muscle, Percutaneous Endoscopic Approach	0KSW4ZZ	Reposition Left Foot Muscle, Percutaneous Endoscopic Approach

0KT – Muscles, Resection

Review Coding Guideline B3.8

0KT00ZZ	Resection of Head Muscle, Open Approach	0KT84ZZ	Resection of Left Upper Arm Muscle, Percutaneous Endoscopic Approach
0KT04ZZ	Resection of Head Muscle, Percutaneous Endoscopic Approach	0KT90ZZ	Resection of Right Lower Arm and Wrist Muscle, Open Approach
0KT10ZZ	Resection of Facial Muscle, Open Approach	0KT94ZZ	Resection of Right Lower Arm and Wrist Muscle, Percutaneous Endoscopic Approach
0KT14ZZ	Resection of Facial Muscle, Percutaneous Endoscopic Approach		
0KT20ZZ	Resection of Right Neck Muscle, Open Approach	0KTB0ZZ	Resection of Left Lower Arm and Wrist Muscle, Open Approach
0KT24ZZ	Resection of Right Neck Muscle, Percutaneous Endoscopic Approach	0KTB4ZZ	Resection of Left Lower Arm and Wrist Muscle, Percutaneous Endoscopic Approach
0KT30ZZ	Resection of Left Neck Muscle, Open Approach	0KTC0ZZ	Resection of Right Hand Muscle, Open Approach
0KT34ZZ	Resection of Left Neck Muscle, Percutaneous Endoscopic Approach	0KTC4ZZ	Resection of Right Hand Muscle, Percutaneous Endoscopic Approach
0KT40ZZ	Resection of Tongue, Palate, Pharynx Muscle, Open Approach	0KTD0ZZ	Resection of Left Hand Muscle, Open Approach
0KT44ZZ	Resection of Tongue, Palate, Pharynx Muscle, Percutaneous Endoscopic Approach	0KTD4ZZ	Resection of Left Hand Muscle, Percutaneous Endoscopic Approach
0KT50ZZ	Resection of Right Shoulder Muscle, Open Approach	0KTF0ZZ	Resection of Right Trunk Muscle, Open Approach
0KT54ZZ	Resection of Right Shoulder Muscle, Percutaneous Endoscopic Approach	0KTF4ZZ	Resection of Right Trunk Muscle, Percutaneous Endoscopic Approach
0KT60ZZ	Resection of Left Shoulder Muscle, Open Approach	0KTG0ZZ	Resection of Left Trunk Muscle, Open Approach
0KT64ZZ	Resection of Left Shoulder Muscle, Percutaneous Endoscopic Approach	0KTG4ZZ	Resection of Left Trunk Muscle, Percutaneous Endoscopic Approach
0KT70ZZ	Resection of Right Upper Arm Muscle, Open Approach	0KTH0ZZ	Resection of Right Thorax Muscle, Open Approach
0KT74ZZ	Resection of Right Upper Arm Muscle, Percutaneous Endoscopic Approach	0KTH4ZZ	Resection of Right Thorax Muscle, Percutaneous Endoscopic Approach
0KT80ZZ	Resection of Left Upper Arm Muscle, Open Approach		

♀ Female-only   ♂ Male-only   ● Limited Coverage   ● Non-OR   ᴴᴬᶜ HAC-associated procedure   ● Non-covered procedures   ✚ Combination

0KTJ0ZZ   Resection of Left Thorax Muscle, Open Approach

0KTJ4ZZ   Resection of Left Thorax Muscle, Percutaneous Endoscopic Approach

0KTK0ZZ   Resection of Right Abdomen Muscle, Open Approach

0KTK4ZZ   Resection of Right Abdomen Muscle, Percutaneous Endoscopic Approach

0KTL0ZZ   Resection of Left Abdomen Muscle, Open Approach

0KTL4ZZ   Resection of Left Abdomen Muscle, Percutaneous Endoscopic Approach

0KTM0ZZ   Resection of Perineum Muscle, Open Approach

0KTM4ZZ   Resection of Perineum Muscle, Percutaneous Endoscopic Approach

0KTN0ZZ   Resection of Right Hip Muscle, Open Approach

0KTN4ZZ   Resection of Right Hip Muscle, Percutaneous Endoscopic Approach

0KTP0ZZ   Resection of Left Hip Muscle, Open Approach

0KTP4ZZ   Resection of Left Hip Muscle, Percutaneous Endoscopic Approach

0KTQ0ZZ   Resection of Right Upper Leg Muscle, Open Approach

0KTQ4ZZ   Resection of Right Upper Leg Muscle, Percutaneous Endoscopic Approach

0KTR0ZZ   Resection of Left Upper Leg Muscle, Open Approach

0KTR4ZZ   Resection of Left Upper Leg Muscle, Percutaneous Endoscopic Approach

0KTS0ZZ   Resection of Right Lower Leg Muscle, Open Approach

0KTS4ZZ   Resection of Right Lower Leg Muscle, Percutaneous Endoscopic Approach

0KTT0ZZ   Resection of Left Lower Leg Muscle, Open Approach

0KTT4ZZ   Resection of Left Lower Leg Muscle, Percutaneous Endoscopic Approach

0KTV0ZZ   Resection of Right Foot Muscle, Open Approach

0KTV4ZZ   Resection of Right Foot Muscle, Percutaneous Endoscopic Approach

0KTW0ZZ   Resection of Left Foot Muscle, Open Approach

0KTW4ZZ   Resection of Left Foot Muscle, Percutaneous Endoscopic Approach

0KU – Muscles, Supplement

0KU007Z   Supplement Head Muscle with Autologous Tissue Substitute, Open Approach

0KU00JZ   Supplement Head Muscle with Synthetic Substitute, Open Approach

0KU00KZ   Supplement Head Muscle with Nonautologous Tissue Substitute, Open Approach

0KU047Z   Supplement Head Muscle with Autologous Tissue Substitute, Percutaneous Endoscopic Approach

0KU04JZ   Supplement Head Muscle with Synthetic Substitute, Percutaneous Endoscopic Approach

0KU04KZ   Supplement Head Muscle with Nonautologous Tissue Substitute, Percutaneous Endoscopic Approach

0KU107Z   Supplement Facial Muscle with Autologous Tissue Substitute, Open Approach

0KU10JZ   Supplement Facial Muscle with Synthetic Substitute, Open Approach

0KU10KZ   Supplement Facial Muscle with Nonautologous Tissue Substitute, Open Approach

0KU147Z   Supplement Facial Muscle with Autologous Tissue Substitute, Percutaneous Endoscopic Approach

0KU14JZ   Supplement Facial Muscle with Synthetic Substitute, Percutaneous Endoscopic Approach

0KU14KZ   Supplement Facial Muscle with Nonautologous Tissue Substitute, Percutaneous Endoscopic Approach

0KU207Z   Supplement Right Neck Muscle with Autologous Tissue Substitute, Open Approach

0KU20JZ   Supplement Right Neck Muscle with Synthetic Substitute, Open Approach

0KU20KZ   Supplement Right Neck Muscle with Nonautologous Tissue Substitute, Open Approach

0KU247Z   Supplement Right Neck Muscle with Autologous Tissue Substitute, Percutaneous Endoscopic Approach

0KU24JZ   Supplement Right Neck Muscle with Synthetic Substitute, Percutaneous Endoscopic Approach

0KU24KZ   Supplement Right Neck Muscle with Nonautologous Tissue Substitute, Percutaneous Endoscopic Approach

0KU307Z   Supplement Left Neck Muscle with Autologous Tissue Substitute, Open Approach

0KU30JZ   Supplement Left Neck Muscle with Synthetic Substitute, Open Approach

0KU30KZ   Supplement Left Neck Muscle with Nonautologous Tissue Substitute, Open Approach

0KU347Z   Supplement Left Neck Muscle with Autologous Tissue Substitute, Percutaneous Endoscopic Approach

0KU34JZ   Supplement Left Neck Muscle with Synthetic Substitute, Percutaneous Endoscopic Approach

0KU34KZ   Supplement Left Neck Muscle with Nonautologous Tissue Substitute, Percutaneous Endoscopic Approach

0KU407Z   Supplement Tongue, Palate, Pharynx Muscle with Autologous Tissue Substitute, Open Approach

0KU40JZ   Supplement Tongue, Palate, Pharynx Muscle with Synthetic Substitute, Open Approach

0KU40KZ   Supplement Tongue, Palate, Pharynx Muscle with Nonautologous Tissue Substitute, Open Approach

0KU447Z   Supplement Tongue, Palate, Pharynx Muscle with Autologous Tissue Substitute, Percutaneous Endoscopic Approach

0KU44JZ   Supplement Tongue, Palate, Pharynx Muscle with Synthetic Substitute, Percutaneous Endoscopic Approach

0KU44KZ   Supplement Tongue, Palate, Pharynx Muscle with Nonautologous Tissue Substitute, Percutaneous Endoscopic Approach

0KU507Z   Supplement Right Shoulder Muscle with Autologous Tissue Substitute, Open Approach

0KU50JZ   Supplement Right Shoulder Muscle with Synthetic Substitute, Open Approach

0KU50KZ   Supplement Right Shoulder Muscle with Nonautologous Tissue Substitute, Open Approach

0KU547Z   Supplement Right Shoulder Muscle with Autologous Tissue Substitute, Percutaneous Endoscopic Approach

0KU54JZ   Supplement Right Shoulder Muscle with Synthetic Substitute, Percutaneous Endoscopic Approach

0KU54KZ   Supplement Right Shoulder Muscle with Nonautologous Tissue Substitute, Percutaneous Endoscopic Approach

0KU607Z   Supplement Left Shoulder Muscle with Autologous Tissue Substitute, Open Approach

0KU60JZ   Supplement Left Shoulder Muscle with Synthetic Substitute, Open Approach

0KU60KZ   Supplement Left Shoulder Muscle with Nonautologous Tissue Substitute, Open Approach

0KU647Z   Supplement Left Shoulder Muscle with Autologous Tissue Substitute, Percutaneous Endoscopic Approach

0KU64JZ   Supplement Left Shoulder Muscle with Synthetic Substitute, Percutaneous Endoscopic Approach

0KU64KZ   Supplement Left Shoulder Muscle with Nonautologous Tissue Substitute, Percutaneous Endoscopic Approach

0KU707Z   Supplement Right Upper Arm Muscle with Autologous Tissue Substitute, Open Approach

0KU70JZ   Supplement Right Upper Arm Muscle with Synthetic Substitute, Open Approach

0KU70KZ   Supplement Right Upper Arm Muscle with Nonautologous Tissue Substitute, Open Approach

0KU747Z   Supplement Right Upper Arm Muscle with Autologous Tissue Substitute, Percutaneous Endoscopic Approach

0KU74JZ   Supplement Right Upper Arm Muscle with Synthetic Substitute, Percutaneous Endoscopic Approach

0KU74KZ   Supplement Right Upper Arm Muscle with Nonautologous Tissue Substitute, Percutaneous Endoscopic Approach

0KU807Z   Supplement Left Upper Arm Muscle with Autologous Tissue Substitute, Open Approach

0KU80JZ   Supplement Left Upper Arm Muscle with Synthetic Substitute, Open Approach

0KU80KZ   Supplement Left Upper Arm Muscle with Nonautologous Tissue Substitute, Open Approach

0KU847Z   Supplement Left Upper Arm Muscle with Autologous Tissue Substitute, Percutaneous Endoscopic Approach

0KU84JZ   Supplement Left Upper Arm Muscle with Synthetic Substitute, Percutaneous Endoscopic Approach

0KU84KZ Supplement Left Upper Arm Muscle with Nonautologous Tissue Substitute, Percutaneous Endoscopic Approach

0KU907Z Supplement Right Lower Arm and Wrist Muscle with Autologous Tissue Substitute, Open Approach

0KU90JZ Supplement Right Lower Arm and Wrist Muscle with Synthetic Substitute, Open Approach

0KU90KZ Supplement Right Lower Arm and Wrist Muscle with Nonautologous Tissue Substitute, Open Approach

0KU947Z Supplement Right Lower Arm and Wrist Muscle with Autologous Tissue Substitute, Percutaneous Endoscopic Approach

0KU94JZ Supplement Right Lower Arm and Wrist Muscle with Synthetic Substitute, Percutaneous Endoscopic Approach

0KU94KZ Supplement Right Lower Arm and Wrist Muscle with Nonautologous Tissue Substitute, Percutaneous Endoscopic Approach

0KUB07Z Supplement Left Lower Arm and Wrist Muscle with Autologous Tissue Substitute, Open Approach

0KUB0JZ Supplement Left Lower Arm and Wrist Muscle with Synthetic Substitute, Open Approach

0KUB0KZ Supplement Left Lower Arm and Wrist Muscle with Nonautologous Tissue Substitute, Open Approach

0KUB47Z Supplement Left Lower Arm and Wrist Muscle with Autologous Tissue Substitute, Percutaneous Endoscopic Approach

0KUB4JZ Supplement Left Lower Arm and Wrist Muscle with Synthetic Substitute, Percutaneous Endoscopic Approach

0KUB4KZ Supplement Left Lower Arm and Wrist Muscle with Nonautologous Tissue Substitute, Percutaneous Endoscopic Approach

0KUC07Z Supplement Right Hand Muscle with Autologous Tissue Substitute, Open Approach

0KUC0JZ Supplement Right Hand Muscle with Synthetic Substitute, Open Approach

0KUC0KZ Supplement Right Hand Muscle with Nonautologous Tissue Substitute, Open Approach

0KUC47Z Supplement Right Hand Muscle with Autologous Tissue Substitute, Percutaneous Endoscopic Approach

0KUC4JZ Supplement Right Hand Muscle with Synthetic Substitute, Percutaneous Endoscopic Approach

0KUC4KZ Supplement Right Hand Muscle with Nonautologous Tissue Substitute, Percutaneous Endoscopic Approach

0KUD07Z Supplement Left Hand Muscle with Autologous Tissue Substitute, Open Approach

0KUD0JZ Supplement Left Hand Muscle with Synthetic Substitute, Open Approach

0KUD0KZ Supplement Left Hand Muscle with Nonautologous Tissue Substitute, Open Approach

0KUD47Z Supplement Left Hand Muscle with Autologous Tissue Substitute, Percutaneous Endoscopic Approach

0KUD4JZ Supplement Left Hand Muscle with Synthetic Substitute, Percutaneous Endoscopic Approach

0KUD4KZ Supplement Left Hand Muscle with Nonautologous Tissue Substitute, Percutaneous Endoscopic Approach

0KUF07Z Supplement Right Trunk Muscle with Autologous Tissue Substitute, Open Approach

0KUF0JZ Supplement Right Trunk Muscle with Synthetic Substitute, Open Approach

0KUF0KZ Supplement Right Trunk Muscle with Nonautologous Tissue Substitute, Open Approach

0KUF47Z Supplement Right Trunk Muscle with Autologous Tissue Substitute, Percutaneous Endoscopic Approach

0KUF4JZ Supplement Right Trunk Muscle with Synthetic Substitute, Percutaneous Endoscopic Approach

0KUF4KZ Supplement Right Trunk Muscle with Nonautologous Tissue Substitute, Percutaneous Endoscopic Approach

0KUG07Z Supplement Left Trunk Muscle with Autologous Tissue Substitute, Open Approach

0KUG0JZ Supplement Left Trunk Muscle with Synthetic Substitute, Open Approach

0KUG0KZ Supplement Left Trunk Muscle with Nonautologous Tissue Substitute, Open Approach

0KUG47Z Supplement Left Trunk Muscle with Autologous Tissue Substitute, Percutaneous Endoscopic Approach

0KUG4JZ Supplement Left Trunk Muscle with Synthetic Substitute, Percutaneous Endoscopic Approach

0KUG4KZ Supplement Left Trunk Muscle with Nonautologous Tissue Substitute, Percutaneous Endoscopic Approach

0KUH07Z Supplement Right Thorax Muscle with Autologous Tissue Substitute, Open Approach

0KUH0JZ Supplement Right Thorax Muscle with Synthetic Substitute, Open Approach

0KUH0KZ Supplement Right Thorax Muscle with Nonautologous Tissue Substitute, Open Approach

0KUH47Z Supplement Right Thorax Muscle with Autologous Tissue Substitute, Percutaneous Endoscopic Approach

0KUH4JZ Supplement Right Thorax Muscle with Synthetic Substitute, Percutaneous Endoscopic Approach

0KUH4KZ Supplement Right Thorax Muscle with Nonautologous Tissue Substitute, Percutaneous Endoscopic Approach

0KUJ07Z Supplement Left Thorax Muscle with Autologous Tissue Substitute, Open Approach

0KUJ0JZ Supplement Left Thorax Muscle with Synthetic Substitute, Open Approach

0KUJ0KZ Supplement Left Thorax Muscle with Nonautologous Tissue Substitute, Open Approach

0KUJ47Z Supplement Left Thorax Muscle with Autologous Tissue Substitute, Percutaneous Endoscopic Approach

0KUJ4JZ Supplement Left Thorax Muscle with Synthetic Substitute, Percutaneous Endoscopic Approach

0KUJ4KZ Supplement Left Thorax Muscle with Nonautologous Tissue Substitute, Percutaneous Endoscopic Approach

0KUK07Z Supplement Right Abdomen Muscle with Autologous Tissue Substitute, Open Approach

0KUK0JZ Supplement Right Abdomen Muscle with Synthetic Substitute, Open Approach

0KUK0KZ Supplement Right Abdomen Muscle with Nonautologous Tissue Substitute, Open Approach

0KUK47Z Supplement Right Abdomen Muscle with Autologous Tissue Substitute, Percutaneous Endoscopic Approach

0KUK4JZ Supplement Right Abdomen Muscle with Synthetic Substitute, Percutaneous Endoscopic Approach

0KUK4KZ Supplement Right Abdomen Muscle with Nonautologous Tissue Substitute, Percutaneous Endoscopic Approach

0KUL07Z Supplement Left Abdomen Muscle with Autologous Tissue Substitute, Open Approach

0KUL0JZ Supplement Left Abdomen Muscle with Synthetic Substitute, Open Approach

0KUL0KZ Supplement Left Abdomen Muscle with Nonautologous Tissue Substitute, Open Approach

0KUL47Z Supplement Left Abdomen Muscle with Autologous Tissue Substitute, Percutaneous Endoscopic Approach

0KUL4JZ Supplement Left Abdomen Muscle with Synthetic Substitute, Percutaneous Endoscopic Approach

0KUL4KZ Supplement Left Abdomen Muscle with Nonautologous Tissue Substitute, Percutaneous Endoscopic Approach

0KUM07Z Supplement Perineum Muscle with Autologous Tissue Substitute, Open Approach

0KUM0JZ Supplement Perineum Muscle with Synthetic Substitute, Open Approach

0KUM0KZ Supplement Perineum Muscle with Nonautologous Tissue Substitute, Open Approach

0KUM47Z Supplement Perineum Muscle with Autologous Tissue Substitute, Percutaneous Endoscopic Approach

0KUM4JZ Supplement Perineum Muscle with Synthetic Substitute, Percutaneous Endoscopic Approach

0KUM4KZ Supplement Perineum Muscle with Nonautologous Tissue Substitute, Percutaneous Endoscopic Approach

0KUN07Z Supplement Right Hip Muscle with Autologous Tissue Substitute, Open Approach

0KUN0JZ Supplement Right Hip Muscle with Synthetic Substitute, Open Approach

0KUN0KZ Supplement Right Hip Muscle with Nonautologous Tissue Substitute, Open Approach

0KUN47Z Supplement Right Hip Muscle with Autologous Tissue Substitute, Percutaneous Endoscopic Approach

0KUN4JZ Supplement Right Hip Muscle with Synthetic Substitute, Percutaneous Endoscopic Approach

0KUN4KZ Supplement Right Hip Muscle with Nonautologous Tissue Substitute, Percutaneous Endoscopic Approach

0KUP07Z Supplement Left Hip Muscle with Autologous Tissue Substitute, Open Approach

0KUP0JZ Supplement Left Hip Muscle with Synthetic Substitute, Open Approach

0KUP0KZ Supplement Left Hip Muscle with Nonautologous Tissue Substitute, Open Approach

0KUP47Z Supplement Left Hip Muscle with Autologous Tissue Substitute, Percutaneous Endoscopic Approach

0KUP4JZ Supplement Left Hip Muscle with Synthetic Substitute, Percutaneous Endoscopic Approach

0KUP4KZ Supplement Left Hip Muscle with Nonautologous Tissue Substitute, Percutaneous Endoscopic Approach

0KUQ07Z Supplement Right Upper Leg Muscle with Autologous Tissue Substitute, Open Approach

0KUQ0JZ Supplement Right Upper Leg Muscle with Synthetic Substitute, Open Approach

0KUQ0KZ Supplement Right Upper Leg Muscle with Nonautologous Tissue Substitute, Open Approach

0KUQ47Z Supplement Right Upper Leg Muscle with Autologous Tissue Substitute, Percutaneous Endoscopic Approach

0KUQ4JZ Supplement Right Upper Leg Muscle with Synthetic Substitute, Percutaneous Endoscopic Approach

0KUQ4KZ Supplement Right Upper Leg Muscle with Nonautologous Tissue Substitute, Percutaneous Endoscopic Approach

0KUR07Z Supplement Left Upper Leg Muscle with Autologous Tissue Substitute, Open Approach

0KUR0JZ Supplement Left Upper Leg Muscle with Synthetic Substitute, Open Approach

0KUR0KZ Supplement Left Upper Leg Muscle with Nonautologous Tissue Substitute, Open Approach

0KUR47Z Supplement Left Upper Leg Muscle with Autologous Tissue Substitute, Percutaneous Endoscopic Approach

0KUR4JZ Supplement Left Upper Leg Muscle with Synthetic Substitute, Percutaneous Endoscopic Approach

0KUR4KZ Supplement Left Upper Leg Muscle with Nonautologous Tissue Substitute, Percutaneous Endoscopic Approach

0KUS07Z Supplement Right Lower Leg Muscle with Autologous Tissue Substitute, Open Approach

0KUS0JZ Supplement Right Lower Leg Muscle with Synthetic Substitute, Open Approach

0KUS0KZ Supplement Right Lower Leg Muscle with Nonautologous Tissue Substitute, Open Approach

0KUS47Z Supplement Right Lower Leg Muscle with Autologous Tissue Substitute, Percutaneous Endoscopic Approach

0KUS4JZ Supplement Right Lower Leg Muscle with Synthetic Substitute, Percutaneous Endoscopic Approach

0KUS4KZ Supplement Right Lower Leg Muscle with Nonautologous Tissue Substitute, Percutaneous Endoscopic Approach

0KUT07Z Supplement Left Lower Leg Muscle with Autologous Tissue Substitute, Open Approach

0KUT0JZ Supplement Left Lower Leg Muscle with Synthetic Substitute, Open Approach

0KUT0KZ Supplement Left Lower Leg Muscle with Nonautologous Tissue Substitute, Open Approach

0KUT47Z Supplement Left Lower Leg Muscle with Autologous Tissue Substitute, Percutaneous Endoscopic Approach

0KUT4JZ Supplement Left Lower Leg Muscle with Synthetic Substitute, Percutaneous Endoscopic Approach

0KUT4KZ Supplement Left Lower Leg Muscle with Nonautologous Tissue Substitute, Percutaneous Endoscopic Approach

0KUV07Z Supplement Right Foot Muscle with Autologous Tissue Substitute, Open Approach

0KUV0JZ Supplement Right Foot Muscle with Synthetic Substitute, Open Approach

0KUV0KZ Supplement Right Foot Muscle with Nonautologous Tissue Substitute, Open Approach

0KUV47Z Supplement Right Foot Muscle with Autologous Tissue Substitute, Percutaneous Endoscopic Approach

0KUV4JZ Supplement Right Foot Muscle with Synthetic Substitute, Percutaneous Endoscopic Approach

0KUV4KZ Supplement Right Foot Muscle with Nonautologous Tissue Substitute, Percutaneous Endoscopic Approach

0KUW07Z Supplement Left Foot Muscle with Autologous Tissue Substitute, Open Approach

0KUW0JZ Supplement Left Foot Muscle with Synthetic Substitute, Open Approach

0KUW0KZ Supplement Left Foot Muscle with Nonautologous Tissue Substitute, Open Approach

0KUW47Z Supplement Left Foot Muscle with Autologous Tissue Substitute, Percutaneous Endoscopic Approach

0KUW4JZ Supplement Left Foot Muscle with Synthetic Substitute, Percutaneous Endoscopic Approach

0KUW4KZ Supplement Left Foot Muscle with Nonautologous Tissue Substitute, Percutaneous Endoscopic Approach

0KW – Muscles, Revision

Review Coding Guideline B6.1c

0KWX00Z Revision of Drainage Device in Upper Muscle, Open Approach

0KWX07Z Revision of Autologous Tissue Substitute in Upper Muscle, Open Approach

0KWX0JZ Revision of Synthetic Substitute in Upper Muscle, Open Approach

0KWX0KZ Revision of Nonautologous Tissue Substitute in Upper Muscle, Open Approach

0KWX0MZ Revision of Stimulator Lead in Upper Muscle, Open Approach

0KWX30Z Revision of Drainage Device in Upper Muscle, Percutaneous Approach

0KWX37Z Revision of Autologous Tissue Substitute in Upper Muscle, Percutaneous Approach

0KWX3JZ Revision of Synthetic Substitute in Upper Muscle, Percutaneous Approach

0KWX3KZ Revision of Nonautologous Tissue Substitute in Upper Muscle, Percutaneous Approach

0KWX3MZ Revision of Stimulator Lead in Upper Muscle, Percutaneous Approach

0KWX40Z Revision of Drainage Device in Upper Muscle, Percutaneous Endoscopic Approach

0KWX47Z Revision of Autologous Tissue Substitute in Upper Muscle, Percutaneous Endoscopic Approach

0KWX4JZ Revision of Synthetic Substitute in Upper Muscle, Percutaneous Endoscopic Approach

0KWX4KZ Revision of Nonautologous Tissue Substitute in Upper Muscle, Percutaneous Endoscopic Approach

0KWX4MZ Revision of Stimulator Lead in Upper Muscle, Percutaneous Endoscopic Approach

0KWXX0Z Revision of Drainage Device in Upper Muscle, External Approach

0KWXX7Z Revision of Autologous Tissue Substitute in Upper Muscle, External Approach

0KWXXJZ Revision of Synthetic Substitute in Upper Muscle, External Approach

0KWXXKZ Revision of Nonautologous Tissue Substitute in Upper Muscle, External Approach

0KWXXMZ Revision of Stimulator Lead in Upper Muscle, External Approach

0KWY00Z Revision of Drainage Device in Lower Muscle, Open Approach

0KWY07Z Revision of Autologous Tissue Substitute in Lower Muscle, Open Approach

0KWY0JZ Revision of Synthetic Substitute in Lower Muscle, Open Approach

0KWY0KZ Revision of Nonautologous Tissue Substitute in Lower Muscle, Open Approach

0KWY0MZ Revision of Stimulator Lead in Lower Muscle, Open Approach

0KWY30Z Revision of Drainage Device in Lower Muscle, Percutaneous Approach

0KWY37Z Revision of Autologous Tissue Substitute in Lower Muscle, Percutaneous Approach

0KWY3JZ Revision of Synthetic Substitute in Lower Muscle, Percutaneous Approach

0KWY3KZ Revision of Nonautologous Tissue Substitute in Lower Muscle, Percutaneous Approach

0KWY3MZ Revision of Stimulator Lead in Lower Muscle, Percutaneous Approach

0KWY40Z Revision of Drainage Device in Lower Muscle, Percutaneous Endoscopic Approach

0KWY47Z Revision of Autologous Tissue Substitute in Lower Muscle, Percutaneous Endoscopic Approach

0KWY4JZ Revision of Synthetic Substitute in Lower Muscle, Percutaneous Endoscopic Approach

0KWY4KZ Revision of Nonautologous Tissue Substitute in Lower Muscle, Percutaneous Endoscopic Approach

0KWY4MZ Revision of Stimulator Lead in Lower Muscle, Percutaneous Endoscopic Approach

0KWYX0Z Revision of Drainage Device in Lower Muscle, External Approach

0KWYX7Z Revision of Autologous Tissue Substitute in Lower Muscle, External Approach

0KWYXJZ Revision of Synthetic Substitute in Lower Muscle, External Approach

0KWYXKZ Revision of Nonautologous Tissue Substitute in Lower Muscle, External Approach

0KWYXMZ Revision of Stimulator Lead in Lower Muscle, External Approach

0KX – Muscles, Transfer

0KX00Z0 Transfer Head Muscle with Skin, Open Approach
0KX00Z1 Transfer Head Muscle with Subcutaneous Tissue, Open Approach
0KX00Z2 Transfer Head Muscle with Skin and Subcutaneous Tissue, Open Approach
0KX00ZZ Transfer Head Muscle, Open Approach
0KX04Z0 Transfer Head Muscle with Skin, Percutaneous Endoscopic Approach
0KX04Z1 Transfer Head Muscle with Subcutaneous Tissue, Percutaneous Endoscopic Approach
0KX04Z2 Transfer Head Muscle with Skin and Subcutaneous Tissue, Percutaneous Endoscopic Approach
0KX04ZZ Transfer Head Muscle, Percutaneous Endoscopic Approach
0KX10Z0 Transfer Facial Muscle with Skin, Open Approach
0KX10Z1 Transfer Facial Muscle with Subcutaneous Tissue, Open Approach
0KX10Z2 Transfer Facial Muscle with Skin and Subcutaneous Tissue, Open Approach
0KX10ZZ Transfer Facial Muscle, Open Approach
0KX14Z0 Transfer Facial Muscle with Skin, Percutaneous Endoscopic Approach
0KX14Z1 Transfer Facial Muscle with Subcutaneous Tissue, Percutaneous Endoscopic Approach
0KX14Z2 Transfer Facial Muscle with Skin and Subcutaneous Tissue, Percutaneous Endoscopic Approach
0KX14ZZ Transfer Facial Muscle, Percutaneous Endoscopic Approach
0KX20Z0 Transfer Right Neck Muscle with Skin, Open Approach
0KX20Z1 Transfer Right Neck Muscle with Subcutaneous Tissue, Open Approach
0KX20Z2 Transfer Right Neck Muscle with Skin and Subcutaneous Tissue, Open Approach
0KX20ZZ Transfer Right Neck Muscle, Open Approach
0KX24Z0 Transfer Right Neck Muscle with Skin, Percutaneous Endoscopic Approach
0KX24Z1 Transfer Right Neck Muscle with Subcutaneous Tissue, Percutaneous Endoscopic Approach
0KX24Z2 Transfer Right Neck Muscle with Skin and Subcutaneous Tissue, Percutaneous Endoscopic Approach
0KX24ZZ Transfer Right Neck Muscle, Percutaneous Endoscopic Approach
0KX30Z0 Transfer Left Neck Muscle with Skin, Open Approach
0KX30Z1 Transfer Left Neck Muscle with Subcutaneous Tissue, Open Approach
0KX30Z2 Transfer Left Neck Muscle with Skin and Subcutaneous Tissue, Open Approach
0KX30ZZ Transfer Left Neck Muscle, Open Approach
0KX34Z0 Transfer Left Neck Muscle with Skin, Percutaneous Endoscopic Approach
0KX34Z1 Transfer Left Neck Muscle with Subcutaneous Tissue, Percutaneous Endoscopic Approach
0KX34Z2 Transfer Left Neck Muscle with Skin and Subcutaneous Tissue, Percutaneous Endoscopic Approach
0KX34ZZ Transfer Left Neck Muscle, Percutaneous Endoscopic Approach
0KX40Z0 Transfer Tongue, Palate, Pharynx Muscle with Skin, Open Approach
0KX40Z1 Transfer Tongue, Palate, Pharynx Muscle with Subcutaneous Tissue, Open Approach
0KX40Z2 Transfer Tongue, Palate, Pharynx Muscle with Skin and Subcutaneous Tissue, Open Approach
0KX40ZZ Transfer Tongue, Palate, Pharynx Muscle, Open Approach
0KX44Z0 Transfer Tongue, Palate, Pharynx Muscle with Skin, Percutaneous Endoscopic Approach

0KX44Z1 Transfer Tongue, Palate, Pharynx Muscle with Subcutaneous Tissue, Percutaneous Endoscopic Approach
0KX44Z2 Transfer Tongue, Palate, Pharynx Muscle with Skin and Subcutaneous Tissue, Percutaneous Endoscopic Approach
0KX44ZZ Transfer Tongue, Palate, Pharynx Muscle, Percutaneous Endoscopic Approach
0KX50Z0 Transfer Right Shoulder Muscle with Skin, Open Approach
0KX50Z1 Transfer Right Shoulder Muscle with Subcutaneous Tissue, Open Approach
0KX50Z2 Transfer Right Shoulder Muscle with Skin and Subcutaneous Tissue, Open Approach
0KX50ZZ Transfer Right Shoulder Muscle, Open Approach
0KX54Z0 Transfer Right Shoulder Muscle with Skin, Percutaneous Endoscopic Approach
0KX54Z1 Transfer Right Shoulder Muscle with Subcutaneous Tissue, Percutaneous Endoscopic Approach
0KX54Z2 Transfer Right Shoulder Muscle with Skin and Subcutaneous Tissue, Percutaneous Endoscopic Approach
0KX54ZZ Transfer Right Shoulder Muscle, Percutaneous Endoscopic Approach
0KX60Z0 Transfer Left Shoulder Muscle with Skin, Open Approach
0KX60Z1 Transfer Left Shoulder Muscle with Subcutaneous Tissue, Open Approach
0KX60Z2 Transfer Left Shoulder Muscle with Skin and Subcutaneous Tissue, Open Approach
0KX60ZZ Transfer Left Shoulder Muscle, Open Approach
0KX64Z0 Transfer Left Shoulder Muscle with Skin, Percutaneous Endoscopic Approach
0KX64Z1 Transfer Left Shoulder Muscle with Subcutaneous Tissue, Percutaneous Endoscopic Approach
0KX64Z2 Transfer Left Shoulder Muscle with Skin and Subcutaneous Tissue, Percutaneous Endoscopic Approach
0KX64ZZ Transfer Left Shoulder Muscle, Percutaneous Endoscopic Approach
0KX70Z0 Transfer Right Upper Arm Muscle with Skin, Open Approach
0KX70Z1 Transfer Right Upper Arm Muscle with Subcutaneous Tissue, Open Approach
0KX70Z2 Transfer Right Upper Arm Muscle with Skin and Subcutaneous Tissue, Open Approach
0KX70ZZ Transfer Right Upper Arm Muscle, Open Approach
0KX74Z0 Transfer Right Upper Arm Muscle with Skin, Percutaneous Endoscopic Approach
0KX74Z1 Transfer Right Upper Arm Muscle with Subcutaneous Tissue, Percutaneous Endoscopic Approach
0KX74Z2 Transfer Right Upper Arm Muscle with Skin and Subcutaneous Tissue, Percutaneous Endoscopic Approach
0KX74ZZ Transfer Right Upper Arm Muscle, Percutaneous Endoscopic Approach
0KX80Z0 Transfer Left Upper Arm Muscle with Skin, Open Approach
0KX80Z1 Transfer Left Upper Arm Muscle with Subcutaneous Tissue, Open Approach
0KX80Z2 Transfer Left Upper Arm Muscle with Skin and Subcutaneous Tissue, Open Approach
0KX80ZZ Transfer Left Upper Arm Muscle, Open Approach
0KX84Z0 Transfer Left Upper Arm Muscle with Skin, Percutaneous Endoscopic Approach
0KX84Z1 Transfer Left Upper Arm Muscle with Subcutaneous Tissue, Percutaneous Endoscopic Approach

0KX84Z2 Transfer Left Upper Arm Muscle with Skin and Subcutaneous Tissue, Percutaneous Endoscopic Approach

0KX84ZZ Transfer Left Upper Arm Muscle, Percutaneous Endoscopic Approach

0KX90Z0 Transfer Right Lower Arm and Wrist Muscle with Skin, Open Approach

0KX90Z1 Transfer Right Lower Arm and Wrist Muscle with Subcutaneous Tissue, Open Approach

0KX90Z2 Transfer Right Lower Arm and Wrist Muscle with Skin and Subcutaneous Tissue, Open Approach

0KX90ZZ Transfer Right Lower Arm and Wrist Muscle, Open Approach

0KX94Z0 Transfer Right Lower Arm and Wrist Muscle with Skin, Percutaneous Endoscopic Approach

0KX94Z1 Transfer Right Lower Arm and Wrist Muscle with Subcutaneous Tissue, Percutaneous Endoscopic Approach

0KX94Z2 Transfer Right Lower Arm and Wrist Muscle with Skin and Subcutaneous Tissue, Percutaneous Endoscopic Approach

0KX94ZZ Transfer Right Lower Arm and Wrist Muscle, Percutaneous Endoscopic Approach

0KXB0Z0 Transfer Left Lower Arm and Wrist Muscle with Skin, Open Approach

0KXB0Z1 Transfer Left Lower Arm and Wrist Muscle with Subcutaneous Tissue, Open Approach

0KXB0Z2 Transfer Left Lower Arm and Wrist Muscle with Skin and Subcutaneous Tissue, Open Approach

0KXB0ZZ Transfer Left Lower Arm and Wrist Muscle, Open Approach

0KXB4Z0 Transfer Left Lower Arm and Wrist Muscle with Skin, Percutaneous Endoscopic Approach

0KXB4Z1 Transfer Left Lower Arm and Wrist Muscle with Subcutaneous Tissue, Percutaneous Endoscopic Approach

0KXB4Z2 Transfer Left Lower Arm and Wrist Muscle with Skin and Subcutaneous Tissue, Percutaneous Endoscopic Approach

0KXB4ZZ Transfer Left Lower Arm and Wrist Muscle, Percutaneous Endoscopic Approach

0KXC0Z0 Transfer Right Hand Muscle with Skin, Open Approach

0KXC0Z1 Transfer Right Hand Muscle with Subcutaneous Tissue, Open Approach

0KXC0Z2 Transfer Right Hand Muscle with Skin and Subcutaneous Tissue, Open Approach

0KXC0ZZ Transfer Right Hand Muscle, Open Approach

0KXC4Z0 Transfer Right Hand Muscle with Skin, Percutaneous Endoscopic Approach

0KXC4Z1 Transfer Right Hand Muscle with Subcutaneous Tissue, Percutaneous Endoscopic Approach

0KXC4Z2 Transfer Right Hand Muscle with Skin and Subcutaneous Tissue, Percutaneous Endoscopic Approach

0KXC4ZZ Transfer Right Hand Muscle, Percutaneous Endoscopic Approach

0KXD0Z0 Transfer Left Hand Muscle with Skin, Open Approach

0KXD0Z1 Transfer Left Hand Muscle with Subcutaneous Tissue, Open Approach

0KXD0Z2 Transfer Left Hand Muscle with Skin and Subcutaneous Tissue, Open Approach

0KXD0ZZ Transfer Left Hand Muscle, Open Approach

0KXD4Z0 Transfer Left Hand Muscle with Skin, Percutaneous Endoscopic Approach

0KXD4Z1 Transfer Left Hand Muscle with Subcutaneous Tissue, Percutaneous Endoscopic Approach

0KXD4Z2 Transfer Left Hand Muscle with Skin and Subcutaneous Tissue, Percutaneous Endoscopic Approach

0KXD4ZZ Transfer Left Hand Muscle, Percutaneous Endoscopic Approach

0KXF0Z0 Transfer Right Trunk Muscle with Skin, Open Approach

0KXF0Z1 Transfer Right Trunk Muscle with Subcutaneous Tissue, Open Approach

0KXF0Z2 Transfer Right Trunk Muscle with Skin and Subcutaneous Tissue, Open Approach

0KXF0ZZ Transfer Right Trunk Muscle, Open Approach

0KXF4Z0 Transfer Right Trunk Muscle with Skin, Percutaneous Endoscopic Approach

0KXF4Z1 Transfer Right Trunk Muscle with Subcutaneous Tissue, Percutaneous Endoscopic Approach

0KXF4Z2 Transfer Right Trunk Muscle with Skin and Subcutaneous Tissue, Percutaneous Endoscopic Approach

0KXF4ZZ Transfer Right Trunk Muscle, Percutaneous Endoscopic Approach

0KXG0Z0 Transfer Left Trunk Muscle with Skin, Open Approach

0KXG0Z1 Transfer Left Trunk Muscle with Subcutaneous Tissue, Open Approach

0KXG0Z2 Transfer Left Trunk Muscle with Skin and Subcutaneous Tissue, Open Approach

0KXG0ZZ Transfer Left Trunk Muscle, Open Approach

0KXG4Z0 Transfer Left Trunk Muscle with Skin, Percutaneous Endoscopic Approach

0KXG4Z1 Transfer Left Trunk Muscle with Subcutaneous Tissue, Percutaneous Endoscopic Approach

0KXG4Z2 Transfer Left Trunk Muscle with Skin and Subcutaneous Tissue, Percutaneous Endoscopic Approach

0KXG4ZZ Transfer Left Trunk Muscle, Percutaneous Endoscopic Approach

0KXH0Z0 Transfer Right Thorax Muscle with Skin, Open Approach

0KXH0Z1 Transfer Right Thorax Muscle with Subcutaneous Tissue, Open Approach

0KXH0Z2 Transfer Right Thorax Muscle with Skin and Subcutaneous Tissue, Open Approach

0KXH0ZZ Transfer Right Thorax Muscle, Open Approach

0KXH4Z0 Transfer Right Thorax Muscle with Skin, Percutaneous Endoscopic Approach

0KXH4Z1 Transfer Right Thorax Muscle with Subcutaneous Tissue, Percutaneous Endoscopic Approach

0KXH4Z2 Transfer Right Thorax Muscle with Skin and Subcutaneous Tissue, Percutaneous Endoscopic Approach

0KXH4ZZ Transfer Right Thorax Muscle, Percutaneous Endoscopic Approach

0KXJ0Z0 Transfer Left Thorax Muscle with Skin, Open Approach

0KXJ0Z1 Transfer Left Thorax Muscle with Subcutaneous Tissue, Open Approach

0KXJ0Z2 Transfer Left Thorax Muscle with Skin and Subcutaneous Tissue, Open Approach

0KXJ0ZZ Transfer Left Thorax Muscle, Open Approach

0KXJ4Z0 Transfer Left Thorax Muscle with Skin, Percutaneous Endoscopic Approach

0KXJ4Z1 Transfer Left Thorax Muscle with Subcutaneous Tissue, Percutaneous Endoscopic Approach

0KXJ4Z2 Transfer Left Thorax Muscle with Skin and Subcutaneous Tissue, Percutaneous Endoscopic Approach

0KXJ4ZZ Transfer Left Thorax Muscle, Percutaneous Endoscopic Approach

0KXK0Z0 Transfer Right Abdomen Muscle with Skin, Open Approach

0KXK0Z1 Transfer Right Abdomen Muscle with Subcutaneous Tissue, Open Approach

0KXK0Z2 Transfer Right Abdomen Muscle with Skin and Subcutaneous Tissue, Open Approach

0KXK0Z6 Transfer Right Abdomen Muscle, Transverse Rectus Abdominis Myocutaneous Flap, Open Approach

0KXK0ZZ Transfer Right Abdomen Muscle, Open Approach

0KXK4Z0 Transfer Right Abdomen Muscle with Skin, Percutaneous Endoscopic Approach

0KXK4Z1 Transfer Right Abdomen Muscle with Subcutaneous Tissue, Percutaneous Endoscopic Approach

0KXK4Z2 Transfer Right Abdomen Muscle with Skin and Subcutaneous Tissue, Percutaneous Endoscopic Approach

0KXK4Z6 Transfer Right Abdomen Muscle, Transverse Rectus Abdominis Myocutaneous Flap, Percutaneous Endoscopic Approach

0KXK4ZZ Transfer Right Abdomen Muscle, Percutaneous Endoscopic Approach

0KXL0Z0 Transfer Left Abdomen Muscle with Skin, Open Approach

0KXL0Z1 Transfer Left Abdomen Muscle with Subcutaneous Tissue, Open Approach

0KXL0Z2 Transfer Left Abdomen Muscle with Skin and Subcutaneous Tissue, Open Approach

0KXL0Z6 Transfer Left Abdomen Muscle, Transverse Rectus Abdominis Myocutaneous Flap, Open Approach

0KXL0ZZ Transfer Left Abdomen Muscle, Open Approach

0KXL4Z0 Transfer Left Abdomen Muscle with Skin, Percutaneous Endoscopic Approach

0KXL4Z1 Transfer Left Abdomen Muscle with Subcutaneous Tissue, Percutaneous Endoscopic Approach

0KXL4Z2 Transfer Left Abdomen Muscle with Skin and Subcutaneous Tissue, Percutaneous Endoscopic Approach

0KXL4Z6 Transfer Left Abdomen Muscle, Transverse Rectus Abdominis Myocutaneous Flap, Percutaneous Endoscopic Approach

0KXL4ZZ Transfer Left Abdomen Muscle, Percutaneous Endoscopic Approach

0KXM0Z0 Transfer Perineum Muscle with Skin, Open Approach

0KXM0Z1 Transfer Perineum Muscle with Subcutaneous Tissue, Open Approach

0KXM0Z2 Transfer Perineum Muscle with Skin and Subcutaneous Tissue, Open Approach

0KXM0ZZ Transfer Perineum Muscle, Open Approach

0KXM4Z0 Transfer Perineum Muscle with Skin, Percutaneous Endoscopic Approach

0KXM4Z1 Transfer Perineum Muscle with Subcutaneous Tissue, Percutaneous Endoscopic Approach

0KXM4Z2 Transfer Perineum Muscle with Skin and Subcutaneous Tissue, Percutaneous Endoscopic Approach

0KXM4ZZ Transfer Perineum Muscle, Percutaneous Endoscopic Approach

0KXN0Z0 Transfer Right Hip Muscle with Skin, Open Approach

0KXN0Z1 Transfer Right Hip Muscle with Subcutaneous Tissue, Open Approach

0KXN0Z2 Transfer Right Hip Muscle with Skin and Subcutaneous Tissue, Open Approach

0KXN0ZZ Transfer Right Hip Muscle, Open Approach

0KXN4Z0 Transfer Right Hip Muscle with Skin, Percutaneous Endoscopic Approach

0KXN4Z1 Transfer Right Hip Muscle with Subcutaneous Tissue, Percutaneous Endoscopic Approach

0KXN4Z2 Transfer Right Hip Muscle with Skin and Subcutaneous Tissue, Percutaneous Endoscopic Approach

0KXN4ZZ Transfer Right Hip Muscle, Percutaneous Endoscopic Approach

0KXP0Z0 Transfer Left Hip Muscle with Skin, Open Approach

0KXP0Z1 Transfer Left Hip Muscle with Subcutaneous Tissue, Open Approach

0KXP0Z2 Transfer Left Hip Muscle with Skin and Subcutaneous Tissue, Open Approach

0KXP0ZZ Transfer Left Hip Muscle, Open Approach

0KXP4Z0 Transfer Left Hip Muscle with Skin, Percutaneous Endoscopic Approach

0KXP4Z1 Transfer Left Hip Muscle with Subcutaneous Tissue, Percutaneous Endoscopic Approach

0KXP4Z2 Transfer Left Hip Muscle with Skin and Subcutaneous Tissue, Percutaneous Endoscopic Approach

0KXP4ZZ Transfer Left Hip Muscle, Percutaneous Endoscopic Approach

0KXQ0Z0 Transfer Right Upper Leg Muscle with Skin, Open Approach

0KXQ0Z1 Transfer Right Upper Leg Muscle with Subcutaneous Tissue, Open Approach

0KXQ0Z2 Transfer Right Upper Leg Muscle with Skin and Subcutaneous Tissue, Open Approach

0KXQ0ZZ Transfer Right Upper Leg Muscle, Open Approach

0KXQ4Z0 Transfer Right Upper Leg Muscle with Skin, Percutaneous Endoscopic Approach

0KXQ4Z1 Transfer Right Upper Leg Muscle with Subcutaneous Tissue, Percutaneous Endoscopic Approach

0KXQ4Z2 Transfer Right Upper Leg Muscle with Skin and Subcutaneous Tissue, Percutaneous Endoscopic Approach

0KXQ4ZZ Transfer Right Upper Leg Muscle, Percutaneous Endoscopic Approach

0KXR0Z0 Transfer Left Upper Leg Muscle with Skin, Open Approach

0KXR0Z1 Transfer Left Upper Leg Muscle with Subcutaneous Tissue, Open Approach

0KXR0Z2 Transfer Left Upper Leg Muscle with Skin and Subcutaneous Tissue, Open Approach

0KXR0ZZ Transfer Left Upper Leg Muscle, Open Approach

0KXR4Z0 Transfer Left Upper Leg Muscle with Skin, Percutaneous Endoscopic Approach

0KXR4Z1 Transfer Left Upper Leg Muscle with Subcutaneous Tissue, Percutaneous Endoscopic Approach

0KXR4Z2 Transfer Left Upper Leg Muscle with Skin and Subcutaneous Tissue, Percutaneous Endoscopic Approach

0KXR4ZZ Transfer Left Upper Leg Muscle, Percutaneous Endoscopic Approach

0KXS0Z0 Transfer Right Lower Leg Muscle with Skin, Open Approach

0KXS0Z1 Transfer Right Lower Leg Muscle with Subcutaneous Tissue, Open Approach

0KXS0Z2 Transfer Right Lower Leg Muscle with Skin and Subcutaneous Tissue, Open Approach

0KXS0ZZ Transfer Right Lower Leg Muscle, Open Approach

0KXS4Z0 Transfer Right Lower Leg Muscle with Skin, Percutaneous Endoscopic Approach

0KXS4Z1 Transfer Right Lower Leg Muscle with Subcutaneous Tissue, Percutaneous Endoscopic Approach

0KXS4Z2 Transfer Right Lower Leg Muscle with Skin and Subcutaneous Tissue, Percutaneous Endoscopic Approach

0KXS4ZZ Transfer Right Lower Leg Muscle, Percutaneous Endoscopic Approach

0KXT0Z0 Transfer Left Lower Leg Muscle with Skin, Open Approach

0KXT0Z1 Transfer Left Lower Leg Muscle with Subcutaneous Tissue, Open Approach

0KXT0Z2 Transfer Left Lower Leg Muscle with Skin and Subcutaneous Tissue, Open Approach

0KXT0ZZ Transfer Left Lower Leg Muscle, Open Approach

0KXT4Z0 Transfer Left Lower Leg Muscle with Skin, Percutaneous Endoscopic Approach

0KXT4Z1 Transfer Left Lower Leg Muscle with Subcutaneous Tissue, Percutaneous Endoscopic Approach

0KXT4Z2 Transfer Left Lower Leg Muscle with Skin and Subcutaneous Tissue, Percutaneous Endoscopic Approach

0KXT4ZZ Transfer Left Lower Leg Muscle, Percutaneous Endoscopic Approach

0KXV0Z0 Transfer Right Foot Muscle with Skin, Open Approach

0KXV0Z1 Transfer Right Foot Muscle with Subcutaneous Tissue, Open Approach

0KXV0Z2 Transfer Right Foot Muscle with Skin and Subcutaneous Tissue, Open Approach

0KXV0ZZ Transfer Right Foot Muscle, Open Approach

0KXV4Z0 Transfer Right Foot Muscle with Skin, Percutaneous Endoscopic Approach

0KXV4Z1 Transfer Right Foot Muscle with Subcutaneous Tissue, Percutaneous Endoscopic Approach

0KXV4Z2 Transfer Right Foot Muscle with Skin and Subcutaneous Tissue, Percutaneous Endoscopic Approach

0KXV4ZZ Transfer Right Foot Muscle, Percutaneous Endoscopic Approach

0KXW0Z0 Transfer Left Foot Muscle with Skin, Open Approach

0KXW0Z1 Transfer Left Foot Muscle with Subcutaneous Tissue, Open Approach

0KXW0Z2 Transfer Left Foot Muscle with Skin and Subcutaneous Tissue, Open Approach

0KXW0ZZ Transfer Left Foot Muscle, Open Approach

0KXW4Z0 Transfer Left Foot Muscle with Skin, Percutaneous Endoscopic Approach

0KXW4Z1 Transfer Left Foot Muscle with Subcutaneous Tissue, Percutaneous Endoscopic Approach

0KXW4Z2 Transfer Left Foot Muscle with Skin and Subcutaneous Tissue, Percutaneous Endoscopic Approach

0KXW4ZZ Transfer Left Foot Muscle, Percutaneous Endoscopic Approach

Tendons

Shoulder Tendons and Ligaments

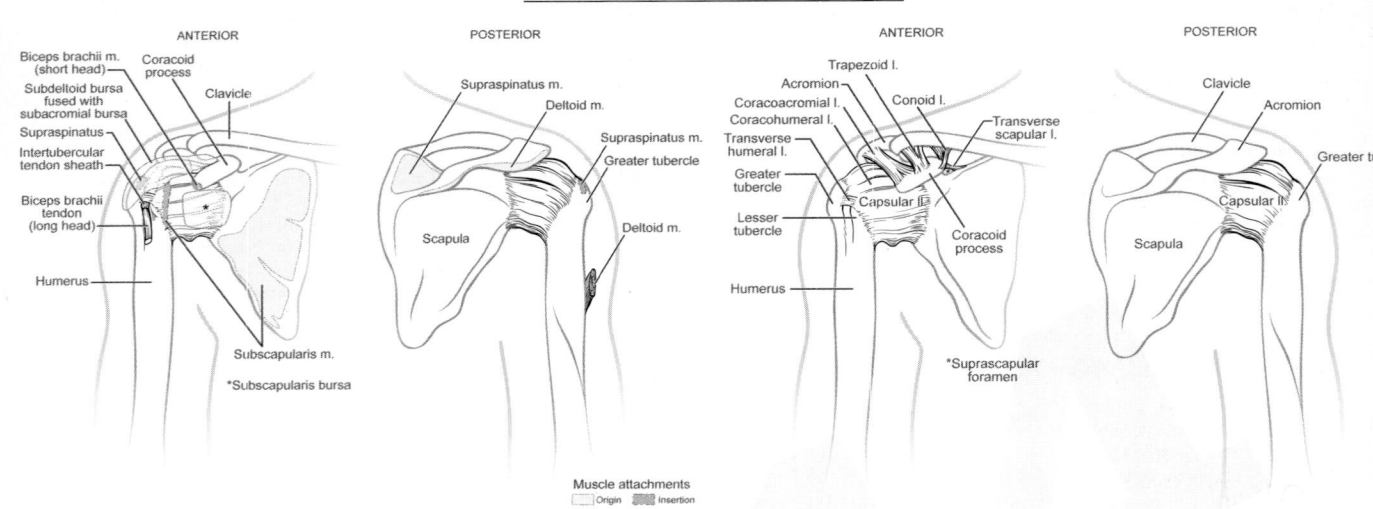

Muscle attachments
☐ Origin ▨ Insertion

Hip Tendons and Ligaments

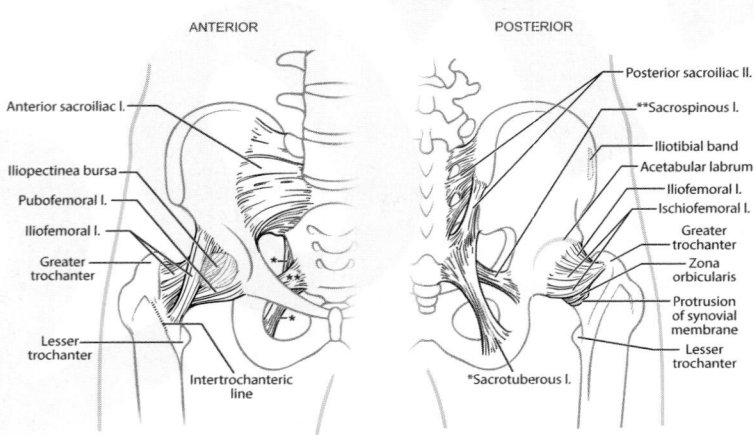

Knee Tendons and Ligaments

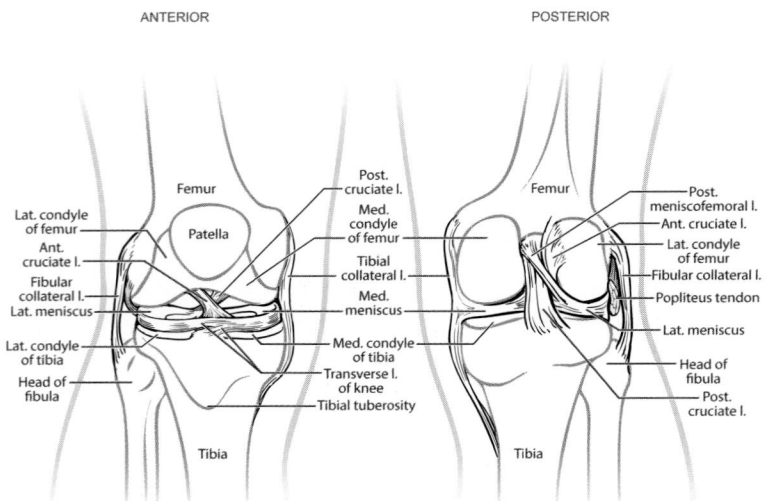

Tendons Tables 0L2–0LX

Section	0	**Medical and Surgical**
Body System	L	Tendons
Operation	2	**Change:** Taking out or off a device from a body part and putting back an identical or similar device in or on the same body part without cutting or puncturing the skin or a mucous membrane

Body Part (4th)	Approach (5th)	Device (6th)	Qualifier (7th)
X Upper Tendon Y Lower Tendon	X External	0 Drainage Device Y Other Device	Z No Qualifier

Section	0	**Medical and Surgical**
Body System	L	Tendons
Operation	5	**Destruction:** Physical eradication of all or a portion of a body part by the direct use of energy, force, or a destructive agent

Body Part (4th)	Approach (5th)	Device (6th)	Qualifier (7th)
0 Head and Neck Tendon 1 Shoulder Tendon, Right 2 Shoulder Tendon, Left 3 Upper Arm Tendon, Right 4 Upper Arm Tendon, Left 5 Lower Arm and Wrist Tendon, Right 6 Lower Arm and Wrist Tendon, Left 7 Hand Tendon, Right 8 Hand Tendon, Left 9 Trunk Tendon, Right B Trunk Tendon, Left C Thorax Tendon, Right D Thorax Tendon, Left F Abdomen Tendon, Right G Abdomen Tendon, Left H Perineum Tendon J Hip Tendon, Right K Hip Tendon, Left L Upper Leg Tendon, Right M Upper Leg Tendon, Left N Lower Leg Tendon, Right P Lower Leg Tendon, Left Q Knee Tendon, Right R Knee Tendon, Left S Ankle Tendon, Right T Ankle Tendon, Left V Foot Tendon, Right W Foot Tendon, Left	0 Open 3 Percutaneous 4 Percutaneous Endoscopic	Z No Device	Z No Qualifier

Section	0	Medical and Surgical
Body System	L	Tendons
Operation	8	**Division:** Cutting into a body part, without draining fluids and/or gases from the body part, in order to separate or transect a body part

Body Part (4ᵗʰ)	Approach (5ᵗʰ)	Device (6ᵗʰ)	Qualifier (7ᵗʰ)
0 Head and Neck Tendon 1 Shoulder Tendon, Right 2 Shoulder Tendon, Left 3 Upper Arm Tendon, Right 4 Upper Arm Tendon, Left 5 Lower Arm and Wrist Tendon, Right 6 Lower Arm and Wrist Tendon, Left 7 Hand Tendon, Right 8 Hand Tendon, Left 9 Trunk Tendon, Right B Trunk Tendon, Left C Thorax Tendon, Right D Thorax Tendon, Left F Abdomen Tendon, Right G Abdomen Tendon, Left H Perineum Tendon J Hip Tendon, Right K Hip Tendon, Left L Upper Leg Tendon, Right M Upper Leg Tendon, Left N Lower Leg Tendon, Right P Lower Leg Tendon, Left Q Knee Tendon, Right R Knee Tendon, Left S Ankle Tendon, Right T Ankle Tendon, Left V Foot Tendon, Right W Foot Tendon, Left	0 Open 3 Percutaneous 4 Percutaneous Endoscopic	Z No Device	Z No Qualifier

	Section	0	**Medical and Surgical**
	Body System	L	**Tendons**
	Operation	9	**Drainage:** Taking or letting out fluids and/or gases from a body part

Body Part (4th)	Approach (5th)	Device (6th)	Qualifier (7th)
0 Head and Neck Tendon 1 Shoulder Tendon, Right 2 Shoulder Tendon, Left 3 Upper Arm Tendon, Right 4 Upper Arm Tendon, Left 5 Lower Arm and Wrist Tendon, Right 6 Lower Arm and Wrist Tendon, Left 7 Hand Tendon, Right 8 Hand Tendon, Left 9 Trunk Tendon, Right B Trunk Tendon, Left C Thorax Tendon, Right D Thorax Tendon, Left F Abdomen Tendon, Right G Abdomen Tendon, Left H Perineum Tendon J Hip Tendon, Right K Hip Tendon, Left L Upper Leg Tendon, Right M Upper Leg Tendon, Left N Lower Leg Tendon, Right P Lower Leg Tendon, Left Q Knee Tendon, Right R Knee Tendon, Left S Ankle Tendon, Right T Ankle Tendon, Left V Foot Tendon, Right W Foot Tendon, Left	0 Open 3 Percutaneous 4 Percutaneous Endoscopic	0 Drainage Device	Z No Qualifier
0 Head and Neck Tendon 1 Shoulder Tendon, Right 2 Shoulder Tendon, Left 3 Upper Arm Tendon, Right 4 Upper Arm Tendon, Left 5 Lower Arm and Wrist Tendon, Right 6 Lower Arm and Wrist Tendon, Left 7 Hand Tendon, Right 8 Hand Tendon, Left 9 Trunk Tendon, Right B Trunk Tendon, Left C Thorax Tendon, Right D Thorax Tendon, Left F Abdomen Tendon, Right G Abdomen Tendon, Left H Perineum Tendon J Hip Tendon, Right K Hip Tendon, Left L Upper Leg Tendon, Right M Upper Leg Tendon, Left N Lower Leg Tendon, Right P Lower Leg Tendon, Left Q Knee Tendon, Right R Knee Tendon, Left S Ankle Tendon, Right T Ankle Tendon, Left V Foot Tendon, Right W Foot Tendon, Left	0 Open 3 Percutaneous 4 Percutaneous Endoscopic	Z No Device	X Diagnostic Z No Qualifier

Section	0	Medical and Surgical
Body System	L	Tendons
Operation	B	**Excision:** Cutting out or off, without replacement, a portion of a body part

Body Part (4th)	Approach (5th)	Device (6th)	Qualifier (7th)
0 Head and Neck Tendon	0 Open	Z No Device	X Diagnostic
1 Shoulder Tendon, Right	3 Percutaneous		Z No Qualifier
2 Shoulder Tendon, Left	4 Percutaneous Endoscopic		
3 Upper Arm Tendon, Right			
4 Upper Arm Tendon, Left			
5 Lower Arm and Wrist Tendon, Right			
6 Lower Arm and Wrist Tendon, Left			
7 Hand Tendon, Right			
8 Hand Tendon, Left			
9 Trunk Tendon, Right			
B Trunk Tendon, Left			
C Thorax Tendon, Right			
D Thorax Tendon, Left			
F Abdomen Tendon, Right			
G Abdomen Tendon, Left			
H Perineum Tendon			
J Hip Tendon, Right			
K Hip Tendon, Left			
L Upper Leg Tendon, Right			
M Upper Leg Tendon, Left			
N Lower Leg Tendon, Right			
P Lower Leg Tendon, Left			
Q Knee Tendon, Right			
R Knee Tendon, Left			
S Ankle Tendon, Right			
T Ankle Tendon, Left			
V Foot Tendon, Right			
W Foot Tendon, Left			

Section	0	Medical and Surgical
Body System	L	Tendons
Operation	C	**Extirpation:** Taking or cutting out solid matter from a body part

Body Part (4th)	Approach (5th)	Device (6th)	Qualifier (7th)
0 Head and Neck Tendon	0 Open	Z No Device	Z No Qualifier
1 Shoulder Tendon, Right	3 Percutaneous		
2 Shoulder Tendon, Left	4 Percutaneous Endoscopic		
3 Upper Arm Tendon, Right			
4 Upper Arm Tendon, Left			
5 Lower Arm and Wrist Tendon, Right			
6 Lower Arm and Wrist Tendon, Left			
7 Hand Tendon, Right			
8 Hand Tendon, Left			
9 Trunk Tendon, Right			
B Trunk Tendon, Left			
C Thorax Tendon, Right			
D Thorax Tendon, Left			
F Abdomen Tendon, Right			
G Abdomen Tendon, Left			
H Perineum Tendon			
J Hip Tendon, Right			
K Hip Tendon, Left			
L Upper Leg Tendon, Right			
M Upper Leg Tendon, Left			
N Lower Leg Tendon, Right			
P Lower Leg Tendon, Left			
Q Knee Tendon, Right			
R Knee Tendon, Left			
S Ankle Tendon, Right			
T Ankle Tendon, Left			
V Foot Tendon, Right			
W Foot Tendon, Left			

Section	0	Medical and Surgical
Body System	L	Tendons
Operation	J	**Inspection:** Visually and/or manually exploring a body part

Body Part (4th)	Approach (5th)	Device (6th)	Qualifier (7th)
X Upper Tendon Y Lower Tendon	0 Open 3 Percutaneous 4 Percutaneous Endoscopic X External	Z No Device	Z No Qualifier

Section	0	Medical and Surgical
Body System	L	Tendons
Operation	M	**Reattachment:** Putting back in or on all or a portion of a separated body part to its normal location or other suitable location

Body Part (4th)	Approach (5th)	Device (6th)	Qualifier (7th)
0 Head and Neck Tendon 1 Shoulder Tendon, Right 2 Shoulder Tendon, Left 3 Upper Arm Tendon, Right 4 Upper Arm Tendon, Left 5 Lower Arm and Wrist Tendon, Right 6 Lower Arm and Wrist Tendon, Left 7 Hand Tendon, Right 8 Hand Tendon, Left 9 Trunk Tendon, Right B Trunk Tendon, Left C Thorax Tendon, Right D Thorax Tendon, Left F Abdomen Tendon, Right G Abdomen Tendon, Left H Perineum Tendon J Hip Tendon, Right K Hip Tendon, Left L Upper Leg Tendon, Right M Upper Leg Tendon, Left N Lower Leg Tendon, Right P Lower Leg Tendon, Left Q Knee Tendon, Right R Knee Tendon, Left S Ankle Tendon, Right T Ankle Tendon, Left V Foot Tendon, Right W Foot Tendon, Left	0 Open 4 Percutaneous Endoscopic	Z No Device	Z No Qualifier

Section	0	Medical and Surgical
Body System	L	Tendons
Operation	N	**Release:** Freeing a body part from an abnormal physical constraint by cutting or by the use of force

Body Part (4th)	Approach (5th)	Device (6th)	Qualifier (7th)
0 Head and Neck Tendon 1 Shoulder Tendon, Right 2 Shoulder Tendon, Left 3 Upper Arm Tendon, Right 4 Upper Arm Tendon, Left 5 Lower Arm and Wrist Tendon, Right 6 Lower Arm and Wrist Tendon, Left 7 Hand Tendon, Right 8 Hand Tendon, Left 9 Trunk Tendon, Right B Trunk Tendon, Left C Thorax Tendon, Right D Thorax Tendon, Left F Abdomen Tendon, Right G Abdomen Tendon, Left H Perineum Tendon J Hip Tendon, Right K Hip Tendon, Left L Upper Leg Tendon, Right M Upper Leg Tendon, Left N Lower Leg Tendon, Right P Lower Leg Tendon, Left Q Knee Tendon, Right R Knee Tendon, Left S Ankle Tendon, Right T Ankle Tendon, Left V Foot Tendon, Right W Foot Tendon, Left	0 Open 3 Percutaneous 4 Percutaneous Endoscopic X External	Z No Device	Z No Qualifier

Section	0	Medical and Surgical
Body System	L	Tendons
Operation	P	**Removal:** Taking out or off a device from a body part

Body Part (4th)	Approach (5th)	Device (6th)	Qualifier (7th)
X Upper Tendon Y Lower Tendon	0 Open 3 Percutaneous 4 Percutaneous Endoscopic	0 Drainage Device 7 Autologous Tissue Substitute J Synthetic Substitute K Nonautologous Tissue Substitute	Z No Qualifier
X Upper Tendon Y Lower Tendon	X External	0 Drainage Device	Z No Qualifier

Section	0	**Medical and Surgical**
Body System	L	**Tendons**
Operation	Q	**Repair:** Restoring, to the extent possible, a body part to its normal anatomic structure and function

Body Part (4th)	Approach (5th)	Device (6th)	Qualifier (7th)
0 Head and Neck Tendon	0 Open	**Z** No Device	**Z** No Qualifier
1 Shoulder Tendon, Right	3 Percutaneous		
2 Shoulder Tendon, Left	4 Percutaneous Endoscopic		
3 Upper Arm Tendon, Right			
4 Upper Arm Tendon, Left			
5 Lower Arm and Wrist Tendon, Right			
6 Lower Arm and Wrist Tendon, Left			
7 Hand Tendon, Right			
8 Hand Tendon, Left			
9 Trunk Tendon, Right			
B Trunk Tendon, Left			
C Thorax Tendon, Right			
D Thorax Tendon, Left			
F Abdomen Tendon, Right			
G Abdomen Tendon, Left			
H Perineum Tendon			
J Hip Tendon, Right			
K Hip Tendon, Left			
L Upper Leg Tendon, Right			
M Upper Leg Tendon, Left			
N Lower Leg Tendon, Right			
P Lower Leg Tendon, Left			
Q Knee Tendon, Right			
R Knee Tendon, Left			
S Ankle Tendon, Right			
T Ankle Tendon, Left			
V Foot Tendon, Right			
W Foot Tendon, Left			

Section	0	**Medical and Surgical**
Body System	L	**Tendons**
Operation	R	**Replacement:** Putting in or on biological or synthetic material that physically takes the place and/or function of all or a portion of a body part

Body Part (4th)	Approach (5th)	Device (6th)	Qualifier (7th)
0 Head and Neck Tendon	0 Open	7 Autologous Tissue Substitute	Z No Qualifier
1 Shoulder Tendon, Right	4 Percutaneous Endoscopic	J Synthetic Substitute	
2 Shoulder Tendon, Left		K Nonautologous Tissue Substitute	
3 Upper Arm Tendon, Right			
4 Upper Arm Tendon, Left			
5 Lower Arm and Wrist Tendon, Right			
6 Lower Arm and Wrist Tendon, Left			
7 Hand Tendon, Right			
8 Hand Tendon, Left			
9 Trunk Tendon, Right			
B Trunk Tendon, Left			
C Thorax Tendon, Right			
D Thorax Tendon, Left			
F Abdomen Tendon, Right			
G Abdomen Tendon, Left			
H Perineum Tendon			
J Hip Tendon, Right			
K Hip Tendon, Left			
L Upper Leg Tendon, Right			
M Upper Leg Tendon, Left			
N Lower Leg Tendon, Right			
P Lower Leg Tendon, Left			
Q Knee Tendon, Right			
R Knee Tendon, Left			
S Ankle Tendon, Right			
T Ankle Tendon, Left			
V Foot Tendon, Right			
W Foot Tendon, Left			

Section	0	Medical and Surgical
Body System	L	Tendons
Operation	S	Reposition: Moving to its normal location, or other suitable location, all or a portion of a body part

Body Part (4th)	Approach (5th)	Device (6th)	Qualifier (7th)
0 Head and Neck Tendon 1 Shoulder Tendon, Right 2 Shoulder Tendon, Left 3 Upper Arm Tendon, Right 4 Upper Arm Tendon, Left 5 Lower Arm and Wrist Tendon, Right 6 Lower Arm and Wrist Tendon, Left 7 Hand Tendon, Right 8 Hand Tendon, Left 9 Trunk Tendon, Right B Trunk Tendon, Left C Thorax Tendon, Right D Thorax Tendon, Left F Abdomen Tendon, Right G Abdomen Tendon, Left H Perineum Tendon J Hip Tendon, Right K Hip Tendon, Left L Upper Leg Tendon, Right M Upper Leg Tendon, Left N Lower Leg Tendon, Right P Lower Leg Tendon, Left Q Knee Tendon, Right R Knee Tendon, Left S Ankle Tendon, Right T Ankle Tendon, Left V Foot Tendon, Right W Foot Tendon, Left	0 Open 4 Percutaneous Endoscopic	Z No Device	Z No Qualifier

Section	0	Medical and Surgical
Body System	L	Tendons
Operation	T	Resection: Cutting out or off, without replacement, all of a body part

Body Part (4th)	Approach (5th)	Device (6th)	Qualifier (7th)
0 Head and Neck Tendon 1 Shoulder Tendon, Right 2 Shoulder Tendon, Left 3 Upper Arm Tendon, Right 4 Upper Arm Tendon, Left 5 Lower Arm and Wrist Tendon, Right 6 Lower Arm and Wrist Tendon, Left 7 Hand Tendon, Right 8 Hand Tendon, Left 9 Trunk Tendon, Right B Trunk Tendon, Left C Thorax Tendon, Right D Thorax Tendon, Left F Abdomen Tendon, Right G Abdomen Tendon, Left H Perineum Tendon J Hip Tendon, Right K Hip Tendon, Left L Upper Leg Tendon, Right M Upper Leg Tendon, Left N Lower Leg Tendon, Right P Lower Leg Tendon, Left Q Knee Tendon, Right R Knee Tendon, Left S Ankle Tendon, Right T Ankle Tendon, Left V Foot Tendon, Right W Foot Tendon, Left	0 Open 4 Percutaneous Endoscopic	Z No Device	Z No Qualifier

Section	0	Medical and Surgical
Body System	L	Tendons
Operation	U	**Supplement:** Putting in or on biological or synthetic material that physically reinforces and/or augments the function of a portion of a body part

Body Part (4th)	Approach (5th)	Device (6th)	Qualifier (7th)
0 Head and Neck Tendon 1 Shoulder Tendon, Right 2 Shoulder Tendon, Left 3 Upper Arm Tendon, Right 4 Upper Arm Tendon, Left 5 Lower Arm and Wrist Tendon, Right 6 Lower Arm and Wrist Tendon, Left 7 Hand Tendon, Right 8 Hand Tendon, Left 9 Trunk Tendon, Right B Trunk Tendon, Left C Thorax Tendon, Right D Thorax Tendon, Left F Abdomen Tendon, Right G Abdomen Tendon, Left H Perineum Tendon J Hip Tendon, Right K Hip Tendon, Left L Upper Leg Tendon, Right M Upper Leg Tendon, Left N Lower Leg Tendon, Right P Lower Leg Tendon, Left Q Knee Tendon, Right R Knee Tendon, Left S Ankle Tendon, Right T Ankle Tendon, Left V Foot Tendon, Right W Foot Tendon, Left	0 Open 4 Percutaneous Endoscopic	7 Autologous Tissue Substitute J Synthetic Substitute K Nonautologous Tissue Substitute	Z No Qualifier

Section	0	Medical and Surgical
Body System	L	Tendons
Operation	W	**Revision:** Correcting, to the extent possible, a portion of a malfunctioning device or the position of a displaced device

Body Part (4th)	Approach (5th)	Device (6th)	Qualifier (7th)
X Upper Tendon Y Lower Tendon	0 Open 3 Percutaneous 4 Percutaneous Endoscopic X External	0 Drainage Device 7 Autologous Tissue Substitute J Synthetic Substitute K Nonautologous Tissue Substitute	Z No Qualifier

Section	0	**Medical and Surgical**
Body System	L	**Tendons**
Operation	X	**Transfer:** Moving, without taking out, all or a portion of a body part to another location to take over the function of all or a portion of a body part

Body Part (4ᵗʰ)	Approach (5ᵗʰ)	Device (6ᵗʰ)	Qualifier (7ᵗʰ)
0 Head and Neck Tendon	0 Open	Z No Device	Z No Qualifier
1 Shoulder Tendon, Right	4 Percutaneous Endoscopic		
2 Shoulder Tendon, Left			
3 Upper Arm Tendon, Right			
4 Upper Arm Tendon, Left			
5 Lower Arm and Wrist Tendon, Right			
6 Lower Arm and Wrist Tendon, Left			
7 Hand Tendon, Right			
8 Hand Tendon, Left			
9 Trunk Tendon, Right			
B Trunk Tendon, Left			
C Thorax Tendon, Right			
D Thorax Tendon, Left			
F Abdomen Tendon, Right			
G Abdomen Tendon, Left			
H Perineum Tendon			
J Hip Tendon, Right			
K Hip Tendon, Left			
L Upper Leg Tendon, Right			
M Upper Leg Tendon, Left			
N Lower Leg Tendon, Right			
P Lower Leg Tendon, Left			
Q Knee Tendon, Right			
R Knee Tendon, Left			
S Ankle Tendon, Right			
T Ankle Tendon, Left			
V Foot Tendon, Right			
W Foot Tendon, Left			

Tendons Code Listing 0L2–0LX

Review Coding Guideline B4.5

0L2 – Tendons, Change

Review Coding Guideline B6.1c

0L2XX0Z	Change Drainage Device in Upper Tendon, External Approach	0L2YX0Z	Change Drainage Device in Lower Tendon, External Approach
0L2XXYZ	Change Other Device in Upper Tendon, External Approach	0L2YXYZ	Change Other Device in Lower Tendon, External Approach

0L5 – Tendons, Destruction

0L500ZZ	Destruction of Head and Neck Tendon, Open Approach	0L540ZZ	Destruction of Left Upper Arm Tendon, Open Approach
0L503ZZ	Destruction of Head and Neck Tendon, Percutaneous Approach	0L543ZZ	Destruction of Left Upper Arm Tendon, Percutaneous Approach
0L504ZZ	Destruction of Head and Neck Tendon, Percutaneous Endoscopic Approach	0L544ZZ	Destruction of Left Upper Arm Tendon, Percutaneous Endoscopic Approach
0L510ZZ	Destruction of Right Shoulder Tendon, Open Approach	0L550ZZ	Destruction of Right Lower Arm and Wrist Tendon, Open Approach
0L513ZZ	Destruction of Right Shoulder Tendon, Percutaneous Approach	0L553ZZ	Destruction of Right Lower Arm and Wrist Tendon, Percutaneous Approach
0L514ZZ	Destruction of Right Shoulder Tendon, Percutaneous Endoscopic Approach	0L554ZZ	Destruction of Right Lower Arm and Wrist Tendon, Percutaneous Endoscopic Approach
0L520ZZ	Destruction of Left Shoulder Tendon, Open Approach	0L560ZZ	Destruction of Left Lower Arm and Wrist Tendon, Open Approach
0L523ZZ	Destruction of Left Shoulder Tendon, Percutaneous Approach	0L563ZZ	Destruction of Left Lower Arm and Wrist Tendon, Percutaneous Approach
0L524ZZ	Destruction of Left Shoulder Tendon, Percutaneous Endoscopic Approach	0L564ZZ	Destruction of Left Lower Arm and Wrist Tendon, Percutaneous Endoscopic Approach
0L530ZZ	Destruction of Right Upper Arm Tendon, Open Approach	0L570ZZ	Destruction of Right Hand Tendon, Open Approach
0L533ZZ	Destruction of Right Upper Arm Tendon, Percutaneous Approach	0L573ZZ	Destruction of Right Hand Tendon, Percutaneous Approach
0L534ZZ	Destruction of Right Upper Arm Tendon, Percutaneous Endoscopic Approach		

0L574ZZ Destruction of Right Hand Tendon, Percutaneous Endoscopic Approach
0L580ZZ Destruction of Left Hand Tendon, Open Approach
0L583ZZ Destruction of Left Hand Tendon, Percutaneous Approach
0L584ZZ Destruction of Left Hand Tendon, Percutaneous Endoscopic Approach
0L590ZZ Destruction of Right Trunk Tendon, Open Approach
0L593ZZ Destruction of Right Trunk Tendon, Percutaneous Approach
0L594ZZ Destruction of Right Trunk Tendon, Percutaneous Endoscopic Approach
0L5B0ZZ Destruction of Left Trunk Tendon, Open Approach
0L5B3ZZ Destruction of Left Trunk Tendon, Percutaneous Approach
0L5B4ZZ Destruction of Left Trunk Tendon, Percutaneous Endoscopic Approach
0L5C0ZZ Destruction of Right Thorax Tendon, Open Approach
0L5C3ZZ Destruction of Right Thorax Tendon, Percutaneous Approach
0L5C4ZZ Destruction of Right Thorax Tendon, Percutaneous Endoscopic Approach
0L5D0ZZ Destruction of Left Thorax Tendon, Open Approach
0L5D3ZZ Destruction of Left Thorax Tendon, Percutaneous Approach
0L5D4ZZ Destruction of Left Thorax Tendon, Percutaneous Endoscopic Approach
0L5F0ZZ Destruction of Right Abdomen Tendon, Open Approach
0L5F3ZZ Destruction of Right Abdomen Tendon, Percutaneous Approach
0L5F4ZZ Destruction of Right Abdomen Tendon, Percutaneous Endoscopic Approach
0L5G0ZZ Destruction of Left Abdomen Tendon, Open Approach
0L5G3ZZ Destruction of Left Abdomen Tendon, Percutaneous Approach
0L5G4ZZ Destruction of Left Abdomen Tendon, Percutaneous Endoscopic Approach
0L5H0ZZ Destruction of Perineum Tendon, Open Approach
0L5H3ZZ Destruction of Perineum Tendon, Percutaneous Approach
0L5H4ZZ Destruction of Perineum Tendon, Percutaneous Endoscopic Approach
0L5J0ZZ Destruction of Right Hip Tendon, Open Approach
0L5J3ZZ Destruction of Right Hip Tendon, Percutaneous Approach
0L5J4ZZ Destruction of Right Hip Tendon, Percutaneous Endoscopic Approach
0L5K0ZZ Destruction of Left Hip Tendon, Open Approach
0L5K3ZZ Destruction of Left Hip Tendon, Percutaneous Approach
0L5K4ZZ Destruction of Left Hip Tendon, Percutaneous Endoscopic Approach

0L5L0ZZ Destruction of Right Upper Leg Tendon, Open Approach
0L5L3ZZ Destruction of Right Upper Leg Tendon, Percutaneous Approach
0L5L4ZZ Destruction of Right Upper Leg Tendon, Percutaneous Endoscopic Approach
0L5M0ZZ Destruction of Left Upper Leg Tendon, Open Approach
0L5M3ZZ Destruction of Left Upper Leg Tendon, Percutaneous Approach
0L5M4ZZ Destruction of Left Upper Leg Tendon, Percutaneous Endoscopic Approach
0L5N0ZZ Destruction of Right Lower Leg Tendon, Open Approach
0L5N3ZZ Destruction of Right Lower Leg Tendon, Percutaneous Approach
0L5N4ZZ Destruction of Right Lower Leg Tendon, Percutaneous Endoscopic Approach
0L5P0ZZ Destruction of Left Lower Leg Tendon, Open Approach
0L5P3ZZ Destruction of Left Lower Leg Tendon, Percutaneous Approach
0L5P4ZZ Destruction of Left Lower Leg Tendon, Percutaneous Endoscopic Approach
0L5Q0ZZ Destruction of Right Knee Tendon, Open Approach
0L5Q3ZZ Destruction of Right Knee Tendon, Percutaneous Approach
0L5Q4ZZ Destruction of Right Knee Tendon, Percutaneous Endoscopic Approach
0L5R0ZZ Destruction of Left Knee Tendon, Open Approach
0L5R3ZZ Destruction of Left Knee Tendon, Percutaneous Approach
0L5R4ZZ Destruction of Left Knee Tendon, Percutaneous Endoscopic Approach
0L5S0ZZ Destruction of Right Ankle Tendon, Open Approach
0L5S3ZZ Destruction of Right Ankle Tendon, Percutaneous Approach
0L5S4ZZ Destruction of Right Ankle Tendon, Percutaneous Endoscopic Approach
0L5T0ZZ Destruction of Left Ankle Tendon, Open Approach
0L5T3ZZ Destruction of Left Ankle Tendon, Percutaneous Approach
0L5T4ZZ Destruction of Left Ankle Tendon, Percutaneous Endoscopic Approach
0L5V0ZZ Destruction of Right Foot Tendon, Open Approach
0L5V3ZZ Destruction of Right Foot Tendon, Percutaneous Approach
0L5V4ZZ Destruction of Right Foot Tendon, Percutaneous Endoscopic Approach
0L5W0ZZ Destruction of Left Foot Tendon, Open Approach
0L5W3ZZ Destruction of Left Foot Tendon, Percutaneous Approach
0L5W4ZZ Destruction of Left Foot Tendon, Percutaneous Endoscopic Approach

0L8 – Tendons, Division

Review Coding Guideline B3.14

0L800ZZ Division of Head and Neck Tendon, Open Approach
0L803ZZ Division of Head and Neck Tendon, Percutaneous Approach
0L804ZZ Division of Head and Neck Tendon, Percutaneous Endoscopic Approach
0L810ZZ Division of Right Shoulder Tendon, Open Approach
0L813ZZ Division of Right Shoulder Tendon, Percutaneous Approach
0L814ZZ Division of Right Shoulder Tendon, Percutaneous Endoscopic Approach
0L820ZZ Division of Left Shoulder Tendon, Open Approach
0L823ZZ Division of Left Shoulder Tendon, Percutaneous Approach
0L824ZZ Division of Left Shoulder Tendon, Percutaneous Endoscopic Approach
0L830ZZ Division of Right Upper Arm Tendon, Open Approach
0L833ZZ Division of Right Upper Arm Tendon, Percutaneous Approach
0L834ZZ Division of Right Upper Arm Tendon, Percutaneous Endoscopic Approach
0L840ZZ Division of Left Upper Arm Tendon, Open Approach
0L843ZZ Division of Left Upper Arm Tendon, Percutaneous Approach
0L844ZZ Division of Left Upper Arm Tendon, Percutaneous Endoscopic Approach
0L850ZZ Division of Right Lower Arm and Wrist Tendon, Open Approach
0L853ZZ Division of Right Lower Arm and Wrist Tendon, Percutaneous Approach
0L854ZZ Division of Right Lower Arm and Wrist Tendon, Percutaneous Endoscopic Approach
0L860ZZ Division of Left Lower Arm and Wrist Tendon, Open Approach

0L863ZZ Division of Left Lower Arm and Wrist Tendon, Percutaneous Approach
0L864ZZ Division of Left Lower Arm and Wrist Tendon, Percutaneous Endoscopic Approach
0L870ZZ Division of Right Hand Tendon, Open Approach
0L873ZZ Division of Right Hand Tendon, Percutaneous Approach
0L874ZZ Division of Right Hand Tendon, Percutaneous Endoscopic Approach
0L880ZZ Division of Left Hand Tendon, Open Approach
0L883ZZ Division of Left Hand Tendon, Percutaneous Approach
0L884ZZ Division of Left Hand Tendon, Percutaneous Endoscopic Approach
0L890ZZ Division of Right Trunk Tendon, Open Approach
0L893ZZ Division of Right Trunk Tendon, Percutaneous Approach
0L894ZZ Division of Right Trunk Tendon, Percutaneous Endoscopic Approach
0L8B0ZZ Division of Left Trunk Tendon, Open Approach
0L8B3ZZ Division of Left Trunk Tendon, Percutaneous Approach
0L8B4ZZ Division of Left Trunk Tendon, Percutaneous Endoscopic Approach
0L8C0ZZ Division of Right Thorax Tendon, Open Approach
0L8C3ZZ Division of Right Thorax Tendon, Percutaneous Approach
0L8C4ZZ Division of Right Thorax Tendon, Percutaneous Endoscopic Approach
0L8D0ZZ Division of Left Thorax Tendon, Open Approach
0L8D3ZZ Division of Left Thorax Tendon, Percutaneous Approach
0L8D4ZZ Division of Left Thorax Tendon, Percutaneous Endoscopic Approach

0L8F0ZZ	Division of Right Abdomen Tendon, Open Approach
0L8F3ZZ	Division of Right Abdomen Tendon, Percutaneous Approach
0L8F4ZZ	Division of Right Abdomen Tendon, Percutaneous Endoscopic Approach
0L8G0ZZ	Division of Left Abdomen Tendon, Open Approach
0L8G3ZZ	Division of Left Abdomen Tendon, Percutaneous Approach
0L8G4ZZ	Division of Left Abdomen Tendon, Percutaneous Endoscopic Approach
0L8H0ZZ	Division of Perineum Tendon, Open Approach
0L8H3ZZ	Division of Perineum Tendon, Percutaneous Approach
0L8H4ZZ	Division of Perineum Tendon, Percutaneous Endoscopic Approach
0L8J0ZZ	Division of Right Hip Tendon, Open Approach
0L8J3ZZ	Division of Right Hip Tendon, Percutaneous Approach
0L8J4ZZ	Division of Right Hip Tendon, Percutaneous Endoscopic Approach
0L8K0ZZ	Division of Left Hip Tendon, Open Approach
0L8K3ZZ	Division of Left Hip Tendon, Percutaneous Approach
0L8K4ZZ	Division of Left Hip Tendon, Percutaneous Endoscopic Approach
0L8L0ZZ	Division of Right Upper Leg Tendon, Open Approach
0L8L3ZZ	Division of Right Upper Leg Tendon, Percutaneous Approach
0L8L4ZZ	Division of Right Upper Leg Tendon, Percutaneous Endoscopic Approach
0L8M0ZZ	Division of Left Upper Leg Tendon, Open Approach
0L8M3ZZ	Division of Left Upper Leg Tendon, Percutaneous Approach
0L8M4ZZ	Division of Left Upper Leg Tendon, Percutaneous Endoscopic Approach
0L8N0ZZ	Division of Right Lower Leg Tendon, Open Approach

0L8N3ZZ	Division of Right Lower Leg Tendon, Percutaneous Approach
0L8N4ZZ	Division of Right Lower Leg Tendon, Percutaneous Endoscopic Approach
0L8P0ZZ	Division of Left Lower Leg Tendon, Open Approach
0L8P3ZZ	Division of Left Lower Leg Tendon, Percutaneous Approach
0L8P4ZZ	Division of Left Lower Leg Tendon, Percutaneous Endoscopic Approach
0L8Q0ZZ	Division of Right Knee Tendon, Open Approach
0L8Q3ZZ	Division of Right Knee Tendon, Percutaneous Approach
0L8Q4ZZ	Division of Right Knee Tendon, Percutaneous Endoscopic Approach
0L8R0ZZ	Division of Left Knee Tendon, Open Approach
0L8R3ZZ	Division of Left Knee Tendon, Percutaneous Approach
0L8R4ZZ	Division of Left Knee Tendon, Percutaneous Endoscopic Approach
0L8S0ZZ	Division of Right Ankle Tendon, Open Approach
0L8S3ZZ	Division of Right Ankle Tendon, Percutaneous Approach
0L8S4ZZ	Division of Right Ankle Tendon, Percutaneous Endoscopic Approach
0L8T0ZZ	Division of Left Ankle Tendon, Open Approach
0L8T3ZZ	Division of Left Ankle Tendon, Percutaneous Approach
0L8T4ZZ	Division of Left Ankle Tendon, Percutaneous Endoscopic Approach
0L8V0ZZ	Division of Right Foot Tendon, Open Approach
0L8V3ZZ	Division of Right Foot Tendon, Percutaneous Approach
0L8V4ZZ	Division of Right Foot Tendon, Percutaneous Endoscopic Approach
0L8W0ZZ	Division of Left Foot Tendon, Open Approach
0L8W3ZZ	Division of Left Foot Tendon, Percutaneous Approach
0L8W4ZZ	Division of Left Foot Tendon, Percutaneous Endoscopic Approach

0L9 – Tendons, Drainage

Review Coding Guidelines B3.4a and B3.4b

Review Coding Guideline B6.2

0L9000Z	Drainage of Head and Neck Tendon with Drainage Device, Open Approach
0L900ZX	Drainage of Head and Neck Tendon, Open Approach, Diagnostic
0L900ZZ	Drainage of Head and Neck Tendon, Open Approach
0L9030Z	Drainage of Head and Neck Tendon with Drainage Device, Percutaneous Approach
0L903ZX	Drainage of Head and Neck Tendon, Percutaneous Approach, Diagnostic
0L903ZZ	Drainage of Head and Neck Tendon, Percutaneous Approach
0L9040Z	Drainage of Head and Neck Tendon with Drainage Device, Percutaneous Endoscopic Approach
0L904ZX	Drainage of Head and Neck Tendon, Percutaneous Endoscopic Approach, Diagnostic
0L904ZZ	Drainage of Head and Neck Tendon, Percutaneous Endoscopic Approach
0L9100Z	Drainage of Right Shoulder Tendon with Drainage Device, Open Approach
0L910ZX	Drainage of Right Shoulder Tendon, Open Approach, Diagnostic
0L910ZZ	Drainage of Right Shoulder Tendon, Open Approach
0L9130Z	Drainage of Right Shoulder Tendon with Drainage Device, Percutaneous Approach
0L913ZX	Drainage of Right Shoulder Tendon, Percutaneous Approach, Diagnostic
0L913ZZ	Drainage of Right Shoulder Tendon, Percutaneous Approach
0L9140Z	Drainage of Right Shoulder Tendon with Drainage Device, Percutaneous Endoscopic Approach
0L914ZX	Drainage of Right Shoulder Tendon, Percutaneous Endoscopic Approach, Diagnostic
0L914ZZ	Drainage of Right Shoulder Tendon, Percutaneous Endoscopic Approach
0L9200Z	Drainage of Left Shoulder Tendon with Drainage Device, Open Approach
0L920ZX	Drainage of Left Shoulder Tendon, Open Approach, Diagnostic
0L920ZZ	Drainage of Left Shoulder Tendon, Open Approach
0L9230Z	Drainage of Left Shoulder Tendon with Drainage Device, Percutaneous Approach
0L923ZX	Drainage of Left Shoulder Tendon, Percutaneous Approach, Diagnostic
0L923ZZ	Drainage of Left Shoulder Tendon, Percutaneous Approach

0L9240Z	Drainage of Left Shoulder Tendon with Drainage Device, Percutaneous Endoscopic Approach
0L924ZX	Drainage of Left Shoulder Tendon, Percutaneous Endoscopic Approach, Diagnostic
0L924ZZ	Drainage of Left Shoulder Tendon, Percutaneous Endoscopic Approach
0L9300Z	Drainage of Right Upper Arm Tendon with Drainage Device, Open Approach
0L930ZX	Drainage of Right Upper Arm Tendon, Open Approach, Diagnostic
0L930ZZ	Drainage of Right Upper Arm Tendon, Open Approach
0L9330Z	Drainage of Right Upper Arm Tendon with Drainage Device, Percutaneous Approach
0L933ZX	Drainage of Right Upper Arm Tendon, Percutaneous Approach, Diagnostic
0L933ZZ	Drainage of Right Upper Arm Tendon, Percutaneous Approach
0L9340Z	Drainage of Right Upper Arm Tendon with Drainage Device, Percutaneous Endoscopic Approach
0L934ZX	Drainage of Right Upper Arm Tendon, Percutaneous Endoscopic Approach, Diagnostic
0L934ZZ	Drainage of Right Upper Arm Tendon, Percutaneous Endoscopic Approach
0L9400Z	Drainage of Left Upper Arm Tendon with Drainage Device, Open Approach
0L940ZX	Drainage of Left Upper Arm Tendon, Open Approach, Diagnostic
0L940ZZ	Drainage of Left Upper Arm Tendon, Open Approach
0L9430Z	Drainage of Left Upper Arm Tendon with Drainage Device, Percutaneous Approach
0L943ZX	Drainage of Left Upper Arm Tendon, Percutaneous Approach, Diagnostic
0L943ZZ	Drainage of Left Upper Arm Tendon, Percutaneous Approach
0L9440Z	Drainage of Left Upper Arm Tendon with Drainage Device, Percutaneous Endoscopic Approach
0L944ZX	Drainage of Left Upper Arm Tendon, Percutaneous Endoscopic Approach, Diagnostic
0L944ZZ	Drainage of Left Upper Arm Tendon, Percutaneous Endoscopic Approach
0L9500Z	Drainage of Right Lower Arm and Wrist Tendon with Drainage Device, Open Approach
0L950ZX	Drainage of Right Lower Arm and Wrist Tendon, Open Approach, Diagnostic

---

♀ Female-only   ♂ Male-only   ● Limited Coverage   ● Non-OR   ▨ HAC-associated procedure   ⬣ Non-covered procedures   ➕ Combination

0L950ZZ	Drainage of Right Lower Arm and Wrist Tendon, Open Approach
0L9530Z	Drainage of Right Lower Arm and Wrist Tendon with Drainage Device, Percutaneous Approach
0L953ZX	Drainage of Right Lower Arm and Wrist Tendon, Percutaneous Approach, Diagnostic
0L953ZZ	Drainage of Right Lower Arm and Wrist Tendon, Percutaneous Approach
0L9540Z	Drainage of Right Lower Arm and Wrist Tendon with Drainage Device, Percutaneous Endoscopic Approach
0L954ZX	Drainage of Right Lower Arm and Wrist Tendon, Percutaneous Endoscopic Approach, Diagnostic
0L954ZZ	Drainage of Right Lower Arm and Wrist Tendon, Percutaneous Endoscopic Approach
0L9600Z	Drainage of Left Lower Arm and Wrist Tendon with Drainage Device, Open Approach
0L960ZX	Drainage of Left Lower Arm and Wrist Tendon, Open Approach, Diagnostic
0L960ZZ	Drainage of Left Lower Arm and Wrist Tendon, Open Approach
0L9630Z	Drainage of Left Lower Arm and Wrist Tendon with Drainage Device, Percutaneous Approach
0L963ZX	Drainage of Left Lower Arm and Wrist Tendon, Percutaneous Approach, Diagnostic
0L963ZZ	Drainage of Left Lower Arm and Wrist Tendon, Percutaneous Approach
0L9640Z	Drainage of Left Lower Arm and Wrist Tendon with Drainage Device, Percutaneous Endoscopic Approach
0L964ZX	Drainage of Left Lower Arm and Wrist Tendon, Percutaneous Endoscopic Approach, Diagnostic
0L964ZZ	Drainage of Left Lower Arm and Wrist Tendon, Percutaneous Endoscopic Approach
0L9700Z	Drainage of Right Hand Tendon with Drainage Device, Open Approach
0L970ZX	Drainage of Right Hand Tendon, Open Approach, Diagnostic
0L970ZZ	Drainage of Right Hand Tendon, Open Approach
0L9730Z	Drainage of Right Hand Tendon with Drainage Device, Percutaneous Approach
0L973ZX	Drainage of Right Hand Tendon, Percutaneous Approach, Diagnostic
0L973ZZ	Drainage of Right Hand Tendon, Percutaneous Approach
0L9740Z	Drainage of Right Hand Tendon with Drainage Device, Percutaneous Endoscopic Approach
0L974ZX	Drainage of Right Hand Tendon, Percutaneous Endoscopic Approach, Diagnostic
0L974ZZ	Drainage of Right Hand Tendon, Percutaneous Endoscopic Approach
0L9800Z	Drainage of Left Hand Tendon with Drainage Device, Open Approach
0L980ZX	Drainage of Left Hand Tendon, Open Approach, Diagnostic
0L980ZZ	Drainage of Left Hand Tendon, Open Approach
0L9830Z	Drainage of Left Hand Tendon with Drainage Device, Percutaneous Approach
0L983ZX	Drainage of Left Hand Tendon, Percutaneous Approach, Diagnostic
0L983ZZ	Drainage of Left Hand Tendon, Percutaneous Approach
0L9840Z	Drainage of Left Hand Tendon with Drainage Device, Percutaneous Endoscopic Approach
0L984ZX	Drainage of Left Hand Tendon, Percutaneous Endoscopic Approach, Diagnostic
0L984ZZ	Drainage of Left Hand Tendon, Percutaneous Endoscopic Approach
0L9900Z	Drainage of Right Trunk Tendon with Drainage Device, Open Approach
0L990ZX	Drainage of Right Trunk Tendon, Open Approach, Diagnostic
0L990ZZ	Drainage of Right Trunk Tendon, Open Approach
0L9930Z	Drainage of Right Trunk Tendon with Drainage Device, Percutaneous Approach
0L993ZX	Drainage of Right Trunk Tendon, Percutaneous Approach, Diagnostic
0L993ZZ	Drainage of Right Trunk Tendon, Percutaneous Approach
0L9940Z	Drainage of Right Trunk Tendon with Drainage Device, Percutaneous Endoscopic Approach
0L994ZX	Drainage of Right Trunk Tendon, Percutaneous Endoscopic Approach, Diagnostic
0L994ZZ	Drainage of Right Trunk Tendon, Percutaneous Endoscopic Approach
0L9B00Z	Drainage of Left Trunk Tendon with Drainage Device, Open Approach
0L9B0ZX	Drainage of Left Trunk Tendon, Open Approach, Diagnostic
0L9B0ZZ	Drainage of Left Trunk Tendon, Open Approach
0L9B30Z	Drainage of Left Trunk Tendon with Drainage Device, Percutaneous Approach
0L9B3ZX	Drainage of Left Trunk Tendon, Percutaneous Approach, Diagnostic
0L9B3ZZ	Drainage of Left Trunk Tendon, Percutaneous Approach
0L9B40Z	Drainage of Left Trunk Tendon with Drainage Device, Percutaneous Endoscopic Approach
0L9B4ZX	Drainage of Left Trunk Tendon, Percutaneous Endoscopic Approach, Diagnostic
0L9B4ZZ	Drainage of Left Trunk Tendon, Percutaneous Endoscopic Approach
0L9C00Z	Drainage of Right Thorax Tendon with Drainage Device, Open Approach
0L9C0ZX	Drainage of Right Thorax Tendon, Open Approach, Diagnostic
0L9C0ZZ	Drainage of Right Thorax Tendon, Open Approach
0L9C30Z	Drainage of Right Thorax Tendon with Drainage Device, Percutaneous Approach
0L9C3ZX	Drainage of Right Thorax Tendon, Percutaneous Approach, Diagnostic
0L9C3ZZ	Drainage of Right Thorax Tendon, Percutaneous Approach
0L9C40Z	Drainage of Right Thorax Tendon with Drainage Device, Percutaneous Endoscopic Approach
0L9C4ZX	Drainage of Right Thorax Tendon, Percutaneous Endoscopic Approach, Diagnostic
0L9C4ZZ	Drainage of Right Thorax Tendon, Percutaneous Endoscopic Approach
0L9D00Z	Drainage of Left Thorax Tendon with Drainage Device, Open Approach
0L9D0ZX	Drainage of Left Thorax Tendon, Open Approach, Diagnostic
0L9D0ZZ	Drainage of Left Thorax Tendon, Open Approach
0L9D30Z	Drainage of Left Thorax Tendon with Drainage Device, Percutaneous Approach
0L9D3ZX	Drainage of Left Thorax Tendon, Percutaneous Approach, Diagnostic
0L9D3ZZ	Drainage of Left Thorax Tendon, Percutaneous Approach
0L9D40Z	Drainage of Left Thorax Tendon with Drainage Device, Percutaneous Endoscopic Approach
0L9D4ZX	Drainage of Left Thorax Tendon, Percutaneous Endoscopic Approach, Diagnostic
0L9D4ZZ	Drainage of Left Thorax Tendon, Percutaneous Endoscopic Approach
0L9F00Z	Drainage of Right Abdomen Tendon with Drainage Device, Open Approach
0L9F0ZX	Drainage of Right Abdomen Tendon, Open Approach, Diagnostic
0L9F0ZZ	Drainage of Right Abdomen Tendon, Open Approach
0L9F30Z	Drainage of Right Abdomen Tendon with Drainage Device, Percutaneous Approach
0L9F3ZX	Drainage of Right Abdomen Tendon, Percutaneous Approach, Diagnostic
0L9F3ZZ	Drainage of Right Abdomen Tendon, Percutaneous Approach
0L9F40Z	Drainage of Right Abdomen Tendon with Drainage Device, Percutaneous Endoscopic Approach
0L9F4ZX	Drainage of Right Abdomen Tendon, Percutaneous Endoscopic Approach, Diagnostic
0L9F4ZZ	Drainage of Right Abdomen Tendon, Percutaneous Endoscopic Approach
0L9G00Z	Drainage of Left Abdomen Tendon with Drainage Device, Open Approach
0L9G0ZX	Drainage of Left Abdomen Tendon, Open Approach, Diagnostic
0L9G0ZZ	Drainage of Left Abdomen Tendon, Open Approach
0L9G30Z	Drainage of Left Abdomen Tendon with Drainage Device, Percutaneous Approach
0L9G3ZX	Drainage of Left Abdomen Tendon, Percutaneous Approach, Diagnostic
0L9G3ZZ	Drainage of Left Abdomen Tendon, Percutaneous Approach
0L9G40Z	Drainage of Left Abdomen Tendon with Drainage Device, Percutaneous Endoscopic Approach
0L9G4ZX	Drainage of Left Abdomen Tendon, Percutaneous Endoscopic Approach, Diagnostic
0L9G4ZZ	Drainage of Left Abdomen Tendon, Percutaneous Endoscopic Approach

0L9H00Z Drainage of Perineum Tendon with Drainage Device, Open Approach

0L9H0ZX Drainage of Perineum Tendon, Open Approach, Diagnostic

0L9H0ZZ Drainage of Perineum Tendon, Open Approach

0L9H30Z Drainage of Perineum Tendon with Drainage Device, Percutaneous Approach

0L9H3ZX Drainage of Perineum Tendon, Percutaneous Approach, Diagnostic

0L9H3ZZ Drainage of Perineum Tendon, Percutaneous Approach

0L9H40Z Drainage of Perineum Tendon with Drainage Device, Percutaneous Endoscopic Approach

0L9H4ZX Drainage of Perineum Tendon, Percutaneous Endoscopic Approach, Diagnostic

0L9H4ZZ Drainage of Perineum Tendon, Percutaneous Endoscopic Approach

0L9J00Z Drainage of Right Hip Tendon with Drainage Device, Open Approach

0L9J0ZX Drainage of Right Hip Tendon, Open Approach, Diagnostic

0L9J0ZZ Drainage of Right Hip Tendon, Open Approach

0L9J30Z Drainage of Right Hip Tendon with Drainage Device, Percutaneous Approach

0L9J3ZX Drainage of Right Hip Tendon, Percutaneous Approach, Diagnostic

0L9J3ZZ Drainage of Right Hip Tendon, Percutaneous Approach

0L9J40Z Drainage of Right Hip Tendon with Drainage Device, Percutaneous Endoscopic Approach

0L9J4ZX Drainage of Right Hip Tendon, Percutaneous Endoscopic Approach, Diagnostic

0L9J4ZZ Drainage of Right Hip Tendon, Percutaneous Endoscopic Approach

0L9K00Z Drainage of Left Hip Tendon with Drainage Device, Open Approach

0L9K0ZX Drainage of Left Hip Tendon, Open Approach, Diagnostic

0L9K0ZZ Drainage of Left Hip Tendon, Open Approach

0L9K30Z Drainage of Left Hip Tendon with Drainage Device, Percutaneous Approach

0L9K3ZX Drainage of Left Hip Tendon, Percutaneous Approach, Diagnostic

0L9K3ZZ Drainage of Left Hip Tendon, Percutaneous Approach

0L9K40Z Drainage of Left Hip Tendon with Drainage Device, Percutaneous Endoscopic Approach

0L9K4ZX Drainage of Left Hip Tendon, Percutaneous Endoscopic Approach, Diagnostic

0L9K4ZZ Drainage of Left Hip Tendon, Percutaneous Endoscopic Approach

0L9L00Z Drainage of Right Upper Leg Tendon with Drainage Device, Open Approach

0L9L0ZX Drainage of Right Upper Leg Tendon, Open Approach, Diagnostic

0L9L0ZZ Drainage of Right Upper Leg Tendon, Open Approach

0L9L30Z Drainage of Right Upper Leg Tendon with Drainage Device, Percutaneous Approach

0L9L3ZX Drainage of Right Upper Leg Tendon, Percutaneous Approach, Diagnostic

0L9L3ZZ Drainage of Right Upper Leg Tendon, Percutaneous Approach

0L9L40Z Drainage of Right Upper Leg Tendon with Drainage Device, Percutaneous Endoscopic Approach

0L9L4ZX Drainage of Right Upper Leg Tendon, Percutaneous Endoscopic Approach, Diagnostic

0L9L4ZZ Drainage of Right Upper Leg Tendon, Percutaneous Endoscopic Approach

0L9M00Z Drainage of Left Upper Leg Tendon with Drainage Device, Open Approach

0L9M0ZX Drainage of Left Upper Leg Tendon, Open Approach, Diagnostic

0L9M0ZZ Drainage of Left Upper Leg Tendon, Open Approach

0L9M30Z Drainage of Left Upper Leg Tendon with Drainage Device, Percutaneous Approach

0L9M3ZX Drainage of Left Upper Leg Tendon, Percutaneous Approach, Diagnostic

0L9M3ZZ Drainage of Left Upper Leg Tendon, Percutaneous Approach

0L9M40Z Drainage of Left Upper Leg Tendon with Drainage Device, Percutaneous Endoscopic Approach

0L9M4ZX Drainage of Left Upper Leg Tendon, Percutaneous Endoscopic Approach, Diagnostic

0L9M4ZZ Drainage of Left Upper Leg Tendon, Percutaneous Endoscopic Approach

0L9N00Z Drainage of Right Lower Leg Tendon with Drainage Device, Open Approach

0L9N0ZX Drainage of Right Lower Leg Tendon, Open Approach, Diagnostic

0L9N0ZZ Drainage of Right Lower Leg Tendon, Open Approach

0L9N30Z Drainage of Right Lower Leg Tendon with Drainage Device, Percutaneous Approach

0L9N3ZX Drainage of Right Lower Leg Tendon, Percutaneous Approach, Diagnostic

0L9N3ZZ Drainage of Right Lower Leg Tendon, Percutaneous Approach

0L9N40Z Drainage of Right Lower Leg Tendon with Drainage Device, Percutaneous Endoscopic Approach

0L9N4ZX Drainage of Right Lower Leg Tendon, Percutaneous Endoscopic Approach, Diagnostic

0L9N4ZZ Drainage of Right Lower Leg Tendon, Percutaneous Endoscopic Approach

0L9P00Z Drainage of Left Lower Leg Tendon with Drainage Device, Open Approach

0L9P0ZX Drainage of Left Lower Leg Tendon, Open Approach, Diagnostic

0L9P0ZZ Drainage of Left Lower Leg Tendon, Open Approach

0L9P30Z Drainage of Left Lower Leg Tendon with Drainage Device, Percutaneous Approach

0L9P3ZX Drainage of Left Lower Leg Tendon, Percutaneous Approach, Diagnostic

0L9P3ZZ Drainage of Left Lower Leg Tendon, Percutaneous Approach

0L9P40Z Drainage of Left Lower Leg Tendon with Drainage Device, Percutaneous Endoscopic Approach

0L9P4ZX Drainage of Left Lower Leg Tendon, Percutaneous Endoscopic Approach, Diagnostic

0L9P4ZZ Drainage of Left Lower Leg Tendon, Percutaneous Endoscopic Approach

0L9Q00Z Drainage of Right Knee Tendon with Drainage Device, Open Approach

0L9Q0ZX Drainage of Right Knee Tendon, Open Approach, Diagnostic

0L9Q0ZZ Drainage of Right Knee Tendon, Open Approach

0L9Q30Z Drainage of Right Knee Tendon with Drainage Device, Percutaneous Approach

0L9Q3ZX Drainage of Right Knee Tendon, Percutaneous Approach, Diagnostic

0L9Q3ZZ Drainage of Right Knee Tendon, Percutaneous Approach

0L9Q40Z Drainage of Right Knee Tendon with Drainage Device, Percutaneous Endoscopic Approach

0L9Q4ZX Drainage of Right Knee Tendon, Percutaneous Endoscopic Approach, Diagnostic

0L9Q4ZZ Drainage of Right Knee Tendon, Percutaneous Endoscopic Approach

0L9R00Z Drainage of Left Knee Tendon with Drainage Device, Open Approach

0L9R0ZX Drainage of Left Knee Tendon, Open Approach, Diagnostic

0L9R0ZZ Drainage of Left Knee Tendon, Open Approach

0L9R30Z Drainage of Left Knee Tendon with Drainage Device, Percutaneous Approach

0L9R3ZX Drainage of Left Knee Tendon, Percutaneous Approach, Diagnostic

0L9R3ZZ Drainage of Left Knee Tendon, Percutaneous Approach

0L9R40Z Drainage of Left Knee Tendon with Drainage Device, Percutaneous Endoscopic Approach

0L9R4ZX Drainage of Left Knee Tendon, Percutaneous Endoscopic Approach, Diagnostic

0L9R4ZZ Drainage of Left Knee Tendon, Percutaneous Endoscopic Approach

0L9S00Z Drainage of Right Ankle Tendon with Drainage Device, Open Approach

0L9S0ZX Drainage of Right Ankle Tendon, Open Approach, Diagnostic

0L9S0ZZ Drainage of Right Ankle Tendon, Open Approach

0L9S30Z Drainage of Right Ankle Tendon with Drainage Device, Percutaneous Approach

0L9S3ZX Drainage of Right Ankle Tendon, Percutaneous Approach, Diagnostic

0L9S3ZZ Drainage of Right Ankle Tendon, Percutaneous Approach

0L9S40Z Drainage of Right Ankle Tendon with Drainage Device, Percutaneous Endoscopic Approach

0L9S4ZX Drainage of Right Ankle Tendon, Percutaneous Endoscopic Approach, Diagnostic

0L9S4ZZ Drainage of Right Ankle Tendon, Percutaneous Endoscopic Approach

0L9T00Z Drainage of Left Ankle Tendon with Drainage Device, Open Approach

0L9T0ZX Drainage of Left Ankle Tendon, Open Approach, Diagnostic

0L9T0ZZ Drainage of Left Ankle Tendon, Open Approach

0L9T30Z	Drainage of Left Ankle Tendon with Drainage Device, Percutaneous Approach
0L9T3ZX	Drainage of Left Ankle Tendon, Percutaneous Approach, Diagnostic
0L9T3ZZ	Drainage of Left Ankle Tendon, Percutaneous Approach
0L9T40Z	Drainage of Left Ankle Tendon with Drainage Device, Percutaneous Endoscopic Approach
0L9T4ZX	Drainage of Left Ankle Tendon, Percutaneous Endoscopic Approach, Diagnostic
0L9T4ZZ	Drainage of Left Ankle Tendon, Percutaneous Endoscopic Approach
0L9V00Z	Drainage of Right Foot Tendon with Drainage Device, Open Approach
0L9V0ZX	Drainage of Right Foot Tendon, Open Approach, Diagnostic
0L9V0ZZ	Drainage of Right Foot Tendon, Open Approach
0L9V30Z	Drainage of Right Foot Tendon with Drainage Device, Percutaneous Approach
0L9V3ZX	Drainage of Right Foot Tendon, Percutaneous Approach, Diagnostic
0L9V3ZZ	Drainage of Right Foot Tendon, Percutaneous Approach
0L9V40Z	Drainage of Right Foot Tendon with Drainage Device, Percutaneous Endoscopic Approach
0L9V4ZX	Drainage of Right Foot Tendon, Percutaneous Endoscopic Approach, Diagnostic
0L9V4ZZ	Drainage of Right Foot Tendon, Percutaneous Endoscopic Approach
0L9W00Z	Drainage of Left Foot Tendon with Drainage Device, Open Approach
0L9W0ZX	Drainage of Left Foot Tendon, Open Approach, Diagnostic
0L9W0ZZ	Drainage of Left Foot Tendon, Open Approach
0L9W30Z	Drainage of Left Foot Tendon with Drainage Device, Percutaneous Approach
0L9W3ZX	Drainage of Left Foot Tendon, Percutaneous Approach, Diagnostic
0L9W3ZZ	Drainage of Left Foot Tendon, Percutaneous Approach
0L9W40Z	Drainage of Left Foot Tendon with Drainage Device, Percutaneous Endoscopic Approach
0L9W4ZX	Drainage of Left Foot Tendon, Percutaneous Endoscopic Approach, Diagnostic
0L9W4ZZ	Drainage of Left Foot Tendon, Percutaneous Endoscopic Approach

0LB – Tendons, Excision

Review Coding Guidelines B3.4a and B3.4b

Review Coding Guideline B3.5

Review Coding Guideline B3.8

0LB00ZX	Excision of Head and Neck Tendon, Open Approach, Diagnostic
0LB00ZZ	Excision of Head and Neck Tendon, Open Approach
0LB03ZX	Excision of Head and Neck Tendon, Percutaneous Approach, Diagnostic
0LB03ZZ	Excision of Head and Neck Tendon, Percutaneous Approach
0LB04ZX	Excision of Head and Neck Tendon, Percutaneous Endoscopic Approach, Diagnostic
0LB04ZZ	Excision of Head and Neck Tendon, Percutaneous Endoscopic Approach
0LB10ZX	Excision of Right Shoulder Tendon, Open Approach, Diagnostic
0LB10ZZ	Excision of Right Shoulder Tendon, Open Approach
0LB13ZX	Excision of Right Shoulder Tendon, Percutaneous Approach, Diagnostic
0LB13ZZ	Excision of Right Shoulder Tendon, Percutaneous Approach
0LB14ZX	Excision of Right Shoulder Tendon, Percutaneous Endoscopic Approach, Diagnostic
0LB14ZZ	Excision of Right Shoulder Tendon, Percutaneous Endoscopic Approach
0LB20ZX	Excision of Left Shoulder Tendon, Open Approach, Diagnostic
0LB20ZZ	Excision of Left Shoulder Tendon, Open Approach
0LB23ZX	Excision of Left Shoulder Tendon, Percutaneous Approach, Diagnostic
0LB23ZZ	Excision of Left Shoulder Tendon, Percutaneous Approach
0LB24ZX	Excision of Left Shoulder Tendon, Percutaneous Endoscopic Approach, Diagnostic
0LB24ZZ	Excision of Left Shoulder Tendon, Percutaneous Endoscopic Approach
0LB30ZX	Excision of Right Upper Arm Tendon, Open Approach, Diagnostic
0LB30ZZ	Excision of Right Upper Arm Tendon, Open Approach
0LB33ZX	Excision of Right Upper Arm Tendon, Percutaneous Approach, Diagnostic
0LB33ZZ	Excision of Right Upper Arm Tendon, Percutaneous Approach
0LB34ZX	Excision of Right Upper Arm Tendon, Percutaneous Endoscopic Approach, Diagnostic
0LB34ZZ	Excision of Right Upper Arm Tendon, Percutaneous Endoscopic Approach
0LB40ZX	Excision of Left Upper Arm Tendon, Open Approach, Diagnostic
0LB40ZZ	Excision of Left Upper Arm Tendon, Open Approach
0LB43ZX	Excision of Left Upper Arm Tendon, Percutaneous Approach, Diagnostic
0LB43ZZ	Excision of Left Upper Arm Tendon, Percutaneous Approach
0LB44ZX	Excision of Left Upper Arm Tendon, Percutaneous Endoscopic Approach, Diagnostic
0LB44ZZ	Excision of Left Upper Arm Tendon, Percutaneous Endoscopic Approach
0LB50ZX	Excision of Right Lower Arm and Wrist Tendon, Open Approach, Diagnostic
0LB50ZZ	Excision of Right Lower Arm and Wrist Tendon, Open Approach
0LB53ZX	Excision of Right Lower Arm and Wrist Tendon, Percutaneous Approach, Diagnostic
0LB53ZZ	Excision of Right Lower Arm and Wrist Tendon, Percutaneous Approach
0LB54ZX	Excision of Right Lower Arm and Wrist Tendon, Percutaneous Endoscopic Approach, Diagnostic
0LB54ZZ	Excision of Right Lower Arm and Wrist Tendon, Percutaneous Endoscopic Approach
0LB60ZX	Excision of Left Lower Arm and Wrist Tendon, Open Approach, Diagnostic
0LB60ZZ	Excision of Left Lower Arm and Wrist Tendon, Open Approach
0LB63ZX	Excision of Left Lower Arm and Wrist Tendon, Percutaneous Approach, Diagnostic
0LB63ZZ	Excision of Left Lower Arm and Wrist Tendon, Percutaneous Approach
0LB64ZX	Excision of Left Lower Arm and Wrist Tendon, Percutaneous Endoscopic Approach, Diagnostic
0LB64ZZ	Excision of Left Lower Arm and Wrist Tendon, Percutaneous Endoscopic Approach
0LB70ZX	Excision of Right Hand Tendon, Open Approach, Diagnostic
0LB70ZZ	Excision of Right Hand Tendon, Open Approach
0LB73ZX	Excision of Right Hand Tendon, Percutaneous Approach, Diagnostic
0LB73ZZ	Excision of Right Hand Tendon, Percutaneous Approach
0LB74ZX	Excision of Right Hand Tendon, Percutaneous Endoscopic Approach, Diagnostic
0LB74ZZ	Excision of Right Hand Tendon, Percutaneous Endoscopic Approach
0LB80ZX	Excision of Left Hand Tendon, Open Approach, Diagnostic
0LB80ZZ	Excision of Left Hand Tendon, Open Approach
0LB83ZX	Excision of Left Hand Tendon, Percutaneous Approach, Diagnostic
0LB83ZZ	Excision of Left Hand Tendon, Percutaneous Approach
0LB84ZX	Excision of Left Hand Tendon, Percutaneous Endoscopic Approach, Diagnostic
0LB84ZZ	Excision of Left Hand Tendon, Percutaneous Endoscopic Approach
0LB90ZX	Excision of Right Trunk Tendon, Open Approach, Diagnostic
0LB90ZZ	Excision of Right Trunk Tendon, Open Approach
0LB93ZX	Excision of Right Trunk Tendon, Percutaneous Approach, Diagnostic
0LB93ZZ	Excision of Right Trunk Tendon, Percutaneous Approach
0LB94ZX	Excision of Right Trunk Tendon, Percutaneous Endoscopic Approach, Diagnostic

0LB94ZZ　Excision of Right Trunk Tendon, Percutaneous Endoscopic Approach

0LBB0ZX　Excision of Left Trunk Tendon, Open Approach, Diagnostic

0LBB0ZZ　Excision of Left Trunk Tendon, Open Approach

0LBB3ZX　Excision of Left Trunk Tendon, Percutaneous Approach, Diagnostic

0LBB3ZZ　Excision of Left Trunk Tendon, Percutaneous Approach

0LBB4ZX　Excision of Left Trunk Tendon, Percutaneous Endoscopic Approach, Diagnostic

0LBB4ZZ　Excision of Left Trunk Tendon, Percutaneous Endoscopic Approach

0LBC0ZX　Excision of Right Thorax Tendon, Open Approach, Diagnostic

0LBC0ZZ　Excision of Right Thorax Tendon, Open Approach

0LBC3ZX　Excision of Right Thorax Tendon, Percutaneous Approach, Diagnostic

0LBC3ZZ　Excision of Right Thorax Tendon, Percutaneous Approach

0LBC4ZX　Excision of Right Thorax Tendon, Percutaneous Endoscopic Approach, Diagnostic

0LBC4ZZ　Excision of Right Thorax Tendon, Percutaneous Endoscopic Approach

0LBD0ZX　Excision of Left Thorax Tendon, Open Approach, Diagnostic

0LBD0ZZ　Excision of Left Thorax Tendon, Open Approach

0LBD3ZX　Excision of Left Thorax Tendon, Percutaneous Approach, Diagnostic

0LBD3ZZ　Excision of Left Thorax Tendon, Percutaneous Approach

0LBD4ZX　Excision of Left Thorax Tendon, Percutaneous Endoscopic Approach, Diagnostic

0LBD4ZZ　Excision of Left Thorax Tendon, Percutaneous Endoscopic Approach

0LBF0ZX　Excision of Right Abdomen Tendon, Open Approach, Diagnostic

0LBF0ZZ　Excision of Right Abdomen Tendon, Open Approach

0LBF3ZX　Excision of Right Abdomen Tendon, Percutaneous Approach, Diagnostic

0LBF3ZZ　Excision of Right Abdomen Tendon, Percutaneous Approach

0LBF4ZX　Excision of Right Abdomen Tendon, Percutaneous Endoscopic Approach, Diagnostic

0LBF4ZZ　Excision of Right Abdomen Tendon, Percutaneous Endoscopic Approach

0LBG0ZX　Excision of Left Abdomen Tendon, Open Approach, Diagnostic

0LBG0ZZ　Excision of Left Abdomen Tendon, Open Approach

0LBG3ZX　Excision of Left Abdomen Tendon, Percutaneous Approach, Diagnostic

0LBG3ZZ　Excision of Left Abdomen Tendon, Percutaneous Approach

0LBG4ZX　Excision of Left Abdomen Tendon, Percutaneous Endoscopic Approach, Diagnostic

0LBG4ZZ　Excision of Left Abdomen Tendon, Percutaneous Endoscopic Approach

0LBH0ZX　Excision of Perineum Tendon, Open Approach, Diagnostic

0LBH0ZZ　Excision of Perineum Tendon, Open Approach

0LBH3ZX　Excision of Perineum Tendon, Percutaneous Approach, Diagnostic

0LBH3ZZ　Excision of Perineum Tendon, Percutaneous Approach

0LBH4ZX　Excision of Perineum Tendon, Percutaneous Endoscopic Approach, Diagnostic

0LBH4ZZ　Excision of Perineum Tendon, Percutaneous Endoscopic Approach

0LBJ0ZX　Excision of Right Hip Tendon, Open Approach, Diagnostic

0LBJ0ZZ　Excision of Right Hip Tendon, Open Approach

0LBJ3ZX　Excision of Right Hip Tendon, Percutaneous Approach, Diagnostic

0LBJ3ZZ　Excision of Right Hip Tendon, Percutaneous Approach

0LBJ4ZX　Excision of Right Hip Tendon, Percutaneous Endoscopic Approach, Diagnostic

0LBJ4ZZ　Excision of Right Hip Tendon, Percutaneous Endoscopic Approach

0LBK0ZX　Excision of Left Hip Tendon, Open Approach, Diagnostic

0LBK0ZZ　Excision of Left Hip Tendon, Open Approach

0LBK3ZX　Excision of Left Hip Tendon, Percutaneous Approach, Diagnostic

0LBK3ZZ　Excision of Left Hip Tendon, Percutaneous Approach

0LBK4ZX　Excision of Left Hip Tendon, Percutaneous Endoscopic Approach, Diagnostic

0LBK4ZZ　Excision of Left Hip Tendon, Percutaneous Endoscopic Approach

0LBL0ZX　Excision of Right Upper Leg Tendon, Open Approach, Diagnostic

0LBL0ZZ　Excision of Right Upper Leg Tendon, Open Approach

0LBL3ZX　Excision of Right Upper Leg Tendon, Percutaneous Approach, Diagnostic

0LBL3ZZ　Excision of Right Upper Leg Tendon, Percutaneous Approach

0LBL4ZX　Excision of Right Upper Leg Tendon, Percutaneous Endoscopic Approach, Diagnostic

0LBL4ZZ　Excision of Right Upper Leg Tendon, Percutaneous Endoscopic Approach

0LBM0ZX　Excision of Left Upper Leg Tendon, Open Approach, Diagnostic

0LBM0ZZ　Excision of Left Upper Leg Tendon, Open Approach

0LBM3ZX　Excision of Left Upper Leg Tendon, Percutaneous Approach, Diagnostic

0LBM3ZZ　Excision of Left Upper Leg Tendon, Percutaneous Approach

0LBM4ZX　Excision of Left Upper Leg Tendon, Percutaneous Endoscopic Approach, Diagnostic

0LBM4ZZ　Excision of Left Upper Leg Tendon, Percutaneous Endoscopic Approach

0LBN0ZX　Excision of Right Lower Leg Tendon, Open Approach, Diagnostic

0LBN0ZZ　Excision of Right Lower Leg Tendon, Open Approach

0LBN3ZX　Excision of Right Lower Leg Tendon, Percutaneous Approach, Diagnostic

0LBN3ZZ　Excision of Right Lower Leg Tendon, Percutaneous Approach

0LBN4ZX　Excision of Right Lower Leg Tendon, Percutaneous Endoscopic Approach, Diagnostic

0LBN4ZZ　Excision of Right Lower Leg Tendon, Percutaneous Endoscopic Approach

0LBP0ZX　Excision of Left Lower Leg Tendon, Open Approach, Diagnostic

0LBP0ZZ　Excision of Left Lower Leg Tendon, Open Approach

0LBP3ZX　Excision of Left Lower Leg Tendon, Percutaneous Approach, Diagnostic

0LBP3ZZ　Excision of Left Lower Leg Tendon, Percutaneous Approach

0LBP4ZX　Excision of Left Lower Leg Tendon, Percutaneous Endoscopic Approach, Diagnostic

0LBP4ZZ　Excision of Left Lower Leg Tendon, Percutaneous Endoscopic Approach

0LBQ0ZX　Excision of Right Knee Tendon, Open Approach, Diagnostic

0LBQ0ZZ　Excision of Right Knee Tendon, Open Approach

0LBQ3ZX　Excision of Right Knee Tendon, Percutaneous Approach, Diagnostic

0LBQ3ZZ　Excision of Right Knee Tendon, Percutaneous Approach

0LBQ4ZX　Excision of Right Knee Tendon, Percutaneous Endoscopic Approach, Diagnostic

0LBQ4ZZ　Excision of Right Knee Tendon, Percutaneous Endoscopic Approach

0LBR0ZX　Excision of Left Knee Tendon, Open Approach, Diagnostic

0LBR0ZZ　Excision of Left Knee Tendon, Open Approach

0LBR3ZX　Excision of Left Knee Tendon, Percutaneous Approach, Diagnostic

0LBR3ZZ　Excision of Left Knee Tendon, Percutaneous Approach

0LBR4ZX　Excision of Left Knee Tendon, Percutaneous Endoscopic Approach, Diagnostic

0LBR4ZZ　Excision of Left Knee Tendon, Percutaneous Endoscopic Approach

0LBS0ZX　Excision of Right Ankle Tendon, Open Approach, Diagnostic

0LBS0ZZ　Excision of Right Ankle Tendon, Open Approach

0LBS3ZX　Excision of Right Ankle Tendon, Percutaneous Approach, Diagnostic

0LBS3ZZ　Excision of Right Ankle Tendon, Percutaneous Approach

0LBS4ZX　Excision of Right Ankle Tendon, Percutaneous Endoscopic Approach, Diagnostic

0LBS4ZZ　Excision of Right Ankle Tendon, Percutaneous Endoscopic Approach

0LBT0ZX　Excision of Left Ankle Tendon, Open Approach, Diagnostic

0LBT0ZZ　Excision of Left Ankle Tendon, Open Approach

0LBT3ZX　Excision of Left Ankle Tendon, Percutaneous Approach, Diagnostic

0LBT3ZZ　Excision of Left Ankle Tendon, Percutaneous Approach

0LBT4ZX　Excision of Left Ankle Tendon, Percutaneous Endoscopic Approach, Diagnostic

0LBT4ZZ　Excision of Left Ankle Tendon, Percutaneous Endoscopic Approach

0LBV0ZX　Excision of Right Foot Tendon, Open Approach, Diagnostic

0LBV0ZZ　Excision of Right Foot Tendon, Open Approach

0LBV3ZX　Excision of Right Foot Tendon, Percutaneous Approach, Diagnostic

0LBV3ZZ　Excision of Right Foot Tendon, Percutaneous Approach

0LBV4ZX　Excision of Right Foot Tendon, Percutaneous Endoscopic Approach, Diagnostic

0LBV4ZZ　Excision of Right Foot Tendon, Percutaneous Endoscopic Approach

0LBW0ZX　Excision of Left Foot Tendon, Open Approach, Diagnostic

0LBW0ZZ　Excision of Left Foot Tendon, Open Approach

0LBW3ZX　Excision of Left Foot Tendon, Percutaneous Approach, Diagnostic

0LBW3ZZ　Excision of Left Foot Tendon, Percutaneous Approach

0LBW4ZX　Excision of Left Foot Tendon, Percutaneous Endoscopic Approach, Diagnostic

0LBW4ZZ　Excision of Left Foot Tendon, Percutaneous Endoscopic Approach

0LC – Tendons, Extirpation

0LC00ZZ	Extirpation of Matter from Head and Neck Tendon, Open Approach
0LC03ZZ	Extirpation of Matter from Head and Neck Tendon, Percutaneous Approach
0LC04ZZ	Extirpation of Matter from Head and Neck Tendon, Percutaneous Endoscopic Approach
0LC10ZZ	Extirpation of Matter from Right Shoulder Tendon, Open Approach
0LC13ZZ	Extirpation of Matter from Right Shoulder Tendon, Percutaneous Approach
0LC14ZZ	Extirpation of Matter from Right Shoulder Tendon, Percutaneous Endoscopic Approach
0LC20ZZ	Extirpation of Matter from Left Shoulder Tendon, Open Approach
0LC23ZZ	Extirpation of Matter from Left Shoulder Tendon, Percutaneous Approach
0LC24ZZ	Extirpation of Matter from Left Shoulder Tendon, Percutaneous Endoscopic Approach
0LC30ZZ	Extirpation of Matter from Right Upper Arm Tendon, Open Approach
0LC33ZZ	Extirpation of Matter from Right Upper Arm Tendon, Percutaneous Approach
0LC34ZZ	Extirpation of Matter from Right Upper Arm Tendon, Percutaneous Endoscopic Approach
0LC40ZZ	Extirpation of Matter from Left Upper Arm Tendon, Open Approach
0LC43ZZ	Extirpation of Matter from Left Upper Arm Tendon, Percutaneous Approach
0LC44ZZ	Extirpation of Matter from Left Upper Arm Tendon, Percutaneous Endoscopic Approach
0LC50ZZ	Extirpation of Matter from Right Lower Arm and Wrist Tendon, Open Approach
0LC53ZZ	Extirpation of Matter from Right Lower Arm and Wrist Tendon, Percutaneous Approach
0LC54ZZ	Extirpation of Matter from Right Lower Arm and Wrist Tendon, Percutaneous Endoscopic Approach
0LC60ZZ	Extirpation of Matter from Left Lower Arm and Wrist Tendon, Open Approach
0LC63ZZ	Extirpation of Matter from Left Lower Arm and Wrist Tendon, Percutaneous Approach
0LC64ZZ	Extirpation of Matter from Left Lower Arm and Wrist Tendon, Percutaneous Endoscopic Approach
0LC70ZZ	Extirpation of Matter from Right Hand Tendon, Open Approach
0LC73ZZ	Extirpation of Matter from Right Hand Tendon, Percutaneous Approach
0LC74ZZ	Extirpation of Matter from Right Hand Tendon, Percutaneous Endoscopic Approach
0LC80ZZ	Extirpation of Matter from Left Hand Tendon, Open Approach
0LC83ZZ	Extirpation of Matter from Left Hand Tendon, Percutaneous Approach
0LC84ZZ	Extirpation of Matter from Left Hand Tendon, Percutaneous Endoscopic Approach
0LC90ZZ	Extirpation of Matter from Right Trunk Tendon, Open Approach
0LC93ZZ	Extirpation of Matter from Right Trunk Tendon, Percutaneous Approach
0LC94ZZ	Extirpation of Matter from Right Trunk Tendon, Percutaneous Endoscopic Approach
0LCB0ZZ	Extirpation of Matter from Left Trunk Tendon, Open Approach
0LCB3ZZ	Extirpation of Matter from Left Trunk Tendon, Percutaneous Approach
0LCB4ZZ	Extirpation of Matter from Left Trunk Tendon, Percutaneous Endoscopic Approach
0LCC0ZZ	Extirpation of Matter from Right Thorax Tendon, Open Approach
0LCC3ZZ	Extirpation of Matter from Right Thorax Tendon, Percutaneous Approach
0LCC4ZZ	Extirpation of Matter from Right Thorax Tendon, Percutaneous Endoscopic Approach
0LCD0ZZ	Extirpation of Matter from Left Thorax Tendon, Open Approach
0LCD3ZZ	Extirpation of Matter from Left Thorax Tendon, Percutaneous Approach
0LCD4ZZ	Extirpation of Matter from Left Thorax Tendon, Percutaneous Endoscopic Approach
0LCF0ZZ	Extirpation of Matter from Right Abdomen Tendon, Open Approach
0LCF3ZZ	Extirpation of Matter from Right Abdomen Tendon, Percutaneous Approach
0LCF4ZZ	Extirpation of Matter from Right Abdomen Tendon, Percutaneous Endoscopic Approach
0LCG0ZZ	Extirpation of Matter from Left Abdomen Tendon, Open Approach
0LCG3ZZ	Extirpation of Matter from Left Abdomen Tendon, Percutaneous Approach
0LCG4ZZ	Extirpation of Matter from Left Abdomen Tendon, Percutaneous Endoscopic Approach
0LCH0ZZ	Extirpation of Matter from Perineum Tendon, Open Approach
0LCH3ZZ	Extirpation of Matter from Perineum Tendon, Percutaneous Approach
0LCH4ZZ	Extirpation of Matter from Perineum Tendon, Percutaneous Endoscopic Approach
0LCJ0ZZ	Extirpation of Matter from Right Hip Tendon, Open Approach
0LCJ3ZZ	Extirpation of Matter from Right Hip Tendon, Percutaneous Approach
0LCJ4ZZ	Extirpation of Matter from Right Hip Tendon, Percutaneous Endoscopic Approach
0LCK0ZZ	Extirpation of Matter from Left Hip Tendon, Open Approach
0LCK3ZZ	Extirpation of Matter from Left Hip Tendon, Percutaneous Approach
0LCK4ZZ	Extirpation of Matter from Left Hip Tendon, Percutaneous Endoscopic Approach
0LCL0ZZ	Extirpation of Matter from Right Upper Leg Tendon, Open Approach
0LCL3ZZ	Extirpation of Matter from Right Upper Leg Tendon, Percutaneous Approach
0LCL4ZZ	Extirpation of Matter from Right Upper Leg Tendon, Percutaneous Endoscopic Approach
0LCM0ZZ	Extirpation of Matter from Left Upper Leg Tendon, Open Approach
0LCM3ZZ	Extirpation of Matter from Left Upper Leg Tendon, Percutaneous Approach
0LCM4ZZ	Extirpation of Matter from Left Upper Leg Tendon, Percutaneous Endoscopic Approach
0LCN0ZZ	Extirpation of Matter from Right Lower Leg Tendon, Open Approach
0LCN3ZZ	Extirpation of Matter from Right Lower Leg Tendon, Percutaneous Approach
0LCN4ZZ	Extirpation of Matter from Right Lower Leg Tendon, Percutaneous Endoscopic Approach
0LCP0ZZ	Extirpation of Matter from Left Lower Leg Tendon, Open Approach
0LCP3ZZ	Extirpation of Matter from Left Lower Leg Tendon, Percutaneous Approach
0LCP4ZZ	Extirpation of Matter from Left Lower Leg Tendon, Percutaneous Endoscopic Approach
0LCQ0ZZ	Extirpation of Matter from Right Knee Tendon, Open Approach
0LCQ3ZZ	Extirpation of Matter from Right Knee Tendon, Percutaneous Approach
0LCQ4ZZ	Extirpation of Matter from Right Knee Tendon, Percutaneous Endoscopic Approach
0LCR0ZZ	Extirpation of Matter from Left Knee Tendon, Open Approach
0LCR3ZZ	Extirpation of Matter from Left Knee Tendon, Percutaneous Approach
0LCR4ZZ	Extirpation of Matter from Left Knee Tendon, Percutaneous Endoscopic Approach
0LCS0ZZ	Extirpation of Matter from Right Ankle Tendon, Open Approach
0LCS3ZZ	Extirpation of Matter from Right Ankle Tendon, Percutaneous Approach
0LCS4ZZ	Extirpation of Matter from Right Ankle Tendon, Percutaneous Endoscopic Approach
0LCT0ZZ	Extirpation of Matter from Left Ankle Tendon, Open Approach
0LCT3ZZ	Extirpation of Matter from Left Ankle Tendon, Percutaneous Approach
0LCT4ZZ	Extirpation of Matter from Left Ankle Tendon, Percutaneous Endoscopic Approach
0LCV0ZZ	Extirpation of Matter from Right Foot Tendon, Open Approach
0LCV3ZZ	Extirpation of Matter from Right Foot Tendon, Percutaneous Approach
0LCV4ZZ	Extirpation of Matter from Right Foot Tendon, Percutaneous Endoscopic Approach
0LCW0ZZ	Extirpation of Matter from Left Foot Tendon, Open Approach
0LCW3ZZ	Extirpation of Matter from Left Foot Tendon, Percutaneous Approach
0LCW4ZZ	Extirpation of Matter from Left Foot Tendon, Percutaneous Endoscopic Approach

---

♀ Female-only   ♂ Male-only   ● Limited Coverage   ● Non-OR   ᴴᴬᶜ HAC-associated procedure   ● Non-covered procedures   ➕ Combination

0LJ – Tendons, Inspection

Review Coding Guidelines B3.5

Review Coding Guidelines B3.11a, B3.11b and B3.11c

0LJX0ZZ	Inspection of Upper Tendon, Open Approach
0LJX3ZZ	Inspection of Upper Tendon, Percutaneous Approach
0LJX4ZZ	Inspection of Upper Tendon, Percutaneous Endoscopic Approach
0LJXXZZ	Inspection of Upper Tendon, External Approach
0LJY0ZZ	Inspection of Lower Tendon, Open Approach
0LJY3ZZ	Inspection of Lower Tendon, Percutaneous Approach
0LJY4ZZ	Inspection of Lower Tendon, Percutaneous Endoscopic Approach
0LJYXZZ	Inspection of Lower Tendon, External Approach

0LM – Tendons, Reattachment

0LM00ZZ	Reattachment of Head and Neck Tendon, Open Approach
0LM04ZZ	Reattachment of Head and Neck Tendon, Percutaneous Endoscopic Approach
0LM10ZZ	Reattachment of Right Shoulder Tendon, Open Approach
0LM14ZZ	Reattachment of Right Shoulder Tendon, Percutaneous Endoscopic Approach
0LM20ZZ	Reattachment of Left Shoulder Tendon, Open Approach
0LM24ZZ	Reattachment of Left Shoulder Tendon, Percutaneous Endoscopic Approach
0LM30ZZ	Reattachment of Right Upper Arm Tendon, Open Approach
0LM34ZZ	Reattachment of Right Upper Arm Tendon, Percutaneous Endoscopic Approach
0LM40ZZ	Reattachment of Left Upper Arm Tendon, Open Approach
0LM44ZZ	Reattachment of Left Upper Arm Tendon, Percutaneous Endoscopic Approach
0LM50ZZ	Reattachment of Right Lower Arm and Wrist Tendon, Open Approach
0LM54ZZ	Reattachment of Right Lower Arm and Wrist Tendon, Percutaneous Endoscopic Approach
0LM60ZZ	Reattachment of Left Lower Arm and Wrist Tendon, Open Approach
0LM64ZZ	Reattachment of Left Lower Arm and Wrist Tendon, Percutaneous Endoscopic Approach
0LM70ZZ	Reattachment of Right Hand Tendon, Open Approach
0LM74ZZ	Reattachment of Right Hand Tendon, Percutaneous Endoscopic Approach
0LM80ZZ	Reattachment of Left Hand Tendon, Open Approach
0LM84ZZ	Reattachment of Left Hand Tendon, Percutaneous Endoscopic Approach
0LM90ZZ	Reattachment of Right Trunk Tendon, Open Approach
0LM94ZZ	Reattachment of Right Trunk Tendon, Percutaneous Endoscopic Approach
0LMB0ZZ	Reattachment of Left Trunk Tendon, Open Approach
0LMB4ZZ	Reattachment of Left Trunk Tendon, Percutaneous Endoscopic Approach
0LMC0ZZ	Reattachment of Right Thorax Tendon, Open Approach
0LMC4ZZ	Reattachment of Right Thorax Tendon, Percutaneous Endoscopic Approach
0LMD0ZZ	Reattachment of Left Thorax Tendon, Open Approach
0LMD4ZZ	Reattachment of Left Thorax Tendon, Percutaneous Endoscopic Approach
0LMF0ZZ	Reattachment of Right Abdomen Tendon, Open Approach
0LMF4ZZ	Reattachment of Right Abdomen Tendon, Percutaneous Endoscopic Approach
0LMG0ZZ	Reattachment of Left Abdomen Tendon, Open Approach
0LMG4ZZ	Reattachment of Left Abdomen Tendon, Percutaneous Endoscopic Approach
0LMH0ZZ	Reattachment of Perineum Tendon, Open Approach
0LMH4ZZ	Reattachment of Perineum Tendon, Percutaneous Endoscopic Approach
0LMJ0ZZ	Reattachment of Right Hip Tendon, Open Approach
0LMJ4ZZ	Reattachment of Right Hip Tendon, Percutaneous Endoscopic Approach
0LMK0ZZ	Reattachment of Left Hip Tendon, Open Approach
0LMK4ZZ	Reattachment of Left Hip Tendon, Percutaneous Endoscopic Approach
0LML0ZZ	Reattachment of Right Upper Leg Tendon, Open Approach
0LML4ZZ	Reattachment of Right Upper Leg Tendon, Percutaneous Endoscopic Approach
0LMM0ZZ	Reattachment of Left Upper Leg Tendon, Open Approach
0LMM4ZZ	Reattachment of Left Upper Leg Tendon, Percutaneous Endoscopic Approach
0LMN0ZZ	Reattachment of Right Lower Leg Tendon, Open Approach
0LMN4ZZ	Reattachment of Right Lower Leg Tendon, Percutaneous Endoscopic Approach
0LMP0ZZ	Reattachment of Left Lower Leg Tendon, Open Approach
0LMP4ZZ	Reattachment of Left Lower Leg Tendon, Percutaneous Endoscopic Approach
0LMQ0ZZ	Reattachment of Right Knee Tendon, Open Approach
0LMQ4ZZ	Reattachment of Right Knee Tendon, Percutaneous Endoscopic Approach
0LMR0ZZ	Reattachment of Left Knee Tendon, Open Approach
0LMR4ZZ	Reattachment of Left Knee Tendon, Percutaneous Endoscopic Approach
0LMS0ZZ	Reattachment of Right Ankle Tendon, Open Approach
0LMS4ZZ	Reattachment of Right Ankle Tendon, Percutaneous Endoscopic Approach
0LMT0ZZ	Reattachment of Left Ankle Tendon, Open Approach
0LMT4ZZ	Reattachment of Left Ankle Tendon, Percutaneous Endoscopic Approach
0LMV0ZZ	Reattachment of Right Foot Tendon, Open Approach
0LMV4ZZ	Reattachment of Right Foot Tendon, Percutaneous Endoscopic Approach
0LMW0ZZ	Reattachment of Left Foot Tendon, Open Approach
0LMW4ZZ	Reattachment of Left Foot Tendon, Percutaneous Endoscopic Approach

0LN – Tendons, Release

Review Coding Guideline B3.13

Review Coding Guideline B3.14

0LN00ZZ	Release Head and Neck Tendon, Open Approach
0LN03ZZ	Release Head and Neck Tendon, Percutaneous Approach
0LN04ZZ	Release Head and Neck Tendon, Percutaneous Endoscopic Approach
0LN0XZZ	Release Head and Neck Tendon, External Approach
0LN10ZZ	Release Right Shoulder Tendon, Open Approach
0LN13ZZ	Release Right Shoulder Tendon, Percutaneous Approach
0LN14ZZ	Release Right Shoulder Tendon, Percutaneous Endoscopic Approach
0LN1XZZ	Release Right Shoulder Tendon, External Approach
0LN20ZZ	Release Left Shoulder Tendon, Open Approach
0LN23ZZ	Release Left Shoulder Tendon, Percutaneous Approach
0LN24ZZ	Release Left Shoulder Tendon, Percutaneous Endoscopic Approach
0LN2XZZ	Release Left Shoulder Tendon, External Approach
0LN30ZZ	Release Right Upper Arm Tendon, Open Approach
0LN33ZZ	Release Right Upper Arm Tendon, Percutaneous Approach

0LN34ZZ	Release Right Upper Arm Tendon, Percutaneous Endoscopic Approach
0LN3XZZ	Release Right Upper Arm Tendon, External Approach
0LN40ZZ	Release Left Upper Arm Tendon, Open Approach
0LN43ZZ	Release Left Upper Arm Tendon, Percutaneous Approach
0LN44ZZ	Release Left Upper Arm Tendon, Percutaneous Endoscopic Approach
0LN4XZZ	Release Left Upper Arm Tendon, External Approach
0LN50ZZ	Release Right Lower Arm and Wrist Tendon, Open Approach
0LN53ZZ	Release Right Lower Arm and Wrist Tendon, Percutaneous Approach
0LN54ZZ	Release Right Lower Arm and Wrist Tendon, Percutaneous Endoscopic Approach
0LN5XZZ	Release Right Lower Arm and Wrist Tendon, External Approach
0LN60ZZ	Release Left Lower Arm and Wrist Tendon, Open Approach
0LN63ZZ	Release Left Lower Arm and Wrist Tendon, Percutaneous Approach
0LN64ZZ	Release Left Lower Arm and Wrist Tendon, Percutaneous Endoscopic Approach
0LN6XZZ	Release Left Lower Arm and Wrist Tendon, External Approach
0LN70ZZ	Release Right Hand Tendon, Open Approach
0LN73ZZ	Release Right Hand Tendon, Percutaneous Approach
0LN74ZZ	Release Right Hand Tendon, Percutaneous Endoscopic Approach
0LN7XZZ	Release Right Hand Tendon, External Approach
0LN80ZZ	Release Left Hand Tendon, Open Approach
0LN83ZZ	Release Left Hand Tendon, Percutaneous Approach
0LN84ZZ	Release Left Hand Tendon, Percutaneous Endoscopic Approach
0LN8XZZ	Release Left Hand Tendon, External Approach
0LN90ZZ	Release Right Trunk Tendon, Open Approach
0LN93ZZ	Release Right Trunk Tendon, Percutaneous Approach
0LN94ZZ	Release Right Trunk Tendon, Percutaneous Endoscopic Approach
0LN9XZZ	Release Right Trunk Tendon, External Approach
0LNB0ZZ	Release Left Trunk Tendon, Open Approach
0LNB3ZZ	Release Left Trunk Tendon, Percutaneous Approach
0LNB4ZZ	Release Left Trunk Tendon, Percutaneous Endoscopic Approach
0LNBXZZ	Release Left Trunk Tendon, External Approach
0LNC0ZZ	Release Right Thorax Tendon, Open Approach
0LNC3ZZ	Release Right Thorax Tendon, Percutaneous Approach
0LNC4ZZ	Release Right Thorax Tendon, Percutaneous Endoscopic Approach
0LNCXZZ	Release Right Thorax Tendon, External Approach
0LND0ZZ	Release Left Thorax Tendon, Open Approach
0LND3ZZ	Release Left Thorax Tendon, Percutaneous Approach
0LND4ZZ	Release Left Thorax Tendon, Percutaneous Endoscopic Approach
0LNDXZZ	Release Left Thorax Tendon, External Approach
0LNF0ZZ	Release Right Abdomen Tendon, Open Approach
0LNF3ZZ	Release Right Abdomen Tendon, Percutaneous Approach
0LNF4ZZ	Release Right Abdomen Tendon, Percutaneous Endoscopic Approach
0LNFXZZ	Release Right Abdomen Tendon, External Approach
0LNG0ZZ	Release Left Abdomen Tendon, Open Approach
0LNG3ZZ	Release Left Abdomen Tendon, Percutaneous Approach
0LNG4ZZ	Release Left Abdomen Tendon, Percutaneous Endoscopic Approach
0LNGXZZ	Release Left Abdomen Tendon, External Approach
0LNH0ZZ	Release Perineum Tendon, Open Approach
0LNH3ZZ	Release Perineum Tendon, Percutaneous Approach
0LNH4ZZ	Release Perineum Tendon, Percutaneous Endoscopic Approach
0LNHXZZ	Release Perineum Tendon, External Approach
0LNJ0ZZ	Release Right Hip Tendon, Open Approach
0LNJ3ZZ	Release Right Hip Tendon, Percutaneous Approach
0LNJ4ZZ	Release Right Hip Tendon, Percutaneous Endoscopic Approach
0LNJXZZ	Release Right Hip Tendon, External Approach
0LNK0ZZ	Release Left Hip Tendon, Open Approach
0LNK3ZZ	Release Left Hip Tendon, Percutaneous Approach
0LNK4ZZ	Release Left Hip Tendon, Percutaneous Endoscopic Approach
0LNKXZZ	Release Left Hip Tendon, External Approach
0LNL0ZZ	Release Right Upper Leg Tendon, Open Approach
0LNL3ZZ	Release Right Upper Leg Tendon, Percutaneous Approach
0LNL4ZZ	Release Right Upper Leg Tendon, Percutaneous Endoscopic Approach
0LNLXZZ	Release Right Upper Leg Tendon, External Approach
0LNM0ZZ	Release Left Upper Leg Tendon, Open Approach
0LNM3ZZ	Release Left Upper Leg Tendon, Percutaneous Approach
0LNM4ZZ	Release Left Upper Leg Tendon, Percutaneous Endoscopic Approach
0LNMXZZ	Release Left Upper Leg Tendon, External Approach
0LNN0ZZ	Release Right Lower Leg Tendon, Open Approach
0LNN3ZZ	Release Right Lower Leg Tendon, Percutaneous Approach
0LNN4ZZ	Release Right Lower Leg Tendon, Percutaneous Endoscopic Approach
0LNNXZZ	Release Right Lower Leg Tendon, External Approach
0LNP0ZZ	Release Left Lower Leg Tendon, Open Approach
0LNP3ZZ	Release Left Lower Leg Tendon, Percutaneous Approach
0LNP4ZZ	Release Left Lower Leg Tendon, Percutaneous Endoscopic Approach
0LNPXZZ	Release Left Lower Leg Tendon, External Approach
0LNQ0ZZ	Release Right Knee Tendon, Open Approach
0LNQ3ZZ	Release Right Knee Tendon, Percutaneous Approach
0LNQ4ZZ	Release Right Knee Tendon, Percutaneous Endoscopic Approach
0LNQXZZ	Release Right Knee Tendon, External Approach
0LNR0ZZ	Release Left Knee Tendon, Open Approach
0LNR3ZZ	Release Left Knee Tendon, Percutaneous Approach
0LNR4ZZ	Release Left Knee Tendon, Percutaneous Endoscopic Approach
0LNRXZZ	Release Left Knee Tendon, External Approach
0LNS0ZZ	Release Right Ankle Tendon, Open Approach
0LNS3ZZ	Release Right Ankle Tendon, Percutaneous Approach
0LNS4ZZ	Release Right Ankle Tendon, Percutaneous Endoscopic Approach
0LNSXZZ	Release Right Ankle Tendon, External Approach
0LNT0ZZ	Release Left Ankle Tendon, Open Approach
0LNT3ZZ	Release Left Ankle Tendon, Percutaneous Approach
0LNT4ZZ	Release Left Ankle Tendon, Percutaneous Endoscopic Approach
0LNTXZZ	Release Left Ankle Tendon, External Approach
0LNV0ZZ	Release Right Foot Tendon, Open Approach
0LNV3ZZ	Release Right Foot Tendon, Percutaneous Approach
0LNV4ZZ	Release Right Foot Tendon, Percutaneous Endoscopic Approach
0LNVXZZ	Release Right Foot Tendon, External Approach
0LNW0ZZ	Release Left Foot Tendon, Open Approach
0LNW3ZZ	Release Left Foot Tendon, Percutaneous Approach
0LNW4ZZ	Release Left Foot Tendon, Percutaneous Endoscopic Approach
0LNWXZZ	Release Left Foot Tendon, External Approach

0LP – Tendons, Removal

Review Coding Guideline B6.1c

0LPX00Z	Removal of Drainage Device from Upper Tendon, Open Approach
0LPX07Z	Removal of Autologous Tissue Substitute from Upper Tendon, Open Approach
0LPX0JZ	Removal of Synthetic Substitute from Upper Tendon, Open Approach
0LPX0KZ	Removal of Nonautologous Tissue Substitute from Upper Tendon, Open Approach
0LPX30Z	Removal of Drainage Device from Upper Tendon, Percutaneous Approach
0LPX37Z	Removal of Autologous Tissue Substitute from Upper Tendon, Percutaneous Approach
0LPX3JZ	Removal of Synthetic Substitute from Upper Tendon, Percutaneous Approach
0LPX3KZ	Removal of Nonautologous Tissue Substitute from Upper Tendon, Percutaneous Approach
0LPX40Z	Removal of Drainage Device from Upper Tendon, Percutaneous Endoscopic Approach
0LPX47Z	Removal of Autologous Tissue Substitute from Upper Tendon, Percutaneous Endoscopic Approach
0LPX4JZ	Removal of Synthetic Substitute from Upper Tendon, Percutaneous Endoscopic Approach
0LPX4KZ	Removal of Nonautologous Tissue Substitute from Upper Tendon, Percutaneous Endoscopic Approach
0LPXX0Z	Removal of Drainage Device from Upper Tendon, External Approach
0LPY00Z	Removal of Drainage Device from Lower Tendon, Open Approach

♀ Female-only   ♂ Male-only   ● Limited Coverage   ● Non-OR   HAC HAC-associated procedure   ● Non-covered procedures   ✚ Combination

0LPY07Z Removal of Autologous Tissue Substitute from Lower Tendon, Open Approach
0LPY0JZ Removal of Synthetic Substitute from Lower Tendon, Open Approach
0LPY0KZ Removal of Nonautologous Tissue Substitute from Lower Tendon, Open Approach
0LPY30Z Removal of Drainage Device from Lower Tendon, Percutaneous Approach
0LPY37Z Removal of Autologous Tissue Substitute from Lower Tendon, Percutaneous Approach
0LPY3JZ Removal of Synthetic Substitute from Lower Tendon, Percutaneous Approach

0LPY3KZ Removal of Nonautologous Tissue Substitute from Lower Tendon, Percutaneous Approach
0LPY40Z Removal of Drainage Device from Lower Tendon, Percutaneous Endoscopic Approach
0LPY47Z Removal of Autologous Tissue Substitute from Lower Tendon, Percutaneous Endoscopic Approach
0LPY4JZ Removal of Synthetic Substitute from Lower Tendon, Percutaneous Endoscopic Approach
0LPY4KZ Removal of Nonautologous Tissue Substitute from Lower Tendon, Percutaneous Endoscopic Approach
0LPYX0Z Removal of Drainage Device from Lower Tendon, External Approach

0LQ – Tendons, Repair

Review Coding Guideline B3.5

0LQ00ZZ Repair Head and Neck Tendon, Open Approach
0LQ03ZZ Repair Head and Neck Tendon, Percutaneous Approach
0LQ04ZZ Repair Head and Neck Tendon, Percutaneous Endoscopic Approach
0LQ10ZZ Repair Right Shoulder Tendon, Open Approach
0LQ13ZZ Repair Right Shoulder Tendon, Percutaneous Approach
0LQ14ZZ Repair Right Shoulder Tendon, Percutaneous Endoscopic Approach
0LQ20ZZ Repair Left Shoulder Tendon, Open Approach
0LQ23ZZ Repair Left Shoulder Tendon, Percutaneous Approach
0LQ24ZZ Repair Left Shoulder Tendon, Percutaneous Endoscopic Approach
0LQ30ZZ Repair Right Upper Arm Tendon, Open Approach
0LQ33ZZ Repair Right Upper Arm Tendon, Percutaneous Approach
0LQ34ZZ Repair Right Upper Arm Tendon, Percutaneous Endoscopic Approach
0LQ40ZZ Repair Left Upper Arm Tendon, Open Approach
0LQ43ZZ Repair Left Upper Arm Tendon, Percutaneous Approach
0LQ44ZZ Repair Left Upper Arm Tendon, Percutaneous Endoscopic Approach
0LQ50ZZ Repair Right Lower Arm and Wrist Tendon, Open Approach
0LQ53ZZ Repair Right Lower Arm and Wrist Tendon, Percutaneous Approach
0LQ54ZZ Repair Right Lower Arm and Wrist Tendon, Percutaneous Endoscopic Approach
0LQ60ZZ Repair Left Lower Arm and Wrist Tendon, Open Approach
0LQ63ZZ Repair Left Lower Arm and Wrist Tendon, Percutaneous Approach
0LQ64ZZ Repair Left Lower Arm and Wrist Tendon, Percutaneous Endoscopic Approach
0LQ70ZZ Repair Right Hand Tendon, Open Approach
0LQ73ZZ Repair Right Hand Tendon, Percutaneous Approach
0LQ74ZZ Repair Right Hand Tendon, Percutaneous Endoscopic Approach
0LQ80ZZ Repair Left Hand Tendon, Open Approach
0LQ83ZZ Repair Left Hand Tendon, Percutaneous Approach
0LQ84ZZ Repair Left Hand Tendon, Percutaneous Endoscopic Approach
0LQ90ZZ Repair Right Trunk Tendon, Open Approach
0LQ93ZZ Repair Right Trunk Tendon, Percutaneous Approach
0LQ94ZZ Repair Right Trunk Tendon, Percutaneous Endoscopic Approach
0LQB0ZZ Repair Left Trunk Tendon, Open Approach
0LQB3ZZ Repair Left Trunk Tendon, Percutaneous Approach
0LQB4ZZ Repair Left Trunk Tendon, Percutaneous Endoscopic Approach
0LQC0ZZ Repair Right Thorax Tendon, Open Approach
0LQC3ZZ Repair Right Thorax Tendon, Percutaneous Approach
0LQC4ZZ Repair Right Thorax Tendon, Percutaneous Endoscopic Approach
0LQD0ZZ Repair Left Thorax Tendon, Open Approach
0LQD3ZZ Repair Left Thorax Tendon, Percutaneous Approach
0LQD4ZZ Repair Left Thorax Tendon, Percutaneous Endoscopic Approach
0LQF0ZZ Repair Right Abdomen Tendon, Open Approach
0LQF3ZZ Repair Right Abdomen Tendon, Percutaneous Approach
0LQF4ZZ Repair Right Abdomen Tendon, Percutaneous Endoscopic Approach

0LQG0ZZ Repair Left Abdomen Tendon, Open Approach
0LQG3ZZ Repair Left Abdomen Tendon, Percutaneous Approach
0LQG4ZZ Repair Left Abdomen Tendon, Percutaneous Endoscopic Approach
0LQH0ZZ Repair Perineum Tendon, Open Approach
0LQH3ZZ Repair Perineum Tendon, Percutaneous Approach
0LQH4ZZ Repair Perineum Tendon, Percutaneous Endoscopic Approach
0LQJ0ZZ Repair Right Hip Tendon, Open Approach
0LQJ3ZZ Repair Right Hip Tendon, Percutaneous Approach
0LQJ4ZZ Repair Right Hip Tendon, Percutaneous Endoscopic Approach
0LQK0ZZ Repair Left Hip Tendon, Open Approach
0LQK3ZZ Repair Left Hip Tendon, Percutaneous Approach
0LQK4ZZ Repair Left Hip Tendon, Percutaneous Endoscopic Approach
0LQL0ZZ Repair Right Upper Leg Tendon, Open Approach
0LQL3ZZ Repair Right Upper Leg Tendon, Percutaneous Approach
0LQL4ZZ Repair Right Upper Leg Tendon, Percutaneous Endoscopic Approach
0LQM0ZZ Repair Left Upper Leg Tendon, Open Approach
0LQM3ZZ Repair Left Upper Leg Tendon, Percutaneous Approach
0LQM4ZZ Repair Left Upper Leg Tendon, Percutaneous Endoscopic Approach
0LQN0ZZ Repair Right Lower Leg Tendon, Open Approach
0LQN3ZZ Repair Right Lower Leg Tendon, Percutaneous Approach
0LQN4ZZ Repair Right Lower Leg Tendon, Percutaneous Endoscopic Approach
0LQP0ZZ Repair Left Lower Leg Tendon, Open Approach
0LQP3ZZ Repair Left Lower Leg Tendon, Percutaneous Approach
0LQP4ZZ Repair Left Lower Leg Tendon, Percutaneous Endoscopic Approach
0LQQ0ZZ Repair Right Knee Tendon, Open Approach
0LQQ3ZZ Repair Right Knee Tendon, Percutaneous Approach
0LQQ4ZZ Repair Right Knee Tendon, Percutaneous Endoscopic Approach
0LQR0ZZ Repair Left Knee Tendon, Open Approach
0LQR3ZZ Repair Left Knee Tendon, Percutaneous Approach
0LQR4ZZ Repair Left Knee Tendon, Percutaneous Endoscopic Approach
0LQS0ZZ Repair Right Ankle Tendon, Open Approach
0LQS3ZZ Repair Right Ankle Tendon, Percutaneous Approach
0LQS4ZZ Repair Right Ankle Tendon, Percutaneous Endoscopic Approach
0LQT0ZZ Repair Left Ankle Tendon, Open Approach
0LQT3ZZ Repair Left Ankle Tendon, Percutaneous Approach
0LQT4ZZ Repair Left Ankle Tendon, Percutaneous Endoscopic Approach
0LQV0ZZ Repair Right Foot Tendon, Open Approach
0LQV3ZZ Repair Right Foot Tendon, Percutaneous Approach
0LQV4ZZ Repair Right Foot Tendon, Percutaneous Endoscopic Approach
0LQW0ZZ Repair Left Foot Tendon, Open Approach
0LQW3ZZ Repair Left Foot Tendon, Percutaneous Approach
0LQW4ZZ Repair Left Foot Tendon, Percutaneous Endoscopic Approach

0LR – Tendons, Replacement

0LR007Z Replacement of Head and Neck Tendon with Autologous Tissue Substitute, Open Approach
0LR00JZ Replacement of Head and Neck Tendon with Synthetic Substitute, Open Approach
0LR00KZ Replacement of Head and Neck Tendon with Nonautologous Tissue Substitute, Open Approach
0LR047Z Replacement of Head and Neck Tendon with Autologous Tissue Substitute, Percutaneous Endoscopic Approach

0LR04JZ Replacement of Head and Neck Tendon with Synthetic Substitute, Percutaneous Endoscopic Approach
0LR04KZ Replacement of Head and Neck Tendon with Nonautologous Tissue Substitute, Percutaneous Endoscopic Approach
0LR107Z Replacement of Right Shoulder Tendon with Autologous Tissue Substitute, Open Approach
0LR10JZ Replacement of Right Shoulder Tendon with Synthetic Substitute, Open Approach

0LR10KZ   Replacement of Right Shoulder Tendon with Nonautologous Tissue Substitute, Open Approach

0LR147Z   Replacement of Right Shoulder Tendon with Autologous Tissue Substitute, Percutaneous Endoscopic Approach

0LR14JZ   Replacement of Right Shoulder Tendon with Synthetic Substitute, Percutaneous Endoscopic Approach

0LR14KZ   Replacement of Right Shoulder Tendon with Nonautologous Tissue Substitute, Percutaneous Endoscopic Approach

0LR207Z   Replacement of Left Shoulder Tendon with Autologous Tissue Substitute, Open Approach

0LR20JZ   Replacement of Left Shoulder Tendon with Synthetic Substitute, Open Approach

0LR20KZ   Replacement of Left Shoulder Tendon with Nonautologous Tissue Substitute, Open Approach

0LR247Z   Replacement of Left Shoulder Tendon with Autologous Tissue Substitute, Percutaneous Endoscopic Approach

0LR24JZ   Replacement of Left Shoulder Tendon with Synthetic Substitute, Percutaneous Endoscopic Approach

0LR24KZ   Replacement of Left Shoulder Tendon with Nonautologous Tissue Substitute, Percutaneous Endoscopic Approach

0LR307Z   Replacement of Right Upper Arm Tendon with Autologous Tissue Substitute, Open Approach

0LR30JZ   Replacement of Right Upper Arm Tendon with Synthetic Substitute, Open Approach

0LR30KZ   Replacement of Right Upper Arm Tendon with Nonautologous Tissue Substitute, Open Approach

0LR347Z   Replacement of Right Upper Arm Tendon with Autologous Tissue Substitute, Percutaneous Endoscopic Approach

0LR34JZ   Replacement of Right Upper Arm Tendon with Synthetic Substitute, Percutaneous Endoscopic Approach

0LR34KZ   Replacement of Right Upper Arm Tendon with Nonautologous Tissue Substitute, Percutaneous Endoscopic Approach

0LR407Z   Replacement of Left Upper Arm Tendon with Autologous Tissue Substitute, Open Approach

0LR40JZ   Replacement of Left Upper Arm Tendon with Synthetic Substitute, Open Approach

0LR40KZ   Replacement of Left Upper Arm Tendon with Nonautologous Tissue Substitute, Open Approach

0LR447Z   Replacement of Left Upper Arm Tendon with Autologous Tissue Substitute, Percutaneous Endoscopic Approach

0LR44JZ   Replacement of Left Upper Arm Tendon with Synthetic Substitute, Percutaneous Endoscopic Approach

0LR44KZ   Replacement of Left Upper Arm Tendon with Nonautologous Tissue Substitute, Percutaneous Endoscopic Approach

0LR507Z   Replacement of Right Lower Arm and Wrist Tendon with Autologous Tissue Substitute, Open Approach

0LR50JZ   Replacement of Right Lower Arm and Wrist Tendon with Synthetic Substitute, Open Approach

0LR50KZ   Replacement of Right Lower Arm and Wrist Tendon with Nonautologous Tissue Substitute, Open Approach

0LR547Z   Replacement of Right Lower Arm and Wrist Tendon with Autologous Tissue Substitute, Percutaneous Endoscopic Approach

0LR54JZ   Replacement of Right Lower Arm and Wrist Tendon with Synthetic Substitute, Percutaneous Endoscopic Approach

0LR54KZ   Replacement of Right Lower Arm and Wrist Tendon with Nonautologous Tissue Substitute, Percutaneous Endoscopic Approach

0LR607Z   Replacement of Left Lower Arm and Wrist Tendon with Autologous Tissue Substitute, Open Approach

0LR60JZ   Replacement of Left Lower Arm and Wrist Tendon with Synthetic Substitute, Open Approach

0LR60KZ   Replacement of Left Lower Arm and Wrist Tendon with Nonautologous Tissue Substitute, Open Approach

0LR647Z   Replacement of Left Lower Arm and Wrist Tendon with Autologous Tissue Substitute, Percutaneous Endoscopic Approach

0LR64JZ   Replacement of Left Lower Arm and Wrist Tendon with Synthetic Substitute, Percutaneous Endoscopic Approach

0LR64KZ   Replacement of Left Lower Arm and Wrist Tendon with Nonautologous Tissue Substitute, Percutaneous Endoscopic Approach

0LR707Z   Replacement of Right Hand Tendon with Autologous Tissue Substitute, Open Approach

0LR70JZ   Replacement of Right Hand Tendon with Synthetic Substitute, Open Approach

0LR70KZ   Replacement of Right Hand Tendon with Nonautologous Tissue Substitute, Open Approach

0LR747Z   Replacement of Right Hand Tendon with Autologous Tissue Substitute, Percutaneous Endoscopic Approach

0LR74JZ   Replacement of Right Hand Tendon with Synthetic Substitute, Percutaneous Endoscopic Approach

0LR74KZ   Replacement of Right Hand Tendon with Nonautologous Tissue Substitute, Percutaneous Endoscopic Approach

0LR807Z   Replacement of Left Hand Tendon with Autologous Tissue Substitute, Open Approach

0LR80JZ   Replacement of Left Hand Tendon with Synthetic Substitute, Open Approach

0LR80KZ   Replacement of Left Hand Tendon with Nonautologous Tissue Substitute, Open Approach

0LR847Z   Replacement of Left Hand Tendon with Autologous Tissue Substitute, Percutaneous Endoscopic Approach

0LR84JZ   Replacement of Left Hand Tendon with Synthetic Substitute, Percutaneous Endoscopic Approach

0LR84KZ   Replacement of Left Hand Tendon with Nonautologous Tissue Substitute, Percutaneous Endoscopic Approach

0LR907Z   Replacement of Right Trunk Tendon with Autologous Tissue Substitute, Open Approach

0LR90JZ   Replacement of Right Trunk Tendon with Synthetic Substitute, Open Approach

0LR90KZ   Replacement of Right Trunk Tendon with Nonautologous Tissue Substitute, Open Approach

0LR947Z   Replacement of Right Trunk Tendon with Autologous Tissue Substitute, Percutaneous Endoscopic Approach

0LR94JZ   Replacement of Right Trunk Tendon with Synthetic Substitute, Percutaneous Endoscopic Approach

0LR94KZ   Replacement of Right Trunk Tendon with Nonautologous Tissue Substitute, Percutaneous Endoscopic Approach

0LRB07Z   Replacement of Left Trunk Tendon with Autologous Tissue Substitute, Open Approach

0LRB0JZ   Replacement of Left Trunk Tendon with Synthetic Substitute, Open Approach

0LRB0KZ   Replacement of Left Trunk Tendon with Nonautologous Tissue Substitute, Open Approach

0LRB47Z   Replacement of Left Trunk Tendon with Autologous Tissue Substitute, Percutaneous Endoscopic Approach

0LRB4JZ   Replacement of Left Trunk Tendon with Synthetic Substitute, Percutaneous Endoscopic Approach

0LRB4KZ   Replacement of Left Trunk Tendon with Nonautologous Tissue Substitute, Percutaneous Endoscopic Approach

0LRC07Z   Replacement of Right Thorax Tendon with Autologous Tissue Substitute, Open Approach

0LRC0JZ   Replacement of Right Thorax Tendon with Synthetic Substitute, Open Approach

0LRC0KZ   Replacement of Right Thorax Tendon with Nonautologous Tissue Substitute, Open Approach

0LRC47Z   Replacement of Right Thorax Tendon with Autologous Tissue Substitute, Percutaneous Endoscopic Approach

0LRC4JZ   Replacement of Right Thorax Tendon with Synthetic Substitute, Percutaneous Endoscopic Approach

0LRC4KZ   Replacement of Right Thorax Tendon with Nonautologous Tissue Substitute, Percutaneous Endoscopic Approach

0LRD07Z   Replacement of Left Thorax Tendon with Autologous Tissue Substitute, Open Approach

0LRD0JZ   Replacement of Left Thorax Tendon with Synthetic Substitute, Open Approach

0LRD0KZ   Replacement of Left Thorax Tendon with Nonautologous Tissue Substitute, Open Approach

0LRD47Z   Replacement of Left Thorax Tendon with Autologous Tissue Substitute, Percutaneous Endoscopic Approach

0LRD4JZ   Replacement of Left Thorax Tendon with Synthetic Substitute, Percutaneous Endoscopic Approach

0LRD4KZ   Replacement of Left Thorax Tendon with Nonautologous Tissue Substitute, Percutaneous Endoscopic Approach

0LRF07Z   Replacement of Right Abdomen Tendon with Autologous Tissue Substitute, Open Approach

0LRF0JZ Replacement of Right Abdomen Tendon with Synthetic Substitute, Open Approach

0LRF0KZ Replacement of Right Abdomen Tendon with Nonautologous Tissue Substitute, Open Approach

0LRF47Z Replacement of Right Abdomen Tendon with Autologous Tissue Substitute, Percutaneous Endoscopic Approach

0LRF4JZ Replacement of Right Abdomen Tendon with Synthetic Substitute, Percutaneous Endoscopic Approach

0LRF4KZ Replacement of Right Abdomen Tendon with Nonautologous Tissue Substitute, Percutaneous Endoscopic Approach

0LRG07Z Replacement of Left Abdomen Tendon with Autologous Tissue Substitute, Open Approach

0LRG0JZ Replacement of Left Abdomen Tendon with Synthetic Substitute, Open Approach

0LRG0KZ Replacement of Left Abdomen Tendon with Nonautologous Tissue Substitute, Open Approach

0LRG47Z Replacement of Left Abdomen Tendon with Autologous Tissue Substitute, Percutaneous Endoscopic Approach

0LRG4JZ Replacement of Left Abdomen Tendon with Synthetic Substitute, Percutaneous Endoscopic Approach

0LRG4KZ Replacement of Left Abdomen Tendon with Nonautologous Tissue Substitute, Percutaneous Endoscopic Approach

0LRH07Z Replacement of Perineum Tendon with Autologous Tissue Substitute, Open Approach

0LRH0JZ Replacement of Perineum Tendon with Synthetic Substitute, Open Approach

0LRH0KZ Replacement of Perineum Tendon with Nonautologous Tissue Substitute, Open Approach

0LRH47Z Replacement of Perineum Tendon with Autologous Tissue Substitute, Percutaneous Endoscopic Approach

0LRH4JZ Replacement of Perineum Tendon with Synthetic Substitute, Percutaneous Endoscopic Approach

0LRH4KZ Replacement of Perineum Tendon with Nonautologous Tissue Substitute, Percutaneous Endoscopic Approach

0LRJ07Z Replacement of Right Hip Tendon with Autologous Tissue Substitute, Open Approach

0LRJ0JZ Replacement of Right Hip Tendon with Synthetic Substitute, Open Approach

0LRJ0KZ Replacement of Right Hip Tendon with Nonautologous Tissue Substitute, Open Approach

0LRJ47Z Replacement of Right Hip Tendon with Autologous Tissue Substitute, Percutaneous Endoscopic Approach

0LRJ4JZ Replacement of Right Hip Tendon with Synthetic Substitute, Percutaneous Endoscopic Approach

0LRJ4KZ Replacement of Right Hip Tendon with Nonautologous Tissue Substitute, Percutaneous Endoscopic Approach

0LRK07Z Replacement of Left Hip Tendon with Autologous Tissue Substitute, Open Approach

0LRK0JZ Replacement of Left Hip Tendon with Synthetic Substitute, Open Approach

0LRK0KZ Replacement of Left Hip Tendon with Nonautologous Tissue Substitute, Open Approach

0LRK47Z Replacement of Left Hip Tendon with Autologous Tissue Substitute, Percutaneous Endoscopic Approach

0LRK4JZ Replacement of Left Hip Tendon with Synthetic Substitute, Percutaneous Endoscopic Approach

0LRK4KZ Replacement of Left Hip Tendon with Nonautologous Tissue Substitute, Percutaneous Endoscopic Approach

0LRL07Z Replacement of Right Upper Leg Tendon with Autologous Tissue Substitute, Open Approach

0LRL0JZ Replacement of Right Upper Leg Tendon with Synthetic Substitute, Open Approach

0LRL0KZ Replacement of Right Upper Leg Tendon with Nonautologous Tissue Substitute, Open Approach

0LRL47Z Replacement of Right Upper Leg Tendon with Autologous Tissue Substitute, Percutaneous Endoscopic Approach

0LRL4JZ Replacement of Right Upper Leg Tendon with Synthetic Substitute, Percutaneous Endoscopic Approach

0LRL4KZ Replacement of Right Upper Leg Tendon with Nonautologous Tissue Substitute, Percutaneous Endoscopic Approach

0LRM07Z Replacement of Left Upper Leg Tendon with Autologous Tissue Substitute, Open Approach

0LRM0JZ Replacement of Left Upper Leg Tendon with Synthetic Substitute, Open Approach

0LRM0KZ Replacement of Left Upper Leg Tendon with Nonautologous Tissue Substitute, Open Approach

0LRM47Z Replacement of Left Upper Leg Tendon with Autologous Tissue Substitute, Percutaneous Endoscopic Approach

0LRM4JZ Replacement of Left Upper Leg Tendon with Synthetic Substitute, Percutaneous Endoscopic Approach

0LRM4KZ Replacement of Left Upper Leg Tendon with Nonautologous Tissue Substitute, Percutaneous Endoscopic Approach

0LRN07Z Replacement of Right Lower Leg Tendon with Autologous Tissue Substitute, Open Approach

0LRN0JZ Replacement of Right Lower Leg Tendon with Synthetic Substitute, Open Approach

0LRN0KZ Replacement of Right Lower Leg Tendon with Nonautologous Tissue Substitute, Open Approach

0LRN47Z Replacement of Right Lower Leg Tendon with Autologous Tissue Substitute, Percutaneous Endoscopic Approach

0LRN4JZ Replacement of Right Lower Leg Tendon with Synthetic Substitute, Percutaneous Endoscopic Approach

0LRN4KZ Replacement of Right Lower Leg Tendon with Nonautologous Tissue Substitute, Percutaneous Endoscopic Approach

0LRP07Z Replacement of Left Lower Leg Tendon with Autologous Tissue Substitute, Open Approach

0LRP0JZ Replacement of Left Lower Leg Tendon with Synthetic Substitute, Open Approach

0LRP0KZ Replacement of Left Lower Leg Tendon with Nonautologous Tissue Substitute, Open Approach

0LRP47Z Replacement of Left Lower Leg Tendon with Autologous Tissue Substitute, Percutaneous Endoscopic Approach

0LRP4JZ Replacement of Left Lower Leg Tendon with Synthetic Substitute, Percutaneous Endoscopic Approach

0LRP4KZ Replacement of Left Lower Leg Tendon with Nonautologous Tissue Substitute, Percutaneous Endoscopic Approach

0LRQ07Z Replacement of Right Knee Tendon with Autologous Tissue Substitute, Open Approach

0LRQ0JZ Replacement of Right Knee Tendon with Synthetic Substitute, Open Approach

0LRQ0KZ Replacement of Right Knee Tendon with Nonautologous Tissue Substitute, Open Approach

0LRQ47Z Replacement of Right Knee Tendon with Autologous Tissue Substitute, Percutaneous Endoscopic Approach

0LRQ4JZ Replacement of Right Knee Tendon with Synthetic Substitute, Percutaneous Endoscopic Approach

0LRQ4KZ Replacement of Right Knee Tendon with Nonautologous Tissue Substitute, Percutaneous Endoscopic Approach

0LRR07Z Replacement of Left Knee Tendon with Autologous Tissue Substitute, Open Approach

0LRR0JZ Replacement of Left Knee Tendon with Synthetic Substitute, Open Approach

0LRR0KZ Replacement of Left Knee Tendon with Nonautologous Tissue Substitute, Open Approach

0LRR47Z Replacement of Left Knee Tendon with Autologous Tissue Substitute, Percutaneous Endoscopic Approach

0LRR4JZ Replacement of Left Knee Tendon with Synthetic Substitute, Percutaneous Endoscopic Approach

0LRR4KZ Replacement of Left Knee Tendon with Nonautologous Tissue Substitute, Percutaneous Endoscopic Approach

0LRS07Z Replacement of Right Ankle Tendon with Autologous Tissue Substitute, Open Approach

0LRS0JZ Replacement of Right Ankle Tendon with Synthetic Substitute, Open Approach

0LRS0KZ Replacement of Right Ankle Tendon with Nonautologous Tissue Substitute, Open Approach

0LRS47Z Replacement of Right Ankle Tendon with Autologous Tissue Substitute, Percutaneous Endoscopic Approach

0LRS4JZ Replacement of Right Ankle Tendon with Synthetic Substitute, Percutaneous Endoscopic Approach

0LRS4KZ Replacement of Right Ankle Tendon with Nonautologous Tissue Substitute, Percutaneous Endoscopic Approach

0LRT07Z Replacement of Left Ankle Tendon with Autologous Tissue Substitute, Open Approach

0LRT0JZ — Replacement of Left Ankle Tendon with Synthetic Substitute, Open Approach

0LRT0KZ — Replacement of Left Ankle Tendon with Nonautologous Tissue Substitute, Open Approach

0LRT47Z — Replacement of Left Ankle Tendon with Autologous Tissue Substitute, Percutaneous Endoscopic Approach

0LRT4JZ — Replacement of Left Ankle Tendon with Synthetic Substitute, Percutaneous Endoscopic Approach

0LRT4KZ — Replacement of Left Ankle Tendon with Nonautologous Tissue Substitute, Percutaneous Endoscopic Approach

0LRV07Z — Replacement of Right Foot Tendon with Autologous Tissue Substitute, Open Approach

0LRV0JZ — Replacement of Right Foot Tendon with Synthetic Substitute, Open Approach

0LRV0KZ — Replacement of Right Foot Tendon with Nonautologous Tissue Substitute, Open Approach

0LRV47Z — Replacement of Right Foot Tendon with Autologous Tissue Substitute, Percutaneous Endoscopic Approach

0LRV4JZ — Replacement of Right Foot Tendon with Synthetic Substitute, Percutaneous Endoscopic Approach

0LRV4KZ — Replacement of Right Foot Tendon with Nonautologous Tissue Substitute, Percutaneous Endoscopic Approach

0LRW07Z — Replacement of Left Foot Tendon with Autologous Tissue Substitute, Open Approach

0LRW0JZ — Replacement of Left Foot Tendon with Synthetic Substitute, Open Approach

0LRW0KZ — Replacement of Left Foot Tendon with Nonautologous Tissue Substitute, Open Approach

0LRW47Z — Replacement of Left Foot Tendon with Autologous Tissue Substitute, Percutaneous Endoscopic Approach

0LRW4JZ — Replacement of Left Foot Tendon with Synthetic Substitute, Percutaneous Endoscopic Approach

0LRW4KZ — Replacement of Left Foot Tendon with Nonautologous Tissue Substitute, Percutaneous Endoscopic Approach

0LS – Tendons, Reposition

0LS00ZZ — Reposition Head and Neck Tendon, Open Approach

0LS04ZZ — Reposition Head and Neck Tendon, Percutaneous Endoscopic Approach

0LS10ZZ — Reposition Right Shoulder Tendon, Open Approach

0LS14ZZ — Reposition Right Shoulder Tendon, Percutaneous Endoscopic Approach

0LS20ZZ — Reposition Left Shoulder Tendon, Open Approach

0LS24ZZ — Reposition Left Shoulder Tendon, Percutaneous Endoscopic Approach

0LS30ZZ — Reposition Right Upper Arm Tendon, Open Approach

0LS34ZZ — Reposition Right Upper Arm Tendon, Percutaneous Endoscopic Approach

0LS40ZZ — Reposition Left Upper Arm Tendon, Open Approach

0LS44ZZ — Reposition Left Upper Arm Tendon, Percutaneous Endoscopic Approach

0LS50ZZ — Reposition Right Lower Arm and Wrist Tendon, Open Approach

0LS54ZZ — Reposition Right Lower Arm and Wrist Tendon, Percutaneous Endoscopic Approach

0LS60ZZ — Reposition Left Lower Arm and Wrist Tendon, Open Approach

0LS64ZZ — Reposition Left Lower Arm and Wrist Tendon, Percutaneous Endoscopic Approach

0LS70ZZ — Reposition Right Hand Tendon, Open Approach

0LS74ZZ — Reposition Right Hand Tendon, Percutaneous Endoscopic Approach

0LS80ZZ — Reposition Left Hand Tendon, Open Approach

0LS84ZZ — Reposition Left Hand Tendon, Percutaneous Endoscopic Approach

0LS90ZZ — Reposition Right Trunk Tendon, Open Approach

0LS94ZZ — Reposition Right Trunk Tendon, Percutaneous Endoscopic Approach

0LSB0ZZ — Reposition Left Trunk Tendon, Open Approach

0LSB4ZZ — Reposition Left Trunk Tendon, Percutaneous Endoscopic Approach

0LSC0ZZ — Reposition Right Thorax Tendon, Open Approach

0LSC4ZZ — Reposition Right Thorax Tendon, Percutaneous Endoscopic Approach

0LSD0ZZ — Reposition Left Thorax Tendon, Open Approach

0LSD4ZZ — Reposition Left Thorax Tendon, Percutaneous Endoscopic Approach

0LSF0ZZ — Reposition Right Abdomen Tendon, Open Approach

0LSF4ZZ — Reposition Right Abdomen Tendon, Percutaneous Endoscopic Approach

0LSG0ZZ — Reposition Left Abdomen Tendon, Open Approach

0LSG4ZZ — Reposition Left Abdomen Tendon, Percutaneous Endoscopic Approach

0LSH0ZZ — Reposition Perineum Tendon, Open Approach

0LSH4ZZ — Reposition Perineum Tendon, Percutaneous Endoscopic Approach

0LSJ0ZZ — Reposition Right Hip Tendon, Open Approach

0LSJ4ZZ — Reposition Right Hip Tendon, Percutaneous Endoscopic Approach

0LSK0ZZ — Reposition Left Hip Tendon, Open Approach

0LSK4ZZ — Reposition Left Hip Tendon, Percutaneous Endoscopic Approach

0LSL0ZZ — Reposition Right Upper Leg Tendon, Open Approach

0LSL4ZZ — Reposition Right Upper Leg Tendon, Percutaneous Endoscopic Approach

0LSM0ZZ — Reposition Left Upper Leg Tendon, Open Approach

0LSM4ZZ — Reposition Left Upper Leg Tendon, Percutaneous Endoscopic Approach

0LSN0ZZ — Reposition Right Lower Leg Tendon, Open Approach

0LSN4ZZ — Reposition Right Lower Leg Tendon, Percutaneous Endoscopic Approach

0LSP0ZZ — Reposition Left Lower Leg Tendon, Open Approach

0LSP4ZZ — Reposition Left Lower Leg Tendon, Percutaneous Endoscopic Approach

0LSQ0ZZ — Reposition Right Knee Tendon, Open Approach

0LSQ4ZZ — Reposition Right Knee Tendon, Percutaneous Endoscopic Approach

0LSR0ZZ — Reposition Left Knee Tendon, Open Approach

0LSR4ZZ — Reposition Left Knee Tendon, Percutaneous Endoscopic Approach

0LSS0ZZ — Reposition Right Ankle Tendon, Open Approach

0LSS4ZZ — Reposition Right Ankle Tendon, Percutaneous Endoscopic Approach

0LST0ZZ — Reposition Left Ankle Tendon, Open Approach

0LST4ZZ — Reposition Left Ankle Tendon, Percutaneous Endoscopic Approach

0LSV0ZZ — Reposition Right Foot Tendon, Open Approach

0LSV4ZZ — Reposition Right Foot Tendon, Percutaneous Endoscopic Approach

0LSW0ZZ — Reposition Left Foot Tendon, Open Approach

0LSW4ZZ — Reposition Left Foot Tendon, Percutaneous Endoscopic Approach

0LT – Tendons, Resection

Review Coding Guideline B3.8

0LT00ZZ — Resection of Head and Neck Tendon, Open Approach

0LT04ZZ — Resection of Head and Neck Tendon, Percutaneous Endoscopic Approach

0LT10ZZ — Resection of Right Shoulder Tendon, Open Approach

0LT14ZZ — Resection of Right Shoulder Tendon, Percutaneous Endoscopic Approach

0LT20ZZ — Resection of Left Shoulder Tendon, Open Approach

0LT24ZZ — Resection of Left Shoulder Tendon, Percutaneous Endoscopic Approach

0LT30ZZ — Resection of Right Upper Arm Tendon, Open Approach

0LT34ZZ — Resection of Right Upper Arm Tendon, Percutaneous Endoscopic Approach

0LT40ZZ — Resection of Left Upper Arm Tendon, Open Approach

0LT44ZZ — Resection of Left Upper Arm Tendon, Percutaneous Endoscopic Approach

0LT50ZZ — Resection of Right Lower Arm and Wrist Tendon, Open Approach

0LT54ZZ — Resection of Right Lower Arm and Wrist Tendon, Percutaneous Endoscopic Approach

0LT60ZZ — Resection of Left Lower Arm and Wrist Tendon, Open Approach

0LT64ZZ   Resection of Left Lower Arm and Wrist Tendon, Percutaneous Endoscopic Approach

0LT70ZZ   Resection of Right Hand Tendon, Open Approach

0LT74ZZ   Resection of Right Hand Tendon, Percutaneous Endoscopic Approach

0LT80ZZ   Resection of Left Hand Tendon, Open Approach

0LT84ZZ   Resection of Left Hand Tendon, Percutaneous Endoscopic Approach

0LT90ZZ   Resection of Right Trunk Tendon, Open Approach

0LT94ZZ   Resection of Right Trunk Tendon, Percutaneous Endoscopic Approach

0LTB0ZZ   Resection of Left Trunk Tendon, Open Approach

0LTB4ZZ   Resection of Left Trunk Tendon, Percutaneous Endoscopic Approach

0LTC0ZZ   Resection of Right Thorax Tendon, Open Approach

0LTC4ZZ   Resection of Right Thorax Tendon, Percutaneous Endoscopic Approach

0LTD0ZZ   Resection of Left Thorax Tendon, Open Approach

0LTD4ZZ   Resection of Left Thorax Tendon, Percutaneous Endoscopic Approach

0LTF0ZZ   Resection of Right Abdomen Tendon, Open Approach

0LTF4ZZ   Resection of Right Abdomen Tendon, Percutaneous Endoscopic Approach

0LTG0ZZ   Resection of Left Abdomen Tendon, Open Approach

0LTG4ZZ   Resection of Left Abdomen Tendon, Percutaneous Endoscopic Approach

0LTH0ZZ   Resection of Perineum Tendon, Open Approach

0LTH4ZZ   Resection of Perineum Tendon, Percutaneous Endoscopic Approach

0LTJ0ZZ   Resection of Right Hip Tendon, Open Approach

0LTJ4ZZ   Resection of Right Hip Tendon, Percutaneous Endoscopic Approach

0LTK0ZZ   Resection of Left Hip Tendon, Open Approach

0LTK4ZZ   Resection of Left Hip Tendon, Percutaneous Endoscopic Approach

0LTL0ZZ   Resection of Right Upper Leg Tendon, Open Approach

0LTL4ZZ   Resection of Right Upper Leg Tendon, Percutaneous Endoscopic Approach

0LTM0ZZ   Resection of Left Upper Leg Tendon, Open Approach

0LTM4ZZ   Resection of Left Upper Leg Tendon, Percutaneous Endoscopic Approach

0LTN0ZZ   Resection of Right Lower Leg Tendon, Open Approach

0LTN4ZZ   Resection of Right Lower Leg Tendon, Percutaneous Endoscopic Approach

0LTP0ZZ   Resection of Left Lower Leg Tendon, Open Approach

0LTP4ZZ   Resection of Left Lower Leg Tendon, Percutaneous Endoscopic Approach

0LTQ0ZZ   Resection of Right Knee Tendon, Open Approach

0LTQ4ZZ   Resection of Right Knee Tendon, Percutaneous Endoscopic Approach

0LTR0ZZ   Resection of Left Knee Tendon, Open Approach

0LTR4ZZ   Resection of Left Knee Tendon, Percutaneous Endoscopic Approach

0LTS0ZZ   Resection of Right Ankle Tendon, Open Approach

0LTS4ZZ   Resection of Right Ankle Tendon, Percutaneous Endoscopic Approach

0LTT0ZZ   Resection of Left Ankle Tendon, Open Approach

0LTT4ZZ   Resection of Left Ankle Tendon, Percutaneous Endoscopic Approach

0LTV0ZZ   Resection of Right Foot Tendon, Open Approach

0LTV4ZZ   Resection of Right Foot Tendon, Percutaneous Endoscopic Approach

0LTW0ZZ   Resection of Left Foot Tendon, Open Approach

0LTW4ZZ   Resection of Left Foot Tendon, Percutaneous Endoscopic Approach

0LU – Tendons, Supplement

0LU007Z   Supplement Head and Neck Tendon with Autologous Tissue Substitute, Open Approach

0LU00JZ   Supplement Head and Neck Tendon with Synthetic Substitute, Open Approach

0LU00KZ   Supplement Head and Neck Tendon with Nonautologous Tissue Substitute, Open Approach

0LU047Z   Supplement Head and Neck Tendon with Autologous Tissue Substitute, Percutaneous Endoscopic Approach

0LU04JZ   Supplement Head and Neck Tendon with Synthetic Substitute, Percutaneous Endoscopic Approach

0LU04KZ   Supplement Head and Neck Tendon with Nonautologous Tissue Substitute, Percutaneous Endoscopic Approach

0LU107Z   Supplement Right Shoulder Tendon with Autologous Tissue Substitute, Open Approach

0LU10JZ   Supplement Right Shoulder Tendon with Synthetic Substitute, Open Approach

0LU10KZ   Supplement Right Shoulder Tendon with Nonautologous Tissue Substitute, Open Approach

0LU147Z   Supplement Right Shoulder Tendon with Autologous Tissue Substitute, Percutaneous Endoscopic Approach

0LU14JZ   Supplement Right Shoulder Tendon with Synthetic Substitute, Percutaneous Endoscopic Approach

0LU14KZ   Supplement Right Shoulder Tendon with Nonautologous Tissue Substitute, Percutaneous Endoscopic Approach

0LU207Z   Supplement Left Shoulder Tendon with Autologous Tissue Substitute, Open Approach

0LU20JZ   Supplement Left Shoulder Tendon with Synthetic Substitute, Open Approach

0LU20KZ   Supplement Left Shoulder Tendon with Nonautologous Tissue Substitute, Open Approach

0LU247Z   Supplement Left Shoulder Tendon with Autologous Tissue Substitute, Percutaneous Endoscopic Approach

0LU24JZ   Supplement Left Shoulder Tendon with Synthetic Substitute, Percutaneous Endoscopic Approach

0LU24KZ   Supplement Left Shoulder Tendon with Nonautologous Tissue Substitute, Percutaneous Endoscopic Approach

0LU307Z   Supplement Right Upper Arm Tendon with Autologous Tissue Substitute, Open Approach

0LU30JZ   Supplement Right Upper Arm Tendon with Synthetic Substitute, Open Approach

0LU30KZ   Supplement Right Upper Arm Tendon with Nonautologous Tissue Substitute, Open Approach

0LU347Z   Supplement Right Upper Arm Tendon with Autologous Tissue Substitute, Percutaneous Endoscopic Approach

0LU34JZ   Supplement Right Upper Arm Tendon with Synthetic Substitute, Percutaneous Endoscopic Approach

0LU34KZ   Supplement Right Upper Arm Tendon with Nonautologous Tissue Substitute, Percutaneous Endoscopic Approach

0LU407Z   Supplement Left Upper Arm Tendon with Autologous Tissue Substitute, Open Approach

0LU40JZ   Supplement Left Upper Arm Tendon with Synthetic Substitute, Open Approach

0LU40KZ   Supplement Left Upper Arm Tendon with Nonautologous Tissue Substitute, Open Approach

0LU447Z   Supplement Left Upper Arm Tendon with Autologous Tissue Substitute, Percutaneous Endoscopic Approach

0LU44JZ   Supplement Left Upper Arm Tendon with Synthetic Substitute, Percutaneous Endoscopic Approach

0LU44KZ   Supplement Left Upper Arm Tendon with Nonautologous Tissue Substitute, Percutaneous Endoscopic Approach

0LU507Z   Supplement Right Lower Arm and Wrist Tendon with Autologous Tissue Substitute, Open Approach

0LU50JZ   Supplement Right Lower Arm and Wrist Tendon with Synthetic Substitute, Open Approach

0LU50KZ   Supplement Right Lower Arm and Wrist Tendon with Nonautologous Tissue Substitute, Open Approach

0LU547Z   Supplement Right Lower Arm and Wrist Tendon with Autologous Tissue Substitute, Percutaneous Endoscopic Approach

0LU54JZ   Supplement Right Lower Arm and Wrist Tendon with Synthetic Substitute, Percutaneous Endoscopic Approach

0LU54KZ   Supplement Right Lower Arm and Wrist Tendon with Nonautologous Tissue Substitute, Percutaneous Endoscopic Approach

0LU607Z   Supplement Left Lower Arm and Wrist Tendon with Autologous Tissue Substitute, Open Approach

0LU60JZ   Supplement Left Lower Arm and Wrist Tendon with Synthetic Substitute, Open Approach

0LU60KZ   Supplement Left Lower Arm and Wrist Tendon with Nonautologous Tissue Substitute, Open Approach

0LU647Z   Supplement Left Lower Arm and Wrist Tendon with Autologous Tissue Substitute, Percutaneous Endoscopic Approach

0LU64JZ Supplement Left Lower Arm and Wrist Tendon with Synthetic Substitute, Percutaneous Endoscopic Approach

0LU64KZ Supplement Left Lower Arm and Wrist Tendon with Nonautologous Tissue Substitute, Percutaneous Endoscopic Approach

0LU707Z Supplement Right Hand Tendon with Autologous Tissue Substitute, Open Approach

0LU70JZ Supplement Right Hand Tendon with Synthetic Substitute, Open Approach

0LU70KZ Supplement Right Hand Tendon with Nonautologous Tissue Substitute, Open Approach

0LU747Z Supplement Right Hand Tendon with Autologous Tissue Substitute, Percutaneous Endoscopic Approach

0LU74JZ Supplement Right Hand Tendon with Synthetic Substitute, Percutaneous Endoscopic Approach

0LU74KZ Supplement Right Hand Tendon with Nonautologous Tissue Substitute, Percutaneous Endoscopic Approach

0LU807Z Supplement Left Hand Tendon with Autologous Tissue Substitute, Open Approach

0LU80JZ Supplement Left Hand Tendon with Synthetic Substitute, Open Approach

0LU80KZ Supplement Left Hand Tendon with Nonautologous Tissue Substitute, Open Approach

0LU847Z Supplement Left Hand Tendon with Autologous Tissue Substitute, Percutaneous Endoscopic Approach

0LU84JZ Supplement Left Hand Tendon with Synthetic Substitute, Percutaneous Endoscopic Approach

0LU84KZ Supplement Left Hand Tendon with Nonautologous Tissue Substitute, Percutaneous Endoscopic Approach

0LU907Z Supplement Right Trunk Tendon with Autologous Tissue Substitute, Open Approach

0LU90JZ Supplement Right Trunk Tendon with Synthetic Substitute, Open Approach

0LU90KZ Supplement Right Trunk Tendon with Nonautologous Tissue Substitute, Open Approach

0LU947Z Supplement Right Trunk Tendon with Autologous Tissue Substitute, Percutaneous Endoscopic Approach

0LU94JZ Supplement Right Trunk Tendon with Synthetic Substitute, Percutaneous Endoscopic Approach

0LU94KZ Supplement Right Trunk Tendon with Nonautologous Tissue Substitute, Percutaneous Endoscopic Approach

0LUB07Z Supplement Left Trunk Tendon with Autologous Tissue Substitute, Open Approach

0LUB0JZ Supplement Left Trunk Tendon with Synthetic Substitute, Open Approach

0LUB0KZ Supplement Left Trunk Tendon with Nonautologous Tissue Substitute, Open Approach

0LUB47Z Supplement Left Trunk Tendon with Autologous Tissue Substitute, Percutaneous Endoscopic Approach

0LUB4JZ Supplement Left Trunk Tendon with Synthetic Substitute, Percutaneous Endoscopic Approach

0LUB4KZ Supplement Left Trunk Tendon with Nonautologous Tissue Substitute, Percutaneous Endoscopic Approach

0LUC07Z Supplement Right Thorax Tendon with Autologous Tissue Substitute, Open Approach

0LUC0JZ Supplement Right Thorax Tendon with Synthetic Substitute, Open Approach

0LUC0KZ Supplement Right Thorax Tendon with Nonautologous Tissue Substitute, Open Approach

0LUC47Z Supplement Right Thorax Tendon with Autologous Tissue Substitute, Percutaneous Endoscopic Approach

0LUC4JZ Supplement Right Thorax Tendon with Synthetic Substitute, Percutaneous Endoscopic Approach

0LUC4KZ Supplement Right Thorax Tendon with Nonautologous Tissue Substitute, Percutaneous Endoscopic Approach

0LUD07Z Supplement Left Thorax Tendon with Autologous Tissue Substitute, Open Approach

0LUD0JZ Supplement Left Thorax Tendon with Synthetic Substitute, Open Approach

0LUD0KZ Supplement Left Thorax Tendon with Nonautologous Tissue Substitute, Open Approach

0LUD47Z Supplement Left Thorax Tendon with Autologous Tissue Substitute, Percutaneous Endoscopic Approach

0LUD4JZ Supplement Left Thorax Tendon with Synthetic Substitute, Percutaneous Endoscopic Approach

0LUD4KZ Supplement Left Thorax Tendon with Nonautologous Tissue Substitute, Percutaneous Endoscopic Approach

0LUF07Z Supplement Right Abdomen Tendon with Autologous Tissue Substitute, Open Approach

0LUF0JZ Supplement Right Abdomen Tendon with Synthetic Substitute, Open Approach

0LUF0KZ Supplement Right Abdomen Tendon with Nonautologous Tissue Substitute, Open Approach

0LUF47Z Supplement Right Abdomen Tendon with Autologous Tissue Substitute, Percutaneous Endoscopic Approach

0LUF4JZ Supplement Right Abdomen Tendon with Synthetic Substitute, Percutaneous Endoscopic Approach

0LUF4KZ Supplement Right Abdomen Tendon with Nonautologous Tissue Substitute, Percutaneous Endoscopic Approach

0LUG07Z Supplement Left Abdomen Tendon with Autologous Tissue Substitute, Open Approach

0LUG0JZ Supplement Left Abdomen Tendon with Synthetic Substitute, Open Approach

0LUG0KZ Supplement Left Abdomen Tendon with Nonautologous Tissue Substitute, Open Approach

0LUG47Z Supplement Left Abdomen Tendon with Autologous Tissue Substitute, Percutaneous Endoscopic Approach

0LUG4JZ Supplement Left Abdomen Tendon with Synthetic Substitute, Percutaneous Endoscopic Approach

0LUG4KZ Supplement Left Abdomen Tendon with Nonautologous Tissue Substitute, Percutaneous Endoscopic Approach

0LUH07Z Supplement Perineum Tendon with Autologous Tissue Substitute, Open Approach

0LUH0JZ Supplement Perineum Tendon with Synthetic Substitute, Open Approach

0LUH0KZ Supplement Perineum Tendon with Nonautologous Tissue Substitute, Open Approach

0LUH47Z Supplement Perineum Tendon with Autologous Tissue Substitute, Percutaneous Endoscopic Approach

0LUH4JZ Supplement Perineum Tendon with Synthetic Substitute, Percutaneous Endoscopic Approach

0LUH4KZ Supplement Perineum Tendon with Nonautologous Tissue Substitute, Percutaneous Endoscopic Approach

0LUJ07Z Supplement Right Hip Tendon with Autologous Tissue Substitute, Open Approach

0LUJ0JZ Supplement Right Hip Tendon with Synthetic Substitute, Open Approach

0LUJ0KZ Supplement Right Hip Tendon with Nonautologous Tissue Substitute, Open Approach

0LUJ47Z Supplement Right Hip Tendon with Autologous Tissue Substitute, Percutaneous Endoscopic Approach

0LUJ4JZ Supplement Right Hip Tendon with Synthetic Substitute, Percutaneous Endoscopic Approach

0LUJ4KZ Supplement Right Hip Tendon with Nonautologous Tissue Substitute, Percutaneous Endoscopic Approach

0LUK07Z Supplement Left Hip Tendon with Autologous Tissue Substitute, Open Approach

0LUK0JZ Supplement Left Hip Tendon with Synthetic Substitute, Open Approach

0LUK0KZ Supplement Left Hip Tendon with Nonautologous Tissue Substitute, Open Approach

0LUK47Z Supplement Left Hip Tendon with Autologous Tissue Substitute, Percutaneous Endoscopic Approach

0LUK4JZ Supplement Left Hip Tendon with Synthetic Substitute, Percutaneous Endoscopic Approach

0LUK4KZ Supplement Left Hip Tendon with Nonautologous Tissue Substitute, Percutaneous Endoscopic Approach

0LUL07Z Supplement Right Upper Leg Tendon with Autologous Tissue Substitute, Open Approach

0LUL0JZ Supplement Right Upper Leg Tendon with Synthetic Substitute, Open Approach

0LUL0KZ Supplement Right Upper Leg Tendon with Nonautologous Tissue Substitute, Open Approach

0LUL47Z Supplement Right Upper Leg Tendon with Autologous Tissue Substitute, Percutaneous Endoscopic Approach

0LUL4JZ Supplement Right Upper Leg Tendon with Synthetic Substitute, Percutaneous Endoscopic Approach

0LUL4KZ Supplement Right Upper Leg Tendon with Nonautologous Tissue Substitute, Percutaneous Endoscopic Approach

0LUM07Z Supplement Left Upper Leg Tendon with Autologous Tissue Substitute, Open Approach

0LUM0JZ Supplement Left Upper Leg Tendon with Synthetic Substitute, Open Approach

0LUM0KZ Supplement Left Upper Leg Tendon with Nonautologous Tissue Substitute, Open Approach

0LUM47Z Supplement Left Upper Leg Tendon with Autologous Tissue Substitute, Percutaneous Endoscopic Approach

0LUM4JZ Supplement Left Upper Leg Tendon with Synthetic Substitute, Percutaneous Endoscopic Approach

0LUM4KZ Supplement Left Upper Leg Tendon with Nonautologous Tissue Substitute, Percutaneous Endoscopic Approach

0LUN07Z Supplement Right Lower Leg Tendon with Autologous Tissue Substitute, Open Approach

0LUN0JZ Supplement Right Lower Leg Tendon with Synthetic Substitute, Open Approach

0LUN0KZ Supplement Right Lower Leg Tendon with Nonautologous Tissue Substitute, Open Approach

0LUN47Z Supplement Right Lower Leg Tendon with Autologous Tissue Substitute, Percutaneous Endoscopic Approach

0LUN4JZ Supplement Right Lower Leg Tendon with Synthetic Substitute, Percutaneous Endoscopic Approach

0LUN4KZ Supplement Right Lower Leg Tendon with Nonautologous Tissue Substitute, Percutaneous Endoscopic Approach

0LUP07Z Supplement Left Lower Leg Tendon with Autologous Tissue Substitute, Open Approach

0LUP0JZ Supplement Left Lower Leg Tendon with Synthetic Substitute, Open Approach

0LUP0KZ Supplement Left Lower Leg Tendon with Nonautologous Tissue Substitute, Open Approach

0LUP47Z Supplement Left Lower Leg Tendon with Autologous Tissue Substitute, Percutaneous Endoscopic Approach

0LUP4JZ Supplement Left Lower Leg Tendon with Synthetic Substitute, Percutaneous Endoscopic Approach

0LUP4KZ Supplement Left Lower Leg Tendon with Nonautologous Tissue Substitute, Percutaneous Endoscopic Approach

0LUQ07Z Supplement Right Knee Tendon with Autologous Tissue Substitute, Open Approach

0LUQ0JZ Supplement Right Knee Tendon with Synthetic Substitute, Open Approach

0LUQ0KZ Supplement Right Knee Tendon with Nonautologous Tissue Substitute, Open Approach

0LUQ47Z Supplement Right Knee Tendon with Autologous Tissue Substitute, Percutaneous Endoscopic Approach

0LUQ4JZ Supplement Right Knee Tendon with Synthetic Substitute, Percutaneous Endoscopic Approach

0LUQ4KZ Supplement Right Knee Tendon with Nonautologous Tissue Substitute, Percutaneous Endoscopic Approach

0LUR07Z Supplement Left Knee Tendon with Autologous Tissue Substitute, Open Approach

0LUR0JZ Supplement Left Knee Tendon with Synthetic Substitute, Open Approach

0LUR0KZ Supplement Left Knee Tendon with Nonautologous Tissue Substitute, Open Approach

0LUR47Z Supplement Left Knee Tendon with Autologous Tissue Substitute, Percutaneous Endoscopic Approach

0LUR4JZ Supplement Left Knee Tendon with Synthetic Substitute, Percutaneous Endoscopic Approach

0LUR4KZ Supplement Left Knee Tendon with Nonautologous Tissue Substitute, Percutaneous Endoscopic Approach

0LUS07Z Supplement Right Ankle Tendon with Autologous Tissue Substitute, Open Approach

0LUS0JZ Supplement Right Ankle Tendon with Synthetic Substitute, Open Approach

0LUS0KZ Supplement Right Ankle Tendon with Nonautologous Tissue Substitute, Open Approach

0LUS47Z Supplement Right Ankle Tendon with Autologous Tissue Substitute, Percutaneous Endoscopic Approach

0LUS4JZ Supplement Right Ankle Tendon with Synthetic Substitute, Percutaneous Endoscopic Approach

0LUS4KZ Supplement Right Ankle Tendon with Nonautologous Tissue Substitute, Percutaneous Endoscopic Approach

0LUT07Z Supplement Left Ankle Tendon with Autologous Tissue Substitute, Open Approach

0LUT0JZ Supplement Left Ankle Tendon with Synthetic Substitute, Open Approach

0LUT0KZ Supplement Left Ankle Tendon with Nonautologous Tissue Substitute, Open Approach

0LUT47Z Supplement Left Ankle Tendon with Autologous Tissue Substitute, Percutaneous Endoscopic Approach

0LUT4JZ Supplement Left Ankle Tendon with Synthetic Substitute, Percutaneous Endoscopic Approach

0LUT4KZ Supplement Left Ankle Tendon with Nonautologous Tissue Substitute, Percutaneous Endoscopic Approach

0LUV07Z Supplement Right Foot Tendon with Autologous Tissue Substitute, Open Approach

0LUV0JZ Supplement Right Foot Tendon with Synthetic Substitute, Open Approach

0LUV0KZ Supplement Right Foot Tendon with Nonautologous Tissue Substitute, Open Approach

0LUV47Z Supplement Right Foot Tendon with Autologous Tissue Substitute, Percutaneous Endoscopic Approach

0LUV4JZ Supplement Right Foot Tendon with Synthetic Substitute, Percutaneous Endoscopic Approach

0LUV4KZ Supplement Right Foot Tendon with Nonautologous Tissue Substitute, Percutaneous Endoscopic Approach

0LUW07Z Supplement Left Foot Tendon with Autologous Tissue Substitute, Open Approach

0LUW0JZ Supplement Left Foot Tendon with Synthetic Substitute, Open Approach

0LUW0KZ Supplement Left Foot Tendon with Nonautologous Tissue Substitute, Open Approach

0LUW47Z Supplement Left Foot Tendon with Autologous Tissue Substitute, Percutaneous Endoscopic Approach

0LUW4JZ Supplement Left Foot Tendon with Synthetic Substitute, Percutaneous Endoscopic Approach

0LUW4KZ Supplement Left Foot Tendon with Nonautologous Tissue Substitute, Percutaneous Endoscopic Approach

0LW – Tendons, Revision

Review Coding Guideline B6.1c

0LWX00Z Revision of Drainage Device in Upper Tendon, Open Approach

0LWX07Z Revision of Autologous Tissue Substitute in Upper Tendon, Open Approach

0LWX0JZ Revision of Synthetic Substitute in Upper Tendon, Open Approach

0LWX0KZ Revision of Nonautologous Tissue Substitute in Upper Tendon, Open Approach

0LWX30Z Revision of Drainage Device in Upper Tendon, Percutaneous Approach

0LWX37Z Revision of Autologous Tissue Substitute in Upper Tendon, Percutaneous Approach

0LWX3JZ Revision of Synthetic Substitute in Upper Tendon, Percutaneous Approach

0LWX3KZ Revision of Nonautologous Tissue Substitute in Upper Tendon, Percutaneous Approach

0LWX40Z Revision of Drainage Device in Upper Tendon, Percutaneous Endoscopic Approach

0LWX47Z Revision of Autologous Tissue Substitute in Upper Tendon, Percutaneous Endoscopic Approach

0LWX4JZ Revision of Synthetic Substitute in Upper Tendon, Percutaneous Endoscopic Approach

0LWX4KZ Revision of Nonautologous Tissue Substitute in Upper Tendon, Percutaneous Endoscopic Approach

0LWXX0Z Revision of Drainage Device in Upper Tendon, External Approach

0LWXX7Z Revision of Autologous Tissue Substitute in Upper Tendon, External Approach

0LWXXJZ Revision of Synthetic Substitute in Upper Tendon, External Approach

---

♀ Female-only   ♂ Male-only   ● Limited Coverage   ● Non-OR   ▦ HAC-associated procedure   ● Non-covered procedures   ✚ Combination

0LWXXKZ Revision of Nonautologous Tissue Substitute in Upper Tendon, External Approach
0LWY00Z Revision of Drainage Device in Lower Tendon, Open Approach
0LWY07Z Revision of Autologous Tissue Substitute in Lower Tendon, Open Approach
0LWY0JZ Revision of Synthetic Substitute in Lower Tendon, Open Approach
0LWY0KZ Revision of Nonautologous Tissue Substitute in Lower Tendon, Open Approach
0LWY30Z Revision of Drainage Device in Lower Tendon, Percutaneous Approach
0LWY37Z Revision of Autologous Tissue Substitute in Lower Tendon, Percutaneous Approach
0LWY3JZ Revision of Synthetic Substitute in Lower Tendon, Percutaneous Approach
0LWY3KZ Revision of Nonautologous Tissue Substitute in Lower Tendon, Percutaneous Approach

0LWY40Z Revision of Drainage Device in Lower Tendon, Percutaneous Endoscopic Approach
0LWY47Z Revision of Autologous Tissue Substitute in Lower Tendon, Percutaneous Endoscopic Approach
0LWY4JZ Revision of Synthetic Substitute in Lower Tendon, Percutaneous Endoscopic Approach
0LWY4KZ Revision of Nonautologous Tissue Substitute in Lower Tendon, Percutaneous Endoscopic Approach
0LWYX0Z Revision of Drainage Device in Lower Tendon, External Approach
0LWYX7Z Revision of Autologous Tissue Substitute in Lower Tendon, External Approach
0LWYXJZ Revision of Synthetic Substitute in Lower Tendon, External Approach
0LWYXKZ Revision of Nonautologous Tissue Substitute in Lower Tendon, External Approach

0LX – Tendons, Transfer

0LX00ZZ Transfer Head and Neck Tendon, Open Approach
0LX04ZZ Transfer Head and Neck Tendon, Percutaneous Endoscopic Approach
0LX10ZZ Transfer Right Shoulder Tendon, Open Approach
0LX14ZZ Transfer Right Shoulder Tendon, Percutaneous Endoscopic Approach
0LX20ZZ Transfer Left Shoulder Tendon, Open Approach
0LX24ZZ Transfer Left Shoulder Tendon, Percutaneous Endoscopic Approach
0LX30ZZ Transfer Right Upper Arm Tendon, Open Approach
0LX34ZZ Transfer Right Upper Arm Tendon, Percutaneous Endoscopic Approach
0LX40ZZ Transfer Left Upper Arm Tendon, Open Approach
0LX44ZZ Transfer Left Upper Arm Tendon, Percutaneous Endoscopic Approach
0LX50ZZ Transfer Right Lower Arm and Wrist Tendon, Open Approach
0LX54ZZ Transfer Right Lower Arm and Wrist Tendon, Percutaneous Endoscopic Approach
0LX60ZZ Transfer Left Lower Arm and Wrist Tendon, Open Approach
0LX64ZZ Transfer Left Lower Arm and Wrist Tendon, Percutaneous Endoscopic Approach
0LX70ZZ Transfer Right Hand Tendon, Open Approach
0LX74ZZ Transfer Right Hand Tendon, Percutaneous Endoscopic Approach
0LX80ZZ Transfer Left Hand Tendon, Open Approach
0LX84ZZ Transfer Left Hand Tendon, Percutaneous Endoscopic Approach
0LX90ZZ Transfer Right Trunk Tendon, Open Approach
0LX94ZZ Transfer Right Trunk Tendon, Percutaneous Endoscopic Approach
0LXB0ZZ Transfer Left Trunk Tendon, Open Approach
0LXB4ZZ Transfer Left Trunk Tendon, Percutaneous Endoscopic Approach
0LXC0ZZ Transfer Right Thorax Tendon, Open Approach
0LXC4ZZ Transfer Right Thorax Tendon, Percutaneous Endoscopic Approach
0LXD0ZZ Transfer Left Thorax Tendon, Open Approach
0LXD4ZZ Transfer Left Thorax Tendon, Percutaneous Endoscopic Approach
0LXF0ZZ Transfer Right Abdomen Tendon, Open Approach

0LXF4ZZ Transfer Right Abdomen Tendon, Percutaneous Endoscopic Approach
0LXG0ZZ Transfer Left Abdomen Tendon, Open Approach
0LXG4ZZ Transfer Left Abdomen Tendon, Percutaneous Endoscopic Approach
0LXH0ZZ Transfer Perineum Tendon, Open Approach
0LXH4ZZ Transfer Perineum Tendon, Percutaneous Endoscopic Approach
0LXJ0ZZ Transfer Right Hip Tendon, Open Approach
0LXJ4ZZ Transfer Right Hip Tendon, Percutaneous Endoscopic Approach
0LXK0ZZ Transfer Left Hip Tendon, Open Approach
0LXK4ZZ Transfer Left Hip Tendon, Percutaneous Endoscopic Approach
0LXL0ZZ Transfer Right Upper Leg Tendon, Open Approach
0LXL4ZZ Transfer Right Upper Leg Tendon, Percutaneous Endoscopic Approach
0LXM0ZZ Transfer Left Upper Leg Tendon, Open Approach
0LXM4ZZ Transfer Left Upper Leg Tendon, Percutaneous Endoscopic Approach
0LXN0ZZ Transfer Right Lower Leg Tendon, Open Approach
0LXN4ZZ Transfer Right Lower Leg Tendon, Percutaneous Endoscopic Approach
0LXP0ZZ Transfer Left Lower Leg Tendon, Open Approach
0LXP4ZZ Transfer Left Lower Leg Tendon, Percutaneous Endoscopic Approach
0LXQ0ZZ Transfer Right Knee Tendon, Open Approach
0LXQ4ZZ Transfer Right Knee Tendon, Percutaneous Endoscopic Approach
0LXR0ZZ Transfer Left Knee Tendon, Open Approach
0LXR4ZZ Transfer Left Knee Tendon, Percutaneous Endoscopic Approach
0LXS0ZZ Transfer Right Ankle Tendon, Open Approach
0LXS4ZZ Transfer Right Ankle Tendon, Percutaneous Endoscopic Approach
0LXT0ZZ Transfer Left Ankle Tendon, Open Approach
0LXT4ZZ Transfer Left Ankle Tendon, Percutaneous Endoscopic Approach
0LXV0ZZ Transfer Right Foot Tendon, Open Approach
0LXV4ZZ Transfer Right Foot Tendon, Percutaneous Endoscopic Approach
0LXW0ZZ Transfer Left Foot Tendon, Open Approach
0LXW4ZZ Transfer Left Foot Tendon, Percutaneous Endoscopic Approach

Bursae and Ligaments

Bursa of the Knee

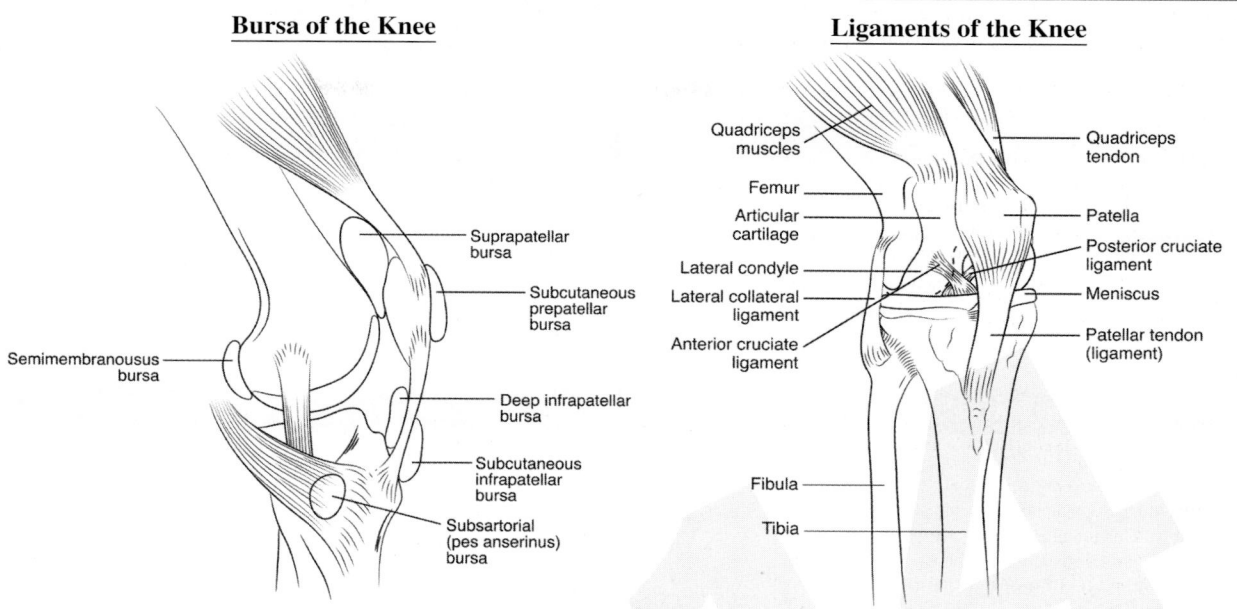

Suprapatellar bursa

Subcutaneous prepatellar bursa

Semimembranousus bursa

Deep infrapatellar bursa

Subcutaneous infrapatellar bursa

Subsartorial (pes anserinus) bursa

Ligaments of the Knee

Quadriceps muscles

Femur

Articular cartilage

Lateral condyle

Lateral collateral ligament

Anterior cruciate ligament

Fibula

Tibia

Quadriceps tendon

Patella

Posterior cruciate ligament

Meniscus

Patellar tendon (ligament)

Shoulder Tendons and Ligaments

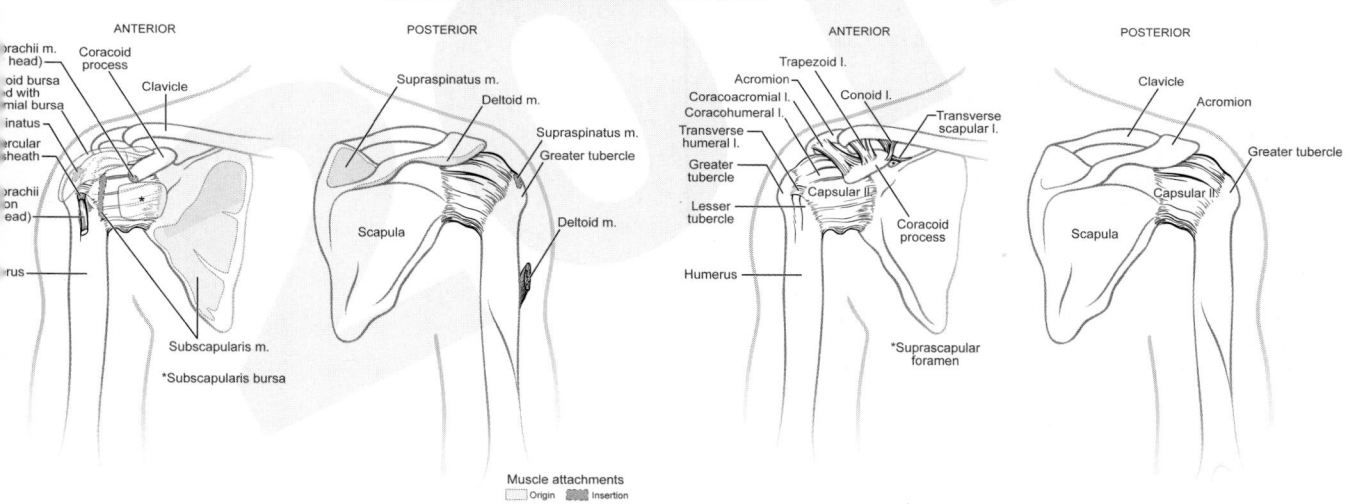

ANTERIOR

rachii m. head)

Coracoid process

oid bursa d with mial bursa

Clavicle

inatus

ercular heath

rachii on ead)

Subscapularis m.

*Subscapularis bursa

POSTERIOR

Supraspinatus m.

Deltoid m.

Supraspinatus m.

Greater tubercle

Scapula

Deltoid m.

ANTERIOR

Trapezoid I.

Acromion

Coracoacromial I.

Coracohumeral I.

Transverse humeral I.

Greater tubercle

Lesser tubercle

Humerus

Conoid I.

Transverse scapular I.

Capsular I.

Coracoid process

*Suprascapular foramen

POSTERIOR

Clavicle

Acromion

Greater tubercle

Scapula

Capsular I.

Muscle attachments
☐ Origin ▨ Insertion

Knee Tendons and Ligaments

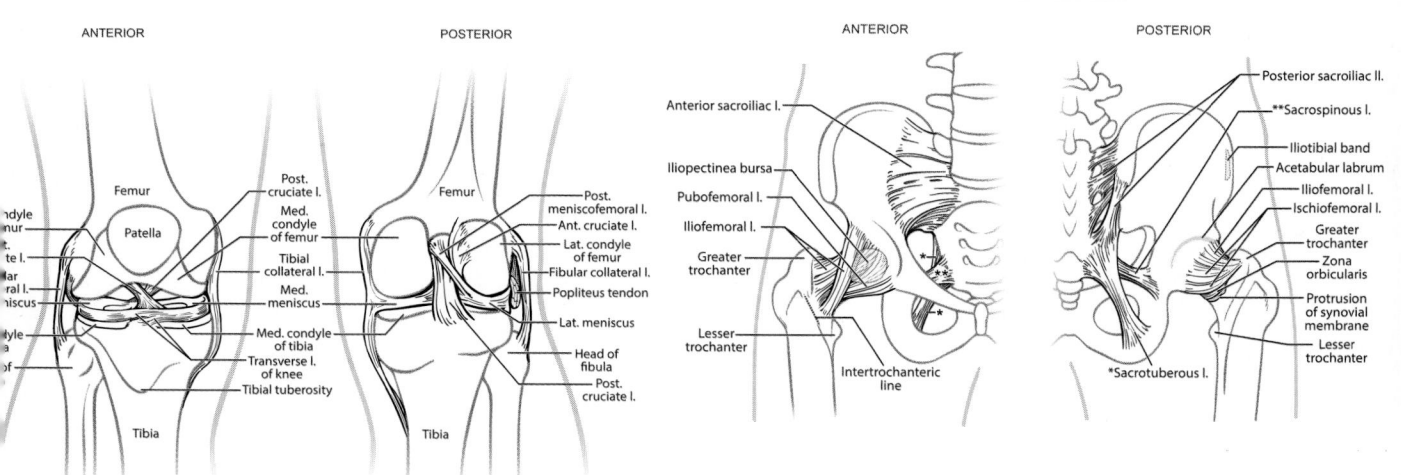

ANTERIOR

Femur

Patella

ndyle ur t. te I.

lar ral I. iscus

dyle a f

Tibia

Post. cruciate I.

Med. condyle of femur

Tibial collateral I.

Med. meniscus

Med. condyle of tibia

Transverse I. of knee

Tibial tuberosity

POSTERIOR

Femur

Tibia

Post. meniscofemoral I.

Ant. cruciate I.

Lat. condyle of femur

Fibular collateral I.

Popliteus tendon

Lat. meniscus

Head of fibula

Post. cruciate I.

Hip Tendons and Ligaments

ANTERIOR

Anterior sacroiliac I.

Iliopectinea bursa

Pubofemoral I.

Iliofemoral I.

Greater trochanter

Lesser trochanter

Intertrochanteric line

POSTERIOR

Posterior sacroiliac II.

**Sacrospinous I.

Iliotibial band

Acetabular labrum

Iliofemoral I.

Ischiofemoral I.

Greater trochanter

Zona orbicularis

Protrusion of synovial membrane

Lesser trochanter

*Sacrotuberous I.

Bursae and Ligaments Tables 0M2–0MX

Section	0	Medical and Surgical
Body System	M	Bursae and Ligaments
Operation	2	**Change:** Taking out or off a device from a body part and putting back an identical or similar device in or on the same body part without cutting or puncturing the skin or a mucous membrane

Body Part (4th)	Approach (5th)	Device (6th)	Qualifier (7th)
X Upper Bursa and Ligament **Y** Lower Bursa and Ligament	**X** External	**0** Drainage Device **Y** Other Device	**Z** No Qualifier

Section	0	Medical and Surgical
Body System	M	Bursae and Ligaments
Operation	5	**Destruction:** Physical eradication of all or a portion of a body part by the direct use of energy, force, or a destructive agent

Body Part (4th)	Approach (5th)	Device (6th)	Qualifier (7th)
0 Head and Neck Bursa and Ligament **1** Shoulder Bursa and Ligament, Right **2** Shoulder Bursa and Ligament, Left **3** Elbow Bursa and Ligament, Right **4** Elbow Bursa and Ligament, Left **5** Wrist Bursa and Ligament, Right **6** Wrist Bursa and Ligament, Left **7** Hand Bursa and Ligament, Right **8** Hand Bursa and Ligament, Left **9** Upper Extremity Bursa and Ligament, Right **B** Upper Extremity Bursa and Ligament, Left **C** Trunk Bursa and Ligament, Right **D** Trunk Bursa and Ligament, Left **F** Thorax Bursa and Ligament, Right **G** Thorax Bursa and Ligament, Left **H** Abdomen Bursa and Ligament, Right **J** Abdomen Bursa and Ligament, Left **K** Perineum Bursa and Ligament **L** Hip Bursa and Ligament, Right **M** Hip Bursa and Ligament, Left **N** Knee Bursa and Ligament, Right **P** Knee Bursa and Ligament, Left **Q** Ankle Bursa and Ligament, Right **R** Ankle Bursa and Ligament, Left **S** Foot Bursa and Ligament, Right **T** Foot Bursa and Ligament, Left **V** Lower Extremity Bursa and Ligament, Right **W** Lower Extremity Bursa and Ligament, Left	**0** Open **3** Percutaneous **4** Percutaneous Endoscopic	**Z** No Device	**Z** No Qualifier

Section	0	Medical and Surgical
Body System	M	Bursae and Ligaments
Operation	8	**Division:** Cutting into a body part, without draining fluids and/or gases from the body part, in order to separate or transect a body part

Body Part (4th)	Approach (5th)	Device (6th)	Qualifier (7th)
0 Head and Neck Bursa and Ligament 1 Shoulder Bursa and Ligament, Right 2 Shoulder Bursa and Ligament, Left 3 Elbow Bursa and Ligament, Right 4 Elbow Bursa and Ligament, Left 5 Wrist Bursa and Ligament, Right 6 Wrist Bursa and Ligament, Left 7 Hand Bursa and Ligament, Right 8 Hand Bursa and Ligament, Left 9 Upper Extremity Bursa and Ligament, Right B Upper Extremity Bursa and Ligament, Left C Trunk Bursa and Ligament, Right D Trunk Bursa and Ligament, Left F Thorax Bursa and Ligament, Right G Thorax Bursa and Ligament, Left H Abdomen Bursa and Ligament, Right J Abdomen Bursa and Ligament, Left K Perineum Bursa and Ligament L Hip Bursa and Ligament, Right M Hip Bursa and Ligament, Left N Knee Bursa and Ligament, Right P Knee Bursa and Ligament, Left Q Ankle Bursa and Ligament, Right R Ankle Bursa and Ligament, Left S Foot Bursa and Ligament, Right T Foot Bursa and Ligament, Left V Lower Extremity Bursa and Ligament, Right W Lower Extremity Bursa and Ligament, Left	0 Open 3 Percutaneous 4 Percutaneous Endoscopic	Z No Device	Z No Qualifier

Section	0	Medical and Surgical
Body System	M	Bursae and Ligaments
Operation	9	**Drainage:** Taking or letting out fluids and/or gases from a body part

Body Part (4th)	Approach (5th)	Device (6th)	Qualifier (7th)
0 Head and Neck Bursa and Ligament 1 Shoulder Bursa and Ligament, Right 2 Shoulder Bursa and Ligament, Left 3 Elbow Bursa and Ligament, Right 4 Elbow Bursa and Ligament, Left 5 Wrist Bursa and Ligament, Right 6 Wrist Bursa and Ligament, Left 7 Hand Bursa and Ligament, Right 8 Hand Bursa and Ligament, Left 9 Upper Extremity Bursa and Ligament, Right B Upper Extremity Bursa and Ligament, Left C Trunk Bursa and Ligament, Right D Trunk Bursa and Ligament, Left F Thorax Bursa and Ligament, Right G Thorax Bursa and Ligament, Left H Abdomen Bursa and Ligament, Right J Abdomen Bursa and Ligament, Left K Perineum Bursa and Ligament L Hip Bursa and Ligament, Right M Hip Bursa and Ligament, Left N Knee Bursa and Ligament, Right P Knee Bursa and Ligament, Left Q Ankle Bursa and Ligament, Right R Ankle Bursa and Ligament, Left S Foot Bursa and Ligament, Right T Foot Bursa and Ligament, Left V Lower Extremity Bursa and Ligament, Right W Lower Extremity Bursa and Ligament, Left	0 Open 3 Percutaneous 4 Percutaneous Endoscopic	0 Drainage Device	Z No Qualifier
0 Head and Neck Bursa and Ligament 1 Shoulder Bursa and Ligament, Right 2 Shoulder Bursa and Ligament, Left 3 Elbow Bursa and Ligament, Right 4 Elbow Bursa and Ligament, Left 5 Wrist Bursa and Ligament, Right 6 Wrist Bursa and Ligament, Left 7 Hand Bursa and Ligament, Right 8 Hand Bursa and Ligament, Left 9 Upper Extremity Bursa and Ligament, Right B Upper Extremity Bursa and Ligament, Left C Trunk Bursa and Ligament, Right D Trunk Bursa and Ligament, Left F Thorax Bursa and Ligament, Right G Thorax Bursa and Ligament, Left H Abdomen Bursa and Ligament, Right J Abdomen Bursa and Ligament, Left K Perineum Bursa and Ligament L Hip Bursa and Ligament, Right M Hip Bursa and Ligament, Left N Knee Bursa and Ligament, Right P Knee Bursa and Ligament, Left Q Ankle Bursa and Ligament, Right R Ankle Bursa and Ligament, Left S Foot Bursa and Ligament, Right T Foot Bursa and Ligament, Left V Lower Extremity Bursa and Ligament, Right W Lower Extremity Bursa and Ligament, Left	0 Open 3 Percutaneous 4 Percutaneous Endoscopic	Z No Device	X Diagnostic Z No Qualifier

Section	0	Medical and Surgical
Body System	M	Bursae and Ligaments
Operation	B	Excision: Cutting out or off, without replacement, a portion of a body part

Body Part (4th)	Approach (5th)	Device (6th)	Qualifier (7th)
0 Head and Neck Bursa and Ligament 1 Shoulder Bursa and Ligament, Right 2 Shoulder Bursa and Ligament, Left 3 Elbow Bursa and Ligament, Right 4 Elbow Bursa and Ligament, Left 5 Wrist Bursa and Ligament, Right 6 Wrist Bursa and Ligament, Left 7 Hand Bursa and Ligament, Right 8 Hand Bursa and Ligament, Left 9 Upper Extremity Bursa and Ligament, Right B Upper Extremity Bursa and Ligament, Left C Trunk Bursa and Ligament, Right D Trunk Bursa and Ligament, Left F Thorax Bursa and Ligament, Right G Thorax Bursa and Ligament, Left H Abdomen Bursa and Ligament, Right J Abdomen Bursa and Ligament, Left K Perineum Bursa and Ligament L Hip Bursa and Ligament, Right M Hip Bursa and Ligament, Left N Knee Bursa and Ligament, Right P Knee Bursa and Ligament, Left Q Ankle Bursa and Ligament, Right R Ankle Bursa and Ligament, Left S Foot Bursa and Ligament, Right T Foot Bursa and Ligament, Left V Lower Extremity Bursa and Ligament, Right W Lower Extremity Bursa and Ligament, Left	0 Open 3 Percutaneous 4 Percutaneous Endoscopic	Z No Device	X Diagnostic Z No Qualifier

Section	0	Medical and Surgical
Body System	M	Bursae and Ligaments
Operation	C	Extirpation: Taking or cutting out solid matter from a body part

Body Part (4th)	Approach (5th)	Device (6th)	Qualifier (7th)
0 Head and Neck Bursa and Ligament 1 Shoulder Bursa and Ligament, Right 2 Shoulder Bursa and Ligament, Left 3 Elbow Bursa and Ligament, Right 4 Elbow Bursa and Ligament, Left 5 Wrist Bursa and Ligament, Right 6 Wrist Bursa and Ligament, Left 7 Hand Bursa and Ligament, Right 8 Hand Bursa and Ligament, Left 9 Upper Extremity Bursa and Ligament, Right B Upper Extremity Bursa and Ligament, Left C Trunk Bursa and Ligament, Right D Trunk Bursa and Ligament, Left F Thorax Bursa and Ligament, Right G Thorax Bursa and Ligament, Left H Abdomen Bursa and Ligament, Right J Abdomen Bursa and Ligament, Left K Perineum Bursa and Ligament L Hip Bursa and Ligament, Right M Hip Bursa and Ligament, Left N Knee Bursa and Ligament, Right P Knee Bursa and Ligament, Left Q Ankle Bursa and Ligament, Right R Ankle Bursa and Ligament, Left S Foot Bursa and Ligament, Right T Foot Bursa and Ligament, Left V Lower Extremity Bursa and Ligament, Right W Lower Extremity Bursa and Ligament, Left	0 Open 3 Percutaneous 4 Percutaneous Endoscopic	Z No Device	Z No Qualifier

Section	0	Medical and Surgical
Body System	M	Bursae and Ligaments
Operation	D	Extraction: Pulling or stripping out or off all or a portion of a body part by the use of force

Body Part (4th)	Approach (5th)	Device (6th)	Qualifier (7th)
0 Head and Neck Bursa and Ligament 1 Shoulder Bursa and Ligament, Right 2 Shoulder Bursa and Ligament, Left 3 Elbow Bursa and Ligament, Right 4 Elbow Bursa and Ligament, Left 5 Wrist Bursa and Ligament, Right 6 Wrist Bursa and Ligament, Left 7 Hand Bursa and Ligament, Right 8 Hand Bursa and Ligament, Left 9 Upper Extremity Bursa and Ligament, Right B Upper Extremity Bursa and Ligament, Left C Trunk Bursa and Ligament, Right D Trunk Bursa and Ligament, Left F Thorax Bursa and Ligament, Right G Thorax Bursa and Ligament, Left H Abdomen Bursa and Ligament, Right J Abdomen Bursa and Ligament, Left K Perineum Bursa and Ligament L Hip Bursa and Ligament, Right M Hip Bursa and Ligament, Left N Knee Bursa and Ligament, Right P Knee Bursa and Ligament, Left Q Ankle Bursa and Ligament, Right R Ankle Bursa and Ligament, Left S Foot Bursa and Ligament, Right T Foot Bursa and Ligament, Left V Lower Extremity Bursa and Ligament, Right W Lower Extremity Bursa and Ligament, Left	0 Open 3 Percutaneous 4 Percutaneous Endoscopic	Z No Device	Z No Qualifier

Section	0	Medical and Surgical
Body System	M	Bursae and Ligaments
Operation	J	Inspection: Visually and/or manually exploring a body part

Body Part (4th)	Approach (5th)	Device (6th)	Qualifier (7th)
X Upper Bursa and Ligament Y Lower Bursa and Ligament	0 Open 3 Percutaneous 4 Percutaneous Endoscopic X External	Z No Device	Z No Qualifier

Section	0	**Medical and Surgical**
Body System	M	**Bursae and Ligaments**
Operation	M	**Reattachment:** Putting back in or on all or a portion of a separated body part to its normal location or other suitable location

Body Part (4th)	Approach (5th)	Device (6th)	Qualifier (7th)
0 Head and Neck Bursa and Ligament	0 Open	Z No Device	Z No Qualifier
1 Shoulder Bursa and Ligament, Right	4 Percutaneous Endoscopic		
2 Shoulder Bursa and Ligament, Left			
3 Elbow Bursa and Ligament, Right			
4 Elbow Bursa and Ligament, Left			
5 Wrist Bursa and Ligament, Right			
6 Wrist Bursa and Ligament, Left			
7 Hand Bursa and Ligament, Right			
8 Hand Bursa and Ligament, Left			
9 Upper Extremity Bursa and Ligament, Right			
B Upper Extremity Bursa and Ligament, Left			
C Trunk Bursa and Ligament, Right			
D Trunk Bursa and Ligament, Left			
F Thorax Bursa and Ligament, Right			
G Thorax Bursa and Ligament, Left			
H Abdomen Bursa and Ligament, Right			
J Abdomen Bursa and Ligament, Left			
K Perineum Bursa and Ligament			
L Hip Bursa and Ligament, Right			
M Hip Bursa and Ligament, Left			
N Knee Bursa and Ligament, Right			
P Knee Bursa and Ligament, Left			
Q Ankle Bursa and Ligament, Right			
R Ankle Bursa and Ligament, Left			
S Foot Bursa and Ligament, Right			
T Foot Bursa and Ligament, Left			
V Lower Extremity Bursa and Ligament, Right			
W Lower Extremity Bursa and Ligament, Left			

Section **0** Medical and Surgical
Body System **M** Bursae and Ligaments
Operation **N** Release: Freeing a body part from an abnormal physical constraint by cutting or by the use of force

Body Part (4th)	Approach (5th)	Device (6th)	Qualifier (7th)
0 Head and Neck Bursa and Ligament	0 Open	Z No Device	Z No Qualifier
1 Shoulder Bursa and Ligament, Right	3 Percutaneous		
2 Shoulder Bursa and Ligament, Left	4 Percutaneous		
3 Elbow Bursa and Ligament, Right	Endoscopic		
4 Elbow Bursa and Ligament, Left	X External		
5 Wrist Bursa and Ligament, Right			
6 Wrist Bursa and Ligament, Left			
7 Hand Bursa and Ligament, Right			
8 Hand Bursa and Ligament, Left			
9 Upper Extremity Bursa and Ligament, Right			
B Upper Extremity Bursa and Ligament, Left			
C Trunk Bursa and Ligament, Right			
D Trunk Bursa and Ligament, Left			
F Thorax Bursa and Ligament, Right			
G Thorax Bursa and Ligament, Left			
H Abdomen Bursa and Ligament, Right			
J Abdomen Bursa and Ligament, Left			
K Perineum Bursa and Ligament			
L Hip Bursa and Ligament, Right			
M Hip Bursa and Ligament, Left			
N Knee Bursa and Ligament, Right			
P Knee Bursa and Ligament, Left			
Q Ankle Bursa and Ligament, Right			
R Ankle Bursa and Ligament, Left			
S Foot Bursa and Ligament, Right			
T Foot Bursa and Ligament, Left			
V Lower Extremity Bursa and Ligament, Right			
W Lower Extremity Bursa and Ligament, Left			

Section **0** Medical and Surgical
Body System **M** Bursae and Ligaments
Operation **P** Removal: Taking out or off a device from a body part

Body Part (4th)	Approach (5th)	Device (6th)	Qualifier (7th)

X Upper Bursa and Ligament
Y Lower Bursa and Ligament
	0 Open
	3 Percutaneous
	4 Percutaneous
	  Endoscopic
		0 Drainage Device
		7 Autologous Tissue
		  Substitute
		J Synthetic Substitute
		K Nonautologous Tissue
		  Substitute
			Z No Qualifier

X Upper Bursa and Ligament Y Lower Bursa and Ligament	X External	0 Drainage Device	Z No Qualifier

Section	0	Medical and Surgical
Body System	M	Bursae and Ligaments
Operation	Q	**Repair:** Restoring, to the extent possible, a body part to its normal anatomic structure and function

Body Part (4th)	Approach (5th)	Device (6th)	Qualifier (7th)
0 Head and Neck Bursa and Ligament	0 Open	Z No Device	Z No Qualifier
1 Shoulder Bursa and Ligament, Right	3 Percutaneous		
2 Shoulder Bursa and Ligament, Left	4 Percutaneous Endoscopic		
3 Elbow Bursa and Ligament, Right			
4 Elbow Bursa and Ligament, Left			
5 Wrist Bursa and Ligament, Right			
6 Wrist Bursa and Ligament, Left			
7 Hand Bursa and Ligament, Right			
8 Hand Bursa and Ligament, Left			
9 Upper Extremity Bursa and Ligament, Right			
B Upper Extremity Bursa and Ligament, Left			
C Trunk Bursa and Ligament, Right			
D Trunk Bursa and Ligament, Left			
F Thorax Bursa and Ligament, Right			
G Thorax Bursa and Ligament, Left			
H Abdomen Bursa and Ligament, Right			
J Abdomen Bursa and Ligament, Left			
K Perineum Bursa and Ligament			
L Hip Bursa and Ligament, Right			
M Hip Bursa and Ligament, Left			
N Knee Bursa and Ligaxment, Right			
P Knee Bursa and Ligament, Left			
Q Ankle Bursa and Ligament, Right			
R Ankle Bursa and Ligament, Left			
S Foot Bursa and Ligament, Right			
T Foot Bursa and Ligament, Left			
V Lower Extremity Bursa and Ligament, Right			
W Lower Extremity Bursa and Ligament, Left			

Medical and Surgical Section (0)

0MQ

Section	0	Medical and Surgical
Body System	M	Bursae and Ligaments
Operation	S	**Reposition:** Moving to its normal location, or other suitable location, all or a portion of a body part

Body Part (4th)	Approach (5th)	Device (6th)	Qualifier (7th)
0 Head and Neck Bursa and Ligament 1 Shoulder Bursa and Ligament, Right 2 Shoulder Bursa and Ligament, Left 3 Elbow Bursa and Ligament, Right 4 Elbow Bursa and Ligament, Left 5 Wrist Bursa and Ligament, Right 6 Wrist Bursa and Ligament, Left 7 Hand Bursa and Ligament, Right 8 Hand Bursa and Ligament, Left 9 Upper Extremity Bursa and Ligament, Right B Upper Extremity Bursa and Ligament, Left C Trunk Bursa and Ligament, Right D Trunk Bursa and Ligament, Left F Thorax Bursa and Ligament, Right G Thorax Bursa and Ligament, Left H Abdomen Bursa and Ligament, Right J Abdomen Bursa and Ligament, Left K Perineum Bursa and Ligament L Hip Bursa and Ligament, Right M Hip Bursa and Ligament, Left N Knee Bursa and Ligament, Right P Knee Bursa and Ligament, Left Q Ankle Bursa and Ligament, Right R Ankle Bursa and Ligament, Left S Foot Bursa and Ligament, Right T Foot Bursa and Ligament, Left V Lower Extremity Bursa and Ligament, Right W Lower Extremity Bursa and Ligament, Left	0 Open 4 Percutaneous Endoscopic	Z No Device	Z No Qualifier

Section	0	Medical and Surgical
Body System	M	Bursae and Ligaments
Operation	T	**Resection:** Cutting out or off, without replacement, all of a body part

Body Part (4th)	Approach (5th)	Device (6th)	Qualifier (7th)
0 Head and Neck Bursa and Ligament 1 Shoulder Bursa and Ligament, Right 2 Shoulder Bursa and Ligament, Left 3 Elbow Bursa and Ligament, Right 4 Elbow Bursa and Ligament, Left 5 Wrist Bursa and Ligament, Right 6 Wrist Bursa and Ligament, Left 7 Hand Bursa and Ligament, Right 8 Hand Bursa and Ligament, Left 9 Upper Extremity Bursa and Ligament, Right B Upper Extremity Bursa and Ligament, Left C Trunk Bursa and Ligament, Right D Trunk Bursa and Ligament, Left F Thorax Bursa and Ligament, Right G Thorax Bursa and Ligament, Left H Abdomen Bursa and Ligament, Right J Abdomen Bursa and Ligament, Left K Perineum Bursa and Ligament L Hip Bursa and Ligament, Right M Hip Bursa and Ligament, Left N Knee Bursa and Ligament, Right P Knee Bursa and Ligament, Left Q Ankle Bursa and Ligament, Right R Ankle Bursa and Ligament, Left S Foot Bursa and Ligament, Right T Foot Bursa and Ligament, Left V Lower Extremity Bursa and Ligament, Right W Lower Extremity Bursa and Ligament, Left	0 Open 4 Percutaneous Endoscopic	Z No Device	Z No Qualifier

Section   0   **Medical and Surgical**
Body System   M   **Bursae and Ligaments**
Operation   U   **Supplement:** Putting in or on biological or synthetic material that physically reinforces and/or augments the function of a portion of a body part

Body Part (4th)	Approach (5th)	Device (6th)	Qualifier (7th)
0 Head and Neck Bursa and Ligament 1 Shoulder Bursa and Ligament, Right 2 Shoulder Bursa and Ligament, Left 3 Elbow Bursa and Ligament, Right 4 Elbow Bursa and Ligament, Left 5 Wrist Bursa and Ligament, Right 6 Wrist Bursa and Ligament, Left 7 Hand Bursa and Ligament, Right 8 Hand Bursa and Ligament, Left 9 Upper Extremity Bursa and Ligament, Right B Upper Extremity Bursa and Ligament, Left C Trunk Bursa and Ligament, Right D Trunk Bursa and Ligament, Left F Thorax Bursa and Ligament, Right G Thorax Bursa and Ligament, Left H Abdomen Bursa and Ligament, Right J Abdomen Bursa and Ligament, Left K Perineum Bursa and Ligament L Hip Bursa and Ligament, Right M Hip Bursa and Ligament, Left N Knee Bursa and Ligament, Right P Knee Bursa and Ligament, Left Q Ankle Bursa and Ligament, Right R Ankle Bursa and Ligament, Left S Foot Bursa and Ligament, Right T Foot Bursa and Ligament, Left V Lower Extremity Bursa and Ligament, Right W Lower Extremity Bursa and Ligament, Left	0 Open 4 Percutaneous Endoscopic	7 Autologous Tissue Substitute J Synthetic Substitute K Nonautologous Tissue Substitute	Z No Qualifier

Section   0   **Medical and Surgical**
Body System   M   **Bursae and Ligaments**
Operation   W   **Revision:** Correcting, to the extent possible, a portion of a malfunctioning device or the position of a displaced device

Body Part (4th)	Approach (5th)	Device (6th)	Qualifier (7th)
X Upper Bursa and Ligament Y Lower Bursa and Ligament	0 Open 3 Percutaneous 4 Percutaneous Endoscopic X External	0 Drainage Device 7 Autologous Tissue Substitute J Synthetic Substitute K Nonautologous Tissue Substitute	Z No Qualifier

Medical and Surgical Section (0)

0MX

Section	0	Medical and Surgical
Body System	M	Bursae and Ligaments
Operation	X	Transfer: Moving, without taking out, all or a portion of a body part to another location to take over the function of all or a portion of a body part

Body Part (4th)	Approach (5th)	Device (6th)	Qualifier (7th)
0 Head and Neck Bursa and Ligament 1 Shoulder Bursa and Ligament, Right 2 Shoulder Bursa and Ligament, Left 3 Elbow Bursa and Ligament, Right 4 Elbow Bursa and Ligament, Left 5 Wrist Bursa and Ligament, Right 6 Wrist Bursa and Ligament, Left 7 Hand Bursa and Ligament, Right 8 Hand Bursa and Ligament, Left 9 Upper Extremity Bursa and Ligament, Right B Upper Extremity Bursa and Ligament, Left C Trunk Bursa and Ligament, Right D Trunk Bursa and Ligament, Left F Thorax Bursa and Ligament, Right G Thorax Bursa and Ligament, Left H Abdomen Bursa and Ligament, Right J Abdomen Bursa and Ligament, Left K Perineum Bursa and Ligament L Hip Bursa and Ligament, Right M Hip Bursa and Ligament, Left N Knee Bursa and Ligament, Right P Knee Bursa and Ligament, Left Q Ankle Bursa and Ligament, Right R Ankle Bursa and Ligament, Left S Foot Bursa and Ligament, Right T Foot Bursa and Ligament, Left V Lower Extremity Bursa and Ligament, Right W Lower Extremity Bursa and Ligament, Left	0 Open 4 Percutaneous Endoscopic	Z No Device	Z No Qualifier

Bursae and Ligaments Code Listing 0M2–0MX

Review Coding Guideline B4.5

0M2 – Bursae and Ligaments, Change

0M2XX0Z Change Drainage Device in Upper Bursa and Ligament, External Approach
0M2XXYZ Change Other Device in Upper Bursa and Ligament, External Approach

0M2YX0Z Change Drainage Device in Lower Bursa and Ligament, External Approach
0M2YXYZ Change Other Device in Lower Bursa and Ligament, External Approach

0M5 – Bursae and Ligaments, Destruction

Review Coding Guideline B6.1c

0M500ZZ Destruction of Head and Neck Bursa and Ligament, Open Approach
0M503ZZ Destruction of Head and Neck Bursa and Ligament, Percutaneous Approach
0M504ZZ Destruction of Head and Neck Bursa and Ligament, Percutaneous Endoscopic Approach
0M510ZZ Destruction of Right Shoulder Bursa and Ligament, Open Approach
0M513ZZ Destruction of Right Shoulder Bursa and Ligament, Percutaneous Approach
0M514ZZ Destruction of Right Shoulder Bursa and Ligament, Percutaneous Endoscopic Approach
0M520ZZ Destruction of Left Shoulder Bursa and Ligament, Open Approach
0M523ZZ Destruction of Left Shoulder Bursa and Ligament, Percutaneous Approach

0M524ZZ Destruction of Left Shoulder Bursa and Ligament, Percutaneous Endoscopic Approach
0M530ZZ Destruction of Right Elbow Bursa and Ligament, Open Approach
0M533ZZ Destruction of Right Elbow Bursa and Ligament, Percutaneous Approach
0M534ZZ Destruction of Right Elbow Bursa and Ligament, Percutaneous Endoscopic Approach
0M540ZZ Destruction of Left Elbow Bursa and Ligament, Open Approach
0M543ZZ Destruction of Left Elbow Bursa and Ligament, Percutaneous Approach
0M544ZZ Destruction of Left Elbow Bursa and Ligament, Percutaneous Endoscopic Approach
0M550ZZ Destruction of Right Wrist Bursa and Ligament, Open Approach

0M553ZZ Destruction of Right Wrist Bursa and Ligament, Percutaneous Approach

0M554ZZ Destruction of Right Wrist Bursa and Ligament, Percutaneous Endoscopic Approach

0M560ZZ Destruction of Left Wrist Bursa and Ligament, Open Approach

0M563ZZ Destruction of Left Wrist Bursa and Ligament, Percutaneous Approach

0M564ZZ Destruction of Left Wrist Bursa and Ligament, Percutaneous Endoscopic Approach

0M570ZZ Destruction of Right Hand Bursa and Ligament, Open Approach

0M573ZZ Destruction of Right Hand Bursa and Ligament, Percutaneous Approach

0M574ZZ Destruction of Right Hand Bursa and Ligament, Percutaneous Endoscopic Approach

0M580ZZ Destruction of Left Hand Bursa and Ligament, Open Approach

0M583ZZ Destruction of Left Hand Bursa and Ligament, Percutaneous Approach

0M584ZZ Destruction of Left Hand Bursa and Ligament, Percutaneous Endoscopic Approach

0M590ZZ Destruction of Right Upper Extremity Bursa and Ligament, Open Approach

0M593ZZ Destruction of Right Upper Extremity Bursa and Ligament, Percutaneous Approach

0M594ZZ Destruction of Right Upper Extremity Bursa and Ligament, Percutaneous Endoscopic Approach

0M5B0ZZ Destruction of Left Upper Extremity Bursa and Ligament, Open Approach

0M5B3ZZ Destruction of Left Upper Extremity Bursa and Ligament, Percutaneous Approach

0M5B4ZZ Destruction of Left Upper Extremity Bursa and Ligament, Percutaneous Endoscopic Approach

0M5C0ZZ Destruction of Right Trunk Bursa and Ligament, Open Approach

0M5C3ZZ Destruction of Right Trunk Bursa and Ligament, Percutaneous Approach

0M5C4ZZ Destruction of Right Trunk Bursa and Ligament, Percutaneous Endoscopic Approach

0M5D0ZZ Destruction of Left Trunk Bursa and Ligament, Open Approach

0M5D3ZZ Destruction of Left Trunk Bursa and Ligament, Percutaneous Approach

0M5D4ZZ Destruction of Left Trunk Bursa and Ligament, Percutaneous Endoscopic Approach

0M5F0ZZ Destruction of Right Thorax Bursa and Ligament, Open Approach

0M5F3ZZ Destruction of Right Thorax Bursa and Ligament, Percutaneous Approach

0M5F4ZZ Destruction of Right Thorax Bursa and Ligament, Percutaneous Endoscopic Approach

0M5G0ZZ Destruction of Left Thorax Bursa and Ligament, Open Approach

0M5G3ZZ Destruction of Left Thorax Bursa and Ligament, Percutaneous Approach

0M5G4ZZ Destruction of Left Thorax Bursa and Ligament, Percutaneous Endoscopic Approach

0M5H0ZZ Destruction of Right Abdomen Bursa and Ligament, Open Approach

0M5H3ZZ Destruction of Right Abdomen Bursa and Ligament, Percutaneous Approach

0M5H4ZZ Destruction of Right Abdomen Bursa and Ligament, Percutaneous Endoscopic Approach

0M5J0ZZ Destruction of Left Abdomen Bursa and Ligament, Open Approach

0M5J3ZZ Destruction of Left Abdomen Bursa and Ligament, Percutaneous Approach

0M5J4ZZ Destruction of Left Abdomen Bursa and Ligament, Percutaneous Endoscopic Approach

0M5K0ZZ Destruction of Perineum Bursa and Ligament, Open Approach

0M5K3ZZ Destruction of Perineum Bursa and Ligament, Percutaneous Approach

0M5K4ZZ Destruction of Perineum Bursa and Ligament, Percutaneous Endoscopic Approach

0M5L0ZZ Destruction of Right Hip Bursa and Ligament, Open Approach

0M5L3ZZ Destruction of Right Hip Bursa and Ligament, Percutaneous Approach

0M5L4ZZ Destruction of Right Hip Bursa and Ligament, Percutaneous Endoscopic Approach

0M5M0ZZ Destruction of Left Hip Bursa and Ligament, Open Approach

0M5M3ZZ Destruction of Left Hip Bursa and Ligament, Percutaneous Approach

0M5M4ZZ Destruction of Left Hip Bursa and Ligament, Percutaneous Endoscopic Approach

0M5N0ZZ Destruction of Right Knee Bursa and Ligament, Open Approach

0M5N3ZZ Destruction of Right Knee Bursa and Ligament, Percutaneous Approach

0M5N4ZZ Destruction of Right Knee Bursa and Ligament, Percutaneous Endoscopic Approach

0M5P0ZZ Destruction of Left Knee Bursa and Ligament, Open Approach

0M5P3ZZ Destruction of Left Knee Bursa and Ligament, Percutaneous Approach

0M5P4ZZ Destruction of Left Knee Bursa and Ligament, Percutaneous Endoscopic Approach

0M5Q0ZZ Destruction of Right Ankle Bursa and Ligament, Open Approach

0M5Q3ZZ Destruction of Right Ankle Bursa and Ligament, Percutaneous Approach

0M5Q4ZZ Destruction of Right Ankle Bursa and Ligament, Percutaneous Endoscopic Approach

0M5R0ZZ Destruction of Left Ankle Bursa and Ligament, Open Approach

0M5R3ZZ Destruction of Left Ankle Bursa and Ligament, Percutaneous Approach

0M5R4ZZ Destruction of Left Ankle Bursa and Ligament, Percutaneous Endoscopic Approach

0M5S0ZZ Destruction of Right Foot Bursa and Ligament, Open Approach

0M5S3ZZ Destruction of Right Foot Bursa and Ligament, Percutaneous Approach

0M5S4ZZ Destruction of Right Foot Bursa and Ligament, Percutaneous Endoscopic Approach

0M5T0ZZ Destruction of Left Foot Bursa and Ligament, Open Approach

0M5T3ZZ Destruction of Left Foot Bursa and Ligament, Percutaneous Approach

0M5T4ZZ Destruction of Left Foot Bursa and Ligament, Percutaneous Endoscopic Approach

0M5V0ZZ Destruction of Right Lower Extremity Bursa and Ligament, Open Approach

0M5V3ZZ Destruction of Right Lower Extremity Bursa and Ligament, Percutaneous Approach

0M5V4ZZ Destruction of Right Lower Extremity Bursa and Ligament, Percutaneous Endoscopic Approach

0M5W0ZZ Destruction of Left Lower Extremity Bursa and Ligament, Open Approach

0M5W3ZZ Destruction of Left Lower Extremity Bursa and Ligament, Percutaneous Approach

0M5W4ZZ Destruction of Left Lower Extremity Bursa and Ligament, Percutaneous Endoscopic Approach

0M8 – Bursae and Ligaments, Division

Review Coding Guideline B3.14

0M800ZZ Division of Head and Neck Bursa and Ligament, Open Approach

0M803ZZ Division of Head and Neck Bursa and Ligament, Percutaneous Approach

0M804ZZ Division of Head and Neck Bursa and Ligament, Percutaneous Endoscopic Approach

0M810ZZ Division of Right Shoulder Bursa and Ligament, Open Approach

0M813ZZ Division of Right Shoulder Bursa and Ligament, Percutaneous Approach

0M814ZZ Division of Right Shoulder Bursa and Ligament, Percutaneous Endoscopic Approach

0M820ZZ Division of Left Shoulder Bursa and Ligament, Open Approach

0M823ZZ Division of Left Shoulder Bursa and Ligament, Percutaneous Approach

0M824ZZ Division of Left Shoulder Bursa and Ligament, Percutaneous Endoscopic Approach

0M830ZZ Division of Right Elbow Bursa and Ligament, Open Approach

0M833ZZ Division of Right Elbow Bursa and Ligament, Percutaneous Approach

0M834ZZ Division of Right Elbow Bursa and Ligament, Percutaneous Endoscopic Approach

0M840ZZ Division of Left Elbow Bursa and Ligament, Open Approach

0M843ZZ Division of Left Elbow Bursa and Ligament, Percutaneous Approach

0M844ZZ Division of Left Elbow Bursa and Ligament, Percutaneous Endoscopic Approach

0M850ZZ Division of Right Wrist Bursa and Ligament, Open Approach

0M853ZZ Division of Right Wrist Bursa and Ligament, Percutaneous Approach

0M854ZZ Division of Right Wrist Bursa and Ligament, Percutaneous Endoscopic Approach

0M860ZZ Division of Left Wrist Bursa and Ligament, Open Approach

0M863ZZ Division of Left Wrist Bursa and Ligament, Percutaneous Approach

0M864ZZ Division of Left Wrist Bursa and Ligament, Percutaneous Endoscopic Approach

0M870ZZ Division of Right Hand Bursa and Ligament, Open Approach

0M873ZZ Division of Right Hand Bursa and Ligament, Percutaneous Approach

0M874ZZ Division of Right Hand Bursa and Ligament, Percutaneous Endoscopic Approach

0M880ZZ Division of Left Hand Bursa and Ligament, Open Approach

0M883ZZ Division of Left Hand Bursa and Ligament, Percutaneous Approach

0M884ZZ Division of Left Hand Bursa and Ligament, Percutaneous Endoscopic Approach

0M890ZZ Division of Right Upper Extremity Bursa and Ligament, Open Approach

0M893ZZ Division of Right Upper Extremity Bursa and Ligament, Percutaneous Approach

0M894ZZ Division of Right Upper Extremity Bursa and Ligament, Percutaneous Endoscopic Approach

0M8B0ZZ Division of Left Upper Extremity Bursa and Ligament, Open Approach

0M8B3ZZ Division of Left Upper Extremity Bursa and Ligament, Percutaneous Approach

0M8B4ZZ Division of Left Upper Extremity Bursa and Ligament, Percutaneous Endoscopic Approach

0M8C0ZZ Division of Right Trunk Bursa and Ligament, Open Approach

0M8C3ZZ Division of Right Trunk Bursa and Ligament, Percutaneous Approach

0M8C4ZZ Division of Right Trunk Bursa and Ligament, Percutaneous Endoscopic Approach

0M8D0ZZ Division of Left Trunk Bursa and Ligament, Open Approach

0M8D3ZZ Division of Left Trunk Bursa and Ligament, Percutaneous Approach

0M8D4ZZ Division of Left Trunk Bursa and Ligament, Percutaneous Endoscopic Approach

0M8F0ZZ Division of Right Thorax Bursa and Ligament, Open Approach

0M8F3ZZ Division of Right Thorax Bursa and Ligament, Percutaneous Approach

0M8F4ZZ Division of Right Thorax Bursa and Ligament, Percutaneous Endoscopic Approach

0M8G0ZZ Division of Left Thorax Bursa and Ligament, Open Approach

0M8G3ZZ Division of Left Thorax Bursa and Ligament, Percutaneous Approach

0M8G4ZZ Division of Left Thorax Bursa and Ligament, Percutaneous Endoscopic Approach

0M8H0ZZ Division of Right Abdomen Bursa and Ligament, Open Approach

0M8H3ZZ Division of Right Abdomen Bursa and Ligament, Percutaneous Approach

0M8H4ZZ Division of Right Abdomen Bursa and Ligament, Percutaneous Endoscopic Approach

0M8J0ZZ Division of Left Abdomen Bursa and Ligament, Open Approach

0M8J3ZZ Division of Left Abdomen Bursa and Ligament, Percutaneous Approach

0M8J4ZZ Division of Left Abdomen Bursa and Ligament, Percutaneous Endoscopic Approach

0M8K0ZZ Division of Perineum Bursa and Ligament, Open Approach

0M8K3ZZ Division of Perineum Bursa and Ligament, Percutaneous Approach

0M8K4ZZ Division of Perineum Bursa and Ligament, Percutaneous Endoscopic Approach

0M8L0ZZ Division of Right Hip Bursa and Ligament, Open Approach

0M8L3ZZ Division of Right Hip Bursa and Ligament, Percutaneous Approach

0M8L4ZZ Division of Right Hip Bursa and Ligament, Percutaneous Endoscopic Approach

0M8M0ZZ Division of Left Hip Bursa and Ligament, Open Approach

0M8M3ZZ Division of Left Hip Bursa and Ligament, Percutaneous Approach

0M8M4ZZ Division of Left Hip Bursa and Ligament, Percutaneous Endoscopic Approach

0M8N0ZZ Division of Right Knee Bursa and Ligament, Open Approach

0M8N3ZZ Division of Right Knee Bursa and Ligament, Percutaneous Approach

0M8N4ZZ Division of Right Knee Bursa and Ligament, Percutaneous Endoscopic Approach

0M8P0ZZ Division of Left Knee Bursa and Ligament, Open Approach

0M8P3ZZ Division of Left Knee Bursa and Ligament, Percutaneous Approach

0M8P4ZZ Division of Left Knee Bursa and Ligament, Percutaneous Endoscopic Approach

0M8Q0ZZ Division of Right Ankle Bursa and Ligament, Open Approach

0M8Q3ZZ Division of Right Ankle Bursa and Ligament, Percutaneous Approach

0M8Q4ZZ Division of Right Ankle Bursa and Ligament, Percutaneous Endoscopic Approach

0M8R0ZZ Division of Left Ankle Bursa and Ligament, Open Approach

0M8R3ZZ Division of Left Ankle Bursa and Ligament, Percutaneous Approach

0M8R4ZZ Division of Left Ankle Bursa and Ligament, Percutaneous Endoscopic Approach

0M8S0ZZ Division of Right Foot Bursa and Ligament, Open Approach

0M8S3ZZ Division of Right Foot Bursa and Ligament, Percutaneous Approach

0M8S4ZZ Division of Right Foot Bursa and Ligament, Percutaneous Endoscopic Approach

0M8T0ZZ Division of Left Foot Bursa and Ligament, Open Approach

0M8T3ZZ Division of Left Foot Bursa and Ligament, Percutaneous Approach

0M8T4ZZ Division of Left Foot Bursa and Ligament, Percutaneous Approach

0M8V0ZZ Division of Right Lower Extremity Bursa and Ligament, Open Approach

0M8V3ZZ Division of Right Lower Extremity Bursa and Ligament, Percutaneous Approach

0M8V4ZZ Division of Right Lower Extremity Bursa and Ligament, Percutaneous Endoscopic Approach

0M8W0ZZ Division of Left Lower Extremity Bursa and Ligament, Open Approach

0M8W3ZZ Division of Left Lower Extremity Bursa and Ligament, Percutaneous Approach

0M8W4ZZ Division of Left Lower Extremity Bursa and Ligament, Percutaneous Endoscopic Approach

0M9 – Bursae and Ligaments, Drainage

Review Coding Guidelines B3.4a and B3.4b

Review Coding Guideline B6.2

0M9000Z Drainage of Head and Neck Bursa and Ligament with Drainage Device, Open Approach

0M900ZX Drainage of Head and Neck Bursa and Ligament, Open Approach, Diagnostic

0M900ZZ Drainage of Head and Neck Bursa and Ligament, Open Approach

0M9030Z Drainage of Head and Neck Bursa and Ligament with Drainage Device, Percutaneous Approach

0M903ZX Drainage of Head and Neck Bursa and Ligament, Percutaneous Approach, Diagnostic

0M903ZZ Drainage of Head and Neck Bursa and Ligament, Percutaneous Approach

---

0M9040Z Drainage of Head and Neck Bursa and Ligament with Drainage Device, Percutaneous Endoscopic Approach

0M904ZX Drainage of Head and Neck Bursa and Ligament, Percutaneous Endoscopic Approach, Diagnostic

0M904ZZ Drainage of Head and Neck Bursa and Ligament, Percutaneous Endoscopic Approach

0M9100Z Drainage of Right Shoulder Bursa and Ligament with Drainage Device, Open Approach

0M910ZX Drainage of Right Shoulder Bursa and Ligament, Open Approach, Diagnostic

0M910ZZ Drainage of Right Shoulder Bursa and Ligament, Open Approach

0M9130Z Drainage of Right Shoulder Bursa and Ligament with Drainage Device, Percutaneous Approach

0M913ZX Drainage of Right Shoulder Bursa and Ligament, Percutaneous Approach, Diagnostic

0M913ZZ Drainage of Right Shoulder Bursa and Ligament, Percutaneous Approach

0M9140Z Drainage of Right Shoulder Bursa and Ligament with Drainage Device, Percutaneous Endoscopic Approach

0M914ZX Drainage of Right Shoulder Bursa and Ligament, Percutaneous Endoscopic Approach, Diagnostic

0M914ZZ Drainage of Right Shoulder Bursa and Ligament, Percutaneous Endoscopic Approach

0M9200Z Drainage of Left Shoulder Bursa and Ligament with Drainage Device, Open Approach

0M920ZX Drainage of Left Shoulder Bursa and Ligament, Open Approach, Diagnostic

0M920ZZ Drainage of Left Shoulder Bursa and Ligament, Open Approach

0M9230Z Drainage of Left Shoulder Bursa and Ligament with Drainage Device, Percutaneous Approach

0M923ZX Drainage of Left Shoulder Bursa and Ligament, Percutaneous Approach, Diagnostic

0M923ZZ Drainage of Left Shoulder Bursa and Ligament, Percutaneous Approach

0M9240Z Drainage of Left Shoulder Bursa and Ligament with Drainage Device, Percutaneous Endoscopic Approach

0M924ZX Drainage of Left Shoulder Bursa and Ligament, Percutaneous Endoscopic Approach, Diagnostic

0M924ZZ Drainage of Left Shoulder Bursa and Ligament, Percutaneous Endoscopic Approach

0M9300Z Drainage of Right Elbow Bursa and Ligament with Drainage Device, Open Approach

0M930ZX Drainage of Right Elbow Bursa and Ligament, Open Approach, Diagnostic

0M930ZZ Drainage of Right Elbow Bursa and Ligament, Open Approach

0M9330Z Drainage of Right Elbow Bursa and Ligament with Drainage Device, Percutaneous Approach

0M933ZX Drainage of Right Elbow Bursa and Ligament, Percutaneous Approach, Diagnostic

0M933ZZ Drainage of Right Elbow Bursa and Ligament, Percutaneous Approach

0M9340Z Drainage of Right Elbow Bursa and Ligament with Drainage Device, Percutaneous Endoscopic Approach

0M934ZX Drainage of Right Elbow Bursa and Ligament, Percutaneous Endoscopic Approach, Diagnostic

0M934ZZ Drainage of Right Elbow Bursa and Ligament, Percutaneous Endoscopic Approach

0M9400Z Drainage of Left Elbow Bursa and Ligament with Drainage Device, Open Approach

0M940ZX Drainage of Left Elbow Bursa and Ligament, Open Approach, Diagnostic

0M940ZZ Drainage of Left Elbow Bursa and Ligament, Open Approach

0M9430Z Drainage of Left Elbow Bursa and Ligament with Drainage Device, Percutaneous Approach

0M943ZX Drainage of Left Elbow Bursa and Ligament, Percutaneous Approach, Diagnostic

0M943ZZ Drainage of Left Elbow Bursa and Ligament, Percutaneous Approach

0M9440Z Drainage of Left Elbow Bursa and Ligament with Drainage Device, Percutaneous Endoscopic Approach

0M944ZX Drainage of Left Elbow Bursa and Ligament, Percutaneous Endoscopic Approach, Diagnostic

0M944ZZ Drainage of Left Elbow Bursa and Ligament, Percutaneous Endoscopic Approach

0M9500Z Drainage of Right Wrist Bursa and Ligament with Drainage Device, Open Approach

0M950ZX Drainage of Right Wrist Bursa and Ligament, Open Approach, Diagnostic

0M950ZZ Drainage of Right Wrist Bursa and Ligament, Open Approach

0M9530Z Drainage of Right Wrist Bursa and Ligament with Drainage Device, Percutaneous Approach

0M953ZX Drainage of Right Wrist Bursa and Ligament, Percutaneous Approach, Diagnostic

0M953ZZ Drainage of Right Wrist Bursa and Ligament, Percutaneous Approach

0M9540Z Drainage of Right Wrist Bursa and Ligament with Drainage Device, Percutaneous Endoscopic Approach

0M954ZX Drainage of Right Wrist Bursa and Ligament, Percutaneous Endoscopic Approach, Diagnostic

0M954ZZ Drainage of Right Wrist Bursa and Ligament, Percutaneous Endoscopic Approach

0M9600Z Drainage of Left Wrist Bursa and Ligament with Drainage Device, Open Approach

0M960ZX Drainage of Left Wrist Bursa and Ligament, Open Approach, Diagnostic

0M960ZZ Drainage of Left Wrist Bursa and Ligament, Open Approach

0M9630Z Drainage of Left Wrist Bursa and Ligament with Drainage Device, Percutaneous Approach

0M963ZX Drainage of Left Wrist Bursa and Ligament, Percutaneous Approach, Diagnostic

0M963ZZ Drainage of Left Wrist Bursa and Ligament, Percutaneous Approach

0M9640Z Drainage of Left Wrist Bursa and Ligament with Drainage Device, Percutaneous Endoscopic Approach

0M964ZX Drainage of Left Wrist Bursa and Ligament, Percutaneous Endoscopic Approach, Diagnostic

0M964ZZ Drainage of Left Wrist Bursa and Ligament, Percutaneous Endoscopic Approach

0M9700Z Drainage of Right Hand Bursa and Ligament with Drainage Device, Open Approach

0M970ZX Drainage of Right Hand Bursa and Ligament, Open Approach, Diagnostic

0M970ZZ Drainage of Right Hand Bursa and Ligament, Open Approach

0M9730Z Drainage of Right Hand Bursa and Ligament with Drainage Device, Percutaneous Approach

0M973ZX Drainage of Right Hand Bursa and Ligament, Percutaneous Approach, Diagnostic

0M973ZZ Drainage of Right Hand Bursa and Ligament, Percutaneous Approach

0M9740Z Drainage of Right Hand Bursa and Ligament with Drainage Device, Percutaneous Endoscopic Approach

0M974ZX Drainage of Right Hand Bursa and Ligament, Percutaneous Endoscopic Approach, Diagnostic

0M974ZZ Drainage of Right Hand Bursa and Ligament, Percutaneous Endoscopic Approach

0M9800Z Drainage of Left Hand Bursa and Ligament with Drainage Device, Open Approach

0M980ZX Drainage of Left Hand Bursa and Ligament, Open Approach, Diagnostic

0M980ZZ Drainage of Left Hand Bursa and Ligament, Open Approach

0M9830Z Drainage of Left Hand Bursa and Ligament with Drainage Device, Percutaneous Approach

0M983ZX Drainage of Left Hand Bursa and Ligament, Percutaneous Approach, Diagnostic

0M983ZZ Drainage of Left Hand Bursa and Ligament, Percutaneous Approach

0M9840Z Drainage of Left Hand Bursa and Ligament with Drainage Device, Percutaneous Endoscopic Approach

0M984ZX Drainage of Left Hand Bursa and Ligament, Percutaneous Endoscopic Approach, Diagnostic

0M984ZZ Drainage of Left Hand Bursa and Ligament, Percutaneous Endoscopic Approach

0M9900Z Drainage of Right Upper Extremity Bursa and Ligament with Drainage Device, Open Approach

0M990ZX Drainage of Right Upper Extremity Bursa and Ligament, Open Approach, Diagnostic

0M990ZZ Drainage of Right Upper Extremity Bursa and Ligament, Open Approach

0M9930Z Drainage of Right Upper Extremity Bursa and Ligament with Drainage Device, Percutaneous Approach

0M993ZX   Drainage of Right Upper Extremity Bursa and Ligament, Percutaneous Approach, Diagnostic

0M993ZZ   Drainage of Right Upper Extremity Bursa and Ligament, Percutaneous Approach

0M9940Z   Drainage of Right Upper Extremity Bursa and Ligament with Drainage Device, Percutaneous Endoscopic Approach

0M994ZX   Drainage of Right Upper Extremity Bursa and Ligament, Percutaneous Endoscopic Approach, Diagnostic

0M994ZZ   Drainage of Right Upper Extremity Bursa and Ligament, Percutaneous Endoscopic Approach

0M9B00Z   Drainage of Left Upper Extremity Bursa and Ligament with Drainage Device, Open Approach

0M9B0ZX   Drainage of Left Upper Extremity Bursa and Ligament, Open Approach, Diagnostic

0M9B0ZZ   Drainage of Left Upper Extremity Bursa and Ligament, Open Approach

0M9B30Z   Drainage of Left Upper Extremity Bursa and Ligament with Drainage Device, Percutaneous Approach

0M9B3ZX   Drainage of Left Upper Extremity Bursa and Ligament, Percutaneous Approach, Diagnostic

0M9B3ZZ   Drainage of Left Upper Extremity Bursa and Ligament, Percutaneous Approach

0M9B40Z   Drainage of Left Upper Extremity Bursa and Ligament with Drainage Device, Percutaneous Endoscopic Approach

0M9B4ZX   Drainage of Left Upper Extremity Bursa and Ligament, Percutaneous Endoscopic Approach, Diagnostic

0M9B4ZZ   Drainage of Left Upper Extremity Bursa and Ligament, Percutaneous Endoscopic Approach

0M9C00Z   Drainage of Right Trunk Bursa and Ligament with Drainage Device, Open Approach

0M9C0ZX   Drainage of Right Trunk Bursa and Ligament, Open Approach, Diagnostic

0M9C0ZZ   Drainage of Right Trunk Bursa and Ligament, Open Approach

0M9C30Z   Drainage of Right Trunk Bursa and Ligament with Drainage Device, Percutaneous Approach

0M9C3ZX   Drainage of Right Trunk Bursa and Ligament, Percutaneous Approach, Diagnostic

0M9C3ZZ   Drainage of Right Trunk Bursa and Ligament, Percutaneous Approach

0M9C40Z   Drainage of Right Trunk Bursa and Ligament with Drainage Device, Percutaneous Endoscopic Approach

0M9C4ZX   Drainage of Right Trunk Bursa and Ligament, Percutaneous Endoscopic Approach, Diagnostic

0M9C4ZZ   Drainage of Right Trunk Bursa and Ligament, Percutaneous Endoscopic Approach

0M9D00Z   Drainage of Left Trunk Bursa and Ligament with Drainage Device, Open Approach

0M9D0ZX   Drainage of Left Trunk Bursa and Ligament, Open Approach, Diagnostic

0M9D0ZZ   Drainage of Left Trunk Bursa and Ligament, Open Approach

0M9D30Z   Drainage of Left Trunk Bursa and Ligament with Drainage Device, Percutaneous Approach

0M9D3ZX   Drainage of Left Trunk Bursa and Ligament, Percutaneous Approach, Diagnostic

0M9D3ZZ   Drainage of Left Trunk Bursa and Ligament, Percutaneous Approach

0M9D40Z   Drainage of Left Trunk Bursa and Ligament with Drainage Device, Percutaneous Endoscopic Approach

0M9D4ZX   Drainage of Left Trunk Bursa and Ligament, Percutaneous Endoscopic Approach, Diagnostic

0M9D4ZZ   Drainage of Left Trunk Bursa and Ligament, Percutaneous Endoscopic Approach

0M9F00Z   Drainage of Right Thorax Bursa and Ligament with Drainage Device, Open Approach

0M9F0ZX   Drainage of Right Thorax Bursa and Ligament, Open Approach, Diagnostic

0M9F0ZZ   Drainage of Right Thorax Bursa and Ligament, Open Approach

0M9F30Z   Drainage of Right Thorax Bursa and Ligament with Drainage Device, Percutaneous Approach

0M9F3ZX   Drainage of Right Thorax Bursa and Ligament, Percutaneous Approach, Diagnostic

0M9F3ZZ   Drainage of Right Thorax Bursa and Ligament, Percutaneous Approach

0M9F40Z   Drainage of Right Thorax Bursa and Ligament with Drainage Device, Percutaneous Endoscopic Approach

0M9F4ZX   Drainage of Right Thorax Bursa and Ligament, Percutaneous Endoscopic Approach, Diagnostic

0M9F4ZZ   Drainage of Right Thorax Bursa and Ligament, Percutaneous Endoscopic Approach

0M9G00Z   Drainage of Left Thorax Bursa and Ligament with Drainage Device, Open Approach

0M9G0ZX   Drainage of Left Thorax Bursa and Ligament, Open Approach, Diagnostic

0M9G0ZZ   Drainage of Left Thorax Bursa and Ligament, Open Approach

0M9G30Z   Drainage of Left Thorax Bursa and Ligament with Drainage Device, Percutaneous Approach

0M9G3ZX   Drainage of Left Thorax Bursa and Ligament, Percutaneous Approach, Diagnostic

0M9G3ZZ   Drainage of Left Thorax Bursa and Ligament, Percutaneous Approach

0M9G40Z   Drainage of Left Thorax Bursa and Ligament with Drainage Device, Percutaneous Endoscopic Approach

0M9G4ZX   Drainage of Left Thorax Bursa and Ligament, Percutaneous Endoscopic Approach, Diagnostic

0M9G4ZZ   Drainage of Left Thorax Bursa and Ligament, Percutaneous Endoscopic Approach

0M9H00Z   Drainage of Right Abdomen Bursa and Ligament with Drainage Device, Open Approach

0M9H0ZX   Drainage of Right Abdomen Bursa and Ligament, Open Approach, Diagnostic

0M9H0ZZ   Drainage of Right Abdomen Bursa and Ligament, Open Approach

0M9H30Z   Drainage of Right Abdomen Bursa and Ligament with Drainage Device, Percutaneous Approach

0M9H3ZX   Drainage of Right Abdomen Bursa and Ligament, Percutaneous Approach, Diagnostic

0M9H3ZZ   Drainage of Right Abdomen Bursa and Ligament, Percutaneous Approach

0M9H40Z   Drainage of Right Abdomen Bursa and Ligament with Drainage Device, Percutaneous Endoscopic Approach

0M9H4ZX   Drainage of Right Abdomen Bursa and Ligament, Percutaneous Endoscopic Approach, Diagnostic

0M9H4ZZ   Drainage of Right Abdomen Bursa and Ligament, Percutaneous Endoscopic Approach

0M9J00Z   Drainage of Left Abdomen Bursa and Ligament with Drainage Device, Open Approach

0M9J0ZX   Drainage of Left Abdomen Bursa and Ligament, Open Approach, Diagnostic

0M9J0ZZ   Drainage of Left Abdomen Bursa and Ligament, Open Approach

0M9J30Z   Drainage of Left Abdomen Bursa and Ligament with Drainage Device, Percutaneous Approach

0M9J3ZX   Drainage of Left Abdomen Bursa and Ligament, Percutaneous Approach, Diagnostic

0M9J3ZZ   Drainage of Left Abdomen Bursa and Ligament, Percutaneous Approach

0M9J40Z   Drainage of Left Abdomen Bursa and Ligament with Drainage Device, Percutaneous Endoscopic Approach

0M9J4ZX   Drainage of Left Abdomen Bursa and Ligament, Percutaneous Endoscopic Approach, Diagnostic

0M9J4ZZ   Drainage of Left Abdomen Bursa and Ligament, Percutaneous Endoscopic Approach

0M9K00Z   Drainage of Perineum Bursa and Ligament with Drainage Device, Open Approach

0M9K0ZX   Drainage of Perineum Bursa and Ligament, Open Approach, Diagnostic

0M9K0ZZ   Drainage of Perineum Bursa and Ligament, Open Approach

0M9K30Z   Drainage of Perineum Bursa and Ligament with Drainage Device, Percutaneous Approach

0M9K3ZX   Drainage of Perineum Bursa and Ligament, Percutaneous Approach, Diagnostic

0M9K3ZZ   Drainage of Perineum Bursa and Ligament, Percutaneous Approach

0M9K40Z   Drainage of Perineum Bursa and Ligament with Drainage Device, Percutaneous Endoscopic Approach

0M9K4ZX   Drainage of Perineum Bursa and Ligament, Percutaneous Endoscopic Approach, Diagnostic

0M9K4ZZ   Drainage of Perineum Bursa and Ligament, Percutaneous Endoscopic Approach

0M9L00Z Drainage of Right Hip Bursa and Ligament with Drainage Device, Open Approach

0M9L0ZX Drainage of Right Hip Bursa and Ligament, Open Approach, Diagnostic

0M9L0ZZ Drainage of Right Hip Bursa and Ligament, Open Approach

0M9L30Z Drainage of Right Hip Bursa and Ligament with Drainage Device, Percutaneous Approach

0M9L3ZX Drainage of Right Hip Bursa and Ligament, Percutaneous Approach, Diagnostic

0M9L3ZZ Drainage of Right Hip Bursa and Ligament, Percutaneous Approach

0M9L40Z Drainage of Right Hip Bursa and Ligament with Drainage Device, Percutaneous Endoscopic Approach

0M9L4ZX Drainage of Right Hip Bursa and Ligament, Percutaneous Endoscopic Approach, Diagnostic

0M9L4ZZ Drainage of Right Hip Bursa and Ligament, Percutaneous Endoscopic Approach

0M9M00Z Drainage of Left Hip Bursa and Ligament with Drainage Device, Open Approach

0M9M0ZX Drainage of Left Hip Bursa and Ligament, Open Approach, Diagnostic

0M9M0ZZ Drainage of Left Hip Bursa and Ligament, Open Approach

0M9M30Z Drainage of Left Hip Bursa and Ligament with Drainage Device, Percutaneous Approach

0M9M3ZX Drainage of Left Hip Bursa and Ligament, Percutaneous Approach, Diagnostic

0M9M3ZZ Drainage of Left Hip Bursa and Ligament, Percutaneous Approach

0M9M40Z Drainage of Left Hip Bursa and Ligament with Drainage Device, Percutaneous Endoscopic Approach

0M9M4ZX Drainage of Left Hip Bursa and Ligament, Percutaneous Endoscopic Approach, Diagnostic

0M9M4ZZ Drainage of Left Hip Bursa and Ligament, Percutaneous Endoscopic Approach

0M9N00Z Drainage of Right Knee Bursa and Ligament with Drainage Device, Open Approach

0M9N0ZX Drainage of Right Knee Bursa and Ligament, Open Approach, Diagnostic

0M9N0ZZ Drainage of Right Knee Bursa and Ligament, Open Approach

0M9N30Z Drainage of Right Knee Bursa and Ligament with Drainage Device, Percutaneous Approach

0M9N3ZX Drainage of Right Knee Bursa and Ligament, Percutaneous Approach, Diagnostic

0M9N3ZZ Drainage of Right Knee Bursa and Ligament, Percutaneous Approach

0M9N40Z Drainage of Right Knee Bursa and Ligament with Drainage Device, Percutaneous Endoscopic Approach

0M9N4ZX Drainage of Right Knee Bursa and Ligament, Percutaneous Endoscopic Approach, Diagnostic

0M9N4ZZ Drainage of Right Knee Bursa and Ligament, Percutaneous Endoscopic Approach

0M9P00Z Drainage of Left Knee Bursa and Ligament with Drainage Device, Open Approach

0M9P0ZX Drainage of Left Knee Bursa and Ligament, Open Approach, Diagnostic

0M9P0ZZ Drainage of Left Knee Bursa and Ligament, Open Approach

0M9P30Z Drainage of Left Knee Bursa and Ligament with Drainage Device, Percutaneous Approach

0M9P3ZX Drainage of Left Knee Bursa and Ligament, Percutaneous Approach, Diagnostic

0M9P3ZZ Drainage of Left Knee Bursa and Ligament, Percutaneous Approach

0M9P40Z Drainage of Left Knee Bursa and Ligament with Drainage Device, Percutaneous Endoscopic Approach

0M9P4ZX Drainage of Left Knee Bursa and Ligament, Percutaneous Endoscopic Approach, Diagnostic

0M9P4ZZ Drainage of Left Knee Bursa and Ligament, Percutaneous Endoscopic Approach

0M9Q00Z Drainage of Right Ankle Bursa and Ligament with Drainage Device, Open Approach

0M9Q0ZX Drainage of Right Ankle Bursa and Ligament, Open Approach, Diagnostic

0M9Q0ZZ Drainage of Right Ankle Bursa and Ligament, Open Approach

0M9Q30Z Drainage of Right Ankle Bursa and Ligament with Drainage Device, Percutaneous Approach

0M9Q3ZX Drainage of Right Ankle Bursa and Ligament, Percutaneous Approach, Diagnostic

0M9Q3ZZ Drainage of Right Ankle Bursa and Ligament, Percutaneous Approach

0M9Q40Z Drainage of Right Ankle Bursa and Ligament with Drainage Device, Percutaneous Endoscopic Approach

0M9Q4ZX Drainage of Right Ankle Bursa and Ligament, Percutaneous Endoscopic Approach, Diagnostic

0M9Q4ZZ Drainage of Right Ankle Bursa and Ligament, Percutaneous Endoscopic Approach

0M9R00Z Drainage of Left Ankle Bursa and Ligament with Drainage Device, Open Approach

0M9R0ZX Drainage of Left Ankle Bursa and Ligament, Open Approach, Diagnostic

0M9R0ZZ Drainage of Left Ankle Bursa and Ligament, Open Approach

0M9R30Z Drainage of Left Ankle Bursa and Ligament with Drainage Device, Percutaneous Approach

0M9R3ZX Drainage of Left Ankle Bursa and Ligament, Percutaneous Approach, Diagnostic

0M9R3ZZ Drainage of Left Ankle Bursa and Ligament, Percutaneous Approach

0M9R40Z Drainage of Left Ankle Bursa and Ligament with Drainage Device, Percutaneous Endoscopic Approach

0M9R4ZX Drainage of Left Ankle Bursa and Ligament, Percutaneous Endoscopic Approach, Diagnostic

0M9R4ZZ Drainage of Left Ankle Bursa and Ligament, Percutaneous Endoscopic Approach

0M9S00Z Drainage of Right Foot Bursa and Ligament with Drainage Device, Open Approach

0M9S0ZX Drainage of Right Foot Bursa and Ligament, Open Approach, Diagnostic

0M9S0ZZ Drainage of Right Foot Bursa and Ligament, Open Approach

0M9S30Z Drainage of Right Foot Bursa and Ligament with Drainage Device, Percutaneous Approach

0M9S3ZX Drainage of Right Foot Bursa and Ligament, Percutaneous Approach, Diagnostic

0M9S3ZZ Drainage of Right Foot Bursa and Ligament, Percutaneous Approach

0M9S40Z Drainage of Right Foot Bursa and Ligament with Drainage Device, Percutaneous Endoscopic Approach

0M9S4ZX Drainage of Right Foot Bursa and Ligament, Percutaneous Endoscopic Approach, Diagnostic

0M9S4ZZ Drainage of Right Foot Bursa and Ligament, Percutaneous Endoscopic Approach

0M9T00Z Drainage of Left Foot Bursa and Ligament with Drainage Device, Open Approach

0M9T0ZX Drainage of Left Foot Bursa and Ligament, Open Approach, Diagnostic

0M9T0ZZ Drainage of Left Foot Bursa and Ligament, Open Approach

0M9T30Z Drainage of Left Foot Bursa and Ligament with Drainage Device, Percutaneous Approach

0M9T3ZX Drainage of Left Foot Bursa and Ligament, Percutaneous Approach, Diagnostic

0M9T3ZZ Drainage of Left Foot Bursa and Ligament, Percutaneous Approach

0M9T40Z Drainage of Left Foot Bursa and Ligament with Drainage Device, Percutaneous Endoscopic Approach

0M9T4ZX Drainage of Left Foot Bursa and Ligament, Percutaneous Endoscopic Approach, Diagnostic

0M9T4ZZ Drainage of Left Foot Bursa and Ligament, Percutaneous Endoscopic Approach

0M9V00Z Drainage of Right Lower Extremity Bursa and Ligament with Drainage Device, Open Approach

0M9V0ZX Drainage of Right Lower Extremity Bursa and Ligament, Open Approach, Diagnostic

0M9V0ZZ Drainage of Right Lower Extremity Bursa and Ligament, Open Approach

0M9V30Z Drainage of Right Lower Extremity Bursa and Ligament with Drainage Device, Percutaneous Approach

0M9V3ZX Drainage of Right Lower Extremity Bursa and Ligament, Percutaneous Approach, Diagnostic

0M9V3ZZ Drainage of Right Lower Extremity Bursa and Ligament, Percutaneous Approach

0M9V40Z Drainage of Right Lower Extremity Bursa and Ligament with Drainage Device, Percutaneous Endoscopic Approach

0M9V4ZX Drainage of Right Lower Extremity Bursa and Ligament, Percutaneous Endoscopic Approach, Diagnostic

0M9V4ZZ Drainage of Right Lower Extremity Bursa and Ligament, Percutaneous Endoscopic Approach

0M9W00Z Drainage of Left Lower Extremity Bursa and Ligament with Drainage Device, Open Approach

0M9W0ZX Drainage of Left Lower Extremity Bursa and Ligament, Open Approach, Diagnostic

0M9W0ZZ Drainage of Left Lower Extremity Bursa and Ligament, Open Approach

0M9W30Z Drainage of Left Lower Extremity Bursa and Ligament with Drainage Device, Percutaneous Approach

0M9W3ZX Drainage of Left Lower Extremity Bursa and Ligament, Percutaneous Approach, Diagnostic

0M9W3ZZ Drainage of Left Lower Extremity Bursa and Ligament, Percutaneous Approach

0M9W40Z Drainage of Left Lower Extremity Bursa and Ligament with Drainage Device, Percutaneous Endoscopic Approach

0M9W4ZX Drainage of Left Lower Extremity Bursa and Ligament, Percutaneous Endoscopic Approach, Diagnostic

0M9W4ZZ Drainage of Left Lower Extremity Bursa and Ligament, Percutaneous Endoscopic Approach

0MB – Bursae and Ligaments, Excision

Review Coding Guidelines B3.4a and B3.4b

Review Coding Guideline B3.5

Review Coding Guideline B3.8

0MB00ZX Excision of Head and Neck Bursa and Ligament, Open Approach, Diagnostic

0MB00ZZ Excision of Head and Neck Bursa and Ligament, Open Approach

0MB03ZX Excision of Head and Neck Bursa and Ligament, Percutaneous Approach, Diagnostic

0MB03ZZ Excision of Head and Neck Bursa and Ligament, Percutaneous Approach

0MB04ZX Excision of Head and Neck Bursa and Ligament, Percutaneous Endoscopic Approach, Diagnostic

0MB04ZZ Excision of Head and Neck Bursa and Ligament, Percutaneous Endoscopic Approach

0MB10ZX Excision of Right Shoulder Bursa and Ligament, Open Approach, Diagnostic

0MB10ZZ Excision of Right Shoulder Bursa and Ligament, Open Approach

0MB13ZX Excision of Right Shoulder Bursa and Ligament, Percutaneous Approach, Diagnostic

0MB13ZZ Excision of Right Shoulder Bursa and Ligament, Percutaneous Approach

0MB14ZX Excision of Right Shoulder Bursa and Ligament, Percutaneous Endoscopic Approach, Diagnostic

0MB14ZZ Excision of Right Shoulder Bursa and Ligament, Percutaneous Endoscopic Approach

0MB20ZX Excision of Left Shoulder Bursa and Ligament, Open Approach, Diagnostic

0MB20ZZ Excision of Left Shoulder Bursa and Ligament, Open Approach

0MB23ZX Excision of Left Shoulder Bursa and Ligament, Percutaneous Approach, Diagnostic

0MB23ZZ Excision of Left Shoulder Bursa and Ligament, Percutaneous Approach

0MB24ZX Excision of Left Shoulder Bursa and Ligament, Percutaneous Endoscopic Approach, Diagnostic

0MB24ZZ Excision of Left Shoulder Bursa and Ligament, Percutaneous Endoscopic Approach

0MB30ZX Excision of Right Elbow Bursa and Ligament, Open Approach, Diagnostic

0MB30ZZ Excision of Right Elbow Bursa and Ligament, Open Approach

0MB33ZX Excision of Right Elbow Bursa and Ligament, Percutaneous Approach, Diagnostic

0MB33ZZ Excision of Right Elbow Bursa and Ligament, Percutaneous Approach

0MB34ZX Excision of Right Elbow Bursa and Ligament, Percutaneous Endoscopic Approach, Diagnostic

0MB34ZZ Excision of Right Elbow Bursa and Ligament, Percutaneous Endoscopic Approach

0MB40ZX Excision of Left Elbow Bursa and Ligament, Open Approach, Diagnostic

0MB40ZZ Excision of Left Elbow Bursa and Ligament, Open Approach

0MB43ZX Excision of Left Elbow Bursa and Ligament, Percutaneous Approach, Diagnostic

0MB43ZZ Excision of Left Elbow Bursa and Ligament, Percutaneous Approach

0MB44ZX Excision of Left Elbow Bursa and Ligament, Percutaneous Endoscopic Approach, Diagnostic

0MB44ZZ Excision of Left Elbow Bursa and Ligament, Percutaneous Endoscopic Approach

0MB50ZX Excision of Right Wrist Bursa and Ligament, Open Approach, Diagnostic

0MB50ZZ Excision of Right Wrist Bursa and Ligament, Open Approach

0MB53ZX Excision of Right Wrist Bursa and Ligament, Percutaneous Approach, Diagnostic

0MB53ZZ Excision of Right Wrist Bursa and Ligament, Percutaneous Approach

0MB54ZX Excision of Right Wrist Bursa and Ligament, Percutaneous Endoscopic Approach, Diagnostic

0MB54ZZ Excision of Right Wrist Bursa and Ligament, Percutaneous Endoscopic Approach

0MB60ZX Excision of Left Wrist Bursa and Ligament, Open Approach, Diagnostic

0MB60ZZ Excision of Left Wrist Bursa and Ligament, Open Approach

0MB63ZX Excision of Left Wrist Bursa and Ligament, Percutaneous Approach, Diagnostic

0MB63ZZ Excision of Left Wrist Bursa and Ligament, Percutaneous Approach

0MB64ZX Excision of Left Wrist Bursa and Ligament, Percutaneous Endoscopic Approach, Diagnostic

0MB64ZZ Excision of Left Wrist Bursa and Ligament, Percutaneous Endoscopic Approach

0MB70ZX Excision of Right Hand Bursa and Ligament, Open Approach, Diagnostic

0MB70ZZ Excision of Right Hand Bursa and Ligament, Open Approach

0MB73ZX Excision of Right Hand Bursa and Ligament, Percutaneous Approach, Diagnostic

0MB73ZZ Excision of Right Hand Bursa and Ligament, Percutaneous Approach

0MB74ZX Excision of Right Hand Bursa and Ligament, Percutaneous Endoscopic Approach, Diagnostic

0MB74ZZ Excision of Right Hand Bursa and Ligament, Percutaneous Endoscopic Approach

0MB80ZX Excision of Left Hand Bursa and Ligament, Open Approach, Diagnostic

0MB80ZZ Excision of Left Hand Bursa and Ligament, Open Approach

0MB83ZX Excision of Left Hand Bursa and Ligament, Percutaneous Approach, Diagnostic

0MB83ZZ Excision of Left Hand Bursa and Ligament, Percutaneous Approach

0MB84ZX Excision of Left Hand Bursa and Ligament, Percutaneous Endoscopic Approach, Diagnostic

0MB84ZZ Excision of Left Hand Bursa and Ligament, Percutaneous Endoscopic Approach

0MB90ZX Excision of Right Upper Extremity Bursa and Ligament, Open Approach, Diagnostic

0MB90ZZ Excision of Right Upper Extremity Bursa and Ligament, Open Approach

0MB93ZX Excision of Right Upper Extremity Bursa and Ligament, Percutaneous Approach, Diagnostic

0MB93ZZ Excision of Right Upper Extremity Bursa and Ligament, Percutaneous Approach

0MB94ZX Excision of Right Upper Extremity Bursa and Ligament, Percutaneous Endoscopic Approach, Diagnostic

0MB94ZZ Excision of Right Upper Extremity Bursa and Ligament, Percutaneous Endoscopic Approach

0MBB0ZX Excision of Left Upper Extremity Bursa and Ligament, Open Approach, Diagnostic

0MBB0ZZ Excision of Left Upper Extremity Bursa and Ligament, Open Approach

0MBB3ZX Excision of Left Upper Extremity Bursa and Ligament, Percutaneous Approach, Diagnostic

0MBB3ZZ Excision of Left Upper Extremity Bursa and Ligament, Percutaneous Approach

0MBB4ZX Excision of Left Upper Extremity Bursa and Ligament, Percutaneous Endoscopic Approach, Diagnostic

0MBB4ZZ Excision of Left Upper Extremity Bursa and Ligament, Percutaneous Endoscopic Approach

0MBC0ZX Excision of Right Trunk Bursa and Ligament, Open Approach, Diagnostic

0MBC0ZZ Excision of Right Trunk Bursa and Ligament, Open Approach

0MBC3ZX Excision of Right Trunk Bursa and Ligament, Percutaneous Approach, Diagnostic

0MBC3ZZ Excision of Right Trunk Bursa and Ligament, Percutaneous Approach

0MBC4ZX Excision of Right Trunk Bursa and Ligament, Percutaneous Endoscopic Approach, Diagnostic

0MBC4ZZ Excision of Right Trunk Bursa and Ligament, Percutaneous Endoscopic Approach

0MBD0ZX Excision of Left Trunk Bursa and Ligament, Open Approach, Diagnostic

0MBD0ZZ Excision of Left Trunk Bursa and Ligament, Open Approach

0MBD3ZX Excision of Left Trunk Bursa and Ligament, Percutaneous Approach, Diagnostic

0MBD3ZZ Excision of Left Trunk Bursa and Ligament, Percutaneous Approach

0MBD4ZX Excision of Left Trunk Bursa and Ligament, Percutaneous Endoscopic Approach, Diagnostic

0MBD4ZZ Excision of Left Trunk Bursa and Ligament, Percutaneous Endoscopic Approach

0MBF0ZX Excision of Right Thorax Bursa and Ligament, Open Approach, Diagnostic

0MBF0ZZ Excision of Right Thorax Bursa and Ligament, Open Approach

0MBF3ZX Excision of Right Thorax Bursa and Ligament, Percutaneous Approach, Diagnostic

0MBF3ZZ Excision of Right Thorax Bursa and Ligament, Percutaneous Approach

0MBF4ZX Excision of Right Thorax Bursa and Ligament, Percutaneous Endoscopic Approach, Diagnostic

0MBF4ZZ Excision of Right Thorax Bursa and Ligament, Percutaneous Endoscopic Approach

0MBG0ZX Excision of Left Thorax Bursa and Ligament, Open Approach, Diagnostic

0MBG0ZZ Excision of Left Thorax Bursa and Ligament, Open Approach

0MBG3ZX Excision of Left Thorax Bursa and Ligament, Percutaneous Approach, Diagnostic

0MBG3ZZ Excision of Left Thorax Bursa and Ligament, Percutaneous Approach

0MBG4ZX Excision of Left Thorax Bursa and Ligament, Percutaneous Endoscopic Approach, Diagnostic

0MBG4ZZ Excision of Left Thorax Bursa and Ligament, Percutaneous Endoscopic Approach

0MBH0ZX Excision of Right Abdomen Bursa and Ligament, Open Approach, Diagnostic

0MBH0ZZ Excision of Right Abdomen Bursa and Ligament, Open Approach

0MBH3ZX Excision of Right Abdomen Bursa and Ligament, Percutaneous Approach, Diagnostic

0MBH3ZZ Excision of Right Abdomen Bursa and Ligament, Percutaneous Approach

0MBH4ZX Excision of Right Abdomen Bursa and Ligament, Percutaneous Endoscopic Approach, Diagnostic

0MBH4ZZ Excision of Right Abdomen Bursa and Ligament, Percutaneous Endoscopic Approach

0MBJ0ZX Excision of Left Abdomen Bursa and Ligament, Open Approach, Diagnostic

0MBJ0ZZ Excision of Left Abdomen Bursa and Ligament, Open Approach

0MBJ3ZX Excision of Left Abdomen Bursa and Ligament, Percutaneous Approach, Diagnostic

0MBJ3ZZ Excision of Left Abdomen Bursa and Ligament, Percutaneous Approach

0MBJ4ZX Excision of Left Abdomen Bursa and Ligament, Percutaneous Endoscopic Approach, Diagnostic

0MBJ4ZZ Excision of Left Abdomen Bursa and Ligament, Percutaneous Endoscopic Approach

0MBK0ZX Excision of Perineum Bursa and Ligament, Open Approach, Diagnostic

0MBK0ZZ Excision of Perineum Bursa and Ligament, Open Approach

0MBK3ZX Excision of Perineum Bursa and Ligament, Percutaneous Approach, Diagnostic

0MBK3ZZ Excision of Perineum Bursa and Ligament, Percutaneous Approach

0MBK4ZX Excision of Perineum Bursa and Ligament, Percutaneous Endoscopic Approach, Diagnostic

0MBK4ZZ Excision of Perineum Bursa and Ligament, Percutaneous Endoscopic Approach

0MBL0ZX Excision of Right Hip Bursa and Ligament, Open Approach, Diagnostic

0MBL0ZZ Excision of Right Hip Bursa and Ligament, Open Approach

0MBL3ZX Excision of Right Hip Bursa and Ligament, Percutaneous Approach, Diagnostic

0MBL3ZZ Excision of Right Hip Bursa and Ligament, Percutaneous Approach

0MBL4ZX Excision of Right Hip Bursa and Ligament, Percutaneous Endoscopic Approach, Diagnostic

0MBL4ZZ Excision of Right Hip Bursa and Ligament, Percutaneous Endoscopic Approach

0MBM0ZX Excision of Left Hip Bursa and Ligament, Open Approach, Diagnostic

0MBM0ZZ Excision of Left Hip Bursa and Ligament, Open Approach

0MBM3ZX Excision of Left Hip Bursa and Ligament, Percutaneous Approach, Diagnostic

0MBM3ZZ Excision of Left Hip Bursa and Ligament, Percutaneous Approach

0MBM4ZX Excision of Left Hip Bursa and Ligament, Percutaneous Endoscopic Approach, Diagnostic

0MBM4ZZ Excision of Left Hip Bursa and Ligament, Percutaneous Endoscopic Approach

0MBN0ZX Excision of Right Knee Bursa and Ligament, Open Approach, Diagnostic

0MBN0ZZ Excision of Right Knee Bursa and Ligament, Open Approach

0MBN3ZX Excision of Right Knee Bursa and Ligament, Percutaneous Approach, Diagnostic

0MBN3ZZ Excision of Right Knee Bursa and Ligament, Percutaneous Approach

0MBN4ZX Excision of Right Knee Bursa and Ligament, Percutaneous Endoscopic Approach, Diagnostic

0MBN4ZZ Excision of Right Knee Bursa and Ligament, Percutaneous Endoscopic Approach

0MBP0ZX Excision of Left Knee Bursa and Ligament, Open Approach, Diagnostic

0MBP0ZZ Excision of Left Knee Bursa and Ligament, Open Approach

0MBP3ZX Excision of Left Knee Bursa and Ligament, Percutaneous Approach, Diagnostic

0MBP3ZZ Excision of Left Knee Bursa and Ligament, Percutaneous Approach

0MBP4ZX Excision of Left Knee Bursa and Ligament, Percutaneous Endoscopic Approach, Diagnostic

0MBP4ZZ Excision of Left Knee Bursa and Ligament, Percutaneous Endoscopic Approach

0MBQ0ZX Excision of Right Ankle Bursa and Ligament, Open Approach, Diagnostic

0MBQ0ZZ Excision of Right Ankle Bursa and Ligament, Open Approach

0MBQ3ZX Excision of Right Ankle Bursa and Ligament, Percutaneous Approach, Diagnostic

0MBQ3ZZ Excision of Right Ankle Bursa and Ligament, Percutaneous Approach

0MBQ4ZX Excision of Right Ankle Bursa and Ligament, Percutaneous Endoscopic Approach, Diagnostic

0MBQ4ZZ Excision of Right Ankle Bursa and Ligament, Percutaneous Endoscopic Approach

0MBR0ZX Excision of Left Ankle Bursa and Ligament, Open Approach, Diagnostic

0MBR0ZZ Excision of Left Ankle Bursa and Ligament, Open Approach

0MBR3ZX Excision of Left Ankle Bursa and Ligament, Percutaneous Approach, Diagnostic

0MBR3ZZ Excision of Left Ankle Bursa and Ligament, Percutaneous Approach

0MBR4ZX Excision of Left Ankle Bursa and Ligament, Percutaneous Endoscopic Approach, Diagnostic

0MBR4ZZ Excision of Left Ankle Bursa and Ligament, Percutaneous Endoscopic Approach

0MBS0ZX Excision of Right Foot Bursa and Ligament, Open Approach, Diagnostic

0MBS0ZZ Excision of Right Foot Bursa and Ligament, Open Approach

0MBS3ZX Excision of Right Foot Bursa and Ligament, Percutaneous Approach, Diagnostic

0MBS3ZZ Excision of Right Foot Bursa and Ligament, Percutaneous Approach

0MBS4ZX Excision of Right Foot Bursa and Ligament, Percutaneous Endoscopic Approach, Diagnostic

0MBS4ZZ Excision of Right Foot Bursa and Ligament, Percutaneous Endoscopic Approach

0MBT0ZX Excision of Left Foot Bursa and Ligament, Open Approach, Diagnostic

0MBT0ZZ Excision of Left Foot Bursa and Ligament, Open Approach

0MBT3ZX Excision of Left Foot Bursa and Ligament, Percutaneous Approach, Diagnostic

0MBT3ZZ Excision of Left Foot Bursa and Ligament, Percutaneous Approach

0MBT4ZX Excision of Left Foot Bursa and Ligament, Percutaneous Endoscopic Approach, Diagnostic

0MBT4ZZ Excision of Left Foot Bursa and Ligament, Percutaneous Endoscopic Approach

0MBV0ZX Excision of Right Lower Extremity Bursa and Ligament, Open Approach, Diagnostic

0MBV0ZZ Excision of Right Lower Extremity Bursa and Ligament, Open Approach

0MBV3ZX Excision of Right Lower Extremity Bursa and Ligament, Percutaneous Approach, Diagnostic

0MBV3ZZ Excision of Right Lower Extremity Bursa and Ligament, Percutaneous Approach

0MBV4ZX Excision of Right Lower Extremity Bursa and Ligament, Percutaneous Endoscopic Approach, Diagnostic

0MBV4ZZ Excision of Right Lower Extremity Bursa and Ligament, Percutaneous Endoscopic Approach

0MBW0ZX Excision of Left Lower Extremity Bursa and Ligament, Open Approach, Diagnostic

0MBW0ZZ Excision of Left Lower Extremity Bursa and Ligament, Open Approach

0MBW3ZX Excision of Left Lower Extremity Bursa and Ligament, Percutaneous Approach, Diagnostic

0MBW3ZZ Excision of Left Lower Extremity Bursa and Ligament, Percutaneous Approach

0MBW4ZX Excision of Left Lower Extremity Bursa and Ligament, Percutaneous Endoscopic Approach, Diagnostic

0MBW4ZZ Excision of Left Lower Extremity Bursa and Ligament, Percutaneous Endoscopic Approach

0MC – Bursae and Ligaments, Extirpation

0MC00ZZ Extirpation of Matter from Head and Neck Bursa and Ligament, Open Approach

0MC03ZZ Extirpation of Matter from Head and Neck Bursa and Ligament, Percutaneous Approach

0MC04ZZ Extirpation of Matter from Head and Neck Bursa and Ligament, Percutaneous Endoscopic Approach

0MC10ZZ Extirpation of Matter from Right Shoulder Bursa and Ligament, Open Approach

0MC13ZZ Extirpation of Matter from Right Shoulder Bursa and Ligament, Percutaneous Approach

0MC14ZZ Extirpation of Matter from Right Shoulder Bursa and Ligament, Percutaneous Endoscopic Approach

0MC20ZZ Extirpation of Matter from Left Shoulder Bursa and Ligament, Open Approach

0MC23ZZ Extirpation of Matter from Left Shoulder Bursa and Ligament, Percutaneous Approach

0MC24ZZ Extirpation of Matter from Left Shoulder Bursa and Ligament, Percutaneous Endoscopic Approach

0MC30ZZ Extirpation of Matter from Right Elbow Bursa and Ligament, Open Approach

0MC33ZZ Extirpation of Matter from Right Elbow Bursa and Ligament, Percutaneous Approach

0MC34ZZ Extirpation of Matter from Right Elbow Bursa and Ligament, Percutaneous Endoscopic Approach

0MC40ZZ Extirpation of Matter from Left Elbow Bursa and Ligament, Open Approach

0MC43ZZ Extirpation of Matter from Left Elbow Bursa and Ligament, Percutaneous Approach

0MC44ZZ Extirpation of Matter from Left Elbow Bursa and Ligament, Percutaneous Endoscopic Approach

0MC50ZZ Extirpation of Matter from Right Wrist Bursa and Ligament, Open Approach

0MC53ZZ Extirpation of Matter from Right Wrist Bursa and Ligament, Percutaneous Approach

0MC54ZZ Extirpation of Matter from Right Wrist Bursa and Ligament, Percutaneous Endoscopic Approach

0MC60ZZ Extirpation of Matter from Left Wrist Bursa and Ligament, Open Approach

0MC63ZZ Extirpation of Matter from Left Wrist Bursa and Ligament, Percutaneous Approach

0MC64ZZ Extirpation of Matter from Left Wrist Bursa and Ligament, Percutaneous Endoscopic Approach

0MC70ZZ Extirpation of Matter from Right Hand Bursa and Ligament, Open Approach

0MC73ZZ Extirpation of Matter from Right Hand Bursa and Ligament, Percutaneous Approach

0MC74ZZ Extirpation of Matter from Right Hand Bursa and Ligament, Percutaneous Endoscopic Approach

0MC80ZZ Extirpation of Matter from Left Hand Bursa and Ligament, Open Approach

0MC83ZZ Extirpation of Matter from Left Hand Bursa and Ligament, Percutaneous Approach

0MC84ZZ Extirpation of Matter from Left Hand Bursa and Ligament, Percutaneous Endoscopic Approach

0MC90ZZ Extirpation of Matter from Right Upper Extremity Bursa and Ligament, Open Approach

0MC93ZZ Extirpation of Matter from Right Upper Extremity Bursa and Ligament, Percutaneous Approach

0MC94ZZ Extirpation of Matter from Right Upper Extremity Bursa and Ligament, Percutaneous Endoscopic Approach

0MCB0ZZ Extirpation of Matter from Left Upper Extremity Bursa and Ligament, Open Approach

0MCB3ZZ Extirpation of Matter from Left Upper Extremity Bursa and Ligament, Percutaneous Approach

0MCB4ZZ Extirpation of Matter from Left Upper Extremity Bursa and Ligament, Percutaneous Endoscopic Approach

0MCC0ZZ Extirpation of Matter from Right Trunk Bursa and Ligament, Open Approach

0MCC3ZZ Extirpation of Matter from Right Trunk Bursa and Ligament, Percutaneous Approach

0MCC4ZZ Extirpation of Matter from Right Trunk Bursa and Ligament, Percutaneous Endoscopic Approach

0MCD0ZZ Extirpation of Matter from Left Trunk Bursa and Ligament, Open Approach

0MCD3ZZ Extirpation of Matter from Left Trunk Bursa and Ligament, Percutaneous Approach

0MCD4ZZ Extirpation of Matter from Left Trunk Bursa and Ligament, Percutaneous Endoscopic Approach

0MCF0ZZ Extirpation of Matter from Right Thorax Bursa and Ligament, Open Approach

0MCF3ZZ Extirpation of Matter from Right Thorax Bursa and Ligament, Percutaneous Approach

0MCF4ZZ Extirpation of Matter from Right Thorax Bursa and Ligament, Percutaneous Endoscopic Approach

0MCG0ZZ Extirpation of Matter from Left Thorax Bursa and Ligament, Open Approach

0MCG3ZZ Extirpation of Matter from Left Thorax Bursa and Ligament, Percutaneous Approach

0MCG4ZZ Extirpation of Matter from Left Thorax Bursa and Ligament, Percutaneous Endoscopic Approach

0MCH0ZZ Extirpation of Matter from Right Abdomen Bursa and Ligament, Open Approach

0MCH3ZZ Extirpation of Matter from Right Abdomen Bursa and Ligament, Percutaneous Approach

0MCH4ZZ Extirpation of Matter from Right Abdomen Bursa and Ligament, Percutaneous Endoscopic Approach

0MCJ0ZZ Extirpation of Matter from Left Abdomen Bursa and Ligament, Open Approach

0MCJ3ZZ Extirpation of Matter from Left Abdomen Bursa and Ligament, Percutaneous Approach

0MCJ4ZZ Extirpation of Matter from Left Abdomen Bursa and Ligament, Percutaneous Endoscopic Approach

0MCK0ZZ Extirpation of Matter from Perineum Bursa and Ligament, Open Approach

0MCK3ZZ Extirpation of Matter from Perineum Bursa and Ligament, Percutaneous Approach

0MCK4ZZ Extirpation of Matter from Perineum Bursa and Ligament, Percutaneous Endoscopic Approach

0MCL0ZZ Extirpation of Matter from Right Hip Bursa and Ligament, Open Approach

0MCL3ZZ Extirpation of Matter from Right Hip Bursa and Ligament, Percutaneous Approach

0MCL4ZZ Extirpation of Matter from Right Hip Bursa and Ligament, Percutaneous Endoscopic Approach

0MCM0ZZ Extirpation of Matter from Left Hip Bursa and Ligament, Open Approach

0MCM3ZZ Extirpation of Matter from Left Hip Bursa and Ligament, Percutaneous Approach

0MCM4ZZ Extirpation of Matter from Left Hip Bursa and Ligament, Percutaneous Endoscopic Approach

0MCN0ZZ Extirpation of Matter from Right Knee Bursa and Ligament, Open Approach

0MCN3ZZ Extirpation of Matter from Right Knee Bursa and Ligament, Percutaneous Approach

0MCN4ZZ Extirpation of Matter from Right Knee Bursa and Ligament, Percutaneous Endoscopic Approach

0MCP0ZZ Extirpation of Matter from Left Knee Bursa and Ligament, Open Approach

0MCP3ZZ Extirpation of Matter from Left Knee Bursa and Ligament, Percutaneous Approach

0MCP4ZZ Extirpation of Matter from Left Knee Bursa and Ligament, Percutaneous Endoscopic Approach

0MCQ0ZZ Extirpation of Matter from Right Ankle Bursa and Ligament, Open Approach

0MCQ3ZZ Extirpation of Matter from Right Ankle Bursa and Ligament, Percutaneous Approach

0MCQ4ZZ Extirpation of Matter from Right Ankle Bursa and Ligament, Percutaneous Endoscopic Approach

0MCR0ZZ Extirpation of Matter from Left Ankle Bursa and Ligament, Open Approach

0MCR3ZZ Extirpation of Matter from Left Ankle Bursa and Ligament, Percutaneous Approach

0MCR4ZZ Extirpation of Matter from Left Ankle Bursa and Ligament, Percutaneous Endoscopic Approach

0MCS0ZZ Extirpation of Matter from Right Foot Bursa and Ligament, Open Approach

0MCS3ZZ Extirpation of Matter from Right Foot Bursa and Ligament, Percutaneous Approach

0MCS4ZZ Extirpation of Matter from Right Foot Bursa and Ligament, Percutaneous Endoscopic Approach

0MCT0ZZ Extirpation of Matter from Left Foot Bursa and Ligament, Open Approach

0MCT3ZZ Extirpation of Matter from Left Foot Bursa and Ligament, Percutaneous Approach

0MCT4ZZ Extirpation of Matter from Left Foot Bursa and Ligament, Percutaneous Endoscopic Approach

0MCV0ZZ Extirpation of Matter from Right Lower Extremity Bursa and Ligament, Open Approach

0MCV3ZZ Extirpation of Matter from Right Lower Extremity Bursa and Ligament, Percutaneous Approach

0MCV4ZZ Extirpation of Matter from Right Lower Extremity Bursa and Ligament, Percutaneous Endoscopic Approach

0MCW0ZZ Extirpation of Matter from Left Lower Extremity Bursa and Ligament, Open Approach

0MCW3ZZ Extirpation of Matter from Left Lower Extremity Bursa and Ligament, Percutaneous Approach

0MCW4ZZ Extirpation of Matter from Left Lower Extremity Bursa and Ligament, Percutaneous Endoscopic Approach

0MD – Bursae and Ligaments, Extraction

0MD00ZZ Extraction of Head and Neck Bursa and Ligament, Open Approach

0MD03ZZ Extraction of Head and Neck Bursa and Ligament, Percutaneous Approach

0MD04ZZ Extraction of Head and Neck Bursa and Ligament, Percutaneous Endoscopic Approach

0MD10ZZ Extraction of Right Shoulder Bursa and Ligament, Open Approach

0MD13ZZ Extraction of Right Shoulder Bursa and Ligament, Percutaneous Approach

0MD14ZZ Extraction of Right Shoulder Bursa and Ligament, Percutaneous Endoscopic Approach

0MD20ZZ Extraction of Left Shoulder Bursa and Ligament, Open Approach

0MD23ZZ Extraction of Left Shoulder Bursa and Ligament, Percutaneous Approach

0MD24ZZ Extraction of Left Shoulder Bursa and Ligament, Percutaneous Endoscopic Approach

0MD30ZZ Extraction of Right Elbow Bursa and Ligament, Open Approach

0MD33ZZ Extraction of Right Elbow Bursa and Ligament, Percutaneous Approach

0MD34ZZ Extraction of Right Elbow Bursa and Ligament, Percutaneous Endoscopic Approach

0MD40ZZ Extraction of Left Elbow Bursa and Ligament, Open Approach

0MD43ZZ Extraction of Left Elbow Bursa and Ligament, Percutaneous Approach

0MD44ZZ Extraction of Left Elbow Bursa and Ligament, Percutaneous Endoscopic Approach

0MD50ZZ Extraction of Right Wrist Bursa and Ligament, Open Approach

0MD53ZZ Extraction of Right Wrist Bursa and Ligament, Percutaneous Approach

0MD54ZZ Extraction of Right Wrist Bursa and Ligament, Percutaneous Endoscopic Approach

0MD60ZZ Extraction of Left Wrist Bursa and Ligament, Open Approach

0MD63ZZ Extraction of Left Wrist Bursa and Ligament, Percutaneous Approach

0MD64ZZ Extraction of Left Wrist Bursa and Ligament, Percutaneous Endoscopic Approach

0MD70ZZ Extraction of Right Hand Bursa and Ligament, Open Approach

0MD73ZZ Extraction of Right Hand Bursa and Ligament, Percutaneous Approach

0MD74ZZ Extraction of Right Hand Bursa and Ligament, Percutaneous Endoscopic Approach

0MD80ZZ Extraction of Left Hand Bursa and Ligament, Open Approach

0MD83ZZ Extraction of Left Hand Bursa and Ligament, Percutaneous Approach

0MD84ZZ Extraction of Left Hand Bursa and Ligament, Percutaneous Endoscopic Approach

0MD90ZZ Extraction of Right Upper Extremity Bursa and Ligament, Open Approach

0MD93ZZ Extraction of Right Upper Extremity Bursa and Ligament, Percutaneous Approach

0MD94ZZ Extraction of Right Upper Extremity Bursa and Ligament, Percutaneous Endoscopic Approach

0MDB0ZZ Extraction of Left Upper Extremity Bursa and Ligament, Open Approach

0MDB3ZZ Extraction of Left Upper Extremity Bursa and Ligament, Percutaneous Approach

0MDB4ZZ Extraction of Left Upper Extremity Bursa and Ligament, Percutaneous Endoscopic Approach

0MDC0ZZ Extraction of Right Trunk Bursa and Ligament, Open Approach

0MDC3ZZ Extraction of Right Trunk Bursa and Ligament, Percutaneous Approach

0MDC4ZZ Extraction of Right Trunk Bursa and Ligament, Percutaneous Endoscopic Approach

0MDD0ZZ Extraction of Left Trunk Bursa and Ligament, Open Approach

0MDD3ZZ Extraction of Left Trunk Bursa and Ligament, Percutaneous Approach

0MDD4ZZ Extraction of Left Trunk Bursa and Ligament, Percutaneous Endoscopic Approach

0MDF0ZZ Extraction of Right Thorax Bursa and Ligament, Open Approach

0MDF3ZZ Extraction of Right Thorax Bursa and Ligament, Percutaneous Approach

0MDF4ZZ Extraction of Right Thorax Bursa and Ligament, Percutaneous Endoscopic Approach

0MDG0ZZ Extraction of Left Thorax Bursa and Ligament, Open Approach

0MDG3ZZ Extraction of Left Thorax Bursa and Ligament, Percutaneous Approach

0MDG4ZZ Extraction of Left Thorax Bursa and Ligament, Percutaneous Endoscopic Approach

0MDH0ZZ Extraction of Right Abdomen Bursa and Ligament, Open Approach

0MDH3ZZ Extraction of Right Abdomen Bursa and Ligament, Percutaneous Approach

0MDH4ZZ Extraction of Right Abdomen Bursa and Ligament, Percutaneous Endoscopic Approach

0MDJ0ZZ Extraction of Left Abdomen Bursa and Ligament, Open Approach

0MDJ3ZZ Extraction of Left Abdomen Bursa and Ligament, Percutaneous Approach

0MDJ4ZZ Extraction of Left Abdomen Bursa and Ligament, Percutaneous Endoscopic Approach

0MDK0ZZ Extraction of Perineum Bursa and Ligament, Open Approach

0MDK3ZZ Extraction of Perineum Bursa and Ligament, Percutaneous Approach

0MDK4ZZ Extraction of Perineum Bursa and Ligament, Percutaneous Endoscopic Approach

0MDL0ZZ Extraction of Right Hip Bursa and Ligament, Open Approach

0MDL3ZZ Extraction of Right Hip Bursa and Ligament, Percutaneous Approach

0MDL4ZZ Extraction of Right Hip Bursa and Ligament, Percutaneous Endoscopic Approach

0MDM0ZZ Extraction of Left Hip Bursa and Ligament, Open Approach

0MDM3ZZ Extraction of Left Hip Bursa and Ligament, Percutaneous Approach

0MDM4ZZ Extraction of Left Hip Bursa and Ligament, Percutaneous Endoscopic Approach

0MDN0ZZ Extraction of Right Knee Bursa and Ligament, Open Approach

0MDN3ZZ Extraction of Right Knee Bursa and Ligament, Percutaneous Approach

0MDN4ZZ Extraction of Right Knee Bursa and Ligament, Percutaneous Endoscopic Approach

0MDP0ZZ Extraction of Left Knee Bursa and Ligament, Open Approach

0MDP3ZZ Extraction of Left Knee Bursa and Ligament, Percutaneous Approach

0MDP4ZZ Extraction of Left Knee Bursa and Ligament, Percutaneous Endoscopic Approach

0MDQ0ZZ Extraction of Right Ankle Bursa and Ligament, Open Approach

0MDQ3ZZ Extraction of Right Ankle Bursa and Ligament, Percutaneous Approach

0MDQ4ZZ Extraction of Right Ankle Bursa and Ligament, Percutaneous Endoscopic Approach

0MDR0ZZ Extraction of Left Ankle Bursa and Ligament, Open Approach

0MDR3ZZ Extraction of Left Ankle Bursa and Ligament, Percutaneous Approach

0MDR4ZZ Extraction of Left Ankle Bursa and Ligament, Percutaneous Endoscopic Approach

0MDS0ZZ Extraction of Right Foot Bursa and Ligament, Open Approach

0MDS3ZZ Extraction of Right Foot Bursa and Ligament, Percutaneous Approach

0MDS4ZZ Extraction of Right Foot Bursa and Ligament, Percutaneous Endoscopic Approach

0MDT0ZZ Extraction of Left Foot Bursa and Ligament, Open Approach

0MDT3ZZ Extraction of Left Foot Bursa and Ligament, Percutaneous Approach

0MDT4ZZ Extraction of Left Foot Bursa and Ligament, Percutaneous Endoscopic Approach

0MDV0ZZ Extraction of Right Lower Extremity Bursa and Ligament, Open Approach

0MDV3ZZ Extraction of Right Lower Extremity Bursa and Ligament, Percutaneous Approach

0MDV4ZZ Extraction of Right Lower Extremity Bursa and Ligament, Percutaneous Endoscopic Approach

0MDW0ZZ Extraction of Left Lower Extremity Bursa and Ligament, Open Approach

0MDW3ZZ Extraction of Left Lower Extremity Bursa and Ligament, Percutaneous Approach

0MDW4ZZ Extraction of Left Lower Extremity Bursa and Ligament, Percutaneous Endoscopic Approach

0MJ – Bursae and Ligaments, Inspection

Review Coding Guideline B3.5

Review Coding Guidelines B3.11a, B3.11b and B3.11c

0MJX0ZZ Inspection of Upper Bursa and Ligament, Open Approach

0MJX3ZZ Inspection of Upper Bursa and Ligament, Percutaneous Approach

0MJX4ZZ Inspection of Upper Bursa and Ligament, Percutaneous Endoscopic Approach

0MJXXZZ Inspection of Upper Bursa and Ligament, External Approach

0MJY0ZZ Inspection of Lower Bursa and Ligament, Open Approach

0MJY3ZZ Inspection of Lower Bursa and Ligament, Percutaneous Approach

0MJY4ZZ Inspection of Lower Bursa and Ligament, Percutaneous Endoscopic Approach

0MJYXZZ Inspection of Lower Bursa and Ligament, External Approach

0MM – Bursae and Ligaments, Reattachment

0MM00ZZ Reattachment of Head and Neck Bursa and Ligament, Open Approach

0MM04ZZ Reattachment of Head and Neck Bursa and Ligament, Percutaneous Endoscopic Approach

0MM10ZZ Reattachment of Right Shoulder Bursa and Ligament, Open Approach

0MM14ZZ Reattachment of Right Shoulder Bursa and Ligament, Percutaneous Endoscopic Approach

0MM20ZZ Reattachment of Left Shoulder Bursa and Ligament, Open Approach

0MM24ZZ Reattachment of Left Shoulder Bursa and Ligament, Percutaneous Endoscopic Approach

0MM30ZZ Reattachment of Right Elbow Bursa and Ligament, Open Approach

0MM34ZZ Reattachment of Right Elbow Bursa and Ligament, Percutaneous Endoscopic Approach

0MM40ZZ Reattachment of Left Elbow Bursa and Ligament, Open Approach

0MM44ZZ Reattachment of Left Elbow Bursa and Ligament, Percutaneous Endoscopic Approach

0MM50ZZ Reattachment of Right Wrist Bursa and Ligament, Open Approach

0MM54ZZ Reattachment of Right Wrist Bursa and Ligament, Percutaneous Endoscopic Approach

0MM60ZZ Reattachment of Left Wrist Bursa and Ligament, Open Approach

0MM64ZZ Reattachment of Left Wrist Bursa and Ligament, Percutaneous Endoscopic Approach
0MM70ZZ Reattachment of Right Hand Bursa and Ligament, Open Approach
0MM74ZZ Reattachment of Right Hand Bursa and Ligament, Percutaneous Endoscopic Approach
0MM80ZZ Reattachment of Left Hand Bursa and Ligament, Open Approach
0MM84ZZ Reattachment of Left Hand Bursa and Ligament, Percutaneous Endoscopic Approach
0MM90ZZ Reattachment of Right Upper Extremity Bursa and Ligament, Open Approach
0MM94ZZ Reattachment of Right Upper Extremity Bursa and Ligament, Percutaneous Endoscopic Approach
0MMB0ZZ Reattachment of Left Upper Extremity Bursa and Ligament, Open Approach
0MMB4ZZ Reattachment of Left Upper Extremity Bursa and Ligament, Percutaneous Endoscopic Approach
0MMC0ZZ Reattachment of Right Trunk Bursa and Ligament, Open Approach
0MMC4ZZ Reattachment of Right Trunk Bursa and Ligament, Percutaneous Endoscopic Approach
0MMD0ZZ Reattachment of Left Trunk Bursa and Ligament, Open Approach
0MMD4ZZ Reattachment of Left Trunk Bursa and Ligament, Percutaneous Endoscopic Approach
0MMF0ZZ Reattachment of Right Thorax Bursa and Ligament, Open Approach
0MMF4ZZ Reattachment of Right Thorax Bursa and Ligament, Percutaneous Endoscopic Approach
0MMG0ZZ Reattachment of Left Thorax Bursa and Ligament, Open Approach
0MMG4ZZ Reattachment of Left Thorax Bursa and Ligament, Percutaneous Endoscopic Approach
0MMH0ZZ Reattachment of Right Abdomen Bursa and Ligament, Open Approach
0MMH4ZZ Reattachment of Right Abdomen Bursa and Ligament, Percutaneous Endoscopic Approach
0MMJ0ZZ Reattachment of Left Abdomen Bursa and Ligament, Open Approach
0MMJ4ZZ Reattachment of Left Abdomen Bursa and Ligament, Percutaneous Endoscopic Approach

0MMK0ZZ Reattachment of Perineum Bursa and Ligament, Open Approach
0MMK4ZZ Reattachment of Perineum Bursa and Ligament, Percutaneous Endoscopic Approach
0MML0ZZ Reattachment of Right Hip Bursa and Ligament, Open Approach
0MML4ZZ Reattachment of Right Hip Bursa and Ligament, Percutaneous Endoscopic Approach
0MMM0ZZ Reattachment of Left Hip Bursa and Ligament, Open Approach
0MMM4ZZ Reattachment of Left Hip Bursa and Ligament, Percutaneous Endoscopic Approach
0MMN0ZZ Reattachment of Right Knee Bursa and Ligament, Open Approach
0MMN4ZZ Reattachment of Right Knee Bursa and Ligament, Percutaneous Endoscopic Approach
0MMP0ZZ Reattachment of Left Knee Bursa and Ligament, Open Approach
0MMP4ZZ Reattachment of Left Knee Bursa and Ligament, Percutaneous Endoscopic Approach
0MMQ0ZZ Reattachment of Right Ankle Bursa and Ligament, Open Approach
0MMQ4ZZ Reattachment of Right Ankle Bursa and Ligament, Percutaneous Endoscopic Approach
0MMR0ZZ Reattachment of Left Ankle Bursa and Ligament, Open Approach
0MMR4ZZ Reattachment of Left Ankle Bursa and Ligament, Percutaneous Endoscopic Approach
0MMS0ZZ Reattachment of Right Foot Bursa and Ligament, Open Approach
0MMS4ZZ Reattachment of Right Foot Bursa and Ligament, Percutaneous Endoscopic Approach
0MMT0ZZ Reattachment of Left Foot Bursa and Ligament, Open Approach
0MMT4ZZ Reattachment of Left Foot Bursa and Ligament, Percutaneous Endoscopic Approach
0MMV0ZZ Reattachment of Right Lower Extremity Bursa and Ligament, Open Approach
0MMV4ZZ Reattachment of Right Lower Extremity Bursa and Ligament, Percutaneous Endoscopic Approach
0MMW0ZZ Reattachment of Left Lower Extremity Bursa and Ligament, Open Approach
0MMW4ZZ Reattachment of Left Lower Extremity Bursa and Ligament, Percutaneous Endoscopic Approach

0MN – Bursae and Ligaments, Release

Review Coding Guideline B3.13

Review Coding Guideline B3.14

0MN00ZZ Release Head and Neck Bursa and Ligament, Open Approach
0MN03ZZ Release Head and Neck Bursa and Ligament, Percutaneous Approach
0MN04ZZ Release Head and Neck Bursa and Ligament, Percutaneous Endoscopic Approach
0MN0XZZ Release Head and Neck Bursa and Ligament, External Approach
0MN10ZZ Release Right Shoulder Bursa and Ligament, Open Approach
0MN13ZZ Release Right Shoulder Bursa and Ligament, Percutaneous Approach
0MN14ZZ Release Right Shoulder Bursa and Ligament, Percutaneous Endoscopic Approach
0MN1XZZ Release Right Shoulder Bursa and Ligament, External Approach
0MN20ZZ Release Left Shoulder Bursa and Ligament, Open Approach
0MN23ZZ Release Left Shoulder Bursa and Ligament, Percutaneous Approach
0MN24ZZ Release Left Shoulder Bursa and Ligament, Percutaneous Endoscopic Approach
0MN2XZZ Release Left Shoulder Bursa and Ligament, External Approach
0MN30ZZ Release Right Elbow Bursa and Ligament, Open Approach
0MN33ZZ Release Right Elbow Bursa and Ligament, Percutaneous Approach
0MN34ZZ Release Right Elbow Bursa and Ligament, Percutaneous Endoscopic Approach
0MN3XZZ Release Right Elbow Bursa and Ligament, External Approach
0MN40ZZ Release Left Elbow Bursa and Ligament, Open Approach
0MN43ZZ Release Left Elbow Bursa and Ligament, Percutaneous Approach
0MN44ZZ Release Left Elbow Bursa and Ligament, Percutaneous Endoscopic Approach
0MN4XZZ Release Left Elbow Bursa and Ligament, External Approach
0MN50ZZ Release Right Wrist Bursa and Ligament, Open Approach

0MN53ZZ Release Right Wrist Bursa and Ligament, Percutaneous Approach
0MN54ZZ Release Right Wrist Bursa and Ligament, Percutaneous Endoscopic Approach
0MN5XZZ Release Right Wrist Bursa and Ligament, External Approach
0MN60ZZ Release Left Wrist Bursa and Ligament, Open Approach
0MN63ZZ Release Left Wrist Bursa and Ligament, Percutaneous Approach
0MN64ZZ Release Left Wrist Bursa and Ligament, Percutaneous Endoscopic Approach
0MN6XZZ Release Left Wrist Bursa and Ligament, External Approach
0MN70ZZ Release Right Hand Bursa and Ligament, Open Approach
0MN73ZZ Release Right Hand Bursa and Ligament, Percutaneous Approach
0MN74ZZ Release Right Hand Bursa and Ligament, Percutaneous Endoscopic Approach
0MN7XZZ Release Right Hand Bursa and Ligament, External Approach
0MN80ZZ Release Left Hand Bursa and Ligament, Open Approach
0MN83ZZ Release Left Hand Bursa and Ligament, Percutaneous Approach
0MN84ZZ Release Left Hand Bursa and Ligament, Percutaneous Endoscopic Approach
0MN8XZZ Release Left Hand Bursa and Ligament, External Approach
0MN90ZZ Release Right Upper Extremity Bursa and Ligament, Open Approach
0MN93ZZ Release Right Upper Extremity Bursa and Ligament, Percutaneous Approach
0MN94ZZ Release Right Upper Extremity Bursa and Ligament, Percutaneous Endoscopic Approach
0MN9XZZ Release Right Upper Extremity Bursa and Ligament, External Approach

0MNB0ZZ	Release Left Upper Extremity Bursa and Ligament, Open Approach
0MNB3ZZ	Release Left Upper Extremity Bursa and Ligament, Percutaneous Approach
0MNB4ZZ	Release Left Upper Extremity Bursa and Ligament, Percutaneous Endoscopic Approach
0MNBXZZ	Release Left Upper Extremity Bursa and Ligament, External Approach
0MNC0ZZ	Release Right Trunk Bursa and Ligament, Open Approach
0MNC3ZZ	Release Right Trunk Bursa and Ligament, Percutaneous Approach
0MNC4ZZ	Release Right Trunk Bursa and Ligament, Percutaneous Endoscopic Approach
0MNCXZZ	Release Right Trunk Bursa and Ligament, External Approach
0MND0ZZ	Release Left Trunk Bursa and Ligament, Open Approach
0MND3ZZ	Release Left Trunk Bursa and Ligament, Percutaneous Approach
0MND4ZZ	Release Left Trunk Bursa and Ligament, Percutaneous Endoscopic Approach
0MNDXZZ	Release Left Trunk Bursa and Ligament, External Approach
0MNF0ZZ	Release Right Thorax Bursa and Ligament, Open Approach
0MNF3ZZ	Release Right Thorax Bursa and Ligament, Percutaneous Approach
0MNF4ZZ	Release Right Thorax Bursa and Ligament, Percutaneous Endoscopic Approach
0MNFXZZ	Release Right Thorax Bursa and Ligament, External Approach
0MNG0ZZ	Release Left Thorax Bursa and Ligament, Open Approach
0MNG3ZZ	Release Left Thorax Bursa and Ligament, Percutaneous Approach
0MNG4ZZ	Release Left Thorax Bursa and Ligament, Percutaneous Endoscopic Approach
0MNGXZZ	Release Left Thorax Bursa and Ligament, External Approach
0MNH0ZZ	Release Right Abdomen Bursa and Ligament, Open Approach
0MNH3ZZ	Release Right Abdomen Bursa and Ligament, Percutaneous Approach
0MNH4ZZ	Release Right Abdomen Bursa and Ligament, Percutaneous Endoscopic Approach
0MNHXZZ	Release Right Abdomen Bursa and Ligament, External Approach
0MNJ0ZZ	Release Left Abdomen Bursa and Ligament, Open Approach
0MNJ3ZZ	Release Left Abdomen Bursa and Ligament, Percutaneous Approach
0MNJ4ZZ	Release Left Abdomen Bursa and Ligament, Percutaneous Endoscopic Approach
0MNJXZZ	Release Left Abdomen Bursa and Ligament, External Approach
0MNK0ZZ	Release Perineum Bursa and Ligament, Open Approach
0MNK3ZZ	Release Perineum Bursa and Ligament, Percutaneous Approach
0MNK4ZZ	Release Perineum Bursa and Ligament, Percutaneous Endoscopic Approach
0MNKXZZ	Release Perineum Bursa and Ligament, External Approach
0MNL0ZZ	Release Right Hip Bursa and Ligament, Open Approach
0MNL3ZZ	Release Right Hip Bursa and Ligament, Percutaneous Approach
0MNL4ZZ	Release Right Hip Bursa and Ligament, Percutaneous Endoscopic Approach
0MNLXZZ	Release Right Hip Bursa and Ligament, External Approach

0MNM0ZZ	Release Left Hip Bursa and Ligament, Open Approach
0MNM3ZZ	Release Left Hip Bursa and Ligament, Percutaneous Approach
0MNM4ZZ	Release Left Hip Bursa and Ligament, Percutaneous Endoscopic Approach
0MNMXZZ	Release Left Hip Bursa and Ligament, External Approach
0MNN0ZZ	Release Right Knee Bursa and Ligament, Open Approach
0MNN3ZZ	Release Right Knee Bursa and Ligament, Percutaneous Approach
0MNN4ZZ	Release Right Knee Bursa and Ligament, Percutaneous Endoscopic Approach
0MNNXZZ	Release Right Knee Bursa and Ligament, External Approach
0MNP0ZZ	Release Left Knee Bursa and Ligament, Open Approach
0MNP3ZZ	Release Left Knee Bursa and Ligament, Percutaneous Approach
0MNP4ZZ	Release Left Knee Bursa and Ligament, Percutaneous Endoscopic Approach
0MNPXZZ	Release Left Knee Bursa and Ligament, External Approach
0MNQ0ZZ	Release Right Ankle Bursa and Ligament, Open Approach
0MNQ3ZZ	Release Right Ankle Bursa and Ligament, Percutaneous Approach
0MNQ4ZZ	Release Right Ankle Bursa and Ligament, Percutaneous Endoscopic Approach
0MNQXZZ	Release Right Ankle Bursa and Ligament, External Approach
0MNR0ZZ	Release Left Ankle Bursa and Ligament, Open Approach
0MNR3ZZ	Release Left Ankle Bursa and Ligament, Percutaneous Approach
0MNR4ZZ	Release Left Ankle Bursa and Ligament, Percutaneous Endoscopic Approach
0MNRXZZ	Release Left Ankle Bursa and Ligament, External Approach
0MNS0ZZ	Release Right Foot Bursa and Ligament, Open Approach
0MNS3ZZ	Release Right Foot Bursa and Ligament, Percutaneous Approach
0MNS4ZZ	Release Right Foot Bursa and Ligament, Percutaneous Endoscopic Approach
0MNSXZZ	Release Right Foot Bursa and Ligament, External Approach
0MNT0ZZ	Release Left Foot Bursa and Ligament, Open Approach
0MNT3ZZ	Release Left Foot Bursa and Ligament, Percutaneous Approach
0MNT4ZZ	Release Left Foot Bursa and Ligament, Percutaneous Endoscopic Approach
0MNTXZZ	Release Left Foot Bursa and Ligament, External Approach
0MNV0ZZ	Release Right Lower Extremity Bursa and Ligament, Open Approach
0MNV3ZZ	Release Right Lower Extremity Bursa and Ligament, Percutaneous Approach
0MNV4ZZ	Release Right Lower Extremity Bursa and Ligament, Percutaneous Endoscopic Approach
0MNVXZZ	Release Right Lower Extremity Bursa and Ligament, External Approach
0MNW0ZZ	Release Left Lower Extremity Bursa and Ligament, Open Approach
0MNW3ZZ	Release Left Lower Extremity Bursa and Ligament, Percutaneous Approach
0MNW4ZZ	Release Left Lower Extremity Bursa and Ligament, Percutaneous Endoscopic Approach
0MNWXZZ	Release Left Lower Extremity Bursa and Ligament, External Approach

0MP – Bursae and Ligaments, Removal

Review Coding Guideline B6.1c

0MPX00Z	Removal of Drainage Device from Upper Bursa and Ligament, Open Approach
0MPX07Z	Removal of Autologous Tissue Substitute from Upper Bursa and Ligament, Open Approach
0MPX0JZ	Removal of Synthetic Substitute from Upper Bursa and Ligament, Open Approach
0MPX0KZ	Removal of Nonautologous Tissue Substitute from Upper Bursa and Ligament, Open Approach
0MPX30Z	Removal of Drainage Device from Upper Bursa and Ligament, Percutaneous Approach
0MPX37Z	Removal of Autologous Tissue Substitute from Upper Bursa and Ligament, Percutaneous Approach
0MPX3JZ	Removal of Synthetic Substitute from Upper Bursa and Ligament, Percutaneous Approach
0MPX3KZ	Removal of Nonautologous Tissue Substitute from Upper Bursa and Ligament, Percutaneous Approach
0MPX40Z	Removal of Drainage Device from Upper Bursa and Ligament, Percutaneous Endoscopic Approach

0MPX47Z	Removal of Autologous Tissue Substitute from Upper Bursa and Ligament, Percutaneous Endoscopic Approach
0MPX4JZ	Removal of Synthetic Substitute from Upper Bursa and Ligament, Percutaneous Endoscopic Approach
0MPX4KZ	Removal of Nonautologous Tissue Substitute from Upper Bursa and Ligament, Percutaneous Endoscopic Approach
0MPXX0Z	Removal of Drainage Device from Upper Bursa and Ligament, External Approach
0MPY00Z	Removal of Drainage Device from Lower Bursa and Ligament, Open Approach
0MPY07Z	Removal of Autologous Tissue Substitute from Lower Bursa and Ligament, Open Approach
0MPY0JZ	Removal of Synthetic Substitute from Lower Bursa and Ligament, Open Approach
0MPY0KZ	Removal of Nonautologous Tissue Substitute from Lower Bursa and Ligament, Open Approach
0MPY30Z	Removal of Drainage Device from Lower Bursa and Ligament, Percutaneous Approach

---

♀ Female-only　　♂ Male-only　　● Limited Coverage　　● Non-OR　　HAC HAC-associated procedure　　⬡ Non-covered procedures　　✚ Combination

0MPY37Z Removal of Autologous Tissue Substitute from Lower Bursa and Ligament, Percutaneous Approach
0MPY3JZ Removal of Synthetic Substitute from Lower Bursa and Ligament, Percutaneous Approach
0MPY3KZ Removal of Nonautologous Tissue Substitute from Lower Bursa and Ligament, Percutaneous Approach
0MPY40Z Removal of Drainage Device from Lower Bursa and Ligament, Percutaneous Endoscopic Approach

0MPY47Z Removal of Autologous Tissue Substitute from Lower Bursa and Ligament, Percutaneous Endoscopic Approach
0MPY4JZ Removal of Synthetic Substitute from Lower Bursa and Ligament, Percutaneous Endoscopic Approach
0MPY4KZ Removal of Nonautologous Tissue Substitute from Lower Bursa and Ligament, Percutaneous Endoscopic Approach
0MPYX0Z Removal of Drainage Device from Lower Bursa and Ligament, External Approach

0MQ – Bursae and Ligaments, Repair

Review Coding Guideline B3.5

0MQ00ZZ Repair Head and Neck Bursa and Ligament, Open Approach
0MQ03ZZ Repair Head and Neck Bursa and Ligament, Percutaneous Approach
0MQ04ZZ Repair Head and Neck Bursa and Ligament, Percutaneous Endoscopic Approach
0MQ10ZZ Repair Right Shoulder Bursa and Ligament, Open Approach
0MQ13ZZ Repair Right Shoulder Bursa and Ligament, Percutaneous Approach
0MQ14ZZ Repair Right Shoulder Bursa and Ligament, Percutaneous Endoscopic Approach
0MQ20ZZ Repair Left Shoulder Bursa and Ligament, Open Approach
0MQ23ZZ Repair Left Shoulder Bursa and Ligament, Percutaneous Approach
0MQ24ZZ Repair Left Shoulder Bursa and Ligament, Percutaneous Endoscopic Approach
0MQ30ZZ Repair Right Elbow Bursa and Ligament, Open Approach
0MQ33ZZ Repair Right Elbow Bursa and Ligament, Percutaneous Approach
0MQ34ZZ Repair Right Elbow Bursa and Ligament, Percutaneous Endoscopic Approach
0MQ40ZZ Repair Left Elbow Bursa and Ligament, Open Approach
0MQ43ZZ Repair Left Elbow Bursa and Ligament, Percutaneous Approach
0MQ44ZZ Repair Left Elbow Bursa and Ligament, Percutaneous Endoscopic Approach
0MQ50ZZ Repair Right Wrist Bursa and Ligament, Open Approach
0MQ53ZZ Repair Right Wrist Bursa and Ligament, Percutaneous Approach
0MQ54ZZ Repair Right Wrist Bursa and Ligament, Percutaneous Endoscopic Approach
0MQ60ZZ Repair Left Wrist Bursa and Ligament, Open Approach
0MQ63ZZ Repair Left Wrist Bursa and Ligament, Percutaneous Approach
0MQ64ZZ Repair Left Wrist Bursa and Ligament, Percutaneous Endoscopic Approach
0MQ70ZZ Repair Right Hand Bursa and Ligament, Open Approach
0MQ73ZZ Repair Right Hand Bursa and Ligament, Percutaneous Approach
0MQ74ZZ Repair Right Hand Bursa and Ligament, Percutaneous Endoscopic Approach
0MQ80ZZ Repair Left Hand Bursa and Ligament, Open Approach
0MQ83ZZ Repair Left Hand Bursa and Ligament, Percutaneous Approach
0MQ84ZZ Repair Left Hand Bursa and Ligament, Percutaneous Endoscopic Approach
0MQ90ZZ Repair Right Upper Extremity Bursa and Ligament, Open Approach
0MQ93ZZ Repair Right Upper Extremity Bursa and Ligament, Percutaneous Approach
0MQ94ZZ Repair Right Upper Extremity Bursa and Ligament, Percutaneous Endoscopic Approach
0MQB0ZZ Repair Left Upper Extremity Bursa and Ligament, Open Approach
0MQB3ZZ Repair Left Upper Extremity Bursa and Ligament, Percutaneous Approach
0MQB4ZZ Repair Left Upper Extremity Bursa and Ligament, Percutaneous Endoscopic Approach
0MQC0ZZ Repair Right Trunk Bursa and Ligament, Open Approach
0MQC3ZZ Repair Right Trunk Bursa and Ligament, Percutaneous Approach
0MQC4ZZ Repair Right Trunk Bursa and Ligament, Percutaneous Endoscopic Approach
0MQD0ZZ Repair Left Trunk Bursa and Ligament, Open Approach
0MQD3ZZ Repair Left Trunk Bursa and Ligament, Percutaneous Approach
0MQD4ZZ Repair Left Trunk Bursa and Ligament, Percutaneous Endoscopic Approach
0MQF0ZZ Repair Right Thorax Bursa and Ligament, Open Approach
0MQF3ZZ Repair Right Thorax Bursa and Ligament, Percutaneous Approach
0MQF4ZZ Repair Right Thorax Bursa and Ligament, Percutaneous Endoscopic Approach

0MQG0ZZ Repair Left Thorax Bursa and Ligament, Open Approach
0MQG3ZZ Repair Left Thorax Bursa and Ligament, Percutaneous Approach
0MQG4ZZ Repair Left Thorax Bursa and Ligament, Percutaneous Endoscopic Approach
0MQH0ZZ Repair Right Abdomen Bursa and Ligament, Open Approach
0MQH3ZZ Repair Right Abdomen Bursa and Ligament, Percutaneous Approach
0MQH4ZZ Repair Right Abdomen Bursa and Ligament, Percutaneous Endoscopic Approach
0MQJ0ZZ Repair Left Abdomen Bursa and Ligament, Open Approach
0MQJ3ZZ Repair Left Abdomen Bursa and Ligament, Percutaneous Approach
0MQJ4ZZ Repair Left Abdomen Bursa and Ligament, Percutaneous Endoscopic Approach
0MQK0ZZ Repair Perineum Bursa and Ligament, Open Approach
0MQK3ZZ Repair Perineum Bursa and Ligament, Percutaneous Approach
0MQK4ZZ Repair Perineum Bursa and Ligament, Percutaneous Endoscopic Approach
0MQL0ZZ Repair Right Hip Bursa and Ligament, Open Approach
0MQL3ZZ Repair Right Hip Bursa and Ligament, Percutaneous Approach
0MQL4ZZ Repair Right Hip Bursa and Ligament, Percutaneous Endoscopic Approach
0MQM0ZZ Repair Left Hip Bursa and Ligament, Open Approach
0MQM3ZZ Repair Left Hip Bursa and Ligament, Percutaneous Approach
0MQM4ZZ Repair Left Hip Bursa and Ligament, Percutaneous Endoscopic Approach
0MQN0ZZ Repair Right Knee Bursa and Ligament, Open Approach
0MQN3ZZ Repair Right Knee Bursa and Ligament, Percutaneous Approach
0MQN4ZZ Repair Right Knee Bursa and Ligament, Percutaneous Endoscopic Approach
0MQP0ZZ Repair Left Knee Bursa and Ligament, Open Approach
0MQP3ZZ Repair Left Knee Bursa and Ligament, Percutaneous Approach
0MQP4ZZ Repair Left Knee Bursa and Ligament, Percutaneous Endoscopic Approach
0MQQ0ZZ Repair Right Ankle Bursa and Ligament, Open Approach
0MQQ3ZZ Repair Right Ankle Bursa and Ligament, Percutaneous Approach
0MQQ4ZZ Repair Right Ankle Bursa and Ligament, Percutaneous Endoscopic Approach
0MQR0ZZ Repair Left Ankle Bursa and Ligament, Open Approach
0MQR3ZZ Repair Left Ankle Bursa and Ligament, Percutaneous Approach
0MQR4ZZ Repair Left Ankle Bursa and Ligament, Percutaneous Endoscopic Approach
0MQS0ZZ Repair Right Foot Bursa and Ligament, Open Approach
0MQS3ZZ Repair Right Foot Bursa and Ligament, Percutaneous Approach
0MQS4ZZ Repair Right Foot Bursa and Ligament, Percutaneous Endoscopic Approach
0MQT0ZZ Repair Left Foot Bursa and Ligament, Open Approach
0MQT3ZZ Repair Left Foot Bursa and Ligament, Percutaneous Approach
0MQT4ZZ Repair Left Foot Bursa and Ligament, Percutaneous Endoscopic Approach
0MQV0ZZ Repair Right Lower Extremity Bursa and Ligament, Open Approach
0MQV3ZZ Repair Right Lower Extremity Bursa and Ligament, Percutaneous Approach
0MQV4ZZ Repair Right Lower Extremity Bursa and Ligament, Percutaneous Endoscopic Approach
0MQW0ZZ Repair Left Lower Extremity Bursa and Ligament, Open Approach
0MQW3ZZ Repair Left Lower Extremity Bursa and Ligament, Percutaneous Approach
0MQW4ZZ Repair Left Lower Extremity Bursa and Ligament, Percutaneous Endoscopic Approach

0MS – Bursae and Ligaments, Reposition

0MS00ZZ	Reposition Head and Neck Bursa and Ligament, Open Approach
0MS04ZZ	Reposition Head and Neck Bursa and Ligament, Percutaneous Endoscopic Approach
0MS10ZZ	Reposition Right Shoulder Bursa and Ligament, Open Approach
0MS14ZZ	Reposition Right Shoulder Bursa and Ligament, Percutaneous Endoscopic Approach
0MS20ZZ	Reposition Left Shoulder Bursa and Ligament, Open Approach
0MS24ZZ	Reposition Left Shoulder Bursa and Ligament, Percutaneous Endoscopic Approach
0MS30ZZ	Reposition Right Elbow Bursa and Ligament, Open Approach
0MS34ZZ	Reposition Right Elbow Bursa and Ligament, Percutaneous Endoscopic Approach
0MS40ZZ	Reposition Left Elbow Bursa and Ligament, Open Approach
0MS44ZZ	Reposition Left Elbow Bursa and Ligament, Percutaneous Endoscopic Approach
0MS50ZZ	Reposition Right Wrist Bursa and Ligament, Open Approach
0MS54ZZ	Reposition Right Wrist Bursa and Ligament, Percutaneous Endoscopic Approach
0MS60ZZ	Reposition Left Wrist Bursa and Ligament, Open Approach
0MS64ZZ	Reposition Left Wrist Bursa and Ligament, Percutaneous Endoscopic Approach
0MS70ZZ	Reposition Right Hand Bursa and Ligament, Open Approach
0MS74ZZ	Reposition Right Hand Bursa and Ligament, Percutaneous Endoscopic Approach
0MS80ZZ	Reposition Left Hand Bursa and Ligament, Open Approach
0MS84ZZ	Reposition Left Hand Bursa and Ligament, Percutaneous Endoscopic Approach
0MS90ZZ	Reposition Right Upper Extremity Bursa and Ligament, Open Approach
0MS94ZZ	Reposition Right Upper Extremity Bursa and Ligament, Percutaneous Endoscopic Approach
0MSB0ZZ	Reposition Left Upper Extremity Bursa and Ligament, Open Approach
0MSB4ZZ	Reposition Left Upper Extremity Bursa and Ligament, Percutaneous Endoscopic Approach
0MSC0ZZ	Reposition Right Trunk Bursa and Ligament, Open Approach
0MSC4ZZ	Reposition Right Trunk Bursa and Ligament, Percutaneous Endoscopic Approach
0MSD0ZZ	Reposition Left Trunk Bursa and Ligament, Open Approach
0MSD4ZZ	Reposition Left Trunk Bursa and Ligament, Percutaneous Endoscopic Approach
0MSF0ZZ	Reposition Right Thorax Bursa and Ligament, Open Approach
0MSF4ZZ	Reposition Right Thorax Bursa and Ligament, Percutaneous Endoscopic Approach
0MSG0ZZ	Reposition Left Thorax Bursa and Ligament, Open Approach
0MSG4ZZ	Reposition Left Thorax Bursa and Ligament, Percutaneous Endoscopic Approach
0MSH0ZZ	Reposition Right Abdomen Bursa and Ligament, Open Approach
0MSH4ZZ	Reposition Right Abdomen Bursa and Ligament, Percutaneous Endoscopic Approach
0MSJ0ZZ	Reposition Left Abdomen Bursa and Ligament, Open Approach
0MSJ4ZZ	Reposition Left Abdomen Bursa and Ligament, Percutaneous Endoscopic Approach
0MSK0ZZ	Reposition Perineum Bursa and Ligament, Open Approach
0MSK4ZZ	Reposition Perineum Bursa and Ligament, Percutaneous Endoscopic Approach
0MSL0ZZ	Reposition Right Hip Bursa and Ligament, Open Approach
0MSL4ZZ	Reposition Right Hip Bursa and Ligament, Percutaneous Endoscopic Approach
0MSM0ZZ	Reposition Left Hip Bursa and Ligament, Open Approach
0MSM4ZZ	Reposition Left Hip Bursa and Ligament, Percutaneous Endoscopic Approach
0MSN0ZZ	Reposition Right Knee Bursa and Ligament, Open Approach
0MSN4ZZ	Reposition Right Knee Bursa and Ligament, Percutaneous Endoscopic Approach
0MSP0ZZ	Reposition Left Knee Bursa and Ligament, Open Approach
0MSP4ZZ	Reposition Left Knee Bursa and Ligament, Percutaneous Endoscopic Approach
0MSQ0ZZ	Reposition Right Ankle Bursa and Ligament, Open Approach
0MSQ4ZZ	Reposition Right Ankle Bursa and Ligament, Percutaneous Endoscopic Approach
0MSR0ZZ	Reposition Left Ankle Bursa and Ligament, Open Approach
0MSR4ZZ	Reposition Left Ankle Bursa and Ligament, Percutaneous Endoscopic Approach
0MSS0ZZ	Reposition Right Foot Bursa and Ligament, Open Approach
0MSS4ZZ	Reposition Right Foot Bursa and Ligament, Percutaneous Endoscopic Approach
0MST0ZZ	Reposition Left Foot Bursa and Ligament, Open Approach
0MST4ZZ	Reposition Left Foot Bursa and Ligament, Percutaneous Endoscopic Approach
0MSV0ZZ	Reposition Right Lower Extremity Bursa and Ligament, Open Approach
0MSV4ZZ	Reposition Right Lower Extremity Bursa and Ligament, Percutaneous Endoscopic Approach
0MSW0ZZ	Reposition Left Lower Extremity Bursa and Ligament, Open Approach
0MSW4ZZ	Reposition Left Lower Extremity Bursa and Ligament, Percutaneous Endoscopic Approach

0MT – Bursae and Ligaments, Resection

Review Coding Guideline B3.8

0MT00ZZ	Resection of Head and Neck Bursa and Ligament, Open Approach
0MT04ZZ	Resection of Head and Neck Bursa and Ligament, Percutaneous Endoscopic Approach
0MT10ZZ	Resection of Right Shoulder Bursa and Ligament, Open Approach
0MT14ZZ	Resection of Right Shoulder Bursa and Ligament, Percutaneous Endoscopic Approach
0MT20ZZ	Resection of Left Shoulder Bursa and Ligament, Open Approach
0MT24ZZ	Resection of Left Shoulder Bursa and Ligament, Percutaneous Endoscopic Approach
0MT30ZZ	Resection of Right Elbow Bursa and Ligament, Open Approach
0MT34ZZ	Resection of Right Elbow Bursa and Ligament, Percutaneous Endoscopic Approach
0MT40ZZ	Resection of Left Elbow Bursa and Ligament, Open Approach
0MT44ZZ	Resection of Left Elbow Bursa and Ligament, Percutaneous Endoscopic Approach
0MT50ZZ	Resection of Right Wrist Bursa and Ligament, Open Approach
0MT54ZZ	Resection of Right Wrist Bursa and Ligament, Percutaneous Endoscopic Approach
0MT60ZZ	Resection of Left Wrist Bursa and Ligament, Open Approach
0MT64ZZ	Resection of Left Wrist Bursa and Ligament, Percutaneous Endoscopic Approach
0MT70ZZ	Resection of Right Hand Bursa and Ligament, Open Approach
0MT74ZZ	Resection of Right Hand Bursa and Ligament, Percutaneous Endoscopic Approach
0MT80ZZ	Resection of Left Hand Bursa and Ligament, Open Approach
0MT84ZZ	Resection of Left Hand Bursa and Ligament, Percutaneous Endoscopic Approach
0MT90ZZ	Resection of Right Upper Extremity Bursa and Ligament, Open Approach
0MT94ZZ	Resection of Right Upper Extremity Bursa and Ligament, Percutaneous Endoscopic Approach
0MTB0ZZ	Resection of Left Upper Extremity Bursa and Ligament, Open Approach
0MTB4ZZ	Resection of Left Upper Extremity Bursa and Ligament, Percutaneous Endoscopic Approach
0MTC0ZZ	Resection of Right Trunk Bursa and Ligament, Open Approach
0MTC4ZZ	Resection of Right Trunk Bursa and Ligament, Percutaneous Endoscopic Approach
0MTD0ZZ	Resection of Left Trunk Bursa and Ligament, Open Approach
0MTD4ZZ	Resection of Left Trunk Bursa and Ligament, Percutaneous Endoscopic Approach
0MTF0ZZ	Resection of Right Thorax Bursa and Ligament, Open Approach
0MTF4ZZ	Resection of Right Thorax Bursa and Ligament, Percutaneous Endoscopic Approach

♀ Female-only   ♂ Male-only   ● Limited Coverage   ● Non-OR   🅗🅐🅒 HAC-associated procedure   ● Non-covered procedures   ✚ Combination

0MTG0ZZ Resection of Left Thorax Bursa and Ligament, Open Approach
0MTG4ZZ Resection of Left Thorax Bursa and Ligament, Percutaneous Endoscopic Approach
0MTH0ZZ Resection of Right Abdomen Bursa and Ligament, Open Approach
0MTH4ZZ Resection of Right Abdomen Bursa and Ligament, Percutaneous Endoscopic Approach
0MTJ0ZZ Resection of Left Abdomen Bursa and Ligament, Open Approach
0MTJ4ZZ Resection of Left Abdomen Bursa and Ligament, Percutaneous Endoscopic Approach
0MTK0ZZ Resection of Perineum Bursa and Ligament, Open Approach
0MTK4ZZ Resection of Perineum Bursa and Ligament, Percutaneous Endoscopic Approach
0MTL0ZZ Resection of Right Hip Bursa and Ligament, Open Approach
0MTL4ZZ Resection of Right Hip Bursa and Ligament, Percutaneous Endoscopic Approach
0MTM0ZZ Resection of Left Hip Bursa and Ligament, Open Approach
0MTM4ZZ Resection of Left Hip Bursa and Ligament, Percutaneous Endoscopic Approach
0MTN0ZZ Resection of Right Knee Bursa and Ligament, Open Approach
0MTN4ZZ Resection of Right Knee Bursa and Ligament, Percutaneous Endoscopic Approach
0MTP0ZZ Resection of Left Knee Bursa and Ligament, Open Approach

0MTP4ZZ Resection of Left Knee Bursa and Ligament, Percutaneous Endoscopic Approach
0MTQ0ZZ Resection of Right Ankle Bursa and Ligament, Open Approach
0MTQ4ZZ Resection of Right Ankle Bursa and Ligament, Percutaneous Endoscopic Approach
0MTR0ZZ Resection of Left Ankle Bursa and Ligament, Open Approach
0MTR4ZZ Resection of Left Ankle Bursa and Ligament, Percutaneous Endoscopic Approach
0MTS0ZZ Resection of Right Foot Bursa and Ligament, Open Approach
0MTS4ZZ Resection of Right Foot Bursa and Ligament, Percutaneous Endoscopic Approach
0MTT0ZZ Resection of Left Foot Bursa and Ligament, Open Approach
0MTT4ZZ Resection of Left Foot Bursa and Ligament, Percutaneous Endoscopic Approach
0MTV0ZZ Resection of Right Lower Extremity Bursa and Ligament, Open Approach
0MTV4ZZ Resection of Right Lower Extremity Bursa and Ligament, Percutaneous Endoscopic Approach
0MTW0ZZ Resection of Left Lower Extremity Bursa and Ligament, Open Approach
0MTW4ZZ Resection of Left Lower Extremity Bursa and Ligament, Percutaneous Endoscopic Approach

0MU – Bursae and Ligaments, Supplement

0MU007Z Supplement Head and Neck Bursa and Ligament with Autologous Tissue Substitute, Open Approach
0MU00JZ Supplement Head and Neck Bursa and Ligament with Synthetic Substitute, Open Approach
0MU00KZ Supplement Head and Neck Bursa and Ligament with Nonautologous Tissue Substitute, Open Approach
0MU047Z Supplement Head and Neck Bursa and Ligament with Autologous Tissue Substitute, Percutaneous Endoscopic Approach
0MU04JZ Supplement Head and Neck Bursa and Ligament with Synthetic Substitute, Percutaneous Endoscopic Approach
0MU04KZ Supplement Head and Neck Bursa and Ligament with Nonautologous Tissue Substitute, Percutaneous Endoscopic Approach
0MU107Z Supplement Right Shoulder Bursa and Ligament with Autologous Tissue Substitute, Open Approach
0MU10JZ Supplement Right Shoulder Bursa and Ligament with Synthetic Substitute, Open Approach
0MU10KZ Supplement Right Shoulder Bursa and Ligament with Nonautologous Tissue Substitute, Open Approach
0MU147Z Supplement Right Shoulder Bursa and Ligament with Autologous Tissue Substitute, Percutaneous Endoscopic Approach
0MU14JZ Supplement Right Shoulder Bursa and Ligament with Synthetic Substitute, Percutaneous Endoscopic Approach
0MU14KZ Supplement Right Shoulder Bursa and Ligament with Nonautologous Tissue Substitute, Percutaneous Endoscopic Approach
0MU207Z Supplement Left Shoulder Bursa and Ligament with Autologous Tissue Substitute, Open Approach
0MU20JZ Supplement Left Shoulder Bursa and Ligament with Synthetic Substitute, Open Approach
0MU20KZ Supplement Left Shoulder Bursa and Ligament with Nonautologous Tissue Substitute, Open Approach
0MU247Z Supplement Left Shoulder Bursa and Ligament with Autologous Tissue Substitute, Percutaneous Endoscopic Approach
0MU24JZ Supplement Left Shoulder Bursa and Ligament with Synthetic Substitute, Percutaneous Endoscopic Approach
0MU24KZ Supplement Left Shoulder Bursa and Ligament with Nonautologous Tissue Substitute, Percutaneous Endoscopic Approach
0MU307Z Supplement Right Elbow Bursa and Ligament with Autologous Tissue Substitute, Open Approach
0MU30JZ Supplement Right Elbow Bursa and Ligament with Synthetic Substitute, Open Approach
0MU30KZ Supplement Right Elbow Bursa and Ligament with Nonautologous Tissue Substitute, Open Approach
0MU347Z Supplement Right Elbow Bursa and Ligament with Autologous Tissue Substitute, Percutaneous Endoscopic Approach
0MU34JZ Supplement Right Elbow Bursa and Ligament with Synthetic Substitute, Percutaneous Endoscopic Approach

0MU34KZ Supplement Right Elbow Bursa and Ligament with Nonautologous Tissue Substitute, Percutaneous Endoscopic Approach
0MU407Z Supplement Left Elbow Bursa and Ligament with Autologous Tissue Substitute, Open Approach
0MU40JZ Supplement Left Elbow Bursa and Ligament with Synthetic Substitute, Open Approach
0MU40KZ Supplement Left Elbow Bursa and Ligament with Nonautologous Tissue Substitute, Open Approach
0MU447Z Supplement Left Elbow Bursa and Ligament with Autologous Tissue Substitute, Percutaneous Endoscopic Approach
0MU44JZ Supplement Left Elbow Bursa and Ligament with Synthetic Substitute, Percutaneous Endoscopic Approach
0MU44KZ Supplement Left Elbow Bursa and Ligament with Nonautologous Tissue Substitute, Percutaneous Endoscopic Approach
0MU507Z Supplement Right Wrist Bursa and Ligament with Autologous Tissue Substitute, Open Approach
0MU50JZ Supplement Right Wrist Bursa and Ligament with Synthetic Substitute, Open Approach
0MU50KZ Supplement Right Wrist Bursa and Ligament with Nonautologous Tissue Substitute, Open Approach
0MU547Z Supplement Right Wrist Bursa and Ligament with Autologous Tissue Substitute, Percutaneous Endoscopic Approach
0MU54JZ Supplement Right Wrist Bursa and Ligament with Synthetic Substitute, Percutaneous Endoscopic Approach
0MU54KZ Supplement Right Wrist Bursa and Ligament with Nonautologous Tissue Substitute, Percutaneous Endoscopic Approach
0MU607Z Supplement Left Wrist Bursa and Ligament with Autologous Tissue Substitute, Open Approach
0MU60JZ Supplement Left Wrist Bursa and Ligament with Synthetic Substitute, Open Approach
0MU60KZ Supplement Left Wrist Bursa and Ligament with Nonautologous Tissue Substitute, Open Approach
0MU647Z Supplement Left Wrist Bursa and Ligament with Autologous Tissue Substitute, Percutaneous Endoscopic Approach
0MU64JZ Supplement Left Wrist Bursa and Ligament with Synthetic Substitute, Percutaneous Endoscopic Approach
0MU64KZ Supplement Left Wrist Bursa and Ligament with Nonautologous Tissue Substitute, Percutaneous Endoscopic Approach
0MU707Z Supplement Right Hand Bursa and Ligament with Autologous Tissue Substitute, Open Approach
0MU70JZ Supplement Right Hand Bursa and Ligament with Synthetic Substitute, Open Approach
0MU70KZ Supplement Right Hand Bursa and Ligament with Nonautologous Tissue Substitute, Open Approach
0MU747Z Supplement Right Hand Bursa and Ligament with Autologous Tissue Substitute, Percutaneous Endoscopic Approach
0MU74JZ Supplement Right Hand Bursa and Ligament with Synthetic Substitute, Percutaneous Endoscopic Approach

0MU74KZ Supplement Right Hand Bursa and Ligament with Nonautologous Tissue Substitute, Percutaneous Endoscopic Approach

0MU807Z Supplement Left Hand Bursa and Ligament with Autologous Tissue Substitute, Open Approach

0MU80JZ Supplement Left Hand Bursa and Ligament with Synthetic Substitute, Open Approach

0MU80KZ Supplement Left Hand Bursa and Ligament with Nonautologous Tissue Substitute, Open Approach

0MU847Z Supplement Left Hand Bursa and Ligament with Autologous Tissue Substitute, Percutaneous Endoscopic Approach

0MU84JZ Supplement Left Hand Bursa and Ligament with Synthetic Substitute, Percutaneous Endoscopic Approach

0MU84KZ Supplement Left Hand Bursa and Ligament with Nonautologous Tissue Substitute, Percutaneous Endoscopic Approach

0MU907Z Supplement Right Upper Extremity Bursa and Ligament with Autologous Tissue Substitute, Open Approach

0MU90JZ Supplement Right Upper Extremity Bursa and Ligament with Synthetic Substitute, Open Approach

0MU90KZ Supplement Right Upper Extremity Bursa and Ligament with Nonautologous Tissue Substitute, Open Approach

0MU947Z Supplement Right Upper Extremity Bursa and Ligament with Autologous Tissue Substitute, Percutaneous Endoscopic Approach

0MU94JZ Supplement Right Upper Extremity Bursa and Ligament with Synthetic Substitute, Percutaneous Endoscopic Approach

0MU94KZ Supplement Right Upper Extremity Bursa and Ligament with Nonautologous Tissue Substitute, Percutaneous Endoscopic Approach

0MUB07Z Supplement Left Upper Extremity Bursa and Ligament with Autologous Tissue Substitute, Open Approach

0MUB0JZ Supplement Left Upper Extremity Bursa and Ligament with Synthetic Substitute, Open Approach

0MUB0KZ Supplement Left Upper Extremity Bursa and Ligament with Nonautologous Tissue Substitute, Open Approach

0MUB47Z Supplement Left Upper Extremity Bursa and Ligament with Autologous Tissue Substitute, Percutaneous Endoscopic Approach

0MUB4JZ Supplement Left Upper Extremity Bursa and Ligament with Synthetic Substitute, Percutaneous Endoscopic Approach

0MUB4KZ Supplement Left Upper Extremity Bursa and Ligament with Nonautologous Tissue Substitute, Percutaneous Endoscopic Approach

0MUC07Z Supplement Right Trunk Bursa and Ligament with Autologous Tissue Substitute, Open Approach

0MUC0JZ Supplement Right Trunk Bursa and Ligament with Synthetic Substitute, Open Approach

0MUC0KZ Supplement Right Trunk Bursa and Ligament with Nonautologous Tissue Substitute, Open Approach

0MUC47Z Supplement Right Trunk Bursa and Ligament with Autologous Tissue Substitute, Percutaneous Endoscopic Approach

0MUC4JZ Supplement Right Trunk Bursa and Ligament with Synthetic Substitute, Percutaneous Endoscopic Approach

0MUC4KZ Supplement Right Trunk Bursa and Ligament with Nonautologous Tissue Substitute, Percutaneous Endoscopic Approach

0MUD07Z Supplement Left Trunk Bursa and Ligament with Autologous Tissue Substitute, Open Approach

0MUD0JZ Supplement Left Trunk Bursa and Ligament with Synthetic Substitute, Open Approach

0MUD0KZ Supplement Left Trunk Bursa and Ligament with Nonautologous Tissue Substitute, Open Approach

0MUD47Z Supplement Left Trunk Bursa and Ligament with Autologous Tissue Substitute, Percutaneous Endoscopic Approach

0MUD4JZ Supplement Left Trunk Bursa and Ligament with Synthetic Substitute, Percutaneous Endoscopic Approach

0MUD4KZ Supplement Left Trunk Bursa and Ligament with Nonautologous Tissue Substitute, Percutaneous Endoscopic Approach

0MUF07Z Supplement Right Thorax Bursa and Ligament with Autologous Tissue Substitute, Open Approach

0MUF0JZ Supplement Right Thorax Bursa and Ligament with Synthetic Substitute, Open Approach

0MUF0KZ Supplement Right Thorax Bursa and Ligament with Nonautologous Tissue Substitute, Open Approach

0MUF47Z Supplement Right Thorax Bursa and Ligament with Autologous Tissue Substitute, Percutaneous Endoscopic Approach

0MUF4JZ Supplement Right Thorax Bursa and Ligament with Synthetic Substitute, Percutaneous Endoscopic Approach

0MUF4KZ Supplement Right Thorax Bursa and Ligament with Nonautologous Tissue Substitute, Percutaneous Endoscopic Approach

0MUG07Z Supplement Left Thorax Bursa and Ligament with Autologous Tissue Substitute, Open Approach

0MUG0JZ Supplement Left Thorax Bursa and Ligament with Synthetic Substitute, Open Approach

0MUG0KZ Supplement Left Thorax Bursa and Ligament with Nonautologous Tissue Substitute, Open Approach

0MUG47Z Supplement Left Thorax Bursa and Ligament with Autologous Tissue Substitute, Percutaneous Endoscopic Approach

0MUG4JZ Supplement Left Thorax Bursa and Ligament with Synthetic Substitute, Percutaneous Endoscopic Approach

0MUG4KZ Supplement Left Thorax Bursa and Ligament with Nonautologous Tissue Substitute, Percutaneous Endoscopic Approach

0MUH07Z Supplement Right Abdomen Bursa and Ligament with Autologous Tissue Substitute, Open Approach

0MUH0JZ Supplement Right Abdomen Bursa and Ligament with Synthetic Substitute, Open Approach

0MUH0KZ Supplement Right Abdomen Bursa and Ligament with Nonautologous Tissue Substitute, Open Approach

0MUH47Z Supplement Right Abdomen Bursa and Ligament with Autologous Tissue Substitute, Percutaneous Endoscopic Approach

0MUH4JZ Supplement Right Abdomen Bursa and Ligament with Synthetic Substitute, Percutaneous Endoscopic Approach

0MUH4KZ Supplement Right Abdomen Bursa and Ligament with Nonautologous Tissue Substitute, Percutaneous Endoscopic Approach

0MUJ07Z Supplement Left Abdomen Bursa and Ligament with Autologous Tissue Substitute, Open Approach

0MUJ0JZ Supplement Left Abdomen Bursa and Ligament with Synthetic Substitute, Open Approach

0MUJ0KZ Supplement Left Abdomen Bursa and Ligament with Nonautologous Tissue Substitute, Open Approach

0MUJ47Z Supplement Left Abdomen Bursa and Ligament with Autologous Tissue Substitute, Percutaneous Endoscopic Approach

0MUJ4JZ Supplement Left Abdomen Bursa and Ligament with Synthetic Substitute, Percutaneous Endoscopic Approach

0MUJ4KZ Supplement Left Abdomen Bursa and Ligament with Nonautologous Tissue Substitute, Percutaneous Endoscopic Approach

0MUK07Z Supplement Perineum Bursa and Ligament with Autologous Tissue Substitute, Open Approach

0MUK0JZ Supplement Perineum Bursa and Ligament with Synthetic Substitute, Open Approach

0MUK0KZ Supplement Perineum Bursa and Ligament with Nonautologous Tissue Substitute, Open Approach

0MUK47Z Supplement Perineum Bursa and Ligament with Autologous Tissue Substitute, Percutaneous Endoscopic Approach

0MUK4JZ Supplement Perineum Bursa and Ligament with Synthetic Substitute, Percutaneous Endoscopic Approach

0MUK4KZ Supplement Perineum Bursa and Ligament with Nonautologous Tissue Substitute, Percutaneous Endoscopic Approach

0MUL07Z Supplement Right Hip Bursa and Ligament with Autologous Tissue Substitute, Open Approach

0MUL0JZ Supplement Right Hip Bursa and Ligament with Synthetic Substitute, Open Approach

0MUL0KZ Supplement Right Hip Bursa and Ligament with Nonautologous Tissue Substitute, Open Approach

0MUL47Z Supplement Right Hip Bursa and Ligament with Autologous Tissue Substitute, Percutaneous Endoscopic Approach

0MUL4JZ Supplement Right Hip Bursa and Ligament with Synthetic Substitute, Percutaneous Endoscopic Approach

0MUL4KZ Supplement Right Hip Bursa and Ligament with Nonautologous Tissue Substitute, Percutaneous Endoscopic Approach

0MUM07Z Supplement Left Hip Bursa and Ligament with Autologous Tissue Substitute, Open Approach

0MUM0JZ Supplement Left Hip Bursa and Ligament with Synthetic Substitute, Open Approach

0MUM0KZ Supplement Left Hip Bursa and Ligament with Nonautologous Tissue Substitute, Open Approach

0MUM47Z Supplement Left Hip Bursa and Ligament with Autologous Tissue Substitute, Percutaneous Endoscopic Approach

0MUM4JZ Supplement Left Hip Bursa and Ligament with Synthetic Substitute, Percutaneous Endoscopic Approach

0MUM4KZ Supplement Left Hip Bursa and Ligament with Nonautologous Tissue Substitute, Percutaneous Endoscopic Approach

0MUN07Z Supplement Right Knee Bursa and Ligament with Autologous Tissue Substitute, Open Approach

0MUN0JZ Supplement Right Knee Bursa and Ligament with Synthetic Substitute, Open Approach

0MUN0KZ Supplement Right Knee Bursa and Ligament with Nonautologous Tissue Substitute, Open Approach

0MUN47Z Supplement Right Knee Bursa and Ligament with Autologous Tissue Substitute, Percutaneous Endoscopic Approach

0MUN4JZ Supplement Right Knee Bursa and Ligament with Synthetic Substitute, Percutaneous Endoscopic Approach

0MUN4KZ Supplement Right Knee Bursa and Ligament with Nonautologous Tissue Substitute, Percutaneous Endoscopic Approach

0MUP07Z Supplement Left Knee Bursa and Ligament with Autologous Tissue Substitute, Open Approach

0MUP0JZ Supplement Left Knee Bursa and Ligament with Synthetic Substitute, Open Approach

0MUP0KZ Supplement Left Knee Bursa and Ligament with Nonautologous Tissue Substitute, Open Approach

0MUP47Z Supplement Left Knee Bursa and Ligament with Autologous Tissue Substitute, Percutaneous Endoscopic Approach

0MUP4JZ Supplement Left Knee Bursa and Ligament with Synthetic Substitute, Percutaneous Endoscopic Approach

0MUP4KZ Supplement Left Knee Bursa and Ligament with Nonautologous Tissue Substitute, Percutaneous Endoscopic Approach

0MUQ07Z Supplement Right Ankle Bursa and Ligament with Autologous Tissue Substitute, Open Approach

0MUQ0JZ Supplement Right Ankle Bursa and Ligament with Synthetic Substitute, Open Approach

0MUQ0KZ Supplement Right Ankle Bursa and Ligament with Nonautologous Tissue Substitute, Open Approach

0MUQ47Z Supplement Right Ankle Bursa and Ligament with Autologous Tissue Substitute, Percutaneous Endoscopic Approach

0MUQ4JZ Supplement Right Ankle Bursa and Ligament with Synthetic Substitute, Percutaneous Endoscopic Approach

0MUQ4KZ Supplement Right Ankle Bursa and Ligament with Nonautologous Tissue Substitute, Percutaneous Endoscopic Approach

0MUR07Z Supplement Left Ankle Bursa and Ligament with Autologous Tissue Substitute, Open Approach

0MUR0JZ Supplement Left Ankle Bursa and Ligament with Synthetic Substitute, Open Approach

0MUR0KZ Supplement Left Ankle Bursa and Ligament with Nonautologous Tissue Substitute, Open Approach

0MUR47Z Supplement Left Ankle Bursa and Ligament with Autologous Tissue Substitute, Percutaneous Endoscopic Approach

0MUR4JZ Supplement Left Ankle Bursa and Ligament with Synthetic Substitute, Percutaneous Endoscopic Approach

0MUR4KZ Supplement Left Ankle Bursa and Ligament with Nonautologous Tissue Substitute, Percutaneous Endoscopic Approach

0MUS07Z Supplement Right Foot Bursa and Ligament with Autologous Tissue Substitute, Open Approach

0MUS0JZ Supplement Right Foot Bursa and Ligament with Synthetic Substitute, Open Approach

0MUS0KZ Supplement Right Foot Bursa and Ligament with Nonautologous Tissue Substitute, Open Approach

0MUS47Z Supplement Right Foot Bursa and Ligament with Autologous Tissue Substitute, Percutaneous Endoscopic Approach

0MUS4JZ Supplement Right Foot Bursa and Ligament with Synthetic Substitute, Percutaneous Endoscopic Approach

0MUS4KZ Supplement Right Foot Bursa and Ligament with Nonautologous Tissue Substitute, Percutaneous Endoscopic Approach

0MUT07Z Supplement Left Foot Bursa and Ligament with Autologous Tissue Substitute, Open Approach

0MUT0JZ Supplement Left Foot Bursa and Ligament with Synthetic Substitute, Open Approach

0MUT0KZ Supplement Left Foot Bursa and Ligament with Nonautologous Tissue Substitute, Open Approach

0MUT47Z Supplement Left Foot Bursa and Ligament with Autologous Tissue Substitute, Percutaneous Endoscopic Approach

0MUT4JZ Supplement Left Foot Bursa and Ligament with Synthetic Substitute, Percutaneous Endoscopic Approach

0MUT4KZ Supplement Left Foot Bursa and Ligament with Nonautologous Tissue Substitute, Percutaneous Endoscopic Approach

0MUV07Z Supplement Right Lower Extremity Bursa and Ligament with Autologous Tissue Substitute, Open Approach

0MUV0JZ Supplement Right Lower Extremity Bursa and Ligament with Synthetic Substitute, Open Approach

0MUV0KZ Supplement Right Lower Extremity Bursa and Ligament with Nonautologous Tissue Substitute, Open Approach

0MUV47Z Supplement Right Lower Extremity Bursa and Ligament with Autologous Tissue Substitute, Percutaneous Endoscopic Approach

0MUV4JZ Supplement Right Lower Extremity Bursa and Ligament with Synthetic Substitute, Percutaneous Endoscopic Approach

0MUV4KZ Supplement Right Lower Extremity Bursa and Ligament with Nonautologous Tissue Substitute, Percutaneous Endoscopic Approach

0MUW07Z Supplement Left Lower Extremity Bursa and Ligament with Autologous Tissue Substitute, Open Approach

0MUW0JZ Supplement Left Lower Extremity Bursa and Ligament with Synthetic Substitute, Open Approach

0MUW0KZ Supplement Left Lower Extremity Bursa and Ligament with Nonautologous Tissue Substitute, Open Approach

0MUW47Z Supplement Left Lower Extremity Bursa and Ligament with Autologous Tissue Substitute, Percutaneous Endoscopic Approach

0MUW4JZ Supplement Left Lower Extremity Bursa and Ligament with Synthetic Substitute, Percutaneous Endoscopic Approach

0MUW4KZ Supplement Left Lower Extremity Bursa and Ligament with Nonautologous Tissue Substitute, Percutaneous Endoscopic Approach

0MW – Bursae and Ligaments, Revision

Review Coding Guideline B6.1c

0MWX00Z Revision of Drainage Device in Upper Bursa and Ligament, Open Approach

0MWX07Z Revision of Autologous Tissue Substitute in Upper Bursa and Ligament, Open Approach

0MWX0JZ Revision of Synthetic Substitute in Upper Bursa and Ligament, Open Approach

0MWX0KZ Revision of Nonautologous Tissue Substitute in Upper Bursa and Ligament, Open Approach

0MWX30Z Revision of Drainage Device in Upper Bursa and Ligament, Percutaneous Approach

0MWX37Z Revision of Autologous Tissue Substitute in Upper Bursa and Ligament, Percutaneous Approach

0MWX3JZ Revision of Synthetic Substitute in Upper Bursa and Ligament, Percutaneous Approach

0MWX3KZ Revision of Nonautologous Tissue Substitute in Upper Bursa and Ligament, Percutaneous Approach

0MWX40Z Revision of Drainage Device in Upper Bursa and Ligament, Percutaneous Endoscopic Approach

0MWX47Z Revision of Autologous Tissue Substitute in Upper Bursa and Ligament, Percutaneous Endoscopic Approach

0MWX4JZ Revision of Synthetic Substitute in Upper Bursa and Ligament, Percutaneous Endoscopic Approach

0MWX4KZ Revision of Nonautologous Tissue Substitute in Upper Bursa and Ligament, Percutaneous Endoscopic Approach

0MWXX0Z Revision of Drainage Device in Upper Bursa and Ligament, External Approach

0MWXX7Z Revision of Autologous Tissue Substitute in Upper Bursa and Ligament, External Approach

0MWXXJZ Revision of Synthetic Substitute in Upper Bursa and Ligament, External Approach

0MWXXKZ Revision of Nonautologous Tissue Substitute in Upper Bursa and Ligament, External Approach

0MWY00Z Revision of Drainage Device in Lower Bursa and Ligament, Open Approach

0MWY07Z Revision of Autologous Tissue Substitute in Lower Bursa and Ligament, Open Approach

0MWY0JZ   Revision of Synthetic Substitute in Lower Bursa and Ligament, Open Approach

0MWY0KZ   Revision of Nonautologous Tissue Substitute in Lower Bursa and Ligament, Open Approach

0MWY30Z   Revision of Drainage Device in Lower Bursa and Ligament, Percutaneous Approach

0MWY37Z   Revision of Autologous Tissue Substitute in Lower Bursa and Ligament, Percutaneous Approach

0MWY3JZ   Revision of Synthetic Substitute in Lower Bursa and Ligament, Percutaneous Approach

0MWY3KZ   Revision of Nonautologous Tissue Substitute in Lower Bursa and Ligament, Percutaneous Approach

0MWY40Z   Revision of Drainage Device in Lower Bursa and Ligament, Percutaneous Endoscopic Approach

0MWY47Z   Revision of Autologous Tissue Substitute in Lower Bursa and Ligament, Percutaneous Endoscopic Approach

0MWY4JZ   Revision of Synthetic Substitute in Lower Bursa and Ligament, Percutaneous Endoscopic Approach

0MWY4KZ   Revision of Nonautologous Tissue Substitute in Lower Bursa and Ligament, Percutaneous Endoscopic Approach

0MWYX0Z   Revision of Drainage Device in Lower Bursa and Ligament, External Approach

0MWYX7Z   Revision of Autologous Tissue Substitute in Lower Bursa and Ligament, External Approach

0MWYXJZ   Revision of Synthetic Substitute in Lower Bursa and Ligament, External Approach

0MWYXKZ   Revision of Nonautologous Tissue Substitute in Lower Bursa and Ligament, External Approach

0MX – Bursae and Ligaments, Transfer

0MX00ZZ   Transfer Head and Neck Bursa and Ligament, Open Approach

0MX04ZZ   Transfer Head and Neck Bursa and Ligament, Percutaneous Endoscopic Approach

0MX10ZZ   Transfer Right Shoulder Bursa and Ligament, Open Approach

0MX14ZZ   Transfer Right Shoulder Bursa and Ligament, Percutaneous Endoscopic Approach

0MX20ZZ   Transfer Left Shoulder Bursa and Ligament, Open Approach

0MX24ZZ   Transfer Left Shoulder Bursa and Ligament, Percutaneous Endoscopic Approach

0MX30ZZ   Transfer Right Elbow Bursa and Ligament, Open Approach

0MX34ZZ   Transfer Right Elbow Bursa and Ligament, Percutaneous Endoscopic Approach

0MX40ZZ   Transfer Left Elbow Bursa and Ligament, Open Approach

0MX44ZZ   Transfer Left Elbow Bursa and Ligament, Percutaneous Endoscopic Approach

0MX50ZZ   Transfer Right Wrist Bursa and Ligament, Open Approach

0MX54ZZ   Transfer Right Wrist Bursa and Ligament, Percutaneous Endoscopic Approach

0MX60ZZ   Transfer Left Wrist Bursa and Ligament, Open Approach

0MX64ZZ   Transfer Left Wrist Bursa and Ligament, Percutaneous Endoscopic Approach

0MX70ZZ   Transfer Right Hand Bursa and Ligament, Open Approach

0MX74ZZ   Transfer Right Hand Bursa and Ligament, Percutaneous Endoscopic Approach

0MX80ZZ   Transfer Left Hand Bursa and Ligament, Open Approach

0MX84ZZ   Transfer Left Hand Bursa and Ligament, Percutaneous Endoscopic Approach

0MX90ZZ   Transfer Right Upper Extremity Bursa and Ligament, Open Approach

0MX94ZZ   Transfer Right Upper Extremity Bursa and Ligament, Percutaneous Endoscopic Approach

0MXB0ZZ   Transfer Left Upper Extremity Bursa and Ligament, Open Approach

0MXB4ZZ   Transfer Left Upper Extremity Bursa and Ligament, Percutaneous Endoscopic Approach

0MXC0ZZ   Transfer Right Trunk Bursa and Ligament, Open Approach

0MXC4ZZ   Transfer Right Trunk Bursa and Ligament, Percutaneous Endoscopic Approach

0MXD0ZZ   Transfer Left Trunk Bursa and Ligament, Open Approach

0MXD4ZZ   Transfer Left Trunk Bursa and Ligament, Percutaneous Endoscopic Approach

0MXF0ZZ   Transfer Right Thorax Bursa and Ligament, Open Approach

0MXF4ZZ   Transfer Right Thorax Bursa and Ligament, Percutaneous Endoscopic Approach

0MXG0ZZ   Transfer Left Thorax Bursa and Ligament, Open Approach

0MXG4ZZ   Transfer Left Thorax Bursa and Ligament, Percutaneous Endoscopic Approach

0MXH0ZZ   Transfer Right Abdomen Bursa and Ligament, Open Approach

0MXH4ZZ   Transfer Right Abdomen Bursa and Ligament, Percutaneous Endoscopic Approach

0MXJ0ZZ   Transfer Left Abdomen Bursa and Ligament, Open Approach

0MXJ4ZZ   Transfer Left Abdomen Bursa and Ligament, Percutaneous Endoscopic Approach

0MXK0ZZ   Transfer Perineum Bursa and Ligament, Open Approach

0MXK4ZZ   Transfer Perineum Bursa and Ligament, Percutaneous Endoscopic Approach

0MXL0ZZ   Transfer Right Hip Bursa and Ligament, Open Approach

0MXL4ZZ   Transfer Right Hip Bursa and Ligament, Percutaneous Endoscopic Approach

0MXM0ZZ   Transfer Left Hip Bursa and Ligament, Open Approach

0MXM4ZZ   Transfer Left Hip Bursa and Ligament, Percutaneous Endoscopic Approach

0MXN0ZZ   Transfer Right Knee Bursa and Ligament, Open Approach

0MXN4ZZ   Transfer Right Knee Bursa and Ligament, Percutaneous Endoscopic Approach

0MXP0ZZ   Transfer Left Knee Bursa and Ligament, Open Approach

0MXP4ZZ   Transfer Left Knee Bursa and Ligament, Percutaneous Endoscopic Approach

0MXQ0ZZ   Transfer Right Ankle Bursa and Ligament, Open Approach

0MXQ4ZZ   Transfer Right Ankle Bursa and Ligament, Percutaneous Endoscopic Approach

0MXR0ZZ   Transfer Left Ankle Bursa and Ligament, Open Approach

0MXR4ZZ   Transfer Left Ankle Bursa and Ligament, Percutaneous Endoscopic Approach

0MXS0ZZ   Transfer Right Foot Bursa and Ligament, Open Approach

0MXS4ZZ   Transfer Right Foot Bursa and Ligament, Percutaneous Endoscopic Approach

0MXT0ZZ   Transfer Left Foot Bursa and Ligament, Open Approach

0MXT4ZZ   Transfer Left Foot Bursa and Ligament, Percutaneous Endoscopic Approach

0MXV0ZZ   Transfer Right Lower Extremity Bursa and Ligament, Open Approach

0MXV4ZZ   Transfer Right Lower Extremity Bursa and Ligament, Percutaneous Endoscopic Approach

0MXW0ZZ   Transfer Left Lower Extremity Bursa and Ligament, Open Approach

0MXW4ZZ   Transfer Left Lower Extremity Bursa and Ligament, Percutaneous Endoscopic Approach

Head and Facial Bones

Head and Facial Bones

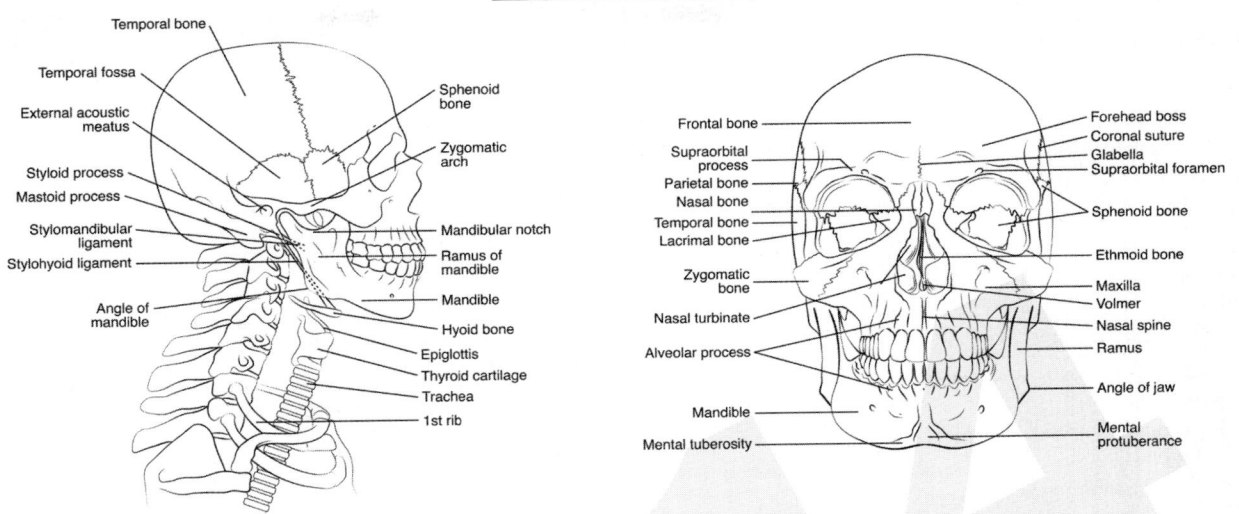

Head and Facial Bones Tables 0N2–0NW

Section	0	**Medical and Surgical**
Body System	N	**Head and Facial Bones**
Operation	2	**Change:** Taking out or off a device from a body part and putting back an identical or similar device in or on the same body part without cutting or puncturing the skin or a mucous membrane

Body Part (4th)	Approach (5th)	Device (6th)	Qualifier (7th)
0 Skull **B** Nasal Bone **W** Facial Bone	**X** External	**0** Drainage Device **Y** Other Device	**Z** No Qualifier

Section	0	Medical and Surgical
Body System	N	Head and Facial Bones
Operation	5	**Destruction:** Physical eradication of all or a portion of a body part by the direct use of energy, force, or a destructive agent

Body Part (4th)	Approach (5th)	Device (6th)	Qualifier (7th)
0 Skull	0 Open	Z No Device	Z No Qualifier
1 Frontal Bone, Right	3 Percutaneous		
2 Frontal Bone, Left	4 Percutaneous Endoscopic		
3 Parietal Bone, Right			
4 Parietal Bone, Left			
5 Temporal Bone, Right			
6 Temporal Bone, Left			
7 Occipital Bone, Right			
8 Occipital Bone, Left			
B Nasal Bone			
C Sphenoid Bone, Right			
D Sphenoid Bone, Left			
F Ethmoid Bone, Right			
G Ethmoid Bone, Left			
H Lacrimal Bone, Right			
J Lacrimal Bone, Left			
K Palatine Bone, Right			
L Palatine Bone, Left			
M Zygomatic Bone, Right			
N Zygomatic Bone, Left			
P Orbit, Right			
Q Orbit, Left			
R Maxilla, Right			
S Maxilla, Left			
T Mandible, Right			
V Mandible, Left			
X Hyoid Bone			

Section	0	Medical and Surgical
Body System	N	Head and Facial Bones
Operation	8	**Division:** Cutting into a body part, without draining fluids and/or gases from the body part, in order to separate or transect a body part

Body Part (4th)	Approach (5th)	Device (6th)	Qualifier (7th)
0 Skull	0 Open	Z No Device	Z No Qualifier
1 Frontal Bone, Right	3 Percutaneous		
2 Frontal Bone, Left	4 Percutaneous Endoscopic		
3 Parietal Bone, Right			
4 Parietal Bone, Left			
5 Temporal Bone, Right			
6 Temporal Bone, Left			
7 Occipital Bone, Right			
8 Occipital Bone, Left			
B Nasal Bone			
C Sphenoid Bone, Right			
D Sphenoid Bone, Left			
F Ethmoid Bone, Right			
G Ethmoid Bone, Left			
H Lacrimal Bone, Right			
J Lacrimal Bone, Left			
K Palatine Bone, Right			
L Palatine Bone, Left			
M Zygomatic Bone, Right			
N Zygomatic Bone, Left			
P Orbit, Right			
Q Orbit, Left			
R Maxilla, Right			
S Maxilla, Left			
T Mandible, Right			
V Mandible, Left			
X Hyoid Bone			

Section	0	**Medical and Surgical**
Body System	N	**Head and Facial Bones**
Operation	9	**Drainage:** Taking or letting out fluids and/or gases from a body part

Body Part (4th)	Approach (5th)	Device (6th)	Qualifier (7th)
0 Skull 1 Frontal Bone, Right 2 Frontal Bone, Left 3 Parietal Bone, Right 4 Parietal Bone, Left 5 Temporal Bone, Right 6 Temporal Bone, Left 7 Occipital Bone, Right 8 Occipital Bone, Left B Nasal Bone C Sphenoid Bone, Right D Sphenoid Bone, Left F Ethmoid Bone, Right G Ethmoid Bone, Left H Lacrimal Bone, Right J Lacrimal Bone, Left K Palatine Bone, Right L Palatine Bone, Left M Zygomatic Bone, Right N Zygomatic Bone, Left P Orbit, Right Q Orbit, Left R Maxilla, Right S Maxilla, Left T Mandible, Right V Mandible, Left X Hyoid Bone	0 Open 3 Percutaneous 4 Percutaneous Endoscopic	0 Drainage Device	Z No Qualifier
0 Skull 1 Frontal Bone, Right 2 Frontal Bone, Left 3 Parietal Bone, Right 4 Parietal Bone, Left 5 Temporal Bone, Right 6 Temporal Bone, Left 7 Occipital Bone, Right 8 Occipital Bone, Left B Nasal Bone C Sphenoid Bone, Right D Sphenoid Bone, Left F Ethmoid Bone, Right G Ethmoid Bone, Left H Lacrimal Bone, Right J Lacrimal Bone, Left K Palatine Bone, Right L Palatine Bone, Left M Zygomatic Bone, Right N Zygomatic Bone, Left P Orbit, Right Q Orbit, Left R Maxilla, Right S Maxilla, Left T Mandible, Right V Mandible, Left X Hyoid Bone	0 Open 3 Percutaneous 4 Percutaneous Endoscopic	Z No Device	X Diagnostic Z No Qualifier

Section	0	Medical and Surgical
Body System	N	Head and Facial Bones
Operation	B	Excision: Cutting out or off, without replacement, a portion of a body part

Body Part (4th)	Approach (5th)	Device (6th)	Qualifier (7th)
0 Skull 1 Frontal Bone, Right 2 Frontal Bone, Left 3 Parietal Bone, Right 4 Parietal Bone, Left 5 Temporal Bone, Right 6 Temporal Bone, Left 7 Occipital Bone, Right 8 Occipital Bone, Left B Nasal Bone C Sphenoid Bone, Right D Sphenoid Bone, Left F Ethmoid Bone, Right G Ethmoid Bone, Left H Lacrimal Bone, Right J Lacrimal Bone, Left K Palatine Bone, Right L Palatine Bone, Left M Zygomatic Bone, Right N Zygomatic Bone, Left P Orbit, Right Q Orbit, Left R Maxilla, Right S Maxilla, Left T Mandible, Right V Mandible, Left X Hyoid Bone	0 Open 3 Percutaneous 4 Percutaneous Endoscopic	Z No Device	X Diagnostic Z No Qualifier

Section	0	Medical and Surgical
Body System	N	Head and Facial Bones
Operation	C	Extirpation: Taking or cutting out solid matter from a body part

Body Part (4th)	Approach (5th)	Device (6th)	Qualifier (7th)
1 Frontal Bone, Right 2 Frontal Bone, Left 3 Parietal Bone, Right 4 Parietal Bone, Left 5 Temporal Bone, Right 6 Temporal Bone, Left 7 Occipital Bone, Right 8 Occipital Bone, Left B Nasal Bone C Sphenoid Bone, Right D Sphenoid Bone, Left F Ethmoid Bone, Right G Ethmoid Bone, Left H Lacrimal Bone, Right J Lacrimal Bone, Left K Palatine Bone, Right L Palatine Bone, Left M Zygomatic Bone, Right N Zygomatic Bone, Left P Orbit, Right Q Orbit, Left R Maxilla, Right S Maxilla, Left T Mandible, Right V Mandible, Left X Hyoid Bone	0 Open 3 Percutaneous 4 Percutaneous Endoscopic	Z No Device	Z No Qualifier

Section	0	Medical and Surgical
Body System	N	Head and Facial Bones
Operation	H	Insertion: Putting in a nonbiological appliance that monitors, assists, performs, or prevents a physiological function but does not physically take the place of a body part

Body Part (4th)	Approach (5th)	Device (6th)	Qualifier (7th)
0 Skull	0 Open	4 Internal Fixation Device 5 External Fixation Device M Bone Growth Stimulator N Neurostimulator Generator	Z No Qualifier
0 Skull	3 Percutaneous 4 Percutaneous Endoscopic	4 Internal Fixation Device 5 External Fixation Device M Bone Growth Stimulator	Z No Qualifier
1 Frontal Bone, Right 2 Frontal Bone, Left 3 Parietal Bone, Right 4 Parietal Bone, Left 7 Occipital Bone, Right 8 Occipital Bone, Left C Sphenoid Bone, Right D Sphenoid Bone, Left F Ethmoid Bone, Right G Ethmoid Bone, Left H Lacrimal Bone, Right J Lacrimal Bone, Left K Palatine Bone, Right L Palatine Bone, Left M Zygomatic Bone, Right N Zygomatic Bone, Left P Orbit, Right Q Orbit, Left X Hyoid Bone	0 Open 3 Percutaneous 4 Percutaneous Endoscopic	4 Internal Fixation Device	Z No Qualifier
5 Temporal Bone, Right 6 Temporal Bone, Left	0 Open 3 Percutaneous 4 Percutaneous Endoscopic	4 Internal Fixation Device S Hearing Device	Z No Qualifier
B Nasal Bone	0 Open 3 Percutaneous 4 Percutaneous Endoscopic	4 Internal Fixation Device M Bone Growth Stimulator	Z No Qualifier
R Maxilla, Right S Maxilla, Left T Mandible, Right V Mandible, Left	0 Open 3 Percutaneous 4 Percutaneous Endoscopic	4 Internal Fixation Device 5 External Fixation Device	Z No Qualifier
W Facial Bone	0 Open 3 Percutaneous 4 Percutaneous Endoscopic	M Bone Growth Stimulator	Z No Qualifier

Section	0	Medical and Surgical
Body System	N	Head and Facial Bones
Operation	J	Inspection: Visually and/or manually exploring a body part

Body Part (4th)	Approach (5th)	Device (6th)	Qualifier (7th)
0 Skull B Nasal Bone W Facial Bone	0 Open 3 Percutaneous 4 Percutaneous Endoscopic X External	Z No Device	Z No Qualifier

Section	0	Medical and Surgical
Body System	N	Head and Facial Bones
Operation	N	Release: Freeing a body part from an abnormal physical constraint by cutting or by the use of force

Body Part (4th)	Approach (5th)	Device (6th)	Qualifier (7th)
1 Frontal Bone, Right 2 Frontal Bone, Left 3 Parietal Bone, Right 4 Parietal Bone, Left 5 Temporal Bone, Right 6 Temporal Bone, Left 7 Occipital Bone, Right 8 Occipital Bone, Left B Nasal Bone C Sphenoid Bone, Right D Sphenoid Bone, Left F Ethmoid Bone, Right G Ethmoid Bone, Left H Lacrimal Bone, Right J Lacrimal Bone, Left K Palatine Bone, Right L Palatine Bone, Left M Zygomatic Bone, Right N Zygomatic Bone, Left P Orbit, Right Q Orbit, Left R Maxilla, Right S Maxilla, Left T Mandible, Right V Mandible, Left X Hyoid Bone	0 Open 3 Percutaneous 4 Percutaneous Endoscopic	Z No Device	Z No Qualifier

Section	0	Medical and Surgical
Body System	N	Head and Facial Bones
Operation	P	Removal: Taking out or off a device from a body part

Body Part (4th)	Approach (5th)	Device (6th)	Qualifier (7th)
0 Skull	0 Open	0 Drainage Device 4 Internal Fixation Device 5 External Fixation Device 7 Autologous Tissue Substitute J Synthetic Substitute K Nonautologous Tissue Substitute M Bone Growth Stimulator N Neurostimulator Generator S Hearing Device	Z No Qualifier
0 Skull	3 Percutaneous 4 Percutaneous Endoscopic	0 Drainage Device 4 Internal Fixation Device 5 External Fixation Device 7 Autologous Tissue Substitute J Synthetic Substitute K Nonautologous Tissue Substitute M Bone Growth Stimulator S Hearing Device	Z No Qualifier
0 Skull	X External	0 Drainage Device 4 Internal Fixation Device 5 External Fixation Device M Bone Growth Stimulator S Hearing Device	Z No Qualifier

Continued

0NP *Continued*

Section	0	Medical and Surgical
Body System	N	Head and Facial Bones
Operation	P	**Removal:** Taking out or off a device from a body part

Body Part (4th)	Approach (5th)	Device (6th)	Qualifier (7th)
B Nasal Bone **W** Facial Bone	**0** Open **3** Percutaneous **4** Percutaneous Endoscopic	**0** Drainage Device **4** Internal Fixation Device **7** Autologous Tissue Substitute **J** Synthetic Substitute **K** Nonautologous Tissue Substitute **M** Bone Growth Stimulator	**Z** No Qualifier
B Nasal Bone **W** Facial Bone	**X** External	**0** Drainage Device **4** Internal Fixation Device **M** Bone Growth Stimulator	**Z** No Qualifier

Section	0	Medical and Surgical
Body System	N	Head and Facial Bones
Operation	Q	**Repair:** Restoring, to the extent possible, a body part to its normal anatomic structure and function

Body Part (4th)	Approach (5th)	Device (6th)	Qualifier (7th)
0 Skull **1** Frontal Bone, Right **2** Frontal Bone, Left **3** Parietal Bone, Right **4** Parietal Bone, Left **5** Temporal Bone, Right **6** Temporal Bone, Left **7** Occipital Bone, Right **8** Occipital Bone, Left **B** Nasal Bone **C** Sphenoid Bone, Right **D** Sphenoid Bone, Left **F** Ethmoid Bone, Right **G** Ethmoid Bone, Left **H** Lacrimal Bone, Right **J** Lacrimal Bone, Left **K** Palatine Bone, Right **L** Palatine Bone, Left **M** Zygomatic Bone, Right **N** Zygomatic Bone, Left **P** Orbit, Right **Q** Orbit, Left **R** Maxilla, Right **S** Maxilla, Left **T** Mandible, Right **V** Mandible, Left **X** Hyoid Bone	**0** Open **3** Percutaneous **4** Percutaneous Endoscopic **X** External	**Z** No Device	**Z** No Qualifier

Section	0	Medical and Surgical
Body System	N	Head and Facial Bones
Operation	R	Replacement: Putting in or on biological or synthetic material that physically takes the place and/or function of all or a portion of a body part

Body Part (4th)	Approach (5th)	Device (6th)	Qualifier (7th)
0 Skull	0 Open	7 Autologous Tissue Substitute	Z No Qualifier
1 Frontal Bone, Right	3 Percutaneous	J Synthetic Substitute	
2 Frontal Bone, Left	4 Percutaneous Endoscopic	K Nonautologous Tissue Substitute	
3 Parietal Bone, Right			
4 Parietal Bone, Left			
5 Temporal Bone, Right			
6 Temporal Bone, Left			
7 Occipital Bone, Right			
8 Occipital Bone, Left			
B Nasal Bone			
C Sphenoid Bone, Right			
D Sphenoid Bone, Left			
F Ethmoid Bone, Right			
G Ethmoid Bone, Left			
H Lacrimal Bone, Right			
J Lacrimal Bone, Left			
K Palatine Bone, Right			
L Palatine Bone, Left			
M Zygomatic Bone, Right			
N Zygomatic Bone, Left			
P Orbit, Right			
Q Orbit, Left			
R Maxilla, Right			
S Maxilla, Left			
T Mandible, Right			
V Mandible, Left			
X Hyoid Bone			

Section	0	Medical and Surgical
Body System	N	Head and Facial Bones
Operation	S	Reposition: Moving to its normal location, or other suitable location, all or a portion of a body part

Body Part (4th)	Approach (5th)	Device (6th)	Qualifier (7th)
0 Skull	0 Open	4 Internal Fixation Device	Z No Qualifier
R Maxilla, Right	3 Percutaneous	5 External Fixation Device	
S Maxilla, Left	4 Percutaneous Endoscopic	Z No Device	
T Mandible, Right			
V Mandible, Left			
0 Skull	X External	Z No Device	Z No Qualifier
R Maxilla, Right			
S Maxilla, Left			
T Mandible, Right			
V Mandible, Left			

Continued

Section	0	Medical and Surgical
Body System	N	Head and Facial Bones
Operation	S	**Reposition:** Moving to its normal location, or other suitable location, all or a portion of a body part

Body Part (4th)	Approach (5th)	Device (6th)	Qualifier (7th)
1 Frontal Bone, Right 2 Frontal Bone, Left 3 Parietal Bone, Right 4 Parietal Bone, Left 5 Temporal Bone, Right 6 Temporal Bone, Left 7 Occipital Bone, Right 8 Occipital Bone, Left B Nasal Bone C Sphenoid Bone, Right D Sphenoid Bone, Left F Ethmoid Bone, Right G Ethmoid Bone, Left H Lacrimal Bone, Right J Lacrimal Bone, Left K Palatine Bone, Right L Palatine Bone, Left M Zygomatic Bone, Right N Zygomatic Bone, Left P Orbit, Right Q Orbit, Left X Hyoid Bone	0 Open 3 Percutaneous 4 Percutaneous Endoscopic	4 Internal Fixation Device Z No Device	Z No Qualifier
1 Frontal Bone, Right 2 Frontal Bone, Left 3 Parietal Bone, Right 4 Parietal Bone, Left 5 Temporal Bone, Right 6 Temporal Bone, Left 7 Occipital Bone, Right 8 Occipital Bone, Left B Nasal Bone C Sphenoid Bone, Right D Sphenoid Bone, Left F Ethmoid Bone, Right G Ethmoid Bone, Left H Lacrimal Bone, Right J Lacrimal Bone, Left K Palatine Bone, Right L Palatine Bone, Left M Zygomatic Bone, Right N Zygomatic Bone, Left P Orbit, Right Q Orbit, Left X Hyoid Bone	X External	Z No Device	Z No Qualifier

Section	0	Medical and Surgical
Body System	N	Head and Facial Bones
Operation	T	Resection: Cutting out or off, without replacement, all of a body part

Body Part (4th)	Approach (5th)	Device (6th)	Qualifier (7th)
1 Frontal Bone, Right 2 Frontal Bone, Left 3 Parietal Bone, Right 4 Parietal Bone, Left 5 Temporal Bone, Right 6 Temporal Bone, Left 7 Occipital Bone, Right 8 Occipital Bone, Left B Nasal Bone C Sphenoid Bone, Right D Sphenoid Bone, Left F Ethmoid Bone, Right G Ethmoid Bone, Left H Lacrimal Bone, Right J Lacrimal Bone, Left K Palatine Bone, Right L Palatine Bone, Left M Zygomatic Bone, Right N Zygomatic Bone, Left P Orbit, Right Q Orbit, Left R Maxilla, Right S Maxilla, Left T Mandible, Right V Mandible, Left X Hyoid Bone	0 Open	Z No Device	Z No Qualifier

Section	0	Medical and Surgical
Body System	N	Head and Facial Bones
Operation	U	Supplement: Putting in or on biological or synthetic material that physically reinforces and/or augments the function of a portion of a body part

Body Part (4th)	Approach (5th)	Device (6th)	Qualifier (7th)
0 Skull 1 Frontal Bone, Right 2 Frontal Bone, Left 3 Parietal Bone, Right 4 Parietal Bone, Left 5 Temporal Bone, Right 6 Temporal Bone, Left 7 Occipital Bone, Right 8 Occipital Bone, Left B Nasal Bone C Sphenoid Bone, Right D Sphenoid Bone, Left F Ethmoid Bone, Right G Ethmoid Bone, Left H Lacrimal Bone, Right J Lacrimal Bone, Left K Palatine Bone, Right L Palatine Bone, Left M Zygomatic Bone, Right N Zygomatic Bone, Left P Orbit, Right Q Orbit, Left R Maxilla, Right S Maxilla, Left T Mandible, Right V Mandible, Left X Hyoid Bone	0 Open 3 Percutaneous 4 Percutaneous Endoscopic	7 Autologous Tissue Substitute J Synthetic Substitute K Nonautologous Tissue Substitute	Z No Qualifier

Section	0	**Medical and Surgical**
Body System	N	**Head and Facial Bones**
Operation	W	**Revision:** Correcting, to the extent possible, a portion of a malfunctioning device or the position of a displaced device

Body Part (4th)	Approach (5th)	Device (6th)	Qualifier (7th)
0 Skull	0 Open	0 Drainage Device 4 Internal Fixation Device 5 External Fixation Device 7 Autologous Tissue Substitute J Synthetic Substitute K Nonautologous Tissue Substitute M Bone Growth Stimulator N Neurostimulator Generator S Hearing Device	Z No Qualifier
0 Skull	3 Percutaneous 4 Percutaneous Endoscopic X External	0 Drainage Device 4 Internal Fixation Device 5 External Fixation Device 7 Autologous Tissue Substitute J Synthetic Substitute K Nonautologous Tissue Substitute M Bone Growth Stimulator S Hearing Device	Z No Qualifier
B Nasal Bone W Facial Bone	0 Open 3 Percutaneous 4 Percutaneous Endoscopic X External	0 Drainage Device 4 Internal Fixation Device 7 Autologous Tissue Substitute J Synthetic Substitute K Nonautologous Tissue Substitute M Bone Growth Stimulator	Z No Qualifier

Head and Facial Bones Code Listing 0N2–0NW

0N2 – Head and Facial Bones, Change

Review Coding Guideline B6.1c

0N20X0Z	Change Drainage Device in Skull, External Approach
0N20XYZ	Change Other Device in Skull, External Approach
0N2BX0Z	Change Drainage Device in Nasal Bone, External Approach
0N2BXYZ	Change Other Device in Nasal Bone, External Approach
0N2WX0Z	Change Drainage Device in Facial Bone, External Approach
0N2WXYZ	Change Other Device in Facial Bone, External Approach

0N5 – Head and Facial Bones, Destruction

0N500ZZ	Destruction of Skull, Open Approach
0N503ZZ	Destruction of Skull, Percutaneous Approach
0N504ZZ	Destruction of Skull, Percutaneous Endoscopic Approach
0N510ZZ	Destruction of Right Frontal Bone, Open Approach
0N513ZZ	Destruction of Right Frontal Bone, Percutaneous Approach
0N514ZZ	Destruction of Right Frontal Bone, Percutaneous Endoscopic Approach
0N520ZZ	Destruction of Left Frontal Bone, Open Approach
0N523ZZ	Destruction of Left Frontal Bone, Percutaneous Approach
0N524ZZ	Destruction of Left Frontal Bone, Percutaneous Endoscopic Approach
0N530ZZ	Destruction of Right Parietal Bone, Open Approach
0N533ZZ	Destruction of Right Parietal Bone, Percutaneous Approach
0N534ZZ	Destruction of Right Parietal Bone, Percutaneous Endoscopic Approach
0N540ZZ	Destruction of Left Parietal Bone, Open Approach
0N543ZZ	Destruction of Left Parietal Bone, Percutaneous Approach
0N544ZZ	Destruction of Left Parietal Bone, Percutaneous Endoscopic Approach
0N550ZZ	Destruction of Right Temporal Bone, Open Approach
0N553ZZ	Destruction of Right Temporal Bone, Percutaneous Approach
0N554ZZ	Destruction of Right Temporal Bone, Percutaneous Endoscopic Approach
0N560ZZ	Destruction of Left Temporal Bone, Open Approach
0N563ZZ	Destruction of Left Temporal Bone, Percutaneous Approach
0N564ZZ	Destruction of Left Temporal Bone, Percutaneous Endoscopic Approach
0N570ZZ	Destruction of Right Occipital Bone, Open Approach
0N573ZZ	Destruction of Right Occipital Bone, Percutaneous Approach
0N574ZZ	Destruction of Right Occipital Bone, Percutaneous Endoscopic Approach
0N580ZZ	Destruction of Left Occipital Bone, Open Approach
0N583ZZ	Destruction of Left Occipital Bone, Percutaneous Approach
0N584ZZ	Destruction of Left Occipital Bone, Percutaneous Endoscopic Approach
0N5B0ZZ	Destruction of Nasal Bone, Open Approach
0N5B3ZZ	Destruction of Nasal Bone, Percutaneous Approach
0N5B4ZZ	Destruction of Nasal Bone, Percutaneous Endoscopic Approach
0N5C0ZZ	Destruction of Right Sphenoid Bone, Open Approach
0N5C3ZZ	Destruction of Right Sphenoid Bone, Percutaneous Approach
0N5C4ZZ	Destruction of Right Sphenoid Bone, Percutaneous Endoscopic Approach
0N5D0ZZ	Destruction of Left Sphenoid Bone, Open Approach
0N5D3ZZ	Destruction of Left Sphenoid Bone, Percutaneous Approach
0N5D4ZZ	Destruction of Left Sphenoid Bone, Percutaneous Endoscopic Approach
0N5F0ZZ	Destruction of Right Ethmoid Bone, Open Approach
0N5F3ZZ	Destruction of Right Ethmoid Bone, Percutaneous Approach
0N5F4ZZ	Destruction of Right Ethmoid Bone, Percutaneous Endoscopic Approach

♀ Female-only   ♂ Male-only   ● Limited Coverage   ● Non-OR   HAC HAC-associated procedure   ● Non-covered procedures   + Combination

0N5G0ZZ	Destruction of Left Ethmoid Bone, Open Approach
0N5G3ZZ	Destruction of Left Ethmoid Bone, Percutaneous Approach
0N5G4ZZ	Destruction of Left Ethmoid Bone, Percutaneous Endoscopic Approach
0N5H0ZZ	Destruction of Right Lacrimal Bone, Open Approach
0N5H3ZZ	Destruction of Right Lacrimal Bone, Percutaneous Approach
0N5H4ZZ	Destruction of Right Lacrimal Bone, Percutaneous Endoscopic Approach
0N5J0ZZ	Destruction of Left Lacrimal Bone, Open Approach
0N5J3ZZ	Destruction of Left Lacrimal Bone, Percutaneous Approach
0N5J4ZZ	Destruction of Left Lacrimal Bone, Percutaneous Endoscopic Approach
0N5K0ZZ	Destruction of Right Palatine Bone, Open Approach
0N5K3ZZ	Destruction of Right Palatine Bone, Percutaneous Approach
0N5K4ZZ	Destruction of Right Palatine Bone, Percutaneous Endoscopic Approach
0N5L0ZZ	Destruction of Left Palatine Bone, Open Approach
0N5L3ZZ	Destruction of Left Palatine Bone, Percutaneous Approach
0N5L4ZZ	Destruction of Left Palatine Bone, Percutaneous Endoscopic Approach
0N5M0ZZ	Destruction of Right Zygomatic Bone, Open Approach
0N5M3ZZ	Destruction of Right Zygomatic Bone, Percutaneous Approach
0N5M4ZZ	Destruction of Right Zygomatic Bone, Percutaneous Endoscopic Approach
0N5N0ZZ	Destruction of Left Zygomatic Bone, Open Approach
0N5N3ZZ	Destruction of Left Zygomatic Bone, Percutaneous Approach
0N5N4ZZ	Destruction of Left Zygomatic Bone, Percutaneous Endoscopic Approach
0N5P0ZZ	Destruction of Right Orbit, Open Approach
0N5P3ZZ	Destruction of Right Orbit, Percutaneous Approach
0N5P4ZZ	Destruction of Right Orbit, Percutaneous Endoscopic Approach
0N5Q0ZZ	Destruction of Left Orbit, Open Approach
0N5Q3ZZ	Destruction of Left Orbit, Percutaneous Approach
0N5Q4ZZ	Destruction of Left Orbit, Percutaneous Endoscopic Approach
0N5R0ZZ	Destruction of Right Maxilla, Open Approach
0N5R3ZZ	Destruction of Right Maxilla, Percutaneous Approach
0N5R4ZZ	Destruction of Right Maxilla, Percutaneous Endoscopic Approach
0N5S0ZZ	Destruction of Left Maxilla, Open Approach
0N5S3ZZ	Destruction of Left Maxilla, Percutaneous Approach
0N5S4ZZ	Destruction of Left Maxilla, Percutaneous Endoscopic Approach
0N5T0ZZ	Destruction of Right Mandible, Open Approach
0N5T3ZZ	Destruction of Right Mandible, Percutaneous Approach
0N5T4ZZ	Destruction of Right Mandible, Percutaneous Endoscopic Approach
0N5V0ZZ	Destruction of Left Mandible, Open Approach
0N5V3ZZ	Destruction of Left Mandible, Percutaneous Approach
0N5V4ZZ	Destruction of Left Mandible, Percutaneous Endoscopic Approach
0N5X0ZZ	Destruction of Hyoid Bone, Open Approach
0N5X3ZZ	Destruction of Hyoid Bone, Percutaneous Approach
0N5X4ZZ	Destruction of Hyoid Bone, Percutaneous Endoscopic Approach

0N8 – Head and Facial Bones, Division

Review Coding Guideline B3.14

0N800ZZ	Division of Skull, Open Approach
0N803ZZ	Division of Skull, Percutaneous Approach
0N804ZZ	Division of Skull, Percutaneous Endoscopic Approach
0N810ZZ	Division of Right Frontal Bone, Open Approach
0N813ZZ	Division of Right Frontal Bone, Percutaneous Approach
0N814ZZ	Division of Right Frontal Bone, Percutaneous Endoscopic Approach
0N820ZZ	Division of Left Frontal Bone, Open Approach
0N823ZZ	Division of Left Frontal Bone, Percutaneous Approach
0N824ZZ	Division of Left Frontal Bone, Percutaneous Endoscopic Approach
0N830ZZ	Division of Right Parietal Bone, Open Approach
0N833ZZ	Division of Right Parietal Bone, Percutaneous Approach
0N834ZZ	Division of Right Parietal Bone, Percutaneous Endoscopic Approach
0N840ZZ	Division of Left Parietal Bone, Open Approach
0N843ZZ	Division of Left Parietal Bone, Percutaneous Approach
0N844ZZ	Division of Left Parietal Bone, Percutaneous Endoscopic Approach
0N850ZZ	Division of Right Temporal Bone, Open Approach
0N853ZZ	Division of Right Temporal Bone, Percutaneous Approach
0N854ZZ	Division of Right Temporal Bone, Percutaneous Endoscopic Approach
0N860ZZ	Division of Left Temporal Bone, Open Approach
0N863ZZ	Division of Left Temporal Bone, Percutaneous Approach
0N864ZZ	Division of Left Temporal Bone, Percutaneous Endoscopic Approach
0N870ZZ	Division of Right Occipital Bone, Open Approach
0N873ZZ	Division of Right Occipital Bone, Percutaneous Approach
0N874ZZ	Division of Right Occipital Bone, Percutaneous Endoscopic Approach
0N880ZZ	Division of Left Occipital Bone, Open Approach
0N883ZZ	Division of Left Occipital Bone, Percutaneous Approach
0N884ZZ	Division of Left Occipital Bone, Percutaneous Endoscopic Approach
0N8B0ZZ	Division of Nasal Bone, Open Approach
0N8B3ZZ	Division of Nasal Bone, Percutaneous Approach
0N8B4ZZ	Division of Nasal Bone, Percutaneous Endoscopic Approach
0N8C0ZZ	Division of Right Sphenoid Bone, Open Approach
0N8C3ZZ	Division of Right Sphenoid Bone, Percutaneous Approach
0N8C4ZZ	Division of Right Sphenoid Bone, Percutaneous Endoscopic Approach
0N8D0ZZ	Division of Left Sphenoid Bone, Open Approach
0N8D3ZZ	Division of Left Sphenoid Bone, Percutaneous Approach
0N8D4ZZ	Division of Left Sphenoid Bone, Percutaneous Endoscopic Approach
0N8F0ZZ	Division of Right Ethmoid Bone, Open Approach
0N8F3ZZ	Division of Right Ethmoid Bone, Percutaneous Approach
0N8F4ZZ	Division of Right Ethmoid Bone, Percutaneous Endoscopic Approach
0N8G0ZZ	Division of Left Ethmoid Bone, Open Approach
0N8G3ZZ	Division of Left Ethmoid Bone, Percutaneous Approach
0N8G4ZZ	Division of Left Ethmoid Bone, Percutaneous Endoscopic Approach
0N8H0ZZ	Division of Right Lacrimal Bone, Open Approach
0N8H3ZZ	Division of Right Lacrimal Bone, Percutaneous Approach
0N8H4ZZ	Division of Right Lacrimal Bone, Percutaneous Endoscopic Approach
0N8J0ZZ	Division of Left Lacrimal Bone, Open Approach
0N8J3ZZ	Division of Left Lacrimal Bone, Percutaneous Approach
0N8J4ZZ	Division of Left Lacrimal Bone, Percutaneous Endoscopic Approach
0N8K0ZZ	Division of Right Palatine Bone, Open Approach
0N8K3ZZ	Division of Right Palatine Bone, Percutaneous Approach
0N8K4ZZ	Division of Right Palatine Bone, Percutaneous Endoscopic Approach
0N8L0ZZ	Division of Left Palatine Bone, Open Approach
0N8L3ZZ	Division of Left Palatine Bone, Percutaneous Approach
0N8L4ZZ	Division of Left Palatine Bone, Percutaneous Endoscopic Approach
0N8M0ZZ	Division of Right Zygomatic Bone, Open Approach
0N8M3ZZ	Division of Right Zygomatic Bone, Percutaneous Approach
0N8M4ZZ	Division of Right Zygomatic Bone, Percutaneous Endoscopic Approach
0N8N0ZZ	Division of Left Zygomatic Bone, Open Approach
0N8N3ZZ	Division of Left Zygomatic Bone, Percutaneous Approach
0N8N4ZZ	Division of Left Zygomatic Bone, Percutaneous Endoscopic Approach
0N8P0ZZ	Division of Right Orbit, Open Approach
0N8P3ZZ	Division of Right Orbit, Percutaneous Approach
0N8P4ZZ	Division of Right Orbit, Percutaneous Endoscopic Approach
0N8Q0ZZ	Division of Left Orbit, Open Approach
0N8Q3ZZ	Division of Left Orbit, Percutaneous Approach
0N8Q4ZZ	Division of Left Orbit, Percutaneous Endoscopic Approach
0N8R0ZZ	Division of Right Maxilla, Open Approach
0N8R3ZZ	Division of Right Maxilla, Percutaneous Approach
0N8R4ZZ	Division of Right Maxilla, Percutaneous Endoscopic Approach
0N8S0ZZ	Division of Left Maxilla, Open Approach
0N8S3ZZ	Division of Left Maxilla, Percutaneous Approach
0N8S4ZZ	Division of Left Maxilla, Percutaneous Endoscopic Approach
0N8T0ZZ	Division of Right Mandible, Open Approach

0N8T3ZZ	Division of Right Mandible, Percutaneous Approach
0N8T4ZZ	Division of Right Mandible, Percutaneous Endoscopic Approach
0N8V0ZZ	Division of Left Mandible, Open Approach
0N8V3ZZ	Division of Left Mandible, Percutaneous Approach

0N8V4ZZ	Division of Left Mandible, Percutaneous Endoscopic Approach
0N8X0ZZ	Division of Hyoid Bone, Open Approach
0N8X3ZZ	Division of Hyoid Bone, Percutaneous Approach
0N8X4ZZ	Division of Hyoid Bone, Percutaneous Endoscopic Approach

0N9 – Head and Facial Bones, Drainage

Review Coding Guidelines B3.4a and B3.4b

Review Coding Guideline B6.2

0N9000Z	Drainage of Skull with Drainage Device, Open Approach
0N900ZX	Drainage of Skull, Open Approach, Diagnostic
0N900ZZ	Drainage of Skull, Open Approach
0N9030Z	Drainage of Skull with Drainage Device, Percutaneous Approach
0N903ZX	Drainage of Skull, Percutaneous Approach, Diagnostic
0N903ZZ	Drainage of Skull, Percutaneous Approach
0N9040Z	Drainage of Skull with Drainage Device, Percutaneous Endoscopic Approach
0N904ZX	Drainage of Skull, Percutaneous Endoscopic Approach, Diagnostic
0N904ZZ	Drainage of Skull, Percutaneous Endoscopic Approach
0N9100Z	Drainage of Right Frontal Bone with Drainage Device, Open Approach
0N910ZX	Drainage of Right Frontal Bone, Open Approach, Diagnostic
0N910ZZ	Drainage of Right Frontal Bone, Open Approach
0N9130Z	Drainage of Right Frontal Bone with Drainage Device, Percutaneous Approach
0N913ZX	Drainage of Right Frontal Bone, Percutaneous Approach, Diagnostic
0N913ZZ	Drainage of Right Frontal Bone, Percutaneous Approach
0N9140Z	Drainage of Right Frontal Bone with Drainage Device, Percutaneous Endoscopic Approach
0N914ZX	Drainage of Right Frontal Bone, Percutaneous Endoscopic Approach, Diagnostic
0N914ZZ	Drainage of Right Frontal Bone, Percutaneous Endoscopic Approach
0N9200Z	Drainage of Left Frontal Bone with Drainage Device, Open Approach
0N920ZX	Drainage of Left Frontal Bone, Open Approach, Diagnostic
0N920ZZ	Drainage of Left Frontal Bone, Open Approach
0N9230Z	Drainage of Left Frontal Bone with Drainage Device, Percutaneous Approach
0N923ZX	Drainage of Left Frontal Bone, Percutaneous Approach, Diagnostic
0N923ZZ	Drainage of Left Frontal Bone, Percutaneous Approach
0N9240Z	Drainage of Left Frontal Bone with Drainage Device, Percutaneous Endoscopic Approach
0N924ZX	Drainage of Left Frontal Bone, Percutaneous Endoscopic Approach, Diagnostic
0N924ZZ	Drainage of Left Frontal Bone, Percutaneous Endoscopic Approach
0N9300Z	Drainage of Right Parietal Bone with Drainage Device, Open Approach
0N930ZX	Drainage of Right Parietal Bone, Open Approach, Diagnostic
0N930ZZ	Drainage of Right Parietal Bone, Open Approach
0N9330Z	Drainage of Right Parietal Bone with Drainage Device, Percutaneous Approach
0N933ZX	Drainage of Right Parietal Bone, Percutaneous Approach, Diagnostic
0N933ZZ	Drainage of Right Parietal Bone, Percutaneous Approach
0N9340Z	Drainage of Right Parietal Bone with Drainage Device, Percutaneous Endoscopic Approach
0N934ZX	Drainage of Right Parietal Bone, Percutaneous Endoscopic Approach, Diagnostic
0N934ZZ	Drainage of Right Parietal Bone, Percutaneous Endoscopic Approach
0N9400Z	Drainage of Left Parietal Bone with Drainage Device, Open Approach
0N940ZX	Drainage of Left Parietal Bone, Open Approach, Diagnostic
0N940ZZ	Drainage of Left Parietal Bone, Open Approach
0N9430Z	Drainage of Left Parietal Bone with Drainage Device, Percutaneous Approach
0N943ZX	Drainage of Left Parietal Bone, Percutaneous Approach, Diagnostic
0N943ZZ	Drainage of Left Parietal Bone, Percutaneous Approach
0N9440Z	Drainage of Left Parietal Bone with Drainage Device, Percutaneous Endoscopic Approach

0N944ZX	Drainage of Left Parietal Bone, Percutaneous Endoscopic Approach, Diagnostic
0N944ZZ	Drainage of Left Parietal Bone, Percutaneous Endoscopic Approach
0N9500Z	Drainage of Right Temporal Bone with Drainage Device, Open Approach
0N950ZX	Drainage of Right Temporal Bone, Open Approach, Diagnostic
0N950ZZ	Drainage of Right Temporal Bone, Open Approach
0N9530Z	Drainage of Right Temporal Bone with Drainage Device, Percutaneous Approach
0N953ZX	Drainage of Right Temporal Bone, Percutaneous Approach, Diagnostic
0N953ZZ	Drainage of Right Temporal Bone, Percutaneous Approach
0N9540Z	Drainage of Right Temporal Bone with Drainage Device, Percutaneous Endoscopic Approach
0N954ZX	Drainage of Right Temporal Bone, Percutaneous Endoscopic Approach, Diagnostic
0N954ZZ	Drainage of Right Temporal Bone, Percutaneous Endoscopic Approach
0N9600Z	Drainage of Left Temporal Bone with Drainage Device, Open Approach
0N960ZX	Drainage of Left Temporal Bone, Open Approach, Diagnostic
0N960ZZ	Drainage of Left Temporal Bone, Open Approach
0N9630Z	Drainage of Left Temporal Bone with Drainage Device, Percutaneous Approach
0N963ZX	Drainage of Left Temporal Bone, Percutaneous Approach, Diagnostic
0N963ZZ	Drainage of Left Temporal Bone, Percutaneous Approach
0N9640Z	Drainage of Left Temporal Bone with Drainage Device, Percutaneous Endoscopic Approach
0N964ZX	Drainage of Left Temporal Bone, Percutaneous Endoscopic Approach, Diagnostic
0N964ZZ	Drainage of Left Temporal Bone, Percutaneous Endoscopic Approach
0N9700Z	Drainage of Right Occipital Bone with Drainage Device, Open Approach
0N970ZX	Drainage of Right Occipital Bone, Open Approach, Diagnostic
0N970ZZ	Drainage of Right Occipital Bone, Open Approach
0N9730Z	Drainage of Right Occipital Bone with Drainage Device, Percutaneous Approach
0N973ZX	Drainage of Right Occipital Bone, Percutaneous Approach, Diagnostic
0N973ZZ	Drainage of Right Occipital Bone, Percutaneous Approach
0N9740Z	Drainage of Right Occipital Bone with Drainage Device, Percutaneous Endoscopic Approach
0N974ZX	Drainage of Right Occipital Bone, Percutaneous Endoscopic Approach, Diagnostic
0N974ZZ	Drainage of Right Occipital Bone, Percutaneous Endoscopic Approach
0N9800Z	Drainage of Left Occipital Bone with Drainage Device, Open Approach
0N980ZX	Drainage of Left Occipital Bone, Open Approach, Diagnostic
0N980ZZ	Drainage of Left Occipital Bone, Open Approach
0N9830Z	Drainage of Left Occipital Bone with Drainage Device, Percutaneous Approach
0N983ZX	Drainage of Left Occipital Bone, Percutaneous Approach, Diagnostic
0N983ZZ	Drainage of Left Occipital Bone, Percutaneous Approach
0N9840Z	Drainage of Left Occipital Bone with Drainage Device, Percutaneous Endoscopic Approach
0N984ZX	Drainage of Left Occipital Bone, Percutaneous Endoscopic Approach, Diagnostic
0N984ZZ	Drainage of Left Occipital Bone, Percutaneous Endoscopic Approach

0N9B00Z	Drainage of Nasal Bone with Drainage Device, Open Approach
0N9B0ZX	Drainage of Nasal Bone, Open Approach, Diagnostic
0N9B0ZZ	Drainage of Nasal Bone, Open Approach
0N9B30Z	Drainage of Nasal Bone with Drainage Device, Percutaneous Approach
0N9B3ZX	Drainage of Nasal Bone, Percutaneous Approach, Diagnostic
0N9B3ZZ	Drainage of Nasal Bone, Percutaneous Approach
0N9B40Z	Drainage of Nasal Bone with Drainage Device, Percutaneous Endoscopic Approach
0N9B4ZX	Drainage of Nasal Bone, Percutaneous Endoscopic Approach, Diagnostic
0N9B4ZZ	Drainage of Nasal Bone, Percutaneous Endoscopic Approach
0N9C00Z	Drainage of Right Sphenoid Bone with Drainage Device, Open Approach
0N9C0ZX	Drainage of Right Sphenoid Bone, Open Approach, Diagnostic
0N9C0ZZ	Drainage of Right Sphenoid Bone, Open Approach
0N9C30Z	Drainage of Right Sphenoid Bone with Drainage Device, Percutaneous Approach
0N9C3ZX	Drainage of Right Sphenoid Bone, Percutaneous Approach, Diagnostic
0N9C3ZZ	Drainage of Right Sphenoid Bone, Percutaneous Approach
0N9C40Z	Drainage of Right Sphenoid Bone with Drainage Device, Percutaneous Endoscopic Approach
0N9C4ZX	Drainage of Right Sphenoid Bone, Percutaneous Endoscopic Approach, Diagnostic
0N9C4ZZ	Drainage of Right Sphenoid Bone, Percutaneous Endoscopic Approach
0N9D00Z	Drainage of Left Sphenoid Bone with Drainage Device, Open Approach
0N9D0ZX	Drainage of Left Sphenoid Bone, Open Approach, Diagnostic
0N9D0ZZ	Drainage of Left Sphenoid Bone, Open Approach
0N9D30Z	Drainage of Left Sphenoid Bone with Drainage Device, Percutaneous Approach
0N9D3ZX	Drainage of Left Sphenoid Bone, Percutaneous Approach, Diagnostic
0N9D3ZZ	Drainage of Left Sphenoid Bone, Percutaneous Approach
0N9D40Z	Drainage of Left Sphenoid Bone with Drainage Device, Percutaneous Endoscopic Approach
0N9D4ZX	Drainage of Left Sphenoid Bone, Percutaneous Endoscopic Approach, Diagnostic
0N9D4ZZ	Drainage of Left Sphenoid Bone, Percutaneous Endoscopic Approach
0N9F00Z	Drainage of Right Ethmoid Bone with Drainage Device, Open Approach
0N9F0ZX	Drainage of Right Ethmoid Bone, Open Approach, Diagnostic
0N9F0ZZ	Drainage of Right Ethmoid Bone, Open Approach
0N9F30Z	Drainage of Right Ethmoid Bone with Drainage Device, Percutaneous Approach
0N9F3ZX	Drainage of Right Ethmoid Bone, Percutaneous Approach, Diagnostic
0N9F3ZZ	Drainage of Right Ethmoid Bone, Percutaneous Approach
0N9F40Z	Drainage of Right Ethmoid Bone with Drainage Device, Percutaneous Endoscopic Approach
0N9F4ZX	Drainage of Right Ethmoid Bone, Percutaneous Endoscopic Approach, Diagnostic
0N9F4ZZ	Drainage of Right Ethmoid Bone, Percutaneous Endoscopic Approach
0N9G00Z	Drainage of Left Ethmoid Bone with Drainage Device, Open Approach
0N9G0ZX	Drainage of Left Ethmoid Bone, Open Approach, Diagnostic
0N9G0ZZ	Drainage of Left Ethmoid Bone, Open Approach
0N9G30Z	Drainage of Left Ethmoid Bone with Drainage Device, Percutaneous Approach
0N9G3ZX	Drainage of Left Ethmoid Bone, Percutaneous Approach, Diagnostic
0N9G3ZZ	Drainage of Left Ethmoid Bone, Percutaneous Approach
0N9G40Z	Drainage of Left Ethmoid Bone with Drainage Device, Percutaneous Endoscopic Approach
0N9G4ZX	Drainage of Left Ethmoid Bone, Percutaneous Endoscopic Approach, Diagnostic
0N9G4ZZ	Drainage of Left Ethmoid Bone, Percutaneous Endoscopic Approach
0N9H00Z	Drainage of Right Lacrimal Bone with Drainage Device, Open Approach
0N9H0ZX	Drainage of Right Lacrimal Bone, Open Approach, Diagnostic
0N9H0ZZ	Drainage of Right Lacrimal Bone, Open Approach
0N9H30Z	Drainage of Right Lacrimal Bone with Drainage Device, Percutaneous Approach
0N9H3ZX	Drainage of Right Lacrimal Bone, Percutaneous Approach, Diagnostic
0N9H3ZZ	Drainage of Right Lacrimal Bone, Percutaneous Approach
0N9H40Z	Drainage of Right Lacrimal Bone with Drainage Device, Percutaneous Endoscopic Approach
0N9H4ZX	Drainage of Right Lacrimal Bone, Percutaneous Endoscopic Approach, Diagnostic
0N9H4ZZ	Drainage of Right Lacrimal Bone, Percutaneous Endoscopic Approach
0N9J00Z	Drainage of Left Lacrimal Bone with Drainage Device, Open Approach
0N9J0ZX	Drainage of Left Lacrimal Bone, Open Approach, Diagnostic
0N9J0ZZ	Drainage of Left Lacrimal Bone, Open Approach
0N9J30Z	Drainage of Left Lacrimal Bone with Drainage Device, Percutaneous Approach
0N9J3ZX	Drainage of Left Lacrimal Bone, Percutaneous Approach, Diagnostic
0N9J3ZZ	Drainage of Left Lacrimal Bone, Percutaneous Approach
0N9J40Z	Drainage of Left Lacrimal Bone with Drainage Device, Percutaneous Endoscopic Approach
0N9J4ZX	Drainage of Left Lacrimal Bone, Percutaneous Endoscopic Approach, Diagnostic
0N9J4ZZ	Drainage of Left Lacrimal Bone, Percutaneous Endoscopic Approach
0N9K00Z	Drainage of Right Palatine Bone with Drainage Device, Open Approach
0N9K0ZX	Drainage of Right Palatine Bone, Open Approach, Diagnostic
0N9K0ZZ	Drainage of Right Palatine Bone, Open Approach
0N9K30Z	Drainage of Right Palatine Bone with Drainage Device, Percutaneous Approach
0N9K3ZX	Drainage of Right Palatine Bone, Percutaneous Approach, Diagnostic
0N9K3ZZ	Drainage of Right Palatine Bone, Percutaneous Approach
0N9K40Z	Drainage of Right Palatine Bone with Drainage Device, Percutaneous Endoscopic Approach
0N9K4ZX	Drainage of Right Palatine Bone, Percutaneous Endoscopic Approach, Diagnostic
0N9K4ZZ	Drainage of Right Palatine Bone, Percutaneous Endoscopic Approach
0N9L00Z	Drainage of Left Palatine Bone with Drainage Device, Open Approach
0N9L0ZX	Drainage of Left Palatine Bone, Open Approach, Diagnostic
0N9L0ZZ	Drainage of Left Palatine Bone, Open Approach
0N9L30Z	Drainage of Left Palatine Bone with Drainage Device, Percutaneous Approach
0N9L3ZX	Drainage of Left Palatine Bone, Percutaneous Approach, Diagnostic
0N9L3ZZ	Drainage of Left Palatine Bone, Percutaneous Approach
0N9L40Z	Drainage of Left Palatine Bone with Drainage Device, Percutaneous Endoscopic Approach
0N9L4ZX	Drainage of Left Palatine Bone, Percutaneous Endoscopic Approach, Diagnostic
0N9L4ZZ	Drainage of Left Palatine Bone, Percutaneous Endoscopic Approach
0N9M00Z	Drainage of Right Zygomatic Bone with Drainage Device, Open Approach
0N9M0ZX	Drainage of Right Zygomatic Bone, Open Approach, Diagnostic
0N9M0ZZ	Drainage of Right Zygomatic Bone, Open Approach
0N9M30Z	Drainage of Right Zygomatic Bone with Drainage Device, Percutaneous Approach
0N9M3ZX	Drainage of Right Zygomatic Bone, Percutaneous Approach, Diagnostic
0N9M3ZZ	Drainage of Right Zygomatic Bone, Percutaneous Approach
0N9M40Z	Drainage of Right Zygomatic Bone with Drainage Device, Percutaneous Endoscopic Approach
0N9M4ZX	Drainage of Right Zygomatic Bone, Percutaneous Endoscopic Approach, Diagnostic
0N9M4ZZ	Drainage of Right Zygomatic Bone, Percutaneous Endoscopic Approach
0N9N00Z	Drainage of Left Zygomatic Bone with Drainage Device, Open Approach
0N9N0ZX	Drainage of Left Zygomatic Bone, Open Approach, Diagnostic

0N9N0ZZ	Drainage of Left Zygomatic Bone, Open Approach
0N9N30Z	Drainage of Left Zygomatic Bone with Drainage Device, Percutaneous Approach
0N9N3ZX	Drainage of Left Zygomatic Bone, Percutaneous Approach, Diagnostic
0N9N3ZZ	Drainage of Left Zygomatic Bone, Percutaneous Approach
0N9N40Z	Drainage of Left Zygomatic Bone with Drainage Device, Percutaneous Endoscopic Approach
0N9N4ZX	Drainage of Left Zygomatic Bone, Percutaneous Endoscopic Approach, Diagnostic
0N9N4ZZ	Drainage of Left Zygomatic Bone, Percutaneous Endoscopic Approach
0N9P00Z	Drainage of Right Orbit with Drainage Device, Open Approach
0N9P0ZX	Drainage of Right Orbit, Open Approach, Diagnostic
0N9P0ZZ	Drainage of Right Orbit, Open Approach
0N9P30Z	Drainage of Right Orbit with Drainage Device, Percutaneous Approach
0N9P3ZX	Drainage of Right Orbit, Percutaneous Approach, Diagnostic
0N9P3ZZ	Drainage of Right Orbit, Percutaneous Approach
0N9P40Z	Drainage of Right Orbit with Drainage Device, Percutaneous Endoscopic Approach
0N9P4ZX	Drainage of Right Orbit, Percutaneous Endoscopic Approach, Diagnostic
0N9P4ZZ	Drainage of Right Orbit, Percutaneous Endoscopic Approach
0N9Q00Z	Drainage of Left Orbit with Drainage Device, Open Approach
0N9Q0ZX	Drainage of Left Orbit, Open Approach, Diagnostic
0N9Q0ZZ	Drainage of Left Orbit, Open Approach
0N9Q30Z	Drainage of Left Orbit with Drainage Device, Percutaneous Approach
0N9Q3ZX	Drainage of Left Orbit, Percutaneous Approach, Diagnostic
0N9Q3ZZ	Drainage of Left Orbit, Percutaneous Approach
0N9Q40Z	Drainage of Left Orbit with Drainage Device, Percutaneous Endoscopic Approach
0N9Q4ZX	Drainage of Left Orbit, Percutaneous Endoscopic Approach, Diagnostic
0N9Q4ZZ	Drainage of Left Orbit, Percutaneous Endoscopic Approach
0N9R00Z	Drainage of Right Maxilla with Drainage Device, Open Approach
0N9R0ZX	Drainage of Right Maxilla, Open Approach, Diagnostic
0N9R0ZZ	Drainage of Right Maxilla, Open Approach
0N9R30Z	Drainage of Right Maxilla with Drainage Device, Percutaneous Approach
0N9R3ZX	Drainage of Right Maxilla, Percutaneous Approach, Diagnostic
0N9R3ZZ	Drainage of Right Maxilla, Percutaneous Approach
0N9R40Z	Drainage of Right Maxilla with Drainage Device, Percutaneous Endoscopic Approach
0N9R4ZX	Drainage of Right Maxilla, Percutaneous Endoscopic Approach, Diagnostic
0N9R4ZZ	Drainage of Right Maxilla, Percutaneous Endoscopic Approach

0N9S00Z	Drainage of Left Maxilla with Drainage Device, Open Approach
0N9S0ZX	Drainage of Left Maxilla, Open Approach, Diagnostic
0N9S0ZZ	Drainage of Left Maxilla, Open Approach
0N9S30Z	Drainage of Left Maxilla with Drainage Device, Percutaneous Approach
0N9S3ZX	Drainage of Left Maxilla, Percutaneous Approach, Diagnostic
0N9S3ZZ	Drainage of Left Maxilla, Percutaneous Approach
0N9S40Z	Drainage of Left Maxilla with Drainage Device, Percutaneous Endoscopic Approach
0N9S4ZX	Drainage of Left Maxilla, Percutaneous Endoscopic Approach, Diagnostic
0N9S4ZZ	Drainage of Left Maxilla, Percutaneous Endoscopic Approach
0N9T00Z	Drainage of Right Mandible with Drainage Device, Open Approach
0N9T0ZX	Drainage of Right Mandible, Open Approach, Diagnostic
0N9T0ZZ	Drainage of Right Mandible, Open Approach
0N9T30Z	Drainage of Right Mandible with Drainage Device, Percutaneous Approach
0N9T3ZX	Drainage of Right Mandible, Percutaneous Approach, Diagnostic
0N9T3ZZ	Drainage of Right Mandible, Percutaneous Approach
0N9T40Z	Drainage of Right Mandible with Drainage Device, Percutaneous Endoscopic Approach
0N9T4ZX	Drainage of Right Mandible, Percutaneous Endoscopic Approach, Diagnostic
0N9T4ZZ	Drainage of Right Mandible, Percutaneous Endoscopic Approach
0N9V00Z	Drainage of Left Mandible with Drainage Device, Open Approach
0N9V0ZX	Drainage of Left Mandible, Open Approach, Diagnostic
0N9V0ZZ	Drainage of Left Mandible, Open Approach
0N9V30Z	Drainage of Left Mandible with Drainage Device, Percutaneous Approach
0N9V3ZX	Drainage of Left Mandible, Percutaneous Approach, Diagnostic
0N9V3ZZ	Drainage of Left Mandible, Percutaneous Approach
0N9V40Z	Drainage of Left Mandible with Drainage Device, Percutaneous Endoscopic Approach
0N9V4ZX	Drainage of Left Mandible, Percutaneous Endoscopic Approach, Diagnostic
0N9V4ZZ	Drainage of Left Mandible, Percutaneous Endoscopic Approach
0N9X00Z	Drainage of Hyoid Bone with Drainage Device, Open Approach
0N9X0ZX	Drainage of Hyoid Bone, Open Approach, Diagnostic
0N9X0ZZ	Drainage of Hyoid Bone, Open Approach
0N9X30Z	Drainage of Hyoid Bone with Drainage Device, Percutaneous Approach
0N9X3ZX	Drainage of Hyoid Bone, Percutaneous Approach, Diagnostic
0N9X3ZZ	Drainage of Hyoid Bone, Percutaneous Approach
0N9X40Z	Drainage of Hyoid Bone with Drainage Device, Percutaneous Endoscopic Approach
0N9X4ZX	Drainage of Hyoid Bone, Percutaneous Endoscopic Approach, Diagnostic
0N9X4ZZ	Drainage of Hyoid Bone, Percutaneous Endoscopic Approach

0NB – Head and Facial Bones, Excision

Review Coding Guidelines B3.4a and B3.4b

Review Coding Guideline B3.5

Review Coding Guideline B3.8

0NB00ZX	Excision of Skull, Open Approach, Diagnostic
0NB00ZZ	Excision of Skull, Open Approach
0NB03ZX	Excision of Skull, Percutaneous Approach, Diagnostic
0NB03ZZ	Excision of Skull, Percutaneous Approach
0NB04ZX	Excision of Skull, Percutaneous Endoscopic Approach, Diagnostic
0NB04ZZ	Excision of Skull, Percutaneous Endoscopic Approach
0NB10ZX	Excision of Right Frontal Bone, Open Approach, Diagnostic
0NB10ZZ	Excision of Right Frontal Bone, Open Approach
0NB13ZX	Excision of Right Frontal Bone, Percutaneous Approach, Diagnostic
0NB13ZZ	Excision of Right Frontal Bone, Percutaneous Approach
0NB14ZX	Excision of Right Frontal Bone, Percutaneous Endoscopic Approach, Diagnostic
0NB14ZZ	Excision of Right Frontal Bone, Percutaneous Endoscopic Approach
0NB20ZX	Excision of Left Frontal Bone, Open Approach, Diagnostic
0NB20ZZ	Excision of Left Frontal Bone, Open Approach
0NB23ZX	Excision of Left Frontal Bone, Percutaneous Approach, Diagnostic

0NB23ZZ	Excision of Left Frontal Bone, Percutaneous Approach
0NB24ZX	Excision of Left Frontal Bone, Percutaneous Endoscopic Approach, Diagnostic
0NB24ZZ	Excision of Left Frontal Bone, Percutaneous Endoscopic Approach
0NB30ZX	Excision of Right Parietal Bone, Open Approach, Diagnostic
0NB30ZZ	Excision of Right Parietal Bone, Open Approach
0NB33ZX	Excision of Right Parietal Bone, Percutaneous Approach, Diagnostic
0NB33ZZ	Excision of Right Parietal Bone, Percutaneous Approach
0NB34ZX	Excision of Right Parietal Bone, Percutaneous Endoscopic Approach, Diagnostic
0NB34ZZ	Excision of Right Parietal Bone, Percutaneous Endoscopic Approach
0NB40ZX	Excision of Left Parietal Bone, Open Approach, Diagnostic
0NB40ZZ	Excision of Left Parietal Bone, Open Approach
0NB43ZX	Excision of Left Parietal Bone, Percutaneous Approach, Diagnostic

♀ Female-only   ♂ Male-only   ● Limited Coverage   ● Non-OR   ■ HAC-associated procedure   ● Non-covered procedures   ✚ Combination

0NB43ZZ	Excision of Left Parietal Bone, Percutaneous Approach
0NB44ZX	Excision of Left Parietal Bone, Percutaneous Endoscopic Approach, Diagnostic
0NB44ZZ	Excision of Left Parietal Bone, Percutaneous Endoscopic Approach
0NB50ZX	Excision of Right Temporal Bone, Open Approach, Diagnostic
0NB50ZZ	Excision of Right Temporal Bone, Open Approach
0NB53ZX	Excision of Right Temporal Bone, Percutaneous Approach, Diagnostic
0NB53ZZ	Excision of Right Temporal Bone, Percutaneous Approach
0NB54ZX	Excision of Right Temporal Bone, Percutaneous Endoscopic Approach, Diagnostic
0NB54ZZ	Excision of Right Temporal Bone, Percutaneous Endoscopic Approach
0NB60ZX	Excision of Left Temporal Bone, Open Approach, Diagnostic
0NB60ZZ	Excision of Left Temporal Bone, Open Approach
0NB63ZX	Excision of Left Temporal Bone, Percutaneous Approach, Diagnostic
0NB63ZZ	Excision of Left Temporal Bone, Percutaneous Approach
0NB64ZX	Excision of Left Temporal Bone, Percutaneous Endoscopic Approach, Diagnostic
0NB64ZZ	Excision of Left Temporal Bone, Percutaneous Endoscopic Approach
0NB70ZX	Excision of Right Occipital Bone, Open Approach, Diagnostic
0NB70ZZ	Excision of Right Occipital Bone, Open Approach
0NB73ZX	Excision of Right Occipital Bone, Percutaneous Approach, Diagnostic
0NB73ZZ	Excision of Right Occipital Bone, Percutaneous Approach
0NB74ZX	Excision of Right Occipital Bone, Percutaneous Endoscopic Approach, Diagnostic
0NB74ZZ	Excision of Right Occipital Bone, Percutaneous Endoscopic Approach
0NB80ZX	Excision of Left Occipital Bone, Open Approach, Diagnostic
0NB80ZZ	Excision of Left Occipital Bone, Open Approach
0NB83ZX	Excision of Left Occipital Bone, Percutaneous Approach, Diagnostic
0NB83ZZ	Excision of Left Occipital Bone, Percutaneous Approach
0NB84ZX	Excision of Left Occipital Bone, Percutaneous Endoscopic Approach, Diagnostic
0NB84ZZ	Excision of Left Occipital Bone, Percutaneous Endoscopic Approach
0NBB0ZX	Excision of Nasal Bone, Open Approach, Diagnostic
0NBB0ZZ	Excision of Nasal Bone, Open Approach
0NBB3ZX	Excision of Nasal Bone, Percutaneous Approach, Diagnostic
0NBB3ZZ	Excision of Nasal Bone, Percutaneous Approach
0NBB4ZX	Excision of Nasal Bone, Percutaneous Endoscopic Approach, Diagnostic
0NBB4ZZ	Excision of Nasal Bone, Percutaneous Endoscopic Approach
0NBC0ZX	Excision of Right Sphenoid Bone, Open Approach, Diagnostic
0NBC0ZZ	Excision of Right Sphenoid Bone, Open Approach
0NBC3ZX	Excision of Right Sphenoid Bone, Percutaneous Approach, Diagnostic
0NBC3ZZ	Excision of Right Sphenoid Bone, Percutaneous Approach
0NBC4ZX	Excision of Right Sphenoid Bone, Percutaneous Endoscopic Approach, Diagnostic
0NBC4ZZ	Excision of Right Sphenoid Bone, Percutaneous Endoscopic Approach
0NBD0ZX	Excision of Left Sphenoid Bone, Open Approach, Diagnostic
0NBD0ZZ	Excision of Left Sphenoid Bone, Open Approach
0NBD3ZX	Excision of Left Sphenoid Bone, Percutaneous Approach, Diagnostic
0NBD3ZZ	Excision of Left Sphenoid Bone, Percutaneous Approach
0NBD4ZX	Excision of Left Sphenoid Bone, Percutaneous Endoscopic Approach, Diagnostic
0NBD4ZZ	Excision of Left Sphenoid Bone, Percutaneous Endoscopic Approach
0NBF0ZX	Excision of Right Ethmoid Bone, Open Approach, Diagnostic
0NBF0ZZ	Excision of Right Ethmoid Bone, Open Approach
0NBF3ZX	Excision of Right Ethmoid Bone, Percutaneous Approach, Diagnostic
0NBF3ZZ	Excision of Right Ethmoid Bone, Percutaneous Approach
0NBF4ZX	Excision of Right Ethmoid Bone, Percutaneous Endoscopic Approach, Diagnostic
0NBF4ZZ	Excision of Right Ethmoid Bone, Percutaneous Endoscopic Approach
0NBG0ZX	Excision of Left Ethmoid Bone, Open Approach, Diagnostic
0NBG0ZZ	Excision of Left Ethmoid Bone, Open Approach
0NBG3ZX	Excision of Left Ethmoid Bone, Percutaneous Approach, Diagnostic
0NBG3ZZ	Excision of Left Ethmoid Bone, Percutaneous Approach
0NBG4ZX	Excision of Left Ethmoid Bone, Percutaneous Endoscopic Approach, Diagnostic
0NBG4ZZ	Excision of Left Ethmoid Bone, Percutaneous Endoscopic Approach
0NBH0ZX	Excision of Right Lacrimal Bone, Open Approach, Diagnostic
0NBH0ZZ	Excision of Right Lacrimal Bone, Open Approach
0NBH3ZX	Excision of Right Lacrimal Bone, Percutaneous Approach, Diagnostic
0NBH3ZZ	Excision of Right Lacrimal Bone, Percutaneous Approach
0NBH4ZX	Excision of Right Lacrimal Bone, Percutaneous Endoscopic Approach, Diagnostic
0NBH4ZZ	Excision of Right Lacrimal Bone, Percutaneous Endoscopic Approach
0NBJ0ZX	Excision of Left Lacrimal Bone, Open Approach, Diagnostic
0NBJ0ZZ	Excision of Left Lacrimal Bone, Open Approach
0NBJ3ZX	Excision of Left Lacrimal Bone, Percutaneous Approach, Diagnostic
0NBJ3ZZ	Excision of Left Lacrimal Bone, Percutaneous Approach
0NBJ4ZX	Excision of Left Lacrimal Bone, Percutaneous Endoscopic Approach, Diagnostic
0NBJ4ZZ	Excision of Left Lacrimal Bone, Percutaneous Endoscopic Approach
0NBK0ZX	Excision of Right Palatine Bone, Open Approach, Diagnostic
0NBK0ZZ	Excision of Right Palatine Bone, Open Approach
0NBK3ZX	Excision of Right Palatine Bone, Percutaneous Approach, Diagnostic
0NBK3ZZ	Excision of Right Palatine Bone, Percutaneous Approach
0NBK4ZX	Excision of Right Palatine Bone, Percutaneous Endoscopic Approach, Diagnostic
0NBK4ZZ	Excision of Right Palatine Bone, Percutaneous Endoscopic Approach
0NBL0ZX	Excision of Left Palatine Bone, Open Approach, Diagnostic
0NBL0ZZ	Excision of Left Palatine Bone, Open Approach
0NBL3ZX	Excision of Left Palatine Bone, Percutaneous Approach, Diagnostic
0NBL3ZZ	Excision of Left Palatine Bone, Percutaneous Approach
0NBL4ZX	Excision of Left Palatine Bone, Percutaneous Endoscopic Approach, Diagnostic
0NBL4ZZ	Excision of Left Palatine Bone, Percutaneous Endoscopic Approach
0NBM0ZX	Excision of Right Zygomatic Bone, Open Approach, Diagnostic
0NBM0ZZ	Excision of Right Zygomatic Bone, Open Approach
0NBM3ZX	Excision of Right Zygomatic Bone, Percutaneous Approach, Diagnostic
0NBM3ZZ	Excision of Right Zygomatic Bone, Percutaneous Approach
0NBM4ZX	Excision of Right Zygomatic Bone, Percutaneous Endoscopic Approach, Diagnostic
0NBM4ZZ	Excision of Right Zygomatic Bone, Percutaneous Endoscopic Approach
0NBN0ZX	Excision of Left Zygomatic Bone, Open Approach, Diagnostic
0NBN0ZZ	Excision of Left Zygomatic Bone, Open Approach
0NBN3ZX	Excision of Left Zygomatic Bone, Percutaneous Approach, Diagnostic
0NBN3ZZ	Excision of Left Zygomatic Bone, Percutaneous Approach
0NBN4ZX	Excision of Left Zygomatic Bone, Percutaneous Endoscopic Approach, Diagnostic
0NBN4ZZ	Excision of Left Zygomatic Bone, Percutaneous Endoscopic Approach
0NBP0ZX	Excision of Right Orbit, Open Approach, Diagnostic
0NBP0ZZ	Excision of Right Orbit, Open Approach
0NBP3ZX	Excision of Right Orbit, Percutaneous Approach, Diagnostic
0NBP3ZZ	Excision of Right Orbit, Percutaneous Approach
0NBP4ZX	Excision of Right Orbit, Percutaneous Endoscopic Approach, Diagnostic
0NBP4ZZ	Excision of Right Orbit, Percutaneous Endoscopic Approach
0NBQ0ZX	Excision of Left Orbit, Open Approach, Diagnostic
0NBQ0ZZ	Excision of Left Orbit, Open Approach
0NBQ3ZX	Excision of Left Orbit, Percutaneous Approach, Diagnostic
0NBQ3ZZ	Excision of Left Orbit, Percutaneous Approach

0NBQ4ZX Excision of Left Orbit, Percutaneous Endoscopic Approach, Diagnostic
0NBQ4ZZ Excision of Left Orbit, Percutaneous Endoscopic Approach
0NBR0ZX Excision of Right Maxilla, Open Approach, Diagnostic
0NBR0ZZ Excision of Right Maxilla, Open Approach
0NBR3ZX Excision of Right Maxilla, Percutaneous Approach, Diagnostic
0NBR3ZZ Excision of Right Maxilla, Percutaneous Approach
0NBR4ZX Excision of Right Maxilla, Percutaneous Endoscopic Approach, Diagnostic
0NBR4ZZ Excision of Right Maxilla, Percutaneous Endoscopic Approach
0NBS0ZX Excision of Left Maxilla, Open Approach, Diagnostic
0NBS0ZZ Excision of Left Maxilla, Open Approach
0NBS3ZX Excision of Left Maxilla, Percutaneous Approach, Diagnostic
0NBS3ZZ Excision of Left Maxilla, Percutaneous Approach
0NBS4ZX Excision of Left Maxilla, Percutaneous Endoscopic Approach, Diagnostic
0NBS4ZZ Excision of Left Maxilla, Percutaneous Endoscopic Approach
0NBT0ZX Excision of Right Mandible, Open Approach, Diagnostic
0NBT0ZZ Excision of Right Mandible, Open Approach

0NBT3ZX Excision of Right Mandible, Percutaneous Approach, Diagnostic
0NBT3ZZ Excision of Right Mandible, Percutaneous Approach
0NBT4ZX Excision of Right Mandible, Percutaneous Endoscopic Approach, Diagnostic
0NBT4ZZ Excision of Right Mandible, Percutaneous Endoscopic Approach
0NBV0ZX Excision of Left Mandible, Open Approach, Diagnostic
0NBV0ZZ Excision of Left Mandible, Open Approach
0NBV3ZX Excision of Left Mandible, Percutaneous Approach, Diagnostic
0NBV3ZZ Excision of Left Mandible, Percutaneous Approach
0NBV4ZX Excision of Left Mandible, Percutaneous Endoscopic Approach, Diagnostic
0NBV4ZZ Excision of Left Mandible, Percutaneous Endoscopic Approach
0NBX0ZX Excision of Hyoid Bone, Open Approach, Diagnostic
0NBX0ZZ Excision of Hyoid Bone, Open Approach
0NBX3ZX Excision of Hyoid Bone, Percutaneous Approach, Diagnostic
0NBX3ZZ Excision of Hyoid Bone, Percutaneous Approach
0NBX4ZX Excision of Hyoid Bone, Percutaneous Endoscopic Approach, Diagnostic
0NBX4ZZ Excision of Hyoid Bone, Percutaneous Endoscopic Approach

0NC – Head and Facial Bones, Extirpation

0NC10ZZ Extirpation of Matter from Right Frontal Bone, Open Approach
0NC13ZZ Extirpation of Matter from Right Frontal Bone, Percutaneous Approach
0NC14ZZ Extirpation of Matter from Right Frontal Bone, Percutaneous Endoscopic Approach
0NC20ZZ Extirpation of Matter from Left Frontal Bone, Open Approach
0NC23ZZ Extirpation of Matter from Left Frontal Bone, Percutaneous Approach
0NC24ZZ Extirpation of Matter from Left Frontal Bone, Percutaneous Endoscopic Approach
0NC30ZZ Extirpation of Matter from Right Parietal Bone, Open Approach
0NC33ZZ Extirpation of Matter from Right Parietal Bone, Percutaneous Approach
0NC34ZZ Extirpation of Matter from Right Parietal Bone, Percutaneous Endoscopic Approach
0NC40ZZ Extirpation of Matter from Left Parietal Bone, Open Approach
0NC43ZZ Extirpation of Matter from Left Parietal Bone, Percutaneous Approach
0NC44ZZ Extirpation of Matter from Left Parietal Bone, Percutaneous Endoscopic Approach
0NC50ZZ Extirpation of Matter from Right Temporal Bone, Open Approach
0NC53ZZ Extirpation of Matter from Right Temporal Bone, Percutaneous Approach
0NC54ZZ Extirpation of Matter from Right Temporal Bone, Percutaneous Endoscopic Approach
0NC60ZZ Extirpation of Matter from Left Temporal Bone, Open Approach
0NC63ZZ Extirpation of Matter from Left Temporal Bone, Percutaneous Approach
0NC64ZZ Extirpation of Matter from Left Temporal Bone, Percutaneous Endoscopic Approach
0NC70ZZ Extirpation of Matter from Right Occipital Bone, Open Approach
0NC73ZZ Extirpation of Matter from Right Occipital Bone, Percutaneous Approach
0NC74ZZ Extirpation of Matter from Right Occipital Bone, Percutaneous Endoscopic Approach
0NC80ZZ Extirpation of Matter from Left Occipital Bone, Open Approach
0NC83ZZ Extirpation of Matter from Left Occipital Bone, Percutaneous Approach
0NC84ZZ Extirpation of Matter from Left Occipital Bone, Percutaneous Endoscopic Approach
0NCB0ZZ Extirpation of Matter from Nasal Bone, Open Approach
0NCB3ZZ Extirpation of Matter from Nasal Bone, Percutaneous Approach
0NCB4ZZ Extirpation of Matter from Nasal Bone, Percutaneous Endoscopic Approach
0NCC0ZZ Extirpation of Matter from Right Sphenoid Bone, Open Approach
0NCC3ZZ Extirpation of Matter from Right Sphenoid Bone, Percutaneous Approach
0NCC4ZZ Extirpation of Matter from Right Sphenoid Bone, Percutaneous Endoscopic Approach
0NCD0ZZ Extirpation of Matter from Left Sphenoid Bone, Open Approach

0NCD3ZZ Extirpation of Matter from Left Sphenoid Bone, Percutaneous Approach
0NCD4ZZ Extirpation of Matter from Left Sphenoid Bone, Percutaneous Endoscopic Approach
0NCF0ZZ Extirpation of Matter from Right Ethmoid Bone, Open Approach
0NCF3ZZ Extirpation of Matter from Right Ethmoid Bone, Percutaneous Approach
0NCF4ZZ Extirpation of Matter from Right Ethmoid Bone, Percutaneous Endoscopic Approach
0NCG0ZZ Extirpation of Matter from Left Ethmoid Bone, Open Approach
0NCG3ZZ Extirpation of Matter from Left Ethmoid Bone, Percutaneous Approach
0NCG4ZZ Extirpation of Matter from Left Ethmoid Bone, Percutaneous Endoscopic Approach
0NCH0ZZ Extirpation of Matter from Right Lacrimal Bone, Open Approach
0NCH3ZZ Extirpation of Matter from Right Lacrimal Bone, Percutaneous Approach
0NCH4ZZ Extirpation of Matter from Right Lacrimal Bone, Percutaneous Endoscopic Approach
0NCJ0ZZ Extirpation of Matter from Left Lacrimal Bone, Open Approach
0NCJ3ZZ Extirpation of Matter from Left Lacrimal Bone, Percutaneous Approach
0NCJ4ZZ Extirpation of Matter from Left Lacrimal Bone, Percutaneous Endoscopic Approach
0NCK0ZZ Extirpation of Matter from Right Palatine Bone, Open Approach
0NCK3ZZ Extirpation of Matter from Right Palatine Bone, Percutaneous Approach
0NCK4ZZ Extirpation of Matter from Right Palatine Bone, Percutaneous Endoscopic Approach
0NCL0ZZ Extirpation of Matter from Left Palatine Bone, Open Approach
0NCL3ZZ Extirpation of Matter from Left Palatine Bone, Percutaneous Approach
0NCL4ZZ Extirpation of Matter from Left Palatine Bone, Percutaneous Endoscopic Approach
0NCM0ZZ Extirpation of Matter from Right Zygomatic Bone, Open Approach
0NCM3ZZ Extirpation of Matter from Right Zygomatic Bone, Percutaneous Approach
0NCM4ZZ Extirpation of Matter from Right Zygomatic Bone, Percutaneous Endoscopic Approach
0NCN0ZZ Extirpation of Matter from Left Zygomatic Bone, Open Approach
0NCN3ZZ Extirpation of Matter from Left Zygomatic Bone, Percutaneous Approach
0NCN4ZZ Extirpation of Matter from Left Zygomatic Bone, Percutaneous Endoscopic Approach
0NCP0ZZ Extirpation of Matter from Right Orbit, Open Approach
0NCP3ZZ Extirpation of Matter from Right Orbit, Percutaneous Approach
0NCP4ZZ Extirpation of Matter from Right Orbit, Percutaneous Endoscopic Approach
0NCQ0ZZ Extirpation of Matter from Left Orbit, Open Approach
0NCQ3ZZ Extirpation of Matter from Left Orbit, Percutaneous Approach

0NCQ4ZZ Extirpation of Matter from Left Orbit, Percutaneous Endoscopic Approach

0NCR0ZZ Extirpation of Matter from Right Maxilla, Open Approach

0NCR3ZZ Extirpation of Matter from Right Maxilla, Percutaneous Approach

0NCR4ZZ Extirpation of Matter from Right Maxilla, Percutaneous Endoscopic Approach

0NCS0ZZ Extirpation of Matter from Left Maxilla, Open Approach

0NCS3ZZ Extirpation of Matter from Left Maxilla, Percutaneous Approach

0NCS4ZZ Extirpation of Matter from Left Maxilla, Percutaneous Endoscopic Approach

0NCT0ZZ Extirpation of Matter from Right Mandible, Open Approach

0NCT3ZZ Extirpation of Matter from Right Mandible, Percutaneous Approach

0NCT4ZZ Extirpation of Matter from Right Mandible, Percutaneous Endoscopic Approach

0NCV0ZZ Extirpation of Matter from Left Mandible, Open Approach

0NCV3ZZ Extirpation of Matter from Left Mandible, Percutaneous Approach

0NCV4ZZ Extirpation of Matter from Left Mandible, Percutaneous Endoscopic Approach

0NCX0ZZ Extirpation of Matter from Hyoid Bone, Open Approach

0NCX3ZZ Extirpation of Matter from Hyoid Bone, Percutaneous Approach

0NCX4ZZ Extirpation of Matter from Hyoid Bone, Percutaneous Endoscopic Approach

0NH – Head and Facial Bones, Insertion

0NH004Z Insertion of Internal Fixation Device into Skull, Open Approach

0NH005Z Insertion of External Fixation Device into Skull, Open Approach

0NH00MZ Insertion of Bone Growth Stimulator into Skull, Open Approach

0NH00NZ Insertion of Neurostimulator Generator into Skull, Open Approach

➕ Major brain device implant when reported with an Insertion of a neurostimulator lead (6th character M) into the brain or cerebral ventricle. *See table 00H to construct the Insertion code.*

0NH034Z Insertion of Internal Fixation Device into Skull, Percutaneous Approach

0NH035Z Insertion of External Fixation Device into Skull, Percutaneous Approach

0NH03MZ Insertion of Bone Growth Stimulator into Skull, Percutaneous Approach

0NH044Z Insertion of Internal Fixation Device into Skull, Percutaneous Endoscopic Approach

0NH045Z Insertion of External Fixation Device into Skull, Percutaneous Endoscopic Approach

0NH04MZ Insertion of Bone Growth Stimulator into Skull, Percutaneous Endoscopic Approach

0NH104Z Insertion of Internal Fixation Device into Right Frontal Bone, Open Approach

0NH134Z Insertion of Internal Fixation Device into Right Frontal Bone, Percutaneous Approach

0NH144Z Insertion of Internal Fixation Device into Right Frontal Bone, Percutaneous Endoscopic Approach

0NH204Z Insertion of Internal Fixation Device into Left Frontal Bone, Open Approach

0NH234Z Insertion of Internal Fixation Device into Left Frontal Bone, Percutaneous Approach

0NH244Z Insertion of Internal Fixation Device into Left Frontal Bone, Percutaneous Endoscopic Approach

0NH304Z Insertion of Internal Fixation Device into Right Parietal Bone, Open Approach

0NH334Z Insertion of Internal Fixation Device into Right Parietal Bone, Percutaneous Approach

0NH344Z Insertion of Internal Fixation Device into Right Parietal Bone, Percutaneous Endoscopic Approach

0NH404Z Insertion of Internal Fixation Device into Left Parietal Bone, Open Approach

0NH434Z Insertion of Internal Fixation Device into Left Parietal Bone, Percutaneous Approach

0NH444Z Insertion of Internal Fixation Device into Left Parietal Bone, Percutaneous Endoscopic Approach

0NH504Z Insertion of Internal Fixation Device into Right Temporal Bone, Open Approach

0NH50SZ Insertion of Hearing Device into Right Temporal Bone, Open Approach

0NH534Z Insertion of Internal Fixation Device into Right Temporal Bone, Percutaneous Approach

0NH53SZ Insertion of Hearing Device into Right Temporal Bone, Percutaneous Approach

0NH544Z Insertion of Internal Fixation Device into Right Temporal Bone, Percutaneous Endoscopic Approach

0NH54SZ Insertion of Hearing Device into Right Temporal Bone, Percutaneous Endoscopic Approach

0NH604Z Insertion of Internal Fixation Device into Left Temporal Bone, Open Approach

0NH60SZ Insertion of Hearing Device into Left Temporal Bone, Open Approach

0NH634Z Insertion of Internal Fixation Device into Left Temporal Bone, Percutaneous Approach

0NH63SZ Insertion of Hearing Device into Left Temporal Bone, Percutaneous Approach

0NH644Z Insertion of Internal Fixation Device into Left Temporal Bone, Percutaneous Endoscopic Approach

0NH64SZ Insertion of Hearing Device into Left Temporal Bone, Percutaneous Endoscopic Approach

0NH704Z Insertion of Internal Fixation Device into Right Occipital Bone, Open Approach

0NH734Z Insertion of Internal Fixation Device into Right Occipital Bone, Percutaneous Approach

0NH744Z Insertion of Internal Fixation Device into Right Occipital Bone, Percutaneous Endoscopic Approach

0NH804Z Insertion of Internal Fixation Device into Left Occipital Bone, Open Approach

0NH834Z Insertion of Internal Fixation Device into Left Occipital Bone, Percutaneous Approach

0NH844Z Insertion of Internal Fixation Device into Left Occipital Bone, Percutaneous Endoscopic Approach

0NHB04Z Insertion of Internal Fixation Device into Nasal Bone, Open Approach

0NHB0MZ Insertion of Bone Growth Stimulator into Nasal Bone, Open Approach

0NHB34Z Insertion of Internal Fixation Device into Nasal Bone, Percutaneous Approach

0NHB3MZ Insertion of Bone Growth Stimulator into Nasal Bone, Percutaneous Approach

0NHB44Z Insertion of Internal Fixation Device into Nasal Bone, Percutaneous Endoscopic Approach

0NHB4MZ Insertion of Bone Growth Stimulator into Nasal Bone, Percutaneous Endoscopic Approach

0NHC04Z Insertion of Internal Fixation Device into Right Sphenoid Bone, Open Approach

0NHC34Z Insertion of Internal Fixation Device into Right Sphenoid Bone, Percutaneous Approach

0NHC44Z Insertion of Internal Fixation Device into Right Sphenoid Bone, Percutaneous Endoscopic Approach

0NHD04Z Insertion of Internal Fixation Device into Left Sphenoid Bone, Open Approach

0NHD34Z Insertion of Internal Fixation Device into Left Sphenoid Bone, Percutaneous Approach

0NHD44Z Insertion of Internal Fixation Device into Left Sphenoid Bone, Percutaneous Endoscopic Approach

0NHF04Z Insertion of Internal Fixation Device into Right Ethmoid Bone, Open Approach

0NHF34Z Insertion of Internal Fixation Device into Right Ethmoid Bone, Percutaneous Approach

0NHF44Z Insertion of Internal Fixation Device into Right Ethmoid Bone, Percutaneous Endoscopic Approach

0NHG04Z Insertion of Internal Fixation Device into Left Ethmoid Bone, Open Approach

0NHG34Z Insertion of Internal Fixation Device into Left Ethmoid Bone, Percutaneous Approach

0NHG44Z Insertion of Internal Fixation Device into Left Ethmoid Bone, Percutaneous Endoscopic Approach

0NHH04Z Insertion of Internal Fixation Device into Right Lacrimal Bone, Open Approach

0NHH34Z Insertion of Internal Fixation Device into Right Lacrimal Bone, Percutaneous Approach

0NHH44Z	Insertion of Internal Fixation Device into Right Lacrimal Bone, Percutaneous Endoscopic Approach	**0NHR44Z**	Insertion of Internal Fixation Device into Right Maxilla, Percutaneous Endoscopic Approach
0NHJ04Z	Insertion of Internal Fixation Device into Left Lacrimal Bone, Open Approach	**0NHR45Z**	Insertion of External Fixation Device into Right Maxilla, Percutaneous Endoscopic Approach
0NHJ34Z	Insertion of Internal Fixation Device into Left Lacrimal Bone, Percutaneous Approach	**0NHS04Z**	Insertion of Internal Fixation Device into Left Maxilla, Open Approach
0NHJ44Z	Insertion of Internal Fixation Device into Left Lacrimal Bone, Percutaneous Endoscopic Approach	**0NHS05Z**	Insertion of External Fixation Device into Left Maxilla, Open Approach
0NHK04Z	Insertion of Internal Fixation Device into Right Palatine Bone, Open Approach	**0NHS34Z**	Insertion of Internal Fixation Device into Left Maxilla, Percutaneous Approach
0NHK34Z	Insertion of Internal Fixation Device into Right Palatine Bone, Percutaneous Approach	**0NHS35Z**	Insertion of External Fixation Device into Left Maxilla, Percutaneous Approach
0NHK44Z	Insertion of Internal Fixation Device into Right Palatine Bone, Percutaneous Endoscopic Approach	**0NHS44Z**	Insertion of Internal Fixation Device into Left Maxilla, Percutaneous Endoscopic Approach
0NHL04Z	Insertion of Internal Fixation Device into Left Palatine Bone, Open Approach	**0NHS45Z**	Insertion of External Fixation Device into Left Maxilla, Percutaneous Endoscopic Approach
0NHL34Z	Insertion of Internal Fixation Device into Left Palatine Bone, Percutaneous Approach	**0NHT04Z**	Insertion of Internal Fixation Device into Right Mandible, Open Approach
0NHL44Z	Insertion of Internal Fixation Device into Left Palatine Bone, Percutaneous Endoscopic Approach	**0NHT05Z**	Insertion of External Fixation Device into Right Mandible, Open Approach
0NHM04Z	Insertion of Internal Fixation Device into Right Zygomatic Bone, Open Approach	**0NHT34Z**	Insertion of Internal Fixation Device into Right Mandible, Percutaneous Approach
0NHM34Z	Insertion of Internal Fixation Device into Right Zygomatic Bone, Percutaneous Approach	**0NHT35Z**	Insertion of External Fixation Device into Right Mandible, Percutaneous Approach
0NHM44Z	Insertion of Internal Fixation Device into Right Zygomatic Bone, Percutaneous Endoscopic Approach	**0NHT44Z**	Insertion of Internal Fixation Device into Right Mandible, Percutaneous Endoscopic Approach
0NHN04Z	Insertion of Internal Fixation Device into Left Zygomatic Bone, Open Approach	**0NHT45Z**	Insertion of External Fixation Device into Right Mandible, Percutaneous Endoscopic Approach
0NHN34Z	Insertion of Internal Fixation Device into Left Zygomatic Bone, Percutaneous Approach	**0NHV04Z**	Insertion of Internal Fixation Device into Left Mandible, Open Approach
0NHN44Z	Insertion of Internal Fixation Device into Left Zygomatic Bone, Percutaneous Endoscopic Approach	**0NHV05Z**	Insertion of External Fixation Device into Left Mandible, Open Approach
0NHP04Z	Insertion of Internal Fixation Device into Right Orbit, Open Approach	**0NHV34Z**	Insertion of Internal Fixation Device into Left Mandible, Percutaneous Approach
0NHP34Z	Insertion of Internal Fixation Device into Right Orbit, Percutaneous Approach	**0NHV35Z**	Insertion of External Fixation Device into Left Mandible, Percutaneous Approach
0NHP44Z	Insertion of Internal Fixation Device into Right Orbit, Percutaneous Endoscopic Approach	**0NHV44Z**	Insertion of Internal Fixation Device into Left Mandible, Percutaneous Endoscopic Approach
0NHQ04Z	Insertion of Internal Fixation Device into Left Orbit, Open Approach	**0NHV45Z**	Insertion of External Fixation Device into Left Mandible, Percutaneous Endoscopic Approach
0NHQ34Z	Insertion of Internal Fixation Device into Left Orbit, Percutaneous Approach	**0NHW0MZ**	Insertion of Bone Growth Stimulator into Facial Bone, Open Approach
0NHQ44Z	Insertion of Internal Fixation Device into Left Orbit, Percutaneous Endoscopic Approach	**0NHW3MZ**	Insertion of Bone Growth Stimulator into Facial Bone, Percutaneous Approach
0NHR04Z	Insertion of Internal Fixation Device into Right Maxilla, Open Approach	**0NHW4MZ**	Insertion of Bone Growth Stimulator into Facial Bone, Percutaneous Endoscopic Approach
0NHR05Z	Insertion of External Fixation Device into Right Maxilla, Open Approach	**0NHX04Z**	Insertion of Internal Fixation Device into Hyoid Bone, Open Approach
0NHR34Z	Insertion of Internal Fixation Device into Right Maxilla, Percutaneous Approach	**0NHX34Z**	Insertion of Internal Fixation Device into Hyoid Bone, Percutaneous Approach
0NHR35Z	Insertion of External Fixation Device into Right Maxilla, Percutaneous Approach	**0NHX44Z**	Insertion of Internal Fixation Device into Hyoid Bone, Percutaneous Endoscopic Approach

0NJ – Head and Facial Bones, Inspection

Review Coding Guideline B3.5

Review Coding Guidelines B3.11a, B3.11b and B3.11c

0NJ00ZZ	Inspection of Skull, Open Approach	**0NJB4ZZ**	Inspection of Nasal Bone, Percutaneous Endoscopic Approach
0NJ03ZZ	Inspection of Skull, Percutaneous Approach	**0NJBXZZ**	Inspection of Nasal Bone, External Approach
0NJ04ZZ	Inspection of Skull, Percutaneous Endoscopic Approach	**0NJW0ZZ**	Inspection of Facial Bone, Open Approach
0NJ0XZZ	Inspection of Skull, External Approach	**0NJW3ZZ**	Inspection of Facial Bone, Percutaneous Approach
0NJB0ZZ	Inspection of Nasal Bone, Open Approach	**0NJW4ZZ**	Inspection of Facial Bone, Percutaneous Endoscopic Approach
0NJB3ZZ	Inspection of Nasal Bone, Percutaneous Approach	**0NJWXZZ**	Inspection of Facial Bone, External Approach

0NN – Head and Facial Bones, Release

Review Coding Guideline B3.13

Review Coding Guideline B3.14

0NN10ZZ	Release Right Frontal Bone, Open Approach	**0NN14ZZ**	Release Right Frontal Bone, Percutaneous Endoscopic Approach
0NN13ZZ	Release Right Frontal Bone, Percutaneous Approach	**0NN20ZZ**	Release Left Frontal Bone, Open Approach

---

♀ Female-only   ♂ Male-only   ◯ Limited Coverage   ● Non-OR   🄷🄰🄲 HAC-associated procedure   ● Non-covered procedures   ✚ Combination

0NN23ZZ	Release Left Frontal Bone, Percutaneous Approach
0NN24ZZ	Release Left Frontal Bone, Percutaneous Endoscopic Approach
0NN30ZZ	Release Right Parietal Bone, Open Approach
0NN33ZZ	Release Right Parietal Bone, Percutaneous Approach
0NN34ZZ	Release Right Parietal Bone, Percutaneous Endoscopic Approach
0NN40ZZ	Release Left Parietal Bone, Open Approach
0NN43ZZ	Release Left Parietal Bone, Percutaneous Approach
0NN44ZZ	Release Left Parietal Bone, Percutaneous Endoscopic Approach
0NN50ZZ	Release Right Temporal Bone, Open Approach
0NN53ZZ	Release Right Temporal Bone, Percutaneous Approach
0NN54ZZ	Release Right Temporal Bone, Percutaneous Endoscopic Approach
0NN60ZZ	Release Left Temporal Bone, Open Approach
0NN63ZZ	Release Left Temporal Bone, Percutaneous Approach
0NN64ZZ	Release Left Temporal Bone, Percutaneous Endoscopic Approach
0NN70ZZ	Release Right Occipital Bone, Open Approach
0NN73ZZ	Release Right Occipital Bone, Percutaneous Approach
0NN74ZZ	Release Right Occipital Bone, Percutaneous Endoscopic Approach
0NN80ZZ	Release Left Occipital Bone, Open Approach
0NN83ZZ	Release Left Occipital Bone, Percutaneous Approach
0NN84ZZ	Release Left Occipital Bone, Percutaneous Endoscopic Approach
0NNB0ZZ	Release Nasal Bone, Open Approach
0NNB3ZZ	Release Nasal Bone, Percutaneous Approach
0NNB4ZZ	Release Nasal Bone, Percutaneous Endoscopic Approach
0NNC0ZZ	Release Right Sphenoid Bone, Open Approach
0NNC3ZZ	Release Right Sphenoid Bone, Percutaneous Approach
0NNC4ZZ	Release Right Sphenoid Bone, Percutaneous Endoscopic Approach
0NND0ZZ	Release Left Sphenoid Bone, Open Approach
0NND3ZZ	Release Left Sphenoid Bone, Percutaneous Approach
0NND4ZZ	Release Left Sphenoid Bone, Percutaneous Endoscopic Approach
0NNF0ZZ	Release Right Ethmoid Bone, Open Approach
0NNF3ZZ	Release Right Ethmoid Bone, Percutaneous Approach
0NNF4ZZ	Release Right Ethmoid Bone, Percutaneous Endoscopic Approach
0NNG0ZZ	Release Left Ethmoid Bone, Open Approach
0NNG3ZZ	Release Left Ethmoid Bone, Percutaneous Approach
0NNG4ZZ	Release Left Ethmoid Bone, Percutaneous Endoscopic Approach
0NNH0ZZ	Release Right Lacrimal Bone, Open Approach
0NNH3ZZ	Release Right Lacrimal Bone, Percutaneous Approach
0NNH4ZZ	Release Right Lacrimal Bone, Percutaneous Endoscopic Approach

0NNJ0ZZ	Release Left Lacrimal Bone, Open Approach
0NNJ3ZZ	Release Left Lacrimal Bone, Percutaneous Approach
0NNJ4ZZ	Release Left Lacrimal Bone, Percutaneous Endoscopic Approach
0NNK0ZZ	Release Right Palatine Bone, Open Approach
0NNK3ZZ	Release Right Palatine Bone, Percutaneous Approach
0NNK4ZZ	Release Right Palatine Bone, Percutaneous Endoscopic Approach
0NNL0ZZ	Release Left Palatine Bone, Open Approach
0NNL3ZZ	Release Left Palatine Bone, Percutaneous Approach
0NNL4ZZ	Release Left Palatine Bone, Percutaneous Endoscopic Approach
0NNM0ZZ	Release Right Zygomatic Bone, Open Approach
0NNM3ZZ	Release Right Zygomatic Bone, Percutaneous Approach
0NNM4ZZ	Release Right Zygomatic Bone, Percutaneous Endoscopic Approach
0NNN0ZZ	Release Left Zygomatic Bone, Open Approach
0NNN3ZZ	Release Left Zygomatic Bone, Percutaneous Approach
0NNN4ZZ	Release Left Zygomatic Bone, Percutaneous Endoscopic Approach
0NNP0ZZ	Release Right Orbit, Open Approach
0NNP3ZZ	Release Right Orbit, Percutaneous Approach
0NNP4ZZ	Release Right Orbit, Percutaneous Endoscopic Approach
0NNQ0ZZ	Release Left Orbit, Open Approach
0NNQ3ZZ	Release Left Orbit, Percutaneous Approach
0NNQ4ZZ	Release Left Orbit, Percutaneous Endoscopic Approach
0NNR0ZZ	Release Right Maxilla, Open Approach
0NNR3ZZ	Release Right Maxilla, Percutaneous Approach
0NNR4ZZ	Release Right Maxilla, Percutaneous Endoscopic Approach
0NNS0ZZ	Release Left Maxilla, Open Approach
0NNS3ZZ	Release Left Maxilla, Percutaneous Approach
0NNS4ZZ	Release Left Maxilla, Percutaneous Endoscopic Approach
0NNT0ZZ	Release Right Mandible, Open Approach
0NNT3ZZ	Release Right Mandible, Percutaneous Approach
0NNT4ZZ	Release Right Mandible, Percutaneous Endoscopic Approach
0NNV0ZZ	Release Left Mandible, Open Approach
0NNV3ZZ	Release Left Mandible, Percutaneous Approach
0NNV4ZZ	Release Left Mandible, Percutaneous Endoscopic Approach
0NNX0ZZ	Release Hyoid Bone, Open Approach
0NNX3ZZ	Release Hyoid Bone, Percutaneous Approach
0NNX4ZZ	Release Hyoid Bone, Percutaneous Endoscopic Approach

0NP – Head and Facial Bones, Removal

Review Coding Guideline B6.1c

0NP000Z	Removal of Drainage Device from Skull, Open Approach
0NP004Z	Removal of Internal Fixation Device from Skull, Open Approach
0NP005Z	Removal of External Fixation Device from Skull, Open Approach
0NP007Z	Removal of Autologous Tissue Substitute from Skull, Open Approach
0NP00JZ	Removal of Synthetic Substitute from Skull, Open Approach
0NP00KZ	Removal of Nonautologous Tissue Substitute from Skull, Open Approach
0NP00MZ	Removal of Bone Growth Stimulator from Skull, Open Approach
0NP00NZ	Removal of Neurostimulator Generator from Skull, Open Approach
0NP00SZ	Removal of Hearing Device from Skull, Open Approach
0NP030Z	Removal of Drainage Device from Skull, Percutaneous Approach
0NP034Z	Removal of Internal Fixation Device from Skull, Percutaneous Approach
0NP035Z	Removal of External Fixation Device from Skull, Percutaneous Approach
0NP037Z	Removal of Autologous Tissue Substitute from Skull, Percutaneous Approach
0NP03JZ	Removal of Synthetic Substitute from Skull, Percutaneous Approach
0NP03KZ	Removal of Nonautologous Tissue Substitute from Skull, Percutaneous Approach
0NP03MZ	Removal of Bone Growth Stimulator from Skull, Percutaneous Approach
0NP03SZ	Removal of Hearing Device from Skull, Percutaneous Approach
0NP040Z	Removal of Drainage Device from Skull, Percutaneous Endoscopic Approach
0NP044Z	Removal of Internal Fixation Device from Skull, Percutaneous Endoscopic Approach

0NP045Z	Removal of External Fixation Device from Skull, Percutaneous Endoscopic Approach
0NP047Z	Removal of Autologous Tissue Substitute from Skull, Percutaneous Endoscopic Approach
0NP04JZ	Removal of Synthetic Substitute from Skull, Percutaneous Endoscopic Approach
0NP04KZ	Removal of Nonautologous Tissue Substitute from Skull, Percutaneous Endoscopic Approach
0NP04MZ	Removal of Bone Growth Stimulator from Skull, Percutaneous Endoscopic Approach
0NP04SZ	Removal of Hearing Device from Skull, Percutaneous Endoscopic Approach
0NP0X0Z	Removal of Drainage Device from Skull, External Approach
0NP0X4Z	Removal of Internal Fixation Device from Skull, External Approach
0NP0X5Z	Removal of External Fixation Device from Skull, External Approach
0NP0XMZ	Removal of Bone Growth Stimulator from Skull, External Approach
0NP0XSZ	Removal of Hearing Device from Skull, External Approach
0NPB00Z	Removal of Drainage Device from Nasal Bone, Open Approach
0NPB04Z	Removal of Internal Fixation Device from Nasal Bone, Open Approach
0NPB07Z	Removal of Autologous Tissue Substitute from Nasal Bone, Open Approach
0NPB0JZ	Removal of Synthetic Substitute from Nasal Bone, Open Approach
0NPB0KZ	Removal of Nonautologous Tissue Substitute from Nasal Bone, Open Approach
0NPB0MZ	Removal of Bone Growth Stimulator from Nasal Bone, Open Approach

---

♀ Female-only   ♂ Male-only   ● Limited Coverage   ● Non-OR   🅷🅰🅲 HAC-associated procedure   ● Non-covered procedures   ➕ Combination

0NPB30Z   Removal of Drainage Device from Nasal Bone, Percutaneous Approach
0NPB34Z   Removal of Internal Fixation Device from Nasal Bone, Percutaneous Approach
0NPB37Z   Removal of Autologous Tissue Substitute from Nasal Bone, Percutaneous Approach
0NPB3JZ   Removal of Synthetic Substitute from Nasal Bone, Percutaneous Approach
0NPB3KZ   Removal of Nonautologous Tissue Substitute from Nasal Bone, Percutaneous Approach
0NPB3MZ   Removal of Bone Growth Stimulator from Nasal Bone, Percutaneous Approach
0NPB40Z   Removal of Drainage Device from Nasal Bone, Percutaneous Endoscopic Approach
0NPB44Z   Removal of Internal Fixation Device from Nasal Bone, Percutaneous Endoscopic Approach
0NPB47Z   Removal of Autologous Tissue Substitute from Nasal Bone, Percutaneous Endoscopic Approach
0NPB4JZ   Removal of Synthetic Substitute from Nasal Bone, Percutaneous Endoscopic Approach
0NPB4KZ   Removal of Nonautologous Tissue Substitute from Nasal Bone, Percutaneous Endoscopic Approach
0NPB4MZ   Removal of Bone Growth Stimulator from Nasal Bone, Percutaneous Endoscopic Approach
0NPBX0Z   Removal of Drainage Device from Nasal Bone, External Approach
0NPBX4Z   Removal of Internal Fixation Device from Nasal Bone, External Approach
0NPBXMZ   Removal of Bone Growth Stimulator from Nasal Bone, External Approach
0NPW00Z   Removal of Drainage Device from Facial Bone, Open Approach
0NPW04Z   Removal of Internal Fixation Device from Facial Bone, Open Approach
0NPW07Z   Removal of Autologous Tissue Substitute from Facial Bone, Open Approach

0NPW0JZ   Removal of Synthetic Substitute from Facial Bone, Open Approach
0NPW0KZ   Removal of Nonautologous Tissue Substitute from Facial Bone, Open Approach
0NPW0MZ   Removal of Bone Growth Stimulator from Facial Bone, Open Approach
0NPW30Z   Removal of Drainage Device from Facial Bone, Percutaneous Approach
0NPW34Z   Removal of Internal Fixation Device from Facial Bone, Percutaneous Approach
0NPW37Z   Removal of Autologous Tissue Substitute from Facial Bone, Percutaneous Approach
0NPW3JZ   Removal of Synthetic Substitute from Facial Bone, Percutaneous Approach
0NPW3KZ   Removal of Nonautologous Tissue Substitute from Facial Bone, Percutaneous Approach
0NPW3MZ   Removal of Bone Growth Stimulator from Facial Bone, Percutaneous Approach
0NPW40Z   Removal of Drainage Device from Facial Bone, Percutaneous Endoscopic Approach
0NPW44Z   Removal of Internal Fixation Device from Facial Bone, Percutaneous Endoscopic Approach
0NPW47Z   Removal of Autologous Tissue Substitute from Facial Bone, Percutaneous Endoscopic Approach
0NPW4JZ   Removal of Synthetic Substitute from Facial Bone, Percutaneous Endoscopic Approach
0NPW4KZ   Removal of Nonautologous Tissue Substitute from Facial Bone, Percutaneous Endoscopic Approach
0NPW4MZ   Removal of Bone Growth Stimulator from Facial Bone, Percutaneous Endoscopic Approach
0NPWX0Z   Removal of Drainage Device from Facial Bone, External Approach
0NPWX4Z   Removal of Internal Fixation Device from Facial Bone, External Approach
0NPWXMZ   Removal of Bone Growth Stimulator from Facial Bone, External Approach

0NQ – Head and Facial Bones, Repair

Review Coding Guideline B3.5

0NQ00ZZ   Repair Skull, Open Approach
0NQ03ZZ   Repair Skull, Percutaneous Approach
0NQ04ZZ   Repair Skull, Percutaneous Endoscopic Approach
0NQ0XZZ   Repair Skull, External Approach
0NQ10ZZ   Repair Right Frontal Bone, Open Approach
0NQ13ZZ   Repair Right Frontal Bone, Percutaneous Approach
0NQ14ZZ   Repair Right Frontal Bone, Percutaneous Endoscopic Approach
0NQ1XZZ   Repair Right Frontal Bone, External Approach
0NQ20ZZ   Repair Left Frontal Bone, Open Approach
0NQ23ZZ   Repair Left Frontal Bone, Percutaneous Approach
0NQ24ZZ   Repair Left Frontal Bone, Percutaneous Endoscopic Approach
0NQ2XZZ   Repair Left Frontal Bone, External Approach
0NQ30ZZ   Repair Right Parietal Bone, Open Approach
0NQ33ZZ   Repair Right Parietal Bone, Percutaneous Approach
0NQ34ZZ   Repair Right Parietal Bone, Percutaneous Endoscopic Approach
0NQ3XZZ   Repair Right Parietal Bone, External Approach
0NQ40ZZ   Repair Left Parietal Bone, Open Approach
0NQ43ZZ   Repair Left Parietal Bone, Percutaneous Approach
0NQ44ZZ   Repair Left Parietal Bone, Percutaneous Endoscopic Approach
0NQ4XZZ   Repair Left Parietal Bone, External Approach
0NQ50ZZ   Repair Right Temporal Bone, Open Approach
0NQ53ZZ   Repair Right Temporal Bone, Percutaneous Approach
0NQ54ZZ   Repair Right Temporal Bone, Percutaneous Endoscopic Approach
0NQ5XZZ   Repair Right Temporal Bone, External Approach
0NQ60ZZ   Repair Left Temporal Bone, Open Approach
0NQ63ZZ   Repair Left Temporal Bone, Percutaneous Approach
0NQ64ZZ   Repair Left Temporal Bone, Percutaneous Endoscopic Approach
0NQ6XZZ   Repair Left Temporal Bone, External Approach
0NQ70ZZ   Repair Right Occipital Bone, Open Approach
0NQ73ZZ   Repair Right Occipital Bone, Percutaneous Approach
0NQ74ZZ   Repair Right Occipital Bone, Percutaneous Endoscopic Approach
0NQ7XZZ   Repair Right Occipital Bone, External Approach

0NQ80ZZ   Repair Left Occipital Bone, Open Approach
0NQ83ZZ   Repair Left Occipital Bone, Percutaneous Approach
0NQ84ZZ   Repair Left Occipital Bone, Percutaneous Endoscopic Approach
0NQ8XZZ   Repair Left Occipital Bone, External Approach
0NQB0ZZ   Repair Nasal Bone, Open Approach
0NQB3ZZ   Repair Nasal Bone, Percutaneous Approach
0NQB4ZZ   Repair Nasal Bone, Percutaneous Endoscopic Approach
0NQBXZZ   Repair Nasal Bone, External Approach
0NQC0ZZ   Repair Right Sphenoid Bone, Open Approach
0NQC3ZZ   Repair Right Sphenoid Bone, Percutaneous Approach
0NQC4ZZ   Repair Right Sphenoid Bone, Percutaneous Endoscopic Approach
0NQCXZZ   Repair Right Sphenoid Bone, External Approach
0NQD0ZZ   Repair Left Sphenoid Bone, Open Approach
0NQD3ZZ   Repair Left Sphenoid Bone, Percutaneous Approach
0NQD4ZZ   Repair Left Sphenoid Bone, Percutaneous Endoscopic Approach
0NQDXZZ   Repair Left Sphenoid Bone, External Approach
0NQF0ZZ   Repair Right Ethmoid Bone, Open Approach
0NQF3ZZ   Repair Right Ethmoid Bone, Percutaneous Approach
0NQF4ZZ   Repair Right Ethmoid Bone, Percutaneous Endoscopic Approach
0NQFXZZ   Repair Right Ethmoid Bone, External Approach
0NQG0ZZ   Repair Left Ethmoid Bone, Open Approach
0NQG3ZZ   Repair Left Ethmoid Bone, Percutaneous Approach
0NQG4ZZ   Repair Left Ethmoid Bone, Percutaneous Endoscopic Approach
0NQGXZZ   Repair Left Ethmoid Bone, External Approach
0NQH0ZZ   Repair Right Lacrimal Bone, Open Approach
0NQH3ZZ   Repair Right Lacrimal Bone, Percutaneous Approach
0NQH4ZZ   Repair Right Lacrimal Bone, Percutaneous Endoscopic Approach
0NQHXZZ   Repair Right Lacrimal Bone, External Approach
0NQJ0ZZ   Repair Left Lacrimal Bone, Open Approach
0NQJ3ZZ   Repair Left Lacrimal Bone, Percutaneous Approach
0NQJ4ZZ   Repair Left Lacrimal Bone, Percutaneous Endoscopic Approach
0NQJXZZ   Repair Left Lacrimal Bone, External Approach

0NQK0ZZ	Repair Right Palatine Bone, Open Approach
0NQK3ZZ	Repair Right Palatine Bone, Percutaneous Approach
0NQK4ZZ	Repair Right Palatine Bone, Percutaneous Endoscopic Approach
0NQKXZZ	Repair Right Palatine Bone, External Approach
0NQL0ZZ	Repair Left Palatine Bone, Open Approach
0NQL3ZZ	Repair Left Palatine Bone, Percutaneous Approach
0NQL4ZZ	Repair Left Palatine Bone, Percutaneous Endoscopic Approach
0NQLXZZ	Repair Left Palatine Bone, External Approach
0NQM0ZZ	Repair Right Zygomatic Bone, Open Approach
0NQM3ZZ	Repair Right Zygomatic Bone, Percutaneous Approach
0NQM4ZZ	Repair Right Zygomatic Bone, Percutaneous Endoscopic Approach
0NQMXZZ	Repair Right Zygomatic Bone, External Approach
0NQN0ZZ	Repair Left Zygomatic Bone, Open Approach
0NQN3ZZ	Repair Left Zygomatic Bone, Percutaneous Approach
0NQN4ZZ	Repair Left Zygomatic Bone, Percutaneous Endoscopic Approach
0NQNXZZ	Repair Left Zygomatic Bone, External Approach
0NQP0ZZ	Repair Right Orbit, Open Approach
0NQP3ZZ	Repair Right Orbit, Percutaneous Approach
0NQP4ZZ	Repair Right Orbit, Percutaneous Endoscopic Approach
0NQPXZZ	Repair Right Orbit, External Approach
0NQQ0ZZ	Repair Left Orbit, Open Approach
0NQQ3ZZ	Repair Left Orbit, Percutaneous Approach
0NQQ4ZZ	Repair Left Orbit, Percutaneous Endoscopic Approach
0NQQXZZ	Repair Left Orbit, External Approach
0NQR0ZZ	Repair Right Maxilla, Open Approach
0NQR3ZZ	Repair Right Maxilla, Percutaneous Approach
0NQR4ZZ	Repair Right Maxilla, Percutaneous Endoscopic Approach
0NQRXZZ	Repair Right Maxilla, External Approach
0NQS0ZZ	Repair Left Maxilla, Open Approach
0NQS3ZZ	Repair Left Maxilla, Percutaneous Approach
0NQS4ZZ	Repair Left Maxilla, Percutaneous Endoscopic Approach
0NQSXZZ	Repair Left Maxilla, External Approach
0NQT0ZZ	Repair Right Mandible, Open Approach
0NQT3ZZ	Repair Right Mandible, Percutaneous Approach
0NQT4ZZ	Repair Right Mandible, Percutaneous Endoscopic Approach
0NQTXZZ	Repair Right Mandible, External Approach
0NQV0ZZ	Repair Left Mandible, Open Approach
0NQV3ZZ	Repair Left Mandible, Percutaneous Approach
0NQV4ZZ	Repair Left Mandible, Percutaneous Endoscopic Approach
0NQVXZZ	Repair Left Mandible, External Approach
0NQX0ZZ	Repair Hyoid Bone, Open Approach
0NQX3ZZ	Repair Hyoid Bone, Percutaneous Approach
0NQX4ZZ	Repair Hyoid Bone, Percutaneous Endoscopic Approach
0NQXXZZ	Repair Hyoid Bone, External Approach

0NR – Head and Facial Bones, Replacement

0NR007Z	Replacement of Skull with Autologous Tissue Substitute, Open Approach
0NR00JZ	Replacement of Skull with Synthetic Substitute, Open Approach
0NR00KZ	Replacement of Skull with Nonautologous Tissue Substitute, Open Approach
0NR037Z	Replacement of Skull with Autologous Tissue Substitute, Percutaneous Approach
0NR03JZ	Replacement of Skull with Synthetic Substitute, Percutaneous Approach
0NR03KZ	Replacement of Skull with Nonautologous Tissue Substitute, Percutaneous Approach
0NR047Z	Replacement of Skull with Autologous Tissue Substitute, Percutaneous Endoscopic Approach
0NR04JZ	Replacement of Skull with Synthetic Substitute, Percutaneous Endoscopic Approach
0NR04KZ	Replacement of Skull with Nonautologous Tissue Substitute, Percutaneous Endoscopic Approach
0NR107Z	Replacement of Right Frontal Bone with Autologous Tissue Substitute, Open Approach
0NR10JZ	Replacement of Right Frontal Bone with Synthetic Substitute, Open Approach
0NR10KZ	Replacement of Right Frontal Bone with Nonautologous Tissue Substitute, Open Approach
0NR137Z	Replacement of Right Frontal Bone with Autologous Tissue Substitute, Percutaneous Approach
0NR13JZ	Replacement of Right Frontal Bone with Synthetic Substitute, Percutaneous Approach
0NR13KZ	Replacement of Right Frontal Bone with Nonautologous Tissue Substitute, Percutaneous Approach
0NR147Z	Replacement of Right Frontal Bone with Autologous Tissue Substitute, Percutaneous Endoscopic Approach
0NR14JZ	Replacement of Right Frontal Bone with Synthetic Substitute, Percutaneous Endoscopic Approach
0NR14KZ	Replacement of Right Frontal Bone with Nonautologous Tissue Substitute, Percutaneous Endoscopic Approach
0NR207Z	Replacement of Left Frontal Bone with Autologous Tissue Substitute, Open Approach
0NR20JZ	Replacement of Left Frontal Bone with Synthetic Substitute, Open Approach
0NR20KZ	Replacement of Left Frontal Bone with Nonautologous Tissue Substitute, Open Approach
0NR237Z	Replacement of Left Frontal Bone with Autologous Tissue Substitute, Percutaneous Approach
0NR23JZ	Replacement of Left Frontal Bone with Synthetic Substitute, Percutaneous Approach
0NR23KZ	Replacement of Left Frontal Bone with Nonautologous Tissue Substitute, Percutaneous Approach
0NR247Z	Replacement of Left Frontal Bone with Autologous Tissue Substitute, Percutaneous Endoscopic Approach
0NR24JZ	Replacement of Left Frontal Bone with Synthetic Substitute, Percutaneous Endoscopic Approach
0NR24KZ	Replacement of Left Frontal Bone with Nonautologous Tissue Substitute, Percutaneous Endoscopic Approach
0NR307Z	Replacement of Right Parietal Bone with Autologous Tissue Substitute, Open Approach
0NR30JZ	Replacement of Right Parietal Bone with Synthetic Substitute, Open Approach
0NR30KZ	Replacement of Right Parietal Bone with Nonautologous Tissue Substitute, Open Approach
0NR337Z	Replacement of Right Parietal Bone with Autologous Tissue Substitute, Percutaneous Approach
0NR33JZ	Replacement of Right Parietal Bone with Synthetic Substitute, Percutaneous Approach
0NR33KZ	Replacement of Right Parietal Bone with Nonautologous Tissue Substitute, Percutaneous Approach
0NR347Z	Replacement of Right Parietal Bone with Autologous Tissue Substitute, Percutaneous Endoscopic Approach
0NR34JZ	Replacement of Right Parietal Bone with Synthetic Substitute, Percutaneous Endoscopic Approach
0NR34KZ	Replacement of Right Parietal Bone with Nonautologous Tissue Substitute, Percutaneous Endoscopic Approach
0NR407Z	Replacement of Left Parietal Bone with Autologous Tissue Substitute, Open Approach
0NR40JZ	Replacement of Left Parietal Bone with Synthetic Substitute, Open Approach
0NR40KZ	Replacement of Left Parietal Bone with Nonautologous Tissue Substitute, Open Approach
0NR437Z	Replacement of Left Parietal Bone with Autologous Tissue Substitute, Percutaneous Approach
0NR43JZ	Replacement of Left Parietal Bone with Synthetic Substitute, Percutaneous Approach
0NR43KZ	Replacement of Left Parietal Bone with Nonautologous Tissue Substitute, Percutaneous Approach
0NR447Z	Replacement of Left Parietal Bone with Autologous Tissue Substitute, Percutaneous Endoscopic Approach
0NR44JZ	Replacement of Left Parietal Bone with Synthetic Substitute, Percutaneous Endoscopic Approach
0NR44KZ	Replacement of Left Parietal Bone with Nonautologous Tissue Substitute, Percutaneous Endoscopic Approach
0NR507Z	Replacement of Right Temporal Bone with Autologous Tissue Substitute, Open Approach
0NR50JZ	Replacement of Right Temporal Bone with Synthetic Substitute, Open Approach
0NR50KZ	Replacement of Right Temporal Bone with Nonautologous Tissue Substitute, Open Approach

0NR537Z   Replacement of Right Temporal Bone with Autologous Tissue Substitute, Percutaneous Approach

0NR53JZ   Replacement of Right Temporal Bone with Synthetic Substitute, Percutaneous Approach

0NR53KZ   Replacement of Right Temporal Bone with Nonautologous Tissue Substitute, Percutaneous Approach

0NR547Z   Replacement of Right Temporal Bone with Autologous Tissue Substitute, Percutaneous Endoscopic Approach

0NR54JZ   Replacement of Right Temporal Bone with Synthetic Substitute, Percutaneous Endoscopic Approach

0NR54KZ   Replacement of Right Temporal Bone with Nonautologous Tissue Substitute, Percutaneous Endoscopic Approach

0NR607Z   Replacement of Left Temporal Bone with Autologous Tissue Substitute, Open Approach

0NR60JZ   Replacement of Left Temporal Bone with Synthetic Substitute, Open Approach

0NR60KZ   Replacement of Left Temporal Bone with Nonautologous Tissue Substitute, Open Approach

0NR637Z   Replacement of Left Temporal Bone with Autologous Tissue Substitute, Percutaneous Approach

0NR63JZ   Replacement of Left Temporal Bone with Synthetic Substitute, Percutaneous Approach

0NR63KZ   Replacement of Left Temporal Bone with Nonautologous Tissue Substitute, Percutaneous Approach

0NR647Z   Replacement of Left Temporal Bone with Autologous Tissue Substitute, Percutaneous Endoscopic Approach

0NR64JZ   Replacement of Left Temporal Bone with Synthetic Substitute, Percutaneous Endoscopic Approach

0NR64KZ   Replacement of Left Temporal Bone with Nonautologous Tissue Substitute, Percutaneous Endoscopic Approach

0NR707Z   Replacement of Right Occipital Bone with Autologous Tissue Substitute, Open Approach

0NR70JZ   Replacement of Right Occipital Bone with Synthetic Substitute, Open Approach

0NR70KZ   Replacement of Right Occipital Bone with Nonautologous Tissue Substitute, Open Approach

0NR737Z   Replacement of Right Occipital Bone with Autologous Tissue Substitute, Percutaneous Approach

0NR73JZ   Replacement of Right Occipital Bone with Synthetic Substitute, Percutaneous Approach

0NR73KZ   Replacement of Right Occipital Bone with Nonautologous Tissue Substitute, Percutaneous Approach

0NR747Z   Replacement of Right Occipital Bone with Autologous Tissue Substitute, Percutaneous Endoscopic Approach

0NR74JZ   Replacement of Right Occipital Bone with Synthetic Substitute, Percutaneous Endoscopic Approach

0NR74KZ   Replacement of Right Occipital Bone with Nonautologous Tissue Substitute, Percutaneous Endoscopic Approach

0NR807Z   Replacement of Left Occipital Bone with Autologous Tissue Substitute, Open Approach

0NR80JZ   Replacement of Left Occipital Bone with Synthetic Substitute, Open Approach

0NR80KZ   Replacement of Left Occipital Bone with Nonautologous Tissue Substitute, Open Approach

0NR837Z   Replacement of Left Occipital Bone with Autologous Tissue Substitute, Percutaneous Approach

0NR83JZ   Replacement of Left Occipital Bone with Synthetic Substitute, Percutaneous Approach

0NR83KZ   Replacement of Left Occipital Bone with Nonautologous Tissue Substitute, Percutaneous Approach

0NR847Z   Replacement of Left Occipital Bone with Autologous Tissue Substitute, Percutaneous Endoscopic Approach

0NR84JZ   Replacement of Left Occipital Bone with Synthetic Substitute, Percutaneous Endoscopic Approach

0NR84KZ   Replacement of Left Occipital Bone with Nonautologous Tissue Substitute, Percutaneous Endoscopic Approach

0NRB07Z   Replacement of Nasal Bone with Autologous Tissue Substitute, Open Approach

0NRB0JZ   Replacement of Nasal Bone with Synthetic Substitute, Open Approach

0NRB0KZ   Replacement of Nasal Bone with Nonautologous Tissue Substitute, Open Approach

0NRB37Z   Replacement of Nasal Bone with Autologous Tissue Substitute, Percutaneous Approach

0NRB3JZ   Replacement of Nasal Bone with Synthetic Substitute, Percutaneous Approach

0NRB3KZ   Replacement of Nasal Bone with Nonautologous Tissue Substitute, Percutaneous Approach

0NRB47Z   Replacement of Nasal Bone with Autologous Tissue Substitute, Percutaneous Endoscopic Approach

0NRB4JZ   Replacement of Nasal Bone with Synthetic Substitute, Percutaneous Endoscopic Approach

0NRB4KZ   Replacement of Nasal Bone with Nonautologous Tissue Substitute, Percutaneous Endoscopic Approach

0NRC07Z   Replacement of Right Sphenoid Bone with Autologous Tissue Substitute, Open Approach

0NRC0JZ   Replacement of Right Sphenoid Bone with Synthetic Substitute, Open Approach

0NRC0KZ   Replacement of Right Sphenoid Bone with Nonautologous Tissue Substitute, Open Approach

0NRC37Z   Replacement of Right Sphenoid Bone with Autologous Tissue Substitute, Percutaneous Approach

0NRC3JZ   Replacement of Right Sphenoid Bone with Synthetic Substitute, Percutaneous Approach

0NRC3KZ   Replacement of Right Sphenoid Bone with Nonautologous Tissue Substitute, Percutaneous Approach

0NRC47Z   Replacement of Right Sphenoid Bone with Autologous Tissue Substitute, Percutaneous Endoscopic Approach

0NRC4JZ   Replacement of Right Sphenoid Bone with Synthetic Substitute, Percutaneous Endoscopic Approach

0NRC4KZ   Replacement of Right Sphenoid Bone with Nonautologous Tissue Substitute, Percutaneous Endoscopic Approach

0NRD07Z   Replacement of Left Sphenoid Bone with Autologous Tissue Substitute, Open Approach

0NRD0JZ   Replacement of Left Sphenoid Bone with Synthetic Substitute, Open Approach

0NRD0KZ   Replacement of Left Sphenoid Bone with Nonautologous Tissue Substitute, Open Approach

0NRD37Z   Replacement of Left Sphenoid Bone with Autologous Tissue Substitute, Percutaneous Approach

0NRD3JZ   Replacement of Left Sphenoid Bone with Synthetic Substitute, Percutaneous Approach

0NRD3KZ   Replacement of Left Sphenoid Bone with Nonautologous Tissue Substitute, Percutaneous Approach

0NRD47Z   Replacement of Left Sphenoid Bone with Autologous Tissue Substitute, Percutaneous Endoscopic Approach

0NRD4JZ   Replacement of Left Sphenoid Bone with Synthetic Substitute, Percutaneous Endoscopic Approach

0NRD4KZ   Replacement of Left Sphenoid Bone with Nonautologous Tissue Substitute, Percutaneous Endoscopic Approach

0NRF07Z   Replacement of Right Ethmoid Bone with Autologous Tissue Substitute, Open Approach

0NRF0JZ   Replacement of Right Ethmoid Bone with Synthetic Substitute, Open Approach

0NRF0KZ   Replacement of Right Ethmoid Bone with Nonautologous Tissue Substitute, Open Approach

0NRF37Z   Replacement of Right Ethmoid Bone with Autologous Tissue Substitute, Percutaneous Approach

0NRF3JZ   Replacement of Right Ethmoid Bone with Synthetic Substitute, Percutaneous Approach

0NRF3KZ   Replacement of Right Ethmoid Bone with Nonautologous Tissue Substitute, Percutaneous Approach

0NRF47Z   Replacement of Right Ethmoid Bone with Autologous Tissue Substitute, Percutaneous Endoscopic Approach

0NRF4JZ   Replacement of Right Ethmoid Bone with Synthetic Substitute, Percutaneous Endoscopic Approach

0NRF4KZ   Replacement of Right Ethmoid Bone with Nonautologous Tissue Substitute, Percutaneous Endoscopic Approach

0NRG07Z   Replacement of Left Ethmoid Bone with Autologous Tissue Substitute, Open Approach

0NRG0JZ   Replacement of Left Ethmoid Bone with Synthetic Substitute, Open Approach

0NRG0KZ   Replacement of Left Ethmoid Bone with Nonautologous Tissue Substitute, Open Approach

0NRG37Z   Replacement of Left Ethmoid Bone with Autologous Tissue Substitute, Percutaneous Approach

0NRG3JZ   Replacement of Left Ethmoid Bone with Synthetic Substitute, Percutaneous Approach

0NRG3KZ Replacement of Left Ethmoid Bone with Nonautologous Tissue Substitute, Percutaneous Approach

0NRG47Z Replacement of Left Ethmoid Bone with Autologous Tissue Substitute, Percutaneous Endoscopic Approach

0NRG4JZ Replacement of Left Ethmoid Bone with Synthetic Substitute, Percutaneous Endoscopic Approach

0NRG4KZ Replacement of Left Ethmoid Bone with Nonautologous Tissue Substitute, Percutaneous Endoscopic Approach

0NRH07Z Replacement of Right Lacrimal Bone with Autologous Tissue Substitute, Open Approach

0NRH0JZ Replacement of Right Lacrimal Bone with Synthetic Substitute, Open Approach

0NRH0KZ Replacement of Right Lacrimal Bone with Nonautologous Tissue Substitute, Open Approach

0NRH37Z Replacement of Right Lacrimal Bone with Autologous Tissue Substitute, Percutaneous Approach

0NRH3JZ Replacement of Right Lacrimal Bone with Synthetic Substitute, Percutaneous Approach

0NRH3KZ Replacement of Right Lacrimal Bone with Nonautologous Tissue Substitute, Percutaneous Approach

0NRH47Z Replacement of Right Lacrimal Bone with Autologous Tissue Substitute, Percutaneous Endoscopic Approach

0NRH4JZ Replacement of Right Lacrimal Bone with Synthetic Substitute, Percutaneous Endoscopic Approach

0NRH4KZ Replacement of Right Lacrimal Bone with Nonautologous Tissue Substitute, Percutaneous Endoscopic Approach

0NRJ07Z Replacement of Left Lacrimal Bone with Autologous Tissue Substitute, Open Approach

0NRJ0JZ Replacement of Left Lacrimal Bone with Synthetic Substitute, Open Approach

0NRJ0KZ Replacement of Left Lacrimal Bone with Nonautologous Tissue Substitute, Open Approach

0NRJ37Z Replacement of Left Lacrimal Bone with Autologous Tissue Substitute, Percutaneous Approach

0NRJ3JZ Replacement of Left Lacrimal Bone with Synthetic Substitute, Percutaneous Approach

0NRJ3KZ Replacement of Left Lacrimal Bone with Nonautologous Tissue Substitute, Percutaneous Approach

0NRJ47Z Replacement of Left Lacrimal Bone with Autologous Tissue Substitute, Percutaneous Endoscopic Approach

0NRJ4JZ Replacement of Left Lacrimal Bone with Synthetic Substitute, Percutaneous Endoscopic Approach

0NRJ4KZ Replacement of Left Lacrimal Bone with Nonautologous Tissue Substitute, Percutaneous Endoscopic Approach

0NRK07Z Replacement of Right Palatine Bone with Autologous Tissue Substitute, Open Approach

0NRK0JZ Replacement of Right Palatine Bone with Synthetic Substitute, Open Approach

0NRK0KZ Replacement of Right Palatine Bone with Nonautologous Tissue Substitute, Open Approach

0NRK37Z Replacement of Right Palatine Bone with Autologous Tissue Substitute, Percutaneous Approach

0NRK3JZ Replacement of Right Palatine Bone with Synthetic Substitute, Percutaneous Approach

0NRK3KZ Replacement of Right Palatine Bone with Nonautologous Tissue Substitute, Percutaneous Approach

0NRK47Z Replacement of Right Palatine Bone with Autologous Tissue Substitute, Percutaneous Endoscopic Approach

0NRK4JZ Replacement of Right Palatine Bone with Synthetic Substitute, Percutaneous Endoscopic Approach

0NRK4KZ Replacement of Right Palatine Bone with Nonautologous Tissue Substitute, Percutaneous Endoscopic Approach

0NRL07Z Replacement of Left Palatine Bone with Autologous Tissue Substitute, Open Approach

0NRL0JZ Replacement of Left Palatine Bone with Synthetic Substitute, Open Approach

0NRL0KZ Replacement of Left Palatine Bone with Nonautologous Tissue Substitute, Open Approach

0NRL37Z Replacement of Left Palatine Bone with Autologous Tissue Substitute, Percutaneous Approach

0NRL3JZ Replacement of Left Palatine Bone with Synthetic Substitute, Percutaneous Approach

0NRL3KZ Replacement of Left Palatine Bone with Nonautologous Tissue Substitute, Percutaneous Approach

0NRL47Z Replacement of Left Palatine Bone with Autologous Tissue Substitute, Percutaneous Endoscopic Approach

0NRL4JZ Replacement of Left Palatine Bone with Synthetic Substitute, Percutaneous Endoscopic Approach

0NRL4KZ Replacement of Left Palatine Bone with Nonautologous Tissue Substitute, Percutaneous Endoscopic Approach

0NRM07Z Replacement of Right Zygomatic Bone with Autologous Tissue Substitute, Open Approach

0NRM0JZ Replacement of Right Zygomatic Bone with Synthetic Substitute, Open Approach

0NRM0KZ Replacement of Right Zygomatic Bone with Nonautologous Tissue Substitute, Open Approach

0NRM37Z Replacement of Right Zygomatic Bone with Autologous Tissue Substitute, Percutaneous Approach

0NRM3JZ Replacement of Right Zygomatic Bone with Synthetic Substitute, Percutaneous Approach

0NRM3KZ Replacement of Right Zygomatic Bone with Nonautologous Tissue Substitute, Percutaneous Approach

0NRM47Z Replacement of Right Zygomatic Bone with Autologous Tissue Substitute, Percutaneous Endoscopic Approach

0NRM4JZ Replacement of Right Zygomatic Bone with Synthetic Substitute, Percutaneous Endoscopic Approach

0NRM4KZ Replacement of Right Zygomatic Bone with Nonautologous Tissue Substitute, Percutaneous Endoscopic Approach

0NRN07Z Replacement of Left Zygomatic Bone with Autologous Tissue Substitute, Open Approach

0NRN0JZ Replacement of Left Zygomatic Bone with Synthetic Substitute, Open Approach

0NRN0KZ Replacement of Left Zygomatic Bone with Nonautologous Tissue Substitute, Open Approach

0NRN37Z Replacement of Left Zygomatic Bone with Autologous Tissue Substitute, Percutaneous Approach

0NRN3JZ Replacement of Left Zygomatic Bone with Synthetic Substitute, Percutaneous Approach

0NRN3KZ Replacement of Left Zygomatic Bone with Nonautologous Tissue Substitute, Percutaneous Approach

0NRN47Z Replacement of Left Zygomatic Bone with Autologous Tissue Substitute, Percutaneous Endoscopic Approach

0NRN4JZ Replacement of Left Zygomatic Bone with Synthetic Substitute, Percutaneous Endoscopic Approach

0NRN4KZ Replacement of Left Zygomatic Bone with Nonautologous Tissue Substitute, Percutaneous Endoscopic Approach

0NRP07Z Replacement of Right Orbit with Autologous Tissue Substitute, Open Approach

0NRP0JZ Replacement of Right Orbit with Synthetic Substitute, Open Approach

0NRP0KZ Replacement of Right Orbit with Nonautologous Tissue Substitute, Open Approach

0NRP37Z Replacement of Right Orbit with Autologous Tissue Substitute, Percutaneous Approach

0NRP3JZ Replacement of Right Orbit with Synthetic Substitute, Percutaneous Approach

0NRP3KZ Replacement of Right Orbit with Nonautologous Tissue Substitute, Percutaneous Approach

0NRP47Z Replacement of Right Orbit with Autologous Tissue Substitute, Percutaneous Endoscopic Approach

0NRP4JZ Replacement of Right Orbit with Synthetic Substitute, Percutaneous Endoscopic Approach

0NRP4KZ Replacement of Right Orbit with Nonautologous Tissue Substitute, Percutaneous Endoscopic Approach

0NRQ07Z Replacement of Left Orbit with Autologous Tissue Substitute, Open Approach

0NRQ0JZ Replacement of Left Orbit with Synthetic Substitute, Open Approach

0NRQ0KZ Replacement of Left Orbit with Nonautologous Tissue Substitute, Open Approach

0NRQ37Z Replacement of Left Orbit with Autologous Tissue Substitute, Percutaneous Approach

0NRQ3JZ Replacement of Left Orbit with Synthetic Substitute, Percutaneous Approach

0NRQ3KZ Replacement of Left Orbit with Nonautologous Tissue Substitute, Percutaneous Approach

0NRQ47Z Replacement of Left Orbit with Autologous Tissue Substitute, Percutaneous Endoscopic Approach

0NRQ4JZ Replacement of Left Orbit with Synthetic Substitute, Percutaneous Endoscopic Approach

0NRQ4KZ Replacement of Left Orbit with Nonautologous Tissue Substitute, Percutaneous Endoscopic Approach

0NRR07Z Replacement of Right Maxilla with Autologous Tissue Substitute, Open Approach

0NRR0JZ Replacement of Right Maxilla with Synthetic Substitute, Open Approach

0NRR0KZ Replacement of Right Maxilla with Nonautologous Tissue Substitute, Open Approach

0NRR37Z Replacement of Right Maxilla with Autologous Tissue Substitute, Percutaneous Approach

0NRR3JZ Replacement of Right Maxilla with Synthetic Substitute, Percutaneous Approach

0NRR3KZ Replacement of Right Maxilla with Nonautologous Tissue Substitute, Percutaneous Approach

0NRR47Z Replacement of Right Maxilla with Autologous Tissue Substitute, Percutaneous Endoscopic Approach

0NRR4JZ Replacement of Right Maxilla with Synthetic Substitute, Percutaneous Endoscopic Approach

0NRR4KZ Replacement of Right Maxilla with Nonautologous Tissue Substitute, Percutaneous Endoscopic Approach

0NRS07Z Replacement of Left Maxilla with Autologous Tissue Substitute, Open Approach

0NRS0JZ Replacement of Left Maxilla with Synthetic Substitute, Open Approach

0NRS0KZ Replacement of Left Maxilla with Nonautologous Tissue Substitute, Open Approach

0NRS37Z Replacement of Left Maxilla with Autologous Tissue Substitute, Percutaneous Approach

0NRS3JZ Replacement of Left Maxilla with Synthetic Substitute, Percutaneous Approach

0NRS3KZ Replacement of Left Maxilla with Nonautologous Tissue Substitute, Percutaneous Approach

0NRS47Z Replacement of Left Maxilla with Autologous Tissue Substitute, Percutaneous Endoscopic Approach

0NRS4JZ Replacement of Left Maxilla with Synthetic Substitute, Percutaneous Endoscopic Approach

0NRS4KZ Replacement of Left Maxilla with Nonautologous Tissue Substitute, Percutaneous Endoscopic Approach

0NRT07Z Replacement of Right Mandible with Autologous Tissue Substitute, Open Approach

0NRT0JZ Replacement of Right Mandible with Synthetic Substitute, Open Approach

0NRT0KZ Replacement of Right Mandible with Nonautologous Tissue Substitute, Open Approach

0NRT37Z Replacement of Right Mandible with Autologous Tissue Substitute, Percutaneous Approach

0NRT3JZ Replacement of Right Mandible with Synthetic Substitute, Percutaneous Approach

0NRT3KZ Replacement of Right Mandible with Nonautologous Tissue Substitute, Percutaneous Approach

0NRT47Z Replacement of Right Mandible with Autologous Tissue Substitute, Percutaneous Endoscopic Approach

0NRT4JZ Replacement of Right Mandible with Synthetic Substitute, Percutaneous Endoscopic Approach

0NRT4KZ Replacement of Right Mandible with Nonautologous Tissue Substitute, Percutaneous Endoscopic Approach

0NRV07Z Replacement of Left Mandible with Autologous Tissue Substitute, Open Approach

0NRV0JZ Replacement of Left Mandible with Synthetic Substitute, Open Approach

0NRV0KZ Replacement of Left Mandible with Nonautologous Tissue Substitute, Open Approach

0NRV37Z Replacement of Left Mandible with Autologous Tissue Substitute, Percutaneous Approach

0NRV3JZ Replacement of Left Mandible with Synthetic Substitute, Percutaneous Approach

0NRV3KZ Replacement of Left Mandible with Nonautologous Tissue Substitute, Percutaneous Approach

0NRV47Z Replacement of Left Mandible with Autologous Tissue Substitute, Percutaneous Endoscopic Approach

0NRV4JZ Replacement of Left Mandible with Synthetic Substitute, Percutaneous Endoscopic Approach

0NRV4KZ Replacement of Left Mandible with Nonautologous Tissue Substitute, Percutaneous Endoscopic Approach

0NRX07Z Replacement of Hyoid Bone with Autologous Tissue Substitute, Open Approach

0NRX0JZ Replacement of Hyoid Bone with Synthetic Substitute, Open Approach

0NRX0KZ Replacement of Hyoid Bone with Nonautologous Tissue Substitute, Open Approach

0NRX37Z Replacement of Hyoid Bone with Autologous Tissue Substitute, Percutaneous Approach

0NRX3JZ Replacement of Hyoid Bone with Synthetic Substitute, Percutaneous Approach

0NRX3KZ Replacement of Hyoid Bone with Nonautologous Tissue Substitute, Percutaneous Approach

0NRX47Z Replacement of Hyoid Bone with Autologous Tissue Substitute, Percutaneous Endoscopic Approach

0NRX4JZ Replacement of Hyoid Bone with Synthetic Substitute, Percutaneous Endoscopic Approach

0NRX4KZ Replacement of Hyoid Bone with Nonautologous Tissue Substitute, Percutaneous Endoscopic Approach

0NS – Head and Facial Bones, Reposition

Review Coding Guideline B3.15

0NS004Z Reposition Skull with Internal Fixation Device, Open Approach

0NS005Z Reposition Skull with External Fixation Device, Open Approach

0NS00ZZ Reposition Skull, Open Approach

0NS034Z Reposition Skull with Internal Fixation Device, Percutaneous Approach

0NS035Z Reposition Skull with External Fixation Device, Percutaneous Approach

0NS03ZZ Reposition Skull, Percutaneous Approach

0NS044Z Reposition Skull with Internal Fixation Device, Percutaneous Endoscopic Approach

0NS045Z Reposition Skull with External Fixation Device, Percutaneous Endoscopic Approach

0NS04ZZ Reposition Skull, Percutaneous Endoscopic Approach

0NS0XZZ Reposition Skull, External Approach

0NS104Z Reposition Right Frontal Bone with Internal Fixation Device, Open Approach

0NS10ZZ Reposition Right Frontal Bone, Open Approach

0NS134Z Reposition Right Frontal Bone with Internal Fixation Device, Percutaneous Approach

0NS13ZZ Reposition Right Frontal Bone, Percutaneous Approach

0NS144Z Reposition Right Frontal Bone with Internal Fixation Device, Percutaneous Endoscopic Approach

0NS14ZZ Reposition Right Frontal Bone, Percutaneous Endoscopic Approach

0NS1XZZ Reposition Right Frontal Bone, External Approach

0NS204Z Reposition Left Frontal Bone with Internal Fixation Device, Open Approach

0NS20ZZ Reposition Left Frontal Bone, Open Approach

0NS234Z Reposition Left Frontal Bone with Internal Fixation Device, Percutaneous Approach

0NS23ZZ Reposition Left Frontal Bone, Percutaneous Approach

0NS244Z Reposition Left Frontal Bone with Internal Fixation Device, Percutaneous Endoscopic Approach

0NS24ZZ Reposition Left Frontal Bone, Percutaneous Endoscopic Approach

0NS2XZZ Reposition Left Frontal Bone, External Approach

0NS304Z   Reposition Right Parietal Bone with Internal Fixation Device, Open Approach

0NS30ZZ   Reposition Right Parietal Bone, Open Approach

0NS334Z   Reposition Right Parietal Bone with Internal Fixation Device, Percutaneous Approach

0NS33ZZ   Reposition Right Parietal Bone, Percutaneous Approach

0NS344Z   Reposition Right Parietal Bone with Internal Fixation Device, Percutaneous Endoscopic Approach

0NS34ZZ   Reposition Right Parietal Bone, Percutaneous Endoscopic Approach

0NS3XZZ   Reposition Right Parietal Bone, External Approach

0NS404Z   Reposition Left Parietal Bone with Internal Fixation Device, Open Approach

0NS40ZZ   Reposition Left Parietal Bone, Open Approach

0NS434Z   Reposition Left Parietal Bone with Internal Fixation Device, Percutaneous Approach

0NS43ZZ   Reposition Left Parietal Bone, Percutaneous Approach

0NS444Z   Reposition Left Parietal Bone with Internal Fixation Device, Percutaneous Endoscopic Approach

0NS44ZZ   Reposition Left Parietal Bone, Percutaneous Endoscopic Approach

0NS4XZZ   Reposition Left Parietal Bone, External Approach

0NS504Z   Reposition Right Temporal Bone with Internal Fixation Device, Open Approach

0NS50ZZ   Reposition Right Temporal Bone, Open Approach

0NS534Z   Reposition Right Temporal Bone with Internal Fixation Device, Percutaneous Approach

0NS53ZZ   Reposition Right Temporal Bone, Percutaneous Approach

0NS544Z   Reposition Right Temporal Bone with Internal Fixation Device, Percutaneous Endoscopic Approach

0NS54ZZ   Reposition Right Temporal Bone, Percutaneous Endoscopic Approach

0NS5XZZ   Reposition Right Temporal Bone, External Approach

0NS604Z   Reposition Left Temporal Bone with Internal Fixation Device, Open Approach

0NS60ZZ   Reposition Left Temporal Bone, Open Approach

0NS634Z   Reposition Left Temporal Bone with Internal Fixation Device, Percutaneous Approach

0NS63ZZ   Reposition Left Temporal Bone, Percutaneous Approach

0NS644Z   Reposition Left Temporal Bone with Internal Fixation Device, Percutaneous Endoscopic Approach

0NS64ZZ   Reposition Left Temporal Bone, Percutaneous Endoscopic Approach

0NS6XZZ   Reposition Left Temporal Bone, External Approach

0NS704Z   Reposition Right Occipital Bone with Internal Fixation Device, Open Approach

0NS70ZZ   Reposition Right Occipital Bone, Open Approach

0NS734Z   Reposition Right Occipital Bone with Internal Fixation Device, Percutaneous Approach

0NS73ZZ   Reposition Right Occipital Bone, Percutaneous Approach

0NS744Z   Reposition Right Occipital Bone with Internal Fixation Device, Percutaneous Endoscopic Approach

0NS74ZZ   Reposition Right Occipital Bone, Percutaneous Endoscopic Approach

0NS7XZZ   Reposition Right Occipital Bone, External Approach

0NS804Z   Reposition Left Occipital Bone with Internal Fixation Device, Open Approach

0NS80ZZ   Reposition Left Occipital Bone, Open Approach

0NS834Z   Reposition Left Occipital Bone with Internal Fixation Device, Percutaneous Approach

0NS83ZZ   Reposition Left Occipital Bone, Percutaneous Approach

0NS844Z   Reposition Left Occipital Bone with Internal Fixation Device, Percutaneous Endoscopic Approach

0NS84ZZ   Reposition Left Occipital Bone, Percutaneous Endoscopic Approach

0NS8XZZ   Reposition Left Occipital Bone, External Approach

0NSB04Z   Reposition Nasal Bone with Internal Fixation Device, Open Approach

0NSB0ZZ   Reposition Nasal Bone, Open Approach

0NSB34Z   Reposition Nasal Bone with Internal Fixation Device, Percutaneous Approach

0NSB3ZZ   Reposition Nasal Bone, Percutaneous Approach

0NSB44Z   Reposition Nasal Bone with Internal Fixation Device, Percutaneous Endoscopic Approach

0NSB4ZZ   Reposition Nasal Bone, Percutaneous Endoscopic Approach

0NSBXZZ   Reposition Nasal Bone, External Approach

0NSC04Z   Reposition Right Sphenoid Bone with Internal Fixation Device, Open Approach

0NSC0ZZ   Reposition Right Sphenoid Bone, Open Approach

0NSC34Z   Reposition Right Sphenoid Bone with Internal Fixation Device, Percutaneous Approach

0NSC3ZZ   Reposition Right Sphenoid Bone, Percutaneous Approach

0NSC44Z   Reposition Right Sphenoid Bone with Internal Fixation Device, Percutaneous Endoscopic Approach

0NSC4ZZ   Reposition Right Sphenoid Bone, Percutaneous Endoscopic Approach

0NSCXZZ   Reposition Right Sphenoid Bone, External Approach

0NSD04Z   Reposition Left Sphenoid Bone with Internal Fixation Device, Open Approach

0NSD0ZZ   Reposition Left Sphenoid Bone, Open Approach

0NSD34Z   Reposition Left Sphenoid Bone with Internal Fixation Device, Percutaneous Approach

0NSD3ZZ   Reposition Left Sphenoid Bone, Percutaneous Approach

0NSD44Z   Reposition Left Sphenoid Bone with Internal Fixation Device, Percutaneous Endoscopic Approach

0NSD4ZZ   Reposition Left Sphenoid Bone, Percutaneous Endoscopic Approach

0NSDXZZ   Reposition Left Sphenoid Bone, External Approach

0NSF04Z   Reposition Right Ethmoid Bone with Internal Fixation Device, Open Approach

0NSF0ZZ   Reposition Right Ethmoid Bone, Open Approach

0NSF34Z   Reposition Right Ethmoid Bone with Internal Fixation Device, Percutaneous Approach

0NSF3ZZ   Reposition Right Ethmoid Bone, Percutaneous Approach

0NSF44Z   Reposition Right Ethmoid Bone with Internal Fixation Device, Percutaneous Endoscopic Approach

0NSF4ZZ   Reposition Right Ethmoid Bone, Percutaneous Endoscopic Approach

0NSFXZZ   Reposition Right Ethmoid Bone, External Approach

0NSG04Z   Reposition Left Ethmoid Bone with Internal Fixation Device, Open Approach

0NSG0ZZ   Reposition Left Ethmoid Bone, Open Approach

0NSG34Z   Reposition Left Ethmoid Bone with Internal Fixation Device, Percutaneous Approach

0NSG3ZZ   Reposition Left Ethmoid Bone, Percutaneous Approach

0NSG44Z   Reposition Left Ethmoid Bone with Internal Fixation Device, Percutaneous Endoscopic Approach

0NSG4ZZ   Reposition Left Ethmoid Bone, Percutaneous Endoscopic Approach

0NSGXZZ   Reposition Left Ethmoid Bone, External Approach

0NSH04Z   Reposition Right Lacrimal Bone with Internal Fixation Device, Open Approach

0NSH0ZZ   Reposition Right Lacrimal Bone, Open Approach

0NSH34Z   Reposition Right Lacrimal Bone with Internal Fixation Device, Percutaneous Approach

0NSH3ZZ   Reposition Right Lacrimal Bone, Percutaneous Approach

0NSH44Z   Reposition Right Lacrimal Bone with Internal Fixation Device, Percutaneous Endoscopic Approach

0NSH4ZZ   Reposition Right Lacrimal Bone, Percutaneous Endoscopic Approach

0NSHXZZ   Reposition Right Lacrimal Bone, External Approach

0NSJ04Z   Reposition Left Lacrimal Bone with Internal Fixation Device, Open Approach

0NSJ0ZZ   Reposition Left Lacrimal Bone, Open Approach

0NSJ34Z   Reposition Left Lacrimal Bone with Internal Fixation Device, Percutaneous Approach

0NSJ3ZZ   Reposition Left Lacrimal Bone, Percutaneous Approach

0NSJ44Z   Reposition Left Lacrimal Bone with Internal Fixation Device, Percutaneous Endoscopic Approach

0NSJ4ZZ   Reposition Left Lacrimal Bone, Percutaneous Endoscopic Approach

0NSJXZZ   Reposition Left Lacrimal Bone, External Approach

0NSK04Z   Reposition Right Palatine Bone with Internal Fixation Device, Open Approach

0NSK0ZZ   Reposition Right Palatine Bone, Open Approach

0NSK34Z   Reposition Right Palatine Bone with Internal Fixation Device, Percutaneous Approach

0NSK3ZZ   Reposition Right Palatine Bone, Percutaneous Approach

0NSK44Z   Reposition Right Palatine Bone with Internal Fixation Device, Percutaneous Endoscopic Approach

0NSK4ZZ	Reposition Right Palatine Bone, Percutaneous Endoscopic Approach
0NSKXZZ	Reposition Right Palatine Bone, External Approach
0NSL04Z	Reposition Left Palatine Bone with Internal Fixation Device, Open Approach
0NSL0ZZ	Reposition Left Palatine Bone, Open Approach
0NSL34Z	Reposition Left Palatine Bone with Internal Fixation Device, Percutaneous Approach
0NSL3ZZ	Reposition Left Palatine Bone, Percutaneous Approach
0NSL44Z	Reposition Left Palatine Bone with Internal Fixation Device, Percutaneous Endoscopic Approach
0NSL4ZZ	Reposition Left Palatine Bone, Percutaneous Endoscopic Approach
0NSLXZZ	Reposition Left Palatine Bone, External Approach
0NSM04Z	Reposition Right Zygomatic Bone with Internal Fixation Device, Open Approach
0NSM0ZZ	Reposition Right Zygomatic Bone, Open Approach
0NSM34Z	Reposition Right Zygomatic Bone with Internal Fixation Device, Percutaneous Approach
0NSM3ZZ	Reposition Right Zygomatic Bone, Percutaneous Approach
0NSM44Z	Reposition Right Zygomatic Bone with Internal Fixation Device, Percutaneous Endoscopic Approach
0NSM4ZZ	Reposition Right Zygomatic Bone, Percutaneous Endoscopic Approach
0NSMXZZ	Reposition Right Zygomatic Bone, External Approach
0NSN04Z	Reposition Left Zygomatic Bone with Internal Fixation Device, Open Approach
0NSN0ZZ	Reposition Left Zygomatic Bone, Open Approach
0NSN34Z	Reposition Left Zygomatic Bone with Internal Fixation Device, Percutaneous Approach
0NSN3ZZ	Reposition Left Zygomatic Bone, Percutaneous Approach
0NSN44Z	Reposition Left Zygomatic Bone with Internal Fixation Device, Percutaneous Endoscopic Approach
0NSN4ZZ	Reposition Left Zygomatic Bone, Percutaneous Endoscopic Approach
0NSNXZZ	Reposition Left Zygomatic Bone, External Approach
0NSP04Z	Reposition Right Orbit with Internal Fixation Device, Open Approach
0NSP0ZZ	Reposition Right Orbit, Open Approach
0NSP34Z	Reposition Right Orbit with Internal Fixation Device, Percutaneous Approach
0NSP3ZZ	Reposition Right Orbit, Percutaneous Approach
0NSP44Z	Reposition Right Orbit with Internal Fixation Device, Percutaneous Endoscopic Approach
0NSP4ZZ	Reposition Right Orbit, Percutaneous Endoscopic Approach
0NSPXZZ	Reposition Right Orbit, External Approach
0NSQ04Z	Reposition Left Orbit with Internal Fixation Device, Open Approach
0NSQ0ZZ	Reposition Left Orbit, Open Approach
0NSQ34Z	Reposition Left Orbit with Internal Fixation Device, Percutaneous Approach
0NSQ3ZZ	Reposition Left Orbit, Percutaneous Approach
0NSQ44Z	Reposition Left Orbit with Internal Fixation Device, Percutaneous Endoscopic Approach
0NSQ4ZZ	Reposition Left Orbit, Percutaneous Endoscopic Approach
0NSQXZZ	Reposition Left Orbit, External Approach
0NSR04Z	Reposition Right Maxilla with Internal Fixation Device, Open Approach
0NSR05Z	Reposition Right Maxilla with External Fixation Device, Open Approach
0NSR0ZZ	Reposition Right Maxilla, Open Approach
0NSR34Z	Reposition Right Maxilla with Internal Fixation Device, Percutaneous Approach
0NSR35Z	Reposition Right Maxilla with External Fixation Device, Percutaneous Approach
0NSR3ZZ	Reposition Right Maxilla, Percutaneous Approach
0NSR44Z	Reposition Right Maxilla with Internal Fixation Device, Percutaneous Endoscopic Approach
0NSR45Z	Reposition Right Maxilla with External Fixation Device, Percutaneous Endoscopic Approach
0NSR4ZZ	Reposition Right Maxilla, Percutaneous Endoscopic Approach
0NSRXZZ	Reposition Right Maxilla, External Approach
0NSS04Z	Reposition Left Maxilla with Internal Fixation Device, Open Approach
0NSS05Z	Reposition Left Maxilla with External Fixation Device, Open Approach
0NSS0ZZ	Reposition Left Maxilla, Open Approach
0NSS34Z	Reposition Left Maxilla with Internal Fixation Device, Percutaneous Approach
0NSS35Z	Reposition Left Maxilla with External Fixation Device, Percutaneous Approach
0NSS3ZZ	Reposition Left Maxilla, Percutaneous Approach
0NSS44Z	Reposition Left Maxilla with Internal Fixation Device, Percutaneous Endoscopic Approach
0NSS45Z	Reposition Left Maxilla with External Fixation Device, Percutaneous Endoscopic Approach
0NSS4ZZ	Reposition Left Maxilla, Percutaneous Endoscopic Approach
0NSSXZZ	Reposition Left Maxilla, External Approach
0NST04Z	Reposition Right Mandible with Internal Fixation Device, Open Approach
0NST05Z	Reposition Right Mandible with External Fixation Device, Open Approach
0NST0ZZ	Reposition Right Mandible, Open Approach
0NST34Z	Reposition Right Mandible with Internal Fixation Device, Percutaneous Approach
0NST35Z	Reposition Right Mandible with External Fixation Device, Percutaneous Approach
0NST3ZZ	Reposition Right Mandible, Percutaneous Approach
0NST44Z	Reposition Right Mandible with Internal Fixation Device, Percutaneous Endoscopic Approach
0NST45Z	Reposition Right Mandible with External Fixation Device, Percutaneous Endoscopic Approach
0NST4ZZ	Reposition Right Mandible, Percutaneous Endoscopic Approach
0NSTXZZ	Reposition Right Mandible, External Approach
0NSV04Z	Reposition Left Mandible with Internal Fixation Device, Open Approach
0NSV05Z	Reposition Left Mandible with External Fixation Device, Open Approach
0NSV0ZZ	Reposition Left Mandible, Open Approach
0NSV34Z	Reposition Left Mandible with Internal Fixation Device, Percutaneous Approach
0NSV35Z	Reposition Left Mandible with External Fixation Device, Percutaneous Approach
0NSV3ZZ	Reposition Left Mandible, Percutaneous Approach
0NSV44Z	Reposition Left Mandible with Internal Fixation Device, Percutaneous Endoscopic Approach
0NSV45Z	Reposition Left Mandible with External Fixation Device, Percutaneous Endoscopic Approach
0NSV4ZZ	Reposition Left Mandible, Percutaneous Endoscopic Approach
0NSVXZZ	Reposition Left Mandible, External Approach
0NSX04Z	Reposition Hyoid Bone with Internal Fixation Device, Open Approach
0NSX0ZZ	Reposition Hyoid Bone, Open Approach
0NSX34Z	Reposition Hyoid Bone with Internal Fixation Device, Percutaneous Approach
0NSX3ZZ	Reposition Hyoid Bone, Percutaneous Approach
0NSX44Z	Reposition Hyoid Bone with Internal Fixation Device, Percutaneous Endoscopic Approach
0NSX4ZZ	Reposition Hyoid Bone, Percutaneous Endoscopic Approach
0NSXXZZ	Reposition Hyoid Bone, External Approach

0NT – Head and Facial Bones, Resection

Review Coding Guideline B3.8

0NT10ZZ	Resection of Right Frontal Bone, Open Approach
0NT20ZZ	Resection of Left Frontal Bone, Open Approach
0NT30ZZ	Resection of Right Parietal Bone, Open Approach
0NT40ZZ	Resection of Left Parietal Bone, Open Approach
0NT50ZZ	Resection of Right Temporal Bone, Open Approach
0NT60ZZ	Resection of Left Temporal Bone, Open Approach
0NT70ZZ	Resection of Right Occipital Bone, Open Approach
0NT80ZZ	Resection of Left Occipital Bone, Open Approach

♀ Female-only   ♂ Male-only   ⬤ Limited Coverage   ● Non-OR   ᴴᴬᶜ HAC-associated procedure   ● Non-covered procedures   ✚ Combination

0NTB0ZZ	Resection of Nasal Bone, Open Approach
0NTC0ZZ	Resection of Right Sphenoid Bone, Open Approach
0NTD0ZZ	Resection of Left Sphenoid Bone, Open Approach
0NTF0ZZ	Resection of Right Ethmoid Bone, Open Approach
0NTG0ZZ	Resection of Left Ethmoid Bone, Open Approach
0NTH0ZZ	Resection of Right Lacrimal Bone, Open Approach
0NTJ0ZZ	Resection of Left Lacrimal Bone, Open Approach
0NTK0ZZ	Resection of Right Palatine Bone, Open Approach
0NTL0ZZ	Resection of Left Palatine Bone, Open Approach

0NTM0ZZ	Resection of Right Zygomatic Bone, Open Approach
0NTN0ZZ	Resection of Left Zygomatic Bone, Open Approach
0NTP0ZZ	Resection of Right Orbit, Open Approach
0NTQ0ZZ	Resection of Left Orbit, Open Approach
0NTR0ZZ	Resection of Right Maxilla, Open Approach
0NTS0ZZ	Resection of Left Maxilla, Open Approach
0NTT0ZZ	Resection of Right Mandible, Open Approach
0NTV0ZZ	Resection of Left Mandible, Open Approach
0NTX0ZZ	Resection of Hyoid Bone, Open Approach

0NU – Head and Facial Bones, Supplement

0NU007Z	Supplement Skull with Autologous Tissue Substitute, Open Approach
0NU00JZ	Supplement Skull with Synthetic Substitute, Open Approach
0NU00KZ	Supplement Skull with Nonautologous Tissue Substitute, Open Approach
0NU037Z	Supplement Skull with Autologous Tissue Substitute, Percutaneous Approach
0NU03JZ	Supplement Skull with Synthetic Substitute, Percutaneous Approach
0NU03KZ	Supplement Skull with Nonautologous Tissue Substitute, Percutaneous Approach
0NU047Z	Supplement Skull with Autologous Tissue Substitute, Percutaneous Endoscopic Approach
0NU04JZ	Supplement Skull with Synthetic Substitute, Percutaneous Endoscopic Approach
0NU04KZ	Supplement Skull with Nonautologous Tissue Substitute, Percutaneous Endoscopic Approach
0NU107Z	Supplement Right Frontal Bone with Autologous Tissue Substitute, Open Approach
0NU10JZ	Supplement Right Frontal Bone with Synthetic Substitute, Open Approach
0NU10KZ	Supplement Right Frontal Bone with Nonautologous Tissue Substitute, Open Approach
0NU137Z	Supplement Right Frontal Bone with Autologous Tissue Substitute, Percutaneous Approach
0NU13JZ	Supplement Right Frontal Bone with Synthetic Substitute, Percutaneous Approach
0NU13KZ	Supplement Right Frontal Bone with Nonautologous Tissue Substitute, Percutaneous Approach
0NU147Z	Supplement Right Frontal Bone with Autologous Tissue Substitute, Percutaneous Endoscopic Approach
0NU14JZ	Supplement Right Frontal Bone with Synthetic Substitute, Percutaneous Endoscopic Approach
0NU14KZ	Supplement Right Frontal Bone with Nonautologous Tissue Substitute, Percutaneous Endoscopic Approach
0NU207Z	Supplement Left Frontal Bone with Autologous Tissue Substitute, Open Approach
0NU20JZ	Supplement Left Frontal Bone with Synthetic Substitute, Open Approach
0NU20KZ	Supplement Left Frontal Bone with Nonautologous Tissue Substitute, Open Approach
0NU237Z	Supplement Left Frontal Bone with Autologous Tissue Substitute, Percutaneous Approach
0NU23JZ	Supplement Left Frontal Bone with Synthetic Substitute, Percutaneous Approach
0NU23KZ	Supplement Left Frontal Bone with Nonautologous Tissue Substitute, Percutaneous Approach
0NU247Z	Supplement Left Frontal Bone with Autologous Tissue Substitute, Percutaneous Endoscopic Approach
0NU24JZ	Supplement Left Frontal Bone with Synthetic Substitute, Percutaneous Endoscopic Approach
0NU24KZ	Supplement Left Frontal Bone with Nonautologous Tissue Substitute, Percutaneous Endoscopic Approach
0NU307Z	Supplement Right Parietal Bone with Autologous Tissue Substitute, Open Approach
0NU30JZ	Supplement Right Parietal Bone with Synthetic Substitute, Open Approach
0NU30KZ	Supplement Right Parietal Bone with Nonautologous Tissue Substitute, Open Approach
0NU337Z	Supplement Right Parietal Bone with Autologous Tissue Substitute, Percutaneous Approach
0NU33JZ	Supplement Right Parietal Bone with Synthetic Substitute, Percutaneous Approach

0NU33KZ	Supplement Right Parietal Bone with Nonautologous Tissue Substitute, Percutaneous Approach
0NU347Z	Supplement Right Parietal Bone with Autologous Tissue Substitute, Percutaneous Endoscopic Approach
0NU34JZ	Supplement Right Parietal Bone with Synthetic Substitute, Percutaneous Endoscopic Approach
0NU34KZ	Supplement Right Parietal Bone with Nonautologous Tissue Substitute, Percutaneous Endoscopic Approach
0NU407Z	Supplement Left Parietal Bone with Autologous Tissue Substitute, Open Approach
0NU40JZ	Supplement Left Parietal Bone with Synthetic Substitute, Open Approach
0NU40KZ	Supplement Left Parietal Bone with Nonautologous Tissue Substitute, Open Approach
0NU437Z	Supplement Left Parietal Bone with Autologous Tissue Substitute, Percutaneous Approach
0NU43JZ	Supplement Left Parietal Bone with Synthetic Substitute, Percutaneous Approach
0NU43KZ	Supplement Left Parietal Bone with Nonautologous Tissue Substitute, Percutaneous Approach
0NU447Z	Supplement Left Parietal Bone with Autologous Tissue Substitute, Percutaneous Endoscopic Approach
0NU44JZ	Supplement Left Parietal Bone with Synthetic Substitute, Percutaneous Endoscopic Approach
0NU44KZ	Supplement Left Parietal Bone with Nonautologous Tissue Substitute, Percutaneous Endoscopic Approach
0NU507Z	Supplement Right Temporal Bone with Autologous Tissue Substitute, Open Approach
0NU50JZ	Supplement Right Temporal Bone with Synthetic Substitute, Open Approach
0NU50KZ	Supplement Right Temporal Bone with Nonautologous Tissue Substitute, Open Approach
0NU537Z	Supplement Right Temporal Bone with Autologous Tissue Substitute, Percutaneous Approach
0NU53JZ	Supplement Right Temporal Bone with Synthetic Substitute, Percutaneous Approach
0NU53KZ	Supplement Right Temporal Bone with Nonautologous Tissue Substitute, Percutaneous Approach
0NU547Z	Supplement Right Temporal Bone with Autologous Tissue Substitute, Percutaneous Endoscopic Approach
0NU54JZ	Supplement Right Temporal Bone with Synthetic Substitute, Percutaneous Endoscopic Approach
0NU54KZ	Supplement Right Temporal Bone with Nonautologous Tissue Substitute, Percutaneous Endoscopic Approach
0NU607Z	Supplement Left Temporal Bone with Autologous Tissue Substitute, Open Approach
0NU60JZ	Supplement Left Temporal Bone with Synthetic Substitute, Open Approach
0NU60KZ	Supplement Left Temporal Bone with Nonautologous Tissue Substitute, Open Approach
0NU637Z	Supplement Left Temporal Bone with Autologous Tissue Substitute, Percutaneous Approach
0NU63JZ	Supplement Left Temporal Bone with Synthetic Substitute, Percutaneous Approach
0NU63KZ	Supplement Left Temporal Bone with Nonautologous Tissue Substitute, Percutaneous Approach
0NU647Z	Supplement Left Temporal Bone with Autologous Tissue Substitute, Percutaneous Endoscopic Approach
0NU64JZ	Supplement Left Temporal Bone with Synthetic Substitute, Percutaneous Endoscopic Approach
0NU64KZ	Supplement Left Temporal Bone with Nonautologous Tissue Substitute, Percutaneous Endoscopic Approach

0NU707Z Supplement Right Occipital Bone with Autologous Tissue Substitute, Open Approach

0NU70JZ Supplement Right Occipital Bone with Synthetic Substitute, Open Approach

0NU70KZ Supplement Right Occipital Bone with Nonautologous Tissue Substitute, Open Approach

0NU737Z Supplement Right Occipital Bone with Autologous Tissue Substitute, Percutaneous Approach

0NU73JZ Supplement Right Occipital Bone with Synthetic Substitute, Percutaneous Approach

0NU73KZ Supplement Right Occipital Bone with Nonautologous Tissue Substitute, Percutaneous Approach

0NU747Z Supplement Right Occipital Bone with Autologous Tissue Substitute, Percutaneous Endoscopic Approach

0NU74JZ Supplement Right Occipital Bone with Synthetic Substitute, Percutaneous Endoscopic Approach

0NU74KZ Supplement Right Occipital Bone with Nonautologous Tissue Substitute, Percutaneous Endoscopic Approach

0NU807Z Supplement Left Occipital Bone with Autologous Tissue Substitute, Open Approach

0NU80JZ Supplement Left Occipital Bone with Synthetic Substitute, Open Approach

0NU80KZ Supplement Left Occipital Bone with Nonautologous Tissue Substitute, Open Approach

0NU837Z Supplement Left Occipital Bone with Autologous Tissue Substitute, Percutaneous Approach

0NU83JZ Supplement Left Occipital Bone with Synthetic Substitute, Percutaneous Approach

0NU83KZ Supplement Left Occipital Bone with Nonautologous Tissue Substitute, Percutaneous Approach

0NU847Z Supplement Left Occipital Bone with Autologous Tissue Substitute, Percutaneous Endoscopic Approach

0NU84JZ Supplement Left Occipital Bone with Synthetic Substitute, Percutaneous Endoscopic Approach

0NU84KZ Supplement Left Occipital Bone with Nonautologous Tissue Substitute, Percutaneous Endoscopic Approach

0NUB07Z Supplement Nasal Bone with Autologous Tissue Substitute, Open Approach

0NUB0JZ Supplement Nasal Bone with Synthetic Substitute, Open Approach

0NUB0KZ Supplement Nasal Bone with Nonautologous Tissue Substitute, Open Approach

0NUB37Z Supplement Nasal Bone with Autologous Tissue Substitute, Percutaneous Approach

0NUB3JZ Supplement Nasal Bone with Synthetic Substitute, Percutaneous Approach

0NUB3KZ Supplement Nasal Bone with Nonautologous Tissue Substitute, Percutaneous Approach

0NUB47Z Supplement Nasal Bone with Autologous Tissue Substitute, Percutaneous Endoscopic Approach

0NUB4JZ Supplement Nasal Bone with Synthetic Substitute, Percutaneous Endoscopic Approach

0NUB4KZ Supplement Nasal Bone with Nonautologous Tissue Substitute, Percutaneous Endoscopic Approach

0NUC07Z Supplement Right Sphenoid Bone with Autologous Tissue Substitute, Open Approach

0NUC0JZ Supplement Right Sphenoid Bone with Synthetic Substitute, Open Approach

0NUC0KZ Supplement Right Sphenoid Bone with Nonautologous Tissue Substitute, Open Approach

0NUC37Z Supplement Right Sphenoid Bone with Autologous Tissue Substitute, Percutaneous Approach

0NUC3JZ Supplement Right Sphenoid Bone with Synthetic Substitute, Percutaneous Approach

0NUC3KZ Supplement Right Sphenoid Bone with Nonautologous Tissue Substitute, Percutaneous Approach

0NUC47Z Supplement Right Sphenoid Bone with Autologous Tissue Substitute, Percutaneous Endoscopic Approach

0NUC4JZ Supplement Right Sphenoid Bone with Synthetic Substitute, Percutaneous Endoscopic Approach

0NUC4KZ Supplement Right Sphenoid Bone with Nonautologous Tissue Substitute, Percutaneous Endoscopic Approach

0NUD07Z Supplement Left Sphenoid Bone with Autologous Tissue Substitute, Open Approach

0NUD0JZ Supplement Left Sphenoid Bone with Synthetic Substitute, Open Approach

0NUD0KZ Supplement Left Sphenoid Bone with Nonautologous Tissue Substitute, Open Approach

0NUD37Z Supplement Left Sphenoid Bone with Autologous Tissue Substitute, Percutaneous Approach

0NUD3JZ Supplement Left Sphenoid Bone with Synthetic Substitute, Percutaneous Approach

0NUD3KZ Supplement Left Sphenoid Bone with Nonautologous Tissue Substitute, Percutaneous Approach

0NUD47Z Supplement Left Sphenoid Bone with Autologous Tissue Substitute, Percutaneous Endoscopic Approach

0NUD4JZ Supplement Left Sphenoid Bone with Synthetic Substitute, Percutaneous Endoscopic Approach

0NUD4KZ Supplement Left Sphenoid Bone with Nonautologous Tissue Substitute, Percutaneous Endoscopic Approach

0NUF07Z Supplement Right Ethmoid Bone with Autologous Tissue Substitute, Open Approach

0NUF0JZ Supplement Right Ethmoid Bone with Synthetic Substitute, Open Approach

0NUF0KZ Supplement Right Ethmoid Bone with Nonautologous Tissue Substitute, Open Approach

0NUF37Z Supplement Right Ethmoid Bone with Autologous Tissue Substitute, Percutaneous Approach

0NUF3JZ Supplement Right Ethmoid Bone with Synthetic Substitute, Percutaneous Approach

0NUF3KZ Supplement Right Ethmoid Bone with Nonautologous Tissue Substitute, Percutaneous Approach

0NUF47Z Supplement Right Ethmoid Bone with Autologous Tissue Substitute, Percutaneous Endoscopic Approach

0NUF4JZ Supplement Right Ethmoid Bone with Synthetic Substitute, Percutaneous Endoscopic Approach

0NUF4KZ Supplement Right Ethmoid Bone with Nonautologous Tissue Substitute, Percutaneous Endoscopic Approach

0NUG07Z Supplement Left Ethmoid Bone with Autologous Tissue Substitute, Open Approach

0NUG0JZ Supplement Left Ethmoid Bone with Synthetic Substitute, Open Approach

0NUG0KZ Supplement Left Ethmoid Bone with Nonautologous Tissue Substitute, Open Approach

0NUG37Z Supplement Left Ethmoid Bone with Autologous Tissue Substitute, Percutaneous Approach

0NUG3JZ Supplement Left Ethmoid Bone with Synthetic Substitute, Percutaneous Approach

0NUG3KZ Supplement Left Ethmoid Bone with Nonautologous Tissue Substitute, Percutaneous Approach

0NUG47Z Supplement Left Ethmoid Bone with Autologous Tissue Substitute, Percutaneous Endoscopic Approach

0NUG4JZ Supplement Left Ethmoid Bone with Synthetic Substitute, Percutaneous Endoscopic Approach

0NUG4KZ Supplement Left Ethmoid Bone with Nonautologous Tissue Substitute, Percutaneous Endoscopic Approach

0NUH07Z Supplement Right Lacrimal Bone with Autologous Tissue Substitute, Open Approach

0NUH0JZ Supplement Right Lacrimal Bone with Synthetic Substitute, Open Approach

0NUH0KZ Supplement Right Lacrimal Bone with Nonautologous Tissue Substitute, Open Approach

0NUH37Z Supplement Right Lacrimal Bone with Autologous Tissue Substitute, Percutaneous Approach

0NUH3JZ Supplement Right Lacrimal Bone with Synthetic Substitute, Percutaneous Approach

0NUH3KZ Supplement Right Lacrimal Bone with Nonautologous Tissue Substitute, Percutaneous Approach

0NUH47Z Supplement Right Lacrimal Bone with Autologous Tissue Substitute, Percutaneous Endoscopic Approach

0NUH4JZ Supplement Right Lacrimal Bone with Synthetic Substitute, Percutaneous Endoscopic Approach

0NUH4KZ Supplement Right Lacrimal Bone with Nonautologous Tissue Substitute, Percutaneous Endoscopic Approach

0NUJ07Z Supplement Left Lacrimal Bone with Autologous Tissue Substitute, Open Approach

0NUJ0JZ Supplement Left Lacrimal Bone with Synthetic Substitute, Open Approach

♀ Female-only   ♂ Male-only   ● Limited Coverage   ● Non-OR   [HAC] HAC-associated procedure   ● Non-covered procedures   ✚ Combination

0NUJ0KZ   Supplement Left Lacrimal Bone with Nonautologous Tissue Substitute, Open Approach

0NUJ37Z   Supplement Left Lacrimal Bone with Autologous Tissue Substitute, Percutaneous Approach

0NUJ3JZ   Supplement Left Lacrimal Bone with Synthetic Substitute, Percutaneous Approach

0NUJ3KZ   Supplement Left Lacrimal Bone with Nonautologous Tissue Substitute, Percutaneous Approach

0NUJ47Z   Supplement Left Lacrimal Bone with Autologous Tissue Substitute, Percutaneous Endoscopic Approach

0NUJ4JZ   Supplement Left Lacrimal Bone with Synthetic Substitute, Percutaneous Endoscopic Approach

0NUJ4KZ   Supplement Left Lacrimal Bone with Nonautologous Tissue Substitute, Percutaneous Endoscopic Approach

0NUK07Z   Supplement Right Palatine Bone with Autologous Tissue Substitute, Open Approach

0NUK0JZ   Supplement Right Palatine Bone with Synthetic Substitute, Open Approach

0NUK0KZ   Supplement Right Palatine Bone with Nonautologous Tissue Substitute, Open Approach

0NUK37Z   Supplement Right Palatine Bone with Autologous Tissue Substitute, Percutaneous Approach

0NUK3JZ   Supplement Right Palatine Bone with Synthetic Substitute, Percutaneous Approach

0NUK3KZ   Supplement Right Palatine Bone with Nonautologous Tissue Substitute, Percutaneous Approach

0NUK47Z   Supplement Right Palatine Bone with Autologous Tissue Substitute, Percutaneous Endoscopic Approach

0NUK4JZ   Supplement Right Palatine Bone with Synthetic Substitute, Percutaneous Endoscopic Approach

0NUK4KZ   Supplement Right Palatine Bone with Nonautologous Tissue Substitute, Percutaneous Endoscopic Approach

0NUL07Z   Supplement Left Palatine Bone with Autologous Tissue Substitute, Open Approach

0NUL0JZ   Supplement Left Palatine Bone with Synthetic Substitute, Open Approach

0NUL0KZ   Supplement Left Palatine Bone with Nonautologous Tissue Substitute, Open Approach

0NUL37Z   Supplement Left Palatine Bone with Autologous Tissue Substitute, Percutaneous Approach

0NUL3JZ   Supplement Left Palatine Bone with Synthetic Substitute, Percutaneous Approach

0NUL3KZ   Supplement Left Palatine Bone with Nonautologous Tissue Substitute, Percutaneous Approach

0NUL47Z   Supplement Left Palatine Bone with Autologous Tissue Substitute, Percutaneous Endoscopic Approach

0NUL4JZ   Supplement Left Palatine Bone with Synthetic Substitute, Percutaneous Endoscopic Approach

0NUL4KZ   Supplement Left Palatine Bone with Nonautologous Tissue Substitute, Percutaneous Endoscopic Approach

0NUM07Z   Supplement Right Zygomatic Bone with Autologous Tissue Substitute, Open Approach

0NUM0JZ   Supplement Right Zygomatic Bone with Synthetic Substitute, Open Approach

0NUM0KZ   Supplement Right Zygomatic Bone with Nonautologous Tissue Substitute, Open Approach

0NUM37Z   Supplement Right Zygomatic Bone with Autologous Tissue Substitute, Percutaneous Approach

0NUM3JZ   Supplement Right Zygomatic Bone with Synthetic Substitute, Percutaneous Approach

0NUM3KZ   Supplement Right Zygomatic Bone with Nonautologous Tissue Substitute, Percutaneous Approach

0NUM47Z   Supplement Right Zygomatic Bone with Autologous Tissue Substitute, Percutaneous Endoscopic Approach

0NUM4JZ   Supplement Right Zygomatic Bone with Synthetic Substitute, Percutaneous Endoscopic Approach

0NUM4KZ   Supplement Right Zygomatic Bone with Nonautologous Tissue Substitute, Percutaneous Endoscopic Approach

0NUN07Z   Supplement Left Zygomatic Bone with Autologous Tissue Substitute, Open Approach

0NUN0JZ   Supplement Left Zygomatic Bone with Synthetic Substitute, Open Approach

0NUN0KZ   Supplement Left Zygomatic Bone with Nonautologous Tissue Substitute, Open Approach

0NUN37Z   Supplement Left Zygomatic Bone with Autologous Tissue Substitute, Percutaneous Approach

0NUN3JZ   Supplement Left Zygomatic Bone with Synthetic Substitute, Percutaneous Approach

0NUN3KZ   Supplement Left Zygomatic Bone with Nonautologous Tissue Substitute, Percutaneous Approach

0NUN47Z   Supplement Left Zygomatic Bone with Autologous Tissue Substitute, Percutaneous Endoscopic Approach

0NUN4JZ   Supplement Left Zygomatic Bone with Synthetic Substitute, Percutaneous Endoscopic Approach

0NUN4KZ   Supplement Left Zygomatic Bone with Nonautologous Tissue Substitute, Percutaneous Endoscopic Approach

0NUP07Z   Supplement Right Orbit with Autologous Tissue Substitute, Open Approach

0NUP0JZ   Supplement Right Orbit with Synthetic Substitute, Open Approach

0NUP0KZ   Supplement Right Orbit with Nonautologous Tissue Substitute, Open Approach

0NUP37Z   Supplement Right Orbit with Autologous Tissue Substitute, Percutaneous Approach

0NUP3JZ   Supplement Right Orbit with Synthetic Substitute, Percutaneous Approach

0NUP3KZ   Supplement Right Orbit with Nonautologous Tissue Substitute, Percutaneous Approach

0NUP47Z   Supplement Right Orbit with Autologous Tissue Substitute, Percutaneous Endoscopic Approach

0NUP4JZ   Supplement Right Orbit with Synthetic Substitute, Percutaneous Endoscopic Approach

0NUP4KZ   Supplement Right Orbit with Nonautologous Tissue Substitute, Percutaneous Endoscopic Approach

0NUQ07Z   Supplement Left Orbit with Autologous Tissue Substitute, Open Approach

0NUQ0JZ   Supplement Left Orbit with Synthetic Substitute, Open Approach

0NUQ0KZ   Supplement Left Orbit with Nonautologous Tissue Substitute, Open Approach

0NUQ37Z   Supplement Left Orbit with Autologous Tissue Substitute, Percutaneous Approach

0NUQ3JZ   Supplement Left Orbit with Synthetic Substitute, Percutaneous Approach

0NUQ3KZ   Supplement Left Orbit with Nonautologous Tissue Substitute, Percutaneous Approach

0NUQ47Z   Supplement Left Orbit with Autologous Tissue Substitute, Percutaneous Endoscopic Approach

0NUQ4JZ   Supplement Left Orbit with Synthetic Substitute, Percutaneous Endoscopic Approach

0NUQ4KZ   Supplement Left Orbit with Nonautologous Tissue Substitute, Percutaneous Endoscopic Approach

0NUR07Z   Supplement Right Maxilla with Autologous Tissue Substitute, Open Approach

0NUR0JZ   Supplement Right Maxilla with Synthetic Substitute, Open Approach

0NUR0KZ   Supplement Right Maxilla with Nonautologous Tissue Substitute, Open Approach

0NUR37Z   Supplement Right Maxilla with Autologous Tissue Substitute, Percutaneous Approach

0NUR3JZ   Supplement Right Maxilla with Synthetic Substitute, Percutaneous Approach

0NUR3KZ   Supplement Right Maxilla with Nonautologous Tissue Substitute, Percutaneous Approach

0NUR47Z   Supplement Right Maxilla with Autologous Tissue Substitute, Percutaneous Endoscopic Approach

0NUR4JZ   Supplement Right Maxilla with Synthetic Substitute, Percutaneous Endoscopic Approach

0NUR4KZ   Supplement Right Maxilla with Nonautologous Tissue Substitute, Percutaneous Endoscopic Approach

0NUS07Z   Supplement Left Maxilla with Autologous Tissue Substitute, Open Approach

0NUS0JZ   Supplement Left Maxilla with Synthetic Substitute, Open Approach

0NUS0KZ   Supplement Left Maxilla with Nonautologous Tissue Substitute, Open Approach

0NUS37Z	Supplement Left Maxilla with Autologous Tissue Substitute, Percutaneous Approach
0NUS3JZ	Supplement Left Maxilla with Synthetic Substitute, Percutaneous Approach
0NUS3KZ	Supplement Left Maxilla with Nonautologous Tissue Substitute, Percutaneous Approach
0NUS47Z	Supplement Left Maxilla with Autologous Tissue Substitute, Percutaneous Endoscopic Approach
0NUS4JZ	Supplement Left Maxilla with Synthetic Substitute, Percutaneous Endoscopic Approach
0NUS4KZ	Supplement Left Maxilla with Nonautologous Tissue Substitute, Percutaneous Endoscopic Approach
0NUT07Z	Supplement Right Mandible with Autologous Tissue Substitute, Open Approach
0NUT0JZ	Supplement Right Mandible with Synthetic Substitute, Open Approach
0NUT0KZ	Supplement Right Mandible with Nonautologous Tissue Substitute, Open Approach
0NUT37Z	Supplement Right Mandible with Autologous Tissue Substitute, Percutaneous Approach
0NUT3JZ	Supplement Right Mandible with Synthetic Substitute, Percutaneous Approach
0NUT3KZ	Supplement Right Mandible with Nonautologous Tissue Substitute, Percutaneous Approach
0NUT47Z	Supplement Right Mandible with Autologous Tissue Substitute, Percutaneous Endoscopic Approach
0NUT4JZ	Supplement Right Mandible with Synthetic Substitute, Percutaneous Endoscopic Approach
0NUT4KZ	Supplement Right Mandible with Nonautologous Tissue Substitute, Percutaneous Endoscopic Approach
0NUV07Z	Supplement Left Mandible with Autologous Tissue Substitute, Open Approach
0NUV0JZ	Supplement Left Mandible with Synthetic Substitute, Open Approach
0NUV0KZ	Supplement Left Mandible with Nonautologous Tissue Substitute, Open Approach
0NUV37Z	Supplement Left Mandible with Autologous Tissue Substitute, Percutaneous Approach
0NUV3JZ	Supplement Left Mandible with Synthetic Substitute, Percutaneous Approach
0NUV3KZ	Supplement Left Mandible with Nonautologous Tissue Substitute, Percutaneous Approach
0NUV47Z	Supplement Left Mandible with Autologous Tissue Substitute, Percutaneous Endoscopic Approach
0NUV4JZ	Supplement Left Mandible with Synthetic Substitute, Percutaneous Endoscopic Approach
0NUV4KZ	Supplement Left Mandible with Nonautologous Tissue Substitute, Percutaneous Endoscopic Approach
0NUX07Z	Supplement Hyoid Bone with Autologous Tissue Substitute, Open Approach
0NUX0JZ	Supplement Hyoid Bone with Synthetic Substitute, Open Approach
0NUX0KZ	Supplement Hyoid Bone with Nonautologous Tissue Substitute, Open Approach
0NUX37Z	Supplement Hyoid Bone with Autologous Tissue Substitute, Percutaneous Approach
0NUX3JZ	Supplement Hyoid Bone with Synthetic Substitute, Percutaneous Approach
0NUX3KZ	Supplement Hyoid Bone with Nonautologous Tissue Substitute, Percutaneous Approach
0NUX47Z	Supplement Hyoid Bone with Autologous Tissue Substitute, Percutaneous Endoscopic Approach
0NUX4JZ	Supplement Hyoid Bone with Synthetic Substitute, Percutaneous Endoscopic Approach
0NUX4KZ	Supplement Hyoid Bone with Nonautologous Tissue Substitute, Percutaneous Endoscopic Approach

0NW – Head and Facial Bones, Revision

Review Coding Guideline B6.1c

0NW000Z	Revision of Drainage Device in Skull, Open Approach
0NW004Z	Revision of Internal Fixation Device in Skull, Open Approach
0NW005Z	Revision of External Fixation Device in Skull, Open Approach
0NW007Z	Revision of Autologous Tissue Substitute in Skull, Open Approach
0NW00JZ	Revision of Synthetic Substitute in Skull, Open Approach
0NW00KZ	Revision of Nonautologous Tissue Substitute in Skull, Open Approach
0NW00MZ	Revision of Bone Growth Stimulator in Skull, Open Approach
0NW00NZ	Revision of Neurostimulator Generator in Skull, Open Approach
0NW00SZ	Revision of Hearing Device in Skull, Open Approach
0NW030Z	Revision of Drainage Device in Skull, Percutaneous Approach
0NW034Z	Revision of Internal Fixation Device in Skull, Percutaneous Approach
0NW035Z	Revision of External Fixation Device in Skull, Percutaneous Approach
0NW037Z	Revision of Autologous Tissue Substitute in Skull, Percutaneous Approach
0NW03JZ	Revision of Synthetic Substitute in Skull, Percutaneous Approach
0NW03KZ	Revision of Nonautologous Tissue Substitute in Skull, Percutaneous Approach
0NW03MZ	Revision of Bone Growth Stimulator in Skull, Percutaneous Approach
0NW03SZ	Revision of Hearing Device in Skull, Percutaneous Approach
0NW040Z	Revision of Drainage Device in Skull, Percutaneous Endoscopic Approach
0NW044Z	Revision of Internal Fixation Device in Skull, Percutaneous Endoscopic Approach
0NW045Z	Revision of External Fixation Device in Skull, Percutaneous Endoscopic Approach
0NW047Z	Revision of Autologous Tissue Substitute in Skull, Percutaneous Endoscopic Approach
0NW04JZ	Revision of Synthetic Substitute in Skull, Percutaneous Endoscopic Approach
0NW04KZ	Revision of Nonautologous Tissue Substitute in Skull, Percutaneous Endoscopic Approach
0NW04MZ	Revision of Bone Growth Stimulator in Skull, Percutaneous Endoscopic Approach
0NW04SZ	Revision of Hearing Device in Skull, Percutaneous Endoscopic Approach
0NW0X0Z	Revision of Drainage Device in Skull, External Approach
0NW0X4Z	Revision of Internal Fixation Device in Skull, External Approach
0NW0X5Z	Revision of External Fixation Device in Skull, External Approach
0NW0X7Z	Revision of Autologous Tissue Substitute in Skull, External Approach
0NW0XJZ	Revision of Synthetic Substitute in Skull, External Approach
0NW0XKZ	Revision of Nonautologous Tissue Substitute in Skull, External Approach
0NW0XMZ	Revision of Bone Growth Stimulator in Skull, External Approach
0NW0XSZ	Revision of Hearing Device in Skull, External Approach
0NWB00Z	Revision of Drainage Device in Nasal Bone, Open Approach
0NWB04Z	Revision of Internal Fixation Device in Nasal Bone, Open Approach
0NWB07Z	Revision of Autologous Tissue Substitute in Nasal Bone, Open Approach
0NWB0JZ	Revision of Synthetic Substitute in Nasal Bone, Open Approach
0NWB0KZ	Revision of Nonautologous Tissue Substitute in Nasal Bone, Open Approach
0NWB0MZ	Revision of Bone Growth Stimulator in Nasal Bone, Open Approach
0NWB30Z	Revision of Drainage Device in Nasal Bone, Percutaneous Approach
0NWB34Z	Revision of Internal Fixation Device in Nasal Bone, Percutaneous Approach
0NWB37Z	Revision of Autologous Tissue Substitute in Nasal Bone, Percutaneous Approach
0NWB3JZ	Revision of Synthetic Substitute in Nasal Bone, Percutaneous Approach

0NWB3KZ	Revision of Nonautologous Tissue Substitute in Nasal Bone, Percutaneous Approach
0NWB3MZ	Revision of Bone Growth Stimulator in Nasal Bone, Percutaneous Approach
0NWB40Z	Revision of Drainage Device in Nasal Bone, Percutaneous Endoscopic Approach
0NWB44Z	Revision of Internal Fixation Device in Nasal Bone, Percutaneous Endoscopic Approach
0NWB47Z	Revision of Autologous Tissue Substitute in Nasal Bone, Percutaneous Endoscopic Approach
0NWB4JZ	Revision of Synthetic Substitute in Nasal Bone, Percutaneous Endoscopic Approach
0NWB4KZ	Revision of Nonautologous Tissue Substitute in Nasal Bone, Percutaneous Endoscopic Approach
0NWB4MZ	Revision of Bone Growth Stimulator in Nasal Bone, Percutaneous Endoscopic Approach
0NWBX0Z	Revision of Drainage Device in Nasal Bone, External Approach
0NWBX4Z	Revision of Internal Fixation Device in Nasal Bone, External Approach
0NWBX7Z	Revision of Autologous Tissue Substitute in Nasal Bone, External Approach
0NWBXJZ	Revision of Synthetic Substitute in Nasal Bone, External Approach
0NWBXKZ	Revision of Nonautologous Tissue Substitute in Nasal Bone, External Approach
0NWBXMZ	Revision of Bone Growth Stimulator in Nasal Bone, External Approach
0NWW00Z	Revision of Drainage Device in Facial Bone, Open Approach
0NWW04Z	Revision of Internal Fixation Device in Facial Bone, Open Approach
0NWW07Z	Revision of Autologous Tissue Substitute in Facial Bone, Open Approach
0NWW0JZ	Revision of Synthetic Substitute in Facial Bone, Open Approach
0NWW0KZ	Revision of Nonautologous Tissue Substitute in Facial Bone, Open Approach
0NWW0MZ	Revision of Bone Growth Stimulator in Facial Bone, Open Approach
0NWW30Z	Revision of Drainage Device in Facial Bone, Percutaneous Approach
0NWW34Z	Revision of Internal Fixation Device in Facial Bone, Percutaneous Approach
0NWW37Z	Revision of Autologous Tissue Substitute in Facial Bone, Percutaneous Approach
0NWW3JZ	Revision of Synthetic Substitute in Facial Bone, Percutaneous Approach
0NWW3KZ	Revision of Nonautologous Tissue Substitute in Facial Bone, Percutaneous Approach
0NWW3MZ	Revision of Bone Growth Stimulator in Facial Bone, Percutaneous Approach
0NWW40Z	Revision of Drainage Device in Facial Bone, Percutaneous Endoscopic Approach
0NWW44Z	Revision of Internal Fixation Device in Facial Bone, Percutaneous Endoscopic Approach
0NWW47Z	Revision of Autologous Tissue Substitute in Facial Bone, Percutaneous Endoscopic Approach
0NWW4JZ	Revision of Synthetic Substitute in Facial Bone, Percutaneous Endoscopic Approach
0NWW4KZ	Revision of Nonautologous Tissue Substitute in Facial Bone, Percutaneous Endoscopic Approach
0NWW4MZ	Revision of Bone Growth Stimulator in Facial Bone, Percutaneous Endoscopic Approach
0NWWX0Z	Revision of Drainage Device in Facial Bone, External Approach
0NWWX4Z	Revision of Internal Fixation Device in Facial Bone, External Approach
0NWWX7Z	Revision of Autologous Tissue Substitute in Facial Bone, External Approach
0NWWXJZ	Revision of Synthetic Substitute in Facial Bone, External Approach
0NWWXKZ	Revision of Nonautologous Tissue Substitute in Facial Bone, External Approach
0NWWXMZ	Revision of Bone Growth Stimulator in Facial Bone, External Approach

Upper Bones

Bones - Front and Back Views

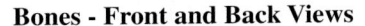

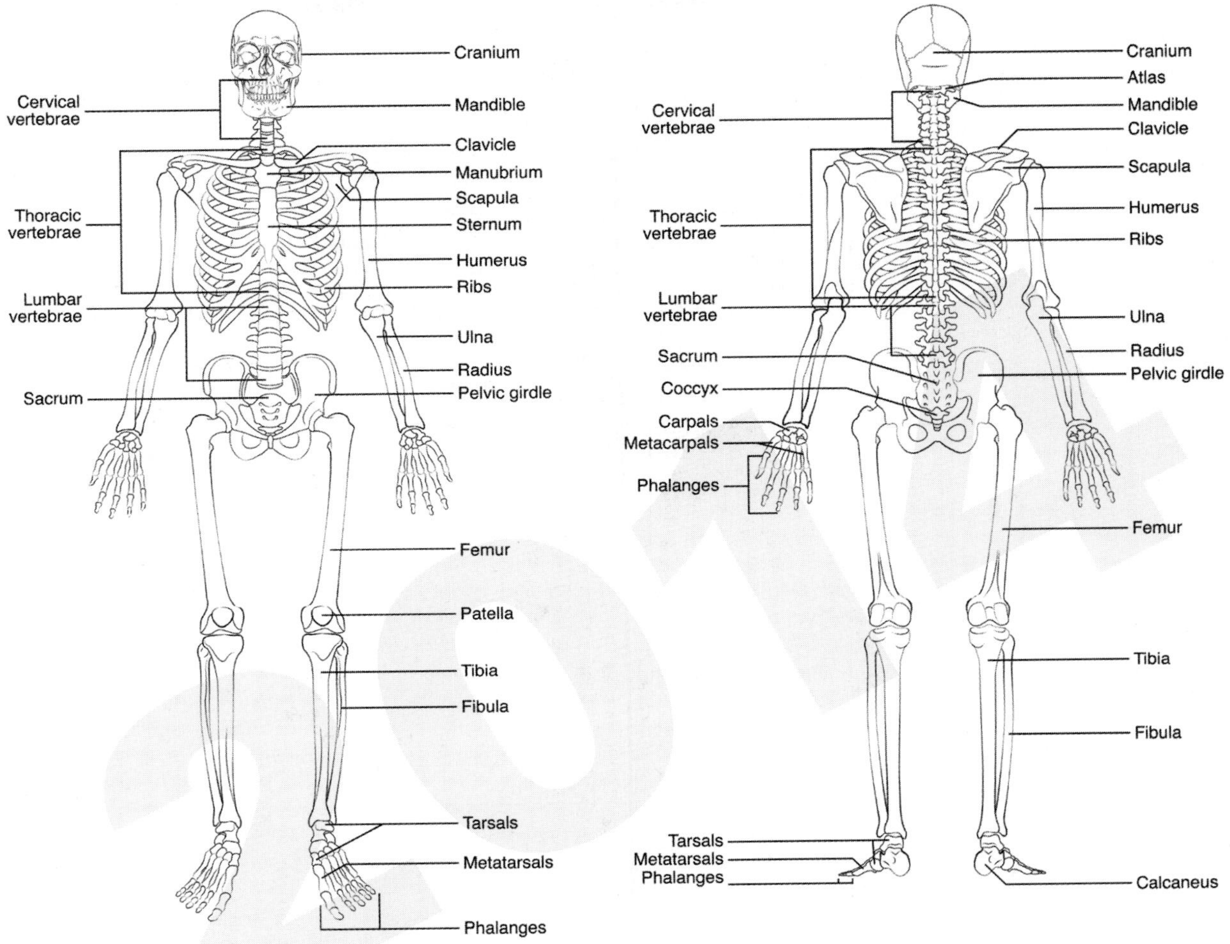

Cranium
Mandible
Cervical vertebrae
Clavicle
Manubrium
Scapula
Sternum
Thoracic vertebrae
Humerus
Ribs
Lumbar vertebrae
Ulna
Radius
Pelvic girdle
Sacrum
Femur
Patella
Tibia
Fibula
Tarsals
Metatarsals
Phalanges

Cranium
Atlas
Cervical vertebrae
Mandible
Clavicle
Scapula
Humerus
Thoracic vertebrae
Ribs
Lumbar vertebrae
Ulna
Radius
Sacrum
Pelvic girdle
Coccyx
Carpals
Metacarpals
Phalanges
Femur
Tibia
Fibula
Tarsals
Metatarsals
Phalanges
Calcaneus

Vertebrae

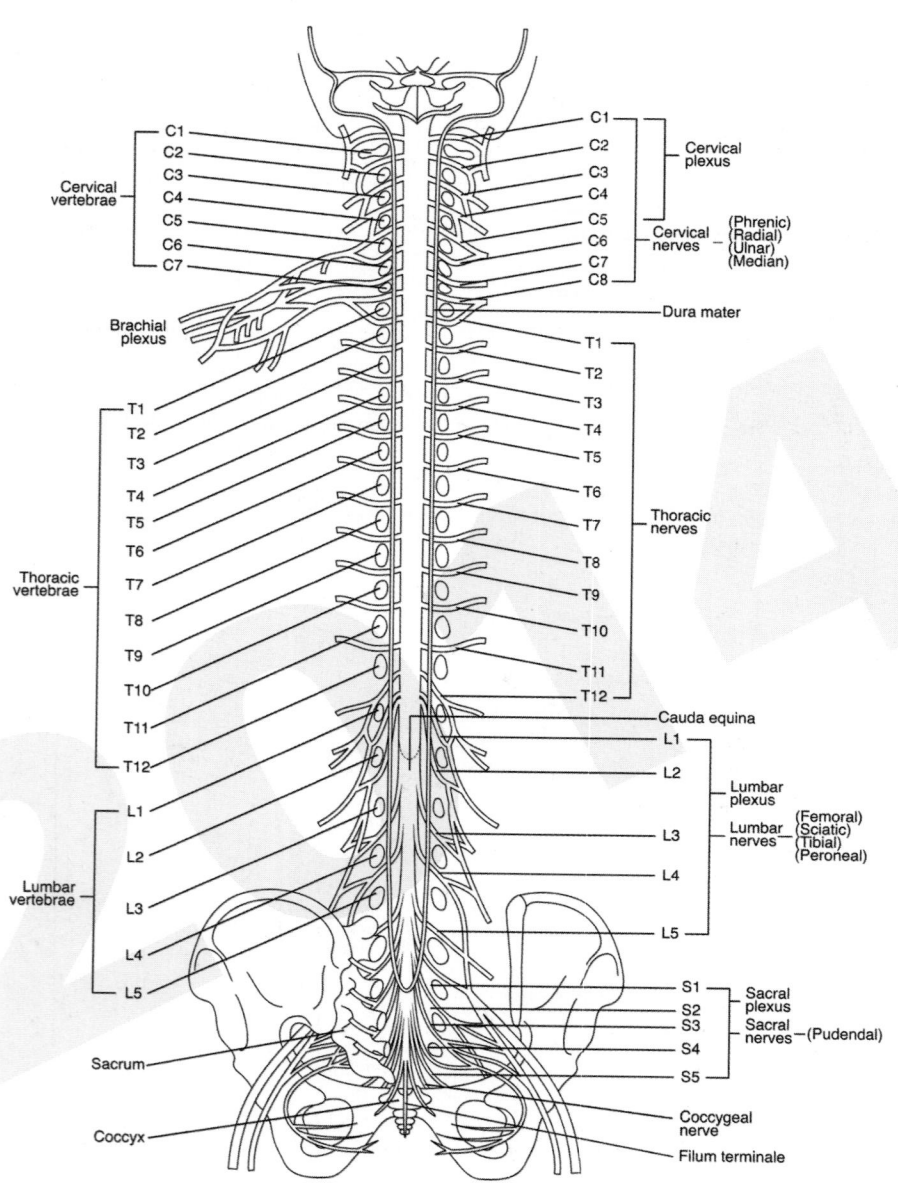

Cervical vertebrae
C1
C2
C3
C4
C5
C6
C7

Brachial plexus

Thoracic vertebrae
T1
T2
T3
T4
T5
T6
T7
T8
T9
T10
T11
T12

Lumbar vertebrae
L1
L2
L3
L4
L5

Sacrum

Coccyx

C1
C2
C3
C4
C5
C6
C7
C8

Cervical plexus

Cervical nerves — (Phrenic) (Radial) (Ulnar) (Median)

Dura mater

T1
T2
T3
T4
T5
T6
T7
T8
T9
T10
T11
T12

Thoracic nerves

Cauda equina
L1
L2
L3
L4
L5

Lumbar plexus
Lumbar nerves — (Femoral) (Sciatic) (Tibial) (Peroneal)

S1
S2
S3
S4
S5

Sacral plexus
Sacral nerves — (Pudendal)

Coccygeal nerve

Filum terminale

Cross-section Spine

Spinous process

Superior articular facet

Lamina

Transverse process

Pedicle

Spinal canal (intravertebral foramen)

Spinal cord in spinal canal

Body

Hand Bones

Ulna

Radius

Lunate (semilunar)

Scaphoid (navicular)

Triangular (triquetrum)

Capitate

Carpals

Pisiform

Trapezoid (lesser multangular)

Carpals

Hamate (unciform)

Trapezium (greater multangular)

Metacarpals

1

5 4 3 2

Phalanges

Proimal phalanx

Middle phalanx

Distal phalanx

Upper Bones Tables 0P2–0PW

Section	0	Medical and Surgical
Body System	P	Upper Bones
Operation	2	Change: Taking out or off a device from a body part and putting back an identical or similar device in or on the same body part without cutting or puncturing the skin or a mucous membrane

Body Part (4th)	Approach (5th)	Device (6th)	Qualifier (7th)
Y Upper Bone	X External	0 Drainage Device Y Other Device	Z No Qualifier

Section	0	Medical and Surgical
Body System	P	Upper Bones
Operation	5	Destruction: Physical eradication of all or a portion of a body part by the direct use of energy, force, or a destructive agent

Body Part (4th)	Approach (5th)	Device (6th)	Qualifier (7th)
0 Sternum 1 Rib, Right 2 Rib, Left 3 Cervical Vertebra 4 Thoracic Vertebra 5 Scapula, Right 6 Scapula, Left 7 Glenoid Cavity, Right 8 Glenoid Cavity, Left 9 Clavicle, Right B Clavicle, Left C Humeral Head, Right D Humeral Head, Left F Humeral Shaft, Right G Humeral Shaft, Left H Radius, Right J Radius, Left K Ulna, Right L Ulna, Left M Carpal, Right N Carpal, Left P Metacarpal, Right Q Metacarpal, Left R Thumb Phalanx, Right S Thumb Phalanx, Left T Finger Phalanx, Right V Finger Phalanx, Left	0 Open 3 Percutaneous 4 Percutaneous Endoscopic	Z No Device	Z No Qualifier

Section	0	Medical and Surgical
Body System	P	Upper Bones
Operation	8	Division: Cutting into a body part, without draining fluids and/or gases from the body part, in order to separate or transect a body part

Body Part (4th)	Approach (5th)	Device (6th)	Qualifier (7th)
0 Sternum 1 Rib, Right 2 Rib, Left 3 Cervical Vertebra 4 Thoracic Vertebra 5 Scapula, Right 6 Scapula, Left 7 Glenoid Cavity, Right 8 Glenoid Cavity, Left 9 Clavicle, Right B Clavicle, Left C Humeral Head, Right D Humeral Head, Left F Humeral Shaft, Right G Humeral Shaft, Left H Radius, Right J Radius, Left K Ulna, Right L Ulna, Left M Carpal, Right N Carpal, Left P Metacarpal, Right Q Metacarpal, Left R Thumb Phalanx, Right S Thumb Phalanx, Left T Finger Phalanx, Right V Finger Phalanx, Left	0 Open 3 Percutaneous 4 Percutaneous Endoscopic	Z No Device	Z No Qualifier

Section	0	Medical and Surgical
Body System	P	Upper Bones
Operation	9	Drainage: Taking or letting out fluids and/or gases from a body part

Body Part (4th)	Approach (5th)	Device (6th)	Qualifier (7th)
0 Sternum 1 Rib, Right 2 Rib, Left 3 Cervical Vertebra 4 Thoracic Vertebra 5 Scapula, Right 6 Scapula, Left 7 Glenoid Cavity, Right 8 Glenoid Cavity, Left 9 Clavicle, Right B Clavicle, Left C Humeral Head, Right D Humeral Head, Left F Humeral Shaft, Right G Humeral Shaft, Left H Radius, Right J Radius, Left K Ulna, Right L Ulna, Left M Carpal, Right N Carpal, Left P Metacarpal, Right Q Metacarpal, Left R Thumb Phalanx, Right S Thumb Phalanx, Left T Finger Phalanx, Right V Finger Phalanx, Left	0 Open 3 Percutaneous 4 Percutaneous Endoscopic	0 Drainage Device	Z No Qualifier

Continued

0P9 *Continued*

Section	0	**Medical and Surgical**
Body System	P	**Upper Bones**
Operation	9	**Drainage:** Taking or letting out fluids and/or gases from a body part

Body Part (4th)	Approach (5th)	Device (6th)	Qualifier (7th)
0 Sternum 1 Rib, Right 2 Rib, Left 3 Cervical Vertebra 4 Thoracic Vertebra 5 Scapula, Right 6 Scapula, Left 7 Glenoid Cavity, Right 8 Glenoid Cavity, Left 9 Clavicle, Right B Clavicle, Left C Humeral Head, Right D Humeral Head, Left F Humeral Shaft, Right G Humeral Shaft, Left H Radius, Right J Radius, Left K Ulna, Right L Ulna, Left M Carpal, Right N Carpal, Left P Metacarpal, Right Q Metacarpal, Left R Thumb Phalanx, Right S Thumb Phalanx, Left T Finger Phalanx, Right V Finger Phalanx, Left	0 Open 3 Percutaneous 4 Percutaneous Endoscopic	Z No Device	X Diagnostic Z No Qualifier

Section	0	**Medical and Surgical**
Body System	P	**Upper Bones**
Operation	B	**Excision:** Cutting out or off, without replacement, a portion of a body part

Body Part (4th)	Approach (5th)	Device (6th)	Qualifier (7th)
0 Sternum 1 Rib, Right 2 Rib, Left 3 Cervical Vertebra 4 Thoracic Vertebra 5 Scapula, Right 6 Scapula, Left 7 Glenoid Cavity, Right 8 Glenoid Cavity, Left 9 Clavicle, Right B Clavicle, Left C Humeral Head, Right D Humeral Head, Left F Humeral Shaft, Right G Humeral Shaft, Left H Radius, Right J Radius, Left K Ulna, Right L Ulna, Left M Carpal, Right N Carpal, Left P Metacarpal, Right Q Metacarpal, Left R Thumb Phalanx, Right S Thumb Phalanx, Left T Finger Phalanx, Right V Finger Phalanx, Left	0 Open 3 Percutaneous 4 Percutaneous Endoscopic	Z No Device	X Diagnostic Z No Qualifier

Section	0	Medical and Surgical
Body System	P	Upper Bones
Operation	C	**Extirpation:** Taking or cutting out solid matter from a body part

Body Part (4th)	Approach (5th)	Device (6th)	Qualifier (7th)
0 Sternum 1 Rib, Right 2 Rib, Left 3 Cervical Vertebra 4 Thoracic Vertebra 5 Scapula, Right 6 Scapula, Left 7 Glenoid Cavity, Right 8 Glenoid Cavity, Left 9 Clavicle, Right B Clavicle, Left C Humeral Head, Right D Humeral Head, Left F Humeral Shaft, Right G Humeral Shaft, Left H Radius, Right J Radius, Left K Ulna, Right L Ulna, Left M Carpal, Right N Carpal, Left P Metacarpal, Right Q Metacarpal, Left R Thumb Phalanx, Right S Thumb Phalanx, Left T Finger Phalanx, Right V Finger Phalanx, Left	0 Open 3 Percutaneous 4 Percutaneous Endoscopic	Z No Device	Z No Qualifier

Section	0	Medical and Surgical
Body System	P	Upper Bones
Operation	H	**Insertion:** Putting in a nonbiological appliance that monitors, assists, performs, or prevents a physiological function but does not physically take the place of a body part

Body Part (4th)	Approach (5th)	Device (6th)	Qualifier (7th)
0 Sternum	0 Open 3 Percutaneous 4 Percutaneous Endoscopic	0 Internal Fixation Device, Rigid Plate 4 Internal Fixation Device	Z No Qualifier
1 Rib, Right 2 Rib, Left 3 Cervical Vertebra 4 Thoracic Vertebra 5 Scapula, Right 6 Scapula, Left 7 Glenoid Cavity, Right 8 Glenoid Cavity, Left 9 Clavicle, Right B Clavicle, Left	0 Open 3 Percutaneous 4 Percutaneous Endoscopic	4 Internal Fixation Device	Z No Qualifier
C Humeral Head, Right D Humeral Head, Left F Humeral Shaft, Right G Humeral Shaft, Left H Radius, Right J Radius, Left K Ulna, Right L Ulna, Left	0 Open 3 Percutaneous 4 Percutaneous Endoscopic	4 Internal Fixation Device 5 External Fixation Device 6 Internal Fixation Device, Intramedullary 8 External Fixation Device, Limb Lengthening B External Fixation Device, Monoplanar C External Fixation Device, Ring D External Fixation Device, Hybrid	Z No Qualifier

Continued

Section	0	Medical and Surgical		0PH *Continued*
Body System	P	Upper Bones		
Operation	H	Insertion: Putting in a nonbiological appliance that monitors, assists, performs, or prevents a physiological function but does not physically take the place of a body part		

Body Part (4th)	Approach (5th)	Device (6th)	Qualifier (7th)
M Carpal, Right N Carpal, Left P Metacarpal, Right Q Metacarpal, Left R Thumb Phalanx, Right S Thumb Phalanx, Left T Finger Phalanx, Right V Finger Phalanx, Left	0 Open 3 Percutaneous 4 Percutaneous Endoscopic	4 Internal Fixation Device 5 External Fixation Device	Z No Qualifier
Y Upper Bone	0 Open 3 Percutaneous 4 Percutaneous Endoscopic	M Bone Growth Stimulator	Z No Qualifier

Section	0	Medical and Surgical
Body System	P	Upper Bones
Operation	J	Inspection: Visually and/or manually exploring a body part

Body Part (4th)	Approach (5th)	Device (6th)	Qualifier (7th)
Y Upper Bone	0 Open 3 Percutaneous 4 Percutaneous Endoscopic X External	Z No Device	Z No Qualifier

Section	0	Medical and Surgical
Body System	P	Upper Bones
Operation	N	Release: Freeing a body part from an abnormal physical constraint by cutting or by the use of force

Body Part (4th)	Approach (5th)	Device (6th)	Qualifier (7th)
0 Sternum 1 Rib, Right 2 Rib, Left 3 Cervical Vertebra 4 Thoracic Vertebra 5 Scapula, Right 6 Scapula, Left 7 Glenoid Cavity, Right 8 Glenoid Cavity, Left 9 Clavicle, Right B Clavicle, Left C Humeral Head, Right D Humeral Head, Left F Humeral Shaft, Right G Humeral Shaft, Left H Radius, Right J Radius, Left K Ulna, Right L Ulna, Left M Carpal, Right N Carpal, Left P Metacarpal, Right Q Metacarpal, Left R Thumb Phalanx, Right S Thumb Phalanx, Left T Finger Phalanx, Right V Finger Phalanx, Left	0 Open 3 Percutaneous 4 Percutaneous Endoscopic	Z No Device	Z No Qualifier

Section	0	Medical and Surgical
Body System	P	Upper Bones
Operation	P	**Removal:** Taking out or off a device from a body part

Body Part (4th)	Approach (5th)	Device (6th)	Qualifier (7th)
0 Sternum 1 Rib, Right 2 Rib, Left 3 Cervical Vertebra 4 Thoracic Vertebra 5 Scapula, Right 6 Scapula, Left 7 Glenoid Cavity, Right 8 Glenoid Cavity, Left 9 Clavicle, Right B Clavicle, Left	0 Open 3 Percutaneous 4 Percutaneous Endoscopic	4 Internal Fixation Device 7 Autologous Tissue Substitute J Synthetic Substitute K Nonautologous Tissue Substitute	Z No Qualifier
0 Sternum 1 Rib, Right 2 Rib, Left 3 Cervical Vertebra 4 Thoracic Vertebra 5 Scapula, Right 6 Scapula, Left 7 Glenoid Cavity, Right 8 Glenoid Cavity, Left 9 Clavicle, Right B Clavicle, Left	X External	4 Internal Fixation Device	Z No Qualifier
C Humeral Head, Right D Humeral Head, Left F Humeral Shaft, Right G Humeral Shaft, Left H Radius, Right J Radius, Left K Ulna, Right L Ulna, Left M Carpal, Right N Carpal, Left P Metacarpal, Right Q Metacarpal, Left R Thumb Phalanx, Right S Thumb Phalanx, Left T Finger Phalanx, Right V Finger Phalanx, Left	0 Open 3 Percutaneous 4 Percutaneous Endoscopic	4 Internal Fixation Device 5 External Fixation Device 7 Autologous Tissue Substitute J Synthetic Substitute K Nonautologous Tissue Substitute	Z No Qualifier

Continued

Section	0	Medical and Surgical		0PP *Continued*
Body System	P	Upper Bones		
Operation	P	**Removal:** Taking out or off a device from a body part		

Body Part (4th)	Approach (5th)	Device (6th)	Qualifier (7th)
C Humeral Head, Right D Humeral Head, Left F Humeral Shaft, Right G Humeral Shaft, Left H Radius, Right J Radius, Left K Ulna, Right L Ulna, Left M Carpal, Right N Carpal, Left P Metacarpal, Right Q Metacarpal, Left R Thumb Phalanx, Right S Thumb Phalanx, Left T Finger Phalanx, Right V Finger Phalanx, Left	X External	4 Internal Fixation Device 5 External Fixation Device	Z No Qualifier
Y Upper Bone	0 Open 3 Percutaneous 4 Percutaneous Endoscopic X External	0 Drainage Device M Bone Growth Stimulator	Z No Qualifier

Section	0	Medical and Surgical
Body System	P	Upper Bones
Operation	Q	**Repair:** Restoring, to the extent possible, a body part to its normal anatomic structure and function

Body Part (4th)	Approach (5th)	Device (6th)	Qualifier (7th)
0 Sternum 1 Rib, Right 2 Rib, Left 3 Cervical Vertebra 4 Thoracic Vertebra 5 Scapula, Right 6 Scapula, Left 7 Glenoid Cavity, Right 8 Glenoid Cavity, Left 9 Clavicle, Right B Clavicle, Left C Humeral Head, Right D Humeral Head, Left F Humeral Shaft, Right G Humeral Shaft, Left H Radius, Right J Radius, Left K Ulna, Right L Ulna, Left M Carpal, Right N Carpal, Left P Metacarpal, Right Q Metacarpal, Left R Thumb Phalanx, Right S Thumb Phalanx, Left T Finger Phalanx, Right V Finger Phalanx, Left	0 Open 3 Percutaneous 4 Percutaneous Endoscopic X External	Z No Device	Z No Qualifier

Section	0	Medical and Surgical	
Body System	P	Upper Bones	
Operation	R	Replacement: Putting in or on biological or synthetic material that physically takes the place and/or function of all or a portion of a body part	

Body Part (4th)	Approach (5th)	Device (6th)	Qualifier (7th)
0 Sternum 1 Rib, Right 2 Rib, Left 3 Cervical Vertebra 4 Thoracic Vertebra 5 Scapula, Right 6 Scapula, Left 7 Glenoid Cavity, Right 8 Glenoid Cavity, Left 9 Clavicle, Right B Clavicle, Left C Humeral Head, Right D Humeral Head, Left F Humeral Shaft, Right G Humeral Shaft, Left H Radius, Right J Radius, Left K Ulna, Right L Ulna, Left M Carpal, Right N Carpal, Left P Metacarpal, Right Q Metacarpal, Left R Thumb Phalanx, Right S Thumb Phalanx, Left T Finger Phalanx, Right V Finger Phalanx, Left	0 Open 3 Percutaneous 4 Percutaneous Endoscopic	7 Autologous Tissue Substitute J Synthetic Substitute K Nonautologous Tissue Substitute	Z No Qualifier

Section	0	Medical and Surgical	
Body System	P	Upper Bones	
Operation	S	Reposition: Moving to its normal location, or other suitable location, all or a portion of a body part	

Body Part (4th)	Approach (5th)	Device (6th)	Qualifier (7th)
0 Sternum	0 Open 3 Percutaneous 4 Percutaneous Endoscopic	0 Internal Fixation Device, Rigid Plate 4 Internal Fixation Device Z No Device	Z No Qualifier
0 Sternum	X External	Z No Device	Z No Qualifier
1 Rib, Right 2 Rib, Left 3 Cervical Vertebra 4 Thoracic Vertebra 5 Scapula, Right 6 Scapula, Left 7 Glenoid Cavity, Right 8 Glenoid Cavity, Left 9 Clavicle, Right B Clavicle, Left	0 Open 3 Percutaneous 4 Percutaneous Endoscopic	4 Internal Fixation Device Z No Device	Z No Qualifier

Continued

Section	0	**Medical and Surgical**
Body System	P	**Upper Bones**
Operation	S	**Reposition:** Moving to its normal location, or other suitable location, all or a portion of a body part

Body Part (4th)	Approach (5th)	Device (6th)	Qualifier (7th)
1 Rib, Right 2 Rib, Left 3 Cervical Vertebra 4 Thoracic Vertebra 5 Scapula, Right 6 Scapula, Left 7 Glenoid Cavity, Right 8 Glenoid Cavity, Left 9 Clavicle, Right B Clavicle, Left	X External	Z No Device	Z No Qualifier
C Humeral Head, Right D Humeral Head, Left F Humeral Shaft, Right G Humeral Shaft, Left H Radius, Right J Radius, Left K Ulna, Right L Ulna, Left	0 Open 3 Percutaneous 4 Percutaneous Endoscopic	4 Internal Fixation Device 5 External Fixation Device 6 Internal Fixation Device, Intramedullary B External Fixation Device, Monoplanar C External Fixation Device, Ring D External Fixation Device, Hybrid Z No Device	Z No Qualifier
C Humeral Head, Right D Humeral Head, Left F Humeral Shaft, Right G Humeral Shaft, Left H Radius, Right J Radius, Left K Ulna, Right L Ulna, Left	X External	Z No Device	Z No Qualifier
M Carpal, Right N Carpal, Left P Metacarpal, Right Q Metacarpal, Left R Thumb Phalanx, Right S Thumb Phalanx, Left T Finger Phalanx, Right V Finger Phalanx, Left	0 Open 3 Percutaneous 4 Percutaneous Endoscopic	4 Internal Fixation Device 5 External Fixation Device Z No Device	Z No Qualifier
M Carpal, Right N Carpal, Left P Metacarpal, Right Q Metacarpal, Left R Thumb Phalanx, Right S Thumb Phalanx, Left T Finger Phalanx, Right V Finger Phalanx, Left	X External	Z No Device	Z No Qualifier

Section	0	Medical and Surgical
Body System	P	Upper Bones
Operation	T	Resection: Cutting out or off, without replacement, all of a body part

Body Part (4th)	Approach (5th)	Device (6th)	Qualifier (7th)
0 Sternum	0 Open	Z No Device	Z No Qualifier
1 Rib, Right			
2 Rib, Left			
5 Scapula, Right			
6 Scapula, Left			
7 Glenoid Cavity, Right			
8 Glenoid Cavity, Left			
9 Clavicle, Right			
B Clavicle, Left			
C Humeral Head, Right			
D Humeral Head, Left			
F Humeral Shaft, Right			
G Humeral Shaft, Left			
H Radius, Right			
J Radius, Left			
K Ulna, Right			
L Ulna, Left			
M Carpal, Right			
N Carpal, Left			
P Metacarpal, Right			
Q Metacarpal, Left			
R Thumb Phalanx, Right			
S Thumb Phalanx, Left			
T Finger Phalanx, Right			
V Finger Phalanx, Left			

Section	0	Medical and Surgical
Body System	P	Upper Bones
Operation	U	Supplement: Putting in or on biological or synthetic material that physically reinforces and/or augments the function of a portion of a body part

Body Part (4th)	Approach (5th)	Device (6th)	Qualifier (7th)
0 Sternum	0 Open	7 Autologous Tissue Substitute	Z No Qualifier
1 Rib, Right	3 Percutaneous	J Synthetic Substitute	
2 Rib, Left	4 Percutaneous Endoscopic	K Nonautologous Tissue Substitute	
3 Cervical Vertebra			
4 Thoracic Vertebra			
5 Scapula, Right			
6 Scapula, Left			
7 Glenoid Cavity, Right			
8 Glenoid Cavity, Left			
9 Clavicle, Right			
B Clavicle, Left			
C Humeral Head, Right			
D Humeral Head, Left			
F Humeral Shaft, Right			
G Humeral Shaft, Left			
H Radius, Right			
J Radius, Left			
K Ulna, Right			
L Ulna, Left			
M Carpal, Right			
N Carpal, Left			
P Metacarpal, Right			
Q Metacarpal, Left			
R Thumb Phalanx, Right			
S Thumb Phalanx, Left			
T Finger Phalanx, Right			
V Finger Phalanx, Left			

Section	0	Medical and Surgical
Body System	P	Upper Bones
Operation	W	Revision: Correcting, to the extent possible, a portion of a malfunctioning device or the position of a displaced device

Body Part (4th)	Approach (5th)	Device (6th)	Qualifier (7th)
0 Sternum 1 Rib, Right 2 Rib, Left 3 Cervical Vertebra 4 Thoracic Vertebra 5 Scapula, Right 6 Scapula, Left 7 Glenoid Cavity, Right 8 Glenoid Cavity, Left 9 Clavicle, Right B Clavicle, Left	0 Open 3 Percutaneous 4 Percutaneous Endoscopic X External	4 Internal Fixation Device 7 Autologous Tissue Substitute J Synthetic Substitute K Nonautologous Tissue Substitute	Z No Qualifier
C Humeral Head, Right D Humeral Head, Left F Humeral Shaft, Right G Humeral Shaft, Left H Radius, Right J Radius, Left K Ulna, Right L Ulna, Left M Carpal, Right N Carpal, Left P Metacarpal, Right Q Metacarpal, Left R Thumb Phalanx, Right S Thumb Phalanx, Left T Finger Phalanx, Right V Finger Phalanx, Left	0 Open 3 Percutaneous 4 Percutaneous Endoscopic X External	4 Internal Fixation Device 5 External Fixation Device 7 Autologous Tissue Substitute J Synthetic Substitute K Nonautologous Tissue Substitute	Z No Qualifier
Y Upper Bone	0 Open 3 Percutaneous 4 Percutaneous Endoscopic X External	0 Drainage Device M Bone Growth Stimulator	Z No Qualifier

Upper Bones Code Listing 0P2–0PW

0P2 – Upper Bones, Change

Review Coding Guideline B6.1c

0P2YX0Z   Change Drainage Device in Upper Bone, External Approach
0P2YXYZ   Change Other Device in Upper Bone, External Approach

0P5 – Upper Bones, Destruction

0P500ZZ   Destruction of Sternum, Open Approach
0P503ZZ   Destruction of Sternum, Percutaneous Approach
0P504ZZ   Destruction of Sternum, Percutaneous Endoscopic Approach
0P510ZZ   Destruction of Right Rib, Open Approach
0P513ZZ   Destruction of Right Rib, Percutaneous Approach
0P514ZZ   Destruction of Right Rib, Percutaneous Endoscopic Approach
0P520ZZ   Destruction of Left Rib, Open Approach
0P523ZZ   Destruction of Left Rib, Percutaneous Approach
0P524ZZ   Destruction of Left Rib, Percutaneous Endoscopic Approach
0P530ZZ   Destruction of Cervical Vertebra, Open Approach
0P533ZZ   Destruction of Cervical Vertebra, Percutaneous Approach
0P534ZZ   Destruction of Cervical Vertebra, Percutaneous Endoscopic Approach
0P540ZZ   Destruction of Thoracic Vertebra, Open Approach

0P543ZZ   Destruction of Thoracic Vertebra, Percutaneous Approach
0P544ZZ   Destruction of Thoracic Vertebra, Percutaneous Endoscopic Approach
0P550ZZ   Destruction of Right Scapula, Open Approach
0P553ZZ   Destruction of Right Scapula, Percutaneous Approach
0P554ZZ   Destruction of Right Scapula, Percutaneous Endoscopic Approach
0P560ZZ   Destruction of Left Scapula, Open Approach
0P563ZZ   Destruction of Left Scapula, Percutaneous Approach
0P564ZZ   Destruction of Left Scapula, Percutaneous Endoscopic Approach
0P570ZZ   Destruction of Right Glenoid Cavity, Open Approach
0P573ZZ   Destruction of Right Glenoid Cavity, Percutaneous Approach
0P574ZZ   Destruction of Right Glenoid Cavity, Percutaneous Endoscopic Approach
0P580ZZ   Destruction of Left Glenoid Cavity, Open Approach

0P583ZZ   Destruction of Left Glenoid Cavity, Percutaneous Approach
0P584ZZ   Destruction of Left Glenoid Cavity, Percutaneous Endoscopic Approach
0P590ZZ   Destruction of Right Clavicle, Open Approach
0P593ZZ   Destruction of Right Clavicle, Percutaneous Approach
0P594ZZ   Destruction of Right Clavicle, Percutaneous Endoscopic Approach
0P5B0ZZ   Destruction of Left Clavicle, Open Approach
0P5B3ZZ   Destruction of Left Clavicle, Percutaneous Approach
0P5B4ZZ   Destruction of Left Clavicle, Percutaneous Endoscopic Approach
0P5C0ZZ   Destruction of Right Humeral Head, Open Approach
0P5C3ZZ   Destruction of Right Humeral Head, Percutaneous Approach
0P5C4ZZ   Destruction of Right Humeral Head, Percutaneous Endoscopic Approach
0P5D0ZZ   Destruction of Left Humeral Head, Open Approach
0P5D3ZZ   Destruction of Left Humeral Head, Percutaneous Approach
0P5D4ZZ   Destruction of Left Humeral Head, Percutaneous Endoscopic Approach
0P5F0ZZ   Destruction of Right Humeral Shaft, Open Approach
0P5F3ZZ   Destruction of Right Humeral Shaft, Percutaneous Approach
0P5F4ZZ   Destruction of Right Humeral Shaft, Percutaneous Endoscopic Approach
0P5G0ZZ   Destruction of Left Humeral Shaft, Open Approach
0P5G3ZZ   Destruction of Left Humeral Shaft, Percutaneous Approach
0P5G4ZZ   Destruction of Left Humeral Shaft, Percutaneous Endoscopic Approach
0P5H0ZZ   Destruction of Right Radius, Open Approach
0P5H3ZZ   Destruction of Right Radius, Percutaneous Approach
0P5H4ZZ   Destruction of Right Radius, Percutaneous Endoscopic Approach
0P5J0ZZ   Destruction of Left Radius, Open Approach
0P5J3ZZ   Destruction of Left Radius, Percutaneous Approach
0P5J4ZZ   Destruction of Left Radius, Percutaneous Endoscopic Approach
0P5K0ZZ   Destruction of Right Ulna, Open Approach
0P5K3ZZ   Destruction of Right Ulna, Percutaneous Approach

0P5K4ZZ   Destruction of Right Ulna, Percutaneous Endoscopic Approach
0P5L0ZZ   Destruction of Left Ulna, Open Approach
0P5L3ZZ   Destruction of Left Ulna, Percutaneous Approach
0P5L4ZZ   Destruction of Left Ulna, Percutaneous Endoscopic Approach
0P5M0ZZ   Destruction of Right Carpal, Open Approach
0P5M3ZZ   Destruction of Right Carpal, Percutaneous Approach
0P5M4ZZ   Destruction of Right Carpal, Percutaneous Endoscopic Approach
0P5N0ZZ   Destruction of Left Carpal, Open Approach
0P5N3ZZ   Destruction of Left Carpal, Percutaneous Approach
0P5N4ZZ   Destruction of Left Carpal, Percutaneous Endoscopic Approach
0P5P0ZZ   Destruction of Right Metacarpal, Open Approach
0P5P3ZZ   Destruction of Right Metacarpal, Percutaneous Approach
0P5P4ZZ   Destruction of Right Metacarpal, Percutaneous Endoscopic Approach
0P5Q0ZZ   Destruction of Left Metacarpal, Open Approach
0P5Q3ZZ   Destruction of Left Metacarpal, Percutaneous Approach
0P5Q4ZZ   Destruction of Left Metacarpal, Percutaneous Endoscopic Approach
0P5R0ZZ   Destruction of Right Thumb Phalanx, Open Approach
0P5R3ZZ   Destruction of Right Thumb Phalanx, Percutaneous Approach
0P5R4ZZ   Destruction of Right Thumb Phalanx, Percutaneous Endoscopic Approach
0P5S0ZZ   Destruction of Left Thumb Phalanx, Open Approach
0P5S3ZZ   Destruction of Left Thumb Phalanx, Percutaneous Approach
0P5S4ZZ   Destruction of Left Thumb Phalanx, Percutaneous Endoscopic Approach
0P5T0ZZ   Destruction of Right Finger Phalanx, Open Approach
0P5T3ZZ   Destruction of Right Finger Phalanx, Percutaneous Approach
0P5T4ZZ   Destruction of Right Finger Phalanx, Percutaneous Endoscopic Approach
0P5V0ZZ   Destruction of Left Finger Phalanx, Open Approach
0P5V3ZZ   Destruction of Left Finger Phalanx, Percutaneous Approach
0P5V4ZZ   Destruction of Left Finger Phalanx, Percutaneous Endoscopic Approach

0P8 – Upper Bones, Division

Review Coding Guideline B3.14

0P800ZZ   Division of Sternum, Open Approach
0P803ZZ   Division of Sternum, Percutaneous Approach
0P804ZZ   Division of Sternum, Percutaneous Endoscopic Approach
0P810ZZ   Division of Right Rib, Open Approach
0P813ZZ   Division of Right Rib, Percutaneous Approach
0P814ZZ   Division of Right Rib, Percutaneous Endoscopic Approach
0P820ZZ   Division of Left Rib, Open Approach
0P823ZZ   Division of Left Rib, Percutaneous Approach
0P824ZZ   Division of Left Rib, Percutaneous Endoscopic Approach
0P830ZZ   Division of Cervical Vertebra, Open Approach
0P833ZZ   Division of Cervical Vertebra, Percutaneous Approach
0P834ZZ   Division of Cervical Vertebra, Percutaneous Endoscopic Approach
0P840ZZ   Division of Thoracic Vertebra, Open Approach
0P843ZZ   Division of Thoracic Vertebra, Percutaneous Approach
0P844ZZ   Division of Thoracic Vertebra, Percutaneous Endoscopic Approach
0P850ZZ   Division of Right Scapula, Open Approach
0P853ZZ   Division of Right Scapula, Percutaneous Approach
0P854ZZ   Division of Right Scapula, Percutaneous Endoscopic Approach
0P860ZZ   Division of Left Scapula, Open Approach
0P863ZZ   Division of Left Scapula, Percutaneous Approach
0P864ZZ   Division of Left Scapula, Percutaneous Endoscopic Approach
0P870ZZ   Division of Right Glenoid Cavity, Open Approach
0P873ZZ   Division of Right Glenoid Cavity, Percutaneous Approach
0P874ZZ   Division of Right Glenoid Cavity, Percutaneous Endoscopic Approach
0P880ZZ   Division of Left Glenoid Cavity, Open Approach
0P883ZZ   Division of Left Glenoid Cavity, Percutaneous Approach
0P884ZZ   Division of Left Glenoid Cavity, Percutaneous Endoscopic Approach
0P890ZZ   Division of Right Clavicle, Open Approach
0P893ZZ   Division of Right Clavicle, Percutaneous Approach
0P894ZZ   Division of Right Clavicle, Percutaneous Endoscopic Approach
0P8B0ZZ   Division of Left Clavicle, Open Approach
0P8B3ZZ   Division of Left Clavicle, Percutaneous Approach
0P8B4ZZ   Division of Left Clavicle, Percutaneous Endoscopic Approach

0P8C0ZZ   Division of Right Humeral Head, Open Approach
0P8C3ZZ   Division of Right Humeral Head, Percutaneous Approach
0P8C4ZZ   Division of Right Humeral Head, Percutaneous Endoscopic Approach
0P8D0ZZ   Division of Left Humeral Head, Open Approach
0P8D3ZZ   Division of Left Humeral Head, Percutaneous Approach
0P8D4ZZ   Division of Left Humeral Head, Percutaneous Endoscopic Approach
0P8F0ZZ   Division of Right Humeral Shaft, Open Approach
0P8F3ZZ   Division of Right Humeral Shaft, Percutaneous Approach
0P8F4ZZ   Division of Right Humeral Shaft, Percutaneous Endoscopic Approach
0P8G0ZZ   Division of Left Humeral Shaft, Open Approach
0P8G3ZZ   Division of Left Humeral Shaft, Percutaneous Approach
0P8G4ZZ   Division of Left Humeral Shaft, Percutaneous Endoscopic Approach
0P8H0ZZ   Division of Right Radius, Open Approach
0P8H3ZZ   Division of Right Radius, Percutaneous Approach
0P8H4ZZ   Division of Right Radius, Percutaneous Endoscopic Approach
0P8J0ZZ   Division of Left Radius, Open Approach
0P8J3ZZ   Division of Left Radius, Percutaneous Approach
0P8J4ZZ   Division of Left Radius, Percutaneous Endoscopic Approach
0P8K0ZZ   Division of Right Ulna, Open Approach
0P8K3ZZ   Division of Right Ulna, Percutaneous Approach
0P8K4ZZ   Division of Right Ulna, Percutaneous Endoscopic Approach
0P8L0ZZ   Division of Left Ulna, Open Approach
0P8L3ZZ   Division of Left Ulna, Percutaneous Approach
0P8L4ZZ   Division of Left Ulna, Percutaneous Endoscopic Approach
0P8M0ZZ   Division of Right Carpal, Open Approach
0P8M3ZZ   Division of Right Carpal, Percutaneous Approach
0P8M4ZZ   Division of Right Carpal, Percutaneous Endoscopic Approach
0P8N0ZZ   Division of Left Carpal, Open Approach
0P8N3ZZ   Division of Left Carpal, Percutaneous Approach
0P8N4ZZ   Division of Left Carpal, Percutaneous Endoscopic Approach
0P8P0ZZ   Division of Right Metacarpal, Open Approach
0P8P3ZZ   Division of Right Metacarpal, Percutaneous Approach
0P8P4ZZ   Division of Right Metacarpal, Percutaneous Endoscopic Approach

0P8Q0ZZ	Division of Left Metacarpal, Open Approach
0P8Q3ZZ	Division of Left Metacarpal, Percutaneous Approach
0P8Q4ZZ	Division of Left Metacarpal, Percutaneous Endoscopic Approach
0P8R0ZZ	Division of Right Thumb Phalanx, Open Approach
0P8R3ZZ	Division of Right Thumb Phalanx, Percutaneous Approach
0P8R4ZZ	Division of Right Thumb Phalanx, Percutaneous Endoscopic Approach
0P8S0ZZ	Division of Left Thumb Phalanx, Open Approach
0P8S3ZZ	Division of Left Thumb Phalanx, Percutaneous Approach
0P8S4ZZ	Division of Left Thumb Phalanx, Percutaneous Endoscopic Approach
0P8T0ZZ	Division of Right Finger Phalanx, Open Approach
0P8T3ZZ	Division of Right Finger Phalanx, Percutaneous Approach
0P8T4ZZ	Division of Right Finger Phalanx, Percutaneous Endoscopic Approach
0P8V0ZZ	Division of Left Finger Phalanx, Open Approach
0P8V3ZZ	Division of Left Finger Phalanx, Percutaneous Approach
0P8V4ZZ	Division of Left Finger Phalanx, Percutaneous Endoscopic Approach

0P9 – Upper Bones, Drainage

Review Coding Guidelines B3.4a and B3.4b

Review Coding Guideline B6.2

0P9000Z	Drainage of Sternum with Drainage Device, Open Approach
0P900ZX	Drainage of Sternum, Open Approach, Diagnostic
0P900ZZ	Drainage of Sternum, Open Approach
0P9030Z	Drainage of Sternum with Drainage Device, Percutaneous Approach
0P903ZX	Drainage of Sternum, Percutaneous Approach, Diagnostic
0P903ZZ	Drainage of Sternum, Percutaneous Approach
0P9040Z	Drainage of Sternum with Drainage Device, Percutaneous Endoscopic Approach
0P904ZX	Drainage of Sternum, Percutaneous Endoscopic Approach, Diagnostic
0P904ZZ	Drainage of Sternum, Percutaneous Endoscopic Approach
0P9100Z	Drainage of Right Rib with Drainage Device, Open Approach
0P910ZX	Drainage of Right Rib, Open Approach, Diagnostic
0P910ZZ	Drainage of Right Rib, Open Approach
0P9130Z	Drainage of Right Rib with Drainage Device, Percutaneous Approach
0P913ZX	Drainage of Right Rib, Percutaneous Approach, Diagnostic
0P913ZZ	Drainage of Right Rib, Percutaneous Approach
0P9140Z	Drainage of Right Rib with Drainage Device, Percutaneous Endoscopic Approach
0P914ZX	Drainage of Right Rib, Percutaneous Endoscopic Approach, Diagnostic
0P914ZZ	Drainage of Right Rib, Percutaneous Endoscopic Approach
0P9200Z	Drainage of Left Rib with Drainage Device, Open Approach
0P920ZX	Drainage of Left Rib, Open Approach, Diagnostic
0P920ZZ	Drainage of Left Rib, Open Approach
0P9230Z	Drainage of Left Rib with Drainage Device, Percutaneous Approach
0P923ZX	Drainage of Left Rib, Percutaneous Approach, Diagnostic
0P923ZZ	Drainage of Left Rib, Percutaneous Approach
0P9240Z	Drainage of Left Rib with Drainage Device, Percutaneous Endoscopic Approach
0P924ZX	Drainage of Left Rib, Percutaneous Endoscopic Approach, Diagnostic
0P924ZZ	Drainage of Left Rib, Percutaneous Endoscopic Approach
0P9300Z	Drainage of Cervical Vertebra with Drainage Device, Open Approach
0P930ZX	Drainage of Cervical Vertebra, Open Approach, Diagnostic
0P930ZZ	Drainage of Cervical Vertebra, Open Approach
0P9330Z	Drainage of Cervical Vertebra with Drainage Device, Percutaneous Approach
0P933ZX	Drainage of Cervical Vertebra, Percutaneous Approach, Diagnostic
0P933ZZ	Drainage of Cervical Vertebra, Percutaneous Approach
0P9340Z	Drainage of Cervical Vertebra with Drainage Device, Percutaneous Endoscopic Approach
0P934ZX	Drainage of Cervical Vertebra, Percutaneous Endoscopic Approach, Diagnostic
0P934ZZ	Drainage of Cervical Vertebra, Percutaneous Endoscopic Approach
0P9400Z	Drainage of Thoracic Vertebra with Drainage Device, Open Approach
0P940ZX	Drainage of Thoracic Vertebra, Open Approach, Diagnostic
0P940ZZ	Drainage of Thoracic Vertebra, Open Approach
0P9430Z	Drainage of Thoracic Vertebra with Drainage Device, Percutaneous Approach
0P943ZX	Drainage of Thoracic Vertebra, Percutaneous Approach, Diagnostic
0P943ZZ	Drainage of Thoracic Vertebra, Percutaneous Approach
0P9440Z	Drainage of Thoracic Vertebra with Drainage Device, Percutaneous Endoscopic Approach
0P944ZX	Drainage of Thoracic Vertebra, Percutaneous Endoscopic Approach, Diagnostic
0P944ZZ	Drainage of Thoracic Vertebra, Percutaneous Endoscopic Approach
0P9500Z	Drainage of Right Scapula with Drainage Device, Open Approach
0P950ZX	Drainage of Right Scapula, Open Approach, Diagnostic
0P950ZZ	Drainage of Right Scapula, Open Approach
0P9530Z	Drainage of Right Scapula with Drainage Device, Percutaneous Approach
0P953ZX	Drainage of Right Scapula, Percutaneous Approach, Diagnostic
0P953ZZ	Drainage of Right Scapula, Percutaneous Approach
0P9540Z	Drainage of Right Scapula with Drainage Device, Percutaneous Endoscopic Approach
0P954ZX	Drainage of Right Scapula, Percutaneous Endoscopic Approach, Diagnostic
0P954ZZ	Drainage of Right Scapula, Percutaneous Endoscopic Approach
0P9600Z	Drainage of Left Scapula with Drainage Device, Open Approach
0P960ZX	Drainage of Left Scapula, Open Approach, Diagnostic
0P960ZZ	Drainage of Left Scapula, Open Approach
0P9630Z	Drainage of Left Scapula with Drainage Device, Percutaneous Approach
0P963ZX	Drainage of Left Scapula, Percutaneous Approach, Diagnostic
0P963ZZ	Drainage of Left Scapula, Percutaneous Approach
0P9640Z	Drainage of Left Scapula with Drainage Device, Percutaneous Endoscopic Approach
0P964ZX	Drainage of Left Scapula, Percutaneous Endoscopic Approach, Diagnostic
0P964ZZ	Drainage of Left Scapula, Percutaneous Endoscopic Approach
0P9700Z	Drainage of Right Glenoid Cavity with Drainage Device, Open Approach
0P970ZX	Drainage of Right Glenoid Cavity, Open Approach, Diagnostic
0P970ZZ	Drainage of Right Glenoid Cavity, Open Approach
0P9730Z	Drainage of Right Glenoid Cavity with Drainage Device, Percutaneous Approach
0P973ZX	Drainage of Right Glenoid Cavity, Percutaneous Approach, Diagnostic
0P973ZZ	Drainage of Right Glenoid Cavity, Percutaneous Approach
0P9740Z	Drainage of Right Glenoid Cavity with Drainage Device, Percutaneous Endoscopic Approach
0P974ZX	Drainage of Right Glenoid Cavity, Percutaneous Endoscopic Approach, Diagnostic
0P974ZZ	Drainage of Right Glenoid Cavity, Percutaneous Endoscopic Approach
0P9800Z	Drainage of Left Glenoid Cavity with Drainage Device, Open Approach
0P980ZX	Drainage of Left Glenoid Cavity, Open Approach, Diagnostic
0P980ZZ	Drainage of Left Glenoid Cavity, Open Approach
0P9830Z	Drainage of Left Glenoid Cavity with Drainage Device, Percutaneous Approach
0P983ZX	Drainage of Left Glenoid Cavity, Percutaneous Approach, Diagnostic
0P983ZZ	Drainage of Left Glenoid Cavity, Percutaneous Approach
0P9840Z	Drainage of Left Glenoid Cavity with Drainage Device, Percutaneous Endoscopic Approach
0P984ZX	Drainage of Left Glenoid Cavity, Percutaneous Endoscopic Approach, Diagnostic
0P984ZZ	Drainage of Left Glenoid Cavity, Percutaneous Endoscopic Approach

---

♀ Female-only   ♂ Male-only   ◐ Limited Coverage   ● Non-OR   ▨ HAC-associated procedure   ⬤ Non-covered procedures   ➕ Combination

0P9900Z	Drainage of Right Clavicle with Drainage Device, Open Approach
0P990ZX	Drainage of Right Clavicle, Open Approach, Diagnostic
0P990ZZ	Drainage of Right Clavicle, Open Approach
0P9930Z	Drainage of Right Clavicle with Drainage Device, Percutaneous Approach
0P993ZX	Drainage of Right Clavicle, Percutaneous Approach, Diagnostic
0P993ZZ	Drainage of Right Clavicle, Percutaneous Approach
0P9940Z	Drainage of Right Clavicle with Drainage Device, Percutaneous Endoscopic Approach
0P994ZX	Drainage of Right Clavicle, Percutaneous Endoscopic Approach, Diagnostic
0P994ZZ	Drainage of Right Clavicle, Percutaneous Endoscopic Approach
0P9B00Z	Drainage of Left Clavicle with Drainage Device, Open Approach
0P9B0ZX	Drainage of Left Clavicle, Open Approach, Diagnostic
0P9B0ZZ	Drainage of Left Clavicle, Open Approach
0P9B30Z	Drainage of Left Clavicle with Drainage Device, Percutaneous Approach
0P9B3ZX	Drainage of Left Clavicle, Percutaneous Approach, Diagnostic
0P9B3ZZ	Drainage of Left Clavicle, Percutaneous Approach
0P9B40Z	Drainage of Left Clavicle with Drainage Device, Percutaneous Endoscopic Approach
0P9B4ZX	Drainage of Left Clavicle, Percutaneous Endoscopic Approach, Diagnostic
0P9B4ZZ	Drainage of Left Clavicle, Percutaneous Endoscopic Approach
0P9C00Z	Drainage of Right Humeral Head with Drainage Device, Open Approach
0P9C0ZX	Drainage of Right Humeral Head, Open Approach, Diagnostic
0P9C0ZZ	Drainage of Right Humeral Head, Open Approach
0P9C30Z	Drainage of Right Humeral Head with Drainage Device, Percutaneous Approach
0P9C3ZX	Drainage of Right Humeral Head, Percutaneous Approach, Diagnostic
0P9C3ZZ	Drainage of Right Humeral Head, Percutaneous Approach
0P9C40Z	Drainage of Right Humeral Head with Drainage Device, Percutaneous Endoscopic Approach
0P9C4ZX	Drainage of Right Humeral Head, Percutaneous Endoscopic Approach, Diagnostic
0P9C4ZZ	Drainage of Right Humeral Head, Percutaneous Endoscopic Approach
0P9D00Z	Drainage of Left Humeral Head with Drainage Device, Open Approach
0P9D0ZX	Drainage of Left Humeral Head, Open Approach, Diagnostic
0P9D0ZZ	Drainage of Left Humeral Head, Open Approach
0P9D30Z	Drainage of Left Humeral Head with Drainage Device, Percutaneous Approach
0P9D3ZX	Drainage of Left Humeral Head, Percutaneous Approach, Diagnostic
0P9D3ZZ	Drainage of Left Humeral Head, Percutaneous Approach
0P9D40Z	Drainage of Left Humeral Head with Drainage Device, Percutaneous Endoscopic Approach
0P9D4ZX	Drainage of Left Humeral Head, Percutaneous Endoscopic Approach, Diagnostic
0P9D4ZZ	Drainage of Left Humeral Head, Percutaneous Endoscopic Approach
0P9F00Z	Drainage of Right Humeral Shaft with Drainage Device, Open Approach
0P9F0ZX	Drainage of Right Humeral Shaft, Open Approach, Diagnostic
0P9F0ZZ	Drainage of Right Humeral Shaft, Open Approach
0P9F30Z	Drainage of Right Humeral Shaft with Drainage Device, Percutaneous Approach
0P9F3ZX	Drainage of Right Humeral Shaft, Percutaneous Approach, Diagnostic
0P9F3ZZ	Drainage of Right Humeral Shaft, Percutaneous Approach
0P9F40Z	Drainage of Right Humeral Shaft with Drainage Device, Percutaneous Endoscopic Approach
0P9F4ZX	Drainage of Right Humeral Shaft, Percutaneous Endoscopic Approach, Diagnostic
0P9F4ZZ	Drainage of Right Humeral Shaft, Percutaneous Endoscopic Approach
0P9G00Z	Drainage of Left Humeral Shaft with Drainage Device, Open Approach
0P9G0ZX	Drainage of Left Humeral Shaft, Open Approach, Diagnostic
0P9G0ZZ	Drainage of Left Humeral Shaft, Open Approach
0P9G30Z	Drainage of Left Humeral Shaft with Drainage Device, Percutaneous Approach
0P9G3ZX	Drainage of Left Humeral Shaft, Percutaneous Approach, Diagnostic
0P9G3ZZ	Drainage of Left Humeral Shaft, Percutaneous Approach
0P9G40Z	Drainage of Left Humeral Shaft with Drainage Device, Percutaneous Endoscopic Approach
0P9G4ZX	Drainage of Left Humeral Shaft, Percutaneous Endoscopic Approach, Diagnostic
0P9G4ZZ	Drainage of Left Humeral Shaft, Percutaneous Endoscopic Approach
0P9H00Z	Drainage of Right Radius with Drainage Device, Open Approach
0P9H0ZX	Drainage of Right Radius, Open Approach, Diagnostic
0P9H0ZZ	Drainage of Right Radius, Open Approach
0P9H30Z	Drainage of Right Radius with Drainage Device, Percutaneous Approach
0P9H3ZX	Drainage of Right Radius, Percutaneous Approach, Diagnostic
0P9H3ZZ	Drainage of Right Radius, Percutaneous Approach
0P9H40Z	Drainage of Right Radius with Drainage Device, Percutaneous Endoscopic Approach
0P9H4ZX	Drainage of Right Radius, Percutaneous Endoscopic Approach, Diagnostic
0P9H4ZZ	Drainage of Right Radius, Percutaneous Endoscopic Approach
0P9J00Z	Drainage of Left Radius with Drainage Device, Open Approach
0P9J0ZX	Drainage of Left Radius, Open Approach, Diagnostic
0P9J0ZZ	Drainage of Left Radius, Open Approach
0P9J30Z	Drainage of Left Radius with Drainage Device, Percutaneous Approach
0P9J3ZX	Drainage of Left Radius, Percutaneous Approach, Diagnostic
0P9J3ZZ	Drainage of Left Radius, Percutaneous Approach
0P9J40Z	Drainage of Left Radius with Drainage Device, Percutaneous Endoscopic Approach
0P9J4ZX	Drainage of Left Radius, Percutaneous Endoscopic Approach, Diagnostic
0P9J4ZZ	Drainage of Left Radius, Percutaneous Endoscopic Approach
0P9K00Z	Drainage of Right Ulna with Drainage Device, Open Approach
0P9K0ZX	Drainage of Right Ulna, Open Approach, Diagnostic
0P9K0ZZ	Drainage of Right Ulna, Open Approach
0P9K30Z	Drainage of Right Ulna with Drainage Device, Percutaneous Approach
0P9K3ZX	Drainage of Right Ulna, Percutaneous Approach, Diagnostic
0P9K3ZZ	Drainage of Right Ulna, Percutaneous Approach
0P9K40Z	Drainage of Right Ulna with Drainage Device, Percutaneous Endoscopic Approach
0P9K4ZX	Drainage of Right Ulna, Percutaneous Endoscopic Approach, Diagnostic
0P9K4ZZ	Drainage of Right Ulna, Percutaneous Endoscopic Approach
0P9L00Z	Drainage of Left Ulna with Drainage Device, Open Approach
0P9L0ZX	Drainage of Left Ulna, Open Approach, Diagnostic
0P9L0ZZ	Drainage of Left Ulna, Open Approach
0P9L30Z	Drainage of Left Ulna with Drainage Device, Percutaneous Approach
0P9L3ZX	Drainage of Left Ulna, Percutaneous Approach, Diagnostic
0P9L3ZZ	Drainage of Left Ulna, Percutaneous Approach
0P9L40Z	Drainage of Left Ulna with Drainage Device, Percutaneous Endoscopic Approach
0P9L4ZX	Drainage of Left Ulna, Percutaneous Endoscopic Approach, Diagnostic
0P9L4ZZ	Drainage of Left Ulna, Percutaneous Endoscopic Approach
0P9M00Z	Drainage of Right Carpal with Drainage Device, Open Approach
0P9M0ZX	Drainage of Right Carpal, Open Approach, Diagnostic
0P9M0ZZ	Drainage of Right Carpal, Open Approach
0P9M30Z	Drainage of Right Carpal with Drainage Device, Percutaneous Approach
0P9M3ZX	Drainage of Right Carpal, Percutaneous Approach, Diagnostic
0P9M3ZZ	Drainage of Right Carpal, Percutaneous Approach
0P9M40Z	Drainage of Right Carpal with Drainage Device, Percutaneous Endoscopic Approach
0P9M4ZX	Drainage of Right Carpal, Percutaneous Endoscopic Approach, Diagnostic
0P9M4ZZ	Drainage of Right Carpal, Percutaneous Endoscopic Approach
0P9N00Z	Drainage of Left Carpal with Drainage Device, Open Approach
0P9N0ZX	Drainage of Left Carpal, Open Approach, Diagnostic

0P9N0ZZ Drainage of Left Carpal, Open Approach
0P9N30Z Drainage of Left Carpal with Drainage Device, Percutaneous Approach
0P9N3ZX Drainage of Left Carpal, Percutaneous Approach, Diagnostic
0P9N3ZZ Drainage of Left Carpal, Percutaneous Approach
0P9N40Z Drainage of Left Carpal with Drainage Device, Percutaneous Endoscopic Approach
0P9N4ZX Drainage of Left Carpal, Percutaneous Endoscopic Approach, Diagnostic
0P9N4ZZ Drainage of Left Carpal, Percutaneous Endoscopic Approach
0P9P00Z Drainage of Right Metacarpal with Drainage Device, Open Approach
0P9P0ZX Drainage of Right Metacarpal, Open Approach, Diagnostic
0P9P0ZZ Drainage of Right Metacarpal, Open Approach
0P9P30Z Drainage of Right Metacarpal with Drainage Device, Percutaneous Approach
0P9P3ZX Drainage of Right Metacarpal, Percutaneous Approach, Diagnostic
0P9P3ZZ Drainage of Right Metacarpal, Percutaneous Approach
0P9P40Z Drainage of Right Metacarpal with Drainage Device, Percutaneous Endoscopic Approach
0P9P4ZX Drainage of Right Metacarpal, Percutaneous Endoscopic Approach, Diagnostic
0P9P4ZZ Drainage of Right Metacarpal, Percutaneous Endoscopic Approach
0P9Q00Z Drainage of Left Metacarpal with Drainage Device, Open Approach
0P9Q0ZX Drainage of Left Metacarpal, Open Approach, Diagnostic
0P9Q0ZZ Drainage of Left Metacarpal, Open Approach
0P9Q30Z Drainage of Left Metacarpal with Drainage Device, Percutaneous Approach
0P9Q3ZX Drainage of Left Metacarpal, Percutaneous Approach, Diagnostic
0P9Q3ZZ Drainage of Left Metacarpal, Percutaneous Approach
0P9Q40Z Drainage of Left Metacarpal with Drainage Device, Percutaneous Endoscopic Approach
0P9Q4ZX Drainage of Left Metacarpal, Percutaneous Endoscopic Approach, Diagnostic
0P9Q4ZZ Drainage of Left Metacarpal, Percutaneous Endoscopic Approach
0P9R00Z Drainage of Right Thumb Phalanx with Drainage Device, Open Approach
0P9R0ZX Drainage of Right Thumb Phalanx, Open Approach, Diagnostic
0P9R0ZZ Drainage of Right Thumb Phalanx, Open Approach
0P9R30Z Drainage of Right Thumb Phalanx with Drainage Device, Percutaneous Approach
0P9R3ZX Drainage of Right Thumb Phalanx, Percutaneous Approach, Diagnostic
0P9R3ZZ Drainage of Right Thumb Phalanx, Percutaneous Approach
0P9R40Z Drainage of Right Thumb Phalanx with Drainage Device, Percutaneous Endoscopic Approach
0P9R4ZX Drainage of Right Thumb Phalanx, Percutaneous Endoscopic Approach, Diagnostic

0P9R4ZZ Drainage of Right Thumb Phalanx, Percutaneous Endoscopic Approach
0P9S00Z Drainage of Left Thumb Phalanx with Drainage Device, Open Approach
0P9S0ZX Drainage of Left Thumb Phalanx, Open Approach, Diagnostic
0P9S0ZZ Drainage of Left Thumb Phalanx, Open Approach
0P9S30Z Drainage of Left Thumb Phalanx with Drainage Device, Percutaneous Approach
0P9S3ZX Drainage of Left Thumb Phalanx, Percutaneous Approach, Diagnostic
0P9S3ZZ Drainage of Left Thumb Phalanx, Percutaneous Approach
0P9S40Z Drainage of Left Thumb Phalanx with Drainage Device, Percutaneous Endoscopic Approach
0P9S4ZX Drainage of Left Thumb Phalanx, Percutaneous Endoscopic Approach, Diagnostic
0P9S4ZZ Drainage of Left Thumb Phalanx, Percutaneous Endoscopic Approach
0P9T00Z Drainage of Right Finger Phalanx with Drainage Device, Open Approach
0P9T0ZX Drainage of Right Finger Phalanx, Open Approach, Diagnostic
0P9T0ZZ Drainage of Right Finger Phalanx, Open Approach
0P9T30Z Drainage of Right Finger Phalanx with Drainage Device, Percutaneous Approach
0P9T3ZX Drainage of Right Finger Phalanx, Percutaneous Approach, Diagnostic
0P9T3ZZ Drainage of Right Finger Phalanx, Percutaneous Approach
0P9T40Z Drainage of Right Finger Phalanx with Drainage Device, Percutaneous Endoscopic Approach
0P9T4ZX Drainage of Right Finger Phalanx, Percutaneous Endoscopic Approach, Diagnostic
0P9T4ZZ Drainage of Right Finger Phalanx, Percutaneous Endoscopic Approach
0P9V00Z Drainage of Left Finger Phalanx with Drainage Device, Open Approach
0P9V0ZX Drainage of Left Finger Phalanx, Open Approach, Diagnostic
0P9V0ZZ Drainage of Left Finger Phalanx, Open Approach
0P9V30Z Drainage of Left Finger Phalanx with Drainage Device, Percutaneous Approach
0P9V3ZX Drainage of Left Finger Phalanx, Percutaneous Approach, Diagnostic
0P9V3ZZ Drainage of Left Finger Phalanx, Percutaneous Approach
0P9V40Z Drainage of Left Finger Phalanx with Drainage Device, Percutaneous Endoscopic Approach
0P9V4ZX Drainage of Left Finger Phalanx, Percutaneous Endoscopic Approach, Diagnostic
0P9V4ZZ Drainage of Left Finger Phalanx, Percutaneous Endoscopic Approach

0PB – Upper Bones, Excision

Review Coding Guideline B3.5

Review Coding Guidelines B3.4a and B3.4b

Review Coding Guideline B3.8

0PB00ZX Excision of Sternum, Open Approach, Diagnostic
0PB00ZZ Excision of Sternum, Open Approach
0PB03ZX Excision of Sternum, Percutaneous Approach, Diagnostic
0PB03ZZ Excision of Sternum, Percutaneous Approach
0PB04ZX Excision of Sternum, Percutaneous Endoscopic Approach, Diagnostic
0PB04ZZ Excision of Sternum, Percutaneous Endoscopic Approach
0PB10ZX Excision of Right Rib, Open Approach, Diagnostic
0PB10ZZ Excision of Right Rib, Open Approach
0PB13ZX Excision of Right Rib, Percutaneous Approach, Diagnostic
0PB13ZZ Excision of Right Rib, Percutaneous Approach
0PB14ZX Excision of Right Rib, Percutaneous Endoscopic Approach, Diagnostic
0PB14ZZ Excision of Right Rib, Percutaneous Endoscopic Approach
0PB20ZX Excision of Left Rib, Open Approach, Diagnostic
0PB20ZZ Excision of Left Rib, Open Approach
0PB23ZX Excision of Left Rib, Percutaneous Approach, Diagnostic
0PB23ZZ Excision of Left Rib, Percutaneous Approach
0PB24ZX Excision of Left Rib, Percutaneous Endoscopic Approach, Diagnostic
0PB24ZZ Excision of Left Rib, Percutaneous Endoscopic Approach
0PB30ZX Excision of Cervical Vertebra, Open Approach, Diagnostic
0PB30ZZ Excision of Cervical Vertebra, Open Approach
0PB33ZX Excision of Cervical Vertebra, Percutaneous Approach, Diagnostic
0PB33ZZ Excision of Cervical Vertebra, Percutaneous Approach
0PB34ZX Excision of Cervical Vertebra, Percutaneous Endoscopic Approach, Diagnostic
0PB34ZZ Excision of Cervical Vertebra, Percutaneous Endoscopic Approach
0PB40ZX Excision of Thoracic Vertebra, Open Approach, Diagnostic
0PB40ZZ Excision of Thoracic Vertebra, Open Approach
0PB43ZX Excision of Thoracic Vertebra, Percutaneous Approach, Diagnostic
0PB43ZZ Excision of Thoracic Vertebra, Percutaneous Approach

0PB44ZX	Excision of Thoracic Vertebra, Percutaneous Endoscopic Approach, Diagnostic
0PB44ZZ	Excision of Thoracic Vertebra, Percutaneous Endoscopic Approach
0PB50ZX	Excision of Right Scapula, Open Approach, Diagnostic
0PB50ZZ	Excision of Right Scapula, Open Approach
0PB53ZX	Excision of Right Scapula, Percutaneous Approach, Diagnostic
0PB53ZZ	Excision of Right Scapula, Percutaneous Approach
0PB54ZX	Excision of Right Scapula, Percutaneous Endoscopic Approach, Diagnostic
0PB54ZZ	Excision of Right Scapula, Percutaneous Endoscopic Approach
0PB60ZX	Excision of Left Scapula, Open Approach, Diagnostic
0PB60ZZ	Excision of Left Scapula, Open Approach
0PB63ZX	Excision of Left Scapula, Percutaneous Approach, Diagnostic
0PB63ZZ	Excision of Left Scapula, Percutaneous Approach
0PB64ZX	Excision of Left Scapula, Percutaneous Endoscopic Approach, Diagnostic
0PB64ZZ	Excision of Left Scapula, Percutaneous Endoscopic Approach
0PB70ZX	Excision of Right Glenoid Cavity, Open Approach, Diagnostic
0PB70ZZ	Excision of Right Glenoid Cavity, Open Approach
0PB73ZX	Excision of Right Glenoid Cavity, Percutaneous Approach, Diagnostic
0PB73ZZ	Excision of Right Glenoid Cavity, Percutaneous Approach
0PB74ZX	Excision of Right Glenoid Cavity, Percutaneous Endoscopic Approach, Diagnostic
0PB74ZZ	Excision of Right Glenoid Cavity, Percutaneous Endoscopic Approach
0PB80ZX	Excision of Left Glenoid Cavity, Open Approach, Diagnostic
0PB80ZZ	Excision of Left Glenoid Cavity, Open Approach
0PB83ZX	Excision of Left Glenoid Cavity, Percutaneous Approach, Diagnostic
0PB83ZZ	Excision of Left Glenoid Cavity, Percutaneous Approach
0PB84ZX	Excision of Left Glenoid Cavity, Percutaneous Endoscopic Approach, Diagnostic
0PB84ZZ	Excision of Left Glenoid Cavity, Percutaneous Endoscopic Approach
0PB90ZX	Excision of Right Clavicle, Open Approach, Diagnostic
0PB90ZZ	Excision of Right Clavicle, Open Approach
0PB93ZX	Excision of Right Clavicle, Percutaneous Approach, Diagnostic
0PB93ZZ	Excision of Right Clavicle, Percutaneous Approach
0PB94ZX	Excision of Right Clavicle, Percutaneous Endoscopic Approach, Diagnostic
0PB94ZZ	Excision of Right Clavicle, Percutaneous Endoscopic Approach
0PBB0ZX	Excision of Left Clavicle, Open Approach, Diagnostic
0PBB0ZZ	Excision of Left Clavicle, Open Approach
0PBB3ZX	Excision of Left Clavicle, Percutaneous Approach, Diagnostic
0PBB3ZZ	Excision of Left Clavicle, Percutaneous Approach
0PBB4ZX	Excision of Left Clavicle, Percutaneous Endoscopic Approach, Diagnostic
0PBB4ZZ	Excision of Left Clavicle, Percutaneous Endoscopic Approach
0PBC0ZX	Excision of Right Humeral Head, Open Approach, Diagnostic
0PBC0ZZ	Excision of Right Humeral Head, Open Approach
0PBC3ZX	Excision of Right Humeral Head, Percutaneous Approach, Diagnostic
0PBC3ZZ	Excision of Right Humeral Head, Percutaneous Approach
0PBC4ZX	Excision of Right Humeral Head, Percutaneous Endoscopic Approach, Diagnostic
0PBC4ZZ	Excision of Right Humeral Head, Percutaneous Endoscopic Approach
0PBD0ZX	Excision of Left Humeral Head, Open Approach, Diagnostic
0PBD0ZZ	Excision of Left Humeral Head, Open Approach
0PBD3ZX	Excision of Left Humeral Head, Percutaneous Approach, Diagnostic
0PBD3ZZ	Excision of Left Humeral Head, Percutaneous Approach
0PBD4ZX	Excision of Left Humeral Head, Percutaneous Endoscopic Approach, Diagnostic
0PBD4ZZ	Excision of Left Humeral Head, Percutaneous Endoscopic Approach
0PBF0ZX	Excision of Right Humeral Shaft, Open Approach, Diagnostic
0PBF0ZZ	Excision of Right Humeral Shaft, Open Approach
0PBF3ZX	Excision of Right Humeral Shaft, Percutaneous Approach, Diagnostic
0PBF3ZZ	Excision of Right Humeral Shaft, Percutaneous Approach
0PBF4ZX	Excision of Right Humeral Shaft, Percutaneous Endoscopic Approach, Diagnostic
0PBF4ZZ	Excision of Right Humeral Shaft, Percutaneous Endoscopic Approach
0PBG0ZX	Excision of Left Humeral Shaft, Open Approach, Diagnostic
0PBG0ZZ	Excision of Left Humeral Shaft, Open Approach
0PBG3ZX	Excision of Left Humeral Shaft, Percutaneous Approach, Diagnostic
0PBG3ZZ	Excision of Left Humeral Shaft, Percutaneous Approach
0PBG4ZX	Excision of Left Humeral Shaft, Percutaneous Endoscopic Approach, Diagnostic
0PBG4ZZ	Excision of Left Humeral Shaft, Percutaneous Endoscopic Approach
0PBH0ZX	Excision of Right Radius, Open Approach, Diagnostic
0PBH0ZZ	Excision of Right Radius, Open Approach
0PBH3ZX	Excision of Right Radius, Percutaneous Approach, Diagnostic
0PBH3ZZ	Excision of Right Radius, Percutaneous Approach
0PBH4ZX	Excision of Right Radius, Percutaneous Endoscopic Approach, Diagnostic
0PBH4ZZ	Excision of Right Radius, Percutaneous Endoscopic Approach
0PBJ0ZX	Excision of Left Radius, Open Approach, Diagnostic
0PBJ0ZZ	Excision of Left Radius, Open Approach
0PBJ3ZX	Excision of Left Radius, Percutaneous Approach, Diagnostic
0PBJ3ZZ	Excision of Left Radius, Percutaneous Approach
0PBJ4ZX	Excision of Left Radius, Percutaneous Endoscopic Approach, Diagnostic
0PBJ4ZZ	Excision of Left Radius, Percutaneous Endoscopic Approach
0PBK0ZX	Excision of Right Ulna, Open Approach, Diagnostic
0PBK0ZZ	Excision of Right Ulna, Open Approach
0PBK3ZX	Excision of Right Ulna, Percutaneous Approach, Diagnostic
0PBK3ZZ	Excision of Right Ulna, Percutaneous Approach
0PBK4ZX	Excision of Right Ulna, Percutaneous Endoscopic Approach, Diagnostic
0PBK4ZZ	Excision of Right Ulna, Percutaneous Endoscopic Approach
0PBL0ZX	Excision of Left Ulna, Open Approach, Diagnostic
0PBL0ZZ	Excision of Left Ulna, Open Approach
0PBL3ZX	Excision of Left Ulna, Percutaneous Approach, Diagnostic
0PBL3ZZ	Excision of Left Ulna, Percutaneous Approach
0PBL4ZX	Excision of Left Ulna, Percutaneous Endoscopic Approach, Diagnostic
0PBL4ZZ	Excision of Left Ulna, Percutaneous Endoscopic Approach
0PBM0ZX	Excision of Right Carpal, Open Approach, Diagnostic
0PBM0ZZ	Excision of Right Carpal, Open Approach
0PBM3ZX	Excision of Right Carpal, Percutaneous Approach, Diagnostic
0PBM3ZZ	Excision of Right Carpal, Percutaneous Approach
0PBM4ZX	Excision of Right Carpal, Percutaneous Endoscopic Approach, Diagnostic
0PBM4ZZ	Excision of Right Carpal, Percutaneous Endoscopic Approach
0PBN0ZX	Excision of Left Carpal, Open Approach, Diagnostic
0PBN0ZZ	Excision of Left Carpal, Open Approach
0PBN3ZX	Excision of Left Carpal, Percutaneous Approach, Diagnostic
0PBN3ZZ	Excision of Left Carpal, Percutaneous Approach
0PBN4ZX	Excision of Left Carpal, Percutaneous Endoscopic Approach, Diagnostic
0PBN4ZZ	Excision of Left Carpal, Percutaneous Endoscopic Approach
0PBP0ZX	Excision of Right Metacarpal, Open Approach, Diagnostic
0PBP0ZZ	Excision of Right Metacarpal, Open Approach
0PBP3ZX	Excision of Right Metacarpal, Percutaneous Approach, Diagnostic
0PBP3ZZ	Excision of Right Metacarpal, Percutaneous Approach
0PBP4ZX	Excision of Right Metacarpal, Percutaneous Endoscopic Approach, Diagnostic
0PBP4ZZ	Excision of Right Metacarpal, Percutaneous Endoscopic Approach
0PBQ0ZX	Excision of Left Metacarpal, Open Approach, Diagnostic
0PBQ0ZZ	Excision of Left Metacarpal, Open Approach
0PBQ3ZX	Excision of Left Metacarpal, Percutaneous Approach, Diagnostic
0PBQ3ZZ	Excision of Left Metacarpal, Percutaneous Approach
0PBQ4ZX	Excision of Left Metacarpal, Percutaneous Endoscopic Approach, Diagnostic
0PBQ4ZZ	Excision of Left Metacarpal, Percutaneous Endoscopic Approach
0PBR0ZX	Excision of Right Thumb Phalanx, Open Approach, Diagnostic
0PBR0ZZ	Excision of Right Thumb Phalanx, Open Approach
0PBR3ZX	Excision of Right Thumb Phalanx, Percutaneous Approach, Diagnostic
0PBR3ZZ	Excision of Right Thumb Phalanx, Percutaneous Approach
0PBR4ZX	Excision of Right Thumb Phalanx, Percutaneous Endoscopic Approach, Diagnostic

0PBR4ZZ Excision of Right Thumb Phalanx, Percutaneous Endoscopic Approach
0PBS0ZX Excision of Left Thumb Phalanx, Open Approach, Diagnostic
0PBS0ZZ Excision of Left Thumb Phalanx, Open Approach
0PBS3ZX Excision of Left Thumb Phalanx, Percutaneous Approach, Diagnostic
0PBS3ZZ Excision of Left Thumb Phalanx, Percutaneous Approach
0PBS4ZX Excision of Left Thumb Phalanx, Percutaneous Endoscopic Approach, Diagnostic
0PBS4ZZ Excision of Left Thumb Phalanx, Percutaneous Endoscopic Approach
0PBT0ZX Excision of Right Finger Phalanx, Open Approach, Diagnostic
0PBT0ZZ Excision of Right Finger Phalanx, Open Approach
0PBT3ZX Excision of Right Finger Phalanx, Percutaneous Approach, Diagnostic

0PBT3ZZ Excision of Right Finger Phalanx, Percutaneous Approach
0PBT4ZX Excision of Right Finger Phalanx, Percutaneous Endoscopic Approach, Diagnostic
0PBT4ZZ Excision of Right Finger Phalanx, Percutaneous Endoscopic Approach
0PBV0ZX Excision of Left Finger Phalanx, Open Approach, Diagnostic
0PBV0ZZ Excision of Left Finger Phalanx, Open Approach
0PBV3ZX Excision of Left Finger Phalanx, Percutaneous Approach, Diagnostic
0PBV3ZZ Excision of Left Finger Phalanx, Percutaneous Approach
0PBV4ZX Excision of Left Finger Phalanx, Percutaneous Endoscopic Approach, Diagnostic
0PBV4ZZ Excision of Left Finger Phalanx, Percutaneous Endoscopic Approach

0PC – Upper Bones, Extirpation

0PC00ZZ Extirpation of Matter from Sternum, Open Approach
0PC03ZZ Extirpation of Matter from Sternum, Percutaneous Approach
0PC04ZZ Extirpation of Matter from Sternum, Percutaneous Endoscopic Approach
0PC10ZZ Extirpation of Matter from Right Rib, Open Approach
0PC13ZZ Extirpation of Matter from Right Rib, Percutaneous Approach
0PC14ZZ Extirpation of Matter from Right Rib, Percutaneous Endoscopic Approach
0PC20ZZ Extirpation of Matter from Left Rib, Open Approach
0PC23ZZ Extirpation of Matter from Left Rib, Percutaneous Approach
0PC24ZZ Extirpation of Matter from Left Rib, Percutaneous Endoscopic Approach
0PC30ZZ Extirpation of Matter from Cervical Vertebra, Open Approach
0PC33ZZ Extirpation of Matter from Cervical Vertebra, Percutaneous Approach
0PC34ZZ Extirpation of Matter from Cervical Vertebra, Percutaneous Endoscopic Approach
0PC40ZZ Extirpation of Matter from Thoracic Vertebra, Open Approach
0PC43ZZ Extirpation of Matter from Thoracic Vertebra, Percutaneous Approach
0PC44ZZ Extirpation of Matter from Thoracic Vertebra, Percutaneous Endoscopic Approach
0PC50ZZ Extirpation of Matter from Right Scapula, Open Approach
0PC53ZZ Extirpation of Matter from Right Scapula, Percutaneous Approach
0PC54ZZ Extirpation of Matter from Right Scapula, Percutaneous Endoscopic Approach
0PC60ZZ Extirpation of Matter from Left Scapula, Open Approach
0PC63ZZ Extirpation of Matter from Left Scapula, Percutaneous Approach
0PC64ZZ Extirpation of Matter from Left Scapula, Percutaneous Endoscopic Approach
0PC70ZZ Extirpation of Matter from Right Glenoid Cavity, Open Approach
0PC73ZZ Extirpation of Matter from Right Glenoid Cavity, Percutaneous Approach
0PC74ZZ Extirpation of Matter from Right Glenoid Cavity, Percutaneous Endoscopic Approach
0PC80ZZ Extirpation of Matter from Left Glenoid Cavity, Open Approach
0PC83ZZ Extirpation of Matter from Left Glenoid Cavity, Percutaneous Approach
0PC84ZZ Extirpation of Matter from Left Glenoid Cavity, Percutaneous Endoscopic Approach
0PC90ZZ Extirpation of Matter from Right Clavicle, Open Approach
0PC93ZZ Extirpation of Matter from Right Clavicle, Percutaneous Approach
0PC94ZZ Extirpation of Matter from Right Clavicle, Percutaneous Endoscopic Approach
0PCB0ZZ Extirpation of Matter from Left Clavicle, Open Approach
0PCB3ZZ Extirpation of Matter from Left Clavicle, Percutaneous Approach
0PCB4ZZ Extirpation of Matter from Left Clavicle, Percutaneous Endoscopic Approach
0PCC0ZZ Extirpation of Matter from Right Humeral Head, Open Approach
0PCC3ZZ Extirpation of Matter from Right Humeral Head, Percutaneous Approach
0PCC4ZZ Extirpation of Matter from Right Humeral Head, Percutaneous Endoscopic Approach
0PCD0ZZ Extirpation of Matter from Left Humeral Head, Open Approach

0PCD3ZZ Extirpation of Matter from Left Humeral Head, Percutaneous Approach
0PCD4ZZ Extirpation of Matter from Left Humeral Head, Percutaneous Endoscopic Approach
0PCF0ZZ Extirpation of Matter from Right Humeral Shaft, Open Approach
0PCF3ZZ Extirpation of Matter from Right Humeral Shaft, Percutaneous Approach
0PCF4ZZ Extirpation of Matter from Right Humeral Shaft, Percutaneous Endoscopic Approach
0PCG0ZZ Extirpation of Matter from Left Humeral Shaft, Open Approach
0PCG3ZZ Extirpation of Matter from Left Humeral Shaft, Percutaneous Approach
0PCG4ZZ Extirpation of Matter from Left Humeral Shaft, Percutaneous Endoscopic Approach
0PCH0ZZ Extirpation of Matter from Right Radius, Open Approach
0PCH3ZZ Extirpation of Matter from Right Radius, Percutaneous Approach
0PCH4ZZ Extirpation of Matter from Right Radius, Percutaneous Endoscopic Approach
0PCJ0ZZ Extirpation of Matter from Left Radius, Open Approach
0PCJ3ZZ Extirpation of Matter from Left Radius, Percutaneous Approach
0PCJ4ZZ Extirpation of Matter from Left Radius, Percutaneous Endoscopic Approach
0PCK0ZZ Extirpation of Matter from Right Ulna, Open Approach
0PCK3ZZ Extirpation of Matter from Right Ulna, Percutaneous Approach
0PCK4ZZ Extirpation of Matter from Right Ulna, Percutaneous Endoscopic Approach
0PCL0ZZ Extirpation of Matter from Left Ulna, Open Approach
0PCL3ZZ Extirpation of Matter from Left Ulna, Percutaneous Approach
0PCL4ZZ Extirpation of Matter from Left Ulna, Percutaneous Endoscopic Approach
0PCM0ZZ Extirpation of Matter from Right Carpal, Open Approach
0PCM3ZZ Extirpation of Matter from Right Carpal, Percutaneous Approach
0PCM4ZZ Extirpation of Matter from Right Carpal, Percutaneous Endoscopic Approach
0PCN0ZZ Extirpation of Matter from Left Carpal, Open Approach
0PCN3ZZ Extirpation of Matter from Left Carpal, Percutaneous Approach
0PCN4ZZ Extirpation of Matter from Left Carpal, Percutaneous Endoscopic Approach
0PCP0ZZ Extirpation of Matter from Right Metacarpal, Open Approach
0PCP3ZZ Extirpation of Matter from Right Metacarpal, Percutaneous Approach
0PCP4ZZ Extirpation of Matter from Right Metacarpal, Percutaneous Endoscopic Approach
0PCQ0ZZ Extirpation of Matter from Left Metacarpal, Open Approach
0PCQ3ZZ Extirpation of Matter from Left Metacarpal, Percutaneous Approach
0PCQ4ZZ Extirpation of Matter from Left Metacarpal, Percutaneous Endoscopic Approach
0PCR0ZZ Extirpation of Matter from Right Thumb Phalanx, Open Approach
0PCR3ZZ Extirpation of Matter from Right Thumb Phalanx, Percutaneous Approach
0PCR4ZZ Extirpation of Matter from Right Thumb Phalanx, Percutaneous Endoscopic Approach
0PCS0ZZ Extirpation of Matter from Left Thumb Phalanx, Open Approach
0PCS3ZZ Extirpation of Matter from Left Thumb Phalanx, Percutaneous Approach

0PCS4ZZ   Extirpation of Matter from Left Thumb Phalanx, Percutaneous Endoscopic Approach

0PCT0ZZ   Extirpation of Matter from Right Finger Phalanx, Open Approach

0PCT3ZZ   Extirpation of Matter from Right Finger Phalanx, Percutaneous Approach

0PCT4ZZ   Extirpation of Matter from Right Finger Phalanx, Percutaneous Endoscopic Approach

0PCV0ZZ   Extirpation of Matter from Left Finger Phalanx, Open Approach

0PCV3ZZ   Extirpation of Matter from Left Finger Phalanx, Percutaneous Approach

0PCV4ZZ   Extirpation of Matter from Left Finger Phalanx, Percutaneous Endoscopic Approach

0PH – Upper Bones, Insertion

0PH000Z   Insertion of Rigid Plate Internal Fixation Device into Sternum, Open Approach

0PH004Z   Insertion of Internal Fixation Device into Sternum, Open Approach

0PH030Z   Insertion of Rigid Plate Internal Fixation Device into Sternum, Percutaneous Approach

0PH034Z   Insertion of Internal Fixation Device into Sternum, Percutaneous Approach

0PH040Z   Insertion of Rigid Plate Internal Fixation Device into Sternum, Percutaneous Endoscopic Approach

0PH044Z   Insertion of Internal Fixation Device into Sternum, Percutaneous Endoscopic Approach

0PH104Z   Insertion of Internal Fixation Device into Right Rib, Open Approach

0PH134Z   Insertion of Internal Fixation Device into Right Rib, Percutaneous Approach

0PH144Z   Insertion of Internal Fixation Device into Right Rib, Percutaneous Endoscopic Approach

0PH204Z   Insertion of Internal Fixation Device into Left Rib, Open Approach

0PH234Z   Insertion of Internal Fixation Device into Left Rib, Percutaneous Approach

0PH244Z   Insertion of Internal Fixation Device into Left Rib, Percutaneous Endoscopic Approach

0PH304Z   Insertion of Internal Fixation Device into Cervical Vertebra, Open Approach

0PH334Z   Insertion of Internal Fixation Device into Cervical Vertebra, Percutaneous Approach

0PH344Z   Insertion of Internal Fixation Device into Cervical Vertebra, Percutaneous Endoscopic Approach

0PH404Z   Insertion of Internal Fixation Device into Thoracic Vertebra, Open Approach

0PH434Z   Insertion of Internal Fixation Device into Thoracic Vertebra, Percutaneous Approach

0PH444Z   Insertion of Internal Fixation Device into Thoracic Vertebra, Percutaneous Endoscopic Approach

0PH504Z   Insertion of Internal Fixation Device into Right Scapula, Open Approach

0PH534Z   Insertion of Internal Fixation Device into Right Scapula, Percutaneous Approach

0PH544Z   Insertion of Internal Fixation Device into Right Scapula, Percutaneous Endoscopic Approach

0PH604Z   Insertion of Internal Fixation Device into Left Scapula, Open Approach

0PH634Z   Insertion of Internal Fixation Device into Left Scapula, Percutaneous Approach

0PH644Z   Insertion of Internal Fixation Device into Left Scapula, Percutaneous Endoscopic Approach

0PH704Z   Insertion of Internal Fixation Device into Right Glenoid Cavity, Open Approach

0PH734Z   Insertion of Internal Fixation Device into Right Glenoid Cavity, Percutaneous Approach

0PH744Z   Insertion of Internal Fixation Device into Right Glenoid Cavity, Percutaneous Endoscopic Approach

0PH804Z   Insertion of Internal Fixation Device into Left Glenoid Cavity, Open Approach

0PH834Z   Insertion of Internal Fixation Device into Left Glenoid Cavity, Percutaneous Approach

0PH844Z   Insertion of Internal Fixation Device into Left Glenoid Cavity, Percutaneous Endoscopic Approach

0PH904Z   Insertion of Internal Fixation Device into Right Clavicle, Open Approach

0PH934Z   Insertion of Internal Fixation Device into Right Clavicle, Percutaneous Approach

0PH944Z   Insertion of Internal Fixation Device into Right Clavicle, Percutaneous Endoscopic Approach

0PHB04Z   Insertion of Internal Fixation Device into Left Clavicle, Open Approach

0PHB34Z   Insertion of Internal Fixation Device into Left Clavicle, Percutaneous Approach

0PHB44Z   Insertion of Internal Fixation Device into Left Clavicle, Percutaneous Endoscopic Approach

0PHC04Z   Insertion of Internal Fixation Device into Right Humeral Head, Open Approach

0PHC05Z   Insertion of External Fixation Device into Right Humeral Head, Open Approach

0PHC06Z   Insertion of Intramedullary Internal Fixation Device into Right Humeral Head, Open Approach

0PHC08Z   Insertion of Limb Lengthening External Fixation Device into Right Humeral Head, Open Approach

0PHC0BZ   Insertion of Monoplanar External Fixation Device into Right Humeral Head, Open Approach

0PHC0CZ   Insertion of Ring External Fixation Device into Right Humeral Head, Open Approach

0PHC0DZ   Insertion of Hybrid External Fixation Device into Right Humeral Head, Open Approach

0PHC34Z   Insertion of Internal Fixation Device into Right Humeral Head, Percutaneous Approach

0PHC35Z   Insertion of External Fixation Device into Right Humeral Head, Percutaneous Approach

0PHC36Z   Insertion of Intramedullary Internal Fixation Device into Right Humeral Head, Percutaneous Approach

0PHC38Z   Insertion of Limb Lengthening External Fixation Device into Right Humeral Head, Percutaneous Approach

0PHC3BZ   Insertion of Monoplanar External Fixation Device into Right Humeral Head, Percutaneous Approach

0PHC3CZ   Insertion of Ring External Fixation Device into Right Humeral Head, Percutaneous Approach

0PHC3DZ   Insertion of Hybrid External Fixation Device into Right Humeral Head, Percutaneous Approach

0PHC44Z   Insertion of Internal Fixation Device into Right Humeral Head, Percutaneous Endoscopic Approach

0PHC45Z   Insertion of External Fixation Device into Right Humeral Head, Percutaneous Endoscopic Approach

0PHC46Z   Insertion of Intramedullary Internal Fixation Device into Right Humeral Head, Percutaneous Endoscopic Approach

0PHC48Z   Insertion of Limb Lengthening External Fixation Device into Right Humeral Head, Percutaneous Endoscopic Approach

0PHC4BZ   Insertion of Monoplanar External Fixation Device into Right Humeral Head, Percutaneous Endoscopic Approach

0PHC4CZ   Insertion of Ring External Fixation Device into Right Humeral Head, Percutaneous Endoscopic Approach

0PHC4DZ   Insertion of Hybrid External Fixation Device into Right Humeral Head, Percutaneous Endoscopic Approach

0PHD04Z   Insertion of Internal Fixation Device into Left Humeral Head, Open Approach

0PHD05Z   Insertion of External Fixation Device into Left Humeral Head, Open Approach

0PHD06Z   Insertion of Intramedullary Internal Fixation Device into Left Humeral Head, Open Approach

0PHD08Z   Insertion of Limb Lengthening External Fixation Device into Left Humeral Head, Open Approach

0PHD0BZ   Insertion of Monoplanar External Fixation Device into Left Humeral Head, Open Approach

0PHD0CZ   Insertion of Ring External Fixation Device into Left Humeral Head, Open Approach

0PHD0DZ   Insertion of Hybrid External Fixation Device into Left Humeral Head, Open Approach

0PHD34Z   Insertion of Internal Fixation Device into Left Humeral Head, Percutaneous Approach

0PHD35Z Insertion of External Fixation Device into Left Humeral Head, Percutaneous Approach

0PHD36Z Insertion of Intramedullary Internal Fixation Device into Left Humeral Head, Percutaneous Approach

0PHD38Z Insertion of Limb Lengthening External Fixation Device into Left Humeral Head, Percutaneous Approach

0PHD3BZ Insertion of Monoplanar External Fixation Device into Left Humeral Head, Percutaneous Approach

0PHD3CZ Insertion of Ring External Fixation Device into Left Humeral Head, Percutaneous Approach

0PHD3DZ Insertion of Hybrid External Fixation Device into Left Humeral Head, Percutaneous Approach

0PHD44Z Insertion of Internal Fixation Device into Left Humeral Head, Percutaneous Endoscopic Approach

0PHD45Z Insertion of External Fixation Device into Left Humeral Head, Percutaneous Endoscopic Approach

0PHD46Z Insertion of Intramedullary Internal Fixation Device into Left Humeral Head, Percutaneous Endoscopic Approach

0PHD48Z Insertion of Limb Lengthening External Fixation Device into Left Humeral Head, Percutaneous Endoscopic Approach

0PHD4BZ Insertion of Monoplanar External Fixation Device into Left Humeral Head, Percutaneous Endoscopic Approach

0PHD4CZ Insertion of Ring External Fixation Device into Left Humeral Head, Percutaneous Endoscopic Approach

0PHD4DZ Insertion of Hybrid External Fixation Device into Left Humeral Head, Percutaneous Endoscopic Approach

0PHF04Z Insertion of Internal Fixation Device into Right Humeral Shaft, Open Approach

0PHF05Z Insertion of External Fixation Device into Right Humeral Shaft, Open Approach

0PHF06Z Insertion of Intramedullary Internal Fixation Device into Right Humeral Shaft, Open Approach

0PHF08Z Insertion of Limb Lengthening External Fixation Device into Right Humeral Shaft, Open Approach

0PHF0BZ Insertion of Monoplanar External Fixation Device into Right Humeral Shaft, Open Approach

0PHF0CZ Insertion of Ring External Fixation Device into Right Humeral Shaft, Open Approach

0PHF0DZ Insertion of Hybrid External Fixation Device into Right Humeral Shaft, Open Approach

0PHF34Z Insertion of Internal Fixation Device into Right Humeral Shaft, Percutaneous Approach

0PHF35Z Insertion of External Fixation Device into Right Humeral Shaft, Percutaneous Approach

0PHF36Z Insertion of Intramedullary Internal Fixation Device into Right Humeral Shaft, Percutaneous Approach

0PHF38Z Insertion of Limb Lengthening External Fixation Device into Right Humeral Shaft, Percutaneous Approach

0PHF3BZ Insertion of Monoplanar External Fixation Device into Right Humeral Shaft, Percutaneous Approach

0PHF3CZ Insertion of Ring External Fixation Device into Right Humeral Shaft, Percutaneous Approach

0PHF3DZ Insertion of Hybrid External Fixation Device into Right Humeral Shaft, Percutaneous Approach

0PHF44Z Insertion of Internal Fixation Device into Right Humeral Shaft, Percutaneous Endoscopic Approach

0PHF45Z Insertion of External Fixation Device into Right Humeral Shaft, Percutaneous Endoscopic Approach

0PHF46Z Insertion of Intramedullary Internal Fixation Device into Right Humeral Shaft, Percutaneous Endoscopic Approach

0PHF48Z Insertion of Limb Lengthening External Fixation Device into Right Humeral Shaft, Percutaneous Endoscopic Approach

0PHF4BZ Insertion of Monoplanar External Fixation Device into Right Humeral Shaft, Percutaneous Endoscopic Approach

0PHF4CZ Insertion of Ring External Fixation Device into Right Humeral Shaft, Percutaneous Endoscopic Approach

0PHF4DZ Insertion of Hybrid External Fixation Device into Right Humeral Shaft, Percutaneous Endoscopic Approach

0PHG04Z Insertion of Internal Fixation Device into Left Humeral Shaft, Open Approach

0PHG05Z Insertion of External Fixation Device into Left Humeral Shaft, Open Approach

0PHG06Z Insertion of Intramedullary Internal Fixation Device into Left Humeral Shaft, Open Approach

0PHG08Z Insertion of Limb Lengthening External Fixation Device into Left Humeral Shaft, Open Approach

0PHG0BZ Insertion of Monoplanar External Fixation Device into Left Humeral Shaft, Open Approach

0PHG0CZ Insertion of Ring External Fixation Device into Left Humeral Shaft, Open Approach

0PHG0DZ Insertion of Hybrid External Fixation Device into Left Humeral Shaft, Open Approach

0PHG34Z Insertion of Internal Fixation Device into Left Humeral Shaft, Percutaneous Approach

0PHG35Z Insertion of External Fixation Device into Left Humeral Shaft, Percutaneous Approach

0PHG36Z Insertion of Intramedullary Internal Fixation Device into Left Humeral Shaft, Percutaneous Approach

0PHG38Z Insertion of Limb Lengthening External Fixation Device into Left Humeral Shaft, Percutaneous Approach

0PHG3BZ Insertion of Monoplanar External Fixation Device into Left Humeral Shaft, Percutaneous Approach

0PHG3CZ Insertion of Ring External Fixation Device into Left Humeral Shaft, Percutaneous Approach

0PHG3DZ Insertion of Hybrid External Fixation Device into Left Humeral Shaft, Percutaneous Approach

0PHG44Z Insertion of Internal Fixation Device into Left Humeral Shaft, Percutaneous Endoscopic Approach

0PHG45Z Insertion of External Fixation Device into Left Humeral Shaft, Percutaneous Endoscopic Approach

0PHG46Z Insertion of Intramedullary Internal Fixation Device into Left Humeral Shaft, Percutaneous Endoscopic Approach

0PHG48Z Insertion of Limb Lengthening External Fixation Device into Left Humeral Shaft, Percutaneous Endoscopic Approach

0PHG4BZ Insertion of Monoplanar External Fixation Device into Left Humeral Shaft, Percutaneous Endoscopic Approach

0PHG4CZ Insertion of Ring External Fixation Device into Left Humeral Shaft, Percutaneous Endoscopic Approach

0PHG4DZ Insertion of Hybrid External Fixation Device into Left Humeral Shaft, Percutaneous Endoscopic Approach

0PHH04Z Insertion of Internal Fixation Device into Right Radius, Open Approach

0PHH05Z Insertion of External Fixation Device into Right Radius, Open Approach

0PHH06Z Insertion of Intramedullary Internal Fixation Device into Right Radius, Open Approach

0PHH08Z Insertion of Limb Lengthening External Fixation Device into Right Radius, Open Approach

0PHH0BZ Insertion of Monoplanar External Fixation Device into Right Radius, Open Approach

0PHH0CZ Insertion of Ring External Fixation Device into Right Radius, Open Approach

0PHH0DZ Insertion of Hybrid External Fixation Device into Right Radius, Open Approach

0PHH34Z Insertion of Internal Fixation Device into Right Radius, Percutaneous Approach

0PHH35Z Insertion of External Fixation Device into Right Radius, Percutaneous Approach

0PHH36Z Insertion of Intramedullary Internal Fixation Device into Right Radius, Percutaneous Approach

0PHH38Z Insertion of Limb Lengthening External Fixation Device into Right Radius, Percutaneous Approach

0PHH3BZ Insertion of Monoplanar External Fixation Device into Right Radius, Percutaneous Approach

0PHH3CZ Insertion of Ring External Fixation Device into Right Radius, Percutaneous Approach

0PHH3DZ Insertion of Hybrid External Fixation Device into Right Radius, Percutaneous Approach

0PHH44Z Insertion of Internal Fixation Device into Right Radius, Percutaneous Endoscopic Approach

0PHH45Z Insertion of External Fixation Device into Right Radius, Percutaneous Endoscopic Approach

0PHH46Z Insertion of Intramedullary Internal Fixation Device into Right Radius, Percutaneous Endoscopic Approach

0PHH48Z Insertion of Limb Lengthening External Fixation Device into Right Radius, Percutaneous Endoscopic Approach

0PHH4BZ Insertion of Monoplanar External Fixation Device into Right Radius, Percutaneous Endoscopic Approach

0PHH4CZ Insertion of Ring External Fixation Device into Right Radius, Percutaneous Endoscopic Approach

0PHH4DZ Insertion of Hybrid External Fixation Device into Right Radius, Percutaneous Endoscopic Approach

0PHJ04Z Insertion of Internal Fixation Device into Left Radius, Open Approach

0PHJ05Z Insertion of External Fixation Device into Left Radius, Open Approach

0PHJ06Z Insertion of Intramedullary Internal Fixation Device into Left Radius, Open Approach

0PHJ08Z Insertion of Limb Lengthening External Fixation Device into Left Radius, Open Approach

0PHJ0BZ Insertion of Monoplanar External Fixation Device into Left Radius, Open Approach

0PHJ0CZ Insertion of Ring External Fixation Device into Left Radius, Open Approach

0PHJ0DZ Insertion of Hybrid External Fixation Device into Left Radius, Open Approach

0PHJ34Z Insertion of Internal Fixation Device into Left Radius, Percutaneous Approach

0PHJ35Z Insertion of External Fixation Device into Left Radius, Percutaneous Approach

0PHJ36Z Insertion of Intramedullary Internal Fixation Device into Left Radius, Percutaneous Approach

0PHJ38Z Insertion of Limb Lengthening External Fixation Device into Left Radius, Percutaneous Approach

0PHJ3BZ Insertion of Monoplanar External Fixation Device into Left Radius, Percutaneous Approach

0PHJ3CZ Insertion of Ring External Fixation Device into Left Radius, Percutaneous Approach

0PHJ3DZ Insertion of Hybrid External Fixation Device into Left Radius, Percutaneous Approach

0PHJ44Z Insertion of Internal Fixation Device into Left Radius, Percutaneous Endoscopic Approach

0PHJ45Z Insertion of External Fixation Device into Left Radius, Percutaneous Endoscopic Approach

0PHJ46Z Insertion of Intramedullary Internal Fixation Device into Left Radius, Percutaneous Endoscopic Approach

0PHJ48Z Insertion of Limb Lengthening External Fixation Device into Left Radius, Percutaneous Endoscopic Approach

0PHJ4BZ Insertion of Monoplanar External Fixation Device into Left Radius, Percutaneous Endoscopic Approach

0PHJ4CZ Insertion of Ring External Fixation Device into Left Radius, Percutaneous Endoscopic Approach

0PHJ4DZ Insertion of Hybrid External Fixation Device into Left Radius, Percutaneous Endoscopic Approach

0PHK04Z Insertion of Internal Fixation Device into Right Ulna, Open Approach

0PHK05Z Insertion of External Fixation Device into Right Ulna, Open Approach

0PHK06Z Insertion of Intramedullary Internal Fixation Device into Right Ulna, Open Approach

0PHK08Z Insertion of Limb Lengthening External Fixation Device into Right Ulna, Open Approach

0PHK0BZ Insertion of Monoplanar External Fixation Device into Right Ulna, Open Approach

0PHK0CZ Insertion of Ring External Fixation Device into Right Ulna, Open Approach

0PHK0DZ Insertion of Hybrid External Fixation Device into Right Ulna, Open Approach

0PHK34Z Insertion of Internal Fixation Device into Right Ulna, Percutaneous Approach

0PHK35Z Insertion of External Fixation Device into Right Ulna, Percutaneous Approach

0PHK36Z Insertion of Intramedullary Internal Fixation Device into Right Ulna, Percutaneous Approach

0PHK38Z Insertion of Limb Lengthening External Fixation Device into Right Ulna, Percutaneous Approach

0PHK3BZ Insertion of Monoplanar External Fixation Device into Right Ulna, Percutaneous Approach

0PHK3CZ Insertion of Ring External Fixation Device into Right Ulna, Percutaneous Approach

0PHK3DZ Insertion of Hybrid External Fixation Device into Right Ulna, Percutaneous Approach

0PHK44Z Insertion of Internal Fixation Device into Right Ulna, Percutaneous Endoscopic Approach

0PHK45Z Insertion of External Fixation Device into Right Ulna, Percutaneous Endoscopic Approach

0PHK46Z Insertion of Intramedullary Internal Fixation Device into Right Ulna, Percutaneous Endoscopic Approach

0PHK48Z Insertion of Limb Lengthening External Fixation Device into Right Ulna, Percutaneous Endoscopic Approach

0PHK4BZ Insertion of Monoplanar External Fixation Device into Right Ulna, Percutaneous Endoscopic Approach

0PHK4CZ Insertion of Ring External Fixation Device into Right Ulna, Percutaneous Endoscopic Approach

0PHK4DZ Insertion of Hybrid External Fixation Device into Right Ulna, Percutaneous Endoscopic Approach

0PHL04Z Insertion of Internal Fixation Device into Left Ulna, Open Approach

0PHL05Z Insertion of External Fixation Device into Left Ulna, Open Approach

0PHL06Z Insertion of Intramedullary Internal Fixation Device into Left Ulna, Open Approach

0PHL08Z Insertion of Limb Lengthening External Fixation Device into Left Ulna, Open Approach

0PHL0BZ Insertion of Monoplanar External Fixation Device into Left Ulna, Open Approach

0PHL0CZ Insertion of Ring External Fixation Device into Left Ulna, Open Approach

0PHL0DZ Insertion of Hybrid External Fixation Device into Left Ulna, Open Approach

0PHL34Z Insertion of Internal Fixation Device into Left Ulna, Percutaneous Approach

0PHL35Z Insertion of External Fixation Device into Left Ulna, Percutaneous Approach

0PHL36Z Insertion of Intramedullary Internal Fixation Device into Left Ulna, Percutaneous Approach

0PHL38Z Insertion of Limb Lengthening External Fixation Device into Left Ulna, Percutaneous Approach

0PHL3BZ Insertion of Monoplanar External Fixation Device into Left Ulna, Percutaneous Approach

0PHL3CZ Insertion of Ring External Fixation Device into Left Ulna, Percutaneous Approach

0PHL3DZ Insertion of Hybrid External Fixation Device into Left Ulna, Percutaneous Approach

0PHL44Z Insertion of Internal Fixation Device into Left Ulna, Percutaneous Endoscopic Approach

0PHL45Z Insertion of External Fixation Device into Left Ulna, Percutaneous Endoscopic Approach

0PHL46Z Insertion of Intramedullary Internal Fixation Device into Left Ulna, Percutaneous Endoscopic Approach

0PHL48Z Insertion of Limb Lengthening External Fixation Device into Left Ulna, Percutaneous Endoscopic Approach

0PHL4BZ Insertion of Monoplanar External Fixation Device into Left Ulna, Percutaneous Endoscopic Approach

0PHL4CZ Insertion of Ring External Fixation Device into Left Ulna, Percutaneous Endoscopic Approach

0PHL4DZ Insertion of Hybrid External Fixation Device into Left Ulna, Percutaneous Endoscopic Approach

0PHM04Z Insertion of Internal Fixation Device into Right Carpal, Open Approach

0PHM05Z Insertion of External Fixation Device into Right Carpal, Open Approach

0PHM34Z Insertion of Internal Fixation Device into Right Carpal, Percutaneous Approach

0PHM35Z Insertion of External Fixation Device into Right Carpal, Percutaneous Approach

0PHM44Z Insertion of Internal Fixation Device into Right Carpal, Percutaneous Endoscopic Approach

0PHM45Z Insertion of External Fixation Device into Right Carpal, Percutaneous Endoscopic Approach

---

♀ Female-only ♂ Male-only ● Limited Coverage ● Non-OR 🅷🅰🅲 HAC-associated procedure ● Non-covered procedures ✚ Combination

0PHN04Z	Insertion of Internal Fixation Device into Left Carpal, Open Approach	0PHR45Z	Insertion of External Fixation Device into Right Thumb Phalanx, Percutaneous Endoscopic Approach
0PHN05Z	Insertion of External Fixation Device into Left Carpal, Open Approach	0PHS04Z	Insertion of Internal Fixation Device into Left Thumb Phalanx, Open Approach
0PHN34Z	Insertion of Internal Fixation Device into Left Carpal, Percutaneous Approach	0PHS05Z	Insertion of External Fixation Device into Left Thumb Phalanx, Open Approach
0PHN35Z	Insertion of External Fixation Device into Left Carpal, Percutaneous Approach	0PHS34Z	Insertion of Internal Fixation Device into Left Thumb Phalanx, Percutaneous Approach
0PHN44Z	Insertion of Internal Fixation Device into Left Carpal, Percutaneous Endoscopic Approach	0PHS35Z	Insertion of External Fixation Device into Left Thumb Phalanx, Percutaneous Approach
0PHN45Z	Insertion of External Fixation Device into Left Carpal, Percutaneous Endoscopic Approach	0PHS44Z	Insertion of Internal Fixation Device into Left Thumb Phalanx, Percutaneous Endoscopic Approach
0PHP04Z	Insertion of Internal Fixation Device into Right Metacarpal, Open Approach	0PHS45Z	Insertion of External Fixation Device into Left Thumb Phalanx, Percutaneous Endoscopic Approach
0PHP05Z	Insertion of External Fixation Device into Right Metacarpal, Open Approach	0PHT04Z	Insertion of Internal Fixation Device into Right Finger Phalanx, Open Approach
0PHP34Z	Insertion of Internal Fixation Device into Right Metacarpal, Percutaneous Approach	0PHT05Z	Insertion of External Fixation Device into Right Finger Phalanx, Open Approach
0PHP35Z	Insertion of External Fixation Device into Right Metacarpal, Percutaneous Approach	0PHT34Z	Insertion of Internal Fixation Device into Right Finger Phalanx, Percutaneous Approach
0PHP44Z	Insertion of Internal Fixation Device into Right Metacarpal, Percutaneous Endoscopic Approach	0PHT35Z	Insertion of External Fixation Device into Right Finger Phalanx, Percutaneous Approach
0PHP45Z	Insertion of External Fixation Device into Right Metacarpal, Percutaneous Endoscopic Approach	0PHT44Z	Insertion of Internal Fixation Device into Right Finger Phalanx, Percutaneous Endoscopic Approach
0PHQ04Z	Insertion of Internal Fixation Device into Left Metacarpal, Open Approach	0PHT45Z	Insertion of External Fixation Device into Right Finger Phalanx, Percutaneous Endoscopic Approach
0PHQ05Z	Insertion of External Fixation Device into Left Metacarpal, Open Approach	0PHV04Z	Insertion of Internal Fixation Device into Left Finger Phalanx, Open Approach
0PHQ34Z	Insertion of Internal Fixation Device into Left Metacarpal, Percutaneous Approach	0PHV05Z	Insertion of External Fixation Device into Left Finger Phalanx, Open Approach
0PHQ35Z	Insertion of External Fixation Device into Left Metacarpal, Percutaneous Approach	0PHV34Z	Insertion of Internal Fixation Device into Left Finger Phalanx, Percutaneous Approach
0PHQ44Z	Insertion of Internal Fixation Device into Left Metacarpal, Percutaneous Endoscopic Approach	0PHV35Z	Insertion of External Fixation Device into Left Finger Phalanx, Percutaneous Approach
0PHQ45Z	Insertion of External Fixation Device into Left Metacarpal, Percutaneous Endoscopic Approach	0PHV44Z	Insertion of Internal Fixation Device into Left Finger Phalanx, Percutaneous Endoscopic Approach
0PHR04Z	Insertion of Internal Fixation Device into Right Thumb Phalanx, Open Approach	0PHV45Z	Insertion of External Fixation Device into Left Finger Phalanx, Percutaneous Endoscopic Approach
0PHR05Z	Insertion of External Fixation Device into Right Thumb Phalanx, Open Approach	0PHY0MZ	Insertion of Bone Growth Stimulator into Upper Bone, Open Approach
0PHR34Z	Insertion of Internal Fixation Device into Right Thumb Phalanx, Percutaneous Approach	0PHY3MZ	Insertion of Bone Growth Stimulator into Upper Bone, Percutaneous Approach
0PHR35Z	Insertion of External Fixation Device into Right Thumb Phalanx, Percutaneous Approach	0PHY4MZ	Insertion of Bone Growth Stimulator into Upper Bone, Percutaneous Endoscopic Approach
0PHR44Z	Insertion of Internal Fixation Device into Right Thumb Phalanx, Percutaneous Endoscopic Approach		

0PJ – Upper Bones, Inspection

Review Coding Guideline B3.5

Review Coding Guidelines B3.11a, B3.11b and B3.11c

0PJY0ZZ	Inspection of Upper Bone, Open Approach	0PJY4ZZ	Inspection of Upper Bone, Percutaneous Endoscopic Approach
0PJY3ZZ	Inspection of Upper Bone, Percutaneous Approach	0PJYXZZ	Inspection of Upper Bone, External Approach

0PN – Upper Bones, Release

Review Coding Guideline B3.13

Review Coding Guideline B3.14

0PN00ZZ	Release Sternum, Open Approach	0PN33ZZ	Release Cervical Vertebra, Percutaneous Approach
0PN03ZZ	Release Sternum, Percutaneous Approach	0PN34ZZ	Release Cervical Vertebra, Percutaneous Endoscopic Approach
0PN04ZZ	Release Sternum, Percutaneous Endoscopic Approach	0PN40ZZ	Release Thoracic Vertebra, Open Approach
0PN10ZZ	Release Right Rib, Open Approach	0PN43ZZ	Release Thoracic Vertebra, Percutaneous Approach
0PN13ZZ	Release Right Rib, Percutaneous Approach	0PN44ZZ	Release Thoracic Vertebra, Percutaneous Endoscopic Approach
0PN14ZZ	Release Right Rib, Percutaneous Endoscopic Approach	0PN50ZZ	Release Right Scapula, Open Approach
0PN20ZZ	Release Left Rib, Open Approach	0PN53ZZ	Release Right Scapula, Percutaneous Approach
0PN23ZZ	Release Left Rib, Percutaneous Approach	0PN54ZZ	Release Right Scapula, Percutaneous Endoscopic Approach
0PN24ZZ	Release Left Rib, Percutaneous Endoscopic Approach	0PN60ZZ	Release Left Scapula, Open Approach
0PN30ZZ	Release Cervical Vertebra, Open Approach	0PN63ZZ	Release Left Scapula, Percutaneous Approach

0PN64ZZ	Release Left Scapula, Percutaneous Endoscopic Approach
0PN70ZZ	Release Right Glenoid Cavity, Open Approach
0PN73ZZ	Release Right Glenoid Cavity, Percutaneous Approach
0PN74ZZ	Release Right Glenoid Cavity, Percutaneous Endoscopic Approach
0PN80ZZ	Release Left Glenoid Cavity, Open Approach
0PN83ZZ	Release Left Glenoid Cavity, Percutaneous Approach
0PN84ZZ	Release Left Glenoid Cavity, Percutaneous Endoscopic Approach
0PN90ZZ	Release Right Clavicle, Open Approach
0PN93ZZ	Release Right Clavicle, Percutaneous Approach
0PN94ZZ	Release Right Clavicle, Percutaneous Endoscopic Approach
0PNB0ZZ	Release Left Clavicle, Open Approach
0PNB3ZZ	Release Left Clavicle, Percutaneous Approach
0PNB4ZZ	Release Left Clavicle, Percutaneous Endoscopic Approach
0PNC0ZZ	Release Right Humeral Head, Open Approach
0PNC3ZZ	Release Right Humeral Head, Percutaneous Approach
0PNC4ZZ	Release Right Humeral Head, Percutaneous Endoscopic Approach
0PND0ZZ	Release Left Humeral Head, Open Approach
0PND3ZZ	Release Left Humeral Head, Percutaneous Approach
0PND4ZZ	Release Left Humeral Head, Percutaneous Endoscopic Approach
0PNF0ZZ	Release Right Humeral Shaft, Open Approach
0PNF3ZZ	Release Right Humeral Shaft, Percutaneous Approach
0PNF4ZZ	Release Right Humeral Shaft, Percutaneous Endoscopic Approach
0PNG0ZZ	Release Left Humeral Shaft, Open Approach
0PNG3ZZ	Release Left Humeral Shaft, Percutaneous Approach
0PNG4ZZ	Release Left Humeral Shaft, Percutaneous Endoscopic Approach
0PNH0ZZ	Release Right Radius, Open Approach
0PNH3ZZ	Release Right Radius, Percutaneous Approach
0PNH4ZZ	Release Right Radius, Percutaneous Endoscopic Approach
0PNJ0ZZ	Release Left Radius, Open Approach
0PNJ3ZZ	Release Left Radius, Percutaneous Approach
0PNJ4ZZ	Release Left Radius, Percutaneous Endoscopic Approach

0PNK0ZZ	Release Right Ulna, Open Approach
0PNK3ZZ	Release Right Ulna, Percutaneous Approach
0PNK4ZZ	Release Right Ulna, Percutaneous Endoscopic Approach
0PNL0ZZ	Release Left Ulna, Open Approach
0PNL3ZZ	Release Left Ulna, Percutaneous Approach
0PNL4ZZ	Release Left Ulna, Percutaneous Endoscopic Approach
0PNM0ZZ	Release Right Carpal, Open Approach
0PNM3ZZ	Release Right Carpal, Percutaneous Approach
0PNM4ZZ	Release Right Carpal, Percutaneous Endoscopic Approach
0PNN0ZZ	Release Left Carpal, Open Approach
0PNN3ZZ	Release Left Carpal, Percutaneous Approach
0PNN4ZZ	Release Left Carpal, Percutaneous Endoscopic Approach
0PNP0ZZ	Release Right Metacarpal, Open Approach
0PNP3ZZ	Release Right Metacarpal, Percutaneous Approach
0PNP4ZZ	Release Right Metacarpal, Percutaneous Endoscopic Approach
0PNQ0ZZ	Release Left Metacarpal, Open Approach
0PNQ3ZZ	Release Left Metacarpal, Percutaneous Approach
0PNQ4ZZ	Release Left Metacarpal, Percutaneous Endoscopic Approach
0PNR0ZZ	Release Right Thumb Phalanx, Open Approach
0PNR3ZZ	Release Right Thumb Phalanx, Percutaneous Approach
0PNR4ZZ	Release Right Thumb Phalanx, Percutaneous Endoscopic Approach
0PNS0ZZ	Release Left Thumb Phalanx, Open Approach
0PNS3ZZ	Release Left Thumb Phalanx, Percutaneous Approach
0PNS4ZZ	Release Left Thumb Phalanx, Percutaneous Endoscopic Approach
0PNT0ZZ	Release Right Finger Phalanx, Open Approach
0PNT3ZZ	Release Right Finger Phalanx, Percutaneous Approach
0PNT4ZZ	Release Right Finger Phalanx, Percutaneous Endoscopic Approach
0PNV0ZZ	Release Left Finger Phalanx, Open Approach
0PNV3ZZ	Release Left Finger Phalanx, Percutaneous Approach
0PNV4ZZ	Release Left Finger Phalanx, Percutaneous Endoscopic Approach

0PP – Upper Bones, Removal

Review Coding Guideline B6.1c

0PP004Z	Removal of Internal Fixation Device from Sternum, Open Approach
0PP007Z	Removal of Autologous Tissue Substitute from Sternum, Open Approach
0PP00JZ	Removal of Synthetic Substitute from Sternum, Open Approach
0PP00KZ	Removal of Nonautologous Tissue Substitute from Sternum, Open Approach
0PP034Z	Removal of Internal Fixation Device from Sternum, Percutaneous Approach
0PP037Z	Removal of Autologous Tissue Substitute from Sternum, Percutaneous Approach
0PP03JZ	Removal of Synthetic Substitute from Sternum, Percutaneous Approach
0PP03KZ	Removal of Nonautologous Tissue Substitute from Sternum, Percutaneous Approach
0PP044Z	Removal of Internal Fixation Device from Sternum, Percutaneous Endoscopic Approach
0PP047Z	Removal of Autologous Tissue Substitute from Sternum, Percutaneous Endoscopic Approach
0PP04JZ	Removal of Synthetic Substitute from Sternum, Percutaneous Endoscopic Approach
0PP04KZ	Removal of Nonautologous Tissue Substitute from Sternum, Percutaneous Endoscopic Approach
0PP0X4Z	Removal of Internal Fixation Device from Sternum, External Approach
0PP104Z	Removal of Internal Fixation Device from Right Rib, Open Approach
0PP107Z	Removal of Autologous Tissue Substitute from Right Rib, Open Approach
0PP10JZ	Removal of Synthetic Substitute from Right Rib, Open Approach
0PP10KZ	Removal of Nonautologous Tissue Substitute from Right Rib, Open Approach
0PP134Z	Removal of Internal Fixation Device from Right Rib, Percutaneous Approach
0PP137Z	Removal of Autologous Tissue Substitute from Right Rib, Percutaneous Approach
0PP13JZ	Removal of Synthetic Substitute from Right Rib, Percutaneous Approach

0PP13KZ	Removal of Nonautologous Tissue Substitute from Right Rib, Percutaneous Approach
0PP144Z	Removal of Internal Fixation Device from Right Rib, Percutaneous Endoscopic Approach
0PP147Z	Removal of Autologous Tissue Substitute from Right Rib, Percutaneous Endoscopic Approach
0PP14JZ	Removal of Synthetic Substitute from Right Rib, Percutaneous Endoscopic Approach
0PP14KZ	Removal of Nonautologous Tissue Substitute from Right Rib, Percutaneous Endoscopic Approach
0PP1X4Z	Removal of Internal Fixation Device from Right Rib, External Approach
0PP204Z	Removal of Internal Fixation Device from Left Rib, Open Approach
0PP207Z	Removal of Autologous Tissue Substitute from Left Rib, Open Approach
0PP20JZ	Removal of Synthetic Substitute from Left Rib, Open Approach
0PP20KZ	Removal of Nonautologous Tissue Substitute from Left Rib, Open Approach
0PP234Z	Removal of Internal Fixation Device from Left Rib, Percutaneous Approach
0PP237Z	Removal of Autologous Tissue Substitute from Left Rib, Percutaneous Approach
0PP23JZ	Removal of Synthetic Substitute from Left Rib, Percutaneous Approach
0PP23KZ	Removal of Nonautologous Tissue Substitute from Left Rib, Percutaneous Approach
0PP244Z	Removal of Internal Fixation Device from Left Rib, Percutaneous Endoscopic Approach
0PP247Z	Removal of Autologous Tissue Substitute from Left Rib, Percutaneous Endoscopic Approach
0PP24JZ	Removal of Synthetic Substitute from Left Rib, Percutaneous Endoscopic Approach
0PP24KZ	Removal of Nonautologous Tissue Substitute from Left Rib, Percutaneous Endoscopic Approach
0PP2X4Z	Removal of Internal Fixation Device from Left Rib, External Approach

0PP304Z	Removal of Internal Fixation Device from Cervical Vertebra, Open Approach
0PP307Z	Removal of Autologous Tissue Substitute from Cervical Vertebra, Open Approach
0PP30JZ	Removal of Synthetic Substitute from Cervical Vertebra, Open Approach
0PP30KZ	Removal of Nonautologous Tissue Substitute from Cervical Vertebra, Open Approach
0PP334Z	Removal of Internal Fixation Device from Cervical Vertebra, Percutaneous Approach
0PP337Z	Removal of Autologous Tissue Substitute from Cervical Vertebra, Percutaneous Approach
0PP33JZ	Removal of Synthetic Substitute from Cervical Vertebra, Percutaneous Approach
0PP33KZ	Removal of Nonautologous Tissue Substitute from Cervical Vertebra, Percutaneous Approach
0PP344Z	Removal of Internal Fixation Device from Cervical Vertebra, Percutaneous Endoscopic Approach
0PP347Z	Removal of Autologous Tissue Substitute from Cervical Vertebra, Percutaneous Endoscopic Approach
0PP34JZ	Removal of Synthetic Substitute from Cervical Vertebra, Percutaneous Endoscopic Approach
0PP34KZ	Removal of Nonautologous Tissue Substitute from Cervical Vertebra, Percutaneous Endoscopic Approach
0PP3X4Z	Removal of Internal Fixation Device from Cervical Vertebra, External Approach
0PP404Z	Removal of Internal Fixation Device from Thoracic Vertebra, Open Approach
0PP407Z	Removal of Autologous Tissue Substitute from Thoracic Vertebra, Open Approach
0PP40JZ	Removal of Synthetic Substitute from Thoracic Vertebra, Open Approach
0PP40KZ	Removal of Nonautologous Tissue Substitute from Thoracic Vertebra, Open Approach
0PP434Z	Removal of Internal Fixation Device from Thoracic Vertebra, Percutaneous Approach
0PP437Z	Removal of Autologous Tissue Substitute from Thoracic Vertebra, Percutaneous Approach
0PP43JZ	Removal of Synthetic Substitute from Thoracic Vertebra, Percutaneous Approach
0PP43KZ	Removal of Nonautologous Tissue Substitute from Thoracic Vertebra, Percutaneous Approach
0PP444Z	Removal of Internal Fixation Device from Thoracic Vertebra, Percutaneous Endoscopic Approach
0PP447Z	Removal of Autologous Tissue Substitute from Thoracic Vertebra, Percutaneous Endoscopic Approach
0PP44JZ	Removal of Synthetic Substitute from Thoracic Vertebra, Percutaneous Endoscopic Approach
0PP44KZ	Removal of Nonautologous Tissue Substitute from Thoracic Vertebra, Percutaneous Endoscopic Approach
0PP4X4Z	Removal of Internal Fixation Device from Thoracic Vertebra, External Approach
0PP504Z	Removal of Internal Fixation Device from Right Scapula, Open Approach
0PP507Z	Removal of Autologous Tissue Substitute from Right Scapula, Open Approach
0PP50JZ	Removal of Synthetic Substitute from Right Scapula, Open Approach
0PP50KZ	Removal of Nonautologous Tissue Substitute from Right Scapula, Open Approach
0PP534Z	Removal of Internal Fixation Device from Right Scapula, Percutaneous Approach
0PP537Z	Removal of Autologous Tissue Substitute from Right Scapula, Percutaneous Approach
0PP53JZ	Removal of Synthetic Substitute from Right Scapula, Percutaneous Approach
0PP53KZ	Removal of Nonautologous Tissue Substitute from Right Scapula, Percutaneous Approach
0PP544Z	Removal of Internal Fixation Device from Right Scapula, Percutaneous Endoscopic Approach
0PP547Z	Removal of Autologous Tissue Substitute from Right Scapula, Percutaneous Endoscopic Approach
0PP54JZ	Removal of Synthetic Substitute from Right Scapula, Percutaneous Endoscopic Approach
0PP54KZ	Removal of Nonautologous Tissue Substitute from Right Scapula, Percutaneous Endoscopic Approach
0PP5X4Z	Removal of Internal Fixation Device from Right Scapula, External Approach
0PP604Z	Removal of Internal Fixation Device from Left Scapula, Open Approach
0PP607Z	Removal of Autologous Tissue Substitute from Left Scapula, Open Approach
0PP60JZ	Removal of Synthetic Substitute from Left Scapula, Open Approach
0PP60KZ	Removal of Nonautologous Tissue Substitute from Left Scapula, Open Approach
0PP634Z	Removal of Internal Fixation Device from Left Scapula, Percutaneous Approach
0PP637Z	Removal of Autologous Tissue Substitute from Left Scapula, Percutaneous Approach
0PP63JZ	Removal of Synthetic Substitute from Left Scapula, Percutaneous Approach
0PP63KZ	Removal of Nonautologous Tissue Substitute from Left Scapula, Percutaneous Approach
0PP644Z	Removal of Internal Fixation Device from Left Scapula, Percutaneous Endoscopic Approach
0PP647Z	Removal of Autologous Tissue Substitute from Left Scapula, Percutaneous Endoscopic Approach
0PP64JZ	Removal of Synthetic Substitute from Left Scapula, Percutaneous Endoscopic Approach
0PP64KZ	Removal of Nonautologous Tissue Substitute from Left Scapula, Percutaneous Endoscopic Approach
0PP6X4Z	Removal of Internal Fixation Device from Left Scapula, External Approach
0PP704Z	Removal of Internal Fixation Device from Right Glenoid Cavity, Open Approach
0PP707Z	Removal of Autologous Tissue Substitute from Right Glenoid Cavity, Open Approach
0PP70JZ	Removal of Synthetic Substitute from Right Glenoid Cavity, Open Approach
0PP70KZ	Removal of Nonautologous Tissue Substitute from Right Glenoid Cavity, Open Approach
0PP734Z	Removal of Internal Fixation Device from Right Glenoid Cavity, Percutaneous Approach
0PP737Z	Removal of Autologous Tissue Substitute from Right Glenoid Cavity, Percutaneous Approach
0PP73JZ	Removal of Synthetic Substitute from Right Glenoid Cavity, Percutaneous Approach
0PP73KZ	Removal of Nonautologous Tissue Substitute from Right Glenoid Cavity, Percutaneous Approach
0PP744Z	Removal of Internal Fixation Device from Right Glenoid Cavity, Percutaneous Endoscopic Approach
0PP747Z	Removal of Autologous Tissue Substitute from Right Glenoid Cavity, Percutaneous Endoscopic Approach
0PP74JZ	Removal of Synthetic Substitute from Right Glenoid Cavity, Percutaneous Endoscopic Approach
0PP74KZ	Removal of Nonautologous Tissue Substitute from Right Glenoid Cavity, Percutaneous Endoscopic Approach
0PP7X4Z	Removal of Internal Fixation Device from Right Glenoid Cavity, External Approach
0PP804Z	Removal of Internal Fixation Device from Left Glenoid Cavity, Open Approach
0PP807Z	Removal of Autologous Tissue Substitute from Left Glenoid Cavity, Open Approach
0PP80JZ	Removal of Synthetic Substitute from Left Glenoid Cavity, Open Approach
0PP80KZ	Removal of Nonautologous Tissue Substitute from Left Glenoid Cavity, Open Approach
0PP834Z	Removal of Internal Fixation Device from Left Glenoid Cavity, Percutaneous Approach
0PP837Z	Removal of Autologous Tissue Substitute from Left Glenoid Cavity, Percutaneous Approach
0PP83JZ	Removal of Synthetic Substitute from Left Glenoid Cavity, Percutaneous Approach
0PP83KZ	Removal of Nonautologous Tissue Substitute from Left Glenoid Cavity, Percutaneous Approach

0PP844Z Removal of Internal Fixation Device from Left Glenoid Cavity, Percutaneous Endoscopic Approach

0PP847Z Removal of Autologous Tissue Substitute from Left Glenoid Cavity, Percutaneous Endoscopic Approach

0PP84JZ Removal of Synthetic Substitute from Left Glenoid Cavity, Percutaneous Endoscopic Approach

0PP84KZ Removal of Nonautologous Tissue Substitute from Left Glenoid Cavity, Percutaneous Endoscopic Approach

0PP8X4Z Removal of Internal Fixation Device from Left Glenoid Cavity, External Approach

0PP904Z Removal of Internal Fixation Device from Right Clavicle, Open Approach

0PP907Z Removal of Autologous Tissue Substitute from Right Clavicle, Open Approach

0PP90JZ Removal of Synthetic Substitute from Right Clavicle, Open Approach

0PP90KZ Removal of Nonautologous Tissue Substitute from Right Clavicle, Open Approach

0PP934Z Removal of Internal Fixation Device from Right Clavicle, Percutaneous Approach

0PP937Z Removal of Autologous Tissue Substitute from Right Clavicle, Percutaneous Approach

0PP93JZ Removal of Synthetic Substitute from Right Clavicle, Percutaneous Approach

0PP93KZ Removal of Nonautologous Tissue Substitute from Right Clavicle, Percutaneous Approach

0PP944Z Removal of Internal Fixation Device from Right Clavicle, Percutaneous Endoscopic Approach

0PP947Z Removal of Autologous Tissue Substitute from Right Clavicle, Percutaneous Endoscopic Approach

0PP94JZ Removal of Synthetic Substitute from Right Clavicle, Percutaneous Endoscopic Approach

0PP94KZ Removal of Nonautologous Tissue Substitute from Right Clavicle, Percutaneous Endoscopic Approach

0PP9X4Z Removal of Internal Fixation Device from Right Clavicle, External Approach

0PPB04Z Removal of Internal Fixation Device from Left Clavicle, Open Approach

0PPB07Z Removal of Autologous Tissue Substitute from Left Clavicle, Open Approach

0PPB0JZ Removal of Synthetic Substitute from Left Clavicle, Open Approach

0PPB0KZ Removal of Nonautologous Tissue Substitute from Left Clavicle, Open Approach

0PPB34Z Removal of Internal Fixation Device from Left Clavicle, Percutaneous Approach

0PPB37Z Removal of Autologous Tissue Substitute from Left Clavicle, Percutaneous Approach

0PPB3JZ Removal of Synthetic Substitute from Left Clavicle, Percutaneous Approach

0PPB3KZ Removal of Nonautologous Tissue Substitute from Left Clavicle, Percutaneous Approach

0PPB44Z Removal of Internal Fixation Device from Left Clavicle, Percutaneous Endoscopic Approach

0PPB47Z Removal of Autologous Tissue Substitute from Left Clavicle, Percutaneous Endoscopic Approach

0PPB4JZ Removal of Synthetic Substitute from Left Clavicle, Percutaneous Endoscopic Approach

0PPB4KZ Removal of Nonautologous Tissue Substitute from Left Clavicle, Percutaneous Endoscopic Approach

0PPBX4Z Removal of Internal Fixation Device from Left Clavicle, External Approach

0PPC04Z Removal of Internal Fixation Device from Right Humeral Head, Open Approach

0PPC05Z Removal of External Fixation Device from Right Humeral Head, Open Approach

0PPC07Z Removal of Autologous Tissue Substitute from Right Humeral Head, Open Approach

0PPC0JZ Removal of Synthetic Substitute from Right Humeral Head, Open Approach

0PPC0KZ Removal of Nonautologous Tissue Substitute from Right Humeral Head, Open Approach

0PPC34Z Removal of Internal Fixation Device from Right Humeral Head, Percutaneous Approach

0PPC35Z Removal of External Fixation Device from Right Humeral Head, Percutaneous Approach

0PPC37Z Removal of Autologous Tissue Substitute from Right Humeral Head, Percutaneous Approach

0PPC3JZ Removal of Synthetic Substitute from Right Humeral Head, Percutaneous Approach

0PPC3KZ Removal of Nonautologous Tissue Substitute from Right Humeral Head, Percutaneous Approach

0PPC44Z Removal of Internal Fixation Device from Right Humeral Head, Percutaneous Endoscopic Approach

0PPC45Z Removal of External Fixation Device from Right Humeral Head, Percutaneous Endoscopic Approach

0PPC47Z Removal of Autologous Tissue Substitute from Right Humeral Head, Percutaneous Endoscopic Approach

0PPC4JZ Removal of Synthetic Substitute from Right Humeral Head, Percutaneous Endoscopic Approach

0PPC4KZ Removal of Nonautologous Tissue Substitute from Right Humeral Head, Percutaneous Endoscopic Approach

0PPCX4Z Removal of Internal Fixation Device from Right Humeral Head, External Approach

0PPCX5Z Removal of External Fixation Device from Right Humeral Head, External Approach

0PPD04Z Removal of Internal Fixation Device from Left Humeral Head, Open Approach

0PPD05Z Removal of External Fixation Device from Left Humeral Head, Open Approach

0PPD07Z Removal of Autologous Tissue Substitute from Left Humeral Head, Open Approach

0PPD0JZ Removal of Synthetic Substitute from Left Humeral Head, Open Approach

0PPD0KZ Removal of Nonautologous Tissue Substitute from Left Humeral Head, Open Approach

0PPD34Z Removal of Internal Fixation Device from Left Humeral Head, Percutaneous Approach

0PPD35Z Removal of External Fixation Device from Left Humeral Head, Percutaneous Approach

0PPD37Z Removal of Autologous Tissue Substitute from Left Humeral Head, Percutaneous Approach

0PPD3JZ Removal of Synthetic Substitute from Left Humeral Head, Percutaneous Approach

0PPD3KZ Removal of Nonautologous Tissue Substitute from Left Humeral Head, Percutaneous Approach

0PPD44Z Removal of Internal Fixation Device from Left Humeral Head, Percutaneous Endoscopic Approach

0PPD45Z Removal of External Fixation Device from Left Humeral Head, Percutaneous Endoscopic Approach

0PPD47Z Removal of Autologous Tissue Substitute from Left Humeral Head, Percutaneous Endoscopic Approach

0PPD4JZ Removal of Synthetic Substitute from Left Humeral Head, Percutaneous Endoscopic Approach

0PPD4KZ Removal of Nonautologous Tissue Substitute from Left Humeral Head, Percutaneous Endoscopic Approach

0PPDX4Z Removal of Internal Fixation Device from Left Humeral Head, External Approach

0PPDX5Z Removal of External Fixation Device from Left Humeral Head, External Approach

0PPF04Z Removal of Internal Fixation Device from Right Humeral Shaft, Open Approach

0PPF05Z Removal of External Fixation Device from Right Humeral Shaft, Open Approach

0PPF07Z Removal of Autologous Tissue Substitute from Right Humeral Shaft, Open Approach

0PPF0JZ Removal of Synthetic Substitute from Right Humeral Shaft, Open Approach

0PPF0KZ Removal of Nonautologous Tissue Substitute from Right Humeral Shaft, Open Approach

0PPF34Z Removal of Internal Fixation Device from Right Humeral Shaft, Percutaneous Approach

0PPF35Z Removal of External Fixation Device from Right Humeral Shaft, Percutaneous Approach

0PPF37Z Removal of Autologous Tissue Substitute from Right Humeral Shaft, Percutaneous Approach

0PPF3JZ Removal of Synthetic Substitute from Right Humeral Shaft, Percutaneous Approach

0PPF3KZ Removal of Nonautologous Tissue Substitute from Right Humeral Shaft, Percutaneous Approach

0PPF44Z Removal of Internal Fixation Device from Right Humeral Shaft, Percutaneous Endoscopic Approach

0PPF45Z Removal of External Fixation Device from Right Humeral Shaft, Percutaneous Endoscopic Approach

0PPF47Z Removal of Autologous Tissue Substitute from Right Humeral Shaft, Percutaneous Endoscopic Approach

0PPF4JZ Removal of Synthetic Substitute from Right Humeral Shaft, Percutaneous Endoscopic Approach

0PPF4KZ Removal of Nonautologous Tissue Substitute from Right Humeral Shaft, Percutaneous Endoscopic Approach

0PPFX4Z Removal of Internal Fixation Device from Right Humeral Shaft, External Approach

0PPFX5Z Removal of External Fixation Device from Right Humeral Shaft, External Approach

0PPG04Z Removal of Internal Fixation Device from Left Humeral Shaft, Open Approach

0PPG05Z Removal of External Fixation Device from Left Humeral Shaft, Open Approach

0PPG07Z Removal of Autologous Tissue Substitute from Left Humeral Shaft, Open Approach

0PPG0JZ Removal of Synthetic Substitute from Left Humeral Shaft, Open Approach

0PPG0KZ Removal of Nonautologous Tissue Substitute from Left Humeral Shaft, Open Approach

0PPG34Z Removal of Internal Fixation Device from Left Humeral Shaft, Percutaneous Approach

0PPG35Z Removal of External Fixation Device from Left Humeral Shaft, Percutaneous Approach

0PPG37Z Removal of Autologous Tissue Substitute from Left Humeral Shaft, Percutaneous Approach

0PPG3JZ Removal of Synthetic Substitute from Left Humeral Shaft, Percutaneous Approach

0PPG3KZ Removal of Nonautologous Tissue Substitute from Left Humeral Shaft, Percutaneous Approach

0PPG44Z Removal of Internal Fixation Device from Left Humeral Shaft, Percutaneous Endoscopic Approach

0PPG45Z Removal of External Fixation Device from Left Humeral Shaft, Percutaneous Endoscopic Approach

0PPG47Z Removal of Autologous Tissue Substitute from Left Humeral Shaft, Percutaneous Endoscopic Approach

0PPG4JZ Removal of Synthetic Substitute from Left Humeral Shaft, Percutaneous Endoscopic Approach

0PPG4KZ Removal of Nonautologous Tissue Substitute from Left Humeral Shaft, Percutaneous Endoscopic Approach

0PPGX4Z Removal of Internal Fixation Device from Left Humeral Shaft, External Approach

0PPGX5Z Removal of External Fixation Device from Left Humeral Shaft, External Approach

0PPH04Z Removal of Internal Fixation Device from Right Radius, Open Approach

0PPH05Z Removal of External Fixation Device from Right Radius, Open Approach

0PPH07Z Removal of Autologous Tissue Substitute from Right Radius, Open Approach

0PPH0JZ Removal of Synthetic Substitute from Right Radius, Open Approach

0PPH0KZ Removal of Nonautologous Tissue Substitute from Right Radius, Open Approach

0PPH34Z Removal of Internal Fixation Device from Right Radius, Percutaneous Approach

0PPH35Z Removal of External Fixation Device from Right Radius, Percutaneous Approach

0PPH37Z Removal of Autologous Tissue Substitute from Right Radius, Percutaneous Approach

0PPH3JZ Removal of Synthetic Substitute from Right Radius, Percutaneous Approach

0PPH3KZ Removal of Nonautologous Tissue Substitute from Right Radius, Percutaneous Approach

0PPH44Z Removal of Internal Fixation Device from Right Radius, Percutaneous Endoscopic Approach

0PPH45Z Removal of External Fixation Device from Right Radius, Percutaneous Endoscopic Approach

0PPH47Z Removal of Autologous Tissue Substitute from Right Radius, Percutaneous Endoscopic Approach

0PPH4JZ Removal of Synthetic Substitute from Right Radius, Percutaneous Endoscopic Approach

0PPH4KZ Removal of Nonautologous Tissue Substitute from Right Radius, Percutaneous Endoscopic Approach

0PPHX4Z Removal of Internal Fixation Device from Right Radius, External Approach

0PPHX5Z Removal of External Fixation Device from Right Radius, External Approach

0PPJ04Z Removal of Internal Fixation Device from Left Radius, Open Approach

0PPJ05Z Removal of External Fixation Device from Left Radius, Open Approach

0PPJ07Z Removal of Autologous Tissue Substitute from Left Radius, Open Approach

0PPJ0JZ Removal of Synthetic Substitute from Left Radius, Open Approach

0PPJ0KZ Removal of Nonautologous Tissue Substitute from Left Radius, Open Approach

0PPJ34Z Removal of Internal Fixation Device from Left Radius, Percutaneous Approach

0PPJ35Z Removal of External Fixation Device from Left Radius, Percutaneous Approach

0PPJ37Z Removal of Autologous Tissue Substitute from Left Radius, Percutaneous Approach

0PPJ3JZ Removal of Synthetic Substitute from Left Radius, Percutaneous Approach

0PPJ3KZ Removal of Nonautologous Tissue Substitute from Left Radius, Percutaneous Approach

0PPJ44Z Removal of Internal Fixation Device from Left Radius, Percutaneous Endoscopic Approach

0PPJ45Z Removal of External Fixation Device from Left Radius, Percutaneous Endoscopic Approach

0PPJ47Z Removal of Autologous Tissue Substitute from Left Radius, Percutaneous Endoscopic Approach

0PPJ4JZ Removal of Synthetic Substitute from Left Radius, Percutaneous Endoscopic Approach

0PPJ4KZ Removal of Nonautologous Tissue Substitute from Left Radius, Percutaneous Endoscopic Approach

0PPJX4Z Removal of Internal Fixation Device from Left Radius, External Approach

0PPJX5Z Removal of External Fixation Device from Left Radius, External Approach

0PPK04Z Removal of Internal Fixation Device from Right Ulna, Open Approach

0PPK05Z Removal of External Fixation Device from Right Ulna, Open Approach

0PPK07Z Removal of Autologous Tissue Substitute from Right Ulna, Open Approach

0PPK0JZ Removal of Synthetic Substitute from Right Ulna, Open Approach

0PPK0KZ Removal of Nonautologous Tissue Substitute from Right Ulna, Open Approach

0PPK34Z Removal of Internal Fixation Device from Right Ulna, Percutaneous Approach

0PPK35Z Removal of External Fixation Device from Right Ulna, Percutaneous Approach

0PPK37Z Removal of Autologous Tissue Substitute from Right Ulna, Percutaneous Approach

0PPK3JZ Removal of Synthetic Substitute from Right Ulna, Percutaneous Approach

0PPK3KZ Removal of Nonautologous Tissue Substitute from Right Ulna, Percutaneous Approach

0PPK44Z Removal of Internal Fixation Device from Right Ulna, Percutaneous Endoscopic Approach

0PPK45Z Removal of External Fixation Device from Right Ulna, Percutaneous Endoscopic Approach

0PPK47Z Removal of Autologous Tissue Substitute from Right Ulna, Percutaneous Endoscopic Approach

0PPK4JZ Removal of Synthetic Substitute from Right Ulna, Percutaneous Endoscopic Approach

0PPK4KZ Removal of Nonautologous Tissue Substitute from Right Ulna, Percutaneous Endoscopic Approach

0PPKX4Z Removal of Internal Fixation Device from Right Ulna, External Approach

0PPKX5Z   Removal of External Fixation Device from Right Ulna, External Approach

0PPL04Z   Removal of Internal Fixation Device from Left Ulna, Open Approach

0PPL05Z   Removal of External Fixation Device from Left Ulna, Open Approach

0PPL07Z   Removal of Autologous Tissue Substitute from Left Ulna, Open Approach

0PPL0JZ   Removal of Synthetic Substitute from Left Ulna, Open Approach

0PPL0KZ   Removal of Nonautologous Tissue Substitute from Left Ulna, Open Approach

0PPL34Z   Removal of Internal Fixation Device from Left Ulna, Percutaneous Approach

0PPL35Z   Removal of External Fixation Device from Left Ulna, Percutaneous Approach

0PPL37Z   Removal of Autologous Tissue Substitute from Left Ulna, Percutaneous Approach

0PPL3JZ   Removal of Synthetic Substitute from Left Ulna, Percutaneous Approach

0PPL3KZ   Removal of Nonautologous Tissue Substitute from Left Ulna, Percutaneous Approach

0PPL44Z   Removal of Internal Fixation Device from Left Ulna, Percutaneous Endoscopic Approach

0PPL45Z   Removal of External Fixation Device from Left Ulna, Percutaneous Endoscopic Approach

0PPL47Z   Removal of Autologous Tissue Substitute from Left Ulna, Percutaneous Endoscopic Approach

0PPL4JZ   Removal of Synthetic Substitute from Left Ulna, Percutaneous Endoscopic Approach

0PPL4KZ   Removal of Nonautologous Tissue Substitute from Left Ulna, Percutaneous Endoscopic Approach

0PPLX4Z   Removal of Internal Fixation Device from Left Ulna, External Approach

0PPLX5Z   Removal of External Fixation Device from Left Ulna, External Approach

0PPM04Z   Removal of Internal Fixation Device from Right Carpal, Open Approach

0PPM05Z   Removal of External Fixation Device from Right Carpal, Open Approach

0PPM07Z   Removal of Autologous Tissue Substitute from Right Carpal, Open Approach

0PPM0JZ   Removal of Synthetic Substitute from Right Carpal, Open Approach

0PPM0KZ   Removal of Nonautologous Tissue Substitute from Right Carpal, Open Approach

0PPM34Z   Removal of Internal Fixation Device from Right Carpal, Percutaneous Approach

0PPM35Z   Removal of External Fixation Device from Right Carpal, Percutaneous Approach

0PPM37Z   Removal of Autologous Tissue Substitute from Right Carpal, Percutaneous Approach

0PPM3JZ   Removal of Synthetic Substitute from Right Carpal, Percutaneous Approach

0PPM3KZ   Removal of Nonautologous Tissue Substitute from Right Carpal, Percutaneous Approach

0PPM44Z   Removal of Internal Fixation Device from Right Carpal, Percutaneous Endoscopic Approach

0PPM45Z   Removal of External Fixation Device from Right Carpal, Percutaneous Endoscopic Approach

0PPM47Z   Removal of Autologous Tissue Substitute from Right Carpal, Percutaneous Endoscopic Approach

0PPM4JZ   Removal of Synthetic Substitute from Right Carpal, Percutaneous Endoscopic Approach

0PPM4KZ   Removal of Nonautologous Tissue Substitute from Right Carpal, Percutaneous Endoscopic Approach

0PPMX4Z   Removal of Internal Fixation Device from Right Carpal, External Approach

0PPMX5Z   Removal of External Fixation Device from Right Carpal, External Approach

0PPN04Z   Removal of Internal Fixation Device from Left Carpal, Open Approach

0PPN05Z   Removal of External Fixation Device from Left Carpal, Open Approach

0PPN07Z   Removal of Autologous Tissue Substitute from Left Carpal, Open Approach

0PPN0JZ   Removal of Synthetic Substitute from Left Carpal, Open Approach

0PPN0KZ   Removal of Nonautologous Tissue Substitute from Left Carpal, Open Approach

0PPN34Z   Removal of Internal Fixation Device from Left Carpal, Percutaneous Approach

0PPN35Z   Removal of External Fixation Device from Left Carpal, Percutaneous Approach

0PPN37Z   Removal of Autologous Tissue Substitute from Left Carpal, Percutaneous Approach

0PPN3JZ   Removal of Synthetic Substitute from Left Carpal, Percutaneous Approach

0PPN3KZ   Removal of Nonautologous Tissue Substitute from Left Carpal, Percutaneous Approach

0PPN44Z   Removal of Internal Fixation Device from Left Carpal, Percutaneous Endoscopic Approach

0PPN45Z   Removal of External Fixation Device from Left Carpal, Percutaneous Endoscopic Approach

0PPN47Z   Removal of Autologous Tissue Substitute from Left Carpal, Percutaneous Endoscopic Approach

0PPN4JZ   Removal of Synthetic Substitute from Left Carpal, Percutaneous Endoscopic Approach

0PPN4KZ   Removal of Nonautologous Tissue Substitute from Left Carpal, Percutaneous Endoscopic Approach

0PPNX4Z   Removal of Internal Fixation Device from Left Carpal, External Approach

0PPNX5Z   Removal of External Fixation Device from Left Carpal, External Approach

0PPP04Z   Removal of Internal Fixation Device from Right Metacarpal, Open Approach

0PPP05Z   Removal of External Fixation Device from Right Metacarpal, Open Approach

0PPP07Z   Removal of Autologous Tissue Substitute from Right Metacarpal, Open Approach

0PPP0JZ   Removal of Synthetic Substitute from Right Metacarpal, Open Approach

0PPP0KZ   Removal of Nonautologous Tissue Substitute from Right Metacarpal, Open Approach

0PPP34Z   Removal of Internal Fixation Device from Right Metacarpal, Percutaneous Approach

0PPP35Z   Removal of External Fixation Device from Right Metacarpal, Percutaneous Approach

0PPP37Z   Removal of Autologous Tissue Substitute from Right Metacarpal, Percutaneous Approach

0PPP3JZ   Removal of Synthetic Substitute from Right Metacarpal, Percutaneous Approach

0PPP3KZ   Removal of Nonautologous Tissue Substitute from Right Metacarpal, Percutaneous Approach

0PPP44Z   Removal of Internal Fixation Device from Right Metacarpal, Percutaneous Endoscopic Approach

0PPP45Z   Removal of External Fixation Device from Right Metacarpal, Percutaneous Endoscopic Approach

0PPP47Z   Removal of Autologous Tissue Substitute from Right Metacarpal, Percutaneous Endoscopic Approach

0PPP4JZ   Removal of Synthetic Substitute from Right Metacarpal, Percutaneous Endoscopic Approach

0PPP4KZ   Removal of Nonautologous Tissue Substitute from Right Metacarpal, Percutaneous Endoscopic Approach

0PPPX4Z   Removal of Internal Fixation Device from Right Metacarpal, External Approach

0PPPX5Z   Removal of External Fixation Device from Right Metacarpal, External Approach

0PPQ04Z   Removal of Internal Fixation Device from Left Metacarpal, Open Approach

0PPQ05Z   Removal of External Fixation Device from Left Metacarpal, Open Approach

0PPQ07Z   Removal of Autologous Tissue Substitute from Left Metacarpal, Open Approach

0PPQ0JZ   Removal of Synthetic Substitute from Left Metacarpal, Open Approach

0PPQ0KZ   Removal of Nonautologous Tissue Substitute from Left Metacarpal, Open Approach

0PPQ34Z   Removal of Internal Fixation Device from Left Metacarpal, Percutaneous Approach

♀ Female-only   ♂ Male-only   ⬤ Limited Coverage   ⬤ Non-OR   **HAC** HAC-associated procedure   ⬤ Non-covered procedures   ✚ Combination

0PPQ35Z Removal of External Fixation Device from Left Metacarpal, Percutaneous Approach

0PPQ37Z Removal of Autologous Tissue Substitute from Left Metacarpal, Percutaneous Approach

0PPQ3JZ Removal of Synthetic Substitute from Left Metacarpal, Percutaneous Approach

0PPQ3KZ Removal of Nonautologous Tissue Substitute from Left Metacarpal, Percutaneous Approach

0PPQ44Z Removal of Internal Fixation Device from Left Metacarpal, Percutaneous Endoscopic Approach

0PPQ45Z Removal of External Fixation Device from Left Metacarpal, Percutaneous Endoscopic Approach

0PPQ47Z Removal of Autologous Tissue Substitute from Left Metacarpal, Percutaneous Endoscopic Approach

0PPQ4JZ Removal of Synthetic Substitute from Left Metacarpal, Percutaneous Endoscopic Approach

0PPQ4KZ Removal of Nonautologous Tissue Substitute from Left Metacarpal, Percutaneous Endoscopic Approach

0PPQX4Z Removal of Internal Fixation Device from Left Metacarpal, External Approach

0PPQX5Z Removal of External Fixation Device from Left Metacarpal, External Approach

0PPR04Z Removal of Internal Fixation Device from Right Thumb Phalanx, Open Approach

0PPR05Z Removal of External Fixation Device from Right Thumb Phalanx, Open Approach

0PPR07Z Removal of Autologous Tissue Substitute from Right Thumb Phalanx, Open Approach

0PPR0JZ Removal of Synthetic Substitute from Right Thumb Phalanx, Open Approach

0PPR0KZ Removal of Nonautologous Tissue Substitute from Right Thumb Phalanx, Open Approach

0PPR34Z Removal of Internal Fixation Device from Right Thumb Phalanx, Percutaneous Approach

0PPR35Z Removal of External Fixation Device from Right Thumb Phalanx, Percutaneous Approach

0PPR37Z Removal of Autologous Tissue Substitute from Right Thumb Phalanx, Percutaneous Approach

0PPR3JZ Removal of Synthetic Substitute from Right Thumb Phalanx, Percutaneous Approach

0PPR3KZ Removal of Nonautologous Tissue Substitute from Right Thumb Phalanx, Percutaneous Approach

0PPR44Z Removal of Internal Fixation Device from Right Thumb Phalanx, Percutaneous Endoscopic Approach

0PPR45Z Removal of External Fixation Device from Right Thumb Phalanx, Percutaneous Endoscopic Approach

0PPR47Z Removal of Autologous Tissue Substitute from Right Thumb Phalanx, Percutaneous Endoscopic Approach

0PPR4JZ Removal of Synthetic Substitute from Right Thumb Phalanx, Percutaneous Endoscopic Approach

0PPR4KZ Removal of Nonautologous Tissue Substitute from Right Thumb Phalanx, Percutaneous Endoscopic Approach

0PPRX4Z Removal of Internal Fixation Device from Right Thumb Phalanx, External Approach

0PPRX5Z Removal of External Fixation Device from Right Thumb Phalanx, External Approach

0PPS04Z Removal of Internal Fixation Device from Left Thumb Phalanx, Open Approach

0PPS05Z Removal of External Fixation Device from Left Thumb Phalanx, Open Approach

0PPS07Z Removal of Autologous Tissue Substitute from Left Thumb Phalanx, Open Approach

0PPS0JZ Removal of Synthetic Substitute from Left Thumb Phalanx, Open Approach

0PPS0KZ Removal of Nonautologous Tissue Substitute from Left Thumb Phalanx, Open Approach

0PPS34Z Removal of Internal Fixation Device from Left Thumb Phalanx, Percutaneous Approach

0PPS35Z Removal of External Fixation Device from Left Thumb Phalanx, Percutaneous Approach

0PPS37Z Removal of Autologous Tissue Substitute from Left Thumb Phalanx, Percutaneous Approach

0PPS3JZ Removal of Synthetic Substitute from Left Thumb Phalanx, Percutaneous Approach

0PPS3KZ Removal of Nonautologous Tissue Substitute from Left Thumb Phalanx, Percutaneous Approach

0PPS44Z Removal of Internal Fixation Device from Left Thumb Phalanx, Percutaneous Endoscopic Approach

0PPS45Z Removal of External Fixation Device from Left Thumb Phalanx, Percutaneous Endoscopic Approach

0PPS47Z Removal of Autologous Tissue Substitute from Left Thumb Phalanx, Percutaneous Endoscopic Approach

0PPS4JZ Removal of Synthetic Substitute from Left Thumb Phalanx, Percutaneous Endoscopic Approach

0PPS4KZ Removal of Nonautologous Tissue Substitute from Left Thumb Phalanx, Percutaneous Endoscopic Approach

0PPSX4Z Removal of Internal Fixation Device from Left Thumb Phalanx, External Approach

0PPSX5Z Removal of External Fixation Device from Left Thumb Phalanx, External Approach

0PPT04Z Removal of Internal Fixation Device from Right Finger Phalanx, Open Approach

0PPT05Z Removal of External Fixation Device from Right Finger Phalanx, Open Approach

0PPT07Z Removal of Autologous Tissue Substitute from Right Finger Phalanx, Open Approach

0PPT0JZ Removal of Synthetic Substitute from Right Finger Phalanx, Open Approach

0PPT0KZ Removal of Nonautologous Tissue Substitute from Right Finger Phalanx, Open Approach

0PPT34Z Removal of Internal Fixation Device from Right Finger Phalanx, Percutaneous Approach

0PPT35Z Removal of External Fixation Device from Right Finger Phalanx, Percutaneous Approach

0PPT37Z Removal of Autologous Tissue Substitute from Right Finger Phalanx, Percutaneous Approach

0PPT3JZ Removal of Synthetic Substitute from Right Finger Phalanx, Percutaneous Approach

0PPT3KZ Removal of Nonautologous Tissue Substitute from Right Finger Phalanx, Percutaneous Approach

0PPT44Z Removal of Internal Fixation Device from Right Finger Phalanx, Percutaneous Endoscopic Approach

0PPT45Z Removal of External Fixation Device from Right Finger Phalanx, Percutaneous Endoscopic Approach

0PPT47Z Removal of Autologous Tissue Substitute from Right Finger Phalanx, Percutaneous Endoscopic Approach

0PPT4JZ Removal of Synthetic Substitute from Right Finger Phalanx, Percutaneous Endoscopic Approach

0PPT4KZ Removal of Nonautologous Tissue Substitute from Right Finger Phalanx, Percutaneous Endoscopic Approach

0PPTX4Z Removal of Internal Fixation Device from Right Finger Phalanx, External Approach

0PPTX5Z Removal of External Fixation Device from Right Finger Phalanx, External Approach

0PPV04Z Removal of Internal Fixation Device from Left Finger Phalanx, Open Approach

0PPV05Z Removal of External Fixation Device from Left Finger Phalanx, Open Approach

0PPV07Z Removal of Autologous Tissue Substitute from Left Finger Phalanx, Open Approach

0PPV0JZ Removal of Synthetic Substitute from Left Finger Phalanx, Open Approach

0PPV0KZ Removal of Nonautologous Tissue Substitute from Left Finger Phalanx, Open Approach

0PPV34Z Removal of Internal Fixation Device from Left Finger Phalanx, Percutaneous Approach

0PPV35Z Removal of External Fixation Device from Left Finger Phalanx, Percutaneous Approach

0PPV37Z Removal of Autologous Tissue Substitute from Left Finger Phalanx, Percutaneous Approach

0PPV3JZ Removal of Synthetic Substitute from Left Finger Phalanx, Percutaneous Approach

0PPV3KZ Removal of Nonautologous Tissue Substitute from Left Finger Phalanx, Percutaneous Approach

0PPV44Z Removal of Internal Fixation Device from Left Finger Phalanx, Percutaneous Endoscopic Approach

0PPV45Z Removal of External Fixation Device from Left Finger Phalanx, Percutaneous Endoscopic Approach

0PPV47Z Removal of Autologous Tissue Substitute from Left Finger Phalanx, Percutaneous Endoscopic Approach

0PPV4JZ Removal of Synthetic Substitute from Left Finger Phalanx, Percutaneous Endoscopic Approach

0PPV4KZ Removal of Nonautologous Tissue Substitute from Left Finger Phalanx, Percutaneous Endoscopic Approach

0PPVX4Z Removal of Internal Fixation Device from Left Finger Phalanx, External Approach

0PPVX5Z Removal of External Fixation Device from Left Finger Phalanx, External Approach

0PPY00Z Removal of Drainage Device from Upper Bone, Open Approach

0PPY0MZ Removal of Bone Growth Stimulator from Upper Bone, Open Approach

0PPY30Z Removal of Drainage Device from Upper Bone, Percutaneous Approach

0PPY3MZ Removal of Bone Growth Stimulator from Upper Bone, Percutaneous Approach

0PPY40Z Removal of Drainage Device from Upper Bone, Percutaneous Endoscopic Approach

0PPY4MZ Removal of Bone Growth Stimulator from Upper Bone, Percutaneous Endoscopic Approach

0PPYX0Z Removal of Drainage Device from Upper Bone, External Approach

0PPYXMZ Removal of Bone Growth Stimulator from Upper Bone, External Approach

0PQ – Upper Bones, Repair

Review Coding Guideline B3.5

0PQ00ZZ Repair Sternum, Open Approach
0PQ03ZZ Repair Sternum, Percutaneous Approach
0PQ04ZZ Repair Sternum, Percutaneous Endoscopic Approach
0PQ0XZZ Repair Sternum, External Approach
0PQ10ZZ Repair Right Rib, Open Approach
0PQ13ZZ Repair Right Rib, Percutaneous Approach
0PQ14ZZ Repair Right Rib, Percutaneous Endoscopic Approach
0PQ1XZZ Repair Right Rib, External Approach
0PQ20ZZ Repair Left Rib, Open Approach
0PQ23ZZ Repair Left Rib, Percutaneous Approach
0PQ24ZZ Repair Left Rib, Percutaneous Endoscopic Approach
0PQ2XZZ Repair Left Rib, External Approach
0PQ30ZZ Repair Cervical Vertebra, Open Approach
0PQ33ZZ Repair Cervical Vertebra, Percutaneous Approach
0PQ34ZZ Repair Cervical Vertebra, Percutaneous Endoscopic Approach
0PQ3XZZ Repair Cervical Vertebra, External Approach
0PQ40ZZ Repair Thoracic Vertebra, Open Approach
0PQ43ZZ Repair Thoracic Vertebra, Percutaneous Approach
0PQ44ZZ Repair Thoracic Vertebra, Percutaneous Endoscopic Approach
0PQ4XZZ Repair Thoracic Vertebra, External Approach
0PQ50ZZ Repair Right Scapula, Open Approach
0PQ53ZZ Repair Right Scapula, Percutaneous Approach
0PQ54ZZ Repair Right Scapula, Percutaneous Endoscopic Approach
0PQ5XZZ Repair Right Scapula, External Approach
0PQ60ZZ Repair Left Scapula, Open Approach
0PQ63ZZ Repair Left Scapula, Percutaneous Approach
0PQ64ZZ Repair Left Scapula, Percutaneous Endoscopic Approach
0PQ6XZZ Repair Left Scapula, External Approach
0PQ70ZZ Repair Right Glenoid Cavity, Open Approach
0PQ73ZZ Repair Right Glenoid Cavity, Percutaneous Approach
0PQ74ZZ Repair Right Glenoid Cavity, Percutaneous Endoscopic Approach
0PQ7XZZ Repair Right Glenoid Cavity, External Approach
0PQ80ZZ Repair Left Glenoid Cavity, Open Approach
0PQ83ZZ Repair Left Glenoid Cavity, Percutaneous Approach
0PQ84ZZ Repair Left Glenoid Cavity, Percutaneous Endoscopic Approach
0PQ8XZZ Repair Left Glenoid Cavity, External Approach
0PQ90ZZ Repair Right Clavicle, Open Approach
0PQ93ZZ Repair Right Clavicle, Percutaneous Approach
0PQ94ZZ Repair Right Clavicle, Percutaneous Endoscopic Approach
0PQ9XZZ Repair Right Clavicle, External Approach
0PQB0ZZ Repair Left Clavicle, Open Approach
0PQB3ZZ Repair Left Clavicle, Percutaneous Approach
0PQB4ZZ Repair Left Clavicle, Percutaneous Endoscopic Approach
0PQBXZZ Repair Left Clavicle, External Approach
0PQC0ZZ Repair Right Humeral Head, Open Approach
0PQC3ZZ Repair Right Humeral Head, Percutaneous Approach
0PQC4ZZ Repair Right Humeral Head, Percutaneous Endoscopic Approach
0PQCXZZ Repair Right Humeral Head, External Approach
0PQD0ZZ Repair Left Humeral Head, Open Approach
0PQD3ZZ Repair Left Humeral Head, Percutaneous Approach
0PQD4ZZ Repair Left Humeral Head, Percutaneous Endoscopic Approach
0PQDXZZ Repair Left Humeral Head, External Approach
0PQF0ZZ Repair Right Humeral Shaft, Open Approach
0PQF3ZZ Repair Right Humeral Shaft, Percutaneous Approach

0PQF4ZZ Repair Right Humeral Shaft, Percutaneous Endoscopic Approach
0PQFXZZ Repair Right Humeral Shaft, External Approach
0PQG0ZZ Repair Left Humeral Shaft, Open Approach
0PQG3ZZ Repair Left Humeral Shaft, Percutaneous Approach
0PQG4ZZ Repair Left Humeral Shaft, Percutaneous Endoscopic Approach
0PQGXZZ Repair Left Humeral Shaft, External Approach
0PQH0ZZ Repair Right Radius, Open Approach
0PQH3ZZ Repair Right Radius, Percutaneous Approach
0PQH4ZZ Repair Right Radius, Percutaneous Endoscopic Approach
0PQHXZZ Repair Right Radius, External Approach
0PQJ0ZZ Repair Left Radius, Open Approach
0PQJ3ZZ Repair Left Radius, Percutaneous Approach
0PQJ4ZZ Repair Left Radius, Percutaneous Endoscopic Approach
0PQJXZZ Repair Left Radius, External Approach
0PQK0ZZ Repair Right Ulna, Open Approach
0PQK3ZZ Repair Right Ulna, Percutaneous Approach
0PQK4ZZ Repair Right Ulna, Percutaneous Endoscopic Approach
0PQKXZZ Repair Right Ulna, External Approach
0PQL0ZZ Repair Left Ulna, Open Approach
0PQL3ZZ Repair Left Ulna, Percutaneous Approach
0PQL4ZZ Repair Left Ulna, Percutaneous Endoscopic Approach
0PQLXZZ Repair Left Ulna, External Approach
0PQM0ZZ Repair Right Carpal, Open Approach
0PQM3ZZ Repair Right Carpal, Percutaneous Approach
0PQM4ZZ Repair Right Carpal, Percutaneous Endoscopic Approach
0PQMXZZ Repair Right Carpal, External Approach
0PQN0ZZ Repair Left Carpal, Open Approach
0PQN3ZZ Repair Left Carpal, Percutaneous Approach
0PQN4ZZ Repair Left Carpal, Percutaneous Endoscopic Approach
0PQNXZZ Repair Left Carpal, External Approach
0PQP0ZZ Repair Right Metacarpal, Open Approach
0PQP3ZZ Repair Right Metacarpal, Percutaneous Approach
0PQP4ZZ Repair Right Metacarpal, Percutaneous Endoscopic Approach
0PQPXZZ Repair Right Metacarpal, External Approach
0PQQ0ZZ Repair Left Metacarpal, Open Approach
0PQQ3ZZ Repair Left Metacarpal, Percutaneous Approach
0PQQ4ZZ Repair Left Metacarpal, Percutaneous Endoscopic Approach
0PQQXZZ Repair Left Metacarpal, External Approach
0PQR0ZZ Repair Right Thumb Phalanx, Open Approach
0PQR3ZZ Repair Right Thumb Phalanx, Percutaneous Approach
0PQR4ZZ Repair Right Thumb Phalanx, Percutaneous Endoscopic Approach
0PQRXZZ Repair Right Thumb Phalanx, External Approach
0PQS0ZZ Repair Left Thumb Phalanx, Open Approach
0PQS3ZZ Repair Left Thumb Phalanx, Percutaneous Approach
0PQS4ZZ Repair Left Thumb Phalanx, Percutaneous Endoscopic Approach
0PQSXZZ Repair Left Thumb Phalanx, External Approach
0PQT0ZZ Repair Right Finger Phalanx, Open Approach
0PQT3ZZ Repair Right Finger Phalanx, Percutaneous Approach
0PQT4ZZ Repair Right Finger Phalanx, Percutaneous Endoscopic Approach
0PQTXZZ Repair Right Finger Phalanx, External Approach
0PQV0ZZ Repair Left Finger Phalanx, Open Approach
0PQV3ZZ Repair Left Finger Phalanx, Percutaneous Approach
0PQV4ZZ Repair Left Finger Phalanx, Percutaneous Endoscopic Approach
0PQVXZZ Repair Left Finger Phalanx, External Approach

0PR – Upper Bones, Replacement

0PR007Z   Replacement of Sternum with Autologous Tissue Substitute, Open Approach

0PR00JZ   Replacement of Sternum with Synthetic Substitute, Open Approach

0PR00KZ   Replacement of Sternum with Nonautologous Tissue Substitute, Open Approach

0PR037Z   Replacement of Sternum with Autologous Tissue Substitute, Percutaneous Approach

0PR03JZ   Replacement of Sternum with Synthetic Substitute, Percutaneous Approach

0PR03KZ   Replacement of Sternum with Nonautologous Tissue Substitute, Percutaneous Approach

0PR047Z   Replacement of Sternum with Autologous Tissue Substitute, Percutaneous Endoscopic Approach

0PR04JZ   Replacement of Sternum with Synthetic Substitute, Percutaneous Endoscopic Approach

0PR04KZ   Replacement of Sternum with Nonautologous Tissue Substitute, Percutaneous Endoscopic Approach

0PR107Z   Replacement of Right Rib with Autologous Tissue Substitute, Open Approach

0PR10JZ   Replacement of Right Rib with Synthetic Substitute, Open Approach

0PR10KZ   Replacement of Right Rib with Nonautologous Tissue Substitute, Open Approach

0PR137Z   Replacement of Right Rib with Autologous Tissue Substitute, Percutaneous Approach

0PR13JZ   Replacement of Right Rib with Synthetic Substitute, Percutaneous Approach

0PR13KZ   Replacement of Right Rib with Nonautologous Tissue Substitute, Percutaneous Approach

0PR147Z   Replacement of Right Rib with Autologous Tissue Substitute, Percutaneous Endoscopic Approach

0PR14JZ   Replacement of Right Rib with Synthetic Substitute, Percutaneous Endoscopic Approach

0PR14KZ   Replacement of Right Rib with Nonautologous Tissue Substitute, Percutaneous Endoscopic Approach

0PR207Z   Replacement of Left Rib with Autologous Tissue Substitute, Open Approach

0PR20JZ   Replacement of Left Rib with Synthetic Substitute, Open Approach

0PR20KZ   Replacement of Left Rib with Nonautologous Tissue Substitute, Open Approach

0PR237Z   Replacement of Left Rib with Autologous Tissue Substitute, Percutaneous Approach

0PR23JZ   Replacement of Left Rib with Synthetic Substitute, Percutaneous Approach

0PR23KZ   Replacement of Left Rib with Nonautologous Tissue Substitute, Percutaneous Approach

0PR247Z   Replacement of Left Rib with Autologous Tissue Substitute, Percutaneous Endoscopic Approach

0PR24JZ   Replacement of Left Rib with Synthetic Substitute, Percutaneous Endoscopic Approach

0PR24KZ   Replacement of Left Rib with Nonautologous Tissue Substitute, Percutaneous Endoscopic Approach

0PR307Z   Replacement of Cervical Vertebra with Autologous Tissue Substitute, Open Approach

0PR30JZ   Replacement of Cervical Vertebra with Synthetic Substitute, Open Approach

0PR30KZ   Replacement of Cervical Vertebra with Nonautologous Tissue Substitute, Open Approach

0PR337Z   Replacement of Cervical Vertebra with Autologous Tissue Substitute, Percutaneous Approach

0PR33JZ   Replacement of Cervical Vertebra with Synthetic Substitute, Percutaneous Approach

0PR33KZ   Replacement of Cervical Vertebra with Nonautologous Tissue Substitute, Percutaneous Approach

0PR347Z   Replacement of Cervical Vertebra with Autologous Tissue Substitute, Percutaneous Endoscopic Approach

0PR34JZ   Replacement of Cervical Vertebra with Synthetic Substitute, Percutaneous Endoscopic Approach

0PR34KZ   Replacement of Cervical Vertebra with Nonautologous Tissue Substitute, Percutaneous Endoscopic Approach

0PR407Z   Replacement of Thoracic Vertebra with Autologous Tissue Substitute, Open Approach

0PR40JZ   Replacement of Thoracic Vertebra with Synthetic Substitute, Open Approach

0PR40KZ   Replacement of Thoracic Vertebra with Nonautologous Tissue Substitute, Open Approach

0PR437Z   Replacement of Thoracic Vertebra with Autologous Tissue Substitute, Percutaneous Approach

0PR43JZ   Replacement of Thoracic Vertebra with Synthetic Substitute, Percutaneous Approach

0PR43KZ   Replacement of Thoracic Vertebra with Nonautologous Tissue Substitute, Percutaneous Approach

0PR447Z   Replacement of Thoracic Vertebra with Autologous Tissue Substitute, Percutaneous Endoscopic Approach

0PR44JZ   Replacement of Thoracic Vertebra with Synthetic Substitute, Percutaneous Endoscopic Approach

0PR44KZ   Replacement of Thoracic Vertebra with Nonautologous Tissue Substitute, Percutaneous Endoscopic Approach

0PR507Z   Replacement of Right Scapula with Autologous Tissue Substitute, Open Approach

0PR50JZ   Replacement of Right Scapula with Synthetic Substitute, Open Approach

0PR50KZ   Replacement of Right Scapula with Nonautologous Tissue Substitute, Open Approach

0PR537Z   Replacement of Right Scapula with Autologous Tissue Substitute, Percutaneous Approach

0PR53JZ   Replacement of Right Scapula with Synthetic Substitute, Percutaneous Approach

0PR53KZ   Replacement of Right Scapula with Nonautologous Tissue Substitute, Percutaneous Approach

0PR547Z   Replacement of Right Scapula with Autologous Tissue Substitute, Percutaneous Endoscopic Approach

0PR54JZ   Replacement of Right Scapula with Synthetic Substitute, Percutaneous Endoscopic Approach

0PR54KZ   Replacement of Right Scapula with Nonautologous Tissue Substitute, Percutaneous Endoscopic Approach

0PR607Z   Replacement of Left Scapula with Autologous Tissue Substitute, Open Approach

0PR60JZ   Replacement of Left Scapula with Synthetic Substitute, Open Approach

0PR60KZ   Replacement of Left Scapula with Nonautologous Tissue Substitute, Open Approach

0PR637Z   Replacement of Left Scapula with Autologous Tissue Substitute, Percutaneous Approach

0PR63JZ   Replacement of Left Scapula with Synthetic Substitute, Percutaneous Approach

0PR63KZ   Replacement of Left Scapula with Nonautologous Tissue Substitute, Percutaneous Approach

0PR647Z   Replacement of Left Scapula with Autologous Tissue Substitute, Percutaneous Endoscopic Approach

0PR64JZ   Replacement of Left Scapula with Synthetic Substitute, Percutaneous Endoscopic Approach

0PR64KZ   Replacement of Left Scapula with Nonautologous Tissue Substitute, Percutaneous Endoscopic Approach

0PR707Z   Replacement of Right Glenoid Cavity with Autologous Tissue Substitute, Open Approach

0PR70JZ   Replacement of Right Glenoid Cavity with Synthetic Substitute, Open Approach

0PR70KZ   Replacement of Right Glenoid Cavity with Nonautologous Tissue Substitute, Open Approach

0PR737Z   Replacement of Right Glenoid Cavity with Autologous Tissue Substitute, Percutaneous Approach

0PR73JZ   Replacement of Right Glenoid Cavity with Synthetic Substitute, Percutaneous Approach

0PR73KZ   Replacement of Right Glenoid Cavity with Nonautologous Tissue Substitute, Percutaneous Approach

0PR747Z   Replacement of Right Glenoid Cavity with Autologous Tissue Substitute, Percutaneous Endoscopic Approach

0PR74JZ   Replacement of Right Glenoid Cavity with Synthetic Substitute, Percutaneous Endoscopic Approach

0PR74KZ   Replacement of Right Glenoid Cavity with Nonautologous Tissue Substitute, Percutaneous Endoscopic Approach

0PR807Z   Replacement of Left Glenoid Cavity with Autologous Tissue Substitute, Open Approach

0PR80JZ Replacement of Left Glenoid Cavity with Synthetic Substitute, Open Approach

0PR80KZ Replacement of Left Glenoid Cavity with Nonautologous Tissue Substitute, Open Approach

0PR837Z Replacement of Left Glenoid Cavity with Autologous Tissue Substitute, Percutaneous Approach

0PR83JZ Replacement of Left Glenoid Cavity with Synthetic Substitute, Percutaneous Approach

0PR83KZ Replacement of Left Glenoid Cavity with Nonautologous Tissue Substitute, Percutaneous Approach

0PR847Z Replacement of Left Glenoid Cavity with Autologous Tissue Substitute, Percutaneous Endoscopic Approach

0PR84JZ Replacement of Left Glenoid Cavity with Synthetic Substitute, Percutaneous Endoscopic Approach

0PR84KZ Replacement of Left Glenoid Cavity with Nonautologous Tissue Substitute, Percutaneous Endoscopic Approach

0PR907Z Replacement of Right Clavicle with Autologous Tissue Substitute, Open Approach

0PR90JZ Replacement of Right Clavicle with Synthetic Substitute, Open Approach

0PR90KZ Replacement of Right Clavicle with Nonautologous Tissue Substitute, Open Approach

0PR937Z Replacement of Right Clavicle with Autologous Tissue Substitute, Percutaneous Approach

0PR93JZ Replacement of Right Clavicle with Synthetic Substitute, Percutaneous Approach

0PR93KZ Replacement of Right Clavicle with Nonautologous Tissue Substitute, Percutaneous Approach

0PR947Z Replacement of Right Clavicle with Autologous Tissue Substitute, Percutaneous Endoscopic Approach

0PR94JZ Replacement of Right Clavicle with Synthetic Substitute, Percutaneous Endoscopic Approach

0PR94KZ Replacement of Right Clavicle with Nonautologous Tissue Substitute, Percutaneous Endoscopic Approach

0PRB07Z Replacement of Left Clavicle with Autologous Tissue Substitute, Open Approach

0PRB0JZ Replacement of Left Clavicle with Synthetic Substitute, Open Approach

0PRB0KZ Replacement of Left Clavicle with Nonautologous Tissue Substitute, Open Approach

0PRB37Z Replacement of Left Clavicle with Autologous Tissue Substitute, Percutaneous Approach

0PRB3JZ Replacement of Left Clavicle with Synthetic Substitute, Percutaneous Approach

0PRB3KZ Replacement of Left Clavicle with Nonautologous Tissue Substitute, Percutaneous Approach

0PRB47Z Replacement of Left Clavicle with Autologous Tissue Substitute, Percutaneous Endoscopic Approach

0PRB4JZ Replacement of Left Clavicle with Synthetic Substitute, Percutaneous Endoscopic Approach

0PRB4KZ Replacement of Left Clavicle with Nonautologous Tissue Substitute, Percutaneous Endoscopic Approach

0PRC07Z Replacement of Right Humeral Head with Autologous Tissue Substitute, Open Approach

0PRC0JZ Replacement of Right Humeral Head with Synthetic Substitute, Open Approach

0PRC0KZ Replacement of Right Humeral Head with Nonautologous Tissue Substitute, Open Approach

0PRC37Z Replacement of Right Humeral Head with Autologous Tissue Substitute, Percutaneous Approach

0PRC3JZ Replacement of Right Humeral Head with Synthetic Substitute, Percutaneous Approach

0PRC3KZ Replacement of Right Humeral Head with Nonautologous Tissue Substitute, Percutaneous Approach

0PRC47Z Replacement of Right Humeral Head with Autologous Tissue Substitute, Percutaneous Endoscopic Approach

0PRC4JZ Replacement of Right Humeral Head with Synthetic Substitute, Percutaneous Endoscopic Approach

0PRC4KZ Replacement of Right Humeral Head with Nonautologous Tissue Substitute, Percutaneous Endoscopic Approach

0PRD07Z Replacement of Left Humeral Head with Autologous Tissue Substitute, Open Approach

0PRD0JZ Replacement of Left Humeral Head with Synthetic Substitute, Open Approach

0PRD0KZ Replacement of Left Humeral Head with Nonautologous Tissue Substitute, Open Approach

0PRD37Z Replacement of Left Humeral Head with Autologous Tissue Substitute, Percutaneous Approach

0PRD3JZ Replacement of Left Humeral Head with Synthetic Substitute, Percutaneous Approach

0PRD3KZ Replacement of Left Humeral Head with Nonautologous Tissue Substitute, Percutaneous Approach

0PRD47Z Replacement of Left Humeral Head with Autologous Tissue Substitute, Percutaneous Endoscopic Approach

0PRD4JZ Replacement of Left Humeral Head with Synthetic Substitute, Percutaneous Endoscopic Approach

0PRD4KZ Replacement of Left Humeral Head with Nonautologous Tissue Substitute, Percutaneous Endoscopic Approach

0PRF07Z Replacement of Right Humeral Shaft with Autologous Tissue Substitute, Open Approach

0PRF0JZ Replacement of Right Humeral Shaft with Synthetic Substitute, Open Approach

0PRF0KZ Replacement of Right Humeral Shaft with Nonautologous Tissue Substitute, Open Approach

0PRF37Z Replacement of Right Humeral Shaft with Autologous Tissue Substitute, Percutaneous Approach

0PRF3JZ Replacement of Right Humeral Shaft with Synthetic Substitute, Percutaneous Approach

0PRF3KZ Replacement of Right Humeral Shaft with Nonautologous Tissue Substitute, Percutaneous Approach

0PRF47Z Replacement of Right Humeral Shaft with Autologous Tissue Substitute, Percutaneous Endoscopic Approach

0PRF4JZ Replacement of Right Humeral Shaft with Synthetic Substitute, Percutaneous Endoscopic Approach

0PRF4KZ Replacement of Right Humeral Shaft with Nonautologous Tissue Substitute, Percutaneous Endoscopic Approach

0PRG07Z Replacement of Left Humeral Shaft with Autologous Tissue Substitute, Open Approach

0PRG0JZ Replacement of Left Humeral Shaft with Synthetic Substitute, Open Approach

0PRG0KZ Replacement of Left Humeral Shaft with Nonautologous Tissue Substitute, Open Approach

0PRG37Z Replacement of Left Humeral Shaft with Autologous Tissue Substitute, Percutaneous Approach

0PRG3JZ Replacement of Left Humeral Shaft with Synthetic Substitute, Percutaneous Approach

0PRG3KZ Replacement of Left Humeral Shaft with Nonautologous Tissue Substitute, Percutaneous Approach

0PRG47Z Replacement of Left Humeral Shaft with Autologous Tissue Substitute, Percutaneous Endoscopic Approach

0PRG4JZ Replacement of Left Humeral Shaft with Synthetic Substitute, Percutaneous Endoscopic Approach

0PRG4KZ Replacement of Left Humeral Shaft with Nonautologous Tissue Substitute, Percutaneous Endoscopic Approach

0PRH07Z Replacement of Right Radius with Autologous Tissue Substitute, Open Approach

0PRH0JZ Replacement of Right Radius with Synthetic Substitute, Open Approach

0PRH0KZ Replacement of Right Radius with Nonautologous Tissue Substitute, Open Approach

0PRH37Z Replacement of Right Radius with Autologous Tissue Substitute, Percutaneous Approach

0PRH3JZ Replacement of Right Radius with Synthetic Substitute, Percutaneous Approach

0PRH3KZ Replacement of Right Radius with Nonautologous Tissue Substitute, Percutaneous Approach

0PRH47Z Replacement of Right Radius with Autologous Tissue Substitute, Percutaneous Endoscopic Approach

0PRH4JZ Replacement of Right Radius with Synthetic Substitute, Percutaneous Endoscopic Approach

0PRH4KZ Replacement of Right Radius with Nonautologous Tissue Substitute, Percutaneous Endoscopic Approach

0PRJ07Z Replacement of Left Radius with Autologous Tissue Substitute, Open Approach

0PRJ0JZ Replacement of Left Radius with Synthetic Substitute, Open Approach

0PRJ0KZ Replacement of Left Radius with Nonautologous Tissue Substitute, Open Approach

0PRJ37Z Replacement of Left Radius with Autologous Tissue Substitute, Percutaneous Approach

0PRJ3JZ Replacement of Left Radius with Synthetic Substitute, Percutaneous Approach

0PRJ3KZ Replacement of Left Radius with Nonautologous Tissue Substitute, Percutaneous Approach

0PRJ47Z Replacement of Left Radius with Autologous Tissue Substitute, Percutaneous Endoscopic Approach

0PRJ4JZ Replacement of Left Radius with Synthetic Substitute, Percutaneous Endoscopic Approach

0PRJ4KZ Replacement of Left Radius with Nonautologous Tissue Substitute, Percutaneous Endoscopic Approach

0PRK07Z Replacement of Right Ulna with Autologous Tissue Substitute, Open Approach

0PRK0JZ Replacement of Right Ulna with Synthetic Substitute, Open Approach

0PRK0KZ Replacement of Right Ulna with Nonautologous Tissue Substitute, Open Approach

0PRK37Z Replacement of Right Ulna with Autologous Tissue Substitute, Percutaneous Approach

0PRK3JZ Replacement of Right Ulna with Synthetic Substitute, Percutaneous Approach

0PRK3KZ Replacement of Right Ulna with Nonautologous Tissue Substitute, Percutaneous Approach

0PRK47Z Replacement of Right Ulna with Autologous Tissue Substitute, Percutaneous Endoscopic Approach

0PRK4JZ Replacement of Right Ulna with Synthetic Substitute, Percutaneous Endoscopic Approach

0PRK4KZ Replacement of Right Ulna with Nonautologous Tissue Substitute, Percutaneous Endoscopic Approach

0PRL07Z Replacement of Left Ulna with Autologous Tissue Substitute, Open Approach

0PRL0JZ Replacement of Left Ulna with Synthetic Substitute, Open Approach

0PRL0KZ Replacement of Left Ulna with Nonautologous Tissue Substitute, Open Approach

0PRL37Z Replacement of Left Ulna with Autologous Tissue Substitute, Percutaneous Approach

0PRL3JZ Replacement of Left Ulna with Synthetic Substitute, Percutaneous Approach

0PRL3KZ Replacement of Left Ulna with Nonautologous Tissue Substitute, Percutaneous Approach

0PRL47Z Replacement of Left Ulna with Autologous Tissue Substitute, Percutaneous Endoscopic Approach

0PRL4JZ Replacement of Left Ulna with Synthetic Substitute, Percutaneous Endoscopic Approach

0PRL4KZ Replacement of Left Ulna with Nonautologous Tissue Substitute, Percutaneous Endoscopic Approach

0PRM07Z Replacement of Right Carpal with Autologous Tissue Substitute, Open Approach

0PRM0JZ Replacement of Right Carpal with Synthetic Substitute, Open Approach

0PRM0KZ Replacement of Right Carpal with Nonautologous Tissue Substitute, Open Approach

0PRM37Z Replacement of Right Carpal with Autologous Tissue Substitute, Percutaneous Approach

0PRM3JZ Replacement of Right Carpal with Synthetic Substitute, Percutaneous Approach

0PRM3KZ Replacement of Right Carpal with Nonautologous Tissue Substitute, Percutaneous Approach

0PRM47Z Replacement of Right Carpal with Autologous Tissue Substitute, Percutaneous Endoscopic Approach

0PRM4JZ Replacement of Right Carpal with Synthetic Substitute, Percutaneous Endoscopic Approach

0PRM4KZ Replacement of Right Carpal with Nonautologous Tissue Substitute, Percutaneous Endoscopic Approach

0PRN07Z Replacement of Left Carpal with Autologous Tissue Substitute, Open Approach

0PRN0JZ Replacement of Left Carpal with Synthetic Substitute, Open Approach

0PRN0KZ Replacement of Left Carpal with Nonautologous Tissue Substitute, Open Approach

0PRN37Z Replacement of Left Carpal with Autologous Tissue Substitute, Percutaneous Approach

0PRN3JZ Replacement of Left Carpal with Synthetic Substitute, Percutaneous Approach

0PRN3KZ Replacement of Left Carpal with Nonautologous Tissue Substitute, Percutaneous Approach

0PRN47Z Replacement of Left Carpal with Autologous Tissue Substitute, Percutaneous Endoscopic Approach

0PRN4JZ Replacement of Left Carpal with Synthetic Substitute, Percutaneous Endoscopic Approach

0PRN4KZ Replacement of Left Carpal with Nonautologous Tissue Substitute, Percutaneous Endoscopic Approach

0PRP07Z Replacement of Right Metacarpal with Autologous Tissue Substitute, Open Approach

0PRP0JZ Replacement of Right Metacarpal with Synthetic Substitute, Open Approach

0PRP0KZ Replacement of Right Metacarpal with Nonautologous Tissue Substitute, Open Approach

0PRP37Z Replacement of Right Metacarpal with Autologous Tissue Substitute, Percutaneous Approach

0PRP3JZ Replacement of Right Metacarpal with Synthetic Substitute, Percutaneous Approach

0PRP3KZ Replacement of Right Metacarpal with Nonautologous Tissue Substitute, Percutaneous Approach

0PRP47Z Replacement of Right Metacarpal with Autologous Tissue Substitute, Percutaneous Endoscopic Approach

0PRP4JZ Replacement of Right Metacarpal with Synthetic Substitute, Percutaneous Endoscopic Approach

0PRP4KZ Replacement of Right Metacarpal with Nonautologous Tissue Substitute, Percutaneous Endoscopic Approach

0PRQ07Z Replacement of Left Metacarpal with Autologous Tissue Substitute, Open Approach

0PRQ0JZ Replacement of Left Metacarpal with Synthetic Substitute, Open Approach

0PRQ0KZ Replacement of Left Metacarpal with Nonautologous Tissue Substitute, Open Approach

0PRQ37Z Replacement of Left Metacarpal with Autologous Tissue Substitute, Percutaneous Approach

0PRQ3JZ Replacement of Left Metacarpal with Synthetic Substitute, Percutaneous Approach

0PRQ3KZ Replacement of Left Metacarpal with Nonautologous Tissue Substitute, Percutaneous Approach

0PRQ47Z Replacement of Left Metacarpal with Autologous Tissue Substitute, Percutaneous Endoscopic Approach

0PRQ4JZ Replacement of Left Metacarpal with Synthetic Substitute, Percutaneous Endoscopic Approach

0PRQ4KZ Replacement of Left Metacarpal with Nonautologous Tissue Substitute, Percutaneous Endoscopic Approach

0PRR07Z Replacement of Right Thumb Phalanx with Autologous Tissue Substitute, Open Approach

0PRR0JZ Replacement of Right Thumb Phalanx with Synthetic Substitute, Open Approach

0PRR0KZ Replacement of Right Thumb Phalanx with Nonautologous Tissue Substitute, Open Approach

0PRR37Z Replacement of Right Thumb Phalanx with Autologous Tissue Substitute, Percutaneous Approach

0PRR3JZ Replacement of Right Thumb Phalanx with Synthetic Substitute, Percutaneous Approach

0PRR3KZ Replacement of Right Thumb Phalanx with Nonautologous Tissue Substitute, Percutaneous Approach

0PRR47Z Replacement of Right Thumb Phalanx with Autologous Tissue Substitute, Percutaneous Endoscopic Approach

0PRR4JZ Replacement of Right Thumb Phalanx with Synthetic Substitute, Percutaneous Endoscopic Approach

0PRR4KZ Replacement of Right Thumb Phalanx with Nonautologous Tissue Substitute, Percutaneous Endoscopic Approach

0PRS07Z Replacement of Left Thumb Phalanx with Autologous Tissue Substitute, Open Approach

0PRS0JZ Replacement of Left Thumb Phalanx with Synthetic Substitute, Open Approach

0PRS0KZ Replacement of Left Thumb Phalanx with Nonautologous Tissue Substitute, Open Approach

0PRS37Z Replacement of Left Thumb Phalanx with Autologous Tissue Substitute, Percutaneous Approach

0PRS3JZ Replacement of Left Thumb Phalanx with Synthetic Substitute, Percutaneous Approach

0PRS3KZ   Replacement of Left Thumb Phalanx with Nonautologous Tissue Substitute, Percutaneous Approach

0PRS47Z   Replacement of Left Thumb Phalanx with Autologous Tissue Substitute, Percutaneous Endoscopic Approach

0PRS4JZ   Replacement of Left Thumb Phalanx with Synthetic Substitute, Percutaneous Endoscopic Approach

0PRS4KZ   Replacement of Left Thumb Phalanx with Nonautologous Tissue Substitute, Percutaneous Endoscopic Approach

0PRT07Z   Replacement of Right Finger Phalanx with Autologous Tissue Substitute, Open Approach

0PRT0JZ   Replacement of Right Finger Phalanx with Synthetic Substitute, Open Approach

0PRT0KZ   Replacement of Right Finger Phalanx with Nonautologous Tissue Substitute, Open Approach

0PRT37Z   Replacement of Right Finger Phalanx with Autologous Tissue Substitute, Percutaneous Approach

0PRT3JZ   Replacement of Right Finger Phalanx with Synthetic Substitute, Percutaneous Approach

0PRT3KZ   Replacement of Right Finger Phalanx with Nonautologous Tissue Substitute, Percutaneous Approach

0PRT47Z   Replacement of Right Finger Phalanx with Autologous Tissue Substitute, Percutaneous Endoscopic Approach

0PRT4JZ   Replacement of Right Finger Phalanx with Synthetic Substitute, Percutaneous Endoscopic Approach

0PRT4KZ   Replacement of Right Finger Phalanx with Nonautologous Tissue Substitute, Percutaneous Endoscopic Approach

0PRV07Z   Replacement of Left Finger Phalanx with Autologous Tissue Substitute, Open Approach

0PRV0JZ   Replacement of Left Finger Phalanx with Synthetic Substitute, Open Approach

0PRV0KZ   Replacement of Left Finger Phalanx with Nonautologous Tissue Substitute, Open Approach

0PRV37Z   Replacement of Left Finger Phalanx with Autologous Tissue Substitute, Percutaneous Approach

0PRV3JZ   Replacement of Left Finger Phalanx with Synthetic Substitute, Percutaneous Approach

0PRV3KZ   Replacement of Left Finger Phalanx with Nonautologous Tissue Substitute, Percutaneous Approach

0PRV47Z   Replacement of Left Finger Phalanx with Autologous Tissue Substitute, Percutaneous Endoscopic Approach

0PRV4JZ   Replacement of Left Finger Phalanx with Synthetic Substitute, Percutaneous Endoscopic Approach

0PRV4KZ   Replacement of Left Finger Phalanx with Nonautologous Tissue Substitute, Percutaneous Endoscopic Approach

0PS – Upper Bones, Reposition

Review Coding Guideline B3.15

0PS000Z   Reposition Sternum with Rigid Plate Internal Fixation Device, Open Approach

0PS004Z   Reposition Sternum with Internal Fixation Device, Open Approach

0PS00ZZ   Reposition Sternum, Open Approach

0PS030Z   Reposition Sternum with Rigid Plate Internal Fixation Device, Percutaneous Approach

0PS034Z   Reposition Sternum with Internal Fixation Device, Percutaneous Approach

0PS03ZZ   Reposition Sternum, Percutaneous Approach

0PS040Z   Reposition Sternum with Rigid Plate Internal Fixation Device, Percutaneous Endoscopic Approach

0PS044Z   Reposition Sternum with Internal Fixation Device, Percutaneous Endoscopic Approach

0PS04ZZ   Reposition Sternum, Percutaneous Endoscopic Approach

0PS0XZZ   Reposition Sternum, External Approach

0PS104Z   Reposition Right Rib with Internal Fixation Device, Open Approach

0PS10ZZ   Reposition Right Rib, Open Approach

0PS134Z   Reposition Right Rib with Internal Fixation Device, Percutaneous Approach

0PS13ZZ   Reposition Right Rib, Percutaneous Approach

0PS144Z   Reposition Right Rib with Internal Fixation Device, Percutaneous Endoscopic Approach

0PS14ZZ   Reposition Right Rib, Percutaneous Endoscopic Approach

0PS1XZZ   Reposition Right Rib, External Approach

0PS204Z   Reposition Left Rib with Internal Fixation Device, Open Approach

0PS20ZZ   Reposition Left Rib, Open Approach

0PS234Z   Reposition Left Rib with Internal Fixation Device, Percutaneous Approach

0PS23ZZ   Reposition Left Rib, Percutaneous Approach

0PS244Z   Reposition Left Rib with Internal Fixation Device, Percutaneous Endoscopic Approach

0PS24ZZ   Reposition Left Rib, Percutaneous Endoscopic Approach

0PS2XZZ   Reposition Left Rib, External Approach

0PS304Z   Reposition Cervical Vertebra with Internal Fixation Device, Open Approach

0PS30ZZ   Reposition Cervical Vertebra, Open Approach

0PS334Z   Reposition Cervical Vertebra with Internal Fixation Device, Percutaneous Approach

0PS33ZZ   Reposition Cervical Vertebra, Percutaneous Approach

0PS344Z   Reposition Cervical Vertebra with Internal Fixation Device, Percutaneous Endoscopic Approach

0PS34ZZ   Reposition Cervical Vertebra, Percutaneous Endoscopic Approach

0PS3XZZ   Reposition Cervical Vertebra, External Approach

0PS404Z   Reposition Thoracic Vertebra with Internal Fixation Device, Open Approach

0PS40ZZ   Reposition Thoracic Vertebra, Open Approach

0PS434Z   Reposition Thoracic Vertebra with Internal Fixation Device, Percutaneous Approach

0PS43ZZ   Reposition Thoracic Vertebra, Percutaneous Approach

0PS444Z   Reposition Thoracic Vertebra with Internal Fixation Device, Percutaneous Endoscopic Approach

0PS44ZZ   Reposition Thoracic Vertebra, Percutaneous Endoscopic Approach

0PS4XZZ   Reposition Thoracic Vertebra, External Approach

0PS504Z   Reposition Right Scapula with Internal Fixation Device, Open Approach

0PS50ZZ   Reposition Right Scapula, Open Approach

0PS534Z   Reposition Right Scapula with Internal Fixation Device, Percutaneous Approach

0PS53ZZ   Reposition Right Scapula, Percutaneous Approach

0PS544Z   Reposition Right Scapula with Internal Fixation Device, Percutaneous Endoscopic Approach

0PS54ZZ   Reposition Right Scapula, Percutaneous Endoscopic Approach

0PS5XZZ   Reposition Right Scapula, External Approach

0PS604Z   Reposition Left Scapula with Internal Fixation Device, Open Approach

0PS60ZZ   Reposition Left Scapula, Open Approach

0PS634Z   Reposition Left Scapula with Internal Fixation Device, Percutaneous Approach

0PS63ZZ   Reposition Left Scapula, Percutaneous Approach

0PS644Z   Reposition Left Scapula with Internal Fixation Device, Percutaneous Endoscopic Approach

0PS64ZZ   Reposition Left Scapula, Percutaneous Endoscopic Approach

0PS6XZZ   Reposition Left Scapula, External Approach

0PS704Z   Reposition Right Glenoid Cavity with Internal Fixation Device, Open Approach

0PS70ZZ   Reposition Right Glenoid Cavity, Open Approach

0PS734Z   Reposition Right Glenoid Cavity with Internal Fixation Device, Percutaneous Approach

0PS73ZZ   Reposition Right Glenoid Cavity, Percutaneous Approach

0PS744Z   Reposition Right Glenoid Cavity with Internal Fixation Device, Percutaneous Endoscopic Approach

0PS74ZZ   Reposition Right Glenoid Cavity, Percutaneous Endoscopic Approach

0PS7XZZ   Reposition Right Glenoid Cavity, External Approach

0PS804Z   Reposition Left Glenoid Cavity with Internal Fixation Device, Open Approach

0PS80ZZ   Reposition Left Glenoid Cavity, Open Approach

0PS834Z   Reposition Left Glenoid Cavity with Internal Fixation Device, Percutaneous Approach

0PS83ZZ   Reposition Left Glenoid Cavity, Percutaneous Approach

0PS844Z   Reposition Left Glenoid Cavity with Internal Fixation Device, Percutaneous Endoscopic Approach

0PS84ZZ   Reposition Left Glenoid Cavity, Percutaneous Endoscopic Approach

0PS8XZZ   Reposition Left Glenoid Cavity, External Approach

0PS904Z   Reposition Right Clavicle with Internal Fixation Device, Open Approach

0PS90ZZ   Reposition Right Clavicle, Open Approach

0PS934Z   Reposition Right Clavicle with Internal Fixation Device, Percutaneous Approach

0PS93ZZ   Reposition Right Clavicle, Percutaneous Approach

0PS944Z   Reposition Right Clavicle with Internal Fixation Device, Percutaneous Endoscopic Approach

0PS94ZZ   Reposition Right Clavicle, Percutaneous Endoscopic Approach

0PS9XZZ   Reposition Right Clavicle, External Approach

0PSB04Z   Reposition Left Clavicle with Internal Fixation Device, Open Approach

0PSB0ZZ   Reposition Left Clavicle, Open Approach

0PSB34Z   Reposition Left Clavicle with Internal Fixation Device, Percutaneous Approach

0PSB3ZZ   Reposition Left Clavicle, Percutaneous Approach

0PSB44Z   Reposition Left Clavicle with Internal Fixation Device, Percutaneous Endoscopic Approach

0PSB4ZZ   Reposition Left Clavicle, Percutaneous Endoscopic Approach

0PSBXZZ   Reposition Left Clavicle, External Approach

0PSC04Z   Reposition Right Humeral Head with Internal Fixation Device, Open Approach

0PSC05Z   Reposition Right Humeral Head with External Fixation Device, Open Approach

0PSC06Z   Reposition Right Humeral Head with Intramedullary Internal Fixation Device, Open Approach

0PSC0BZ   Reposition Right Humeral Head with Monoplanar External Fixation Device, Open Approach

0PSC0CZ   Reposition Right Humeral Head with Ring External Fixation Device, Open Approach

0PSC0DZ   Reposition Right Humeral Head with Hybrid External Fixation Device, Open Approach

0PSC0ZZ   Reposition Right Humeral Head, Open Approach

0PSC34Z   Reposition Right Humeral Head with Internal Fixation Device, Percutaneous Approach

0PSC35Z   Reposition Right Humeral Head with External Fixation Device, Percutaneous Approach

0PSC36Z   Reposition Right Humeral Head with Intramedullary Internal Fixation Device, Percutaneous Approach

0PSC3BZ   Reposition Right Humeral Head with Monoplanar External Fixation Device, Percutaneous Approach

0PSC3CZ   Reposition Right Humeral Head with Ring External Fixation Device, Percutaneous Approach

0PSC3DZ   Reposition Right Humeral Head with Hybrid External Fixation Device, Percutaneous Approach

0PSC3ZZ   Reposition Right Humeral Head, Percutaneous Approach

0PSC44Z   Reposition Right Humeral Head with Internal Fixation Device, Percutaneous Endoscopic Approach

0PSC45Z   Reposition Right Humeral Head with External Fixation Device, Percutaneous Endoscopic Approach

0PSC46Z   Reposition Right Humeral Head with Intramedullary Internal Fixation Device, Percutaneous Endoscopic Approach

0PSC4BZ   Reposition Right Humeral Head with Monoplanar External Fixation Device, Percutaneous Endoscopic Approach

0PSC4CZ   Reposition Right Humeral Head with Ring External Fixation Device, Percutaneous Endoscopic Approach

0PSC4DZ   Reposition Right Humeral Head with Hybrid External Fixation Device, Percutaneous Endoscopic Approach

0PSC4ZZ   Reposition Right Humeral Head, Percutaneous Endoscopic Approach

0PSCXZZ   Reposition Right Humeral Head, External Approach

0PSD04Z   Reposition Left Humeral Head with Internal Fixation Device, Open Approach

0PSD05Z   Reposition Left Humeral Head with External Fixation Device, Open Approach

0PSD06Z   Reposition Left Humeral Head with Intramedullary Internal Fixation Device, Open Approach

0PSD0BZ   Reposition Left Humeral Head with Monoplanar External Fixation Device, Open Approach

0PSD0CZ   Reposition Left Humeral Head with Ring External Fixation Device, Open Approach

0PSD0DZ   Reposition Left Humeral Head with Hybrid External Fixation Device, Open Approach

0PSD0ZZ   Reposition Left Humeral Head, Open Approach

0PSD34Z   Reposition Left Humeral Head with Internal Fixation Device, Percutaneous Approach

0PSD35Z   Reposition Left Humeral Head with External Fixation Device, Percutaneous Approach

0PSD36Z   Reposition Left Humeral Head with Intramedullary Internal Fixation Device, Percutaneous Approach

0PSD3BZ   Reposition Left Humeral Head with Monoplanar External Fixation Device, Percutaneous Approach

0PSD3CZ   Reposition Left Humeral Head with Ring External Fixation Device, Percutaneous Approach

0PSD3DZ   Reposition Left Humeral Head with Hybrid External Fixation Device, Percutaneous Approach

0PSD3ZZ   Reposition Left Humeral Head, Percutaneous Approach

0PSD44Z   Reposition Left Humeral Head with Internal Fixation Device, Percutaneous Endoscopic Approach

0PSD45Z   Reposition Left Humeral Head with External Fixation Device, Percutaneous Endoscopic Approach

0PSD46Z   Reposition Left Humeral Head with Intramedullary Internal Fixation Device, Percutaneous Endoscopic Approach

0PSD4BZ   Reposition Left Humeral Head with Monoplanar External Fixation Device, Percutaneous Endoscopic Approach

0PSD4CZ   Reposition Left Humeral Head with Ring External Fixation Device, Percutaneous Endoscopic Approach

0PSD4DZ   Reposition Left Humeral Head with Hybrid External Fixation Device, Percutaneous Endoscopic Approach

0PSD4ZZ   Reposition Left Humeral Head, Percutaneous Endoscopic Approach

0PSDXZZ   Reposition Left Humeral Head, External Approach

0PSF04Z   Reposition Right Humeral Shaft with Internal Fixation Device, Open Approach

0PSF05Z   Reposition Right Humeral Shaft with External Fixation Device, Open Approach

0PSF06Z   Reposition Right Humeral Shaft with Intramedullary Internal Fixation Device, Open Approach

0PSF0BZ   Reposition Right Humeral Shaft with Monoplanar External Fixation Device, Open Approach

0PSF0CZ   Reposition Right Humeral Shaft with Ring External Fixation Device, Open Approach

0PSF0DZ   Reposition Right Humeral Shaft with Hybrid External Fixation Device, Open Approach

0PSF0ZZ   Reposition Right Humeral Shaft, Open Approach

0PSF34Z   Reposition Right Humeral Shaft with Internal Fixation Device, Percutaneous Approach

0PSF35Z   Reposition Right Humeral Shaft with External Fixation Device, Percutaneous Approach

0PSF36Z   Reposition Right Humeral Shaft with Intramedullary Internal Fixation Device, Percutaneous Approach

0PSF3BZ   Reposition Right Humeral Shaft with Monoplanar External Fixation Device, Percutaneous Approach

0PSF3CZ   Reposition Right Humeral Shaft with Ring External Fixation Device, Percutaneous Approach

0PSF3DZ   Reposition Right Humeral Shaft with Hybrid External Fixation Device, Percutaneous Approach

0PSF3ZZ   Reposition Right Humeral Shaft, Percutaneous Approach

0PSF44Z   Reposition Right Humeral Shaft with Internal Fixation Device, Percutaneous Endoscopic Approach

0PSF45Z   Reposition Right Humeral Shaft with External Fixation Device, Percutaneous Endoscopic Approach

0PSF46Z   Reposition Right Humeral Shaft with Intramedullary Internal Fixation Device, Percutaneous Endoscopic Approach

0PSF4BZ   Reposition Right Humeral Shaft with Monoplanar External Fixation Device, Percutaneous Endoscopic Approach

0PSF4CZ   Reposition Right Humeral Shaft with Ring External Fixation Device, Percutaneous Endoscopic Approach

0PSF4DZ   Reposition Right Humeral Shaft with Hybrid External Fixation Device, Percutaneous Endoscopic Approach

0PSF4ZZ   Reposition Right Humeral Shaft, Percutaneous Endoscopic Approach

0PSFXZZ   Reposition Right Humeral Shaft, External Approach

0PSG04Z   Reposition Left Humeral Shaft with Internal Fixation Device, Open Approach

0PSG05Z Reposition Left Humeral Shaft with External Fixation Device, Open Approach

0PSG06Z Reposition Left Humeral Shaft with Intramedullary Internal Fixation Device, Open Approach

0PSG0BZ Reposition Left Humeral Shaft with Monoplanar External Fixation Device, Open Approach

0PSG0CZ Reposition Left Humeral Shaft with Ring External Fixation Device, Open Approach

0PSG0DZ Reposition Left Humeral Shaft with Hybrid External Fixation Device, Open Approach

0PSG0ZZ Reposition Left Humeral Shaft, Open Approach

0PSG34Z Reposition Left Humeral Shaft with Internal Fixation Device, Percutaneous Approach

0PSG35Z Reposition Left Humeral Shaft with External Fixation Device, Percutaneous Approach

0PSG36Z Reposition Left Humeral Shaft with Intramedullary Internal Fixation Device, Percutaneous Approach

0PSG3BZ Reposition Left Humeral Shaft with Monoplanar External Fixation Device, Percutaneous Approach

0PSG3CZ Reposition Left Humeral Shaft with Ring External Fixation Device, Percutaneous Approach

0PSG3DZ Reposition Left Humeral Shaft with Hybrid External Fixation Device, Percutaneous Approach

0PSG3ZZ Reposition Left Humeral Shaft, Percutaneous Approach

0PSG44Z Reposition Left Humeral Shaft with Internal Fixation Device, Percutaneous Endoscopic Approach

0PSG45Z Reposition Left Humeral Shaft with External Fixation Device, Percutaneous Endoscopic Approach

0PSG46Z Reposition Left Humeral Shaft with Intramedullary Internal Fixation Device, Percutaneous Endoscopic Approach

0PSG4BZ Reposition Left Humeral Shaft with Monoplanar External Fixation Device, Percutaneous Endoscopic Approach

0PSG4CZ Reposition Left Humeral Shaft with Ring External Fixation Device, Percutaneous Endoscopic Approach

0PSG4DZ Reposition Left Humeral Shaft with Hybrid External Fixation Device, Percutaneous Endoscopic Approach

0PSG4ZZ Reposition Left Humeral Shaft, Percutaneous Endoscopic Approach

0PSGXZZ Reposition Left Humeral Shaft, External Approach

0PSH04Z Reposition Right Radius with Internal Fixation Device, Open Approach

0PSH05Z Reposition Right Radius with External Fixation Device, Open Approach

0PSH06Z Reposition Right Radius with Intramedullary Internal Fixation Device, Open Approach

0PSH0BZ Reposition Right Radius with Monoplanar External Fixation Device, Open Approach

0PSH0CZ Reposition Right Radius with Ring External Fixation Device, Open Approach

0PSH0DZ Reposition Right Radius with Hybrid External Fixation Device, Open Approach

0PSH0ZZ Reposition Right Radius, Open Approach

0PSH34Z Reposition Right Radius with Internal Fixation Device, Percutaneous Approach

0PSH35Z Reposition Right Radius with External Fixation Device, Percutaneous Approach

0PSH36Z Reposition Right Radius with Intramedullary Internal Fixation Device, Percutaneous Approach

0PSH3BZ Reposition Right Radius with Monoplanar External Fixation Device, Percutaneous Approach

0PSH3CZ Reposition Right Radius with Ring External Fixation Device, Percutaneous Approach

0PSH3DZ Reposition Right Radius with Hybrid External Fixation Device, Percutaneous Approach

0PSH3ZZ Reposition Right Radius, Percutaneous Approach

0PSH44Z Reposition Right Radius with Internal Fixation Device, Percutaneous Endoscopic Approach

0PSH45Z Reposition Right Radius with External Fixation Device, Percutaneous Endoscopic Approach

0PSH46Z Reposition Right Radius with Intramedullary Internal Fixation Device, Percutaneous Endoscopic Approach

0PSH4BZ Reposition Right Radius with Monoplanar External Fixation Device, Percutaneous Endoscopic Approach

0PSH4CZ Reposition Right Radius with Ring External Fixation Device, Percutaneous Endoscopic Approach

0PSH4DZ Reposition Right Radius with Hybrid External Fixation Device, Percutaneous Endoscopic Approach

0PSH4ZZ Reposition Right Radius, Percutaneous Endoscopic Approach

0PSHXZZ Reposition Right Radius, External Approach

0PSJ04Z Reposition Left Radius with Internal Fixation Device, Open Approach

0PSJ05Z Reposition Left Radius with External Fixation Device, Open Approach

0PSJ06Z Reposition Left Radius with Intramedullary Internal Fixation Device, Open Approach

0PSJ0BZ Reposition Left Radius with Monoplanar External Fixation Device, Open Approach

0PSJ0CZ Reposition Left Radius with Ring External Fixation Device, Open Approach

0PSJ0DZ Reposition Left Radius with Hybrid External Fixation Device, Open Approach

0PSJ0ZZ Reposition Left Radius, Open Approach

0PSJ34Z Reposition Left Radius with Internal Fixation Device, Percutaneous Approach

0PSJ35Z Reposition Left Radius with External Fixation Device, Percutaneous Approach

0PSJ36Z Reposition Left Radius with Intramedullary Internal Fixation Device, Percutaneous Approach

0PSJ3BZ Reposition Left Radius with Monoplanar External Fixation Device, Percutaneous Approach

0PSJ3CZ Reposition Left Radius with Ring External Fixation Device, Percutaneous Approach

0PSJ3DZ Reposition Left Radius with Hybrid External Fixation Device, Percutaneous Approach

0PSJ3ZZ Reposition Left Radius, Percutaneous Approach

0PSJ44Z Reposition Left Radius with Internal Fixation Device, Percutaneous Endoscopic Approach

0PSJ45Z Reposition Left Radius with External Fixation Device, Percutaneous Endoscopic Approach

0PSJ46Z Reposition Left Radius with Intramedullary Internal Fixation Device, Percutaneous Endoscopic Approach

0PSJ4BZ Reposition Left Radius with Monoplanar External Fixation Device, Percutaneous Endoscopic Approach

0PSJ4CZ Reposition Left Radius with Ring External Fixation Device, Percutaneous Endoscopic Approach

0PSJ4DZ Reposition Left Radius with Hybrid External Fixation Device, Percutaneous Endoscopic Approach

0PSJ4ZZ Reposition Left Radius, Percutaneous Endoscopic Approach

0PSJXZZ Reposition Left Radius, External Approach

0PSK04Z Reposition Right Ulna with Internal Fixation Device, Open Approach

0PSK05Z Reposition Right Ulna with External Fixation Device, Open Approach

0PSK06Z Reposition Right Ulna with Intramedullary Internal Fixation Device, Open Approach

0PSK0BZ Reposition Right Ulna with Monoplanar External Fixation Device, Open Approach

0PSK0CZ Reposition Right Ulna with Ring External Fixation Device, Open Approach

0PSK0DZ Reposition Right Ulna with Hybrid External Fixation Device, Open Approach

0PSK0ZZ Reposition Right Ulna, Open Approach

0PSK34Z Reposition Right Ulna with Internal Fixation Device, Percutaneous Approach

0PSK35Z Reposition Right Ulna with External Fixation Device, Percutaneous Approach

0PSK36Z Reposition Right Ulna with Intramedullary Internal Fixation Device, Percutaneous Approach

0PSK3BZ Reposition Right Ulna with Monoplanar External Fixation Device, Percutaneous Approach

0PSK3CZ Reposition Right Ulna with Ring External Fixation Device, Percutaneous Approach

0PSK3DZ Reposition Right Ulna with Hybrid External Fixation Device, Percutaneous Approach

0PSK3ZZ Reposition Right Ulna, Percutaneous Approach

0PSK44Z Reposition Right Ulna with Internal Fixation Device, Percutaneous Endoscopic Approach

0PSK45Z Reposition Right Ulna with External Fixation Device, Percutaneous Endoscopic Approach

0PSK46Z Reposition Right Ulna with Intramedullary Internal Fixation Device, Percutaneous Endoscopic Approach

0PSK4BZ Reposition Right Ulna with Monoplanar External Fixation Device, Percutaneous Endoscopic Approach

0PSK4CZ Reposition Right Ulna with Ring External Fixation Device, Percutaneous Endoscopic Approach

0PSK4DZ Reposition Right Ulna with Hybrid External Fixation Device, Percutaneous Endoscopic Approach

0PSK4ZZ Reposition Right Ulna, Percutaneous Endoscopic Approach

0PSKXZZ Reposition Right Ulna, External Approach

0PSL04Z Reposition Left Ulna with Internal Fixation Device, Open Approach

0PSL05Z Reposition Left Ulna with External Fixation Device, Open Approach

0PSL06Z Reposition Left Ulna with Intramedullary Internal Fixation Device, Open Approach

0PSL0BZ Reposition Left Ulna with Monoplanar External Fixation Device, Open Approach

0PSL0CZ Reposition Left Ulna with Ring External Fixation Device, Open Approach

0PSL0DZ Reposition Left Ulna with Hybrid External Fixation Device, Open Approach

0PSL0ZZ Reposition Left Ulna, Open Approach

0PSL34Z Reposition Left Ulna with Internal Fixation Device, Percutaneous Approach

0PSL35Z Reposition Left Ulna with External Fixation Device, Percutaneous Approach

0PSL36Z Reposition Left Ulna with Intramedullary Internal Fixation Device, Percutaneous Approach

0PSL3BZ Reposition Left Ulna with Monoplanar External Fixation Device, Percutaneous Approach

0PSL3CZ Reposition Left Ulna with Ring External Fixation Device, Percutaneous Approach

0PSL3DZ Reposition Left Ulna with Hybrid External Fixation Device, Percutaneous Approach

0PSL3ZZ Reposition Left Ulna, Percutaneous Approach

0PSL44Z Reposition Left Ulna with Internal Fixation Device, Percutaneous Endoscopic Approach

0PSL45Z Reposition Left Ulna with External Fixation Device, Percutaneous Endoscopic Approach

0PSL46Z Reposition Left Ulna with Intramedullary Internal Fixation Device, Percutaneous Endoscopic Approach

0PSL4BZ Reposition Left Ulna with Monoplanar External Fixation Device, Percutaneous Endoscopic Approach

0PSL4CZ Reposition Left Ulna with Ring External Fixation Device, Percutaneous Endoscopic Approach

0PSL4DZ Reposition Left Ulna with Hybrid External Fixation Device, Percutaneous Endoscopic Approach

0PSL4ZZ Reposition Left Ulna, Percutaneous Endoscopic Approach

0PSLXZZ Reposition Left Ulna, External Approach

0PSM04Z Reposition Right Carpal with Internal Fixation Device, Open Approach

0PSM05Z Reposition Right Carpal with External Fixation Device, Open Approach

0PSM0ZZ Reposition Right Carpal, Open Approach

0PSM34Z Reposition Right Carpal with Internal Fixation Device, Percutaneous Approach

0PSM35Z Reposition Right Carpal with External Fixation Device, Percutaneous Approach

0PSM3ZZ Reposition Right Carpal, Percutaneous Approach

0PSM44Z Reposition Right Carpal with Internal Fixation Device, Percutaneous Endoscopic Approach

0PSM45Z Reposition Right Carpal with External Fixation Device, Percutaneous Endoscopic Approach

0PSM4ZZ Reposition Right Carpal, Percutaneous Endoscopic Approach

0PSMXZZ Reposition Right Carpal, External Approach

0PSN04Z Reposition Left Carpal with Internal Fixation Device, Open Approach

0PSN05Z Reposition Left Carpal with External Fixation Device, Open Approach

0PSN0ZZ Reposition Left Carpal, Open Approach

0PSN34Z Reposition Left Carpal with Internal Fixation Device, Percutaneous Approach

0PSN35Z Reposition Left Carpal with External Fixation Device, Percutaneous Approach

0PSN3ZZ Reposition Left Carpal, Percutaneous Approach

0PSN44Z Reposition Left Carpal with Internal Fixation Device, Percutaneous Endoscopic Approach

0PSN45Z Reposition Left Carpal with External Fixation Device, Percutaneous Endoscopic Approach

0PSN4ZZ Reposition Left Carpal, Percutaneous Endoscopic Approach

0PSNXZZ Reposition Left Carpal, External Approach

0PSP04Z Reposition Right Metacarpal with Internal Fixation Device, Open Approach

0PSP05Z Reposition Right Metacarpal with External Fixation Device, Open Approach

0PSP0ZZ Reposition Right Metacarpal, Open Approach

0PSP34Z Reposition Right Metacarpal with Internal Fixation Device, Percutaneous Approach

0PSP35Z Reposition Right Metacarpal with External Fixation Device, Percutaneous Approach

0PSP3ZZ Reposition Right Metacarpal, Percutaneous Approach

0PSP44Z Reposition Right Metacarpal with Internal Fixation Device, Percutaneous Endoscopic Approach

0PSP45Z Reposition Right Metacarpal with External Fixation Device, Percutaneous Endoscopic Approach

0PSP4ZZ Reposition Right Metacarpal, Percutaneous Endoscopic Approach

0PSPXZZ Reposition Right Metacarpal, External Approach

0PSQ04Z Reposition Left Metacarpal with Internal Fixation Device, Open Approach

0PSQ05Z Reposition Left Metacarpal with External Fixation Device, Open Approach

0PSQ0ZZ Reposition Left Metacarpal, Open Approach

0PSQ34Z Reposition Left Metacarpal with Internal Fixation Device, Percutaneous Approach

0PSQ35Z Reposition Left Metacarpal with External Fixation Device, Percutaneous Approach

0PSQ3ZZ Reposition Left Metacarpal, Percutaneous Approach

0PSQ44Z Reposition Left Metacarpal with Internal Fixation Device, Percutaneous Endoscopic Approach

0PSQ45Z Reposition Left Metacarpal with External Fixation Device, Percutaneous Endoscopic Approach

0PSQ4ZZ Reposition Left Metacarpal, Percutaneous Endoscopic Approach

0PSQXZZ Reposition Left Metacarpal, External Approach

0PSR04Z Reposition Right Thumb Phalanx with Internal Fixation Device, Open Approach

0PSR05Z Reposition Right Thumb Phalanx with External Fixation Device, Open Approach

0PSR0ZZ Reposition Right Thumb Phalanx, Open Approach

0PSR34Z Reposition Right Thumb Phalanx with Internal Fixation Device, Percutaneous Approach

0PSR35Z Reposition Right Thumb Phalanx with External Fixation Device, Percutaneous Approach

0PSR3ZZ Reposition Right Thumb Phalanx, Percutaneous Approach

0PSR44Z Reposition Right Thumb Phalanx with Internal Fixation Device, Percutaneous Endoscopic Approach

0PSR45Z Reposition Right Thumb Phalanx with External Fixation Device, Percutaneous Endoscopic Approach

0PSR4ZZ Reposition Right Thumb Phalanx, Percutaneous Endoscopic Approach

0PSRXZZ Reposition Right Thumb Phalanx, External Approach

0PSS04Z Reposition Left Thumb Phalanx with Internal Fixation Device, Open Approach

0PSS05Z Reposition Left Thumb Phalanx with External Fixation Device, Open Approach

0PSS0ZZ Reposition Left Thumb Phalanx, Open Approach

0PSS34Z Reposition Left Thumb Phalanx with Internal Fixation Device, Percutaneous Approach

0PSS35Z Reposition Left Thumb Phalanx with External Fixation Device, Percutaneous Approach

0PSS3ZZ Reposition Left Thumb Phalanx, Percutaneous Approach

0PSS44Z Reposition Left Thumb Phalanx with Internal Fixation Device, Percutaneous Endoscopic Approach

0PSS45Z	Reposition Left Thumb Phalanx with External Fixation Device, Percutaneous Endoscopic Approach
0PSS4ZZ	Reposition Left Thumb Phalanx, Percutaneous Endoscopic Approach
0PSSXZZ	Reposition Left Thumb Phalanx, External Approach
0PST04Z	Reposition Right Finger Phalanx with Internal Fixation Device, Open Approach
0PST05Z	Reposition Right Finger Phalanx with External Fixation Device, Open Approach
0PST0ZZ	Reposition Right Finger Phalanx, Open Approach
0PST34Z	Reposition Right Finger Phalanx with Internal Fixation Device, Percutaneous Approach
0PST35Z	Reposition Right Finger Phalanx with External Fixation Device, Percutaneous Approach
0PST3ZZ	Reposition Right Finger Phalanx, Percutaneous Approach
0PST44Z	Reposition Right Finger Phalanx with Internal Fixation Device, Percutaneous Endoscopic Approach
0PST45Z	Reposition Right Finger Phalanx with External Fixation Device, Percutaneous Endoscopic Approach

0PST4ZZ	Reposition Right Finger Phalanx, Percutaneous Endoscopic Approach
0PSTXZZ	Reposition Right Finger Phalanx, External Approach
0PSV04Z	Reposition Left Finger Phalanx with Internal Fixation Device, Open Approach
0PSV05Z	Reposition Left Finger Phalanx with External Fixation Device, Open Approach
0PSV0ZZ	Reposition Left Finger Phalanx, Open Approach
0PSV34Z	Reposition Left Finger Phalanx with Internal Fixation Device, Percutaneous Approach
0PSV35Z	Reposition Left Finger Phalanx with External Fixation Device, Percutaneous Approach
0PSV3ZZ	Reposition Left Finger Phalanx, Percutaneous Approach
0PSV44Z	Reposition Left Finger Phalanx with Internal Fixation Device, Percutaneous Endoscopic Approach
0PSV45Z	Reposition Left Finger Phalanx with External Fixation Device, Percutaneous Endoscopic Approach
0PSV4ZZ	Reposition Left Finger Phalanx, Percutaneous Endoscopic Approach
0PSVXZZ	Reposition Left Finger Phalanx, External Approach

0PT – Upper Bones, Resection

Review Coding Guideline B3.8

0PT00ZZ	Resection of Sternum, Open Approach
0PT10ZZ	Resection of Right Rib, Open Approach
0PT20ZZ	Resection of Left Rib, Open Approach
0PT50ZZ	Resection of Right Scapula, Open Approach
0PT60ZZ	Resection of Left Scapula, Open Approach
0PT70ZZ	Resection of Right Glenoid Cavity, Open Approach
0PT80ZZ	Resection of Left Glenoid Cavity, Open Approach
0PT90ZZ	Resection of Right Clavicle, Open Approach
0PTB0ZZ	Resection of Left Clavicle, Open Approach
0PTC0ZZ	Resection of Right Humeral Head, Open Approach
0PTD0ZZ	Resection of Left Humeral Head, Open Approach
0PTF0ZZ	Resection of Right Humeral Shaft, Open Approach
0PTG0ZZ	Resection of Left Humeral Shaft, Open Approach

0PTH0ZZ	Resection of Right Radius, Open Approach
0PTJ0ZZ	Resection of Left Radius, Open Approach
0PTK0ZZ	Resection of Right Ulna, Open Approach
0PTL0ZZ	Resection of Left Ulna, Open Approach
0PTM0ZZ	Resection of Right Carpal, Open Approach
0PTN0ZZ	Resection of Left Carpal, Open Approach
0PTP0ZZ	Resection of Right Metacarpal, Open Approach
0PTQ0ZZ	Resection of Left Metacarpal, Open Approach
0PTR0ZZ	Resection of Right Thumb Phalanx, Open Approach
0PTS0ZZ	Resection of Left Thumb Phalanx, Open Approach
0PTT0ZZ	Resection of Right Finger Phalanx, Open Approach
0PTV0ZZ	Resection of Left Finger Phalanx, Open Approach

0PU – Upper Bones, Supplement

0PU007Z	Supplement Sternum with Autologous Tissue Substitute, Open Approach
0PU00JZ	Supplement Sternum with Synthetic Substitute, Open Approach
0PU00KZ	Supplement Sternum with Nonautologous Tissue Substitute, Open Approach
0PU037Z	Supplement Sternum with Autologous Tissue Substitute, Percutaneous Approach
0PU03JZ	Supplement Sternum with Synthetic Substitute, Percutaneous Approach
0PU03KZ	Supplement Sternum with Nonautologous Tissue Substitute, Percutaneous Approach
0PU047Z	Supplement Sternum with Autologous Tissue Substitute, Percutaneous Endoscopic Approach
0PU04JZ	Supplement Sternum with Synthetic Substitute, Percutaneous Endoscopic Approach
0PU04KZ	Supplement Sternum with Nonautologous Tissue Substitute, Percutaneous Endoscopic Approach
0PU107Z	Supplement Right Rib with Autologous Tissue Substitute, Open Approach
0PU10JZ	Supplement Right Rib with Synthetic Substitute, Open Approach
0PU10KZ	Supplement Right Rib with Nonautologous Tissue Substitute, Open Approach
0PU137Z	Supplement Right Rib with Autologous Tissue Substitute, Percutaneous Approach
0PU13JZ	Supplement Right Rib with Synthetic Substitute, Percutaneous Approach
0PU13KZ	Supplement Right Rib with Nonautologous Tissue Substitute, Percutaneous Approach
0PU147Z	Supplement Right Rib with Autologous Tissue Substitute, Percutaneous Endoscopic Approach
0PU14JZ	Supplement Right Rib with Synthetic Substitute, Percutaneous Endoscopic Approach

0PU14KZ	Supplement Right Rib with Nonautologous Tissue Substitute, Percutaneous Endoscopic Approach
0PU207Z	Supplement Left Rib with Autologous Tissue Substitute, Open Approach
0PU20JZ	Supplement Left Rib with Synthetic Substitute, Open Approach
0PU20KZ	Supplement Left Rib with Nonautologous Tissue Substitute, Open Approach
0PU237Z	Supplement Left Rib with Autologous Tissue Substitute, Percutaneous Approach
0PU23JZ	Supplement Left Rib with Synthetic Substitute, Percutaneous Approach
0PU23KZ	Supplement Left Rib with Nonautologous Tissue Substitute, Percutaneous Approach
0PU247Z	Supplement Left Rib with Autologous Tissue Substitute, Percutaneous Endoscopic Approach
0PU24JZ	Supplement Left Rib with Synthetic Substitute, Percutaneous Endoscopic Approach
0PU24KZ	Supplement Left Rib with Nonautologous Tissue Substitute, Percutaneous Endoscopic Approach
0PU307Z	Supplement Cervical Vertebra with Autologous Tissue Substitute, Open Approach
0PU30JZ	Supplement Cervical Vertebra with Synthetic Substitute, Open Approach
0PU30KZ	Supplement Cervical Vertebra with Nonautologous Tissue Substitute, Open Approach
0PU337Z	Supplement Cervical Vertebra with Autologous Tissue Substitute, Percutaneous Approach
0PU33JZ	Supplement Cervical Vertebra with Synthetic Substitute, Percutaneous Approach
0PU33KZ	Supplement Cervical Vertebra with Nonautologous Tissue Substitute, Percutaneous Approach
0PU347Z	Supplement Cervical Vertebra with Autologous Tissue Substitute, Percutaneous Endoscopic Approach

0PU34JZ Supplement Cervical Vertebra with Synthetic Substitute, Percutaneous Endoscopic Approach

0PU34KZ Supplement Cervical Vertebra with Nonautologous Tissue Substitute, Percutaneous Endoscopic Approach

0PU407Z Supplement Thoracic Vertebra with Autologous Tissue Substitute, Open Approach

0PU40JZ Supplement Thoracic Vertebra with Synthetic Substitute, Open Approach

0PU40KZ Supplement Thoracic Vertebra with Nonautologous Tissue Substitute, Open Approach

0PU437Z Supplement Thoracic Vertebra with Autologous Tissue Substitute, Percutaneous Approach

0PU43JZ Supplement Thoracic Vertebra with Synthetic Substitute, Percutaneous Approach

0PU43KZ Supplement Thoracic Vertebra with Nonautologous Tissue Substitute, Percutaneous Approach

0PU447Z Supplement Thoracic Vertebra with Autologous Tissue Substitute, Percutaneous Endoscopic Approach

0PU44JZ Supplement Thoracic Vertebra with Synthetic Substitute, Percutaneous Endoscopic Approach

0PU44KZ Supplement Thoracic Vertebra with Nonautologous Tissue Substitute, Percutaneous Endoscopic Approach

0PU507Z Supplement Right Scapula with Autologous Tissue Substitute, Open Approach

0PU50JZ Supplement Right Scapula with Synthetic Substitute, Open Approach

0PU50KZ Supplement Right Scapula with Nonautologous Tissue Substitute, Open Approach

0PU537Z Supplement Right Scapula with Autologous Tissue Substitute, Percutaneous Approach

0PU53JZ Supplement Right Scapula with Synthetic Substitute, Percutaneous Approach

0PU53KZ Supplement Right Scapula with Nonautologous Tissue Substitute, Percutaneous Approach

0PU547Z Supplement Right Scapula with Autologous Tissue Substitute, Percutaneous Endoscopic Approach

0PU54JZ Supplement Right Scapula with Synthetic Substitute, Percutaneous Endoscopic Approach

0PU54KZ Supplement Right Scapula with Nonautologous Tissue Substitute, Percutaneous Endoscopic Approach

0PU607Z Supplement Left Scapula with Autologous Tissue Substitute, Open Approach

0PU60JZ Supplement Left Scapula with Synthetic Substitute, Open Approach

0PU60KZ Supplement Left Scapula with Nonautologous Tissue Substitute, Open Approach

0PU637Z Supplement Left Scapula with Autologous Tissue Substitute, Percutaneous Approach

0PU63JZ Supplement Left Scapula with Synthetic Substitute, Percutaneous Approach

0PU63KZ Supplement Left Scapula with Nonautologous Tissue Substitute, Percutaneous Approach

0PU647Z Supplement Left Scapula with Autologous Tissue Substitute, Percutaneous Endoscopic Approach

0PU64JZ Supplement Left Scapula with Synthetic Substitute, Percutaneous Endoscopic Approach

0PU64KZ Supplement Left Scapula with Nonautologous Tissue Substitute, Percutaneous Endoscopic Approach

0PU707Z Supplement Right Glenoid Cavity with Autologous Tissue Substitute, Open Approach

0PU70JZ Supplement Right Glenoid Cavity with Synthetic Substitute, Open Approach

0PU70KZ Supplement Right Glenoid Cavity with Nonautologous Tissue Substitute, Open Approach

0PU737Z Supplement Right Glenoid Cavity with Autologous Tissue Substitute, Percutaneous Approach

0PU73JZ Supplement Right Glenoid Cavity with Synthetic Substitute, Percutaneous Approach

0PU73KZ Supplement Right Glenoid Cavity with Nonautologous Tissue Substitute, Percutaneous Approach

0PU747Z Supplement Right Glenoid Cavity with Autologous Tissue Substitute, Percutaneous Endoscopic Approach

0PU74JZ Supplement Right Glenoid Cavity with Synthetic Substitute, Percutaneous Endoscopic Approach

0PU74KZ Supplement Right Glenoid Cavity with Nonautologous Tissue Substitute, Percutaneous Endoscopic Approach

0PU807Z Supplement Left Glenoid Cavity with Autologous Tissue Substitute, Open Approach

0PU80JZ Supplement Left Glenoid Cavity with Synthetic Substitute, Open Approach

0PU80KZ Supplement Left Glenoid Cavity with Nonautologous Tissue Substitute, Open Approach

0PU837Z Supplement Left Glenoid Cavity with Autologous Tissue Substitute, Percutaneous Approach

0PU83JZ Supplement Left Glenoid Cavity with Synthetic Substitute, Percutaneous Approach

0PU83KZ Supplement Left Glenoid Cavity with Nonautologous Tissue Substitute, Percutaneous Approach

0PU847Z Supplement Left Glenoid Cavity with Autologous Tissue Substitute, Percutaneous Endoscopic Approach

0PU84JZ Supplement Left Glenoid Cavity with Synthetic Substitute, Percutaneous Endoscopic Approach

0PU84KZ Supplement Left Glenoid Cavity with Nonautologous Tissue Substitute, Percutaneous Endoscopic Approach

0PU907Z Supplement Right Clavicle with Autologous Tissue Substitute, Open Approach

0PU90JZ Supplement Right Clavicle with Synthetic Substitute, Open Approach

0PU90KZ Supplement Right Clavicle with Nonautologous Tissue Substitute, Open Approach

0PU937Z Supplement Right Clavicle with Autologous Tissue Substitute, Percutaneous Approach

0PU93JZ Supplement Right Clavicle with Synthetic Substitute, Percutaneous Approach

0PU93KZ Supplement Right Clavicle with Nonautologous Tissue Substitute, Percutaneous Approach

0PU947Z Supplement Right Clavicle with Autologous Tissue Substitute, Percutaneous Endoscopic Approach

0PU94JZ Supplement Right Clavicle with Synthetic Substitute, Percutaneous Endoscopic Approach

0PU94KZ Supplement Right Clavicle with Nonautologous Tissue Substitute, Percutaneous Endoscopic Approach

0PUB07Z Supplement Left Clavicle with Autologous Tissue Substitute, Open Approach

0PUB0JZ Supplement Left Clavicle with Synthetic Substitute, Open Approach

0PUB0KZ Supplement Left Clavicle with Nonautologous Tissue Substitute, Open Approach

0PUB37Z Supplement Left Clavicle with Autologous Tissue Substitute, Percutaneous Approach

0PUB3JZ Supplement Left Clavicle with Synthetic Substitute, Percutaneous Approach

0PUB3KZ Supplement Left Clavicle with Nonautologous Tissue Substitute, Percutaneous Approach

0PUB47Z Supplement Left Clavicle with Autologous Tissue Substitute, Percutaneous Endoscopic Approach

0PUB4JZ Supplement Left Clavicle with Synthetic Substitute, Percutaneous Endoscopic Approach

0PUB4KZ Supplement Left Clavicle with Nonautologous Tissue Substitute, Percutaneous Endoscopic Approach

0PUC07Z Supplement Right Humeral Head with Autologous Tissue Substitute, Open Approach

0PUC0JZ Supplement Right Humeral Head with Synthetic Substitute, Open Approach

0PUC0KZ Supplement Right Humeral Head with Nonautologous Tissue Substitute, Open Approach

0PUC37Z Supplement Right Humeral Head with Autologous Tissue Substitute, Percutaneous Approach

0PUC3JZ Supplement Right Humeral Head with Synthetic Substitute, Percutaneous Approach

0PUC3KZ Supplement Right Humeral Head with Nonautologous Tissue Substitute, Percutaneous Approach

0PUC47Z Supplement Right Humeral Head with Autologous Tissue Substitute, Percutaneous Endoscopic Approach

0PUC4JZ Supplement Right Humeral Head with Synthetic Substitute, Percutaneous Endoscopic Approach

0PUC4KZ Supplement Right Humeral Head with Nonautologous Tissue Substitute, Percutaneous Endoscopic Approach

0PUD07Z   Supplement Left Humeral Head with Autologous Tissue Substitute, Open Approach

0PUD0JZ   Supplement Left Humeral Head with Synthetic Substitute, Open Approach

0PUD0KZ   Supplement Left Humeral Head with Nonautologous Tissue Substitute, Open Approach

0PUD37Z   Supplement Left Humeral Head with Autologous Tissue Substitute, Percutaneous Approach

0PUD3JZ   Supplement Left Humeral Head with Synthetic Substitute, Percutaneous Approach

0PUD3KZ   Supplement Left Humeral Head with Nonautologous Tissue Substitute, Percutaneous Approach

0PUD47Z   Supplement Left Humeral Head with Autologous Tissue Substitute, Percutaneous Endoscopic Approach

0PUD4JZ   Supplement Left Humeral Head with Synthetic Substitute, Percutaneous Endoscopic Approach

0PUD4KZ   Supplement Left Humeral Head with Nonautologous Tissue Substitute, Percutaneous Endoscopic Approach

0PUF07Z   Supplement Right Humeral Shaft with Autologous Tissue Substitute, Open Approach

0PUF0JZ   Supplement Right Humeral Shaft with Synthetic Substitute, Open Approach

0PUF0KZ   Supplement Right Humeral Shaft with Nonautologous Tissue Substitute, Open Approach

0PUF37Z   Supplement Right Humeral Shaft with Autologous Tissue Substitute, Percutaneous Approach

0PUF3JZ   Supplement Right Humeral Shaft with Synthetic Substitute, Percutaneous Approach

0PUF3KZ   Supplement Right Humeral Shaft with Nonautologous Tissue Substitute, Percutaneous Approach

0PUF47Z   Supplement Right Humeral Shaft with Autologous Tissue Substitute, Percutaneous Endoscopic Approach

0PUF4JZ   Supplement Right Humeral Shaft with Synthetic Substitute, Percutaneous Endoscopic Approach

0PUF4KZ   Supplement Right Humeral Shaft with Nonautologous Tissue Substitute, Percutaneous Endoscopic Approach

0PUG07Z   Supplement Left Humeral Shaft with Autologous Tissue Substitute, Open Approach

0PUG0JZ   Supplement Left Humeral Shaft with Synthetic Substitute, Open Approach

0PUG0KZ   Supplement Left Humeral Shaft with Nonautologous Tissue Substitute, Open Approach

0PUG37Z   Supplement Left Humeral Shaft with Autologous Tissue Substitute, Percutaneous Approach

0PUG3JZ   Supplement Left Humeral Shaft with Synthetic Substitute, Percutaneous Approach

0PUG3KZ   Supplement Left Humeral Shaft with Nonautologous Tissue Substitute, Percutaneous Approach

0PUG47Z   Supplement Left Humeral Shaft with Autologous Tissue Substitute, Percutaneous Endoscopic Approach

0PUG4JZ   Supplement Left Humeral Shaft with Synthetic Substitute, Percutaneous Endoscopic Approach

0PUG4KZ   Supplement Left Humeral Shaft with Nonautologous Tissue Substitute, Percutaneous Endoscopic Approach

0PUH07Z   Supplement Right Radius with Autologous Tissue Substitute, Open Approach

0PUH0JZ   Supplement Right Radius with Synthetic Substitute, Open Approach

0PUH0KZ   Supplement Right Radius with Nonautologous Tissue Substitute, Open Approach

0PUH37Z   Supplement Right Radius with Autologous Tissue Substitute, Percutaneous Approach

0PUH3JZ   Supplement Right Radius with Synthetic Substitute, Percutaneous Approach

0PUH3KZ   Supplement Right Radius with Nonautologous Tissue Substitute, Percutaneous Approach

0PUH47Z   Supplement Right Radius with Autologous Tissue Substitute, Percutaneous Endoscopic Approach

0PUH4JZ   Supplement Right Radius with Synthetic Substitute, Percutaneous Endoscopic Approach

0PUH4KZ   Supplement Right Radius with Nonautologous Tissue Substitute, Percutaneous Endoscopic Approach

0PUJ07Z   Supplement Left Radius with Autologous Tissue Substitute, Open Approach

0PUJ0JZ   Supplement Left Radius with Synthetic Substitute, Open Approach

0PUJ0KZ   Supplement Left Radius with Nonautologous Tissue Substitute, Open Approach

0PUJ37Z   Supplement Left Radius with Autologous Tissue Substitute, Percutaneous Approach

0PUJ3JZ   Supplement Left Radius with Synthetic Substitute, Percutaneous Approach

0PUJ3KZ   Supplement Left Radius with Nonautologous Tissue Substitute, Percutaneous Approach

0PUJ47Z   Supplement Left Radius with Autologous Tissue Substitute, Percutaneous Endoscopic Approach

0PUJ4JZ   Supplement Left Radius with Synthetic Substitute, Percutaneous Endoscopic Approach

0PUJ4KZ   Supplement Left Radius with Nonautologous Tissue Substitute, Percutaneous Endoscopic Approach

0PUK07Z   Supplement Right Ulna with Autologous Tissue Substitute, Open Approach

0PUK0JZ   Supplement Right Ulna with Synthetic Substitute, Open Approach

0PUK0KZ   Supplement Right Ulna with Nonautologous Tissue Substitute, Open Approach

0PUK37Z   Supplement Right Ulna with Autologous Tissue Substitute, Percutaneous Approach

0PUK3JZ   Supplement Right Ulna with Synthetic Substitute, Percutaneous Approach

0PUK3KZ   Supplement Right Ulna with Nonautologous Tissue Substitute, Percutaneous Approach

0PUK47Z   Supplement Right Ulna with Autologous Tissue Substitute, Percutaneous Endoscopic Approach

0PUK4JZ   Supplement Right Ulna with Synthetic Substitute, Percutaneous Endoscopic Approach

0PUK4KZ   Supplement Right Ulna with Nonautologous Tissue Substitute, Percutaneous Endoscopic Approach

0PUL07Z   Supplement Left Ulna with Autologous Tissue Substitute, Open Approach

0PUL0JZ   Supplement Left Ulna with Synthetic Substitute, Open Approach

0PUL0KZ   Supplement Left Ulna with Nonautologous Tissue Substitute, Open Approach

0PUL37Z   Supplement Left Ulna with Autologous Tissue Substitute, Percutaneous Approach

0PUL3JZ   Supplement Left Ulna with Synthetic Substitute, Percutaneous Approach

0PUL3KZ   Supplement Left Ulna with Nonautologous Tissue Substitute, Percutaneous Approach

0PUL47Z   Supplement Left Ulna with Autologous Tissue Substitute, Percutaneous Endoscopic Approach

0PUL4JZ   Supplement Left Ulna with Synthetic Substitute, Percutaneous Endoscopic Approach

0PUL4KZ   Supplement Left Ulna with Nonautologous Tissue Substitute, Percutaneous Endoscopic Approach

0PUM07Z   Supplement Right Carpal with Autologous Tissue Substitute, Open Approach

0PUM0JZ   Supplement Right Carpal with Synthetic Substitute, Open Approach

0PUM0KZ   Supplement Right Carpal with Nonautologous Tissue Substitute, Open Approach

0PUM37Z   Supplement Right Carpal with Autologous Tissue Substitute, Percutaneous Approach

0PUM3JZ   Supplement Right Carpal with Synthetic Substitute, Percutaneous Approach

0PUM3KZ   Supplement Right Carpal with Nonautologous Tissue Substitute, Percutaneous Approach

0PUM47Z   Supplement Right Carpal with Autologous Tissue Substitute, Percutaneous Endoscopic Approach

0PUM4JZ   Supplement Right Carpal with Synthetic Substitute, Percutaneous Endoscopic Approach

0PUM4KZ   Supplement Right Carpal with Nonautologous Tissue Substitute, Percutaneous Endoscopic Approach

0PUN07Z   Supplement Left Carpal with Autologous Tissue Substitute, Open Approach

0PUN0JZ   Supplement Left Carpal with Synthetic Substitute, Open Approach

0PUN0KZ   Supplement Left Carpal with Nonautologous Tissue Substitute, Open Approach

0PUN37Z   Supplement Left Carpal with Autologous Tissue Substitute, Percutaneous Approach

0PUN3JZ	Supplement Left Carpal with Synthetic Substitute, Percutaneous Approach
0PUN3KZ	Supplement Left Carpal with Nonautologous Tissue Substitute, Percutaneous Approach
0PUN47Z	Supplement Left Carpal with Autologous Tissue Substitute, Percutaneous Endoscopic Approach
0PUN4JZ	Supplement Left Carpal with Synthetic Substitute, Percutaneous Endoscopic Approach
0PUN4KZ	Supplement Left Carpal with Nonautologous Tissue Substitute, Percutaneous Endoscopic Approach
0PUP07Z	Supplement Right Metacarpal with Autologous Tissue Substitute, Open Approach
0PUP0JZ	Supplement Right Metacarpal with Synthetic Substitute, Open Approach
0PUP0KZ	Supplement Right Metacarpal with Nonautologous Tissue Substitute, Open Approach
0PUP37Z	Supplement Right Metacarpal with Autologous Tissue Substitute, Percutaneous Approach
0PUP3JZ	Supplement Right Metacarpal with Synthetic Substitute, Percutaneous Approach
0PUP3KZ	Supplement Right Metacarpal with Nonautologous Tissue Substitute, Percutaneous Approach
0PUP47Z	Supplement Right Metacarpal with Autologous Tissue Substitute, Percutaneous Endoscopic Approach
0PUP4JZ	Supplement Right Metacarpal with Synthetic Substitute, Percutaneous Endoscopic Approach
0PUP4KZ	Supplement Right Metacarpal with Nonautologous Tissue Substitute, Percutaneous Endoscopic Approach
0PUQ07Z	Supplement Left Metacarpal with Autologous Tissue Substitute, Open Approach
0PUQ0JZ	Supplement Left Metacarpal with Synthetic Substitute, Open Approach
0PUQ0KZ	Supplement Left Metacarpal with Nonautologous Tissue Substitute, Open Approach
0PUQ37Z	Supplement Left Metacarpal with Autologous Tissue Substitute, Percutaneous Approach
0PUQ3JZ	Supplement Left Metacarpal with Synthetic Substitute, Percutaneous Approach
0PUQ3KZ	Supplement Left Metacarpal with Nonautologous Tissue Substitute, Percutaneous Approach
0PUQ47Z	Supplement Left Metacarpal with Autologous Tissue Substitute, Percutaneous Endoscopic Approach
0PUQ4JZ	Supplement Left Metacarpal with Synthetic Substitute, Percutaneous Endoscopic Approach
0PUQ4KZ	Supplement Left Metacarpal with Nonautologous Tissue Substitute, Percutaneous Endoscopic Approach
0PUR07Z	Supplement Right Thumb Phalanx with Autologous Tissue Substitute, Open Approach
0PUR0JZ	Supplement Right Thumb Phalanx with Synthetic Substitute, Open Approach
0PUR0KZ	Supplement Right Thumb Phalanx with Nonautologous Tissue Substitute, Open Approach
0PUR37Z	Supplement Right Thumb Phalanx with Autologous Tissue Substitute, Percutaneous Approach
0PUR3JZ	Supplement Right Thumb Phalanx with Synthetic Substitute, Percutaneous Approach
0PUR3KZ	Supplement Right Thumb Phalanx with Nonautologous Tissue Substitute, Percutaneous Approach
0PUR47Z	Supplement Right Thumb Phalanx with Autologous Tissue Substitute, Percutaneous Endoscopic Approach

0PUR4JZ	Supplement Right Thumb Phalanx with Synthetic Substitute, Percutaneous Endoscopic Approach
0PUR4KZ	Supplement Right Thumb Phalanx with Nonautologous Tissue Substitute, Percutaneous Endoscopic Approach
0PUS07Z	Supplement Left Thumb Phalanx with Autologous Tissue Substitute, Open Approach
0PUS0JZ	Supplement Left Thumb Phalanx with Synthetic Substitute, Open Approach
0PUS0KZ	Supplement Left Thumb Phalanx with Nonautologous Tissue Substitute, Open Approach
0PUS37Z	Supplement Left Thumb Phalanx with Autologous Tissue Substitute, Percutaneous Approach
0PUS3JZ	Supplement Left Thumb Phalanx with Synthetic Substitute, Percutaneous Approach
0PUS3KZ	Supplement Left Thumb Phalanx with Nonautologous Tissue Substitute, Percutaneous Approach
0PUS47Z	Supplement Left Thumb Phalanx with Autologous Tissue Substitute, Percutaneous Endoscopic Approach
0PUS4JZ	Supplement Left Thumb Phalanx with Synthetic Substitute, Percutaneous Endoscopic Approach
0PUS4KZ	Supplement Left Thumb Phalanx with Nonautologous Tissue Substitute, Percutaneous Endoscopic Approach
0PUT07Z	Supplement Right Finger Phalanx with Autologous Tissue Substitute, Open Approach
0PUT0JZ	Supplement Right Finger Phalanx with Synthetic Substitute, Open Approach
0PUT0KZ	Supplement Right Finger Phalanx with Nonautologous Tissue Substitute, Open Approach
0PUT37Z	Supplement Right Finger Phalanx with Autologous Tissue Substitute, Percutaneous Approach
0PUT3JZ	Supplement Right Finger Phalanx with Synthetic Substitute, Percutaneous Approach
0PUT3KZ	Supplement Right Finger Phalanx with Nonautologous Tissue Substitute, Percutaneous Approach
0PUT47Z	Supplement Right Finger Phalanx with Autologous Tissue Substitute, Percutaneous Endoscopic Approach
0PUT4JZ	Supplement Right Finger Phalanx with Synthetic Substitute, Percutaneous Endoscopic Approach
0PUT4KZ	Supplement Right Finger Phalanx with Nonautologous Tissue Substitute, Percutaneous Endoscopic Approach
0PUV07Z	Supplement Left Finger Phalanx with Autologous Tissue Substitute, Open Approach
0PUV0JZ	Supplement Left Finger Phalanx with Synthetic Substitute, Open Approach
0PUV0KZ	Supplement Left Finger Phalanx with Nonautologous Tissue Substitute, Open Approach
0PUV37Z	Supplement Left Finger Phalanx with Autologous Tissue Substitute, Percutaneous Approach
0PUV3JZ	Supplement Left Finger Phalanx with Synthetic Substitute, Percutaneous Approach
0PUV3KZ	Supplement Left Finger Phalanx with Nonautologous Tissue Substitute, Percutaneous Approach
0PUV47Z	Supplement Left Finger Phalanx with Autologous Tissue Substitute, Percutaneous Endoscopic Approach
0PUV4JZ	Supplement Left Finger Phalanx with Synthetic Substitute, Percutaneous Endoscopic Approach
0PUV4KZ	Supplement Left Finger Phalanx with Nonautologous Tissue Substitute, Percutaneous Endoscopic Approach

0PW – Upper Bones, Revision

Review Coding Guideline B6.1c

0PW004Z	Revision of Internal Fixation Device in Sternum, Open Approach
0PW007Z	Revision of Autologous Tissue Substitute in Sternum, Open Approach
0PW00JZ	Revision of Synthetic Substitute in Sternum, Open Approach
0PW00KZ	Revision of Nonautologous Tissue Substitute in Sternum, Open Approach
0PW034Z	Revision of Internal Fixation Device in Sternum, Percutaneous Approach

0PW037Z	Revision of Autologous Tissue Substitute in Sternum, Percutaneous Approach
0PW03JZ	Revision of Synthetic Substitute in Sternum, Percutaneous Approach
0PW03KZ	Revision of Nonautologous Tissue Substitute in Sternum, Percutaneous Approach
0PW044Z	Revision of Internal Fixation Device in Sternum, Percutaneous Endoscopic Approach

0PW047Z Revision of Autologous Tissue Substitute in Sternum, Percutaneous Endoscopic Approach

0PW04JZ Revision of Synthetic Substitute in Sternum, Percutaneous Endoscopic Approach

0PW04KZ Revision of Nonautologous Tissue Substitute in Sternum, Percutaneous Endoscopic Approach

0PW0X4Z Revision of Internal Fixation Device in Sternum, External Approach

0PW0X7Z Revision of Autologous Tissue Substitute in Sternum, External Approach

0PW0XJZ Revision of Synthetic Substitute in Sternum, External Approach

0PW0XKZ Revision of Nonautologous Tissue Substitute in Sternum, External Approach

0PW104Z Revision of Internal Fixation Device in Right Rib, Open Approach

0PW107Z Revision of Autologous Tissue Substitute in Right Rib, Open Approach

0PW10JZ Revision of Synthetic Substitute in Right Rib, Open Approach

0PW10KZ Revision of Nonautologous Tissue Substitute in Right Rib, Open Approach

0PW134Z Revision of Internal Fixation Device in Right Rib, Percutaneous Approach

0PW137Z Revision of Autologous Tissue Substitute in Right Rib, Percutaneous Approach

0PW13JZ Revision of Synthetic Substitute in Right Rib, Percutaneous Approach

0PW13KZ Revision of Nonautologous Tissue Substitute in Right Rib, Percutaneous Approach

0PW144Z Revision of Internal Fixation Device in Right Rib, Percutaneous Endoscopic Approach

0PW147Z Revision of Autologous Tissue Substitute in Right Rib, Percutaneous Endoscopic Approach

0PW14JZ Revision of Synthetic Substitute in Right Rib, Percutaneous Endoscopic Approach

0PW14KZ Revision of Nonautologous Tissue Substitute in Right Rib, Percutaneous Endoscopic Approach

0PW1X4Z Revision of Internal Fixation Device in Right Rib, External Approach

0PW1X7Z Revision of Autologous Tissue Substitute in Right Rib, External Approach

0PW1XJZ Revision of Synthetic Substitute in Right Rib, External Approach

0PW1XKZ Revision of Nonautologous Tissue Substitute in Right Rib, External Approach

0PW204Z Revision of Internal Fixation Device in Left Rib, Open Approach

0PW207Z Revision of Autologous Tissue Substitute in Left Rib, Open Approach

0PW20JZ Revision of Synthetic Substitute in Left Rib, Open Approach

0PW20KZ Revision of Nonautologous Tissue Substitute in Left Rib, Open Approach

0PW234Z Revision of Internal Fixation Device in Left Rib, Percutaneous Approach

0PW237Z Revision of Autologous Tissue Substitute in Left Rib, Percutaneous Approach

0PW23JZ Revision of Synthetic Substitute in Left Rib, Percutaneous Approach

0PW23KZ Revision of Nonautologous Tissue Substitute in Left Rib, Percutaneous Approach

0PW244Z Revision of Internal Fixation Device in Left Rib, Percutaneous Endoscopic Approach

0PW247Z Revision of Autologous Tissue Substitute in Left Rib, Percutaneous Endoscopic Approach

0PW24JZ Revision of Synthetic Substitute in Left Rib, Percutaneous Endoscopic Approach

0PW24KZ Revision of Nonautologous Tissue Substitute in Left Rib, Percutaneous Endoscopic Approach

0PW2X4Z Revision of Internal Fixation Device in Left Rib, External Approach

0PW2X7Z Revision of Autologous Tissue Substitute in Left Rib, External Approach

0PW2XJZ Revision of Synthetic Substitute in Left Rib, External Approach

0PW2XKZ Revision of Nonautologous Tissue Substitute in Left Rib, External Approach

0PW304Z Revision of Internal Fixation Device in Cervical Vertebra, Open Approach

0PW307Z Revision of Autologous Tissue Substitute in Cervical Vertebra, Open Approach

0PW30JZ Revision of Synthetic Substitute in Cervical Vertebra, Open Approach

0PW30KZ Revision of Nonautologous Tissue Substitute in Cervical Vertebra, Open Approach

0PW334Z Revision of Internal Fixation Device in Cervical Vertebra, Percutaneous Approach

0PW337Z Revision of Autologous Tissue Substitute in Cervical Vertebra, Percutaneous Approach

0PW33JZ Revision of Synthetic Substitute in Cervical Vertebra, Percutaneous Approach

0PW33KZ Revision of Nonautologous Tissue Substitute in Cervical Vertebra, Percutaneous Approach

0PW344Z Revision of Internal Fixation Device in Cervical Vertebra, Percutaneous Endoscopic Approach

0PW347Z Revision of Autologous Tissue Substitute in Cervical Vertebra, Percutaneous Endoscopic Approach

0PW34JZ Revision of Synthetic Substitute in Cervical Vertebra, Percutaneous Endoscopic Approach

0PW34KZ Revision of Nonautologous Tissue Substitute in Cervical Vertebra, Percutaneous Endoscopic Approach

0PW3X4Z Revision of Internal Fixation Device in Cervical Vertebra, External Approach

0PW3X7Z Revision of Autologous Tissue Substitute in Cervical Vertebra, External Approach

0PW3XJZ Revision of Synthetic Substitute in Cervical Vertebra, External Approach

0PW3XKZ Revision of Nonautologous Tissue Substitute in Cervical Vertebra, External Approach

0PW404Z Revision of Internal Fixation Device in Thoracic Vertebra, Open Approach

0PW407Z Revision of Autologous Tissue Substitute in Thoracic Vertebra, Open Approach

0PW40JZ Revision of Synthetic Substitute in Thoracic Vertebra, Open Approach

0PW40KZ Revision of Nonautologous Tissue Substitute in Thoracic Vertebra, Open Approach

0PW434Z Revision of Internal Fixation Device in Thoracic Vertebra, Percutaneous Approach

0PW437Z Revision of Autologous Tissue Substitute in Thoracic Vertebra, Percutaneous Approach

0PW43JZ Revision of Synthetic Substitute in Thoracic Vertebra, Percutaneous Approach

0PW43KZ Revision of Nonautologous Tissue Substitute in Thoracic Vertebra, Percutaneous Approach

0PW444Z Revision of Internal Fixation Device in Thoracic Vertebra, Percutaneous Endoscopic Approach

0PW447Z Revision of Autologous Tissue Substitute in Thoracic Vertebra, Percutaneous Endoscopic Approach

0PW44JZ Revision of Synthetic Substitute in Thoracic Vertebra, Percutaneous Endoscopic Approach

0PW44KZ Revision of Nonautologous Tissue Substitute in Thoracic Vertebra, Percutaneous Endoscopic Approach

0PW4X4Z Revision of Internal Fixation Device in Thoracic Vertebra, External Approach

0PW4X7Z Revision of Autologous Tissue Substitute in Thoracic Vertebra, External Approach

0PW4XJZ Revision of Synthetic Substitute in Thoracic Vertebra, External Approach

0PW4XKZ Revision of Nonautologous Tissue Substitute in Thoracic Vertebra, External Approach

0PW504Z Revision of Internal Fixation Device in Right Scapula, Open Approach

0PW507Z Revision of Autologous Tissue Substitute in Right Scapula, Open Approach

0PW50JZ Revision of Synthetic Substitute in Right Scapula, Open Approach

0PW50KZ Revision of Nonautologous Tissue Substitute in Right Scapula, Open Approach

0PW534Z Revision of Internal Fixation Device in Right Scapula, Percutaneous Approach

0PW537Z Revision of Autologous Tissue Substitute in Right Scapula, Percutaneous Approach

0PW53JZ Revision of Synthetic Substitute in Right Scapula, Percutaneous Approach

---

♀ Female-only   ♂ Male-only   ● Limited Coverage   ● Non-OR   ▩ HAC-associated procedure   ● Non-covered procedures   ➕ Combination

0PW53KZ Revision of Nonautologous Tissue Substitute in Right Scapula, Percutaneous Approach

0PW544Z Revision of Internal Fixation Device in Right Scapula, Percutaneous Endoscopic Approach

0PW547Z Revision of Autologous Tissue Substitute in Right Scapula, Percutaneous Endoscopic Approach

0PW54JZ Revision of Synthetic Substitute in Right Scapula, Percutaneous Endoscopic Approach

0PW54KZ Revision of Nonautologous Tissue Substitute in Right Scapula, Percutaneous Endoscopic Approach

0PW5X4Z Revision of Internal Fixation Device in Right Scapula, External Approach

0PW5X7Z Revision of Autologous Tissue Substitute in Right Scapula, External Approach

0PW5XJZ Revision of Synthetic Substitute in Right Scapula, External Approach

0PW5XKZ Revision of Nonautologous Tissue Substitute in Right Scapula, External Approach

0PW604Z Revision of Internal Fixation Device in Left Scapula, Open Approach

0PW607Z Revision of Autologous Tissue Substitute in Left Scapula, Open Approach

0PW60JZ Revision of Synthetic Substitute in Left Scapula, Open Approach

0PW60KZ Revision of Nonautologous Tissue Substitute in Left Scapula, Open Approach

0PW634Z Revision of Internal Fixation Device in Left Scapula, Percutaneous Approach

0PW637Z Revision of Autologous Tissue Substitute in Left Scapula, Percutaneous Approach

0PW63JZ Revision of Synthetic Substitute in Left Scapula, Percutaneous Approach

0PW63KZ Revision of Nonautologous Tissue Substitute in Left Scapula, Percutaneous Approach

0PW644Z Revision of Internal Fixation Device in Left Scapula, Percutaneous Endoscopic Approach

0PW647Z Revision of Autologous Tissue Substitute in Left Scapula, Percutaneous Endoscopic Approach

0PW64JZ Revision of Synthetic Substitute in Left Scapula, Percutaneous Endoscopic Approach

0PW64KZ Revision of Nonautologous Tissue Substitute in Left Scapula, Percutaneous Endoscopic Approach

0PW6X4Z Revision of Internal Fixation Device in Left Scapula, External Approach

0PW6X7Z Revision of Autologous Tissue Substitute in Left Scapula, External Approach

0PW6XJZ Revision of Synthetic Substitute in Left Scapula, External Approach

0PW6XKZ Revision of Nonautologous Tissue Substitute in Left Scapula, External Approach

0PW704Z Revision of Internal Fixation Device in Right Glenoid Cavity, Open Approach

0PW707Z Revision of Autologous Tissue Substitute in Right Glenoid Cavity, Open Approach

0PW70JZ Revision of Synthetic Substitute in Right Glenoid Cavity, Open Approach

0PW70KZ Revision of Nonautologous Tissue Substitute in Right Glenoid Cavity, Open Approach

0PW734Z Revision of Internal Fixation Device in Right Glenoid Cavity, Percutaneous Approach

0PW737Z Revision of Autologous Tissue Substitute in Right Glenoid Cavity, Percutaneous Approach

0PW73JZ Revision of Synthetic Substitute in Right Glenoid Cavity, Percutaneous Approach

0PW73KZ Revision of Nonautologous Tissue Substitute in Right Glenoid Cavity, Percutaneous Approach

0PW744Z Revision of Internal Fixation Device in Right Glenoid Cavity, Percutaneous Endoscopic Approach

0PW747Z Revision of Autologous Tissue Substitute in Right Glenoid Cavity, Percutaneous Endoscopic Approach

0PW74JZ Revision of Synthetic Substitute in Right Glenoid Cavity, Percutaneous Endoscopic Approach

0PW74KZ Revision of Nonautologous Tissue Substitute in Right Glenoid Cavity, Percutaneous Endoscopic Approach

0PW7X4Z Revision of Internal Fixation Device in Right Glenoid Cavity, External Approach

0PW7X7Z Revision of Autologous Tissue Substitute in Right Glenoid Cavity, External Approach

0PW7XJZ Revision of Synthetic Substitute in Right Glenoid Cavity, External Approach

0PW7XKZ Revision of Nonautologous Tissue Substitute in Right Glenoid Cavity, External Approach

0PW804Z Revision of Internal Fixation Device in Left Glenoid Cavity, Open Approach

0PW807Z Revision of Autologous Tissue Substitute in Left Glenoid Cavity, Open Approach

0PW80JZ Revision of Synthetic Substitute in Left Glenoid Cavity, Open Approach

0PW80KZ Revision of Nonautologous Tissue Substitute in Left Glenoid Cavity, Open Approach

0PW834Z Revision of Internal Fixation Device in Left Glenoid Cavity, Percutaneous Approach

0PW837Z Revision of Autologous Tissue Substitute in Left Glenoid Cavity, Percutaneous Approach

0PW83JZ Revision of Synthetic Substitute in Left Glenoid Cavity, Percutaneous Approach

0PW83KZ Revision of Nonautologous Tissue Substitute in Left Glenoid Cavity, Percutaneous Approach

0PW844Z Revision of Internal Fixation Device in Left Glenoid Cavity, Percutaneous Endoscopic Approach

0PW847Z Revision of Autologous Tissue Substitute in Left Glenoid Cavity, Percutaneous Endoscopic Approach

0PW84JZ Revision of Synthetic Substitute in Left Glenoid Cavity, Percutaneous Endoscopic Approach

0PW84KZ Revision of Nonautologous Tissue Substitute in Left Glenoid Cavity, Percutaneous Endoscopic Approach

0PW8X4Z Revision of Internal Fixation Device in Left Glenoid Cavity, External Approach

0PW8X7Z Revision of Autologous Tissue Substitute in Left Glenoid Cavity, External Approach

0PW8XJZ Revision of Synthetic Substitute in Left Glenoid Cavity, External Approach

0PW8XKZ Revision of Nonautologous Tissue Substitute in Left Glenoid Cavity, External Approach

0PW904Z Revision of Internal Fixation Device in Right Clavicle, Open Approach

0PW907Z Revision of Autologous Tissue Substitute in Right Clavicle, Open Approach

0PW90JZ Revision of Synthetic Substitute in Right Clavicle, Open Approach

0PW90KZ Revision of Nonautologous Tissue Substitute in Right Clavicle, Open Approach

0PW934Z Revision of Internal Fixation Device in Right Clavicle, Percutaneous Approach

0PW937Z Revision of Autologous Tissue Substitute in Right Clavicle, Percutaneous Approach

0PW93JZ Revision of Synthetic Substitute in Right Clavicle, Percutaneous Approach

0PW93KZ Revision of Nonautologous Tissue Substitute in Right Clavicle, Percutaneous Approach

0PW944Z Revision of Internal Fixation Device in Right Clavicle, Percutaneous Endoscopic Approach

0PW947Z Revision of Autologous Tissue Substitute in Right Clavicle, Percutaneous Endoscopic Approach

0PW94JZ Revision of Synthetic Substitute in Right Clavicle, Percutaneous Endoscopic Approach

0PW94KZ Revision of Nonautologous Tissue Substitute in Right Clavicle, Percutaneous Endoscopic Approach

0PW9X4Z Revision of Internal Fixation Device in Right Clavicle, External Approach

0PW9X7Z Revision of Autologous Tissue Substitute in Right Clavicle, External Approach

0PW9XJZ Revision of Synthetic Substitute in Right Clavicle, External Approach

0PW9XKZ Revision of Nonautologous Tissue Substitute in Right Clavicle, External Approach

0PWB04Z Revision of Internal Fixation Device in Left Clavicle, Open Approach

0PWB07Z Revision of Autologous Tissue Substitute in Left Clavicle, Open Approach

0PWB0JZ Revision of Synthetic Substitute in Left Clavicle, Open Approach

0PWB0KZ Revision of Nonautologous Tissue Substitute in Left Clavicle, Open Approach

0PWB34Z Revision of Internal Fixation Device in Left Clavicle, Percutaneous Approach

0PWB37Z Revision of Autologous Tissue Substitute in Left Clavicle, Percutaneous Approach

0PWB3JZ Revision of Synthetic Substitute in Left Clavicle, Percutaneous Approach

0PWB3KZ Revision of Nonautologous Tissue Substitute in Left Clavicle, Percutaneous Approach

0PWB44Z Revision of Internal Fixation Device in Left Clavicle, Percutaneous Endoscopic Approach

0PWB47Z Revision of Autologous Tissue Substitute in Left Clavicle, Percutaneous Endoscopic Approach

0PWB4JZ Revision of Synthetic Substitute in Left Clavicle, Percutaneous Endoscopic Approach

0PWB4KZ Revision of Nonautologous Tissue Substitute in Left Clavicle, Percutaneous Endoscopic Approach

0PWBX4Z Revision of Internal Fixation Device in Left Clavicle, External Approach

0PWBX7Z Revision of Autologous Tissue Substitute in Left Clavicle, External Approach

0PWBXJZ Revision of Synthetic Substitute in Left Clavicle, External Approach

0PWBXKZ Revision of Nonautologous Tissue Substitute in Left Clavicle, External Approach

0PWC04Z Revision of Internal Fixation Device in Right Humeral Head, Open Approach

0PWC05Z Revision of External Fixation Device in Right Humeral Head, Open Approach

0PWC07Z Revision of Autologous Tissue Substitute in Right Humeral Head, Open Approach

0PWC0JZ Revision of Synthetic Substitute in Right Humeral Head, Open Approach

0PWC0KZ Revision of Nonautologous Tissue Substitute in Right Humeral Head, Open Approach

0PWC34Z Revision of Internal Fixation Device in Right Humeral Head, Percutaneous Approach

0PWC35Z Revision of External Fixation Device in Right Humeral Head, Percutaneous Approach

0PWC37Z Revision of Autologous Tissue Substitute in Right Humeral Head, Percutaneous Approach

0PWC3JZ Revision of Synthetic Substitute in Right Humeral Head, Percutaneous Approach

0PWC3KZ Revision of Nonautologous Tissue Substitute in Right Humeral Head, Percutaneous Approach

0PWC44Z Revision of Internal Fixation Device in Right Humeral Head, Percutaneous Endoscopic Approach

0PWC45Z Revision of External Fixation Device in Right Humeral Head, Percutaneous Endoscopic Approach

0PWC47Z Revision of Autologous Tissue Substitute in Right Humeral Head, Percutaneous Endoscopic Approach

0PWC4JZ Revision of Synthetic Substitute in Right Humeral Head, Percutaneous Endoscopic Approach

0PWC4KZ Revision of Nonautologous Tissue Substitute in Right Humeral Head, Percutaneous Endoscopic Approach

0PWCX4Z Revision of Internal Fixation Device in Right Humeral Head, External Approach

0PWCX5Z Revision of External Fixation Device in Right Humeral Head, External Approach

0PWCX7Z Revision of Autologous Tissue Substitute in Right Humeral Head, External Approach

0PWCXJZ Revision of Synthetic Substitute in Right Humeral Head, External Approach

0PWCXKZ Revision of Nonautologous Tissue Substitute in Right Humeral Head, External Approach

0PWD04Z Revision of Internal Fixation Device in Left Humeral Head, Open Approach

0PWD05Z Revision of External Fixation Device in Left Humeral Head, Open Approach

0PWD07Z Revision of Autologous Tissue Substitute in Left Humeral Head, Open Approach

0PWD0JZ Revision of Synthetic Substitute in Left Humeral Head, Open Approach

0PWD0KZ Revision of Nonautologous Tissue Substitute in Left Humeral Head, Open Approach

0PWD34Z Revision of Internal Fixation Device in Left Humeral Head, Percutaneous Approach

0PWD35Z Revision of External Fixation Device in Left Humeral Head, Percutaneous Approach

0PWD37Z Revision of Autologous Tissue Substitute in Left Humeral Head, Percutaneous Approach

0PWD3JZ Revision of Synthetic Substitute in Left Humeral Head, Percutaneous Approach

0PWD3KZ Revision of Nonautologous Tissue Substitute in Left Humeral Head, Percutaneous Approach

0PWD44Z Revision of Internal Fixation Device in Left Humeral Head, Percutaneous Endoscopic Approach

0PWD45Z Revision of External Fixation Device in Left Humeral Head, Percutaneous Endoscopic Approach

0PWD47Z Revision of Autologous Tissue Substitute in Left Humeral Head, Percutaneous Endoscopic Approach

0PWD4JZ Revision of Synthetic Substitute in Left Humeral Head, Percutaneous Endoscopic Approach

0PWD4KZ Revision of Nonautologous Tissue Substitute in Left Humeral Head, Percutaneous Endoscopic Approach

0PWDX4Z Revision of Internal Fixation Device in Left Humeral Head, External Approach

0PWDX5Z Revision of External Fixation Device in Left Humeral Head, External Approach

0PWDX7Z Revision of Autologous Tissue Substitute in Left Humeral Head, External Approach

0PWDXJZ Revision of Synthetic Substitute in Left Humeral Head, External Approach

0PWDXKZ Revision of Nonautologous Tissue Substitute in Left Humeral Head, External Approach

0PWF04Z Revision of Internal Fixation Device in Right Humeral Shaft, Open Approach

0PWF05Z Revision of External Fixation Device in Right Humeral Shaft, Open Approach

0PWF07Z Revision of Autologous Tissue Substitute in Right Humeral Shaft, Open Approach

0PWF0JZ Revision of Synthetic Substitute in Right Humeral Shaft, Open Approach

0PWF0KZ Revision of Nonautologous Tissue Substitute in Right Humeral Shaft, Open Approach

0PWF34Z Revision of Internal Fixation Device in Right Humeral Shaft, Percutaneous Approach

0PWF35Z Revision of External Fixation Device in Right Humeral Shaft, Percutaneous Approach

0PWF37Z Revision of Autologous Tissue Substitute in Right Humeral Shaft, Percutaneous Approach

0PWF3JZ Revision of Synthetic Substitute in Right Humeral Shaft, Percutaneous Approach

0PWF3KZ Revision of Nonautologous Tissue Substitute in Right Humeral Shaft, Percutaneous Approach

0PWF44Z Revision of Internal Fixation Device in Right Humeral Shaft, Percutaneous Endoscopic Approach

0PWF45Z Revision of External Fixation Device in Right Humeral Shaft, Percutaneous Endoscopic Approach

0PWF47Z Revision of Autologous Tissue Substitute in Right Humeral Shaft, Percutaneous Endoscopic Approach

0PWF4JZ Revision of Synthetic Substitute in Right Humeral Shaft, Percutaneous Endoscopic Approach

0PWF4KZ Revision of Nonautologous Tissue Substitute in Right Humeral Shaft, Percutaneous Endoscopic Approach

0PWFX4Z Revision of Internal Fixation Device in Right Humeral Shaft, External Approach

0PWFX5Z Revision of External Fixation Device in Right Humeral Shaft, External Approach

0PWFX7Z Revision of Autologous Tissue Substitute in Right Humeral Shaft, External Approach

0PWFXJZ Revision of Synthetic Substitute in Right Humeral Shaft, External Approach

0PWFXKZ Revision of Nonautologous Tissue Substitute in Right Humeral Shaft, External Approach

0PWG04Z Revision of Internal Fixation Device in Left Humeral Shaft, Open Approach

0PWG05Z Revision of External Fixation Device in Left Humeral Shaft, Open Approach

0PWG07Z Revision of Autologous Tissue Substitute in Left Humeral Shaft, Open Approach

0PWG0JZ Revision of Synthetic Substitute in Left Humeral Shaft, Open Approach

0PWG0KZ Revision of Nonautologous Tissue Substitute in Left Humeral Shaft, Open Approach

0PWG34Z Revision of Internal Fixation Device in Left Humeral Shaft, Percutaneous Approach

0PWG35Z Revision of External Fixation Device in Left Humeral Shaft, Percutaneous Approach

0PWG37Z Revision of Autologous Tissue Substitute in Left Humeral Shaft, Percutaneous Approach

0PWG3JZ Revision of Synthetic Substitute in Left Humeral Shaft, Percutaneous Approach

0PWG3KZ Revision of Nonautologous Tissue Substitute in Left Humeral Shaft, Percutaneous Approach

0PWG44Z Revision of Internal Fixation Device in Left Humeral Shaft, Percutaneous Endoscopic Approach

0PWG45Z Revision of External Fixation Device in Left Humeral Shaft, Percutaneous Endoscopic Approach

0PWG47Z Revision of Autologous Tissue Substitute in Left Humeral Shaft, Percutaneous Endoscopic Approach

0PWG4JZ Revision of Synthetic Substitute in Left Humeral Shaft, Percutaneous Endoscopic Approach

0PWG4KZ Revision of Nonautologous Tissue Substitute in Left Humeral Shaft, Percutaneous Endoscopic Approach

0PWGX4Z Revision of Internal Fixation Device in Left Humeral Shaft, External Approach

0PWGX5Z Revision of External Fixation Device in Left Humeral Shaft, External Approach

0PWGX7Z Revision of Autologous Tissue Substitute in Left Humeral Shaft, External Approach

0PWGXJZ Revision of Synthetic Substitute in Left Humeral Shaft, External Approach

0PWGXKZ Revision of Nonautologous Tissue Substitute in Left Humeral Shaft, External Approach

0PWH04Z Revision of Internal Fixation Device in Right Radius, Open Approach

0PWH05Z Revision of External Fixation Device in Right Radius, Open Approach

0PWH07Z Revision of Autologous Tissue Substitute in Right Radius, Open Approach

0PWH0JZ Revision of Synthetic Substitute in Right Radius, Open Approach

0PWH0KZ Revision of Nonautologous Tissue Substitute in Right Radius, Open Approach

0PWH34Z Revision of Internal Fixation Device in Right Radius, Percutaneous Approach

0PWH35Z Revision of External Fixation Device in Right Radius, Percutaneous Approach

0PWH37Z Revision of Autologous Tissue Substitute in Right Radius, Percutaneous Approach

0PWH3JZ Revision of Synthetic Substitute in Right Radius, Percutaneous Approach

0PWH3KZ Revision of Nonautologous Tissue Substitute in Right Radius, Percutaneous Approach

0PWH44Z Revision of Internal Fixation Device in Right Radius, Percutaneous Endoscopic Approach

0PWH45Z Revision of External Fixation Device in Right Radius, Percutaneous Endoscopic Approach

0PWH47Z Revision of Autologous Tissue Substitute in Right Radius, Percutaneous Endoscopic Approach

0PWH4JZ Revision of Synthetic Substitute in Right Radius, Percutaneous Endoscopic Approach

0PWH4KZ Revision of Nonautologous Tissue Substitute in Right Radius, Percutaneous Endoscopic Approach

0PWHX4Z Revision of Internal Fixation Device in Right Radius, External Approach

0PWHX5Z Revision of External Fixation Device in Right Radius, External Approach

0PWHX7Z Revision of Autologous Tissue Substitute in Right Radius, External Approach

0PWHXJZ Revision of Synthetic Substitute in Right Radius, External Approach

0PWHXKZ Revision of Nonautologous Tissue Substitute in Right Radius, External Approach

0PWJ04Z Revision of Internal Fixation Device in Left Radius, Open Approach

0PWJ05Z Revision of External Fixation Device in Left Radius, Open Approach

0PWJ07Z Revision of Autologous Tissue Substitute in Left Radius, Open Approach

0PWJ0JZ Revision of Synthetic Substitute in Left Radius, Open Approach

0PWJ0KZ Revision of Nonautologous Tissue Substitute in Left Radius, Open Approach

0PWJ34Z Revision of Internal Fixation Device in Left Radius, Percutaneous Approach

0PWJ35Z Revision of External Fixation Device in Left Radius, Percutaneous Approach

0PWJ37Z Revision of Autologous Tissue Substitute in Left Radius, Percutaneous Approach

0PWJ3JZ Revision of Synthetic Substitute in Left Radius, Percutaneous Approach

0PWJ3KZ Revision of Nonautologous Tissue Substitute in Left Radius, Percutaneous Approach

0PWJ44Z Revision of Internal Fixation Device in Left Radius, Percutaneous Endoscopic Approach

0PWJ45Z Revision of External Fixation Device in Left Radius, Percutaneous Endoscopic Approach

0PWJ47Z Revision of Autologous Tissue Substitute in Left Radius, Percutaneous Endoscopic Approach

0PWJ4JZ Revision of Synthetic Substitute in Left Radius, Percutaneous Endoscopic Approach

0PWJ4KZ Revision of Nonautologous Tissue Substitute in Left Radius, Percutaneous Endoscopic Approach

0PWJX4Z Revision of Internal Fixation Device in Left Radius, External Approach

0PWJX5Z Revision of External Fixation Device in Left Radius, External Approach

0PWJX7Z Revision of Autologous Tissue Substitute in Left Radius, External Approach

0PWJXJZ Revision of Synthetic Substitute in Left Radius, External Approach

0PWJXKZ Revision of Nonautologous Tissue Substitute in Left Radius, External Approach

0PWK04Z Revision of Internal Fixation Device in Right Ulna, Open Approach

0PWK05Z Revision of External Fixation Device in Right Ulna, Open Approach

0PWK07Z Revision of Autologous Tissue Substitute in Right Ulna, Open Approach

0PWK0JZ Revision of Synthetic Substitute in Right Ulna, Open Approach

0PWK0KZ Revision of Nonautologous Tissue Substitute in Right Ulna, Open Approach

0PWK34Z Revision of Internal Fixation Device in Right Ulna, Percutaneous Approach

0PWK35Z Revision of External Fixation Device in Right Ulna, Percutaneous Approach

0PWK37Z Revision of Autologous Tissue Substitute in Right Ulna, Percutaneous Approach

0PWK3JZ Revision of Synthetic Substitute in Right Ulna, Percutaneous Approach

0PWK3KZ Revision of Nonautologous Tissue Substitute in Right Ulna, Percutaneous Approach

0PWK44Z Revision of Internal Fixation Device in Right Ulna, Percutaneous Endoscopic Approach

0PWK45Z Revision of External Fixation Device in Right Ulna, Percutaneous Endoscopic Approach

0PWK47Z Revision of Autologous Tissue Substitute in Right Ulna, Percutaneous Endoscopic Approach

0PWK4JZ Revision of Synthetic Substitute in Right Ulna, Percutaneous Endoscopic Approach

0PWK4KZ Revision of Nonautologous Tissue Substitute in Right Ulna, Percutaneous Endoscopic Approach

0PWKX4Z Revision of Internal Fixation Device in Right Ulna, External Approach

0PWKX5Z Revision of External Fixation Device in Right Ulna, External Approach

0PWKX7Z Revision of Autologous Tissue Substitute in Right Ulna, External Approach
0PWKXJZ Revision of Synthetic Substitute in Right Ulna, External Approach
0PWKXKZ Revision of Nonautologous Tissue Substitute in Right Ulna, External Approach
0PWL04Z Revision of Internal Fixation Device in Left Ulna, Open Approach
0PWL05Z Revision of External Fixation Device in Left Ulna, Open Approach
0PWL07Z Revision of Autologous Tissue Substitute in Left Ulna, Open Approach
0PWL0JZ Revision of Synthetic Substitute in Left Ulna, Open Approach
0PWL0KZ Revision of Nonautologous Tissue Substitute in Left Ulna, Open Approach
0PWL34Z Revision of Internal Fixation Device in Left Ulna, Percutaneous Approach
0PWL35Z Revision of External Fixation Device in Left Ulna, Percutaneous Approach
0PWL37Z Revision of Autologous Tissue Substitute in Left Ulna, Percutaneous Approach
0PWL3JZ Revision of Synthetic Substitute in Left Ulna, Percutaneous Approach
0PWL3KZ Revision of Nonautologous Tissue Substitute in Left Ulna, Percutaneous Approach
0PWL44Z Revision of Internal Fixation Device in Left Ulna, Percutaneous Endoscopic Approach
0PWL45Z Revision of External Fixation Device in Left Ulna, Percutaneous Endoscopic Approach
0PWL47Z Revision of Autologous Tissue Substitute in Left Ulna, Percutaneous Endoscopic Approach
0PWL4JZ Revision of Synthetic Substitute in Left Ulna, Percutaneous Endoscopic Approach
0PWL4KZ Revision of Nonautologous Tissue Substitute in Left Ulna, Percutaneous Endoscopic Approach
0PWLX4Z Revision of Internal Fixation Device in Left Ulna, External Approach
0PWLX5Z Revision of External Fixation Device in Left Ulna, External Approach
0PWLX7Z Revision of Autologous Tissue Substitute in Left Ulna, External Approach
0PWLXJZ Revision of Synthetic Substitute in Left Ulna, External Approach
0PWLXKZ Revision of Nonautologous Tissue Substitute in Left Ulna, External Approach
0PWM04Z Revision of Internal Fixation Device in Right Carpal, Open Approach
0PWM05Z Revision of External Fixation Device in Right Carpal, Open Approach
0PWM07Z Revision of Autologous Tissue Substitute in Right Carpal, Open Approach
0PWM0JZ Revision of Synthetic Substitute in Right Carpal, Open Approach
0PWM0KZ Revision of Nonautologous Tissue Substitute in Right Carpal, Open Approach
0PWM34Z Revision of Internal Fixation Device in Right Carpal, Percutaneous Approach
0PWM35Z Revision of External Fixation Device in Right Carpal, Percutaneous Approach
0PWM37Z Revision of Autologous Tissue Substitute in Right Carpal, Percutaneous Approach
0PWM3JZ Revision of Synthetic Substitute in Right Carpal, Percutaneous Approach
0PWM3KZ Revision of Nonautologous Tissue Substitute in Right Carpal, Percutaneous Approach
0PWM44Z Revision of Internal Fixation Device in Right Carpal, Percutaneous Endoscopic Approach
0PWM45Z Revision of External Fixation Device in Right Carpal, Percutaneous Endoscopic Approach
0PWM47Z Revision of Autologous Tissue Substitute in Right Carpal, Percutaneous Endoscopic Approach
0PWM4JZ Revision of Synthetic Substitute in Right Carpal, Percutaneous Endoscopic Approach
0PWM4KZ Revision of Nonautologous Tissue Substitute in Right Carpal, Percutaneous Endoscopic Approach
0PWMX4Z Revision of Internal Fixation Device in Right Carpal, External Approach
0PWMX5Z Revision of External Fixation Device in Right Carpal, External Approach

0PWMX7Z Revision of Autologous Tissue Substitute in Right Carpal, External Approach
0PWMXJZ Revision of Synthetic Substitute in Right Carpal, External Approach
0PWMXKZ Revision of Nonautologous Tissue Substitute in Right Carpal, External Approach
0PWN04Z Revision of Internal Fixation Device in Left Carpal, Open Approach
0PWN05Z Revision of External Fixation Device in Left Carpal, Open Approach
0PWN07Z Revision of Autologous Tissue Substitute in Left Carpal, Open Approach
0PWN0JZ Revision of Synthetic Substitute in Left Carpal, Open Approach
0PWN0KZ Revision of Nonautologous Tissue Substitute in Left Carpal, Open Approach
0PWN34Z Revision of Internal Fixation Device in Left Carpal, Percutaneous Approach
0PWN35Z Revision of External Fixation Device in Left Carpal, Percutaneous Approach
0PWN37Z Revision of Autologous Tissue Substitute in Left Carpal, Percutaneous Approach
0PWN3JZ Revision of Synthetic Substitute in Left Carpal, Percutaneous Approach
0PWN3KZ Revision of Nonautologous Tissue Substitute in Left Carpal, Percutaneous Approach
0PWN44Z Revision of Internal Fixation Device in Left Carpal, Percutaneous Endoscopic Approach
0PWN45Z Revision of External Fixation Device in Left Carpal, Percutaneous Endoscopic Approach
0PWN47Z Revision of Autologous Tissue Substitute in Left Carpal, Percutaneous Endoscopic Approach
0PWN4JZ Revision of Synthetic Substitute in Left Carpal, Percutaneous Endoscopic Approach
0PWN4KZ Revision of Nonautologous Tissue Substitute in Left Carpal, Percutaneous Endoscopic Approach
0PWNX4Z Revision of Internal Fixation Device in Left Carpal, External Approach
0PWNX5Z Revision of External Fixation Device in Left Carpal, External Approach
0PWNX7Z Revision of Autologous Tissue Substitute in Left Carpal, External Approach
0PWNXJZ Revision of Synthetic Substitute in Left Carpal, External Approach
0PWNXKZ Revision of Nonautologous Tissue Substitute in Left Carpal, External Approach
0PWP04Z Revision of Internal Fixation Device in Right Metacarpal, Open Approach
0PWP05Z Revision of External Fixation Device in Right Metacarpal, Open Approach
0PWP07Z Revision of Autologous Tissue Substitute in Right Metacarpal, Open Approach
0PWP0JZ Revision of Synthetic Substitute in Right Metacarpal, Open Approach
0PWP0KZ Revision of Nonautologous Tissue Substitute in Right Metacarpal, Open Approach
0PWP34Z Revision of Internal Fixation Device in Right Metacarpal, Percutaneous Approach
0PWP35Z Revision of External Fixation Device in Right Metacarpal, Percutaneous Approach
0PWP37Z Revision of Autologous Tissue Substitute in Right Metacarpal, Percutaneous Approach
0PWP3JZ Revision of Synthetic Substitute in Right Metacarpal, Percutaneous Approach
0PWP3KZ Revision of Nonautologous Tissue Substitute in Right Metacarpal, Percutaneous Approach
0PWP44Z Revision of Internal Fixation Device in Right Metacarpal, Percutaneous Endoscopic Approach
0PWP45Z Revision of External Fixation Device in Right Metacarpal, Percutaneous Endoscopic Approach
0PWP47Z Revision of Autologous Tissue Substitute in Right Metacarpal, Percutaneous Endoscopic Approach
0PWP4JZ Revision of Synthetic Substitute in Right Metacarpal, Percutaneous Endoscopic Approach
0PWP4KZ Revision of Nonautologous Tissue Substitute in Right Metacarpal, Percutaneous Endoscopic Approach

0PWPX4Z   Revision of Internal Fixation Device in Right Metacarpal, External Approach

0PWPX5Z   Revision of External Fixation Device in Right Metacarpal, External Approach

0PWPX7Z   Revision of Autologous Tissue Substitute in Right Metacarpal, External Approach

0PWPXJZ   Revision of Synthetic Substitute in Right Metacarpal, External Approach

0PWPXKZ   Revision of Nonautologous Tissue Substitute in Right Metacarpal, External Approach

0PWQ04Z   Revision of Internal Fixation Device in Left Metacarpal, Open Approach

0PWQ05Z   Revision of External Fixation Device in Left Metacarpal, Open Approach

0PWQ07Z   Revision of Autologous Tissue Substitute in Left Metacarpal, Open Approach

0PWQ0JZ   Revision of Synthetic Substitute in Left Metacarpal, Open Approach

0PWQ0KZ   Revision of Nonautologous Tissue Substitute in Left Metacarpal, Open Approach

0PWQ34Z   Revision of Internal Fixation Device in Left Metacarpal, Percutaneous Approach

0PWQ35Z   Revision of External Fixation Device in Left Metacarpal, Percutaneous Approach

0PWQ37Z   Revision of Autologous Tissue Substitute in Left Metacarpal, Percutaneous Approach

0PWQ3JZ   Revision of Synthetic Substitute in Left Metacarpal, Percutaneous Approach

0PWQ3KZ   Revision of Nonautologous Tissue Substitute in Left Metacarpal, Percutaneous Approach

0PWQ44Z   Revision of Internal Fixation Device in Left Metacarpal, Percutaneous Endoscopic Approach

0PWQ45Z   Revision of External Fixation Device in Left Metacarpal, Percutaneous Endoscopic Approach

0PWQ47Z   Revision of Autologous Tissue Substitute in Left Metacarpal, Percutaneous Endoscopic Approach

0PWQ4JZ   Revision of Synthetic Substitute in Left Metacarpal, Percutaneous Endoscopic Approach

0PWQ4KZ   Revision of Nonautologous Tissue Substitute in Left Metacarpal, Percutaneous Endoscopic Approach

0PWQX4Z   Revision of Internal Fixation Device in Left Metacarpal, External Approach

0PWQX5Z   Revision of External Fixation Device in Left Metacarpal, External Approach

0PWQX7Z   Revision of Autologous Tissue Substitute in Left Metacarpal, External Approach

0PWQXJZ   Revision of Synthetic Substitute in Left Metacarpal, External Approach

0PWQXKZ   Revision of Nonautologous Tissue Substitute in Left Metacarpal, External Approach

0PWR04Z   Revision of Internal Fixation Device in Right Thumb Phalanx, Open Approach

0PWR05Z   Revision of External Fixation Device in Right Thumb Phalanx, Open Approach

0PWR07Z   Revision of Autologous Tissue Substitute in Right Thumb Phalanx, Open Approach

0PWR0JZ   Revision of Synthetic Substitute in Right Thumb Phalanx, Open Approach

0PWR0KZ   Revision of Nonautologous Tissue Substitute in Right Thumb Phalanx, Open Approach

0PWR34Z   Revision of Internal Fixation Device in Right Thumb Phalanx, Percutaneous Approach

0PWR35Z   Revision of External Fixation Device in Right Thumb Phalanx, Percutaneous Approach

0PWR37Z   Revision of Autologous Tissue Substitute in Right Thumb Phalanx, Percutaneous Approach

0PWR3JZ   Revision of Synthetic Substitute in Right Thumb Phalanx, Percutaneous Approach

0PWR3KZ   Revision of Nonautologous Tissue Substitute in Right Thumb Phalanx, Percutaneous Approach

0PWR44Z   Revision of Internal Fixation Device in Right Thumb Phalanx, Percutaneous Endoscopic Approach

0PWR45Z   Revision of External Fixation Device in Right Thumb Phalanx, Percutaneous Endoscopic Approach

0PWR47Z   Revision of Autologous Tissue Substitute in Right Thumb Phalanx, Percutaneous Endoscopic Approach

0PWR4JZ   Revision of Synthetic Substitute in Right Thumb Phalanx, Percutaneous Endoscopic Approach

0PWR4KZ   Revision of Nonautologous Tissue Substitute in Right Thumb Phalanx, Percutaneous Endoscopic Approach

0PWRX4Z   Revision of Internal Fixation Device in Right Thumb Phalanx, External Approach

0PWRX5Z   Revision of External Fixation Device in Right Thumb Phalanx, External Approach

0PWRX7Z   Revision of Autologous Tissue Substitute in Right Thumb Phalanx, External Approach

0PWRXJZ   Revision of Synthetic Substitute in Right Thumb Phalanx, External Approach

0PWRXKZ   Revision of Nonautologous Tissue Substitute in Right Thumb Phalanx, External Approach

0PWS04Z   Revision of Internal Fixation Device in Left Thumb Phalanx, Open Approach

0PWS05Z   Revision of External Fixation Device in Left Thumb Phalanx, Open Approach

0PWS07Z   Revision of Autologous Tissue Substitute in Left Thumb Phalanx, Open Approach

0PWS0JZ   Revision of Synthetic Substitute in Left Thumb Phalanx, Open Approach

0PWS0KZ   Revision of Nonautologous Tissue Substitute in Left Thumb Phalanx, Open Approach

0PWS34Z   Revision of Internal Fixation Device in Left Thumb Phalanx, Percutaneous Approach

0PWS35Z   Revision of External Fixation Device in Left Thumb Phalanx, Percutaneous Approach

0PWS37Z   Revision of Autologous Tissue Substitute in Left Thumb Phalanx, Percutaneous Approach

0PWS3JZ   Revision of Synthetic Substitute in Left Thumb Phalanx, Percutaneous Approach

0PWS3KZ   Revision of Nonautologous Tissue Substitute in Left Thumb Phalanx, Percutaneous Approach

0PWS44Z   Revision of Internal Fixation Device in Left Thumb Phalanx, Percutaneous Endoscopic Approach

0PWS45Z   Revision of External Fixation Device in Left Thumb Phalanx, Percutaneous Endoscopic Approach

0PWS47Z   Revision of Autologous Tissue Substitute in Left Thumb Phalanx, Percutaneous Endoscopic Approach

0PWS4JZ   Revision of Synthetic Substitute in Left Thumb Phalanx, Percutaneous Endoscopic Approach

0PWS4KZ   Revision of Nonautologous Tissue Substitute in Left Thumb Phalanx, Percutaneous Endoscopic Approach

0PWSX4Z   Revision of Internal Fixation Device in Left Thumb Phalanx, External Approach

0PWSX5Z   Revision of External Fixation Device in Left Thumb Phalanx, External Approach

0PWSX7Z   Revision of Autologous Tissue Substitute in Left Thumb Phalanx, External Approach

0PWSXJZ   Revision of Synthetic Substitute in Left Thumb Phalanx, External Approach

0PWSXKZ   Revision of Nonautologous Tissue Substitute in Left Thumb Phalanx, External Approach

0PWT04Z   Revision of Internal Fixation Device in Right Finger Phalanx, Open Approach

0PWT05Z   Revision of External Fixation Device in Right Finger Phalanx, Open Approach

0PWT07Z   Revision of Autologous Tissue Substitute in Right Finger Phalanx, Open Approach

0PWT0JZ   Revision of Synthetic Substitute in Right Finger Phalanx, Open Approach

0PWT0KZ   Revision of Nonautologous Tissue Substitute in Right Finger Phalanx, Open Approach

0PWT34Z   Revision of Internal Fixation Device in Right Finger Phalanx, Percutaneous Approach

0PWT35Z   Revision of External Fixation Device in Right Finger Phalanx, Percutaneous Approach

0PWT37Z   Revision of Autologous Tissue Substitute in Right Finger Phalanx, Percutaneous Approach

0PWT3JZ   Revision of Synthetic Substitute in Right Finger Phalanx, Percutaneous Approach

---

♀ Female-only   ♂ Male-only   ● Limited Coverage   ● Non-OR   ▨ HAC-associated procedure   ● Non-covered procedures   ✚ Combination

0PWT3KZ   Revision of Nonautologous Tissue Substitute in Right Finger Phalanx, Percutaneous Approach

0PWT44Z   Revision of Internal Fixation Device in Right Finger Phalanx, Percutaneous Endoscopic Approach

0PWT45Z   Revision of External Fixation Device in Right Finger Phalanx, Percutaneous Endoscopic Approach

0PWT47Z   Revision of Autologous Tissue Substitute in Right Finger Phalanx, Percutaneous Endoscopic Approach

0PWT4JZ   Revision of Synthetic Substitute in Right Finger Phalanx, Percutaneous Endoscopic Approach

0PWT4KZ   Revision of Nonautologous Tissue Substitute in Right Finger Phalanx, Percutaneous Endoscopic Approach

0PWTX4Z   Revision of Internal Fixation Device in Right Finger Phalanx, External Approach

0PWTX5Z   Revision of External Fixation Device in Right Finger Phalanx, External Approach

0PWTX7Z   Revision of Autologous Tissue Substitute in Right Finger Phalanx, External Approach

0PWTXJZ   Revision of Synthetic Substitute in Right Finger Phalanx, External Approach

0PWTXKZ   Revision of Nonautologous Tissue Substitute in Right Finger Phalanx, External Approach

0PWV04Z   Revision of Internal Fixation Device in Left Finger Phalanx, Open Approach

0PWV05Z   Revision of External Fixation Device in Left Finger Phalanx, Open Approach

0PWV07Z   Revision of Autologous Tissue Substitute in Left Finger Phalanx, Open Approach

0PWV0JZ   Revision of Synthetic Substitute in Left Finger Phalanx, Open Approach

0PWV0KZ   Revision of Nonautologous Tissue Substitute in Left Finger Phalanx, Open Approach

0PWV34Z   Revision of Internal Fixation Device in Left Finger Phalanx, Percutaneous Approach

0PWV35Z   Revision of External Fixation Device in Left Finger Phalanx, Percutaneous Approach

0PWV37Z   Revision of Autologous Tissue Substitute in Left Finger Phalanx, Percutaneous Approach

0PWV3JZ   Revision of Synthetic Substitute in Left Finger Phalanx, Percutaneous Approach

0PWV3KZ   Revision of Nonautologous Tissue Substitute in Left Finger Phalanx, Percutaneous Approach

0PWV44Z   Revision of Internal Fixation Device in Left Finger Phalanx, Percutaneous Endoscopic Approach

0PWV45Z   Revision of External Fixation Device in Left Finger Phalanx, Percutaneous Endoscopic Approach

0PWV47Z   Revision of Autologous Tissue Substitute in Left Finger Phalanx, Percutaneous Endoscopic Approach

0PWV4JZ   Revision of Synthetic Substitute in Left Finger Phalanx, Percutaneous Endoscopic Approach

0PWV4KZ   Revision of Nonautologous Tissue Substitute in Left Finger Phalanx, Percutaneous Endoscopic Approach

0PWVX4Z   Revision of Internal Fixation Device in Left Finger Phalanx, External Approach

0PWVX5Z   Revision of External Fixation Device in Left Finger Phalanx, External Approach

0PWVX7Z   Revision of Autologous Tissue Substitute in Left Finger Phalanx, External Approach

0PWVXJZ   Revision of Synthetic Substitute in Left Finger Phalanx, External Approach

0PWVXKZ   Revision of Nonautologous Tissue Substitute in Left Finger Phalanx, External Approach

0PWY00Z   Revision of Drainage Device in Upper Bone, Open Approach

0PWY0MZ   Revision of Bone Growth Stimulator in Upper Bone, Open Approach

0PWY30Z   Revision of Drainage Device in Upper Bone, Percutaneous Approach

0PWY3MZ   Revision of Bone Growth Stimulator in Upper Bone, Percutaneous Approach

0PWY40Z   Revision of Drainage Device in Upper Bone, Percutaneous Endoscopic Approach

0PWY4MZ   Revision of Bone Growth Stimulator in Upper Bone, Percutaneous Endoscopic Approach

0PWYX0Z   Revision of Drainage Device in Upper Bone, External Approach

0PWYXMZ   Revision of Bone Growth Stimulator in Upper Bone, External Approach

Lower Bones

Bones - Front and Back Views

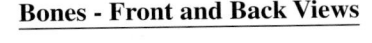

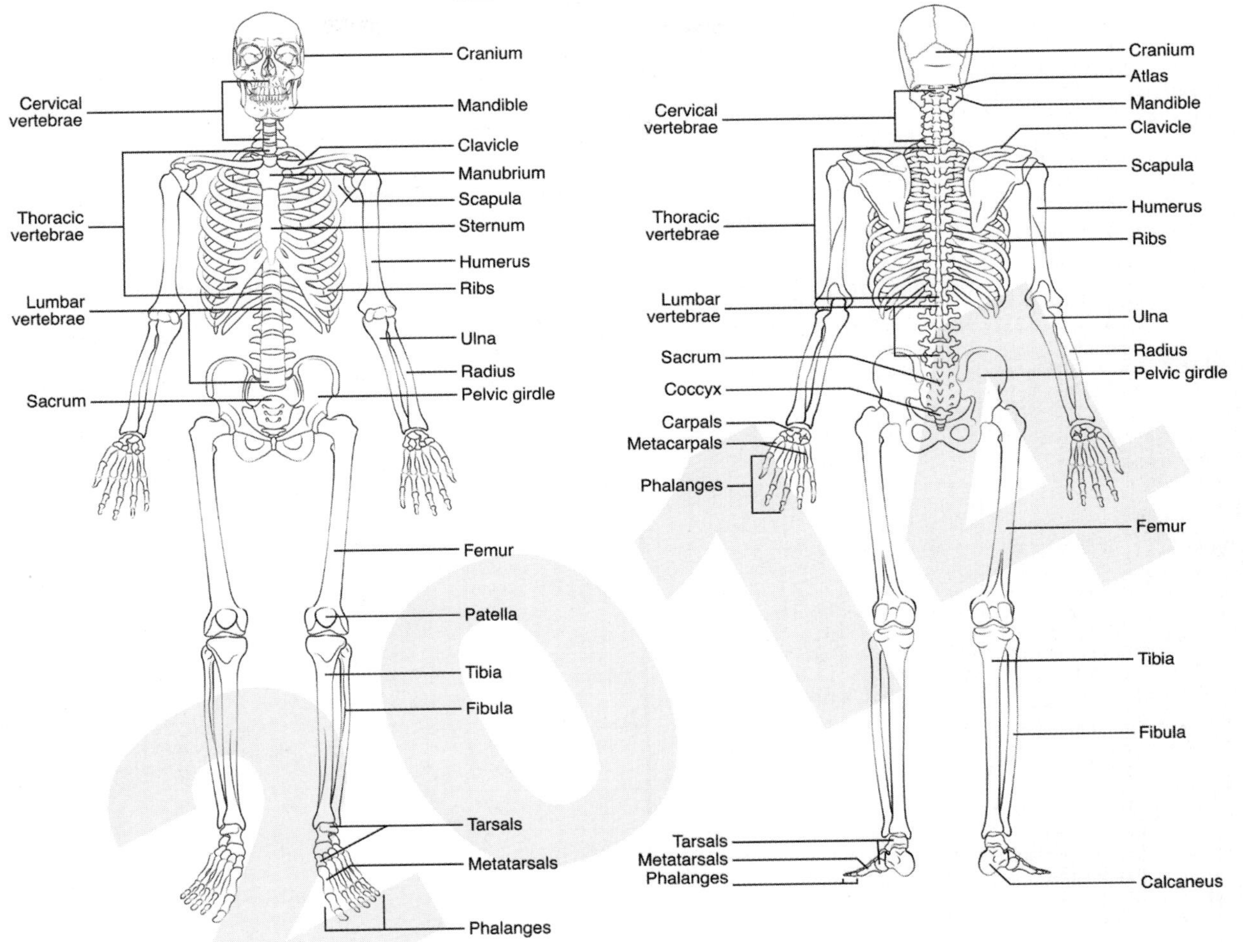

Cranium

Cervical vertebrae

Mandible

Clavicle

Manubrium

Scapula

Sternum

Thoracic vertebrae

Humerus

Ribs

Lumbar vertebrae

Ulna

Radius

Sacrum

Pelvic girdle

Femur

Patella

Tibia

Fibula

Tarsals

Metatarsals

Phalanges

Cranium

Atlas

Cervical vertebrae

Mandible

Clavicle

Scapula

Humerus

Thoracic vertebrae

Ribs

Lumbar vertebrae

Ulna

Radius

Sacrum

Pelvic girdle

Coccyx

Carpals

Metacarpals

Phalanges

Femur

Tibia

Fibula

Tarsals

Metatarsals

Phalanges

Calcaneus

Vertebrae

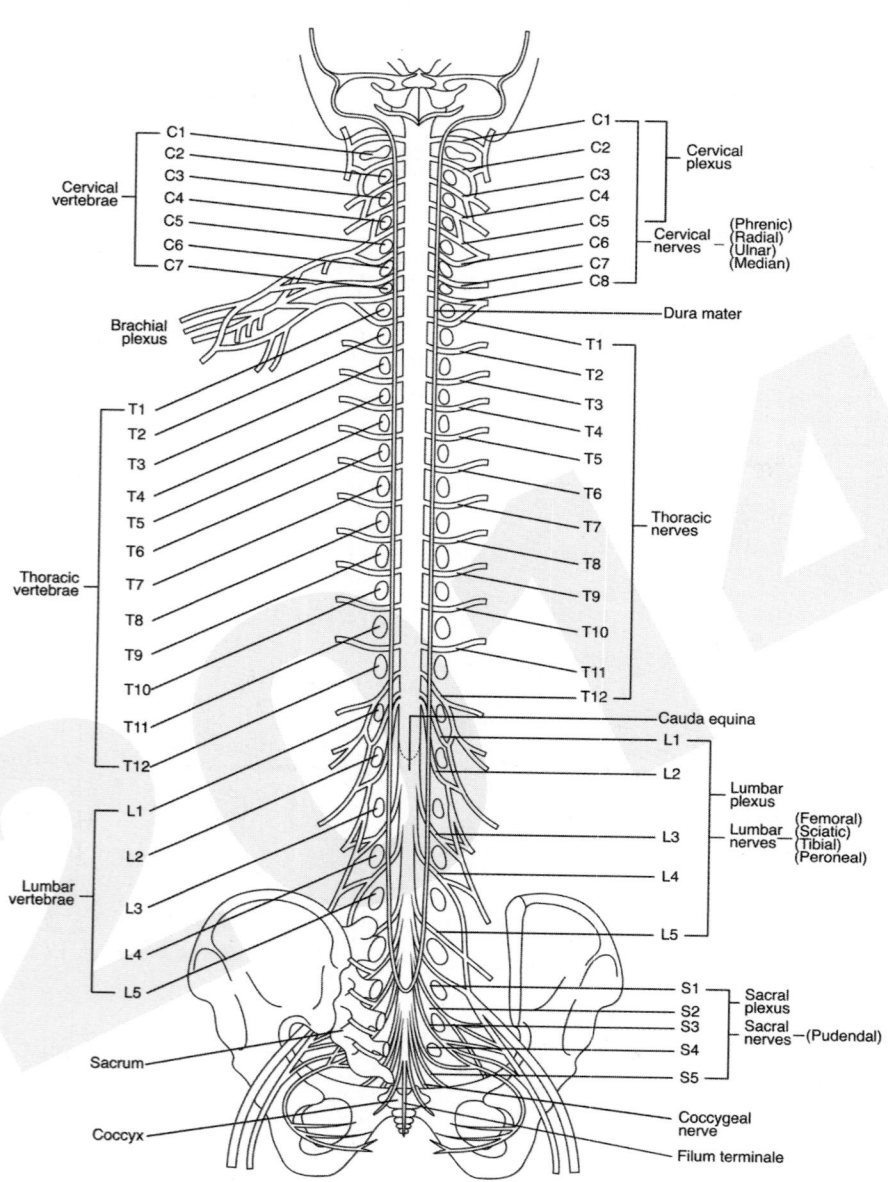

Lower Bones Tables 0Q2–0QW

Section	0	Medical and Surgical
Body System	Q	Lower Bones
Operation	2	Change: Taking out or off a device from a body part and putting back an identical or similar device in or on the same body part without cutting or puncturing the skin or a mucous membrane

Body Part (4th)	Approach (5th)	Device (6th)	Qualifier (7th)
Y Lower Bone	**X** External	**0** Drainage Device **Y** Other Device	**Z** No Qualifier

Section	0	Medical and Surgical
Body System	Q	Lower Bones
Operation	5	**Destruction:** Physical eradication of all or a portion of a body part by the direct use of energy, force, or a destructive agent

Body Part (4th)	Approach (5th)	Device (6th)	Qualifier (7th)
0 Lumbar Vertebra 1 Sacrum 2 Pelvic Bone, Right 3 Pelvic Bone, Left 4 Acetabulum, Right 5 Acetabulum, Left 6 Upper Femur, Right 7 Upper Femur, Left 8 Femoral Shaft, Right 9 Femoral Shaft, Left B Lower Femur, Right C Lower Femur, Left D Patella, Right F Patella, Left G Tibia, Right H Tibia, Left J Fibula, Right K Fibula, Left L Tarsal, Right M Tarsal, Left N Metatarsal, Right P Metatarsal, Left Q Toe Phalanx, Right R Toe Phalanx, Left S Coccyx	0 Open 3 Percutaneous 4 Percutaneous Endoscopic	Z No Device	Z No Qualifier

Section	0	Medical and Surgical
Body System	Q	Lower Bones
Operation	8	**Division:** Cutting into a body part, without draining fluids and/or gases from the body part, in order to separate or transect a body part

Body Part (4th)	Approach (5th)	Device (6th)	Qualifier (7th)
0 Lumbar Vertebra 1 Sacrum 2 Pelvic Bone, Right 3 Pelvic Bone, Left 4 Acetabulum, Right 5 Acetabulum, Left 6 Upper Femur, Right 7 Upper Femur, Left 8 Femoral Shaft, Right 9 Femoral Shaft, Left B Lower Femur, Right C Lower Femur, Left D Patella, Right F Patella, Left G Tibia, Right H Tibia, Left J Fibula, Right K Fibula, Left L Tarsal, Right M Tarsal, Left N Metatarsal, Right P Metatarsal, Left Q Toe Phalanx, Right R Toe Phalanx, Left S Coccyx	0 Open 3 Percutaneous 4 Percutaneous Endoscopic	Z No Device	Z No Qualifier

Section	0	Medical and Surgical
Body System	Q	Lower Bones
Operation	9	**Drainage:** Taking or letting out fluids and/or gases from a body part

Body Part (4th)	Approach (5th)	Device (6th)	Qualifier (7th)
0 Lumbar Vertebra 1 Sacrum 2 Pelvic Bone, Right 3 Pelvic Bone, Left 4 Acetabulum, Right 5 Acetabulum, Left 6 Upper Femur, Right 7 Upper Femur, Left 8 Femoral Shaft, Right 9 Femoral Shaft, Left B Lower Femur, Right C Lower Femur, Left D Patella, Right F Patella, Left G Tibia, Right H Tibia, Left J Fibula, Right K Fibula, Left L Tarsal, Right M Tarsal, Left N Metatarsal, Right P Metatarsal, Left Q Toe Phalanx, Right R Toe Phalanx, Left S Coccyx	0 Open 3 Percutaneous 4 Percutaneous Endoscopic	0 Drainage Device	Z No Qualifier
0 Lumbar Vertebra 1 Sacrum 2 Pelvic Bone, Right 3 Pelvic Bone, Left 4 Acetabulum, Right 5 Acetabulum, Left 6 Upper Femur, Right 7 Upper Femur, Left 8 Femoral Shaft, Right 9 Femoral Shaft, Left B Lower Femur, Right C Lower Femur, Left D Patella, Right F Patella, Left G Tibia, Right H Tibia, Left J Fibula, Right K Fibula, Left L Tarsal, Right M Tarsal, Left N Metatarsal, Right P Metatarsal, Left Q Toe Phalanx, Right R Toe Phalanx, Left S Coccyx	0 Open 3 Percutaneous 4 Percutaneous Endoscopic	Z No Device	X Diagnostic Z No Qualifier

Section	0	Medical and Surgical
Body System	Q	Lower Bones
Operation	B	Excision: Cutting out or off, without replacement, a portion of a body part

Body Part (4th)	Approach (5th)	Device (6th)	Qualifier (7th)
0 Lumbar Vertebra 1 Sacrum 2 Pelvic Bone, Right 3 Pelvic Bone, Left 4 Acetabulum, Right 5 Acetabulum, Left 6 Upper Femur, Right 7 Upper Femur, Left 8 Femoral Shaft, Right 9 Femoral Shaft, Left B Lower Femur, Right C Lower Femur, Left D Patella, Right F Patella, Left G Tibia, Right H Tibia, Left J Fibula, Right K Fibula, Left L Tarsal, Right M Tarsal, Left N Metatarsal, Right P Metatarsal, Left Q Toe Phalanx, Right R Toe Phalanx, Left S Coccyx	0 Open 3 Percutaneous 4 Percutaneous Endoscopic	Z No Device	X Diagnostic Z No Qualifier

Section	0	Medical and Surgical
Body System	Q	Lower Bones
Operation	C	Extirpation: Taking or cutting out solid matter from a body part

Body Part (4th)	Approach (5th)	Device (6th)	Qualifier (7th)
0 Lumbar Vertebra 1 Sacrum 2 Pelvic Bone, Right 3 Pelvic Bone, Left 4 Acetabulum, Right 5 Acetabulum, Left 6 Upper Femur, Right 7 Upper Femur, Left 8 Femoral Shaft, Right 9 Femoral Shaft, Left B Lower Femur, Right C Lower Femur, Left D Patella, Right F Patella, Left G Tibia, Right H Tibia, Left J Fibula, Right K Fibula, Left L Tarsal, Right M Tarsal, Left N Metatarsal, Right P Metatarsal, Left Q Toe Phalanx, Right R Toe Phalanx, Left S Coccyx	0 Open 3 Percutaneous 4 Percutaneous Endoscopic	Z No Device	Z No Qualifier

Section	0	Medical and Surgical
Body System	Q	Lower Bones
Operation	H	Insertion: Putting in a nonbiological appliance that monitors, assists, performs, or prevents a physiological function but does not physically take the place of a body part

Body Part (4th)	Approach (5th)	Device (6th)	Qualifier (7th)
0 Lumbar Vertebra 1 Sacrum 2 Pelvic Bone, Right 3 Pelvic Bone, Left 4 Acetabulum, Right 5 Acetabulum, Left D Patella, Right F Patella, Left L Tarsal, Right M Tarsal, Left N Metatarsal, Right P Metatarsal, Left Q Toe Phalanx, Right R Toe Phalanx, Left S Coccyx	0 Open 3 Percutaneous 4 Percutaneous Endoscopic	4 Internal Fixation Device 5 External Fixation Device	Z No Qualifier
6 Upper Femur, Right 7 Upper Femur, Left 8 Femoral Shaft, Right 9 Femoral Shaft, Left B Lower Femur, Right C Lower Femur, Left G Tibia, Right H Tibia, Left J Fibula, Right K Fibula, Left	0 Open 3 Percutaneous 4 Percutaneous Endoscopic	4 Internal Fixation Device 5 External Fixation Device 6 Internal Fixation Device, Intramedullary 8 External Fixation Device, Limb Lengthening B External Fixation Device, Monoplanar C External Fixation Device, Ring D External Fixation Device, Hybrid	Z No Qualifier
Y Lower Bone	0 Open 3 Percutaneous 4 Percutaneous Endoscopic	M Bone Growth Stimulator	Z No Qualifier

Section	0	Medical and Surgical
Body System	Q	Lower Bones
Operation	J	Inspection: Visually and/or manually exploring a body part

Body Part (4th)	Approach (5th)	Device (6th)	Qualifier (7th)
Y Lower Bone	0 Open 3 Percutaneous 4 Percutaneous Endoscopic X External	Z No Device	Z No Qualifier

Section	0	Medical and Surgical
Body System	Q	Lower Bones
Operation	N	Release: Freeing a body part from an abnormal physical constraint by cutting or by the use of force

Body Part (4th)	Approach (5th)	Device (6th)	Qualifier (7th)
0 Lumbar Vertebra 1 Sacrum 2 Pelvic Bone, Right 3 Pelvic Bone, Left 4 Acetabulum, Right 5 Acetabulum, Left 6 Upper Femur, Right 7 Upper Femur, Left 8 Femoral Shaft, Right 9 Femoral Shaft, Left B Lower Femur, Right C Lower Femur, Left D Patella, Right F Patella, Left G Tibia, Right H Tibia, Left J Fibula, Right K Fibula, Left L Tarsal, Right M Tarsal, Left N Metatarsal, Right P Metatarsal, Left Q Toe Phalanx, Right R Toe Phalanx, Left S Coccyx	0 Open 3 Percutaneous 4 Percutaneous Endoscopic	Z No Device	Z No Qualifier

Section	0	Medical and Surgical
Body System	Q	Lower Bones
Operation	P	Removal: Taking out or off a device from a body part

Body Part (4th)	Approach (5th)	Device (6th)	Qualifier (7th)
0 Lumbar Vertebra 1 Sacrum 4 Acetabulum, Right 5 Acetabulum, Left S Coccyx	0 Open 3 Percutaneous 4 Percutaneous Endoscopic	4 Internal Fixation Device 7 Autologous Tissue Substitute J Synthetic Substitute K Nonautologous Tissue Substitute	Z No Qualifier
0 Lumbar Vertebra 1 Sacrum 4 Acetabulum, Right 5 Acetabulum, Left S Coccyx	X External	4 Internal Fixation Device	Z No Qualifier

Continued

Section	0	Medical and Surgical
Body System	Q	Lower Bones
Operation	P	Removal: Taking out or off a device from a body part

Body Part (4th)	Approach (5th)	Device (6th)	Qualifier (7th)
2 Pelvic Bone, Right 3 Pelvic Bone, Left 6 Upper Femur, Right 7 Upper Femur, Left 8 Femoral Shaft, Right 9 Femoral Shaft, Left B Lower Femur, Right C Lower Femur, Left D Patella, Right F Patella, Left G Tibia, Right H Tibia, Left J Fibula, Right K Fibula, Left L Tarsal, Right M Tarsal, Left N Metatarsal, Right P Metatarsal, Left Q Toe Phalanx, Right R Toe Phalanx, Left	0 Open 3 Percutaneous 4 Percutaneous Endoscopic	4 Internal Fixation Device 5 External Fixation Device 7 Autologous Tissue Substitute J Synthetic Substitute K Nonautologous Tissue Substitute	Z No Qualifier
2 Pelvic Bone, Right 3 Pelvic Bone, Left 6 Upper Femur, Right 7 Upper Femur, Left 8 Femoral Shaft, Right 9 Femoral Shaft, Left B Lower Femur, Right C Lower Femur, Left D Patella, Right F Patella, Left G Tibia, Right H Tibia, Left J Fibula, Right K Fibula, Left L Tarsal, Right M Tarsal, Left N Metatarsal, Right P Metatarsal, Left Q Toe Phalanx, Right R Toe Phalanx, Left	X External	4 Internal Fixation Device 5 External Fixation Device	Z No Qualifier
Y Lower Bone	0 Open 3 Percutaneous 4 Percutaneous Endoscopic X External	0 Drainage Device M Bone Growth Stimulator	Z No Qualifier

Section	0	Medical and Surgical
Body System	Q	Lower Bones
Operation	Q	**Repair:** Restoring, to the extent possible, a body part to its normal anatomic structure and function

Body Part (4ᵗʰ)	Approach (5ᵗʰ)	Device (6ᵗʰ)	Qualifier (7ᵗʰ)
0 Lumbar Vertebra 1 Sacrum 2 Pelvic Bone, Right 3 Pelvic Bone, Left 4 Acetabulum, Right 5 Acetabulum, Left 6 Upper Femur, Right 7 Upper Femur, Left 8 Femoral Shaft, Right 9 Femoral Shaft, Left B Lower Femur, Right C Lower Femur, Left D Patella, Right F Patella, Left G Tibia, Right H Tibia, Left J Fibula, Right K Fibula, Left L Tarsal, Right M Tarsal, Left N Metatarsal, Right P Metatarsal, Left Q Toe Phalanx, Right R Toe Phalanx, Left S Coccyx	0 Open 3 Percutaneous 4 Percutaneous Endoscopic X External	Z No Device	Z No Qualifier

Section	0	Medical and Surgical
Body System	Q	Lower Bones
Operation	R	**Replacement:** Putting in or on biological or synthetic material that physically takes the place and/or function of all or a portion of a body part

Body Part (4ᵗʰ)	Approach (5ᵗʰ)	Device (6ᵗʰ)	Qualifier (7ᵗʰ)

0 Lumbar Vertebra
1 Sacrum
2 Pelvic Bone, Right
3 Pelvic Bone, Left
4 Acetabulum, Right
5 Acetabulum, Left
6 Upper Femur, Right
7 Upper Femur, Left
8 Femoral Shaft, Right
9 Femoral Shaft, Left
B Lower Femur, Right
C Lower Femur, Left
D Patella, Right
F Patella, Left
G Tibia, Right
H Tibia, Left
J Fibula, Right
K Fibula, Left
L Tarsal, Right
M Tarsal, Left
N Metatarsal, Right
P Metatarsal, Left
Q Toe Phalanx, Right
R Toe Phalanx, Left
S Coccyx
	0 Open
	3 Percutaneous
	4 Percutaneous
	   Endoscopic
		7 Autologous Tissue
		   Substitute
		J Synthetic Substitute
		K Nonautologous Tissue
		   Substitute
			Z No Qualifier

Section	0	Medical and Surgical
Body System	Q	Lower Bones
Operation	S	Reposition: Moving to its normal location, or other suitable location, all or a portion of a body part

Body Part (4th)	Approach (5th)	Device (6th)	Qualifier (7th)
0 Lumbar Vertebra 1 Sacrum 4 Acetabulum, Right 5 Acetabulum, Left S Coccyx	0 Open 3 Percutaneous 4 Percutaneous Endoscopic	4 Internal Fixation Device Z No Device	Z No Qualifier
0 Lumbar Vertebra 1 Sacrum 4 Acetabulum, Right 5 Acetabulum, Left S Coccyx	X External	Z No Device	Z No Qualifier
2 Pelvic Bone, Right 3 Pelvic Bone, Left D Patella, Right F Patella, Left L Tarsal, Right M Tarsal, Left N Metatarsal, Right P Metatarsal, Left Q Toe Phalanx, Right R Toe Phalanx, Left	0 Open 3 Percutaneous 4 Percutaneous Endoscopic	4 Internal Fixation Device 5 External Fixation Device Z No Device	Z No Qualifier
2 Pelvic Bone, Right 3 Pelvic Bone, Left D Patella, Right F Patella, Left L Tarsal, Right M Tarsal, Left N Metatarsal, Right P Metatarsal, Left Q Toe Phalanx, Right R Toe Phalanx, Left	X External	Z No Device	Z No Qualifier
6 Upper Femur, Right 7 Upper Femur, Left 8 Femoral Shaft, Right 9 Femoral Shaft, Left B Lower Femur, Right C Lower Femur, Left G Tibia, Right H Tibia, Left J Fibula, Right K Fibula, Left	0 Open 3 Percutaneous 4 Percutaneous Endoscopic	4 Internal Fixation Device 5 External Fixation Device 6 Internal Fixation Device, Intramedullary B External Fixation Device, Monoplanar C External Fixation Device, Ring D External Fixation Device, Hybrid Z No Device	Z No Qualifier
6 Upper Femur, Right 7 Upper Femur, Left 8 Femoral Shaft, Right 9 Femoral Shaft, Left B Lower Femur, Right C Lower Femur, Left G Tibia, Right H Tibia, Left J Fibula, Right K Fibula, Left	X External	Z No Device	Z No Qualifier

Section	0	Medical and Surgical
Body System	Q	Lower Bones
Operation	T	**Resection:** Cutting out or off, without replacement, all of a body part

Body Part (4ᵗʰ)	Approach (5ᵗʰ)	Device (6ᵗʰ)	Qualifier (7ᵗʰ)
2 Pelvic Bone, Right **3** Pelvic Bone, Left **4** Acetabulum, Right **5** Acetabulum, Left **6** Upper Femur, Right **7** Upper Femur, Left **8** Femoral Shaft, Right **9** Femoral Shaft, Left **B** Lower Femur, Right **C** Lower Femur, Left **D** Patella, Right **F** Patella, Left **G** Tibia, Right **H** Tibia, Left **J** Fibula, Right **K** Fibula, Left **L** Tarsal, Right **M** Tarsal, Left **N** Metatarsal, Right **P** Metatarsal, Left **Q** Toe Phalanx, Right **R** Toe Phalanx, Left **S** Coccyx	**0** Open	**Z** No Device	**Z** No Qualifier

Section	0	Medical and Surgical
Body System	Q	Lower Bones
Operation	U	**Supplement:** Putting in or on biological or synthetic material that physically reinforces and/or augments the function of a portion of a body part

Body Part (4ᵗʰ)	Approach (5ᵗʰ)	Device (6ᵗʰ)	Qualifier (7ᵗʰ)
0 Lumbar Vertebra **1** Sacrum **2** Pelvic Bone, Right **3** Pelvic Bone, Left **4** Acetabulum, Right **5** Acetabulum, Left **6** Upper Femur, Right **7** Upper Femur, Left **8** Femoral Shaft, Right **9** Femoral Shaft, Left **B** Lower Femur, Right **C** Lower Femur, Left **D** Patella, Right **F** Patella, Left **G** Tibia, Right **H** Tibia, Left **J** Fibula, Right **K** Fibula, Left **L** Tarsal, Right **M** Tarsal, Left **N** Metatarsal, Right **P** Metatarsal, Left **Q** Toe Phalanx, Right **R** Toe Phalanx, Left **S** Coccyx	**0** Open **3** Percutaneous **4** Percutaneous Endoscopic	**7** Autologous Tissue Substitute **J** Synthetic Substitute **K** Nonautologous Tissue Substitute	**Z** No Qualifier

Section	0	Medical and Surgical
Body System	Q	Lower Bones
Operation	W	**Revision:** Correcting, to the extent possible, a portion of a malfunctioning device or the position of a displaced device

Body Part (4th)	Approach (5th)	Device (6th)	Qualifier (7th)
0 Lumbar Vertebra 1 Sacrum 4 Acetabulum, Right 5 Acetabulum, Left S Coccyx	0 Open 3 Percutaneous 4 Percutaneous Endoscopic X External	4 Internal Fixation Device 7 Autologous Tissue Substitute J Synthetic Substitute K Nonautologous Tissue Substitute	Z No Qualifier
2 Pelvic Bone, Right 3 Pelvic Bone, Left 6 Upper Femur, Right 7 Upper Femur, Left 8 Femoral Shaft, Right 9 Femoral Shaft, Left B Lower Femur, Right C Lower Femur, Left D Patella, Right F Patella, Left G Tibia, Right H Tibia, Left J Fibula, Right K Fibula, Left L Tarsal, Right M Tarsal, Left N Metatarsal, Right P Metatarsal, Left Q Toe Phalanx, Right R Toe Phalanx, Left	0 Open 3 Percutaneous 4 Percutaneous Endoscopic X External	4 Internal Fixation Device 5 External Fixation Device 7 Autologous Tissue Substitute J Synthetic Substitute K Nonautologous Tissue Substitute	Z No Qualifier
Y Lower Bone	0 Open 3 Percutaneous 4 Percutaneous Endoscopic X External	0 Drainage Device M Bone Growth Stimulator	Z No Qualifier

Lower Bones Code Listing 0Q2–0QW

0Q2 – Lower Bones, Change

Review Coding Guideline B6.1c

0Q2YX0Z Change Drainage Device in Lower Bone, External Approach

0Q2YXYZ Change Other Device in Lower Bone, External Approach

0Q5 – Lower Bones, Destruction

0Q500ZZ Destruction of Lumbar Vertebra, Open Approach
0Q503ZZ Destruction of Lumbar Vertebra, Percutaneous Approach
0Q504ZZ Destruction of Lumbar Vertebra, Percutaneous Endoscopic Approach
0Q510ZZ Destruction of Sacrum, Open Approach
0Q513ZZ Destruction of Sacrum, Percutaneous Approach
0Q514ZZ Destruction of Sacrum, Percutaneous Endoscopic Approach
0Q520ZZ Destruction of Right Pelvic Bone, Open Approach
0Q523ZZ Destruction of Right Pelvic Bone, Percutaneous Approach
0Q524ZZ Destruction of Right Pelvic Bone, Percutaneous Endoscopic Approach
0Q530ZZ Destruction of Left Pelvic Bone, Open Approach
0Q533ZZ Destruction of Left Pelvic Bone, Percutaneous Approach
0Q534ZZ Destruction of Left Pelvic Bone, Percutaneous Endoscopic Approach
0Q540ZZ Destruction of Right Acetabulum, Open Approach
0Q543ZZ Destruction of Right Acetabulum, Percutaneous Approach

0Q544ZZ Destruction of Right Acetabulum, Percutaneous Endoscopic Approach
0Q550ZZ Destruction of Left Acetabulum, Open Approach
0Q553ZZ Destruction of Left Acetabulum, Percutaneous Approach
0Q554ZZ Destruction of Left Acetabulum, Percutaneous Endoscopic Approach
0Q560ZZ Destruction of Right Upper Femur, Open Approach
0Q563ZZ Destruction of Right Upper Femur, Percutaneous Approach
0Q564ZZ Destruction of Right Upper Femur, Percutaneous Endoscopic Approach
0Q570ZZ Destruction of Left Upper Femur, Open Approach
0Q573ZZ Destruction of Left Upper Femur, Percutaneous Approach
0Q574ZZ Destruction of Left Upper Femur, Percutaneous Endoscopic Approach
0Q580ZZ Destruction of Right Femoral Shaft, Open Approach
0Q583ZZ Destruction of Right Femoral Shaft, Percutaneous Approach

0Q584ZZ Destruction of Right Femoral Shaft, Percutaneous Endoscopic Approach
0Q590ZZ Destruction of Left Femoral Shaft, Open Approach
0Q593ZZ Destruction of Left Femoral Shaft, Percutaneous Approach
0Q594ZZ Destruction of Left Femoral Shaft, Percutaneous Endoscopic Approach
0Q5B0ZZ Destruction of Right Lower Femur, Open Approach
0Q5B3ZZ Destruction of Right Lower Femur, Percutaneous Approach
0Q5B4ZZ Destruction of Right Lower Femur, Percutaneous Endoscopic Approach
0Q5C0ZZ Destruction of Left Lower Femur, Open Approach
0Q5C3ZZ Destruction of Left Lower Femur, Percutaneous Approach
0Q5C4ZZ Destruction of Left Lower Femur, Percutaneous Endoscopic Approach
0Q5D0ZZ Destruction of Right Patella, Open Approach
0Q5D3ZZ Destruction of Right Patella, Percutaneous Approach
0Q5D4ZZ Destruction of Right Patella, Percutaneous Endoscopic Approach
0Q5F0ZZ Destruction of Left Patella, Open Approach
0Q5F3ZZ Destruction of Left Patella, Percutaneous Approach
0Q5F4ZZ Destruction of Left Patella, Percutaneous Endoscopic Approach
0Q5G0ZZ Destruction of Right Tibia, Open Approach
0Q5G3ZZ Destruction of Right Tibia, Percutaneous Approach
0Q5G4ZZ Destruction of Right Tibia, Percutaneous Endoscopic Approach
0Q5H0ZZ Destruction of Left Tibia, Open Approach
0Q5H3ZZ Destruction of Left Tibia, Percutaneous Approach
0Q5H4ZZ Destruction of Left Tibia, Percutaneous Endoscopic Approach
0Q5J0ZZ Destruction of Right Fibula, Open Approach
0Q5J3ZZ Destruction of Right Fibula, Percutaneous Approach
0Q5J4ZZ Destruction of Right Fibula, Percutaneous Endoscopic Approach
0Q5K0ZZ Destruction of Left Fibula, Open Approach
0Q5K3ZZ Destruction of Left Fibula, Percutaneous Approach
0Q5K4ZZ Destruction of Left Fibula, Percutaneous Endoscopic Approach
0Q5L0ZZ Destruction of Right Tarsal, Open Approach
0Q5L3ZZ Destruction of Right Tarsal, Percutaneous Approach
0Q5L4ZZ Destruction of Right Tarsal, Percutaneous Endoscopic Approach
0Q5M0ZZ Destruction of Left Tarsal, Open Approach
0Q5M3ZZ Destruction of Left Tarsal, Percutaneous Approach
0Q5M4ZZ Destruction of Left Tarsal, Percutaneous Endoscopic Approach
0Q5N0ZZ Destruction of Right Metatarsal, Open Approach
0Q5N3ZZ Destruction of Right Metatarsal, Percutaneous Approach
0Q5N4ZZ Destruction of Right Metatarsal, Percutaneous Endoscopic Approach
0Q5P0ZZ Destruction of Left Metatarsal, Open Approach
0Q5P3ZZ Destruction of Left Metatarsal, Percutaneous Approach
0Q5P4ZZ Destruction of Left Metatarsal, Percutaneous Endoscopic Approach
0Q5Q0ZZ Destruction of Right Toe Phalanx, Open Approach
0Q5Q3ZZ Destruction of Right Toe Phalanx, Percutaneous Approach
0Q5Q4ZZ Destruction of Right Toe Phalanx, Percutaneous Endoscopic Approach
0Q5R0ZZ Destruction of Left Toe Phalanx, Open Approach
0Q5R3ZZ Destruction of Left Toe Phalanx, Percutaneous Approach
0Q5R4ZZ Destruction of Left Toe Phalanx, Percutaneous Endoscopic Approach
0Q5S0ZZ Destruction of Coccyx, Open Approach
0Q5S3ZZ Destruction of Coccyx, Percutaneous Approach
0Q5S4ZZ Destruction of Coccyx, Percutaneous Endoscopic Approach

0Q8 – Lower Bones, Division

Review Coding Guideline B3.14

0Q800ZZ Division of Lumbar Vertebra, Open Approach
0Q803ZZ Division of Lumbar Vertebra, Percutaneous Approach
0Q804ZZ Division of Lumbar Vertebra, Percutaneous Endoscopic Approach
0Q810ZZ Division of Sacrum, Open Approach
0Q813ZZ Division of Sacrum, Percutaneous Approach
0Q814ZZ Division of Sacrum, Percutaneous Endoscopic Approach
0Q820ZZ Division of Right Pelvic Bone, Open Approach
0Q823ZZ Division of Right Pelvic Bone, Percutaneous Approach
0Q824ZZ Division of Right Pelvic Bone, Percutaneous Endoscopic Approach
0Q830ZZ Division of Left Pelvic Bone, Open Approach
0Q833ZZ Division of Left Pelvic Bone, Percutaneous Approach
0Q834ZZ Division of Left Pelvic Bone, Percutaneous Endoscopic Approach
0Q840ZZ Division of Right Acetabulum, Open Approach
0Q843ZZ Division of Right Acetabulum, Percutaneous Approach
0Q844ZZ Division of Right Acetabulum, Percutaneous Endoscopic Approach
0Q850ZZ Division of Left Acetabulum, Open Approach
0Q853ZZ Division of Left Acetabulum, Percutaneous Approach
0Q854ZZ Division of Left Acetabulum, Percutaneous Endoscopic Approach
0Q860ZZ Division of Right Upper Femur, Open Approach
0Q863ZZ Division of Right Upper Femur, Percutaneous Approach
0Q864ZZ Division of Right Upper Femur, Percutaneous Endoscopic Approach
0Q870ZZ Division of Left Upper Femur, Open Approach
0Q873ZZ Division of Left Upper Femur, Percutaneous Approach
0Q874ZZ Division of Left Upper Femur, Percutaneous Endoscopic Approach
0Q880ZZ Division of Right Femoral Shaft, Open Approach
0Q883ZZ Division of Right Femoral Shaft, Percutaneous Approach
0Q884ZZ Division of Right Femoral Shaft, Percutaneous Endoscopic Approach
0Q890ZZ Division of Left Femoral Shaft, Open Approach
0Q893ZZ Division of Left Femoral Shaft, Percutaneous Approach
0Q894ZZ Division of Left Femoral Shaft, Percutaneous Endoscopic Approach
0Q8B0ZZ Division of Right Lower Femur, Open Approach
0Q8B3ZZ Division of Right Lower Femur, Percutaneous Approach
0Q8B4ZZ Division of Right Lower Femur, Percutaneous Endoscopic Approach
0Q8C0ZZ Division of Left Lower Femur, Open Approach
0Q8C3ZZ Division of Left Lower Femur, Percutaneous Approach
0Q8C4ZZ Division of Left Lower Femur, Percutaneous Endoscopic Approach
0Q8D0ZZ Division of Right Patella, Open Approach
0Q8D3ZZ Division of Right Patella, Percutaneous Approach
0Q8D4ZZ Division of Right Patella, Percutaneous Endoscopic Approach
0Q8F0ZZ Division of Left Patella, Open Approach
0Q8F3ZZ Division of Left Patella, Percutaneous Approach
0Q8F4ZZ Division of Left Patella, Percutaneous Endoscopic Approach
0Q8G0ZZ Division of Right Tibia, Open Approach
0Q8G3ZZ Division of Right Tibia, Percutaneous Approach
0Q8G4ZZ Division of Right Tibia, Percutaneous Endoscopic Approach
0Q8H0ZZ Division of Left Tibia, Open Approach
0Q8H3ZZ Division of Left Tibia, Percutaneous Approach
0Q8H4ZZ Division of Left Tibia, Percutaneous Endoscopic Approach
0Q8J0ZZ Division of Right Fibula, Open Approach
0Q8J3ZZ Division of Right Fibula, Percutaneous Approach
0Q8J4ZZ Division of Right Fibula, Percutaneous Endoscopic Approach
0Q8K0ZZ Division of Left Fibula, Open Approach
0Q8K3ZZ Division of Left Fibula, Percutaneous Approach
0Q8K4ZZ Division of Left Fibula, Percutaneous Endoscopic Approach
0Q8L0ZZ Division of Right Tarsal, Open Approach
0Q8L3ZZ Division of Right Tarsal, Percutaneous Approach
0Q8L4ZZ Division of Right Tarsal, Percutaneous Endoscopic Approach
0Q8M0ZZ Division of Left Tarsal, Open Approach
0Q8M3ZZ Division of Left Tarsal, Percutaneous Approach
0Q8M4ZZ Division of Left Tarsal, Percutaneous Endoscopic Approach
0Q8N0ZZ Division of Right Metatarsal, Open Approach
0Q8N3ZZ Division of Right Metatarsal, Percutaneous Approach
0Q8N4ZZ Division of Right Metatarsal, Percutaneous Endoscopic Approach
0Q8P0ZZ Division of Left Metatarsal, Open Approach
0Q8P3ZZ Division of Left Metatarsal, Percutaneous Approach
0Q8P4ZZ Division of Left Metatarsal, Percutaneous Endoscopic Approach
0Q8Q0ZZ Division of Right Toe Phalanx, Open Approach
0Q8Q3ZZ Division of Right Toe Phalanx, Percutaneous Approach
0Q8Q4ZZ Division of Right Toe Phalanx, Percutaneous Endoscopic Approach
0Q8R0ZZ Division of Left Toe Phalanx, Open Approach
0Q8R3ZZ Division of Left Toe Phalanx, Percutaneous Approach
0Q8R4ZZ Division of Left Toe Phalanx, Percutaneous Endoscopic Approach
0Q8S0ZZ Division of Coccyx, Open Approach
0Q8S3ZZ Division of Coccyx, Percutaneous Approach
0Q8S4ZZ Division of Coccyx, Percutaneous Endoscopic Approach

0Q9 – Lower Bones, Drainage

Review Coding Guidelines B3.4a and B3.4b

Review Coding Guideline B6.2

0Q9000Z	Drainage of Lumbar Vertebra with Drainage Device, Open Approach
0Q900ZX	Drainage of Lumbar Vertebra, Open Approach, Diagnostic
0Q900ZZ	Drainage of Lumbar Vertebra, Open Approach
0Q9030Z	Drainage of Lumbar Vertebra with Drainage Device, Percutaneous Approach
0Q903ZX	Drainage of Lumbar Vertebra, Percutaneous Approach, Diagnostic
0Q903ZZ	Drainage of Lumbar Vertebra, Percutaneous Approach
0Q9040Z	Drainage of Lumbar Vertebra with Drainage Device, Percutaneous Endoscopic Approach
0Q904ZX	Drainage of Lumbar Vertebra, Percutaneous Endoscopic Approach, Diagnostic
0Q904ZZ	Drainage of Lumbar Vertebra, Percutaneous Endoscopic Approach
0Q9100Z	Drainage of Sacrum with Drainage Device, Open Approach
0Q910ZX	Drainage of Sacrum, Open Approach, Diagnostic
0Q910ZZ	Drainage of Sacrum, Open Approach
0Q9130Z	Drainage of Sacrum with Drainage Device, Percutaneous Approach
0Q913ZX	Drainage of Sacrum, Percutaneous Approach, Diagnostic
0Q913ZZ	Drainage of Sacrum, Percutaneous Approach
0Q9140Z	Drainage of Sacrum with Drainage Device, Percutaneous Endoscopic Approach
0Q914ZX	Drainage of Sacrum, Percutaneous Endoscopic Approach, Diagnostic
0Q914ZZ	Drainage of Sacrum, Percutaneous Endoscopic Approach
0Q9200Z	Drainage of Right Pelvic Bone with Drainage Device, Open Approach
0Q920ZX	Drainage of Right Pelvic Bone, Open Approach, Diagnostic
0Q920ZZ	Drainage of Right Pelvic Bone, Open Approach
0Q9230Z	Drainage of Right Pelvic Bone with Drainage Device, Percutaneous Approach
0Q923ZX	Drainage of Right Pelvic Bone, Percutaneous Approach, Diagnostic
0Q923ZZ	Drainage of Right Pelvic Bone, Percutaneous Approach
0Q9240Z	Drainage of Right Pelvic Bone with Drainage Device, Percutaneous Endoscopic Approach
0Q924ZX	Drainage of Right Pelvic Bone, Percutaneous Endoscopic Approach, Diagnostic
0Q924ZZ	Drainage of Right Pelvic Bone, Percutaneous Endoscopic Approach
0Q9300Z	Drainage of Left Pelvic Bone with Drainage Device, Open Approach
0Q930ZX	Drainage of Left Pelvic Bone, Open Approach, Diagnostic
0Q930ZZ	Drainage of Left Pelvic Bone, Open Approach
0Q9330Z	Drainage of Left Pelvic Bone with Drainage Device, Percutaneous Approach
0Q933ZX	Drainage of Left Pelvic Bone, Percutaneous Approach, Diagnostic
0Q933ZZ	Drainage of Left Pelvic Bone, Percutaneous Approach
0Q9340Z	Drainage of Left Pelvic Bone with Drainage Device, Percutaneous Endoscopic Approach
0Q934ZX	Drainage of Left Pelvic Bone, Percutaneous Endoscopic Approach, Diagnostic
0Q934ZZ	Drainage of Left Pelvic Bone, Percutaneous Endoscopic Approach
0Q9400Z	Drainage of Right Acetabulum with Drainage Device, Open Approach
0Q940ZX	Drainage of Right Acetabulum, Open Approach, Diagnostic
0Q940ZZ	Drainage of Right Acetabulum, Open Approach
0Q9430Z	Drainage of Right Acetabulum with Drainage Device, Percutaneous Approach
0Q943ZX	Drainage of Right Acetabulum, Percutaneous Approach, Diagnostic
0Q943ZZ	Drainage of Right Acetabulum, Percutaneous Approach
0Q9440Z	Drainage of Right Acetabulum with Drainage Device, Percutaneous Endoscopic Approach
0Q944ZX	Drainage of Right Acetabulum, Percutaneous Endoscopic Approach, Diagnostic
0Q944ZZ	Drainage of Right Acetabulum, Percutaneous Endoscopic Approach
0Q9500Z	Drainage of Left Acetabulum with Drainage Device, Open Approach
0Q950ZX	Drainage of Left Acetabulum, Open Approach, Diagnostic
0Q950ZZ	Drainage of Left Acetabulum, Open Approach
0Q9530Z	Drainage of Left Acetabulum with Drainage Device, Percutaneous Approach
0Q953ZX	Drainage of Left Acetabulum, Percutaneous Approach, Diagnostic
0Q953ZZ	Drainage of Left Acetabulum, Percutaneous Approach
0Q9540Z	Drainage of Left Acetabulum with Drainage Device, Percutaneous Endoscopic Approach
0Q954ZX	Drainage of Left Acetabulum, Percutaneous Endoscopic Approach, Diagnostic
0Q954ZZ	Drainage of Left Acetabulum, Percutaneous Endoscopic Approach
0Q9600Z	Drainage of Right Upper Femur with Drainage Device, Open Approach
0Q960ZX	Drainage of Right Upper Femur, Open Approach, Diagnostic
0Q960ZZ	Drainage of Right Upper Femur, Open Approach
0Q9630Z	Drainage of Right Upper Femur with Drainage Device, Percutaneous Approach
0Q963ZX	Drainage of Right Upper Femur, Percutaneous Approach, Diagnostic
0Q963ZZ	Drainage of Right Upper Femur, Percutaneous Approach
0Q9640Z	Drainage of Right Upper Femur with Drainage Device, Percutaneous Endoscopic Approach
0Q964ZX	Drainage of Right Upper Femur, Percutaneous Endoscopic Approach, Diagnostic
0Q964ZZ	Drainage of Right Upper Femur, Percutaneous Endoscopic Approach
0Q9700Z	Drainage of Left Upper Femur with Drainage Device, Open Approach
0Q970ZX	Drainage of Left Upper Femur, Open Approach, Diagnostic
0Q970ZZ	Drainage of Left Upper Femur, Open Approach
0Q9730Z	Drainage of Left Upper Femur with Drainage Device, Percutaneous Approach
0Q973ZX	Drainage of Left Upper Femur, Percutaneous Approach, Diagnostic
0Q973ZZ	Drainage of Left Upper Femur, Percutaneous Approach
0Q9740Z	Drainage of Left Upper Femur with Drainage Device, Percutaneous Endoscopic Approach
0Q974ZX	Drainage of Left Upper Femur, Percutaneous Endoscopic Approach, Diagnostic
0Q974ZZ	Drainage of Left Upper Femur, Percutaneous Endoscopic Approach
0Q9800Z	Drainage of Right Femoral Shaft with Drainage Device, Open Approach
0Q980ZX	Drainage of Right Femoral Shaft, Open Approach, Diagnostic
0Q980ZZ	Drainage of Right Femoral Shaft, Open Approach
0Q9830Z	Drainage of Right Femoral Shaft with Drainage Device, Percutaneous Approach
0Q983ZX	Drainage of Right Femoral Shaft, Percutaneous Approach, Diagnostic
0Q983ZZ	Drainage of Right Femoral Shaft, Percutaneous Approach
0Q9840Z	Drainage of Right Femoral Shaft with Drainage Device, Percutaneous Endoscopic Approach
0Q984ZX	Drainage of Right Femoral Shaft, Percutaneous Endoscopic Approach, Diagnostic
0Q984ZZ	Drainage of Right Femoral Shaft, Percutaneous Endoscopic Approach
0Q9900Z	Drainage of Left Femoral Shaft with Drainage Device, Open Approach
0Q990ZX	Drainage of Left Femoral Shaft, Open Approach, Diagnostic
0Q990ZZ	Drainage of Left Femoral Shaft, Open Approach
0Q9930Z	Drainage of Left Femoral Shaft with Drainage Device, Percutaneous Approach
0Q993ZX	Drainage of Left Femoral Shaft, Percutaneous Approach, Diagnostic
0Q993ZZ	Drainage of Left Femoral Shaft, Percutaneous Approach
0Q9940Z	Drainage of Left Femoral Shaft with Drainage Device, Percutaneous Endoscopic Approach
0Q994ZX	Drainage of Left Femoral Shaft, Percutaneous Endoscopic Approach, Diagnostic
0Q994ZZ	Drainage of Left Femoral Shaft, Percutaneous Endoscopic Approach
0Q9B00Z	Drainage of Right Lower Femur with Drainage Device, Open Approach

0Q9B0ZX	Drainage of Right Lower Femur, Open Approach, Diagnostic
0Q9B0ZZ	Drainage of Right Lower Femur, Open Approach
0Q9B30Z	Drainage of Right Lower Femur with Drainage Device, Percutaneous Approach
0Q9B3ZX	Drainage of Right Lower Femur, Percutaneous Approach, Diagnostic
0Q9B3ZZ	Drainage of Right Lower Femur, Percutaneous Approach
0Q9B40Z	Drainage of Right Lower Femur with Drainage Device, Percutaneous Endoscopic Approach
0Q9B4ZX	Drainage of Right Lower Femur, Percutaneous Endoscopic Approach, Diagnostic
0Q9B4ZZ	Drainage of Right Lower Femur, Percutaneous Endoscopic Approach
0Q9C00Z	Drainage of Left Lower Femur with Drainage Device, Open Approach
0Q9C0ZX	Drainage of Left Lower Femur, Open Approach, Diagnostic
0Q9C0ZZ	Drainage of Left Lower Femur, Open Approach
0Q9C30Z	Drainage of Left Lower Femur with Drainage Device, Percutaneous Approach
0Q9C3ZX	Drainage of Left Lower Femur, Percutaneous Approach, Diagnostic
0Q9C3ZZ	Drainage of Left Lower Femur, Percutaneous Approach
0Q9C40Z	Drainage of Left Lower Femur with Drainage Device, Percutaneous Endoscopic Approach
0Q9C4ZX	Drainage of Left Lower Femur, Percutaneous Endoscopic Approach, Diagnostic
0Q9C4ZZ	Drainage of Left Lower Femur, Percutaneous Endoscopic Approach
0Q9D00Z	Drainage of Right Patella with Drainage Device, Open Approach
0Q9D0ZX	Drainage of Right Patella, Open Approach, Diagnostic
0Q9D0ZZ	Drainage of Right Patella, Open Approach
0Q9D30Z	Drainage of Right Patella with Drainage Device, Percutaneous Approach
0Q9D3ZX	Drainage of Right Patella, Percutaneous Approach, Diagnostic
0Q9D3ZZ	Drainage of Right Patella, Percutaneous Approach
0Q9D40Z	Drainage of Right Patella with Drainage Device, Percutaneous Endoscopic Approach
0Q9D4ZX	Drainage of Right Patella, Percutaneous Endoscopic Approach, Diagnostic
0Q9D4ZZ	Drainage of Right Patella, Percutaneous Endoscopic Approach
0Q9F00Z	Drainage of Left Patella with Drainage Device, Open Approach
0Q9F0ZX	Drainage of Left Patella, Open Approach, Diagnostic
0Q9F0ZZ	Drainage of Left Patella, Open Approach
0Q9F30Z	Drainage of Left Patella with Drainage Device, Percutaneous Approach
0Q9F3ZX	Drainage of Left Patella, Percutaneous Approach, Diagnostic
0Q9F3ZZ	Drainage of Left Patella, Percutaneous Approach
0Q9F40Z	Drainage of Left Patella with Drainage Device, Percutaneous Endoscopic Approach
0Q9F4ZX	Drainage of Left Patella, Percutaneous Endoscopic Approach, Diagnostic
0Q9F4ZZ	Drainage of Left Patella, Percutaneous Endoscopic Approach
0Q9G00Z	Drainage of Right Tibia with Drainage Device, Open Approach
0Q9G0ZX	Drainage of Right Tibia, Open Approach, Diagnostic
0Q9G0ZZ	Drainage of Right Tibia, Open Approach
0Q9G30Z	Drainage of Right Tibia with Drainage Device, Percutaneous Approach
0Q9G3ZX	Drainage of Right Tibia, Percutaneous Approach, Diagnostic
0Q9G3ZZ	Drainage of Right Tibia, Percutaneous Approach
0Q9G40Z	Drainage of Right Tibia with Drainage Device, Percutaneous Endoscopic Approach
0Q9G4ZX	Drainage of Right Tibia, Percutaneous Endoscopic Approach, Diagnostic
0Q9G4ZZ	Drainage of Right Tibia, Percutaneous Endoscopic Approach
0Q9H00Z	Drainage of Left Tibia with Drainage Device, Open Approach
0Q9H0ZX	Drainage of Left Tibia, Open Approach, Diagnostic
0Q9H0ZZ	Drainage of Left Tibia, Open Approach
0Q9H30Z	Drainage of Left Tibia with Drainage Device, Percutaneous Approach
0Q9H3ZX	Drainage of Left Tibia, Percutaneous Approach, Diagnostic
0Q9H3ZZ	Drainage of Left Tibia, Percutaneous Approach
0Q9H40Z	Drainage of Left Tibia with Drainage Device, Percutaneous Endoscopic Approach
0Q9H4ZX	Drainage of Left Tibia, Percutaneous Endoscopic Approach, Diagnostic
0Q9H4ZZ	Drainage of Left Tibia, Percutaneous Endoscopic Approach
0Q9J00Z	Drainage of Right Fibula with Drainage Device, Open Approach
0Q9J0ZX	Drainage of Right Fibula, Open Approach, Diagnostic
0Q9J0ZZ	Drainage of Right Fibula, Open Approach
0Q9J30Z	Drainage of Right Fibula with Drainage Device, Percutaneous Approach
0Q9J3ZX	Drainage of Right Fibula, Percutaneous Approach, Diagnostic
0Q9J3ZZ	Drainage of Right Fibula, Percutaneous Approach
0Q9J40Z	Drainage of Right Fibula with Drainage Device, Percutaneous Endoscopic Approach
0Q9J4ZX	Drainage of Right Fibula, Percutaneous Endoscopic Approach, Diagnostic
0Q9J4ZZ	Drainage of Right Fibula, Percutaneous Endoscopic Approach
0Q9K00Z	Drainage of Left Fibula with Drainage Device, Open Approach
0Q9K0ZX	Drainage of Left Fibula, Open Approach, Diagnostic
0Q9K0ZZ	Drainage of Left Fibula, Open Approach
0Q9K30Z	Drainage of Left Fibula with Drainage Device, Percutaneous Approach
0Q9K3ZX	Drainage of Left Fibula, Percutaneous Approach, Diagnostic
0Q9K3ZZ	Drainage of Left Fibula, Percutaneous Approach
0Q9K40Z	Drainage of Left Fibula with Drainage Device, Percutaneous Endoscopic Approach
0Q9K4ZX	Drainage of Left Fibula, Percutaneous Endoscopic Approach, Diagnostic
0Q9K4ZZ	Drainage of Left Fibula, Percutaneous Endoscopic Approach
0Q9L00Z	Drainage of Right Tarsal with Drainage Device, Open Approach
0Q9L0ZX	Drainage of Right Tarsal, Open Approach, Diagnostic
0Q9L0ZZ	Drainage of Right Tarsal, Open Approach
0Q9L30Z	Drainage of Right Tarsal with Drainage Device, Percutaneous Approach
0Q9L3ZX	Drainage of Right Tarsal, Percutaneous Approach, Diagnostic
0Q9L3ZZ	Drainage of Right Tarsal, Percutaneous Approach
0Q9L40Z	Drainage of Right Tarsal with Drainage Device, Percutaneous Endoscopic Approach
0Q9L4ZX	Drainage of Right Tarsal, Percutaneous Endoscopic Approach, Diagnostic
0Q9L4ZZ	Drainage of Right Tarsal, Percutaneous Endoscopic Approach
0Q9M00Z	Drainage of Left Tarsal with Drainage Device, Open Approach
0Q9M0ZX	Drainage of Left Tarsal, Open Approach, Diagnostic
0Q9M0ZZ	Drainage of Left Tarsal, Open Approach
0Q9M30Z	Drainage of Left Tarsal with Drainage Device, Percutaneous Approach
0Q9M3ZX	Drainage of Left Tarsal, Percutaneous Approach, Diagnostic
0Q9M3ZZ	Drainage of Left Tarsal, Percutaneous Approach
0Q9M40Z	Drainage of Left Tarsal with Drainage Device, Percutaneous Endoscopic Approach
0Q9M4ZX	Drainage of Left Tarsal, Percutaneous Endoscopic Approach, Diagnostic
0Q9M4ZZ	Drainage of Left Tarsal, Percutaneous Endoscopic Approach
0Q9N00Z	Drainage of Right Metatarsal with Drainage Device, Open Approach
0Q9N0ZX	Drainage of Right Metatarsal, Open Approach, Diagnostic
0Q9N0ZZ	Drainage of Right Metatarsal, Open Approach
0Q9N30Z	Drainage of Right Metatarsal with Drainage Device, Percutaneous Approach
0Q9N3ZX	Drainage of Right Metatarsal, Percutaneous Approach, Diagnostic
0Q9N3ZZ	Drainage of Right Metatarsal, Percutaneous Approach
0Q9N40Z	Drainage of Right Metatarsal with Drainage Device, Percutaneous Endoscopic Approach
0Q9N4ZX	Drainage of Right Metatarsal, Percutaneous Endoscopic Approach, Diagnostic
0Q9N4ZZ	Drainage of Right Metatarsal, Percutaneous Endoscopic Approach
0Q9P00Z	Drainage of Left Metatarsal with Drainage Device, Open Approach
0Q9P0ZX	Drainage of Left Metatarsal, Open Approach, Diagnostic
0Q9P0ZZ	Drainage of Left Metatarsal, Open Approach
0Q9P30Z	Drainage of Left Metatarsal with Drainage Device, Percutaneous Approach
0Q9P3ZX	Drainage of Left Metatarsal, Percutaneous Approach, Diagnostic
0Q9P3ZZ	Drainage of Left Metatarsal, Percutaneous Approach
0Q9P40Z	Drainage of Left Metatarsal with Drainage Device, Percutaneous Endoscopic Approach
0Q9P4ZX	Drainage of Left Metatarsal, Percutaneous Endoscopic Approach, Diagnostic
0Q9P4ZZ	Drainage of Left Metatarsal, Percutaneous Endoscopic Approach

0Q9Q00Z Drainage of Right Toe Phalanx with Drainage Device, Open Approach
0Q9Q0ZX Drainage of Right Toe Phalanx, Open Approach, Diagnostic
0Q9Q0ZZ Drainage of Right Toe Phalanx, Open Approach
0Q9Q30Z Drainage of Right Toe Phalanx with Drainage Device, Percutaneous Approach
0Q9Q3ZX Drainage of Right Toe Phalanx, Percutaneous Approach, Diagnostic
0Q9Q3ZZ Drainage of Right Toe Phalanx, Percutaneous Approach
0Q9Q40Z Drainage of Right Toe Phalanx with Drainage Device, Percutaneous Endoscopic Approach
0Q9Q4ZX Drainage of Right Toe Phalanx, Percutaneous Endoscopic Approach, Diagnostic
0Q9Q4ZZ Drainage of Right Toe Phalanx, Percutaneous Endoscopic Approach
0Q9R00Z Drainage of Left Toe Phalanx with Drainage Device, Open Approach
0Q9R0ZX Drainage of Left Toe Phalanx, Open Approach, Diagnostic
0Q9R0ZZ Drainage of Left Toe Phalanx, Open Approach
0Q9R30Z Drainage of Left Toe Phalanx with Drainage Device, Percutaneous Approach

0Q9R3ZX Drainage of Left Toe Phalanx, Percutaneous Approach, Diagnostic
0Q9R3ZZ Drainage of Left Toe Phalanx, Percutaneous Approach
0Q9R40Z Drainage of Left Toe Phalanx with Drainage Device, Percutaneous Endoscopic Approach
0Q9R4ZX Drainage of Left Toe Phalanx, Percutaneous Endoscopic Approach, Diagnostic
0Q9R4ZZ Drainage of Left Toe Phalanx, Percutaneous Endoscopic Approach
0Q9S00Z Drainage of Coccyx with Drainage Device, Open Approach
0Q9S0ZX Drainage of Coccyx, Open Approach, Diagnostic
0Q9S0ZZ Drainage of Coccyx, Open Approach
0Q9S30Z Drainage of Coccyx with Drainage Device, Percutaneous Approach
0Q9S3ZX Drainage of Coccyx, Percutaneous Approach, Diagnostic
0Q9S3ZZ Drainage of Coccyx, Percutaneous Approach
0Q9S40Z Drainage of Coccyx with Drainage Device, Percutaneous Endoscopic Approach
0Q9S4ZX Drainage of Coccyx, Percutaneous Endoscopic Approach, Diagnostic
0Q9S4ZZ Drainage of Coccyx, Percutaneous Endoscopic Approach

0QB – Lower Bones, Excision

Review Coding Guidelines B3.4a and B3.4b

Review Coding Guideline B3.5

Review Coding Guideline B3.8

0QB00ZX Excision of Lumbar Vertebra, Open Approach, Diagnostic
0QB00ZZ Excision of Lumbar Vertebra, Open Approach
0QB03ZX Excision of Lumbar Vertebra, Percutaneous Approach, Diagnostic
0QB03ZZ Excision of Lumbar Vertebra, Percutaneous Approach
0QB04ZX Excision of Lumbar Vertebra, Percutaneous Endoscopic Approach, Diagnostic
0QB04ZZ Excision of Lumbar Vertebra, Percutaneous Endoscopic Approach
0QB10ZX Excision of Sacrum, Open Approach, Diagnostic
0QB10ZZ Excision of Sacrum, Open Approach
0QB13ZX Excision of Sacrum, Percutaneous Approach, Diagnostic
0QB13ZZ Excision of Sacrum, Percutaneous Approach
0QB14ZX Excision of Sacrum, Percutaneous Endoscopic Approach, Diagnostic
0QB14ZZ Excision of Sacrum, Percutaneous Endoscopic Approach
0QB20ZX Excision of Right Pelvic Bone, Open Approach, Diagnostic
0QB20ZZ Excision of Right Pelvic Bone, Open Approach
0QB23ZX Excision of Right Pelvic Bone, Percutaneous Approach, Diagnostic
0QB23ZZ Excision of Right Pelvic Bone, Percutaneous Approach
0QB24ZX Excision of Right Pelvic Bone, Percutaneous Endoscopic Approach, Diagnostic
0QB24ZZ Excision of Right Pelvic Bone, Percutaneous Endoscopic Approach
0QB30ZX Excision of Left Pelvic Bone, Open Approach, Diagnostic
0QB30ZZ Excision of Left Pelvic Bone, Open Approach
0QB33ZX Excision of Left Pelvic Bone, Percutaneous Approach, Diagnostic
0QB33ZZ Excision of Left Pelvic Bone, Percutaneous Approach
0QB34ZX Excision of Left Pelvic Bone, Percutaneous Endoscopic Approach, Diagnostic
0QB34ZZ Excision of Left Pelvic Bone, Percutaneous Endoscopic Approach
0QB40ZX Excision of Right Acetabulum, Open Approach, Diagnostic
0QB40ZZ Excision of Right Acetabulum, Open Approach
0QB43ZX Excision of Right Acetabulum, Percutaneous Approach, Diagnostic
0QB43ZZ Excision of Right Acetabulum, Percutaneous Approach
0QB44ZX Excision of Right Acetabulum, Percutaneous Endoscopic Approach, Diagnostic
0QB44ZZ Excision of Right Acetabulum, Percutaneous Endoscopic Approach
0QB50ZX Excision of Left Acetabulum, Open Approach, Diagnostic
0QB50ZZ Excision of Left Acetabulum, Open Approach
0QB53ZX Excision of Left Acetabulum, Percutaneous Approach, Diagnostic
0QB53ZZ Excision of Left Acetabulum, Percutaneous Approach
0QB54ZX Excision of Left Acetabulum, Percutaneous Endoscopic Approach, Diagnostic
0QB54ZZ Excision of Left Acetabulum, Percutaneous Endoscopic Approach
0QB60ZX Excision of Right Upper Femur, Open Approach, Diagnostic
0QB60ZZ Excision of Right Upper Femur, Open Approach
0QB63ZX Excision of Right Upper Femur, Percutaneous Approach, Diagnostic
0QB63ZZ Excision of Right Upper Femur, Percutaneous Approach

0QB64ZX Excision of Right Upper Femur, Percutaneous Endoscopic Approach, Diagnostic
0QB64ZZ Excision of Right Upper Femur, Percutaneous Endoscopic Approach
0QB70ZX Excision of Left Upper Femur, Open Approach, Diagnostic
0QB70ZZ Excision of Left Upper Femur, Open Approach
0QB73ZX Excision of Left Upper Femur, Percutaneous Approach, Diagnostic
0QB73ZZ Excision of Left Upper Femur, Percutaneous Approach
0QB74ZX Excision of Left Upper Femur, Percutaneous Endoscopic Approach, Diagnostic
0QB74ZZ Excision of Left Upper Femur, Percutaneous Endoscopic Approach
0QB80ZX Excision of Right Femoral Shaft, Open Approach, Diagnostic
0QB80ZZ Excision of Right Femoral Shaft, Open Approach
0QB83ZX Excision of Right Femoral Shaft, Percutaneous Approach, Diagnostic
0QB83ZZ Excision of Right Femoral Shaft, Percutaneous Approach
0QB84ZX Excision of Right Femoral Shaft, Percutaneous Endoscopic Approach, Diagnostic
0QB84ZZ Excision of Right Femoral Shaft, Percutaneous Endoscopic Approach
0QB90ZX Excision of Left Femoral Shaft, Open Approach, Diagnostic
0QB90ZZ Excision of Left Femoral Shaft, Open Approach
0QB93ZX Excision of Left Femoral Shaft, Percutaneous Approach, Diagnostic
0QB93ZZ Excision of Left Femoral Shaft, Percutaneous Approach
0QB94ZX Excision of Left Femoral Shaft, Percutaneous Endoscopic Approach, Diagnostic
0QB94ZZ Excision of Left Femoral Shaft, Percutaneous Endoscopic Approach
0QBB0ZX Excision of Right Lower Femur, Open Approach, Diagnostic
0QBB0ZZ Excision of Right Lower Femur, Open Approach
0QBB3ZX Excision of Right Lower Femur, Percutaneous Approach, Diagnostic
0QBB3ZZ Excision of Right Lower Femur, Percutaneous Approach
0QBB4ZX Excision of Right Lower Femur, Percutaneous Endoscopic Approach, Diagnostic
0QBB4ZZ Excision of Right Lower Femur, Percutaneous Endoscopic Approach
0QBC0ZX Excision of Left Lower Femur, Open Approach, Diagnostic
0QBC0ZZ Excision of Left Lower Femur, Open Approach
0QBC3ZX Excision of Left Lower Femur, Percutaneous Approach, Diagnostic
0QBC3ZZ Excision of Left Lower Femur, Percutaneous Approach
0QBC4ZX Excision of Left Lower Femur, Percutaneous Endoscopic Approach, Diagnostic
0QBC4ZZ Excision of Left Lower Femur, Percutaneous Endoscopic Approach
0QBD0ZX Excision of Right Patella, Open Approach, Diagnostic
0QBD0ZZ Excision of Right Patella, Open Approach
0QBD3ZX Excision of Right Patella, Percutaneous Approach, Diagnostic

0QBD3ZZ Excision of Right Patella, Percutaneous Approach
0QBD4ZX Excision of Right Patella, Percutaneous Endoscopic Approach, Diagnostic
0QBD4ZZ Excision of Right Patella, Percutaneous Endoscopic Approach
0QBF0ZX Excision of Left Patella, Open Approach, Diagnostic
0QBF0ZZ Excision of Left Patella, Open Approach
0QBF3ZX Excision of Left Patella, Percutaneous Approach, Diagnostic
0QBF3ZZ Excision of Left Patella, Percutaneous Approach
0QBF4ZX Excision of Left Patella, Percutaneous Endoscopic Approach, Diagnostic
0QBF4ZZ Excision of Left Patella, Percutaneous Endoscopic Approach
0QBG0ZX Excision of Right Tibia, Open Approach, Diagnostic
0QBG0ZZ Excision of Right Tibia, Open Approach
0QBG3ZX Excision of Right Tibia, Percutaneous Approach, Diagnostic
0QBG3ZZ Excision of Right Tibia, Percutaneous Approach
0QBG4ZX Excision of Right Tibia, Percutaneous Endoscopic Approach, Diagnostic
0QBG4ZZ Excision of Right Tibia, Percutaneous Endoscopic Approach
0QBH0ZX Excision of Left Tibia, Open Approach, Diagnostic
0QBH0ZZ Excision of Left Tibia, Open Approach
0QBH3ZX Excision of Left Tibia, Percutaneous Approach, Diagnostic
0QBH3ZZ Excision of Left Tibia, Percutaneous Approach
0QBH4ZX Excision of Left Tibia, Percutaneous Endoscopic Approach, Diagnostic
0QBH4ZZ Excision of Left Tibia, Percutaneous Endoscopic Approach
0QBJ0ZX Excision of Right Fibula, Open Approach, Diagnostic
0QBJ0ZZ Excision of Right Fibula, Open Approach
0QBJ3ZX Excision of Right Fibula, Percutaneous Approach, Diagnostic
0QBJ3ZZ Excision of Right Fibula, Percutaneous Approach
0QBJ4ZX Excision of Right Fibula, Percutaneous Endoscopic Approach, Diagnostic
0QBJ4ZZ Excision of Right Fibula, Percutaneous Endoscopic Approach
0QBK0ZX Excision of Left Fibula, Open Approach, Diagnostic
0QBK0ZZ Excision of Left Fibula, Open Approach
0QBK3ZX Excision of Left Fibula, Percutaneous Approach, Diagnostic
0QBK3ZZ Excision of Left Fibula, Percutaneous Approach
0QBK4ZX Excision of Left Fibula, Percutaneous Endoscopic Approach, Diagnostic
0QBK4ZZ Excision of Left Fibula, Percutaneous Endoscopic Approach
0QBL0ZX Excision of Right Tarsal, Open Approach, Diagnostic
0QBL0ZZ Excision of Right Tarsal, Open Approach
0QBL3ZX Excision of Right Tarsal, Percutaneous Approach, Diagnostic
0QBL3ZZ Excision of Right Tarsal, Percutaneous Approach
0QBL4ZX Excision of Right Tarsal, Percutaneous Endoscopic Approach, Diagnostic

0QBL4ZZ Excision of Right Tarsal, Percutaneous Endoscopic Approach
0QBM0ZX Excision of Left Tarsal, Open Approach, Diagnostic
0QBM0ZZ Excision of Left Tarsal, Open Approach
0QBM3ZX Excision of Left Tarsal, Percutaneous Approach, Diagnostic
0QBM3ZZ Excision of Left Tarsal, Percutaneous Approach
0QBM4ZX Excision of Left Tarsal, Percutaneous Endoscopic Approach, Diagnostic
0QBM4ZZ Excision of Left Tarsal, Percutaneous Endoscopic Approach
0QBN0ZX Excision of Right Metatarsal, Open Approach, Diagnostic
0QBN0ZZ Excision of Right Metatarsal, Open Approach
0QBN3ZX Excision of Right Metatarsal, Percutaneous Approach, Diagnostic
0QBN3ZZ Excision of Right Metatarsal, Percutaneous Approach
0QBN4ZX Excision of Right Metatarsal, Percutaneous Endoscopic Approach, Diagnostic
0QBN4ZZ Excision of Right Metatarsal, Percutaneous Endoscopic Approach
0QBP0ZX Excision of Left Metatarsal, Open Approach, Diagnostic
0QBP0ZZ Excision of Left Metatarsal, Open Approach
0QBP3ZX Excision of Left Metatarsal, Percutaneous Approach, Diagnostic
0QBP3ZZ Excision of Left Metatarsal, Percutaneous Approach
0QBP4ZX Excision of Left Metatarsal, Percutaneous Endoscopic Approach, Diagnostic
0QBP4ZZ Excision of Left Metatarsal, Percutaneous Endoscopic Approach
0QBQ0ZX Excision of Right Toe Phalanx, Open Approach, Diagnostic
0QBQ0ZZ Excision of Right Toe Phalanx, Open Approach
0QBQ3ZX Excision of Right Toe Phalanx, Percutaneous Approach, Diagnostic
0QBQ3ZZ Excision of Right Toe Phalanx, Percutaneous Approach
0QBQ4ZX Excision of Right Toe Phalanx, Percutaneous Endoscopic Approach, Diagnostic
0QBQ4ZZ Excision of Right Toe Phalanx, Percutaneous Endoscopic Approach
0QBR0ZX Excision of Left Toe Phalanx, Open Approach, Diagnostic
0QBR0ZZ Excision of Left Toe Phalanx, Open Approach
0QBR3ZX Excision of Left Toe Phalanx, Percutaneous Approach, Diagnostic
0QBR3ZZ Excision of Left Toe Phalanx, Percutaneous Approach
0QBR4ZX Excision of Left Toe Phalanx, Percutaneous Endoscopic Approach, Diagnostic
0QBR4ZZ Excision of Left Toe Phalanx, Percutaneous Endoscopic Approach
0QBS0ZX Excision of Coccyx, Open Approach, Diagnostic
0QBS0ZZ Excision of Coccyx, Open Approach
0QBS3ZX Excision of Coccyx, Percutaneous Approach, Diagnostic
0QBS3ZZ Excision of Coccyx, Percutaneous Approach
0QBS4ZX Excision of Coccyx, Percutaneous Endoscopic Approach, Diagnostic
0QBS4ZZ Excision of Coccyx, Percutaneous Endoscopic Approach

0QC – Lower Bones, Extirpation

0QC00ZZ Extirpation of Matter from Lumbar Vertebra, Open Approach
0QC03ZZ Extirpation of Matter from Lumbar Vertebra, Percutaneous Approach
0QC04ZZ Extirpation of Matter from Lumbar Vertebra, Percutaneous Endoscopic Approach
0QC10ZZ Extirpation of Matter from Sacrum, Open Approach
0QC13ZZ Extirpation of Matter from Sacrum, Percutaneous Approach
0QC14ZZ Extirpation of Matter from Sacrum, Percutaneous Endoscopic Approach
0QC20ZZ Extirpation of Matter from Right Pelvic Bone, Open Approach
0QC23ZZ Extirpation of Matter from Right Pelvic Bone, Percutaneous Approach
0QC24ZZ Extirpation of Matter from Right Pelvic Bone, Percutaneous Endoscopic Approach
0QC30ZZ Extirpation of Matter from Left Pelvic Bone, Open Approach
0QC33ZZ Extirpation of Matter from Left Pelvic Bone, Percutaneous Approach
0QC34ZZ Extirpation of Matter from Left Pelvic Bone, Percutaneous Endoscopic Approach
0QC40ZZ Extirpation of Matter from Right Acetabulum, Open Approach
0QC43ZZ Extirpation of Matter from Right Acetabulum, Percutaneous Approach
0QC44ZZ Extirpation of Matter from Right Acetabulum, Percutaneous Endoscopic Approach
0QC50ZZ Extirpation of Matter from Left Acetabulum, Open Approach
0QC53ZZ Extirpation of Matter from Left Acetabulum, Percutaneous Approach

0QC54ZZ Extirpation of Matter from Left Acetabulum, Percutaneous Endoscopic Approach
0QC60ZZ Extirpation of Matter from Right Upper Femur, Open Approach
0QC63ZZ Extirpation of Matter from Right Upper Femur, Percutaneous Approach
0QC64ZZ Extirpation of Matter from Right Upper Femur, Percutaneous Endoscopic Approach
0QC70ZZ Extirpation of Matter from Left Upper Femur, Open Approach
0QC73ZZ Extirpation of Matter from Left Upper Femur, Percutaneous Approach
0QC74ZZ Extirpation of Matter from Left Upper Femur, Percutaneous Endoscopic Approach
0QC80ZZ Extirpation of Matter from Right Femoral Shaft, Open Approach
0QC83ZZ Extirpation of Matter from Right Femoral Shaft, Percutaneous Approach
0QC84ZZ Extirpation of Matter from Right Femoral Shaft, Percutaneous Endoscopic Approach
0QC90ZZ Extirpation of Matter from Left Femoral Shaft, Open Approach
0QC93ZZ Extirpation of Matter from Left Femoral Shaft, Percutaneous Approach
0QC94ZZ Extirpation of Matter from Left Femoral Shaft, Percutaneous Endoscopic Approach
0QCB0ZZ Extirpation of Matter from Right Lower Femur, Open Approach
0QCB3ZZ Extirpation of Matter from Right Lower Femur, Percutaneous Approach
0QCB4ZZ Extirpation of Matter from Right Lower Femur, Percutaneous Endoscopic Approach

♀ Female-only   ♂ Male-only   ● Limited Coverage   ● Non-OR   🅷🅰🅲 HAC-associated procedure   ◆ Non-covered procedures   ➕ Combination

0QCC0ZZ Extirpation of Matter from Left Lower Femur, Open Approach
0QCC3ZZ Extirpation of Matter from Left Lower Femur, Percutaneous Approach
0QCC4ZZ Extirpation of Matter from Left Lower Femur, Percutaneous Endoscopic Approach
0QCD0ZZ Extirpation of Matter from Right Patella, Open Approach
0QCD3ZZ Extirpation of Matter from Right Patella, Percutaneous Approach
0QCD4ZZ Extirpation of Matter from Right Patella, Percutaneous Endoscopic Approach
0QCF0ZZ Extirpation of Matter from Left Patella, Open Approach
0QCF3ZZ Extirpation of Matter from Left Patella, Percutaneous Approach
0QCF4ZZ Extirpation of Matter from Left Patella, Percutaneous Endoscopic Approach
0QCG0ZZ Extirpation of Matter from Right Tibia, Open Approach
0QCG3ZZ Extirpation of Matter from Right Tibia, Percutaneous Approach
0QCG4ZZ Extirpation of Matter from Right Tibia, Percutaneous Endoscopic Approach
0QCH0ZZ Extirpation of Matter from Left Tibia, Open Approach
0QCH3ZZ Extirpation of Matter from Left Tibia, Percutaneous Approach
0QCH4ZZ Extirpation of Matter from Left Tibia, Percutaneous Endoscopic Approach
0QCJ0ZZ Extirpation of Matter from Right Fibula, Open Approach
0QCJ3ZZ Extirpation of Matter from Right Fibula, Percutaneous Approach
0QCJ4ZZ Extirpation of Matter from Right Fibula, Percutaneous Endoscopic Approach
0QCK0ZZ Extirpation of Matter from Left Fibula, Open Approach
0QCK3ZZ Extirpation of Matter from Left Fibula, Percutaneous Approach
0QCK4ZZ Extirpation of Matter from Left Fibula, Percutaneous Endoscopic Approach
0QCL0ZZ Extirpation of Matter from Right Tarsal, Open Approach

0QCL3ZZ Extirpation of Matter from Right Tarsal, Percutaneous Approach
0QCL4ZZ Extirpation of Matter from Right Tarsal, Percutaneous Endoscopic Approach
0QCM0ZZ Extirpation of Matter from Left Tarsal, Open Approach
0QCM3ZZ Extirpation of Matter from Left Tarsal, Percutaneous Approach
0QCM4ZZ Extirpation of Matter from Left Tarsal, Percutaneous Endoscopic Approach
0QCN0ZZ Extirpation of Matter from Right Metatarsal, Open Approach
0QCN3ZZ Extirpation of Matter from Right Metatarsal, Percutaneous Approach
0QCN4ZZ Extirpation of Matter from Right Metatarsal, Percutaneous Endoscopic Approach
0QCP0ZZ Extirpation of Matter from Left Metatarsal, Open Approach
0QCP3ZZ Extirpation of Matter from Left Metatarsal, Percutaneous Approach
0QCP4ZZ Extirpation of Matter from Left Metatarsal, Percutaneous Endoscopic Approach
0QCQ0ZZ Extirpation of Matter from Right Toe Phalanx, Open Approach
0QCQ3ZZ Extirpation of Matter from Right Toe Phalanx, Percutaneous Approach
0QCQ4ZZ Extirpation of Matter from Right Toe Phalanx, Percutaneous Endoscopic Approach
0QCR0ZZ Extirpation of Matter from Left Toe Phalanx, Open Approach
0QCR3ZZ Extirpation of Matter from Left Toe Phalanx, Percutaneous Approach
0QCR4ZZ Extirpation of Matter from Left Toe Phalanx, Percutaneous Endoscopic Approach
0QCS0ZZ Extirpation of Matter from Coccyx, Open Approach
0QCS3ZZ Extirpation of Matter from Coccyx, Percutaneous Approach
0QCS4ZZ Extirpation of Matter from Coccyx, Percutaneous Endoscopic Approach

0QH – Lower Bones, Insertion

0QH004Z Insertion of Internal Fixation Device into Lumbar Vertebra, Open Approach
0QH005Z Insertion of External Fixation Device into Lumbar Vertebra, Open Approach
0QH034Z Insertion of Internal Fixation Device into Lumbar Vertebra, Percutaneous Approach
0QH035Z Insertion of External Fixation Device into Lumbar Vertebra, Percutaneous Approach
0QH044Z Insertion of Internal Fixation Device into Lumbar Vertebra, Percutaneous Endoscopic Approach
0QH045Z Insertion of External Fixation Device into Lumbar Vertebra, Percutaneous Endoscopic Approach
0QH104Z Insertion of Internal Fixation Device into Sacrum, Open Approach
0QH105Z Insertion of External Fixation Device into Sacrum, Open Approach
0QH134Z Insertion of Internal Fixation Device into Sacrum, Percutaneous Approach
0QH135Z Insertion of External Fixation Device into Sacrum, Percutaneous Approach
0QH144Z Insertion of Internal Fixation Device into Sacrum, Percutaneous Endoscopic Approach
0QH145Z Insertion of External Fixation Device into Sacrum, Percutaneous Endoscopic Approach
0QH204Z Insertion of Internal Fixation Device into Right Pelvic Bone, Open Approach
0QH205Z Insertion of External Fixation Device into Right Pelvic Bone, Open Approach
0QH234Z Insertion of Internal Fixation Device into Right Pelvic Bone, Percutaneous Approach
0QH235Z Insertion of External Fixation Device into Right Pelvic Bone, Percutaneous Approach
0QH244Z Insertion of Internal Fixation Device into Right Pelvic Bone, Percutaneous Endoscopic Approach
0QH245Z Insertion of External Fixation Device into Right Pelvic Bone, Percutaneous Endoscopic Approach
0QH304Z Insertion of Internal Fixation Device into Left Pelvic Bone, Open Approach
0QH305Z Insertion of External Fixation Device into Left Pelvic Bone, Open Approach
0QH334Z Insertion of Internal Fixation Device into Left Pelvic Bone, Percutaneous Approach

0QH335Z Insertion of External Fixation Device into Left Pelvic Bone, Percutaneous Approach
0QH344Z Insertion of Internal Fixation Device into Left Pelvic Bone, Percutaneous Endoscopic Approach
0QH345Z Insertion of External Fixation Device into Left Pelvic Bone, Percutaneous Endoscopic Approach
0QH404Z Insertion of Internal Fixation Device into Right Acetabulum, Open Approach
0QH405Z Insertion of External Fixation Device into Right Acetabulum, Open Approach
0QH434Z Insertion of Internal Fixation Device into Right Acetabulum, Percutaneous Approach
0QH435Z Insertion of External Fixation Device into Right Acetabulum, Percutaneous Approach
0QH444Z Insertion of Internal Fixation Device into Right Acetabulum, Percutaneous Endoscopic Approach
0QH445Z Insertion of External Fixation Device into Right Acetabulum, Percutaneous Endoscopic Approach
0QH504Z Insertion of Internal Fixation Device into Left Acetabulum, Open Approach
0QH505Z Insertion of External Fixation Device into Left Acetabulum, Open Approach
0QH534Z Insertion of Internal Fixation Device into Left Acetabulum, Percutaneous Approach
0QH535Z Insertion of External Fixation Device into Left Acetabulum, Percutaneous Approach
0QH544Z Insertion of Internal Fixation Device into Left Acetabulum, Percutaneous Endoscopic Approach
0QH545Z Insertion of External Fixation Device into Left Acetabulum, Percutaneous Endoscopic Approach
0QH604Z Insertion of Internal Fixation Device into Right Upper Femur, Open Approach
0QH605Z Insertion of External Fixation Device into Right Upper Femur, Open Approach
0QH606Z Insertion of Intramedullary Internal Fixation Device into Right Upper Femur, Open Approach
0QH608Z Insertion of Limb Lengthening External Fixation Device into Right Upper Femur, Open Approach
0QH60BZ Insertion of Monoplanar External Fixation Device into Right Upper Femur, Open Approach

0QH60CZ Insertion of Ring External Fixation Device into Right Upper Femur, Open Approach

0QH60DZ Insertion of Hybrid External Fixation Device into Right Upper Femur, Open Approach

0QH634Z Insertion of Internal Fixation Device into Right Upper Femur, Percutaneous Approach

0QH635Z Insertion of External Fixation Device into Right Upper Femur, Percutaneous Approach

0QH636Z Insertion of Intramedullary Internal Fixation Device into Right Upper Femur, Percutaneous Approach

0QH638Z Insertion of Limb Lengthening External Fixation Device into Right Upper Femur, Percutaneous Approach

0QH63BZ Insertion of Monoplanar External Fixation Device into Right Upper Femur, Percutaneous Approach

0QH63CZ Insertion of Ring External Fixation Device into Right Upper Femur, Percutaneous Approach

0QH63DZ Insertion of Hybrid External Fixation Device into Right Upper Femur, Percutaneous Approach

0QH644Z Insertion of Internal Fixation Device into Right Upper Femur, Percutaneous Endoscopic Approach

0QH645Z Insertion of External Fixation Device into Right Upper Femur, Percutaneous Endoscopic Approach

0QH646Z Insertion of Intramedullary Internal Fixation Device into Right Upper Femur, Percutaneous Endoscopic Approach

0QH648Z Insertion of Limb Lengthening External Fixation Device into Right Upper Femur, Percutaneous Endoscopic Approach

0QH64BZ Insertion of Monoplanar External Fixation Device into Right Upper Femur, Percutaneous Endoscopic Approach

0QH64CZ Insertion of Ring External Fixation Device into Right Upper Femur, Percutaneous Endoscopic Approach

0QH64DZ Insertion of Hybrid External Fixation Device into Right Upper Femur, Percutaneous Endoscopic Approach

0QH704Z Insertion of Internal Fixation Device into Left Upper Femur, Open Approach

0QH705Z Insertion of External Fixation Device into Left Upper Femur, Open Approach

0QH706Z Insertion of Intramedullary Internal Fixation Device into Left Upper Femur, Open Approach

0QH708Z Insertion of Limb Lengthening External Fixation Device into Left Upper Femur, Open Approach

0QH70BZ Insertion of Monoplanar External Fixation Device into Left Upper Femur, Open Approach

0QH70CZ Insertion of Ring External Fixation Device into Left Upper Femur, Open Approach

0QH70DZ Insertion of Hybrid External Fixation Device into Left Upper Femur, Open Approach

0QH734Z Insertion of Internal Fixation Device into Left Upper Femur, Percutaneous Approach

0QH735Z Insertion of External Fixation Device into Left Upper Femur, Percutaneous Approach

0QH736Z Insertion of Intramedullary Internal Fixation Device into Left Upper Femur, Percutaneous Approach

0QH738Z Insertion of Limb Lengthening External Fixation Device into Left Upper Femur, Percutaneous Approach

0QH73BZ Insertion of Monoplanar External Fixation Device into Left Upper Femur, Percutaneous Approach

0QH73CZ Insertion of Ring External Fixation Device into Left Upper Femur, Percutaneous Approach

0QH73DZ Insertion of Hybrid External Fixation Device into Left Upper Femur, Percutaneous Approach

0QH744Z Insertion of Internal Fixation Device into Left Upper Femur, Percutaneous Endoscopic Approach

0QH745Z Insertion of External Fixation Device into Left Upper Femur, Percutaneous Endoscopic Approach

0QH746Z Insertion of Intramedullary Internal Fixation Device into Left Upper Femur, Percutaneous Endoscopic Approach

0QH748Z Insertion of Limb Lengthening External Fixation Device into Left Upper Femur, Percutaneous Endoscopic Approach

0QH74BZ Insertion of Monoplanar External Fixation Device into Left Upper Femur, Percutaneous Endoscopic Approach

0QH74CZ Insertion of Ring External Fixation Device into Left Upper Femur, Percutaneous Endoscopic Approach

0QH74DZ Insertion of Hybrid External Fixation Device into Left Upper Femur, Percutaneous Endoscopic Approach

0QH804Z Insertion of Internal Fixation Device into Right Femoral Shaft, Open Approach

0QH805Z Insertion of External Fixation Device into Right Femoral Shaft, Open Approach

0QH806Z Insertion of Intramedullary Internal Fixation Device into Right Femoral Shaft, Open Approach

0QH808Z Insertion of Limb Lengthening External Fixation Device into Right Femoral Shaft, Open Approach

0QH80BZ Insertion of Monoplanar External Fixation Device into Right Femoral Shaft, Open Approach

0QH80CZ Insertion of Ring External Fixation Device into Right Femoral Shaft, Open Approach

0QH80DZ Insertion of Hybrid External Fixation Device into Right Femoral Shaft, Open Approach

0QH834Z Insertion of Internal Fixation Device into Right Femoral Shaft, Percutaneous Approach

0QH835Z Insertion of External Fixation Device into Right Femoral Shaft, Percutaneous Approach

0QH836Z Insertion of Intramedullary Internal Fixation Device into Right Femoral Shaft, Percutaneous Approach

0QH838Z Insertion of Limb Lengthening External Fixation Device into Right Femoral Shaft, Percutaneous Approach

0QH83BZ Insertion of Monoplanar External Fixation Device into Right Femoral Shaft, Percutaneous Approach

0QH83CZ Insertion of Ring External Fixation Device into Right Femoral Shaft, Percutaneous Approach

0QH83DZ Insertion of Hybrid External Fixation Device into Right Femoral Shaft, Percutaneous Approach

0QH844Z Insertion of Internal Fixation Device into Right Femoral Shaft, Percutaneous Endoscopic Approach

0QH845Z Insertion of External Fixation Device into Right Femoral Shaft, Percutaneous Endoscopic Approach

0QH846Z Insertion of Intramedullary Internal Fixation Device into Right Femoral Shaft, Percutaneous Endoscopic Approach

0QH848Z Insertion of Limb Lengthening External Fixation Device into Right Femoral Shaft, Percutaneous Endoscopic Approach

0QH84BZ Insertion of Monoplanar External Fixation Device into Right Femoral Shaft, Percutaneous Endoscopic Approach

0QH84CZ Insertion of Ring External Fixation Device into Right Femoral Shaft, Percutaneous Endoscopic Approach

0QH84DZ Insertion of Hybrid External Fixation Device into Right Femoral Shaft, Percutaneous Endoscopic Approach

0QH904Z Insertion of Internal Fixation Device into Left Femoral Shaft, Open Approach

0QH905Z Insertion of External Fixation Device into Left Femoral Shaft, Open Approach

0QH906Z Insertion of Intramedullary Internal Fixation Device into Left Femoral Shaft, Open Approach

0QH908Z Insertion of Limb Lengthening External Fixation Device into Left Femoral Shaft, Open Approach

0QH90BZ Insertion of Monoplanar External Fixation Device into Left Femoral Shaft, Open Approach

0QH90CZ Insertion of Ring External Fixation Device into Left Femoral Shaft, Open Approach

0QH90DZ Insertion of Hybrid External Fixation Device into Left Femoral Shaft, Open Approach

0QH934Z Insertion of Internal Fixation Device into Left Femoral Shaft, Percutaneous Approach

0QH935Z Insertion of External Fixation Device into Left Femoral Shaft, Percutaneous Approach

0QH936Z Insertion of Intramedullary Internal Fixation Device into Left Femoral Shaft, Percutaneous Approach

0QH938Z Insertion of Limb Lengthening External Fixation Device into Left Femoral Shaft, Percutaneous Approach

0QH93BZ Insertion of Monoplanar External Fixation Device into Left Femoral Shaft, Percutaneous Approach

0QH93CZ Insertion of Ring External Fixation Device into Left Femoral Shaft, Percutaneous Approach

0QH93DZ Insertion of Hybrid External Fixation Device into Left Femoral Shaft, Percutaneous Approach

0QH944Z Insertion of Internal Fixation Device into Left Femoral Shaft, Percutaneous Endoscopic Approach

0QH945Z Insertion of External Fixation Device into Left Femoral Shaft, Percutaneous Endoscopic Approach

---

0QH946Z Insertion of Intramedullary Internal Fixation Device into Left Femoral Shaft, Percutaneous Endoscopic Approach

0QH948Z Insertion of Limb Lengthening External Fixation Device into Left Femoral Shaft, Percutaneous Endoscopic Approach

0QH94BZ Insertion of Monoplanar External Fixation Device into Left Femoral Shaft, Percutaneous Endoscopic Approach

0QH94CZ Insertion of Ring External Fixation Device into Left Femoral Shaft, Percutaneous Endoscopic Approach

0QH94DZ Insertion of Hybrid External Fixation Device into Left Femoral Shaft, Percutaneous Endoscopic Approach

0QHB04Z Insertion of Internal Fixation Device into Right Lower Femur, Open Approach

0QHB05Z Insertion of External Fixation Device into Right Lower Femur, Open Approach

0QHB06Z Insertion of Intramedullary Internal Fixation Device into Right Lower Femur, Open Approach

0QHB08Z Insertion of Limb Lengthening External Fixation Device into Right Lower Femur, Open Approach

0QHB0BZ Insertion of Monoplanar External Fixation Device into Right Lower Femur, Open Approach

0QHB0CZ Insertion of Ring External Fixation Device into Right Lower Femur, Open Approach

0QHB0DZ Insertion of Hybrid External Fixation Device into Right Lower Femur, Open Approach

0QHB34Z Insertion of Internal Fixation Device into Right Lower Femur, Percutaneous Approach

0QHB35Z Insertion of External Fixation Device into Right Lower Femur, Percutaneous Approach

0QHB36Z Insertion of Intramedullary Internal Fixation Device into Right Lower Femur, Percutaneous Approach

0QHB38Z Insertion of Limb Lengthening External Fixation Device into Right Lower Femur, Percutaneous Approach

0QHB3BZ Insertion of Monoplanar External Fixation Device into Right Lower Femur, Percutaneous Approach

0QHB3CZ Insertion of Ring External Fixation Device into Right Lower Femur, Percutaneous Approach

0QHB3DZ Insertion of Hybrid External Fixation Device into Right Lower Femur, Percutaneous Approach

0QHB44Z Insertion of Internal Fixation Device into Right Lower Femur, Percutaneous Endoscopic Approach

0QHB45Z Insertion of External Fixation Device into Right Lower Femur, Percutaneous Endoscopic Approach

0QHB46Z Insertion of Intramedullary Internal Fixation Device into Right Lower Femur, Percutaneous Endoscopic Approach

0QHB48Z Insertion of Limb Lengthening External Fixation Device into Right Lower Femur, Percutaneous Endoscopic Approach

0QHB4BZ Insertion of Monoplanar External Fixation Device into Right Lower Femur, Percutaneous Endoscopic Approach

0QHB4CZ Insertion of Ring External Fixation Device into Right Lower Femur, Percutaneous Endoscopic Approach

0QHB4DZ Insertion of Hybrid External Fixation Device into Right Lower Femur, Percutaneous Endoscopic Approach

0QHC04Z Insertion of Internal Fixation Device into Left Lower Femur, Open Approach

0QHC05Z Insertion of External Fixation Device into Left Lower Femur, Open Approach

0QHC06Z Insertion of Intramedullary Internal Fixation Device into Left Lower Femur, Open Approach

0QHC08Z Insertion of Limb Lengthening External Fixation Device into Left Lower Femur, Open Approach

0QHC0BZ Insertion of Monoplanar External Fixation Device into Left Lower Femur, Open Approach

0QHC0CZ Insertion of Ring External Fixation Device into Left Lower Femur, Open Approach

0QHC0DZ Insertion of Hybrid External Fixation Device into Left Lower Femur, Open Approach

0QHC34Z Insertion of Internal Fixation Device into Left Lower Femur, Percutaneous Approach

0QHC35Z Insertion of External Fixation Device into Left Lower Femur, Percutaneous Approach

0QHC36Z Insertion of Intramedullary Internal Fixation Device into Left Lower Femur, Percutaneous Approach

0QHC38Z Insertion of Limb Lengthening External Fixation Device into Left Lower Femur, Percutaneous Approach

0QHC3BZ Insertion of Monoplanar External Fixation Device into Left Lower Femur, Percutaneous Approach

0QHC3CZ Insertion of Ring External Fixation Device into Left Lower Femur, Percutaneous Approach

0QHC3DZ Insertion of Hybrid External Fixation Device into Left Lower Femur, Percutaneous Approach

0QHC44Z Insertion of Internal Fixation Device into Left Lower Femur, Percutaneous Endoscopic Approach

0QHC45Z Insertion of External Fixation Device into Left Lower Femur, Percutaneous Endoscopic Approach

0QHC46Z Insertion of Intramedullary Internal Fixation Device into Left Lower Femur, Percutaneous Endoscopic Approach

0QHC48Z Insertion of Limb Lengthening External Fixation Device into Left Lower Femur, Percutaneous Endoscopic Approach

0QHC4BZ Insertion of Monoplanar External Fixation Device into Left Lower Femur, Percutaneous Endoscopic Approach

0QHC4CZ Insertion of Ring External Fixation Device into Left Lower Femur, Percutaneous Endoscopic Approach

0QHC4DZ Insertion of Hybrid External Fixation Device into Left Lower Femur, Percutaneous Endoscopic Approach

0QHD04Z Insertion of Internal Fixation Device into Right Patella, Open Approach

0QHD05Z Insertion of External Fixation Device into Right Patella, Open Approach

0QHD34Z Insertion of Internal Fixation Device into Right Patella, Percutaneous Approach

0QHD35Z Insertion of External Fixation Device into Right Patella, Percutaneous Approach

0QHD44Z Insertion of Internal Fixation Device into Right Patella, Percutaneous Endoscopic Approach

0QHD45Z Insertion of External Fixation Device into Right Patella, Percutaneous Endoscopic Approach

0QHF04Z Insertion of Internal Fixation Device into Left Patella, Open Approach

0QHF05Z Insertion of External Fixation Device into Left Patella, Open Approach

0QHF34Z Insertion of Internal Fixation Device into Left Patella, Percutaneous Approach

0QHF35Z Insertion of External Fixation Device into Left Patella, Percutaneous Approach

0QHF44Z Insertion of Internal Fixation Device into Left Patella, Percutaneous Endoscopic Approach

0QHF45Z Insertion of External Fixation Device into Left Patella, Percutaneous Endoscopic Approach

0QHG04Z Insertion of Internal Fixation Device into Right Tibia, Open Approach

0QHG05Z Insertion of External Fixation Device into Right Tibia, Open Approach

0QHG06Z Insertion of Intramedullary Internal Fixation Device into Right Tibia, Open Approach

0QHG08Z Insertion of Limb Lengthening External Fixation Device into Right Tibia, Open Approach

0QHG0BZ Insertion of Monoplanar External Fixation Device into Right Tibia, Open Approach

0QHG0CZ Insertion of Ring External Fixation Device into Right Tibia, Open Approach

0QHG0DZ Insertion of Hybrid External Fixation Device into Right Tibia, Open Approach

0QHG34Z Insertion of Internal Fixation Device into Right Tibia, Percutaneous Approach

0QHG35Z Insertion of External Fixation Device into Right Tibia, Percutaneous Approach

0QHG36Z Insertion of Intramedullary Internal Fixation Device into Right Tibia, Percutaneous Approach

0QHG38Z Insertion of Limb Lengthening External Fixation Device into Right Tibia, Percutaneous Approach

0QHG3BZ Insertion of Monoplanar External Fixation Device into Right Tibia, Percutaneous Approach

0QHG3CZ Insertion of Ring External Fixation Device into Right Tibia, Percutaneous Approach

0QHG3DZ Insertion of Hybrid External Fixation Device into Right Tibia, Percutaneous Approach

0QHG44Z Insertion of Internal Fixation Device into Right Tibia, Percutaneous Endoscopic Approach

0QHG45Z Insertion of External Fixation Device into Right Tibia, Percutaneous Endoscopic Approach

0QHG46Z Insertion of Intramedullary Internal Fixation Device into Right Tibia, Percutaneous Endoscopic Approach

0QHG48Z Insertion of Limb Lengthening External Fixation Device into Right Tibia, Percutaneous Endoscopic Approach

0QHG4BZ Insertion of Monoplanar External Fixation Device into Right Tibia, Percutaneous Endoscopic Approach

0QHG4CZ Insertion of Ring External Fixation Device into Right Tibia, Percutaneous Endoscopic Approach

0QHG4DZ Insertion of Hybrid External Fixation Device into Right Tibia, Percutaneous Endoscopic Approach

0QHH04Z Insertion of Internal Fixation Device into Left Tibia, Open Approach

0QHH05Z Insertion of External Fixation Device into Left Tibia, Open Approach

0QHH06Z Insertion of Intramedullary Internal Fixation Device into Left Tibia, Open Approach

0QHH08Z Insertion of Limb Lengthening External Fixation Device into Left Tibia, Open Approach

0QHH0BZ Insertion of Monoplanar External Fixation Device into Left Tibia, Open Approach

0QHH0CZ Insertion of Ring External Fixation Device into Left Tibia, Open Approach

0QHH0DZ Insertion of Hybrid External Fixation Device into Left Tibia, Open Approach

0QHH34Z Insertion of Internal Fixation Device into Left Tibia, Percutaneous Approach

0QHH35Z Insertion of External Fixation Device into Left Tibia, Percutaneous Approach

0QHH36Z Insertion of Intramedullary Internal Fixation Device into Left Tibia, Percutaneous Approach

0QHH38Z Insertion of Limb Lengthening External Fixation Device into Left Tibia, Percutaneous Approach

0QHH3BZ Insertion of Monoplanar External Fixation Device into Left Tibia, Percutaneous Approach

0QHH3CZ Insertion of Ring External Fixation Device into Left Tibia, Percutaneous Approach

0QHH3DZ Insertion of Hybrid External Fixation Device into Left Tibia, Percutaneous Approach

0QHH44Z Insertion of Internal Fixation Device into Left Tibia, Percutaneous Endoscopic Approach

0QHH45Z Insertion of External Fixation Device into Left Tibia, Percutaneous Endoscopic Approach

0QHH46Z Insertion of Intramedullary Internal Fixation Device into Left Tibia, Percutaneous Endoscopic Approach

0QHH48Z Insertion of Limb Lengthening External Fixation Device into Left Tibia, Percutaneous Endoscopic Approach

0QHH4BZ Insertion of Monoplanar External Fixation Device into Left Tibia, Percutaneous Endoscopic Approach

0QHH4CZ Insertion of Ring External Fixation Device into Left Tibia, Percutaneous Endoscopic Approach

0QHH4DZ Insertion of Hybrid External Fixation Device into Left Tibia, Percutaneous Endoscopic Approach

0QHJ04Z Insertion of Internal Fixation Device into Right Fibula, Open Approach

0QHJ05Z Insertion of External Fixation Device into Right Fibula, Open Approach

0QHJ06Z Insertion of Intramedullary Internal Fixation Device into Right Fibula, Open Approach

0QHJ08Z Insertion of Limb Lengthening External Fixation Device into Right Fibula, Open Approach

0QHJ0BZ Insertion of Monoplanar External Fixation Device into Right Fibula, Open Approach

0QHJ0CZ Insertion of Ring External Fixation Device into Right Fibula, Open Approach

0QHJ0DZ Insertion of Hybrid External Fixation Device into Right Fibula, Open Approach

0QHJ34Z Insertion of Internal Fixation Device into Right Fibula, Percutaneous Approach

0QHJ35Z Insertion of External Fixation Device into Right Fibula, Percutaneous Approach

0QHJ36Z Insertion of Intramedullary Internal Fixation Device into Right Fibula, Percutaneous Approach

0QHJ38Z Insertion of Limb Lengthening External Fixation Device into Right Fibula, Percutaneous Approach

0QHJ3BZ Insertion of Monoplanar External Fixation Device into Right Fibula, Percutaneous Approach

0QHJ3CZ Insertion of Ring External Fixation Device into Right Fibula, Percutaneous Approach

0QHJ3DZ Insertion of Hybrid External Fixation Device into Right Fibula, Percutaneous Approach

0QHJ44Z Insertion of Internal Fixation Device into Right Fibula, Percutaneous Endoscopic Approach

0QHJ45Z Insertion of External Fixation Device into Right Fibula, Percutaneous Endoscopic Approach

0QHJ46Z Insertion of Intramedullary Internal Fixation Device into Right Fibula, Percutaneous Endoscopic Approach

0QHJ48Z Insertion of Limb Lengthening External Fixation Device into Right Fibula, Percutaneous Endoscopic Approach

0QHJ4BZ Insertion of Monoplanar External Fixation Device into Right Fibula, Percutaneous Endoscopic Approach

0QHJ4CZ Insertion of Ring External Fixation Device into Right Fibula, Percutaneous Endoscopic Approach

0QHJ4DZ Insertion of Hybrid External Fixation Device into Right Fibula, Percutaneous Endoscopic Approach

0QHK04Z Insertion of Internal Fixation Device into Left Fibula, Open Approach

0QHK05Z Insertion of External Fixation Device into Left Fibula, Open Approach

0QHK06Z Insertion of Intramedullary Internal Fixation Device into Left Fibula, Open Approach

0QHK08Z Insertion of Limb Lengthening External Fixation Device into Left Fibula, Open Approach

0QHK0BZ Insertion of Monoplanar External Fixation Device into Left Fibula, Open Approach

0QHK0CZ Insertion of Ring External Fixation Device into Left Fibula, Open Approach

0QHK0DZ Insertion of Hybrid External Fixation Device into Left Fibula, Open Approach

0QHK34Z Insertion of Internal Fixation Device into Left Fibula, Percutaneous Approach

0QHK35Z Insertion of External Fixation Device into Left Fibula, Percutaneous Approach

0QHK36Z Insertion of Intramedullary Internal Fixation Device into Left Fibula, Percutaneous Approach

0QHK38Z Insertion of Limb Lengthening External Fixation Device into Left Fibula, Percutaneous Approach

0QHK3BZ Insertion of Monoplanar External Fixation Device into Left Fibula, Percutaneous Approach

0QHK3CZ Insertion of Ring External Fixation Device into Left Fibula, Percutaneous Approach

0QHK3DZ Insertion of Hybrid External Fixation Device into Left Fibula, Percutaneous Approach

0QHK44Z Insertion of Internal Fixation Device into Left Fibula, Percutaneous Endoscopic Approach

0QHK45Z Insertion of External Fixation Device into Left Fibula, Percutaneous Endoscopic Approach

0QHK46Z Insertion of Intramedullary Internal Fixation Device into Left Fibula, Percutaneous Endoscopic Approach

0QHK48Z Insertion of Limb Lengthening External Fixation Device into Left Fibula, Percutaneous Endoscopic Approach

0QHK4BZ Insertion of Monoplanar External Fixation Device into Left Fibula, Percutaneous Endoscopic Approach

0QHK4CZ Insertion of Ring External Fixation Device into Left Fibula, Percutaneous Endoscopic Approach

0QHK4DZ Insertion of Hybrid External Fixation Device into Left Fibula, Percutaneous Endoscopic Approach

0QHL04Z Insertion of Internal Fixation Device into Right Tarsal, Open Approach

0QHL05Z Insertion of External Fixation Device into Right Tarsal, Open Approach

0QHL34Z Insertion of Internal Fixation Device into Right Tarsal, Percutaneous Approach

0QHL35Z Insertion of External Fixation Device into Right Tarsal, Percutaneous Approach

0QHL44Z Insertion of Internal Fixation Device into Right Tarsal, Percutaneous Endoscopic Approach

---

♀ Female-only   ♂ Male-only   ◐ Limited Coverage   ● Non-OR   ▣ HAC-associated procedure   ⬣ Non-covered procedures   ✚ Combination

0QHL45Z Insertion of External Fixation Device into Right Tarsal, Percutaneous Endoscopic Approach

0QHM04Z Insertion of Internal Fixation Device into Left Tarsal, Open Approach

0QHM05Z Insertion of External Fixation Device into Left Tarsal, Open Approach

0QHM34Z Insertion of Internal Fixation Device into Left Tarsal, Percutaneous Approach

0QHM35Z Insertion of External Fixation Device into Left Tarsal, Percutaneous Approach

0QHM44Z Insertion of Internal Fixation Device into Left Tarsal, Percutaneous Endoscopic Approach

0QHM45Z Insertion of External Fixation Device into Left Tarsal, Percutaneous Endoscopic Approach

0QHN04Z Insertion of Internal Fixation Device into Right Metatarsal, Open Approach

0QHN05Z Insertion of External Fixation Device into Right Metatarsal, Open Approach

0QHN34Z Insertion of Internal Fixation Device into Right Metatarsal, Percutaneous Approach

0QHN35Z Insertion of External Fixation Device into Right Metatarsal, Percutaneous Approach

0QHN44Z Insertion of Internal Fixation Device into Right Metatarsal, Percutaneous Endoscopic Approach

0QHN45Z Insertion of External Fixation Device into Right Metatarsal, Percutaneous Endoscopic Approach

0QHP04Z Insertion of Internal Fixation Device into Left Metatarsal, Open Approach

0QHP05Z Insertion of External Fixation Device into Left Metatarsal, Open Approach

0QHP34Z Insertion of Internal Fixation Device into Left Metatarsal, Percutaneous Approach

0QHP35Z Insertion of External Fixation Device into Left Metatarsal, Percutaneous Approach

0QHP44Z Insertion of Internal Fixation Device into Left Metatarsal, Percutaneous Endoscopic Approach

0QHP45Z Insertion of External Fixation Device into Left Metatarsal, Percutaneous Endoscopic Approach

0QHQ04Z Insertion of Internal Fixation Device into Right Toe Phalanx, Open Approach

0QHQ05Z Insertion of External Fixation Device into Right Toe Phalanx, Open Approach

0QHQ34Z Insertion of Internal Fixation Device into Right Toe Phalanx, Percutaneous Approach

0QHQ35Z Insertion of External Fixation Device into Right Toe Phalanx, Percutaneous Approach

0QHQ44Z Insertion of Internal Fixation Device into Right Toe Phalanx, Percutaneous Endoscopic Approach

0QHQ45Z Insertion of External Fixation Device into Right Toe Phalanx, Percutaneous Endoscopic Approach

0QHR04Z Insertion of Internal Fixation Device into Left Toe Phalanx, Open Approach

0QHR05Z Insertion of External Fixation Device into Left Toe Phalanx, Open Approach

0QHR34Z Insertion of Internal Fixation Device into Left Toe Phalanx, Percutaneous Approach

0QHR35Z Insertion of External Fixation Device into Left Toe Phalanx, Percutaneous Approach

0QHR44Z Insertion of Internal Fixation Device into Left Toe Phalanx, Percutaneous Endoscopic Approach

0QHR45Z Insertion of External Fixation Device into Left Toe Phalanx, Percutaneous Endoscopic Approach

0QHS04Z Insertion of Internal Fixation Device into Coccyx, Open Approach

0QHS05Z Insertion of External Fixation Device into Coccyx, Open Approach

0QHS34Z Insertion of Internal Fixation Device into Coccyx, Percutaneous Approach

0QHS35Z Insertion of External Fixation Device into Coccyx, Percutaneous Approach

0QHS44Z Insertion of Internal Fixation Device into Coccyx, Percutaneous Endoscopic Approach

0QHS45Z Insertion of External Fixation Device into Coccyx, Percutaneous Endoscopic Approach

0QHY0MZ Insertion of Bone Growth Stimulator into Lower Bone, Open Approach

0QHY3MZ Insertion of Bone Growth Stimulator into Lower Bone, Percutaneous Approach

0QHY4MZ Insertion of Bone Growth Stimulator into Lower Bone, Percutaneous Endoscopic Approach

0QJ – Lower Bones, Inspection

Review Coding Guideline B3.5

Review Coding Guidelines B3.11a, B3.11b and B3.11c

0QJY0ZZ Inspection of Lower Bone, Open Approach
0QJY3ZZ Inspection of Lower Bone, Percutaneous Approach

0QJY4ZZ Inspection of Lower Bone, Percutaneous Endoscopic Approach
0QJYXZZ Inspection of Lower Bone, External Approach

0QN – Lower Bones, Release

Review Coding Guideline B3.13

Review Coding Guideline B3.14

0QN00ZZ Release Lumbar Vertebra, Open Approach
0QN03ZZ Release Lumbar Vertebra, Percutaneous Approach
0QN04ZZ Release Lumbar Vertebra, Percutaneous Endoscopic Approach
0QN10ZZ Release Sacrum, Open Approach
0QN13ZZ Release Sacrum, Percutaneous Approach
0QN14ZZ Release Sacrum, Percutaneous Endoscopic Approach
0QN20ZZ Release Right Pelvic Bone, Open Approach
0QN23ZZ Release Right Pelvic Bone, Percutaneous Approach
0QN24ZZ Release Right Pelvic Bone, Percutaneous Endoscopic Approach
0QN30ZZ Release Left Pelvic Bone, Open Approach
0QN33ZZ Release Left Pelvic Bone, Percutaneous Approach
0QN34ZZ Release Left Pelvic Bone, Percutaneous Endoscopic Approach
0QN40ZZ Release Right Acetabulum, Open Approach
0QN43ZZ Release Right Acetabulum, Percutaneous Approach
0QN44ZZ Release Right Acetabulum, Percutaneous Endoscopic Approach
0QN50ZZ Release Left Acetabulum, Open Approach
0QN53ZZ Release Left Acetabulum, Percutaneous Approach
0QN54ZZ Release Left Acetabulum, Percutaneous Endoscopic Approach
0QN60ZZ Release Right Upper Femur, Open Approach
0QN63ZZ Release Right Upper Femur, Percutaneous Approach

0QN64ZZ Release Right Upper Femur, Percutaneous Endoscopic Approach
0QN70ZZ Release Left Upper Femur, Open Approach
0QN73ZZ Release Left Upper Femur, Percutaneous Approach
0QN74ZZ Release Left Upper Femur, Percutaneous Endoscopic Approach
0QN80ZZ Release Right Femoral Shaft, Open Approach
0QN83ZZ Release Right Femoral Shaft, Percutaneous Approach
0QN84ZZ Release Right Femoral Shaft, Percutaneous Endoscopic Approach
0QN90ZZ Release Left Femoral Shaft, Open Approach
0QN93ZZ Release Left Femoral Shaft, Percutaneous Approach
0QN94ZZ Release Left Femoral Shaft, Percutaneous Endoscopic Approach
0QNB0ZZ Release Right Lower Femur, Open Approach
0QNB3ZZ Release Right Lower Femur, Percutaneous Approach
0QNB4ZZ Release Right Lower Femur, Percutaneous Endoscopic Approach
0QNC0ZZ Release Left Lower Femur, Open Approach
0QNC3ZZ Release Left Lower Femur, Percutaneous Approach
0QNC4ZZ Release Left Lower Femur, Percutaneous Endoscopic Approach
0QND0ZZ Release Right Patella, Open Approach
0QND3ZZ Release Right Patella, Percutaneous Approach
0QND4ZZ Release Right Patella, Percutaneous Endoscopic Approach
0QNF0ZZ Release Left Patella, Open Approach

0QNF3ZZ Release Left Patella, Percutaneous Approach
0QNF4ZZ Release Left Patella, Percutaneous Endoscopic Approach
0QNG0ZZ Release Right Tibia, Open Approach
0QNG3ZZ Release Right Tibia, Percutaneous Approach
0QNG4ZZ Release Right Tibia, Percutaneous Endoscopic Approach
0QNH0ZZ Release Left Tibia, Open Approach
0QNH3ZZ Release Left Tibia, Percutaneous Approach
0QNH4ZZ Release Left Tibia, Percutaneous Endoscopic Approach
0QNJ0ZZ Release Right Fibula, Open Approach
0QNJ3ZZ Release Right Fibula, Percutaneous Approach
0QNJ4ZZ Release Right Fibula, Percutaneous Endoscopic Approach
0QNK0ZZ Release Left Fibula, Open Approach
0QNK3ZZ Release Left Fibula, Percutaneous Approach
0QNK4ZZ Release Left Fibula, Percutaneous Endoscopic Approach
0QNL0ZZ Release Right Tarsal, Open Approach
0QNL3ZZ Release Right Tarsal, Percutaneous Approach
0QNL4ZZ Release Right Tarsal, Percutaneous Endoscopic Approach
0QNM0ZZ Release Left Tarsal, Open Approach

0QNM3ZZ Release Left Tarsal, Percutaneous Approach
0QNM4ZZ Release Left Tarsal, Percutaneous Endoscopic Approach
0QNN0ZZ Release Right Metatarsal, Open Approach
0QNN3ZZ Release Right Metatarsal, Percutaneous Approach
0QNN4ZZ Release Right Metatarsal, Percutaneous Endoscopic Approach
0QNP0ZZ Release Left Metatarsal, Open Approach
0QNP3ZZ Release Left Metatarsal, Percutaneous Approach
0QNP4ZZ Release Left Metatarsal, Percutaneous Endoscopic Approach
0QNQ0ZZ Release Right Toe Phalanx, Open Approach
0QNQ3ZZ Release Right Toe Phalanx, Percutaneous Approach
0QNQ4ZZ Release Right Toe Phalanx, Percutaneous Endoscopic Approach
0QNR0ZZ Release Left Toe Phalanx, Open Approach
0QNR3ZZ Release Left Toe Phalanx, Percutaneous Approach
0QNR4ZZ Release Left Toe Phalanx, Percutaneous Endoscopic Approach
0QNS0ZZ Release Coccyx, Open Approach
0QNS3ZZ Release Coccyx, Percutaneous Approach
0QNS4ZZ Release Coccyx, Percutaneous Endoscopic Approach

0QP – Lower Bones, Removal

Review Coding Guideline B6.1c

0QP004Z Removal of Internal Fixation Device from Lumbar Vertebra, Open Approach
0QP007Z Removal of Autologous Tissue Substitute from Lumbar Vertebra, Open Approach
0QP00JZ Removal of Synthetic Substitute from Lumbar Vertebra, Open Approach
0QP00KZ Removal of Nonautologous Tissue Substitute from Lumbar Vertebra, Open Approach
0QP034Z Removal of Internal Fixation Device from Lumbar Vertebra, Percutaneous Approach
0QP037Z Removal of Autologous Tissue Substitute from Lumbar Vertebra, Percutaneous Approach
0QP03JZ Removal of Synthetic Substitute from Lumbar Vertebra, Percutaneous Approach
0QP03KZ Removal of Nonautologous Tissue Substitute from Lumbar Vertebra, Percutaneous Approach
0QP044Z Removal of Internal Fixation Device from Lumbar Vertebra, Percutaneous Endoscopic Approach
0QP047Z Removal of Autologous Tissue Substitute from Lumbar Vertebra, Percutaneous Endoscopic Approach
0QP04JZ Removal of Synthetic Substitute from Lumbar Vertebra, Percutaneous Endoscopic Approach
0QP04KZ Removal of Nonautologous Tissue Substitute from Lumbar Vertebra, Percutaneous Endoscopic Approach
0QP0X4Z Removal of Internal Fixation Device from Lumbar Vertebra, External Approach
0QP104Z Removal of Internal Fixation Device from Sacrum, Open Approach
0QP107Z Removal of Autologous Tissue Substitute from Sacrum, Open Approach
0QP10JZ Removal of Synthetic Substitute from Sacrum, Open Approach
0QP10KZ Removal of Nonautologous Tissue Substitute from Sacrum, Open Approach
0QP134Z Removal of Internal Fixation Device from Sacrum, Percutaneous Approach
0QP137Z Removal of Autologous Tissue Substitute from Sacrum, Percutaneous Approach
0QP13JZ Removal of Synthetic Substitute from Sacrum, Percutaneous Approach
0QP13KZ Removal of Nonautologous Tissue Substitute from Sacrum, Percutaneous Approach
0QP144Z Removal of Internal Fixation Device from Sacrum, Percutaneous Endoscopic Approach
0QP147Z Removal of Autologous Tissue Substitute from Sacrum, Percutaneous Endoscopic Approach
0QP14JZ Removal of Synthetic Substitute from Sacrum, Percutaneous Endoscopic Approach
0QP14KZ Removal of Nonautologous Tissue Substitute from Sacrum, Percutaneous Endoscopic Approach
0QP1X4Z Removal of Internal Fixation Device from Sacrum, External Approach
0QP204Z Removal of Internal Fixation Device from Right Pelvic Bone, Open Approach

0QP205Z Removal of External Fixation Device from Right Pelvic Bone, Open Approach
0QP207Z Removal of Autologous Tissue Substitute from Right Pelvic Bone, Open Approach
0QP20JZ Removal of Synthetic Substitute from Right Pelvic Bone, Open Approach
0QP20KZ Removal of Nonautologous Tissue Substitute from Right Pelvic Bone, Open Approach
0QP234Z Removal of Internal Fixation Device from Right Pelvic Bone, Percutaneous Approach
0QP235Z Removal of External Fixation Device from Right Pelvic Bone, Percutaneous Approach
0QP237Z Removal of Autologous Tissue Substitute from Right Pelvic Bone, Percutaneous Approach
0QP23JZ Removal of Synthetic Substitute from Right Pelvic Bone, Percutaneous Approach
0QP23KZ Removal of Nonautologous Tissue Substitute from Right Pelvic Bone, Percutaneous Approach
0QP244Z Removal of Internal Fixation Device from Right Pelvic Bone, Percutaneous Endoscopic Approach
0QP245Z Removal of External Fixation Device from Right Pelvic Bone, Percutaneous Endoscopic Approach
0QP247Z Removal of Autologous Tissue Substitute from Right Pelvic Bone, Percutaneous Endoscopic Approach
0QP24JZ Removal of Synthetic Substitute from Right Pelvic Bone, Percutaneous Endoscopic Approach
0QP24KZ Removal of Nonautologous Tissue Substitute from Right Pelvic Bone, Percutaneous Endoscopic Approach
0QP2X4Z Removal of Internal Fixation Device from Right Pelvic Bone, External Approach
0QP2X5Z Removal of External Fixation Device from Right Pelvic Bone, External Approach
0QP304Z Removal of Internal Fixation Device from Left Pelvic Bone, Open Approach
0QP305Z Removal of External Fixation Device from Left Pelvic Bone, Open Approach
0QP307Z Removal of Autologous Tissue Substitute from Left Pelvic Bone, Open Approach
0QP30JZ Removal of Synthetic Substitute from Left Pelvic Bone, Open Approach
0QP30KZ Removal of Nonautologous Tissue Substitute from Left Pelvic Bone, Open Approach
0QP334Z Removal of Internal Fixation Device from Left Pelvic Bone, Percutaneous Approach
0QP335Z Removal of External Fixation Device from Left Pelvic Bone, Percutaneous Approach
0QP337Z Removal of Autologous Tissue Substitute from Left Pelvic Bone, Percutaneous Approach
0QP33JZ Removal of Synthetic Substitute from Left Pelvic Bone, Percutaneous Approach
0QP33KZ Removal of Nonautologous Tissue Substitute from Left Pelvic Bone, Percutaneous Approach

0QP344Z   Removal of Internal Fixation Device from Left Pelvic Bone, Percutaneous Endoscopic Approach

0QP345Z   Removal of External Fixation Device from Left Pelvic Bone, Percutaneous Endoscopic Approach

0QP347Z   Removal of Autologous Tissue Substitute from Left Pelvic Bone, Percutaneous Endoscopic Approach

0QP34JZ   Removal of Synthetic Substitute from Left Pelvic Bone, Percutaneous Endoscopic Approach

0QP34KZ   Removal of Nonautologous Tissue Substitute from Left Pelvic Bone, Percutaneous Endoscopic Approach

0QP3X4Z   Removal of Internal Fixation Device from Left Pelvic Bone, External Approach

0QP3X5Z   Removal of External Fixation Device from Left Pelvic Bone, External Approach

0QP404Z   Removal of Internal Fixation Device from Right Acetabulum, Open Approach

0QP407Z   Removal of Autologous Tissue Substitute from Right Acetabulum, Open Approach

0QP40JZ   Removal of Synthetic Substitute from Right Acetabulum, Open Approach

0QP40KZ   Removal of Nonautologous Tissue Substitute from Right Acetabulum, Open Approach

0QP434Z   Removal of Internal Fixation Device from Right Acetabulum, Percutaneous Approach

0QP437Z   Removal of Autologous Tissue Substitute from Right Acetabulum, Percutaneous Approach

0QP43JZ   Removal of Synthetic Substitute from Right Acetabulum, Percutaneous Approach

0QP43KZ   Removal of Nonautologous Tissue Substitute from Right Acetabulum, Percutaneous Approach

0QP444Z   Removal of Internal Fixation Device from Right Acetabulum, Percutaneous Endoscopic Approach

0QP447Z   Removal of Autologous Tissue Substitute from Right Acetabulum, Percutaneous Endoscopic Approach

0QP44JZ   Removal of Synthetic Substitute from Right Acetabulum, Percutaneous Endoscopic Approach

0QP44KZ   Removal of Nonautologous Tissue Substitute from Right Acetabulum, Percutaneous Endoscopic Approach

0QP4X4Z   Removal of Internal Fixation Device from Right Acetabulum, External Approach

0QP504Z   Removal of Internal Fixation Device from Left Acetabulum, Open Approach

0QP507Z   Removal of Autologous Tissue Substitute from Left Acetabulum, Open Approach

0QP50JZ   Removal of Synthetic Substitute from Left Acetabulum, Open Approach

0QP50KZ   Removal of Nonautologous Tissue Substitute from Left Acetabulum, Open Approach

0QP534Z   Removal of Internal Fixation Device from Left Acetabulum, Percutaneous Approach

0QP537Z   Removal of Autologous Tissue Substitute from Left Acetabulum, Percutaneous Approach

0QP53JZ   Removal of Synthetic Substitute from Left Acetabulum, Percutaneous Approach

0QP53KZ   Removal of Nonautologous Tissue Substitute from Left Acetabulum, Percutaneous Approach

0QP544Z   Removal of Internal Fixation Device from Left Acetabulum, Percutaneous Endoscopic Approach

0QP547Z   Removal of Autologous Tissue Substitute from Left Acetabulum, Percutaneous Endoscopic Approach

0QP54JZ   Removal of Synthetic Substitute from Left Acetabulum, Percutaneous Endoscopic Approach

0QP54KZ   Removal of Nonautologous Tissue Substitute from Left Acetabulum, Percutaneous Endoscopic Approach

0QP5X4Z   Removal of Internal Fixation Device from Left Acetabulum, External Approach

0QP604Z   Removal of Internal Fixation Device from Right Upper Femur, Open Approach

0QP605Z   Removal of External Fixation Device from Right Upper Femur, Open Approach

0QP607Z   Removal of Autologous Tissue Substitute from Right Upper Femur, Open Approach

0QP60JZ   Removal of Synthetic Substitute from Right Upper Femur, Open Approach

0QP60KZ   Removal of Nonautologous Tissue Substitute from Right Upper Femur, Open Approach

0QP634Z   Removal of Internal Fixation Device from Right Upper Femur, Percutaneous Approach

0QP635Z   Removal of External Fixation Device from Right Upper Femur, Percutaneous Approach

0QP637Z   Removal of Autologous Tissue Substitute from Right Upper Femur, Percutaneous Approach

0QP63JZ   Removal of Synthetic Substitute from Right Upper Femur, Percutaneous Approach

0QP63KZ   Removal of Nonautologous Tissue Substitute from Right Upper Femur, Percutaneous Approach

0QP644Z   Removal of Internal Fixation Device from Right Upper Femur, Percutaneous Endoscopic Approach

0QP645Z   Removal of External Fixation Device from Right Upper Femur, Percutaneous Endoscopic Approach

0QP647Z   Removal of Autologous Tissue Substitute from Right Upper Femur, Percutaneous Endoscopic Approach

0QP64JZ   Removal of Synthetic Substitute from Right Upper Femur, Percutaneous Endoscopic Approach

0QP64KZ   Removal of Nonautologous Tissue Substitute from Right Upper Femur, Percutaneous Endoscopic Approach

0QP6X4Z   Removal of Internal Fixation Device from Right Upper Femur, External Approach

0QP6X5Z   Removal of External Fixation Device from Right Upper Femur, External Approach

0QP704Z   Removal of Internal Fixation Device from Left Upper Femur, Open Approach

0QP705Z   Removal of External Fixation Device from Left Upper Femur, Open Approach

0QP707Z   Removal of Autologous Tissue Substitute from Left Upper Femur, Open Approach

0QP70JZ   Removal of Synthetic Substitute from Left Upper Femur, Open Approach

0QP70KZ   Removal of Nonautologous Tissue Substitute from Left Upper Femur, Open Approach

0QP734Z   Removal of Internal Fixation Device from Left Upper Femur, Percutaneous Approach

0QP735Z   Removal of External Fixation Device from Left Upper Femur, Percutaneous Approach

0QP737Z   Removal of Autologous Tissue Substitute from Left Upper Femur, Percutaneous Approach

0QP73JZ   Removal of Synthetic Substitute from Left Upper Femur, Percutaneous Approach

0QP73KZ   Removal of Nonautologous Tissue Substitute from Left Upper Femur, Percutaneous Approach

0QP744Z   Removal of Internal Fixation Device from Left Upper Femur, Percutaneous Endoscopic Approach

0QP745Z   Removal of External Fixation Device from Left Upper Femur, Percutaneous Endoscopic Approach

0QP747Z   Removal of Autologous Tissue Substitute from Left Upper Femur, Percutaneous Endoscopic Approach

0QP74JZ   Removal of Synthetic Substitute from Left Upper Femur, Percutaneous Endoscopic Approach

0QP74KZ   Removal of Nonautologous Tissue Substitute from Left Upper Femur, Percutaneous Endoscopic Approach

0QP7X4Z   Removal of Internal Fixation Device from Left Upper Femur, External Approach

0QP7X5Z   Removal of External Fixation Device from Left Upper Femur, External Approach

0QP804Z   Removal of Internal Fixation Device from Right Femoral Shaft, Open Approach

0QP805Z   Removal of External Fixation Device from Right Femoral Shaft, Open Approach

0QP807Z   Removal of Autologous Tissue Substitute from Right Femoral Shaft, Open Approach

0QP80JZ   Removal of Synthetic Substitute from Right Femoral Shaft, Open Approach

0QP80KZ   Removal of Nonautologous Tissue Substitute from Right Femoral Shaft, Open Approach

0QP834Z   Removal of Internal Fixation Device from Right Femoral Shaft, Percutaneous Approach

0QP835Z   Removal of External Fixation Device from Right Femoral Shaft, Percutaneous Approach

0QP837Z   Removal of Autologous Tissue Substitute from Right Femoral Shaft, Percutaneous Approach

0QP83JZ   Removal of Synthetic Substitute from Right Femoral Shaft, Percutaneous Approach

0QP83KZ   Removal of Nonautologous Tissue Substitute from Right Femoral Shaft, Percutaneous Approach

0QP844Z   Removal of Internal Fixation Device from Right Femoral Shaft, Percutaneous Endoscopic Approach

0QP845Z   Removal of External Fixation Device from Right Femoral Shaft, Percutaneous Endoscopic Approach

0QP847Z   Removal of Autologous Tissue Substitute from Right Femoral Shaft, Percutaneous Endoscopic Approach

0QP84JZ   Removal of Synthetic Substitute from Right Femoral Shaft, Percutaneous Endoscopic Approach

0QP84KZ   Removal of Nonautologous Tissue Substitute from Right Femoral Shaft, Percutaneous Endoscopic Approach

0QP8X4Z   Removal of Internal Fixation Device from Right Femoral Shaft, External Approach

0QP8X5Z   Removal of External Fixation Device from Right Femoral Shaft, External Approach

0QP904Z   Removal of Internal Fixation Device from Left Femoral Shaft, Open Approach

0QP905Z   Removal of External Fixation Device from Left Femoral Shaft, Open Approach

0QP907Z   Removal of Autologous Tissue Substitute from Left Femoral Shaft, Open Approach

0QP90JZ   Removal of Synthetic Substitute from Left Femoral Shaft, Open Approach

0QP90KZ   Removal of Nonautologous Tissue Substitute from Left Femoral Shaft, Open Approach

0QP934Z   Removal of Internal Fixation Device from Left Femoral Shaft, Percutaneous Approach

0QP935Z   Removal of External Fixation Device from Left Femoral Shaft, Percutaneous Approach

0QP937Z   Removal of Autologous Tissue Substitute from Left Femoral Shaft, Percutaneous Approach

0QP93JZ   Removal of Synthetic Substitute from Left Femoral Shaft, Percutaneous Approach

0QP93KZ   Removal of Nonautologous Tissue Substitute from Left Femoral Shaft, Percutaneous Approach

0QP944Z   Removal of Internal Fixation Device from Left Femoral Shaft, Percutaneous Endoscopic Approach

0QP945Z   Removal of External Fixation Device from Left Femoral Shaft, Percutaneous Endoscopic Approach

0QP947Z   Removal of Autologous Tissue Substitute from Left Femoral Shaft, Percutaneous Endoscopic Approach

0QP94JZ   Removal of Synthetic Substitute from Left Femoral Shaft, Percutaneous Endoscopic Approach

0QP94KZ   Removal of Nonautologous Tissue Substitute from Left Femoral Shaft, Percutaneous Endoscopic Approach

0QP9X4Z   Removal of Internal Fixation Device from Left Femoral Shaft, External Approach

0QP9X5Z   Removal of External Fixation Device from Left Femoral Shaft, External Approach

0QPB04Z   Removal of Internal Fixation Device from Right Lower Femur, Open Approach

0QPB05Z   Removal of External Fixation Device from Right Lower Femur, Open Approach

0QPB07Z   Removal of Autologous Tissue Substitute from Right Lower Femur, Open Approach

0QPB0JZ   Removal of Synthetic Substitute from Right Lower Femur, Open Approach

0QPB0KZ   Removal of Nonautologous Tissue Substitute from Right Lower Femur, Open Approach

0QPB34Z   Removal of Internal Fixation Device from Right Lower Femur, Percutaneous Approach

0QPB35Z   Removal of External Fixation Device from Right Lower Femur, Percutaneous Approach

0QPB37Z   Removal of Autologous Tissue Substitute from Right Lower Femur, Percutaneous Approach

0QPB3JZ   Removal of Synthetic Substitute from Right Lower Femur, Percutaneous Approach

0QPB3KZ   Removal of Nonautologous Tissue Substitute from Right Lower Femur, Percutaneous Approach

0QPB44Z   Removal of Internal Fixation Device from Right Lower Femur, Percutaneous Endoscopic Approach

0QPB45Z   Removal of External Fixation Device from Right Lower Femur, Percutaneous Endoscopic Approach

0QPB47Z   Removal of Autologous Tissue Substitute from Right Lower Femur, Percutaneous Endoscopic Approach

0QPB4JZ   Removal of Synthetic Substitute from Right Lower Femur, Percutaneous Endoscopic Approach

0QPB4KZ   Removal of Nonautologous Tissue Substitute from Right Lower Femur, Percutaneous Endoscopic Approach

0QPBX4Z   Removal of Internal Fixation Device from Right Lower Femur, External Approach

0QPBX5Z   Removal of External Fixation Device from Right Lower Femur, External Approach

0QPC04Z   Removal of Internal Fixation Device from Left Lower Femur, Open Approach

0QPC05Z   Removal of External Fixation Device from Left Lower Femur, Open Approach

0QPC07Z   Removal of Autologous Tissue Substitute from Left Lower Femur, Open Approach

0QPC0JZ   Removal of Synthetic Substitute from Left Lower Femur, Open Approach

0QPC0KZ   Removal of Nonautologous Tissue Substitute from Left Lower Femur, Open Approach

0QPC34Z   Removal of Internal Fixation Device from Left Lower Femur, Percutaneous Approach

0QPC35Z   Removal of External Fixation Device from Left Lower Femur, Percutaneous Approach

0QPC37Z   Removal of Autologous Tissue Substitute from Left Lower Femur, Percutaneous Approach

0QPC3JZ   Removal of Synthetic Substitute from Left Lower Femur, Percutaneous Approach

0QPC3KZ   Removal of Nonautologous Tissue Substitute from Left Lower Femur, Percutaneous Approach

0QPC44Z   Removal of Internal Fixation Device from Left Lower Femur, Percutaneous Endoscopic Approach

0QPC45Z   Removal of External Fixation Device from Left Lower Femur, Percutaneous Endoscopic Approach

0QPC47Z   Removal of Autologous Tissue Substitute from Left Lower Femur, Percutaneous Endoscopic Approach

0QPC4JZ   Removal of Synthetic Substitute from Left Lower Femur, Percutaneous Endoscopic Approach

0QPC4KZ   Removal of Nonautologous Tissue Substitute from Left Lower Femur, Percutaneous Endoscopic Approach

0QPCX4Z   Removal of Internal Fixation Device from Left Lower Femur, External Approach

0QPCX5Z   Removal of External Fixation Device from Left Lower Femur, External Approach

0QPD04Z   Removal of Internal Fixation Device from Right Patella, Open Approach

0QPD05Z   Removal of External Fixation Device from Right Patella, Open Approach

0QPD07Z   Removal of Autologous Tissue Substitute from Right Patella, Open Approach

0QPD0JZ   Removal of Synthetic Substitute from Right Patella, Open Approach

0QPD0KZ   Removal of Nonautologous Tissue Substitute from Right Patella, Open Approach

0QPD34Z   Removal of Internal Fixation Device from Right Patella, Percutaneous Approach

0QPD35Z   Removal of External Fixation Device from Right Patella, Percutaneous Approach

0QPD37Z   Removal of Autologous Tissue Substitute from Right Patella, Percutaneous Approach

0QPD3JZ   Removal of Synthetic Substitute from Right Patella, Percutaneous Approach

0QPD3KZ   Removal of Nonautologous Tissue Substitute from Right Patella, Percutaneous Approach

0QPD44Z   Removal of Internal Fixation Device from Right Patella, Percutaneous Endoscopic Approach

0QPD45Z   Removal of External Fixation Device from Right Patella, Percutaneous Endoscopic Approach

0QPD47Z   Removal of Autologous Tissue Substitute from Right Patella, Percutaneous Endoscopic Approach

0QPD4JZ Removal of Synthetic Substitute from Right Patella, Percutaneous Endoscopic Approach

0QPD4KZ Removal of Nonautologous Tissue Substitute from Right Patella, Percutaneous Endoscopic Approach

0QPDX4Z Removal of Internal Fixation Device from Right Patella, External Approach

0QPDX5Z Removal of External Fixation Device from Right Patella, External Approach

0QPF04Z Removal of Internal Fixation Device from Left Patella, Open Approach

0QPF05Z Removal of External Fixation Device from Left Patella, Open Approach

0QPF07Z Removal of Autologous Tissue Substitute from Left Patella, Open Approach

0QPF0JZ Removal of Synthetic Substitute from Left Patella, Open Approach

0QPF0KZ Removal of Nonautologous Tissue Substitute from Left Patella, Open Approach

0QPF34Z Removal of Internal Fixation Device from Left Patella, Percutaneous Approach

0QPF35Z Removal of External Fixation Device from Left Patella, Percutaneous Approach

0QPF37Z Removal of Autologous Tissue Substitute from Left Patella, Percutaneous Approach

0QPF3JZ Removal of Synthetic Substitute from Left Patella, Percutaneous Approach

0QPF3KZ Removal of Nonautologous Tissue Substitute from Left Patella, Percutaneous Approach

0QPF44Z Removal of Internal Fixation Device from Left Patella, Percutaneous Endoscopic Approach

0QPF45Z Removal of External Fixation Device from Left Patella, Percutaneous Endoscopic Approach

0QPF47Z Removal of Autologous Tissue Substitute from Left Patella, Percutaneous Endoscopic Approach

0QPF4JZ Removal of Synthetic Substitute from Left Patella, Percutaneous Endoscopic Approach

0QPF4KZ Removal of Nonautologous Tissue Substitute from Left Patella, Percutaneous Endoscopic Approach

0QPFX4Z Removal of Internal Fixation Device from Left Patella, External Approach

0QPFX5Z Removal of External Fixation Device from Left Patella, External Approach

0QPG04Z Removal of Internal Fixation Device from Right Tibia, Open Approach

0QPG05Z Removal of External Fixation Device from Right Tibia, Open Approach

0QPG07Z Removal of Autologous Tissue Substitute from Right Tibia, Open Approach

0QPG0JZ Removal of Synthetic Substitute from Right Tibia, Open Approach

0QPG0KZ Removal of Nonautologous Tissue Substitute from Right Tibia, Open Approach

0QPG34Z Removal of Internal Fixation Device from Right Tibia, Percutaneous Approach

0QPG35Z Removal of External Fixation Device from Right Tibia, Percutaneous Approach

0QPG37Z Removal of Autologous Tissue Substitute from Right Tibia, Percutaneous Approach

0QPG3JZ Removal of Synthetic Substitute from Right Tibia, Percutaneous Approach

0QPG3KZ Removal of Nonautologous Tissue Substitute from Right Tibia, Percutaneous Approach

0QPG44Z Removal of Internal Fixation Device from Right Tibia, Percutaneous Endoscopic Approach

0QPG45Z Removal of External Fixation Device from Right Tibia, Percutaneous Endoscopic Approach

0QPG47Z Removal of Autologous Tissue Substitute from Right Tibia, Percutaneous Endoscopic Approach

0QPG4JZ Removal of Synthetic Substitute from Right Tibia, Percutaneous Endoscopic Approach

0QPG4KZ Removal of Nonautologous Tissue Substitute from Right Tibia, Percutaneous Endoscopic Approach

0QPGX4Z Removal of Internal Fixation Device from Right Tibia, External Approach

0QPGX5Z Removal of External Fixation Device from Right Tibia, External Approach

0QPH04Z Removal of Internal Fixation Device from Left Tibia, Open Approach

0QPH05Z Removal of External Fixation Device from Left Tibia, Open Approach

0QPH07Z Removal of Autologous Tissue Substitute from Left Tibia, Open Approach

0QPH0JZ Removal of Synthetic Substitute from Left Tibia, Open Approach

0QPH0KZ Removal of Nonautologous Tissue Substitute from Left Tibia, Open Approach

0QPH34Z Removal of Internal Fixation Device from Left Tibia, Percutaneous Approach

0QPH35Z Removal of External Fixation Device from Left Tibia, Percutaneous Approach

0QPH37Z Removal of Autologous Tissue Substitute from Left Tibia, Percutaneous Approach

0QPH3JZ Removal of Synthetic Substitute from Left Tibia, Percutaneous Approach

0QPH3KZ Removal of Nonautologous Tissue Substitute from Left Tibia, Percutaneous Approach

0QPH44Z Removal of Internal Fixation Device from Left Tibia, Percutaneous Endoscopic Approach

0QPH45Z Removal of External Fixation Device from Left Tibia, Percutaneous Endoscopic Approach

0QPH47Z Removal of Autologous Tissue Substitute from Left Tibia, Percutaneous Endoscopic Approach

0QPH4JZ Removal of Synthetic Substitute from Left Tibia, Percutaneous Endoscopic Approach

0QPH4KZ Removal of Nonautologous Tissue Substitute from Left Tibia, Percutaneous Endoscopic Approach

0QPHX4Z Removal of Internal Fixation Device from Left Tibia, External Approach

0QPHX5Z Removal of External Fixation Device from Left Tibia, External Approach

0QPJ04Z Removal of Internal Fixation Device from Right Fibula, Open Approach

0QPJ05Z Removal of External Fixation Device from Right Fibula, Open Approach

0QPJ07Z Removal of Autologous Tissue Substitute from Right Fibula, Open Approach

0QPJ0JZ Removal of Synthetic Substitute from Right Fibula, Open Approach

0QPJ0KZ Removal of Nonautologous Tissue Substitute from Right Fibula, Open Approach

0QPJ34Z Removal of Internal Fixation Device from Right Fibula, Percutaneous Approach

0QPJ35Z Removal of External Fixation Device from Right Fibula, Percutaneous Approach

0QPJ37Z Removal of Autologous Tissue Substitute from Right Fibula, Percutaneous Approach

0QPJ3JZ Removal of Synthetic Substitute from Right Fibula, Percutaneous Approach

0QPJ3KZ Removal of Nonautologous Tissue Substitute from Right Fibula, Percutaneous Approach

0QPJ44Z Removal of Internal Fixation Device from Right Fibula, Percutaneous Endoscopic Approach

0QPJ45Z Removal of External Fixation Device from Right Fibula, Percutaneous Endoscopic Approach

0QPJ47Z Removal of Autologous Tissue Substitute from Right Fibula, Percutaneous Endoscopic Approach

0QPJ4JZ Removal of Synthetic Substitute from Right Fibula, Percutaneous Endoscopic Approach

0QPJ4KZ Removal of Nonautologous Tissue Substitute from Right Fibula, Percutaneous Endoscopic Approach

0QPJX4Z Removal of Internal Fixation Device from Right Fibula, External Approach

0QPJX5Z Removal of External Fixation Device from Right Fibula, External Approach

0QPK04Z Removal of Internal Fixation Device from Left Fibula, Open Approach

0QPK05Z Removal of External Fixation Device from Left Fibula, Open Approach

0QPK07Z Removal of Autologous Tissue Substitute from Left Fibula, Open Approach

0QPK0JZ Removal of Synthetic Substitute from Left Fibula, Open Approach

0QPK0KZ Removal of Nonautologous Tissue Substitute from Left Fibula, Open Approach

0QPK34Z Removal of Internal Fixation Device from Left Fibula, Percutaneous Approach

0QPK35Z Removal of External Fixation Device from Left Fibula, Percutaneous Approach

0QPK37Z Removal of Autologous Tissue Substitute from Left Fibula, Percutaneous Approach

0QPK3JZ Removal of Synthetic Substitute from Left Fibula, Percutaneous Approach

0QPK3KZ Removal of Nonautologous Tissue Substitute from Left Fibula, Percutaneous Approach

0QPK44Z Removal of Internal Fixation Device from Left Fibula, Percutaneous Endoscopic Approach

0QPK45Z Removal of External Fixation Device from Left Fibula, Percutaneous Endoscopic Approach

0QPK47Z Removal of Autologous Tissue Substitute from Left Fibula, Percutaneous Endoscopic Approach

0QPK4JZ Removal of Synthetic Substitute from Left Fibula, Percutaneous Endoscopic Approach

0QPK4KZ Removal of Nonautologous Tissue Substitute from Left Fibula, Percutaneous Endoscopic Approach

0QPKX4Z Removal of Internal Fixation Device from Left Fibula, External Approach

0QPKX5Z Removal of External Fixation Device from Left Fibula, External Approach

0QPL04Z Removal of Internal Fixation Device from Right Tarsal, Open Approach

0QPL05Z Removal of External Fixation Device from Right Tarsal, Open Approach

0QPL07Z Removal of Autologous Tissue Substitute from Right Tarsal, Open Approach

0QPL0JZ Removal of Synthetic Substitute from Right Tarsal, Open Approach

0QPL0KZ Removal of Nonautologous Tissue Substitute from Right Tarsal, Open Approach

0QPL34Z Removal of Internal Fixation Device from Right Tarsal, Percutaneous Approach

0QPL35Z Removal of External Fixation Device from Right Tarsal, Percutaneous Approach

0QPL37Z Removal of Autologous Tissue Substitute from Right Tarsal, Percutaneous Approach

0QPL3JZ Removal of Synthetic Substitute from Right Tarsal, Percutaneous Approach

0QPL3KZ Removal of Nonautologous Tissue Substitute from Right Tarsal, Percutaneous Approach

0QPL44Z Removal of Internal Fixation Device from Right Tarsal, Percutaneous Endoscopic Approach

0QPL45Z Removal of External Fixation Device from Right Tarsal, Percutaneous Endoscopic Approach

0QPL47Z Removal of Autologous Tissue Substitute from Right Tarsal, Percutaneous Endoscopic Approach

0QPL4JZ Removal of Synthetic Substitute from Right Tarsal, Percutaneous Endoscopic Approach

0QPL4KZ Removal of Nonautologous Tissue Substitute from Right Tarsal, Percutaneous Endoscopic Approach

0QPLX4Z Removal of Internal Fixation Device from Right Tarsal, External Approach

0QPLX5Z Removal of External Fixation Device from Right Tarsal, External Approach

0QPM04Z Removal of Internal Fixation Device from Left Tarsal, Open Approach

0QPM05Z Removal of External Fixation Device from Left Tarsal, Open Approach

0QPM07Z Removal of Autologous Tissue Substitute from Left Tarsal, Open Approach

0QPM0JZ Removal of Synthetic Substitute from Left Tarsal, Open Approach

0QPM0KZ Removal of Nonautologous Tissue Substitute from Left Tarsal, Open Approach

0QPM34Z Removal of Internal Fixation Device from Left Tarsal, Percutaneous Approach

0QPM35Z Removal of External Fixation Device from Left Tarsal, Percutaneous Approach

0QPM37Z Removal of Autologous Tissue Substitute from Left Tarsal, Percutaneous Approach

0QPM3JZ Removal of Synthetic Substitute from Left Tarsal, Percutaneous Approach

0QPM3KZ Removal of Nonautologous Tissue Substitute from Left Tarsal, Percutaneous Approach

0QPM44Z Removal of Internal Fixation Device from Left Tarsal, Percutaneous Endoscopic Approach

0QPM45Z Removal of External Fixation Device from Left Tarsal, Percutaneous Endoscopic Approach

0QPM47Z Removal of Autologous Tissue Substitute from Left Tarsal, Percutaneous Endoscopic Approach

0QPM4JZ Removal of Synthetic Substitute from Left Tarsal, Percutaneous Endoscopic Approach

0QPM4KZ Removal of Nonautologous Tissue Substitute from Left Tarsal, Percutaneous Endoscopic Approach

0QPMX4Z Removal of Internal Fixation Device from Left Tarsal, External Approach

0QPMX5Z Removal of External Fixation Device from Left Tarsal, External Approach

0QPN04Z Removal of Internal Fixation Device from Right Metatarsal, Open Approach

0QPN05Z Removal of External Fixation Device from Right Metatarsal, Open Approach

0QPN07Z Removal of Autologous Tissue Substitute from Right Metatarsal, Open Approach

0QPN0JZ Removal of Synthetic Substitute from Right Metatarsal, Open Approach

0QPN0KZ Removal of Nonautologous Tissue Substitute from Right Metatarsal, Open Approach

0QPN34Z Removal of Internal Fixation Device from Right Metatarsal, Percutaneous Approach

0QPN35Z Removal of External Fixation Device from Right Metatarsal, Percutaneous Approach

0QPN37Z Removal of Autologous Tissue Substitute from Right Metatarsal, Percutaneous Approach

0QPN3JZ Removal of Synthetic Substitute from Right Metatarsal, Percutaneous Approach

0QPN3KZ Removal of Nonautologous Tissue Substitute from Right Metatarsal, Percutaneous Approach

0QPN44Z Removal of Internal Fixation Device from Right Metatarsal, Percutaneous Endoscopic Approach

0QPN45Z Removal of External Fixation Device from Right Metatarsal, Percutaneous Endoscopic Approach

0QPN47Z Removal of Autologous Tissue Substitute from Right Metatarsal, Percutaneous Endoscopic Approach

0QPN4JZ Removal of Synthetic Substitute from Right Metatarsal, Percutaneous Endoscopic Approach

0QPN4KZ Removal of Nonautologous Tissue Substitute from Right Metatarsal, Percutaneous Endoscopic Approach

0QPNX4Z Removal of Internal Fixation Device from Right Metatarsal, External Approach

0QPNX5Z Removal of External Fixation Device from Right Metatarsal, External Approach

0QPP04Z Removal of Internal Fixation Device from Left Metatarsal, Open Approach

0QPP05Z Removal of External Fixation Device from Left Metatarsal, Open Approach

0QPP07Z Removal of Autologous Tissue Substitute from Left Metatarsal, Open Approach

0QPP0JZ Removal of Synthetic Substitute from Left Metatarsal, Open Approach

0QPP0KZ Removal of Nonautologous Tissue Substitute from Left Metatarsal, Open Approach

0QPP34Z Removal of Internal Fixation Device from Left Metatarsal, Percutaneous Approach

0QPP35Z Removal of External Fixation Device from Left Metatarsal, Percutaneous Approach

0QPP37Z Removal of Autologous Tissue Substitute from Left Metatarsal, Percutaneous Approach

0QPP3JZ Removal of Synthetic Substitute from Left Metatarsal, Percutaneous Approach

0QPP3KZ Removal of Nonautologous Tissue Substitute from Left Metatarsal, Percutaneous Approach

0QPP44Z Removal of Internal Fixation Device from Left Metatarsal, Percutaneous Endoscopic Approach

0QPP45Z Removal of External Fixation Device from Left Metatarsal, Percutaneous Endoscopic Approach

0QPP47Z Removal of Autologous Tissue Substitute from Left Metatarsal, Percutaneous Endoscopic Approach

0QPP4JZ Removal of Synthetic Substitute from Left Metatarsal, Percutaneous Endoscopic Approach

0QPP4KZ Removal of Nonautologous Tissue Substitute from Left Metatarsal, Percutaneous Endoscopic Approach

0QPPX4Z Removal of Internal Fixation Device from Left Metatarsal, External Approach

0QPPX5Z Removal of External Fixation Device from Left Metatarsal, External Approach

0QPQ04Z Removal of Internal Fixation Device from Right Toe Phalanx, Open Approach

0QPQ05Z Removal of External Fixation Device from Right Toe Phalanx, Open Approach

0QPQ07Z Removal of Autologous Tissue Substitute from Right Toe Phalanx, Open Approach

0QPQ0JZ Removal of Synthetic Substitute from Right Toe Phalanx, Open Approach

0QPQ0KZ Removal of Nonautologous Tissue Substitute from Right Toe Phalanx, Open Approach

0QPQ34Z Removal of Internal Fixation Device from Right Toe Phalanx, Percutaneous Approach

0QPQ35Z Removal of External Fixation Device from Right Toe Phalanx, Percutaneous Approach

0QPQ37Z Removal of Autologous Tissue Substitute from Right Toe Phalanx, Percutaneous Approach

0QPQ3JZ Removal of Synthetic Substitute from Right Toe Phalanx, Percutaneous Approach

0QPQ3KZ Removal of Nonautologous Tissue Substitute from Right Toe Phalanx, Percutaneous Approach

0QPQ44Z Removal of Internal Fixation Device from Right Toe Phalanx, Percutaneous Endoscopic Approach

0QPQ45Z Removal of External Fixation Device from Right Toe Phalanx, Percutaneous Endoscopic Approach

0QPQ47Z Removal of Autologous Tissue Substitute from Right Toe Phalanx, Percutaneous Endoscopic Approach

0QPQ4JZ Removal of Synthetic Substitute from Right Toe Phalanx, Percutaneous Endoscopic Approach

0QPQ4KZ Removal of Nonautologous Tissue Substitute from Right Toe Phalanx, Percutaneous Endoscopic Approach

0QPQX4Z Removal of Internal Fixation Device from Right Toe Phalanx, External Approach

0QPQX5Z Removal of External Fixation Device from Right Toe Phalanx, External Approach

0QPR04Z Removal of Internal Fixation Device from Left Toe Phalanx, Open Approach

0QPR05Z Removal of External Fixation Device from Left Toe Phalanx, Open Approach

0QPR07Z Removal of Autologous Tissue Substitute from Left Toe Phalanx, Open Approach

0QPR0JZ Removal of Synthetic Substitute from Left Toe Phalanx, Open Approach

0QPR0KZ Removal of Nonautologous Tissue Substitute from Left Toe Phalanx, Open Approach

0QPR34Z Removal of Internal Fixation Device from Left Toe Phalanx, Percutaneous Approach

0QPR35Z Removal of External Fixation Device from Left Toe Phalanx, Percutaneous Approach

0QPR37Z Removal of Autologous Tissue Substitute from Left Toe Phalanx, Percutaneous Approach

0QPR3JZ Removal of Synthetic Substitute from Left Toe Phalanx, Percutaneous Approach

0QPR3KZ Removal of Nonautologous Tissue Substitute from Left Toe Phalanx, Percutaneous Approach

0QPR44Z Removal of Internal Fixation Device from Left Toe Phalanx, Percutaneous Endoscopic Approach

0QPR45Z Removal of External Fixation Device from Left Toe Phalanx, Percutaneous Endoscopic Approach

0QPR47Z Removal of Autologous Tissue Substitute from Left Toe Phalanx, Percutaneous Endoscopic Approach

0QPR4JZ Removal of Synthetic Substitute from Left Toe Phalanx, Percutaneous Endoscopic Approach

0QPR4KZ Removal of Nonautologous Tissue Substitute from Left Toe Phalanx, Percutaneous Endoscopic Approach

0QPRX4Z Removal of Internal Fixation Device from Left Toe Phalanx, External Approach

0QPRX5Z Removal of External Fixation Device from Left Toe Phalanx, External Approach

0QPS04Z Removal of Internal Fixation Device from Coccyx, Open Approach

0QPS07Z Removal of Autologous Tissue Substitute from Coccyx, Open Approach

0QPS0JZ Removal of Synthetic Substitute from Coccyx, Open Approach

0QPS0KZ Removal of Nonautologous Tissue Substitute from Coccyx, Open Approach

0QPS34Z Removal of Internal Fixation Device from Coccyx, Percutaneous Approach

0QPS37Z Removal of Autologous Tissue Substitute from Coccyx, Percutaneous Approach

0QPS3JZ Removal of Synthetic Substitute from Coccyx, Percutaneous Approach

0QPS3KZ Removal of Nonautologous Tissue Substitute from Coccyx, Percutaneous Approach

0QPS44Z Removal of Internal Fixation Device from Coccyx, Percutaneous Endoscopic Approach

0QPS47Z Removal of Autologous Tissue Substitute from Coccyx, Percutaneous Endoscopic Approach

0QPS4JZ Removal of Synthetic Substitute from Coccyx, Percutaneous Endoscopic Approach

0QPS4KZ Removal of Nonautologous Tissue Substitute from Coccyx, Percutaneous Endoscopic Approach

0QPSX4Z Removal of Internal Fixation Device from Coccyx, External Approach

0QPY00Z Removal of Drainage Device from Lower Bone, Open Approach

0QPY0MZ Removal of Bone Growth Stimulator from Lower Bone, Open Approach

0QPY30Z Removal of Drainage Device from Lower Bone, Percutaneous Approach

0QPY3MZ Removal of Bone Growth Stimulator from Lower Bone, Percutaneous Approach

0QPY40Z Removal of Drainage Device from Lower Bone, Percutaneous Endoscopic Approach

0QPY4MZ Removal of Bone Growth Stimulator from Lower Bone, Percutaneous Endoscopic Approach

0QPYX0Z Removal of Drainage Device from Lower Bone, External Approach

0QPYXMZ Removal of Bone Growth Stimulator from Lower Bone, External Approach

0QQ – Lower Bones, Repair

Review Coding Guideline B3.5

0QQ00ZZ Repair Lumbar Vertebra, Open Approach
0QQ03ZZ Repair Lumbar Vertebra, Percutaneous Approach
0QQ04ZZ Repair Lumbar Vertebra, Percutaneous Endoscopic Approach
0QQ0XZZ Repair Lumbar Vertebra, External Approach
0QQ10ZZ Repair Sacrum, Open Approach
0QQ13ZZ Repair Sacrum, Percutaneous Approach
0QQ14ZZ Repair Sacrum, Percutaneous Endoscopic Approach
0QQ1XZZ Repair Sacrum, External Approach
0QQ20ZZ Repair Right Pelvic Bone, Open Approach
0QQ23ZZ Repair Right Pelvic Bone, Percutaneous Approach
0QQ24ZZ Repair Right Pelvic Bone, Percutaneous Endoscopic Approach
0QQ2XZZ Repair Right Pelvic Bone, External Approach

♀ Female-only   ♂ Male-only   ● Limited Coverage   ● Non-OR   **HAC** HAC-associated procedure   ● Non-covered procedures   ✚ Combination

0QQ30ZZ	Repair Left Pelvic Bone, Open Approach
0QQ33ZZ	Repair Left Pelvic Bone, Percutaneous Approach
0QQ34ZZ	Repair Left Pelvic Bone, Percutaneous Endoscopic Approach
0QQ3XZZ	Repair Left Pelvic Bone, External Approach
0QQ40ZZ	Repair Right Acetabulum, Open Approach
0QQ43ZZ	Repair Right Acetabulum, Percutaneous Approach
0QQ44ZZ	Repair Right Acetabulum, Percutaneous Endoscopic Approach
0QQ4XZZ	Repair Right Acetabulum, External Approach
0QQ50ZZ	Repair Left Acetabulum, Open Approach
0QQ53ZZ	Repair Left Acetabulum, Percutaneous Approach
0QQ54ZZ	Repair Left Acetabulum, Percutaneous Endoscopic Approach
0QQ5XZZ	Repair Left Acetabulum, External Approach
0QQ60ZZ	Repair Right Upper Femur, Open Approach
0QQ63ZZ	Repair Right Upper Femur, Percutaneous Approach
0QQ64ZZ	Repair Right Upper Femur, Percutaneous Endoscopic Approach
0QQ6XZZ	Repair Right Upper Femur, External Approach
0QQ70ZZ	Repair Left Upper Femur, Open Approach
0QQ73ZZ	Repair Left Upper Femur, Percutaneous Approach
0QQ74ZZ	Repair Left Upper Femur, Percutaneous Endoscopic Approach
0QQ7XZZ	Repair Left Upper Femur, External Approach
0QQ80ZZ	Repair Right Femoral Shaft, Open Approach
0QQ83ZZ	Repair Right Femoral Shaft, Percutaneous Approach
0QQ84ZZ	Repair Right Femoral Shaft, Percutaneous Endoscopic Approach
0QQ8XZZ	Repair Right Femoral Shaft, External Approach
0QQ90ZZ	Repair Left Femoral Shaft, Open Approach
0QQ93ZZ	Repair Left Femoral Shaft, Percutaneous Approach
0QQ94ZZ	Repair Left Femoral Shaft, Percutaneous Endoscopic Approach
0QQ9XZZ	Repair Left Femoral Shaft, External Approach
0QQB0ZZ	Repair Right Lower Femur, Open Approach
0QQB3ZZ	Repair Right Lower Femur, Percutaneous Approach
0QQB4ZZ	Repair Right Lower Femur, Percutaneous Endoscopic Approach
0QQBXZZ	Repair Right Lower Femur, External Approach
0QQC0ZZ	Repair Left Lower Femur, Open Approach
0QQC3ZZ	Repair Left Lower Femur, Percutaneous Approach
0QQC4ZZ	Repair Left Lower Femur, Percutaneous Endoscopic Approach
0QQCXZZ	Repair Left Lower Femur, External Approach
0QQD0ZZ	Repair Right Patella, Open Approach
0QQD3ZZ	Repair Right Patella, Percutaneous Approach
0QQD4ZZ	Repair Right Patella, Percutaneous Endoscopic Approach
0QQDXZZ	Repair Right Patella, External Approach
0QQF0ZZ	Repair Left Patella, Open Approach
0QQF3ZZ	Repair Left Patella, Percutaneous Approach
0QQF4ZZ	Repair Left Patella, Percutaneous Endoscopic Approach
0QQFXZZ	Repair Left Patella, External Approach
0QQG0ZZ	Repair Right Tibia, Open Approach
0QQG3ZZ	Repair Right Tibia, Percutaneous Approach
0QQG4ZZ	Repair Right Tibia, Percutaneous Endoscopic Approach
0QQGXZZ	Repair Right Tibia, External Approach
0QQH0ZZ	Repair Left Tibia, Open Approach
0QQH3ZZ	Repair Left Tibia, Percutaneous Approach
0QQH4ZZ	Repair Left Tibia, Percutaneous Endoscopic Approach
0QQHXZZ	Repair Left Tibia, External Approach
0QQJ0ZZ	Repair Right Fibula, Open Approach
0QQJ3ZZ	Repair Right Fibula, Percutaneous Approach
0QQJ4ZZ	Repair Right Fibula, Percutaneous Endoscopic Approach
0QQJXZZ	Repair Right Fibula, External Approach
0QQK0ZZ	Repair Left Fibula, Open Approach
0QQK3ZZ	Repair Left Fibula, Percutaneous Approach
0QQK4ZZ	Repair Left Fibula, Percutaneous Endoscopic Approach
0QQKXZZ	Repair Left Fibula, External Approach
0QQL0ZZ	Repair Right Tarsal, Open Approach
0QQL3ZZ	Repair Right Tarsal, Percutaneous Approach
0QQL4ZZ	Repair Right Tarsal, Percutaneous Endoscopic Approach
0QQLXZZ	Repair Right Tarsal, External Approach
0QQM0ZZ	Repair Left Tarsal, Open Approach
0QQM3ZZ	Repair Left Tarsal, Percutaneous Approach
0QQM4ZZ	Repair Left Tarsal, Percutaneous Endoscopic Approach
0QQMXZZ	Repair Left Tarsal, External Approach
0QQN0ZZ	Repair Right Metatarsal, Open Approach
0QQN3ZZ	Repair Right Metatarsal, Percutaneous Approach
0QQN4ZZ	Repair Right Metatarsal, Percutaneous Endoscopic Approach
0QQNXZZ	Repair Right Metatarsal, External Approach
0QQP0ZZ	Repair Left Metatarsal, Open Approach
0QQP3ZZ	Repair Left Metatarsal, Percutaneous Approach
0QQP4ZZ	Repair Left Metatarsal, Percutaneous Endoscopic Approach
0QQPXZZ	Repair Left Metatarsal, External Approach
0QQQ0ZZ	Repair Right Toe Phalanx, Open Approach
0QQQ3ZZ	Repair Right Toe Phalanx, Percutaneous Approach
0QQQ4ZZ	Repair Right Toe Phalanx, Percutaneous Endoscopic Approach
0QQQXZZ	Repair Right Toe Phalanx, External Approach
0QQR0ZZ	Repair Left Toe Phalanx, Open Approach
0QQR3ZZ	Repair Left Toe Phalanx, Percutaneous Approach
0QQR4ZZ	Repair Left Toe Phalanx, Percutaneous Endoscopic Approach
0QQRXZZ	Repair Left Toe Phalanx, External Approach
0QQS0ZZ	Repair Coccyx, Open Approach
0QQS3ZZ	Repair Coccyx, Percutaneous Approach
0QQS4ZZ	Repair Coccyx, Percutaneous Endoscopic Approach
0QQSXZZ	Repair Coccyx, External Approach

0QR – Lower Bones, Replacement

0QR007Z	Replacement of Lumbar Vertebra with Autologous Tissue Substitute, Open Approach
0QR00JZ	Replacement of Lumbar Vertebra with Synthetic Substitute, Open Approach
0QR00KZ	Replacement of Lumbar Vertebra with Nonautologous Tissue Substitute, Open Approach
0QR037Z	Replacement of Lumbar Vertebra with Autologous Tissue Substitute, Percutaneous Approach
0QR03JZ	Replacement of Lumbar Vertebra with Synthetic Substitute, Percutaneous Approach
0QR03KZ	Replacement of Lumbar Vertebra with Nonautologous Tissue Substitute, Percutaneous Approach
0QR047Z	Replacement of Lumbar Vertebra with Autologous Tissue Substitute, Percutaneous Endoscopic Approach
0QR04JZ	Replacement of Lumbar Vertebra with Synthetic Substitute, Percutaneous Endoscopic Approach
0QR04KZ	Replacement of Lumbar Vertebra with Nonautologous Tissue Substitute, Percutaneous Endoscopic Approach
0QR107Z	Replacement of Sacrum with Autologous Tissue Substitute, Open Approach
0QR10JZ	Replacement of Sacrum with Synthetic Substitute, Open Approach
0QR10KZ	Replacement of Sacrum with Nonautologous Tissue Substitute, Open Approach
0QR137Z	Replacement of Sacrum with Autologous Tissue Substitute, Percutaneous Approach
0QR13JZ	Replacement of Sacrum with Synthetic Substitute, Percutaneous Approach
0QR13KZ	Replacement of Sacrum with Nonautologous Tissue Substitute, Percutaneous Approach
0QR147Z	Replacement of Sacrum with Autologous Tissue Substitute, Percutaneous Endoscopic Approach
0QR14JZ	Replacement of Sacrum with Synthetic Substitute, Percutaneous Endoscopic Approach
0QR14KZ	Replacement of Sacrum with Nonautologous Tissue Substitute, Percutaneous Endoscopic Approach
0QR207Z	Replacement of Right Pelvic Bone with Autologous Tissue Substitute, Open Approach
0QR20JZ	Replacement of Right Pelvic Bone with Synthetic Substitute, Open Approach
0QR20KZ	Replacement of Right Pelvic Bone with Nonautologous Tissue Substitute, Open Approach
0QR237Z	Replacement of Right Pelvic Bone with Autologous Tissue Substitute, Percutaneous Approach
0QR23JZ	Replacement of Right Pelvic Bone with Synthetic Substitute, Percutaneous Approach
0QR23KZ	Replacement of Right Pelvic Bone with Nonautologous Tissue Substitute, Percutaneous Approach
0QR247Z	Replacement of Right Pelvic Bone with Autologous Tissue Substitute, Percutaneous Endoscopic Approach
0QR24JZ	Replacement of Right Pelvic Bone with Synthetic Substitute, Percutaneous Endoscopic Approach

♀ Female-only   ♂ Male-only   ● Limited Coverage   ● Non-OR   HAC HAC-associated procedure   ● Non-covered procedures   ➕ Combination

0QR24KZ Replacement of Right Pelvic Bone with Nonautologous Tissue Substitute, Percutaneous Endoscopic Approach

0QR307Z Replacement of Left Pelvic Bone with Autologous Tissue Substitute, Open Approach

0QR30JZ Replacement of Left Pelvic Bone with Synthetic Substitute, Open Approach

0QR30KZ Replacement of Left Pelvic Bone with Nonautologous Tissue Substitute, Open Approach

0QR337Z Replacement of Left Pelvic Bone with Autologous Tissue Substitute, Percutaneous Approach

0QR33JZ Replacement of Left Pelvic Bone with Synthetic Substitute, Percutaneous Approach

0QR33KZ Replacement of Left Pelvic Bone with Nonautologous Tissue Substitute, Percutaneous Approach

0QR347Z Replacement of Left Pelvic Bone with Autologous Tissue Substitute, Percutaneous Endoscopic Approach

0QR34JZ Replacement of Left Pelvic Bone with Synthetic Substitute, Percutaneous Endoscopic Approach

0QR34KZ Replacement of Left Pelvic Bone with Nonautologous Tissue Substitute, Percutaneous Endoscopic Approach

0QR407Z Replacement of Right Acetabulum with Autologous Tissue Substitute, Open Approach

0QR40JZ Replacement of Right Acetabulum with Synthetic Substitute, Open Approach

0QR40KZ Replacement of Right Acetabulum with Nonautologous Tissue Substitute, Open Approach

0QR437Z Replacement of Right Acetabulum with Autologous Tissue Substitute, Percutaneous Approach

0QR43JZ Replacement of Right Acetabulum with Synthetic Substitute, Percutaneous Approach

0QR43KZ Replacement of Right Acetabulum with Nonautologous Tissue Substitute, Percutaneous Approach

0QR447Z Replacement of Right Acetabulum with Autologous Tissue Substitute, Percutaneous Endoscopic Approach

0QR44JZ Replacement of Right Acetabulum with Synthetic Substitute, Percutaneous Endoscopic Approach

0QR44KZ Replacement of Right Acetabulum with Nonautologous Tissue Substitute, Percutaneous Endoscopic Approach

0QR507Z Replacement of Left Acetabulum with Autologous Tissue Substitute, Open Approach

0QR50JZ Replacement of Left Acetabulum with Synthetic Substitute, Open Approach

0QR50KZ Replacement of Left Acetabulum with Nonautologous Tissue Substitute, Open Approach

0QR537Z Replacement of Left Acetabulum with Autologous Tissue Substitute, Percutaneous Approach

0QR53JZ Replacement of Left Acetabulum with Synthetic Substitute, Percutaneous Approach

0QR53KZ Replacement of Left Acetabulum with Nonautologous Tissue Substitute, Percutaneous Approach

0QR547Z Replacement of Left Acetabulum with Autologous Tissue Substitute, Percutaneous Endoscopic Approach

0QR54JZ Replacement of Left Acetabulum with Synthetic Substitute, Percutaneous Endoscopic Approach

0QR54KZ Replacement of Left Acetabulum with Nonautologous Tissue Substitute, Percutaneous Endoscopic Approach

0QR607Z Replacement of Right Upper Femur with Autologous Tissue Substitute, Open Approach

0QR60JZ Replacement of Right Upper Femur with Synthetic Substitute, Open Approach

0QR60KZ Replacement of Right Upper Femur with Nonautologous Tissue Substitute, Open Approach

0QR637Z Replacement of Right Upper Femur with Autologous Tissue Substitute, Percutaneous Approach

0QR63JZ Replacement of Right Upper Femur with Synthetic Substitute, Percutaneous Approach

0QR63KZ Replacement of Right Upper Femur with Nonautologous Tissue Substitute, Percutaneous Approach

0QR647Z Replacement of Right Upper Femur with Autologous Tissue Substitute, Percutaneous Endoscopic Approach

0QR64JZ Replacement of Right Upper Femur with Synthetic Substitute, Percutaneous Endoscopic Approach

0QR64KZ Replacement of Right Upper Femur with Nonautologous Tissue Substitute, Percutaneous Endoscopic Approach

0QR707Z Replacement of Left Upper Femur with Autologous Tissue Substitute, Open Approach

0QR70JZ Replacement of Left Upper Femur with Synthetic Substitute, Open Approach

0QR70KZ Replacement of Left Upper Femur with Nonautologous Tissue Substitute, Open Approach

0QR737Z Replacement of Left Upper Femur with Autologous Tissue Substitute, Percutaneous Approach

0QR73JZ Replacement of Left Upper Femur with Synthetic Substitute, Percutaneous Approach

0QR73KZ Replacement of Left Upper Femur with Nonautologous Tissue Substitute, Percutaneous Approach

0QR747Z Replacement of Left Upper Femur with Autologous Tissue Substitute, Percutaneous Endoscopic Approach

0QR74JZ Replacement of Left Upper Femur with Synthetic Substitute, Percutaneous Endoscopic Approach

0QR74KZ Replacement of Left Upper Femur with Nonautologous Tissue Substitute, Percutaneous Endoscopic Approach

0QR807Z Replacement of Right Femoral Shaft with Autologous Tissue Substitute, Open Approach

0QR80JZ Replacement of Right Femoral Shaft with Synthetic Substitute, Open Approach

0QR80KZ Replacement of Right Femoral Shaft with Nonautologous Tissue Substitute, Open Approach

0QR837Z Replacement of Right Femoral Shaft with Autologous Tissue Substitute, Percutaneous Approach

0QR83JZ Replacement of Right Femoral Shaft with Synthetic Substitute, Percutaneous Approach

0QR83KZ Replacement of Right Femoral Shaft with Nonautologous Tissue Substitute, Percutaneous Approach

0QR847Z Replacement of Right Femoral Shaft with Autologous Tissue Substitute, Percutaneous Endoscopic Approach

0QR84JZ Replacement of Right Femoral Shaft with Synthetic Substitute, Percutaneous Endoscopic Approach

0QR84KZ Replacement of Right Femoral Shaft with Nonautologous Tissue Substitute, Percutaneous Endoscopic Approach

0QR907Z Replacement of Left Femoral Shaft with Autologous Tissue Substitute, Open Approach

0QR90JZ Replacement of Left Femoral Shaft with Synthetic Substitute, Open Approach

0QR90KZ Replacement of Left Femoral Shaft with Nonautologous Tissue Substitute, Open Approach

0QR937Z Replacement of Left Femoral Shaft with Autologous Tissue Substitute, Percutaneous Approach

0QR93JZ Replacement of Left Femoral Shaft with Synthetic Substitute, Percutaneous Approach

0QR93KZ Replacement of Left Femoral Shaft with Nonautologous Tissue Substitute, Percutaneous Approach

0QR947Z Replacement of Left Femoral Shaft with Autologous Tissue Substitute, Percutaneous Endoscopic Approach

0QR94JZ Replacement of Left Femoral Shaft with Synthetic Substitute, Percutaneous Endoscopic Approach

0QR94KZ Replacement of Left Femoral Shaft with Nonautologous Tissue Substitute, Percutaneous Endoscopic Approach

0QRB07Z Replacement of Right Lower Femur with Autologous Tissue Substitute, Open Approach

0QRB0JZ Replacement of Right Lower Femur with Synthetic Substitute, Open Approach

0QRB0KZ Replacement of Right Lower Femur with Nonautologous Tissue Substitute, Open Approach

0QRB37Z Replacement of Right Lower Femur with Autologous Tissue Substitute, Percutaneous Approach

0QRB3JZ Replacement of Right Lower Femur with Synthetic Substitute, Percutaneous Approach

0QRB3KZ Replacement of Right Lower Femur with Nonautologous Tissue Substitute, Percutaneous Approach

0QRB47Z Replacement of Right Lower Femur with Autologous Tissue Substitute, Percutaneous Endoscopic Approach

0QRB4JZ Replacement of Right Lower Femur with Synthetic Substitute, Percutaneous Endoscopic Approach

0QRB4KZ Replacement of Right Lower Femur with Nonautologous Tissue Substitute, Percutaneous Endoscopic Approach

0QRC07Z Replacement of Left Lower Femur with Autologous Tissue Substitute, Open Approach

0QRC0JZ Replacement of Left Lower Femur with Synthetic Substitute, Open Approach

0QRC0KZ Replacement of Left Lower Femur with Nonautologous Tissue Substitute, Open Approach

0QRC37Z Replacement of Left Lower Femur with Autologous Tissue Substitute, Percutaneous Approach

0QRC3JZ Replacement of Left Lower Femur with Synthetic Substitute, Percutaneous Approach

0QRC3KZ Replacement of Left Lower Femur with Nonautologous Tissue Substitute, Percutaneous Approach

0QRC47Z Replacement of Left Lower Femur with Autologous Tissue Substitute, Percutaneous Endoscopic Approach

0QRC4JZ Replacement of Left Lower Femur with Synthetic Substitute, Percutaneous Endoscopic Approach

0QRC4KZ Replacement of Left Lower Femur with Nonautologous Tissue Substitute, Percutaneous Endoscopic Approach

0QRD07Z Replacement of Right Patella with Autologous Tissue Substitute, Open Approach

0QRD0JZ Replacement of Right Patella with Synthetic Substitute, Open Approach

0QRD0KZ Replacement of Right Patella with Nonautologous Tissue Substitute, Open Approach

0QRD37Z Replacement of Right Patella with Autologous Tissue Substitute, Percutaneous Approach

0QRD3JZ Replacement of Right Patella with Synthetic Substitute, Percutaneous Approach

0QRD3KZ Replacement of Right Patella with Nonautologous Tissue Substitute, Percutaneous Approach

0QRD47Z Replacement of Right Patella with Autologous Tissue Substitute, Percutaneous Endoscopic Approach

0QRD4JZ Replacement of Right Patella with Synthetic Substitute, Percutaneous Endoscopic Approach

0QRD4KZ Replacement of Right Patella with Nonautologous Tissue Substitute, Percutaneous Endoscopic Approach

0QRF07Z Replacement of Left Patella with Autologous Tissue Substitute, Open Approach

0QRF0JZ Replacement of Left Patella with Synthetic Substitute, Open Approach

0QRF0KZ Replacement of Left Patella with Nonautologous Tissue Substitute, Open Approach

0QRF37Z Replacement of Left Patella with Autologous Tissue Substitute, Percutaneous Approach

0QRF3JZ Replacement of Left Patella with Synthetic Substitute, Percutaneous Approach

0QRF3KZ Replacement of Left Patella with Nonautologous Tissue Substitute, Percutaneous Approach

0QRF47Z Replacement of Left Patella with Autologous Tissue Substitute, Percutaneous Endoscopic Approach

0QRF4JZ Replacement of Left Patella with Synthetic Substitute, Percutaneous Endoscopic Approach

0QRF4KZ Replacement of Left Patella with Nonautologous Tissue Substitute, Percutaneous Endoscopic Approach

0QRG07Z Replacement of Right Tibia with Autologous Tissue Substitute, Open Approach

0QRG0JZ Replacement of Right Tibia with Synthetic Substitute, Open Approach

0QRG0KZ Replacement of Right Tibia with Nonautologous Tissue Substitute, Open Approach

0QRG37Z Replacement of Right Tibia with Autologous Tissue Substitute, Percutaneous Approach

0QRG3JZ Replacement of Right Tibia with Synthetic Substitute, Percutaneous Approach

0QRG3KZ Replacement of Right Tibia with Nonautologous Tissue Substitute, Percutaneous Approach

0QRG47Z Replacement of Right Tibia with Autologous Tissue Substitute, Percutaneous Endoscopic Approach

0QRG4JZ Replacement of Right Tibia with Synthetic Substitute, Percutaneous Endoscopic Approach

0QRG4KZ Replacement of Right Tibia with Nonautologous Tissue Substitute, Percutaneous Endoscopic Approach

0QRH07Z Replacement of Left Tibia with Autologous Tissue Substitute, Open Approach

0QRH0JZ Replacement of Left Tibia with Synthetic Substitute, Open Approach

0QRH0KZ Replacement of Left Tibia with Nonautologous Tissue Substitute, Open Approach

0QRH37Z Replacement of Left Tibia with Autologous Tissue Substitute, Percutaneous Approach

0QRH3JZ Replacement of Left Tibia with Synthetic Substitute, Percutaneous Approach

0QRH3KZ Replacement of Left Tibia with Nonautologous Tissue Substitute, Percutaneous Approach

0QRH47Z Replacement of Left Tibia with Autologous Tissue Substitute, Percutaneous Endoscopic Approach

0QRH4JZ Replacement of Left Tibia with Synthetic Substitute, Percutaneous Endoscopic Approach

0QRH4KZ Replacement of Left Tibia with Nonautologous Tissue Substitute, Percutaneous Endoscopic Approach

0QRJ07Z Replacement of Right Fibula with Autologous Tissue Substitute, Open Approach

0QRJ0JZ Replacement of Right Fibula with Synthetic Substitute, Open Approach

0QRJ0KZ Replacement of Right Fibula with Nonautologous Tissue Substitute, Open Approach

0QRJ37Z Replacement of Right Fibula with Autologous Tissue Substitute, Percutaneous Approach

0QRJ3JZ Replacement of Right Fibula with Synthetic Substitute, Percutaneous Approach

0QRJ3KZ Replacement of Right Fibula with Nonautologous Tissue Substitute, Percutaneous Approach

0QRJ47Z Replacement of Right Fibula with Autologous Tissue Substitute, Percutaneous Endoscopic Approach

0QRJ4JZ Replacement of Right Fibula with Synthetic Substitute, Percutaneous Endoscopic Approach

0QRJ4KZ Replacement of Right Fibula with Nonautologous Tissue Substitute, Percutaneous Endoscopic Approach

0QRK07Z Replacement of Left Fibula with Autologous Tissue Substitute, Open Approach

0QRK0JZ Replacement of Left Fibula with Synthetic Substitute, Open Approach

0QRK0KZ Replacement of Left Fibula with Nonautologous Tissue Substitute, Open Approach

0QRK37Z Replacement of Left Fibula with Autologous Tissue Substitute, Percutaneous Approach

0QRK3JZ Replacement of Left Fibula with Synthetic Substitute, Percutaneous Approach

0QRK3KZ Replacement of Left Fibula with Nonautologous Tissue Substitute, Percutaneous Approach

0QRK47Z Replacement of Left Fibula with Autologous Tissue Substitute, Percutaneous Endoscopic Approach

0QRK4JZ Replacement of Left Fibula with Synthetic Substitute, Percutaneous Endoscopic Approach

0QRK4KZ Replacement of Left Fibula with Nonautologous Tissue Substitute, Percutaneous Endoscopic Approach

0QRL07Z Replacement of Right Tarsal with Autologous Tissue Substitute, Open Approach

0QRL0JZ Replacement of Right Tarsal with Synthetic Substitute, Open Approach

0QRL0KZ Replacement of Right Tarsal with Nonautologous Tissue Substitute, Open Approach

0QRL37Z Replacement of Right Tarsal with Autologous Tissue Substitute, Percutaneous Approach

0QRL3JZ Replacement of Right Tarsal with Synthetic Substitute, Percutaneous Approach

0QRL3KZ Replacement of Right Tarsal with Nonautologous Tissue Substitute, Percutaneous Approach

0QRL47Z Replacement of Right Tarsal with Autologous Tissue Substitute, Percutaneous Endoscopic Approach

0QRL4JZ Replacement of Right Tarsal with Synthetic Substitute, Percutaneous Endoscopic Approach

0QRL4KZ Replacement of Right Tarsal with Nonautologous Tissue Substitute, Percutaneous Endoscopic Approach

0QRM07Z Replacement of Left Tarsal with Autologous Tissue Substitute, Open Approach

0QRM0JZ Replacement of Left Tarsal with Synthetic Substitute, Open Approach

0QRM0KZ   Replacement of Left Tarsal with Nonautologous Tissue Substitute, Open Approach

0QRM37Z   Replacement of Left Tarsal with Autologous Tissue Substitute, Percutaneous Approach

0QRM3JZ   Replacement of Left Tarsal with Synthetic Substitute, Percutaneous Approach

0QRM3KZ   Replacement of Left Tarsal with Nonautologous Tissue Substitute, Percutaneous Approach

0QRM47Z   Replacement of Left Tarsal with Autologous Tissue Substitute, Percutaneous Endoscopic Approach

0QRM4JZ   Replacement of Left Tarsal with Synthetic Substitute, Percutaneous Endoscopic Approach

0QRM4KZ   Replacement of Left Tarsal with Nonautologous Tissue Substitute, Percutaneous Endoscopic Approach

0QRN07Z   Replacement of Right Metatarsal with Autologous Tissue Substitute, Open Approach

0QRN0JZ   Replacement of Right Metatarsal with Synthetic Substitute, Open Approach

0QRN0KZ   Replacement of Right Metatarsal with Nonautologous Tissue Substitute, Open Approach

0QRN37Z   Replacement of Right Metatarsal with Autologous Tissue Substitute, Percutaneous Approach

0QRN3JZ   Replacement of Right Metatarsal with Synthetic Substitute, Percutaneous Approach

0QRN3KZ   Replacement of Right Metatarsal with Nonautologous Tissue Substitute, Percutaneous Approach

0QRN47Z   Replacement of Right Metatarsal with Autologous Tissue Substitute, Percutaneous Endoscopic Approach

0QRN4JZ   Replacement of Right Metatarsal with Synthetic Substitute, Percutaneous Endoscopic Approach

0QRN4KZ   Replacement of Right Metatarsal with Nonautologous Tissue Substitute, Percutaneous Endoscopic Approach

0QRP07Z   Replacement of Left Metatarsal with Autologous Tissue Substitute, Open Approach

0QRP0JZ   Replacement of Left Metatarsal with Synthetic Substitute, Open Approach

0QRP0KZ   Replacement of Left Metatarsal with Nonautologous Tissue Substitute, Open Approach

0QRP37Z   Replacement of Left Metatarsal with Autologous Tissue Substitute, Percutaneous Approach

0QRP3JZ   Replacement of Left Metatarsal with Synthetic Substitute, Percutaneous Approach

0QRP3KZ   Replacement of Left Metatarsal with Nonautologous Tissue Substitute, Percutaneous Approach

0QRP47Z   Replacement of Left Metatarsal with Autologous Tissue Substitute, Percutaneous Endoscopic Approach

0QRP4JZ   Replacement of Left Metatarsal with Synthetic Substitute, Percutaneous Endoscopic Approach

0QRP4KZ   Replacement of Left Metatarsal with Nonautologous Tissue Substitute, Percutaneous Endoscopic Approach

0QRQ07Z   Replacement of Right Toe Phalanx with Autologous Tissue Substitute, Open Approach

0QRQ0JZ   Replacement of Right Toe Phalanx with Synthetic Substitute, Open Approach

0QRQ0KZ   Replacement of Right Toe Phalanx with Nonautologous Tissue Substitute, Open Approach

0QRQ37Z   Replacement of Right Toe Phalanx with Autologous Tissue Substitute, Percutaneous Approach

0QRQ3JZ   Replacement of Right Toe Phalanx with Synthetic Substitute, Percutaneous Approach

0QRQ3KZ   Replacement of Right Toe Phalanx with Nonautologous Tissue Substitute, Percutaneous Approach

0QRQ47Z   Replacement of Right Toe Phalanx with Autologous Tissue Substitute, Percutaneous Endoscopic Approach

0QRQ4JZ   Replacement of Right Toe Phalanx with Synthetic Substitute, Percutaneous Endoscopic Approach

0QRQ4KZ   Replacement of Right Toe Phalanx with Nonautologous Tissue Substitute, Percutaneous Endoscopic Approach

0QRR07Z   Replacement of Left Toe Phalanx with Autologous Tissue Substitute, Open Approach

0QRR0JZ   Replacement of Left Toe Phalanx with Synthetic Substitute, Open Approach

0QRR0KZ   Replacement of Left Toe Phalanx with Nonautologous Tissue Substitute, Open Approach

0QRR37Z   Replacement of Left Toe Phalanx with Autologous Tissue Substitute, Percutaneous Approach

0QRR3JZ   Replacement of Left Toe Phalanx with Synthetic Substitute, Percutaneous Approach

0QRR3KZ   Replacement of Left Toe Phalanx with Nonautologous Tissue Substitute, Percutaneous Approach

0QRR47Z   Replacement of Left Toe Phalanx with Autologous Tissue Substitute, Percutaneous Endoscopic Approach

0QRR4JZ   Replacement of Left Toe Phalanx with Synthetic Substitute, Percutaneous Endoscopic Approach

0QRR4KZ   Replacement of Left Toe Phalanx with Nonautologous Tissue Substitute, Percutaneous Endoscopic Approach

0QRS07Z   Replacement of Coccyx with Autologous Tissue Substitute, Open Approach

0QRS0JZ   Replacement of Coccyx with Synthetic Substitute, Open Approach

0QRS0KZ   Replacement of Coccyx with Nonautologous Tissue Substitute, Open Approach

0QRS37Z   Replacement of Coccyx with Autologous Tissue Substitute, Percutaneous Approach

0QRS3JZ   Replacement of Coccyx with Synthetic Substitute, Percutaneous Approach

0QRS3KZ   Replacement of Coccyx with Nonautologous Tissue Substitute, Percutaneous Approach

0QRS47Z   Replacement of Coccyx with Autologous Tissue Substitute, Percutaneous Endoscopic Approach

0QRS4JZ   Replacement of Coccyx with Synthetic Substitute, Percutaneous Endoscopic Approach

0QRS4KZ   Replacement of Coccyx with Nonautologous Tissue Substitute, Percutaneous Endoscopic Approach

0QS – Lower Bones, Reposition

Review Coding Guideline B3.15

0QS004Z   Reposition Lumbar Vertebra with Internal Fixation Device, Open Approach

0QS00ZZ   Reposition Lumbar Vertebra, Open Approach

0QS034Z   Reposition Lumbar Vertebra with Internal Fixation Device, Percutaneous Approach

0QS03ZZ   Reposition Lumbar Vertebra, Percutaneous Approach

0QS044Z   Reposition Lumbar Vertebra with Internal Fixation Device, Percutaneous Endoscopic Approach

0QS04ZZ   Reposition Lumbar Vertebra, Percutaneous Endoscopic Approach

0QS0XZZ   Reposition Lumbar Vertebra, External Approach

0QS104Z   Reposition Sacrum with Internal Fixation Device, Open Approach

0QS10ZZ   Reposition Sacrum, Open Approach

0QS134Z   Reposition Sacrum with Internal Fixation Device, Percutaneous Approach

0QS13ZZ   Reposition Sacrum, Percutaneous Approach

0QS144Z   Reposition Sacrum with Internal Fixation Device, Percutaneous Endoscopic Approach

0QS14ZZ   Reposition Sacrum, Percutaneous Endoscopic Approach

0QS1XZZ   Reposition Sacrum, External Approach

0QS204Z   Reposition Right Pelvic Bone with Internal Fixation Device, Open Approach

0QS205Z   Reposition Right Pelvic Bone with External Fixation Device, Open Approach

0QS20ZZ   Reposition Right Pelvic Bone, Open Approach

0QS234Z   Reposition Right Pelvic Bone with Internal Fixation Device, Percutaneous Approach

0QS235Z   Reposition Right Pelvic Bone with External Fixation Device, Percutaneous Approach

0QS23ZZ   Reposition Right Pelvic Bone, Percutaneous Approach

0QS244Z   Reposition Right Pelvic Bone with Internal Fixation Device, Percutaneous Endoscopic Approach

0QS245Z Reposition Right Pelvic Bone with External Fixation Device, Percutaneous Endoscopic Approach

0QS24ZZ Reposition Right Pelvic Bone, Percutaneous Endoscopic Approach

0QS2XZZ Reposition Right Pelvic Bone, External Approach

0QS304Z Reposition Left Pelvic Bone with Internal Fixation Device, Open Approach

0QS305Z Reposition Left Pelvic Bone with External Fixation Device, Open Approach

0QS30ZZ Reposition Left Pelvic Bone, Open Approach

0QS334Z Reposition Left Pelvic Bone with Internal Fixation Device, Percutaneous Approach

0QS335Z Reposition Left Pelvic Bone with External Fixation Device, Percutaneous Approach

0QS33ZZ Reposition Left Pelvic Bone, Percutaneous Approach

0QS344Z Reposition Left Pelvic Bone with Internal Fixation Device, Percutaneous Endoscopic Approach

0QS345Z Reposition Left Pelvic Bone with External Fixation Device, Percutaneous Endoscopic Approach

0QS34ZZ Reposition Left Pelvic Bone, Percutaneous Endoscopic Approach

0QS3XZZ Reposition Left Pelvic Bone, External Approach

0QS404Z Reposition Right Acetabulum with Internal Fixation Device, Open Approach

0QS40ZZ Reposition Right Acetabulum, Open Approach

0QS434Z Reposition Right Acetabulum with Internal Fixation Device, Percutaneous Approach

0QS43ZZ Reposition Right Acetabulum, Percutaneous Approach

0QS444Z Reposition Right Acetabulum with Internal Fixation Device, Percutaneous Endoscopic Approach

0QS44ZZ Reposition Right Acetabulum, Percutaneous Endoscopic Approach

0QS4XZZ Reposition Right Acetabulum, External Approach

0QS504Z Reposition Left Acetabulum with Internal Fixation Device, Open Approach

0QS50ZZ Reposition Left Acetabulum, Open Approach

0QS534Z Reposition Left Acetabulum with Internal Fixation Device, Percutaneous Approach

0QS53ZZ Reposition Left Acetabulum, Percutaneous Approach

0QS544Z Reposition Left Acetabulum with Internal Fixation Device, Percutaneous Endoscopic Approach

0QS54ZZ Reposition Left Acetabulum, Percutaneous Endoscopic Approach

0QS5XZZ Reposition Left Acetabulum, External Approach

0QS604Z Reposition Right Upper Femur with Internal Fixation Device, Open Approach

0QS605Z Reposition Right Upper Femur with External Fixation Device, Open Approach

0QS606Z Reposition Right Upper Femur with Intramedullary Internal Fixation Device, Open Approach

0QS60BZ Reposition Right Upper Femur with Monoplanar External Fixation Device, Open Approach

0QS60CZ Reposition Right Upper Femur with Ring External Fixation Device, Open Approach

0QS60DZ Reposition Right Upper Femur with Hybrid External Fixation Device, Open Approach

0QS60ZZ Reposition Right Upper Femur, Open Approach

0QS634Z Reposition Right Upper Femur with Internal Fixation Device, Percutaneous Approach

0QS635Z Reposition Right Upper Femur with External Fixation Device, Percutaneous Approach

0QS636Z Reposition Right Upper Femur with Intramedullary Internal Fixation Device, Percutaneous Approach

0QS63BZ Reposition Right Upper Femur with Monoplanar External Fixation Device, Percutaneous Approach

0QS63CZ Reposition Right Upper Femur with Ring External Fixation Device, Percutaneous Approach

0QS63DZ Reposition Right Upper Femur with Hybrid External Fixation Device, Percutaneous Approach

0QS63ZZ Reposition Right Upper Femur, Percutaneous Approach

0QS644Z Reposition Right Upper Femur with Internal Fixation Device, Percutaneous Endoscopic Approach

0QS645Z Reposition Right Upper Femur with External Fixation Device, Percutaneous Endoscopic Approach

0QS646Z Reposition Right Upper Femur with Intramedullary Internal Fixation Device, Percutaneous Endoscopic Approach

0QS64BZ Reposition Right Upper Femur with Monoplanar External Fixation Device, Percutaneous Endoscopic Approach

0QS64CZ Reposition Right Upper Femur with Ring External Fixation Device, Percutaneous Endoscopic Approach

0QS64DZ Reposition Right Upper Femur with Hybrid External Fixation Device, Percutaneous Endoscopic Approach

0QS64ZZ Reposition Right Upper Femur, Percutaneous Endoscopic Approach

0QS6XZZ Reposition Right Upper Femur, External Approach

0QS704Z Reposition Left Upper Femur with Internal Fixation Device, Open Approach

0QS705Z Reposition Left Upper Femur with External Fixation Device, Open Approach

0QS706Z Reposition Left Upper Femur with Intramedullary Internal Fixation Device, Open Approach

0QS70BZ Reposition Left Upper Femur with Monoplanar External Fixation Device, Open Approach

0QS70CZ Reposition Left Upper Femur with Ring External Fixation Device, Open Approach

0QS70DZ Reposition Left Upper Femur with Hybrid External Fixation Device, Open Approach

0QS70ZZ Reposition Left Upper Femur, Open Approach

0QS734Z Reposition Left Upper Femur with Internal Fixation Device, Percutaneous Approach

0QS735Z Reposition Left Upper Femur with External Fixation Device, Percutaneous Approach

0QS736Z Reposition Left Upper Femur with Intramedullary Internal Fixation Device, Percutaneous Approach

0QS73BZ Reposition Left Upper Femur with Monoplanar External Fixation Device, Percutaneous Approach

0QS73CZ Reposition Left Upper Femur with Ring External Fixation Device, Percutaneous Approach

0QS73DZ Reposition Left Upper Femur with Hybrid External Fixation Device, Percutaneous Approach

0QS73ZZ Reposition Left Upper Femur, Percutaneous Approach

0QS744Z Reposition Left Upper Femur with Internal Fixation Device, Percutaneous Endoscopic Approach

0QS745Z Reposition Left Upper Femur with External Fixation Device, Percutaneous Endoscopic Approach

0QS746Z Reposition Left Upper Femur with Intramedullary Internal Fixation Device, Percutaneous Endoscopic Approach

0QS74BZ Reposition Left Upper Femur with Monoplanar External Fixation Device, Percutaneous Endoscopic Approach

0QS74CZ Reposition Left Upper Femur with Ring External Fixation Device, Percutaneous Endoscopic Approach

0QS74DZ Reposition Left Upper Femur with Hybrid External Fixation Device, Percutaneous Endoscopic Approach

0QS74ZZ Reposition Left Upper Femur, Percutaneous Endoscopic Approach

0QS7XZZ Reposition Left Upper Femur, External Approach

0QS804Z Reposition Right Femoral Shaft with Internal Fixation Device, Open Approach

0QS805Z Reposition Right Femoral Shaft with External Fixation Device, Open Approach

0QS806Z Reposition Right Femoral Shaft with Intramedullary Internal Fixation Device, Open Approach

0QS80BZ Reposition Right Femoral Shaft with Monoplanar External Fixation Device, Open Approach

0QS80CZ Reposition Right Femoral Shaft with Ring External Fixation Device, Open Approach

0QS80DZ Reposition Right Femoral Shaft with Hybrid External Fixation Device, Open Approach

0QS80ZZ Reposition Right Femoral Shaft, Open Approach

0QS834Z Reposition Right Femoral Shaft with Internal Fixation Device, Percutaneous Approach

0QS835Z Reposition Right Femoral Shaft with External Fixation Device, Percutaneous Approach

0QS836Z Reposition Right Femoral Shaft with Intramedullary Internal Fixation Device, Percutaneous Approach

0QS83BZ Reposition Right Femoral Shaft with Monoplanar External Fixation Device, Percutaneous Approach

0QS83CZ Reposition Right Femoral Shaft with Ring External Fixation Device, Percutaneous Approach

0QS83DZ Reposition Right Femoral Shaft with Hybrid External Fixation Device, Percutaneous Approach

---

♀ Female-only   ♂ Male-only   ⬤ Limited Coverage   ● Non-OR   HAC HAC-associated procedure   ⬣ Non-covered procedures   ✚ Combination

0QS83ZZ Reposition Right Femoral Shaft, Percutaneous Approach

0QS844Z Reposition Right Femoral Shaft with Internal Fixation Device, Percutaneous Endoscopic Approach

0QS845Z Reposition Right Femoral Shaft with External Fixation Device, Percutaneous Endoscopic Approach

0QS846Z Reposition Right Femoral Shaft with Intramedullary Internal Fixation Device, Percutaneous Endoscopic Approach

0QS84BZ Reposition Right Femoral Shaft with Monoplanar External Fixation Device, Percutaneous Endoscopic Approach

0QS84CZ Reposition Right Femoral Shaft with Ring External Fixation Device, Percutaneous Endoscopic Approach

0QS84DZ Reposition Right Femoral Shaft with Hybrid External Fixation Device, Percutaneous Endoscopic Approach

0QS84ZZ Reposition Right Femoral Shaft, Percutaneous Endoscopic Approach

0QS8XZZ Reposition Right Femoral Shaft, External Approach

0QS904Z Reposition Left Femoral Shaft with Internal Fixation Device, Open Approach

0QS905Z Reposition Left Femoral Shaft with External Fixation Device, Open Approach

0QS906Z Reposition Left Femoral Shaft with Intramedullary Internal Fixation Device, Open Approach

0QS90BZ Reposition Left Femoral Shaft with Monoplanar External Fixation Device, Open Approach

0QS90CZ Reposition Left Femoral Shaft with Ring External Fixation Device, Open Approach

0QS90DZ Reposition Left Femoral Shaft with Hybrid External Fixation Device, Open Approach

0QS90ZZ Reposition Left Femoral Shaft, Open Approach

0QS934Z Reposition Left Femoral Shaft with Internal Fixation Device, Percutaneous Approach

0QS935Z Reposition Left Femoral Shaft with External Fixation Device, Percutaneous Approach

0QS936Z Reposition Left Femoral Shaft with Intramedullary Internal Fixation Device, Percutaneous Approach

0QS93BZ Reposition Left Femoral Shaft with Monoplanar External Fixation Device, Percutaneous Approach

0QS93CZ Reposition Left Femoral Shaft with Ring External Fixation Device, Percutaneous Approach

0QS93DZ Reposition Left Femoral Shaft with Hybrid External Fixation Device, Percutaneous Approach

0QS93ZZ Reposition Left Femoral Shaft, Percutaneous Approach

0QS944Z Reposition Left Femoral Shaft with Internal Fixation Device, Percutaneous Endoscopic Approach

0QS945Z Reposition Left Femoral Shaft with External Fixation Device, Percutaneous Endoscopic Approach

0QS946Z Reposition Left Femoral Shaft with Intramedullary Internal Fixation Device, Percutaneous Endoscopic Approach

0QS94BZ Reposition Left Femoral Shaft with Monoplanar External Fixation Device, Percutaneous Endoscopic Approach

0QS94CZ Reposition Left Femoral Shaft with Ring External Fixation Device, Percutaneous Endoscopic Approach

0QS94DZ Reposition Left Femoral Shaft with Hybrid External Fixation Device, Percutaneous Endoscopic Approach

0QS94ZZ Reposition Left Femoral Shaft, Percutaneous Endoscopic Approach

0QS9XZZ Reposition Left Femoral Shaft, External Approach

0QSB04Z Reposition Right Lower Femur with Internal Fixation Device, Open Approach

0QSB05Z Reposition Right Lower Femur with External Fixation Device, Open Approach

0QSB06Z Reposition Right Lower Femur with Intramedullary Internal Fixation Device, Open Approach

0QSB0BZ Reposition Right Lower Femur with Monoplanar External Fixation Device, Open Approach

0QSB0CZ Reposition Right Lower Femur with Ring External Fixation Device, Open Approach

0QSB0DZ Reposition Right Lower Femur with Hybrid External Fixation Device, Open Approach

0QSB0ZZ Reposition Right Lower Femur, Open Approach

0QSB34Z Reposition Right Lower Femur with Internal Fixation Device, Percutaneous Approach

0QSB35Z Reposition Right Lower Femur with External Fixation Device, Percutaneous Approach

0QSB36Z Reposition Right Lower Femur with Intramedullary Internal Fixation Device, Percutaneous Approach

0QSB3BZ Reposition Right Lower Femur with Monoplanar External Fixation Device, Percutaneous Approach

0QSB3CZ Reposition Right Lower Femur with Ring External Fixation Device, Percutaneous Approach

0QSB3DZ Reposition Right Lower Femur with Hybrid External Fixation Device, Percutaneous Approach

0QSB3ZZ Reposition Right Lower Femur, Percutaneous Approach

0QSB44Z Reposition Right Lower Femur with Internal Fixation Device, Percutaneous Endoscopic Approach

0QSB45Z Reposition Right Lower Femur with External Fixation Device, Percutaneous Endoscopic Approach

0QSB46Z Reposition Right Lower Femur with Intramedullary Internal Fixation Device, Percutaneous Endoscopic Approach

0QSB4BZ Reposition Right Lower Femur with Monoplanar External Fixation Device, Percutaneous Endoscopic Approach

0QSB4CZ Reposition Right Lower Femur with Ring External Fixation Device, Percutaneous Endoscopic Approach

0QSB4DZ Reposition Right Lower Femur with Hybrid External Fixation Device, Percutaneous Endoscopic Approach

0QSB4ZZ Reposition Right Lower Femur, Percutaneous Endoscopic Approach

0QSBXZZ Reposition Right Lower Femur, External Approach

0QSC04Z Reposition Left Lower Femur with Internal Fixation Device, Open Approach

0QSC05Z Reposition Left Lower Femur with External Fixation Device, Open Approach

0QSC06Z Reposition Left Lower Femur with Intramedullary Internal Fixation Device, Open Approach

0QSC0BZ Reposition Left Lower Femur with Monoplanar External Fixation Device, Open Approach

0QSC0CZ Reposition Left Lower Femur with Ring External Fixation Device, Open Approach

0QSC0DZ Reposition Left Lower Femur with Hybrid External Fixation Device, Open Approach

0QSC0ZZ Reposition Left Lower Femur, Open Approach

0QSC34Z Reposition Left Lower Femur with Internal Fixation Device, Percutaneous Approach

0QSC35Z Reposition Left Lower Femur with External Fixation Device, Percutaneous Approach

0QSC36Z Reposition Left Lower Femur with Intramedullary Internal Fixation Device, Percutaneous Approach

0QSC3BZ Reposition Left Lower Femur with Monoplanar External Fixation Device, Percutaneous Approach

0QSC3CZ Reposition Left Lower Femur with Ring External Fixation Device, Percutaneous Approach

0QSC3DZ Reposition Left Lower Femur with Hybrid External Fixation Device, Percutaneous Approach

0QSC3ZZ Reposition Left Lower Femur, Percutaneous Approach

0QSC44Z Reposition Left Lower Femur with Internal Fixation Device, Percutaneous Endoscopic Approach

0QSC45Z Reposition Left Lower Femur with External Fixation Device, Percutaneous Endoscopic Approach

0QSC46Z Reposition Left Lower Femur with Intramedullary Internal Fixation Device, Percutaneous Endoscopic Approach

0QSC4BZ Reposition Left Lower Femur with Monoplanar External Fixation Device, Percutaneous Endoscopic Approach

0QSC4CZ Reposition Left Lower Femur with Ring External Fixation Device, Percutaneous Endoscopic Approach

0QSC4DZ Reposition Left Lower Femur with Hybrid External Fixation Device, Percutaneous Endoscopic Approach

0QSC4ZZ Reposition Left Lower Femur, Percutaneous Endoscopic Approach

0QSCXZZ Reposition Left Lower Femur, External Approach

0QSD04Z Reposition Right Patella with Internal Fixation Device, Open Approach

0QSD05Z Reposition Right Patella with External Fixation Device, Open Approach

0QSD0ZZ Reposition Right Patella, Open Approach

0QSD34Z Reposition Right Patella with Internal Fixation Device, Percutaneous Approach

0QSD35Z Reposition Right Patella with External Fixation Device, Percutaneous Approach

0QSD3ZZ	Reposition Right Patella, Percutaneous Approach
0QSD44Z	Reposition Right Patella with Internal Fixation Device, Percutaneous Endoscopic Approach
0QSD45Z	Reposition Right Patella with External Fixation Device, Percutaneous Endoscopic Approach
0QSD4ZZ	Reposition Right Patella, Percutaneous Endoscopic Approach
0QSDXZZ	Reposition Right Patella, External Approach
0QSF04Z	Reposition Left Patella with Internal Fixation Device, Open Approach
0QSF05Z	Reposition Left Patella with External Fixation Device, Open Approach
0QSF0ZZ	Reposition Left Patella, Open Approach
0QSF34Z	Reposition Left Patella with Internal Fixation Device, Percutaneous Approach
0QSF35Z	Reposition Left Patella with External Fixation Device, Percutaneous Approach
0QSF3ZZ	Reposition Left Patella, Percutaneous Approach
0QSF44Z	Reposition Left Patella with Internal Fixation Device, Percutaneous Endoscopic Approach
0QSF45Z	Reposition Left Patella with External Fixation Device, Percutaneous Endoscopic Approach
0QSF4ZZ	Reposition Left Patella, Percutaneous Endoscopic Approach
0QSFXZZ	Reposition Left Patella, External Approach
0QSG04Z	Reposition Right Tibia with Internal Fixation Device, Open Approach
0QSG05Z	Reposition Right Tibia with External Fixation Device, Open Approach
0QSG06Z	Reposition Right Tibia with Intramedullary Internal Fixation Device, Open Approach
0QSG0BZ	Reposition Right Tibia with Monoplanar External Fixation Device, Open Approach
0QSG0CZ	Reposition Right Tibia with Ring External Fixation Device, Open Approach
0QSG0DZ	Reposition Right Tibia with Hybrid External Fixation Device, Open Approach
0QSG0ZZ	Reposition Right Tibia, Open Approach
0QSG34Z	Reposition Right Tibia with Internal Fixation Device, Percutaneous Approach
0QSG35Z	Reposition Right Tibia with External Fixation Device, Percutaneous Approach
0QSG36Z	Reposition Right Tibia with Intramedullary Internal Fixation Device, Percutaneous Approach
0QSG3BZ	Reposition Right Tibia with Monoplanar External Fixation Device, Percutaneous Approach
0QSG3CZ	Reposition Right Tibia with Ring External Fixation Device, Percutaneous Approach
0QSG3DZ	Reposition Right Tibia with Hybrid External Fixation Device, Percutaneous Approach
0QSG3ZZ	Reposition Right Tibia, Percutaneous Approach
0QSG44Z	Reposition Right Tibia with Internal Fixation Device, Percutaneous Endoscopic Approach
0QSG45Z	Reposition Right Tibia with External Fixation Device, Percutaneous Endoscopic Approach
0QSG46Z	Reposition Right Tibia with Intramedullary Internal Fixation Device, Percutaneous Endoscopic Approach
0QSG4BZ	Reposition Right Tibia with Monoplanar External Fixation Device, Percutaneous Endoscopic Approach
0QSG4CZ	Reposition Right Tibia with Ring External Fixation Device, Percutaneous Endoscopic Approach
0QSG4DZ	Reposition Right Tibia with Hybrid External Fixation Device, Percutaneous Endoscopic Approach
0QSG4ZZ	Reposition Right Tibia, Percutaneous Endoscopic Approach
0QSGXZZ	Reposition Right Tibia, External Approach
0QSH04Z	Reposition Left Tibia with Internal Fixation Device, Open Approach
0QSH05Z	Reposition Left Tibia with External Fixation Device, Open Approach
0QSH06Z	Reposition Left Tibia with Intramedullary Internal Fixation Device, Open Approach
0QSH0BZ	Reposition Left Tibia with Monoplanar External Fixation Device, Open Approach
0QSH0CZ	Reposition Left Tibia with Ring External Fixation Device, Open Approach
0QSH0DZ	Reposition Left Tibia with Hybrid External Fixation Device, Open Approach
0QSH0ZZ	Reposition Left Tibia, Open Approach
0QSH34Z	Reposition Left Tibia with Internal Fixation Device, Percutaneous Approach
0QSH35Z	Reposition Left Tibia with External Fixation Device, Percutaneous Approach
0QSH36Z	Reposition Left Tibia with Intramedullary Internal Fixation Device, Percutaneous Approach
0QSH3BZ	Reposition Left Tibia with Monoplanar External Fixation Device, Percutaneous Approach
0QSH3CZ	Reposition Left Tibia with Ring External Fixation Device, Percutaneous Approach
0QSH3DZ	Reposition Left Tibia with Hybrid External Fixation Device, Percutaneous Approach
0QSH3ZZ	Reposition Left Tibia, Percutaneous Approach
0QSH44Z	Reposition Left Tibia with Internal Fixation Device, Percutaneous Endoscopic Approach
0QSH45Z	Reposition Left Tibia with External Fixation Device, Percutaneous Endoscopic Approach
0QSH46Z	Reposition Left Tibia with Intramedullary Internal Fixation Device, Percutaneous Endoscopic Approach
0QSH4BZ	Reposition Left Tibia with Monoplanar External Fixation Device, Percutaneous Endoscopic Approach
0QSH4CZ	Reposition Left Tibia with Ring External Fixation Device, Percutaneous Endoscopic Approach
0QSH4DZ	Reposition Left Tibia with Hybrid External Fixation Device, Percutaneous Endoscopic Approach
0QSH4ZZ	Reposition Left Tibia, Percutaneous Endoscopic Approach
0QSHXZZ	Reposition Left Tibia, External Approach
0QSJ04Z	Reposition Right Fibula with Internal Fixation Device, Open Approach
0QSJ05Z	Reposition Right Fibula with External Fixation Device, Open Approach
0QSJ06Z	Reposition Right Fibula with Intramedullary Internal Fixation Device, Open Approach
0QSJ0BZ	Reposition Right Fibula with Monoplanar External Fixation Device, Open Approach
0QSJ0CZ	Reposition Right Fibula with Ring External Fixation Device, Open Approach
0QSJ0DZ	Reposition Right Fibula with Hybrid External Fixation Device, Open Approach
0QSJ0ZZ	Reposition Right Fibula, Open Approach
0QSJ34Z	Reposition Right Fibula with Internal Fixation Device, Percutaneous Approach
0QSJ35Z	Reposition Right Fibula with External Fixation Device, Percutaneous Approach
0QSJ36Z	Reposition Right Fibula with Intramedullary Internal Fixation Device, Percutaneous Approach
0QSJ3BZ	Reposition Right Fibula with Monoplanar External Fixation Device, Percutaneous Approach
0QSJ3CZ	Reposition Right Fibula with Ring External Fixation Device, Percutaneous Approach
0QSJ3DZ	Reposition Right Fibula with Hybrid External Fixation Device, Percutaneous Approach
0QSJ3ZZ	Reposition Right Fibula, Percutaneous Approach
0QSJ44Z	Reposition Right Fibula with Internal Fixation Device, Percutaneous Endoscopic Approach
0QSJ45Z	Reposition Right Fibula with External Fixation Device, Percutaneous Endoscopic Approach
0QSJ46Z	Reposition Right Fibula with Intramedullary Internal Fixation Device, Percutaneous Endoscopic Approach
0QSJ4BZ	Reposition Right Fibula with Monoplanar External Fixation Device, Percutaneous Endoscopic Approach
0QSJ4CZ	Reposition Right Fibula with Ring External Fixation Device, Percutaneous Endoscopic Approach
0QSJ4DZ	Reposition Right Fibula with Hybrid External Fixation Device, Percutaneous Endoscopic Approach
0QSJ4ZZ	Reposition Right Fibula, Percutaneous Endoscopic Approach
0QSJXZZ	Reposition Right Fibula, External Approach
0QSK04Z	Reposition Left Fibula with Internal Fixation Device, Open Approach
0QSK05Z	Reposition Left Fibula with External Fixation Device, Open Approach

0QSK06Z Reposition Left Fibula with Intramedullary Internal Fixation Device, Open Approach

0QSK0BZ Reposition Left Fibula with Monoplanar External Fixation Device, Open Approach

0QSK0CZ Reposition Left Fibula with Ring External Fixation Device, Open Approach

0QSK0DZ Reposition Left Fibula with Hybrid External Fixation Device, Open Approach

0QSK0ZZ Reposition Left Fibula, Open Approach

0QSK34Z Reposition Left Fibula with Internal Fixation Device, Percutaneous Approach

0QSK35Z Reposition Left Fibula with External Fixation Device, Percutaneous Approach

0QSK36Z Reposition Left Fibula with Intramedullary Internal Fixation Device, Percutaneous Approach

0QSK3BZ Reposition Left Fibula with Monoplanar External Fixation Device, Percutaneous Approach

0QSK3CZ Reposition Left Fibula with Ring External Fixation Device, Percutaneous Approach

0QSK3DZ Reposition Left Fibula with Hybrid External Fixation Device, Percutaneous Approach

0QSK3ZZ Reposition Left Fibula, Percutaneous Approach

0QSK44Z Reposition Left Fibula with Internal Fixation Device, Percutaneous Endoscopic Approach

0QSK45Z Reposition Left Fibula with External Fixation Device, Percutaneous Endoscopic Approach

0QSK46Z Reposition Left Fibula with Intramedullary Internal Fixation Device, Percutaneous Endoscopic Approach

0QSK4BZ Reposition Left Fibula with Monoplanar External Fixation Device, Percutaneous Endoscopic Approach

0QSK4CZ Reposition Left Fibula with Ring External Fixation Device, Percutaneous Endoscopic Approach

0QSK4DZ Reposition Left Fibula with Hybrid External Fixation Device, Percutaneous Endoscopic Approach

0QSK4ZZ Reposition Left Fibula, Percutaneous Endoscopic Approach

0QSKXZZ Reposition Left Fibula, External Approach

0QSL04Z Reposition Right Tarsal with Internal Fixation Device, Open Approach

0QSL05Z Reposition Right Tarsal with External Fixation Device, Open Approach

0QSL0ZZ Reposition Right Tarsal, Open Approach

0QSL34Z Reposition Right Tarsal with Internal Fixation Device, Percutaneous Approach

0QSL35Z Reposition Right Tarsal with External Fixation Device, Percutaneous Approach

0QSL3ZZ Reposition Right Tarsal, Percutaneous Approach

0QSL44Z Reposition Right Tarsal with Internal Fixation Device, Percutaneous Endoscopic Approach

0QSL45Z Reposition Right Tarsal with External Fixation Device, Percutaneous Endoscopic Approach

0QSL4ZZ Reposition Right Tarsal, Percutaneous Endoscopic Approach

0QSLXZZ Reposition Right Tarsal, External Approach

0QSM04Z Reposition Left Tarsal with Internal Fixation Device, Open Approach

0QSM05Z Reposition Left Tarsal with External Fixation Device, Open Approach

0QSM0ZZ Reposition Left Tarsal, Open Approach

0QSM34Z Reposition Left Tarsal with Internal Fixation Device, Percutaneous Approach

0QSM35Z Reposition Left Tarsal with External Fixation Device, Percutaneous Approach

0QSM3ZZ Reposition Left Tarsal, Percutaneous Approach

0QSM44Z Reposition Left Tarsal with Internal Fixation Device, Percutaneous Endoscopic Approach

0QSM45Z Reposition Left Tarsal with External Fixation Device, Percutaneous Endoscopic Approach

0QSM4ZZ Reposition Left Tarsal, Percutaneous Endoscopic Approach

0QSMXZZ Reposition Left Tarsal, External Approach

0QSN04Z Reposition Right Metatarsal with Internal Fixation Device, Open Approach

0QSN05Z Reposition Right Metatarsal with External Fixation Device, Open Approach

0QSN0ZZ Reposition Right Metatarsal, Open Approach

0QSN34Z Reposition Right Metatarsal with Internal Fixation Device, Percutaneous Approach

0QSN35Z Reposition Right Metatarsal with External Fixation Device, Percutaneous Approach

0QSN3ZZ Reposition Right Metatarsal, Percutaneous Approach

0QSN44Z Reposition Right Metatarsal with Internal Fixation Device, Percutaneous Endoscopic Approach

0QSN45Z Reposition Right Metatarsal with External Fixation Device, Percutaneous Endoscopic Approach

0QSN4ZZ Reposition Right Metatarsal, Percutaneous Endoscopic Approach

0QSNXZZ Reposition Right Metatarsal, External Approach

0QSP04Z Reposition Left Metatarsal with Internal Fixation Device, Open Approach

0QSP05Z Reposition Left Metatarsal with External Fixation Device, Open Approach

0QSP0ZZ Reposition Left Metatarsal, Open Approach

0QSP34Z Reposition Left Metatarsal with Internal Fixation Device, Percutaneous Approach

0QSP35Z Reposition Left Metatarsal with External Fixation Device, Percutaneous Approach

0QSP3ZZ Reposition Left Metatarsal, Percutaneous Approach

0QSP44Z Reposition Left Metatarsal with Internal Fixation Device, Percutaneous Endoscopic Approach

0QSP45Z Reposition Left Metatarsal with External Fixation Device, Percutaneous Endoscopic Approach

0QSP4ZZ Reposition Left Metatarsal, Percutaneous Endoscopic Approach

0QSPXZZ Reposition Left Metatarsal, External Approach

0QSQ04Z Reposition Right Toe Phalanx with Internal Fixation Device, Open Approach

0QSQ05Z Reposition Right Toe Phalanx with External Fixation Device, Open Approach

0QSQ0ZZ Reposition Right Toe Phalanx, Open Approach

0QSQ34Z Reposition Right Toe Phalanx with Internal Fixation Device, Percutaneous Approach

0QSQ35Z Reposition Right Toe Phalanx with External Fixation Device, Percutaneous Approach

0QSQ3ZZ Reposition Right Toe Phalanx, Percutaneous Approach

0QSQ44Z Reposition Right Toe Phalanx with Internal Fixation Device, Percutaneous Endoscopic Approach

0QSQ45Z Reposition Right Toe Phalanx with External Fixation Device, Percutaneous Endoscopic Approach

0QSQ4ZZ Reposition Right Toe Phalanx, Percutaneous Endoscopic Approach

0QSQXZZ Reposition Right Toe Phalanx, External Approach

0QSR04Z Reposition Left Toe Phalanx with Internal Fixation Device, Open Approach

0QSR05Z Reposition Left Toe Phalanx with External Fixation Device, Open Approach

0QSR0ZZ Reposition Left Toe Phalanx, Open Approach

0QSR34Z Reposition Left Toe Phalanx with Internal Fixation Device, Percutaneous Approach

0QSR35Z Reposition Left Toe Phalanx with External Fixation Device, Percutaneous Approach

0QSR3ZZ Reposition Left Toe Phalanx, Percutaneous Approach

0QSR44Z Reposition Left Toe Phalanx with Internal Fixation Device, Percutaneous Endoscopic Approach

0QSR45Z Reposition Left Toe Phalanx with External Fixation Device, Percutaneous Endoscopic Approach

0QSR4ZZ Reposition Left Toe Phalanx, Percutaneous Endoscopic Approach

0QSRXZZ Reposition Left Toe Phalanx, External Approach

0QSS04Z Reposition Coccyx with Internal Fixation Device, Open Approach

0QSS0ZZ Reposition Coccyx, Open Approach

0QSS34Z Reposition Coccyx with Internal Fixation Device, Percutaneous Approach

0QSS3ZZ Reposition Coccyx, Percutaneous Approach

0QSS44Z Reposition Coccyx with Internal Fixation Device, Percutaneous Endoscopic Approach

0QSS4ZZ Reposition Coccyx, Percutaneous Endoscopic Approach

0QSSXZZ Reposition Coccyx, External Approach

0QT – Lower Bones, Resection

Review Coding Guideline B3.8

0QT20ZZ	Resection of Right Pelvic Bone, Open Approach
0QT30ZZ	Resection of Left Pelvic Bone, Open Approach
0QT40ZZ	Resection of Right Acetabulum, Open Approach
0QT50ZZ	Resection of Left Acetabulum, Open Approach
0QT60ZZ	Resection of Right Upper Femur, Open Approach
0QT70ZZ	Resection of Left Upper Femur, Open Approach
0QT80ZZ	Resection of Right Femoral Shaft, Open Approach
0QT90ZZ	Resection of Left Femoral Shaft, Open Approach
0QTB0ZZ	Resection of Right Lower Femur, Open Approach
0QTC0ZZ	Resection of Left Lower Femur, Open Approach
0QTD0ZZ	Resection of Right Patella, Open Approach
0QTF0ZZ	Resection of Left Patella, Open Approach

0QTG0ZZ	Resection of Right Tibia, Open Approach
0QTH0ZZ	Resection of Left Tibia, Open Approach
0QTJ0ZZ	Resection of Right Fibula, Open Approach
0QTK0ZZ	Resection of Left Fibula, Open Approach
0QTL0ZZ	Resection of Right Tarsal, Open Approach
0QTM0ZZ	Resection of Left Tarsal, Open Approach
0QTN0ZZ	Resection of Right Metatarsal, Open Approach
0QTP0ZZ	Resection of Left Metatarsal, Open Approach
0QTQ0ZZ	Resection of Right Toe Phalanx, Open Approach
0QTR0ZZ	Resection of Left Toe Phalanx, Open Approach
0QTS0ZZ	Resection of Coccyx, Open Approach

0QU – Lower Bones, Supplement

0QU007Z	Supplement Lumbar Vertebra with Autologous Tissue Substitute, Open Approach
0QU00JZ	Supplement Lumbar Vertebra with Synthetic Substitute, Open Approach
0QU00KZ	Supplement Lumbar Vertebra with Nonautologous Tissue Substitute, Open Approach
0QU037Z	Supplement Lumbar Vertebra with Autologous Tissue Substitute, Percutaneous Approach
0QU03JZ	Supplement Lumbar Vertebra with Synthetic Substitute, Percutaneous Approach
0QU03KZ	Supplement Lumbar Vertebra with Nonautologous Tissue Substitute, Percutaneous Approach
0QU047Z	Supplement Lumbar Vertebra with Autologous Tissue Substitute, Percutaneous Endoscopic Approach
0QU04JZ	Supplement Lumbar Vertebra with Synthetic Substitute, Percutaneous Endoscopic Approach
0QU04KZ	Supplement Lumbar Vertebra with Nonautologous Tissue Substitute, Percutaneous Endoscopic Approach
0QU107Z	Supplement Sacrum with Autologous Tissue Substitute, Open Approach
0QU10JZ	Supplement Sacrum with Synthetic Substitute, Open Approach
0QU10KZ	Supplement Sacrum with Nonautologous Tissue Substitute, Open Approach
0QU137Z	Supplement Sacrum with Autologous Tissue Substitute, Percutaneous Approach
0QU13JZ	Supplement Sacrum with Synthetic Substitute, Percutaneous Approach
0QU13KZ	Supplement Sacrum with Nonautologous Tissue Substitute, Percutaneous Approach
0QU147Z	Supplement Sacrum with Autologous Tissue Substitute, Percutaneous Endoscopic Approach
0QU14JZ	Supplement Sacrum with Synthetic Substitute, Percutaneous Endoscopic Approach
0QU14KZ	Supplement Sacrum with Nonautologous Tissue Substitute, Percutaneous Endoscopic Approach
0QU207Z	Supplement Right Pelvic Bone with Autologous Tissue Substitute, Open Approach
0QU20JZ	Supplement Right Pelvic Bone with Synthetic Substitute, Open Approach
0QU20KZ	Supplement Right Pelvic Bone with Nonautologous Tissue Substitute, Open Approach
0QU237Z	Supplement Right Pelvic Bone with Autologous Tissue Substitute, Percutaneous Approach
0QU23JZ	Supplement Right Pelvic Bone with Synthetic Substitute, Percutaneous Approach
0QU23KZ	Supplement Right Pelvic Bone with Nonautologous Tissue Substitute, Percutaneous Approach
0QU247Z	Supplement Right Pelvic Bone with Autologous Tissue Substitute, Percutaneous Endoscopic Approach
0QU24JZ	Supplement Right Pelvic Bone with Synthetic Substitute, Percutaneous Endoscopic Approach
0QU24KZ	Supplement Right Pelvic Bone with Nonautologous Tissue Substitute, Percutaneous Endoscopic Approach
0QU307Z	Supplement Left Pelvic Bone with Autologous Tissue Substitute, Open Approach

0QU30JZ	Supplement Left Pelvic Bone with Synthetic Substitute, Open Approach
0QU30KZ	Supplement Left Pelvic Bone with Nonautologous Tissue Substitute, Open Approach
0QU337Z	Supplement Left Pelvic Bone with Autologous Tissue Substitute, Percutaneous Approach
0QU33JZ	Supplement Left Pelvic Bone with Synthetic Substitute, Percutaneous Approach
0QU33KZ	Supplement Left Pelvic Bone with Nonautologous Tissue Substitute, Percutaneous Approach
0QU347Z	Supplement Left Pelvic Bone with Autologous Tissue Substitute, Percutaneous Endoscopic Approach
0QU34JZ	Supplement Left Pelvic Bone with Synthetic Substitute, Percutaneous Endoscopic Approach
0QU34KZ	Supplement Left Pelvic Bone with Nonautologous Tissue Substitute, Percutaneous Endoscopic Approach
0QU407Z	Supplement Right Acetabulum with Autologous Tissue Substitute, Open Approach
0QU40JZ	Supplement Right Acetabulum with Synthetic Substitute, Open Approach
0QU40KZ	Supplement Right Acetabulum with Nonautologous Tissue Substitute, Open Approach
0QU437Z	Supplement Right Acetabulum with Autologous Tissue Substitute, Percutaneous Approach
0QU43JZ	Supplement Right Acetabulum with Synthetic Substitute, Percutaneous Approach
0QU43KZ	Supplement Right Acetabulum with Nonautologous Tissue Substitute, Percutaneous Approach
0QU447Z	Supplement Right Acetabulum with Autologous Tissue Substitute, Percutaneous Endoscopic Approach
0QU44JZ	Supplement Right Acetabulum with Synthetic Substitute, Percutaneous Endoscopic Approach
0QU44KZ	Supplement Right Acetabulum with Nonautologous Tissue Substitute, Percutaneous Endoscopic Approach
0QU507Z	Supplement Left Acetabulum with Autologous Tissue Substitute, Open Approach
0QU50JZ	Supplement Left Acetabulum with Synthetic Substitute, Open Approach
0QU50KZ	Supplement Left Acetabulum with Nonautologous Tissue Substitute, Open Approach
0QU537Z	Supplement Left Acetabulum with Autologous Tissue Substitute, Percutaneous Approach
0QU53JZ	Supplement Left Acetabulum with Synthetic Substitute, Percutaneous Approach
0QU53KZ	Supplement Left Acetabulum with Nonautologous Tissue Substitute, Percutaneous Approach
0QU547Z	Supplement Left Acetabulum with Autologous Tissue Substitute, Percutaneous Endoscopic Approach
0QU54JZ	Supplement Left Acetabulum with Synthetic Substitute, Percutaneous Endoscopic Approach
0QU54KZ	Supplement Left Acetabulum with Nonautologous Tissue Substitute, Percutaneous Endoscopic Approach
0QU607Z	Supplement Right Upper Femur with Autologous Tissue Substitute, Open Approach

0QU60JZ Supplement Right Upper Femur with Synthetic Substitute, Open Approach

0QU60KZ Supplement Right Upper Femur with Nonautologous Tissue Substitute, Open Approach

0QU637Z Supplement Right Upper Femur with Autologous Tissue Substitute, Percutaneous Approach

0QU63JZ Supplement Right Upper Femur with Synthetic Substitute, Percutaneous Approach

0QU63KZ Supplement Right Upper Femur with Nonautologous Tissue Substitute, Percutaneous Approach

0QU647Z Supplement Right Upper Femur with Autologous Tissue Substitute, Percutaneous Endoscopic Approach

0QU64JZ Supplement Right Upper Femur with Synthetic Substitute, Percutaneous Endoscopic Approach

0QU64KZ Supplement Right Upper Femur with Nonautologous Tissue Substitute, Percutaneous Endoscopic Approach

0QU707Z Supplement Left Upper Femur with Autologous Tissue Substitute, Open Approach

0QU70JZ Supplement Left Upper Femur with Synthetic Substitute, Open Approach

0QU70KZ Supplement Left Upper Femur with Nonautologous Tissue Substitute, Open Approach

0QU737Z Supplement Left Upper Femur with Autologous Tissue Substitute, Percutaneous Approach

0QU73JZ Supplement Left Upper Femur with Synthetic Substitute, Percutaneous Approach

0QU73KZ Supplement Left Upper Femur with Nonautologous Tissue Substitute, Percutaneous Approach

0QU747Z Supplement Left Upper Femur with Autologous Tissue Substitute, Percutaneous Endoscopic Approach

0QU74JZ Supplement Left Upper Femur with Synthetic Substitute, Percutaneous Endoscopic Approach

0QU74KZ Supplement Left Upper Femur with Nonautologous Tissue Substitute, Percutaneous Endoscopic Approach

0QU807Z Supplement Right Femoral Shaft with Autologous Tissue Substitute, Open Approach

0QU80JZ Supplement Right Femoral Shaft with Synthetic Substitute, Open Approach

0QU80KZ Supplement Right Femoral Shaft with Nonautologous Tissue Substitute, Open Approach

0QU837Z Supplement Right Femoral Shaft with Autologous Tissue Substitute, Percutaneous Approach

0QU83JZ Supplement Right Femoral Shaft with Synthetic Substitute, Percutaneous Approach

0QU83KZ Supplement Right Femoral Shaft with Nonautologous Tissue Substitute, Percutaneous Approach

0QU847Z Supplement Right Femoral Shaft with Autologous Tissue Substitute, Percutaneous Endoscopic Approach

0QU84JZ Supplement Right Femoral Shaft with Synthetic Substitute, Percutaneous Endoscopic Approach

0QU84KZ Supplement Right Femoral Shaft with Nonautologous Tissue Substitute, Percutaneous Endoscopic Approach

0QU907Z Supplement Left Femoral Shaft with Autologous Tissue Substitute, Open Approach

0QU90JZ Supplement Left Femoral Shaft with Synthetic Substitute, Open Approach

0QU90KZ Supplement Left Femoral Shaft with Nonautologous Tissue Substitute, Open Approach

0QU937Z Supplement Left Femoral Shaft with Autologous Tissue Substitute, Percutaneous Approach

0QU93JZ Supplement Left Femoral Shaft with Synthetic Substitute, Percutaneous Approach

0QU93KZ Supplement Left Femoral Shaft with Nonautologous Tissue Substitute, Percutaneous Approach

0QU947Z Supplement Left Femoral Shaft with Autologous Tissue Substitute, Percutaneous Endoscopic Approach

0QU94JZ Supplement Left Femoral Shaft with Synthetic Substitute, Percutaneous Endoscopic Approach

0QU94KZ Supplement Left Femoral Shaft with Nonautologous Tissue Substitute, Percutaneous Endoscopic Approach

0QUB07Z Supplement Right Lower Femur with Autologous Tissue Substitute, Open Approach

0QUB0JZ Supplement Right Lower Femur with Synthetic Substitute, Open Approach

0QUB0KZ Supplement Right Lower Femur with Nonautologous Tissue Substitute, Open Approach

0QUB37Z Supplement Right Lower Femur with Autologous Tissue Substitute, Percutaneous Approach

0QUB3JZ Supplement Right Lower Femur with Synthetic Substitute, Percutaneous Approach

0QUB3KZ Supplement Right Lower Femur with Nonautologous Tissue Substitute, Percutaneous Approach

0QUB47Z Supplement Right Lower Femur with Autologous Tissue Substitute, Percutaneous Endoscopic Approach

0QUB4JZ Supplement Right Lower Femur with Synthetic Substitute, Percutaneous Endoscopic Approach

0QUB4KZ Supplement Right Lower Femur with Nonautologous Tissue Substitute, Percutaneous Endoscopic Approach

0QUC07Z Supplement Left Lower Femur with Autologous Tissue Substitute, Open Approach

0QUC0JZ Supplement Left Lower Femur with Synthetic Substitute, Open Approach

0QUC0KZ Supplement Left Lower Femur with Nonautologous Tissue Substitute, Open Approach

0QUC37Z Supplement Left Lower Femur with Autologous Tissue Substitute, Percutaneous Approach

0QUC3JZ Supplement Left Lower Femur with Synthetic Substitute, Percutaneous Approach

0QUC3KZ Supplement Left Lower Femur with Nonautologous Tissue Substitute, Percutaneous Approach

0QUC47Z Supplement Left Lower Femur with Autologous Tissue Substitute, Percutaneous Endoscopic Approach

0QUC4JZ Supplement Left Lower Femur with Synthetic Substitute, Percutaneous Endoscopic Approach

0QUC4KZ Supplement Left Lower Femur with Nonautologous Tissue Substitute, Percutaneous Endoscopic Approach

0QUD07Z Supplement Right Patella with Autologous Tissue Substitute, Open Approach

0QUD0JZ Supplement Right Patella with Synthetic Substitute, Open Approach

0QUD0KZ Supplement Right Patella with Nonautologous Tissue Substitute, Open Approach

0QUD37Z Supplement Right Patella with Autologous Tissue Substitute, Percutaneous Approach

0QUD3JZ Supplement Right Patella with Synthetic Substitute, Percutaneous Approach

0QUD3KZ Supplement Right Patella with Nonautologous Tissue Substitute, Percutaneous Approach

0QUD47Z Supplement Right Patella with Autologous Tissue Substitute, Percutaneous Endoscopic Approach

0QUD4JZ Supplement Right Patella with Synthetic Substitute, Percutaneous Endoscopic Approach

0QUD4KZ Supplement Right Patella with Nonautologous Tissue Substitute, Percutaneous Endoscopic Approach

0QUF07Z Supplement Left Patella with Autologous Tissue Substitute, Open Approach

0QUF0JZ Supplement Left Patella with Synthetic Substitute, Open Approach

0QUF0KZ Supplement Left Patella with Nonautologous Tissue Substitute, Open Approach

0QUF37Z Supplement Left Patella with Autologous Tissue Substitute, Percutaneous Approach

0QUF3JZ Supplement Left Patella with Synthetic Substitute, Percutaneous Approach

0QUF3KZ Supplement Left Patella with Nonautologous Tissue Substitute, Percutaneous Approach

0QUF47Z Supplement Left Patella with Autologous Tissue Substitute, Percutaneous Endoscopic Approach

0QUF4JZ Supplement Left Patella with Synthetic Substitute, Percutaneous Endoscopic Approach

0QUF4KZ Supplement Left Patella with Nonautologous Tissue Substitute, Percutaneous Endoscopic Approach

0QUG07Z Supplement Right Tibia with Autologous Tissue Substitute, Open Approach

0QUG0JZ Supplement Right Tibia with Synthetic Substitute, Open Approach

0QUG0KZ Supplement Right Tibia with Nonautologous Tissue Substitute, Open Approach

0QUG37Z Supplement Right Tibia with Autologous Tissue Substitute, Percutaneous Approach

0QUG3JZ Supplement Right Tibia with Synthetic Substitute, Percutaneous Approach

0QUG3KZ Supplement Right Tibia with Nonautologous Tissue Substitute, Percutaneous Approach

0QUG47Z Supplement Right Tibia with Autologous Tissue Substitute, Percutaneous Endoscopic Approach

0QUG4JZ Supplement Right Tibia with Synthetic Substitute, Percutaneous Endoscopic Approach

0QUG4KZ Supplement Right Tibia with Nonautologous Tissue Substitute, Percutaneous Endoscopic Approach

0QUH07Z Supplement Left Tibia with Autologous Tissue Substitute, Open Approach

0QUH0JZ Supplement Left Tibia with Synthetic Substitute, Open Approach

0QUH0KZ Supplement Left Tibia with Nonautologous Tissue Substitute, Open Approach

0QUH37Z Supplement Left Tibia with Autologous Tissue Substitute, Percutaneous Approach

0QUH3JZ Supplement Left Tibia with Synthetic Substitute, Percutaneous Approach

0QUH3KZ Supplement Left Tibia with Nonautologous Tissue Substitute, Percutaneous Approach

0QUH47Z Supplement Left Tibia with Autologous Tissue Substitute, Percutaneous Endoscopic Approach

0QUH4JZ Supplement Left Tibia with Synthetic Substitute, Percutaneous Endoscopic Approach

0QUH4KZ Supplement Left Tibia with Nonautologous Tissue Substitute, Percutaneous Endoscopic Approach

0QUJ07Z Supplement Right Fibula with Autologous Tissue Substitute, Open Approach

0QUJ0JZ Supplement Right Fibula with Synthetic Substitute, Open Approach

0QUJ0KZ Supplement Right Fibula with Nonautologous Tissue Substitute, Open Approach

0QUJ37Z Supplement Right Fibula with Autologous Tissue Substitute, Percutaneous Approach

0QUJ3JZ Supplement Right Fibula with Synthetic Substitute, Percutaneous Approach

0QUJ3KZ Supplement Right Fibula with Nonautologous Tissue Substitute, Percutaneous Approach

0QUJ47Z Supplement Right Fibula with Autologous Tissue Substitute, Percutaneous Endoscopic Approach

0QUJ4JZ Supplement Right Fibula with Synthetic Substitute, Percutaneous Endoscopic Approach

0QUJ4KZ Supplement Right Fibula with Nonautologous Tissue Substitute, Percutaneous Endoscopic Approach

0QUK07Z Supplement Left Fibula with Autologous Tissue Substitute, Open Approach

0QUK0JZ Supplement Left Fibula with Synthetic Substitute, Open Approach

0QUK0KZ Supplement Left Fibula with Nonautologous Tissue Substitute, Open Approach

0QUK37Z Supplement Left Fibula with Autologous Tissue Substitute, Percutaneous Approach

0QUK3JZ Supplement Left Fibula with Synthetic Substitute, Percutaneous Approach

0QUK3KZ Supplement Left Fibula with Nonautologous Tissue Substitute, Percutaneous Approach

0QUK47Z Supplement Left Fibula with Autologous Tissue Substitute, Percutaneous Endoscopic Approach

0QUK4JZ Supplement Left Fibula with Synthetic Substitute, Percutaneous Endoscopic Approach

0QUK4KZ Supplement Left Fibula with Nonautologous Tissue Substitute, Percutaneous Endoscopic Approach

0QUL07Z Supplement Right Tarsal with Autologous Tissue Substitute, Open Approach

0QUL0JZ Supplement Right Tarsal with Synthetic Substitute, Open Approach

0QUL0KZ Supplement Right Tarsal with Nonautologous Tissue Substitute, Open Approach

0QUL37Z Supplement Right Tarsal with Autologous Tissue Substitute, Percutaneous Approach

0QUL3JZ Supplement Right Tarsal with Synthetic Substitute, Percutaneous Approach

0QUL3KZ Supplement Right Tarsal with Nonautologous Tissue Substitute, Percutaneous Approach

0QUL47Z Supplement Right Tarsal with Autologous Tissue Substitute, Percutaneous Endoscopic Approach

0QUL4JZ Supplement Right Tarsal with Synthetic Substitute, Percutaneous Endoscopic Approach

0QUL4KZ Supplement Right Tarsal with Nonautologous Tissue Substitute, Percutaneous Endoscopic Approach

0QUM07Z Supplement Left Tarsal with Autologous Tissue Substitute, Open Approach

0QUM0JZ Supplement Left Tarsal with Synthetic Substitute, Open Approach

0QUM0KZ Supplement Left Tarsal with Nonautologous Tissue Substitute, Open Approach

0QUM37Z Supplement Left Tarsal with Autologous Tissue Substitute, Percutaneous Approach

0QUM3JZ Supplement Left Tarsal with Synthetic Substitute, Percutaneous Approach

0QUM3KZ Supplement Left Tarsal with Nonautologous Tissue Substitute, Percutaneous Approach

0QUM47Z Supplement Left Tarsal with Autologous Tissue Substitute, Percutaneous Endoscopic Approach

0QUM4JZ Supplement Left Tarsal with Synthetic Substitute, Percutaneous Endoscopic Approach

0QUM4KZ Supplement Left Tarsal with Nonautologous Tissue Substitute, Percutaneous Endoscopic Approach

0QUN07Z Supplement Right Metatarsal with Autologous Tissue Substitute, Open Approach

0QUN0JZ Supplement Right Metatarsal with Synthetic Substitute, Open Approach

0QUN0KZ Supplement Right Metatarsal with Nonautologous Tissue Substitute, Open Approach

0QUN37Z Supplement Right Metatarsal with Autologous Tissue Substitute, Percutaneous Approach

0QUN3JZ Supplement Right Metatarsal with Synthetic Substitute, Percutaneous Approach

0QUN3KZ Supplement Right Metatarsal with Nonautologous Tissue Substitute, Percutaneous Approach

0QUN47Z Supplement Right Metatarsal with Autologous Tissue Substitute, Percutaneous Endoscopic Approach

0QUN4JZ Supplement Right Metatarsal with Synthetic Substitute, Percutaneous Endoscopic Approach

0QUN4KZ Supplement Right Metatarsal with Nonautologous Tissue Substitute, Percutaneous Endoscopic Approach

0QUP07Z Supplement Left Metatarsal with Autologous Tissue Substitute, Open Approach

0QUP0JZ Supplement Left Metatarsal with Synthetic Substitute, Open Approach

0QUP0KZ Supplement Left Metatarsal with Nonautologous Tissue Substitute, Open Approach

0QUP37Z Supplement Left Metatarsal with Autologous Tissue Substitute, Percutaneous Approach

0QUP3JZ Supplement Left Metatarsal with Synthetic Substitute, Percutaneous Approach

0QUP3KZ Supplement Left Metatarsal with Nonautologous Tissue Substitute, Percutaneous Approach

0QUP47Z Supplement Left Metatarsal with Autologous Tissue Substitute, Percutaneous Endoscopic Approach

0QUP4JZ Supplement Left Metatarsal with Synthetic Substitute, Percutaneous Endoscopic Approach

0QUP4KZ Supplement Left Metatarsal with Nonautologous Tissue Substitute, Percutaneous Endoscopic Approach

0QUQ07Z Supplement Right Toe Phalanx with Autologous Tissue Substitute, Open Approach

0QUQ0JZ Supplement Right Toe Phalanx with Synthetic Substitute, Open Approach

0QUQ0KZ Supplement Right Toe Phalanx with Nonautologous Tissue Substitute, Open Approach

0QUQ37Z Supplement Right Toe Phalanx with Autologous Tissue Substitute, Percutaneous Approach

0QUQ3JZ Supplement Right Toe Phalanx with Synthetic Substitute, Percutaneous Approach

0QUQ3KZ Supplement Right Toe Phalanx with Nonautologous Tissue Substitute, Percutaneous Approach

0QUQ47Z Supplement Right Toe Phalanx with Autologous Tissue Substitute, Percutaneous Endoscopic Approach

0QUQ4JZ Supplement Right Toe Phalanx with Synthetic Substitute, Percutaneous Endoscopic Approach

0QUQ4KZ Supplement Right Toe Phalanx with Nonautologous Tissue Substitute, Percutaneous Endoscopic Approach

0QUR07Z Supplement Left Toe Phalanx with Autologous Tissue Substitute, Open Approach

0QUR0JZ Supplement Left Toe Phalanx with Synthetic Substitute, Open Approach

0QUR0KZ Supplement Left Toe Phalanx with Nonautologous Tissue Substitute, Open Approach

0QUR37Z Supplement Left Toe Phalanx with Autologous Tissue Substitute, Percutaneous Approach

0QUR3JZ Supplement Left Toe Phalanx with Synthetic Substitute, Percutaneous Approach

0QUR3KZ Supplement Left Toe Phalanx with Nonautologous Tissue Substitute, Percutaneous Approach

0QUR47Z Supplement Left Toe Phalanx with Autologous Tissue Substitute, Percutaneous Endoscopic Approach

0QUR4JZ Supplement Left Toe Phalanx with Synthetic Substitute, Percutaneous Endoscopic Approach

0QUR4KZ Supplement Left Toe Phalanx with Nonautologous Tissue Substitute, Percutaneous Endoscopic Approach

0QUS07Z Supplement Coccyx with Autologous Tissue Substitute, Open Approach

0QUS0JZ Supplement Coccyx with Synthetic Substitute, Open Approach

0QUS0KZ Supplement Coccyx with Nonautologous Tissue Substitute, Open Approach

0QUS37Z Supplement Coccyx with Autologous Tissue Substitute, Percutaneous Approach

0QUS3JZ Supplement Coccyx with Synthetic Substitute, Percutaneous Approach

0QUS3KZ Supplement Coccyx with Nonautologous Tissue Substitute, Percutaneous Approach

0QUS47Z Supplement Coccyx with Autologous Tissue Substitute, Percutaneous Endoscopic Approach

0QUS4JZ Supplement Coccyx with Synthetic Substitute, Percutaneous Endoscopic Approach

0QUS4KZ Supplement Coccyx with Nonautologous Tissue Substitute, Percutaneous Endoscopic Approach

0QW – Lower Bones, Revision

Review Coding Guideline B6.1c

0QW004Z Revision of Internal Fixation Device in Lumbar Vertebra, Open Approach

0QW007Z Revision of Autologous Tissue Substitute in Lumbar Vertebra, Open Approach

0QW00JZ Revision of Synthetic Substitute in Lumbar Vertebra, Open Approach

0QW00KZ Revision of Nonautologous Tissue Substitute in Lumbar Vertebra, Open Approach

0QW034Z Revision of Internal Fixation Device in Lumbar Vertebra, Percutaneous Approach

0QW037Z Revision of Autologous Tissue Substitute in Lumbar Vertebra, Percutaneous Approach

0QW03JZ Revision of Synthetic Substitute in Lumbar Vertebra, Percutaneous Approach

0QW03KZ Revision of Nonautologous Tissue Substitute in Lumbar Vertebra, Percutaneous Approach

0QW044Z Revision of Internal Fixation Device in Lumbar Vertebra, Percutaneous Endoscopic Approach

0QW047Z Revision of Autologous Tissue Substitute in Lumbar Vertebra, Percutaneous Endoscopic Approach

0QW04JZ Revision of Synthetic Substitute in Lumbar Vertebra, Percutaneous Endoscopic Approach

0QW04KZ Revision of Nonautologous Tissue Substitute in Lumbar Vertebra, Percutaneous Endoscopic Approach

0QW0X4Z Revision of Internal Fixation Device in Lumbar Vertebra, External Approach

0QW0X7Z Revision of Autologous Tissue Substitute in Lumbar Vertebra, External Approach

0QW0XJZ Revision of Synthetic Substitute in Lumbar Vertebra, External Approach

0QW0XKZ Revision of Nonautologous Tissue Substitute in Lumbar Vertebra, External Approach

0QW104Z Revision of Internal Fixation Device in Sacrum, Open Approach

0QW107Z Revision of Autologous Tissue Substitute in Sacrum, Open Approach

0QW10JZ Revision of Synthetic Substitute in Sacrum, Open Approach

0QW10KZ Revision of Nonautologous Tissue Substitute in Sacrum, Open Approach

0QW134Z Revision of Internal Fixation Device in Sacrum, Percutaneous Approach

0QW137Z Revision of Autologous Tissue Substitute in Sacrum, Percutaneous Approach

0QW13JZ Revision of Synthetic Substitute in Sacrum, Percutaneous Approach

0QW13KZ Revision of Nonautologous Tissue Substitute in Sacrum, Percutaneous Approach

0QW144Z Revision of Internal Fixation Device in Sacrum, Percutaneous Endoscopic Approach

0QW147Z Revision of Autologous Tissue Substitute in Sacrum, Percutaneous Endoscopic Approach

0QW14JZ Revision of Synthetic Substitute in Sacrum, Percutaneous Endoscopic Approach

0QW14KZ Revision of Nonautologous Tissue Substitute in Sacrum, Percutaneous Endoscopic Approach

0QW1X4Z Revision of Internal Fixation Device in Sacrum, External Approach

0QW1X7Z Revision of Autologous Tissue Substitute in Sacrum, External Approach

0QW1XJZ Revision of Synthetic Substitute in Sacrum, External Approach

0QW1XKZ Revision of Nonautologous Tissue Substitute in Sacrum, External Approach

0QW204Z Revision of Internal Fixation Device in Right Pelvic Bone, Open Approach

0QW205Z Revision of External Fixation Device in Right Pelvic Bone, Open Approach

0QW207Z Revision of Autologous Tissue Substitute in Right Pelvic Bone, Open Approach

0QW20JZ Revision of Synthetic Substitute in Right Pelvic Bone, Open Approach

0QW20KZ Revision of Nonautologous Tissue Substitute in Right Pelvic Bone, Open Approach

0QW234Z Revision of Internal Fixation Device in Right Pelvic Bone, Percutaneous Approach

0QW235Z Revision of External Fixation Device in Right Pelvic Bone, Percutaneous Approach

0QW237Z Revision of Autologous Tissue Substitute in Right Pelvic Bone, Percutaneous Approach

0QW23JZ Revision of Synthetic Substitute in Right Pelvic Bone, Percutaneous Approach

0QW23KZ Revision of Nonautologous Tissue Substitute in Right Pelvic Bone, Percutaneous Approach

0QW244Z Revision of Internal Fixation Device in Right Pelvic Bone, Percutaneous Endoscopic Approach

0QW245Z Revision of External Fixation Device in Right Pelvic Bone, Percutaneous Endoscopic Approach

0QW247Z Revision of Autologous Tissue Substitute in Right Pelvic Bone, Percutaneous Endoscopic Approach

0QW24JZ Revision of Synthetic Substitute in Right Pelvic Bone, Percutaneous Endoscopic Approach

0QW24KZ Revision of Nonautologous Tissue Substitute in Right Pelvic Bone, Percutaneous Endoscopic Approach

0QW2X4Z Revision of Internal Fixation Device in Right Pelvic Bone, External Approach

0QW2X5Z Revision of External Fixation Device in Right Pelvic Bone, External Approach

0QW2X7Z Revision of Autologous Tissue Substitute in Right Pelvic Bone, External Approach

0QW2XJZ Revision of Synthetic Substitute in Right Pelvic Bone, External Approach

0QW2XKZ Revision of Nonautologous Tissue Substitute in Right Pelvic Bone, External Approach

0QW304Z Revision of Internal Fixation Device in Left Pelvic Bone, Open Approach

0QW305Z Revision of External Fixation Device in Left Pelvic Bone, Open Approach

0QW307Z Revision of Autologous Tissue Substitute in Left Pelvic Bone, Open Approach

0QW30JZ Revision of Synthetic Substitute in Left Pelvic Bone, Open Approach

0QW30KZ Revision of Nonautologous Tissue Substitute in Left Pelvic Bone, Open Approach

0QW334Z Revision of Internal Fixation Device in Left Pelvic Bone, Percutaneous Approach

0QW335Z Revision of External Fixation Device in Left Pelvic Bone, Percutaneous Approach

0QW337Z Revision of Autologous Tissue Substitute in Left Pelvic Bone, Percutaneous Approach

0QW33JZ Revision of Synthetic Substitute in Left Pelvic Bone, Percutaneous Approach

0QW33KZ Revision of Nonautologous Tissue Substitute in Left Pelvic Bone, Percutaneous Approach

0QW344Z Revision of Internal Fixation Device in Left Pelvic Bone, Percutaneous Endoscopic Approach

0QW345Z Revision of External Fixation Device in Left Pelvic Bone, Percutaneous Endoscopic Approach

0QW347Z Revision of Autologous Tissue Substitute in Left Pelvic Bone, Percutaneous Endoscopic Approach

0QW34JZ Revision of Synthetic Substitute in Left Pelvic Bone, Percutaneous Endoscopic Approach

0QW34KZ Revision of Nonautologous Tissue Substitute in Left Pelvic Bone, Percutaneous Endoscopic Approach

0QW3X4Z Revision of Internal Fixation Device in Left Pelvic Bone, External Approach

0QW3X5Z Revision of External Fixation Device in Left Pelvic Bone, External Approach

0QW3X7Z Revision of Autologous Tissue Substitute in Left Pelvic Bone, External Approach

0QW3XJZ Revision of Synthetic Substitute in Left Pelvic Bone, External Approach

0QW3XKZ Revision of Nonautologous Tissue Substitute in Left Pelvic Bone, External Approach

0QW404Z Revision of Internal Fixation Device in Right Acetabulum, Open Approach

0QW407Z Revision of Autologous Tissue Substitute in Right Acetabulum, Open Approach

0QW40JZ Revision of Synthetic Substitute in Right Acetabulum, Open Approach

0QW40KZ Revision of Nonautologous Tissue Substitute in Right Acetabulum, Open Approach

0QW434Z Revision of Internal Fixation Device in Right Acetabulum, Percutaneous Approach

0QW437Z Revision of Autologous Tissue Substitute in Right Acetabulum, Percutaneous Approach

0QW43JZ Revision of Synthetic Substitute in Right Acetabulum, Percutaneous Approach

0QW43KZ Revision of Nonautologous Tissue Substitute in Right Acetabulum, Percutaneous Approach

0QW444Z Revision of Internal Fixation Device in Right Acetabulum, Percutaneous Endoscopic Approach

0QW447Z Revision of Autologous Tissue Substitute in Right Acetabulum, Percutaneous Endoscopic Approach

0QW44JZ Revision of Synthetic Substitute in Right Acetabulum, Percutaneous Endoscopic Approach

0QW44KZ Revision of Nonautologous Tissue Substitute in Right Acetabulum, Percutaneous Endoscopic Approach

0QW4X4Z Revision of Internal Fixation Device in Right Acetabulum, External Approach

0QW4X7Z Revision of Autologous Tissue Substitute in Right Acetabulum, External Approach

0QW4XJZ Revision of Synthetic Substitute in Right Acetabulum, External Approach

0QW4XKZ Revision of Nonautologous Tissue Substitute in Right Acetabulum, External Approach

0QW504Z Revision of Internal Fixation Device in Left Acetabulum, Open Approach

0QW507Z Revision of Autologous Tissue Substitute in Left Acetabulum, Open Approach

0QW50JZ Revision of Synthetic Substitute in Left Acetabulum, Open Approach

0QW50KZ Revision of Nonautologous Tissue Substitute in Left Acetabulum, Open Approach

0QW534Z Revision of Internal Fixation Device in Left Acetabulum, Percutaneous Approach

0QW537Z Revision of Autologous Tissue Substitute in Left Acetabulum, Percutaneous Approach

0QW53JZ Revision of Synthetic Substitute in Left Acetabulum, Percutaneous Approach

0QW53KZ Revision of Nonautologous Tissue Substitute in Left Acetabulum, Percutaneous Approach

0QW544Z Revision of Internal Fixation Device in Left Acetabulum, Percutaneous Endoscopic Approach

0QW547Z Revision of Autologous Tissue Substitute in Left Acetabulum, Percutaneous Endoscopic Approach

0QW54JZ Revision of Synthetic Substitute in Left Acetabulum, Percutaneous Endoscopic Approach

0QW54KZ Revision of Nonautologous Tissue Substitute in Left Acetabulum, Percutaneous Endoscopic Approach

0QW5X4Z Revision of Internal Fixation Device in Left Acetabulum, External Approach

0QW5X7Z Revision of Autologous Tissue Substitute in Left Acetabulum, External Approach

0QW5XJZ Revision of Synthetic Substitute in Left Acetabulum, External Approach

0QW5XKZ Revision of Nonautologous Tissue Substitute in Left Acetabulum, External Approach

0QW604Z Revision of Internal Fixation Device in Right Upper Femur, Open Approach

0QW605Z Revision of External Fixation Device in Right Upper Femur, Open Approach

0QW607Z Revision of Autologous Tissue Substitute in Right Upper Femur, Open Approach

0QW60JZ Revision of Synthetic Substitute in Right Upper Femur, Open Approach

0QW60KZ Revision of Nonautologous Tissue Substitute in Right Upper Femur, Open Approach

0QW634Z Revision of Internal Fixation Device in Right Upper Femur, Percutaneous Approach

0QW635Z Revision of External Fixation Device in Right Upper Femur, Percutaneous Approach

0QW637Z Revision of Autologous Tissue Substitute in Right Upper Femur, Percutaneous Approach

0QW63JZ Revision of Synthetic Substitute in Right Upper Femur, Percutaneous Approach

0QW63KZ Revision of Nonautologous Tissue Substitute in Right Upper Femur, Percutaneous Approach

0QW644Z Revision of Internal Fixation Device in Right Upper Femur, Percutaneous Endoscopic Approach

0QW645Z Revision of External Fixation Device in Right Upper Femur, Percutaneous Endoscopic Approach

0QW647Z Revision of Autologous Tissue Substitute in Right Upper Femur, Percutaneous Endoscopic Approach

0QW64JZ Revision of Synthetic Substitute in Right Upper Femur, Percutaneous Endoscopic Approach

0QW64KZ Revision of Nonautologous Tissue Substitute in Right Upper Femur, Percutaneous Endoscopic Approach

0QW6X4Z Revision of Internal Fixation Device in Right Upper Femur, External Approach

0QW6X5Z Revision of External Fixation Device in Right Upper Femur, External Approach

0QW6X7Z Revision of Autologous Tissue Substitute in Right Upper Femur, External Approach

0QW6XJZ Revision of Synthetic Substitute in Right Upper Femur, External Approach

0QW6XKZ Revision of Nonautologous Tissue Substitute in Right Upper Femur, External Approach

0QW704Z Revision of Internal Fixation Device in Left Upper Femur, Open Approach

0QW705Z Revision of External Fixation Device in Left Upper Femur, Open Approach

0QW707Z Revision of Autologous Tissue Substitute in Left Upper Femur, Open Approach

0QW70JZ Revision of Synthetic Substitute in Left Upper Femur, Open Approach

0QW70KZ Revision of Nonautologous Tissue Substitute in Left Upper Femur, Open Approach

0QW734Z Revision of Internal Fixation Device in Left Upper Femur, Percutaneous Approach

0QW735Z Revision of External Fixation Device in Left Upper Femur, Percutaneous Approach

0QW737Z Revision of Autologous Tissue Substitute in Left Upper Femur, Percutaneous Approach

0QW73JZ Revision of Synthetic Substitute in Left Upper Femur, Percutaneous Approach

0QW73KZ Revision of Nonautologous Tissue Substitute in Left Upper Femur, Percutaneous Approach

0QW744Z Revision of Internal Fixation Device in Left Upper Femur, Percutaneous Endoscopic Approach

0QW745Z Revision of External Fixation Device in Left Upper Femur, Percutaneous Endoscopic Approach

0QW747Z Revision of Autologous Tissue Substitute in Left Upper Femur, Percutaneous Endoscopic Approach

0QW74JZ Revision of Synthetic Substitute in Left Upper Femur, Percutaneous Endoscopic Approach

0QW74KZ Revision of Nonautologous Tissue Substitute in Left Upper Femur, Percutaneous Endoscopic Approach

0QW7X4Z Revision of Internal Fixation Device in Left Upper Femur, External Approach

0QW7X5Z Revision of External Fixation Device in Left Upper Femur, External Approach

0QW7X7Z Revision of Autologous Tissue Substitute in Left Upper Femur, External Approach

0QW7XJZ Revision of Synthetic Substitute in Left Upper Femur, External Approach

0QW7XKZ Revision of Nonautologous Tissue Substitute in Left Upper Femur, External Approach

0QW804Z Revision of Internal Fixation Device in Right Femoral Shaft, Open Approach

0QW805Z Revision of External Fixation Device in Right Femoral Shaft, Open Approach

0QW807Z Revision of Autologous Tissue Substitute in Right Femoral Shaft, Open Approach

0QW80JZ Revision of Synthetic Substitute in Right Femoral Shaft, Open Approach

0QW80KZ Revision of Nonautologous Tissue Substitute in Right Femoral Shaft, Open Approach

0QW834Z Revision of Internal Fixation Device in Right Femoral Shaft, Percutaneous Approach

0QW835Z Revision of External Fixation Device in Right Femoral Shaft, Percutaneous Approach

0QW837Z Revision of Autologous Tissue Substitute in Right Femoral Shaft, Percutaneous Approach

0QW83JZ Revision of Synthetic Substitute in Right Femoral Shaft, Percutaneous Approach

0QW83KZ Revision of Nonautologous Tissue Substitute in Right Femoral Shaft, Percutaneous Approach

0QW844Z Revision of Internal Fixation Device in Right Femoral Shaft, Percutaneous Endoscopic Approach

0QW845Z Revision of External Fixation Device in Right Femoral Shaft, Percutaneous Endoscopic Approach

0QW847Z Revision of Autologous Tissue Substitute in Right Femoral Shaft, Percutaneous Endoscopic Approach

0QW84JZ Revision of Synthetic Substitute in Right Femoral Shaft, Percutaneous Endoscopic Approach

0QW84KZ Revision of Nonautologous Tissue Substitute in Right Femoral Shaft, Percutaneous Endoscopic Approach

0QW8X4Z Revision of Internal Fixation Device in Right Femoral Shaft, External Approach

0QW8X5Z Revision of External Fixation Device in Right Femoral Shaft, External Approach

0QW8X7Z Revision of Autologous Tissue Substitute in Right Femoral Shaft, External Approach

0QW8XJZ Revision of Synthetic Substitute in Right Femoral Shaft, External Approach

0QW8XKZ Revision of Nonautologous Tissue Substitute in Right Femoral Shaft, External Approach

0QW904Z Revision of Internal Fixation Device in Left Femoral Shaft, Open Approach

0QW905Z Revision of External Fixation Device in Left Femoral Shaft, Open Approach

0QW907Z Revision of Autologous Tissue Substitute in Left Femoral Shaft, Open Approach

0QW90JZ Revision of Synthetic Substitute in Left Femoral Shaft, Open Approach

0QW90KZ Revision of Nonautologous Tissue Substitute in Left Femoral Shaft, Open Approach

0QW934Z Revision of Internal Fixation Device in Left Femoral Shaft, Percutaneous Approach

0QW935Z Revision of External Fixation Device in Left Femoral Shaft, Percutaneous Approach

0QW937Z Revision of Autologous Tissue Substitute in Left Femoral Shaft, Percutaneous Approach

0QW93JZ Revision of Synthetic Substitute in Left Femoral Shaft, Percutaneous Approach

0QW93KZ Revision of Nonautologous Tissue Substitute in Left Femoral Shaft, Percutaneous Approach

0QW944Z Revision of Internal Fixation Device in Left Femoral Shaft, Percutaneous Endoscopic Approach

0QW945Z Revision of External Fixation Device in Left Femoral Shaft, Percutaneous Endoscopic Approach

0QW947Z Revision of Autologous Tissue Substitute in Left Femoral Shaft, Percutaneous Endoscopic Approach

0QW94JZ Revision of Synthetic Substitute in Left Femoral Shaft, Percutaneous Endoscopic Approach

0QW94KZ Revision of Nonautologous Tissue Substitute in Left Femoral Shaft, Percutaneous Endoscopic Approach

0QW9X4Z Revision of Internal Fixation Device in Left Femoral Shaft, External Approach

0QW9X5Z Revision of External Fixation Device in Left Femoral Shaft, External Approach

0QW9X7Z Revision of Autologous Tissue Substitute in Left Femoral Shaft, External Approach

0QW9XJZ Revision of Synthetic Substitute in Left Femoral Shaft, External Approach

0QW9XKZ Revision of Nonautologous Tissue Substitute in Left Femoral Shaft, External Approach

0QWB04Z Revision of Internal Fixation Device in Right Lower Femur, Open Approach

0QWB05Z Revision of External Fixation Device in Right Lower Femur, Open Approach

0QWB07Z Revision of Autologous Tissue Substitute in Right Lower Femur, Open Approach

0QWB0JZ Revision of Synthetic Substitute in Right Lower Femur, Open Approach

0QWB0KZ Revision of Nonautologous Tissue Substitute in Right Lower Femur, Open Approach

0QWB34Z Revision of Internal Fixation Device in Right Lower Femur, Percutaneous Approach

0QWB35Z Revision of External Fixation Device in Right Lower Femur, Percutaneous Approach

0QWB37Z Revision of Autologous Tissue Substitute in Right Lower Femur, Percutaneous Approach

0QWB3JZ Revision of Synthetic Substitute in Right Lower Femur, Percutaneous Approach

0QWB3KZ   Revision of Nonautologous Tissue Substitute in Right Lower Femur, Percutaneous Approach

0QWB44Z   Revision of Internal Fixation Device in Right Lower Femur, Percutaneous Endoscopic Approach

0QWB45Z   Revision of External Fixation Device in Right Lower Femur, Percutaneous Endoscopic Approach

0QWB47Z   Revision of Autologous Tissue Substitute in Right Lower Femur, Percutaneous Endoscopic Approach

0QWB4JZ   Revision of Synthetic Substitute in Right Lower Femur, Percutaneous Endoscopic Approach

0QWB4KZ   Revision of Nonautologous Tissue Substitute in Right Lower Femur, Percutaneous Endoscopic Approach

0QWBX4Z   Revision of Internal Fixation Device in Right Lower Femur, External Approach

0QWBX5Z   Revision of External Fixation Device in Right Lower Femur, External Approach

0QWBX7Z   Revision of Autologous Tissue Substitute in Right Lower Femur, External Approach

0QWBXJZ   Revision of Synthetic Substitute in Right Lower Femur, External Approach

0QWBXKZ   Revision of Nonautologous Tissue Substitute in Right Lower Femur, External Approach

0QWC04Z   Revision of Internal Fixation Device in Left Lower Femur, Open Approach

0QWC05Z   Revision of External Fixation Device in Left Lower Femur, Open Approach

0QWC07Z   Revision of Autologous Tissue Substitute in Left Lower Femur, Open Approach

0QWC0JZ   Revision of Synthetic Substitute in Left Lower Femur, Open Approach

0QWC0KZ   Revision of Nonautologous Tissue Substitute in Left Lower Femur, Open Approach

0QWC34Z   Revision of Internal Fixation Device in Left Lower Femur, Percutaneous Approach

0QWC35Z   Revision of External Fixation Device in Left Lower Femur, Percutaneous Approach

0QWC37Z   Revision of Autologous Tissue Substitute in Left Lower Femur, Percutaneous Approach

0QWC3JZ   Revision of Synthetic Substitute in Left Lower Femur, Percutaneous Approach

0QWC3KZ   Revision of Nonautologous Tissue Substitute in Left Lower Femur, Percutaneous Approach

0QWC44Z   Revision of Internal Fixation Device in Left Lower Femur, Percutaneous Endoscopic Approach

0QWC45Z   Revision of External Fixation Device in Left Lower Femur, Percutaneous Endoscopic Approach

0QWC47Z   Revision of Autologous Tissue Substitute in Left Lower Femur, Percutaneous Endoscopic Approach

0QWC4JZ   Revision of Synthetic Substitute in Left Lower Femur, Percutaneous Endoscopic Approach

0QWC4KZ   Revision of Nonautologous Tissue Substitute in Left Lower Femur, Percutaneous Endoscopic Approach

0QWCX4Z   Revision of Internal Fixation Device in Left Lower Femur, External Approach

0QWCX5Z   Revision of External Fixation Device in Left Lower Femur, External Approach

0QWCX7Z   Revision of Autologous Tissue Substitute in Left Lower Femur, External Approach

0QWCXJZ   Revision of Synthetic Substitute in Left Lower Femur, External Approach

0QWCXKZ   Revision of Nonautologous Tissue Substitute in Left Lower Femur, External Approach

0QWD04Z   Revision of Internal Fixation Device in Right Patella, Open Approach

0QWD05Z   Revision of External Fixation Device in Right Patella, Open Approach

0QWD07Z   Revision of Autologous Tissue Substitute in Right Patella, Open Approach

0QWD0JZ   Revision of Synthetic Substitute in Right Patella, Open Approach

0QWD0KZ   Revision of Nonautologous Tissue Substitute in Right Patella, Open Approach

0QWD34Z   Revision of Internal Fixation Device in Right Patella, Percutaneous Approach

0QWD35Z   Revision of External Fixation Device in Right Patella, Percutaneous Approach

0QWD37Z   Revision of Autologous Tissue Substitute in Right Patella, Percutaneous Approach

0QWD3JZ   Revision of Synthetic Substitute in Right Patella, Percutaneous Approach

0QWD3KZ   Revision of Nonautologous Tissue Substitute in Right Patella, Percutaneous Approach

0QWD44Z   Revision of Internal Fixation Device in Right Patella, Percutaneous Endoscopic Approach

0QWD45Z   Revision of External Fixation Device in Right Patella, Percutaneous Endoscopic Approach

0QWD47Z   Revision of Autologous Tissue Substitute in Right Patella, Percutaneous Endoscopic Approach

0QWD4JZ   Revision of Synthetic Substitute in Right Patella, Percutaneous Endoscopic Approach

0QWD4KZ   Revision of Nonautologous Tissue Substitute in Right Patella, Percutaneous Endoscopic Approach

0QWDX4Z   Revision of Internal Fixation Device in Right Patella, External Approach

0QWDX5Z   Revision of External Fixation Device in Right Patella, External Approach

0QWDX7Z   Revision of Autologous Tissue Substitute in Right Patella, External Approach

0QWDXJZ   Revision of Synthetic Substitute in Right Patella, External Approach

0QWDXKZ   Revision of Nonautologous Tissue Substitute in Right Patella, External Approach

0QWF04Z   Revision of Internal Fixation Device in Left Patella, Open Approach

0QWF05Z   Revision of External Fixation Device in Left Patella, Open Approach

0QWF07Z   Revision of Autologous Tissue Substitute in Left Patella, Open Approach

0QWF0JZ   Revision of Synthetic Substitute in Left Patella, Open Approach

0QWF0KZ   Revision of Nonautologous Tissue Substitute in Left Patella, Open Approach

0QWF34Z   Revision of Internal Fixation Device in Left Patella, Percutaneous Approach

0QWF35Z   Revision of External Fixation Device in Left Patella, Percutaneous Approach

0QWF37Z   Revision of Autologous Tissue Substitute in Left Patella, Percutaneous Approach

0QWF3JZ   Revision of Synthetic Substitute in Left Patella, Percutaneous Approach

0QWF3KZ   Revision of Nonautologous Tissue Substitute in Left Patella, Percutaneous Approach

0QWF44Z   Revision of Internal Fixation Device in Left Patella, Percutaneous Endoscopic Approach

0QWF45Z   Revision of External Fixation Device in Left Patella, Percutaneous Endoscopic Approach

0QWF47Z   Revision of Autologous Tissue Substitute in Left Patella, Percutaneous Endoscopic Approach

0QWF4JZ   Revision of Synthetic Substitute in Left Patella, Percutaneous Endoscopic Approach

0QWF4KZ   Revision of Nonautologous Tissue Substitute in Left Patella, Percutaneous Endoscopic Approach

0QWFX4Z   Revision of Internal Fixation Device in Left Patella, External Approach

0QWFX5Z   Revision of External Fixation Device in Left Patella, External Approach

0QWFX7Z   Revision of Autologous Tissue Substitute in Left Patella, External Approach

0QWFXJZ   Revision of Synthetic Substitute in Left Patella, External Approach

0QWFXKZ   Revision of Nonautologous Tissue Substitute in Left Patella, External Approach

0QWG04Z   Revision of Internal Fixation Device in Right Tibia, Open Approach

0QWG05Z   Revision of External Fixation Device in Right Tibia, Open Approach

0QWG07Z   Revision of Autologous Tissue Substitute in Right Tibia, Open Approach

0QWG0JZ   Revision of Synthetic Substitute in Right Tibia, Open Approach

0QWG0KZ Revision of Nonautologous Tissue Substitute in Right Tibia, Open Approach

0QWG34Z Revision of Internal Fixation Device in Right Tibia, Percutaneous Approach

0QWG35Z Revision of External Fixation Device in Right Tibia, Percutaneous Approach

0QWG37Z Revision of Autologous Tissue Substitute in Right Tibia, Percutaneous Approach

0QWG3JZ Revision of Synthetic Substitute in Right Tibia, Percutaneous Approach

0QWG3KZ Revision of Nonautologous Tissue Substitute in Right Tibia, Percutaneous Approach

0QWG44Z Revision of Internal Fixation Device in Right Tibia, Percutaneous Endoscopic Approach

0QWG45Z Revision of External Fixation Device in Right Tibia, Percutaneous Endoscopic Approach

0QWG47Z Revision of Autologous Tissue Substitute in Right Tibia, Percutaneous Endoscopic Approach

0QWG4JZ Revision of Synthetic Substitute in Right Tibia, Percutaneous Endoscopic Approach

0QWG4KZ Revision of Nonautologous Tissue Substitute in Right Tibia, Percutaneous Endoscopic Approach

0QWGX4Z Revision of Internal Fixation Device in Right Tibia, External Approach

0QWGX5Z Revision of External Fixation Device in Right Tibia, External Approach

0QWGX7Z Revision of Autologous Tissue Substitute in Right Tibia, External Approach

0QWGXJZ Revision of Synthetic Substitute in Right Tibia, External Approach

0QWGXKZ Revision of Nonautologous Tissue Substitute in Right Tibia, External Approach

0QWH04Z Revision of Internal Fixation Device in Left Tibia, Open Approach

0QWH05Z Revision of External Fixation Device in Left Tibia, Open Approach

0QWH07Z Revision of Autologous Tissue Substitute in Left Tibia, Open Approach

0QWH0JZ Revision of Synthetic Substitute in Left Tibia, Open Approach

0QWH0KZ Revision of Nonautologous Tissue Substitute in Left Tibia, Open Approach

0QWH34Z Revision of Internal Fixation Device in Left Tibia, Percutaneous Approach

0QWH35Z Revision of External Fixation Device in Left Tibia, Percutaneous Approach

0QWH37Z Revision of Autologous Tissue Substitute in Left Tibia, Percutaneous Approach

0QWH3JZ Revision of Synthetic Substitute in Left Tibia, Percutaneous Approach

0QWH3KZ Revision of Nonautologous Tissue Substitute in Left Tibia, Percutaneous Approach

0QWH44Z Revision of Internal Fixation Device in Left Tibia, Percutaneous Endoscopic Approach

0QWH45Z Revision of External Fixation Device in Left Tibia, Percutaneous Endoscopic Approach

0QWH47Z Revision of Autologous Tissue Substitute in Left Tibia, Percutaneous Endoscopic Approach

0QWH4JZ Revision of Synthetic Substitute in Left Tibia, Percutaneous Endoscopic Approach

0QWH4KZ Revision of Nonautologous Tissue Substitute in Left Tibia, Percutaneous Endoscopic Approach

0QWHX4Z Revision of Internal Fixation Device in Left Tibia, External Approach

0QWHX5Z Revision of External Fixation Device in Left Tibia, External Approach

0QWHX7Z Revision of Autologous Tissue Substitute in Left Tibia, External Approach

0QWHXJZ Revision of Synthetic Substitute in Left Tibia, External Approach

0QWHXKZ Revision of Nonautologous Tissue Substitute in Left Tibia, External Approach

0QWJ04Z Revision of Internal Fixation Device in Right Fibula, Open Approach

0QWJ05Z Revision of External Fixation Device in Right Fibula, Open Approach

0QWJ07Z Revision of Autologous Tissue Substitute in Right Fibula, Open Approach

0QWJ0JZ Revision of Synthetic Substitute in Right Fibula, Open Approach

0QWJ0KZ Revision of Nonautologous Tissue Substitute in Right Fibula, Open Approach

0QWJ34Z Revision of Internal Fixation Device in Right Fibula, Percutaneous Approach

0QWJ35Z Revision of External Fixation Device in Right Fibula, Percutaneous Approach

0QWJ37Z Revision of Autologous Tissue Substitute in Right Fibula, Percutaneous Approach

0QWJ3JZ Revision of Synthetic Substitute in Right Fibula, Percutaneous Approach

0QWJ3KZ Revision of Nonautologous Tissue Substitute in Right Fibula, Percutaneous Approach

0QWJ44Z Revision of Internal Fixation Device in Right Fibula, Percutaneous Endoscopic Approach

0QWJ45Z Revision of External Fixation Device in Right Fibula, Percutaneous Endoscopic Approach

0QWJ47Z Revision of Autologous Tissue Substitute in Right Fibula, Percutaneous Endoscopic Approach

0QWJ4JZ Revision of Synthetic Substitute in Right Fibula, Percutaneous Endoscopic Approach

0QWJ4KZ Revision of Nonautologous Tissue Substitute in Right Fibula, Percutaneous Endoscopic Approach

0QWJX4Z Revision of Internal Fixation Device in Right Fibula, External Approach

0QWJX5Z Revision of External Fixation Device in Right Fibula, External Approach

0QWJX7Z Revision of Autologous Tissue Substitute in Right Fibula, External Approach

0QWJXJZ Revision of Synthetic Substitute in Right Fibula, External Approach

0QWJXKZ Revision of Nonautologous Tissue Substitute in Right Fibula, External Approach

0QWK04Z Revision of Internal Fixation Device in Left Fibula, Open Approach

0QWK05Z Revision of External Fixation Device in Left Fibula, Open Approach

0QWK07Z Revision of Autologous Tissue Substitute in Left Fibula, Open Approach

0QWK0JZ Revision of Synthetic Substitute in Left Fibula, Open Approach

0QWK0KZ Revision of Nonautologous Tissue Substitute in Left Fibula, Open Approach

0QWK34Z Revision of Internal Fixation Device in Left Fibula, Percutaneous Approach

0QWK35Z Revision of External Fixation Device in Left Fibula, Percutaneous Approach

0QWK37Z Revision of Autologous Tissue Substitute in Left Fibula, Percutaneous Approach

0QWK3JZ Revision of Synthetic Substitute in Left Fibula, Percutaneous Approach

0QWK3KZ Revision of Nonautologous Tissue Substitute in Left Fibula, Percutaneous Approach

0QWK44Z Revision of Internal Fixation Device in Left Fibula, Percutaneous Endoscopic Approach

0QWK45Z Revision of External Fixation Device in Left Fibula, Percutaneous Endoscopic Approach

0QWK47Z Revision of Autologous Tissue Substitute in Left Fibula, Percutaneous Endoscopic Approach

0QWK4JZ Revision of Synthetic Substitute in Left Fibula, Percutaneous Endoscopic Approach

0QWK4KZ Revision of Nonautologous Tissue Substitute in Left Fibula, Percutaneous Endoscopic Approach

0QWKX4Z Revision of Internal Fixation Device in Left Fibula, External Approach

0QWKX5Z Revision of External Fixation Device in Left Fibula, External Approach

0QWKX7Z Revision of Autologous Tissue Substitute in Left Fibula, External Approach

0QWKXJZ Revision of Synthetic Substitute in Left Fibula, External Approach

0QWKXKZ Revision of Nonautologous Tissue Substitute in Left Fibula, External Approach

---

♀ Female-only   ♂ Male-only   ● Limited Coverage   ● Non-OR   HAC HAC-associated procedure   ⬢ Non-covered procedures   + Combination

0QWL04Z   Revision of Internal Fixation Device in Right Tarsal, Open Approach

0QWL05Z   Revision of External Fixation Device in Right Tarsal, Open Approach

0QWL07Z   Revision of Autologous Tissue Substitute in Right Tarsal, Open Approach

0QWL0JZ   Revision of Synthetic Substitute in Right Tarsal, Open Approach

0QWL0KZ   Revision of Nonautologous Tissue Substitute in Right Tarsal, Open Approach

0QWL34Z   Revision of Internal Fixation Device in Right Tarsal, Percutaneous Approach

0QWL35Z   Revision of External Fixation Device in Right Tarsal, Percutaneous Approach

0QWL37Z   Revision of Autologous Tissue Substitute in Right Tarsal, Percutaneous Approach

0QWL3JZ   Revision of Synthetic Substitute in Right Tarsal, Percutaneous Approach

0QWL3KZ   Revision of Nonautologous Tissue Substitute in Right Tarsal, Percutaneous Approach

0QWL44Z   Revision of Internal Fixation Device in Right Tarsal, Percutaneous Endoscopic Approach

0QWL45Z   Revision of External Fixation Device in Right Tarsal, Percutaneous Endoscopic Approach

0QWL47Z   Revision of Autologous Tissue Substitute in Right Tarsal, Percutaneous Endoscopic Approach

0QWL4JZ   Revision of Synthetic Substitute in Right Tarsal, Percutaneous Endoscopic Approach

0QWL4KZ   Revision of Nonautologous Tissue Substitute in Right Tarsal, Percutaneous Endoscopic Approach

0QWLX4Z   Revision of Internal Fixation Device in Right Tarsal, External Approach

0QWLX5Z   Revision of External Fixation Device in Right Tarsal, External Approach

0QWLX7Z   Revision of Autologous Tissue Substitute in Right Tarsal, External Approach

0QWLXJZ   Revision of Synthetic Substitute in Right Tarsal, External Approach

0QWLXKZ   Revision of Nonautologous Tissue Substitute in Right Tarsal, External Approach

0QWM04Z   Revision of Internal Fixation Device in Left Tarsal, Open Approach

0QWM05Z   Revision of External Fixation Device in Left Tarsal, Open Approach

0QWM07Z   Revision of Autologous Tissue Substitute in Left Tarsal, Open Approach

0QWM0JZ   Revision of Synthetic Substitute in Left Tarsal, Open Approach

0QWM0KZ   Revision of Nonautologous Tissue Substitute in Left Tarsal, Open Approach

0QWM34Z   Revision of Internal Fixation Device in Left Tarsal, Percutaneous Approach

0QWM35Z   Revision of External Fixation Device in Left Tarsal, Percutaneous Approach

0QWM37Z   Revision of Autologous Tissue Substitute in Left Tarsal, Percutaneous Approach

0QWM3JZ   Revision of Synthetic Substitute in Left Tarsal, Percutaneous Approach

0QWM3KZ   Revision of Nonautologous Tissue Substitute in Left Tarsal, Percutaneous Approach

0QWM44Z   Revision of Internal Fixation Device in Left Tarsal, Percutaneous Endoscopic Approach

0QWM45Z   Revision of External Fixation Device in Left Tarsal, Percutaneous Endoscopic Approach

0QWM47Z   Revision of Autologous Tissue Substitute in Left Tarsal, Percutaneous Endoscopic Approach

0QWM4JZ   Revision of Synthetic Substitute in Left Tarsal, Percutaneous Endoscopic Approach

0QWM4KZ   Revision of Nonautologous Tissue Substitute in Left Tarsal, Percutaneous Endoscopic Approach

0QWMX4Z   Revision of Internal Fixation Device in Left Tarsal, External Approach

0QWMX5Z   Revision of External Fixation Device in Left Tarsal, External Approach

0QWMX7Z   Revision of Autologous Tissue Substitute in Left Tarsal, External Approach

0QWMXJZ   Revision of Synthetic Substitute in Left Tarsal, External Approach

0QWMXKZ   Revision of Nonautologous Tissue Substitute in Left Tarsal, External Approach

0QWN04Z   Revision of Internal Fixation Device in Right Metatarsal, Open Approach

0QWN05Z   Revision of External Fixation Device in Right Metatarsal, Open Approach

0QWN07Z   Revision of Autologous Tissue Substitute in Right Metatarsal, Open Approach

0QWN0JZ   Revision of Synthetic Substitute in Right Metatarsal, Open Approach

0QWN0KZ   Revision of Nonautologous Tissue Substitute in Right Metatarsal, Open Approach

0QWN34Z   Revision of Internal Fixation Device in Right Metatarsal, Percutaneous Approach

0QWN35Z   Revision of External Fixation Device in Right Metatarsal, Percutaneous Approach

0QWN37Z   Revision of Autologous Tissue Substitute in Right Metatarsal, Percutaneous Approach

0QWN3JZ   Revision of Synthetic Substitute in Right Metatarsal, Percutaneous Approach

0QWN3KZ   Revision of Nonautologous Tissue Substitute in Right Metatarsal, Percutaneous Approach

0QWN44Z   Revision of Internal Fixation Device in Right Metatarsal, Percutaneous Endoscopic Approach

0QWN45Z   Revision of External Fixation Device in Right Metatarsal, Percutaneous Endoscopic Approach

0QWN47Z   Revision of Autologous Tissue Substitute in Right Metatarsal, Percutaneous Endoscopic Approach

0QWN4JZ   Revision of Synthetic Substitute in Right Metatarsal, Percutaneous Endoscopic Approach

0QWN4KZ   Revision of Nonautologous Tissue Substitute in Right Metatarsal, Percutaneous Endoscopic Approach

0QWNX4Z   Revision of Internal Fixation Device in Right Metatarsal, External Approach

0QWNX5Z   Revision of External Fixation Device in Right Metatarsal, External Approach

0QWNX7Z   Revision of Autologous Tissue Substitute in Right Metatarsal, External Approach

0QWNXJZ   Revision of Synthetic Substitute in Right Metatarsal, External Approach

0QWNXKZ   Revision of Nonautologous Tissue Substitute in Right Metatarsal, External Approach

0QWP04Z   Revision of Internal Fixation Device in Left Metatarsal, Open Approach

0QWP05Z   Revision of External Fixation Device in Left Metatarsal, Open Approach

0QWP07Z   Revision of Autologous Tissue Substitute in Left Metatarsal, Open Approach

0QWP0JZ   Revision of Synthetic Substitute in Left Metatarsal, Open Approach

0QWP0KZ   Revision of Nonautologous Tissue Substitute in Left Metatarsal, Open Approach

0QWP34Z   Revision of Internal Fixation Device in Left Metatarsal, Percutaneous Approach

0QWP35Z   Revision of External Fixation Device in Left Metatarsal, Percutaneous Approach

0QWP37Z   Revision of Autologous Tissue Substitute in Left Metatarsal, Percutaneous Approach

0QWP3JZ   Revision of Synthetic Substitute in Left Metatarsal, Percutaneous Approach

0QWP3KZ   Revision of Nonautologous Tissue Substitute in Left Metatarsal, Percutaneous Approach

0QWP44Z   Revision of Internal Fixation Device in Left Metatarsal, Percutaneous Endoscopic Approach

0QWP45Z   Revision of External Fixation Device in Left Metatarsal, Percutaneous Endoscopic Approach

0QWP47Z   Revision of Autologous Tissue Substitute in Left Metatarsal, Percutaneous Endoscopic Approach

0QWP4JZ   Revision of Synthetic Substitute in Left Metatarsal, Percutaneous Endoscopic Approach

0QWP4KZ   Revision of Nonautologous Tissue Substitute in Left Metatarsal, Percutaneous Endoscopic Approach

0QWPX4Z   Revision of Internal Fixation Device in Left Metatarsal, External Approach

0QWPX5Z   Revision of External Fixation Device in Left Metatarsal, External Approach

0QWPX7Z   Revision of Autologous Tissue Substitute in Left Metatarsal, External Approach

0QWPXJZ   Revision of Synthetic Substitute in Left Metatarsal, External Approach

0QWPXKZ   Revision of Nonautologous Tissue Substitute in Left Metatarsal, External Approach

0QWQ04Z   Revision of Internal Fixation Device in Right Toe Phalanx, Open Approach

0QWQ05Z   Revision of External Fixation Device in Right Toe Phalanx, Open Approach

0QWQ07Z   Revision of Autologous Tissue Substitute in Right Toe Phalanx, Open Approach

0QWQ0JZ   Revision of Synthetic Substitute in Right Toe Phalanx, Open Approach

0QWQ0KZ   Revision of Nonautologous Tissue Substitute in Right Toe Phalanx, Open Approach

0QWQ34Z   Revision of Internal Fixation Device in Right Toe Phalanx, Percutaneous Approach

0QWQ35Z   Revision of External Fixation Device in Right Toe Phalanx, Percutaneous Approach

0QWQ37Z   Revision of Autologous Tissue Substitute in Right Toe Phalanx, Percutaneous Approach

0QWQ3JZ   Revision of Synthetic Substitute in Right Toe Phalanx, Percutaneous Approach

0QWQ3KZ   Revision of Nonautologous Tissue Substitute in Right Toe Phalanx, Percutaneous Approach

0QWQ44Z   Revision of Internal Fixation Device in Right Toe Phalanx, Percutaneous Endoscopic Approach

0QWQ45Z   Revision of External Fixation Device in Right Toe Phalanx, Percutaneous Endoscopic Approach

0QWQ47Z   Revision of Autologous Tissue Substitute in Right Toe Phalanx, Percutaneous Endoscopic Approach

0QWQ4JZ   Revision of Synthetic Substitute in Right Toe Phalanx, Percutaneous Endoscopic Approach

0QWQ4KZ   Revision of Nonautologous Tissue Substitute in Right Toe Phalanx, Percutaneous Endoscopic Approach

0QWQX4Z   Revision of Internal Fixation Device in Right Toe Phalanx, External Approach

0QWQX5Z   Revision of External Fixation Device in Right Toe Phalanx, External Approach

0QWQX7Z   Revision of Autologous Tissue Substitute in Right Toe Phalanx, External Approach

0QWQXJZ   Revision of Synthetic Substitute in Right Toe Phalanx, External Approach

0QWQXKZ   Revision of Nonautologous Tissue Substitute in Right Toe Phalanx, External Approach

0QWR04Z   Revision of Internal Fixation Device in Left Toe Phalanx, Open Approach

0QWR05Z   Revision of External Fixation Device in Left Toe Phalanx, Open Approach

0QWR07Z   Revision of Autologous Tissue Substitute in Left Toe Phalanx, Open Approach

0QWR0JZ   Revision of Synthetic Substitute in Left Toe Phalanx, Open Approach

0QWR0KZ   Revision of Nonautologous Tissue Substitute in Left Toe Phalanx, Open Approach

0QWR34Z   Revision of Internal Fixation Device in Left Toe Phalanx, Percutaneous Approach

0QWR35Z   Revision of External Fixation Device in Left Toe Phalanx, Percutaneous Approach

0QWR37Z   Revision of Autologous Tissue Substitute in Left Toe Phalanx, Percutaneous Approach

0QWR3JZ   Revision of Synthetic Substitute in Left Toe Phalanx, Percutaneous Approach

0QWR3KZ   Revision of Nonautologous Tissue Substitute in Left Toe Phalanx, Percutaneous Approach

0QWR44Z   Revision of Internal Fixation Device in Left Toe Phalanx, Percutaneous Endoscopic Approach

0QWR45Z   Revision of External Fixation Device in Left Toe Phalanx, Percutaneous Endoscopic Approach

0QWR47Z   Revision of Autologous Tissue Substitute in Left Toe Phalanx, Percutaneous Endoscopic Approach

0QWR4JZ   Revision of Synthetic Substitute in Left Toe Phalanx, Percutaneous Endoscopic Approach

0QWR4KZ   Revision of Nonautologous Tissue Substitute in Left Toe Phalanx, Percutaneous Endoscopic Approach

0QWRX4Z   Revision of Internal Fixation Device in Left Toe Phalanx, External Approach

0QWRX5Z   Revision of External Fixation Device in Left Toe Phalanx, External Approach

0QWRX7Z   Revision of Autologous Tissue Substitute in Left Toe Phalanx, External Approach

0QWRXJZ   Revision of Synthetic Substitute in Left Toe Phalanx, External Approach

0QWRXKZ   Revision of Nonautologous Tissue Substitute in Left Toe Phalanx, External Approach

0QWS04Z   Revision of Internal Fixation Device in Coccyx, Open Approach

0QWS07Z   Revision of Autologous Tissue Substitute in Coccyx, Open Approach

0QWS0JZ   Revision of Synthetic Substitute in Coccyx, Open Approach

0QWS0KZ   Revision of Nonautologous Tissue Substitute in Coccyx, Open Approach

0QWS34Z   Revision of Internal Fixation Device in Coccyx, Percutaneous Approach

0QWS37Z   Revision of Autologous Tissue Substitute in Coccyx, Percutaneous Approach

0QWS3JZ   Revision of Synthetic Substitute in Coccyx, Percutaneous Approach

0QWS3KZ   Revision of Nonautologous Tissue Substitute in Coccyx, Percutaneous Approach

0QWS44Z   Revision of Internal Fixation Device in Coccyx, Percutaneous Endoscopic Approach

0QWS47Z   Revision of Autologous Tissue Substitute in Coccyx, Percutaneous Endoscopic Approach

0QWS4JZ   Revision of Synthetic Substitute in Coccyx, Percutaneous Endoscopic Approach

0QWS4KZ   Revision of Nonautologous Tissue Substitute in Coccyx, Percutaneous Endoscopic Approach

0QWSX4Z   Revision of Internal Fixation Device in Coccyx, External Approach

0QWSX7Z   Revision of Autologous Tissue Substitute in Coccyx, External Approach

0QWSXJZ   Revision of Synthetic Substitute in Coccyx, External Approach

0QWSXKZ   Revision of Nonautologous Tissue Substitute in Coccyx, External Approach

0QWY00Z   Revision of Drainage Device in Lower Bone, Open Approach

0QWY0MZ   Revision of Bone Growth Stimulator in Lower Bone, Open Approach

0QWY30Z   Revision of Drainage Device in Lower Bone, Percutaneous Approach

0QWY3MZ   Revision of Bone Growth Stimulator in Lower Bone, Percutaneous Approach

0QWY40Z   Revision of Drainage Device in Lower Bone, Percutaneous Endoscopic Approach

0QWY4MZ   Revision of Bone Growth Stimulator in Lower Bone, Percutaneous Endoscopic Approach

0QWYX0Z   Revision of Drainage Device in Lower Bone, External Approach

0QWYXMZ   Revision of Bone Growth Stimulator in Lower Bone, External Approach

Upper Joints

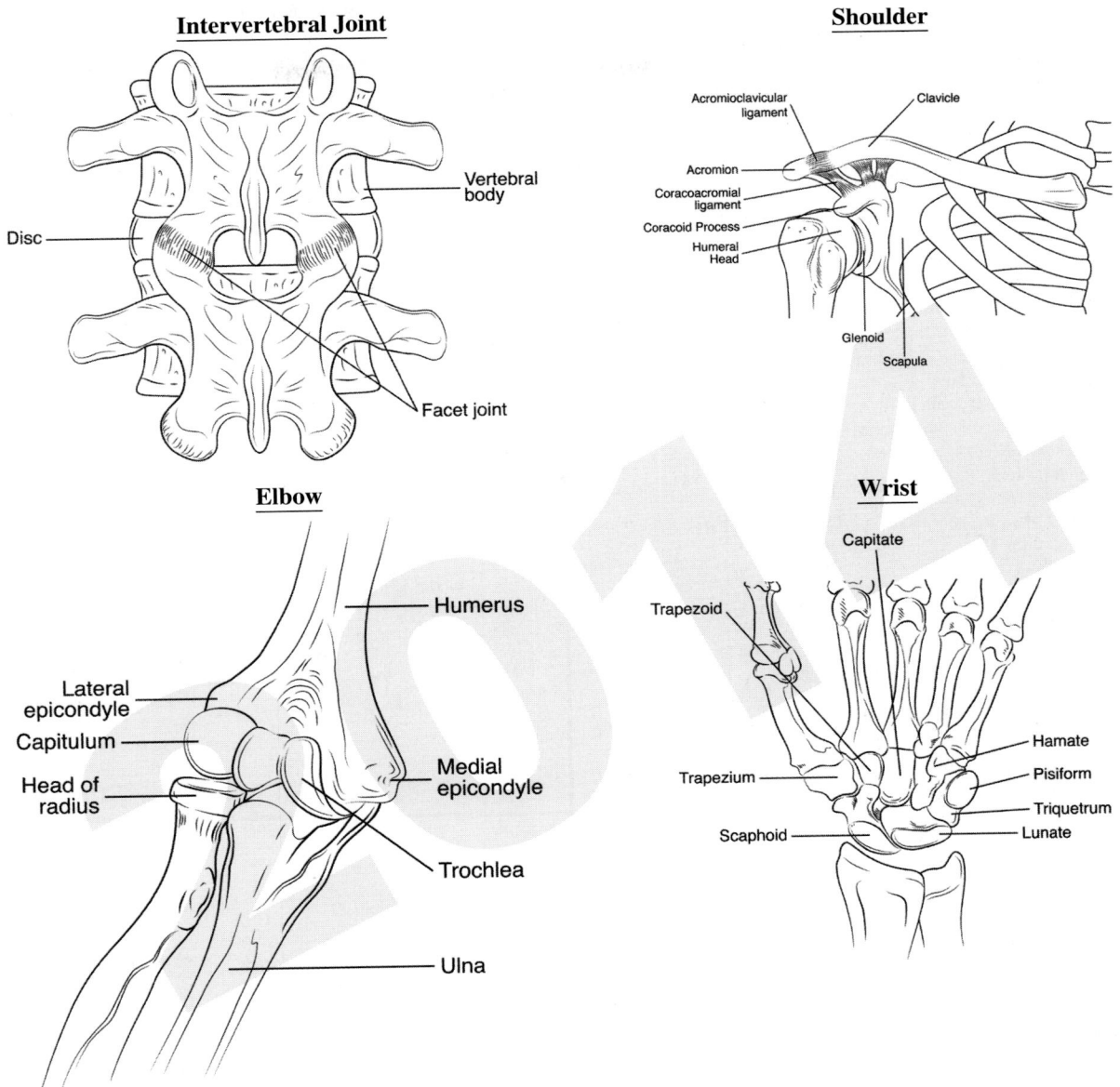

Intervertebral Joint

Vertebral body

Disc

Facet joint

Shoulder

Acromioclavicular ligament

Clavicle

Acromion

Coracoacromial ligament

Coracoid Process

Humeral Head

Glenoid

Scapula

Elbow

Humerus

Lateral epicondyle

Capitulum

Head of radius

Medial epicondyle

Trochlea

Ulna

Wrist

Capitate

Trapezoid

Trapezium

Scaphoid

Hamate

Pisiform

Triquetrum

Lunate

Upper Joints Tables 0R2–0RW

Section	0	Medical and Surgical
Body System	R	Upper Joints
Operation	2	**Change:** Taking out or off a device from a body part and putting back an identical or similar device in or on the same body part without cutting or puncturing the skin or a mucous membrane

Body Part (4th)	Approach (5th)	Device (6th)	Qualifier (7th)
Y Upper Joint	X External	0 Drainage Device Y Other Device	Z No Qualifier

Section	0	Medical and Surgical
Body System	R	Upper Joints
Operation	5	Destruction: Physical eradication of all or a portion of a body part by the direct use of energy, force, or a destructive agent

Body Part (4th)	Approach (5th)	Device (6th)	Qualifier (7th)
0 Occipital-cervical Joint	0 Open	Z No Device	Z No Qualifier
1 Cervical Vertebral Joint	3 Percutaneous		
3 Cervical Vertebral Disc	4 Percutaneous Endoscopic		
4 Cervicothoracic Vertebral Joint			
5 Cervicothoracic Vertebral Disc			
6 Thoracic Vertebral Joint			
9 Thoracic Vertebral Disc			
A Thoracolumbar Vertebral Joint			
B Thoracolumbar Vertebral Disc			
C Temporomandibular Joint, Right			
D Temporomandibular Joint, Left			
E Sternoclavicular Joint, Right			
F Sternoclavicular Joint, Left			
G Acromioclavicular Joint, Right			
H Acromioclavicular Joint, Left			
J Shoulder Joint, Right			
K Shoulder Joint, Left			
L Elbow Joint, Right			
M Elbow Joint, Left			
N Wrist Joint, Right			
P Wrist Joint, Left			
Q Carpal Joint, Right			
R Carpal Joint, Left			
S Metacarpocarpal Joint, Right			
T Metacarpocarpal Joint, Left			
U Metacarpophalangeal Joint, Right			
V Metacarpophalangeal Joint, Left			
W Finger Phalangeal Joint, Right			
X Finger Phalangeal Joint, Left			

Section	0	Medical and Surgical
Body System	R	Upper Joints
Operation	9	Drainage: Taking or letting out fluids and/or gases from a body part

Body Part (4th)	Approach (5th)	Device (6th)	Qualifier (7th)
0 Occipital-cervical Joint 1 Cervical Vertebral Joint 3 Cervical Vertebral Disc 4 Cervicothoracic Vertebral Joint 5 Cervicothoracic Vertebral Disc 6 Thoracic Vertebral Joint 9 Thoracic Vertebral Disc A Thoracolumbar Vertebral Joint B Thoracolumbar Vertebral Disc C Temporomandibular Joint, Right D Temporomandibular Joint, Left E Sternoclavicular Joint, Right F Sternoclavicular Joint, Left G Acromioclavicular Joint, Right H Acromioclavicular Joint, Left J Shoulder Joint, Right K Shoulder Joint, Left L Elbow Joint, Right M Elbow Joint, Left N Wrist Joint, Right P Wrist Joint, Left Q Carpal Joint, Right R Carpal Joint, Left S Metacarpocarpal Joint, Right T Metacarpocarpal Joint, Left U Metacarpophalangeal Joint, Right V Metacarpophalangeal Joint, Left W Finger Phalangeal Joint, Right X Finger Phalangeal Joint, Left	0 Open 3 Percutaneous 4 Percutaneous Endoscopic	0 Drainage Device	Z No Qualifier
0 Occipital-cervical Joint 1 Cervical Vertebral Joint 3 Cervical Vertebral Disc 4 Cervicothoracic Vertebral Joint 5 Cervicothoracic Vertebral Disc 6 Thoracic Vertebral Joint 9 Thoracic Vertebral Disc A Thoracolumbar Vertebral Joint B Thoracolumbar Vertebral Disc C Temporomandibular Joint, Right D Temporomandibular Joint, Left E Sternoclavicular Joint, Right F Sternoclavicular Joint, Left G Acromioclavicular Joint, Right H Acromioclavicular Joint, Left J Shoulder Joint, Right K Shoulder Joint, Left L Elbow Joint, Right M Elbow Joint, Left N Wrist Joint, Right P Wrist Joint, Left Q Carpal Joint, Right R Carpal Joint, Left S Metacarpocarpal Joint, Right T Metacarpocarpal Joint, Left U Metacarpophalangeal Joint, Right V Metacarpophalangeal Joint, Left W Finger Phalangeal Joint, Right X Finger Phalangeal Joint, Left	0 Open 3 Percutaneous 4 Percutaneous Endoscopic	Z No Device	X Diagnostic Z No Qualifier

Section	0	Medical and Surgical
Body System	R	Upper Joints
Operation	B	Excision: Cutting out or off, without replacement, a portion of a body part

Body Part (4th)	Approach (5th)	Device (6th)	Qualifier (7th)
0 Occipital-cervical Joint 1 Cervical Vertebral Joint 3 Cervical Vertebral Disc 4 Cervicothoracic Vertebral Joint 5 Cervicothoracic Vertebral Disc 6 Thoracic Vertebral Joint 9 Thoracic Vertebral Disc A Thoracolumbar Vertebral Joint B Thoracolumbar Vertebral Disc C Temporomandibular Joint, Right D Temporomandibular Joint, Left E Sternoclavicular Joint, Right F Sternoclavicular Joint, Left G Acromioclavicular Joint, Right H Acromioclavicular Joint, Left J Shoulder Joint, Right K Shoulder Joint, Left L Elbow Joint, Right M Elbow Joint, Left N Wrist Joint, Right P Wrist Joint, Left Q Carpal Joint, Right R Carpal Joint, Left S Metacarpocarpal Joint, Right T Metacarpocarpal Joint, Left U Metacarpophalangeal Joint, Right V Metacarpophalangeal Joint, Left W Finger Phalangeal Joint, Right X Finger Phalangeal Joint, Left	0 Open 3 Percutaneous 4 Percutaneous Endoscopic	Z No Device	X Diagnostic Z No Qualifier

Section	0	Medical and Surgical
Body System	R	Upper Joints
Operation	C	Extirpation: Taking or cutting out solid matter from a body part

Body Part (4th)	Approach (5th)	Device (6th)	Qualifier (7th)
0 Occipital-cervical Joint	0 Open	Z No Device	Z No Qualifier
1 Cervical Vertebral Joint	3 Percutaneous		
3 Cervical Vertebral Disc	4 Percutaneous		
4 Cervicothoracic Vertebral Joint	Endoscopic		
5 Cervicothoracic Vertebral Disc			
6 Thoracic Vertebral Joint			
9 Thoracic Vertebral Disc			
A Thoracolumbar Vertebral Joint			
B Thoracolumbar Vertebral Disc			
C Temporomandibular Joint, Right			
D Temporomandibular Joint, Left			
E Sternoclavicular Joint, Right			
F Sternoclavicular Joint, Left			
G Acromioclavicular Joint, Right			
H Acromioclavicular Joint, Left			
J Shoulder Joint, Right			
K Shoulder Joint, Left			
L Elbow Joint, Right			
M Elbow Joint, Left			
N Wrist Joint, Right			
P Wrist Joint, Left			
Q Carpal Joint, Right			
R Carpal Joint, Left			
S Metacarpocarpal Joint, Right			
T Metacarpocarpal Joint, Left			
U Metacarpophalangeal Joint, Right			
V Metacarpophalangeal Joint, Left			
W Finger Phalangeal Joint, Right			
X Finger Phalangeal Joint, Left			

Section	0	Medical and Surgical
Body System	R	Upper Joints
Operation	G	Fusion: Joining together portions of an articular body part rendering the articular body part immobile

Body Part (4th)	Approach (5th)	Device (6th)	Qualifier (7th)
0 Occipital-cervical Joint	0 Open	7 Autologous Tissue Substitute	0 Anterior Approach, Anterior Column
1 Cervical Vertebral Joint	3 Percutaneous	A Interbody Fusion Device	1 Posterior Approach, Posterior Column
2 Cervical Vertebral Joints, 2 or more	4 Percutaneous Endoscopic	J Synthetic Substitute	J Posterior Approach, Anterior Column
4 Cervicothoracic Vertebral Joint		K Nonautologous Tissue Substitute	
6 Thoracic Vertebral Joint		Z No Device	
7 Thoracic Vertebral Joints, 2 to 7			
8 Thoracic Vertebral Joints, 8 or more			
A Thoracolumbar Vertebral Joint			
C Temporomandibular Joint, Right	0 Open	4 Internal Fixation Device	Z No Qualifier
D Temporomandibular Joint, Left	3 Percutaneous	7 Autologous Tissue Substitute	
E Sternoclavicular Joint, Right	4 Percutaneous Endoscopic	J Synthetic Substitute	
F Sternoclavicular Joint, Left		K Nonautologous Tissue Substitute	
G Acromioclavicular Joint, Right		Z No Device	
H Acromioclavicular Joint, Left			
J Shoulder Joint, Right			
K Shoulder Joint, Left			

Continued

Section	0	Medical and Surgical
Body System	R	Upper Joints
Operation	G	Fusion: Joining together portions of an articular body part rendering the articular body part immobile

Body Part (4th)	Approach (5th)	Device (6th)	Qualifier (7th)
L Elbow Joint, Right M Elbow Joint, Left N Wrist Joint, Right P Wrist Joint, Left Q Carpal Joint, Right R Carpal Joint, Left S Metacarpocarpal Joint, Right T Metacarpocarpal Joint, Left U Metacarpophalangeal Joint, Right V Metacarpophalangeal Joint, Left W Finger Phalangeal Joint, Right X Finger Phalangeal Joint, Left	0 Open 3 Percutaneous 4 Percutaneous Endoscopic	4 Internal Fixation Device 5 External Fixation Device 7 Autologous Tissue Substitute J Synthetic Substitute K Nonautologous Tissue Substitute Z No Device	Z No Qualifier

Section	0	Medical and Surgical
Body System	R	Upper Joints
Operation	H	Insertion: Putting in a nonbiological appliance that monitors, assists, performs, or prevents a physiological function but does not physically take the place of a body part

Body Part (4th)	Approach (5th)	Device (6th)	Qualifier (7th)
0 Occipital-cervical Joint 1 Cervical Vertebral Joint 4 Cervicothoracic Vertebral Joint 6 Thoracic Vertebral Joint A Thoracolumbar Vertebral Joint	0 Open 3 Percutaneous 4 Percutaneous Endoscopic	3 Infusion Device 4 Internal Fixation Device 8 Spacer B Spinal Stabilization Device, Interspinous Process C Spinal Stabilization Device, Pedicle-Based D Spinal Stabilization Device, Facet Replacement	Z No Qualifier
3 Cervical Vertebral Disc 5 Cervicothoracic Vertebral Disc 9 Thoracic Vertebral Disc B Thoracolumbar Vertebral Disc	0 Open 3 Percutaneous 4 Percutaneous Endoscopic	3 Infusion Device	Z No Qualifier
C Temporomandibular Joint, Right D Temporomandibular Joint, Left E Sternoclavicular Joint, Right F Sternoclavicular Joint, Left G Acromioclavicular Joint, Right H Acromioclavicular Joint, Left J Shoulder Joint, Right K Shoulder Joint, Left	0 Open 3 Percutaneous 4 Percutaneous Endoscopic	3 Infusion Device 4 Internal Fixation Device 8 Spacer	Z No Qualifier
L Elbow Joint, Right M Elbow Joint, Left N Wrist Joint, Right P Wrist Joint, Left Q Carpal Joint, Right R Carpal Joint, Left S Metacarpocarpal Joint, Right T Metacarpocarpal Joint, Left U Metacarpophalangeal Joint, Right V Metacarpophalangeal Joint, Left W Finger Phalangeal Joint, Right X Finger Phalangeal Joint, Left	0 Open 3 Percutaneous 4 Percutaneous Endoscopic	3 Infusion Device 4 Internal Fixation Device 5 External Fixation Device 8 Spacer	Z No Qualifier

Section	0	Medical and Surgical
Body System	R	Upper Joints
Operation	J	Inspection: Visually and/or manually exploring a body part

Body Part (4th)	Approach (5th)	Device (6th)	Qualifier (7th)
0 Occipital-cervical Joint 1 Cervical Vertebral Joint 3 Cervical Vertebral Disc 4 Cervicothoracic Vertebral Joint 5 Cervicothoracic Vertebral Disc 6 Thoracic Vertebral Joint 9 Thoracic Vertebral Disc A Thoracolumbar Vertebral Joint B Thoracolumbar Vertebral Disc C Temporomandibular Joint, Right D Temporomandibular Joint, Left E Sternoclavicular Joint, Right F Sternoclavicular Joint, Left G Acromioclavicular Joint, Right H Acromioclavicular Joint, Left J Shoulder Joint, Right K Shoulder Joint, Left L Elbow Joint, Right M Elbow Joint, Left N Wrist Joint, Right P Wrist Joint, Left Q Carpal Joint, Right R Carpal Joint, Left S Metacarpocarpal Joint, Right T Metacarpocarpal Joint, Left U Metacarpophalangeal Joint, Right V Metacarpophalangeal Joint, Left W Finger Phalangeal Joint, Right X Finger Phalangeal Joint, Left	0 Open 3 Percutaneous 4 Percutaneous Endoscopic X External	Z No Device	Z No Qualifier

Section	0	Medical and Surgical
Body System	R	Upper Joints
Operation	N	Release: Freeing a body part from an abnormal physical constraint by cutting or by the use of force

Body Part (4th)	Approach (5th)	Device (6th)	Qualifier (7th)
0 Occipital-cervical Joint	0 Open	Z No Device	Z No Qualifier
1 Cervical Vertebral Joint	3 Percutaneous		
3 Cervical Vertebral Disc	4 Percutaneous		
4 Cervicothoracic Vertebral Joint	Endoscopic		
5 Cervicothoracic Vertebral Disc	X External		
6 Thoracic Vertebral Joint			
9 Thoracic Vertebral Disc			
A Thoracolumbar Vertebral Joint			
B Thoracolumbar Vertebral Disc			
C Temporomandibular Joint, Right			
D Temporomandibular Joint, Left			
E Sternoclavicular Joint, Right			
F Sternoclavicular Joint, Left			
G Acromioclavicular Joint, Right			
H Acromioclavicular Joint, Left			
J Shoulder Joint, Right			
K Shoulder Joint, Left			
L Elbow Joint, Right			
M Elbow Joint, Left			
N Wrist Joint, Right			
P Wrist Joint, Left			
Q Carpal Joint, Right			
R Carpal Joint, Left			
S Metacarpocarpal Joint, Right			
T Metacarpocarpal Joint, Left			
U Metacarpophalangeal Joint, Right			
V Metacarpophalangeal Joint, Left			
W Finger Phalangeal Joint, Right			
X Finger Phalangeal Joint, Left			

Section	0	Medical and Surgical
Body System	R	Upper Joints
Operation	P	Removal: Taking out or off a device from a body part

Body Part (4th)	Approach (5th)	Device (6th)	Qualifier (7th)
0 Occipital-cervical Joint 1 Cervical Vertebral Joint 4 Cervicothoracic Vertebral Joint 6 Thoracic Vertebral Joint A Thoracolumbar Vertebral Joint	0 Open 3 Percutaneous 4 Percutaneous Endoscopic	0 Drainage Device 3 Infusion Device 4 Internal Fixation Device 7 Autologous Tissue Substitute 8 Spacer A Interbody Fusion Device J Synthetic Substitute K Nonautologous Tissue Substitute	Z No Qualifier
0 Occipital-cervical Joint 1 Cervical Vertebral Joint 4 Cervicothoracic Vertebral Joint 6 Thoracic Vertebral Joint A Thoracolumbar Vertebral Joint	X External	0 Drainage Device 3 Infusion Device 4 Internal Fixation Device	Z No Qualifier
3 Cervical Vertebral Disc 5 Cervicothoracic Vertebral Disc 9 Thoracic Vertebral Disc B Thoracolumbar Vertebral Disc	0 Open 3 Percutaneous 4 Percutaneous Endoscopic	0 Drainage Device 3 Infusion Device 7 Autologous Tissue Substitute J Synthetic Substitute K Nonautologous Tissue Substitute	Z No Qualifier
3 Cervical Vertebral Disc 5 Cervicothoracic Vertebral Disc 9 Thoracic Vertebral Disc B Thoracolumbar Vertebral Disc	X External	0 Drainage Device 3 Infusion Device	Z No Qualifier

Continued

Section	0	Medical and Surgical	
Body System	R	Upper Joints	
Operation	P	**Removal:** Taking out or off a device from a body part	0RP *Continued*

Body Part (4th)	Approach (5th)	Device (6th)	Qualifier (7th)
C Temporomandibular Joint, Right **D** Temporomandibular Joint, Left **E** Sternoclavicular Joint, Right **F** Sternoclavicular Joint, Left **G** Acromioclavicular Joint, Right **H** Acromioclavicular Joint, Left **J** Shoulder Joint, Right **K** Shoulder Joint, Left	**0** Open **3** Percutaneous **4** Percutaneous Endoscopic	**0** Drainage Device **3** Infusion Device **4** Internal Fixation Device **7** Autologous Tissue Substitute **8** Spacer **J** Synthetic Substitute **K** Nonautologous Tissue Substitute	**Z** No Qualifier
C Temporomandibular Joint, Right **D** Temporomandibular Joint, Left **E** Sternoclavicular Joint, Right **F** Sternoclavicular Joint, Left **G** Acromioclavicular Joint, Right **H** Acromioclavicular Joint, Left **J** Shoulder Joint, Right **K** Shoulder Joint, Left	**X** External	**0** Drainage Device **3** Infusion Device **4** Internal Fixation Device	**Z** No Qualifier
L Elbow Joint, Right **M** Elbow Joint, Left **N** Wrist Joint, Right **P** Wrist Joint, Left **Q** Carpal Joint, Right **R** Carpal Joint, Left **S** Metacarpocarpal Joint, Right **T** Metacarpocarpal Joint, Left **U** Metacarpophalangeal Joint, Right **V** Metacarpophalangeal Joint, Left **W** Finger Phalangeal Joint, Right **X** Finger Phalangeal Joint, Left	**0** Open **3** Percutaneous **4** Percutaneous Endoscopic	**0** Drainage Device **3** Infusion Device **4** Internal Fixation Device **5** External Fixation Device **7** Autologous Tissue Substitute **8** Spacer **J** Synthetic Substitute **K** Nonautologous Tissue Substitute	**Z** No Qualifier
L Elbow Joint, Right **M** Elbow Joint, Left **N** Wrist Joint, Right **P** Wrist Joint, Left **Q** Carpal Joint, Right **R** Carpal Joint, Left **S** Metacarpocarpal Joint, Right **T** Metacarpocarpal Joint, Left **U** Metacarpophalangeal Joint, Right **V** Metacarpophalangeal Joint, Left **W** Finger Phalangeal Joint, Right **X** Finger Phalangeal Joint, Left	**X** External	**0** Drainage Device **3** Infusion Device **4** Internal Fixation Device **5** External Fixation Device	**Z** No Qualifier

Section	0	Medical and Surgical
Body System	R	Upper Joints
Operation	Q	**Repair:** Restoring, to the extent possible, a body part to its normal anatomic structure and function

Body Part (4th)	Approach (5th)	Device (6th)	Qualifier (7th)
0 Occipital-cervical Joint	0 Open	Z No Device	Z No Qualifier
1 Cervical Vertebral Joint	3 Percutaneous		
3 Cervical Vertebral Disc	4 Percutaneous		
4 Cervicothoracic Vertebral Joint	Endoscopic		
5 Cervicothoracic Vertebral Disc	X External		
6 Thoracic Vertebral Joint			
9 Thoracic Vertebral Disc			
A Thoracolumbar Vertebral Joint			
B Thoracolumbar Vertebral Disc			
C Temporomandibular Joint, Right			
D Temporomandibular Joint, Left			
E Sternoclavicular Joint, Right			
F Sternoclavicular Joint, Left			
G Acromioclavicular Joint, Right			
H Acromioclavicular Joint, Left			
J Shoulder Joint, Right			
K Shoulder Joint, Left			
L Elbow Joint, Right			
M Elbow Joint, Left			
N Wrist Joint, Right			
P Wrist Joint, Left			
Q Carpal Joint, Right			
R Carpal Joint, Left			
S Metacarpocarpal Joint, Right			
T Metacarpocarpal Joint, Left			
U Metacarpophalangeal Joint, Right			
V Metacarpophalangeal Joint, Left			
W Finger Phalangeal Joint, Right			
X Finger Phalangeal Joint, Left			

Section	0	Medical and Surgical
Body System	R	Upper Joints
Operation	R	**Replacement:** Putting in or on biological or synthetic material that physically takes the place and/or function of all or a portion of a body part

Body Part (4th)	Approach (5th)	Device (6th)	Qualifier (7th)
0 Occipital-cervical Joint 1 Cervical Vertebral Joint 3 Cervical Vertebral Disc 4 Cervicothoracic Vertebral Joint 5 Cervicothoracic Vertebral Disc 6 Thoracic Vertebral Joint 9 Thoracic Vertebral Disc A Thoracolumbar Vertebral Joint B Thoracolumbar Vertebral Disc C Temporomandibular Joint, Right D Temporomandibular Joint, Left E Sternoclavicular Joint, Right F Sternoclavicular Joint, Left G Acromioclavicular Joint, Right H Acromioclavicular Joint, Left L Elbow Joint, Right M Elbow Joint, Left N Wrist Joint, Right P Wrist Joint, Left Q Carpal Joint, Right R Carpal Joint, Left S Metacarpocarpal Joint, Right T Metacarpocarpal Joint, Left U Metacarpophalangeal Joint, Right V Metacarpophalangeal Joint, Left W Finger Phalangeal Joint, Right X Finger Phalangeal Joint, Left	0 Open	7 Autologous Tissue Substitute J Synthetic Substitute K Nonautologous Tissue Substitute	Z No Qualifier
J Shoulder Joint, Right K Shoulder Joint, Left	0 Open	0 Synthetic Substitute, Reverse Ball and Socket 7 Autologous Tissue Substitute K Nonautologous Tissue Substitute	Z No Qualifier
J Shoulder Joint, Right K Shoulder Joint, Left	0 Open	J Synthetic Substitute	6 Humeral Surface 7 Glenoid Surface Z No Qualifier

Section	0	Medical and Surgical
Body System	R	Upper Joints
Operation	S	Reposition: Moving to its normal location, or other suitable location, all or a portion of a body part

Body Part (4th)	Approach (5th)	Device (6th)	Qualifier (7th)
0 Occipital-cervical Joint 1 Cervical Vertebral Joint 4 Cervicothoracic Vertebral Joint 6 Thoracic Vertebral Joint A Thoracolumbar Vertebral Joint C Temporomandibular Joint, Right D Temporomandibular Joint, Left E Sternoclavicular Joint, Right F Sternoclavicular Joint, Left G Acromioclavicular Joint, Right H Acromioclavicular Joint, Left J Shoulder Joint, Right K Shoulder Joint, Left	0 Open 3 Percutaneous 4 Percutaneous Endoscopic X External	4 Internal Fixation Device Z No Device	Z No Qualifier
L Elbow Joint, Right M Elbow Joint, Left N Wrist Joint, Right P Wrist Joint, Left Q Carpal Joint, Right R Carpal Joint, Left S Metacarpocarpal Joint, Right T Metacarpocarpal Joint, Left U Metacarpophalangeal Joint, Right V Metacarpophalangeal Joint, Left W Finger Phalangeal Joint, Right X Finger Phalangeal Joint, Left	0 Open 3 Percutaneous 4 Percutaneous Endoscopic X External	4 Internal Fixation Device 5 External Fixation Device Z No Device	Z No Qualifier

Section	0	Medical and Surgical
Body System	R	Upper Joints
Operation	T	Resection: Cutting out or off, without replacement, all of a body part

Body Part (4th)	Approach (5th)	Device (6th)	Qualifier (7th)
3 Cervical Vertebral Disc 4 Cervicothoracic Vertebral Joint 5 Cervicothoracic Vertebral Disc 9 Thoracic Vertebral Disc B Thoracolumbar Vertebral Disc C Temporomandibular Joint, Right D Temporomandibular Joint, Left E Sternoclavicular Joint, Right F Sternoclavicular Joint, Left G Acromioclavicular Joint, Right H Acromioclavicular Joint, Left J Shoulder Joint, Right K Shoulder Joint, Left L Elbow Joint, Right M Elbow Joint, Left N Wrist Joint, Right P Wrist Joint, Left Q Carpal Joint, Right R Carpal Joint, Left S Metacarpocarpal Joint, Right T Metacarpocarpal Joint, Left U Metacarpophalangeal Joint, Right V Metacarpophalangeal Joint, Left W Finger Phalangeal Joint, Right X Finger Phalangeal Joint, Left	0 Open	Z No Device	Z No Qualifier

Section	0	Medical and Surgical
Body System	R	Upper Joints
Operation	U	**Supplement:** Putting in or on biological or synthetic material that physically reinforces and/or augments the function of a portion of a body part

Body Part (4th)	Approach (5th)	Device (6th)	Qualifier (7th)
0 Occipital-cervical Joint 1 Cervical Vertebral Joint 3 Cervical Vertebral Disc 4 Cervicothoracic Vertebral Joint 5 Cervicothoracic Vertebral Disc 6 Thoracic Vertebral Joint 9 Thoracic Vertebral Disc A Thoracolumbar Vertebral Joint B Thoracolumbar Vertebral Disc C Temporomandibular Joint, Right D Temporomandibular Joint, Left E Sternoclavicular Joint, Right F Sternoclavicular Joint, Left G Acromioclavicular Joint, Right H Acromioclavicular Joint, Left J Shoulder Joint, Right K Shoulder Joint, Left L Elbow Joint, Right M Elbow Joint, Left N Wrist Joint, Right P Wrist Joint, Left Q Carpal Joint, Right R Carpal Joint, Left S Metacarpocarpal Joint, Right T Metacarpocarpal Joint, Left U Metacarpophalangeal Joint, Right V Metacarpophalangeal Joint, Left W Finger Phalangeal Joint, Right X Finger Phalangeal Joint, Left	0 Open 3 Percutaneous 4 Percutaneous Endoscopic	7 Autologous Tissue Substitute J Synthetic Substitute K Nonautologous Tissue Substitute	Z No Qualifier

Section	0	Medical and Surgical
Body System	R	Upper Joints
Operation	W	**Revision:** Correcting, to the extent possible, a portion of a malfunctioning device or the position of a displaced device

Body Part (4th)	Approach (5th)	Device (6th)	Qualifier (7th)
0 Occipital-cervical Joint 1 Cervical Vertebral Joint 4 Cervicothoracic Vertebral Joint 6 Thoracic Vertebral Joint A Thoracolumbar Vertebral Joint	0 Open 3 Percutaneous 4 Percutaneous Endoscopic X External	0 Drainage Device 3 Infusion Device 4 Internal Fixation Device 7 Autologous Tissue Substitute 8 Spacer A Interbody Fusion Device J Synthetic Substitute K Nonautologous Tissue Substitute	Z No Qualifier
3 Cervical Vertebral Disc 5 Cervicothoracic Vertebral Disc 9 Thoracic Vertebral Disc B Thoracolumbar Vertebral Disc	0 Open 3 Percutaneous 4 Percutaneous Endoscopic X External	0 Drainage Device 3 Infusion Device 7 Autologous Tissue Substitute J Synthetic Substitute K Nonautologous Tissue Substitute	Z No Qualifier
C Temporomandibular Joint, Right D Temporomandibular Joint, Left E Sternoclavicular Joint, Right F Sternoclavicular Joint, Left G Acromioclavicular Joint, Right H Acromioclavicular Joint, Left J Shoulder Joint, Right K Shoulder Joint, Left	0 Open 3 Percutaneous 4 Percutaneous Endoscopic X External	0 Drainage Device 3 Infusion Device 4 Internal Fixation Device 7 Autologous Tissue Substitute 8 Spacer J Synthetic Substitute K Nonautologous Tissue Substitute	Z No Qualifier

Continued

Section	0	Medical and Surgical
Body System	R	Upper Joints
Operation	W	Revision: Correcting, to the extent possible, a portion of a malfunctioning device or the position of a displaced device

0RW Continued

Body Part (4th)	Approach (5th)	Device (6th)	Qualifier (7th)
L Elbow Joint, Right M Elbow Joint, Left N Wrist Joint, Right P Wrist Joint, Left Q Carpal Joint, Right R Carpal Joint, Left S Metacarpocarpal Joint, Right T Metacarpocarpal Joint, Left U Metacarpophalangeal Joint, Right V Metacarpophalangeal Joint, Left W Finger Phalangeal Joint, Right X Finger Phalangeal Joint, Left	0 Open 3 Percutaneous 4 Percutaneous Endoscopic X External	0 Drainage Device 3 Infusion Device 4 Internal Fixation Device 5 External Fixation Device 7 Autologous Tissue Substitute 8 Spacer J Synthetic Substitute K Nonautologous Tissue Substitute	Z No Qualifier

Upper Joints Code Listing 0R2–0RW

Review Coding Guideline B4.5

0R2 – Upper Joints, Change

Review Coding Guideline B6.1c

0R2YX0Z Change Drainage Device in Upper Joint, External Approach

0R2YXYZ Change Other Device in Upper Joint, External Approach

0R5 – Upper Joints, Destruction

0R500ZZ Destruction of Occipital-cervical Joint, Open Approach
0R503ZZ Destruction of Occipital-cervical Joint, Percutaneous Approach
0R504ZZ Destruction of Occipital-cervical Joint, Percutaneous Endoscopic Approach
0R510ZZ Destruction of Cervical Vertebral Joint, Open Approach
0R513ZZ Destruction of Cervical Vertebral Joint, Percutaneous Approach
0R514ZZ Destruction of Cervical Vertebral Joint, Percutaneous Endoscopic Approach
0R530ZZ Destruction of Cervical Vertebral Disc, Open Approach
0R533ZZ Destruction of Cervical Vertebral Disc, Percutaneous Approach
0R534ZZ Destruction of Cervical Vertebral Disc, Percutaneous Endoscopic Approach
0R540ZZ Destruction of Cervicothoracic Vertebral Joint, Open Approach
0R543ZZ Destruction of Cervicothoracic Vertebral Joint, Percutaneous Approach
0R544ZZ Destruction of Cervicothoracic Vertebral Joint, Percutaneous Endoscopic Approach
0R550ZZ Destruction of Cervicothoracic Vertebral Disc, Open Approach
0R553ZZ Destruction of Cervicothoracic Vertebral Disc, Percutaneous Approach
0R554ZZ Destruction of Cervicothoracic Vertebral Disc, Percutaneous Endoscopic Approach
0R560ZZ Destruction of Thoracic Vertebral Joint, Open Approach
0R563ZZ Destruction of Thoracic Vertebral Joint, Percutaneous Approach
0R564ZZ Destruction of Thoracic Vertebral Joint, Percutaneous Endoscopic Approach
0R590ZZ Destruction of Thoracic Vertebral Disc, Open Approach
0R593ZZ Destruction of Thoracic Vertebral Disc, Percutaneous Approach
0R594ZZ Destruction of Thoracic Vertebral Disc, Percutaneous Endoscopic Approach
0R5A0ZZ Destruction of Thoracolumbar Vertebral Joint, Open Approach

0R5A3ZZ Destruction of Thoracolumbar Vertebral Joint, Percutaneous Approach
0R5A4ZZ Destruction of Thoracolumbar Vertebral Joint, Percutaneous Endoscopic Approach
0R5B0ZZ Destruction of Thoracolumbar Vertebral Disc, Open Approach
0R5B3ZZ Destruction of Thoracolumbar Vertebral Disc, Percutaneous Approach
0R5B4ZZ Destruction of Thoracolumbar Vertebral Disc, Percutaneous Endoscopic Approach
0R5C0ZZ Destruction of Right Temporomandibular Joint, Open Approach
0R5C3ZZ Destruction of Right Temporomandibular Joint, Percutaneous Approach
0R5C4ZZ Destruction of Right Temporomandibular Joint, Percutaneous Endoscopic Approach
0R5D0ZZ Destruction of Left Temporomandibular Joint, Open Approach
0R5D3ZZ Destruction of Left Temporomandibular Joint, Percutaneous Approach
0R5D4ZZ Destruction of Left Temporomandibular Joint, Percutaneous Endoscopic Approach
0R5E0ZZ Destruction of Right Sternoclavicular Joint, Open Approach
0R5E3ZZ Destruction of Right Sternoclavicular Joint, Percutaneous Approach
0R5E4ZZ Destruction of Right Sternoclavicular Joint, Percutaneous Endoscopic Approach
0R5F0ZZ Destruction of Left Sternoclavicular Joint, Open Approach
0R5F3ZZ Destruction of Left Sternoclavicular Joint, Percutaneous Approach
0R5F4ZZ Destruction of Left Sternoclavicular Joint, Percutaneous Endoscopic Approach
0R5G0ZZ Destruction of Right Acromioclavicular Joint, Open Approach
0R5G3ZZ Destruction of Right Acromioclavicular Joint, Percutaneous Approach

0R5G4ZZ	Destruction of Right Acromioclavicular Joint, Percutaneous Endoscopic Approach
0R5H0ZZ	Destruction of Left Acromioclavicular Joint, Open Approach
0R5H3ZZ	Destruction of Left Acromioclavicular Joint, Percutaneous Approach
0R5H4ZZ	Destruction of Left Acromioclavicular Joint, Percutaneous Endoscopic Approach
0R5J0ZZ	Destruction of Right Shoulder Joint, Open Approach
0R5J3ZZ	Destruction of Right Shoulder Joint, Percutaneous Approach
0R5J4ZZ	Destruction of Right Shoulder Joint, Percutaneous Endoscopic Approach
0R5K0ZZ	Destruction of Left Shoulder Joint, Open Approach
0R5K3ZZ	Destruction of Left Shoulder Joint, Percutaneous Approach
0R5K4ZZ	Destruction of Left Shoulder Joint, Percutaneous Endoscopic Approach
0R5L0ZZ	Destruction of Right Elbow Joint, Open Approach
0R5L3ZZ	Destruction of Right Elbow Joint, Percutaneous Approach
0R5L4ZZ	Destruction of Right Elbow Joint, Percutaneous Endoscopic Approach
0R5M0ZZ	Destruction of Left Elbow Joint, Open Approach
0R5M3ZZ	Destruction of Left Elbow Joint, Percutaneous Approach
0R5M4ZZ	Destruction of Left Elbow Joint, Percutaneous Endoscopic Approach
0R5N0ZZ	Destruction of Right Wrist Joint, Open Approach
0R5N3ZZ	Destruction of Right Wrist Joint, Percutaneous Approach
0R5N4ZZ	Destruction of Right Wrist Joint, Percutaneous Endoscopic Approach
0R5P0ZZ	Destruction of Left Wrist Joint, Open Approach
0R5P3ZZ	Destruction of Left Wrist Joint, Percutaneous Approach
0R5P4ZZ	Destruction of Left Wrist Joint, Percutaneous Endoscopic Approach
0R5Q0ZZ	Destruction of Right Carpal Joint, Open Approach
0R5Q3ZZ	Destruction of Right Carpal Joint, Percutaneous Approach
0R5Q4ZZ	Destruction of Right Carpal Joint, Percutaneous Endoscopic Approach
0R5R0ZZ	Destruction of Left Carpal Joint, Open Approach
0R5R3ZZ	Destruction of Left Carpal Joint, Percutaneous Approach
0R5R4ZZ	Destruction of Left Carpal Joint, Percutaneous Endoscopic Approach
0R5S0ZZ	Destruction of Right Metacarpocarpal Joint, Open Approach
0R5S3ZZ	Destruction of Right Metacarpocarpal Joint, Percutaneous Approach
0R5S4ZZ	Destruction of Right Metacarpocarpal Joint, Percutaneous Endoscopic Approach
0R5T0ZZ	Destruction of Left Metacarpocarpal Joint, Open Approach
0R5T3ZZ	Destruction of Left Metacarpocarpal Joint, Percutaneous Approach
0R5T4ZZ	Destruction of Left Metacarpocarpal Joint, Percutaneous Endoscopic Approach
0R5U0ZZ	Destruction of Right Metacarpophalangeal Joint, Open Approach
0R5U3ZZ	Destruction of Right Metacarpophalangeal Joint, Percutaneous Approach
0R5U4ZZ	Destruction of Right Metacarpophalangeal Joint, Percutaneous Endoscopic Approach
0R5V0ZZ	Destruction of Left Metacarpophalangeal Joint, Open Approach
0R5V3ZZ	Destruction of Left Metacarpophalangeal Joint, Percutaneous Approach
0R5V4ZZ	Destruction of Left Metacarpophalangeal Joint, Percutaneous Endoscopic Approach
0R5W0ZZ	Destruction of Right Finger Phalangeal Joint, Open Approach
0R5W3ZZ	Destruction of Right Finger Phalangeal Joint, Percutaneous Approach
0R5W4ZZ	Destruction of Right Finger Phalangeal Joint, Percutaneous Endoscopic Approach
0R5X0ZZ	Destruction of Left Finger Phalangeal Joint, Open Approach
0R5X3ZZ	Destruction of Left Finger Phalangeal Joint, Percutaneous Approach
0R5X4ZZ	Destruction of Left Finger Phalangeal Joint, Percutaneous Endoscopic Approach

0R9 – Upper Joints, Drainage

Review Coding Guidelines B3.4a and B3.4b

Review Coding Guideline B6.2

0R9000Z	Drainage of Occipital-cervical Joint with Drainage Device, Open Approach
0R900ZX	Drainage of Occipital-cervical Joint, Open Approach, Diagnostic
0R900ZZ	Drainage of Occipital-cervical Joint, Open Approach
0R9030Z	Drainage of Occipital-cervical Joint with Drainage Device, Percutaneous Approach
0R903ZX	Drainage of Occipital-cervical Joint, Percutaneous Approach, Diagnostic
0R903ZZ	Drainage of Occipital-cervical Joint, Percutaneous Approach
0R9040Z	Drainage of Occipital-cervical Joint with Drainage Device, Percutaneous Endoscopic Approach
0R904ZX	Drainage of Occipital-cervical Joint, Percutaneous Endoscopic Approach, Diagnostic
0R904ZZ	Drainage of Occipital-cervical Joint, Percutaneous Endoscopic Approach
0R9100Z	Drainage of Cervical Vertebral Joint with Drainage Device, Open Approach
0R910ZX	Drainage of Cervical Vertebral Joint, Open Approach, Diagnostic
0R910ZZ	Drainage of Cervical Vertebral Joint, Open Approach
0R9130Z	Drainage of Cervical Vertebral Joint with Drainage Device, Percutaneous Approach
0R913ZX	Drainage of Cervical Vertebral Joint, Percutaneous Approach, Diagnostic
0R913ZZ	Drainage of Cervical Vertebral Joint, Percutaneous Approach
0R9140Z	Drainage of Cervical Vertebral Joint with Drainage Device, Percutaneous Endoscopic Approach
0R914ZX	Drainage of Cervical Vertebral Joint, Percutaneous Endoscopic Approach, Diagnostic
0R914ZZ	Drainage of Cervical Vertebral Joint, Percutaneous Endoscopic Approach
0R9300Z	Drainage of Cervical Vertebral Disc with Drainage Device, Open Approach
0R930ZX	Drainage of Cervical Vertebral Disc, Open Approach, Diagnostic
0R930ZZ	Drainage of Cervical Vertebral Disc, Open Approach
0R9330Z	Drainage of Cervical Vertebral Disc with Drainage Device, Percutaneous Approach
0R933ZX	Drainage of Cervical Vertebral Disc, Percutaneous Approach, Diagnostic
0R933ZZ	Drainage of Cervical Vertebral Disc, Percutaneous Approach
0R9340Z	Drainage of Cervical Vertebral Disc with Drainage Device, Percutaneous Endoscopic Approach
0R934ZX	Drainage of Cervical Vertebral Disc, Percutaneous Endoscopic Approach, Diagnostic
0R934ZZ	Drainage of Cervical Vertebral Disc, Percutaneous Endoscopic Approach
0R9400Z	Drainage of Cervicothoracic Vertebral Joint with Drainage Device, Open Approach
0R940ZX	Drainage of Cervicothoracic Vertebral Joint, Open Approach, Diagnostic
0R940ZZ	Drainage of Cervicothoracic Vertebral Joint, Open Approach
0R9430Z	Drainage of Cervicothoracic Vertebral Joint with Drainage Device, Percutaneous Approach
0R943ZX	Drainage of Cervicothoracic Vertebral Joint, Percutaneous Approach, Diagnostic
0R943ZZ	Drainage of Cervicothoracic Vertebral Joint, Percutaneous Approach
0R9440Z	Drainage of Cervicothoracic Vertebral Joint with Drainage Device, Percutaneous Endoscopic Approach
0R944ZX	Drainage of Cervicothoracic Vertebral Joint, Percutaneous Endoscopic Approach, Diagnostic

0R944ZZ   Drainage of Cervicothoracic Vertebral Joint, Percutaneous Endoscopic Approach

0R9500Z   Drainage of Cervicothoracic Vertebral Disc with Drainage Device, Open Approach

0R950ZX   Drainage of Cervicothoracic Vertebral Disc, Open Approach, Diagnostic

0R950ZZ   Drainage of Cervicothoracic Vertebral Disc, Open Approach

0R9530Z   Drainage of Cervicothoracic Vertebral Disc with Drainage Device, Percutaneous Approach

0R953ZX   Drainage of Cervicothoracic Vertebral Disc, Percutaneous Approach, Diagnostic

0R953ZZ   Drainage of Cervicothoracic Vertebral Disc, Percutaneous Approach

0R9540Z   Drainage of Cervicothoracic Vertebral Disc with Drainage Device, Percutaneous Endoscopic Approach

0R954ZX   Drainage of Cervicothoracic Vertebral Disc, Percutaneous Endoscopic Approach, Diagnostic

0R954ZZ   Drainage of Cervicothoracic Vertebral Disc, Percutaneous Endoscopic Approach

0R9600Z   Drainage of Thoracic Vertebral Joint with Drainage Device, Open Approach

0R960ZX   Drainage of Thoracic Vertebral Joint, Open Approach, Diagnostic

0R960ZZ   Drainage of Thoracic Vertebral Joint, Open Approach

0R9630Z   Drainage of Thoracic Vertebral Joint with Drainage Device, Percutaneous Approach

0R963ZX   Drainage of Thoracic Vertebral Joint, Percutaneous Approach, Diagnostic

0R963ZZ   Drainage of Thoracic Vertebral Joint, Percutaneous Approach

0R9640Z   Drainage of Thoracic Vertebral Joint with Drainage Device, Percutaneous Endoscopic Approach

0R964ZX   Drainage of Thoracic Vertebral Joint, Percutaneous Endoscopic Approach, Diagnostic

0R964ZZ   Drainage of Thoracic Vertebral Joint, Percutaneous Endoscopic Approach

0R9900Z   Drainage of Thoracic Vertebral Disc with Drainage Device, Open Approach

0R990ZX   Drainage of Thoracic Vertebral Disc, Open Approach, Diagnostic

0R990ZZ   Drainage of Thoracic Vertebral Disc, Open Approach

0R9930Z   Drainage of Thoracic Vertebral Disc with Drainage Device, Percutaneous Approach

0R993ZX   Drainage of Thoracic Vertebral Disc, Percutaneous Approach, Diagnostic

0R993ZZ   Drainage of Thoracic Vertebral Disc, Percutaneous Approach

0R9940Z   Drainage of Thoracic Vertebral Disc with Drainage Device, Percutaneous Endoscopic Approach

0R994ZX   Drainage of Thoracic Vertebral Disc, Percutaneous Endoscopic Approach, Diagnostic

0R994ZZ   Drainage of Thoracic Vertebral Disc, Percutaneous Endoscopic Approach

0R9A00Z   Drainage of Thoracolumbar Vertebral Joint with Drainage Device, Open Approach

0R9A0ZX   Drainage of Thoracolumbar Vertebral Joint, Open Approach, Diagnostic

0R9A0ZZ   Drainage of Thoracolumbar Vertebral Joint, Open Approach

0R9A30Z   Drainage of Thoracolumbar Vertebral Joint with Drainage Device, Percutaneous Approach

0R9A3ZX   Drainage of Thoracolumbar Vertebral Joint, Percutaneous Approach, Diagnostic

0R9A3ZZ   Drainage of Thoracolumbar Vertebral Joint, Percutaneous Approach

0R9A40Z   Drainage of Thoracolumbar Vertebral Joint with Drainage Device, Percutaneous Endoscopic Approach

0R9A4ZX   Drainage of Thoracolumbar Vertebral Joint, Percutaneous Endoscopic Approach, Diagnostic

0R9A4ZZ   Drainage of Thoracolumbar Vertebral Joint, Percutaneous Endoscopic Approach

0R9B00Z   Drainage of Thoracolumbar Vertebral Disc with Drainage Device, Open Approach

0R9B0ZX   Drainage of Thoracolumbar Vertebral Disc, Open Approach, Diagnostic

0R9B0ZZ   Drainage of Thoracolumbar Vertebral Disc, Open Approach

0R9B30Z   Drainage of Thoracolumbar Vertebral Disc with Drainage Device, Percutaneous Approach

0R9B3ZX   Drainage of Thoracolumbar Vertebral Disc, Percutaneous Approach, Diagnostic

0R9B3ZZ   Drainage of Thoracolumbar Vertebral Disc, Percutaneous Approach

0R9B40Z   Drainage of Thoracolumbar Vertebral Disc with Drainage Device, Percutaneous Endoscopic Approach

0R9B4ZX   Drainage of Thoracolumbar Vertebral Disc, Percutaneous Endoscopic Approach, Diagnostic

0R9B4ZZ   Drainage of Thoracolumbar Vertebral Disc, Percutaneous Endoscopic Approach

0R9C00Z   Drainage of Right Temporomandibular Joint with Drainage Device, Open Approach

0R9C0ZX   Drainage of Right Temporomandibular Joint, Open Approach, Diagnostic

0R9C0ZZ   Drainage of Right Temporomandibular Joint, Open Approach

0R9C30Z   Drainage of Right Temporomandibular Joint with Drainage Device, Percutaneous Approach

0R9C3ZX   Drainage of Right Temporomandibular Joint, Percutaneous Approach, Diagnostic

0R9C3ZZ   Drainage of Right Temporomandibular Joint, Percutaneous Approach

0R9C40Z   Drainage of Right Temporomandibular Joint with Drainage Device, Percutaneous Endoscopic Approach

0R9C4ZX   Drainage of Right Temporomandibular Joint, Percutaneous Endoscopic Approach, Diagnostic

0R9C4ZZ   Drainage of Right Temporomandibular Joint, Percutaneous Endoscopic Approach

0R9D00Z   Drainage of Left Temporomandibular Joint with Drainage Device, Open Approach

0R9D0ZX   Drainage of Left Temporomandibular Joint, Open Approach, Diagnostic

0R9D0ZZ   Drainage of Left Temporomandibular Joint, Open Approach

0R9D30Z   Drainage of Left Temporomandibular Joint with Drainage Device, Percutaneous Approach

0R9D3ZX   Drainage of Left Temporomandibular Joint, Percutaneous Approach, Diagnostic

0R9D3ZZ   Drainage of Left Temporomandibular Joint, Percutaneous Approach

0R9D40Z   Drainage of Left Temporomandibular Joint with Drainage Device, Percutaneous Endoscopic Approach

0R9D4ZX   Drainage of Left Temporomandibular Joint, Percutaneous Endoscopic Approach, Diagnostic

0R9D4ZZ   Drainage of Left Temporomandibular Joint, Percutaneous Endoscopic Approach

0R9E00Z   Drainage of Right Sternoclavicular Joint with Drainage Device, Open Approach

0R9E0ZX   Drainage of Right Sternoclavicular Joint, Open Approach, Diagnostic

0R9E0ZZ   Drainage of Right Sternoclavicular Joint, Open Approach

0R9E30Z   Drainage of Right Sternoclavicular Joint with Drainage Device, Percutaneous Approach

0R9E3ZX   Drainage of Right Sternoclavicular Joint, Percutaneous Approach, Diagnostic

0R9E3ZZ   Drainage of Right Sternoclavicular Joint, Percutaneous Approach

0R9E40Z   Drainage of Right Sternoclavicular Joint with Drainage Device, Percutaneous Endoscopic Approach

0R9E4ZX   Drainage of Right Sternoclavicular Joint, Percutaneous Endoscopic Approach, Diagnostic

0R9E4ZZ   Drainage of Right Sternoclavicular Joint, Percutaneous Endoscopic Approach

0R9F00Z   Drainage of Left Sternoclavicular Joint with Drainage Device, Open Approach

0R9F0ZX   Drainage of Left Sternoclavicular Joint, Open Approach, Diagnostic

0R9F0ZZ   Drainage of Left Sternoclavicular Joint, Open Approach

0R9F30Z   Drainage of Left Sternoclavicular Joint with Drainage Device, Percutaneous Approach

0R9F3ZX   Drainage of Left Sternoclavicular Joint, Percutaneous Approach, Diagnostic

0R9F3ZZ   Drainage of Left Sternoclavicular Joint, Percutaneous Approach

0R9F40Z   Drainage of Left Sternoclavicular Joint with Drainage Device, Percutaneous Endoscopic Approach

0R9F4ZX   Drainage of Left Sternoclavicular Joint, Percutaneous Endoscopic Approach, Diagnostic

0R9F4ZZ   Drainage of Left Sternoclavicular Joint, Percutaneous Endoscopic Approach

0R9G00Z   Drainage of Right Acromioclavicular Joint with Drainage Device, Open Approach

0R9G0ZX Drainage of Right Acromioclavicular Joint, Open Approach, Diagnostic

0R9G0ZZ Drainage of Right Acromioclavicular Joint, Open Approach

0R9G30Z Drainage of Right Acromioclavicular Joint with Drainage Device, Percutaneous Approach

0R9G3ZX Drainage of Right Acromioclavicular Joint, Percutaneous Approach, Diagnostic

0R9G3ZZ Drainage of Right Acromioclavicular Joint, Percutaneous Approach

0R9G40Z Drainage of Right Acromioclavicular Joint with Drainage Device, Percutaneous Endoscopic Approach

0R9G4ZX Drainage of Right Acromioclavicular Joint, Percutaneous Endoscopic Approach, Diagnostic

0R9G4ZZ Drainage of Right Acromioclavicular Joint, Percutaneous Endoscopic Approach

0R9H00Z Drainage of Left Acromioclavicular Joint with Drainage Device, Open Approach

0R9H0ZX Drainage of Left Acromioclavicular Joint, Open Approach, Diagnostic

0R9H0ZZ Drainage of Left Acromioclavicular Joint, Open Approach

0R9H30Z Drainage of Left Acromioclavicular Joint with Drainage Device, Percutaneous Approach

0R9H3ZX Drainage of Left Acromioclavicular Joint, Percutaneous Approach, Diagnostic

0R9H3ZZ Drainage of Left Acromioclavicular Joint, Percutaneous Approach

0R9H40Z Drainage of Left Acromioclavicular Joint with Drainage Device, Percutaneous Endoscopic Approach

0R9H4ZX Drainage of Left Acromioclavicular Joint, Percutaneous Endoscopic Approach, Diagnostic

0R9H4ZZ Drainage of Left Acromioclavicular Joint, Percutaneous Endoscopic Approach

0R9J00Z Drainage of Right Shoulder Joint with Drainage Device, Open Approach

0R9J0ZX Drainage of Right Shoulder Joint, Open Approach, Diagnostic

0R9J0ZZ Drainage of Right Shoulder Joint, Open Approach

0R9J30Z Drainage of Right Shoulder Joint with Drainage Device, Percutaneous Approach

0R9J3ZX Drainage of Right Shoulder Joint, Percutaneous Approach, Diagnostic

0R9J3ZZ Drainage of Right Shoulder Joint, Percutaneous Approach

0R9J40Z Drainage of Right Shoulder Joint with Drainage Device, Percutaneous Endoscopic Approach

0R9J4ZX Drainage of Right Shoulder Joint, Percutaneous Endoscopic Approach, Diagnostic

0R9J4ZZ Drainage of Right Shoulder Joint, Percutaneous Endoscopic Approach

0R9K00Z Drainage of Left Shoulder Joint with Drainage Device, Open Approach

0R9K0ZX Drainage of Left Shoulder Joint, Open Approach, Diagnostic

0R9K0ZZ Drainage of Left Shoulder Joint, Open Approach

0R9K30Z Drainage of Left Shoulder Joint with Drainage Device, Percutaneous Approach

0R9K3ZX Drainage of Left Shoulder Joint, Percutaneous Approach, Diagnostic

0R9K3ZZ Drainage of Left Shoulder Joint, Percutaneous Approach

0R9K40Z Drainage of Left Shoulder Joint with Drainage Device, Percutaneous Endoscopic Approach

0R9K4ZX Drainage of Left Shoulder Joint, Percutaneous Endoscopic Approach, Diagnostic

0R9K4ZZ Drainage of Left Shoulder Joint, Percutaneous Endoscopic Approach

0R9L00Z Drainage of Right Elbow Joint with Drainage Device, Open Approach

0R9L0ZX Drainage of Right Elbow Joint, Open Approach, Diagnostic

0R9L0ZZ Drainage of Right Elbow Joint, Open Approach

0R9L30Z Drainage of Right Elbow Joint with Drainage Device, Percutaneous Approach

0R9L3ZX Drainage of Right Elbow Joint, Percutaneous Approach, Diagnostic

0R9L3ZZ Drainage of Right Elbow Joint, Percutaneous Approach

0R9L40Z Drainage of Right Elbow Joint with Drainage Device, Percutaneous Endoscopic Approach

0R9L4ZX Drainage of Right Elbow Joint, Percutaneous Endoscopic Approach, Diagnostic

0R9L4ZZ Drainage of Right Elbow Joint, Percutaneous Endoscopic Approach

0R9M00Z Drainage of Left Elbow Joint with Drainage Device, Open Approach

0R9M0ZX Drainage of Left Elbow Joint, Open Approach, Diagnostic

0R9M0ZZ Drainage of Left Elbow Joint, Open Approach

0R9M30Z Drainage of Left Elbow Joint with Drainage Device, Percutaneous Approach

0R9M3ZX Drainage of Left Elbow Joint, Percutaneous Approach, Diagnostic

0R9M3ZZ Drainage of Left Elbow Joint, Percutaneous Approach

0R9M40Z Drainage of Left Elbow Joint with Drainage Device, Percutaneous Endoscopic Approach

0R9M4ZX Drainage of Left Elbow Joint, Percutaneous Endoscopic Approach, Diagnostic

0R9M4ZZ Drainage of Left Elbow Joint, Percutaneous Endoscopic Approach

0R9N00Z Drainage of Right Wrist Joint with Drainage Device, Open Approach

0R9N0ZX Drainage of Right Wrist Joint, Open Approach, Diagnostic

0R9N0ZZ Drainage of Right Wrist Joint, Open Approach

0R9N30Z Drainage of Right Wrist Joint with Drainage Device, Percutaneous Approach

0R9N3ZX Drainage of Right Wrist Joint, Percutaneous Approach, Diagnostic

0R9N3ZZ Drainage of Right Wrist Joint, Percutaneous Approach

0R9N40Z Drainage of Right Wrist Joint with Drainage Device, Percutaneous Endoscopic Approach

0R9N4ZX Drainage of Right Wrist Joint, Percutaneous Endoscopic Approach, Diagnostic

0R9N4ZZ Drainage of Right Wrist Joint, Percutaneous Endoscopic Approach

0R9P00Z Drainage of Left Wrist Joint with Drainage Device, Open Approach

0R9P0ZX Drainage of Left Wrist Joint, Open Approach, Diagnostic

0R9P0ZZ Drainage of Left Wrist Joint, Open Approach

0R9P30Z Drainage of Left Wrist Joint with Drainage Device, Percutaneous Approach

0R9P3ZX Drainage of Left Wrist Joint, Percutaneous Approach, Diagnostic

0R9P3ZZ Drainage of Left Wrist Joint, Percutaneous Approach

0R9P40Z Drainage of Left Wrist Joint with Drainage Device, Percutaneous Endoscopic Approach

0R9P4ZX Drainage of Left Wrist Joint, Percutaneous Endoscopic Approach, Diagnostic

0R9P4ZZ Drainage of Left Wrist Joint, Percutaneous Endoscopic Approach

0R9Q00Z Drainage of Right Carpal Joint with Drainage Device, Open Approach

0R9Q0ZX Drainage of Right Carpal Joint, Open Approach, Diagnostic

0R9Q0ZZ Drainage of Right Carpal Joint, Open Approach

0R9Q30Z Drainage of Right Carpal Joint with Drainage Device, Percutaneous Approach

0R9Q3ZX Drainage of Right Carpal Joint, Percutaneous Approach, Diagnostic

0R9Q3ZZ Drainage of Right Carpal Joint, Percutaneous Approach

0R9Q40Z Drainage of Right Carpal Joint with Drainage Device, Percutaneous Endoscopic Approach

0R9Q4ZX Drainage of Right Carpal Joint, Percutaneous Endoscopic Approach, Diagnostic

0R9Q4ZZ Drainage of Right Carpal Joint, Percutaneous Endoscopic Approach

0R9R00Z Drainage of Left Carpal Joint with Drainage Device, Open Approach

0R9R0ZX Drainage of Left Carpal Joint, Open Approach, Diagnostic

0R9R0ZZ Drainage of Left Carpal Joint, Open Approach

0R9R30Z Drainage of Left Carpal Joint with Drainage Device, Percutaneous Approach

0R9R3ZX Drainage of Left Carpal Joint, Percutaneous Approach, Diagnostic

0R9R3ZZ Drainage of Left Carpal Joint, Percutaneous Approach

0R9R40Z Drainage of Left Carpal Joint with Drainage Device, Percutaneous Endoscopic Approach

0R9R4ZX Drainage of Left Carpal Joint, Percutaneous Endoscopic Approach, Diagnostic

0R9R4ZZ Drainage of Left Carpal Joint, Percutaneous Endoscopic Approach

0R9S00Z Drainage of Right Metacarpocarpal Joint with Drainage Device, Open Approach

0R9S0ZX Drainage of Right Metacarpocarpal Joint, Open Approach, Diagnostic

0R9S0ZZ Drainage of Right Metacarpocarpal Joint, Open Approach

0R9S30Z Drainage of Right Metacarpocarpal Joint with Drainage Device, Percutaneous Approach

0R9S3ZX Drainage of Right Metacarpocarpal Joint, Percutaneous Approach, Diagnostic

0R9S3ZZ	Drainage of Right Metacarpocarpal Joint, Percutaneous Approach
0R9S40Z	Drainage of Right Metacarpocarpal Joint with Drainage Device, Percutaneous Endoscopic Approach
0R9S4ZX	Drainage of Right Metacarpocarpal Joint, Percutaneous Endoscopic Approach, Diagnostic
0R9S4ZZ	Drainage of Right Metacarpocarpal Joint, Percutaneous Endoscopic Approach
0R9T00Z	Drainage of Left Metacarpocarpal Joint with Drainage Device, Open Approach
0R9T0ZX	Drainage of Left Metacarpocarpal Joint, Open Approach, Diagnostic
0R9T0ZZ	Drainage of Left Metacarpocarpal Joint, Open Approach
0R9T30Z	Drainage of Left Metacarpocarpal Joint with Drainage Device, Percutaneous Approach
0R9T3ZX	Drainage of Left Metacarpocarpal Joint, Percutaneous Approach, Diagnostic
0R9T3ZZ	Drainage of Left Metacarpocarpal Joint, Percutaneous Approach
0R9T40Z	Drainage of Left Metacarpocarpal Joint with Drainage Device, Percutaneous Endoscopic Approach
0R9T4ZX	Drainage of Left Metacarpocarpal Joint, Percutaneous Endoscopic Approach, Diagnostic
0R9T4ZZ	Drainage of Left Metacarpocarpal Joint, Percutaneous Endoscopic Approach
0R9U00Z	Drainage of Right Metacarpophalangeal Joint with Drainage Device, Open Approach
0R9U0ZX	Drainage of Right Metacarpophalangeal Joint, Open Approach, Diagnostic
0R9U0ZZ	Drainage of Right Metacarpophalangeal Joint, Open Approach
0R9U30Z	Drainage of Right Metacarpophalangeal Joint with Drainage Device, Percutaneous Approach
0R9U3ZX	Drainage of Right Metacarpophalangeal Joint, Percutaneous Approach, Diagnostic
0R9U3ZZ	Drainage of Right Metacarpophalangeal Joint, Percutaneous Approach
0R9U40Z	Drainage of Right Metacarpophalangeal Joint with Drainage Device, Percutaneous Endoscopic Approach
0R9U4ZX	Drainage of Right Metacarpophalangeal Joint, Percutaneous Endoscopic Approach, Diagnostic
0R9U4ZZ	Drainage of Right Metacarpophalangeal Joint, Percutaneous Endoscopic Approach
0R9V00Z	Drainage of Left Metacarpophalangeal Joint with Drainage Device, Open Approach
0R9V0ZX	Drainage of Left Metacarpophalangeal Joint, Open Approach, Diagnostic
0R9V0ZZ	Drainage of Left Metacarpophalangeal Joint, Open Approach
0R9V30Z	Drainage of Left Metacarpophalangeal Joint with Drainage Device, Percutaneous Approach
0R9V3ZX	Drainage of Left Metacarpophalangeal Joint, Percutaneous Approach, Diagnostic
0R9V3ZZ	Drainage of Left Metacarpophalangeal Joint, Percutaneous Approach
0R9V40Z	Drainage of Left Metacarpophalangeal Joint with Drainage Device, Percutaneous Endoscopic Approach
0R9V4ZX	Drainage of Left Metacarpophalangeal Joint, Percutaneous Endoscopic Approach, Diagnostic
0R9V4ZZ	Drainage of Left Metacarpophalangeal Joint, Percutaneous Endoscopic Approach
0R9W00Z	Drainage of Right Finger Phalangeal Joint with Drainage Device, Open Approach
0R9W0ZX	Drainage of Right Finger Phalangeal Joint, Open Approach, Diagnostic
0R9W0ZZ	Drainage of Right Finger Phalangeal Joint, Open Approach
0R9W30Z	Drainage of Right Finger Phalangeal Joint with Drainage Device, Percutaneous Approach
0R9W3ZX	Drainage of Right Finger Phalangeal Joint, Percutaneous Approach, Diagnostic
0R9W3ZZ	Drainage of Right Finger Phalangeal Joint, Percutaneous Approach
0R9W40Z	Drainage of Right Finger Phalangeal Joint with Drainage Device, Percutaneous Endoscopic Approach
0R9W4ZX	Drainage of Right Finger Phalangeal Joint, Percutaneous Endoscopic Approach, Diagnostic
0R9W4ZZ	Drainage of Right Finger Phalangeal Joint, Percutaneous Endoscopic Approach
0R9X00Z	Drainage of Left Finger Phalangeal Joint with Drainage Device, Open Approach
0R9X0ZX	Drainage of Left Finger Phalangeal Joint, Open Approach, Diagnostic
0R9X0ZZ	Drainage of Left Finger Phalangeal Joint, Open Approach
0R9X30Z	Drainage of Left Finger Phalangeal Joint with Drainage Device, Percutaneous Approach
0R9X3ZX	Drainage of Left Finger Phalangeal Joint, Percutaneous Approach, Diagnostic
0R9X3ZZ	Drainage of Left Finger Phalangeal Joint, Percutaneous Approach
0R9X40Z	Drainage of Left Finger Phalangeal Joint with Drainage Device, Percutaneous Endoscopic Approach
0R9X4ZX	Drainage of Left Finger Phalangeal Joint, Percutaneous Endoscopic Approach, Diagnostic
0R9X4ZZ	Drainage of Left Finger Phalangeal Joint, Percutaneous Endoscopic Approach

0RB – Upper Joints, Excision

Review Coding Guidelines B3.4a and B3.4b

Review Coding Guideline B3.5

Review Coding Guideline B3.8

0RB00ZX	Excision of Occipital-cervical Joint, Open Approach, Diagnostic
0RB00ZZ	Excision of Occipital-cervical Joint, Open Approach
0RB03ZX	Excision of Occipital-cervical Joint, Percutaneous Approach, Diagnostic
0RB03ZZ	Excision of Occipital-cervical Joint, Percutaneous Approach
0RB04ZX	Excision of Occipital-cervical Joint, Percutaneous Endoscopic Approach, Diagnostic
0RB04ZZ	Excision of Occipital-cervical Joint, Percutaneous Endoscopic Approach
0RB10ZX	Excision of Cervical Vertebral Joint, Open Approach, Diagnostic
0RB10ZZ	Excision of Cervical Vertebral Joint, Open Approach
0RB13ZX	Excision of Cervical Vertebral Joint, Percutaneous Approach, Diagnostic
0RB13ZZ	Excision of Cervical Vertebral Joint, Percutaneous Approach
0RB14ZX	Excision of Cervical Vertebral Joint, Percutaneous Endoscopic Approach, Diagnostic
0RB14ZZ	Excision of Cervical Vertebral Joint, Percutaneous Endoscopic Approach
0RB30ZX	Excision of Cervical Vertebral Disc, Open Approach, Diagnostic
0RB30ZZ	Excision of Cervical Vertebral Disc, Open Approach
0RB33ZX	Excision of Cervical Vertebral Disc, Percutaneous Approach, Diagnostic
0RB33ZZ	Excision of Cervical Vertebral Disc, Percutaneous Approach
0RB34ZX	Excision of Cervical Vertebral Disc, Percutaneous Endoscopic Approach, Diagnostic
0RB34ZZ	Excision of Cervical Vertebral Disc, Percutaneous Endoscopic Approach
0RB40ZX	Excision of Cervicothoracic Vertebral Joint, Open Approach, Diagnostic
0RB40ZZ	Excision of Cervicothoracic Vertebral Joint, Open Approach
0RB43ZX	Excision of Cervicothoracic Vertebral Joint, Percutaneous Approach, Diagnostic
0RB43ZZ	Excision of Cervicothoracic Vertebral Joint, Percutaneous Approach
0RB44ZX	Excision of Cervicothoracic Vertebral Joint, Percutaneous Endoscopic Approach, Diagnostic
0RB44ZZ	Excision of Cervicothoracic Vertebral Joint, Percutaneous Endoscopic Approach
0RB50ZX	Excision of Cervicothoracic Vertebral Disc, Open Approach, Diagnostic
0RB50ZZ	Excision of Cervicothoracic Vertebral Disc, Open Approach

0RB53ZX Excision of Cervicothoracic Vertebral Disc, Percutaneous Approach, Diagnostic

0RB53ZZ Excision of Cervicothoracic Vertebral Disc, Percutaneous Approach

0RB54ZX Excision of Cervicothoracic Vertebral Disc, Percutaneous Endoscopic Approach, Diagnostic

0RB54ZZ Excision of Cervicothoracic Vertebral Disc, Percutaneous Endoscopic Approach

0RB60ZX Excision of Thoracic Vertebral Joint, Open Approach, Diagnostic

0RB60ZZ Excision of Thoracic Vertebral Joint, Open Approach

0RB63ZX Excision of Thoracic Vertebral Joint, Percutaneous Approach, Diagnostic

0RB63ZZ Excision of Thoracic Vertebral Joint, Percutaneous Approach

0RB64ZX Excision of Thoracic Vertebral Joint, Percutaneous Endoscopic Approach, Diagnostic

0RB64ZZ Excision of Thoracic Vertebral Joint, Percutaneous Endoscopic Approach

0RB90ZX Excision of Thoracic Vertebral Disc, Open Approach, Diagnostic

0RB90ZZ Excision of Thoracic Vertebral Disc, Open Approach

0RB93ZX Excision of Thoracic Vertebral Disc, Percutaneous Approach, Diagnostic

0RB93ZZ Excision of Thoracic Vertebral Disc, Percutaneous Approach

0RB94ZX Excision of Thoracic Vertebral Disc, Percutaneous Endoscopic Approach, Diagnostic

0RB94ZZ Excision of Thoracic Vertebral Disc, Percutaneous Endoscopic Approach

0RBA0ZX Excision of Thoracolumbar Vertebral Joint, Open Approach, Diagnostic

0RBA0ZZ Excision of Thoracolumbar Vertebral Joint, Open Approach

0RBA3ZX Excision of Thoracolumbar Vertebral Joint, Percutaneous Approach, Diagnostic

0RBA3ZZ Excision of Thoracolumbar Vertebral Joint, Percutaneous Approach

0RBA4ZX Excision of Thoracolumbar Vertebral Joint, Percutaneous Endoscopic Approach, Diagnostic

0RBA4ZZ Excision of Thoracolumbar Vertebral Joint, Percutaneous Endoscopic Approach

0RBB0ZX Excision of Thoracolumbar Vertebral Disc, Open Approach, Diagnostic

0RBB0ZZ Excision of Thoracolumbar Vertebral Disc, Open Approach

0RBB3ZX Excision of Thoracolumbar Vertebral Disc, Percutaneous Approach, Diagnostic

0RBB3ZZ Excision of Thoracolumbar Vertebral Disc, Percutaneous Approach

0RBB4ZX Excision of Thoracolumbar Vertebral Disc, Percutaneous Endoscopic Approach, Diagnostic

0RBB4ZZ Excision of Thoracolumbar Vertebral Disc, Percutaneous Endoscopic Approach

0RBC0ZX Excision of Right Temporomandibular Joint, Open Approach, Diagnostic

0RBC0ZZ Excision of Right Temporomandibular Joint, Open Approach

0RBC3ZX Excision of Right Temporomandibular Joint, Percutaneous Approach, Diagnostic

0RBC3ZZ Excision of Right Temporomandibular Joint, Percutaneous Approach

0RBC4ZX Excision of Right Temporomandibular Joint, Percutaneous Endoscopic Approach, Diagnostic

0RBC4ZZ Excision of Right Temporomandibular Joint, Percutaneous Endoscopic Approach

0RBD0ZX Excision of Left Temporomandibular Joint, Open Approach, Diagnostic

0RBD0ZZ Excision of Left Temporomandibular Joint, Open Approach

0RBD3ZX Excision of Left Temporomandibular Joint, Percutaneous Approach, Diagnostic

0RBD3ZZ Excision of Left Temporomandibular Joint, Percutaneous Approach

0RBD4ZX Excision of Left Temporomandibular Joint, Percutaneous Endoscopic Approach, Diagnostic

0RBD4ZZ Excision of Left Temporomandibular Joint, Percutaneous Endoscopic Approach

0RBE0ZX Excision of Right Sternoclavicular Joint, Open Approach, Diagnostic

0RBE0ZZ Excision of Right Sternoclavicular Joint, Open Approach

0RBE3ZX Excision of Right Sternoclavicular Joint, Percutaneous Approach, Diagnostic

0RBE3ZZ Excision of Right Sternoclavicular Joint, Percutaneous Approach

0RBE4ZX Excision of Right Sternoclavicular Joint, Percutaneous Endoscopic Approach, Diagnostic

0RBE4ZZ Excision of Right Sternoclavicular Joint, Percutaneous Endoscopic Approach

0RBF0ZX Excision of Left Sternoclavicular Joint, Open Approach, Diagnostic

0RBF0ZZ Excision of Left Sternoclavicular Joint, Open Approach

0RBF3ZX Excision of Left Sternoclavicular Joint, Percutaneous Approach, Diagnostic

0RBF3ZZ Excision of Left Sternoclavicular Joint, Percutaneous Approach

0RBF4ZX Excision of Left Sternoclavicular Joint, Percutaneous Endoscopic Approach, Diagnostic

0RBF4ZZ Excision of Left Sternoclavicular Joint, Percutaneous Endoscopic Approach

0RBG0ZX Excision of Right Acromioclavicular Joint, Open Approach, Diagnostic

0RBG0ZZ Excision of Right Acromioclavicular Joint, Open Approach

0RBG3ZX Excision of Right Acromioclavicular Joint, Percutaneous Approach, Diagnostic

0RBG3ZZ Excision of Right Acromioclavicular Joint, Percutaneous Approach

0RBG4ZX Excision of Right Acromioclavicular Joint, Percutaneous Endoscopic Approach, Diagnostic

0RBG4ZZ Excision of Right Acromioclavicular Joint, Percutaneous Endoscopic Approach

0RBH0ZX Excision of Left Acromioclavicular Joint, Open Approach, Diagnostic

0RBH0ZZ Excision of Left Acromioclavicular Joint, Open Approach

0RBH3ZX Excision of Left Acromioclavicular Joint, Percutaneous Approach, Diagnostic

0RBH3ZZ Excision of Left Acromioclavicular Joint, Percutaneous Approach

0RBH4ZX Excision of Left Acromioclavicular Joint, Percutaneous Endoscopic Approach, Diagnostic

0RBH4ZZ Excision of Left Acromioclavicular Joint, Percutaneous Endoscopic Approach

0RBJ0ZX Excision of Right Shoulder Joint, Open Approach, Diagnostic

0RBJ0ZZ Excision of Right Shoulder Joint, Open Approach

0RBJ3ZX Excision of Right Shoulder Joint, Percutaneous Approach, Diagnostic

0RBJ3ZZ Excision of Right Shoulder Joint, Percutaneous Approach

0RBJ4ZX Excision of Right Shoulder Joint, Percutaneous Endoscopic Approach, Diagnostic

0RBJ4ZZ Excision of Right Shoulder Joint, Percutaneous Endoscopic Approach

0RBK0ZX Excision of Left Shoulder Joint, Open Approach, Diagnostic

0RBK0ZZ Excision of Left Shoulder Joint, Open Approach

0RBK3ZX Excision of Left Shoulder Joint, Percutaneous Approach, Diagnostic

0RBK3ZZ Excision of Left Shoulder Joint, Percutaneous Approach

0RBK4ZX Excision of Left Shoulder Joint, Percutaneous Endoscopic Approach, Diagnostic

0RBK4ZZ Excision of Left Shoulder Joint, Percutaneous Endoscopic Approach

0RBL0ZX Excision of Right Elbow Joint, Open Approach, Diagnostic

0RBL0ZZ Excision of Right Elbow Joint, Open Approach

0RBL3ZX Excision of Right Elbow Joint, Percutaneous Approach, Diagnostic

0RBL3ZZ Excision of Right Elbow Joint, Percutaneous Approach

0RBL4ZX Excision of Right Elbow Joint, Percutaneous Endoscopic Approach, Diagnostic

0RBL4ZZ Excision of Right Elbow Joint, Percutaneous Endoscopic Approach

0RBM0ZX Excision of Left Elbow Joint, Open Approach, Diagnostic

0RBM0ZZ Excision of Left Elbow Joint, Open Approach

0RBM3ZX Excision of Left Elbow Joint, Percutaneous Approach, Diagnostic

0RBM3ZZ Excision of Left Elbow Joint, Percutaneous Approach

0RBM4ZX Excision of Left Elbow Joint, Percutaneous Endoscopic Approach, Diagnostic

0RBM4ZZ Excision of Left Elbow Joint, Percutaneous Endoscopic Approach

0RBN0ZX Excision of Right Wrist Joint, Open Approach, Diagnostic

0RBN0ZZ Excision of Right Wrist Joint, Open Approach

0RBN3ZX Excision of Right Wrist Joint, Percutaneous Approach, Diagnostic

0RBN3ZZ Excision of Right Wrist Joint, Percutaneous Approach

0RBN4ZX Excision of Right Wrist Joint, Percutaneous Endoscopic Approach, Diagnostic

0RBN4ZZ Excision of Right Wrist Joint, Percutaneous Endoscopic Approach

0RBP0ZX Excision of Left Wrist Joint, Open Approach, Diagnostic

0RBP0ZZ Excision of Left Wrist Joint, Open Approach

0RBP3ZX Excision of Left Wrist Joint, Percutaneous Approach, Diagnostic

---

♀ Female-only   ♂ Male-only   ● Limited Coverage   ● Non-OR   ▧ HAC-associated procedure   ⬣ Non-covered procedures   ✚ Combination

0RBP3ZZ Excision of Left Wrist Joint, Percutaneous Approach
0RBP4ZX Excision of Left Wrist Joint, Percutaneous Endoscopic Approach, Diagnostic
0RBP4ZZ Excision of Left Wrist Joint, Percutaneous Endoscopic Approach
0RBQ0ZX Excision of Right Carpal Joint, Open Approach, Diagnostic
0RBQ0ZZ Excision of Right Carpal Joint, Open Approach
0RBQ3ZX Excision of Right Carpal Joint, Percutaneous Approach, Diagnostic
0RBQ3ZZ Excision of Right Carpal Joint, Percutaneous Approach
0RBQ4ZX Excision of Right Carpal Joint, Percutaneous Endoscopic Approach, Diagnostic
0RBQ4ZZ Excision of Right Carpal Joint, Percutaneous Endoscopic Approach
0RBR0ZX Excision of Left Carpal Joint, Open Approach, Diagnostic
0RBR0ZZ Excision of Left Carpal Joint, Open Approach
0RBR3ZX Excision of Left Carpal Joint, Percutaneous Approach, Diagnostic
0RBR3ZZ Excision of Left Carpal Joint, Percutaneous Approach
0RBR4ZX Excision of Left Carpal Joint, Percutaneous Endoscopic Approach, Diagnostic
0RBR4ZZ Excision of Left Carpal Joint, Percutaneous Endoscopic Approach
0RBS0ZX Excision of Right Metacarpocarpal Joint, Open Approach, Diagnostic
0RBS0ZZ Excision of Right Metacarpocarpal Joint, Open Approach
0RBS3ZX Excision of Right Metacarpocarpal Joint, Percutaneous Approach, Diagnostic
0RBS3ZZ Excision of Right Metacarpocarpal Joint, Percutaneous Approach
0RBS4ZX Excision of Right Metacarpocarpal Joint, Percutaneous Endoscopic Approach, Diagnostic
0RBS4ZZ Excision of Right Metacarpocarpal Joint, Percutaneous Endoscopic Approach
0RBT0ZX Excision of Left Metacarpocarpal Joint, Open Approach, Diagnostic
0RBT0ZZ Excision of Left Metacarpocarpal Joint, Open Approach
0RBT3ZX Excision of Left Metacarpocarpal Joint, Percutaneous Approach, Diagnostic
0RBT3ZZ Excision of Left Metacarpocarpal Joint, Percutaneous Approach
0RBT4ZX Excision of Left Metacarpocarpal Joint, Percutaneous Endoscopic Approach, Diagnostic
0RBT4ZZ Excision of Left Metacarpocarpal Joint, Percutaneous Endoscopic Approach
0RBU0ZX Excision of Right Metacarpophalangeal Joint, Open Approach, Diagnostic
0RBU0ZZ Excision of Right Metacarpophalangeal Joint, Open Approach

0RBU3ZX Excision of Right Metacarpophalangeal Joint, Percutaneous Approach, Diagnostic
0RBU3ZZ Excision of Right Metacarpophalangeal Joint, Percutaneous Approach
0RBU4ZX Excision of Right Metacarpophalangeal Joint, Percutaneous Endoscopic Approach, Diagnostic
0RBU4ZZ Excision of Right Metacarpophalangeal Joint, Percutaneous Endoscopic Approach
0RBV0ZX Excision of Left Metacarpophalangeal Joint, Open Approach, Diagnostic
0RBV0ZZ Excision of Left Metacarpophalangeal Joint, Open Approach
0RBV3ZX Excision of Left Metacarpophalangeal Joint, Percutaneous Approach, Diagnostic
0RBV3ZZ Excision of Left Metacarpophalangeal Joint, Percutaneous Approach
0RBV4ZX Excision of Left Metacarpophalangeal Joint, Percutaneous Endoscopic Approach, Diagnostic
0RBV4ZZ Excision of Left Metacarpophalangeal Joint, Percutaneous Endoscopic Approach
0RBW0ZX Excision of Right Finger Phalangeal Joint, Open Approach, Diagnostic
0RBW0ZZ Excision of Right Finger Phalangeal Joint, Open Approach
0RBW3ZX Excision of Right Finger Phalangeal Joint, Percutaneous Approach, Diagnostic
0RBW3ZZ Excision of Right Finger Phalangeal Joint, Percutaneous Approach
0RBW4ZX Excision of Right Finger Phalangeal Joint, Percutaneous Endoscopic Approach, Diagnostic
0RBW4ZZ Excision of Right Finger Phalangeal Joint, Percutaneous Endoscopic Approach
0RBX0ZX Excision of Left Finger Phalangeal Joint, Open Approach, Diagnostic
0RBX0ZZ Excision of Left Finger Phalangeal Joint, Open Approach
0RBX3ZX Excision of Left Finger Phalangeal Joint, Percutaneous Approach, Diagnostic
0RBX3ZZ Excision of Left Finger Phalangeal Joint, Percutaneous Approach
0RBX4ZX Excision of Left Finger Phalangeal Joint, Percutaneous Endoscopic Approach, Diagnostic
0RBX4ZZ Excision of Left Finger Phalangeal Joint, Percutaneous Endoscopic Approach

0RC – Upper Joints, Extirpation

0RC00ZZ Extirpation of Matter from Occipital-cervical Joint, Open Approach
0RC03ZZ Extirpation of Matter from Occipital-cervical Joint, Percutaneous Approach
0RC04ZZ Extirpation of Matter from Occipital-cervical Joint, Percutaneous Endoscopic Approach
0RC10ZZ Extirpation of Matter from Cervical Vertebral Joint, Open Approach
0RC13ZZ Extirpation of Matter from Cervical Vertebral Joint, Percutaneous Approach
0RC14ZZ Extirpation of Matter from Cervical Vertebral Joint, Percutaneous Endoscopic Approach
0RC30ZZ Extirpation of Matter from Cervical Vertebral Disc, Open Approach
0RC33ZZ Extirpation of Matter from Cervical Vertebral Disc, Percutaneous Approach
0RC34ZZ Extirpation of Matter from Cervical Vertebral Disc, Percutaneous Endoscopic Approach
0RC40ZZ Extirpation of Matter from Cervicothoracic Vertebral Joint, Open Approach
0RC43ZZ Extirpation of Matter from Cervicothoracic Vertebral Joint, Percutaneous Approach
0RC44ZZ Extirpation of Matter from Cervicothoracic Vertebral Joint, Percutaneous Endoscopic Approach
0RC50ZZ Extirpation of Matter from Cervicothoracic Vertebral Disc, Open Approach
0RC53ZZ Extirpation of Matter from Cervicothoracic Vertebral Disc, Percutaneous Approach
0RC54ZZ Extirpation of Matter from Cervicothoracic Vertebral Disc, Percutaneous Endoscopic Approach
0RC60ZZ Extirpation of Matter from Thoracic Vertebral Joint, Open Approach

0RC63ZZ Extirpation of Matter from Thoracic Vertebral Joint, Percutaneous Approach
0RC64ZZ Extirpation of Matter from Thoracic Vertebral Joint, Percutaneous Endoscopic Approach
0RC90ZZ Extirpation of Matter from Thoracic Vertebral Disc, Open Approach
0RC93ZZ Extirpation of Matter from Thoracic Vertebral Disc, Percutaneous Approach
0RC94ZZ Extirpation of Matter from Thoracic Vertebral Disc, Percutaneous Endoscopic Approach
0RCA0ZZ Extirpation of Matter from Thoracolumbar Vertebral Joint, Open Approach
0RCA3ZZ Extirpation of Matter from Thoracolumbar Vertebral Joint, Percutaneous Approach
0RCA4ZZ Extirpation of Matter from Thoracolumbar Vertebral Joint, Percutaneous Endoscopic Approach
0RCB0ZZ Extirpation of Matter from Thoracolumbar Vertebral Disc, Open Approach
0RCB3ZZ Extirpation of Matter from Thoracolumbar Vertebral Disc, Percutaneous Approach
0RCB4ZZ Extirpation of Matter from Thoracolumbar Vertebral Disc, Percutaneous Endoscopic Approach
0RCC0ZZ Extirpation of Matter from Right Temporomandibular Joint, Open Approach
0RCC3ZZ Extirpation of Matter from Right Temporomandibular Joint, Percutaneous Approach
0RCC4ZZ Extirpation of Matter from Right Temporomandibular Joint, Percutaneous Endoscopic Approach

0RCD0ZZ Extirpation of Matter from Left Temporomandibular Joint, Open Approach

0RCD3ZZ Extirpation of Matter from Left Temporomandibular Joint, Percutaneous Approach

0RCD4ZZ Extirpation of Matter from Left Temporomandibular Joint, Percutaneous Endoscopic Approach

0RCE0ZZ Extirpation of Matter from Right Sternoclavicular Joint, Open Approach

0RCE3ZZ Extirpation of Matter from Right Sternoclavicular Joint, Percutaneous Approach

0RCE4ZZ Extirpation of Matter from Right Sternoclavicular Joint, Percutaneous Endoscopic Approach

0RCF0ZZ Extirpation of Matter from Left Sternoclavicular Joint, Open Approach

0RCF3ZZ Extirpation of Matter from Left Sternoclavicular Joint, Percutaneous Approach

0RCF4ZZ Extirpation of Matter from Left Sternoclavicular Joint, Percutaneous Endoscopic Approach

0RCG0ZZ Extirpation of Matter from Right Acromioclavicular Joint, Open Approach

0RCG3ZZ Extirpation of Matter from Right Acromioclavicular Joint, Percutaneous Approach

0RCG4ZZ Extirpation of Matter from Right Acromioclavicular Joint, Percutaneous Endoscopic Approach

0RCH0ZZ Extirpation of Matter from Left Acromioclavicular Joint, Open Approach

0RCH3ZZ Extirpation of Matter from Left Acromioclavicular Joint, Percutaneous Approach

0RCH4ZZ Extirpation of Matter from Left Acromioclavicular Joint, Percutaneous Endoscopic Approach

0RCJ0ZZ Extirpation of Matter from Right Shoulder Joint, Open Approach

0RCJ3ZZ Extirpation of Matter from Right Shoulder Joint, Percutaneous Approach

0RCJ4ZZ Extirpation of Matter from Right Shoulder Joint, Percutaneous Endoscopic Approach

0RCK0ZZ Extirpation of Matter from Left Shoulder Joint, Open Approach

0RCK3ZZ Extirpation of Matter from Left Shoulder Joint, Percutaneous Approach

0RCK4ZZ Extirpation of Matter from Left Shoulder Joint, Percutaneous Endoscopic Approach

0RCL0ZZ Extirpation of Matter from Right Elbow Joint, Open Approach

0RCL3ZZ Extirpation of Matter from Right Elbow Joint, Percutaneous Approach

0RCL4ZZ Extirpation of Matter from Right Elbow Joint, Percutaneous Endoscopic Approach

0RCM0ZZ Extirpation of Matter from Left Elbow Joint, Open Approach

0RCM3ZZ Extirpation of Matter from Left Elbow Joint, Percutaneous Approach

0RCM4ZZ Extirpation of Matter from Left Elbow Joint, Percutaneous Endoscopic Approach

0RCN0ZZ Extirpation of Matter from Right Wrist Joint, Open Approach

0RCN3ZZ Extirpation of Matter from Right Wrist Joint, Percutaneous Approach

0RCN4ZZ Extirpation of Matter from Right Wrist Joint, Percutaneous Endoscopic Approach

0RCP0ZZ Extirpation of Matter from Left Wrist Joint, Open Approach

0RCP3ZZ Extirpation of Matter from Left Wrist Joint, Percutaneous Approach

0RCP4ZZ Extirpation of Matter from Left Wrist Joint, Percutaneous Endoscopic Approach

0RCQ0ZZ Extirpation of Matter from Right Carpal Joint, Open Approach

0RCQ3ZZ Extirpation of Matter from Right Carpal Joint, Percutaneous Approach

0RCQ4ZZ Extirpation of Matter from Right Carpal Joint, Percutaneous Endoscopic Approach

0RCR0ZZ Extirpation of Matter from Left Carpal Joint, Open Approach

0RCR3ZZ Extirpation of Matter from Left Carpal Joint, Percutaneous Approach

0RCR4ZZ Extirpation of Matter from Left Carpal Joint, Percutaneous Endoscopic Approach

0RCS0ZZ Extirpation of Matter from Right Metacarpocarpal Joint, Open Approach

0RCS3ZZ Extirpation of Matter from Right Metacarpocarpal Joint, Percutaneous Approach

0RCS4ZZ Extirpation of Matter from Right Metacarpocarpal Joint, Percutaneous Endoscopic Approach

0RCT0ZZ Extirpation of Matter from Left Metacarpocarpal Joint, Open Approach

0RCT3ZZ Extirpation of Matter from Left Metacarpocarpal Joint, Percutaneous Approach

0RCT4ZZ Extirpation of Matter from Left Metacarpocarpal Joint, Percutaneous Endoscopic Approach

0RCU0ZZ Extirpation of Matter from Right Metacarpophalangeal Joint, Open Approach

0RCU3ZZ Extirpation of Matter from Right Metacarpophalangeal Joint, Percutaneous Approach

0RCU4ZZ Extirpation of Matter from Right Metacarpophalangeal Joint, Percutaneous Endoscopic Approach

0RCV0ZZ Extirpation of Matter from Left Metacarpophalangeal Joint, Open Approach

0RCV3ZZ Extirpation of Matter from Left Metacarpophalangeal Joint, Percutaneous Approach

0RCV4ZZ Extirpation of Matter from Left Metacarpophalangeal Joint, Percutaneous Endoscopic Approach

0RCW0ZZ Extirpation of Matter from Right Finger Phalangeal Joint, Open Approach

0RCW3ZZ Extirpation of Matter from Right Finger Phalangeal Joint, Percutaneous Approach

0RCW4ZZ Extirpation of Matter from Right Finger Phalangeal Joint, Percutaneous Endoscopic Approach

0RCX0ZZ Extirpation of Matter from Left Finger Phalangeal Joint, Open Approach

0RCX3ZZ Extirpation of Matter from Left Finger Phalangeal Joint, Percutaneous Approach

0RCX4ZZ Extirpation of Matter from Left Finger Phalangeal Joint, Percutaneous Endoscopic Approach

0RG – Upper Joints, Fusion

For Fusion procedures involving the vertebral joints Review Coding Guidelines B3.10a, B3.10b and B3.10c

0RG0070 Fusion of Occipital-cervical Joint with Autologous Tissue Substitute, Anterior Approach, Anterior Column, Open Approach

HAC When reported with secondary diagnosis code T84.60XA, T84.610A, T84.611A, T84.612A, T84.613A, T84.614A, T84.615A, T84.619A, T84.63XA, T84.69XA, T84.7XXA

0RG0071 Fusion of Occipital-cervical Joint with Autologous Tissue Substitute, Posterior Approach, Posterior Column, Open Approach

HAC When reported with secondary diagnosis code T84.60XA, T84.610A, T84.611A, T84.612A, T84.613A, T84.614A, T84.615A, T84.619A, T84.63XA, T84.69XA, T84.7XXA

0RG007J Fusion of Occipital-cervical Joint with Autologous Tissue Substitute, Posterior Approach, Anterior Column, Open Approach

HAC When reported with secondary diagnosis code T84.60XA, T84.610A, T84.611A, T84.612A, T84.613A, T84.614A, T84.615A, T84.619A, T84.63XA, T84.69XA, T84.7XXA

0RG00A0 Fusion of Occipital-cervical Joint with Interbody Fusion Device, Anterior Approach, Anterior Column, Open Approach

HAC When reported with secondary diagnosis code T84.60XA, T84.610A, T84.611A, T84.612A, T84.613A, T84.614A, T84.615A, T84.619A, T84.63XA, T84.69XA, T84.7XXA

0RG00A1 Fusion of Occipital-cervical Joint with Interbody Fusion Device, Posterior Approach, Posterior Column, Open Approach

HAC When reported with secondary diagnosis code T84.60XA, T84.610A, T84.611A, T84.612A, T84.613A, T84.614A, T84.615A, T84.619A, T84.63XA, T84.69XA, T84.7XXA

0RG00AJ Fusion of Occipital-cervical Joint with Interbody Fusion Device, Posterior Approach, Anterior Column, Open Approach

HAC When reported with secondary diagnosis code T84.60XA, T84.610A, T84.611A, T84.612A, T84.613A, T84.614A, T84.615A, T84.619A, T84.63XA, T84.69XA, T84.7XXA

♀ Female-only   ♂ Male-only   ● Limited Coverage   ● Non-OR   HAC HAC-associated procedure   ● Non-covered procedures   ➕ Combination

0RG00J0 Fusion of Occipital-cervical Joint with Synthetic Substitute, Anterior Approach, Anterior Column, Open Approach
HAC When reported with secondary diagnosis code T84.60XA, T84.610A, T84.611A, T84.612A, T84.613A, T84.614A, T84.615A, T84.619A, T84.63XA, T84.69XA, T84.7XXA

0RG00J1 Fusion of Occipital-cervical Joint with Synthetic Substitute, Posterior Approach, Posterior Column, Open Approach
HAC When reported with secondary diagnosis code T84.60XA, T84.610A, T84.611A, T84.612A, T84.613A, T84.614A, T84.615A, T84.619A, T84.63XA, T84.69XA, T84.7XXA

0RG00JJ Fusion of Occipital-cervical Joint with Synthetic Substitute, Posterior Approach, Anterior Column, Open Approach
HAC When reported with secondary diagnosis code T84.60XA, T84.610A, T84.611A, T84.612A, T84.613A, T84.614A, T84.615A, T84.619A, T84.63XA, T84.69XA, T84.7XXA

0RG00K0 Fusion of Occipital-cervical Joint with Nonautologous Tissue Substitute, Anterior Approach, Anterior Column, Open Approach
HAC When reported with secondary diagnosis code T84.60XA, T84.610A, T84.611A, T84.612A, T84.613A, T84.614A, T84.615A, T84.619A, T84.63XA, T84.69XA, T84.7XXA

0RG00K1 Fusion of Occipital-cervical Joint with Nonautologous Tissue Substitute, Posterior Approach, Posterior Column, Open Approach
HAC When reported with secondary diagnosis code T84.60XA, T84.610A, T84.611A, T84.612A, T84.613A, T84.614A, T84.615A, T84.619A, T84.63XA, T84.69XA, T84.7XXA

0RG00KJ Fusion of Occipital-cervical Joint with Nonautologous Tissue Substitute, Posterior Approach, Anterior Column, Open Approach
HAC When reported with secondary diagnosis code T84.60XA, T84.610A, T84.611A, T84.612A, T84.613A, T84.614A, T84.615A, T84.619A, T84.63XA, T84.69XA, T84.7XXA

0RG00Z0 Fusion of Occipital-cervical Joint, Anterior Approach, Anterior Column, Open Approach
HAC When reported with secondary diagnosis code T84.60XA, T84.610A, T84.611A, T84.612A, T84.613A, T84.614A, T84.615A, T84.619A, T84.63XA, T84.69XA, T84.7XXA

0RG00Z1 Fusion of Occipital-cervical Joint, Posterior Approach, Posterior Column, Open Approach
HAC When reported with secondary diagnosis code T84.60XA, T84.610A, T84.611A, T84.612A, T84.613A, T84.614A, T84.615A, T84.619A, T84.63XA, T84.69XA, T84.7XXA

0RG00ZJ Fusion of Occipital-cervical Joint, Posterior Approach, Anterior Column, Open Approach
HAC When reported with secondary diagnosis code T84.60XA, T84.610A, T84.611A, T84.612A, T84.613A, T84.614A, T84.615A, T84.619A, T84.63XA, T84.69XA, T84.7XXA

0RG0370 Fusion of Occipital-cervical Joint with Autologous Tissue Substitute, Anterior Approach, Anterior Column, Percutaneous Approach
HAC When reported with secondary diagnosis code T84.60XA, T84.610A, T84.611A, T84.612A, T84.613A, T84.614A, T84.615A, T84.619A, T84.63XA, T84.69XA, T84.7XXA

0RG0371 Fusion of Occipital-cervical Joint with Autologous Tissue Substitute, Posterior Approach, Posterior Column, Percutaneous Approach
HAC When reported with secondary diagnosis code T84.60XA, T84.610A, T84.611A, T84.612A, T84.613A, T84.614A, T84.615A, T84.619A, T84.63XA, T84.69XA, T84.7XXA

0RG037J Fusion of Occipital-cervical Joint with Autologous Tissue Substitute, Posterior Approach, Anterior Column, Percutaneous Approach
HAC When reported with secondary diagnosis code T84.60XA, T84.610A, T84.611A, T84.612A, T84.613A, T84.614A, T84.615A, T84.619A, T84.63XA, T84.69XA, T84.7XXA

0RG03A0 Fusion of Occipital-cervical Joint with Interbody Fusion Device, Anterior Approach, Anterior Column, Percutaneous Approach
HAC When reported with secondary diagnosis code T84.60XA, T84.610A, T84.611A, T84.612A, T84.613A, T84.614A, T84.615A, T84.619A, T84.63XA, T84.69XA, T84.7XXA

0RG03A1 Fusion of Occipital-cervical Joint with Interbody Fusion Device, Posterior Approach, Posterior Column, Percutaneous Approach
HAC When reported with secondary diagnosis code T84.60XA, T84.610A, T84.611A, T84.612A, T84.613A, T84.614A, T84.615A, T84.619A, T84.63XA, T84.69XA, T84.7XXA

0RG03AJ Fusion of Occipital-cervical Joint with Interbody Fusion Device, Posterior Approach, Anterior Column, Percutaneous Approach
HAC When reported with secondary diagnosis code T84.60XA, T84.610A, T84.611A, T84.612A, T84.613A, T84.614A, T84.615A, T84.619A, T84.63XA, T84.69XA, T84.7XXA

0RG03J0 Fusion of Occipital-cervical Joint with Synthetic Substitute, Anterior Approach, Anterior Column, Percutaneous Approach
HAC When reported with secondary diagnosis code T84.60XA, T84.610A, T84.611A, T84.612A, T84.613A, T84.614A, T84.615A, T84.619A, T84.63XA, T84.69XA, T84.7XXA

0RG03J1 Fusion of Occipital-cervical Joint with Synthetic Substitute, Posterior Approach, Posterior Column, Percutaneous Approach
HAC When reported with secondary diagnosis code T84.60XA, T84.610A, T84.611A, T84.612A, T84.613A, T84.614A, T84.615A, T84.619A, T84.63XA, T84.69XA, T84.7XXA

0RG03JJ Fusion of Occipital-cervical Joint with Synthetic Substitute, Posterior Approach, Anterior Column, Percutaneous Approach
HAC When reported with secondary diagnosis code T84.60XA, T84.610A, T84.611A, T84.612A, T84.613A, T84.614A, T84.615A, T84.619A, T84.63XA, T84.69XA, T84.7XXA

0RG03K0 Fusion of Occipital-cervical Joint with Nonautologous Tissue Substitute, Anterior Approach, Anterior Column, Percutaneous Approach
HAC When reported with secondary diagnosis code T84.60XA, T84.610A, T84.611A, T84.612A, T84.613A, T84.614A, T84.615A, T84.619A, T84.63XA, T84.69XA, T84.7XXA

0RG03K1 Fusion of Occipital-cervical Joint with Nonautologous Tissue Substitute, Posterior Approach, Posterior Column, Percutaneous Approach
HAC When reported with secondary diagnosis code T84.60XA, T84.610A, T84.611A, T84.612A, T84.613A, T84.614A, T84.615A, T84.619A, T84.63XA, T84.69XA, T84.7XXA

0RG03KJ Fusion of Occipital-cervical Joint with Nonautologous Tissue Substitute, Posterior Approach, Anterior Column, Percutaneous Approach
HAC When reported with secondary diagnosis code T84.60XA, T84.610A, T84.611A, T84.612A, T84.613A, T84.614A, T84.615A, T84.619A, T84.63XA, T84.69XA, T84.7XXA

0RG03Z0 Fusion of Occipital-cervical Joint, Anterior Approach, Anterior Column, Percutaneous Approach
HAC When reported with secondary diagnosis code T84.60XA, T84.610A, T84.611A, T84.612A, T84.613A, T84.614A, T84.615A, T84.619A, T84.63XA, T84.69XA, T84.7XXA

0RG03Z1 Fusion of Occipital-cervical Joint, Posterior Approach, Posterior Column, Percutaneous Approach
HAC When reported with secondary diagnosis code T84.60XA, T84.610A, T84.611A, T84.612A, T84.613A, T84.614A, T84.615A, T84.619A, T84.63XA, T84.69XA, T84.7XXA

0RG03ZJ Fusion of Occipital-cervical Joint, Posterior Approach, Anterior Column, Percutaneous Approach
HAC When reported with secondary diagnosis code T84.60XA, T84.610A, T84.611A, T84.612A, T84.613A, T84.614A, T84.615A, T84.619A, T84.63XA, T84.69XA, T84.7XXA

0RG0470 Fusion of Occipital-cervical Joint with Autologous Tissue Substitute, Anterior Approach, Anterior Column, Percutaneous Endoscopic Approach
HAC When reported with secondary diagnosis code T84.60XA, T84.610A, T84.611A, T84.612A, T84.613A, T84.614A, T84.615A, T84.619A, T84.63XA, T84.69XA, T84.7XXA

0RG0471 Fusion of Occipital-cervical Joint with Autologous Tissue Substitute, Posterior Approach, Posterior Column, Percutaneous Endoscopic Approach
HAC When reported with secondary diagnosis code T84.60XA, T84.610A, T84.611A, T84.612A, T84.613A, T84.614A, T84.615A, T84.619A, T84.63XA, T84.69XA, T84.7XXA

0RG047J Fusion of Occipital-cervical Joint with Autologous Tissue Substitute, Posterior Approach, Anterior Column, Percutaneous Endoscopic Approach
HAC When reported with secondary diagnosis code T84.60XA, T84.610A, T84.611A, T84.612A, T84.613A, T84.614A, T84.615A, T84.619A, T84.63XA, T84.69XA, T84.7XXA

♀ Female-only   ♂ Male-only   ◐ Limited Coverage   ● Non-OR   HAC HAC-associated procedure   ⬣ Non-covered procedures   ✚ Combination

0RG04A0   Fusion of Occipital-cervical Joint with Interbody Fusion Device, Anterior Approach, Anterior Column, Percutaneous Endoscopic Approach
    HAC   When reported with secondary diagnosis code T84.60XA, T84.610A, T84.611A, T84.612A, T84.613A, T84.614A, T84.615A, T84.619A, T84.63XA, T84.69XA, T84.7XXA

0RG04A1   Fusion of Occipital-cervical Joint with Interbody Fusion Device, Posterior Approach, Posterior Column, Percutaneous Endoscopic Approach
    HAC   When reported with secondary diagnosis code T84.60XA, T84.610A, T84.611A, T84.612A, T84.613A, T84.614A, T84.615A, T84.619A, T84.63XA, T84.69XA, T84.7XXA

0RG04AJ   Fusion of Occipital-cervical Joint with Interbody Fusion Device, Posterior Approach, Anterior Column, Percutaneous Endoscopic Approach
    HAC   When reported with secondary diagnosis code T84.60XA, T84.610A, T84.611A, T84.612A, T84.613A, T84.614A, T84.615A, T84.619A, T84.63XA, T84.69XA, T84.7XXA

0RG04J0   Fusion of Occipital-cervical Joint with Synthetic Substitute, Anterior Approach, Anterior Column, Percutaneous Endoscopic Approach
    HAC   When reported with secondary diagnosis code T84.60XA, T84.610A, T84.611A, T84.612A, T84.613A, T84.614A, T84.615A, T84.619A, T84.63XA, T84.69XA, T84.7XXA

0RG04J1   Fusion of Occipital-cervical Joint with Synthetic Substitute, Posterior Approach, Posterior Column, Percutaneous Endoscopic Approach
    HAC   When reported with secondary diagnosis code T84.60XA, T84.610A, T84.611A, T84.612A, T84.613A, T84.614A, T84.615A, T84.619A, T84.63XA, T84.69XA, T84.7XXA

0RG04JJ   Fusion of Occipital-cervical Joint with Synthetic Substitute, Posterior Approach, Anterior Column, Percutaneous Endoscopic Approach
    HAC   When reported with secondary diagnosis code T84.60XA, T84.610A, T84.611A, T84.612A, T84.613A, T84.614A, T84.615A, T84.619A, T84.63XA, T84.69XA, T84.7XXA

0RG04K0   Fusion of Occipital-cervical Joint with Nonautologous Tissue Substitute, Anterior Approach, Anterior Column, Percutaneous Endoscopic Approach
    HAC   When reported with secondary diagnosis code T84.60XA, T84.610A, T84.611A, T84.612A, T84.613A, T84.614A, T84.615A, T84.619A, T84.63XA, T84.69XA, T84.7XXA

0RG04K1   Fusion of Occipital-cervical Joint with Nonautologous Tissue Substitute, Posterior Approach, Posterior Column, Percutaneous Endoscopic Approach
    HAC   When reported with secondary diagnosis code T84.60XA, T84.610A, T84.611A, T84.612A, T84.613A, T84.614A, T84.615A, T84.619A, T84.63XA, T84.69XA, T84.7XXA

0RG04KJ   Fusion of Occipital-cervical Joint with Nonautologous Tissue Substitute, Posterior Approach, Anterior Column, Percutaneous Endoscopic Approach
    HAC   When reported with secondary diagnosis code T84.60XA, T84.610A, T84.611A, T84.612A, T84.613A, T84.614A, T84.615A, T84.619A, T84.63XA, T84.69XA, T84.7XXA

0RG04Z0   Fusion of Occipital-cervical Joint, Anterior Approach, Anterior Column, Percutaneous Endoscopic Approach
    HAC   When reported with secondary diagnosis code T84.60XA, T84.610A, T84.611A, T84.612A, T84.613A, T84.614A, T84.615A, T84.619A, T84.63XA, T84.69XA, T84.7XXA

0RG04Z1   Fusion of Occipital-cervical Joint, Posterior Approach, Posterior Column, Percutaneous Endoscopic Approach
    HAC   When reported with secondary diagnosis code T84.60XA, T84.610A, T84.611A, T84.612A, T84.613A, T84.614A, T84.615A, T84.619A, T84.63XA, T84.69XA, T84.7XXA

0RG04ZJ   Fusion of Occipital-cervical Joint, Posterior Approach, Anterior Column, Percutaneous Endoscopic Approach
    HAC   When reported with secondary diagnosis code T84.60XA, T84.610A, T84.611A, T84.612A, T84.613A, T84.614A, T84.615A, T84.619A, T84.63XA, T84.69XA, T84.7XXA

0RG1070   Fusion of Cervical Vertebral Joint with Autologous Tissue Substitute, Anterior Approach, Anterior Column, Open Approach
    HAC   When reported with secondary diagnosis code T84.60XA, T84.610A, T84.611A, T84.612A, T84.613A, T84.614A, T84.615A, T84.619A, T84.63XA, T84.69XA, T84.7XXA

0RG1071   Fusion of Cervical Vertebral Joint with Autologous Tissue Substitute, Posterior Approach, Posterior Column, Open Approach
    HAC   When reported with secondary diagnosis code T84.60XA, T84.610A, T84.611A, T84.612A, T84.613A, T84.614A, T84.615A, T84.619A, T84.63XA, T84.69XA, T84.7XXA

0RG107J   Fusion of Cervical Vertebral Joint with Autologous Tissue Substitute, Posterior Approach, Anterior Column, Open Approach
    HAC   When reported with secondary diagnosis code T84.60XA, T84.610A, T84.611A, T84.612A, T84.613A, T84.614A, T84.615A, T84.619A, T84.63XA, T84.69XA, T84.7XXA

0RG10A0   Fusion of Cervical Vertebral Joint with Interbody Fusion Device, Anterior Approach, Anterior Column, Open Approach
    HAC   When reported with secondary diagnosis code T84.60XA, T84.610A, T84.611A, T84.612A, T84.613A, T84.614A, T84.615A, T84.619A, T84.63XA, T84.69XA, T84.7XXA

0RG10A1   Fusion of Cervical Vertebral Joint with Interbody Fusion Device, Posterior Approach, Posterior Column, Open Approach
    HAC   When reported with secondary diagnosis code T84.60XA, T84.610A, T84.611A, T84.612A, T84.613A, T84.614A, T84.615A, T84.619A, T84.63XA, T84.69XA, T84.7XXA

v0RG10AJ   Fusion of Cervical Vertebral Joint with Interbody Fusion Device, Posterior Approach, Anterior Column, Open Approach
    HAC   When reported with secondary diagnosis code T84.60XA, T84.610A, T84.611A, T84.612A, T84.613A, T84.614A, T84.615A, T84.619A, T84.63XA, T84.69XA, T84.7XXA

0RG10J0   Fusion of Cervical Vertebral Joint with Synthetic Substitute, Anterior Approach, Anterior Column, Open Approach
    HAC   When reported with secondary diagnosis code T84.60XA, T84.610A, T84.611A, T84.612A, T84.613A, T84.614A, T84.615A, T84.619A, T84.63XA, T84.69XA, T84.7XXA

0RG10J1   Fusion of Cervical Vertebral Joint with Synthetic Substitute, Posterior Approach, Posterior Column, Open Approach
    HAC   When reported with secondary diagnosis code T84.60XA, T84.610A, T84.611A, T84.612A, T84.613A, T84.614A, T84.615A, T84.619A, T84.63XA, T84.69XA, T84.7XXA

0RG10JJ   Fusion of Cervical Vertebral Joint with Synthetic Substitute, Posterior Approach, Anterior Column, Open Approach
    HAC   When reported with secondary diagnosis code T84.60XA, T84.610A, T84.611A, T84.612A, T84.613A, T84.614A, T84.615A, T84.619A, T84.63XA, T84.69XA, T84.7XXA

0RG10K0   Fusion of Cervical Vertebral Joint with Nonautologous Tissue Substitute, Anterior Approach, Anterior Column, Open Approach
    HAC   When reported with secondary diagnosis code T84.60XA, T84.610A, T84.611A, T84.612A, T84.613A, T84.614A, T84.615A, T84.619A, T84.63XA, T84.69XA, T84.7XXA

0RG10K1   Fusion of Cervical Vertebral Joint with Nonautologous Tissue Substitute, Posterior Approach, Posterior Column, Open Approach
    HAC   When reported with secondary diagnosis code T84.60XA, T84.610A, T84.611A, T84.612A, T84.613A, T84.614A, T84.615A, T84.619A, T84.63XA, T84.69XA, T84.7XXA

0RG10KJ   Fusion of Cervical Vertebral Joint with Nonautologous Tissue Substitute, Posterior Approach, Anterior Column, Open Approach
    HAC   When reported with secondary diagnosis code T84.60XA, T84.610A, T84.611A, T84.612A, T84.613A, T84.614A, T84.615A, T84.619A, T84.63XA, T84.69XA, T84.7XXA

0RG10Z0   Fusion of Cervical Vertebral Joint, Anterior Approach, Anterior Column, Open Approach
    HAC   When reported with secondary diagnosis code T84.60XA, T84.610A, T84.611A, T84.612A, T84.613A, T84.614A, T84.615A, T84.619A, T84.63XA, T84.69XA, T84.7XXA

0RG10Z1   Fusion of Cervical Vertebral Joint, Posterior Approach, Posterior Column, Open Approach
    HAC   When reported with secondary diagnosis code T84.60XA, T84.610A, T84.611A, T84.612A, T84.613A, T84.614A, T84.615A, T84.619A, T84.63XA, T84.69XA, T84.7XXA

0RG10ZJ   Fusion of Cervical Vertebral Joint, Posterior Approach, Anterior Column, Open Approach
    HAC   When reported with secondary diagnosis code T84.60XA, T84.610A, T84.611A, T84.612A, T84.613A, T84.614A, T84.615A, T84.619A, T84.63XA, T84.69XA, T84.7XXA

0RG1370   Fusion of Cervical Vertebral Joint with Autologous Tissue Substitute, Anterior Approach, Anterior Column, Percutaneous Approach
> HAC   When reported with secondary diagnosis code T84.60XA, T84.610A, T84.611A, T84.612A, T84.613A, T84.614A, T84.615A, T84.619A, T84.63XA, T84.69XA, T84.7XXA

0RG1371   Fusion of Cervical Vertebral Joint with Autologous Tissue Substitute, Posterior Approach, Posterior Column, Percutaneous Approach
> HAC   When reported with secondary diagnosis code T84.60XA, T84.610A, T84.611A, T84.612A, T84.613A, T84.614A, T84.615A, T84.619A, T84.63XA, T84.69XA, T84.7XXA

0RG137J   Fusion of Cervical Vertebral Joint with Autologous Tissue Substitute, Posterior Approach, Anterior Column, Percutaneous Approach
> HAC   When reported with secondary diagnosis code T84.60XA, T84.610A, T84.611A, T84.612A, T84.613A, T84.614A, T84.615A, T84.619A, T84.63XA, T84.69XA, T84.7XXA

0RG13A0   Fusion of Cervical Vertebral Joint with Interbody Fusion Device, Anterior Approach, Anterior Column, Percutaneous Approach
> HAC   When reported with secondary diagnosis code T84.60XA, T84.610A, T84.611A, T84.612A, T84.613A, T84.614A, T84.615A, T84.619A, T84.63XA, T84.69XA, T84.7XXA

0RG13A1   Fusion of Cervical Vertebral Joint with Interbody Fusion Device, Posterior Approach, Posterior Column, Percutaneous Approach
> HAC   When reported with secondary diagnosis code T84.60XA, T84.610A, T84.611A, T84.612A, T84.613A, T84.614A, T84.615A, T84.619A, T84.63XA, T84.69XA, T84.7XXA

0RG13AJ   Fusion of Cervical Vertebral Joint with Interbody Fusion Device, Posterior Approach, Anterior Column, Percutaneous Approach
> HAC   When reported with secondary diagnosis code T84.60XA, T84.610A, T84.611A, T84.612A, T84.613A, T84.614A, T84.615A, T84.619A, T84.63XA, T84.69XA, T84.7XXA

0RG13J0   Fusion of Cervical Vertebral Joint with Synthetic Substitute, Anterior Approach, Anterior Column, Percutaneous Approach
> HAC   When reported with secondary diagnosis code T84.60XA, T84.610A, T84.611A, T84.612A, T84.613A, T84.614A, T84.615A, T84.619A, T84.63XA, T84.69XA, T84.7XXA

0RG13J1   Fusion of Cervical Vertebral Joint with Synthetic Substitute, Posterior Approach, Posterior Column, Percutaneous Approach
> HAC   When reported with secondary diagnosis code T84.60XA, T84.610A, T84.611A, T84.612A, T84.613A, T84.614A, T84.615A, T84.619A, T84.63XA, T84.69XA, T84.7XXA

0RG13JJ   Fusion of Cervical Vertebral Joint with Synthetic Substitute, Posterior Approach, Anterior Column, Percutaneous Approach
> HAC   When reported with secondary diagnosis code T84.60XA, T84.610A, T84.611A, T84.612A, T84.613A, T84.614A, T84.615A, T84.619A, T84.63XA, T84.69XA, T84.7XXA

0RG13K0   Fusion of Cervical Vertebral Joint with Nonautologous Tissue Substitute, Anterior Approach, Anterior Column, Percutaneous Approach
> HAC   When reported with secondary diagnosis code T84.60XA, T84.610A, T84.611A, T84.612A, T84.613A, T84.614A, T84.615A, T84.619A, T84.63XA, T84.69XA, T84.7XXA

0RG13K1   Fusion of Cervical Vertebral Joint with Nonautologous Tissue Substitute, Posterior Approach, Posterior Column, Percutaneous Approach
> HAC   When reported with secondary diagnosis code T84.60XA, T84.610A, T84.611A, T84.612A, T84.613A, T84.614A, T84.615A, T84.619A, T84.63XA, T84.69XA, T84.7XXA

0RG13KJ   Fusion of Cervical Vertebral Joint with Nonautologous Tissue Substitute, Posterior Approach, Anterior Column, Percutaneous Approach
> HAC   When reported with secondary diagnosis code T84.60XA, T84.610A, T84.611A, T84.612A, T84.613A, T84.614A, T84.615A, T84.619A, T84.63XA, T84.69XA, T84.7XXA

0RG13Z0   Fusion of Cervical Vertebral Joint, Anterior Approach, Anterior Column, Percutaneous Approach
> HAC   When reported with secondary diagnosis code T84.60XA, T84.610A, T84.611A, T84.612A, T84.613A, T84.614A, T84.615A, T84.619A, T84.63XA, T84.69XA, T84.7XXA

0RG13Z1   Fusion of Cervical Vertebral Joint, Posterior Approach, Posterior Column, Percutaneous Approach
> HAC   When reported with secondary diagnosis code T84.60XA, T84.610A, T84.611A, T84.612A, T84.613A, T84.614A, T84.615A, T84.619A, T84.63XA, T84.69XA, T84.7XXA

0RG13ZJ   Fusion of Cervical Vertebral Joint, Posterior Approach, Anterior Column, Percutaneous Approach
> HAC   When reported with secondary diagnosis code T84.60XA, T84.610A, T84.611A, T84.612A, T84.613A, T84.614A, T84.615A, T84.619A, T84.63XA, T84.69XA, T84.7XXA

0RG1470   Fusion of Cervical Vertebral Joint with Autologous Tissue Substitute, Anterior Approach, Anterior Column, Percutaneous Endoscopic Approach
> HAC   When reported with secondary diagnosis code T84.60XA, T84.610A, T84.611A, T84.612A, T84.613A, T84.614A, T84.615A, T84.619A, T84.63XA, T84.69XA, T84.7XXA

0RG1471   Fusion of Cervical Vertebral Joint with Autologous Tissue Substitute, Posterior Approach, Posterior Column, Percutaneous Endoscopic Approach
> HAC   When reported with secondary diagnosis code T84.60XA, T84.610A, T84.611A, T84.612A, T84.613A, T84.614A, T84.615A, T84.619A, T84.63XA, T84.69XA, T84.7XXA

0RG147J   Fusion of Cervical Vertebral Joint with Autologous Tissue Substitute, Posterior Approach, Anterior Column, Percutaneous Endoscopic Approach
> HAC   When reported with secondary diagnosis code T84.60XA, T84.610A, T84.611A, T84.612A, T84.613A, T84.614A, T84.615A, T84.619A, T84.63XA, T84.69XA, T84.7XXA

0RG14A0   Fusion of Cervical Vertebral Joint with Interbody Fusion Device, Anterior Approach, Anterior Column, Percutaneous Endoscopic Approach
> HAC   When reported with secondary diagnosis code T84.60XA, T84.610A, T84.611A, T84.612A, T84.613A, T84.614A, T84.615A, T84.619A, T84.63XA, T84.69XA, T84.7XXA

0RG14A1   Fusion of Cervical Vertebral Joint with Interbody Fusion Device, Posterior Approach, Posterior Column, Percutaneous Endoscopic Approach
> HAC   When reported with secondary diagnosis code T84.60XA, T84.610A, T84.611A, T84.612A, T84.613A, T84.614A, T84.615A, T84.619A, T84.63XA, T84.69XA, T84.7XXA

0RG14AJ   Fusion of Cervical Vertebral Joint with Interbody Fusion Device, Posterior Approach, Anterior Column, Percutaneous Endoscopic Approach
> HAC   When reported with secondary diagnosis code T84.60XA, T84.610A, T84.611A, T84.612A, T84.613A, T84.614A, T84.615A, T84.619A, T84.63XA, T84.69XA, T84.7XXA

0RG14J0   Fusion of Cervical Vertebral Joint with Synthetic Substitute, Anterior Approach, Anterior Column, Percutaneous Endoscopic Approach
> HAC   When reported with secondary diagnosis code T84.60XA, T84.610A, T84.611A, T84.612A, T84.613A, T84.614A, T84.615A, T84.619A, T84.63XA, T84.69XA, T84.7XXA

0RG14J1   Fusion of Cervical Vertebral Joint with Synthetic Substitute, Posterior Approach, Posterior Column, Percutaneous Endoscopic Approach
> HAC   When reported with secondary diagnosis code T84.60XA, T84.610A, T84.611A, T84.612A, T84.613A, T84.614A, T84.615A, T84.619A, T84.63XA, T84.69XA, T84.7XXA

0RG14JJ   Fusion of Cervical Vertebral Joint with Synthetic Substitute, Posterior Approach, Anterior Column, Percutaneous Endoscopic Approach
> HAC   When reported with secondary diagnosis code T84.60XA, T84.610A, T84.611A, T84.612A, T84.613A, T84.614A, T84.615A, T84.619A, T84.63XA, T84.69XA, T84.7XXA

0RG14K0   Fusion of Cervical Vertebral Joint with Nonautologous Tissue Substitute, Anterior Approach, Anterior Column, Percutaneous Endoscopic Approach
> HAC   When reported with secondary diagnosis code T84.60XA, T84.610A, T84.611A, T84.612A, T84.613A, T84.614A, T84.615A, T84.619A, T84.63XA, T84.69XA, T84.7XXA

0RG14K1   Fusion of Cervical Vertebral Joint with Nonautologous Tissue Substitute, Posterior Approach, Posterior Column, Percutaneous Endoscopic Approach
> HAC   When reported with secondary diagnosis code T84.60XA, T84.610A, T84.611A, T84.612A, T84.613A, T84.614A, T84.615A, T84.619A, T84.63XA, T84.69XA, T84.7XXA

0RG14KJ   Fusion of Cervical Vertebral Joint with Nonautologous Tissue Substitute, Posterior Approach, Anterior Column, Percutaneous Endoscopic Approach
> HAC   When reported with secondary diagnosis code T84.60XA, T84.610A, T84.611A, T84.612A, T84.613A, T84.614A, T84.615A, T84.619A, T84.63XA, T84.69XA, T84.7XXA

0RG14Z0 Fusion of Cervical Vertebral Joint, Anterior Approach, Anterior Column, Percutaneous Endoscopic Approach

HAC When reported with secondary diagnosis code T84.60XA, T84.610A, T84.611A, T84.612A, T84.613A, T84.614A, T84.615A, T84.619A, T84.63XA, T84.69XA, T84.7XXA

0RG14Z1 Fusion of Cervical Vertebral Joint, Posterior Approach, Posterior Column, Percutaneous Endoscopic Approach

HAC When reported with secondary diagnosis code T84.60XA, T84.610A, T84.611A, T84.612A, T84.613A, T84.614A, T84.615A, T84.619A, T84.63XA, T84.69XA, T84.7XXA

0RG14ZJ Fusion of Cervical Vertebral Joint, Posterior Approach, Anterior Column, Percutaneous Endoscopic Approach

HAC When reported with secondary diagnosis code T84.60XA, T84.610A, T84.611A, T84.612A, T84.613A, T84.614A, T84.615A, T84.619A, T84.63XA, T84.69XA, T84.7XXA

0RG2070 Fusion of 2 or more Cervical Vertebral Joints with Autologous Tissue Substitute, Anterior Approach, Anterior Column, Open Approach

HAC When reported with secondary diagnosis code T84.60XA, T84.610A, T84.611A, T84.612A, T84.613A, T84.614A, T84.615A, T84.619A, T84.63XA, T84.69XA, T84.7XXA

0RG2071 Fusion of 2 or more Cervical Vertebral Joints with Autologous Tissue Substitute, Posterior Approach, Posterior Column, Open Approach

HAC When reported with secondary diagnosis code T84.60XA, T84.610A, T84.611A, T84.612A, T84.613A, T84.614A, T84.615A, T84.619A, T84.63XA, T84.69XA, T84.7XXA

0RG207J Fusion of 2 or more Cervical Vertebral Joints with Autologous Tissue Substitute, Posterior Approach, Anterior Column, Open Approach

HAC When reported with secondary diagnosis code T84.60XA, T84.610A, T84.611A, T84.612A, T84.613A, T84.614A, T84.615A, T84.619A, T84.63XA, T84.69XA, T84.7XXA

0RG20A0 Fusion of 2 or more Cervical Vertebral Joints with Interbody Fusion Device, Anterior Approach, Anterior Column, Open Approach

HAC When reported with secondary diagnosis code T84.60XA, T84.610A, T84.611A, T84.612A, T84.613A, T84.614A, T84.615A, T84.619A, T84.63XA, T84.69XA, T84.7XXA

0RG20A1 Fusion of 2 or more Cervical Vertebral Joints with Interbody Fusion Device, Posterior Approach, Posterior Column, Open Approach

HAC When reported with secondary diagnosis code T84.60XA, T84.610A, T84.611A, T84.612A, T84.613A, T84.614A, T84.615A, T84.619A, T84.63XA, T84.69XA, T84.7XXA

0RG20AJ Fusion of 2 or more Cervical Vertebral Joints with Interbody Fusion Device, Posterior Approach, Anterior Column, Open Approach

HAC When reported with secondary diagnosis code T84.60XA, T84.610A, T84.611A, T84.612A, T84.613A, T84.614A, T84.615A, T84.619A, T84.63XA, T84.69XA, T84.7XXA

0RG20J0 Fusion of 2 or more Cervical Vertebral Joints with Synthetic Substitute, Anterior Approach, Anterior Column, Open Approach

HAC When reported with secondary diagnosis code T84.60XA, T84.610A, T84.611A, T84.612A, T84.613A, T84.614A, T84.615A, T84.619A, T84.63XA, T84.69XA, T84.7XXA

0RG20J1 Fusion of 2 or more Cervical Vertebral Joints with Synthetic Substitute, Posterior Approach, Posterior Column, Open Approach

HAC When reported with secondary diagnosis code T84.60XA, T84.610A, T84.611A, T84.612A, T84.613A, T84.614A, T84.615A, T84.619A, T84.63XA, T84.69XA, T84.7XXA

0RG20JJ Fusion of 2 or more Cervical Vertebral Joints with Synthetic Substitute, Posterior Approach, Anterior Column, Open Approach

HAC When reported with secondary diagnosis code T84.60XA, T84.610A, T84.611A, T84.612A, T84.613A, T84.614A, T84.615A, T84.619A, T84.63XA, T84.69XA, T84.7XXA

0RG20K0 Fusion of 2 or more Cervical Vertebral Joints with Nonautologous Tissue Substitute, Anterior Approach, Anterior Column, Open Approach

HAC When reported with secondary diagnosis code T84.60XA, T84.610A, T84.611A, T84.612A, T84.613A, T84.614A, T84.615A, T84.619A, T84.63XA, T84.69XA, T84.7XXA

0RG20K1 Fusion of 2 or more Cervical Vertebral Joints with Nonautologous Tissue Substitute, Posterior Approach, Posterior Column, Open Approach

HAC When reported with secondary diagnosis code T84.60XA, T84.610A, T84.611A, T84.612A, T84.613A, T84.614A, T84.615A, T84.619A, T84.63XA, T84.69XA, T84.7XXA

0RG20KJ Fusion of 2 or more Cervical Vertebral Joints with Nonautologous Tissue Substitute, Posterior Approach, Anterior Column, Open Approach

HAC When reported with secondary diagnosis code T84.60XA, T84.610A, T84.611A, T84.612A, T84.613A, T84.614A, T84.615A, T84.619A, T84.63XA, T84.69XA, T84.7XXA

0RG20Z0 Fusion of 2 or more Cervical Vertebral Joints, Anterior Approach, Anterior Column, Open Approach

HAC When reported with secondary diagnosis code T84.60XA, T84.610A, T84.611A, T84.612A, T84.613A, T84.614A, T84.615A, T84.619A, T84.63XA, T84.69XA, T84.7XXA

0RG20Z1 Fusion of 2 or more Cervical Vertebral Joints, Posterior Approach, Posterior Column, Open Approach

HAC When reported with secondary diagnosis code T84.60XA, T84.610A, T84.611A, T84.612A, T84.613A, T84.614A, T84.615A, T84.619A, T84.63XA, T84.69XA, T84.7XXA

0RG20ZJ Fusion of 2 or more Cervical Vertebral Joints, Posterior Approach, Anterior Column, Open Approach

HAC When reported with secondary diagnosis code T84.60XA, T84.610A, T84.611A, T84.612A, T84.613A, T84.614A, T84.615A, T84.619A, T84.63XA, T84.69XA, T84.7XXA

0RG2370 Fusion of 2 or more Cervical Vertebral Joints with Autologous Tissue Substitute, Anterior Approach, Anterior Column, Percutaneous Approach

HAC When reported with secondary diagnosis code T84.60XA, T84.610A, T84.611A, T84.612A, T84.613A, T84.614A, T84.615A, T84.619A, T84.63XA, T84.69XA, T84.7XXA

0RG2371 Fusion of 2 or more Cervical Vertebral Joints with Autologous Tissue Substitute, Posterior Approach, Posterior Column, Percutaneous Approach

HAC When reported with secondary diagnosis code T84.60XA, T84.610A, T84.611A, T84.612A, T84.613A, T84.614A, T84.615A, T84.619A, T84.63XA, T84.69XA, T84.7XXA

0RG237J Fusion of 2 or more Cervical Vertebral Joints with Autologous Tissue Substitute, Posterior Approach, Anterior Column, Percutaneous Approach

HAC When reported with secondary diagnosis code T84.60XA, T84.610A, T84.611A, T84.612A, T84.613A, T84.614A, T84.615A, T84.619A, T84.63XA, T84.69XA, T84.7XXA

0RG23A0 Fusion of 2 or more Cervical Vertebral Joints with Interbody Fusion Device, Anterior Approach, Anterior Column, Percutaneous Approach

HAC When reported with secondary diagnosis code T84.60XA, T84.610A, T84.611A, T84.612A, T84.613A, T84.614A, T84.615A, T84.619A, T84.63XA, T84.69XA, T84.7XXA

0RG23A1 Fusion of 2 or more Cervical Vertebral Joints with Interbody Fusion Device, Posterior Approach, Posterior Column, Percutaneous Approach

HAC When reported with secondary diagnosis code T84.60XA, T84.610A, T84.611A, T84.612A, T84.613A, T84.614A, T84.615A, T84.619A, T84.63XA, T84.69XA, T84.7XXA

0RG23AJ Fusion of 2 or more Cervical Vertebral Joints with Interbody Fusion Device, Posterior Approach, Anterior Column, Percutaneous Approach

HAC When reported with secondary diagnosis code T84.60XA, T84.610A, T84.611A, T84.612A, T84.613A, T84.614A, T84.615A, T84.619A, T84.63XA, T84.69XA, T84.7XXA

0RG23J0 Fusion of 2 or more Cervical Vertebral Joints with Synthetic Substitute, Anterior Approach, Anterior Column, Percutaneous Approach

HAC When reported with secondary diagnosis code T84.60XA, T84.610A, T84.611A, T84.612A, T84.613A, T84.614A, T84.615A, T84.619A, T84.63XA, T84.69XA, T84.7XXA

0RG23J1 Fusion of 2 or more Cervical Vertebral Joints with Synthetic Substitute, Posterior Approach, Posterior Column, Percutaneous Approach

HAC When reported with secondary diagnosis code T84.60XA, T84.610A, T84.611A, T84.612A, T84.613A, T84.614A, T84.615A, T84.619A, T84.63XA, T84.69XA, T84.7XXA

0RG23JJ Fusion of 2 or more Cervical Vertebral Joints with Synthetic Substitute, Posterior Approach, Anterior Column, Percutaneous Approach

HAC When reported with secondary diagnosis code T84.60XA, T84.610A, T84.611A, T84.612A, T84.613A, T84.614A, T84.615A, T84.619A, T84.63XA, T84.69XA, T84.7XXA

♀ Female-only   ♂ Male-only   ● Limited Coverage   ● Non-OR   HAC HAC-associated procedure   ● Non-covered procedures   ✚ Combination

0RG23K0 Fusion of 2 or more Cervical Vertebral Joints with Nonautologous Tissue Substitute, Anterior Approach, Anterior Column, Percutaneous Approach

HAC When reported with secondary diagnosis code T84.60XA, T84.610A, T84.611A, T84.612A, T84.613A, T84.614A, T84.615A, T84.619A, T84.63XA, T84.69XA, T84.7XXA

0RG23K1 Fusion of 2 or more Cervical Vertebral Joints with Nonautologous Tissue Substitute, Posterior Approach, Posterior Column, Percutaneous Approach

HAC When reported with secondary diagnosis code T84.60XA, T84.610A, T84.611A, T84.612A, T84.613A, T84.614A, T84.615A, T84.619A, T84.63XA, T84.69XA, T84.7XXA

0RG23KJ Fusion of 2 or more Cervical Vertebral Joints with Nonautologous Tissue Substitute, Posterior Approach, Anterior Column, Percutaneous Approach

HAC When reported with secondary diagnosis code T84.60XA, T84.610A, T84.611A, T84.612A, T84.613A, T84.614A, T84.615A, T84.619A, T84.63XA, T84.69XA, T84.7XXA

0RG23Z0 Fusion of 2 or more Cervical Vertebral Joints, Anterior Approach, Anterior Column, Percutaneous Approach

HAC When reported with secondary diagnosis code T84.60XA, T84.610A, T84.611A, T84.612A, T84.613A, T84.614A, T84.615A, T84.619A, T84.63XA, T84.69XA, T84.7XXA

0RG23Z1 Fusion of 2 or more Cervical Vertebral Joints, Posterior Approach, Posterior Column, Percutaneous Approach

HAC When reported with secondary diagnosis code T84.60XA, T84.610A, T84.611A, T84.612A, T84.613A, T84.614A, T84.615A, T84.619A, T84.63XA, T84.69XA, T84.7XXA

0RG23ZJ Fusion of 2 or more Cervical Vertebral Joints, Posterior Approach, Anterior Column, Percutaneous Approach

HAC When reported with secondary diagnosis code T84.60XA, T84.610A, T84.611A, T84.612A, T84.613A, T84.614A, T84.615A, T84.619A, T84.63XA, T84.69XA, T84.7XXA

0RG2470 Fusion of 2 or more Cervical Vertebral Joints with Autologous Tissue Substitute, Anterior Approach, Anterior Column, Percutaneous Endoscopic Approach

HAC When reported with secondary diagnosis code T84.60XA, T84.610A, T84.611A, T84.612A, T84.613A, T84.614A, T84.615A, T84.619A, T84.63XA, T84.69XA, T84.7XXA

0RG2471 Fusion of 2 or more Cervical Vertebral Joints with Autologous Tissue Substitute, Posterior Approach, Posterior Column, Percutaneous Endoscopic Approach

HAC When reported with secondary diagnosis code T84.60XA, T84.610A, T84.611A, T84.612A, T84.613A, T84.614A, T84.615A, T84.619A, T84.63XA, T84.69XA, T84.7XXA

0RG247J Fusion of 2 or more Cervical Vertebral Joints with Autologous Tissue Substitute, Posterior Approach, Anterior Column, Percutaneous Endoscopic Approach

HAC When reported with secondary diagnosis code T84.60XA, T84.610A, T84.611A, T84.612A, T84.613A, T84.614A, T84.615A, T84.619A, T84.63XA, T84.69XA, T84.7XXA

0RG24A0 Fusion of 2 or more Cervical Vertebral Joints with Interbody Fusion Device, Anterior Approach, Anterior Column, Percutaneous Endoscopic Approach

HAC When reported with secondary diagnosis code T84.60XA, T84.610A, T84.611A, T84.612A, T84.613A, T84.614A, T84.615A, T84.619A, T84.63XA, T84.69XA, T84.7XXA

0RG24A1 Fusion of 2 or more Cervical Vertebral Joints with Interbody Fusion Device, Posterior Approach, Posterior Column, Percutaneous Endoscopic Approach

HAC When reported with secondary diagnosis code T84.60XA, T84.610A, T84.611A, T84.612A, T84.613A, T84.614A, T84.615A, T84.619A, T84.63XA, T84.69XA, T84.7XXA

0RG24AJ Fusion of 2 or more Cervical Vertebral Joints with Interbody Fusion Device, Posterior Approach, Anterior Column, Percutaneous Endoscopic Approach

HAC When reported with secondary diagnosis code T84.60XA, T84.610A, T84.611A, T84.612A, T84.613A, T84.614A, T84.615A, T84.619A, T84.63XA, T84.69XA, T84.7XXA

0RG24J0 Fusion of 2 or more Cervical Vertebral Joints with Synthetic Substitute, Anterior Approach, Anterior Column, Percutaneous Endoscopic Approach

HAC When reported with secondary diagnosis code T84.60XA, T84.610A, T84.611A, T84.612A, T84.613A, T84.614A, T84.615A, T84.619A, T84.63XA, T84.69XA, T84.7XXA

0RG24J1 Fusion of 2 or more Cervical Vertebral Joints with Synthetic Substitute, Posterior Approach, Posterior Column, Percutaneous Endoscopic Approach

HAC When reported with secondary diagnosis code T84.60XA, T84.610A, T84.611A, T84.612A, T84.613A, T84.614A, T84.615A, T84.619A, T84.63XA, T84.69XA, T84.7XXA

0RG24JJ Fusion of 2 or more Cervical Vertebral Joints with Synthetic Substitute, Posterior Approach, Anterior Column, Percutaneous Endoscopic Approach

HAC When reported with secondary diagnosis code T84.60XA, T84.610A, T84.611A, T84.612A, T84.613A, T84.614A, T84.615A, T84.619A, T84.63XA, T84.69XA, T84.7XXA

0RG24K0 Fusion of 2 or more Cervical Vertebral Joints with Nonautologous Tissue Substitute, Anterior Approach, Anterior Column, Percutaneous Endoscopic Approach

HAC When reported with secondary diagnosis code T84.60XA, T84.610A, T84.611A, T84.612A, T84.613A, T84.614A, T84.615A, T84.619A, T84.63XA, T84.69XA, T84.7XXA

0RG24K1 Fusion of 2 or more Cervical Vertebral Joints with Nonautologous Tissue Substitute, Posterior Approach, Posterior Column, Percutaneous Endoscopic Approach

HAC When reported with secondary diagnosis code T84.60XA, T84.610A, T84.611A, T84.612A, T84.613A, T84.614A, T84.615A, T84.619A, T84.63XA, T84.69XA, T84.7XXA

0RG24KJ Fusion of 2 or more Cervical Vertebral Joints with Nonautologous Tissue Substitute, Posterior Approach, Anterior Column, Percutaneous Endoscopic Approach

HAC When reported with secondary diagnosis code T84.60XA, T84.610A, T84.611A, T84.612A, T84.613A, T84.614A, T84.615A, T84.619A, T84.63XA, T84.69XA, T84.7XXA

0RG24Z0 Fusion of 2 or more Cervical Vertebral Joints, Anterior Approach, Anterior Column, Percutaneous Endoscopic Approach

HAC When reported with secondary diagnosis code T84.60XA, T84.610A, T84.611A, T84.612A, T84.613A, T84.614A, T84.615A, T84.619A, T84.63XA, T84.69XA, T84.7XXA

0RG24Z1 Fusion of 2 or more Cervical Vertebral Joints, Posterior Approach, Posterior Column, Percutaneous Endoscopic Approach

HAC When reported with secondary diagnosis code T84.60XA, T84.610A, T84.611A, T84.612A, T84.613A, T84.614A, T84.615A, T84.619A, T84.63XA, T84.69XA, T84.7XXA

0RG24ZJ Fusion of 2 or more Cervical Vertebral Joints, Posterior Approach, Anterior Column, Percutaneous Endoscopic Approach

HAC When reported with secondary diagnosis code T84.60XA, T84.610A, T84.611A, T84.612A, T84.613A, T84.614A, T84.615A, T84.619A, T84.63XA, T84.69XA, T84.7XXA

0RG4070 Fusion of Cervicothoracic Vertebral Joint with Autologous Tissue Substitute, Anterior Approach, Anterior Column, Open Approach

HAC When reported with secondary diagnosis code T84.60XA, T84.610A, T84.611A, T84.612A, T84.613A, T84.614A, T84.615A, T84.619A, T84.63XA, T84.69XA, T84.7XXA

0RG4071 Fusion of Cervicothoracic Vertebral Joint with Autologous Tissue Substitute, Posterior Approach, Posterior Column, Open Approach

HAC When reported with secondary diagnosis code T84.60XA, T84.610A, T84.611A, T84.612A, T84.613A, T84.614A, T84.615A, T84.619A, T84.63XA, T84.69XA, T84.7XXA

0RG407J Fusion of Cervicothoracic Vertebral Joint with Autologous Tissue Substitute, Posterior Approach, Anterior Column, Open Approach

HAC When reported with secondary diagnosis code T84.60XA, T84.610A, T84.611A, T84.612A, T84.613A, T84.614A, T84.615A, T84.619A, T84.63XA, T84.69XA, T84.7XXA

0RG40A0 Fusion of Cervicothoracic Vertebral Joint with Interbody Fusion Device, Anterior Approach, Anterior Column, Open Approach

HAC When reported with secondary diagnosis code T84.60XA, T84.610A, T84.611A, T84.612A, T84.613A, T84.614A, T84.615A, T84.619A, T84.63XA, T84.69XA, T84.7XXA

0RG40A1 Fusion of Cervicothoracic Vertebral Joint with Interbody Fusion Device, Posterior Approach, Posterior Column, Open Approach

HAC When reported with secondary diagnosis code T84.60XA, T84.610A, T84.611A, T84.612A, T84.613A, T84.614A, T84.615A, T84.619A, T84.63XA, T84.69XA, T84.7XXA

0RG40AJ Fusion of Cervicothoracic Vertebral Joint with Interbody Fusion Device, Posterior Approach, Anterior Column, Open Approach

HAC When reported with secondary diagnosis code T84.60XA, T84.610A, T84.611A, T84.612A, T84.613A, T84.614A, T84.615A, T84.619A, T84.63XA, T84.69XA, T84.7XXA

♀ Female-only   ♂ Male-only   ● Limited Coverage   ● Non-OR   HAC HAC-associated procedure   ● Non-covered procedures   ✚ Combination

0RG40J0   Fusion of Cervicothoracic Vertebral Joint with Synthetic Substitute, Anterior Approach, Anterior Column, Open Approach

HAC   When reported with secondary diagnosis code T84.60XA, T84.610A, T84.611A, T84.612A, T84.613A, T84.614A, T84.615A, T84.619A, T84.63XA, T84.69XA, T84.7XXA

0RG40J1   Fusion of Cervicothoracic Vertebral Joint with Synthetic Substitute, Posterior Approach, Posterior Column, Open Approach

HAC   When reported with secondary diagnosis code T84.60XA, T84.610A, T84.611A, T84.612A, T84.613A, T84.614A, T84.615A, T84.619A, T84.63XA, T84.69XA, T84.7XXA

0RG40JJ   Fusion of Cervicothoracic Vertebral Joint with Synthetic Substitute, Posterior Approach, Anterior Column, Open Approach

HAC   When reported with secondary diagnosis code T84.60XA, T84.610A, T84.611A, T84.612A, T84.613A, T84.614A, T84.615A, T84.619A, T84.63XA, T84.69XA, T84.7XXA

0RG40K0   Fusion of Cervicothoracic Vertebral Joint with Nonautologous Tissue Substitute, Anterior Approach, Anterior Column, Open Approach

HAC   When reported with secondary diagnosis code T84.60XA, T84.610A, T84.611A, T84.612A, T84.613A, T84.614A, T84.615A, T84.619A, T84.63XA, T84.69XA, T84.7XXA

0RG40K1   Fusion of Cervicothoracic Vertebral Joint with Nonautologous Tissue Substitute, Posterior Approach, Posterior Column, Open Approach

HAC   When reported with secondary diagnosis code T84.60XA, T84.610A, T84.611A, T84.612A, T84.613A, T84.614A, T84.615A, T84.619A, T84.63XA, T84.69XA, T84.7XXA

0RG40KJ   Fusion of Cervicothoracic Vertebral Joint with Nonautologous Tissue Substitute, Posterior Approach, Anterior Column, Open Approach

HAC   When reported with secondary diagnosis code T84.60XA, T84.610A, T84.611A, T84.612A, T84.613A, T84.614A, T84.615A, T84.619A, T84.63XA, T84.69XA, T84.7XXA

0RG40Z0   Fusion of Cervicothoracic Vertebral Joint, Anterior Approach, Anterior Column, Open Approach

HAC   When reported with secondary diagnosis code T84.60XA, T84.610A, T84.611A, T84.612A, T84.613A, T84.614A, T84.615A, T84.619A, T84.63XA, T84.69XA, T84.7XXA

0RG40Z1   Fusion of Cervicothoracic Vertebral Joint, Posterior Approach, Posterior Column, Open Approach

HAC   When reported with secondary diagnosis code T84.60XA, T84.610A, T84.611A, T84.612A, T84.613A, T84.614A, T84.615A, T84.619A, T84.63XA, T84.69XA, T84.7XXA

0RG40ZJ   Fusion of Cervicothoracic Vertebral Joint, Posterior Approach, Anterior Column, Open Approach

HAC   When reported with secondary diagnosis code T84.60XA, T84.610A, T84.611A, T84.612A, T84.613A, T84.614A, T84.615A, T84.619A, T84.63XA, T84.69XA, T84.7XXA

0RG4370   Fusion of Cervicothoracic Vertebral Joint with Autologous Tissue Substitute, Anterior Approach, Anterior Column, Percutaneous Approach

HAC   When reported with secondary diagnosis code T84.60XA, T84.610A, T84.611A, T84.612A, T84.613A, T84.614A, T84.615A, T84.619A, T84.63XA, T84.69XA, T84.7XXA

0RG4371   Fusion of Cervicothoracic Vertebral Joint with Autologous Tissue Substitute, Posterior Approach, Posterior Column, Percutaneous Approach

HAC   When reported with secondary diagnosis code T84.60XA, T84.610A, T84.611A, T84.612A, T84.613A, T84.614A, T84.615A, T84.619A, T84.63XA, T84.69XA, T84.7XXA

0RG437J   Fusion of Cervicothoracic Vertebral Joint with Autologous Tissue Substitute, Posterior Approach, Anterior Column, Percutaneous Approach

HAC   When reported with secondary diagnosis code T84.60XA, T84.610A, T84.611A, T84.612A, T84.613A, T84.614A, T84.615A, T84.619A, T84.63XA, T84.69XA, T84.7XXA

0RG43A0   Fusion of Cervicothoracic Vertebral Joint with Interbody Fusion Device, Anterior Approach, Anterior Column, Percutaneous Approach

HAC   When reported with secondary diagnosis code T84.60XA, T84.610A, T84.611A, T84.612A, T84.613A, T84.614A, T84.615A, T84.619A, T84.63XA, T84.69XA, T84.7XXA

0RG43A1   Fusion of Cervicothoracic Vertebral Joint with Interbody Fusion Device, Posterior Approach, Posterior Column, Percutaneous Approach

HAC   When reported with secondary diagnosis code T84.60XA, T84.610A, T84.611A, T84.612A, T84.613A, T84.614A, T84.615A, T84.619A, T84.63XA, T84.69XA, T84.7XXA

0RG43AJ   Fusion of Cervicothoracic Vertebral Joint with Interbody Fusion Device, Posterior Approach, Anterior Column, Percutaneous Approach

HAC   When reported with secondary diagnosis code T84.60XA, T84.610A, T84.611A, T84.612A, T84.613A, T84.614A, T84.615A, T84.619A, T84.63XA, T84.69XA, T84.7XXA

0RG43J0   Fusion of Cervicothoracic Vertebral Joint with Synthetic Substitute, Anterior Approach, Anterior Column, Percutaneous Approach

HAC   When reported with secondary diagnosis code T84.60XA, T84.610A, T84.611A, T84.612A, T84.613A, T84.614A, T84.615A, T84.619A, T84.63XA, T84.69XA, T84.7XXA

0RG43J1   Fusion of Cervicothoracic Vertebral Joint with Synthetic Substitute, Posterior Approach, Posterior Column, Percutaneous Approach

HAC   When reported with secondary diagnosis code T84.60XA, T84.610A, T84.611A, T84.612A, T84.613A, T84.614A, T84.615A, T84.619A, T84.63XA, T84.69XA, T84.7XXA

0RG43JJ   Fusion of Cervicothoracic Vertebral Joint with Synthetic Substitute, Posterior Approach, Anterior Column, Percutaneous Approach

HAC   When reported with secondary diagnosis code T84.60XA, T84.610A, T84.611A, T84.612A, T84.613A, T84.614A, T84.615A, T84.619A, T84.63XA, T84.69XA, T84.7XXA

0RG43K0   Fusion of Cervicothoracic Vertebral Joint with Nonautologous Tissue Substitute, Anterior Approach, Anterior Column, Percutaneous Approach

HAC   When reported with secondary diagnosis code T84.60XA, T84.610A, T84.611A, T84.612A, T84.613A, T84.614A, T84.615A, T84.619A, T84.63XA, T84.69XA, T84.7XXA

0RG43K1   Fusion of Cervicothoracic Vertebral Joint with Nonautologous Tissue Substitute, Posterior Approach, Posterior Column, Percutaneous Approach

HAC   When reported with secondary diagnosis code T84.60XA, T84.610A, T84.611A, T84.612A, T84.613A, T84.614A, T84.615A, T84.619A, T84.63XA, T84.69XA, T84.7XXA

0RG43KJ   Fusion of Cervicothoracic Vertebral Joint with Nonautologous Tissue Substitute, Posterior Approach, Anterior Column, Percutaneous Approach

HAC   When reported with secondary diagnosis code T84.60XA, T84.610A, T84.611A, T84.612A, T84.613A, T84.614A, T84.615A, T84.619A, T84.63XA, T84.69XA, T84.7XXA

0RG43Z0   Fusion of Cervicothoracic Vertebral Joint, Anterior Approach, Anterior Column, Percutaneous Approach

HAC   When reported with secondary diagnosis code T84.60XA, T84.610A, T84.611A, T84.612A, T84.613A, T84.614A, T84.615A, T84.619A, T84.63XA, T84.69XA, T84.7XXA

0RG43Z1   Fusion of Cervicothoracic Vertebral Joint, Posterior Approach, Posterior Column, Percutaneous Approach

HAC   When reported with secondary diagnosis code T84.60XA, T84.610A, T84.611A, T84.612A, T84.613A, T84.614A, T84.615A, T84.619A, T84.63XA, T84.69XA, T84.7XXA

0RG43ZJ   Fusion of Cervicothoracic Vertebral Joint, Posterior Approach, Anterior Column, Percutaneous Approach

HAC   When reported with secondary diagnosis code T84.60XA, T84.610A, T84.611A, T84.612A, T84.613A, T84.614A, T84.615A, T84.619A, T84.63XA, T84.69XA, T84.7XXA

0RG4470   Fusion of Cervicothoracic Vertebral Joint with Autologous Tissue Substitute, Anterior Approach, Anterior Column, Percutaneous Endoscopic Approach

HAC   When reported with secondary diagnosis code T84.60XA, T84.610A, T84.611A, T84.612A, T84.613A, T84.614A, T84.615A, T84.619A, T84.63XA, T84.69XA, T84.7XXA

0RG4471   Fusion of Cervicothoracic Vertebral Joint with Autologous Tissue Substitute, Posterior Approach, Posterior Column, Percutaneous Endoscopic Approach

HAC   When reported with secondary diagnosis code T84.60XA, T84.610A, T84.611A, T84.612A, T84.613A, T84.614A, T84.615A, T84.619A, T84.63XA, T84.69XA, T84.7XXA

0RG447J   Fusion of Cervicothoracic Vertebral Joint with Autologous Tissue Substitute, Posterior Approach, Anterior Column, Percutaneous Endoscopic Approach
- HAC   When reported with secondary diagnosis code T84.60XA, T84.610A. T84.611A, T84.612A, T84.613A, T84.614A, T84.615A, T84.619A. T84.63XA, T84.69XA, T84.7XXA

0RG44A0   Fusion of Cervicothoracic Vertebral Joint with Interbody Fusion Device, Anterior Approach, Anterior Column, Percutaneous Endoscopic Approach
- HAC   When reported with secondary diagnosis code T84.60XA, T84.610A, T84.611A, T84.612A, T84.613A, T84.614A, T84.615A, T84.619A, T84.63XA, T84.69XA, T84.7XXA

0RG44A1   Fusion of Cervicothoracic Vertebral Joint with Interbody Fusion Device, Posterior Approach, Posterior Column, Percutaneous Endoscopic Approach
- HAC   When reported with secondary diagnosis code T84.60XA, T84.610A, T84.611A, T84.612A, T84.613A, T84.614A, T84.615A, T84.619A, T84.63XA, T84.69XA, T84.7XXA

0RG44AJ   Fusion of Cervicothoracic Vertebral Joint with Interbody Fusion Device, Posterior Approach, Anterior Column, Percutaneous Endoscopic Approach
- HAC   When reported with secondary diagnosis code T84.60XA, T84.610A, T84.611A, T84.612A, T84.613A, T84.614A, T84.615A, T84.619A, T84.63XA, T84.69XA, T84.7XXA

0RG44J0   Fusion of Cervicothoracic Vertebral Joint with Synthetic Substitute, Anterior Approach, Anterior Column, Percutaneous Endoscopic Approach
- HAC   When reported with secondary diagnosis code T84.60XA, T84.610A, T84.611A, T84.612A, T84.613A, T84.614A, T84.615A, T84.619A, T84.63XA, T84.69XA, T84.7XXA

0RG44J1   Fusion of Cervicothoracic Vertebral Joint with Synthetic Substitute, Posterior Approach, Posterior Column, Percutaneous Endoscopic Approach
- HAC   When reported with secondary diagnosis code T84.60XA, T84.610A, T84.611A, T84.612A, T84.613A, T84.614A, T84.615A, T84.619A, T84.63XA, T84.69XA, T84.7XXA

0RG44JJ   Fusion of Cervicothoracic Vertebral Joint with Synthetic Substitute, Posterior Approach, Anterior Column, Percutaneous Endoscopic Approach
- HAC   When reported with secondary diagnosis code T84.60XA, T84.610A, T84.611A, T84.612A, T84.613A, T84.614A, T84.615A, T84.619A, T84.63XA, T84.69XA, T84.7XXA

0RG44K0   Fusion of Cervicothoracic Vertebral Joint with Nonautologous Tissue Substitute, Anterior Approach, Anterior Column, Percutaneous Endoscopic Approach
- HAC   When reported with secondary diagnosis code T84.60XA, T84.610A, T84.611A, T84.612A, T84.613A, T84.614A, T84.615A, T84.619A, T84.63XA, T84.69XA, T84.7XXA

0RG44K1   Fusion of Cervicothoracic Vertebral Joint with Nonautologous Tissue Substitute, Posterior Approach, Posterior Column, Percutaneous Endoscopic Approach
- HAC   When reported with secondary diagnosis code T84.60XA, T84.610A, T84.611A, T84.612A, T84.613A, T84.614A, T84.615A, T84.619A, T84.63XA, T84.69XA, T84.7XXA

0RG44KJ   Fusion of Cervicothoracic Vertebral Joint with Nonautologous Tissue Substitute, Posterior Approach, Anterior Column, Percutaneous Endoscopic Approach
- HAC   When reported with secondary diagnosis code T84.60XA, T84.610A, T84.611A, T84.612A, T84.613A, T84.614A, T84.615A, T84.619A, T84.63XA, T84.69XA, T84.7XXA

0RG44Z0   Fusion of Cervicothoracic Vertebral Joint, Anterior Approach, Anterior Column, Percutaneous Endoscopic Approach
- HAC   When reported with secondary diagnosis code T84.60XA, T84.610A, T84.611A, T84.612A, T84.613A, T84.614A, T84.615A, T84.619A, T84.63XA, T84.69XA, T84.7XXA

0RG44Z1   Fusion of Cervicothoracic Vertebral Joint, Posterior Approach, Posterior Column, Percutaneous Endoscopic Approach
- HAC   When reported with secondary diagnosis code T84.60XA, T84.610A, T84.611A, T84.612A, T84.613A, T84.614A, T84.615A, T84.619A, T84.63XA, T84.69XA, T84.7XXA

0RG44ZJ   Fusion of Cervicothoracic Vertebral Joint, Posterior Approach, Anterior Column, Percutaneous Endoscopic Approach
- HAC   When reported with secondary diagnosis code T84.60XA, T84.610A, T84.611A, T84.612A, T84.613A, T84.614A, T84.615A, T84.619A, T84.63XA, T84.69XA, T84.7XXA

0RG6070   Fusion of Thoracic Vertebral Joint with Autologous Tissue Substitute, Anterior Approach, Anterior Column, Open Approach
- HAC   When reported with secondary diagnosis code T84.60XA, T84.610A, T84.611A, T84.612A, T84.613A, T84.614A, T84.615A, T84.619A, T84.63XA, T84.69XA, T84.7XXA

0RG6071   Fusion of Thoracic Vertebral Joint with Autologous Tissue Substitute, Posterior Approach, Posterior Column, Open Approach
- HAC   When reported with secondary diagnosis code T84.60XA, T84.610A, T84.611A, T84.612A, T84.613A, T84.614A, T84.615A, T84.619A, T84.63XA, T84.69XA, T84.7XXA

0RG607J   Fusion of Thoracic Vertebral Joint with Autologous Tissue Substitute, Posterior Approach, Anterior Column, Open Approach
- HAC   When reported with secondary diagnosis code T84.60XA, T84.610A, T84.611A, T84.612A, T84.613A, T84.614A, T84.615A, T84.619A, T84.63XA, T84.69XA, T84.7XXA

0RG60A0   Fusion of Thoracic Vertebral Joint with Interbody Fusion Device, Anterior Approach, Anterior Column, Open Approach
- HAC   When reported with secondary diagnosis code T84.60XA, T84.610A, T84.611A, T84.612A, T84.613A, T84.614A, T84.615A, T84.619A, T84.63XA, T84.69XA, T84.7XXA

0RG60A1   Fusion of Thoracic Vertebral Joint with Interbody Fusion Device, Posterior Approach, Posterior Column, Open Approach
- HAC   When reported with secondary diagnosis code T84.60XA, T84.610A, T84.611A, T84.612A, T84.613A, T84.614A, T84.615A, T84.619A, T84.63XA, T84.69XA, T84.7XXA

0RG60AJ   Fusion of Thoracic Vertebral Joint with Interbody Fusion Device, Posterior Approach, Anterior Column, Open Approach
- HAC   When reported with secondary diagnosis code T84.60XA, T84.610A, T84.611A, T84.612A, T84.613A, T84.614A, T84.615A, T84.619A, T84.63XA, T84.69XA, T84.7XXA

0RG60J0   Fusion of Thoracic Vertebral Joint with Synthetic Substitute, Anterior Approach, Anterior Column, Open Approach
- HAC   When reported with secondary diagnosis code T84.60XA, T84.610A, T84.611A, T84.612A, T84.613A, T84.614A, T84.615A, T84.619A, T84.63XA, T84.69XA, T84.7XXA

0RG60J1   Fusion of Thoracic Vertebral Joint with Synthetic Substitute, Posterior Approach, Posterior Column, Open Approach
- HAC   When reported with secondary diagnosis code T84.60XA, T84.610A, T84.611A, T84.612A, T84.613A, T84.614A, T84.615A, T84.619A, T84.63XA, T84.69XA, T84.7XXA

0RG60JJ   Fusion of Thoracic Vertebral Joint with Synthetic Substitute, Posterior Approach, Anterior Column, Open Approach
- HAC   When reported with secondary diagnosis code T84.60XA, T84.610A, T84.611A, T84.612A, T84.613A, T84.614A, T84.615A, T84.619A, T84.63XA, T84.69XA, T84.7XXA

0RG60K0   Fusion of Thoracic Vertebral Joint with Nonautologous Tissue Substitute, Anterior Approach, Anterior Column, Open Approach
- HAC   When reported with secondary diagnosis code T84.60XA, T84.610A, T84.611A, T84.612A, T84.613A, T84.614A, T84.615A, T84.619A, T84.63XA, T84.69XA, T84.7XXA

0RG60K1   Fusion of Thoracic Vertebral Joint with Nonautologous Tissue Substitute, Posterior Approach, Posterior Column, Open Approach
- HAC   When reported with secondary diagnosis code T84.60XA, T84.610A, T84.611A, T84.612A, T84.613A, T84.614A, T84.615A, T84.619A, T84.63XA, T84.69XA, T84.7XXA

0RG60KJ   Fusion of Thoracic Vertebral Joint with Nonautologous Tissue Substitute, Posterior Approach, Anterior Column, Open Approach
- HAC   When reported with secondary diagnosis code T84.60XA, T84.610A, T84.611A, T84.612A, T84.613A, T84.614A, T84.615A, T84.619A, T84.63XA, T84.69XA, T84.7XXA

0RG60Z0   Fusion of Thoracic Vertebral Joint, Anterior Approach, Anterior Column, Open Approach
- HAC   When reported with secondary diagnosis code T84.60XA, T84.610A, T84.611A, T84.612A, T84.613A, T84.614A, T84.615A, T84.619A, T84.63XA, T84.69XA, T84.7XXA

0RG60Z1   Fusion of Thoracic Vertebral Joint, Posterior Approach, Posterior Column, Open Approach
- HAC   When reported with secondary diagnosis code T84.60XA, T84.610A, T84.611A, T84.612A, T84.613A, T84.614A, T84.615A, T84.619A, T84.63XA, T84.69XA, T84.7XXA

0RG60ZJ   Fusion of Thoracic Vertebral Joint, Posterior Approach, Anterior Column, Open Approach
- HAC   When reported with secondary diagnosis code T84.60XA, T84.610A, T84.611A, T84.612A, T84.613A, T84.614A, T84.615A, T84.619A, T84.63XA, T84.69XA, T84.7XXA

♀ Female-only   ♂ Male-only   ● Limited Coverage   ● Non-OR   HAC HAC-associated procedure   ● Non-covered procedures   + Combination

0RG6370 Fusion of Thoracic Vertebral Joint with Autologous Tissue Substitute, Anterior Approach, Anterior Column, Percutaneous Approach
- HAC When reported with secondary diagnosis code T84.60XA, T84.610A, T84.611A, T84.612A, T84.613A, T84.614A, T84.615A, T84.619A, T84.63XA, T84.69XA, T84.7XXA

0RG6371 Fusion of Thoracic Vertebral Joint with Autologous Tissue Substitute, Posterior Approach, Posterior Column, Percutaneous Approach
- HAC When reported with secondary diagnosis code T84.60XA, T84.610A, T84.611A, T84.612A, T84.613A, T84.614A, T84.615A, T84.619A, T84.63XA, T84.69XA, T84.7XXA

0RG637J Fusion of Thoracic Vertebral Joint with Autologous Tissue Substitute, Posterior Approach, Anterior Column, Percutaneous Approach
- HAC When reported with secondary diagnosis code T84.60XA, T84.610A, T84.611A, T84.612A, T84.613A, T84.614A, T84.615A, T84.619A, T84.63XA, T84.69XA, T84.7XXA

0RG63A0 Fusion of Thoracic Vertebral Joint with Interbody Fusion Device, Anterior Approach, Anterior Column, Percutaneous Approach
- HAC When reported with secondary diagnosis code T84.60XA, T84.610A, T84.611A, T84.612A, T84.613A, T84.614A, T84.615A, T84.619A, T84.63XA, T84.69XA, T84.7XXA

0RG63A1 Fusion of Thoracic Vertebral Joint with Interbody Fusion Device, Posterior Approach, Posterior Column, Percutaneous Approach
- HAC When reported with secondary diagnosis code T84.60XA, T84.610A, T84.611A, T84.612A, T84.613A, T84.614A, T84.615A, T84.619A, T84.63XA, T84.69XA, T84.7XXA

0RG63AJ Fusion of Thoracic Vertebral Joint with Interbody Fusion Device, Posterior Approach, Anterior Column, Percutaneous Approach
- HAC When reported with secondary diagnosis code T84.60XA, T84.610A, T84.611A, T84.612A, T84.613A, T84.614A, T84.615A, T84.619A, T84.63XA, T84.69XA, T84.7XXA

0RG63J0 Fusion of Thoracic Vertebral Joint with Synthetic Substitute, Anterior Approach, Anterior Column, Percutaneous Approach
- HAC When reported with secondary diagnosis code T84.60XA, T84.610A, T84.611A, T84.612A, T84.613A, T84.614A, T84.615A, T84.619A, T84.63XA, T84.69XA, T84.7XXA

0RG63J1 Fusion of Thoracic Vertebral Joint with Synthetic Substitute, Posterior Approach, Posterior Column, Percutaneous Approach
- HAC When reported with secondary diagnosis code T84.60XA, T84.610A, T84.611A, T84.612A, T84.613A, T84.614A, T84.615A, T84.619A, T84.63XA, T84.69XA, T84.7XXA

0RG63JJ Fusion of Thoracic Vertebral Joint with Synthetic Substitute, Posterior Approach, Anterior Column, Percutaneous Approach
- HAC When reported with secondary diagnosis code T84.60XA, T84.610A, T84.611A, T84.612A, T84.613A, T84.614A, T84.615A, T84.619A, T84.63XA, T84.69XA, T84.7XXA

0RG63K0 Fusion of Thoracic Vertebral Joint with Nonautologous Tissue Substitute, Anterior Approach, Anterior Column, Percutaneous Approach
- HAC When reported with secondary diagnosis code T84.60XA, T84.610A, T84.611A, T84.612A, T84.613A, T84.614A, T84.615A, T84.619A, T84.63XA, T84.69XA, T84.7XXA

0RG63K1 Fusion of Thoracic Vertebral Joint with Nonautologous Tissue Substitute, Posterior Approach, Posterior Column, Percutaneous Approach
- HAC When reported with secondary diagnosis code T84.60XA, T84.610A, T84.611A, T84.612A, T84.613A, T84.614A, T84.615A, T84.619A, T84.63XA, T84.69XA, T84.7XXA

0RG63KJ Fusion of Thoracic Vertebral Joint with Nonautologous Tissue Substitute, Posterior Approach, Anterior Column, Percutaneous Approach
- HAC When reported with secondary diagnosis code T84.60XA, T84.610A, T84.611A, T84.612A, T84.613A, T84.614A, T84.615A, T84.619A, T84.63XA, T84.69XA, T84.7XXA

0RG63Z0 Fusion of Thoracic Vertebral Joint, Anterior Approach, Anterior Column, Percutaneous Approach
- HAC When reported with secondary diagnosis code T84.60XA, T84.610A, T84.611A, T84.612A, T84.613A, T84.614A, T84.615A, T84.619A, T84.63XA, T84.69XA, T84.7XXA

0RG63Z1 Fusion of Thoracic Vertebral Joint, Posterior Approach, Posterior Column, Percutaneous Approach
- HAC When reported with secondary diagnosis code T84.60XA, T84.610A, T84.611A, T84.612A, T84.613A, T84.614A, T84.615A, T84.619A, T84.63XA, T84.69XA, T84.7XXA

0RG63ZJ Fusion of Thoracic Vertebral Joint, Posterior Approach, Anterior Column, Percutaneous Approach
- HAC When reported with secondary diagnosis code T84.60XA, T84.610A, T84.611A, T84.612A, T84.613A, T84.614A, T84.615A, T84.619A, T84.63XA, T84.69XA, T84.7XXA

0RG6470 Fusion of Thoracic Vertebral Joint with Autologous Tissue Substitute, Anterior Approach, Anterior Column, Percutaneous Endoscopic Approach
- HAC When reported with secondary diagnosis code T84.60XA, T84.610A, T84.611A, T84.612A, T84.613A, T84.614A, T84.615A, T84.619A, T84.63XA, T84.69XA, T84.7XXA

0RG6471 Fusion of Thoracic Vertebral Joint with Autologous Tissue Substitute, Posterior Approach, Posterior Column, Percutaneous Endoscopic Approach
- HAC When reported with secondary diagnosis code T84.60XA, T84.610A, T84.611A, T84.612A, T84.613A, T84.614A, T84.615A, T84.619A, T84.63XA, T84.69XA, T84.7XXA

0RG647J Fusion of Thoracic Vertebral Joint with Autologous Tissue Substitute, Posterior Approach, Anterior Column, Percutaneous Endoscopic Approach
- HAC When reported with secondary diagnosis code T84.60XA, T84.610A, T84.611A, T84.612A, T84.613A, T84.614A, T84.615A, T84.619A, T84.63XA, T84.69XA, T84.7XXA

0RG64A0 Fusion of Thoracic Vertebral Joint with Interbody Fusion Device, Anterior Approach, Anterior Column, Percutaneous Endoscopic Approach
- HAC When reported with secondary diagnosis code T84.60XA, T84.610A, T84.611A, T84.612A, T84.613A, T84.614A, T84.615A, T84.619A, T84.63XA, T84.69XA, T84.7XXA

0RG64A1 Fusion of Thoracic Vertebral Joint with Interbody Fusion Device, Posterior Approach, Posterior Column, Percutaneous Endoscopic Approach
- HAC When reported with secondary diagnosis code T84.60XA, T84.610A, T84.611A, T84.612A, T84.613A, T84.614A, T84.615A, T84.619A, T84.63XA, T84.69XA, T84.7XXA

0RG64AJ Fusion of Thoracic Vertebral Joint with Interbody Fusion Device, Posterior Approach, Anterior Column, Percutaneous Endoscopic Approach
- HAC When reported with secondary diagnosis code T84.60XA, T84.610A, T84.611A, T84.612A, T84.613A, T84.614A, T84.615A, T84.619A, T84.63XA, T84.69XA, T84.7XXA

0RG64J0 Fusion of Thoracic Vertebral Joint with Synthetic Substitute, Anterior Approach, Anterior Column, Percutaneous Endoscopic Approach
- HAC When reported with secondary diagnosis code T84.60XA, T84.610A, T84.611A, T84.612A, T84.613A, T84.614A, T84.615A, T84.619A, T84.63XA, T84.69XA, T84.7XXA

0RG64J1 Fusion of Thoracic Vertebral Joint with Synthetic Substitute, Posterior Approach, Posterior Column, Percutaneous Endoscopic Approach
- HAC When reported with secondary diagnosis code T84.60XA, T84.610A, T84.611A, T84.612A, T84.613A, T84.614A, T84.615A, T84.619A, T84.63XA, T84.69XA, T84.7XXA

0RG64JJ Fusion of Thoracic Vertebral Joint with Synthetic Substitute, Posterior Approach, Anterior Column, Percutaneous Endoscopic Approach
- HAC When reported with secondary diagnosis code T84.60XA, T84.610A, T84.611A, T84.612A, T84.613A, T84.614A, T84.615A, T84.619A, T84.63XA, T84.69XA, T84.7XXA

0RG64K0 Fusion of Thoracic Vertebral Joint with Nonautologous Tissue Substitute, Anterior Approach, Anterior Column, Percutaneous Endoscopic Approach
- HAC When reported with secondary diagnosis code T84.60XA, T84.610A, T84.611A, T84.612A, T84.613A, T84.614A, T84.615A, T84.619A, T84.63XA, T84.69XA, T84.7XXA

0RG64K1 Fusion of Thoracic Vertebral Joint with Nonautologous Tissue Substitute, Posterior Approach, Posterior Column, Percutaneous Endoscopic Approach
- HAC When reported with secondary diagnosis code T84.60XA, T84.610A, T84.611A, T84.612A, T84.613A, T84.614A, T84.615A, T84.619A, T84.63XA, T84.69XA, T84.7XXA

0RG64KJ Fusion of Thoracic Vertebral Joint with Nonautologous Tissue Substitute, Posterior Approach, Anterior Column, Percutaneous Endoscopic Approach
- HAC When reported with secondary diagnosis code T84.60XA, T84.610A, T84.611A, T84.612A, T84.613A, T84.614A, T84.615A, T84.619A, T84.63XA, T84.69XA, T84.7XXA

0RG64Z0   Fusion of Thoracic Vertebral Joint, Anterior Approach, Anterior Column, Percutaneous Endoscopic Approach
> HAC   When reported with secondary diagnosis code T84.60XA, T84.610A, T84.611A, T84.612A, T84.613A, T84.614A, T84.615A, T84.619A, T84.63XA, T84.69XA, T84.7XXA

0RG64Z1   Fusion of Thoracic Vertebral Joint, Posterior Approach, Posterior Column, Percutaneous Endoscopic Approach
> HAC   When reported with secondary diagnosis code T84.60XA, T84.610A, T84.611A, T84.612A, T84.613A, T84.614A, T84.615A, T84.619A, T84.63XA, T84.69XA, T84.7XXA

0RG64ZJ   Fusion of Thoracic Vertebral Joint, Posterior Approach, Anterior Column, Percutaneous Endoscopic Approach
> HAC   When reported with secondary diagnosis code T84.60XA, T84.610A, T84.611A, T84.612A, T84.613A, T84.614A, T84.615A, T84.619A, T84.63XA, T84.69XA, T84.7XXA

0RG7070   Fusion of 2 to 7 Thoracic Vertebral Joints with Autologous Tissue Substitute, Anterior Approach, Anterior Column, Open Approach
> HAC   When reported with secondary diagnosis code T84.60XA, T84.610A, T84.611A, T84.612A, T84.613A, T84.614A, T84.615A, T84.619A, T84.63XA, T84.69XA, T84.7XXA

0RG7071   Fusion of 2 to 7 Thoracic Vertebral Joints with Autologous Tissue Substitute, Posterior Approach, Posterior Column, Open Approach
> HAC   When reported with secondary diagnosis code T84.60XA, T84.610A, T84.611A, T84.612A, T84.613A, T84.614A, T84.615A, T84.619A, T84.63XA, T84.69XA, T84.7XXA

0RG707J   Fusion of 2 to 7 Thoracic Vertebral Joints with Autologous Tissue Substitute, Posterior Approach, Anterior Column, Open Approach
> HAC   When reported with secondary diagnosis code T84.60XA, T84.610A, T84.611A, T84.612A, T84.613A, T84.614A, T84.615A, T84.619A, T84.63XA, T84.69XA, T84.7XXA

0RG70A0   Fusion of 2 to 7 Thoracic Vertebral Joints with Interbody Fusion Device, Anterior Approach, Anterior Column, Open Approach
> HAC   When reported with secondary diagnosis code T84.60XA, T84.610A, T84.611A, T84.612A, T84.613A, T84.614A, T84.615A, T84.619A, T84.63XA, T84.69XA, T84.7XXA

0RG70A1   Fusion of 2 to 7 Thoracic Vertebral Joints with Interbody Fusion Device, Posterior Approach, Posterior Column, Open Approach
> HAC   When reported with secondary diagnosis code T84.60XA, T84.610A, T84.611A, T84.612A, T84.613A, T84.614A, T84.615A, T84.619A, T84.63XA, T84.69XA, T84.7XXA

0RG70AJ   Fusion of 2 to 7 Thoracic Vertebral Joints with Interbody Fusion Device, Posterior Approach, Anterior Column, Open Approach
> HAC   When reported with secondary diagnosis code T84.60XA, T84.610A, T84.611A, T84.612A, T84.613A, T84.614A, T84.615A, T84.619A, T84.63XA, T84.69XA, T84.7XXA

0RG70J0   Fusion of 2 to 7 Thoracic Vertebral Joints with Synthetic Substitute, Anterior Approach, Anterior Column, Open Approach
> HAC   When reported with secondary diagnosis code T84.60XA, T84.610A, T84.611A, T84.612A, T84.613A, T84.614A, T84.615A, T84.619A, T84.63XA, T84.69XA, T84.7XXA

0RG70J1   Fusion of 2 to 7 Thoracic Vertebral Joints with Synthetic Substitute, Posterior Approach, Posterior Column, Open Approach
> HAC   When reported with secondary diagnosis code T84.60XA, T84.610A, T84.611A, T84.612A, T84.613A, T84.614A, T84.615A, T84.619A, T84.63XA, T84.69XA, T84.7XXA

0RG70JJ   Fusion of 2 to 7 Thoracic Vertebral Joints with Synthetic Substitute, Posterior Approach, Anterior Column, Open Approach
> HAC   When reported with secondary diagnosis code T84.60XA, T84.610A, T84.611A, T84.612A, T84.613A, T84.614A, T84.615A, T84.619A, T84.63XA, T84.69XA, T84.7XXA

0RG70K0   Fusion of 2 to 7 Thoracic Vertebral Joints with Nonautologous Tissue Substitute, Anterior Approach, Anterior Column, Open Approach
> HAC   When reported with secondary diagnosis code T84.60XA, T84.610A, T84.611A, T84.612A, T84.613A, T84.614A, T84.615A, T84.619A, T84.63XA, T84.69XA, T84.7XXA

0RG70K1   Fusion of 2 to 7 Thoracic Vertebral Joints with Nonautologous Tissue Substitute, Posterior Approach, Posterior Column, Open Approach
> HAC   When reported with secondary diagnosis code T84.60XA, T84.610A, T84.611A, T84.612A, T84.613A, T84.614A, T84.615A, T84.619A, T84.63XA, T84.69XA, T84.7XXA

0RG70KJ   Fusion of 2 to 7 Thoracic Vertebral Joints with Nonautologous Tissue Substitute, Posterior Approach, Anterior Column, Open Approach
> HAC   When reported with secondary diagnosis code T84.60XA, T84.610A, T84.611A, T84.612A, T84.613A, T84.614A, T84.615A, T84.619A, T84.63XA, T84.69XA, T84.7XXA

0RG70Z0   Fusion of 2 to 7 Thoracic Vertebral Joints, Anterior Approach, Anterior Column, Open Approach
> HAC   When reported with secondary diagnosis code T84.60XA, T84.610A, T84.611A, T84.612A, T84.613A, T84.614A, T84.615A, T84.619A, T84.63XA, T84.69XA, T84.7XXA

0RG70Z1   Fusion of 2 to 7 Thoracic Vertebral Joints, Posterior Approach, Posterior Column, Open Approach
> HAC   When reported with secondary diagnosis code T84.60XA, T84.610A, T84.611A, T84.612A, T84.613A, T84.614A, T84.615A, T84.619A, T84.63XA, T84.69XA, T84.7XXA

0RG70ZJ   Fusion of 2 to 7 Thoracic Vertebral Joints, Posterior Approach, Anterior Column, Open Approach
> HAC   When reported with secondary diagnosis code T84.60XA, T84.610A, T84.611A, T84.612A, T84.613A, T84.614A, T84.615A, T84.619A, T84.63XA, T84.69XA, T84.7XXA

0RG7370   Fusion of 2 to 7 Thoracic Vertebral Joints with Autologous Tissue Substitute, Anterior Approach, Anterior Column, Percutaneous Approach
> HAC   When reported with secondary diagnosis code T84.60XA, T84.610A, T84.611A, T84.612A, T84.613A, T84.614A, T84.615A, T84.619A, T84.63XA, T84.69XA, T84.7XXA

0RG7371   Fusion of 2 to 7 Thoracic Vertebral Joints with Autologous Tissue Substitute, Posterior Approach, Posterior Column, Percutaneous Approach
> HAC   When reported with secondary diagnosis code T84.60XA, T84.610A, T84.611A, T84.612A, T84.613A, T84.614A, T84.615A, T84.619A, T84.63XA, T84.69XA, T84.7XXA

0RG737J   Fusion of 2 to 7 Thoracic Vertebral Joints with Autologous Tissue Substitute, Posterior Approach, Anterior Column, Percutaneous Approach
> HAC   When reported with secondary diagnosis code T84.60XA, T84.610A, T84.611A, T84.612A, T84.613A, T84.614A, T84.615A, T84.619A, T84.63XA, T84.69XA, T84.7XXA

0RG73A0   Fusion of 2 to 7 Thoracic Vertebral Joints with Interbody Fusion Device, Anterior Approach, Anterior Column, Percutaneous Approach
> HAC   When reported with secondary diagnosis code T84.60XA, T84.610A, T84.611A, T84.612A, T84.613A, T84.614A, T84.615A, T84.619A, T84.63XA, T84.69XA, T84.7XXA

0RG73A1   Fusion of 2 to 7 Thoracic Vertebral Joints with Interbody Fusion Device, Posterior Approach, Posterior Column, Percutaneous Approach
> HAC   When reported with secondary diagnosis code T84.60XA, T84.610A, T84.611A, T84.612A, T84.613A, T84.614A, T84.615A, T84.619A, T84.63XA, T84.69XA, T84.7XXA

0RG73AJ   Fusion of 2 to 7 Thoracic Vertebral Joints with Interbody Fusion Device, Posterior Approach, Anterior Column, Percutaneous Approach
> HAC   When reported with secondary diagnosis code T84.60XA, T84.610A, T84.611A, T84.612A, T84.613A, T84.614A, T84.615A, T84.619A, T84.63XA, T84.69XA, T84.7XXA

0RG73J0   Fusion of 2 to 7 Thoracic Vertebral Joints with Synthetic Substitute, Anterior Approach, Anterior Column, Percutaneous Approach
> HAC   When reported with secondary diagnosis code T84.60XA, T84.610A, T84.611A, T84.612A, T84.613A, T84.614A, T84.615A, T84.619A, T84.63XA, T84.69XA, T84.7XXA

0RG73J1   Fusion of 2 to 7 Thoracic Vertebral Joints with Synthetic Substitute, Posterior Approach, Posterior Column, Percutaneous Approach
> HAC   When reported with secondary diagnosis code T84.60XA, T84.610A, T84.611A, T84.612A, T84.613A, T84.614A, T84.615A, T84.619A, T84.63XA, T84.69XA, T84.7XXA

0RG73JJ   Fusion of 2 to 7 Thoracic Vertebral Joints with Synthetic Substitute, Posterior Approach, Anterior Column, Percutaneous Approach
> HAC   When reported with secondary diagnosis code T84.60XA, T84.610A, T84.611A, T84.612A, T84.613A, T84.614A, T84.615A, T84.619A, T84.63XA, T84.69XA, T84.7XXA

0RG73K0 Fusion of 2 to 7 Thoracic Vertebral Joints with Nonautologous Tissue Substitute, Anterior Approach, Anterior Column, Percutaneous Approach
HAC When reported with secondary diagnosis code T84.60XA, T84.610A, T84.611A, T84.612A, T84.613A, T84.614A, T84.615A, T84.619A, T84.63XA, T84.69XA, T84.7XXA

0RG73K1 Fusion of 2 to 7 Thoracic Vertebral Joints with Nonautologous Tissue Substitute, Posterior Approach, Posterior Column, Percutaneous Approach
HAC When reported with secondary diagnosis code T84.60XA, T84.610A, T84.611A, T84.612A, T84.613A, T84.614A, T84.615A, T84.619A, T84.63XA, T84.69XA, T84.7XXA

0RG73KJ Fusion of 2 to 7 Thoracic Vertebral Joints with Nonautologous Tissue Substitute, Posterior Approach, Anterior Column, Percutaneous Approach
HAC When reported with secondary diagnosis code T84.60XA, T84.610A, T84.611A, T84.612A, T84.613A, T84.614A, T84.615A, T84.619A, T84.63XA, T84.69XA, T84.7XXA

0RG73Z0 Fusion of 2 to 7 Thoracic Vertebral Joints, Anterior Approach, Anterior Column, Percutaneous Approach
HAC When reported with secondary diagnosis code T84.60XA, T84.610A, T84.611A, T84.612A, T84.613A, T84.614A, T84.615A, T84.619A, T84.63XA, T84.69XA, T84.7XXA

0RG73Z1 Fusion of 2 to 7 Thoracic Vertebral Joints, Posterior Approach, Posterior Column, Percutaneous Approach
HAC When reported with secondary diagnosis code T84.60XA, T84.610A, T84.611A, T84.612A, T84.613A, T84.614A, T84.615A, T84.619A, T84.63XA, T84.69XA, T84.7XXA

0RG73ZJ Fusion of 2 to 7 Thoracic Vertebral Joints, Posterior Approach, Anterior Column, Percutaneous Approach
HAC When reported with secondary diagnosis code T84.60XA, T84.610A, T84.611A, T84.612A, T84.613A, T84.614A, T84.615A, T84.619A, T84.63XA, T84.69XA, T84.7XXA

0RG7470 Fusion of 2 to 7 Thoracic Vertebral Joints with Autologous Tissue Substitute, Anterior Approach, Anterior Column, Percutaneous Endoscopic Approach
HAC When reported with secondary diagnosis code T84.60XA, T84.610A, T84.611A, T84.612A, T84.613A, T84.614A, T84.615A, T84.619A, T84.63XA, T84.69XA, T84.7XXA

0RG7471 Fusion of 2 to 7 Thoracic Vertebral Joints with Autologous Tissue Substitute, Posterior Approach, Posterior Column, Percutaneous Endoscopic Approach
HAC When reported with secondary diagnosis code T84.60XA, T84.610A, T84.611A, T84.612A, T84.613A, T84.614A, T84.615A, T84.619A, T84.63XA, T84.69XA, T84.7XXA

0RG747J Fusion of 2 to 7 Thoracic Vertebral Joints with Autologous Tissue Substitute, Posterior Approach, Anterior Column, Percutaneous Endoscopic Approach
HAC When reported with secondary diagnosis code T84.60XA, T84.610A, T84.611A, T84.612A, T84.613A, T84.614A, T84.615A, T84.619A, T84.63XA, T84.69XA, T84.7XXA

0RG74A0 Fusion of 2 to 7 Thoracic Vertebral Joints with Interbody Fusion Device, Anterior Approach, Anterior Column, Percutaneous Endoscopic Approach
HAC When reported with secondary diagnosis code T84.60XA, T84.610A, T84.611A, T84.612A, T84.613A, T84.614A, T84.615A, T84.619A, T84.63XA, T84.69XA, T84.7XXA

0RG74A1 Fusion of 2 to 7 Thoracic Vertebral Joints with Interbody Fusion Device, Posterior Approach, Posterior Column, Percutaneous Endoscopic Approach
HAC When reported with secondary diagnosis code T84.60XA, T84.610A, T84.611A, T84.612A, T84.613A, T84.614A, T84.615A, T84.619A, T84.63XA, T84.69XA, T84.7XXA

0RG74AJ Fusion of 2 to 7 Thoracic Vertebral Joints with Interbody Fusion Device, Posterior Approach, Anterior Column, Percutaneous Endoscopic Approach
HAC When reported with secondary diagnosis code T84.60XA, T84.610A, T84.611A, T84.612A, T84.613A, T84.614A, T84.615A, T84.619A, T84.63XA, T84.69XA, T84.7XXA

0RG74J0 Fusion of 2 to 7 Thoracic Vertebral Joints with Synthetic Substitute, Anterior Approach, Anterior Column, Percutaneous Endoscopic Approach
HAC When reported with secondary diagnosis code T84.60XA, T84.610A, T84.611A, T84.612A, T84.613A, T84.614A, T84.615A, T84.619A, T84.63XA, T84.69XA, T84.7XXA

0RG74J1 Fusion of 2 to 7 Thoracic Vertebral Joints with Synthetic Substitute, Posterior Approach, Posterior Column, Percutaneous Endoscopic Approach
HAC When reported with secondary diagnosis code T84.60XA, T84.610A, T84.611A, T84.612A, T84.613A, T84.614A, T84.615A, T84.619A, T84.63XA, T84.69XA, T84.7XXA

0RG74JJ Fusion of 2 to 7 Thoracic Vertebral Joints with Synthetic Substitute, Posterior Approach, Anterior Column, Percutaneous Endoscopic Approach
HAC When reported with secondary diagnosis code T84.60XA, T84.610A, T84.611A, T84.612A, T84.613A, T84.614A, T84.615A, T84.619A, T84.63XA, T84.69XA, T84.7XXA

0RG74K0 Fusion of 2 to 7 Thoracic Vertebral Joints with Nonautologous Tissue Substitute, Anterior Approach, Anterior Column, Percutaneous Endoscopic Approach
HAC When reported with secondary diagnosis code T84.60XA, T84.610A, T84.611A, T84.612A, T84.613A, T84.614A, T84.615A, T84.619A, T84.63XA, T84.69XA, T84.7XXA

0RG74K1 Fusion of 2 to 7 Thoracic Vertebral Joints with Nonautologous Tissue Substitute, Posterior Approach, Posterior Column, Percutaneous Endoscopic Approach
HAC When reported with secondary diagnosis code T84.60XA, T84.610A, T84.611A, T84.612A, T84.613A, T84.614A, T84.615A, T84.619A, T84.63XA, T84.69XA, T84.7XXA

0RG74KJ Fusion of 2 to 7 Thoracic Vertebral Joints with Nonautologous Tissue Substitute, Posterior Approach, Anterior Column, Percutaneous Endoscopic Approach
HAC When reported with secondary diagnosis code T84.60XA, T84.610A, T84.611A, T84.612A, T84.613A, T84.614A, T84.615A, T84.619A, T84.63XA, T84.69XA, T84.7XXA

0RG74Z0 Fusion of 2 to 7 Thoracic Vertebral Joints, Anterior Approach, Anterior Column, Percutaneous Endoscopic Approach
HAC When reported with secondary diagnosis code T84.60XA, T84.610A, T84.611A, T84.612A, T84.613A, T84.614A, T84.615A, T84.619A, T84.63XA, T84.69XA, T84.7XXA

0RG74Z1 Fusion of 2 to 7 Thoracic Vertebral Joints, Posterior Approach, Posterior Column, Percutaneous Endoscopic Approach
HAC When reported with secondary diagnosis code T84.60XA, T84.610A, T84.611A, T84.612A, T84.613A, T84.614A, T84.615A, T84.619A, T84.63XA, T84.69XA, T84.7XXA

0RG74ZJ Fusion of 2 to 7 Thoracic Vertebral Joints, Posterior Approach, Anterior Column, Percutaneous Endoscopic Approach
HAC When reported with secondary diagnosis code T84.60XA, T84.610A, T84.611A, T84.612A, T84.613A, T84.614A, T84.615A, T84.619A, T84.63XA, T84.69XA, T84.7XXA

0RG8070 Fusion of 8 or more Thoracic Vertebral Joints with Autologous Tissue Substitute, Anterior Approach, Anterior Column, Open Approach
HAC When reported with secondary diagnosis code T84.60XA, T84.610A, T84.611A, T84.612A, T84.613A, T84.614A, T84.615A, T84.619A, T84.63XA, T84.69XA, T84.7XXA

0RG8071 Fusion of 8 or more Thoracic Vertebral Joints with Autologous Tissue Substitute, Posterior Approach, Posterior Column, Open Approach
HAC When reported with secondary diagnosis code T84.60XA, T84.610A, T84.611A, T84.612A, T84.613A, T84.614A, T84.615A, T84.619A, T84.63XA, T84.69XA, T84.7XXA

0RG807J Fusion of 8 or more Thoracic Vertebral Joints with Autologous Tissue Substitute, Posterior Approach, Anterior Column, Open Approach
HAC When reported with secondary diagnosis code T84.60XA, T84.610A, T84.611A, T84.612A, T84.613A, T84.614A, T84.615A, T84.619A, T84.63XA, T84.69XA, T84.7XXA

0RG80A0 Fusion of 8 or more Thoracic Vertebral Joints with Interbody Fusion Device, Anterior Approach, Anterior Column, Open Approach
HAC When reported with secondary diagnosis code T84.60XA, T84.610A, T84.611A, T84.612A, T84.613A, T84.614A, T84.615A, T84.619A, T84.63XA, T84.69XA, T84.7XXA

0RG80A1 Fusion of 8 or more Thoracic Vertebral Joints with Interbody Fusion Device, Posterior Approach, Posterior Column, Open Approach
HAC When reported with secondary diagnosis code T84.60XA, T84.610A, T84.611A, T84.612A, T84.613A, T84.614A, T84.615A, T84.619A, T84.63XA, T84.69XA, T84.7XXA

♀ Female-only   ♂ Male-only   ● Limited Coverage   ● Non-OR   HAC HAC-associated procedure   ● Non-covered procedures   + Combination

0RG80AJ Fusion of 8 or more Thoracic Vertebral Joints with Interbody Fusion Device, Posterior Approach, Anterior Column, Open Approach
HAC When reported with secondary diagnosis code T84.60XA, T84.610A, T84.611A, T84.612A, T84.613A, T84.614A, T84.615A, T84.619A, T84.63XA, T84.69XA, T84.7XXA

0RG80J0 Fusion of 8 or more Thoracic Vertebral Joints with Synthetic Substitute, Anterior Approach, Anterior Column, Open Approach
HAC When reported with secondary diagnosis code T84.60XA, T84.610A, T84.611A, T84.612A, T84.613A, T84.614A, T84.615A, T84.619A, T84.63XA, T84.69XA, T84.7XXA

0RG80J1 Fusion of 8 or more Thoracic Vertebral Joints with Synthetic Substitute, Posterior Approach, Posterior Column, Open Approach
HAC When reported with secondary diagnosis code T84.60XA, T84.610A, T84.611A, T84.612A, T84.613A, T84.614A, T84.615A, T84.619A, T84.63XA, T84.69XA, T84.7XXA

0RG80JJ Fusion of 8 or more Thoracic Vertebral Joints with Synthetic Substitute, Posterior Approach, Anterior Column, Open Approach
HAC When reported with secondary diagnosis code T84.60XA, T84.610A, T84.611A, T84.612A, T84.613A, T84.614A, T84.615A, T84.619A, T84.63XA, T84.69XA, T84.7XXA

0RG80K0 Fusion of 8 or more Thoracic Vertebral Joints with Nonautologous Tissue Substitute, Anterior Approach, Anterior Column, Open Approach
HAC When reported with secondary diagnosis code T84.60XA, T84.610A, T84.611A, T84.612A, T84.613A, T84.614A, T84.615A, T84.619A, T84.63XA, T84.69XA, T84.7XXA

0RG80K1 Fusion of 8 or more Thoracic Vertebral Joints with Nonautologous Tissue Substitute, Posterior Approach, Posterior Column, Open Approach
HAC When reported with secondary diagnosis code T84.60XA, T84.610A, T84.611A, T84.612A, T84.613A, T84.614A, T84.615A, T84.619A, T84.63XA, T84.69XA, T84.7XXA

0RG80KJ Fusion of 8 or more Thoracic Vertebral Joints with Nonautologous Tissue Substitute, Posterior Approach, Anterior Column, Open Approach
HAC When reported with secondary diagnosis code T84.60XA, T84.610A, T84.611A, T84.612A, T84.613A, T84.614A, T84.615A, T84.619A, T84.63XA, T84.69XA, T84.7XXA

0RG80Z0 Fusion of 8 or more Thoracic Vertebral Joints, Anterior Approach, Anterior Column, Open Approach
HAC When reported with secondary diagnosis code T84.60XA, T84.610A, T84.611A, T84.612A, T84.613A, T84.614A, T84.615A, T84.619A, T84.63XA, T84.69XA, T84.7XXA

0RG80Z1 Fusion of 8 or more Thoracic Vertebral Joints, Posterior Approach, Posterior Column, Open Approach
HAC When reported with secondary diagnosis code T84.60XA, T84.610A, T84.611A, T84.612A, T84.613A, T84.614A, T84.615A, T84.619A, T84.63XA, T84.69XA, T84.7XXA

0RG80ZJ Fusion of 8 or more Thoracic Vertebral Joints, Posterior Approach, Anterior Column, Open Approach
HAC When reported with secondary diagnosis code T84.60XA, T84.610A, T84.611A, T84.612A, T84.613A, T84.614A, T84.615A, T84.619A, T84.63XA, T84.69XA, T84.7XXA

0RG8370 Fusion of 8 or more Thoracic Vertebral Joints with Autologous Tissue Substitute, Anterior Approach, Anterior Column, Percutaneous Approach
HAC When reported with secondary diagnosis code T84.60XA, T84.610A, T84.611A, T84.612A, T84.613A, T84.614A, T84.615A, T84.619A, T84.63XA, T84.69XA, T84.7XXA

0RG8371 Fusion of 8 or more Thoracic Vertebral Joints with Autologous Tissue Substitute, Posterior Approach, Posterior Column, Percutaneous Approach
HAC When reported with secondary diagnosis code T84.60XA, T84.610A, T84.611A, T84.612A, T84.613A, T84.614A, T84.615A, T84.619A, T84.63XA, T84.69XA, T84.7XXA

0RG837J Fusion of 8 or more Thoracic Vertebral Joints with Autologous Tissue Substitute, Posterior Approach, Anterior Column, Percutaneous Approach
HAC When reported with secondary diagnosis code T84.60XA, T84.610A, T84.611A, T84.612A, T84.613A, T84.614A, T84.615A, T84.619A, T84.63XA, T84.69XA, T84.7XXA

0RG83A0 Fusion of 8 or more Thoracic Vertebral Joints with Interbody Fusion Device, Anterior Approach, Anterior Column, Percutaneous Approach
HAC When reported with secondary diagnosis code T84.60XA, T84.610A, T84.611A, T84.612A, T84.613A, T84.614A, T84.615A, T84.619A, T84.63XA, T84.69XA, T84.7XXA

0RG83A1 Fusion of 8 or more Thoracic Vertebral Joints with Interbody Fusion Device, Posterior Approach, Posterior Column, Percutaneous Approach
HAC When reported with secondary diagnosis code T84.60XA, T84.610A, T84.611A, T84.612A, T84.613A, T84.614A, T84.615A, T84.619A, T84.63XA, T84.69XA, T84.7XXA

0RG83AJ Fusion of 8 or more Thoracic Vertebral Joints with Interbody Fusion Device, Posterior Approach, Anterior Column, Percutaneous Approach
HAC When reported with secondary diagnosis code T84.60XA, T84.610A, T84.611A, T84.612A, T84.613A, T84.614A, T84.615A, T84.619A, T84.63XA, T84.69XA, T84.7XXA

0RG83J0 Fusion of 8 or more Thoracic Vertebral Joints with Synthetic Substitute, Anterior Approach, Anterior Column, Percutaneous Approach
HAC When reported with secondary diagnosis code T84.60XA, T84.610A, T84.611A, T84.612A, T84.613A, T84.614A, T84.615A, T84.619A, T84.63XA, T84.69XA, T84.7XXA

0RG83J1 Fusion of 8 or more Thoracic Vertebral Joints with Synthetic Substitute, Posterior Approach, Posterior Column, Percutaneous Approach
HAC When reported with secondary diagnosis code T84.60XA, T84.610A, T84.611A, T84.612A, T84.613A, T84.614A, T84.615A, T84.619A, T84.63XA, T84.69XA, T84.7XXA

0RG83JJ Fusion of 8 or more Thoracic Vertebral Joints with Synthetic Substitute, Posterior Approach, Anterior Column, Percutaneous Approach
HAC When reported with secondary diagnosis code T84.60XA, T84.610A, T84.611A, T84.612A, T84.613A, T84.614A, T84.615A, T84.619A, T84.63XA, T84.69XA, T84.7XXA

0RG83K0 Fusion of 8 or more Thoracic Vertebral Joints with Nonautologous Tissue Substitute, Anterior Approach, Anterior Column, Percutaneous Approach
HAC When reported with secondary diagnosis code T84.60XA, T84.610A, T84.611A, T84.612A, T84.613A, T84.614A, T84.615A, T84.619A, T84.63XA, T84.69XA, T84.7XXA

0RG83K1 Fusion of 8 or more Thoracic Vertebral Joints with Nonautologous Tissue Substitute, Posterior Approach, Posterior Column, Percutaneous Approach
HAC When reported with secondary diagnosis code T84.60XA, T84.610A, T84.611A, T84.612A, T84.613A, T84.614A, T84.615A, T84.619A, T84.63XA, T84.69XA, T84.7XXA

0RG83KJ Fusion of 8 or more Thoracic Vertebral Joints with Nonautologous Tissue Substitute, Posterior Approach, Anterior Column, Percutaneous Approach
HAC When reported with secondary diagnosis code T84.60XA, T84.610A, T84.611A, T84.612A, T84.613A, T84.614A, T84.615A, T84.619A, T84.63XA, T84.69XA, T84.7XXA

0RG83Z0 Fusion of 8 or more Thoracic Vertebral Joints, Anterior Approach, Anterior Column, Percutaneous Approach
HAC When reported with secondary diagnosis code T84.60XA, T84.610A, T84.611A, T84.612A, T84.613A, T84.614A, T84.615A, T84.619A, T84.63XA, T84.69XA, T84.7XXA

0RG83Z1 Fusion of 8 or more Thoracic Vertebral Joints, Posterior Approach, Posterior Column, Percutaneous Approach
HAC When reported with secondary diagnosis code T84.60XA, T84.610A, T84.611A, T84.612A, T84.613A, T84.614A, T84.615A, T84.619A, T84.63XA, T84.69XA, T84.7XXA

0RG83ZJ Fusion of 8 or more Thoracic Vertebral Joints, Posterior Approach, Anterior Column, Percutaneous Approach
HAC When reported with secondary diagnosis code T84.60XA, T84.610A, T84.611A, T84.612A, T84.613A, T84.614A, T84.615A, T84.619A, T84.63XA, T84.69XA, T84.7XXA

0RG8470 Fusion of 8 or more Thoracic Vertebral Joints with Autologous Tissue Substitute, Anterior Approach, Anterior Column, Percutaneous Endoscopic Approach
HAC When reported with secondary diagnosis code T84.60XA, T84.610A, T84.611A, T84.612A, T84.613A, T84.614A, T84.615A, T84.619A, T84.63XA, T84.69XA, T84.7XXA

0RG8471 Fusion of 8 or more Thoracic Vertebral Joints with Autologous Tissue Substitute, Posterior Approach, Posterior Column, Percutaneous Endoscopic Approach

HAC When reported with secondary diagnosis code T84.60XA, T84.610A, T84.611A, T84.612A, T84.613A, T84.614A, T84.615A, T84.619A, T84.63XA, T84.69XA, T84.7XXA

0RG847J Fusion of 8 or more Thoracic Vertebral Joints with Autologous Tissue Substitute, Posterior Approach, Anterior Column, Percutaneous Endoscopic Approach

HAC When reported with secondary diagnosis code T84.60XA, T84.610A, T84.611A, T84.612A, T84.613A, T84.614A, T84.615A, T84.619A, T84.63XA, T84.69XA, T84.7XXA

0RG84A0 Fusion of 8 or more Thoracic Vertebral Joints with Interbody Fusion Device, Anterior Approach, Anterior Column, Percutaneous Endoscopic Approach

HAC When reported with secondary diagnosis code T84.60XA, T84.610A, T84.611A, T84.612A, T84.613A, T84.614A, T84.615A, T84.619A, T84.63XA, T84.69XA, T84.7XXA

0RG84A1 Fusion of 8 or more Thoracic Vertebral Joints with Interbody Fusion Device, Posterior Approach, Posterior Column, Percutaneous Endoscopic Approach

HAC When reported with secondary diagnosis code T84.60XA, T84.610A, T84.611A, T84.612A, T84.613A, T84.614A, T84.615A, T84.619A, T84.63XA, T84.69XA, T84.7XXA

0RG84AJ Fusion of 8 or more Thoracic Vertebral Joints with Interbody Fusion Device, Posterior Approach, Anterior Column, Percutaneous Endoscopic Approach

HAC When reported with secondary diagnosis code T84.60XA, T84.610A, T84.611A, T84.612A, T84.613A, T84.614A, T84.615A, T84.619A, T84.63XA, T84.69XA, T84.7XXA

0RG84J0 Fusion of 8 or more Thoracic Vertebral Joints with Synthetic Substitute, Anterior Approach, Anterior Column, Percutaneous Endoscopic Approach

HAC When reported with secondary diagnosis code T84.60XA, T84.610A, T84.611A, T84.612A, T84.613A, T84.614A, T84.615A, T84.619A, T84.63XA, T84.69XA, T84.7XXA

0RG84J1 Fusion of 8 or more Thoracic Vertebral Joints with Synthetic Substitute, Posterior Approach, Posterior Column, Percutaneous Endoscopic Approach

HAC When reported with secondary diagnosis code T84.60XA, T84.610A, T84.611A, T84.612A, T84.613A, T84.614A, T84.615A, T84.619A, T84.63XA, T84.69XA, T84.7XXA

0RG84JJ Fusion of 8 or more Thoracic Vertebral Joints with Synthetic Substitute, Posterior Approach, Anterior Column, Percutaneous Endoscopic Approach

HAC When reported with secondary diagnosis code T84.60XA, T84.610A, T84.611A, T84.612A, T84.613A, T84.614A, T84.615A, T84.619A, T84.63XA, T84.69XA, T84.7XXA

0RG84K0 Fusion of 8 or more Thoracic Vertebral Joints with Nonautologous Tissue Substitute, Anterior Approach, Anterior Column, Percutaneous Endoscopic Approach

HAC When reported with secondary diagnosis code T84.60XA, T84.610A, T84.611A, T84.612A, T84.613A, T84.614A, T84.615A, T84.619A, T84.63XA, T84.69XA, T84.7XXA

0RG84K1 Fusion of 8 or more Thoracic Vertebral Joints with Nonautologous Tissue Substitute, Posterior Approach, Posterior Column, Percutaneous Endoscopic Approach

HAC When reported with secondary diagnosis code T84.60XA, T84.610A, T84.611A, T84.612A, T84.613A, T84.614A, T84.615A, T84.619A, T84.63XA, T84.69XA, T84.7XXA

0RG84KJ Fusion of 8 or more Thoracic Vertebral Joints with Nonautologous Tissue Substitute, Posterior Approach, Anterior Column, Percutaneous Endoscopic Approach

HAC When reported with secondary diagnosis code T84.60XA, T84.610A, T84.611A, T84.612A, T84.613A, T84.614A, T84.615A, T84.619A, T84.63XA, T84.69XA, T84.7XXA

0RG84Z0 Fusion of 8 or more Thoracic Vertebral Joints, Anterior Approach, Anterior Column, Percutaneous Endoscopic Approach

HAC When reported with secondary diagnosis code T84.60XA, T84.610A, T84.611A, T84.612A, T84.613A, T84.614A, T84.615A, T84.619A, T84.63XA, T84.69XA, T84.7XXA

0RG84Z1 Fusion of 8 or more Thoracic Vertebral Joints, Posterior Approach, Posterior Column, Percutaneous Endoscopic Approach

HAC When reported with secondary diagnosis code T84.60XA, T84.610A, T84.611A, T84.612A, T84.613A, T84.614A, T84.615A, T84.619A, T84.63XA, T84.69XA, T84.7XXA

0RG84ZJ Fusion of 8 or more Thoracic Vertebral Joints, Posterior Approach, Anterior Column, Percutaneous Endoscopic Approach

HAC When reported with secondary diagnosis code T84.60XA, T84.610A, T84.611A, T84.612A, T84.613A, T84.614A, T84.615A, T84.619A, T84.63XA, T84.69XA, T84.7XXA

0RGA070 Fusion of Thoracolumbar Vertebral Joint with Autologous Tissue Substitute, Anterior Approach, Anterior Column, Open Approach

HAC When reported with secondary diagnosis code T84.60XA, T84.610A, T84.611A, T84.612A, T84.613A, T84.614A, T84.615A, T84.619A, T84.63XA, T84.69XA, T84.7XXA

0RGA071 Fusion of Thoracolumbar Vertebral Joint with Autologous Tissue Substitute, Posterior Approach, Posterior Column, Open Approach

HAC When reported with secondary diagnosis code T84.60XA, T84.610A, T84.611A, T84.612A, T84.613A, T84.614A, T84.615A, T84.619A, T84.63XA, T84.69XA, T84.7XXA

0RGA07J Fusion of Thoracolumbar Vertebral Joint with Autologous Tissue Substitute, Posterior Approach, Anterior Column, Open Approach

HAC When reported with secondary diagnosis code T84.60XA, T84.610A, T84.611A, T84.612A, T84.613A, T84.614A, T84.615A, T84.619A, T84.63XA, T84.69XA, T84.7XXA

0RGA0A0 Fusion of Thoracolumbar Vertebral Joint with Interbody Fusion Device, Anterior Approach, Anterior Column, Open Approach

HAC When reported with secondary diagnosis code T84.60XA, T84.610A, T84.611A, T84.612A, T84.613A, T84.614A, T84.615A, T84.619A, T84.63XA, T84.69XA, T84.7XXA

0RGA0A1 Fusion of Thoracolumbar Vertebral Joint with Interbody Fusion Device, Posterior Approach, Posterior Column, Open Approach

HAC When reported with secondary diagnosis code T84.60XA, T84.610A, T84.611A, T84.612A, T84.613A, T84.614A, T84.615A, T84.619A, T84.63XA, T84.69XA, T84.7XXA

0RGA0AJ Fusion of Thoracolumbar Vertebral Joint with Interbody Fusion Device, Posterior Approach, Anterior Column, Open Approach

HAC When reported with secondary diagnosis code T84.60XA, T84.610A, T84.611A, T84.612A, T84.613A, T84.614A, T84.615A, T84.619A, T84.63XA, T84.69XA, T84.7XXA

0RGA0J0 Fusion of Thoracolumbar Vertebral Joint with Synthetic Substitute, Anterior Approach, Anterior Column, Open Approach

HAC When reported with secondary diagnosis code T84.60XA, T84.610A, T84.611A, T84.612A, T84.613A, T84.614A, T84.615A, T84.619A, T84.63XA, T84.69XA, T84.7XXA

0RGA0J1 Fusion of Thoracolumbar Vertebral Joint with Synthetic Substitute, Posterior Approach, Posterior Column, Open Approach

HAC When reported with secondary diagnosis code T84.60XA, T84.610A, T84.611A, T84.612A, T84.613A, T84.614A, T84.615A, T84.619A, T84.63XA, T84.69XA, T84.7XXA

0RGA0JJ Fusion of Thoracolumbar Vertebral Joint with Synthetic Substitute, Posterior Approach, Anterior Column, Open Approach

HAC When reported with secondary diagnosis code T84.60XA, T84.610A, T84.611A, T84.612A, T84.613A, T84.614A, T84.615A, T84.619A, T84.63XA, T84.69XA, T84.7XXA

0RGA0K0 Fusion of Thoracolumbar Vertebral Joint with Nonautologous Tissue Substitute, Anterior Approach, Anterior Column, Open Approach

HAC When reported with secondary diagnosis code T84.60XA, T84.610A, T84.611A, T84.612A, T84.613A, T84.614A, T84.615A, T84.619A, T84.63XA, T84.69XA, T84.7XXA

0RGA0K1 Fusion of Thoracolumbar Vertebral Joint with Nonautologous Tissue Substitute, Posterior Approach, Posterior Column, Open Approach

HAC When reported with secondary diagnosis code T84.60XA, T84.610A, T84.611A, T84.612A, T84.613A, T84.614A, T84.615A, T84.619A, T84.63XA, T84.69XA, T84.7XXA

0RGA0KJ Fusion of Thoracolumbar Vertebral Joint with Nonautologous Tissue Substitute, Posterior Approach, Anterior Column, Open Approach

HAC When reported with secondary diagnosis code T84.60XA, T84.610A, T84.611A, T84.612A, T84.613A, T84.614A, T84.615A, T84.619A, T84.63XA, T84.69XA, T84.7XXA

0RGA0Z0 Fusion of Thoracolumbar Vertebral Joint, Anterior Approach, Anterior Column, Open Approach
  HAC When reported with secondary diagnosis code T84.60XA, T84.610A, T84.611A, T84.612A, T84.613A, T84.614A, T84.615A, T84.619A, T84.63XA, T84.69XA, T84.7XXA

0RGA0Z1 Fusion of Thoracolumbar Vertebral Joint, Posterior Approach, Posterior Column, Open Approach
  HAC When reported with secondary diagnosis code T84.60XA, T84.610A, T84.611A, T84.612A, T84.613A, T84.614A, T84.615A, T84.619A, T84.63XA, T84.69XA, T84.7XXA

0RGA0ZJ Fusion of Thoracolumbar Vertebral Joint, Posterior Approach, Anterior Column, Open Approach
  HAC When reported with secondary diagnosis code T84.60XA, T84.610A, T84.611A, T84.612A, T84.613A, T84.614A, T84.615A, T84.619A, T84.63XA, T84.69XA, T84.7XXA

0RGA370 Fusion of Thoracolumbar Vertebral Joint with Autologous Tissue Substitute, Anterior Approach, Anterior Column, Percutaneous Approach
  HAC When reported with secondary diagnosis code T84.60XA, T84.610A, T84.611A, T84.612A, T84.613A, T84.614A, T84.615A, T84.619A, T84.63XA, T84.69XA, T84.7XXA

0RGA371 Fusion of Thoracolumbar Vertebral Joint with Autologous Tissue Substitute, Posterior Approach, Posterior Column, Percutaneous Approach
  HAC When reported with secondary diagnosis code T84.60XA, T84.610A, T84.611A, T84.612A, T84.613A, T84.614A, T84.615A, T84.619A, T84.63XA, T84.69XA, T84.7XXA

0RGA37J Fusion of Thoracolumbar Vertebral Joint with Autologous Tissue Substitute, Posterior Approach, Anterior Column, Percutaneous Approach
  HAC When reported with secondary diagnosis code T84.60XA, T84.610A, T84.611A, T84.612A, T84.613A, T84.614A, T84.615A, T84.619A, T84.63XA, T84.69XA, T84.7XXA

0RGA3A0 Fusion of Thoracolumbar Vertebral Joint with Interbody Fusion Device, Anterior Approach, Anterior Column, Percutaneous Approach
  HAC When reported with secondary diagnosis code T84.60XA, T84.610A, T84.611A, T84.612A, T84.613A, T84.614A, T84.615A, T84.619A, T84.63XA, T84.69XA, T84.7XXA

0RGA3A1 Fusion of Thoracolumbar Vertebral Joint with Interbody Fusion Device, Posterior Approach, Posterior Column, Percutaneous Approach
  HAC When reported with secondary diagnosis code T84.60XA, T84.610A, T84.611A, T84.612A, T84.613A, T84.614A, T84.615A, T84.619A, T84.63XA, T84.69XA, T84.7XXA

0RGA3AJ Fusion of Thoracolumbar Vertebral Joint with Interbody Fusion Device, Posterior Approach, Anterior Column, Percutaneous Approach
  HAC When reported with secondary diagnosis code T84.60XA, T84.610A, T84.611A, T84.612A, T84.613A, T84.614A, T84.615A, T84.619A, T84.63XA, T84.69XA, T84.7XXA

0RGA3J0 Fusion of Thoracolumbar Vertebral Joint with Synthetic Substitute, Anterior Approach, Anterior Column, Percutaneous Approach
  HAC When reported with secondary diagnosis code T84.60XA, T84.610A, T84.611A, T84.612A, T84.613A, T84.614A, T84.615A, T84.619A, T84.63XA, T84.69XA, T84.7XXA

0RGA3J1 Fusion of Thoracolumbar Vertebral Joint with Synthetic Substitute, Posterior Approach, Posterior Column, Percutaneous Approach
  HAC When reported with secondary diagnosis code T84.60XA, T84.610A, T84.611A, T84.612A, T84.613A, T84.614A, T84.615A, T84.619A, T84.63XA, T84.69XA, T84.7XXA

0RGA3JJ Fusion of Thoracolumbar Vertebral Joint with Synthetic Substitute, Posterior Approach, Anterior Column, Percutaneous Approach
  HAC When reported with secondary diagnosis code T84.60XA, T84.610A, T84.611A, T84.612A, T84.613A, T84.614A, T84.615A, T84.619A, T84.63XA, T84.69XA, T84.7XXA

0RGA3K0 Fusion of Thoracolumbar Vertebral Joint with Nonautologous Tissue Substitute, Anterior Approach, Anterior Column, Percutaneous Approach
  HAC When reported with secondary diagnosis code T84.60XA, T84.610A, T84.611A, T84.612A, T84.613A, T84.614A, T84.615A, T84.619A, T84.63XA, T84.69XA, T84.7XXA

0RGA3K1 Fusion of Thoracolumbar Vertebral Joint with Nonautologous Tissue Substitute, Posterior Approach, Posterior Column, Percutaneous Approach
  HAC When reported with secondary diagnosis code T84.60XA, T84.610A, T84.611A, T84.612A, T84.613A, T84.614A, T84.615A, T84.619A, T84.63XA, T84.69XA, T84.7XXA

0RGA3KJ Fusion of Thoracolumbar Vertebral Joint with Nonautologous Tissue Substitute, Posterior Approach, Anterior Column, Percutaneous Approach
  HAC When reported with secondary diagnosis code T84.60XA, T84.610A, T84.611A, T84.612A, T84.613A, T84.614A, T84.615A, T84.619A, T84.63XA, T84.69XA, T84.7XXA

0RGA3Z0 Fusion of Thoracolumbar Vertebral Joint, Anterior Approach, Anterior Column, Percutaneous Approach
  HAC When reported with secondary diagnosis code T84.60XA, T84.610A, T84.611A, T84.612A, T84.613A, T84.614A, T84.615A, T84.619A, T84.63XA, T84.69XA, T84.7XXA

0RGA3Z1 Fusion of Thoracolumbar Vertebral Joint, Posterior Approach, Posterior Column, Percutaneous Approach
  HAC When reported with secondary diagnosis code T84.60XA, T84.610A, T84.611A, T84.612A, T84.613A, T84.614A, T84.615A, T84.619A, T84.63XA, T84.69XA, T84.7XXA

0RGA3ZJ Fusion of Thoracolumbar Vertebral Joint, Posterior Approach, Anterior Column, Percutaneous Approach
  HAC When reported with secondary diagnosis code T84.60XA, T84.610A, T84.611A, T84.612A, T84.613A, T84.614A, T84.615A, T84.619A, T84.63XA, T84.69XA, T84.7XXA

0RGA470 Fusion of Thoracolumbar Vertebral Joint with Autologous Tissue Substitute, Anterior Approach, Anterior Column, Percutaneous Endoscopic Approach
  HAC When reported with secondary diagnosis code T84.60XA, T84.610A, T84.611A, T84.612A, T84.613A, T84.614A, T84.615A, T84.619A, T84.63XA, T84.69XA, T84.7XXA

0RGA471 Fusion of Thoracolumbar Vertebral Joint with Autologous Tissue Substitute, Posterior Approach, Posterior Column, Percutaneous Endoscopic Approach
  HAC When reported with secondary diagnosis code T84.60XA, T84.610A, T84.611A, T84.612A, T84.613A, T84.614A, T84.615A, T84.619A, T84.63XA, T84.69XA, T84.7XXA

0RGA47J Fusion of Thoracolumbar Vertebral Joint with Autologous Tissue Substitute, Posterior Approach, Anterior Column, Percutaneous Endoscopic Approach
  HAC When reported with secondary diagnosis code T84.60XA, T84.610A, T84.611A, T84.612A, T84.613A, T84.614A, T84.615A, T84.619A, T84.63XA, T84.69XA, T84.7XXA

0RGA4A0 Fusion of Thoracolumbar Vertebral Joint with Interbody Fusion Device, Anterior Approach, Anterior Column, Percutaneous Endoscopic Approach
  HAC When reported with secondary diagnosis code T84.60XA, T84.610A, T84.611A, T84.612A, T84.613A, T84.614A, T84.615A, T84.619A, T84.63XA, T84.69XA, T84.7XXA

0RGA4A1 Fusion of Thoracolumbar Vertebral Joint with Interbody Fusion Device, Posterior Approach, Posterior Column, Percutaneous Endoscopic Approach
  HAC When reported with secondary diagnosis code T84.60XA, T84.610A, T84.611A, T84.612A, T84.613A, T84.614A, T84.615A, T84.619A, T84.63XA, T84.69XA, T84.7XXA

0RGA4AJ Fusion of Thoracolumbar Vertebral Joint with Interbody Fusion Device, Posterior Approach, Anterior Column, Percutaneous Endoscopic Approach
  HAC When reported with secondary diagnosis code T84.60XA, T84.610A, T84.611A, T84.612A, T84.613A, T84.614A, T84.615A, T84.619A, T84.63XA, T84.69XA, T84.7XXA

0RGA4J0 Fusion of Thoracolumbar Vertebral Joint with Synthetic Substitute, Anterior Approach, Anterior Column, Percutaneous Endoscopic Approach
  HAC When reported with secondary diagnosis code T84.60XA, T84.610A, T84.611A, T84.612A, T84.613A, T84.614A, T84.615A, T84.619A, T84.63XA, T84.69XA, T84.7XXA

0RGA4J1 Fusion of Thoracolumbar Vertebral Joint with Synthetic Substitute, Posterior Approach, Posterior Column, Percutaneous Endoscopic Approach
  HAC When reported with secondary diagnosis code T84.60XA, T84.610A, T84.611A, T84.612A, T84.613A, T84.614A, T84.615A, T84.619A, T84.63XA, T84.69XA, T84.7XXA

0RGA4JJ Fusion of Thoracolumbar Vertebral Joint with Synthetic Substitute, Posterior Approach, Anterior Column, Percutaneous Endoscopic Approach
- HAC When reported with secondary diagnosis code T84.60XA, T84.610A, T84.611A, T84.612A, T84.613A, T84.614A, T84.615A, T84.619A, T84.63XA, T84.69XA, T84.7XXA

0RGA4K0 Fusion of Thoracolumbar Vertebral Joint with Nonautologous Tissue Substitute, Anterior Approach, Anterior Column, Percutaneous Endoscopic Approach
- HAC When reported with secondary diagnosis code T84.60XA, T84.610A, T84.611A, T84.612A, T84.613A, T84.614A, T84.615A, T84.619A, T84.63XA, T84.69XA, T84.7XXA

0RGA4K1 Fusion of Thoracolumbar Vertebral Joint with Nonautologous Tissue Substitute, Posterior Approach, Posterior Column, Percutaneous Endoscopic Approach
- HAC When reported with secondary diagnosis code T84.60XA, T84.610A, T84.611A, T84.612A, T84.613A, T84.614A, T84.615A, T84.619A, T84.63XA, T84.69XA, T84.7XXA

0RGA4KJ Fusion of Thoracolumbar Vertebral Joint with Nonautologous Tissue Substitute, Posterior Approach, Anterior Column, Percutaneous Endoscopic Approach
- HAC When reported with secondary diagnosis code T84.60XA, T84.610A, T84.611A, T84.612A, T84.613A, T84.614A, T84.615A, T84.619A, T84.63XA, T84.69XA, T84.7XXA

0RGA4Z0 Fusion of Thoracolumbar Vertebral Joint, Anterior Approach, Anterior Column, Percutaneous Endoscopic Approach
- HAC When reported with secondary diagnosis code T84.60XA, T84.610A, T84.611A, T84.612A, T84.613A, T84.614A, T84.615A, T84.619A, T84.63XA, T84.69XA, T84.7XXA

0RGA4Z1 Fusion of Thoracolumbar Vertebral Joint, Posterior Approach, Posterior Column, Percutaneous Endoscopic Approach
- HAC When reported with secondary diagnosis code T84.60XA, T84.610A, T84.611A, T84.612A, T84.613A, T84.614A, T84.615A, T84.619A, T84.63XA, T84.69XA, T84.7XXA

0RGA4ZJ Fusion of Thoracolumbar Vertebral Joint, Posterior Approach, Anterior Column, Percutaneous Endoscopic Approach
- HAC When reported with secondary diagnosis code T84.60XA, T84.611A, T84.612A, T84.613A, T84.614A, T84.615A, T84.619A, T84.63XA, T84.69XA, T84.7XXA

0RGC04Z Fusion of Right Temporomandibular Joint with Internal Fixation Device, Open Approach

0RGC07Z Fusion of Right Temporomandibular Joint with Autologous Tissue Substitute, Open Approach

0RGC0JZ Fusion of Right Temporomandibular Joint with Synthetic Substitute, Open Approach

0RGC0KZ Fusion of Right Temporomandibular Joint with Nonautologous Tissue Substitute, Open Approach

0RGC0ZZ Fusion of Right Temporomandibular Joint, Open Approach

0RGC34Z Fusion of Right Temporomandibular Joint with Internal Fixation Device, Percutaneous Approach

0RGC37Z Fusion of Right Temporomandibular Joint with Autologous Tissue Substitute, Percutaneous Approach

0RGC3JZ Fusion of Right Temporomandibular Joint with Synthetic Substitute, Percutaneous Approach

0RGC3KZ Fusion of Right Temporomandibular Joint with Nonautologous Tissue Substitute, Percutaneous Approach

0RGC3ZZ Fusion of Right Temporomandibular Joint, Percutaneous Approach

0RGC44Z Fusion of Right Temporomandibular Joint with Internal Fixation Device, Percutaneous Endoscopic Approach

0RGC47Z Fusion of Right Temporomandibular Joint with Autologous Tissue Substitute, Percutaneous Endoscopic Approach

0RGC4JZ Fusion of Right Temporomandibular Joint with Synthetic Substitute, Percutaneous Endoscopic Approach

0RGC4KZ Fusion of Right Temporomandibular Joint with Nonautologous Tissue Substitute, Percutaneous Endoscopic Approach

0RGC4ZZ Fusion of Right Temporomandibular Joint, Percutaneous Endoscopic Approach

0RGD04Z Fusion of Left Temporomandibular Joint with Internal Fixation Device, Open Approach

0RGD07Z Fusion of Left Temporomandibular Joint with Autologous Tissue Substitute, Open Approach

0RGD0JZ Fusion of Left Temporomandibular Joint with Synthetic Substitute, Open Approach

0RGD0KZ Fusion of Left Temporomandibular Joint with Nonautologous Tissue Substitute, Open Approach

0RGD0ZZ Fusion of Left Temporomandibular Joint, Open Approach

0RGD34Z Fusion of Left Temporomandibular Joint with Internal Fixation Device, Percutaneous Approach

0RGD37Z Fusion of Left Temporomandibular Joint with Autologous Tissue Substitute, Percutaneous Approach

0RGD3JZ Fusion of Left Temporomandibular Joint with Synthetic Substitute, Percutaneous Approach

0RGD3KZ Fusion of Left Temporomandibular Joint with Nonautologous Tissue Substitute, Percutaneous Approach

0RGD3ZZ Fusion of Left Temporomandibular Joint, Percutaneous Approach

0RGD44Z Fusion of Left Temporomandibular Joint with Internal Fixation Device, Percutaneous Endoscopic Approach

0RGD47Z Fusion of Left Temporomandibular Joint with Autologous Tissue Substitute, Percutaneous Endoscopic Approach

0RGD4JZ Fusion of Left Temporomandibular Joint with Synthetic Substitute, Percutaneous Endoscopic Approach

0RGD4KZ Fusion of Left Temporomandibular Joint with Nonautologous Tissue Substitute, Percutaneous Endoscopic Approach

0RGD4ZZ Fusion of Left Temporomandibular Joint, Percutaneous Endoscopic Approach

0RGE04Z Fusion of Right Sternoclavicular Joint with Internal Fixation Device, Open Approach
- HAC When reported with secondary diagnosis code T84.60XA, T84.610A, T84.611A, T84.612A, T84.613A, T84.614A, T84.615A, T84.619A, T84.63XA, T84.69XA, T84.7XXA

0RGE07Z Fusion of Right Sternoclavicular Joint with Autologous Tissue Substitute, Open Approach
- HAC When reported with secondary diagnosis code T84.60XA, T84.610A, T84.611A, T84.612A, T84.613A, T84.614A, T84.615A, T84.619A, T84.63XA, T84.69XA, T84.7XXA

0RGE0JZ Fusion of Right Sternoclavicular Joint with Synthetic Substitute, Open Approach
- HAC When reported with secondary diagnosis code T84.60XA, T84.610A, T84.611A, T84.612A, T84.613A, T84.614A, T84.615A, T84.619A, T84.63XA, T84.69XA, T84.7XXA

0RGE0KZ Fusion of Right Sternoclavicular Joint with Nonautologous Tissue Substitute, Open Approach
- HAC When reported with secondary diagnosis code T84.60XA, T84.610A, T84.611A, T84.612A, T84.613A, T84.614A, T84.615A, T84.619A, T84.63XA, T84.69XA, T84.7XXA

0RGE0ZZ Fusion of Right Sternoclavicular Joint, Open Approach
- HAC When reported with secondary diagnosis code T84.60XA, T84.610A, T84.611A, T84.612A, T84.613A, T84.614A, T84.615A, T84.619A, T84.63XA, T84.69XA, T84.7XXA

0RGE34Z Fusion of Right Sternoclavicular Joint with Internal Fixation Device, Percutaneous Approach
- HAC When reported with secondary diagnosis code T84.60XA, T84.610A, T84.611A, T84.612A, T84.613A, T84.614A, T84.615A, T84.619A, T84.63XA, T84.69XA, T84.7XXA

0RGE37Z Fusion of Right Sternoclavicular Joint with Autologous Tissue Substitute, Percutaneous Approach
- HAC When reported with secondary diagnosis code T84.60XA, T84.610A, T84.611A, T84.612A, T84.613A, T84.614A, T84.615A, T84.619A, T84.63XA, T84.69XA, T84.7XXA

0RGE3JZ Fusion of Right Sternoclavicular Joint with Synthetic Substitute, Percutaneous Approach
- HAC When reported with secondary diagnosis code T84.60XA, T84.610A, T84.611A, T84.612A, T84.613A, T84.614A, T84.615A, T84.619A, T84.63XA, T84.69XA, T84.7XXA

0RGE3KZ Fusion of Right Sternoclavicular Joint with Nonautologous Tissue Substitute, Percutaneous Approach
- HAC When reported with secondary diagnosis code T84.60XA, T84.611A, T84.612A, T84.613A, T84.614A, T84.615A, T84.619A, T84.63XA, T84.69XA, T84.7XXA

0RGE3ZZ Fusion of Right Sternoclavicular Joint, Percutaneous Approach
- HAC When reported with secondary diagnosis code T84.60XA, T84.610A, T84.611A, T84.612A, T84.613A, T84.614A, T84.615A, T84.619A, T84.63XA, T84.69XA, T84.7XXA

0RGE44Z Fusion of Right Sternoclavicular Joint with Internal Fixation Device, Percutaneous Endoscopic Approach

HAC When reported with secondary diagnosis code T84.60XA, T84.610A, T84.611A, T84.612A, T84.613A, T84.614A, T84.615A, T84.619A, T84.63XA, T84.69XA, T84.7XXA

0RGE47Z Fusion of Right Sternoclavicular Joint with Autologous Tissue Substitute, Percutaneous Endoscopic Approach

HAC When reported with secondary diagnosis code T84.60XA, T84.610A, T84.611A, T84.612A, T84.613A, T84.614A, T84.615A, T84.619A, T84.63XA, T84.69XA, T84.7XXA

0RGE4JZ Fusion of Right Sternoclavicular Joint with Synthetic Substitute, Percutaneous Endoscopic Approach

HAC When reported with secondary diagnosis code T84.60XA, T84.610A, T84.611A, T84.612A, T84.613A, T84.614A, T84.615A, T84.619A, T84.63XA, T84.69XA, T84.7XXA

0RGE4KZ Fusion of Right Sternoclavicular Joint with Nonautologous Tissue Substitute, Percutaneous Endoscopic Approach

HAC When reported with secondary diagnosis code T84.60XA, T84.610A, T84.611A, T84.612A, T84.613A, T84.614A, T84.615A, T84.619A, T84.63XA, T84.69XA, T84.7XXA

0RGE4ZZ Fusion of Right Sternoclavicular Joint, Percutaneous Endoscopic Approach

HAC When reported with secondary diagnosis code T84.60XA, T84.610A, T84.611A, T84.612A, T84.613A, T84.614A, T84.615A, T84.619A, T84.63XA, T84.69XA, T84.7XXA

0RGF04Z Fusion of Left Sternoclavicular Joint with Internal Fixation Device, Open Approach

HAC When reported with secondary diagnosis code T84.60XA, T84.610A, T84.611A, T84.612A, T84.613A, T84.614A, T84.615A, T84.619A, T84.63XA, T84.69XA, T84.7XXA

0RGF07Z Fusion of Left Sternoclavicular Joint with Autologous Tissue Substitute, Open Approach

HAC When reported with secondary diagnosis code T84.60XA, T84.610A, T84.611A, T84.612A, T84.613A, T84.614A, T84.615A, T84.619A, T84.63XA, T84.69XA, T84.7XXA

0RGF0JZ Fusion of Left Sternoclavicular Joint with Synthetic Substitute, Open Approach

HAC When reported with secondary diagnosis code T84.60XA, T84.610A, T84.611A, T84.612A, T84.613A, T84.614A, T84.615A, T84.619A, T84.63XA, T84.69XA, T84.7XXA

0RGF0KZ Fusion of Left Sternoclavicular Joint with Nonautologous Tissue Substitute, Open Approach

HAC When reported with secondary diagnosis code T84.60XA, T84.610A, T84.611A, T84.612A, T84.613A, T84.614A, T84.615A, T84.619A, T84.63XA, T84.69XA, T84.7XXA

0RGF0ZZ Fusion of Left Sternoclavicular Joint, Open Approach

HAC When reported with secondary diagnosis code T84.60XA, T84.610A, T84.611A, T84.612A, T84.613A, T84.614A, T84.615A, T84.619A, T84.63XA, T84.69XA, T84.7XXA

0RGF34Z Fusion of Left Sternoclavicular Joint with Internal Fixation Device, Percutaneous Approach

HAC When reported with secondary diagnosis code T84.60XA, T84.610A, T84.611A, T84.612A, T84.613A, T84.614A, T84.615A, T84.619A, T84.63XA, T84.69XA, T84.7XXA

0RGF37Z Fusion of Left Sternoclavicular Joint with Autologous Tissue Substitute, Percutaneous Approach

HAC When reported with secondary diagnosis code T84.60XA, T84.610A, T84.611A, T84.612A, T84.613A, T84.614A, T84.615A, T84.619A, T84.63XA, T84.69XA, T84.7XXA

0RGF3JZ Fusion of Left Sternoclavicular Joint with Synthetic Substitute, Percutaneous Approach

HAC When reported with secondary diagnosis code T84.60XA, T84.610A, T84.611A, T84.612A, T84.613A, T84.614A, T84.615A, T84.619A, T84.63XA, T84.69XA, T84.7XXA

0RGF3KZ Fusion of Left Sternoclavicular Joint with Nonautologous Tissue Substitute, Percutaneous Approach

HAC When reported with secondary diagnosis code T84.60XA, T84.610A, T84.611A, T84.612A, T84.613A, T84.614A, T84.615A, T84.619A, T84.63XA, T84.69XA, T84.7XXA

0RGF3ZZ Fusion of Left Sternoclavicular Joint, Percutaneous Approach

HAC When reported with secondary diagnosis code T84.60XA, T84.610A, T84.611A, T84.612A, T84.613A, T84.614A, T84.615A, T84.619A, T84.63XA, T84.69XA, T84.7XXA

0RGF44Z Fusion of Left Sternoclavicular Joint with Internal Fixation Device, Percutaneous Endoscopic Approach

HAC When reported with secondary diagnosis code T84.60XA, T84.610A, T84.611A, T84.612A, T84.613A, T84.614A, T84.615A, T84.619A, T84.63XA, T84.69XA, T84.7XXA

0RGF47Z Fusion of Left Sternoclavicular Joint with Autologous Tissue Substitute, Percutaneous Endoscopic Approach

HAC When reported with secondary diagnosis code T84.60XA, T84.610A, T84.611A, T84.612A, T84.613A, T84.614A, T84.615A, T84.619A, T84.63XA, T84.69XA, T84.7XXA

0RGF4JZ Fusion of Left Sternoclavicular Joint with Synthetic Substitute, Percutaneous Endoscopic Approach

HAC When reported with secondary diagnosis code T84.60XA, T84.610A, T84.611A, T84.612A, T84.613A, T84.614A, T84.615A, T84.619A, T84.63XA, T84.69XA, T84.7XXA

0RGF4KZ Fusion of Left Sternoclavicular Joint with Nonautologous Tissue Substitute, Percutaneous Endoscopic Approach

HAC When reported with secondary diagnosis code T84.60XA, T84.610A, T84.611A, T84.612A, T84.613A, T84.614A, T84.615A, T84.619A, T84.63XA, T84.69XA, T84.7XXA

0RGF4ZZ Fusion of Left Sternoclavicular Joint, Percutaneous Endoscopic Approach

HAC When reported with secondary diagnosis code T84.60XA, T84.610A, T84.611A, T84.612A, T84.613A, T84.614A, T84.615A, T84.619A, T84.63XA, T84.69XA, T84.7XXA

0RGG04Z Fusion of Right Acromioclavicular Joint with Internal Fixation Device, Open Approach

HAC When reported with secondary diagnosis code T84.60XA, T84.610A, T84.611A, T84.612A, T84.613A, T84.614A, T84.615A, T84.619A, T84.63XA, T84.69XA, T84.7XXA

0RGG07Z Fusion of Right Acromioclavicular Joint with Autologous Tissue Substitute, Open Approach

HAC When reported with secondary diagnosis code T84.60XA, T84.610A, T84.611A, T84.612A, T84.613A, T84.614A, T84.615A, T84.619A, T84.63XA, T84.69XA, T84.7XXA

0RGG0JZ Fusion of Right Acromioclavicular Joint with Synthetic Substitute, Open Approach

HAC When reported with secondary diagnosis code T84.60XA, T84.610A, T84.611A, T84.612A, T84.613A, T84.614A, T84.615A, T84.619A, T84.63XA, T84.69XA, T84.7XXA

0RGG0KZ Fusion of Right Acromioclavicular Joint with Nonautologous Tissue Substitute, Open Approach

HAC When reported with secondary diagnosis code T84.60XA, T84.610A, T84.611A, T84.612A, T84.613A, T84.614A, T84.615A, T84.619A, T84.63XA, T84.69XA, T84.7XXA

0RGG0ZZ Fusion of Right Acromioclavicular Joint, Open Approach

HAC When reported with secondary diagnosis code T84.60XA, T84.610A, T84.611A, T84.612A, T84.613A, T84.614A, T84.615A, T84.619A, T84.63XA, T84.69XA, T84.7XXA

0RGG34Z Fusion of Right Acromioclavicular Joint with Internal Fixation Device, Percutaneous Approach

HAC When reported with secondary diagnosis code T84.60XA, T84.610A, T84.611A, T84.612A, T84.613A, T84.614A, T84.615A, T84.619A, T84.63XA, T84.69XA, T84.7XXA

0RGG37Z Fusion of Right Acromioclavicular Joint with Autologous Tissue Substitute, Percutaneous Approach

HAC When reported with secondary diagnosis code T84.60XA, T84.610A, T84.611A, T84.612A, T84.613A, T84.614A, T84.615A, T84.619A, T84.63XA, T84.69XA, T84.7XXA

0RGG3JZ Fusion of Right Acromioclavicular Joint with Synthetic Substitute, Percutaneous Approach

HAC When reported with secondary diagnosis code T84.60XA, T84.610A, T84.611A, T84.612A, T84.613A, T84.614A, T84.615A, T84.619A, T84.63XA, T84.69XA, T84.7XXA

0RGG3KZ Fusion of Right Acromioclavicular Joint with Nonautologous Tissue Substitute, Percutaneous Approach

HAC When reported with secondary diagnosis code T84.60XA, T84.610A, T84.611A, T84.612A, T84.613A, T84.614A, T84.615A, T84.619A, T84.63XA, T84.69XA, T84.7XXA

0RGG3ZZ Fusion of Right Acromioclavicular Joint, Percutaneous Approach

HAC When reported with secondary diagnosis code T84.60XA, T84.610A, T84.611A, T84.612A, T84.613A, T84.614A, T84.615A, T84.619A, T84.63XA, T84.69XA, T84.7XXA

0RGG44Z Fusion of Right Acromioclavicular Joint with Internal Fixation Device, Percutaneous Endoscopic Approach
- HAC When reported with secondary diagnosis code T84.60XA, T84.610A, T84.611A, T84.612A, T84.613A, T84.614A, T84.615A, T84.619A, T84.63XA, T84.69XA, T84.7XXA

0RGG47Z Fusion of Right Acromioclavicular Joint with Autologous Tissue Substitute, Percutaneous Endoscopic Approach
- HAC When reported with secondary diagnosis code T84.60XA, T84.610A, T84.611A, T84.612A, T84.613A, T84.614A, T84.615A, T84.619A, T84.63XA, T84.69XA, T84.7XXA

0RGG4JZ Fusion of Right Acromioclavicular Joint with Synthetic Substitute, Percutaneous Endoscopic Approach
- HAC When reported with secondary diagnosis code T84.60XA, T84.610A, T84.611A, T84.612A, T84.613A, T84.614A, T84.615A, T84.619A, T84.63XA, T84.69XA, T84.7XXA

0RGG4KZ Fusion of Right Acromioclavicular Joint with Nonautologous Tissue Substitute, Percutaneous Endoscopic Approach
- HAC When reported with secondary diagnosis code T84.60XA, T84.610A, T84.611A, T84.612A, T84.613A, T84.614A, T84.615A, T84.619A, T84.63XA, T84.69XA, T84.7XXA

0RGG4ZZ Fusion of Right Acromioclavicular Joint, Percutaneous Endoscopic Approach
- HAC When reported with secondary diagnosis code T84.60XA, T84.610A, T84.611A, T84.612A, T84.613A, T84.614A, T84.615A, T84.619A, T84.63XA, T84.69XA, T84.7XXA

0RGH04Z Fusion of Left Acromioclavicular Joint with Internal Fixation Device, Open Approach
- HAC When reported with secondary diagnosis code T84.60XA, T84.610A, T84.611A, T84.612A, T84.613A, T84.614A, T84.615A, T84.619A, T84.63XA, T84.69XA, T84.7XXA

0RGH07Z Fusion of Left Acromioclavicular Joint with Autologous Tissue Substitute, Open Approach
- HAC When reported with secondary diagnosis code T84.60XA, T84.610A, T84.611A, T84.612A, T84.613A, T84.614A, T84.615A, T84.619A, T84.63XA, T84.69XA, T84.7XXA

0RGH0JZ Fusion of Left Acromioclavicular Joint with Synthetic Substitute, Open Approach
- HAC When reported with secondary diagnosis code T84.60XA, T84.610A, T84.611A, T84.612A, T84.613A, T84.614A, T84.615A, T84.619A, T84.63XA, T84.69XA, T84.7XXA

0RGH0KZ Fusion of Left Acromioclavicular Joint with Nonautologous Tissue Substitute, Open Approach
- HAC When reported with secondary diagnosis code T84.60XA, T84.610A, T84.611A, T84.612A, T84.613A, T84.614A, T84.615A, T84.619A, T84.63XA, T84.69XA, T84.7XXA

0RGH0ZZ Fusion of Left Acromioclavicular Joint, Open Approach
- HAC When reported with secondary diagnosis code T84.60XA, T84.610A, T84.611A, T84.612A, T84.613A, T84.614A, T84.615A, T84.619A, T84.63XA, T84.69XA, T84.7XXA

0RGH34Z Fusion of Left Acromioclavicular Joint with Internal Fixation Device, Percutaneous Approach
- HAC When reported with secondary diagnosis code T84.60XA, T84.610A, T84.611A, T84.612A, T84.613A, T84.614A, T84.615A, T84.619A, T84.63XA, T84.69XA, T84.7XXA

0RGH37Z Fusion of Left Acromioclavicular Joint with Autologous Tissue Substitute, Percutaneous Approach
- HAC When reported with secondary diagnosis code T84.60XA, T84.610A, T84.611A, T84.612A, T84.613A, T84.614A, T84.615A, T84.619A, T84.63XA, T84.69XA, T84.7XXA

0RGH3JZ Fusion of Left Acromioclavicular Joint with Synthetic Substitute, Percutaneous Approach
- HAC When reported with secondary diagnosis code T84.60XA, T84.610A, T84.611A, T84.612A, T84.613A, T84.614A, T84.615A, T84.619A, T84.63XA, T84.69XA, T84.7XXA

0RGH3KZ Fusion of Left Acromioclavicular Joint with Nonautologous Tissue Substitute, Percutaneous Approach
- HAC When reported with secondary diagnosis code T84.60XA, T84.610A, T84.611A, T84.612A, T84.613A, T84.614A, T84.615A, T84.619A, T84.63XA, T84.69XA, T84.7XXA

0RGH3ZZ Fusion of Left Acromioclavicular Joint, Percutaneous Approach
- HAC When reported with secondary diagnosis code T84.60XA, T84.610A, T84.611A, T84.612A, T84.613A, T84.614A, T84.615A, T84.619A, T84.63XA, T84.69XA, T84.7XXA

0RGH44Z Fusion of Left Acromioclavicular Joint with Internal Fixation Device, Percutaneous Endoscopic Approach
- HAC When reported with secondary diagnosis code T84.60XA, T84.610A, T84.611A, T84.612A, T84.613A, T84.614A, T84.615A, T84.619A, T84.63XA, T84.69XA, T84.7XXA

0RGH47Z Fusion of Left Acromioclavicular Joint with Autologous Tissue Substitute, Percutaneous Endoscopic Approach
- HAC When reported with secondary diagnosis code T84.60XA, T84.610A, T84.611A, T84.612A, T84.613A, T84.614A, T84.615A, T84.619A, T84.63XA, T84.69XA, T84.7XXA

0RGH4JZ Fusion of Left Acromioclavicular Joint with Synthetic Substitute, Percutaneous Endoscopic Approach
- HAC When reported with secondary diagnosis code T84.60XA, T84.610A, T84.611A, T84.612A, T84.613A, T84.614A, T84.615A, T84.619A, T84.63XA, T84.69XA, T84.7XXA

0RGH4KZ Fusion of Left Acromioclavicular Joint with Nonautologous Tissue Substitute, Percutaneous Endoscopic Approach
- HAC When reported with secondary diagnosis code T84.60XA, T84.610A, T84.611A, T84.612A, T84.613A, T84.614A, T84.615A, T84.619A, T84.63XA, T84.69XA, T84.7XXA

0RGH4ZZ Fusion of Left Acromioclavicular Joint, Percutaneous Endoscopic Approach
- HAC When reported with secondary diagnosis code T84.60XA, T84.610A, T84.611A, T84.612A, T84.613A, T84.614A, T84.615A, T84.619A, T84.63XA, T84.69XA, T84.7XXA

0RGJ04Z Fusion of Right Shoulder Joint with Internal Fixation Device, Open Approach
- HAC When reported with secondary diagnosis code T84.60XA, T84.610A, T84.611A, T84.612A, T84.613A, T84.614A, T84.615A, T84.619A, T84.63XA, T84.69XA, T84.7XXA

0RGJ07Z Fusion of Right Shoulder Joint with Autologous Tissue Substitute, Open Approach
- HAC When reported with secondary diagnosis code T84.60XA, T84.610A, T84.611A, T84.612A, T84.613A, T84.614A, T84.615A, T84.619A, T84.63XA, T84.69XA, T84.7XXA

0RGJ0JZ Fusion of Right Shoulder Joint with Synthetic Substitute, Open Approach
- HAC When reported with secondary diagnosis code T84.60XA, T84.610A, T84.611A, T84.612A, T84.613A, T84.614A, T84.615A, T84.619A, T84.63XA, T84.69XA, T84.7XXA

0RGJ0KZ Fusion of Right Shoulder Joint with Nonautologous Tissue Substitute, Open Approach
- HAC When reported with secondary diagnosis code T84.60XA, T84.610A, T84.611A, T84.612A, T84.613A, T84.614A, T84.615A, T84.619A, T84.63XA, T84.69XA, T84.7XXA

0RGJ0ZZ Fusion of Right Shoulder Joint, Open Approach
- HAC When reported with secondary diagnosis code T84.60XA, T84.610A, T84.611A, T84.612A, T84.613A, T84.614A, T84.615A, T84.619A, T84.63XA, T84.69XA, T84.7XXA

0RGJ34Z Fusion of Right Shoulder Joint with Internal Fixation Device, Percutaneous Approach
- HAC When reported with secondary diagnosis code T84.60XA, T84.610A, T84.611A, T84.612A, T84.613A, T84.614A, T84.615A, T84.619A, T84.63XA, T84.69XA, T84.7XXA

0RGJ37Z Fusion of Right Shoulder Joint with Autologous Tissue Substitute, Percutaneous Approach
- HAC When reported with secondary diagnosis code T84.60XA, T84.610A, T84.611A, T84.612A, T84.613A, T84.614A, T84.615A, T84.619A, T84.63XA, T84.69XA, T84.7XXA

0RGJ3JZ Fusion of Right Shoulder Joint with Synthetic Substitute, Percutaneous Approach
- HAC When reported with secondary diagnosis code T84.60XA, T84.610A, T84.611A, T84.612A, T84.613A, T84.614A, T84.615A, T84.619A, T84.63XA, T84.69XA, T84.7XXA

0RGJ3KZ Fusion of Right Shoulder Joint with Nonautologous Tissue Substitute, Percutaneous Approach
- HAC When reported with secondary diagnosis code T84.60XA, T84.610A, T84.611A, T84.612A, T84.613A, T84.614A, T84.615A, T84.619A, T84.63XA, T84.69XA, T84.7XXA

0RGJ3ZZ Fusion of Right Shoulder Joint, Percutaneous Approach
- HAC When reported with secondary diagnosis code T84.60XA, T84.610A, T84.611A, T84.612A, T84.613A, T84.614A, T84.615A, T84.619A, T84.63XA, T84.69XA, T84.7XXA

0RGJ44Z   Fusion of Right Shoulder Joint with Internal Fixation Device, Percutaneous Endoscopic Approach

HAC   When reported with secondary diagnosis code T84.60XA, T84.610A, T84.611A, T84.612A, T84.613A, T84.614A, T84.615A, T84.619A, T84.63XA, T84.69XA, T84.7XXA

0RGJ47Z   Fusion of Right Shoulder Joint with Autologous Tissue Substitute, Percutaneous Endoscopic Approach

HAC   When reported with secondary diagnosis code T84.60XA, T84.610A, T84.611A, T84.612A, T84.613A, T84.614A, T84.615A, T84.619A, T84.63XA, T84.69XA, T84.7XXA

0RGJ4JZ   Fusion of Right Shoulder Joint with Synthetic Substitute, Percutaneous Endoscopic Approach

HAC   When reported with secondary diagnosis code T84.60XA, T84.610A, T84.611A, T84.612A, T84.613A, T84.614A, T84.615A, T84.619A, T84.63XA, T84.69XA, T84.7XXA

0RGJ4KZ   Fusion of Right Shoulder Joint with Nonautologous Tissue Substitute, Percutaneous Endoscopic Approach

HAC   When reported with secondary diagnosis code T84.60XA, T84.610A, T84.611A, T84.612A, T84.613A, T84.614A, T84.615A, T84.619A, T84.63XA, T84.69XA, T84.7XXA

0RGJ4ZZ   Fusion of Right Shoulder Joint, Percutaneous Endoscopic Approach

HAC   When reported with secondary diagnosis code T84.60XA, T84.610A, T84.611A, T84.612A, T84.613A, T84.614A, T84.615A, T84.619A, T84.63XA, T84.69XA, T84.7XXA

0RGK04Z   Fusion of Left Shoulder Joint with Internal Fixation Device, Open Approach

HAC   When reported with secondary diagnosis code T84.60XA, T84.610A, T84.611A, T84.612A, T84.613A, T84.614A, T84.615A, T84.619A, T84.63XA, T84.69XA, T84.7XXA

0RGK07Z   Fusion of Left Shoulder Joint with Autologous Tissue Substitute, Open Approach

HAC   When reported with secondary diagnosis code T84.60XA, T84.610A, T84.611A, T84.612A, T84.613A, T84.614A, T84.615A, T84.619A, T84.63XA, T84.69XA, T84.7XXA

0RGK0JZ   Fusion of Left Shoulder Joint with Synthetic Substitute, Open Approach

HAC   When reported with secondary diagnosis code T84.60XA, T84.610A, T84.611A, T84.612A, T84.613A, T84.614A, T84.615A, T84.619A, T84.63XA, T84.69XA, T84.7XXA

0RGK0KZ   Fusion of Left Shoulder Joint with Nonautologous Tissue Substitute, Open Approach

HAC   When reported with secondary diagnosis code T84.60XA, T84.610A, T84.611A, T84.612A, T84.613A, T84.614A, T84.615A, T84.619A, T84.63XA, T84.69XA, T84.7XXA

0RGK0ZZ   Fusion of Left Shoulder Joint, Open Approach

HAC   When reported with secondary diagnosis code T84.60XA, T84.610A, T84.611A, T84.612A, T84.613A, T84.614A, T84.615A, T84.619A, T84.63XA, T84.69XA, T84.7XXA

0RGK34Z   Fusion of Left Shoulder Joint with Internal Fixation Device, Percutaneous Approach

HAC   When reported with secondary diagnosis code T84.60XA, T84.610A, T84.611A, T84.612A, T84.613A, T84.614A, T84.615A, T84.619A, T84.63XA, T84.69XA, T84.7XXA

0RGK37Z   Fusion of Left Shoulder Joint with Autologous Tissue Substitute, Percutaneous Approach

HAC   When reported with secondary diagnosis code T84.60XA, T84.610A, T84.611A, T84.612A, T84.613A, T84.614A, T84.615A, T84.619A, T84.63XA, T84.69XA, T84.7XXA

0RGK3JZ   Fusion of Left Shoulder Joint with Synthetic Substitute, Percutaneous Approach

HAC   When reported with secondary diagnosis code T84.60XA, T84.610A, T84.611A, T84.612A, T84.613A, T84.614A, T84.615A, T84.619A, T84.63XA, T84.69XA, T84.7XXA

0RGK3KZ   Fusion of Left Shoulder Joint with Nonautologous Tissue Substitute, Percutaneous Approach

HAC   When reported with secondary diagnosis code T84.60XA, T84.610A, T84.611A, T84.612A, T84.613A, T84.614A, T84.615A, T84.619A, T84.63XA, T84.69XA, T84.7XXA

0RGK3ZZ   Fusion of Left Shoulder Joint, Percutaneous Approach

HAC   When reported with secondary diagnosis code T84.60XA, T84.610A, T84.611A, T84.612A, T84.613A, T84.614A, T84.615A, T84.619A, T84.63XA, T84.69XA, T84.7XXA

0RGK44Z   Fusion of Left Shoulder Joint with Internal Fixation Device, Percutaneous Endoscopic Approach

HAC   When reported with secondary diagnosis code T84.60XA, T84.610A, T84.611A, T84.612A, T84.613A, T84.614A, T84.615A, T84.619A, T84.63XA, T84.69XA, T84.7XXA

0RGK47Z   Fusion of Left Shoulder Joint with Autologous Tissue Substitute, Percutaneous Endoscopic Approach

HAC   When reported with secondary diagnosis code T84.60XA, T84.610A, T84.611A, T84.612A, T84.613A, T84.614A, T84.615A, T84.619A, T84.63XA, T84.69XA, T84.7XXA

0RGK4JZ   Fusion of Left Shoulder Joint with Synthetic Substitute, Percutaneous Endoscopic Approach

HAC   When reported with secondary diagnosis code T84.60XA, T84.610A, T84.611A, T84.612A, T84.613A, T84.614A, T84.615A, T84.619A, T84.63XA, T84.69XA, T84.7XXA

0RGK4KZ   Fusion of Left Shoulder Joint with Nonautologous Tissue Substitute, Percutaneous Endoscopic Approach

HAC   When reported with secondary diagnosis code T84.60XA, T84.610A, T84.611A, T84.612A, T84.613A, T84.614A, T84.615A, T84.619A, T84.63XA, T84.69XA, T84.7XXA

0RGK4ZZ   Fusion of Left Shoulder Joint, Percutaneous Endoscopic Approach

HAC   When reported with secondary diagnosis code T84.60XA, T84.610A, T84.611A, T84.612A, T84.613A, T84.614A, T84.615A, T84.619A, T84.63XA, T84.69XA, T84.7XXA

0RGL04Z   Fusion of Right Elbow Joint with Internal Fixation Device, Open Approach

HAC   When reported with secondary diagnosis code T84.60XA, T84.610A, T84.611A, T84.612A, T84.613A, T84.614A, T84.615A, T84.619A, T84.63XA, T84.69XA, T84.7XXA

0RGL05Z   Fusion of Right Elbow Joint with External Fixation Device, Open Approach

HAC   When reported with secondary diagnosis code T84.60XA, T84.610A, T84.611A, T84.612A, T84.613A, T84.614A, T84.615A, T84.619A, T84.63XA, T84.69XA, T84.7XXA

0RGL07Z   Fusion of Right Elbow Joint with Autologous Tissue Substitute, Open Approach

HAC   When reported with secondary diagnosis code T84.60XA, T84.610A, T84.611A, T84.612A, T84.613A, T84.614A, T84.615A, T84.619A, T84.63XA, T84.69XA, T84.7XXA

0RGL0JZ   Fusion of Right Elbow Joint with Synthetic Substitute, Open Approach

HAC   When reported with secondary diagnosis code T84.60XA, T84.610A, T84.611A, T84.612A, T84.613A, T84.614A, T84.615A, T84.619A, T84.63XA, T84.69XA, T84.7XXA

0RGL0KZ   Fusion of Right Elbow Joint with Nonautologous Tissue Substitute, Open Approach

HAC   When reported with secondary diagnosis code T84.60XA, T84.610A, T84.611A, T84.612A, T84.613A, T84.614A, T84.615A, T84.619A, T84.63XA, T84.69XA, T84.7XXA

0RGL0ZZ   Fusion of Right Elbow Joint, Open Approach

HAC   When reported with secondary diagnosis code T84.60XA, T84.610A, T84.611A, T84.612A, T84.613A, T84.614A, T84.615A, T84.619A, T84.63XA, T84.69XA, T84.7XXA

0RGL34Z   Fusion of Right Elbow Joint with Internal Fixation Device, Percutaneous Approach

HAC   When reported with secondary diagnosis code T84.60XA, T84.610A, T84.611A, T84.612A, T84.613A, T84.614A, T84.615A, T84.619A, T84.63XA, T84.69XA, T84.7XXA

0RGL35Z   Fusion of Right Elbow Joint with External Fixation Device, Percutaneous Approach

HAC   When reported with secondary diagnosis code T84.60XA, T84.610A, T84.611A, T84.612A, T84.613A, T84.614A, T84.615A, T84.619A, T84.63XA, T84.69XA, T84.7XXA

0RGL37Z   Fusion of Right Elbow Joint with Autologous Tissue Substitute, Percutaneous Approach

HAC   When reported with secondary diagnosis code T84.60XA, T84.610A, T84.611A, T84.612A, T84.613A, T84.614A, T84.615A, T84.619A, T84.63XA, T84.69XA, T84.7XXA

0RGL3JZ   Fusion of Right Elbow Joint with Synthetic Substitute, Percutaneous Approach

HAC   When reported with secondary diagnosis code T84.60XA, T84.610A, T84.611A, T84.612A, T84.613A, T84.614A, T84.615A, T84.619A, T84.63XA, T84.69XA, T84.7XXA

0RGL3KZ Fusion of Right Elbow Joint with Nonautologous Tissue Substitute, Percutaneous Approach

HAC When reported with secondary diagnosis code T84.60XA, T84.610A, T84.611A, T84.612A, T84.613A, T84.614A, T84.615A, T84.619A, T84.63XA, T84.69XA, T84.7XXA

0RGL3ZZ Fusion of Right Elbow Joint, Percutaneous Approach

HAC When reported with secondary diagnosis code T84.60XA, T84.610A, T84.611A, T84.612A, T84.613A, T84.614A, T84.615A, T84.619A, T84.63XA, T84.69XA, T84.7XXA

0RGL44Z Fusion of Right Elbow Joint with Internal Fixation Device, Percutaneous Endoscopic Approach

HAC When reported with secondary diagnosis code T84.60XA, T84.610A, T84.611A, T84.612A, T84.613A, T84.614A, T84.615A, T84.619A, T84.63XA, T84.69XA, T84.7XXA

0RGL45Z Fusion of Right Elbow Joint with External Fixation Device, Percutaneous Endoscopic Approach

HAC When reported with secondary diagnosis code T84.60XA, T84.610A, T84.611A, T84.612A, T84.613A, T84.614A, T84.615A, T84.619A, T84.63XA, T84.69XA, T84.7XXA

0RGL47Z Fusion of Right Elbow Joint with Autologous Tissue Substitute, Percutaneous Endoscopic Approach

HAC When reported with secondary diagnosis code T84.60XA, T84.610A, T84.611A, T84.612A, T84.613A, T84.614A, T84.615A, T84.619A, T84.63XA, T84.69XA, T84.7XXA

0RGL4JZ Fusion of Right Elbow Joint with Synthetic Substitute, Percutaneous Endoscopic Approach

HAC When reported with secondary diagnosis code T84.60XA, T84.610A, T84.611A, T84.612A, T84.613A, T84.614A, T84.615A, T84.619A, T84.63XA, T84.69XA, T84.7XXA

0RGL4KZ Fusion of Right Elbow Joint with Nonautologous Tissue Substitute, Percutaneous Endoscopic Approach

HAC When reported with secondary diagnosis code T84.60XA, T84.610A, T84.611A, T84.612A, T84.613A, T84.614A, T84.615A, T84.619A, T84.63XA, T84.69XA, T84.7XXA

0RGL4ZZ Fusion of Right Elbow Joint, Percutaneous Endoscopic Approach

HAC When reported with secondary diagnosis code T84.60XA, T84.610A, T84.611A, T84.612A, T84.613A, T84.614A, T84.615A, T84.619A, T84.63XA, T84.69XA, T84.7XXA

0RGM04Z Fusion of Left Elbow Joint with Internal Fixation Device, Open Approach

HAC When reported with secondary diagnosis code T84.60XA, T84.610A, T84.611A, T84.612A, T84.613A, T84.614A, T84.615A, T84.619A, T84.63XA, T84.69XA, T84.7XXA

0RGM05Z Fusion of Left Elbow Joint with External Fixation Device, Open Approach

HAC When reported with secondary diagnosis code T84.60XA, T84.610A, T84.611A, T84.612A, T84.613A, T84.614A, T84.615A, T84.619A, T84.63XA, T84.69XA, T84.7XXA

0RGM07Z Fusion of Left Elbow Joint with Autologous Tissue Substitute, Open Approach

HAC When reported with secondary diagnosis code T84.60XA, T84.610A, T84.611A, T84.612A, T84.613A, T84.614A, T84.615A, T84.619A, T84.63XA, T84.69XA, T84.7XXA

0RGM0JZ Fusion of Left Elbow Joint with Synthetic Substitute, Open Approach

HAC When reported with secondary diagnosis code T84.60XA, T84.610A, T84.611A, T84.612A, T84.613A, T84.614A, T84.615A, T84.619A, T84.63XA, T84.69XA, T84.7XXA

0RGM0KZ Fusion of Left Elbow Joint with Nonautologous Tissue Substitute, Open Approach

HAC When reported with secondary diagnosis code T84.60XA, T84.610A, T84.611A, T84.612A, T84.613A, T84.614A, T84.615A, T84.619A, T84.63XA, T84.69XA, T84.7XXA

0RGM0ZZ Fusion of Left Elbow Joint, Open Approach

HAC When reported with secondary diagnosis code T84.60XA, T84.610A, T84.611A, T84.612A, T84.613A, T84.614A, T84.615A, T84.619A, T84.63XA, T84.69XA, T84.7XXA

0RGM34Z Fusion of Left Elbow Joint with Internal Fixation Device, Percutaneous Approach

HAC When reported with secondary diagnosis code T84.60XA, T84.610A, T84.611A, T84.612A, T84.613A, T84.614A, T84.615A, T84.619A, T84.63XA, T84.69XA, T84.7XXA

0RGM35Z Fusion of Left Elbow Joint with External Fixation Device, Percutaneous Approach

HAC When reported with secondary diagnosis code T84.60XA, T84.610A, T84.611A, T84.612A, T84.613A, T84.614A, T84.615A, T84.619A, T84.63XA, T84.69XA, T84.7XXA

0RGM37Z Fusion of Left Elbow Joint with Autologous Tissue Substitute, Percutaneous Approach

HAC When reported with secondary diagnosis code T84.60XA, T84.610A, T84.611A, T84.612A, T84.613A, T84.614A, T84.615A, T84.619A, T84.63XA, T84.69XA, T84.7XXA

0RGM3JZ Fusion of Left Elbow Joint with Synthetic Substitute, Percutaneous Approach

HAC When reported with secondary diagnosis code T84.60XA, T84.610A, T84.611A, T84.612A, T84.613A, T84.614A, T84.615A, T84.619A, T84.63XA, T84.69XA, T84.7XXA

0RGM3KZ Fusion of Left Elbow Joint with Nonautologous Tissue Substitute, Percutaneous Approach

HAC When reported with secondary diagnosis code T84.60XA, T84.610A, T84.611A, T84.612A, T84.613A, T84.614A, T84.615A, T84.619A, T84.63XA, T84.69XA, T84.7XXA

0RGM3ZZ Fusion of Left Elbow Joint, Percutaneous Approach

HAC When reported with secondary diagnosis code T84.60XA, T84.610A, T84.611A, T84.612A, T84.613A, T84.614A, T84.615A, T84.619A, T84.63XA, T84.69XA, T84.7XXA

0RGM44Z Fusion of Left Elbow Joint with Internal Fixation Device, Percutaneous Endoscopic Approach

HAC When reported with secondary diagnosis code T84.60XA, T84.610A, T84.611A, T84.612A, T84.613A, T84.614A, T84.615A, T84.619A, T84.63XA, T84.69XA, T84.7XXA

0RGM45Z Fusion of Left Elbow Joint with External Fixation Device, Percutaneous Endoscopic Approach

HAC When reported with secondary diagnosis code T84.60XA, T84.610A, T84.611A, T84.612A, T84.613A, T84.614A, T84.615A, T84.619A, T84.63XA, T84.69XA, T84.7XXA

0RGM47Z Fusion of Left Elbow Joint with Autologous Tissue Substitute, Percutaneous Endoscopic Approach

HAC When reported with secondary diagnosis code T84.60XA, T84.610A, T84.611A, T84.612A, T84.613A, T84.614A, T84.615A, T84.619A, T84.63XA, T84.69XA, T84.7XXA

0RGM4JZ Fusion of Left Elbow Joint with Synthetic Substitute, Percutaneous Endoscopic Approach

HAC When reported with secondary diagnosis code T84.60XA, T84.610A, T84.611A, T84.612A, T84.613A, T84.614A, T84.615A, T84.619A, T84.63XA, T84.69XA, T84.7XXA

0RGM4KZ Fusion of Left Elbow Joint with Nonautologous Tissue Substitute, Percutaneous Endoscopic Approach

HAC When reported with secondary diagnosis code T84.60XA, T84.610A, T84.611A, T84.612A, T84.613A, T84.614A, T84.615A, T84.619A, T84.63XA, T84.69XA, T84.7XXA

0RGM4ZZ Fusion of Left Elbow Joint, Percutaneous Endoscopic Approach

HAC When reported with secondary diagnosis code T84.60XA, T84.610A, T84.611A, T84.612A, T84.613A, T84.614A, T84.615A, T84.619A, T84.63XA, T84.69XA, T84.7XXA

0RGN04Z Fusion of Right Wrist Joint with Internal Fixation Device, Open Approach

0RGN05Z Fusion of Right Wrist Joint with External Fixation Device, Open Approach

0RGN07Z Fusion of Right Wrist Joint with Autologous Tissue Substitute, Open Approach

0RGN0JZ Fusion of Right Wrist Joint with Synthetic Substitute, Open Approach

0RGN0KZ Fusion of Right Wrist Joint with Nonautologous Tissue Substitute, Open Approach

0RGN0ZZ Fusion of Right Wrist Joint, Open Approach

0RGN34Z Fusion of Right Wrist Joint with Internal Fixation Device, Percutaneous Approach

0RGN35Z Fusion of Right Wrist Joint with External Fixation Device, Percutaneous Approach

0RGN37Z Fusion of Right Wrist Joint with Autologous Tissue Substitute, Percutaneous Approach

0RGN3JZ Fusion of Right Wrist Joint with Synthetic Substitute, Percutaneous Approach

0RGN3KZ Fusion of Right Wrist Joint with Nonautologous Tissue Substitute, Percutaneous Approach

0RGN3ZZ Fusion of Right Wrist Joint, Percutaneous Approach

0RGN44Z Fusion of Right Wrist Joint with Internal Fixation Device, Percutaneous Endoscopic Approach

0RGN45Z Fusion of Right Wrist Joint with External Fixation Device, Percutaneous Endoscopic Approach

0RGN47Z Fusion of Right Wrist Joint with Autologous Tissue Substitute, Percutaneous Endoscopic Approach

0RGN4JZ Fusion of Right Wrist Joint with Synthetic Substitute, Percutaneous Endoscopic Approach

0RGN4KZ Fusion of Right Wrist Joint with Nonautologous Tissue Substitute, Percutaneous Endoscopic Approach

0RGN4ZZ Fusion of Right Wrist Joint, Percutaneous Endoscopic Approach

0RGP04Z Fusion of Left Wrist Joint with Internal Fixation Device, Open Approach

0RGP05Z Fusion of Left Wrist Joint with External Fixation Device, Open Approach

0RGP07Z Fusion of Left Wrist Joint with Autologous Tissue Substitute, Open Approach

0RGP0JZ Fusion of Left Wrist Joint with Synthetic Substitute, Open Approach

0RGP0KZ Fusion of Left Wrist Joint with Nonautologous Tissue Substitute, Open Approach

0RGP0ZZ Fusion of Left Wrist Joint, Open Approach

0RGP34Z Fusion of Left Wrist Joint with Internal Fixation Device, Percutaneous Approach

0RGP35Z Fusion of Left Wrist Joint with External Fixation Device, Percutaneous Approach

0RGP37Z Fusion of Left Wrist Joint with Autologous Tissue Substitute, Percutaneous Approach

0RGP3JZ Fusion of Left Wrist Joint with Synthetic Substitute, Percutaneous Approach

0RGP3KZ Fusion of Left Wrist Joint with Nonautologous Tissue Substitute, Percutaneous Approach

0RGP3ZZ Fusion of Left Wrist Joint, Percutaneous Approach

0RGP44Z Fusion of Left Wrist Joint with Internal Fixation Device, Percutaneous Endoscopic Approach

0RGP45Z Fusion of Left Wrist Joint with External Fixation Device, Percutaneous Endoscopic Approach

0RGP47Z Fusion of Left Wrist Joint with Autologous Tissue Substitute, Percutaneous Endoscopic Approach

0RGP4JZ Fusion of Left Wrist Joint with Synthetic Substitute, Percutaneous Endoscopic Approach

0RGP4KZ Fusion of Left Wrist Joint with Nonautologous Tissue Substitute, Percutaneous Endoscopic Approach

0RGP4ZZ Fusion of Left Wrist Joint, Percutaneous Endoscopic Approach

0RGQ04Z Fusion of Right Carpal Joint with Internal Fixation Device, Open Approach

0RGQ05Z Fusion of Right Carpal Joint with External Fixation Device, Open Approach

0RGQ07Z Fusion of Right Carpal Joint with Autologous Tissue Substitute, Open Approach

0RGQ0JZ Fusion of Right Carpal Joint with Synthetic Substitute, Open Approach

0RGQ0KZ Fusion of Right Carpal Joint with Nonautologous Tissue Substitute, Open Approach

0RGQ0ZZ Fusion of Right Carpal Joint, Open Approach

0RGQ34Z Fusion of Right Carpal Joint with Internal Fixation Device, Percutaneous Approach

0RGQ35Z Fusion of Right Carpal Joint with External Fixation Device, Percutaneous Approach

0RGQ37Z Fusion of Right Carpal Joint with Autologous Tissue Substitute, Percutaneous Approach

0RGQ3JZ Fusion of Right Carpal Joint with Synthetic Substitute, Percutaneous Approach

0RGQ3KZ Fusion of Right Carpal Joint with Nonautologous Tissue Substitute, Percutaneous Approach

0RGQ3ZZ Fusion of Right Carpal Joint, Percutaneous Approach

0RGQ44Z Fusion of Right Carpal Joint with Internal Fixation Device, Percutaneous Endoscopic Approach

0RGQ45Z Fusion of Right Carpal Joint with External Fixation Device, Percutaneous Endoscopic Approach

0RGQ47Z Fusion of Right Carpal Joint with Autologous Tissue Substitute, Percutaneous Endoscopic Approach

0RGQ4JZ Fusion of Right Carpal Joint with Synthetic Substitute, Percutaneous Endoscopic Approach

0RGQ4KZ Fusion of Right Carpal Joint with Nonautologous Tissue Substitute, Percutaneous Endoscopic Approach

0RGQ4ZZ Fusion of Right Carpal Joint, Percutaneous Endoscopic Approach

0RGR04Z Fusion of Left Carpal Joint with Internal Fixation Device, Open Approach

0RGR05Z Fusion of Left Carpal Joint with External Fixation Device, Open Approach

0RGR07Z Fusion of Left Carpal Joint with Autologous Tissue Substitute, Open Approach

0RGR0JZ Fusion of Left Carpal Joint with Synthetic Substitute, Open Approach

0RGR0KZ Fusion of Left Carpal Joint with Nonautologous Tissue Substitute, Open Approach

0RGR0ZZ Fusion of Left Carpal Joint, Open Approach

0RGR34Z Fusion of Left Carpal Joint with Internal Fixation Device, Percutaneous Approach

0RGR35Z Fusion of Left Carpal Joint with External Fixation Device, Percutaneous Approach

0RGR37Z Fusion of Left Carpal Joint with Autologous Tissue Substitute, Percutaneous Approach

0RGR3JZ Fusion of Left Carpal Joint with Synthetic Substitute, Percutaneous Approach

0RGR3KZ Fusion of Left Carpal Joint with Nonautologous Tissue Substitute, Percutaneous Approach

0RGR3ZZ Fusion of Left Carpal Joint, Percutaneous Approach

0RGR44Z Fusion of Left Carpal Joint with Internal Fixation Device, Percutaneous Endoscopic Approach

0RGR45Z Fusion of Left Carpal Joint with External Fixation Device, Percutaneous Endoscopic Approach

0RGR47Z Fusion of Left Carpal Joint with Autologous Tissue Substitute, Percutaneous Endoscopic Approach

0RGR4JZ Fusion of Left Carpal Joint with Synthetic Substitute, Percutaneous Endoscopic Approach

0RGR4KZ Fusion of Left Carpal Joint with Nonautologous Tissue Substitute, Percutaneous Endoscopic Approach

0RGR4ZZ Fusion of Left Carpal Joint, Percutaneous Endoscopic Approach

0RGS04Z Fusion of Right Metacarpocarpal Joint with Internal Fixation Device, Open Approach

0RGS05Z Fusion of Right Metacarpocarpal Joint with External Fixation Device, Open Approach

0RGS07Z Fusion of Right Metacarpocarpal Joint with Autologous Tissue Substitute, Open Approach

0RGS0JZ Fusion of Right Metacarpocarpal Joint with Synthetic Substitute, Open Approach

0RGS0KZ Fusion of Right Metacarpocarpal Joint with Nonautologous Tissue Substitute, Open Approach

0RGS0ZZ Fusion of Right Metacarpocarpal Joint, Open Approach

0RGS34Z Fusion of Right Metacarpocarpal Joint with Internal Fixation Device, Percutaneous Approach

0RGS35Z Fusion of Right Metacarpocarpal Joint with External Fixation Device, Percutaneous Approach

0RGS37Z Fusion of Right Metacarpocarpal Joint with Autologous Tissue Substitute, Percutaneous Approach

0RGS3JZ Fusion of Right Metacarpocarpal Joint with Synthetic Substitute, Percutaneous Approach

0RGS3KZ Fusion of Right Metacarpocarpal Joint with Nonautologous Tissue Substitute, Percutaneous Approach

0RGS3ZZ Fusion of Right Metacarpocarpal Joint, Percutaneous Approach

0RGS44Z Fusion of Right Metacarpocarpal Joint with Internal Fixation Device, Percutaneous Endoscopic Approach

0RGS45Z Fusion of Right Metacarpocarpal Joint with External Fixation Device, Percutaneous Endoscopic Approach

0RGS47Z Fusion of Right Metacarpocarpal Joint with Autologous Tissue Substitute, Percutaneous Endoscopic Approach

0RGS4JZ Fusion of Right Metacarpocarpal Joint with Synthetic Substitute, Percutaneous Endoscopic Approach

0RGS4KZ Fusion of Right Metacarpocarpal Joint with Nonautologous Tissue Substitute, Percutaneous Endoscopic Approach

0RGS4ZZ Fusion of Right Metacarpocarpal Joint, Percutaneous Endoscopic Approach

---

♀ Female-only   ♂ Male-only   ● Limited Coverage   ● Non-OR   **HAC** HAC-associated procedure   ● Non-covered procedures   ➕ Combination

0RGT04Z Fusion of Left Metacarpocarpal Joint with Internal Fixation Device, Open Approach

0RGT05Z Fusion of Left Metacarpocarpal Joint with External Fixation Device, Open Approach

0RGT07Z Fusion of Left Metacarpocarpal Joint with Autologous Tissue Substitute, Open Approach

0RGT0JZ Fusion of Left Metacarpocarpal Joint with Synthetic Substitute, Open Approach

0RGT0KZ Fusion of Left Metacarpocarpal Joint with Nonautologous Tissue Substitute, Open Approach

0RGT0ZZ Fusion of Left Metacarpocarpal Joint, Open Approach

0RGT34Z Fusion of Left Metacarpocarpal Joint with Internal Fixation Device, Percutaneous Approach

0RGT35Z Fusion of Left Metacarpocarpal Joint with External Fixation Device, Percutaneous Approach

0RGT37Z Fusion of Left Metacarpocarpal Joint with Autologous Tissue Substitute, Percutaneous Approach

0RGT3JZ Fusion of Left Metacarpocarpal Joint with Synthetic Substitute, Percutaneous Approach

0RGT3KZ Fusion of Left Metacarpocarpal Joint with Nonautologous Tissue Substitute, Percutaneous Approach

0RGT3ZZ Fusion of Left Metacarpocarpal Joint, Percutaneous Approach

0RGT44Z Fusion of Left Metacarpocarpal Joint with Internal Fixation Device, Percutaneous Endoscopic Approach

0RGT45Z Fusion of Left Metacarpocarpal Joint with External Fixation Device, Percutaneous Endoscopic Approach

0RGT47Z Fusion of Left Metacarpocarpal Joint with Autologous Tissue Substitute, Percutaneous Endoscopic Approach

0RGT4JZ Fusion of Left Metacarpocarpal Joint with Synthetic Substitute, Percutaneous Endoscopic Approach

0RGT4KZ Fusion of Left Metacarpocarpal Joint with Nonautologous Tissue Substitute, Percutaneous Endoscopic Approach

0RGT4ZZ Fusion of Left Metacarpocarpal Joint, Percutaneous Endoscopic Approach

0RGU04Z Fusion of Right Metacarpophalangeal Joint with Internal Fixation Device, Open Approach

0RGU05Z Fusion of Right Metacarpophalangeal Joint with External Fixation Device, Open Approach

0RGU07Z Fusion of Right Metacarpophalangeal Joint with Autologous Tissue Substitute, Open Approach

0RGU0JZ Fusion of Right Metacarpophalangeal Joint with Synthetic Substitute, Open Approach

0RGU0KZ Fusion of Right Metacarpophalangeal Joint with Nonautologous Tissue Substitute, Open Approach

0RGU0ZZ Fusion of Right Metacarpophalangeal Joint, Open Approach

0RGU34Z Fusion of Right Metacarpophalangeal Joint with Internal Fixation Device, Percutaneous Approach

0RGU35Z Fusion of Right Metacarpophalangeal Joint with External Fixation Device, Percutaneous Approach

0RGU37Z Fusion of Right Metacarpophalangeal Joint with Autologous Tissue Substitute, Percutaneous Approach

0RGU3JZ Fusion of Right Metacarpophalangeal Joint with Synthetic Substitute, Percutaneous Approach

0RGU3KZ Fusion of Right Metacarpophalangeal Joint with Nonautologous Tissue Substitute, Percutaneous Approach

0RGU3ZZ Fusion of Right Metacarpophalangeal Joint, Percutaneous Approach

0RGU44Z Fusion of Right Metacarpophalangeal Joint with Internal Fixation Device, Percutaneous Endoscopic Approach

0RGU45Z Fusion of Right Metacarpophalangeal Joint with External Fixation Device, Percutaneous Endoscopic Approach

0RGU47Z Fusion of Right Metacarpophalangeal Joint with Autologous Tissue Substitute, Percutaneous Endoscopic Approach

0RGU4JZ Fusion of Right Metacarpophalangeal Joint with Synthetic Substitute, Percutaneous Endoscopic Approach

0RGU4KZ Fusion of Right Metacarpophalangeal Joint with Nonautologous Tissue Substitute, Percutaneous Endoscopic Approach

0RGU4ZZ Fusion of Right Metacarpophalangeal Joint, Percutaneous Endoscopic Approach

0RGV04Z Fusion of Left Metacarpophalangeal Joint with Internal Fixation Device, Open Approach

0RGV05Z Fusion of Left Metacarpophalangeal Joint with External Fixation Device, Open Approach

0RGV07Z Fusion of Left Metacarpophalangeal Joint with Autologous Tissue Substitute, Open Approach

0RGV0JZ Fusion of Left Metacarpophalangeal Joint with Synthetic Substitute, Open Approach

0RGV0KZ Fusion of Left Metacarpophalangeal Joint with Nonautologous Tissue Substitute, Open Approach

0RGV0ZZ Fusion of Left Metacarpophalangeal Joint, Open Approach

0RGV34Z Fusion of Left Metacarpophalangeal Joint with Internal Fixation Device, Percutaneous Approach

0RGV35Z Fusion of Left Metacarpophalangeal Joint with External Fixation Device, Percutaneous Approach

0RGV37Z Fusion of Left Metacarpophalangeal Joint with Autologous Tissue Substitute, Percutaneous Approach

0RGV3JZ Fusion of Left Metacarpophalangeal Joint with Synthetic Substitute, Percutaneous Approach

0RGV3KZ Fusion of Left Metacarpophalangeal Joint with Nonautologous Tissue Substitute, Percutaneous Approach

0RGV3ZZ Fusion of Left Metacarpophalangeal Joint, Percutaneous Approach

0RGV44Z Fusion of Left Metacarpophalangeal Joint with Internal Fixation Device, Percutaneous Endoscopic Approach

0RGV45Z Fusion of Left Metacarpophalangeal Joint with External Fixation Device, Percutaneous Endoscopic Approach

0RGV47Z Fusion of Left Metacarpophalangeal Joint with Autologous Tissue Substitute, Percutaneous Endoscopic Approach

0RGV4JZ Fusion of Left Metacarpophalangeal Joint with Synthetic Substitute, Percutaneous Endoscopic Approach

0RGV4KZ Fusion of Left Metacarpophalangeal Joint with Nonautologous Tissue Substitute, Percutaneous Endoscopic Approach

0RGV4ZZ Fusion of Left Metacarpophalangeal Joint, Percutaneous Endoscopic Approach

0RGW04Z Fusion of Right Finger Phalangeal Joint with Internal Fixation Device, Open Approach

0RGW05Z Fusion of Right Finger Phalangeal Joint with External Fixation Device, Open Approach

0RGW07Z Fusion of Right Finger Phalangeal Joint with Autologous Tissue Substitute, Open Approach

0RGW0JZ Fusion of Right Finger Phalangeal Joint with Synthetic Substitute, Open Approach

0RGW0KZ Fusion of Right Finger Phalangeal Joint with Nonautologous Tissue Substitute, Open Approach

0RGW0ZZ Fusion of Right Finger Phalangeal Joint, Open Approach

0RGW34Z Fusion of Right Finger Phalangeal Joint with Internal Fixation Device, Percutaneous Approach

0RGW35Z Fusion of Right Finger Phalangeal Joint with External Fixation Device, Percutaneous Approach

0RGW37Z Fusion of Right Finger Phalangeal Joint with Autologous Tissue Substitute, Percutaneous Approach

0RGW3JZ Fusion of Right Finger Phalangeal Joint with Synthetic Substitute, Percutaneous Approach

0RGW3KZ Fusion of Right Finger Phalangeal Joint with Nonautologous Tissue Substitute, Percutaneous Approach

0RGW3ZZ Fusion of Right Finger Phalangeal Joint, Percutaneous Approach

0RGW44Z Fusion of Right Finger Phalangeal Joint with Internal Fixation Device, Percutaneous Endoscopic Approach

0RGW45Z Fusion of Right Finger Phalangeal Joint with External Fixation Device, Percutaneous Endoscopic Approach

0RGW47Z Fusion of Right Finger Phalangeal Joint with Autologous Tissue Substitute, Percutaneous Endoscopic Approach

0RGW4JZ Fusion of Right Finger Phalangeal Joint with Synthetic Substitute, Percutaneous Endoscopic Approach

0RGW4KZ Fusion of Right Finger Phalangeal Joint with Nonautologous Tissue Substitute, Percutaneous Endoscopic Approach

0RGW4ZZ Fusion of Right Finger Phalangeal Joint, Percutaneous Endoscopic Approach

0RGX04Z Fusion of Left Finger Phalangeal Joint with Internal Fixation Device, Open Approach

0RGX05Z Fusion of Left Finger Phalangeal Joint with External Fixation Device, Open Approach

0RGX07Z Fusion of Left Finger Phalangeal Joint with Autologous Tissue Substitute, Open Approach

0RGX0JZ Fusion of Left Finger Phalangeal Joint with Synthetic Substitute, Open Approach

0RGX0KZ Fusion of Left Finger Phalangeal Joint with Nonautologous Tissue Substitute, Open Approach

0RGX0ZZ Fusion of Left Finger Phalangeal Joint, Open Approach

0RGX34Z Fusion of Left Finger Phalangeal Joint with Internal Fixation Device, Percutaneous Approach

0RGX35Z Fusion of Left Finger Phalangeal Joint with External Fixation Device, Percutaneous Approach

0RGX37Z Fusion of Left Finger Phalangeal Joint with Autologous Tissue Substitute, Percutaneous Approach

0RGX3JZ Fusion of Left Finger Phalangeal Joint with Synthetic Substitute, Percutaneous Approach

0RGX3KZ Fusion of Left Finger Phalangeal Joint with Nonautologous Tissue Substitute, Percutaneous Approach

0RGX3ZZ Fusion of Left Finger Phalangeal Joint, Percutaneous Approach

0RGX44Z Fusion of Left Finger Phalangeal Joint with Internal Fixation Device, Percutaneous Endoscopic Approach

0RGX45Z Fusion of Left Finger Phalangeal Joint with External Fixation Device, Percutaneous Endoscopic Approach

0RGX47Z Fusion of Left Finger Phalangeal Joint with Autologous Tissue Substitute, Percutaneous Endoscopic Approach

0RGX4JZ Fusion of Left Finger Phalangeal Joint with Synthetic Substitute, Percutaneous Endoscopic Approach

0RGX4KZ Fusion of Left Finger Phalangeal Joint with Nonautologous Tissue Substitute, Percutaneous Endoscopic Approach

0RGX4ZZ Fusion of Left Finger Phalangeal Joint, Percutaneous Endoscopic Approach

0RH – Upper Joints, Insertion

0RH003Z Insertion of Infusion Device into Occipital-cervical Joint, Open Approach

0RH004Z Insertion of Internal Fixation Device into Occipital-cervical Joint, Open Approach

0RH008Z Insertion of Spacer into Occipital-cervical Joint, Open Approach

0RH00BZ Insertion of Interspinous Process Spinal Stabilization Device into Occipital-cervical Joint, Open Approach

0RH00CZ Insertion of Pedicle-Based Spinal Stabilization Device into Occipital-cervical Joint, Open Approach

0RH00DZ Insertion of Facet Replacement Spinal Stabilization Device into Occipital-cervical Joint, Open Approach

0RH033Z Insertion of Infusion Device into Occipital-cervical Joint, Percutaneous Approach

0RH034Z Insertion of Internal Fixation Device into Occipital-cervical Joint, Percutaneous Approach

0RH038Z Insertion of Spacer into Occipital-cervical Joint, Percutaneous Approach

0RH03BZ Insertion of Interspinous Process Spinal Stabilization Device into Occipital-cervical Joint, Percutaneous Approach

0RH03CZ Insertion of Pedicle-Based Spinal Stabilization Device into Occipital-cervical Joint, Percutaneous Approach

0RH03DZ Insertion of Facet Replacement Spinal Stabilization Device into Occipital-cervical Joint, Percutaneous Approach

0RH043Z Insertion of Infusion Device into Occipital-cervical Joint, Percutaneous Endoscopic Approach

0RH044Z Insertion of Internal Fixation Device into Occipital-cervical Joint, Percutaneous Endoscopic Approach

0RH048Z Insertion of Spacer into Occipital-cervical Joint, Percutaneous Endoscopic Approach

0RH04BZ Insertion of Interspinous Process Spinal Stabilization Device into Occipital-cervical Joint, Percutaneous Endoscopic Approach

0RH04CZ Insertion of Pedicle-Based Spinal Stabilization Device into Occipital-cervical Joint, Percutaneous Endoscopic Approach

0RH04DZ Insertion of Facet Replacement Spinal Stabilization Device into Occipital-cervical Joint, Percutaneous Endoscopic Approach

0RH103Z Insertion of Infusion Device into Cervical Vertebral Joint, Open Approach

0RH104Z Insertion of Internal Fixation Device into Cervical Vertebral Joint, Open Approach

0RH108Z Insertion of Spacer into Cervical Vertebral Joint, Open Approach

0RH10BZ Insertion of Interspinous Process Spinal Stabilization Device into Cervical Vertebral Joint, Open Approach

0RH10CZ Insertion of Pedicle-Based Spinal Stabilization Device into Cervical Vertebral Joint, Open Approach

0RH10DZ Insertion of Facet Replacement Spinal Stabilization Device into Cervical Vertebral Joint, Open Approach

0RH133Z Insertion of Infusion Device into Cervical Vertebral Joint, Percutaneous Approach

0RH134Z Insertion of Internal Fixation Device into Cervical Vertebral Joint, Percutaneous Approach

0RH138Z Insertion of Spacer into Cervical Vertebral Joint, Percutaneous Approach

0RH13BZ Insertion of Interspinous Process Spinal Stabilization Device into Cervical Vertebral Joint, Percutaneous Approach

0RH13CZ Insertion of Pedicle-Based Spinal Stabilization Device into Cervical Vertebral Joint, Percutaneous Approach

0RH13DZ Insertion of Facet Replacement Spinal Stabilization Device into Cervical Vertebral Joint, Percutaneous Approach

0RH143Z Insertion of Infusion Device into Cervical Vertebral Joint, Percutaneous Endoscopic Approach

0RH144Z Insertion of Internal Fixation Device into Cervical Vertebral Joint, Percutaneous Endoscopic Approach

0RH148Z Insertion of Spacer into Cervical Vertebral Joint, Percutaneous Endoscopic Approach

0RH14BZ Insertion of Interspinous Process Spinal Stabilization Device into Cervical Vertebral Joint, Percutaneous Endoscopic Approach

0RH14CZ Insertion of Pedicle-Based Spinal Stabilization Device into Cervical Vertebral Joint, Percutaneous Endoscopic Approach

0RH14DZ Insertion of Facet Replacement Spinal Stabilization Device into Cervical Vertebral Joint, Percutaneous Endoscopic Approach

0RH303Z Insertion of Infusion Device into Cervical Vertebral Disc, Open Approach

0RH333Z Insertion of Infusion Device into Cervical Vertebral Disc, Percutaneous Approach

0RH343Z Insertion of Infusion Device into Cervical Vertebral Disc, Percutaneous Endoscopic Approach

0RH403Z Insertion of Infusion Device into Cervicothoracic Vertebral Joint, Open Approach

0RH404Z Insertion of Internal Fixation Device into Cervicothoracic Vertebral Joint, Open Approach

0RH408Z Insertion of Spacer into Cervicothoracic Vertebral Joint, Open Approach

0RH40BZ Insertion of Interspinous Process Spinal Stabilization Device into Cervicothoracic Vertebral Joint, Open Approach

0RH40CZ Insertion of Pedicle-Based Spinal Stabilization Device into Cervicothoracic Vertebral Joint, Open Approach

0RH40DZ Insertion of Facet Replacement Spinal Stabilization Device into Cervicothoracic Vertebral Joint, Open Approach

0RH433Z Insertion of Infusion Device into Cervicothoracic Vertebral Joint, Percutaneous Approach

0RH434Z Insertion of Internal Fixation Device into Cervicothoracic Vertebral Joint, Percutaneous Approach

0RH438Z Insertion of Spacer into Cervicothoracic Vertebral Joint, Percutaneous Approach

0RH43BZ Insertion of Interspinous Process Spinal Stabilization Device into Cervicothoracic Vertebral Joint, Percutaneous Approach

0RH43CZ Insertion of Pedicle-Based Spinal Stabilization Device into Cervicothoracic Vertebral Joint, Percutaneous Approach

0RH43DZ Insertion of Facet Replacement Spinal Stabilization Device into Cervicothoracic Vertebral Joint, Percutaneous Approach

0RH443Z Insertion of Infusion Device into Cervicothoracic Vertebral Joint, Percutaneous Endoscopic Approach

0RH444Z Insertion of Internal Fixation Device into Cervicothoracic Vertebral Joint, Percutaneous Endoscopic Approach

0RH448Z Insertion of Spacer into Cervicothoracic Vertebral Joint, Percutaneous Endoscopic Approach

0RH44BZ Insertion of Interspinous Process Spinal Stabilization Device into Cervicothoracic Vertebral Joint, Percutaneous Endoscopic Approach

0RH44CZ Insertion of Pedicle-Based Spinal Stabilization Device into Cervicothoracic Vertebral Joint, Percutaneous Endoscopic Approach

0RH44DZ Insertion of Facet Replacement Spinal Stabilization Device into Cervicothoracic Vertebral Joint, Percutaneous Endoscopic Approach

0RH503Z Insertion of Infusion Device into Cervicothoracic Vertebral Disc, Open Approach

0RH533Z Insertion of Infusion Device into Cervicothoracic Vertebral Disc, Percutaneous Approach

0RH543Z Insertion of Infusion Device into Cervicothoracic Vertebral Disc, Percutaneous Endoscopic Approach

0RH603Z Insertion of Infusion Device into Thoracic Vertebral Joint, Open Approach

0RH604Z Insertion of Internal Fixation Device into Thoracic Vertebral Joint, Open Approach

0RH608Z Insertion of Spacer into Thoracic Vertebral Joint, Open Approach

0RH60BZ Insertion of Interspinous Process Spinal Stabilization Device into Thoracic Vertebral Joint, Open Approach

0RH60CZ Insertion of Pedicle-Based Spinal Stabilization Device into Thoracic Vertebral Joint, Open Approach

0RH60DZ Insertion of Facet Replacement Spinal Stabilization Device into Thoracic Vertebral Joint, Open Approach

0RH633Z Insertion of Infusion Device into Thoracic Vertebral Joint, Percutaneous Approach

0RH634Z Insertion of Internal Fixation Device into Thoracic Vertebral Joint, Percutaneous Approach

0RH638Z Insertion of Spacer into Thoracic Vertebral Joint, Percutaneous Approach

0RH63BZ Insertion of Interspinous Process Spinal Stabilization Device into Thoracic Vertebral Joint, Percutaneous Approach

0RH63CZ Insertion of Pedicle-Based Spinal Stabilization Device into Thoracic Vertebral Joint, Percutaneous Approach

0RH63DZ Insertion of Facet Replacement Spinal Stabilization Device into Thoracic Vertebral Joint, Percutaneous Approach

0RH643Z Insertion of Infusion Device into Thoracic Vertebral Joint, Percutaneous Endoscopic Approach

0RH644Z Insertion of Internal Fixation Device into Thoracic Vertebral Joint, Percutaneous Endoscopic Approach

0RH648Z Insertion of Spacer into Thoracic Vertebral Joint, Percutaneous Endoscopic Approach

0RH64BZ Insertion of Interspinous Process Spinal Stabilization Device into Thoracic Vertebral Joint, Percutaneous Endoscopic Approach

0RH64CZ Insertion of Pedicle-Based Spinal Stabilization Device into Thoracic Vertebral Joint, Percutaneous Endoscopic Approach

0RH64DZ Insertion of Facet Replacement Spinal Stabilization Device into Thoracic Vertebral Joint, Percutaneous Endoscopic Approach

0RH903Z Insertion of Infusion Device into Thoracic Vertebral Disc, Open Approach

0RH933Z Insertion of Infusion Device into Thoracic Vertebral Disc, Percutaneous Approach

0RH943Z Insertion of Infusion Device into Thoracic Vertebral Disc, Percutaneous Endoscopic Approach

0RHA03Z Insertion of Infusion Device into Thoracolumbar Vertebral Joint, Open Approach

0RHA04Z Insertion of Internal Fixation Device into Thoracolumbar Vertebral Joint, Open Approach

0RHA08Z Insertion of Spacer into Thoracolumbar Vertebral Joint, Open Approach

0RHA0BZ Insertion of Interspinous Process Spinal Stabilization Device into Thoracolumbar Vertebral Joint, Open Approach

0RHA0CZ Insertion of Pedicle-Based Spinal Stabilization Device into Thoracolumbar Vertebral Joint, Open Approach

0RHA0DZ Insertion of Facet Replacement Spinal Stabilization Device into Thoracolumbar Vertebral Joint, Open Approach

0RHA33Z Insertion of Infusion Device into Thoracolumbar Vertebral Joint, Percutaneous Approach

0RHA34Z Insertion of Internal Fixation Device into Thoracolumbar Vertebral Joint, Percutaneous Approach

0RHA38Z Insertion of Spacer into Thoracolumbar Vertebral Joint, Percutaneous Approach

0RHA3BZ Insertion of Interspinous Process Spinal Stabilization Device into Thoracolumbar Vertebral Joint, Percutaneous Approach

0RHA3CZ Insertion of Pedicle-Based Spinal Stabilization Device into Thoracolumbar Vertebral Joint, Percutaneous Approach

0RHA3DZ Insertion of Facet Replacement Spinal Stabilization Device into Thoracolumbar Vertebral Joint, Percutaneous Approach

0RHA43Z Insertion of Infusion Device into Thoracolumbar Vertebral Joint, Percutaneous Endoscopic Approach

0RHA44Z Insertion of Internal Fixation Device into Thoracolumbar Vertebral Joint, Percutaneous Endoscopic Approach

0RHA48Z Insertion of Spacer into Thoracolumbar Vertebral Joint, Percutaneous Endoscopic Approach

0RHA4BZ Insertion of Interspinous Process Spinal Stabilization Device into Thoracolumbar Vertebral Joint, Percutaneous Endoscopic Approach

0RHA4CZ Insertion of Pedicle-Based Spinal Stabilization Device into Thoracolumbar Vertebral Joint, Percutaneous Endoscopic Approach

0RHA4DZ Insertion of Facet Replacement Spinal Stabilization Device into Thoracolumbar Vertebral Joint, Percutaneous Endoscopic Approach

0RHB03Z Insertion of Infusion Device into Thoracolumbar Vertebral Disc, Open Approach

0RHB33Z Insertion of Infusion Device into Thoracolumbar Vertebral Disc, Percutaneous Approach

0RHB43Z Insertion of Infusion Device into Thoracolumbar Vertebral Disc, Percutaneous Endoscopic Approach

0RHC03Z Insertion of Infusion Device into Right Temporomandibular Joint, Open Approach

0RHC04Z Insertion of Internal Fixation Device into Right Temporomandibular Joint, Open Approach

0RHC08Z Insertion of Spacer into Right Temporomandibular Joint, Open Approach

0RHC33Z Insertion of Infusion Device into Right Temporomandibular Joint, Percutaneous Approach

0RHC34Z Insertion of Internal Fixation Device into Right Temporomandibular Joint, Percutaneous Approach

0RHC38Z Insertion of Spacer into Right Temporomandibular Joint, Percutaneous Approach

0RHC43Z Insertion of Infusion Device into Right Temporomandibular Joint, Percutaneous Endoscopic Approach

0RHC44Z Insertion of Internal Fixation Device into Right Temporomandibular Joint, Percutaneous Endoscopic Approach

0RHC48Z Insertion of Spacer into Right Temporomandibular Joint, Percutaneous Endoscopic Approach

0RHD03Z Insertion of Infusion Device into Left Temporomandibular Joint, Open Approach

0RHD04Z Insertion of Internal Fixation Device into Left Temporomandibular Joint, Open Approach

0RHD08Z Insertion of Spacer into Left Temporomandibular Joint, Open Approach

0RHD33Z Insertion of Infusion Device into Left Temporomandibular Joint, Percutaneous Approach

0RHD34Z Insertion of Internal Fixation Device into Left Temporomandibular Joint, Percutaneous Approach

0RHD38Z Insertion of Spacer into Left Temporomandibular Joint, Percutaneous Approach

0RHD43Z Insertion of Infusion Device into Left Temporomandibular Joint, Percutaneous Endoscopic Approach

0RHD44Z Insertion of Internal Fixation Device into Left Temporomandibular Joint, Percutaneous Endoscopic Approach

0RHD48Z Insertion of Spacer into Left Temporomandibular Joint, Percutaneous Endoscopic Approach

0RHE03Z Insertion of Infusion Device into Right Sternoclavicular Joint, Open Approach

0RHE04Z Insertion of Internal Fixation Device into Right Sternoclavicular Joint, Open Approach

0RHE08Z Insertion of Spacer into Right Sternoclavicular Joint, Open Approach

0RHE33Z Insertion of Infusion Device into Right Sternoclavicular Joint, Percutaneous Approach

0RHE34Z Insertion of Internal Fixation Device into Right Sternoclavicular Joint, Percutaneous Approach

0RHE38Z Insertion of Spacer into Right Sternoclavicular Joint, Percutaneous Approach

0RHE43Z Insertion of Infusion Device into Right Sternoclavicular Joint, Percutaneous Endoscopic Approach

0RHE44Z Insertion of Internal Fixation Device into Right Sternoclavicular Joint, Percutaneous Endoscopic Approach

0RHE48Z Insertion of Spacer into Right Sternoclavicular Joint, Percutaneous Endoscopic Approach

0RHF03Z Insertion of Infusion Device into Left Sternoclavicular Joint, Open Approach

0RHF04Z Insertion of Internal Fixation Device into Left Sternoclavicular Joint, Open Approach

0RHF08Z Insertion of Spacer into Left Sternoclavicular Joint, Open Approach

0RHF33Z Insertion of Infusion Device into Left Sternoclavicular Joint, Percutaneous Approach

0RHF34Z Insertion of Internal Fixation Device into Left Sternoclavicular Joint, Percutaneous Approach

0RHF38Z Insertion of Spacer into Left Sternoclavicular Joint, Percutaneous Approach

0RHF43Z Insertion of Infusion Device into Left Sternoclavicular Joint, Percutaneous Endoscopic Approach

0RHF44Z Insertion of Internal Fixation Device into Left Sternoclavicular Joint, Percutaneous Endoscopic Approach

0RHF48Z Insertion of Spacer into Left Sternoclavicular Joint, Percutaneous Endoscopic Approach

0RHG03Z Insertion of Infusion Device into Right Acromioclavicular Joint, Open Approach

0RHG04Z Insertion of Internal Fixation Device into Right Acromioclavicular Joint, Open Approach

0RHG08Z Insertion of Spacer into Right Acromioclavicular Joint, Open Approach

0RHG33Z Insertion of Infusion Device into Right Acromioclavicular Joint, Percutaneous Approach

0RHG34Z Insertion of Internal Fixation Device into Right Acromioclavicular Joint, Percutaneous Approach

0RHG38Z Insertion of Spacer into Right Acromioclavicular Joint, Percutaneous Approach

0RHG43Z Insertion of Infusion Device into Right Acromioclavicular Joint, Percutaneous Endoscopic Approach

0RHG44Z Insertion of Internal Fixation Device into Right Acromioclavicular Joint, Percutaneous Endoscopic Approach

0RHG48Z Insertion of Spacer into Right Acromioclavicular Joint, Percutaneous Endoscopic Approach

0RHH03Z Insertion of Infusion Device into Left Acromioclavicular Joint, Open Approach

0RHH04Z Insertion of Internal Fixation Device into Left Acromioclavicular Joint, Open Approach

0RHH08Z Insertion of Spacer into Left Acromioclavicular Joint, Open Approach

0RHH33Z Insertion of Infusion Device into Left Acromioclavicular Joint, Percutaneous Approach

0RHH34Z Insertion of Internal Fixation Device into Left Acromioclavicular Joint, Percutaneous Approach

0RHH38Z Insertion of Spacer into Left Acromioclavicular Joint, Percutaneous Approach

0RHH43Z Insertion of Infusion Device into Left Acromioclavicular Joint, Percutaneous Endoscopic Approach

0RHH44Z Insertion of Internal Fixation Device into Left Acromioclavicular Joint, Percutaneous Endoscopic Approach

0RHH48Z Insertion of Spacer into Left Acromioclavicular Joint, Percutaneous Endoscopic Approach

0RHJ03Z Insertion of Infusion Device into Right Shoulder Joint, Open Approach

0RHJ04Z Insertion of Internal Fixation Device into Right Shoulder Joint, Open Approach

0RHJ08Z Insertion of Spacer into Right Shoulder Joint, Open Approach

0RHJ33Z Insertion of Infusion Device into Right Shoulder Joint, Percutaneous Approach

0RHJ34Z Insertion of Internal Fixation Device into Right Shoulder Joint, Percutaneous Approach

0RHJ38Z Insertion of Spacer into Right Shoulder Joint, Percutaneous Approach

0RHJ43Z Insertion of Infusion Device into Right Shoulder Joint, Percutaneous Endoscopic Approach

0RHJ44Z Insertion of Internal Fixation Device into Right Shoulder Joint, Percutaneous Endoscopic Approach

0RHJ48Z Insertion of Spacer into Right Shoulder Joint, Percutaneous Endoscopic Approach

0RHK03Z Insertion of Infusion Device into Left Shoulder Joint, Open Approach

0RHK04Z Insertion of Internal Fixation Device into Left Shoulder Joint, Open Approach

0RHK08Z Insertion of Spacer into Left Shoulder Joint, Open Approach

0RHK33Z Insertion of Infusion Device into Left Shoulder Joint, Percutaneous Approach

0RHK34Z Insertion of Internal Fixation Device into Left Shoulder Joint, Percutaneous Approach

0RHK38Z Insertion of Spacer into Left Shoulder Joint, Percutaneous Approach

0RHK43Z Insertion of Infusion Device into Left Shoulder Joint, Percutaneous Endoscopic Approach

0RHK44Z Insertion of Internal Fixation Device into Left Shoulder Joint, Percutaneous Endoscopic Approach

0RHK48Z Insertion of Spacer into Left Shoulder Joint, Percutaneous Endoscopic Approach

0RHL03Z Insertion of Infusion Device into Right Elbow Joint, Open Approach

0RHL04Z Insertion of Internal Fixation Device into Right Elbow Joint, Open Approach

0RHL05Z Insertion of External Fixation Device into Right Elbow Joint, Open Approach

0RHL08Z Insertion of Spacer into Right Elbow Joint, Open Approach

0RHL33Z Insertion of Infusion Device into Right Elbow Joint, Percutaneous Approach

0RHL34Z Insertion of Internal Fixation Device into Right Elbow Joint, Percutaneous Approach

0RHL35Z Insertion of External Fixation Device into Right Elbow Joint, Percutaneous Approach

0RHL38Z Insertion of Spacer into Right Elbow Joint, Percutaneous Approach

0RHL43Z Insertion of Infusion Device into Right Elbow Joint, Percutaneous Endoscopic Approach

0RHL44Z Insertion of Internal Fixation Device into Right Elbow Joint, Percutaneous Endoscopic Approach

0RHL45Z Insertion of External Fixation Device into Right Elbow Joint, Percutaneous Endoscopic Approach

0RHL48Z Insertion of Spacer into Right Elbow Joint, Percutaneous Endoscopic Approach

0RHM03Z Insertion of Infusion Device into Left Elbow Joint, Open Approach

0RHM04Z Insertion of Internal Fixation Device into Left Elbow Joint, Open Approach

0RHM05Z Insertion of External Fixation Device into Left Elbow Joint, Open Approach

0RHM08Z Insertion of Spacer into Left Elbow Joint, Open Approach

0RHM33Z Insertion of Infusion Device into Left Elbow Joint, Percutaneous Approach

0RHM34Z Insertion of Internal Fixation Device into Left Elbow Joint, Percutaneous Approach

0RHM35Z Insertion of External Fixation Device into Left Elbow Joint, Percutaneous Approach

0RHM38Z Insertion of Spacer into Left Elbow Joint, Percutaneous Approach

0RHM43Z Insertion of Infusion Device into Left Elbow Joint, Percutaneous Endoscopic Approach

0RHM44Z Insertion of Internal Fixation Device into Left Elbow Joint, Percutaneous Endoscopic Approach

0RHM45Z Insertion of External Fixation Device into Left Elbow Joint, Percutaneous Endoscopic Approach

0RHM48Z Insertion of Spacer into Left Elbow Joint, Percutaneous Endoscopic Approach

0RHN03Z Insertion of Infusion Device into Right Wrist Joint, Open Approach

0RHN04Z Insertion of Internal Fixation Device into Right Wrist Joint, Open Approach

0RHN05Z Insertion of External Fixation Device into Right Wrist Joint, Open Approach

0RHN08Z Insertion of Spacer into Right Wrist Joint, Open Approach

0RHN33Z Insertion of Infusion Device into Right Wrist Joint, Percutaneous Approach

0RHN34Z Insertion of Internal Fixation Device into Right Wrist Joint, Percutaneous Approach

0RHN35Z Insertion of External Fixation Device into Right Wrist Joint, Percutaneous Approach

0RHN38Z Insertion of Spacer into Right Wrist Joint, Percutaneous Approach

0RHN43Z Insertion of Infusion Device into Right Wrist Joint, Percutaneous Endoscopic Approach

0RHN44Z Insertion of Internal Fixation Device into Right Wrist Joint, Percutaneous Endoscopic Approach

0RHN45Z Insertion of External Fixation Device into Right Wrist Joint, Percutaneous Endoscopic Approach

0RHN48Z Insertion of Spacer into Right Wrist Joint, Percutaneous Endoscopic Approach

0RHP03Z Insertion of Infusion Device into Left Wrist Joint, Open Approach

0RHP04Z Insertion of Internal Fixation Device into Left Wrist Joint, Open Approach

0RHP05Z Insertion of External Fixation Device into Left Wrist Joint, Open Approach

0RHP08Z Insertion of Spacer into Left Wrist Joint, Open Approach

0RHP33Z Insertion of Infusion Device into Left Wrist Joint, Percutaneous Approach

0RHP34Z Insertion of Internal Fixation Device into Left Wrist Joint, Percutaneous Approach

0RHP35Z Insertion of External Fixation Device into Left Wrist Joint, Percutaneous Approach

0RHP38Z Insertion of Spacer into Left Wrist Joint, Percutaneous Approach

0RHP43Z Insertion of Infusion Device into Left Wrist Joint, Percutaneous Endoscopic Approach

0RHP44Z Insertion of Internal Fixation Device into Left Wrist Joint, Percutaneous Endoscopic Approach

0RHP45Z Insertion of External Fixation Device into Left Wrist Joint, Percutaneous Endoscopic Approach

0RHP48Z Insertion of Spacer into Left Wrist Joint, Percutaneous Endoscopic Approach

0RHQ03Z Insertion of Infusion Device into Right Carpal Joint, Open Approach

0RHQ04Z Insertion of Internal Fixation Device into Right Carpal Joint, Open Approach

0RHQ05Z Insertion of External Fixation Device into Right Carpal Joint, Open Approach

0RHQ08Z Insertion of Spacer into Right Carpal Joint, Open Approach

0RHQ33Z Insertion of Infusion Device into Right Carpal Joint, Percutaneous Approach

0RHQ34Z Insertion of Internal Fixation Device into Right Carpal Joint, Percutaneous Approach

0RHQ35Z Insertion of External Fixation Device into Right Carpal Joint, Percutaneous Approach

0RHQ38Z Insertion of Spacer into Right Carpal Joint, Percutaneous Approach

0RHQ43Z Insertion of Infusion Device into Right Carpal Joint, Percutaneous Endoscopic Approach

0RHQ44Z Insertion of Internal Fixation Device into Right Carpal Joint, Percutaneous Endoscopic Approach

0RHQ45Z Insertion of External Fixation Device into Right Carpal Joint, Percutaneous Endoscopic Approach

0RHQ48Z Insertion of Spacer into Right Carpal Joint, Percutaneous Endoscopic Approach

0RHR03Z Insertion of Infusion Device into Left Carpal Joint, Open Approach

0RHR04Z Insertion of Internal Fixation Device into Left Carpal Joint, Open Approach

0RHR05Z Insertion of External Fixation Device into Left Carpal Joint, Open Approach

0RHR08Z Insertion of Spacer into Left Carpal Joint, Open Approach

0RHR33Z Insertion of Infusion Device into Left Carpal Joint, Percutaneous Approach

0RHR34Z Insertion of Internal Fixation Device into Left Carpal Joint, Percutaneous Approach

0RHR35Z Insertion of External Fixation Device into Left Carpal Joint, Percutaneous Approach

0RHR38Z Insertion of Spacer into Left Carpal Joint, Percutaneous Approach

0RHR43Z Insertion of Infusion Device into Left Carpal Joint, Percutaneous Endoscopic Approach

0RHR44Z Insertion of Internal Fixation Device into Left Carpal Joint, Percutaneous Endoscopic Approach

0RHR45Z Insertion of External Fixation Device into Left Carpal Joint, Percutaneous Endoscopic Approach

0RHR48Z Insertion of Spacer into Left Carpal Joint, Percutaneous Endoscopic Approach

0RHS03Z Insertion of Infusion Device into Right Metacarpocarpal Joint, Open Approach

0RHS04Z Insertion of Internal Fixation Device into Right Metacarpocarpal Joint, Open Approach

0RHS05Z Insertion of External Fixation Device into Right Metacarpocarpal Joint, Open Approach

0RHS08Z Insertion of Spacer into Right Metacarpocarpal Joint, Open Approach

0RHS33Z Insertion of Infusion Device into Right Metacarpocarpal Joint, Percutaneous Approach

0RHS34Z Insertion of Internal Fixation Device into Right Metacarpocarpal Joint, Percutaneous Approach

0RHS35Z Insertion of External Fixation Device into Right Metacarpocarpal Joint, Percutaneous Approach

0RHS38Z Insertion of Spacer into Right Metacarpocarpal Joint, Percutaneous Approach

0RHS43Z Insertion of Infusion Device into Right Metacarpocarpal Joint, Percutaneous Endoscopic Approach

0RHS44Z Insertion of Internal Fixation Device into Right Metacarpocarpal Joint, Percutaneous Endoscopic Approach

0RHS45Z Insertion of External Fixation Device into Right Metacarpocarpal Joint, Percutaneous Endoscopic Approach

0RHS48Z Insertion of Spacer into Right Metacarpocarpal Joint, Percutaneous Endoscopic Approach

0RHT03Z Insertion of Infusion Device into Left Metacarpocarpal Joint, Open Approach

0RHT04Z Insertion of Internal Fixation Device into Left Metacarpocarpal Joint, Open Approach

0RHT05Z Insertion of External Fixation Device into Left Metacarpocarpal Joint, Open Approach

0RHT08Z Insertion of Spacer into Left Metacarpocarpal Joint, Open Approach

0RHT33Z Insertion of Infusion Device into Left Metacarpocarpal Joint, Percutaneous Approach

0RHT34Z Insertion of Internal Fixation Device into Left Metacarpocarpal Joint, Percutaneous Approach

0RHT35Z Insertion of External Fixation Device into Left Metacarpocarpal Joint, Percutaneous Approach

0RHT38Z Insertion of Spacer into Left Metacarpocarpal Joint, Percutaneous Approach

0RHT43Z Insertion of Infusion Device into Left Metacarpocarpal Joint, Percutaneous Endoscopic Approach

0RHT44Z Insertion of Internal Fixation Device into Left Metacarpocarpal Joint, Percutaneous Endoscopic Approach

0RHT45Z Insertion of External Fixation Device into Left Metacarpocarpal Joint, Percutaneous Endoscopic Approach

0RHT48Z Insertion of Spacer into Left Metacarpocarpal Joint, Percutaneous Endoscopic Approach

0RHU03Z Insertion of Infusion Device into Right Metacarpophalangeal Joint, Open Approach

0RHU04Z Insertion of Internal Fixation Device into Right Metacarpophalangeal Joint, Open Approach

0RHU05Z Insertion of External Fixation Device into Right Metacarpophalangeal Joint, Open Approach

0RHU08Z Insertion of Spacer into Right Metacarpophalangeal Joint, Open Approach

0RHU33Z Insertion of Infusion Device into Right Metacarpophalangeal Joint, Percutaneous Approach

0RHU34Z Insertion of Internal Fixation Device into Right Metacarpophalangeal Joint, Percutaneous Approach

0RHU35Z Insertion of External Fixation Device into Right Metacarpophalangeal Joint, Percutaneous Approach

0RHU38Z Insertion of Spacer into Right Metacarpophalangeal Joint, Percutaneous Approach

0RHU43Z Insertion of Infusion Device into Right Metacarpophalangeal Joint, Percutaneous Endoscopic Approach

0RHU44Z Insertion of Internal Fixation Device into Right Metacarpophalangeal Joint, Percutaneous Endoscopic Approach

0RHU45Z Insertion of External Fixation Device into Right Metacarpophalangeal Joint, Percutaneous Endoscopic Approach

0RHU48Z Insertion of Spacer into Right Metacarpophalangeal Joint, Percutaneous Endoscopic Approach

0RHV03Z Insertion of Infusion Device into Left Metacarpophalangeal Joint, Open Approach

0RHV04Z Insertion of Internal Fixation Device into Left Metacarpophalangeal Joint, Open Approach

0RHV05Z Insertion of External Fixation Device into Left Metacarpophalangeal Joint, Open Approach

0RHV08Z Insertion of Spacer into Left Metacarpophalangeal Joint, Open Approach

0RHV33Z Insertion of Infusion Device into Left Metacarpophalangeal Joint, Percutaneous Approach

0RHV34Z Insertion of Internal Fixation Device into Left Metacarpophalangeal Joint, Percutaneous Approach

0RHV35Z Insertion of External Fixation Device into Left Metacarpophalangeal Joint, Percutaneous Approach

0RHV38Z Insertion of Spacer into Left Metacarpophalangeal Joint, Percutaneous Approach

0RHV43Z Insertion of Infusion Device into Left Metacarpophalangeal Joint, Percutaneous Endoscopic Approach

0RHV44Z Insertion of Internal Fixation Device into Left Metacarpophalangeal Joint, Percutaneous Endoscopic Approach

0RHV45Z Insertion of External Fixation Device into Left Metacarpophalangeal Joint, Percutaneous Endoscopic Approach

0RHV48Z Insertion of Spacer into Left Metacarpophalangeal Joint, Percutaneous Endoscopic Approach

0RHW03Z Insertion of Infusion Device into Right Finger Phalangeal Joint, Open Approach

0RHW04Z Insertion of Internal Fixation Device into Right Finger Phalangeal Joint, Open Approach

0RHW05Z Insertion of External Fixation Device into Right Finger Phalangeal Joint, Open Approach

0RHW08Z Insertion of Spacer into Right Finger Phalangeal Joint, Open Approach

0RHW33Z Insertion of Infusion Device into Right Finger Phalangeal Joint, Percutaneous Approach

0RHW34Z Insertion of Internal Fixation Device into Right Finger Phalangeal Joint, Percutaneous Approach

0RHW35Z Insertion of External Fixation Device into Right Finger Phalangeal Joint, Percutaneous Approach

0RHW38Z Insertion of Spacer into Right Finger Phalangeal Joint, Percutaneous Approach

0RHW43Z Insertion of Infusion Device into Right Finger Phalangeal Joint, Percutaneous Endoscopic Approach

0RHW44Z Insertion of Internal Fixation Device into Right Finger Phalangeal Joint, Percutaneous Endoscopic Approach

0RHW45Z Insertion of External Fixation Device into Right Finger Phalangeal Joint, Percutaneous Endoscopic Approach

0RHW48Z Insertion of Spacer into Right Finger Phalangeal Joint, Percutaneous Endoscopic Approach

0RHX03Z Insertion of Infusion Device into Left Finger Phalangeal Joint, Open Approach

0RHX04Z Insertion of Internal Fixation Device into Left Finger Phalangeal Joint, Open Approach

0RHX05Z Insertion of External Fixation Device into Left Finger Phalangeal Joint, Open Approach

0RHX08Z Insertion of Spacer into Left Finger Phalangeal Joint, Open Approach

0RHX33Z Insertion of Infusion Device into Left Finger Phalangeal Joint, Percutaneous Approach

0RHX34Z Insertion of Internal Fixation Device into Left Finger Phalangeal Joint, Percutaneous Approach

0RHX35Z Insertion of External Fixation Device into Left Finger Phalangeal Joint, Percutaneous Approach

0RHX38Z Insertion of Spacer into Left Finger Phalangeal Joint, Percutaneous Approach

0RHX43Z Insertion of Infusion Device into Left Finger Phalangeal Joint, Percutaneous Endoscopic Approach

0RHX44Z Insertion of Internal Fixation Device into Left Finger Phalangeal Joint, Percutaneous Endoscopic Approach

0RHX45Z Insertion of External Fixation Device into Left Finger Phalangeal Joint, Percutaneous Endoscopic Approach

0RHX48Z Insertion of Spacer into Left Finger Phalangeal Joint, Percutaneous Endoscopic Approach

0RJ – Upper Joints, Inspection

Review Coding Guideline B3.5

Review Coding Guidelines B3.11a, B3.11b and B3.11c

0RJ00ZZ Inspection of Occipital-cervical Joint, Open Approach

0RJ03ZZ Inspection of Occipital-cervical Joint, Percutaneous Approach

0RJ04ZZ Inspection of Occipital-cervical Joint, Percutaneous Endoscopic Approach

0RJ0XZZ Inspection of Occipital-cervical Joint, External Approach

0RJ10ZZ Inspection of Cervical Vertebral Joint, Open Approach

0RJ13ZZ Inspection of Cervical Vertebral Joint, Percutaneous Approach

0RJ14ZZ Inspection of Cervical Vertebral Joint, Percutaneous Endoscopic Approach

0RJ1XZZ Inspection of Cervical Vertebral Joint, External Approach

0RJ30ZZ Inspection of Cervical Vertebral Disc, Open Approach

0RJ33ZZ Inspection of Cervical Vertebral Disc, Percutaneous Approach

0RJ34ZZ Inspection of Cervical Vertebral Disc, Percutaneous Endoscopic Approach

0RJ3XZZ Inspection of Cervical Vertebral Disc, External Approach

0RJ40ZZ Inspection of Cervicothoracic Vertebral Joint, Open Approach

0RJ43ZZ Inspection of Cervicothoracic Vertebral Joint, Percutaneous Approach

0RJ44ZZ Inspection of Cervicothoracic Vertebral Joint, Percutaneous Endoscopic Approach

0RJ4XZZ Inspection of Cervicothoracic Vertebral Joint, External Approach

0RJ50ZZ Inspection of Cervicothoracic Vertebral Disc, Open Approach

0RJ53ZZ Inspection of Cervicothoracic Vertebral Disc, Percutaneous Approach

0RJ54ZZ Inspection of Cervicothoracic Vertebral Disc, Percutaneous Endoscopic Approach

0RJ5XZZ Inspection of Cervicothoracic Vertebral Disc, External Approach

0RJ60ZZ Inspection of Thoracic Vertebral Joint, Open Approach

0RJ63ZZ Inspection of Thoracic Vertebral Joint, Percutaneous Approach

0RJ64ZZ Inspection of Thoracic Vertebral Joint, Percutaneous Endoscopic Approach

0RJ6XZZ Inspection of Thoracic Vertebral Joint, External Approach

0RJ90ZZ Inspection of Thoracic Vertebral Disc, Open Approach

0RJ93ZZ Inspection of Thoracic Vertebral Disc, Percutaneous Approach

0RJ94ZZ Inspection of Thoracic Vertebral Disc, Percutaneous Endoscopic Approach

0RJ9XZZ Inspection of Thoracic Vertebral Disc, External Approach

0RJA0ZZ Inspection of Thoracolumbar Vertebral Joint, Open Approach

0RJA3ZZ Inspection of Thoracolumbar Vertebral Joint, Percutaneous Approach

0RJA4ZZ Inspection of Thoracolumbar Vertebral Joint, Percutaneous Endoscopic Approach

0RJAXZZ Inspection of Thoracolumbar Vertebral Joint, External Approach

0RJB0ZZ Inspection of Thoracolumbar Vertebral Disc, Open Approach

0RJB3ZZ Inspection of Thoracolumbar Vertebral Disc, Percutaneous Approach

0RJB4ZZ Inspection of Thoracolumbar Vertebral Disc, Percutaneous Endoscopic Approach

0RJBXZZ Inspection of Thoracolumbar Vertebral Disc, External Approach

0RJC0ZZ Inspection of Right Temporomandibular Joint, Open Approach

0RJC3ZZ Inspection of Right Temporomandibular Joint, Percutaneous Approach

0RJC4ZZ Inspection of Right Temporomandibular Joint, Percutaneous Endoscopic Approach

0RJCXZZ Inspection of Right Temporomandibular Joint, External Approach

0RJD0ZZ Inspection of Left Temporomandibular Joint, Open Approach

0RJD3ZZ Inspection of Left Temporomandibular Joint, Percutaneous Approach

0RJD4ZZ Inspection of Left Temporomandibular Joint, Percutaneous Endoscopic Approach

0RJDXZZ Inspection of Left Temporomandibular Joint, External Approach

0RJE0ZZ Inspection of Right Sternoclavicular Joint, Open Approach

0RJE3ZZ Inspection of Right Sternoclavicular Joint, Percutaneous Approach

0RJE4ZZ Inspection of Right Sternoclavicular Joint, Percutaneous Endoscopic Approach

0RJEXZZ Inspection of Right Sternoclavicular Joint, External Approach

0RJF0ZZ Inspection of Left Sternoclavicular Joint, Open Approach

0RJF3ZZ Inspection of Left Sternoclavicular Joint, Percutaneous Approach

0RJF4ZZ Inspection of Left Sternoclavicular Joint, Percutaneous Endoscopic Approach

0RJFXZZ Inspection of Left Sternoclavicular Joint, External Approach

0RJG0ZZ Inspection of Right Acromioclavicular Joint, Open Approach

0RJG3ZZ   Inspection of Right Acromioclavicular Joint, Percutaneous Approach
0RJG4ZZ   Inspection of Right Acromioclavicular Joint, Percutaneous Endoscopic Approach
0RJGXZZ   Inspection of Right Acromioclavicular Joint, External Approach
0RJH0ZZ   Inspection of Left Acromioclavicular Joint, Open Approach
0RJH3ZZ   Inspection of Left Acromioclavicular Joint, Percutaneous Approach
0RJH4ZZ   Inspection of Left Acromioclavicular Joint, Percutaneous Endoscopic Approach
0RJHXZZ   Inspection of Left Acromioclavicular Joint, External Approach
0RJJ0ZZ   Inspection of Right Shoulder Joint, Open Approach
0RJJ3ZZ   Inspection of Right Shoulder Joint, Percutaneous Approach
0RJJ4ZZ   Inspection of Right Shoulder Joint, Percutaneous Endoscopic Approach
0RJJXZZ   Inspection of Right Shoulder Joint, External Approach
0RJK0ZZ   Inspection of Left Shoulder Joint, Open Approach
0RJK3ZZ   Inspection of Left Shoulder Joint, Percutaneous Approach
0RJK4ZZ   Inspection of Left Shoulder Joint, Percutaneous Endoscopic Approach
0RJKXZZ   Inspection of Left Shoulder Joint, External Approach
0RJL0ZZ   Inspection of Right Elbow Joint, Open Approach
0RJL3ZZ   Inspection of Right Elbow Joint, Percutaneous Approach
0RJL4ZZ   Inspection of Right Elbow Joint, Percutaneous Endoscopic Approach
0RJLXZZ   Inspection of Right Elbow Joint, External Approach
0RJM0ZZ   Inspection of Left Elbow Joint, Open Approach
0RJM3ZZ   Inspection of Left Elbow Joint, Percutaneous Approach
0RJM4ZZ   Inspection of Left Elbow Joint, Percutaneous Endoscopic Approach
0RJMXZZ   Inspection of Left Elbow Joint, External Approach
0RJN0ZZ   Inspection of Right Wrist Joint, Open Approach
0RJN3ZZ   Inspection of Right Wrist Joint, Percutaneous Approach
0RJN4ZZ   Inspection of Right Wrist Joint, Percutaneous Endoscopic Approach
0RJNXZZ   Inspection of Right Wrist Joint, External Approach
0RJP0ZZ   Inspection of Left Wrist Joint, Open Approach
0RJP3ZZ   Inspection of Left Wrist Joint, Percutaneous Approach
0RJP4ZZ   Inspection of Left Wrist Joint, Percutaneous Endoscopic Approach
0RJPXZZ   Inspection of Left Wrist Joint, External Approach
0RJQ0ZZ   Inspection of Right Carpal Joint, Open Approach
0RJQ3ZZ   Inspection of Right Carpal Joint, Percutaneous Approach

0RJQ4ZZ   Inspection of Right Carpal Joint, Percutaneous Endoscopic Approach
0RJQXZZ   Inspection of Right Carpal Joint, External Approach
0RJR0ZZ   Inspection of Left Carpal Joint, Open Approach
0RJR3ZZ   Inspection of Left Carpal Joint, Percutaneous Approach
0RJR4ZZ   Inspection of Left Carpal Joint, Percutaneous Endoscopic Approach
0RJRXZZ   Inspection of Left Carpal Joint, External Approach
0RJS0ZZ   Inspection of Right Metacarpocarpal Joint, Open Approach
0RJS3ZZ   Inspection of Right Metacarpocarpal Joint, Percutaneous Approach
0RJS4ZZ   Inspection of Right Metacarpocarpal Joint, Percutaneous Endoscopic Approach
0RJSXZZ   Inspection of Right Metacarpocarpal Joint, External Approach
0RJT0ZZ   Inspection of Left Metacarpocarpal Joint, Open Approach
0RJT3ZZ   Inspection of Left Metacarpocarpal Joint, Percutaneous Approach
0RJT4ZZ   Inspection of Left Metacarpocarpal Joint, Percutaneous Endoscopic Approach
0RJTXZZ   Inspection of Left Metacarpocarpal Joint, External Approach
0RJU0ZZ   Inspection of Right Metacarpophalangeal Joint, Open Approach
0RJU3ZZ   Inspection of Right Metacarpophalangeal Joint, Percutaneous Approach
0RJU4ZZ   Inspection of Right Metacarpophalangeal Joint, Percutaneous Endoscopic Approach
0RJUXZZ   Inspection of Right Metacarpophalangeal Joint, External Approach
0RJV0ZZ   Inspection of Left Metacarpophalangeal Joint, Open Approach
0RJV3ZZ   Inspection of Left Metacarpophalangeal Joint, Percutaneous Approach
0RJV4ZZ   Inspection of Left Metacarpophalangeal Joint, Percutaneous Endoscopic Approach
0RJVXZZ   Inspection of Left Metacarpophalangeal Joint, External Approach
0RJW0ZZ   Inspection of Right Finger Phalangeal Joint, Open Approach
0RJW3ZZ   Inspection of Right Finger Phalangeal Joint, Percutaneous Approach
0RJW4ZZ   Inspection of Right Finger Phalangeal Joint, Percutaneous Endoscopic Approach
0RJWXZZ   Inspection of Right Finger Phalangeal Joint, External Approach
0RJX0ZZ   Inspection of Left Finger Phalangeal Joint, Open Approach
0RJX3ZZ   Inspection of Left Finger Phalangeal Joint, Percutaneous Approach
0RJX4ZZ   Inspection of Left Finger Phalangeal Joint, Percutaneous Endoscopic Approach
0RJXXZZ   Inspection of Left Finger Phalangeal Joint, External Approach

0RN – Upper Joints, Release

Review Coding Guideline B3.13

0RN00ZZ   Release Occipital-cervical Joint, Open Approach
0RN03ZZ   Release Occipital-cervical Joint, Percutaneous Approach
0RN04ZZ   Release Occipital-cervical Joint, Percutaneous Endoscopic Approach
0RN0XZZ   Release Occipital-cervical Joint, External Approach
0RN10ZZ   Release Cervical Vertebral Joint, Open Approach
0RN13ZZ   Release Cervical Vertebral Joint, Percutaneous Approach
0RN14ZZ   Release Cervical Vertebral Joint, Percutaneous Endoscopic Approach
0RN1XZZ   Release Cervical Vertebral Joint, External Approach
0RN30ZZ   Release Cervical Vertebral Disc, Open Approach
0RN33ZZ   Release Cervical Vertebral Disc, Percutaneous Approach
0RN34ZZ   Release Cervical Vertebral Disc, Percutaneous Endoscopic Approach
0RN3XZZ   Release Cervical Vertebral Disc, External Approach
0RN40ZZ   Release Cervicothoracic Vertebral Joint, Open Approach
0RN43ZZ   Release Cervicothoracic Vertebral Joint, Percutaneous Approach
0RN44ZZ   Release Cervicothoracic Vertebral Joint, Percutaneous Endoscopic Approach
0RN4XZZ   Release Cervicothoracic Vertebral Joint, External Approach
0RN50ZZ   Release Cervicothoracic Vertebral Disc, Open Approach
0RN53ZZ   Release Cervicothoracic Vertebral Disc, Percutaneous Approach
0RN54ZZ   Release Cervicothoracic Vertebral Disc, Percutaneous Endoscopic Approach
0RN5XZZ   Release Cervicothoracic Vertebral Disc, External Approach
0RN60ZZ   Release Thoracic Vertebral Joint, Open Approach
0RN63ZZ   Release Thoracic Vertebral Joint, Percutaneous Approach
0RN64ZZ   Release Thoracic Vertebral Joint, Percutaneous Endoscopic Approach

0RN6XZZ   Release Thoracic Vertebral Joint, External Approach
0RN90ZZ   Release Thoracic Vertebral Disc, Open Approach
0RN93ZZ   Release Thoracic Vertebral Disc, Percutaneous Approach
0RN94ZZ   Release Thoracic Vertebral Disc, Percutaneous Endoscopic Approach
0RN9XZZ   Release Thoracic Vertebral Disc, External Approach
0RNA0ZZ   Release Thoracolumbar Vertebral Joint, Open Approach
0RNA3ZZ   Release Thoracolumbar Vertebral Joint, Percutaneous Approach
0RNA4ZZ   Release Thoracolumbar Vertebral Joint, Percutaneous Endoscopic Approach
0RNAXZZ   Release Thoracolumbar Vertebral Joint, External Approach
0RNB0ZZ   Release Thoracolumbar Vertebral Disc, Open Approach
0RNB3ZZ   Release Thoracolumbar Vertebral Disc, Percutaneous Approach
0RNB4ZZ   Release Thoracolumbar Vertebral Disc, Percutaneous Endoscopic Approach
0RNBXZZ   Release Thoracolumbar Vertebral Disc, External Approach
0RNC0ZZ   Release Right Temporomandibular Joint, Open Approach
0RNC3ZZ   Release Right Temporomandibular Joint, Percutaneous Approach
0RNC4ZZ   Release Right Temporomandibular Joint, Percutaneous Endoscopic Approach
0RNCXZZ   Release Right Temporomandibular Joint, External Approach
0RND0ZZ   Release Left Temporomandibular Joint, Open Approach
0RND3ZZ   Release Left Temporomandibular Joint, Percutaneous Approach
0RND4ZZ   Release Left Temporomandibular Joint, Percutaneous Endoscopic Approach
0RNDXZZ   Release Left Temporomandibular Joint, External Approach
0RNE0ZZ   Release Right Sternoclavicular Joint, Open Approach
0RNE3ZZ   Release Right Sternoclavicular Joint, Percutaneous Approach

0RNE4ZZ Release Right Sternoclavicular Joint, Percutaneous Endoscopic Approach
0RNEXZZ Release Right Sternoclavicular Joint, External Approach
0RNF0ZZ Release Left Sternoclavicular Joint, Open Approach
0RNF3ZZ Release Left Sternoclavicular Joint, Percutaneous Approach
0RNF4ZZ Release Left Sternoclavicular Joint, Percutaneous Endoscopic Approach
0RNFXZZ Release Left Sternoclavicular Joint, External Approach
0RNG0ZZ Release Right Acromioclavicular Joint, Open Approach
0RNG3ZZ Release Right Acromioclavicular Joint, Percutaneous Approach
0RNG4ZZ Release Right Acromioclavicular Joint, Percutaneous Endoscopic Approach
0RNGXZZ Release Right Acromioclavicular Joint, External Approach
0RNH0ZZ Release Left Acromioclavicular Joint, Open Approach
0RNH3ZZ Release Left Acromioclavicular Joint, Percutaneous Approach
0RNH4ZZ Release Left Acromioclavicular Joint, Percutaneous Endoscopic Approach
0RNHXZZ Release Left Acromioclavicular Joint, External Approach
0RNJ0ZZ Release Right Shoulder Joint, Open Approach
0RNJ3ZZ Release Right Shoulder Joint, Percutaneous Approach
0RNJ4ZZ Release Right Shoulder Joint, Percutaneous Endoscopic Approach
0RNJXZZ Release Right Shoulder Joint, External Approach
0RNK0ZZ Release Left Shoulder Joint, Open Approach
0RNK3ZZ Release Left Shoulder Joint, Percutaneous Approach
0RNK4ZZ Release Left Shoulder Joint, Percutaneous Endoscopic Approach
0RNKXZZ Release Left Shoulder Joint, External Approach
0RNL0ZZ Release Right Elbow Joint, Open Approach
0RNL3ZZ Release Right Elbow Joint, Percutaneous Approach
0RNL4ZZ Release Right Elbow Joint, Percutaneous Endoscopic Approach
0RNLXZZ Release Right Elbow Joint, External Approach
0RNM0ZZ Release Left Elbow Joint, Open Approach
0RNM3ZZ Release Left Elbow Joint, Percutaneous Approach
0RNM4ZZ Release Left Elbow Joint, Percutaneous Endoscopic Approach
0RNMXZZ Release Left Elbow Joint, External Approach
0RNN0ZZ Release Right Wrist Joint, Open Approach
0RNN3ZZ Release Right Wrist Joint, Percutaneous Approach
0RNN4ZZ Release Right Wrist Joint, Percutaneous Endoscopic Approach
0RNNXZZ Release Right Wrist Joint, External Approach
0RNP0ZZ Release Left Wrist Joint, Open Approach
0RNP3ZZ Release Left Wrist Joint, Percutaneous Approach
0RNP4ZZ Release Left Wrist Joint, Percutaneous Endoscopic Approach

0RNPXZZ Release Left Wrist Joint, External Approach
0RNQ0ZZ Release Right Carpal Joint, Open Approach
0RNQ3ZZ Release Right Carpal Joint, Percutaneous Approach
0RNQ4ZZ Release Right Carpal Joint, Percutaneous Endoscopic Approach
0RNQXZZ Release Right Carpal Joint, External Approach
0RNR0ZZ Release Left Carpal Joint, Open Approach
0RNR3ZZ Release Left Carpal Joint, Percutaneous Approach
0RNR4ZZ Release Left Carpal Joint, Percutaneous Endoscopic Approach
0RNRXZZ Release Left Carpal Joint, External Approach
0RNS0ZZ Release Right Metacarpocarpal Joint, Open Approach
0RNS3ZZ Release Right Metacarpocarpal Joint, Percutaneous Approach
0RNS4ZZ Release Right Metacarpocarpal Joint, Percutaneous Endoscopic Approach
0RNSXZZ Release Right Metacarpocarpal Joint, External Approach
0RNT0ZZ Release Left Metacarpocarpal Joint, Open Approach
0RNT3ZZ Release Left Metacarpocarpal Joint, Percutaneous Approach
0RNT4ZZ Release Left Metacarpocarpal Joint, Percutaneous Endoscopic Approach
0RNTXZZ Release Left Metacarpocarpal Joint, External Approach
0RNU0ZZ Release Right Metacarpophalangeal Joint, Open Approach
0RNU3ZZ Release Right Metacarpophalangeal Joint, Percutaneous Approach
0RNU4ZZ Release Right Metacarpophalangeal Joint, Percutaneous Endoscopic Approach
0RNUXZZ Release Right Metacarpophalangeal Joint, External Approach
0RNV0ZZ Release Left Metacarpophalangeal Joint, Open Approach
0RNV3ZZ Release Left Metacarpophalangeal Joint, Percutaneous Approach
0RNV4ZZ Release Left Metacarpophalangeal Joint, Percutaneous Endoscopic Approach
0RNVXZZ Release Left Metacarpophalangeal Joint, External Approach
0RNW0ZZ Release Right Finger Phalangeal Joint, Open Approach
0RNW3ZZ Release Right Finger Phalangeal Joint, Percutaneous Approach
0RNW4ZZ Release Right Finger Phalangeal Joint, Percutaneous Endoscopic Approach
0RNWXZZ Release Right Finger Phalangeal Joint, External Approach
0RNX0ZZ Release Left Finger Phalangeal Joint, Open Approach
0RNX3ZZ Release Left Finger Phalangeal Joint, Percutaneous Approach
0RNX4ZZ Release Left Finger Phalangeal Joint, Percutaneous Endoscopic Approach
0RNXXZZ Release Left Finger Phalangeal Joint, External Approach

0RP – Upper Joints, Removal

Review Coding Guideline B6.1c

0RP000Z Removal of Drainage Device from Occipital-cervical Joint, Open Approach
0RP003Z Removal of Infusion Device from Occipital-cervical Joint, Open Approach
0RP004Z Removal of Internal Fixation Device from Occipital-cervical Joint, Open Approach
0RP007Z Removal of Autologous Tissue Substitute from Occipital-cervical Joint, Open Approach
0RP008Z Removal of Spacer from Occipital-cervical Joint, Open Approach
0RP00AZ Removal of Interbody Fusion Device from Occipital-cervical Joint, Open Approach
0RP00JZ Removal of Synthetic Substitute from Occipital-cervical Joint, Open Approach
0RP00KZ Removal of Nonautologous Tissue Substitute from Occipital-cervical Joint, Open Approach
0RP030Z Removal of Drainage Device from Occipital-cervical Joint, Percutaneous Approach
0RP033Z Removal of Infusion Device from Occipital-cervical Joint, Percutaneous Approach
0RP034Z Removal of Internal Fixation Device from Occipital-cervical Joint, Percutaneous Approach
0RP037Z Removal of Autologous Tissue Substitute from Occipital-cervical Joint, Percutaneous Approach
0RP038Z Removal of Spacer from Occipital-cervical Joint, Percutaneous Approach

0RP03AZ Removal of Interbody Fusion Device from Occipital-cervical Joint, Percutaneous Approach
0RP03JZ Removal of Synthetic Substitute from Occipital-cervical Joint, Percutaneous Approach
0RP03KZ Removal of Nonautologous Tissue Substitute from Occipital-cervical Joint, Percutaneous Approach
0RP040Z Removal of Drainage Device from Occipital-cervical Joint, Percutaneous Endoscopic Approach
0RP043Z Removal of Infusion Device from Occipital-cervical Joint, Percutaneous Endoscopic Approach
0RP044Z Removal of Internal Fixation Device from Occipital-cervical Joint, Percutaneous Endoscopic Approach
0RP047Z Removal of Autologous Tissue Substitute from Occipital-cervical Joint, Percutaneous Endoscopic Approach
0RP048Z Removal of Spacer from Occipital-cervical Joint, Percutaneous Endoscopic Approach
0RP04AZ Removal of Interbody Fusion Device from Occipital-cervical Joint, Percutaneous Endoscopic Approach
0RP04JZ Removal of Synthetic Substitute from Occipital-cervical Joint, Percutaneous Endoscopic Approach
0RP04KZ Removal of Nonautologous Tissue Substitute from Occipital-cervical Joint, Percutaneous Endoscopic Approach
0RP0X0Z Removal of Drainage Device from Occipital-cervical Joint, External Approach
0RP0X3Z Removal of Infusion Device from Occipital-cervical Joint, External Approach

0RP0X4Z Removal of Internal Fixation Device from Occipital-cervical Joint, External Approach

0RP100Z Removal of Drainage Device from Cervical Vertebral Joint, Open Approach

0RP103Z Removal of Infusion Device from Cervical Vertebral Joint, Open Approach

0RP104Z Removal of Internal Fixation Device from Cervical Vertebral Joint, Open Approach

0RP107Z Removal of Autologous Tissue Substitute from Cervical Vertebral Joint, Open Approach

0RP108Z Removal of Spacer from Cervical Vertebral Joint, Open Approach

0RP10AZ Removal of Interbody Fusion Device from Cervical Vertebral Joint, Open Approach

0RP10JZ Removal of Synthetic Substitute from Cervical Vertebral Joint, Open Approach

0RP10KZ Removal of Nonautologous Tissue Substitute from Cervical Vertebral Joint, Open Approach

0RP130Z Removal of Drainage Device from Cervical Vertebral Joint, Percutaneous Approach

0RP133Z Removal of Infusion Device from Cervical Vertebral Joint, Percutaneous Approach

0RP134Z Removal of Internal Fixation Device from Cervical Vertebral Joint, Percutaneous Approach

0RP137Z Removal of Autologous Tissue Substitute from Cervical Vertebral Joint, Percutaneous Approach

0RP138Z Removal of Spacer from Cervical Vertebral Joint, Percutaneous Approach

0RP13AZ Removal of Interbody Fusion Device from Cervical Vertebral Joint, Percutaneous Approach

0RP13JZ Removal of Synthetic Substitute from Cervical Vertebral Joint, Percutaneous Approach

0RP13KZ Removal of Nonautologous Tissue Substitute from Cervical Vertebral Joint, Percutaneous Approach

0RP140Z Removal of Drainage Device from Cervical Vertebral Joint, Percutaneous Endoscopic Approach

0RP143Z Removal of Infusion Device from Cervical Vertebral Joint, Percutaneous Endoscopic Approach

0RP144Z Removal of Internal Fixation Device from Cervical Vertebral Joint, Percutaneous Endoscopic Approach

0RP147Z Removal of Autologous Tissue Substitute from Cervical Vertebral Joint, Percutaneous Endoscopic Approach

0RP148Z Removal of Spacer from Cervical Vertebral Joint, Percutaneous Endoscopic Approach

0RP14AZ Removal of Interbody Fusion Device from Cervical Vertebral Joint, Percutaneous Endoscopic Approach

0RP14JZ Removal of Synthetic Substitute from Cervical Vertebral Joint, Percutaneous Endoscopic Approach

0RP14KZ Removal of Nonautologous Tissue Substitute from Cervical Vertebral Joint, Percutaneous Endoscopic Approach

0RP1X0Z Removal of Drainage Device from Cervical Vertebral Joint, External Approach

0RP1X3Z Removal of Infusion Device from Cervical Vertebral Joint, External Approach

0RP1X4Z Removal of Internal Fixation Device from Cervical Vertebral Joint, External Approach

0RP300Z Removal of Drainage Device from Cervical Vertebral Disc, Open Approach

0RP303Z Removal of Infusion Device from Cervical Vertebral Disc, Open Approach

0RP307Z Removal of Autologous Tissue Substitute from Cervical Vertebral Disc, Open Approach

0RP30JZ Removal of Synthetic Substitute from Cervical Vertebral Disc, Open Approach

0RP30KZ Removal of Nonautologous Tissue Substitute from Cervical Vertebral Disc, Open Approach

0RP330Z Removal of Drainage Device from Cervical Vertebral Disc, Percutaneous Approach

0RP333Z Removal of Infusion Device from Cervical Vertebral Disc, Percutaneous Approach

0RP337Z Removal of Autologous Tissue Substitute from Cervical Vertebral Disc, Percutaneous Approach

0RP33JZ Removal of Synthetic Substitute from Cervical Vertebral Disc, Percutaneous Approach

0RP33KZ Removal of Nonautologous Tissue Substitute from Cervical Vertebral Disc, Percutaneous Approach

0RP340Z Removal of Drainage Device from Cervical Vertebral Disc, Percutaneous Endoscopic Approach

0RP343Z Removal of Infusion Device from Cervical Vertebral Disc, Percutaneous Endoscopic Approach

0RP347Z Removal of Autologous Tissue Substitute from Cervical Vertebral Disc, Percutaneous Endoscopic Approach

0RP34JZ Removal of Synthetic Substitute from Cervical Vertebral Disc, Percutaneous Endoscopic Approach

0RP34KZ Removal of Nonautologous Tissue Substitute from Cervical Vertebral Disc, Percutaneous Endoscopic Approach

0RP3X0Z Removal of Drainage Device from Cervical Vertebral Disc, External Approach

0RP3X3Z Removal of Infusion Device from Cervical Vertebral Disc, External Approach

0RP400Z Removal of Drainage Device from Cervicothoracic Vertebral Joint, Open Approach

0RP403Z Removal of Infusion Device from Cervicothoracic Vertebral Joint, Open Approach

0RP404Z Removal of Internal Fixation Device from Cervicothoracic Vertebral Joint, Open Approach

0RP407Z Removal of Autologous Tissue Substitute from Cervicothoracic Vertebral Joint, Open Approach

0RP408Z Removal of Spacer from Cervicothoracic Vertebral Joint, Open Approach

0RP40AZ Removal of Interbody Fusion Device from Cervicothoracic Vertebral Joint, Open Approach

0RP40JZ Removal of Synthetic Substitute from Cervicothoracic Vertebral Joint, Open Approach

0RP40KZ Removal of Nonautologous Tissue Substitute from Cervicothoracic Vertebral Joint, Open Approach

0RP430Z Removal of Drainage Device from Cervicothoracic Vertebral Joint, Percutaneous Approach

0RP433Z Removal of Infusion Device from Cervicothoracic Vertebral Joint, Percutaneous Approach

0RP434Z Removal of Internal Fixation Device from Cervicothoracic Vertebral Joint, Percutaneous Approach

0RP437Z Removal of Autologous Tissue Substitute from Cervicothoracic Vertebral Joint, Percutaneous Approach

0RP438Z Removal of Spacer from Cervicothoracic Vertebral Joint, Percutaneous Approach

0RP43AZ Removal of Interbody Fusion Device from Cervicothoracic Vertebral Joint, Percutaneous Approach

0RP43JZ Removal of Synthetic Substitute from Cervicothoracic Vertebral Joint, Percutaneous Approach

0RP43KZ Removal of Nonautologous Tissue Substitute from Cervicothoracic Vertebral Joint, Percutaneous Approach

0RP440Z Removal of Drainage Device from Cervicothoracic Vertebral Joint, Percutaneous Endoscopic Approach

0RP443Z Removal of Infusion Device from Cervicothoracic Vertebral Joint, Percutaneous Endoscopic Approach

0RP444Z Removal of Internal Fixation Device from Cervicothoracic Vertebral Joint, Percutaneous Endoscopic Approach

0RP447Z Removal of Autologous Tissue Substitute from Cervicothoracic Vertebral Joint, Percutaneous Endoscopic Approach

0RP448Z Removal of Spacer from Cervicothoracic Vertebral Joint, Percutaneous Endoscopic Approach

0RP44AZ Removal of Interbody Fusion Device from Cervicothoracic Vertebral Joint, Percutaneous Endoscopic Approach

0RP44JZ Removal of Synthetic Substitute from Cervicothoracic Vertebral Joint, Percutaneous Endoscopic Approach

0RP44KZ Removal of Nonautologous Tissue Substitute from Cervicothoracic Vertebral Joint, Percutaneous Endoscopic Approach

0RP4X0Z Removal of Drainage Device from Cervicothoracic Vertebral Joint, External Approach

0RP4X3Z Removal of Infusion Device from Cervicothoracic Vertebral Joint, External Approach

0RP4X4Z Removal of Internal Fixation Device from Cervicothoracic Vertebral Joint, External Approach

0RP500Z Removal of Drainage Device from Cervicothoracic Vertebral Disc, Open Approach

0RP503Z Removal of Infusion Device from Cervicothoracic Vertebral Disc, Open Approach

0RP507Z Removal of Autologous Tissue Substitute from Cervicothoracic Vertebral Disc, Open Approach

0RP50JZ Removal of Synthetic Substitute from Cervicothoracic Vertebral Disc, Open Approach

0RP50KZ Removal of Nonautologous Tissue Substitute from Cervicothoracic Vertebral Disc, Open Approach

0RP530Z Removal of Drainage Device from Cervicothoracic Vertebral Disc, Percutaneous Approach

0RP533Z Removal of Infusion Device from Cervicothoracic Vertebral Disc, Percutaneous Approach

0RP537Z Removal of Autologous Tissue Substitute from Cervicothoracic Vertebral Disc, Percutaneous Approach

0RP53JZ Removal of Synthetic Substitute from Cervicothoracic Vertebral Disc, Percutaneous Approach

0RP53KZ Removal of Nonautologous Tissue Substitute from Cervicothoracic Vertebral Disc, Percutaneous Approach

0RP540Z Removal of Drainage Device from Cervicothoracic Vertebral Disc, Percutaneous Endoscopic Approach

0RP543Z Removal of Infusion Device from Cervicothoracic Vertebral Disc, Percutaneous Endoscopic Approach

0RP547Z Removal of Autologous Tissue Substitute from Cervicothoracic Vertebral Disc, Percutaneous Endoscopic Approach

0RP54JZ Removal of Synthetic Substitute from Cervicothoracic Vertebral Disc, Percutaneous Endoscopic Approach

0RP54KZ Removal of Nonautologous Tissue Substitute from Cervicothoracic Vertebral Disc, Percutaneous Endoscopic Approach

0RP5X0Z Removal of Drainage Device from Cervicothoracic Vertebral Disc, External Approach

0RP5X3Z Removal of Infusion Device from Cervicothoracic Vertebral Disc, External Approach

0RP600Z Removal of Drainage Device from Thoracic Vertebral Joint, Open Approach

0RP603Z Removal of Infusion Device from Thoracic Vertebral Joint, Open Approach

0RP604Z Removal of Internal Fixation Device from Thoracic Vertebral Joint, Open Approach

0RP607Z Removal of Autologous Tissue Substitute from Thoracic Vertebral Joint, Open Approach

0RP608Z Removal of Spacer from Thoracic Vertebral Joint, Open Approach

0RP60AZ Removal of Interbody Fusion Device from Thoracic Vertebral Joint, Open Approach

0RP60JZ Removal of Synthetic Substitute from Thoracic Vertebral Joint, Open Approach

0RP60KZ Removal of Nonautologous Tissue Substitute from Thoracic Vertebral Joint, Open Approach

0RP630Z Removal of Drainage Device from Thoracic Vertebral Joint, Percutaneous Approach

0RP633Z Removal of Infusion Device from Thoracic Vertebral Joint, Percutaneous Approach

0RP634Z Removal of Internal Fixation Device from Thoracic Vertebral Joint, Percutaneous Approach

0RP637Z Removal of Autologous Tissue Substitute from Thoracic Vertebral Joint, Percutaneous Approach

0RP638Z Removal of Spacer from Thoracic Vertebral Joint, Percutaneous Approach

0RP63AZ Removal of Interbody Fusion Device from Thoracic Vertebral Joint, Percutaneous Approach

0RP63JZ Removal of Synthetic Substitute from Thoracic Vertebral Joint, Percutaneous Approach

0RP63KZ Removal of Nonautologous Tissue Substitute from Thoracic Vertebral Joint, Percutaneous Approach

0RP640Z Removal of Drainage Device from Thoracic Vertebral Joint, Percutaneous Endoscopic Approach

0RP643Z Removal of Infusion Device from Thoracic Vertebral Joint, Percutaneous Endoscopic Approach

0RP644Z Removal of Internal Fixation Device from Thoracic Vertebral Joint, Percutaneous Endoscopic Approach

0RP647Z Removal of Autologous Tissue Substitute from Thoracic Vertebral Joint, Percutaneous Endoscopic Approach

0RP648Z Removal of Spacer from Thoracic Vertebral Joint, Percutaneous Endoscopic Approach

0RP64AZ Removal of Interbody Fusion Device from Thoracic Vertebral Joint, Percutaneous Endoscopic Approach

0RP64JZ Removal of Synthetic Substitute from Thoracic Vertebral Joint, Percutaneous Endoscopic Approach

0RP64KZ Removal of Nonautologous Tissue Substitute from Thoracic Vertebral Joint, Percutaneous Endoscopic Approach

0RP6X0Z Removal of Drainage Device from Thoracic Vertebral Joint, External Approach

0RP6X3Z Removal of Infusion Device from Thoracic Vertebral Joint, External Approach

0RP6X4Z Removal of Internal Fixation Device from Thoracic Vertebral Joint, External Approach

0RP900Z Removal of Drainage Device from Thoracic Vertebral Disc, Open Approach

0RP903Z Removal of Infusion Device from Thoracic Vertebral Disc, Open Approach

0RP907Z Removal of Autologous Tissue Substitute from Thoracic Vertebral Disc, Open Approach

0RP90JZ Removal of Synthetic Substitute from Thoracic Vertebral Disc, Open Approach

0RP90KZ Removal of Nonautologous Tissue Substitute from Thoracic Vertebral Disc, Open Approach

0RP930Z Removal of Drainage Device from Thoracic Vertebral Disc, Percutaneous Approach

0RP933Z Removal of Infusion Device from Thoracic Vertebral Disc, Percutaneous Approach

0RP937Z Removal of Autologous Tissue Substitute from Thoracic Vertebral Disc, Percutaneous Approach

0RP93JZ Removal of Synthetic Substitute from Thoracic Vertebral Disc, Percutaneous Approach

0RP93KZ Removal of Nonautologous Tissue Substitute from Thoracic Vertebral Disc, Percutaneous Approach

0RP940Z Removal of Drainage Device from Thoracic Vertebral Disc, Percutaneous Endoscopic Approach

0RP943Z Removal of Infusion Device from Thoracic Vertebral Disc, Percutaneous Endoscopic Approach

0RP947Z Removal of Autologous Tissue Substitute from Thoracic Vertebral Disc, Percutaneous Endoscopic Approach

0RP94JZ Removal of Synthetic Substitute from Thoracic Vertebral Disc, Percutaneous Endoscopic Approach

0RP94KZ Removal of Nonautologous Tissue Substitute from Thoracic Vertebral Disc, Percutaneous Endoscopic Approach

0RP9X0Z Removal of Drainage Device from Thoracic Vertebral Disc, External Approach

0RP9X3Z Removal of Infusion Device from Thoracic Vertebral Disc, External Approach

0RPA00Z Removal of Drainage Device from Thoracolumbar Vertebral Joint, Open Approach

0RPA03Z Removal of Infusion Device from Thoracolumbar Vertebral Joint, Open Approach

0RPA04Z Removal of Internal Fixation Device from Thoracolumbar Vertebral Joint, Open Approach

0RPA07Z Removal of Autologous Tissue Substitute from Thoracolumbar Vertebral Joint, Open Approach

0RPA08Z Removal of Spacer from Thoracolumbar Vertebral Joint, Open Approach

0RPA0AZ Removal of Interbody Fusion Device from Thoracolumbar Vertebral Joint, Open Approach

0RPA0JZ Removal of Synthetic Substitute from Thoracolumbar Vertebral Joint, Open Approach

0RPA0KZ Removal of Nonautologous Tissue Substitute from Thoracolumbar Vertebral Joint, Open Approach

0RPA30Z Removal of Drainage Device from Thoracolumbar Vertebral Joint, Percutaneous Approach

0RPA33Z Removal of Infusion Device from Thoracolumbar Vertebral Joint, Percutaneous Approach

0RPA34Z Removal of Internal Fixation Device from Thoracolumbar Vertebral Joint, Percutaneous Approach

0RPA37Z Removal of Autologous Tissue Substitute from Thoracolumbar Vertebral Joint, Percutaneous Approach

0RPA38Z Removal of Spacer from Thoracolumbar Vertebral Joint, Percutaneous Approach

0RPA3AZ Removal of Interbody Fusion Device from Thoracolumbar Vertebral Joint, Percutaneous Approach

0RPA3JZ Removal of Synthetic Substitute from Thoracolumbar Vertebral Joint, Percutaneous Approach

0RPA3KZ Removal of Nonautologous Tissue Substitute from Thoracolumbar Vertebral Joint, Percutaneous Approach

0RPA40Z Removal of Drainage Device from Thoracolumbar Vertebral Joint, Percutaneous Endoscopic Approach

0RPA43Z Removal of Infusion Device from Thoracolumbar Vertebral Joint, Percutaneous Endoscopic Approach

0RPA44Z Removal of Internal Fixation Device from Thoracolumbar Vertebral Joint, Percutaneous Endoscopic Approach

0RPA47Z Removal of Autologous Tissue Substitute from Thoracolumbar Vertebral Joint, Percutaneous Endoscopic Approach

0RPA48Z Removal of Spacer from Thoracolumbar Vertebral Joint, Percutaneous Endoscopic Approach

0RPA4AZ Removal of Interbody Fusion Device from Thoracolumbar Vertebral Joint, Percutaneous Endoscopic Approach

0RPA4JZ Removal of Synthetic Substitute from Thoracolumbar Vertebral Joint, Percutaneous Endoscopic Approach

0RPA4KZ Removal of Nonautologous Tissue Substitute from Thoracolumbar Vertebral Joint, Percutaneous Endoscopic Approach

0RPAX0Z Removal of Drainage Device from Thoracolumbar Vertebral Joint, External Approach

0RPAX3Z Removal of Infusion Device from Thoracolumbar Vertebral Joint, External Approach

0RPAX4Z Removal of Internal Fixation Device from Thoracolumbar Vertebral Joint, External Approach

0RPB00Z Removal of Drainage Device from Thoracolumbar Vertebral Disc, Open Approach

0RPB03Z Removal of Infusion Device from Thoracolumbar Vertebral Disc, Open Approach

0RPB07Z Removal of Autologous Tissue Substitute from Thoracolumbar Vertebral Disc, Open Approach

0RPB0JZ Removal of Synthetic Substitute from Thoracolumbar Vertebral Disc, Open Approach

0RPB0KZ Removal of Nonautologous Tissue Substitute from Thoracolumbar Vertebral Disc, Open Approach

0RPB30Z Removal of Drainage Device from Thoracolumbar Vertebral Disc, Percutaneous Approach

0RPB33Z Removal of Infusion Device from Thoracolumbar Vertebral Disc, Percutaneous Approach

0RPB37Z Removal of Autologous Tissue Substitute from Thoracolumbar Vertebral Disc, Percutaneous Approach

0RPB3JZ Removal of Synthetic Substitute from Thoracolumbar Vertebral Disc, Percutaneous Approach

0RPB3KZ Removal of Nonautologous Tissue Substitute from Thoracolumbar Vertebral Disc, Percutaneous Approach

0RPB40Z Removal of Drainage Device from Thoracolumbar Vertebral Disc, Percutaneous Endoscopic Approach

0RPB43Z Removal of Infusion Device from Thoracolumbar Vertebral Disc, Percutaneous Endoscopic Approach

0RPB47Z Removal of Autologous Tissue Substitute from Thoracolumbar Vertebral Disc, Percutaneous Endoscopic Approach

0RPB4JZ Removal of Synthetic Substitute from Thoracolumbar Vertebral Disc, Percutaneous Endoscopic Approach

0RPB4KZ Removal of Nonautologous Tissue Substitute from Thoracolumbar Vertebral Disc, Percutaneous Endoscopic Approach

0RPBX0Z Removal of Drainage Device from Thoracolumbar Vertebral Disc, External Approach

0RPBX3Z Removal of Infusion Device from Thoracolumbar Vertebral Disc, External Approach

0RPC00Z Removal of Drainage Device from Right Temporomandibular Joint, Open Approach

0RPC03Z Removal of Infusion Device from Right Temporomandibular Joint, Open Approach

0RPC04Z Removal of Internal Fixation Device from Right Temporomandibular Joint, Open Approach

0RPC07Z Removal of Autologous Tissue Substitute from Right Temporomandibular Joint, Open Approach

0RPC08Z Removal of Spacer from Right Temporomandibular Joint, Open Approach

0RPC0JZ Removal of Synthetic Substitute from Right Temporomandibular Joint, Open Approach

0RPC0KZ Removal of Nonautologous Tissue Substitute from Right Temporomandibular Joint, Open Approach

0RPC30Z Removal of Drainage Device from Right Temporomandibular Joint, Percutaneous Approach

0RPC33Z Removal of Infusion Device from Right Temporomandibular Joint, Percutaneous Approach

0RPC34Z Removal of Internal Fixation Device from Right Temporomandibular Joint, Percutaneous Approach

0RPC37Z Removal of Autologous Tissue Substitute from Right Temporomandibular Joint, Percutaneous Approach

0RPC38Z Removal of Spacer from Right Temporomandibular Joint, Percutaneous Approach

0RPC3JZ Removal of Synthetic Substitute from Right Temporomandibular Joint, Percutaneous Approach

0RPC3KZ Removal of Nonautologous Tissue Substitute from Right Temporomandibular Joint, Percutaneous Approach

0RPC40Z Removal of Drainage Device from Right Temporomandibular Joint, Percutaneous Endoscopic Approach

0RPC43Z Removal of Infusion Device from Right Temporomandibular Joint, Percutaneous Endoscopic Approach

0RPC44Z Removal of Internal Fixation Device from Right Temporomandibular Joint, Percutaneous Endoscopic Approach

0RPC47Z Removal of Autologous Tissue Substitute from Right Temporomandibular Joint, Percutaneous Endoscopic Approach

0RPC48Z Removal of Spacer from Right Temporomandibular Joint, Percutaneous Endoscopic Approach

0RPC4JZ Removal of Synthetic Substitute from Right Temporomandibular Joint, Percutaneous Endoscopic Approach

0RPC4KZ Removal of Nonautologous Tissue Substitute from Right Temporomandibular Joint, Percutaneous Endoscopic Approach

0RPCX0Z Removal of Drainage Device from Right Temporomandibular Joint, External Approach

0RPCX3Z Removal of Infusion Device from Right Temporomandibular Joint, External Approach

0RPCX4Z Removal of Internal Fixation Device from Right Temporomandibular Joint, External Approach

0RPD00Z Removal of Drainage Device from Left Temporomandibular Joint, Open Approach

0RPD03Z Removal of Infusion Device from Left Temporomandibular Joint, Open Approach

0RPD04Z Removal of Internal Fixation Device from Left Temporomandibular Joint, Open Approach

0RPD07Z Removal of Autologous Tissue Substitute from Left Temporomandibular Joint, Open Approach

0RPD08Z Removal of Spacer from Left Temporomandibular Joint, Open Approach

0RPD0JZ Removal of Synthetic Substitute from Left Temporomandibular Joint, Open Approach

0RPD0KZ Removal of Nonautologous Tissue Substitute from Left Temporomandibular Joint, Open Approach

0RPD30Z Removal of Drainage Device from Left Temporomandibular Joint, Percutaneous Approach

0RPD33Z Removal of Infusion Device from Left Temporomandibular Joint, Percutaneous Approach

0RPD34Z Removal of Internal Fixation Device from Left Temporomandibular Joint, Percutaneous Approach

0RPD37Z Removal of Autologous Tissue Substitute from Left Temporomandibular Joint, Percutaneous Approach

0RPD38Z Removal of Spacer from Left Temporomandibular Joint, Percutaneous Approach

0RPD3JZ Removal of Synthetic Substitute from Left Temporomandibular Joint, Percutaneous Approach

0RPD3KZ Removal of Nonautologous Tissue Substitute from Left Temporomandibular Joint, Percutaneous Approach

0RPD40Z Removal of Drainage Device from Left Temporomandibular Joint, Percutaneous Endoscopic Approach

0RPD43Z Removal of Infusion Device from Left Temporomandibular Joint, Percutaneous Endoscopic Approach

0RPD44Z Removal of Internal Fixation Device from Left Temporomandibular Joint, Percutaneous Endoscopic Approach

0RPD47Z Removal of Autologous Tissue Substitute from Left Temporomandibular Joint, Percutaneous Endoscopic Approach

0RPD48Z Removal of Spacer from Left Temporomandibular Joint, Percutaneous Endoscopic Approach

0RPD4JZ Removal of Synthetic Substitute from Left Temporomandibular Joint, Percutaneous Endoscopic Approach

0RPD4KZ Removal of Nonautologous Tissue Substitute from Left Temporomandibular Joint, Percutaneous Endoscopic Approach

---

♀ Female-only   ♂ Male-only   ◐ Limited Coverage   ● Non-OR   ▨ HAC-associated procedure   ⬤ Non-covered procedures   ✚ Combination

0RPDX0Z Removal of Drainage Device from Left Temporomandibular Joint, External Approach

0RPDX3Z Removal of Infusion Device from Left Temporomandibular Joint, External Approach

0RPDX4Z Removal of Internal Fixation Device from Left Temporomandibular Joint, External Approach

0RPE00Z Removal of Drainage Device from Right Sternoclavicular Joint, Open Approach

0RPE03Z Removal of Infusion Device from Right Sternoclavicular Joint, Open Approach

0RPE04Z Removal of Internal Fixation Device from Right Sternoclavicular Joint, Open Approach

0RPE07Z Removal of Autologous Tissue Substitute from Right Sternoclavicular Joint, Open Approach

0RPE08Z Removal of Spacer from Right Sternoclavicular Joint, Open Approach

0RPE0JZ Removal of Synthetic Substitute from Right Sternoclavicular Joint, Open Approach

0RPE0KZ Removal of Nonautologous Tissue Substitute from Right Sternoclavicular Joint, Open Approach

0RPE30Z Removal of Drainage Device from Right Sternoclavicular Joint, Percutaneous Approach

0RPE33Z Removal of Infusion Device from Right Sternoclavicular Joint, Percutaneous Approach

0RPE34Z Removal of Internal Fixation Device from Right Sternoclavicular Joint, Percutaneous Approach

0RPE37Z Removal of Autologous Tissue Substitute from Right Sternoclavicular Joint, Percutaneous Approach

0RPE38Z Removal of Spacer from Right Sternoclavicular Joint, Percutaneous Approach

0RPE3JZ Removal of Synthetic Substitute from Right Sternoclavicular Joint, Percutaneous Approach

0RPE3KZ Removal of Nonautologous Tissue Substitute from Right Sternoclavicular Joint, Percutaneous Approach

0RPE40Z Removal of Drainage Device from Right Sternoclavicular Joint, Percutaneous Endoscopic Approach

0RPE43Z Removal of Infusion Device from Right Sternoclavicular Joint, Percutaneous Endoscopic Approach

0RPE44Z Removal of Internal Fixation Device from Right Sternoclavicular Joint, Percutaneous Endoscopic Approach

0RPE47Z Removal of Autologous Tissue Substitute from Right Sternoclavicular Joint, Percutaneous Endoscopic Approach

0RPE48Z Removal of Spacer from Right Sternoclavicular Joint, Percutaneous Endoscopic Approach

0RPE4JZ Removal of Synthetic Substitute from Right Sternoclavicular Joint, Percutaneous Endoscopic Approach

0RPE4KZ Removal of Nonautologous Tissue Substitute from Right Sternoclavicular Joint, Percutaneous Endoscopic Approach

0RPEX0Z Removal of Drainage Device from Right Sternoclavicular Joint, External Approach

0RPEX3Z Removal of Infusion Device from Right Sternoclavicular Joint, External Approach

0RPEX4Z Removal of Internal Fixation Device from Right Sternoclavicular Joint, External Approach

0RPF00Z Removal of Drainage Device from Left Sternoclavicular Joint, Open Approach

0RPF03Z Removal of Infusion Device from Left Sternoclavicular Joint, Open Approach

0RPF04Z Removal of Internal Fixation Device from Left Sternoclavicular Joint, Open Approach

0RPF07Z Removal of Autologous Tissue Substitute from Left Sternoclavicular Joint, Open Approach

0RPF08Z Removal of Spacer from Left Sternoclavicular Joint, Open Approach

0RPF0JZ Removal of Synthetic Substitute from Left Sternoclavicular Joint, Open Approach

0RPF0KZ Removal of Nonautologous Tissue Substitute from Left Sternoclavicular Joint, Open Approach

0RPF30Z Removal of Drainage Device from Left Sternoclavicular Joint, Percutaneous Approach

0RPF33Z Removal of Infusion Device from Left Sternoclavicular Joint, Percutaneous Approach

0RPF34Z Removal of Internal Fixation Device from Left Sternoclavicular Joint, Percutaneous Approach

0RPF37Z Removal of Autologous Tissue Substitute from Left Sternoclavicular Joint, Percutaneous Approach

0RPF38Z Removal of Spacer from Left Sternoclavicular Joint, Percutaneous Approach

0RPF3JZ Removal of Synthetic Substitute from Left Sternoclavicular Joint, Percutaneous Approach

0RPF3KZ Removal of Nonautologous Tissue Substitute from Left Sternoclavicular Joint, Percutaneous Approach

0RPF40Z Removal of Drainage Device from Left Sternoclavicular Joint, Percutaneous Endoscopic Approach

0RPF43Z Removal of Infusion Device from Left Sternoclavicular Joint, Percutaneous Endoscopic Approach

0RPF44Z Removal of Internal Fixation Device from Left Sternoclavicular Joint, Percutaneous Endoscopic Approach

0RPF47Z Removal of Autologous Tissue Substitute from Left Sternoclavicular Joint, Percutaneous Endoscopic Approach

0RPF48Z Removal of Spacer from Left Sternoclavicular Joint, Percutaneous Endoscopic Approach

0RPF4JZ Removal of Synthetic Substitute from Left Sternoclavicular Joint, Percutaneous Endoscopic Approach

0RPF4KZ Removal of Nonautologous Tissue Substitute from Left Sternoclavicular Joint, Percutaneous Endoscopic Approach

0RPFX0Z Removal of Drainage Device from Left Sternoclavicular Joint, External Approach

0RPFX3Z Removal of Infusion Device from Left Sternoclavicular Joint, External Approach

0RPFX4Z Removal of Internal Fixation Device from Left Sternoclavicular Joint, External Approach

0RPG00Z Removal of Drainage Device from Right Acromioclavicular Joint, Open Approach

0RPG03Z Removal of Infusion Device from Right Acromioclavicular Joint, Open Approach

0RPG04Z Removal of Internal Fixation Device from Right Acromioclavicular Joint, Open Approach

0RPG07Z Removal of Autologous Tissue Substitute from Right Acromioclavicular Joint, Open Approach

0RPG08Z Removal of Spacer from Right Acromioclavicular Joint, Open Approach

0RPG0JZ Removal of Synthetic Substitute from Right Acromioclavicular Joint, Open Approach

0RPG0KZ Removal of Nonautologous Tissue Substitute from Right Acromioclavicular Joint, Open Approach

0RPG30Z Removal of Drainage Device from Right Acromioclavicular Joint, Percutaneous Approach

0RPG33Z Removal of Infusion Device from Right Acromioclavicular Joint, Percutaneous Approach

0RPG34Z Removal of Internal Fixation Device from Right Acromioclavicular Joint, Percutaneous Approach

0RPG37Z Removal of Autologous Tissue Substitute from Right Acromioclavicular Joint, Percutaneous Approach

0RPG38Z Removal of Spacer from Right Acromioclavicular Joint, Percutaneous Approach

0RPG3JZ Removal of Synthetic Substitute from Right Acromioclavicular Joint, Percutaneous Approach

0RPG3KZ Removal of Nonautologous Tissue Substitute from Right Acromioclavicular Joint, Percutaneous Approach

0RPG40Z Removal of Drainage Device from Right Acromioclavicular Joint, Percutaneous Endoscopic Approach

0RPG43Z Removal of Infusion Device from Right Acromioclavicular Joint, Percutaneous Endoscopic Approach

0RPG44Z Removal of Internal Fixation Device from Right Acromioclavicular Joint, Percutaneous Endoscopic Approach

0RPG47Z Removal of Autologous Tissue Substitute from Right Acromioclavicular Joint, Percutaneous Endoscopic Approach

0RPG48Z Removal of Spacer from Right Acromioclavicular Joint, Percutaneous Endoscopic Approach

0RPG4JZ Removal of Synthetic Substitute from Right Acromioclavicular Joint, Percutaneous Endoscopic Approach

0RPG4KZ Removal of Nonautologous Tissue Substitute from Right Acromioclavicular Joint, Percutaneous Endoscopic Approach

0RPGX0Z Removal of Drainage Device from Right Acromioclavicular Joint, External Approach

0RPGX3Z Removal of Infusion Device from Right Acromioclavicular Joint, External Approach

0RPGX4Z Removal of Internal Fixation Device from Right Acromioclavicular Joint, External Approach

0RPH00Z Removal of Drainage Device from Left Acromioclavicular Joint, Open Approach

0RPH03Z Removal of Infusion Device from Left Acromioclavicular Joint, Open Approach

0RPH04Z Removal of Internal Fixation Device from Left Acromioclavicular Joint, Open Approach

0RPH07Z Removal of Autologous Tissue Substitute from Left Acromioclavicular Joint, Open Approach

0RPH08Z Removal of Spacer from Left Acromioclavicular Joint, Open Approach

0RPH0JZ Removal of Synthetic Substitute from Left Acromioclavicular Joint, Open Approach

0RPH0KZ Removal of Nonautologous Tissue Substitute from Left Acromioclavicular Joint, Open Approach

0RPH30Z Removal of Drainage Device from Left Acromioclavicular Joint, Percutaneous Approach

0RPH33Z Removal of Infusion Device from Left Acromioclavicular Joint, Percutaneous Approach

0RPH34Z Removal of Internal Fixation Device from Left Acromioclavicular Joint, Percutaneous Approach

0RPH37Z Removal of Autologous Tissue Substitute from Left Acromioclavicular Joint, Percutaneous Approach

0RPH38Z Removal of Spacer from Left Acromioclavicular Joint, Percutaneous Approach

0RPH3JZ Removal of Synthetic Substitute from Left Acromioclavicular Joint, Percutaneous Approach

0RPH3KZ Removal of Nonautologous Tissue Substitute from Left Acromioclavicular Joint, Percutaneous Approach

0RPH40Z Removal of Drainage Device from Left Acromioclavicular Joint, Percutaneous Endoscopic Approach

0RPH43Z Removal of Infusion Device from Left Acromioclavicular Joint, Percutaneous Endoscopic Approach

0RPH44Z Removal of Internal Fixation Device from Left Acromioclavicular Joint, Percutaneous Endoscopic Approach

0RPH47Z Removal of Autologous Tissue Substitute from Left Acromioclavicular Joint, Percutaneous Endoscopic Approach

0RPH48Z Removal of Spacer from Left Acromioclavicular Joint, Percutaneous Endoscopic Approach

0RPH4JZ Removal of Synthetic Substitute from Left Acromioclavicular Joint, Percutaneous Endoscopic Approach

0RPH4KZ Removal of Nonautologous Tissue Substitute from Left Acromioclavicular Joint, Percutaneous Endoscopic Approach

0RPHX0Z Removal of Drainage Device from Left Acromioclavicular Joint, External Approach

0RPHX3Z Removal of Infusion Device from Left Acromioclavicular Joint, External Approach

0RPHX4Z Removal of Internal Fixation Device from Left Acromioclavicular Joint, External Approach

0RPJ00Z Removal of Drainage Device from Right Shoulder Joint, Open Approach

0RPJ03Z Removal of Infusion Device from Right Shoulder Joint, Open Approach

0RPJ04Z Removal of Internal Fixation Device from Right Shoulder Joint, Open Approach

0RPJ07Z Removal of Autologous Tissue Substitute from Right Shoulder Joint, Open Approach

0RPJ08Z Removal of Spacer from Right Shoulder Joint, Open Approach

0RPJ0JZ Removal of Synthetic Substitute from Right Shoulder Joint, Open Approach

0RPJ0KZ Removal of Nonautologous Tissue Substitute from Right Shoulder Joint, Open Approach

0RPJ30Z Removal of Drainage Device from Right Shoulder Joint, Percutaneous Approach

0RPJ33Z Removal of Infusion Device from Right Shoulder Joint, Percutaneous Approach

0RPJ34Z Removal of Internal Fixation Device from Right Shoulder Joint, Percutaneous Approach

0RPJ37Z Removal of Autologous Tissue Substitute from Right Shoulder Joint, Percutaneous Approach

0RPJ38Z Removal of Spacer from Right Shoulder Joint, Percutaneous Approach

0RPJ3JZ Removal of Synthetic Substitute from Right Shoulder Joint, Percutaneous Approach

0RPJ3KZ Removal of Nonautologous Tissue Substitute from Right Shoulder Joint, Percutaneous Approach

0RPJ40Z Removal of Drainage Device from Right Shoulder Joint, Percutaneous Endoscopic Approach

0RPJ43Z Removal of Infusion Device from Right Shoulder Joint, Percutaneous Endoscopic Approach

0RPJ44Z Removal of Internal Fixation Device from Right Shoulder Joint, Percutaneous Endoscopic Approach

0RPJ47Z Removal of Autologous Tissue Substitute from Right Shoulder Joint, Percutaneous Endoscopic Approach

0RPJ48Z Removal of Spacer from Right Shoulder Joint, Percutaneous Endoscopic Approach

0RPJ4JZ Removal of Synthetic Substitute from Right Shoulder Joint, Percutaneous Endoscopic Approach

0RPJ4KZ Removal of Nonautologous Tissue Substitute from Right Shoulder Joint, Percutaneous Endoscopic Approach

0RPJX0Z Removal of Drainage Device from Right Shoulder Joint, External Approach

0RPJX3Z Removal of Infusion Device from Right Shoulder Joint, External Approach

0RPJX4Z Removal of Internal Fixation Device from Right Shoulder Joint, External Approach

0RPK00Z Removal of Drainage Device from Left Shoulder Joint, Open Approach

0RPK03Z Removal of Infusion Device from Left Shoulder Joint, Open Approach

0RPK04Z Removal of Internal Fixation Device from Left Shoulder Joint, Open Approach

0RPK07Z Removal of Autologous Tissue Substitute from Left Shoulder Joint, Open Approach

0RPK08Z Removal of Spacer from Left Shoulder Joint, Open Approach

0RPK0JZ Removal of Synthetic Substitute from Left Shoulder Joint, Open Approach

0RPK0KZ Removal of Nonautologous Tissue Substitute from Left Shoulder Joint, Open Approach

0RPK30Z Removal of Drainage Device from Left Shoulder Joint, Percutaneous Approach

0RPK33Z Removal of Infusion Device from Left Shoulder Joint, Percutaneous Approach

0RPK34Z Removal of Internal Fixation Device from Left Shoulder Joint, Percutaneous Approach

0RPK37Z Removal of Autologous Tissue Substitute from Left Shoulder Joint, Percutaneous Approach

0RPK38Z Removal of Spacer from Left Shoulder Joint, Percutaneous Approach

0RPK3JZ Removal of Synthetic Substitute from Left Shoulder Joint, Percutaneous Approach

0RPK3KZ Removal of Nonautologous Tissue Substitute from Left Shoulder Joint, Percutaneous Approach

0RPK40Z Removal of Drainage Device from Left Shoulder Joint, Percutaneous Endoscopic Approach

0RPK43Z Removal of Infusion Device from Left Shoulder Joint, Percutaneous Endoscopic Approach

0RPK44Z Removal of Internal Fixation Device from Left Shoulder Joint, Percutaneous Endoscopic Approach

0RPK47Z Removal of Autologous Tissue Substitute from Left Shoulder Joint, Percutaneous Endoscopic Approach

0RPK48Z Removal of Spacer from Left Shoulder Joint, Percutaneous Endoscopic Approach

0RPK4JZ Removal of Synthetic Substitute from Left Shoulder Joint, Percutaneous Endoscopic Approach

0RPK4KZ Removal of Nonautologous Tissue Substitute from Left Shoulder Joint, Percutaneous Endoscopic Approach

0RPKX0Z Removal of Drainage Device from Left Shoulder Joint, External Approach

0RPKX3Z Removal of Infusion Device from Left Shoulder Joint, External Approach

0RPKX4Z Removal of Internal Fixation Device from Left Shoulder Joint, External Approach

0RPL00Z Removal of Drainage Device from Right Elbow Joint, Open Approach

0RPL03Z Removal of Infusion Device from Right Elbow Joint, Open Approach

0RPL04Z Removal of Internal Fixation Device from Right Elbow Joint, Open Approach

0RPL05Z Removal of External Fixation Device from Right Elbow Joint, Open Approach

0RPL07Z Removal of Autologous Tissue Substitute from Right Elbow Joint, Open Approach

0RPL08Z Removal of Spacer from Right Elbow Joint, Open Approach

0RPL0JZ Removal of Synthetic Substitute from Right Elbow Joint, Open Approach

0RPL0KZ Removal of Nonautologous Tissue Substitute from Right Elbow Joint, Open Approach

0RPL30Z Removal of Drainage Device from Right Elbow Joint, Percutaneous Approach

0RPL33Z Removal of Infusion Device from Right Elbow Joint, Percutaneous Approach

0RPL34Z Removal of Internal Fixation Device from Right Elbow Joint, Percutaneous Approach

0RPL35Z Removal of External Fixation Device from Right Elbow Joint, Percutaneous Approach

0RPL37Z Removal of Autologous Tissue Substitute from Right Elbow Joint, Percutaneous Approach

0RPL38Z Removal of Spacer from Right Elbow Joint, Percutaneous Approach

0RPL3JZ Removal of Synthetic Substitute from Right Elbow Joint, Percutaneous Approach

0RPL3KZ Removal of Nonautologous Tissue Substitute from Right Elbow Joint, Percutaneous Approach

0RPL40Z Removal of Drainage Device from Right Elbow Joint, Percutaneous Endoscopic Approach

0RPL43Z Removal of Infusion Device from Right Elbow Joint, Percutaneous Endoscopic Approach

0RPL44Z Removal of Internal Fixation Device from Right Elbow Joint, Percutaneous Endoscopic Approach

0RPL45Z Removal of External Fixation Device from Right Elbow Joint, Percutaneous Endoscopic Approach

0RPL47Z Removal of Autologous Tissue Substitute from Right Elbow Joint, Percutaneous Endoscopic Approach

0RPL48Z Removal of Spacer from Right Elbow Joint, Percutaneous Endoscopic Approach

0RPL4JZ Removal of Synthetic Substitute from Right Elbow Joint, Percutaneous Endoscopic Approach

0RPL4KZ Removal of Nonautologous Tissue Substitute from Right Elbow Joint, Percutaneous Endoscopic Approach

0RPLX0Z Removal of Drainage Device from Right Elbow Joint, External Approach

0RPLX3Z Removal of Infusion Device from Right Elbow Joint, External Approach

0RPLX4Z Removal of Internal Fixation Device from Right Elbow Joint, External Approach

0RPLX5Z Removal of External Fixation Device from Right Elbow Joint, External Approach

0RPM00Z Removal of Drainage Device from Left Elbow Joint, Open Approach

0RPM03Z Removal of Infusion Device from Left Elbow Joint, Open Approach

0RPM04Z Removal of Internal Fixation Device from Left Elbow Joint, Open Approach

0RPM05Z Removal of External Fixation Device from Left Elbow Joint, Open Approach

0RPM07Z Removal of Autologous Tissue Substitute from Left Elbow Joint, Open Approach

0RPM08Z Removal of Spacer from Left Elbow Joint, Open Approach

0RPM0JZ Removal of Synthetic Substitute from Left Elbow Joint, Open Approach

0RPM0KZ Removal of Nonautologous Tissue Substitute from Left Elbow Joint, Open Approach

0RPM30Z Removal of Drainage Device from Left Elbow Joint, Percutaneous Approach

0RPM33Z Removal of Infusion Device from Left Elbow Joint, Percutaneous Approach

0RPM34Z Removal of Internal Fixation Device from Left Elbow Joint, Percutaneous Approach

0RPM35Z Removal of External Fixation Device from Left Elbow Joint, Percutaneous Approach

0RPM37Z Removal of Autologous Tissue Substitute from Left Elbow Joint, Percutaneous Approach

0RPM38Z Removal of Spacer from Left Elbow Joint, Percutaneous Approach

0RPM3JZ Removal of Synthetic Substitute from Left Elbow Joint, Percutaneous Approach

0RPM3KZ Removal of Nonautologous Tissue Substitute from Left Elbow Joint, Percutaneous Approach

0RPM40Z Removal of Drainage Device from Left Elbow Joint, Percutaneous Endoscopic Approach

0RPM43Z Removal of Infusion Device from Left Elbow Joint, Percutaneous Endoscopic Approach

0RPM44Z Removal of Internal Fixation Device from Left Elbow Joint, Percutaneous Endoscopic Approach

0RPM45Z Removal of External Fixation Device from Left Elbow Joint, Percutaneous Endoscopic Approach

0RPM47Z Removal of Autologous Tissue Substitute from Left Elbow Joint, Percutaneous Endoscopic Approach

0RPM48Z Removal of Spacer from Left Elbow Joint, Percutaneous Endoscopic Approach

0RPM4JZ Removal of Synthetic Substitute from Left Elbow Joint, Percutaneous Endoscopic Approach

0RPM4KZ Removal of Nonautologous Tissue Substitute from Left Elbow Joint, Percutaneous Endoscopic Approach

0RPMX0Z Removal of Drainage Device from Left Elbow Joint, External Approach

0RPMX3Z Removal of Infusion Device from Left Elbow Joint, External Approach

0RPMX4Z Removal of Internal Fixation Device from Left Elbow Joint, External Approach

0RPMX5Z Removal of External Fixation Device from Left Elbow Joint, External Approach

0RPN00Z Removal of Drainage Device from Right Wrist Joint, Open Approach

0RPN03Z Removal of Infusion Device from Right Wrist Joint, Open Approach

0RPN04Z Removal of Internal Fixation Device from Right Wrist Joint, Open Approach

0RPN05Z Removal of External Fixation Device from Right Wrist Joint, Open Approach

0RPN07Z Removal of Autologous Tissue Substitute from Right Wrist Joint, Open Approach

0RPN08Z Removal of Spacer from Right Wrist Joint, Open Approach

0RPN0JZ Removal of Synthetic Substitute from Right Wrist Joint, Open Approach

0RPN0KZ Removal of Nonautologous Tissue Substitute from Right Wrist Joint, Open Approach

0RPN30Z Removal of Drainage Device from Right Wrist Joint, Percutaneous Approach

0RPN33Z Removal of Infusion Device from Right Wrist Joint, Percutaneous Approach

0RPN34Z Removal of Internal Fixation Device from Right Wrist Joint, Percutaneous Approach

0RPN35Z Removal of External Fixation Device from Right Wrist Joint, Percutaneous Approach

0RPN37Z Removal of Autologous Tissue Substitute from Right Wrist Joint, Percutaneous Approach

0RPN38Z Removal of Spacer from Right Wrist Joint, Percutaneous Approach

0RPN3JZ Removal of Synthetic Substitute from Right Wrist Joint, Percutaneous Approach

0RPN3KZ Removal of Nonautologous Tissue Substitute from Right Wrist Joint, Percutaneous Approach

0RPN40Z Removal of Drainage Device from Right Wrist Joint, Percutaneous Endoscopic Approach

0RPN43Z Removal of Infusion Device from Right Wrist Joint, Percutaneous Endoscopic Approach

0RPN44Z Removal of Internal Fixation Device from Right Wrist Joint, Percutaneous Endoscopic Approach

0RPN45Z Removal of External Fixation Device from Right Wrist Joint, Percutaneous Endoscopic Approach

0RPN47Z Removal of Autologous Tissue Substitute from Right Wrist Joint, Percutaneous Endoscopic Approach

0RPN48Z Removal of Spacer from Right Wrist Joint, Percutaneous Endoscopic Approach

0RPN4JZ Removal of Synthetic Substitute from Right Wrist Joint, Percutaneous Endoscopic Approach

0RPN4KZ Removal of Nonautologous Tissue Substitute from Right Wrist Joint, Percutaneous Endoscopic Approach

0RPNX0Z Removal of Drainage Device from Right Wrist Joint, External Approach

0RPNX3Z Removal of Infusion Device from Right Wrist Joint, External Approach

0RPNX4Z Removal of Internal Fixation Device from Right Wrist Joint, External Approach

0RPNX5Z Removal of External Fixation Device from Right Wrist Joint, External Approach

0RPP00Z Removal of Drainage Device from Left Wrist Joint, Open Approach

0RPP03Z Removal of Infusion Device from Left Wrist Joint, Open Approach

0RPP04Z Removal of Internal Fixation Device from Left Wrist Joint, Open Approach

0RPP05Z Removal of External Fixation Device from Left Wrist Joint, Open Approach

0RPP07Z Removal of Autologous Tissue Substitute from Left Wrist Joint, Open Approach

0RPP08Z Removal of Spacer from Left Wrist Joint, Open Approach

0RPP0JZ Removal of Synthetic Substitute from Left Wrist Joint, Open Approach

0RPP0KZ Removal of Nonautologous Tissue Substitute from Left Wrist Joint, Open Approach

0RPP30Z Removal of Drainage Device from Left Wrist Joint, Percutaneous Approach

0RPP33Z Removal of Infusion Device from Left Wrist Joint, Percutaneous Approach

0RPP34Z Removal of Internal Fixation Device from Left Wrist Joint, Percutaneous Approach

0RPP35Z Removal of External Fixation Device from Left Wrist Joint, Percutaneous Approach

0RPP37Z Removal of Autologous Tissue Substitute from Left Wrist Joint, Percutaneous Approach

0RPP38Z Removal of Spacer from Left Wrist Joint, Percutaneous Approach

0RPP3JZ Removal of Synthetic Substitute from Left Wrist Joint, Percutaneous Approach

0RPP3KZ Removal of Nonautologous Tissue Substitute from Left Wrist Joint, Percutaneous Approach

0RPP40Z Removal of Drainage Device from Left Wrist Joint, Percutaneous Endoscopic Approach

0RPP43Z Removal of Infusion Device from Left Wrist Joint, Percutaneous Endoscopic Approach

0RPP44Z Removal of Internal Fixation Device from Left Wrist Joint, Percutaneous Endoscopic Approach

0RPP45Z Removal of External Fixation Device from Left Wrist Joint, Percutaneous Endoscopic Approach

0RPP47Z Removal of Autologous Tissue Substitute from Left Wrist Joint, Percutaneous Endoscopic Approach

0RPP48Z Removal of Spacer from Left Wrist Joint, Percutaneous Endoscopic Approach

0RPP4JZ Removal of Synthetic Substitute from Left Wrist Joint, Percutaneous Endoscopic Approach

0RPP4KZ Removal of Nonautologous Tissue Substitute from Left Wrist Joint, Percutaneous Endoscopic Approach

0RPPX0Z Removal of Drainage Device from Left Wrist Joint, External Approach

0RPPX3Z Removal of Infusion Device from Left Wrist Joint, External Approach

0RPPX4Z Removal of Internal Fixation Device from Left Wrist Joint, External Approach

0RPPX5Z Removal of External Fixation Device from Left Wrist Joint, External Approach

0RPQ00Z Removal of Drainage Device from Right Carpal Joint, Open Approach

0RPQ03Z Removal of Infusion Device from Right Carpal Joint, Open Approach

0RPQ04Z Removal of Internal Fixation Device from Right Carpal Joint, Open Approach

0RPQ05Z Removal of External Fixation Device from Right Carpal Joint, Open Approach

0RPQ07Z Removal of Autologous Tissue Substitute from Right Carpal Joint, Open Approach

0RPQ08Z Removal of Spacer from Right Carpal Joint, Open Approach

0RPQ0JZ Removal of Synthetic Substitute from Right Carpal Joint, Open Approach

0RPQ0KZ Removal of Nonautologous Tissue Substitute from Right Carpal Joint, Open Approach

0RPQ30Z Removal of Drainage Device from Right Carpal Joint, Percutaneous Approach

0RPQ33Z Removal of Infusion Device from Right Carpal Joint, Percutaneous Approach

0RPQ34Z Removal of Internal Fixation Device from Right Carpal Joint, Percutaneous Approach

0RPQ35Z Removal of External Fixation Device from Right Carpal Joint, Percutaneous Approach

0RPQ37Z Removal of Autologous Tissue Substitute from Right Carpal Joint, Percutaneous Approach

0RPQ38Z Removal of Spacer from Right Carpal Joint, Percutaneous Approach

0RPQ3JZ Removal of Synthetic Substitute from Right Carpal Joint, Percutaneous Approach

0RPQ3KZ Removal of Nonautologous Tissue Substitute from Right Carpal Joint, Percutaneous Approach

0RPQ40Z Removal of Drainage Device from Right Carpal Joint, Percutaneous Endoscopic Approach

0RPQ43Z Removal of Infusion Device from Right Carpal Joint, Percutaneous Endoscopic Approach

0RPQ44Z Removal of Internal Fixation Device from Right Carpal Joint, Percutaneous Endoscopic Approach

0RPQ45Z Removal of External Fixation Device from Right Carpal Joint, Percutaneous Endoscopic Approach

0RPQ47Z Removal of Autologous Tissue Substitute from Right Carpal Joint, Percutaneous Endoscopic Approach

0RPQ48Z Removal of Spacer from Right Carpal Joint, Percutaneous Endoscopic Approach

0RPQ4JZ Removal of Synthetic Substitute from Right Carpal Joint, Percutaneous Endoscopic Approach

0RPQ4KZ Removal of Nonautologous Tissue Substitute from Right Carpal Joint, Percutaneous Endoscopic Approach

0RPQX0Z Removal of Drainage Device from Right Carpal Joint, External Approach

0RPQX3Z Removal of Infusion Device from Right Carpal Joint, External Approach

0RPQX4Z Removal of Internal Fixation Device from Right Carpal Joint, External Approach

0RPQX5Z Removal of External Fixation Device from Right Carpal Joint, External Approach

0RPR00Z Removal of Drainage Device from Left Carpal Joint, Open Approach

0RPR03Z Removal of Infusion Device from Left Carpal Joint, Open Approach

0RPR04Z Removal of Internal Fixation Device from Left Carpal Joint, Open Approach

0RPR05Z Removal of External Fixation Device from Left Carpal Joint, Open Approach

0RPR07Z Removal of Autologous Tissue Substitute from Left Carpal Joint, Open Approach

0RPR08Z Removal of Spacer from Left Carpal Joint, Open Approach

0RPR0JZ Removal of Synthetic Substitute from Left Carpal Joint, Open Approach

0RPR0KZ Removal of Nonautologous Tissue Substitute from Left Carpal Joint, Open Approach

0RPR30Z Removal of Drainage Device from Left Carpal Joint, Percutaneous Approach

0RPR33Z Removal of Infusion Device from Left Carpal Joint, Percutaneous Approach

0RPR34Z Removal of Internal Fixation Device from Left Carpal Joint, Percutaneous Approach

0RPR35Z Removal of External Fixation Device from Left Carpal Joint, Percutaneous Approach

0RPR37Z Removal of Autologous Tissue Substitute from Left Carpal Joint, Percutaneous Approach

0RPR38Z Removal of Spacer from Left Carpal Joint, Percutaneous Approach

0RPR3JZ Removal of Synthetic Substitute from Left Carpal Joint, Percutaneous Approach

0RPR3KZ Removal of Nonautologous Tissue Substitute from Left Carpal Joint, Percutaneous Approach

0RPR40Z Removal of Drainage Device from Left Carpal Joint, Percutaneous Endoscopic Approach

0RPR43Z Removal of Infusion Device from Left Carpal Joint, Percutaneous Endoscopic Approach

0RPR44Z Removal of Internal Fixation Device from Left Carpal Joint, Percutaneous Endoscopic Approach

0RPR45Z Removal of External Fixation Device from Left Carpal Joint, Percutaneous Endoscopic Approach

0RPR47Z Removal of Autologous Tissue Substitute from Left Carpal Joint, Percutaneous Endoscopic Approach

0RPR48Z Removal of Spacer from Left Carpal Joint, Percutaneous Endoscopic Approach

0RPR4JZ Removal of Synthetic Substitute from Left Carpal Joint, Percutaneous Endoscopic Approach

0RPR4KZ Removal of Nonautologous Tissue Substitute from Left Carpal Joint, Percutaneous Endoscopic Approach

0RPRX0Z Removal of Drainage Device from Left Carpal Joint, External Approach

0RPRX3Z Removal of Infusion Device from Left Carpal Joint, External Approach

0RPRX4Z Removal of Internal Fixation Device from Left Carpal Joint, External Approach

0RPRX5Z Removal of External Fixation Device from Left Carpal Joint, External Approach

0RPS00Z Removal of Drainage Device from Right Metacarpocarpal Joint, Open Approach

0RPS03Z Removal of Infusion Device from Right Metacarpocarpal Joint, Open Approach

0RPS04Z Removal of Internal Fixation Device from Right Metacarpocarpal Joint, Open Approach

0RPS05Z Removal of External Fixation Device from Right Metacarpocarpal Joint, Open Approach

0RPS07Z Removal of Autologous Tissue Substitute from Right Metacarpocarpal Joint, Open Approach

0RPS08Z Removal of Spacer from Right Metacarpocarpal Joint, Open Approach

0RPS0JZ Removal of Synthetic Substitute from Right Metacarpocarpal Joint, Open Approach

0RPS0KZ Removal of Nonautologous Tissue Substitute from Right Metacarpocarpal Joint, Open Approach

0RPS30Z Removal of Drainage Device from Right Metacarpocarpal Joint, Percutaneous Approach

0RPS33Z Removal of Infusion Device from Right Metacarpocarpal Joint, Percutaneous Approach

0RPS34Z Removal of Internal Fixation Device from Right Metacarpocarpal Joint, Percutaneous Approach

0RPS35Z Removal of External Fixation Device from Right Metacarpocarpal Joint, Percutaneous Approach

0RPS37Z Removal of Autologous Tissue Substitute from Right Metacarpocarpal Joint, Percutaneous Approach

0RPS38Z Removal of Spacer from Right Metacarpocarpal Joint, Percutaneous Approach

0RPS3JZ Removal of Synthetic Substitute from Right Metacarpocarpal Joint, Percutaneous Approach

0RPS3KZ Removal of Nonautologous Tissue Substitute from Right Metacarpocarpal Joint, Percutaneous Approach

0RPS40Z Removal of Drainage Device from Right Metacarpocarpal Joint, Percutaneous Endoscopic Approach

0RPS43Z Removal of Infusion Device from Right Metacarpocarpal Joint, Percutaneous Endoscopic Approach

0RPS44Z Removal of Internal Fixation Device from Right Metacarpocarpal Joint, Percutaneous Endoscopic Approach

0RPS45Z Removal of External Fixation Device from Right Metacarpocarpal Joint, Percutaneous Endoscopic Approach

0RPS47Z Removal of Autologous Tissue Substitute from Right Metacarpocarpal Joint, Percutaneous Endoscopic Approach

0RPS48Z Removal of Spacer from Right Metacarpocarpal Joint, Percutaneous Endoscopic Approach

0RPS4JZ Removal of Synthetic Substitute from Right Metacarpocarpal Joint, Percutaneous Endoscopic Approach

0RPS4KZ Removal of Nonautologous Tissue Substitute from Right Metacarpocarpal Joint, Percutaneous Endoscopic Approach

0RPSX0Z Removal of Drainage Device from Right Metacarpocarpal Joint, External Approach

0RPSX3Z Removal of Infusion Device from Right Metacarpocarpal Joint, External Approach

0RPSX4Z Removal of Internal Fixation Device from Right Metacarpocarpal Joint, External Approach

0RPSX5Z Removal of External Fixation Device from Right Metacarpocarpal Joint, External Approach

0RPT00Z Removal of Drainage Device from Left Metacarpocarpal Joint, Open Approach

0RPT03Z Removal of Infusion Device from Left Metacarpocarpal Joint, Open Approach

0RPT04Z Removal of Internal Fixation Device from Left Metacarpocarpal Joint, Open Approach

0RPT05Z Removal of External Fixation Device from Left Metacarpocarpal Joint, Open Approach

0RPT07Z Removal of Autologous Tissue Substitute from Left Metacarpocarpal Joint, Open Approach

0RPT08Z Removal of Spacer from Left Metacarpocarpal Joint, Open Approach

0RPT0JZ Removal of Synthetic Substitute from Left Metacarpocarpal Joint, Open Approach

0RPT0KZ Removal of Nonautologous Tissue Substitute from Left Metacarpocarpal Joint, Open Approach

0RPT30Z Removal of Drainage Device from Left Metacarpocarpal Joint, Percutaneous Approach

0RPT33Z Removal of Infusion Device from Left Metacarpocarpal Joint, Percutaneous Approach

0RPT34Z Removal of Internal Fixation Device from Left Metacarpocarpal Joint, Percutaneous Approach

0RPT35Z Removal of External Fixation Device from Left Metacarpocarpal Joint, Percutaneous Approach

0RPT37Z Removal of Autologous Tissue Substitute from Left Metacarpocarpal Joint, Percutaneous Approach

0RPT38Z Removal of Spacer from Left Metacarpocarpal Joint, Percutaneous Approach

0RPT3JZ Removal of Synthetic Substitute from Left Metacarpocarpal Joint, Percutaneous Approach

0RPT3KZ Removal of Nonautologous Tissue Substitute from Left Metacarpocarpal Joint, Percutaneous Approach

0RPT40Z Removal of Drainage Device from Left Metacarpocarpal Joint, Percutaneous Endoscopic Approach

0RPT43Z Removal of Infusion Device from Left Metacarpocarpal Joint, Percutaneous Endoscopic Approach

0RPT44Z Removal of Internal Fixation Device from Left Metacarpocarpal Joint, Percutaneous Endoscopic Approach

0RPT45Z Removal of External Fixation Device from Left Metacarpocarpal Joint, Percutaneous Endoscopic Approach

0RPT47Z Removal of Autologous Tissue Substitute from Left Metacarpocarpal Joint, Percutaneous Endoscopic Approach

0RPT48Z Removal of Spacer from Left Metacarpocarpal Joint, Percutaneous Endoscopic Approach

0RPT4JZ Removal of Synthetic Substitute from Left Metacarpocarpal Joint, Percutaneous Endoscopic Approach

0RPT4KZ Removal of Nonautologous Tissue Substitute from Left Metacarpocarpal Joint, Percutaneous Endoscopic Approach

0RPTX0Z Removal of Drainage Device from Left Metacarpocarpal Joint, External Approach

0RPTX3Z Removal of Infusion Device from Left Metacarpocarpal Joint, External Approach

0RPTX4Z Removal of Internal Fixation Device from Left Metacarpocarpal Joint, External Approach

0RPTX5Z Removal of External Fixation Device from Left Metacarpocarpal Joint, External Approach

0RPU00Z Removal of Drainage Device from Right Metacarpophalangeal Joint, Open Approach

0RPU03Z Removal of Infusion Device from Right Metacarpophalangeal Joint, Open Approach

0RPU04Z Removal of Internal Fixation Device from Right Metacarpophalangeal Joint, Open Approach

0RPU05Z Removal of External Fixation Device from Right Metacarpophalangeal Joint, Open Approach

0RPU07Z Removal of Autologous Tissue Substitute from Right Metacarpophalangeal Joint, Open Approach

0RPU08Z Removal of Spacer from Right Metacarpophalangeal Joint, Open Approach

0RPU0JZ Removal of Synthetic Substitute from Right Metacarpophalangeal Joint, Open Approach

0RPU0KZ Removal of Nonautologous Tissue Substitute from Right Metacarpophalangeal Joint, Open Approach

0RPU30Z Removal of Drainage Device from Right Metacarpophalangeal Joint, Percutaneous Approach

0RPU33Z Removal of Infusion Device from Right Metacarpophalangeal Joint, Percutaneous Approach

0RPU34Z Removal of Internal Fixation Device from Right Metacarpophalangeal Joint, Percutaneous Approach

0RPU35Z Removal of External Fixation Device from Right Metacarpophalangeal Joint, Percutaneous Approach

0RPU37Z Removal of Autologous Tissue Substitute from Right Metacarpophalangeal Joint, Percutaneous Approach

0RPU38Z Removal of Spacer from Right Metacarpophalangeal Joint, Percutaneous Approach

0RPU3JZ Removal of Synthetic Substitute from Right Metacarpophalangeal Joint, Percutaneous Approach

0RPU3KZ Removal of Nonautologous Tissue Substitute from Right Metacarpophalangeal Joint, Percutaneous Approach

0RPU40Z Removal of Drainage Device from Right Metacarpophalangeal Joint, Percutaneous Endoscopic Approach

0RPU43Z Removal of Infusion Device from Right Metacarpophalangeal Joint, Percutaneous Endoscopic Approach

0RPU44Z Removal of Internal Fixation Device from Right Metacarpophalangeal Joint, Percutaneous Endoscopic Approach

0RPU45Z Removal of External Fixation Device from Right Metacarpophalangeal Joint, Percutaneous Endoscopic Approach

0RPU47Z Removal of Autologous Tissue Substitute from Right Metacarpophalangeal Joint, Percutaneous Endoscopic Approach

0RPU48Z Removal of Spacer from Right Metacarpophalangeal Joint, Percutaneous Endoscopic Approach

0RPU4JZ Removal of Synthetic Substitute from Right Metacarpophalangeal Joint, Percutaneous Endoscopic Approach

0RPU4KZ Removal of Nonautologous Tissue Substitute from Right Metacarpophalangeal Joint, Percutaneous Endoscopic Approach

0RPUX0Z Removal of Drainage Device from Right Metacarpophalangeal Joint, External Approach

0RPUX3Z Removal of Infusion Device from Right Metacarpophalangeal Joint, External Approach

0RPUX4Z Removal of Internal Fixation Device from Right Metacarpophalangeal Joint, External Approach

0RPUX5Z Removal of External Fixation Device from Right Metacarpophalangeal Joint, External Approach

0RPV00Z Removal of Drainage Device from Left Metacarpophalangeal Joint, Open Approach

0RPV03Z Removal of Infusion Device from Left Metacarpophalangeal Joint, Open Approach

0RPV04Z Removal of Internal Fixation Device from Left Metacarpophalangeal Joint, Open Approach

0RPV05Z Removal of External Fixation Device from Left Metacarpophalangeal Joint, Open Approach

0RPV07Z Removal of Autologous Tissue Substitute from Left Metacarpophalangeal Joint, Open Approach

0RPV08Z Removal of Spacer from Left Metacarpophalangeal Joint, Open Approach

0RPV0JZ Removal of Synthetic Substitute from Left Metacarpophalangeal Joint, Open Approach

0RPV0KZ Removal of Nonautologous Tissue Substitute from Left Metacarpophalangeal Joint, Open Approach

0RPV30Z Removal of Drainage Device from Left Metacarpophalangeal Joint, Percutaneous Approach

0RPV33Z Removal of Infusion Device from Left Metacarpophalangeal Joint, Percutaneous Approach

0RPV34Z Removal of Internal Fixation Device from Left Metacarpophalangeal Joint, Percutaneous Approach

0RPV35Z Removal of External Fixation Device from Left Metacarpophalangeal Joint, Percutaneous Approach

0RPV37Z Removal of Autologous Tissue Substitute from Left Metacarpophalangeal Joint, Percutaneous Approach

0RPV38Z Removal of Spacer from Left Metacarpophalangeal Joint, Percutaneous Approach

0RPV3JZ Removal of Synthetic Substitute from Left Metacarpophalangeal Joint, Percutaneous Approach

0RPV3KZ Removal of Nonautologous Tissue Substitute from Left Metacarpophalangeal Joint, Percutaneous Approach

0RPV40Z Removal of Drainage Device from Left Metacarpophalangeal Joint, Percutaneous Endoscopic Approach

0RPV43Z Removal of Infusion Device from Left Metacarpophalangeal Joint, Percutaneous Endoscopic Approach

0RPV44Z Removal of Internal Fixation Device from Left Metacarpophalangeal Joint, Percutaneous Endoscopic Approach

0RPV45Z Removal of External Fixation Device from Left Metacarpophalangeal Joint, Percutaneous Endoscopic Approach

0RPV47Z Removal of Autologous Tissue Substitute from Left Metacarpophalangeal Joint, Percutaneous Endoscopic Approach

0RPV48Z Removal of Spacer from Left Metacarpophalangeal Joint, Percutaneous Endoscopic Approach

0RPV4JZ Removal of Synthetic Substitute from Left Metacarpophalangeal Joint, Percutaneous Endoscopic Approach

0RPV4KZ Removal of Nonautologous Tissue Substitute from Left Metacarpophalangeal Joint, Percutaneous Endoscopic Approach

0RPVX0Z Removal of Drainage Device from Left Metacarpophalangeal Joint, External Approach

0RPVX3Z Removal of Infusion Device from Left Metacarpophalangeal Joint, External Approach

0RPVX4Z Removal of Internal Fixation Device from Left Metacarpophalangeal Joint, External Approach

0RPVX5Z Removal of External Fixation Device from Left Metacarpophalangeal Joint, External Approach

0RPW00Z Removal of Drainage Device from Right Finger Phalangeal Joint, Open Approach

0RPW03Z Removal of Infusion Device from Right Finger Phalangeal Joint, Open Approach

0RPW04Z Removal of Internal Fixation Device from Right Finger Phalangeal Joint, Open Approach

0RPW05Z Removal of External Fixation Device from Right Finger Phalangeal Joint, Open Approach

0RPW07Z Removal of Autologous Tissue Substitute from Right Finger Phalangeal Joint, Open Approach

0RPW08Z Removal of Spacer from Right Finger Phalangeal Joint, Open Approach

0RPW0JZ Removal of Synthetic Substitute from Right Finger Phalangeal Joint, Open Approach

0RPW0KZ Removal of Nonautologous Tissue Substitute from Right Finger Phalangeal Joint, Open Approach

0RPW30Z Removal of Drainage Device from Right Finger Phalangeal Joint, Percutaneous Approach

0RPW33Z Removal of Infusion Device from Right Finger Phalangeal Joint, Percutaneous Approach

0RPW34Z Removal of Internal Fixation Device from Right Finger Phalangeal Joint, Percutaneous Approach

0RPW35Z Removal of External Fixation Device from Right Finger Phalangeal Joint, Percutaneous Approach

0RPW37Z Removal of Autologous Tissue Substitute from Right Finger Phalangeal Joint, Percutaneous Approach

0RPW38Z Removal of Spacer from Right Finger Phalangeal Joint, Percutaneous Approach

0RPW3JZ Removal of Synthetic Substitute from Right Finger Phalangeal Joint, Percutaneous Approach

0RPW3KZ Removal of Nonautologous Tissue Substitute from Right Finger Phalangeal Joint, Percutaneous Approach

0RPW40Z Removal of Drainage Device from Right Finger Phalangeal Joint, Percutaneous Endoscopic Approach

0RPW43Z Removal of Infusion Device from Right Finger Phalangeal Joint, Percutaneous Endoscopic Approach

0RPW44Z Removal of Internal Fixation Device from Right Finger Phalangeal Joint, Percutaneous Endoscopic Approach

0RPW45Z Removal of External Fixation Device from Right Finger Phalangeal Joint, Percutaneous Endoscopic Approach

0RPW47Z Removal of Autologous Tissue Substitute from Right Finger Phalangeal Joint, Percutaneous Endoscopic Approach

0RPW48Z Removal of Spacer from Right Finger Phalangeal Joint, Percutaneous Endoscopic Approach

0RPW4JZ Removal of Synthetic Substitute from Right Finger Phalangeal Joint, Percutaneous Endoscopic Approach

0RPW4KZ Removal of Nonautologous Tissue Substitute from Right Finger Phalangeal Joint, Percutaneous Endoscopic Approach

0RPWX0Z Removal of Drainage Device from Right Finger Phalangeal Joint, External Approach

0RPWX3Z Removal of Infusion Device from Right Finger Phalangeal Joint, External Approach

0RPWX4Z Removal of Internal Fixation Device from Right Finger Phalangeal Joint, External Approach

0RPWX5Z Removal of External Fixation Device from Right Finger Phalangeal Joint, External Approach

0RPX00Z Removal of Drainage Device from Left Finger Phalangeal Joint, Open Approach

0RPX03Z Removal of Infusion Device from Left Finger Phalangeal Joint, Open Approach

0RPX04Z Removal of Internal Fixation Device from Left Finger Phalangeal Joint, Open Approach

0RPX05Z Removal of External Fixation Device from Left Finger Phalangeal Joint, Open Approach

0RPX07Z Removal of Autologous Tissue Substitute from Left Finger Phalangeal Joint, Open Approach

0RPX08Z Removal of Spacer from Left Finger Phalangeal Joint, Open Approach

0RPX0JZ Removal of Synthetic Substitute from Left Finger Phalangeal Joint, Open Approach

0RPX0KZ Removal of Nonautologous Tissue Substitute from Left Finger Phalangeal Joint, Open Approach

0RPX30Z Removal of Drainage Device from Left Finger Phalangeal Joint, Percutaneous Approach

0RPX33Z Removal of Infusion Device from Left Finger Phalangeal Joint, Percutaneous Approach

0RPX34Z Removal of Internal Fixation Device from Left Finger Phalangeal Joint, Percutaneous Approach

0RPX35Z Removal of External Fixation Device from Left Finger Phalangeal Joint, Percutaneous Approach

0RPX37Z Removal of Autologous Tissue Substitute from Left Finger Phalangeal Joint, Percutaneous Approach

0RPX38Z Removal of Spacer from Left Finger Phalangeal Joint, Percutaneous Approach

0RPX3JZ Removal of Synthetic Substitute from Left Finger Phalangeal Joint, Percutaneous Approach

0RPX3KZ Removal of Nonautologous Tissue Substitute from Left Finger Phalangeal Joint, Percutaneous Approach

0RPX40Z Removal of Drainage Device from Left Finger Phalangeal Joint, Percutaneous Endoscopic Approach

0RPX43Z Removal of Infusion Device from Left Finger Phalangeal Joint, Percutaneous Endoscopic Approach

0RPX44Z Removal of Internal Fixation Device from Left Finger Phalangeal Joint, Percutaneous Endoscopic Approach

0RPX45Z Removal of External Fixation Device from Left Finger Phalangeal Joint, Percutaneous Endoscopic Approach

0RPX47Z Removal of Autologous Tissue Substitute from Left Finger Phalangeal Joint, Percutaneous Endoscopic Approach

0RPX48Z Removal of Spacer from Left Finger Phalangeal Joint, Percutaneous Endoscopic Approach

0RPX4JZ Removal of Synthetic Substitute from Left Finger Phalangeal Joint, Percutaneous Endoscopic Approach

0RPX4KZ Removal of Nonautologous Tissue Substitute from Left Finger Phalangeal Joint, Percutaneous Endoscopic Approach

0RPXX0Z Removal of Drainage Device from Left Finger Phalangeal Joint, External Approach

0RPXX3Z Removal of Infusion Device from Left Finger Phalangeal Joint, External Approach

0RPXX4Z Removal of Internal Fixation Device from Left Finger Phalangeal Joint, External Approach

0RPXX5Z Removal of External Fixation Device from Left Finger Phalangeal Joint, External Approach

0RQ – Upper Joints, Repair

Review Coding Guideline B3.5

0RQ00ZZ Repair Occipital-cervical Joint, Open Approach

0RQ03ZZ Repair Occipital-cervical Joint, Percutaneous Approach

0RQ04ZZ Repair Occipital-cervical Joint, Percutaneous Endoscopic Approach

0RQ0XZZ Repair Occipital-cervical Joint, External Approach

0RQ10ZZ Repair Cervical Vertebral Joint, Open Approach

0RQ13ZZ Repair Cervical Vertebral Joint, Percutaneous Approach

0RQ14ZZ Repair Cervical Vertebral Joint, Percutaneous Endoscopic Approach

0RQ1XZZ Repair Cervical Vertebral Joint, External Approach

0RQ30ZZ Repair Cervical Vertebral Disc, Open Approach

0RQ33ZZ Repair Cervical Vertebral Disc, Percutaneous Approach

0RQ34ZZ Repair Cervical Vertebral Disc, Percutaneous Endoscopic Approach

0RQ3XZZ Repair Cervical Vertebral Disc, External Approach

0RQ40ZZ Repair Cervicothoracic Vertebral Joint, Open Approach

0RQ43ZZ Repair Cervicothoracic Vertebral Joint, Percutaneous Approach

0RQ44ZZ Repair Cervicothoracic Vertebral Joint, Percutaneous Endoscopic Approach

0RQ4XZZ Repair Cervicothoracic Vertebral Joint, External Approach

0RQ50ZZ Repair Cervicothoracic Vertebral Disc, Open Approach

0RQ53ZZ Repair Cervicothoracic Vertebral Disc, Percutaneous Approach

0RQ54ZZ Repair Cervicothoracic Vertebral Disc, Percutaneous Endoscopic Approach

0RQ5XZZ Repair Cervicothoracic Vertebral Disc, External Approach

0RQ60ZZ Repair Thoracic Vertebral Joint, Open Approach

0RQ63ZZ Repair Thoracic Vertebral Joint, Percutaneous Approach

0RQ64ZZ Repair Thoracic Vertebral Joint, Percutaneous Endoscopic Approach

0RQ6XZZ Repair Thoracic Vertebral Joint, External Approach

0RQ90ZZ Repair Thoracic Vertebral Disc, Open Approach

0RQ93ZZ Repair Thoracic Vertebral Disc, Percutaneous Approach

0RQ94ZZ Repair Thoracic Vertebral Disc, Percutaneous Endoscopic Approach

0RQ9XZZ Repair Thoracic Vertebral Disc, External Approach

0RQA0ZZ Repair Thoracolumbar Vertebral Joint, Open Approach

0RQA3ZZ Repair Thoracolumbar Vertebral Joint, Percutaneous Approach

0RQA4ZZ Repair Thoracolumbar Vertebral Joint, Percutaneous Endoscopic Approach

0RQAXZZ Repair Thoracolumbar Vertebral Joint, External Approach

0RQB0ZZ Repair Thoracolumbar Vertebral Disc, Open Approach

0RQB3ZZ Repair Thoracolumbar Vertebral Disc, Percutaneous Approach

0RQB4ZZ Repair Thoracolumbar Vertebral Disc, Percutaneous Endoscopic Approach

0RQBXZZ Repair Thoracolumbar Vertebral Disc, External Approach

0RQC0ZZ Repair Right Temporomandibular Joint, Open Approach

0RQC3ZZ Repair Right Temporomandibular Joint, Percutaneous Approach

0RQC4ZZ Repair Right Temporomandibular Joint, Percutaneous Endoscopic Approach

0RQCXZZ Repair Right Temporomandibular Joint, External Approach

0RQD0ZZ Repair Left Temporomandibular Joint, Open Approach

0RQD3ZZ Repair Left Temporomandibular Joint, Percutaneous Approach

0RQD4ZZ Repair Left Temporomandibular Joint, Percutaneous Endoscopic Approach

0RQDXZZ Repair Left Temporomandibular Joint, External Approach

0RQE0ZZ Repair Right Sternoclavicular Joint, Open Approach
    HAC When reported with secondary diagnosis code T84.60XA, T84.610A, T84.611A, T84.612A, T84.613A, T84.614A, T84.615A, T84.619A, T84.63XA, T84.69XA, T84.7XXA

0RQE3ZZ Repair Right Sternoclavicular Joint, Percutaneous Approach
    HAC When reported with secondary diagnosis code T84.60XA, T84.610A, T84.611A, T84.612A, T84.613A, T84.614A, T84.615A, T84.619A, T84.63XA, T84.69XA, T84.7XXA

0RQE4ZZ Repair Right Sternoclavicular Joint, Percutaneous Endoscopic Approach
    HAC When reported with secondary diagnosis code T84.60XA, T84.610A, T84.611A, T84.612A, T84.613A, T84.614A, T84.615A, T84.619A, T84.63XA, T84.69XA, T84.7XXA

0RQEXZZ Repair Right Sternoclavicular Joint, External Approach
    HAC When reported with secondary diagnosis code T84.60XA, T84.610A, T84.611A, T84.612A, T84.613A, T84.614A, T84.615A, T84.619A, T84.63XA, T84.69XA, T84.7XXA

0RQF0ZZ Repair Left Sternoclavicular Joint, Open Approach
    HAC When reported with secondary diagnosis code T84.60XA, T84.610A, T84.611A, T84.612A, T84.613A, T84.614A, T84.615A, T84.619A, T84.63XA, T84.69XA, T84.7XXA

0RQF3ZZ Repair Left Sternoclavicular Joint, Percutaneous Approach
    HAC When reported with secondary diagnosis code T84.60XA, T84.610A, T84.611A, T84.612A, T84.613A, T84.614A, T84.615A, T84.619A, T84.63XA, T84.69XA, T84.7XXA

0RQF4ZZ Repair Left Sternoclavicular Joint, Percutaneous Endoscopic Approach
HAC When reported with secondary diagnosis code T84.60XA,
T84.610A, T84.611A, T84.612A, T84.613A, T84.614A, T84.615A,
T84.619A, T84.63XA, T84.69XA, T84.7XXA

0RQFXZZ Repair Left Sternoclavicular Joint, External Approach
HAC When reported with secondary diagnosis code T84.60XA,
T84.610A, T84.611A, T84.612A, T84.613A, T84.614A, T84.615A,
T84.619A, T84.63XA, T84.69XA, T84.7XXA

0RQG0ZZ Repair Right Acromioclavicular Joint, Open Approach
HAC When reported with secondary diagnosis code T84.60XA,
T84.610A, T84.611A, T84.612A, T84.613A, T84.614A, T84.615A,
T84.619A, T84.63XA, T84.69XA, T84.7XXA

0RQG3ZZ Repair Right Acromioclavicular Joint, Percutaneous Approach
HAC When reported with secondary diagnosis code T84.60XA,
T84.610A, T84.611A, T84.612A, T84.613A, T84.614A, T84.615A,
T84.619A, T84.63XA, T84.69XA, T84.7XXA

0RQG4ZZ Repair Right Acromioclavicular Joint, Percutaneous Endoscopic
Approach
HAC When reported with secondary diagnosis code T84.60XA,
T84.610A, T84.611A, T84.612A, T84.613A, T84.614A, T84.615A,
T84.619A, T84.63XA, T84.69XA, T84.7XXA

0RQGXZZ Repair Right Acromioclavicular Joint, External Approach
HAC When reported with secondary diagnosis code T84.60XA,
T84.610A, T84.611A, T84.612A, T84.613A, T84.614A, T84.615A,
T84.619A, T84.63XA, T84.69XA, T84.7XXA

0RQH0ZZ Repair Left Acromioclavicular Joint, Open Approach
HAC When reported with secondary diagnosis code T84.60XA,
T84.610A, T84.611A, T84.612A, T84.613A, T84.614A, T84.615A,
T84.619A, T84.63XA, T84.69XA, T84.7XXA

0RQH3ZZ Repair Left Acromioclavicular Joint, Percutaneous Approach
HAC When reported with secondary diagnosis code T84.60XA,
T84.610A, T84.611A, T84.612A, T84.613A, T84.614A, T84.615A,
T84.619A, T84.63XA, T84.69XA, T84.7XXA

0RQH4ZZ Repair Left Acromioclavicular Joint, Percutaneous Endoscopic
Approach
HAC When reported with secondary diagnosis code T84.60XA,
T84.610A, T84.611A, T84.612A, T84.613A, T84.614A, T84.615A,
T84.619A, T84.63XA, T84.69XA, T84.7XXA

0RQHXZZ Repair Left Acromioclavicular Joint, External Approach
HAC When reported with secondary diagnosis code T84.60XA,
T84.610A, T84.611A, T84.612A, T84.613A, T84.614A, T84.615A,
T84.619A, T84.63XA, T84.69XA, T84.7XXA

0RQJ0ZZ Repair Right Shoulder Joint, Open Approach
HAC When reported with secondary diagnosis code T84.60XA,
T84.610A, T84.611A, T84.612A, T84.613A, T84.614A, T84.615A,
T84.619A, T84.63XA, T84.69XA, T84.7XXA

0RQJ3ZZ Repair Right Shoulder Joint, Percutaneous Approach
HAC When reported with secondary diagnosis code T84.60XA,
T84.610A, T84.611A, T84.612A, T84.613A, T84.614A, T84.615A,
T84.619A, T84.63XA, T84.69XA, T84.7XXA

0RQJ4ZZ Repair Right Shoulder Joint, Percutaneous Endoscopic Approach
HAC When reported with secondary diagnosis code T84.60XA,
T84.610A, T84.611A, T84.612A, T84.613A, T84.614A, T84.615A,
T84.619A, T84.63XA, T84.69XA, T84.7XXA

0RQJXZZ Repair Right Shoulder Joint, External Approach
HAC When reported with secondary diagnosis code T84.60XA,
T84.610A, T84.611A, T84.612A, T84.613A, T84.614A, T84.615A,
T84.619A, T84.63XA, T84.69XA, T84.7XXA

0RQK0ZZ Repair Left Shoulder Joint, Open Approach
HAC When reported with secondary diagnosis code T84.60XA,
T84.610A, T84.611A, T84.612A, T84.613A, T84.614A, T84.615A,
T84.619A, T84.63XA, T84.69XA, T84.7XXA

0RQK3ZZ Repair Left Shoulder Joint, Percutaneous Approach
HAC When reported with secondary diagnosis code T84.60XA,
T84.610A, T84.611A, T84.612A, T84.613A, T84.614A, T84.615A,
T84.619A, T84.63XA, T84.69XA, T84.7XXA

0RQK4ZZ Repair Left Shoulder Joint, Percutaneous Endoscopic Approach
HAC When reported with secondary diagnosis code T84.60XA,
T84.610A, T84.611A, T84.612A, T84.613A, T84.614A, T84.615A,
T84.619A, T84.63XA, T84.69XA, T84.7XXA

0RQKXZZ Repair Left Shoulder Joint, External Approach
HAC When reported with secondary diagnosis code T84.60XA,
T84.610A, T84.611A, T84.612A, T84.613A, T84.614A, T84.615A,
T84.619A, T84.63XA, T84.69XA, T84.7XXA

0RQL0ZZ Repair Right Elbow Joint, Open Approach
HAC When reported with secondary diagnosis code T84.60XA,
T84.610A, T84.611A, T84.612A, T84.613A, T84.614A, T84.615A,
T84.619A, T84.63XA, T84.69XA, T84.7XXA

0RQL3ZZ Repair Right Elbow Joint, Percutaneous Approach
HAC When reported with secondary diagnosis code T84.60XA,
T84.610A, T84.611A, T84.612A, T84.613A, T84.614A, T84.615A,
T84.619A, T84.63XA, T84.69XA, T84.7XXA

0RQL4ZZ Repair Right Elbow Joint, Percutaneous Endoscopic Approach
HAC When reported with secondary diagnosis code T84.60XA,
T84.610A, T84.611A, T84.612A, T84.613A, T84.614A, T84.615A,
T84.619A, T84.63XA, T84.69XA, T84.7XXA

0RQLXZZ Repair Right Elbow Joint, External Approach
HAC When reported with secondary diagnosis code T84.60XA,
T84.610A, T84.611A, T84.612A, T84.613A, T84.614A, T84.615A,
T84.619A, T84.63XA, T84.69XA, T84.7XXA

0RQM0ZZ Repair Left Elbow Joint, Open Approach
HAC When reported with secondary diagnosis code T84.60XA,
T84.610A, T84.611A, T84.612A, T84.613A, T84.614A, T84.615A,
T84.619A, T84.63XA, T84.69XA, T84.7XXA

0RQM3ZZ Repair Left Elbow Joint, Percutaneous Approach
HAC When reported with secondary diagnosis code T84.60XA,
T84.610A, T84.611A, T84.612A, T84.613A, T84.614A, T84.615A,
T84.619A, T84.63XA, T84.69XA, T84.7XXA

0RQM4ZZ Repair Left Elbow Joint, Percutaneous Endoscopic Approach
HAC When reported with secondary diagnosis code T84.60XA,
T84.610A, T84.611A, T84.612A, T84.613A, T84.614A, T84.615A,
T84.619A, T84.63XA, T84.69XA, T84.7XXA

0RQMXZZ Repair Left Elbow Joint, External Approach
HAC When reported with secondary diagnosis code T84.60XA,
T84.610A, T84.611A, T84.612A, T84.613A, T84.614A, T84.615A,
T84.619A, T84.63XA, T84.69XA, T84.7XXA

0RQN0ZZ Repair Right Wrist Joint, Open Approach
0RQN3ZZ Repair Right Wrist Joint, Percutaneous Approach
0RQN4ZZ Repair Right Wrist Joint, Percutaneous Endoscopic Approach
0RQNXZZ Repair Right Wrist Joint, External Approach
0RQP0ZZ Repair Left Wrist Joint, Open Approach
0RQP3ZZ Repair Left Wrist Joint, Percutaneous Approach
0RQP4ZZ Repair Left Wrist Joint, Percutaneous Endoscopic Approach
0RQPXZZ Repair Left Wrist Joint, External Approach
0RQQ0ZZ Repair Right Carpal Joint, Open Approach
0RQQ3ZZ Repair Right Carpal Joint, Percutaneous Approach
0RQQ4ZZ Repair Right Carpal Joint, Percutaneous Endoscopic Approach
0RQQXZZ Repair Right Carpal Joint, External Approach
0RQR0ZZ Repair Left Carpal Joint, Open Approach
0RQR3ZZ Repair Left Carpal Joint, Percutaneous Approach
0RQR4ZZ Repair Left Carpal Joint, Percutaneous Endoscopic Approach
0RQRXZZ Repair Left Carpal Joint, External Approach
0RQS0ZZ Repair Right Metacarpocarpal Joint, Open Approach
0RQS3ZZ Repair Right Metacarpocarpal Joint, Percutaneous Approach
0RQS4ZZ Repair Right Metacarpocarpal Joint, Percutaneous Endoscopic
Approach
0RQSXZZ Repair Right Metacarpocarpal Joint, External Approach
0RQT0ZZ Repair Left Metacarpocarpal Joint, Open Approach
0RQT3ZZ Repair Left Metacarpocarpal Joint, Percutaneous Approach
0RQT4ZZ Repair Left Metacarpocarpal Joint, Percutaneous Endoscopic
Approach
0RQTXZZ Repair Left Metacarpocarpal Joint, External Approach
0RQU0ZZ Repair Right Metacarpophalangeal Joint, Open Approach
0RQU3ZZ Repair Right Metacarpophalangeal Joint, Percutaneous
Approach
0RQU4ZZ Repair Right Metacarpophalangeal Joint, Percutaneous Endoscopic
Approach
0RQUXZZ Repair Right Metacarpophalangeal Joint, External Approach
0RQV0ZZ Repair Left Metacarpophalangeal Joint, Open Approach
0RQV3ZZ Repair Left Metacarpophalangeal Joint, Percutaneous Approach
0RQV4ZZ Repair Left Metacarpophalangeal Joint, Percutaneous Endoscopic
Approach
0RQVXZZ Repair Left Metacarpophalangeal Joint, External Approach
0RQW0ZZ Repair Right Finger Phalangeal Joint, Open Approach
0RQW3ZZ Repair Right Finger Phalangeal Joint, Percutaneous Approach
0RQW4ZZ Repair Right Finger Phalangeal Joint, Percutaneous Endoscopic
Approach
0RQWXZZ Repair Right Finger Phalangeal Joint, External Approach

---

0RQX0ZZ Repair Left Finger Phalangeal Joint, Open Approach

0RQX3ZZ Repair Left Finger Phalangeal Joint, Percutaneous Approach

0RQX4ZZ Repair Left Finger Phalangeal Joint, Percutaneous Endoscopic Approach

0RQXXZZ Repair Left Finger Phalangeal Joint, External Approach

0RR – Upper Joints, Replacement

0RR007Z Replacement of Occipital-cervical Joint with Autologous Tissue Substitute, Open Approach

0RR00JZ Replacement of Occipital-cervical Joint with Synthetic Substitute, Open Approach

0RR00KZ Replacement of Occipital-cervical Joint with Nonautologous Tissue Substitute, Open Approach

0RR107Z Replacement of Cervical Vertebral Joint with Autologous Tissue Substitute, Open Approach

0RR10JZ Replacement of Cervical Vertebral Joint with Synthetic Substitute, Open Approach

0RR10KZ Replacement of Cervical Vertebral Joint with Nonautologous Tissue Substitute, Open Approach

0RR307Z Replacement of Cervical Vertebral Disc with Autologous Tissue Substitute, Open Approach

0RR30JZ Replacement of Cervical Vertebral Disc with Synthetic Substitute, Open Approach

0RR30KZ Replacement of Cervical Vertebral Disc with Nonautologous Tissue Substitute, Open Approach

0RR407Z Replacement of Cervicothoracic Vertebral Joint with Autologous Tissue Substitute, Open Approach

0RR40JZ Replacement of Cervicothoracic Vertebral Joint with Synthetic Substitute, Open Approach

0RR40KZ Replacement of Cervicothoracic Vertebral Joint with Nonautologous Tissue Substitute, Open Approach

0RR507Z Replacement of Cervicothoracic Vertebral Disc with Autologous Tissue Substitute, Open Approach

0RR50JZ Replacement of Cervicothoracic Vertebral Disc with Synthetic Substitute, Open Approach

0RR50KZ Replacement of Cervicothoracic Vertebral Disc with Nonautologous Tissue Substitute, Open Approach

0RR607Z Replacement of Thoracic Vertebral Joint with Autologous Tissue Substitute, Open Approach

0RR60JZ Replacement of Thoracic Vertebral Joint with Synthetic Substitute, Open Approach

0RR60KZ Replacement of Thoracic Vertebral Joint with Nonautologous Tissue Substitute, Open Approach

0RR907Z Replacement of Thoracic Vertebral Disc with Autologous Tissue Substitute, Open Approach

0RR90JZ Replacement of Thoracic Vertebral Disc with Synthetic Substitute, Open Approach

0RR90KZ Replacement of Thoracic Vertebral Disc with Nonautologous Tissue Substitute, Open Approach

0RRA07Z Replacement of Thoracolumbar Vertebral Joint with Autologous Tissue Substitute, Open Approach

0RRA0JZ Replacement of Thoracolumbar Vertebral Joint with Synthetic Substitute, Open Approach

0RRA0KZ Replacement of Thoracolumbar Vertebral Joint with Nonautologous Tissue Substitute, Open Approach

0RRB07Z Replacement of Thoracolumbar Vertebral Disc with Autologous Tissue Substitute, Open Approach

0RRB0JZ Replacement of Thoracolumbar Vertebral Disc with Synthetic Substitute, Open Approach

0RRB0KZ Replacement of Thoracolumbar Vertebral Disc with Nonautologous Tissue Substitute, Open Approach

0RRC07Z Replacement of Right Temporomandibular Joint with Autologous Tissue Substitute, Open Approach

0RRC0JZ Replacement of Right Temporomandibular Joint with Synthetic Substitute, Open Approach

0RRC0KZ Replacement of Right Temporomandibular Joint with Nonautologous Tissue Substitute, Open Approach

0RRD07Z Replacement of Left Temporomandibular Joint with Autologous Tissue Substitute, Open Approach

0RRD0JZ Replacement of Left Temporomandibular Joint with Synthetic Substitute, Open Approach

0RRD0KZ Replacement of Left Temporomandibular Joint with Nonautologous Tissue Substitute, Open Approach

0RRE07Z Replacement of Right Sternoclavicular Joint with Autologous Tissue Substitute, Open Approach

0RRE0JZ Replacement of Right Sternoclavicular Joint with Synthetic Substitute, Open Approach

0RRE0KZ Replacement of Right Sternoclavicular Joint with Nonautologous Tissue Substitute, Open Approach

0RRF07Z Replacement of Left Sternoclavicular Joint with Autologous Tissue Substitute, Open Approach

0RRF0JZ Replacement of Left Sternoclavicular Joint with Synthetic Substitute, Open Approach

0RRF0KZ Replacement of Left Sternoclavicular Joint with Nonautologous Tissue Substitute, Open Approach

0RRG07Z Replacement of Right Acromioclavicular Joint with Autologous Tissue Substitute, Open Approach

0RRG0JZ Replacement of Right Acromioclavicular Joint with Synthetic Substitute, Open Approach

0RRG0KZ Replacement of Right Acromioclavicular Joint with Nonautologous Tissue Substitute, Open Approach

0RRH07Z Replacement of Left Acromioclavicular Joint with Autologous Tissue Substitute, Open Approach

0RRH0JZ Replacement of Left Acromioclavicular Joint with Synthetic Substitute, Open Approach

0RRH0KZ Replacement of Left Acromioclavicular Joint with Nonautologous Tissue Substitute, Open Approach

0RRJ00Z Replacement of Right Shoulder Joint with Reverse Ball and Socket Synthetic Substitute, Open Approach

0RRJ07Z Replacement of Right Shoulder Joint with Autologous Tissue Substitute, Open Approach

0RRJ0J6 Replacement of Right Shoulder Joint with Synthetic Substitute, Humeral Surface, Open Approach

0RRJ0J7 Replacement of Right Shoulder Joint with Synthetic Substitute, Glenoid Surface, Open Approach

0RRJ0JZ Replacement of Right Shoulder Joint with Synthetic Substitute, Open Approach

0RRJ0KZ Replacement of Right Shoulder Joint with Nonautologous Tissue Substitute, Open Approach

0RRK00Z Replacement of Left Shoulder Joint with Reverse Ball and Socket Synthetic Substitute, Open Approach

0RRK07Z Replacement of Left Shoulder Joint with Autologous Tissue Substitute, Open Approach

0RRK0J6 Replacement of Left Shoulder Joint with Synthetic Substitute, Humeral Surface, Open Approach

0RRK0J7 Replacement of Left Shoulder Joint with Synthetic Substitute, Glenoid Surface, Open Approach

0RRK0JZ Replacement of Left Shoulder Joint with Synthetic Substitute, Open Approach

0RRK0KZ Replacement of Left Shoulder Joint with Nonautologous Tissue Substitute, Open Approach

0RRL07Z Replacement of Right Elbow Joint with Autologous Tissue Substitute, Open Approach

0RRL0JZ Replacement of Right Elbow Joint with Synthetic Substitute, Open Approach

0RRL0KZ Replacement of Right Elbow Joint with Nonautologous Tissue Substitute, Open Approach

0RRM07Z Replacement of Left Elbow Joint with Autologous Tissue Substitute, Open Approach

0RRM0JZ Replacement of Left Elbow Joint with Synthetic Substitute, Open Approach

0RRM0KZ Replacement of Left Elbow Joint with Nonautologous Tissue Substitute, Open Approach

0RRN07Z Replacement of Right Wrist Joint with Autologous Tissue Substitute, Open Approach

0RRN0JZ Replacement of Right Wrist Joint with Synthetic Substitute, Open Approach

0RRN0KZ Replacement of Right Wrist Joint with Nonautologous Tissue Substitute, Open Approach

0RRP07Z Replacement of Left Wrist Joint with Autologous Tissue Substitute, Open Approach

0RRP0JZ Replacement of Left Wrist Joint with Synthetic Substitute, Open Approach

0RRP0KZ Replacement of Left Wrist Joint with Nonautologous Tissue Substitute, Open Approach

0RRQ07Z Replacement of Right Carpal Joint with Autologous Tissue Substitute, Open Approach

0RRQ0JZ Replacement of Right Carpal Joint with Synthetic Substitute, Open Approach

0RRQ0KZ Replacement of Right Carpal Joint with Nonautologous Tissue Substitute, Open Approach

0RRR07Z Replacement of Left Carpal Joint with Autologous Tissue Substitute, Open Approach

0RRR0JZ Replacement of Left Carpal Joint with Synthetic Substitute, Open Approach

0RRR0KZ Replacement of Left Carpal Joint with Nonautologous Tissue Substitute, Open Approach

0RRS07Z Replacement of Right Metacarpocarpal Joint with Autologous Tissue Substitute, Open Approach

0RRS0JZ Replacement of Right Metacarpocarpal Joint with Synthetic Substitute, Open Approach

0RRS0KZ Replacement of Right Metacarpocarpal Joint with Nonautologous Tissue Substitute, Open Approach

0RRT07Z Replacement of Left Metacarpocarpal Joint with Autologous Tissue Substitute, Open Approach

0RRT0JZ Replacement of Left Metacarpocarpal Joint with Synthetic Substitute, Open Approach

0RRT0KZ Replacement of Left Metacarpocarpal Joint with Nonautologous Tissue Substitute, Open Approach

0RRU07Z Replacement of Right Metacarpophalangeal Joint with Autologous Tissue Substitute, Open Approach

0RRU0JZ Replacement of Right Metacarpophalangeal Joint with Synthetic Substitute, Open Approach

0RRU0KZ Replacement of Right Metacarpophalangeal Joint with Nonautologous Tissue Substitute, Open Approach

0RRV07Z Replacement of Left Metacarpophalangeal Joint with Autologous Tissue Substitute, Open Approach

0RRV0JZ Replacement of Left Metacarpophalangeal Joint with Synthetic Substitute, Open Approach

0RRV0KZ Replacement of Left Metacarpophalangeal Joint with Nonautologous Tissue Substitute, Open Approach

0RRW07Z Replacement of Right Finger Phalangeal Joint with Autologous Tissue Substitute, Open Approach

0RRW0JZ Replacement of Right Finger Phalangeal Joint with Synthetic Substitute, Open Approach

0RRW0KZ Replacement of Right Finger Phalangeal Joint with Nonautologous Tissue Substitute, Open Approach

0RRX07Z Replacement of Left Finger Phalangeal Joint with Autologous Tissue Substitute, Open Approach

0RRX0JZ Replacement of Left Finger Phalangeal Joint with Synthetic Substitute, Open Approach

0RRX0KZ Replacement of Left Finger Phalangeal Joint with Nonautologous Tissue Substitute, Open Approach

0RS – Upper Joints, Reposition

0RS004Z Reposition Occipital-cervical Joint with Internal Fixation Device, Open Approach

0RS00ZZ Reposition Occipital-cervical Joint, Open Approach

0RS034Z Reposition Occipital-cervical Joint with Internal Fixation Device, Percutaneous Approach

0RS03ZZ Reposition Occipital-cervical Joint, Percutaneous Approach

0RS044Z Reposition Occipital-cervical Joint with Internal Fixation Device, Percutaneous Endoscopic Approach

0RS04ZZ Reposition Occipital-cervical Joint, Percutaneous Endoscopic Approach

0RS0X4Z Reposition Occipital-cervical Joint with Internal Fixation Device, External Approach

0RS0XZZ Reposition Occipital-cervical Joint, External Approach

0RS104Z Reposition Cervical Vertebral Joint with Internal Fixation Device, Open Approach

0RS10ZZ Reposition Cervical Vertebral Joint, Open Approach

0RS134Z Reposition Cervical Vertebral Joint with Internal Fixation Device, Percutaneous Approach

0RS13ZZ Reposition Cervical Vertebral Joint, Percutaneous Approach

0RS144Z Reposition Cervical Vertebral Joint with Internal Fixation Device, Percutaneous Endoscopic Approach

0RS14ZZ Reposition Cervical Vertebral Joint, Percutaneous Endoscopic Approach

0RS1X4Z Reposition Cervical Vertebral Joint with Internal Fixation Device, External Approach

0RS1XZZ Reposition Cervical Vertebral Joint, External Approach

0RS404Z Reposition Cervicothoracic Vertebral Joint with Internal Fixation Device, Open Approach

0RS40ZZ Reposition Cervicothoracic Vertebral Joint, Open Approach

0RS434Z Reposition Cervicothoracic Vertebral Joint with Internal Fixation Device, Percutaneous Approach

0RS43ZZ Reposition Cervicothoracic Vertebral Joint, Percutaneous Approach

0RS444Z Reposition Cervicothoracic Vertebral Joint with Internal Fixation Device, Percutaneous Endoscopic Approach

0RS44ZZ Reposition Cervicothoracic Vertebral Joint, Percutaneous Endoscopic Approach

0RS4X4Z Reposition Cervicothoracic Vertebral Joint with Internal Fixation Device, External Approach

0RS4XZZ Reposition Cervicothoracic Vertebral Joint, External Approach

0RS604Z Reposition Thoracic Vertebral Joint with Internal Fixation Device, Open Approach

0RS60ZZ Reposition Thoracic Vertebral Joint, Open Approach

0RS634Z Reposition Thoracic Vertebral Joint with Internal Fixation Device, Percutaneous Approach

0RS63ZZ Reposition Thoracic Vertebral Joint, Percutaneous Approach

0RS644Z Reposition Thoracic Vertebral Joint with Internal Fixation Device, Percutaneous Endoscopic Approach

0RS64ZZ Reposition Thoracic Vertebral Joint, Percutaneous Endoscopic Approach

0RS6X4Z Reposition Thoracic Vertebral Joint with Internal Fixation Device, External Approach

0RS6XZZ Reposition Thoracic Vertebral Joint, External Approach

0RSA04Z Reposition Thoracolumbar Vertebral Joint with Internal Fixation Device, Open Approach

0RSA0ZZ Reposition Thoracolumbar Vertebral Joint, Open Approach

0RSA34Z Reposition Thoracolumbar Vertebral Joint with Internal Fixation Device, Percutaneous Approach

0RSA3ZZ Reposition Thoracolumbar Vertebral Joint, Percutaneous Approach

0RSA44Z Reposition Thoracolumbar Vertebral Joint with Internal Fixation Device, Percutaneous Endoscopic Approach

0RSA4ZZ Reposition Thoracolumbar Vertebral Joint, Percutaneous Endoscopic Approach

0RSAX4Z Reposition Thoracolumbar Vertebral Joint with Internal Fixation Device, External Approach

0RSAXZZ Reposition Thoracolumbar Vertebral Joint, External Approach

0RSC04Z Reposition Right Temporomandibular Joint with Internal Fixation Device, Open Approach

0RSC0ZZ Reposition Right Temporomandibular Joint, Open Approach

0RSC34Z Reposition Right Temporomandibular Joint with Internal Fixation Device, Percutaneous Approach

0RSC3ZZ Reposition Right Temporomandibular Joint, Percutaneous Approach

0RSC44Z Reposition Right Temporomandibular Joint with Internal Fixation Device, Percutaneous Endoscopic Approach

0RSC4ZZ Reposition Right Temporomandibular Joint, Percutaneous Endoscopic Approach

0RSCX4Z Reposition Right Temporomandibular Joint with Internal Fixation Device, External Approach

0RSCXZZ Reposition Right Temporomandibular Joint, External Approach

0RSD04Z Reposition Left Temporomandibular Joint with Internal Fixation Device, Open Approach

0RSD0ZZ Reposition Left Temporomandibular Joint, Open Approach

0RSD34Z Reposition Left Temporomandibular Joint with Internal Fixation Device, Percutaneous Approach

0RSD3ZZ Reposition Left Temporomandibular Joint, Percutaneous Approach

0RSD44Z Reposition Left Temporomandibular Joint with Internal Fixation Device, Percutaneous Endoscopic Approach

0RSD4ZZ Reposition Left Temporomandibular Joint, Percutaneous Endoscopic Approach

0RSDX4Z Reposition Left Temporomandibular Joint with Internal Fixation Device, External Approach

0RSDXZZ Reposition Left Temporomandibular Joint, External Approach

0RSE04Z Reposition Right Sternoclavicular Joint with Internal Fixation Device, Open Approach

0RSE0ZZ Reposition Right Sternoclavicular Joint, Open Approach

0RSE34Z Reposition Right Sternoclavicular Joint with Internal Fixation Device, Percutaneous Approach

0RSE3ZZ Reposition Right Sternoclavicular Joint, Percutaneous Approach

0RSE44Z Reposition Right Sternoclavicular Joint with Internal Fixation Device, Percutaneous Endoscopic Approach

0RSE4ZZ Reposition Right Sternoclavicular Joint, Percutaneous Endoscopic Approach

0RSEX4Z Reposition Right Sternoclavicular Joint with Internal Fixation Device, External Approach

0RSEXZZ Reposition Right Sternoclavicular Joint, External Approach

0RSF04Z Reposition Left Sternoclavicular Joint with Internal Fixation Device, Open Approach

0RSF0ZZ Reposition Left Sternoclavicular Joint, Open Approach

0RSF34Z Reposition Left Sternoclavicular Joint with Internal Fixation Device, Percutaneous Approach

0RSF3ZZ Reposition Left Sternoclavicular Joint, Percutaneous Approach

0RSF44Z Reposition Left Sternoclavicular Joint with Internal Fixation Device, Percutaneous Endoscopic Approach

0RSF4ZZ Reposition Left Sternoclavicular Joint, Percutaneous Endoscopic Approach

0RSFX4Z Reposition Left Sternoclavicular Joint with Internal Fixation Device, External Approach

0RSFXZZ Reposition Left Sternoclavicular Joint, External Approach

0RSG04Z Reposition Right Acromioclavicular Joint with Internal Fixation Device, Open Approach

0RSG0ZZ Reposition Right Acromioclavicular Joint, Open Approach

0RSG34Z Reposition Right Acromioclavicular Joint with Internal Fixation Device, Percutaneous Approach

0RSG3ZZ Reposition Right Acromioclavicular Joint, Percutaneous Approach

0RSG44Z Reposition Right Acromioclavicular Joint with Internal Fixation Device, Percutaneous Endoscopic Approach

0RSG4ZZ Reposition Right Acromioclavicular Joint, Percutaneous Endoscopic Approach

0RSGX4Z Reposition Right Acromioclavicular Joint with Internal Fixation Device, External Approach

0RSGXZZ Reposition Right Acromioclavicular Joint, External Approach

0RSH04Z Reposition Left Acromioclavicular Joint with Internal Fixation Device, Open Approach

0RSH0ZZ Reposition Left Acromioclavicular Joint, Open Approach

0RSH34Z Reposition Left Acromioclavicular Joint with Internal Fixation Device, Percutaneous Approach

0RSH3ZZ Reposition Left Acromioclavicular Joint, Percutaneous Approach

0RSH44Z Reposition Left Acromioclavicular Joint with Internal Fixation Device, Percutaneous Endoscopic Approach

0RSH4ZZ Reposition Left Acromioclavicular Joint, Percutaneous Endoscopic Approach

0RSHX4Z Reposition Left Acromioclavicular Joint with Internal Fixation Device, External Approach

0RSHXZZ Reposition Left Acromioclavicular Joint, External Approach

0RSJ04Z Reposition Right Shoulder Joint with Internal Fixation Device, Open Approach

0RSJ0ZZ Reposition Right Shoulder Joint, Open Approach

0RSJ34Z Reposition Right Shoulder Joint with Internal Fixation Device, Percutaneous Approach

0RSJ3ZZ Reposition Right Shoulder Joint, Percutaneous Approach

0RSJ44Z Reposition Right Shoulder Joint with Internal Fixation Device, Percutaneous Endoscopic Approach

0RSJ4ZZ Reposition Right Shoulder Joint, Percutaneous Endoscopic Approach

0RSJX4Z Reposition Right Shoulder Joint with Internal Fixation Device, External Approach

0RSJXZZ Reposition Right Shoulder Joint, External Approach

0RSK04Z Reposition Left Shoulder Joint with Internal Fixation Device, Open Approach

0RSK0ZZ Reposition Left Shoulder Joint, Open Approach

0RSK34Z Reposition Left Shoulder Joint with Internal Fixation Device, Percutaneous Approach

0RSK3ZZ Reposition Left Shoulder Joint, Percutaneous Approach

0RSK44Z Reposition Left Shoulder Joint with Internal Fixation Device, Percutaneous Endoscopic Approach

0RSK4ZZ Reposition Left Shoulder Joint, Percutaneous Endoscopic Approach

0RSKX4Z Reposition Left Shoulder Joint with Internal Fixation Device, External Approach

0RSKXZZ Reposition Left Shoulder Joint, External Approach

0RSL04Z Reposition Right Elbow Joint with Internal Fixation Device, Open Approach

0RSL05Z Reposition Right Elbow Joint with External Fixation Device, Open Approach

0RSL0ZZ Reposition Right Elbow Joint, Open Approach

0RSL34Z Reposition Right Elbow Joint with Internal Fixation Device, Percutaneous Approach

0RSL35Z Reposition Right Elbow Joint with External Fixation Device, Percutaneous Approach

0RSL3ZZ Reposition Right Elbow Joint, Percutaneous Approach

0RSL44Z Reposition Right Elbow Joint with Internal Fixation Device, Percutaneous Endoscopic Approach

0RSL45Z Reposition Right Elbow Joint with External Fixation Device, Percutaneous Endoscopic Approach

0RSL4ZZ Reposition Right Elbow Joint, Percutaneous Endoscopic Approach

0RSLX4Z Reposition Right Elbow Joint with Internal Fixation Device, External Approach

0RSLX5Z Reposition Right Elbow Joint with External Fixation Device, External Approach

0RSLXZZ Reposition Right Elbow Joint, External Approach

0RSM04Z Reposition Left Elbow Joint with Internal Fixation Device, Open Approach

0RSM05Z Reposition Left Elbow Joint with External Fixation Device, Open Approach

0RSM0ZZ Reposition Left Elbow Joint, Open Approach

0RSM34Z Reposition Left Elbow Joint with Internal Fixation Device, Percutaneous Approach

0RSM35Z Reposition Left Elbow Joint with External Fixation Device, Percutaneous Approach

0RSM3ZZ Reposition Left Elbow Joint, Percutaneous Approach

0RSM44Z Reposition Left Elbow Joint with Internal Fixation Device, Percutaneous Endoscopic Approach

0RSM45Z Reposition Left Elbow Joint with External Fixation Device, Percutaneous Endoscopic Approach

0RSM4ZZ Reposition Left Elbow Joint, Percutaneous Endoscopic Approach

0RSMX4Z Reposition Left Elbow Joint with Internal Fixation Device, External Approach

0RSMX5Z Reposition Left Elbow Joint with External Fixation Device, External Approach

0RSMXZZ Reposition Left Elbow Joint, External Approach

0RSN04Z Reposition Right Wrist Joint with Internal Fixation Device, Open Approach

0RSN05Z Reposition Right Wrist Joint with External Fixation Device, Open Approach

0RSN0ZZ Reposition Right Wrist Joint, Open Approach

0RSN34Z Reposition Right Wrist Joint with Internal Fixation Device, Percutaneous Approach

0RSN35Z Reposition Right Wrist Joint with External Fixation Device, Percutaneous Approach

0RSN3ZZ Reposition Right Wrist Joint, Percutaneous Approach

0RSN44Z Reposition Right Wrist Joint with Internal Fixation Device, Percutaneous Endoscopic Approach

0RSN45Z Reposition Right Wrist Joint with External Fixation Device, Percutaneous Endoscopic Approach

0RSN4ZZ Reposition Right Wrist Joint, Percutaneous Endoscopic Approach

0RSNX4Z Reposition Right Wrist Joint with Internal Fixation Device, External Approach

0RSNX5Z Reposition Right Wrist Joint with External Fixation Device, External Approach

0RSNXZZ Reposition Right Wrist Joint, External Approach

0RSP04Z Reposition Left Wrist Joint with Internal Fixation Device, Open Approach

0RSP05Z Reposition Left Wrist Joint with External Fixation Device, Open Approach

0RSP0ZZ Reposition Left Wrist Joint, Open Approach

0RSP34Z Reposition Left Wrist Joint with Internal Fixation Device, Percutaneous Approach

0RSP35Z   Reposition Left Wrist Joint with External Fixation Device, Percutaneous Approach

0RSP3ZZ   Reposition Left Wrist Joint, Percutaneous Approach

0RSP44Z   Reposition Left Wrist Joint with Internal Fixation Device, Percutaneous Endoscopic Approach

0RSP45Z   Reposition Left Wrist Joint with External Fixation Device, Percutaneous Endoscopic Approach

0RSP4ZZ   Reposition Left Wrist Joint, Percutaneous Endoscopic Approach

0RSPX4Z   Reposition Left Wrist Joint with Internal Fixation Device, External Approach

0RSPX5Z   Reposition Left Wrist Joint with External Fixation Device, External Approach

0RSPXZZ   Reposition Left Wrist Joint, External Approach

0RSQ04Z   Reposition Right Carpal Joint with Internal Fixation Device, Open Approach

0RSQ05Z   Reposition Right Carpal Joint with External Fixation Device, Open Approach

0RSQ0ZZ   Reposition Right Carpal Joint, Open Approach

0RSQ34Z   Reposition Right Carpal Joint with Internal Fixation Device, Percutaneous Approach

0RSQ35Z   Reposition Right Carpal Joint with External Fixation Device, Percutaneous Approach

0RSQ3ZZ   Reposition Right Carpal Joint, Percutaneous Approach

0RSQ44Z   Reposition Right Carpal Joint with Internal Fixation Device, Percutaneous Endoscopic Approach

0RSQ45Z   Reposition Right Carpal Joint with External Fixation Device, Percutaneous Endoscopic Approach

0RSQ4ZZ   Reposition Right Carpal Joint, Percutaneous Endoscopic Approach

0RSQX4Z   Reposition Right Carpal Joint with Internal Fixation Device, External Approach

0RSQX5Z   Reposition Right Carpal Joint with External Fixation Device, External Approach

0RSQXZZ   Reposition Right Carpal Joint, External Approach

0RSR04Z   Reposition Left Carpal Joint with Internal Fixation Device, Open Approach

0RSR05Z   Reposition Left Carpal Joint with External Fixation Device, Open Approach

0RSR0ZZ   Reposition Left Carpal Joint, Open Approach

0RSR34Z   Reposition Left Carpal Joint with Internal Fixation Device, Percutaneous Approach

0RSR35Z   Reposition Left Carpal Joint with External Fixation Device, Percutaneous Approach

0RSR3ZZ   Reposition Left Carpal Joint, Percutaneous Approach

0RSR44Z   Reposition Left Carpal Joint with Internal Fixation Device, Percutaneous Endoscopic Approach

0RSR45Z   Reposition Left Carpal Joint with External Fixation Device, Percutaneous Endoscopic Approach

0RSR4ZZ   Reposition Left Carpal Joint, Percutaneous Endoscopic Approach

0RSRX4Z   Reposition Left Carpal Joint with Internal Fixation Device, External Approach

0RSRX5Z   Reposition Left Carpal Joint with External Fixation Device, External Approach

0RSRXZZ   Reposition Left Carpal Joint, External Approach

0RSS04Z   Reposition Right Metacarpocarpal Joint with Internal Fixation Device, Open Approach

0RSS05Z   Reposition Right Metacarpocarpal Joint with External Fixation Device, Open Approach

0RSS0ZZ   Reposition Right Metacarpocarpal Joint, Open Approach

0RSS34Z   Reposition Right Metacarpocarpal Joint with Internal Fixation Device, Percutaneous Approach

0RSS35Z   Reposition Right Metacarpocarpal Joint with External Fixation Device, Percutaneous Approach

0RSS3ZZ   Reposition Right Metacarpocarpal Joint, Percutaneous Approach

0RSS44Z   Reposition Right Metacarpocarpal Joint with Internal Fixation Device, Percutaneous Endoscopic Approach

0RSS45Z   Reposition Right Metacarpocarpal Joint with External Fixation Device, Percutaneous Endoscopic Approach

0RSS4ZZ   Reposition Right Metacarpocarpal Joint, Percutaneous Endoscopic Approach

0RSSX4Z   Reposition Right Metacarpocarpal Joint with Internal Fixation Device, External Approach

0RSSX5Z   Reposition Right Metacarpocarpal Joint with External Fixation Device, External Approach

0RSSXZZ   Reposition Right Metacarpocarpal Joint, External Approach

0RST04Z   Reposition Left Metacarpocarpal Joint with Internal Fixation Device, Open Approach

0RST05Z   Reposition Left Metacarpocarpal Joint with External Fixation Device, Open Approach

0RST0ZZ   Reposition Left Metacarpocarpal Joint, Open Approach

0RST34Z   Reposition Left Metacarpocarpal Joint with Internal Fixation Device, Percutaneous Approach

0RST35Z   Reposition Left Metacarpocarpal Joint with External Fixation Device, Percutaneous Approach

0RST3ZZ   Reposition Left Metacarpocarpal Joint, Percutaneous Approach

0RST44Z   Reposition Left Metacarpocarpal Joint with Internal Fixation Device, Percutaneous Endoscopic Approach

0RST45Z   Reposition Left Metacarpocarpal Joint with External Fixation Device, Percutaneous Endoscopic Approach

0RST4ZZ   Reposition Left Metacarpocarpal Joint, Percutaneous Endoscopic Approach

0RSTX4Z   Reposition Left Metacarpocarpal Joint with Internal Fixation Device, External Approach

0RSTX5Z   Reposition Left Metacarpocarpal Joint with External Fixation Device, External Approach

0RSTXZZ   Reposition Left Metacarpocarpal Joint, External Approach

0RSU04Z   Reposition Right Metacarpophalangeal Joint with Internal Fixation Device, Open Approach

0RSU05Z   Reposition Right Metacarpophalangeal Joint with External Fixation Device, Open Approach

0RSU0ZZ   Reposition Right Metacarpophalangeal Joint, Open Approach

0RSU34Z   Reposition Right Metacarpophalangeal Joint with Internal Fixation Device, Percutaneous Approach

0RSU35Z   Reposition Right Metacarpophalangeal Joint with External Fixation Device, Percutaneous Approach

0RSU3ZZ   Reposition Right Metacarpophalangeal Joint, Percutaneous Approach

0RSU44Z   Reposition Right Metacarpophalangeal Joint with Internal Fixation Device, Percutaneous Endoscopic Approach

0RSU45Z   Reposition Right Metacarpophalangeal Joint with External Fixation Device, Percutaneous Endoscopic Approach

0RSU4ZZ   Reposition Right Metacarpophalangeal Joint, Percutaneous Endoscopic Approach

0RSUX4Z   Reposition Right Metacarpophalangeal Joint with Internal Fixation Device, External Approach

0RSUX5Z   Reposition Right Metacarpophalangeal Joint with External Fixation Device, External Approach

0RSUXZZ   Reposition Right Metacarpophalangeal Joint, External Approach

0RSV04Z   Reposition Left Metacarpophalangeal Joint with Internal Fixation Device, Open Approach

0RSV05Z   Reposition Left Metacarpophalangeal Joint with External Fixation Device, Open Approach

0RSV0ZZ   Reposition Left Metacarpophalangeal Joint, Open Approach

0RSV34Z   Reposition Left Metacarpophalangeal Joint with Internal Fixation Device, Percutaneous Approach

0RSV35Z   Reposition Left Metacarpophalangeal Joint with External Fixation Device, Percutaneous Approach

0RSV3ZZ   Reposition Left Metacarpophalangeal Joint, Percutaneous Approach

0RSV44Z   Reposition Left Metacarpophalangeal Joint with Internal Fixation Device, Percutaneous Endoscopic Approach

0RSV45Z   Reposition Left Metacarpophalangeal Joint with External Fixation Device, Percutaneous Endoscopic Approach

0RSV4ZZ   Reposition Left Metacarpophalangeal Joint, Percutaneous Endoscopic Approach

0RSVX4Z   Reposition Left Metacarpophalangeal Joint with Internal Fixation Device, External Approach

0RSVX5Z   Reposition Left Metacarpophalangeal Joint with External Fixation Device, External Approach

0RSVXZZ   Reposition Left Metacarpophalangeal Joint, External Approach

0RSW04Z   Reposition Right Finger Phalangeal Joint with Internal Fixation Device, Open Approach

0RSW05Z   Reposition Right Finger Phalangeal Joint with External Fixation Device, Open Approach

0RSW0ZZ   Reposition Right Finger Phalangeal Joint, Open Approach

0RSW34Z   Reposition Right Finger Phalangeal Joint with Internal Fixation Device, Percutaneous Approach

---

♀ Female-only   ♂ Male-only   ● Limited Coverage   ● Non-OR   🄷🄰🄲 HAC-associated procedure   ⬣ Non-covered procedures   ✚ Combination

0RSW35Z   Reposition Right Finger Phalangeal Joint with External Fixation Device, Percutaneous Approach

0RSW3ZZ   Reposition Right Finger Phalangeal Joint, Percutaneous Approach

0RSW44Z   Reposition Right Finger Phalangeal Joint with Internal Fixation Device, Percutaneous Endoscopic Approach

0RSW45Z   Reposition Right Finger Phalangeal Joint with External Fixation Device, Percutaneous Endoscopic Approach

0RSW4ZZ   Reposition Right Finger Phalangeal Joint, Percutaneous Endoscopic Approach

0RSWX4Z   Reposition Right Finger Phalangeal Joint with Internal Fixation Device, External Approach

0RSWX5Z   Reposition Right Finger Phalangeal Joint with External Fixation Device, External Approach

0RSWXZZ   Reposition Right Finger Phalangeal Joint, External Approach

0RSX04Z   Reposition Left Finger Phalangeal Joint with Internal Fixation Device, Open Approach

0RSX05Z   Reposition Left Finger Phalangeal Joint with External Fixation Device, Open Approach

0RSX0ZZ   Reposition Left Finger Phalangeal Joint, Open Approach

0RSX34Z   Reposition Left Finger Phalangeal Joint with Internal Fixation Device, Percutaneous Approach

0RSX35Z   Reposition Left Finger Phalangeal Joint with External Fixation Device, Percutaneous Approach

0RSX3ZZ   Reposition Left Finger Phalangeal Joint, Percutaneous Approach

0RSX44Z   Reposition Left Finger Phalangeal Joint with Internal Fixation Device, Percutaneous Endoscopic Approach

0RSX45Z   Reposition Left Finger Phalangeal Joint with External Fixation Device, Percutaneous Endoscopic Approach

0RSX4ZZ   Reposition Left Finger Phalangeal Joint, Percutaneous Endoscopic Approach

0RSXX4Z   Reposition Left Finger Phalangeal Joint with Internal Fixation Device, External Approach

0RSXX5Z   Reposition Left Finger Phalangeal Joint with External Fixation Device, External Approach

0RSXXZZ   Reposition Left Finger Phalangeal Joint, External Approach

0RT – Upper Joints, Resection

Review Coding Guideline B3.8

0RT30ZZ   Resection of Cervical Vertebral Disc, Open Approach

0RT40ZZ   Resection of Cervicothoracic Vertebral Joint, Open Approach

0RT50ZZ   Resection of Cervicothoracic Vertebral Disc, Open Approach

0RT90ZZ   Resection of Thoracic Vertebral Disc, Open Approach

0RTB0ZZ   Resection of Thoracolumbar Vertebral Disc, Open Approach

0RTC0ZZ   Resection of Right Temporomandibular Joint, Open Approach

0RTD0ZZ   Resection of Left Temporomandibular Joint, Open Approach

0RTE0ZZ   Resection of Right Sternoclavicular Joint, Open Approach

0RTF0ZZ   Resection of Left Sternoclavicular Joint, Open Approach

0RTG0ZZ   Resection of Right Acromioclavicular Joint, Open Approach

0RTH0ZZ   Resection of Left Acromioclavicular Joint, Open Approach

0RTJ0ZZ   Resection of Right Shoulder Joint, Open Approach

0RTK0ZZ   Resection of Left Shoulder Joint, Open Approach

0RTL0ZZ   Resection of Right Elbow Joint, Open Approach

0RTM0ZZ   Resection of Left Elbow Joint, Open Approach

0RTN0ZZ   Resection of Right Wrist Joint, Open Approach

0RTP0ZZ   Resection of Left Wrist Joint, Open Approach

0RTQ0ZZ   Resection of Right Carpal Joint, Open Approach

0RTR0ZZ   Resection of Left Carpal Joint, Open Approach

0RTS0ZZ   Resection of Right Metacarpocarpal Joint, Open Approach

0RTT0ZZ   Resection of Left Metacarpocarpal Joint, Open Approach

0RTU0ZZ   Resection of Right Metacarpophalangeal Joint, Open Approach

0RTV0ZZ   Resection of Left Metacarpophalangeal Joint, Open Approach

0RTW0ZZ   Resection of Right Finger Phalangeal Joint, Open Approach

0RTX0ZZ   Resection of Left Finger Phalangeal Joint, Open Approach

0RU – Upper Joints, Supplement

0RU007Z   Supplement Occipital-cervical Joint with Autologous Tissue Substitute, Open Approach

0RU00JZ   Supplement Occipital-cervical Joint with Synthetic Substitute, Open Approach

0RU00KZ   Supplement Occipital-cervical Joint with Nonautologous Tissue Substitute, Open Approach

0RU037Z   Supplement Occipital-cervical Joint with Autologous Tissue Substitute, Percutaneous Approach

0RU03JZ   Supplement Occipital-cervical Joint with Synthetic Substitute, Percutaneous Approach

0RU03KZ   Supplement Occipital-cervical Joint with Nonautologous Tissue Substitute, Percutaneous Approach

0RU047Z   Supplement Occipital-cervical Joint with Autologous Tissue Substitute, Percutaneous Endoscopic Approach

0RU04JZ   Supplement Occipital-cervical Joint with Synthetic Substitute, Percutaneous Endoscopic Approach

0RU04KZ   Supplement Occipital-cervical Joint with Nonautologous Tissue Substitute, Percutaneous Endoscopic Approach

0RU107Z   Supplement Cervical Vertebral Joint with Autologous Tissue Substitute, Open Approach

0RU10JZ   Supplement Cervical Vertebral Joint with Synthetic Substitute, Open Approach

0RU10KZ   Supplement Cervical Vertebral Joint with Nonautologous Tissue Substitute, Open Approach

0RU137Z   Supplement Cervical Vertebral Joint with Autologous Tissue Substitute, Percutaneous Approach

0RU13JZ   Supplement Cervical Vertebral Joint with Synthetic Substitute, Percutaneous Approach

0RU13KZ   Supplement Cervical Vertebral Joint with Nonautologous Tissue Substitute, Percutaneous Approach

0RU147Z   Supplement Cervical Vertebral Joint with Autologous Tissue Substitute, Percutaneous Endoscopic Approach

0RU14JZ   Supplement Cervical Vertebral Joint with Synthetic Substitute, Percutaneous Endoscopic Approach

0RU14KZ   Supplement Cervical Vertebral Joint with Nonautologous Tissue Substitute, Percutaneous Endoscopic Approach

0RU307Z   Supplement Cervical Vertebral Disc with Autologous Tissue Substitute, Open Approach

0RU30JZ   Supplement Cervical Vertebral Disc with Synthetic Substitute, Open Approach

0RU30KZ   Supplement Cervical Vertebral Disc with Nonautologous Tissue Substitute, Open Approach

0RU337Z   Supplement Cervical Vertebral Disc with Autologous Tissue Substitute, Percutaneous Approach

0RU33JZ   Supplement Cervical Vertebral Disc with Synthetic Substitute, Percutaneous Approach

0RU33KZ   Supplement Cervical Vertebral Disc with Nonautologous Tissue Substitute, Percutaneous Approach

0RU347Z   Supplement Cervical Vertebral Disc with Autologous Tissue Substitute, Percutaneous Endoscopic Approach

0RU34JZ   Supplement Cervical Vertebral Disc with Synthetic Substitute, Percutaneous Endoscopic Approach

0RU34KZ   Supplement Cervical Vertebral Disc with Nonautologous Tissue Substitute, Percutaneous Endoscopic Approach

0RU407Z   Supplement Cervicothoracic Vertebral Joint with Autologous Tissue Substitute, Open Approach

0RU40JZ   Supplement Cervicothoracic Vertebral Joint with Synthetic Substitute, Open Approach

0RU40KZ   Supplement Cervicothoracic Vertebral Joint with Nonautologous Tissue Substitute, Open Approach

0RU437Z   Supplement Cervicothoracic Vertebral Joint with Autologous Tissue Substitute, Percutaneous Approach

0RU43JZ   Supplement Cervicothoracic Vertebral Joint with Synthetic Substitute, Percutaneous Approach

0RU43KZ   Supplement Cervicothoracic Vertebral Joint with Nonautologous Tissue Substitute, Percutaneous Approach

0RU447Z   Supplement Cervicothoracic Vertebral Joint with Autologous Tissue Substitute, Percutaneous Endoscopic Approach

0RU44JZ Supplement Cervicothoracic Vertebral Joint with Synthetic Substitute, Percutaneous Endoscopic Approach

0RU44KZ Supplement Cervicothoracic Vertebral Joint with Nonautologous Tissue Substitute, Percutaneous Endoscopic Approach

0RU507Z Supplement Cervicothoracic Vertebral Disc with Autologous Tissue Substitute, Open Approach

0RU50JZ Supplement Cervicothoracic Vertebral Disc with Synthetic Substitute, Open Approach

0RU50KZ Supplement Cervicothoracic Vertebral Disc with Nonautologous Tissue Substitute, Open Approach

0RU537Z Supplement Cervicothoracic Vertebral Disc with Autologous Tissue Substitute, Percutaneous Approach

0RU53JZ Supplement Cervicothoracic Vertebral Disc with Synthetic Substitute, Percutaneous Approach

0RU53KZ Supplement Cervicothoracic Vertebral Disc with Nonautologous Tissue Substitute, Percutaneous Approach

0RU547Z Supplement Cervicothoracic Vertebral Disc with Autologous Tissue Substitute, Percutaneous Endoscopic Approach

0RU54JZ Supplement Cervicothoracic Vertebral Disc with Synthetic Substitute, Percutaneous Endoscopic Approach

0RU54KZ Supplement Cervicothoracic Vertebral Disc with Nonautologous Tissue Substitute, Percutaneous Endoscopic Approach

0RU607Z Supplement Thoracic Vertebral Joint with Autologous Tissue Substitute, Open Approach

0RU60JZ Supplement Thoracic Vertebral Joint with Synthetic Substitute, Open Approach

0RU60KZ Supplement Thoracic Vertebral Joint with Nonautologous Tissue Substitute, Open Approach

0RU637Z Supplement Thoracic Vertebral Joint with Autologous Tissue Substitute, Percutaneous Approach

0RU63JZ Supplement Thoracic Vertebral Joint with Synthetic Substitute, Percutaneous Approach

0RU63KZ Supplement Thoracic Vertebral Joint with Nonautologous Tissue Substitute, Percutaneous Approach

0RU647Z Supplement Thoracic Vertebral Joint with Autologous Tissue Substitute, Percutaneous Endoscopic Approach

0RU64JZ Supplement Thoracic Vertebral Joint with Synthetic Substitute, Percutaneous Endoscopic Approach

0RU64KZ Supplement Thoracic Vertebral Joint with Nonautologous Tissue Substitute, Percutaneous Endoscopic Approach

0RU907Z Supplement Thoracic Vertebral Disc with Autologous Tissue Substitute, Open Approach

0RU90JZ Supplement Thoracic Vertebral Disc with Synthetic Substitute, Open Approach

0RU90KZ Supplement Thoracic Vertebral Disc with Nonautologous Tissue Substitute, Open Approach

0RU937Z Supplement Thoracic Vertebral Disc with Autologous Tissue Substitute, Percutaneous Approach

0RU93JZ Supplement Thoracic Vertebral Disc with Synthetic Substitute, Percutaneous Approach

0RU93KZ Supplement Thoracic Vertebral Disc with Nonautologous Tissue Substitute, Percutaneous Approach

0RU947Z Supplement Thoracic Vertebral Disc with Autologous Tissue Substitute, Percutaneous Endoscopic Approach

0RU94JZ Supplement Thoracic Vertebral Disc with Synthetic Substitute, Percutaneous Endoscopic Approach

0RU94KZ Supplement Thoracic Vertebral Disc with Nonautologous Tissue Substitute, Percutaneous Endoscopic Approach

0RUA07Z Supplement Thoracolumbar Vertebral Joint with Autologous Tissue Substitute, Open Approach

0RUA0JZ Supplement Thoracolumbar Vertebral Joint with Synthetic Substitute, Open Approach

0RUA0KZ Supplement Thoracolumbar Vertebral Joint with Nonautologous Tissue Substitute, Open Approach

0RUA37Z Supplement Thoracolumbar Vertebral Joint with Autologous Tissue Substitute, Percutaneous Approach

0RUA3JZ Supplement Thoracolumbar Vertebral Joint with Synthetic Substitute, Percutaneous Approach

0RUA3KZ Supplement Thoracolumbar Vertebral Joint with Nonautologous Tissue Substitute, Percutaneous Approach

0RUA47Z Supplement Thoracolumbar Vertebral Joint with Autologous Tissue Substitute, Percutaneous Endoscopic Approach

0RUA4JZ Supplement Thoracolumbar Vertebral Joint with Synthetic Substitute, Percutaneous Endoscopic Approach

0RUA4KZ Supplement Thoracolumbar Vertebral Joint with Nonautologous Tissue Substitute, Percutaneous Endoscopic Approach

0RUB07Z Supplement Thoracolumbar Vertebral Disc with Autologous Tissue Substitute, Open Approach

0RUB0JZ Supplement Thoracolumbar Vertebral Disc with Synthetic Substitute, Open Approach

0RUB0KZ Supplement Thoracolumbar Vertebral Disc with Nonautologous Tissue Substitute, Open Approach

0RUB37Z Supplement Thoracolumbar Vertebral Disc with Autologous Tissue Substitute, Percutaneous Approach

0RUB3JZ Supplement Thoracolumbar Vertebral Disc with Synthetic Substitute, Percutaneous Approach

0RUB3KZ Supplement Thoracolumbar Vertebral Disc with Nonautologous Tissue Substitute, Percutaneous Approach

0RUB47Z Supplement Thoracolumbar Vertebral Disc with Autologous Tissue Substitute, Percutaneous Endoscopic Approach

0RUB4JZ Supplement Thoracolumbar Vertebral Disc with Synthetic Substitute, Percutaneous Endoscopic Approach

0RUB4KZ Supplement Thoracolumbar Vertebral Disc with Nonautologous Tissue Substitute, Percutaneous Endoscopic Approach

0RUC07Z Supplement Right Temporomandibular Joint with Autologous Tissue Substitute, Open Approach

0RUC0JZ Supplement Right Temporomandibular Joint with Synthetic Substitute, Open Approach

0RUC0KZ Supplement Right Temporomandibular Joint with Nonautologous Tissue Substitute, Open Approach

0RUC37Z Supplement Right Temporomandibular Joint with Autologous Tissue Substitute, Percutaneous Approach

0RUC3JZ Supplement Right Temporomandibular Joint with Synthetic Substitute, Percutaneous Approach

0RUC3KZ Supplement Right Temporomandibular Joint with Nonautologous Tissue Substitute, Percutaneous Approach

0RUC47Z Supplement Right Temporomandibular Joint with Autologous Tissue Substitute, Percutaneous Endoscopic Approach

0RUC4JZ Supplement Right Temporomandibular Joint with Synthetic Substitute, Percutaneous Endoscopic Approach

0RUC4KZ Supplement Right Temporomandibular Joint with Nonautologous Tissue Substitute, Percutaneous Endoscopic Approach

0RUD07Z Supplement Left Temporomandibular Joint with Autologous Tissue Substitute, Open Approach

0RUD0JZ Supplement Left Temporomandibular Joint with Synthetic Substitute, Open Approach

0RUD0KZ Supplement Left Temporomandibular Joint with Nonautologous Tissue Substitute, Open Approach

0RUD37Z Supplement Left Temporomandibular Joint with Autologous Tissue Substitute, Percutaneous Approach

0RUD3JZ Supplement Left Temporomandibular Joint with Synthetic Substitute, Percutaneous Approach

0RUD3KZ Supplement Left Temporomandibular Joint with Nonautologous Tissue Substitute, Percutaneous Approach

0RUD47Z Supplement Left Temporomandibular Joint with Autologous Tissue Substitute, Percutaneous Endoscopic Approach

0RUD4JZ Supplement Left Temporomandibular Joint with Synthetic Substitute, Percutaneous Endoscopic Approach

0RUD4KZ Supplement Left Temporomandibular Joint with Nonautologous Tissue Substitute, Percutaneous Endoscopic Approach

0RUE07Z Supplement Right Sternoclavicular Joint with Autologous Tissue Substitute, Open Approach

HAC When reported with secondary diagnosis code T84.60XA, T84.610A, T84.611A, T84.612A, T84.613A, T84.614A, T84.615A, T84.619A, T84.63XA, T84.69XA, T84.7XXA

0RUE0JZ Supplement Right Sternoclavicular Joint with Synthetic Substitute, Open Approach

HAC When reported with secondary diagnosis code T84.60XA, T84.610A, T84.611A, T84.612A, T84.613A, T84.614A, T84.615A, T84.619A, T84.63XA, T84.69XA, T84.7XXA

0RUE0KZ Supplement Right Sternoclavicular Joint with Nonautologous Tissue Substitute, Open Approach

HAC When reported with secondary diagnosis code T84.60XA, T84.610A, T84.611A, T84.612A, T84.613A, T84.614A, T84.615A, T84.619A, T84.63XA, T84.69XA, T84.7XXA

♀ Female-only   ♂ Male-only   ⬤ Limited Coverage   ● Non-OR   HAC HAC-associated procedure   ⬤ Non-covered procedures   ✛ Combination

0RUE37Z   Supplement Right Sternoclavicular Joint with Autologous Tissue Substitute, Percutaneous Approach
- HAC   When reported with secondary diagnosis code T84.60XA, T84.610A, T84.611A, T84.612A, T84.613A, T84.614A, T84.615A, T84.619A, T84.63XA, T84.69XA, T84.7XXA

0RUE3JZ   Supplement Right Sternoclavicular Joint with Synthetic Substitute, Percutaneous Approach
- HAC   When reported with secondary diagnosis code T84.60XA, T84.610A, T84.611A, T84.612A, T84.613A, T84.614A, T84.615A, T84.619A, T84.63XA, T84.69XA, T84.7XXA

0RUE3KZ   Supplement Right Sternoclavicular Joint with Nonautologous Tissue Substitute, Percutaneous Approach
- HAC   When reported with secondary diagnosis code T84.60XA, T84.610A, T84.611A, T84.612A, T84.613A, T84.614A, T84.615A, T84.619A, T84.63XA, T84.69XA, T84.7XXA

0RUE47Z   Supplement Right Sternoclavicular Joint with Autologous Tissue Substitute, Percutaneous Endoscopic Approach
- HAC   When reported with secondary diagnosis code T84.60XA, T84.610A, T84.611A, T84.612A, T84.613A, T84.614A, T84.615A, T84.619A, T84.63XA, T84.69XA, T84.7XXA

0RUE4JZ   Supplement Right Sternoclavicular Joint with Synthetic Substitute, Percutaneous Endoscopic Approach
- HAC   When reported with secondary diagnosis code T84.60XA, T84.610A, T84.611A, T84.612A, T84.613A, T84.614A, T84.615A, T84.619A, T84.63XA, T84.69XA, T84.7XXA

0RUE4KZ   Supplement Right Sternoclavicular Joint with Nonautologous Tissue Substitute, Percutaneous Endoscopic Approach
- HAC   When reported with secondary diagnosis code T84.60XA, T84.610A, T84.611A, T84.612A, T84.613A, T84.614A, T84.615A, T84.619A, T84.63XA, T84.69XA, T84.7XXA

0RUF07Z   Supplement Left Sternoclavicular Joint with Autologous Tissue Substitute, Open Approach
- HAC   When reported with secondary diagnosis code T84.60XA, T84.610A, T84.611A, T84.612A, T84.613A, T84.614A, T84.615A, T84.619A, T84.63XA, T84.69XA, T84.7XXA

0RUF0JZ   Supplement Left Sternoclavicular Joint with Synthetic Substitute, Open Approach
- HAC   When reported with secondary diagnosis code T84.60XA, T84.610A, T84.611A, T84.612A, T84.613A, T84.614A, T84.615A, T84.619A, T84.63XA, T84.69XA, T84.7XXA

0RUF0KZ   Supplement Left Sternoclavicular Joint with Nonautologous Tissue Substitute, Open Approach
- HAC   When reported with secondary diagnosis code T84.60XA, T84.610A, T84.611A, T84.612A, T84.613A, T84.614A, T84.615A, T84.619A, T84.63XA, T84.69XA, T84.7XXA

0RUF37Z   Supplement Left Sternoclavicular Joint with Autologous Tissue Substitute, Percutaneous Approach
- HAC   When reported with secondary diagnosis code T84.60XA, T84.610A, T84.611A, T84.612A, T84.613A, T84.614A, T84.615A, T84.619A, T84.63XA, T84.69XA, T84.7XXA

0RUF3JZ   Supplement Left Sternoclavicular Joint with Synthetic Substitute, Percutaneous Approach
- HAC   When reported with secondary diagnosis code T84.60XA, T84.610A, T84.611A, T84.612A, T84.613A, T84.614A, T84.615A, T84.619A, T84.63XA, T84.69XA, T84.7XXA

0RUF3KZ   Supplement Left Sternoclavicular Joint with Nonautologous Tissue Substitute, Percutaneous Approach
- HAC   When reported with secondary diagnosis code T84.60XA, T84.610A, T84.611A, T84.612A, T84.613A, T84.614A, T84.615A, T84.619A, T84.63XA, T84.69XA, T84.7XXA

0RUF47Z   Supplement Left Sternoclavicular Joint with Autologous Tissue Substitute, Percutaneous Endoscopic Approach
- HAC   When reported with secondary diagnosis code T84.60XA, T84.610A, T84.611A, T84.612A, T84.613A, T84.614A, T84.615A, T84.619A, T84.63XA, T84.69XA, T84.7XXA

0RUF4JZ   Supplement Left Sternoclavicular Joint with Synthetic Substitute, Percutaneous Endoscopic Approach
- HAC   When reported with secondary diagnosis code T84.60XA, T84.610A, T84.611A, T84.612A, T84.613A, T84.614A, T84.615A, T84.619A, T84.63XA, T84.69XA, T84.7XXA

0RUF4KZ   Supplement Left Sternoclavicular Joint with Nonautologous Tissue Substitute, Percutaneous Endoscopic Approach
- HAC   When reported with secondary diagnosis code T84.60XA, T84.610A, T84.611A, T84.612A, T84.613A, T84.614A, T84.615A, T84.619A, T84.63XA, T84.69XA, T84.7XXA

0RUG07Z   Supplement Right Acromioclavicular Joint with Autologous Tissue Substitute, Open Approach
- HAC   When reported with secondary diagnosis code T84.60XA, T84.610A, T84.611A, T84.612A, T84.613A, T84.614A, T84.615A, T84.619A, T84.63XA, T84.69XA, T84.7XXA

0RUG0JZ   Supplement Right Acromioclavicular Joint with Synthetic Substitute, Open Approach
- HAC   When reported with secondary diagnosis code T84.60XA, T84.610A, T84.611A, T84.612A, T84.613A, T84.614A, T84.615A, T84.619A, T84.63XA, T84.69XA, T84.7XXA

0RUG0KZ   Supplement Right Acromioclavicular Joint with Nonautologous Tissue Substitute, Open Approach
- HAC   When reported with secondary diagnosis code T84.60XA, T84.610A, T84.611A, T84.612A, T84.613A, T84.614A, T84.615A, T84.619A, T84.63XA, T84.69XA, T84.7XXA

0RUG37Z   Supplement Right Acromioclavicular Joint with Autologous Tissue Substitute, Percutaneous Approach
- HAC   When reported with secondary diagnosis code T84.60XA, T84.610A, T84.611A, T84.612A, T84.613A, T84.614A, T84.615A, T84.619A, T84.63XA, T84.69XA, T84.7XXA

0RUG3JZ   Supplement Right Acromioclavicular Joint with Synthetic Substitute, Percutaneous Approach
- HAC   When reported with secondary diagnosis code T84.60XA, T84.610A, T84.611A, T84.612A, T84.613A, T84.614A, T84.615A, T84.619A, T84.63XA, T84.69XA, T84.7XXA

0RUG3KZ   Supplement Right Acromioclavicular Joint with Nonautologous Tissue Substitute, Percutaneous Approach
- HAC   When reported with secondary diagnosis code T84.60XA, T84.610A, T84.611A, T84.612A, T84.613A, T84.614A, T84.615A, T84.619A, T84.63XA, T84.69XA, T84.7XXA

0RUG47Z   Supplement Right Acromioclavicular Joint with Autologous Tissue Substitute, Percutaneous Endoscopic Approach
- HAC   When reported with secondary diagnosis code T84.60XA, T84.610A, T84.611A, T84.612A, T84.613A, T84.614A, T84.615A, T84.619A, T84.63XA, T84.69XA, T84.7XXA

0RUG4JZ   Supplement Right Acromioclavicular Joint with Synthetic Substitute, Percutaneous Endoscopic Approach
- HAC   When reported with secondary diagnosis code T84.60XA, T84.610A, T84.611A, T84.612A, T84.613A, T84.614A, T84.615A, T84.619A, T84.63XA, T84.69XA, T84.7XXA

0RUG4KZ   Supplement Right Acromioclavicular Joint with Nonautologous Tissue Substitute, Percutaneous Endoscopic Approach
- HAC   When reported with secondary diagnosis code T84.60XA, T84.610A, T84.611A, T84.612A, T84.613A, T84.614A, T84.615A, T84.619A, T84.63XA, T84.69XA, T84.7XXA

0RUH07Z   Supplement Left Acromioclavicular Joint with Autologous Tissue Substitute, Open Approach
- HAC   When reported with secondary diagnosis code T84.60XA, T84.610A, T84.611A, T84.612A, T84.613A, T84.614A, T84.615A, T84.619A, T84.63XA, T84.69XA, T84.7XXA

0RUH0JZ   Supplement Left Acromioclavicular Joint with Synthetic Substitute, Open Approach
- HAC   When reported with secondary diagnosis code T84.60XA, T84.610A, T84.611A, T84.612A, T84.613A, T84.614A, T84.615A, T84.619A, T84.63XA, T84.69XA, T84.7XXA

0RUH0KZ   Supplement Left Acromioclavicular Joint with Nonautologous Tissue Substitute, Open Approach
- HAC   When reported with secondary diagnosis code T84.60XA, T84.610A, T84.611A, T84.612A, T84.613A, T84.614A, T84.615A, T84.619A, T84.63XA, T84.69XA, T84.7XXA

0RUH37Z   Supplement Left Acromioclavicular Joint with Autologous Tissue Substitute, Percutaneous Approach
- HAC   When reported with secondary diagnosis code T84.60XA, T84.610A, T84.611A, T84.612A, T84.613A, T84.614A, T84.615A, T84.619A, T84.63XA, T84.69XA, T84.7XXA

0RUH3JZ   Supplement Left Acromioclavicular Joint with Synthetic Substitute, Percutaneous Approach
- HAC   When reported with secondary diagnosis code T84.60XA, T84.610A, T84.611A, T84.612A, T84.613A, T84.614A, T84.615A, T84.619A, T84.63XA, T84.69XA, T84.7XXA

0RUH3KZ   Supplement Left Acromioclavicular Joint with Nonautologous Tissue Substitute, Percutaneous Approach
- HAC   When reported with secondary diagnosis code T84.60XA, T84.610A, T84.611A, T84.612A, T84.613A, T84.614A, T84.615A, T84.619A, T84.63XA, T84.69XA, T84.7XXA

♀ Female-only   ♂ Male-only   ● Limited Coverage   ● Non-OR   HAC HAC-associated procedure   ⬣ Non-covered procedures   ✚ Combination

0RUH47Z Supplement Left Acromioclavicular Joint with Autologous Tissue Substitute, Percutaneous Endoscopic Approach
> **HAC** When reported with secondary diagnosis code T84.60XA, T84.610A, T84.611A, T84.612A, T84.613A, T84.614A, T84.615A, T84.619A, T84.63XA, T84.69XA, T84.7XXA

0RUH4JZ Supplement Left Acromioclavicular Joint with Synthetic Substitute, Percutaneous Endoscopic Approach
> **HAC** When reported with secondary diagnosis code T84.60XA, T84.610A, T84.611A, T84.612A, T84.613A, T84.614A, T84.615A, T84.619A, T84.63XA, T84.69XA, T84.7XXA

0RUH4KZ Supplement Left Acromioclavicular Joint with Nonautologous Tissue Substitute, Percutaneous Endoscopic Approach
> **HAC** When reported with secondary diagnosis code T84.60XA, T84.610A, T84.611A, T84.612A, T84.613A, T84.614A, T84.615A, T84.619A, T84.63XA, T84.69XA, T84.7XXA

0RUJ07Z Supplement Right Shoulder Joint with Autologous Tissue Substitute, Open Approach
> **HAC** When reported with secondary diagnosis code T84.60XA, T84.610A, T84.611A, T84.612A, T84.613A, T84.614A, T84.615A, T84.619A, T84.63XA, T84.69XA, T84.7XXA

0RUJ0JZ Supplement Right Shoulder Joint with Synthetic Substitute, Open Approach
> **HAC** When reported with secondary diagnosis code T84.60XA, T84.610A, T84.611A, T84.612A, T84.613A, T84.614A, T84.615A, T84.619A, T84.63XA, T84.69XA, T84.7XXA

0RUJ0KZ Supplement Right Shoulder Joint with Nonautologous Tissue Substitute, Open Approach
> **HAC** When reported with secondary diagnosis code T84.60XA, T84.610A, T84.611A, T84.612A, T84.613A, T84.614A, T84.615A, T84.619A, T84.63XA, T84.69XA, T84.7XXA

0RUJ37Z Supplement Right Shoulder Joint with Autologous Tissue Substitute, Percutaneous Approach
> **HAC** When reported with secondary diagnosis code T84.60XA, T84.610A, T84.611A, T84.612A, T84.613A, T84.614A, T84.615A, T84.619A, T84.63XA, T84.69XA, T84.7XXA

0RUJ3JZ Supplement Right Shoulder Joint with Synthetic Substitute, Percutaneous Approach
> **HAC** When reported with secondary diagnosis code T84.60XA, T84.610A, T84.611A, T84.612A, T84.613A, T84.614A, T84.615A, T84.619A, T84.63XA, T84.69XA, T84.7XXA

0RUJ3KZ Supplement Right Shoulder Joint with Nonautologous Tissue Substitute, Percutaneous Approach
> **HAC** When reported with secondary diagnosis code T84.60XA, T84.610A, T84.611A, T84.612A, T84.613A, T84.614A, T84.615A, T84.619A, T84.63XA, T84.69XA, T84.7XXA

0RUJ47Z Supplement Right Shoulder Joint with Autologous Tissue Substitute, Percutaneous Endoscopic Approach
> **HAC** When reported with secondary diagnosis code T84.60XA, T84.610A, T84.611A, T84.612A, T84.613A, T84.614A, T84.615A, T84.619A, T84.63XA, T84.69XA, T84.7XXA

0RUJ4JZ Supplement Right Shoulder Joint with Synthetic Substitute, Percutaneous Endoscopic Approach
> **HAC** When reported with secondary diagnosis code T84.60XA, T84.610A, T84.611A, T84.612A, T84.613A, T84.614A, T84.615A, T84.619A, T84.63XA, T84.69XA, T84.7XXA

0RUJ4KZ Supplement Right Shoulder Joint with Nonautologous Tissue Substitute, Percutaneous Endoscopic Approach
> **HAC** When reported with secondary diagnosis code T84.60XA, T84.610A, T84.611A, T84.612A, T84.613A, T84.614A, T84.615A, T84.619A, T84.63XA, T84.69XA, T84.7XXA

0RUK07Z Supplement Left Shoulder Joint with Autologous Tissue Substitute, Open Approach
> **HAC** When reported with secondary diagnosis code T84.60XA, T84.610A, T84.611A, T84.612A, T84.613A, T84.614A, T84.615A, T84.619A, T84.63XA, T84.69XA, T84.7XXA

0RUK0JZ Supplement Left Shoulder Joint with Synthetic Substitute, Open Approach
> **HAC** When reported with secondary diagnosis code T84.60XA, T84.610A, T84.611A, T84.612A, T84.613A, T84.614A, T84.615A, T84.619A, T84.63XA, T84.69XA, T84.7XXA

0RUK0KZ Supplement Left Shoulder Joint with Nonautologous Tissue Substitute, Open Approach
> **HAC** When reported with secondary diagnosis code T84.60XA, T84.610A, T84.611A, T84.612A, T84.613A, T84.614A, T84.615A, T84.619A, T84.63XA, T84.69XA, T84.7XXA

0RUK37Z Supplement Left Shoulder Joint with Autologous Tissue Substitute, Percutaneous Approach
> **HAC** When reported with secondary diagnosis code T84.60XA, T84.610A, T84.611A, T84.612A, T84.613A, T84.614A, T84.615A, T84.619A, T84.63XA, T84.69XA, T84.7XXA

0RUK3JZ Supplement Left Shoulder Joint with Synthetic Substitute, Percutaneous Approach
> **HAC** When reported with secondary diagnosis code T84.60XA, T84.610A, T84.611A, T84.612A, T84.613A, T84.614A, T84.615A, T84.619A, T84.63XA, T84.69XA, T84.7XXA

0RUK3KZ Supplement Left Shoulder Joint with Nonautologous Tissue Substitute, Percutaneous Approach
> **HAC** When reported with secondary diagnosis code T84.60XA, T84.610A, T84.611A, T84.612A, T84.613A, T84.614A, T84.615A, T84.619A, T84.63XA, T84.69XA, T84.7XXA

0RUK47Z Supplement Left Shoulder Joint with Autologous Tissue Substitute, Percutaneous Endoscopic Approach
> **HAC** When reported with secondary diagnosis code T84.60XA, T84.610A, T84.611A, T84.612A, T84.613A, T84.614A, T84.615A, T84.619A, T84.63XA, T84.69XA, T84.7XXA

0RUK4JZ Supplement Left Shoulder Joint with Synthetic Substitute, Percutaneous Endoscopic Approach
> **HAC** When reported with secondary diagnosis code T84.60XA, T84.610A, T84.611A, T84.612A, T84.613A, T84.614A, T84.615A, T84.619A, T84.63XA, T84.69XA, T84.7XXA

0RUK4KZ Supplement Left Shoulder Joint with Nonautologous Tissue Substitute, Percutaneous Endoscopic Approach
> **HAC** When reported with secondary diagnosis code T84.60XA, T84.610A, T84.611A, T84.612A, T84.613A, T84.614A, T84.615A, T84.619A, T84.63XA, T84.69XA, T84.7XXA

0RUL07Z Supplement Right Elbow Joint with Autologous Tissue Substitute, Open Approach
> **HAC** When reported with secondary diagnosis code T84.60XA, T84.610A, T84.611A, T84.612A, T84.613A, T84.614A, T84.615A, T84.619A, T84.63XA, T84.69XA, T84.7XXA

0RUL0JZ Supplement Right Elbow Joint with Synthetic Substitute, Open Approach
> **HAC** When reported with secondary diagnosis code T84.60XA, T84.610A, T84.611A, T84.612A, T84.613A, T84.614A, T84.615A, T84.619A, T84.63XA, T84.69XA, T84.7XXA

0RUL0KZ Supplement Right Elbow Joint with Nonautologous Tissue Substitute, Open Approach
> **HAC** When reported with secondary diagnosis code T84.60XA, T84.610A, T84.611A, T84.612A, T84.613A, T84.614A, T84.615A, T84.619A, T84.63XA, T84.69XA, T84.7XXA

0RUL37Z Supplement Right Elbow Joint with Autologous Tissue Substitute, Percutaneous Approach
> **HAC** When reported with secondary diagnosis code T84.60XA, T84.610A, T84.611A, T84.612A, T84.613A, T84.614A, T84.615A, T84.619A, T84.63XA, T84.69XA, T84.7XXA

0RUL3JZ Supplement Right Elbow Joint with Synthetic Substitute, Percutaneous Approach
> **HAC** When reported with secondary diagnosis code T84.60XA, T84.610A, T84.611A, T84.612A, T84.613A, T84.614A, T84.615A, T84.619A, T84.63XA, T84.69XA, T84.7XXA

0RUL3KZ Supplement Right Elbow Joint with Nonautologous Tissue Substitute, Percutaneous Approach
> **HAC** When reported with secondary diagnosis code T84.60XA, T84.610A, T84.611A, T84.612A, T84.613A, T84.614A, T84.615A, T84.619A, T84.63XA, T84.69XA, T84.7XXA

0RUL47Z Supplement Right Elbow Joint with Autologous Tissue Substitute, Percutaneous Endoscopic Approach
> **HAC** When reported with secondary diagnosis code T84.60XA, T84.610A, T84.611A, T84.612A, T84.613A, T84.614A, T84.615A, T84.619A, T84.63XA, T84.69XA, T84.7XXA

0RUL4JZ Supplement Right Elbow Joint with Synthetic Substitute, Percutaneous Endoscopic Approach
> **HAC** When reported with secondary diagnosis code T84.60XA, T84.610A, T84.611A, T84.612A, T84.613A, T84.614A, T84.615A, T84.619A, T84.63XA, T84.69XA, T84.7XXA

0RUL4KZ Supplement Right Elbow Joint with Nonautologous Tissue Substitute, Percutaneous Endoscopic Approach
> **HAC** When reported with secondary diagnosis code T84.60XA, T84.610A, T84.611A, T84.612A, T84.613A, T84.614A, T84.615A, T84.619A, T84.63XA, T84.69XA, T84.7XXA

♀ Female-only   ♂ Male-only   ◐ Limited Coverage   ● Non-OR   **HAC** HAC-associated procedure   ⬤ Non-covered procedures   ➕ Combination

0RUM07Z Supplement Left Elbow Joint with Autologous Tissue Substitute, Open Approach
   HAC When reported with secondary diagnosis code T84.60XA, T84.610A, T84.611A, T84.612A, T84.613A, T84.614A, T84.615A, T84.619A, T84.63XA, T84.69XA, T84.7XXA

0RUM0JZ Supplement Left Elbow Joint with Synthetic Substitute, Open Approach
   HAC When reported with secondary diagnosis code T84.60XA, T84.610A, T84.611A, T84.612A, T84.613A, T84.614A, T84.615A, T84.619A, T84.63XA, T84.69XA, T84.7XXA

0RUM0KZ Supplement Left Elbow Joint with Nonautologous Tissue Substitute, Open Approach
   HAC When reported with secondary diagnosis code T84.60XA, T84.610A, T84.611A, T84.612A, T84.613A, T84.614A, T84.615A, T84.619A, T84.63XA, T84.69XA, T84.7XXA

0RUM37Z Supplement Left Elbow Joint with Autologous Tissue Substitute, Percutaneous Approach
   HAC When reported with secondary diagnosis code T84.60XA, T84.610A, T84.611A, T84.612A, T84.613A, T84.614A, T84.615A, T84.619A, T84.63XA, T84.69XA, T84.7XXA

0RUM3JZ Supplement Left Elbow Joint with Synthetic Substitute, Percutaneous Approach
   HAC When reported with secondary diagnosis code T84.60XA, T84.610A, T84.611A, T84.612A, T84.613A, T84.614A, T84.615A, T84.619A, T84.63XA, T84.69XA, T84.7XXA

0RUM3KZ Supplement Left Elbow Joint with Nonautologous Tissue Substitute, Percutaneous Approach
   HAC When reported with secondary diagnosis code T84.60XA, T84.610A, T84.611A, T84.612A, T84.613A, T84.614A, T84.615A, T84.619A, T84.63XA, T84.69XA, T84.7XXA

0RUM47Z Supplement Left Elbow Joint with Autologous Tissue Substitute, Percutaneous Endoscopic Approach
   HAC When reported with secondary diagnosis code T84.60XA, T84.610A, T84.611A, T84.612A, T84.613A, T84.614A, T84.615A, T84.619A, T84.63XA, T84.69XA, T84.7XXA

0RUM4JZ Supplement Left Elbow Joint with Synthetic Substitute, Percutaneous Endoscopic Approach
   HAC When reported with secondary diagnosis code T84.60XA, T84.610A, T84.611A, T84.612A, T84.613A, T84.614A, T84.615A, T84.619A, T84.63XA, T84.69XA, T84.7XXA

0RUM4KZ Supplement Left Elbow Joint with Nonautologous Tissue Substitute, Percutaneous Endoscopic Approach
   HAC When reported with secondary diagnosis code T84.60XA, T84.610A, T84.611A, T84.612A, T84.613A, T84.614A, T84.615A, T84.619A, T84.63XA, T84.69XA, T84.7XXA

0RUN07Z Supplement Right Wrist Joint with Autologous Tissue Substitute, Open Approach

0RUN0JZ Supplement Right Wrist Joint with Synthetic Substitute, Open Approach

0RUN0KZ Supplement Right Wrist Joint with Nonautologous Tissue Substitute, Open Approach

0RUN37Z Supplement Right Wrist Joint with Autologous Tissue Substitute, Percutaneous Approach

0RUN3JZ Supplement Right Wrist Joint with Synthetic Substitute, Percutaneous Approach

0RUN3KZ Supplement Right Wrist Joint with Nonautologous Tissue Substitute, Percutaneous Approach

0RUN47Z Supplement Right Wrist Joint with Autologous Tissue Substitute, Percutaneous Endoscopic Approach

0RUN4JZ Supplement Right Wrist Joint with Synthetic Substitute, Percutaneous Endoscopic Approach

0RUN4KZ Supplement Right Wrist Joint with Nonautologous Tissue Substitute, Percutaneous Endoscopic Approach

0RUP07Z Supplement Left Wrist Joint with Autologous Tissue Substitute, Open Approach

0RUP0JZ Supplement Left Wrist Joint with Synthetic Substitute, Open Approach

0RUP0KZ Supplement Left Wrist Joint with Nonautologous Tissue Substitute, Open Approach

0RUP37Z Supplement Left Wrist Joint with Autologous Tissue Substitute, Percutaneous Approach

0RUP3JZ Supplement Left Wrist Joint with Synthetic Substitute, Percutaneous Approach

0RUP3KZ Supplement Left Wrist Joint with Nonautologous Tissue Substitute, Percutaneous Approach

0RUP47Z Supplement Left Wrist Joint with Autologous Tissue Substitute, Percutaneous Endoscopic Approach

0RUP4JZ Supplement Left Wrist Joint with Synthetic Substitute, Percutaneous Endoscopic Approach

0RUP4KZ Supplement Left Wrist Joint with Nonautologous Tissue Substitute, Percutaneous Endoscopic Approach

0RUQ07Z Supplement Right Carpal Joint with Autologous Tissue Substitute, Open Approach

0RUQ0JZ Supplement Right Carpal Joint with Synthetic Substitute, Open Approach

0RUQ0KZ Supplement Right Carpal Joint with Nonautologous Tissue Substitute, Open Approach

0RUQ37Z Supplement Right Carpal Joint with Autologous Tissue Substitute, Percutaneous Approach

0RUQ3JZ Supplement Right Carpal Joint with Synthetic Substitute, Percutaneous Approach

0RUQ3KZ Supplement Right Carpal Joint with Nonautologous Tissue Substitute, Percutaneous Approach

0RUQ47Z Supplement Right Carpal Joint with Autologous Tissue Substitute, Percutaneous Endoscopic Approach

0RUQ4JZ Supplement Right Carpal Joint with Synthetic Substitute, Percutaneous Endoscopic Approach

0RUQ4KZ Supplement Right Carpal Joint with Nonautologous Tissue Substitute, Percutaneous Endoscopic Approach

0RUR07Z Supplement Left Carpal Joint with Autologous Tissue Substitute, Open Approach

0RUR0JZ Supplement Left Carpal Joint with Synthetic Substitute, Open Approach

0RUR0KZ Supplement Left Carpal Joint with Nonautologous Tissue Substitute, Open Approach

0RUR37Z Supplement Left Carpal Joint with Autologous Tissue Substitute, Percutaneous Approach

0RUR3JZ Supplement Left Carpal Joint with Synthetic Substitute, Percutaneous Approach

0RUR3KZ Supplement Left Carpal Joint with Nonautologous Tissue Substitute, Percutaneous Approach

0RUR47Z Supplement Left Carpal Joint with Autologous Tissue Substitute, Percutaneous Endoscopic Approach

0RUR4JZ Supplement Left Carpal Joint with Synthetic Substitute, Percutaneous Endoscopic Approach

0RUR4KZ Supplement Left Carpal Joint with Nonautologous Tissue Substitute, Percutaneous Endoscopic Approach

0RUS07Z Supplement Right Metacarpocarpal Joint with Autologous Tissue Substitute, Open Approach

0RUS0JZ Supplement Right Metacarpocarpal Joint with Synthetic Substitute, Open Approach

0RUS0KZ Supplement Right Metacarpocarpal Joint with Nonautologous Tissue Substitute, Open Approach

0RUS37Z Supplement Right Metacarpocarpal Joint with Autologous Tissue Substitute, Percutaneous Approach

0RUS3JZ Supplement Right Metacarpocarpal Joint with Synthetic Substitute, Percutaneous Approach

0RUS3KZ Supplement Right Metacarpocarpal Joint with Nonautologous Tissue Substitute, Percutaneous Approach

0RUS47Z Supplement Right Metacarpocarpal Joint with Autologous Tissue Substitute, Percutaneous Endoscopic Approach

0RUS4JZ Supplement Right Metacarpocarpal Joint with Synthetic Substitute, Percutaneous Endoscopic Approach

0RUS4KZ Supplement Right Metacarpocarpal Joint with Nonautologous Tissue Substitute, Percutaneous Endoscopic Approach

0RUT07Z Supplement Left Metacarpocarpal Joint with Autologous Tissue Substitute, Open Approach

0RUT0JZ Supplement Left Metacarpocarpal Joint with Synthetic Substitute, Open Approach

0RUT0KZ Supplement Left Metacarpocarpal Joint with Nonautologous Tissue Substitute, Open Approach

0RUT37Z Supplement Left Metacarpocarpal Joint with Autologous Tissue Substitute, Percutaneous Approach

0RUT3JZ Supplement Left Metacarpocarpal Joint with Synthetic Substitute, Percutaneous Approach

0RUT3KZ Supplement Left Metacarpocarpal Joint with Nonautologous Tissue Substitute, Percutaneous Approach

0RUT47Z Supplement Left Metacarpocarpal Joint with Autologous Tissue Substitute, Percutaneous Endoscopic Approach

0RUT4JZ Supplement Left Metacarpocarpal Joint with Synthetic Substitute, Percutaneous Endoscopic Approach

0RUT4KZ Supplement Left Metacarpocarpal Joint with Nonautologous Tissue Substitute, Percutaneous Endoscopic Approach

0RUU07Z Supplement Right Metacarpophalangeal Joint with Autologous Tissue Substitute, Open Approach

0RUU0JZ Supplement Right Metacarpophalangeal Joint with Synthetic Substitute, Open Approach

0RUU0KZ Supplement Right Metacarpophalangeal Joint with Nonautologous Tissue Substitute, Open Approach

0RUU37Z Supplement Right Metacarpophalangeal Joint with Autologous Tissue Substitute, Percutaneous Approach

0RUU3JZ Supplement Right Metacarpophalangeal Joint with Synthetic Substitute, Percutaneous Approach

0RUU3KZ Supplement Right Metacarpophalangeal Joint with Nonautologous Tissue Substitute, Percutaneous Approach

0RUU47Z Supplement Right Metacarpophalangeal Joint with Autologous Tissue Substitute, Percutaneous Endoscopic Approach

0RUU4JZ Supplement Right Metacarpophalangeal Joint with Synthetic Substitute, Percutaneous Endoscopic Approach

0RUU4KZ Supplement Right Metacarpophalangeal Joint with Nonautologous Tissue Substitute, Percutaneous Endoscopic Approach

0RUV07Z Supplement Left Metacarpophalangeal Joint with Autologous Tissue Substitute, Open Approach

0RUV0JZ Supplement Left Metacarpophalangeal Joint with Synthetic Substitute, Open Approach

0RUV0KZ Supplement Left Metacarpophalangeal Joint with Nonautologous Tissue Substitute, Open Approach

0RUV37Z Supplement Left Metacarpophalangeal Joint with Autologous Tissue Substitute, Percutaneous Approach

0RUV3JZ Supplement Left Metacarpophalangeal Joint with Synthetic Substitute, Percutaneous Approach

0RUV3KZ Supplement Left Metacarpophalangeal Joint with Nonautologous Tissue Substitute, Percutaneous Approach

0RUV47Z Supplement Left Metacarpophalangeal Joint with Autologous Tissue Substitute, Percutaneous Endoscopic Approach

0RUV4JZ Supplement Left Metacarpophalangeal Joint with Synthetic Substitute, Percutaneous Endoscopic Approach

0RUV4KZ Supplement Left Metacarpophalangeal Joint with Nonautologous Tissue Substitute, Percutaneous Endoscopic Approach

0RUW07Z Supplement Right Finger Phalangeal Joint with Autologous Tissue Substitute, Open Approach

0RUW0JZ Supplement Right Finger Phalangeal Joint with Synthetic Substitute, Open Approach

0RUW0KZ Supplement Right Finger Phalangeal Joint with Nonautologous Tissue Substitute, Open Approach

0RUW37Z Supplement Right Finger Phalangeal Joint with Autologous Tissue Substitute, Percutaneous Approach

0RUW3JZ Supplement Right Finger Phalangeal Joint with Synthetic Substitute, Percutaneous Approach

0RUW3KZ Supplement Right Finger Phalangeal Joint with Nonautologous Tissue Substitute, Percutaneous Approach

0RUW47Z Supplement Right Finger Phalangeal Joint with Autologous Tissue Substitute, Percutaneous Endoscopic Approach

0RUW4JZ Supplement Right Finger Phalangeal Joint with Synthetic Substitute, Percutaneous Endoscopic Approach

0RUW4KZ Supplement Right Finger Phalangeal Joint with Nonautologous Tissue Substitute, Percutaneous Endoscopic Approach

0RUX07Z Supplement Left Finger Phalangeal Joint with Autologous Tissue Substitute, Open Approach

0RUX0JZ Supplement Left Finger Phalangeal Joint with Synthetic Substitute, Open Approach

0RUX0KZ Supplement Left Finger Phalangeal Joint with Nonautologous Tissue Substitute, Open Approach

0RUX37Z Supplement Left Finger Phalangeal Joint with Autologous Tissue Substitute, Percutaneous Approach

0RUX3JZ Supplement Left Finger Phalangeal Joint with Synthetic Substitute, Percutaneous Approach

0RUX3KZ Supplement Left Finger Phalangeal Joint with Nonautologous Tissue Substitute, Percutaneous Approach

0RUX47Z Supplement Left Finger Phalangeal Joint with Autologous Tissue Substitute, Percutaneous Endoscopic Approach

0RUX4JZ Supplement Left Finger Phalangeal Joint with Synthetic Substitute, Percutaneous Endoscopic Approach

0RUX4KZ Supplement Left Finger Phalangeal Joint with Nonautologous Tissue Substitute, Percutaneous Endoscopic Approach

0RW – Upper Joints, Revision

Review Coding Guideline B6.1c

0RW000Z Revision of Drainage Device in Occipital-cervical Joint, Open Approach

0RW003Z Revision of Infusion Device in Occipital-cervical Joint, Open Approach

0RW004Z Revision of Internal Fixation Device in Occipital-cervical Joint, Open Approach

0RW007Z Revision of Autologous Tissue Substitute in Occipital-cervical Joint, Open Approach

0RW008Z Revision of Spacer in Occipital-cervical Joint, Open Approach

0RW00AZ Revision of Interbody Fusion Device in Occipital-cervical Joint, Open Approach

0RW00JZ Revision of Synthetic Substitute in Occipital-cervical Joint, Open Approach

0RW00KZ Revision of Nonautologous Tissue Substitute in Occipital-cervical Joint, Open Approach

0RW030Z Revision of Drainage Device in Occipital-cervical Joint, Percutaneous Approach

0RW033Z Revision of Infusion Device in Occipital-cervical Joint, Percutaneous Approach

0RW034Z Revision of Internal Fixation Device in Occipital-cervical Joint, Percutaneous Approach

0RW037Z Revision of Autologous Tissue Substitute in Occipital-cervical Joint, Percutaneous Approach

0RW038Z Revision of Spacer in Occipital-cervical Joint, Percutaneous Approach

0RW03AZ Revision of Interbody Fusion Device in Occipital-cervical Joint, Percutaneous Approach

0RW03JZ Revision of Synthetic Substitute in Occipital-cervical Joint, Percutaneous Approach

0RW03KZ Revision of Nonautologous Tissue Substitute in Occipital-cervical Joint, Percutaneous Approach

0RW040Z Revision of Drainage Device in Occipital-cervical Joint, Percutaneous Endoscopic Approach

0RW043Z Revision of Infusion Device in Occipital-cervical Joint, Percutaneous Endoscopic Approach

0RW044Z Revision of Internal Fixation Device in Occipital-cervical Joint, Percutaneous Endoscopic Approach

0RW047Z Revision of Autologous Tissue Substitute in Occipital-cervical Joint, Percutaneous Endoscopic Approach

0RW048Z Revision of Spacer in Occipital-cervical Joint, Percutaneous Endoscopic Approach

0RW04AZ Revision of Interbody Fusion Device in Occipital-cervical Joint, Percutaneous Endoscopic Approach

0RW04JZ Revision of Synthetic Substitute in Occipital-cervical Joint, Percutaneous Endoscopic Approach

0RW04KZ Revision of Nonautologous Tissue Substitute in Occipital-cervical Joint, Percutaneous Endoscopic Approach

0RW0X0Z Revision of Drainage Device in Occipital-cervical Joint, External Approach

0RW0X3Z Revision of Infusion Device in Occipital-cervical Joint, External Approach

0RW0X4Z Revision of Internal Fixation Device in Occipital-cervical Joint, External Approach

0RW0X7Z Revision of Autologous Tissue Substitute in Occipital-cervical Joint, External Approach

0RW0X8Z Revision of Spacer in Occipital-cervical Joint, External Approach

0RW0XAZ Revision of Interbody Fusion Device in Occipital-cervical Joint, External Approach

0RW0XJZ Revision of Synthetic Substitute in Occipital-cervical Joint, External Approach

---

♀ Female-only   ♂ Male-only   ● Limited Coverage   ● Non-OR   🅷🅰🅲 HAC-associated procedure   ● Non-covered procedures   ➕ Combination

0RW0XKZ Revision of Nonautologous Tissue Substitute in Occipital-cervical Joint, External Approach

0RW100Z Revision of Drainage Device in Cervical Vertebral Joint, Open Approach

0RW103Z Revision of Infusion Device in Cervical Vertebral Joint, Open Approach

0RW104Z Revision of Internal Fixation Device in Cervical Vertebral Joint, Open Approach

0RW107Z Revision of Autologous Tissue Substitute in Cervical Vertebral Joint, Open Approach

0RW108Z Revision of Spacer in Cervical Vertebral Joint, Open Approach

0RW10AZ Revision of Interbody Fusion Device in Cervical Vertebral Joint, Open Approach

0RW10JZ Revision of Synthetic Substitute in Cervical Vertebral Joint, Open Approach

0RW10KZ Revision of Nonautologous Tissue Substitute in Cervical Vertebral Joint, Open Approach

0RW130Z Revision of Drainage Device in Cervical Vertebral Joint, Percutaneous Approach

0RW133Z Revision of Infusion Device in Cervical Vertebral Joint, Percutaneous Approach

0RW134Z Revision of Internal Fixation Device in Cervical Vertebral Joint, Percutaneous Approach

0RW137Z Revision of Autologous Tissue Substitute in Cervical Vertebral Joint, Percutaneous Approach

0RW138Z Revision of Spacer in Cervical Vertebral Joint, Percutaneous Approach

0RW13AZ Revision of Interbody Fusion Device in Cervical Vertebral Joint, Percutaneous Approach

0RW13JZ Revision of Synthetic Substitute in Cervical Vertebral Joint, Percutaneous Approach

0RW13KZ Revision of Nonautologous Tissue Substitute in Cervical Vertebral Joint, Percutaneous Approach

0RW140Z Revision of Drainage Device in Cervical Vertebral Joint, Percutaneous Endoscopic Approach

0RW143Z Revision of Infusion Device in Cervical Vertebral Joint, Percutaneous Endoscopic Approach

0RW144Z Revision of Internal Fixation Device in Cervical Vertebral Joint, Percutaneous Endoscopic Approach

0RW147Z Revision of Autologous Tissue Substitute in Cervical Vertebral Joint, Percutaneous Endoscopic Approach

0RW148Z Revision of Spacer in Cervical Vertebral Joint, Percutaneous Endoscopic Approach

0RW14AZ Revision of Interbody Fusion Device in Cervical Vertebral Joint, Percutaneous Endoscopic Approach

0RW14JZ Revision of Synthetic Substitute in Cervical Vertebral Joint, Percutaneous Endoscopic Approach

0RW14KZ Revision of Nonautologous Tissue Substitute in Cervical Vertebral Joint, Percutaneous Endoscopic Approach

0RW1X0Z Revision of Drainage Device in Cervical Vertebral Joint, External Approach

0RW1X3Z Revision of Infusion Device in Cervical Vertebral Joint, External Approach

0RW1X4Z Revision of Internal Fixation Device in Cervical Vertebral Joint, External Approach

0RW1X7Z Revision of Autologous Tissue Substitute in Cervical Vertebral Joint, External Approach

0RW1X8Z Revision of Spacer in Cervical Vertebral Joint, External Approach

0RW1XAZ Revision of Interbody Fusion Device in Cervical Vertebral Joint, External Approach

0RW1XJZ Revision of Synthetic Substitute in Cervical Vertebral Joint, External Approach

0RW1XKZ Revision of Nonautologous Tissue Substitute in Cervical Vertebral Joint, External Approach

0RW300Z Revision of Drainage Device in Cervical Vertebral Disc, Open Approach

0RW303Z Revision of Infusion Device in Cervical Vertebral Disc, Open Approach

0RW307Z Revision of Autologous Tissue Substitute in Cervical Vertebral Disc, Open Approach

0RW30JZ Revision of Synthetic Substitute in Cervical Vertebral Disc, Open Approach

0RW30KZ Revision of Nonautologous Tissue Substitute in Cervical Vertebral Disc, Open Approach

0RW330Z Revision of Drainage Device in Cervical Vertebral Disc, Percutaneous Approach

0RW333Z Revision of Infusion Device in Cervical Vertebral Disc, Percutaneous Approach

0RW337Z Revision of Autologous Tissue Substitute in Cervical Vertebral Disc, Percutaneous Approach

0RW33JZ Revision of Synthetic Substitute in Cervical Vertebral Disc, Percutaneous Approach

0RW33KZ Revision of Nonautologous Tissue Substitute in Cervical Vertebral Disc, Percutaneous Approach

0RW340Z Revision of Drainage Device in Cervical Vertebral Disc, Percutaneous Endoscopic Approach

0RW343Z Revision of Infusion Device in Cervical Vertebral Disc, Percutaneous Endoscopic Approach

0RW347Z Revision of Autologous Tissue Substitute in Cervical Vertebral Disc, Percutaneous Endoscopic Approach

0RW34JZ Revision of Synthetic Substitute in Cervical Vertebral Disc, Percutaneous Endoscopic Approach

0RW34KZ Revision of Nonautologous Tissue Substitute in Cervical Vertebral Disc, Percutaneous Endoscopic Approach

0RW3X0Z Revision of Drainage Device in Cervical Vertebral Disc, External Approach

0RW3X3Z Revision of Infusion Device in Cervical Vertebral Disc, External Approach

0RW3X7Z Revision of Autologous Tissue Substitute in Cervical Vertebral Disc, External Approach

0RW3XJZ Revision of Synthetic Substitute in Cervical Vertebral Disc, External Approach

0RW3XKZ Revision of Nonautologous Tissue Substitute in Cervical Vertebral Disc, External Approach

0RW400Z Revision of Drainage Device in Cervicothoracic Vertebral Joint, Open Approach

0RW403Z Revision of Infusion Device in Cervicothoracic Vertebral Joint, Open Approach

0RW404Z Revision of Internal Fixation Device in Cervicothoracic Vertebral Joint, Open Approach

0RW407Z Revision of Autologous Tissue Substitute in Cervicothoracic Vertebral Joint, Open Approach

0RW408Z Revision of Spacer in Cervicothoracic Vertebral Joint, Open Approach

0RW40AZ Revision of Interbody Fusion Device in Cervicothoracic Vertebral Joint, Open Approach

0RW40JZ Revision of Synthetic Substitute in Cervicothoracic Vertebral Joint, Open Approach

0RW40KZ Revision of Nonautologous Tissue Substitute in Cervicothoracic Vertebral Joint, Open Approach

0RW430Z Revision of Drainage Device in Cervicothoracic Vertebral Joint, Percutaneous Approach

0RW433Z Revision of Infusion Device in Cervicothoracic Vertebral Joint, Percutaneous Approach

0RW434Z Revision of Internal Fixation Device in Cervicothoracic Vertebral Joint, Percutaneous Approach

0RW437Z Revision of Autologous Tissue Substitute in Cervicothoracic Vertebral Joint, Percutaneous Approach

0RW438Z Revision of Spacer in Cervicothoracic Vertebral Joint, Percutaneous Approach

0RW43AZ Revision of Interbody Fusion Device in Cervicothoracic Vertebral Joint, Percutaneous Approach

0RW43JZ Revision of Synthetic Substitute in Cervicothoracic Vertebral Joint, Percutaneous Approach

0RW43KZ Revision of Nonautologous Tissue Substitute in Cervicothoracic Vertebral Joint, Percutaneous Approach

0RW440Z Revision of Drainage Device in Cervicothoracic Vertebral Joint, Percutaneous Endoscopic Approach

0RW443Z Revision of Infusion Device in Cervicothoracic Vertebral Joint, Percutaneous Endoscopic Approach

0RW444Z Revision of Internal Fixation Device in Cervicothoracic Vertebral Joint, Percutaneous Endoscopic Approach

0RW447Z Revision of Autologous Tissue Substitute in Cervicothoracic Vertebral Joint, Percutaneous Endoscopic Approach

0RW448Z Revision of Spacer in Cervicothoracic Vertebral Joint, Percutaneous Endoscopic Approach

0RW44AZ Revision of Interbody Fusion Device in Cervicothoracic Vertebral Joint, Percutaneous Endoscopic Approach

0RW44JZ Revision of Synthetic Substitute in Cervicothoracic Vertebral Joint, Percutaneous Endoscopic Approach

0RW44KZ Revision of Nonautologous Tissue Substitute in Cervicothoracic Vertebral Joint, Percutaneous Endoscopic Approach

0RW4X0Z Revision of Drainage Device in Cervicothoracic Vertebral Joint, External Approach

0RW4X3Z Revision of Infusion Device in Cervicothoracic Vertebral Joint, External Approach

0RW4X4Z Revision of Internal Fixation Device in Cervicothoracic Vertebral Joint, External Approach

0RW4X7Z Revision of Autologous Tissue Substitute in Cervicothoracic Vertebral Joint, External Approach

0RW4X8Z Revision of Spacer in Cervicothoracic Vertebral Joint, External Approach

0RW4XAZ Revision of Interbody Fusion Device in Cervicothoracic Vertebral Joint, External Approach

0RW4XJZ Revision of Synthetic Substitute in Cervicothoracic Vertebral Joint, External Approach

0RW4XKZ Revision of Nonautologous Tissue Substitute in Cervicothoracic Vertebral Joint, External Approach

0RW500Z Revision of Drainage Device in Cervicothoracic Vertebral Disc, Open Approach

0RW503Z Revision of Infusion Device in Cervicothoracic Vertebral Disc, Open Approach

0RW507Z Revision of Autologous Tissue Substitute in Cervicothoracic Vertebral Disc, Open Approach

0RW50JZ Revision of Synthetic Substitute in Cervicothoracic Vertebral Disc, Open Approach

0RW50KZ Revision of Nonautologous Tissue Substitute in Cervicothoracic Vertebral Disc, Open Approach

0RW530Z Revision of Drainage Device in Cervicothoracic Vertebral Disc, Percutaneous Approach

0RW533Z Revision of Infusion Device in Cervicothoracic Vertebral Disc, Percutaneous Approach

0RW537Z Revision of Autologous Tissue Substitute in Cervicothoracic Vertebral Disc, Percutaneous Approach

0RW53JZ Revision of Synthetic Substitute in Cervicothoracic Vertebral Disc, Percutaneous Approach

0RW53KZ Revision of Nonautologous Tissue Substitute in Cervicothoracic Vertebral Disc, Percutaneous Approach

0RW540Z Revision of Drainage Device in Cervicothoracic Vertebral Disc, Percutaneous Endoscopic Approach

0RW543Z Revision of Infusion Device in Cervicothoracic Vertebral Disc, Percutaneous Endoscopic Approach

0RW547Z Revision of Autologous Tissue Substitute in Cervicothoracic Vertebral Disc, Percutaneous Endoscopic Approach

0RW54JZ Revision of Synthetic Substitute in Cervicothoracic Vertebral Disc, Percutaneous Endoscopic Approach

0RW54KZ Revision of Nonautologous Tissue Substitute in Cervicothoracic Vertebral Disc, Percutaneous Endoscopic Approach

0RW5X0Z Revision of Drainage Device in Cervicothoracic Vertebral Disc, External Approach

0RW5X3Z Revision of Infusion Device in Cervicothoracic Vertebral Disc, External Approach

0RW5X7Z Revision of Autologous Tissue Substitute in Cervicothoracic Vertebral Disc, External Approach

0RW5XJZ Revision of Synthetic Substitute in Cervicothoracic Vertebral Disc, External Approach

0RW5XKZ Revision of Nonautologous Tissue Substitute in Cervicothoracic Vertebral Disc, External Approach

0RW600Z Revision of Drainage Device in Thoracic Vertebral Joint, Open Approach

0RW603Z Revision of Infusion Device in Thoracic Vertebral Joint, Open Approach

0RW604Z Revision of Internal Fixation Device in Thoracic Vertebral Joint, Open Approach

0RW607Z Revision of Autologous Tissue Substitute in Thoracic Vertebral Joint, Open Approach

0RW608Z Revision of Spacer in Thoracic Vertebral Joint, Open Approach

0RW60AZ Revision of Interbody Fusion Device in Thoracic Vertebral Joint, Open Approach

0RW60JZ Revision of Synthetic Substitute in Thoracic Vertebral Joint, Open Approach

0RW60KZ Revision of Nonautologous Tissue Substitute in Thoracic Vertebral Joint, Open Approach

0RW630Z Revision of Drainage Device in Thoracic Vertebral Joint, Percutaneous Approach

0RW633Z Revision of Infusion Device in Thoracic Vertebral Joint, Percutaneous Approach

0RW634Z Revision of Internal Fixation Device in Thoracic Vertebral Joint, Percutaneous Approach

0RW637Z Revision of Autologous Tissue Substitute in Thoracic Vertebral Joint, Percutaneous Approach

0RW638Z Revision of Spacer in Thoracic Vertebral Joint, Percutaneous Approach

0RW63AZ Revision of Interbody Fusion Device in Thoracic Vertebral Joint, Percutaneous Approach

0RW63JZ Revision of Synthetic Substitute in Thoracic Vertebral Joint, Percutaneous Approach

0RW63KZ Revision of Nonautologous Tissue Substitute in Thoracic Vertebral Joint, Percutaneous Approach

0RW640Z Revision of Drainage Device in Thoracic Vertebral Joint, Percutaneous Endoscopic Approach

0RW643Z Revision of Infusion Device in Thoracic Vertebral Joint, Percutaneous Endoscopic Approach

0RW644Z Revision of Internal Fixation Device in Thoracic Vertebral Joint, Percutaneous Endoscopic Approach

0RW647Z Revision of Autologous Tissue Substitute in Thoracic Vertebral Joint, Percutaneous Endoscopic Approach

0RW648Z Revision of Spacer in Thoracic Vertebral Joint, Percutaneous Endoscopic Approach

0RW64AZ Revision of Interbody Fusion Device in Thoracic Vertebral Joint, Percutaneous Endoscopic Approach

0RW64JZ Revision of Synthetic Substitute in Thoracic Vertebral Joint, Percutaneous Endoscopic Approach

0RW64KZ Revision of Nonautologous Tissue Substitute in Thoracic Vertebral Joint, Percutaneous Endoscopic Approach

0RW6X0Z Revision of Drainage Device in Thoracic Vertebral Joint, External Approach

0RW6X3Z Revision of Infusion Device in Thoracic Vertebral Joint, External Approach

0RW6X4Z Revision of Internal Fixation Device in Thoracic Vertebral Joint, External Approach

0RW6X7Z Revision of Autologous Tissue Substitute in Thoracic Vertebral Joint, External Approach

0RW6X8Z Revision of Spacer in Thoracic Vertebral Joint, External Approach

0RW6XAZ Revision of Interbody Fusion Device in Thoracic Vertebral Joint, External Approach

0RW6XJZ Revision of Synthetic Substitute in Thoracic Vertebral Joint, External Approach

0RW6XKZ Revision of Nonautologous Tissue Substitute in Thoracic Vertebral Joint, External Approach

0RW900Z Revision of Drainage Device in Thoracic Vertebral Disc, Open Approach

0RW903Z Revision of Infusion Device in Thoracic Vertebral Disc, Open Approach

0RW907Z Revision of Autologous Tissue Substitute in Thoracic Vertebral Disc, Open Approach

0RW90JZ Revision of Synthetic Substitute in Thoracic Vertebral Disc, Open Approach

0RW90KZ Revision of Nonautologous Tissue Substitute in Thoracic Vertebral Disc, Open Approach

0RW930Z Revision of Drainage Device in Thoracic Vertebral Disc, Percutaneous Approach

0RW933Z Revision of Infusion Device in Thoracic Vertebral Disc, Percutaneous Approach

0RW937Z Revision of Autologous Tissue Substitute in Thoracic Vertebral Disc, Percutaneous Approach

0RW93JZ Revision of Synthetic Substitute in Thoracic Vertebral Disc, Percutaneous Approach

0RW93KZ Revision of Nonautologous Tissue Substitute in Thoracic Vertebral Disc, Percutaneous Approach

0RW940Z Revision of Drainage Device in Thoracic Vertebral Disc, Percutaneous Endoscopic Approach

0RW943Z Revision of Infusion Device in Thoracic Vertebral Disc, Percutaneous Endoscopic Approach

0RW947Z Revision of Autologous Tissue Substitute in Thoracic Vertebral Disc, Percutaneous Endoscopic Approach

0RW94JZ Revision of Synthetic Substitute in Thoracic Vertebral Disc, Percutaneous Endoscopic Approach

0RW94KZ Revision of Nonautologous Tissue Substitute in Thoracic Vertebral Disc, Percutaneous Endoscopic Approach

0RW9X0Z Revision of Drainage Device in Thoracic Vertebral Disc, External Approach

0RW9X3Z Revision of Infusion Device in Thoracic Vertebral Disc, External Approach

0RW9X7Z Revision of Autologous Tissue Substitute in Thoracic Vertebral Disc, External Approach

0RW9XJZ Revision of Synthetic Substitute in Thoracic Vertebral Disc, External Approach

0RW9XKZ Revision of Nonautologous Tissue Substitute in Thoracic Vertebral Disc, External Approach

0RWA00Z Revision of Drainage Device in Thoracolumbar Vertebral Joint, Open Approach

0RWA03Z Revision of Infusion Device in Thoracolumbar Vertebral Joint, Open Approach

0RWA04Z Revision of Internal Fixation Device in Thoracolumbar Vertebral Joint, Open Approach

0RWA07Z Revision of Autologous Tissue Substitute in Thoracolumbar Vertebral Joint, Open Approach

0RWA08Z Revision of Spacer in Thoracolumbar Vertebral Joint, Open Approach

0RWA0AZ Revision of Interbody Fusion Device in Thoracolumbar Vertebral Joint, Open Approach

0RWA0JZ Revision of Synthetic Substitute in Thoracolumbar Vertebral Joint, Open Approach

0RWA0KZ Revision of Nonautologous Tissue Substitute in Thoracolumbar Vertebral Joint, Open Approach

0RWA30Z Revision of Drainage Device in Thoracolumbar Vertebral Joint, Percutaneous Approach

0RWA33Z Revision of Infusion Device in Thoracolumbar Vertebral Joint, Percutaneous Approach

0RWA34Z Revision of Internal Fixation Device in Thoracolumbar Vertebral Joint, Percutaneous Approach

0RWA37Z Revision of Autologous Tissue Substitute in Thoracolumbar Vertebral Joint, Percutaneous Approach

0RWA38Z Revision of Spacer in Thoracolumbar Vertebral Joint, Percutaneous Approach

0RWA3AZ Revision of Interbody Fusion Device in Thoracolumbar Vertebral Joint, Percutaneous Approach

0RWA3JZ Revision of Synthetic Substitute in Thoracolumbar Vertebral Joint, Percutaneous Approach

0RWA3KZ Revision of Nonautologous Tissue Substitute in Thoracolumbar Vertebral Joint, Percutaneous Approach

0RWA40Z Revision of Drainage Device in Thoracolumbar Vertebral Joint, Percutaneous Endoscopic Approach

0RWA43Z Revision of Infusion Device in Thoracolumbar Vertebral Joint, Percutaneous Endoscopic Approach

0RWA44Z Revision of Internal Fixation Device in Thoracolumbar Vertebral Joint, Percutaneous Endoscopic Approach

0RWA47Z Revision of Autologous Tissue Substitute in Thoracolumbar Vertebral Joint, Percutaneous Endoscopic Approach

0RWA48Z Revision of Spacer in Thoracolumbar Vertebral Joint, Percutaneous Endoscopic Approach

0RWA4AZ Revision of Interbody Fusion Device in Thoracolumbar Vertebral Joint, Percutaneous Endoscopic Approach

0RWA4JZ Revision of Synthetic Substitute in Thoracolumbar Vertebral Joint, Percutaneous Endoscopic Approach

0RWA4KZ Revision of Nonautologous Tissue Substitute in Thoracolumbar Vertebral Joint, Percutaneous Endoscopic Approach

0RWAX0Z Revision of Drainage Device in Thoracolumbar Vertebral Joint, External Approach

0RWAX3Z Revision of Infusion Device in Thoracolumbar Vertebral Joint, External Approach

0RWAX4Z Revision of Internal Fixation Device in Thoracolumbar Vertebral Joint, External Approach

0RWAX7Z Revision of Autologous Tissue Substitute in Thoracolumbar Vertebral Joint, External Approach

0RWAX8Z Revision of Spacer in Thoracolumbar Vertebral Joint, External Approach

0RWAXAZ Revision of Interbody Fusion Device in Thoracolumbar Vertebral Joint, External Approach

0RWAXJZ Revision of Synthetic Substitute in Thoracolumbar Vertebral Joint, External Approach

0RWAXKZ Revision of Nonautologous Tissue Substitute in Thoracolumbar Vertebral Joint, External Approach

0RWB00Z Revision of Drainage Device in Thoracolumbar Vertebral Disc, Open Approach

0RWB03Z Revision of Infusion Device in Thoracolumbar Vertebral Disc, Open Approach

0RWB07Z Revision of Autologous Tissue Substitute in Thoracolumbar Vertebral Disc, Open Approach

0RWB0JZ Revision of Synthetic Substitute in Thoracolumbar Vertebral Disc, Open Approach

0RWB0KZ Revision of Nonautologous Tissue Substitute in Thoracolumbar Vertebral Disc, Open Approach

0RWB30Z Revision of Drainage Device in Thoracolumbar Vertebral Disc, Percutaneous Approach

0RWB33Z Revision of Infusion Device in Thoracolumbar Vertebral Disc, Percutaneous Approach

0RWB37Z Revision of Autologous Tissue Substitute in Thoracolumbar Vertebral Disc, Percutaneous Approach

0RWB3JZ Revision of Synthetic Substitute in Thoracolumbar Vertebral Disc, Percutaneous Approach

0RWB3KZ Revision of Nonautologous Tissue Substitute in Thoracolumbar Vertebral Disc, Percutaneous Approach

0RWB40Z Revision of Drainage Device in Thoracolumbar Vertebral Disc, Percutaneous Endoscopic Approach

0RWB43Z Revision of Infusion Device in Thoracolumbar Vertebral Disc, Percutaneous Endoscopic Approach

0RWB47Z Revision of Autologous Tissue Substitute in Thoracolumbar Vertebral Disc, Percutaneous Endoscopic Approach

0RWB4JZ Revision of Synthetic Substitute in Thoracolumbar Vertebral Disc, Percutaneous Endoscopic Approach

0RWB4KZ Revision of Nonautologous Tissue Substitute in Thoracolumbar Vertebral Disc, Percutaneous Endoscopic Approach

0RWBX0Z Revision of Drainage Device in Thoracolumbar Vertebral Disc, External Approach

0RWBX3Z Revision of Infusion Device in Thoracolumbar Vertebral Disc, External Approach

0RWBX7Z Revision of Autologous Tissue Substitute in Thoracolumbar Vertebral Disc, External Approach

0RWBXJZ Revision of Synthetic Substitute in Thoracolumbar Vertebral Disc, External Approach

0RWBXKZ Revision of Nonautologous Tissue Substitute in Thoracolumbar Vertebral Disc, External Approach

0RWC00Z Revision of Drainage Device in Right Temporomandibular Joint, Open Approach

0RWC03Z Revision of Infusion Device in Right Temporomandibular Joint, Open Approach

0RWC04Z Revision of Internal Fixation Device in Right Temporomandibular Joint, Open Approach

0RWC07Z Revision of Autologous Tissue Substitute in Right Temporomandibular Joint, Open Approach

0RWC08Z Revision of Spacer in Right Temporomandibular Joint, Open Approach

0RWC0JZ Revision of Synthetic Substitute in Right Temporomandibular Joint, Open Approach

0RWC0KZ Revision of Nonautologous Tissue Substitute in Right Temporomandibular Joint, Open Approach

0RWC30Z Revision of Drainage Device in Right Temporomandibular Joint, Percutaneous Approach

0RWC33Z Revision of Infusion Device in Right Temporomandibular Joint, Percutaneous Approach

0RWC34Z Revision of Internal Fixation Device in Right Temporomandibular Joint, Percutaneous Approach

0RWC37Z Revision of Autologous Tissue Substitute in Right Temporomandibular Joint, Percutaneous Approach

0RWC38Z Revision of Spacer in Right Temporomandibular Joint, Percutaneous Approach

0RWC3JZ Revision of Synthetic Substitute in Right Temporomandibular Joint, Percutaneous Approach

0RWC3KZ Revision of Nonautologous Tissue Substitute in Right Temporomandibular Joint, Percutaneous Approach

♀ Female-only   ♂ Male-only   ● Limited Coverage   ● Non-OR   **HAC** HAC-associated procedure   ● Non-covered procedures   **+** Combination

0RWC40Z Revision of Drainage Device in Right Temporomandibular Joint, Percutaneous Endoscopic Approach

0RWC43Z Revision of Infusion Device in Right Temporomandibular Joint, Percutaneous Endoscopic Approach

0RWC44Z Revision of Internal Fixation Device in Right Temporomandibular Joint, Percutaneous Endoscopic Approach

0RWC47Z Revision of Autologous Tissue Substitute in Right Temporomandibular Joint, Percutaneous Endoscopic Approach

0RWC48Z Revision of Spacer in Right Temporomandibular Joint, Percutaneous Endoscopic Approach

0RWC4JZ Revision of Synthetic Substitute in Right Temporomandibular Joint, Percutaneous Endoscopic Approach

0RWC4KZ Revision of Nonautologous Tissue Substitute in Right Temporomandibular Joint, Percutaneous Endoscopic Approach

0RWCX0Z Revision of Drainage Device in Right Temporomandibular Joint, External Approach

0RWCX3Z Revision of Infusion Device in Right Temporomandibular Joint, External Approach

0RWCX4Z Revision of Internal Fixation Device in Right Temporomandibular Joint, External Approach

0RWCX7Z Revision of Autologous Tissue Substitute in Right Temporomandibular Joint, External Approach

0RWCX8Z Revision of Spacer in Right Temporomandibular Joint, External Approach

0RWCXJZ Revision of Synthetic Substitute in Right Temporomandibular Joint, External Approach

0RWCXKZ Revision of Nonautologous Tissue Substitute in Right Temporomandibular Joint, External Approach

0RWD00Z Revision of Drainage Device in Left Temporomandibular Joint, Open Approach

0RWD03Z Revision of Infusion Device in Left Temporomandibular Joint, Open Approach

0RWD04Z Revision of Internal Fixation Device in Left Temporomandibular Joint, Open Approach

0RWD07Z Revision of Autologous Tissue Substitute in Left Temporomandibular Joint, Open Approach

0RWD08Z Revision of Spacer in Left Temporomandibular Joint, Open Approach

0RWD0JZ Revision of Synthetic Substitute in Left Temporomandibular Joint, Open Approach

0RWD0KZ Revision of Nonautologous Tissue Substitute in Left Temporomandibular Joint, Open Approach

0RWD30Z Revision of Drainage Device in Left Temporomandibular Joint, Percutaneous Approach

0RWD33Z Revision of Infusion Device in Left Temporomandibular Joint, Percutaneous Approach

0RWD34Z Revision of Internal Fixation Device in Left Temporomandibular Joint, Percutaneous Approach

0RWD37Z Revision of Autologous Tissue Substitute in Left Temporomandibular Joint, Percutaneous Approach

0RWD38Z Revision of Spacer in Left Temporomandibular Joint, Percutaneous Approach

0RWD3JZ Revision of Synthetic Substitute in Left Temporomandibular Joint, Percutaneous Approach

0RWD3KZ Revision of Nonautologous Tissue Substitute in Left Temporomandibular Joint, Percutaneous Approach

0RWD40Z Revision of Drainage Device in Left Temporomandibular Joint, Percutaneous Endoscopic Approach

0RWD43Z Revision of Infusion Device in Left Temporomandibular Joint, Percutaneous Endoscopic Approach

0RWD44Z Revision of Internal Fixation Device in Left Temporomandibular Joint, Percutaneous Endoscopic Approach

0RWD47Z Revision of Autologous Tissue Substitute in Left Temporomandibular Joint, Percutaneous Endoscopic Approach

0RWD48Z Revision of Spacer in Left Temporomandibular Joint, Percutaneous Endoscopic Approach

0RWD4JZ Revision of Synthetic Substitute in Left Temporomandibular Joint, Percutaneous Endoscopic Approach

0RWD4KZ Revision of Nonautologous Tissue Substitute in Left Temporomandibular Joint, Percutaneous Endoscopic Approach

0RWDX0Z Revision of Drainage Device in Left Temporomandibular Joint, External Approach

0RWDX3Z Revision of Infusion Device in Left Temporomandibular Joint, External Approach

0RWDX4Z Revision of Internal Fixation Device in Left Temporomandibular Joint, External Approach

0RWDX7Z Revision of Autologous Tissue Substitute in Left Temporomandibular Joint, External Approach

0RWDX8Z Revision of Spacer in Left Temporomandibular Joint, External Approach

0RWDXJZ Revision of Synthetic Substitute in Left Temporomandibular Joint, External Approach

0RWDXKZ Revision of Nonautologous Tissue Substitute in Left Temporomandibular Joint, External Approach

0RWE00Z Revision of Drainage Device in Right Sternoclavicular Joint, Open Approach

0RWE03Z Revision of Infusion Device in Right Sternoclavicular Joint, Open Approach

0RWE04Z Revision of Internal Fixation Device in Right Sternoclavicular Joint, Open Approach

0RWE07Z Revision of Autologous Tissue Substitute in Right Sternoclavicular Joint, Open Approach

0RWE08Z Revision of Spacer in Right Sternoclavicular Joint, Open Approach

0RWE0JZ Revision of Synthetic Substitute in Right Sternoclavicular Joint, Open Approach

0RWE0KZ Revision of Nonautologous Tissue Substitute in Right Sternoclavicular Joint, Open Approach

0RWE30Z Revision of Drainage Device in Right Sternoclavicular Joint, Percutaneous Approach

0RWE33Z Revision of Infusion Device in Right Sternoclavicular Joint, Percutaneous Approach

0RWE34Z Revision of Internal Fixation Device in Right Sternoclavicular Joint, Percutaneous Approach

0RWE37Z Revision of Autologous Tissue Substitute in Right Sternoclavicular Joint, Percutaneous Approach

0RWE38Z Revision of Spacer in Right Sternoclavicular Joint, Percutaneous Approach

0RWE3JZ Revision of Synthetic Substitute in Right Sternoclavicular Joint, Percutaneous Approach

0RWE3KZ Revision of Nonautologous Tissue Substitute in Right Sternoclavicular Joint, Percutaneous Approach

0RWE40Z Revision of Drainage Device in Right Sternoclavicular Joint, Percutaneous Endoscopic Approach

0RWE43Z Revision of Infusion Device in Right Sternoclavicular Joint, Percutaneous Endoscopic Approach

0RWE44Z Revision of Internal Fixation Device in Right Sternoclavicular Joint, Percutaneous Endoscopic Approach

0RWE47Z Revision of Autologous Tissue Substitute in Right Sternoclavicular Joint, Percutaneous Endoscopic Approach

0RWE48Z Revision of Spacer in Right Sternoclavicular Joint, Percutaneous Endoscopic Approach

0RWE4JZ Revision of Synthetic Substitute in Right Sternoclavicular Joint, Percutaneous Endoscopic Approach

0RWE4KZ Revision of Nonautologous Tissue Substitute in Right Sternoclavicular Joint, Percutaneous Endoscopic Approach

0RWEX0Z Revision of Drainage Device in Right Sternoclavicular Joint, External Approach

0RWEX3Z Revision of Infusion Device in Right Sternoclavicular Joint, External Approach

0RWEX4Z Revision of Internal Fixation Device in Right Sternoclavicular Joint, External Approach

0RWEX7Z Revision of Autologous Tissue Substitute in Right Sternoclavicular Joint, External Approach

0RWEX8Z Revision of Spacer in Right Sternoclavicular Joint, External Approach

0RWEXJZ Revision of Synthetic Substitute in Right Sternoclavicular Joint, External Approach

0RWEXKZ Revision of Nonautologous Tissue Substitute in Right Sternoclavicular Joint, External Approach

0RWF00Z Revision of Drainage Device in Left Sternoclavicular Joint, Open Approach

0RWF03Z Revision of Infusion Device in Left Sternoclavicular Joint, Open Approach

0RWF04Z Revision of Internal Fixation Device in Left Sternoclavicular Joint, Open Approach

0RWF07Z Revision of Autologous Tissue Substitute in Left Sternoclavicular Joint, Open Approach

0RWF08Z Revision of Spacer in Left Sternoclavicular Joint, Open Approach

0RWF0JZ Revision of Synthetic Substitute in Left Sternoclavicular Joint, Open Approach

0RWF0KZ Revision of Nonautologous Tissue Substitute in Left Sternoclavicular Joint, Open Approach

0RWF30Z Revision of Drainage Device in Left Sternoclavicular Joint, Percutaneous Approach

0RWF33Z Revision of Infusion Device in Left Sternoclavicular Joint, Percutaneous Approach

0RWF34Z Revision of Internal Fixation Device in Left Sternoclavicular Joint, Percutaneous Approach

0RWF37Z Revision of Autologous Tissue Substitute in Left Sternoclavicular Joint, Percutaneous Approach

0RWF38Z Revision of Spacer in Left Sternoclavicular Joint, Percutaneous Approach

0RWF3JZ Revision of Synthetic Substitute in Left Sternoclavicular Joint, Percutaneous Approach

0RWF3KZ Revision of Nonautologous Tissue Substitute in Left Sternoclavicular Joint, Percutaneous Approach

0RWF40Z Revision of Drainage Device in Left Sternoclavicular Joint, Percutaneous Endoscopic Approach

0RWF43Z Revision of Infusion Device in Left Sternoclavicular Joint, Percutaneous Endoscopic Approach

0RWF44Z Revision of Internal Fixation Device in Left Sternoclavicular Joint, Percutaneous Endoscopic Approach

0RWF47Z Revision of Autologous Tissue Substitute in Left Sternoclavicular Joint, Percutaneous Endoscopic Approach

0RWF48Z Revision of Spacer in Left Sternoclavicular Joint, Percutaneous Endoscopic Approach

0RWF4JZ Revision of Synthetic Substitute in Left Sternoclavicular Joint, Percutaneous Endoscopic Approach

0RWF4KZ Revision of Nonautologous Tissue Substitute in Left Sternoclavicular Joint, Percutaneous Endoscopic Approach

0RWFX0Z Revision of Drainage Device in Left Sternoclavicular Joint, External Approach

0RWFX3Z Revision of Infusion Device in Left Sternoclavicular Joint, External Approach

0RWFX4Z Revision of Internal Fixation Device in Left Sternoclavicular Joint, External Approach

0RWFX7Z Revision of Autologous Tissue Substitute in Left Sternoclavicular Joint, External Approach

0RWFX8Z Revision of Spacer in Left Sternoclavicular Joint, External Approach

0RWFXJZ Revision of Synthetic Substitute in Left Sternoclavicular Joint, External Approach

0RWFXKZ Revision of Nonautologous Tissue Substitute in Left Sternoclavicular Joint, External Approach

0RWG00Z Revision of Drainage Device in Right Acromioclavicular Joint, Open Approach

0RWG03Z Revision of Infusion Device in Right Acromioclavicular Joint, Open Approach

0RWG04Z Revision of Internal Fixation Device in Right Acromioclavicular Joint, Open Approach

0RWG07Z Revision of Autologous Tissue Substitute in Right Acromioclavicular Joint, Open Approach

0RWG08Z Revision of Spacer in Right Acromioclavicular Joint, Open Approach

0RWG0JZ Revision of Synthetic Substitute in Right Acromioclavicular Joint, Open Approach

0RWG0KZ Revision of Nonautologous Tissue Substitute in Right Acromioclavicular Joint, Open Approach

0RWG30Z Revision of Drainage Device in Right Acromioclavicular Joint, Percutaneous Approach

0RWG33Z Revision of Infusion Device in Right Acromioclavicular Joint, Percutaneous Approach

0RWG34Z Revision of Internal Fixation Device in Right Acromioclavicular Joint, Percutaneous Approach

0RWG37Z Revision of Autologous Tissue Substitute in Right Acromioclavicular Joint, Percutaneous Approach

0RWG38Z Revision of Spacer in Right Acromioclavicular Joint, Percutaneous Approach

0RWG3JZ Revision of Synthetic Substitute in Right Acromioclavicular Joint, Percutaneous Approach

0RWG3KZ Revision of Nonautologous Tissue Substitute in Right Acromioclavicular Joint, Percutaneous Approach

0RWG40Z Revision of Drainage Device in Right Acromioclavicular Joint, Percutaneous Endoscopic Approach

0RWG43Z Revision of Infusion Device in Right Acromioclavicular Joint, Percutaneous Endoscopic Approach

0RWG44Z Revision of Internal Fixation Device in Right Acromioclavicular Joint, Percutaneous Endoscopic Approach

0RWG47Z Revision of Autologous Tissue Substitute in Right Acromioclavicular Joint, Percutaneous Endoscopic Approach

0RWG48Z Revision of Spacer in Right Acromioclavicular Joint, Percutaneous Endoscopic Approach

0RWG4JZ Revision of Synthetic Substitute in Right Acromioclavicular Joint, Percutaneous Endoscopic Approach

0RWG4KZ Revision of Nonautologous Tissue Substitute in Right Acromioclavicular Joint, Percutaneous Endoscopic Approach

0RWGX0Z Revision of Drainage Device in Right Acromioclavicular Joint, External Approach

0RWGX3Z Revision of Infusion Device in Right Acromioclavicular Joint, External Approach

0RWGX4Z Revision of Internal Fixation Device in Right Acromioclavicular Joint, External Approach

0RWGX7Z Revision of Autologous Tissue Substitute in Right Acromioclavicular Joint, External Approach

0RWGX8Z Revision of Spacer in Right Acromioclavicular Joint, External Approach

0RWGXJZ Revision of Synthetic Substitute in Right Acromioclavicular Joint, External Approach

0RWGXKZ Revision of Nonautologous Tissue Substitute in Right Acromioclavicular Joint, External Approach

0RWH00Z Revision of Drainage Device in Left Acromioclavicular Joint, Open Approach

0RWH03Z Revision of Infusion Device in Left Acromioclavicular Joint, Open Approach

0RWH04Z Revision of Internal Fixation Device in Left Acromioclavicular Joint, Open Approach

0RWH07Z Revision of Autologous Tissue Substitute in Left Acromioclavicular Joint, Open Approach

0RWH08Z Revision of Spacer in Left Acromioclavicular Joint, Open Approach

0RWH0JZ Revision of Synthetic Substitute in Left Acromioclavicular Joint, Open Approach

0RWH0KZ Revision of Nonautologous Tissue Substitute in Left Acromioclavicular Joint, Open Approach

0RWH30Z Revision of Drainage Device in Left Acromioclavicular Joint, Percutaneous Approach

0RWH33Z Revision of Infusion Device in Left Acromioclavicular Joint, Percutaneous Approach

0RWH34Z Revision of Internal Fixation Device in Left Acromioclavicular Joint, Percutaneous Approach

0RWH37Z Revision of Autologous Tissue Substitute in Left Acromioclavicular Joint, Percutaneous Approach

0RWH38Z Revision of Spacer in Left Acromioclavicular Joint, Percutaneous Approach

0RWH3JZ Revision of Synthetic Substitute in Left Acromioclavicular Joint, Percutaneous Approach

0RWH3KZ Revision of Nonautologous Tissue Substitute in Left Acromioclavicular Joint, Percutaneous Approach

0RWH40Z Revision of Drainage Device in Left Acromioclavicular Joint, Percutaneous Endoscopic Approach

0RWH43Z Revision of Infusion Device in Left Acromioclavicular Joint, Percutaneous Endoscopic Approach

0RWH44Z Revision of Internal Fixation Device in Left Acromioclavicular Joint, Percutaneous Endoscopic Approach

0RWH47Z Revision of Autologous Tissue Substitute in Left Acromioclavicular Joint, Percutaneous Endoscopic Approach

0RWH48Z Revision of Spacer in Left Acromioclavicular Joint, Percutaneous Endoscopic Approach

0RWH4JZ Revision of Synthetic Substitute in Left Acromioclavicular Joint, Percutaneous Endoscopic Approach

0RWH4KZ Revision of Nonautologous Tissue Substitute in Left Acromioclavicular Joint, Percutaneous Endoscopic Approach

0RWHX0Z Revision of Drainage Device in Left Acromioclavicular Joint, External Approach

0RWHX3Z Revision of Infusion Device in Left Acromioclavicular Joint, External Approach

0RWHX4Z Revision of Internal Fixation Device in Left Acromioclavicular Joint, External Approach

0RWHX7Z Revision of Autologous Tissue Substitute in Left Acromioclavicular Joint, External Approach

0RWHX8Z Revision of Spacer in Left Acromioclavicular Joint, External Approach

0RWHXJZ Revision of Synthetic Substitute in Left Acromioclavicular Joint, External Approach

0RWHXKZ Revision of Nonautologous Tissue Substitute in Left Acromioclavicular Joint, External Approach

0RWJ00Z Revision of Drainage Device in Right Shoulder Joint, Open Approach

0RWJ03Z Revision of Infusion Device in Right Shoulder Joint, Open Approach

0RWJ04Z Revision of Internal Fixation Device in Right Shoulder Joint, Open Approach

0RWJ07Z Revision of Autologous Tissue Substitute in Right Shoulder Joint, Open Approach

0RWJ08Z Revision of Spacer in Right Shoulder Joint, Open Approach

0RWJ0JZ Revision of Synthetic Substitute in Right Shoulder Joint, Open Approach

0RWJ0KZ Revision of Nonautologous Tissue Substitute in Right Shoulder Joint, Open Approach

0RWJ30Z Revision of Drainage Device in Right Shoulder Joint, Percutaneous Approach

0RWJ33Z Revision of Infusion Device in Right Shoulder Joint, Percutaneous Approach

0RWJ34Z Revision of Internal Fixation Device in Right Shoulder Joint, Percutaneous Approach

0RWJ37Z Revision of Autologous Tissue Substitute in Right Shoulder Joint, Percutaneous Approach

0RWJ38Z Revision of Spacer in Right Shoulder Joint, Percutaneous Approach

0RWJ3JZ Revision of Synthetic Substitute in Right Shoulder Joint, Percutaneous Approach

0RWJ3KZ Revision of Nonautologous Tissue Substitute in Right Shoulder Joint, Percutaneous Approach

0RWJ40Z Revision of Drainage Device in Right Shoulder Joint, Percutaneous Endoscopic Approach

0RWJ43Z Revision of Infusion Device in Right Shoulder Joint, Percutaneous Endoscopic Approach

0RWJ44Z Revision of Internal Fixation Device in Right Shoulder Joint, Percutaneous Endoscopic Approach

0RWJ47Z Revision of Autologous Tissue Substitute in Right Shoulder Joint, Percutaneous Endoscopic Approach

0RWJ48Z Revision of Spacer in Right Shoulder Joint, Percutaneous Endoscopic Approach

0RWJ4JZ Revision of Synthetic Substitute in Right Shoulder Joint, Percutaneous Endoscopic Approach

0RWJ4KZ Revision of Nonautologous Tissue Substitute in Right Shoulder Joint, Percutaneous Endoscopic Approach

0RWJX0Z Revision of Drainage Device in Right Shoulder Joint, External Approach

0RWJX3Z Revision of Infusion Device in Right Shoulder Joint, External Approach

0RWJX4Z Revision of Internal Fixation Device in Right Shoulder Joint, External Approach

0RWJX7Z Revision of Autologous Tissue Substitute in Right Shoulder Joint, External Approach

0RWJX8Z Revision of Spacer in Right Shoulder Joint, External Approach

0RWJXJZ Revision of Synthetic Substitute in Right Shoulder Joint, External Approach

0RWJXKZ Revision of Nonautologous Tissue Substitute in Right Shoulder Joint, External Approach

0RWK00Z Revision of Drainage Device in Left Shoulder Joint, Open Approach

0RWK03Z Revision of Infusion Device in Left Shoulder Joint, Open Approach

0RWK04Z Revision of Internal Fixation Device in Left Shoulder Joint, Open Approach

0RWK07Z Revision of Autologous Tissue Substitute in Left Shoulder Joint, Open Approach

0RWK08Z Revision of Spacer in Left Shoulder Joint, Open Approach

0RWK0JZ Revision of Synthetic Substitute in Left Shoulder Joint, Open Approach

0RWK0KZ Revision of Nonautologous Tissue Substitute in Left Shoulder Joint, Open Approach

0RWK30Z Revision of Drainage Device in Left Shoulder Joint, Percutaneous Approach

0RWK33Z Revision of Infusion Device in Left Shoulder Joint, Percutaneous Approach

0RWK34Z Revision of Internal Fixation Device in Left Shoulder Joint, Percutaneous Approach

0RWK37Z Revision of Autologous Tissue Substitute in Left Shoulder Joint, Percutaneous Approach

0RWK38Z Revision of Spacer in Left Shoulder Joint, Percutaneous Approach

0RWK3JZ Revision of Synthetic Substitute in Left Shoulder Joint, Percutaneous Approach

0RWK3KZ Revision of Nonautologous Tissue Substitute in Left Shoulder Joint, Percutaneous Approach

0RWK40Z Revision of Drainage Device in Left Shoulder Joint, Percutaneous Endoscopic Approach

0RWK43Z Revision of Infusion Device in Left Shoulder Joint, Percutaneous Endoscopic Approach

0RWK44Z Revision of Internal Fixation Device in Left Shoulder Joint, Percutaneous Endoscopic Approach

0RWK47Z Revision of Autologous Tissue Substitute in Left Shoulder Joint, Percutaneous Endoscopic Approach

0RWK48Z Revision of Spacer in Left Shoulder Joint, Percutaneous Endoscopic Approach

0RWK4JZ Revision of Synthetic Substitute in Left Shoulder Joint, Percutaneous Endoscopic Approach

0RWK4KZ Revision of Nonautologous Tissue Substitute in Left Shoulder Joint, Percutaneous Endoscopic Approach

0RWKX0Z Revision of Drainage Device in Left Shoulder Joint, External Approach

0RWKX3Z Revision of Infusion Device in Left Shoulder Joint, External Approach

0RWKX4Z Revision of Internal Fixation Device in Left Shoulder Joint, External Approach

0RWKX7Z Revision of Autologous Tissue Substitute in Left Shoulder Joint, External Approach

0RWKX8Z Revision of Spacer in Left Shoulder Joint, External Approach

0RWKXJZ Revision of Synthetic Substitute in Left Shoulder Joint, External Approach

0RWKXKZ Revision of Nonautologous Tissue Substitute in Left Shoulder Joint, External Approach

0RWL00Z Revision of Drainage Device in Right Elbow Joint, Open Approach

0RWL03Z Revision of Infusion Device in Right Elbow Joint, Open Approach

0RWL04Z Revision of Internal Fixation Device in Right Elbow Joint, Open Approach

0RWL05Z Revision of External Fixation Device in Right Elbow Joint, Open Approach

0RWL07Z Revision of Autologous Tissue Substitute in Right Elbow Joint, Open Approach

0RWL08Z Revision of Spacer in Right Elbow Joint, Open Approach

0RWL0JZ Revision of Synthetic Substitute in Right Elbow Joint, Open Approach

0RWL0KZ Revision of Nonautologous Tissue Substitute in Right Elbow Joint, Open Approach

0RWL30Z Revision of Drainage Device in Right Elbow Joint, Percutaneous Approach

0RWL33Z Revision of Infusion Device in Right Elbow Joint, Percutaneous Approach

0RWL34Z Revision of Internal Fixation Device in Right Elbow Joint, Percutaneous Approach

0RWL35Z Revision of External Fixation Device in Right Elbow Joint, Percutaneous Approach

0RWL37Z Revision of Autologous Tissue Substitute in Right Elbow Joint, Percutaneous Approach

0RWL38Z Revision of Spacer in Right Elbow Joint, Percutaneous Approach

0RWL3JZ Revision of Synthetic Substitute in Right Elbow Joint, Percutaneous Approach

0RWL3KZ Revision of Nonautologous Tissue Substitute in Right Elbow Joint, Percutaneous Approach

0RWL40Z Revision of Drainage Device in Right Elbow Joint, Percutaneous Endoscopic Approach

0RWL43Z Revision of Infusion Device in Right Elbow Joint, Percutaneous Endoscopic Approach

0RWL44Z Revision of Internal Fixation Device in Right Elbow Joint, Percutaneous Endoscopic Approach

0RWL45Z Revision of External Fixation Device in Right Elbow Joint, Percutaneous Endoscopic Approach

0RWL47Z Revision of Autologous Tissue Substitute in Right Elbow Joint, Percutaneous Endoscopic Approach

0RWL48Z Revision of Spacer in Right Elbow Joint, Percutaneous Endoscopic Approach

0RWL4JZ Revision of Synthetic Substitute in Right Elbow Joint, Percutaneous Endoscopic Approach

0RWL4KZ Revision of Nonautologous Tissue Substitute in Right Elbow Joint, Percutaneous Endoscopic Approach

0RWLX0Z Revision of Drainage Device in Right Elbow Joint, External Approach

0RWLX3Z Revision of Infusion Device in Right Elbow Joint, External Approach

0RWLX4Z Revision of Internal Fixation Device in Right Elbow Joint, External Approach

0RWLX5Z Revision of External Fixation Device in Right Elbow Joint, External Approach

0RWLX7Z Revision of Autologous Tissue Substitute in Right Elbow Joint, External Approach

0RWLX8Z Revision of Spacer in Right Elbow Joint, External Approach

0RWLXJZ Revision of Synthetic Substitute in Right Elbow Joint, External Approach

0RWLXKZ Revision of Nonautologous Tissue Substitute in Right Elbow Joint, External Approach

0RWM00Z Revision of Drainage Device in Left Elbow Joint, Open Approach

0RWM03Z Revision of Infusion Device in Left Elbow Joint, Open Approach

0RWM04Z Revision of Internal Fixation Device in Left Elbow Joint, Open Approach

0RWM05Z Revision of External Fixation Device in Left Elbow Joint, Open Approach

0RWM07Z Revision of Autologous Tissue Substitute in Left Elbow Joint, Open Approach

0RWM08Z Revision of Spacer in Left Elbow Joint, Open Approach

0RWM0JZ Revision of Synthetic Substitute in Left Elbow Joint, Open Approach

0RWM0KZ Revision of Nonautologous Tissue Substitute in Left Elbow Joint, Open Approach

0RWM30Z Revision of Drainage Device in Left Elbow Joint, Percutaneous Approach

0RWM33Z Revision of Infusion Device in Left Elbow Joint, Percutaneous Approach

0RWM34Z Revision of Internal Fixation Device in Left Elbow Joint, Percutaneous Approach

0RWM35Z Revision of External Fixation Device in Left Elbow Joint, Percutaneous Approach

0RWM37Z Revision of Autologous Tissue Substitute in Left Elbow Joint, Percutaneous Approach

0RWM38Z Revision of Spacer in Left Elbow Joint, Percutaneous Approach

0RWM3JZ Revision of Synthetic Substitute in Left Elbow Joint, Percutaneous Approach

0RWM3KZ Revision of Nonautologous Tissue Substitute in Left Elbow Joint, Percutaneous Approach

0RWM40Z Revision of Drainage Device in Left Elbow Joint, Percutaneous Endoscopic Approach

0RWM43Z Revision of Infusion Device in Left Elbow Joint, Percutaneous Endoscopic Approach

0RWM44Z Revision of Internal Fixation Device in Left Elbow Joint, Percutaneous Endoscopic Approach

0RWM45Z Revision of External Fixation Device in Left Elbow Joint, Percutaneous Endoscopic Approach

0RWM47Z Revision of Autologous Tissue Substitute in Left Elbow Joint, Percutaneous Endoscopic Approach

0RWM48Z Revision of Spacer in Left Elbow Joint, Percutaneous Endoscopic Approach

0RWM4JZ Revision of Synthetic Substitute in Left Elbow Joint, Percutaneous Endoscopic Approach

0RWM4KZ Revision of Nonautologous Tissue Substitute in Left Elbow Joint, Percutaneous Endoscopic Approach

0RWMX0Z Revision of Drainage Device in Left Elbow Joint, External Approach

0RWMX3Z Revision of Infusion Device in Left Elbow Joint, External Approach

0RWMX4Z Revision of Internal Fixation Device in Left Elbow Joint, External Approach

0RWMX5Z Revision of External Fixation Device in Left Elbow Joint, External Approach

0RWMX7Z Revision of Autologous Tissue Substitute in Left Elbow Joint, External Approach

0RWMX8Z Revision of Spacer in Left Elbow Joint, External Approach

0RWMXJZ Revision of Synthetic Substitute in Left Elbow Joint, External Approach

0RWMXKZ Revision of Nonautologous Tissue Substitute in Left Elbow Joint, External Approach

0RWN00Z Revision of Drainage Device in Right Wrist Joint, Open Approach

0RWN03Z Revision of Infusion Device in Right Wrist Joint, Open Approach

0RWN04Z Revision of Internal Fixation Device in Right Wrist Joint, Open Approach

0RWN05Z Revision of External Fixation Device in Right Wrist Joint, Open Approach

0RWN07Z Revision of Autologous Tissue Substitute in Right Wrist Joint, Open Approach

0RWN08Z Revision of Spacer in Right Wrist Joint, Open Approach

0RWN0JZ Revision of Synthetic Substitute in Right Wrist Joint, Open Approach

0RWN0KZ Revision of Nonautologous Tissue Substitute in Right Wrist Joint, Open Approach

0RWN30Z Revision of Drainage Device in Right Wrist Joint, Percutaneous Approach

0RWN33Z Revision of Infusion Device in Right Wrist Joint, Percutaneous Approach

0RWN34Z Revision of Internal Fixation Device in Right Wrist Joint, Percutaneous Approach

0RWN35Z Revision of External Fixation Device in Right Wrist Joint, Percutaneous Approach

0RWN37Z Revision of Autologous Tissue Substitute in Right Wrist Joint, Percutaneous Approach

0RWN38Z Revision of Spacer in Right Wrist Joint, Percutaneous Approach

0RWN3JZ Revision of Synthetic Substitute in Right Wrist Joint, Percutaneous Approach

0RWN3KZ Revision of Nonautologous Tissue Substitute in Right Wrist Joint, Percutaneous Approach

0RWN40Z Revision of Drainage Device in Right Wrist Joint, Percutaneous Endoscopic Approach

0RWN43Z Revision of Infusion Device in Right Wrist Joint, Percutaneous Endoscopic Approach

0RWN44Z Revision of Internal Fixation Device in Right Wrist Joint, Percutaneous Endoscopic Approach

0RWN45Z Revision of External Fixation Device in Right Wrist Joint, Percutaneous Endoscopic Approach

0RWN47Z Revision of Autologous Tissue Substitute in Right Wrist Joint, Percutaneous Endoscopic Approach

0RWN48Z Revision of Spacer in Right Wrist Joint, Percutaneous Endoscopic Approach

0RWN4JZ Revision of Synthetic Substitute in Right Wrist Joint, Percutaneous Endoscopic Approach

0RWN4KZ Revision of Nonautologous Tissue Substitute in Right Wrist Joint, Percutaneous Endoscopic Approach

0RWNX0Z Revision of Drainage Device in Right Wrist Joint, External Approach

0RWNX3Z Revision of Infusion Device in Right Wrist Joint, External Approach

0RWNX4Z Revision of Internal Fixation Device in Right Wrist Joint, External Approach

0RWNX5Z Revision of External Fixation Device in Right Wrist Joint, External Approach

0RWNX7Z Revision of Autologous Tissue Substitute in Right Wrist Joint, External Approach

0RWNX8Z Revision of Spacer in Right Wrist Joint, External Approach

0RWNXJZ Revision of Synthetic Substitute in Right Wrist Joint, External Approach

---

0RWNXKZ Revision of Nonautologous Tissue Substitute in Right Wrist Joint, External Approach

0RWP00Z Revision of Drainage Device in Left Wrist Joint, Open Approach

0RWP03Z Revision of Infusion Device in Left Wrist Joint, Open Approach

0RWP04Z Revision of Internal Fixation Device in Left Wrist Joint, Open Approach

0RWP05Z Revision of External Fixation Device in Left Wrist Joint, Open Approach

0RWP07Z Revision of Autologous Tissue Substitute in Left Wrist Joint, Open Approach

0RWP08Z Revision of Spacer in Left Wrist Joint, Open Approach

0RWP0JZ Revision of Synthetic Substitute in Left Wrist Joint, Open Approach

0RWP0KZ Revision of Nonautologous Tissue Substitute in Left Wrist Joint, Open Approach

0RWP30Z Revision of Drainage Device in Left Wrist Joint, Percutaneous Approach

0RWP33Z Revision of Infusion Device in Left Wrist Joint, Percutaneous Approach

0RWP34Z Revision of Internal Fixation Device in Left Wrist Joint, Percutaneous Approach

0RWP35Z Revision of External Fixation Device in Left Wrist Joint, Percutaneous Approach

0RWP37Z Revision of Autologous Tissue Substitute in Left Wrist Joint, Percutaneous Approach

0RWP38Z Revision of Spacer in Left Wrist Joint, Percutaneous Approach

0RWP3JZ Revision of Synthetic Substitute in Left Wrist Joint, Percutaneous Approach

0RWP3KZ Revision of Nonautologous Tissue Substitute in Left Wrist Joint, Percutaneous Approach

0RWP40Z Revision of Drainage Device in Left Wrist Joint, Percutaneous Endoscopic Approach

0RWP43Z Revision of Infusion Device in Left Wrist Joint, Percutaneous Endoscopic Approach

0RWP44Z Revision of Internal Fixation Device in Left Wrist Joint, Percutaneous Endoscopic Approach

0RWP45Z Revision of External Fixation Device in Left Wrist Joint, Percutaneous Endoscopic Approach

0RWP47Z Revision of Autologous Tissue Substitute in Left Wrist Joint, Percutaneous Endoscopic Approach

0RWP48Z Revision of Spacer in Left Wrist Joint, Percutaneous Endoscopic Approach

0RWP4JZ Revision of Synthetic Substitute in Left Wrist Joint, Percutaneous Endoscopic Approach

0RWP4KZ Revision of Nonautologous Tissue Substitute in Left Wrist Joint, Percutaneous Endoscopic Approach

0RWPX0Z Revision of Drainage Device in Left Wrist Joint, External Approach

0RWPX3Z Revision of Infusion Device in Left Wrist Joint, External Approach

0RWPX4Z Revision of Internal Fixation Device in Left Wrist Joint, External Approach

0RWPX5Z Revision of External Fixation Device in Left Wrist Joint, External Approach

0RWPX7Z Revision of Autologous Tissue Substitute in Left Wrist Joint, External Approach

0RWPX8Z Revision of Spacer in Left Wrist Joint, External Approach

0RWPXJZ Revision of Synthetic Substitute in Left Wrist Joint, External Approach

0RWPXKZ Revision of Nonautologous Tissue Substitute in Left Wrist Joint, External Approach

0RWQ00Z Revision of Drainage Device in Right Carpal Joint, Open Approach

0RWQ03Z Revision of Infusion Device in Right Carpal Joint, Open Approach

0RWQ04Z Revision of Internal Fixation Device in Right Carpal Joint, Open Approach

0RWQ05Z Revision of External Fixation Device in Right Carpal Joint, Open Approach

0RWQ07Z Revision of Autologous Tissue Substitute in Right Carpal Joint, Open Approach

0RWQ08Z Revision of Spacer in Right Carpal Joint, Open Approach

0RWQ0JZ Revision of Synthetic Substitute in Right Carpal Joint, Open Approach

0RWQ0KZ Revision of Nonautologous Tissue Substitute in Right Carpal Joint, Open Approach

0RWQ30Z Revision of Drainage Device in Right Carpal Joint, Percutaneous Approach

0RWQ33Z Revision of Infusion Device in Right Carpal Joint, Percutaneous Approach

0RWQ34Z Revision of Internal Fixation Device in Right Carpal Joint, Percutaneous Approach

0RWQ35Z Revision of External Fixation Device in Right Carpal Joint, Percutaneous Approach

0RWQ37Z Revision of Autologous Tissue Substitute in Right Carpal Joint, Percutaneous Approach

0RWQ38Z Revision of Spacer in Right Carpal Joint, Percutaneous Approach

0RWQ3JZ Revision of Synthetic Substitute in Right Carpal Joint, Percutaneous Approach

0RWQ3KZ Revision of Nonautologous Tissue Substitute in Right Carpal Joint, Percutaneous Approach

0RWQ40Z Revision of Drainage Device in Right Carpal Joint, Percutaneous Endoscopic Approach

0RWQ43Z Revision of Infusion Device in Right Carpal Joint, Percutaneous Endoscopic Approach

0RWQ44Z Revision of Internal Fixation Device in Right Carpal Joint, Percutaneous Endoscopic Approach

0RWQ45Z Revision of External Fixation Device in Right Carpal Joint, Percutaneous Endoscopic Approach

0RWQ47Z Revision of Autologous Tissue Substitute in Right Carpal Joint, Percutaneous Endoscopic Approach

0RWQ48Z Revision of Spacer in Right Carpal Joint, Percutaneous Endoscopic Approach

0RWQ4JZ Revision of Synthetic Substitute in Right Carpal Joint, Percutaneous Endoscopic Approach

0RWQ4KZ Revision of Nonautologous Tissue Substitute in Right Carpal Joint, Percutaneous Endoscopic Approach

0RWQX0Z Revision of Drainage Device in Right Carpal Joint, External Approach

0RWQX3Z Revision of Infusion Device in Right Carpal Joint, External Approach

0RWQX4Z Revision of Internal Fixation Device in Right Carpal Joint, External Approach

0RWQX5Z Revision of External Fixation Device in Right Carpal Joint, External Approach

0RWQX7Z Revision of Autologous Tissue Substitute in Right Carpal Joint, External Approach

0RWQX8Z Revision of Spacer in Right Carpal Joint, External Approach

0RWQXJZ Revision of Synthetic Substitute in Right Carpal Joint, External Approach

0RWQXKZ Revision of Nonautologous Tissue Substitute in Right Carpal Joint, External Approach

0RWR00Z Revision of Drainage Device in Left Carpal Joint, Open Approach

0RWR03Z Revision of Infusion Device in Left Carpal Joint, Open Approach

0RWR04Z Revision of Internal Fixation Device in Left Carpal Joint, Open Approach

0RWR05Z Revision of External Fixation Device in Left Carpal Joint, Open Approach

0RWR07Z Revision of Autologous Tissue Substitute in Left Carpal Joint, Open Approach

0RWR08Z Revision of Spacer in Left Carpal Joint, Open Approach

0RWR0JZ Revision of Synthetic Substitute in Left Carpal Joint, Open Approach

0RWR0KZ Revision of Nonautologous Tissue Substitute in Left Carpal Joint, Open Approach

0RWR30Z Revision of Drainage Device in Left Carpal Joint, Percutaneous Approach

0RWR33Z Revision of Infusion Device in Left Carpal Joint, Percutaneous Approach

0RWR34Z Revision of Internal Fixation Device in Left Carpal Joint, Percutaneous Approach

0RWR35Z Revision of External Fixation Device in Left Carpal Joint, Percutaneous Approach

0RWR37Z Revision of Autologous Tissue Substitute in Left Carpal Joint, Percutaneous Approach

0RWR38Z Revision of Spacer in Left Carpal Joint, Percutaneous Approach

0RWR3JZ Revision of Synthetic Substitute in Left Carpal Joint, Percutaneous Approach

0RWR3KZ Revision of Nonautologous Tissue Substitute in Left Carpal Joint, Percutaneous Approach

0RWR40Z Revision of Drainage Device in Left Carpal Joint, Percutaneous Endoscopic Approach

0RWR43Z Revision of Infusion Device in Left Carpal Joint, Percutaneous Endoscopic Approach

0RWR44Z Revision of Internal Fixation Device in Left Carpal Joint, Percutaneous Endoscopic Approach

0RWR45Z Revision of External Fixation Device in Left Carpal Joint, Percutaneous Endoscopic Approach

0RWR47Z Revision of Autologous Tissue Substitute in Left Carpal Joint, Percutaneous Endoscopic Approach

0RWR48Z Revision of Spacer in Left Carpal Joint, Percutaneous Endoscopic Approach

0RWR4JZ Revision of Synthetic Substitute in Left Carpal Joint, Percutaneous Endoscopic Approach

0RWR4KZ Revision of Nonautologous Tissue Substitute in Left Carpal Joint, Percutaneous Endoscopic Approach

0RWRX0Z Revision of Drainage Device in Left Carpal Joint, External Approach

0RWRX3Z Revision of Infusion Device in Left Carpal Joint, External Approach

0RWRX4Z Revision of Internal Fixation Device in Left Carpal Joint, External Approach

0RWRX5Z Revision of External Fixation Device in Left Carpal Joint, External Approach

0RWRX7Z Revision of Autologous Tissue Substitute in Left Carpal Joint, External Approach

0RWRX8Z Revision of Spacer in Left Carpal Joint, External Approach

0RWRXJZ Revision of Synthetic Substitute in Left Carpal Joint, External Approach

0RWRXKZ Revision of Nonautologous Tissue Substitute in Left Carpal Joint, External Approach

0RWS00Z Revision of Drainage Device in Right Metacarpocarpal Joint, Open Approach

0RWS03Z Revision of Infusion Device in Right Metacarpocarpal Joint, Open Approach

0RWS04Z Revision of Internal Fixation Device in Right Metacarpocarpal Joint, Open Approach

0RWS05Z Revision of External Fixation Device in Right Metacarpocarpal Joint, Open Approach

0RWS07Z Revision of Autologous Tissue Substitute in Right Metacarpocarpal Joint, Open Approach

0RWS08Z Revision of Spacer in Right Metacarpocarpal Joint, Open Approach

0RWS0JZ Revision of Synthetic Substitute in Right Metacarpocarpal Joint, Open Approach

0RWS0KZ Revision of Nonautologous Tissue Substitute in Right Metacarpocarpal Joint, Open Approach

0RWS30Z Revision of Drainage Device in Right Metacarpocarpal Joint, Percutaneous Approach

0RWS33Z Revision of Infusion Device in Right Metacarpocarpal Joint, Percutaneous Approach

0RWS34Z Revision of Internal Fixation Device in Right Metacarpocarpal Joint, Percutaneous Approach

0RWS35Z Revision of External Fixation Device in Right Metacarpocarpal Joint, Percutaneous Approach

0RWS37Z Revision of Autologous Tissue Substitute in Right Metacarpocarpal Joint, Percutaneous Approach

0RWS38Z Revision of Spacer in Right Metacarpocarpal Joint, Percutaneous Approach

0RWS3JZ Revision of Synthetic Substitute in Right Metacarpocarpal Joint, Percutaneous Approach

0RWS3KZ Revision of Nonautologous Tissue Substitute in Right Metacarpocarpal Joint, Percutaneous Approach

0RWS40Z Revision of Drainage Device in Right Metacarpocarpal Joint, Percutaneous Endoscopic Approach

0RWS43Z Revision of Infusion Device in Right Metacarpocarpal Joint, Percutaneous Endoscopic Approach

0RWS44Z Revision of Internal Fixation Device in Right Metacarpocarpal Joint, Percutaneous Endoscopic Approach

0RWS45Z Revision of External Fixation Device in Right Metacarpocarpal Joint, Percutaneous Endoscopic Approach

0RWS47Z Revision of Autologous Tissue Substitute in Right Metacarpocarpal Joint, Percutaneous Endoscopic Approach

0RWS48Z Revision of Spacer in Right Metacarpocarpal Joint, Percutaneous Endoscopic Approach

0RWS4JZ Revision of Synthetic Substitute in Right Metacarpocarpal Joint, Percutaneous Endoscopic Approach

0RWS4KZ Revision of Nonautologous Tissue Substitute in Right Metacarpocarpal Joint, Percutaneous Endoscopic Approach

0RWSX0Z Revision of Drainage Device in Right Metacarpocarpal Joint, External Approach

0RWSX3Z Revision of Infusion Device in Right Metacarpocarpal Joint, External Approach

0RWSX4Z Revision of Internal Fixation Device in Right Metacarpocarpal Joint, External Approach

0RWSX5Z Revision of External Fixation Device in Right Metacarpocarpal Joint, External Approach

0RWSX7Z Revision of Autologous Tissue Substitute in Right Metacarpocarpal Joint, External Approach

0RWSX8Z Revision of Spacer in Right Metacarpocarpal Joint, External Approach

0RWSXJZ Revision of Synthetic Substitute in Right Metacarpocarpal Joint, External Approach

0RWSXKZ Revision of Nonautologous Tissue Substitute in Right Metacarpocarpal Joint, External Approach

0RWT00Z Revision of Drainage Device in Left Metacarpocarpal Joint, Open Approach

0RWT03Z Revision of Infusion Device in Left Metacarpocarpal Joint, Open Approach

0RWT04Z Revision of Internal Fixation Device in Left Metacarpocarpal Joint, Open Approach

0RWT05Z Revision of External Fixation Device in Left Metacarpocarpal Joint, Open Approach

0RWT07Z Revision of Autologous Tissue Substitute in Left Metacarpocarpal Joint, Open Approach

0RWT08Z Revision of Spacer in Left Metacarpocarpal Joint, Open Approach

0RWT0JZ Revision of Synthetic Substitute in Left Metacarpocarpal Joint, Open Approach

0RWT0KZ Revision of Nonautologous Tissue Substitute in Left Metacarpocarpal Joint, Open Approach

0RWT30Z Revision of Drainage Device in Left Metacarpocarpal Joint, Percutaneous Approach

0RWT33Z Revision of Infusion Device in Left Metacarpocarpal Joint, Percutaneous Approach

0RWT34Z Revision of Internal Fixation Device in Left Metacarpocarpal Joint, Percutaneous Approach

0RWT35Z Revision of External Fixation Device in Left Metacarpocarpal Joint, Percutaneous Approach

0RWT37Z Revision of Autologous Tissue Substitute in Left Metacarpocarpal Joint, Percutaneous Approach

0RWT38Z Revision of Spacer in Left Metacarpocarpal Joint, Percutaneous Approach

0RWT3JZ Revision of Synthetic Substitute in Left Metacarpocarpal Joint, Percutaneous Approach

0RWT3KZ Revision of Nonautologous Tissue Substitute in Left Metacarpocarpal Joint, Percutaneous Approach

0RWT40Z Revision of Drainage Device in Left Metacarpocarpal Joint, Percutaneous Endoscopic Approach

0RWT43Z Revision of Infusion Device in Left Metacarpocarpal Joint, Percutaneous Endoscopic Approach

0RWT44Z Revision of Internal Fixation Device in Left Metacarpocarpal Joint, Percutaneous Endoscopic Approach

0RWT45Z Revision of External Fixation Device in Left Metacarpocarpal Joint, Percutaneous Endoscopic Approach

0RWT47Z Revision of Autologous Tissue Substitute in Left Metacarpocarpal Joint, Percutaneous Endoscopic Approach

0RWT48Z Revision of Spacer in Left Metacarpocarpal Joint, Percutaneous Endoscopic Approach

0RWT4JZ Revision of Synthetic Substitute in Left Metacarpocarpal Joint, Percutaneous Endoscopic Approach

0RWT4KZ Revision of Nonautologous Tissue Substitute in Left Metacarpocarpal Joint, Percutaneous Endoscopic Approach

0RWTX0Z Revision of Drainage Device in Left Metacarpocarpal Joint, External Approach

0RWTX3Z Revision of Infusion Device in Left Metacarpocarpal Joint, External Approach

0RWTX4Z Revision of Internal Fixation Device in Left Metacarpocarpal Joint, External Approach

0RWTX5Z Revision of External Fixation Device in Left Metacarpocarpal Joint, External Approach

0RWTX7Z Revision of Autologous Tissue Substitute in Left Metacarpocarpal Joint, External Approach

0RWTX8Z Revision of Spacer in Left Metacarpocarpal Joint, External Approach

0RWTXJZ Revision of Synthetic Substitute in Left Metacarpocarpal Joint, External Approach

0RWTXKZ Revision of Nonautologous Tissue Substitute in Left Metacarpocarpal Joint, External Approach

0RWU00Z Revision of Drainage Device in Right Metacarpophalangeal Joint, Open Approach

0RWU03Z Revision of Infusion Device in Right Metacarpophalangeal Joint, Open Approach

0RWU04Z Revision of Internal Fixation Device in Right Metacarpophalangeal Joint, Open Approach

0RWU05Z Revision of External Fixation Device in Right Metacarpophalangeal Joint, Open Approach

0RWU07Z Revision of Autologous Tissue Substitute in Right Metacarpophalangeal Joint, Open Approach

0RWU08Z Revision of Spacer in Right Metacarpophalangeal Joint, Open Approach

0RWU0JZ Revision of Synthetic Substitute in Right Metacarpophalangeal Joint, Open Approach

0RWU0KZ Revision of Nonautologous Tissue Substitute in Right Metacarpophalangeal Joint, Open Approach

0RWU30Z Revision of Drainage Device in Right Metacarpophalangeal Joint, Percutaneous Approach

0RWU33Z Revision of Infusion Device in Right Metacarpophalangeal Joint, Percutaneous Approach

0RWU34Z Revision of Internal Fixation Device in Right Metacarpophalangeal Joint, Percutaneous Approach

0RWU35Z Revision of External Fixation Device in Right Metacarpophalangeal Joint, Percutaneous Approach

0RWU37Z Revision of Autologous Tissue Substitute in Right Metacarpophalangeal Joint, Percutaneous Approach

0RWU38Z Revision of Spacer in Right Metacarpophalangeal Joint, Percutaneous Approach

0RWU3JZ Revision of Synthetic Substitute in Right Metacarpophalangeal Joint, Percutaneous Approach

0RWU3KZ Revision of Nonautologous Tissue Substitute in Right Metacarpophalangeal Joint, Percutaneous Approach

0RWU40Z Revision of Drainage Device in Right Metacarpophalangeal Joint, Percutaneous Endoscopic Approach

0RWU43Z Revision of Infusion Device in Right Metacarpophalangeal Joint, Percutaneous Endoscopic Approach

0RWU44Z Revision of Internal Fixation Device in Right Metacarpophalangeal Joint, Percutaneous Endoscopic Approach

0RWU45Z Revision of External Fixation Device in Right Metacarpophalangeal Joint, Percutaneous Endoscopic Approach

0RWU47Z Revision of Autologous Tissue Substitute in Right Metacarpophalangeal Joint, Percutaneous Endoscopic Approach

0RWU48Z Revision of Spacer in Right Metacarpophalangeal Joint, Percutaneous Endoscopic Approach

0RWU4JZ Revision of Synthetic Substitute in Right Metacarpophalangeal Joint, Percutaneous Endoscopic Approach

0RWU4KZ Revision of Nonautologous Tissue Substitute in Right Metacarpophalangeal Joint, Percutaneous Endoscopic Approach

0RWUX0Z Revision of Drainage Device in Right Metacarpophalangeal Joint, External Approach

0RWUX3Z Revision of Infusion Device in Right Metacarpophalangeal Joint, External Approach

0RWUX4Z Revision of Internal Fixation Device in Right Metacarpophalangeal Joint, External Approach

0RWUX5Z Revision of External Fixation Device in Right Metacarpophalangeal Joint, External Approach

0RWUX7Z Revision of Autologous Tissue Substitute in Right Metacarpophalangeal Joint, External Approach

0RWUX8Z Revision of Spacer in Right Metacarpophalangeal Joint, External Approach

0RWUXJZ Revision of Synthetic Substitute in Right Metacarpophalangeal Joint, External Approach

0RWUXKZ Revision of Nonautologous Tissue Substitute in Right Metacarpophalangeal Joint, External Approach

0RWV00Z Revision of Drainage Device in Left Metacarpophalangeal Joint, Open Approach

0RWV03Z Revision of Infusion Device in Left Metacarpophalangeal Joint, Open Approach

0RWV04Z Revision of Internal Fixation Device in Left Metacarpophalangeal Joint, Open Approach

0RWV05Z Revision of External Fixation Device in Left Metacarpophalangeal Joint, Open Approach

0RWV07Z Revision of Autologous Tissue Substitute in Left Metacarpophalangeal Joint, Open Approach

0RWV08Z Revision of Spacer in Left Metacarpophalangeal Joint, Open Approach

0RWV0JZ Revision of Synthetic Substitute in Left Metacarpophalangeal Joint, Open Approach

0RWV0KZ Revision of Nonautologous Tissue Substitute in Left Metacarpophalangeal Joint, Open Approach

0RWV30Z Revision of Drainage Device in Left Metacarpophalangeal Joint, Percutaneous Approach

0RWV33Z Revision of Infusion Device in Left Metacarpophalangeal Joint, Percutaneous Approach

0RWV34Z Revision of Internal Fixation Device in Left Metacarpophalangeal Joint, Percutaneous Approach

0RWV35Z Revision of External Fixation Device in Left Metacarpophalangeal Joint, Percutaneous Approach

0RWV37Z Revision of Autologous Tissue Substitute in Left Metacarpophalangeal Joint, Percutaneous Approach

0RWV38Z Revision of Spacer in Left Metacarpophalangeal Joint, Percutaneous Approach

0RWV3JZ Revision of Synthetic Substitute in Left Metacarpophalangeal Joint, Percutaneous Approach

0RWV3KZ Revision of Nonautologous Tissue Substitute in Left Metacarpophalangeal Joint, Percutaneous Approach

0RWV40Z Revision of Drainage Device in Left Metacarpophalangeal Joint, Percutaneous Endoscopic Approach

0RWV43Z Revision of Infusion Device in Left Metacarpophalangeal Joint, Percutaneous Endoscopic Approach

0RWV44Z Revision of Internal Fixation Device in Left Metacarpophalangeal Joint, Percutaneous Endoscopic Approach

0RWV45Z Revision of External Fixation Device in Left Metacarpophalangeal Joint, Percutaneous Endoscopic Approach

0RWV47Z Revision of Autologous Tissue Substitute in Left Metacarpophalangeal Joint, Percutaneous Endoscopic Approach

0RWV48Z Revision of Spacer in Left Metacarpophalangeal Joint, Percutaneous Endoscopic Approach

0RWV4JZ Revision of Synthetic Substitute in Left Metacarpophalangeal Joint, Percutaneous Endoscopic Approach

0RWV4KZ Revision of Nonautologous Tissue Substitute in Left Metacarpophalangeal Joint, Percutaneous Endoscopic Approach

0RWVX0Z Revision of Drainage Device in Left Metacarpophalangeal Joint, External Approach

0RWVX3Z Revision of Infusion Device in Left Metacarpophalangeal Joint, External Approach

0RWVX4Z Revision of Internal Fixation Device in Left Metacarpophalangeal Joint, External Approach

0RWVX5Z Revision of External Fixation Device in Left Metacarpophalangeal Joint, External Approach

0RWVX7Z Revision of Autologous Tissue Substitute in Left Metacarpophalangeal Joint, External Approach

0RWVX8Z Revision of Spacer in Left Metacarpophalangeal Joint, External Approach

0RWVXJZ Revision of Synthetic Substitute in Left Metacarpophalangeal Joint, External Approach

0RWVXKZ Revision of Nonautologous Tissue Substitute in Left Metacarpophalangeal Joint, External Approach

0RWW00Z Revision of Drainage Device in Right Finger Phalangeal Joint, Open Approach

0RWW03Z Revision of Infusion Device in Right Finger Phalangeal Joint, Open Approach

0RWW04Z Revision of Internal Fixation Device in Right Finger Phalangeal Joint, Open Approach

0RWW05Z Revision of External Fixation Device in Right Finger Phalangeal Joint, Open Approach

0RWW07Z Revision of Autologous Tissue Substitute in Right Finger Phalangeal Joint, Open Approach

0RWW08Z Revision of Spacer in Right Finger Phalangeal Joint, Open Approach

0RWW0JZ Revision of Synthetic Substitute in Right Finger Phalangeal Joint, Open Approach

0RWW0KZ Revision of Nonautologous Tissue Substitute in Right Finger Phalangeal Joint, Open Approach

0RWW30Z Revision of Drainage Device in Right Finger Phalangeal Joint, Percutaneous Approach

0RWW33Z Revision of Infusion Device in Right Finger Phalangeal Joint, Percutaneous Approach

0RWW34Z Revision of Internal Fixation Device in Right Finger Phalangeal Joint, Percutaneous Approach

0RWW35Z Revision of External Fixation Device in Right Finger Phalangeal Joint, Percutaneous Approach

0RWW37Z Revision of Autologous Tissue Substitute in Right Finger Phalangeal Joint, Percutaneous Approach

0RWW38Z Revision of Spacer in Right Finger Phalangeal Joint, Percutaneous Approach

0RWW3JZ Revision of Synthetic Substitute in Right Finger Phalangeal Joint, Percutaneous Approach

0RWW3KZ Revision of Nonautologous Tissue Substitute in Right Finger Phalangeal Joint, Percutaneous Approach

0RWW40Z Revision of Drainage Device in Right Finger Phalangeal Joint, Percutaneous Endoscopic Approach

0RWW43Z Revision of Infusion Device in Right Finger Phalangeal Joint, Percutaneous Endoscopic Approach

0RWW44Z Revision of Internal Fixation Device in Right Finger Phalangeal Joint, Percutaneous Endoscopic Approach

0RWW45Z Revision of External Fixation Device in Right Finger Phalangeal Joint, Percutaneous Endoscopic Approach

0RWW47Z Revision of Autologous Tissue Substitute in Right Finger Phalangeal Joint, Percutaneous Endoscopic Approach

0RWW48Z Revision of Spacer in Right Finger Phalangeal Joint, Percutaneous Endoscopic Approach

0RWW4JZ Revision of Synthetic Substitute in Right Finger Phalangeal Joint, Percutaneous Endoscopic Approach

0RWW4KZ Revision of Nonautologous Tissue Substitute in Right Finger Phalangeal Joint, Percutaneous Endoscopic Approach

0RWWX0Z Revision of Drainage Device in Right Finger Phalangeal Joint, External Approach

0RWWX3Z Revision of Infusion Device in Right Finger Phalangeal Joint, External Approach

0RWWX4Z Revision of Internal Fixation Device in Right Finger Phalangeal Joint, External Approach

0RWWX5Z Revision of External Fixation Device in Right Finger Phalangeal Joint, External Approach

0RWWX7Z Revision of Autologous Tissue Substitute in Right Finger Phalangeal Joint, External Approach

0RWWX8Z Revision of Spacer in Right Finger Phalangeal Joint, External Approach

0RWWXJZ Revision of Synthetic Substitute in Right Finger Phalangeal Joint, External Approach

0RWWXKZ Revision of Nonautologous Tissue Substitute in Right Finger Phalangeal Joint, External Approach

0RWX00Z Revision of Drainage Device in Left Finger Phalangeal Joint, Open Approach

0RWX03Z Revision of Infusion Device in Left Finger Phalangeal Joint, Open Approach

0RWX04Z Revision of Internal Fixation Device in Left Finger Phalangeal Joint, Open Approach

0RWX05Z Revision of External Fixation Device in Left Finger Phalangeal Joint, Open Approach

0RWX07Z Revision of Autologous Tissue Substitute in Left Finger Phalangeal Joint, Open Approach

0RWX08Z Revision of Spacer in Left Finger Phalangeal Joint, Open Approach

0RWX0JZ Revision of Synthetic Substitute in Left Finger Phalangeal Joint, Open Approach

0RWX0KZ Revision of Nonautologous Tissue Substitute in Left Finger Phalangeal Joint, Open Approach

0RWX30Z Revision of Drainage Device in Left Finger Phalangeal Joint, Percutaneous Approach

0RWX33Z Revision of Infusion Device in Left Finger Phalangeal Joint, Percutaneous Approach

0RWX34Z Revision of Internal Fixation Device in Left Finger Phalangeal Joint, Percutaneous Approach

0RWX35Z Revision of External Fixation Device in Left Finger Phalangeal Joint, Percutaneous Approach

0RWX37Z Revision of Autologous Tissue Substitute in Left Finger Phalangeal Joint, Percutaneous Approach

0RWX38Z Revision of Spacer in Left Finger Phalangeal Joint, Percutaneous Approach

0RWX3JZ Revision of Synthetic Substitute in Left Finger Phalangeal Joint, Percutaneous Approach

0RWX3KZ Revision of Nonautologous Tissue Substitute in Left Finger Phalangeal Joint, Percutaneous Approach

0RWX40Z Revision of Drainage Device in Left Finger Phalangeal Joint, Percutaneous Endoscopic Approach

0RWX43Z Revision of Infusion Device in Left Finger Phalangeal Joint, Percutaneous Endoscopic Approach

0RWX44Z Revision of Internal Fixation Device in Left Finger Phalangeal Joint, Percutaneous Endoscopic Approach

0RWX45Z Revision of External Fixation Device in Left Finger Phalangeal Joint, Percutaneous Endoscopic Approach

0RWX47Z Revision of Autologous Tissue Substitute in Left Finger Phalangeal Joint, Percutaneous Endoscopic Approach

0RWX48Z Revision of Spacer in Left Finger Phalangeal Joint, Percutaneous Endoscopic Approach

0RWX4JZ Revision of Synthetic Substitute in Left Finger Phalangeal Joint, Percutaneous Endoscopic Approach

0RWX4KZ Revision of Nonautologous Tissue Substitute in Left Finger Phalangeal Joint, Percutaneous Endoscopic Approach

0RWXX0Z Revision of Drainage Device in Left Finger Phalangeal Joint, External Approach

0RWXX3Z Revision of Infusion Device in Left Finger Phalangeal Joint, External Approach

0RWXX4Z Revision of Internal Fixation Device in Left Finger Phalangeal Joint, External Approach

0RWXX5Z Revision of External Fixation Device in Left Finger Phalangeal Joint, External Approach

0RWXX7Z Revision of Autologous Tissue Substitute in Left Finger Phalangeal Joint, External Approach

0RWXX8Z Revision of Spacer in Left Finger Phalangeal Joint, External Approach

0RWXXJZ Revision of Synthetic Substitute in Left Finger Phalangeal Joint, External Approach

0RWXXKZ Revision of Nonautologous Tissue Substitute in Left Finger Phalangeal Joint, External Approach

Lower Joints

Intervertebral Joint

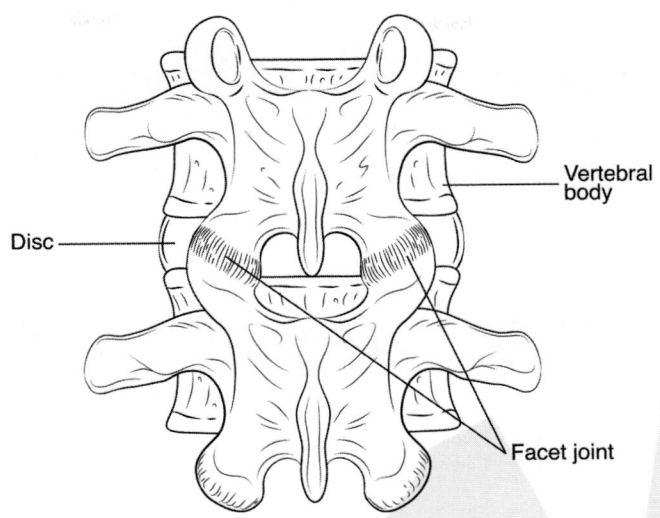

Disc

Vertebral body

Facet joint

Hip

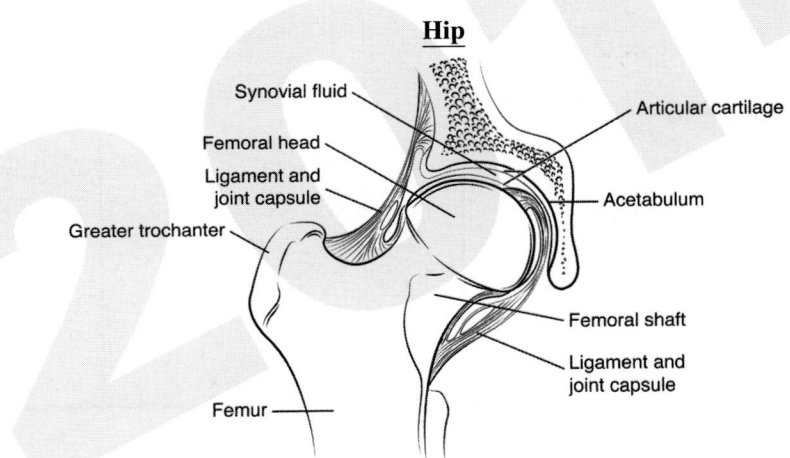

Synovial fluid

Femoral head

Ligament and joint capsule

Greater trochanter

Femur

Articular cartilage

Acetabulum

Femoral shaft

Ligament and joint capsule

Knee

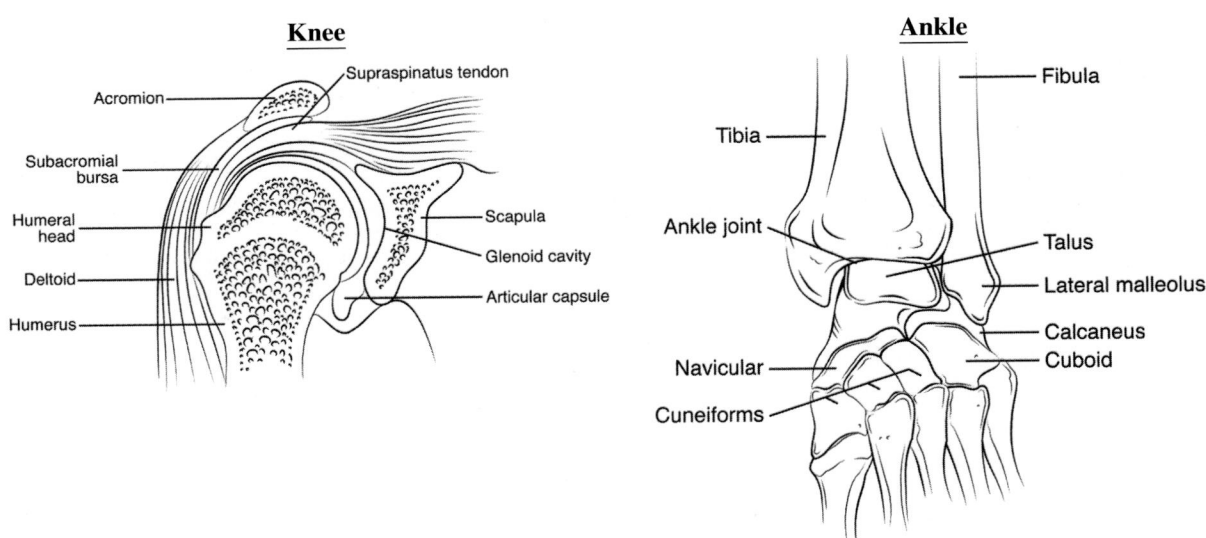

Supraspinatus tendon

Acromion

Subacromial bursa

Humeral head

Deltoid

Humerus

Scapula

Glenoid cavity

Articular capsule

Ankle

Fibula

Tibia

Ankle joint

Navicular

Cuneiforms

Talus

Lateral malleolus

Calcaneus

Cuboid

Lower Joints Tables 0S2–0SW

Section	0	Medical and Surgical
Body System	S	Lower Joints
Operation	2	**Change:** Taking out or off a device from a body part and putting back an identical or similar device in or on the same body part without cutting or puncturing the skin or a mucous membrane

Body Part (4th)	Approach (5th)	Device (6th)	Qualifier (7th)
Y Lower Joint	X External	0 Drainage Device Y Other Device	Z No Qualifier

Section	0	Medical and Surgical
Body System	S	Lower Joints
Operation	5	**Destruction:** Physical eradication of all or a portion of a body part by the direct use of energy, force, or a destructive agent

Body Part (4th)	Approach (5th)	Device (6th)	Qualifier (7th)
0 Lumbar Vertebral Joint 2 Lumbar Vertebral Disc 3 Lumbosacral Joint 4 Lumbosacral Disc 5 Sacrococcygeal Joint 6 Coccygeal Joint 7 Sacroiliac Joint, Right 8 Sacroiliac Joint, Left 9 Hip Joint, Right B Hip Joint, Left C Knee Joint, Right D Knee Joint, Left F Ankle Joint, Right G Ankle Joint, Left H Tarsal Joint, Right J Tarsal Joint, Left K Metatarsal-Tarsal Joint, Right L Metatarsal-Tarsal Joint, Left M Metatarsal-Phalangeal Joint, Right N Metatarsal-Phalangeal Joint, Left P Toe Phalangeal Joint, Right Q Toe Phalangeal Joint, Left	0 Open 3 Percutaneous 4 Percutaneous Endoscopic	Z No Device	Z No Qualifier

Section	0	Medical and Surgical
Body System	S	Lower Joints
Operation	9	**Drainage:** Taking or letting out fluids and/or gases from a body part

Body Part (4th)	Approach (5th)	Device (6th)	Qualifier (7th)
0 Lumbar Vertebral Joint 2 Lumbar Vertebral Disc 3 Lumbosacral Joint 4 Lumbosacral Disc 5 Sacrococcygeal Joint 6 Coccygeal Joint 7 Sacroiliac Joint, Right 8 Sacroiliac Joint, Left 9 Hip Joint, Right B Hip Joint, Left C Knee Joint, Right D Knee Joint, Left F Ankle Joint, Right G Ankle Joint, Left H Tarsal Joint, Right J Tarsal Joint, Left K Metatarsal-Tarsal Joint, Right L Metatarsal-Tarsal Joint, Left M Metatarsal-Phalangeal Joint, Right N Metatarsal-Phalangeal Joint, Left P Toe Phalangeal Joint, Right Q Toe Phalangeal Joint, Left	0 Open 3 Percutaneous 4 Percutaneous Endoscopic	0 Drainage Device	Z No Qualifier
0 Lumbar Vertebral Joint 2 Lumbar Vertebral Disc 3 Lumbosacral Joint 4 Lumbosacral Disc 5 Sacrococcygeal Joint 6 Coccygeal Joint 7 Sacroiliac Joint, Right 8 Sacroiliac Joint, Left 9 Hip Joint, Right B Hip Joint, Left C Knee Joint, Right D Knee Joint, Left F Ankle Joint, Right G Ankle Joint, Left H Tarsal Joint, Right J Tarsal Joint, Left K Metatarsal-Tarsal Joint, Right L Metatarsal-Tarsal Joint, Left M Metatarsal-Phalangeal Joint, Right N Metatarsal-Phalangeal Joint, Left P Toe Phalangeal Joint, Right Q Toe Phalangeal Joint, Left	0 Open 3 Percutaneous 4 Percutaneous Endoscopic	Z No Device	X Diagnostic Z No Qualifier

Section	0	Medical and Surgical
Body System	S	Lower Joints
Operation	B	Excision: Cutting out or off, without replacement, a portion of a body part

Body Part (4th)	Approach (5th)	Device (6th)	Qualifier (7th)
0 Lumbar Vertebral Joint 2 Lumbar Vertebral Disc 3 Lumbosacral Joint 4 Lumbosacral Disc 5 Sacrococcygeal Joint 6 Coccygeal Joint 7 Sacroiliac Joint, Right 8 Sacroiliac Joint, Left 9 Hip Joint, Right B Hip Joint, Left C Knee Joint, Right D Knee Joint, Left F Ankle Joint, Right G Ankle Joint, Left H Tarsal Joint, Right J Tarsal Joint, Left K Metatarsal-Tarsal Joint, Right L Metatarsal-Tarsal Joint, Left M Metatarsal-Phalangeal Joint, Right N Metatarsal-Phalangeal Joint, Left P Toe Phalangeal Joint, Right Q Toe Phalangeal Joint, Left	0 Open 3 Percutaneous 4 Percutaneous Endoscopic	Z No Device	X Diagnostic Z No Qualifier

Section	0	Medical and Surgical
Body System	S	Lower Joints
Operation	C	Extirpation: Taking or cutting out solid matter from a body part

Body Part (4th)	Approach (5th)	Device (6th)	Qualifier (7th)
0 Lumbar Vertebral Joint 2 Lumbar Vertebral Disc 3 Lumbosacral Joint 4 Lumbosacral Disc 5 Sacrococcygeal Joint 6 Coccygeal Joint 7 Sacroiliac Joint, Right 8 Sacroiliac Joint, Left 9 Hip Joint, Right B Hip Joint, Left C Knee Joint, Right D Knee Joint, Left F Ankle Joint, Right G Ankle Joint, Left H Tarsal Joint, Right J Tarsal Joint, Left K Metatarsal-Tarsal Joint, Right L Metatarsal-Tarsal Joint, Left M Metatarsal-Phalangeal Joint, Right N Metatarsal-Phalangeal Joint, Left P Toe Phalangeal Joint, Right Q Toe Phalangeal Joint, Left	0 Open 3 Percutaneous 4 Percutaneous Endoscopic	Z No Device	Z No Qualifier

Section	0	Medical and Surgical
Body System	S	Lower Joints
Operation	G	**Fusion:** Joining together portions of an articular body part rendering the articular body part immobile

Body Part (4th)	Approach (5th)	Device (6th)	Qualifier (7th)
0 Lumbar Vertebral Joint 1 Lumbar Vertebral Joints, 2 or more 3 Lumbosacral Joint	0 Open 3 Percutaneous 4 Percutaneous Endoscopic	7 Autologous Tissue Substitute A Interbody Fusion Device J Synthetic Substitute K Nonautologous Tissue Substitute Z No Device	0 Anterior Approach, Anterior Column 1 Posterior Approach, Posterior Column J Posterior Approach, Anterior Column
5 Sacrococcygeal Joint 6 Coccygeal Joint 7 Sacroiliac Joint, Right 8 Sacroiliac Joint, Left	0 Open 3 Percutaneous 4 Percutaneous Endoscopic	4 Internal Fixation Device 7 Autologous Tissue Substitute J Synthetic Substitute K Nonautologous Tissue Substitute Z No Device	Z No Qualifier
9 Hip Joint, Right B Hip Joint, Left C Knee Joint, Right D Knee Joint, Left F Ankle Joint, Right G Ankle Joint, Left H Tarsal Joint, Right J Tarsal Joint, Left K Metatarsal-Tarsal Joint, Right L Metatarsal-Tarsal Joint, Left M Metatarsal-Phalangeal Joint, Right N Metatarsal-Phalangeal Joint, Left P Toe Phalangeal Joint, Right Q Toe Phalangeal Joint, Left	0 Open 3 Percutaneous 4 Percutaneous Endoscopic	4 Internal Fixation Device 5 External Fixation Device 7 Autologous Tissue Substitute J Synthetic Substitute K Nonautologous Tissue Substitute Z No Device	Z No Qualifier

Section	0	Medical and Surgical
Body System	S	Lower Joints
Operation	H	**Insertion:** Putting in a nonbiological appliance that monitors, assists, performs, or prevents a physiological function but does not physically take the place of a body part

Body Part (4th)	Approach (5th)	Device (6th)	Qualifier (7th)
0 Lumbar Vertebral Joint 3 Lumbosacral Joint	0 Open 3 Percutaneous 4 Percutaneous Endoscopic	3 Infusion Device 4 Internal Fixation Device 8 Spacer B Spinal Stabilization Device, Interspinous Process C Spinal Stabilization Device, Pedicle-Based D Spinal Stabilization Device, Facet Replacement	Z No Qualifier
2 Lumbar Vertebral Disc 4 Lumbosacral Disc	0 Open 3 Percutaneous 4 Percutaneous Endoscopic	3 Infusion Device 8 Spacer	Z No Qualifier
5 Sacrococcygeal Joint 6 Coccygeal Joint 7 Sacroiliac Joint, Right 8 Sacroiliac Joint, Left	0 Open 3 Percutaneous 4 Percutaneous Endoscopic	3 Infusion Device 4 Internal Fixation Device 8 Spacer	Z No Qualifier

Continued

0SH *Continued*

Section	0	Medical and Surgical
Body System	S	Lower Joints
Operation	H	**Insertion:** Putting in a nonbiological appliance that monitors, assists, performs, or prevents a physiological function but does not physically take the place of a body part

Body Part (4ᵗʰ)	Approach (5ᵗʰ)	Device (6ᵗʰ)	Qualifier (7ᵗʰ)
9 Hip Joint, Right B Hip Joint, Left C Knee Joint, Right D Knee Joint, Left F Ankle Joint, Right G Ankle Joint, Left H Tarsal Joint, Right J Tarsal Joint, Left K Metatarsal-Tarsal Joint, Right L Metatarsal-Tarsal Joint, Left M Metatarsal-Phalangeal Joint, Right N Metatarsal-Phalangeal Joint, Left P Toe Phalangeal Joint, Right Q Toe Phalangeal Joint, Left	0 Open 3 Percutaneous 4 Percutaneous Endoscopic	3 Infusion Device 4 Internal Fixation Device 5 External Fixation Device 8 Spacer	Z No Qualifier

Section	0	Medical and Surgical
Body System	S	Lower Joints
Operation	J	**Inspection:** Visually and/or manually exploring a body part

Body Part (4ᵗʰ)	Approach (5ᵗʰ)	Device (6ᵗʰ)	Qualifier (7ᵗʰ)
0 Lumbar Vertebral Joint 2 Lumbar Vertebral Disc 3 Lumbosacral Joint 4 Lumbosacral Disc 5 Sacrococcygeal Joint 6 Coccygeal Joint 7 Sacroiliac Joint, Right 8 Sacroiliac Joint, Left 9 Hip Joint, Right B Hip Joint, Left C Knee Joint, Right D Knee Joint, Left F Ankle Joint, Right G Ankle Joint, Left H Tarsal Joint, Right J Tarsal Joint, Left K Metatarsal-Tarsal Joint, Right L Metatarsal-Tarsal Joint, Left M Metatarsal-Phalangeal Joint, Right N Metatarsal-Phalangeal Joint, Left P Toe Phalangeal Joint, Right Q Toe Phalangeal Joint, Left	0 Open 3 Percutaneous 4 Percutaneous Endoscopic X External	Z No Device	Z No Qualifier

Section   **0**   **Medical and Surgical**
Body System   **S**   **Lower Joints**
Operation   **N**   **Release:** Freeing a body part from an abnormal physical constraint by cutting or by the use of force

Body Part (4ᵗʰ)	Approach (5ᵗʰ)	Device (6ᵗʰ)	Qualifier (7ᵗʰ)
0 Lumbar Vertebral Joint 2 Lumbar Vertebral Disc 3 Lumbosacral Joint 4 Lumbosacral Disc 5 Sacrococcygeal Joint 6 Coccygeal Joint 7 Sacroiliac Joint, Right 8 Sacroiliac Joint, Left 9 Hip Joint, Right B Hip Joint, Left C Knee Joint, Right D Knee Joint, Left F Ankle Joint, Right G Ankle Joint, Left H Tarsal Joint, Right J Tarsal Joint, Left K Metatarsal-Tarsal Joint, Right L Metatarsal-Tarsal Joint, Left M Metatarsal-Phalangeal Joint, Right N Metatarsal-Phalangeal Joint, Left P Toe Phalangeal Joint, Right Q Toe Phalangeal Joint, Left	0 Open 3 Percutaneous 4 Percutaneous Endoscopic X External	Z No Device	Z No Qualifier

Section   **0**   **Medical and Surgical**
Body System   **S**   **Lower Joints**
Operation   **P**   **Removal:** Taking out or off a device from a body part

Body Part (4ᵗʰ)	Approach (5ᵗʰ)	Device (6ᵗʰ)	Qualifier (7ᵗʰ)
0 Lumbar Vertebral Joint 3 Lumbosacral Joint	0 Open 3 Percutaneous 4 Percutaneous Endoscopic	0 Drainage Device 3 Infusion Device 4 Internal Fixation Device 7 Autologous Tissue Substitute 8 Spacer A Interbody Fusion Device J Synthetic Substitute K Nonautologous Tissue Substitute	Z No Qualifier
0 Lumbar Vertebral Joint 3 Lumbosacral Joint	X External	0 Drainage Device 3 Infusion Device 4 Internal Fixation Device	Z No Qualifier
2 Lumbar Vertebral Disc 4 Lumbosacral Disc	0 Open 3 Percutaneous 4 Percutaneous Endoscopic	0 Drainage Device 3 Infusion Device 7 Autologous Tissue Substitute J Synthetic Substitute K Nonautologous Tissue Substitute	Z No Qualifier
2 Lumbar Vertebral Disc 4 Lumbosacral Disc	X External	0 Drainage Device 3 Infusion Device	Z No Qualifier
5 Sacrococcygeal Joint 6 Coccygeal Joint 7 Sacroiliac Joint, Right 8 Sacroiliac Joint, Left	0 Open 3 Percutaneous 4 Percutaneous Endoscopic	0 Drainage Device 3 Infusion Device 4 Internal Fixation Device 7 Autologous Tissue Substitute 8 Spacer J Synthetic Substitute K Nonautologous Tissue Substitute	Z No Qualifier

Continued

Section	0	Medical and Surgical
Body System	S	Lower Joints
Operation	P	Removal: Taking out or off a device from a body part

Body Part (4th)	Approach (5th)	Device (6th)	Qualifier (7th)
5 Sacrococcygeal Joint 6 Coccygeal Joint 7 Sacroiliac Joint, Right 8 Sacroiliac Joint, Left	X External	0 Drainage Device 3 Infusion Device 4 Internal Fixation Device	Z No Qualifier
9 Hip Joint, Right B Hip Joint, Left	0 Open	0 Drainage Device 3 Infusion Device 4 Internal Fixation Device 5 External Fixation Device 7 Autologous Tissue Substitute 8 Spacer 9 Liner B Resurfacing Device J Synthetic Substitute K Nonautologous Tissue Substitute	Z No Qualifier
9 Hip Joint, Right B Hip Joint, Left	3 Percutaneous 4 Percutaneous Endoscopic	0 Drainage Device 3 Infusion Device 4 Internal Fixation Device 5 External Fixation Device 7 Autologous Tissue Substitute 8 Spacer J Synthetic Substitute K Nonautologous Tissue Substitute	Z No Qualifier
9 Hip Joint, Right B Hip Joint, Left	X External	0 Drainage Device 3 Infusion Device 4 Internal Fixation Device 5 External Fixation Device	Z No Qualifier
C Knee Joint, Right D Knee Joint, Left	0 Open	0 Drainage Device 3 Infusion Device 4 Internal Fixation Device 5 External Fixation Device 7 Autologous Tissue Substitute 8 Spacer 9 Liner J Synthetic Substitute K Nonautologous Tissue Substitute	Z No Qualifier
C Knee Joint, Right D Knee Joint, Left	3 Percutaneous 4 Percutaneous Endoscopic	0 Drainage Device 3 Infusion Device 4 Internal Fixation Device 5 External Fixation Device 7 Autologous Tissue Substitute 8 Spacer J Synthetic Substitute K Nonautologous Tissue Substitute	Z No Qualifier
C Knee Joint, Right D Knee Joint, Left	X External	0 Drainage Device 3 Infusion Device 4 Internal Fixation Device 5 External Fixation Device	Z No Qualifier

Continued

0SP *Continued*

Section	0	Medical and Surgical
Body System	S	Lower Joints
Operation	P	**Removal:** Taking out or off a device from a body part

Body Part (4th)	Approach (5th)	Device (6th)	Qualifier (7th)
F Ankle Joint, Right G Ankle Joint, Left H Tarsal Joint, Right J Tarsal Joint, Left K Metatarsal-Tarsal Joint, Right L Metatarsal-Tarsal Joint, Left M Metatarsal-Phalangeal Joint, Right N Metatarsal-Phalangeal Joint, Left P Toe Phalangeal Joint, Right Q Toe Phalangeal Joint, Left	0 Open 3 Percutaneous 4 Percutaneous Endoscopic	0 Drainage Device 3 Infusion Device 4 Internal Fixation Device 5 External Fixation Device 7 Autologous Tissue Substitute 8 Spacer J Synthetic Substitute K Nonautologous Tissue Substitute	Z No Qualifier
F Ankle Joint, Right G Ankle Joint, Left H Tarsal Joint, Right J Tarsal Joint, Left K Metatarsal-Tarsal Joint, Right L Metatarsal-Tarsal Joint, Left M Metatarsal-Phalangeal Joint, Right N Metatarsal-Phalangeal Joint, Left P Toe Phalangeal Joint, Right Q Toe Phalangeal Joint, Left	X External	0 Drainage Device 3 Infusion Device 4 Internal Fixation Device 5 External Fixation Device	Z No Qualifier

Section	0	Medical and Surgical
Body System	S	Lower Joints
Operation	Q	**Repair:** Restoring, to the extent possible, a body part to its normal anatomic structure and function

Body Part (4th)	Approach (5th)	Device (6th)	Qualifier (7th)
0 Lumbar Vertebral Joint 2 Lumbar Vertebral Disc 3 Lumbosacral Joint 4 Lumbosacral Disc 5 Sacrococcygeal Joint 6 Coccygeal Joint 7 Sacroiliac Joint, Right 8 Sacroiliac Joint, Left 9 Hip Joint, Right B Hip Joint, Left C Knee Joint, Right D Knee Joint, Left F Ankle Joint, Right G Ankle Joint, Left H Tarsal Joint, Right J Tarsal Joint, Left K Metatarsal-Tarsal Joint, Right L Metatarsal-Tarsal Joint, Left M Metatarsal-Phalangeal Joint, Right N Metatarsal-Phalangeal Joint, Left P Toe Phalangeal Joint, Right Q Toe Phalangeal Joint, Left	0 Open 3 Percutaneous 4 Percutaneous Endoscopic X External	Z No Device	Z No Qualifier

Section	0	Medical and Surgical
Body System	S	Lower Joints
Operation	R	Replacement: Putting in or on biological or synthetic material that physically takes the place and/or function of all or a portion of a body part

Body Part (4th)	Approach (5th)	Device (6th)	Qualifier (7th)
0 Lumbar Vertebral Joint 2 Lumbar Vertebral Disc 3 Lumbosacral Joint 4 Lumbosacral Disc 5 Sacrococcygeal Joint 6 Coccygeal Joint 7 Sacroiliac Joint, Right 8 Sacroiliac Joint, Left H Tarsal Joint, Right J Tarsal Joint, Left K Metatarsal-Tarsal Joint, Right L Metatarsal-Tarsal Joint, Left M Metatarsal-Phalangeal Joint, Right N Metatarsal-Phalangeal Joint, Left P Toe Phalangeal Joint, Right Q Toe Phalangeal Joint, Left	0 Open	7 Autologous Tissue Substitute J Synthetic Substitute K Nonautologous Tissue Substitute	Z No Qualifier
9 Hip Joint, Right B Hip Joint, Left	0 Open	1 Synthetic Substitute, Metal 2 Synthetic Substitute, Metal on Polyethylene 3 Synthetic Substitute, Ceramic 4 Synthetic Substitute, Ceramic on Polyethylene J Synthetic Substitute	9 Cemented A Uncemented Z No Qualifier
9 Hip Joint, Right B Hip Joint, Left	0 Open	7 Autologous Tissue Substitute K Nonautologous Tissue Substitute	Z No Qualifier
A Hip Joint, Acetabular Surface, Right E Hip Joint, Acetabular Surface, Left	0 Open	0 Synthetic Substitute, Polyethylene 1 Synthetic Substitute, Metal 3 Synthetic Substitute, Ceramic J Synthetic Substitute	9 Cemented A Uncemented Z No Qualifier
A Hip Joint, Acetabular Surface, Right E Hip Joint, Acetabular Surface, Left	0 Open	7 Autologous Tissue Substitute K Nonautologous Tissue Substitute	Z No Qualifier
C Knee Joint, Right D Knee Joint, Left F Ankle Joint, Right G Ankle Joint, Left T Knee Joint, Femoral Surface, Right U Knee Joint, Femoral Surface, Left V Knee Joint, Tibial Surface, Right W Knee Joint, Tibial Surface, Left	0 Open	7 Autologous Tissue Substitute K Nonautologous Tissue Substitute	Z No Qualifier
C Knee Joint, Right D Knee Joint, Left F Ankle Joint, Right G Ankle Joint, Left T Knee Joint, Femoral Surface, Right U Knee Joint, Femoral Surface, Left V Knee Joint, Tibial Surface, Right W Knee Joint, Tibial Surface, Left	0 Open	J Synthetic Substitute	9 Cemented A Uncemented Z No Qualifier

Continued

0SR *Continued*

Section	0	**Medical and Surgical**
Body System	S	**Lower Joints**
Operation	R	**Replacement:** Putting in or on biological or synthetic material that physically takes the place and/or function of all or a portion of a body part

Body Part (4th)	Approach (5th)	Device (6th)	Qualifier (7th)
R Hip Joint, Femoral Surface, Right **S** Hip Joint, Femoral Surface, Left	**0** Open	**1** Synthetic Substitute, Metal **3** Synthetic Substitute, Ceramic **J** Synthetic Substitute	**9** Cemented **A** Uncemented **Z** No Qualifier
R Hip Joint, Femoral Surface, Right **S** Hip Joint, Femoral Surface, Left	**0** Open	**7** Autologous Tissue Substitute **K** Nonautologous Tissue Substitute	**Z** No Qualifier

Section	0	**Medical and Surgical**
Body System	S	**Lower Joints**
Operation	S	**Reposition:** Moving to its normal location, or other suitable location, all or a portion of a body part

Body Part (4th)	Approach (5th)	Device (6th)	Qualifier (7th)
0 Lumbar Vertebral Joint **3** Lumbosacral Joint **5** Sacrococcygeal Joint **6** Coccygeal Joint **7** Sacroiliac Joint, Right **8** Sacroiliac Joint, Left	**0** Open **3** Percutaneous **4** Percutaneous Endoscopic **X** External	**4** Internal Fixation Device **Z** No Device	**Z** No Qualifier
9 Hip Joint, Right **B** Hip Joint, Left **C** Knee Joint, Right **D** Knee Joint, Left **F** Ankle Joint, Right **G** Ankle Joint, Left **H** Tarsal Joint, Right **J** Tarsal Joint, Left **K** Metatarsal-Tarsal Joint, Right **L** Metatarsal-Tarsal Joint, Left **M** Metatarsal-Phalangeal Joint, Right **N** Metatarsal-Phalangeal Joint, Left **P** Toe Phalangeal Joint, Right **Q** Toe Phalangeal Joint, Left	**0** Open **3** Percutaneous **4** Percutaneous Endoscopic **X** External	**4** Internal Fixation Device **5** External Fixation Device **Z** No Device	**Z** No Qualifier

Section	0	Medical and Surgical
Body System	S	Lower Joints
Operation	T	**Resection:** Cutting out or off, without replacement, all of a body part

Body Part (4th)	Approach (5th)	Device (6th)	Qualifier (7th)
2 Lumbar Vertebral Disc 4 Lumbosacral Disc 5 Sacrococcygeal Joint 6 Coccygeal Joint 7 Sacroiliac Joint, Right 8 Sacroiliac Joint, Left 9 Hip Joint, Right B Hip Joint, Left C Knee Joint, Right D Knee Joint, Left F Ankle Joint, Right G Ankle Joint, Left H Tarsal Joint, Right J Tarsal Joint, Left K Metatarsal-Tarsal Joint, Right L Metatarsal-Tarsal Joint, Left M Metatarsal-Phalangeal Joint, Right N Metatarsal-Phalangeal Joint, Left P Toe Phalangeal Joint, Right Q Toe Phalangeal Joint, Left	0 Open	Z No Device	Z No Qualifier

Section	0	Medical and Surgical
Body System	S	Lower Joints
Operation	U	**Supplement:** Putting in or on biological or synthetic material that physically reinforces and/or augments the function of a portion of a body part

Body Part (4th)	Approach (5th)	Device (6th)	Qualifier (7th)
0 Lumbar Vertebral Joint 2 Lumbar Vertebral Disc 3 Lumbosacral Joint 4 Lumbosacral Disc 5 Sacrococcygeal Joint 6 Coccygeal Joint 7 Sacroiliac Joint, Right 8 Sacroiliac Joint, Left F Ankle Joint, Right G Ankle Joint, Left H Tarsal Joint, Right J Tarsal Joint, Left K Metatarsal-Tarsal Joint, Right L Metatarsal-Tarsal Joint, Left M Metatarsal-Phalangeal Joint, Right N Metatarsal-Phalangeal Joint, Left P Toe Phalangeal Joint, Right Q Toe Phalangeal Joint, Left	0 Open 3 Percutaneous 4 Percutaneous Endoscopic	7 Autologous Tissue Substitute J Synthetic Substitute K Nonautologous Tissue Substitute	Z No Qualifier
9 Hip Joint, Right B Hip Joint, Left	0 Open	7 Autologous Tissue Substitute 9 Liner B Resurfacing Device J Synthetic Substitute K Nonautologous Tissue Substitute	Z No Qualifier
9 Hip Joint, Right B Hip Joint, Left	3 Percutaneous 4 Percutaneous Endoscopic	7 Autologous Tissue Substitute J Synthetic Substitute K Nonautologous Tissue Substitute	Z No Qualifier
A Hip Joint, Acetabular Surface, Right E Hip Joint, Acetabular Surface, Left R Hip Joint, Femoral Surface, Right S Hip Joint, Femoral Surface, Left	0 Open	9 Liner B Resurfacing Device	Z No Qualifier

Continued

Section	0	Medical and Surgical
Body System	S	Lower Joints
Operation	U	**Supplement:** Putting in or on biological or synthetic material that physically reinforces and/or augments the function of a portion of a body part

Body Part (4ᵗʰ)	Approach (5ᵗʰ)	Device (6ᵗʰ)	Qualifier (7ᵗʰ)
C Knee Joint, Right D Knee Joint, Left	0 Open	7 Autologous Tissue Substitute J Synthetic Substitute K Nonautologous Tissue Substitute	Z No Qualifier
C Knee Joint, Right D Knee Joint, Left	0 Open	9 Liner	C Patellar Surface Z No Qualifier
C Knee Joint, Right D Knee Joint, Left	3 Percutaneous 4 Percutaneous Endoscopic	7 Autologous Tissue Substitute J Synthetic Substitute K Nonautologous Tissue Substitute	Z No Qualifier
T Knee Joint, Femoral Surface, Right U Knee Joint, Femoral Surface, Left V Knee Joint, Tibial Surface, Right W Knee Joint, Tibial Surface, Left	0 Open	9 Liner	Z No Qualifier

Section	0	Medical and Surgical
Body System	S	Lower Joints
Operation	W	**Revision:** Correcting, to the extent possible, a portion of a malfunctioning device or the position of a displaced device

Body Part (4ᵗʰ)	Approach (5ᵗʰ)	Device (6ᵗʰ)	Qualifier (7ᵗʰ)
0 Lumbar Vertebral Joint 3 Lumbosacral Joint	0 Open 3 Percutaneous 4 Percutaneous Endoscopic X External	0 Drainage Device 3 Infusion Device 4 Internal Fixation Device 7 Autologous Tissue Substitute 8 Spacer A Interbody Fusion Device J Synthetic Substitute K Nonautologous Tissue Substitute	Z No Qualifier
2 Lumbar Vertebral Disc 4 Lumbosacral Disc	0 Open 3 Percutaneous 4 Percutaneous Endoscopic X External	0 Drainage Device 3 Infusion Device 7 Autologous Tissue Substitute J Synthetic Substitute K Nonautologous Tissue Substitute	Z No Qualifier
5 Sacrococcygeal Joint 6 Coccygeal Joint 7 Sacroiliac Joint, Right 8 Sacroiliac Joint, Left	0 Open 3 Percutaneous 4 Percutaneous Endoscopic X External	0 Drainage Device 3 Infusion Device 4 Internal Fixation Device 7 Autologous Tissue Substitute 8 Spacer J Synthetic Substitute K Nonautologous Tissue Substitute	Z No Qualifier
9 Hip Joint, Right B Hip Joint, Left	0 Open	0 Drainage Device 3 Infusion Device 4 Internal Fixation Device 5 External Fixation Device 7 Autologous Tissue Substitute 8 Spacer 9 Liner B Resurfacing Device J Synthetic Substitute K Nonautologous Tissue Substitute	Z No Qualifier

Continued

Medical and Surgical Section (0)

0SW

Section	0	Medical and Surgical
Body System	S	Lower Joints
Operation	W	Revision: Correcting, to the extent possible, a portion of a malfunctioning device or the position of a displaced device

Body Part (4th)	Approach (5th)	Device (6th)	Qualifier (7th)
9 Hip Joint, Right B Hip Joint, Left	3 Percutaneous 4 Percutaneous Endoscopic X External	0 Drainage Device 3 Infusion Device 4 Internal Fixation Device 5 External Fixation Device 7 Autologous Tissue Substitute 8 Spacer J Synthetic Substitute K Nonautologous Tissue Substitute	Z No Qualifier
C Knee Joint, Right D Knee Joint, Left	0 Open	0 Drainage Device 3 Infusion Device 4 Internal Fixation Device 5 External Fixation Device 7 Autologous Tissue Substitute 8 Spacer 9 Liner J Synthetic Substitute K Nonautologous Tissue Substitute	Z No Qualifier
C Knee Joint, Right D Knee Joint, Left	3 Percutaneous 4 Percutaneous Endoscopic X External	0 Drainage Device 3 Infusion Device 4 Internal Fixation Device 5 External Fixation Device 7 Autologous Tissue Substitute 8 Spacer J Synthetic Substitute K Nonautologous Tissue Substitute	Z No Qualifier
F Ankle Joint, Right G Ankle Joint, Left H Tarsal Joint, Right J Tarsal Joint, Left K Metatarsal-Tarsal Joint, Right L Metatarsal-Tarsal Joint, Left M Metatarsal-Phalangeal Joint, Right N Metatarsal-Phalangeal Joint, Left P Toe Phalangeal Joint, Right Q Toe Phalangeal Joint, Left	0 Open 3 Percutaneous 4 Percutaneous Endoscopic X External	0 Drainage Device 3 Infusion Device 4 Internal Fixation Device 5 External Fixation Device 7 Autologous Tissue Substitute 8 Spacer J Synthetic Substitute K Nonautologous Tissue Substitute	Z No Qualifier

Lower Joints Code Listing 0S2–0SW

Review Coding Guideline B4.5

0S2 – Lower Joints, Change

Review Coding Guideline B6.1c

0S2YX0Z   Change Drainage Device in Lower Joint, External Approach

0S2YXYZ   Change Other Device in Lower Joint, External Approach

0S5 – Lower Joints, Destruction

0S500ZZ Destruction of Lumbar Vertebral Joint, Open Approach	**0S520ZZ** Destruction of Lumbar Vertebral Disc, Open Approach
0S503ZZ Destruction of Lumbar Vertebral Joint, Percutaneous Approach	**0S523ZZ** Destruction of Lumbar Vertebral Disc, Percutaneous Approach
0S504ZZ Destruction of Lumbar Vertebral Joint, Percutaneous Endoscopic Approach	**0S524ZZ** Destruction of Lumbar Vertebral Disc, Percutaneous Endoscopic Approach

0S530ZZ	Destruction of Lumbosacral Joint, Open Approach
0S533ZZ	Destruction of Lumbosacral Joint, Percutaneous Approach
0S534ZZ	Destruction of Lumbosacral Joint, Percutaneous Endoscopic Approach
0S540ZZ	Destruction of Lumbosacral Disc, Open Approach
0S543ZZ	Destruction of Lumbosacral Disc, Percutaneous Approach
0S544ZZ	Destruction of Lumbosacral Disc, Percutaneous Endoscopic Approach
0S550ZZ	Destruction of Sacrococcygeal Joint, Open Approach
0S553ZZ	Destruction of Sacrococcygeal Joint, Percutaneous Approach
0S554ZZ	Destruction of Sacrococcygeal Joint, Percutaneous Endoscopic Approach
0S560ZZ	Destruction of Coccygeal Joint, Open Approach
0S563ZZ	Destruction of Coccygeal Joint, Percutaneous Approach
0S564ZZ	Destruction of Coccygeal Joint, Percutaneous Endoscopic Approach
0S570ZZ	Destruction of Right Sacroiliac Joint, Open Approach
0S573ZZ	Destruction of Right Sacroiliac Joint, Percutaneous Approach
0S574ZZ	Destruction of Right Sacroiliac Joint, Percutaneous Endoscopic Approach
0S580ZZ	Destruction of Left Sacroiliac Joint, Open Approach
0S583ZZ	Destruction of Left Sacroiliac Joint, Percutaneous Approach
0S584ZZ	Destruction of Left Sacroiliac Joint, Percutaneous Endoscopic Approach
0S590ZZ	Destruction of Right Hip Joint, Open Approach
0S593ZZ	Destruction of Right Hip Joint, Percutaneous Approach
0S594ZZ	Destruction of Right Hip Joint, Percutaneous Endoscopic Approach
0S5B0ZZ	Destruction of Left Hip Joint, Open Approach
0S5B3ZZ	Destruction of Left Hip Joint, Percutaneous Approach
0S5B4ZZ	Destruction of Left Hip Joint, Percutaneous Endoscopic Approach
0S5C0ZZ	Destruction of Right Knee Joint, Open Approach
0S5C3ZZ	Destruction of Right Knee Joint, Percutaneous Approach
0S5C4ZZ	Destruction of Right Knee Joint, Percutaneous Endoscopic Approach
0S5D0ZZ	Destruction of Left Knee Joint, Open Approach
0S5D3ZZ	Destruction of Left Knee Joint, Percutaneous Approach
0S5D4ZZ	Destruction of Left Knee Joint, Percutaneous Endoscopic Approach
0S5F0ZZ	Destruction of Right Ankle Joint, Open Approach
0S5F3ZZ	Destruction of Right Ankle Joint, Percutaneous Approach
0S5F4ZZ	Destruction of Right Ankle Joint, Percutaneous Endoscopic Approach
0S5G0ZZ	Destruction of Left Ankle Joint, Open Approach
0S5G3ZZ	Destruction of Left Ankle Joint, Percutaneous Approach
0S5G4ZZ	Destruction of Left Ankle Joint, Percutaneous Endoscopic Approach
0S5H0ZZ	Destruction of Right Tarsal Joint, Open Approach
0S5H3ZZ	Destruction of Right Tarsal Joint, Percutaneous Approach
0S5H4ZZ	Destruction of Right Tarsal Joint, Percutaneous Endoscopic Approach
0S5J0ZZ	Destruction of Left Tarsal Joint, Open Approach
0S5J3ZZ	Destruction of Left Tarsal Joint, Percutaneous Approach
0S5J4ZZ	Destruction of Left Tarsal Joint, Percutaneous Endoscopic Approach
0S5K0ZZ	Destruction of Right Metatarsal-Tarsal Joint, Open Approach
0S5K3ZZ	Destruction of Right Metatarsal-Tarsal Joint, Percutaneous Approach
0S5K4ZZ	Destruction of Right Metatarsal-Tarsal Joint, Percutaneous Endoscopic Approach
0S5L0ZZ	Destruction of Left Metatarsal-Tarsal Joint, Open Approach
0S5L3ZZ	Destruction of Left Metatarsal-Tarsal Joint, Percutaneous Approach
0S5L4ZZ	Destruction of Left Metatarsal-Tarsal Joint, Percutaneous Endoscopic Approach
0S5M0ZZ	Destruction of Right Metatarsal-Phalangeal Joint, Open Approach
0S5M3ZZ	Destruction of Right Metatarsal-Phalangeal Joint, Percutaneous Approach
0S5M4ZZ	Destruction of Right Metatarsal-Phalangeal Joint, Percutaneous Endoscopic Approach
0S5N0ZZ	Destruction of Left Metatarsal-Phalangeal Joint, Open Approach
0S5N3ZZ	Destruction of Left Metatarsal-Phalangeal Joint, Percutaneous Approach
0S5N4ZZ	Destruction of Left Metatarsal-Phalangeal Joint, Percutaneous Endoscopic Approach
0S5P0ZZ	Destruction of Right Toe Phalangeal Joint, Open Approach
0S5P3ZZ	Destruction of Right Toe Phalangeal Joint, Percutaneous Approach
0S5P4ZZ	Destruction of Right Toe Phalangeal Joint, Percutaneous Endoscopic Approach
0S5Q0ZZ	Destruction of Left Toe Phalangeal Joint, Open Approach
0S5Q3ZZ	Destruction of Left Toe Phalangeal Joint, Percutaneous Approach
0S5Q4ZZ	Destruction of Left Toe Phalangeal Joint, Percutaneous Endoscopic Approach

0S9 – Lower Joints, Drainage

Review Coding Guidelines B3.4a and B3.4b

Review Coding Guideline B6.2

0S9000Z	Drainage of Lumbar Vertebral Joint with Drainage Device, Open Approach
0S900ZX	Drainage of Lumbar Vertebral Joint, Open Approach, Diagnostic
0S900ZZ	Drainage of Lumbar Vertebral Joint, Open Approach
0S9030Z	Drainage of Lumbar Vertebral Joint with Drainage Device, Percutaneous Approach
0S903ZX	Drainage of Lumbar Vertebral Joint, Percutaneous Approach, Diagnostic
0S903ZZ	Drainage of Lumbar Vertebral Joint, Percutaneous Approach
0S9040Z	Drainage of Lumbar Vertebral Joint with Drainage Device, Percutaneous Endoscopic Approach
0S904ZX	Drainage of Lumbar Vertebral Joint, Percutaneous Endoscopic Approach, Diagnostic
0S904ZZ	Drainage of Lumbar Vertebral Joint, Percutaneous Endoscopic Approach
0S9200Z	Drainage of Lumbar Vertebral Disc with Drainage Device, Open Approach
0S920ZX	Drainage of Lumbar Vertebral Disc, Open Approach, Diagnostic
0S920ZZ	Drainage of Lumbar Vertebral Disc, Open Approach
0S9230Z	Drainage of Lumbar Vertebral Disc with Drainage Device, Percutaneous Approach
0S923ZX	Drainage of Lumbar Vertebral Disc, Percutaneous Approach, Diagnostic
0S923ZZ	Drainage of Lumbar Vertebral Disc, Percutaneous Approach
0S9240Z	Drainage of Lumbar Vertebral Disc with Drainage Device, Percutaneous Endoscopic Approach
0S924ZX	Drainage of Lumbar Vertebral Disc, Percutaneous Endoscopic Approach, Diagnostic
0S924ZZ	Drainage of Lumbar Vertebral Disc, Percutaneous Endoscopic Approach
0S9300Z	Drainage of Lumbosacral Joint with Drainage Device, Open Approach
0S930ZX	Drainage of Lumbosacral Joint, Open Approach, Diagnostic
0S930ZZ	Drainage of Lumbosacral Joint, Open Approach
0S9330Z	Drainage of Lumbosacral Joint with Drainage Device, Percutaneous Approach
0S933ZX	Drainage of Lumbosacral Joint, Percutaneous Approach, Diagnostic
0S933ZZ	Drainage of Lumbosacral Joint, Percutaneous Approach
0S9340Z	Drainage of Lumbosacral Joint with Drainage Device, Percutaneous Endoscopic Approach
0S934ZX	Drainage of Lumbosacral Joint, Percutaneous Endoscopic Approach, Diagnostic
0S934ZZ	Drainage of Lumbosacral Joint, Percutaneous Endoscopic Approach
0S9400Z	Drainage of Lumbosacral Disc with Drainage Device, Open Approach
0S940ZX	Drainage of Lumbosacral Disc, Open Approach, Diagnostic
0S940ZZ	Drainage of Lumbosacral Disc, Open Approach
0S9430Z	Drainage of Lumbosacral Disc with Drainage Device, Percutaneous Approach
0S943ZX	Drainage of Lumbosacral Disc, Percutaneous Approach, Diagnostic
0S943ZZ	Drainage of Lumbosacral Disc, Percutaneous Approach
0S9440Z	Drainage of Lumbosacral Disc with Drainage Device, Percutaneous Endoscopic Approach
0S944ZX	Drainage of Lumbosacral Disc, Percutaneous Endoscopic Approach, Diagnostic
0S944ZZ	Drainage of Lumbosacral Disc, Percutaneous Endoscopic Approach

0S9500Z	Drainage of Sacrococcygeal Joint with Drainage Device, Open Approach
0S950ZX	Drainage of Sacrococcygeal Joint, Open Approach, Diagnostic
0S950ZZ	Drainage of Sacrococcygeal Joint, Open Approach
0S9530Z	Drainage of Sacrococcygeal Joint with Drainage Device, Percutaneous Approach
0S953ZX	Drainage of Sacrococcygeal Joint, Percutaneous Approach, Diagnostic
0S953ZZ	Drainage of Sacrococcygeal Joint, Percutaneous Approach
0S9540Z	Drainage of Sacrococcygeal Joint with Drainage Device, Percutaneous Endoscopic Approach
0S954ZX	Drainage of Sacrococcygeal Joint, Percutaneous Endoscopic Approach, Diagnostic
0S954ZZ	Drainage of Sacrococcygeal Joint, Percutaneous Endoscopic Approach
0S9600Z	Drainage of Coccygeal Joint with Drainage Device, Open Approach
0S960ZX	Drainage of Coccygeal Joint, Open Approach, Diagnostic
0S960ZZ	Drainage of Coccygeal Joint, Open Approach
0S9630Z	Drainage of Coccygeal Joint with Drainage Device, Percutaneous Approach
0S963ZX	Drainage of Coccygeal Joint, Percutaneous Approach, Diagnostic
0S963ZZ	Drainage of Coccygeal Joint, Percutaneous Approach
0S9640Z	Drainage of Coccygeal Joint with Drainage Device, Percutaneous Endoscopic Approach
0S964ZX	Drainage of Coccygeal Joint, Percutaneous Endoscopic Approach, Diagnostic
0S964ZZ	Drainage of Coccygeal Joint, Percutaneous Endoscopic Approach
0S9700Z	Drainage of Right Sacroiliac Joint with Drainage Device, Open Approach
0S970ZX	Drainage of Right Sacroiliac Joint, Open Approach, Diagnostic
0S970ZZ	Drainage of Right Sacroiliac Joint, Open Approach
0S9730Z	Drainage of Right Sacroiliac Joint with Drainage Device, Percutaneous Approach
0S973ZX	Drainage of Right Sacroiliac Joint, Percutaneous Approach, Diagnostic
0S973ZZ	Drainage of Right Sacroiliac Joint, Percutaneous Approach
0S9740Z	Drainage of Right Sacroiliac Joint with Drainage Device, Percutaneous Endoscopic Approach
0S974ZX	Drainage of Right Sacroiliac Joint, Percutaneous Endoscopic Approach, Diagnostic
0S974ZZ	Drainage of Right Sacroiliac Joint, Percutaneous Endoscopic Approach
0S9800Z	Drainage of Left Sacroiliac Joint with Drainage Device, Open Approach
0S980ZX	Drainage of Left Sacroiliac Joint, Open Approach, Diagnostic
0S980ZZ	Drainage of Left Sacroiliac Joint, Open Approach
0S9830Z	Drainage of Left Sacroiliac Joint with Drainage Device, Percutaneous Approach
0S983ZX	Drainage of Left Sacroiliac Joint, Percutaneous Approach, Diagnostic
0S983ZZ	Drainage of Left Sacroiliac Joint, Percutaneous Approach
0S9840Z	Drainage of Left Sacroiliac Joint with Drainage Device, Percutaneous Endoscopic Approach
0S984ZX	Drainage of Left Sacroiliac Joint, Percutaneous Endoscopic Approach, Diagnostic
0S984ZZ	Drainage of Left Sacroiliac Joint, Percutaneous Endoscopic Approach
0S9900Z	Drainage of Right Hip Joint with Drainage Device, Open Approach
0S990ZX	Drainage of Right Hip Joint, Open Approach, Diagnostic
0S990ZZ	Drainage of Right Hip Joint, Open Approach
0S9930Z	Drainage of Right Hip Joint with Drainage Device, Percutaneous Approach
0S993ZX	Drainage of Right Hip Joint, Percutaneous Approach, Diagnostic
0S993ZZ	Drainage of Right Hip Joint, Percutaneous Approach
0S9940Z	Drainage of Right Hip Joint with Drainage Device, Percutaneous Endoscopic Approach
0S994ZX	Drainage of Right Hip Joint, Percutaneous Endoscopic Approach, Diagnostic
0S994ZZ	Drainage of Right Hip Joint, Percutaneous Endoscopic Approach
0S9B00Z	Drainage of Left Hip Joint with Drainage Device, Open Approach
0S9B0ZX	Drainage of Left Hip Joint, Open Approach, Diagnostic
0S9B0ZZ	Drainage of Left Hip Joint, Open Approach
0S9B30Z	Drainage of Left Hip Joint with Drainage Device, Percutaneous Approach
0S9B3ZX	Drainage of Left Hip Joint, Percutaneous Approach, Diagnostic
0S9B3ZZ	Drainage of Left Hip Joint, Percutaneous Approach
0S9B40Z	Drainage of Left Hip Joint with Drainage Device, Percutaneous Endoscopic Approach
0S9B4ZX	Drainage of Left Hip Joint, Percutaneous Endoscopic Approach, Diagnostic
0S9B4ZZ	Drainage of Left Hip Joint, Percutaneous Endoscopic Approach
0S9C00Z	Drainage of Right Knee Joint with Drainage Device, Open Approach
0S9C0ZX	Drainage of Right Knee Joint, Open Approach, Diagnostic
0S9C0ZZ	Drainage of Right Knee Joint, Open Approach
0S9C30Z	Drainage of Right Knee Joint with Drainage Device, Percutaneous Approach
0S9C3ZX	Drainage of Right Knee Joint, Percutaneous Approach, Diagnostic
0S9C3ZZ	Drainage of Right Knee Joint, Percutaneous Approach
0S9C40Z	Drainage of Right Knee Joint with Drainage Device, Percutaneous Endoscopic Approach
0S9C4ZX	Drainage of Right Knee Joint, Percutaneous Endoscopic Approach, Diagnostic
0S9C4ZZ	Drainage of Right Knee Joint, Percutaneous Endoscopic Approach
0S9D00Z	Drainage of Left Knee Joint with Drainage Device, Open Approach
0S9D0ZX	Drainage of Left Knee Joint, Open Approach, Diagnostic
0S9D0ZZ	Drainage of Left Knee Joint, Open Approach
0S9D30Z	Drainage of Left Knee Joint with Drainage Device, Percutaneous Approach
0S9D3ZX	Drainage of Left Knee Joint, Percutaneous Approach, Diagnostic
0S9D3ZZ	Drainage of Left Knee Joint, Percutaneous Approach
0S9D40Z	Drainage of Left Knee Joint with Drainage Device, Percutaneous Endoscopic Approach
0S9D4ZX	Drainage of Left Knee Joint, Percutaneous Endoscopic Approach, Diagnostic
0S9D4ZZ	Drainage of Left Knee Joint, Percutaneous Endoscopic Approach
0S9F00Z	Drainage of Right Ankle Joint with Drainage Device, Open Approach
0S9F0ZX	Drainage of Right Ankle Joint, Open Approach, Diagnostic
0S9F0ZZ	Drainage of Right Ankle Joint, Open Approach
0S9F30Z	Drainage of Right Ankle Joint with Drainage Device, Percutaneous Approach
0S9F3ZX	Drainage of Right Ankle Joint, Percutaneous Approach, Diagnostic
0S9F3ZZ	Drainage of Right Ankle Joint, Percutaneous Approach
0S9F40Z	Drainage of Right Ankle Joint with Drainage Device, Percutaneous Endoscopic Approach
0S9F4ZX	Drainage of Right Ankle Joint, Percutaneous Endoscopic Approach, Diagnostic
0S9F4ZZ	Drainage of Right Ankle Joint, Percutaneous Endoscopic Approach
0S9G00Z	Drainage of Left Ankle Joint with Drainage Device, Open Approach
0S9G0ZX	Drainage of Left Ankle Joint, Open Approach, Diagnostic
0S9G0ZZ	Drainage of Left Ankle Joint, Open Approach
0S9G30Z	Drainage of Left Ankle Joint with Drainage Device, Percutaneous Approach
0S9G3ZX	Drainage of Left Ankle Joint, Percutaneous Approach, Diagnostic
0S9G3ZZ	Drainage of Left Ankle Joint, Percutaneous Approach
0S9G40Z	Drainage of Left Ankle Joint with Drainage Device, Percutaneous Endoscopic Approach
0S9G4ZX	Drainage of Left Ankle Joint, Percutaneous Endoscopic Approach, Diagnostic
0S9G4ZZ	Drainage of Left Ankle Joint, Percutaneous Endoscopic Approach
0S9H00Z	Drainage of Right Tarsal Joint with Drainage Device, Open Approach
0S9H0ZX	Drainage of Right Tarsal Joint, Open Approach, Diagnostic
0S9H0ZZ	Drainage of Right Tarsal Joint, Open Approach
0S9H30Z	Drainage of Right Tarsal Joint with Drainage Device, Percutaneous Approach
0S9H3ZX	Drainage of Right Tarsal Joint, Percutaneous Approach, Diagnostic
0S9H3ZZ	Drainage of Right Tarsal Joint, Percutaneous Approach
0S9H40Z	Drainage of Right Tarsal Joint with Drainage Device, Percutaneous Endoscopic Approach
0S9H4ZX	Drainage of Right Tarsal Joint, Percutaneous Endoscopic Approach, Diagnostic
0S9H4ZZ	Drainage of Right Tarsal Joint, Percutaneous Endoscopic Approach
0S9J00Z	Drainage of Left Tarsal Joint with Drainage Device, Open Approach
0S9J0ZX	Drainage of Left Tarsal Joint, Open Approach, Diagnostic
0S9J0ZZ	Drainage of Left Tarsal Joint, Open Approach
0S9J30Z	Drainage of Left Tarsal Joint with Drainage Device, Percutaneous Approach

---

♀ Female-only   ♂ Male-only   ● Limited Coverage   ● Non-OR   **HAC** HAC-associated procedure   ● Non-covered procedures   ✚ Combination

0S9J3ZX	Drainage of Left Tarsal Joint, Percutaneous Approach, Diagnostic
0S9J3ZZ	Drainage of Left Tarsal Joint, Percutaneous Approach
0S9J40Z	Drainage of Left Tarsal Joint with Drainage Device, Percutaneous Endoscopic Approach
0S9J4ZX	Drainage of Left Tarsal Joint, Percutaneous Endoscopic Approach, Diagnostic
0S9J4ZZ	Drainage of Left Tarsal Joint, Percutaneous Endoscopic Approach
0S9K00Z	Drainage of Right Metatarsal-Tarsal Joint with Drainage Device, Open Approach
0S9K0ZX	Drainage of Right Metatarsal-Tarsal Joint, Open Approach, Diagnostic
0S9K0ZZ	Drainage of Right Metatarsal-Tarsal Joint, Open Approach
0S9K30Z	Drainage of Right Metatarsal-Tarsal Joint with Drainage Device, Percutaneous Approach
0S9K3ZX	Drainage of Right Metatarsal-Tarsal Joint, Percutaneous Approach, Diagnostic
0S9K3ZZ	Drainage of Right Metatarsal-Tarsal Joint, Percutaneous Approach
0S9K40Z	Drainage of Right Metatarsal-Tarsal Joint with Drainage Device, Percutaneous Endoscopic Approach
0S9K4ZX	Drainage of Right Metatarsal-Tarsal Joint, Percutaneous Endoscopic Approach, Diagnostic
0S9K4ZZ	Drainage of Right Metatarsal-Tarsal Joint, Percutaneous Endoscopic Approach
0S9L00Z	Drainage of Left Metatarsal-Tarsal Joint with Drainage Device, Open Approach
0.0S9L0ZZ	Drainage of Left Metatarsal-Tarsal Joint, Open Approach
0S9L30Z	Drainage of Left Metatarsal-Tarsal Joint with Drainage Device, Percutaneous Approach
0S9L3ZX	Drainage of Left Metatarsal-Tarsal Joint, Percutaneous Approach, Diagnostic
0S9L3ZZ	Drainage of Left Metatarsal-Tarsal Joint, Percutaneous Approach
0S9L40Z	Drainage of Left Metatarsal-Tarsal Joint with Drainage Device, Percutaneous Endoscopic Approach
0S9L4ZX	Drainage of Left Metatarsal-Tarsal Joint, Percutaneous Endoscopic Approach, Diagnostic
0S9L4ZZ	Drainage of Left Metatarsal-Tarsal Joint, Percutaneous Endoscopic Approach
0S9M00Z	Drainage of Right Metatarsal-Phalangeal Joint with Drainage Device, Open Approach
0S9M0ZX	Drainage of Right Metatarsal-Phalangeal Joint, Open Approach, Diagnostic
0S9M0ZZ	Drainage of Right Metatarsal-Phalangeal Joint, Open Approach
0S9M30Z	Drainage of Right Metatarsal-Phalangeal Joint with Drainage Device, Percutaneous Approach
0S9M3ZX	Drainage of Right Metatarsal-Phalangeal Joint, Percutaneous Approach, Diagnostic
0S9M3ZZ	Drainage of Right Metatarsal-Phalangeal Joint, Percutaneous Approach
0S9M40Z	Drainage of Right Metatarsal-Phalangeal Joint with Drainage Device, Percutaneous Endoscopic Approach
0S9M4ZX	Drainage of Right Metatarsal-Phalangeal Joint, Percutaneous Endoscopic Approach, Diagnostic
0S9M4ZZ	Drainage of Right Metatarsal-Phalangeal Joint, Percutaneous Endoscopic Approach
0S9N00Z	Drainage of Left Metatarsal-Phalangeal Joint with Drainage Device, Open Approach
0S9N0ZX	Drainage of Left Metatarsal-Phalangeal Joint, Open Approach, Diagnostic
0S9N0ZZ	Drainage of Left Metatarsal-Phalangeal Joint, Open Approach
0S9N30Z	Drainage of Left Metatarsal-Phalangeal Joint with Drainage Device, Percutaneous Approach
0S9N3ZX	Drainage of Left Metatarsal-Phalangeal Joint, Percutaneous Approach, Diagnostic
0S9N3ZZ	Drainage of Left Metatarsal-Phalangeal Joint, Percutaneous Approach
0S9N40Z	Drainage of Left Metatarsal-Phalangeal Joint with Drainage Device, Percutaneous Endoscopic Approach
0S9N4ZX	Drainage of Left Metatarsal-Phalangeal Joint, Percutaneous Endoscopic Approach, Diagnostic
0S9N4ZZ	Drainage of Left Metatarsal-Phalangeal Joint, Percutaneous Endoscopic Approach
0S9P00Z	Drainage of Right Toe Phalangeal Joint with Drainage Device, Open Approach
0S9P0ZX	Drainage of Right Toe Phalangeal Joint, Open Approach, Diagnostic
0S9P0ZZ	Drainage of Right Toe Phalangeal Joint, Open Approach
0S9P30Z	Drainage of Right Toe Phalangeal Joint with Drainage Device, Percutaneous Approach
0S9P3ZX	Drainage of Right Toe Phalangeal Joint, Percutaneous Approach, Diagnostic
0S9P3ZZ	Drainage of Right Toe Phalangeal Joint, Percutaneous Approach
0S9P40Z	Drainage of Right Toe Phalangeal Joint with Drainage Device, Percutaneous Endoscopic Approach
0S9P4ZX	Drainage of Right Toe Phalangeal Joint, Percutaneous Endoscopic Approach, Diagnostic
0S9P4ZZ	Drainage of Right Toe Phalangeal Joint, Percutaneous Endoscopic Approach
0S9Q00Z	Drainage of Left Toe Phalangeal Joint with Drainage Device, Open Approach
0S9Q0ZX	Drainage of Left Toe Phalangeal Joint, Open Approach, Diagnostic
0S9Q0ZZ	Drainage of Left Toe Phalangeal Joint, Open Approach
0S9Q30Z	Drainage of Left Toe Phalangeal Joint with Drainage Device, Percutaneous Approach
0S9Q3ZX	Drainage of Left Toe Phalangeal Joint, Percutaneous Approach, Diagnostic
0S9Q3ZZ	Drainage of Left Toe Phalangeal Joint, Percutaneous Approach
0S9Q40Z	Drainage of Left Toe Phalangeal Joint with Drainage Device, Percutaneous Endoscopic Approach
0S9Q4ZX	Drainage of Left Toe Phalangeal Joint, Percutaneous Endoscopic Approach, Diagnostic
0S9Q4ZZ	Drainage of Left Toe Phalangeal Joint, Percutaneous Endoscopic Approach

0SB – Lower Joints, Excision

Review Coding Guidelines B3.4a and B3.4b

Review Coding Guideline B3.5

Review Coding Guideline B3.8

0SB00ZX	Excision of Lumbar Vertebral Joint, Open Approach, Diagnostic
0SB00ZZ	Excision of Lumbar Vertebral Joint, Open Approach
0SB03ZX	Excision of Lumbar Vertebral Joint, Percutaneous Approach, Diagnostic
0SB03ZZ	Excision of Lumbar Vertebral Joint, Percutaneous Approach
0SB04ZX	Excision of Lumbar Vertebral Joint, Percutaneous Endoscopic Approach, Diagnostic
0SB04ZZ	Excision of Lumbar Vertebral Joint, Percutaneous Endoscopic Approach
0SB20ZX	Excision of Lumbar Vertebral Disc, Open Approach, Diagnostic
0SB20ZZ	Excision of Lumbar Vertebral Disc, Open Approach
0SB23ZX	Excision of Lumbar Vertebral Disc, Percutaneous Approach, Diagnostic
0SB23ZZ	Excision of Lumbar Vertebral Disc, Percutaneous Approach
0SB24ZX	Excision of Lumbar Vertebral Disc, Percutaneous Endoscopic Approach, Diagnostic
0SB24ZZ	Excision of Lumbar Vertebral Disc, Percutaneous Endoscopic Approach
0SB30ZX	Excision of Lumbosacral Joint, Open Approach, Diagnostic
0SB30ZZ	Excision of Lumbosacral Joint, Open Approach
0SB33ZX	Excision of Lumbosacral Joint, Percutaneous Approach, Diagnostic
0SB33ZZ	Excision of Lumbosacral Joint, Percutaneous Approach
0SB34ZX	Excision of Lumbosacral Joint, Percutaneous Endoscopic Approach, Diagnostic
0SB34ZZ	Excision of Lumbosacral Joint, Percutaneous Endoscopic Approach
0SB40ZX	Excision of Lumbosacral Disc, Open Approach, Diagnostic

0SB40ZZ   Excision of Lumbosacral Disc, Open Approach
0SB43ZX   Excision of Lumbosacral Disc, Percutaneous Approach, Diagnostic
0SB43ZZ   Excision of Lumbosacral Disc, Percutaneous Approach
0SB44ZX   Excision of Lumbosacral Disc, Percutaneous Endoscopic Approach, Diagnostic
0SB44ZZ   Excision of Lumbosacral Disc, Percutaneous Endoscopic Approach
0SB50ZX   Excision of Sacrococcygeal Joint, Open Approach, Diagnostic
0SB50ZZ   Excision of Sacrococcygeal Joint, Open Approach
0SB53ZX   Excision of Sacrococcygeal Joint, Percutaneous Approach, Diagnostic
0SB53ZZ   Excision of Sacrococcygeal Joint, Percutaneous Approach
0SB54ZX   Excision of Sacrococcygeal Joint, Percutaneous Endoscopic Approach, Diagnostic
0SB54ZZ   Excision of Sacrococcygeal Joint, Percutaneous Endoscopic Approach
0SB60ZX   Excision of Coccygeal Joint, Open Approach, Diagnostic
0SB60ZZ   Excision of Coccygeal Joint, Open Approach
0SB63ZX   Excision of Coccygeal Joint, Percutaneous Approach, Diagnostic
0SB63ZZ   Excision of Coccygeal Joint, Percutaneous Approach
0SB64ZX   Excision of Coccygeal Joint, Percutaneous Endoscopic Approach, Diagnostic
0SB64ZZ   Excision of Coccygeal Joint, Percutaneous Endoscopic Approach
0SB70ZX   Excision of Right Sacroiliac Joint, Open Approach, Diagnostic
0SB70ZZ   Excision of Right Sacroiliac Joint, Open Approach
0SB73ZX   Excision of Right Sacroiliac Joint, Percutaneous Approach, Diagnostic
0SB73ZZ   Excision of Right Sacroiliac Joint, Percutaneous Approach
0SB74ZX   Excision of Right Sacroiliac Joint, Percutaneous Endoscopic Approach, Diagnostic
0SB74ZZ   Excision of Right Sacroiliac Joint, Percutaneous Endoscopic Approach
0SB80ZX   Excision of Left Sacroiliac Joint, Open Approach, Diagnostic
0SB80ZZ   Excision of Left Sacroiliac Joint, Open Approach
0SB83ZX   Excision of Left Sacroiliac Joint, Percutaneous Approach, Diagnostic
0SB83ZZ   Excision of Left Sacroiliac Joint, Percutaneous Approach
0SB84ZX   Excision of Left Sacroiliac Joint, Percutaneous Endoscopic Approach, Diagnostic
0SB84ZZ   Excision of Left Sacroiliac Joint, Percutaneous Endoscopic Approach
0SB90ZX   Excision of Right Hip Joint, Open Approach, Diagnostic
0SB90ZZ   Excision of Right Hip Joint, Open Approach
0SB93ZX   Excision of Right Hip Joint, Percutaneous Approach, Diagnostic
0SB93ZZ   Excision of Right Hip Joint, Percutaneous Approach
0SB94ZX   Excision of Right Hip Joint, Percutaneous Endoscopic Approach, Diagnostic
0SB94ZZ   Excision of Right Hip Joint, Percutaneous Endoscopic Approach
0SBB0ZX   Excision of Left Hip Joint, Open Approach, Diagnostic
0SBB0ZZ   Excision of Left Hip Joint, Open Approach
0SBB3ZX   Excision of Left Hip Joint, Percutaneous Approach, Diagnostic
0SBB3ZZ   Excision of Left Hip Joint, Percutaneous Approach
0SBB4ZX   Excision of Left Hip Joint, Percutaneous Endoscopic Approach, Diagnostic
0SBB4ZZ   Excision of Left Hip Joint, Percutaneous Endoscopic Approach
0SBC0ZX   Excision of Right Knee Joint, Open Approach, Diagnostic
0SBC0ZZ   Excision of Right Knee Joint, Open Approach
0SBC3ZX   Excision of Right Knee Joint, Percutaneous Approach, Diagnostic
0SBC3ZZ   Excision of Right Knee Joint, Percutaneous Approach
0SBC4ZX   Excision of Right Knee Joint, Percutaneous Endoscopic Approach, Diagnostic
0SBC4ZZ   Excision of Right Knee Joint, Percutaneous Endoscopic Approach
0SBD0ZX   Excision of Left Knee Joint, Open Approach, Diagnostic
0SBD0ZZ   Excision of Left Knee Joint, Open Approach
0SBD3ZX   Excision of Left Knee Joint, Percutaneous Approach, Diagnostic
0SBD3ZZ   Excision of Left Knee Joint, Percutaneous Approach
0SBD4ZX   Excision of Left Knee Joint, Percutaneous Endoscopic Approach, Diagnostic
0SBD4ZZ   Excision of Left Knee Joint, Percutaneous Endoscopic Approach
0SBF0ZX   Excision of Right Ankle Joint, Open Approach, Diagnostic
0SBF0ZZ   Excision of Right Ankle Joint, Open Approach
0SBF3ZX   Excision of Right Ankle Joint, Percutaneous Approach, Diagnostic
0SBF3ZZ   Excision of Right Ankle Joint, Percutaneous Approach
0SBF4ZX   Excision of Right Ankle Joint, Percutaneous Endoscopic Approach, Diagnostic

0SBF4ZZ   Excision of Right Ankle Joint, Percutaneous Endoscopic Approach
0SBG0ZX   Excision of Left Ankle Joint, Open Approach, Diagnostic
0SBG0ZZ   Excision of Left Ankle Joint, Open Approach
0SBG3ZX   Excision of Left Ankle Joint, Percutaneous Approach, Diagnostic
0SBG3ZZ   Excision of Left Ankle Joint, Percutaneous Approach
0SBG4ZX   Excision of Left Ankle Joint, Percutaneous Endoscopic Approach, Diagnostic
0SBG4ZZ   Excision of Left Ankle Joint, Percutaneous Endoscopic Approach
0SBH0ZX   Excision of Right Tarsal Joint, Open Approach, Diagnostic
0SBH0ZZ   Excision of Right Tarsal Joint, Open Approach
0SBH3ZX   Excision of Right Tarsal Joint, Percutaneous Approach, Diagnostic
0SBH3ZZ   Excision of Right Tarsal Joint, Percutaneous Approach
0SBH4ZX   Excision of Right Tarsal Joint, Percutaneous Endoscopic Approach, Diagnostic
0SBH4ZZ   Excision of Right Tarsal Joint, Percutaneous Endoscopic Approach
0SBJ0ZX   Excision of Left Tarsal Joint, Open Approach, Diagnostic
0SBJ0ZZ   Excision of Left Tarsal Joint, Open Approach
0SBJ3ZX   Excision of Left Tarsal Joint, Percutaneous Approach, Diagnostic
0SBJ3ZZ   Excision of Left Tarsal Joint, Percutaneous Approach
0SBJ4ZX   Excision of Left Tarsal Joint, Percutaneous Endoscopic Approach, Diagnostic
0SBJ4ZZ   Excision of Left Tarsal Joint, Percutaneous Endoscopic Approach
0SBK0ZX   Excision of Right Metatarsal-Tarsal Joint, Open Approach, Diagnostic
0SBK0ZZ   Excision of Right Metatarsal-Tarsal Joint, Open Approach
0SBK3ZX   Excision of Right Metatarsal-Tarsal Joint, Percutaneous Approach, Diagnostic
0SBK3ZZ   Excision of Right Metatarsal-Tarsal Joint, Percutaneous Approach
0SBK4ZX   Excision of Right Metatarsal-Tarsal Joint, Percutaneous Endoscopic Approach, Diagnostic
0SBK4ZZ   Excision of Right Metatarsal-Tarsal Joint, Percutaneous Endoscopic Approach
0SBL0ZX   Excision of Left Metatarsal-Tarsal Joint, Open Approach, Diagnostic
0SBL0ZZ   Excision of Left Metatarsal-Tarsal Joint, Open Approach
0SBL3ZX   Excision of Left Metatarsal-Tarsal Joint, Percutaneous Approach, Diagnostic
0SBL3ZZ   Excision of Left Metatarsal-Tarsal Joint, Percutaneous Approach
0SBL4ZX   Excision of Left Metatarsal-Tarsal Joint, Percutaneous Endoscopic Approach, Diagnostic
0SBL4ZZ   Excision of Left Metatarsal-Tarsal Joint, Percutaneous Endoscopic Approach
0SBM0ZX   Excision of Right Metatarsal-Phalangeal Joint, Open Approach, Diagnostic
0SBM0ZZ   Excision of Right Metatarsal-Phalangeal Joint, Open Approach
0SBM3ZX   Excision of Right Metatarsal-Phalangeal Joint, Percutaneous Approach, Diagnostic
0SBM3ZZ   Excision of Right Metatarsal-Phalangeal Joint, Percutaneous Approach
0SBM4ZX   Excision of Right Metatarsal-Phalangeal Joint, Percutaneous Endoscopic Approach, Diagnostic
0SBM4ZZ   Excision of Right Metatarsal-Phalangeal Joint, Percutaneous Endoscopic Approach
0SBN0ZX   Excision of Left Metatarsal-Phalangeal Joint, Open Approach, Diagnostic
0SBN0ZZ   Excision of Left Metatarsal-Phalangeal Joint, Open Approach
0SBN3ZX   Excision of Left Metatarsal-Phalangeal Joint, Percutaneous Approach, Diagnostic
0SBN3ZZ   Excision of Left Metatarsal-Phalangeal Joint, Percutaneous Approach
0SBN4ZX   Excision of Left Metatarsal-Phalangeal Joint, Percutaneous Endoscopic Approach, Diagnostic
0SBN4ZZ   Excision of Left Metatarsal-Phalangeal Joint, Percutaneous Endoscopic Approach
0SBP0ZX   Excision of Right Toe Phalangeal Joint, Open Approach, Diagnostic
0SBP0ZZ   Excision of Right Toe Phalangeal Joint, Open Approach
0SBP3ZX   Excision of Right Toe Phalangeal Joint, Percutaneous Approach, Diagnostic
0SBP3ZZ   Excision of Right Toe Phalangeal Joint, Percutaneous Approach
0SBP4ZX   Excision of Right Toe Phalangeal Joint, Percutaneous Endoscopic Approach, Diagnostic
0SBP4ZZ   Excision of Right Toe Phalangeal Joint, Percutaneous Endoscopic Approach
0SBQ0ZX   Excision of Left Toe Phalangeal Joint, Open Approach, Diagnostic

---

♀ Female-only   ♂ Male-only   ● Limited Coverage   ● Non-OR   [HAC] HAC-associated procedure   ◆ Non-covered procedures   ✚ Combination

0SBQ0ZZ   Excision of Left Toe Phalangeal Joint, Open Approach
0SBQ3ZX   Excision of Left Toe Phalangeal Joint, Percutaneous Approach, Diagnostic
0SBQ3ZZ   Excision of Left Toe Phalangeal Joint, Percutaneous Approach

0SBQ4ZX   Excision of Left Toe Phalangeal Joint, Percutaneous Endoscopic Approach, Diagnostic
0SBQ4ZZ   Excision of Left Toe Phalangeal Joint, Percutaneous Endoscopic Approach

0SC – Lower Joints, Extirpation

0SC00ZZ   Extirpation of Matter from Lumbar Vertebral Joint, Open Approach
0SC03ZZ   Extirpation of Matter from Lumbar Vertebral Joint, Percutaneous Approach
0SC04ZZ   Extirpation of Matter from Lumbar Vertebral Joint, Percutaneous Endoscopic Approach
0SC20ZZ   Extirpation of Matter from Lumbar Vertebral Disc, Open Approach
0SC23ZZ   Extirpation of Matter from Lumbar Vertebral Disc, Percutaneous Approach
0SC24ZZ   Extirpation of Matter from Lumbar Vertebral Disc, Percutaneous Endoscopic Approach
0SC30ZZ   Extirpation of Matter from Lumbosacral Joint, Open Approach
0SC33ZZ   Extirpation of Matter from Lumbosacral Joint, Percutaneous Approach
0SC34ZZ   Extirpation of Matter from Lumbosacral Joint, Percutaneous Endoscopic Approach
0SC40ZZ   Extirpation of Matter from Lumbosacral Disc, Open Approach
0SC43ZZ   Extirpation of Matter from Lumbosacral Disc, Percutaneous Approach
0SC44ZZ   Extirpation of Matter from Lumbosacral Disc, Percutaneous Endoscopic Approach
0SC50ZZ   Extirpation of Matter from Sacrococcygeal Joint, Open Approach
0SC53ZZ   Extirpation of Matter from Sacrococcygeal Joint, Percutaneous Approach
0SC54ZZ   Extirpation of Matter from Sacrococcygeal Joint, Percutaneous Endoscopic Approach
0SC60ZZ   Extirpation of Matter from Coccygeal Joint, Open Approach
0SC63ZZ   Extirpation of Matter from Coccygeal Joint, Percutaneous Approach
0SC64ZZ   Extirpation of Matter from Coccygeal Joint, Percutaneous Endoscopic Approach
0SC70ZZ   Extirpation of Matter from Right Sacroiliac Joint, Open Approach
0SC73ZZ   Extirpation of Matter from Right Sacroiliac Joint, Percutaneous Approach
0SC74ZZ   Extirpation of Matter from Right Sacroiliac Joint, Percutaneous Endoscopic Approach
0SC80ZZ   Extirpation of Matter from Left Sacroiliac Joint, Open Approach
0SC83ZZ   Extirpation of Matter from Left Sacroiliac Joint, Percutaneous Approach
0SC84ZZ   Extirpation of Matter from Left Sacroiliac Joint, Percutaneous Endoscopic Approach
0SC90ZZ   Extirpation of Matter from Right Hip Joint, Open Approach
0SC93ZZ   Extirpation of Matter from Right Hip Joint, Percutaneous Approach
0SC94ZZ   Extirpation of Matter from Right Hip Joint, Percutaneous Endoscopic Approach
0SCB0ZZ   Extirpation of Matter from Left Hip Joint, Open Approach
0SCB3ZZ   Extirpation of Matter from Left Hip Joint, Percutaneous Approach
0SCB4ZZ   Extirpation of Matter from Left Hip Joint, Percutaneous Endoscopic Approach
0SCC0ZZ   Extirpation of Matter from Right Knee Joint, Open Approach
0SCC3ZZ   Extirpation of Matter from Right Knee Joint, Percutaneous Approach
0SCC4ZZ   Extirpation of Matter from Right Knee Joint, Percutaneous Endoscopic Approach
0SCD0ZZ   Extirpation of Matter from Left Knee Joint, Open Approach
0SCD3ZZ   Extirpation of Matter from Left Knee Joint, Percutaneous Approach
0SCD4ZZ   Extirpation of Matter from Left Knee Joint, Percutaneous Endoscopic Approach

0SCF0ZZ   Extirpation of Matter from Right Ankle Joint, Open Approach
0SCF3ZZ   Extirpation of Matter from Right Ankle Joint, Percutaneous Approach
0SCF4ZZ   Extirpation of Matter from Right Ankle Joint, Percutaneous Endoscopic Approach
0SCG0ZZ   Extirpation of Matter from Left Ankle Joint, Open Approach
0SCG3ZZ   Extirpation of Matter from Left Ankle Joint, Percutaneous Approach
0SCG4ZZ   Extirpation of Matter from Left Ankle Joint, Percutaneous Endoscopic Approach
0SCH0ZZ   Extirpation of Matter from Right Tarsal Joint, Open Approach
0SCH3ZZ   Extirpation of Matter from Right Tarsal Joint, Percutaneous Approach
0SCH4ZZ   Extirpation of Matter from Right Tarsal Joint, Percutaneous Endoscopic Approach
0SCJ0ZZ   Extirpation of Matter from Left Tarsal Joint, Open Approach
0SCJ3ZZ   Extirpation of Matter from Left Tarsal Joint, Percutaneous Approach
0SCJ4ZZ   Extirpation of Matter from Left Tarsal Joint, Percutaneous Endoscopic Approach
0SCK0ZZ   Extirpation of Matter from Right Metatarsal-Tarsal Joint, Open Approach
0SCK3ZZ   Extirpation of Matter from Right Metatarsal-Tarsal Joint, Percutaneous Approach
0SCK4ZZ   Extirpation of Matter from Right Metatarsal-Tarsal Joint, Percutaneous Endoscopic Approach
0SCL0ZZ   Extirpation of Matter from Left Metatarsal-Tarsal Joint, Open Approach
0SCL3ZZ   Extirpation of Matter from Left Metatarsal-Tarsal Joint, Percutaneous Approach
0SCL4ZZ   Extirpation of Matter from Left Metatarsal-Tarsal Joint, Percutaneous Endoscopic Approach
0SCM0ZZ   Extirpation of Matter from Right Metatarsal-Phalangeal Joint, Open Approach
0SCM3ZZ   Extirpation of Matter from Right Metatarsal-Phalangeal Joint, Percutaneous Approach
0SCM4ZZ   Extirpation of Matter from Right Metatarsal-Phalangeal Joint, Percutaneous Endoscopic Approach
0SCN0ZZ   Extirpation of Matter from Left Metatarsal-Phalangeal Joint, Open Approach
0SCN3ZZ   Extirpation of Matter from Left Metatarsal-Phalangeal Joint, Percutaneous Approach
0SCN4ZZ   Extirpation of Matter from Left Metatarsal-Phalangeal Joint, Percutaneous Endoscopic Approach
0SCP0ZZ   Extirpation of Matter from Right Toe Phalangeal Joint, Open Approach
0SCP3ZZ   Extirpation of Matter from Right Toe Phalangeal Joint, Percutaneous Approach
0SCP4ZZ   Extirpation of Matter from Right Toe Phalangeal Joint, Percutaneous Endoscopic Approach
0SCQ0ZZ   Extirpation of Matter from Left Toe Phalangeal Joint, Open Approach
0SCQ3ZZ   Extirpation of Matter from Left Toe Phalangeal Joint, Percutaneous Approach
0SCQ4ZZ   Extirpation of Matter from Left Toe Phalangeal Joint, Percutaneous Endoscopic Approach

0SG – Lower Joints, Fusion

For Fusion procedures involving the vertebral joints Review Coding Guidelines B3.10a, B3.10b and B3.10c

0SG0070   Fusion of Lumbar Vertebral Joint with Autologous Tissue Substitute, Anterior Approach, Anterior Column, Open Approach
   HAC   When reported with secondary diagnosis code T84.60XA, T84.610A, T84.611A, T84.612A, T84.613A, T84.614A, T84.615A, T84.619A, T84.63XA, T84.69XA, T84.7XXA

0SG0071   Fusion of Lumbar Vertebral Joint with Autologous Tissue Substitute, Posterior Approach, Posterior Column, Open Approach
   HAC   When reported with secondary diagnosis code T84.60XA, T84.610A, T84.611A, T84.612A, T84.613A, T84.614A, T84.615A, T84.619A, T84.63XA, T84.69XA, T84.7XXA

♀ Female-only   ♂ Male-only   ● Limited Coverage   ● Non-OR   HAC HAC-associated procedure   ● Non-covered procedures   ✚ Combination

0SG007J   Fusion of Lumbar Vertebral Joint with Autologous Tissue Substitute, Posterior Approach, Anterior Column, Open Approach
  HAC   When reported with secondary diagnosis code T84.60XA, T84.610A, T84.611A, T84.612A, T84.613A, T84.614A, T84.615A, T84.619A, T84.63XA, T84.69XA, T84.7XXA

0SG00A0   Fusion of Lumbar Vertebral Joint with Interbody Fusion Device, Anterior Approach, Anterior Column, Open Approach
  HAC   When reported with secondary diagnosis code T84.60XA, T84.610A, T84.611A, T84.612A, T84.613A, T84.614A, T84.615A, T84.619A, T84.63XA, T84.69XA, T84.7XXA

0SG00A1   Fusion of Lumbar Vertebral Joint with Interbody Fusion Device, Posterior Approach, Posterior Column, Open Approach
  HAC   When reported with secondary diagnosis code T84.60XA, T84.610A, T84.611A, T84.612A, T84.613A, T84.614A, T84.615A, T84.619A, T84.63XA, T84.69XA, T84.7XXA

0SG00AJ   Fusion of Lumbar Vertebral Joint with Interbody Fusion Device, Posterior Approach, Anterior Column, Open Approach
  HAC   When reported with secondary diagnosis code T84.60XA, T84.610A, T84.611A, T84.612A, T84.613A, T84.614A, T84.615A, T84.619A, T84.63XA, T84.69XA, T84.7XXA

0SG00J0   Fusion of Lumbar Vertebral Joint with Synthetic Substitute, Anterior Approach, Anterior Column, Open Approach
  HAC   When reported with secondary diagnosis code T84.60XA, T84.610A, T84.611A, T84.612A, T84.613A, T84.614A, T84.615A, T84.619A, T84.63XA, T84.69XA, T84.7XXA

0SG00J1   Fusion of Lumbar Vertebral Joint with Synthetic Substitute, Posterior Approach, Posterior Column, Open Approach
  HAC   When reported with secondary diagnosis code T84.60XA, T84.610A, T84.611A, T84.612A, T84.613A, T84.614A, T84.615A, T84.619A, T84.63XA, T84.69XA, T84.7XXA

0SG00JJ   Fusion of Lumbar Vertebral Joint with Synthetic Substitute, Posterior Approach, Anterior Column, Open Approach
  HAC   When reported with secondary diagnosis code T84.60XA, T84.610A, T84.611A, T84.612A, T84.613A, T84.614A, T84.615A, T84.619A, T84.63XA, T84.69XA, T84.7XXA

0SG00K0   Fusion of Lumbar Vertebral Joint with Nonautologous Tissue Substitute, Anterior Approach, Anterior Column, Open Approach
  HAC   When reported with secondary diagnosis code T84.60XA, T84.610A, T84.611A, T84.612A, T84.613A, T84.614A, T84.615A, T84.619A, T84.63XA, T84.69XA, T84.7XXA

0SG00K1   Fusion of Lumbar Vertebral Joint with Nonautologous Tissue Substitute, Posterior Approach, Posterior Column, Open Approach
  HAC   When reported with secondary diagnosis code T84.60XA, T84.610A, T84.611A, T84.612A, T84.613A, T84.614A, T84.615A, T84.619A, T84.63XA, T84.69XA, T84.7XXA

0SG00KJ   Fusion of Lumbar Vertebral Joint with Nonautologous Tissue Substitute, Posterior Approach, Anterior Column, Open Approach
  HAC   When reported with secondary diagnosis code T84.60XA, T84.610A, T84.611A, T84.612A, T84.613A, T84.614A, T84.615A, T84.619A, T84.63XA, T84.69XA, T84.7XXA

0SG00Z0   Fusion of Lumbar Vertebral Joint, Anterior Approach, Anterior Column, Open Approach
  HAC   When reported with secondary diagnosis code T84.60XA, T84.610A, T84.611A, T84.612A, T84.613A, T84.614A, T84.615A, T84.619A, T84.63XA, T84.69XA, T84.7XXA

0SG00Z1   Fusion of Lumbar Vertebral Joint, Posterior Approach, Posterior Column, Open Approach
  HAC   When reported with secondary diagnosis code T84.60XA, T84.610A, T84.611A, T84.612A, T84.613A, T84.614A, T84.615A, T84.619A, T84.63XA, T84.69XA, T84.7XXA

0SG00ZJ   Fusion of Lumbar Vertebral Joint, Posterior Approach, Anterior Column, Open Approach
  HAC   When reported with secondary diagnosis code T84.60XA, T84.610A, T84.611A, T84.612A, T84.613A, T84.614A, T84.615A, T84.619A, T84.63XA, T84.69XA, T84.7XXA

0SG0370   Fusion of Lumbar Vertebral Joint with Autologous Tissue Substitute, Anterior Approach, Anterior Column, Percutaneous Approach
  HAC   When reported with secondary diagnosis code T84.60XA, T84.610A, T84.611A, T84.612A, T84.613A, T84.614A, T84.615A, T84.619A, T84.63XA, T84.69XA, T84.7XXA

0SG0371   Fusion of Lumbar Vertebral Joint with Autologous Tissue Substitute, Posterior Approach, Posterior Column, Percutaneous Approach
  HAC   When reported with secondary diagnosis code T84.60XA, T84.610A, T84.611A, T84.612A, T84.613A, T84.614A, T84.615A, T84.619A, T84.63XA, T84.69XA, T84.7XXA

0SG037J   Fusion of Lumbar Vertebral Joint with Autologous Tissue Substitute, Posterior Approach, Anterior Column, Percutaneous Approach
  HAC   When reported with secondary diagnosis code T84.60XA, T84.610A, T84.611A, T84.612A, T84.613A, T84.614A, T84.615A, T84.619A, T84.63XA, T84.69XA, T84.7XXA

0SG03A0   Fusion of Lumbar Vertebral Joint with Interbody Fusion Device, Anterior Approach, Anterior Column, Percutaneous Approach
  HAC   When reported with secondary diagnosis code T84.60XA, T84.610A, T84.611A, T84.612A, T84.613A, T84.614A, T84.615A, T84.619A, T84.63XA, T84.69XA, T84.7XXA

0SG03A1   Fusion of Lumbar Vertebral Joint with Interbody Fusion Device, Posterior Approach, Posterior Column, Percutaneous Approach
  HAC   When reported with secondary diagnosis code T84.60XA, T84.610A, T84.611A, T84.612A, T84.613A, T84.614A, T84.615A, T84.619A, T84.63XA, T84.69XA, T84.7XXA

0SG03AJ   Fusion of Lumbar Vertebral Joint with Interbody Fusion Device, Posterior Approach, Anterior Column, Percutaneous Approach
  HAC   When reported with secondary diagnosis code T84.60XA, T84.610A, T84.611A, T84.612A, T84.613A, T84.614A, T84.615A, T84.619A, T84.63XA, T84.69XA, T84.7XXA

0SG03J0   Fusion of Lumbar Vertebral Joint with Synthetic Substitute, Anterior Approach, Anterior Column, Percutaneous Approach
  HAC   When reported with secondary diagnosis code T84.60XA, T84.610A, T84.611A, T84.612A, T84.613A, T84.614A, T84.615A, T84.619A, T84.63XA, T84.69XA, T84.7XXA

0SG03J1   Fusion of Lumbar Vertebral Joint with Synthetic Substitute, Posterior Approach, Posterior Column, Percutaneous Approach
  HAC   When reported with secondary diagnosis code T84.60XA, T84.610A, T84.611A, T84.612A, T84.613A, T84.614A, T84.615A, T84.619A, T84.63XA, T84.69XA, T84.7XXA

0SG03JJ   Fusion of Lumbar Vertebral Joint with Synthetic Substitute, Posterior Approach, Anterior Column, Percutaneous Approach
  HAC   When reported with secondary diagnosis code T84.60XA, T84.610A, T84.611A, T84.612A, T84.613A, T84.614A, T84.615A, T84.619A, T84.63XA, T84.69XA, T84.7XXA

0SG03K0   Fusion of Lumbar Vertebral Joint with Nonautologous Tissue Substitute, Anterior Approach, Anterior Column, Percutaneous Approach
  HAC   When reported with secondary diagnosis code T84.60XA, T84.610A, T84.611A, T84.612A, T84.613A, T84.614A, T84.615A, T84.619A, T84.63XA, T84.69XA, T84.7XXA

0SG03K1   Fusion of Lumbar Vertebral Joint with Nonautologous Tissue Substitute, Posterior Approach, Posterior Column, Percutaneous Approach
  HAC   When reported with secondary diagnosis code T84.60XA, T84.610A, T84.611A, T84.612A, T84.613A, T84.614A, T84.615A, T84.619A, T84.63XA, T84.69XA, T84.7XXA

0SG03KJ   Fusion of Lumbar Vertebral Joint with Nonautologous Tissue Substitute, Posterior Approach, Anterior Column, Percutaneous Approach
  HAC   When reported with secondary diagnosis code T84.60XA, T84.610A, T84.611A, T84.612A, T84.613A, T84.614A, T84.615A, T84.619A, T84.63XA, T84.69XA, T84.7XXA

0SG03Z0   Fusion of Lumbar Vertebral Joint, Anterior Approach, Anterior Column, Percutaneous Approach
  HAC   When reported with secondary diagnosis code T84.60XA, T84.610A, T84.611A, T84.612A, T84.613A, T84.614A, T84.615A, T84.619A, T84.63XA, T84.69XA, T84.7XXA

0SG03Z1   Fusion of Lumbar Vertebral Joint, Posterior Approach, Posterior Column, Percutaneous Approach
  HAC   When reported with secondary diagnosis code T84.60XA, T84.610A, T84.611A, T84.612A, T84.613A, T84.614A, T84.615A, T84.619A, T84.63XA, T84.69XA, T84.7XXA

0SG03ZJ   Fusion of Lumbar Vertebral Joint, Posterior Approach, Anterior Column, Percutaneous Approach
  HAC   When reported with secondary diagnosis code T84.60XA, T84.610A, T84.611A, T84.612A, T84.613A, T84.614A, T84.615A, T84.619A, T84.63XA, T84.69XA, T84.7XXA

0SG0470   Fusion of Lumbar Vertebral Joint with Autologous Tissue Substitute, Anterior Approach, Anterior Column, Percutaneous Endoscopic Approach
  HAC   When reported with secondary diagnosis code T84.60XA, T84.610A, T84.611A, T84.612A, T84.613A, T84.614A, T84.615A, T84.619A, T84.63XA, T84.69XA, T84.7XXA

♀ Female-only   ♂ Male-only   ● Limited Coverage   ● Non-OR   HAC HAC-associated procedure   ● Non-covered procedures   + Combination

0SG0471 Fusion of Lumbar Vertebral Joint with Autologous Tissue Substitute, Posterior Approach, Posterior Column, Percutaneous Endoscopic Approach
- HAC When reported with secondary diagnosis code T84.60XA, T84.610A, T84.611A, T84.612A, T84.613A, T84.614A, T84.615A, T84.619A, T84.63XA, T84.69XA, T84.7XXA

0SG047J Fusion of Lumbar Vertebral Joint with Autologous Tissue Substitute, Posterior Approach, Anterior Column, Percutaneous Endoscopic Approach
- HAC When reported with secondary diagnosis code T84.60XA, T84.610A, T84.611A, T84.612A, T84.613A, T84.614A, T84.615A, T84.619A, T84.63XA, T84.69XA, T84.7XXA

0SG04A0 Fusion of Lumbar Vertebral Joint with Interbody Fusion Device, Anterior Approach, Anterior Column, Percutaneous Endoscopic Approach
- HAC When reported with secondary diagnosis code T84.60XA, T84.610A, T84.611A, T84.612A, T84.613A, T84.614A, T84.615A, T84.619A, T84.63XA, T84.69XA, T84.7XXA

0SG04A1 Fusion of Lumbar Vertebral Joint with Interbody Fusion Device, Posterior Approach, Posterior Column, Percutaneous Endoscopic Approach
- HAC When reported with secondary diagnosis code T84.60XA, T84.610A, T84.611A, T84.612A, T84.613A, T84.614A, T84.615A, T84.619A, T84.63XA, T84.69XA, T84.7XXA

0SG04AJ Fusion of Lumbar Vertebral Joint with Interbody Fusion Device, Posterior Approach, Anterior Column, Percutaneous Endoscopic Approach
- HAC When reported with secondary diagnosis code T84.60XA, T84.610A, T84.611A, T84.612A, T84.613A, T84.614A, T84.615A, T84.619A, T84.63XA, T84.69XA, T84.7XXA

0SG04J0 Fusion of Lumbar Vertebral Joint with Synthetic Substitute, Anterior Approach, Anterior Column, Percutaneous Endoscopic Approach
- HAC When reported with secondary diagnosis code T84.60XA, T84.610A, T84.611A, T84.612A, T84.613A, T84.614A, T84.615A, T84.619A, T84.63XA, T84.69XA, T84.7XXA

0SG04J1 Fusion of Lumbar Vertebral Joint with Synthetic Substitute, Posterior Approach, Posterior Column, Percutaneous Endoscopic Approach
- HAC When reported with secondary diagnosis code T84.60XA, T84.610A, T84.611A, T84.612A, T84.613A, T84.614A, T84.615A, T84.619A, T84.63XA, T84.69XA, T84.7XXA

0SG04JJ Fusion of Lumbar Vertebral Joint with Synthetic Substitute, Posterior Approach, Anterior Column, Percutaneous Endoscopic Approach
- HAC When reported with secondary diagnosis code T84.60XA, T84.610A, T84.611A, T84.612A, T84.613A, T84.614A, T84.615A, T84.619A, T84.63XA, T84.69XA, T84.7XXA

0SG04K0 Fusion of Lumbar Vertebral Joint with Nonautologous Tissue Substitute, Anterior Approach, Anterior Column, Percutaneous Endoscopic Approach
- HAC When reported with secondary diagnosis code T84.60XA, T84.610A, T84.611A, T84.612A, T84.613A, T84.614A, T84.615A, T84.619A, T84.63XA, T84.69XA, T84.7XXA

0SG04K1 Fusion of Lumbar Vertebral Joint with Nonautologous Tissue Substitute, Posterior Approach, Posterior Column, Percutaneous Endoscopic Approach
- HAC When reported with secondary diagnosis code T84.60XA, T84.610A, T84.611A, T84.612A, T84.613A, T84.614A, T84.615A, T84.619A, T84.63XA, T84.69XA, T84.7XXA

0SG04KJ Fusion of Lumbar Vertebral Joint with Nonautologous Tissue Substitute, Posterior Approach, Anterior Column, Percutaneous Endoscopic Approach
- HAC When reported with secondary diagnosis code T84.60XA, T84.610A, T84.611A, T84.612A, T84.613A, T84.614A, T84.615A, T84.619A, T84.63XA, T84.69XA, T84.7XXA

0SG04Z0 Fusion of Lumbar Vertebral Joint, Anterior Approach, Anterior Column, Percutaneous Endoscopic Approach
- HAC When reported with secondary diagnosis code T84.60XA, T84.610A, T84.611A, T84.612A, T84.613A, T84.614A, T84.615A, T84.619A, T84.63XA, T84.69XA, T84.7XXA

0SG04Z1 Fusion of Lumbar Vertebral Joint, Posterior Approach, Posterior Column, Percutaneous Endoscopic Approach
- HAC When reported with secondary diagnosis code T84.60XA, T84.610A, T84.611A, T84.612A, T84.613A, T84.614A, T84.615A, T84.619A, T84.63XA, T84.69XA, T84.7XXA

0SG04ZJ Fusion of Lumbar Vertebral Joint, Posterior Approach, Anterior Column, Percutaneous Endoscopic Approach
- HAC When reported with secondary diagnosis code T84.60XA, T84.610A, T84.611A, T84.612A, T84.613A, T84.614A, T84.615A, T84.619A, T84.63XA, T84.69XA, T84.7XXA

0SG1070 Fusion of 2 or more Lumbar Vertebral Joints with Autologous Tissue Substitute, Anterior Approach, Anterior Column, Open Approach
- HAC When reported with secondary diagnosis code T84.60XA, T84.610A, T84.611A, T84.612A, T84.613A, T84.614A, T84.615A, T84.619A, T84.63XA, T84.69XA, T84.7XXA

0SG1071 Fusion of 2 or more Lumbar Vertebral Joints with Autologous Tissue Substitute, Posterior Approach, Posterior Column, Open Approach
- HAC When reported with secondary diagnosis code T84.60XA, T84.610A, T84.611A, T84.612A, T84.613A, T84.614A, T84.615A, T84.619A, T84.63XA, T84.69XA, T84.7XXA

0SG107J Fusion of 2 or more Lumbar Vertebral Joints with Autologous Tissue Substitute, Posterior Approach, Anterior Column, Open Approach
- HAC When reported with secondary diagnosis code T84.60XA, T84.610A, T84.611A, T84.612A, T84.613A, T84.614A, T84.615A, T84.619A, T84.63XA, T84.69XA, T84.7XXA

0SG10A0 Fusion of 2 or more Lumbar Vertebral Joints with Interbody Fusion Device, Anterior Approach, Anterior Column, Open Approach
- HAC When reported with secondary diagnosis code T84.60XA, T84.610A, T84.611A, T84.612A, T84.613A, T84.614A, T84.615A, T84.619A, T84.63XA, T84.69XA, T84.7XXA

0SG10A1 Fusion of 2 or more Lumbar Vertebral Joints with Interbody Fusion Device, Posterior Approach, Posterior Column, Open Approach
- HAC When reported with secondary diagnosis code T84.60XA, T84.610A, T84.611A, T84.612A, T84.613A, T84.614A, T84.615A, T84.619A, T84.63XA, T84.69XA, T84.7XXA

0SG10AJ Fusion of 2 or more Lumbar Vertebral Joints with Interbody Fusion Device, Posterior Approach, Anterior Column, Open Approach
- HAC When reported with secondary diagnosis code T84.60XA, T84.610A, T84.611A, T84.612A, T84.613A, T84.614A, T84.615A, T84.619A, T84.63XA, T84.69XA, T84.7XXA

0SG10J0 Fusion of 2 or more Lumbar Vertebral Joints with Synthetic Substitute, Anterior Approach, Anterior Column, Open Approach
- HAC When reported with secondary diagnosis code T84.60XA, T84.610A, T84.611A, T84.612A, T84.613A, T84.614A, T84.615A, T84.619A, T84.63XA, T84.69XA, T84.7XXA

0SG10J1 Fusion of 2 or more Lumbar Vertebral Joints with Synthetic Substitute, Posterior Approach, Posterior Column, Open Approach
- HAC When reported with secondary diagnosis code T84.60XA, T84.610A, T84.611A, T84.612A, T84.613A, T84.614A, T84.615A, T84.619A, T84.63XA, T84.69XA, T84.7XXA

0SG10JJ Fusion of 2 or more Lumbar Vertebral Joints with Synthetic Substitute, Posterior Approach, Anterior Column, Open Approach
- HAC When reported with secondary diagnosis code T84.60XA, T84.610A, T84.611A, T84.612A, T84.613A, T84.614A, T84.615A, T84.619A, T84.63XA, T84.69XA, T84.7XXA

0SG10K0 Fusion of 2 or more Lumbar Vertebral Joints with Nonautologous Tissue Substitute, Anterior Approach, Anterior Column, Open Approach
- HAC When reported with secondary diagnosis code T84.60XA, T84.610A, T84.611A, T84.612A, T84.613A, T84.614A, T84.615A, T84.619A, T84.63XA, T84.69XA, T84.7XXA

0SG10K1 Fusion of 2 or more Lumbar Vertebral Joints with Nonautologous Tissue Substitute, Posterior Approach, Posterior Column, Open Approach
- HAC When reported with secondary diagnosis code T84.60XA, T84.610A, T84.611A, T84.612A, T84.613A, T84.614A, T84.615A, T84.619A, T84.63XA, T84.69XA, T84.7XXA

0SG10KJ Fusion of 2 or more Lumbar Vertebral Joints with Nonautologous Tissue Substitute, Posterior Approach, Anterior Column, Open Approach
- HAC When reported with secondary diagnosis code T84.60XA, T84.610A, T84.611A, T84.612A, T84.613A, T84.614A, T84.615A, T84.619A, T84.63XA, T84.69XA, T84.7XXA

0SG10Z0 Fusion of 2 or more Lumbar Vertebral Joints, Anterior Approach, Anterior Column, Open Approach
- HAC When reported with secondary diagnosis code T84.60XA, T84.610A, T84.611A, T84.612A, T84.613A, T84.614A, T84.615A, T84.619A, T84.63XA, T84.69XA, T84.7XXA

0SG10Z1 Fusion of 2 or more Lumbar Vertebral Joints, Posterior Approach, Posterior Column, Open Approach
> HAC When reported with secondary diagnosis code T84.60XA, T84.610A, T84.611A, T84.612A, T84.613A, T84.614A, T84.615A, T84.619A, T84.63XA, T84.69XA, T84.7XXA

0SG10ZJ Fusion of 2 or more Lumbar Vertebral Joints, Posterior Approach, Anterior Column, Open Approach
> HAC When reported with secondary diagnosis code T84.60XA, T84.610A, T84.611A, T84.612A, T84.613A, T84.614A, T84.615A, T84.619A, T84.63XA, T84.69XA, T84.7XXA

0SG1370 Fusion of 2 or more Lumbar Vertebral Joints with Autologous Tissue Substitute, Anterior Approach, Anterior Column, Percutaneous Approach
> HAC When reported with secondary diagnosis code T84.60XA, T84.610A, T84.611A, T84.612A, T84.613A, T84.614A, T84.615A, T84.619A, T84.63XA, T84.69XA, T84.7XXA

0SG1371 Fusion of 2 or more Lumbar Vertebral Joints with Autologous Tissue Substitute, Posterior Approach, Posterior Column, Percutaneous Approach
> HAC When reported with secondary diagnosis code T84.60XA, T84.610A, T84.611A, T84.612A, T84.613A, T84.614A, T84.615A, T84.619A, T84.63XA, T84.69XA, T84.7XXA

0SG137J Fusion of 2 or more Lumbar Vertebral Joints with Autologous Tissue Substitute, Posterior Approach, Anterior Column, Percutaneous Approach
> HAC When reported with secondary diagnosis code T84.60XA, T84.610A, T84.611A, T84.612A, T84.613A, T84.614A, T84.615A, T84.619A, T84.63XA, T84.69XA, T84.7XXA

0SG13A0 Fusion of 2 or more Lumbar Vertebral Joints with Interbody Fusion Device, Anterior Approach, Anterior Column, Percutaneous Approach
> HAC When reported with secondary diagnosis code T84.60XA, T84.610A, T84.611A, T84.612A, T84.613A, T84.614A, T84.615A, T84.619A, T84.63XA, T84.69XA, T84.7XXA

0SG13A1 Fusion of 2 or more Lumbar Vertebral Joints with Interbody Fusion Device, Posterior Approach, Posterior Column, Percutaneous Approach
> HAC When reported with secondary diagnosis code T84.60XA, T84.610A, T84.611A, T84.612A, T84.613A, T84.614A, T84.615A, T84.619A, T84.63XA, T84.69XA, T84.7XXA

0SG13AJ Fusion of 2 or more Lumbar Vertebral Joints with Interbody Fusion Device, Posterior Approach, Anterior Column, Percutaneous Approach
> HAC When reported with secondary diagnosis code T84.60XA, T84.610A, T84.611A, T84.612A, T84.613A, T84.614A, T84.615A, T84.619A, T84.63XA, T84.69XA, T84.7XXA

0SG13J0 Fusion of 2 or more Lumbar Vertebral Joints with Synthetic Substitute, Anterior Approach, Anterior Column, Percutaneous Approach
> HAC When reported with secondary diagnosis code T84.60XA, T84.610A, T84.611A, T84.612A, T84.613A, T84.614A, T84.615A, T84.619A, T84.63XA, T84.69XA, T84.7XXA

0SG13J1 Fusion of 2 or more Lumbar Vertebral Joints with Synthetic Substitute, Posterior Approach, Posterior Column, Percutaneous Approach
> HAC When reported with secondary diagnosis code T84.60XA, T84.610A, T84.611A, T84.612A, T84.613A, T84.614A, T84.615A, T84.619A, T84.63XA, T84.69XA, T84.7XXA

0SG13JJ Fusion of 2 or more Lumbar Vertebral Joints with Synthetic Substitute, Posterior Approach, Anterior Column, Percutaneous Approach
> HAC When reported with secondary diagnosis code T84.60XA, T84.610A, T84.611A, T84.612A, T84.613A, T84.614A, T84.615A, T84.619A, T84.63XA, T84.69XA, T84.7XXA

0SG13K0 Fusion of 2 or more Lumbar Vertebral Joints with Nonautologous Tissue Substitute, Anterior Approach, Anterior Column, Percutaneous Approach
> HAC When reported with secondary diagnosis code T84.60XA, T84.610A, T84.611A, T84.612A, T84.613A, T84.614A, T84.615A, T84.619A, T84.63XA, T84.69XA, T84.7XXA

0SG13K1 Fusion of 2 or more Lumbar Vertebral Joints with Nonautologous Tissue Substitute, Posterior Approach, Posterior Column, Percutaneous Approach
> HAC When reported with secondary diagnosis code T84.60XA, T84.610A, T84.611A, T84.612A, T84.613A, T84.614A, T84.615A, T84.619A, T84.63XA, T84.69XA, T84.7XXA

0SG13KJ Fusion of 2 or more Lumbar Vertebral Joints with Nonautologous Tissue Substitute, Posterior Approach, Anterior Column, Percutaneous Approach
> HAC When reported with secondary diagnosis code T84.60XA, T84.610A, T84.611A, T84.612A, T84.613A, T84.614A, T84.615A, T84.619A, T84.63XA, T84.69XA, T84.7XXA

0SG13Z0 Fusion of 2 or more Lumbar Vertebral Joints, Anterior Approach, Anterior Column, Percutaneous Approach
> HAC When reported with secondary diagnosis code T84.60XA, T84.610A, T84.611A, T84.612A, T84.613A, T84.614A, T84.615A, T84.619A, T84.63XA, T84.69XA, T84.7XXA

0SG13Z1 Fusion of 2 or more Lumbar Vertebral Joints, Posterior Approach, Posterior Column, Percutaneous Approach
> HAC When reported with secondary diagnosis code T84.60XA, T84.610A, T84.611A, T84.612A, T84.613A, T84.614A, T84.615A, T84.619A, T84.63XA, T84.69XA, T84.7XXA

0SG13ZJ Fusion of 2 or more Lumbar Vertebral Joints, Posterior Approach, Anterior Column, Percutaneous Approach
> HAC When reported with secondary diagnosis code T84.60XA, T84.610A, T84.611A, T84.612A, T84.613A, T84.614A, T84.615A, T84.619A, T84.63XA, T84.69XA, T84.7XXA

0SG1470 Fusion of 2 or more Lumbar Vertebral Joints with Autologous Tissue Substitute, Anterior Approach, Anterior Column, Percutaneous Endoscopic Approach
> HAC When reported with secondary diagnosis code T84.60XA, T84.610A, T84.611A, T84.612A, T84.613A, T84.614A, T84.615A, T84.619A, T84.63XA, T84.69XA, T84.7XXA

0SG1471 Fusion of 2 or more Lumbar Vertebral Joints with Autologous Tissue Substitute, Posterior Approach, Posterior Column, Percutaneous Endoscopic Approach
> HAC When reported with secondary diagnosis code T84.60XA, T84.610A, T84.611A, T84.612A, T84.613A, T84.614A, T84.615A, T84.619A, T84.63XA, T84.69XA, T84.7XXA

0SG147J Fusion of 2 or more Lumbar Vertebral Joints with Autologous Tissue Substitute, Posterior Approach, Anterior Column, Percutaneous Endoscopic Approach
> HAC When reported with secondary diagnosis code T84.60XA, T84.610A, T84.611A, T84.612A, T84.613A, T84.614A, T84.615A, T84.619A, T84.63XA, T84.69XA, T84.7XXA

0SG14A0 Fusion of 2 or more Lumbar Vertebral Joints with Interbody Fusion Device, Anterior Approach, Anterior Column, Percutaneous Endoscopic Approach
> HAC When reported with secondary diagnosis code T84.60XA, T84.610A, T84.611A, T84.612A, T84.613A, T84.614A, T84.615A, T84.619A, T84.63XA, T84.69XA, T84.7XXA

0SG14A1 Fusion of 2 or more Lumbar Vertebral Joints with Interbody Fusion Device, Posterior Approach, Posterior Column, Percutaneous Endoscopic Approach
> HAC When reported with secondary diagnosis code T84.60XA, T84.610A, T84.611A, T84.612A, T84.613A, T84.614A, T84.615A, T84.619A, T84.63XA, T84.69XA, T84.7XXA

0SG14AJ Fusion of 2 or more Lumbar Vertebral Joints with Interbody Fusion Device, Posterior Approach, Anterior Column, Percutaneous Endoscopic Approach
> HAC When reported with secondary diagnosis code T84.60XA, T84.610A, T84.611A, T84.612A, T84.613A, T84.614A, T84.615A, T84.619A, T84.63XA, T84.69XA, T84.7XXA

0SG14J0 Fusion of 2 or more Lumbar Vertebral Joints with Synthetic Substitute, Anterior Approach, Anterior Column, Percutaneous Endoscopic Approach
> HAC When reported with secondary diagnosis code T84.60XA, T84.610A, T84.611A, T84.612A, T84.613A, T84.614A, T84.615A, T84.619A, T84.63XA, T84.69XA, T84.7XXA

0SG14J1 Fusion of 2 or more Lumbar Vertebral Joints with Synthetic Substitute, Posterior Approach, Posterior Column, Percutaneous Endoscopic Approach
> HAC When reported with secondary diagnosis code T84.60XA, T84.610A, T84.611A, T84.612A, T84.613A, T84.614A, T84.615A, T84.619A, T84.63XA, T84.69XA, T84.7XXA

0SG14JJ Fusion of 2 or more Lumbar Vertebral Joints with Synthetic Substitute, Posterior Approach, Anterior Column, Percutaneous Endoscopic Approach
> HAC When reported with secondary diagnosis code T84.60XA, T84.610A, T84.611A, T84.612A, T84.613A, T84.614A, T84.615A, T84.619A, T84.63XA, T84.69XA, T84.7XXA

0SG14K0   Fusion of 2 or more Lumbar Vertebral Joints with Nonautologous Tissue Substitute, Anterior Approach, Anterior Column, Percutaneous Endoscopic Approach
HAC   When reported with secondary diagnosis code T84.60XA, T84.610A, T84.611A, T84.612A, T84.613A, T84.614A, T84.615A, T84.619A, T84.63XA, T84.69XA, T84.7XXA

0SG14K1   Fusion of 2 or more Lumbar Vertebral Joints with Nonautologous Tissue Substitute, Posterior Approach, Posterior Column, Percutaneous Endoscopic Approach
HAC   When reported with secondary diagnosis code T84.60XA, T84.610A, T84.611A, T84.612A, T84.613A, T84.614A, T84.615A, T84.619A, T84.63XA, T84.69XA, T84.7XXA

0SG14KJ   Fusion of 2 or more Lumbar Vertebral Joints with Nonautologous Tissue Substitute, Posterior Approach, Anterior Column, Percutaneous Endoscopic Approach
HAC   When reported with secondary diagnosis code T84.60XA, T84.610A, T84.611A, T84.612A, T84.613A, T84.614A, T84.615A, T84.619A, T84.63XA, T84.69XA, T84.7XXA

0SG14Z0   Fusion of 2 or more Lumbar Vertebral Joints, Anterior Approach, Anterior Column, Percutaneous Endoscopic Approach
HAC   When reported with secondary diagnosis code T84.60XA, T84.610A, T84.611A, T84.612A, T84.613A, T84.614A, T84.615A, T84.619A, T84.63XA, T84.69XA, T84.7XXA

0SG14Z1   Fusion of 2 or more Lumbar Vertebral Joints, Posterior Approach, Posterior Column, Percutaneous Endoscopic Approach
HAC   When reported with secondary diagnosis code T84.60XA, T84.610A, T84.611A, T84.612A, T84.613A, T84.614A, T84.615A, T84.619A, T84.63XA, T84.69XA, T84.7XXA

0SG14ZJ   Fusion of 2 or more Lumbar Vertebral Joints, Posterior Approach, Anterior Column, Percutaneous Endoscopic Approach
HAC   When reported with secondary diagnosis code T84.60XA, T84.610A, T84.611A, T84.612A, T84.613A, T84.614A, T84.615A, T84.619A, T84.63XA, T84.69XA, T84.7XXA

0SG3070   Fusion of Lumbosacral Joint with Autologous Tissue Substitute, Anterior Approach, Anterior Column, Open Approach
HAC   When reported with secondary diagnosis code T84.60XA, T84.610A, T84.611A, T84.612A, T84.613A, T84.614A, T84.615A, T84.619A, T84.63XA, T84.69XA, T84.7XXA

0SG3071   Fusion of Lumbosacral Joint with Autologous Tissue Substitute, Posterior Approach, Posterior Column, Open Approach
HAC   When reported with secondary diagnosis code T84.60XA, T84.610A, T84.611A, T84.612A, T84.613A, T84.614A, T84.615A, T84.619A, T84.63XA, T84.69XA, T84.7XXA

0SG307J   Fusion of Lumbosacral Joint with Autologous Tissue Substitute, Posterior Approach, Anterior Column, Open Approach
HAC   When reported with secondary diagnosis code T84.60XA, T84.610A, T84.611A, T84.612A, T84.613A, T84.614A, T84.615A, T84.619A, T84.63XA, T84.69XA, T84.7XXA

0SG30A0   Fusion of Lumbosacral Joint with Interbody Fusion Device, Anterior Approach, Anterior Column, Open Approach
HAC   When reported with secondary diagnosis code T84.60XA, T84.610A, T84.611A, T84.612A, T84.613A, T84.614A, T84.615A, T84.619A, T84.63XA, T84.69XA, T84.7XXA

0SG30A1   Fusion of Lumbosacral Joint with Interbody Fusion Device, Posterior Approach, Posterior Column, Open Approach
HAC   When reported with secondary diagnosis code T84.60XA, T84.610A, T84.611A, T84.612A, T84.613A, T84.614A, T84.615A, T84.619A, T84.63XA, T84.69XA, T84.7XXA

0SG30AJ   Fusion of Lumbosacral Joint with Interbody Fusion Device, Posterior Approach, Anterior Column, Open Approach
HAC   When reported with secondary diagnosis code T84.60XA, T84.610A, T84.611A, T84.612A, T84.613A, T84.614A, T84.615A, T84.619A, T84.63XA, T84.69XA, T84.7XXA

0SG30J0   Fusion of Lumbosacral Joint with Synthetic Substitute, Anterior Approach, Anterior Column, Open Approach
HAC   When reported with secondary diagnosis code T84.60XA, T84.610A, T84.611A, T84.612A, T84.613A, T84.614A, T84.615A, T84.619A, T84.63XA, T84.69XA, T84.7XXA

0SG30J1   Fusion of Lumbosacral Joint with Synthetic Substitute, Posterior Approach, Posterior Column, Open Approach
HAC   When reported with secondary diagnosis code T84.60XA, T84.610A, T84.611A, T84.612A, T84.613A, T84.614A, T84.615A, T84.619A, T84.63XA, T84.69XA, T84.7XXA

0SG30JJ   Fusion of Lumbosacral Joint with Synthetic Substitute, Posterior Approach, Anterior Column, Open Approach
HAC   When reported with secondary diagnosis code T84.60XA, T84.610A, T84.611A, T84.612A, T84.613A, T84.614A, T84.615A, T84.619A, T84.63XA, T84.69XA, T84.7XXA

0SG30K0   Fusion of Lumbosacral Joint with Nonautologous Tissue Substitute, Anterior Approach, Anterior Column, Open Approach
HAC   When reported with secondary diagnosis code T84.60XA, T84.610A, T84.611A, T84.612A, T84.613A, T84.614A, T84.615A, T84.619A, T84.63XA, T84.69XA, T84.7XXA

0SG30K1   Fusion of Lumbosacral Joint with Nonautologous Tissue Substitute, Posterior Approach, Posterior Column, Open Approach
HAC   When reported with secondary diagnosis code T84.60XA, T84.610A, T84.611A, T84.612A, T84.613A, T84.614A, T84.615A, T84.619A, T84.63XA, T84.69XA, T84.7XXA

0SG30KJ   Fusion of Lumbosacral Joint with Nonautologous Tissue Substitute, Posterior Approach, Anterior Column, Open Approach
HAC   When reported with secondary diagnosis code T84.60XA, T84.610A, T84.611A, T84.612A, T84.613A, T84.614A, T84.615A, T84.619A, T84.63XA, T84.69XA, T84.7XXA

0SG30Z0   Fusion of Lumbosacral Joint, Anterior Approach, Anterior Column, Open Approach
HAC   When reported with secondary diagnosis code T84.60XA, T84.610A, T84.611A, T84.612A, T84.613A, T84.614A, T84.615A, T84.619A, T84.63XA, T84.69XA, T84.7XXA

0SG30Z1   Fusion of Lumbosacral Joint, Posterior Approach, Posterior Column, Open Approach
HAC   When reported with secondary diagnosis code T84.60XA, T84.610A, T84.611A, T84.612A, T84.613A, T84.614A, T84.615A, T84.619A, T84.63XA, T84.69XA, T84.7XXA

0SG30ZJ   Fusion of Lumbosacral Joint, Posterior Approach, Anterior Column, Open Approach
HAC   When reported with secondary diagnosis code T84.60XA, T84.610A, T84.611A, T84.612A, T84.613A, T84.614A, T84.615A, T84.619A, T84.63XA, T84.69XA, T84.7XXA

0SG3370   Fusion of Lumbosacral Joint with Autologous Tissue Substitute, Anterior Approach, Anterior Column, Percutaneous Approach
HAC   When reported with secondary diagnosis code T84.60XA, T84.610A, T84.611A, T84.612A, T84.613A, T84.614A, T84.615A, T84.619A, T84.63XA, T84.69XA, T84.7XXA

0SG3371   Fusion of Lumbosacral Joint with Autologous Tissue Substitute, Posterior Approach, Posterior Column, Percutaneous Approach
HAC   When reported with secondary diagnosis code T84.60XA, T84.610A, T84.611A, T84.612A, T84.613A, T84.614A, T84.615A, T84.619A, T84.63XA, T84.69XA, T84.7XXA

0SG337J   Fusion of Lumbosacral Joint with Autologous Tissue Substitute, Posterior Approach, Anterior Column, Percutaneous Approach
HAC   When reported with secondary diagnosis code T84.60XA, T84.610A, T84.611A, T84.612A, T84.613A, T84.614A, T84.615A, T84.619A, T84.63XA, T84.69XA, T84.7XXA

0SG33A0   Fusion of Lumbosacral Joint with Interbody Fusion Device, Anterior Approach, Anterior Column, Percutaneous Approach
HAC   When reported with secondary diagnosis code T84.60XA, T84.610A, T84.611A, T84.612A, T84.613A, T84.614A, T84.615A, T84.619A, T84.63XA, T84.69XA, T84.7XXA

0SG33A1   Fusion of Lumbosacral Joint with Interbody Fusion Device, Posterior Approach, Posterior Column, Percutaneous Approach
HAC   When reported with secondary diagnosis code T84.60XA, T84.610A, T84.611A, T84.612A, T84.613A, T84.614A, T84.615A, T84.619A, T84.63XA, T84.69XA, T84.7XXA

0SG33AJ   Fusion of Lumbosacral Joint with Interbody Fusion Device, Posterior Approach, Anterior Column, Percutaneous Approach
HAC   When reported with secondary diagnosis code T84.60XA, T84.610A, T84.611A, T84.612A, T84.613A, T84.614A, T84.615A, T84.619A, T84.63XA, T84.69XA, T84.7XXA

0SG33J0   Fusion of Lumbosacral Joint with Synthetic Substitute, Anterior Approach, Anterior Column, Percutaneous Approach
HAC   When reported with secondary diagnosis code T84.60XA, T84.610A, T84.611A, T84.612A, T84.613A, T84.614A, T84.615A, T84.619A, T84.63XA, T84.69XA, T84.7XXA

0SG33J1   Fusion of Lumbosacral Joint with Synthetic Substitute, Posterior Approach, Posterior Column, Percutaneous Approach
HAC   When reported with secondary diagnosis code T84.60XA, T84.610A, T84.611A, T84.612A, T84.613A, T84.614A, T84.615A, T84.619A, T84.63XA, T84.69XA, T84.7XXA

0SG33JJ Fusion of Lumbosacral Joint with Synthetic Substitute, Posterior Approach, Anterior Column, Percutaneous Approach
> HAC When reported with secondary diagnosis code T84.60XA, T84.610A, T84.611A, T84.612A, T84.613A, T84.614A, T84.615A, T84.619A, T84.63XA, T84.69XA, T84.7XXA

0SG33K0 Fusion of Lumbosacral Joint with Nonautologous Tissue Substitute, Anterior Approach, Anterior Column, Percutaneous Approach
> HAC When reported with secondary diagnosis code T84.60XA, T84.610A, T84.611A, T84.612A, T84.613A, T84.614A, T84.615A, T84.619A, T84.63XA, T84.69XA, T84.7XXA

0SG33K1 Fusion of Lumbosacral Joint with Nonautologous Tissue Substitute, Posterior Approach, Posterior Column, Percutaneous Approach
> HAC When reported with secondary diagnosis code T84.60XA, T84.610A, T84.611A, T84.612A, T84.613A, T84.614A, T84.615A, T84.619A, T84.63XA, T84.69XA, T84.7XXA

0SG33KJ Fusion of Lumbosacral Joint with Nonautologous Tissue Substitute, Posterior Approach, Anterior Column, Percutaneous Approach
> HAC When reported with secondary diagnosis code T84.60XA, T84.610A, T84.611A, T84.612A, T84.613A, T84.614A, T84.615A, T84.619A, T84.63XA, T84.69XA, T84.7XXA

0SG33Z0 Fusion of Lumbosacral Joint, Anterior Approach, Anterior Column, Percutaneous Approach
> HAC When reported with secondary diagnosis code T84.60XA, T84.610A, T84.611A, T84.612A, T84.613A, T84.614A, T84.615A, T84.619A, T84.63XA, T84.69XA, T84.7XXA

0SG33Z1 Fusion of Lumbosacral Joint, Posterior Approach, Posterior Column, Percutaneous Approach
> HAC When reported with secondary diagnosis code T84.60XA, T84.610A, T84.611A, T84.612A, T84.613A, T84.614A, T84.615A, T84.619A, T84.63XA, T84.69XA, T84.7XXA

0SG33ZJ Fusion of Lumbosacral Joint, Posterior Approach, Anterior Column, Percutaneous Approach
> HAC When reported with secondary diagnosis code T84.60XA, T84.610A, T84.611A, T84.612A, T84.613A, T84.614A, T84.615A, T84.619A, T84.63XA, T84.69XA, T84.7XXA

0SG3470 Fusion of Lumbosacral Joint with Autologous Tissue Substitute, Anterior Approach, Anterior Column, Percutaneous Endoscopic Approach
> HAC When reported with secondary diagnosis code T84.60XA, T84.610A, T84.611A, T84.612A, T84.613A, T84.614A, T84.615A, T84.619A, T84.63XA, T84.69XA, T84.7XXA

0SG3471 Fusion of Lumbosacral Joint with Autologous Tissue Substitute, Posterior Approach, Posterior Column, Percutaneous Endoscopic Approach
> HAC When reported with secondary diagnosis code T84.60XA, T84.610A, T84.611A, T84.612A, T84.613A, T84.614A, T84.615A, T84.619A, T84.63XA, T84.69XA, T84.7XXA

0SG347J Fusion of Lumbosacral Joint with Autologous Tissue Substitute, Posterior Approach, Anterior Column, Percutaneous Endoscopic Approach
> HAC When reported with secondary diagnosis code T84.60XA, T84.610A, T84.611A, T84.612A, T84.613A, T84.614A, T84.615A, T84.619A, T84.63XA, T84.69XA, T84.7XXA

0SG34A0 Fusion of Lumbosacral Joint with Interbody Fusion Device, Anterior Approach, Anterior Column, Percutaneous Endoscopic Approach
> HAC When reported with secondary diagnosis code T84.60XA, T84.610A, T84.611A, T84.612A, T84.613A, T84.614A, T84.615A, T84.619A, T84.63XA, T84.69XA, T84.7XXA

0SG34A1 Fusion of Lumbosacral Joint with Interbody Fusion Device, Posterior Approach, Posterior Column, Percutaneous Endoscopic Approach
> HAC When reported with secondary diagnosis code T84.60XA, T84.610A, T84.611A, T84.612A, T84.613A, T84.614A, T84.615A, T84.619A, T84.63XA, T84.69XA, T84.7XXA

0SG34AJ Fusion of Lumbosacral Joint with Interbody Fusion Device, Posterior Approach, Anterior Column, Percutaneous Endoscopic Approach
> HAC When reported with secondary diagnosis code T84.60XA, T84.610A, T84.611A, T84.612A, T84.613A, T84.614A, T84.615A, T84.619A, T84.63XA, T84.69XA, T84.7XXA

0SG34J0 Fusion of Lumbosacral Joint with Synthetic Substitute, Anterior Approach, Anterior Column, Percutaneous Endoscopic Approach
> HAC When reported with secondary diagnosis code T84.60XA, T84.610A, T84.611A, T84.612A, T84.613A, T84.614A, T84.615A, T84.619A, T84.63XA, T84.69XA, T84.7XXA

0SG34J1 Fusion of Lumbosacral Joint with Synthetic Substitute, Posterior Approach, Posterior Column, Percutaneous Endoscopic Approach
> HAC When reported with secondary diagnosis code T84.60XA, T84.610A, T84.611A, T84.612A, T84.613A, T84.614A, T84.615A, T84.619A, T84.63XA, T84.69XA, T84.7XXA

0SG34JJ Fusion of Lumbosacral Joint with Synthetic Substitute, Posterior Approach, Anterior Column, Percutaneous Endoscopic Approach
> HAC **When** reported with secondary diagnosis code T84.60XA, T84.610A, T84.611A, T84.612A, T84.613A, T84.614A, T84.615A, T84.619A, T84.63XA, T84.69XA, T84.7XXA

0SG34K0 Fusion of Lumbosacral Joint with Nonautologous Tissue Substitute, Anterior Approach, Anterior Column, Percutaneous Endoscopic Approach
> HAC When reported with secondary diagnosis code T84.60XA, T84.610A, T84.611A, T84.612A, T84.613A, T84.614A, T84.615A, T84.619A, T84.63XA, T84.69XA, T84.7XXA

0SG34K1 Fusion of Lumbosacral Joint with Nonautologous Tissue Substitute, Posterior Approach, Posterior Column, Percutaneous Endoscopic Approach
> HAC When reported with secondary diagnosis code T84.60XA, T84.610A, T84.611A, T84.612A, T84.613A, T84.614A, T84.615A, T84.619A, T84.63XA, T84.69XA, T84.7XXA

0SG34KJ Fusion of Lumbosacral Joint with Nonautologous Tissue Substitute, Posterior Approach, Anterior Column, Percutaneous Endoscopic Approach
> HAC When reported with secondary diagnosis code T84.60XA, T84.610A, T84.611A, T84.612A, T84.613A, T84.614A, T84.615A, T84.619A, T84.63XA, T84.69XA, T84.7XXA

0SG34Z0 Fusion of Lumbosacral Joint, Anterior Approach, Anterior Column, Percutaneous Endoscopic Approach
> HAC When reported with secondary diagnosis code T84.60XA, T84.610A, T84.611A, T84.612A, T84.613A, T84.614A, T84.615A, T84.619A, T84.63XA, T84.69XA, T84.7XXA

0SG34Z1 Fusion of Lumbosacral Joint, Posterior Approach, Posterior Column, Percutaneous Endoscopic Approach
> HAC When reported with secondary diagnosis code T84.60XA, T84.610A, T84.611A, T84.612A, T84.613A, T84.614A, T84.615A, T84.619A, T84.63XA, T84.69XA, T84.7XXA

0SG34ZJ Fusion of Lumbosacral Joint, Posterior Approach, Anterior Column, Percutaneous Endoscopic Approach
> HAC When reported with secondary diagnosis code T84.60XA, T84.610A, T84.611A, T84.612A, T84.613A, T84.614A, T84.615A, T84.619A, T84.63XA, T84.69XA, T84.7XXA

0SG504Z Fusion of Sacrococcygeal Joint with Internal Fixation Device, Open Approach

0SG507Z Fusion of Sacrococcygeal Joint with Autologous Tissue Substitute, Open Approach

0SG50JZ Fusion of Sacrococcygeal Joint with Synthetic Substitute, Open Approach

0SG50KZ Fusion of Sacrococcygeal Joint with Nonautologous Tissue Substitute, Open Approach

0SG50ZZ Fusion of Sacrococcygeal Joint, Open Approach

0SG534Z Fusion of Sacrococcygeal Joint with Internal Fixation Device, Percutaneous Approach

0SG537Z Fusion of Sacrococcygeal Joint with Autologous Tissue Substitute, Percutaneous Approach

0SG53JZ Fusion of Sacrococcygeal Joint with Synthetic Substitute, Percutaneous Approach

0SG53KZ Fusion of Sacrococcygeal Joint with Nonautologous Tissue Substitute, Percutaneous Approach

0SG53ZZ Fusion of Sacrococcygeal Joint, Percutaneous Approach

0SG544Z Fusion of Sacrococcygeal Joint with Internal Fixation Device, Percutaneous Endoscopic Approach

0SG547Z Fusion of Sacrococcygeal Joint with Autologous Tissue Substitute, Percutaneous Endoscopic Approach

0SG54JZ Fusion of Sacrococcygeal Joint with Synthetic Substitute, Percutaneous Endoscopic Approach

0SG54KZ Fusion of Sacrococcygeal Joint with Nonautologous Tissue Substitute, Percutaneous Endoscopic Approach

0SG54ZZ Fusion of Sacrococcygeal Joint, Percutaneous Endoscopic Approach

0SG604Z Fusion of Coccygeal Joint with Internal Fixation Device, Open Approach

0SG607Z Fusion of Coccygeal Joint with Autologous Tissue Substitute, Open Approach

---

♀ Female-only   ♂ Male-only   ● Limited Coverage   ● Non-OR   HAC HAC-associated procedure   ● Non-covered procedures   ✚ Combination

0SG60JZ Fusion of Coccygeal Joint with Synthetic Substitute, Open Approach

0SG60KZ Fusion of Coccygeal Joint with Nonautologous Tissue Substitute, Open Approach

0SG60ZZ Fusion of Coccygeal Joint, Open Approach

0SG634Z Fusion of Coccygeal Joint with Internal Fixation Device, Percutaneous Approach

0SG637Z Fusion of Coccygeal Joint with Autologous Tissue Substitute, Percutaneous Approach

0SG63JZ Fusion of Coccygeal Joint with Synthetic Substitute, Percutaneous Approach

0SG63KZ Fusion of Coccygeal Joint with Nonautologous Tissue Substitute, Percutaneous Approach

0SG63ZZ Fusion of Coccygeal Joint, Percutaneous Approach

0SG644Z Fusion of Coccygeal Joint with Internal Fixation Device, Percutaneous Endoscopic Approach

0SG647Z Fusion of Coccygeal Joint with Autologous Tissue Substitute, Percutaneous Endoscopic Approach

0SG64JZ Fusion of Coccygeal Joint with Synthetic Substitute, Percutaneous Endoscopic Approach

0SG64KZ Fusion of Coccygeal Joint with Nonautologous Tissue Substitute, Percutaneous Endoscopic Approach

0SG64ZZ Fusion of Coccygeal Joint, Percutaneous Endoscopic Approach

0SG704Z Fusion of Right Sacroiliac Joint with Internal Fixation Device, Open Approach

0SG707Z Fusion of Right Sacroiliac Joint with Autologous Tissue Substitute, Open Approach

0SG70JZ Fusion of Right Sacroiliac Joint with Synthetic Substitute, Open Approach

0SG70KZ Fusion of Right Sacroiliac Joint with Nonautologous Tissue Substitute, Open Approach

0SG70ZZ Fusion of Right Sacroiliac Joint, Open Approach

0SG734Z Fusion of Right Sacroiliac Joint with Internal Fixation Device, Percutaneous Approach

0SG737Z Fusion of Right Sacroiliac Joint with Autologous Tissue Substitute, Percutaneous Approach

0SG73JZ Fusion of Right Sacroiliac Joint with Synthetic Substitute, Percutaneous Approach

0SG73KZ Fusion of Right Sacroiliac Joint with Nonautologous Tissue Substitute, Percutaneous Approach

0SG73ZZ Fusion of Right Sacroiliac Joint, Percutaneous Approach

0SG744Z Fusion of Right Sacroiliac Joint with Internal Fixation Device, Percutaneous Endoscopic Approach

0SG747Z Fusion of Right Sacroiliac Joint with Autologous Tissue Substitute, Percutaneous Endoscopic Approach

0SG74JZ Fusion of Right Sacroiliac Joint with Synthetic Substitute, Percutaneous Endoscopic Approach

0SG74KZ Fusion of Right Sacroiliac Joint with Nonautologous Tissue Substitute, Percutaneous Endoscopic Approach

0SG74ZZ Fusion of Right Sacroiliac Joint, Percutaneous Endoscopic Approach

0SG804Z Fusion of Left Sacroiliac Joint with Internal Fixation Device, Open Approach

0SG807Z Fusion of Left Sacroiliac Joint with Autologous Tissue Substitute, Open Approach

0SG80JZ Fusion of Left Sacroiliac Joint with Synthetic Substitute, Open Approach

0SG80KZ Fusion of Left Sacroiliac Joint with Nonautologous Tissue Substitute, Open Approach

0SG80ZZ Fusion of Left Sacroiliac Joint, Open Approach

0SG834Z Fusion of Left Sacroiliac Joint with Internal Fixation Device, Percutaneous Approach

0SG837Z Fusion of Left Sacroiliac Joint with Autologous Tissue Substitute, Percutaneous Approach

0SG83JZ Fusion of Left Sacroiliac Joint with Synthetic Substitute, Percutaneous Approach

0SG83KZ Fusion of Left Sacroiliac Joint with Nonautologous Tissue Substitute, Percutaneous Approach

0SG83ZZ Fusion of Left Sacroiliac Joint, Percutaneous Approach

0SG844Z Fusion of Left Sacroiliac Joint with Internal Fixation Device, Percutaneous Endoscopic Approach

0SG847Z Fusion of Left Sacroiliac Joint with Autologous Tissue Substitute, Percutaneous Endoscopic Approach

0SG84JZ Fusion of Left Sacroiliac Joint with Synthetic Substitute, Percutaneous Endoscopic Approach

0SG84KZ Fusion of Left Sacroiliac Joint with Nonautologous Tissue Substitute, Percutaneous Endoscopic Approach

0SG84ZZ Fusion of Left Sacroiliac Joint, Percutaneous Endoscopic Approach

0SG904Z Fusion of Right Hip Joint with Internal Fixation Device, Open Approach

0SG905Z Fusion of Right Hip Joint with External Fixation Device, Open Approach

0SG907Z Fusion of Right Hip Joint with Autologous Tissue Substitute, Open Approach

0SG90JZ Fusion of Right Hip Joint with Synthetic Substitute, Open Approach

0SG90KZ Fusion of Right Hip Joint with Nonautologous Tissue Substitute, Open Approach

0SG90ZZ Fusion of Right Hip Joint, Open Approach

0SG934Z Fusion of Right Hip Joint with Internal Fixation Device, Percutaneous Approach

0SG935Z Fusion of Right Hip Joint with External Fixation Device, Percutaneous Approach

0SG937Z Fusion of Right Hip Joint with Autologous Tissue Substitute, Percutaneous Approach

0SG93JZ Fusion of Right Hip Joint with Synthetic Substitute, Percutaneous Approach

0SG93KZ Fusion of Right Hip Joint with Nonautologous Tissue Substitute, Percutaneous Approach

0SG93ZZ Fusion of Right Hip Joint, Percutaneous Approach

0SG944Z Fusion of Right Hip Joint with Internal Fixation Device, Percutaneous Endoscopic Approach

0SG945Z Fusion of Right Hip Joint with External Fixation Device, Percutaneous Endoscopic Approach

0SG947Z Fusion of Right Hip Joint with Autologous Tissue Substitute, Percutaneous Endoscopic Approach

0SG94JZ Fusion of Right Hip Joint with Synthetic Substitute, Percutaneous Endoscopic Approach

0SG94KZ Fusion of Right Hip Joint with Nonautologous Tissue Substitute, Percutaneous Endoscopic Approach

0SG94ZZ Fusion of Right Hip Joint, Percutaneous Endoscopic Approach

0SGB04Z Fusion of Left Hip Joint with Internal Fixation Device, Open Approach

0SGB05Z Fusion of Left Hip Joint with External Fixation Device, Open Approach

0SGB07Z Fusion of Left Hip Joint with Autologous Tissue Substitute, Open Approach

0SGB0JZ Fusion of Left Hip Joint with Synthetic Substitute, Open Approach

0SGB0KZ Fusion of Left Hip Joint with Nonautologous Tissue Substitute, Open Approach

0SGB0ZZ Fusion of Left Hip Joint, Open Approach

0SGB34Z Fusion of Left Hip Joint with Internal Fixation Device, Percutaneous Approach

0SGB35Z Fusion of Left Hip Joint with External Fixation Device, Percutaneous Approach

0SGB37Z Fusion of Left Hip Joint with Autologous Tissue Substitute, Percutaneous Approach

0SGB3JZ Fusion of Left Hip Joint with Synthetic Substitute, Percutaneous Approach

0SGB3KZ Fusion of Left Hip Joint with Nonautologous Tissue Substitute, Percutaneous Approach

0SGB3ZZ Fusion of Left Hip Joint, Percutaneous Approach

0SGB44Z Fusion of Left Hip Joint with Internal Fixation Device, Percutaneous Endoscopic Approach

0SGB45Z Fusion of Left Hip Joint with External Fixation Device, Percutaneous Endoscopic Approach

0SGB47Z Fusion of Left Hip Joint with Autologous Tissue Substitute, Percutaneous Endoscopic Approach

0SGB4JZ Fusion of Left Hip Joint with Synthetic Substitute, Percutaneous Endoscopic Approach

0SGB4KZ Fusion of Left Hip Joint with Nonautologous Tissue Substitute, Percutaneous Endoscopic Approach

0SGB4ZZ Fusion of Left Hip Joint, Percutaneous Endoscopic Approach

0SGC04Z Fusion of Right Knee Joint with Internal Fixation Device, Open Approach

0SGC05Z Fusion of Right Knee Joint with External Fixation Device, Open Approach

0SGC07Z Fusion of Right Knee Joint with Autologous Tissue Substitute, Open Approach

---

♀ Female-only   ♂ Male-only   ● Limited Coverage   ● Non-OR   █ HAC-associated procedure   ◆ Non-covered procedures   ➕ Combination

0SGC0JZ Fusion of Right Knee Joint with Synthetic Substitute, Open Approach

0SGC0KZ Fusion of Right Knee Joint with Nonautologous Tissue Substitute, Open Approach

0SGC0ZZ Fusion of Right Knee Joint, Open Approach

0SGC34Z Fusion of Right Knee Joint with Internal Fixation Device, Percutaneous Approach

0SGC35Z Fusion of Right Knee Joint with External Fixation Device, Percutaneous Approach

0SGC37Z Fusion of Right Knee Joint with Autologous Tissue Substitute, Percutaneous Approach

0SGC3JZ Fusion of Right Knee Joint with Synthetic Substitute, Percutaneous Approach

0SGC3KZ Fusion of Right Knee Joint with Nonautologous Tissue Substitute, Percutaneous Approach

0SGC3ZZ Fusion of Right Knee Joint, Percutaneous Approach

0SGC44Z Fusion of Right Knee Joint with Internal Fixation Device, Percutaneous Endoscopic Approach

0SGC45Z Fusion of Right Knee Joint with External Fixation Device, Percutaneous Endoscopic Approach

0SGC47Z Fusion of Right Knee Joint with Autologous Tissue Substitute, Percutaneous Endoscopic Approach

0SGC4JZ Fusion of Right Knee Joint with Synthetic Substitute, Percutaneous Endoscopic Approach

0SGC4KZ Fusion of Right Knee Joint with Nonautologous Tissue Substitute, Percutaneous Endoscopic Approach

0SGC4ZZ Fusion of Right Knee Joint, Percutaneous Endoscopic Approach

0SGD04Z Fusion of Left Knee Joint with Internal Fixation Device, Open Approach

0SGD05Z Fusion of Left Knee Joint with External Fixation Device, Open Approach

0SGD07Z Fusion of Left Knee Joint with Autologous Tissue Substitute, Open Approach

0SGD0JZ Fusion of Left Knee Joint with Synthetic Substitute, Open Approach

0SGD0KZ Fusion of Left Knee Joint with Nonautologous Tissue Substitute, Open Approach

0SGD0ZZ Fusion of Left Knee Joint, Open Approach

0SGD34Z Fusion of Left Knee Joint with Internal Fixation Device, Percutaneous Approach

0SGD35Z Fusion of Left Knee Joint with External Fixation Device, Percutaneous Approach

0SGD37Z Fusion of Left Knee Joint with Autologous Tissue Substitute, Percutaneous Approach

0SGD3JZ Fusion of Left Knee Joint with Synthetic Substitute, Percutaneous Approach

0SGD3KZ Fusion of Left Knee Joint with Nonautologous Tissue Substitute, Percutaneous Approach

0SGD3ZZ Fusion of Left Knee Joint, Percutaneous Approach

0SGD44Z Fusion of Left Knee Joint with Internal Fixation Device, Percutaneous Endoscopic Approach

0SGD45Z Fusion of Left Knee Joint with External Fixation Device, Percutaneous Endoscopic Approach

0SGD47Z Fusion of Left Knee Joint with Autologous Tissue Substitute, Percutaneous Endoscopic Approach

0SGD4JZ Fusion of Left Knee Joint with Synthetic Substitute, Percutaneous Endoscopic Approach

0SGD4KZ Fusion of Left Knee Joint with Nonautologous Tissue Substitute, Percutaneous Endoscopic Approach

0SGD4ZZ Fusion of Left Knee Joint, Percutaneous Endoscopic Approach

0SGF04Z Fusion of Right Ankle Joint with Internal Fixation Device, Open Approach

0SGF05Z Fusion of Right Ankle Joint with External Fixation Device, Open Approach

0SGF07Z Fusion of Right Ankle Joint with Autologous Tissue Substitute, Open Approach

0SGF0JZ Fusion of Right Ankle Joint with Synthetic Substitute, Open Approach

0SGF0KZ Fusion of Right Ankle Joint with Nonautologous Tissue Substitute, Open Approach

0SGF0ZZ Fusion of Right Ankle Joint, Open Approach

0SGF34Z Fusion of Right Ankle Joint with Internal Fixation Device, Percutaneous Approach

0SGF35Z Fusion of Right Ankle Joint with External Fixation Device, Percutaneous Approach

0SGF37Z Fusion of Right Ankle Joint with Autologous Tissue Substitute, Percutaneous Approach

0SGF3JZ Fusion of Right Ankle Joint with Synthetic Substitute, Percutaneous Approach

0SGF3KZ Fusion of Right Ankle Joint with Nonautologous Tissue Substitute, Percutaneous Approach

0SGF3ZZ Fusion of Right Ankle Joint, Percutaneous Approach

0SGF44Z Fusion of Right Ankle Joint with Internal Fixation Device, Percutaneous Endoscopic Approach

0SGF45Z Fusion of Right Ankle Joint with External Fixation Device, Percutaneous Endoscopic Approach

0SGF47Z Fusion of Right Ankle Joint with Autologous Tissue Substitute, Percutaneous Endoscopic Approach

0SGF4JZ Fusion of Right Ankle Joint with Synthetic Substitute, Percutaneous Endoscopic Approach

0SGF4KZ Fusion of Right Ankle Joint with Nonautologous Tissue Substitute, Percutaneous Endoscopic Approach

0SGF4ZZ Fusion of Right Ankle Joint, Percutaneous Endoscopic Approach

0SGG04Z Fusion of Left Ankle Joint with Internal Fixation Device, Open Approach

0SGG05Z Fusion of Left Ankle Joint with External Fixation Device, Open Approach

0SGG07Z Fusion of Left Ankle Joint with Autologous Tissue Substitute, Open Approach

0SGG0JZ Fusion of Left Ankle Joint with Synthetic Substitute, Open Approach

0SGG0KZ Fusion of Left Ankle Joint with Nonautologous Tissue Substitute, Open Approach

0SGG0ZZ Fusion of Left Ankle Joint, Open Approach

0SGG34Z Fusion of Left Ankle Joint with Internal Fixation Device, Percutaneous Approach

0SGG35Z Fusion of Left Ankle Joint with External Fixation Device, Percutaneous Approach

0SGG37Z Fusion of Left Ankle Joint with Autologous Tissue Substitute, Percutaneous Approach

0SGG3JZ Fusion of Left Ankle Joint with Synthetic Substitute, Percutaneous Approach

0SGG3KZ Fusion of Left Ankle Joint with Nonautologous Tissue Substitute, Percutaneous Approach

0SGG3ZZ Fusion of Left Ankle Joint, Percutaneous Approach

0SGG44Z Fusion of Left Ankle Joint with Internal Fixation Device, Percutaneous Endoscopic Approach

0SGG45Z Fusion of Left Ankle Joint with External Fixation Device, Percutaneous Endoscopic Approach

0SGG47Z Fusion of Left Ankle Joint with Autologous Tissue Substitute, Percutaneous Endoscopic Approach

0SGG4JZ Fusion of Left Ankle Joint with Synthetic Substitute, Percutaneous Endoscopic Approach

0SGG4KZ Fusion of Left Ankle Joint with Nonautologous Tissue Substitute, Percutaneous Endoscopic Approach

0SGG4ZZ Fusion of Left Ankle Joint, Percutaneous Endoscopic Approach

0SGH04Z Fusion of Right Tarsal Joint with Internal Fixation Device, Open Approach

0SGH05Z Fusion of Right Tarsal Joint with External Fixation Device, Open Approach

0SGH07Z Fusion of Right Tarsal Joint with Autologous Tissue Substitute, Open Approach

0SGH0JZ Fusion of Right Tarsal Joint with Synthetic Substitute, Open Approach

0SGH0KZ Fusion of Right Tarsal Joint with Nonautologous Tissue Substitute, Open Approach

0SGH0ZZ Fusion of Right Tarsal Joint, Open Approach

0SGH34Z Fusion of Right Tarsal Joint with Internal Fixation Device, Percutaneous Approach

0SGH35Z Fusion of Right Tarsal Joint with External Fixation Device, Percutaneous Approach

0SGH37Z Fusion of Right Tarsal Joint with Autologous Tissue Substitute, Percutaneous Approach

0SGH3JZ Fusion of Right Tarsal Joint with Synthetic Substitute, Percutaneous Approach

0SGH3KZ Fusion of Right Tarsal Joint with Nonautologous Tissue Substitute, Percutaneous Approach

0SGH3ZZ Fusion of Right Tarsal Joint, Percutaneous Approach

0SGH44Z Fusion of Right Tarsal Joint with Internal Fixation Device, Percutaneous Endoscopic Approach

0SGH45Z Fusion of Right Tarsal Joint with External Fixation Device, Percutaneous Endoscopic Approach

0SGH47Z Fusion of Right Tarsal Joint with Autologous Tissue Substitute, Percutaneous Endoscopic Approach

0SGH4JZ Fusion of Right Tarsal Joint with Synthetic Substitute, Percutaneous Endoscopic Approach

0SGH4KZ Fusion of Right Tarsal Joint with Nonautologous Tissue Substitute, Percutaneous Endoscopic Approach

0SGH4ZZ Fusion of Right Tarsal Joint, Percutaneous Endoscopic Approach

0SGJ04Z Fusion of Left Tarsal Joint with Internal Fixation Device, Open Approach

0SGJ05Z Fusion of Left Tarsal Joint with External Fixation Device, Open Approach

0SGJ07Z Fusion of Left Tarsal Joint with Autologous Tissue Substitute, Open Approach

0SGJ0JZ Fusion of Left Tarsal Joint with Synthetic Substitute, Open Approach

0SGJ0KZ Fusion of Left Tarsal Joint with Nonautologous Tissue Substitute, Open Approach

0SGJ0ZZ Fusion of Left Tarsal Joint, Open Approach

0SGJ34Z Fusion of Left Tarsal Joint with Internal Fixation Device, Percutaneous Approach

0SGJ35Z Fusion of Left Tarsal Joint with External Fixation Device, Percutaneous Approach

0SGJ37Z Fusion of Left Tarsal Joint with Autologous Tissue Substitute, Percutaneous Approach

0SGJ3JZ Fusion of Left Tarsal Joint with Synthetic Substitute, Percutaneous Approach

0SGJ3KZ Fusion of Left Tarsal Joint with Nonautologous Tissue Substitute, Percutaneous Approach

0SGJ3ZZ Fusion of Left Tarsal Joint, Percutaneous Approach

0SGJ44Z Fusion of Left Tarsal Joint with Internal Fixation Device, Percutaneous Endoscopic Approach

0SGJ45Z Fusion of Left Tarsal Joint with External Fixation Device, Percutaneous Endoscopic Approach

0SGJ47Z Fusion of Left Tarsal Joint with Autologous Tissue Substitute, Percutaneous Endoscopic Approach

0SGJ4JZ Fusion of Left Tarsal Joint with Synthetic Substitute, Percutaneous Endoscopic Approach

0SGJ4KZ Fusion of Left Tarsal Joint with Nonautologous Tissue Substitute, Percutaneous Endoscopic Approach

0SGJ4ZZ Fusion of Left Tarsal Joint, Percutaneous Endoscopic Approach

0SGK04Z Fusion of Right Metatarsal-Tarsal Joint with Internal Fixation Device, Open Approach

0SGK05Z Fusion of Right Metatarsal-Tarsal Joint with External Fixation Device, Open Approach

0SGK07Z Fusion of Right Metatarsal-Tarsal Joint with Autologous Tissue Substitute, Open Approach

0SGK0JZ Fusion of Right Metatarsal-Tarsal Joint with Synthetic Substitute, Open Approach

0SGK0KZ Fusion of Right Metatarsal-Tarsal Joint with Nonautologous Tissue Substitute, Open Approach

0SGK0ZZ Fusion of Right Metatarsal-Tarsal Joint, Open Approach

0SGK34Z Fusion of Right Metatarsal-Tarsal Joint with Internal Fixation Device, Percutaneous Approach

0SGK35Z Fusion of Right Metatarsal-Tarsal Joint with External Fixation Device, Percutaneous Approach

0SGK37Z Fusion of Right Metatarsal-Tarsal Joint with Autologous Tissue Substitute, Percutaneous Approach

0SGK3JZ Fusion of Right Metatarsal-Tarsal Joint with Synthetic Substitute, Percutaneous Approach

0SGK3KZ Fusion of Right Metatarsal-Tarsal Joint with Nonautologous Tissue Substitute, Percutaneous Approach

0SGK3ZZ Fusion of Right Metatarsal-Tarsal Joint, Percutaneous Approach

0SGK44Z Fusion of Right Metatarsal-Tarsal Joint with Internal Fixation Device, Percutaneous Endoscopic Approach

0SGK45Z Fusion of Right Metatarsal-Tarsal Joint with External Fixation Device, Percutaneous Endoscopic Approach

0SGK47Z Fusion of Right Metatarsal-Tarsal Joint with Autologous Tissue Substitute, Percutaneous Endoscopic Approach

0SGK4JZ Fusion of Right Metatarsal-Tarsal Joint with Synthetic Substitute, Percutaneous Endoscopic Approach

0SGK4KZ Fusion of Right Metatarsal-Tarsal Joint with Nonautologous Tissue Substitute, Percutaneous Endoscopic Approach

0SGK4ZZ Fusion of Right Metatarsal-Tarsal Joint, Percutaneous Endoscopic Approach

0SGL04Z Fusion of Left Metatarsal-Tarsal Joint with Internal Fixation Device, Open Approach

0SGL05Z Fusion of Left Metatarsal-Tarsal Joint with External Fixation Device, Open Approach

0SGL07Z Fusion of Left Metatarsal-Tarsal Joint with Autologous Tissue Substitute, Open Approach

0SGL0JZ Fusion of Left Metatarsal-Tarsal Joint with Synthetic Substitute, Open Approach

0SGL0KZ Fusion of Left Metatarsal-Tarsal Joint with Nonautologous Tissue Substitute, Open Approach

0SGL0ZZ Fusion of Left Metatarsal-Tarsal Joint, Open Approach

0SGL34Z Fusion of Left Metatarsal-Tarsal Joint with Internal Fixation Device, Percutaneous Approach

0SGL35Z Fusion of Left Metatarsal-Tarsal Joint with External Fixation Device, Percutaneous Approach

0SGL37Z Fusion of Left Metatarsal-Tarsal Joint with Autologous Tissue Substitute, Percutaneous Approach

0SGL3JZ Fusion of Left Metatarsal-Tarsal Joint with Synthetic Substitute, Percutaneous Approach

0SGL3KZ Fusion of Left Metatarsal-Tarsal Joint with Nonautologous Tissue Substitute, Percutaneous Approach

0SGL3ZZ Fusion of Left Metatarsal-Tarsal Joint, Percutaneous Approach

0SGL44Z Fusion of Left Metatarsal-Tarsal Joint with Internal Fixation Device, Percutaneous Endoscopic Approach

0SGL45Z Fusion of Left Metatarsal-Tarsal Joint with External Fixation Device, Percutaneous Endoscopic Approach

0SGL47Z Fusion of Left Metatarsal-Tarsal Joint with Autologous Tissue Substitute, Percutaneous Endoscopic Approach

0SGL4JZ Fusion of Left Metatarsal-Tarsal Joint with Synthetic Substitute, Percutaneous Endoscopic Approach

0SGL4KZ Fusion of Left Metatarsal-Tarsal Joint with Nonautologous Tissue Substitute, Percutaneous Endoscopic Approach

0SGL4ZZ Fusion of Left Metatarsal-Tarsal Joint, Percutaneous Endoscopic Approach

0SGM04Z Fusion of Right Metatarsal-Phalangeal Joint with Internal Fixation Device, Open Approach

0SGM05Z Fusion of Right Metatarsal-Phalangeal Joint with External Fixation Device, Open Approach

0SGM07Z Fusion of Right Metatarsal-Phalangeal Joint with Autologous Tissue Substitute, Open Approach

0SGM0JZ Fusion of Right Metatarsal-Phalangeal Joint with Synthetic Substitute, Open Approach

0SGM0KZ Fusion of Right Metatarsal-Phalangeal Joint with Nonautologous Tissue Substitute, Open Approach

0SGM0ZZ Fusion of Right Metatarsal-Phalangeal Joint, Open Approach

0SGM34Z Fusion of Right Metatarsal-Phalangeal Joint with Internal Fixation Device, Percutaneous Approach

0SGM35Z Fusion of Right Metatarsal-Phalangeal Joint with External Fixation Device, Percutaneous Approach

0SGM37Z Fusion of Right Metatarsal-Phalangeal Joint with Autologous Tissue Substitute, Percutaneous Approach

0SGM3JZ Fusion of Right Metatarsal-Phalangeal Joint with Synthetic Substitute, Percutaneous Approach

0SGM3KZ Fusion of Right Metatarsal-Phalangeal Joint with Nonautologous Tissue Substitute, Percutaneous Approach

0SGM3ZZ Fusion of Right Metatarsal-Phalangeal Joint, Percutaneous Approach

0SGM44Z Fusion of Right Metatarsal-Phalangeal Joint with Internal Fixation Device, Percutaneous Endoscopic Approach

0SGM45Z Fusion of Right Metatarsal-Phalangeal Joint with External Fixation Device, Percutaneous Endoscopic Approach

0SGM47Z Fusion of Right Metatarsal-Phalangeal Joint with Autologous Tissue Substitute, Percutaneous Endoscopic Approach

0SGM4JZ Fusion of Right Metatarsal-Phalangeal Joint with Synthetic Substitute, Percutaneous Endoscopic Approach

0SGM4KZ Fusion of Right Metatarsal-Phalangeal Joint with Nonautologous Tissue Substitute, Percutaneous Endoscopic Approach

0SGM4ZZ Fusion of Right Metatarsal-Phalangeal Joint, Percutaneous Endoscopic Approach

0SGN04Z Fusion of Left Metatarsal-Phalangeal Joint with Internal Fixation Device, Open Approach

0SGN05Z Fusion of Left Metatarsal-Phalangeal Joint with External Fixation Device, Open Approach

0SGN07Z Fusion of Left Metatarsal-Phalangeal Joint with Autologous Tissue Substitute, Open Approach

0SGN0JZ Fusion of Left Metatarsal-Phalangeal Joint with Synthetic Substitute, Open Approach

0SGN0KZ Fusion of Left Metatarsal-Phalangeal Joint with Nonautologous Tissue Substitute, Open Approach

0SGN0ZZ Fusion of Left Metatarsal-Phalangeal Joint, Open Approach

0SGN34Z Fusion of Left Metatarsal-Phalangeal Joint with Internal Fixation Device, Percutaneous Approach

0SGN35Z Fusion of Left Metatarsal-Phalangeal Joint with External Fixation Device, Percutaneous Approach

0SGN37Z Fusion of Left Metatarsal-Phalangeal Joint with Autologous Tissue Substitute, Percutaneous Approach

0SGN3JZ Fusion of Left Metatarsal-Phalangeal Joint with Synthetic Substitute, Percutaneous Approach

0SGN3KZ Fusion of Left Metatarsal-Phalangeal Joint with Nonautologous Tissue Substitute, Percutaneous Approach

0SGN3ZZ Fusion of Left Metatarsal-Phalangeal Joint, Percutaneous Approach

0SGN44Z Fusion of Left Metatarsal-Phalangeal Joint with Internal Fixation Device, Percutaneous Endoscopic Approach

0SGN45Z Fusion of Left Metatarsal-Phalangeal Joint with External Fixation Device, Percutaneous Endoscopic Approach

0SGN47Z Fusion of Left Metatarsal-Phalangeal Joint with Autologous Tissue Substitute, Percutaneous Endoscopic Approach

0SGN4JZ Fusion of Left Metatarsal-Phalangeal Joint with Synthetic Substitute, Percutaneous Endoscopic Approach

0SGN4KZ Fusion of Left Metatarsal-Phalangeal Joint with Nonautologous Tissue Substitute, Percutaneous Endoscopic Approach

0SGN4ZZ Fusion of Left Metatarsal-Phalangeal Joint, Percutaneous Endoscopic Approach

0SGP04Z Fusion of Right Toe Phalangeal Joint with Internal Fixation Device, Open Approach

0SGP05Z Fusion of Right Toe Phalangeal Joint with External Fixation Device, Open Approach

0SGP07Z Fusion of Right Toe Phalangeal Joint with Autologous Tissue Substitute, Open Approach

0SGP0JZ Fusion of Right Toe Phalangeal Joint with Synthetic Substitute, Open Approach

0SGP0KZ Fusion of Right Toe Phalangeal Joint with Nonautologous Tissue Substitute, Open Approach

0SGP0ZZ Fusion of Right Toe Phalangeal Joint, Open Approach

0SGP34Z Fusion of Right Toe Phalangeal Joint with Internal Fixation Device, Percutaneous Approach

0SGP35Z Fusion of Right Toe Phalangeal Joint with External Fixation Device, Percutaneous Approach

0SGP37Z Fusion of Right Toe Phalangeal Joint with Autologous Tissue Substitute, Percutaneous Approach

0SGP3JZ Fusion of Right Toe Phalangeal Joint with Synthetic Substitute, Percutaneous Approach

0SGP3KZ Fusion of Right Toe Phalangeal Joint with Nonautologous Tissue Substitute, Percutaneous Approach

0SGP3ZZ Fusion of Right Toe Phalangeal Joint, Percutaneous Approach

0SGP44Z Fusion of Right Toe Phalangeal Joint with Internal Fixation Device, Percutaneous Endoscopic Approach

0SGP45Z Fusion of Right Toe Phalangeal Joint with External Fixation Device, Percutaneous Endoscopic Approach

0SGP47Z Fusion of Right Toe Phalangeal Joint with Autologous Tissue Substitute, Percutaneous Endoscopic Approach

0SGP4JZ Fusion of Right Toe Phalangeal Joint with Synthetic Substitute, Percutaneous Endoscopic Approach

0SGP4KZ Fusion of Right Toe Phalangeal Joint with Nonautologous Tissue Substitute, Percutaneous Endoscopic Approach

0SGP4ZZ Fusion of Right Toe Phalangeal Joint, Percutaneous Endoscopic Approach

0SGQ04Z Fusion of Left Toe Phalangeal Joint with Internal Fixation Device, Open Approach

0SGQ05Z Fusion of Left Toe Phalangeal Joint with External Fixation Device, Open Approach

0SGQ07Z Fusion of Left Toe Phalangeal Joint with Autologous Tissue Substitute, Open Approach

0SGQ0JZ Fusion of Left Toe Phalangeal Joint with Synthetic Substitute, Open Approach

0SGQ0KZ Fusion of Left Toe Phalangeal Joint with Nonautologous Tissue Substitute, Open Approach

0SGQ0ZZ Fusion of Left Toe Phalangeal Joint, Open Approach

0SGQ34Z Fusion of Left Toe Phalangeal Joint with Internal Fixation Device, Percutaneous Approach

0SGQ35Z Fusion of Left Toe Phalangeal Joint with External Fixation Device, Percutaneous Approach

0SGQ37Z Fusion of Left Toe Phalangeal Joint with Autologous Tissue Substitute, Percutaneous Approach

0SGQ3JZ Fusion of Left Toe Phalangeal Joint with Synthetic Substitute, Percutaneous Approach

0SGQ3KZ Fusion of Left Toe Phalangeal Joint with Nonautologous Tissue Substitute, Percutaneous Approach

0SGQ3ZZ Fusion of Left Toe Phalangeal Joint, Percutaneous Approach

0SGQ44Z Fusion of Left Toe Phalangeal Joint with Internal Fixation Device, Percutaneous Endoscopic Approach

0SGQ45Z Fusion of Left Toe Phalangeal Joint with External Fixation Device, Percutaneous Endoscopic Approach

0SGQ47Z Fusion of Left Toe Phalangeal Joint with Autologous Tissue Substitute, Percutaneous Endoscopic Approach

0SGQ4JZ Fusion of Left Toe Phalangeal Joint with Synthetic Substitute, Percutaneous Endoscopic Approach

0SGQ4KZ Fusion of Left Toe Phalangeal Joint with Nonautologous Tissue Substitute, Percutaneous Endoscopic Approach

0SGQ4ZZ Fusion of Left Toe Phalangeal Joint, Percutaneous Endoscopic Approach

0SH – Lower Joints, Insertion

0SH003Z Insertion of Infusion Device into Lumbar Vertebral Joint, Open Approach

0SH004Z Insertion of Internal Fixation Device into Lumbar Vertebral Joint, Open Approach

0SH008Z Insertion of Spacer into Lumbar Vertebral Joint, Open Approach

0SH00BZ Insertion of Interspinous Process Spinal Stabilization Device into Lumbar Vertebral Joint, Open Approach

0SH00CZ Insertion of Pedicle-Based Spinal Stabilization Device into Lumbar Vertebral Joint, Open Approach

0SH00DZ Insertion of Facet Replacement Spinal Stabilization Device into Lumbar Vertebral Joint, Open Approach

0SH033Z Insertion of Infusion Device into Lumbar Vertebral Joint, Percutaneous Approach

0SH034Z Insertion of Internal Fixation Device into Lumbar Vertebral Joint, Percutaneous Approach

0SH038Z Insertion of Spacer into Lumbar Vertebral Joint, Percutaneous Approach

0SH03BZ Insertion of Interspinous Process Spinal Stabilization Device into Lumbar Vertebral Joint, Percutaneous Approach

0SH03CZ Insertion of Pedicle-Based Spinal Stabilization Device into Lumbar Vertebral Joint, Percutaneous Approach

0SH03DZ Insertion of Facet Replacement Spinal Stabilization Device into Lumbar Vertebral Joint, Percutaneous Approach

0SH043Z Insertion of Infusion Device into Lumbar Vertebral Joint, Percutaneous Endoscopic Approach

0SH044Z Insertion of Internal Fixation Device into Lumbar Vertebral Joint, Percutaneous Endoscopic Approach

0SH048Z Insertion of Spacer into Lumbar Vertebral Joint, Percutaneous Endoscopic Approach

0SH04BZ Insertion of Interspinous Process Spinal Stabilization Device into Lumbar Vertebral Joint, Percutaneous Endoscopic Approach

0SH04CZ Insertion of Pedicle-Based Spinal Stabilization Device into Lumbar Vertebral Joint, Percutaneous Endoscopic Approach

0SH04DZ Insertion of Facet Replacement Spinal Stabilization Device into Lumbar Vertebral Joint, Percutaneous Endoscopic Approach

0SH203Z Insertion of Infusion Device into Lumbar Vertebral Disc, Open Approach

0SH208Z Insertion of Spacer into Lumbar Vertebral Disc, Open Approach

0SH233Z Insertion of Infusion Device into Lumbar Vertebral Disc, Percutaneous Approach

0SH238Z Insertion of Spacer into Lumbar Vertebral Disc, Percutaneous Approach

0SH243Z Insertion of Infusion Device into Lumbar Vertebral Disc, Percutaneous Endoscopic Approach

0SH248Z Insertion of Spacer into Lumbar Vertebral Disc, Percutaneous Endoscopic Approach

0SH303Z Insertion of Infusion Device into Lumbosacral Joint, Open Approach

0SH304Z Insertion of Internal Fixation Device into Lumbosacral Joint, Open Approach

0SH308Z Insertion of Spacer into Lumbosacral Joint, Open Approach

0SH30BZ Insertion of Interspinous Process Spinal Stabilization Device into Lumbosacral Joint, Open Approach

0SH30CZ Insertion of Pedicle-Based Spinal Stabilization Device into Lumbosacral Joint, Open Approach

0SH30DZ Insertion of Facet Replacement Spinal Stabilization Device into Lumbosacral Joint, Open Approach

0SH333Z Insertion of Infusion Device into Lumbosacral Joint, Percutaneous Approach

0SH334Z Insertion of Internal Fixation Device into Lumbosacral Joint, Percutaneous Approach

0SH338Z Insertion of Spacer into Lumbosacral Joint, Percutaneous Approach

0SH33BZ Insertion of Interspinous Process Spinal Stabilization Device into Lumbosacral Joint, Percutaneous Approach

0SH33CZ Insertion of Pedicle-Based Spinal Stabilization Device into Lumbosacral Joint, Percutaneous Approach

0SH33DZ Insertion of Facet Replacement Spinal Stabilization Device into Lumbosacral Joint, Percutaneous Approach

0SH343Z Insertion of Infusion Device into Lumbosacral Joint, Percutaneous Endoscopic Approach

0SH344Z Insertion of Internal Fixation Device into Lumbosacral Joint, Percutaneous Endoscopic Approach

0SH348Z Insertion of Spacer into Lumbosacral Joint, Percutaneous Endoscopic Approach

0SH34BZ Insertion of Interspinous Process Spinal Stabilization Device into Lumbosacral Joint, Percutaneous Endoscopic Approach

0SH34CZ Insertion of Pedicle-Based Spinal Stabilization Device into Lumbosacral Joint, Percutaneous Endoscopic Approach

0SH34DZ Insertion of Facet Replacement Spinal Stabilization Device into Lumbosacral Joint, Percutaneous Endoscopic Approach

0SH403Z Insertion of Infusion Device into Lumbosacral Disc, Open Approach

0SH408Z Insertion of Spacer into Lumbosacral Disc, Open Approach

0SH433Z Insertion of Infusion Device into Lumbosacral Disc, Percutaneous Approach

0SH438Z Insertion of Spacer into Lumbosacral Disc, Percutaneous Approach

0SH443Z Insertion of Infusion Device into Lumbosacral Disc, Percutaneous Endoscopic Approach

0SH448Z Insertion of Spacer into Lumbosacral Disc, Percutaneous Endoscopic Approach

0SH503Z Insertion of Infusion Device into Sacrococcygeal Joint, Open Approach

0SH504Z Insertion of Internal Fixation Device into Sacrococcygeal Joint, Open Approach

0SH508Z Insertion of Spacer into Sacrococcygeal Joint, Open Approach

0SH533Z Insertion of Infusion Device into Sacrococcygeal Joint, Percutaneous Approach

0SH534Z Insertion of Internal Fixation Device into Sacrococcygeal Joint, Percutaneous Approach

0SH538Z Insertion of Spacer into Sacrococcygeal Joint, Percutaneous Approach

0SH543Z Insertion of Infusion Device into Sacrococcygeal Joint, Percutaneous Endoscopic Approach

0SH544Z Insertion of Internal Fixation Device into Sacrococcygeal Joint, Percutaneous Endoscopic Approach

0SH548Z Insertion of Spacer into Sacrococcygeal Joint, Percutaneous Endoscopic Approach

0SH603Z Insertion of Infusion Device into Coccygeal Joint, Open Approach

0SH604Z Insertion of Internal Fixation Device into Coccygeal Joint, Open Approach

0SH608Z Insertion of Spacer into Coccygeal Joint, Open Approach

0SH633Z Insertion of Infusion Device into Coccygeal Joint, Percutaneous Approach

0SH634Z Insertion of Internal Fixation Device into Coccygeal Joint, Percutaneous Approach

0SH638Z Insertion of Spacer into Coccygeal Joint, Percutaneous Approach

0SH643Z Insertion of Infusion Device into Coccygeal Joint, Percutaneous Endoscopic Approach

0SH644Z Insertion of Internal Fixation Device into Coccygeal Joint, Percutaneous Endoscopic Approach

0SH648Z Insertion of Spacer into Coccygeal Joint, Percutaneous Endoscopic Approach

0SH703Z Insertion of Infusion Device into Right Sacroiliac Joint, Open Approach

0SH704Z Insertion of Internal Fixation Device into Right Sacroiliac Joint, Open Approach

0SH708Z Insertion of Spacer into Right Sacroiliac Joint, Open Approach

0SH733Z Insertion of Infusion Device into Right Sacroiliac Joint, Percutaneous Approach

0SH734Z Insertion of Internal Fixation Device into Right Sacroiliac Joint, Percutaneous Approach

0SH738Z Insertion of Spacer into Right Sacroiliac Joint, Percutaneous Approach

0SH743Z Insertion of Infusion Device into Right Sacroiliac Joint, Percutaneous Endoscopic Approach

0SH744Z Insertion of Internal Fixation Device into Right Sacroiliac Joint, Percutaneous Endoscopic Approach

0SH748Z Insertion of Spacer into Right Sacroiliac Joint, Percutaneous Endoscopic Approach

0SH803Z Insertion of Infusion Device into Left Sacroiliac Joint, Open Approach

0SH804Z Insertion of Internal Fixation Device into Left Sacroiliac Joint, Open Approach

0SH808Z Insertion of Spacer into Left Sacroiliac Joint, Open Approach

0SH833Z Insertion of Infusion Device into Left Sacroiliac Joint, Percutaneous Approach

0SH834Z Insertion of Internal Fixation Device into Left Sacroiliac Joint, Percutaneous Approach

0SH838Z Insertion of Spacer into Left Sacroiliac Joint, Percutaneous Approach

0SH843Z Insertion of Infusion Device into Left Sacroiliac Joint, Percutaneous Endoscopic Approach

0SH844Z Insertion of Internal Fixation Device into Left Sacroiliac Joint, Percutaneous Endoscopic Approach

0SH848Z Insertion of Spacer into Left Sacroiliac Joint, Percutaneous Endoscopic Approach

0SH903Z Insertion of Infusion Device into Right Hip Joint, Open Approach

0SH904Z Insertion of Internal Fixation Device into Right Hip Joint, Open Approach

0SH905Z Insertion of External Fixation Device into Right Hip Joint, Open Approach

0SH908Z Insertion of Spacer into Right Hip Joint, Open Approach

0SH933Z Insertion of Infusion Device into Right Hip Joint, Percutaneous Approach

0SH934Z Insertion of Internal Fixation Device into Right Hip Joint, Percutaneous Approach

0SH935Z Insertion of External Fixation Device into Right Hip Joint, Percutaneous Approach

0SH938Z Insertion of Spacer into Right Hip Joint, Percutaneous Approach

0SH943Z Insertion of Infusion Device into Right Hip Joint, Percutaneous Endoscopic Approach

0SH944Z Insertion of Internal Fixation Device into Right Hip Joint, Percutaneous Endoscopic Approach

0SH945Z Insertion of External Fixation Device into Right Hip Joint, Percutaneous Endoscopic Approach

0SH948Z Insertion of Spacer into Right Hip Joint, Percutaneous Endoscopic Approach

0SHB03Z Insertion of Infusion Device into Left Hip Joint, Open Approach

0SHB04Z Insertion of Internal Fixation Device into Left Hip Joint, Open Approach

0SHB05Z Insertion of External Fixation Device into Left Hip Joint, Open Approach

0SHB08Z Insertion of Spacer into Left Hip Joint, Open Approach

0SHB33Z Insertion of Infusion Device into Left Hip Joint, Percutaneous Approach

0SHB34Z Insertion of Internal Fixation Device into Left Hip Joint, Percutaneous Approach

0SHB35Z Insertion of External Fixation Device into Left Hip Joint, Percutaneous Approach

0SHB38Z Insertion of Spacer into Left Hip Joint, Percutaneous Approach

0SHB43Z Insertion of Infusion Device into Left Hip Joint, Percutaneous Endoscopic Approach

---

♀ Female-only   ♂ Male-only   ● Limited Coverage   ● Non-OR   🅷🅰🅲 HAC-associated procedure   ● Non-covered procedures   ➕ Combination

0SHB44Z Insertion of Internal Fixation Device into Left Hip Joint, Percutaneous Endoscopic Approach

0SHB45Z Insertion of External Fixation Device into Left Hip Joint, Percutaneous Endoscopic Approach

0SHB48Z Insertion of Spacer into Left Hip Joint, Percutaneous Endoscopic Approach

0SHC03Z Insertion of Infusion Device into Right Knee Joint, Open Approach

0SHC04Z Insertion of Internal Fixation Device into Right Knee Joint, Open Approach

0SHC05Z Insertion of External Fixation Device into Right Knee Joint, Open Approach

0SHC08Z Insertion of Spacer into Right Knee Joint, Open Approach

0SHC33Z Insertion of Infusion Device into Right Knee Joint, Percutaneous Approach

0SHC34Z Insertion of Internal Fixation Device into Right Knee Joint, Percutaneous Approach

0SHC35Z Insertion of External Fixation Device into Right Knee Joint, Percutaneous Approach

0SHC38Z Insertion of Spacer into Right Knee Joint, Percutaneous Approach

0SHC43Z Insertion of Infusion Device into Right Knee Joint, Percutaneous Endoscopic Approach

0SHC44Z Insertion of Internal Fixation Device into Right Knee Joint, Percutaneous Endoscopic Approach

0SHC45Z Insertion of External Fixation Device into Right Knee Joint, Percutaneous Endoscopic Approach

0SHC48Z Insertion of Spacer into Right Knee Joint, Percutaneous Endoscopic Approach

0SHD03Z Insertion of Infusion Device into Left Knee Joint, Open Approach

0SHD04Z Insertion of Internal Fixation Device into Left Knee Joint, Open Approach

0SHD05Z Insertion of External Fixation Device into Left Knee Joint, Open Approach

0SHD08Z Insertion of Spacer into Left Knee Joint, Open Approach

0SHD33Z Insertion of Infusion Device into Left Knee Joint, Percutaneous Approach

0SHD34Z Insertion of Internal Fixation Device into Left Knee Joint, Percutaneous Approach

0SHD35Z Insertion of External Fixation Device into Left Knee Joint, Percutaneous Approach

0SHD38Z Insertion of Spacer into Left Knee Joint, Percutaneous Approach

0SHD43Z Insertion of Infusion Device into Left Knee Joint, Percutaneous Endoscopic Approach

0SHD44Z Insertion of Internal Fixation Device into Left Knee Joint, Percutaneous Endoscopic Approach

0SHD45Z Insertion of External Fixation Device into Left Knee Joint, Percutaneous Endoscopic Approach

0SHD48Z Insertion of Spacer into Left Knee Joint, Percutaneous Endoscopic Approach

0SHF03Z Insertion of Infusion Device into Right Ankle Joint, Open Approach

0SHF04Z Insertion of Internal Fixation Device into Right Ankle Joint, Open Approach

0SHF05Z Insertion of External Fixation Device into Right Ankle Joint, Open Approach

0SHF08Z Insertion of Spacer into Right Ankle Joint, Open Approach

0SHF33Z Insertion of Infusion Device into Right Ankle Joint, Percutaneous Approach

0SHF34Z Insertion of Internal Fixation Device into Right Ankle Joint, Percutaneous Approach

0SHF35Z Insertion of External Fixation Device into Right Ankle Joint, Percutaneous Approach

0SHF38Z Insertion of Spacer into Right Ankle Joint, Percutaneous Approach

0SHF43Z Insertion of Infusion Device into Right Ankle Joint, Percutaneous Endoscopic Approach

0SHF44Z Insertion of Internal Fixation Device into Right Ankle Joint, Percutaneous Endoscopic Approach

0SHF45Z Insertion of External Fixation Device into Right Ankle Joint, Percutaneous Endoscopic Approach

0SHF48Z Insertion of Spacer into Right Ankle Joint, Percutaneous Endoscopic Approach

0SHG03Z Insertion of Infusion Device into Left Ankle Joint, Open Approach

0SHG04Z Insertion of Internal Fixation Device into Left Ankle Joint, Open Approach

0SHG05Z Insertion of External Fixation Device into Left Ankle Joint, Open Approach

0SHG08Z Insertion of Spacer into Left Ankle Joint, Open Approach

0SHG33Z Insertion of Infusion Device into Left Ankle Joint, Percutaneous Approach

0SHG34Z Insertion of Internal Fixation Device into Left Ankle Joint, Percutaneous Approach

0SHG35Z Insertion of External Fixation Device into Left Ankle Joint, Percutaneous Approach

0SHG38Z Insertion of Spacer into Left Ankle Joint, Percutaneous Approach

0SHG43Z Insertion of Infusion Device into Left Ankle Joint, Percutaneous Endoscopic Approach

0SHG44Z Insertion of Internal Fixation Device into Left Ankle Joint, Percutaneous Endoscopic Approach

0SHG45Z Insertion of External Fixation Device into Left Ankle Joint, Percutaneous Endoscopic Approach

0SHG48Z Insertion of Spacer into Left Ankle Joint, Percutaneous Endoscopic Approach

0SHH03Z Insertion of Infusion Device into Right Tarsal Joint, Open Approach

0SHH04Z Insertion of Internal Fixation Device into Right Tarsal Joint, Open Approach

0SHH05Z Insertion of External Fixation Device into Right Tarsal Joint, Open Approach

0SHH08Z Insertion of Spacer into Right Tarsal Joint, Open Approach

0SHH33Z Insertion of Infusion Device into Right Tarsal Joint, Percutaneous Approach

0SHH34Z Insertion of Internal Fixation Device into Right Tarsal Joint, Percutaneous Approach

0SHH35Z Insertion of External Fixation Device into Right Tarsal Joint, Percutaneous Approach

0SHH38Z Insertion of Spacer into Right Tarsal Joint, Percutaneous Approach

0SHH43Z Insertion of Infusion Device into Right Tarsal Joint, Percutaneous Endoscopic Approach

0SHH44Z Insertion of Internal Fixation Device into Right Tarsal Joint, Percutaneous Endoscopic Approach

0SHH45Z Insertion of External Fixation Device into Right Tarsal Joint, Percutaneous Endoscopic Approach

0SHH48Z Insertion of Spacer into Right Tarsal Joint, Percutaneous Endoscopic Approach

0SHJ03Z Insertion of Infusion Device into Left Tarsal Joint, Open Approach

0SHJ04Z Insertion of Internal Fixation Device into Left Tarsal Joint, Open Approach

0SHJ05Z Insertion of External Fixation Device into Left Tarsal Joint, Open Approach

0SHJ08Z Insertion of Spacer into Left Tarsal Joint, Open Approach

0SHJ33Z Insertion of Infusion Device into Left Tarsal Joint, Percutaneous Approach

0SHJ34Z Insertion of Internal Fixation Device into Left Tarsal Joint, Percutaneous Approach

0SHJ35Z Insertion of External Fixation Device into Left Tarsal Joint, Percutaneous Approach

0SHJ38Z Insertion of Spacer into Left Tarsal Joint, Percutaneous Approach

0SHJ43Z Insertion of Infusion Device into Left Tarsal Joint, Percutaneous Endoscopic Approach

0SHJ44Z Insertion of Internal Fixation Device into Left Tarsal Joint, Percutaneous Endoscopic Approach

0SHJ45Z Insertion of External Fixation Device into Left Tarsal Joint, Percutaneous Endoscopic Approach

0SHJ48Z Insertion of Spacer into Left Tarsal Joint, Percutaneous Endoscopic Approach

0SHK03Z Insertion of Infusion Device into Right Metatarsal-Tarsal Joint, Open Approach

0SHK04Z Insertion of Internal Fixation Device into Right Metatarsal-Tarsal Joint, Open Approach

0SHK05Z Insertion of External Fixation Device into Right Metatarsal-Tarsal Joint, Open Approach

0SHK08Z Insertion of Spacer into Right Metatarsal-Tarsal Joint, Open Approach

0SHK33Z Insertion of Infusion Device into Right Metatarsal-Tarsal Joint, Percutaneous Approach

0SHK34Z Insertion of Internal Fixation Device into Right Metatarsal-Tarsal Joint, Percutaneous Approach

0SHK35Z Insertion of External Fixation Device into Right Metatarsal-Tarsal Joint, Percutaneous Approach

0SHK38Z Insertion of Spacer into Right Metatarsal-Tarsal Joint, Percutaneous Approach

0SHK43Z Insertion of Infusion Device into Right Metatarsal-Tarsal Joint, Percutaneous Endoscopic Approach

0SHK44Z Insertion of Internal Fixation Device into Right Metatarsal-Tarsal Joint, Percutaneous Endoscopic Approach

0SHK45Z Insertion of External Fixation Device into Right Metatarsal-Tarsal Joint, Percutaneous Endoscopic Approach

0SHK48Z Insertion of Spacer into Right Metatarsal-Tarsal Joint, Percutaneous Endoscopic Approach

0SHL03Z Insertion of Infusion Device into Left Metatarsal-Tarsal Joint, Open Approach

0SHL04Z Insertion of Internal Fixation Device into Left Metatarsal-Tarsal Joint, Open Approach

0SHL05Z Insertion of External Fixation Device into Left Metatarsal-Tarsal Joint, Open Approach

0SHL08Z Insertion of Spacer into Left Metatarsal-Tarsal Joint, Open Approach

0SHL33Z Insertion of Infusion Device into Left Metatarsal-Tarsal Joint, Percutaneous Approach

0SHL34Z Insertion of Internal Fixation Device into Left Metatarsal-Tarsal Joint, Percutaneous Approach

0SHL35Z Insertion of External Fixation Device into Left Metatarsal-Tarsal Joint, Percutaneous Approach

0SHL38Z Insertion of Spacer into Left Metatarsal-Tarsal Joint, Percutaneous Approach

0SHL43Z Insertion of Infusion Device into Left Metatarsal-Tarsal Joint, Percutaneous Endoscopic Approach

0SHL44Z Insertion of Internal Fixation Device into Left Metatarsal-Tarsal Joint, Percutaneous Endoscopic Approach

0SHL45Z Insertion of External Fixation Device into Left Metatarsal-Tarsal Joint, Percutaneous Endoscopic Approach

0SHL48Z Insertion of Spacer into Left Metatarsal-Tarsal Joint, Percutaneous Endoscopic Approach

0SHM03Z Insertion of Infusion Device into Right Metatarsal-Phalangeal Joint, Open Approach

0SHM04Z Insertion of Internal Fixation Device into Right Metatarsal-Phalangeal Joint, Open Approach

0SHM05Z Insertion of External Fixation Device into Right Metatarsal-Phalangeal Joint, Open Approach

0SHM08Z Insertion of Spacer into Right Metatarsal-Phalangeal Joint, Open Approach

0SHM33Z Insertion of Infusion Device into Right Metatarsal-Phalangeal Joint, Percutaneous Approach

0SHM34Z Insertion of Internal Fixation Device into Right Metatarsal-Phalangeal Joint, Percutaneous Approach

0SHM35Z Insertion of External Fixation Device into Right Metatarsal-Phalangeal Joint, Percutaneous Approach

0SHM38Z Insertion of Spacer into Right Metatarsal-Phalangeal Joint, Percutaneous Approach

0SHM43Z Insertion of Infusion Device into Right Metatarsal-Phalangeal Joint, Percutaneous Endoscopic Approach

0SHM44Z Insertion of Internal Fixation Device into Right Metatarsal-Phalangeal Joint, Percutaneous Endoscopic Approach

0SHM45Z Insertion of External Fixation Device into Right Metatarsal-Phalangeal Joint, Percutaneous Endoscopic Approach

0SHM48Z Insertion of Spacer into Right Metatarsal-Phalangeal Joint, Percutaneous Endoscopic Approach

0SHN03Z Insertion of Infusion Device into Left Metatarsal-Phalangeal Joint, Open Approach

0SHN04Z Insertion of Internal Fixation Device into Left Metatarsal-Phalangeal Joint, Open Approach

0SHN05Z Insertion of External Fixation Device into Left Metatarsal-Phalangeal Joint, Open Approach

0SHN08Z Insertion of Spacer into Left Metatarsal-Phalangeal Joint, Open Approach

0SHN33Z Insertion of Infusion Device into Left Metatarsal-Phalangeal Joint, Percutaneous Approach

0SHN34Z Insertion of Internal Fixation Device into Left Metatarsal-Phalangeal Joint, Percutaneous Approach

0SHN35Z Insertion of External Fixation Device into Left Metatarsal-Phalangeal Joint, Percutaneous Approach

0SHN38Z Insertion of Spacer into Left Metatarsal-Phalangeal Joint, Percutaneous Approach

0SHN43Z Insertion of Infusion Device into Left Metatarsal-Phalangeal Joint, Percutaneous Endoscopic Approach

0SHN44Z Insertion of Internal Fixation Device into Left Metatarsal-Phalangeal Joint, Percutaneous Endoscopic Approach

0SHN45Z Insertion of External Fixation Device into Left Metatarsal-Phalangeal Joint, Percutaneous Endoscopic Approach

0SHN48Z Insertion of Spacer into Left Metatarsal-Phalangeal Joint, Percutaneous Endoscopic Approach

0SHP03Z Insertion of Infusion Device into Right Toe Phalangeal Joint, Open Approach

0SHP04Z Insertion of Internal Fixation Device into Right Toe Phalangeal Joint, Open Approach

0SHP05Z Insertion of External Fixation Device into Right Toe Phalangeal Joint, Open Approach

0SHP08Z Insertion of Spacer into Right Toe Phalangeal Joint, Open Approach

0SHP33Z Insertion of Infusion Device into Right Toe Phalangeal Joint, Percutaneous Approach

0SHP34Z Insertion of Internal Fixation Device into Right Toe Phalangeal Joint, Percutaneous Approach

0SHP35Z Insertion of External Fixation Device into Right Toe Phalangeal Joint, Percutaneous Approach

0SHP38Z Insertion of Spacer into Right Toe Phalangeal Joint, Percutaneous Approach

0SHP43Z Insertion of Infusion Device into Right Toe Phalangeal Joint, Percutaneous Endoscopic Approach

0SHP44Z Insertion of Internal Fixation Device into Right Toe Phalangeal Joint, Percutaneous Endoscopic Approach

0SHP45Z Insertion of External Fixation Device into Right Toe Phalangeal Joint, Percutaneous Endoscopic Approach

0SHP48Z Insertion of Spacer into Right Toe Phalangeal Joint, Percutaneous Endoscopic Approach

0SHQ03Z Insertion of Infusion Device into Left Toe Phalangeal Joint, Open Approach

0SHQ04Z Insertion of Internal Fixation Device into Left Toe Phalangeal Joint, Open Approach

0SHQ05Z Insertion of External Fixation Device into Left Toe Phalangeal Joint, Open Approach

0SHQ08Z Insertion of Spacer into Left Toe Phalangeal Joint, Open Approach

0SHQ33Z Insertion of Infusion Device into Left Toe Phalangeal Joint, Percutaneous Approach

0SHQ34Z Insertion of Internal Fixation Device into Left Toe Phalangeal Joint, Percutaneous Approach

0SHQ35Z Insertion of External Fixation Device into Left Toe Phalangeal Joint, Percutaneous Approach

0SHQ38Z Insertion of Spacer into Left Toe Phalangeal Joint, Percutaneous Approach

0SHQ43Z Insertion of Infusion Device into Left Toe Phalangeal Joint, Percutaneous Endoscopic Approach

0SHQ44Z Insertion of Internal Fixation Device into Left Toe Phalangeal Joint, Percutaneous Endoscopic Approach

0SHQ45Z Insertion of External Fixation Device into Left Toe Phalangeal Joint, Percutaneous Endoscopic Approach

0SHQ48Z Insertion of Spacer into Left Toe Phalangeal Joint, Percutaneous Endoscopic Approach

0SJ – Lower Joints, Inspection

Review Coding Guideline B3.5

Review Coding Guidelines B3.11a, B3.11b and B3.11c

0SJ00ZZ Inspection of Lumbar Vertebral Joint, Open Approach
0SJ03ZZ Inspection of Lumbar Vertebral Joint, Percutaneous Approach
0SJ04ZZ Inspection of Lumbar Vertebral Joint, Percutaneous Endoscopic Approach

0SJ0XZZ Inspection of Lumbar Vertebral Joint, External Approach
0SJ20ZZ Inspection of Lumbar Vertebral Disc, Open Approach
0SJ23ZZ Inspection of Lumbar Vertebral Disc, Percutaneous Approach

0SJ24ZZ	Inspection of Lumbar Vertebral Disc, Percutaneous Endoscopic Approach
0SJ2XZZ	Inspection of Lumbar Vertebral Disc, External Approach
0SJ30ZZ	Inspection of Lumbosacral Joint, Open Approach
0SJ33ZZ	Inspection of Lumbosacral Joint, Percutaneous Approach
0SJ34ZZ	Inspection of Lumbosacral Joint, Percutaneous Endoscopic Approach
0SJ3XZZ	Inspection of Lumbosacral Joint, External Approach
0SJ40ZZ	Inspection of Lumbosacral Disc, Open Approach
0SJ43ZZ	Inspection of Lumbosacral Disc, Percutaneous Approach
0SJ44ZZ	Inspection of Lumbosacral Disc, Percutaneous Endoscopic Approach
0SJ4XZZ	Inspection of Lumbosacral Disc, External Approach
0SJ50ZZ	Inspection of Sacrococcygeal Joint, Open Approach
0SJ53ZZ	Inspection of Sacrococcygeal Joint, Percutaneous Approach
0SJ54ZZ	Inspection of Sacrococcygeal Joint, Percutaneous Endoscopic Approach
0SJ5XZZ	Inspection of Sacrococcygeal Joint, External Approach
0SJ60ZZ	Inspection of Coccygeal Joint, Open Approach
0SJ63ZZ	Inspection of Coccygeal Joint, Percutaneous Approach
0SJ64ZZ	Inspection of Coccygeal Joint, Percutaneous Endoscopic Approach
0SJ6XZZ	Inspection of Coccygeal Joint, External Approach
0SJ70ZZ	Inspection of Right Sacroiliac Joint, Open Approach
0SJ73ZZ	Inspection of Right Sacroiliac Joint, Percutaneous Approach
0SJ74ZZ	Inspection of Right Sacroiliac Joint, Percutaneous Endoscopic Approach
0SJ7XZZ	Inspection of Right Sacroiliac Joint, External Approach
0SJ80ZZ	Inspection of Left Sacroiliac Joint, Open Approach
0SJ83ZZ	Inspection of Left Sacroiliac Joint, Percutaneous Approach
0SJ84ZZ	Inspection of Left Sacroiliac Joint, Percutaneous Endoscopic Approach
0SJ8XZZ	Inspection of Left Sacroiliac Joint, External Approach
0SJ90ZZ	Inspection of Right Hip Joint, Open Approach
0SJ93ZZ	Inspection of Right Hip Joint, Percutaneous Approach
0SJ94ZZ	Inspection of Right Hip Joint, Percutaneous Endoscopic Approach
0SJ9XZZ	Inspection of Right Hip Joint, External Approach
0SJB0ZZ	Inspection of Left Hip Joint, Open Approach
0SJB3ZZ	Inspection of Left Hip Joint, Percutaneous Approach
0SJB4ZZ	Inspection of Left Hip Joint, Percutaneous Endoscopic Approach
0SJBXZZ	Inspection of Left Hip Joint, External Approach
0SJC0ZZ	Inspection of Right Knee Joint, Open Approach
0SJC3ZZ	Inspection of Right Knee Joint, Percutaneous Approach
0SJC4ZZ	Inspection of Right Knee Joint, Percutaneous Endoscopic Approach
0SJCXZZ	Inspection of Right Knee Joint, External Approach
0SJD0ZZ	Inspection of Left Knee Joint, Open Approach
0SJD3ZZ	Inspection of Left Knee Joint, Percutaneous Approach
0SJD4ZZ	Inspection of Left Knee Joint, Percutaneous Endoscopic Approach
0SJDXZZ	Inspection of Left Knee Joint, External Approach
0SJF0ZZ	Inspection of Right Ankle Joint, Open Approach
0SJF3ZZ	Inspection of Right Ankle Joint, Percutaneous Approach
0SJF4ZZ	Inspection of Right Ankle Joint, Percutaneous Endoscopic Approach
0SJFXZZ	Inspection of Right Ankle Joint, External Approach
0SJG0ZZ	Inspection of Left Ankle Joint, Open Approach
0SJG3ZZ	Inspection of Left Ankle Joint, Percutaneous Approach
0SJG4ZZ	Inspection of Left Ankle Joint, Percutaneous Endoscopic Approach
0SJGXZZ	Inspection of Left Ankle Joint, External Approach
0SJH0ZZ	Inspection of Right Tarsal Joint, Open Approach
0SJH3ZZ	Inspection of Right Tarsal Joint, Percutaneous Approach
0SJH4ZZ	Inspection of Right Tarsal Joint, Percutaneous Endoscopic Approach
0SJHXZZ	Inspection of Right Tarsal Joint, External Approach
0SJJ0ZZ	Inspection of Left Tarsal Joint, Open Approach
0SJJ3ZZ	Inspection of Left Tarsal Joint, Percutaneous Approach
0SJJ4ZZ	Inspection of Left Tarsal Joint, Percutaneous Endoscopic Approach
0SJJXZZ	Inspection of Left Tarsal Joint, External Approach
0SJK0ZZ	Inspection of Right Metatarsal-Tarsal Joint, Open Approach
0SJK3ZZ	Inspection of Right Metatarsal-Tarsal Joint, Percutaneous Approach
0SJK4ZZ	Inspection of Right Metatarsal-Tarsal Joint, Percutaneous Endoscopic Approach
0SJKXZZ	Inspection of Right Metatarsal-Tarsal Joint, External Approach
0SJL0ZZ	Inspection of Left Metatarsal-Tarsal Joint, Open Approach
0SJL3ZZ	Inspection of Left Metatarsal-Tarsal Joint, Percutaneous Approach
0SJL4ZZ	Inspection of Left Metatarsal-Tarsal Joint, Percutaneous Endoscopic Approach
0SJLXZZ	Inspection of Left Metatarsal-Tarsal Joint, External Approach
0SJM0ZZ	Inspection of Right Metatarsal-Phalangeal Joint, Open Approach
0SJM3ZZ	Inspection of Right Metatarsal-Phalangeal Joint, Percutaneous Approach
0SJM4ZZ	Inspection of Right Metatarsal-Phalangeal Joint, Percutaneous Endoscopic Approach
0SJMXZZ	Inspection of Right Metatarsal-Phalangeal Joint, External Approach
0SJN0ZZ	Inspection of Left Metatarsal-Phalangeal Joint, Open Approach
0SJN3ZZ	Inspection of Left Metatarsal-Phalangeal Joint, Percutaneous Approach
0SJN4ZZ	Inspection of Left Metatarsal-Phalangeal Joint, Percutaneous Endoscopic Approach
0SJNXZZ	Inspection of Left Metatarsal-Phalangeal Joint, External Approach
0SJP0ZZ	Inspection of Right Toe Phalangeal Joint, Open Approach
0SJP3ZZ	Inspection of Right Toe Phalangeal Joint, Percutaneous Approach
0SJP4ZZ	Inspection of Right Toe Phalangeal Joint, Percutaneous Endoscopic Approach
0SJPXZZ	Inspection of Right Toe Phalangeal Joint, External Approach
0SJQ0ZZ	Inspection of Left Toe Phalangeal Joint, Open Approach
0SJQ3ZZ	Inspection of Left Toe Phalangeal Joint, Percutaneous Approach
0SJQ4ZZ	Inspection of Left Toe Phalangeal Joint, Percutaneous Endoscopic Approach
0SJQXZZ	Inspection of Left Toe Phalangeal Joint, External Approach

0SN – Lower Joints, Release

Review Coding Guideline B3.13

0SN00ZZ	Release Lumbar Vertebral Joint, Open Approach
0SN03ZZ	Release Lumbar Vertebral Joint, Percutaneous Approach
0SN04ZZ	Release Lumbar Vertebral Joint, Percutaneous Endoscopic Approach
0SN0XZZ	Release Lumbar Vertebral Joint, External Approach
0SN20ZZ	Release Lumbar Vertebral Disc, Open Approach
0SN23ZZ	Release Lumbar Vertebral Disc, Percutaneous Approach
0SN24ZZ	Release Lumbar Vertebral Disc, Percutaneous Endoscopic Approach
0SN2XZZ	Release Lumbar Vertebral Disc, External Approach
0SN30ZZ	Release Lumbosacral Joint, Open Approach
0SN33ZZ	Release Lumbosacral Joint, Percutaneous Approach
0SN34ZZ	Release Lumbosacral Joint, Percutaneous Endoscopic Approach
0SN3XZZ	Release Lumbosacral Joint, External Approach
0SN40ZZ	Release Lumbosacral Disc, Open Approach
0SN43ZZ	Release Lumbosacral Disc, Percutaneous Approach
0SN44ZZ	Release Lumbosacral Disc, Percutaneous Endoscopic Approach
0SN4XZZ	Release Lumbosacral Disc, External Approach
0SN50ZZ	Release Sacrococcygeal Joint, Open Approach
0SN53ZZ	Release Sacrococcygeal Joint, Percutaneous Approach
0SN54ZZ	Release Sacrococcygeal Joint, Percutaneous Endoscopic Approach
0SN5XZZ	Release Sacrococcygeal Joint, External Approach
0SN60ZZ	Release Coccygeal Joint, Open Approach
0SN63ZZ	Release Coccygeal Joint, Percutaneous Approach
0SN64ZZ	Release Coccygeal Joint, Percutaneous Endoscopic Approach
0SN6XZZ	Release Coccygeal Joint, External Approach
0SN70ZZ	Release Right Sacroiliac Joint, Open Approach
0SN73ZZ	Release Right Sacroiliac Joint, Percutaneous Approach
0SN74ZZ	Release Right Sacroiliac Joint, Percutaneous Endoscopic Approach
0SN7XZZ	Release Right Sacroiliac Joint, External Approach
0SN80ZZ	Release Left Sacroiliac Joint, Open Approach
0SN83ZZ	Release Left Sacroiliac Joint, Percutaneous Approach
0SN84ZZ	Release Left Sacroiliac Joint, Percutaneous Endoscopic Approach
0SN8XZZ	Release Left Sacroiliac Joint, External Approach
0SN90ZZ	Release Right Hip Joint, Open Approach
0SN93ZZ	Release Right Hip Joint, Percutaneous Approach
0SN94ZZ	Release Right Hip Joint, Percutaneous Endoscopic Approach
0SN9XZZ	Release Right Hip Joint, External Approach
0SNB0ZZ	Release Left Hip Joint, Open Approach
0SNB3ZZ	Release Left Hip Joint, Percutaneous Approach
0SNB4ZZ	Release Left Hip Joint, Percutaneous Endoscopic Approach
0SNBXZZ	Release Left Hip Joint, External Approach
0SNC0ZZ	Release Right Knee Joint, Open Approach
0SNC3ZZ	Release Right Knee Joint, Percutaneous Approach
0SNC4ZZ	Release Right Knee Joint, Percutaneous Endoscopic Approach

0SNCXZZ Release Right Knee Joint, External Approach
0SND0ZZ Release Left Knee Joint, Open Approach
0SND3ZZ Release Left Knee Joint, Percutaneous Approach
0SND4ZZ Release Left Knee Joint, Percutaneous Endoscopic Approach
0SNDXZZ Release Left Knee Joint, External Approach
0SNF0ZZ Release Right Ankle Joint, Open Approach
0SNF3ZZ Release Right Ankle Joint, Percutaneous Approach
0SNF4ZZ Release Right Ankle Joint, Percutaneous Endoscopic Approach
0SNFXZZ Release Right Ankle Joint, External Approach
0SNG0ZZ Release Left Ankle Joint, Open Approach
0SNG3ZZ Release Left Ankle Joint, Percutaneous Approach
0SNG4ZZ Release Left Ankle Joint, Percutaneous Endoscopic Approach
0SNGXZZ Release Left Ankle Joint, External Approach
0SNH0ZZ Release Right Tarsal Joint, Open Approach
0SNH3ZZ Release Right Tarsal Joint, Percutaneous Approach
0SNH4ZZ Release Right Tarsal Joint, Percutaneous Endoscopic Approach
0SNHXZZ Release Right Tarsal Joint, External Approach
0SNJ0ZZ Release Left Tarsal Joint, Open Approach
0SNJ3ZZ Release Left Tarsal Joint, Percutaneous Approach
0SNJ4ZZ Release Left Tarsal Joint, Percutaneous Endoscopic Approach
0SNJXZZ Release Left Tarsal Joint, External Approach
0SNK0ZZ Release Right Metatarsal-Tarsal Joint, Open Approach
0SNK3ZZ Release Right Metatarsal-Tarsal Joint, Percutaneous Approach
0SNK4ZZ Release Right Metatarsal-Tarsal Joint, Percutaneous Endoscopic Approach

0SNKXZZ Release Right Metatarsal-Tarsal Joint, External Approach
0SNL0ZZ Release Left Metatarsal-Tarsal Joint, Open Approach
0SNL3ZZ Release Left Metatarsal-Tarsal Joint, Percutaneous Approach
0SNL4ZZ Release Left Metatarsal-Tarsal Joint, Percutaneous Endoscopic Approach
0SNLXZZ Release Left Metatarsal-Tarsal Joint, External Approach
0SNM0ZZ Release Right Metatarsal-Phalangeal Joint, Open Approach
0SNM3ZZ Release Right Metatarsal-Phalangeal Joint, Percutaneous Approach
0SNM4ZZ Release Right Metatarsal-Phalangeal Joint, Percutaneous Endoscopic Approach
0SNMXZZ Release Right Metatarsal-Phalangeal Joint, External Approach
0SNN0ZZ Release Left Metatarsal-Phalangeal Joint, Open Approach
0SNN3ZZ Release Left Metatarsal-Phalangeal Joint, Percutaneous Approach
0SNN4ZZ Release Left Metatarsal-Phalangeal Joint, Percutaneous Endoscopic Approach
0SNNXZZ Release Left Metatarsal-Phalangeal Joint, External Approach
0SNP0ZZ Release Right Toe Phalangeal Joint, Open Approach
0SNP3ZZ Release Right Toe Phalangeal Joint, Percutaneous Approach
0SNP4ZZ Release Right Toe Phalangeal Joint, Percutaneous Endoscopic Approach
0SNPXZZ Release Right Toe Phalangeal Joint, External Approach
0SNQ0ZZ Release Left Toe Phalangeal Joint, Open Approach
0SNQ3ZZ Release Left Toe Phalangeal Joint, Percutaneous Approach
0SNQ4ZZ Release Left Toe Phalangeal Joint, Percutaneous Endoscopic Approach
0SNQXZZ Release Left Toe Phalangeal Joint, External Approach

0SP – Lower Joints, Removal

Review Coding Guideline B6.1c

0SP000Z Removal of Drainage Device from Lumbar Vertebral Joint, Open Approach
0SP003Z Removal of Infusion Device from Lumbar Vertebral Joint, Open Approach
0SP004Z Removal of Internal Fixation Device from Lumbar Vertebral Joint, Open Approach
0SP007Z Removal of Autologous Tissue Substitute from Lumbar Vertebral Joint, Open Approach
0SP008Z Removal of Spacer from Lumbar Vertebral Joint, Open Approach
0SP00AZ Removal of Interbody Fusion Device from Lumbar Vertebral Joint, Open Approach
0SP00JZ Removal of Synthetic Substitute from Lumbar Vertebral Joint, Open Approach
0SP00KZ Removal of Nonautologous Tissue Substitute from Lumbar Vertebral Joint, Open Approach
0SP030Z Removal of Drainage Device from Lumbar Vertebral Joint, Percutaneous Approach
0SP033Z Removal of Infusion Device from Lumbar Vertebral Joint, Percutaneous Approach
0SP034Z Removal of Internal Fixation Device from Lumbar Vertebral Joint, Percutaneous Approach
0SP037Z Removal of Autologous Tissue Substitute from Lumbar Vertebral Joint, Percutaneous Approach
0SP038Z Removal of Spacer from Lumbar Vertebral Joint, Percutaneous Approach
0SP03AZ Removal of Interbody Fusion Device from Lumbar Vertebral Joint, Percutaneous Approach
0SP03JZ Removal of Synthetic Substitute from Lumbar Vertebral Joint, Percutaneous Approach
0SP03KZ Removal of Nonautologous Tissue Substitute from Lumbar Vertebral Joint, Percutaneous Approach
0SP040Z Removal of Drainage Device from Lumbar Vertebral Joint, Percutaneous Endoscopic Approach
0SP043Z Removal of Infusion Device from Lumbar Vertebral Joint, Percutaneous Endoscopic Approach
0SP044Z Removal of Internal Fixation Device from Lumbar Vertebral Joint, Percutaneous Endoscopic Approach
0SP047Z Removal of Autologous Tissue Substitute from Lumbar Vertebral Joint, Percutaneous Endoscopic Approach
0SP048Z Removal of Spacer from Lumbar Vertebral Joint, Percutaneous Endoscopic Approach
0SP04AZ Removal of Interbody Fusion Device from Lumbar Vertebral Joint, Percutaneous Endoscopic Approach
0SP04JZ Removal of Synthetic Substitute from Lumbar Vertebral Joint, Percutaneous Endoscopic Approach

0SP04KZ Removal of Nonautologous Tissue Substitute from Lumbar Vertebral Joint, Percutaneous Endoscopic Approach
0SP0X0Z Removal of Drainage Device from Lumbar Vertebral Joint, External Approach
0SP0X3Z Removal of Infusion Device from Lumbar Vertebral Joint, External Approach
0SP0X4Z Removal of Internal Fixation Device from Lumbar Vertebral Joint, External Approach
0SP200Z Removal of Drainage Device from Lumbar Vertebral Disc, Open Approach
0SP203Z Removal of Infusion Device from Lumbar Vertebral Disc, Open Approach
0SP207Z Removal of Autologous Tissue Substitute from Lumbar Vertebral Disc, Open Approach
0SP20JZ Removal of Synthetic Substitute from Lumbar Vertebral Disc, Open Approach
0SP20KZ Removal of Nonautologous Tissue Substitute from Lumbar Vertebral Disc, Open Approach
0SP230Z Removal of Drainage Device from Lumbar Vertebral Disc, Percutaneous Approach
0SP233Z Removal of Infusion Device from Lumbar Vertebral Disc, Percutaneous Approach
0SP237Z Removal of Autologous Tissue Substitute from Lumbar Vertebral Disc, Percutaneous Approach
0SP23JZ Removal of Synthetic Substitute from Lumbar Vertebral Disc, Percutaneous Approach
0SP23KZ Removal of Nonautologous Tissue Substitute from Lumbar Vertebral Disc, Percutaneous Approach
0SP240Z Removal of Drainage Device from Lumbar Vertebral Disc, Percutaneous Endoscopic Approach
0SP243Z Removal of Infusion Device from Lumbar Vertebral Disc, Percutaneous Endoscopic Approach
0SP247Z Removal of Autologous Tissue Substitute from Lumbar Vertebral Disc, Percutaneous Endoscopic Approach
0SP24JZ Removal of Synthetic Substitute from Lumbar Vertebral Disc, Percutaneous Endoscopic Approach
0SP24KZ Removal of Nonautologous Tissue Substitute from Lumbar Vertebral Disc, Percutaneous Endoscopic Approach
0SP2X0Z Removal of Drainage Device from Lumbar Vertebral Disc, External Approach
0SP2X3Z Removal of Infusion Device from Lumbar Vertebral Disc, External Approach
0SP300Z Removal of Drainage Device from Lumbosacral Joint, Open Approach
0SP303Z Removal of Infusion Device from Lumbosacral Joint, Open Approach

0SP304Z   Removal of Internal Fixation Device from Lumbosacral Joint, Open Approach

0SP307Z   Removal of Autologous Tissue Substitute from Lumbosacral Joint, Open Approach

0SP308Z   Removal of Spacer from Lumbosacral Joint, Open Approach

0SP30AZ   Removal of Interbody Fusion Device from Lumbosacral Joint, Open Approach

0SP30JZ   Removal of Synthetic Substitute from Lumbosacral Joint, Open Approach

0SP30KZ   Removal of Nonautologous Tissue Substitute from Lumbosacral Joint, Open Approach

0SP330Z   Removal of Drainage Device from Lumbosacral Joint, Percutaneous Approach

0SP333Z   Removal of Infusion Device from Lumbosacral Joint, Percutaneous Approach

0SP334Z   Removal of Internal Fixation Device from Lumbosacral Joint, Percutaneous Approach

0SP337Z   Removal of Autologous Tissue Substitute from Lumbosacral Joint, Percutaneous Approach

0SP338Z   Removal of Spacer from Lumbosacral Joint, Percutaneous Approach

0SP33AZ   Removal of Interbody Fusion Device from Lumbosacral Joint, Percutaneous Approach

0SP33JZ   Removal of Synthetic Substitute from Lumbosacral Joint, Percutaneous Approach

0SP33KZ   Removal of Nonautologous Tissue Substitute from Lumbosacral Joint, Percutaneous Approach

0SP340Z   Removal of Drainage Device from Lumbosacral Joint, Percutaneous Endoscopic Approach

0SP343Z   Removal of Infusion Device from Lumbosacral Joint, Percutaneous Endoscopic Approach

0SP344Z   Removal of Internal Fixation Device from Lumbosacral Joint, Percutaneous Endoscopic Approach

0SP347Z   Removal of Autologous Tissue Substitute from Lumbosacral Joint, Percutaneous Endoscopic Approach

0SP348Z   Removal of Spacer from Lumbosacral Joint, Percutaneous Endoscopic Approach

0SP34AZ   Removal of Interbody Fusion Device from Lumbosacral Joint, Percutaneous Endoscopic Approach

0SP34JZ   Removal of Synthetic Substitute from Lumbosacral Joint, Percutaneous Endoscopic Approach

0SP34KZ   Removal of Nonautologous Tissue Substitute from Lumbosacral Joint, Percutaneous Endoscopic Approach

0SP3X0Z   Removal of Drainage Device from Lumbosacral Joint, External Approach

0SP3X3Z   Removal of Infusion Device from Lumbosacral Joint, External Approach

0SP3X4Z   Removal of Internal Fixation Device from Lumbosacral Joint, External Approach

0SP400Z   Removal of Drainage Device from Lumbosacral Disc, Open Approach

0SP403Z   Removal of Infusion Device from Lumbosacral Disc, Open Approach

0SP407Z   Removal of Autologous Tissue Substitute from Lumbosacral Disc, Open Approach

0SP40JZ   Removal of Synthetic Substitute from Lumbosacral Disc, Open Approach

0SP40KZ   Removal of Nonautologous Tissue Substitute from Lumbosacral Disc, Open Approach

0SP430Z   Removal of Drainage Device from Lumbosacral Disc, Percutaneous Approach

0SP433Z   Removal of Infusion Device from Lumbosacral Disc, Percutaneous Approach

0SP437Z   Removal of Autologous Tissue Substitute from Lumbosacral Disc, Percutaneous Approach

0SP43JZ   Removal of Synthetic Substitute from Lumbosacral Disc, Percutaneous Approach

0SP43KZ   Removal of Nonautologous Tissue Substitute from Lumbosacral Disc, Percutaneous Approach

0SP440Z   Removal of Drainage Device from Lumbosacral Disc, Percutaneous Endoscopic Approach

0SP443Z   Removal of Infusion Device from Lumbosacral Disc, Percutaneous Endoscopic Approach

0SP447Z   Removal of Autologous Tissue Substitute from Lumbosacral Disc, Percutaneous Endoscopic Approach

0SP44JZ   Removal of Synthetic Substitute from Lumbosacral Disc, Percutaneous Endoscopic Approach

0SP44KZ   Removal of Nonautologous Tissue Substitute from Lumbosacral Disc, Percutaneous Endoscopic Approach

0SP4X0Z   Removal of Drainage Device from Lumbosacral Disc, External Approach

0SP4X3Z   Removal of Infusion Device from Lumbosacral Disc, External Approach

0SP500Z   Removal of Drainage Device from Sacrococcygeal Joint, Open Approach

0SP503Z   Removal of Infusion Device from Sacrococcygeal Joint, Open Approach

0SP504Z   Removal of Internal Fixation Device from Sacrococcygeal Joint, Open Approach

0SP507Z   Removal of Autologous Tissue Substitute from Sacrococcygeal Joint, Open Approach

0SP508Z   Removal of Spacer from Sacrococcygeal Joint, Open Approach

0SP50JZ   Removal of Synthetic Substitute from Sacrococcygeal Joint, Open Approach

0SP50KZ   Removal of Nonautologous Tissue Substitute from Sacrococcygeal Joint, Open Approach

0SP530Z   Removal of Drainage Device from Sacrococcygeal Joint, Percutaneous Approach

0SP533Z   Removal of Infusion Device from Sacrococcygeal Joint, Percutaneous Approach

0SP534Z   Removal of Internal Fixation Device from Sacrococcygeal Joint, Percutaneous Approach

0SP537Z   Removal of Autologous Tissue Substitute from Sacrococcygeal Joint, Percutaneous Approach

0SP538Z   Removal of Spacer from Sacrococcygeal Joint, Percutaneous Approach

0SP53JZ   Removal of Synthetic Substitute from Sacrococcygeal Joint, Percutaneous Approach

0SP53KZ   Removal of Nonautologous Tissue Substitute from Sacrococcygeal Joint, Percutaneous Approach

0SP540Z   Removal of Drainage Device from Sacrococcygeal Joint, Percutaneous Endoscopic Approach

0SP543Z   Removal of Infusion Device from Sacrococcygeal Joint, Percutaneous Endoscopic Approach

0SP544Z   Removal of Internal Fixation Device from Sacrococcygeal Joint, Percutaneous Endoscopic Approach

0SP547Z   Removal of Autologous Tissue Substitute from Sacrococcygeal Joint, Percutaneous Endoscopic Approach

0SP548Z   Removal of Spacer from Sacrococcygeal Joint, Percutaneous Endoscopic Approach

0SP54JZ   Removal of Synthetic Substitute from Sacrococcygeal Joint, Percutaneous Endoscopic Approach

0SP54KZ   Removal of Nonautologous Tissue Substitute from Sacrococcygeal Joint, Percutaneous Endoscopic Approach

0SP5X0Z   Removal of Drainage Device from Sacrococcygeal Joint, External Approach

0SP5X3Z   Removal of Infusion Device from Sacrococcygeal Joint, External Approach

0SP5X4Z   Removal of Internal Fixation Device from Sacrococcygeal Joint, External Approach

0SP600Z   Removal of Drainage Device from Coccygeal Joint, Open Approach

0SP603Z   Removal of Infusion Device from Coccygeal Joint, Open Approach

0SP604Z   Removal of Internal Fixation Device from Coccygeal Joint, Open Approach

0SP607Z   Removal of Autologous Tissue Substitute from Coccygeal Joint, Open Approach

0SP608Z   Removal of Spacer from Coccygeal Joint, Open Approach

0SP60JZ   Removal of Synthetic Substitute from Coccygeal Joint, Open Approach

0SP60KZ   Removal of Nonautologous Tissue Substitute from Coccygeal Joint, Open Approach

0SP630Z   Removal of Drainage Device from Coccygeal Joint, Percutaneous Approach

0SP633Z   Removal of Infusion Device from Coccygeal Joint, Percutaneous Approach

0SP634Z   Removal of Internal Fixation Device from Coccygeal Joint, Percutaneous Approach

0SP637Z   Removal of Autologous Tissue Substitute from Coccygeal Joint, Percutaneous Approach

---

♀ Female-only   ♂ Male-only   ◐ Limited Coverage   ● Non-OR   ▦ HAC-associated procedure   ⬤ Non-covered procedures   ⊞ Combination

0SP638Z Removal of Spacer from Coccygeal Joint, Percutaneous Approach

0SP63JZ Removal of Synthetic Substitute from Coccygeal Joint, Percutaneous Approach

0SP63KZ Removal of Nonautologous Tissue Substitute from Coccygeal Joint, Percutaneous Approach

0SP640Z Removal of Drainage Device from Coccygeal Joint, Percutaneous Endoscopic Approach

0SP643Z Removal of Infusion Device from Coccygeal Joint, Percutaneous Endoscopic Approach

0SP644Z Removal of Internal Fixation Device from Coccygeal Joint, Percutaneous Endoscopic Approach

0SP647Z Removal of Autologous Tissue Substitute from Coccygeal Joint, Percutaneous Endoscopic Approach

0SP648Z Removal of Spacer from Coccygeal Joint, Percutaneous Endoscopic Approach

0SP64JZ Removal of Synthetic Substitute from Coccygeal Joint, Percutaneous Endoscopic Approach

0SP64KZ Removal of Nonautologous Tissue Substitute from Coccygeal Joint, Percutaneous Endoscopic Approach

0SP6X0Z Removal of Drainage Device from Coccygeal Joint, External Approach

0SP6X3Z Removal of Infusion Device from Coccygeal Joint, External Approach

0SP6X4Z Removal of Internal Fixation Device from Coccygeal Joint, External Approach

0SP700Z Removal of Drainage Device from Right Sacroiliac Joint, Open Approach

0SP703Z Removal of Infusion Device from Right Sacroiliac Joint, Open Approach

0SP704Z Removal of Internal Fixation Device from Right Sacroiliac Joint, Open Approach

0SP707Z Removal of Autologous Tissue Substitute from Right Sacroiliac Joint, Open Approach

0SP708Z Removal of Spacer from Right Sacroiliac Joint, Open Approach

0SP70JZ Removal of Synthetic Substitute from Right Sacroiliac Joint, Open Approach

0SP70KZ Removal of Nonautologous Tissue Substitute from Right Sacroiliac Joint, Open Approach

0SP730Z Removal of Drainage Device from Right Sacroiliac Joint, Percutaneous Approach

0SP733Z Removal of Infusion Device from Right Sacroiliac Joint, Percutaneous Approach

0SP734Z Removal of Internal Fixation Device from Right Sacroiliac Joint, Percutaneous Approach

0SP737Z Removal of Autologous Tissue Substitute from Right Sacroiliac Joint, Percutaneous Approach

0SP738Z Removal of Spacer from Right Sacroiliac Joint, Percutaneous Approach

0SP73JZ Removal of Synthetic Substitute from Right Sacroiliac Joint, Percutaneous Approach

0SP73KZ Removal of Nonautologous Tissue Substitute from Right Sacroiliac Joint, Percutaneous Approach

0SP740Z Removal of Drainage Device from Right Sacroiliac Joint, Percutaneous Endoscopic Approach

0SP743Z Removal of Infusion Device from Right Sacroiliac Joint, Percutaneous Endoscopic Approach

0SP744Z Removal of Internal Fixation Device from Right Sacroiliac Joint, Percutaneous Endoscopic Approach

0SP747Z Removal of Autologous Tissue Substitute from Right Sacroiliac Joint, Percutaneous Endoscopic Approach

0SP748Z Removal of Spacer from Right Sacroiliac Joint, Percutaneous Endoscopic Approach

0SP74JZ Removal of Synthetic Substitute from Right Sacroiliac Joint, Percutaneous Endoscopic Approach

0SP74KZ Removal of Nonautologous Tissue Substitute from Right Sacroiliac Joint, Percutaneous Endoscopic Approach

0SP7X0Z Removal of Drainage Device from Right Sacroiliac Joint, External Approach

0SP7X3Z Removal of Infusion Device from Right Sacroiliac Joint, External Approach

0SP7X4Z Removal of Internal Fixation Device from Right Sacroiliac Joint, External Approach

0SP800Z Removal of Drainage Device from Left Sacroiliac Joint, Open Approach

0SP803Z Removal of Infusion Device from Left Sacroiliac Joint, Open Approach

0SP804Z Removal of Internal Fixation Device from Left Sacroiliac Joint, Open Approach

0SP807Z Removal of Autologous Tissue Substitute from Left Sacroiliac Joint, Open Approach

0SP808Z Removal of Spacer from Left Sacroiliac Joint, Open Approach

0SP80JZ Removal of Synthetic Substitute from Left Sacroiliac Joint, Open Approach

0SP80KZ Removal of Nonautologous Tissue Substitute from Left Sacroiliac Joint, Open Approach

0SP830Z Removal of Drainage Device from Left Sacroiliac Joint, Percutaneous Approach

0SP833Z Removal of Infusion Device from Left Sacroiliac Joint, Percutaneous Approach

0SP834Z Removal of Internal Fixation Device from Left Sacroiliac Joint, Percutaneous Approach

0SP837Z Removal of Autologous Tissue Substitute from Left Sacroiliac Joint, Percutaneous Approach

0SP838Z Removal of Spacer from Left Sacroiliac Joint, Percutaneous Approach

0SP83JZ Removal of Synthetic Substitute from Left Sacroiliac Joint, Percutaneous Approach

0SP83KZ Removal of Nonautologous Tissue Substitute from Left Sacroiliac Joint, Percutaneous Approach

0SP840Z Removal of Drainage Device from Left Sacroiliac Joint, Percutaneous Endoscopic Approach

0SP843Z Removal of Infusion Device from Left Sacroiliac Joint, Percutaneous Endoscopic Approach

0SP844Z Removal of Internal Fixation Device from Left Sacroiliac Joint, Percutaneous Endoscopic Approach

0SP847Z Removal of Autologous Tissue Substitute from Left Sacroiliac Joint, Percutaneous Endoscopic Approach

0SP848Z Removal of Spacer from Left Sacroiliac Joint, Percutaneous Endoscopic Approach

0SP84JZ Removal of Synthetic Substitute from Left Sacroiliac Joint, Percutaneous Endoscopic Approach

0SP84KZ Removal of Nonautologous Tissue Substitute from Left Sacroiliac Joint, Percutaneous Endoscopic Approach

0SP8X0Z Removal of Drainage Device from Left Sacroiliac Joint, External Approach

0SP8X3Z Removal of Infusion Device from Left Sacroiliac Joint, External Approach

0SP8X4Z Removal of Internal Fixation Device from Left Sacroiliac Joint, External Approach

0SP900Z Removal of Drainage Device from Right Hip Joint, Open Approach

0SP903Z Removal of Infusion Device from Right Hip Joint, Open Approach

0SP904Z Removal of Internal Fixation Device from Right Hip Joint, Open Approach

0SP905Z Removal of External Fixation Device from Right Hip Joint, Open Approach

0SP907Z Removal of Autologous Tissue Substitute from Right Hip Joint, Open Approach

0SP908Z Removal of Spacer from Right Hip Joint, Open Approach

0SP909Z Removal of Liner from Right Hip Joint, Open Approach

0SP90BZ Removal of Resurfacing Device from Right Hip Joint, Open Approach

0SP90JZ Removal of Synthetic Substitute from Right Hip Joint, Open Approach

0SP90KZ Removal of Nonautologous Tissue Substitute from Right Hip Joint, Open Approach

0SP930Z Removal of Drainage Device from Right Hip Joint, Percutaneous Approach

0SP933Z Removal of Infusion Device from Right Hip Joint, Percutaneous Approach

0SP934Z Removal of Internal Fixation Device from Right Hip Joint, Percutaneous Approach

0SP935Z Removal of External Fixation Device from Right Hip Joint, Percutaneous Approach

0SP937Z Removal of Autologous Tissue Substitute from Right Hip Joint, Percutaneous Approach

0SP938Z Removal of Spacer from Right Hip Joint, Percutaneous Approach

0SP93JZ Removal of Synthetic Substitute from Right Hip Joint, Percutaneous Approach

0SP93KZ Removal of Nonautologous Tissue Substitute from Right Hip Joint, Percutaneous Approach

0SP940Z Removal of Drainage Device from Right Hip Joint, Percutaneous Endoscopic Approach

0SP943Z Removal of Infusion Device from Right Hip Joint, Percutaneous Endoscopic Approach

0SP944Z Removal of Internal Fixation Device from Right Hip Joint, Percutaneous Endoscopic Approach

0SP945Z Removal of External Fixation Device from Right Hip Joint, Percutaneous Endoscopic Approach

0SP947Z Removal of Autologous Tissue Substitute from Right Hip Joint, Percutaneous Endoscopic Approach

0SP948Z Removal of Spacer from Right Hip Joint, Percutaneous Endoscopic Approach

0SP94JZ Removal of Synthetic Substitute from Right Hip Joint, Percutaneous Endoscopic Approach

0SP94KZ Removal of Nonautologous Tissue Substitute from Right Hip Joint, Percutaneous Endoscopic Approach

0SP9X0Z Removal of Drainage Device from Right Hip Joint, External Approach

0SP9X3Z Removal of Infusion Device from Right Hip Joint, External Approach

0SP9X4Z Removal of Internal Fixation Device from Right Hip Joint, External Approach

0SP9X5Z Removal of External Fixation Device from Right Hip Joint, External Approach

0SPB00Z Removal of Drainage Device from Left Hip Joint, Open Approach

0SPB03Z Removal of Infusion Device from Left Hip Joint, Open Approach

0SPB04Z Removal of Internal Fixation Device from Left Hip Joint, Open Approach

0SPB05Z Removal of External Fixation Device from Left Hip Joint, Open Approach

0SPB07Z Removal of Autologous Tissue Substitute from Left Hip Joint, Open Approach

0SPB08Z Removal of Spacer from Left Hip Joint, Open Approach

0SPB09Z Removal of Liner from Left Hip Joint, Open Approach

0SPB0BZ Removal of Resurfacing Device from Left Hip Joint, Open Approach

0SPB0JZ Removal of Synthetic Substitute from Left Hip Joint, Open Approach

0SPB0KZ Removal of Nonautologous Tissue Substitute from Left Hip Joint, Open Approach

0SPB30Z Removal of Drainage Device from Left Hip Joint, Percutaneous Approach

0SPB33Z Removal of Infusion Device from Left Hip Joint, Percutaneous Approach

0SPB34Z Removal of Internal Fixation Device from Left Hip Joint, Percutaneous Approach

0SPB35Z Removal of External Fixation Device from Left Hip Joint, Percutaneous Approach

0SPB37Z Removal of Autologous Tissue Substitute from Left Hip Joint, Percutaneous Approach

0SPB38Z Removal of Spacer from Left Hip Joint, Percutaneous Approach

0SPB3JZ Removal of Synthetic Substitute from Left Hip Joint, Percutaneous Approach

0SPB3KZ Removal of Nonautologous Tissue Substitute from Left Hip Joint, Percutaneous Approach

0SPB40Z Removal of Drainage Device from Left Hip Joint, Percutaneous Endoscopic Approach

0SPB43Z Removal of Infusion Device from Left Hip Joint, Percutaneous Endoscopic Approach

0SPB44Z Removal of Internal Fixation Device from Left Hip Joint, Percutaneous Endoscopic Approach

0SPB45Z Removal of External Fixation Device from Left Hip Joint, Percutaneous Endoscopic Approach

0SPB47Z Removal of Autologous Tissue Substitute from Left Hip Joint, Percutaneous Endoscopic Approach

0SPB48Z Removal of Spacer from Left Hip Joint, Percutaneous Endoscopic Approach

0SPB4JZ Removal of Synthetic Substitute from Left Hip Joint, Percutaneous Endoscopic Approach

0SPB4KZ Removal of Nonautologous Tissue Substitute from Left Hip Joint, Percutaneous Endoscopic Approach

0SPBX0Z Removal of Drainage Device from Left Hip Joint, External Approach

0SPBX3Z Removal of Infusion Device from Left Hip Joint, External Approach

0SPBX4Z Removal of Internal Fixation Device from Left Hip Joint, External Approach

0SPBX5Z Removal of External Fixation Device from Left Hip Joint, External Approach

0SPC00Z Removal of Drainage Device from Right Knee Joint, Open Approach

0SPC03Z Removal of Infusion Device from Right Knee Joint, Open Approach

0SPC04Z Removal of Internal Fixation Device from Right Knee Joint, Open Approach

0SPC05Z Removal of External Fixation Device from Right Knee Joint, Open Approach

0SPC07Z Removal of Autologous Tissue Substitute from Right Knee Joint, Open Approach

0SPC08Z Removal of Spacer from Right Knee Joint, Open Approach

0SPC09Z Removal of Liner from Right Knee Joint, Open Approach

0SPC0JZ Removal of Synthetic Substitute from Right Knee Joint, Open Approach

0SPC0KZ Removal of Nonautologous Tissue Substitute from Right Knee Joint, Open Approach

0SPC30Z Removal of Drainage Device from Right Knee Joint, Percutaneous Approach

0SPC33Z Removal of Infusion Device from Right Knee Joint, Percutaneous Approach

0SPC34Z Removal of Internal Fixation Device from Right Knee Joint, Percutaneous Approach

0SPC35Z Removal of External Fixation Device from Right Knee Joint, Percutaneous Approach

0SPC37Z Removal of Autologous Tissue Substitute from Right Knee Joint, Percutaneous Approach

0SPC38Z Removal of Spacer from Right Knee Joint, Percutaneous Approach

0SPC3JZ Removal of Synthetic Substitute from Right Knee Joint, Percutaneous Approach

0SPC3KZ Removal of Nonautologous Tissue Substitute from Right Knee Joint, Percutaneous Approach

0SPC40Z Removal of Drainage Device from Right Knee Joint, Percutaneous Endoscopic Approach

0SPC43Z Removal of Infusion Device from Right Knee Joint, Percutaneous Endoscopic Approach

0SPC44Z Removal of Internal Fixation Device from Right Knee Joint, Percutaneous Endoscopic Approach

0SPC45Z Removal of External Fixation Device from Right Knee Joint, Percutaneous Endoscopic Approach

0SPC47Z Removal of Autologous Tissue Substitute from Right Knee Joint, Percutaneous Endoscopic Approach

0SPC48Z Removal of Spacer from Right Knee Joint, Percutaneous Endoscopic Approach

0SPC4JZ Removal of Synthetic Substitute from Right Knee Joint, Percutaneous Endoscopic Approach

0SPC4KZ Removal of Nonautologous Tissue Substitute from Right Knee Joint, Percutaneous Endoscopic Approach

0SPCX0Z Removal of Drainage Device from Right Knee Joint, External Approach

0SPCX3Z Removal of Infusion Device from Right Knee Joint, External Approach

0SPCX4Z Removal of Internal Fixation Device from Right Knee Joint, External Approach

0SPCX5Z Removal of External Fixation Device from Right Knee Joint, External Approach

0SPD00Z Removal of Drainage Device from Left Knee Joint, Open Approach

0SPD03Z Removal of Infusion Device from Left Knee Joint, Open Approach

0SPD04Z Removal of Internal Fixation Device from Left Knee Joint, Open Approach

0SPD05Z Removal of External Fixation Device from Left Knee Joint, Open Approach

0SPD07Z Removal of Autologous Tissue Substitute from Left Knee Joint, Open Approach

0SPD08Z Removal of Spacer from Left Knee Joint, Open Approach

0SPD09Z Removal of Liner from Left Knee Joint, Open Approach

0SPD0JZ Removal of Synthetic Substitute from Left Knee Joint, Open Approach

0SPD0KZ Removal of Nonautologous Tissue Substitute from Left Knee Joint, Open Approach

0SPD30Z Removal of Drainage Device from Left Knee Joint, Percutaneous Approach

0SPD33Z Removal of Infusion Device from Left Knee Joint, Percutaneous Approach

0SPD34Z Removal of Internal Fixation Device from Left Knee Joint, Percutaneous Approach

0SPD35Z Removal of External Fixation Device from Left Knee Joint, Percutaneous Approach

0SPD37Z Removal of Autologous Tissue Substitute from Left Knee Joint, Percutaneous Approach

---

♀ Female-only   ♂ Male-only   ● Limited Coverage   ● Non-OR   ᴴᴬᶜ HAC-associated procedure   ● Non-covered procedures   ➕ Combination

0SPD38Z   Removal of Spacer from Left Knee Joint, Percutaneous Approach

0SPD3JZ   Removal of Synthetic Substitute from Left Knee Joint, Percutaneous Approach

0SPD3KZ   Removal of Nonautologous Tissue Substitute from Left Knee Joint, Percutaneous Approach

0SPD40Z   Removal of Drainage Device from Left Knee Joint, Percutaneous Endoscopic Approach

0SPD43Z   Removal of Infusion Device from Left Knee Joint, Percutaneous Endoscopic Approach

0SPD44Z   Removal of Internal Fixation Device from Left Knee Joint, Percutaneous Endoscopic Approach

0SPD45Z   Removal of External Fixation Device from Left Knee Joint, Percutaneous Endoscopic Approach

0SPD47Z   Removal of Autologous Tissue Substitute from Left Knee Joint, Percutaneous Endoscopic Approach

0SPD48Z   Removal of Spacer from Left Knee Joint, Percutaneous Endoscopic Approach

0SPD4JZ   Removal of Synthetic Substitute from Left Knee Joint, Percutaneous Endoscopic Approach

0SPD4KZ   Removal of Nonautologous Tissue Substitute from Left Knee Joint, Percutaneous Endoscopic Approach

0SPDX0Z   Removal of Drainage Device from Left Knee Joint, External Approach

0SPDX3Z   Removal of Infusion Device from Left Knee Joint, External Approach

0SPDX4Z   Removal of Internal Fixation Device from Left Knee Joint, External Approach

0SPDX5Z   Removal of External Fixation Device from Left Knee Joint, External Approach

0SPF00Z   Removal of Drainage Device from Right Ankle Joint, Open Approach

0SPF03Z   Removal of Infusion Device from Right Ankle Joint, Open Approach

0SPF04Z   Removal of Internal Fixation Device from Right Ankle Joint, Open Approach

0SPF05Z   Removal of External Fixation Device from Right Ankle Joint, Open Approach

0SPF07Z   Removal of Autologous Tissue Substitute from Right Ankle Joint, Open Approach

0SPF08Z   Removal of Spacer from Right Ankle Joint, Open Approach

0SPF0JZ   Removal of Synthetic Substitute from Right Ankle Joint, Open Approach

0SPF0KZ   Removal of Nonautologous Tissue Substitute from Right Ankle Joint, Open Approach

0SPF30Z   Removal of Drainage Device from Right Ankle Joint, Percutaneous Approach

0SPF33Z   Removal of Infusion Device from Right Ankle Joint, Percutaneous Approach

0SPF34Z   Removal of Internal Fixation Device from Right Ankle Joint, Percutaneous Approach

0SPF35Z   Removal of External Fixation Device from Right Ankle Joint, Percutaneous Approach

0SPF37Z   Removal of Autologous Tissue Substitute from Right Ankle Joint, Percutaneous Approach

0SPF38Z   Removal of Spacer from Right Ankle Joint, Percutaneous Approach

0SPF3JZ   Removal of Synthetic Substitute from Right Ankle Joint, Percutaneous Approach

0SPF3KZ   Removal of Nonautologous Tissue Substitute from Right Ankle Joint, Percutaneous Approach

0SPF40Z   Removal of Drainage Device from Right Ankle Joint, Percutaneous Endoscopic Approach

0SPF43Z   Removal of Infusion Device from Right Ankle Joint, Percutaneous Endoscopic Approach

0SPF44Z   Removal of Internal Fixation Device from Right Ankle Joint, Percutaneous Endoscopic Approach

0SPF45Z   Removal of External Fixation Device from Right Ankle Joint, Percutaneous Endoscopic Approach

0SPF47Z   Removal of Autologous Tissue Substitute from Right Ankle Joint, Percutaneous Endoscopic Approach

0SPF48Z   Removal of Spacer from Right Ankle Joint, Percutaneous Endoscopic Approach

0SPF4JZ   Removal of Synthetic Substitute from Right Ankle Joint, Percutaneous Endoscopic Approach

0SPF4KZ   Removal of Nonautologous Tissue Substitute from Right Ankle Joint, Percutaneous Endoscopic Approach

0SPFX0Z   Removal of Drainage Device from Right Ankle Joint, External Approach

0SPFX3Z   Removal of Infusion Device from Right Ankle Joint, External Approach

0SPFX4Z   Removal of Internal Fixation Device from Right Ankle Joint, External Approach

0SPFX5Z   Removal of External Fixation Device from Right Ankle Joint, External Approach

0SPG00Z   Removal of Drainage Device from Left Ankle Joint, Open Approach

0SPG03Z   Removal of Infusion Device from Left Ankle Joint, Open Approach

0SPG04Z   Removal of Internal Fixation Device from Left Ankle Joint, Open Approach

0SPG05Z   Removal of External Fixation Device from Left Ankle Joint, Open Approach

0SPG07Z   Removal of Autologous Tissue Substitute from Left Ankle Joint, Open Approach

0SPG08Z   Removal of Spacer from Left Ankle Joint, Open Approach

0SPG0JZ   Removal of Synthetic Substitute from Left Ankle Joint, Open Approach

0SPG0KZ   Removal of Nonautologous Tissue Substitute from Left Ankle Joint, Open Approach

0SPG30Z   Removal of Drainage Device from Left Ankle Joint, Percutaneous Approach

0SPG33Z   Removal of Infusion Device from Left Ankle Joint, Percutaneous Approach

0SPG34Z   Removal of Internal Fixation Device from Left Ankle Joint, Percutaneous Approach

0SPG35Z   Removal of External Fixation Device from Left Ankle Joint, Percutaneous Approach

0SPG37Z   Removal of Autologous Tissue Substitute from Left Ankle Joint, Percutaneous Approach

0SPG38Z   Removal of Spacer from Left Ankle Joint, Percutaneous Approach

0SPG3JZ   Removal of Synthetic Substitute from Left Ankle Joint, Percutaneous Approach

0SPG3KZ   Removal of Nonautologous Tissue Substitute from Left Ankle Joint, Percutaneous Approach

0SPG40Z   Removal of Drainage Device from Left Ankle Joint, Percutaneous Endoscopic Approach

0SPG43Z   Removal of Infusion Device from Left Ankle Joint, Percutaneous Endoscopic Approach

0SPG44Z   Removal of Internal Fixation Device from Left Ankle Joint, Percutaneous Endoscopic Approach

0SPG45Z   Removal of External Fixation Device from Left Ankle Joint, Percutaneous Endoscopic Approach

0SPG47Z   Removal of Autologous Tissue Substitute from Left Ankle Joint, Percutaneous Endoscopic Approach

0SPG48Z   Removal of Spacer from Left Ankle Joint, Percutaneous Endoscopic Approach

0SPG4JZ   Removal of Synthetic Substitute from Left Ankle Joint, Percutaneous Endoscopic Approach

0SPG4KZ   Removal of Nonautologous Tissue Substitute from Left Ankle Joint, Percutaneous Endoscopic Approach

0SPGX0Z   Removal of Drainage Device from Left Ankle Joint, External Approach

0SPGX3Z   Removal of Infusion Device from Left Ankle Joint, External Approach

0SPGX4Z   Removal of Internal Fixation Device from Left Ankle Joint, External Approach

0SPGX5Z   Removal of External Fixation Device from Left Ankle Joint, External Approach

0SPH00Z   Removal of Drainage Device from Right Tarsal Joint, Open Approach

0SPH03Z   Removal of Infusion Device from Right Tarsal Joint, Open Approach

0SPH04Z   Removal of Internal Fixation Device from Right Tarsal Joint, Open Approach

0SPH05Z   Removal of External Fixation Device from Right Tarsal Joint, Open Approach

0SPH07Z   Removal of Autologous Tissue Substitute from Right Tarsal Joint, Open Approach

0SPH08Z   Removal of Spacer from Right Tarsal Joint, Open Approach

0SPH0JZ   Removal of Synthetic Substitute from Right Tarsal Joint, Open Approach

0SPH0KZ   Removal of Nonautologous Tissue Substitute from Right Tarsal Joint, Open Approach

0SPH30Z   Removal of Drainage Device from Right Tarsal Joint, Percutaneous Approach

0SPH33Z Removal of Infusion Device from Right Tarsal Joint, Percutaneous Approach

0SPH34Z Removal of Internal Fixation Device from Right Tarsal Joint, Percutaneous Approach

0SPH35Z Removal of External Fixation Device from Right Tarsal Joint, Percutaneous Approach

0SPH37Z Removal of Autologous Tissue Substitute from Right Tarsal Joint, Percutaneous Approach

0SPH38Z Removal of Spacer from Right Tarsal Joint, Percutaneous Approach

0SPH3JZ Removal of Synthetic Substitute from Right Tarsal Joint, Percutaneous Approach

0SPH3KZ Removal of Nonautologous Tissue Substitute from Right Tarsal Joint, Percutaneous Approach

0SPH40Z Removal of Drainage Device from Right Tarsal Joint, Percutaneous Endoscopic Approach

0SPH43Z Removal of Infusion Device from Right Tarsal Joint, Percutaneous Endoscopic Approach

0SPH44Z Removal of Internal Fixation Device from Right Tarsal Joint, Percutaneous Endoscopic Approach

0SPH45Z Removal of External Fixation Device from Right Tarsal Joint, Percutaneous Endoscopic Approach

0SPH47Z Removal of Autologous Tissue Substitute from Right Tarsal Joint, Percutaneous Endoscopic Approach

0SPH48Z Removal of Spacer from Right Tarsal Joint, Percutaneous Endoscopic Approach

0SPH4JZ Removal of Synthetic Substitute from Right Tarsal Joint, Percutaneous Endoscopic Approach

0SPH4KZ Removal of Nonautologous Tissue Substitute from Right Tarsal Joint, Percutaneous Endoscopic Approach

0SPHX0Z Removal of Drainage Device from Right Tarsal Joint, External Approach

0SPHX3Z Removal of Infusion Device from Right Tarsal Joint, External Approach

0SPHX4Z Removal of Internal Fixation Device from Right Tarsal Joint, External Approach

0SPHX5Z Removal of External Fixation Device from Right Tarsal Joint, External Approach

0SPJ00Z Removal of Drainage Device from Left Tarsal Joint, Open Approach

0SPJ03Z Removal of Infusion Device from Left Tarsal Joint, Open Approach

0SPJ04Z Removal of Internal Fixation Device from Left Tarsal Joint, Open Approach

0SPJ05Z Removal of External Fixation Device from Left Tarsal Joint, Open Approach

0SPJ07Z Removal of Autologous Tissue Substitute from Left Tarsal Joint, Open Approach

0SPJ08Z Removal of Spacer from Left Tarsal Joint, Open Approach

0SPJ0JZ Removal of Synthetic Substitute from Left Tarsal Joint, Open Approach

0SPJ0KZ Removal of Nonautologous Tissue Substitute from Left Tarsal Joint, Open Approach

0SPJ30Z Removal of Drainage Device from Left Tarsal Joint, Percutaneous Approach

0SPJ33Z Removal of Infusion Device from Left Tarsal Joint, Percutaneous Approach

0SPJ34Z Removal of Internal Fixation Device from Left Tarsal Joint, Percutaneous Approach

0SPJ35Z Removal of External Fixation Device from Left Tarsal Joint, Percutaneous Approach

0SPJ37Z Removal of Autologous Tissue Substitute from Left Tarsal Joint, Percutaneous Approach

0SPJ38Z Removal of Spacer from Left Tarsal Joint, Percutaneous Approach

0SPJ3JZ Removal of Synthetic Substitute from Left Tarsal Joint, Percutaneous Approach

0SPJ3KZ Removal of Nonautologous Tissue Substitute from Left Tarsal Joint, Percutaneous Approach

0SPJ40Z Removal of Drainage Device from Left Tarsal Joint, Percutaneous Endoscopic Approach

0SPJ43Z Removal of Infusion Device from Left Tarsal Joint, Percutaneous Endoscopic Approach

0SPJ44Z Removal of Internal Fixation Device from Left Tarsal Joint, Percutaneous Endoscopic Approach

0SPJ45Z Removal of External Fixation Device from Left Tarsal Joint, Percutaneous Endoscopic Approach

0SPJ47Z Removal of Autologous Tissue Substitute from Left Tarsal Joint, Percutaneous Endoscopic Approach

0SPJ48Z Removal of Spacer from Left Tarsal Joint, Percutaneous Endoscopic Approach

0SPJ4JZ Removal of Synthetic Substitute from Left Tarsal Joint, Percutaneous Endoscopic Approach

0SPJ4KZ Removal of Nonautologous Tissue Substitute from Left Tarsal Joint, Percutaneous Endoscopic Approach

0SPJX0Z Removal of Drainage Device from Left Tarsal Joint, External Approach

0SPJX3Z Removal of Infusion Device from Left Tarsal Joint, External Approach

0SPJX4Z Removal of Internal Fixation Device from Left Tarsal Joint, External Approach

0SPJX5Z Removal of External Fixation Device from Left Tarsal Joint, External Approach

0SPK00Z Removal of Drainage Device from Right Metatarsal-Tarsal Joint, Open Approach

0SPK03Z Removal of Infusion Device from Right Metatarsal-Tarsal Joint, Open Approach

0SPK04Z Removal of Internal Fixation Device from Right Metatarsal-Tarsal Joint, Open Approach

0SPK05Z Removal of External Fixation Device from Right Metatarsal-Tarsal Joint, Open Approach

0SPK07Z Removal of Autologous Tissue Substitute from Right Metatarsal-Tarsal Joint, Open Approach

0SPK08Z Removal of Spacer from Right Metatarsal-Tarsal Joint, Open Approach

0SPK0JZ Removal of Synthetic Substitute from Right Metatarsal-Tarsal Joint, Open Approach

0SPK0KZ Removal of Nonautologous Tissue Substitute from Right Metatarsal-Tarsal Joint, Open Approach

0SPK30Z Removal of Drainage Device from Right Metatarsal-Tarsal Joint, Percutaneous Approach

0SPK33Z Removal of Infusion Device from Right Metatarsal-Tarsal Joint, Percutaneous Approach

0SPK34Z Removal of Internal Fixation Device from Right Metatarsal-Tarsal Joint, Percutaneous Approach

0SPK35Z Removal of External Fixation Device from Right Metatarsal-Tarsal Joint, Percutaneous Approach

0SPK37Z Removal of Autologous Tissue Substitute from Right Metatarsal-Tarsal Joint, Percutaneous Approach

0SPK38Z Removal of Spacer from Right Metatarsal-Tarsal Joint, Percutaneous Approach

0SPK3JZ Removal of Synthetic Substitute from Right Metatarsal-Tarsal Joint, Percutaneous Approach

0SPK3KZ Removal of Nonautologous Tissue Substitute from Right Metatarsal-Tarsal Joint, Percutaneous Approach

0SPK40Z Removal of Drainage Device from Right Metatarsal-Tarsal Joint, Percutaneous Endoscopic Approach

0SPK43Z Removal of Infusion Device from Right Metatarsal-Tarsal Joint, Percutaneous Endoscopic Approach

0SPK44Z Removal of Internal Fixation Device from Right Metatarsal-Tarsal Joint, Percutaneous Endoscopic Approach

0SPK45Z Removal of External Fixation Device from Right Metatarsal-Tarsal Joint, Percutaneous Endoscopic Approach

0SPK47Z Removal of Autologous Tissue Substitute from Right Metatarsal-Tarsal Joint, Percutaneous Endoscopic Approach

0SPK48Z Removal of Spacer from Right Metatarsal-Tarsal Joint, Percutaneous Endoscopic Approach

0SPK4JZ Removal of Synthetic Substitute from Right Metatarsal-Tarsal Joint, Percutaneous Endoscopic Approach

0SPK4KZ Removal of Nonautologous Tissue Substitute from Right Metatarsal-Tarsal Joint, Percutaneous Endoscopic Approach

0SPKX0Z Removal of Drainage Device from Right Metatarsal-Tarsal Joint, External Approach

0SPKX3Z Removal of Infusion Device from Right Metatarsal-Tarsal Joint, External Approach

0SPKX4Z Removal of Internal Fixation Device from Right Metatarsal-Tarsal Joint, External Approach

0SPKX5Z Removal of External Fixation Device from Right Metatarsal-Tarsal Joint, External Approach

0SPL00Z Removal of Drainage Device from Left Metatarsal-Tarsal Joint, Open Approach

0SPL03Z Removal of Infusion Device from Left Metatarsal-Tarsal Joint, Open Approach

0SPL04Z Removal of Internal Fixation Device from Left Metatarsal-Tarsal Joint, Open Approach

0SPL05Z Removal of External Fixation Device from Left Metatarsal-Tarsal Joint, Open Approach

0SPL07Z Removal of Autologous Tissue Substitute from Left Metatarsal-Tarsal Joint, Open Approach

0SPL08Z Removal of Spacer from Left Metatarsal-Tarsal Joint, Open Approach

0SPL0JZ Removal of Synthetic Substitute from Left Metatarsal-Tarsal Joint, Open Approach

0SPL0KZ Removal of Nonautologous Tissue Substitute from Left Metatarsal-Tarsal Joint, Open Approach

0SPL30Z Removal of Drainage Device from Left Metatarsal-Tarsal Joint, Percutaneous Approach

0SPL33Z Removal of Infusion Device from Left Metatarsal-Tarsal Joint, Percutaneous Approach

0SPL34Z Removal of Internal Fixation Device from Left Metatarsal-Tarsal Joint, Percutaneous Approach

0SPL35Z Removal of External Fixation Device from Left Metatarsal-Tarsal Joint, Percutaneous Approach

0SPL37Z Removal of Autologous Tissue Substitute from Left Metatarsal-Tarsal Joint, Percutaneous Approach

0SPL38Z Removal of Spacer from Left Metatarsal-Tarsal Joint, Percutaneous Approach

0SPL3JZ Removal of Synthetic Substitute from Left Metatarsal-Tarsal Joint, Percutaneous Approach

0SPL3KZ Removal of Nonautologous Tissue Substitute from Left Metatarsal-Tarsal Joint, Percutaneous Approach

0SPL40Z Removal of Drainage Device from Left Metatarsal-Tarsal Joint, Percutaneous Endoscopic Approach

0SPL43Z Removal of Infusion Device from Left Metatarsal-Tarsal Joint, Percutaneous Endoscopic Approach

0SPL44Z Removal of Internal Fixation Device from Left Metatarsal-Tarsal Joint, Percutaneous Endoscopic Approach

0SPL45Z Removal of External Fixation Device from Left Metatarsal-Tarsal Joint, Percutaneous Endoscopic Approach

0SPL47Z Removal of Autologous Tissue Substitute from Left Metatarsal-Tarsal Joint, Percutaneous Endoscopic Approach

0SPL48Z Removal of Spacer from Left Metatarsal-Tarsal Joint, Percutaneous Endoscopic Approach

0SPL4JZ Removal of Synthetic Substitute from Left Metatarsal-Tarsal Joint, Percutaneous Endoscopic Approach

0SPL4KZ Removal of Nonautologous Tissue Substitute from Left Metatarsal-Tarsal Joint, Percutaneous Endoscopic Approach

0SPLX0Z Removal of Drainage Device from Left Metatarsal-Tarsal Joint, External Approach

0SPLX3Z Removal of Infusion Device from Left Metatarsal-Tarsal Joint, External Approach

0SPLX4Z Removal of Internal Fixation Device from Left Metatarsal-Tarsal Joint, External Approach

0SPLX5Z Removal of External Fixation Device from Left Metatarsal-Tarsal Joint, External Approach

0SPM00Z Removal of Drainage Device from Right Metatarsal-Phalangeal Joint, Open Approach

0SPM03Z Removal of Infusion Device from Right Metatarsal-Phalangeal Joint, Open Approach

0SPM04Z Removal of Internal Fixation Device from Right Metatarsal-Phalangeal Joint, Open Approach

0SPM05Z Removal of External Fixation Device from Right Metatarsal-Phalangeal Joint, Open Approach

0SPM07Z Removal of Autologous Tissue Substitute from Right Metatarsal-Phalangeal Joint, Open Approach

0SPM08Z Removal of Spacer from Right Metatarsal-Phalangeal Joint, Open Approach

0SPM0JZ Removal of Synthetic Substitute from Right Metatarsal-Phalangeal Joint, Open Approach

0SPM0KZ Removal of Nonautologous Tissue Substitute from Right Metatarsal-Phalangeal Joint, Open Approach

0SPM30Z Removal of Drainage Device from Right Metatarsal-Phalangeal Joint, Percutaneous Approach

0SPM33Z Removal of Infusion Device from Right Metatarsal-Phalangeal Joint, Percutaneous Approach

0SPM34Z Removal of Internal Fixation Device from Right Metatarsal-Phalangeal Joint, Percutaneous Approach

0SPM35Z Removal of External Fixation Device from Right Metatarsal-Phalangeal Joint, Percutaneous Approach

0SPM37Z Removal of Autologous Tissue Substitute from Right Metatarsal-Phalangeal Joint, Percutaneous Approach

0SPM38Z Removal of Spacer from Right Metatarsal-Phalangeal Joint, Percutaneous Approach

0SPM3JZ Removal of Synthetic Substitute from Right Metatarsal-Phalangeal Joint, Percutaneous Approach

0SPM3KZ Removal of Nonautologous Tissue Substitute from Right Metatarsal-Phalangeal Joint, Percutaneous Approach

0SPM40Z Removal of Drainage Device from Right Metatarsal-Phalangeal Joint, Percutaneous Endoscopic Approach

0SPM43Z Removal of Infusion Device from Right Metatarsal-Phalangeal Joint, Percutaneous Endoscopic Approach

0SPM44Z Removal of Internal Fixation Device from Right Metatarsal-Phalangeal Joint, Percutaneous Endoscopic Approach

0SPM45Z Removal of External Fixation Device from Right Metatarsal-Phalangeal Joint, Percutaneous Endoscopic Approach

0SPM47Z Removal of Autologous Tissue Substitute from Right Metatarsal-Phalangeal Joint, Percutaneous Endoscopic Approach

0SPM48Z Removal of Spacer from Right Metatarsal-Phalangeal Joint, Percutaneous Endoscopic Approach

0SPM4JZ Removal of Synthetic Substitute from Right Metatarsal-Phalangeal Joint, Percutaneous Endoscopic Approach

0SPM4KZ Removal of Nonautologous Tissue Substitute from Right Metatarsal-Phalangeal Joint, Percutaneous Endoscopic Approach

0SPMX0Z Removal of Drainage Device from Right Metatarsal-Phalangeal Joint, External Approach

0SPMX3Z Removal of Infusion Device from Right Metatarsal-Phalangeal Joint, External Approach

0SPMX4Z Removal of Internal Fixation Device from Right Metatarsal-Phalangeal Joint, External Approach

0SPMX5Z Removal of External Fixation Device from Right Metatarsal-Phalangeal Joint, External Approach

0SPN00Z Removal of Drainage Device from Left Metatarsal-Phalangeal Joint, Open Approach

0SPN03Z Removal of Infusion Device from Left Metatarsal-Phalangeal Joint, Open Approach

0SPN04Z Removal of Internal Fixation Device from Left Metatarsal-Phalangeal Joint, Open Approach

0SPN05Z Removal of External Fixation Device from Left Metatarsal-Phalangeal Joint, Open Approach

0SPN07Z Removal of Autologous Tissue Substitute from Left Metatarsal-Phalangeal Joint, Open Approach

0SPN08Z Removal of Spacer from Left Metatarsal-Phalangeal Joint, Open Approach

0SPN0JZ Removal of Synthetic Substitute from Left Metatarsal-Phalangeal Joint, Open Approach

0SPN0KZ Removal of Nonautologous Tissue Substitute from Left Metatarsal-Phalangeal Joint, Open Approach

0SPN30Z Removal of Drainage Device from Left Metatarsal-Phalangeal Joint, Percutaneous Approach

0SPN33Z Removal of Infusion Device from Left Metatarsal-Phalangeal Joint, Percutaneous Approach

0SPN34Z Removal of Internal Fixation Device from Left Metatarsal-Phalangeal Joint, Percutaneous Approach

0SPN35Z Removal of External Fixation Device from Left Metatarsal-Phalangeal Joint, Percutaneous Approach

0SPN37Z Removal of Autologous Tissue Substitute from Left Metatarsal-Phalangeal Joint, Percutaneous Approach

0SPN38Z Removal of Spacer from Left Metatarsal-Phalangeal Joint, Percutaneous Approach

0SPN3JZ Removal of Synthetic Substitute from Left Metatarsal-Phalangeal Joint, Percutaneous Approach

0SPN3KZ Removal of Nonautologous Tissue Substitute from Left Metatarsal-Phalangeal Joint, Percutaneous Approach

0SPN40Z Removal of Drainage Device from Left Metatarsal-Phalangeal Joint, Percutaneous Endoscopic Approach

0SPN43Z Removal of Infusion Device from Left Metatarsal-Phalangeal Joint, Percutaneous Endoscopic Approach

0SPN44Z Removal of Internal Fixation Device from Left Metatarsal-Phalangeal Joint, Percutaneous Endoscopic Approach

0SPN45Z Removal of External Fixation Device from Left Metatarsal-Phalangeal Joint, Percutaneous Endoscopic Approach

0SPN47Z Removal of Autologous Tissue Substitute from Left Metatarsal-Phalangeal Joint, Percutaneous Endoscopic Approach

0SPN48Z Removal of Spacer from Left Metatarsal-Phalangeal Joint, Percutaneous Endoscopic Approach

---

0SPN4JZ Removal of Synthetic Substitute from Left Metatarsal-Phalangeal Joint, Percutaneous Endoscopic Approach
0SPN4KZ Removal of Nonautologous Tissue Substitute from Left Metatarsal-Phalangeal Joint, Percutaneous Endoscopic Approach
0SPNX0Z Removal of Drainage Device from Left Metatarsal-Phalangeal Joint, External Approach
0SPNX3Z Removal of Infusion Device from Left Metatarsal-Phalangeal Joint, External Approach
0SPNX4Z Removal of Internal Fixation Device from Left Metatarsal-Phalangeal Joint, External Approach
0SPNX5Z Removal of External Fixation Device from Left Metatarsal-Phalangeal Joint, External Approach
0SPP00Z Removal of Drainage Device from Right Toe Phalangeal Joint, Open Approach
0SPP03Z Removal of Infusion Device from Right Toe Phalangeal Joint, Open Approach
0SPP04Z Removal of Internal Fixation Device from Right Toe Phalangeal Joint, Open Approach
0SPP05Z Removal of External Fixation Device from Right Toe Phalangeal Joint, Open Approach
0SPP07Z Removal of Autologous Tissue Substitute from Right Toe Phalangeal Joint, Open Approach
0SPP08Z Removal of Spacer from Right Toe Phalangeal Joint, Open Approach
0SPP0JZ Removal of Synthetic Substitute from Right Toe Phalangeal Joint, Open Approach
0SPP0KZ Removal of Nonautologous Tissue Substitute from Right Toe Phalangeal Joint, Open Approach
0SPP30Z Removal of Drainage Device from Right Toe Phalangeal Joint, Percutaneous Approach
0SPP33Z Removal of Infusion Device from Right Toe Phalangeal Joint, Percutaneous Approach
0SPP34Z Removal of Internal Fixation Device from Right Toe Phalangeal Joint, Percutaneous Approach
0SPP35Z Removal of External Fixation Device from Right Toe Phalangeal Joint, Percutaneous Approach
0SPP37Z Removal of Autologous Tissue Substitute from Right Toe Phalangeal Joint, Percutaneous Approach
0SPP38Z Removal of Spacer from Right Toe Phalangeal Joint, Percutaneous Approach
0SPP3JZ Removal of Synthetic Substitute from Right Toe Phalangeal Joint, Percutaneous Approach
0SPP3KZ Removal of Nonautologous Tissue Substitute from Right Toe Phalangeal Joint, Percutaneous Approach
0SPP40Z Removal of Drainage Device from Right Toe Phalangeal Joint, Percutaneous Endoscopic Approach
0SPP43Z Removal of Infusion Device from Right Toe Phalangeal Joint, Percutaneous Endoscopic Approach
0SPP44Z Removal of Internal Fixation Device from Right Toe Phalangeal Joint, Percutaneous Endoscopic Approach
0SPP45Z Removal of External Fixation Device from Right Toe Phalangeal Joint, Percutaneous Endoscopic Approach
0SPP47Z Removal of Autologous Tissue Substitute from Right Toe Phalangeal Joint, Percutaneous Endoscopic Approach
0SPP48Z Removal of Spacer from Right Toe Phalangeal Joint, Percutaneous Endoscopic Approach
0SPP4JZ Removal of Synthetic Substitute from Right Toe Phalangeal Joint, Percutaneous Endoscopic Approach
0SPP4KZ Removal of Nonautologous Tissue Substitute from Right Toe Phalangeal Joint, Percutaneous Endoscopic Approach
0SPPX0Z Removal of Drainage Device from Right Toe Phalangeal Joint, External Approach

0SPPX3Z Removal of Infusion Device from Right Toe Phalangeal Joint, External Approach
0SPPX4Z Removal of Internal Fixation Device from Right Toe Phalangeal Joint, External Approach
0SPPX5Z Removal of External Fixation Device from Right Toe Phalangeal Joint, External Approach
0SPQ00Z Removal of Drainage Device from Left Toe Phalangeal Joint, Open Approach
0SPQ03Z Removal of Infusion Device from Left Toe Phalangeal Joint, Open Approach
0SPQ04Z Removal of Internal Fixation Device from Left Toe Phalangeal Joint, Open Approach
0SPQ05Z Removal of External Fixation Device from Left Toe Phalangeal Joint, Open Approach
0SPQ07Z Removal of Autologous Tissue Substitute from Left Toe Phalangeal Joint, Open Approach
0SPQ08Z Removal of Spacer from Left Toe Phalangeal Joint, Open Approach
0SPQ0JZ Removal of Synthetic Substitute from Left Toe Phalangeal Joint, Open Approach
0SPQ0KZ Removal of Nonautologous Tissue Substitute from Left Toe Phalangeal Joint, Open Approach
0SPQ30Z Removal of Drainage Device from Left Toe Phalangeal Joint, Percutaneous Approach
0SPQ33Z Removal of Infusion Device from Left Toe Phalangeal Joint, Percutaneous Approach
0SPQ34Z Removal of Internal Fixation Device from Left Toe Phalangeal Joint, Percutaneous Approach
0SPQ35Z Removal of External Fixation Device from Left Toe Phalangeal Joint, Percutaneous Approach
0SPQ37Z Removal of Autologous Tissue Substitute from Left Toe Phalangeal Joint, Percutaneous Approach
0SPQ38Z Removal of Spacer from Left Toe Phalangeal Joint, Percutaneous Approach
0SPQ3JZ Removal of Synthetic Substitute from Left Toe Phalangeal Joint, Percutaneous Approach
0SPQ3KZ Removal of Nonautologous Tissue Substitute from Left Toe Phalangeal Joint, Percutaneous Approach
0SPQ40Z Removal of Drainage Device from Left Toe Phalangeal Joint, Percutaneous Endoscopic Approach
0SPQ43Z Removal of Infusion Device from Left Toe Phalangeal Joint, Percutaneous Endoscopic Approach
0SPQ44Z Removal of Internal Fixation Device from Left Toe Phalangeal Joint, Percutaneous Endoscopic Approach
0SPQ45Z Removal of External Fixation Device from Left Toe Phalangeal Joint, Percutaneous Endoscopic Approach
0SPQ47Z Removal of Autologous Tissue Substitute from Left Toe Phalangeal Joint, Percutaneous Endoscopic Approach
0SPQ48Z Removal of Spacer from Left Toe Phalangeal Joint, Percutaneous Endoscopic Approach
0SPQ4JZ Removal of Synthetic Substitute from Left Toe Phalangeal Joint, Percutaneous Endoscopic Approach
0SPQ4KZ Removal of Nonautologous Tissue Substitute from Left Toe Phalangeal Joint, Percutaneous Endoscopic Approach
0SPQX0Z Removal of Drainage Device from Left Toe Phalangeal Joint, External Approach
0SPQX3Z Removal of Infusion Device from Left Toe Phalangeal Joint, External Approach
0SPQX4Z Removal of Internal Fixation Device from Left Toe Phalangeal Joint, External Approach
0SPQX5Z Removal of External Fixation Device from Left Toe Phalangeal Joint, External Approach

0SQ – Lower Joints, Repair

Review Coding Guideline B3.5

0SQ00ZZ Repair Lumbar Vertebral Joint, Open Approach
0SQ03ZZ Repair Lumbar Vertebral Joint, Percutaneous Approach
0SQ04ZZ Repair Lumbar Vertebral Joint, Percutaneous Endoscopic Approach
0SQ0XZZ Repair Lumbar Vertebral Joint, External Approach
0SQ20ZZ Repair Lumbar Vertebral Disc, Open Approach
0SQ23ZZ Repair Lumbar Vertebral Disc, Percutaneous Approach
0SQ24ZZ Repair Lumbar Vertebral Disc, Percutaneous Endoscopic Approach
0SQ2XZZ Repair Lumbar Vertebral Disc, External Approach

0SQ30ZZ Repair Lumbosacral Joint, Open Approach
0SQ33ZZ Repair Lumbosacral Joint, Percutaneous Approach
0SQ34ZZ Repair Lumbosacral Joint, Percutaneous Endoscopic Approach
0SQ3XZZ Repair Lumbosacral Joint, External Approach
0SQ40ZZ Repair Lumbosacral Disc, Open Approach
0SQ43ZZ Repair Lumbosacral Disc, Percutaneous Approach
0SQ44ZZ Repair Lumbosacral Disc, Percutaneous Endoscopic Approach
0SQ4XZZ Repair Lumbosacral Disc, External Approach

0SQ50ZZ	Repair Sacrococcygeal Joint, Open Approach
0SQ53ZZ	Repair Sacrococcygeal Joint, Percutaneous Approach
0SQ54ZZ	Repair Sacrococcygeal Joint, Percutaneous Endoscopic Approach
0SQ5XZZ	Repair Sacrococcygeal Joint, External Approach
0SQ60ZZ	Repair Coccygeal Joint, Open Approach
0SQ63ZZ	Repair Coccygeal Joint, Percutaneous Approach
0SQ64ZZ	Repair Coccygeal Joint, Percutaneous Endoscopic Approach
0SQ6XZZ	Repair Coccygeal Joint, External Approach
0SQ70ZZ	Repair Right Sacroiliac Joint, Open Approach
0SQ73ZZ	Repair Right Sacroiliac Joint, Percutaneous Approach
0SQ74ZZ	Repair Right Sacroiliac Joint, Percutaneous Endoscopic Approach
0SQ7XZZ	Repair Right Sacroiliac Joint, External Approach
0SQ80ZZ	Repair Left Sacroiliac Joint, Open Approach
0SQ83ZZ	Repair Left Sacroiliac Joint, Percutaneous Approach
0SQ84ZZ	Repair Left Sacroiliac Joint, Percutaneous Endoscopic Approach
0SQ8XZZ	Repair Left Sacroiliac Joint, External Approach
0SQ90ZZ	Repair Right Hip Joint, Open Approach
0SQ93ZZ	Repair Right Hip Joint, Percutaneous Approach
0SQ94ZZ	Repair Right Hip Joint, Percutaneous Endoscopic Approach
0SQ9XZZ	Repair Right Hip Joint, External Approach
0SQB0ZZ	Repair Left Hip Joint, Open Approach
0SQB3ZZ	Repair Left Hip Joint, Percutaneous Approach
0SQB4ZZ	Repair Left Hip Joint, Percutaneous Endoscopic Approach
0SQBXZZ	Repair Left Hip Joint, External Approach
0SQC0ZZ	Repair Right Knee Joint, Open Approach
0SQC3ZZ	Repair Right Knee Joint, Percutaneous Approach
0SQC4ZZ	Repair Right Knee Joint, Percutaneous Endoscopic Approach
0SQCXZZ	Repair Right Knee Joint, External Approach
0SQD0ZZ	Repair Left Knee Joint, Open Approach
0SQD3ZZ	Repair Left Knee Joint, Percutaneous Approach
0SQD4ZZ	Repair Left Knee Joint, Percutaneous Endoscopic Approach
0SQDXZZ	Repair Left Knee Joint, External Approach
0SQF0ZZ	Repair Right Ankle Joint, Open Approach
0SQF3ZZ	Repair Right Ankle Joint, Percutaneous Approach
0SQF4ZZ	Repair Right Ankle Joint, Percutaneous Endoscopic Approach
0SQFXZZ	Repair Right Ankle Joint, External Approach
0SQG0ZZ	Repair Left Ankle Joint, Open Approach
0SQG3ZZ	Repair Left Ankle Joint, Percutaneous Approach
0SQG4ZZ	Repair Left Ankle Joint, Percutaneous Endoscopic Approach

0SQGXZZ	Repair Left Ankle Joint, External Approach
0SQH0ZZ	Repair Right Tarsal Joint, Open Approach
0SQH3ZZ	Repair Right Tarsal Joint, Percutaneous Approach
0SQH4ZZ	Repair Right Tarsal Joint, Percutaneous Endoscopic Approach
0SQHXZZ	Repair Right Tarsal Joint, External Approach
0SQJ0ZZ	Repair Left Tarsal Joint, Open Approach
0SQJ3ZZ	Repair Left Tarsal Joint, Percutaneous Approach
0SQJ4ZZ	Repair Left Tarsal Joint, Percutaneous Endoscopic Approach
0SQJXZZ	Repair Left Tarsal Joint, External Approach
0SQK0ZZ	Repair Right Metatarsal-Tarsal Joint, Open Approach
0SQK3ZZ	Repair Right Metatarsal-Tarsal Joint, Percutaneous Approach
0SQK4ZZ	Repair Right Metatarsal-Tarsal Joint, Percutaneous Endoscopic Approach
0SQKXZZ	Repair Right Metatarsal-Tarsal Joint, External Approach
0SQL0ZZ	Repair Left Metatarsal-Tarsal Joint, Open Approach
0SQL3ZZ	Repair Left Metatarsal-Tarsal Joint, Percutaneous Approach
0SQL4ZZ	Repair Left Metatarsal-Tarsal Joint, Percutaneous Endoscopic Approach
0SQLXZZ	Repair Left Metatarsal-Tarsal Joint, External Approach
0SQM0ZZ	Repair Right Metatarsal-Phalangeal Joint, Open Approach
0SQM3ZZ	Repair Right Metatarsal-Phalangeal Joint, Percutaneous Approach
0SQM4ZZ	Repair Right Metatarsal-Phalangeal Joint, Percutaneous Endoscopic Approach
0SQMXZZ	Repair Right Metatarsal-Phalangeal Joint, External Approach
0SQN0ZZ	Repair Left Metatarsal-Phalangeal Joint, Open Approach
0SQN3ZZ	Repair Left Metatarsal-Phalangeal Joint, Percutaneous Approach
0SQN4ZZ	Repair Left Metatarsal-Phalangeal Joint, Percutaneous Endoscopic Approach
0SQNXZZ	Repair Left Metatarsal-Phalangeal Joint, External Approach
0SQP0ZZ	Repair Right Toe Phalangeal Joint, Open Approach
0SQP3ZZ	Repair Right Toe Phalangeal Joint, Percutaneous Approach
0SQP4ZZ	Repair Right Toe Phalangeal Joint, Percutaneous Endoscopic Approach
0SQPXZZ	Repair Right Toe Phalangeal Joint, External Approach
0SQQ0ZZ	Repair Left Toe Phalangeal Joint, Open Approach
0SQQ3ZZ	Repair Left Toe Phalangeal Joint, Percutaneous Approach
0SQQ4ZZ	Repair Left Toe Phalangeal Joint, Percutaneous Endoscopic Approach
0SQQXZZ	Repair Left Toe Phalangeal Joint, External Approach

0SR – Lower Joints, Replacement

0SR007Z	Replacement of Lumbar Vertebral Joint with Autologous Tissue Substitute, Open Approach
0SR00JZ	Replacement of Lumbar Vertebral Joint with Synthetic Substitute, Open Approach
0SR00KZ	Replacement of Lumbar Vertebral Joint with Nonautologous Tissue Substitute, Open Approach
0SR207Z	Replacement of Lumbar Vertebral Disc with Autologous Tissue Substitute, Open Approach
0SR20JZ	Replacement of Lumbar Vertebral Disc with Synthetic Substitute, Open Approach
●	*When the patients age is greater than 60 years old*
0SR20KZ	Replacement of Lumbar Vertebral Disc with Nonautologous Tissue Substitute, Open Approach
0SR307Z	Replacement of Lumbosacral Joint with Autologous Tissue Substitute, Open Approach
0SR30JZ	Replacement of Lumbosacral Joint with Synthetic Substitute, Open Approach
0SR30KZ	Replacement of Lumbosacral Joint with Nonautologous Tissue Substitute, Open Approach
0SR407Z	Replacement of Lumbosacral Disc with Autologous Tissue Substitute, Open Approach
0SR40JZ	Replacement of Lumbosacral Disc with Synthetic Substitute, Open Approach
●	*When the patients age is greater than 60 years old*
0SR40KZ	Replacement of Lumbosacral Disc with Nonautologous Tissue Substitute, Open Approach
0SR507Z	Replacement of Sacrococcygeal Joint with Autologous Tissue Substitute, Open Approach
0SR50JZ	Replacement of Sacrococcygeal Joint with Synthetic Substitute, Open Approach
0SR50KZ	Replacement of Sacrococcygeal Joint with Nonautologous Tissue Substitute, Open Approach

0SR607Z	Replacement of Coccygeal Joint with Autologous Tissue Substitute, Open Approach
0SR60JZ	Replacement of Coccygeal Joint with Synthetic Substitute, Open Approach
0SR60KZ	Replacement of Coccygeal Joint with Nonautologous Tissue Substitute, Open Approach
0SR707Z	Replacement of Right Sacroiliac Joint with Autologous Tissue Substitute, Open Approach
0SR70JZ	Replacement of Right Sacroiliac Joint with Synthetic Substitute, Open Approach
0SR70KZ	Replacement of Right Sacroiliac Joint with Nonautologous Tissue Substitute, Open Approach
0SR807Z	Replacement of Left Sacroiliac Joint with Autologous Tissue Substitute, Open Approach
0SR80JZ	Replacement of Left Sacroiliac Joint with Synthetic Substitute, Open Approach
0SR80KZ	Replacement of Left Sacroiliac Joint with Nonautologous Tissue Substitute, Open Approach
0SR9019	Replacement of Right Hip Joint with Metal Synthetic Substitute, Cemented, Open Approach
0SR901A	Replacement of Right Hip Joint with Metal Synthetic Substitute, Uncemented, Open Approach
0SR901Z	Replacement of Right Hip Joint with Metal Synthetic Substitute, Open Approach
0SR9029	Replacement of Right Hip Joint with Metal on Polyethylene Synthetic Substitute, Cemented, Open Approach
0SR902A	Replacement of Right Hip Joint with Metal on Polyethylene Synthetic Substitute, Uncemented, Open Approach
0SR902Z	Replacement of Right Hip Joint with Metal on Polyethylene Synthetic Substitute, Open Approach
0SR9039	Replacement of Right Hip Joint with Ceramic Synthetic Substitute, Cemented, Open Approach

---

♀ Female-only   ♂ Male-only   ○ Limited Coverage   ● Non-OR   ▦ HAC-associated procedure   ● Non-covered procedures   ✚ Combination

0SR903A Replacement of Right Hip Joint with Ceramic Synthetic Substitute, Uncemented, Open Approach

0SR903Z Replacement of Right Hip Joint with Ceramic Synthetic Substitute, Open Approach

0SR9049 Replacement of Right Hip Joint with Ceramic on Polyethylene Synthetic Substitute, Cemented, Open Approach

0SR904A Replacement of Right Hip Joint with Ceramic on Polyethylene Synthetic Substitute, Uncemented, Open Approach

0SR904Z Replacement of Right Hip Joint with Ceramic on Polyethylene Synthetic Substitute, Open Approach

0SR907Z Replacement of Right Hip Joint with Autologous Tissue Substitute, Open Approach

0SR90J9 Replacement of Right Hip Joint with Synthetic Substitute, Cemented, Open Approach

0SR90JA Replacement of Right Hip Joint with Synthetic Substitute, Uncemented, Open Approach

0SR90JZ Replacement of Right Hip Joint with Synthetic Substitute, Open Approach

0SR90KZ Replacement of Right Hip Joint with Nonautologous Tissue Substitute, Open Approach

0SRA009 Replacement of Right Hip Joint, Acetabular Surface with Polyethylene Synthetic Substitute, Cemented, Open Approach

0SRA00A Replacement of Right Hip Joint, Acetabular Surface with Polyethylene Synthetic Substitute, Uncemented, Open Approach

0SRA00Z Replacement of Right Hip Joint, Acetabular Surface with Polyethylene Synthetic Substitute, Open Approach

0SRA019 Replacement of Right Hip Joint, Acetabular Surface with Metal Synthetic Substitute, Cemented, Open Approach

0SRA01A Replacement of Right Hip Joint, Acetabular Surface with Metal Synthetic Substitute, Uncemented, Open Approach

0SRA01Z Replacement of Right Hip Joint, Acetabular Surface with Metal Synthetic Substitute, Open Approach

0SRA039 Replacement of Right Hip Joint, Acetabular Surface with Ceramic Synthetic Substitute, Cemented, Open Approach

0SRA03A Replacement of Right Hip Joint, Acetabular Surface with Ceramic Synthetic Substitute, Uncemented, Open Approach

0SRA03Z Replacement of Right Hip Joint, Acetabular Surface with Ceramic Synthetic Substitute, Open Approach

0SRA07Z Replacement of Right Hip Joint, Acetabular Surface with Autologous Tissue Substitute, Open Approach

0SRA0J9 Replacement of Right Hip Joint, Acetabular Surface with Synthetic Substitute, Cemented, Open Approach

0SRA0JA Replacement of Right Hip Joint, Acetabular Surface with Synthetic Substitute, Uncemented, Open Approach

0SRA0JZ Replacement of Right Hip Joint, Acetabular Surface with Synthetic Substitute, Open Approach

0SRA0KZ Replacement of Right Hip Joint, Acetabular Surface with Nonautologous Tissue Substitute, Open Approach

0SRB019 Replacement of Left Hip Joint with Metal Synthetic Substitute, Cemented, Open Approach

0SRB01A Replacement of Left Hip Joint with Metal Synthetic Substitute, Uncemented, Open Approach

0SRB01Z Replacement of Left Hip Joint with Metal Synthetic Substitute, Open Approach

0SRB029 Replacement of Left Hip Joint with Metal on Polyethylene Synthetic Substitute, Cemented, Open Approach

0SRB02A Replacement of Left Hip Joint with Metal on Polyethylene Synthetic Substitute, Uncemented, Open Approach

0SRB02Z Replacement of Left Hip Joint with Metal on Polyethylene Synthetic Substitute, Open Approach

0SRB039 Replacement of Left Hip Joint with Ceramic Synthetic Substitute, Cemented, Open Approach

0SRB03A Replacement of Left Hip Joint with Ceramic Synthetic Substitute, Uncemented, Open Approach

0SRB03Z Replacement of Left Hip Joint with Ceramic Synthetic Substitute, Open Approach

0SRB049 Replacement of Left Hip Joint with Ceramic on Polyethylene Synthetic Substitute, Cemented, Open Approach

0SRB04A Replacement of Left Hip Joint with Ceramic on Polyethylene Synthetic Substitute, Uncemented, Open Approach

0SRB04Z Replacement of Left Hip Joint with Ceramic on Polyethylene Synthetic Substitute, Open Approach

0SRB07Z Replacement of Left Hip Joint with Autologous Tissue Substitute, Open Approach

0SRB0J9 Replacement of Left Hip Joint with Synthetic Substitute, Cemented, Open Approach

0SRB0JA Replacement of Left Hip Joint with Synthetic Substitute, Uncemented, Open Approach

0SRB0JZ Replacement of Left Hip Joint with Synthetic Substitute, Open Approach

0SRB0KZ Replacement of Left Hip Joint with Nonautologous Tissue Substitute, Open Approach

0SRC07Z Replacement of Right Knee Joint with Autologous Tissue Substitute, Open Approach

0SRC0J9 Replacement of Right Knee Joint with Synthetic Substitute, Cemented, Open Approach

0SRC0JA Replacement of Right Knee Joint with Synthetic Substitute, Uncemented, Open Approach

0SRC0JZ Replacement of Right Knee Joint with Synthetic Substitute, Open Approach

0SRC0KZ Replacement of Right Knee Joint with Nonautologous Tissue Substitute, Open Approach

0SRD07Z Replacement of Left Knee Joint with Autologous Tissue Substitute, Open Approach

0SRD0J9 Replacement of Left Knee Joint with Synthetic Substitute, Cemented, Open Approach

0SRD0JA Replacement of Left Knee Joint with Synthetic Substitute, Uncemented, Open Approach

0SRD0JZ Replacement of Left Knee Joint with Synthetic Substitute, Open Approach

0SRD0KZ Replacement of Left Knee Joint with Nonautologous Tissue Substitute, Open Approach

0SRE009 Replacement of Left Hip Joint, Acetabular Surface with Polyethylene Synthetic Substitute, Cemented, Open Approach

0SRE00A Replacement of Left Hip Joint, Acetabular Surface with Polyethylene Synthetic Substitute, Uncemented, Open Approach

0SRE00Z Replacement of Left Hip Joint, Acetabular Surface with Polyethylene Synthetic Substitute, Open Approach

0SRE019 Replacement of Left Hip Joint, Acetabular Surface with Metal Synthetic Substitute, Cemented, Open Approach

0SRE01A Replacement of Left Hip Joint, Acetabular Surface with Metal Synthetic Substitute, Uncemented, Open Approach

0SRE01Z Replacement of Left Hip Joint, Acetabular Surface with Metal Synthetic Substitute, Open Approach

0SRE039 Replacement of Left Hip Joint, Acetabular Surface with Ceramic Synthetic Substitute, Cemented, Open Approach

0SRE03A Replacement of Left Hip Joint, Acetabular Surface with Ceramic Synthetic Substitute, Uncemented, Open Approach

0SRE03Z Replacement of Left Hip Joint, Acetabular Surface with Ceramic Synthetic Substitute, Open Approach

0SRE07Z Replacement of Left Hip Joint, Acetabular Surface with Autologous Tissue Substitute, Open Approach

0SRE0J9 Replacement of Left Hip Joint, Acetabular Surface with Synthetic Substitute, Cemented, Open Approach

0SRE0JA Replacement of Left Hip Joint, Acetabular Surface with Synthetic Substitute, Uncemented, Open Approach

0SRE0JZ Replacement of Left Hip Joint, Acetabular Surface with Synthetic Substitute, Open Approach

0SRE0KZ Replacement of Left Hip Joint, Acetabular Surface with Nonautologous Tissue Substitute, Open Approach

0SRF07Z Replacement of Right Ankle Joint with Autologous Tissue Substitute, Open Approach

0SRF0J9 Replacement of Right Ankle Joint with Synthetic Substitute, Cemented, Open Approach

0SRF0JA Replacement of Right Ankle Joint with Synthetic Substitute, Uncemented, Open Approach

0SRF0JZ Replacement of Right Ankle Joint with Synthetic Substitute, Open Approach

0SRF0KZ Replacement of Right Ankle Joint with Nonautologous Tissue Substitute, Open Approach

0SRG07Z Replacement of Left Ankle Joint with Autologous Tissue Substitute, Open Approach

0SRG0J9 Replacement of Left Ankle Joint with Synthetic Substitute, Cemented, Open Approach

0SRG0JA Replacement of Left Ankle Joint with Synthetic Substitute, Uncemented, Open Approach

0SRG0JZ Replacement of Left Ankle Joint with Synthetic Substitute, Open Approach

0SRG0KZ   Replacement of Left Ankle Joint with Nonautologous Tissue Substitute, Open Approach

0SRH07Z   Replacement of Right Tarsal Joint with Autologous Tissue Substitute, Open Approach

0SRH0JZ   Replacement of Right Tarsal Joint with Synthetic Substitute, Open Approach

0SRH0KZ   Replacement of Right Tarsal Joint with Nonautologous Tissue Substitute, Open Approach

0SRJ07Z   Replacement of Left Tarsal Joint with Autologous Tissue Substitute, Open Approach

0SRJ0JZ   Replacement of Left Tarsal Joint with Synthetic Substitute, Open Approach

0SRJ0KZ   Replacement of Left Tarsal Joint with Nonautologous Tissue Substitute, Open Approach

0SRK07Z   Replacement of Right Metatarsal-Tarsal Joint with Autologous Tissue Substitute, Open Approach

0SRK0JZ   Replacement of Right Metatarsal-Tarsal Joint with Synthetic Substitute, Open Approach

0SRK0KZ   Replacement of Right Metatarsal-Tarsal Joint with Nonautologous Tissue Substitute, Open Approach

0SRL07Z   Replacement of Left Metatarsal-Tarsal Joint with Autologous Tissue Substitute, Open Approach

0SRL0JZ   Replacement of Left Metatarsal-Tarsal Joint with Synthetic Substitute, Open Approach

0SRL0KZ   Replacement of Left Metatarsal-Tarsal Joint with Nonautologous Tissue Substitute, Open Approach

0SRM07Z   Replacement of Right Metatarsal-Phalangeal Joint with Autologous Tissue Substitute, Open Approach

0SRM0JZ   Replacement of Right Metatarsal-Phalangeal Joint with Synthetic Substitute, Open Approach

0SRM0KZ   Replacement of Right Metatarsal-Phalangeal Joint with Nonautologous Tissue Substitute, Open Approach

0SRN07Z   Replacement of Left Metatarsal-Phalangeal Joint with Autologous Tissue Substitute, Open Approach

0SRN0JZ   Replacement of Left Metatarsal-Phalangeal Joint with Synthetic Substitute, Open Approach

0SRN0KZ   Replacement of Left Metatarsal-Phalangeal Joint with Nonautologous Tissue Substitute, Open Approach

0SRP07Z   Replacement of Right Toe Phalangeal Joint with Autologous Tissue Substitute, Open Approach

0SRP0JZ   Replacement of Right Toe Phalangeal Joint with Synthetic Substitute, Open Approach

0SRP0KZ   Replacement of Right Toe Phalangeal Joint with Nonautologous Tissue Substitute, Open Approach

0SRQ07Z   Replacement of Left Toe Phalangeal Joint with Autologous Tissue Substitute, Open Approach

0SRQ0JZ   Replacement of Left Toe Phalangeal Joint with Synthetic Substitute, Open Approach

0SRQ0KZ   Replacement of Left Toe Phalangeal Joint with Nonautologous Tissue Substitute, Open Approach

0SRR019   Replacement of Right Hip Joint, Femoral Surface with Metal Synthetic Substitute, Cemented, Open Approach

0SRR01A   Replacement of Right Hip Joint, Femoral Surface with Metal Synthetic Substitute, Uncemented, Open Approach

0SRR01Z   Replacement of Right Hip Joint, Femoral Surface with Metal Synthetic Substitute, Open Approach

0SRR039   Replacement of Right Hip Joint, Femoral Surface with Ceramic Synthetic Substitute, Cemented, Open Approach

0SRR03A   Replacement of Right Hip Joint, Femoral Surface with Ceramic Synthetic Substitute, Uncemented, Open Approach

0SRR03Z   Replacement of Right Hip Joint, Femoral Surface with Ceramic Synthetic Substitute, Open Approach

0SRR07Z   Replacement of Right Hip Joint, Femoral Surface with Autologous Tissue Substitute, Open Approach

0SRR0J9   Replacement of Right Hip Joint, Femoral Surface with Synthetic Substitute, Cemented, Open Approach

0SRR0JA   Replacement of Right Hip Joint, Femoral Surface with Synthetic Substitute, Uncemented, Open Approach

0SRR0JZ   Replacement of Right Hip Joint, Femoral Surface with Synthetic Substitute, Open Approach

0SRR0KZ   Replacement of Right Hip Joint, Femoral Surface with Nonautologous Tissue Substitute, Open Approach

0SRS019   Replacement of Left Hip Joint, Femoral Surface with Metal Synthetic Substitute, Cemented, Open Approach

0SRS01A   Replacement of Left Hip Joint, Femoral Surface with Metal Synthetic Substitute, Uncemented, Open Approach

0SRS01Z   Replacement of Left Hip Joint, Femoral Surface with Metal Synthetic Substitute, Open Approach

0SRS039   Replacement of Left Hip Joint, Femoral Surface with Ceramic Synthetic Substitute, Cemented, Open Approach

0SRS03A   Replacement of Left Hip Joint, Femoral Surface with Ceramic Synthetic Substitute, Uncemented, Open Approach

0SRS03Z   Replacement of Left Hip Joint, Femoral Surface with Ceramic Synthetic Substitute, Open Approach

0SRS07Z   Replacement of Left Hip Joint, Femoral Surface with Autologous Tissue Substitute, Open Approach

0SRS0J9   Replacement of Left Hip Joint, Femoral Surface with Synthetic Substitute, Cemented, Open Approach

0SRS0JA   Replacement of Left Hip Joint, Femoral Surface with Synthetic Substitute, Uncemented, Open Approach

0SRS0JZ   Replacement of Left Hip Joint, Femoral Surface with Synthetic Substitute, Open Approach

0SRS0KZ   Replacement of Left Hip Joint, Femoral Surface with Nonautologous Tissue Substitute, Open Approach

0SRT07Z   Replacement of Right Knee Joint, Femoral Surface with Autologous Tissue Substitute, Open Approach

0SRT0J9   Replacement of Right Knee Joint, Femoral Surface with Synthetic Substitute, Cemented, Open Approach

0SRT0JA   Replacement of Right Knee Joint, Femoral Surface with Synthetic Substitute, Uncemented, Open Approach

0SRT0JZ   Replacement of Right Knee Joint, Femoral Surface with Synthetic Substitute, Open Approach

0SRT0KZ   Replacement of Right Knee Joint, Femoral Surface with Nonautologous Tissue Substitute, Open Approach

0SRU07Z   Replacement of Left Knee Joint, Femoral Surface with Autologous Tissue Substitute, Open Approach

0SRU0J9   Replacement of Left Knee Joint, Femoral Surface with Synthetic Substitute, Cemented, Open Approach

0SRU0JA   Replacement of Left Knee Joint, Femoral Surface with Synthetic Substitute, Uncemented, Open Approach

0SRU0JZ   Replacement of Left Knee Joint, Femoral Surface with Synthetic Substitute, Open Approach

0SRU0KZ   Replacement of Left Knee Joint, Femoral Surface with Nonautologous Tissue Substitute, Open Approach

0SRV07Z   Replacement of Right Knee Joint, Tibial Surface with Autologous Tissue Substitute, Open Approach

0SRV0J9   Replacement of Right Knee Joint, Tibial Surface with Synthetic Substitute, Cemented, Open Approach

0SRV0JA   Replacement of Right Knee Joint, Tibial Surface with Synthetic Substitute, Uncemented, Open Approach

0SRV0JZ   Replacement of Right Knee Joint, Tibial Surface with Synthetic Substitute, Open Approach

0SRV0KZ   Replacement of Right Knee Joint, Tibial Surface with Nonautologous Tissue Substitute, Open Approach

0SRW07Z   Replacement of Left Knee Joint, Tibial Surface with Autologous Tissue Substitute, Open Approach

0SRW0J9   Replacement of Left Knee Joint, Tibial Surface with Synthetic Substitute, Cemented, Open Approach

0SRW0JA   Replacement of Left Knee Joint, Tibial Surface with Synthetic Substitute, Uncemented, Open Approach

0SRW0JZ   Replacement of Left Knee Joint, Tibial Surface with Synthetic Substitute, Open Approach

0SRW0KZ   Replacement of Left Knee Joint, Tibial Surface with Nonautologous Tissue Substitute, Open Approach

0SS – Lower Joints, Reposition

0SS004Z   Reposition Lumbar Vertebral Joint with Internal Fixation Device, Open Approach

0SS00ZZ   Reposition Lumbar Vertebral Joint, Open Approach

0SS034Z   Reposition Lumbar Vertebral Joint with Internal Fixation Device, Percutaneous Approach

0SS03ZZ   Reposition Lumbar Vertebral Joint, Percutaneous Approach

---

♀ Female-only   ♂ Male-only   ● Limited Coverage   ● Non-OR   ▥ HAC-associated procedure   ● Non-covered procedures   ✚ Combination

0SS044Z   Reposition Lumbar Vertebral Joint with Internal Fixation Device, Percutaneous Endoscopic Approach

0SS04ZZ   Reposition Lumbar Vertebral Joint, Percutaneous Endoscopic Approach

0SS0X4Z   Reposition Lumbar Vertebral Joint with Internal Fixation Device, External Approach

0SS0XZZ   Reposition Lumbar Vertebral Joint, External Approach

0SS304Z   Reposition Lumbosacral Joint with Internal Fixation Device, Open Approach

0SS30ZZ   Reposition Lumbosacral Joint, Open Approach

0SS334Z   Reposition Lumbosacral Joint with Internal Fixation Device, Percutaneous Approach

0SS33ZZ   Reposition Lumbosacral Joint, Percutaneous Approach

0SS344Z   Reposition Lumbosacral Joint with Internal Fixation Device, Percutaneous Endoscopic Approach

0SS34ZZ   Reposition Lumbosacral Joint, Percutaneous Endoscopic Approach

0SS3X4Z   Reposition Lumbosacral Joint with Internal Fixation Device, External Approach

0SS3XZZ   Reposition Lumbosacral Joint, External Approach

0SS504Z   Reposition Sacrococcygeal Joint with Internal Fixation Device, Open Approach

0SS50ZZ   Reposition Sacrococcygeal Joint, Open Approach

0SS534Z   Reposition Sacrococcygeal Joint with Internal Fixation Device, Percutaneous Approach

0SS53ZZ   Reposition Sacrococcygeal Joint, Percutaneous Approach

0SS544Z   Reposition Sacrococcygeal Joint with Internal Fixation Device, Percutaneous Endoscopic Approach

0SS54ZZ   Reposition Sacrococcygeal Joint, Percutaneous Endoscopic Approach

0SS5X4Z   Reposition Sacrococcygeal Joint with Internal Fixation Device, External Approach

0SS5XZZ   Reposition Sacrococcygeal Joint, External Approach

0SS604Z   Reposition Coccygeal Joint with Internal Fixation Device, Open Approach

0SS60ZZ   Reposition Coccygeal Joint, Open Approach

0SS634Z   Reposition Coccygeal Joint with Internal Fixation Device, Percutaneous Approach

0SS63ZZ   Reposition Coccygeal Joint, Percutaneous Approach

0SS644Z   Reposition Coccygeal Joint with Internal Fixation Device, Percutaneous Endoscopic Approach

0SS64ZZ   Reposition Coccygeal Joint, Percutaneous Endoscopic Approach

0SS6X4Z   Reposition Coccygeal Joint with Internal Fixation Device, External Approach

0SS6XZZ   Reposition Coccygeal Joint, External Approach

0SS704Z   Reposition Right Sacroiliac Joint with Internal Fixation Device, Open Approach

0SS70ZZ   Reposition Right Sacroiliac Joint, Open Approach

0SS734Z   Reposition Right Sacroiliac Joint with Internal Fixation Device, Percutaneous Approach

0SS73ZZ   Reposition Right Sacroiliac Joint, Percutaneous Approach

0SS744Z   Reposition Right Sacroiliac Joint with Internal Fixation Device, Percutaneous Endoscopic Approach

0SS74ZZ   Reposition Right Sacroiliac Joint, Percutaneous Endoscopic Approach

0SS7X4Z   Reposition Right Sacroiliac Joint with Internal Fixation Device, External Approach

0SS7XZZ   Reposition Right Sacroiliac Joint, External Approach

0SS804Z   Reposition Left Sacroiliac Joint with Internal Fixation Device, Open Approach

0SS80ZZ   Reposition Left Sacroiliac Joint, Open Approach

0SS834Z   Reposition Left Sacroiliac Joint with Internal Fixation Device, Percutaneous Approach

0SS83ZZ   Reposition Left Sacroiliac Joint, Percutaneous Approach

0SS844Z   Reposition Left Sacroiliac Joint with Internal Fixation Device, Percutaneous Endoscopic Approach

0SS84ZZ   Reposition Left Sacroiliac Joint, Percutaneous Endoscopic Approach

0SS8X4Z   Reposition Left Sacroiliac Joint with Internal Fixation Device, External Approach

0SS8XZZ   Reposition Left Sacroiliac Joint, External Approach

0SS904Z   Reposition Right Hip Joint with Internal Fixation Device, Open Approach

0SS905Z   Reposition Right Hip Joint with External Fixation Device, Open Approach

0SS90ZZ   Reposition Right Hip Joint, Open Approach

0SS934Z   Reposition Right Hip Joint with Internal Fixation Device, Percutaneous Approach

0SS935Z   Reposition Right Hip Joint with External Fixation Device, Percutaneous Approach

0SS93ZZ   Reposition Right Hip Joint, Percutaneous Approach

0SS944Z   Reposition Right Hip Joint with Internal Fixation Device, Percutaneous Endoscopic Approach

0SS945Z   Reposition Right Hip Joint with External Fixation Device, Percutaneous Endoscopic Approach

0SS94ZZ   Reposition Right Hip Joint, Percutaneous Endoscopic Approach

0SS9X4Z   Reposition Right Hip Joint with Internal Fixation Device, External Approach

0SS9X5Z   Reposition Right Hip Joint with External Fixation Device, External Approach

0SS9XZZ   Reposition Right Hip Joint, External Approach

0SSB04Z   Reposition Left Hip Joint with Internal Fixation Device, Open Approach

0SSB05Z   Reposition Left Hip Joint with External Fixation Device, Open Approach

0SSB0ZZ   Reposition Left Hip Joint, Open Approach

0SSB34Z   Reposition Left Hip Joint with Internal Fixation Device, Percutaneous Approach

0SSB35Z   Reposition Left Hip Joint with External Fixation Device, Percutaneous Approach

0SSB3ZZ   Reposition Left Hip Joint, Percutaneous Approach

0SSB44Z   Reposition Left Hip Joint with Internal Fixation Device, Percutaneous Endoscopic Approach

0SSB45Z   Reposition Left Hip Joint with External Fixation Device, Percutaneous Endoscopic Approach

0SSB4ZZ   Reposition Left Hip Joint, Percutaneous Endoscopic Approach

0SSBX4Z   Reposition Left Hip Joint with Internal Fixation Device, External Approach

0SSBX5Z   Reposition Left Hip Joint with External Fixation Device, External Approach

0SSBXZZ   Reposition Left Hip Joint, External Approach

0SSC04Z   Reposition Right Knee Joint with Internal Fixation Device, Open Approach

0SSC05Z   Reposition Right Knee Joint with External Fixation Device, Open Approach

0SSC0ZZ   Reposition Right Knee Joint, Open Approach

0SSC34Z   Reposition Right Knee Joint with Internal Fixation Device, Percutaneous Approach

0SSC35Z   Reposition Right Knee Joint with External Fixation Device, Percutaneous Approach

0SSC3ZZ   Reposition Right Knee Joint, Percutaneous Approach

0SSC44Z   Reposition Right Knee Joint with Internal Fixation Device, Percutaneous Endoscopic Approach

0SSC45Z   Reposition Right Knee Joint with External Fixation Device, Percutaneous Endoscopic Approach

0SSC4ZZ   Reposition Right Knee Joint, Percutaneous Endoscopic Approach

0SSCX4Z   Reposition Right Knee Joint with Internal Fixation Device, External Approach

0SSCX5Z   Reposition Right Knee Joint with External Fixation Device, External Approach

0SSCXZZ   Reposition Right Knee Joint, External Approach

0SSD04Z   Reposition Left Knee Joint with Internal Fixation Device, Open Approach

0SSD05Z   Reposition Left Knee Joint with External Fixation Device, Open Approach

0SSD0ZZ   Reposition Left Knee Joint, Open Approach

0SSD34Z   Reposition Left Knee Joint with Internal Fixation Device, Percutaneous Approach

0SSD35Z   Reposition Left Knee Joint with External Fixation Device, Percutaneous Approach

0SSD3ZZ   Reposition Left Knee Joint, Percutaneous Approach

0SSD44Z   Reposition Left Knee Joint with Internal Fixation Device, Percutaneous Endoscopic Approach

0SSD45Z   Reposition Left Knee Joint with External Fixation Device, Percutaneous Endoscopic Approach

0SSD4ZZ   Reposition Left Knee Joint, Percutaneous Endoscopic Approach

0SSDX4Z   Reposition Left Knee Joint with Internal Fixation Device, External Approach

0SSDX5Z   Reposition Left Knee Joint with External Fixation Device, External Approach

0SSDXZZ   Reposition Left Knee Joint, External Approach

0SSF04Z   Reposition Right Ankle Joint with Internal Fixation Device, Open Approach

0SSF05Z   Reposition Right Ankle Joint with External Fixation Device, Open Approach

0SSF0ZZ   Reposition Right Ankle Joint, Open Approach

0SSF34Z   Reposition Right Ankle Joint with Internal Fixation Device, Percutaneous Approach

0SSF35Z   Reposition Right Ankle Joint with External Fixation Device, Percutaneous Approach

0SSF3ZZ   Reposition Right Ankle Joint, Percutaneous Approach

0SSF44Z   Reposition Right Ankle Joint with Internal Fixation Device, Percutaneous Endoscopic Approach

0SSF45Z   Reposition Right Ankle Joint with External Fixation Device, Percutaneous Endoscopic Approach

0SSF4ZZ   Reposition Right Ankle Joint, Percutaneous Endoscopic Approach

0SSFX4Z   Reposition Right Ankle Joint with Internal Fixation Device, External Approach

0SSFX5Z   Reposition Right Ankle Joint with External Fixation Device, External Approach

0SSFXZZ   Reposition Right Ankle Joint, External Approach

0SSG04Z   Reposition Left Ankle Joint with Internal Fixation Device, Open Approach

0SSG05Z   Reposition Left Ankle Joint with External Fixation Device, Open Approach

0SSG0ZZ   Reposition Left Ankle Joint, Open Approach

0SSG34Z   Reposition Left Ankle Joint with Internal Fixation Device, Percutaneous Approach

0SSG35Z   Reposition Left Ankle Joint with External Fixation Device, Percutaneous Approach

0SSG3ZZ   Reposition Left Ankle Joint, Percutaneous Approach

0SSG44Z   Reposition Left Ankle Joint with Internal Fixation Device, Percutaneous Endoscopic Approach

0SSG45Z   Reposition Left Ankle Joint with External Fixation Device, Percutaneous Endoscopic Approach

0SSG4ZZ   Reposition Left Ankle Joint, Percutaneous Endoscopic Approach

0SSGX4Z   Reposition Left Ankle Joint with Internal Fixation Device, External Approach

0SSGX5Z   Reposition Left Ankle Joint with External Fixation Device, External Approach

0SSGXZZ   Reposition Left Ankle Joint, External Approach

0SSH04Z   Reposition Right Tarsal Joint with Internal Fixation Device, Open Approach

0SSH05Z   Reposition Right Tarsal Joint with External Fixation Device, Open Approach

0SSH0ZZ   Reposition Right Tarsal Joint, Open Approach

0SSH34Z   Reposition Right Tarsal Joint with Internal Fixation Device, Percutaneous Approach

0SSH35Z   Reposition Right Tarsal Joint with External Fixation Device, Percutaneous Approach

0SSH3ZZ   Reposition Right Tarsal Joint, Percutaneous Approach

0SSH44Z   Reposition Right Tarsal Joint with Internal Fixation Device, Percutaneous Endoscopic Approach

0SSH45Z   Reposition Right Tarsal Joint with External Fixation Device, Percutaneous Endoscopic Approach

0SSH4ZZ   Reposition Right Tarsal Joint, Percutaneous Endoscopic Approach

0SSHX4Z   Reposition Right Tarsal Joint with Internal Fixation Device, External Approach

0SSHX5Z   Reposition Right Tarsal Joint with External Fixation Device, External Approach

0SSHXZZ   Reposition Right Tarsal Joint, External Approach

0SSJ04Z   Reposition Left Tarsal Joint with Internal Fixation Device, Open Approach

0SSJ05Z   Reposition Left Tarsal Joint with External Fixation Device, Open Approach

0SSJ0ZZ   Reposition Left Tarsal Joint, Open Approach

0SSJ34Z   Reposition Left Tarsal Joint with Internal Fixation Device, Percutaneous Approach

0SSJ35Z   Reposition Left Tarsal Joint with External Fixation Device, Percutaneous Approach

0SSJ3ZZ   Reposition Left Tarsal Joint, Percutaneous Approach

0SSJ44Z   Reposition Left Tarsal Joint with Internal Fixation Device, Percutaneous Endoscopic Approach

0SSJ45Z   Reposition Left Tarsal Joint with External Fixation Device, Percutaneous Endoscopic Approach

0SSJ4ZZ   Reposition Left Tarsal Joint, Percutaneous Endoscopic Approach

0SSJX4Z   Reposition Left Tarsal Joint with Internal Fixation Device, External Approach

0SSJX5Z   Reposition Left Tarsal Joint with External Fixation Device, External Approach

0SSJXZZ   Reposition Left Tarsal Joint, External Approach

0SSK04Z   Reposition Right Metatarsal-Tarsal Joint with Internal Fixation Device, Open Approach

0SSK05Z   Reposition Right Metatarsal-Tarsal Joint with External Fixation Device, Open Approach

0SSK0ZZ   Reposition Right Metatarsal-Tarsal Joint, Open Approach

0SSK34Z   Reposition Right Metatarsal-Tarsal Joint with Internal Fixation Device, Percutaneous Approach

0SSK35Z   Reposition Right Metatarsal-Tarsal Joint with External Fixation Device, Percutaneous Approach

0SSK3ZZ   Reposition Right Metatarsal-Tarsal Joint, Percutaneous Approach

0SSK44Z   Reposition Right Metatarsal-Tarsal Joint with Internal Fixation Device, Percutaneous Endoscopic Approach

0SSK45Z   Reposition Right Metatarsal-Tarsal Joint with External Fixation Device, Percutaneous Endoscopic Approach

0SSK4ZZ   Reposition Right Metatarsal-Tarsal Joint, Percutaneous Endoscopic Approach

0SSKX4Z   Reposition Right Metatarsal-Tarsal Joint with Internal Fixation Device, External Approach

0SSKX5Z   Reposition Right Metatarsal-Tarsal Joint with External Fixation Device, External Approach

0SSKXZZ   Reposition Right Metatarsal-Tarsal Joint, External Approach

0SSL04Z   Reposition Left Metatarsal-Tarsal Joint with Internal Fixation Device, Open Approach

0SSL05Z   Reposition Left Metatarsal-Tarsal Joint with External Fixation Device, Open Approach

0SSL0ZZ   Reposition Left Metatarsal-Tarsal Joint, Open Approach

0SSL34Z   Reposition Left Metatarsal-Tarsal Joint with Internal Fixation Device, Percutaneous Approach

0SSL35Z   Reposition Left Metatarsal-Tarsal Joint with External Fixation Device, Percutaneous Approach

0SSL3ZZ   Reposition Left Metatarsal-Tarsal Joint, Percutaneous Approach

0SSL44Z   Reposition Left Metatarsal-Tarsal Joint with Internal Fixation Device, Percutaneous Endoscopic Approach

0SSL45Z   Reposition Left Metatarsal-Tarsal Joint with External Fixation Device, Percutaneous Endoscopic Approach

0SSL4ZZ   Reposition Left Metatarsal-Tarsal Joint, Percutaneous Endoscopic Approach

0SSLX4Z   Reposition Left Metatarsal-Tarsal Joint with Internal Fixation Device, External Approach

0SSLX5Z   Reposition Left Metatarsal-Tarsal Joint with External Fixation Device, External Approach

0SSLXZZ   Reposition Left Metatarsal-Tarsal Joint, External Approach

0SSM04Z   Reposition Right Metatarsal-Phalangeal Joint with Internal Fixation Device, Open Approach

0SSM05Z   Reposition Right Metatarsal-Phalangeal Joint with External Fixation Device, Open Approach

0SSM0ZZ   Reposition Right Metatarsal-Phalangeal Joint, Open Approach

0SSM34Z   Reposition Right Metatarsal-Phalangeal Joint with Internal Fixation Device, Percutaneous Approach

0SSM35Z   Reposition Right Metatarsal-Phalangeal Joint with External Fixation Device, Percutaneous Approach

0SSM3ZZ   Reposition Right Metatarsal-Phalangeal Joint, Percutaneous Approach

0SSM44Z   Reposition Right Metatarsal-Phalangeal Joint with Internal Fixation Device, Percutaneous Endoscopic Approach

0SSM45Z   Reposition Right Metatarsal-Phalangeal Joint with External Fixation Device, Percutaneous Endoscopic Approach

0SSM4ZZ   Reposition Right Metatarsal-Phalangeal Joint, Percutaneous Endoscopic Approach

0SSMX4Z Reposition Right Metatarsal-Phalangeal Joint with Internal Fixation Device, External Approach
0SSMX5Z Reposition Right Metatarsal-Phalangeal Joint with External Fixation Device, External Approach
0SSMXZZ Reposition Right Metatarsal-Phalangeal Joint, External Approach
0SSN04Z Reposition Left Metatarsal-Phalangeal Joint with Internal Fixation Device, Open Approach
0SSN05Z Reposition Left Metatarsal-Phalangeal Joint with External Fixation Device, Open Approach
0SSN0ZZ Reposition Left Metatarsal-Phalangeal Joint, Open Approach
0SSN34Z Reposition Left Metatarsal-Phalangeal Joint with Internal Fixation Device, Percutaneous Approach
0SSN35Z Reposition Left Metatarsal-Phalangeal Joint with External Fixation Device, Percutaneous Approach
0SSN3ZZ Reposition Left Metatarsal-Phalangeal Joint, Percutaneous Approach
0SSN44Z Reposition Left Metatarsal-Phalangeal Joint with Internal Fixation Device, Percutaneous Endoscopic Approach
0SSN45Z Reposition Left Metatarsal-Phalangeal Joint with External Fixation Device, Percutaneous Endoscopic Approach
0SSN4ZZ Reposition Left Metatarsal-Phalangeal Joint, Percutaneous Endoscopic Approach
0SSNX4Z Reposition Left Metatarsal-Phalangeal Joint with Internal Fixation Device, External Approach
0SSNX5Z Reposition Left Metatarsal-Phalangeal Joint with External Fixation Device, External Approach
0SSNXZZ Reposition Left Metatarsal-Phalangeal Joint, External Approach
0SSP04Z Reposition Right Toe Phalangeal Joint with Internal Fixation Device, Open Approach
0SSP05Z Reposition Right Toe Phalangeal Joint with External Fixation Device, Open Approach
0SSP0ZZ Reposition Right Toe Phalangeal Joint, Open Approach
0SSP34Z Reposition Right Toe Phalangeal Joint with Internal Fixation Device, Percutaneous Approach
0SSP35Z Reposition Right Toe Phalangeal Joint with External Fixation Device, Percutaneous Approach

0SSP3ZZ Reposition Right Toe Phalangeal Joint, Percutaneous Approach
0SSP44Z Reposition Right Toe Phalangeal Joint with Internal Fixation Device, Percutaneous Endoscopic Approach
0SSP45Z Reposition Right Toe Phalangeal Joint with External Fixation Device, Percutaneous Endoscopic Approach
0SSP4ZZ Reposition Right Toe Phalangeal Joint, Percutaneous Endoscopic Approach
0SSPX4Z Reposition Right Toe Phalangeal Joint with Internal Fixation Device, External Approach
0SSPX5Z Reposition Right Toe Phalangeal Joint with External Fixation Device, External Approach
0SSPXZZ Reposition Right Toe Phalangeal Joint, External Approach
0SSQ04Z Reposition Left Toe Phalangeal Joint with Internal Fixation Device, Open Approach
0SSQ05Z Reposition Left Toe Phalangeal Joint with External Fixation Device, Open Approach
0SSQ0ZZ Reposition Left Toe Phalangeal Joint, Open Approach
0SSQ34Z Reposition Left Toe Phalangeal Joint with Internal Fixation Device, Percutaneous Approach
0SSQ35Z Reposition Left Toe Phalangeal Joint with External Fixation Device, Percutaneous Approach
0SSQ3ZZ Reposition Left Toe Phalangeal Joint, Percutaneous Approach
0SSQ44Z Reposition Left Toe Phalangeal Joint with Internal Fixation Device, Percutaneous Endoscopic Approach
0SSQ45Z Reposition Left Toe Phalangeal Joint with External Fixation Device, Percutaneous Endoscopic Approach
0SSQ4ZZ Reposition Left Toe Phalangeal Joint, Percutaneous Endoscopic Approach
0SSQX4Z Reposition Left Toe Phalangeal Joint with Internal Fixation Device, External Approach
0SSQX5Z Reposition Left Toe Phalangeal Joint with External Fixation Device, External Approach
0SSQXZZ Reposition Left Toe Phalangeal Joint, External Approach

0ST – Lower Joints, Resection

Review Coding Guideline B3.8

0ST20ZZ Resection of Lumbar Vertebral Disc, Open Approach
0ST40ZZ Resection of Lumbosacral Disc, Open Approach
0ST50ZZ Resection of Sacrococcygeal Joint, Open Approach
0ST60ZZ Resection of Coccygeal Joint, Open Approach
0ST70ZZ Resection of Right Sacroiliac Joint, Open Approach
0ST80ZZ Resection of Left Sacroiliac Joint, Open Approach
0ST90ZZ Resection of Right Hip Joint, Open Approach
0STB0ZZ Resection of Left Hip Joint, Open Approach
0STC0ZZ Resection of Right Knee Joint, Open Approach
0STD0ZZ Resection of Left Knee Joint, Open Approach

0STF0ZZ Resection of Right Ankle Joint, Open Approach
0STG0ZZ Resection of Left Ankle Joint, Open Approach
0STH0ZZ Resection of Right Tarsal Joint, Open Approach
0STJ0ZZ Resection of Left Tarsal Joint, Open Approach
0STK0ZZ Resection of Right Metatarsal-Tarsal Joint, Open Approach
0STL0ZZ Resection of Left Metatarsal-Tarsal Joint, Open Approach
0STM0ZZ Resection of Right Metatarsal-Phalangeal Joint, Open Approach
0STN0ZZ Resection of Left Metatarsal-Phalangeal Joint, Open Approach
0STP0ZZ Resection of Right Toe Phalangeal Joint, Open Approach
0STQ0ZZ Resection of Left Toe Phalangeal Joint, Open Approach

0SU – Lower Joints, Supplement

0SU007Z Supplement Lumbar Vertebral Joint with Autologous Tissue Substitute, Open Approach
0SU00JZ Supplement Lumbar Vertebral Joint with Synthetic Substitute, Open Approach
0SU00KZ Supplement Lumbar Vertebral Joint with Nonautologous Tissue Substitute, Open Approach
0SU037Z Supplement Lumbar Vertebral Joint with Autologous Tissue Substitute, Percutaneous Approach
0SU03JZ Supplement Lumbar Vertebral Joint with Synthetic Substitute, Percutaneous Approach
0SU03KZ Supplement Lumbar Vertebral Joint with Nonautologous Tissue Substitute, Percutaneous Approach
0SU047Z Supplement Lumbar Vertebral Joint with Autologous Tissue Substitute, Percutaneous Endoscopic Approach
0SU04JZ Supplement Lumbar Vertebral Joint with Synthetic Substitute, Percutaneous Endoscopic Approach
0SU04KZ Supplement Lumbar Vertebral Joint with Nonautologous Tissue Substitute, Percutaneous Endoscopic Approach
0SU207Z Supplement Lumbar Vertebral Disc with Autologous Tissue Substitute, Open Approach

0SU20JZ Supplement Lumbar Vertebral Disc with Synthetic Substitute, Open Approach
0SU20KZ Supplement Lumbar Vertebral Disc with Nonautologous Tissue Substitute, Open Approach
0SU237Z Supplement Lumbar Vertebral Disc with Autologous Tissue Substitute, Percutaneous Approach
0SU23JZ Supplement Lumbar Vertebral Disc with Synthetic Substitute, Percutaneous Approach
0SU23KZ Supplement Lumbar Vertebral Disc with Nonautologous Tissue Substitute, Percutaneous Approach
0SU247Z Supplement Lumbar Vertebral Disc with Autologous Tissue Substitute, Percutaneous Endoscopic Approach
0SU24JZ Supplement Lumbar Vertebral Disc with Synthetic Substitute, Percutaneous Endoscopic Approach
0SU24KZ Supplement Lumbar Vertebral Disc with Nonautologous Tissue Substitute, Percutaneous Endoscopic Approach
0SU307Z Supplement Lumbosacral Joint with Autologous Tissue Substitute, Open Approach
0SU30JZ Supplement Lumbosacral Joint with Synthetic Substitute, Open Approach

0SU30KZ Supplement Lumbosacral Joint with Nonautologous Tissue Substitute, Open Approach

0SU337Z Supplement Lumbosacral Joint with Autologous Tissue Substitute, Percutaneous Approach

0SU33JZ Supplement Lumbosacral Joint with Synthetic Substitute, Percutaneous Approach

0SU33KZ Supplement Lumbosacral Joint with Nonautologous Tissue Substitute, Percutaneous Approach

0SU347Z Supplement Lumbosacral Joint with Autologous Tissue Substitute, Percutaneous Endoscopic Approach

0SU34JZ Supplement Lumbosacral Joint with Synthetic Substitute, Percutaneous Endoscopic Approach

0SU34KZ Supplement Lumbosacral Joint with Nonautologous Tissue Substitute, Percutaneous Endoscopic Approach

0SU407Z Supplement Lumbosacral Disc with Autologous Tissue Substitute, Open Approach

0SU40JZ Supplement Lumbosacral Disc with Synthetic Substitute, Open Approach

0SU40KZ Supplement Lumbosacral Disc with Nonautologous Tissue Substitute, Open Approach

0SU437Z Supplement Lumbosacral Disc with Autologous Tissue Substitute, Percutaneous Approach

0SU43JZ Supplement Lumbosacral Disc with Synthetic Substitute, Percutaneous Approach

0SU43KZ Supplement Lumbosacral Disc with Nonautologous Tissue Substitute, Percutaneous Approach

0SU447Z Supplement Lumbosacral Disc with Autologous Tissue Substitute, Percutaneous Endoscopic Approach

0SU44JZ Supplement Lumbosacral Disc with Synthetic Substitute, Percutaneous Endoscopic Approach

0SU44KZ Supplement Lumbosacral Disc with Nonautologous Tissue Substitute, Percutaneous Endoscopic Approach

0SU507Z Supplement Sacrococcygeal Joint with Autologous Tissue Substitute, Open Approach

0SU50JZ Supplement Sacrococcygeal Joint with Synthetic Substitute, Open Approach

0SU50KZ Supplement Sacrococcygeal Joint with Nonautologous Tissue Substitute, Open Approach

0SU537Z Supplement Sacrococcygeal Joint with Autologous Tissue Substitute, Percutaneous Approach

0SU53JZ Supplement Sacrococcygeal Joint with Synthetic Substitute, Percutaneous Approach

0SU53KZ Supplement Sacrococcygeal Joint with Nonautologous Tissue Substitute, Percutaneous Approach

0SU547Z Supplement Sacrococcygeal Joint with Autologous Tissue Substitute, Percutaneous Endoscopic Approach

0SU54JZ Supplement Sacrococcygeal Joint with Synthetic Substitute, Percutaneous Endoscopic Approach

0SU54KZ Supplement Sacrococcygeal Joint with Nonautologous Tissue Substitute, Percutaneous Endoscopic Approach

0SU607Z Supplement Coccygeal Joint with Autologous Tissue Substitute, Open Approach

0SU60JZ Supplement Coccygeal Joint with Synthetic Substitute, Open Approach

0SU60KZ Supplement Coccygeal Joint with Nonautologous Tissue Substitute, Open Approach

0SU637Z Supplement Coccygeal Joint with Autologous Tissue Substitute, Percutaneous Approach

0SU63JZ Supplement Coccygeal Joint with Synthetic Substitute, Percutaneous Approach

0SU63KZ Supplement Coccygeal Joint with Nonautologous Tissue Substitute, Percutaneous Approach

0SU647Z Supplement Coccygeal Joint with Autologous Tissue Substitute, Percutaneous Endoscopic Approach

0SU64JZ Supplement Coccygeal Joint with Synthetic Substitute, Percutaneous Endoscopic Approach

0SU64KZ Supplement Coccygeal Joint with Nonautologous Tissue Substitute, Percutaneous Endoscopic Approach

0SU707Z Supplement Right Sacroiliac Joint with Autologous Tissue Substitute, Open Approach

0SU70JZ Supplement Right Sacroiliac Joint with Synthetic Substitute, Open Approach

0SU70KZ Supplement Right Sacroiliac Joint with Nonautologous Tissue Substitute, Open Approach

0SU737Z Supplement Right Sacroiliac Joint with Autologous Tissue Substitute, Percutaneous Approach

0SU73JZ Supplement Right Sacroiliac Joint with Synthetic Substitute, Percutaneous Approach

0SU73KZ Supplement Right Sacroiliac Joint with Nonautologous Tissue Substitute, Percutaneous Approach

0SU747Z Supplement Right Sacroiliac Joint with Autologous Tissue Substitute, Percutaneous Endoscopic Approach

0SU74JZ Supplement Right Sacroiliac Joint with Synthetic Substitute, Percutaneous Endoscopic Approach

0SU74KZ Supplement Right Sacroiliac Joint with Nonautologous Tissue Substitute, Percutaneous Endoscopic Approach

0SU807Z Supplement Left Sacroiliac Joint with Autologous Tissue Substitute, Open Approach

0SU80JZ Supplement Left Sacroiliac Joint with Synthetic Substitute, Open Approach

0SU80KZ Supplement Left Sacroiliac Joint with Nonautologous Tissue Substitute, Open Approach

0SU837Z Supplement Left Sacroiliac Joint with Autologous Tissue Substitute, Percutaneous Approach

0SU83JZ Supplement Left Sacroiliac Joint with Synthetic Substitute, Percutaneous Approach

0SU83KZ Supplement Left Sacroiliac Joint with Nonautologous Tissue Substitute, Percutaneous Approach

0SU847Z Supplement Left Sacroiliac Joint with Autologous Tissue Substitute, Percutaneous Endoscopic Approach

0SU84JZ Supplement Left Sacroiliac Joint with Synthetic Substitute, Percutaneous Endoscopic Approach

0SU84KZ Supplement Left Sacroiliac Joint with Nonautologous Tissue Substitute, Percutaneous Endoscopic Approach

0SU907Z Supplement Right Hip Joint with Autologous Tissue Substitute, Open Approach

0SU909Z Supplement Right Hip Joint with Liner, Open Approach

0SU90BZ Supplement Right Hip Joint with Resurfacing Device, Open Approach

    HAC   When reported with secondary diagnosis code I26.02, I26.09, I26.92, I26.99, I82.401-I82.4Z9

0SU90JZ Supplement Right Hip Joint with Synthetic Substitute, Open Approach

0SU90KZ Supplement Right Hip Joint with Nonautologous Tissue Substitute, Open Approach

0SU937Z Supplement Right Hip Joint with Autologous Tissue Substitute, Percutaneous Approach

0SU93JZ Supplement Right Hip Joint with Synthetic Substitute, Percutaneous Approach

0SU93KZ Supplement Right Hip Joint with Nonautologous Tissue Substitute, Percutaneous Approach

0SU947Z Supplement Right Hip Joint with Autologous Tissue Substitute, Percutaneous Endoscopic Approach

0SU94JZ Supplement Right Hip Joint with Synthetic Substitute, Percutaneous Endoscopic Approach

0SU94KZ Supplement Right Hip Joint with Nonautologous Tissue Substitute, Percutaneous Endoscopic Approach

0SUA09Z Supplement Right Hip Joint, Acetabular Surface with Liner, Open Approach

0SUA0BZ Supplement Right Hip Joint, Acetabular Surface with Resurfacing Device, Open Approach

    HAC   When reported with secondary diagnosis code I26.02, I26.09, I26.92, I26.99, I82.401-I82.4Z9

0SUB07Z Supplement Left Hip Joint with Autologous Tissue Substitute, Open Approach

0SUB09Z Supplement Left Hip Joint with Liner, Open Approach

0SUB0BZ Supplement Left Hip Joint with Resurfacing Device, Open Approach

    HAC   When reported with secondary diagnosis code I26.02, I26.09, I26.92, I26.99, I82.401-I82.4Z9

0SUB0JZ Supplement Left Hip Joint with Synthetic Substitute, Open Approach

0SUB0KZ Supplement Left Hip Joint with Nonautologous Tissue Substitute, Open Approach

0SUB37Z Supplement Left Hip Joint with Autologous Tissue Substitute, Percutaneous Approach

0SUB3JZ Supplement Left Hip Joint with Synthetic Substitute, Percutaneous Approach

---

♀ Female-only   ♂ Male-only   ◐ Limited Coverage   ● Non-OR   HAC HAC-associated procedure   ⬤ Non-covered procedures   ✚ Combination

0SUB3KZ Supplement Left Hip Joint with Nonautologous Tissue Substitute, Percutaneous Approach

0SUB47Z Supplement Left Hip Joint with Autologous Tissue Substitute, Percutaneous Endoscopic Approach

0SUB4JZ Supplement Left Hip Joint with Synthetic Substitute, Percutaneous Endoscopic Approach

0SUB4KZ Supplement Left Hip Joint with Nonautologous Tissue Substitute, Percutaneous Endoscopic Approach

0SUC07Z Supplement Right Knee Joint with Autologous Tissue Substitute, Open Approach

0SUC09C Supplement Right Knee Joint with Liner, Patellar Surface, Open Approach

0SUC09Z Supplement Right Knee Joint with Liner, Open Approach

0SUC0JZ Supplement Right Knee Joint with Synthetic Substitute, Open Approach

0SUC0KZ Supplement Right Knee Joint with Nonautologous Tissue Substitute, Open Approach

0SUC37Z Supplement Right Knee Joint with Autologous Tissue Substitute, Percutaneous Approach

0SUC3JZ Supplement Right Knee Joint with Synthetic Substitute, Percutaneous Approach

0SUC3KZ Supplement Right Knee Joint with Nonautologous Tissue Substitute, Percutaneous Approach

0SUC47Z Supplement Right Knee Joint with Autologous Tissue Substitute, Percutaneous Endoscopic Approach

0SUC4JZ Supplement Right Knee Joint with Synthetic Substitute, Percutaneous Endoscopic Approach

0SUC4KZ Supplement Right Knee Joint with Nonautologous Tissue Substitute, Percutaneous Endoscopic Approach

0SUD07Z Supplement Left Knee Joint with Autologous Tissue Substitute, Open Approach

0SUD09C Supplement Left Knee Joint with Liner, Patellar Surface, Open Approach

0SUD09Z Supplement Left Knee Joint with Liner, Open Approach

0SUD0JZ Supplement Left Knee Joint with Synthetic Substitute, Open Approach

0SUD0KZ Supplement Left Knee Joint with Nonautologous Tissue Substitute, Open Approach

0SUD37Z Supplement Left Knee Joint with Autologous Tissue Substitute, Percutaneous Approach

0SUD3JZ Supplement Left Knee Joint with Synthetic Substitute, Percutaneous Approach

0SUD3KZ Supplement Left Knee Joint with Nonautologous Tissue Substitute, Percutaneous Approach

0SUD47Z Supplement Left Knee Joint with Autologous Tissue Substitute, Percutaneous Endoscopic Approach

0SUD4JZ Supplement Left Knee Joint with Synthetic Substitute, Percutaneous Endoscopic Approach

0SUD4KZ Supplement Left Knee Joint with Nonautologous Tissue Substitute, Percutaneous Endoscopic Approach

0SUE09Z Supplement Left Hip Joint, Acetabular Surface with Liner, Open Approach

0SUE0BZ Supplement Left Hip Joint, Acetabular Surface with Resurfacing Device, Open Approach

  HAC When reported with secondary diagnosis code I26.02, I26.09, I26.92, I26.99, I82.401-I82.4Z9

0SUF07Z Supplement Right Ankle Joint with Autologous Tissue Substitute, Open Approach

0SUF0JZ Supplement Right Ankle Joint with Synthetic Substitute, Open Approach

0SUF0KZ Supplement Right Ankle Joint with Nonautologous Tissue Substitute, Open Approach

0SUF37Z Supplement Right Ankle Joint with Autologous Tissue Substitute, Percutaneous Approach

0SUF3JZ Supplement Right Ankle Joint with Synthetic Substitute, Percutaneous Approach

0SUF3KZ Supplement Right Ankle Joint with Nonautologous Tissue Substitute, Percutaneous Approach

0SUF47Z Supplement Right Ankle Joint with Autologous Tissue Substitute, Percutaneous Endoscopic Approach

0SUF4JZ Supplement Right Ankle Joint with Synthetic Substitute, Percutaneous Endoscopic Approach

0SUF4KZ Supplement Right Ankle Joint with Nonautologous Tissue Substitute, Percutaneous Endoscopic Approach

0SUG07Z Supplement Left Ankle Joint with Autologous Tissue Substitute, Open Approach

0SUG0JZ Supplement Left Ankle Joint with Synthetic Substitute, Open Approach

0SUG0KZ Supplement Left Ankle Joint with Nonautologous Tissue Substitute, Open Approach

0SUG37Z Supplement Left Ankle Joint with Autologous Tissue Substitute, Percutaneous Approach

0SUG3JZ Supplement Left Ankle Joint with Synthetic Substitute, Percutaneous Approach

0SUG3KZ Supplement Left Ankle Joint with Nonautologous Tissue Substitute, Percutaneous Approach

0SUG47Z Supplement Left Ankle Joint with Autologous Tissue Substitute, Percutaneous Endoscopic Approach

0SUG4JZ Supplement Left Ankle Joint with Synthetic Substitute, Percutaneous Endoscopic Approach

0SUG4KZ Supplement Left Ankle Joint with Nonautologous Tissue Substitute, Percutaneous Endoscopic Approach

0SUH07Z Supplement Right Tarsal Joint with Autologous Tissue Substitute, Open Approach

0SUH0JZ Supplement Right Tarsal Joint with Synthetic Substitute, Open Approach

0SUH0KZ Supplement Right Tarsal Joint with Nonautologous Tissue Substitute, Open Approach

0SUH37Z Supplement Right Tarsal Joint with Autologous Tissue Substitute, Percutaneous Approach

0SUH3JZ Supplement Right Tarsal Joint with Synthetic Substitute, Percutaneous Approach

0SUH3KZ Supplement Right Tarsal Joint with Nonautologous Tissue Substitute, Percutaneous Approach

0SUH47Z Supplement Right Tarsal Joint with Autologous Tissue Substitute, Percutaneous Endoscopic Approach

0SUH4JZ Supplement Right Tarsal Joint with Synthetic Substitute, Percutaneous Endoscopic Approach

0SUH4KZ Supplement Right Tarsal Joint with Nonautologous Tissue Substitute, Percutaneous Endoscopic Approach

0SUJ07Z Supplement Left Tarsal Joint with Autologous Tissue Substitute, Open Approach

0SUJ0JZ Supplement Left Tarsal Joint with Synthetic Substitute, Open Approach

0SUJ0KZ Supplement Left Tarsal Joint with Nonautologous Tissue Substitute, Open Approach

0SUJ37Z Supplement Left Tarsal Joint with Autologous Tissue Substitute, Percutaneous Approach

0SUJ3JZ Supplement Left Tarsal Joint with Synthetic Substitute, Percutaneous Approach

0SUJ3KZ Supplement Left Tarsal Joint with Nonautologous Tissue Substitute, Percutaneous Approach

0SUJ47Z Supplement Left Tarsal Joint with Autologous Tissue Substitute, Percutaneous Endoscopic Approach

0SUJ4JZ Supplement Left Tarsal Joint with Synthetic Substitute, Percutaneous Endoscopic Approach

0SUJ4KZ Supplement Left Tarsal Joint with Nonautologous Tissue Substitute, Percutaneous Endoscopic Approach

0SUK07Z Supplement Right Metatarsal-Tarsal Joint with Autologous Tissue Substitute, Open Approach

0SUK0JZ Supplement Right Metatarsal-Tarsal Joint with Synthetic Substitute, Open Approach

0SUK0KZ Supplement Right Metatarsal-Tarsal Joint with Nonautologous Tissue Substitute, Open Approach

0SUK37Z Supplement Right Metatarsal-Tarsal Joint with Autologous Tissue Substitute, Percutaneous Approach

0SUK3JZ Supplement Right Metatarsal-Tarsal Joint with Synthetic Substitute, Percutaneous Approach

0SUK3KZ Supplement Right Metatarsal-Tarsal Joint with Nonautologous Tissue Substitute, Percutaneous Approach

0SUK47Z Supplement Right Metatarsal-Tarsal Joint with Autologous Tissue Substitute, Percutaneous Endoscopic Approach

0SUK4JZ Supplement Right Metatarsal-Tarsal Joint with Synthetic Substitute, Percutaneous Endoscopic Approach

0SUK4KZ Supplement Right Metatarsal-Tarsal Joint with Nonautologous Tissue Substitute, Percutaneous Endoscopic Approach

0SUL07Z Supplement Left Metatarsal-Tarsal Joint with Autologous Tissue Substitute, Open Approach

---

♀ Female-only   ♂ Male-only   ● Limited Coverage   ● Non-OR   HAC HAC-associated procedure   ● Non-covered procedures   ✚ Combination

0SUL0JZ Supplement Left Metatarsal-Tarsal Joint with Synthetic Substitute, Open Approach

0SUL0KZ Supplement Left Metatarsal-Tarsal Joint with Nonautologous Tissue Substitute, Open Approach

0SUL37Z Supplement Left Metatarsal-Tarsal Joint with Autologous Tissue Substitute, Percutaneous Approach

0SUL3JZ Supplement Left Metatarsal-Tarsal Joint with Synthetic Substitute, Percutaneous Approach

0SUL3KZ Supplement Left Metatarsal-Tarsal Joint with Nonautologous Tissue Substitute, Percutaneous Approach

0SUL47Z Supplement Left Metatarsal-Tarsal Joint with Autologous Tissue Substitute, Percutaneous Endoscopic Approach

0SUL4JZ Supplement Left Metatarsal-Tarsal Joint with Synthetic Substitute, Percutaneous Endoscopic Approach

0SUL4KZ Supplement Left Metatarsal-Tarsal Joint with Nonautologous Tissue Substitute, Percutaneous Endoscopic Approach

0SUM07Z Supplement Right Metatarsal-Phalangeal Joint with Autologous Tissue Substitute, Open Approach

0SUM0JZ Supplement Right Metatarsal-Phalangeal Joint with Synthetic Substitute, Open Approach

0SUM0KZ Supplement Right Metatarsal-Phalangeal Joint with Nonautologous Tissue Substitute, Open Approach

0SUM37Z Supplement Right Metatarsal-Phalangeal Joint with Autologous Tissue Substitute, Percutaneous Approach

0SUM3JZ Supplement Right Metatarsal-Phalangeal Joint with Synthetic Substitute, Percutaneous Approach

0SUM3KZ Supplement Right Metatarsal-Phalangeal Joint with Nonautologous Tissue Substitute, Percutaneous Approach

0SUM47Z Supplement Right Metatarsal-Phalangeal Joint with Autologous Tissue Substitute, Percutaneous Endoscopic Approach

0SUM4JZ Supplement Right Metatarsal-Phalangeal Joint with Synthetic Substitute, Percutaneous Endoscopic Approach

0SUM4KZ Supplement Right Metatarsal-Phalangeal Joint with Nonautologous Tissue Substitute, Percutaneous Endoscopic Approach

0SUN07Z Supplement Left Metatarsal-Phalangeal Joint with Autologous Tissue Substitute, Open Approach

0SUN0JZ Supplement Left Metatarsal-Phalangeal Joint with Synthetic Substitute, Open Approach

0SUN0KZ Supplement Left Metatarsal-Phalangeal Joint with Nonautologous Tissue Substitute, Open Approach

0SUN37Z Supplement Left Metatarsal-Phalangeal Joint with Autologous Tissue Substitute, Percutaneous Approach

0SUN3JZ Supplement Left Metatarsal-Phalangeal Joint with Synthetic Substitute, Percutaneous Approach

0SUN3KZ Supplement Left Metatarsal-Phalangeal Joint with Nonautologous Tissue Substitute, Percutaneous Approach

0SUN47Z Supplement Left Metatarsal-Phalangeal Joint with Autologous Tissue Substitute, Percutaneous Endoscopic Approach

0SUN4JZ Supplement Left Metatarsal-Phalangeal Joint with Synthetic Substitute, Percutaneous Endoscopic Approach

0SUN4KZ Supplement Left Metatarsal-Phalangeal Joint with Nonautologous Tissue Substitute, Percutaneous Endoscopic Approach

0SUP07Z Supplement Right Toe Phalangeal Joint with Autologous Tissue Substitute, Open Approach

0SUP0JZ Supplement Right Toe Phalangeal Joint with Synthetic Substitute, Open Approach

0SUP0KZ Supplement Right Toe Phalangeal Joint with Nonautologous Tissue Substitute, Open Approach

0SUP37Z Supplement Right Toe Phalangeal Joint with Autologous Tissue Substitute, Percutaneous Approach

0SUP3JZ Supplement Right Toe Phalangeal Joint with Synthetic Substitute, Percutaneous Approach

0SUP3KZ Supplement Right Toe Phalangeal Joint with Nonautologous Tissue Substitute, Percutaneous Approach

0SUP47Z Supplement Right Toe Phalangeal Joint with Autologous Tissue Substitute, Percutaneous Endoscopic Approach

0SUP4JZ Supplement Right Toe Phalangeal Joint with Synthetic Substitute, Percutaneous Endoscopic Approach

0SUP4KZ Supplement Right Toe Phalangeal Joint with Nonautologous Tissue Substitute, Percutaneous Endoscopic Approach

0SUQ07Z Supplement Left Toe Phalangeal Joint with Autologous Tissue Substitute, Open Approach

0SUQ0JZ Supplement Left Toe Phalangeal Joint with Synthetic Substitute, Open Approach

0SUQ0KZ Supplement Left Toe Phalangeal Joint with Nonautologous Tissue Substitute, Open Approach

0SUQ37Z Supplement Left Toe Phalangeal Joint with Autologous Tissue Substitute, Percutaneous Approach

0SUQ3JZ Supplement Left Toe Phalangeal Joint with Synthetic Substitute, Percutaneous Approach

0SUQ3KZ Supplement Left Toe Phalangeal Joint with Nonautologous Tissue Substitute, Percutaneous Approach

0SUQ47Z Supplement Left Toe Phalangeal Joint with Autologous Tissue Substitute, Percutaneous Endoscopic Approach

0SUQ4JZ Supplement Left Toe Phalangeal Joint with Synthetic Substitute, Percutaneous Endoscopic Approach

0SUQ4KZ Supplement Left Toe Phalangeal Joint with Nonautologous Tissue Substitute, Percutaneous Endoscopic Approach

0SUR09Z Supplement Right Hip Joint, Femoral Surface with Liner, Open Approach

0SUR0BZ Supplement Right Hip Joint, Femoral Surface with Resurfacing Device, Open Approach

HAC   When reported with secondary diagnosis code I26.02, I26.09, I26.92, I26.99, I82.401-I82.4Z9

0SUS09Z Supplement Left Hip Joint, Femoral Surface with Liner, Open Approach

0SUS0BZ Supplement Left Hip Joint, Femoral Surface with Resurfacing Device, Open Approach

HAC   When reported with secondary diagnosis code I26.02, I26.09, I26.92, I26.99, I82.401-I82.4Z9

0SUT09Z Supplement Right Knee Joint, Femoral Surface with Liner, Open Approach

0SUU09Z Supplement Left Knee Joint, Femoral Surface with Liner, Open Approach

0SUV09Z Supplement Right Knee Joint, Tibial Surface with Liner, Open Approach

0SUW09Z Supplement Left Knee Joint, Tibial Surface with Liner, Open Approach

0SW – Lower Joints, Revision

Review Coding Guideline B6.1c

0SW000Z Revision of Drainage Device in Lumbar Vertebral Joint, Open Approach

0SW003Z Revision of Infusion Device in Lumbar Vertebral Joint, Open Approach

0SW004Z Revision of Internal Fixation Device in Lumbar Vertebral Joint, Open Approach

0SW007Z Revision of Autologous Tissue Substitute in Lumbar Vertebral Joint, Open Approach

0SW008Z Revision of Spacer in Lumbar Vertebral Joint, Open Approach

0SW00AZ Revision of Interbody Fusion Device in Lumbar Vertebral Joint, Open Approach

0SW00JZ Revision of Synthetic Substitute in Lumbar Vertebral Joint, Open Approach

0SW00KZ Revision of Nonautologous Tissue Substitute in Lumbar Vertebral Joint, Open Approach

0SW030Z Revision of Drainage Device in Lumbar Vertebral Joint, Percutaneous Approach

0SW033Z Revision of Infusion Device in Lumbar Vertebral Joint, Percutaneous Approach

0SW034Z Revision of Internal Fixation Device in Lumbar Vertebral Joint, Percutaneous Approach

0SW037Z Revision of Autologous Tissue Substitute in Lumbar Vertebral Joint, Percutaneous Approach

0SW038Z Revision of Spacer in Lumbar Vertebral Joint, Percutaneous Approach

0SW03AZ Revision of Interbody Fusion Device in Lumbar Vertebral Joint, Percutaneous Approach

0SW03JZ Revision of Synthetic Substitute in Lumbar Vertebral Joint, Percutaneous Approach

0SW03KZ Revision of Nonautologous Tissue Substitute in Lumbar Vertebral Joint, Percutaneous Approach

0SW040Z Revision of Drainage Device in Lumbar Vertebral Joint, Percutaneous Endoscopic Approach

0SW043Z Revision of Infusion Device in Lumbar Vertebral Joint, Percutaneous Endoscopic Approach

0SW044Z Revision of Internal Fixation Device in Lumbar Vertebral Joint, Percutaneous Endoscopic Approach

0SW047Z Revision of Autologous Tissue Substitute in Lumbar Vertebral Joint, Percutaneous Endoscopic Approach

0SW048Z Revision of Spacer in Lumbar Vertebral Joint, Percutaneous Endoscopic Approach

0SW04AZ Revision of Interbody Fusion Device in Lumbar Vertebral Joint, Percutaneous Endoscopic Approach

0SW04JZ Revision of Synthetic Substitute in Lumbar Vertebral Joint, Percutaneous Endoscopic Approach

0SW04KZ Revision of Nonautologous Tissue Substitute in Lumbar Vertebral Joint, Percutaneous Endoscopic Approach

0SW0X0Z Revision of Drainage Device in Lumbar Vertebral Joint, External Approach

0SW0X3Z Revision of Infusion Device in Lumbar Vertebral Joint, External Approach

0SW0X4Z Revision of Internal Fixation Device in Lumbar Vertebral Joint, External Approach

0SW0X7Z Revision of Autologous Tissue Substitute in Lumbar Vertebral Joint, External Approach

0SW0X8Z Revision of Spacer in Lumbar Vertebral Joint, External Approach

0SW0XAZ Revision of Interbody Fusion Device in Lumbar Vertebral Joint, External Approach

0SW0XJZ Revision of Synthetic Substitute in Lumbar Vertebral Joint, External Approach

0SW0XKZ Revision of Nonautologous Tissue Substitute in Lumbar Vertebral Joint, External Approach

0SW200Z Revision of Drainage Device in Lumbar Vertebral Disc, Open Approach

0SW203Z Revision of Infusion Device in Lumbar Vertebral Disc, Open Approach

0SW207Z Revision of Autologous Tissue Substitute in Lumbar Vertebral Disc, Open Approach

0SW20JZ Revision of Synthetic Substitute in Lumbar Vertebral Disc, Open Approach

0SW20KZ Revision of Nonautologous Tissue Substitute in Lumbar Vertebral Disc, Open Approach

0SW230Z Revision of Drainage Device in Lumbar Vertebral Disc, Percutaneous Approach

0SW233Z Revision of Infusion Device in Lumbar Vertebral Disc, Percutaneous Approach

0SW237Z Revision of Autologous Tissue Substitute in Lumbar Vertebral Disc, Percutaneous Approach

0SW23JZ Revision of Synthetic Substitute in Lumbar Vertebral Disc, Percutaneous Approach

0SW23KZ Revision of Nonautologous Tissue Substitute in Lumbar Vertebral Disc, Percutaneous Approach

0SW240Z Revision of Drainage Device in Lumbar Vertebral Disc, Percutaneous Endoscopic Approach

0SW243Z Revision of Infusion Device in Lumbar Vertebral Disc, Percutaneous Endoscopic Approach

0SW247Z Revision of Autologous Tissue Substitute in Lumbar Vertebral Disc, Percutaneous Endoscopic Approach

0SW24JZ Revision of Synthetic Substitute in Lumbar Vertebral Disc, Percutaneous Endoscopic Approach

0SW24KZ Revision of Nonautologous Tissue Substitute in Lumbar Vertebral Disc, Percutaneous Endoscopic Approach

0SW2X0Z Revision of Drainage Device in Lumbar Vertebral Disc, External Approach

0SW2X3Z Revision of Infusion Device in Lumbar Vertebral Disc, External Approach

0SW2X7Z Revision of Autologous Tissue Substitute in Lumbar Vertebral Disc, External Approach

0SW2XJZ Revision of Synthetic Substitute in Lumbar Vertebral Disc, External Approach

0SW2XKZ Revision of Nonautologous Tissue Substitute in Lumbar Vertebral Disc, External Approach

0SW300Z Revision of Drainage Device in Lumbosacral Joint, Open Approach

0SW303Z Revision of Infusion Device in Lumbosacral Joint, Open Approach

0SW304Z Revision of Internal Fixation Device in Lumbosacral Joint, Open Approach

0SW307Z Revision of Autologous Tissue Substitute in Lumbosacral Joint, Open Approach

0SW308Z Revision of Spacer in Lumbosacral Joint, Open Approach

0SW30AZ Revision of Interbody Fusion Device in Lumbosacral Joint, Open Approach

0SW30JZ Revision of Synthetic Substitute in Lumbosacral Joint, Open Approach

0SW30KZ Revision of Nonautologous Tissue Substitute in Lumbosacral Joint, Open Approach

0SW330Z Revision of Drainage Device in Lumbosacral Joint, Percutaneous Approach

0SW333Z Revision of Infusion Device in Lumbosacral Joint, Percutaneous Approach

0SW334Z Revision of Internal Fixation Device in Lumbosacral Joint, Percutaneous Approach

0SW337Z Revision of Autologous Tissue Substitute in Lumbosacral Joint, Percutaneous Approach

0SW338Z Revision of Spacer in Lumbosacral Joint, Percutaneous Approach

0SW33AZ Revision of Interbody Fusion Device in Lumbosacral Joint, Percutaneous Approach

0SW33JZ Revision of Synthetic Substitute in Lumbosacral Joint, Percutaneous Approach

0SW33KZ Revision of Nonautologous Tissue Substitute in Lumbosacral Joint, Percutaneous Approach

0SW340Z Revision of Drainage Device in Lumbosacral Joint, Percutaneous Endoscopic Approach

0SW343Z Revision of Infusion Device in Lumbosacral Joint, Percutaneous Endoscopic Approach

0SW344Z Revision of Internal Fixation Device in Lumbosacral Joint, Percutaneous Endoscopic Approach

0SW347Z Revision of Autologous Tissue Substitute in Lumbosacral Joint, Percutaneous Endoscopic Approach

0SW348Z Revision of Spacer in Lumbosacral Joint, Percutaneous Endoscopic Approach

0SW34AZ Revision of Interbody Fusion Device in Lumbosacral Joint, Percutaneous Endoscopic Approach

0SW34JZ Revision of Synthetic Substitute in Lumbosacral Joint, Percutaneous Endoscopic Approach

0SW34KZ Revision of Nonautologous Tissue Substitute in Lumbosacral Joint, Percutaneous Endoscopic Approach

0SW3X0Z Revision of Drainage Device in Lumbosacral Joint, External Approach

0SW3X3Z Revision of Infusion Device in Lumbosacral Joint, External Approach

0SW3X4Z Revision of Internal Fixation Device in Lumbosacral Joint, External Approach

0SW3X7Z Revision of Autologous Tissue Substitute in Lumbosacral Joint, External Approach

0SW3X8Z Revision of Spacer in Lumbosacral Joint, External Approach

0SW3XAZ Revision of Interbody Fusion Device in Lumbosacral Joint, External Approach

0SW3XJZ Revision of Synthetic Substitute in Lumbosacral Joint, External Approach

0SW3XKZ Revision of Nonautologous Tissue Substitute in Lumbosacral Joint, External Approach

0SW400Z Revision of Drainage Device in Lumbosacral Disc, Open Approach

0SW403Z Revision of Infusion Device in Lumbosacral Disc, Open Approach

0SW407Z Revision of Autologous Tissue Substitute in Lumbosacral Disc, Open Approach

0SW40JZ Revision of Synthetic Substitute in Lumbosacral Disc, Open Approach

0SW40KZ Revision of Nonautologous Tissue Substitute in Lumbosacral Disc, Open Approach

0SW430Z Revision of Drainage Device in Lumbosacral Disc, Percutaneous Approach

0SW433Z Revision of Infusion Device in Lumbosacral Disc, Percutaneous Approach

0SW437Z Revision of Autologous Tissue Substitute in Lumbosacral Disc, Percutaneous Approach

0SW43JZ Revision of Synthetic Substitute in Lumbosacral Disc, Percutaneous Approach

0SW43KZ Revision of Nonautologous Tissue Substitute in Lumbosacral Disc, Percutaneous Approach

0SW440Z Revision of Drainage Device in Lumbosacral Disc, Percutaneous Endoscopic Approach

0SW443Z Revision of Infusion Device in Lumbosacral Disc, Percutaneous Endoscopic Approach

0SW447Z Revision of Autologous Tissue Substitute in Lumbosacral Disc, Percutaneous Endoscopic Approach

0SW44JZ Revision of Synthetic Substitute in Lumbosacral Disc, Percutaneous Endoscopic Approach

0SW44KZ Revision of Nonautologous Tissue Substitute in Lumbosacral Disc, Percutaneous Endoscopic Approach

0SW4X0Z Revision of Drainage Device in Lumbosacral Disc, External Approach

0SW4X3Z Revision of Infusion Device in Lumbosacral Disc, External Approach

0SW4X7Z Revision of Autologous Tissue Substitute in Lumbosacral Disc, External Approach

0SW4XJZ Revision of Synthetic Substitute in Lumbosacral Disc, External Approach

0SW4XKZ Revision of Nonautologous Tissue Substitute in Lumbosacral Disc, External Approach

0SW500Z Revision of Drainage Device in Sacrococcygeal Joint, Open Approach

0SW503Z Revision of Infusion Device in Sacrococcygeal Joint, Open Approach

0SW504Z Revision of Internal Fixation Device in Sacrococcygeal Joint, Open Approach

0SW507Z Revision of Autologous Tissue Substitute in Sacrococcygeal Joint, Open Approach

0SW508Z Revision of Spacer in Sacrococcygeal Joint, Open Approach

0SW50JZ Revision of Synthetic Substitute in Sacrococcygeal Joint, Open Approach

0SW50KZ Revision of Nonautologous Tissue Substitute in Sacrococcygeal Joint, Open Approach

0SW530Z Revision of Drainage Device in Sacrococcygeal Joint, Percutaneous Approach

0SW533Z Revision of Infusion Device in Sacrococcygeal Joint, Percutaneous Approach

0SW534Z Revision of Internal Fixation Device in Sacrococcygeal Joint, Percutaneous Approach

0SW537Z Revision of Autologous Tissue Substitute in Sacrococcygeal Joint, Percutaneous Approach

0SW538Z Revision of Spacer in Sacrococcygeal Joint, Percutaneous Approach

0SW53JZ Revision of Synthetic Substitute in Sacrococcygeal Joint, Percutaneous Approach

0SW53KZ Revision of Nonautologous Tissue Substitute in Sacrococcygeal Joint, Percutaneous Approach

0SW540Z Revision of Drainage Device in Sacrococcygeal Joint, Percutaneous Endoscopic Approach

0SW543Z Revision of Infusion Device in Sacrococcygeal Joint, Percutaneous Endoscopic Approach

0SW544Z Revision of Internal Fixation Device in Sacrococcygeal Joint, Percutaneous Endoscopic Approach

0SW547Z Revision of Autologous Tissue Substitute in Sacrococcygeal Joint, Percutaneous Endoscopic Approach

0SW548Z Revision of Spacer in Sacrococcygeal Joint, Percutaneous Endoscopic Approach

0SW54JZ Revision of Synthetic Substitute in Sacrococcygeal Joint, Percutaneous Endoscopic Approach

0SW54KZ Revision of Nonautologous Tissue Substitute in Sacrococcygeal Joint, Percutaneous Endoscopic Approach

0SW5X0Z Revision of Drainage Device in Sacrococcygeal Joint, External Approach

0SW5X3Z Revision of Infusion Device in Sacrococcygeal Joint, External Approach

0SW5X4Z Revision of Internal Fixation Device in Sacrococcygeal Joint, External Approach

0SW5X7Z Revision of Autologous Tissue Substitute in Sacrococcygeal Joint, External Approach

0SW5X8Z Revision of Spacer in Sacrococcygeal Joint, External Approach

0SW5XJZ Revision of Synthetic Substitute in Sacrococcygeal Joint, External Approach

0SW5XKZ Revision of Nonautologous Tissue Substitute in Sacrococcygeal Joint, External Approach

0SW600Z Revision of Drainage Device in Coccygeal Joint, Open Approach

0SW603Z Revision of Infusion Device in Coccygeal Joint, Open Approach

0SW604Z Revision of Internal Fixation Device in Coccygeal Joint, Open Approach

0SW607Z Revision of Autologous Tissue Substitute in Coccygeal Joint, Open Approach

0SW608Z Revision of Spacer in Coccygeal Joint, Open Approach

0SW60JZ Revision of Synthetic Substitute in Coccygeal Joint, Open Approach

0SW60KZ Revision of Nonautologous Tissue Substitute in Coccygeal Joint, Open Approach

0SW630Z Revision of Drainage Device in Coccygeal Joint, Percutaneous Approach

0SW633Z Revision of Infusion Device in Coccygeal Joint, Percutaneous Approach

0SW634Z Revision of Internal Fixation Device in Coccygeal Joint, Percutaneous Approach

0SW637Z Revision of Autologous Tissue Substitute in Coccygeal Joint, Percutaneous Approach

0SW638Z Revision of Spacer in Coccygeal Joint, Percutaneous Approach

0SW63JZ Revision of Synthetic Substitute in Coccygeal Joint, Percutaneous Approach

0SW63KZ Revision of Nonautologous Tissue Substitute in Coccygeal Joint, Percutaneous Approach

0SW640Z Revision of Drainage Device in Coccygeal Joint, Percutaneous Endoscopic Approach

0SW643Z Revision of Infusion Device in Coccygeal Joint, Percutaneous Endoscopic Approach

0SW644Z Revision of Internal Fixation Device in Coccygeal Joint, Percutaneous Endoscopic Approach

0SW647Z Revision of Autologous Tissue Substitute in Coccygeal Joint, Percutaneous Endoscopic Approach

0SW648Z Revision of Spacer in Coccygeal Joint, Percutaneous Endoscopic Approach

0SW64JZ Revision of Synthetic Substitute in Coccygeal Joint, Percutaneous Endoscopic Approach

0SW64KZ Revision of Nonautologous Tissue Substitute in Coccygeal Joint, Percutaneous Endoscopic Approach

0SW6X0Z Revision of Drainage Device in Coccygeal Joint, External Approach

0SW6X3Z Revision of Infusion Device in Coccygeal Joint, External Approach

0SW6X4Z Revision of Internal Fixation Device in Coccygeal Joint, External Approach

0SW6X7Z Revision of Autologous Tissue Substitute in Coccygeal Joint, External Approach

0SW6X8Z Revision of Spacer in Coccygeal Joint, External Approach

0SW6XJZ Revision of Synthetic Substitute in Coccygeal Joint, External Approach

0SW6XKZ Revision of Nonautologous Tissue Substitute in Coccygeal Joint, External Approach

0SW700Z Revision of Drainage Device in Right Sacroiliac Joint, Open Approach

0SW703Z Revision of Infusion Device in Right Sacroiliac Joint, Open Approach

0SW704Z Revision of Internal Fixation Device in Right Sacroiliac Joint, Open Approach

0SW707Z Revision of Autologous Tissue Substitute in Right Sacroiliac Joint, Open Approach

0SW708Z Revision of Spacer in Right Sacroiliac Joint, Open Approach

0SW70JZ Revision of Synthetic Substitute in Right Sacroiliac Joint, Open Approach

0SW70KZ Revision of Nonautologous Tissue Substitute in Right Sacroiliac Joint, Open Approach

0SW730Z Revision of Drainage Device in Right Sacroiliac Joint, Percutaneous Approach

0SW733Z Revision of Infusion Device in Right Sacroiliac Joint, Percutaneous Approach

0SW734Z Revision of Internal Fixation Device in Right Sacroiliac Joint, Percutaneous Approach

0SW737Z Revision of Autologous Tissue Substitute in Right Sacroiliac Joint, Percutaneous Approach

0SW738Z Revision of Spacer in Right Sacroiliac Joint, Percutaneous Approach

0SW73JZ Revision of Synthetic Substitute in Right Sacroiliac Joint, Percutaneous Approach

0SW73KZ Revision of Nonautologous Tissue Substitute in Right Sacroiliac Joint, Percutaneous Approach

0SW740Z Revision of Drainage Device in Right Sacroiliac Joint, Percutaneous Endoscopic Approach

0SW743Z Revision of Infusion Device in Right Sacroiliac Joint, Percutaneous Endoscopic Approach

0SW744Z Revision of Internal Fixation Device in Right Sacroiliac Joint, Percutaneous Endoscopic Approach

0SW747Z Revision of Autologous Tissue Substitute in Right Sacroiliac Joint, Percutaneous Endoscopic Approach

0SW748Z Revision of Spacer in Right Sacroiliac Joint, Percutaneous Endoscopic Approach

0SW74JZ Revision of Synthetic Substitute in Right Sacroiliac Joint, Percutaneous Endoscopic Approach

0SW74KZ Revision of Nonautologous Tissue Substitute in Right Sacroiliac Joint, Percutaneous Endoscopic Approach

0SW7X0Z Revision of Drainage Device in Right Sacroiliac Joint, External Approach

0SW7X3Z Revision of Infusion Device in Right Sacroiliac Joint, External Approach

0SW7X4Z Revision of Internal Fixation Device in Right Sacroiliac Joint, External Approach

0SW7X7Z Revision of Autologous Tissue Substitute in Right Sacroiliac Joint, External Approach

0SW7X8Z Revision of Spacer in Right Sacroiliac Joint, External Approach

0SW7XJZ Revision of Synthetic Substitute in Right Sacroiliac Joint, External Approach

0SW7XKZ Revision of Nonautologous Tissue Substitute in Right Sacroiliac Joint, External Approach

0SW800Z Revision of Drainage Device in Left Sacroiliac Joint, Open Approach

0SW803Z Revision of Infusion Device in Left Sacroiliac Joint, Open Approach

0SW804Z Revision of Internal Fixation Device in Left Sacroiliac Joint, Open Approach

0SW807Z Revision of Autologous Tissue Substitute in Left Sacroiliac Joint, Open Approach

0SW808Z Revision of Spacer in Left Sacroiliac Joint, Open Approach

0SW80JZ Revision of Synthetic Substitute in Left Sacroiliac Joint, Open Approach

0SW80KZ Revision of Nonautologous Tissue Substitute in Left Sacroiliac Joint, Open Approach

0SW830Z Revision of Drainage Device in Left Sacroiliac Joint, Percutaneous Approach

0SW833Z Revision of Infusion Device in Left Sacroiliac Joint, Percutaneous Approach

0SW834Z Revision of Internal Fixation Device in Left Sacroiliac Joint, Percutaneous Approach

0SW837Z Revision of Autologous Tissue Substitute in Left Sacroiliac Joint, Percutaneous Approach

0SW838Z Revision of Spacer in Left Sacroiliac Joint, Percutaneous Approach

0SW83JZ Revision of Synthetic Substitute in Left Sacroiliac Joint, Percutaneous Approach

0SW83KZ Revision of Nonautologous Tissue Substitute in Left Sacroiliac Joint, Percutaneous Approach

0SW840Z Revision of Drainage Device in Left Sacroiliac Joint, Percutaneous Endoscopic Approach

0SW843Z Revision of Infusion Device in Left Sacroiliac Joint, Percutaneous Endoscopic Approach

0SW844Z Revision of Internal Fixation Device in Left Sacroiliac Joint, Percutaneous Endoscopic Approach

0SW847Z Revision of Autologous Tissue Substitute in Left Sacroiliac Joint, Percutaneous Endoscopic Approach

0SW848Z Revision of Spacer in Left Sacroiliac Joint, Percutaneous Endoscopic Approach

0SW84JZ Revision of Synthetic Substitute in Left Sacroiliac Joint, Percutaneous Endoscopic Approach

0SW84KZ Revision of Nonautologous Tissue Substitute in Left Sacroiliac Joint, Percutaneous Endoscopic Approach

0SW8X0Z Revision of Drainage Device in Left Sacroiliac Joint, External Approach

0SW8X3Z Revision of Infusion Device in Left Sacroiliac Joint, External Approach

0SW8X4Z Revision of Internal Fixation Device in Left Sacroiliac Joint, External Approach

0SW8X7Z Revision of Autologous Tissue Substitute in Left Sacroiliac Joint, External Approach

0SW8X8Z Revision of Spacer in Left Sacroiliac Joint, External Approach

0SW8XJZ Revision of Synthetic Substitute in Left Sacroiliac Joint, External Approach

0SW8XKZ Revision of Nonautologous Tissue Substitute in Left Sacroiliac Joint, External Approach

0SW900Z Revision of Drainage Device in Right Hip Joint, Open Approach

0SW903Z Revision of Infusion Device in Right Hip Joint, Open Approach

0SW904Z Revision of Internal Fixation Device in Right Hip Joint, Open Approach

0SW905Z Revision of External Fixation Device in Right Hip Joint, Open Approach

0SW907Z Revision of Autologous Tissue Substitute in Right Hip Joint, Open Approach

0SW908Z Revision of Spacer in Right Hip Joint, Open Approach

0SW909Z Revision of Liner in Right Hip Joint, Open Approach

0SW90BZ Revision of Resurfacing Device in Right Hip Joint, Open Approach

0SW90JZ Revision of Synthetic Substitute in Right Hip Joint, Open Approach

0SW90KZ Revision of Nonautologous Tissue Substitute in Right Hip Joint, Open Approach

0SW930Z Revision of Drainage Device in Right Hip Joint, Percutaneous Approach

0SW933Z Revision of Infusion Device in Right Hip Joint, Percutaneous Approach

0SW934Z Revision of Internal Fixation Device in Right Hip Joint, Percutaneous Approach

0SW935Z Revision of External Fixation Device in Right Hip Joint, Percutaneous Approach

0SW937Z Revision of Autologous Tissue Substitute in Right Hip Joint, Percutaneous Approach

0SW938Z Revision of Spacer in Right Hip Joint, Percutaneous Approach

0SW93JZ Revision of Synthetic Substitute in Right Hip Joint, Percutaneous Approach

0SW93KZ Revision of Nonautologous Tissue Substitute in Right Hip Joint, Percutaneous Approach

0SW940Z Revision of Drainage Device in Right Hip Joint, Percutaneous Endoscopic Approach

0SW943Z Revision of Infusion Device in Right Hip Joint, Percutaneous Endoscopic Approach

0SW944Z Revision of Internal Fixation Device in Right Hip Joint, Percutaneous Endoscopic Approach

0SW945Z Revision of External Fixation Device in Right Hip Joint, Percutaneous Endoscopic Approach

0SW947Z Revision of Autologous Tissue Substitute in Right Hip Joint, Percutaneous Endoscopic Approach

0SW948Z Revision of Spacer in Right Hip Joint, Percutaneous Endoscopic Approach

0SW94JZ Revision of Synthetic Substitute in Right Hip Joint, Percutaneous Endoscopic Approach

0SW94KZ Revision of Nonautologous Tissue Substitute in Right Hip Joint, Percutaneous Endoscopic Approach

0SW9X0Z Revision of Drainage Device in Right Hip Joint, External Approach

0SW9X3Z Revision of Infusion Device in Right Hip Joint, External Approach

0SW9X4Z Revision of Internal Fixation Device in Right Hip Joint, External Approach

0SW9X5Z Revision of External Fixation Device in Right Hip Joint, External Approach

0SW9X7Z Revision of Autologous Tissue Substitute in Right Hip Joint, External Approach

0SW9X8Z Revision of Spacer in Right Hip Joint, External Approach

0SW9XJZ Revision of Synthetic Substitute in Right Hip Joint, External Approach

0SW9XKZ Revision of Nonautologous Tissue Substitute in Right Hip Joint, External Approach

0SWB00Z Revision of Drainage Device in Left Hip Joint, Open Approach

0SWB03Z Revision of Infusion Device in Left Hip Joint, Open Approach

0SWB04Z Revision of Internal Fixation Device in Left Hip Joint, Open Approach

---

♀ Female-only   ♂ Male-only   ● Limited Coverage   ● Non-OR   ▩ HAC-associated procedure   ● Non-covered procedures   ✚ Combination

0SWB05Z Revision of External Fixation Device in Left Hip Joint, Open Approach

0SWB07Z Revision of Autologous Tissue Substitute in Left Hip Joint, Open Approach

0SWB08Z Revision of Spacer in Left Hip Joint, Open Approach

0SWB09Z Revision of Liner in Left Hip Joint, Open Approach

0SWB0BZ Revision of Resurfacing Device in Left Hip Joint, Open Approach

0SWB0JZ Revision of Synthetic Substitute in Left Hip Joint, Open Approach

0SWB0KZ Revision of Nonautologous Tissue Substitute in Left Hip Joint, Open Approach

0SWB30Z Revision of Drainage Device in Left Hip Joint, Percutaneous Approach

0SWB33Z Revision of Infusion Device in Left Hip Joint, Percutaneous Approach

0SWB34Z Revision of Internal Fixation Device in Left Hip Joint, Percutaneous Approach

0SWB35Z Revision of External Fixation Device in Left Hip Joint, Percutaneous Approach

0SWB37Z Revision of Autologous Tissue Substitute in Left Hip Joint, Percutaneous Approach

0SWB38Z Revision of Spacer in Left Hip Joint, Percutaneous Approach

0SWB3JZ Revision of Synthetic Substitute in Left Hip Joint, Percutaneous Approach

0SWB3KZ Revision of Nonautologous Tissue Substitute in Left Hip Joint, Percutaneous Approach

0SWB40Z Revision of Drainage Device in Left Hip Joint, Percutaneous Endoscopic Approach

0SWB43Z Revision of Infusion Device in Left Hip Joint, Percutaneous Endoscopic Approach

0SWB44Z Revision of Internal Fixation Device in Left Hip Joint, Percutaneous Endoscopic Approach

0SWB45Z Revision of External Fixation Device in Left Hip Joint, Percutaneous Endoscopic Approach

0SWB47Z Revision of Autologous Tissue Substitute in Left Hip Joint, Percutaneous Endoscopic Approach

0SWB48Z Revision of Spacer in Left Hip Joint, Percutaneous Endoscopic Approach

0SWB4JZ Revision of Synthetic Substitute in Left Hip Joint, Percutaneous Endoscopic Approach

0SWB4KZ Revision of Nonautologous Tissue Substitute in Left Hip Joint, Percutaneous Endoscopic Approach

0SWBX0Z Revision of Drainage Device in Left Hip Joint, External Approach

0SWBX3Z Revision of Infusion Device in Left Hip Joint, External Approach

0SWBX4Z Revision of Internal Fixation Device in Left Hip Joint, External Approach

0SWBX5Z Revision of External Fixation Device in Left Hip Joint, External Approach

0SWBX7Z Revision of Autologous Tissue Substitute in Left Hip Joint, External Approach

0SWBX8Z Revision of Spacer in Left Hip Joint, External Approach

0SWBXJZ Revision of Synthetic Substitute in Left Hip Joint, External Approach

0SWBXKZ Revision of Nonautologous Tissue Substitute in Left Hip Joint, External Approach

0SWC00Z Revision of Drainage Device in Right Knee Joint, Open Approach

0SWC03Z Revision of Infusion Device in Right Knee Joint, Open Approach

0SWC04Z Revision of Internal Fixation Device in Right Knee Joint, Open Approach

0SWC05Z Revision of External Fixation Device in Right Knee Joint, Open Approach

0SWC07Z Revision of Autologous Tissue Substitute in Right Knee Joint, Open Approach

0SWC08Z Revision of Spacer in Right Knee Joint, Open Approach

0SWC09Z Revision of Liner in Right Knee Joint, Open Approach

0SWC0JZ Revision of Synthetic Substitute in Right Knee Joint, Open Approach

0SWC0KZ Revision of Nonautologous Tissue Substitute in Right Knee Joint, Open Approach

0SWC30Z Revision of Drainage Device in Right Knee Joint, Percutaneous Approach

0SWC33Z Revision of Infusion Device in Right Knee Joint, Percutaneous Approach

0SWC34Z Revision of Internal Fixation Device in Right Knee Joint, Percutaneous Approach

0SWC35Z Revision of External Fixation Device in Right Knee Joint, Percutaneous Approach

0SWC37Z Revision of Autologous Tissue Substitute in Right Knee Joint, Percutaneous Approach

0SWC38Z Revision of Spacer in Right Knee Joint, Percutaneous Approach

0SWC3JZ Revision of Synthetic Substitute in Right Knee Joint, Percutaneous Approach

0SWC3KZ Revision of Nonautologous Tissue Substitute in Right Knee Joint, Percutaneous Approach

0SWC40Z Revision of Drainage Device in Right Knee Joint, Percutaneous Endoscopic Approach

0SWC43Z Revision of Infusion Device in Right Knee Joint, Percutaneous Endoscopic Approach

0SWC44Z Revision of Internal Fixation Device in Right Knee Joint, Percutaneous Endoscopic Approach

0SWC45Z Revision of External Fixation Device in Right Knee Joint, Percutaneous Endoscopic Approach

0SWC47Z Revision of Autologous Tissue Substitute in Right Knee Joint, Percutaneous Endoscopic Approach

0SWC48Z Revision of Spacer in Right Knee Joint, Percutaneous Endoscopic Approach

0SWC4JZ Revision of Synthetic Substitute in Right Knee Joint, Percutaneous Endoscopic Approach

0SWC4KZ Revision of Nonautologous Tissue Substitute in Right Knee Joint, Percutaneous Endoscopic Approach

0SWCX0Z Revision of Drainage Device in Right Knee Joint, External Approach

0SWCX3Z Revision of Infusion Device in Right Knee Joint, External Approach

0SWCX4Z Revision of Internal Fixation Device in Right Knee Joint, External Approach

0SWCX5Z Revision of External Fixation Device in Right Knee Joint, External Approach

0SWCX7Z Revision of Autologous Tissue Substitute in Right Knee Joint, External Approach

0SWCX8Z Revision of Spacer in Right Knee Joint, External Approach

0SWCXJZ Revision of Synthetic Substitute in Right Knee Joint, External Approach

0SWCXKZ Revision of Nonautologous Tissue Substitute in Right Knee Joint, External Approach

0SWD00Z Revision of Drainage Device in Left Knee Joint, Open Approach

0SWD03Z Revision of Infusion Device in Left Knee Joint, Open Approach

0SWD04Z Revision of Internal Fixation Device in Left Knee Joint, Open Approach

0SWD05Z Revision of External Fixation Device in Left Knee Joint, Open Approach

0SWD07Z Revision of Autologous Tissue Substitute in Left Knee Joint, Open Approach

0SWD08Z Revision of Spacer in Left Knee Joint, Open Approach

0SWD09Z Revision of Liner in Left Knee Joint, Open Approach

0SWD0JZ Revision of Synthetic Substitute in Left Knee Joint, Open Approach

0SWD0KZ Revision of Nonautologous Tissue Substitute in Left Knee Joint, Open Approach

0SWD30Z Revision of Drainage Device in Left Knee Joint, Percutaneous Approach

0SWD33Z Revision of Infusion Device in Left Knee Joint, Percutaneous Approach

0SWD34Z Revision of Internal Fixation Device in Left Knee Joint, Percutaneous Approach

0SWD35Z Revision of External Fixation Device in Left Knee Joint, Percutaneous Approach

0SWD37Z Revision of Autologous Tissue Substitute in Left Knee Joint, Percutaneous Approach

0SWD38Z Revision of Spacer in Left Knee Joint, Percutaneous Approach

0SWD3JZ Revision of Synthetic Substitute in Left Knee Joint, Percutaneous Approach

0SWD3KZ Revision of Nonautologous Tissue Substitute in Left Knee Joint, Percutaneous Approach

0SWD40Z Revision of Drainage Device in Left Knee Joint, Percutaneous Endoscopic Approach

0SWD43Z   Revision of Infusion Device in Left Knee Joint, Percutaneous Endoscopic Approach

0SWD44Z   Revision of Internal Fixation Device in Left Knee Joint, Percutaneous Endoscopic Approach

0SWD45Z   Revision of External Fixation Device in Left Knee Joint, Percutaneous Endoscopic Approach

0SWD47Z   Revision of Autologous Tissue Substitute in Left Knee Joint, Percutaneous Endoscopic Approach

0SWD48Z   Revision of Spacer in Left Knee Joint, Percutaneous Endoscopic Approach

0SWD4JZ   Revision of Synthetic Substitute in Left Knee Joint, Percutaneous Endoscopic Approach

0SWD4KZ   Revision of Nonautologous Tissue Substitute in Left Knee Joint, Percutaneous Endoscopic Approach

0SWDX0Z   Revision of Drainage Device in Left Knee Joint, External Approach

0SWDX3Z   Revision of Infusion Device in Left Knee Joint, External Approach

0SWDX4Z   Revision of Internal Fixation Device in Left Knee Joint, External Approach

0SWDX5Z   Revision of External Fixation Device in Left Knee Joint, External Approach

0SWDX7Z   Revision of Autologous Tissue Substitute in Left Knee Joint, External Approach

0SWDX8Z   Revision of Spacer in Left Knee Joint, External Approach

0SWDXJZ   Revision of Synthetic Substitute in Left Knee Joint, External Approach

0SWDXKZ   Revision of Nonautologous Tissue Substitute in Left Knee Joint, External Approach

0SWF00Z   Revision of Drainage Device in Right Ankle Joint, Open Approach

0SWF03Z   Revision of Infusion Device in Right Ankle Joint, Open Approach

0SWF04Z   Revision of Internal Fixation Device in Right Ankle Joint, Open Approach

0SWF05Z   Revision of External Fixation Device in Right Ankle Joint, Open Approach

0SWF07Z   Revision of Autologous Tissue Substitute in Right Ankle Joint, Open Approach

0SWF08Z   Revision of Spacer in Right Ankle Joint, Open Approach

0SWF0JZ   Revision of Synthetic Substitute in Right Ankle Joint, Open Approach

0SWF0KZ   Revision of Nonautologous Tissue Substitute in Right Ankle Joint, Open Approach

0SWF30Z   Revision of Drainage Device in Right Ankle Joint, Percutaneous Approach

0SWF33Z   Revision of Infusion Device in Right Ankle Joint, Percutaneous Approach

0SWF34Z   Revision of Internal Fixation Device in Right Ankle Joint, Percutaneous Approach

0SWF35Z   Revision of External Fixation Device in Right Ankle Joint, Percutaneous Approach

0SWF37Z   Revision of Autologous Tissue Substitute in Right Ankle Joint, Percutaneous Approach

0SWF38Z   Revision of Spacer in Right Ankle Joint, Percutaneous Approach

0SWF3JZ   Revision of Synthetic Substitute in Right Ankle Joint, Percutaneous Approach

0SWF3KZ   Revision of Nonautologous Tissue Substitute in Right Ankle Joint, Percutaneous Approach

0SWF40Z   Revision of Drainage Device in Right Ankle Joint, Percutaneous Endoscopic Approach

0SWF43Z   Revision of Infusion Device in Right Ankle Joint, Percutaneous Endoscopic Approach

0SWF44Z   Revision of Internal Fixation Device in Right Ankle Joint, Percutaneous Endoscopic Approach

0SWF45Z   Revision of External Fixation Device in Right Ankle Joint, Percutaneous Endoscopic Approach

0SWF47Z   Revision of Autologous Tissue Substitute in Right Ankle Joint, Percutaneous Endoscopic Approach

0SWF48Z   Revision of Spacer in Right Ankle Joint, Percutaneous Endoscopic Approach

0SWF4JZ   Revision of Synthetic Substitute in Right Ankle Joint, Percutaneous Endoscopic Approach

0SWF4KZ   Revision of Nonautologous Tissue Substitute in Right Ankle Joint, Percutaneous Endoscopic Approach

0SWFX0Z   Revision of Drainage Device in Right Ankle Joint, External Approach

0SWFX3Z   Revision of Infusion Device in Right Ankle Joint, External Approach

0SWFX4Z   Revision of Internal Fixation Device in Right Ankle Joint, External Approach

0SWFX5Z   Revision of External Fixation Device in Right Ankle Joint, External Approach

0SWFX7Z   Revision of Autologous Tissue Substitute in Right Ankle Joint, External Approach

0SWFX8Z   Revision of Spacer in Right Ankle Joint, External Approach

0SWFXJZ   Revision of Synthetic Substitute in Right Ankle Joint, External Approach

0SWFXKZ   Revision of Nonautologous Tissue Substitute in Right Ankle Joint, External Approach

0SWG00Z   Revision of Drainage Device in Left Ankle Joint, Open Approach

0SWG03Z   Revision of Infusion Device in Left Ankle Joint, Open Approach

0SWG04Z   Revision of Internal Fixation Device in Left Ankle Joint, Open Approach

0SWG05Z   Revision of External Fixation Device in Left Ankle Joint, Open Approach

0SWG07Z   Revision of Autologous Tissue Substitute in Left Ankle Joint, Open Approach

0SWG08Z   Revision of Spacer in Left Ankle Joint, Open Approach

0SWG0JZ   Revision of Synthetic Substitute in Left Ankle Joint, Open Approach

0SWG0KZ   Revision of Nonautologous Tissue Substitute in Left Ankle Joint, Open Approach

0SWG30Z   Revision of Drainage Device in Left Ankle Joint, Percutaneous Approach

0SWG33Z   Revision of Infusion Device in Left Ankle Joint, Percutaneous Approach

0SWG34Z   Revision of Internal Fixation Device in Left Ankle Joint, Percutaneous Approach

0SWG35Z   Revision of External Fixation Device in Left Ankle Joint, Percutaneous Approach

0SWG37Z   Revision of Autologous Tissue Substitute in Left Ankle Joint, Percutaneous Approach

0SWG38Z   Revision of Spacer in Left Ankle Joint, Percutaneous Approach

0SWG3JZ   Revision of Synthetic Substitute in Left Ankle Joint, Percutaneous Approach

0SWG3KZ   Revision of Nonautologous Tissue Substitute in Left Ankle Joint, Percutaneous Approach

0SWG40Z   Revision of Drainage Device in Left Ankle Joint, Percutaneous Endoscopic Approach

0SWG43Z   Revision of Infusion Device in Left Ankle Joint, Percutaneous Endoscopic Approach

0SWG44Z   Revision of Internal Fixation Device in Left Ankle Joint, Percutaneous Endoscopic Approach

0SWG45Z   Revision of External Fixation Device in Left Ankle Joint, Percutaneous Endoscopic Approach

0SWG47Z   Revision of Autologous Tissue Substitute in Left Ankle Joint, Percutaneous Endoscopic Approach

0SWG48Z   Revision of Spacer in Left Ankle Joint, Percutaneous Endoscopic Approach

0SWG4JZ   Revision of Synthetic Substitute in Left Ankle Joint, Percutaneous Endoscopic Approach

0SWG4KZ   Revision of Nonautologous Tissue Substitute in Left Ankle Joint, Percutaneous Endoscopic Approach

0SWGX0Z   Revision of Drainage Device in Left Ankle Joint, External Approach

0SWGX3Z   Revision of Infusion Device in Left Ankle Joint, External Approach

0SWGX4Z   Revision of Internal Fixation Device in Left Ankle Joint, External Approach

0SWGX5Z   Revision of External Fixation Device in Left Ankle Joint, External Approach

0SWGX7Z   Revision of Autologous Tissue Substitute in Left Ankle Joint, External Approach

0SWGX8Z   Revision of Spacer in Left Ankle Joint, External Approach

0SWGXJZ   Revision of Synthetic Substitute in Left Ankle Joint, External Approach

0SWGXKZ   Revision of Nonautologous Tissue Substitute in Left Ankle Joint, External Approach

0SWH00Z   Revision of Drainage Device in Right Tarsal Joint, Open Approach

0SWH03Z Revision of Infusion Device in Right Tarsal Joint, Open Approach

0SWH04Z Revision of Internal Fixation Device in Right Tarsal Joint, Open Approach

0SWH05Z Revision of External Fixation Device in Right Tarsal Joint, Open Approach

0SWH07Z Revision of Autologous Tissue Substitute in Right Tarsal Joint, Open Approach

0SWH08Z Revision of Spacer in Right Tarsal Joint, Open Approach

0SWH0JZ Revision of Synthetic Substitute in Right Tarsal Joint, Open Approach

0SWH0KZ Revision of Nonautologous Tissue Substitute in Right Tarsal Joint, Open Approach

0SWH30Z Revision of Drainage Device in Right Tarsal Joint, Percutaneous Approach

0SWH33Z Revision of Infusion Device in Right Tarsal Joint, Percutaneous Approach

0SWH34Z Revision of Internal Fixation Device in Right Tarsal Joint, Percutaneous Approach

0SWH35Z Revision of External Fixation Device in Right Tarsal Joint, Percutaneous Approach

0SWH37Z Revision of Autologous Tissue Substitute in Right Tarsal Joint, Percutaneous Approach

0SWH38Z Revision of Spacer in Right Tarsal Joint, Percutaneous Approach

0SWH3JZ Revision of Synthetic Substitute in Right Tarsal Joint, Percutaneous Approach

0SWH3KZ Revision of Nonautologous Tissue Substitute in Right Tarsal Joint, Percutaneous Approach

0SWH40Z Revision of Drainage Device in Right Tarsal Joint, Percutaneous Endoscopic Approach

0SWH43Z Revision of Infusion Device in Right Tarsal Joint, Percutaneous Endoscopic Approach

0SWH44Z Revision of Internal Fixation Device in Right Tarsal Joint, Percutaneous Endoscopic Approach

0SWH45Z Revision of External Fixation Device in Right Tarsal Joint, Percutaneous Endoscopic Approach

0SWH47Z Revision of Autologous Tissue Substitute in Right Tarsal Joint, Percutaneous Endoscopic Approach

0SWH48Z Revision of Spacer in Right Tarsal Joint, Percutaneous Endoscopic Approach

0SWH4JZ Revision of Synthetic Substitute in Right Tarsal Joint, Percutaneous Endoscopic Approach

0SWH4KZ Revision of Nonautologous Tissue Substitute in Right Tarsal Joint, Percutaneous Endoscopic Approach

0SWHX0Z Revision of Drainage Device in Right Tarsal Joint, External Approach

0SWHX3Z Revision of Infusion Device in Right Tarsal Joint, External Approach

0SWHX4Z Revision of Internal Fixation Device in Right Tarsal Joint, External Approach

0SWHX5Z Revision of External Fixation Device in Right Tarsal Joint, External Approach

0SWHX7Z Revision of Autologous Tissue Substitute in Right Tarsal Joint, External Approach

0SWHX8Z Revision of Spacer in Right Tarsal Joint, External Approach

0SWHXJZ Revision of Synthetic Substitute in Right Tarsal Joint, External Approach

0SWHXKZ Revision of Nonautologous Tissue Substitute in Right Tarsal Joint, External Approach

0SWJ00Z Revision of Drainage Device in Left Tarsal Joint, Open Approach

0SWJ03Z Revision of Infusion Device in Left Tarsal Joint, Open Approach

0SWJ04Z Revision of Internal Fixation Device in Left Tarsal Joint, Open Approach

0SWJ05Z Revision of External Fixation Device in Left Tarsal Joint, Open Approach

0SWJ07Z Revision of Autologous Tissue Substitute in Left Tarsal Joint, Open Approach

0SWJ08Z Revision of Spacer in Left Tarsal Joint, Open Approach

0SWJ0JZ Revision of Synthetic Substitute in Left Tarsal Joint, Open Approach

0SWJ0KZ Revision of Nonautologous Tissue Substitute in Left Tarsal Joint, Open Approach

0SWJ30Z Revision of Drainage Device in Left Tarsal Joint, Percutaneous Approach

0SWJ33Z Revision of Infusion Device in Left Tarsal Joint, Percutaneous Approach

0SWJ34Z Revision of Internal Fixation Device in Left Tarsal Joint, Percutaneous Approach

0SWJ35Z Revision of External Fixation Device in Left Tarsal Joint, Percutaneous Approach

0SWJ37Z Revision of Autologous Tissue Substitute in Left Tarsal Joint, Percutaneous Approach

0SWJ38Z Revision of Spacer in Left Tarsal Joint, Percutaneous Approach

0SWJ3JZ Revision of Synthetic Substitute in Left Tarsal Joint, Percutaneous Approach

0SWJ3KZ Revision of Nonautologous Tissue Substitute in Left Tarsal Joint, Percutaneous Approach

0SWJ40Z Revision of Drainage Device in Left Tarsal Joint, Percutaneous Endoscopic Approach

0SWJ43Z Revision of Infusion Device in Left Tarsal Joint, Percutaneous Endoscopic Approach

0SWJ44Z Revision of Internal Fixation Device in Left Tarsal Joint, Percutaneous Endoscopic Approach

0SWJ45Z Revision of External Fixation Device in Left Tarsal Joint, Percutaneous Endoscopic Approach

0SWJ47Z Revision of Autologous Tissue Substitute in Left Tarsal Joint, Percutaneous Endoscopic Approach

0SWJ48Z Revision of Spacer in Left Tarsal Joint, Percutaneous Endoscopic Approach

0SWJ4JZ Revision of Synthetic Substitute in Left Tarsal Joint, Percutaneous Endoscopic Approach

0SWJ4KZ Revision of Nonautologous Tissue Substitute in Left Tarsal Joint, Percutaneous Endoscopic Approach

0SWJX0Z Revision of Drainage Device in Left Tarsal Joint, External Approach

0SWJX3Z Revision of Infusion Device in Left Tarsal Joint, External Approach

0SWJX4Z Revision of Internal Fixation Device in Left Tarsal Joint, External Approach

0SWJX5Z Revision of External Fixation Device in Left Tarsal Joint, External Approach

0SWJX7Z Revision of Autologous Tissue Substitute in Left Tarsal Joint, External Approach

0SWJX8Z Revision of Spacer in Left Tarsal Joint, External Approach

0SWJXJZ Revision of Synthetic Substitute in Left Tarsal Joint, External Approach

0SWJXKZ Revision of Nonautologous Tissue Substitute in Left Tarsal Joint, External Approach

0SWK00Z Revision of Drainage Device in Right Metatarsal-Tarsal Joint, Open Approach

0SWK03Z Revision of Infusion Device in Right Metatarsal-Tarsal Joint, Open Approach

0SWK04Z Revision of Internal Fixation Device in Right Metatarsal-Tarsal Joint, Open Approach

0SWK05Z Revision of External Fixation Device in Right Metatarsal-Tarsal Joint, Open Approach

0SWK07Z Revision of Autologous Tissue Substitute in Right Metatarsal-Tarsal Joint, Open Approach

0SWK08Z Revision of Spacer in Right Metatarsal-Tarsal Joint, Open Approach

0SWK0JZ Revision of Synthetic Substitute in Right Metatarsal-Tarsal Joint, Open Approach

0SWK0KZ Revision of Nonautologous Tissue Substitute in Right Metatarsal-Tarsal Joint, Open Approach

0SWK30Z Revision of Drainage Device in Right Metatarsal-Tarsal Joint, Percutaneous Approach

0SWK33Z Revision of Infusion Device in Right Metatarsal-Tarsal Joint, Percutaneous Approach

0SWK34Z Revision of Internal Fixation Device in Right Metatarsal-Tarsal Joint, Percutaneous Approach

0SWK35Z Revision of External Fixation Device in Right Metatarsal-Tarsal Joint, Percutaneous Approach

0SWK37Z Revision of Autologous Tissue Substitute in Right Metatarsal-Tarsal Joint, Percutaneous Approach

0SWK38Z Revision of Spacer in Right Metatarsal-Tarsal Joint, Percutaneous Approach

0SWK3JZ Revision of Synthetic Substitute in Right Metatarsal-Tarsal Joint, Percutaneous Approach

0SWK3KZ   Revision of Nonautologous Tissue Substitute in Right Metatarsal-Tarsal Joint, Percutaneous Approach

0SWK40Z   Revision of Drainage Device in Right Metatarsal-Tarsal Joint, Percutaneous Endoscopic Approach

0SWK43Z   Revision of Infusion Device in Right Metatarsal-Tarsal Joint, Percutaneous Endoscopic Approach

0SWK44Z   Revision of Internal Fixation Device in Right Metatarsal-Tarsal Joint, Percutaneous Endoscopic Approach

0SWK45Z   Revision of External Fixation Device in Right Metatarsal-Tarsal Joint, Percutaneous Endoscopic Approach

0SWK47Z   Revision of Autologous Tissue Substitute in Right Metatarsal-Tarsal Joint, Percutaneous Endoscopic Approach

0SWK48Z   Revision of Spacer in Right Metatarsal-Tarsal Joint, Percutaneous Endoscopic Approach

0SWK4JZ   Revision of Synthetic Substitute in Right Metatarsal-Tarsal Joint, Percutaneous Endoscopic Approach

0SWK4KZ   Revision of Nonautologous Tissue Substitute in Right Metatarsal-Tarsal Joint, Percutaneous Endoscopic Approach

0SWKX0Z   Revision of Drainage Device in Right Metatarsal-Tarsal Joint, External Approach

0SWKX3Z   Revision of Infusion Device in Right Metatarsal-Tarsal Joint, External Approach

0SWKX4Z   Revision of Internal Fixation Device in Right Metatarsal-Tarsal Joint, External Approach

0SWKX5Z   Revision of External Fixation Device in Right Metatarsal-Tarsal Joint, External Approach

0SWKX7Z   Revision of Autologous Tissue Substitute in Right Metatarsal-Tarsal Joint, External Approach

0SWKX8Z   Revision of Spacer in Right Metatarsal-Tarsal Joint, External Approach

0SWKXJZ   Revision of Synthetic Substitute in Right Metatarsal-Tarsal Joint, External Approach

0SWKXKZ   Revision of Nonautologous Tissue Substitute in Right Metatarsal-Tarsal Joint, External Approach

0SWL00Z   Revision of Drainage Device in Left Metatarsal-Tarsal Joint, Open Approach

0SWL03Z   Revision of Infusion Device in Left Metatarsal-Tarsal Joint, Open Approach

0SWL04Z   Revision of Internal Fixation Device in Left Metatarsal-Tarsal Joint, Open Approach

0SWL05Z   Revision of External Fixation Device in Left Metatarsal-Tarsal Joint, Open Approach

0SWL07Z   Revision of Autologous Tissue Substitute in Left Metatarsal-Tarsal Joint, Open Approach

0SWL08Z   Revision of Spacer in Left Metatarsal-Tarsal Joint, Open Approach

0SWL0JZ   Revision of Synthetic Substitute in Left Metatarsal-Tarsal Joint, Open Approach

0SWL0KZ   Revision of Nonautologous Tissue Substitute in Left Metatarsal-Tarsal Joint, Open Approach

0SWL30Z   Revision of Drainage Device in Left Metatarsal-Tarsal Joint, Percutaneous Approach

0SWL33Z   Revision of Infusion Device in Left Metatarsal-Tarsal Joint, Percutaneous Approach

0SWL34Z   Revision of Internal Fixation Device in Left Metatarsal-Tarsal Joint, Percutaneous Approach

0SWL35Z   Revision of External Fixation Device in Left Metatarsal-Tarsal Joint, Percutaneous Approach

0SWL37Z   Revision of Autologous Tissue Substitute in Left Metatarsal-Tarsal Joint, Percutaneous Approach

0SWL38Z   Revision of Spacer in Left Metatarsal-Tarsal Joint, Percutaneous Approach

0SWL3JZ   Revision of Synthetic Substitute in Left Metatarsal-Tarsal Joint, Percutaneous Approach

0SWL3KZ   Revision of Nonautologous Tissue Substitute in Left Metatarsal-Tarsal Joint, Percutaneous Approach

0SWL40Z   Revision of Drainage Device in Left Metatarsal-Tarsal Joint, Percutaneous Endoscopic Approach

0SWL43Z   Revision of Infusion Device in Left Metatarsal-Tarsal Joint, Percutaneous Endoscopic Approach

0SWL44Z   Revision of Internal Fixation Device in Left Metatarsal-Tarsal Joint, Percutaneous Endoscopic Approach

0SWL45Z   Revision of External Fixation Device in Left Metatarsal-Tarsal Joint, Percutaneous Endoscopic Approach

0SWL47Z   Revision of Autologous Tissue Substitute in Left Metatarsal-Tarsal Joint, Percutaneous Endoscopic Approach

0SWL48Z   Revision of Spacer in Left Metatarsal-Tarsal Joint, Percutaneous Endoscopic Approach

0SWL4JZ   Revision of Synthetic Substitute in Left Metatarsal-Tarsal Joint, Percutaneous Endoscopic Approach

0SWL4KZ   Revision of Nonautologous Tissue Substitute in Left Metatarsal-Tarsal Joint, Percutaneous Endoscopic Approach

0SWLX0Z   Revision of Drainage Device in Left Metatarsal-Tarsal Joint, External Approach

0SWLX3Z   Revision of Infusion Device in Left Metatarsal-Tarsal Joint, External Approach

0SWLX4Z   Revision of Internal Fixation Device in Left Metatarsal-Tarsal Joint, External Approach

0SWLX5Z   Revision of External Fixation Device in Left Metatarsal-Tarsal Joint, External Approach

0SWLX7Z   Revision of Autologous Tissue Substitute in Left Metatarsal-Tarsal Joint, External Approach

0SWLX8Z   Revision of Spacer in Left Metatarsal-Tarsal Joint, External Approach

0SWLXJZ   Revision of Synthetic Substitute in Left Metatarsal-Tarsal Joint, External Approach

0SWLXKZ   Revision of Nonautologous Tissue Substitute in Left Metatarsal-Tarsal Joint, External Approach

0SWM00Z   Revision of Drainage Device in Right Metatarsal-Phalangeal Joint, Open Approach

0SWM03Z   Revision of Infusion Device in Right Metatarsal-Phalangeal Joint, Open Approach

0SWM04Z   Revision of Internal Fixation Device in Right Metatarsal-Phalangeal Joint, Open Approach

0SWM05Z   Revision of External Fixation Device in Right Metatarsal-Phalangeal Joint, Open Approach

0SWM07Z   Revision of Autologous Tissue Substitute in Right Metatarsal-Phalangeal Joint, Open Approach

0SWM08Z   Revision of Spacer in Right Metatarsal-Phalangeal Joint, Open Approach

0SWM0JZ   Revision of Synthetic Substitute in Right Metatarsal-Phalangeal Joint, Open Approach

0SWM0KZ   Revision of Nonautologous Tissue Substitute in Right Metatarsal-Phalangeal Joint, Open Approach

0SWM30Z   Revision of Drainage Device in Right Metatarsal-Phalangeal Joint, Percutaneous Approach

0SWM33Z   Revision of Infusion Device in Right Metatarsal-Phalangeal Joint, Percutaneous Approach

0SWM34Z   Revision of Internal Fixation Device in Right Metatarsal-Phalangeal Joint, Percutaneous Approach

0SWM35Z   Revision of External Fixation Device in Right Metatarsal-Phalangeal Joint, Percutaneous Approach

0SWM37Z   Revision of Autologous Tissue Substitute in Right Metatarsal-Phalangeal Joint, Percutaneous Approach

0SWM38Z   Revision of Spacer in Right Metatarsal-Phalangeal Joint, Percutaneous Approach

0SWM3JZ   Revision of Synthetic Substitute in Right Metatarsal-Phalangeal Joint, Percutaneous Approach

0SWM3KZ   Revision of Nonautologous Tissue Substitute in Right Metatarsal-Phalangeal Joint, Percutaneous Approach

0SWM40Z   Revision of Drainage Device in Right Metatarsal-Phalangeal Joint, Percutaneous Endoscopic Approach

0SWM43Z   Revision of Infusion Device in Right Metatarsal-Phalangeal Joint, Percutaneous Endoscopic Approach

0SWM44Z   Revision of Internal Fixation Device in Right Metatarsal-Phalangeal Joint, Percutaneous Endoscopic Approach

0SWM45Z   Revision of External Fixation Device in Right Metatarsal-Phalangeal Joint, Percutaneous Endoscopic Approach

0SWM47Z   Revision of Autologous Tissue Substitute in Right Metatarsal-Phalangeal Joint, Percutaneous Endoscopic Approach

0SWM48Z   Revision of Spacer in Right Metatarsal-Phalangeal Joint, Percutaneous Endoscopic Approach

0SWM4JZ   Revision of Synthetic Substitute in Right Metatarsal-Phalangeal Joint, Percutaneous Endoscopic Approach

0SWM4KZ   Revision of Nonautologous Tissue Substitute in Right Metatarsal-Phalangeal Joint, Percutaneous Endoscopic Approach

0SWMX0Z   Revision of Drainage Device in Right Metatarsal-Phalangeal Joint, External Approach

---

♀ Female-only   ♂ Male-only   ◕ Limited Coverage   ● Non-OR   ▨ HAC-associated procedure   ⬤ Non-covered procedures   ✚ Combination

0SWMX3Z Revision of Infusion Device in Right Metatarsal-Phalangeal Joint, External Approach

0SWMX4Z Revision of Internal Fixation Device in Right Metatarsal-Phalangeal Joint, External Approach

0SWMX5Z Revision of External Fixation Device in Right Metatarsal-Phalangeal Joint, External Approach

0SWMX7Z Revision of Autologous Tissue Substitute in Right Metatarsal-Phalangeal Joint, External Approach

0SWMX8Z Revision of Spacer in Right Metatarsal-Phalangeal Joint, External Approach

0SWMXJZ Revision of Synthetic Substitute in Right Metatarsal-Phalangeal Joint, External Approach

0SWMXKZ Revision of Nonautologous Tissue Substitute in Right Metatarsal-Phalangeal Joint, External Approach

0SWN00Z Revision of Drainage Device in Left Metatarsal-Phalangeal Joint, Open Approach

0SWN03Z Revision of Infusion Device in Left Metatarsal-Phalangeal Joint, Open Approach

0SWN04Z Revision of Internal Fixation Device in Left Metatarsal-Phalangeal Joint, Open Approach

0SWN05Z Revision of External Fixation Device in Left Metatarsal-Phalangeal Joint, Open Approach

0SWN07Z Revision of Autologous Tissue Substitute in Left Metatarsal-Phalangeal Joint, Open Approach

0SWN08Z Revision of Spacer in Left Metatarsal-Phalangeal Joint, Open Approach

0SWN0JZ Revision of Synthetic Substitute in Left Metatarsal-Phalangeal Joint, Open Approach

0SWN0KZ Revision of Nonautologous Tissue Substitute in Left Metatarsal-Phalangeal Joint, Open Approach

0SWN30Z Revision of Drainage Device in Left Metatarsal-Phalangeal Joint, Percutaneous Approach

0SWN33Z Revision of Infusion Device in Left Metatarsal-Phalangeal Joint, Percutaneous Approach

0SWN34Z Revision of Internal Fixation Device in Left Metatarsal-Phalangeal Joint, Percutaneous Approach

0SWN35Z Revision of External Fixation Device in Left Metatarsal-Phalangeal Joint, Percutaneous Approach

0SWN37Z Revision of Autologous Tissue Substitute in Left Metatarsal-Phalangeal Joint, Percutaneous Approach

0SWN38Z Revision of Spacer in Left Metatarsal-Phalangeal Joint, Percutaneous Approach

0SWN3JZ Revision of Synthetic Substitute in Left Metatarsal-Phalangeal Joint, Percutaneous Approach

0SWN3KZ Revision of Nonautologous Tissue Substitute in Left Metatarsal-Phalangeal Joint, Percutaneous Approach

0SWN40Z Revision of Drainage Device in Left Metatarsal-Phalangeal Joint, Percutaneous Endoscopic Approach

0SWN43Z Revision of Infusion Device in Left Metatarsal-Phalangeal Joint, Percutaneous Endoscopic Approach

0SWN44Z Revision of Internal Fixation Device in Left Metatarsal-Phalangeal Joint, Percutaneous Endoscopic Approach

0SWN45Z Revision of External Fixation Device in Left Metatarsal-Phalangeal Joint, Percutaneous Endoscopic Approach

0SWN47Z Revision of Autologous Tissue Substitute in Left Metatarsal-Phalangeal Joint, Percutaneous Endoscopic Approach

0SWN48Z Revision of Spacer in Left Metatarsal-Phalangeal Joint, Percutaneous Endoscopic Approach

0SWN4JZ Revision of Synthetic Substitute in Left Metatarsal-Phalangeal Joint, Percutaneous Endoscopic Approach

0SWN4KZ Revision of Nonautologous Tissue Substitute in Left Metatarsal-Phalangeal Joint, Percutaneous Endoscopic Approach

0SWNX0Z Revision of Drainage Device in Left Metatarsal-Phalangeal Joint, External Approach

0SWNX3Z Revision of Infusion Device in Left Metatarsal-Phalangeal Joint, External Approach

0SWNX4Z Revision of Internal Fixation Device in Left Metatarsal-Phalangeal Joint, External Approach

0SWNX5Z Revision of External Fixation Device in Left Metatarsal-Phalangeal Joint, External Approach

0SWNX7Z Revision of Autologous Tissue Substitute in Left Metatarsal-Phalangeal Joint, External Approach

0SWNX8Z Revision of Spacer in Left Metatarsal-Phalangeal Joint, External Approach

0SWNXJZ Revision of Synthetic Substitute in Left Metatarsal-Phalangeal Joint, External Approach

0SWNXKZ Revision of Nonautologous Tissue Substitute in Left Metatarsal-Phalangeal Joint, External Approach

0SWP00Z Revision of Drainage Device in Right Toe Phalangeal Joint, Open Approach

0SWP03Z Revision of Infusion Device in Right Toe Phalangeal Joint, Open Approach

0SWP04Z Revision of Internal Fixation Device in Right Toe Phalangeal Joint, Open Approach

0SWP05Z Revision of External Fixation Device in Right Toe Phalangeal Joint, Open Approach

0SWP07Z Revision of Autologous Tissue Substitute in Right Toe Phalangeal Joint, Open Approach

0SWP08Z Revision of Spacer in Right Toe Phalangeal Joint, Open Approach

0SWP0JZ Revision of Synthetic Substitute in Right Toe Phalangeal Joint, Open Approach

0SWP0KZ Revision of Nonautologous Tissue Substitute in Right Toe Phalangeal Joint, Open Approach

0SWP30Z Revision of Drainage Device in Right Toe Phalangeal Joint, Percutaneous Approach

0SWP33Z Revision of Infusion Device in Right Toe Phalangeal Joint, Percutaneous Approach

0SWP34Z Revision of Internal Fixation Device in Right Toe Phalangeal Joint, Percutaneous Approach

0SWP35Z Revision of External Fixation Device in Right Toe Phalangeal Joint, Percutaneous Approach

0SWP37Z Revision of Autologous Tissue Substitute in Right Toe Phalangeal Joint, Percutaneous Approach

0SWP38Z Revision of Spacer in Right Toe Phalangeal Joint, Percutaneous Approach

0SWP3JZ Revision of Synthetic Substitute in Right Toe Phalangeal Joint, Percutaneous Approach

0SWP3KZ Revision of Nonautologous Tissue Substitute in Right Toe Phalangeal Joint, Percutaneous Approach

0SWP40Z Revision of Drainage Device in Right Toe Phalangeal Joint, Percutaneous Endoscopic Approach

0SWP43Z Revision of Infusion Device in Right Toe Phalangeal Joint, Percutaneous Endoscopic Approach

0SWP44Z Revision of Internal Fixation Device in Right Toe Phalangeal Joint, Percutaneous Endoscopic Approach

0SWP45Z Revision of External Fixation Device in Right Toe Phalangeal Joint, Percutaneous Endoscopic Approach

0SWP47Z Revision of Autologous Tissue Substitute in Right Toe Phalangeal Joint, Percutaneous Endoscopic Approach

0SWP48Z Revision of Spacer in Right Toe Phalangeal Joint, Percutaneous Endoscopic Approach

0SWP4JZ Revision of Synthetic Substitute in Right Toe Phalangeal Joint, Percutaneous Endoscopic Approach

0SWP4KZ Revision of Nonautologous Tissue Substitute in Right Toe Phalangeal Joint, Percutaneous Endoscopic Approach

0SWPX0Z Revision of Drainage Device in Right Toe Phalangeal Joint, External Approach

0SWPX3Z Revision of Infusion Device in Right Toe Phalangeal Joint, External Approach

0SWPX4Z Revision of Internal Fixation Device in Right Toe Phalangeal Joint, External Approach

0SWPX5Z Revision of External Fixation Device in Right Toe Phalangeal Joint, External Approach

0SWPX7Z Revision of Autologous Tissue Substitute in Right Toe Phalangeal Joint, External Approach

0SWPX8Z Revision of Spacer in Right Toe Phalangeal Joint, External Approach

0SWPXJZ Revision of Synthetic Substitute in Right Toe Phalangeal Joint, External Approach

0SWPXKZ Revision of Nonautologous Tissue Substitute in Right Toe Phalangeal Joint, External Approach

0SWQ00Z Revision of Drainage Device in Left Toe Phalangeal Joint, Open Approach

0SWQ03Z Revision of Infusion Device in Left Toe Phalangeal Joint, Open Approach

0SWQ04Z Revision of Internal Fixation Device in Left Toe Phalangeal Joint, Open Approach

---

 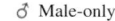

0SWQ05Z Revision of External Fixation Device in Left Toe Phalangeal Joint, Open Approach

0SWQ07Z Revision of Autologous Tissue Substitute in Left Toe Phalangeal Joint, Open Approach

0SWQ08Z Revision of Spacer in Left Toe Phalangeal Joint, Open Approach

0SWQ0JZ Revision of Synthetic Substitute in Left Toe Phalangeal Joint, Open Approach

0SWQ0KZ Revision of Nonautologous Tissue Substitute in Left Toe Phalangeal Joint, Open Approach

0SWQ30Z Revision of Drainage Device in Left Toe Phalangeal Joint, Percutaneous Approach

0SWQ33Z Revision of Infusion Device in Left Toe Phalangeal Joint, Percutaneous Approach

0SWQ34Z Revision of Internal Fixation Device in Left Toe Phalangeal Joint, Percutaneous Approach

0SWQ35Z Revision of External Fixation Device in Left Toe Phalangeal Joint, Percutaneous Approach

0SWQ37Z Revision of Autologous Tissue Substitute in Left Toe Phalangeal Joint, Percutaneous Approach

0SWQ38Z Revision of Spacer in Left Toe Phalangeal Joint, Percutaneous Approach

0SWQ3JZ Revision of Synthetic Substitute in Left Toe Phalangeal Joint, Percutaneous Approach

0SWQ3KZ Revision of Nonautologous Tissue Substitute in Left Toe Phalangeal Joint, Percutaneous Approach

0SWQ40Z Revision of Drainage Device in Left Toe Phalangeal Joint, Percutaneous Endoscopic Approach

0SWQ43Z Revision of Infusion Device in Left Toe Phalangeal Joint, Percutaneous Endoscopic Approach

0SWQ44Z Revision of Internal Fixation Device in Left Toe Phalangeal Joint, Percutaneous Endoscopic Approach

0SWQ45Z Revision of External Fixation Device in Left Toe Phalangeal Joint, Percutaneous Endoscopic Approach

0SWQ47Z Revision of Autologous Tissue Substitute in Left Toe Phalangeal Joint, Percutaneous Endoscopic Approach

0SWQ48Z Revision of Spacer in Left Toe Phalangeal Joint, Percutaneous Endoscopic Approach

0SWQ4JZ Revision of Synthetic Substitute in Left Toe Phalangeal Joint, Percutaneous Endoscopic Approach

0SWQ4KZ Revision of Nonautologous Tissue Substitute in Left Toe Phalangeal Joint, Percutaneous Endoscopic Approach

0SWQX0Z Revision of Drainage Device in Left Toe Phalangeal Joint, External Approach

0SWQX3Z Revision of Infusion Device in Left Toe Phalangeal Joint, External Approach

0SWQX4Z Revision of Internal Fixation Device in Left Toe Phalangeal Joint, External Approach

0SWQX5Z Revision of External Fixation Device in Left Toe Phalangeal Joint, External Approach

0SWQX7Z Revision of Autologous Tissue Substitute in Left Toe Phalangeal Joint, External Approach

0SWQX8Z Revision of Spacer in Left Toe Phalangeal Joint, External Approach

0SWQXJZ Revision of Synthetic Substitute in Left Toe Phalangeal Joint, External Approach

0SWQXKZ Revision of Nonautologous Tissue Substitute in Left Toe Phalangeal Joint, External Approach

Urinary System

Urinary System

- Diaphragm
- Adrenal gland
- Kidney
- Renal artery
- Renl vein
- Inferior vena cava
- Abdominal aorta
- Ureter
- Urinary bladder
- Urethra

Lower Urinary Tract

- Median umbilical ligament
- Ureter
- Peritoneum
- Ureteral openings
- Trigone
- Bladder neck
- Internal urethral sphincter
- External urethral sphincter

Kidney

- Renal cortex
- Blood vessels
- Renal medulla (renal pyramid)
- Renal sinus
- Renal papilla
- Renal column (of Bertin)
- Medullary rays
- Base of renal pyramid
- Fibrous capsule
- Minor calyces
- Major calyces
- Renal pelvis
- Fat in renal sinus
- Ureter

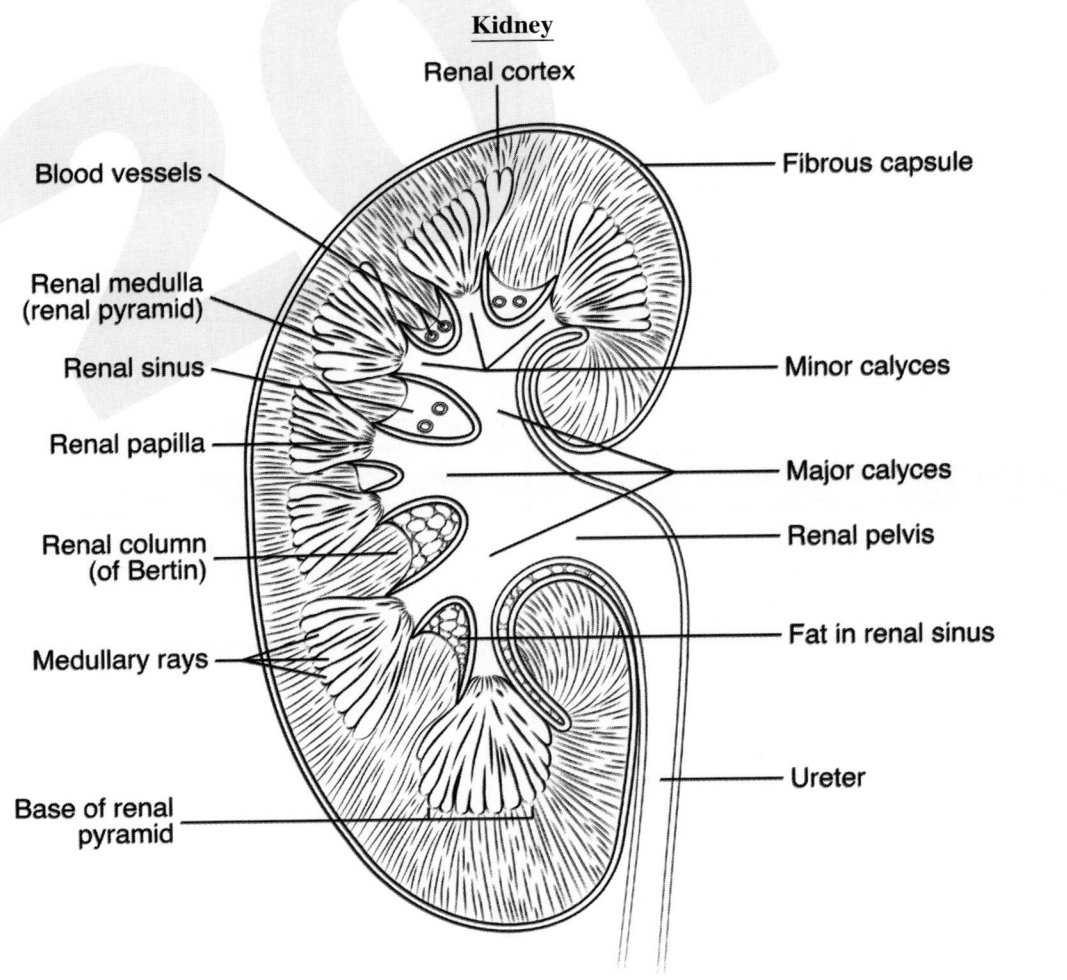

Urinary System Tables 0T1–0TY

Section	**0**	**Medical and Surgical**
Body System	**T**	**Urinary System**
Operation	**1**	**Bypass:** Altering the route of passage of the contents of a tubular body part

Body Part (4ᵗʰ)	Approach (5ᵗʰ)	Device (6ᵗʰ)	Qualifier (7ᵗʰ)
3 Kidney Pelvis, Right **4** Kidney Pelvis, Left	**0** Open **4** Percutaneous Endoscopic	**7** Autologous Tissue Substitute **J** Synthetic Substitute **K** Nonautologous Tissue Substitute **Z** No Device	**3** Kidney Pelvis, Right **4** Kidney Pelvis, Left **6** Ureter, Right **7** Ureter, Left **8** Colon **9** Colocutaneous **A** Ileum **B** Bladder **C** Ileocutaneous **D** Cutaneous
3 Kidney Pelvis, Right **4** Kidney Pelvis, Left	**3** Percutaneous	**J** Synthetic Substitute	**D** Cutaneous
6 Ureter, Right **7** Ureter, Left **8** Ureters, Bilateral	**0** Open **4** Percutaneous Endoscopic	**7** Autologous Tissue Substitute **J** Synthetic Substitute **K** Nonautologous Tissue Substitute **Z** No Device	**6** Ureter, Right **7** Ureter, Left **8** Colon **9** Colocutaneous **A** Ileum **B** Bladder **C** Ileocutaneous **D** Cutaneous
6 Ureter, Right **7** Ureter, Left **8** Ureters, Bilateral	**3** Percutaneous	**J** Synthetic Substitute	**D** Cutaneous
B Bladder	**0** Open **4** Percutaneous Endoscopic	**7** Autologous Tissue Substitute **J** Synthetic Substitute **K** Nonautologous Tissue Substitute **Z** No Device	**9** Colocutaneous **C** Ileocutaneous **D** Cutaneous
B Bladder	**3** Percutaneous	**J** Synthetic Substitute	**D** Cutaneous

Section	**0**	**Medical and Surgical**
Body System	**T**	**Urinary System**
Operation	**2**	**Change:** Taking out or off a device from a body part and putting back an identical or similar device in or on the same body part without cutting or puncturing the skin or a mucous membrane

Body Part (4ᵗʰ)	Approach (5ᵗʰ)	Device (6ᵗʰ)	Qualifier (7ᵗʰ)
5 Kidney **9** Ureter **B** Bladder **D** Urethra	**X** External	**0** Drainage Device **Y** Other Device	**Z** No Qualifier

Section	0	Medical and Surgical
Body System	T	Urinary System
Operation	5	Destruction: Physical eradication of all or a portion of a body part by the direct use of energy, force, or a destructive agent

Body Part (4th)	Approach (5th)	Device (6th)	Qualifier (7th)
0 Kidney, Right 1 Kidney, Left 3 Kidney Pelvis, Right 4 Kidney Pelvis, Left 6 Ureter, Right 7 Ureter, Left B Bladder C Bladder Neck	0 Open 3 Percutaneous 4 Percutaneous Endoscopic 7 Via Natural or Artificial Opening 8 Via Natural or Artificial Opening Endoscopic	Z No Device	Z No Qualifier
D Urethra	0 Open 3 Percutaneous 4 Percutaneous Endoscopic 7 Via Natural or Artificial Opening 8 Via Natural or Artificial Opening Endoscopic X External	Z No Device	Z No Qualifier

Section	0	Medical and Surgical
Body System	T	Urinary System
Operation	7	Dilation: Expanding an orifice or the lumen of a tubular body part

Body Part (4th)	Approach (5th)	Device (6th)	Qualifier (7th)
3 Kidney Pelvis, Right 4 Kidney Pelvis, Left 6 Ureter, Right 7 Ureter, Left 8 Ureters, Bilateral B Bladder C Bladder Neck D Urethra	0 Open 3 Percutaneous 4 Percutaneous Endoscopic 7 Via Natural or Artificial Opening 8 Via Natural or Artificial Opening Endoscopic	D Intraluminal Device Z No Device	Z No Qualifier

Section	0	Medical and Surgical
Body System	T	Urinary System
Operation	8	Division: Cutting into a body part, without draining fluids and/or gases from the body part, in order to separate or transect a body part

Body Part (4th)	Approach (5th)	Device (6th)	Qualifier (7th)
2 Kidneys, Bilateral C Bladder Neck	0 Open 3 Percutaneous 4 Percutaneous Endoscopic	Z No Device	Z No Qualifier

Section	0	Medical and Surgical
Body System	T	Urinary System
Operation	9	Drainage: Taking or letting out fluids and/or gases from a body part

Body Part (4th)	Approach (5th)	Device (6th)	Qualifier (7th)
0 Kidney, Right 1 Kidney, Left 3 Kidney Pelvis, Right 4 Kidney Pelvis, Left 6 Ureter, Right 7 Ureter, Left 8 Ureters, Bilateral B Bladder C Bladder Neck	0 Open 3 Percutaneous 4 Percutaneous Endoscopic 7 Via Natural or Artificial Opening 8 Via Natural or Artificial Opening Endoscopic	0 Drainage Device	Z No Qualifier

Continued

Section	0	Medical and Surgical			0T9 *Continued*
Body System	T	Urinary System			
Operation	9	**Drainage:** Taking or letting out fluids and/or gases from a body part			

Body Part (4th)	Approach (5th)	Device (6th)	Qualifier (7th)
0 Kidney, Right 1 Kidney, Left 3 Kidney Pelvis, Right 4 Kidney Pelvis, Left 6 Ureter, Right 7 Ureter, Left 8 Ureters, Bilateral B Bladder C Bladder Neck	0 Open 3 Percutaneous 4 Percutaneous Endoscopic 7 Via Natural or Artificial Opening 8 Via Natural or Artificial Opening Endoscopic	Z No Device	X Diagnostic Z No Qualifier
D Urethra	0 Open 3 Percutaneous 4 Percutaneous Endoscopic 7 Via Natural or Artificial Opening 8 Via Natural or Artificial Opening Endoscopic X External	0 Drainage Device	Z No Qualifier
D Urethra	0 Open 3 Percutaneous 4 Percutaneous Endoscopic 7 Via Natural or Artificial Opening 8 Via Natural or Artificial Opening Endoscopic X External	Z No Device	X Diagnostic Z No Qualifier

Section	0	Medical and Surgical			
Body System	T	Urinary System			
Operation	B	**Excision:** Cutting out or off, without replacement, a portion of a body part			

Body Part (4th)	Approach (5th)	Device (6th)	Qualifier (7th)
0 Kidney, Right 1 Kidney, Left 3 Kidney Pelvis, Right 4 Kidney Pelvis, Left 6 Ureter, Right 7 Ureter, Left B Bladder C Bladder Neck	0 Open 3 Percutaneous 4 Percutaneous Endoscopic 7 Via Natural or Artificial Opening 8 Via Natural or Artificial Opening Endoscopic	Z No Device	X Diagnostic Z No Qualifier
D Urethra	0 Open 3 Percutaneous 4 Percutaneous Endoscopic 7 Via Natural or Artificial Opening 8 Via Natural or Artificial Opening Endoscopic X External	Z No Device	X Diagnostic Z No Qualifier

Section	0	**Medical and Surgical**
Body System	T	**Urinary System**
Operation	C	**Extirpation:** Taking or cutting out solid matter from a body part

Body Part (4ᵗʰ)	Approach (5ᵗʰ)	Device (6ᵗʰ)	Qualifier (7ᵗʰ)
0 Kidney, Right 1 Kidney, Left 3 Kidney Pelvis, Right 4 Kidney Pelvis, Left 6 Ureter, Right 7 Ureter, Left B Bladder C Bladder Neck	0 Open 3 Percutaneous 4 Percutaneous Endoscopic 7 Via Natural or Artificial Opening 8 Via Natural or Artificial Opening Endoscopic	Z No Device	Z No Qualifier
D Urethra	0 Open 3 Percutaneous 4 Percutaneous Endoscopic 7 Via Natural or Artificial Opening 8 Via Natural or Artificial Opening Endoscopic X External	Z No Device	Z No Qualifier

Section	0	**Medical and Surgical**
Body System	T	**Urinary System**
Operation	D	**Extraction:** Pulling or stripping out or off all or a portion of a body part by the use of force

Body Part (4ᵗʰ)	Approach (5ᵗʰ)	Device (6ᵗʰ)	Qualifier (7ᵗʰ)
0 Kidney, Right 1 Kidney, Left	0 Open 3 Percutaneous 4 Percutaneous Endoscopic	Z No Device	Z No Qualifier

Section	0	**Medical and Surgical**
Body System	T	**Urinary System**
Operation	F	**Fragmentation:** Breaking solid matter in a body part into pieces

Body Part (4ᵗʰ)	Approach (5ᵗʰ)	Device (6ᵗʰ)	Qualifier (7ᵗʰ)
3 Kidney Pelvis, Right 4 Kidney Pelvis, Left 6 Ureter, Right 7 Ureter, Left B Bladder C Bladder Neck D Urethra	0 Open 3 Percutaneous 4 Percutaneous Endoscopic 7 Via Natural or Artificial Opening 8 Via Natural or Artificial Opening Endoscopic X External	Z No Device	Z No Qualifier

Section	0	**Medical and Surgical**
Body System	T	**Urinary System**
Operation	H	**Insertion:** Putting in a nonbiological appliance that monitors, assists, performs, or prevents a physiological function but does not physically take the place of a body part

Body Part (4ᵗʰ)	Approach (5ᵗʰ)	Device (6ᵗʰ)	Qualifier (7ᵗʰ)
5 Kidney	0 Open 3 Percutaneous 4 Percutaneous Endoscopic 7 Via Natural or Artificial Opening 8 Via Natural or Artificial Opening Endoscopic	2 Monitoring Device 3 Infusion Device	Z No Qualifier
9 Ureter	0 Open 3 Percutaneous 4 Percutaneous Endoscopic 7 Via Natural or Artificial Opening 8 Via Natural or Artificial Opening Endoscopic	2 Monitoring Device 3 Infusion Device M Stimulator Lead	Z No Qualifier

Continued

Section	0	Medical and Surgical
Body System	T	Urinary System
Operation	H	Insertion: Putting in a nonbiological appliance that monitors, assists, performs, or prevents a physiological function but does not physically take the place of a body part

Body Part (4th)	Approach (5th)	Device (6th)	Qualifier (7th)
B Bladder	**0** Open **3** Percutaneous **4** Percutaneous Endoscopic **7** Via Natural or Artificial Opening **8** Via Natural or Artificial Opening Endoscopic	**2** Monitoring Device **3** Infusion Device **L** Artificial Sphincter **M** Stimulator Lead	**Z** No Qualifier
C Bladder Neck	**0** Open **3** Percutaneous **4** Percutaneous Endoscopic **7** Via Natural or Artificial Opening **8** Via Natural or Artificial Opening Endoscopic	**L** Artificial Sphincter	**Z** No Qualifier
D Urethra	**0** Open **3** Percutaneous **4** Percutaneous Endoscopic **7** Via Natural or Artificial Opening **8** Via Natural or Artificial Opening Endoscopic **X** External	**2** Monitoring Device **3** Infusion Device **L** Artificial Sphincter	**Z** No Qualifier

Section	0	Medical and Surgical
Body System	T	Urinary System
Operation	J	Inspection: Visually and/or manually exploring a body part

Body Part (4th)	Approach (5th)	Device (6th)	Qualifier (7th)
5 Kidney **9** Ureter **B** Bladder **D** Urethra	**0** Open **3** Percutaneous **4** Percutaneous Endoscopic **7** Via Natural or Artificial Opening **8** Via Natural or Artificial Opening Endoscopic **X** External	**Z** No Device	**Z** No Qualifier

Section	0	Medical and Surgical
Body System	T	Urinary System
Operation	L	Occlusion: Completely closing an orifice or the lumen of a tubular body part

Body Part (4th)	Approach (5th)	Device (6th)	Qualifier (7th)
3 Kidney Pelvis, Right **4** Kidney Pelvis, Left **6** Ureter, Right **7** Ureter, Left **B** Bladder **C** Bladder Neck	**0** Open **3** Percutaneous **4** Percutaneous Endoscopic	**C** Extraluminal Device **D** Intraluminal Device **Z** No Device	**Z** No Qualifier
3 Kidney Pelvis, Right **4** Kidney Pelvis, Left **6** Ureter, Right **7** Ureter, Left **B** Bladder **C** Bladder Neck	**7** Via Natural or Artificial Opening **8** Via Natural or Artificial Opening Endoscopic	**D** Intraluminal Device **Z** No Device	**Z** No Qualifier

Continued

Section	0	Medical and Surgical
Body System	T	Urinary System
Operation	L	**Occlusion:** Completely closing an orifice or the lumen of a tubular body part

Body Part (4th)	Approach (5th)	Device (6th)	Qualifier (7th)
D Urethra	0 Open 3 Percutaneous 4 Percutaneous Endoscopic X External	C Extraluminal Device D Intraluminal Device Z No Device	Z No Qualifier
D Urethra	7 Via Natural or Artificial Opening 8 Via Natural or Artificial Opening Endoscopic	D Intraluminal Device Z No Device	Z No Qualifier

Section	0	Medical and Surgical
Body System	T	Urinary System
Operation	M	**Reattachment:** Putting back in or on all or a portion of a separated body part to its normal location or other suitable location

Body Part (4th)	Approach (5th)	Device (6th)	Qualifier (7th)
0 Kidney, Right 1 Kidney, Left 2 Kidneys, Bilateral 3 Kidney Pelvis, Right 4 Kidney Pelvis, Left 6 Ureter, Right 7 Ureter, Left 8 Ureters, Bilateral B Bladder C Bladder Neck D Urethra	0 Open 4 Percutaneous Endoscopic	Z No Device	Z No Qualifier

Section	0	Medical and Surgical
Body System	T	Urinary System
Operation	N	**Release:** Freeing a body part from an abnormal physical constraint by cutting or by the use of force

Body Part (4th)	Approach (5th)	Device (6th)	Qualifier (7th)
0 Kidney, Right 1 Kidney, Left 3 Kidney Pelvis, Right 4 Kidney Pelvis, Left 6 Ureter, Right 7 Ureter, Left B Bladder C Bladder Neck	0 Open 3 Percutaneous 4 Percutaneous Endoscopic 7 Via Natural or Artificial Opening 8 Via Natural or Artificial Opening Endoscopic	Z No Device	Z No Qualifier
D Urethra	0 Open 3 Percutaneous 4 Percutaneous Endoscopic 7 Via Natural or Artificial Opening 8 Via Natural or Artificial Opening Endoscopic X External	Z No Device	Z No Qualifier

Section	0	**Medical and Surgical**
Body System	**T**	**Urinary System**
Operation	**P**	**Removal:** Taking out or off a device from a body part

Body Part (4ᵗʰ)	Approach (5ᵗʰ)	Device (6ᵗʰ)	Qualifier (7ᵗʰ)
5 Kidney	0 Open 3 Percutaneous 4 Percutaneous Endoscopic 7 Via Natural or Artificial Opening 8 Via Natural or Artificial Opening Endoscopic	0 Drainage Device 2 Monitoring Device 3 Infusion Device 7 Autologous Tissue Substitute C Extraluminal Device D Intraluminal Device J Synthetic Substitute K Nonautologous Tissue Substitute	Z No Qualifier
5 Kidney	X External	0 Drainage Device 2 Monitoring Device 3 Infusion Device D Intraluminal Device	Z No Qualifier
9 Ureter	0 Open 3 Percutaneous 4 Percutaneous Endoscopic 7 Via Natural or Artificial Opening 8 Via Natural or Artificial Opening Endoscopic	0 Drainage Device 2 Monitoring Device 3 Infusion Device 7 Autologous Tissue Substitute C Extraluminal Device D Intraluminal Device J Synthetic Substitute K Nonautologous Tissue Substitute M Stimulator Lead	Z No Qualifier
9 Ureter	X External	0 Drainage Device 2 Monitoring Device 3 Infusion Device D Intraluminal Device M Stimulator Lead	Z No Qualifier
B Bladder	0 Open 3 Percutaneous 4 Percutaneous Endoscopic 7 Via Natural or Artificial Opening 8 Via Natural or Artificial Opening Endoscopic	0 Drainage Device 2 Monitoring Device 3 Infusion Device 7 Autologous Tissue Substitute C Extraluminal Device D Intraluminal Device J Synthetic Substitute K Nonautologous Tissue Substitute L Artificial Sphincter M Stimulator Lead	Z No Qualifier
B Bladder	X External	0 Drainage Device 2 Monitoring Device 3 Infusion Device D Intraluminal Device L Artificial Sphincter M Stimulator Lead	Z No Qualifier
D Urethra	0 Open 3 Percutaneous 4 Percutaneous Endoscopic 7 Via Natural or Artificial Opening 8 Via Natural or Artificial Opening Endoscopic	0 Drainage Device 2 Monitoring Device 3 Infusion Device 7 Autologous Tissue Substitute C Extraluminal Device D Intraluminal Device J Synthetic Substitute K Nonautologous Tissue Substitute L Artificial Sphincter	Z No Qualifier
D Urethra	X External	0 Drainage Device 2 Monitoring Device 3 Infusion Device D Intraluminal Device L Artificial Sphincter	Z No Qualifier

Section	0	Medical and Surgical
Body System	T	Urinary System
Operation	Q	**Repair:** Restoring, to the extent possible, a body part to its normal anatomic structure and function

Body Part (4ᵗʰ)	Approach (5ᵗʰ)	Device (6ᵗʰ)	Qualifier (7ᵗʰ)
0 Kidney, Right 1 Kidney, Left 3 Kidney Pelvis, Right 4 Kidney Pelvis, Left 6 Ureter, Right 7 Ureter, Left B Bladder C Bladder Neck	0 Open 3 Percutaneous 4 Percutaneous Endoscopic 7 Via Natural or Artificial Opening 8 Via Natural or Artificial Opening Endoscopic	Z No Device	Z No Qualifier
D Urethra	0 Open 3 Percutaneous 4 Percutaneous Endoscopic 7 Via Natural or Artificial Opening 8 Via Natural or Artificial Opening Endoscopic X External	Z No Device	Z No Qualifier

Section	0	Medical and Surgical
Body System	T	Urinary System
Operation	R	**Replacement:** Putting in or on biological or synthetic material that physically takes the place and/or function of all or a portion of a body part

Body Part (4ᵗʰ)	Approach (5ᵗʰ)	Device (6ᵗʰ)	Qualifier (7ᵗʰ)
3 Kidney Pelvis, Right 4 Kidney Pelvis, Left 6 Ureter, Right 7 Ureter, Left B Bladder C Bladder Neck	0 Open 4 Percutaneous Endoscopic 7 Via Natural or Artificial Opening 8 Via Natural or Artificial Opening Endoscopic	7 Autologous Tissue Substitute J Synthetic Substitute K Nonautologous Tissue Substitute	Z No Qualifier
D Urethra	0 Open 4 Percutaneous Endoscopic 7 Via Natural or Artificial Opening 8 Via Natural or Artificial Opening Endoscopic X External	7 Autologous Tissue Substitute J Synthetic Substitute K Nonautologous Tissue Substitute	Z No Qualifier

Section	0	Medical and Surgical
Body System	T	Urinary System
Operation	S	Reposition: Moving to its normal location, or other suitable location, all or a portion of a body part

Body Part (4th)	Approach (5th)	Device (6th)	Qualifier (7th)
0 Kidney, Right 1 Kidney, Left 2 Kidneys, Bilateral 3 Kidney Pelvis, Right 4 Kidney Pelvis, Left 6 Ureter, Right 7 Ureter, Left 8 Ureters, Bilateral B Bladder C Bladder Neck D Urethra	0 Open 4 Percutaneous Endoscopic	Z No Device	Z No Qualifier

Section	0	Medical and Surgical
Body System	T	Urinary System
Operation	T	Resection: Cutting out or off, without replacement, all of a body part

Body Part (4th)	Approach (5th)	Device (6th)	Qualifier (7th)
0 Kidney, Right 1 Kidney, Left 2 Kidneys, Bilateral	0 Open 4 Percutaneous Endoscopic	Z No Device	Z No Qualifier
3 Kidney Pelvis, Right 4 Kidney Pelvis, Left 6 Ureter, Right 7 Ureter, Left B Bladder C Bladder Neck D Urethra	0 Open 4 Percutaneous Endoscopic 7 Via Natural or Artificial Opening 8 Via Natural or Artificial Opening Endoscopic	Z No Device	Z No Qualifier

Section	0	Medical and Surgical
Body System	T	Urinary System
Operation	U	Supplement: Putting in or on biological or synthetic material that physically reinforces and/or augments the function of a portion of a body part

Body Part (4th)	Approach (5th)	Device (6th)	Qualifier (7th)
3 Kidney Pelvis, Right 4 Kidney Pelvis, Left 6 Ureter, Right 7 Ureter, Left B Bladder C Bladder Neck	0 Open 4 Percutaneous Endoscopic 7 Via Natural or Artificial Opening 8 Via Natural or Artificial Opening Endoscopic	7 Autologous Tissue Substitute J Synthetic Substitute K Nonautologous Tissue Substitute	Z No Qualifier
D Urethra	0 Open 4 Percutaneous Endoscopic 7 Via Natural or Artificial Opening 8 Via Natural or Artificial Opening Endoscopic X External	7 Autologous Tissue Substitute J Synthetic Substitute K Nonautologous Tissue Substitute	Z No Qualifier

Section	0	Medical and Surgical
Body System	T	Urinary System
Operation	V	**Restriction:** Partially closing an orifice or the lumen of a tubular body part

Body Part (4th)	Approach (5th)	Device (6th)	Qualifier (7th)
3 Kidney Pelvis, Right 4 Kidney Pelvis, Left 6 Ureter, Right 7 Ureter, Left B Bladder C Bladder Neck	0 Open 3 Percutaneous 4 Percutaneous Endoscopic	C Extraluminal Device D Intraluminal Device Z No Device	Z No Qualifier
3 Kidney Pelvis, Right 4 Kidney Pelvis, Left 6 Ureter, Right 7 Ureter, Left B Bladder C Bladder Neck	7 Via Natural or Artificial Opening 8 Via Natural or Artificial Opening Endoscopic	D Intraluminal Device Z No Device	Z No Qualifier
D Urethra	0 Open 3 Percutaneous 4 Percutaneous Endoscopic	C Extraluminal Device D Intraluminal Device Z No Device	Z No Qualifier
D Urethra	7 Via Natural or Artificial Opening 8 Via Natural or Artificial Opening Endoscopic	D Intraluminal Device Z No Device	Z No Qualifier
D Urethra	X External	Z No Device	Z No Qualifier

Section	0	Medical and Surgical
Body System	T	Urinary System
Operation	W	**Revision:** Correcting, to the extent possible, a portion of a malfunctioning device or the position of a displaced device

Body Part (4th)	Approach (5th)	Device (6th)	Qualifier (7th)
5 Kidney	0 Open 3 Percutaneous 4 Percutaneous Endoscopic 7 Via Natural or Artificial Opening 8 Via Natural or Artificial Opening Endoscopic X External	0 Drainage Device 2 Monitoring Device 3 Infusion Device 7 Autologous Tissue Substitute C Extraluminal Device D Intraluminal Device J Synthetic Substitute K Nonautologous Tissue Substitute	Z No Qualifier
9 Ureter	0 Open 3 Percutaneous 4 Percutaneous Endoscopic 7 Via Natural or Artificial Opening 8 Via Natural or Artificial Opening Endoscopic X External	0 Drainage Device 2 Monitoring Device 3 Infusion Device 7 Autologous Tissue Substitute C Extraluminal Device D Intraluminal Device J Synthetic Substitute K Nonautologous Tissue Substitute M Stimulator Lead	Z No Qualifier

Continued

Section	0	Medical and Surgical
Body System	T	Urinary System
Operation	W	**Revision:** Correcting, to the extent possible, a portion of a malfunctioning device or the position of a displaced device

Body Part (4th)	Approach (5th)	Device (6th)	Qualifier (7th)
B Bladder	0 Open 3 Percutaneous 4 Percutaneous Endoscopic 7 Via Natural or Artificial Opening 8 Via Natural or Artificial Opening Endoscopic X External	0 Drainage Device 2 Monitoring Device 3 Infusion Device 7 Autologous Tissue Substitute C Extraluminal Device D Intraluminal Device J Synthetic Substitute K Nonautologous Tissue Substitute L Artificial Sphincter M Stimulator Lead	Z No Qualifier
D Urethra	0 Open 3 Percutaneous 4 Percutaneous Endoscopic 7 Via Natural or Artificial Opening 8 Via Natural or Artificial Opening Endoscopic X External	0 Drainage Device 2 Monitoring Device 3 Infusion Device 7 Autologous Tissue Substitute C Extraluminal Device D Intraluminal Device J Synthetic Substitute K Nonautologous Tissue Substitute L Artificial Sphincter	Z No Qualifier

Section	0	Medical and Surgical
Body System	T	Urinary System
Operation	Y	**Transplantation:** Putting in or on all or a portion of a living body part taken from another individual or animal to physically take the place and/or function of all or a portion of a similar body part

Body Part (4th)	Approach (5th)	Device (6th)	Qualifier (7th)
0 Kidney, Right 1 Kidney, Left	0 Open	Z No Device	0 Allogeneic 1 Syngeneic 2 Zooplastic

Urinary System Code Listing 0T1–0TY

0T1 – Urinary System, Bypass

Review Coding Guideline B3.6a

0T13073 Bypass Right Kidney Pelvis to Right Kidney Pelvis with Autologous Tissue Substitute, Open Approach

0T13074 Bypass Right Kidney Pelvis to Left Kidney Pelvis with Autologous Tissue Substitute, Open Approach

0T13076 Bypass Right Kidney Pelvis to Right Ureter with Autologous Tissue Substitute, Open Approach

0T13077 Bypass Right Kidney Pelvis to Left Ureter with Autologous Tissue Substitute, Open Approach

0T13078 Bypass Right Kidney Pelvis to Colon with Autologous Tissue Substitute, Open Approach

0T13079 Bypass Right Kidney Pelvis to Colocutaneous with Autologous Tissue Substitute, Open Approach

0T1307A Bypass Right Kidney Pelvis to Ileum with Autologous Tissue Substitute, Open Approach

0T1307B Bypass Right Kidney Pelvis to Bladder with Autologous Tissue Substitute, Open Approach

0T1307C Bypass Right Kidney Pelvis to Ileocutaneous with Autologous Tissue Substitute, Open Approach

0T1307D Bypass Right Kidney Pelvis to Cutaneous with Autologous Tissue Substitute, Open Approach

0T130J3 Bypass Right Kidney Pelvis to Right Kidney Pelvis with Synthetic Substitute, Open Approach

0T130J4 Bypass Right Kidney Pelvis to Left Kidney Pelvis with Synthetic Substitute, Open Approach

0T130J6 Bypass Right Kidney Pelvis to Right Ureter with Synthetic Substitute, Open Approach

0T130J7 Bypass Right Kidney Pelvis to Left Ureter with Synthetic Substitute, Open Approach

0T130J8 Bypass Right Kidney Pelvis to Colon with Synthetic Substitute, Open Approach

0T130J9 Bypass Right Kidney Pelvis to Colocutaneous with Synthetic Substitute, Open Approach

0T130JA	Bypass Right Kidney Pelvis to Ileum with Synthetic Substitute, Open Approach
0T130JB	Bypass Right Kidney Pelvis to Bladder with Synthetic Substitute, Open Approach
0T130JC	Bypass Right Kidney Pelvis to Ileocutaneous with Synthetic Substitute, Open Approach
0T130JD	Bypass Right Kidney Pelvis to Cutaneous with Synthetic Substitute, Open Approach
0T130K3	Bypass Right Kidney Pelvis to Right Kidney Pelvis with Nonautologous Tissue Substitute, Open Approach
0T130K4	Bypass Right Kidney Pelvis to Left Kidney Pelvis with Nonautologous Tissue Substitute, Open Approach
0T130K6	Bypass Right Kidney Pelvis to Right Ureter with Nonautologous Tissue Substitute, Open Approach
0T130K7	Bypass Right Kidney Pelvis to Left Ureter with Nonautologous Tissue Substitute, Open Approach
0T130K8	Bypass Right Kidney Pelvis to Colon with Nonautologous Tissue Substitute, Open Approach
0T130K9	Bypass Right Kidney Pelvis to Colocutaneous with Nonautologous Tissue Substitute, Open Approach
0T130KA	Bypass Right Kidney Pelvis to Ileum with Nonautologous Tissue Substitute, Open Approach
0T130KB	Bypass Right Kidney Pelvis to Bladder with Nonautologous Tissue Substitute, Open Approach
0T130KC	Bypass Right Kidney Pelvis to Ileocutaneous with Nonautologous Tissue Substitute, Open Approach
0T130KD	Bypass Right Kidney Pelvis to Cutaneous with Nonautologous Tissue Substitute, Open Approach
0T130Z3	Bypass Right Kidney Pelvis to Right Kidney Pelvis, Open Approach
0T130Z4	Bypass Right Kidney Pelvis to Left Kidney Pelvis, Open Approach
0T130Z6	Bypass Right Kidney Pelvis to Right Ureter, Open Approach
0T130Z7	Bypass Right Kidney Pelvis to Left Ureter, Open Approach
0T130Z8	Bypass Right Kidney Pelvis to Colon, Open Approach
0T130Z9	Bypass Right Kidney Pelvis to Colocutaneous, Open Approach
0T130ZA	Bypass Right Kidney Pelvis to Ileum, Open Approach
0T130ZB	Bypass Right Kidney Pelvis to Bladder, Open Approach
0T130ZC	Bypass Right Kidney Pelvis to Ileocutaneous, Open Approach
0T130ZD	Bypass Right Kidney Pelvis to Cutaneous, Open Approach
0T133JD	Bypass Right Kidney Pelvis to Cutaneous with Synthetic Substitute, Percutaneous Approach
0T13473	Bypass Right Kidney Pelvis to Right Kidney Pelvis with Autologous Tissue Substitute, Percutaneous Endoscopic Approach
0T13474	Bypass Right Kidney Pelvis to Left Kidney Pelvis with Autologous Tissue Substitute, Percutaneous Endoscopic Approach
0T13476	Bypass Right Kidney Pelvis to Right Ureter with Autologous Tissue Substitute, Percutaneous Endoscopic Approach
0T13477	Bypass Right Kidney Pelvis to Left Ureter with Autologous Tissue Substitute, Percutaneous Endoscopic Approach
0T13478	Bypass Right Kidney Pelvis to Colon with Autologous Tissue Substitute, Percutaneous Endoscopic Approach
0T13479	Bypass Right Kidney Pelvis to Colocutaneous with Autologous Tissue Substitute, Percutaneous Endoscopic Approach
0T1347A	Bypass Right Kidney Pelvis to Ileum with Autologous Tissue Substitute, Percutaneous Endoscopic Approach
0T1347B	Bypass Right Kidney Pelvis to Bladder with Autologous Tissue Substitute, Percutaneous Endoscopic Approach
0T1347C	Bypass Right Kidney Pelvis to Ileocutaneous with Autologous Tissue Substitute, Percutaneous Endoscopic Approach
0T1347D	Bypass Right Kidney Pelvis to Cutaneous with Autologous Tissue Substitute, Percutaneous Endoscopic Approach
0T134J3	Bypass Right Kidney Pelvis to Right Kidney Pelvis with Synthetic Substitute, Percutaneous Endoscopic Approach
0T134J4	Bypass Right Kidney Pelvis to Left Kidney Pelvis with Synthetic Substitute, Percutaneous Endoscopic Approach
0T134J6	Bypass Right Kidney Pelvis to Right Ureter with Synthetic Substitute, Percutaneous Endoscopic Approach
0T134J7	Bypass Right Kidney Pelvis to Left Ureter with Synthetic Substitute, Percutaneous Endoscopic Approach
0T134J8	Bypass Right Kidney Pelvis to Colon with Synthetic Substitute, Percutaneous Endoscopic Approach
0T134J9	Bypass Right Kidney Pelvis to Colocutaneous with Synthetic Substitute, Percutaneous Endoscopic Approach

0T134JA	Bypass Right Kidney Pelvis to Ileum with Synthetic Substitute, Percutaneous Endoscopic Approach
0T134JB	Bypass Right Kidney Pelvis to Bladder with Synthetic Substitute, Percutaneous Endoscopic Approach
0T134JC	Bypass Right Kidney Pelvis to Ileocutaneous with Synthetic Substitute, Percutaneous Endoscopic Approach
0T134JD	Bypass Right Kidney Pelvis to Cutaneous with Synthetic Substitute, Percutaneous Endoscopic Approach
0T134K3	Bypass Right Kidney Pelvis to Right Kidney Pelvis with Nonautologous Tissue Substitute, Percutaneous Endoscopic Approach
0T134K4	Bypass Right Kidney Pelvis to Left Kidney Pelvis with Nonautologous Tissue Substitute, Percutaneous Endoscopic Approach
0T134K6	Bypass Right Kidney Pelvis to Right Ureter with Nonautologous Tissue Substitute, Percutaneous Endoscopic Approach
0T134K7	Bypass Right Kidney Pelvis to Left Ureter with Nonautologous Tissue Substitute, Percutaneous Endoscopic Approach
0T134K8	Bypass Right Kidney Pelvis to Colon with Nonautologous Tissue Substitute, Percutaneous Endoscopic Approach
0T134K9	Bypass Right Kidney Pelvis to Colocutaneous with Nonautologous Tissue Substitute, Percutaneous Endoscopic Approach
0T134KA	Bypass Right Kidney Pelvis to Ileum with Nonautologous Tissue Substitute, Percutaneous Endoscopic Approach
0T134KB	Bypass Right Kidney Pelvis to Bladder with Nonautologous Tissue Substitute, Percutaneous Endoscopic Approach
0T134KC	Bypass Right Kidney Pelvis to Ileocutaneous with Nonautologous Tissue Substitute, Percutaneous Endoscopic Approach
0T134KD	Bypass Right Kidney Pelvis to Cutaneous with Nonautologous Tissue Substitute, Percutaneous Endoscopic Approach
0T134Z3	Bypass Right Kidney Pelvis to Right Kidney Pelvis, Percutaneous Endoscopic Approach
0T134Z4	Bypass Right Kidney Pelvis to Left Kidney Pelvis, Percutaneous Endoscopic Approach
0T134Z6	Bypass Right Kidney Pelvis to Right Ureter, Percutaneous Endoscopic Approach
0T134Z7	Bypass Right Kidney Pelvis to Left Ureter, Percutaneous Endoscopic Approach
0T134Z8	Bypass Right Kidney Pelvis to Colon, Percutaneous Endoscopic Approach
0T134Z9	Bypass Right Kidney Pelvis to Colocutaneous, Percutaneous Endoscopic Approach
0T134ZA	Bypass Right Kidney Pelvis to Ileum, Percutaneous Endoscopic Approach
0T134ZB	Bypass Right Kidney Pelvis to Bladder, Percutaneous Endoscopic Approach
0T134ZC	Bypass Right Kidney Pelvis to Ileocutaneous, Percutaneous Endoscopic Approach
0T134ZD	Bypass Right Kidney Pelvis to Cutaneous, Percutaneous Endoscopic Approach
0T14073	Bypass Left Kidney Pelvis to Right Kidney Pelvis with Autologous Tissue Substitute, Open Approach
0T14074	Bypass Left Kidney Pelvis to Left Kidney Pelvis with Autologous Tissue Substitute, Open Approach
0T14076	Bypass Left Kidney Pelvis to Right Ureter with Autologous Tissue Substitute, Open Approach
0T14077	Bypass Left Kidney Pelvis to Left Ureter with Autologous Tissue Substitute, Open Approach
0T14078	Bypass Left Kidney Pelvis to Colon with Autologous Tissue Substitute, Open Approach
0T14079	Bypass Left Kidney Pelvis to Colocutaneous with Autologous Tissue Substitute, Open Approach
0T1407A	Bypass Left Kidney Pelvis to Ileum with Autologous Tissue Substitute, Open Approach
0T1407B	Bypass Left Kidney Pelvis to Bladder with Autologous Tissue Substitute, Open Approach
0T1407C	Bypass Left Kidney Pelvis to Ileocutaneous with Autologous Tissue Substitute, Open Approach
0T1407D	Bypass Left Kidney Pelvis to Cutaneous with Autologous Tissue Substitute, Open Approach
0T140J3	Bypass Left Kidney Pelvis to Right Kidney Pelvis with Synthetic Substitute, Open Approach

0T140J4 Bypass Left Kidney Pelvis to Left Kidney Pelvis with Synthetic Substitute, Open Approach

0T140J6 Bypass Left Kidney Pelvis to Right Ureter with Synthetic Substitute, Open Approach

0T140J7 Bypass Left Kidney Pelvis to Left Ureter with Synthetic Substitute, Open Approach

0T140J8 Bypass Left Kidney Pelvis to Colon with Synthetic Substitute, Open Approach

0T140J9 Bypass Left Kidney Pelvis to Colocutaneous with Synthetic Substitute, Open Approach

0T140JA Bypass Left Kidney Pelvis to Ileum with Synthetic Substitute, Open Approach

0T140JB Bypass Left Kidney Pelvis to Bladder with Synthetic Substitute, Open Approach

0T140JC Bypass Left Kidney Pelvis to Ileocutaneous with Synthetic Substitute, Open Approach

0T140JD Bypass Left Kidney Pelvis to Cutaneous with Synthetic Substitute, Open Approach

0T140K3 Bypass Left Kidney Pelvis to Right Kidney Pelvis with Nonautologous Tissue Substitute, Open Approach

0T140K4 Bypass Left Kidney Pelvis to Left Kidney Pelvis with Nonautologous Tissue Substitute, Open Approach

0T140K6 Bypass Left Kidney Pelvis to Right Ureter with Nonautologous Tissue Substitute, Open Approach

0T140K7 Bypass Left Kidney Pelvis to Left Ureter with Nonautologous Tissue Substitute, Open Approach

0T140K8 Bypass Left Kidney Pelvis to Colon with Nonautologous Tissue Substitute, Open Approach

0T140K9 Bypass Left Kidney Pelvis to Colocutaneous with Nonautologous Tissue Substitute, Open Approach

0T140KA Bypass Left Kidney Pelvis to Ileum with Nonautologous Tissue Substitute, Open Approach

0T140KB Bypass Left Kidney Pelvis to Bladder with Nonautologous Tissue Substitute, Open Approach

0T140KC Bypass Left Kidney Pelvis to Ileocutaneous with Nonautologous Tissue Substitute, Open Approach

0T140KD Bypass Left Kidney Pelvis to Cutaneous with Nonautologous Tissue Substitute, Open Approach

0T140Z3 Bypass Left Kidney Pelvis to Right Kidney Pelvis, Open Approach

0T140Z4 Bypass Left Kidney Pelvis to Left Kidney Pelvis, Open Approach

0T140Z6 Bypass Left Kidney Pelvis to Right Ureter, Open Approach

0T140Z7 Bypass Left Kidney Pelvis to Left Ureter, Open Approach

0T140Z8 Bypass Left Kidney Pelvis to Colon, Open Approach

0T140Z9 Bypass Left Kidney Pelvis to Colocutaneous, Open Approach

0T140ZA Bypass Left Kidney Pelvis to Ileum, Open Approach

0T140ZB Bypass Left Kidney Pelvis to Bladder, Open Approach

0T140ZC Bypass Left Kidney Pelvis to Ileocutaneous, Open Approach

0T140ZD Bypass Left Kidney Pelvis to Cutaneous, Open Approach

0T143JD Bypass Left Kidney Pelvis to Cutaneous with Synthetic Substitute, Percutaneous Approach

0T14473 Bypass Left Kidney Pelvis to Right Kidney Pelvis with Autologous Tissue Substitute, Percutaneous Endoscopic Approach

0T14474 Bypass Left Kidney Pelvis to Left Kidney Pelvis with Autologous Tissue Substitute, Percutaneous Endoscopic Approach

0T14476 Bypass Left Kidney Pelvis to Right Ureter with Autologous Tissue Substitute, Percutaneous Endoscopic Approach

0T14477 Bypass Left Kidney Pelvis to Left Ureter with Autologous Tissue Substitute, Percutaneous Endoscopic Approach

0T14478 Bypass Left Kidney Pelvis to Colon with Autologous Tissue Substitute, Percutaneous Endoscopic Approach

0T14479 Bypass Left Kidney Pelvis to Colocutaneous with Autologous Tissue Substitute, Percutaneous Endoscopic Approach

0T1447A Bypass Left Kidney Pelvis to Ileum with Autologous Tissue Substitute, Percutaneous Endoscopic Approach

0T1447B Bypass Left Kidney Pelvis to Bladder with Autologous Tissue Substitute, Percutaneous Endoscopic Approach

0T1447C Bypass Left Kidney Pelvis to Ileocutaneous with Autologous Tissue Substitute, Percutaneous Endoscopic Approach

0T1447D Bypass Left Kidney Pelvis to Cutaneous with Autologous Tissue Substitute, Percutaneous Endoscopic Approach

0T144J3 Bypass Left Kidney Pelvis to Right Kidney Pelvis with Synthetic Substitute, Percutaneous Endoscopic Approach

0T144J4 Bypass Left Kidney Pelvis to Left Kidney Pelvis with Synthetic Substitute, Percutaneous Endoscopic Approach

0T144J6 Bypass Left Kidney Pelvis to Right Ureter with Synthetic Substitute, Percutaneous Endoscopic Approach

0T144J7 Bypass Left Kidney Pelvis to Left Ureter with Synthetic Substitute, Percutaneous Endoscopic Approach

0T144J8 Bypass Left Kidney Pelvis to Colon with Synthetic Substitute, Percutaneous Endoscopic Approach

0T144J9 Bypass Left Kidney Pelvis to Colocutaneous with Synthetic Substitute, Percutaneous Endoscopic Approach

0T144JA Bypass Left Kidney Pelvis to Ileum with Synthetic Substitute, Percutaneous Endoscopic Approach

0T144JB Bypass Left Kidney Pelvis to Bladder with Synthetic Substitute, Percutaneous Endoscopic Approach

0T144JC Bypass Left Kidney Pelvis to Ileocutaneous with Synthetic Substitute, Percutaneous Endoscopic Approach

0T144JD Bypass Left Kidney Pelvis to Cutaneous with Synthetic Substitute, Percutaneous Endoscopic Approach

0T144K3 Bypass Left Kidney Pelvis to Right Kidney Pelvis with Nonautologous Tissue Substitute, Percutaneous Endoscopic Approach

0T144K4 Bypass Left Kidney Pelvis to Left Kidney Pelvis with Nonautologous Tissue Substitute, Percutaneous Endoscopic Approach

0T144K6 Bypass Left Kidney Pelvis to Right Ureter with Nonautologous Tissue Substitute, Percutaneous Endoscopic Approach

0T144K7 Bypass Left Kidney Pelvis to Left Ureter with Nonautologous Tissue Substitute, Percutaneous Endoscopic Approach

0T144K8 Bypass Left Kidney Pelvis to Colon with Nonautologous Tissue Substitute, Percutaneous Endoscopic Approach

0T144K9 Bypass Left Kidney Pelvis to Colocutaneous with Nonautologous Tissue Substitute, Percutaneous Endoscopic Approach

0T144KA Bypass Left Kidney Pelvis to Ileum with Nonautologous Tissue Substitute, Percutaneous Endoscopic Approach

0T144KB Bypass Left Kidney Pelvis to Bladder with Nonautologous Tissue Substitute, Percutaneous Endoscopic Approach

0T144KC Bypass Left Kidney Pelvis to Ileocutaneous with Nonautologous Tissue Substitute, Percutaneous Endoscopic Approach

0T144KD Bypass Left Kidney Pelvis to Cutaneous with Nonautologous Tissue Substitute, Percutaneous Endoscopic Approach

0T144Z3 Bypass Left Kidney Pelvis to Right Kidney Pelvis, Percutaneous Endoscopic Approach

0T144Z4 Bypass Left Kidney Pelvis to Left Kidney Pelvis, Percutaneous Endoscopic Approach

0T144Z6 Bypass Left Kidney Pelvis to Right Ureter, Percutaneous Endoscopic Approach

0T144Z7 Bypass Left Kidney Pelvis to Left Ureter, Percutaneous Endoscopic Approach

0T144Z8 Bypass Left Kidney Pelvis to Colon, Percutaneous Endoscopic Approach

0T144Z9 Bypass Left Kidney Pelvis to Colocutaneous, Percutaneous Endoscopic Approach

0T144ZA Bypass Left Kidney Pelvis to Ileum, Percutaneous Endoscopic Approach

0T144ZB Bypass Left Kidney Pelvis to Bladder, Percutaneous Endoscopic Approach

0T144ZC Bypass Left Kidney Pelvis to Ileocutaneous, Percutaneous Endoscopic Approach

0T144ZD Bypass Left Kidney Pelvis to Cutaneous, Percutaneous Endoscopic Approach

0T16076 Bypass Right Ureter to Right Ureter with Autologous Tissue Substitute, Open Approach

0T16077 Bypass Right Ureter to Left Ureter with Autologous Tissue Substitute, Open Approach

0T16078 Bypass Right Ureter to Colon with Autologous Tissue Substitute, Open Approach

0T16079 Bypass Right Ureter to Colocutaneous with Autologous Tissue Substitute, Open Approach

0T1607A Bypass Right Ureter to Ileum with Autologous Tissue Substitute, Open Approach

0T1607B Bypass Right Ureter to Bladder with Autologous Tissue Substitute, Open Approach

0T1607C Bypass Right Ureter to Ileocutaneous with Autologous Tissue Substitute, Open Approach

0T1607D Bypass Right Ureter to Cutaneous with Autologous Tissue Substitute, Open Approach

0T160J6 Bypass Right Ureter to Right Ureter with Synthetic Substitute, Open Approach

0T160J7 Bypass Right Ureter to Left Ureter with Synthetic Substitute, Open Approach

0T160J8 Bypass Right Ureter to Colon with Synthetic Substitute, Open Approach

0T160J9 Bypass Right Ureter to Colocutaneous with Synthetic Substitute, Open Approach

0T160JA Bypass Right Ureter to Ileum with Synthetic Substitute, Open Approach

0T160JB Bypass Right Ureter to Bladder with Synthetic Substitute, Open Approach

0T160JC Bypass Right Ureter to Ileocutaneous with Synthetic Substitute, Open Approach

0T160JD Bypass Right Ureter to Cutaneous with Synthetic Substitute, Open Approach

0T160K6 Bypass Right Ureter to Right Ureter with Nonautologous Tissue Substitute, Open Approach

0T160K7 Bypass Right Ureter to Left Ureter with Nonautologous Tissue Substitute, Open Approach

0T160K8 Bypass Right Ureter to Colon with Nonautologous Tissue Substitute, Open Approach

0T160K9 Bypass Right Ureter to Colocutaneous with Nonautologous Tissue Substitute, Open Approach

0T160KA Bypass Right Ureter to Ileum with Nonautologous Tissue Substitute, Open Approach

0T160KB Bypass Right Ureter to Bladder with Nonautologous Tissue Substitute, Open Approach

0T160KC Bypass Right Ureter to Ileocutaneous with Nonautologous Tissue Substitute, Open Approach

0T160KD Bypass Right Ureter to Cutaneous with Nonautologous Tissue Substitute, Open Approach

0T160Z6 Bypass Right Ureter to Right Ureter, Open Approach

0T160Z7 Bypass Right Ureter to Left Ureter, Open Approach

0T160Z8 Bypass Right Ureter to Colon, Open Approach

0T160Z9 Bypass Right Ureter to Colocutaneous, Open Approach

0T160ZA Bypass Right Ureter to Ileum, Open Approach

0T160ZB Bypass Right Ureter to Bladder, Open Approach

0T160ZC Bypass Right Ureter to Ileocutaneous, Open Approach

0T160ZD Bypass Right Ureter to Cutaneous, Open Approach

0T163JD Bypass Right Ureter to Cutaneous with Synthetic Substitute, Percutaneous Approach

0T16476 Bypass Right Ureter to Right Ureter with Autologous Tissue Substitute, Percutaneous Endoscopic Approach

0T16477 Bypass Right Ureter to Left Ureter with Autologous Tissue Substitute, Percutaneous Endoscopic Approach

0T16478 Bypass Right Ureter to Colon with Autologous Tissue Substitute, Percutaneous Endoscopic Approach

0T16479 Bypass Right Ureter to Colocutaneous with Autologous Tissue Substitute, Percutaneous Endoscopic Approach

0T1647A Bypass Right Ureter to Ileum with Autologous Tissue Substitute, Percutaneous Endoscopic Approach

0T1647B Bypass Right Ureter to Bladder with Autologous Tissue Substitute, Percutaneous Endoscopic Approach

0T1647C Bypass Right Ureter to Ileocutaneous with Autologous Tissue Substitute, Percutaneous Endoscopic Approach

0T1647D Bypass Right Ureter to Cutaneous with Autologous Tissue Substitute, Percutaneous Endoscopic Approach

0T164J6 Bypass Right Ureter to Right Ureter with Synthetic Substitute, Percutaneous Endoscopic Approach

0T164J7 Bypass Right Ureter to Left Ureter with Synthetic Substitute, Percutaneous Endoscopic Approach

0T164J8 Bypass Right Ureter to Colon with Synthetic Substitute, Percutaneous Endoscopic Approach

0T164J9 Bypass Right Ureter to Colocutaneous with Synthetic Substitute, Percutaneous Endoscopic Approach

0T164JA Bypass Right Ureter to Ileum with Synthetic Substitute, Percutaneous Endoscopic Approach

0T164JB Bypass Right Ureter to Bladder with Synthetic Substitute, Percutaneous Endoscopic Approach

0T164JC Bypass Right Ureter to Ileocutaneous with Synthetic Substitute, Percutaneous Endoscopic Approach

0T164JD Bypass Right Ureter to Cutaneous with Synthetic Substitute, Percutaneous Endoscopic Approach

0T164K6 Bypass Right Ureter to Right Ureter with Nonautologous Tissue Substitute, Percutaneous Endoscopic Approach

0T164K7 Bypass Right Ureter to Left Ureter with Nonautologous Tissue Substitute, Percutaneous Endoscopic Approach

0T164K8 Bypass Right Ureter to Colon with Nonautologous Tissue Substitute, Percutaneous Endoscopic Approach

0T164K9 Bypass Right Ureter to Colocutaneous with Nonautologous Tissue Substitute, Percutaneous Endoscopic Approach

0T164KA Bypass Right Ureter to Ileum with Nonautologous Tissue Substitute, Percutaneous Endoscopic Approach

0T164KB Bypass Right Ureter to Bladder with Nonautologous Tissue Substitute, Percutaneous Endoscopic Approach

0T164KC Bypass Right Ureter to Ileocutaneous with Nonautologous Tissue Substitute, Percutaneous Endoscopic Approach

0T164KD Bypass Right Ureter to Cutaneous with Nonautologous Tissue Substitute, Percutaneous Endoscopic Approach

0T164Z6 Bypass Right Ureter to Right Ureter, Percutaneous Endoscopic Approach

0T164Z7 Bypass Right Ureter to Left Ureter, Percutaneous Endoscopic Approach

0T164Z8 Bypass Right Ureter to Colon, Percutaneous Endoscopic Approach

0T164Z9 Bypass Right Ureter to Colocutaneous, Percutaneous Endoscopic Approach

0T164ZA Bypass Right Ureter to Ileum, Percutaneous Endoscopic Approach

0T164ZB Bypass Right Ureter to Bladder, Percutaneous Endoscopic Approach

0T164ZC Bypass Right Ureter to Ileocutaneous, Percutaneous Endoscopic Approach

0T164ZD Bypass Right Ureter to Cutaneous, Percutaneous Endoscopic Approach

0T17076 Bypass Left Ureter to Right Ureter with Autologous Tissue Substitute, Open Approach

0T17077 Bypass Left Ureter to Left Ureter with Autologous Tissue Substitute, Open Approach

0T17078 Bypass Left Ureter to Colon with Autologous Tissue Substitute, Open Approach

0T17079 Bypass Left Ureter to Colocutaneous with Autologous Tissue Substitute, Open Approach

0T1707A Bypass Left Ureter to Ileum with Autologous Tissue Substitute, Open Approach

0T1707B Bypass Left Ureter to Bladder with Autologous Tissue Substitute, Open Approach

0T1707C Bypass Left Ureter to Ileocutaneous with Autologous Tissue Substitute, Open Approach

0T1707D Bypass Left Ureter to Cutaneous with Autologous Tissue Substitute, Open Approach

0T170J6 Bypass Left Ureter to Right Ureter with Synthetic Substitute, Open Approach

0T170J7 Bypass Left Ureter to Left Ureter with Synthetic Substitute, Open Approach

0T170J8 Bypass Left Ureter to Colon with Synthetic Substitute, Open Approach

0T170J9 Bypass Left Ureter to Colocutaneous with Synthetic Substitute, Open Approach

0T170JA Bypass Left Ureter to Ileum with Synthetic Substitute, Open Approach

0T170JB Bypass Left Ureter to Bladder with Synthetic Substitute, Open Approach

0T170JC Bypass Left Ureter to Ileocutaneous with Synthetic Substitute, Open Approach

0T170JD Bypass Left Ureter to Cutaneous with Synthetic Substitute, Open Approach

0T170K6 Bypass Left Ureter to Right Ureter with Nonautologous Tissue Substitute, Open Approach

0T170K7 Bypass Left Ureter to Left Ureter with Nonautologous Tissue Substitute, Open Approach

0T170K8 Bypass Left Ureter to Colon with Nonautologous Tissue Substitute, Open Approach

0T170K9 Bypass Left Ureter to Colocutaneous with Nonautologous Tissue Substitute, Open Approach

0T170KA Bypass Left Ureter to Ileum with Nonautologous Tissue Substitute, Open Approach

0T170KB Bypass Left Ureter to Bladder with Nonautologous Tissue Substitute, Open Approach

---

0T170KC Bypass Left Ureter to Ileocutaneous with Nonautologous Tissue Substitute, Open Approach

0T170KD Bypass Left Ureter to Cutaneous with Nonautologous Tissue Substitute, Open Approach

0T170Z6 Bypass Left Ureter to Right Ureter, Open Approach

0T170Z7 Bypass Left Ureter to Left Ureter, Open Approach

0T170Z8 Bypass Left Ureter to Colon, Open Approach

0T170Z9 Bypass Left Ureter to Colocutaneous, Open Approach

0T170ZA Bypass Left Ureter to Ileum, Open Approach

0T170ZB Bypass Left Ureter to Bladder, Open Approach

0T170ZC Bypass Left Ureter to Ileocutaneous, Open Approach

0T170ZD Bypass Left Ureter to Cutaneous, Open Approach

0T173JD Bypass Left Ureter to Cutaneous with Synthetic Substitute, Percutaneous Approach

0T17476 Bypass Left Ureter to Right Ureter with Autologous Tissue Substitute, Percutaneous Endoscopic Approach

0T17477 Bypass Left Ureter to Left Ureter with Autologous Tissue Substitute, Percutaneous Endoscopic Approach

0T17478 Bypass Left Ureter to Colon with Autologous Tissue Substitute, Percutaneous Endoscopic Approach

0T17479 Bypass Left Ureter to Colocutaneous with Autologous Tissue Substitute, Percutaneous Endoscopic Approach

0T1747A Bypass Left Ureter to Ileum with Autologous Tissue Substitute, Percutaneous Endoscopic Approach

0T1747B Bypass Left Ureter to Bladder with Autologous Tissue Substitute, Percutaneous Endoscopic Approach

0T1747C Bypass Left Ureter to Ileocutaneous with Autologous Tissue Substitute, Percutaneous Endoscopic Approach

0T1747D Bypass Left Ureter to Cutaneous with Autologous Tissue Substitute, Percutaneous Endoscopic Approach

0T174J6 Bypass Left Ureter to Right Ureter with Synthetic Substitute, Percutaneous Endoscopic Approach

0T174J7 Bypass Left Ureter to Left Ureter with Synthetic Substitute, Percutaneous Endoscopic Approach

0T174J8 Bypass Left Ureter to Colon with Synthetic Substitute, Percutaneous Endoscopic Approach

0T174J9 Bypass Left Ureter to Colocutaneous with Synthetic Substitute, Percutaneous Endoscopic Approach

0T174JA Bypass Left Ureter to Ileum with Synthetic Substitute, Percutaneous Endoscopic Approach

0T174JB Bypass Left Ureter to Bladder with Synthetic Substitute, Percutaneous Endoscopic Approach

0T174JC Bypass Left Ureter to Ileocutaneous with Synthetic Substitute, Percutaneous Endoscopic Approach

0T174JD Bypass Left Ureter to Cutaneous with Synthetic Substitute, Percutaneous Endoscopic Approach

0T174K6 Bypass Left Ureter to Right Ureter with Nonautologous Tissue Substitute, Percutaneous Endoscopic Approach

0T174K7 Bypass Left Ureter to Left Ureter with Nonautologous Tissue Substitute, Percutaneous Endoscopic Approach

0T174K8 Bypass Left Ureter to Colon with Nonautologous Tissue Substitute, Percutaneous Endoscopic Approach

0T174K9 Bypass Left Ureter to Colocutaneous with Nonautologous Tissue Substitute, Percutaneous Endoscopic Approach

0T174KA Bypass Left Ureter to Ileum with Nonautologous Tissue Substitute, Percutaneous Endoscopic Approach

0T174KB Bypass Left Ureter to Bladder with Nonautologous Tissue Substitute, Percutaneous Endoscopic Approach

0T174KC Bypass Left Ureter to Ileocutaneous with Nonautologous Tissue Substitute, Percutaneous Endoscopic Approach

0T174KD Bypass Left Ureter to Cutaneous with Nonautologous Tissue Substitute, Percutaneous Endoscopic Approach

0T174Z6 Bypass Left Ureter to Right Ureter, Percutaneous Endoscopic Approach

0T174Z7 Bypass Left Ureter to Left Ureter, Percutaneous Endoscopic Approach

0T174Z8 Bypass Left Ureter to Colon, Percutaneous Endoscopic Approach

0T174Z9 Bypass Left Ureter to Colocutaneous, Percutaneous Endoscopic Approach

0T174ZA Bypass Left Ureter to Ileum, Percutaneous Endoscopic Approach

0T174ZB Bypass Left Ureter to Bladder, Percutaneous Endoscopic Approach

0T174ZC Bypass Left Ureter to Ileocutaneous, Percutaneous Endoscopic Approach

0T174ZD Bypass Left Ureter to Cutaneous, Percutaneous Endoscopic Approach

0T18076 Bypass Bilateral Ureters to Right Ureter with Autologous Tissue Substitute, Open Approach

0T18077 Bypass Bilateral Ureters to Left Ureter with Autologous Tissue Substitute, Open Approach

0T18078 Bypass Bilateral Ureters to Colon with Autologous Tissue Substitute, Open Approach

0T18079 Bypass Bilateral Ureters to Colocutaneous with Autologous Tissue Substitute, Open Approach

0T1807A Bypass Bilateral Ureters to Ileum with Autologous Tissue Substitute, Open Approach

0T1807B Bypass Bilateral Ureters to Bladder with Autologous Tissue Substitute, Open Approach

0T1807C Bypass Bilateral Ureters to Ileocutaneous with Autologous Tissue Substitute, Open Approach

0T1807D Bypass Bilateral Ureters to Cutaneous with Autologous Tissue Substitute, Open Approach

0T180J6 Bypass Bilateral Ureters to Right Ureter with Synthetic Substitute, Open Approach

0T180J7 Bypass Bilateral Ureters to Left Ureter with Synthetic Substitute, Open Approach

0T180J8 Bypass Bilateral Ureters to Colon with Synthetic Substitute, Open Approach

0T180J9 Bypass Bilateral Ureters to Colocutaneous with Synthetic Substitute, Open Approach

0T180JA Bypass Bilateral Ureters to Ileum with Synthetic Substitute, Open Approach

0T180JB Bypass Bilateral Ureters to Bladder with Synthetic Substitute, Open Approach

0T180JC Bypass Bilateral Ureters to Ileocutaneous with Synthetic Substitute, Open Approach

0T180JD Bypass Bilateral Ureters to Cutaneous with Synthetic Substitute, Open Approach

0T180K6 Bypass Bilateral Ureters to Right Ureter with Nonautologous Tissue Substitute, Open Approach

0T180K7 Bypass Bilateral Ureters to Left Ureter with Nonautologous Tissue Substitute, Open Approach

0T180K8 Bypass Bilateral Ureters to Colon with Nonautologous Tissue Substitute, Open Approach

0T180K9 Bypass Bilateral Ureters to Colocutaneous with Nonautologous Tissue Substitute, Open Approach

0T180KA Bypass Bilateral Ureters to Ileum with Nonautologous Tissue Substitute, Open Approach

0T180KB Bypass Bilateral Ureters to Bladder with Nonautologous Tissue Substitute, Open Approach

0T180KC Bypass Bilateral Ureters to Ileocutaneous with Nonautologous Tissue Substitute, Open Approach

0T180KD Bypass Bilateral Ureters to Cutaneous with Nonautologous Tissue Substitute, Open Approach

0T180Z6 Bypass Bilateral Ureters to Right Ureter, Open Approach

0T180Z7 Bypass Bilateral Ureters to Left Ureter, Open Approach

0T180Z8 Bypass Bilateral Ureters to Colon, Open Approach

0T180Z9 Bypass Bilateral Ureters to Colocutaneous, Open Approach

0T180ZA Bypass Bilateral Ureters to Ileum, Open Approach

0T180ZB Bypass Bilateral Ureters to Bladder, Open Approach

0T180ZC Bypass Bilateral Ureters to Ileocutaneous, Open Approach

0T180ZD Bypass Bilateral Ureters to Cutaneous, Open Approach

0T183JD Bypass Bilateral Ureters to Cutaneous with Synthetic Substitute, Percutaneous Approach

0T18476 Bypass Bilateral Ureters to Right Ureter with Autologous Tissue Substitute, Percutaneous Endoscopic Approach

0T18477 Bypass Bilateral Ureters to Left Ureter with Autologous Tissue Substitute, Percutaneous Endoscopic Approach

0T18478 Bypass Bilateral Ureters to Colon with Autologous Tissue Substitute, Percutaneous Endoscopic Approach

0T18479 Bypass Bilateral Ureters to Colocutaneous with Autologous Tissue Substitute, Percutaneous Endoscopic Approach

0T1847A Bypass Bilateral Ureters to Ileum with Autologous Tissue Substitute, Percutaneous Endoscopic Approach

0T1847B Bypass Bilateral Ureters to Bladder with Autologous Tissue Substitute, Percutaneous Endoscopic Approach

0T1847C Bypass Bilateral Ureters to Ileocutaneous with Autologous Tissue Substitute, Percutaneous Endoscopic Approach

0T1847D	Bypass Bilateral Ureters to Cutaneous with Autologous Tissue Substitute, Percutaneous Endoscopic Approach	**0T184ZD**	Bypass Bilateral Ureters to Cutaneous, Percutaneous Endoscopic Approach
0T184J6	Bypass Bilateral Ureters to Right Ureter with Synthetic Substitute, Percutaneous Endoscopic Approach	**0T1B079**	Bypass Bladder to Colocutaneous with Autologous Tissue Substitute, Open Approach
0T184J7	Bypass Bilateral Ureters to Left Ureter with Synthetic Substitute, Percutaneous Endoscopic Approach	**0T1B07C**	Bypass Bladder to Ileocutaneous with Autologous Tissue Substitute, Open Approach
0T184J8	Bypass Bilateral Ureters to Colon with Synthetic Substitute, Percutaneous Endoscopic Approach	**0T1B07D**	Bypass Bladder to Cutaneous with Autologous Tissue Substitute, Open Approach
0T184J9	Bypass Bilateral Ureters to Colocutaneous with Synthetic Substitute, Percutaneous Endoscopic Approach	**0T1B0J9**	Bypass Bladder to Colocutaneous with Synthetic Substitute, Open Approach
0T184JA	Bypass Bilateral Ureters to Ileum with Synthetic Substitute, Percutaneous Endoscopic Approach	**0T1B0JC**	Bypass Bladder to Ileocutaneous with Synthetic Substitute, Open Approach
0T184JB	Bypass Bilateral Ureters to Bladder with Synthetic Substitute, Percutaneous Endoscopic Approach	**0T1B0JD**	Bypass Bladder to Cutaneous with Synthetic Substitute, Open Approach
0T184JC	Bypass Bilateral Ureters to Ileocutaneous with Synthetic Substitute, Percutaneous Endoscopic Approach	**0T1B0K9**	Bypass Bladder to Colocutaneous with Nonautologous Tissue Substitute, Open Approach
0T184JD	Bypass Bilateral Ureters to Cutaneous with Synthetic Substitute, Percutaneous Endoscopic Approach	**0T1B0KC**	Bypass Bladder to Ileocutaneous with Nonautologous Tissue Substitute, Open Approach
0T184K6	Bypass Bilateral Ureters to Right Ureter with Nonautologous Tissue Substitute, Percutaneous Endoscopic Approach	**0T1B0KD**	Bypass Bladder to Cutaneous with Nonautologous Tissue Substitute, Open Approach
0T184K7	Bypass Bilateral Ureters to Left Ureter with Nonautologous Tissue Substitute, Percutaneous Endoscopic Approach	**0T1B0Z9**	Bypass Bladder to Colocutaneous, Open Approach
0T184K8	Bypass Bilateral Ureters to Colon with Nonautologous Tissue Substitute, Percutaneous Endoscopic Approach	**0T1B0ZC**	Bypass Bladder to Ileocutaneous, Open Approach
0T184K9	Bypass Bilateral Ureters to Colocutaneous with Nonautologous Tissue Substitute, Percutaneous Endoscopic Approach	**0T1B0ZD**	Bypass Bladder to Cutaneous, Open Approach
		0T1B3JD	Bypass Bladder to Cutaneous with Synthetic Substitute, Percutaneous Approach
0T184KA	Bypass Bilateral Ureters to Ileum with Nonautologous Tissue Substitute, Percutaneous Endoscopic Approach	**0T1B479**	Bypass Bladder to Colocutaneous with Autologous Tissue Substitute, Percutaneous Endoscopic Approach
0T184KB	Bypass Bilateral Ureters to Bladder with Nonautologous Tissue Substitute, Percutaneous Endoscopic Approach	**0T1B47C**	Bypass Bladder to Ileocutaneous with Autologous Tissue Substitute, Percutaneous Endoscopic Approach
0T184KC	Bypass Bilateral Ureters to Ileocutaneous with Nonautologous Tissue Substitute, Percutaneous Endoscopic Approach	**0T1B47D**	Bypass Bladder to Cutaneous with Autologous Tissue Substitute, Percutaneous Endoscopic Approach
0T184KD	Bypass Bilateral Ureters to Cutaneous with Nonautologous Tissue Substitute, Percutaneous Endoscopic Approach	**0T1B4J9**	Bypass Bladder to Colocutaneous with Synthetic Substitute, Percutaneous Endoscopic Approach
0T184Z6	Bypass Bilateral Ureters to Right Ureter, Percutaneous Endoscopic Approach	**0T1B4JC**	Bypass Bladder to Ileocutaneous with Synthetic Substitute, Percutaneous Endoscopic Approach
0T184Z7	Bypass Bilateral Ureters to Left Ureter, Percutaneous Endoscopic Approach	**0T1B4JD**	Bypass Bladder to Cutaneous with Synthetic Substitute, Percutaneous Endoscopic Approach
0T184Z8	Bypass Bilateral Ureters to Colon, Percutaneous Endoscopic Approach	**0T1B4K9**	Bypass Bladder to Colocutaneous with Nonautologous Tissue Substitute, Percutaneous Endoscopic Approach
0T184Z9	Bypass Bilateral Ureters to Colocutaneous, Percutaneous Endoscopic Approach	**0T1B4KC**	Bypass Bladder to Ileocutaneous with Nonautologous Tissue Substitute, Percutaneous Endoscopic Approach
0T184ZA	Bypass Bilateral Ureters to Ileum, Percutaneous Endoscopic Approach	**0T1B4KD**	Bypass Bladder to Cutaneous with Nonautologous Tissue Substitute, Percutaneous Endoscopic Approach
0T184ZB	Bypass Bilateral Ureters to Bladder, Percutaneous Endoscopic Approach	**0T1B4Z9**	Bypass Bladder to Colocutaneous, Percutaneous Endoscopic Approach
0T184ZC	Bypass Bilateral Ureters to Ileocutaneous, Percutaneous Endoscopic Approach	**0T1B4ZC**	Bypass Bladder to Ileocutaneous, Percutaneous Endoscopic Approach
		0T1B4ZD	Bypass Bladder to Cutaneous, Percutaneous Endoscopic Approach

0T2 – Urinary System, Change

Review Coding Guideline B6.1c

0T25X0Z	Change Drainage Device in Kidney, External Approach	**0T2BX0Z**	Change Drainage Device in Bladder, External Approach
0T25XYZ	Change Other Device in Kidney, External Approach	**0T2BXYZ**	Change Other Device in Bladder, External Approach
0T29X0Z	Change Drainage Device in Ureter, External Approach	**0T2DX0Z**	Change Drainage Device in Urethra, External Approach
0T29XYZ	Change Other Device in Ureter, External Approach	**0T2DXYZ**	Change Other Device in Urethra, External Approach

0T5 – Urinary System, Destruction

0T500ZZ	Destruction of Right Kidney, Open Approach	**0T533ZZ**	Destruction of Right Kidney Pelvis, Percutaneous Approach
0T503ZZ	Destruction of Right Kidney, Percutaneous Approach	**0T534ZZ**	Destruction of Right Kidney Pelvis, Percutaneous Endoscopic Approach
0T504ZZ	Destruction of Right Kidney, Percutaneous Endoscopic Approach		
0T507ZZ	Destruction of Right Kidney, Via Natural or Artificial Opening	**0T537ZZ**	Destruction of Right Kidney Pelvis, Via Natural or Artificial Opening
0T508ZZ	Destruction of Right Kidney, Via Natural or Artificial Opening Endoscopic	**0T538ZZ**	Destruction of Right Kidney Pelvis, Via Natural or Artificial Opening Endoscopic
0T510ZZ	Destruction of Left Kidney, Open Approach	**0T540ZZ**	Destruction of Left Kidney Pelvis, Open Approach
0T513ZZ	Destruction of Left Kidney, Percutaneous Approach	**0T543ZZ**	Destruction of Left Kidney Pelvis, Percutaneous Approach
0T514ZZ	Destruction of Left Kidney, Percutaneous Endoscopic Approach	**0T544ZZ**	Destruction of Left Kidney Pelvis, Percutaneous Endoscopic Approach
0T517ZZ	Destruction of Left Kidney, Via Natural or Artificial Opening		
0T518ZZ	Destruction of Left Kidney, Via Natural or Artificial Opening Endoscopic	**0T547ZZ**	Destruction of Left Kidney Pelvis, Via Natural or Artificial Opening
0T530ZZ	Destruction of Right Kidney Pelvis, Open Approach		

0T548ZZ	Destruction of Left Kidney Pelvis, Via Natural or Artificial Opening Endoscopic
0T560ZZ	Destruction of Right Ureter, Open Approach
0T563ZZ	Destruction of Right Ureter, Percutaneous Approach
0T564ZZ	Destruction of Right Ureter, Percutaneous Endoscopic Approach
0T567ZZ	Destruction of Right Ureter, Via Natural or Artificial Opening
0T568ZZ	Destruction of Right Ureter, Via Natural or Artificial Opening Endoscopic
0T570ZZ	Destruction of Left Ureter, Open Approach
0T573ZZ	Destruction of Left Ureter, Percutaneous Approach
0T574ZZ	Destruction of Left Ureter, Percutaneous Endoscopic Approach
0T577ZZ	Destruction of Left Ureter, Via Natural or Artificial Opening
0T578ZZ	Destruction of Left Ureter, Via Natural or Artificial Opening Endoscopic
0T5B0ZZ	Destruction of Bladder, Open Approach
0T5B3ZZ	Destruction of Bladder, Percutaneous Approach
0T5B4ZZ	Destruction of Bladder, Percutaneous Endoscopic Approach

0T5B7ZZ	Destruction of Bladder, Via Natural or Artificial Opening
0T5B8ZZ	Destruction of Bladder, Via Natural or Artificial Opening Endoscopic
0T5C0ZZ	Destruction of Bladder Neck, Open Approach
0T5C3ZZ	Destruction of Bladder Neck, Percutaneous Approach
0T5C4ZZ	Destruction of Bladder Neck, Percutaneous Endoscopic Approach
0T5C7ZZ	Destruction of Bladder Neck, Via Natural or Artificial Opening
0T5C8ZZ	Destruction of Bladder Neck, Via Natural or Artificial Opening Endoscopic
0T5D0ZZ	Destruction of Urethra, Open Approach
0T5D3ZZ	Destruction of Urethra, Percutaneous Approach
0T5D4ZZ	Destruction of Urethra, Percutaneous Endoscopic Approach
0T5D7ZZ	Destruction of Urethra, Via Natural or Artificial Opening
0T5D8ZZ	Destruction of Urethra, Via Natural or Artificial Opening Endoscopic
0T5DXZZ	Destruction of Urethra, External Approach

0T7 – Urinary System, Dilation

0T730DZ	Dilation of Right Kidney Pelvis with Intraluminal Device, Open Approach
0T730ZZ	Dilation of Right Kidney Pelvis, Open Approach
0T733DZ	Dilation of Right Kidney Pelvis with Intraluminal Device, Percutaneous Approach
0T733ZZ	Dilation of Right Kidney Pelvis, Percutaneous Approach
0T734DZ	Dilation of Right Kidney Pelvis with Intraluminal Device, Percutaneous Endoscopic Approach
0T734ZZ	Dilation of Right Kidney Pelvis, Percutaneous Endoscopic Approach
0T737DZ	Dilation of Right Kidney Pelvis with Intraluminal Device, Via Natural or Artificial Opening
0T737ZZ	Dilation of Right Kidney Pelvis, Via Natural or Artificial Opening
0T738DZ	Dilation of Right Kidney Pelvis with Intraluminal Device, Via Natural or Artificial Opening Endoscopic
0T738ZZ	Dilation of Right Kidney Pelvis, Via Natural or Artificial Opening Endoscopic
0T740DZ	Dilation of Left Kidney Pelvis with Intraluminal Device, Open Approach
0T740ZZ	Dilation of Left Kidney Pelvis, Open Approach
0T743DZ	Dilation of Left Kidney Pelvis with Intraluminal Device, Percutaneous Approach
0T743ZZ	Dilation of Left Kidney Pelvis, Percutaneous Approach
0T744DZ	Dilation of Left Kidney Pelvis with Intraluminal Device, Percutaneous Endoscopic Approach
0T744ZZ	Dilation of Left Kidney Pelvis, Percutaneous Endoscopic Approach
0T747DZ	Dilation of Left Kidney Pelvis with Intraluminal Device, Via Natural or Artificial Opening
0T747ZZ	Dilation of Left Kidney Pelvis, Via Natural or Artificial Opening
0T748DZ	Dilation of Left Kidney Pelvis with Intraluminal Device, Via Natural or Artificial Opening Endoscopic
0T748ZZ	Dilation of Left Kidney Pelvis, Via Natural or Artificial Opening Endoscopic
0T760DZ	Dilation of Right Ureter with Intraluminal Device, Open Approach
0T760ZZ	Dilation of Right Ureter, Open Approach
0T763DZ	Dilation of Right Ureter with Intraluminal Device, Percutaneous Approach
0T763ZZ	Dilation of Right Ureter, Percutaneous Approach
0T764DZ	Dilation of Right Ureter with Intraluminal Device, Percutaneous Endoscopic Approach
0T764ZZ	Dilation of Right Ureter, Percutaneous Endoscopic Approach
0T767DZ	Dilation of Right Ureter with Intraluminal Device, Via Natural or Artificial Opening
0T767ZZ	Dilation of Right Ureter, Via Natural or Artificial Opening
0T768DZ	Dilation of Right Ureter with Intraluminal Device, Via Natural or Artificial Opening Endoscopic
0T768ZZ	Dilation of Right Ureter, Via Natural or Artificial Opening Endoscopic
0T770DZ	Dilation of Left Ureter with Intraluminal Device, Open Approach
0T770ZZ	Dilation of Left Ureter, Open Approach
0T773DZ	Dilation of Left Ureter with Intraluminal Device, Percutaneous Approach
0T773ZZ	Dilation of Left Ureter, Percutaneous Approach
0T774DZ	Dilation of Left Ureter with Intraluminal Device, Percutaneous Endoscopic Approach

0T774ZZ	Dilation of Left Ureter, Percutaneous Endoscopic Approach
0T777DZ	Dilation of Left Ureter with Intraluminal Device, Via Natural or Artificial Opening
0T777ZZ	Dilation of Left Ureter, Via Natural or Artificial Opening
0T778DZ	Dilation of Left Ureter with Intraluminal Device, Via Natural or Artificial Opening Endoscopic
0T778ZZ	Dilation of Left Ureter, Via Natural or Artificial Opening Endoscopic
0T780DZ	Dilation of Bilateral Ureters with Intraluminal Device, Open Approach
0T780ZZ	Dilation of Bilateral Ureters, Open Approach
0T783DZ	Dilation of Bilateral Ureters with Intraluminal Device, Percutaneous Approach
0T783ZZ	Dilation of Bilateral Ureters, Percutaneous Approach
0T784DZ	Dilation of Bilateral Ureters with Intraluminal Device, Percutaneous Endoscopic Approach
0T784ZZ	Dilation of Bilateral Ureters, Percutaneous Endoscopic Approach
0T787DZ	Dilation of Bilateral Ureters with Intraluminal Device, Via Natural or Artificial Opening
0T787ZZ	Dilation of Bilateral Ureters, Via Natural or Artificial Opening
0T788DZ	Dilation of Bilateral Ureters with Intraluminal Device, Via Natural or Artificial Opening Endoscopic
0T788ZZ	Dilation of Bilateral Ureters, Via Natural or Artificial Opening Endoscopic
0T7B0DZ	Dilation of Bladder with Intraluminal Device, Open Approach
0T7B0ZZ	Dilation of Bladder, Open Approach
0T7B3DZ	Dilation of Bladder with Intraluminal Device, Percutaneous Approach
0T7B3ZZ	Dilation of Bladder, Percutaneous Approach
0T7B4DZ	Dilation of Bladder with Intraluminal Device, Percutaneous Endoscopic Approach
0T7B4ZZ	Dilation of Bladder, Percutaneous Endoscopic Approach
0T7B7DZ	Dilation of Bladder with Intraluminal Device, Via Natural or Artificial Opening
0T7B7ZZ	Dilation of Bladder, Via Natural or Artificial Opening
0T7B8DZ	Dilation of Bladder with Intraluminal Device, Via Natural or Artificial Opening Endoscopic
0T7B8ZZ	Dilation of Bladder, Via Natural or Artificial Opening Endoscopic
0T7C0DZ	Dilation of Bladder Neck with Intraluminal Device, Open Approach
0T7C0ZZ	Dilation of Bladder Neck, Open Approach
0T7C3DZ	Dilation of Bladder Neck with Intraluminal Device, Percutaneous Approach
0T7C3ZZ	Dilation of Bladder Neck, Percutaneous Approach
0T7C4DZ	Dilation of Bladder Neck with Intraluminal Device, Percutaneous Endoscopic Approach
0T7C4ZZ	Dilation of Bladder Neck, Percutaneous Endoscopic Approach
0T7C7DZ	Dilation of Bladder Neck with Intraluminal Device, Via Natural or Artificial Opening
0T7C7ZZ	Dilation of Bladder Neck, Via Natural or Artificial Opening
0T7C8DZ	Dilation of Bladder Neck with Intraluminal Device, Via Natural or Artificial Opening Endoscopic
0T7C8ZZ	Dilation of Bladder Neck, Via Natural or Artificial Opening Endoscopic
0T7D0DZ	Dilation of Urethra with Intraluminal Device, Open Approach

0T7D0ZZ	Dilation of Urethra, Open Approach
0T7D3DZ	Dilation of Urethra with Intraluminal Device, Percutaneous Approach
0T7D3ZZ	Dilation of Urethra, Percutaneous Approach
0T7D4DZ	Dilation of Urethra with Intraluminal Device, Percutaneous Endoscopic Approach
0T7D4ZZ	Dilation of Urethra, Percutaneous Endoscopic Approach

0T7D7DZ	Dilation of Urethra with Intraluminal Device, Via Natural or Artificial Opening
0T7D7ZZ	Dilation of Urethra, Via Natural or Artificial Opening
0T7D8DZ	Dilation of Urethra with Intraluminal Device, Via Natural or Artificial Opening Endoscopic
0T7D8ZZ	Dilation of Urethra, Via Natural or Artificial Opening Endoscopic

0T8 – Urinary System, Division

Review Coding Guideline B3.14

0T820ZZ	Division of Bilateral Kidneys, Open Approach
0T823ZZ	Division of Bilateral Kidneys, Percutaneous Approach
0T824ZZ	Division of Bilateral Kidneys, Percutaneous Endoscopic Approach

0T8C0ZZ	Division of Bladder Neck, Open Approach
0T8C3ZZ	Division of Bladder Neck, Percutaneous Approach
0T8C4ZZ	Division of Bladder Neck, Percutaneous Endoscopic Approach

0T9 – Urinary System, Drainage

Review Coding Guidelines B3.4a and B3.4b

Review Coding Guideline B6.2

0T9000Z	Drainage of Right Kidney with Drainage Device, Open Approach
0T900ZX	Drainage of Right Kidney, Open Approach, Diagnostic
0T900ZZ	Drainage of Right Kidney, Open Approach
0T9030Z	Drainage of Right Kidney with Drainage Device, Percutaneous Approach
0T903ZX	Drainage of Right Kidney, Percutaneous Approach, Diagnostic
0T903ZZ	Drainage of Right Kidney, Percutaneous Approach
0T9040Z	Drainage of Right Kidney with Drainage Device, Percutaneous Endoscopic Approach
0T904ZX	Drainage of Right Kidney, Percutaneous Endoscopic Approach, Diagnostic
0T904ZZ	Drainage of Right Kidney, Percutaneous Endoscopic Approach
0T9070Z	Drainage of Right Kidney with Drainage Device, Via Natural or Artificial Opening
0T907ZX	Drainage of Right Kidney, Via Natural or Artificial Opening, Diagnostic
0T907ZZ	Drainage of Right Kidney, Via Natural or Artificial Opening
0T9080Z	Drainage of Right Kidney with Drainage Device, Via Natural or Artificial Opening Endoscopic
0T908ZX	Drainage of Right Kidney, Via Natural or Artificial Opening Endoscopic, Diagnostic
0T908ZZ	Drainage of Right Kidney, Via Natural or Artificial Opening Endoscopic
0T9100Z	Drainage of Left Kidney with Drainage Device, Open Approach
0T910ZX	Drainage of Left Kidney, Open Approach, Diagnostic
0T910ZZ	Drainage of Left Kidney, Open Approach
0T9130Z	Drainage of Left Kidney with Drainage Device, Percutaneous Approach
0T913ZX	Drainage of Left Kidney, Percutaneous Approach, Diagnostic
0T913ZZ	Drainage of Left Kidney, Percutaneous Approach
0T9140Z	Drainage of Left Kidney with Drainage Device, Percutaneous Endoscopic Approach
0T914ZX	Drainage of Left Kidney, Percutaneous Endoscopic Approach, Diagnostic
0T914ZZ	Drainage of Left Kidney, Percutaneous Endoscopic Approach
0T9170Z	Drainage of Left Kidney with Drainage Device, Via Natural or Artificial Opening
0T917ZX	Drainage of Left Kidney, Via Natural or Artificial Opening, Diagnostic
0T917ZZ	Drainage of Left Kidney, Via Natural or Artificial Opening
0T9180Z	Drainage of Left Kidney with Drainage Device, Via Natural or Artificial Opening Endoscopic
0T918ZX	Drainage of Left Kidney, Via Natural or Artificial Opening Endoscopic, Diagnostic
0T918ZZ	Drainage of Left Kidney, Via Natural or Artificial Opening Endoscopic
0T9300Z	Drainage of Right Kidney Pelvis with Drainage Device, Open Approach
0T930ZX	Drainage of Right Kidney Pelvis, Open Approach, Diagnostic
0T930ZZ	Drainage of Right Kidney Pelvis, Open Approach
0T9330Z	Drainage of Right Kidney Pelvis with Drainage Device, Percutaneous Approach

0T933ZX	Drainage of Right Kidney Pelvis, Percutaneous Approach, Diagnostic
0T933ZZ	Drainage of Right Kidney Pelvis, Percutaneous Approach
0T9340Z	Drainage of Right Kidney Pelvis with Drainage Device, Percutaneous Endoscopic Approach
0T934ZX	Drainage of Right Kidney Pelvis, Percutaneous Endoscopic Approach, Diagnostic
0T934ZZ	Drainage of Right Kidney Pelvis, Percutaneous Endoscopic Approach
0T9370Z	Drainage of Right Kidney Pelvis with Drainage Device, Via Natural or Artificial Opening
0T937ZX	Drainage of Right Kidney Pelvis, Via Natural or Artificial Opening, Diagnostic
0T937ZZ	Drainage of Right Kidney Pelvis, Via Natural or Artificial Opening
0T9380Z	Drainage of Right Kidney Pelvis with Drainage Device, Via Natural or Artificial Opening Endoscopic
0T938ZX	Drainage of Right Kidney Pelvis, Via Natural or Artificial Opening Endoscopic, Diagnostic
0T938ZZ	Drainage of Right Kidney Pelvis, Via Natural or Artificial Opening Endoscopic
0T9400Z	Drainage of Left Kidney Pelvis with Drainage Device, Open Approach
0T940ZX	Drainage of Left Kidney Pelvis, Open Approach, Diagnostic
0T940ZZ	Drainage of Left Kidney Pelvis, Open Approach
0T9430Z	Drainage of Left Kidney Pelvis with Drainage Device, Percutaneous Approach
0T943ZX	Drainage of Left Kidney Pelvis, Percutaneous Approach, Diagnostic
0T943ZZ	Drainage of Left Kidney Pelvis, Percutaneous Approach
0T9440Z	Drainage of Left Kidney Pelvis with Drainage Device, Percutaneous Endoscopic Approach
0T944ZX	Drainage of Left Kidney Pelvis, Percutaneous Endoscopic Approach, Diagnostic
0T944ZZ	Drainage of Left Kidney Pelvis, Percutaneous Endoscopic Approach
0T9470Z	Drainage of Left Kidney Pelvis with Drainage Device, Via Natural or Artificial Opening
0T947ZX	Drainage of Left Kidney Pelvis, Via Natural or Artificial Opening, Diagnostic
0T947ZZ	Drainage of Left Kidney Pelvis, Via Natural or Artificial Opening
0T9480Z	Drainage of Left Kidney Pelvis with Drainage Device, Via Natural or Artificial Opening Endoscopic
0T948ZX	Drainage of Left Kidney Pelvis, Via Natural or Artificial Opening Endoscopic, Diagnostic
0T948ZZ	Drainage of Left Kidney Pelvis, Via Natural or Artificial Opening Endoscopic
0T9600Z	Drainage of Right Ureter with Drainage Device, Open Approach
0T960ZX	Drainage of Right Ureter, Open Approach, Diagnostic
0T960ZZ	Drainage of Right Ureter, Open Approach
0T9630Z	Drainage of Right Ureter with Drainage Device, Percutaneous Approach
0T963ZX	Drainage of Right Ureter, Percutaneous Approach, Diagnostic
0T963ZZ	Drainage of Right Ureter, Percutaneous Approach
0T9640Z	Drainage of Right Ureter with Drainage Device, Percutaneous Endoscopic Approach

0T964ZX	Drainage of Right Ureter, Percutaneous Endoscopic Approach, Diagnostic
0T964ZZ	Drainage of Right Ureter, Percutaneous Endoscopic Approach
0T9670Z	Drainage of Right Ureter with Drainage Device, Via Natural or Artificial Opening
0T967ZX	Drainage of Right Ureter, Via Natural or Artificial Opening, Diagnostic
0T967ZZ	Drainage of Right Ureter, Via Natural or Artificial Opening
0T9680Z	Drainage of Right Ureter with Drainage Device, Via Natural or Artificial Opening Endoscopic
0T968ZX	Drainage of Right Ureter, Via Natural or Artificial Opening Endoscopic, Diagnostic
0T968ZZ	Drainage of Right Ureter, Via Natural or Artificial Opening Endoscopic
0T9700Z	Drainage of Left Ureter with Drainage Device, Open Approach
0T970ZX	Drainage of Left Ureter, Open Approach, Diagnostic
0T970ZZ	Drainage of Left Ureter, Open Approach
0T9730Z	Drainage of Left Ureter with Drainage Device, Percutaneous Approach
0T973ZX	Drainage of Left Ureter, Percutaneous Approach, Diagnostic
0T973ZZ	Drainage of Left Ureter, Percutaneous Approach
0T9740Z	Drainage of Left Ureter with Drainage Device, Percutaneous Endoscopic Approach
0T974ZX	Drainage of Left Ureter, Percutaneous Endoscopic Approach, Diagnostic
0T974ZZ	Drainage of Left Ureter, Percutaneous Endoscopic Approach
0T9770Z	Drainage of Left Ureter with Drainage Device, Via Natural or Artificial Opening
0T977ZX	Drainage of Left Ureter, Via Natural or Artificial Opening, Diagnostic
0T977ZZ	Drainage of Left Ureter, Via Natural or Artificial Opening
0T9780Z	Drainage of Left Ureter with Drainage Device, Via Natural or Artificial Opening Endoscopic
0T978ZX	Drainage of Left Ureter, Via Natural or Artificial Opening Endoscopic, Diagnostic
0T978ZZ	Drainage of Left Ureter, Via Natural or Artificial Opening Endoscopic
0T9800Z	Drainage of Bilateral Ureters with Drainage Device, Open Approach
0T980ZX	Drainage of Bilateral Ureters, Open Approach, Diagnostic
0T980ZZ	Drainage of Bilateral Ureters, Open Approach
0T9830Z	Drainage of Bilateral Ureters with Drainage Device, Percutaneous Approach
0T983ZX	Drainage of Bilateral Ureters, Percutaneous Approach, Diagnostic
0T983ZZ	Drainage of Bilateral Ureters, Percutaneous Approach
0T9840Z	Drainage of Bilateral Ureters with Drainage Device, Percutaneous Endoscopic Approach
0T984ZX	Drainage of Bilateral Ureters, Percutaneous Endoscopic Approach, Diagnostic
0T984ZZ	Drainage of Bilateral Ureters, Percutaneous Endoscopic Approach
0T9870Z	Drainage of Bilateral Ureters with Drainage Device, Via Natural or Artificial Opening
0T987ZX	Drainage of Bilateral Ureters, Via Natural or Artificial Opening, Diagnostic
0T987ZZ	Drainage of Bilateral Ureters, Via Natural or Artificial Opening
0T9880Z	Drainage of Bilateral Ureters with Drainage Device, Via Natural or Artificial Opening Endoscopic
0T988ZX	Drainage of Bilateral Ureters, Via Natural or Artificial Opening Endoscopic, Diagnostic
0T988ZZ	Drainage of Bilateral Ureters, Via Natural or Artificial Opening Endoscopic
0T9B00Z	Drainage of Bladder with Drainage Device, Open Approach
0T9B0ZX	Drainage of Bladder, Open Approach, Diagnostic
0T9B0ZZ	Drainage of Bladder, Open Approach
0T9B30Z	Drainage of Bladder with Drainage Device, Percutaneous Approach
0T9B3ZX	Drainage of Bladder, Percutaneous Approach, Diagnostic
0T9B3ZZ	Drainage of Bladder, Percutaneous Approach
0T9B40Z	Drainage of Bladder with Drainage Device, Percutaneous Endoscopic Approach
0T9B4ZX	Drainage of Bladder, Percutaneous Endoscopic Approach, Diagnostic
0T9B4ZZ	Drainage of Bladder, Percutaneous Endoscopic Approach
0T9B70Z	Drainage of Bladder with Drainage Device, Via Natural or Artificial Opening
0T9B7ZX	Drainage of Bladder, Via Natural or Artificial Opening, Diagnostic
0T9B7ZZ	Drainage of Bladder, Via Natural or Artificial Opening
0T9B80Z	Drainage of Bladder with Drainage Device, Via Natural or Artificial Opening Endoscopic
0T9B8ZX	Drainage of Bladder, Via Natural or Artificial Opening Endoscopic, Diagnostic
0T9B8ZZ	Drainage of Bladder, Via Natural or Artificial Opening Endoscopic
0T9C00Z	Drainage of Bladder Neck with Drainage Device, Open Approach
0T9C0ZX	Drainage of Bladder Neck, Open Approach, Diagnostic
0T9C0ZZ	Drainage of Bladder Neck, Open Approach
0T9C30Z	Drainage of Bladder Neck with Drainage Device, Percutaneous Approach
0T9C3ZX	Drainage of Bladder Neck, Percutaneous Approach, Diagnostic
0T9C3ZZ	Drainage of Bladder Neck, Percutaneous Approach
0T9C40Z	Drainage of Bladder Neck with Drainage Device, Percutaneous Endoscopic Approach
0T9C4ZX	Drainage of Bladder Neck, Percutaneous Endoscopic Approach, Diagnostic
0T9C4ZZ	Drainage of Bladder Neck, Percutaneous Endoscopic Approach
0T9C70Z	Drainage of Bladder Neck with Drainage Device, Via Natural or Artificial Opening
0T9C7ZX	Drainage of Bladder Neck, Via Natural or Artificial Opening, Diagnostic
0T9C7ZZ	Drainage of Bladder Neck, Via Natural or Artificial Opening
0T9C80Z	Drainage of Bladder Neck with Drainage Device, Via Natural or Artificial Opening Endoscopic
0T9C8ZX	Drainage of Bladder Neck, Via Natural or Artificial Opening Endoscopic, Diagnostic
0T9C8ZZ	Drainage of Bladder Neck, Via Natural or Artificial Opening Endoscopic
0T9D00Z	Drainage of Urethra with Drainage Device, Open Approach
0T9D0ZX	Drainage of Urethra, Open Approach, Diagnostic
0T9D0ZZ	Drainage of Urethra, Open Approach
0T9D30Z	Drainage of Urethra with Drainage Device, Percutaneous Approach
0T9D3ZX	Drainage of Urethra, Percutaneous Approach, Diagnostic
0T9D3ZZ	Drainage of Urethra, Percutaneous Approach
0T9D40Z	Drainage of Urethra with Drainage Device, Percutaneous Endoscopic Approach
0T9D4ZX	Drainage of Urethra, Percutaneous Endoscopic Approach, Diagnostic
0T9D4ZZ	Drainage of Urethra, Percutaneous Endoscopic Approach
0T9D70Z	Drainage of Urethra with Drainage Device, Via Natural or Artificial Opening
0T9D7ZX	Drainage of Urethra, Via Natural or Artificial Opening, Diagnostic
0T9D7ZZ	Drainage of Urethra, Via Natural or Artificial Opening
0T9D80Z	Drainage of Urethra with Drainage Device, Via Natural or Artificial Opening Endoscopic
0T9D8ZX	Drainage of Urethra, Via Natural or Artificial Opening Endoscopic, Diagnostic
0T9D8ZZ	Drainage of Urethra, Via Natural or Artificial Opening Endoscopic
0T9DX0Z	Drainage of Urethra with Drainage Device, External Approach
0T9DXZX	Drainage of Urethra, External Approach, Diagnostic
0T9DXZZ	Drainage of Urethra, External Approach

0TB – Urinary System, Excision

Review Coding Guidelines B3.4a and B3.4b

Review Coding Guideline B3.8

0TB00ZX	Excision of Right Kidney, Open Approach, Diagnostic
0TB00ZZ	Excision of Right Kidney, Open Approach
0TB03ZX	Excision of Right Kidney, Percutaneous Approach, Diagnostic
0TB03ZZ	Excision of Right Kidney, Percutaneous Approach
0TB04ZX	Excision of Right Kidney, Percutaneous Endoscopic Approach, Diagnostic
0TB04ZZ	Excision of Right Kidney, Percutaneous Endoscopic Approach

♀ Female-only   ♂ Male-only   ● Limited Coverage   ● Non-OR   HAC HAC-associated procedure   ● Non-covered procedures   + Combination

0TB07ZX	Excision of Right Kidney, Via Natural or Artificial Opening, Diagnostic
0TB07ZZ	Excision of Right Kidney, Via Natural or Artificial Opening
0TB08ZX	Excision of Right Kidney, Via Natural or Artificial Opening Endoscopic, Diagnostic
0TB08ZZ	Excision of Right Kidney, Via Natural or Artificial Opening Endoscopic
0TB10ZX	Excision of Left Kidney, Open Approach, Diagnostic
0TB10ZZ	Excision of Left Kidney, Open Approach
0TB13ZX	Excision of Left Kidney, Percutaneous Approach, Diagnostic
0TB13ZZ	Excision of Left Kidney, Percutaneous Approach
0TB14ZX	Excision of Left Kidney, Percutaneous Endoscopic Approach, Diagnostic
0TB14ZZ	Excision of Left Kidney, Percutaneous Endoscopic Approach
0TB17ZX	Excision of Left Kidney, Via Natural or Artificial Opening, Diagnostic
0TB17ZZ	Excision of Left Kidney, Via Natural or Artificial Opening
0TB18ZX	Excision of Left Kidney, Via Natural or Artificial Opening Endoscopic, Diagnostic
0TB18ZZ	Excision of Left Kidney, Via Natural or Artificial Opening Endoscopic
0TB30ZX	Excision of Right Kidney Pelvis, Open Approach, Diagnostic
0TB30ZZ	Excision of Right Kidney Pelvis, Open Approach
0TB33ZX	Excision of Right Kidney Pelvis, Percutaneous Approach, Diagnostic
0TB33ZZ	Excision of Right Kidney Pelvis, Percutaneous Approach
0TB34ZX	Excision of Right Kidney Pelvis, Percutaneous Endoscopic Approach, Diagnostic
0TB34ZZ	Excision of Right Kidney Pelvis, Percutaneous Endoscopic Approach
0TB37ZX	Excision of Right Kidney Pelvis, Via Natural or Artificial Opening, Diagnostic
0TB37ZZ	Excision of Right Kidney Pelvis, Via Natural or Artificial Opening
0TB38ZX	Excision of Right Kidney Pelvis, Via Natural or Artificial Opening Endoscopic, Diagnostic
0TB38ZZ	Excision of Right Kidney Pelvis, Via Natural or Artificial Opening Endoscopic
0TB40ZX	Excision of Left Kidney Pelvis, Open Approach, Diagnostic
0TB40ZZ	Excision of Left Kidney Pelvis, Open Approach
0TB43ZX	Excision of Left Kidney Pelvis, Percutaneous Approach, Diagnostic
0TB43ZZ	Excision of Left Kidney Pelvis, Percutaneous Approach
0TB44ZX	Excision of Left Kidney Pelvis, Percutaneous Endoscopic Approach, Diagnostic
0TB44ZZ	Excision of Left Kidney Pelvis, Percutaneous Endoscopic Approach
0TB47ZX	Excision of Left Kidney Pelvis, Via Natural or Artificial Opening, Diagnostic
0TB47ZZ	Excision of Left Kidney Pelvis, Via Natural or Artificial Opening
0TB48ZX	Excision of Left Kidney Pelvis, Via Natural or Artificial Opening Endoscopic, Diagnostic
0TB48ZZ	Excision of Left Kidney Pelvis, Via Natural or Artificial Opening Endoscopic
0TB60ZX	Excision of Right Ureter, Open Approach, Diagnostic
0TB60ZZ	Excision of Right Ureter, Open Approach
0TB63ZX	Excision of Right Ureter, Percutaneous Approach, Diagnostic
0TB63ZZ	Excision of Right Ureter, Percutaneous Approach
0TB64ZX	Excision of Right Ureter, Percutaneous Endoscopic Approach, Diagnostic
0TB64ZZ	Excision of Right Ureter, Percutaneous Endoscopic Approach
0TB67ZX	Excision of Right Ureter, Via Natural or Artificial Opening, Diagnostic
0TB67ZZ	Excision of Right Ureter, Via Natural or Artificial Opening
0TB68ZX	Excision of Right Ureter, Via Natural or Artificial Opening Endoscopic, Diagnostic
0TB68ZZ	Excision of Right Ureter, Via Natural or Artificial Opening Endoscopic
0TB70ZX	Excision of Left Ureter, Open Approach, Diagnostic
0TB70ZZ	Excision of Left Ureter, Open Approach
0TB73ZX	Excision of Left Ureter, Percutaneous Approach, Diagnostic
0TB73ZZ	Excision of Left Ureter, Percutaneous Approach
0TB74ZX	Excision of Left Ureter, Percutaneous Endoscopic Approach, Diagnostic
0TB74ZZ	Excision of Left Ureter, Percutaneous Endoscopic Approach
0TB77ZX	Excision of Left Ureter, Via Natural or Artificial Opening, Diagnostic
0TB77ZZ	Excision of Left Ureter, Via Natural or Artificial Opening
0TB78ZX	Excision of Left Ureter, Via Natural or Artificial Opening Endoscopic, Diagnostic
0TB78ZZ	Excision of Left Ureter, Via Natural or Artificial Opening Endoscopic
0TBB0ZX	Excision of Bladder, Open Approach, Diagnostic
0TBB0ZZ	Excision of Bladder, Open Approach
0TBB3ZX	Excision of Bladder, Percutaneous Approach, Diagnostic
0TBB3ZZ	Excision of Bladder, Percutaneous Approach
0TBB4ZX	Excision of Bladder, Percutaneous Endoscopic Approach, Diagnostic
0TBB4ZZ	Excision of Bladder, Percutaneous Endoscopic Approach
0TBB7ZX	Excision of Bladder, Via Natural or Artificial Opening, Diagnostic
0TBB7ZZ	Excision of Bladder, Via Natural or Artificial Opening
0TBB8ZX	Excision of Bladder, Via Natural or Artificial Opening Endoscopic, Diagnostic
0TBB8ZZ	Excision of Bladder, Via Natural or Artificial Opening Endoscopic
0TBC0ZX	Excision of Bladder Neck, Open Approach, Diagnostic
0TBC0ZZ	Excision of Bladder Neck, Open Approach
0TBC3ZX	Excision of Bladder Neck, Percutaneous Approach, Diagnostic
0TBC3ZZ	Excision of Bladder Neck, Percutaneous Approach
0TBC4ZX	Excision of Bladder Neck, Percutaneous Endoscopic Approach, Diagnostic
0TBC4ZZ	Excision of Bladder Neck, Percutaneous Endoscopic Approach
0TBC7ZX	Excision of Bladder Neck, Via Natural or Artificial Opening, Diagnostic
0TBC7ZZ	Excision of Bladder Neck, Via Natural or Artificial Opening
0TBC8ZX	Excision of Bladder Neck, Via Natural or Artificial Opening Endoscopic, Diagnostic
0TBC8ZZ	Excision of Bladder Neck, Via Natural or Artificial Opening Endoscopic
0TBD0ZX	Excision of Urethra, Open Approach, Diagnostic
0TBD0ZZ	Excision of Urethra, Open Approach
0TBD3ZX	Excision of Urethra, Percutaneous Approach, Diagnostic
0TBD3ZZ	Excision of Urethra, Percutaneous Approach
0TBD4ZX	Excision of Urethra, Percutaneous Endoscopic Approach, Diagnostic
0TBD4ZZ	Excision of Urethra, Percutaneous Endoscopic Approach
0TBD7ZX	Excision of Urethra, Via Natural or Artificial Opening, Diagnostic
0TBD7ZZ	Excision of Urethra, Via Natural or Artificial Opening
0TBD8ZX	Excision of Urethra, Via Natural or Artificial Opening Endoscopic, Diagnostic
0TBD8ZZ	Excision of Urethra, Via Natural or Artificial Opening Endoscopic
0TBDXZX	Excision of Urethra, External Approach, Diagnostic
0TBDXZZ	Excision of Urethra, External Approach

0TC – Urinary System, Extirpation

0TC00ZZ	Extirpation of Matter from Right Kidney, Open Approach
0TC03ZZ	Extirpation of Matter from Right Kidney, Percutaneous Approach
0TC04ZZ	Extirpation of Matter from Right Kidney, Percutaneous Endoscopic Approach
0TC07ZZ	Extirpation of Matter from Right Kidney, Via Natural or Artificial Opening
0TC08ZZ	Extirpation of Matter from Right Kidney, Via Natural or Artificial Opening Endoscopic
0TC10ZZ	Extirpation of Matter from Left Kidney, Open Approach
0TC13ZZ	Extirpation of Matter from Left Kidney, Percutaneous Approach
0TC14ZZ	Extirpation of Matter from Left Kidney, Percutaneous Endoscopic Approach
0TC17ZZ	Extirpation of Matter from Left Kidney, Via Natural or Artificial Opening
0TC18ZZ	Extirpation of Matter from Left Kidney, Via Natural or Artificial Opening Endoscopic
0TC30ZZ	Extirpation of Matter from Right Kidney Pelvis, Open Approach
0TC33ZZ	Extirpation of Matter from Right Kidney Pelvis, Percutaneous Approach
0TC34ZZ	Extirpation of Matter from Right Kidney Pelvis, Percutaneous Endoscopic Approach
0TC37ZZ	Extirpation of Matter from Right Kidney Pelvis, Via Natural or Artificial Opening

0TC38ZZ	Extirpation of Matter from Right Kidney Pelvis, Via Natural or Artificial Opening Endoscopic
0TC40ZZ	Extirpation of Matter from Left Kidney Pelvis, Open Approach
0TC43ZZ	Extirpation of Matter from Left Kidney Pelvis, Percutaneous Approach
0TC44ZZ	Extirpation of Matter from Left Kidney Pelvis, Percutaneous Endoscopic Approach
0TC47ZZ	Extirpation of Matter from Left Kidney Pelvis, Via Natural or Artificial Opening
0TC48ZZ	Extirpation of Matter from Left Kidney Pelvis, Via Natural or Artificial Opening Endoscopic
0TC60ZZ	Extirpation of Matter from Right Ureter, Open Approach
0TC63ZZ	Extirpation of Matter from Right Ureter, Percutaneous Approach
0TC64ZZ	Extirpation of Matter from Right Ureter, Percutaneous Endoscopic Approach
0TC67ZZ	Extirpation of Matter from Right Ureter, Via Natural or Artificial Opening
0TC68ZZ	Extirpation of Matter from Right Ureter, Via Natural or Artificial Opening Endoscopic
0TC70ZZ	Extirpation of Matter from Left Ureter, Open Approach
0TC73ZZ	Extirpation of Matter from Left Ureter, Percutaneous Approach
0TC74ZZ	Extirpation of Matter from Left Ureter, Percutaneous Endoscopic Approach
0TC77ZZ	Extirpation of Matter from Left Ureter, Via Natural or Artificial Opening
0TC78ZZ	Extirpation of Matter from Left Ureter, Via Natural or Artificial Opening Endoscopic
0TCB0ZZ	Extirpation of Matter from Bladder, Open Approach
0TCB3ZZ	Extirpation of Matter from Bladder, Percutaneous Approach
0TCB4ZZ	Extirpation of Matter from Bladder, Percutaneous Endoscopic Approach
0TCB7ZZ	Extirpation of Matter from Bladder, Via Natural or Artificial Opening
0TCB8ZZ	Extirpation of Matter from Bladder, Via Natural or Artificial Opening Endoscopic
0TCC0ZZ	Extirpation of Matter from Bladder Neck, Open Approach
0TCC3ZZ	Extirpation of Matter from Bladder Neck, Percutaneous Approach
0TCC4ZZ	Extirpation of Matter from Bladder Neck, Percutaneous Endoscopic Approach
0TCC7ZZ	Extirpation of Matter from Bladder Neck, Via Natural or Artificial Opening
0TCC8ZZ	Extirpation of Matter from Bladder Neck, Via Natural or Artificial Opening Endoscopic
0TCD0ZZ	Extirpation of Matter from Urethra, Open Approach
0TCD3ZZ	Extirpation of Matter from Urethra, Percutaneous Approach
0TCD4ZZ	Extirpation of Matter from Urethra, Percutaneous Endoscopic Approach
0TCD7ZZ	Extirpation of Matter from Urethra, Via Natural or Artificial Opening
0TCD8ZZ	Extirpation of Matter from Urethra, Via Natural or Artificial Opening Endoscopic
0TCDXZZ	Extirpation of Matter from Urethra, External Approach

0TD   Urinary System, Extraction

0TD00ZZ	Extraction of Right Kidney, Open Approach
0TD03ZZ	Extraction of Right Kidney, Percutaneous Approach
0TD04ZZ	Extraction of Right Kidney, Percutaneous Endoscopic Approach
0TD10ZZ	Extraction of Left Kidney, Open Approach
0TD13ZZ	Extraction of Left Kidney, Percutaneous Approach
0TD14ZZ	Extraction of Left Kidney, Percutaneous Endoscopic Approach

0TF   Urinary System, Fragmentation

0TF30ZZ	Fragmentation in Right Kidney Pelvis, Open Approach
0TF33ZZ	Fragmentation in Right Kidney Pelvis, Percutaneous Approach
0TF34ZZ	Fragmentation in Right Kidney Pelvis, Percutaneous Endoscopic Approach
0TF37ZZ	Fragmentation in Right Kidney Pelvis, Via Natural or Artificial Opening
0TF38ZZ	Fragmentation in Right Kidney Pelvis, Via Natural or Artificial Opening Endoscopic
● **0TF3XZZ**	Fragmentation in Right Kidney Pelvis, External Approach
0TF40ZZ	Fragmentation in Left Kidney Pelvis, Open Approach
0TF43ZZ	Fragmentation in Left Kidney Pelvis, Percutaneous Approach
0TF44ZZ	Fragmentation in Left Kidney Pelvis, Percutaneous Endoscopic Approach
0TF47ZZ	Fragmentation in Left Kidney Pelvis, Via Natural or Artificial Opening
0TF48ZZ	Fragmentation in Left Kidney Pelvis, Via Natural or Artificial Opening Endoscopic
● **0TF4XZZ**	Fragmentation in Left Kidney Pelvis, External Approach
0TF60ZZ	Fragmentation in Right Ureter, Open Approach
0TF63ZZ	Fragmentation in Right Ureter, Percutaneous Approach
0TF64ZZ	Fragmentation in Right Ureter, Percutaneous Endoscopic Approach
0TF67ZZ	Fragmentation in Right Ureter, Via Natural or Artificial Opening
0TF68ZZ	Fragmentation in Right Ureter, Via Natural or Artificial Opening Endoscopic
● **0TF6XZZ**	Fragmentation in Right Ureter, External Approach
0TF70ZZ	Fragmentation in Left Ureter, Open Approach
0TF73ZZ	Fragmentation in Left Ureter, Percutaneous Approach
0TF74ZZ	Fragmentation in Left Ureter, Percutaneous Endoscopic Approach
0TF77ZZ	Fragmentation in Left Ureter, Via Natural or Artificial Opening
0TF78ZZ	Fragmentation in Left Ureter, Via Natural or Artificial Opening Endoscopic
● **0TF7XZZ**	Fragmentation in Left Ureter, External Approach
0TFB0ZZ	Fragmentation in Bladder, Open Approach
0TFB3ZZ	Fragmentation in Bladder, Percutaneous Approach
0TFB4ZZ	Fragmentation in Bladder, Percutaneous Endoscopic Approach
0TFB7ZZ	Fragmentation in Bladder, Via Natural or Artificial Opening
0TFB8ZZ	Fragmentation in Bladder, Via Natural or Artificial Opening Endoscopic
● **0TFBXZZ**	Fragmentation in Bladder, External Approach
0TFC0ZZ	Fragmentation in Bladder Neck, Open Approach
0TFC3ZZ	Fragmentation in Bladder Neck, Percutaneous Approach
0TFC4ZZ	Fragmentation in Bladder Neck, Percutaneous Endoscopic Approach
0TFC7ZZ	Fragmentation in Bladder Neck, Via Natural or Artificial Opening
0TFC8ZZ	Fragmentation in Bladder Neck, Via Natural or Artificial Opening Endoscopic
● **0TFCXZZ**	Fragmentation in Bladder Neck, External Approach
0TFD0ZZ	Fragmentation in Urethra, Open Approach
0TFD3ZZ	Fragmentation in Urethra, Percutaneous Approach
0TFD4ZZ	Fragmentation in Urethra, Percutaneous Endoscopic Approach
0TFD7ZZ	Fragmentation in Urethra, Via Natural or Artificial Opening
● **0TFD8ZZ**	Fragmentation in Urethra, Via Natural or Artificial Opening Endoscopic
0TFDXZZ	Fragmentation in Urethra, External Approach

0TH – Urinary System, Insertion

0TH502Z	Insertion of Monitoring Device into Kidney, Open Approach
0TH503Z	Insertion of Infusion Device into Kidney, Open Approach
0TH532Z	Insertion of Monitoring Device into Kidney, Percutaneous Approach
0TH533Z	Insertion of Infusion Device into Kidney, Percutaneous Approach
0TH542Z	Insertion of Monitoring Device into Kidney, Percutaneous Endoscopic Approach
0TH543Z	Insertion of Infusion Device into Kidney, Percutaneous Endoscopic Approach
0TH572Z	Insertion of Monitoring Device into Kidney, Via Natural or Artificial Opening
0TH573Z	Insertion of Infusion Device into Kidney, Via Natural or Artificial Opening
0TH582Z	Insertion of Monitoring Device into Kidney, Via Natural or Artificial Opening Endoscopic
0TH583Z	Insertion of Infusion Device into Kidney, Via Natural or Artificial Opening Endoscopic

0TH902Z	Insertion of Monitoring Device into Ureter, Open Approach	● 0THB7MZ	Insertion of Stimulator Lead into Bladder, Via Natural or Artificial Opening
0TH903Z	Insertion of Infusion Device into Ureter, Open Approach	0THB82Z	Insertion of Monitoring Device into Bladder, Via Natural or Artificial Opening Endoscopic
0TH90MZ	Insertion of Stimulator Lead into Ureter, Open Approach	0THB83Z	Insertion of Infusion Device into Bladder, Via Natural or Artificial Opening Endoscopic
0TH932Z	Insertion of Monitoring Device into Ureter, Percutaneous Approach	0THB8LZ	Insertion of Artificial Sphincter into Bladder, Via Natural or Artificial Opening Endoscopic
0TH933Z	Insertion of Infusion Device into Ureter, Percutaneous Approach	● 0THB8MZ	Insertion of Stimulator Lead into Bladder, Via Natural or Artificial Opening Endoscopic
0TH93MZ	Insertion of Stimulator Lead into Ureter, Percutaneous Approach	0THC0LZ	Insertion of Artificial Sphincter into Bladder Neck, Open Approach
0TH942Z	Insertion of Monitoring Device into Ureter, Percutaneous Endoscopic Approach	0THC3LZ	Insertion of Artificial Sphincter into Bladder Neck, Percutaneous Approach
0TH943Z	Insertion of Infusion Device into Ureter, Percutaneous Endoscopic Approach	0THC4LZ	Insertion of Artificial Sphincter into Bladder Neck, Percutaneous Endoscopic Approach
0TH94MZ	Insertion of Stimulator Lead into Ureter, Percutaneous Endoscopic Approach	0THC7LZ	Insertion of Artificial Sphincter into Bladder Neck, Via Natural or Artificial Opening
0TH972Z	Insertion of Monitoring Device into Ureter, Via Natural or Artificial Opening	0THC8LZ	Insertion of Artificial Sphincter into Bladder Neck, Via Natural or Artificial Opening Endoscopic
0TH973Z	Insertion of Infusion Device into Ureter, Via Natural or Artificial Opening	0THD02Z	Insertion of Monitoring Device into Urethra, Open Approach
0TH97MZ	Insertion of Stimulator Lead into Ureter, Via Natural or Artificial Opening	0THD03Z	Insertion of Infusion Device into Urethra, Open Approach
0TH982Z	Insertion of Monitoring Device into Ureter, Via Natural or Artificial Opening Endoscopic	0THD0LZ	Insertion of Artificial Sphincter into Urethra, Open Approach
0TH983Z	Insertion of Infusion Device into Ureter, Via Natural or Artificial Opening Endoscopic	0THD32Z	Insertion of Monitoring Device into Urethra, Percutaneous Approach
0TH98MZ	Insertion of Stimulator Lead into Ureter, Via Natural or Artificial Opening Endoscopic	0THD33Z	Insertion of Infusion Device into Urethra, Percutaneous Approach
0THB02Z	Insertion of Monitoring Device into Bladder, Open Approach	0THD3LZ	Insertion of Artificial Sphincter into Urethra, Percutaneous Approach
0THB03Z	Insertion of Infusion Device into Bladder, Open Approach	0THD42Z	Insertion of Monitoring Device into Urethra, Percutaneous Endoscopic Approach
0THB0LZ	Insertion of Artificial Sphincter into Bladder, Open Approach	0THD43Z	Insertion of Infusion Device into Urethra, Percutaneous Endoscopic Approach
● 0THB0MZ	Insertion of Stimulator Lead into Bladder, Open Approach	0THD4LZ	Insertion of Artificial Sphincter into Urethra, Percutaneous Endoscopic Approach
0THB32Z	Insertion of Monitoring Device into Bladder, Percutaneous Approach	0THD72Z	Insertion of Monitoring Device into Urethra, Via Natural or Artificial Opening
0THB33Z	Insertion of Infusion Device into Bladder, Percutaneous Approach	0THD73Z	Insertion of Infusion Device into Urethra, Via Natural or Artificial Opening
0THB3LZ	Insertion of Artificial Sphincter into Bladder, Percutaneous Approach	0THD7LZ	Insertion of Artificial Sphincter into Urethra, Via Natural or Artificial Opening
● 0THB3MZ	Insertion of Stimulator Lead into Bladder, Percutaneous Approach	0THD82Z	Insertion of Monitoring Device into Urethra, Via Natural or Artificial Opening Endoscopic
0THB42Z	Insertion of Monitoring Device into Bladder, Percutaneous Endoscopic Approach	0THD83Z	Insertion of Infusion Device into Urethra, Via Natural or Artificial Opening Endoscopic
0THB43Z	Insertion of Infusion Device into Bladder, Percutaneous Endoscopic Approach	0THD8LZ	Insertion of Artificial Sphincter into Urethra, Via Natural or Artificial Opening Endoscopic
0THB4LZ	Insertion of Artificial Sphincter into Bladder, Percutaneous Endoscopic Approach	0THDX2Z	Insertion of Monitoring Device into Urethra, External Approach
● 0THB4MZ	Insertion of Stimulator Lead into Bladder, Percutaneous Endoscopic Approach	0THDX3Z	Insertion of Infusion Device into Urethra, External Approach
0THB72Z	Insertion of Monitoring Device into Bladder, Via Natural or Artificial Opening	0THDXLZ	Insertion of Artificial Sphincter into Urethra, External Approach
0THB73Z	Insertion of Infusion Device into Bladder, Via Natural or Artificial Opening		
0THB7LZ	Insertion of Artificial Sphincter into Bladder, Via Natural or Artificial Opening		

0TJ – Urinary System, Inspection

Review Coding Guidelines B3.11a, B3.11b and B3.11c

0TJ50ZZ	Inspection of Kidney, Open Approach	0TJB0ZZ	Inspection of Bladder, Open Approach
0TJ53ZZ	Inspection of Kidney, Percutaneous Approach	0TJB3ZZ	Inspection of Bladder, Percutaneous Approach
0TJ54ZZ	Inspection of Kidney, Percutaneous Endoscopic Approach	0TJB4ZZ	Inspection of Bladder, Percutaneous Endoscopic Approach
0TJ57ZZ	Inspection of Kidney, Via Natural or Artificial Opening	0TJB7ZZ	Inspection of Bladder, Via Natural or Artificial Opening
0TJ58ZZ	Inspection of Kidney, Via Natural or Artificial Opening Endoscopic	0TJB8ZZ	Inspection of Bladder, Via Natural or Artificial Opening Endoscopic
0TJ5XZZ	Inspection of Kidney, External Approach	0TJBXZZ	Inspection of Bladder, External Approach
0TJ90ZZ	Inspection of Ureter, Open Approach	0TJD0ZZ	Inspection of Urethra, Open Approach
0TJ93ZZ	Inspection of Ureter, Percutaneous Approach	0TJD3ZZ	Inspection of Urethra, Percutaneous Approach
0TJ94ZZ	Inspection of Ureter, Percutaneous Endoscopic Approach	0TJD4ZZ	Inspection of Urethra, Percutaneous Endoscopic Approach
0TJ97ZZ	Inspection of Ureter, Via Natural or Artificial Opening	0TJD7ZZ	Inspection of Urethra, Via Natural or Artificial Opening
0TJ98ZZ	Inspection of Ureter, Via Natural or Artificial Opening Endoscopic	0TJD8ZZ	Inspection of Urethra, Via Natural or Artificial Opening Endoscopic
0TJ9XZZ	Inspection of Ureter, External Approach	0TJDXZZ	Inspection of Urethra, External Approach

0TL – Urinary System, Occlusion

0TL30CZ	Occlusion of Right Kidney Pelvis with Extraluminal Device, Open Approach	0TL33CZ	Occlusion of Right Kidney Pelvis with Extraluminal Device, Percutaneous Approach
0TL30DZ	Occlusion of Right Kidney Pelvis with Intraluminal Device, Open Approach	0TL33DZ	Occlusion of Right Kidney Pelvis with Intraluminal Device, Percutaneous Approach
0TL30ZZ	Occlusion of Right Kidney Pelvis, Open Approach	0TL33ZZ	Occlusion of Right Kidney Pelvis, Percutaneous Approach

0TL34CZ Occlusion of Right Kidney Pelvis with Extraluminal Device, Percutaneous Endoscopic Approach

0TL34DZ Occlusion of Right Kidney Pelvis with Intraluminal Device, Percutaneous Endoscopic Approach

0TL34ZZ Occlusion of Right Kidney Pelvis, Percutaneous Endoscopic Approach

0TL37DZ Occlusion of Right Kidney Pelvis with Intraluminal Device, Via Natural or Artificial Opening

0TL37ZZ Occlusion of Right Kidney Pelvis, Via Natural or Artificial Opening

0TL38DZ Occlusion of Right Kidney Pelvis with Intraluminal Device, Via Natural or Artificial Opening Endoscopic

0TL38ZZ Occlusion of Right Kidney Pelvis, Via Natural or Artificial Opening Endoscopic

0TL40CZ Occlusion of Left Kidney Pelvis with Extraluminal Device, Open Approach

0TL40DZ Occlusion of Left Kidney Pelvis with Intraluminal Device, Open Approach

0TL40ZZ Occlusion of Left Kidney Pelvis, Open Approach

0TL43CZ Occlusion of Left Kidney Pelvis with Extraluminal Device, Percutaneous Approach

0TL43DZ Occlusion of Left Kidney Pelvis with Intraluminal Device, Percutaneous Approach

0TL43ZZ Occlusion of Left Kidney Pelvis, Percutaneous Approach

0TL44CZ Occlusion of Left Kidney Pelvis with Extraluminal Device, Percutaneous Endoscopic Approach

0TL44DZ Occlusion of Left Kidney Pelvis with Intraluminal Device, Percutaneous Endoscopic Approach

0TL44ZZ Occlusion of Left Kidney Pelvis, Percutaneous Endoscopic Approach

0TL47DZ Occlusion of Left Kidney Pelvis with Intraluminal Device, Via Natural or Artificial Opening

0TL47ZZ Occlusion of Left Kidney Pelvis, Via Natural or Artificial Opening

0TL48DZ Occlusion of Left Kidney Pelvis with Intraluminal Device, Via Natural or Artificial Opening Endoscopic

0TL48ZZ Occlusion of Left Kidney Pelvis, Via Natural or Artificial Opening Endoscopic

0TL60CZ Occlusion of Right Ureter with Extraluminal Device, Open Approach

0TL60DZ Occlusion of Right Ureter with Intraluminal Device, Open Approach

0TL60ZZ Occlusion of Right Ureter, Open Approach

0TL63CZ Occlusion of Right Ureter with Extraluminal Device, Percutaneous Approach

0TL63DZ Occlusion of Right Ureter with Intraluminal Device, Percutaneous Approach

0TL63ZZ Occlusion of Right Ureter, Percutaneous Approach

0TL64CZ Occlusion of Right Ureter with Extraluminal Device, Percutaneous Endoscopic Approach

0TL64DZ Occlusion of Right Ureter with Intraluminal Device, Percutaneous Endoscopic Approach

0TL64ZZ Occlusion of Right Ureter, Percutaneous Endoscopic Approach

0TL67DZ Occlusion of Right Ureter with Intraluminal Device, Via Natural or Artificial Opening

0TL67ZZ Occlusion of Right Ureter, Via Natural or Artificial Opening

0TL68DZ Occlusion of Right Ureter with Intraluminal Device, Via Natural or Artificial Opening Endoscopic

0TL68ZZ Occlusion of Right Ureter, Via Natural or Artificial Opening Endoscopic

0TL70CZ Occlusion of Left Ureter with Extraluminal Device, Open Approach

0TL70DZ Occlusion of Left Ureter with Intraluminal Device, Open Approach

0TL70ZZ Occlusion of Left Ureter, Open Approach

0TL73CZ Occlusion of Left Ureter with Extraluminal Device, Percutaneous Approach

0TL73DZ Occlusion of Left Ureter with Intraluminal Device, Percutaneous Approach

0TL73ZZ Occlusion of Left Ureter, Percutaneous Approach

0TL74CZ Occlusion of Left Ureter with Extraluminal Device, Percutaneous Endoscopic Approach

0TL74DZ Occlusion of Left Ureter with Intraluminal Device, Percutaneous Endoscopic Approach

0TL74ZZ Occlusion of Left Ureter, Percutaneous Endoscopic Approach

0TL77DZ Occlusion of Left Ureter with Intraluminal Device, Via Natural or Artificial Opening

0TL77ZZ Occlusion of Left Ureter, Via Natural or Artificial Opening

0TL78DZ Occlusion of Left Ureter with Intraluminal Device, Via Natural or Artificial Opening Endoscopic

0TL78ZZ Occlusion of Left Ureter, Via Natural or Artificial Opening Endoscopic

0TLB0CZ Occlusion of Bladder with Extraluminal Device, Open Approach

0TLB0DZ Occlusion of Bladder with Intraluminal Device, Open Approach

0TLB0ZZ Occlusion of Bladder, Open Approach

0TLB3CZ Occlusion of Bladder with Extraluminal Device, Percutaneous Approach

0TLB3DZ Occlusion of Bladder with Intraluminal Device, Percutaneous Approach

0TLB3ZZ Occlusion of Bladder, Percutaneous Approach

0TLB4CZ Occlusion of Bladder with Extraluminal Device, Percutaneous Endoscopic Approach

0TLB4DZ Occlusion of Bladder with Intraluminal Device, Percutaneous Endoscopic Approach

0TLB4ZZ Occlusion of Bladder, Percutaneous Endoscopic Approach

0TLB7DZ Occlusion of Bladder with Intraluminal Device, Via Natural or Artificial Opening

0TLB7ZZ Occlusion of Bladder, Via Natural or Artificial Opening

0TLB8DZ Occlusion of Bladder with Intraluminal Device, Via Natural or Artificial Opening Endoscopic

0TLB8ZZ Occlusion of Bladder, Via Natural or Artificial Opening Endoscopic

0TLC0CZ Occlusion of Bladder Neck with Extraluminal Device, Open Approach

0TLC0DZ Occlusion of Bladder Neck with Intraluminal Device, Open Approach

0TLC0ZZ Occlusion of Bladder Neck, Open Approach

0TLC3CZ Occlusion of Bladder Neck with Extraluminal Device, Percutaneous Approach

0TLC3DZ Occlusion of Bladder Neck with Intraluminal Device, Percutaneous Approach

0TLC3ZZ Occlusion of Bladder Neck, Percutaneous Approach

0TLC4CZ Occlusion of Bladder Neck with Extraluminal Device, Percutaneous Endoscopic Approach

0TLC4DZ Occlusion of Bladder Neck with Intraluminal Device, Percutaneous Endoscopic Approach

0TLC4ZZ Occlusion of Bladder Neck, Percutaneous Endoscopic Approach

0TLC7DZ Occlusion of Bladder Neck with Intraluminal Device, Via Natural or Artificial Opening

0TLC7ZZ Occlusion of Bladder Neck, Via Natural or Artificial Opening

0TLC8DZ Occlusion of Bladder Neck with Intraluminal Device, Via Natural or Artificial Opening Endoscopic

0TLC8ZZ Occlusion of Bladder Neck, Via Natural or Artificial Opening Endoscopic

0TLD0CZ Occlusion of Urethra with Extraluminal Device, Open Approach

0TLD0DZ Occlusion of Urethra with Intraluminal Device, Open Approach

0TLD0ZZ Occlusion of Urethra, Open Approach

0TLD3CZ Occlusion of Urethra with Extraluminal Device, Percutaneous Approach

0TLD3DZ Occlusion of Urethra with Intraluminal Device, Percutaneous Approach

0TLD3ZZ Occlusion of Urethra, Percutaneous Approach

0TLD4CZ Occlusion of Urethra with Extraluminal Device, Percutaneous Endoscopic Approach

0TLD4DZ Occlusion of Urethra with Intraluminal Device, Percutaneous Endoscopic Approach

0TLD4ZZ Occlusion of Urethra, Percutaneous Endoscopic Approach

0TLD7DZ Occlusion of Urethra with Intraluminal Device, Via Natural or Artificial Opening

0TLD7ZZ Occlusion of Urethra, Via Natural or Artificial Opening

0TLD8DZ Occlusion of Urethra with Intraluminal Device, Via Natural or Artificial Opening Endoscopic

0TLD8ZZ Occlusion of Urethra, Via Natural or Artificial Opening Endoscopic

0TLDXCZ Occlusion of Urethra with Extraluminal Device, External Approach

0TLDXDZ Occlusion of Urethra with Intraluminal Device, External Approach

0TLDXZZ Occlusion of Urethra, External Approach

♀ Female-only   ♂ Male-only   ◍ Limited Coverage   ● Non-OR   ⬛ HAC-associated procedure   ⬤ Non-covered procedures   ➕ Combination

0TM – Urinary System, Reattachment

0TM00ZZ	Reattachment of Right Kidney, Open Approach
0TM04ZZ	Reattachment of Right Kidney, Percutaneous Endoscopic Approach
0TM10ZZ	Reattachment of Left Kidney, Open Approach
0TM14ZZ	Reattachment of Left Kidney, Percutaneous Endoscopic Approach
0TM20ZZ	Reattachment of Bilateral Kidneys, Open Approach
0TM24ZZ	Reattachment of Bilateral Kidneys, Percutaneous Endoscopic Approach
0TM30ZZ	Reattachment of Right Kidney Pelvis, Open Approach
0TM34ZZ	Reattachment of Right Kidney Pelvis, Percutaneous Endoscopic Approach
0TM40ZZ	Reattachment of Left Kidney Pelvis, Open Approach
0TM44ZZ	Reattachment of Left Kidney Pelvis, Percutaneous Endoscopic Approach
0TM60ZZ	Reattachment of Right Ureter, Open Approach
0TM64ZZ	Reattachment of Right Ureter, Percutaneous Endoscopic Approach
0TM70ZZ	Reattachment of Left Ureter, Open Approach
0TM74ZZ	Reattachment of Left Ureter, Percutaneous Endoscopic Approach
0TM80ZZ	Reattachment of Bilateral Ureters, Open Approach
0TM84ZZ	Reattachment of Bilateral Ureters, Percutaneous Endoscopic Approach
0TMB0ZZ	Reattachment of Bladder, Open Approach
0TMB4ZZ	Reattachment of Bladder, Percutaneous Endoscopic Approach
0TMC0ZZ	Reattachment of Bladder Neck, Open Approach
0TMC4ZZ	Reattachment of Bladder Neck, Percutaneous Endoscopic Approach
0TMD0ZZ	Reattachment of Urethra, Open Approach
0TMD4ZZ	Reattachment of Urethra, Percutaneous Endoscopic Approach

0TN – Urinary System, Release

Review Coding Guideline B3.13

Review Coding Guideline B3.14

0TN00ZZ	Release Right Kidney, Open Approach
0TN03ZZ	Release Right Kidney, Percutaneous Approach
0TN04ZZ	Release Right Kidney, Percutaneous Endoscopic Approach
0TN07ZZ	Release Right Kidney, Via Natural or Artificial Opening
0TN08ZZ	Release Right Kidney, Via Natural or Artificial Opening Endoscopic
0TN10ZZ	Release Left Kidney, Open Approach
0TN13ZZ	Release Left Kidney, Percutaneous Approach
0TN14ZZ	Release Left Kidney, Percutaneous Endoscopic Approach
0TN17ZZ	Release Left Kidney, Via Natural or Artificial Opening
0TN18ZZ	Release Left Kidney, Via Natural or Artificial Opening Endoscopic
0TN30ZZ	Release Right Kidney Pelvis, Open Approach
0TN33ZZ	Release Right Kidney Pelvis, Percutaneous Approach
0TN34ZZ	Release Right Kidney Pelvis, Percutaneous Endoscopic Approach
0TN37ZZ	Release Right Kidney Pelvis, Via Natural or Artificial Opening
0TN38ZZ	Release Right Kidney Pelvis, Via Natural or Artificial Opening Endoscopic
0TN40ZZ	Release Left Kidney Pelvis, Open Approach
0TN43ZZ	Release Left Kidney Pelvis, Percutaneous Approach
0TN44ZZ	Release Left Kidney Pelvis, Percutaneous Endoscopic Approach
0TN47ZZ	Release Left Kidney Pelvis, Via Natural or Artificial Opening
0TN48ZZ	Release Left Kidney Pelvis, Via Natural or Artificial Opening Endoscopic
0TN60ZZ	Release Right Ureter, Open Approach
0TN63ZZ	Release Right Ureter, Percutaneous Approach
0TN64ZZ	Release Right Ureter, Percutaneous Endoscopic Approach
0TN67ZZ	Release Right Ureter, Via Natural or Artificial Opening
0TN68ZZ	Release Right Ureter, Via Natural or Artificial Opening Endoscopic
0TN70ZZ	Release Left Ureter, Open Approach
0TN73ZZ	Release Left Ureter, Percutaneous Approach
0TN74ZZ	Release Left Ureter, Percutaneous Endoscopic Approach
0TN77ZZ	Release Left Ureter, Via Natural or Artificial Opening
0TN78ZZ	Release Left Ureter, Via Natural or Artificial Opening Endoscopic
0TNB0ZZ	Release Bladder, Open Approach
0TNB3ZZ	Release Bladder, Percutaneous Approach
0TNB4ZZ	Release Bladder, Percutaneous Endoscopic Approach
0TNB7ZZ	Release Bladder, Via Natural or Artificial Opening
0TNB8ZZ	Release Bladder, Via Natural or Artificial Opening Endoscopic
0TNC0ZZ	Release Bladder Neck, Open Approach
0TNC3ZZ	Release Bladder Neck, Percutaneous Approach
0TNC4ZZ	Release Bladder Neck, Percutaneous Endoscopic Approach
0TNC7ZZ	Release Bladder Neck, Via Natural or Artificial Opening
0TNC8ZZ	Release Bladder Neck, Via Natural or Artificial Opening Endoscopic
0TND0ZZ	Release Urethra, Open Approach
0TND3ZZ	Release Urethra, Percutaneous Approach
0TND4ZZ	Release Urethra, Percutaneous Endoscopic Approach
0TND7ZZ	Release Urethra, Via Natural or Artificial Opening
0TND8ZZ	Release Urethra, Via Natural or Artificial Opening Endoscopic
0TNDXZZ	Release Urethra, External Approach

0TP – Urinary System, Removal

Review Coding Guideline B6.1c

0TP500Z	Removal of Drainage Device from Kidney, Open Approach
0TP502Z	Removal of Monitoring Device from Kidney, Open Approach
0TP503Z	Removal of Infusion Device from Kidney, Open Approach
0TP507Z	Removal of Autologous Tissue Substitute from Kidney, Open Approach
0TP50CZ	Removal of Extraluminal Device from Kidney, Open Approach
0TP50DZ	Removal of Intraluminal Device from Kidney, Open Approach
0TP50JZ	Removal of Synthetic Substitute from Kidney, Open Approach
0TP50KZ	Removal of Nonautologous Tissue Substitute from Kidney, Open Approach
0TP530Z	Removal of Drainage Device from Kidney, Percutaneous Approach
0TP532Z	Removal of Monitoring Device from Kidney, Percutaneous Approach
0TP533Z	Removal of Infusion Device from Kidney, Percutaneous Approach
0TP537Z	Removal of Autologous Tissue Substitute from Kidney, Percutaneous Approach
0TP53CZ	Removal of Extraluminal Device from Kidney, Percutaneous Approach
0TP53DZ	Removal of Intraluminal Device from Kidney, Percutaneous Approach
0TP53JZ	Removal of Synthetic Substitute from Kidney, Percutaneous Approach
0TP53KZ	Removal of Nonautologous Tissue Substitute from Kidney, Percutaneous Approach
0TP540Z	Removal of Drainage Device from Kidney, Percutaneous Endoscopic Approach
0TP542Z	Removal of Monitoring Device from Kidney, Percutaneous Endoscopic Approach
0TP543Z	Removal of Infusion Device from Kidney, Percutaneous Endoscopic Approach
0TP547Z	Removal of Autologous Tissue Substitute from Kidney, Percutaneous Endoscopic Approach
0TP54CZ	Removal of Extraluminal Device from Kidney, Percutaneous Endoscopic Approach
0TP54DZ	Removal of Intraluminal Device from Kidney, Percutaneous Endoscopic Approach
0TP54JZ	Removal of Synthetic Substitute from Kidney, Percutaneous Endoscopic Approach
0TP54KZ	Removal of Nonautologous Tissue Substitute from Kidney, Percutaneous Endoscopic Approach
0TP570Z	Removal of Drainage Device from Kidney, Via Natural or Artificial Opening
0TP572Z	Removal of Monitoring Device from Kidney, Via Natural or Artificial Opening

---

♀ Female-only   ♂ Male-only   ● Limited Coverage   ● Non-OR   ▓ HAC-associated procedure   ⬣ Non-covered procedures   ✚ Combination

0TP573Z	Removal of Infusion Device from Kidney, Via Natural or Artificial Opening
0TP577Z	Removal of Autologous Tissue Substitute from Kidney, Via Natural or Artificial Opening
0TP57CZ	Removal of Extraluminal Device from Kidney, Via Natural or Artificial Opening
0TP57DZ	Removal of Intraluminal Device from Kidney, Via Natural or Artificial Opening
0TP57JZ	Removal of Synthetic Substitute from Kidney, Via Natural or Artificial Opening
0TP57KZ	Removal of Nonautologous Tissue Substitute from Kidney, Via Natural or Artificial Opening
0TP580Z	Removal of Drainage Device from Kidney, Via Natural or Artificial Opening Endoscopic
0TP582Z	Removal of Monitoring Device from Kidney, Via Natural or Artificial Opening Endoscopic
0TP583Z	Removal of Infusion Device from Kidney, Via Natural or Artificial Opening Endoscopic
0TP587Z	Removal of Autologous Tissue Substitute from Kidney, Via Natural or Artificial Opening Endoscopic
0TP58CZ	Removal of Extraluminal Device from Kidney, Via Natural or Artificial Opening Endoscopic
0TP58DZ	Removal of Intraluminal Device from Kidney, Via Natural or Artificial Opening Endoscopic
0TP58JZ	Removal of Synthetic Substitute from Kidney, Via Natural or Artificial Opening Endoscopic
0TP58KZ	Removal of Nonautologous Tissue Substitute from Kidney, Via Natural or Artificial Opening Endoscopic
0TP5X0Z	Removal of Drainage Device from Kidney, External Approach
0TP5X2Z	Removal of Monitoring Device from Kidney, External Approach
0TP5X3Z	Removal of Infusion Device from Kidney, External Approach
0TP5XDZ	Removal of Intraluminal Device from Kidney, External Approach
0TP900Z	Removal of Drainage Device from Ureter, Open Approach
0TP902Z	Removal of Monitoring Device from Ureter, Open Approach
0TP903Z	Removal of Infusion Device from Ureter, Open Approach
0TP907Z	Removal of Autologous Tissue Substitute from Ureter, Open Approach
0TP90CZ	Removal of Extraluminal Device from Ureter, Open Approach
0TP90DZ	Removal of Intraluminal Device from Ureter, Open Approach
0TP90JZ	Removal of Synthetic Substitute from Ureter, Open Approach
0TP90KZ	Removal of Nonautologous Tissue Substitute from Ureter, Open Approach
0TP90MZ	Removal of Stimulator Lead from Ureter, Open Approach
0TP930Z	Removal of Drainage Device from Ureter, Percutaneous Approach
0TP932Z	Removal of Monitoring Device from Ureter, Percutaneous Approach
0TP933Z	Removal of Infusion Device from Ureter, Percutaneous Approach
0TP937Z	Removal of Autologous Tissue Substitute from Ureter, Percutaneous Approach
0TP93CZ	Removal of Extraluminal Device from Ureter, Percutaneous Approach
0TP93DZ	Removal of Intraluminal Device from Ureter, Percutaneous Approach
0TP93JZ	Removal of Synthetic Substitute from Ureter, Percutaneous Approach
0TP93KZ	Removal of Nonautologous Tissue Substitute from Ureter, Percutaneous Approach
0TP93MZ	Removal of Stimulator Lead from Ureter, Percutaneous Approach
0TP940Z	Removal of Drainage Device from Ureter, Percutaneous Endoscopic Approach
0TP942Z	Removal of Monitoring Device from Ureter, Percutaneous Endoscopic Approach
0TP943Z	Removal of Infusion Device from Ureter, Percutaneous Endoscopic Approach
0TP947Z	Removal of Autologous Tissue Substitute from Ureter, Percutaneous Endoscopic Approach
0TP94CZ	Removal of Extraluminal Device from Ureter, Percutaneous Endoscopic Approach
0TP94DZ	Removal of Intraluminal Device from Ureter, Percutaneous Endoscopic Approach
0TP94JZ	Removal of Synthetic Substitute from Ureter, Percutaneous Endoscopic Approach
0TP94KZ	Removal of Nonautologous Tissue Substitute from Ureter, Percutaneous Endoscopic Approach
0TP94MZ	Removal of Stimulator Lead from Ureter, Percutaneous Endoscopic Approach
0TP970Z	Removal of Drainage Device from Ureter, Via Natural or Artificial Opening
0TP972Z	Removal of Monitoring Device from Ureter, Via Natural or Artificial Opening
0TP973Z	Removal of Infusion Device from Ureter, Via Natural or Artificial Opening
0TP977Z	Removal of Autologous Tissue Substitute from Ureter, Via Natural or Artificial Opening
0TP97CZ	Removal of Extraluminal Device from Ureter, Via Natural or Artificial Opening
0TP97DZ	Removal of Intraluminal Device from Ureter, Via Natural or Artificial Opening
0TP97JZ	Removal of Synthetic Substitute from Ureter, Via Natural or Artificial Opening
0TP97KZ	Removal of Nonautologous Tissue Substitute from Ureter, Via Natural or Artificial Opening
0TP97MZ	Removal of Stimulator Lead from Ureter, Via Natural or Artificial Opening
0TP980Z	Removal of Drainage Device from Ureter, Via Natural or Artificial Opening Endoscopic
0TP982Z	Removal of Monitoring Device from Ureter, Via Natural or Artificial Opening Endoscopic
0TP983Z	Removal of Infusion Device from Ureter, Via Natural or Artificial Opening Endoscopic
0TP987Z	Removal of Autologous Tissue Substitute from Ureter, Via Natural or Artificial Opening Endoscopic
0TP98CZ	Removal of Extraluminal Device from Ureter, Via Natural or Artificial Opening Endoscopic
0TP98DZ	Removal of Intraluminal Device from Ureter, Via Natural or Artificial Opening Endoscopic
0TP98JZ	Removal of Synthetic Substitute from Ureter, Via Natural or Artificial Opening Endoscopic
0TP98KZ	Removal of Nonautologous Tissue Substitute from Ureter, Via Natural or Artificial Opening Endoscopic
0TP98MZ	Removal of Stimulator Lead from Ureter, Via Natural or Artificial Opening Endoscopic
0TP9X0Z	Removal of Drainage Device from Ureter, External Approach
0TP9X2Z	Removal of Monitoring Device from Ureter, External Approach
0TP9X3Z	Removal of Infusion Device from Ureter, External Approach
0TP9XDZ	Removal of Intraluminal Device from Ureter, External Approach
0TP9XMZ	Removal of Stimulator Lead from Ureter, External Approach
0TPB00Z	Removal of Drainage Device from Bladder, Open Approach
0TPB02Z	Removal of Monitoring Device from Bladder, Open Approach
0TPB03Z	Removal of Infusion Device from Bladder, Open Approach
0TPB07Z	Removal of Autologous Tissue Substitute from Bladder, Open Approach
0TPB0CZ	Removal of Extraluminal Device from Bladder, Open Approach
0TPB0DZ	Removal of Intraluminal Device from Bladder, Open Approach
0TPB0JZ	Removal of Synthetic Substitute from Bladder, Open Approach
0TPB0KZ	Removal of Nonautologous Tissue Substitute from Bladder, Open Approach
0TPB0LZ	Removal of Artificial Sphincter from Bladder, Open Approach
● 0TPB0MZ	Removal of Stimulator Lead from Bladder, Open Approach
0TPB30Z	Removal of Drainage Device from Bladder, Percutaneous Approach
0TPB32Z	Removal of Monitoring Device from Bladder, Percutaneous Approach
0TPB33Z	Removal of Infusion Device from Bladder, Percutaneous Approach
0TPB37Z	Removal of Autologous Tissue Substitute from Bladder, Percutaneous Approach
0TPB3CZ	Removal of Extraluminal Device from Bladder, Percutaneous Approach
0TPB3DZ	Removal of Intraluminal Device from Bladder, Percutaneous Approach
0TPB3JZ	Removal of Synthetic Substitute from Bladder, Percutaneous Approach
0TPB3KZ	Removal of Nonautologous Tissue Substitute from Bladder, Percutaneous Approach
0TPB3LZ	Removal of Artificial Sphincter from Bladder, Percutaneous Approach
● 0TPB3MZ	Removal of Stimulator Lead from Bladder, Percutaneous Approach
0TPB40Z	Removal of Drainage Device from Bladder, Percutaneous Endoscopic Approach
0TPB42Z	Removal of Monitoring Device from Bladder, Percutaneous Endoscopic Approach
0TPB43Z	Removal of Infusion Device from Bladder, Percutaneous Endoscopic Approach

0TPB47Z Removal of Autologous Tissue Substitute from Bladder, Percutaneous Endoscopic Approach

0TPB4CZ Removal of Extraluminal Device from Bladder, Percutaneous Endoscopic Approach

0TPB4DZ Removal of Intraluminal Device from Bladder, Percutaneous Endoscopic Approach

0TPB4JZ Removal of Synthetic Substitute from Bladder, Percutaneous Endoscopic Approach

0TPB4KZ Removal of Nonautologous Tissue Substitute from Bladder, Percutaneous Endoscopic Approach

0TPB4LZ Removal of Artificial Sphincter from Bladder, Percutaneous Endoscopic Approach

● **0TPB4MZ** Removal of Stimulator Lead from Bladder, Percutaneous Endoscopic Approach

0TPB70Z Removal of Drainage Device from Bladder, Via Natural or Artificial Opening

0TPB72Z Removal of Monitoring Device from Bladder, Via Natural or Artificial Opening

0TPB73Z Removal of Infusion Device from Bladder, Via Natural or Artificial Opening

0TPB77Z Removal of Autologous Tissue Substitute from Bladder, Via Natural or Artificial Opening

0TPB7CZ Removal of Extraluminal Device from Bladder, Via Natural or Artificial Opening

0TPB7DZ Removal of Intraluminal Device from Bladder, Via Natural or Artificial Opening

0TPB7JZ Removal of Synthetic Substitute from Bladder, Via Natural or Artificial Opening

0TPB7KZ Removal of Nonautologous Tissue Substitute from Bladder, Via Natural or Artificial Opening

0TPB7LZ Removal of Artificial Sphincter from Bladder, Via Natural or Artificial Opening

● **0TPB7MZ** Removal of Stimulator Lead from Bladder, Via Natural or Artificial Opening

0TPB80Z Removal of Drainage Device from Bladder, Via Natural or Artificial Opening Endoscopic

0TPB82Z Removal of Monitoring Device from Bladder, Via Natural or Artificial Opening Endoscopic

0TPB83Z Removal of Infusion Device from Bladder, Via Natural or Artificial Opening Endoscopic

0TPB87Z Removal of Autologous Tissue Substitute from Bladder, Via Natural or Artificial Opening Endoscopic

0TPB8CZ Removal of Extraluminal Device from Bladder, Via Natural or Artificial Opening Endoscopic

0TPB8DZ Removal of Intraluminal Device from Bladder, Via Natural or Artificial Opening Endoscopic

0TPB8JZ Removal of Synthetic Substitute from Bladder, Via Natural or Artificial Opening Endoscopic

0TPB8KZ Removal of Nonautologous Tissue Substitute from Bladder, Via Natural or Artificial Opening Endoscopic

0TPB8LZ Removal of Artificial Sphincter from Bladder, Via Natural or Artificial Opening Endoscopic

● **0TPB8MZ** Removal of Stimulator Lead from Bladder, Via Natural or Artificial Opening Endoscopic

0TPBX0Z Removal of Drainage Device from Bladder, External Approach

0TPBX2Z Removal of Monitoring Device from Bladder, External Approach

0TPBX3Z Removal of Infusion Device from Bladder, External Approach

0TPBXDZ Removal of Intraluminal Device from Bladder, External Approach

0TPBXLZ Removal of Artificial Sphincter from Bladder, External Approach

0TPBXMZ Removal of Stimulator Lead from Bladder, External Approach

0TPD00Z Removal of Drainage Device from Urethra, Open Approach

0TPD02Z Removal of Monitoring Device from Urethra, Open Approach

0TPD03Z Removal of Infusion Device from Urethra, Open Approach

0TPD07Z Removal of Autologous Tissue Substitute from Urethra, Open Approach

0TPD0CZ Removal of Extraluminal Device from Urethra, Open Approach

0TPD0DZ Removal of Intraluminal Device from Urethra, Open Approach

0TPD0JZ Removal of Synthetic Substitute from Urethra, Open Approach

0TPD0KZ Removal of Nonautologous Tissue Substitute from Urethra, Open Approach

0TPD0LZ Removal of Artificial Sphincter from Urethra, Open Approach

0TPD30Z Removal of Drainage Device from Urethra, Percutaneous Approach

0TPD32Z Removal of Monitoring Device from Urethra, Percutaneous Approach

0TPD33Z Removal of Infusion Device from Urethra, Percutaneous Approach

0TPD37Z Removal of Autologous Tissue Substitute from Urethra, Percutaneous Approach

0TPD3CZ Removal of Extraluminal Device from Urethra, Percutaneous Approach

0TPD3DZ Removal of Intraluminal Device from Urethra, Percutaneous Approach

0TPD3JZ Removal of Synthetic Substitute from Urethra, Percutaneous Approach

0TPD3KZ Removal of Nonautologous Tissue Substitute from Urethra, Percutaneous Approach

0TPD3LZ Removal of Artificial Sphincter from Urethra, Percutaneous Approach

0TPD40Z Removal of Drainage Device from Urethra, Percutaneous Endoscopic Approach

0TPD42Z Removal of Monitoring Device from Urethra, Percutaneous Endoscopic Approach

0TPD43Z Removal of Infusion Device from Urethra, Percutaneous Endoscopic Approach

0TPD47Z Removal of Autologous Tissue Substitute from Urethra, Percutaneous Endoscopic Approach

0TPD4CZ Removal of Extraluminal Device from Urethra, Percutaneous Endoscopic Approach

0TPD4DZ Removal of Intraluminal Device from Urethra, Percutaneous Endoscopic Approach

0TPD4JZ Removal of Synthetic Substitute from Urethra, Percutaneous Endoscopic Approach

0TPD4KZ Removal of Nonautologous Tissue Substitute from Urethra, Percutaneous Endoscopic Approach

0TPD4LZ Removal of Artificial Sphincter from Urethra, Percutaneous Endoscopic Approach

0TPD70Z Removal of Drainage Device from Urethra, Via Natural or Artificial Opening

0TPD72Z Removal of Monitoring Device from Urethra, Via Natural or Artificial Opening

0TPD73Z Removal of Infusion Device from Urethra, Via Natural or Artificial Opening

0TPD77Z Removal of Autologous Tissue Substitute from Urethra, Via Natural or Artificial Opening

0TPD7CZ Removal of Extraluminal Device from Urethra, Via Natural or Artificial Opening

0TPD7DZ Removal of Intraluminal Device from Urethra, Via Natural or Artificial Opening

0TPD7JZ Removal of Synthetic Substitute from Urethra, Via Natural or Artificial Opening

0TPD7KZ Removal of Nonautologous Tissue Substitute from Urethra, Via Natural or Artificial Opening

0TPD7LZ Removal of Artificial Sphincter from Urethra, Via Natural or Artificial Opening

0TPD80Z Removal of Drainage Device from Urethra, Via Natural or Artificial Opening Endoscopic

0TPD82Z Removal of Monitoring Device from Urethra, Via Natural or Artificial Opening Endoscopic

0TPD83Z Removal of Infusion Device from Urethra, Via Natural or Artificial Opening Endoscopic

0TPD87Z Removal of Autologous Tissue Substitute from Urethra, Via Natural or Artificial Opening Endoscopic

0TPD8CZ Removal of Extraluminal Device from Urethra, Via Natural or Artificial Opening Endoscopic

0TPD8DZ Removal of Intraluminal Device from Urethra, Via Natural or Artificial Opening Endoscopic

0TPD8JZ Removal of Synthetic Substitute from Urethra, Via Natural or Artificial Opening Endoscopic

0TPD8KZ Removal of Nonautologous Tissue Substitute from Urethra, Via Natural or Artificial Opening Endoscopic

0TPD8LZ Removal of Artificial Sphincter from Urethra, Via Natural or Artificial Opening Endoscopic

0TPDX0Z Removal of Drainage Device from Urethra, External Approach

0TPDX2Z Removal of Monitoring Device from Urethra, External Approach

0TPDX3Z Removal of Infusion Device from Urethra, External Approach

0TPDXDZ Removal of Intraluminal Device from Urethra, External Approach

0TPDXLZ Removal of Artificial Sphincter from Urethra, External Approach

0TQ – Urinary System, Repair

0TQ00ZZ	Repair Right Kidney, Open Approach
0TQ03ZZ	Repair Right Kidney, Percutaneous Approach
0TQ04ZZ	Repair Right Kidney, Percutaneous Endoscopic Approach
0TQ07ZZ	Repair Right Kidney, Via Natural or Artificial Opening
0TQ08ZZ	Repair Right Kidney, Via Natural or Artificial Opening Endoscopic
0TQ10ZZ	Repair Left Kidney, Open Approach
0TQ13ZZ	Repair Left Kidney, Percutaneous Approach
0TQ14ZZ	Repair Left Kidney, Percutaneous Endoscopic Approach
0TQ17ZZ	Repair Left Kidney, Via Natural or Artificial Opening
0TQ18ZZ	Repair Left Kidney, Via Natural or Artificial Opening Endoscopic
0TQ30ZZ	Repair Right Kidney Pelvis, Open Approach
0TQ33ZZ	Repair Right Kidney Pelvis, Percutaneous Approach
0TQ34ZZ	Repair Right Kidney Pelvis, Percutaneous Endoscopic Approach
0TQ37ZZ	Repair Right Kidney Pelvis, Via Natural or Artificial Opening
0TQ38ZZ	Repair Right Kidney Pelvis, Via Natural or Artificial Opening Endoscopic
0TQ40ZZ	Repair Left Kidney Pelvis, Open Approach
0TQ43ZZ	Repair Left Kidney Pelvis, Percutaneous Approach
0TQ44ZZ	Repair Left Kidney Pelvis, Percutaneous Endoscopic Approach
0TQ47ZZ	Repair Left Kidney Pelvis, Via Natural or Artificial Opening
0TQ48ZZ	Repair Left Kidney Pelvis, Via Natural or Artificial Opening Endoscopic
0TQ60ZZ	Repair Right Ureter, Open Approach
0TQ63ZZ	Repair Right Ureter, Percutaneous Approach
0TQ64ZZ	Repair Right Ureter, Percutaneous Endoscopic Approach
0TQ67ZZ	Repair Right Ureter, Via Natural or Artificial Opening
0TQ68ZZ	Repair Right Ureter, Via Natural or Artificial Opening Endoscopic
0TQ70ZZ	Repair Left Ureter, Open Approach
0TQ73ZZ	Repair Left Ureter, Percutaneous Approach
0TQ74ZZ	Repair Left Ureter, Percutaneous Endoscopic Approach
0TQ77ZZ	Repair Left Ureter, Via Natural or Artificial Opening
0TQ78ZZ	Repair Left Ureter, Via Natural or Artificial Opening Endoscopic
0TQB0ZZ	Repair Bladder, Open Approach
0TQB3ZZ	Repair Bladder, Percutaneous Approach
0TQB4ZZ	Repair Bladder, Percutaneous Endoscopic Approach
0TQB7ZZ	Repair Bladder, Via Natural or Artificial Opening
0TQB8ZZ	Repair Bladder, Via Natural or Artificial Opening Endoscopic
0TQC0ZZ	Repair Bladder Neck, Open Approach
0TQC3ZZ	Repair Bladder Neck, Percutaneous Approach
0TQC4ZZ	Repair Bladder Neck, Percutaneous Endoscopic Approach
0TQC7ZZ	Repair Bladder Neck, Via Natural or Artificial Opening
0TQC8ZZ	Repair Bladder Neck, Via Natural or Artificial Opening Endoscopic
0TQD0ZZ	Repair Urethra, Open Approach
0TQD3ZZ	Repair Urethra, Percutaneous Approach
0TQD4ZZ	Repair Urethra, Percutaneous Endoscopic Approach
0TQD7ZZ	Repair Urethra, Via Natural or Artificial Opening
0TQD8ZZ	Repair Urethra, Via Natural or Artificial Opening Endoscopic
0TQDXZZ	Repair Urethra, External Approach

0TR – Urinary System, Replacement

0TR307Z	Replacement of Right Kidney Pelvis with Autologous Tissue Substitute, Open Approach
0TR30JZ	Replacement of Right Kidney Pelvis with Synthetic Substitute, Open Approach
0TR30KZ	Replacement of Right Kidney Pelvis with Nonautologous Tissue Substitute, Open Approach
0TR347Z	Replacement of Right Kidney Pelvis with Autologous Tissue Substitute, Percutaneous Endoscopic Approach
0TR34JZ	Replacement of Right Kidney Pelvis with Synthetic Substitute, Percutaneous Endoscopic Approach
0TR34KZ	Replacement of Right Kidney Pelvis with Nonautologous Tissue Substitute, Percutaneous Endoscopic Approach
0TR377Z	Replacement of Right Kidney Pelvis with Autologous Tissue Substitute, Via Natural or Artificial Opening
0TR37JZ	Replacement of Right Kidney Pelvis with Synthetic Substitute, Via Natural or Artificial Opening
0TR37KZ	Replacement of Right Kidney Pelvis with Nonautologous Tissue Substitute, Via Natural or Artificial Opening
0TR387Z	Replacement of Right Kidney Pelvis with Autologous Tissue Substitute, Via Natural or Artificial Opening Endoscopic
0TR38JZ	Replacement of Right Kidney Pelvis with Synthetic Substitute, Via Natural or Artificial Opening Endoscopic
0TR38KZ	Replacement of Right Kidney Pelvis with Nonautologous Tissue Substitute, Via Natural or Artificial Opening Endoscopic
0TR407Z	Replacement of Left Kidney Pelvis with Autologous Tissue Substitute, Open Approach
0TR40JZ	Replacement of Left Kidney Pelvis with Synthetic Substitute, Open Approach
0TR40KZ	Replacement of Left Kidney Pelvis with Nonautologous Tissue Substitute, Open Approach
0TR447Z	Replacement of Left Kidney Pelvis with Autologous Tissue Substitute, Percutaneous Endoscopic Approach
0TR44JZ	Replacement of Left Kidney Pelvis with Synthetic Substitute, Percutaneous Endoscopic Approach
0TR44KZ	Replacement of Left Kidney Pelvis with Nonautologous Tissue Substitute, Percutaneous Endoscopic Approach
0TR477Z	Replacement of Left Kidney Pelvis with Autologous Tissue Substitute, Via Natural or Artificial Opening
0TR47JZ	Replacement of Left Kidney Pelvis with Synthetic Substitute, Via Natural or Artificial Opening
0TR47KZ	Replacement of Left Kidney Pelvis with Nonautologous Tissue Substitute, Via Natural or Artificial Opening
0TR487Z	Replacement of Left Kidney Pelvis with Autologous Tissue Substitute, Via Natural or Artificial Opening Endoscopic
0TR48JZ	Replacement of Left Kidney Pelvis with Synthetic Substitute, Via Natural or Artificial Opening Endoscopic
0TR48KZ	Replacement of Left Kidney Pelvis with Nonautologous Tissue Substitute, Via Natural or Artificial Opening Endoscopic
0TR607Z	Replacement of Right Ureter with Autologous Tissue Substitute, Open Approach
0TR60JZ	Replacement of Right Ureter with Synthetic Substitute, Open Approach
0TR60KZ	Replacement of Right Ureter with Nonautologous Tissue Substitute, Open Approach
0TR647Z	Replacement of Right Ureter with Autologous Tissue Substitute, Percutaneous Endoscopic Approach
0TR64JZ	Replacement of Right Ureter with Synthetic Substitute, Percutaneous Endoscopic Approach
0TR64KZ	Replacement of Right Ureter with Nonautologous Tissue Substitute, Percutaneous Endoscopic Approach
0TR677Z	Replacement of Right Ureter with Autologous Tissue Substitute, Via Natural or Artificial Opening
0TR67JZ	Replacement of Right Ureter with Synthetic Substitute, Via Natural or Artificial Opening
0TR67KZ	Replacement of Right Ureter with Nonautologous Tissue Substitute, Via Natural or Artificial Opening
0TR687Z	Replacement of Right Ureter with Autologous Tissue Substitute, Via Natural or Artificial Opening Endoscopic
0TR68JZ	Replacement of Right Ureter with Synthetic Substitute, Via Natural or Artificial Opening Endoscopic
0TR68KZ	Replacement of Right Ureter with Nonautologous Tissue Substitute, Via Natural or Artificial Opening Endoscopic
0TR707Z	Replacement of Left Ureter with Autologous Tissue Substitute, Open Approach
0TR70JZ	Replacement of Left Ureter with Synthetic Substitute, Open Approach
0TR70KZ	Replacement of Left Ureter with Nonautologous Tissue Substitute, Open Approach
0TR747Z	Replacement of Left Ureter with Autologous Tissue Substitute, Percutaneous Endoscopic Approach
0TR74JZ	Replacement of Left Ureter with Synthetic Substitute, Percutaneous Endoscopic Approach
0TR74KZ	Replacement of Left Ureter with Nonautologous Tissue Substitute, Percutaneous Endoscopic Approach
0TR777Z	Replacement of Left Ureter with Autologous Tissue Substitute, Via Natural or Artificial Opening
0TR77JZ	Replacement of Left Ureter with Synthetic Substitute, Via Natural or Artificial Opening

0TR77KZ	Replacement of Left Ureter with Nonautologous Tissue Substitute, Via Natural or Artificial Opening
0TR787Z	Replacement of Left Ureter with Autologous Tissue Substitute, Via Natural or Artificial Opening Endoscopic
0TR78JZ	Replacement of Left Ureter with Synthetic Substitute, Via Natural or Artificial Opening Endoscopic
0TR78KZ	Replacement of Left Ureter with Nonautologous Tissue Substitute, Via Natural or Artificial Opening Endoscopic
0TRB07Z	Replacement of Bladder with Autologous Tissue Substitute, Open Approach
0TRB0JZ	Replacement of Bladder with Synthetic Substitute, Open Approach
0TRB0KZ	Replacement of Bladder with Nonautologous Tissue Substitute, Open Approach
0TRB47Z	Replacement of Bladder with Autologous Tissue Substitute, Percutaneous Endoscopic Approach
0TRB4JZ	Replacement of Bladder with Synthetic Substitute, Percutaneous Endoscopic Approach
0TRB4KZ	Replacement of Bladder with Nonautologous Tissue Substitute, Percutaneous Endoscopic Approach
0TRB77Z	Replacement of Bladder with Autologous Tissue Substitute, Via Natural or Artificial Opening
0TRB7JZ	Replacement of Bladder with Synthetic Substitute, Via Natural or Artificial Opening
0TRB7KZ	Replacement of Bladder with Nonautologous Tissue Substitute, Via Natural or Artificial Opening
0TRB87Z	Replacement of Bladder with Autologous Tissue Substitute, Via Natural or Artificial Opening Endoscopic
0TRB8JZ	Replacement of Bladder with Synthetic Substitute, Via Natural or Artificial Opening Endoscopic
0TRB8KZ	Replacement of Bladder with Nonautologous Tissue Substitute, Via Natural or Artificial Opening Endoscopic
0TRC07Z	Replacement of Bladder Neck with Autologous Tissue Substitute, Open Approach
0TRC0JZ	Replacement of Bladder Neck with Synthetic Substitute, Open Approach
0TRC0KZ	Replacement of Bladder Neck with Nonautologous Tissue Substitute, Open Approach
0TRC47Z	Replacement of Bladder Neck with Autologous Tissue Substitute, Percutaneous Endoscopic Approach
0TRC4JZ	Replacement of Bladder Neck with Synthetic Substitute, Percutaneous Endoscopic Approach
0TRC4KZ	Replacement of Bladder Neck with Nonautologous Tissue Substitute, Percutaneous Endoscopic Approach
0TRC77Z	Replacement of Bladder Neck with Autologous Tissue Substitute, Via Natural or Artificial Opening
0TRC7JZ	Replacement of Bladder Neck with Synthetic Substitute, Via Natural or Artificial Opening
0TRC7KZ	Replacement of Bladder Neck with Nonautologous Tissue Substitute, Via Natural or Artificial Opening
0TRC87Z	Replacement of Bladder Neck with Autologous Tissue Substitute, Via Natural or Artificial Opening Endoscopic
0TRC8JZ	Replacement of Bladder Neck with Synthetic Substitute, Via Natural or Artificial Opening Endoscopic
0TRC8KZ	Replacement of Bladder Neck with Nonautologous Tissue Substitute, Via Natural or Artificial Opening Endoscopic
0TRD07Z	Replacement of Urethra with Autologous Tissue Substitute, Open Approach
0TRD0JZ	Replacement of Urethra with Synthetic Substitute, Open Approach
0TRD0KZ	Replacement of Urethra with Nonautologous Tissue Substitute, Open Approach
0TRD47Z	Replacement of Urethra with Autologous Tissue Substitute, Percutaneous Endoscopic Approach
0TRD4JZ	Replacement of Urethra with Synthetic Substitute, Percutaneous Endoscopic Approach
0TRD4KZ	Replacement of Urethra with Nonautologous Tissue Substitute, Percutaneous Endoscopic Approach
0TRD77Z	Replacement of Urethra with Autologous Tissue Substitute, Via Natural or Artificial Opening
0TRD7JZ	Replacement of Urethra with Synthetic Substitute, Via Natural or Artificial Opening
0TRD7KZ	Replacement of Urethra with Nonautologous Tissue Substitute, Via Natural or Artificial Opening
0TRD87Z	Replacement of Urethra with Autologous Tissue Substitute, Via Natural or Artificial Opening Endoscopic
0TRD8JZ	Replacement of Urethra with Synthetic Substitute, Via Natural or Artificial Opening Endoscopic
0TRD8KZ	Replacement of Urethra with Nonautologous Tissue Substitute, Via Natural or Artificial Opening Endoscopic
0TRDX7Z	Replacement of Urethra with Autologous Tissue Substitute, External Approach
0TRDXJZ	Replacement of Urethra with Synthetic Substitute, External Approach
0TRDXKZ	Replacement of Urethra with Nonautologous Tissue Substitute, External Approach

0TS – Urinary System, Reposition

0TS00ZZ	Reposition Right Kidney, Open Approach
0TS04ZZ	Reposition Right Kidney, Percutaneous Endoscopic Approach
0TS10ZZ	Reposition Left Kidney, Open Approach
0TS14ZZ	Reposition Left Kidney, Percutaneous Endoscopic Approach
0TS20ZZ	Reposition Bilateral Kidneys, Open Approach
0TS24ZZ	Reposition Bilateral Kidneys, Percutaneous Endoscopic Approach
0TS30ZZ	Reposition Right Kidney Pelvis, Open Approach
0TS34ZZ	Reposition Right Kidney Pelvis, Percutaneous Endoscopic Approach
0TS40ZZ	Reposition Left Kidney Pelvis, Open Approach
0TS44ZZ	Reposition Left Kidney Pelvis, Percutaneous Endoscopic Approach
0TS60ZZ	Reposition Right Ureter, Open Approach
0TS64ZZ	Reposition Right Ureter, Percutaneous Endoscopic Approach
0TS70ZZ	Reposition Left Ureter, Open Approach
0TS74ZZ	Reposition Left Ureter, Percutaneous Endoscopic Approach
0TS80ZZ	Reposition Bilateral Ureters, Open Approach
0TS84ZZ	Reposition Bilateral Ureters, Percutaneous Endoscopic Approach
0TSB0ZZ	Reposition Bladder, Open Approach
0TSB4ZZ	Reposition Bladder, Percutaneous Endoscopic Approach
0TSC0ZZ	Reposition Bladder Neck, Open Approach
0TSC4ZZ	Reposition Bladder Neck, Percutaneous Endoscopic Approach
0TSD0ZZ	Reposition Urethra, Open Approach
0TSD4ZZ	Reposition Urethra, Percutaneous Endoscopic Approach

0TT – Urinary System, Resection

Review Coding Guideline B3.8

0TT00ZZ	Resection of Right Kidney, Open Approach
0TT04ZZ	Resection of Right Kidney, Percutaneous Endoscopic Approach
0TT10ZZ	Resection of Left Kidney, Open Approach
0TT14ZZ	Resection of Left Kidney, Percutaneous Endoscopic Approach
0TT20ZZ	Resection of Bilateral Kidneys, Open Approach
0TT24ZZ	Resection of Bilateral Kidneys, Percutaneous Endoscopic Approach
0TT30ZZ	Resection of Right Kidney Pelvis, Open Approach
0TT34ZZ	Resection of Right Kidney Pelvis, Percutaneous Endoscopic Approach
0TT37ZZ	Resection of Right Kidney Pelvis, Via Natural or Artificial Opening
0TT38ZZ	Resection of Right Kidney Pelvis, Via Natural or Artificial Opening Endoscopic
0TT40ZZ	Resection of Left Kidney Pelvis, Open Approach
0TT44ZZ	Resection of Left Kidney Pelvis, Percutaneous Endoscopic Approach
0TT47ZZ	Resection of Left Kidney Pelvis, Via Natural or Artificial Opening
0TT48ZZ	Resection of Left Kidney Pelvis, Via Natural or Artificial Opening Endoscopic
0TT60ZZ	Resection of Right Ureter, Open Approach
0TT64ZZ	Resection of Right Ureter, Percutaneous Endoscopic Approach
0TT67ZZ	Resection of Right Ureter, Via Natural or Artificial Opening

♀ Female-only   ♂ Male-only   ● Limited Coverage   ● Non-OR   ▩ HAC-associated procedure   ⬢ Non-covered procedures   ✚ Combination

0TT68ZZ	Resection of Right Ureter, Via Natural or Artificial Opening Endoscopic
0TT70ZZ	Resection of Left Ureter, Open Approach
0TT74ZZ	Resection of Left Ureter, Percutaneous Endoscopic Approach
0TT77ZZ	Resection of Left Ureter, Via Natural or Artificial Opening
0TT78ZZ	Resection of Left Ureter, Via Natural or Artificial Opening Endoscopic
0TTB0ZZ	Resection of Bladder, Open Approach
0TTB4ZZ	Resection of Bladder, Percutaneous Endoscopic Approach
0TTB7ZZ	Resection of Bladder, Via Natural or Artificial Opening
0TTB8ZZ	Resection of Bladder, Via Natural or Artificial Opening Endoscopic
0TTC0ZZ	Resection of Bladder Neck, Open Approach
0TTC4ZZ	Resection of Bladder Neck, Percutaneous Endoscopic Approach
0TTC7ZZ	Resection of Bladder Neck, Via Natural or Artificial Opening
0TTC8ZZ	Resection of Bladder Neck, Via Natural or Artificial Opening Endoscopic
0TTD0ZZ	Resection of Urethra, Open Approach
0TTD4ZZ	Resection of Urethra, Percutaneous Endoscopic Approach
0TTD7ZZ	Resection of Urethra, Via Natural or Artificial Opening
0TTD8ZZ	Resection of Urethra, Via Natural or Artificial Opening Endoscopic

0TU – Urinary System, Supplement

0TU307Z	Supplement Right Kidney Pelvis with Autologous Tissue Substitute, Open Approach
0TU30JZ	Supplement Right Kidney Pelvis with Synthetic Substitute, Open Approach
0TU30KZ	Supplement Right Kidney Pelvis with Nonautologous Tissue Substitute, Open Approach
0TU347Z	Supplement Right Kidney Pelvis with Autologous Tissue Substitute, Percutaneous Endoscopic Approach
0TU34JZ	Supplement Right Kidney Pelvis with Synthetic Substitute, Percutaneous Endoscopic Approach
0TU34KZ	Supplement Right Kidney Pelvis with Nonautologous Tissue Substitute, Percutaneous Endoscopic Approach
0TU377Z	Supplement Right Kidney Pelvis with Autologous Tissue Substitute, Via Natural or Artificial Opening
0TU37JZ	Supplement Right Kidney Pelvis with Synthetic Substitute, Via Natural or Artificial Opening
0TU37KZ	Supplement Right Kidney Pelvis with Nonautologous Tissue Substitute, Via Natural or Artificial Opening
0TU387Z	Supplement Right Kidney Pelvis with Autologous Tissue Substitute, Via Natural or Artificial Opening Endoscopic
0TU38JZ	Supplement Right Kidney Pelvis with Synthetic Substitute, Via Natural or Artificial Opening Endoscopic
0TU38KZ	Supplement Right Kidney Pelvis with Nonautologous Tissue Substitute, Via Natural or Artificial Opening Endoscopic
0TU407Z	Supplement Left Kidney Pelvis with Autologous Tissue Substitute, Open Approach
0TU40JZ	Supplement Left Kidney Pelvis with Synthetic Substitute, Open Approach
0TU40KZ	Supplement Left Kidney Pelvis with Nonautologous Tissue Substitute, Open Approach
0TU447Z	Supplement Left Kidney Pelvis with Autologous Tissue Substitute, Percutaneous Endoscopic Approach
0TU44JZ	Supplement Left Kidney Pelvis with Synthetic Substitute, Percutaneous Endoscopic Approach
0TU44KZ	Supplement Left Kidney Pelvis with Nonautologous Tissue Substitute, Percutaneous Endoscopic Approach
0TU477Z	Supplement Left Kidney Pelvis with Autologous Tissue Substitute, Via Natural or Artificial Opening
0TU47JZ	Supplement Left Kidney Pelvis with Synthetic Substitute, Via Natural or Artificial Opening
0TU47KZ	Supplement Left Kidney Pelvis with Nonautologous Tissue Substitute, Via Natural or Artificial Opening
0TU487Z	Supplement Left Kidney Pelvis with Autologous Tissue Substitute, Via Natural or Artificial Opening Endoscopic
0TU48JZ	Supplement Left Kidney Pelvis with Synthetic Substitute, Via Natural or Artificial Opening Endoscopic
0TU48KZ	Supplement Left Kidney Pelvis with Nonautologous Tissue Substitute, Via Natural or Artificial Opening Endoscopic
0TU607Z	Supplement Right Ureter with Autologous Tissue Substitute, Open Approach
0TU60JZ	Supplement Right Ureter with Synthetic Substitute, Open Approach
0TU60KZ	Supplement Right Ureter with Nonautologous Tissue Substitute, Open Approach
0TU647Z	Supplement Right Ureter with Autologous Tissue Substitute, Percutaneous Endoscopic Approach
0TU64JZ	Supplement Right Ureter with Synthetic Substitute, Percutaneous Endoscopic Approach
0TU64KZ	Supplement Right Ureter with Nonautologous Tissue Substitute, Percutaneous Endoscopic Approach
0TU677Z	Supplement Right Ureter with Autologous Tissue Substitute, Via Natural or Artificial Opening
0TU67JZ	Supplement Right Ureter with Synthetic Substitute, Via Natural or Artificial Opening
0TU67KZ	Supplement Right Ureter with Nonautologous Tissue Substitute, Via Natural or Artificial Opening
0TU687Z	Supplement Right Ureter with Autologous Tissue Substitute, Via Natural or Artificial Opening Endoscopic
0TU68JZ	Supplement Right Ureter with Synthetic Substitute, Via Natural or Artificial Opening Endoscopic
0TU68KZ	Supplement Right Ureter with Nonautologous Tissue Substitute, Via Natural or Artificial Opening Endoscopic
0TU707Z	Supplement Left Ureter with Autologous Tissue Substitute, Open Approach
0TU70JZ	Supplement Left Ureter with Synthetic Substitute, Open Approach
0TU70KZ	Supplement Left Ureter with Nonautologous Tissue Substitute, Open Approach
0TU747Z	Supplement Left Ureter with Autologous Tissue Substitute, Percutaneous Endoscopic Approach
0TU74JZ	Supplement Left Ureter with Synthetic Substitute, Percutaneous Endoscopic Approach
0TU74KZ	Supplement Left Ureter with Nonautologous Tissue Substitute, Percutaneous Endoscopic Approach
0TU777Z	Supplement Left Ureter with Autologous Tissue Substitute, Via Natural or Artificial Opening
0TU77JZ	Supplement Left Ureter with Synthetic Substitute, Via Natural or Artificial Opening
0TU77KZ	Supplement Left Ureter with Nonautologous Tissue Substitute, Via Natural or Artificial Opening
0TU787Z	Supplement Left Ureter with Autologous Tissue Substitute, Via Natural or Artificial Opening Endoscopic
0TU78JZ	Supplement Left Ureter with Synthetic Substitute, Via Natural or Artificial Opening Endoscopic
0TU78KZ	Supplement Left Ureter with Nonautologous Tissue Substitute, Via Natural or Artificial Opening Endoscopic
0TUB07Z	Supplement Bladder with Autologous Tissue Substitute, Open Approach
0TUB0JZ	Supplement Bladder with Synthetic Substitute, Open Approach
0TUB0KZ	Supplement Bladder with Nonautologous Tissue Substitute, Open Approach
0TUB47Z	Supplement Bladder with Autologous Tissue Substitute, Percutaneous Endoscopic Approach
0TUB4JZ	Supplement Bladder with Synthetic Substitute, Percutaneous Endoscopic Approach
0TUB4KZ	Supplement Bladder with Nonautologous Tissue Substitute, Percutaneous Endoscopic Approach
0TUB77Z	Supplement Bladder with Autologous Tissue Substitute, Via Natural or Artificial Opening
0TUB7JZ	Supplement Bladder with Synthetic Substitute, Via Natural or Artificial Opening
0TUB7KZ	Supplement Bladder with Nonautologous Tissue Substitute, Via Natural or Artificial Opening
0TUB87Z	Supplement Bladder with Autologous Tissue Substitute, Via Natural or Artificial Opening Endoscopic
0TUB8JZ	Supplement Bladder with Synthetic Substitute, Via Natural or Artificial Opening Endoscopic
0TUB8KZ	Supplement Bladder with Nonautologous Tissue Substitute, Via Natural or Artificial Opening Endoscopic
0TUC07Z	Supplement Bladder Neck with Autologous Tissue Substitute, Open Approach
0TUC0JZ	Supplement Bladder Neck with Synthetic Substitute, Open Approach
0TUC0KZ	Supplement Bladder Neck with Nonautologous Tissue Substitute, Open Approach

0TUC47Z Supplement Bladder Neck with Autologous Tissue Substitute, Percutaneous Endoscopic Approach

0TUC4JZ Supplement Bladder Neck with Synthetic Substitute, Percutaneous Endoscopic Approach

0TUC4KZ Supplement Bladder Neck with Nonautologous Tissue Substitute, Percutaneous Endoscopic Approach

0TUC77Z Supplement Bladder Neck with Autologous Tissue Substitute, Via Natural or Artificial Opening

0TUC7JZ Supplement Bladder Neck with Synthetic Substitute, Via Natural or Artificial Opening

0TUC7KZ Supplement Bladder Neck with Nonautologous Tissue Substitute, Via Natural or Artificial Opening

0TUC87Z Supplement Bladder Neck with Autologous Tissue Substitute, Via Natural or Artificial Opening Endoscopic

0TUC8JZ Supplement Bladder Neck with Synthetic Substitute, Via Natural or Artificial Opening Endoscopic

0TUC8KZ Supplement Bladder Neck with Nonautologous Tissue Substitute, Via Natural or Artificial Opening Endoscopic

0TUD07Z Supplement Urethra with Autologous Tissue Substitute, Open Approach

0TUD0JZ Supplement Urethra with Synthetic Substitute, Open Approach

0TUD0KZ Supplement Urethra with Nonautologous Tissue Substitute, Open Approach

0TUD47Z Supplement Urethra with Autologous Tissue Substitute, Percutaneous Endoscopic Approach

0TUD4JZ Supplement Urethra with Synthetic Substitute, Percutaneous Endoscopic Approach

0TUD4KZ Supplement Urethra with Nonautologous Tissue Substitute, Percutaneous Endoscopic Approach

0TUD77Z Supplement Urethra with Autologous Tissue Substitute, Via Natural or Artificial Opening

0TUD7JZ Supplement Urethra with Synthetic Substitute, Via Natural or Artificial Opening

0TUD7KZ Supplement Urethra with Nonautologous Tissue Substitute, Via Natural or Artificial Opening

0TUD87Z Supplement Urethra with Autologous Tissue Substitute, Via Natural or Artificial Opening Endoscopic

0TUD8JZ Supplement Urethra with Synthetic Substitute, Via Natural or Artificial Opening Endoscopic

0TUD8KZ Supplement Urethra with Nonautologous Tissue Substitute, Via Natural or Artificial Opening Endoscopic

0TUDX7Z Supplement Urethra with Autologous Tissue Substitute, External Approach

0TUDXJZ Supplement Urethra with Synthetic Substitute, External Approach

0TUDXKZ Supplement Urethra with Nonautologous Tissue Substitute, External Approach

0TV – Urinary System, Restriction

0TV30CZ Restriction of Right Kidney Pelvis with Extraluminal Device, Open Approach

0TV30DZ Restriction of Right Kidney Pelvis with Intraluminal Device, Open Approach

0TV30ZZ Restriction of Right Kidney Pelvis, Open Approach

0TV33CZ Restriction of Right Kidney Pelvis with Extraluminal Device, Percutaneous Approach

0TV33DZ Restriction of Right Kidney Pelvis with Intraluminal Device, Percutaneous Approach

0TV33ZZ Restriction of Right Kidney Pelvis, Percutaneous Approach

0TV34CZ Restriction of Right Kidney Pelvis with Extraluminal Device, Percutaneous Endoscopic Approach

0TV34DZ Restriction of Right Kidney Pelvis with Intraluminal Device, Percutaneous Endoscopic Approach

0TV34ZZ Restriction of Right Kidney Pelvis, Percutaneous Endoscopic Approach

0TV37DZ Restriction of Right Kidney Pelvis with Intraluminal Device, Via Natural or Artificial Opening

0TV37ZZ Restriction of Right Kidney Pelvis, Via Natural or Artificial Opening

0TV38DZ Restriction of Right Kidney Pelvis with Intraluminal Device, Via Natural or Artificial Opening Endoscopic

0TV38ZZ Restriction of Right Kidney Pelvis, Via Natural or Artificial Opening Endoscopic

0TV40CZ Restriction of Left Kidney Pelvis with Extraluminal Device, Open Approach

0TV40DZ Restriction of Left Kidney Pelvis with Intraluminal Device, Open Approach

0TV40ZZ Restriction of Left Kidney Pelvis, Open Approach

0TV43CZ Restriction of Left Kidney Pelvis with Extraluminal Device, Percutaneous Approach

0TV43DZ Restriction of Left Kidney Pelvis with Intraluminal Device, Percutaneous Approach

0TV43ZZ Restriction of Left Kidney Pelvis, Percutaneous Approach

0TV44CZ Restriction of Left Kidney Pelvis with Extraluminal Device, Percutaneous Endoscopic Approach

0TV44DZ Restriction of Left Kidney Pelvis with Intraluminal Device, Percutaneous Endoscopic Approach

0TV44ZZ Restriction of Left Kidney Pelvis, Percutaneous Endoscopic Approach

0TV47DZ Restriction of Left Kidney Pelvis with Intraluminal Device, Via Natural or Artificial Opening

0TV47ZZ Restriction of Left Kidney Pelvis, Via Natural or Artificial Opening

0TV48DZ Restriction of Left Kidney Pelvis with Intraluminal Device, Via Natural or Artificial Opening Endoscopic

0TV48ZZ Restriction of Left Kidney Pelvis, Via Natural or Artificial Opening Endoscopic

0TV60CZ Restriction of Right Ureter with Extraluminal Device, Open Approach

0TV60DZ Restriction of Right Ureter with Intraluminal Device, Open Approach

0TV60ZZ Restriction of Right Ureter, Open Approach

0TV63CZ Restriction of Right Ureter with Extraluminal Device, Percutaneous Approach

0TV63DZ Restriction of Right Ureter with Intraluminal Device, Percutaneous Approach

0TV63ZZ Restriction of Right Ureter, Percutaneous Approach

0TV64CZ Restriction of Right Ureter with Extraluminal Device, Percutaneous Endoscopic Approach

0TV64DZ Restriction of Right Ureter with Intraluminal Device, Percutaneous Endoscopic Approach

0TV64ZZ Restriction of Right Ureter, Percutaneous Endoscopic Approach

0TV67DZ Restriction of Right Ureter with Intraluminal Device, Via Natural or Artificial Opening

0TV67ZZ Restriction of Right Ureter, Via Natural or Artificial Opening

0TV68DZ Restriction of Right Ureter with Intraluminal Device, Via Natural or Artificial Opening Endoscopic

0TV68ZZ Restriction of Right Ureter, Via Natural or Artificial Opening Endoscopic

0TV70CZ Restriction of Left Ureter with Extraluminal Device, Open Approach

0TV70DZ Restriction of Left Ureter with Intraluminal Device, Open Approach

0TV70ZZ Restriction of Left Ureter, Open Approach

0TV73CZ Restriction of Left Ureter with Extraluminal Device, Percutaneous Approach

0TV73DZ Restriction of Left Ureter with Intraluminal Device, Percutaneous Approach

0TV73ZZ Restriction of Left Ureter, Percutaneous Approach

0TV74CZ Restriction of Left Ureter with Extraluminal Device, Percutaneous Endoscopic Approach

0TV74DZ Restriction of Left Ureter with Intraluminal Device, Percutaneous Endoscopic Approach

0TV74ZZ Restriction of Left Ureter, Percutaneous Endoscopic Approach

0TV77DZ Restriction of Left Ureter with Intraluminal Device, Via Natural or Artificial Opening

0TV77ZZ Restriction of Left Ureter, Via Natural or Artificial Opening

0TV78DZ Restriction of Left Ureter with Intraluminal Device, Via Natural or Artificial Opening Endoscopic

0TV78ZZ Restriction of Left Ureter, Via Natural or Artificial Opening Endoscopic

0TVB0CZ Restriction of Bladder with Extraluminal Device, Open Approach

0TVB0DZ Restriction of Bladder with Intraluminal Device, Open Approach

0TVB0ZZ Restriction of Bladder, Open Approach

0TVB3CZ Restriction of Bladder with Extraluminal Device, Percutaneous Approach

0TVB3DZ Restriction of Bladder with Intraluminal Device, Percutaneous Approach

---

♀ Female-only   ♂ Male-only   ● Limited Coverage   ● Non-OR   ▦ HAC-associated procedure   ⬢ Non-covered procedures   ➕ Combination

0TVB3ZZ Restriction of Bladder, Percutaneous Approach
0TVB4CZ Restriction of Bladder with Extraluminal Device, Percutaneous Endoscopic Approach
0TVB4DZ Restriction of Bladder with Intraluminal Device, Percutaneous Endoscopic Approach
0TVB4ZZ Restriction of Bladder, Percutaneous Endoscopic Approach
0TVB7DZ Restriction of Bladder with Intraluminal Device, Via Natural or Artificial Opening
0TVB7ZZ Restriction of Bladder, Via Natural or Artificial Opening
0TVB8DZ Restriction of Bladder with Intraluminal Device, Via Natural or Artificial Opening Endoscopic
0TVB8ZZ Restriction of Bladder, Via Natural or Artificial Opening Endoscopic
0TVC0CZ Restriction of Bladder Neck with Extraluminal Device, Open Approach
0TVC0DZ Restriction of Bladder Neck with Intraluminal Device, Open Approach
0TVC0ZZ Restriction of Bladder Neck, Open Approach
0TVC3CZ Restriction of Bladder Neck with Extraluminal Device, Percutaneous Approach
0TVC3DZ Restriction of Bladder Neck with Intraluminal Device, Percutaneous Approach
0TVC3ZZ Restriction of Bladder Neck, Percutaneous Approach
0TVC4CZ Restriction of Bladder Neck with Extraluminal Device, Percutaneous Endoscopic Approach
0TVC4DZ Restriction of Bladder Neck with Intraluminal Device, Percutaneous Endoscopic Approach
0TVC4ZZ Restriction of Bladder Neck, Percutaneous Endoscopic Approach
0TVC7DZ Restriction of Bladder Neck with Intraluminal Device, Via Natural or Artificial Opening

0TVC7ZZ Restriction of Bladder Neck, Via Natural or Artificial Opening
0TVC8DZ Restriction of Bladder Neck with Intraluminal Device, Via Natural or Artificial Opening Endoscopic
0TVC8ZZ Restriction of Bladder Neck, Via Natural or Artificial Opening Endoscopic
0TVD0CZ Restriction of Urethra with Extraluminal Device, Open Approach
0TVD0DZ Restriction of Urethra with Intraluminal Device, Open Approach
0TVD0ZZ Restriction of Urethra, Open Approach
0TVD3CZ Restriction of Urethra with Extraluminal Device, Percutaneous Approach
0TVD3DZ Restriction of Urethra with Intraluminal Device, Percutaneous Approach
0TVD3ZZ Restriction of Urethra, Percutaneous Approach
0TVD4CZ Restriction of Urethra with Extraluminal Device, Percutaneous Endoscopic Approach
0TVD4DZ Restriction of Urethra with Intraluminal Device, Percutaneous Endoscopic Approach
0TVD4ZZ Restriction of Urethra, Percutaneous Endoscopic Approach
0TVD7DZ Restriction of Urethra with Intraluminal Device, Via Natural or Artificial Opening
0TVD7ZZ Restriction of Urethra, Via Natural or Artificial Opening
0TVD8DZ Restriction of Urethra with Intraluminal Device, Via Natural or Artificial Opening Endoscopic
0TVD8ZZ Restriction of Urethra, Via Natural or Artificial Opening Endoscopic
0TVDXZZ Restriction of Urethra, External Approach

0TW – Urinary System, Revision

Review Coding Guideline B6.1c

0TW500Z Revision of Drainage Device in Kidney, Open Approach
0TW502Z Revision of Monitoring Device in Kidney, Open Approach
0TW503Z Revision of Infusion Device in Kidney, Open Approach
0TW507Z Revision of Autologous Tissue Substitute in Kidney, Open Approach
0TW50CZ Revision of Extraluminal Device in Kidney, Open Approach
0TW50DZ Revision of Intraluminal Device in Kidney, Open Approach
0TW50JZ Revision of Synthetic Substitute in Kidney, Open Approach
0TW50KZ Revision of Nonautologous Tissue Substitute in Kidney, Open Approach
0TW530Z Revision of Drainage Device in Kidney, Percutaneous Approach
0TW532Z Revision of Monitoring Device in Kidney, Percutaneous Approach
0TW533Z Revision of Infusion Device in Kidney, Percutaneous Approach
0TW537Z Revision of Autologous Tissue Substitute in Kidney, Percutaneous Approach
0TW53CZ Revision of Extraluminal Device in Kidney, Percutaneous Approach
0TW53DZ Revision of Intraluminal Device in Kidney, Percutaneous Approach
0TW53JZ Revision of Synthetic Substitute in Kidney, Percutaneous Approach
0TW53KZ Revision of Nonautologous Tissue Substitute in Kidney, Percutaneous Approach
0TW540Z Revision of Drainage Device in Kidney, Percutaneous Endoscopic Approach
0TW542Z Revision of Monitoring Device in Kidney, Percutaneous Endoscopic Approach
0TW543Z Revision of Infusion Device in Kidney, Percutaneous Endoscopic Approach
0TW547Z Revision of Autologous Tissue Substitute in Kidney, Percutaneous Endoscopic Approach
0TW54CZ Revision of Extraluminal Device in Kidney, Percutaneous Endoscopic Approach
0TW54DZ Revision of Intraluminal Device in Kidney, Percutaneous Endoscopic Approach
0TW54JZ Revision of Synthetic Substitute in Kidney, Percutaneous Endoscopic Approach
0TW54KZ Revision of Nonautologous Tissue Substitute in Kidney, Percutaneous Endoscopic Approach
0TW570Z Revision of Drainage Device in Kidney, Via Natural or Artificial Opening
0TW570Z Revision of Monitoring Device in Kidney, Via Natural or Artificial Opening

0TW573Z Revision of Infusion Device in Kidney, Via Natural or Artificial Opening
0TW577Z Revision of Autologous Tissue Substitute in Kidney, Via Natural or Artificial Opening
0TW57CZ Revision of Extraluminal Device in Kidney, Via Natural or Artificial Opening
0TW57DZ Revision of Intraluminal Device in Kidney, Via Natural or Artificial Opening
0TW57JZ Revision of Synthetic Substitute in Kidney, Via Natural or Artificial Opening
0TW57KZ Revision of Nonautologous Tissue Substitute in Kidney, Via Natural or Artificial Opening
0TW580Z Revision of Drainage Device in Kidney, Via Natural or Artificial Opening Endoscopic
0TW582Z Revision of Monitoring Device in Kidney, Via Natural or Artificial Opening Endoscopic
0TW583Z Revision of Infusion Device in Kidney, Via Natural or Artificial Opening Endoscopic
0TW587Z Revision of Autologous Tissue Substitute in Kidney, Via Natural or Artificial Opening Endoscopic
0TW58CZ Revision of Extraluminal Device in Kidney, Via Natural or Artificial Opening Endoscopic
0TW58DZ Revision of Intraluminal Device in Kidney, Via Natural or Artificial Opening Endoscopic
0TW58JZ Revision of Synthetic Substitute in Kidney, Via Natural or Artificial Opening Endoscopic
0TW58KZ Revision of Nonautologous Tissue Substitute in Kidney, Via Natural or Artificial Opening Endoscopic
0TW5X0Z Revision of Drainage Device in Kidney, External Approach
0TW5X2Z Revision of Monitoring Device in Kidney, External Approach
0TW5X3Z Revision of Infusion Device in Kidney, External Approach
0TW5X7Z Revision of Autologous Tissue Substitute in Kidney, External Approach
0TW5XCZ Revision of Extraluminal Device in Kidney, External Approach
0TW5XDZ Revision of Intraluminal Device in Kidney, External Approach
0TW5XJZ Revision of Synthetic Substitute in Kidney, External Approach
0TW5XKZ Revision of Nonautologous Tissue Substitute in Kidney, External Approach
0TW900Z Revision of Drainage Device in Ureter, Open Approach
0TW902Z Revision of Monitoring Device in Ureter, Open Approach
0TW903Z Revision of Infusion Device in Ureter, Open Approach

0TW907Z Revision of Autologous Tissue Substitute in Ureter, Open Approach
0TW90CZ Revision of Extraluminal Device in Ureter, Open Approach
0TW90DZ Revision of Intraluminal Device in Ureter, Open Approach
0TW90JZ Revision of Synthetic Substitute in Ureter, Open Approach
0TW90KZ Revision of Nonautologous Tissue Substitute in Ureter, Open Approach
0TW90MZ Revision of Stimulator Lead in Ureter, Open Approach
0TW930Z Revision of Drainage Device in Ureter, Percutaneous Approach
0TW932Z Revision of Monitoring Device in Ureter, Percutaneous Approach
0TW933Z Revision of Infusion Device in Ureter, Percutaneous Approach
0TW937Z Revision of Autologous Tissue Substitute in Ureter, Percutaneous Approach
0TW93CZ Revision of Extraluminal Device in Ureter, Percutaneous Approach
0TW93DZ Revision of Intraluminal Device in Ureter, Percutaneous Approach
0TW93JZ Revision of Synthetic Substitute in Ureter, Percutaneous Approach
0TW93KZ Revision of Nonautologous Tissue Substitute in Ureter, Percutaneous Approach
0TW93MZ Revision of Stimulator Lead in Ureter, Percutaneous Approach
0TW940Z Revision of Drainage Device in Ureter, Percutaneous Endoscopic Approach
0TW942Z Revision of Monitoring Device in Ureter, Percutaneous Endoscopic Approach
0TW943Z Revision of Infusion Device in Ureter, Percutaneous Endoscopic Approach
0TW947Z Revision of Autologous Tissue Substitute in Ureter, Percutaneous Endoscopic Approach
0TW94CZ Revision of Extraluminal Device in Ureter, Percutaneous Endoscopic Approach
0TW94DZ Revision of Intraluminal Device in Ureter, Percutaneous Endoscopic Approach
0TW94JZ Revision of Synthetic Substitute in Ureter, Percutaneous Endoscopic Approach
0TW94KZ Revision of Nonautologous Tissue Substitute in Ureter, Percutaneous Endoscopic Approach
0TW94MZ Revision of Stimulator Lead in Ureter, Percutaneous Endoscopic Approach
0TW970Z Revision of Drainage Device in Ureter, Via Natural or Artificial Opening
0TW972Z Revision of Monitoring Device in Ureter, Via Natural or Artificial Opening
0TW973Z Revision of Infusion Device in Ureter, Via Natural or Artificial Opening
0TW977Z Revision of Autologous Tissue Substitute in Ureter, Via Natural or Artificial Opening
0TW97CZ Revision of Extraluminal Device in Ureter, Via Natural or Artificial Opening
0TW97DZ Revision of Intraluminal Device in Ureter, Via Natural or Artificial Opening
0TW97JZ Revision of Synthetic Substitute in Ureter, Via Natural or Artificial Opening
0TW97KZ Revision of Nonautologous Tissue Substitute in Ureter, Via Natural or Artificial Opening
0TW97MZ Revision of Stimulator Lead in Ureter, Via Natural or Artificial Opening
0TW980Z Revision of Drainage Device in Ureter, Via Natural or Artificial Opening Endoscopic
0TW982Z Revision of Monitoring Device in Ureter, Via Natural or Artificial Opening Endoscopic
0TW983Z Revision of Infusion Device in Ureter, Via Natural or Artificial Opening Endoscopic
0TW987Z Revision of Autologous Tissue Substitute in Ureter, Via Natural or Artificial Opening Endoscopic
0TW98CZ Revision of Extraluminal Device in Ureter, Via Natural or Artificial Opening Endoscopic
0TW98DZ Revision of Intraluminal Device in Ureter, Via Natural or Artificial Opening Endoscopic
0TW98JZ Revision of Synthetic Substitute in Ureter, Via Natural or Artificial Opening Endoscopic
0TW98KZ Revision of Nonautologous Tissue Substitute in Ureter, Via Natural or Artificial Opening Endoscopic
0TW98MZ Revision of Stimulator Lead in Ureter, Via Natural or Artificial Opening Endoscopic
0TW9X0Z Revision of Drainage Device in Ureter, External Approach
0TW9X2Z Revision of Monitoring Device in Ureter, External Approach
0TW9X3Z Revision of Infusion Device in Ureter, External Approach

0TW9X7Z Revision of Autologous Tissue Substitute in Ureter, External Approach
0TW9XCZ Revision of Extraluminal Device in Ureter, External Approach
0TW9XDZ Revision of Intraluminal Device in Ureter, External Approach
0TW9XJZ Revision of Synthetic Substitute in Ureter, External Approach
0TW9XKZ Revision of Nonautologous Tissue Substitute in Ureter, External Approach
0TW9XMZ Revision of Stimulator Lead in Ureter, External Approach
0TWB00Z Revision of Drainage Device in Bladder, Open Approach
0TWB02Z Revision of Monitoring Device in Bladder, Open Approach
0TWB03Z Revision of Infusion Device in Bladder, Open Approach
0TWB07Z Revision of Autologous Tissue Substitute in Bladder, Open Approach
0TWB0CZ Revision of Extraluminal Device in Bladder, Open Approach
0TWB0DZ Revision of Intraluminal Device in Bladder, Open Approach
0TWB0JZ Revision of Synthetic Substitute in Bladder, Open Approach
0TWB0KZ Revision of Nonautologous Tissue Substitute in Bladder, Open Approach
0TWB0LZ Revision of Artificial Sphincter in Bladder, Open Approach
0TWB0MZ Revision of Stimulator Lead in Bladder, Open Approach
0TWB30Z Revision of Drainage Device in Bladder, Percutaneous Approach
0TWB32Z Revision of Monitoring Device in Bladder, Percutaneous Approach
0TWB33Z Revision of Infusion Device in Bladder, Percutaneous Approach
0TWB37Z Revision of Autologous Tissue Substitute in Bladder, Percutaneous Approach
0TWB3CZ Revision of Extraluminal Device in Bladder, Percutaneous Approach
0TWB3DZ Revision of Intraluminal Device in Bladder, Percutaneous Approach
0TWB3JZ Revision of Synthetic Substitute in Bladder, Percutaneous Approach
0TWB3KZ Revision of Nonautologous Tissue Substitute in Bladder, Percutaneous Approach
0TWB3LZ Revision of Artificial Sphincter in Bladder, Percutaneous Approach
0TWB3MZ Revision of Stimulator Lead in Bladder, Percutaneous Approach
0TWB40Z Revision of Drainage Device in Bladder, Percutaneous Endoscopic Approach
0TWB42Z Revision of Monitoring Device in Bladder, Percutaneous Endoscopic Approach
0TWB43Z Revision of Infusion Device in Bladder, Percutaneous Endoscopic Approach
0TWB47Z Revision of Autologous Tissue Substitute in Bladder, Percutaneous Endoscopic Approach
0TWB4CZ Revision of Extraluminal Device in Bladder, Percutaneous Endoscopic Approach
0TWB4DZ Revision of Intraluminal Device in Bladder, Percutaneous Endoscopic Approach
0TWB4JZ Revision of Synthetic Substitute in Bladder, Percutaneous Endoscopic Approach
0TWB4KZ Revision of Nonautologous Tissue Substitute in Bladder, Percutaneous Endoscopic Approach
0TWB4LZ Revision of Artificial Sphincter in Bladder, Percutaneous Endoscopic Approach
0TWB4MZ Revision of Stimulator Lead in Bladder, Percutaneous Endoscopic Approach
0TWB70Z Revision of Drainage Device in Bladder, Via Natural or Artificial Opening
0TWB72Z Revision of Monitoring Device in Bladder, Via Natural or Artificial Opening
0TWB73Z Revision of Infusion Device in Bladder, Via Natural or Artificial Opening
0TWB77Z Revision of Autologous Tissue Substitute in Bladder, Via Natural or Artificial Opening
0TWB7CZ Revision of Extraluminal Device in Bladder, Via Natural or Artificial Opening
0TWB7DZ Revision of Intraluminal Device in Bladder, Via Natural or Artificial Opening
0TWB7JZ Revision of Synthetic Substitute in Bladder, Via Natural or Artificial Opening
0TWB7KZ Revision of Nonautologous Tissue Substitute in Bladder, Via Natural or Artificial Opening
0TWB7LZ Revision of Artificial Sphincter in Bladder, Via Natural or Artificial Opening
0TWB7MZ Revision of Stimulator Lead in Bladder, Via Natural or Artificial Opening
0TWB80Z Revision of Drainage Device in Bladder, Via Natural or Artificial Opening Endoscopic

0TWB82Z Revision of Monitoring Device in Bladder, Via Natural or Artificial Opening Endoscopic

0TWB83Z Revision of Infusion Device in Bladder, Via Natural or Artificial Opening Endoscopic

0TWB87Z Revision of Autologous Tissue Substitute in Bladder, Via Natural or Artificial Opening Endoscopic

0TWB8CZ Revision of Extraluminal Device in Bladder, Via Natural or Artificial Opening Endoscopic

0TWB8DZ Revision of Intraluminal Device in Bladder, Via Natural or Artificial Opening Endoscopic

0TWB8JZ Revision of Synthetic Substitute in Bladder, Via Natural or Artificial Opening Endoscopic

0TWB8KZ Revision of Nonautologous Tissue Substitute in Bladder, Via Natural or Artificial Opening Endoscopic

0TWB8LZ Revision of Artificial Sphincter in Bladder, Via Natural or Artificial Opening Endoscopic

0TWB8MZ Revision of Stimulator Lead in Bladder, Via Natural or Artificial Opening Endoscopic

0TWBX0Z Revision of Drainage Device in Bladder, External Approach

0TWBX2Z Revision of Monitoring Device in Bladder, External Approach

0TWBX3Z Revision of Infusion Device in Bladder, External Approach

0TWBX7Z Revision of Autologous Tissue Substitute in Bladder, External Approach

0TWBXCZ Revision of Extraluminal Device in Bladder, External Approach

0TWBXDZ Revision of Intraluminal Device in Bladder, External Approach

0TWBXJZ Revision of Synthetic Substitute in Bladder, External Approach

0TWBXKZ Revision of Nonautologous Tissue Substitute in Bladder, External Approach

0TWBXLZ Revision of Artificial Sphincter in Bladder, External Approach

0TWBXMZ Revision of Stimulator Lead in Bladder, External Approach

0TWD00Z Revision of Drainage Device in Urethra, Open Approach

0TWD02Z Revision of Monitoring Device in Urethra, Open Approach

0TWD03Z Revision of Infusion Device in Urethra, Open Approach

0TWD07Z Revision of Autologous Tissue Substitute in Urethra, Open Approach

0TWD0CZ Revision of Extraluminal Device in Urethra, Open Approach

0TWD0DZ Revision of Intraluminal Device in Urethra, Open Approach

0TWD0JZ Revision of Synthetic Substitute in Urethra, Open Approach

0TWD0KZ Revision of Nonautologous Tissue Substitute in Urethra, Open Approach

0TWD0LZ Revision of Artificial Sphincter in Urethra, Open Approach

0TWD30Z Revision of Drainage Device in Urethra, Percutaneous Approach

0TWD32Z Revision of Monitoring Device in Urethra, Percutaneous Approach

0TWD33Z Revision of Infusion Device in Urethra, Percutaneous Approach

0TWD37Z Revision of Autologous Tissue Substitute in Urethra, Percutaneous Approach

0TWD3CZ Revision of Extraluminal Device in Urethra, Percutaneous Approach

0TWD3DZ Revision of Intraluminal Device in Urethra, Percutaneous Approach

0TWD3JZ Revision of Synthetic Substitute in Urethra, Percutaneous Approach

0TWD3KZ Revision of Nonautologous Tissue Substitute in Urethra, Percutaneous Approach

0TWD3LZ Revision of Artificial Sphincter in Urethra, Percutaneous Approach

0TWD40Z Revision of Drainage Device in Urethra, Percutaneous Endoscopic Approach

0TWD42Z Revision of Monitoring Device in Urethra, Percutaneous Endoscopic Approach

0TWD43Z Revision of Infusion Device in Urethra, Percutaneous Endoscopic Approach

0TWD47Z Revision of Autologous Tissue Substitute in Urethra, Percutaneous Endoscopic Approach

0TWD4CZ Revision of Extraluminal Device in Urethra, Percutaneous Endoscopic Approach

0TWD4DZ Revision of Intraluminal Device in Urethra, Percutaneous Endoscopic Approach

0TWD4JZ Revision of Synthetic Substitute in Urethra, Percutaneous Endoscopic Approach

0TWD4KZ Revision of Nonautologous Tissue Substitute in Urethra, Percutaneous Endoscopic Approach

0TWD4LZ Revision of Artificial Sphincter in Urethra, Percutaneous Endoscopic Approach

0TWD70Z Revision of Drainage Device in Urethra, Via Natural or Artificial Opening

0TWD72Z Revision of Monitoring Device in Urethra, Via Natural or Artificial Opening

0TWD73Z Revision of Infusion Device in Urethra, Via Natural or Artificial Opening

0TWD77Z Revision of Autologous Tissue Substitute in Urethra, Via Natural or Artificial Opening

0TWD7CZ Revision of Extraluminal Device in Urethra, Via Natural or Artificial Opening

0TWD7DZ Revision of Intraluminal Device in Urethra, Via Natural or Artificial Opening

0TWD7JZ Revision of Synthetic Substitute in Urethra, Via Natural or Artificial Opening

0TWD7KZ Revision of Nonautologous Tissue Substitute in Urethra, Via Natural or Artificial Opening

0TWD7LZ Revision of Artificial Sphincter in Urethra, Via Natural or Artificial Opening

0TWD80Z Revision of Drainage Device in Urethra, Via Natural or Artificial Opening Endoscopic

0TWD82Z Revision of Monitoring Device in Urethra, Via Natural or Artificial Opening Endoscopic

0TWD83Z Revision of Infusion Device in Urethra, Via Natural or Artificial Opening Endoscopic

0TWD87Z Revision of Autologous Tissue Substitute in Urethra, Via Natural or Artificial Opening Endoscopic

0TWD8CZ Revision of Extraluminal Device in Urethra, Via Natural or Artificial Opening Endoscopic

0TWD8DZ Revision of Intraluminal Device in Urethra, Via Natural or Artificial Opening Endoscopic

0TWD8JZ Revision of Synthetic Substitute in Urethra, Via Natural or Artificial Opening Endoscopic

0TWD8KZ Revision of Nonautologous Tissue Substitute in Urethra, Via Natural or Artificial Opening Endoscopic

0TWD8LZ Revision of Artificial Sphincter in Urethra, Via Natural or Artificial Opening Endoscopic

0TWDX0Z Revision of Drainage Device in Urethra, External Approach

0TWDX2Z Revision of Monitoring Device in Urethra, External Approach

0TWDX3Z Revision of Infusion Device in Urethra, External Approach

0TWDX7Z Revision of Autologous Tissue Substitute in Urethra, External Approach

0TWDXCZ Revision of Extraluminal Device in Urethra, External Approach

0TWDXDZ Revision of Intraluminal Device in Urethra, External Approach

0TWDXJZ Revision of Synthetic Substitute in Urethra, External Approach

0TWDXKZ Revision of Nonautologous Tissue Substitute in Urethra, External Approach

0TWDXLZ Revision of Artificial Sphincter in Urethra, External Approach

0TY – Urinary System, Transplantation

Review Coding Guideline B3.16

0TY00Z0 Transplantation of Right Kidney, Allogeneic, Open Approach
  ➕ Kidney/Pancreas transplant when reported with Transplant of the Pancreas. *See table 0FY to construct the Transplantation code.*

0TY00Z1 Transplantation of Right Kidney, Syngeneic, Open Approach
  ➕ Kidney/Pancreas transplant when reported with Transplant of the Pancreas. *See table 0FY to construct the Transplantation code.*

0TY00Z2 Transplantation of Right Kidney, Zooplastic, Open Approach
  ➕ Kidney/Pancreas transplant when reported with Transplant of the Pancreas. *See table 0FY to construct the Transplantation code.*

0TY10Z0 Transplantation of Left Kidney, Allogeneic, Open Approach
  ➕ Kidney/Pancreas transplant when reported with Transplant of the Pancreas. *See table 0FY to construct the Transplantation code.*

0TY10Z1 Transplantation of Left Kidney, Syngeneic, Open Approach
  ➕ Kidney/Pancreas transplant when reported with Transplant of the Pancreas. *See table 0FY to construct the Transplantation code.*

0TY10Z2 Transplantation of Left Kidney, Zooplastic, Open Approach
  ➕ Kidney/Pancreas transplant when reported with Transplant of the Pancreas. *See table 0FY to construct the Transplantation code.*

Female Reproductive System

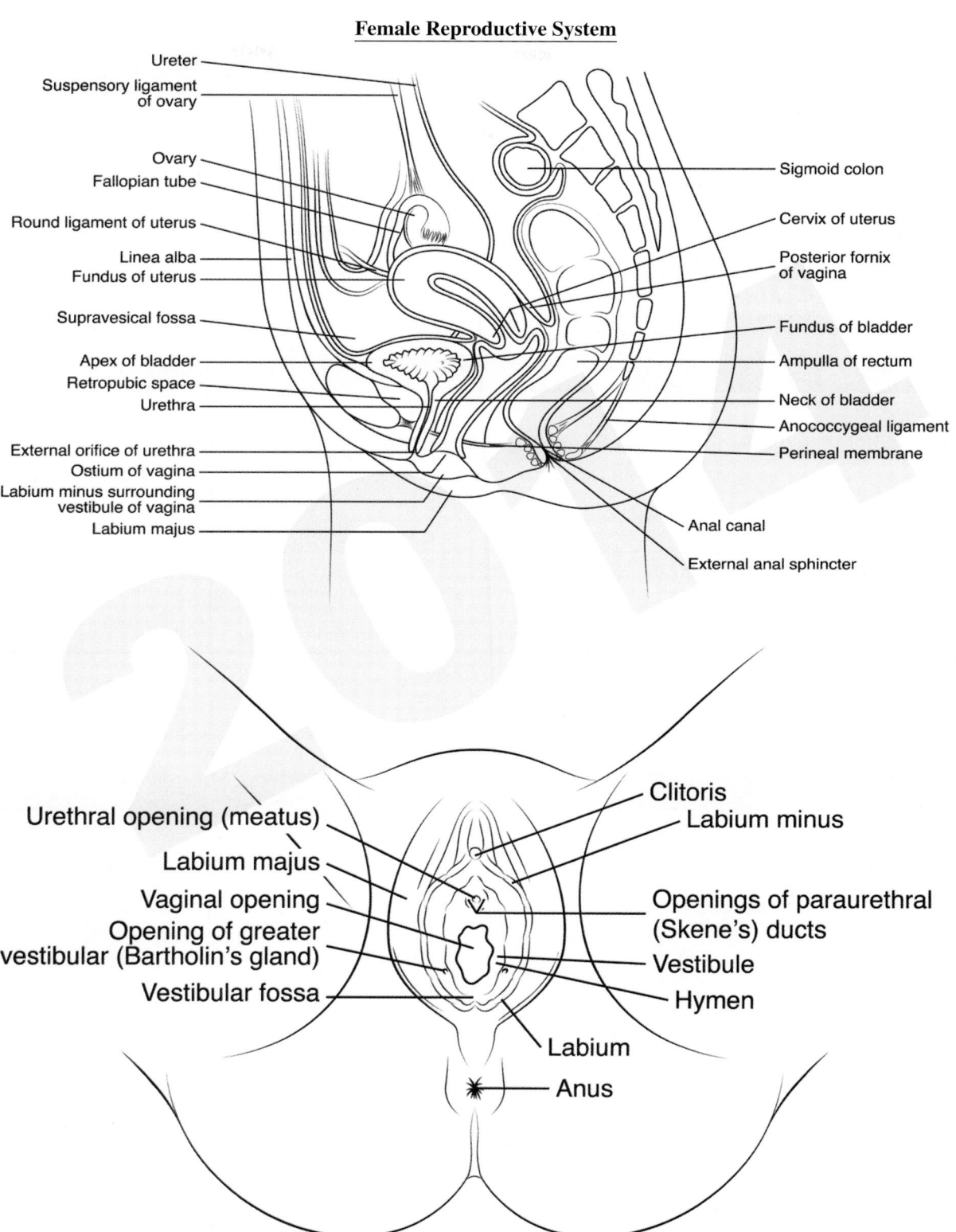

Female Reproductive System

Ureter

Suspensory ligament of ovary

Ovary

Fallopian tube

Round ligament of uterus

Linea alba

Fundus of uterus

Supravesical fossa

Apex of bladder

Retropubic space

Urethra

External orifice of urethra

Ostium of vagina

Labium minus surrounding vestibule of vagina

Labium majus

Sigmoid colon

Cervix of uterus

Posterior fornix of vagina

Fundus of bladder

Ampulla of rectum

Neck of bladder

Anococcygeal ligament

Perineal membrane

Anal canal

External anal sphincter

Urethral opening (meatus)

Labium majus

Vaginal opening

Opening of greater vestibular (Bartholin's gland)

Vestibular fossa

Clitoris

Labium minus

Openings of paraurethral (Skene's) ducts

Vestibule

Hymen

Labium

Anus

Female Reproductive System Tables 0U1–0UY

Section	0	Medical and Surgical
Body System	U	Female Reproductive System
Operation	1	**Bypass:** Altering the route of passage of the contents of a tubular body part

Body Part (4th)	Approach (5th)	Device (6th)	Qualifier (7th)

5 Fallopian Tube, Right
6 Fallopian Tube, Left
	0 Open
	4 Percutaneous Endoscopic
		7 Autologous Tissue
		  Substitute
		J Synthetic Substitute
		K Nonautologous Tissue
		  Substitute
		Z No Device
			5 Fallopian Tube, Right
			6 Fallopian Tube, Left
			9 Uterus

Section	0	Medical and Surgical
Body System	U	Female Reproductive System
Operation	2	**Change:** Taking out or off a device from a body part and putting back an identical or similar device in or on the same body part without cutting or puncturing the skin or a mucous membrane

Body Part (4th)	Approach (5th)	Device (6th)	Qualifier (7th)
3 Ovary 8 Fallopian Tube M Vulva	X External	0 Drainage Device Y Other Device	Z No Qualifier
D Uterus and Cervix	X External	0 Drainage Device H Contraceptive Device Y Other Device	Z No Qualifier
H Vagina and Cul-de-sac	X External	0 Drainage Device G Intraluminal Device, Pessary Y Other Device	Z No Qualifier

Section	0	Medical and Surgical
Body System	U	Female Reproductive System
Operation	5	**Destruction:** Physical eradication of all or a portion of a body part by the direct use of energy, force, or a destructive agent

Body Part (4th)	Approach (5th)	Device (6th)	Qualifier (7th)
0 Ovary, Right 1 Ovary, Left 2 Ovaries, Bilateral 4 Uterine Supporting Structure	0 Open 3 Percutaneous 4 Percutaneous Endoscopic	Z No Device	Z No Qualifier
5 Fallopian Tube, Right 6 Fallopian Tube, Left 7 Fallopian Tubes, Bilateral 9 Uterus B Endometrium C Cervix F Cul-de-sac	0 Open 3 Percutaneous 4 Percutaneous Endoscopic 7 Via Natural or Artificial Opening 8 Via Natural or Artificial Opening Endoscopic	Z No Device	Z No Qualifier
G Vagina K Hymen	0 Open 3 Percutaneous 4 Percutaneous Endoscopic 7 Via Natural or Artificial Opening 8 Via Natural or Artificial Opening Endoscopic X External	Z No Device	Z No Qualifier

Continued

Section	0	Medical and Surgical			0U5 *Continued*
Body System	U	Female Reproductive System			
Operation	5	Destruction: Physical eradication of all or a portion of a body part by the direct use of energy, force, or a destructive agent			

Body Part (4th)	Approach (5th)	Device (6th)	Qualifier (7th)
J Clitoris L Vestibular Gland M Vulva	0 Open X External	Z No Device	Z No Qualifier

Section	0	Medical and Surgical
Body System	U	Female Reproductive System
Operation	7	Dilation: Expanding an orifice or the lumen of a tubular body part

Body Part (4th)	Approach (5th)	Device (6th)	Qualifier (7th)
5 Fallopian Tube, Right 6 Fallopian Tube, Left 7 Fallopian Tubes, Bilateral 9 Uterus C Cervix G Vagina	0 Open 3 Percutaneous 4 Percutaneous Endoscopic 7 Via Natural or Artificial Opening 8 Via Natural or Artificial Opening Endoscopic	D Intraluminal Device Z No Device	Z No Qualifier
K Hymen	0 Open 3 Percutaneous 4 Percutaneous Endoscopic 7 Via Natural or Artificial Opening 8 Via Natural or Artificial Opening Endoscopic X External	D Intraluminal Device Z No Device	Z No Qualifier

Section	0	Medical and Surgical
Body System	U	Female Reproductive System
Operation	8	Division: Cutting into a body part, without draining fluids and/or gases from the body part, in order to separate or transect a body part

Body Part (4th)	Approach (5th)	Device (6th)	Qualifier (7th)
0 Ovary, Right 1 Ovary, Left 2 Ovaries, Bilateral 4 Uterine Supporting Structure	0 Open 3 Percutaneous 4 Percutaneous Endoscopic	Z No Device	Z No Qualifier
K Hymen	7 Via Natural or Artificial Opening 8 Via Natural or Artificial Opening Endoscopic X External	Z No Device	Z No Qualifier

Section	0	Medical and Surgical
Body System	U	Female Reproductive System
Operation	9	**Drainage:** Taking or letting out fluids and/or gases from a body part

Body Part (4ᵗʰ)	Approach (5ᵗʰ)	Device (6ᵗʰ)	Qualifier (7ᵗʰ)
0 Ovary, Right 1 Ovary, Left 2 Ovaries, Bilateral	0 Open 3 Percutaneous 4 Percutaneous Endoscopic	0 Drainage Device	Z No Qualifier
0 Ovary, Right 1 Ovary, Left 2 Ovaries, Bilateral	0 Open 3 Percutaneous 4 Percutaneous Endoscopic	Z No Device	X Diagnostic Z No Qualifier
0 Ovary, Right 1 Ovary, Left 2 Ovaries, Bilateral	X External	Z No Device	Z No Qualifier
4 Uterine Supporting Structure	0 Open 3 Percutaneous 4 Percutaneous Endoscopic	0 Drainage Device	Z No Qualifier
4 Uterine Supporting Structure	0 Open 3 Percutaneous 4 Percutaneous Endoscopic	Z No Device	X Diagnostic Z No Qualifier
5 Fallopian Tube, Right 6 Fallopian Tube, Left 7 Fallopian Tubes, Bilateral 9 Uterus C Cervix F Cul-de-sac	0 Open 3 Percutaneous 4 Percutaneous Endoscopic 7 Via Natural or Artificial Opening 8 Via Natural or Artificial Opening Endoscopic	0 Drainage Device	Z No Qualifier
5 Fallopian Tube, Right 6 Fallopian Tube, Left 7 Fallopian Tubes, Bilateral 9 Uterus C Cervix F Cul-de-sac	0 Open 3 Percutaneous 4 Percutaneous Endoscopic 7 Via Natural or Artificial Opening 8 Via Natural or Artificial Opening Endoscopic	Z No Device	X Diagnostic Z No Qualifier
G Vagina K Hymen	0 Open 3 Percutaneous 4 Percutaneous Endoscopic 7 Via Natural or Artificial Opening 8 Via Natural or Artificial Opening Endoscopic X External	0 Drainage Device	Z No Qualifier
G Vagina K Hymen	0 Open 3 Percutaneous 4 Percutaneous Endoscopic 7 Via Natural or Artificial Opening 8 Via Natural or Artificial Opening Endoscopic X External	Z No Device	X Diagnostic Z No Qualifier
J Clitoris L Vestibular Gland M Vulva	0 Open X External	0 Drainage Device	Z No Qualifier
J Clitoris L Vestibular Gland M Vulva	0 Open X External	Z No Device	X Diagnostic Z No Qualifier

Section	0	Medical and Surgical
Body System	U	Female Reproductive System
Operation	B	Excision: Cutting out or off, without replacement, a portion of a body part

Body Part (4th)	Approach (5th)	Device (6th)	Qualifier (7th)
0 Ovary, Right 1 Ovary, Left 2 Ovaries, Bilateral 4 Uterine Supporting Structure 5 Fallopian Tube, Right 6 Fallopian Tube, Left 7 Fallopian Tubes, Bilateral 9 Uterus C Cervix F Cul-de-sac	0 Open 3 Percutaneous 4 Percutaneous Endoscopic 7 Via Natural or Artificial Opening 8 Via Natural or Artificial Opening Endoscopic	Z No Device	X Diagnostic Z No Qualifier
G Vagina K Hymen	0 Open 3 Percutaneous 4 Percutaneous Endoscopic 7 Via Natural or Artificial Opening 8 Via Natural or Artificial Opening Endoscopic X External	Z No Device	X Diagnostic Z No Qualifier
J Clitoris L Vestibular Gland M Vulva	0 Open X External	Z No Device	X Diagnostic Z No Qualifier

Section	0	Medical and Surgical
Body System	U	Female Reproductive System
Operation	C	Extirpation: Taking or cutting out solid matter from a body part

Body Part (4th)	Approach (5th)	Device (6th)	Qualifier (7th)
0 Ovary, Right 1 Ovary, Left 2 Ovaries, Bilateral 4 Uterine Supporting Structure	0 Open 3 Percutaneous 4 Percutaneous Endoscopic	Z No Device	Z No Qualifier
5 Fallopian Tube, Right 6 Fallopian Tube, Left 7 Fallopian Tubes, Bilateral 9 Uterus B Endometrium C Cervix F Cul-de-sac	0 Open 3 Percutaneous 4 Percutaneous Endoscopic 7 Via Natural or Artificial Opening 8 Via Natural or Artificial Opening Endoscopic	Z No Device	Z No Qualifier
G Vagina K Hymen	0 Open 3 Percutaneous 4 Percutaneous Endoscopic 7 Via Natural or Artificial Opening 8 Via Natural or Artificial Opening Endoscopic X External	Z No Device	Z No Qualifier
J Clitoris L Vestibular Gland M Vulva	0 Open X External	Z No Device	Z No Qualifier

Section	0	Medical and Surgical
Body System	U	Female Reproductive System
Operation	D	Extraction: Pulling or stripping out or off all or a portion of a body part by the use of force

Body Part (4th)	Approach (5th)	Device (6th)	Qualifier (7th)
B Endometrium	**7** Via Natural or Artificial Opening **8** Via Natural or Artificial Opening Endoscopic	**Z** No Device	**X** Diagnostic **Z** No Qualifier
N Ova	**0** Open **3** Percutaneous **4** Percutaneous Endoscopic	**Z** No Device	**Z** No Qualifier

Section	0	Medical and Surgical
Body System	U	Female Reproductive System
Operation	F	Fragmentation: Breaking solid matter in a body part into pieces

Body Part (4th)	Approach (5th)	Device (6th)	Qualifier (7th)
5 Fallopian Tube, Right **6** Fallopian Tube, Left **7** Fallopian Tubes, Bilateral **9** Uterus	**0** Open **3** Percutaneous **4** Percutaneous Endoscopic **7** Via Natural or Artificial Opening **8** Via Natural or Artificial Opening Endoscopic **X** External	**Z** No Device	**Z** No Qualifier

Section	0	Medical and Surgical
Body System	U	Female Reproductive System
Operation	H	Insertion: Putting in a nonbiological appliance that monitors, assists, performs, or prevents a physiological function but does not physically take the place of a body part

Body Part (4th)	Approach (5th)	Device (6th)	Qualifier (7th)
3 Ovary	**0** Open **3** Percutaneous **4** Percutaneous Endoscopic	**3** Infusion Device	**Z** No Qualifier
8 Fallopian Tube **D** Uterus and Cervix **H** Vagina and Cul-de-sac	**0** Open **3** Percutaneous **4** Percutaneous Endoscopic **7** Via Natural or Artificial Opening **8** Via Natural or Artificial Opening Endoscopic	**3** Infusion Device	**Z** No Qualifier
9 Uterus	**7** Via Natural or Artificial Opening **8** Via Natural or Artificial Opening Endoscopic	**H** Contraceptive Device	**Z** No Qualifier
C Cervix	**0** Open **3** Percutaneous **4** Percutaneous Endoscopic	**1** Radioactive Element	**Z** No Qualifier
C Cervix	**7** Via Natural or Artificial Opening **8** Via Natural or Artificial Opening Endoscopic	**1** Radioactive Element **H** Contraceptive Device	**Z** No Qualifier
F Cul-de-sac	**7** Via Natural or Artificial Opening **8** Via Natural or Artificial Opening Endoscopic	**G** Intraluminal Device, Pessary	**Z** No Qualifier

Continued

0UH *Continued*

Section	0	Medical and Surgical
Body System	U	Female Reproductive System
Operation	H	Insertion: Putting in a nonbiological appliance that monitors, assists, performs, or prevents a physiological function but does not physically take the place of a body part

Body Part (4th)	Approach (5th)	Device (6th)	Qualifier (7th)
G Vagina	0 Open 3 Percutaneous 4 Percutaneous Endoscopic X External	1 Radioactive Element	Z No Qualifier
G Vagina	7 Via Natural or Artificial Opening 8 Via Natural or Artificial Opening Endoscopic	1 Radioactive Element G Intraluminal Device, Pessary	Z No Qualifier

Section	0	Medical and Surgical
Body System	U	Female Reproductive System
Operation	J	Inspection: Visually and/or manually exploring a body part

Body Part (4th)	Approach (5th)	Device (6th)	Qualifier (7th)
3 Ovary	0 Open 3 Percutaneous 4 Percutaneous Endoscopic X External	Z No Device	Z No Qualifier
8 Fallopian Tube D Uterus and Cervix H Vagina and Cul-de-sac	0 Open 3 Percutaneous 4 Percutaneous Endoscopic 7 Via Natural or Artificial Opening 8 Via Natural or Artificial Opening Endoscopic X External	Z No Device	Z No Qualifier
M Vulva	0 Open X External	Z No Device	Z No Qualifier

Section	0	Medical and Surgical
Body System	U	Female Reproductive System
Operation	L	Occlusion: Completely closing an orifice or the lumen of a tubular body part

Body Part (4th)	Approach (5th)	Device (6th)	Qualifier (7th)
5 Fallopian Tube, Right 6 Fallopian Tube, Left 7 Fallopian Tubes, Bilateral	0 Open 3 Percutaneous 4 Percutaneous Endoscopic	C Extraluminal Device D Intraluminal Device Z No Device	Z No Qualifier
5 Fallopian Tube, Right 6 Fallopian Tube, Left 7 Fallopian Tubes, Bilateral	7 Via Natural or Artificial Opening 8 Via Natural or Artificial Opening Endoscopic	D Intraluminal Device Z No Device	Z No Qualifier
F Cul-de-sac G Vagina	7 Via Natural or Artificial Opening 8 Via Natural or Artificial Opening Endoscopic	D Intraluminal Device Z No Device	Z No Qualifier

Section	0	Medical and Surgical
Body System	U	Female Reproductive System
Operation	M	**Reattachment:** Putting back in or on all or a portion of a separated body part to its normal location or other suitable location

Body Part (4th)	Approach (5th)	Device (6th)	Qualifier (7th)
0 Ovary, Right 1 Ovary, Left 2 Ovaries, Bilateral 4 Uterine Supporting Structure 5 Fallopian Tube, Right 6 Fallopian Tube, Left 7 Fallopian Tubes, Bilateral 9 Uterus C Cervix F Cul-de-sac G Vagina	0 Open 4 Percutaneous Endoscopic	Z No Device	Z No Qualifier
J Clitoris M Vulva	X External	Z No Device	Z No Qualifier
K Hymen	0 Open 4 Percutaneous Endoscopic X External	Z No Device	Z No Qualifier

Section	0	Medical and Surgical
Body System	U	Female Reproductive System
Operation	N	**Release:** Freeing a body part from an abnormal physical constraint by cutting or by the use of force

Body Part (4th)	Approach (5th)	Device (6th)	Qualifier (7th)
0 Ovary, Right 1 Ovary, Left 2 Ovaries, Bilateral 4 Uterine Supporting Structure	0 Open 3 Percutaneous 4 Percutaneous Endoscopic	Z No Device	Z No Qualifier
5 Fallopian Tube, Right 6 Fallopian Tube, Left 7 Fallopian Tubes, Bilateral 9 Uterus C Cervix F Cul-de-sac	0 Open 3 Percutaneous 4 Percutaneous Endoscopic 7 Via Natural or Artificial Opening 8 Via Natural or Artificial Opening Endoscopic	Z No Device	Z No Qualifier
G Vagina K Hymen	0 Open 3 Percutaneous 4 Percutaneous Endoscopic 7 Via Natural or Artificial Opening 8 Via Natural or Artificial Opening Endoscopic X External	Z No Device	Z No Qualifier
J Clitoris L Vestibular Gland M Vulva	0 Open X External	Z No Device	Z No Qualifier

Section	0	Medical and Surgical
Body System	U	Female Reproductive System
Operation	P	**Removal:** Taking out or off a device from a body part

Body Part (4th)	Approach (5th)	Device (6th)	Qualifier (7th)
3 Ovary	**0** Open **3** Percutaneous **4** Percutaneous Endoscopic **X** External	**0** Drainage Device **3** Infusion Device	**Z** No Qualifier
8 Fallopian Tube	**0** Open **3** Percutaneous **4** Percutaneous Endoscopic **7** Via Natural or Artificial Opening **8** Via Natural or Artificial Opening Endoscopic	**0** Drainage Device **3** Infusion Device **7** Autologous Tissue Substitute **C** Extraluminal Device **D** Intraluminal Device **J** Synthetic Substitute **K** Nonautologous Tissue Substitute	**Z** No Qualifier
8 Fallopian Tube	**X** External	**0** Drainage Device **3** Infusion Device **D** Intraluminal Device	**Z** No Qualifier
D Uterus and Cervix	**0** Open **3** Percutaneous **4** Percutaneous Endoscopic **7** Via Natural or Artificial Opening **8** Via Natural or Artificial Opening Endoscopic	**0** Drainage Device **1** Radioactive Element **3** Infusion Device **7** Autologous Tissue Substitute **C** Extraluminal Device **D** Intraluminal Device **H** Contraceptive Device **J** Synthetic Substitute **K** Nonautologous Tissue Substitute	**Z** No Qualifier
D Uterus and Cervix	**X** External	**0** Drainage Device **3** Infusion Device **D** Intraluminal Device **H** Contraceptive Device	**Z** No Qualifier
H Vagina and Cul-de-sac	**0** Open **3** Percutaneous **4** Percutaneous Endoscopic **7** Via Natural or Artificial Opening **8** Via Natural or Artificial Opening Endoscopic	**0** Drainage Device **1** Radioactive Element **3** Infusion Device **7** Autologous Tissue Substitute **D** Intraluminal Device **J** Synthetic Substitute **K** Nonautologous Tissue Substitute	**Z** No Qualifier
H Vagina and Cul-de-sac	**X** External	**0** Drainage Device **1** Radioactive Element **3** Infusion Device **D** Intraluminal Device	**Z** No Qualifier
M Vulva	**0** Open	**0** Drainage Device **7** Autologous Tissue Substitute **J** Synthetic Substitute **K** Nonautologous Tissue Substitute	**Z** No Qualifier
M Vulva	**X** External	**0** Drainage Device	**Z** No Qualifier

Section	0	Medical and Surgical
Body System	U	Female Reproductive System
Operation	Q	Repair: Restoring, to the extent possible, a body part to its normal anatomic structure and function

Body Part (4th)	Approach (5th)	Device (6th)	Qualifier (7th)
0 Ovary, Right 1 Ovary, Left 2 Ovaries, Bilateral 4 Uterine Supporting Structure	0 Open 3 Percutaneous 4 Percutaneous Endoscopic	Z No Device	Z No Qualifier
5 Fallopian Tube, Right 6 Fallopian Tube, Left 7 Fallopian Tubes, Bilateral 9 Uterus C Cervix F Cul-de-sac	0 Open 3 Percutaneous 4 Percutaneous Endoscopic 7 Via Natural or Artificial Opening 8 Via Natural or Artificial Opening Endoscopic	Z No Device	Z No Qualifier
G Vagina K Hymen	0 Open 3 Percutaneous 4 Percutaneous Endoscopic 7 Via Natural or Artificial Opening 8 Via Natural or Artificial Opening Endoscopic X External	Z No Device	Z No Qualifier
J Clitoris L Vestibular Gland M Vulva	0 Open X External	Z No Device	Z No Qualifier

Section	0	Medical and Surgical
Body System	U	Female Reproductive System
Operation	S	Reposition: Moving to its normal location, or other suitable location, all or a portion of a body part

Body Part (4th)	Approach (5th)	Device (6th)	Qualifier (7th)
0 Ovary, Right 1 Ovary, Left 2 Ovaries, Bilateral 4 Uterine Supporting Structure 5 Fallopian Tube, Right 6 Fallopian Tube, Left 7 Fallopian Tubes, Bilateral C Cervix F Cul-de-sac	0 Open 4 Percutaneous Endoscopic	Z No Device	Z No Qualifier
9 Uterus G Vagina	0 Open 4 Percutaneous Endoscopic X External	Z No Device	Z No Qualifier

Section	0	**Medical and Surgical**
Body System	U	**Female Reproductive System**
Operation	T	**Resection:** Cutting out or off, without replacement, all of a body part

Body Part (4th)	Approach (5th)	Device (6th)	Qualifier (7th)
0 Ovary, Right 1 Ovary, Left 2 Ovaries, Bilateral 5 Fallopian Tube, Right 6 Fallopian Tube, Left 7 Fallopian Tubes, Bilateral 9 Uterus	0 Open 4 Percutaneous Endoscopic 7 Via Natural or Artificial Opening 8 Via Natural or Artificial Opening Endoscopic F Via Natural or Artificial Opening With Percutaneous Endoscopic Assistance	Z No Device	Z No Qualifier
4 Uterine Supporting Structure C Cervix F Cul-de-sac G Vagina	0 Open 4 Percutaneous Endoscopic 7 Via Natural or Artificial Opening 8 Via Natural or Artificial Opening Endoscopic	Z No Device	Z No Qualifier
J Clitoris L Vestibular Gland M Vulva	0 Open X External	Z No Device	Z No Qualifier
K Hymen	0 Open 4 Percutaneous Endoscopic 7 Via Natural or Artificial Opening 8 Via Natural or Artificial Opening Endoscopic X External	Z No Device	Z No Qualifier

Section	0	**Medical and Surgical**
Body System	U	**Female Reproductive System**
Operation	U	**Supplement:** Putting in or on biological or synthetic material that physically reinforces and/or augments the function of a portion of a body part

Body Part (4th)	Approach (5th)	Device (6th)	Qualifier (7th)
4 Uterine Supporting Structure	0 Open 4 Percutaneous Endoscopic	7 Autologous Tissue Substitute J Synthetic Substitute K Nonautologous Tissue Substitute	Z No Qualifier
5 Fallopian Tube, Right 6 Fallopian Tube, Left 7 Fallopian Tubes, Bilateral F Cul-de-sac	0 Open 4 Percutaneous Endoscopic 7 Via Natural or Artificial Opening 8 Via Natural or Artificial Opening Endoscopic	7 Autologous Tissue Substitute J Synthetic Substitute K Nonautologous Tissue Substitute	Z No Qualifier
G Vagina K Hymen	0 Open 4 Percutaneous Endoscopic 7 Via Natural or Artificial Opening 8 Via Natural or Artificial Opening Endoscopic X External	7 Autologous Tissue Substitute J Synthetic Substitute K Nonautologous Tissue Substitute	Z No Qualifier
J Clitoris M Vulva	0 Open X External	7 Autologous Tissue Substitute J Synthetic Substitute K Nonautologous Tissue Substitute	Z No Qualifier

Section	0	Medical and Surgical
Body System	U	Female Reproductive System
Operation	V	**Restriction:** Partially closing an orifice or the lumen of a tubular body part

Body Part (4th)	Approach (5th)	Device (6th)	Qualifier (7th)
C Cervix	0 Open 3 Percutaneous 4 Percutaneous Endoscopic	C Extraluminal Device D Intraluminal Device Z No Device	Z No Qualifier
C Cervix	7 Via Natural or Artificial Opening 8 Via Natural or Artificial Opening Endoscopic	D Intraluminal Device Z No Device	Z No Qualifier

Section	0	Medical and Surgical
Body System	U	Female Reproductive System
Operation	W	**Revision:** Correcting, to the extent possible, a portion of a malfunctioning device or the position of a displaced device

Body Part (4th)	Approach (5th)	Device (6th)	Qualifier (7th)
3 Ovary	0 Open 3 Percutaneous 4 Percutaneous Endoscopic X External	0 Drainage Device 3 Infusion Device	Z No Qualifier
8 Fallopian Tube	0 Open 3 Percutaneous 4 Percutaneous Endoscopic 7 Via Natural or Artificial Opening 8 Via Natural or Artificial Opening Endoscopic X External	0 Drainage Device 3 Infusion Device 7 Autologous Tissue Substitute C Extraluminal Device D Intraluminal Device J Synthetic Substitute K Nonautologous Tissue Substitute	Z No Qualifier
D Uterus and Cervix	0 Open 3 Percutaneous 4 Percutaneous Endoscopic 7 Via Natural or Artificial Opening 8 Via Natural or Artificial Opening Endoscopic	0 Drainage Device 1 Radioactive Element 3 Infusion Device 7 Autologous Tissue Substitute C Extraluminal Device D Intraluminal Device H Contraceptive Device J Synthetic Substitute K Nonautologous Tissue Substitute	Z No Qualifier
D Uterus and Cervix	X External	0 Drainage Device 3 Infusion Device 7 Autologous Tissue Substitute C Extraluminal Device D Intraluminal Device H Contraceptive Device J Synthetic Substitute K Nonautologous Tissue Substitute	Z No Qualifier
H Vagina and Cul-de-sac	0 Open 3 Percutaneous 4 Percutaneous Endoscopic 7 Via Natural or Artificial Opening 8 Via Natural or Artificial Opening Endoscopic	0 Drainage Device 1 Radioactive Element 3 Infusion Device 7 Autologous Tissue Substitute D Intraluminal Device J Synthetic Substitute K Nonautologous Tissue Substitute	Z No Qualifier

Continued

0UW Continued

Section	0	Medical and Surgical
Body System	U	Female Reproductive System
Operation	W	**Revision:** Correcting, to the extent possible, a portion of a malfunctioning device or the position of a displaced device

Body Part (4ᵗʰ)	Approach (5ᵗʰ)	Device (6ᵗʰ)	Qualifier (7ᵗʰ)
H Vagina and Cul-de-sac	X External	0 Drainage Device 3 Infusion Device 7 Autologous Tissue Substitute D Intraluminal Device J Synthetic Substitute K Nonautologous Tissue Substitute	Z No Qualifier
M Vulva	0 Open X External	0 Drainage Device 7 Autologous Tissue Substitute J Synthetic Substitute K Nonautologous Tissue Substitute	Z No Qualifier

Section	0	Medical and Surgical
Body System	U	Female Reproductive System
Operation	Y	**Transplantation:** Putting in or on all or a portion of a living body part taken from another individual or animal to physically take the place and/or function of all or a portion of a similar body part

Body Part (4ᵗʰ)	Approach (5ᵗʰ)	Device (6ᵗʰ)	Qualifier (7ᵗʰ)
0 Ovary, Right 1 Ovary, Left	0 Open	Z No Device	0 Allogeneic 1 Syngeneic 2 Zooplastic

Female Reproductive System Code Listing 0U1–0UY

0U1 – Female Reproductive System, Bypass

Review Coding Guideline B3.6a

♀ **0U15075** Bypass Right Fallopian Tube to Right Fallopian Tube with Autologous Tissue Substitute, Open Approach

♀ **0U15076** Bypass Right Fallopian Tube to Left Fallopian Tube with Autologous Tissue Substitute, Open Approach

♀ **0U15079** Bypass Right Fallopian Tube to Uterus with Autologous Tissue Substitute, Open Approach

♀ **0U150J5** Bypass Right Fallopian Tube to Right Fallopian Tube with Synthetic Substitute, Open Approach

♀ **0U150J6** Bypass Right Fallopian Tube to Left Fallopian Tube with Synthetic Substitute, Open Approach

♀ **0U150J9** Bypass Right Fallopian Tube to Uterus with Synthetic Substitute, Open Approach

♀ **0U150K5** Bypass Right Fallopian Tube to Right Fallopian Tube with Nonautologous Tissue Substitute, Open Approach

♀ **0U150K6** Bypass Right Fallopian Tube to Left Fallopian Tube with Nonautologous Tissue Substitute, Open Approach

♀ **0U150K9** Bypass Right Fallopian Tube to Uterus with Nonautologous Tissue Substitute, Open Approach

♀ **0U150Z5** Bypass Right Fallopian Tube to Right Fallopian Tube, Open Approach

♀ **0U150Z6** Bypass Right Fallopian Tube to Left Fallopian Tube, Open Approach

♀ **0U150Z9** Bypass Right Fallopian Tube to Uterus, Open Approach

♀ **0U15475** Bypass Right Fallopian Tube to Right Fallopian Tube with Autologous Tissue Substitute, Percutaneous Endoscopic Approach

♀ **0U15476** Bypass Right Fallopian Tube to Left Fallopian Tube with Autologous Tissue Substitute, Percutaneous Endoscopic Approach

♀ **0U15479** Bypass Right Fallopian Tube to Uterus with Autologous Tissue Substitute, Percutaneous Endoscopic Approach

♀ **0U154J5** Bypass Right Fallopian Tube to Right Fallopian Tube with Synthetic Substitute, Percutaneous Endoscopic Approach

♀ **0U154J6** Bypass Right Fallopian Tube to Left Fallopian Tube with Synthetic Substitute, Percutaneous Endoscopic Approach

♀ **0U154J9** Bypass Right Fallopian Tube to Uterus with Synthetic Substitute, Percutaneous Endoscopic Approach

♀ **0U154K5** Bypass Right Fallopian Tube to Right Fallopian Tube with Nonautologous Tissue Substitute, Percutaneous Endoscopic Approach

♀ **0U154K6** Bypass Right Fallopian Tube to Left Fallopian Tube with Nonautologous Tissue Substitute, Percutaneous Endoscopic Approach

♀ **0U154K9** Bypass Right Fallopian Tube to Uterus with Nonautologous Tissue Substitute, Percutaneous Endoscopic Approach

♀ **0U154Z5** Bypass Right Fallopian Tube to Right Fallopian Tube, Percutaneous Endoscopic Approach

♀ **0U154Z6** Bypass Right Fallopian Tube to Left Fallopian Tube, Percutaneous Endoscopic Approach

♀ **0U154Z9** Bypass Right Fallopian Tube to Uterus, Percutaneous Endoscopic Approach

♀ **0U16075** Bypass Left Fallopian Tube to Right Fallopian Tube with Autologous Tissue Substitute, Open Approach

♀ **0U16076** Bypass Left Fallopian Tube to Left Fallopian Tube with Autologous Tissue Substitute, Open Approach

♀ **0U16079** Bypass Left Fallopian Tube to Uterus with Autologous Tissue Substitute, Open Approach

♀ **0U160J5** Bypass Left Fallopian Tube to Right Fallopian Tube with Synthetic Substitute, Open Approach

♀ **0U160J6** Bypass Left Fallopian Tube to Left Fallopian Tube with Synthetic Substitute, Open Approach

♀ **0U160J9** Bypass Left Fallopian Tube to Uterus with Synthetic Substitute, Open Approach

♀ 0U160K5 Bypass Left Fallopian Tube to Right Fallopian Tube with Nonautologous Tissue Substitute, Open Approach
♀ 0U160K6 Bypass Left Fallopian Tube to Left Fallopian Tube with Nonautologous Tissue Substitute, Open Approach
♀ 0U160K9 Bypass Left Fallopian Tube to Uterus with Nonautologous Tissue Substitute, Open Approach
♀ 0U160Z5 Bypass Left Fallopian Tube to Right Fallopian Tube, Open Approach
♀ 0U160Z6 Bypass Left Fallopian Tube to Left Fallopian Tube, Open Approach
♀ 0U160Z9 Bypass Left Fallopian Tube to Uterus, Open Approach
♀ 0U16475 Bypass Left Fallopian Tube to Right Fallopian Tube with Autologous Tissue Substitute, Percutaneous Endoscopic Approach
♀ 0U16476 Bypass Left Fallopian Tube to Left Fallopian Tube with Autologous Tissue Substitute, Percutaneous Endoscopic Approach
♀ 0U16479 Bypass Left Fallopian Tube to Uterus with Autologous Tissue Substitute, Percutaneous Endoscopic Approach
♀ 0U164J5 Bypass Left Fallopian Tube to Right Fallopian Tube with Synthetic Substitute, Percutaneous Endoscopic Approach

♀ 0U164J6 Bypass Left Fallopian Tube to Left Fallopian Tube with Synthetic Substitute, Percutaneous Endoscopic Approach
♀ 0U164J9 Bypass Left Fallopian Tube to Uterus with Synthetic Substitute, Percutaneous Endoscopic Approach
♀ 0U164K5 Bypass Left Fallopian Tube to Right Fallopian Tube with Nonautologous Tissue Substitute, Percutaneous Endoscopic Approach
♀ 0U164K6 Bypass Left Fallopian Tube to Left Fallopian Tube with Nonautologous Tissue Substitute, Percutaneous Endoscopic Approach
♀ 0U164K9 Bypass Left Fallopian Tube to Uterus with Nonautologous Tissue Substitute, Percutaneous Endoscopic Approach
♀ 0U164Z5 Bypass Left Fallopian Tube to Right Fallopian Tube, Percutaneous Endoscopic Approach
♀ 0U164Z6 Bypass Left Fallopian Tube to Left Fallopian Tube, Percutaneous Endoscopic Approach
♀ 0U164Z9 Bypass Left Fallopian Tube to Uterus, Percutaneous Endoscopic Approach

0U2 – Female Reproductive System, Change

Review Coding Guideline B6.1c

♀ 0U23X0Z Change Drainage Device in Ovary, External Approach
♀ 0U23XYZ Change Other Device in Ovary, External Approach
♀ 0U28X0Z Change Drainage Device in Fallopian Tube, External Approach
♀ 0U28XYZ Change Other Device in Fallopian Tube, External Approach
♀ 0U2DX0Z Change Drainage Device in Uterus and Cervix, External Approach
♀ 0U2DXHZ Change Contraceptive Device in Uterus and Cervix, External Approach
♀ 0U2DXYZ Change Other Device in Uterus and Cervix, External Approach

♀ 0U2HX0Z Change Drainage Device in Vagina and Cul-de-sac, External Approach
♀ 0U2HXGZ Change Pessary in Vagina and Cul-de-sac, External Approach
♀ 0U2HXYZ Change Other Device in Vagina and Cul-de-sac, External Approach
♀ 0U2MX0Z Change Drainage Device in Vulva, External Approach
♀ 0U2MXYZ Change Other Device in Vulva, External Approach

0U5 – Female Reproductive System, Destruction

♀ 0U500ZZ Destruction of Right Ovary, Open Approach
♀ 0U503ZZ Destruction of Right Ovary, Percutaneous Approach
♀ 0U504ZZ Destruction of Right Ovary, Percutaneous Endoscopic Approach
♀ 0U510ZZ Destruction of Left Ovary, Open Approach
♀ 0U513ZZ Destruction of Left Ovary, Percutaneous Approach
♀ 0U514ZZ Destruction of Left Ovary, Percutaneous Endoscopic Approach
♀ 0U520ZZ Destruction of Bilateral Ovaries, Open Approach
♀ 0U523ZZ Destruction of Bilateral Ovaries, Percutaneous Approach
♀ 0U524ZZ Destruction of Bilateral Ovaries, Percutaneous Endoscopic Approach
♀ 0U540ZZ Destruction of Uterine Supporting Structure, Open Approach
♀ 0U543ZZ Destruction of Uterine Supporting Structure, Percutaneous Approach
♀ 0U544ZZ Destruction of Uterine Supporting Structure, Percutaneous Endoscopic Approach
♀ 0U550ZZ Destruction of Right Fallopian Tube, Open Approach
♀ 0U553ZZ Destruction of Right Fallopian Tube, Percutaneous Approach
♀ 0U554ZZ Destruction of Right Fallopian Tube, Percutaneous Endoscopic Approach
♀ 0U557ZZ Destruction of Right Fallopian Tube, Via Natural or Artificial Opening
♀ 0U558ZZ Destruction of Right Fallopian Tube, Via Natural or Artificial Opening Endoscopic
♀ 0U560ZZ Destruction of Left Fallopian Tube, Open Approach
♀ 0U563ZZ Destruction of Left Fallopian Tube, Percutaneous Approach
♀ 0U564ZZ Destruction of Left Fallopian Tube, Percutaneous Endoscopic Approach
♀ 0U567ZZ Destruction of Left Fallopian Tube, Via Natural or Artificial Opening
♀ 0U568ZZ Destruction of Left Fallopian Tube, Via Natural or Artificial Opening Endoscopic
● ♀ 0U570ZZ Destruction of Bilateral Fallopian Tubes, Open Approach
● ♀ 0U573ZZ Destruction of Bilateral Fallopian Tubes, Percutaneous Approach
● ♀ 0U574ZZ Destruction of Bilateral Fallopian Tubes, Percutaneous Endoscopic Approach
● ♀ 0U577ZZ Destruction of Bilateral Fallopian Tubes, Via Natural or Artificial Opening

● ♀ 0U578ZZ Destruction of Bilateral Fallopian Tubes, Via Natural or Artificial Opening Endoscopic
♀ 0U590ZZ Destruction of Uterus, Open Approach
♀ 0U593ZZ Destruction of Uterus, Percutaneous Approach
♀ 0U594ZZ Destruction of Uterus, Percutaneous Endoscopic Approach
♀ 0U597ZZ Destruction of Uterus, Via Natural or Artificial Opening
♀ 0U598ZZ Destruction of Uterus, Via Natural or Artificial Opening Endoscopic
♀ 0U5B0ZZ Destruction of Endometrium, Open Approach
♀ 0U5B3ZZ Destruction of Endometrium, Percutaneous Approach
♀ 0U5B4ZZ Destruction of Endometrium, Percutaneous Endoscopic Approach
♀ 0U5B7ZZ Destruction of Endometrium, Via Natural or Artificial Opening
♀ 0U5B8ZZ Destruction of Endometrium, Via Natural or Artificial Opening Endoscopic
♀ 0U5C0ZZ Destruction of Cervix, Open Approach
♀ 0U5C3ZZ Destruction of Cervix, Percutaneous Approach
♀ 0U5C4ZZ Destruction of Cervix, Percutaneous Endoscopic Approach
♀ 0U5C7ZZ Destruction of Cervix, Via Natural or Artificial Opening
♀ 0U5C8ZZ Destruction of Cervix, Via Natural or Artificial Opening Endoscopic
♀ 0U5F0ZZ Destruction of Cul-de-sac, Open Approach
♀ 0U5F3ZZ Destruction of Cul-de-sac, Percutaneous Approach
♀ 0U5F4ZZ Destruction of Cul-de-sac, Percutaneous Endoscopic Approach
♀ 0U5F7ZZ Destruction of Cul-de-sac, Via Natural or Artificial Opening
♀ 0U5F8ZZ Destruction of Cul-de-sac, Via Natural or Artificial Opening Endoscopic
♀ 0U5G0ZZ Destruction of Vagina, Open Approach
♀ 0U5G3ZZ Destruction of Vagina, Percutaneous Approach
♀ 0U5G4ZZ Destruction of Vagina, Percutaneous Endoscopic Approach
♀ 0U5G7ZZ Destruction of Vagina, Via Natural or Artificial Opening
♀ 0U5G8ZZ Destruction of Vagina, Via Natural or Artificial Opening Endoscopic
♀ 0U5GXZZ Destruction of Vagina, External Approach
♀ 0U5J0ZZ Destruction of Clitoris, Open Approach
♀ 0U5JXZZ Destruction of Clitoris, External Approach
♀ 0U5K0ZZ Destruction of Hymen, Open Approach
♀ 0U5K3ZZ Destruction of Hymen, Percutaneous Approach
♀ 0U5K4ZZ Destruction of Hymen, Percutaneous Endoscopic Approach
♀ 0U5K7ZZ Destruction of Hymen, Via Natural or Artificial Opening

♀ **0U5K8ZZ** Destruction of Hymen, Via Natural or Artificial Opening Endoscopic
♀ **0U5KXZZ** Destruction of Hymen, External Approach
♀ **0U5L0ZZ** Destruction of Vestibular Gland, Open Approach
♀ **0U5LXZZ** Destruction of Vestibular Gland, External Approach
♀ **0U5M0ZZ** Destruction of Vulva, Open Approach
♀ **0U5MXZZ** Destruction of Vulva, External Approach

0U7 – Female Reproductive System, Dilation

♀ **0U750DZ** Dilation of Right Fallopian Tube with Intraluminal Device, Open Approach
♀ **0U750ZZ** Dilation of Right Fallopian Tube, Open Approach
♀ **0U753DZ** Dilation of Right Fallopian Tube with Intraluminal Device, Percutaneous Approach
♀ **0U753ZZ** Dilation of Right Fallopian Tube, Percutaneous Approach
♀ **0U754DZ** Dilation of Right Fallopian Tube with Intraluminal Device, Percutaneous Endoscopic Approach
♀ **0U754ZZ** Dilation of Right Fallopian Tube, Percutaneous Endoscopic Approach
♀ **0U757DZ** Dilation of Right Fallopian Tube with Intraluminal Device, Via Natural or Artificial Opening
♀ **0U757ZZ** Dilation of Right Fallopian Tube, Via Natural or Artificial Opening
♀ **0U758DZ** Dilation of Right Fallopian Tube with Intraluminal Device, Via Natural or Artificial Opening Endoscopic
♀ **0U758ZZ** Dilation of Right Fallopian Tube, Via Natural or Artificial Opening Endoscopic
♀ **0U760DZ** Dilation of Left Fallopian Tube with Intraluminal Device, Open Approach
♀ **0U760ZZ** Dilation of Left Fallopian Tube, Open Approach
♀ **0U763DZ** Dilation of Left Fallopian Tube with Intraluminal Device, Percutaneous Approach
♀ **0U763ZZ** Dilation of Left Fallopian Tube, Percutaneous Approach
♀ **0U764DZ** Dilation of Left Fallopian Tube with Intraluminal Device, Percutaneous Endoscopic Approach
♀ **0U764ZZ** Dilation of Left Fallopian Tube, Percutaneous Endoscopic Approach
♀ **0U767DZ** Dilation of Left Fallopian Tube with Intraluminal Device, Via Natural or Artificial Opening
♀ **0U767ZZ** Dilation of Left Fallopian Tube, Via Natural or Artificial Opening
♀ **0U768DZ** Dilation of Left Fallopian Tube with Intraluminal Device, Via Natural or Artificial Opening Endoscopic
♀ **0U768ZZ** Dilation of Left Fallopian Tube, Via Natural or Artificial Opening Endoscopic
♀ **0U770DZ** Dilation of Bilateral Fallopian Tubes with Intraluminal Device, Open Approach
♀ **0U770ZZ** Dilation of Bilateral Fallopian Tubes, Open Approach
♀ **0U773DZ** Dilation of Bilateral Fallopian Tubes with Intraluminal Device, Percutaneous Approach
♀ **0U773ZZ** Dilation of Bilateral Fallopian Tubes, Percutaneous Approach
♀ **0U774DZ** Dilation of Bilateral Fallopian Tubes with Intraluminal Device, Percutaneous Endoscopic Approach
♀ **0U774ZZ** Dilation of Bilateral Fallopian Tubes, Percutaneous Endoscopic Approach
♀ **0U777DZ** Dilation of Bilateral Fallopian Tubes with Intraluminal Device, Via Natural or Artificial Opening
♀ **0U777ZZ** Dilation of Bilateral Fallopian Tubes, Via Natural or Artificial Opening
♀ **0U778DZ** Dilation of Bilateral Fallopian Tubes with Intraluminal Device, Via Natural or Artificial Opening Endoscopic
♀ **0U778ZZ** Dilation of Bilateral Fallopian Tubes, Via Natural or Artificial Opening Endoscopic
♀ **0U790DZ** Dilation of Uterus with Intraluminal Device, Open Approach
♀ **0U790ZZ** Dilation of Uterus, Open Approach
♀ **0U793DZ** Dilation of Uterus with Intraluminal Device, Percutaneous Approach

♀ **0U793ZZ** Dilation of Uterus, Percutaneous Approach
♀ **0U794DZ** Dilation of Uterus with Intraluminal Device, Percutaneous Endoscopic Approach
♀ **0U794ZZ** Dilation of Uterus, Percutaneous Endoscopic Approach
♀ **0U797DZ** Dilation of Uterus with Intraluminal Device, Via Natural or Artificial Opening
♀ **0U797ZZ** Dilation of Uterus, Via Natural or Artificial Opening
♀ **0U798DZ** Dilation of Uterus with Intraluminal Device, Via Natural or Artificial Opening Endoscopic
♀ **0U798ZZ** Dilation of Uterus, Via Natural or Artificial Opening Endoscopic
♀ **0U7C0DZ** Dilation of Cervix with Intraluminal Device, Open Approach
♀ **0U7C0ZZ** Dilation of Cervix, Open Approach
♀ **0U7C3DZ** Dilation of Cervix with Intraluminal Device, Percutaneous Approach
♀ **0U7C3ZZ** Dilation of Cervix, Percutaneous Approach
♀ **0U7C4DZ** Dilation of Cervix with Intraluminal Device, Percutaneous Endoscopic Approach
♀ **0U7C4ZZ** Dilation of Cervix, Percutaneous Endoscopic Approach
♀ **0U7C7DZ** Dilation of Cervix with Intraluminal Device, Via Natural or Artificial Opening
♀ **0U7C7ZZ** Dilation of Cervix, Via Natural or Artificial Opening
♀ **0U7C8DZ** Dilation of Cervix with Intraluminal Device, Via Natural or Artificial Opening Endoscopic
♀ **0U7C8ZZ** Dilation of Cervix, Via Natural or Artificial Opening Endoscopic
♀ **0U7G0DZ** Dilation of Vagina with Intraluminal Device, Open Approach
♀ **0U7G0ZZ** Dilation of Vagina, Open Approach
♀ **0U7G3DZ** Dilation of Vagina with Intraluminal Device, Percutaneous Approach
♀ **0U7G3ZZ** Dilation of Vagina, Percutaneous Approach
♀ **0U7G4DZ** Dilation of Vagina with Intraluminal Device, Percutaneous Endoscopic Approach
♀ **0U7G4ZZ** Dilation of Vagina, Percutaneous Endoscopic Approach
♀ **0U7G7DZ** Dilation of Vagina with Intraluminal Device, Via Natural or Artificial Opening
♀ **0U7G7ZZ** Dilation of Vagina, Via Natural or Artificial Opening
♀ **0U7G8DZ** Dilation of Vagina with Intraluminal Device, Via Natural or Artificial Opening Endoscopic
♀ **0U7G8ZZ** Dilation of Vagina, Via Natural or Artificial Opening Endoscopic
♀ **0U7K0DZ** Dilation of Hymen with Intraluminal Device, Open Approach
♀ **0U7K0ZZ** Dilation of Hymen, Open Approach
♀ **0U7K3DZ** Dilation of Hymen with Intraluminal Device, Percutaneous Approach
♀ **0U7K3ZZ** Dilation of Hymen, Percutaneous Approach
♀ **0U7K4DZ** Dilation of Hymen with Intraluminal Device, Percutaneous Endoscopic Approach
♀ **0U7K4ZZ** Dilation of Hymen, Percutaneous Endoscopic Approach
♀ **0U7K7DZ** Dilation of Hymen with Intraluminal Device, Via Natural or Artificial Opening
♀ **0U7K7ZZ** Dilation of Hymen, Via Natural or Artificial Opening
♀ **0U7K8DZ** Dilation of Hymen with Intraluminal Device, Via Natural or Artificial Opening Endoscopic
♀ **0U7K8ZZ** Dilation of Hymen, Via Natural or Artificial Opening Endoscopic
♀ **0U7KXDZ** Dilation of Hymen with Intraluminal Device, External Approach
♀ **0U7KXZZ** Dilation of Hymen, External Approach

0U8 – Female Reproductive System, Division

Review Coding Guideline B3.14

♀ **0U800ZZ** Division of Right Ovary, Open Approach
♀ **0U803ZZ** Division of Right Ovary, Percutaneous Approach
♀ **0U804ZZ** Division of Right Ovary, Percutaneous Endoscopic Approach
♀ **0U810ZZ** Division of Left Ovary, Open Approach
♀ **0U813ZZ** Division of Left Ovary, Percutaneous Approach
♀ **0U814ZZ** Division of Left Ovary, Percutaneous Endoscopic Approach
♀ **0U820ZZ** Division of Bilateral Ovaries, Open Approach
♀ **0U823ZZ** Division of Bilateral Ovaries, Percutaneous Approach

♀ **0U824ZZ** Division of Bilateral Ovaries, Percutaneous Endoscopic Approach
♀ **0U840ZZ** Division of Uterine Supporting Structure, Open Approach
♀ **0U843ZZ** Division of Uterine Supporting Structure, Percutaneous Approach
♀ **0U844ZZ** Division of Uterine Supporting Structure, Percutaneous Endoscopic Approach
♀ **0U8K7ZZ** Division of Hymen, Via Natural or Artificial Opening
♀ **0U8K8ZZ** Division of Hymen, Via Natural or Artificial Opening Endoscopic
♀ **0U8KXZZ** Division of Hymen, External Approach

♀ Female-only   ♂ Male-only   ● Limited Coverage   ● Non-OR   ■ HAC-associated procedure   ● Non-covered procedures   ✚ Combination

0U9 – Female Reproductive System, Drainage

Review Coding Guidelines B3.4a and B3.4b

Review Coding Guideline B6.2

♀ **0U9000Z** Drainage of Right Ovary with Drainage Device, Open Approach
♀ **0U900ZX** Drainage of Right Ovary, Open Approach, Diagnostic
♀ **0U900ZZ** Drainage of Right Ovary, Open Approach
♀ **0U9030Z** Drainage of Right Ovary with Drainage Device, Percutaneous Approach
♀ **0U903ZX** Drainage of Right Ovary, Percutaneous Approach, Diagnostic
♀ **0U903ZZ** Drainage of Right Ovary, Percutaneous Approach
♀ **0U9040Z** Drainage of Right Ovary with Drainage Device, Percutaneous Endoscopic Approach
♀ **0U904ZX** Drainage of Right Ovary, Percutaneous Endoscopic Approach, Diagnostic
♀ **0U904ZZ** Drainage of Right Ovary, Percutaneous Endoscopic Approach
♀ **0U90XZZ** Drainage of Right Ovary, External Approach
♀ **0U9100Z** Drainage of Left Ovary with Drainage Device, Open Approach
♀ **0U910ZX** Drainage of Left Ovary, Open Approach, Diagnostic
♀ **0U910ZZ** Drainage of Left Ovary, Open Approach
♀ **0U9130Z** Drainage of Left Ovary with Drainage Device, Percutaneous Approach
♀ **0U913ZX** Drainage of Left Ovary, Percutaneous Approach, Diagnostic
♀ **0U913ZZ** Drainage of Left Ovary, Percutaneous Approach
♀ **0U9140Z** Drainage of Left Ovary with Drainage Device, Percutaneous Endoscopic Approach
♀ **0U914ZX** Drainage of Left Ovary, Percutaneous Endoscopic Approach, Diagnostic
♀ **0U914ZZ** Drainage of Left Ovary, Percutaneous Endoscopic Approach
♀ **0U91XZZ** Drainage of Left Ovary, External Approach
♀ **0U9200Z** Drainage of Bilateral Ovaries with Drainage Device, Open Approach
♀ **0U920ZX** Drainage of Bilateral Ovaries, Open Approach, Diagnostic
♀ **0U920ZZ** Drainage of Bilateral Ovaries, Open Approach
♀ **0U9230Z** Drainage of Bilateral Ovaries with Drainage Device, Percutaneous Approach
♀ **0U923ZX** Drainage of Bilateral Ovaries, Percutaneous Approach, Diagnostic
♀ **0U923ZZ** Drainage of Bilateral Ovaries, Percutaneous Approach
♀ **0U9240Z** Drainage of Bilateral Ovaries with Drainage Device, Percutaneous Endoscopic Approach
♀ **0U924ZX** Drainage of Bilateral Ovaries, Percutaneous Endoscopic Approach, Diagnostic
♀ **0U924ZZ** Drainage of Bilateral Ovaries, Percutaneous Endoscopic Approach
♀ **0U92XZZ** Drainage of Bilateral Ovaries, External Approach
♀ **0U9400Z** Drainage of Uterine Supporting Structure with Drainage Device, Open Approach
♀ **0U940ZX** Drainage of Uterine Supporting Structure, Open Approach, Diagnostic
♀ **0U940ZZ** Drainage of Uterine Supporting Structure, Open Approach
♀ **0U9430Z** Drainage of Uterine Supporting Structure with Drainage Device, Percutaneous Approach
♀ **0U943ZX** Drainage of Uterine Supporting Structure, Percutaneous Approach, Diagnostic
♀ **0U943ZZ** Drainage of Uterine Supporting Structure, Percutaneous Approach
♀ **0U9440Z** Drainage of Uterine Supporting Structure with Drainage Device, Percutaneous Endoscopic Approach
♀ **0U944ZX** Drainage of Uterine Supporting Structure, Percutaneous Endoscopic Approach, Diagnostic
♀ **0U944ZZ** Drainage of Uterine Supporting Structure, Percutaneous Endoscopic Approach
♀ **0U9500Z** Drainage of Right Fallopian Tube with Drainage Device, Open Approach
♀ **0U950ZX** Drainage of Right Fallopian Tube, Open Approach, Diagnostic
♀ **0U950ZZ** Drainage of Right Fallopian Tube, Open Approach
♀ **0U9530Z** Drainage of Right Fallopian Tube with Drainage Device, Percutaneous Approach
♀ **0U953ZX** Drainage of Right Fallopian Tube, Percutaneous Approach, Diagnostic
♀ **0U953ZZ** Drainage of Right Fallopian Tube, Percutaneous Approach
♀ **0U9540Z** Drainage of Right Fallopian Tube with Drainage Device, Percutaneous Endoscopic Approach

♀ **0U954ZX** Drainage of Right Fallopian Tube, Percutaneous Endoscopic Approach, Diagnostic
♀ **0U954ZZ** Drainage of Right Fallopian Tube, Percutaneous Endoscopic Approach
♀ **0U9570Z** Drainage of Right Fallopian Tube with Drainage Device, Via Natural or Artificial Opening
♀ **0U957ZX** Drainage of Right Fallopian Tube, Via Natural or Artificial Opening, Diagnostic
♀ **0U957ZZ** Drainage of Right Fallopian Tube, Via Natural or Artificial Opening
♀ **0U9580Z** Drainage of Right Fallopian Tube with Drainage Device, Via Natural or Artificial Opening Endoscopic
♀ **0U958ZX** Drainage of Right Fallopian Tube, Via Natural or Artificial Opening Endoscopic, Diagnostic
♀ **0U958ZZ** Drainage of Right Fallopian Tube, Via Natural or Artificial Opening Endoscopic
♀ **0U9600Z** Drainage of Left Fallopian Tube with Drainage Device, Open Approach
♀ **0U960ZX** Drainage of Left Fallopian Tube, Open Approach, Diagnostic
♀ **0U960ZZ** Drainage of Left Fallopian Tube, Open Approach
♀ **0U9630Z** Drainage of Left Fallopian Tube with Drainage Device, Percutaneous Approach
♀ **0U963ZX** Drainage of Left Fallopian Tube, Percutaneous Approach, Diagnostic
♀ **0U963ZZ** Drainage of Left Fallopian Tube, Percutaneous Approach
♀ **0U9640Z** Drainage of Left Fallopian Tube with Drainage Device, Percutaneous Endoscopic Approach
♀ **0U964ZX** Drainage of Left Fallopian Tube, Percutaneous Endoscopic Approach, Diagnostic
♀ **0U964ZZ** Drainage of Left Fallopian Tube, Percutaneous Endoscopic Approach
♀ **0U9670Z** Drainage of Left Fallopian Tube with Drainage Device, Via Natural or Artificial Opening
♀ **0U967ZX** Drainage of Left Fallopian Tube, Via Natural or Artificial Opening, Diagnostic
♀ **0U967ZZ** Drainage of Left Fallopian Tube, Via Natural or Artificial Opening
♀ **0U9680Z** Drainage of Left Fallopian Tube with Drainage Device, Via Natural or Artificial Opening Endoscopic
♀ **0U968ZX** Drainage of Left Fallopian Tube, Via Natural or Artificial Opening Endoscopic, Diagnostic
♀ **0U968ZZ** Drainage of Left Fallopian Tube, Via Natural or Artificial Opening Endoscopic
♀ **0U9700Z** Drainage of Bilateral Fallopian Tubes with Drainage Device, Open Approach
♀ **0U970ZX** Drainage of Bilateral Fallopian Tubes, Open Approach, Diagnostic
♀ **0U970ZZ** Drainage of Bilateral Fallopian Tubes, Open Approach
♀ **0U9730Z** Drainage of Bilateral Fallopian Tubes with Drainage Device, Percutaneous Approach
♀ **0U973ZX** Drainage of Bilateral Fallopian Tubes, Percutaneous Approach, Diagnostic
♀ **0U973ZZ** Drainage of Bilateral Fallopian Tubes, Percutaneous Approach
♀ **0U9740Z** Drainage of Bilateral Fallopian Tubes with Drainage Device, Percutaneous Endoscopic Approach
♀ **0U974ZX** Drainage of Bilateral Fallopian Tubes, Percutaneous Endoscopic Approach, Diagnostic
♀ **0U974ZZ** Drainage of Bilateral Fallopian Tubes, Percutaneous Endoscopic Approach
♀ **0U9770Z** Drainage of Bilateral Fallopian Tubes with Drainage Device, Via Natural or Artificial Opening
♀ **0U977ZX** Drainage of Bilateral Fallopian Tubes, Via Natural or Artificial Opening, Diagnostic
♀ **0U977ZZ** Drainage of Bilateral Fallopian Tubes, Via Natural or Artificial Opening
♀ **0U9780Z** Drainage of Bilateral Fallopian Tubes with Drainage Device, Via Natural or Artificial Opening Endoscopic
♀ **0U978ZX** Drainage of Bilateral Fallopian Tubes, Via Natural or Artificial Opening Endoscopic, Diagnostic

---

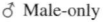 ♀ Female-only   ♂ Male-only   ● Limited Coverage   ● Non-OR   ᴴᴬᶜ HAC-associated procedure   ● Non-covered procedures   ✚ Combination

♀ **0U978ZZ** Drainage of Bilateral Fallopian Tubes, Via Natural or Artificial Opening Endoscopic
♀ **0U9900Z** Drainage of Uterus with Drainage Device, Open Approach
♀ **0U990ZX** Drainage of Uterus, Open Approach, Diagnostic
♀ **0U990ZZ** Drainage of Uterus, Open Approach
♀ **0U9930Z** Drainage of Uterus with Drainage Device, Percutaneous Approach
♀ **0U993ZX** Drainage of Uterus, Percutaneous Approach, Diagnostic
♀ **0U993ZZ** Drainage of Uterus, Percutaneous Approach
♀ **0U9940Z** Drainage of Uterus with Drainage Device, Percutaneous Endoscopic Approach
♀ **0U994ZX** Drainage of Uterus, Percutaneous Endoscopic Approach, Diagnostic
♀ **0U994ZZ** Drainage of Uterus, Percutaneous Endoscopic Approach
♀ **0U9970Z** Drainage of Uterus with Drainage Device, Via Natural or Artificial Opening
♀ **0U997ZX** Drainage of Uterus, Via Natural or Artificial Opening, Diagnostic
♀ **0U997ZZ** Drainage of Uterus, Via Natural or Artificial Opening
♀ **0U9980Z** Drainage of Uterus with Drainage Device, Via Natural or Artificial Opening Endoscopic
♀ **0U998ZX** Drainage of Uterus, Via Natural or Artificial Opening Endoscopic, Diagnostic
♀ **0U998ZZ** Drainage of Uterus, Via Natural or Artificial Opening Endoscopic
♀ **0U9C00Z** Drainage of Cervix with Drainage Device, Open Approach
♀ **0U9C0ZX** Drainage of Cervix, Open Approach, Diagnostic
♀ **0U9C0ZZ** Drainage of Cervix, Open Approach
♀ **0U9C30Z** Drainage of Cervix with Drainage Device, Percutaneous Approach
♀ **0U9C3ZX** Drainage of Cervix, Percutaneous Approach, Diagnostic
♀ **0U9C3ZZ** Drainage of Cervix, Percutaneous Approach
♀ **0U9C40Z** Drainage of Cervix with Drainage Device, Percutaneous Endoscopic Approach
♀ **0U9C4ZX** Drainage of Cervix, Percutaneous Endoscopic Approach, Diagnostic
♀ **0U9C4ZZ** Drainage of Cervix, Percutaneous Endoscopic Approach
♀ **0U9C70Z** Drainage of Cervix with Drainage Device, Via Natural or Artificial Opening
♀ **0U9C7ZX** Drainage of Cervix, Via Natural or Artificial Opening, Diagnostic
♀ **0U9C7ZZ** Drainage of Cervix, Via Natural or Artificial Opening
♀ **0U9C80Z** Drainage of Cervix with Drainage Device, Via Natural or Artificial Opening Endoscopic
♀ **0U9C8ZX** Drainage of Cervix, Via Natural or Artificial Opening Endoscopic, Diagnostic
♀ **0U9C8ZZ** Drainage of Cervix, Via Natural or Artificial Opening Endoscopic
♀ **0U9F00Z** Drainage of Cul-de-sac with Drainage Device, Open Approach
♀ **0U9F0ZX** Drainage of Cul-de-sac, Open Approach, Diagnostic
♀ **0U9F0ZZ** Drainage of Cul-de-sac, Open Approach
♀ **0U9F30Z** Drainage of Cul-de-sac with Drainage Device, Percutaneous Approach
♀ **0U9F3ZX** Drainage of Cul-de-sac, Percutaneous Approach, Diagnostic
♀ **0U9F3ZZ** Drainage of Cul-de-sac, Percutaneous Approach
♀ **0U9F40Z** Drainage of Cul-de-sac with Drainage Device, Percutaneous Endoscopic Approach
♀ **0U9F4ZX** Drainage of Cul-de-sac, Percutaneous Endoscopic Approach, Diagnostic
♀ **0U9F4ZZ** Drainage of Cul-de-sac, Percutaneous Endoscopic Approach
♀ **0U9F70Z** Drainage of Cul-de-sac with Drainage Device, Via Natural or Artificial Opening
♀ **0U9F7ZX** Drainage of Cul-de-sac, Via Natural or Artificial Opening, Diagnostic
♀ **0U9F7ZZ** Drainage of Cul-de-sac, Via Natural or Artificial Opening
♀ **0U9F80Z** Drainage of Cul-de-sac with Drainage Device, Via Natural or Artificial Opening Endoscopic
♀ **0U9F8ZX** Drainage of Cul-de-sac, Via Natural or Artificial Opening Endoscopic, Diagnostic
♀ **0U9F8ZZ** Drainage of Cul-de-sac, Via Natural or Artificial Opening Endoscopic
♀ **0U9G00Z** Drainage of Vagina with Drainage Device, Open Approach

♀ **0U9G0ZX** Drainage of Vagina, Open Approach, Diagnostic
♀ **0U9G0ZZ** Drainage of Vagina, Open Approach
♀ **0U9G30Z** Drainage of Vagina with Drainage Device, Percutaneous Approach
♀ **0U9G3ZX** Drainage of Vagina, Percutaneous Approach, Diagnostic
♀ **0U9G3ZZ** Drainage of Vagina, Percutaneous Approach
♀ **0U9G40Z** Drainage of Vagina with Drainage Device, Percutaneous Endoscopic Approach
♀ **0U9G4ZX** Drainage of Vagina, Percutaneous Endoscopic Approach, Diagnostic
♀ **0U9G4ZZ** Drainage of Vagina, Percutaneous Endoscopic Approach
♀ **0U9G70Z** Drainage of Vagina with Drainage Device, Via Natural or Artificial Opening
♀ **0U9G7ZX** Drainage of Vagina, Via Natural or Artificial Opening, Diagnostic
♀ **0U9G7ZZ** Drainage of Vagina, Via Natural or Artificial Opening
♀ **0U9G80Z** Drainage of Vagina with Drainage Device, Via Natural or Artificial Opening Endoscopic
♀ **0U9G8ZX** Drainage of Vagina, Via Natural or Artificial Opening Endoscopic, Diagnostic
♀ **0U9G8ZZ** Drainage of Vagina, Via Natural or Artificial Opening Endoscopic
♀ **0U9GX0Z** Drainage of Vagina with Drainage Device, External Approach
♀ **0U9GXZX** Drainage of Vagina, External Approach, Diagnostic
♀ **0U9GXZZ** Drainage of Vagina, External Approach
♀ **0U9J00Z** Drainage of Clitoris with Drainage Device, Open Approach
♀ **0U9J0ZX** Drainage of Clitoris, Open Approach, Diagnostic
♀ **0U9J0ZZ** Drainage of Clitoris, Open Approach
♀ **0U9JX0Z** Drainage of Clitoris with Drainage Device, External Approach
♀ **0U9JXZX** Drainage of Clitoris, External Approach, Diagnostic
♀ **0U9JXZZ** Drainage of Clitoris, External Approach
♀ **0U9K00Z** Drainage of Hymen with Drainage Device, Open Approach
♀ **0U9K0ZX** Drainage of Hymen, Open Approach, Diagnostic
♀ **0U9K0ZZ** Drainage of Hymen, Open Approach
♀ **0U9K30Z** Drainage of Hymen with Drainage Device, Percutaneous Approach
♀ **0U9K3ZX** Drainage of Hymen, Percutaneous Approach, Diagnostic
♀ **0U9K3ZZ** Drainage of Hymen, Percutaneous Approach
♀ **0U9K40Z** Drainage of Hymen with Drainage Device, Percutaneous Endoscopic Approach
♀ **0U9K4ZX** Drainage of Hymen, Percutaneous Endoscopic Approach, Diagnostic
♀ **0U9K4ZZ** Drainage of Hymen, Percutaneous Endoscopic Approach
♀ **0U9K70Z** Drainage of Hymen with Drainage Device, Via Natural or Artificial Opening
♀ **0U9K7ZX** Drainage of Hymen, Via Natural or Artificial Opening, Diagnostic
♀ **0U9K7ZZ** Drainage of Hymen, Via Natural or Artificial Opening
♀ **0U9K80Z** Drainage of Hymen with Drainage Device, Via Natural or Artificial Opening Endoscopic
♀ **0U9K8ZX** Drainage of Hymen, Via Natural or Artificial Opening Endoscopic, Diagnostic
♀ **0U9K8ZZ** Drainage of Hymen, Via Natural or Artificial Opening Endoscopic
♀ **0U9KX0Z** Drainage of Hymen with Drainage Device, External Approach
♀ **0U9KXZX** Drainage of Hymen, External Approach, Diagnostic
♀ **0U9KXZZ** Drainage of Hymen, External Approach
♀ **0U9L00Z** Drainage of Vestibular Gland with Drainage Device, Open Approach
♀ **0U9L0ZX** Drainage of Vestibular Gland, Open Approach, Diagnostic
♀ **0U9L0ZZ** Drainage of Vestibular Gland, Open Approach
♀ **0U9LX0Z** Drainage of Vestibular Gland with Drainage Device, External Approach
♀ **0U9LXZX** Drainage of Vestibular Gland, External Approach, Diagnostic
♀ **0U9LXZZ** Drainage of Vestibular Gland, External Approach
♀ **0U9M00Z** Drainage of Vulva with Drainage Device, Open Approach
♀ **0U9M0ZX** Drainage of Vulva, Open Approach, Diagnostic
♀ **0U9M0ZZ** Drainage of Vulva, Open Approach
♀ **0U9MX0Z** Drainage of Vulva with Drainage Device, External Approach
♀ **0U9MXZX** Drainage of Vulva, External Approach, Diagnostic
♀ **0U9MXZZ** Drainage of Vulva, External Approach

0UB – Female Reproductive System, Excision

Review Coding Guidelines B3.4a and B3.4b

Review Coding Guideline B3.8

♀ **0UB00ZX** Excision of Right Ovary, Open Approach, Diagnostic
♀ **0UB00ZZ** Excision of Right Ovary, Open Approach
♀ **0UB03ZX** Excision of Right Ovary, Percutaneous Approach, Diagnostic
♀ **0UB03ZZ** Excision of Right Ovary, Percutaneous Approach
♀ **0UB04ZX** Excision of Right Ovary, Percutaneous Endoscopic Approach, Diagnostic

♀ Female-only　♂ Male-only　● Limited Coverage　● Non-OR　▦ HAC-associated procedure　● Non-covered procedures　＋ Combination

♀ **0UB04ZZ** Excision of Right Ovary, Percutaneous Endoscopic Approach
♀ **0UB07ZX** Excision of Right Ovary, Via Natural or Artificial Opening, Diagnostic
♀ **0UB07ZZ** Excision of Right Ovary, Via Natural or Artificial Opening
♀ **0UB08ZX** Excision of Right Ovary, Via Natural or Artificial Opening Endoscopic, Diagnostic
♀ **0UB08ZZ** Excision of Right Ovary, Via Natural or Artificial Opening Endoscopic
♀ **0UB10ZX** Excision of Left Ovary, Open Approach, Diagnostic
♀ **0UB10ZZ** Excision of Left Ovary, Open Approach
♀ **0UB13ZX** Excision of Left Ovary, Percutaneous Approach, Diagnostic
♀ **0UB13ZZ** Excision of Left Ovary, Percutaneous Approach
♀ **0UB14ZX** Excision of Left Ovary, Percutaneous Endoscopic Approach, Diagnostic
♀ **0UB14ZZ** Excision of Left Ovary, Percutaneous Endoscopic Approach
♀ **0UB17ZX** Excision of Left Ovary, Via Natural or Artificial Opening, Diagnostic
♀ **0UB17ZZ** Excision of Left Ovary, Via Natural or Artificial Opening
♀ **0UB18ZX** Excision of Left Ovary, Via Natural or Artificial Opening Endoscopic, Diagnostic
♀ **0UB18ZZ** Excision of Left Ovary, Via Natural or Artificial Opening Endoscopic
♀ **0UB20ZX** Excision of Bilateral Ovaries, Open Approach, Diagnostic
♀ **0UB20ZZ** Excision of Bilateral Ovaries, Open Approach
♀ **0UB23ZX** Excision of Bilateral Ovaries, Percutaneous Approach, Diagnostic
♀ **0UB23ZZ** Excision of Bilateral Ovaries, Percutaneous Approach
♀ **0UB24ZX** Excision of Bilateral Ovaries, Percutaneous Endoscopic Approach, Diagnostic
♀ **0UB24ZZ** Excision of Bilateral Ovaries, Percutaneous Endoscopic Approach
♀ **0UB27ZX** Excision of Bilateral Ovaries, Via Natural or Artificial Opening, Diagnostic
♀ **0UB27ZZ** Excision of Bilateral Ovaries, Via Natural or Artificial Opening
♀ **0UB28ZX** Excision of Bilateral Ovaries, Via Natural or Artificial Opening Endoscopic, Diagnostic
♀ **0UB28ZZ** Excision of Bilateral Ovaries, Via Natural or Artificial Opening Endoscopic
♀ **0UB40ZX** Excision of Uterine Supporting Structure, Open Approach, Diagnostic
♀ **0UB40ZZ** Excision of Uterine Supporting Structure, Open Approach
♀ **0UB43ZX** Excision of Uterine Supporting Structure, Percutaneous Approach, Diagnostic
♀ **0UB43ZZ** Excision of Uterine Supporting Structure, Percutaneous Approach
♀ **0UB44ZX** Excision of Uterine Supporting Structure, Percutaneous Endoscopic Approach, Diagnostic
♀ **0UB44ZZ** Excision of Uterine Supporting Structure, Percutaneous Endoscopic Approach
♀ **0UB47ZX** Excision of Uterine Supporting Structure, Via Natural or Artificial Opening, Diagnostic
♀ **0UB47ZZ** Excision of Uterine Supporting Structure, Via Natural or Artificial Opening
♀ **0UB48ZX** Excision of Uterine Supporting Structure, Via Natural or Artificial Opening Endoscopic, Diagnostic
♀ **0UB48ZZ** Excision of Uterine Supporting Structure, Via Natural or Artificial Opening Endoscopic
♀ **0UB50ZX** Excision of Right Fallopian Tube, Open Approach, Diagnostic
♀ **0UB50ZZ** Excision of Right Fallopian Tube, Open Approach
♀ **0UB53ZX** Excision of Right Fallopian Tube, Percutaneous Approach, Diagnostic
♀ **0UB53ZZ** Excision of Right Fallopian Tube, Percutaneous Approach
♀ **0UB54ZX** Excision of Right Fallopian Tube, Percutaneous Endoscopic Approach, Diagnostic
♀ **0UB54ZZ** Excision of Right Fallopian Tube, Percutaneous Endoscopic Approach
♀ **0UB57ZX** Excision of Right Fallopian Tube, Via Natural or Artificial Opening, Diagnostic
♀ **0UB57ZZ** Excision of Right Fallopian Tube, Via Natural or Artificial Opening
♀ **0UB58ZX** Excision of Right Fallopian Tube, Via Natural or Artificial Opening Endoscopic, Diagnostic
♀ **0UB58ZZ** Excision of Right Fallopian Tube, Via Natural or Artificial Opening Endoscopic
♀ **0UB60ZX** Excision of Left Fallopian Tube, Open Approach, Diagnostic
♀ **0UB60ZZ** Excision of Left Fallopian Tube, Open Approach

♀ **0UB63ZX** Excision of Left Fallopian Tube, Percutaneous Approach, Diagnostic
♀ **0UB63ZZ** Excision of Left Fallopian Tube, Percutaneous Approach
♀ **0UB64ZX** Excision of Left Fallopian Tube, Percutaneous Endoscopic Approach, Diagnostic
♀ **0UB64ZZ** Excision of Left Fallopian Tube, Percutaneous Endoscopic Approach
♀ **0UB67ZX** Excision of Left Fallopian Tube, Via Natural or Artificial Opening, Diagnostic
♀ **0UB67ZZ** Excision of Left Fallopian Tube, Via Natural or Artificial Opening
♀ **0UB68ZX** Excision of Left Fallopian Tube, Via Natural or Artificial Opening Endoscopic, Diagnostic
♀ **0UB68ZZ** Excision of Left Fallopian Tube, Via Natural or Artificial Opening Endoscopic
♀ **0UB70ZX** Excision of Bilateral Fallopian Tubes, Open Approach, Diagnostic
♀ **0UB70ZZ** Excision of Bilateral Fallopian Tubes, Open Approach
♀ **0UB73ZX** Excision of Bilateral Fallopian Tubes, Percutaneous Approach, Diagnostic
♀ **0UB73ZZ** Excision of Bilateral Fallopian Tubes, Percutaneous Approach
♀ **0UB74ZX** Excision of Bilateral Fallopian Tubes, Percutaneous Endoscopic Approach, Diagnostic
♀ **0UB74ZZ** Excision of Bilateral Fallopian Tubes, Percutaneous Endoscopic Approach
♀ **0UB77ZX** Excision of Bilateral Fallopian Tubes, Via Natural or Artificial Opening, Diagnostic
♀ **0UB77ZZ** Excision of Bilateral Fallopian Tubes, Via Natural or Artificial Opening
♀ **0UB78ZX** Excision of Bilateral Fallopian Tubes, Via Natural or Artificial Opening Endoscopic, Diagnostic
♀ **0UB78ZZ** Excision of Bilateral Fallopian Tubes, Via Natural or Artificial Opening Endoscopic
♀ **0UB90ZX** Excision of Uterus, Open Approach, Diagnostic
♀ **0UB90ZZ** Excision of Uterus, Open Approach
♀ **0UB93ZX** Excision of Uterus, Percutaneous Approach, Diagnostic
♀ **0UB93ZZ** Excision of Uterus, Percutaneous Approach
♀ **0UB94ZX** Excision of Uterus, Percutaneous Endoscopic Approach, Diagnostic
♀ **0UB94ZZ** Excision of Uterus, Percutaneous Endoscopic Approach
♀ **0UB97ZX** Excision of Uterus, Via Natural or Artificial Opening, Diagnostic
♀ **0UB97ZZ** Excision of Uterus, Via Natural or Artificial Opening
♀ **0UB98ZX** Excision of Uterus, Via Natural or Artificial Opening Endoscopic, Diagnostic
♀ **0UB98ZZ** Excision of Uterus, Via Natural or Artificial Opening Endoscopic
♀ **0UBC0ZX** Excision of Cervix, Open Approach, Diagnostic
♀ **0UBC0ZZ** Excision of Cervix, Open Approach
♀ **0UBC3ZX** Excision of Cervix, Percutaneous Approach, Diagnostic
♀ **0UBC3ZZ** Excision of Cervix, Percutaneous Approach
♀ **0UBC4ZX** Excision of Cervix, Percutaneous Endoscopic Approach, Diagnostic
♀ **0UBC4ZZ** Excision of Cervix, Percutaneous Endoscopic Approach
♀ **0UBC7ZX** Excision of Cervix, Via Natural or Artificial Opening, Diagnostic
♀ **0UBC7ZZ** Excision of Cervix, Via Natural or Artificial Opening
♀ **0UBC8ZX** Excision of Cervix, Via Natural or Artificial Opening Endoscopic, Diagnostic
♀ **0UBC8ZZ** Excision of Cervix, Via Natural or Artificial Opening Endoscopic
♀ **0UBF0ZX** Excision of Cul-de-sac, Open Approach, Diagnostic
♀ **0UBF0ZZ** Excision of Cul-de-sac, Open Approach
♀ **0UBF3ZX** Excision of Cul-de-sac, Percutaneous Approach, Diagnostic
♀ **0UBF3ZZ** Excision of Cul-de-sac, Percutaneous Approach
♀ **0UBF4ZX** Excision of Cul-de-sac, Percutaneous Endoscopic Approach, Diagnostic
♀ **0UBF4ZZ** Excision of Cul-de-sac, Percutaneous Endoscopic Approach
♀ **0UBF7ZX** Excision of Cul-de-sac, Via Natural or Artificial Opening, Diagnostic
♀ **0UBF7ZZ** Excision of Cul-de-sac, Via Natural or Artificial Opening
♀ **0UBF8ZX** Excision of Cul-de-sac, Via Natural or Artificial Opening Endoscopic, Diagnostic
♀ **0UBF8ZZ** Excision of Cul-de-sac, Via Natural or Artificial Opening Endoscopic
♀ **0UBG0ZX** Excision of Vagina, Open Approach, Diagnostic
♀ **0UBG0ZZ** Excision of Vagina, Open Approach
♀ **0UBG3ZX** Excision of Vagina, Percutaneous Approach, Diagnostic
♀ **0UBG3ZZ** Excision of Vagina, Percutaneous Approach
♀ **0UBG4ZX** Excision of Vagina, Percutaneous Endoscopic Approach, Diagnostic

♀ **0UBG4ZZ** Excision of Vagina, Percutaneous Endoscopic Approach
♀ **0UBG7ZX** Excision of Vagina, Via Natural or Artificial Opening, Diagnostic
♀ **0UBG7ZZ** Excision of Vagina, Via Natural or Artificial Opening
♀ **0UBG8ZX** Excision of Vagina, Via Natural or Artificial Opening Endoscopic, Diagnostic
♀ **0UBG8ZZ** Excision of Vagina, Via Natural or Artificial Opening Endoscopic
♀ **0UBGXZX** Excision of Vagina, External Approach, Diagnostic
♀ **0UBGXZZ** Excision of Vagina, External Approach
♀ **0UBJ0ZX** Excision of Clitoris, Open Approach, Diagnostic
♀ **0UBJ0ZZ** Excision of Clitoris, Open Approach
♀ **0UBJXZX** Excision of Clitoris, External Approach, Diagnostic
♀ **0UBJXZZ** Excision of Clitoris, External Approach
♀ **0UBK0ZX** Excision of Hymen, Open Approach, Diagnostic
♀ **0UBK0ZZ** Excision of Hymen, Open Approach
♀ **0UBK3ZX** Excision of Hymen, Percutaneous Approach, Diagnostic
♀ **0UBK3ZZ** Excision of Hymen, Percutaneous Approach
♀ **0UBK4ZX** Excision of Hymen, Percutaneous Endoscopic Approach, Diagnostic

♀ **0UBK4ZZ** Excision of Hymen, Percutaneous Endoscopic Approach
♀ **0UBK7ZX** Excision of Hymen, Via Natural or Artificial Opening, Diagnostic
♀ **0UBK7ZZ** Excision of Hymen, Via Natural or Artificial Opening
♀ **0UBK8ZX** Excision of Hymen, Via Natural or Artificial Opening Endoscopic, Diagnostic
♀ **0UBK8ZZ** Excision of Hymen, Via Natural or Artificial Opening Endoscopic
♀ **0UBKXZX** Excision of Hymen, External Approach, Diagnostic
♀ **0UBKXZZ** Excision of Hymen, External Approach
♀ **0UBL0ZX** Excision of Vestibular Gland, Open Approach, Diagnostic
♀ **0UBL0ZZ** Excision of Vestibular Gland, Open Approach
♀ **0UBLXZX** Excision of Vestibular Gland, External Approach, Diagnostic
♀ **0UBLXZZ** Excision of Vestibular Gland, External Approach
♀ **0UBM0ZX** Excision of Vulva, Open Approach, Diagnostic
♀ **0UBM0ZZ** Excision of Vulva, Open Approach
♀ **0UBMXZX** Excision of Vulva, External Approach, Diagnostic
♀ **0UBMXZZ** Excision of Vulva, External Approach

0UC – Female Reproductive System, Extirpation

♀ **0UC00ZZ** Extirpation of Matter from Right Ovary, Open Approach
♀ **0UC03ZZ** Extirpation of Matter from Right Ovary, Percutaneous Approach
♀ **0UC04ZZ** Extirpation of Matter from Right Ovary, Percutaneous Endoscopic Approach
♀ **0UC10ZZ** Extirpation of Matter from Left Ovary, Open Approach
♀ **0UC13ZZ** Extirpation of Matter from Left Ovary, Percutaneous Approach
♀ **0UC14ZZ** Extirpation of Matter from Left Ovary, Percutaneous Endoscopic Approach
♀ **0UC20ZZ** Extirpation of Matter from Bilateral Ovaries, Open Approach
♀ **0UC23ZZ** Extirpation of Matter from Bilateral Ovaries, Percutaneous Approach
♀ **0UC24ZZ** Extirpation of Matter from Bilateral Ovaries, Percutaneous Endoscopic Approach
♀ **0UC40ZZ** Extirpation of Matter from Uterine Supporting Structure, Open Approach
♀ **0UC43ZZ** Extirpation of Matter from Uterine Supporting Structure, Percutaneous Approach
♀ **0UC44ZZ** Extirpation of Matter from Uterine Supporting Structure, Percutaneous Endoscopic Approach
♀ **0UC50ZZ** Extirpation of Matter from Right Fallopian Tube, Open Approach
♀ **0UC53ZZ** Extirpation of Matter from Right Fallopian Tube, Percutaneous Approach
♀ **0UC54ZZ** Extirpation of Matter from Right Fallopian Tube, Percutaneous Endoscopic Approach
♀ **0UC57ZZ** Extirpation of Matter from Right Fallopian Tube, Via Natural or Artificial Opening
♀ **0UC58ZZ** Extirpation of Matter from Right Fallopian Tube, Via Natural or Artificial Opening Endoscopic
♀ **0UC60ZZ** Extirpation of Matter from Left Fallopian Tube, Open Approach
♀ **0UC63ZZ** Extirpation of Matter from Left Fallopian Tube, Percutaneous Approach
♀ **0UC64ZZ** Extirpation of Matter from Left Fallopian Tube, Percutaneous Endoscopic Approach
♀ **0UC67ZZ** Extirpation of Matter from Left Fallopian Tube, Via Natural or Artificial Opening
♀ **0UC68ZZ** Extirpation of Matter from Left Fallopian Tube, Via Natural or Artificial Opening Endoscopic
♀ **0UC70ZZ** Extirpation of Matter from Bilateral Fallopian Tubes, Open Approach
♀ **0UC73ZZ** Extirpation of Matter from Bilateral Fallopian Tubes, Percutaneous Approach
♀ **0UC74ZZ** Extirpation of Matter from Bilateral Fallopian Tubes, Percutaneous Endoscopic Approach
♀ **0UC77ZZ** Extirpation of Matter from Bilateral Fallopian Tubes, Via Natural or Artificial Opening
♀ **0UC78ZZ** Extirpation of Matter from Bilateral Fallopian Tubes, Via Natural or Artificial Opening Endoscopic
♀ **0UC90ZZ** Extirpation of Matter from Uterus, Open Approach
♀ **0UC93ZZ** Extirpation of Matter from Uterus, Percutaneous Approach
♀ **0UC94ZZ** Extirpation of Matter from Uterus, Percutaneous Endoscopic Approach

♀ **0UC97ZZ** Extirpation of Matter from Uterus, Via Natural or Artificial Opening
♀ **0UC98ZZ** Extirpation of Matter from Uterus, Via Natural or Artificial Opening Endoscopic
♀ **0UCB0ZZ** Extirpation of Matter from Endometrium, Open Approach
♀ **0UCB3ZZ** Extirpation of Matter from Endometrium, Percutaneous Approach
♀ **0UCB4ZZ** Extirpation of Matter from Endometrium, Percutaneous Endoscopic Approach
♀ **0UCB7ZZ** Extirpation of Matter from Endometrium, Via Natural or Artificial Opening
♀ **0UCB8ZZ** Extirpation of Matter from Endometrium, Via Natural or Artificial Opening Endoscopic
♀ **0UCC0ZZ** Extirpation of Matter from Cervix, Open Approach
♀ **0UCC3ZZ** Extirpation of Matter from Cervix, Percutaneous Approach
♀ **0UCC4ZZ** Extirpation of Matter from Cervix, Percutaneous Endoscopic Approach
♀ **0UCC7ZZ** Extirpation of Matter from Cervix, Via Natural or Artificial Opening
♀ **0UCC8ZZ** Extirpation of Matter from Cervix, Via Natural or Artificial Opening Endoscopic
♀ **0UCF0ZZ** Extirpation of Matter from Cul-de-sac, Open Approach
♀ **0UCF3ZZ** Extirpation of Matter from Cul-de-sac, Percutaneous Approach
♀ **0UCF4ZZ** Extirpation of Matter from Cul-de-sac, Percutaneous Endoscopic Approach
♀ **0UCF7ZZ** Extirpation of Matter from Cul-de-sac, Via Natural or Artificial Opening
♀ **0UCF8ZZ** Extirpation of Matter from Cul-de-sac, Via Natural or Artificial Opening Endoscopic
♀ **0UCG0ZZ** Extirpation of Matter from Vagina, Open Approach
♀ **0UCG3ZZ** Extirpation of Matter from Vagina, Percutaneous Approach
♀ **0UCG4ZZ** Extirpation of Matter from Vagina, Percutaneous Endoscopic Approach
♀ **0UCG7ZZ** Extirpation of Matter from Vagina, Via Natural or Artificial Opening
♀ **0UCG8ZZ** Extirpation of Matter from Vagina, Via Natural or Artificial Opening Endoscopic
♀ **0UCGXZZ** Extirpation of Matter from Vagina, External Approach
♀ **0UCJ0ZZ** Extirpation of Matter from Clitoris, Open Approach
♀ **0UCJXZZ** Extirpation of Matter from Clitoris, External Approach
♀ **0UCK0ZZ** Extirpation of Matter from Hymen, Open Approach
♀ **0UCK3ZZ** Extirpation of Matter from Hymen, Percutaneous Approach
♀ **0UCK4ZZ** Extirpation of Matter from Hymen, Percutaneous Endoscopic Approach
♀ **0UCK7ZZ** Extirpation of Matter from Hymen, Via Natural or Artificial Opening
♀ **0UCK8ZZ** Extirpation of Matter from Hymen, Via Natural or Artificial Opening Endoscopic
♀ **0UCKXZZ** Extirpation of Matter from Hymen, External Approach
♀ **0UCL0ZZ** Extirpation of Matter from Vestibular Gland, Open Approach
♀ **0UCLXZZ** Extirpation of Matter from Vestibular Gland, External Approach
♀ **0UCM0ZZ** Extirpation of Matter from Vulva, Open Approach
♀ **0UCMXZZ** Extirpation of Matter from Vulva, External Approach

0UD – Female Reproductive System, Extraction

Review Coding Guidelines B3.4a and B3.4b

Review Coding Guideline C2

♀ **0UDB7ZX** Extraction of Endometrium, Via Natural or Artificial Opening, Diagnostic
♀ **0UDB7ZZ** Extraction of Endometrium, Via Natural or Artificial Opening
♀ **0UDB8ZX** Extraction of Endometrium, Via Natural or Artificial Opening Endoscopic, Diagnostic

♀ **0UDB8ZZ** Extraction of Endometrium, Via Natural or Artificial Opening Endoscopic
♀ **0UDN0ZZ** Extraction of Ova, Open
♀ **0UDN3ZZ** Extraction of Ova, Percutaneous
♀ **0UDN4ZZ** Extraction of Ova, Percutaneous Endoscopic

0UF – Female Reproductive System, Fragmentation

♀ **0UF50ZZ** Fragmentation in Right Fallopian Tube, Open Approach
♀ **0UF53ZZ** Fragmentation in Right Fallopian Tube, Percutaneous Approach
♀ **0UF54ZZ** Fragmentation in Right Fallopian Tube, Percutaneous Endoscopic Approach
♀ **0UF57ZZ** Fragmentation in Right Fallopian Tube, Via Natural or Artificial Opening
♀ **0UF58ZZ** Fragmentation in Right Fallopian Tube, Via Natural or Artificial Opening Endoscopic
⬣ **0UF5XZZ** Fragmentation in Right Fallopian Tube, External Approach
♀ **0UF60ZZ** Fragmentation in Left Fallopian Tube, Open Approach
♀ **0UF63ZZ** Fragmentation in Left Fallopian Tube, Percutaneous Approach
♀ **0UF64ZZ** Fragmentation in Left Fallopian Tube, Percutaneous Endoscopic Approach
♀ **0UF67ZZ** Fragmentation in Left Fallopian Tube, Via Natural or Artificial Opening
♀ **0UF68ZZ** Fragmentation in Left Fallopian Tube, Via Natural or Artificial Opening Endoscopic
⬣ ♀ **0UF6XZZ** Fragmentation in Left Fallopian Tube, External Approach

♀ **0UF70ZZ** Fragmentation in Bilateral Fallopian Tubes, Open Approach
♀ **0UF73ZZ** Fragmentation in Bilateral Fallopian Tubes, Percutaneous Approach
♀ **0UF74ZZ** Fragmentation in Bilateral Fallopian Tubes, Percutaneous Endoscopic Approach
♀ **0UF77ZZ** Fragmentation in Bilateral Fallopian Tubes, Via Natural or Artificial Opening
♀ **0UF78ZZ** Fragmentation in Bilateral Fallopian Tubes, Via Natural or Artificial Opening Endoscopic
⬣ **0UF7XZZ** Fragmentation in Bilateral Fallopian Tubes, External Approach
♀ **0UF90ZZ** Fragmentation in Uterus, Open Approach
♀ **0UF93ZZ** Fragmentation in Uterus, Percutaneous Approach
♀ **0UF94ZZ** Fragmentation in Uterus, Percutaneous Endoscopic Approach
♀ **0UF97ZZ** Fragmentation in Uterus, Via Natural or Artificial Opening
♀ **0UF98ZZ** Fragmentation in Uterus, Via Natural or Artificial Opening Endoscopic
⬣ ♀ **0UF9XZZ** Fragmentation in Uterus, External Approach

0UH – Female Reproductive System, Insertion

♀ **0UH303Z** Insertion of Infusion Device into Ovary, Open Approach
♀ **0UH333Z** Insertion of Infusion Device into Ovary, Percutaneous Approach
♀ **0UH343Z** Insertion of Infusion Device into Ovary, Percutaneous Endoscopic Approach
♀ **0UH803Z** Insertion of Infusion Device into Fallopian Tube, Open Approach
♀ **0UH833Z** Insertion of Infusion Device into Fallopian Tube, Percutaneous Approach
♀ **0UH843Z** Insertion of Infusion Device into Fallopian Tube, Percutaneous Endoscopic Approach
♀ **0UH873Z** Insertion of Infusion Device into Fallopian Tube, Via Natural or Artificial Opening
♀ **0UH883Z** Insertion of Infusion Device into Fallopian Tube, Via Natural or Artificial Opening Endoscopic
♀ **0UH97HZ** Insertion of Contraceptive Device into Uterus, Via Natural or Artificial Opening
♀ **0UH98HZ** Insertion of Contraceptive Device into Uterus, Via Natural or Artificial Opening Endoscopic
♀ **0UHC01Z** Insertion of Radioactive Element into Cervix, Open Approach
♀ **0UHC31Z** Insertion of Radioactive Element into Cervix, Percutaneous Approach
♀ **0UHC41Z** Insertion of Radioactive Element into Cervix, Percutaneous Endoscopic Approach
♀ **0UHC71Z** Insertion of Radioactive Element into Cervix, Via Natural or Artificial Opening
♀ **0UHC7HZ** Insertion of Contraceptive Device into Cervix, Via Natural or Artificial Opening
♀ **0UHC81Z** Insertion of Radioactive Element into Cervix, Via Natural or Artificial Opening Endoscopic
♀ **0UHC8HZ** Insertion of Contraceptive Device into Cervix, Via Natural or Artificial Opening Endoscopic
♀ **0UHD03Z** Insertion of Infusion Device into Uterus and Cervix, Open Approach
♀ **0UHD33Z** Insertion of Infusion Device into Uterus and Cervix, Percutaneous Approach

♀ **0UHD43Z** Insertion of Infusion Device into Uterus and Cervix, Percutaneous Endoscopic Approach
♀ **0UHD73Z** Insertion of Infusion Device into Uterus and Cervix, Via Natural or Artificial Opening
♀ **0UHD83Z** Insertion of Infusion Device into Uterus and Cervix, Via Natural or Artificial Opening Endoscopic
♀ **0UHF7GZ** Insertion of Pessary into Cul-de-sac, Via Natural or Artificial Opening
♀ **0UHF8GZ** Insertion of Pessary into Cul-de-sac, Via Natural or Artificial Opening Endoscopic
♀ **0UHG01Z** Insertion of Radioactive Element into Vagina, Open Approach
♀ **0UHG31Z** Insertion of Radioactive Element into Vagina, Percutaneous Approach
♀ **0UHG41Z** Insertion of Radioactive Element into Vagina, Percutaneous Endoscopic Approach
♀ **0UHG71Z** Insertion of Radioactive Element into Vagina, Via Natural or Artificial Opening
♀ **0UHG7GZ** Insertion of Pessary into Vagina, Via Natural or Artificial Opening
♀ **0UHG81Z** Insertion of Radioactive Element into Vagina, Via Natural or Artificial Opening Endoscopic
♀ **0UHG8GZ** Insertion of Pessary into Vagina, Via Natural or Artificial Opening Endoscopic
♀ **0UHGX1Z** Insertion of Radioactive Element into Vagina, External Approach
♀ **0UHH03Z** Insertion of Infusion Device into Vagina and Cul-de-sac, Open Approach
♀ **0UHH33Z** Insertion of Infusion Device into Vagina and Cul-de-sac, Percutaneous Approach
♀ **0UHH43Z** Insertion of Infusion Device into Vagina and Cul-de-sac, Percutaneous Endoscopic Approach
♀ **0UHH73Z** Insertion of Infusion Device into Vagina and Cul-de-sac, Via Natural or Artificial Opening
♀ **0UHH83Z** Insertion of Infusion Device into Vagina and Cul-de-sac, Via Natural or Artificial Opening Endoscopic

0UJ   *Female Reproductive System, Inspection*

Review Coding Guidelines B3.11a, B3.11b and B3.11c

♀ **0UJ30ZZ** Inspection of Ovary, Open Approach
♀ **0UJ33ZZ** Inspection of Ovary, Percutaneous Approach
♀ **0UJ34ZZ** Inspection of Ovary, Percutaneous Endoscopic Approach
♀ **0UJ3XZZ** Inspection of Ovary, External Approach
♀ **0UJ80ZZ** Inspection of Fallopian Tube, Open Approach
♀ **0UJ83ZZ** Inspection of Fallopian Tube, Percutaneous Approach
♀ **0UJ84ZZ** Inspection of Fallopian Tube, Percutaneous Endoscopic Approach
♀ **0UJ87ZZ** Inspection of Fallopian Tube, Via Natural or Artificial Opening
♀ **0UJ88ZZ** Inspection of Fallopian Tube, Via Natural or Artificial Opening Endoscopic
♀ **0UJ8XZZ** Inspection of Fallopian Tube, External Approach
♀ **0UJD0ZZ** Inspection of Uterus and Cervix, Open Approach
♀ **0UJD3ZZ** Inspection of Uterus and Cervix, Percutaneous Approach
♀ **0UJD4ZZ** Inspection of Uterus and Cervix, Percutaneous Endoscopic Approach

♀ **0UJD7ZZ** Inspection of Uterus and Cervix, Via Natural or Artificial Opening
♀ **0UJD8ZZ** Inspection of Uterus and Cervix, Via Natural or Artificial Opening Endoscopic
♀ **0UJDXZZ** Inspection of Uterus and Cervix, External Approach
♀ **0UJH0ZZ** Inspection of Vagina and Cul-de-sac, Open Approach
♀ **0UJH3ZZ** Inspection of Vagina and Cul-de-sac, Percutaneous Approach
♀ **0UJH4ZZ** Inspection of Vagina and Cul-de-sac, Percutaneous Endoscopic Approach
♀ **0UJH7ZZ** Inspection of Vagina and Cul-de-sac, Via Natural or Artificial Opening
♀ **0UJH8ZZ** Inspection of Vagina and Cul-de-sac, Via Natural or Artificial Opening Endoscopic
♀ **0UJHXZZ** Inspection of Vagina and Cul-de-sac, External Approach
♀ **0UJM0ZZ** Inspection of Vulva, Open Approach
♀ **0UJMXZZ** Inspection of Vulva, External Approach

0UL – *Female Reproductive System, Occlusion*

♀ **0UL50CZ** Occlusion of Right Fallopian Tube with Extraluminal Device, Open Approach
♀ **0UL50DZ** Occlusion of Right Fallopian Tube with Intraluminal Device, Open Approach
♀ **0UL50ZZ** Occlusion of Right Fallopian Tube, Open Approach
♀ **0UL53CZ** Occlusion of Right Fallopian Tube with Extraluminal Device, Percutaneous Approach
♀ **0UL53DZ** Occlusion of Right Fallopian Tube with Intraluminal Device, Percutaneous Approach
♀ **0UL53ZZ** Occlusion of Right Fallopian Tube, Percutaneous Approach
♀ **0UL54CZ** Occlusion of Right Fallopian Tube with Extraluminal Device, Percutaneous Endoscopic Approach
♀ **0UL54DZ** Occlusion of Right Fallopian Tube with Intraluminal Device, Percutaneous Endoscopic Approach
♀ **0UL54ZZ** Occlusion of Right Fallopian Tube, Percutaneous Endoscopic Approach
♀ **0UL57DZ** Occlusion of Right Fallopian Tube with Intraluminal Device, Via Natural or Artificial Opening
♀ **0UL57ZZ** Occlusion of Right Fallopian Tube, Via Natural or Artificial Opening
♀ **0UL58DZ** Occlusion of Right Fallopian Tube with Intraluminal Device, Via Natural or Artificial Opening Endoscopic
♀ **0UL58ZZ** Occlusion of Right Fallopian Tube, Via Natural or Artificial Opening Endoscopic
♀ **0UL60CZ** Occlusion of Left Fallopian Tube with Extraluminal Device, Open Approach
♀ **0UL60DZ** Occlusion of Left Fallopian Tube with Intraluminal Device, Open Approach
♀ **0UL60ZZ** Occlusion of Left Fallopian Tube, Open Approach
♀ **0UL63CZ** Occlusion of Left Fallopian Tube with Extraluminal Device, Percutaneous Approach
♀ **0UL63DZ** Occlusion of Left Fallopian Tube with Intraluminal Device, Percutaneous Approach
♀ **0UL63ZZ** Occlusion of Left Fallopian Tube, Percutaneous Approach
♀ **0UL64CZ** Occlusion of Left Fallopian Tube with Extraluminal Device, Percutaneous Endoscopic Approach
♀ **0UL64DZ** Occlusion of Left Fallopian Tube with Intraluminal Device, Percutaneous Endoscopic Approach
♀ **0UL64ZZ** Occlusion of Left Fallopian Tube, Percutaneous Endoscopic Approach
♀ **0UL67DZ** Occlusion of Left Fallopian Tube with Intraluminal Device, Via Natural or Artificial Opening

♀ **0UL67ZZ** Occlusion of Left Fallopian Tube, Via Natural or Artificial Opening
♀ **0UL68DZ** Occlusion of Left Fallopian Tube with Intraluminal Device, Via Natural or Artificial Opening Endoscopic
♀ **0UL68ZZ** Occlusion of Left Fallopian Tube, Via Natural or Artificial Opening Endoscopic
⬤♀ **0UL70CZ** Occlusion of Bilateral Fallopian Tubes with Extraluminal Device, Open Approach
⬤♀ **0UL70DZ** Occlusion of Bilateral Fallopian Tubes with Intraluminal Device, Open Approach
⬤♀ **0UL70ZZ** Occlusion of Bilateral Fallopian Tubes, Open Approach
⬤♀ **0UL73CZ** Occlusion of Bilateral Fallopian Tubes with Extraluminal Device, Percutaneous Approach
⬤♀ **0UL73DZ** Occlusion of Bilateral Fallopian Tubes with Intraluminal Device, Percutaneous Approach
⬤♀ **0UL73ZZ** Occlusion of Bilateral Fallopian Tubes, Percutaneous Approach
⬤♀ **0UL74CZ** Occlusion of Bilateral Fallopian Tubes with Extraluminal Device, Percutaneous Endoscopic Approach
⬤♀ **0UL74DZ** Occlusion of Bilateral Fallopian Tubes with Intraluminal Device, Percutaneous Endoscopic Approach
⬤♀ **0UL74ZZ** Occlusion of Bilateral Fallopian Tubes, Percutaneous Endoscopic Approach
⬤♀ **0UL77DZ** Occlusion of Bilateral Fallopian Tubes with Intraluminal Device, Via Natural or Artificial Opening
⬤♀ **0UL77ZZ** Occlusion of Bilateral Fallopian Tubes, Via Natural or Artificial Opening
⬤♀ **0UL78DZ** Occlusion of Bilateral Fallopian Tubes with Intraluminal Device, Via Natural or Artificial Opening Endoscopic
⬤♀ **0UL78ZZ** Occlusion of Bilateral Fallopian Tubes, Via Natural or Artificial Opening Endoscopic
♀ **0ULF7DZ** Occlusion of Cul-de-sac with Intraluminal Device, Via Natural or Artificial Opening
♀ **0ULF7ZZ** Occlusion of Cul-de-sac, Via Natural or Artificial Opening
♀ **0ULF8DZ** Occlusion of Cul-de-sac with Intraluminal Device, Via Natural or Artificial Opening Endoscopic
♀ **0ULF8ZZ** Occlusion of Cul-de-sac, Via Natural or Artificial Opening Endoscopic
♀ **0ULG7DZ** Occlusion of Vagina with Intraluminal Device, Via Natural or Artificial Opening
♀ **0ULG7ZZ** Occlusion of Vagina, Via Natural or Artificial Opening
♀ **0ULG8DZ** Occlusion of Vagina with Intraluminal Device, Via Natural or Artificial Opening Endoscopic
♀ **0ULG8ZZ** Occlusion of Vagina, Via Natural or Artificial Opening Endoscopic

0UM – *Female Reproductive System, Reattachment*

♀ **0UM00ZZ** Reattachment of Right Ovary, Open Approach
♀ **0UM04ZZ** Reattachment of Right Ovary, Percutaneous Endoscopic Approach
♀ **0UM10ZZ** Reattachment of Left Ovary, Open Approach
♀ **0UM14ZZ** Reattachment of Left Ovary, Percutaneous Endoscopic Approach

♀ **0UM20ZZ** Reattachment of Bilateral Ovaries, Open Approach
♀ **0UM24ZZ** Reattachment of Bilateral Ovaries, Percutaneous Endoscopic Approach
♀ **0UM40ZZ** Reattachment of Uterine Supporting Structure, Open Approach

♀ **0UM44ZZ** Reattachment of Uterine Supporting Structure, Percutaneous Endoscopic Approach
♀ **0UM50ZZ** Reattachment of Right Fallopian Tube, Open Approach
♀ **0UM54ZZ** Reattachment of Right Fallopian Tube, Percutaneous Endoscopic Approach
♀ **0UM60ZZ** Reattachment of Left Fallopian Tube, Open Approach
♀ **0UM64ZZ** Reattachment of Left Fallopian Tube, Percutaneous Endoscopic Approach
♀ **0UM70ZZ** Reattachment of Bilateral Fallopian Tubes, Open Approach
♀ **0UM74ZZ** Reattachment of Bilateral Fallopian Tubes, Percutaneous Endoscopic Approach
♀ **0UM90ZZ** Reattachment of Uterus, Open Approach

♀ **0UM94ZZ** Reattachment of Uterus, Percutaneous Endoscopic Approach
♀ **0UMC0ZZ** Reattachment of Cervix, Open Approach
♀ **0UMC4ZZ** Reattachment of Cervix, Percutaneous Endoscopic Approach
♀ **0UMF0ZZ** Reattachment of Cul-de-sac, Open Approach
♀ **0UMF4ZZ** Reattachment of Cul-de-sac, Percutaneous Endoscopic Approach
♀ **0UMG0ZZ** Reattachment of Vagina, Open Approach
♀ **0UMG4ZZ** Reattachment of Vagina, Percutaneous Endoscopic Approach
♀ **0UMJXZZ** Reattachment of Clitoris, External Approach
♀ **0UMK0ZZ** Reattachment of Hymen, Open Approach
♀ **0UMK4ZZ** Reattachment of Hymen, Percutaneous Endoscopic Approach
♀ **0UMKXZZ** Reattachment of Hymen, External Approach
♀ **0UMMXZZ** Reattachment of Vulva, External Approach

0UN – Female Reproductive System, Release

Review Coding Guideline B3.13

Review Coding Guideline B3.14

♀ **0UN00ZZ** Release Right Ovary, Open Approach
♀ **0UN03ZZ** Release Right Ovary, Percutaneous Approach
♀ **0UN04ZZ** Release Right Ovary, Percutaneous Endoscopic Approach
♀ **0UN10ZZ** Release Left Ovary, Open Approach
♀ **0UN13ZZ** Release Left Ovary, Percutaneous Approach
♀ **0UN14ZZ** Release Left Ovary, Percutaneous Endoscopic Approach
♀ **0UN20ZZ** Release Bilateral Ovaries, Open Approach
♀ **0UN23ZZ** Release Bilateral Ovaries, Percutaneous Approach
♀ **0UN24ZZ** Release Bilateral Ovaries, Percutaneous Endoscopic Approach
♀ **0UN40ZZ** Release Uterine Supporting Structure, Open Approach
♀ **0UN43ZZ** Release Uterine Supporting Structure, Percutaneous Approach
♀ **0UN44ZZ** Release Uterine Supporting Structure, Percutaneous Endoscopic Approach
♀ **0UN50ZZ** Release Right Fallopian Tube, Open Approach
♀ **0UN53ZZ** Release Right Fallopian Tube, Percutaneous Approach
♀ **0UN54ZZ** Release Right Fallopian Tube, Percutaneous Endoscopic Approach
♀ **0UN57ZZ** Release Right Fallopian Tube, Via Natural or Artificial Opening
♀ **0UN58ZZ** Release Right Fallopian Tube, Via Natural or Artificial Opening Endoscopic
♀ **0UN60ZZ** Release Left Fallopian Tube, Open Approach
♀ **0UN63ZZ** Release Left Fallopian Tube, Percutaneous Approach
♀ **0UN64ZZ** Release Left Fallopian Tube, Percutaneous Endoscopic Approach
♀ **0UN67ZZ** Release Left Fallopian Tube, Via Natural or Artificial Opening
♀ **0UN68ZZ** Release Left Fallopian Tube, Via Natural or Artificial Opening Endoscopic
♀ **0UN70ZZ** Release Bilateral Fallopian Tubes, Open Approach
♀ **0UN73ZZ** Release Bilateral Fallopian Tubes, Percutaneous Approach
♀ **0UN74ZZ** Release Bilateral Fallopian Tubes, Percutaneous Endoscopic Approach
♀ **0UN77ZZ** Release Bilateral Fallopian Tubes, Via Natural or Artificial Opening
♀ **0UN78ZZ** Release Bilateral Fallopian Tubes, Via Natural or Artificial Opening Endoscopic

♀ **0UN90ZZ** Release Uterus, Open Approach
♀ **0UN93ZZ** Release Uterus, Percutaneous Approach
♀ **0UN94ZZ** Release Uterus, Percutaneous Endoscopic Approach
♀ **0UN97ZZ** Release Uterus, Via Natural or Artificial Opening
♀ **0UN98ZZ** Release Uterus, Via Natural or Artificial Opening Endoscopic
♀ **0UNC0ZZ** Release Cervix, Open Approach
♀ **0UNC3ZZ** Release Cervix, Percutaneous Approach
♀ **0UNC4ZZ** Release Cervix, Percutaneous Endoscopic Approach
♀ **0UNC7ZZ** Release Cervix, Via Natural or Artificial Opening
♀ **0UNC8ZZ** Release Cervix, Via Natural or Artificial Opening Endoscopic
♀ **0UNF0ZZ** Release Cul-de-sac, Open Approach
♀ **0UNF3ZZ** Release Cul-de-sac, Percutaneous Approach
♀ **0UNF4ZZ** Release Cul-de-sac, Percutaneous Endoscopic Approach
♀ **0UNF7ZZ** Release Cul-de-sac, Via Natural or Artificial Opening
♀ **0UNF8ZZ** Release Cul-de-sac, Via Natural or Artificial Opening Endoscopic
♀ **0UNG0ZZ** Release Vagina, Open Approach
♀ **0UNG3ZZ** Release Vagina, Percutaneous Approach
♀ **0UNG4ZZ** Release Vagina, Percutaneous Endoscopic Approach
♀ **0UNG7ZZ** Release Vagina, Via Natural or Artificial Opening
♀ **0UNG8ZZ** Release Vagina, Via Natural or Artificial Opening Endoscopic
♀ **0UNGXZZ** Release Vagina, External Approach
♀ **0UNJ0ZZ** Release Clitoris, Open Approach
♀ **0UNJXZZ** Release Clitoris, External Approach
♀ **0UNK0ZZ** Release Hymen, Open Approach
♀ **0UNK3ZZ** Release Hymen, Percutaneous Approach
♀ **0UNK4ZZ** Release Hymen, Percutaneous Endoscopic Approach
♀ **0UNK7ZZ** Release Hymen, Via Natural or Artificial Opening
♀ **0UNK8ZZ** Release Hymen, Via Natural or Artificial Opening Endoscopic
♀ **0UNKXZZ** Release Hymen, External Approach
♀ **0UNL0ZZ** Release Vestibular Gland, Open Approach
♀ **0UNLXZZ** Release Vestibular Gland, External Approach
♀ **0UNM0ZZ** Release Vulva, Open Approach
♀ **0UNMXZZ** Release Vulva, External Approach

0UP – Female Reproductive System, Removal

Review Coding Guideline B6.1c

♀ **0UP300Z** Removal of Drainage Device from Ovary, Open Approach
♀ **0UP303Z** Removal of Infusion Device from Ovary, Open Approach
♀ **0UP330Z** Removal of Drainage Device from Ovary, Percutaneous Approach
♀ **0UP333Z** Removal of Infusion Device from Ovary, Percutaneous Approach
♀ **0UP340Z** Removal of Drainage Device from Ovary, Percutaneous Endoscopic Approach
♀ **0UP343Z** Removal of Infusion Device from Ovary, Percutaneous Endoscopic Approach
♀ **0UP3X0Z** Removal of Drainage Device from Ovary, External Approach
♀ **0UP3X3Z** Removal of Infusion Device from Ovary, External Approach
♀ **0UP800Z** Removal of Drainage Device from Fallopian Tube, Open Approach
♀ **0UP803Z** Removal of Infusion Device from Fallopian Tube, Open Approach
♀ **0UP807Z** Removal of Autologous Tissue Substitute from Fallopian Tube, Open Approach
♀ **0UP80CZ** Removal of Extraluminal Device from Fallopian Tube, Open Approach

♀ **0UP80DZ** Removal of Intraluminal Device from Fallopian Tube, Open Approach
♀ **0UP80JZ** Removal of Synthetic Substitute from Fallopian Tube, Open Approach
♀ **0UP80KZ** Removal of Nonautologous Tissue Substitute from Fallopian Tube, Open Approach
♀ **0UP830Z** Removal of Drainage Device from Fallopian Tube, Percutaneous Approach
♀ **0UP833Z** Removal of Infusion Device from Fallopian Tube, Percutaneous Approach
♀ **0UP837Z** Removal of Autologous Tissue Substitute from Fallopian Tube, Percutaneous Approach
♀ **0UP83CZ** Removal of Extraluminal Device from Fallopian Tube, Percutaneous Approach
♀ **0UP83DZ** Removal of Intraluminal Device from Fallopian Tube, Percutaneous Approach

---

♀ Female-only ♂ Male-only ● Limited Coverage ● Non-OR **HAC** HAC-associated procedure ● Non-covered procedures ✚ Combination

♀ **0UP83JZ** Removal of Synthetic Substitute from Fallopian Tube, Percutaneous Approach

♀ **0UP83KZ** Removal of Nonautologous Tissue Substitute from Fallopian Tube, Percutaneous Approach

♀ **0UP840Z** Removal of Drainage Device from Fallopian Tube, Percutaneous Endoscopic Approach

♀ **0UP843Z** Removal of Infusion Device from Fallopian Tube, Percutaneous Endoscopic Approach

♀ **0UP847Z** Removal of Autologous Tissue Substitute from Fallopian Tube, Percutaneous Endoscopic Approach

♀ **0UP84CZ** Removal of Extraluminal Device from Fallopian Tube, Percutaneous Endoscopic Approach

♀ **0UP84DZ** Removal of Intraluminal Device from Fallopian Tube, Percutaneous Endoscopic Approach

♀ **0UP84JZ** Removal of Synthetic Substitute from Fallopian Tube, Percutaneous Endoscopic Approach

♀ **0UP84KZ** Removal of Nonautologous Tissue Substitute from Fallopian Tube, Percutaneous Endoscopic Approach

♀ **0UP870Z** Removal of Drainage Device from Fallopian Tube, Via Natural or Artificial Opening

♀ **0UP873Z** Removal of Infusion Device from Fallopian Tube, Via Natural or Artificial Opening

♀ **0UP877Z** Removal of Autologous Tissue Substitute from Fallopian Tube, Via Natural or Artificial Opening

♀ **0UP87CZ** Removal of Extraluminal Device from Fallopian Tube, Via Natural or Artificial Opening

♀ **0UP87DZ** Removal of Intraluminal Device from Fallopian Tube, Via Natural or Artificial Opening

♀ **0UP87JZ** Removal of Synthetic Substitute from Fallopian Tube, Via Natural or Artificial Opening

♀ **0UP87KZ** Removal of Nonautologous Tissue Substitute from Fallopian Tube, Via Natural or Artificial Opening

♀ **0UP880Z** Removal of Drainage Device from Fallopian Tube, Via Natural or Artificial Opening Endoscopic

♀ **0UP883Z** Removal of Infusion Device from Fallopian Tube, Via Natural or Artificial Opening Endoscopic

♀ **0UP887Z** Removal of Autologous Tissue Substitute from Fallopian Tube, Via Natural or Artificial Opening Endoscopic

♀ **0UP88CZ** Removal of Extraluminal Device from Fallopian Tube, Via Natural or Artificial Opening Endoscopic

♀ **0UP88DZ** Removal of Intraluminal Device from Fallopian Tube, Via Natural or Artificial Opening Endoscopic

♀ **0UP88JZ** Removal of Synthetic Substitute from Fallopian Tube, Via Natural or Artificial Opening Endoscopic

♀ **0UP88KZ** Removal of Nonautologous Tissue Substitute from Fallopian Tube, Via Natural or Artificial Opening Endoscopic

♀ **0UP8X0Z** Removal of Drainage Device from Fallopian Tube, External Approach

♀ **0UP8X3Z** Removal of Infusion Device from Fallopian Tube, External Approach

♀ **0UP8XDZ** Removal of Intraluminal Device from Fallopian Tube, External Approach

♀ **0UPD00Z** Removal of Drainage Device from Uterus and Cervix, Open Approach

♀ **0UPD01Z** Removal of Radioactive Element from Uterus and Cervix, Open Approach

♀ **0UPD03Z** Removal of Infusion Device from Uterus and Cervix, Open Approach

♀ **0UPD07Z** Removal of Autologous Tissue Substitute from Uterus and Cervix, Open Approach

♀ **0UPD0CZ** Removal of Extraluminal Device from Uterus and Cervix, Open Approach

♀ **0UPD0DZ** Removal of Intraluminal Device from Uterus and Cervix, Open Approach

♀ **0UPD0HZ** Removal of Contraceptive Device from Uterus and Cervix, Open Approach

♀ **0UPD0JZ** Removal of Synthetic Substitute from Uterus and Cervix, Open Approach

♀ **0UPD0KZ** Removal of Nonautologous Tissue Substitute from Uterus and Cervix, Open Approach

♀ **0UPD30Z** Removal of Drainage Device from Uterus and Cervix, Percutaneous Approach

♀ **0UPD31Z** Removal of Radioactive Element from Uterus and Cervix, Percutaneous Approach

♀ **0UPD33Z** Removal of Infusion Device from Uterus and Cervix, Percutaneous Approach

♀ **0UPD37Z** Removal of Autologous Tissue Substitute from Uterus and Cervix, Percutaneous Approach

♀ **0UPD3CZ** Removal of Extraluminal Device from Uterus and Cervix, Percutaneous Approach

♀ **0UPD3DZ** Removal of Intraluminal Device from Uterus and Cervix, Percutaneous Approach

♀ **0UPD3HZ** Removal of Contraceptive Device from Uterus and Cervix, Percutaneous Approach

♀ **0UPD3JZ** Removal of Synthetic Substitute from Uterus and Cervix, Percutaneous Approach

♀ **0UPD3KZ** Removal of Nonautologous Tissue Substitute from Uterus and Cervix, Percutaneous Approach

♀ **0UPD40Z** Removal of Drainage Device from Uterus and Cervix, Percutaneous Endoscopic Approach

♀ **0UPD41Z** Removal of Radioactive Element from Uterus and Cervix, Percutaneous Endoscopic Approach

♀ **0UPD43Z** Removal of Infusion Device from Uterus and Cervix, Percutaneous Endoscopic Approach

♀ **0UPD47Z** Removal of Autologous Tissue Substitute from Uterus and Cervix, Percutaneous Endoscopic Approach

♀ **0UPD4CZ** Removal of Extraluminal Device from Uterus and Cervix, Percutaneous Endoscopic Approach

♀ **0UPD4DZ** Removal of Intraluminal Device from Uterus and Cervix, Percutaneous Endoscopic Approach

♀ **0UPD4HZ** Removal of Contraceptive Device from Uterus and Cervix, Percutaneous Endoscopic Approach

♀ **0UPD4JZ** Removal of Synthetic Substitute from Uterus and Cervix, Percutaneous Endoscopic Approach

♀ **0UPD4KZ** Removal of Nonautologous Tissue Substitute from Uterus and Cervix, Percutaneous Endoscopic Approach

♀ **0UPD70Z** Removal of Drainage Device from Uterus and Cervix, Via Natural or Artificial Opening

♀ **0UPD71Z** Removal of Radioactive Element from Uterus and Cervix, Via Natural or Artificial Opening

♀ **0UPD73Z** Removal of Infusion Device from Uterus and Cervix, Via Natural or Artificial Opening

♀ **0UPD77Z** Removal of Autologous Tissue Substitute from Uterus and Cervix, Via Natural or Artificial Opening

♀ **0UPD7CZ** Removal of Extraluminal Device from Uterus and Cervix, Via Natural or Artificial Opening

♀ **0UPD7DZ** Removal of Intraluminal Device from Uterus and Cervix, Via Natural or Artificial Opening

♀ **0UPD7HZ** Removal of Contraceptive Device from Uterus and Cervix, Via Natural or Artificial Opening

♀ **0UPD7JZ** Removal of Synthetic Substitute from Uterus and Cervix, Via Natural or Artificial Opening

♀ **0UPD7KZ** Removal of Nonautologous Tissue Substitute from Uterus and Cervix, Via Natural or Artificial Opening

♀ **0UPD80Z** Removal of Drainage Device from Uterus and Cervix, Via Natural or Artificial Opening Endoscopic

♀ **0UPD81Z** Removal of Radioactive Element from Uterus and Cervix, Via Natural or Artificial Opening Endoscopic

♀ **0UPD83Z** Removal of Infusion Device from Uterus and Cervix, Via Natural or Artificial Opening Endoscopic

♀ **0UPD87Z** Removal of Autologous Tissue Substitute from Uterus and Cervix, Via Natural or Artificial Opening Endoscopic

♀ **0UPD8CZ** Removal of Extraluminal Device from Uterus and Cervix, Via Natural or Artificial Opening Endoscopic

♀ **0UPD8DZ** Removal of Intraluminal Device from Uterus and Cervix, Via Natural or Artificial Opening Endoscopic

♀ **0UPD8HZ** Removal of Contraceptive Device from Uterus and Cervix, Via Natural or Artificial Opening Endoscopic

♀ **0UPD8JZ** Removal of Synthetic Substitute from Uterus and Cervix, Via Natural or Artificial Opening Endoscopic

♀ **0UPD8KZ** Removal of Nonautologous Tissue Substitute from Uterus and Cervix, Via Natural or Artificial Opening Endoscopic

♀ **0UPDX0Z** Removal of Drainage Device from Uterus and Cervix, External Approach

♀ **0UPDX3Z** Removal of Infusion Device from Uterus and Cervix, External Approach

♀ **0UPDXDZ** Removal of Intraluminal Device from Uterus and Cervix, External Approach

---

♀ Female-only   ♂ Male-only   ● Limited Coverage   ● Non-OR   🄷🄰🄲 HAC-associated procedure   ● Non-covered procedures   ✚ Combination

♀ 0UPDXHZ Removal of Contraceptive Device from Uterus and Cervix, External Approach

♀ 0UPH00Z Removal of Drainage Device from Vagina and Cul-de-sac, Open Approach

♀ 0UPH01Z Removal of Radioactive Element from Vagina and Cul-de-sac, Open Approach

♀ 0UPH03Z Removal of Infusion Device from Vagina and Cul-de-sac, Open Approach

♀ 0UPH07Z Removal of Autologous Tissue Substitute from Vagina and Cul-de-sac, Open Approach

♀ 0UPH0DZ Removal of Intraluminal Device from Vagina and Cul-de-sac, Open Approach

♀ 0UPH0JZ Removal of Synthetic Substitute from Vagina and Cul-de-sac, Open Approach

♀ 0UPH0KZ Removal of Nonautologous Tissue Substitute from Vagina and Cul-de-sac, Open Approach

♀ 0UPH30Z Removal of Drainage Device from Vagina and Cul-de-sac, Percutaneous Approach

♀ 0UPH31Z Removal of Radioactive Element from Vagina and Cul-de-sac, Percutaneous Approach

♀ 0UPH33Z Removal of Infusion Device from Vagina and Cul-de-sac, Percutaneous Approach

♀ 0UPH37Z Removal of Autologous Tissue Substitute from Vagina and Cul-de-sac, Percutaneous Approach

♀ 0UPH3DZ Removal of Intraluminal Device from Vagina and Cul-de-sac, Percutaneous Approach

♀ 0UPH3JZ Removal of Synthetic Substitute from Vagina and Cul-de-sac, Percutaneous Approach

♀ 0UPH3KZ Removal of Nonautologous Tissue Substitute from Vagina and Cul-de-sac, Percutaneous Approach

♀ 0UPH40Z Removal of Drainage Device from Vagina and Cul-de-sac, Percutaneous Endoscopic Approach

♀ 0UPH41Z Removal of Radioactive Element from Vagina and Cul-de-sac, Percutaneous Endoscopic Approach

♀ 0UPH43Z Removal of Infusion Device from Vagina and Cul-de-sac, Percutaneous Endoscopic Approach

♀ 0UPH47Z Removal of Autologous Tissue Substitute from Vagina and Cul-de-sac, Percutaneous Endoscopic Approach

♀ 0UPH4DZ Removal of Intraluminal Device from Vagina and Cul-de-sac, Percutaneous Endoscopic Approach

♀ 0UPH4JZ Removal of Synthetic Substitute from Vagina and Cul-de-sac, Percutaneous Endoscopic Approach

♀ 0UPH4KZ Removal of Nonautologous Tissue Substitute from Vagina and Cul-de-sac, Percutaneous Endoscopic Approach

♀ 0UPH70Z Removal of Drainage Device from Vagina and Cul-de-sac, Via Natural or Artificial Opening

♀ 0UPH71Z Removal of Radioactive Element from Vagina and Cul-de-sac, Via Natural or Artificial Opening

♀ 0UPH73Z Removal of Infusion Device from Vagina and Cul-de-sac, Via Natural or Artificial Opening

♀ 0UPH77Z Removal of Autologous Tissue Substitute from Vagina and Cul-de-sac, Via Natural or Artificial Opening

♀ 0UPH7DZ Removal of Intraluminal Device from Vagina and Cul-de-sac, Via Natural or Artificial Opening

♀ 0UPH7JZ Removal of Synthetic Substitute from Vagina and Cul-de-sac, Via Natural or Artificial Opening

♀ 0UPH7KZ Removal of Nonautologous Tissue Substitute from Vagina and Cul-de-sac, Via Natural or Artificial Opening

♀ 0UPH80Z Removal of Drainage Device from Vagina and Cul-de-sac, Via Natural or Artificial Opening Endoscopic

♀ 0UPH81Z Removal of Radioactive Element from Vagina and Cul-de-sac, Via Natural or Artificial Opening Endoscopic

♀ 0UPH83Z Removal of Infusion Device from Vagina and Cul-de-sac, Via Natural or Artificial Opening Endoscopic

♀ 0UPH87Z Removal of Autologous Tissue Substitute from Vagina and Cul-de-sac, Via Natural or Artificial Opening Endoscopic

♀ 0UPH8DZ Removal of Intraluminal Device from Vagina and Cul-de-sac, Via Natural or Artificial Opening Endoscopic

♀ 0UPH8JZ Removal of Synthetic Substitute from Vagina and Cul-de-sac, Via Natural or Artificial Opening Endoscopic

♀ 0UPH8KZ Removal of Nonautologous Tissue Substitute from Vagina and Cul-de-sac, Via Natural or Artificial Opening Endoscopic

♀ 0UPHX0Z Removal of Drainage Device from Vagina and Cul-de-sac, External Approach

♀ 0UPHX1Z Removal of Radioactive Element from Vagina and Cul-de-sac, External Approach

♀ 0UPHX3Z Removal of Infusion Device from Vagina and Cul-de-sac, External Approach

♀ 0UPHXDZ Removal of Intraluminal Device from Vagina and Cul-de-sac, External Approach

♀ 0UPM00Z Removal of Drainage Device from Vulva, Open Approach

♀ 0UPM07Z Removal of Autologous Tissue Substitute from Vulva, Open Approach

♀ 0UPM0JZ Removal of Synthetic Substitute from Vulva, Open Approach

♀ 0UPM0KZ Removal of Nonautologous Tissue Substitute from Vulva, Open Approach

♀ 0UPMX0Z Removal of Drainage Device from Vulva, External Approach

0UQ – Female Reproductive System, Repair

♀ 0UQ00ZZ Repair Right Ovary, Open Approach

♀ 0UQ03ZZ Repair Right Ovary, Percutaneous Approach

♀ 0UQ04ZZ Repair Right Ovary, Percutaneous Endoscopic Approach

♀ 0UQ10ZZ Repair Left Ovary, Open Approach

♀ 0UQ13ZZ Repair Left Ovary, Percutaneous Approach

♀ 0UQ14ZZ Repair Left Ovary, Percutaneous Endoscopic Approach

♀ 0UQ20ZZ Repair Bilateral Ovaries, Open Approach

♀ 0UQ23ZZ Repair Bilateral Ovaries, Percutaneous Approach

♀ 0UQ24ZZ Repair Bilateral Ovaries, Percutaneous Endoscopic Approach

♀ 0UQ40ZZ Repair Uterine Supporting Structure, Open Approach

♀ 0UQ43ZZ Repair Uterine Supporting Structure, Percutaneous Approach

♀ 0UQ44ZZ Repair Uterine Supporting Structure, Percutaneous Endoscopic Approach

♀ 0UQ50ZZ Repair Right Fallopian Tube, Open Approach

♀ 0UQ53ZZ Repair Right Fallopian Tube, Percutaneous Approach

♀ 0UQ54ZZ Repair Right Fallopian Tube, Percutaneous Endoscopic Approach

♀ 0UQ57ZZ Repair Right Fallopian Tube, Via Natural or Artificial Opening

♀ 0UQ58ZZ Repair Right Fallopian Tube, Via Natural or Artificial Opening Endoscopic

♀ 0UQ60ZZ Repair Left Fallopian Tube, Open Approach

♀ 0UQ63ZZ Repair Left Fallopian Tube, Percutaneous Approach

♀ 0UQ64ZZ Repair Left Fallopian Tube, Percutaneous Endoscopic Approach

♀ 0UQ67ZZ Repair Left Fallopian Tube, Via Natural or Artificial Opening

♀ 0UQ68ZZ Repair Left Fallopian Tube, Via Natural or Artificial Opening Endoscopic

♀ 0UQ70ZZ Repair Bilateral Fallopian Tubes, Open Approach

♀ 0UQ73ZZ Repair Bilateral Fallopian Tubes, Percutaneous Approach

♀ 0UQ74ZZ Repair Bilateral Fallopian Tubes, Percutaneous Endoscopic Approach

♀ 0UQ77ZZ Repair Bilateral Fallopian Tubes, Via Natural or Artificial Opening

♀ 0UQ78ZZ Repair Bilateral Fallopian Tubes, Via Natural or Artificial Opening Endoscopic

♀ 0UQ90ZZ Repair Uterus, Open Approach

♀ 0UQ93ZZ Repair Uterus, Percutaneous Approach

♀ 0UQ94ZZ Repair Uterus, Percutaneous Endoscopic Approach

♀ 0UQ97ZZ Repair Uterus, Via Natural or Artificial Opening

♀ 0UQ98ZZ Repair Uterus, Via Natural or Artificial Opening Endoscopic

♀ 0UQC0ZZ Repair Cervix, Open Approach

♀ 0UQC3ZZ Repair Cervix, Percutaneous Approach

♀ 0UQC4ZZ Repair Cervix, Percutaneous Endoscopic Approach

♀ 0UQC7ZZ Repair Cervix, Via Natural or Artificial Opening

♀ 0UQC8ZZ Repair Cervix, Via Natural or Artificial Opening Endoscopic

♀ 0UQF0ZZ Repair Cul-de-sac, Open Approach

♀ 0UQF3ZZ Repair Cul-de-sac, Percutaneous Approach

♀ 0UQF4ZZ Repair Cul-de-sac, Percutaneous Endoscopic Approach

♀ 0UQF7ZZ Repair Cul-de-sac, Via Natural or Artificial Opening

♀ 0UQF8ZZ Repair Cul-de-sac, Via Natural or Artificial Opening Endoscopic

♀ 0UQG0ZZ Repair Vagina, Open Approach

♀ 0UQG3ZZ Repair Vagina, Percutaneous Approach

♀ **0UQG4ZZ**   Repair Vagina, Percutaneous Endoscopic Approach
●♀ **0UQG7ZZ**   Repair Vagina, Via Natural or Artificial Opening
●♀ **0UQG8ZZ**   Repair Vagina, Via Natural or Artificial Opening Endoscopic
●♀ **0UQGXZZ**   Repair Vagina, External Approach
♀ **0UQJ0ZZ**   Repair Clitoris, Open Approach
♀ **0UQJXZZ**   Repair Clitoris, External Approach
♀ **0UQK0ZZ**   Repair Hymen, Open Approach
♀ **0UQK3ZZ**   Repair Hymen, Percutaneous Approach

♀ **0UQK4ZZ**   Repair Hymen, Percutaneous Endoscopic Approach
♀ **0UQK7ZZ**   Repair Hymen, Via Natural or Artificial Opening
♀ **0UQK8ZZ**   Repair Hymen, Via Natural or Artificial Opening Endoscopic
♀ **0UQKXZZ**   Repair Hymen, External Approach
♀ **0UQL0ZZ**   Repair Vestibular Gland, Open Approach
♀ **0UQLXZZ**   Repair Vestibular Gland, External Approach
●♀ **0UQM0ZZ**   Repair Vulva, Open Approach
●♀ **0UQMXZZ**   Repair Vulva, External Approach

0US – Female Reproductive System, Reposition

♀ **0US00ZZ**   Reposition Right Ovary, Open Approach
♀ **0US04ZZ**   Reposition Right Ovary, Percutaneous Endoscopic Approach
♀ **0US10ZZ**   Reposition Left Ovary, Open Approach
♀ **0US14ZZ**   Reposition Left Ovary, Percutaneous Endoscopic Approach
♀ **0US20ZZ**   Reposition Bilateral Ovaries, Open Approach
♀ **0US24ZZ**   Reposition Bilateral Ovaries, Percutaneous Endoscopic Approach
♀ **0US40ZZ**   Reposition Uterine Supporting Structure, Open Approach
♀ **0US44ZZ**   Reposition Uterine Supporting Structure, Percutaneous Endoscopic Approach
♀ **0US50ZZ**   Reposition Right Fallopian Tube, Open Approach
♀ **0US54ZZ**   Reposition Right Fallopian Tube, Percutaneous Endoscopic Approach
♀ **0US60ZZ**   Reposition Left Fallopian Tube, Open Approach
♀ **0US64ZZ**   Reposition Left Fallopian Tube, Percutaneous Endoscopic Approach

♀ **0US70ZZ**   Reposition Bilateral Fallopian Tubes, Open Approach
♀ **0US74ZZ**   Reposition Bilateral Fallopian Tubes, Percutaneous Endoscopic Approach
♀ **0US90ZZ**   Reposition Uterus, Open Approach
♀ **0US94ZZ**   Reposition Uterus, Percutaneous Endoscopic Approach
♀ **0US9XZZ**   Reposition Uterus, External Approach
♀ **0USC0ZZ**   Reposition Cervix, Open Approach
♀ **0USC4ZZ**   Reposition Cervix, Percutaneous Endoscopic Approach
♀ **0USF0ZZ**   Reposition Cul-de-sac, Open Approach
♀ **0USF4ZZ**   Reposition Cul-de-sac, Percutaneous Endoscopic Approach
♀ **0USG0ZZ**   Reposition Vagina, Open Approach
♀ **0USG4ZZ**   Reposition Vagina, Percutaneous Endoscopic Approach
♀ **0USGXZZ**   Reposition Vagina, External Approach

0UT – Female Reproductive System, Resection

Review Coding Guideline B3.8

♀ **0UT00ZZ**   Resection of Right Ovary, Open Approach
♀ **0UT04ZZ**   Resection of Right Ovary, Percutaneous Endoscopic Approach
♀ **0UT07ZZ**   Resection of Right Ovary, Via Natural or Artificial Opening
♀ **0UT08ZZ**   Resection of Right Ovary, Via Natural or Artificial Opening Endoscopic
♀ **0UT0FZZ**   Resection of Right Ovary, Via Natural or Artificial Opening With Percutaneous Endoscopic Assistance
♀ **0UT10ZZ**   Resection of Left Ovary, Open Approach
♀ **0UT14ZZ**   Resection of Left Ovary, Percutaneous Endoscopic Approach
♀ **0UT17ZZ**   Resection of Left Ovary, Via Natural or Artificial Opening
♀ **0UT18ZZ**   Resection of Left Ovary, Via Natural or Artificial Opening Endoscopic
♀ **0UT1FZZ**   Resection of Left Ovary, Via Natural or Artificial Opening With Percutaneous Endoscopic Assistance
♀ **0UT20ZZ**   Resection of Bilateral Ovaries, Open Approach
♀ **0UT24ZZ**   Resection of Bilateral Ovaries, Percutaneous Endoscopic Approach
♀ **0UT27ZZ**   Resection of Bilateral Ovaries, Via Natural or Artificial Opening
♀ **0UT28ZZ**   Resection of Bilateral Ovaries, Via Natural or Artificial Opening Endoscopic
♀ **0UT2FZZ**   Resection of Bilateral Ovaries, Via Natural or Artificial Opening With Percutaneous Endoscopic Assistance
♀ **0UT40ZZ**   Resection of Uterine Supporting Structure, Open Approach
♀ **0UT44ZZ**   Resection of Uterine Supporting Structure, Percutaneous Endoscopic Approach
♀ **0UT47ZZ**   Resection of Uterine Supporting Structure, Via Natural or Artificial Opening
♀ **0UT48ZZ**   Resection of Uterine Supporting Structure, Via Natural or Artificial Opening Endoscopic
♀ **0UT50ZZ**   Resection of Right Fallopian Tube, Open Approach
♀ **0UT54ZZ**   Resection of Right Fallopian Tube, Percutaneous Endoscopic Approach
♀ **0UT57ZZ**   Resection of Right Fallopian Tube, Via Natural or Artificial Opening
♀ **0UT58ZZ**   Resection of Right Fallopian Tube, Via Natural or Artificial Opening Endoscopic
♀ **0UT5FZZ**   Resection of Right Fallopian Tube, Via Natural or Artificial Opening With Percutaneous Endoscopic Assistance
♀ **0UT60ZZ**   Resection of Left Fallopian Tube, Open Approach
♀ **0UT64ZZ**   Resection of Left Fallopian Tube, Percutaneous Endoscopic Approach
♀ **0UT67ZZ**   Resection of Left Fallopian Tube, Via Natural or Artificial Opening

♀ **0UT68ZZ**   Resection of Left Fallopian Tube, Via Natural or Artificial Opening Endoscopic
♀ **0UT6FZZ**   Resection of Left Fallopian Tube, Via Natural or Artificial Opening With Percutaneous Endoscopic Assistance
♀ **0UT70ZZ**   Resection of Bilateral Fallopian Tubes, Open Approach
♀ **0UT74ZZ**   Resection of Bilateral Fallopian Tubes, Percutaneous Endoscopic Approach
♀ **0UT77ZZ**   Resection of Bilateral Fallopian Tubes, Via Natural or Artificial Opening
♀ **0UT78ZZ**   Resection of Bilateral Fallopian Tubes, Via Natural or Artificial Opening Endoscopic
♀ **0UT7FZZ**   Resection of Bilateral Fallopian Tubes, Via Natural or Artificial Opening With Percutaneous Endoscopic Assistance
♀ **0UT90ZZ**   Resection of Uterus, Open Approach
♀ **0UT94ZZ**   Resection of Uterus, Percutaneous Endoscopic Approach
♀ **0UT97ZZ**   Resection of Uterus, Via Natural or Artificial Opening
♀ **0UT98ZZ**   Resection of Uterus, Via Natural or Artificial Opening Endoscopic
♀ **0UT9FZZ**   Resection of Uterus, Via Natural or Artificial Opening With Percutaneous Endoscopic Assistance
♀ **0UTC0ZZ**   Resection of Cervix, Open Approach
♀ **0UTC4ZZ**   Resection of Cervix, Percutaneous Endoscopic Approach
♀ **0UTC7ZZ**   Resection of Cervix, Via Natural or Artificial Opening
♀ **0UTC8ZZ**   Resection of Cervix, Via Natural or Artificial Opening Endoscopic
♀ **0UTF0ZZ**   Resection of Cul-de-sac, Open Approach
♀ **0UTF4ZZ**   Resection of Cul-de-sac, Percutaneous Endoscopic Approach
♀ **0UTF7ZZ**   Resection of Cul-de-sac, Via Natural or Artificial Opening
♀ **0UTF8ZZ**   Resection of Cul-de-sac, Via Natural or Artificial Opening Endoscopic
♀ **0UTG0ZZ**   Resection of Vagina, Open Approach
♀ **0UTG4ZZ**   Resection of Vagina, Percutaneous Endoscopic Approach
♀ **0UTG7ZZ**   Resection of Vagina, Via Natural or Artificial Opening
♀ **0UTG8ZZ**   Resection of Vagina, Via Natural or Artificial Opening Endoscopic
♀ **0UTJ0ZZ**   Resection of Clitoris, Open Approach
♀ **0UTJXZZ**   Resection of Clitoris, External Approach
♀ **0UTK0ZZ**   Resection of Hymen, Open Approach
♀ **0UTK4ZZ**   Resection of Hymen, Percutaneous Endoscopic Approach
♀ **0UTK7ZZ**   Resection of Hymen, Via Natural or Artificial Opening
♀ **0UTK8ZZ**   Resection of Hymen, Via Natural or Artificial Opening Endoscopic
♀ **0UTKXZZ**   Resection of Hymen, External Approach
♀ **0UTL0ZZ**   Resection of Vestibular Gland, Open Approach
♀ **0UTLXZZ**   Resection of Vestibular Gland, External Approach
♀ **0UTM0ZZ**   Resection of Vulva, Open Approach
♀ **0UTMXZZ**   Resection of Vulva, External Approach

♀ Female-only   ♂ Male-only   ● Limited Coverage   ● Non-OR   **HAC** HAC-associated procedure   ● Non-covered procedures   ✚ Combination

0UU – Female Reproductive System, Supplement

♀ **0UU407Z** Supplement Uterine Supporting Structure with Autologous Tissue Substitute, Open Approach

♀ **0UU40JZ** Supplement Uterine Supporting Structure with Synthetic Substitute, Open Approach

♀ **0UU40KZ** Supplement Uterine Supporting Structure with Nonautologous Tissue Substitute, Open Approach

♀ **0UU447Z** Supplement Uterine Supporting Structure with Autologous Tissue Substitute, Percutaneous Endoscopic Approach

♀ **0UU44JZ** Supplement Uterine Supporting Structure with Synthetic Substitute, Percutaneous Endoscopic Approach

♀ **0UU44KZ** Supplement Uterine Supporting Structure with Nonautologous Tissue Substitute, Percutaneous Endoscopic Approach

♀ **0UU507Z** Supplement Right Fallopian Tube with Autologous Tissue Substitute, Open Approach

♀ **0UU50JZ** Supplement Right Fallopian Tube with Synthetic Substitute, Open Approach

♀ **0UU50KZ** Supplement Right Fallopian Tube with Nonautologous Tissue Substitute, Open Approach

♀ **0UU547Z** Supplement Right Fallopian Tube with Autologous Tissue Substitute, Percutaneous Endoscopic Approach

♀ **0UU54JZ** Supplement Right Fallopian Tube with Synthetic Substitute, Percutaneous Endoscopic Approach

♀ **0UU54KZ** Supplement Right Fallopian Tube with Nonautologous Tissue Substitute, Percutaneous Endoscopic Approach

♀ **0UU577Z** Supplement Right Fallopian Tube with Autologous Tissue Substitute, Via Natural or Artificial Opening

♀ **0UU57JZ** Supplement Right Fallopian Tube with Synthetic Substitute, Via Natural or Artificial Opening

♀ **0UU57KZ** Supplement Right Fallopian Tube with Nonautologous Tissue Substitute, Via Natural or Artificial Opening

♀ **0UU587Z** Supplement Right Fallopian Tube with Autologous Tissue Substitute, Via Natural or Artificial Opening Endoscopic

♀ **0UU58JZ** Supplement Right Fallopian Tube with Synthetic Substitute, Via Natural or Artificial Opening Endoscopic

♀ **0UU58KZ** Supplement Right Fallopian Tube with Nonautologous Tissue Substitute, Via Natural or Artificial Opening Endoscopic

♀ **0UU607Z** Supplement Left Fallopian Tube with Autologous Tissue Substitute, Open Approach

♀ **0UU60JZ** Supplement Left Fallopian Tube with Synthetic Substitute, Open Approach

♀ **0UU60KZ** Supplement Left Fallopian Tube with Nonautologous Tissue Substitute, Open Approach

♀ **0UU647Z** Supplement Left Fallopian Tube with Autologous Tissue Substitute, Percutaneous Endoscopic Approach

♀ **0UU64JZ** Supplement Left Fallopian Tube with Synthetic Substitute, Percutaneous Endoscopic Approach

♀ **0UU64KZ** Supplement Left Fallopian Tube with Nonautologous Tissue Substitute, Percutaneous Endoscopic Approach

♀ **0UU677Z** Supplement Left Fallopian Tube with Autologous Tissue Substitute, Via Natural or Artificial Opening

♀ **0UU67JZ** Supplement Left Fallopian Tube with Synthetic Substitute, Via Natural or Artificial Opening

♀ **0UU67KZ** Supplement Left Fallopian Tube with Nonautologous Tissue Substitute, Via Natural or Artificial Opening

♀ **0UU687Z** Supplement Left Fallopian Tube with Autologous Tissue Substitute, Via Natural or Artificial Opening Endoscopic

♀ **0UU68JZ** Supplement Left Fallopian Tube with Synthetic Substitute, Via Natural or Artificial Opening Endoscopic

♀ **0UU68KZ** Supplement Left Fallopian Tube with Nonautologous Tissue Substitute, Via Natural or Artificial Opening Endoscopic

♀ **0UU707Z** Supplement Bilateral Fallopian Tubes with Autologous Tissue Substitute, Open Approach

♀ **0UU70JZ** Supplement Bilateral Fallopian Tubes with Synthetic Substitute, Open Approach

♀ **0UU70KZ** Supplement Bilateral Fallopian Tubes with Nonautologous Tissue Substitute, Open Approach

♀ **0UU747Z** Supplement Bilateral Fallopian Tubes with Autologous Tissue Substitute, Percutaneous Endoscopic Approach

♀ **0UU74JZ** Supplement Bilateral Fallopian Tubes with Synthetic Substitute, Percutaneous Endoscopic Approach

♀ **0UU74KZ** Supplement Bilateral Fallopian Tubes with Nonautologous Tissue Substitute, Percutaneous Endoscopic Approach

♀ **0UU777Z** Supplement Bilateral Fallopian Tubes with Autologous Tissue Substitute, Via Natural or Artificial Opening

♀ **0UU77JZ** Supplement Bilateral Fallopian Tubes with Synthetic Substitute, Via Natural or Artificial Opening

♀ **0UU77KZ** Supplement Bilateral Fallopian Tubes with Nonautologous Tissue Substitute, Via Natural or Artificial Opening

♀ **0UU787Z** Supplement Bilateral Fallopian Tubes with Autologous Tissue Substitute, Via Natural or Artificial Opening Endoscopic

♀ **0UU78JZ** Supplement Bilateral Fallopian Tubes with Synthetic Substitute, Via Natural or Artificial Opening Endoscopic

♀ **0UU78KZ** Supplement Bilateral Fallopian Tubes with Nonautologous Tissue Substitute, Via Natural or Artificial Opening Endoscopic

♀ **0UUF07Z** Supplement Cul-de-sac with Autologous Tissue Substitute, Open Approach

♀ **0UUF0JZ** Supplement Cul-de-sac with Synthetic Substitute, Open Approach

♀ **0UUF0KZ** Supplement Cul-de-sac with Nonautologous Tissue Substitute, Open Approach

♀ **0UUF47Z** Supplement Cul-de-sac with Autologous Tissue Substitute, Percutaneous Endoscopic Approach

♀ **0UUF4JZ** Supplement Cul-de-sac with Synthetic Substitute, Percutaneous Endoscopic Approach

♀ **0UUF4KZ** Supplement Cul-de-sac with Nonautologous Tissue Substitute, Percutaneous Endoscopic Approach

♀ **0UUF77Z** Supplement Cul-de-sac with Autologous Tissue Substitute, Via Natural or Artificial Opening

♀ **0UUF7JZ** Supplement Cul-de-sac with Synthetic Substitute, Via Natural or Artificial Opening

♀ **0UUF7KZ** Supplement Cul-de-sac with Nonautologous Tissue Substitute, Via Natural or Artificial Opening

♀ **0UUF87Z** Supplement Cul-de-sac with Autologous Tissue Substitute, Via Natural or Artificial Opening Endoscopic

♀ **0UUF8JZ** Supplement Cul-de-sac with Synthetic Substitute, Via Natural or Artificial Opening Endoscopic

♀ **0UUF8KZ** Supplement Cul-de-sac with Nonautologous Tissue Substitute, Via Natural or Artificial Opening Endoscopic

♀ **0UUG07Z** Supplement Vagina with Autologous Tissue Substitute, Open Approach

♀ **0UUG0JZ** Supplement Vagina with Synthetic Substitute, Open Approach

♀ **0UUG0KZ** Supplement Vagina with Nonautologous Tissue Substitute, Open Approach

♀ **0UUG47Z** Supplement Vagina with Autologous Tissue Substitute, Percutaneous Endoscopic Approach

♀ **0UUG4JZ** Supplement Vagina with Synthetic Substitute, Percutaneous Endoscopic Approach

♀ **0UUG4KZ** Supplement Vagina with Nonautologous Tissue Substitute, Percutaneous Endoscopic Approach

♀ **0UUG77Z** Supplement Vagina with Autologous Tissue Substitute, Via Natural or Artificial Opening

♀ **0UUG7JZ** Supplement Vagina with Synthetic Substitute, Via Natural or Artificial Opening

♀ **0UUG7KZ** Supplement Vagina with Nonautologous Tissue Substitute, Via Natural or Artificial Opening

♀ **0UUG87Z** Supplement Vagina with Autologous Tissue Substitute, Via Natural or Artificial Opening Endoscopic

♀ **0UUG8JZ** Supplement Vagina with Synthetic Substitute, Via Natural or Artificial Opening Endoscopic

♀ **0UUG8KZ** Supplement Vagina with Nonautologous Tissue Substitute, Via Natural or Artificial Opening Endoscopic

♀ **0UUGX7Z** Supplement Vagina with Autologous Tissue Substitute, External Approach

♀ **0UUGXJZ** Supplement Vagina with Synthetic Substitute, External Approach

♀ **0UUGXKZ** Supplement Vagina with Nonautologous Tissue Substitute, External Approach

♀ **0UUJ07Z** Supplement Clitoris with Autologous Tissue Substitute, Open Approach

♀ **0UUJ0JZ** Supplement Clitoris with Synthetic Substitute, Open Approach

♀ **0UUJ0KZ** Supplement Clitoris with Nonautologous Tissue Substitute, Open Approach

♀ **0UUJX7Z** Supplement Clitoris with Autologous Tissue Substitute, External Approach

♀ **0UUJXJZ** Supplement Clitoris with Synthetic Substitute, External Approach

---

♀ Female-only   ♂ Male-only   ● Limited Coverage   ● Non-OR   HAC HAC-associated procedure   ● Non-covered procedures   ✚ Combination

♀ **0UUJXKZ** Supplement Clitoris with Nonautologous Tissue Substitute, External Approach
♀ **0UUK07Z** Supplement Hymen with Autologous Tissue Substitute, Open Approach
♀ **0UUK0JZ** Supplement Hymen with Synthetic Substitute, Open Approach
♀ **0UUK0KZ** Supplement Hymen with Nonautologous Tissue Substitute, Open Approach
♀ **0UUK47Z** Supplement Hymen with Autologous Tissue Substitute, Percutaneous Endoscopic Approach
♀ **0UUK4JZ** Supplement Hymen with Synthetic Substitute, Percutaneous Endoscopic Approach
♀ **0UUK4KZ** Supplement Hymen with Nonautologous Tissue Substitute, Percutaneous Endoscopic Approach
♀ **0UUK77Z** Supplement Hymen with Autologous Tissue Substitute, Via Natural or Artificial Opening
♀ **0UUK7JZ** Supplement Hymen with Synthetic Substitute, Via Natural or Artificial Opening
♀ **0UUK7KZ** Supplement Hymen with Nonautologous Tissue Substitute, Via Natural or Artificial Opening
♀ **0UUK87Z** Supplement Hymen with Autologous Tissue Substitute, Via Natural or Artificial Opening Endoscopic

♀ **0UUK8JZ** Supplement Hymen with Synthetic Substitute, Via Natural or Artificial Opening Endoscopic
♀ **0UUK8KZ** Supplement Hymen with Nonautologous Tissue Substitute, Via Natural or Artificial Opening Endoscopic
♀ **0UUKX7Z** Supplement Hymen with Autologous Tissue Substitute, External Approach
♀ **0UUKXJZ** Supplement Hymen with Synthetic Substitute, External Approach
♀ **0UUKXKZ** Supplement Hymen with Nonautologous Tissue Substitute, External Approach
♀ **0UUM07Z** Supplement Vulva with Autologous Tissue Substitute, Open Approach
♀ **0UUM0JZ** Supplement Vulva with Synthetic Substitute, Open Approach
♀ **0UUM0KZ** Supplement Vulva with Nonautologous Tissue Substitute, Open Approach
♀ **0UUMX7Z** Supplement Vulva with Autologous Tissue Substitute, External Approach
♀ **0UUMXJZ** Supplement Vulva with Synthetic Substitute, External Approach
♀ **0UUMXKZ** Supplement Vulva with Nonautologous Tissue Substitute, External Approach

0UV – Female Reproductive System, Restriction

♀ **0UVC0CZ** Restriction of Cervix with Extraluminal Device, Open Approach
♀ **0UVC0DZ** Restriction of Cervix with Intraluminal Device, Open Approach
♀ **0UVC0ZZ** Restriction of Cervix, Open Approach
♀ **0UVC3CZ** Restriction of Cervix with Extraluminal Device, Percutaneous Approach
♀ **0UVC3DZ** Restriction of Cervix with Intraluminal Device, Percutaneous Approach
♀ **0UVC3ZZ** Restriction of Cervix, Percutaneous Approach
♀ **0UVC4CZ** Restriction of Cervix with Extraluminal Device, Percutaneous Endoscopic Approach

♀ **0UVC4DZ** Restriction of Cervix with Intraluminal Device, Percutaneous Endoscopic Approach
♀ **0UVC4ZZ** Restriction of Cervix, Percutaneous Endoscopic Approach
♀ **0UVC7DZ** Restriction of Cervix with Intraluminal Device, Via Natural or Artificial Opening
♀ **0UVC7ZZ** Restriction of Cervix, Via Natural or Artificial Opening
♀ **0UVC8DZ** Restriction of Cervix with Intraluminal Device, Via Natural or Artificial Opening Endoscopic
♀ **0UVC8ZZ** Restriction of Cervix, Via Natural or Artificial Opening Endoscopic

0UW – Female Reproductive System, Revision

Review Coding Guideline B6.1c

♀ **0UW300Z** Revision of Drainage Device in Ovary, Open Approach
♀ **0UW303Z** Revision of Infusion Device in Ovary, Open Approach
♀ **0UW330Z** Revision of Drainage Device in Ovary, Percutaneous Approach
♀ **0UW333Z** Revision of Infusion Device in Ovary, Percutaneous Approach
♀ **0UW340Z** Revision of Drainage Device in Ovary, Percutaneous Endoscopic Approach
♀ **0UW343Z** Revision of Infusion Device in Ovary, Percutaneous Endoscopic Approach
♀ **0UW3X0Z** Revision of Drainage Device in Ovary, External Approach
♀ **0UW3X3Z** Revision of Infusion Device in Ovary, External Approach
♀ **0UW800Z** Revision of Drainage Device in Fallopian Tube, Open Approach
♀ **0UW803Z** Revision of Infusion Device in Fallopian Tube, Open Approach
♀ **0UW807Z** Revision of Autologous Tissue Substitute in Fallopian Tube, Open Approach
♀ **0UW80CZ** Revision of Extraluminal Device in Fallopian Tube, Open Approach
♀ **0UW80DZ** Revision of Intraluminal Device in Fallopian Tube, Open Approach
♀ **0UW80JZ** Revision of Synthetic Substitute in Fallopian Tube, Open Approach
♀ **0UW80KZ** Revision of Nonautologous Tissue Substitute in Fallopian Tube, Open Approach
♀ **0UW830Z** Revision of Drainage Device in Fallopian Tube, Percutaneous Approach
♀ **0UW833Z** Revision of Infusion Device in Fallopian Tube, Percutaneous Approach
♀ **0UW837Z** Revision of Autologous Tissue Substitute in Fallopian Tube, Percutaneous Approach
♀ **0UW83CZ** Revision of Extraluminal Device in Fallopian Tube, Percutaneous Approach
♀ **0UW83DZ** Revision of Intraluminal Device in Fallopian Tube, Percutaneous Approach
♀ **0UW83JZ** Revision of Synthetic Substitute in Fallopian Tube, Percutaneous Approach

♀ **0UW83KZ** Revision of Nonautologous Tissue Substitute in Fallopian Tube, Percutaneous Approach
♀ **0UW840Z** Revision of Drainage Device in Fallopian Tube, Percutaneous Endoscopic Approach
♀ **0UW843Z** Revision of Infusion Device in Fallopian Tube, Percutaneous Endoscopic Approach
♀ **0UW847Z** Revision of Autologous Tissue Substitute in Fallopian Tube, Percutaneous Endoscopic Approach
♀ **0UW84CZ** Revision of Extraluminal Device in Fallopian Tube, Percutaneous Endoscopic Approach
♀ **0UW84DZ** Revision of Intraluminal Device in Fallopian Tube, Percutaneous Endoscopic Approach
♀ **0UW84JZ** Revision of Synthetic Substitute in Fallopian Tube, Percutaneous Endoscopic Approach
♀ **0UW84KZ** Revision of Nonautologous Tissue Substitute in Fallopian Tube, Percutaneous Endoscopic Approach
♀ **0UW870Z** Revision of Drainage Device in Fallopian Tube, Via Natural or Artificial Opening
♀ **0UW873Z** Revision of Infusion Device in Fallopian Tube, Via Natural or Artificial Opening
♀ **0UW877Z** Revision of Autologous Tissue Substitute in Fallopian Tube, Via Natural or Artificial Opening
♀ **0UW87CZ** Revision of Extraluminal Device in Fallopian Tube, Via Natural or Artificial Opening
♀ **0UW87DZ** Revision of Intraluminal Device in Fallopian Tube, Via Natural or Artificial Opening
♀ **0UW87JZ** Revision of Synthetic Substitute in Fallopian Tube, Via Natural or Artificial Opening
♀ **0UW87KZ** Revision of Nonautologous Tissue Substitute in Fallopian Tube, Via Natural or Artificial Opening
♀ **0UW880Z** Revision of Drainage Device in Fallopian Tube, Via Natural or Artificial Opening Endoscopic
♀ **0UW883Z** Revision of Infusion Device in Fallopian Tube, Via Natural or Artificial Opening Endoscopic

♀ Female-only   ♂ Male-only   ● Limited Coverage   ● Non-OR   **HAC** HAC-associated procedure   ● Non-covered procedures   **+** Combination

♀ **0UW887Z** Revision of Autologous Tissue Substitute in Fallopian Tube, Via Natural or Artificial Opening Endoscopic

♀ **0UW88CZ** Revision of Extraluminal Device in Fallopian Tube, Via Natural or Artificial Opening Endoscopic

♀ **0UW88DZ** Revision of Intraluminal Device in Fallopian Tube, Via Natural or Artificial Opening Endoscopic

♀ **0UW88JZ** Revision of Synthetic Substitute in Fallopian Tube, Via Natural or Artificial Opening Endoscopic

♀ **0UW88KZ** Revision of Nonautologous Tissue Substitute in Fallopian Tube, Via Natural or Artificial Opening Endoscopic

♀ **0UW8X0Z** Revision of Drainage Device in Fallopian Tube, External Approach

♀ **0UW8X3Z** Revision of Infusion Device in Fallopian Tube, External Approach

♀ **0UW8X7Z** Revision of Autologous Tissue Substitute in Fallopian Tube, External Approach

♀ **0UW8XCZ** Revision of Extraluminal Device in Fallopian Tube, External Approach

♀ **0UW8XDZ** Revision of Intraluminal Device in Fallopian Tube, External Approach

♀ **0UW8XJZ** Revision of Synthetic Substitute in Fallopian Tube, External Approach

♀ **0UW8XKZ** Revision of Nonautologous Tissue Substitute in Fallopian Tube, External Approach

♀ **0UWD00Z** Revision of Drainage Device in Uterus and Cervix, Open Approach

♀ **0UWD01Z** Revision of Radioactive Element in Uterus and Cervix, Open Approach

♀ **0UWD03Z** Revision of Infusion Device in Uterus and Cervix, Open Approach

♀ **0UWD07Z** Revision of Autologous Tissue Substitute in Uterus and Cervix, Open Approach

♀ **0UWD0CZ** Revision of Extraluminal Device in Uterus and Cervix, Open Approach

♀ **0UWD0DZ** Revision of Intraluminal Device in Uterus and Cervix, Open Approach

♀ **0UWD0HZ** Revision of Contraceptive Device in Uterus and Cervix, Open Approach

♀ **0UWD0JZ** Revision of Synthetic Substitute in Uterus and Cervix, Open Approach

♀ **0UWD0KZ** Revision of Nonautologous Tissue Substitute in Uterus and Cervix, Open Approach

♀ **0UWD30Z** Revision of Drainage Device in Uterus and Cervix, Percutaneous Approach

♀ **0UWD31Z** Revision of Radioactive Element in Uterus and Cervix, Percutaneous Approach

♀ **0UWD33Z** Revision of Infusion Device in Uterus and Cervix, Percutaneous Approach

♀ **0UWD37Z** Revision of Autologous Tissue Substitute in Uterus and Cervix, Percutaneous Approach

♀ **0UWD3CZ** Revision of Extraluminal Device in Uterus and Cervix, Percutaneous Approach

♀ **0UWD3DZ** Revision of Intraluminal Device in Uterus and Cervix, Percutaneous Approach

♀ **0UWD3HZ** Revision of Contraceptive Device in Uterus and Cervix, Percutaneous Approach

♀ **0UWD3JZ** Revision of Synthetic Substitute in Uterus and Cervix, Percutaneous Approach

♀ **0UWD3KZ** Revision of Nonautologous Tissue Substitute in Uterus and Cervix, Percutaneous Approach

♀ **0UWD40Z** Revision of Drainage Device in Uterus and Cervix, Percutaneous Endoscopic Approach

♀ **0UWD41Z** Revision of Radioactive Element in Uterus and Cervix, Percutaneous Endoscopic Approach

♀ **0UWD43Z** Revision of Infusion Device in Uterus and Cervix, Percutaneous Endoscopic Approach

♀ **0UWD47Z** Revision of Autologous Tissue Substitute in Uterus and Cervix, Percutaneous Endoscopic Approach

♀ **0UWD4CZ** Revision of Extraluminal Device in Uterus and Cervix, Percutaneous Endoscopic Approach

♀ **0UWD4DZ** Revision of Intraluminal Device in Uterus and Cervix, Percutaneous Endoscopic Approach

♀ **0UWD4HZ** Revision of Contraceptive Device in Uterus and Cervix, Percutaneous Endoscopic Approach

♀ **0UWD4JZ** Revision of Synthetic Substitute in Uterus and Cervix, Percutaneous Endoscopic Approach

♀ **0UWD4KZ** Revision of Nonautologous Tissue Substitute in Uterus and Cervix, Percutaneous Endoscopic Approach

♀ **0UWD70Z** Revision of Drainage Device in Uterus and Cervix, Via Natural or Artificial Opening

♀ **0UWD71Z** Revision of Radioactive Element in Uterus and Cervix, Via Natural or Artificial Opening

♀ **0UWD73Z** Revision of Infusion Device in Uterus and Cervix, Via Natural or Artificial Opening

♀ **0UWD77Z** Revision of Autologous Tissue Substitute in Uterus and Cervix, Via Natural or Artificial Opening

♀ **0UWD7CZ** Revision of Extraluminal Device in Uterus and Cervix, Via Natural or Artificial Opening

♀ **0UWD7DZ** Revision of Intraluminal Device in Uterus and Cervix, Via Natural or Artificial Opening

♀ **0UWD7HZ** Revision of Contraceptive Device in Uterus and Cervix, Via Natural or Artificial Opening

♀ **0UWD7JZ** Revision of Synthetic Substitute in Uterus and Cervix, Via Natural or Artificial Opening

♀ **0UWD7KZ** Revision of Nonautologous Tissue Substitute in Uterus and Cervix, Via Natural or Artificial Opening

♀ **0UWD80Z** Revision of Drainage Device in Uterus and Cervix, Via Natural or Artificial Opening Endoscopic

♀ **0UWD81Z** Revision of Radioactive Element in Uterus and Cervix, Via Natural or Artificial Opening Endoscopic

♀ **0UWD83Z** Revision of Infusion Device in Uterus and Cervix, Via Natural or Artificial Opening Endoscopic

♀ **0UWD87Z** Revision of Autologous Tissue Substitute in Uterus and Cervix, Via Natural or Artificial Opening Endoscopic

♀ **0UWD8CZ** Revision of Extraluminal Device in Uterus and Cervix, Via Natural or Artificial Opening Endoscopic

♀ **0UWD8DZ** Revision of Intraluminal Device in Uterus and Cervix, Via Natural or Artificial Opening Endoscopic

♀ **0UWD8HZ** Revision of Contraceptive Device in Uterus and Cervix, Via Natural or Artificial Opening Endoscopic

♀ **0UWD8JZ** Revision of Synthetic Substitute in Uterus and Cervix, Via Natural or Artificial Opening Endoscopic

♀ **0UWD8KZ** Revision of Nonautologous Tissue Substitute in Uterus and Cervix, Via Natural or Artificial Opening Endoscopic

♀ **0UWDX0Z** Revision of Drainage Device in Uterus and Cervix, External Approach

♀ **0UWDX3Z** Revision of Infusion Device in Uterus and Cervix, External Approach

♀ **0UWDX7Z** Revision of Autologous Tissue Substitute in Uterus and Cervix, External Approach

♀ **0UWDXCZ** Revision of Extraluminal Device in Uterus and Cervix, External Approach

♀ **0UWDXDZ** Revision of Intraluminal Device in Uterus and Cervix, External Approach

♀ **0UWDXHZ** Revision of Contraceptive Device in Uterus and Cervix, External Approach

♀ **0UWDXJZ** Revision of Synthetic Substitute in Uterus and Cervix, External Approach

♀ **0UWDXKZ** Revision of Nonautologous Tissue Substitute in Uterus and Cervix, External Approach

♀ **0UWH00Z** Revision of Drainage Device in Vagina and Cul-de-sac, Open Approach

♀ **0UWH01Z** Revision of Radioactive Element in Vagina and Cul-de-sac, Open Approach

♀ **0UWH03Z** Revision of Infusion Device in Vagina and Cul-de-sac, Open Approach

♀ **0UWH07Z** Revision of Autologous Tissue Substitute in Vagina and Cul-de-sac, Open Approach

♀ **0UWH0DZ** Revision of Intraluminal Device in Vagina and Cul-de-sac, Open Approach

♀ **0UWH0JZ** Revision of Synthetic Substitute in Vagina and Cul-de-sac, Open Approach

♀ **0UWH0KZ** Revision of Nonautologous Tissue Substitute in Vagina and Cul-de-sac, Open Approach

♀ **0UWH30Z** Revision of Drainage Device in Vagina and Cul-de-sac, Percutaneous Approach

♀ **0UWH31Z** Revision of Radioactive Element in Vagina and Cul-de-sac, Percutaneous Approach

♀ **0UWH33Z** Revision of Infusion Device in Vagina and Cul-de-sac, Percutaneous Approach

---

♀ Female-only   ♂ Male-only   ● Limited Coverage   ● Non-OR   **HAC** HAC-associated procedure   ● Non-covered procedures   **+** Combination

♀ **0UWH37Z** Revision of Autologous Tissue Substitute in Vagina and Cul-de-sac, Percutaneous Approach
♀ **0UWH3DZ** Revision of Intraluminal Device in Vagina and Cul-de-sac, Percutaneous Approach
♀ **0UWH3JZ** Revision of Synthetic Substitute in Vagina and Cul-de-sac, Percutaneous Approach
♀ **0UWH3KZ** Revision of Nonautologous Tissue Substitute in Vagina and Cul-de-sac, Percutaneous Approach
♀ **0UWH40Z** Revision of Drainage Device in Vagina and Cul-de-sac, Percutaneous Endoscopic Approach
♀ **0UWH41Z** Revision of Radioactive Element in Vagina and Cul-de-sac, Percutaneous Endoscopic Approach
♀ **0UWH43Z** Revision of Infusion Device in Vagina and Cul-de-sac, Percutaneous Endoscopic Approach
♀ **0UWH47Z** Revision of Autologous Tissue Substitute in Vagina and Cul-de-sac, Percutaneous Endoscopic Approach
♀ **0UWH4DZ** Revision of Intraluminal Device in Vagina and Cul-de-sac, Percutaneous Endoscopic Approach
♀ **0UWH4JZ** Revision of Synthetic Substitute in Vagina and Cul-de-sac, Percutaneous Endoscopic Approach
♀ **0UWH4KZ** Revision of Nonautologous Tissue Substitute in Vagina and Cul-de-sac, Percutaneous Endoscopic Approach
♀ **0UWH70Z** Revision of Drainage Device in Vagina and Cul-de-sac, Via Natural or Artificial Opening
♀ **0UWH71Z** Revision of Radioactive Element in Vagina and Cul-de-sac, Via Natural or Artificial Opening
♀ **0UWH73Z** Revision of Infusion Device in Vagina and Cul-de-sac, Via Natural or Artificial Opening
♀ **0UWH77Z** Revision of Autologous Tissue Substitute in Vagina and Cul-de-sac, Via Natural or Artificial Opening
♀ **0UWH7DZ** Revision of Intraluminal Device in Vagina and Cul-de-sac, Via Natural or Artificial Opening
♀ **0UWH7JZ** Revision of Synthetic Substitute in Vagina and Cul-de-sac, Via Natural or Artificial Opening
♀ **0UWH7KZ** Revision of Nonautologous Tissue Substitute in Vagina and Cul-de-sac, Via Natural or Artificial Opening
♀ **0UWH80Z** Revision of Drainage Device in Vagina and Cul-de-sac, Via Natural or Artificial Opening Endoscopic

♀ **0UWH81Z** Revision of Radioactive Element in Vagina and Cul-de-sac, Via Natural or Artificial Opening Endoscopic
♀ **0UWH83Z** Revision of Infusion Device in Vagina and Cul-de-sac, Via Natural or Artificial Opening Endoscopic
♀ **0UWH87Z** Revision of Autologous Tissue Substitute in Vagina and Cul-de-sac, Via Natural or Artificial Opening Endoscopic
♀ **0UWH8DZ** Revision of Intraluminal Device in Vagina and Cul-de-sac, Via Natural or Artificial Opening Endoscopic
♀ **0UWH8JZ** Revision of Synthetic Substitute in Vagina and Cul-de-sac, Via Natural or Artificial Opening Endoscopic
♀ **0UWH8KZ** Revision of Nonautologous Tissue Substitute in Vagina and Cul-de-sac, Via Natural or Artificial Opening Endoscopic
♀ **0UWHX0Z** Revision of Drainage Device in Vagina and Cul-de-sac, External Approach
♀ **0UWHX3Z** Revision of Infusion Device in Vagina and Cul-de-sac, External Approach
♀ **0UWHX7Z** Revision of Autologous Tissue Substitute in Vagina and Cul-de-sac, External Approach
♀ **0UWHXDZ** Revision of Intraluminal Device in Vagina and Cul-de-sac, External Approach
♀ **0UWHXJZ** Revision of Synthetic Substitute in Vagina and Cul-de-sac, External Approach
♀ **0UWHXKZ** Revision of Nonautologous Tissue Substitute in Vagina and Cul-de-sac, External Approach
♀ **0UWM00Z** Revision of Drainage Device in Vulva, Open Approach
♀ **0UWM07Z** Revision of Autologous Tissue Substitute in Vulva, Open Approach
♀ **0UWM0JZ** Revision of Synthetic Substitute in Vulva, Open Approach
♀ **0UWM0KZ** Revision of Nonautologous Tissue Substitute in Vulva, Open Approach
♀ **0UWMX0Z** Revision of Drainage Device in Vulva, External Approach
♀ **0UWMX7Z** Revision of Autologous Tissue Substitute in Vulva, External Approach
♀ **0UWMXJZ** Revision of Synthetic Substitute in Vulva, External Approach
♀ **0UWMXKZ** Revision of Nonautologous Tissue Substitute in Vulva, External Approach

0UY – Female Reproductive System, Transplantation

Review Coding Guideline B3.16

♀ **0UY00Z0** Transplantation of Right Ovary, Allogeneic, Open Approach
♀ **0UY00Z1** Transplantation of Right Ovary, Syngeneic, Open Approach
♀ **0UY00Z2** Transplantation of Right Ovary, Zooplastic, Open Approach

♀ **0UY10Z0** Transplantation of Left Ovary, Allogeneic, Open Approach
♀ **0UY10Z1** Transplantation of Left Ovary, Syngeneic, Open Approach
♀ **0UY10Z2** Transplantation of Left Ovary, Zooplastic, Open Approach

♀ Female-only   ♂ Male-only   ● Limited Coverage   ● Non-OR   **HAC** HAC-associated procedure   ● Non-covered procedures   ✚ Combination

Male Reproductive System

Male Reproductive System

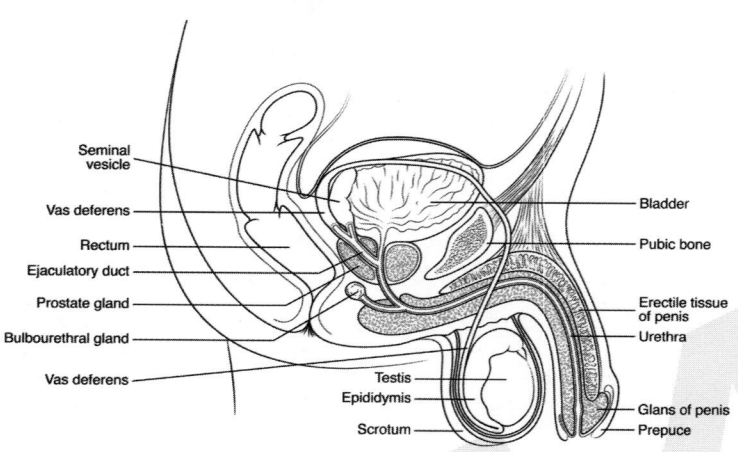

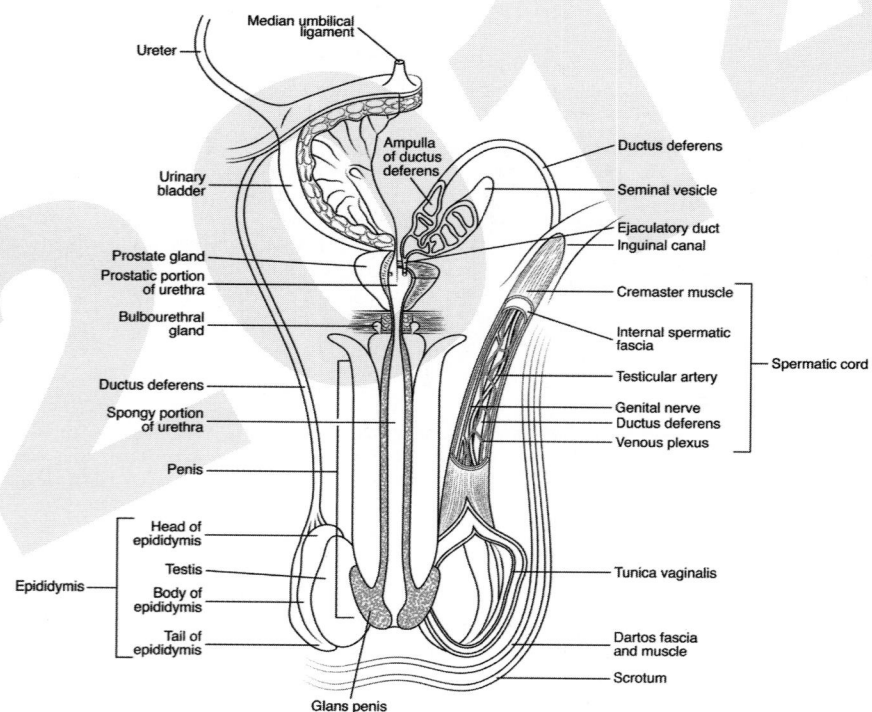

Male Reproductive System Tables 0V1–0VW

Section	0	Medical and Surgical
Body System	V	Male Reproductive System
Operation	1	**Bypass:** Altering the route of passage of the contents of a tubular body part

Body Part (4th)	Approach (5th)	Device (6th)	Qualifier (7th)
N Vas Deferens, Right P Vas Deferens, Left Q Vas Deferens, Bilateral	0 Open 4 Percutaneous Endoscopic	7 Autologous Tissue Substitute J Synthetic Substitute K Nonautologous Tissue Substitute Z No Device	J Epididymis, Right K Epididymis, Left N Vas Deferens, Right P Vas Deferens, Left

Section	0	**Medical and Surgical**
Body System	V	**Male Reproductive System**
Operation	2	**Change:** Taking out or off a device from a body part and putting back an identical or similar device in or on the same body part without cutting or puncturing the skin or a mucous membrane

Body Part (4ᵗʰ)	Approach (5ᵗʰ)	Device (6ᵗʰ)	Qualifier (7ᵗʰ)
4 Prostate and Seminal Vesicles 8 Scrotum and Tunica Vaginalis D Testis M Epididymis and Spermatic Cord R Vas Deferens S Penis	X External	0 Drainage Device Y Other Device	Z No Qualifier

Section	0	**Medical and Surgical**
Body System	V	**Male Reproductive System**
Operation	5	**Destruction:** Physical eradication of all or a portion of a body part by the direct use of energy, force, or a destructive agent

Body Part (4ᵗʰ)	Approach (5ᵗʰ)	Device (6ᵗʰ)	Qualifier (7ᵗʰ)
0 Prostate	0 Open 3 Percutaneous 4 Percutaneous Endoscopic 7 Via Natural or Artificial Opening 8 Via Natural or Artificial Opening Endoscopic	Z No Device	Z No Qualifier
1 Seminal Vesicle, Right 2 Seminal Vesicle, Left 3 Seminal Vesicles, Bilateral 6 Tunica Vaginalis, Right 7 Tunica Vaginalis, Left 9 Testis, Right B Testis, Left C Testes, Bilateral F Spermatic Cord, Right G Spermatic Cord, Left H Spermatic Cords, Bilateral J Epididymis, Right K Epididymis, Left L Epididymis, Bilateral N Vas Deferens, Right P Vas Deferens, Left Q Vas Deferens, Bilateral	0 Open 3 Percutaneous 4 Percutaneous Endoscopic	Z No Device	Z No Qualifier
5 Scrotum S Penis T Prepuce	0 Open 3 Percutaneous 4 Percutaneous Endoscopic X External	Z No Device	Z No Qualifier

Section	0	**Medical and Surgical**
Body System	V	**Male Reproductive System**
Operation	7	**Dilation:** Expanding an orifice or the lumen of a tubular body part

Body Part (4ᵗʰ)	Approach (5ᵗʰ)	Device (6ᵗʰ)	Qualifier (7ᵗʰ)
N Vas Deferens, Right P Vas Deferens, Left Q Vas Deferens, Bilateral	0 Open 3 Percutaneous 4 Percutaneous Endoscopic	D Intraluminal Device Z No Device	Z No Qualifier

Section	0	Medical and Surgical
Body System	V	Male Reproductive System
Operation	9	Drainage: Taking or letting out fluids and/or gases from a body part

Body Part (4th)	Approach (5th)	Device (6th)	Qualifier (7th)
0 Prostate	0 Open 3 Percutaneous 4 Percutaneous Endoscopic 7 Via Natural or Artificial Opening 8 Via Natural or Artificial Opening Endoscopic	0 Drainage Device	Z No Qualifier
0 Prostate	0 Open 3 Percutaneous 4 Percutaneous Endoscopic 7 Via Natural or Artificial Opening 8 Via Natural or Artificial Opening Endoscopic	Z No Device	X Diagnostic Z No Qualifier
1 Seminal Vesicle, Right 2 Seminal Vesicle, Left 3 Seminal Vesicles, Bilateral 6 Tunica Vaginalis, Right 7 Tunica Vaginalis, Left 9 Testis, Right B Testis, Left C Testes, Bilateral F Spermatic Cord, Right G Spermatic Cord, Left H Spermatic Cords, Bilateral J Epididymis, Right K Epididymis, Left L Epididymis, Bilateral N Vas Deferens, Right P Vas Deferens, Left Q Vas Deferens, Bilateral	0 Open 3 Percutaneous 4 Percutaneous Endoscopic	0 Drainage Device	Z No Qualifier
1 Seminal Vesicle, Right 2 Seminal Vesicle, Left 3 Seminal Vesicles, Bilateral 6 Tunica Vaginalis, Right 7 Tunica Vaginalis, Left 9 Testis, Right B Testis, Left C Testes, Bilateral F Spermatic Cord, Right G Spermatic Cord, Left H Spermatic Cords, Bilateral J Epididymis, Right K Epididymis, Left L Epididymis, Bilateral N Vas Deferens, Right P Vas Deferens, Left Q Vas Deferens, Bilateral	0 Open 3 Percutaneous 4 Percutaneous Endoscopic	Z No Device	X Diagnostic Z No Qualifier
5 Scrotum S Penis T Prepuce	0 Open 3 Percutaneous 4 Percutaneous Endoscopic X External	0 Drainage Device	Z No Qualifier
5 Scrotum S Penis T Prepuce	0 Open 3 Percutaneous 4 Percutaneous Endoscopic X External	Z No Device	X Diagnostic Z No Qualifier

Section	0	Medical and Surgical
Body System	V	Male Reproductive System
Operation	B	Excision: Cutting out or off, without replacement, a portion of a body part

Body Part (4th)	Approach (5th)	Device (6th)	Qualifier (7th)
0 Prostate	0 Open 3 Percutaneous 4 Percutaneous Endoscopic 7 Via Natural or Artificial Opening 8 Via Natural or Artificial Opening Endoscopic	Z No Device	X Diagnostic Z No Qualifier
1 Seminal Vesicle, Right 2 Seminal Vesicle, Left 3 Seminal Vesicles, Bilateral 6 Tunica Vaginalis, Right 7 Tunica Vaginalis, Left 9 Testis, Right B Testis, Left C Testes, Bilateral F Spermatic Cord, Right G Spermatic Cord, Left H Spermatic Cords, Bilateral J Epididymis, Right K Epididymis, Left L Epididymis, Bilateral N Vas Deferens, Right P Vas Deferens, Left Q Vas Deferens, Bilateral	0 Open 3 Percutaneous 4 Percutaneous Endoscopic	Z No Device	X Diagnostic Z No Qualifier
5 Scrotum S Penis T Prepuce	0 Open 3 Percutaneous 4 Percutaneous Endoscopic X External	Z No Device	X Diagnostic Z No Qualifier

Section	0	Medical and Surgical
Body System	V	Male Reproductive System
Operation	C	Extirpation: Taking or cutting out solid matter from a body part

Body Part (4th)	Approach (5th)	Device (6th)	Qualifier (7th)
0 Prostate	0 Open 3 Percutaneous 4 Percutaneous Endoscopic 7 Via Natural or Artificial Opening 8 Via Natural or Artificial Opening Endoscopic	Z No Device	Z No Qualifier
1 Seminal Vesicle, Right 2 Seminal Vesicle, Left 3 Seminal Vesicles, Bilateral 6 Tunica Vaginalis, Right 7 Tunica Vaginalis, Left 9 Testis, Right B Testis, Left C Testes, Bilateral F Spermatic Cord, Right G Spermatic Cord, Left H Spermatic Cords, Bilateral J Epididymis, Right K Epididymis, Left L Epididymis, Bilateral N Vas Deferens, Right P Vas Deferens, Left Q Vas Deferens, Bilateral	0 Open 3 Percutaneous 4 Percutaneous Endoscopic	Z No Device	Z No Qualifier
5 Scrotum S Penis T Prepuce	0 Open 3 Percutaneous 4 Percutaneous Endoscopic X External	Z No Device	Z No Qualifier

Section	0	Medical and Surgical
Body System	V	Male Reproductive System
Operation	H	Insertion: Putting in a nonbiological appliance that monitors, assists, performs, or prevents a physiological function but does not physically take the place of a body part

Body Part (4th)	Approach (5th)	Device (6th)	Qualifier (7th)
0 Prostate	0 Open 3 Percutaneous 4 Percutaneous Endoscopic 7 Via Natural or Artificial Opening 8 Via Natural or Artificial Opening Endoscopic	1 Radioactive Element	Z No Qualifier
4 Prostate and Seminal Vesicles 8 Scrotum and Tunica Vaginalis D Testis M Epididymis and Spermatic Cord R Vas Deferens	0 Open 3 Percutaneous 4 Percutaneous Endoscopic 7 Via Natural or Artificial Opening 8 Via Natural or Artificial Opening Endoscopic	3 Infusion Device	Z No Qualifier
S Penis	0 Open 3 Percutaneous 4 Percutaneous Endoscopic X External	3 Infusion Device	Z No Qualifier

Section	0	Medical and Surgical
Body System	V	Male Reproductive System
Operation	J	Inspection: Visually and/or manually exploring a body part

Body Part (4th)	Approach (5th)	Device (6th)	Qualifier (7th)
4 Prostate and Seminal Vesicles 8 Scrotum and Tunica Vaginalis D Testis M Epididymis and Spermatic Cord R Vas Deferens S Penis	0 Open 3 Percutaneous 4 Percutaneous Endoscopic X External	Z No Device	Z No Qualifier

Section	0	Medical and Surgical
Body System	V	Male Reproductive System
Operation	L	Occlusion: Completely closing an orifice or the lumen of a tubular body part

Body Part (4th)	Approach (5th)	Device (6th)	Qualifier (7th)
F Spermatic Cord, Right G Spermatic Cord, Left H Spermatic Cords, Bilateral N Vas Deferens, Right P Vas Deferens, Left Q Vas Deferens, Bilateral	0 Open 3 Percutaneous 4 Percutaneous Endoscopic	C Extraluminal Device D Intraluminal Device Z No Device	Z No Qualifier

Section	0	Medical and Surgical
Body System	V	Male Reproductive System
Operation	M	Reattachment: Putting back in or on all or a portion of a separated body part to its normal location or other suitable location

Body Part (4th)	Approach (5th)	Device (6th)	Qualifier (7th)
5 Scrotum S Penis	X External	Z No Device	Z No Qualifier
6 Tunica Vaginalis, Right 7 Tunica Vaginalis, Left 9 Testis, Right B Testis, Left C Testes, Bilateral F Spermatic Cord, Right G Spermatic Cord, Left H Spermatic Cords, Bilateral	0 Open 4 Percutaneous Endoscopic	Z No Device	Z No Qualifier

Section	0	Medical and Surgical
Body System	V	Male Reproductive System
Operation	N	Release: Freeing a body part from an abnormal physical constraint by cutting or by the use of force

Body Part (4th)	Approach (5th)	Device (6th)	Qualifier (7th)
0 Prostate	0 Open 3 Percutaneous 4 Percutaneous Endoscopic 7 Via Natural or Artificial Opening 8 Via Natural or Artificial Opening Endoscopic	Z No Device	Z No Qualifier
1 Seminal Vesicle, Right 2 Seminal Vesicle, Left 3 Seminal Vesicles, Bilateral 6 Tunica Vaginalis, Right 7 Tunica Vaginalis, Left 9 Testis, Right B Testis, Left C Testes, Bilateral F Spermatic Cord, Right G Spermatic Cord, Left H Spermatic Cords, Bilateral J Epididymis, Right K Epididymis, Left L Epididymis, Bilateral N Vas Deferens, Right P Vas Deferens, Left Q Vas Deferens, Bilateral	0 Open 3 Percutaneous 4 Percutaneous Endoscopic	Z No Device	Z No Qualifier
5 Scrotum S Penis T Prepuce	0 Open 3 Percutaneous 4 Percutaneous Endoscopic X External	Z No Device	Z No Qualifier

Section	0	Medical and Surgical
Body System	V	Male Reproductive System
Operation	P	Removal: Taking out or off a device from a body part

Body Part (4th)	Approach (5th)	Device (6th)	Qualifier (7th)
4 Prostate and Seminal Vesicles	0 Open 3 Percutaneous 4 Percutaneous Endoscopic 7 Via Natural or Artificial Opening 8 Via Natural or Artificial Opening Endoscopic	0 Drainage Device 1 Radioactive Element 3 Infusion Device 7 Autologous Tissue Substitute J Synthetic Substitute K Nonautologous Tissue Substitute	Z No Qualifier
4 Prostate and Seminal Vesicles	X External	0 Drainage Device 1 Radioactive Element 3 Infusion Device	Z No Qualifier
8 Scrotum and Tunica Vaginalis D Testis S Penis	0 Open 3 Percutaneous 4 Percutaneous Endoscopic 7 Via Natural or Artificial Opening 8 Via Natural or Artificial Opening Endoscopic	0 Drainage Device 3 Infusion Device 7 Autologous Tissue Substitute J Synthetic Substitute K Nonautologous Tissue Substitute	Z No Qualifier
8 Scrotum and Tunica Vaginalis D Testis S Penis	X External	0 Drainage Device 3 Infusion Device	Z No Qualifier
M Epididymis and Spermatic Cord	0 Open 3 Percutaneous 4 Percutaneous Endoscopic 7 Via Natural or Artificial Opening 8 Via Natural or Artificial Opening Endoscopic	0 Drainage Device 3 Infusion Device 7 Autologous Tissue Substitute C Extraluminal Device J Synthetic Substitute K Nonautologous Tissue Substitute	Z No Qualifier
M Epididymis and Spermatic Cord	X External	0 Drainage Device 3 Infusion Device	Z No Qualifier
R Vas Deferens	0 Open 3 Percutaneous 4 Percutaneous Endoscopic 7 Via Natural or Artificial Opening 8 Via Natural or Artificial Opening Endoscopic	0 Drainage Device 3 Infusion Device 7 Autologous Tissue Substitute C Extraluminal Device D Intraluminal Device J Synthetic Substitute K Nonautologous Tissue Substitute	Z No Qualifier
R Vas Deferens	X External	0 Drainage Device 3 Infusion Device D Intraluminal Device	Z No Qualifier

Section	0	Medical and Surgical
Body System	V	Male Reproductive System
Operation	Q	**Repair:** Restoring, to the extent possible, a body part to its normal anatomic structure and function

Body Part (4th)	Approach (5th)	Device (6th)	Qualifier (7th)
0 Prostate	0 Open 3 Percutaneous 4 Percutaneous Endoscopic 7 Via Natural or Artificial Opening 8 Via Natural or Artificial Opening Endoscopic	Z No Device	Z No Qualifier
1 Seminal Vesicle, Right 2 Seminal Vesicle, Left 3 Seminal Vesicles, Bilateral 6 Tunica Vaginalis, Right 7 Tunica Vaginalis, Left 9 Testis, Right B Testis, Left C Testes, Bilateral F Spermatic Cord, Right G Spermatic Cord, Left H Spermatic Cords, Bilateral J Epididymis, Right K Epididymis, Left L Epididymis, Bilateral N Vas Deferens, Right P Vas Deferens, Left Q Vas Deferens, Bilateral	0 Open 3 Percutaneous 4 Percutaneous Endoscopic	Z No Device	Z No Qualifier
5 Scrotum S Penis T Prepuce	0 Open 3 Percutaneous 4 Percutaneous Endoscopic X External	Z No Device	Z No Qualifier

Section	0	Medical and Surgical
Body System	V	Male Reproductive System
Operation	R	**Replacement:** Putting in or on biological or synthetic material that physically takes the place and/or function of all or a portion of a body part

Body Part (4th)	Approach (5th)	Device (6th)	Qualifier (7th)
9 Testis, Right B Testis, Left C Testes, Bilateral	0 Open	J Synthetic Substitute	Z No Qualifier

Section	0	Medical and Surgical
Body System	V	Male Reproductive System
Operation	S	**Reposition:** Moving to its normal location, or other suitable location, all or a portion of a body part

Body Part (4th)	Approach (5th)	Device (6th)	Qualifier (7th)
9 Testis, Right B Testis, Left C Testes, Bilateral F Spermatic Cord, Right G Spermatic Cord, Left H Spermatic Cords, Bilateral	0 Open 3 Percutaneous 4 Percutaneous Endoscopic	Z No Device	Z No Qualifier

Section   0   **Medical and Surgical**
Body System   V   **Male Reproductive System**
Operation   T   **Resection:** Cutting out or off, without replacement, all of a body part

Body Part (4th)	Approach (5th)	Device (6th)	Qualifier (7th)
0 Prostate	0 Open 4 Percutaneous Endoscopic 7 Via Natural or Artificial Opening 8 Via Natural or Artificial Opening Endoscopic	Z No Device	Z No Qualifier
1 Seminal Vesicle, Right 2 Seminal Vesicle, Left 3 Seminal Vesicles, Bilateral 6 Tunica Vaginalis, Right 7 Tunica Vaginalis, Left 9 Testis, Right B Testis, Left C Testes, Bilateral F Spermatic Cord, Right G Spermatic Cord, Left H Spermatic Cords, Bilateral J Epididymis, Right K Epididymis, Left L Epididymis, Bilateral N Vas Deferens, Right P Vas Deferens, Left Q Vas Deferens, Bilateral	0 Open 4 Percutaneous Endoscopic	Z No Device	Z No Qualifier
5 Scrotum S Penis T Prepuce	0 Open 4 Percutaneous Endoscopic X External	Z No Device	Z No Qualifier

Section   0   **Medical and Surgical**
Body System   V   **Male Reproductive System**
Operation   U   **Supplement:** Putting in or on biological or synthetic material that physically reinforces and/or augments the function of a portion of a body part

Body Part (4th)	Approach (5th)	Device (6th)	Qualifier (7th)
1 Seminal Vesicle, Right 2 Seminal Vesicle, Left 3 Seminal Vesicles, Bilateral 6 Tunica Vaginalis, Right 7 Tunica Vaginalis, Left F Spermatic Cord, Right G Spermatic Cord, Left H Spermatic Cords, Bilateral J Epididymis, Right K Epididymis, Left L Epididymis, Bilateral N Vas Deferens, Right P Vas Deferens, Left Q Vas Deferens, Bilateral	0 Open 4 Percutaneous Endoscopic	7 Autologous Tissue Substitute J Synthetic Substitute K Nonautologous Tissue Substitute	Z No Qualifier
5 Scrotum S Penis T Prepuce	0 Open 4 Percutaneous Endoscopic X External	7 Autologous Tissue Substitute J Synthetic Substitute K Nonautologous Tissue Substitute	Z No Qualifier
9 Testis, Right B Testis, Left C Testes, Bilateral	0 Open	7 Autologous Tissue Substitute J Synthetic Substitute K Nonautologous Tissue Substitute	Z No Qualifier

Section	0	Medical and Surgical
Body System	V	Male Reproductive System
Operation	W	**Revision:** Correcting, to the extent possible, a portion of a malfunctioning device or the position of a displaced device

Body Part (4ᵗʰ)	Approach (5ᵗʰ)	Device (6ᵗʰ)	Qualifier (7ᵗʰ)
4 Prostate and Seminal Vesicles 8 Scrotum and Tunica Vaginalis D Testis S Penis	0 Open 3 Percutaneous 4 Percutaneous Endoscopic 7 Via Natural or Artificial Opening 8 Via Natural or Artificial Opening Endoscopic X External	0 Drainage Device 3 Infusion Device 7 Autologous Tissue Substitute J Synthetic Substitute K Nonautologous Tissue Substitute	Z No Qualifier
M Epididymis and Spermatic Cord	0 Open 3 Percutaneous 4 Percutaneous Endoscopic 7 Via Natural or Artificial Opening 8 Via Natural or Artificial Opening Endoscopic X External	0 Drainage Device 3 Infusion Device 7 Autologous Tissue Substitute C Extraluminal Device J Synthetic Substitute K Nonautologous Tissue Substitute	Z No Qualifier
R Vas Deferens	0 Open 3 Percutaneous 4 Percutaneous Endoscopic 7 Via Natural or Artificial Opening 8 Via Natural or Artificial Opening Endoscopic X External	0 Drainage Device 3 Infusion Device 7 Autologous Tissue Substitute C Extraluminal Device D Intraluminal Device J Synthetic Substitute K Nonautologous Tissue Substitute	Z No Qualifier

Male Reproductive System Code Listing 0V1–0VW

0V1 – Male Reproductive System, Bypass

Review Coding Guideline B3.6a

♂ **0V1N07J** Bypass Right Vas Deferens to Right Epididymis with Autologous Tissue Substitute, Open Approach

♂ **0V1N07K** Bypass Right Vas Deferens to Left Epididymis with Autologous Tissue Substitute, Open Approach

♂ **0V1N07N** Bypass Right Vas Deferens to Right Vas Deferens with Autologous Tissue Substitute, Open Approach

♂ **0V1N07P** Bypass Right Vas Deferens to Left Vas Deferens with Autologous Tissue Substitute, Open Approach

♂ **0V1N0JJ** Bypass Right Vas Deferens to Right Epididymis with Synthetic Substitute, Open Approach

♂ **0V1N0JK** Bypass Right Vas Deferens to Left Epididymis with Synthetic Substitute, Open Approach

♂ **0V1N0JN** Bypass Right Vas Deferens to Right Vas Deferens with Synthetic Substitute, Open Approach

♂ **0V1N0JP** Bypass Right Vas Deferens to Left Vas Deferens with Synthetic Substitute, Open Approach

♂ **0V1N0KJ** Bypass Right Vas Deferens to Right Epididymis with Nonautologous Tissue Substitute, Open Approach

♂ **0V1N0KK** Bypass Right Vas Deferens to Left Epididymis with Nonautologous Tissue Substitute, Open Approach

♂ **0V1N0KN** Bypass Right Vas Deferens to Right Vas Deferens with Nonautologous Tissue Substitute, Open Approach

♂ **0V1N0KP** Bypass Right Vas Deferens to Left Vas Deferens with Nonautologous Tissue Substitute, Open Approach

♂ **0V1N0ZJ** Bypass Right Vas Deferens to Right Epididymis, Open Approach

♂ **0V1N0ZK** Bypass Right Vas Deferens to Left Epididymis, Open Approach

♂ **0V1N0ZN** Bypass Right Vas Deferens to Right Vas Deferens, Open Approach

♂ **0V1N0ZP** Bypass Right Vas Deferens to Left Vas Deferens, Open Approach

♂ **0V1N47J** Bypass Right Vas Deferens to Right Epididymis with Autologous Tissue Substitute, Percutaneous Endoscopic Approach

♂ **0V1N47K** Bypass Right Vas Deferens to Left Epididymis with Autologous Tissue Substitute, Percutaneous Endoscopic Approach

♂ **0V1N47N** Bypass Right Vas Deferens to Right Vas Deferens with Autologous Tissue Substitute, Percutaneous Endoscopic Approach

♂ **0V1N47P** Bypass Right Vas Deferens to Left Vas Deferens with Autologous Tissue Substitute, Percutaneous Endoscopic Approach

♂ **0V1N4JJ** Bypass Right Vas Deferens to Right Epididymis with Synthetic Substitute, Percutaneous Endoscopic Approach

♂ **0V1N4JK** Bypass Right Vas Deferens to Left Epididymis with Synthetic Substitute, Percutaneous Endoscopic Approach

♂ **0V1N4JN** Bypass Right Vas Deferens to Right Vas Deferens with Synthetic Substitute, Percutaneous Endoscopic Approach

♂ **0V1N4JP** Bypass Right Vas Deferens to Left Vas Deferens with Synthetic Substitute, Percutaneous Endoscopic Approach

♂ **0V1N4KJ** Bypass Right Vas Deferens to Right Epididymis with Nonautologous Tissue Substitute, Percutaneous Endoscopic Approach

♂ **0V1N4KK** Bypass Right Vas Deferens to Left Epididymis with Nonautologous Tissue Substitute, Percutaneous Endoscopic Approach

♂ **0V1N4KN** Bypass Right Vas Deferens to Right Vas Deferens with Nonautologous Tissue Substitute, Percutaneous Endoscopic Approach

♂ **0V1N4KP** Bypass Right Vas Deferens to Left Vas Deferens with Nonautologous Tissue Substitute, Percutaneous Endoscopic Approach

♂ **0V1N4ZJ** Bypass Right Vas Deferens to Right Epididymis, Percutaneous Endoscopic Approach

♀ Female-only   ♂ Male-only   ● Limited Coverage   ● Non-OR   🄷🄰🄲 HAC-associated procedure   ⬢ Non-covered procedures   ➕ Combination

♂ **0V1N4ZK** Bypass Right Vas Deferens to Left Epididymis, Percutaneous Endoscopic Approach

♂ **0V1N4ZN** Bypass Right Vas Deferens to Right Vas Deferens, Percutaneous Endoscopic Approach

♂ **0V1N4ZP** Bypass Right Vas Deferens to Left Vas Deferens, Percutaneous Endoscopic Approach

♂ **0V1P07J** Bypass Left Vas Deferens to Right Epididymis with Autologous Tissue Substitute, Open Approach

♂ **0V1P07K** Bypass Left Vas Deferens to Left Epididymis with Autologous Tissue Substitute, Open Approach

♂ **0V1P07N** Bypass Left Vas Deferens to Right Vas Deferens with Autologous Tissue Substitute, Open Approach

♂ **0V1P07P** Bypass Left Vas Deferens to Left Vas Deferens with Autologous Tissue Substitute, Open Approach

♂ **0V1P0JJ** Bypass Left Vas Deferens to Right Epididymis with Synthetic Substitute, Open Approach

♂ **0V1P0JK** Bypass Left Vas Deferens to Left Epididymis with Synthetic Substitute, Open Approach

♂ **0V1P0JN** Bypass Left Vas Deferens to Right Vas Deferens with Synthetic Substitute, Open Approach

♂ **0V1P0JP** Bypass Left Vas Deferens to Left Vas Deferens with Synthetic Substitute, Open Approach

♂ **0V1P0KJ** Bypass Left Vas Deferens to Right Epididymis with Nonautologous Tissue Substitute, Open Approach

♂ **0V1P0KK** Bypass Left Vas Deferens to Left Epididymis with Nonautologous Tissue Substitute, Open Approach

♂ **0V1P0KN** Bypass Left Vas Deferens to Right Vas Deferens with Nonautologous Tissue Substitute, Open Approach

♂ **0V1P0KP** Bypass Left Vas Deferens to Left Vas Deferens with Nonautologous Tissue Substitute, Open Approach

♂ **0V1P0ZJ** Bypass Left Vas Deferens to Right Epididymis, Open Approach

♂ **0V1P0ZK** Bypass Left Vas Deferens to Left Epididymis, Open Approach

♂ **0V1P0ZN** Bypass Left Vas Deferens to Right Vas Deferens, Open Approach

♂ **0V1P0ZP** Bypass Left Vas Deferens to Left Vas Deferens, Open Approach

♂ **0V1P47J** Bypass Left Vas Deferens to Right Epididymis with Autologous Tissue Substitute, Percutaneous Endoscopic Approach

♂ **0V1P47K** Bypass Left Vas Deferens to Left Epididymis with Autologous Tissue Substitute, Percutaneous Endoscopic Approach

♂ **0V1P47N** Bypass Left Vas Deferens to Right Vas Deferens with Autologous Tissue Substitute, Percutaneous Endoscopic Approach

♂ **0V1P47P** Bypass Left Vas Deferens to Left Vas Deferens with Autologous Tissue Substitute, Percutaneous Endoscopic Approach

♂ **0V1P4JJ** Bypass Left Vas Deferens to Right Epididymis with Synthetic Substitute, Percutaneous Endoscopic Approach

♂ **0V1P4JK** Bypass Left Vas Deferens to Left Epididymis with Synthetic Substitute, Percutaneous Endoscopic Approach

♂ **0V1P4JN** Bypass Left Vas Deferens to Right Vas Deferens with Synthetic Substitute, Percutaneous Endoscopic Approach

♂ **0V1P4JP** Bypass Left Vas Deferens to Left Vas Deferens with Synthetic Substitute, Percutaneous Endoscopic Approach

♂ **0V1P4KJ** Bypass Left Vas Deferens to Right Epididymis with Nonautologous Tissue Substitute, Percutaneous Endoscopic Approach

♂ **0V1P4KK** Bypass Left Vas Deferens to Left Epididymis with Nonautologous Tissue Substitute, Percutaneous Endoscopic Approach

♂ **0V1P4KN** Bypass Left Vas Deferens to Right Vas Deferens with Nonautologous Tissue Substitute, Percutaneous Endoscopic Approach

♂ **0V1P4KP** Bypass Left Vas Deferens to Left Vas Deferens with Nonautologous Tissue Substitute, Percutaneous Endoscopic Approach

♂ **0V1P4ZJ** Bypass Left Vas Deferens to Right Epididymis, Percutaneous Endoscopic Approach

♂ **0V1P4ZK** Bypass Left Vas Deferens to Left Epididymis, Percutaneous Endoscopic Approach

♂ **0V1P4ZN** Bypass Left Vas Deferens to Right Vas Deferens, Percutaneous Endoscopic Approach

♂ **0V1P4ZP** Bypass Left Vas Deferens to Left Vas Deferens, Percutaneous Endoscopic Approach

♂ **0V1Q07J** Bypass Bilateral Vas Deferens to Right Epididymis with Autologous Tissue Substitute, Open Approach

♂ **0V1Q07K** Bypass Bilateral Vas Deferens to Left Epididymis with Autologous Tissue Substitute, Open Approach

♂ **0V1Q07N** Bypass Bilateral Vas Deferens to Right Vas Deferens with Autologous Tissue Substitute, Open Approach

♂ **0V1Q07P** Bypass Bilateral Vas Deferens to Left Vas Deferens with Autologous Tissue Substitute, Open Approach

♂ **0V1Q0JJ** Bypass Bilateral Vas Deferens to Right Epididymis with Synthetic Substitute, Open Approach

♂ **0V1Q0JK** Bypass Bilateral Vas Deferens to Left Epididymis with Synthetic Substitute, Open Approach

♂ **0V1Q0JN** Bypass Bilateral Vas Deferens to Right Vas Deferens with Synthetic Substitute, Open Approach

♂ **0V1Q0JP** Bypass Bilateral Vas Deferens to Left Vas Deferens with Synthetic Substitute, Open Approach

♂ **0V1Q0KJ** Bypass Bilateral Vas Deferens to Right Epididymis with Nonautologous Tissue Substitute, Open Approach

♂ **0V1Q0KK** Bypass Bilateral Vas Deferens to Left Epididymis with Nonautologous Tissue Substitute, Open Approach

♂ **0V1Q0KN** Bypass Bilateral Vas Deferens to Right Vas Deferens with Nonautologous Tissue Substitute, Open Approach

♂ **0V1Q0KP** Bypass Bilateral Vas Deferens to Left Vas Deferens with Nonautologous Tissue Substitute, Open Approach

♂ **0V1Q0ZJ** Bypass Bilateral Vas Deferens to Right Epididymis, Open Approach

♂ **0V1Q0ZK** Bypass Bilateral Vas Deferens to Left Epididymis, Open Approach

♂ **0V1Q0ZN** Bypass Bilateral Vas Deferens to Right Vas Deferens, Open Approach

♂ **0V1Q0ZP** Bypass Bilateral Vas Deferens to Left Vas Deferens, Open Approach

♂ **0V1Q47J** Bypass Bilateral Vas Deferens to Right Epididymis with Autologous Tissue Substitute, Percutaneous Endoscopic Approach

♂ **0V1Q47K** Bypass Bilateral Vas Deferens to Left Epididymis with Autologous Tissue Substitute, Percutaneous Endoscopic Approach

♂ **0V1Q47N** Bypass Bilateral Vas Deferens to Right Vas Deferens with Autologous Tissue Substitute, Percutaneous Endoscopic Approach

♂ **0V1Q47P** Bypass Bilateral Vas Deferens to Left Vas Deferens with Autologous Tissue Substitute, Percutaneous Endoscopic Approach

♂ **0V1Q4JJ** Bypass Bilateral Vas Deferens to Right Epididymis with Synthetic Substitute, Percutaneous Endoscopic Approach

♂ **0V1Q4JK** Bypass Bilateral Vas Deferens to Left Epididymis with Synthetic Substitute, Percutaneous Endoscopic Approach

♂ **0V1Q4JN** Bypass Bilateral Vas Deferens to Right Vas Deferens with Synthetic Substitute, Percutaneous Endoscopic Approach

♂ **0V1Q4JP** Bypass Bilateral Vas Deferens to Left Vas Deferens with Synthetic Substitute, Percutaneous Endoscopic Approach

♂ **0V1Q4KJ** Bypass Bilateral Vas Deferens to Right Epididymis with Nonautologous Tissue Substitute, Percutaneous Endoscopic Approach

♂ **0V1Q4KK** Bypass Bilateral Vas Deferens to Left Epididymis with Nonautologous Tissue Substitute, Percutaneous Endoscopic Approach

♂ **0V1Q4KN** Bypass Bilateral Vas Deferens to Right Vas Deferens with Nonautologous Tissue Substitute, Percutaneous Endoscopic Approach

♂ **0V1Q4KP** Bypass Bilateral Vas Deferens to Left Vas Deferens with Nonautologous Tissue Substitute, Percutaneous Endoscopic Approach

♂ **0V1Q4ZJ** Bypass Bilateral Vas Deferens to Right Epididymis, Percutaneous Endoscopic Approach

♂ **0V1Q4ZK** Bypass Bilateral Vas Deferens to Left Epididymis, Percutaneous Endoscopic Approach

♂ **0V1Q4ZN** Bypass Bilateral Vas Deferens to Right Vas Deferens, Percutaneous Endoscopic Approach

♂ **0V1Q4ZP** Bypass Bilateral Vas Deferens to Left Vas Deferens, Percutaneous Endoscopic Approach

0V2 – Male Reproductive System, Change

Review Coding Guideline B6.1c

♂ **0V24X0Z** Change Drainage Device in Prostate and Seminal Vesicles, External Approach

♂ **0V24XYZ** Change Other Device in Prostate and Seminal Vesicles, External Approach

♂ **0V28X0Z** Change Drainage Device in Scrotum and Tunica Vaginalis, External Approach

♂ **0V28XYZ** Change Other Device in Scrotum and Tunica Vaginalis, External Approach

♂ **0V2DX0Z** Change Drainage Device in Testis, External Approach

♂ **0V2DXYZ** Change Other Device in Testis, External Approach

♂ **0V2MX0Z** Change Drainage Device in Epididymis and Spermatic Cord, External Approach

---

♀ Female-only   ♂ Male-only   ● Limited Coverage   ● Non-OR   HAC HAC-associated procedure   ● Non-covered procedures   + Combination

♂ **0V2MXYZ** Change Other Device in Epididymis and Spermatic Cord, External Approach

♂ **0V2RX0Z** Change Drainage Device in Vas Deferens, External Approach

♂ **0V2RXYZ** Change Other Device in Vas Deferens, External Approach

♂ **0V2SX0Z** Change Drainage Device in Penis, External Approach

♂ **0V2SXYZ** Change Other Device in Penis, External Approach

0V5 – Male Reproductive System, Destruction

♂ **0V500ZZ** Destruction of Prostate, Open Approach

♂ **0V503ZZ** Destruction of Prostate, Percutaneous Approach

♂ **0V504ZZ** Destruction of Prostate, Percutaneous Endoscopic Approach

♂ **0V507ZZ** Destruction of Prostate, Via Natural or Artificial Opening

♂ **0V508ZZ** Destruction of Prostate, Via Natural or Artificial Opening Endoscopic

♂ **0V510ZZ** Destruction of Right Seminal Vesicle, Open Approach

♂ **0V513ZZ** Destruction of Right Seminal Vesicle, Percutaneous Approach

♂ **0V514ZZ** Destruction of Right Seminal Vesicle, Percutaneous Endoscopic Approach

♂ **0V520ZZ** Destruction of Left Seminal Vesicle, Open Approach

♂ **0V523ZZ** Destruction of Left Seminal Vesicle, Percutaneous Approach

♂ **0V524ZZ** Destruction of Left Seminal Vesicle, Percutaneous Endoscopic Approach

♂ **0V530ZZ** Destruction of Bilateral Seminal Vesicles, Open Approach

♂ **0V533ZZ** Destruction of Bilateral Seminal Vesicles, Percutaneous Approach

♂ **0V534ZZ** Destruction of Bilateral Seminal Vesicles, Percutaneous Endoscopic Approach

♂ **0V550ZZ** Destruction of Scrotum, Open Approach

♂ **0V553ZZ** Destruction of Scrotum, Percutaneous Approach

♂ **0V554ZZ** Destruction of Scrotum, Percutaneous Endoscopic Approach

♂ **0V55XZZ** Destruction of Scrotum, External Approach

♂ **0V560ZZ** Destruction of Right Tunica Vaginalis, Open Approach

♂ **0V563ZZ** Destruction of Right Tunica Vaginalis, Percutaneous Approach

♂ **0V564ZZ** Destruction of Right Tunica Vaginalis, Percutaneous Endoscopic Approach

♂ **0V570ZZ** Destruction of Left Tunica Vaginalis, Open Approach

♂ **0V573ZZ** Destruction of Left Tunica Vaginalis, Percutaneous Approach

♂ **0V574ZZ** Destruction of Left Tunica Vaginalis, Percutaneous Endoscopic Approach

♂ **0V590ZZ** Destruction of Right Testis, Open Approach

♂ **0V593ZZ** Destruction of Right Testis, Percutaneous Approach

♂ **0V594ZZ** Destruction of Right Testis, Percutaneous Endoscopic Approach

♂ **0V5B0ZZ** Destruction of Left Testis, Open Approach

♂ **0V5B3ZZ** Destruction of Left Testis, Percutaneous Approach

♂ **0V5B4ZZ** Destruction of Left Testis, Percutaneous Endoscopic Approach

♂ **0V5C0ZZ** Destruction of Bilateral Testes, Open Approach

♂ **0V5C3ZZ** Destruction of Bilateral Testes, Percutaneous Approach

♂ **0V5C4ZZ** Destruction of Bilateral Testes, Percutaneous Endoscopic Approach

♂ **0V5F0ZZ** Destruction of Right Spermatic Cord, Open Approach

♂ **0V5F3ZZ** Destruction of Right Spermatic Cord, Percutaneous Approach

♂ **0V5F4ZZ** Destruction of Right Spermatic Cord, Percutaneous Endoscopic Approach

♂ **0V5G0ZZ** Destruction of Left Spermatic Cord, Open Approach

♂ **0V5G3ZZ** Destruction of Left Spermatic Cord, Percutaneous Approach

♂ **0V5G4ZZ** Destruction of Left Spermatic Cord, Percutaneous Endoscopic Approach

♂ **0V5H0ZZ** Destruction of Bilateral Spermatic Cords, Open Approach

♂ **0V5H3ZZ** Destruction of Bilateral Spermatic Cords, Percutaneous Approach

♂ **0V5H4ZZ** Destruction of Bilateral Spermatic Cords, Percutaneous Endoscopic Approach

♂ **0V5J0ZZ** Destruction of Right Epididymis, Open Approach

♂ **0V5J3ZZ** Destruction of Right Epididymis, Percutaneous Approach

♂ **0V5J4ZZ** Destruction of Right Epididymis, Percutaneous Endoscopic Approach

♂ **0V5K0ZZ** Destruction of Left Epididymis, Open Approach

♂ **0V5K3ZZ** Destruction of Left Epididymis, Percutaneous Approach

♂ **0V5K4ZZ** Destruction of Left Epididymis, Percutaneous Endoscopic Approach

♂ **0V5L0ZZ** Destruction of Bilateral Epididymis, Open Approach

♂ **0V5L3ZZ** Destruction of Bilateral Epididymis, Percutaneous Approach

♂ **0V5L4ZZ** Destruction of Bilateral Epididymis, Percutaneous Endoscopic Approach

●♂ **0V5N0ZZ** Destruction of Right Vas Deferens, Open Approach

●♂ **0V5N3ZZ** Destruction of Right Vas Deferens, Percutaneous Approach

●♂ **0V5N4ZZ** Destruction of Right Vas Deferens, Percutaneous Endoscopic Approach

●♂ **0V5P0ZZ** Destruction of Left Vas Deferens, Open Approach

●♂ **0V5P3ZZ** Destruction of Left Vas Deferens, Percutaneous Approach

●♂ **0V5P4ZZ** Destruction of Left Vas Deferens, Percutaneous Endoscopic Approach

♂ **0V5Q0ZZ** Destruction of Bilateral Vas Deferens, Open Approach

♂ **0V5Q3ZZ** Destruction of Bilateral Vas Deferens, Percutaneous Approach

♂ **0V5Q4ZZ** Destruction of Bilateral Vas Deferens, Percutaneous Endoscopic Approach

♂ **0V5S0ZZ** Destruction of Penis, Open Approach

♂ **0V5S3ZZ** Destruction of Penis, Percutaneous Approach

♂ **0V5S4ZZ** Destruction of Penis, Percutaneous Endoscopic Approach

♂ **0V5SXZZ** Destruction of Penis, External Approach

♂ **0V5T0ZZ** Destruction of Prepuce, Open Approach

♂ **0V5T3ZZ** Destruction of Prepuce, Percutaneous Approach

♂ **0V5T4ZZ** Destruction of Prepuce, Percutaneous Endoscopic Approach

♂ **0V5TXZZ** Destruction of Prepuce, External Approach

0V7 – Male Reproductive System, Dilation

♂ **0V7N0DZ** Dilation of Right Vas Deferens with Intraluminal Device, Open Approach

♂ **0V7N0ZZ** Dilation of Right Vas Deferens, Open Approach

♂ **0V7N3DZ** Dilation of Right Vas Deferens with Intraluminal Device, Percutaneous Approach

♂ **0V7N3ZZ** Dilation of Right Vas Deferens, Percutaneous Approach

♂ **0V7N4DZ** Dilation of Right Vas Deferens with Intraluminal Device, Percutaneous Endoscopic Approach

♂ **0V7N4ZZ** Dilation of Right Vas Deferens, Percutaneous Endoscopic Approach

♂ **0V7P0DZ** Dilation of Left Vas Deferens with Intraluminal Device, Open Approach

♂ **0V7P0ZZ** Dilation of Left Vas Deferens, Open Approach

♂ **0V7P3DZ** Dilation of Left Vas Deferens with Intraluminal Device, Percutaneous Approach

♂ **0V7P3ZZ** Dilation of Left Vas Deferens, Percutaneous Approach

♂ **0V7P4DZ** Dilation of Left Vas Deferens with Intraluminal Device, Percutaneous Endoscopic Approach

♂ **0V7P4ZZ** Dilation of Left Vas Deferens, Percutaneous Endoscopic Approach

♂ **0V7Q0DZ** Dilation of Bilateral Vas Deferens with Intraluminal Device, Open Approach

♂ **0V7Q0ZZ** Dilation of Bilateral Vas Deferens, Open Approach

♂ **0V7Q3DZ** Dilation of Bilateral Vas Deferens with Intraluminal Device, Percutaneous Approach

♂ **0V7Q3ZZ** Dilation of Bilateral Vas Deferens, Percutaneous Approach

♂ **0V7Q4DZ** Dilation of Bilateral Vas Deferens with Intraluminal Device, Percutaneous Endoscopic Approach

♂ **0V7Q4ZZ** Dilation of Bilateral Vas Deferens, Percutaneous Endoscopic Approach

0V9 – Male Reproductive System, Drainage

Review Coding Guidelines B3.4a and B3.4b

Review Coding Guideline B6.2

♂ **0V9000Z** Drainage of Prostate with Drainage Device, Open Approach

♂ **0V900ZX** Drainage of Prostate, Open Approach, Diagnostic

♂ **0V900ZZ** Drainage of Prostate, Open Approach

♂ **0V9030Z** Drainage of Prostate with Drainage Device, Percutaneous Approach

♂ **0V903ZX** Drainage of Prostate, Percutaneous Approach, Diagnostic

♂ **0V903ZZ** Drainage of Prostate, Percutaneous Approach

♂ **0V9040Z** Drainage of Prostate with Drainage Device, Percutaneous Endoscopic Approach

♂ **0V904ZX** Drainage of Prostate, Percutaneous Endoscopic Approach, Diagnostic

---

♀ Female-only   ♂ Male-only   ○ Limited Coverage   ● Non-OR   **HAC** HAC-associated procedure   ● Non-covered procedures   **+** Combination

Medical and Surgical Section (0)

Male Reproductive System Code Listing

♂ **0V904ZZ** Drainage of Prostate, Percutaneous Endoscopic Approach

♂ **0V9070Z** Drainage of Prostate with Drainage Device, Via Natural or Artificial Opening

♂ **0V907ZX** Drainage of Prostate, Via Natural or Artificial Opening, Diagnostic

♂ **0V907ZZ** Drainage of Prostate, Via Natural or Artificial Opening

♂ **0V9080Z** Drainage of Prostate with Drainage Device, Via Natural or Artificial Opening Endoscopic

♂ **0V908ZX** Drainage of Prostate, Via Natural or Artificial Opening Endoscopic, Diagnostic

♂ **0V908ZZ** Drainage of Prostate, Via Natural or Artificial Opening Endoscopic

♂ **0V9100Z** Drainage of Right Seminal Vesicle with Drainage Device, Open Approach

♂ **0V910ZX** Drainage of Right Seminal Vesicle, Open Approach, Diagnostic

♂ **0V910ZZ** Drainage of Right Seminal Vesicle, Open Approach

♂ **0V9130Z** Drainage of Right Seminal Vesicle with Drainage Device, Percutaneous Approach

♂ **0V913ZX** Drainage of Right Seminal Vesicle, Percutaneous Approach, Diagnostic

♂ **0V913ZZ** Drainage of Right Seminal Vesicle, Percutaneous Approach

♂ **0V9140Z** Drainage of Right Seminal Vesicle with Drainage Device, Percutaneous Endoscopic Approach

♂ **0V914ZX** Drainage of Right Seminal Vesicle, Percutaneous Endoscopic Approach, Diagnostic

♂ **0V914ZZ** Drainage of Right Seminal Vesicle, Percutaneous Endoscopic Approach

♂ **0V9200Z** Drainage of Left Seminal Vesicle with Drainage Device, Open Approach

♂ **0V920ZX** Drainage of Left Seminal Vesicle, Open Approach, Diagnostic

♂ **0V920ZZ** Drainage of Left Seminal Vesicle, Open Approach

♂ **0V9230Z** Drainage of Left Seminal Vesicle with Drainage Device, Percutaneous Approach

♂ **0V923ZX** Drainage of Left Seminal Vesicle, Percutaneous Approach, Diagnostic

♂ **0V923ZZ** Drainage of Left Seminal Vesicle, Percutaneous Approach

♂ **0V9240Z** Drainage of Left Seminal Vesicle with Drainage Device, Percutaneous Endoscopic Approach

♂ **0V924ZX** Drainage of Left Seminal Vesicle, Percutaneous Endoscopic Approach, Diagnostic

♂ **0V924ZZ** Drainage of Left Seminal Vesicle, Percutaneous Endoscopic Approach

♂ **0V9300Z** Drainage of Bilateral Seminal Vesicles with Drainage Device, Open Approach

♂ **0V930ZX** Drainage of Bilateral Seminal Vesicles, Open Approach, Diagnostic

♂ **0V930ZZ** Drainage of Bilateral Seminal Vesicles, Open Approach

♂ **0V9330Z** Drainage of Bilateral Seminal Vesicles with Drainage Device, Percutaneous Approach

♂ **0V933ZX** Drainage of Bilateral Seminal Vesicles, Percutaneous Approach, Diagnostic

♂ **0V933ZZ** Drainage of Bilateral Seminal Vesicles, Percutaneous Approach

♂ **0V9340Z** Drainage of Bilateral Seminal Vesicles with Drainage Device, Percutaneous Endoscopic Approach

♂ **0V934ZX** Drainage of Bilateral Seminal Vesicles, Percutaneous Endoscopic Approach, Diagnostic

♂ **0V934ZZ** Drainage of Bilateral Seminal Vesicles, Percutaneous Endoscopic Approach

♂ **0V9500Z** Drainage of Scrotum with Drainage Device, Open Approach

♂ **0V950ZX** Drainage of Scrotum, Open Approach, Diagnostic

♂ **0V950ZZ** Drainage of Scrotum, Open Approach

♂ **0V9530Z** Drainage of Scrotum with Drainage Device, Percutaneous Approach

♂ **0V953ZX** Drainage of Scrotum, Percutaneous Approach, Diagnostic

♂ **0V953ZZ** Drainage of Scrotum, Percutaneous Approach

♂ **0V9540Z** Drainage of Scrotum with Drainage Device, Percutaneous Endoscopic Approach

♂ **0V954ZX** Drainage of Scrotum, Percutaneous Endoscopic Approach, Diagnostic

♂ **0V954ZZ** Drainage of Scrotum, Percutaneous Endoscopic Approach

♂ **0V95X0Z** Drainage of Scrotum with Drainage Device, External Approach

♂ **0V95XZX** Drainage of Scrotum, External Approach, Diagnostic

♂ **0V95XZZ** Drainage of Scrotum, External Approach

♂ **0V9600Z** Drainage of Right Tunica Vaginalis with Drainage Device, Open Approach

♂ **0V960ZX** Drainage of Right Tunica Vaginalis, Open Approach, Diagnostic

♂ **0V960ZZ** Drainage of Right Tunica Vaginalis, Open Approach

♂ **0V9630Z** Drainage of Right Tunica Vaginalis with Drainage Device, Percutaneous Approach

♂ **0V963ZX** Drainage of Right Tunica Vaginalis, Percutaneous Approach, Diagnostic

♂ **0V963ZZ** Drainage of Right Tunica Vaginalis, Percutaneous Approach

♂ **0V9640Z** Drainage of Right Tunica Vaginalis with Drainage Device, Percutaneous Endoscopic Approach

♂ **0V964ZX** Drainage of Right Tunica Vaginalis, Percutaneous Endoscopic Approach, Diagnostic

♂ **0V964ZZ** Drainage of Right Tunica Vaginalis, Percutaneous Endoscopic Approach

♂ **0V9700Z** Drainage of Left Tunica Vaginalis with Drainage Device, Open Approach

♂ **0V970ZX** Drainage of Left Tunica Vaginalis, Open Approach, Diagnostic

♂ **0V970ZZ** Drainage of Left Tunica Vaginalis, Open Approach

♂ **0V9730Z** Drainage of Left Tunica Vaginalis with Drainage Device, Percutaneous Approach

♂ **0V973ZX** Drainage of Left Tunica Vaginalis, Percutaneous Approach, Diagnostic

♂ **0V973ZZ** Drainage of Left Tunica Vaginalis, Percutaneous Approach

♂ **0V9740Z** Drainage of Left Tunica Vaginalis with Drainage Device, Percutaneous Endoscopic Approach

♂ **0V974ZX** Drainage of Left Tunica Vaginalis, Percutaneous Endoscopic Approach, Diagnostic

♂ **0V974ZZ** Drainage of Left Tunica Vaginalis, Percutaneous Endoscopic Approach

♂ **0V9900Z** Drainage of Right Testis with Drainage Device, Open Approach

♂ **0V990ZX** Drainage of Right Testis, Open Approach, Diagnostic

♂ **0V990ZZ** Drainage of Right Testis, Open Approach

♂ **0V9930Z** Drainage of Right Testis with Drainage Device, Percutaneous Approach

♂ **0V993ZX** Drainage of Right Testis, Percutaneous Approach, Diagnostic

♂ **0V993ZZ** Drainage of Right Testis, Percutaneous Approach

♂ **0V9940Z** Drainage of Right Testis with Drainage Device, Percutaneous Endoscopic Approach

♂ **0V994ZX** Drainage of Right Testis, Percutaneous Endoscopic Approach, Diagnostic

♂ **0V994ZZ** Drainage of Right Testis, Percutaneous Endoscopic Approach

♂ **0V9B00Z** Drainage of Left Testis with Drainage Device, Open Approach

♂ **0V9B0ZX** Drainage of Left Testis, Open Approach, Diagnostic

♂ **0V9B0ZZ** Drainage of Left Testis, Open Approach

♂ **0V9B30Z** Drainage of Left Testis with Drainage Device, Percutaneous Approach

♂ **0V9B3ZX** Drainage of Left Testis, Percutaneous Approach, Diagnostic

♂ **0V9B3ZZ** Drainage of Left Testis, Percutaneous Approach

♂ **0V9B40Z** Drainage of Left Testis with Drainage Device, Percutaneous Endoscopic Approach

♂ **0V9B4ZX** Drainage of Left Testis, Percutaneous Endoscopic Approach, Diagnostic

♂ **0V9B4ZZ** Drainage of Left Testis, Percutaneous Endoscopic Approach

♂ **0V9C00Z** Drainage of Bilateral Testes with Drainage Device, Open Approach

♂ **0V9C0ZX** Drainage of Bilateral Testes, Open Approach, Diagnostic

♂ **0V9C0ZZ** Drainage of Bilateral Testes, Open Approach

♂ **0V9C30Z** Drainage of Bilateral Testes with Drainage Device, Percutaneous Approach

♂ **0V9C3ZX** Drainage of Bilateral Testes, Percutaneous Approach, Diagnostic

♂ **0V9C3ZZ** Drainage of Bilateral Testes, Percutaneous Approach

♂ **0V9C40Z** Drainage of Bilateral Testes with Drainage Device, Percutaneous Endoscopic Approach

♂ **0V9C4ZX** Drainage of Bilateral Testes, Percutaneous Endoscopic Approach, Diagnostic

♂ **0V9C4ZZ** Drainage of Bilateral Testes, Percutaneous Endoscopic Approach

♂ **0V9F00Z** Drainage of Right Spermatic Cord with Drainage Device, Open Approach

♂ **0V9F0ZX** Drainage of Right Spermatic Cord, Open Approach, Diagnostic

♂ **0V9F0ZZ** Drainage of Right Spermatic Cord, Open Approach

♂ **0V9F30Z** Drainage of Right Spermatic Cord with Drainage Device, Percutaneous Approach

♂ **0V9F3ZX** Drainage of Right Spermatic Cord, Percutaneous Approach, Diagnostic

♂ **0V9F3ZZ** Drainage of Right Spermatic Cord, Percutaneous Approach

---

♀ Female-only   ♂ Male-only   ◐ Limited Coverage   ● Non-OR   **HAC** HAC-associated procedure   ● Non-covered procedures   ✚ Combination

♂ **0V9F40Z**   Drainage of Right Spermatic Cord with Drainage Device, Percutaneous Endoscopic Approach

♂ **0V9F4ZX**   Drainage of Right Spermatic Cord, Percutaneous Endoscopic Approach, Diagnostic

♂ **0V9F4ZZ**   Drainage of Right Spermatic Cord, Percutaneous Endoscopic Approach

♂ **0V9G00Z**   Drainage of Left Spermatic Cord with Drainage Device, Open Approach

♂ **0V9G0ZX**   Drainage of Left Spermatic Cord, Open Approach, Diagnostic

♂ **0V9G0ZZ**   Drainage of Left Spermatic Cord, Open Approach

♂ **0V9G30Z**   Drainage of Left Spermatic Cord with Drainage Device, Percutaneous Approach

♂ **0V9G3ZX**   Drainage of Left Spermatic Cord, Percutaneous Approach, Diagnostic

♂ **0V9G3ZZ**   Drainage of Left Spermatic Cord, Percutaneous Approach

♂ **0V9G40Z**   Drainage of Left Spermatic Cord with Drainage Device, Percutaneous Endoscopic Approach

♂ **0V9G4ZX**   Drainage of Left Spermatic Cord, Percutaneous Endoscopic Approach, Diagnostic

♂ **0V9G4ZZ**   Drainage of Left Spermatic Cord, Percutaneous Endoscopic Approach

♂ **0V9H00Z**   Drainage of Bilateral Spermatic Cords with Drainage Device, Open Approach

♂ **0V9H0ZX**   Drainage of Bilateral Spermatic Cords, Open Approach, Diagnostic

♂ **0V9H0ZZ**   Drainage of Bilateral Spermatic Cords, Open Approach

♂ **0V9H30Z**   Drainage of Bilateral Spermatic Cords with Drainage Device, Percutaneous Approach

♂ **0V9H3ZX**   Drainage of Bilateral Spermatic Cords, Percutaneous Approach, Diagnostic

♂ **0V9H3ZZ**   Drainage of Bilateral Spermatic Cords, Percutaneous Approach

♂ **0V9H40Z**   Drainage of Bilateral Spermatic Cords with Drainage Device, Percutaneous Endoscopic Approach

♂ **0V9H4ZX**   Drainage of Bilateral Spermatic Cords, Percutaneous Endoscopic Approach, Diagnostic

♂ **0V9H4ZZ**   Drainage of Bilateral Spermatic Cords, Percutaneous Endoscopic Approach

♂ **0V9J00Z**   Drainage of Right Epididymis with Drainage Device, Open Approach

♂ **0V9J0ZX**   Drainage of Right Epididymis, Open Approach, Diagnostic

♂ **0V9J0ZZ**   Drainage of Right Epididymis, Open Approach

♂ **0V9J30Z**   Drainage of Right Epididymis with Drainage Device, Percutaneous Approach

♂ **0V9J3ZX**   Drainage of Right Epididymis, Percutaneous Approach, Diagnostic

♂ **0V9J3ZZ**   Drainage of Right Epididymis, Percutaneous Approach

♂ **0V9J40Z**   Drainage of Right Epididymis with Drainage Device, Percutaneous Endoscopic Approach

♂ **0V9J4ZX**   Drainage of Right Epididymis, Percutaneous Endoscopic Approach, Diagnostic

♂ **0V9J4ZZ**   Drainage of Right Epididymis, Percutaneous Endoscopic Approach

♂ **0V9K00Z**   Drainage of Left Epididymis with Drainage Device, Open Approach

♂ **0V9K0ZX**   Drainage of Left Epididymis, Open Approach, Diagnostic

♂ **0V9K0ZZ**   Drainage of Left Epididymis, Open Approach

♂ **0V9K30Z**   Drainage of Left Epididymis with Drainage Device, Percutaneous Approach

♂ **0V9K3ZX**   Drainage of Left Epididymis, Percutaneous Approach, Diagnostic

♂ **0V9K3ZZ**   Drainage of Left Epididymis, Percutaneous Approach

♂ **0V9K40Z**   Drainage of Left Epididymis with Drainage Device, Percutaneous Endoscopic Approach

♂ **0V9K4ZX**   Drainage of Left Epididymis, Percutaneous Endoscopic Approach, Diagnostic

♂ **0V9K4ZZ**   Drainage of Left Epididymis, Percutaneous Endoscopic Approach

♂ **0V9L00Z**   Drainage of Bilateral Epididymis with Drainage Device, Open Approach

♂ **0V9L0ZX**   Drainage of Bilateral Epididymis, Open Approach, Diagnostic

♂ **0V9L0ZZ**   Drainage of Bilateral Epididymis, Open Approach

♂ **0V9L30Z**   Drainage of Bilateral Epididymis with Drainage Device, Percutaneous Approach

♂ **0V9L3ZX**   Drainage of Bilateral Epididymis, Percutaneous Approach, Diagnostic

♂ **0V9L3ZZ**   Drainage of Bilateral Epididymis, Percutaneous Approach

♂ **0V9L40Z**   Drainage of Bilateral Epididymis with Drainage Device, Percutaneous Endoscopic Approach

♂ **0V9L4ZX**   Drainage of Bilateral Epididymis, Percutaneous Endoscopic Approach, Diagnostic

♂ **0V9L4ZZ**   Drainage of Bilateral Epididymis, Percutaneous Endoscopic Approach

♂ **0V9N00Z**   Drainage of Right Vas Deferens with Drainage Device, Open Approach

♂ **0V9N0ZX**   Drainage of Right Vas Deferens, Open Approach, Diagnostic

♂ **0V9N0ZZ**   Drainage of Right Vas Deferens, Open Approach

♂ **0V9N30Z**   Drainage of Right Vas Deferens with Drainage Device, Percutaneous Approach

♂ **0V9N3ZX**   Drainage of Right Vas Deferens, Percutaneous Approach, Diagnostic

♂ **0V9N3ZZ**   Drainage of Right Vas Deferens, Percutaneous Approach

♂ **0V9N40Z**   Drainage of Right Vas Deferens with Drainage Device, Percutaneous Endoscopic Approach

♂ **0V9N4ZX**   Drainage of Right Vas Deferens, Percutaneous Endoscopic Approach, Diagnostic

♂ **0V9N4ZZ**   Drainage of Right Vas Deferens, Percutaneous Endoscopic Approach

♂ **0V9P00Z**   Drainage of Left Vas Deferens with Drainage Device, Open Approach

♂ **0V9P0ZX**   Drainage of Left Vas Deferens, Open Approach, Diagnostic

♂ **0V9P0ZZ**   Drainage of Left Vas Deferens, Open Approach

♂ **0V9P30Z**   Drainage of Left Vas Deferens with Drainage Device, Percutaneous Approach

♂ **0V9P3ZX**   Drainage of Left Vas Deferens, Percutaneous Approach, Diagnostic

♂ **0V9P3ZZ**   Drainage of Left Vas Deferens, Percutaneous Approach

♂ **0V9P40Z**   Drainage of Left Vas Deferens with Drainage Device, Percutaneous Endoscopic Approach

♂ **0V9P4ZX**   Drainage of Left Vas Deferens, Percutaneous Endoscopic Approach, Diagnostic

♂ **0V9P4ZZ**   Drainage of Left Vas Deferens, Percutaneous Endoscopic Approach

♂ **0V9Q00Z**   Drainage of Bilateral Vas Deferens with Drainage Device, Open Approach

♂ **0V9Q0ZX**   Drainage of Bilateral Vas Deferens, Open Approach, Diagnostic

♂ **0V9Q0ZZ**   Drainage of Bilateral Vas Deferens, Open Approach

♂ **0V9Q30Z**   Drainage of Bilateral Vas Deferens with Drainage Device, Percutaneous Approach

♂ **0V9Q3ZX**   Drainage of Bilateral Vas Deferens, Percutaneous Approach, Diagnostic

♂ **0V9Q3ZZ**   Drainage of Bilateral Vas Deferens, Percutaneous Approach

♂ **0V9Q40Z**   Drainage of Bilateral Vas Deferens with Drainage Device, Percutaneous Endoscopic Approach

♂ **0V9Q4ZX**   Drainage of Bilateral Vas Deferens, Percutaneous Endoscopic Approach, Diagnostic

♂ **0V9Q4ZZ**   Drainage of Bilateral Vas Deferens, Percutaneous Endoscopic Approach

♂ **0V9S00Z**   Drainage of Penis with Drainage Device, Open Approach

♂ **0V9S0ZX**   Drainage of Penis, Open Approach, Diagnostic

♂ **0V9S0ZZ**   Drainage of Penis, Open Approach

♂ **0V9S30Z**   Drainage of Penis with Drainage Device, Percutaneous Approach

♂ **0V9S3ZX**   Drainage of Penis, Percutaneous Approach, Diagnostic

♂ **0V9S3ZZ**   Drainage of Penis, Percutaneous Approach

♂ **0V9S40Z**   Drainage of Penis with Drainage Device, Percutaneous Endoscopic Approach

♂ **0V9S4ZX**   Drainage of Penis, Percutaneous Endoscopic Approach, Diagnostic

♂ **0V9S4ZZ**   Drainage of Penis, Percutaneous Endoscopic Approach

♂ **0V9SX0Z**   Drainage of Penis with Drainage Device, External Approach

♂ **0V9SXZX**   Drainage of Penis, External Approach, Diagnostic

♂ **0V9SXZZ**   Drainage of Penis, External Approach

♂ **0V9T00Z**   Drainage of Prepuce with Drainage Device, Open Approach

♂ **0V9T0ZX**   Drainage of Prepuce, Open Approach, Diagnostic

♂ **0V9T0ZZ**   Drainage of Prepuce, Open Approach

♂ **0V9T30Z**   Drainage of Prepuce with Drainage Device, Percutaneous Approach

♂ **0V9T3ZX**   Drainage of Prepuce, Percutaneous Approach, Diagnostic

♂ **0V9T3ZZ**   Drainage of Prepuce, Percutaneous Approach

♂ **0V9T40Z**   Drainage of Prepuce with Drainage Device, Percutaneous Endoscopic Approach

♂ **0V9T4ZX**   Drainage of Prepuce, Percutaneous Endoscopic Approach, Diagnostic

♂ **0V9T4ZZ**   Drainage of Prepuce, Percutaneous Endoscopic Approach

♂ **0V9TX0Z**   Drainage of Prepuce with Drainage Device, External Approach

♂ **0V9TXZX**   Drainage of Prepuce, External Approach, Diagnostic

♂ **0V9TXZZ**   Drainage of Prepuce, External Approach

♀ Female-only   ♂ Male-only   ⬤ Limited Coverage   ⬤ Non-OR   ▨ HAC-associated procedure   ⬣ Non-covered procedures   ➕ Combination

0VB – Male Reproductive System, Excision

Review Coding Guidelines B3.4a and B3.4b

Review Coding Guideline B3.8

♂ **0VB00ZX** Excision of Prostate, Open Approach, Diagnostic
♂ **0VB00ZZ** Excision of Prostate, Open Approach
♂ **0VB03ZX** Excision of Prostate, Percutaneous Approach, Diagnostic
♂ **0VB03ZZ** Excision of Prostate, Percutaneous Approach
♂ **0VB04ZX** Excision of Prostate, Percutaneous Endoscopic Approach, Diagnostic
♂ **0VB04ZZ** Excision of Prostate, Percutaneous Endoscopic Approach
♂ **0VB07ZX** Excision of Prostate, Via Natural or Artificial Opening, Diagnostic
♂ **0VB07ZZ** Excision of Prostate, Via Natural or Artificial Opening
♂ **0VB08ZX** Excision of Prostate, Via Natural or Artificial Opening Endoscopic, Diagnostic
♂ **0VB08ZZ** Excision of Prostate, Via Natural or Artificial Opening Endoscopic
♂ **0VB10ZX** Excision of Right Seminal Vesicle, Open Approach, Diagnostic
♂ **0VB10ZZ** Excision of Right Seminal Vesicle, Open Approach
♂ **0VB13ZX** Excision of Right Seminal Vesicle, Percutaneous Approach, Diagnostic
♂ **0VB13ZZ** Excision of Right Seminal Vesicle, Percutaneous Approach
♂ **0VB14ZX** Excision of Right Seminal Vesicle, Percutaneous Endoscopic Approach, Diagnostic
♂ **0VB14ZZ** Excision of Right Seminal Vesicle, Percutaneous Endoscopic Approach
♂ **0VB20ZX** Excision of Left Seminal Vesicle, Open Approach, Diagnostic
♂ **0VB20ZZ** Excision of Left Seminal Vesicle, Open Approach
♂ **0VB23ZX** Excision of Left Seminal Vesicle, Percutaneous Approach, Diagnostic
♂ **0VB23ZZ** Excision of Left Seminal Vesicle, Percutaneous Approach
♂ **0VB24ZX** Excision of Left Seminal Vesicle, Percutaneous Endoscopic Approach, Diagnostic
♂ **0VB24ZZ** Excision of Left Seminal Vesicle, Percutaneous Endoscopic Approach
♂ **0VB30ZX** Excision of Bilateral Seminal Vesicles, Open Approach, Diagnostic
♂ **0VB30ZZ** Excision of Bilateral Seminal Vesicles, Open Approach
♂ **0VB33ZX** Excision of Bilateral Seminal Vesicles, Percutaneous Approach, Diagnostic
♂ **0VB33ZZ** Excision of Bilateral Seminal Vesicles, Percutaneous Approach
♂ **0VB34ZX** Excision of Bilateral Seminal Vesicles, Percutaneous Endoscopic Approach, Diagnostic
♂ **0VB34ZZ** Excision of Bilateral Seminal Vesicles, Percutaneous Endoscopic Approach
♂ **0VB50ZX** Excision of Scrotum, Open Approach, Diagnostic
♂ **0VB50ZZ** Excision of Scrotum, Open Approach
♂ **0VB53ZX** Excision of Scrotum, Percutaneous Approach, Diagnostic
♂ **0VB53ZZ** Excision of Scrotum, Percutaneous Approach
♂ **0VB54ZX** Excision of Scrotum, Percutaneous Endoscopic Approach, Diagnostic
♂ **0VB54ZZ** Excision of Scrotum, Percutaneous Endoscopic Approach
♂ **0VB5XZX** Excision of Scrotum, External Approach, Diagnostic
♂ **0VB5XZZ** Excision of Scrotum, External Approach
♂ **0VB60ZX** Excision of Right Tunica Vaginalis, Open Approach, Diagnostic
♂ **0VB60ZZ** Excision of Right Tunica Vaginalis, Open Approach
♂ **0VB63ZX** Excision of Right Tunica Vaginalis, Percutaneous Approach, Diagnostic
♂ **0VB63ZZ** Excision of Right Tunica Vaginalis, Percutaneous Approach
♂ **0VB64ZX** Excision of Right Tunica Vaginalis, Percutaneous Endoscopic Approach, Diagnostic
♂ **0VB64ZZ** Excision of Right Tunica Vaginalis, Percutaneous Endoscopic Approach
♂ **0VB70ZX** Excision of Left Tunica Vaginalis, Open Approach, Diagnostic
♂ **0VB70ZZ** Excision of Left Tunica Vaginalis, Open Approach
♂ **0VB73ZX** Excision of Left Tunica Vaginalis, Percutaneous Approach, Diagnostic
♂ **0VB73ZZ** Excision of Left Tunica Vaginalis, Percutaneous Approach
♂ **0VB74ZX** Excision of Left Tunica Vaginalis, Percutaneous Endoscopic Approach, Diagnostic
♂ **0VB74ZZ** Excision of Left Tunica Vaginalis, Percutaneous Endoscopic Approach
♂ **0VB90ZX** Excision of Right Testis, Open Approach, Diagnostic

♂ **0VB90ZZ** Excision of Right Testis, Open Approach
♂ **0VB93ZX** Excision of Right Testis, Percutaneous Approach, Diagnostic
♂ **0VB93ZZ** Excision of Right Testis, Percutaneous Approach
♂ **0VB94ZX** Excision of Right Testis, Percutaneous Endoscopic Approach, Diagnostic
♂ **0VB94ZZ** Excision of Right Testis, Percutaneous Endoscopic Approach
♂ **0VBB0ZX** Excision of Left Testis, Open Approach, Diagnostic
♂ **0VBB0ZZ** Excision of Left Testis, Open Approach
♂ **0VBB3ZX** Excision of Left Testis, Percutaneous Approach, Diagnostic
♂ **0VBB3ZZ** Excision of Left Testis, Percutaneous Approach
♂ **0VBB4ZX** Excision of Left Testis, Percutaneous Endoscopic Approach, Diagnostic
♂ **0VBB4ZZ** Excision of Left Testis, Percutaneous Endoscopic Approach
♂ **0VBC0ZX** Excision of Bilateral Testes, Open Approach, Diagnostic
♂ **0VBC0ZZ** Excision of Bilateral Testes, Open Approach
♂ **0VBC3ZX** Excision of Bilateral Testes, Percutaneous Approach, Diagnostic
♂ **0VBC3ZZ** Excision of Bilateral Testes, Percutaneous Approach
♂ **0VBC4ZX** Excision of Bilateral Testes, Percutaneous Endoscopic Approach, Diagnostic
♂ **0VBC4ZZ** Excision of Bilateral Testes, Percutaneous Endoscopic Approach
♂ **0VBF0ZX** Excision of Right Spermatic Cord, Open Approach, Diagnostic
♂ **0VBF0ZZ** Excision of Right Spermatic Cord, Open Approach
♂ **0VBF3ZX** Excision of Right Spermatic Cord, Percutaneous Approach, Diagnostic
♂ **0VBF3ZZ** Excision of Right Spermatic Cord, Percutaneous Approach
♂ **0VBF4ZX** Excision of Right Spermatic Cord, Percutaneous Endoscopic Approach, Diagnostic
♂ **0VBF4ZZ** Excision of Right Spermatic Cord, Percutaneous Endoscopic Approach
♂ **0VBG0ZX** Excision of Left Spermatic Cord, Open Approach, Diagnostic
♂ **0VBG0ZZ** Excision of Left Spermatic Cord, Open Approach
♂ **0VBG3ZX** Excision of Left Spermatic Cord, Percutaneous Approach, Diagnostic
♂ **0VBG3ZZ** Excision of Left Spermatic Cord, Percutaneous Approach
♂ **0VBG4ZX** Excision of Left Spermatic Cord, Percutaneous Endoscopic Approach, Diagnostic
♂ **0VBG4ZZ** Excision of Left Spermatic Cord, Percutaneous Endoscopic Approach
♂ **0VBH0ZX** Excision of Bilateral Spermatic Cords, Open Approach, vDiagnostic
♂ **0VBH0ZZ** Excision of Bilateral Spermatic Cords, Open Approach
♂ **0VBH3ZX** Excision of Bilateral Spermatic Cords, Percutaneous Approach, Diagnostic
♂ **0VBH3ZZ** Excision of Bilateral Spermatic Cords, Percutaneous Approach
♂ **0VBH4ZX** Excision of Bilateral Spermatic Cords, Percutaneous Endoscopic Approach, Diagnostic
♂ **0VBH4ZZ** Excision of Bilateral Spermatic Cords, Percutaneous Endoscopic Approach
♂ **0VBJ0ZX** Excision of Right Epididymis, Open Approach, Diagnostic
♂ **0VBJ0ZZ** Excision of Right Epididymis, Open Approach
♂ **0VBJ3ZX** Excision of Right Epididymis, Percutaneous Approach, Diagnostic
♂ **0VBJ3ZZ** Excision of Right Epididymis, Percutaneous Approach
♂ **0VBJ4ZX** Excision of Right Epididymis, Percutaneous Endoscopic Approach, Diagnostic
♂ **0VBJ4ZZ** Excision of Right Epididymis, Percutaneous Endoscopic Approach
♂ **0VBK0ZX** Excision of Left Epididymis, Open Approach, Diagnostic
♂ **0VBK0ZZ** Excision of Left Epididymis, Open Approach
♂ **0VBK3ZX** Excision of Left Epididymis, Percutaneous Approach, Diagnostic
♂ **0VBK3ZZ** Excision of Left Epididymis, Percutaneous Approach
♂ **0VBK4ZX** Excision of Left Epididymis, Percutaneous Endoscopic Approach, Diagnostic
♂ **0VBK4ZZ** Excision of Left Epididymis, Percutaneous Endoscopic Approach
♂ **0VBL0ZX** Excision of Bilateral Epididymis, Open Approach, Diagnostic
♂ **0VBL0ZZ** Excision of Bilateral Epididymis, Open Approach
♂ **0VBL3ZX** Excision of Bilateral Epididymis, Percutaneous Approach, Diagnostic
♂ **0VBL3ZZ** Excision of Bilateral Epididymis, Percutaneous Approach

---

♀ Female-only   ♂ Male-only   ● Limited Coverage   ● Non-OR   **HAC** HAC-associated procedure   ● Non-covered procedures   + Combination

♂ **0VBL4ZX** Excision of Bilateral Epididymis, Percutaneous Endoscopic Approach, Diagnostic

♂ **0VBL4ZZ** Excision of Bilateral Epididymis, Percutaneous Endoscopic Approach

♂ **0VBN0ZX** Excision of Right Vas Deferens, Open Approach, Diagnostic

●♂ **0VBN0ZZ** Excision of Right Vas Deferens, Open Approach

♂ **0VBN3ZX** Excision of Right Vas Deferens, Percutaneous Approach, Diagnostic

●♂ **0VBN3ZZ** Excision of Right Vas Deferens, Percutaneous Approach

♂ **0VBN4ZX** Excision of Right Vas Deferens, Percutaneous Endoscopic Approach, Diagnostic

●♂ **0VBN4ZZ** Excision of Right Vas Deferens, Percutaneous Endoscopic Approach

♂ **0VBP0ZX** Excision of Left Vas Deferens, Open Approach, Diagnostic

♂ **0VBP0ZZ** Excision of Left Vas Deferens, Open Approach

♂ **0VBP3ZX** Excision of Left Vas Deferens, Percutaneous Approach, Diagnostic

●♂ **0VBP3ZZ** Excision of Left Vas Deferens, Percutaneous Approach

♂ **0VBP4ZX** Excision of Left Vas Deferens, Percutaneous Endoscopic Approach, Diagnostic

●♂ **0VBP4ZZ** Excision of Left Vas Deferens, Percutaneous Endoscopic Approach

♂ **0VBQ0ZX** Excision of Bilateral Vas Deferens, Open Approach, Diagnostic

●♂ **0VBQ0ZZ** Excision of Bilateral Vas Deferens, Open Approach

♂ **0VBQ3ZX** Excision of Bilateral Vas Deferens, Percutaneous Approach, Diagnostic

●♂ **0VBQ3ZZ** Excision of Bilateral Vas Deferens, Percutaneous Approach

♂ **0VBQ4ZX** Excision of Bilateral Vas Deferens, Percutaneous Endoscopic Approach, Diagnostic

●♂ **0VBQ4ZZ** Excision of Bilateral Vas Deferens, Percutaneous Endoscopic Approach

♂ **0VBS0ZX** Excision of Penis, Open Approach, Diagnostic

♂ **0VBS0ZZ** Excision of Penis, Open Approach

♂ **0VBS3ZX** Excision of Penis, Percutaneous Approach, Diagnostic

♂ **0VBS3ZZ** Excision of Penis, Percutaneous Approach

♂ **0VBS4ZX** Excision of Penis, Percutaneous Endoscopic Approach, Diagnostic

♂ **0VBS4ZZ** Excision of Penis, Percutaneous Endoscopic Approach

♂ **0VBSXZX** Excision of Penis, External Approach, Diagnostic

♂ **0VBSXZZ** Excision of Penis, External Approach

♂ **0VBT0ZX** Excision of Prepuce, Open Approach, Diagnostic

♂ **0VBT0ZZ** Excision of Prepuce, Open Approach

♂ **0VBT3ZX** Excision of Prepuce, Percutaneous Approach, Diagnostic

♂ **0VBT3ZZ** Excision of Prepuce, Percutaneous Approach

♂ **0VBT4ZX** Excision of Prepuce, Percutaneous Endoscopic Approach, Diagnostic

♂ **0VBT4ZZ** Excision of Prepuce, Percutaneous Endoscopic Approach

♂ **0VBTXZX** Excision of Prepuce, External Approach, Diagnostic

♂ **0VBTXZZ** Excision of Prepuce, External Approach

0VC – Male Reproductive System, Extirpation

♂ **0VC00ZZ** Extirpation of Matter from Prostate, Open Approach

♂ **0VC03ZZ** Extirpation of Matter from Prostate, Percutaneous Approach

♂ **0VC04ZZ** Extirpation of Matter from Prostate, Percutaneous Endoscopic Approach

♂ **0VC07ZZ** Extirpation of Matter from Prostate, Via Natural or Artificial Opening

♂ **0VC08ZZ** Extirpation of Matter from Prostate, Via Natural or Artificial Opening Endoscopic

♂ **0VC10ZZ** Extirpation of Matter from Right Seminal Vesicle, Open Approach

♂ **0VC13ZZ** Extirpation of Matter from Right Seminal Vesicle, Percutaneous Approach

♂ **0VC14ZZ** Extirpation of Matter from Right Seminal Vesicle, Percutaneous Endoscopic Approach

♂ **0VC20ZZ** Extirpation of Matter from Left Seminal Vesicle, Open Approach

♂ **0VC23ZZ** Extirpation of Matter from Left Seminal Vesicle, Percutaneous Approach

♂ **0VC24ZZ** Extirpation of Matter from Left Seminal Vesicle, Percutaneous Endoscopic Approach

♂ **0VC30ZZ** Extirpation of Matter from Bilateral Seminal Vesicles, Open Approach

♂ **0VC33ZZ** Extirpation of Matter from Bilateral Seminal Vesicles, Percutaneous Approach

♂ **0VC34ZZ** Extirpation of Matter from Bilateral Seminal Vesicles, Percutaneous Endoscopic Approach

♂ **0VC50ZZ** Extirpation of Matter from Scrotum, Open Approach

♂ **0VC53ZZ** Extirpation of Matter from Scrotum, Percutaneous Approach

♂ **0VC54ZZ** Extirpation of Matter from Scrotum, Percutaneous Endoscopic Approach

♂ **0VC5XZZ** Extirpation of Matter from Scrotum, External Approach

♂ **0VC60ZZ** Extirpation of Matter from Right Tunica Vaginalis, Open Approach

♂ **0VC63ZZ** Extirpation of Matter from Right Tunica Vaginalis, Percutaneous Approach

♂ **0VC64ZZ** Extirpation of Matter from Right Tunica Vaginalis, Percutaneous Endoscopic Approach

♂ **0VC70ZZ** Extirpation of Matter from Left Tunica Vaginalis, Open Approach

♂ **0VC73ZZ** Extirpation of Matter from Left Tunica Vaginalis, Percutaneous Approach

♂ **0VC74ZZ** Extirpation of Matter from Left Tunica Vaginalis, Percutaneous Endoscopic Approach

♂ **0VC90ZZ** Extirpation of Matter from Right Testis, Open Approach

♂ **0VC93ZZ** Extirpation of Matter from Right Testis, Percutaneous Approach

♂ **0VC94ZZ** Extirpation of Matter from Right Testis, Percutaneous Endoscopic Approach

♂ **0VCB0ZZ** Extirpation of Matter from Left Testis, Open Approach

♂ **0VCB3ZZ** Extirpation of Matter from Left Testis, Percutaneous Approach

♂ **0VCB4ZZ** Extirpation of Matter from Left Testis, Percutaneous Endoscopic Approach

♂ **0VCC0ZZ** Extirpation of Matter from Bilateral Testes, Open Approach

♂ **0VCC3ZZ** Extirpation of Matter from Bilateral Testes, Percutaneous Approach

♂ **0VCC4ZZ** Extirpation of Matter from Bilateral Testes, Percutaneous Endoscopic Approach

♂ **0VCF0ZZ** Extirpation of Matter from Right Spermatic Cord, Open Approach

♂ **0VCF3ZZ** Extirpation of Matter from Right Spermatic Cord, Percutaneous Approach

♂ **0VCF4ZZ** Extirpation of Matter from Right Spermatic Cord, Percutaneous Endoscopic Approach

♂ **0VCG0ZZ** Extirpation of Matter from Left Spermatic Cord, Open Approach

♂ **0VCG3ZZ** Extirpation of Matter from Left Spermatic Cord, Percutaneous Approach

♂ **0VCG4ZZ** Extirpation of Matter from Left Spermatic Cord, Percutaneous Endoscopic Approach

♂ **0VCH0ZZ** Extirpation of Matter from Bilateral Spermatic Cords, Open Approach

♂ **0VCH3ZZ** Extirpation of Matter from Bilateral Spermatic Cords, Percutaneous Approach

♂ **0VCH4ZZ** Extirpation of Matter from Bilateral Spermatic Cords, Percutaneous Endoscopic Approach

♂ **0VCJ0ZZ** Extirpation of Matter from Right Epididymis, Open Approach

♂ **0VCJ3ZZ** Extirpation of Matter from Right Epididymis, Percutaneous Approach

♂ **0VCJ4ZZ** Extirpation of Matter from Right Epididymis, Percutaneous Endoscopic Approach

♂ **0VCK0ZZ** Extirpation of Matter from Left Epididymis, Open Approach

♂ **0VCK3ZZ** Extirpation of Matter from Left Epididymis, Percutaneous Approach

♂ **0VCK4ZZ** Extirpation of Matter from Left Epididymis, Percutaneous Endoscopic Approach

♂ **0VCL0ZZ** Extirpation of Matter from Bilateral Epididymis, Open Approach

♂ **0VCL3ZZ** Extirpation of Matter from Bilateral Epididymis, Percutaneous Approach

♂ **0VCL4ZZ** Extirpation of Matter from Bilateral Epididymis, Percutaneous Endoscopic Approach

♂ **0VCN0ZZ** Extirpation of Matter from Right Vas Deferens, Open Approach

♂ **0VCN3ZZ** Extirpation of Matter from Right Vas Deferens, Percutaneous Approach

♂ **0VCN4ZZ** Extirpation of Matter from Right Vas Deferens, Percutaneous Endoscopic Approach

♂ **0VCP0ZZ** Extirpation of Matter from Left Vas Deferens, Open Approach

♂ **0VCP3ZZ** Extirpation of Matter from Left Vas Deferens, Percutaneous Approach

♂ **0VCP4ZZ** Extirpation of Matter from Left Vas Deferens, Percutaneous Endoscopic Approach

♂ **0VCQ0ZZ** Extirpation of Matter from Bilateral Vas Deferens, Open Approach

♂ **0VCQ3ZZ** Extirpation of Matter from Bilateral Vas Deferens, Percutaneous Approach

♂ **0VCQ4ZZ** Extirpation of Matter from Bilateral Vas Deferens, Percutaneous Endoscopic Approach

♂ **0VCS0ZZ** Extirpation of Matter from Penis, Open Approach
♂ **0VCS3ZZ** Extirpation of Matter from Penis, Percutaneous Approach
♂ **0VCS4ZZ** Extirpation of Matter from Penis, Percutaneous Endoscopic Approach
♂ **0VCSXZZ** Extirpation of Matter from Penis, External Approach

♂ **0VCT0ZZ** Extirpation of Matter from Prepuce, Open Approach
♂ **0VCT3ZZ** Extirpation of Matter from Prepuce, Percutaneous Approach
♂ **0VCT4ZZ** Extirpation of Matter from Prepuce, Percutaneous Endoscopic Approach
♂ **0VCTXZZ** Extirpation of Matter from Prepuce, External Approach

0VH – Male Reproductive System, Insertion

♂ **0VH001Z** Insertion of Radioactive Element into Prostate, Open Approach
♂ **0VH031Z** Insertion of Radioactive Element into Prostate, Percutaneous Approach
♂ **0VH041Z** Insertion of Radioactive Element into Prostate, Percutaneous Endoscopic Approach
♂ **0VH071Z** Insertion of Radioactive Element into Prostate, Via Natural or Artificial Opening
♂ **0VH081Z** Insertion of Radioactive Element into Prostate, Via Natural or Artificial Opening Endoscopic
♂ **0VH403Z** Insertion of Infusion Device into Prostate and Seminal Vesicles, Open Approach
♂ **0VH433Z** Insertion of Infusion Device into Prostate and Seminal Vesicles, Percutaneous Approach
♂ **0VH443Z** Insertion of Infusion Device into Prostate and Seminal Vesicles, Percutaneous Endoscopic Approach
♂ **0VH473Z** Insertion of Infusion Device into Prostate and Seminal Vesicles, Via Natural or Artificial Opening
♂ **0VH483Z** Insertion of Infusion Device into Prostate and Seminal Vesicles, Via Natural or Artificial Opening Endoscopic
♂ **0VH803Z** Insertion of Infusion Device into Scrotum and Tunica Vaginalis, Open Approach
♂ **0VH833Z** Insertion of Infusion Device into Scrotum and Tunica Vaginalis, Percutaneous Approach
♂ **0VH843Z** Insertion of Infusion Device into Scrotum and Tunica Vaginalis, Percutaneous Endoscopic Approach
♂ **0VH873Z** Insertion of Infusion Device into Scrotum and Tunica Vaginalis, Via Natural or Artificial Opening
♂ **0VH883Z** Insertion of Infusion Device into Scrotum and Tunica Vaginalis, Via Natural or Artificial Opening Endoscopic
♂ **0VHD03Z** Insertion of Infusion Device into Testis, Open Approach
♂ **0VHD33Z** Insertion of Infusion Device into Testis, Percutaneous Approach

♂ **0VHD43Z** Insertion of Infusion Device into Testis, Percutaneous Endoscopic Approach
♂ **0VHD73Z** Insertion of Infusion Device into Testis, Via Natural or Artificial Opening
♂ **0VHD83Z** Insertion of Infusion Device into Testis, Via Natural or Artificial Opening Endoscopic
♂ **0VHM03Z** Insertion of Infusion Device into Epididymis and Spermatic Cord, Open Approach
♂ **0VHM33Z** Insertion of Infusion Device into Epididymis and Spermatic Cord, Percutaneous Approach
♂ **0VHM43Z** Insertion of Infusion Device into Epididymis and Spermatic Cord, Percutaneous Endoscopic Approach
♂ **0VHM73Z** Insertion of Infusion Device into Epididymis and Spermatic Cord, Via Natural or Artificial Opening
♂ **0VHM83Z** Insertion of Infusion Device into Epididymis and Spermatic Cord, Via Natural or Artificial Opening Endoscopic
♂ **0VHR03Z** Insertion of Infusion Device into Vas Deferens, Open Approach
♂ **0VHR33Z** Insertion of Infusion Device into Vas Deferens, Percutaneous Approach
♂ **0VHR43Z** Insertion of Infusion Device into Vas Deferens, Percutaneous Endoscopic Approach
♂ **0VHR73Z** Insertion of Infusion Device into Vas Deferens, Via Natural or Artificial Opening
♂ **0VHR83Z** Insertion of Infusion Device into Vas Deferens, Via Natural or Artificial Opening Endoscopic
♂ **0VHS03Z** Insertion of Infusion Device into Penis, Open Approach
♂ **0VHS33Z** Insertion of Infusion Device into Penis, Percutaneous Approach
♂ **0VHS43Z** Insertion of Infusion Device into Penis, Percutaneous Endoscopic Approach
♂ **0VHSX3Z** Insertion of Infusion Device into Penis, External Approach

0VJ – Male Reproductive System, Inspection

Review Coding Guidelines B3.11a, B3.11b and B3.11c

♂ **0VJ40ZZ** Inspection of Prostate and Seminal Vesicles, Open Approach
♂ **0VJ43ZZ** Inspection of Prostate and Seminal Vesicles, Percutaneous Approach
♂ **0VJ44ZZ** Inspection of Prostate and Seminal Vesicles, Percutaneous Endoscopic Approach
♂ **0VJ4XZZ** Inspection of Prostate and Seminal Vesicles, External Approach
♂ **0VJ80ZZ** Inspection of Scrotum and Tunica Vaginalis, Open Approach
♂ **0VJ83ZZ** Inspection of Scrotum and Tunica Vaginalis, Percutaneous Approach
♂ **0VJ84ZZ** Inspection of Scrotum and Tunica Vaginalis, Percutaneous Endoscopic Approach
♂ **0VJ8XZZ** Inspection of Scrotum and Tunica Vaginalis, External Approach
♂ **0VJD0ZZ** Inspection of Testis, Open Approach
♂ **0VJD3ZZ** Inspection of Testis, Percutaneous Approach
♂ **0VJD4ZZ** Inspection of Testis, Percutaneous Endoscopic Approach
♂ **0VJDXZZ** Inspection of Testis, External Approach

♂ **0VJM0ZZ** Inspection of Epididymis and Spermatic Cord, Open Approach
♂ **0VJM3ZZ** Inspection of Epididymis and Spermatic Cord, Percutaneous Approach
♂ **0VJM4ZZ** Inspection of Epididymis and Spermatic Cord, Percutaneous Endoscopic Approach
♂ **0VJMXZZ** Inspection of Epididymis and Spermatic Cord, External Approach
♂ **0VJR0ZZ** Inspection of Vas Deferens, Open Approach
♂ **0VJR3ZZ** Inspection of Vas Deferens, Percutaneous Approach
♂ **0VJR4ZZ** Inspection of Vas Deferens, Percutaneous Endoscopic Approach
♂ **0VJRXZZ** Inspection of Vas Deferens, External Approach
♂ **0VJS0ZZ** Inspection of Penis, Open Approach
♂ **0VJS3ZZ** Inspection of Penis, Percutaneous Approach
♂ **0VJS4ZZ** Inspection of Penis, Percutaneous Endoscopic Approach
♂ **0VJSXZZ** Inspection of Penis, External Approach

0VL – Male Reproductive System, Occlusion

●♂ **0VLF0CZ** Occlusion of Right Spermatic Cord with Extraluminal Device, Open Approach
●♂ **0VLF0DZ** Occlusion of Right Spermatic Cord with Intraluminal Device, Open Approach
●♂ **0VLF0ZZ** Occlusion of Right Spermatic Cord, Open Approach
●♂ **0VLF3CZ** Occlusion of Right Spermatic Cord with Extraluminal Device, Percutaneous Approach
●♂ **0VLF3DZ** Occlusion of Right Spermatic Cord with Intraluminal Device, Percutaneous Approach
●♂ **0VLF3ZZ** Occlusion of Right Spermatic Cord, Percutaneous Approach
●♂ **0VLF4CZ** Occlusion of Right Spermatic Cord with Extraluminal Device, Percutaneous Endoscopic Approach

●♂ **0VLF4DZ** Occlusion of Right Spermatic Cord with Intraluminal Device, Percutaneous Endoscopic Approach
♂ **0VLF4ZZ** Occlusion of Right Spermatic Cord, Percutaneous Endoscopic Approach
●♂ **0VLG0CZ** Occlusion of Left Spermatic Cord with Extraluminal Device, Open Approach
●♂ **0VLG0DZ** Occlusion of Left Spermatic Cord with Intraluminal Device, Open Approach
●♂ **0VLG0ZZ** Occlusion of Left Spermatic Cord, Open Approach
●♂ **0VLG3CZ** Occlusion of Left Spermatic Cord with Extraluminal Device, Percutaneous Approach

---

♀ Female-only   ♂ Male-only   ● Limited Coverage   ● Non-OR   ᴴᴬᶜ HAC-associated procedure   ● Non-covered procedures   ✚ Combination

● ♂ **0VLG3DZ** Occlusion of Left Spermatic Cord with Intraluminal Device, Percutaneous Approach
● ♂ **0VLG3ZZ** Occlusion of Left Spermatic Cord, Percutaneous Approach
● ♂ **0VLG4CZ** Occlusion of Left Spermatic Cord with Extraluminal Device, Percutaneous Endoscopic Approach
● ♂ **0VLG4DZ** Occlusion of Left Spermatic Cord with Intraluminal Device, Percutaneous Endoscopic Approach
● ♂ **0VLG4ZZ** Occlusion of Left Spermatic Cord, Percutaneous Endoscopic Approach
● ♂ **0VLH0CZ** Occlusion of Bilateral Spermatic Cords with Extraluminal Device, Open Approach
● ♂ **0VLH0DZ** Occlusion of Bilateral Spermatic Cords with Intraluminal Device, Open Approach
● ♂ **0VLH0ZZ** Occlusion of Bilateral Spermatic Cords, Open Approach
● ♂ **0VLH3CZ** Occlusion of Bilateral Spermatic Cords with Extraluminal Device, Percutaneous Approach
● ♂ **0VLH3DZ** Occlusion of Bilateral Spermatic Cords with Intraluminal Device, Percutaneous Approach
● ♂ **0VLH3ZZ** Occlusion of Bilateral Spermatic Cords, Percutaneous Approach
● ♂ **0VLH4CZ** Occlusion of Bilateral Spermatic Cords with Extraluminal Device, Percutaneous Endoscopic Approach
● ♂ **0VLH4DZ** Occlusion of Bilateral Spermatic Cords with Intraluminal Device, Percutaneous Endoscopic Approach
● ♂ **0VLH4ZZ** Occlusion of Bilateral Spermatic Cords, Percutaneous Endoscopic Approach
● ♂ **0VLN0CZ** Occlusion of Right Vas Deferens with Extraluminal Device, Open Approach
  ♂ **0VLN0DZ** Occlusion of Right Vas Deferens with Intraluminal Device, Open Approach
● ♂ **0VLN0ZZ** Occlusion of Right Vas Deferens, Open Approach
● ♂ **0VLN3CZ** Occlusion of Right Vas Deferens with Extraluminal Device, Percutaneous Approach
● ♂ **0VLN3DZ** Occlusion of Right Vas Deferens with Intraluminal Device, Percutaneous Approach
● ♂ **0VLN3ZZ** Occlusion of Right Vas Deferens, Percutaneous Approach
● ♂ **0VLN4CZ** Occlusion of Right Vas Deferens with Extraluminal Device, Percutaneous Endoscopic Approach

  ♂ **0VLN4DZ** Occlusion of Right Vas Deferens with Intraluminal Device, Percutaneous Endoscopic Approach
● ♂ **0VLN4ZZ** Occlusion of Right Vas Deferens, Percutaneous Endoscopic Approach
● ♂ **0VLP0CZ** Occlusion of Left Vas Deferens with Extraluminal Device, Open Approach
● ♂ **0VLP0DZ** Occlusion of Left Vas Deferens with Intraluminal Device, Open Approach
● ♂ **0VLP0ZZ** Occlusion of Left Vas Deferens, Open Approach
● ♂ **0VLP3CZ** Occlusion of Left Vas Deferens with Extraluminal Device, Percutaneous Approach
● ♂ **0VLP3DZ** Occlusion of Left Vas Deferens with Intraluminal Device, Percutaneous Approach
● ♂ **0VLP3ZZ** Occlusion of Left Vas Deferens, Percutaneous Approach
● ♂ **0VLP4CZ** Occlusion of Left Vas Deferens with Extraluminal Device, Percutaneous Endoscopic Approach
● ♂ **0VLP4DZ** Occlusion of Left Vas Deferens with Intraluminal Device, Percutaneous Endoscopic Approach
● ♂ **0VLP4ZZ** Occlusion of Left Vas Deferens, Percutaneous Endoscopic Approach
● ♂ **0VLQ0CZ** Occlusion of Bilateral Vas Deferens with Extraluminal Device, Open Approach
● ♂ **0VLQ0DZ** Occlusion of Bilateral Vas Deferens with Intraluminal Device, Open Approach
● ♂ **0VLQ0ZZ** Occlusion of Bilateral Vas Deferens, Open Approach
● ♂ **0VLQ3CZ** Occlusion of Bilateral Vas Deferens with Extraluminal Device, Percutaneous Approach
● ♂ **0VLQ3DZ** Occlusion of Bilateral Vas Deferens with Intraluminal Device, Percutaneous Approach
● ♂ **0VLQ3ZZ** Occlusion of Bilateral Vas Deferens, Percutaneous Approach
● ♂ **0VLQ4CZ** Occlusion of Bilateral Vas Deferens with Extraluminal Device, Percutaneous Endoscopic Approach
  ♂ **0VLQ4DZ** Occlusion of Bilateral Vas Deferens with Intraluminal Device, Percutaneous Endoscopic Approach
● ♂ **0VLQ4ZZ** Occlusion of Bilateral Vas Deferens, Percutaneous Endoscopic Approach

0VM – Male Reproductive System, Reattachment

  ♂ **0VM5XZZ** Reattachment of Scrotum, External Approach
  ♂ **0VM60ZZ** Reattachment of Right Tunica Vaginalis, Open Approach
  ♂ **0VM64ZZ** Reattachment of Right Tunica Vaginalis, Percutaneous Endoscopic Approach
  ♂ **0VM70ZZ** Reattachment of Left Tunica Vaginalis, Open Approach
  ♂ **0VM74ZZ** Reattachment of Left Tunica Vaginalis, Percutaneous Endoscopic Approach
  ♂ **0VM90ZZ** Reattachment of Right Testis, Open Approach
  ♂ **0VM94ZZ** Reattachment of Right Testis, Percutaneous Endoscopic Approach
  ♂ **0VMB0ZZ** Reattachment of Left Testis, Open Approach
  ♂ **0VMB4ZZ** Reattachment of Left Testis, Percutaneous Endoscopic Approach
  ♂ **0VMC0ZZ** Reattachment of Bilateral Testes, Open Approach

  ♂ **0VMC4ZZ** Reattachment of Bilateral Testes, Percutaneous Endoscopic Approach
  ♂ **0VMF0ZZ** Reattachment of Right Spermatic Cord, Open Approach
  ♂ **0VMF4ZZ** Reattachment of Right Spermatic Cord, Percutaneous Endoscopic Approach
  ♂ **0VMG0ZZ** Reattachment of Left Spermatic Cord, Open Approach
  ♂ **0VMG4ZZ** Reattachment of Left Spermatic Cord, Percutaneous Endoscopic Approach
  ♂ **0VMH0ZZ** Reattachment of Bilateral Spermatic Cords, Open Approach
  ♂ **0VMH4ZZ** Reattachment of Bilateral Spermatic Cords, Percutaneous Endoscopic Approach
  ♂ **0VMSXZZ** Reattachment of Penis, External Approach

0VN – Male Reproductive System, Release

Review Coding Guideline B3.13

  ♂ **0VN00ZZ** Release Prostate, Open Approach
  ♂ **0VN03ZZ** Release Prostate, Percutaneous Approach
  ♂ **0VN04ZZ** Release Prostate, Percutaneous Endoscopic Approach
  ♂ **0VN07ZZ** Release Prostate, Via Natural or Artificial Opening
  ♂ **0VN08ZZ** Release Prostate, Via Natural or Artificial Opening Endoscopic
  ♂ **0VN10ZZ** Release Right Seminal Vesicle, Open Approach
  ♂ **0VN13ZZ** Release Right Seminal Vesicle, Percutaneous Approach
  ♂ **0VN14ZZ** Release Right Seminal Vesicle, Percutaneous Endoscopic Approach
  ♂ **0VN20ZZ** Release Left Seminal Vesicle, Open Approach
  ♂ **0VN23ZZ** Release Left Seminal Vesicle, Percutaneous Approach
  ♂ **0VN24ZZ** Release Left Seminal Vesicle, Percutaneous Endoscopic Approach
  ♂ **0VN30ZZ** Release Bilateral Seminal Vesicles, Open Approach
  ♂ **0VN33ZZ** Release Bilateral Seminal Vesicles, Percutaneous Approach
  ♂ **0VN34ZZ** Release Bilateral Seminal Vesicles, Percutaneous Endoscopic Approach
  ♂ **0VN50ZZ** Release Scrotum, Open Approach
  ♂ **0VN53ZZ** Release Scrotum, Percutaneous Approach

  ♂ **0VN54ZZ** Release Scrotum, Percutaneous Endoscopic Approach
  ♂ **0VN5XZZ** Release Scrotum, External Approach
  ♂ **0VN60ZZ** Release Right Tunica Vaginalis, Open Approach
  ♂ **0VN63ZZ** Release Right Tunica Vaginalis, Percutaneous Approach
  ♂ **0VN64ZZ** Release Right Tunica Vaginalis, Percutaneous Endoscopic Approach
  ♂ **0VN70ZZ** Release Left Tunica Vaginalis, Open Approach
  ♂ **0VN73ZZ** Release Left Tunica Vaginalis, Percutaneous Approach
  ♂ **0VN74ZZ** Release Left Tunica Vaginalis, Percutaneous Endoscopic Approach
  ♂ **0VN90ZZ** Release Right Testis, Open Approach
  ♂ **0VN93ZZ** Release Right Testis, Percutaneous Approach
  ♂ **0VN94ZZ** Release Right Testis, Percutaneous Endoscopic Approach
  ♂ **0VNB0ZZ** Release Left Testis, Open Approach
  ♂ **0VNB3ZZ** Release Left Testis, Percutaneous Approach
  ♂ **0VNB4ZZ** Release Left Testis, Percutaneous Endoscopic Approach
  ♂ **0VNC0ZZ** Release Bilateral Testes, Open Approach
  ♂ **0VNC3ZZ** Release Bilateral Testes, Percutaneous Approach
  ♂ **0VNC4ZZ** Release Bilateral Testes, Percutaneous Endoscopic Approach

♀ Female-only   ♂ Male-only   ○ Limited Coverage   ● Non-OR   HAC HAC-associated procedure   ● Non-covered procedures   ✚ Combination

♂ **0VNF0ZZ** Release Right Spermatic Cord, Open Approach
♂ **0VNF3ZZ** Release Right Spermatic Cord, Percutaneous Approach
♂ **0VNF4ZZ** Release Right Spermatic Cord, Percutaneous Endoscopic Approach
♂ **0VNG0ZZ** Release Left Spermatic Cord, Open Approach
♂ **0VNG3ZZ** Release Left Spermatic Cord, Percutaneous Approach
♂ **0VNG4ZZ** Release Left Spermatic Cord, Percutaneous Endoscopic Approach
♂ **0VNH0ZZ** Release Bilateral Spermatic Cords, Open Approach
♂ **0VNH3ZZ** Release Bilateral Spermatic Cords, Percutaneous Approach
♂ **0VNH4ZZ** Release Bilateral Spermatic Cords, Percutaneous Endoscopic Approach
♂ **0VNJ0ZZ** Release Right Epididymis, Open Approach
♂ **0VNJ3ZZ** Release Right Epididymis, Percutaneous Approach
♂ **0VNJ4ZZ** Release Right Epididymis, Percutaneous Endoscopic Approach
♂ **0VNK0ZZ** Release Left Epididymis, Open Approach
♂ **0VNK3ZZ** Release Left Epididymis, Percutaneous Approach
♂ **0VNK4ZZ** Release Left Epididymis, Percutaneous Endoscopic Approach
♂ **0VNL0ZZ** Release Bilateral Epididymis, Open Approach
♂ **0VNL3ZZ** Release Bilateral Epididymis, Percutaneous Approach

♂ **0VNL4ZZ** Release Bilateral Epididymis, Percutaneous Endoscopic Approach
♂ **0VNN0ZZ** Release Right Vas Deferens, Open Approach
♂ **0VNN3ZZ** Release Right Vas Deferens, Percutaneous Approach
♂ **0VNN4ZZ** Release Right Vas Deferens, Percutaneous Endoscopic Approach
♂ **0VNP0ZZ** Release Left Vas Deferens, Open Approach
♂ **0VNP3ZZ** Release Left Vas Deferens, Percutaneous Approach
♂ **0VNP4ZZ** Release Left Vas Deferens, Percutaneous Endoscopic Approach
♂ **0VNQ0ZZ** Release Bilateral Vas Deferens, Open Approach
♂ **0VNQ3ZZ** Release Bilateral Vas Deferens, Percutaneous Approach
♂ **0VNQ4ZZ** Release Bilateral Vas Deferens, Percutaneous Endoscopic Approach
♂ **0VNS0ZZ** Release Penis, Open Approach
♂ **0VNS3ZZ** Release Penis, Percutaneous Approach
♂ **0VNS4ZZ** Release Penis, Percutaneous Endoscopic Approach
♂ **0VNSXZZ** Release Penis, External Approach
♂ **0VNT0ZZ** Release Prepuce, Open Approach
♂ **0VNT3ZZ** Release Prepuce, Percutaneous Approach
♂ **0VNT4ZZ** Release Prepuce, Percutaneous Endoscopic Approach
♂ **0VNTXZZ** Release Prepuce, External Approach

0VP – Male Reproductive System, Removal

Review Coding Guideline B6.1c

♂ **0VP400Z** Removal of Drainage Device from Prostate and Seminal Vesicles, Open Approach
♂ **0VP401Z** Removal of Radioactive Element from Prostate and Seminal Vesicles, Open Approach
♂ **0VP403Z** Removal of Infusion Device from Prostate and Seminal Vesicles, Open Approach
♂ **0VP407Z** Removal of Autologous Tissue Substitute from Prostate and Seminal Vesicles, Open Approach
♂ **0VP40JZ** Removal of Synthetic Substitute from Prostate and Seminal Vesicles, Open Approach
♂ **0VP40KZ** Removal of Nonautologous Tissue Substitute from Prostate and Seminal Vesicles, Open Approach
♂ **0VP430Z** Removal of Drainage Device from Prostate and Seminal Vesicles, Percutaneous Approach
♂ **0VP431Z** Removal of Radioactive Element from Prostate and Seminal Vesicles, Percutaneous Approach
♂ **0VP433Z** Removal of Infusion Device from Prostate and Seminal Vesicles, Percutaneous Approach
♂ **0VP437Z** Removal of Autologous Tissue Substitute from Prostate and Seminal Vesicles, Percutaneous Approach
♂ **0VP43JZ** Removal of Synthetic Substitute from Prostate and Seminal Vesicles, Percutaneous Approach
♂ **0VP43KZ** Removal of Nonautologous Tissue Substitute from Prostate and Seminal Vesicles, Percutaneous Approach
♂ **0VP440Z** Removal of Drainage Device from Prostate and Seminal Vesicles, Percutaneous Endoscopic Approach
♂ **0VP441Z** Removal of Radioactive Element from Prostate and Seminal Vesicles, Percutaneous Endoscopic Approach
♂ **0VP443Z** Removal of Infusion Device from Prostate and Seminal Vesicles, Percutaneous Endoscopic Approach
♂ **0VP447Z** Removal of Autologous Tissue Substitute from Prostate and Seminal Vesicles, Percutaneous Endoscopic Approach
♂ **0VP44JZ** Removal of Synthetic Substitute from Prostate and Seminal Vesicles, Percutaneous Endoscopic Approach
♂ **0VP44KZ** Removal of Nonautologous Tissue Substitute from Prostate and Seminal Vesicles, Percutaneous Endoscopic Approach
♂ **0VP470Z** Removal of Drainage Device from Prostate and Seminal Vesicles, Via Natural or Artificial Opening
♂ **0VP471Z** Removal of Radioactive Element from Prostate and Seminal Vesicles, Via Natural or Artificial Opening
♂ **0VP473Z** Removal of Infusion Device from Prostate and Seminal Vesicles, Via Natural or Artificial Opening
♂ **0VP477Z** Removal of Autologous Tissue Substitute from Prostate and Seminal Vesicles, Via Natural or Artificial Opening
♂ **0VP47JZ** Removal of Synthetic Substitute from Prostate and Seminal Vesicles, Via Natural or Artificial Opening
♂ **0VP47KZ** Removal of Nonautologous Tissue Substitute from Prostate and Seminal Vesicles, Via Natural or Artificial Opening

♂ **0VP480Z** Removal of Drainage Device from Prostate and Seminal Vesicles, Via Natural or Artificial Opening Endoscopic
♂ **0VP481Z** Removal of Radioactive Element from Prostate and Seminal Vesicles, Via Natural or Artificial Opening Endoscopic
♂ **0VP483Z** Removal of Infusion Device from Prostate and Seminal Vesicles, Via Natural or Artificial Opening Endoscopic
♂ **0VP487Z** Removal of Autologous Tissue Substitute from Prostate and Seminal Vesicles, Via Natural or Artificial Opening Endoscopic
♂ **0VP48JZ** Removal of Synthetic Substitute from Prostate and Seminal Vesicles, Via Natural or Artificial Opening Endoscopic
♂ **0VP48KZ** Removal of Nonautologous Tissue Substitute from Prostate and Seminal Vesicles, Via Natural or Artificial Opening Endoscopic
♂ **0VP4X0Z** Removal of Drainage Device from Prostate and Seminal Vesicles, External Approach
♂ **0VP4X1Z** Removal of Radioactive Element from Prostate and Seminal Vesicles, External Approach
♂ **0VP4X3Z** Removal of Infusion Device from Prostate and Seminal Vesicles, External Approach
♂ **0VP800Z** Removal of Drainage Device from Scrotum and Tunica Vaginalis, Open Approach
♂ **0VP803Z** Removal of Infusion Device from Scrotum and Tunica Vaginalis, Open Approach
♂ **0VP807Z** Removal of Autologous Tissue Substitute from Scrotum and Tunica Vaginalis, Open Approach
♂ **0VP80JZ** Removal of Synthetic Substitute from Scrotum and Tunica Vaginalis, Open Approach
♂ **0VP80KZ** Removal of Nonautologous Tissue Substitute from Scrotum and Tunica Vaginalis, Open Approach
♂ **0VP830Z** Removal of Drainage Device from Scrotum and Tunica Vaginalis, Percutaneous Approach
♂ **0VP833Z** Removal of Infusion Device from Scrotum and Tunica Vaginalis, Percutaneous Approach
♂ **0VP837Z** Removal of Autologous Tissue Substitute from Scrotum and Tunica Vaginalis, Percutaneous Approach
♂ **0VP83JZ** Removal of Synthetic Substitute from Scrotum and Tunica Vaginalis, Percutaneous Approach
♂ **0VP83KZ** Removal of Nonautologous Tissue Substitute from Scrotum and Tunica Vaginalis, Percutaneous Approach
♂ **0VP840Z** Removal of Drainage Device from Scrotum and Tunica Vaginalis, Percutaneous Endoscopic Approach
♂ **0VP843Z** Removal of Infusion Device from Scrotum and Tunica Vaginalis, Percutaneous Endoscopic Approach
♂ **0VP847Z** Removal of Autologous Tissue Substitute from Scrotum and Tunica Vaginalis, Percutaneous Endoscopic Approach
♂ **0VP84JZ** Removal of Synthetic Substitute from Scrotum and Tunica Vaginalis, Percutaneous Endoscopic Approach
♂ **0VP84KZ** Removal of Nonautologous Tissue Substitute from Scrotum and Tunica Vaginalis, Percutaneous Endoscopic Approach

♂ **0VP870Z** Removal of Drainage Device from Scrotum and Tunica Vaginalis, Via Natural or Artificial Opening

♂ **0VP873Z** Removal of Infusion Device from Scrotum and Tunica Vaginalis, Via Natural or Artificial Opening

♂ **0VP877Z** Removal of Autologous Tissue Substitute from Scrotum and Tunica Vaginalis, Via Natural or Artificial Opening

♂ **0VP87JZ** Removal of Synthetic Substitute from Scrotum and Tunica Vaginalis, Via Natural or Artificial Opening

♂ **0VP87KZ** Removal of Nonautologous Tissue Substitute from Scrotum and Tunica Vaginalis, Via Natural or Artificial Opening

♂ **0VP880Z** Removal of Drainage Device from Scrotum and Tunica Vaginalis, Via Natural or Artificial Opening Endoscopic

♂ **0VP883Z** Removal of Infusion Device from Scrotum and Tunica Vaginalis, Via Natural or Artificial Opening Endoscopic

♂ **0VP887Z** Removal of Autologous Tissue Substitute from Scrotum and Tunica Vaginalis, Via Natural or Artificial Opening Endoscopic

♂ **0VP88JZ** Removal of Synthetic Substitute from Scrotum and Tunica Vaginalis, Via Natural or Artificial Opening Endoscopic

♂ **0VP88KZ** Removal of Nonautologous Tissue Substitute from Scrotum and Tunica Vaginalis, Via Natural or Artificial Opening Endoscopic

♂ **0VP8X0Z** Removal of Drainage Device from Scrotum and Tunica Vaginalis, External Approach

♂ **0VP8X3Z** Removal of Infusion Device from Scrotum and Tunica Vaginalis, External Approach

♂ **0VPD00Z** Removal of Drainage Device from Testis, Open Approach

♂ **0VPD03Z** Removal of Infusion Device from Testis, Open Approach

♂ **0VPD07Z** Removal of Autologous Tissue Substitute from Testis, Open Approach

♂ **0VPD0JZ** Removal of Synthetic Substitute from Testis, Open Approach

♂ **0VPD0KZ** Removal of Nonautologous Tissue Substitute from Testis, Open Approach

♂ **0VPD30Z** Removal of Drainage Device from Testis, Percutaneous Approach

♂ **0VPD33Z** Removal of Infusion Device from Testis, Percutaneous Approach

♂ **0VPD37Z** Removal of Autologous Tissue Substitute from Testis, Percutaneous Approach

♂ **0VPD3JZ** Removal of Synthetic Substitute from Testis, Percutaneous Approach

♂ **0VPD3KZ** Removal of Nonautologous Tissue Substitute from Testis, Percutaneous Approach

♂ **0VPD40Z** Removal of Drainage Device from Testis, Percutaneous Endoscopic Approach

♂ **0VPD43Z** Removal of Infusion Device from Testis, Percutaneous Endoscopic Approach

♂ **0VPD47Z** Removal of Autologous Tissue Substitute from Testis, Percutaneous Endoscopic Approach

♂ **0VPD4JZ** Removal of Synthetic Substitute from Testis, Percutaneous Endoscopic Approach

♂ **0VPD4KZ** Removal of Nonautologous Tissue Substitute from Testis, Percutaneous Endoscopic Approach

♂ **0VPD70Z** Removal of Drainage Device from Testis, Via Natural or Artificial Opening

♂ **0VPD73Z** Removal of Infusion Device from Testis, Via Natural or Artificial Opening

♂ **0VPD77Z** Removal of Autologous Tissue Substitute from Testis, Via Natural or Artificial Opening

♂ **0VPD7JZ** Removal of Synthetic Substitute from Testis, Via Natural or Artificial Opening

♂ **0VPD7KZ** Removal of Nonautologous Tissue Substitute from Testis, Via Natural or Artificial Opening

♂ **0VPD80Z** Removal of Drainage Device from Testis, Via Natural or Artificial Opening Endoscopic

♂ **0VPD83Z** Removal of Infusion Device from Testis, Via Natural or Artificial Opening Endoscopic

♂ **0VPD87Z** Removal of Autologous Tissue Substitute from Testis, Via Natural or Artificial Opening Endoscopic

♂ **0VPD8JZ** Removal of Synthetic Substitute from Testis, Via Natural or Artificial Opening Endoscopic

♂ **0VPD8KZ** Removal of Nonautologous Tissue Substitute from Testis, Via Natural or Artificial Opening Endoscopic

♂ **0VPDX0Z** Removal of Drainage Device from Testis, External Approach

♂ **0VPDX3Z** Removal of Infusion Device from Testis, External Approach

♂ **0VPM00Z** Removal of Drainage Device from Epididymis and Spermatic Cord, Open Approach

♂ **0VPM03Z** Removal of Infusion Device from Epididymis and Spermatic Cord, Open Approach

♂ **0VPM07Z** Removal of Autologous Tissue Substitute from Epididymis and Spermatic Cord, Open Approach

♂ **0VPM0CZ** Removal of Extraluminal Device from Epididymis and Spermatic Cord, Open Approach

♂ **0VPM0JZ** Removal of Synthetic Substitute from Epididymis and Spermatic Cord, Open Approach

♂ **0VPM0KZ** Removal of Nonautologous Tissue Substitute from Epididymis and Spermatic Cord, Open Approach

♂ **0VPM30Z** Removal of Drainage Device from Epididymis and Spermatic Cord, Percutaneous Approach

♂ **0VPM33Z** Removal of Infusion Device from Epididymis and Spermatic Cord, Percutaneous Approach

♂ **0VPM37Z** Removal of Autologous Tissue Substitute from Epididymis and Spermatic Cord, Percutaneous Approach

♂ **0VPM3CZ** Removal of Extraluminal Device from Epididymis and Spermatic Cord, Percutaneous Approach

♂ **0VPM3JZ** Removal of Synthetic Substitute from Epididymis and Spermatic Cord, Percutaneous Approach

♂ **0VPM3KZ** Removal of Nonautologous Tissue Substitute from Epididymis and Spermatic Cord, Percutaneous Approach

♂ **0VPM40Z** Removal of Drainage Device from Epididymis and Spermatic Cord, Percutaneous Endoscopic Approach

♂ **0VPM43Z** Removal of Infusion Device from Epididymis and Spermatic Cord, Percutaneous Endoscopic Approach

♂ **0VPM47Z** Removal of Autologous Tissue Substitute from Epididymis and Spermatic Cord, Percutaneous Endoscopic Approach

♂ **0VPM4CZ** Removal of Extraluminal Device from Epididymis and Spermatic Cord, Percutaneous Endoscopic Approach

♂ **0VPM4JZ** Removal of Synthetic Substitute from Epididymis and Spermatic Cord, Percutaneous Endoscopic Approach

♂ **0VPM4KZ** Removal of Nonautologous Tissue Substitute from Epididymis and Spermatic Cord, Percutaneous Endoscopic Approach

♂ **0VPM70Z** Removal of Drainage Device from Epididymis and Spermatic Cord, Via Natural or Artificial Opening

♂ **0VPM73Z** Removal of Infusion Device from Epididymis and Spermatic Cord, Via Natural or Artificial Opening

♂ **0VPM77Z** Removal of Autologous Tissue Substitute from Epididymis and Spermatic Cord, Via Natural or Artificial Opening

♂ **0VPM7CZ** Removal of Extraluminal Device from Epididymis and Spermatic Cord, Via Natural or Artificial Opening

♂ **0VPM7JZ** Removal of Synthetic Substitute from Epididymis and Spermatic Cord, Via Natural or Artificial Opening

♂ **0VPM7KZ** Removal of Nonautologous Tissue Substitute from Epididymis and Spermatic Cord, Via Natural or Artificial Opening

♂ **0VPM80Z** Removal of Drainage Device from Epididymis and Spermatic Cord, Via Natural or Artificial Opening Endoscopic

♂ **0VPM83Z** Removal of Infusion Device from Epididymis and Spermatic Cord, Via Natural or Artificial Opening Endoscopic

♂ **0VPM87Z** Removal of Autologous Tissue Substitute from Epididymis and Spermatic Cord, Via Natural or Artificial Opening Endoscopic

♂ **0VPM8CZ** Removal of Extraluminal Device from Epididymis and Spermatic Cord, Via Natural or Artificial Opening Endoscopic

♂ **0VPM8JZ** Removal of Synthetic Substitute from Epididymis and Spermatic Cord, Via Natural or Artificial Opening Endoscopic

♂ **0VPM8KZ** Removal of Nonautologous Tissue Substitute from Epididymis and Spermatic Cord, Via Natural or Artificial Opening Endoscopic

♂ **0VPMX0Z** Removal of Drainage Device from Epididymis and Spermatic Cord, External Approach

♂ **0VPMX3Z** Removal of Infusion Device from Epididymis and Spermatic Cord, External Approach

♂ **0VPR00Z** Removal of Drainage Device from Vas Deferens, Open Approach

♂ **0VPR03Z** Removal of Infusion Device from Vas Deferens, Open Approach

♂ **0VPR07Z** Removal of Autologous Tissue Substitute from Vas Deferens, Open Approach

♂ **0VPR0CZ** Removal of Extraluminal Device from Vas Deferens, Open Approach

♂ **0VPR0DZ** Removal of Intraluminal Device from Vas Deferens, Open Approach

♂ **0VPR0JZ** Removal of Synthetic Substitute from Vas Deferens, Open Approach

♂ **0VPR0KZ** Removal of Nonautologous Tissue Substitute from Vas Deferens, Open Approach

♂ **0VPR30Z** Removal of Drainage Device from Vas Deferens, Percutaneous Approach

♂ **0VPR33Z** Removal of Infusion Device from Vas Deferens, Percutaneous Approach

---

♂ **0VPR37Z** Removal of Autologous Tissue Substitute from Vas Deferens, Percutaneous Approach

♂ **0VPR3CZ** Removal of Extraluminal Device from Vas Deferens, Percutaneous Approach

♂ **0VPR3DZ** Removal of Intraluminal Device from Vas Deferens, Percutaneous Approach

♂ **0VPR3JZ** Removal of Synthetic Substitute from Vas Deferens, Percutaneous Approach

♂ **0VPR3KZ** Removal of Nonautologous Tissue Substitute from Vas Deferens, Percutaneous Approach

♂ **0VPR40Z** Removal of Drainage Device from Vas Deferens, Percutaneous Endoscopic Approach

♂ **0VPR43Z** Removal of Infusion Device from Vas Deferens, Percutaneous Endoscopic Approach

♂ **0VPR47Z** Removal of Autologous Tissue Substitute from Vas Deferens, Percutaneous Endoscopic Approach

♂ **0VPR4CZ** Removal of Extraluminal Device from Vas Deferens, Percutaneous Endoscopic Approach

♂ **0VPR4DZ** Removal of Intraluminal Device from Vas Deferens, Percutaneous Endoscopic Approach

♂ **0VPR4JZ** Removal of Synthetic Substitute from Vas Deferens, Percutaneous Endoscopic Approach

♂ **0VPR4KZ** Removal of Nonautologous Tissue Substitute from Vas Deferens, Percutaneous Endoscopic Approach

♂ **0VPR70Z** Removal of Drainage Device from Vas Deferens, Via Natural or Artificial Opening

♂ **0VPR73Z** Removal of Infusion Device from Vas Deferens, Via Natural or Artificial Opening

♂ **0VPR77Z** Removal of Autologous Tissue Substitute from Vas Deferens, Via Natural or Artificial Opening

♂ **0VPR7CZ** Removal of Extraluminal Device from Vas Deferens, Via Natural or Artificial Opening

♂ **0VPR7DZ** Removal of Intraluminal Device from Vas Deferens, Via Natural or Artificial Opening

♂ **0VPR7JZ** Removal of Synthetic Substitute from Vas Deferens, Via Natural or Artificial Opening

♂ **0VPR7KZ** Removal of Nonautologous Tissue Substitute from Vas Deferens, Via Natural or Artificial Opening

♂ **0VPR80Z** Removal of Drainage Device from Vas Deferens, Via Natural or Artificial Opening Endoscopic

♂ **0VPR83Z** Removal of Infusion Device from Vas Deferens, Via Natural or Artificial Opening Endoscopic

♂ **0VPR87Z** Removal of Autologous Tissue Substitute from Vas Deferens, Via Natural or Artificial Opening Endoscopic

♂ **0VPR8CZ** Removal of Extraluminal Device from Vas Deferens, Via Natural or Artificial Opening Endoscopic

♂ **0VPR8DZ** Removal of Intraluminal Device from Vas Deferens, Via Natural or Artificial Opening Endoscopic

♂ **0VPR8JZ** Removal of Synthetic Substitute from Vas Deferens, Via Natural or Artificial Opening Endoscopic

♂ **0VPR8KZ** Removal of Nonautologous Tissue Substitute from Vas Deferens, Via Natural or Artificial Opening Endoscopic

♂ **0VPRX0Z** Removal of Drainage Device from Vas Deferens, External Approach

♂ **0VPRX3Z** Removal of Infusion Device from Vas Deferens, External Approach

♂ **0VPRXDZ** Removal of Intraluminal Device from Vas Deferens, External Approach

♂ **0VPS00Z** Removal of Drainage Device from Penis, Open Approach

♂ **0VPS03Z** Removal of Infusion Device from Penis, Open Approach

♂ **0VPS07Z** Removal of Autologous Tissue Substitute from Penis, Open Approach

♂ **0VPS0JZ** Removal of Synthetic Substitute from Penis, Open Approach

♂ **0VPS0KZ** Removal of Nonautologous Tissue Substitute from Penis, Open Approach

♂ **0VPS30Z** Removal of Drainage Device from Penis, Percutaneous Approach

♂ **0VPS33Z** Removal of Infusion Device from Penis, Percutaneous Approach

♂ **0VPS37Z** Removal of Autologous Tissue Substitute from Penis, Percutaneous Approach

♂ **0VPS3JZ** Removal of Synthetic Substitute from Penis, Percutaneous Approach

♂ **0VPS3KZ** Removal of Nonautologous Tissue Substitute from Penis, Percutaneous Approach

♂ **0VPS40Z** Removal of Drainage Device from Penis, Percutaneous Endoscopic Approach

♂ **0VPS43Z** Removal of Infusion Device from Penis, Percutaneous Endoscopic Approach

♂ **0VPS47Z** Removal of Autologous Tissue Substitute from Penis, Percutaneous Endoscopic Approach

♂ **0VPS4JZ** Removal of Synthetic Substitute from Penis, Percutaneous Endoscopic Approach

♂ **0VPS4KZ** Removal of Nonautologous Tissue Substitute from Penis, Percutaneous Endoscopic Approach

♂ **0VPS70Z** Removal of Drainage Device from Penis, Via Natural or Artificial Opening

♂ **0VPS73Z** Removal of Infusion Device from Penis, Via Natural or Artificial Opening

♂ **0VPS77Z** Removal of Autologous Tissue Substitute from Penis, Via Natural or Artificial Opening

♂ **0VPS7JZ** Removal of Synthetic Substitute from Penis, Via Natural or Artificial Opening

♂ **0VPS7KZ** Removal of Nonautologous Tissue Substitute from Penis, Via Natural or Artificial Opening

♂ **0VPS80Z** Removal of Drainage Device from Penis, Via Natural or Artificial Opening Endoscopic

♂ **0VPS83Z** Removal of Infusion Device from Penis, Via Natural or Artificial Opening Endoscopic

♂ **0VPS87Z** Removal of Autologous Tissue Substitute from Penis, Via Natural or Artificial Opening Endoscopic

♂ **0VPS8JZ** Removal of Synthetic Substitute from Penis, Via Natural or Artificial Opening Endoscopic

♂ **0VPS8KZ** Removal of Nonautologous Tissue Substitute from Penis, Via Natural or Artificial Opening Endoscopic

♂ **0VPSX0Z** Removal of Drainage Device from Penis, External Approach

♂ **0VPSX3Z** Removal of Infusion Device from Penis, External Approach

0VQ – Male Reproductive System, Repair

♂ **0VQ00ZZ** Repair Prostate, Open Approach

♂ **0VQ03ZZ** Repair Prostate, Percutaneous Approach

♂ **0VQ04ZZ** Repair Prostate, Percutaneous Endoscopic Approach

♂ **0VQ07ZZ** Repair Prostate, Via Natural or Artificial Opening

♂ **0VQ08ZZ** Repair Prostate, Via Natural or Artificial Opening Endoscopic

♂ **0VQ10ZZ** Repair Right Seminal Vesicle, Open Approach

♂ **0VQ13ZZ** Repair Right Seminal Vesicle, Percutaneous Approach

♂ **0VQ14ZZ** Repair Right Seminal Vesicle, Percutaneous Endoscopic Approach

♂ **0VQ20ZZ** Repair Left Seminal Vesicle, Open Approach

♂ **0VQ23ZZ** Repair Left Seminal Vesicle, Percutaneous Approach

♂ **0VQ24ZZ** Repair Left Seminal Vesicle, Percutaneous Endoscopic Approach

♂ **0VQ30ZZ** Repair Bilateral Seminal Vesicles, Open Approach

♂ **0VQ33ZZ** Repair Bilateral Seminal Vesicles, Percutaneous Approach

♂ **0VQ34ZZ** Repair Bilateral Seminal Vesicles, Percutaneous Endoscopic Approach

♂ **0VQ50ZZ** Repair Scrotum, Open Approach

♂ **0VQ53ZZ** Repair Scrotum, Percutaneous Approach

♂ **0VQ54ZZ** Repair Scrotum, Percutaneous Endoscopic Approach

♂ **0VQ5XZZ** Repair Scrotum, External Approach

♂ **0VQ60ZZ** Repair Right Tunica Vaginalis, Open Approach

♂ **0VQ63ZZ** Repair Right Tunica Vaginalis, Percutaneous Approach

♂ **0VQ64ZZ** Repair Right Tunica Vaginalis, Percutaneous Endoscopic Approach

♂ **0VQ70ZZ** Repair Left Tunica Vaginalis, Open Approach

♂ **0VQ73ZZ** Repair Left Tunica Vaginalis, Percutaneous Approach

♂ **0VQ74ZZ** Repair Left Tunica Vaginalis, Percutaneous Endoscopic Approach

♂ **0VQ90ZZ** Repair Right Testis, Open Approach

♂ **0VQ93ZZ** Repair Right Testis, Percutaneous Approach

♂ **0VQ94ZZ** Repair Right Testis, Percutaneous Endoscopic Approach

♂ **0VQB0ZZ** Repair Left Testis, Open Approach

♂ **0VQB3ZZ** Repair Left Testis, Percutaneous Approach

♂ **0VQB4ZZ** Repair Left Testis, Percutaneous Endoscopic Approach

♂ **0VQC0ZZ** Repair Bilateral Testes, Open Approach

♂ **0VQC3ZZ** Repair Bilateral Testes, Percutaneous Approach

♂ **0VQC4ZZ** Repair Bilateral Testes, Percutaneous Endoscopic Approach

♂ **0VQF0ZZ** Repair Right Spermatic Cord, Open Approach

♂ **0VQF3ZZ** Repair Right Spermatic Cord, Percutaneous Approach

♂ **0VQF4ZZ** Repair Right Spermatic Cord, Percutaneous Endoscopic Approach
♂ **0VQG0ZZ** Repair Left Spermatic Cord, Open Approach
♂ **0VQG3ZZ** Repair Left Spermatic Cord, Percutaneous Approach
♂ **0VQG4ZZ** Repair Left Spermatic Cord, Percutaneous Endoscopic Approach
♂ **0VQH0ZZ** Repair Bilateral Spermatic Cords, Open Approach
♂ **0VQH3ZZ** Repair Bilateral Spermatic Cords, Percutaneous Approach
♂ **0VQH4ZZ** Repair Bilateral Spermatic Cords, Percutaneous Endoscopic Approach
♂ **0VQJ0ZZ** Repair Right Epididymis, Open Approach
♂ **0VQJ3ZZ** Repair Right Epididymis, Percutaneous Approach
♂ **0VQJ4ZZ** Repair Right Epididymis, Percutaneous Endoscopic Approach
♂ **0VQK0ZZ** Repair Left Epididymis, Open Approach
♂ **0VQK3ZZ** Repair Left Epididymis, Percutaneous Approach
♂ **0VQK4ZZ** Repair Left Epididymis, Percutaneous Endoscopic Approach
♂ **0VQL0ZZ** Repair Bilateral Epididymis, Open Approach
♂ **0VQL3ZZ** Repair Bilateral Epididymis, Percutaneous Approach
♂ **0VQL4ZZ** Repair Bilateral Epididymis, Percutaneous Endoscopic Approach

♂ **0VQN0ZZ** Repair Right Vas Deferens, Open Approach
♂ **0VQN3ZZ** Repair Right Vas Deferens, Percutaneous Approach
♂ **0VQN4ZZ** Repair Right Vas Deferens, Percutaneous Endoscopic Approach
♂ **0VQP0ZZ** Repair Left Vas Deferens, Open Approach
♂ **0VQP3ZZ** Repair Left Vas Deferens, Percutaneous Approach
♂ **0VQP4ZZ** Repair Left Vas Deferens, Percutaneous Endoscopic Approach
♂ **0VQQ0ZZ** Repair Bilateral Vas Deferens, Open Approach
♂ **0VQQ3ZZ** Repair Bilateral Vas Deferens, Percutaneous Approach
♂ **0VQQ4ZZ** Repair Bilateral Vas Deferens, Percutaneous Endoscopic Approach
♂ **0VQS0ZZ** Repair Penis, Open Approach
♂ **0VQS3ZZ** Repair Penis, Percutaneous Approach
♂ **0VQS4ZZ** Repair Penis, Percutaneous Endoscopic Approach
♂ **0VQSXZZ** Repair Penis, External Approach
♂ **0VQT0ZZ** Repair Prepuce, Open Approach
♂ **0VQT3ZZ** Repair Prepuce, Percutaneous Approach
♂ **0VQT4ZZ** Repair Prepuce, Percutaneous Endoscopic Approach
♂ **0VQTXZZ** Repair Prepuce, External Approach

0VR – Male Reproductive System, Replacement

♂ **0VR90JZ** Replacement of Right Testis with Synthetic Substitute, Open Approach
♂ **0VRB0JZ** Replacement of Left Testis with Synthetic Substitute, Open Approach

♂ **0VRC0JZ** Replacement of Bilateral Testes with Synthetic Substitute, Open Approach

0VS – Male Reproductive System, Reposition

♂ **0VS90ZZ** Reposition Right Testis, Open Approach
♂ **0VS93ZZ** Reposition Right Testis, Percutaneous Approach
♂ **0VS94ZZ** Reposition Right Testis, Percutaneous Endoscopic Approach
♂ **0VSB0ZZ** Reposition Left Testis, Open Approach
♂ **0VSB3ZZ** Reposition Left Testis, Percutaneous Approach
♂ **0VSB4ZZ** Reposition Left Testis, Percutaneous Endoscopic Approach
♂ **0VSC0ZZ** Reposition Bilateral Testes, Open Approach
♂ **0VSC3ZZ** Reposition Bilateral Testes, Percutaneous Approach
♂ **0VSC4ZZ** Reposition Bilateral Testes, Percutaneous Endoscopic Approach
♂ **0VSF0ZZ** Reposition Right Spermatic Cord, Open Approach
♂ **0VSF3ZZ** Reposition Right Spermatic Cord, Percutaneous Approach

♂ **0VSF4ZZ** Reposition Right Spermatic Cord, Percutaneous Endoscopic Approach
♂ **0VSG0ZZ** Reposition Left Spermatic Cord, Open Approach
♂ **0VSG3ZZ** Reposition Left Spermatic Cord, Percutaneous Approach
♂ **0VSG4ZZ** Reposition Left Spermatic Cord, Percutaneous Endoscopic Approach
♂ **0VSH0ZZ** Reposition Bilateral Spermatic Cords, Open Approach
♂ **0VSH3ZZ** Reposition Bilateral Spermatic Cords, Percutaneous Approach
♂ **0VSH4ZZ** Reposition Bilateral Spermatic Cords, Percutaneous Endoscopic Approach

0VT – Male Reproductive System, Resection

Review Coding Guideline B3.8

♂ **0VT00ZZ** Resection of Prostate, Open Approach
♂ **0VT04ZZ** Resection of Prostate, Percutaneous Endoscopic Approach
♂ **0VT07ZZ** Resection of Prostate, Via Natural or Artificial Opening
♂ **0VT08ZZ** Resection of Prostate, Via Natural or Artificial Opening Endoscopic
♂ **0VT10ZZ** Resection of Right Seminal Vesicle, Open Approach
♂ **0VT14ZZ** Resection of Right Seminal Vesicle, Percutaneous Endoscopic Approach
♂ **0VT20ZZ** Resection of Left Seminal Vesicle, Open Approach
♂ **0VT24ZZ** Resection of Left Seminal Vesicle, Percutaneous Endoscopic Approach
♂ **0VT30ZZ** Resection of Bilateral Seminal Vesicles, Open Approach
♂ **0VT34ZZ** Resection of Bilateral Seminal Vesicles, Percutaneous Endoscopic Approach
♂ **0VT50ZZ** Resection of Scrotum, Open Approach
♂ **0VT54ZZ** Resection of Scrotum, Percutaneous Endoscopic Approach
♂ **0VT5XZZ** Resection of Scrotum, External Approach
♂ **0VT60ZZ** Resection of Right Tunica Vaginalis, Open Approach
♂ **0VT64ZZ** Resection of Right Tunica Vaginalis, Percutaneous Endoscopic Approach
♂ **0VT70ZZ** Resection of Left Tunica Vaginalis, Open Approach
♂ **0VT74ZZ** Resection of Left Tunica Vaginalis, Percutaneous Endoscopic Approach
♂ **0VT90ZZ** Resection of Right Testis, Open Approach
♂ **0VT94ZZ** Resection of Right Testis, Percutaneous Endoscopic Approach
♂ **0VTB0ZZ** Resection of Left Testis, Open Approach
♂ **0VTB4ZZ** Resection of Left Testis, Percutaneous Endoscopic Approach
♂ **0VTC0ZZ** Resection of Bilateral Testes, Open Approach
♂ **0VTC4ZZ** Resection of Bilateral Testes, Percutaneous Endoscopic Approach
♂ **0VTF0ZZ** Resection of Right Spermatic Cord, Open Approach

♂ **0VTF4ZZ** Resection of Right Spermatic Cord, Percutaneous Endoscopic Approach
♂ **0VTG0ZZ** Resection of Left Spermatic Cord, Open Approach
♂ **0VTG4ZZ** Resection of Left Spermatic Cord, Percutaneous Endoscopic Approach
♂ **0VTH0ZZ** Resection of Bilateral Spermatic Cords, Open Approach
♂ **0VTH4ZZ** Resection of Bilateral Spermatic Cords, Percutaneous Endoscopic Approach
♂ **0VTJ0ZZ** Resection of Right Epididymis, Open Approach
♂ **0VTJ4ZZ** Resection of Right Epididymis, Percutaneous Endoscopic Approach
♂ **0VTK0ZZ** Resection of Left Epididymis, Open Approach
♂ **0VTK4ZZ** Resection of Left Epididymis, Percutaneous Endoscopic Approach
♂ **0VTL0ZZ** Resection of Bilateral Epididymis, Open Approach
♂ **0VTL4ZZ** Resection of Bilateral Epididymis, Percutaneous Endoscopic Approach
●♂ **0VTN0ZZ** Resection of Right Vas Deferens, Open Approach
●♂ **0VTN4ZZ** Resection of Right Vas Deferens, Percutaneous Endoscopic Approach
⬣♂ **0VTP0ZZ** Resection of Left Vas Deferens, Open Approach
●♂ **0VTP4ZZ** Resection of Left Vas Deferens, Percutaneous Endoscopic Approach
●♂ **0VTQ0ZZ** Resection of Bilateral Vas Deferens, Open Approach
●♂ **0VTQ4ZZ** Resection of Bilateral Vas Deferens, Percutaneous Endoscopic Approach
♂ **0VTS0ZZ** Resection of Penis, Open Approach
♂ **0VTS4ZZ** Resection of Penis, Percutaneous Endoscopic Approach
♂ **0VTSXZZ** Resection of Penis, External Approach
♂ **0VTT0ZZ** Resection of Prepuce, Open Approach
♂ **0VTT4ZZ** Resection of Prepuce, Percutaneous Endoscopic Approach
♂ **0VTTXZZ** Resection of Prepuce, External Approach

0VU – Male Reproductive System, Supplement

♂ **0VU107Z**   Supplement Right Seminal Vesicle with Autologous Tissue Substitute, Open Approach

♂ **0VU10JZ**   Supplement Right Seminal Vesicle with Synthetic Substitute, Open Approach

♂ **0VU10KZ**   Supplement Right Seminal Vesicle with Nonautologous Tissue Substitute, Open Approach

♂ **0VU147Z**   Supplement Right Seminal Vesicle with Autologous Tissue Substitute, Percutaneous Endoscopic Approach

♂ **0VU14JZ**   Supplement Right Seminal Vesicle with Synthetic Substitute, Percutaneous Endoscopic Approach

♂ **0VU14KZ**   Supplement Right Seminal Vesicle with Nonautologous Tissue Substitute, Percutaneous Endoscopic Approach

♂ **0VU207Z**   Supplement Left Seminal Vesicle with Autologous Tissue Substitute, Open Approach

♂ **0VU20JZ**   Supplement Left Seminal Vesicle with Synthetic Substitute, Open Approach

♂ **0VU20KZ**   Supplement Left Seminal Vesicle with Nonautologous Tissue Substitute, Open Approach

♂ **0VU247Z**   Supplement Left Seminal Vesicle with Autologous Tissue Substitute, Percutaneous Endoscopic Approach

♂ **0VU24JZ**   Supplement Left Seminal Vesicle with Synthetic Substitute, Percutaneous Endoscopic Approach

♂ **0VU24KZ**   Supplement Left Seminal Vesicle with Nonautologous Tissue Substitute, Percutaneous Endoscopic Approach

♂ **0VU307Z**   Supplement Bilateral Seminal Vesicles with Autologous Tissue Substitute, Open Approach

♂ **0VU30JZ**   Supplement Bilateral Seminal Vesicles with Synthetic Substitute, Open Approach

♂ **0VU30KZ**   Supplement Bilateral Seminal Vesicles with Nonautologous Tissue Substitute, Open Approach

♂ **0VU347Z**   Supplement Bilateral Seminal Vesicles with Autologous Tissue Substitute, Percutaneous Endoscopic Approach

♂ **0VU34JZ**   Supplement Bilateral Seminal Vesicles with Synthetic Substitute, Percutaneous Endoscopic Approach

♂ **0VU34KZ**   Supplement Bilateral Seminal Vesicles with Nonautologous Tissue Substitute, Percutaneous Endoscopic Approach

♂ **0VU507Z**   Supplement Scrotum with Autologous Tissue Substitute, Open Approach

♂ **0VU50JZ**   Supplement Scrotum with Synthetic Substitute, Open Approach

♂ **0VU50KZ**   Supplement Scrotum with Nonautologous Tissue Substitute, Open Approach

♂ **0VU547Z**   Supplement Scrotum with Autologous Tissue Substitute, Percutaneous Endoscopic Approach

♂ **0VU54JZ**   Supplement Scrotum with Synthetic Substitute, Percutaneous Endoscopic Approach

♂ **0VU54KZ**   Supplement Scrotum with Nonautologous Tissue Substitute, Percutaneous Endoscopic Approach

♂ **0VU5X7Z**   Supplement Scrotum with Autologous Tissue Substitute, External Approach

♂ **0VU5XJZ**   Supplement Scrotum with Synthetic Substitute, External Approach

♂ **0VU5XKZ**   Supplement Scrotum with Nonautologous Tissue Substitute, External Approach

♂ **0VU607Z**   Supplement Right Tunica Vaginalis with Autologous Tissue Substitute, Open Approach

♂ **0VU60JZ**   Supplement Right Tunica Vaginalis with Synthetic Substitute, Open Approach

♂ **0VU60KZ**   Supplement Right Tunica Vaginalis with Nonautologous Tissue Substitute, Open Approach

♂ **0VU647Z**   Supplement Right Tunica Vaginalis with Autologous Tissue Substitute, Percutaneous Endoscopic Approach

♂ **0VU64JZ**   Supplement Right Tunica Vaginalis with Synthetic Substitute, Percutaneous Endoscopic Approach

♂ **0VU64KZ**   Supplement Right Tunica Vaginalis with Nonautologous Tissue Substitute, Percutaneous Endoscopic Approach

♂ **0VU707Z**   Supplement Left Tunica Vaginalis with Autologous Tissue Substitute, Open Approach

♂ **0VU70JZ**   Supplement Left Tunica Vaginalis with Synthetic Substitute, Open Approach

♂ **0VU70KZ**   Supplement Left Tunica Vaginalis with Nonautologous Tissue Substitute, Open Approach

♂ **0VU747Z**   Supplement Left Tunica Vaginalis with Autologous Tissue Substitute, Percutaneous Endoscopic Approach

♂ **0VU74JZ**   Supplement Left Tunica Vaginalis with Synthetic Substitute, Percutaneous Endoscopic Approach

♂ **0VU74KZ**   Supplement Left Tunica Vaginalis with Nonautologous Tissue Substitute, Percutaneous Endoscopic Approach

♂ **0VU907Z**   Supplement Right Testis with Autologous Tissue Substitute, Open Approach

♂ **0VU90JZ**   Supplement Right Testis with Synthetic Substitute, Open Approach

♂ **0VU90KZ**   Supplement Right Testis with Nonautologous Tissue Substitute, Open Approach

♂ **0VUB07Z**   Supplement Left Testis with Autologous Tissue Substitute, Open Approach

♂ **0VUB0JZ**   Supplement Left Testis with Synthetic Substitute, Open Approach

♂ **0VUB0KZ**   Supplement Left Testis with Nonautologous Tissue Substitute, Open Approach

♂ **0VUC07Z**   Supplement Bilateral Testes with Autologous Tissue Substitute, Open Approach

♂ **0VUC0JZ**   Supplement Bilateral Testes with Synthetic Substitute, Open Approach

♂ **0VUC0KZ**   Supplement Bilateral Testes with Nonautologous Tissue Substitute, Open Approach

♂ **0VUF07Z**   Supplement Right Spermatic Cord with Autologous Tissue Substitute, Open Approach

♂ **0VUF0JZ**   Supplement Right Spermatic Cord with Synthetic Substitute, Open Approach

♂ **0VUF0KZ**   Supplement Right Spermatic Cord with Nonautologous Tissue Substitute, Open Approach

♂ **0VUF47Z**   Supplement Right Spermatic Cord with Autologous Tissue Substitute, Percutaneous Endoscopic Approach

♂ **0VUF4JZ**   Supplement Right Spermatic Cord with Synthetic Substitute, Percutaneous Endoscopic Approach

♂ **0VUF4KZ**   Supplement Right Spermatic Cord with Nonautologous Tissue Substitute, Percutaneous Endoscopic Approach

♂ **0VUG07Z**   Supplement Left Spermatic Cord with Autologous Tissue Substitute, Open Approach

♂ **0VUG0JZ**   Supplement Left Spermatic Cord with Synthetic Substitute, Open Approach

♂ **0VUG0KZ**   Supplement Left Spermatic Cord with Nonautologous Tissue Substitute, Open Approach

♂ **0VUG47Z**   Supplement Left Spermatic Cord with Autologous Tissue Substitute, Percutaneous Endoscopic Approach

♂ **0VUG4JZ**   Supplement Left Spermatic Cord with Synthetic Substitute, Percutaneous Endoscopic Approach

♂ **0VUG4KZ**   Supplement Left Spermatic Cord with Nonautologous Tissue Substitute, Percutaneous Endoscopic Approach

♂ **0VUH07Z**   Supplement Bilateral Spermatic Cords with Autologous Tissue Substitute, Open Approach

♂ **0VUH0JZ**   Supplement Bilateral Spermatic Cords with Synthetic Substitute, Open Approach

♂ **0VUH0KZ**   Supplement Bilateral Spermatic Cords with Nonautologous Tissue Substitute, Open Approach

♂ **0VUH47Z**   Supplement Bilateral Spermatic Cords with Autologous Tissue Substitute, Percutaneous Endoscopic Approach

♂ **0VUH4JZ**   Supplement Bilateral Spermatic Cords with Synthetic Substitute, Percutaneous Endoscopic Approach

♂ **0VUH4KZ**   Supplement Bilateral Spermatic Cords with Nonautologous Tissue Substitute, Percutaneous Endoscopic Approach

♂ **0VUJ07Z**   Supplement Right Epididymis with Autologous Tissue Substitute, Open Approach

♂ **0VUJ0JZ**   Supplement Right Epididymis with Synthetic Substitute, Open Approach

♂ **0VUJ0KZ**   Supplement Right Epididymis with Nonautologous Tissue Substitute, Open Approach

♂ **0VUJ47Z**   Supplement Right Epididymis with Autologous Tissue Substitute, Percutaneous Endoscopic Approach

♂ **0VUJ4JZ**   Supplement Right Epididymis with Synthetic Substitute, Percutaneous Endoscopic Approach

♂ **0VUJ4KZ**   Supplement Right Epididymis with Nonautologous Tissue Substitute, Percutaneous Endoscopic Approach

---

♀ Female-only   ♂ Male-only   ● Limited Coverage   ● Non-OR   � HAC-associated procedure   ● Non-covered procedures   ✚ Combination

♂ **0VUK07Z** Supplement Left Epididymis with Autologous Tissue Substitute, Open Approach

♂ **0VUK0JZ** Supplement Left Epididymis with Synthetic Substitute, Open Approach

♂ **0VUK0KZ** Supplement Left Epididymis with Nonautologous Tissue Substitute, Open Approach

♂ **0VUK47Z** Supplement Left Epididymis with Autologous Tissue Substitute, Percutaneous Endoscopic Approach

♂ **0VUK4JZ** Supplement Left Epididymis with Synthetic Substitute, Percutaneous Endoscopic Approach

♂ **0VUK4KZ** Supplement Left Epididymis with Nonautologous Tissue Substitute, Percutaneous Endoscopic Approach

♂ **0VUL07Z** Supplement Bilateral Epididymis with Autologous Tissue Substitute, Open Approach

♂ **0VUL0JZ** Supplement Bilateral Epididymis with Synthetic Substitute, Open Approach

♂ **0VUL0KZ** Supplement Bilateral Epididymis with Nonautologous Tissue Substitute, Open Approach

♂ **0VUL47Z** Supplement Bilateral Epididymis with Autologous Tissue Substitute, Percutaneous Endoscopic Approach

♂ **0VUL4JZ** Supplement Bilateral Epididymis with Synthetic Substitute, Percutaneous Endoscopic Approach

♂ **0VUL4KZ** Supplement Bilateral Epididymis with Nonautologous Tissue Substitute, Percutaneous Endoscopic Approach

♂ **0VUN07Z** Supplement Right Vas Deferens with Autologous Tissue Substitute, Open Approach

♂ **0VUN0JZ** Supplement Right Vas Deferens with Synthetic Substitute, Open Approach

♂ **0VUN0KZ** Supplement Right Vas Deferens with Nonautologous Tissue Substitute, Open Approach

♂ **0VUN47Z** Supplement Right Vas Deferens with Autologous Tissue Substitute, Percutaneous Endoscopic Approach

♂ **0VUN4JZ** Supplement Right Vas Deferens with Synthetic Substitute, Percutaneous Endoscopic Approach

♂ **0VUN4KZ** Supplement Right Vas Deferens with Nonautologous Tissue Substitute, Percutaneous Endoscopic Approach

♂ **0VUP07Z** Supplement Left Vas Deferens with Autologous Tissue Substitute, Open Approach

♂ **0VUP0JZ** Supplement Left Vas Deferens with Synthetic Substitute, Open Approach

♂ **0VUP0KZ** Supplement Left Vas Deferens with Nonautologous Tissue Substitute, Open Approach

♂ **0VUP47Z** Supplement Left Vas Deferens with Autologous Tissue Substitute, Percutaneous Endoscopic Approach

♂ **0VUP4JZ** Supplement Left Vas Deferens with Synthetic Substitute, Percutaneous Endoscopic Approach

♂ **0VUP4KZ** Supplement Left Vas Deferens with Nonautologous Tissue Substitute, Percutaneous Endoscopic Approach

♂ **0VUQ07Z** Supplement Bilateral Vas Deferens with Autologous Tissue Substitute, Open Approach

♂ **0VUQ0JZ** Supplement Bilateral Vas Deferens with Synthetic Substitute, Open Approach

♂ **0VUQ0KZ** Supplement Bilateral Vas Deferens with Nonautologous Tissue Substitute, Open Approach

♂ **0VUQ47Z** Supplement Bilateral Vas Deferens with Autologous Tissue Substitute, Percutaneous Endoscopic Approach

♂ **0VUQ4JZ** Supplement Bilateral Vas Deferens with Synthetic Substitute, Percutaneous Endoscopic Approach

♂ **0VUQ4KZ** Supplement Bilateral Vas Deferens with Nonautologous Tissue Substitute, Percutaneous Endoscopic Approach

♂ **0VUS07Z** Supplement Penis with Autologous Tissue Substitute, Open Approach

♂ **0VUS0JZ** Supplement Penis with Synthetic Substitute, Open Approach

♂ **0VUS0KZ** Supplement Penis with Nonautologous Tissue Substitute, Open Approach

♂ **0VUS47Z** Supplement Penis with Autologous Tissue Substitute, Percutaneous Endoscopic Approach

♂ **0VUS4JZ** Supplement Penis with Synthetic Substitute, Percutaneous Endoscopic Approach

♂ **0VUS4KZ** Supplement Penis with Nonautologous Tissue Substitute, Percutaneous Endoscopic Approach

♂ **0VUSX7Z** Supplement Penis with Autologous Tissue Substitute, External Approach

♂ **0VUSXJZ** Supplement Penis with Synthetic Substitute, External Approach

♂ **0VUSXKZ** Supplement Penis with Nonautologous Tissue Substitute, External Approach

♂ **0VUT07Z** Supplement Prepuce with Autologous Tissue Substitute, Open Approach

♂ **0VUT0JZ** Supplement Prepuce with Synthetic Substitute, Open Approach

♂ **0VUT0KZ** Supplement Prepuce with Nonautologous Tissue Substitute, Open Approach

♂ **0VUT47Z** Supplement Prepuce with Autologous Tissue Substitute, Percutaneous Endoscopic Approach

♂ **0VUT4JZ** Supplement Prepuce with Synthetic Substitute, Percutaneous Endoscopic Approach

♂ **0VUT4KZ** Supplement Prepuce with Nonautologous Tissue Substitute, Percutaneous Endoscopic Approach

♂ **0VUTX7Z** Supplement Prepuce with Autologous Tissue Substitute, External Approach

♂ **0VUTXJZ** Supplement Prepuce with Synthetic Substitute, External Approach

♂ **0VUTXKZ** Supplement Prepuce with Nonautologous Tissue Substitute, External Approach

0VW – Male Reproductive System, Revision

Review Coding Guideline B6.1c

♂ **0VW400Z** Revision of Drainage Device in Prostate and Seminal Vesicles, Open Approach

♂ **0VW403Z** Revision of Infusion Device in Prostate and Seminal Vesicles, Open Approach

♂ **0VW407Z** Revision of Autologous Tissue Substitute in Prostate and Seminal Vesicles, Open Approach

♂ **0VW40JZ** Revision of Synthetic Substitute in Prostate and Seminal Vesicles, Open Approach

♂ **0VW40KZ** Revision of Nonautologous Tissue Substitute in Prostate and Seminal Vesicles, Open Approach

♂ **0VW430Z** Revision of Drainage Device in Prostate and Seminal Vesicles, Percutaneous Approach

♂ **0VW433Z** Revision of Infusion Device in Prostate and Seminal Vesicles, Percutaneous Approach

♂ **0VW437Z** Revision of Autologous Tissue Substitute in Prostate and Seminal Vesicles, Percutaneous Approach

♂ **0VW43JZ** Revision of Synthetic Substitute in Prostate and Seminal Vesicles, Percutaneous Approach

♂ **0VW43KZ** Revision of Nonautologous Tissue Substitute in Prostate and Seminal Vesicles, Percutaneous Approach

♂ **0VW440Z** Revision of Drainage Device in Prostate and Seminal Vesicles, Percutaneous Endoscopic Approach

♂ **0VW443Z** Revision of Infusion Device in Prostate and Seminal Vesicles, Percutaneous Endoscopic Approach

♂ **0VW447Z** Revision of Autologous Tissue Substitute in Prostate and Seminal Vesicles, Percutaneous Endoscopic Approach

♂ **0VW44JZ** Revision of Synthetic Substitute in Prostate and Seminal Vesicles, Percutaneous Endoscopic Approach

♂ **0VW44KZ** Revision of Nonautologous Tissue Substitute in Prostate and Seminal Vesicles, Percutaneous Endoscopic Approach

♂ **0VW470Z** Revision of Drainage Device in Prostate and Seminal Vesicles, Via Natural or Artificial Opening

♂ **0VW473Z** Revision of Infusion Device in Prostate and Seminal Vesicles, Via Natural or Artificial Opening

♂ **0VW477Z** Revision of Autologous Tissue Substitute in Prostate and Seminal Vesicles, Via Natural or Artificial Opening

♂ **0VW47JZ** Revision of Synthetic Substitute in Prostate and Seminal Vesicles, Via Natural or Artificial Opening

♂ **0VW47KZ** Revision of Nonautologous Tissue Substitute in Prostate and Seminal Vesicles, Via Natural or Artificial Opening

---

♀ Female-only   ♂ Male-only   ● Limited Coverage   ● Non-OR   ᴴᴬᶜ HAC-associated procedure   ⬢ Non-covered procedures   ✚ Combination

♂ **0VW480Z** Revision of Drainage Device in Prostate and Seminal Vesicles, Via Natural or Artificial Opening Endoscopic

♂ **0VW483Z** Revision of Infusion Device in Prostate and Seminal Vesicles, Via Natural or Artificial Opening Endoscopic

♂ **0VW487Z** Revision of Autologous Tissue Substitute in Prostate and Seminal Vesicles, Via Natural or Artificial Opening Endoscopic

♂ **0VW48JZ** Revision of Synthetic Substitute in Prostate and Seminal Vesicles, Via Natural or Artificial Opening Endoscopic

♂ **0VW48KZ** Revision of Nonautologous Tissue Substitute in Prostate and Seminal Vesicles, Via Natural or Artificial Opening Endoscopic

♂ **0VW4X0Z** Revision of Drainage Device in Prostate and Seminal Vesicles, External Approach

♂ **0VW4X3Z** Revision of Infusion Device in Prostate and Seminal Vesicles, External Approach

♂ **0VW4X7Z** Revision of Autologous Tissue Substitute in Prostate and Seminal Vesicles, External Approach

♂ **0VW4XJZ** Revision of Synthetic Substitute in Prostate and Seminal Vesicles, External Approach

♂ **0VW4XKZ** Revision of Nonautologous Tissue Substitute in Prostate and Seminal Vesicles, External Approach

♂ **0VW800Z** Revision of Drainage Device in Scrotum and Tunica Vaginalis, Open Approach

♂ **0VW803Z** Revision of Infusion Device in Scrotum and Tunica Vaginalis, Open Approach

♂ **0VW807Z** Revision of Autologous Tissue Substitute in Scrotum and Tunica Vaginalis, Open Approach

♂ **0VW80JZ** Revision of Synthetic Substitute in Scrotum and Tunica Vaginalis, Open Approach

♂ **0VW80KZ** Revision of Nonautologous Tissue Substitute in Scrotum and Tunica Vaginalis, Open Approach

♂ **0VW830Z** Revision of Drainage Device in Scrotum and Tunica Vaginalis, Percutaneous Approach

♂ **0VW833Z** Revision of Infusion Device in Scrotum and Tunica Vaginalis, Percutaneous Approach

♂ **0VW837Z** Revision of Autologous Tissue Substitute in Scrotum and Tunica Vaginalis, Percutaneous Approach

♂ **0VW83JZ** Revision of Synthetic Substitute in Scrotum and Tunica Vaginalis, Percutaneous Approach

♂ **0VW83KZ** Revision of Nonautologous Tissue Substitute in Scrotum and Tunica Vaginalis, Percutaneous Approach

♂ **0VW840Z** Revision of Drainage Device in Scrotum and Tunica Vaginalis, Percutaneous Endoscopic Approach

♂ **0VW843Z** Revision of Infusion Device in Scrotum and Tunica Vaginalis, Percutaneous Endoscopic Approach

♂ **0VW847Z** Revision of Autologous Tissue Substitute in Scrotum and Tunica Vaginalis, Percutaneous Endoscopic Approach

♂ **0VW84JZ** Revision of Synthetic Substitute in Scrotum and Tunica Vaginalis, Percutaneous Endoscopic Approach

♂ **0VW84KZ** Revision of Nonautologous Tissue Substitute in Scrotum and Tunica Vaginalis, Percutaneous Endoscopic Approach

♂ **0VW870Z** Revision of Drainage Device in Scrotum and Tunica Vaginalis, Via Natural or Artificial Opening

♂ **0VW873Z** Revision of Infusion Device in Scrotum and Tunica Vaginalis, Via Natural or Artificial Opening

♂ **0VW877Z** Revision of Autologous Tissue Substitute in Scrotum and Tunica Vaginalis, Via Natural or Artificial Opening

♂ **0VW87JZ** Revision of Synthetic Substitute in Scrotum and Tunica Vaginalis, Via Natural or Artificial Opening

♂ **0VW87KZ** Revision of Nonautologous Tissue Substitute in Scrotum and Tunica Vaginalis, Via Natural or Artificial Opening

♂ **0VW880Z** Revision of Drainage Device in Scrotum and Tunica Vaginalis, Via Natural or Artificial Opening Endoscopic

♂ **0VW883Z** Revision of Infusion Device in Scrotum and Tunica Vaginalis, Via Natural or Artificial Opening Endoscopic

♂ **0VW887Z** Revision of Autologous Tissue Substitute in Scrotum and Tunica Vaginalis, Via Natural or Artificial Opening Endoscopic

♂ **0VW88JZ** Revision of Synthetic Substitute in Scrotum and Tunica Vaginalis, Via Natural or Artificial Opening Endoscopic

♂ **0VW88KZ** Revision of Nonautologous Tissue Substitute in Scrotum and Tunica Vaginalis, Via Natural or Artificial Opening Endoscopic

♂ **0VW8X0Z** Revision of Drainage Device in Scrotum and Tunica Vaginalis, External Approach

♂ **0VW8X3Z** Revision of Infusion Device in Scrotum and Tunica Vaginalis, External Approach

♂ **0VW8X7Z** Revision of Autologous Tissue Substitute in Scrotum and Tunica Vaginalis, External Approach

♂ **0VW8XJZ** Revision of Synthetic Substitute in Scrotum and Tunica Vaginalis, External Approach

♂ **0VW8XKZ** Revision of Nonautologous Tissue Substitute in Scrotum and Tunica Vaginalis, External Approach

♂ **0VWD00Z** Revision of Drainage Device in Testis, Open Approach

♂ **0VWD03Z** Revision of Infusion Device in Testis, Open Approach

♂ **0VWD07Z** Revision of Autologous Tissue Substitute in Testis, Open Approach

♂ **0VWD0JZ** Revision of Synthetic Substitute in Testis, Open Approach

♂ **0VWD0KZ** Revision of Nonautologous Tissue Substitute in Testis, Open Approach

♂ **0VWD30Z** Revision of Drainage Device in Testis, Percutaneous Approach

♂ **0VWD33Z** Revision of Infusion Device in Testis, Percutaneous Approach

♂ **0VWD37Z** Revision of Autologous Tissue Substitute in Testis, Percutaneous Approach

♂ **0VWD3JZ** Revision of Synthetic Substitute in Testis, Percutaneous Approach

♂ **0VWD3KZ** Revision of Nonautologous Tissue Substitute in Testis, Percutaneous Approach

♂ **0VWD40Z** Revision of Drainage Device in Testis, Percutaneous Endoscopic Approach

♂ **0VWD43Z** Revision of Infusion Device in Testis, Percutaneous Endoscopic Approach

♂ **0VWD47Z** Revision of Autologous Tissue Substitute in Testis, Percutaneous Endoscopic Approach

♂ **0VWD4JZ** Revision of Synthetic Substitute in Testis, Percutaneous Endoscopic Approach

♂ **0VWD4KZ** Revision of Nonautologous Tissue Substitute in Testis, Percutaneous Endoscopic Approach

♂ **0VWD70Z** Revision of Drainage Device in Testis, Via Natural or Artificial Opening

♂ **0VWD73Z** Revision of Infusion Device in Testis, Via Natural or Artificial Opening

♂ **0VWD77Z** Revision of Autologous Tissue Substitute in Testis, Via Natural or Artificial Opening

♂ **0VWD7JZ** Revision of Synthetic Substitute in Testis, Via Natural or Artificial Opening

♂ **0VWD7KZ** Revision of Nonautologous Tissue Substitute in Testis, Via Natural or Artificial Opening

♂ **0VWD80Z** Revision of Drainage Device in Testis, Via Natural or Artificial Opening Endoscopic

♂ **0VWD83Z** Revision of Infusion Device in Testis, Via Natural or Artificial Opening Endoscopic

♂ **0VWD87Z** Revision of Autologous Tissue Substitute in Testis, Via Natural or Artificial Opening Endoscopic

♂ **0VWD8JZ** Revision of Synthetic Substitute in Testis, Via Natural or Artificial Opening Endoscopic

♂ **0VWD8KZ** Revision of Nonautologous Tissue Substitute in Testis, Via Natural or Artificial Opening Endoscopic

♂ **0VWDX0Z** Revision of Drainage Device in Testis, External Approach

♂ **0VWDX3Z** Revision of Infusion Device in Testis, External Approach

♂ **0VWDX7Z** Revision of Autologous Tissue Substitute in Testis, External Approach

♂ **0VWDXJZ** Revision of Synthetic Substitute in Testis, External Approach

♂ **0VWDXKZ** Revision of Nonautologous Tissue Substitute in Testis, External Approach

♂ **0VWM00Z** Revision of Drainage Device in Epididymis and Spermatic Cord, Open Approach

♂ **0VWM03Z** Revision of Infusion Device in Epididymis and Spermatic Cord, Open Approach

♂ **0VWM07Z** Revision of Autologous Tissue Substitute in Epididymis and Spermatic Cord, Open Approach

♂ **0VWM0CZ** Revision of Extraluminal Device in Epididymis and Spermatic Cord, Open Approach

♂ **0VWM0JZ** Revision of Synthetic Substitute in Epididymis and Spermatic Cord, Open Approach

♂ **0VWM0KZ** Revision of Nonautologous Tissue Substitute in Epididymis and Spermatic Cord, Open Approach

♂ **0VWM30Z** Revision of Drainage Device in Epididymis and Spermatic Cord, Percutaneous Approach

♂ **0VWM33Z**   Revision of Infusion Device in Epididymis and Spermatic Cord, Percutaneous Approach

♂ **0VWM37Z**   Revision of Autologous Tissue Substitute in Epididymis and Spermatic Cord, Percutaneous Approach

♂ **0VWM3CZ**   Revision of Extraluminal Device in Epididymis and Spermatic Cord, Percutaneous Approach

♂ **0VWM3JZ**   Revision of Synthetic Substitute in Epididymis and Spermatic Cord, Percutaneous Approach

♂ **0VWM3KZ**   Revision of Nonautologous Tissue Substitute in Epididymis and Spermatic Cord, Percutaneous Approach

♂ **0VWM40Z**   Revision of Drainage Device in Epididymis and Spermatic Cord, Percutaneous Endoscopic Approach

♂ **0VWM43Z**   Revision of Infusion Device in Epididymis and Spermatic Cord, Percutaneous Endoscopic Approach

♂ **0VWM47Z**   Revision of Autologous Tissue Substitute in Epididymis and Spermatic Cord, Percutaneous Endoscopic Approach

♂ **0VWM4CZ**   Revision of Extraluminal Device in Epididymis and Spermatic Cord, Percutaneous Endoscopic Approach

♂ **0VWM4JZ**   Revision of Synthetic Substitute in Epididymis and Spermatic Cord, Percutaneous Endoscopic Approach

♂ **0VWM4KZ**   Revision of Nonautologous Tissue Substitute in Epididymis and Spermatic Cord, Percutaneous Endoscopic Approach

♂ **0VWM70Z**   Revision of Drainage Device in Epididymis and Spermatic Cord, Via Natural or Artificial Opening

♂ **0VWM73Z**   Revision of Infusion Device in Epididymis and Spermatic Cord, Via Natural or Artificial Opening

♂ **0VWM77Z**   Revision of Autologous Tissue Substitute in Epididymis and Spermatic Cord, Via Natural or Artificial Opening

♂ **0VWM7CZ**   Revision of Extraluminal Device in Epididymis and Spermatic Cord, Via Natural or Artificial Opening

♂ **0VWM7JZ**   Revision of Synthetic Substitute in Epididymis and Spermatic Cord, Via Natural or Artificial Opening

♂ **0VWM7KZ**   Revision of Nonautologous Tissue Substitute in Epididymis and Spermatic Cord, Via Natural or Artificial Opening

♂ **0VWM80Z**   Revision of Drainage Device in Epididymis and Spermatic Cord, Via Natural or Artificial Opening Endoscopic

♂ **0VWM83Z**   Revision of Infusion Device in Epididymis and Spermatic Cord, Via Natural or Artificial Opening Endoscopic

♂ **0VWM87Z**   Revision of Autologous Tissue Substitute in Epididymis and Spermatic Cord, Via Natural or Artificial Opening Endoscopic

♂ **0VWM8CZ**   Revision of Extraluminal Device in Epididymis and Spermatic Cord, Via Natural or Artificial Opening Endoscopic

♂ **0VWM8JZ**   Revision of Synthetic Substitute in Epididymis and Spermatic Cord, Via Natural or Artificial Opening Endoscopic

♂ **0VWM8KZ**   Revision of Nonautologous Tissue Substitute in Epididymis and Spermatic Cord, Via Natural or Artificial Opening Endoscopic

♂ **0VWMX0Z**   Revision of Drainage Device in Epididymis and Spermatic Cord, External Approach

♂ **0VWMX3Z**   Revision of Infusion Device in Epididymis and Spermatic Cord, External Approach

♂ **0VWMX7Z**   Revision of Autologous Tissue Substitute in Epididymis and Spermatic Cord, External Approach

♂ **0VWMXCZ**   Revision of Extraluminal Device in Epididymis and Spermatic Cord, External Approach

♂ **0VWMXJZ**   Revision of Synthetic Substitute in Epididymis and Spermatic Cord, External Approach

♂ **0VWMXKZ**   Revision of Nonautologous Tissue Substitute in Epididymis and Spermatic Cord, External Approach

♂ **0VWR00Z**   Revision of Drainage Device in Vas Deferens, Open Approach

♂ **0VWR03Z**   Revision of Infusion Device in Vas Deferens, Open Approach

♂ **0VWR07Z**   Revision of Autologous Tissue Substitute in Vas Deferens, Open Approach

♂ **0VWR0CZ**   Revision of Extraluminal Device in Vas Deferens, Open Approach

♂ **0VWR0DZ**   Revision of Intraluminal Device in Vas Deferens, Open Approach

♂ **0VWR0JZ**   Revision of Synthetic Substitute in Vas Deferens, Open Approach

♂ **0VWR0KZ**   Revision of Nonautologous Tissue Substitute in Vas Deferens, Open Approach

♂ **0VWR30Z**   Revision of Drainage Device in Vas Deferens, Percutaneous Approach

♂ **0VWR33Z**   Revision of Infusion Device in Vas Deferens, Percutaneous Approach

♂ **0VWR37Z**   Revision of Autologous Tissue Substitute in Vas Deferens, Percutaneous Approach

♂ **0VWR3CZ**   Revision of Extraluminal Device in Vas Deferens, Percutaneous Approach

♂ **0VWR3DZ**   Revision of Intraluminal Device in Vas Deferens, Percutaneous Approach

♂ **0VWR3JZ**   Revision of Synthetic Substitute in Vas Deferens, Percutaneous Approach

♂ **0VWR3KZ**   Revision of Nonautologous Tissue Substitute in Vas Deferens, Percutaneous Approach

♂ **0VWR40Z**   Revision of Drainage Device in Vas Deferens, Percutaneous Endoscopic Approach

♂ **0VWR43Z**   Revision of Infusion Device in Vas Deferens, Percutaneous Endoscopic Approach

♂ **0VWR47Z**   Revision of Autologous Tissue Substitute in Vas Deferens, Percutaneous Endoscopic Approach

♂ **0VWR4CZ**   Revision of Extraluminal Device in Vas Deferens, Percutaneous Endoscopic Approach

♂ **0VWR4DZ**   Revision of Intraluminal Device in Vas Deferens, Percutaneous Endoscopic Approach

♂ **0VWR4JZ**   Revision of Synthetic Substitute in Vas Deferens, Percutaneous Endoscopic Approach

♂ **0VWR4KZ**   Revision of Nonautologous Tissue Substitute in Vas Deferens, Percutaneous Endoscopic Approach

♂ **0VWR70Z**   Revision of Drainage Device in Vas Deferens, Via Natural or Artificial Opening

♂ **0VWR73Z**   Revision of Infusion Device in Vas Deferens, Via Natural or Artificial Opening

♂ **0VWR77Z**   Revision of Autologous Tissue Substitute in Vas Deferens, Via Natural or Artificial Opening

♂ **0VWR7CZ**   Revision of Extraluminal Device in Vas Deferens, Via Natural or Artificial Opening

♂ **0VWR7DZ**   Revision of Intraluminal Device in Vas Deferens, Via Natural or Artificial Opening

♂ **0VWR7JZ**   Revision of Synthetic Substitute in Vas Deferens, Via Natural or Artificial Opening

♂ **0VWR7KZ**   Revision of Nonautologous Tissue Substitute in Vas Deferens, Via Natural or Artificial Opening

♂ **0VWR80Z**   Revision of Drainage Device in Vas Deferens, Via Natural or Artificial Opening Endoscopic

♂ **0VWR83Z**   Revision of Infusion Device in Vas Deferens, Via Natural or Artificial Opening Endoscopic

♂ **0VWR87Z**   Revision of Autologous Tissue Substitute in Vas Deferens, Via Natural or Artificial Opening Endoscopic

♂ **0VWR8CZ**   Revision of Extraluminal Device in Vas Deferens, Via Natural or Artificial Opening Endoscopic

♂ **0VWR8DZ**   Revision of Intraluminal Device in Vas Deferens, Via Natural or Artificial Opening Endoscopic

♂ **0VWR8JZ**   Revision of Synthetic Substitute in Vas Deferens, Via Natural or Artificial Opening Endoscopic

♂ **0VWR8KZ**   Revision of Nonautologous Tissue Substitute in Vas Deferens, Via Natural or Artificial Opening Endoscopic

♂ **0VWRX0Z**   Revision of Drainage Device in Vas Deferens, External Approach

♂ **0VWRX3Z**   Revision of Infusion Device in Vas Deferens, External Approach

♂ **0VWRX7Z**   Revision of Autologous Tissue Substitute in Vas Deferens, External Approach

♂ **0VWRXCZ**   Revision of Extraluminal Device in Vas Deferens, External Approach

♂ **0VWRXDZ**   Revision of Intraluminal Device in Vas Deferens, External Approach

♂ **0VWRXJZ**   Revision of Synthetic Substitute in Vas Deferens, External Approach

♂ **0VWRXKZ**   Revision of Nonautologous Tissue Substitute in Vas Deferens, External Approach

♂ **0VWS00Z**   Revision of Drainage Device in Penis, Open Approach

♂ **0VWS03Z**   Revision of Infusion Device in Penis, Open Approach

♂ **0VWS07Z**   Revision of Autologous Tissue Substitute in Penis, Open Approach

♂ **0VWS0JZ**   Revision of Synthetic Substitute in Penis, Open Approach

♂ **0VWS0KZ**   Revision of Nonautologous Tissue Substitute in Penis, Open Approach

♂ **0VWS30Z**   Revision of Drainage Device in Penis, Percutaneous Approach

♂ **0VWS33Z**   Revision of Infusion Device in Penis, Percutaneous Approach

♂ **0VWS37Z**   Revision of Autologous Tissue Substitute in Penis, Percutaneous Approach

♂ **0VWS3JZ**   Revision of Synthetic Substitute in Penis, Percutaneous Approach

---

♀ Female-only   ♂ Male-only   ○ Limited Coverage   ● Non-OR   HAC HAC-associated procedure   ⬤ Non-covered procedures   ✚ Combination

♂ **0VWS3KZ**   Revision of Nonautologous Tissue Substitute in Penis, Percutaneous Approach

♂ **0VWS40Z**   Revision of Drainage Device in Penis, Percutaneous Endoscopic Approach

♂ **0VWS43Z**   Revision of Infusion Device in Penis, Percutaneous Endoscopic Approach

♂ **0VWS47Z**   Revision of Autologous Tissue Substitute in Penis, Percutaneous Endoscopic Approach

♂ **0VWS4JZ**   Revision of Synthetic Substitute in Penis, Percutaneous Endoscopic Approach

♂ **0VWS4KZ**   Revision of Nonautologous Tissue Substitute in Penis, Percutaneous Endoscopic Approach

♂ **0VWS70Z**   Revision of Drainage Device in Penis, Via Natural or Artificial Opening

♂ **0VWS73Z**   Revision of Infusion Device in Penis, Via Natural or Artificial Opening

♂ **0VWS77Z**   Revision of Autologous Tissue Substitute in Penis, Via Natural or Artificial Opening

♂ **0VWS7JZ**   Revision of Synthetic Substitute in Penis, Via Natural or Artificial Opening

♂ **0VWS7KZ**   Revision of Nonautologous Tissue Substitute in Penis, Via Natural or Artificial Opening

♂ **0VWS80Z**   Revision of Drainage Device in Penis, Via Natural or Artificial Opening Endoscopic

♂ **0VWS83Z**   Revision of Infusion Device in Penis, Via Natural or Artificial Opening Endoscopic

♂ **0VWS87Z**   Revision of Autologous Tissue Substitute in Penis, Via Natural or Artificial Opening Endoscopic

♂ **0VWS8JZ**   Revision of Synthetic Substitute in Penis, Via Natural or Artificial Opening Endoscopic

♂ **0VWS8KZ**   Revision of Nonautologous Tissue Substitute in Penis, Via Natural or Artificial Opening Endoscopic

♂ **0VWSX0Z**   Revision of Drainage Device in Penis, External Approach

♂ **0VWSX3Z**   Revision of Infusion Device in Penis, External Approach

♂ **0VWSX7Z**   Revision of Autologous Tissue Substitute in Penis, External Approach

♂ **0VWSXJZ**   Revision of Synthetic Substitute in Penis, External Approach

♂ **0VWSXKZ**   Revision of Nonautologous Tissue Substitute in Penis, External Approach

Anatomical Regions, General

Body Cavities

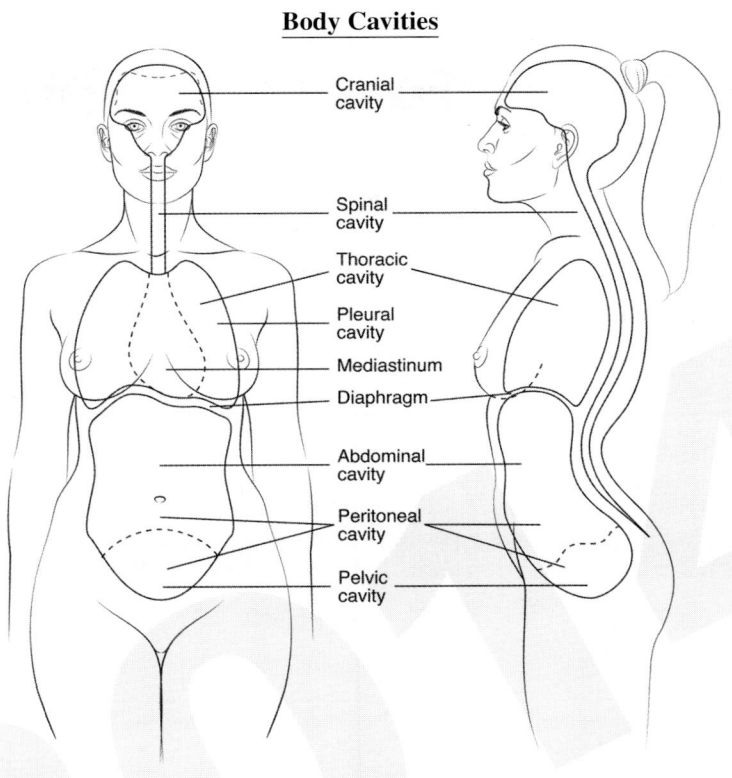

Cranial cavity
Spinal cavity
Thoracic cavity
Pleural cavity
Mediastinum
Diaphragm
Abdominal cavity
Peritoneal cavity
Pelvic cavity

Body Areas

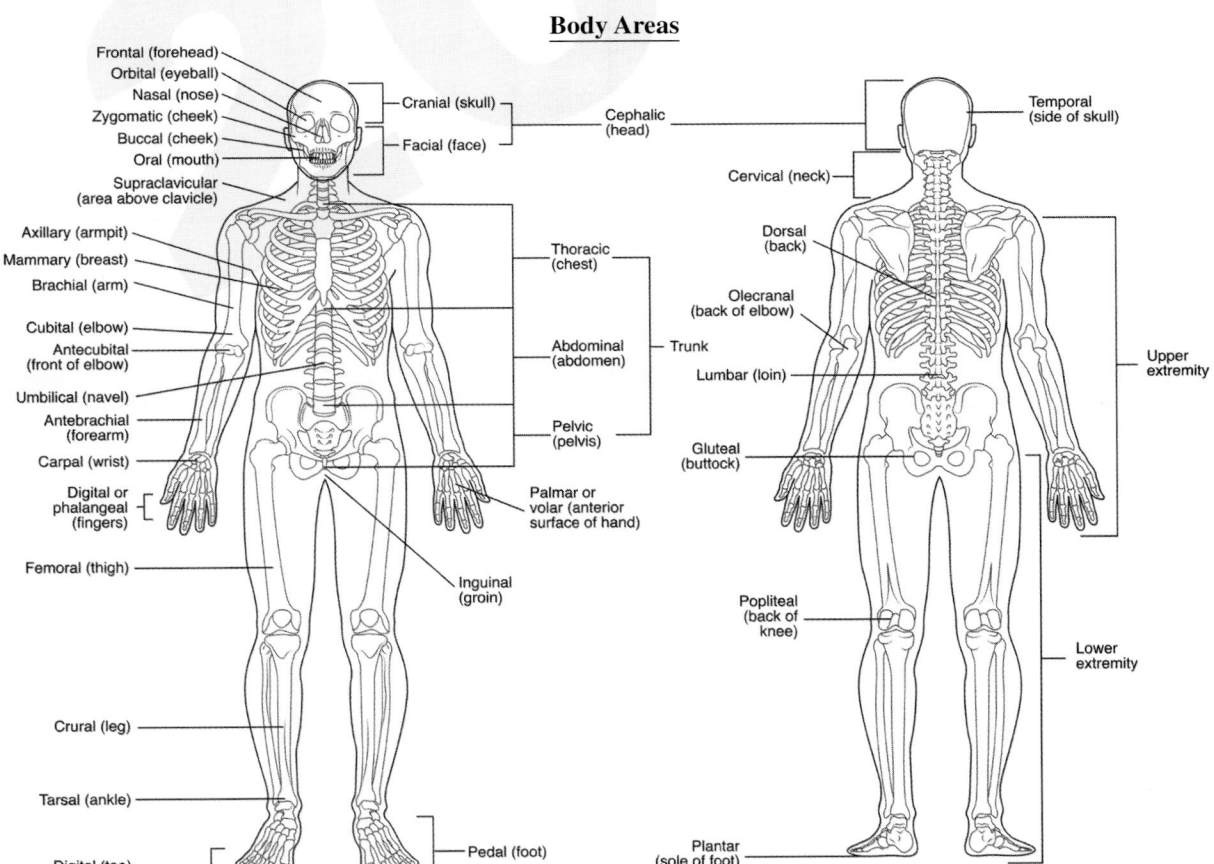

Frontal (forehead)
Orbital (eyeball)
Nasal (nose)
Zygomatic (cheek)
Buccal (cheek)
Oral (mouth)
Supraclavicular (area above clavicle)
Axillary (armpit)
Mammary (breast)
Brachial (arm)
Cubital (elbow)
Antecubital (front of elbow)
Umbilical (navel)
Antebrachial (forearm)
Carpal (wrist)
Digital or phalangeal (fingers)
Femoral (thigh)
Crural (leg)
Tarsal (ankle)
Digital (toe)

Cranial (skull)
Facial (face)
Cephalic (head)

Thoracic (chest)
Abdominal (abdomen)
Pelvic (pelvis)
Trunk

Palmar or volar (anterior surface of hand)
Inguinal (groin)
Pedal (foot)

Temporal (side of skull)
Cervical (neck)
Dorsal (back)
Olecranal (back of elbow)
Lumbar (loin)
Gluteal (buttock)
Popliteal (back of knee)
Plantar (sole of foot)
Upper extremity
Lower extremity

Anatomical Regions, General Tables 0W0–0WW

Section	0	Medical and Surgical
Body System	W	Anatomical Regions, General
Operation	0	Alteration: Modifying the anatomic structure of a body part without affecting the function of the body part

Body Part (4th)	Approach (5th)	Device (6th)	Qualifier (7th)
0 Head 2 Face 4 Upper Jaw 5 Lower Jaw 6 Neck 8 Chest Wall F Abdominal Wall K Upper Back L Lower Back M Perineum, Male N Perineum, Female	0 Open 3 Percutaneous 4 Percutaneous Endoscopic	7 Autologous Tissue Substitute J Synthetic Substitute K Nonautologous Tissue Substitute Z No Device	Z No Qualifier

Section	0	Medical and Surgical
Body System	W	Anatomical Regions, General
Operation	1	Bypass: Altering the route of passage of the contents of a tubular body part

Body Part (4th)	Approach (5th)	Device (6th)	Qualifier (7th)
1 Cranial Cavity	0 Open	J Synthetic Substitute	9 Pleural Cavity, Right B Pleural Cavity, Left G Peritoneal Cavity J Pelvic Cavity
9 Pleural Cavity, Right B Pleural Cavity, Left G Peritoneal Cavity J Pelvic Cavity	0 Open 4 Percutaneous Endoscopic	J Synthetic Substitute	4 Cutaneous 9 Pleural Cavity, Right B Pleural Cavity, Left G Peritoneal Cavity J Pelvic Cavity Y Lower Vein
9 Pleural Cavity, Right B Pleural Cavity, Left G Peritoneal Cavity J Pelvic Cavity	3 Percutaneous	J Synthetic Substitute	4 Cutaneous

Section	0	Medical and Surgical
Body System	W	Anatomical Regions, General
Operation	2	Change: Taking out or off a device from a body part and putting back an identical or similar device in or on the same body part without cutting or puncturing the skin or a mucous membrane

Body Part (4th)	Approach (5th)	Device (6th)	Qualifier (7th)
0 Head 1 Cranial Cavity 2 Face 4 Upper Jaw 5 Lower Jaw 6 Neck 8 Chest Wall 9 Pleural Cavity, Right B Pleural Cavity, Left C Mediastinum D Pericardial Cavity F Abdominal Wall G Peritoneal Cavity H Retroperitoneum J Pelvic Cavity K Upper Back L Lower Back M Perineum, Male N Perineum, Female	X External	0 Drainage Device Y Other Device	Z No Qualifier

Section	0	Medical and Surgical
Body System	W	Anatomical Regions, General
Operation	3	**Control:** Stopping, or attempting to stop, postprocedural bleeding

Body Part (4th)	Approach (5th)	Device (6th)	Qualifier (7th)
0 Head **1** Cranial Cavity **2** Face **4** Upper Jaw **5** Lower Jaw **6** Neck **8** Chest Wall **9** Pleural Cavity, Right **B** Pleural Cavity, Left **C** Mediastinum **D** Pericardial Cavity **F** Abdominal Wall **G** Peritoneal Cavity **H** Retroperitoneum **J** Pelvic Cavity **K** Upper Back **L** Lower Back **M** Perineum, Male **N** Perineum, Female	**0** Open **3** Percutaneous **4** Percutaneous Endoscopic	**Z** No Device	**Z** No Qualifier
3 Oral Cavity and Throat	**0** Open **3** Percutaneous **4** Percutaneous Endoscopic **7** Via Natural or Artificial Opening **8** Via Natural or Artificial Opening Endoscopic **X** External	**Z** No Device	**Z** No Qualifier
P Gastrointestinal Tract **Q** Respiratory Tract **R** Genitourinary Tract	**0** Open **3** Percutaneous **4** Percutaneous Endoscopic **7** Via Natural or Artificial Opening **8** Via Natural or Artificial Opening Endoscopic	**Z** No Device	**Z** No Qualifier

Section	0	Medical and Surgical
Body System	W	Anatomical Regions, General
Operation	4	**Creation:** Making a new genital structure that does not take over the function of a body part

Body Part (4th)	Approach (5th)	Device (6th)	Qualifier (7th)
M Perineum, Male	**0** Open	**7** Autologous Tissue Substitute **J** Synthetic Substitute **K** Nonautologous Tissue Substitute **Z** No Device	**0** Vagina
N Perineum, Female	**0** Open	**7** Autologous Tissue Substitute **J** Synthetic Substitute **K** Nonautologous Tissue Substitute **Z** No Device	**1** Penis

Section   0   **Medical and Surgical**
Body System   W   **Anatomical Regions, General**
Operation   8   **Division:** Cutting into a body part, without draining fluids and/or gases from the body part, in order to separate or transect a body part

Body Part (4th)	Approach (5th)	Device (6th)	Qualifier (7th)
N Perineum, Female	X External	Z No Device	Z No Qualifier

Section   0   **Medical and Surgical**
Body System   W   **Anatomical Regions, General**
Operation   9   **Drainage:** Taking or letting out fluids and/or gases from a body part

Body Part (4th)	Approach (5th)	Device (6th)	Qualifier (7th)
0 Head 1 Cranial Cavity 2 Face 3 Oral Cavity and Throat 4 Upper Jaw 5 Lower Jaw 6 Neck 8 Chest Wall 9 Pleural Cavity, Right B Pleural Cavity, Left C Mediastinum D Pericardial Cavity F Abdominal Wall G Peritoneal Cavity H Retroperitoneum J Pelvic Cavity K Upper Back L Lower Back M Perineum, Male N Perineum, Female	0 Open 3 Percutaneous 4 Percutaneous Endoscopic	0 Drainage Device	Z No Qualifier
0 Head 1 Cranial Cavity 2 Face 3 Oral Cavity and Throat 4 Upper Jaw 5 Lower Jaw 6 Neck 8 Chest Wall 9 Pleural Cavity, Right B Pleural Cavity, Left C Mediastinum D Pericardial Cavity F Abdominal Wall G Peritoneal Cavity H Retroperitoneum J Pelvic Cavity K Upper Back L Lower Back M Perineum, Male N Perineum, Female	0 Open 3 Percutaneous 4 Percutaneous Endoscopic	Z No Device	X Diagnostic Z No Qualifier

Section   **0**   **Medical and Surgical**
Body System   **W**   **Anatomical Regions, General**
Operation   **B**   **Excision:** Cutting out or off, without replacement, a portion of a body part

Body Part (4th)	Approach (5th)	Device (6th)	Qualifier (7th)
0 Head 2 Face 4 Upper Jaw 5 Lower Jaw 8 Chest Wall K Upper Back L Lower Back M Perineum, Male N Perineum, Female	0 Open 3 Percutaneous 4 Percutaneous Endoscopic X External	Z No Device	X Diagnostic Z No Qualifier
6 Neck F Abdominal Wall	0 Open 3 Percutaneous 4 Percutaneous Endoscopic	Z No Device	X Diagnostic Z No Qualifier
6 Neck F Abdominal Wall	X External	Z No Device	2 Stoma X Diagnostic Z No Qualifier
C Mediastinum H Retroperitoneum	0 Open 3 Percutaneous 4 Percutaneous Endoscopic	Z No Device	X Diagnostic Z No Qualifier

Section   **0**   **Medical and Surgical**
Body System   **W**   **Anatomical Regions, General**
Operation   **C**   **Extirpation:** Taking or cutting out solid matter from a body part

Body Part (4th)	Approach (5th)	Device (6th)	Qualifier (7th)
1 Cranial Cavity 3 Oral Cavity and Throat 9 Pleural Cavity, Right B Pleural Cavity, Left C Mediastinum D Pericardial Cavity G Peritoneal Cavity J Pelvic Cavity	0 Open 3 Percutaneous 4 Percutaneous Endoscopic X External	Z No Device	Z No Qualifier
P Gastrointestinal Tract Q Respiratory Tract R Genitourinary Tract	0 Open 3 Percutaneous 4 Percutaneous Endoscopic 7 Via Natural or Artificial Opening 8 Via Natural or Artificial Opening Endoscopic X External	Z No Device	Z No Qualifier

Section	0	Medical and Surgical
Body System	W	Anatomical Regions, General
Operation	F	Fragmentation: Breaking solid matter in a body part into pieces

Body Part (4th)	Approach (5th)	Device (6th)	Qualifier (7th)
1 Cranial Cavity 3 Oral Cavity and Throat 9 Pleural Cavity, Right B Pleural Cavity, Left C Mediastinum D Pericardial Cavity G Peritoneal Cavity J Pelvic Cavity	0 Open 3 Percutaneous 4 Percutaneous Endoscopic X External	Z No Device	Z No Qualifier
P Gastrointestinal Tract Q Respiratory Tract R Genitourinary Tract	0 Open 3 Percutaneous 4 Percutaneous Endoscopic 7 Via Natural or Artificial Opening 8 Via Natural or Artificial Opening Endoscopic X External	Z No Device	Z No Qualifier

Section	0	Medical and Surgical
Body System	W	Anatomical Regions, General
Operation	H	Insertion: Putting in a nonbiological appliance that monitors, assists, performs, or prevents a physiological function but does not physically take the place of a body part

Body Part (4th)	Approach (5th)	Device (6th)	Qualifier (7th)
0 Head 1 Cranial Cavity 2 Face 3 Oral Cavity and Throat 4 Upper Jaw 5 Lower Jaw 6 Neck 8 Chest Wall 9 Pleural Cavity, Right B Pleural Cavity, Left C Mediastinum D Pericardial Cavity F Abdominal Wall G Peritoneal Cavity H Retroperitoneum J Pelvic Cavity K Upper Back L Lower Back M Perineum, Male N Perineum, Female	0 Open 3 Percutaneous 4 Percutaneous Endoscopic	1 Radioactive Element 3 Infusion Device Y Other Device	Z No Qualifier
P Gastrointestinal Tract Q Respiratory Tract R Genitourinary Tract	0 Open 3 Percutaneous 4 Percutaneous Endoscopic 7 Via Natural or Artificial Opening 8 Via Natural or Artificial Opening Endoscopic	1 Radioactive Element 3 Infusion Device Y Other Device	Z No Qualifier

Section	0	Medical and Surgical
Body System	W	Anatomical Regions, General
Operation	J	**Inspection:** Visually and/or manually exploring a body part

Body Part (4th)	Approach (5th)	Device (6th)	Qualifier (7th)
0 Head 2 Face 3 Oral Cavity and Throat 4 Upper Jaw 5 Lower Jaw 6 Neck 8 Chest Wall F Abdominal Wall K Upper Back L Lower Back M Perineum, Male N Perineum, Female	0 Open 3 Percutaneous 4 Percutaneous Endoscopic X External	Z No Device	Z No Qualifier
1 Cranial Cavity 9 Pleural Cavity, Right B Pleural Cavity, Left C Mediastinum D Pericardial Cavity G Peritoneal Cavity H Retroperitoneum J Pelvic Cavity	0 Open 3 Percutaneous 4 Percutaneous Endoscopic	Z No Device	Z No Qualifier
P Gastrointestinal Tract Q Respiratory Tract R Genitourinary Tract	0 Open 3 Percutaneous 4 Percutaneous Endoscopic 7 Via Natural or Artificial Opening 8 Via Natural or Artificial Opening Endoscopic	Z No Device	Z No Qualifier

Section	0	Medical and Surgical
Body System	W	Anatomical Regions, General
Operation	M	**Reattachment:** Putting back in or on all or a portion of a separated body part to its normal location or other suitable location

Body Part (4th)	Approach (5th)	Device (6th)	Qualifier (7th)
2 Face 4 Upper Jaw 5 Lower Jaw 6 Neck 8 Chest Wall F Abdominal Wall K Upper Back L Lower Back M Perineum, Male N Perineum, Female	0 Open	Z No Device	Z No Qualifier

Section	0	Medical and Surgical
Body System	W	Anatomical Regions, General
Operation	P	Removal: Taking out or off a device from a body part

Body Part (4th)	Approach (5th)	Device (6th)	Qualifier (7th)
0 Head 2 Face 4 Upper Jaw 5 Lower Jaw 6 Neck 8 Chest Wall C Mediastinum F Abdominal Wall K Upper Back L Lower Back M Perineum, Male N Perineum, Female	0 Open 3 Percutaneous 4 Percutaneous Endoscopic X External	0 Drainage Device 1 Radioactive Element 3 Infusion Device 7 Autologous Tissue Substitute J Synthetic Substitute K Nonautologous Tissue Substitute Y Other Device	Z No Qualifier
1 Cranial Cavity 9 Pleural Cavity, Right B Pleural Cavity, Left G Peritoneal Cavity J Pelvic Cavity	0 Open 3 Percutaneous 4 Percutaneous Endoscopic	0 Drainage Device 1 Radioactive Element 3 Infusion Device J Synthetic Substitute Y Other Device	Z No Qualifier
1 Cranial Cavity 9 Pleural Cavity, Right B Pleural Cavity, Left G Peritoneal Cavity J Pelvic Cavity	X External	0 Drainage Device 1 Radioactive Element 3 Infusion Device	Z No Qualifier
D Pericardial Cavity H Retroperitoneum	0 Open 3 Percutaneous 4 Percutaneous Endoscopic	0 Drainage Device 1 Radioactive Element 3 Infusion Device Y Other Device	Z No Qualifier
D Pericardial Cavity H Retroperitoneum	X External	0 Drainage Device 1 Radioactive Element 3 Infusion Device	Z No Qualifier
P Gastrointestinal Tract Q Respiratory Tract R Genitourinary Tract	0 Open 3 Percutaneous 4 Percutaneous Endoscopic 7 Via Natural or Artificial Opening 8 Via Natural or Artificial Opening Endoscopic X External	1 Radioactive Element 3 Infusion Device Y Other Device	Z No Qualifier

Section   **0**   **Medical and Surgical**
Body System   **W**   **Anatomical Regions, General**
Operation   **Q**   **Repair:** Restoring, to the extent possible, a body part to its normal anatomic structure and function

Body Part (4th)	Approach (5th)	Device (6th)	Qualifier (7th)
0 Head 2 Face 4 Upper Jaw 5 Lower Jaw 8 Chest Wall K Upper Back L Lower Back M Perineum, Male N Perineum, Female	0 Open 3 Percutaneous 4 Percutaneous Endoscopic X External	Z No Device	Z No Qualifier
6 Neck F Abdominal Wall	0 Open 3 Percutaneous 4 Percutaneous Endoscopic	Z No Device	Z No Qualifier
6 Neck F Abdominal Wall	X External	Z No Device	2 Stoma Z No Qualifier
C Mediastinum	0 Open 3 Percutaneous 4 Percutaneous Endoscopic	Z No Device	Z No Qualifier

Section   **0**   **Medical and Surgical**
Body System   **W**   **Anatomical Regions, General**
Operation   **U**   **Supplement:** Putting in or on biological or synthetic material that physically reinforces and/or augments the function of a portion of a body part

Body Part (4th)	Approach (5th)	Device (6th)	Qualifier (7th)
0 Head 2 Face 4 Upper Jaw 5 Lower Jaw 6 Neck 8 Chest Wall C Mediastinum F Abdominal Wall K Upper Back L Lower Back M Perineum, Male N Perineum, Female	0 Open 4 Percutaneous Endoscopic	7 Autologous Tissue Substitute J Synthetic Substitute K Nonautologous Tissue Substitute	Z No Qualifier

Section	0	Medical and Surgical
Body System	W	Anatomical Regions, General
Operation	W	Revision: Correcting, to the extent possible, a portion of a malfunctioning device or the position of a displaced device

Body Part (4th)	Approach (5th)	Device (6th)	Qualifier (7th)
0 Head 2 Face 4 Upper Jaw 5 Lower Jaw 6 Neck 8 Chest Wall C Mediastinum F Abdominal Wall K Upper Back L Lower Back M Perineum, Male N Perineum, Female	0 Open 3 Percutaneous 4 Percutaneous Endoscopic X External	0 Drainage Device 1 Radioactive Element 3 Infusion Device 7 Autologous Tissue Substitute J Synthetic Substitute K Nonautologous Tissue Substitute Y Other Device	Z No Qualifier
1 Cranial Cavity 9 Pleural Cavity, Right B Pleural Cavity, Left G Peritoneal Cavity J Pelvic Cavity	0 Open 3 Percutaneous 4 Percutaneous Endoscopic X External	0 Drainage Device 1 Radioactive Element 3 Infusion Device J Synthetic Substitute Y Other Device	Z No Qualifier
D Pericardial Cavity H Retroperitoneum	0 Open 3 Percutaneous 4 Percutaneous Endoscopic X External	0 Drainage Device 1 Radioactive Element 3 Infusion Device Y Other Device	Z No Qualifier
P Gastrointestinal Tract Q Respiratory Tract R Genitourinary Tract	0 Open 3 Percutaneous 4 Percutaneous Endoscopic 7 Via Natural or Artificial Opening 8 Via Natural or Artificial Opening Endoscopic X External	1 Radioactive Element 3 Infusion Device Y Other Device	Z No Qualifier

Anatomical Regions, General Code Listing 0W0–0WW

0W0 – Anatomical Regions, General, Alteration

0W0007Z Alteration of Head with Autologous Tissue Substitute, Open Approach

0W000JZ Alteration of Head with Synthetic Substitute, Open Approach

0W000KZ Alteration of Head with Nonautologous Tissue Substitute, Open Approach

0W000ZZ Alteration of Head, Open Approach

0W0037Z Alteration of Head with Autologous Tissue Substitute, Percutaneous Approach

0W003JZ Alteration of Head with Synthetic Substitute, Percutaneous Approach

0W003KZ Alteration of Head with Nonautologous Tissue Substitute, Percutaneous Approach

0W003ZZ Alteration of Head, Percutaneous Approach

0W0047Z Alteration of Head with Autologous Tissue Substitute, Percutaneous Endoscopic Approach

0W004JZ Alteration of Head with Synthetic Substitute, Percutaneous Endoscopic Approach

0W004KZ Alteration of Head with Nonautologous Tissue Substitute, Percutaneous Endoscopic Approach

0W004ZZ Alteration of Head, Percutaneous Endoscopic Approach

0W0207Z Alteration of Face with Autologous Tissue Substitute, Open Approach

0W020JZ Alteration of Face with Synthetic Substitute, Open Approach

0W020KZ Alteration of Face with Nonautologous Tissue Substitute, Open Approach

0W020ZZ Alteration of Face, Open Approach

0W0237Z Alteration of Face with Autologous Tissue Substitute, Percutaneous Approach

0W023JZ Alteration of Face with Synthetic Substitute, Percutaneous Approach

0W023KZ Alteration of Face with Nonautologous Tissue Substitute, Percutaneous Approach

0W023ZZ Alteration of Face, Percutaneous Approach

0W0247Z Alteration of Face with Autologous Tissue Substitute, Percutaneous Endoscopic Approach

0W024JZ Alteration of Face with Synthetic Substitute, Percutaneous Endoscopic Approach

0W024KZ Alteration of Face with Nonautologous Tissue Substitute, Percutaneous Endoscopic Approach

0W024ZZ Alteration of Face, Percutaneous Endoscopic Approach

♀ Female-only   ♂ Male-only   ● Limited Coverage   ● Non-OR   HAC HAC-associated procedure   ● Non-covered procedures   ✚ Combination

0W0407Z Alteration of Upper Jaw with Autologous Tissue Substitute, Open Approach
0W040JZ Alteration of Upper Jaw with Synthetic Substitute, Open Approach
0W040KZ Alteration of Upper Jaw with Nonautologous Tissue Substitute, Open Approach
0W040ZZ Alteration of Upper Jaw, Open Approach
0W0437Z Alteration of Upper Jaw with Autologous Tissue Substitute, Percutaneous Approach
0W043JZ Alteration of Upper Jaw with Synthetic Substitute, Percutaneous Approach
0W043KZ Alteration of Upper Jaw with Nonautologous Tissue Substitute, Percutaneous Approach
0W043ZZ Alteration of Upper Jaw, Percutaneous Approach
0W0447Z Alteration of Upper Jaw with Autologous Tissue Substitute, Percutaneous Endoscopic Approach
0W044JZ Alteration of Upper Jaw with Synthetic Substitute, Percutaneous Endoscopic Approach
0W044KZ Alteration of Upper Jaw with Nonautologous Tissue Substitute, Percutaneous Endoscopic Approach
0W044ZZ Alteration of Upper Jaw, Percutaneous Endoscopic Approach
0W0507Z Alteration of Lower Jaw with Autologous Tissue Substitute, Open Approach
0W050JZ Alteration of Lower Jaw with Synthetic Substitute, Open Approach
0W050KZ Alteration of Lower Jaw with Nonautologous Tissue Substitute, Open Approach
0W050ZZ Alteration of Lower Jaw, Open Approach
0W0537Z Alteration of Lower Jaw with Autologous Tissue Substitute, Percutaneous Approach
0W053JZ Alteration of Lower Jaw with Synthetic Substitute, Percutaneous Approach
0W053KZ Alteration of Lower Jaw with Nonautologous Tissue Substitute, Percutaneous Approach
0W053ZZ Alteration of Lower Jaw, Percutaneous Approach
0W0547Z Alteration of Lower Jaw with Autologous Tissue Substitute, Percutaneous Endoscopic Approach
0W054JZ Alteration of Lower Jaw with Synthetic Substitute, Percutaneous Endoscopic Approach
0W054KZ Alteration of Lower Jaw with Nonautologous Tissue Substitute, Percutaneous Endoscopic Approach
0W054ZZ Alteration of Lower Jaw, Percutaneous Endoscopic Approach
0W0607Z Alteration of Neck with Autologous Tissue Substitute, Open Approach
0W060JZ Alteration of Neck with Synthetic Substitute, Open Approach
0W060KZ Alteration of Neck with Nonautologous Tissue Substitute, Open Approach
0W060ZZ Alteration of Neck, Open Approach
0W0637Z Alteration of Neck with Autologous Tissue Substitute, Percutaneous Approach
0W063JZ Alteration of Neck with Synthetic Substitute, Percutaneous Approach
0W063KZ Alteration of Neck with Nonautologous Tissue Substitute, Percutaneous Approach
0W063ZZ Alteration of Neck, Percutaneous Approach
0W0647Z Alteration of Neck with Autologous Tissue Substitute, Percutaneous Endoscopic Approach
0W064JZ Alteration of Neck with Synthetic Substitute, Percutaneous Endoscopic Approach
0W064KZ Alteration of Neck with Nonautologous Tissue Substitute, Percutaneous Endoscopic Approach
0W064ZZ Alteration of Neck, Percutaneous Endoscopic Approach
0W0807Z Alteration of Chest Wall with Autologous Tissue Substitute, Open Approach
0W080JZ Alteration of Chest Wall with Synthetic Substitute, Open Approach
0W080KZ Alteration of Chest Wall with Nonautologous Tissue Substitute, Open Approach
0W080ZZ Alteration of Chest Wall, Open Approach
0W0837Z Alteration of Chest Wall with Autologous Tissue Substitute, Percutaneous Approach
0W083JZ Alteration of Chest Wall with Synthetic Substitute, Percutaneous Approach
0W083KZ Alteration of Chest Wall with Nonautologous Tissue Substitute, Percutaneous Approach
0W083ZZ Alteration of Chest Wall, Percutaneous Approach

0W0847Z Alteration of Chest Wall with Autologous Tissue Substitute, Percutaneous Endoscopic Approach
0W084JZ Alteration of Chest Wall with Synthetic Substitute, Percutaneous Endoscopic Approach
0W084KZ Alteration of Chest Wall with Nonautologous Tissue Substitute, Percutaneous Endoscopic Approach
0W084ZZ Alteration of Chest Wall, Percutaneous Endoscopic Approach
0W0F07Z Alteration of Abdominal Wall with Autologous Tissue Substitute, Open Approach
0W0F0JZ Alteration of Abdominal Wall with Synthetic Substitute, Open Approach
0W0F0KZ Alteration of Abdominal Wall with Nonautologous Tissue Substitute, Open Approach
0W0F0ZZ Alteration of Abdominal Wall, Open Approach
0W0F37Z Alteration of Abdominal Wall with Autologous Tissue Substitute, Percutaneous Approach
0W0F3JZ Alteration of Abdominal Wall with Synthetic Substitute, Percutaneous Approach
0W0F3KZ Alteration of Abdominal Wall with Nonautologous Tissue Substitute, Percutaneous Approach
0W0F3ZZ Alteration of Abdominal Wall, Percutaneous Approach
0W0F47Z Alteration of Abdominal Wall with Autologous Tissue Substitute, Percutaneous Endoscopic Approach
0W0F4JZ Alteration of Abdominal Wall with Synthetic Substitute, Percutaneous Endoscopic Approach
0W0F4KZ Alteration of Abdominal Wall with Nonautologous Tissue Substitute, Percutaneous Endoscopic Approach
0W0F4ZZ Alteration of Abdominal Wall, Percutaneous Endoscopic Approach
0W0K07Z Alteration of Upper Back with Autologous Tissue Substitute, Open Approach
0W0K0JZ Alteration of Upper Back with Synthetic Substitute, Open Approach
0W0K0KZ Alteration of Upper Back with Nonautologous Tissue Substitute, Open Approach
0W0K0ZZ Alteration of Upper Back, Open Approach
0W0K37Z Alteration of Upper Back with Autologous Tissue Substitute, Percutaneous Approach
0W0K3JZ Alteration of Upper Back with Synthetic Substitute, Percutaneous Approach
0W0K3KZ Alteration of Upper Back with Nonautologous Tissue Substitute, Percutaneous Approach
0W0K3ZZ Alteration of Upper Back, Percutaneous Approach
0W0K47Z Alteration of Upper Back with Autologous Tissue Substitute, Percutaneous Endoscopic Approach
0W0K4JZ Alteration of Upper Back with Synthetic Substitute, Percutaneous Endoscopic Approach
0W0K4KZ Alteration of Upper Back with Nonautologous Tissue Substitute, Percutaneous Endoscopic Approach
0W0K4ZZ Alteration of Upper Back, Percutaneous Endoscopic Approach
0W0L07Z Alteration of Lower Back with Autologous Tissue Substitute, Open Approach
0W0L0JZ Alteration of Lower Back with Synthetic Substitute, Open Approach
0W0L0KZ Alteration of Lower Back with Nonautologous Tissue Substitute, Open Approach
0W0L0ZZ Alteration of Lower Back, Open Approach
0W0L37Z Alteration of Lower Back with Autologous Tissue Substitute, Percutaneous Approach
0W0L3JZ Alteration of Lower Back with Synthetic Substitute, Percutaneous Approach
0W0L3KZ Alteration of Lower Back with Nonautologous Tissue Substitute, Percutaneous Approach
0W0L3ZZ Alteration of Lower Back, Percutaneous Approach
0W0L47Z Alteration of Lower Back with Autologous Tissue Substitute, Percutaneous Endoscopic Approach
0W0L4JZ Alteration of Lower Back with Synthetic Substitute, Percutaneous Endoscopic Approach
0W0L4KZ Alteration of Lower Back with Nonautologous Tissue Substitute, Percutaneous Endoscopic Approach
0W0L4ZZ Alteration of Lower Back, Percutaneous Endoscopic Approach
♂ 0W0M07Z Alteration of Male Perineum with Autologous Tissue Substitute, Open Approach
♂ 0W0M0JZ Alteration of Male Perineum with Synthetic Substitute, Open Approach

♂ **0W0M0KZ** Alteration of Male Perineum with Nonautologous Tissue Substitute, Open Approach

♂ **0W0M0ZZ** Alteration of Male Perineum, Open Approach

♂ **0W0M37Z** Alteration of Male Perineum with Autologous Tissue Substitute, Percutaneous Approach

♂ **0W0M3JZ** Alteration of Male Perineum with Synthetic Substitute, Percutaneous Approach

♂ **0W0M3KZ** Alteration of Male Perineum with Nonautologous Tissue Substitute, Percutaneous Approach

♂ **0W0M3ZZ** Alteration of Male Perineum, Percutaneous Approach

♂ **0W0M47Z** Alteration of Male Perineum with Autologous Tissue Substitute, Percutaneous Endoscopic Approach

♂ **0W0M4JZ** Alteration of Male Perineum with Synthetic Substitute, Percutaneous Endoscopic Approach

♂ **0W0M4KZ** Alteration of Male Perineum with Nonautologous Tissue Substitute, Percutaneous Endoscopic Approach

♂ **0W0M4ZZ** Alteration of Male Perineum, Percutaneous Endoscopic Approach

♀ **0W0N07Z** Alteration of Female Perineum with Autologous Tissue Substitute, Open Approach

♀ **0W0N0JZ** Alteration of Female Perineum with Synthetic Substitute, Open Approach

♀ **0W0N0KZ** Alteration of Female Perineum with Nonautologous Tissue Substitute, Open Approach

♀ **0W0N0ZZ** Alteration of Female Perineum, Open Approach

♀ **0W0N37Z** Alteration of Female Perineum with Autologous Tissue Substitute, Percutaneous Approach

♀ **0W0N3JZ** Alteration of Female Perineum with Synthetic Substitute, Percutaneous Approach

♀ **0W0N3KZ** Alteration of Female Perineum with Nonautologous Tissue Substitute, Percutaneous Approach

♀ **0W0N3ZZ** Alteration of Female Perineum, Percutaneous Approach

♀ **0W0N47Z** Alteration of Female Perineum with Autologous Tissue Substitute, Percutaneous Endoscopic Approach

♀ **0W0N4JZ** Alteration of Female Perineum with Synthetic Substitute, Percutaneous Endoscopic Approach

♀ **0W0N4KZ** Alteration of Female Perineum with Nonautologous Tissue Substitute, Percutaneous Endoscopic Approach

♀ **0W0N4ZZ** Alteration of Female Perineum, Percutaneous Endoscopic Approach

0W1 – Anatomical Regions, General, Bypass

Review Coding Guideline B3.6a

0W110J9 Bypass Cranial Cavity to Right Pleural Cavity with Synthetic Substitute, Open Approach

0W110JB Bypass Cranial Cavity to Left Pleural Cavity with Synthetic Substitute, Open Approach

0W110JG Bypass Cranial Cavity to Peritoneal Cavity with Synthetic Substitute, Open Approach

0W110JJ Bypass Cranial Cavity to Pelvic Cavity with Synthetic Substitute, Open Approach

0W190J4 Bypass Right Pleural Cavity to Cutaneous with Synthetic Substitute, Open Approach

0W190J9 Bypass Right Pleural Cavity to Right Pleural Cavity with Synthetic Substitute, Open Approach

0W190JB Bypass Right Pleural Cavity to Left Pleural Cavity with Synthetic Substitute, Open Approach

0W190JG Bypass Right Pleural Cavity to Peritoneal Cavity with Synthetic Substitute, Open Approach

0W190JJ Bypass Right Pleural Cavity to Pelvic Cavity with Synthetic Substitute, Open Approach

0W190JY Bypass Right Pleural Cavity to Lower Vein with Synthetic Substitute, Open Approach

0W193J4 Bypass Right Pleural Cavity to Cutaneous with Synthetic Substitute, Percutaneous Approach

0W194J4 Bypass Right Pleural Cavity to Cutaneous with Synthetic Substitute, Percutaneous Endoscopic Approach

0W194J9 Bypass Right Pleural Cavity to Right Pleural Cavity with Synthetic Substitute, Percutaneous Endoscopic Approach

0W194JB Bypass Right Pleural Cavity to Left Pleural Cavity with Synthetic Substitute, Percutaneous Endoscopic Approach

0W194JG Bypass Right Pleural Cavity to Peritoneal Cavity with Synthetic Substitute, Percutaneous Endoscopic Approach

0W194JJ Bypass Right Pleural Cavity to Pelvic Cavity with Synthetic Substitute, Percutaneous Endoscopic Approach

0W194JY Bypass Right Pleural Cavity to Lower Vein with Synthetic Substitute, Percutaneous Endoscopic Approach

0W1B0J4 Bypass Left Pleural Cavity to Cutaneous with Synthetic Substitute, Open Approach

0W1B0J9 Bypass Left Pleural Cavity to Right Pleural Cavity with Synthetic Substitute, Open Approach

0W1B0JB Bypass Left Pleural Cavity to Left Pleural Cavity with Synthetic Substitute, Open Approach

0W1B0JG Bypass Left Pleural Cavity to Peritoneal Cavity with Synthetic Substitute, Open Approach

0W1B0JJ Bypass Left Pleural Cavity to Pelvic Cavity with Synthetic Substitute, Open Approach

0W1B0JY Bypass Left Pleural Cavity to Lower Vein with Synthetic Substitute, Open Approach

0W1B3J4 Bypass Left Pleural Cavity to Cutaneous with Synthetic Substitute, Percutaneous Approach

0W1B4J4 Bypass Left Pleural Cavity to Cutaneous with Synthetic Substitute, Percutaneous Endoscopic Approach

0W1B4J9 Bypass Left Pleural Cavity to Right Pleural Cavity with Synthetic Substitute, Percutaneous Endoscopic Approach

0W1B4JB Bypass Left Pleural Cavity to Left Pleural Cavity with Synthetic Substitute, Percutaneous Endoscopic Approach

0W1B4JG Bypass Left Pleural Cavity to Peritoneal Cavity with Synthetic Substitute, Percutaneous Endoscopic Approach

0W1B4JJ Bypass Left Pleural Cavity to Pelvic Cavity with Synthetic Substitute, Percutaneous Endoscopic Approach

0W1B4JY Bypass Left Pleural Cavity to Lower Vein with Synthetic Substitute, Percutaneous Endoscopic Approach

0W1G0J4 Bypass Peritoneal Cavity to Cutaneous with Synthetic Substitute, Open Approach

0W1G0J9 Bypass Peritoneal Cavity to Right Pleural Cavity with Synthetic Substitute, Open Approach

0W1G0JB Bypass Peritoneal Cavity to Left Pleural Cavity with Synthetic Substitute, Open Approach

0W1G0JG Bypass Peritoneal Cavity to Peritoneal Cavity with Synthetic Substitute, Open Approach

0W1G0JJ Bypass Peritoneal Cavity to Pelvic Cavity with Synthetic Substitute, Open Approach

0W1G0JY Bypass Peritoneal Cavity to Lower Vein with Synthetic Substitute, Open Approach

0W1G3J4 Bypass Peritoneal Cavity to Cutaneous with Synthetic Substitute, Percutaneous Approach

0W1G4J4 Bypass Peritoneal Cavity to Cutaneous with Synthetic Substitute, Percutaneous Endoscopic Approach

0W1G4J9 Bypass Peritoneal Cavity to Right Pleural Cavity with Synthetic Substitute, Percutaneous Endoscopic Approach

0W1G4JB Bypass Peritoneal Cavity to Left Pleural Cavity with Synthetic Substitute, Percutaneous Endoscopic Approach

0W1G4JG Bypass Peritoneal Cavity to Peritoneal Cavity with Synthetic Substitute, Percutaneous Endoscopic Approach

0W1G4JJ Bypass Peritoneal Cavity to Pelvic Cavity with Synthetic Substitute, Percutaneous Endoscopic Approach

0W1G4JY Bypass Peritoneal Cavity to Lower Vein with Synthetic Substitute, Percutaneous Endoscopic Approach

♀ **0W1J0J4** Bypass Pelvic Cavity to Cutaneous with Synthetic Substitute, Open Approach

♀ **0W1J0J9** Bypass Pelvic Cavity to Right Pleural Cavity with Synthetic Substitute, Open Approach

♀ **0W1J0JB** Bypass Pelvic Cavity to Left Pleural Cavity with Synthetic Substitute, Open Approach

♀ **0W1J0JG** Bypass Pelvic Cavity to Peritoneal Cavity with Synthetic Substitute, Open Approach

♀ **0W1J0JJ** Bypass Pelvic Cavity to Pelvic Cavity with Synthetic Substitute, Open Approach

---

♀ Female-only   ♂ Male-only   ● Limited Coverage   ● Non-OR   ▥ HAC-associated procedure   ● Non-covered procedures   ✛ Combination

♀ **0W1J0JY** Bypass Pelvic Cavity to Lower Vein with Synthetic Substitute, Open Approach
♀ **0W1J3J4** Bypass Pelvic Cavity to Cutaneous with Synthetic Substitute, Percutaneous Approach
♀ **0W1J4J4** Bypass Pelvic Cavity to Cutaneous with Synthetic Substitute, Percutaneous Endoscopic Approach
♀ **0W1J4J9** Bypass Pelvic Cavity to Right Pleural Cavity with Synthetic Substitute, Percutaneous Endoscopic Approach
♀ **0W1J4JB** Bypass Pelvic Cavity to Left Pleural Cavity with Synthetic Substitute, Percutaneous Endoscopic Approach

♀ **0W1J4JG** Bypass Pelvic Cavity to Peritoneal Cavity with Synthetic Substitute, Percutaneous Endoscopic Approach
♀ **0W1J4JJ** Bypass Pelvic Cavity to Pelvic Cavity with Synthetic Substitute, Percutaneous Endoscopic Approach
♀ **0W1J4JY** Bypass Pelvic Cavity to Lower Vein with Synthetic Substitute, Percutaneous Endoscopic Approach
This is a female-only service, however, it is not included in the female-only edit logic for MCE V30

0W2 – Anatomical Regions, General, Change

Review Coding Guideline B6.1c

0W20X0Z Change Drainage Device in Head, External Approach
0W20XYZ Change Other Device in Head, External Approach
0W21X0Z Change Drainage Device in Cranial Cavity, External Approach
0W21XYZ Change Other Device in Cranial Cavity, External Approach
0W22X0Z Change Drainage Device in Face, External Approach
0W22XYZ Change Other Device in Face, External Approach
0W24X0Z Change Drainage Device in Upper Jaw, External Approach
0W24XYZ Change Other Device in Upper Jaw, External Approach
0W25X0Z Change Drainage Device in Lower Jaw, External Approach
0W25XYZ Change Other Device in Lower Jaw, External Approach
0W26X0Z Change Drainage Device in Neck, External Approach
0W26XYZ Change Other Device in Neck, External Approach
0W28X0Z Change Drainage Device in Chest Wall, External Approach
0W28XYZ Change Other Device in Chest Wall, External Approach
0W29X0Z Change Drainage Device in Right Pleural Cavity, External Approach
0W29XYZ Change Other Device in Right Pleural Cavity, External Approach
0W2BX0Z Change Drainage Device in Left Pleural Cavity, External Approach
0W2BXYZ Change Other Device in Left Pleural Cavity, External Approach
0W2CX0Z Change Drainage Device in Mediastinum, External Approach

0W2CXYZ Change Other Device in Mediastinum, External Approach
0W2DX0Z Change Drainage Device in Pericardial Cavity, External Approach
0W2DXYZ Change Other Device in Pericardial Cavity, External Approach
0W2FX0Z Change Drainage Device in Abdominal Wall, External Approach
0W2FXYZ Change Other Device in Abdominal Wall, External Approach
0W2GX0Z Change Drainage Device in Peritoneal Cavity, External Approach
0W2GXYZ Change Other Device in Peritoneal Cavity, External Approach
0W2HX0Z Change Drainage Device in Retroperitoneum, External Approach
0W2HXYZ Change Other Device in Retroperitoneum, External Approach
0W2JX0Z Change Drainage Device in Pelvic Cavity, External Approach
0W2JXYZ Change Other Device in Pelvic Cavity, External Approach
0W2KX0Z Change Drainage Device in Upper Back, External Approach
0W2KXYZ Change Other Device in Upper Back, External Approach
0W2LX0Z Change Drainage Device in Lower Back, External Approach
0W2LXYZ Change Other Device in Lower Back, External Approach
0W2MX0Z Change Drainage Device in Male Perineum, External Approach
0W2MXYZ Change Other Device in Male Perineum, External Approach
0W2NX0Z Change Drainage Device in Female Perineum, External Approach
0W2NXYZ Change Other Device in Female Perineum, External Approach

0W3 – Anatomical Regions, General, Control

Review Coding Guideline B3.7

0W300ZZ Control Bleeding in Head, Open Approach
0W303ZZ Control Bleeding in Head, Percutaneous Approach
0W304ZZ Control Bleeding in Head, Percutaneous Endoscopic Approach
0W310ZZ Control Bleeding in Cranial Cavity, Open Approach
0W313ZZ Control Bleeding in Cranial Cavity, Percutaneous Approach
0W314ZZ Control Bleeding in Cranial Cavity, Percutaneous Endoscopic Approach
0W320ZZ Control Bleeding in Face, Open Approach
0W323ZZ Control Bleeding in Face, Percutaneous Approach
0W324ZZ Control Bleeding in Face, Percutaneous Endoscopic Approach
0W330ZZ Control Bleeding in Oral Cavity and Throat, Open Approach
0W333ZZ Control Bleeding in Oral Cavity and Throat, Percutaneous Approach
0W334ZZ Control Bleeding in Oral Cavity and Throat, Percutaneous Endoscopic Approach
0W337ZZ Control Bleeding in Oral Cavity and Throat, Via Natural or Artificial Opening
0W338ZZ Control Bleeding in Oral Cavity and Throat, Via Natural or Artificial Opening Endoscopic
0W33XZZ Control Bleeding in Oral Cavity and Throat, External Approach
0W340ZZ Control Bleeding in Upper Jaw, Open Approach
0W343ZZ Control Bleeding in Upper Jaw, Percutaneous Approach
0W344ZZ Control Bleeding in Upper Jaw, Percutaneous Endoscopic Approach
0W350ZZ Control Bleeding in Lower Jaw, Open Approach
0W353ZZ Control Bleeding in Lower Jaw, Percutaneous Approach
0W354ZZ Control Bleeding in Lower Jaw, Percutaneous Endoscopic Approach
0W360ZZ Control Bleeding in Neck, Open Approach
0W363ZZ Control Bleeding in Neck, Percutaneous Approach
0W364ZZ Control Bleeding in Neck, Percutaneous Endoscopic Approach
0W380ZZ Control Bleeding in Chest Wall, Open Approach
0W383ZZ Control Bleeding in Chest Wall, Percutaneous Approach
0W384ZZ Control Bleeding in Chest Wall, Percutaneous Endoscopic Approach
0W390ZZ Control Bleeding in Right Pleural Cavity, Open Approach

0W393ZZ Control Bleeding in Right Pleural Cavity, Percutaneous Approach
0W394ZZ Control Bleeding in Right Pleural Cavity, Percutaneous Endoscopic Approach
0W3B0ZZ Control Bleeding in Left Pleural Cavity, Open Approach
0W3B3ZZ Control Bleeding in Left Pleural Cavity, Percutaneous Approach
0W3B4ZZ Control Bleeding in Left Pleural Cavity, Percutaneous Endoscopic Approach
0W3C0ZZ Control Bleeding in Mediastinum, Open Approach
0W3C3ZZ Control Bleeding in Mediastinum, Percutaneous Approach
0W3C4ZZ Control Bleeding in Mediastinum, Percutaneous Endoscopic Approach
0W3D0ZZ Control Bleeding in Pericardial Cavity, Open Approach
0W3D3ZZ Control Bleeding in Pericardial Cavity, Percutaneous Approach
0W3D4ZZ Control Bleeding in Pericardial Cavity, Percutaneous Endoscopic Approach
0W3F0ZZ Control Bleeding in Abdominal Wall, Open Approach
0W3F3ZZ Control Bleeding in Abdominal Wall, Percutaneous Approach
0W3F4ZZ Control Bleeding in Abdominal Wall, Percutaneous Endoscopic Approach
0W3G0ZZ Control Bleeding in Peritoneal Cavity, Open Approach
0W3G3ZZ Control Bleeding in Peritoneal Cavity, Percutaneous Approach
0W3G4ZZ Control Bleeding in Peritoneal Cavity, Percutaneous Endoscopic Approach
0W3H0ZZ Control Bleeding in Retroperitoneum, Open Approach
0W3H3ZZ Control Bleeding in Retroperitoneum, Percutaneous Approach
0W3H4ZZ Control Bleeding in Retroperitoneum, Percutaneous Endoscopic Approach
0W3J0ZZ Control Bleeding in Pelvic Cavity, Open Approach
0W3J3ZZ Control Bleeding in Pelvic Cavity, Percutaneous Approach
0W3J4ZZ Control Bleeding in Pelvic Cavity, Percutaneous Endoscopic Approach
0W3K0ZZ Control Bleeding in Upper Back, Open Approach
0W3K3ZZ Control Bleeding in Upper Back, Percutaneous Approach

---

♀ Female-only   ♂ Male-only   ⬤ Limited Coverage   ⬤ Non-OR   🅗🅐🅒 HAC-associated procedure   ⬤ Non-covered procedures   ➕ Combination

0W3K4ZZ	Control Bleeding in Upper Back, Percutaneous Endoscopic Approach
0W3L0ZZ	Control Bleeding in Lower Back, Open Approach
0W3L3ZZ	Control Bleeding in Lower Back, Percutaneous Approach
0W3L4ZZ	Control Bleeding in Lower Back, Percutaneous Endoscopic Approach
0W3M0ZZ	Control Bleeding in Male Perineum, Open Approach
0W3M3ZZ	Control Bleeding in Male Perineum, Percutaneous Approach
0W3M4ZZ	Control Bleeding in Male Perineum, Percutaneous Endoscopic Approach
0W3N0ZZ	Control Bleeding in Female Perineum, Open Approach
0W3N3ZZ	Control Bleeding in Female Perineum, Percutaneous Approach
0W3N4ZZ	Control Bleeding in Female Perineum, Percutaneous Endoscopic Approach
0W3P0ZZ	Control Bleeding in Gastrointestinal Tract, Open Approach
0W3P3ZZ	Control Bleeding in Gastrointestinal Tract, Percutaneous Approach
0W3P4ZZ	Control Bleeding in Gastrointestinal Tract, Percutaneous Endoscopic Approach
0W3P7ZZ	Control Bleeding in Gastrointestinal Tract, Via Natural or Artificial Opening
0W3P8ZZ	Control Bleeding in Gastrointestinal Tract, Via Natural or Artificial Opening Endoscopic
0W3Q0ZZ	Control Bleeding in Respiratory Tract, Open Approach
0W3Q3ZZ	Control Bleeding in Respiratory Tract, Percutaneous Approach
0W3Q4ZZ	Control Bleeding in Respiratory Tract, Percutaneous Endoscopic Approach
0W3Q7ZZ	Control Bleeding in Respiratory Tract, Via Natural or Artificial Opening
0W3Q8ZZ	Control Bleeding in Respiratory Tract, Via Natural or Artificial Opening Endoscopic
0W3R0ZZ	Control Bleeding in Genitourinary Tract, Open Approach
0W3R3ZZ	Control Bleeding in Genitourinary Tract, Percutaneous Approach
0W3R4ZZ	Control Bleeding in Genitourinary Tract, Percutaneous Endoscopic Approach
0W3R7ZZ	Control Bleeding in Genitourinary Tract, Via Natural or Artificial Opening
0W3R8ZZ	Control Bleeding in Genitourinary Tract, Via Natural or Artificial Opening Endoscopic

0W4 – Anatomical Regions, General, Creation

● ♂ 0W4M070	Creation of Vagina in Male Perineum with Autologous Tissue Substitute, Open Approach
● ♂ 0W4M0J0	Creation of Vagina in Male Perineum with Synthetic Substitute, Open Approach
● ♂ 0W4M0K0	Creation of Vagina in Male Perineum with Nonautologous Tissue Substitute, Open Approach
● ♂ 0W4M0Z0	Creation of Vagina in Male Perineum, Open Approach
● ♀ 0W4N071	Creation of Penis in Female Perineum with Autologous Tissue Substitute, Open Approach
● ♀ 0W4N0J1	Creation of Penis in Female Perineum with Synthetic Substitute, Open Approach
● ♀ 0W4N0K1	Creation of Penis in Female Perineum with Nonautologous Tissue Substitute, Open Approach
● ♀ 0W4N0Z1	Creation of Penis in Female Perineum, Open Approach

0W8 – Anatomical Regions, General, Division

♀ 0W8NXZZ	Division of Female Perineum, External Approach

0W9 – Anatomical Regions, General, Drainage

Review Coding Guidelines B3.4a and B3.4b

Review Coding Guideline B6.2

0W9000Z	Drainage of Head with Drainage Device, Open Approach
0W900ZX	Drainage of Head, Open Approach, Diagnostic
0W900ZZ	Drainage of Head, Open Approach
0W9030Z	Drainage of Head with Drainage Device, Percutaneous Approach
0W903ZX	Drainage of Head, Percutaneous Approach, Diagnostic
0W903ZZ	Drainage of Head, Percutaneous Approach
0W9040Z	Drainage of Head with Drainage Device, Percutaneous Endoscopic Approach
0W904ZX	Drainage of Head, Percutaneous Endoscopic Approach, Diagnostic
0W904ZZ	Drainage of Head, Percutaneous Endoscopic Approach
0W9100Z	Drainage of Cranial Cavity with Drainage Device, Open Approach
0W910ZX	Drainage of Cranial Cavity, Open Approach, Diagnostic
0W910ZZ	Drainage of Cranial Cavity, Open Approach
0W9130Z	Drainage of Cranial Cavity with Drainage Device, Percutaneous Approach
0W913ZX	Drainage of Cranial Cavity, Percutaneous Approach, Diagnostic
0W913ZZ	Drainage of Cranial Cavity, Percutaneous Approach
0W9140Z	Drainage of Cranial Cavity with Drainage Device, Percutaneous Endoscopic Approach
0W914ZX	Drainage of Cranial Cavity, Percutaneous Endoscopic Approach, Diagnostic
0W914ZZ	Drainage of Cranial Cavity, Percutaneous Endoscopic Approach
0W9200Z	Drainage of Face with Drainage Device, Open Approach
0W920ZX	Drainage of Face, Open Approach, Diagnostic
0W920ZZ	Drainage of Face, Open Approach
0W9230Z	Drainage of Face with Drainage Device, Percutaneous Approach
0W923ZX	Drainage of Face, Percutaneous Approach, Diagnostic
0W923ZZ	Drainage of Face, Percutaneous Approach
0W9240Z	Drainage of Face with Drainage Device, Percutaneous Endoscopic Approach
0W924ZX	Drainage of Face, Percutaneous Endoscopic Approach, Diagnostic
0W924ZZ	Drainage of Face, Percutaneous Endoscopic Approach
0W9300Z	Drainage of Oral Cavity and Throat with Drainage Device, Open Approach
0W930ZX	Drainage of Oral Cavity and Throat, Open Approach, Diagnostic
0W930ZZ	Drainage of Oral Cavity and Throat, Open Approach
0W9330Z	Drainage of Oral Cavity and Throat with Drainage Device, Percutaneous Approach
0W933ZX	Drainage of Oral Cavity and Throat, Percutaneous Approach, Diagnostic
0W933ZZ	Drainage of Oral Cavity and Throat, Percutaneous Approach
0W9340Z	Drainage of Oral Cavity and Throat with Drainage Device, Percutaneous Endoscopic Approach
0W934ZX	Drainage of Oral Cavity and Throat, Percutaneous Endoscopic Approach, Diagnostic
0W934ZZ	Drainage of Oral Cavity and Throat, Percutaneous Endoscopic Approach
0W9400Z	Drainage of Upper Jaw with Drainage Device, Open Approach
0W940ZX	Drainage of Upper Jaw, Open Approach, Diagnostic
0W940ZZ	Drainage of Upper Jaw, Open Approach
0W9430Z	Drainage of Upper Jaw with Drainage Device, Percutaneous Approach
0W943ZX	Drainage of Upper Jaw, Percutaneous Approach, Diagnostic
0W943ZZ	Drainage of Upper Jaw, Percutaneous Approach
0W9440Z	Drainage of Upper Jaw with Drainage Device, Percutaneous Endoscopic Approach
0W944ZX	Drainage of Upper Jaw, Percutaneous Endoscopic Approach, Diagnostic
0W944ZZ	Drainage of Upper Jaw, Percutaneous Endoscopic Approach
0W9500Z	Drainage of Lower Jaw with Drainage Device, Open Approach
0W950ZX	Drainage of Lower Jaw, Open Approach, Diagnostic
0W950ZZ	Drainage of Lower Jaw, Open Approach

0W9530Z	Drainage of Lower Jaw with Drainage Device, Percutaneous Approach
0W953ZX	Drainage of Lower Jaw, Percutaneous Approach, Diagnostic
0W953ZZ	Drainage of Lower Jaw, Percutaneous Approach
0W9540Z	Drainage of Lower Jaw with Drainage Device, Percutaneous Endoscopic Approach
0W954ZX	Drainage of Lower Jaw, Percutaneous Endoscopic Approach, Diagnostic
0W954ZZ	Drainage of Lower Jaw, Percutaneous Endoscopic Approach
0W9600Z	Drainage of Neck with Drainage Device, Open Approach
0W960ZX	Drainage of Neck, Open Approach, Diagnostic
0W960ZZ	Drainage of Neck, Open Approach
0W9630Z	Drainage of Neck with Drainage Device, Percutaneous Approach
0W963ZX	Drainage of Neck, Percutaneous Approach, Diagnostic
0W963ZZ	Drainage of Neck, Percutaneous Approach
0W9640Z	Drainage of Neck with Drainage Device, Percutaneous Endoscopic Approach
0W964ZX	Drainage of Neck, Percutaneous Endoscopic Approach, Diagnostic
0W964ZZ	Drainage of Neck, Percutaneous Endoscopic Approach
0W9800Z	Drainage of Chest Wall with Drainage Device, Open Approach
0W980ZX	Drainage of Chest Wall, Open Approach, Diagnostic
0W980ZZ	Drainage of Chest Wall, Open Approach
0W9830Z	Drainage of Chest Wall with Drainage Device, Percutaneous Approach
0W983ZX	Drainage of Chest Wall, Percutaneous Approach, Diagnostic
0W983ZZ	Drainage of Chest Wall, Percutaneous Approach
0W9840Z	Drainage of Chest Wall with Drainage Device, Percutaneous Endoscopic Approach
0W984ZX	Drainage of Chest Wall, Percutaneous Endoscopic Approach, Diagnostic
0W984ZZ	Drainage of Chest Wall, Percutaneous Endoscopic Approach
0W9900Z	Drainage of Right Pleural Cavity with Drainage Device, Open Approach
0W990ZX	Drainage of Right Pleural Cavity, Open Approach, Diagnostic
0W990ZZ	Drainage of Right Pleural Cavity, Open Approach
0W9930Z	Drainage of Right Pleural Cavity with Drainage Device, Percutaneous Approach
0W993ZX	Drainage of Right Pleural Cavity, Percutaneous Approach, Diagnostic
0W993ZZ	Drainage of Right Pleural Cavity, Percutaneous Approach
0W9940Z	Drainage of Right Pleural Cavity with Drainage Device, Percutaneous Endoscopic Approach
0W994ZX	Drainage of Right Pleural Cavity, Percutaneous Endoscopic Approach, Diagnostic
0W994ZZ	Drainage of Right Pleural Cavity, Percutaneous Endoscopic Approach
0W9B00Z	Drainage of Left Pleural Cavity with Drainage Device, Open Approach
0W9B0ZX	Drainage of Left Pleural Cavity, Open Approach, Diagnostic
0W9B0ZZ	Drainage of Left Pleural Cavity, Open Approach
0W9B30Z	Drainage of Left Pleural Cavity with Drainage Device, Percutaneous Approach
0W9B3ZX	Drainage of Left Pleural Cavity, Percutaneous Approach, Diagnostic
0W9B3ZZ	Drainage of Left Pleural Cavity, Percutaneous Approach
0W9B40Z	Drainage of Left Pleural Cavity with Drainage Device, Percutaneous Endoscopic Approach
0W9B4ZX	Drainage of Left Pleural Cavity, Percutaneous Endoscopic Approach, Diagnostic
0W9B4ZZ	Drainage of Left Pleural Cavity, Percutaneous Endoscopic Approach
0W9C00Z	Drainage of Mediastinum with Drainage Device, Open Approach
0W9C0ZX	Drainage of Mediastinum, Open Approach, Diagnostic
0W9C0ZZ	Drainage of Mediastinum, Open Approach
0W9C30Z	Drainage of Mediastinum with Drainage Device, Percutaneous Approach
0W9C3ZX	Drainage of Mediastinum, Percutaneous Approach, Diagnostic
0W9C3ZZ	Drainage of Mediastinum, Percutaneous Approach
0W9C40Z	Drainage of Mediastinum with Drainage Device, Percutaneous Endoscopic Approach
0W9C4ZX	Drainage of Mediastinum, Percutaneous Endoscopic Approach, Diagnostic
0W9C4ZZ	Drainage of Mediastinum, Percutaneous Endoscopic Approach
0W9D00Z	Drainage of Pericardial Cavity with Drainage Device, Open Approach
0W9D0ZX	Drainage of Pericardial Cavity, Open Approach, Diagnostic
0W9D0ZZ	Drainage of Pericardial Cavity, Open Approach
0W9D30Z	Drainage of Pericardial Cavity with Drainage Device, Percutaneous Approach
0W9D3ZX	Drainage of Pericardial Cavity, Percutaneous Approach, Diagnostic
0W9D3ZZ	Drainage of Pericardial Cavity, Percutaneous Approach
0W9D40Z	Drainage of Pericardial Cavity with Drainage Device, Percutaneous Endoscopic Approach
0W9D4ZX	Drainage of Pericardial Cavity, Percutaneous Endoscopic Approach, Diagnostic
0W9D4ZZ	Drainage of Pericardial Cavity, Percutaneous Endoscopic Approach
0W9F00Z	Drainage of Abdominal Wall with Drainage Device, Open Approach
0W9F0ZX	Drainage of Abdominal Wall, Open Approach, Diagnostic
0W9F0ZZ	Drainage of Abdominal Wall, Open Approach
0W9F30Z	Drainage of Abdominal Wall with Drainage Device, Percutaneous Approach
0W9F3ZX	Drainage of Abdominal Wall, Percutaneous Approach, Diagnostic
0W9F3ZZ	Drainage of Abdominal Wall, Percutaneous Approach
0W9F40Z	Drainage of Abdominal Wall with Drainage Device, Percutaneous Endoscopic Approach
0W9F4ZX	Drainage of Abdominal Wall, Percutaneous Endoscopic Approach, Diagnostic
0W9F4ZZ	Drainage of Abdominal Wall, Percutaneous Endoscopic Approach
0W9G00Z	Drainage of Peritoneal Cavity with Drainage Device, Open Approach
0W9G0ZX	Drainage of Peritoneal Cavity, Open Approach, Diagnostic
0W9G0ZZ	Drainage of Peritoneal Cavity, Open Approach
0W9G30Z	Drainage of Peritoneal Cavity with Drainage Device, Percutaneous Approach
0W9G3ZX	Drainage of Peritoneal Cavity, Percutaneous Approach, Diagnostic
0W9G3ZZ	Drainage of Peritoneal Cavity, Percutaneous Approach
0W9G40Z	Drainage of Peritoneal Cavity with Drainage Device, Percutaneous Endoscopic Approach
0W9G4ZX	Drainage of Peritoneal Cavity, Percutaneous Endoscopic Approach, Diagnostic
0W9G4ZZ	Drainage of Peritoneal Cavity, Percutaneous Endoscopic Approach
0W9H00Z	Drainage of Retroperitoneum with Drainage Device, Open Approach
0W9H0ZX	Drainage of Retroperitoneum, Open Approach, Diagnostic
0W9H0ZZ	Drainage of Retroperitoneum, Open Approach
0W9H30Z	Drainage of Retroperitoneum with Drainage Device, Percutaneous Approach
0W9H3ZX	Drainage of Retroperitoneum, Percutaneous Approach, Diagnostic
0W9H3ZZ	Drainage of Retroperitoneum, Percutaneous Approach
0W9H40Z	Drainage of Retroperitoneum with Drainage Device, Percutaneous Endoscopic Approach
0W9H4ZX	Drainage of Retroperitoneum, Percutaneous Endoscopic Approach, Diagnostic
0W9H4ZZ	Drainage of Retroperitoneum, Percutaneous Endoscopic Approach
0W9J00Z	Drainage of Pelvic Cavity with Drainage Device, Open Approach
0W9J0ZX	Drainage of Pelvic Cavity, Open Approach, Diagnostic
0W9J0ZZ	Drainage of Pelvic Cavity, Open Approach
0W9J30Z	Drainage of Pelvic Cavity with Drainage Device, Percutaneous Approach
0W9J3ZX	Drainage of Pelvic Cavity, Percutaneous Approach, Diagnostic
0W9J3ZZ	Drainage of Pelvic Cavity, Percutaneous Approach
0W9J40Z	Drainage of Pelvic Cavity with Drainage Device, Percutaneous Endoscopic Approach
0W9J4ZX	Drainage of Pelvic Cavity, Percutaneous Endoscopic Approach, Diagnostic
0W9J4ZZ	Drainage of Pelvic Cavity, Percutaneous Endoscopic Approach
0W9K00Z	Drainage of Upper Back with Drainage Device, Open Approach
0W9K0ZX	Drainage of Upper Back, Open Approach, Diagnostic
0W9K0ZZ	Drainage of Upper Back, Open Approach
0W9K30Z	Drainage of Upper Back with Drainage Device, Percutaneous Approach
0W9K3ZX	Drainage of Upper Back, Percutaneous Approach, Diagnostic
0W9K3ZZ	Drainage of Upper Back, Percutaneous Approach

	0W9K40Z	Drainage of Upper Back with Drainage Device, Percutaneous Endoscopic Approach
	0W9K4ZX	Drainage of Upper Back, Percutaneous Endoscopic Approach, Diagnostic
	0W9K4ZZ	Drainage of Upper Back, Percutaneous Endoscopic Approach
	0W9L00Z	Drainage of Lower Back with Drainage Device, Open Approach
	0W9L0ZX	Drainage of Lower Back, Open Approach, Diagnostic
	0W9L0ZZ	Drainage of Lower Back, Open Approach
	0W9L30Z	Drainage of Lower Back with Drainage Device, Percutaneous Approach
	0W9L3ZX	Drainage of Lower Back, Percutaneous Approach, Diagnostic
	0W9L3ZZ	Drainage of Lower Back, Percutaneous Approach
	0W9L40Z	Drainage of Lower Back with Drainage Device, Percutaneous Endoscopic Approach
	0W9L4ZX	Drainage of Lower Back, Percutaneous Endoscopic Approach, Diagnostic
	0W9L4ZZ	Drainage of Lower Back, Percutaneous Endoscopic Approach
♂	**0W9M00Z**	Drainage of Male Perineum with Drainage Device, Open Approach
♂	**0W9M0ZX**	Drainage of Male Perineum, Open Approach, Diagnostic
♂	**0W9M0ZZ**	Drainage of Male Perineum, Open Approach
♂	**0W9M30Z**	Drainage of Male Perineum with Drainage Device, Percutaneous Approach

♂	**0W9M3ZX**	Drainage of Male Perineum, Percutaneous Approach, Diagnostic
♂	**0W9M3ZZ**	Drainage of Male Perineum, Percutaneous Approach
♂	**0W9M40Z**	Drainage of Male Perineum with Drainage Device, Percutaneous Endoscopic Approach
♂	**0W9M4ZX**	Drainage of Male Perineum, Percutaneous Endoscopic Approach, Diagnostic
♂	**0W9M4ZZ**	Drainage of Male Perineum, Percutaneous Endoscopic Approach
♀	**0W9N00Z**	Drainage of Female Perineum with Drainage Device, Open Approach
♀	**0W9N0ZX**	Drainage of Female Perineum, Open Approach, Diagnostic
♀	**0W9N0ZZ**	Drainage of Female Perineum, Open Approach
♀	**0W9N30Z**	Drainage of Female Perineum with Drainage Device, Percutaneous Approach
♀	**0W9N3ZX**	Drainage of Female Perineum, Percutaneous Approach, Diagnostic
♀	**0W9N3ZZ**	Drainage of Female Perineum, Percutaneous Approach
♀	**0W9N40Z**	Drainage of Female Perineum with Drainage Device, Percutaneous Endoscopic Approach
♀	**0W9N4ZX**	Drainage of Female Perineum, Percutaneous Endoscopic Approach, Diagnostic
		This is a female-only service, however, it is not included in the female-only edit logic for MCE V30
♀	**0W9N4ZZ**	Drainage of Female Perineum, Percutaneous Endoscopic Approach

0WB – Anatomical Regions, General, Excision

Review Coding Guidelines B3.4a and B3.4b

0WB00ZX	Excision of Head, Open Approach, Diagnostic
0WB00ZZ	Excision of Head, Open Approach
0WB03ZX	Excision of Head, Percutaneous Approach, Diagnostic
0WB03ZZ	Excision of Head, Percutaneous Approach
0WB04ZX	Excision of Head, Percutaneous Endoscopic Approach, Diagnostic
0WB04ZZ	Excision of Head, Percutaneous Endoscopic Approach
0WB0XZX	Excision of Head, External Approach, Diagnostic
0WB0XZZ	Excision of Head, External Approach
0WB20ZX	Excision of Face, Open Approach, Diagnostic
0WB20ZZ	Excision of Face, Open Approach
0WB23ZX	Excision of Face, Percutaneous Approach, Diagnostic
0WB23ZZ	Excision of Face, Percutaneous Approach
0WB24ZX	Excision of Face, Percutaneous Endoscopic Approach, Diagnostic
0WB24ZZ	Excision of Face, Percutaneous Endoscopic Approach
0WB2XZX	Excision of Face, External Approach, Diagnostic
0WB2XZZ	Excision of Face, External Approach
0WB40ZX	Excision of Upper Jaw, Open Approach, Diagnostic
0WB40ZZ	Excision of Upper Jaw, Open Approach
0WB43ZX	Excision of Upper Jaw, Percutaneous Approach, Diagnostic
0WB43ZZ	Excision of Upper Jaw, Percutaneous Approach
0WB44ZX	Excision of Upper Jaw, Percutaneous Endoscopic Approach, Diagnostic
0WB44ZZ	Excision of Upper Jaw, Percutaneous Endoscopic Approach
0WB4XZX	Excision of Upper Jaw, External Approach, Diagnostic
0WB4XZZ	Excision of Upper Jaw, External Approach
0WB50ZX	Excision of Lower Jaw, Open Approach, Diagnostic
0WB50ZZ	Excision of Lower Jaw, Open Approach
0WB53ZX	Excision of Lower Jaw, Percutaneous Approach, Diagnostic
0WB53ZZ	Excision of Lower Jaw, Percutaneous Approach
0WB54ZX	Excision of Lower Jaw, Percutaneous Endoscopic Approach, Diagnostic
0WB54ZZ	Excision of Lower Jaw, Percutaneous Endoscopic Approach
0WB5XZX	Excision of Lower Jaw, External Approach, Diagnostic
0WB5XZZ	Excision of Lower Jaw, External Approach
0WB60ZX	Excision of Neck, Open Approach, Diagnostic
0WB60ZZ	Excision of Neck, Open Approach
0WB63ZX	Excision of Neck, Percutaneous Approach, Diagnostic
0WB63ZZ	Excision of Neck, Percutaneous Approach
0WB64ZX	Excision of Neck, Percutaneous Endoscopic Approach, Diagnostic
0WB64ZZ	Excision of Neck, Percutaneous Endoscopic Approach
0WB6XZ2	Excision of Neck, Stoma, External Approach
0WB6XZX	Excision of Neck, External Approach, Diagnostic
0WB6XZZ	Excision of Neck, External Approach
0WB80ZX	Excision of Chest Wall, Open Approach, Diagnostic
0WB80ZZ	Excision of Chest Wall, Open Approach
0WB83ZX	Excision of Chest Wall, Percutaneous Approach, Diagnostic

0WB83ZZ	Excision of Chest Wall, Percutaneous Approach
0WB84ZX	Excision of Chest Wall, Percutaneous Endoscopic Approach, Diagnostic
0WB84ZZ	Excision of Chest Wall, Percutaneous Endoscopic Approach
0WB8XZX	Excision of Chest Wall, External Approach, Diagnostic
0WB8XZZ	Excision of Chest Wall, External Approach
0WBC0ZX	Excision of Mediastinum, Open Approach, Diagnostic
0WBC0ZZ	Excision of Mediastinum, Open Approach
0WBC3ZX	Excision of Mediastinum, Percutaneous Approach, Diagnostic
0WBC3ZZ	Excision of Mediastinum, Percutaneous Approach
0WBC4ZX	Excision of Mediastinum, Percutaneous Endoscopic Approach, Diagnostic
0WBC4ZZ	Excision of Mediastinum, Percutaneous Endoscopic Approach
0WBF0ZX	Excision of Abdominal Wall, Open Approach, Diagnostic
0WBF0ZZ	Excision of Abdominal Wall, Open Approach
0WBF3ZX	Excision of Abdominal Wall, Percutaneous Approach, Diagnostic
0WBF3ZZ	Excision of Abdominal Wall, Percutaneous Approach
0WBF4ZX	Excision of Abdominal Wall, Percutaneous Endoscopic Approach, Diagnostic
0WBF4ZZ	Excision of Abdominal Wall, Percutaneous Endoscopic Approach
0WBFXZ2	Excision of Abdominal Wall, Stoma, External Approach
0WBFXZX	Excision of Abdominal Wall, External Approach, Diagnostic
0WBFXZZ	Excision of Abdominal Wall, External Approach
0WBH0ZX	Excision of Retroperitoneum, Open Approach, Diagnostic
0WBH0ZZ	Excision of Retroperitoneum, Open Approach
0WBH3ZX	Excision of Retroperitoneum, Percutaneous Approach, Diagnostic
0WBH3ZZ	Excision of Retroperitoneum, Percutaneous Approach
0WBH4ZX	Excision of Retroperitoneum, Percutaneous Endoscopic Approach, Diagnostic
0WBH4ZZ	Excision of Retroperitoneum, Percutaneous Endoscopic Approach
0WBK0ZX	Excision of Upper Back, Open Approach, Diagnostic
0WBK0ZZ	Excision of Upper Back, Open Approach
0WBK3ZX	Excision of Upper Back, Percutaneous Approach, Diagnostic
0WBK3ZZ	Excision of Upper Back, Percutaneous Approach
0WBK4ZX	Excision of Upper Back, Percutaneous Endoscopic Approach, Diagnostic
0WBK4ZZ	Excision of Upper Back, Percutaneous Endoscopic Approach
0WBKXZX	Excision of Upper Back, External Approach, Diagnostic
0WBKXZZ	Excision of Upper Back, External Approach
0WBL0ZX	Excision of Lower Back, Open Approach, Diagnostic
0WBL0ZZ	Excision of Lower Back, Open Approach
0WBL3ZX	Excision of Lower Back, Percutaneous Approach, Diagnostic
0WBL3ZZ	Excision of Lower Back, Percutaneous Approach
0WBL4ZX	Excision of Lower Back, Percutaneous Endoscopic Approach, Diagnostic
0WBL4ZZ	Excision of Lower Back, Percutaneous Endoscopic Approach

0WBLXZX Excision of Lower Back, External Approach, Diagnostic
0WBLXZZ Excision of Lower Back, External Approach
♂ **0WBM0ZX** Excision of Male Perineum, Open Approach, Diagnostic
♂ **0WBM0ZZ** Excision of Male Perineum, Open Approach
♂ **0WBM3ZX** Excision of Male Perineum, Percutaneous Approach, Diagnostic
♂ **0WBM3ZZ** Excision of Male Perineum, Percutaneous Approach
♂ **0WBM4ZX** Excision of Male Perineum, Percutaneous Endoscopic Approach, Diagnostic
♂ **0WBM4ZZ** Excision of Male Perineum, Percutaneous Endoscopic Approach
♂ **0WBMXZX** Excision of Male Perineum, External Approach, Diagnostic
♂ **0WBMXZZ** Excision of Male Perineum, External Approach

♀ **0WBN0ZX** Excision of Female Perineum, Open Approach, Diagnostic
♀ **0WBN0ZZ** Excision of Female Perineum, Open Approach
♀ **0WBN3ZX** Excision of Female Perineum, Percutaneous Approach, Diagnostic
♀ **0WBN3ZZ** Excision of Female Perineum, Percutaneous Approach
♀ **0WBN4ZX** Excision of Female Perineum, Percutaneous Endoscopic Approach, Diagnostic
♀ **0WBN4ZZ** Excision of Female Perineum, Percutaneous Endoscopic Approach
♀ **0WBNXZX** Excision of Female Perineum, External Approach, Diagnostic
♀ **0WBNXZZ** Excision of Female Perineum, External Approach

0WC – Anatomical Regions, General, Extirpation

0WC10ZZ Extirpation of Matter from Cranial Cavity, Open Approach
0WC13ZZ Extirpation of Matter from Cranial Cavity, Percutaneous Approach
0WC14ZZ Extirpation of Matter from Cranial Cavity, Percutaneous Endoscopic Approach
0WC1XZZ Extirpation of Matter from Cranial Cavity, External Approach
0WC30ZZ Extirpation of Matter from Oral Cavity and Throat, Open Approach
0WC33ZZ Extirpation of Matter from Oral Cavity and Throat, Percutaneous Approach
0WC34ZZ Extirpation of Matter from Oral Cavity and Throat, Percutaneous Endoscopic Approach
0WC3XZZ Extirpation of Matter from Oral Cavity and Throat, External Approach
0WC90ZZ Extirpation of Matter from Right Pleural Cavity, Open Approach
0WC93ZZ Extirpation of Matter from Right Pleural Cavity, Percutaneous Approach
0WC94ZZ Extirpation of Matter from Right Pleural Cavity, Percutaneous Endoscopic Approach
0WC9XZZ Extirpation of Matter from Right Pleural Cavity, External Approach
0WCB0ZZ Extirpation of Matter from Left Pleural Cavity, Open Approach
0WCB3ZZ Extirpation of Matter from Left Pleural Cavity, Percutaneous Approach
0WCB4ZZ Extirpation of Matter from Left Pleural Cavity, Percutaneous Endoscopic Approach
0WCBXZZ Extirpation of Matter from Left Pleural Cavity, External Approach
0WCC0ZZ Extirpation of Matter from Mediastinum, Open Approach
0WCC3ZZ Extirpation of Matter from Mediastinum, Percutaneous Approach
0WCC4ZZ Extirpation of Matter from Mediastinum, Percutaneous Endoscopic Approach
0WCCXZZ Extirpation of Matter from Mediastinum, External Approach
0WCD0ZZ Extirpation of Matter from Pericardial Cavity, Open Approach
0WCD3ZZ Extirpation of Matter from Pericardial Cavity, Percutaneous Approach
0WCD4ZZ Extirpation of Matter from Pericardial Cavity, Percutaneous Endoscopic Approach
0WCDXZZ Extirpation of Matter from Pericardial Cavity, External Approach
0WCG0ZZ Extirpation of Matter from Peritoneal Cavity, Open Approach
0WCG3ZZ Extirpation of Matter from Peritoneal Cavity, Percutaneous Approach

0WCG4ZZ Extirpation of Matter from Peritoneal Cavity, Percutaneous Endoscopic Approach
0WCGXZZ Extirpation of Matter from Peritoneal Cavity, External Approach
0WCJ0ZZ Extirpation of Matter from Pelvic Cavity, Open Approach
0WCJ3ZZ Extirpation of Matter from Pelvic Cavity, Percutaneous Approach
0WCJ4ZZ Extirpation of Matter from Pelvic Cavity, Percutaneous Endoscopic Approach
0WCJXZZ Extirpation of Matter from Pelvic Cavity, External Approach
0WCP0ZZ Extirpation of Matter from Gastrointestinal Tract, Open Approach
0WCP3ZZ Extirpation of Matter from Gastrointestinal Tract, Percutaneous Approach
0WCP4ZZ Extirpation of Matter from Gastrointestinal Tract, Percutaneous Endoscopic Approach
0WCP7ZZ Extirpation of Matter from Gastrointestinal Tract, Via Natural or Artificial Opening
0WCP8ZZ Extirpation of Matter from Gastrointestinal Tract, Via Natural or Artificial Opening Endoscopic
0WCPXZZ Extirpation of Matter from Gastrointestinal Tract, External Approach
0WCQ0ZZ Extirpation of Matter from Respiratory Tract, Open Approach
0WCQ3ZZ Extirpation of Matter from Respiratory Tract, Percutaneous Approach
0WCQ4ZZ Extirpation of Matter from Respiratory Tract, Percutaneous Endoscopic Approach
0WCQ7ZZ Extirpation of Matter from Respiratory Tract, Via Natural or Artificial Opening
0WCQ8ZZ Extirpation of Matter from Respiratory Tract, Via Natural or Artificial Opening Endoscopic
0WCQXZZ Extirpation of Matter from Respiratory Tract, External Approach
0WCR0ZZ Extirpation of Matter from Genitourinary Tract, Open Approach
0WCR3ZZ Extirpation of Matter from Genitourinary Tract, Percutaneous Approach
0WCR4ZZ Extirpation of Matter from Genitourinary Tract, Percutaneous Endoscopic Approach
0WCR7ZZ Extirpation of Matter from Genitourinary Tract, Via Natural or Artificial Opening
0WCR8ZZ Extirpation of Matter from Genitourinary Tract, Via Natural or Artificial Opening Endoscopic
0WCRXZZ Extirpation of Matter from Genitourinary Tract, External Approach

0WF – Anatomical Regions, General, Fragmentation

0WF10ZZ Fragmentation in Cranial Cavity, Open Approach
0WF13ZZ Fragmentation in Cranial Cavity, Percutaneous Approach
0WF14ZZ Fragmentation in Cranial Cavity, Percutaneous Endoscopic Approach
● **0WF1XZZ** Fragmentation in Cranial Cavity, External Approach
0WF30ZZ Fragmentation in Oral Cavity and Throat, Open Approach
0WF33ZZ Fragmentation in Oral Cavity and Throat, Percutaneous Approach
0WF34ZZ Fragmentation in Oral Cavity and Throat, Percutaneous Endoscopic Approach
● **0WF3XZZ** Fragmentation in Oral Cavity and Throat, External Approach
0WF90ZZ Fragmentation in Right Pleural Cavity, Open Approach
0WF93ZZ Fragmentation in Right Pleural Cavity, Percutaneous Approach
0WF94ZZ Fragmentation in Right Pleural Cavity, Percutaneous Endoscopic Approach
● **0WF9XZZ** Fragmentation in Right Pleural Cavity, External Approach

0WFB0ZZ Fragmentation in Left Pleural Cavity, Open Approach
0WFB3ZZ Fragmentation in Left Pleural Cavity, Percutaneous Approach
0WFB4ZZ Fragmentation in Left Pleural Cavity, Percutaneous Endoscopic Approach
● **0WFBXZZ** Fragmentation in Left Pleural Cavity, External Approach
0WFC0ZZ Fragmentation in Mediastinum, Open Approach
0WFC3ZZ Fragmentation in Mediastinum, Percutaneous Approach
0WFC4ZZ Fragmentation in Mediastinum, Percutaneous Endoscopic Approach
● **0WFCXZZ** Fragmentation in Mediastinum, External Approach
0WFD0ZZ Fragmentation in Pericardial Cavity, Open Approach
0WFD3ZZ Fragmentation in Pericardial Cavity, Percutaneous Approach
0WFD4ZZ Fragmentation in Pericardial Cavity, Percutaneous Endoscopic Approach
0WFDXZZ Fragmentation in Pericardial Cavity, External Approach
0WFG0ZZ Fragmentation in Peritoneal Cavity, Open Approach

0WFG3ZZ	Fragmentation in Peritoneal Cavity, Percutaneous Approach
0WFG4ZZ	Fragmentation in Peritoneal Cavity, Percutaneous Endoscopic Approach
● 0WFGXZZ	Fragmentation in Peritoneal Cavity, External Approach
0WFJ0ZZ	Fragmentation in Pelvic Cavity, Open Approach
0WFJ3ZZ	Fragmentation in Pelvic Cavity, Percutaneous Approach
0WFJ4ZZ	Fragmentation in Pelvic Cavity, Percutaneous Endoscopic Approach
● 0WFJXZZ	Fragmentation in Pelvic Cavity, External Approach
0WFP0ZZ	Fragmentation in Gastrointestinal Tract, Open Approach
0WFP3ZZ	Fragmentation in Gastrointestinal Tract, Percutaneous Approach
0WFP4ZZ	Fragmentation in Gastrointestinal Tract, Percutaneous Endoscopic Approach
0WFP7ZZ	Fragmentation in Gastrointestinal Tract, Via Natural or Artificial Opening
0WFP8ZZ	Fragmentation in Gastrointestinal Tract, Via Natural or Artificial Opening Endoscopic
● 0WFPXZZ	Fragmentation in Gastrointestinal Tract, External Approach
0WFQ0ZZ	Fragmentation in Respiratory Tract, Open Approach
0WFQ3ZZ	Fragmentation in Respiratory Tract, Percutaneous Approach
0WFQ4ZZ	Fragmentation in Respiratory Tract, Percutaneous Endoscopic Approach
0WFQ7ZZ	Fragmentation in Respiratory Tract, Via Natural or Artificial Opening
0WFQ8ZZ	Fragmentation in Respiratory Tract, Via Natural or Artificial Opening Endoscopic
● 0WFQXZZ	Fragmentation in Respiratory Tract, External Approach
0WFR0ZZ	Fragmentation in Genitourinary Tract, Open Approach
0WFR3ZZ	Fragmentation in Genitourinary Tract, Percutaneous Approach
0WFR4ZZ	Fragmentation in Genitourinary Tract, Percutaneous Endoscopic Approach
0WFR7ZZ	Fragmentation in Genitourinary Tract, Via Natural or Artificial Opening
0WFR8ZZ	Fragmentation in Genitourinary Tract, Via Natural or Artificial Opening Endoscopic
● 0WFRXZZ	Fragmentation in Genitourinary Tract, External Approach

0WH – Anatomical Regions, General, Insertion

0WH001Z	Insertion of Radioactive Element into Head, Open Approach
● 0WH003Z	Insertion of Infusion Device into Head, Open Approach
● 0WH00YZ	Insertion of Other Device into Head, Open Approach
0WH031Z	Insertion of Radioactive Element into Head, Percutaneous Approach
● 0WH033Z	Insertion of Infusion Device into Head, Percutaneous Approach
● 0WH03YZ	Insertion of Other Device into Head, Percutaneous Approach
0WH041Z	Insertion of Radioactive Element into Head, Percutaneous Endoscopic Approach
● 0WH043Z	Insertion of Infusion Device into Head, Percutaneous Endoscopic Approach
● 0WH04YZ	Insertion of Other Device into Head, Percutaneous Endoscopic Approach
0WH101Z	Insertion of Radioactive Element into Cranial Cavity, Open Approach
0WH103Z	Insertion of Infusion Device into Cranial Cavity, Open Approach
0WH10YZ	Insertion of Other Device into Cranial Cavity, Open Approach
0WH131Z	Insertion of Radioactive Element into Cranial Cavity, Percutaneous Approach
0WH133Z	Insertion of Infusion Device into Cranial Cavity, Percutaneous Approach
0WH13YZ	Insertion of Other Device into Cranial Cavity, Percutaneous Approach
0WH141Z	Insertion of Radioactive Element into Cranial Cavity, Percutaneous Endoscopic Approach
0WH143Z	Insertion of Infusion Device into Cranial Cavity, Percutaneous Endoscopic Approach
0WH14YZ	Insertion of Other Device into Cranial Cavity, Percutaneous Endoscopic Approach
0WH201Z	Insertion of Radioactive Element into Face, Open Approach
● 0WH203Z	Insertion of Infusion Device into Face, Open Approach
● 0WH20YZ	Insertion of Other Device into Face, Open Approach
0WH231Z	Insertion of Radioactive Element into Face, Percutaneous Approach
● 0WH233Z	Insertion of Infusion Device into Face, Percutaneous Approach
● 0WH23YZ	Insertion of Other Device into Face, Percutaneous Approach
0WH241Z	Insertion of Radioactive Element into Face, Percutaneous Endoscopic Approach
● 0WH243Z	Insertion of Infusion Device into Face, Percutaneous Endoscopic Approach
● 0WH24YZ	Insertion of Other Device into Face, Percutaneous Endoscopic Approach
0WH301Z	Insertion of Radioactive Element into Oral Cavity and Throat, Open Approach
0WH303Z	Insertion of Infusion Device into Oral Cavity and Throat, Open Approach
0WH30YZ	Insertion of Other Device into Oral Cavity and Throat, Open Approach
0WH331Z	Insertion of Radioactive Element into Oral Cavity and Throat, Percutaneous Approach
0WH333Z	Insertion of Infusion Device into Oral Cavity and Throat, Percutaneous Approach
0WH33YZ	Insertion of Other Device into Oral Cavity and Throat, Percutaneous Approach
0WH341Z	Insertion of Radioactive Element into Oral Cavity and Throat, Percutaneous Endoscopic Approach
0WH343Z	Insertion of Infusion Device into Oral Cavity and Throat, Percutaneous Endoscopic Approach
0WH34YZ	Insertion of Other Device into Oral Cavity and Throat, Percutaneous Endoscopic Approach
0WH401Z	Insertion of Radioactive Element into Upper Jaw, Open Approach
● 0WH403Z	Insertion of Infusion Device into Upper Jaw, Open Approach
● 0WH40YZ	Insertion of Other Device into Upper Jaw, Open Approach
0WH431Z	Insertion of Radioactive Element into Upper Jaw, Percutaneous Approach
● 0WH433Z	Insertion of Infusion Device into Upper Jaw, Percutaneous Approach
● 0WH43YZ	Insertion of Other Device into Upper Jaw, Percutaneous Approach
0WH441Z	Insertion of Radioactive Element into Upper Jaw, Percutaneous Endoscopic Approach
● 0WH443Z	Insertion of Infusion Device into Upper Jaw, Percutaneous Endoscopic Approach
● 0WH44YZ	Insertion of Other Device into Upper Jaw, Percutaneous Endoscopic Approach
0WH501Z	Insertion of Radioactive Element into Lower Jaw, Open Approach
● 0WH503Z	Insertion of Infusion Device into Lower Jaw, Open Approach
● 0WH50YZ	Insertion of Other Device into Lower Jaw, Open Approach
0WH531Z	Insertion of Radioactive Element into Lower Jaw, Percutaneous Approach
● 0WH533Z	Insertion of Infusion Device into Lower Jaw, Percutaneous Approach
● 0WH53YZ	Insertion of Other Device into Lower Jaw, Percutaneous Approach
0WH541Z	Insertion of Radioactive Element into Lower Jaw, Percutaneous Endoscopic Approach
● 0WH543Z	Insertion of Infusion Device into Lower Jaw, Percutaneous Endoscopic Approach
● 0WH54YZ	Insertion of Other Device into Lower Jaw, Percutaneous Endoscopic Approach
0WH601Z	Insertion of Radioactive Element into Neck, Open Approach
● 0WH603Z	Insertion of Infusion Device into Neck, Open Approach
● 0WH60YZ	Insertion of Other Device into Neck, Open Approach
0WH631Z	Insertion of Radioactive Element into Neck, Percutaneous Approach
● 0WH633Z	Insertion of Infusion Device into Neck, Percutaneous Approach
● 0WH63YZ	Insertion of Other Device into Neck, Percutaneous Approach
0WH641Z	Insertion of Radioactive Element into Neck, Percutaneous Endoscopic Approach
● 0WH643Z	Insertion of Infusion Device into Neck, Percutaneous Endoscopic Approach
● 0WH64YZ	Insertion of Other Device into Neck, Percutaneous Endoscopic Approach

0WH801Z Insertion of Radioactive Element into Chest Wall, Open Approach

0WH803Z Insertion of Infusion Device into Chest Wall, Open Approach

0WH80YZ Insertion of Other Device into Chest Wall, Open Approach

0WH831Z Insertion of Radioactive Element into Chest Wall, Percutaneous Approach

0WH833Z Insertion of Infusion Device into Chest Wall, Percutaneous Approach

0WH83YZ Insertion of Other Device into Chest Wall, Percutaneous Approach

0WH841Z Insertion of Radioactive Element into Chest Wall, Percutaneous Endoscopic Approach

0WH843Z Insertion of Infusion Device into Chest Wall, Percutaneous Endoscopic Approach

0WH84YZ Insertion of Other Device into Chest Wall, Percutaneous Endoscopic Approach

0WH901Z Insertion of Radioactive Element into Right Pleural Cavity, Open Approach

0WH903Z Insertion of Infusion Device into Right Pleural Cavity, Open Approach

0WH90YZ Insertion of Other Device into Right Pleural Cavity, Open Approach

0WH931Z Insertion of Radioactive Element into Right Pleural Cavity, Percutaneous Approach

0WH933Z Insertion of Infusion Device into Right Pleural Cavity, Percutaneous Approach

0WH93YZ Insertion of Other Device into Right Pleural Cavity, Percutaneous Approach

0WH941Z Insertion of Radioactive Element into Right Pleural Cavity, Percutaneous Endoscopic Approach

0WH943Z Insertion of Infusion Device into Right Pleural Cavity, Percutaneous Endoscopic Approach

0WH94YZ Insertion of Other Device into Right Pleural Cavity, Percutaneous Endoscopic Approach

0WHB01Z Insertion of Radioactive Element into Left Pleural Cavity, Open Approach

0WHB03Z Insertion of Infusion Device into Left Pleural Cavity, Open Approach

0WHB0YZ Insertion of Other Device into Left Pleural Cavity, Open Approach

0WHB31Z Insertion of Radioactive Element into Left Pleural Cavity, Percutaneous Approach

0WHB33Z Insertion of Infusion Device into Left Pleural Cavity, Percutaneous Approach

0WHB3YZ Insertion of Other Device into Left Pleural Cavity, Percutaneous Approach

0WHB41Z Insertion of Radioactive Element into Left Pleural Cavity, Percutaneous Endoscopic Approach

0WHB43Z Insertion of Infusion Device into Left Pleural Cavity, Percutaneous Endoscopic Approach

0WHB4YZ Insertion of Other Device into Left Pleural Cavity, Percutaneous Endoscopic Approach

0WHC01Z Insertion of Radioactive Element into Mediastinum, Open Approach

0WHC03Z Insertion of Infusion Device into Mediastinum, Open Approach

0WHC0YZ Insertion of Other Device into Mediastinum, Open Approach

0WHC31Z Insertion of Radioactive Element into Mediastinum, Percutaneous Approach

0WHC33Z Insertion of Infusion Device into Mediastinum, Percutaneous Approach

0WHC3YZ Insertion of Other Device into Mediastinum, Percutaneous Approach

0WHC41Z Insertion of Radioactive Element into Mediastinum, Percutaneous Endoscopic Approach

0WHC43Z Insertion of Infusion Device into Mediastinum, Percutaneous Endoscopic Approach

0WHC4YZ Insertion of Other Device into Mediastinum, Percutaneous Endoscopic Approach

0WHD01Z Insertion of Radioactive Element into Pericardial Cavity, Open Approach

0WHD03Z Insertion of Infusion Device into Pericardial Cavity, Open Approach

0WHD0YZ Insertion of Other Device into Pericardial Cavity, Open Approach

0WHD31Z Insertion of Radioactive Element into Pericardial Cavity, Percutaneous Approach

0WHD33Z Insertion of Infusion Device into Pericardial Cavity, Percutaneous Approach

0WHD3YZ Insertion of Other Device into Pericardial Cavity, Percutaneous Approach

0WHD41Z Insertion of Radioactive Element into Pericardial Cavity, Percutaneous Endoscopic Approach

0WHD43Z Insertion of Infusion Device into Pericardial Cavity, Percutaneous Endoscopic Approach

0WHD4YZ Insertion of Other Device into Pericardial Cavity, Percutaneous Endoscopic Approach

0WHF01Z Insertion of Radioactive Element into Abdominal Wall, Open Approach

0WHF03Z Insertion of Infusion Device into Abdominal Wall, Open Approach

0WHF0YZ Insertion of Other Device into Abdominal Wall, Open Approach

0WHF31Z Insertion of Radioactive Element into Abdominal Wall, Percutaneous Approach

0WHF33Z Insertion of Infusion Device into Abdominal Wall, Percutaneous Approach

0WHF3YZ Insertion of Other Device into Abdominal Wall, Percutaneous Approach

0WHF41Z Insertion of Radioactive Element into Abdominal Wall, Percutaneous Endoscopic Approach

0WHF43Z Insertion of Infusion Device into Abdominal Wall, Percutaneous Endoscopic Approach

0WHF4YZ Insertion of Other Device into Abdominal Wall, Percutaneous Endoscopic Approach

0WHG01Z Insertion of Radioactive Element into Peritoneal Cavity, Open Approach

0WHG03Z Insertion of Infusion Device into Peritoneal Cavity, Open Approach

0WHG0YZ Insertion of Other Device into Peritoneal Cavity, Open Approach

0WHG31Z Insertion of Radioactive Element into Peritoneal Cavity, Percutaneous Approach

0WHG33Z Insertion of Infusion Device into Peritoneal Cavity, Percutaneous Approach

0WHG3YZ Insertion of Other Device into Peritoneal Cavity, Percutaneous Approach

0WHG41Z Insertion of Radioactive Element into Peritoneal Cavity, Percutaneous Endoscopic Approach

0WHG43Z Insertion of Infusion Device into Peritoneal Cavity, Percutaneous Endoscopic Approach

0WHG4YZ Insertion of Other Device into Peritoneal Cavity, Percutaneous Endoscopic Approach

0WHH01Z Insertion of Radioactive Element into Retroperitoneum, Open Approach

0WHH03Z Insertion of Infusion Device into Retroperitoneum, Open Approach

0WHH0YZ Insertion of Other Device into Retroperitoneum, Open Approach

0WHH31Z Insertion of Radioactive Element into Retroperitoneum, Percutaneous Approach

0WHH33Z Insertion of Infusion Device into Retroperitoneum, Percutaneous Approach

0WHH3YZ Insertion of Other Device into Retroperitoneum, Percutaneous Approach

0WHH41Z Insertion of Radioactive Element into Retroperitoneum, Percutaneous Endoscopic Approach

0WHH43Z Insertion of Infusion Device into Retroperitoneum, Percutaneous Endoscopic Approach

0WHH4YZ Insertion of Other Device into Retroperitoneum, Percutaneous Endoscopic Approach

0WHJ01Z Insertion of Radioactive Element into Pelvic Cavity, Open Approach

0WHJ03Z Insertion of Infusion Device into Pelvic Cavity, Open Approach

0WHJ0YZ Insertion of Other Device into Pelvic Cavity, Open Approach

0WHJ31Z Insertion of Radioactive Element into Pelvic Cavity, Percutaneous Approach

0WHJ33Z Insertion of Infusion Device into Pelvic Cavity, Percutaneous Approach

0WHJ3YZ Insertion of Other Device into Pelvic Cavity, Percutaneous Approach

---

0WHJ41Z Insertion of Radioactive Element into Pelvic Cavity, Percutaneous Endoscopic Approach

0WHJ43Z Insertion of Infusion Device into Pelvic Cavity, Percutaneous Endoscopic Approach

0WHJ4YZ Insertion of Other Device into Pelvic Cavity, Percutaneous Endoscopic Approach

0WHK01Z Insertion of Radioactive Element into Upper Back, Open Approach

● **0WHK03Z** Insertion of Infusion Device into Upper Back, Open Approach

● **0WHK0YZ** Insertion of Other Device into Upper Back, Open Approach

0WHK31Z Insertion of Radioactive Element into Upper Back, Percutaneous Approach

● **0WHK33Z** Insertion of Infusion Device into Upper Back, Percutaneous Approach

● **0WHK3YZ** Insertion of Other Device into Upper Back, Percutaneous Approach

0WHK41Z Insertion of Radioactive Element into Upper Back, Percutaneous Endoscopic Approach

● **0WHK43Z** Insertion of Infusion Device into Upper Back, Percutaneous Endoscopic Approach

● **0WHK4YZ** Insertion of Other Device into Upper Back, Percutaneous Endoscopic Approach

0WHL01Z Insertion of Radioactive Element into Lower Back, Open Approach

● **0WHL03Z** Insertion of Infusion Device into Lower Back, Open Approach

● **0WHL0YZ** Insertion of Other Device into Lower Back, Open Approach

0WHL31Z Insertion of Radioactive Element into Lower Back, Percutaneous Approach

● **0WHL33Z** Insertion of Infusion Device into Lower Back, Percutaneous Approach

● **0WHL3YZ** Insertion of Other Device into Lower Back, Percutaneous Approach

0WHL41Z Insertion of Radioactive Element into Lower Back, Percutaneous Endoscopic Approach

● **0WHL43Z** Insertion of Infusion Device into Lower Back, Percutaneous Endoscopic Approach

● **0WHL4YZ** Insertion of Other Device into Lower Back, Percutaneous Endoscopic Approach

♂ **0WHM01Z** Insertion of Radioactive Element into Male Perineum, Open Approach
This is a male-only service, however, it is not included in the male-only edit logic for MCE V30

●♂ **0WHM03Z** Insertion of Infusion Device into Male Perineum, Open Approach
This is a male-only service, however, it is not included in the male-only edit logic for MCE V30

●♂ **0WHM0YZ** Insertion of Other Device into Male Perineum, Open Approach
This is a male-only service, however, it is not included in the male-only edit logic for MCE V30

♂ **0WHM31Z** Insertion of Radioactive Element into Male Perineum, Percutaneous Approach
This is a male-only service, however, it is not included in the male-only edit logic for MCE V30

●♂ **0WHM33Z** Insertion of Infusion Device into Male Perineum, Percutaneous Approach
This is a male-only service, however, it is not included in the male-only edit logic for MCE V30

●♂ **0WHM3YZ** Insertion of Other Device into Male Perineum, Percutaneous Approach
This is a male-only service, however, it is not included in the male-only edit logic for MCE V30

♂ **0WHM41Z** Insertion of Radioactive Element into Male Perineum, Percutaneous Endoscopic Approach
This is a male-only service, however, it is not included in the male-only edit logic for MCE V30

●♂ **0WHM43Z** Insertion of Infusion Device into Male Perineum, Percutaneous Endoscopic Approach
This is a male-only service, however, it is not included in the male-only edit logic for MCE V30

●♂ **0WHM4YZ** Insertion of Other Device into Male Perineum, Percutaneous Endoscopic Approach
This is a male-only service, however, it is not included in the male-only edit logic for MCE V30

♀ **0WHN01Z** Insertion of Radioactive Element into Female Perineum, Open Approach
This is a female-only service, however, it is not included in the female-only edit logic for MCE V30

♀ **0WHN03Z** Insertion of Infusion Device into Female Perineum, Open Approach

♀ **0WHN0YZ** Insertion of Other Device into Female Perineum, Open Approach

♀ **0WHN31Z** Insertion of Radioactive Element into Female Perineum, Percutaneous Approach
This is a female-only service, however, it is not included in the female-only edit logic for MCE V30

♀ **0WHN33Z** Insertion of Infusion Device into Female Perineum, Percutaneous Approach

♀ **0WHN3YZ** Insertion of Other Device into Female Perineum, Percutaneous Approach

♀ **0WHN41Z** Insertion of Radioactive Element into Female Perineum, Percutaneous Endoscopic Approach
This is a female-only service, however, it is not included in the female-only edit logic for MCE V30

♀ **0WHN43Z** Insertion of Infusion Device into Female Perineum, Percutaneous Endoscopic Approach

♀ **0WHN4YZ** Insertion of Other Device into Female Perineum, Percutaneous Endoscopic Approach

0WHP01Z Insertion of Radioactive Element into Gastrointestinal Tract, Open Approach

0WHP03Z Insertion of Infusion Device into Gastrointestinal Tract, Open Approach

0WHP0YZ Insertion of Other Device into Gastrointestinal Tract, Open Approach

0WHP31Z Insertion of Radioactive Element into Gastrointestinal Tract, Percutaneous Approach

0WHP33Z Insertion of Infusion Device into Gastrointestinal Tract, Percutaneous Approach

0WHP3YZ Insertion of Other Device into Gastrointestinal Tract, Percutaneous Approach

0WHP41Z Insertion of Radioactive Element into Gastrointestinal Tract, Percutaneous Endoscopic Approach

0WHP43Z Insertion of Infusion Device into Gastrointestinal Tract, Percutaneous Endoscopic Approach

0WHP4YZ Insertion of Other Device into Gastrointestinal Tract, Percutaneous Endoscopic Approach

0WHP71Z Insertion of Radioactive Element into Gastrointestinal Tract, Via Natural or Artificial Opening

0WHP73Z Insertion of Infusion Device into Gastrointestinal Tract, Via Natural or Artificial Opening

0WHP7YZ Insertion of Other Device into Gastrointestinal Tract, Via Natural or Artificial Opening

0WHP81Z Insertion of Radioactive Element into Gastrointestinal Tract, Via Natural or Artificial Opening Endoscopic

0WHP83Z Insertion of Infusion Device into Gastrointestinal Tract, Via Natural or Artificial Opening Endoscopic

0WHP8YZ Insertion of Other Device into Gastrointestinal Tract, Via Natural or Artificial Opening Endoscopic

0WHQ01Z Insertion of Radioactive Element into Respiratory Tract, Open Approach

0WHQ03Z Insertion of Infusion Device into Respiratory Tract, Open Approach

0WHQ0YZ Insertion of Other Device into Respiratory Tract, Open Approach

0WHQ31Z Insertion of Radioactive Element into Respiratory Tract, Percutaneous Approach

0WHQ33Z Insertion of Infusion Device into Respiratory Tract, Percutaneous Approach

0WHQ3YZ Insertion of Other Device into Respiratory Tract, Percutaneous Approach

0WHQ41Z Insertion of Radioactive Element into Respiratory Tract, Percutaneous Endoscopic Approach

0WHQ43Z Insertion of Infusion Device into Respiratory Tract, Percutaneous Endoscopic Approach

0WHQ4YZ Insertion of Other Device into Respiratory Tract, Percutaneous Endoscopic Approach

0WHQ71Z Insertion of Radioactive Element into Respiratory Tract, Via Natural or Artificial Opening

0WHQ73Z Insertion of Infusion Device into Respiratory Tract, Via Natural or Artificial Opening

0WHQ7YZ Insertion of Other Device into Respiratory Tract, Via Natural or Artificial Opening

0WHQ81Z Insertion of Radioactive Element into Respiratory Tract, Via Natural or Artificial Opening Endoscopic

0WHQ83Z Insertion of Infusion Device into Respiratory Tract, Via Natural or Artificial Opening Endoscopic

0WHQ8YZ Insertion of Other Device into Respiratory Tract, Via Natural or Artificial Opening Endoscopic

0WHR01Z Insertion of Radioactive Element into Genitourinary Tract, Open Approach

0WHR03Z Insertion of Infusion Device into Genitourinary Tract, Open Approach

0WHR0YZ Insertion of Other Device into Genitourinary Tract, Open Approach

0WHR31Z Insertion of Radioactive Element into Genitourinary Tract, Percutaneous Approach

0WHR33Z Insertion of Infusion Device into Genitourinary Tract, Percutaneous Approach

0WHR3YZ Insertion of Other Device into Genitourinary Tract, Percutaneous Approach

0WHR41Z Insertion of Radioactive Element into Genitourinary Tract, Percutaneous Endoscopic Approach

0WHR43Z Insertion of Infusion Device into Genitourinary Tract, Percutaneous Endoscopic Approach

0WHR4YZ Insertion of Other Device into Genitourinary Tract, Percutaneous Endoscopic Approach

0WHR71Z Insertion of Radioactive Element into Genitourinary Tract, Via Natural or Artificial Opening

0WHR73Z Insertion of Infusion Device into Genitourinary Tract, Via Natural or Artificial Opening

0WHR7YZ Insertion of Other Device into Genitourinary Tract, Via Natural or Artificial Opening

0WHR81Z Insertion of Radioactive Element into Genitourinary Tract, Via Natural or Artificial Opening Endoscopic

0WHR83Z Insertion of Infusion Device into Genitourinary Tract, Via Natural or Artificial Opening Endoscopic

0WHR8YZ Insertion of Other Device into Genitourinary Tract, Via Natural or Artificial Opening Endoscopic

0WJ – Anatomical Regions, General, Inspection

Review Coding Guidelines B3.11a, B3.11b and B3.11c

● **0WJ00ZZ** Inspection of Head, Open Approach
0WJ03ZZ Inspection of Head, Percutaneous Approach
0WJ04ZZ Inspection of Head, Percutaneous Endoscopic Approach
0WJ0XZZ Inspection of Head, External Approach
0WJ10ZZ Inspection of Cranial Cavity, Open Approach
0WJ13ZZ Inspection of Cranial Cavity, Percutaneous Approach
0WJ14ZZ Inspection of Cranial Cavity, Percutaneous Endoscopic Approach
● **0WJ20ZZ** Inspection of Face, Open Approach
0WJ23ZZ Inspection of Face, Percutaneous Approach
0WJ24ZZ Inspection of Face, Percutaneous Endoscopic Approach
0WJ2XZZ Inspection of Face, External Approach
0WJ30ZZ Inspection of Oral Cavity and Throat, Open Approach
0WJ33ZZ Inspection of Oral Cavity and Throat, Percutaneous Approach
0WJ34ZZ Inspection of Oral Cavity and Throat, Percutaneous Endoscopic Approach
0WJ3XZZ Inspection of Oral Cavity and Throat, External Approach
● **0WJ40ZZ** Inspection of Upper Jaw, Open Approach
0WJ43ZZ Inspection of Upper Jaw, Percutaneous Approach
0WJ44ZZ Inspection of Upper Jaw, Percutaneous Endoscopic Approach
0WJ4XZZ Inspection of Upper Jaw, External Approach
● **0WJ50ZZ** Inspection of Lower Jaw, Open Approach
0WJ53ZZ Inspection of Lower Jaw, Percutaneous Approach
0WJ54ZZ Inspection of Lower Jaw, Percutaneous Endoscopic Approach
0WJ5XZZ Inspection of Lower Jaw, External Approach
0WJ60ZZ Inspection of Neck, Open Approach
0WJ63ZZ Inspection of Neck, Percutaneous Approach
0WJ64ZZ Inspection of Neck, Percutaneous Endoscopic Approach
0WJ6XZZ Inspection of Neck, External Approach
0WJ80ZZ Inspection of Chest Wall, Open Approach
0WJ83ZZ Inspection of Chest Wall, Percutaneous Approach
0WJ84ZZ Inspection of Chest Wall, Percutaneous Endoscopic Approach
0WJ8XZZ Inspection of Chest Wall, External Approach
0WJ90ZZ Inspection of Right Pleural Cavity, Open Approach
0WJ93ZZ Inspection of Right Pleural Cavity, Percutaneous Approach
0WJ94ZZ Inspection of Right Pleural Cavity, Percutaneous Endoscopic Approach
0WJB0ZZ Inspection of Left Pleural Cavity, Open Approach
0WJB3ZZ Inspection of Left Pleural Cavity, Percutaneous Approach
0WJB4ZZ Inspection of Left Pleural Cavity, Percutaneous Endoscopic Approach
0WJC0ZZ Inspection of Mediastinum, Open Approach
0WJC3ZZ Inspection of Mediastinum, Percutaneous Approach
0WJC4ZZ Inspection of Mediastinum, Percutaneous Endoscopic Approach
0WJD0ZZ Inspection of Pericardial Cavity, Open Approach
0WJD3ZZ Inspection of Pericardial Cavity, Percutaneous Approach
0WJD4ZZ Inspection of Pericardial Cavity, Percutaneous Endoscopic Approach
0WJF0ZZ Inspection of Abdominal Wall, Open Approach
0WJF3ZZ Inspection of Abdominal Wall, Percutaneous Approach
0WJF4ZZ Inspection of Abdominal Wall, Percutaneous Endoscopic Approach
0WJFXZZ Inspection of Abdominal Wall, External Approach
0WJG0ZZ Inspection of Peritoneal Cavity, Open Approach
0WJG3ZZ Inspection of Peritoneal Cavity, Percutaneous Approach

0WJG4ZZ Inspection of Peritoneal Cavity, Percutaneous Endoscopic Approach
0WJH0ZZ Inspection of Retroperitoneum, Open Approach
0WJH3ZZ Inspection of Retroperitoneum, Percutaneous Approach
0WJH4ZZ Inspection of Retroperitoneum, Percutaneous Endoscopic Approach
0WJJ0ZZ Inspection of Pelvic Cavity, Open Approach
0WJJ3ZZ Inspection of Pelvic Cavity, Percutaneous Approach
0WJJ4ZZ Inspection of Pelvic Cavity, Percutaneous Endoscopic Approach
● **0WJK0ZZ** Inspection of Upper Back, Open Approach
0WJK3ZZ Inspection of Upper Back, Percutaneous Approach
0WJK4ZZ Inspection of Upper Back, Percutaneous Endoscopic Approach
0WJKXZZ Inspection of Upper Back, External Approach
● **0WJL0ZZ** Inspection of Lower Back, Open Approach
0WJL3ZZ Inspection of Lower Back, Percutaneous Approach
0WJL4ZZ Inspection of Lower Back, Percutaneous Endoscopic Approach
0WJLXZZ Inspection of Lower Back, External Approach
♂ **0WJM0ZZ** Inspection of Male Perineum, Open Approach
♂ **0WJM3ZZ** Inspection of Male Perineum, Percutaneous Approach
♂ **0WJM4ZZ** Inspection of Male Perineum, Percutaneous Endoscopic Approach
♂ **0WJMXZZ** Inspection of Male Perineum, External Approach
♀ **0WJN0ZZ** Inspection of Female Perineum, Open Approach
♀ **0WJN3ZZ** Inspection of Female Perineum, Percutaneous Approach
♀ **0WJN4ZZ** Inspection of Female Perineum, Percutaneous Endoscopic Approach
♀ **0WJNXZZ** Inspection of Female Perineum, External Approach
0WJP0ZZ Inspection of Gastrointestinal Tract, Open Approach
0WJP3ZZ Inspection of Gastrointestinal Tract, Percutaneous Approach
0WJP4ZZ Inspection of Gastrointestinal Tract, Percutaneous Endoscopic Approach
0WJP7ZZ Inspection of Gastrointestinal Tract, Via Natural or Artificial Opening Approach
0WJP8ZZ Inspection of Gastrointestinal Tract, Via Natural or Artificial Opening Endoscopic Approach
0WJQ0ZZ Inspection of Respiratory Tract, Open Approach
0WJQ3ZZ Inspection of Respiratory Tract, Percutaneous Approach
0WJQ4ZZ Inspection of Respiratory Tract, Percutaneous Endoscopic Approach
0WJQ7ZZ Inspection of Respiratory Tract, Via Natural or Artificial Opening Approach
0WJQ8ZZ Inspection of Respiratory Tract, Via Natural or Artificial Opening Endoscopic Approach
0WJR0ZZ Inspection of Genitourinary Tract, Open Approach
0WJR3ZZ Inspection of Genitourinary Tract, Percutaneous Approach
0WJR4ZZ Inspection of Genitourinary Tract, Percutaneous Endoscopic Approach
0WJR7ZZ Inspection of Genitourinary Tract, Via Natural or Artificial Opening Approach
0WJR8ZZ Inspection of Genitourinary Tract, Via Natural or Artificial Opening Endoscopic Approach

0WM – Anatomical Regions, General, Reattachment

0WM20ZZ	Reattachment of Face, Open Approach
0WM40ZZ	Reattachment of Upper Jaw, Open Approach
0WM50ZZ	Reattachment of Lower Jaw, Open Approach
0WM60ZZ	Reattachment of Neck, Open Approach
0WM80ZZ	Reattachment of Chest Wall, Open Approach

	0WMF0ZZ	Reattachment of Abdominal Wall, Open Approach
	0WMK0ZZ	Reattachment of Upper Back, Open Approach
	0WML0ZZ	Reattachment of Lower Back, Open Approach
♂	**0WMM0ZZ**	Reattachment of Male Perineum, Open Approach
♀	**0WMN0ZZ**	Reattachment of Female Perineum, Open Approach

0WP   Anatomical Regions, General, Removal

Review Coding Guideline B6.1c

0WP000Z	Removal of Drainage Device from Head, Open Approach
0WP001Z	Removal of Radioactive Element from Head, Open Approach
0WP003Z	Removal of Infusion Device from Head, Open Approach
0WP007Z	Removal of Autologous Tissue Substitute from Head, Open Approach
0WP00JZ	Removal of Synthetic Substitute from Head, Open Approach
0WP00KZ	Removal of Nonautologous Tissue Substitute from Head, Open Approach
0WP00YZ	Removal of Other Device from Head, Open Approach
0WP030Z	Removal of Drainage Device from Head, Percutaneous Approach
0WP031Z	Removal of Radioactive Element from Head, Percutaneous Approach
0WP033Z	Removal of Infusion Device from Head, Percutaneous Approach
0WP037Z	Removal of Autologous Tissue Substitute from Head, Percutaneous Approach
0WP03JZ	Removal of Synthetic Substitute from Head, Percutaneous Approach
0WP03KZ	Removal of Nonautologous Tissue Substitute from Head, Percutaneous Approach
0WP03YZ	Removal of Other Device from Head, Percutaneous Approach
0WP040Z	Removal of Drainage Device from Head, Percutaneous Endoscopic Approach
0WP041Z	Removal of Radioactive Element from Head, Percutaneous Endoscopic Approach
0WP043Z	Removal of Infusion Device from Head, Percutaneous Endoscopic Approach
0WP047Z	Removal of Autologous Tissue Substitute from Head, Percutaneous Endoscopic Approach
0WP04JZ	Removal of Synthetic Substitute from Head, Percutaneous Endoscopic Approach
0WP04KZ	Removal of Nonautologous Tissue Substitute from Head, Percutaneous Endoscopic Approach
0WP04YZ	Removal of Other Device from Head, Percutaneous Endoscopic Approach
0WP0X0Z	Removal of Drainage Device from Head, External Approach
0WP0X1Z	Removal of Radioactive Element from Head, External Approach
0WP0X3Z	Removal of Infusion Device from Head, External Approach
0WP0X7Z	Removal of Autologous Tissue Substitute from Head, External Approach
0WP0XJZ	Removal of Synthetic Substitute from Head, External Approach
0WP0XKZ	Removal of Nonautologous Tissue Substitute from Head, External Approach
0WP0XYZ	Removal of Other Device from Head, External Approach
0WP100Z	Removal of Drainage Device from Cranial Cavity, Open Approach
0WP101Z	Removal of Radioactive Element from Cranial Cavity, Open Approach
0WP103Z	Removal of Infusion Device from Cranial Cavity, Open Approach
0WP10JZ	Removal of Synthetic Substitute from Cranial Cavity, Open Approach
0WP10YZ	Removal of Other Device from Cranial Cavity, Open Approach
0WP130Z	Removal of Drainage Device from Cranial Cavity, Percutaneous Approach
0WP131Z	Removal of Radioactive Element from Cranial Cavity, Percutaneous Approach
0WP133Z	Removal of Infusion Device from Cranial Cavity, Percutaneous Approach
0WP13JZ	Removal of Synthetic Substitute from Cranial Cavity, Percutaneous Approach
0WP13YZ	Removal of Other Device from Cranial Cavity, Percutaneous Approach
0WP140Z	Removal of Drainage Device from Cranial Cavity, Percutaneous Endoscopic Approach

0WP141Z	Removal of Radioactive Element from Cranial Cavity, Percutaneous Endoscopic Approach
0WP143Z	Removal of Infusion Device from Cranial Cavity, Percutaneous Endoscopic Approach
0WP14JZ	Removal of Synthetic Substitute from Cranial Cavity, Percutaneous Endoscopic Approach
0WP14YZ	Removal of Other Device from Cranial Cavity, Percutaneous Endoscopic Approach
0WP1X0Z	Removal of Drainage Device from Cranial Cavity, External Approach
0WP1X1Z	Removal of Radioactive Element from Cranial Cavity, External Approach
0WP1X3Z	Removal of Infusion Device from Cranial Cavity, External Approach
0WP200Z	Removal of Drainage Device from Face, Open Approach
0WP201Z	Removal of Radioactive Element from Face, Open Approach
0WP203Z	Removal of Infusion Device from Face, Open Approach
0WP207Z	Removal of Autologous Tissue Substitute from Face, Open Approach
0WP20JZ	Removal of Synthetic Substitute from Face, Open Approach
0WP20KZ	Removal of Nonautologous Tissue Substitute from Face, Open Approach
0WP20YZ	Removal of Other Device from Face, Open Approach
0WP230Z	Removal of Drainage Device from Face, Percutaneous Approach
0WP231Z	Removal of Radioactive Element from Face, Percutaneous Approach
0WP233Z	Removal of Infusion Device from Face, Percutaneous Approach
0WP237Z	Removal of Autologous Tissue Substitute from Face, Percutaneous Approach
0WP23JZ	Removal of Synthetic Substitute from Face, Percutaneous Approach
0WP23KZ	Removal of Nonautologous Tissue Substitute from Face, Percutaneous Approach
0WP23YZ	Removal of Other Device from Face, Percutaneous Approach
0WP240Z	Removal of Drainage Device from Face, Percutaneous Endoscopic Approach
0WP241Z	Removal of Radioactive Element from Face, Percutaneous Endoscopic Approach
0WP243Z	Removal of Infusion Device from Face, Percutaneous Endoscopic Approach
0WP247Z	Removal of Autologous Tissue Substitute from Face, Percutaneous Endoscopic Approach
0WP24JZ	Removal of Synthetic Substitute from Face, Percutaneous Endoscopic Approach
0WP24KZ	Removal of Nonautologous Tissue Substitute from Face, Percutaneous Endoscopic Approach
0WP24YZ	Removal of Other Device from Face, Percutaneous Endoscopic Approach
0WP2X0Z	Removal of Drainage Device from Face, External Approach
0WP2X1Z	Removal of Radioactive Element from Face, External Approach
0WP2X3Z	Removal of Infusion Device from Face, External Approach
0WP2X7Z	Removal of Autologous Tissue Substitute from Face, External Approach
0WP2XJZ	Removal of Synthetic Substitute from Face, External Approach
0WP2XKZ	Removal of Nonautologous Tissue Substitute from Face, External Approach
0WP2XYZ	Removal of Other Device from Face, External Approach
0WP400Z	Removal of Drainage Device from Upper Jaw, Open Approach
0WP401Z	Removal of Radioactive Element from Upper Jaw, Open Approach
0WP403Z	Removal of Infusion Device from Upper Jaw, Open Approach
0WP407Z	Removal of Autologous Tissue Substitute from Upper Jaw, Open Approach

0WP40JZ Removal of Synthetic Substitute from Upper Jaw, Open Approach

0WP40KZ Removal of Nonautologous Tissue Substitute from Upper Jaw, Open Approach

0WP40YZ Removal of Other Device from Upper Jaw, Open Approach

0WP430Z Removal of Drainage Device from Upper Jaw, Percutaneous Approach

0WP431Z Removal of Radioactive Element from Upper Jaw, Percutaneous Approach

0WP433Z Removal of Infusion Device from Upper Jaw, Percutaneous Approach

0WP437Z Removal of Autologous Tissue Substitute from Upper Jaw, Percutaneous Approach

0WP43JZ Removal of Synthetic Substitute from Upper Jaw, Percutaneous Approach

0WP43KZ Removal of Nonautologous Tissue Substitute from Upper Jaw, Percutaneous Approach

0WP43YZ Removal of Other Device from Upper Jaw, Percutaneous Approach

0WP440Z Removal of Drainage Device from Upper Jaw, Percutaneous Endoscopic Approach

0WP441Z Removal of Radioactive Element from Upper Jaw, Percutaneous Endoscopic Approach

0WP443Z Removal of Infusion Device from Upper Jaw, Percutaneous Endoscopic Approach

0WP447Z Removal of Autologous Tissue Substitute from Upper Jaw, Percutaneous Endoscopic Approach

0WP44JZ Removal of Synthetic Substitute from Upper Jaw, Percutaneous Endoscopic Approach

0WP44KZ Removal of Nonautologous Tissue Substitute from Upper Jaw, Percutaneous Endoscopic Approach

0WP44YZ Removal of Other Device from Upper Jaw, Percutaneous Endoscopic Approach

0WP4X0Z Removal of Drainage Device from Upper Jaw, External Approach

0WP4X1Z Removal of Radioactive Element from Upper Jaw, External Approach

0WP4X3Z Removal of Infusion Device from Upper Jaw, External Approach

0WP4X7Z Removal of Autologous Tissue Substitute from Upper Jaw, External Approach

0WP4XJZ Removal of Synthetic Substitute from Upper Jaw, External Approach

0WP4XKZ Removal of Nonautologous Tissue Substitute from Upper Jaw, External Approach

0WP4XYZ Removal of Other Device from Upper Jaw, External Approach

0WP500Z Removal of Drainage Device from Lower Jaw, Open Approach

0WP501Z Removal of Radioactive Element from Lower Jaw, Open Approach

0WP503Z Removal of Infusion Device from Lower Jaw, Open Approach

0WP507Z Removal of Autologous Tissue Substitute from Lower Jaw, Open Approach

0WP50JZ Removal of Synthetic Substitute from Lower Jaw, Open Approach

0WP50KZ Removal of Nonautologous Tissue Substitute from Lower Jaw, Open Approach

0WP50YZ Removal of Other Device from Lower Jaw, Open Approach

0WP530Z Removal of Drainage Device from Lower Jaw, Percutaneous Approach

0WP531Z Removal of Radioactive Element from Lower Jaw, Percutaneous Approach

0WP533Z Removal of Infusion Device from Lower Jaw, Percutaneous Approach

0WP537Z Removal of Autologous Tissue Substitute from Lower Jaw, Percutaneous Approach

0WP53JZ Removal of Synthetic Substitute from Lower Jaw, Percutaneous Approach

0WP53KZ Removal of Nonautologous Tissue Substitute from Lower Jaw, Percutaneous Approach

0WP53YZ Removal of Other Device from Lower Jaw, Percutaneous Approach

0WP540Z Removal of Drainage Device from Lower Jaw, Percutaneous Endoscopic Approach

0WP541Z Removal of Radioactive Element from Lower Jaw, Percutaneous Endoscopic Approach

0WP543Z Removal of Infusion Device from Lower Jaw, Percutaneous Endoscopic Approach

0WP547Z Removal of Autologous Tissue Substitute from Lower Jaw, Percutaneous Endoscopic Approach

0WP54JZ Removal of Synthetic Substitute from Lower Jaw, Percutaneous Endoscopic Approach

0WP54KZ Removal of Nonautologous Tissue Substitute from Lower Jaw, Percutaneous Endoscopic Approach

0WP54YZ Removal of Other Device from Lower Jaw, Percutaneous Endoscopic Approach

0WP5X0Z Removal of Drainage Device from Lower Jaw, External Approach

0WP5X1Z Removal of Radioactive Element from Lower Jaw, External Approach

0WP5X3Z Removal of Infusion Device from Lower Jaw, External Approach

0WP5X7Z Removal of Autologous Tissue Substitute from Lower Jaw, External Approach

0WP5XJZ Removal of Synthetic Substitute from Lower Jaw, External Approach

0WP5XKZ Removal of Nonautologous Tissue Substitute from Lower Jaw, External Approach

0WP5XYZ Removal of Other Device from Lower Jaw, External Approach

0WP600Z Removal of Drainage Device from Neck, Open Approach

0WP601Z Removal of Radioactive Element from Neck, Open Approach

0WP603Z Removal of Infusion Device from Neck, Open Approach

0WP607Z Removal of Autologous Tissue Substitute from Neck, Open Approach

0WP60JZ Removal of Synthetic Substitute from Neck, Open Approach

0WP60KZ Removal of Nonautologous Tissue Substitute from Neck, Open Approach

0WP60YZ Removal of Other Device from Neck, Open Approach

0WP630Z Removal of Drainage Device from Neck, Percutaneous Approach

0WP631Z Removal of Radioactive Element from Neck, Percutaneous Approach

0WP633Z Removal of Infusion Device from Neck, Percutaneous Approach

0WP637Z Removal of Autologous Tissue Substitute from Neck, Percutaneous Approach

0WP63JZ Removal of Synthetic Substitute from Neck, Percutaneous Approach

0WP63KZ Removal of Nonautologous Tissue Substitute from Neck, Percutaneous Approach

0WP63YZ Removal of Other Device from Neck, Percutaneous Approach

0WP640Z Removal of Drainage Device from Neck, Percutaneous Endoscopic Approach

0WP641Z Removal of Radioactive Element from Neck, Percutaneous Endoscopic Approach

0WP643Z Removal of Infusion Device from Neck, Percutaneous Endoscopic Approach

0WP647Z Removal of Autologous Tissue Substitute from Neck, Percutaneous Endoscopic Approach

0WP64JZ Removal of Synthetic Substitute from Neck, Percutaneous Endoscopic Approach

0WP64KZ Removal of Nonautologous Tissue Substitute from Neck, Percutaneous Endoscopic Approach

0WP64YZ Removal of Other Device from Neck, Percutaneous Endoscopic Approach

0WP6X0Z Removal of Drainage Device from Neck, External Approach

0WP6X1Z Removal of Radioactive Element from Neck, External Approach

0WP6X3Z Removal of Infusion Device from Neck, External Approach

0WP6X7Z Removal of Autologous Tissue Substitute from Neck, External Approach

0WP6XJZ Removal of Synthetic Substitute from Neck, External Approach

0WP6XKZ Removal of Nonautologous Tissue Substitute from Neck, External Approach

0WP6XYZ Removal of Other Device from Neck, External Approach

0WP800Z Removal of Drainage Device from Chest Wall, Open Approach

0WP801Z Removal of Radioactive Element from Chest Wall, Open Approach

0WP803Z Removal of Infusion Device from Chest Wall, Open Approach

0WP807Z Removal of Autologous Tissue Substitute from Chest Wall, Open Approach

0WP80JZ Removal of Synthetic Substitute from Chest Wall, Open Approach

0WP80KZ Removal of Nonautologous Tissue Substitute from Chest Wall, Open Approach

0WP80YZ Removal of Other Device from Chest Wall, Open Approach

0WP830Z Removal of Drainage Device from Chest Wall, Percutaneous Approach

0WP831Z Removal of Radioactive Element from Chest Wall, Percutaneous Approach

0WP833Z Removal of Infusion Device from Chest Wall, Percutaneous Approach

0WP837Z Removal of Autologous Tissue Substitute from Chest Wall, Percutaneous Approach

0WP83JZ Removal of Synthetic Substitute from Chest Wall, Percutaneous Approach

0WP83KZ Removal of Nonautologous Tissue Substitute from Chest Wall, Percutaneous Approach

0WP83YZ Removal of Other Device from Chest Wall, Percutaneous Approach

0WP840Z Removal of Drainage Device from Chest Wall, Percutaneous Endoscopic Approach

0WP841Z Removal of Radioactive Element from Chest Wall, Percutaneous Endoscopic Approach

0WP843Z Removal of Infusion Device from Chest Wall, Percutaneous Endoscopic Approach

0WP847Z Removal of Autologous Tissue Substitute from Chest Wall, Percutaneous Endoscopic Approach

0WP84JZ Removal of Synthetic Substitute from Chest Wall, Percutaneous Endoscopic Approach

0WP84KZ Removal of Nonautologous Tissue Substitute from Chest Wall, Percutaneous Endoscopic Approach

0WP84YZ Removal of Other Device from Chest Wall, Percutaneous Endoscopic Approach

0WP8X0Z Removal of Drainage Device from Chest Wall, External Approach

0WP8X1Z Removal of Radioactive Element from Chest Wall, External Approach

0WP8X3Z Removal of Infusion Device from Chest Wall, External Approach

0WP8X7Z Removal of Autologous Tissue Substitute from Chest Wall, External Approach

0WP8XJZ Removal of Synthetic Substitute from Chest Wall, External Approach

0WP8XKZ Removal of Nonautologous Tissue Substitute from Chest Wall, External Approach

0WP8XYZ Removal of Other Device from Chest Wall, External Approach

0WP900Z Removal of Drainage Device from Right Pleural Cavity, Open Approach

0WP901Z Removal of Radioactive Element from Right Pleural Cavity, Open Approach

0WP903Z Removal of Infusion Device from Right Pleural Cavity, Open Approach

0WP90JZ Removal of Synthetic Substitute from Right Pleural Cavity, Open Approach

0WP90YZ Removal of Other Device from Right Pleural Cavity, Open Approach

0WP930Z Removal of Drainage Device from Right Pleural Cavity, Percutaneous Approach

0WP931Z Removal of Radioactive Element from Right Pleural Cavity, Percutaneous Approach

0WP933Z Removal of Infusion Device from Right Pleural Cavity, Percutaneous Approach

0WP93JZ Removal of Synthetic Substitute from Right Pleural Cavity, Percutaneous Approach

0WP93YZ Removal of Other Device from Right Pleural Cavity, Percutaneous Approach

0WP940Z Removal of Drainage Device from Right Pleural Cavity, Percutaneous Endoscopic Approach

0WP941Z Removal of Radioactive Element from Right Pleural Cavity, Percutaneous Endoscopic Approach

0WP943Z Removal of Infusion Device from Right Pleural Cavity, Percutaneous Endoscopic Approach

0WP94JZ Removal of Synthetic Substitute from Right Pleural Cavity, Percutaneous Endoscopic Approach

0WP94YZ Removal of Other Device from Right Pleural Cavity, Percutaneous Endoscopic Approach

0WP9X0Z Removal of Drainage Device from Right Pleural Cavity, External Approach

0WP9X1Z Removal of Radioactive Element from Right Pleural Cavity, External Approach

0WP9X3Z Removal of Infusion Device from Right Pleural Cavity, External Approach

0WPB00Z Removal of Drainage Device from Left Pleural Cavity, Open Approach

0WPB01Z Removal of Radioactive Element from Left Pleural Cavity, Open Approach

0WPB03Z Removal of Infusion Device from Left Pleural Cavity, Open Approach

0WPB0JZ Removal of Synthetic Substitute from Left Pleural Cavity, Open Approach

0WPB0YZ Removal of Other Device from Left Pleural Cavity, Open Approach

0WPB30Z Removal of Drainage Device from Left Pleural Cavity, Percutaneous Approach

0WPB31Z Removal of Radioactive Element from Left Pleural Cavity, Percutaneous Approach

0WPB33Z Removal of Infusion Device from Left Pleural Cavity, Percutaneous Approach

0WPB3JZ Removal of Synthetic Substitute from Left Pleural Cavity, Percutaneous Approach

0WPB3YZ Removal of Other Device from Left Pleural Cavity, Percutaneous Approach

0WPB40Z Removal of Drainage Device from Left Pleural Cavity, Percutaneous Endoscopic Approach

0WPB41Z Removal of Radioactive Element from Left Pleural Cavity, Percutaneous Endoscopic Approach

0WPB43Z Removal of Infusion Device from Left Pleural Cavity, Percutaneous Endoscopic Approach

0WPB4JZ Removal of Synthetic Substitute from Left Pleural Cavity, Percutaneous Endoscopic Approach

0WPB4YZ Removal of Other Device from Left Pleural Cavity, Percutaneous Endoscopic Approach

0WPBX0Z Removal of Drainage Device from Left Pleural Cavity, External Approach

0WPBX1Z Removal of Radioactive Element from Left Pleural Cavity, External Approach

0WPBX3Z Removal of Infusion Device from Left Pleural Cavity, External Approach

0WPC00Z Removal of Drainage Device from Mediastinum, Open Approach

0WPC01Z Removal of Radioactive Element from Mediastinum, Open Approach

0WPC03Z Removal of Infusion Device from Mediastinum, Open Approach

0WPC07Z Removal of Autologous Tissue Substitute from Mediastinum, Open Approach

0WPC0JZ Removal of Synthetic Substitute from Mediastinum, Open Approach

0WPC0KZ Removal of Nonautologous Tissue Substitute from Mediastinum, Open Approach

0WPC0YZ Removal of Other Device from Mediastinum, Open Approach

0WPC30Z Removal of Drainage Device from Mediastinum, Percutaneous Approach

0WPC31Z Removal of Radioactive Element from Mediastinum, Percutaneous Approach

0WPC33Z Removal of Infusion Device from Mediastinum, Percutaneous Approach

0WPC37Z Removal of Autologous Tissue Substitute from Mediastinum, Percutaneous Approach

0WPC3JZ Removal of Synthetic Substitute from Mediastinum, Percutaneous Approach

0WPC3KZ Removal of Nonautologous Tissue Substitute from Mediastinum, Percutaneous Approach

0WPC3YZ Removal of Other Device from Mediastinum, Percutaneous Approach

0WPC40Z Removal of Drainage Device from Mediastinum, Percutaneous Endoscopic Approach

0WPC41Z Removal of Radioactive Element from Mediastinum, Percutaneous Endoscopic Approach

0WPC43Z Removal of Infusion Device from Mediastinum, Percutaneous Endoscopic Approach

0WPC47Z Removal of Autologous Tissue Substitute from Mediastinum, Percutaneous Endoscopic Approach

0WPC4JZ Removal of Synthetic Substitute from Mediastinum, Percutaneous Endoscopic Approach

0WPC4KZ Removal of Nonautologous Tissue Substitute from Mediastinum, Percutaneous Endoscopic Approach

0WPC4YZ Removal of Other Device from Mediastinum, Percutaneous Endoscopic Approach

0WPCX0Z Removal of Drainage Device from Mediastinum, External Approach

0WPCX1Z Removal of Radioactive Element from Mediastinum, External Approach

0WPCX3Z Removal of Infusion Device from Mediastinum, External Approach

0WPCX7Z Removal of Autologous Tissue Substitute from Mediastinum, External Approach

0WPCXJZ Removal of Synthetic Substitute from Mediastinum, External Approach

0WPCXKZ Removal of Nonautologous Tissue Substitute from Mediastinum, External Approach

0WPCXYZ Removal of Other Device from Mediastinum, External Approach

0WPD00Z Removal of Drainage Device from Pericardial Cavity, Open Approach

0WPD01Z Removal of Radioactive Element from Pericardial Cavity, Open Approach

0WPD03Z Removal of Infusion Device from Pericardial Cavity, Open Approach

0WPD0YZ Removal of Other Device from Pericardial Cavity, Open Approach

0WPD30Z Removal of Drainage Device from Pericardial Cavity, Percutaneous Approach

0WPD31Z Removal of Radioactive Element from Pericardial Cavity, Percutaneous Approach

0WPD33Z Removal of Infusion Device from Pericardial Cavity, Percutaneous Approach

0WPD3YZ Removal of Other Device from Pericardial Cavity, Percutaneous Approach

0WPD40Z Removal of Drainage Device from Pericardial Cavity, Percutaneous Endoscopic Approach

0WPD41Z Removal of Radioactive Element from Pericardial Cavity, Percutaneous Endoscopic Approach

0WPD43Z Removal of Infusion Device from Pericardial Cavity, Percutaneous Endoscopic Approach

0WPD4YZ Removal of Other Device from Pericardial Cavity, Percutaneous Endoscopic Approach

0WPDX0Z Removal of Drainage Device from Pericardial Cavity, External Approach

0WPDX1Z Removal of Radioactive Element from Pericardial Cavity, External Approach

0WPDX3Z Removal of Infusion Device from Pericardial Cavity, External Approach

0WPF00Z Removal of Drainage Device from Abdominal Wall, Open Approach

0WPF01Z Removal of Radioactive Element from Abdominal Wall, Open Approach

0WPF03Z Removal of Infusion Device from Abdominal Wall, Open Approach

0WPF07Z Removal of Autologous Tissue Substitute from Abdominal Wall, Open Approach

0WPF0JZ Removal of Synthetic Substitute from Abdominal Wall, Open Approach

0WPF0KZ Removal of Nonautologous Tissue Substitute from Abdominal Wall, Open Approach

0WPF0YZ Removal of Other Device from Abdominal Wall, Open Approach

0WPF30Z Removal of Drainage Device from Abdominal Wall, Percutaneous Approach

0WPF31Z Removal of Radioactive Element from Abdominal Wall, Percutaneous Approach

0WPF33Z Removal of Infusion Device from Abdominal Wall, Percutaneous Approach

0WPF37Z Removal of Autologous Tissue Substitute from Abdominal Wall, Percutaneous Approach

0WPF3JZ Removal of Synthetic Substitute from Abdominal Wall, Percutaneous Approach

0WPF3KZ Removal of Nonautologous Tissue Substitute from Abdominal Wall, Percutaneous Approach

0WPF3YZ Removal of Other Device from Abdominal Wall, Percutaneous Approach

0WPF40Z Removal of Drainage Device from Abdominal Wall, Percutaneous Endoscopic Approach

0WPF41Z Removal of Radioactive Element from Abdominal Wall, Percutaneous Endoscopic Approach

0WPF43Z Removal of Infusion Device from Abdominal Wall, Percutaneous Endoscopic Approach

0WPF47Z Removal of Autologous Tissue Substitute from Abdominal Wall, Percutaneous Endoscopic Approach

0WPF4JZ Removal of Synthetic Substitute from Abdominal Wall, Percutaneous Endoscopic Approach

0WPF4KZ Removal of Nonautologous Tissue Substitute from Abdominal Wall, Percutaneous Endoscopic Approach

0WPF4YZ Removal of Other Device from Abdominal Wall, Percutaneous Endoscopic Approach

0WPFX0Z Removal of Drainage Device from Abdominal Wall, External Approach

0WPFX1Z Removal of Radioactive Element from Abdominal Wall, External Approach

0WPFX3Z Removal of Infusion Device from Abdominal Wall, External Approach

0WPFX7Z Removal of Autologous Tissue Substitute from Abdominal Wall, External Approach

0WPFXJZ Removal of Synthetic Substitute from Abdominal Wall, External Approach

0WPFXKZ Removal of Nonautologous Tissue Substitute from Abdominal Wall, External Approach

0WPFXYZ Removal of Other Device from Abdominal Wall, External Approach

0WPG00Z Removal of Drainage Device from Peritoneal Cavity, Open Approach

0WPG01Z Removal of Radioactive Element from Peritoneal Cavity, Open Approach

0WPG03Z Removal of Infusion Device from Peritoneal Cavity, Open Approach

0WPG0JZ Removal of Synthetic Substitute from Peritoneal Cavity, Open Approach

0WPG0YZ Removal of Other Device from Peritoneal Cavity, Open Approach

0WPG30Z Removal of Drainage Device from Peritoneal Cavity, Percutaneous Approach

0WPG31Z Removal of Radioactive Element from Peritoneal Cavity, Percutaneous Approach

0WPG33Z Removal of Infusion Device from Peritoneal Cavity, Percutaneous Approach

0WPG3JZ Removal of Synthetic Substitute from Peritoneal Cavity, Percutaneous Approach

0WPG3YZ Removal of Other Device from Peritoneal Cavity, Percutaneous Approach

0WPG40Z Removal of Drainage Device from Peritoneal Cavity, Percutaneous Endoscopic Approach

0WPG41Z Removal of Radioactive Element from Peritoneal Cavity, Percutaneous Endoscopic Approach

0WPG43Z Removal of Infusion Device from Peritoneal Cavity, Percutaneous Endoscopic Approach

0WPG4JZ Removal of Synthetic Substitute from Peritoneal Cavity, Percutaneous Endoscopic Approach

0WPG4YZ Removal of Other Device from Peritoneal Cavity, Percutaneous Endoscopic Approach

0WPGX0Z Removal of Drainage Device from Peritoneal Cavity, External Approach

0WPGX1Z Removal of Radioactive Element from Peritoneal Cavity, External Approach

0WPGX3Z Removal of Infusion Device from Peritoneal Cavity, External Approach

0WPH00Z Removal of Drainage Device from Retroperitoneum, Open Approach

0WPH01Z Removal of Radioactive Element from Retroperitoneum, Open Approach

0WPH03Z Removal of Infusion Device from Retroperitoneum, Open Approach

0WPH0YZ Removal of Other Device from Retroperitoneum, Open Approach

0WPH30Z Removal of Drainage Device from Retroperitoneum, Percutaneous Approach

0WPH31Z Removal of Radioactive Element from Retroperitoneum, Percutaneous Approach

0WPH33Z Removal of Infusion Device from Retroperitoneum, Percutaneous Approach

0WPH3YZ Removal of Other Device from Retroperitoneum, Percutaneous Approach

0WPH40Z Removal of Drainage Device from Retroperitoneum, Percutaneous Endoscopic Approach

0WPH41Z Removal of Radioactive Element from Retroperitoneum, Percutaneous Endoscopic Approach

0WPH43Z Removal of Infusion Device from Retroperitoneum, Percutaneous Endoscopic Approach

0WPH4YZ Removal of Other Device from Retroperitoneum, Percutaneous Endoscopic Approach

0WPHX0Z Removal of Drainage Device from Retroperitoneum, External Approach

0WPHX1Z Removal of Radioactive Element from Retroperitoneum, External Approach

0WPHX3Z Removal of Infusion Device from Retroperitoneum, External Approach

0WPJ00Z Removal of Drainage Device from Pelvic Cavity, Open Approach

0WPJ01Z Removal of Radioactive Element from Pelvic Cavity, Open Approach

0WPJ03Z Removal of Infusion Device from Pelvic Cavity, Open Approach

0WPJ0JZ Removal of Synthetic Substitute from Pelvic Cavity, Open Approach

0WPJ0YZ Removal of Other Device from Pelvic Cavity, Open Approach

0WPJ30Z Removal of Drainage Device from Pelvic Cavity, Percutaneous Approach

0WPJ31Z Removal of Radioactive Element from Pelvic Cavity, Percutaneous Approach

0WPJ33Z Removal of Infusion Device from Pelvic Cavity, Percutaneous Approach

0WPJ3JZ Removal of Synthetic Substitute from Pelvic Cavity, Percutaneous Approach

0WPJ3YZ Removal of Other Device from Pelvic Cavity, Percutaneous Approach

0WPJ40Z Removal of Drainage Device from Pelvic Cavity, Percutaneous Endoscopic Approach

0WPJ41Z Removal of Radioactive Element from Pelvic Cavity, Percutaneous Endoscopic Approach

0WPJ43Z Removal of Infusion Device from Pelvic Cavity, Percutaneous Endoscopic Approach

0WPJ4JZ Removal of Synthetic Substitute from Pelvic Cavity, Percutaneous Endoscopic Approach

0WPJ4YZ Removal of Other Device from Pelvic Cavity, Percutaneous Endoscopic Approach

0WPJX0Z Removal of Drainage Device from Pelvic Cavity, External Approach

0WPJX1Z Removal of Radioactive Element from Pelvic Cavity, External Approach

0WPJX3Z Removal of Infusion Device from Pelvic Cavity, External Approach

0WPK00Z Removal of Drainage Device from Upper Back, Open Approach

0WPK01Z Removal of Radioactive Element from Upper Back, Open Approach

0WPK03Z Removal of Infusion Device from Upper Back, Open Approach

0WPK07Z Removal of Autologous Tissue Substitute from Upper Back, Open Approach

0WPK0JZ Removal of Synthetic Substitute from Upper Back, Open Approach

0WPK0KZ Removal of Nonautologous Tissue Substitute from Upper Back, Open Approach

0WPK0YZ Removal of Other Device from Upper Back, Open Approach

0WPK30Z Removal of Drainage Device from Upper Back, Percutaneous Approach

0WPK31Z Removal of Radioactive Element from Upper Back, Percutaneous Approach

0WPK33Z Removal of Infusion Device from Upper Back, Percutaneous Approach

0WPK37Z Removal of Autologous Tissue Substitute from Upper Back, Percutaneous Approach

0WPK3JZ Removal of Synthetic Substitute from Upper Back, Percutaneous Approach

0WPK3KZ Removal of Nonautologous Tissue Substitute from Upper Back, Percutaneous Approach

0WPK3YZ Removal of Other Device from Upper Back, Percutaneous Approach

0WPK40Z Removal of Drainage Device from Upper Back, Percutaneous Endoscopic Approach

0WPK41Z Removal of Radioactive Element from Upper Back, Percutaneous Endoscopic Approach

0WPK43Z Removal of Infusion Device from Upper Back, Percutaneous Endoscopic Approach

0WPK47Z Removal of Autologous Tissue Substitute from Upper Back, Percutaneous Endoscopic Approach

0WPK4JZ Removal of Synthetic Substitute from Upper Back, Percutaneous Endoscopic Approach

0WPK4KZ Removal of Nonautologous Tissue Substitute from Upper Back, Percutaneous Endoscopic Approach

0WPK4YZ Removal of Other Device from Upper Back, Percutaneous Endoscopic Approach

0WPKX0Z Removal of Drainage Device from Upper Back, External Approach

0WPKX1Z Removal of Radioactive Element from Upper Back, External Approach

0WPKX3Z Removal of Infusion Device from Upper Back, External Approach

0WPKX7Z Removal of Autologous Tissue Substitute from Upper Back, External Approach

0WPKXJZ Removal of Synthetic Substitute from Upper Back, External Approach

0WPKXKZ Removal of Nonautologous Tissue Substitute from Upper Back, External Approach

0WPKXYZ Removal of Other Device from Upper Back, External Approach

0WPL00Z Removal of Drainage Device from Lower Back, Open Approach

0WPL01Z Removal of Radioactive Element from Lower Back, Open Approach

0WPL03Z Removal of Infusion Device from Lower Back, Open Approach

0WPL07Z Removal of Autologous Tissue Substitute from Lower Back, Open Approach

0WPL0JZ Removal of Synthetic Substitute from Lower Back, Open Approach

0WPL0KZ Removal of Nonautologous Tissue Substitute from Lower Back, Open Approach

0WPL0YZ Removal of Other Device from Lower Back, Open Approach

0WPL30Z Removal of Drainage Device from Lower Back, Percutaneous Approach

0WPL31Z Removal of Radioactive Element from Lower Back, Percutaneous Approach

0WPL33Z Removal of Infusion Device from Lower Back, Percutaneous Approach

0WPL37Z Removal of Autologous Tissue Substitute from Lower Back, Percutaneous Approach

0WPL3JZ Removal of Synthetic Substitute from Lower Back, Percutaneous Approach

0WPL3KZ Removal of Nonautologous Tissue Substitute from Lower Back, Percutaneous Approach

0WPL3YZ Removal of Other Device from Lower Back, Percutaneous Approach

0WPL40Z Removal of Drainage Device from Lower Back, Percutaneous Endoscopic Approach

0WPL41Z Removal of Radioactive Element from Lower Back, Percutaneous Endoscopic Approach

0WPL43Z Removal of Infusion Device from Lower Back, Percutaneous Endoscopic Approach

0WPL47Z Removal of Autologous Tissue Substitute from Lower Back, Percutaneous Endoscopic Approach

0WPL4JZ Removal of Synthetic Substitute from Lower Back, Percutaneous Endoscopic Approach

0WPL4KZ Removal of Nonautologous Tissue Substitute from Lower Back, Percutaneous Endoscopic Approach

0WPL4YZ Removal of Other Device from Lower Back, Percutaneous Endoscopic Approach

0WPLX0Z Removal of Drainage Device from Lower Back, External Approach

0WPLX1Z Removal of Radioactive Element from Lower Back, External Approach

0WPLX3Z Removal of Infusion Device from Lower Back, External Approach

0WPLX7Z Removal of Autologous Tissue Substitute from Lower Back, External Approach

0WPLXJZ Removal of Synthetic Substitute from Lower Back, External Approach

0WPLXKZ Removal of Nonautologous Tissue Substitute from Lower Back, External Approach

0WPLXYZ Removal of Other Device from Lower Back, External Approach

♂ **0WPM00Z** Removal of Drainage Device from Male Perineum, Open Approach

♂ **0WPM01Z** Removal of Radioactive Element from Male Perineum, Open Approach

♂ **0WPM03Z** Removal of Infusion Device from Male Perineum, Open Approach

♂ **0WPM07Z** Removal of Autologous Tissue Substitute from Male Perineum, Open Approach

♂ **0WPM0JZ** Removal of Synthetic Substitute from Male Perineum, Open Approach

♂ **0WPM0KZ** Removal of Nonautologous Tissue Substitute from Male Perineum, Open Approach

♂ **0WPM0YZ** Removal of Other Device from Male Perineum, Open Approach
♂ **0WPM30Z** Removal of Drainage Device from Male Perineum, Percutaneous Approach
♂ **0WPM31Z** Removal of Radioactive Element from Male Perineum, Percutaneous Approach
♂ **0WPM33Z** Removal of Infusion Device from Male Perineum, Percutaneous Approach
♂ **0WPM37Z** Removal of Autologous Tissue Substitute from Male Perineum, Percutaneous Approach
♂ **0WPM3JZ** Removal of Synthetic Substitute from Male Perineum, Percutaneous Approach
♂ **0WPM3KZ** Removal of Nonautologous Tissue Substitute from Male Perineum, Percutaneous Approach
♂ **0WPM3YZ** Removal of Other Device from Male Perineum, Percutaneous Approach
♂ **0WPM40Z** Removal of Drainage Device from Male Perineum, Percutaneous Endoscopic Approach
♂ **0WPM41Z** Removal of Radioactive Element from Male Perineum, Percutaneous Endoscopic Approach
♂ **0WPM43Z** Removal of Infusion Device from Male Perineum, Percutaneous Endoscopic Approach
♂ **0WPM47Z** Removal of Autologous Tissue Substitute from Male Perineum, Percutaneous Endoscopic Approach
♂ **0WPM4JZ** Removal of Synthetic Substitute from Male Perineum, Percutaneous Endoscopic Approach
♂ **0WPM4KZ** Removal of Nonautologous Tissue Substitute from Male Perineum, Percutaneous Endoscopic Approach
♂ **0WPM4YZ** Removal of Other Device from Male Perineum, Percutaneous Endoscopic Approach
♂ **0WPMX0Z** Removal of Drainage Device from Male Perineum, External Approach
♂ **0WPMX1Z** Removal of Radioactive Element from Male Perineum, External Approach
♂ **0WPMX3Z** Removal of Infusion Device from Male Perineum, External Approach
♂ **0WPMX7Z** Removal of Autologous Tissue Substitute from Male Perineum, External Approach
♂ **0WPMXJZ** Removal of Synthetic Substitute from Male Perineum, External Approach
♂ **0WPMXKZ** Removal of Nonautologous Tissue Substitute from Male Perineum, External Approach
♂ **0WPMXYZ** Removal of Other Device from Male Perineum, External Approach
♀ **0WPN00Z** Removal of Drainage Device from Female Perineum, Open Approach
♀ **0WPN01Z** Removal of Radioactive Element from Female Perineum, Open Approach
♀ **0WPN03Z** Removal of Infusion Device from Female Perineum, Open Approach
♀ **0WPN07Z** Removal of Autologous Tissue Substitute from Female Perineum, Open Approach
♀ **0WPN0JZ** Removal of Synthetic Substitute from Female Perineum, Open Approach
♀ **0WPN0KZ** Removal of Nonautologous Tissue Substitute from Female Perineum, Open Approach
♀ **0WPN0YZ** Removal of Other Device from Female Perineum, Open Approach
♀ **0WPN30Z** Removal of Drainage Device from Female Perineum, Percutaneous Approach
♀ **0WPN31Z** Removal of Radioactive Element from Female Perineum, Percutaneous Approach
♀ **0WPN33Z** Removal of Infusion Device from Female Perineum, Percutaneous Approach
♀ **0WPN37Z** Removal of Autologous Tissue Substitute from Female Perineum, Percutaneous Approach
♀ **0WPN3JZ** Removal of Synthetic Substitute from Female Perineum, Percutaneous Approach
♀ **0WPN3KZ** Removal of Nonautologous Tissue Substitute from Female Perineum, Percutaneous Approach
♀ **0WPN3YZ** Removal of Other Device from Female Perineum, Percutaneous Approach
♀ **0WPN40Z** Removal of Drainage Device from Female Perineum, Percutaneous Endoscopic Approach
♀ **0WPN41Z** Removal of Radioactive Element from Female Perineum, Percutaneous Endoscopic Approach

♀ **0WPN43Z** Removal of Infusion Device from Female Perineum, Percutaneous Endoscopic Approach
♀ **0WPN47Z** Removal of Autologous Tissue Substitute from Female Perineum, Percutaneous Endoscopic Approach
♀ **0WPN4JZ** Removal of Synthetic Substitute from Female Perineum, Percutaneous Endoscopic Approach
♀ **0WPN4KZ** Removal of Nonautologous Tissue Substitute from Female Perineum, Percutaneous Endoscopic Approach
♀ **0WPN4YZ** Removal of Other Device from Female Perineum, Percutaneous Endoscopic Approach
♀ **0WPNX0Z** Removal of Drainage Device from Female Perineum, External Approach
♀ **0WPNX1Z** Removal of Radioactive Element from Female Perineum, External Approach
♀ **0WPNX3Z** Removal of Infusion Device from Female Perineum, External Approach
♀ **0WPNX7Z** Removal of Autologous Tissue Substitute from Female Perineum, External Approach
♀ **0WPNXJZ** Removal of Synthetic Substitute from Female Perineum, External Approach
♀ **0WPNXKZ** Removal of Nonautologous Tissue Substitute from Female Perineum, External Approach
♀ **0WPNXYZ** Removal of Other Device from Female Perineum, External Approach
0WPP01Z Removal of Radioactive Element from Gastrointestinal Tract, Open Approach
0WPP03Z Removal of Infusion Device from Gastrointestinal Tract, Open Approach
0WPP0YZ Removal of Other Device from Gastrointestinal Tract, Open Approach
0WPP31Z Removal of Radioactive Element from Gastrointestinal Tract, Percutaneous Approach
0WPP33Z Removal of Infusion Device from Gastrointestinal Tract, Percutaneous Approach
0WPP3YZ Removal of Other Device from Gastrointestinal Tract, Percutaneous Approach
0WPP41Z Removal of Radioactive Element from Gastrointestinal Tract, Percutaneous Endoscopic Approach
0WPP43Z Removal of Infusion Device from Gastrointestinal Tract, Percutaneous Endoscopic Approach
0WPP4YZ Removal of Other Device from Gastrointestinal Tract, Percutaneous Endoscopic Approach
0WPP71Z Removal of Radioactive Element from Gastrointestinal Tract, Via Natural or Artificial Opening
0WPP73Z Removal of Infusion Device from Gastrointestinal Tract, Via Natural or Artificial Opening
0WPP7YZ Removal of Other Device from Gastrointestinal Tract, Via Natural or Artificial Opening
0WPP81Z Removal of Radioactive Element from Gastrointestinal Tract, Via Natural or Artificial Opening Endoscopic
0WPP83Z Removal of Infusion Device from Gastrointestinal Tract, Via Natural or Artificial Opening Endoscopic
0WPP8YZ Removal of Other Device from Gastrointestinal Tract, Via Natural or Artificial Opening Endoscopic
0WPPX1Z Removal of Radioactive Element from Gastrointestinal Tract, External Approach
0WPPX3Z Removal of Infusion Device from Gastrointestinal Tract, External Approach
0WPPXYZ Removal of Other Device from Gastrointestinal Tract, External Approach
0WPQ01Z Removal of Radioactive Element from Respiratory Tract, Open Approach
0WPQ03Z Removal of Infusion Device from Respiratory Tract, Open Approach
0WPQ0YZ Removal of Other Device from Respiratory Tract, Open Approach
0WPQ31Z Removal of Radioactive Element from Respiratory Tract, Percutaneous Approach
0WPQ33Z Removal of Infusion Device from Respiratory Tract, Percutaneous Approach
0WPQ3YZ Removal of Other Device from Respiratory Tract, Percutaneous Approach
0WPQ41Z Removal of Radioactive Element from Respiratory Tract, Percutaneous Endoscopic Approach

0WPQ43Z	Removal of Infusion Device from Respiratory Tract, Percutaneous Endoscopic Approach
0WPQ4YZ	Removal of Other Device from Respiratory Tract, Percutaneous Endoscopic Approach
0WPQ71Z	Removal of Radioactive Element from Respiratory Tract, Via Natural or Artificial Opening
0WPQ73Z	Removal of Infusion Device from Respiratory Tract, Via Natural or Artificial Opening
0WPQ7YZ	Removal of Other Device from Respiratory Tract, Via Natural or Artificial Opening
0WPQ81Z	Removal of Radioactive Element from Respiratory Tract, Via Natural or Artificial Opening Endoscopic
0WPQ83Z	Removal of Infusion Device from Respiratory Tract, Via Natural or Artificial Opening Endoscopic
0WPQ8YZ	Removal of Other Device from Respiratory Tract, Via Natural or Artificial Opening Endoscopic
0WPQX1Z	Removal of Radioactive Element from Respiratory Tract, External Approach
0WPQX3Z	Removal of Infusion Device from Respiratory Tract, External Approach
0WPQXYZ	Removal of Other Device from Respiratory Tract, External Approach
0WPR01Z	Removal of Radioactive Element from Genitourinary Tract, Open Approach
0WPR03Z	Removal of Infusion Device from Genitourinary Tract, Open Approach
0WPR0YZ	Removal of Other Device from Genitourinary Tract, Open Approach
0WPR31Z	Removal of Radioactive Element from Genitourinary Tract, Percutaneous Approach

0WPR33Z	Removal of Infusion Device from Genitourinary Tract, Percutaneous Approach
0WPR3YZ	Removal of Other Device from Genitourinary Tract, Percutaneous Approach
0WPR41Z	Removal of Radioactive Element from Genitourinary Tract, Percutaneous Endoscopic Approach
0WPR43Z	Removal of Infusion Device from Genitourinary Tract, Percutaneous Endoscopic Approach
0WPR4YZ	Removal of Other Device from Genitourinary Tract, Percutaneous Endoscopic Approach
0WPR71Z	Removal of Radioactive Element from Genitourinary Tract, Via Natural or Artificial Opening
0WPR73Z	Removal of Infusion Device from Genitourinary Tract, Via Natural or Artificial Opening
0WPR7YZ	Removal of Other Device from Genitourinary Tract, Via Natural or Artificial Opening
0WPR81Z	Removal of Radioactive Element from Genitourinary Tract, Via Natural or Artificial Opening Endoscopic
0WPR83Z	Removal of Infusion Device from Genitourinary Tract, Via Natural or Artificial Opening Endoscopic
0WPR8YZ	Removal of Other Device from Genitourinary Tract, Via Natural or Artificial Opening Endoscopic
0WPRX1Z	Removal of Radioactive Element from Genitourinary Tract, External Approach
0WPRX3Z	Removal of Infusion Device from Genitourinary Tract, External Approach
0WPRXYZ	Removal of Other Device from Genitourinary Tract, External Approach

0WQ – Anatomical Regions, General, Repair

0WQ00ZZ	Repair Head, Open Approach
0WQ03ZZ	Repair Head, Percutaneous Approach
0WQ04ZZ	Repair Head, Percutaneous Endoscopic Approach
0WQ0XZZ	Repair Head, External Approach
0WQ20ZZ	Repair Face, Open Approach
0WQ23ZZ	Repair Face, Percutaneous Approach
0WQ24ZZ	Repair Face, Percutaneous Endoscopic Approach
0WQ2XZZ	Repair Face, External Approach
0WQ40ZZ	Repair Upper Jaw, Open Approach
0WQ43ZZ	Repair Upper Jaw, Percutaneous Approach
0WQ44ZZ	Repair Upper Jaw, Percutaneous Endoscopic Approach
0WQ4XZZ	Repair Upper Jaw, External Approach
0WQ50ZZ	Repair Lower Jaw, Open Approach
0WQ53ZZ	Repair Lower Jaw, Percutaneous Approach
0WQ54ZZ	Repair Lower Jaw, Percutaneous Endoscopic Approach
0WQ5XZZ	Repair Lower Jaw, External Approach
0WQ60ZZ	Repair Neck, Open Approach
0WQ63ZZ	Repair Neck, Percutaneous Approach
0WQ64ZZ	Repair Neck, Percutaneous Endoscopic Approach
0WQ6XZ2	Repair Neck, Stoma, External Approach
0WQ6XZZ	Repair Neck, External Approach
0WQ80ZZ	Repair Chest Wall, Open Approach
0WQ83ZZ	Repair Chest Wall, Percutaneous Approach
0WQ84ZZ	Repair Chest Wall, Percutaneous Endoscopic Approach
0WQ8XZZ	Repair Chest Wall, External Approach
0WQC0ZZ	Repair Mediastinum, Open Approach
0WQC3ZZ	Repair Mediastinum, Percutaneous Approach
0WQC4ZZ	Repair Mediastinum, Percutaneous Endoscopic Approach
0WQF0ZZ	Repair Abdominal Wall, Open Approach

0WQF3ZZ	Repair Abdominal Wall, Percutaneous Approach
0WQF4ZZ	Repair Abdominal Wall, Percutaneous Endoscopic Approach
0WQFXZ2	Repair Abdominal Wall, Stoma, External Approach
0WQFXZZ	Repair Abdominal Wall, External Approach
0WQK0ZZ	Repair Upper Back, Open Approach
0WQK3ZZ	Repair Upper Back, Percutaneous Approach
0WQK4ZZ	Repair Upper Back, Percutaneous Endoscopic Approach
0WQKXZZ	Repair Upper Back, External Approach
0WQL0ZZ	Repair Lower Back, Open Approach
0WQL3ZZ	Repair Lower Back, Percutaneous Approach
0WQL4ZZ	Repair Lower Back, Percutaneous Endoscopic Approach
0WQLXZZ	Repair Lower Back, External Approach
♂ **0WQM0ZZ**	Repair Male Perineum, Open Approach *This is a male-only service, however, it is not included in the male-only edit logic for MCE V30*
♂ **0WQM3ZZ**	Repair Male Perineum, Percutaneous Approach *This is a male-only service, however, it is not included in the male-only edit logic for MCE V30*
♂ **0WQM4ZZ**	Repair Male Perineum, Percutaneous Endoscopic Approach *This is a male-only service, however, it is not included in the male-only edit logic for MCE V30*
♂ **0WQMXZZ**	Repair Male Perineum, External Approach *This is a male-only service, however, it is not included in the male-only edit logic for MCE V30*
♀ **0WQN0ZZ**	Repair Female Perineum, Open Approach
♀ **0WQN3ZZ**	Repair Female Perineum, Percutaneous Approach
♀ **0WQN4ZZ**	Repair Female Perineum, Percutaneous Endoscopic Approach
♀ **0WQNXZZ**	Repair Female Perineum, External Approach

0WU – Anatomical Regions, General, Supplement

0WU007Z	Supplement Head with Autologous Tissue Substitute, Open Approach
0WU00JZ	Supplement Head with Synthetic Substitute, Open Approach
0WU00KZ	Supplement Head with Nonautologous Tissue Substitute, Open Approach
0WU047Z	Supplement Head with Autologous Tissue Substitute, Percutaneous Endoscopic Approach

0WU04JZ	Supplement Head with Synthetic Substitute, Percutaneous Endoscopic Approach
0WU04KZ	Supplement Head with Nonautologous Tissue Substitute, Percutaneous Endoscopic Approach
0WU207Z	Supplement Face with Autologous Tissue Substitute, Open Approach
0WU20JZ	Supplement Face with Synthetic Substitute, Open Approach
0WU20KZ	Supplement Face with Nonautologous Tissue Substitute, Open Approach

0WU247Z	Supplement Face with Autologous Tissue Substitute, Percutaneous Endoscopic Approach
0WU24JZ	Supplement Face with Synthetic Substitute, Percutaneous Endoscopic Approach
0WU24KZ	Supplement Face with Nonautologous Tissue Substitute, Percutaneous Endoscopic Approach
0WU407Z	Supplement Upper Jaw with Autologous Tissue Substitute, Open Approach
0WU40JZ	Supplement Upper Jaw with Synthetic Substitute, Open Approach
0WU40KZ	Supplement Upper Jaw with Nonautologous Tissue Substitute, Open Approach
0WU447Z	Supplement Upper Jaw with Autologous Tissue Substitute, Percutaneous Endoscopic Approach
0WU44JZ	Supplement Upper Jaw with Synthetic Substitute, Percutaneous Endoscopic Approach
0WU44KZ	Supplement Upper Jaw with Nonautologous Tissue Substitute, Percutaneous Endoscopic Approach
0WU507Z	Supplement Lower Jaw with Autologous Tissue Substitute, Open Approach
0WU50JZ	Supplement Lower Jaw with Synthetic Substitute, Open Approach
0WU50KZ	Supplement Lower Jaw with Nonautologous Tissue Substitute, Open Approach
0WU547Z	Supplement Lower Jaw with Autologous Tissue Substitute, Percutaneous Endoscopic Approach
0WU54JZ	Supplement Lower Jaw with Synthetic Substitute, Percutaneous Endoscopic Approach
0WU54KZ	Supplement Lower Jaw with Nonautologous Tissue Substitute, Percutaneous Endoscopic Approach
0WU607Z	Supplement Neck with Autologous Tissue Substitute, Open Approach
0WU60JZ	Supplement Neck with Synthetic Substitute, Open Approach
0WU60KZ	Supplement Neck with Nonautologous Tissue Substitute, Open Approach
0WU647Z	Supplement Neck with Autologous Tissue Substitute, Percutaneous Endoscopic Approach
0WU64JZ	Supplement Neck with Synthetic Substitute, Percutaneous Endoscopic Approach
0WU64KZ	Supplement Neck with Nonautologous Tissue Substitute, Percutaneous Endoscopic Approach
0WU807Z	Supplement Chest Wall with Autologous Tissue Substitute, Open Approach
0WU80JZ	Supplement Chest Wall with Synthetic Substitute, Open Approach
0WU80KZ	Supplement Chest Wall with Nonautologous Tissue Substitute, Open Approach
0WU847Z	Supplement Chest Wall with Autologous Tissue Substitute, Percutaneous Endoscopic Approach
0WU84JZ	Supplement Chest Wall with Synthetic Substitute, Percutaneous Endoscopic Approach
0WU84KZ	Supplement Chest Wall with Nonautologous Tissue Substitute, Percutaneous Endoscopic Approach
0WUC07Z	Supplement Mediastinum with Autologous Tissue Substitute, Open Approach
0WUC0JZ	Supplement Mediastinum with Synthetic Substitute, Open Approach
0WUC0KZ	Supplement Mediastinum with Nonautologous Tissue Substitute, Open Approach
0WUC47Z	Supplement Mediastinum with Autologous Tissue Substitute, Percutaneous Endoscopic Approach
0WUC4JZ	Supplement Mediastinum with Synthetic Substitute, Percutaneous Endoscopic Approach

0WUC4KZ	Supplement Mediastinum with Nonautologous Tissue Substitute, Percutaneous Endoscopic Approach
0WUF07Z	Supplement Abdominal Wall with Autologous Tissue Substitute, Open Approach
0WUF0JZ	Supplement Abdominal Wall with Synthetic Substitute, Open Approach
0WUF0KZ	Supplement Abdominal Wall with Nonautologous Tissue Substitute, Open Approach
0WUF47Z	Supplement Abdominal Wall with Autologous Tissue Substitute, Percutaneous Endoscopic Approach
0WUF4JZ	Supplement Abdominal Wall with Synthetic Substitute, Percutaneous Endoscopic Approach
0WUF4KZ	Supplement Abdominal Wall with Nonautologous Tissue Substitute, Percutaneous Endoscopic Approach
0WUK07Z	Supplement Upper Back with Autologous Tissue Substitute, Open Approach
0WUK0JZ	Supplement Upper Back with Synthetic Substitute, Open Approach
0WUK0KZ	Supplement Upper Back with Nonautologous Tissue Substitute, Open Approach
0WUK47Z	Supplement Upper Back with Autologous Tissue Substitute, Percutaneous Endoscopic Approach
0WUK4JZ	Supplement Upper Back with Synthetic Substitute, Percutaneous Endoscopic Approach
0WUK4KZ	Supplement Upper Back with Nonautologous Tissue Substitute, Percutaneous Endoscopic Approach
0WUL07Z	Supplement Lower Back with Autologous Tissue Substitute, Open Approach
0WUL0JZ	Supplement Lower Back with Synthetic Substitute, Open Approach
0WUL0KZ	Supplement Lower Back with Nonautologous Tissue Substitute, Open Approach
0WUL47Z	Supplement Lower Back with Autologous Tissue Substitute, Percutaneous Endoscopic Approach
0WUL4JZ	Supplement Lower Back with Synthetic Substitute, Percutaneous Endoscopic Approach
0WUL4KZ	Supplement Lower Back with Nonautologous Tissue Substitute, Percutaneous Endoscopic Approach
♂ **0WUM07Z**	Supplement Male Perineum with Autologous Tissue Substitute, Open Approach
♂ **0WUM0JZ**	Supplement Male Perineum with Synthetic Substitute, Open Approach
♂ **0WUM0KZ**	Supplement Male Perineum with Nonautologous Tissue Substitute, Open Approach
♂ **0WUM47Z**	Supplement Male Perineum with Autologous Tissue Substitute, Percutaneous Endoscopic Approach
♂ **0WUM4JZ**	Supplement Male Perineum with Synthetic Substitute, Percutaneous Endoscopic Approach
♂ **0WUM4KZ**	Supplement Male Perineum with Nonautologous Tissue Substitute, Percutaneous Endoscopic Approach
♀ **0WUN07Z**	Supplement Female Perineum with Autologous Tissue Substitute, Open Approach
♀ **0WUN0JZ**	Supplement Female Perineum with Synthetic Substitute, Open Approach
♀ **0WUN0KZ**	Supplement Female Perineum with Nonautologous Tissue Substitute, Open Approach
♀ **0WUN47Z**	Supplement Female Perineum with Autologous Tissue Substitute, Percutaneous Endoscopic Approach
♀ **0WUN4JZ**	Supplement Female Perineum with Synthetic Substitute, Percutaneous Endoscopic Approach
♀ **0WUN4KZ**	Supplement Female Perineum with Nonautologous Tissue Substitute, Percutaneous Endoscopic Approach

0WW – Anatomical Regions, General, Revision

Review Coding Guideline B6.1c

● **0WW000Z**	Revision of Drainage Device in Head, Open Approach
● **0WW001Z**	Revision of Radioactive Element in Head, Open Approach
● **0WW003Z**	Revision of Infusion Device in Head, Open Approach
● **0WW007Z**	Revision of Autologous Tissue Substitute in Head, Open Approach
● **0WW00JZ**	Revision of Synthetic Substitute in Head, Open Approach

● **0WW00KZ**	Revision of Nonautologous Tissue Substitute in Head, Open Approach
● **0WW00YZ**	Revision of Other Device in Head, Open Approach
● **0WW030Z**	Revision of Drainage Device in Head, Percutaneous Approach
● **0WW031Z**	Revision of Radioactive Element in Head, Percutaneous Approach

---

♀ Female-only   ♂ Male-only   ● Limited Coverage   ● Non-OR   ▨ HAC-associated procedure   ● Non-covered procedures   ✚ Combination

● 0WW033Z   Revision of Infusion Device in Head, Percutaneous Approach
● 0WW037Z   Revision of Autologous Tissue Substitute in Head, Percutaneous Approach
● 0WW03JZ   Revision of Synthetic Substitute in Head, Percutaneous Approach
● 0WW03KZ   Revision of Nonautologous Tissue Substitute in Head, Percutaneous Approach
● 0WW03YZ   Revision of Other Device in Head, Percutaneous Approach
● 0WW040Z   Revision of Drainage Device in Head, Percutaneous Endoscopic Approach
● 0WW041Z   Revision of Radioactive Element in Head, Percutaneous Endoscopic Approach
● 0WW043Z   Revision of Infusion Device in Head, Percutaneous Endoscopic Approach
● 0WW047Z   Revision of Autologous Tissue Substitute in Head, Percutaneous Endoscopic Approach
● 0WW04JZ   Revision of Synthetic Substitute in Head, Percutaneous Endoscopic Approach
● 0WW04KZ   Revision of Nonautologous Tissue Substitute in Head, Percutaneous Endoscopic Approach
● 0WW04YZ   Revision of Other Device in Head, Percutaneous Endoscopic Approach
0WW0X0Z   Revision of Drainage Device in Head, External Approach
0WW0X1Z   Revision of Radioactive Element in Head, External Approach
0WW0X3Z   Revision of Infusion Device in Head, External Approach
0WW0X7Z   Revision of Autologous Tissue Substitute in Head, External Approach
0WW0XJZ   Revision of Synthetic Substitute in Head, External Approach
0WW0XKZ   Revision of Nonautologous Tissue Substitute in Head, External Approach
0WW0XYZ   Revision of Other Device in Head, External Approach
0WW100Z   Revision of Drainage Device in Cranial Cavity, Open Approach
0WW101Z   Revision of Radioactive Element in Cranial Cavity, Open Approach
0WW103Z   Revision of Infusion Device in Cranial Cavity, Open Approach
0WW10JZ   Revision of Synthetic Substitute in Cranial Cavity, Open Approach
0WW10YZ   Revision of Other Device in Cranial Cavity, Open Approach
0WW130Z   Revision of Drainage Device in Cranial Cavity, Percutaneous Approach
0WW131Z   Revision of Radioactive Element in Cranial Cavity, Percutaneous Approach
0WW133Z   Revision of Infusion Device in Cranial Cavity, Percutaneous Approach
0WW13JZ   Revision of Synthetic Substitute in Cranial Cavity, Percutaneous Approach
0WW13YZ   Revision of Other Device in Cranial Cavity, Percutaneous Approach
0WW140Z   Revision of Drainage Device in Cranial Cavity, Percutaneous Endoscopic Approach
0WW141Z   Revision of Radioactive Element in Cranial Cavity, Percutaneous Endoscopic Approach
0WW143Z   Revision of Infusion Device in Cranial Cavity, Percutaneous Endoscopic Approach
0WW14JZ   Revision of Synthetic Substitute in Cranial Cavity, Percutaneous Endoscopic Approach
0WW14YZ   Revision of Other Device in Cranial Cavity, Percutaneous Endoscopic Approach
0WW1X0Z   Revision of Drainage Device in Cranial Cavity, External Approach
0WW1X1Z   Revision of Radioactive Element in Cranial Cavity, External Approach
0WW1X3Z   Revision of Infusion Device in Cranial Cavity, External Approach
0WW1XJZ   Revision of Synthetic Substitute in Cranial Cavity, External Approach
0WW1XYZ   Revision of Other Device in Cranial Cavity, External Approach
● 0WW200Z   Revision of Drainage Device in Face, Open Approach
● 0WW201Z   Revision of Radioactive Element in Face, Open Approach
● 0WW203Z   Revision of Infusion Device in Face, Open Approach
● 0WW207Z   Revision of Autologous Tissue Substitute in Face, Open Approach
● 0WW20JZ   Revision of Synthetic Substitute in Face, Open Approach
● 0WW20KZ   Revision of Nonautologous Tissue Substitute in Face, Open Approach
● 0WW20YZ   Revision of Other Device in Face, Open Approach
● 0WW230Z   Revision of Drainage Device in Face, Percutaneous Approach
● 0WW231Z   Revision of Radioactive Element in Face, Percutaneous Approach

● 0WW233Z   Revision of Infusion Device in Face, Percutaneous Approach
● 0WW237Z   Revision of Autologous Tissue Substitute in Face, Percutaneous Approach
● 0WW23JZ   Revision of Synthetic Substitute in Face, Percutaneous Approach
● 0WW23KZ   Revision of Nonautologous Tissue Substitute in Face, Percutaneous Approach
● 0WW23YZ   Revision of Other Device in Face, Percutaneous Approach
● 0WW240Z   Revision of Drainage Device in Face, Percutaneous Endoscopic Approach
● 0WW241Z   Revision of Radioactive Element in Face, Percutaneous Endoscopic Approach
● 0WW243Z   Revision of Infusion Device in Face, Percutaneous Endoscopic Approach
● 0WW247Z   Revision of Autologous Tissue Substitute in Face, Percutaneous Endoscopic Approach
● 0WW24JZ   Revision of Synthetic Substitute in Face, Percutaneous Endoscopic Approach
● 0WW24KZ   Revision of Nonautologous Tissue Substitute in Face, Percutaneous Endoscopic Approach
● 0WW24YZ   Revision of Other Device in Face, Percutaneous Endoscopic Approach
0WW2X0Z   Revision of Drainage Device in Face, External Approach
0WW2X1Z   Revision of Radioactive Element in Face, External Approach
0WW2X3Z   Revision of Infusion Device in Face, External Approach
0WW2X7Z   Revision of Autologous Tissue Substitute in Face, External Approach
0WW2XJZ   Revision of Synthetic Substitute in Face, External Approach
0WW2XKZ   Revision of Nonautologous Tissue Substitute in Face, External Approach
0WW2XYZ   Revision of Other Device in Face, External Approach
● 0WW400Z   Revision of Drainage Device in Upper Jaw, Open Approach
● 0WW401Z   Revision of Radioactive Element in Upper Jaw, Open Approach
● 0WW403Z   Revision of Infusion Device in Upper Jaw, Open Approach
● 0WW407Z   Revision of Autologous Tissue Substitute in Upper Jaw, Open Approach
● 0WW40JZ   Revision of Synthetic Substitute in Upper Jaw, Open Approach
● 0WW40KZ   Revision of Nonautologous Tissue Substitute in Upper Jaw, Open Approach
● 0WW40YZ   Revision of Other Device in Upper Jaw, Open Approach
● 0WW430Z   Revision of Drainage Device in Upper Jaw, Percutaneous Approach
● 0WW431Z   Revision of Radioactive Element in Upper Jaw, Percutaneous Approach
● 0WW433Z   Revision of Infusion Device in Upper Jaw, Percutaneous Approach
● 0WW437Z   Revision of Autologous Tissue Substitute in Upper Jaw, Percutaneous Approach
● 0WW43JZ   Revision of Synthetic Substitute in Upper Jaw, Percutaneous Approach
● 0WW43KZ   Revision of Nonautologous Tissue Substitute in Upper Jaw, Percutaneous Approach
● 0WW43YZ   Revision of Other Device in Upper Jaw, Percutaneous Approach
● 0WW440Z   Revision of Drainage Device in Upper Jaw, Percutaneous Endoscopic Approach
● 0WW441Z   Revision of Radioactive Element in Upper Jaw, Percutaneous Endoscopic Approach
● 0WW443Z   Revision of Infusion Device in Upper Jaw, Percutaneous Endoscopic Approach
● 0WW447Z   Revision of Autologous Tissue Substitute in Upper Jaw, Percutaneous Endoscopic Approach
● 0WW44JZ   Revision of Synthetic Substitute in Upper Jaw, Percutaneous Endoscopic Approach
● 0WW44KZ   Revision of Nonautologous Tissue Substitute in Upper Jaw, Percutaneous Endoscopic Approach
● 0WW44YZ   Revision of Other Device in Upper Jaw, Percutaneous Endoscopic Approach
0WW4X0Z   Revision of Drainage Device in Upper Jaw, External Approach
0WW4X1Z   Revision of Radioactive Element in Upper Jaw, External Approach
0WW4X3Z   Revision of Infusion Device in Upper Jaw, External Approach
0WW4X7Z   Revision of Autologous Tissue Substitute in Upper Jaw, External Approach
0WW4XJZ   Revision of Synthetic Substitute in Upper Jaw, External Approach

0WW4XKZ Revision of Nonautologous Tissue Substitute in Upper Jaw, External Approach

0WW4XYZ Revision of Other Device in Upper Jaw, External Approach

● 0WW500Z Revision of Drainage Device in Lower Jaw, Open Approach

● 0WW501Z Revision of Radioactive Element in Lower Jaw, Open Approach

● 0WW503Z Revision of Infusion Device in Lower Jaw, Open Approach

● 0WW507Z Revision of Autologous Tissue Substitute in Lower Jaw, Open Approach

● 0WW50JZ Revision of Synthetic Substitute in Lower Jaw, Open Approach

● 0WW50KZ Revision of Nonautologous Tissue Substitute in Lower Jaw, Open Approach

● 0WW50YZ Revision of Other Device in Lower Jaw, Open Approach

● 0WW530Z Revision of Drainage Device in Lower Jaw, Percutaneous Approach

● 0WW531Z Revision of Radioactive Element in Lower Jaw, Percutaneous Approach

● 0WW533Z Revision of Infusion Device in Lower Jaw, Percutaneous Approach

● 0WW537Z Revision of Autologous Tissue Substitute in Lower Jaw, Percutaneous Approach

● 0WW53JZ Revision of Synthetic Substitute in Lower Jaw, Percutaneous Approach

● 0WW53KZ Revision of Nonautologous Tissue Substitute in Lower Jaw, Percutaneous Approach

● 0WW53YZ Revision of Other Device in Lower Jaw, Percutaneous Approach

● 0WW540Z Revision of Drainage Device in Lower Jaw, Percutaneous Endoscopic Approach

● 0WW541Z Revision of Radioactive Element in Lower Jaw, Percutaneous Endoscopic Approach

● 0WW543Z Revision of Infusion Device in Lower Jaw, Percutaneous Endoscopic Approach

● 0WW547Z Revision of Autologous Tissue Substitute in Lower Jaw, Percutaneous Endoscopic Approach

● 0WW54JZ Revision of Synthetic Substitute in Lower Jaw, Percutaneous Endoscopic Approach

● 0WW54KZ Revision of Nonautologous Tissue Substitute in Lower Jaw, Percutaneous Endoscopic Approach

● 0WW54YZ Revision of Other Device in Lower Jaw, Percutaneous Endoscopic Approach

0WW5X0Z Revision of Drainage Device in Lower Jaw, External Approach

0WW5X1Z Revision of Radioactive Element in Lower Jaw, External Approach

0WW5X3Z Revision of Infusion Device in Lower Jaw, External Approach

0WW5X7Z Revision of Autologous Tissue Substitute in Lower Jaw, External Approach

0WW5XJZ Revision of Synthetic Substitute in Lower Jaw, External Approach

0WW5XKZ Revision of Nonautologous Tissue Substitute in Lower Jaw, External Approach

0WW5XYZ Revision of Other Device in Lower Jaw, External Approach

● 0WW600Z Revision of Drainage Device in Neck, Open Approach

● 0WW601Z Revision of Radioactive Element in Neck, Open Approach

● 0WW603Z Revision of Infusion Device in Neck, Open Approach

● 0WW607Z Revision of Autologous Tissue Substitute in Neck, Open Approach

● 0WW60JZ Revision of Synthetic Substitute in Neck, Open Approach

● 0WW60KZ Revision of Nonautologous Tissue Substitute in Neck, Open Approach

● 0WW60YZ Revision of Other Device in Neck, Open Approach

● 0WW630Z Revision of Drainage Device in Neck, Percutaneous Approach

● 0WW631Z Revision of Radioactive Element in Neck, Percutaneous Approach

● 0WW633Z Revision of Infusion Device in Neck, Percutaneous Approach

● 0WW637Z Revision of Autologous Tissue Substitute in Neck, Percutaneous Approach

● 0WW63JZ Revision of Synthetic Substitute in Neck, Percutaneous Approach

● 0WW63KZ Revision of Nonautologous Tissue Substitute in Neck, Percutaneous Approach

● 0WW63YZ Revision of Other Device in Neck, Percutaneous Approach

● 0WW640Z Revision of Drainage Device in Neck, Percutaneous Endoscopic Approach

● 0WW641Z Revision of Radioactive Element in Neck, Percutaneous Endoscopic Approach

● 0WW643Z Revision of Infusion Device in Neck, Percutaneous Endoscopic Approach

● 0WW647Z Revision of Autologous Tissue Substitute in Neck, Percutaneous Endoscopic Approach

● 0WW64JZ Revision of Synthetic Substitute in Neck, Percutaneous Endoscopic Approach

● 0WW64KZ Revision of Nonautologous Tissue Substitute in Neck, Percutaneous Endoscopic Approach

● 0WW64YZ Revision of Other Device in Neck, Percutaneous Endoscopic Approach

0WW6X0Z Revision of Drainage Device in Neck, External Approach

0WW6X1Z Revision of Radioactive Element in Neck, External Approach

0WW6X3Z Revision of Infusion Device in Neck, External Approach

0WW6X7Z Revision of Autologous Tissue Substitute in Neck, External Approach

0WW6XJZ Revision of Synthetic Substitute in Neck, External Approach

0WW6XKZ Revision of Nonautologous Tissue Substitute in Neck, External Approach

0WW6XYZ Revision of Other Device in Neck, External Approach

0WW800Z Revision of Drainage Device in Chest Wall, Open Approach

0WW801Z Revision of Radioactive Element in Chest Wall, Open Approach

0WW803Z Revision of Infusion Device in Chest Wall, Open Approach

0WW807Z Revision of Autologous Tissue Substitute in Chest Wall, Open Approach

0WW80JZ Revision of Synthetic Substitute in Chest Wall, Open Approach

0WW80KZ Revision of Nonautologous Tissue Substitute in Chest Wall, Open Approach

0WW80YZ Revision of Other Device in Chest Wall, Open Approach

0WW830Z Revision of Drainage Device in Chest Wall, Percutaneous Approach

0WW831Z Revision of Radioactive Element in Chest Wall, Percutaneous Approach

0WW833Z Revision of Infusion Device in Chest Wall, Percutaneous Approach

0WW837Z Revision of Autologous Tissue Substitute in Chest Wall, Percutaneous Approach

0WW83JZ Revision of Synthetic Substitute in Chest Wall, Percutaneous Approach

0WW83KZ Revision of Nonautologous Tissue Substitute in Chest Wall, Percutaneous Approach

0WW83YZ Revision of Other Device in Chest Wall, Percutaneous Approach

0WW840Z Revision of Drainage Device in Chest Wall, Percutaneous Endoscopic Approach

0WW841Z Revision of Radioactive Element in Chest Wall, Percutaneous Endoscopic Approach

0WW843Z Revision of Infusion Device in Chest Wall, Percutaneous Endoscopic Approach

0WW847Z Revision of Autologous Tissue Substitute in Chest Wall, Percutaneous Endoscopic Approach

0WW84JZ Revision of Synthetic Substitute in Chest Wall, Percutaneous Endoscopic Approach

0WW84KZ Revision of Nonautologous Tissue Substitute in Chest Wall, Percutaneous Endoscopic Approach

0WW84YZ Revision of Other Device in Chest Wall, Percutaneous Endoscopic Approach

0WW8X0Z Revision of Drainage Device in Chest Wall, External Approach

0WW8X1Z Revision of Radioactive Element in Chest Wall, External Approach

0WW8X3Z Revision of Infusion Device in Chest Wall, External Approach

0WW8X7Z Revision of Autologous Tissue Substitute in Chest Wall, External Approach

0WW8XJZ Revision of Synthetic Substitute in Chest Wall, External Approach

0WW8XKZ Revision of Nonautologous Tissue Substitute in Chest Wall, External Approach

0WW8XYZ Revision of Other Device in Chest Wall, External Approach

0WW900Z Revision of Drainage Device in Right Pleural Cavity, Open Approach

0WW901Z Revision of Radioactive Element in Right Pleural Cavity, Open Approach

0WW903Z Revision of Infusion Device in Right Pleural Cavity, Open Approach

0WW90JZ Revision of Synthetic Substitute in Right Pleural Cavity, Open Approach

0WW90YZ Revision of Other Device in Right Pleural Cavity, Open Approach

0WW930Z Revision of Drainage Device in Right Pleural Cavity, Percutaneous Approach

0WW931Z Revision of Radioactive Element in Right Pleural Cavity, Percutaneous Approach

0WW933Z Revision of Infusion Device in Right Pleural Cavity, Percutaneous Approach

0WW93JZ Revision of Synthetic Substitute in Right Pleural Cavity, Percutaneous Approach

0WW93YZ Revision of Other Device in Right Pleural Cavity, Percutaneous Approach

0WW940Z Revision of Drainage Device in Right Pleural Cavity, Percutaneous Endoscopic Approach

0WW941Z Revision of Radioactive Element in Right Pleural Cavity, Percutaneous Endoscopic Approach

0WW943Z Revision of Infusion Device in Right Pleural Cavity, Percutaneous Endoscopic Approach

0WW94JZ Revision of Synthetic Substitute in Right Pleural Cavity, Percutaneous Endoscopic Approach

0WW94YZ Revision of Other Device in Right Pleural Cavity, Percutaneous Endoscopic Approach

0WW9X0Z Revision of Drainage Device in Right Pleural Cavity, External Approach

0WW9X1Z Revision of Radioactive Element in Right Pleural Cavity, External Approach

0WW9X3Z Revision of Infusion Device in Right Pleural Cavity, External Approach

0WW9XJZ Revision of Synthetic Substitute in Right Pleural Cavity, External Approach

0WW9XYZ Revision of Other Device in Right Pleural Cavity, External Approach

0WWB00Z Revision of Drainage Device in Left Pleural Cavity, Open Approach

0WWB01Z Revision of Radioactive Element in Left Pleural Cavity, Open Approach

0WWB03Z Revision of Infusion Device in Left Pleural Cavity, Open Approach

0WWB0JZ Revision of Synthetic Substitute in Left Pleural Cavity, Open Approach

0WWB0YZ Revision of Other Device in Left Pleural Cavity, Open Approach

0WWB30Z Revision of Drainage Device in Left Pleural Cavity, Percutaneous Approach

0WWB31Z Revision of Radioactive Element in Left Pleural Cavity, Percutaneous Approach

0WWB33Z Revision of Infusion Device in Left Pleural Cavity, Percutaneous Approach

0WWB3JZ Revision of Synthetic Substitute in Left Pleural Cavity, Percutaneous Approach

0WWB3YZ Revision of Other Device in Left Pleural Cavity, Percutaneous Approach

0WWB40Z Revision of Drainage Device in Left Pleural Cavity, Percutaneous Endoscopic Approach

0WWB41Z Revision of Radioactive Element in Left Pleural Cavity, Percutaneous Endoscopic Approach

0WWB43Z Revision of Infusion Device in Left Pleural Cavity, Percutaneous Endoscopic Approach

0WWB4JZ Revision of Synthetic Substitute in Left Pleural Cavity, Percutaneous Endoscopic Approach

0WWB4YZ Revision of Other Device in Left Pleural Cavity, Percutaneous Endoscopic Approach

0WWBX0Z Revision of Drainage Device in Left Pleural Cavity, External Approach

0WWBX1Z Revision of Radioactive Element in Left Pleural Cavity, External Approach

0WWBX3Z Revision of Infusion Device in Left Pleural Cavity, External Approach

0WWBXJZ Revision of Synthetic Substitute in Left Pleural Cavity, External Approach

0WWBXYZ Revision of Other Device in Left Pleural Cavity, External Approach

0WWC00Z Revision of Drainage Device in Mediastinum, Open Approach

0WWC01Z Revision of Radioactive Element in Mediastinum, Open Approach

0WWC03Z Revision of Infusion Device in Mediastinum, Open Approach

0WWC07Z Revision of Autologous Tissue Substitute in Mediastinum, Open Approach

0WWC0JZ Revision of Synthetic Substitute in Mediastinum, Open Approach

0WWC0KZ Revision of Nonautologous Tissue Substitute in Mediastinum, Open Approach

0WWC0YZ Revision of Other Device in Mediastinum, Open Approach

0WWC30Z Revision of Drainage Device in Mediastinum, Percutaneous Approach

0WWC31Z Revision of Radioactive Element in Mediastinum, Percutaneous Approach

0WWC33Z Revision of Infusion Device in Mediastinum, Percutaneous Approach

0WWC37Z Revision of Autologous Tissue Substitute in Mediastinum, Percutaneous Approach

0WWC3JZ Revision of Synthetic Substitute in Mediastinum, Percutaneous Approach

0WWC3KZ Revision of Nonautologous Tissue Substitute in Mediastinum, Percutaneous Approach

0WWC3YZ Revision of Other Device in Mediastinum, Percutaneous Approach

0WWC40Z Revision of Drainage Device in Mediastinum, Percutaneous Endoscopic Approach

0WWC41Z Revision of Radioactive Element in Mediastinum, Percutaneous Endoscopic Approach

0WWC43Z Revision of Infusion Device in Mediastinum, Percutaneous Endoscopic Approach

0WWC47Z Revision of Autologous Tissue Substitute in Mediastinum, Percutaneous Endoscopic Approach

0WWC4JZ Revision of Synthetic Substitute in Mediastinum, Percutaneous Endoscopic Approach

0WWC4KZ Revision of Nonautologous Tissue Substitute in Mediastinum, Percutaneous Endoscopic Approach

0WWC4YZ Revision of Other Device in Mediastinum, Percutaneous Endoscopic Approach

0WWCX0Z Revision of Drainage Device in Mediastinum, External Approach

0WWCX1Z Revision of Radioactive Element in Mediastinum, External Approach

0WWCX3Z Revision of Infusion Device in Mediastinum, External Approach

0WWCX7Z Revision of Autologous Tissue Substitute in Mediastinum, External Approach

0WWCXJZ Revision of Synthetic Substitute in Mediastinum, External Approach

0WWCXKZ Revision of Nonautologous Tissue Substitute in Mediastinum, External Approach

0WWCXYZ Revision of Other Device in Mediastinum, External Approach

0WWD00Z Revision of Drainage Device in Pericardial Cavity, Open Approach

0WWD01Z Revision of Radioactive Element in Pericardial Cavity, Open Approach

0WWD03Z Revision of Infusion Device in Pericardial Cavity, Open Approach

0WWD0YZ Revision of Other Device in Pericardial Cavity, Open Approach

0WWD30Z Revision of Drainage Device in Pericardial Cavity, Percutaneous Approach

0WWD31Z Revision of Radioactive Element in Pericardial Cavity, Percutaneous Approach

0WWD33Z Revision of Infusion Device in Pericardial Cavity, Percutaneous Approach

0WWD3YZ Revision of Other Device in Pericardial Cavity, Percutaneous Approach

0WWD40Z Revision of Drainage Device in Pericardial Cavity, Percutaneous Endoscopic Approach

0WWD41Z Revision of Radioactive Element in Pericardial Cavity, Percutaneous Endoscopic Approach

0WWD43Z Revision of Infusion Device in Pericardial Cavity, Percutaneous Endoscopic Approach

0WWD4YZ Revision of Other Device in Pericardial Cavity, Percutaneous Endoscopic Approach

0WWDX0Z Revision of Drainage Device in Pericardial Cavity, External Approach

0WWDX1Z Revision of Radioactive Element in Pericardial Cavity, External Approach

0WWDX3Z Revision of Infusion Device in Pericardial Cavity, External Approach

0WWDXYZ Revision of Other Device in Pericardial Cavity, External Approach

0WWF00Z Revision of Drainage Device in Abdominal Wall, Open Approach

0WWF01Z Revision of Radioactive Element in Abdominal Wall, Open Approach

---

0WWF03Z Revision of Infusion Device in Abdominal Wall, Open Approach

0WWF07Z Revision of Autologous Tissue Substitute in Abdominal Wall, Open Approach

0WWF0JZ Revision of Synthetic Substitute in Abdominal Wall, Open Approach

0WWF0KZ Revision of Nonautologous Tissue Substitute in Abdominal Wall, Open Approach

0WWF0YZ Revision of Other Device in Abdominal Wall, Open Approach

0WWF30Z Revision of Drainage Device in Abdominal Wall, Percutaneous Approach

0WWF31Z Revision of Radioactive Element in Abdominal Wall, Percutaneous Approach

0WWF33Z Revision of Infusion Device in Abdominal Wall, Percutaneous Approach

0WWF37Z Revision of Autologous Tissue Substitute in Abdominal Wall, Percutaneous Approach

0WWF3JZ Revision of Synthetic Substitute in Abdominal Wall, Percutaneous Approach

0WWF3KZ Revision of Nonautologous Tissue Substitute in Abdominal Wall, Percutaneous Approach

0WWF3YZ Revision of Other Device in Abdominal Wall, Percutaneous Approach

0WWF40Z Revision of Drainage Device in Abdominal Wall, Percutaneous Endoscopic Approach

0WWF41Z Revision of Radioactive Element in Abdominal Wall, Percutaneous Endoscopic Approach

0WWF43Z Revision of Infusion Device in Abdominal Wall, Percutaneous Endoscopic Approach

0WWF47Z Revision of Autologous Tissue Substitute in Abdominal Wall, Percutaneous Endoscopic Approach

0WWF4JZ Revision of Synthetic Substitute in Abdominal Wall, Percutaneous Endoscopic Approach

0WWF4KZ Revision of Nonautologous Tissue Substitute in Abdominal Wall, Percutaneous Endoscopic Approach

0WWF4YZ Revision of Other Device in Abdominal Wall, Percutaneous Endoscopic Approach

0WWFX0Z Revision of Drainage Device in Abdominal Wall, External Approach

0WWFX1Z Revision of Radioactive Element in Abdominal Wall, External Approach

0WWFX3Z Revision of Infusion Device in Abdominal Wall, External Approach

0WWFX7Z Revision of Autologous Tissue Substitute in Abdominal Wall, External Approach

0WWFXJZ Revision of Synthetic Substitute in Abdominal Wall, External Approach

0WWFXKZ Revision of Nonautologous Tissue Substitute in Abdominal Wall, External Approach

0WWFXYZ Revision of Other Device in Abdominal Wall, External Approach

0WWG00Z Revision of Drainage Device in Peritoneal Cavity, Open Approach

0WWG01Z Revision of Radioactive Element in Peritoneal Cavity, Open Approach

0WWG03Z Revision of Infusion Device in Peritoneal Cavity, Open Approach

0WWG0JZ Revision of Synthetic Substitute in Peritoneal Cavity, Open Approach

0WWG0YZ Revision of Other Device in Peritoneal Cavity, Open Approach

0WWG30Z Revision of Drainage Device in Peritoneal Cavity, Percutaneous Approach

0WWG31Z Revision of Radioactive Element in Peritoneal Cavity, Percutaneous Approach

0WWG33Z Revision of Infusion Device in Peritoneal Cavity, Percutaneous Approach

0WWG3JZ Revision of Synthetic Substitute in Peritoneal Cavity, Percutaneous Approach

0WWG3YZ Revision of Other Device in Peritoneal Cavity, Percutaneous Approach

0WWG40Z Revision of Drainage Device in Peritoneal Cavity, Percutaneous Endoscopic Approach

0WWG41Z Revision of Radioactive Element in Peritoneal Cavity, Percutaneous Endoscopic Approach

0WWG43Z Revision of Infusion Device in Peritoneal Cavity, Percutaneous Endoscopic Approach

0WWG4JZ Revision of Synthetic Substitute in Peritoneal Cavity, Percutaneous Endoscopic Approach

0WWG4YZ Revision of Other Device in Peritoneal Cavity, Percutaneous Endoscopic Approach

0WWGX0Z Revision of Drainage Device in Peritoneal Cavity, External Approach

0WWGX1Z Revision of Radioactive Element in Peritoneal Cavity, External Approach

0WWGX3Z Revision of Infusion Device in Peritoneal Cavity, External Approach

0WWGXJZ Revision of Synthetic Substitute in Peritoneal Cavity, External Approach

0WWGXYZ Revision of Other Device in Peritoneal Cavity, External Approach

0WWH00Z Revision of Drainage Device in Retroperitoneum, Open Approach

0WWH01Z Revision of Radioactive Element in Retroperitoneum, Open Approach

0WWH03Z Revision of Infusion Device in Retroperitoneum, Open Approach

0WWH0YZ Revision of Other Device in Retroperitoneum, Open Approach

0WWH30Z Revision of Drainage Device in Retroperitoneum, Percutaneous Approach

0WWH31Z Revision of Radioactive Element in Retroperitoneum, Percutaneous Approach

0WWH33Z Revision of Infusion Device in Retroperitoneum, Percutaneous Approach

0WWH3YZ Revision of Other Device in Retroperitoneum, Percutaneous Approach

0WWH40Z Revision of Drainage Device in Retroperitoneum, Percutaneous Endoscopic Approach

0WWH41Z Revision of Radioactive Element in Retroperitoneum, Percutaneous Endoscopic Approach

0WWH43Z Revision of Infusion Device in Retroperitoneum, Percutaneous Endoscopic Approach

0WWH4YZ Revision of Other Device in Retroperitoneum, Percutaneous Endoscopic Approach

0WWHX0Z Revision of Drainage Device in Retroperitoneum, External Approach

0WWHX1Z Revision of Radioactive Element in Retroperitoneum, External Approach

0WWHX3Z Revision of Infusion Device in Retroperitoneum, External Approach

0WWHXYZ Revision of Other Device in Retroperitoneum, External Approach

0WWJ00Z Revision of Drainage Device in Pelvic Cavity, Open Approach

0WWJ01Z Revision of Radioactive Element in Pelvic Cavity, Open Approach

0WWJ03Z Revision of Infusion Device in Pelvic Cavity, Open Approach

0WWJ0JZ Revision of Synthetic Substitute in Pelvic Cavity, Open Approach

0WWJ0YZ Revision of Other Device in Pelvic Cavity, Open Approach

0WWJ30Z Revision of Drainage Device in Pelvic Cavity, Percutaneous Approach

0WWJ31Z Revision of Radioactive Element in Pelvic Cavity, Percutaneous Approach

0WWJ33Z Revision of Infusion Device in Pelvic Cavity, Percutaneous Approach

0WWJ3JZ Revision of Synthetic Substitute in Pelvic Cavity, Percutaneous Approach

0WWJ3YZ Revision of Other Device in Pelvic Cavity, Percutaneous Approach

0WWJ40Z Revision of Drainage Device in Pelvic Cavity, Percutaneous Endoscopic Approach

0WWJ41Z Revision of Radioactive Element in Pelvic Cavity, Percutaneous Endoscopic Approach

0WWJ43Z Revision of Infusion Device in Pelvic Cavity, Percutaneous Endoscopic Approach

0WWJ4JZ Revision of Synthetic Substitute in Pelvic Cavity, Percutaneous Endoscopic Approach

0WWJ4YZ Revision of Other Device in Pelvic Cavity, Percutaneous Endoscopic Approach

0WWJX0Z Revision of Drainage Device in Pelvic Cavity, External Approach

0WWJX1Z Revision of Radioactive Element in Pelvic Cavity, External Approach

0WWJX3Z Revision of Infusion Device in Pelvic Cavity, External Approach

0WWJXJZ Revision of Synthetic Substitute in Pelvic Cavity, External Approach

0WWJXYZ Revision of Other Device in Pelvic Cavity, External Approach

● **0WWK00Z** Revision of Drainage Device in Upper Back, Open Approach

● **0WWK01Z** Revision of Radioactive Element in Upper Back, Open Approach

● **0WWK03Z** Revision of Infusion Device in Upper Back, Open Approach

● **0WWK07Z** Revision of Autologous Tissue Substitute in Upper Back, Open Approach

● **0WWK0JZ** Revision of Synthetic Substitute in Upper Back, Open Approach

● **0WWK0KZ** Revision of Nonautologous Tissue Substitute in Upper Back, Open Approach

● **0WWK0YZ** Revision of Other Device in Upper Back, Open Approach

● **0WWK30Z** Revision of Drainage Device in Upper Back, Percutaneous Approach

● **0WWK31Z** Revision of Radioactive Element in Upper Back, Percutaneous Approach

● **0WWK33Z** Revision of Infusion Device in Upper Back, Percutaneous Approach

● **0WWK37Z** Revision of Autologous Tissue Substitute in Upper Back, Percutaneous Approach

● **0WWK3JZ** Revision of Synthetic Substitute in Upper Back, Percutaneous Approach

● **0WWK3KZ** Revision of Nonautologous Tissue Substitute in Upper Back, Percutaneous Approach

● **0WWK3YZ** Revision of Other Device in Upper Back, Percutaneous Approach

● **0WWK40Z** Revision of Drainage Device in Upper Back, Percutaneous Endoscopic Approach

● **0WWK41Z** Revision of Radioactive Element in Upper Back, Percutaneous Endoscopic Approach

● **0WWK43Z** Revision of Infusion Device in Upper Back, Percutaneous Endoscopic Approach

● **0WWK47Z** Revision of Autologous Tissue Substitute in Upper Back, Percutaneous Endoscopic Approach

● **0WWK4JZ** Revision of Synthetic Substitute in Upper Back, Percutaneous Endoscopic Approach

● **0WWK4KZ** Revision of Nonautologous Tissue Substitute in Upper Back, Percutaneous Endoscopic Approach

● **0WWK4YZ** Revision of Other Device in Upper Back, Percutaneous Endoscopic Approach

0WWKX0Z Revision of Drainage Device in Upper Back, External Approach

0WWKX1Z Revision of Radioactive Element in Upper Back, External Approach

0WWKX3Z Revision of Infusion Device in Upper Back, External Approach

0WWKX7Z Revision of Autologous Tissue Substitute in Upper Back, External Approach

0WWKXJZ Revision of Synthetic Substitute in Upper Back, External Approach

0WWKXKZ Revision of Nonautologous Tissue Substitute in Upper Back, External Approach

0WWKXYZ Revision of Other Device in Upper Back, External Approach

● **0WWL00Z** Revision of Drainage Device in Lower Back, Open Approach

● **0WWL01Z** Revision of Radioactive Element in Lower Back, Open Approach

● **0WWL03Z** Revision of Infusion Device in Lower Back, Open Approach

● **0WWL07Z** Revision of Autologous Tissue Substitute in Lower Back, Open Approach

● **0WWL0JZ** Revision of Synthetic Substitute in Lower Back, Open Approach

● **0WWL0KZ** Revision of Nonautologous Tissue Substitute in Lower Back, Open Approach

● **0WWL0YZ** Revision of Other Device in Lower Back, Open Approach

● **0WWL30Z** Revision of Drainage Device in Lower Back, Percutaneous Approach

● **0WWL31Z** Revision of Radioactive Element in Lower Back, Percutaneous Approach

● **0WWL33Z** Revision of Infusion Device in Lower Back, Percutaneous Approach

● **0WWL37Z** Revision of Autologous Tissue Substitute in Lower Back, Percutaneous Approach

● **0WWL3JZ** Revision of Synthetic Substitute in Lower Back, Percutaneous Approach

● **0WWL3KZ** Revision of Nonautologous Tissue Substitute in Lower Back, Percutaneous Approach

● **0WWL3YZ** Revision of Other Device in Lower Back, Percutaneous Approach

● **0WWL40Z** Revision of Drainage Device in Lower Back, Percutaneous Endoscopic Approach

● **0WWL41Z** Revision of Radioactive Element in Lower Back, Percutaneous Endoscopic Approach

● **0WWL43Z** Revision of Infusion Device in Lower Back, Percutaneous Endoscopic Approach

● **0WWL47Z** Revision of Autologous Tissue Substitute in Lower Back, Percutaneous Endoscopic Approach

● **0WWL4JZ** Revision of Synthetic Substitute in Lower Back, Percutaneous Endoscopic Approach

● **0WWL4KZ** Revision of Nonautologous Tissue Substitute in Lower Back, Percutaneous Endoscopic Approach

● **0WWL4YZ** Revision of Other Device in Lower Back, Percutaneous Endoscopic Approach

0WWLX0Z Revision of Drainage Device in Lower Back, External Approach

0WWLX1Z Revision of Radioactive Element in Lower Back, External Approach

0WWLX3Z Revision of Infusion Device in Lower Back, External Approach

0WWLX7Z Revision of Autologous Tissue Substitute in Lower Back, External Approach

0WWLXJZ Revision of Synthetic Substitute in Lower Back, External Approach

0WWLXKZ Revision of Nonautologous Tissue Substitute in Lower Back, External Approach

0WWLXYZ Revision of Other Device in Lower Back, External Approach

●♂ **0WWM00Z** Revision of Drainage Device in Male Perineum, Open Approach

●♂ **0WWM01Z** Revision of Radioactive Element in Male Perineum, Open Approach

●♂ **0WWM03Z** Revision of Infusion Device in Male Perineum, Open Approach

♂ **0WWM07Z** Revision of Autologous Tissue Substitute in Male Perineum, Open Approach

●♂ **0WWM0JZ** Revision of Synthetic Substitute in Male Perineum, Open Approach

♂ **0WWM0KZ** Revision of Nonautologous Tissue Substitute in Male Perineum, Open Approach

●♂ **0WWM0YZ** Revision of Other Device in Male Perineum, Open Approach

●♂ **0WWM30Z** Revision of Drainage Device in Male Perineum, Percutaneous Approach

●♂ **0WWM31Z** Revision of Radioactive Element in Male Perineum, Percutaneous Approach

●♂ **0WWM33Z** Revision of Infusion Device in Male Perineum, Percutaneous Approach

♂ **0WWM37Z** Revision of Autologous Tissue Substitute in Male Perineum, Percutaneous Approach

●♂ **0WWM3JZ** Revision of Synthetic Substitute in Male Perineum, Percutaneous Approach

♂ **0WWM3KZ** Revision of Nonautologous Tissue Substitute in Male Perineum, Percutaneous Approach

●♂ **0WWM3YZ** Revision of Other Device in Male Perineum, Percutaneous Approach

●♂ **0WWM40Z** Revision of Drainage Device in Male Perineum, Percutaneous Endoscopic Approach

●♂ **0WWM41Z** Revision of Radioactive Element in Male Perineum, Percutaneous Endoscopic Approach

●♂ **0WWM43Z** Revision of Infusion Device in Male Perineum, Percutaneous Endoscopic Approach

♂ **0WWM47Z** Revision of Autologous Tissue Substitute in Male Perineum, Percutaneous Endoscopic Approach

●♂ **0WWM4JZ** Revision of Synthetic Substitute in Male Perineum, Percutaneous Endoscopic Approach

♂ **0WWM4KZ** Revision of Nonautologous Tissue Substitute in Male Perineum, Percutaneous Endoscopic Approach

●♂ **0WWM4YZ** Revision of Other Device in Male Perineum, Percutaneous Endoscopic Approach

♂ **0WWMX0Z** Revision of Drainage Device in Male Perineum, External Approach

♂ **0WWMX1Z** Revision of Radioactive Element in Male Perineum, External Approach

♂ **0WWMX3Z** Revision of Infusion Device in Male Perineum, External Approach

---

♀ Female-only   ♂ Male-only   ● Limited Coverage   ● Non-OR   **HAC** HAC-associated procedure   ● Non-covered procedures   **+** Combination

♂ **0WWMX7Z** Revision of Autologous Tissue Substitute in Male Perineum, External Approach

♂ **0WWMXJZ** Revision of Synthetic Substitute in Male Perineum, External Approach

♂ **0WWMXKZ** Revision of Nonautologous Tissue Substitute in Male Perineum, External Approach
This is a male-only service, however, it is not included in the male-only edit logic for MCE V30

♂ **0WWMXYZ** Revision of Other Device in Male Perineum, External Approach
This is a male-only service, however, it is not included in the male-only edit logic for MCE V30

♀ **0WWN00Z** Revision of Drainage Device in Female Perineum, Open Approach

♀ **0WWN01Z** Revision of Radioactive Element in Female Perineum, Open Approach

♀ **0WWN03Z** Revision of Infusion Device in Female Perineum, Open Approach

♀ **0WWN07Z** Revision of Autologous Tissue Substitute in Female Perineum, Open Approach

♀ **0WWN0JZ** Revision of Synthetic Substitute in Female Perineum, Open Approach

♀ **0WWN0KZ** Revision of Nonautologous Tissue Substitute in Female Perineum, Open Approach

♀ **0WWN0YZ** Revision of Other Device in Female Perineum, Open Approach

♀ **0WWN30Z** Revision of Drainage Device in Female Perineum, Percutaneous Approach

♀ **0WWN31Z** Revision of Radioactive Element in Female Perineum, Percutaneous Approach

♀ **0WWN33Z** Revision of Infusion Device in Female Perineum, Percutaneous Approach

♀ **0WWN37Z** Revision of Autologous Tissue Substitute in Female Perineum, Percutaneous Approach

♀ **0WWN3JZ** Revision of Synthetic Substitute in Female Perineum, Percutaneous Approach

♀ **0WWN3KZ** Revision of Nonautologous Tissue Substitute in Female Perineum, Percutaneous Approach

♀ **0WWN3YZ** Revision of Other Device in Female Perineum, Percutaneous Approach

♀ **0WWN40Z** Revision of Drainage Device in Female Perineum, Percutaneous Endoscopic Approach

♀ **0WWN41Z** Revision of Radioactive Element in Female Perineum, Percutaneous Endoscopic Approach

♀ **0WWN43Z** Revision of Infusion Device in Female Perineum, Percutaneous Endoscopic Approach

♀ **0WWN47Z** Revision of Autologous Tissue Substitute in Female Perineum, Percutaneous Endoscopic Approach

♀ **0WWN4JZ** Revision of Synthetic Substitute in Female Perineum, Percutaneous Endoscopic Approach

♀ **0WWN4KZ** Revision of Nonautologous Tissue Substitute in Female Perineum, Percutaneous Endoscopic Approach

♀ **0WWN4YZ** Revision of Other Device in Female Perineum, Percutaneous Endoscopic Approach

♀ **0WWNX0Z** Revision of Drainage Device in Female Perineum, External Approach

♀ **0WWNX1Z** Revision of Radioactive Element in Female Perineum, External Approach

♀ **0WWNX3Z** Revision of Infusion Device in Female Perineum, External Approach

♀ **0WWNX7Z** Revision of Autologous Tissue Substitute in Female Perineum, External Approach

♀ **0WWNXJZ** Revision of Synthetic Substitute in Female Perineum, External Approach

♀ **0WWNXKZ** Revision of Nonautologous Tissue Substitute in Female Perineum, External Approach

♀ **0WWNXYZ** Revision of Other Device in Female Perineum, External Approach

0WWP01Z Revision of Radioactive Element in Gastrointestinal Tract, Open Approach

0WWP03Z Revision of Infusion Device in Gastrointestinal Tract, Open Approach

0WWP0YZ Revision of Other Device in Gastrointestinal Tract, Open Approach

0WWP31Z Revision of Radioactive Element in Gastrointestinal Tract, Percutaneous Approach

0WWP33Z Revision of Infusion Device in Gastrointestinal Tract, Percutaneous Approach

0WWP3YZ Revision of Other Device in Gastrointestinal Tract, Percutaneous Approach

0WWP41Z Revision of Radioactive Element in Gastrointestinal Tract, Percutaneous Endoscopic Approach

0WWP43Z Revision of Infusion Device in Gastrointestinal Tract, Percutaneous Endoscopic Approach

0WWP4YZ Revision of Other Device in Gastrointestinal Tract, Percutaneous Endoscopic Approach

0WWP71Z Revision of Radioactive Element in Gastrointestinal Tract, Via Natural or Artificial Opening

0WWP73Z Revision of Infusion Device in Gastrointestinal Tract, Via Natural or Artificial Opening

0WWP7YZ Revision of Other Device in Gastrointestinal Tract, Via Natural or Artificial Opening

0WWP81Z Revision of Radioactive Element in Gastrointestinal Tract, Via Natural or Artificial Opening Endoscopic

0WWP83Z Revision of Infusion Device in Gastrointestinal Tract, Via Natural or Artificial Opening Endoscopic

0WWP8YZ Revision of Other Device in Gastrointestinal Tract, Via Natural or Artificial Opening Endoscopic

0WWPX1Z Revision of Radioactive Element in Gastrointestinal Tract, External Approach

0WWPX3Z Revision of Infusion Device in Gastrointestinal Tract, External Approach

0WWPXYZ Revision of Other Device in Gastrointestinal Tract, External Approach

0WWQ01Z Revision of Radioactive Element in Respiratory Tract, Open Approach

0WWQ03Z Revision of Infusion Device in Respiratory Tract, Open Approach

0WWQ0YZ Revision of Other Device in Respiratory Tract, Open Approach

0WWQ31Z Revision of Radioactive Element in Respiratory Tract, Percutaneous Approach

0WWQ33Z Revision of Infusion Device in Respiratory Tract, Percutaneous Approach

0WWQ3YZ Revision of Other Device in Respiratory Tract, Percutaneous Approach

0WWQ41Z Revision of Radioactive Element in Respiratory Tract, Percutaneous Endoscopic Approach

0WWQ43Z Revision of Infusion Device in Respiratory Tract, Percutaneous Endoscopic Approach

0WWQ4YZ Revision of Other Device in Respiratory Tract, Percutaneous Endoscopic Approach

0WWQ71Z Revision of Radioactive Element in Respiratory Tract, Via Natural or Artificial Opening

0WWQ73Z Revision of Infusion Device in Respiratory Tract, Via Natural or Artificial Opening

0WWQ7YZ Revision of Other Device in Respiratory Tract, Via Natural or Artificial Opening

0WWQ81Z Revision of Radioactive Element in Respiratory Tract, Via Natural or Artificial Opening Endoscopic

0WWQ83Z Revision of Infusion Device in Respiratory Tract, Via Natural or Artificial Opening Endoscopic

0WWQ8YZ Revision of Other Device in Respiratory Tract, Via Natural or Artificial Opening Endoscopic

0WWQX1Z Revision of Radioactive Element in Respiratory Tract, External Approach

0WWQX3Z Revision of Infusion Device in Respiratory Tract, External Approach

0WWQXYZ Revision of Other Device in Respiratory Tract, External Approach

0WWR01Z Revision of Radioactive Element in Genitourinary Tract, Open Approach

0WWR03Z Revision of Infusion Device in Genitourinary Tract, Open Approach

0WWR0YZ Revision of Other Device in Genitourinary Tract, Open Approach

0WWR31Z Revision of Radioactive Element in Genitourinary Tract, Percutaneous Approach

0WWR33Z Revision of Infusion Device in Genitourinary Tract, Percutaneous Approach

0WWR3YZ Revision of Other Device in Genitourinary Tract, Percutaneous Approach

---

♀ Female-only   ♂ Male-only   ● Limited Coverage   ● Non-OR   ᴴᴬᶜ HAC-associated procedure   ● Non-covered procedures   ➕ Combination

0WWR41Z   Revision of Radioactive Element in Genitourinary Tract, Percutaneous Endoscopic Approach

0WWR43Z   Revision of Infusion Device in Genitourinary Tract, Percutaneous Endoscopic Approach

0WWR4YZ   Revision of Other Device in Genitourinary Tract, Percutaneous Endoscopic Approach

0WWR71Z   Revision of Radioactive Element in Genitourinary Tract, Via Natural or Artificial Opening

0WWR73Z   Revision of Infusion Device in Genitourinary Tract, Via Natural or Artificial Opening

0WWR7YZ   Revision of Other Device in Genitourinary Tract, Via Natural or Artificial Opening

0WWR81Z   Revision of Radioactive Element in Genitourinary Tract, Via Natural or Artificial Opening Endoscopic

0WWR83Z   Revision of Infusion Device in Genitourinary Tract, Via Natural or Artificial Opening Endoscopic

0WWR8YZ   Revision of Other Device in Genitourinary Tract, Via Natural or Artificial Opening Endoscopic

0WWRX1Z   Revision of Radioactive Element in Genitourinary Tract, External Approach

0WWRX3Z   Revision of Infusion Device in Genitourinary Tract, External Approach

0WWRXYZ   Revision of Other Device in Genitourinary Tract, External Approach

Anatomical Regions, Upper Extremities

Anatomical Regions, Upper Extremities Tables 0X0–0XX

Section	0	**Medical and Surgical**
Body System	X	**Anatomical Regions, Upper Extremities**
Operation	0	**Alteration:** Modifying the anatomic structure of a body part without affecting the function of the body part

Body Part (4ᵗʰ)	Approach (5ᵗʰ)	Device (6ᵗʰ)	Qualifier (7ᵗʰ)
2 Shoulder Region, Right 3 Shoulder Region, Left 4 Axilla, Right 5 Axilla, Left 6 Upper Extremity, Right 7 Upper Extremity, Left 8 Upper Arm, Right 9 Upper Arm, Left B Elbow Region, Right C Elbow Region, Left D Lower Arm, Right F Lower Arm, Left G Wrist Region, Right H Wrist Region, Left	0 Open 3 Percutaneous 4 Percutaneous Endoscopic	7 Autologous Tissue Substitute J Synthetic Substitute K Nonautologous Tissue Substitute Z No Device	Z No Qualifier

Section	0	**Medical and Surgical**
Body System	X	**Anatomical Regions, Upper Extremities**
Operation	2	**Change:** Taking out or off a device from a body part and putting back an identical or similar device in or on the same body part without cutting or puncturing the skin or a mucous membrane

Body Part (4ᵗʰ)	Approach (5ᵗʰ)	Device (6ᵗʰ)	Qualifier (7ᵗʰ)
6 Upper Extremity, Right 7 Upper Extremity, Left	X External	0 Drainage Device Y Other Device	Z No Qualifier

Section	0	**Medical and Surgical**
Body System	X	**Anatomical Regions, Upper Extremities**
Operation	3	**Control:** Stopping, or attempting to stop, postprocedural bleeding

Body Part (4ᵗʰ)	Approach (5ᵗʰ)	Device (6ᵗʰ)	Qualifier (7ᵗʰ)
2 Shoulder Region, Right 3 Shoulder Region, Left 4 Axilla, Right 5 Axilla, Left 6 Upper Extremity, Right 7 Upper Extremity, Left 8 Upper Arm, Right 9 Upper Arm, Left B Elbow Region, Right C Elbow Region, Left D Lower Arm, Right F Lower Arm, Left G Wrist Region, Right H Wrist Region, Left J Hand, Right K Hand, Left	0 Open 3 Percutaneous 4 Percutaneous Endoscopic	Z No Device	Z No Qualifier

Section	0	Medical and Surgical
Body System	X	Anatomical Regions, Upper Extremities
Operation	6	Detachment: Cutting off all or a portion of the upper or lower extremities

Body Part (4th)	Approach (5th)	Device (6th)	Qualifier (7th)
0 Forequarter, Right **1** Forequarter, Left **2** Shoulder Region, Right **3** Shoulder Region, Left **B** Elbow Region, Right **C** Elbow Region, Left	**0** Open	**Z** No Device	**Z** No Qualifier
8 Upper Arm, Right **9** Upper Arm, Left **D** Lower Arm, Right **F** Lower Arm, Left	**0** Open	**Z** No Device	**1** High **2** Mid **3** Low
J Hand, Right **K** Hand, Left	**0** Open	**Z** No Device	**0** Complete **4** Complete 1st Ray **5** Complete 2nd Ray **6** Complete 3rd Ray **7** Complete 4th Ray **8** Complete 5th Ray **9** Partial 1st Ray **B** Partial 2nd Ray **C** Partial 3rd Ray **D** Partial 4th Ray **F** Partial 5th Ray
L Thumb, Right **M** Thumb, Left **N** Index Finger, Right **P** Index Finger, Left **Q** Middle Finger, Right **R** Middle Finger, Left **S** Ring Finger, Right **T** Ring Finger, Left **V** Little Finger, Right **W** Little Finger, Left	**0** Open	**Z** No Device	**0** Complete **1** High **2** Mid **3** Low

Section	0	Medical and Surgical
Body System	X	Anatomical Regions, Upper Extremities
Operation	9	Drainage: Taking or letting out fluids and/or gases from a body part

Body Part (4th)	Approach (5th)	Device (6th)	Qualifier (7th)
2 Shoulder Region, Right **3** Shoulder Region, Left **4** Axilla, Right **5** Axilla, Left **6** Upper Extremity, Right **7** Upper Extremity, Left **8** Upper Arm, Right **9** Upper Arm, Left **B** Elbow Region, Right **C** Elbow Region, Left **D** Lower Arm, Right **F** Lower Arm, Left **G** Wrist Region, Right **H** Wrist Region, Left **J** Hand, Right **K** Hand, Left	**0** Open **3** Percutaneous **4** Percutaneous Endoscopic	**0** Drainage Device	**Z** No Qualifier

Continued

0X9 Continued

Section	0	**Medical and Surgical**
Body System	X	**Anatomical Regions, Upper Extremities**
Operation	9	**Drainage:** Taking or letting out fluids and/or gases from a body part

Body Part (4ᵗʰ)	Approach (5ᵗʰ)	Device (6ᵗʰ)	Qualifier (7ᵗʰ)
2 Shoulder Region, Right 3 Shoulder Region, Left 4 Axilla, Right 5 Axilla, Left 6 Upper Extremity, Right 7 Upper Extremity, Left 8 Upper Arm, Right 9 Upper Arm, Left B Elbow Region, Right C Elbow Region, Left D Lower Arm, Right F Lower Arm, Left G Wrist Region, Right H Wrist Region, Left J Hand, Right K Hand, Left	0 Open 3 Percutaneous 4 Percutaneous Endoscopic	Z No Device	X Diagnostic Z No Qualifier

Section	0	**Medical and Surgical**
Body System	X	**Anatomical Regions, Upper Extremities**
Operation	B	**Excision:** Cutting out or off, without replacement, a portion of a body part

Body Part (4ᵗʰ)	Approach (5ᵗʰ)	Device (6ᵗʰ)	Qualifier (7ᵗʰ)
2 Shoulder Region, Right 3 Shoulder Region, Left 4 Axilla, Right 5 Axilla, Left 6 Upper Extremity, Right 7 Upper Extremity, Left 8 Upper Arm, Right 9 Upper Arm, Left B Elbow Region, Right C Elbow Region, Left D Lower Arm, Right F Lower Arm, Left G Wrist Region, Right H Wrist Region, Left J Hand, Right K Hand, Left	0 Open 3 Percutaneous 4 Percutaneous Endoscopic	Z No Device	X Diagnostic Z No Qualifier

Section	0	Medical and Surgical
Body System	X	Anatomical Regions, Upper Extremities
Operation	H	Insertion: Putting in a nonbiological appliance that monitors, assists, performs, or prevents a physiological function but does not physically take the place of a body part

Body Part (4th)	Approach (5th)	Device (6th)	Qualifier (7th)
2 Shoulder Region, Right 3 Shoulder Region, Left 4 Axilla, Right 5 Axilla, Left 6 Upper Extremity, Right 7 Upper Extremity, Left 8 Upper Arm, Right 9 Upper Arm, Left B Elbow Region, Right C Elbow Region, Left D Lower Arm, Right F Lower Arm, Left G Wrist Region, Right H Wrist Region, Left J Hand, Right K Hand, Left	0 Open 3 Percutaneous 4 Percutaneous Endoscopic	1 Radioactive Element 3 Infusion Device Y Other Device	Z No Qualifier

Section	0	Medical and Surgical
Body System	X	Anatomical Regions, Upper Extremities
Operation	J	Inspection: Visually and/or manually exploring a body part

Body Part (4th)	Approach (5th)	Device (6th)	Qualifier (7th)
2 Shoulder Region, Right 3 Shoulder Region, Left 4 Axilla, Right 5 Axilla, Left 6 Upper Extremity, Right 7 Upper Extremity, Left 8 Upper Arm, Right 9 Upper Arm, Left B Elbow Region, Right C Elbow Region, Left D Lower Arm, Right F Lower Arm, Left G Wrist Region, Right H Wrist Region, Left J Hand, Right K Hand, Left	0 Open 3 Percutaneous 4 Percutaneous Endoscopic X External	Z No Device	Z No Qualifier

Section	0	Medical and Surgical
Body System	X	Anatomical Regions, Upper Extremities
Operation	M	Reattachment: Putting back in or on all or a portion of a separated body part to its normal location or other suitable location

Body Part (4th)	Approach (5th)	Device (6th)	Qualifier (7th)
0 Forequarter, Right	0 Open	Z No Device	Z No Qualifier
1 Forequarter, Left			
2 Shoulder Region, Right			
3 Shoulder Region, Left			
4 Axilla, Right			
5 Axilla, Left			
6 Upper Extremity, Right			
7 Upper Extremity, Left			
8 Upper Arm, Right			
9 Upper Arm, Left			
B Elbow Region, Right			
C Elbow Region, Left			
D Lower Arm, Right			
F Lower Arm, Left			
G Wrist Region, Right			
H Wrist Region, Left			
J Hand, Right			
K Hand, Left			
L Thumb, Right			
M Thumb, Left			
N Index Finger, Right			
P Index Finger, Left			
Q Middle Finger, Right			
R Middle Finger, Left			
S Ring Finger, Right			
T Ring Finger, Left			
V Little Finger, Right			
W Little Finger, Left			

Section	0	Medical and Surgical
Body System	X	Anatomical Regions, Upper Extremities
Operation	P	Removal: Taking out or off a device from a body part

Body Part (4th)	Approach (5th)	Device (6th)	Qualifier (7th)
6 Upper Extremity, Right	0 Open	0 Drainage Device	Z No Qualifier
7 Upper Extremity, Left	3 Percutaneous	1 Radioactive Element	
	4 Percutaneous Endoscopic	3 Infusion Device	
	X External	7 Autologous Tissue Substitute	
		J Synthetic Substitute	
		K Nonautologous Tissue Substitute	
		Y Other Device	

Section	0	Medical and Surgical
Body System	X	Anatomical Regions, Upper Extremities
Operation	Q	**Repair:** Restoring, to the extent possible, a body part to its normal anatomic structure and function

Body Part (4th)	Approach (5th)	Device (6th)	Qualifier (7th)
2 Shoulder Region, Right	0 Open	Z No Device	Z No Qualifier
3 Shoulder Region, Left	3 Percutaneous		
4 Axilla, Right	4 Percutaneous Endoscopic		
5 Axilla, Left	X External		
6 Upper Extremity, Right			
7 Upper Extremity, Left			
8 Upper Arm, Right			
9 Upper Arm, Left			
B Elbow Region, Right			
C Elbow Region, Left			
D Lower Arm, Right			
F Lower Arm, Left			
G Wrist Region, Right			
H Wrist Region, Left			
J Hand, Right			
K Hand, Left			
L Thumb, Right			
M Thumb, Left			
N Index Finger, Right			
P Index Finger, Left			
Q Middle Finger, Right			
R Middle Finger, Left			
S Ring Finger, Right			
T Ring Finger, Left			
V Little Finger, Right			
W Little Finger, Left			

Section	0	Medical and Surgical
Body System	X	Anatomical Regions, Upper Extremities
Operation	R	**Replacement:** Putting in or on biological or synthetic material that physically takes the place and/or function of all or a portion of a body part

Body Part (4th)	Approach (5th)	Device (6th)	Qualifier (7th)
L Thumb, Right	0 Open	7 Autologous Tissue Substitute	N Toe, Right
M Thumb, Left	4 Percutaneous Endoscopic		P Toe, Left

Section	0	Medical and Surgical
Body System	X	Anatomical Regions, Upper Extremities
Operation	U	**Supplement:** Putting in or on biological or synthetic material that physically reinforces and/or augments the function of a portion of a body part

Body Part (4th)	Approach (5th)	Device (6th)	Qualifier (7th)

2 Shoulder Region, Right
3 Shoulder Region, Left
4 Axilla, Right
5 Axilla, Left
6 Upper Extremity, Right
7 Upper Extremity, Left
8 Upper Arm, Right
9 Upper Arm, Left
B Elbow Region, Right
C Elbow Region, Left
D Lower Arm, Right
F Lower Arm, Left
G Wrist Region, Right
H Wrist Region, Left
J Hand, Right
K Hand, Left
L Thumb, Right
M Thumb, Left
N Index Finger, Right
P Index Finger, Left
Q Middle Finger, Right
R Middle Finger, Left
S Ring Finger, Right
T Ring Finger, Left
V Little Finger, Right
W Little Finger, Left
	0 Open
	4 Percutaneous Endoscopic
		7 Autologous Tissue
		   Substitute
		J Synthetic Substitute
		K Nonautologous Tissue
		   Substitute
			Z No Qualifier

Section	0	Medical and Surgical
Body System	X	Anatomical Regions, Upper Extremities
Operation	W	**Revision:** Correcting, to the extent possible, a portion of a malfunctioning device or the position of a displaced device

Body Part (4th)	Approach (5th)	Device (6th)	Qualifier (7th)

6 Upper Extremity, Right
7 Upper Extremity, Left
	0 Open
	3 Percutaneous
	4 Percutaneous Endoscopic
	X External
		0 Drainage Device
		3 Infusion Device
		7 Autologous Tissue
		   Substitute
		J Synthetic Substitute
		K Nonautologous Tissue
		   Substitute
		Y Other Device
			Z No Qualifier

Section	0	Medical and Surgical
Body System	X	Anatomical Regions, Upper Extremities
Operation	X	**Transfer:** Moving, without taking out, all or a portion of a body part to another location to take over the function of all or a portion of a body part

Body Part (4th)	Approach (5th)	Device (6th)	Qualifier (7th)
N Index Finger, Right	0 Open	Z No Device	L Thumb, Right
P Index Finger, Left	0 Open	Z No Device	M Thumb, Left

Anatomical Regions, Upper Extremities Code Listing 0X0–0XX

0X0 – Anatomical Regions, Upper Extremities, Alteration

0X0207Z Alteration of Right Shoulder Region with Autologous Tissue Substitute, Open Approach

0X020JZ Alteration of Right Shoulder Region with Synthetic Substitute, Open Approach

0X020KZ Alteration of Right Shoulder Region with Nonautologous Tissue Substitute, Open Approach

0X020ZZ Alteration of Right Shoulder Region, Open Approach

0X0237Z Alteration of Right Shoulder Region with Autologous Tissue Substitute, Percutaneous Approach

0X023JZ Alteration of Right Shoulder Region with Synthetic Substitute, Percutaneous Approach

0X023KZ Alteration of Right Shoulder Region with Nonautologous Tissue Substitute, Percutaneous Approach

0X023ZZ Alteration of Right Shoulder Region, Percutaneous Approach

0X0247Z Alteration of Right Shoulder Region with Autologous Tissue Substitute, Percutaneous Endoscopic Approach

0X024JZ Alteration of Right Shoulder Region with Synthetic Substitute, Percutaneous Endoscopic Approach

0X024KZ Alteration of Right Shoulder Region with Nonautologous Tissue Substitute, Percutaneous Endoscopic Approach

0X024ZZ Alteration of Right Shoulder Region, Percutaneous Endoscopic Approach

0X0307Z Alteration of Left Shoulder Region with Autologous Tissue Substitute, Open Approach

0X030JZ Alteration of Left Shoulder Region with Synthetic Substitute, Open Approach

0X030KZ Alteration of Left Shoulder Region with Nonautologous Tissue Substitute, Open Approach

0X030ZZ Alteration of Left Shoulder Region, Open Approach

0X0337Z Alteration of Left Shoulder Region with Autologous Tissue Substitute, Percutaneous Approach

0X033JZ Alteration of Left Shoulder Region with Synthetic Substitute, Percutaneous Approach

0X033KZ Alteration of Left Shoulder Region with Nonautologous Tissue Substitute, Percutaneous Approach

0X033ZZ Alteration of Left Shoulder Region, Percutaneous Approach

0X0347Z Alteration of Left Shoulder Region with Autologous Tissue Substitute, Percutaneous Endoscopic Approach

0X034JZ Alteration of Left Shoulder Region with Synthetic Substitute, Percutaneous Endoscopic Approach

0X034KZ Alteration of Left Shoulder Region with Nonautologous Tissue Substitute, Percutaneous Endoscopic Approach

0X034ZZ Alteration of Left Shoulder Region, Percutaneous Endoscopic Approach

0X0407Z Alteration of Right Axilla with Autologous Tissue Substitute, Open Approach

0X040JZ Alteration of Right Axilla with Synthetic Substitute, Open Approach

0X040KZ Alteration of Right Axilla with Nonautologous Tissue Substitute, Open Approach

0X040ZZ Alteration of Right Axilla, Open Approach

0X0437Z Alteration of Right Axilla with Autologous Tissue Substitute, Percutaneous Approach

0X043JZ Alteration of Right Axilla with Synthetic Substitute, Percutaneous Approach

0X043KZ Alteration of Right Axilla with Nonautologous Tissue Substitute, Percutaneous Approach

0X043ZZ Alteration of Right Axilla, Percutaneous Approach

0X0447Z Alteration of Right Axilla with Autologous Tissue Substitute, Percutaneous Endoscopic Approach

0X044JZ Alteration of Right Axilla with Synthetic Substitute, Percutaneous Endoscopic Approach

0X044KZ Alteration of Right Axilla with Nonautologous Tissue Substitute, Percutaneous Endoscopic Approach

0X044ZZ Alteration of Right Axilla, Percutaneous Endoscopic Approach

0X0507Z Alteration of Left Axilla with Autologous Tissue Substitute, Open Approach

0X050JZ Alteration of Left Axilla with Synthetic Substitute, Open Approach

0X050KZ Alteration of Left Axilla with Nonautologous Tissue Substitute, Open Approach

0X050ZZ Alteration of Left Axilla, Open Approach

0X0537Z Alteration of Left Axilla with Autologous Tissue Substitute, Percutaneous Approach

0X053JZ Alteration of Left Axilla with Synthetic Substitute, Percutaneous Approach

0X053KZ Alteration of Left Axilla with Nonautologous Tissue Substitute, Percutaneous Approach

0X053ZZ Alteration of Left Axilla, Percutaneous Approach

0X0547Z Alteration of Left Axilla with Autologous Tissue Substitute, Percutaneous Endoscopic Approach

0X054JZ Alteration of Left Axilla with Synthetic Substitute, Percutaneous Endoscopic Approach

0X054KZ Alteration of Left Axilla with Nonautologous Tissue Substitute, Percutaneous Endoscopic Approach

0X054ZZ Alteration of Left Axilla, Percutaneous Endoscopic Approach

0X0607Z Alteration of Right Upper Extremity with Autologous Tissue Substitute, Open Approach

0X060JZ Alteration of Right Upper Extremity with Synthetic Substitute, Open Approach

0X060KZ Alteration of Right Upper Extremity with Nonautologous Tissue Substitute, Open Approach

0X060ZZ Alteration of Right Upper Extremity, Open Approach

0X0637Z Alteration of Right Upper Extremity with Autologous Tissue Substitute, Percutaneous Approach

0X063JZ Alteration of Right Upper Extremity with Synthetic Substitute, Percutaneous Approach

0X063KZ Alteration of Right Upper Extremity with Nonautologous Tissue Substitute, Percutaneous Approach

0X063ZZ Alteration of Right Upper Extremity, Percutaneous Approach

0X0647Z Alteration of Right Upper Extremity with Autologous Tissue Substitute, Percutaneous Endoscopic Approach

0X064JZ Alteration of Right Upper Extremity with Synthetic Substitute, Percutaneous Endoscopic Approach

0X064KZ Alteration of Right Upper Extremity with Nonautologous Tissue Substitute, Percutaneous Endoscopic Approach

0X064ZZ Alteration of Right Upper Extremity, Percutaneous Endoscopic Approach

0X0707Z Alteration of Left Upper Extremity with Autologous Tissue Substitute, Open Approach

0X070JZ Alteration of Left Upper Extremity with Synthetic Substitute, Open Approach

0X070KZ Alteration of Left Upper Extremity with Nonautologous Tissue Substitute, Open Approach

0X070ZZ Alteration of Left Upper Extremity, Open Approach

0X0737Z Alteration of Left Upper Extremity with Autologous Tissue Substitute, Percutaneous Approach

0X073JZ Alteration of Left Upper Extremity with Synthetic Substitute, Percutaneous Approach

0X073KZ Alteration of Left Upper Extremity with Nonautologous Tissue Substitute, Percutaneous Approach

0X073ZZ Alteration of Left Upper Extremity, Percutaneous Approach

0X0747Z Alteration of Left Upper Extremity with Autologous Tissue Substitute, Percutaneous Endoscopic Approach

0X074JZ Alteration of Left Upper Extremity with Synthetic Substitute, Percutaneous Endoscopic Approach

0X074KZ Alteration of Left Upper Extremity with Nonautologous Tissue Substitute, Percutaneous Endoscopic Approach

0X074ZZ Alteration of Left Upper Extremity, Percutaneous Endoscopic Approach

0X0807Z Alteration of Right Upper Arm with Autologous Tissue Substitute, Open Approach

0X080JZ Alteration of Right Upper Arm with Synthetic Substitute, Open Approach

0X080KZ Alteration of Right Upper Arm with Nonautologous Tissue Substitute, Open Approach

0X080ZZ Alteration of Right Upper Arm, Open Approach

0X0837Z Alteration of Right Upper Arm with Autologous Tissue Substitute, Percutaneous Approach

0X083JZ   Alteration of Right Upper Arm with Synthetic Substitute, Percutaneous Approach

0X083KZ   Alteration of Right Upper Arm with Nonautologous Tissue Substitute, Percutaneous Approach

0X083ZZ   Alteration of Right Upper Arm, Percutaneous Approach

0X0847Z   Alteration of Right Upper Arm with Autologous Tissue Substitute, Percutaneous Endoscopic Approach

0X084JZ   Alteration of Right Upper Arm with Synthetic Substitute, Percutaneous Endoscopic Approach

0X084KZ   Alteration of Right Upper Arm with Nonautologous Tissue Substitute, Percutaneous Endoscopic Approach

0X084ZZ   Alteration of Right Upper Arm, Percutaneous Endoscopic Approach

0X0907Z   Alteration of Left Upper Arm with Autologous Tissue Substitute, Open Approach

0X090JZ   Alteration of Left Upper Arm with Synthetic Substitute, Open Approach

0X090KZ   Alteration of Left Upper Arm with Nonautologous Tissue Substitute, Open Approach

0X090ZZ   Alteration of Left Upper Arm, Open Approach

0X0937Z   Alteration of Left Upper Arm with Autologous Tissue Substitute, Percutaneous Approach

0X093JZ   Alteration of Left Upper Arm with Synthetic Substitute, Percutaneous Approach

0X093KZ   Alteration of Left Upper Arm with Nonautologous Tissue Substitute, Percutaneous Approach

0X093ZZ   Alteration of Left Upper Arm, Percutaneous Approach

0X0947Z   Alteration of Left Upper Arm with Autologous Tissue Substitute, Percutaneous Endoscopic Approach

0X094JZ   Alteration of Left Upper Arm with Synthetic Substitute, Percutaneous Endoscopic Approach

0X094KZ   Alteration of Left Upper Arm with Nonautologous Tissue Substitute, Percutaneous Endoscopic Approach

0X094ZZ   Alteration of Left Upper Arm, Percutaneous Endoscopic Approach

0X0B07Z   Alteration of Right Elbow Region with Autologous Tissue Substitute, Open Approach

0X0B0JZ   Alteration of Right Elbow Region with Synthetic Substitute, Open Approach

0X0B0KZ   Alteration of Right Elbow Region with Nonautologous Tissue Substitute, Open Approach

0X0B0ZZ   Alteration of Right Elbow Region, Open Approach

0X0B37Z   Alteration of Right Elbow Region with Autologous Tissue Substitute, Percutaneous Approach

0X0B3JZ   Alteration of Right Elbow Region with Synthetic Substitute, Percutaneous Approach

0X0B3KZ   Alteration of Right Elbow Region with Nonautologous Tissue Substitute, Percutaneous Approach

0X0B3ZZ   Alteration of Right Elbow Region, Percutaneous Approach

0X0B47Z   Alteration of Right Elbow Region with Autologous Tissue Substitute, Percutaneous Endoscopic Approach

0X0B4JZ   Alteration of Right Elbow Region with Synthetic Substitute, Percutaneous Endoscopic Approach

0X0B4KZ   Alteration of Right Elbow Region with Nonautologous Tissue Substitute, Percutaneous Endoscopic Approach

0X0B4ZZ   Alteration of Right Elbow Region, Percutaneous Endoscopic Approach

0X0C07Z   Alteration of Left Elbow Region with Autologous Tissue Substitute, Open Approach

0X0C0JZ   Alteration of Left Elbow Region with Synthetic Substitute, Open Approach

0X0C0KZ   Alteration of Left Elbow Region with Nonautologous Tissue Substitute, Open Approach

0X0C0ZZ   Alteration of Left Elbow Region, Open Approach

0X0C37Z   Alteration of Left Elbow Region with Autologous Tissue Substitute, Percutaneous Approach

0X0C3JZ   Alteration of Left Elbow Region with Synthetic Substitute, Percutaneous Approach

0X0C3KZ   Alteration of Left Elbow Region with Nonautologous Tissue Substitute, Percutaneous Approach

0X0C3ZZ   Alteration of Left Elbow Region, Percutaneous Approach

0X0C47Z   Alteration of Left Elbow Region with Autologous Tissue Substitute, Percutaneous Endoscopic Approach

0X0C4JZ   Alteration of Left Elbow Region with Synthetic Substitute, Percutaneous Endoscopic Approach

0X0C4KZ   Alteration of Left Elbow Region with Nonautologous Tissue Substitute, Percutaneous Endoscopic Approach

0X0C4ZZ   Alteration of Left Elbow Region, Percutaneous Endoscopic Approach

0X0D07Z   Alteration of Right Lower Arm with Autologous Tissue Substitute, Open Approach

0X0D0JZ   Alteration of Right Lower Arm with Synthetic Substitute, Open Approach

0X0D0KZ   Alteration of Right Lower Arm with Nonautologous Tissue Substitute, Open Approach

0X0D0ZZ   Alteration of Right Lower Arm, Open Approach

0X0D37Z   Alteration of Right Lower Arm with Autologous Tissue Substitute, Percutaneous Approach

0X0D3JZ   Alteration of Right Lower Arm with Synthetic Substitute, Percutaneous Approach

0X0D3KZ   Alteration of Right Lower Arm with Nonautologous Tissue Substitute, Percutaneous Approach

0X0D3ZZ   Alteration of Right Lower Arm, Percutaneous Approach

0X0D47Z   Alteration of Right Lower Arm with Autologous Tissue Substitute, Percutaneous Endoscopic Approach

0X0D4JZ   Alteration of Right Lower Arm with Synthetic Substitute, Percutaneous Endoscopic Approach

0X0D4KZ   Alteration of Right Lower Arm with Nonautologous Tissue Substitute, Percutaneous Endoscopic Approach

0X0D4ZZ   Alteration of Right Lower Arm, Percutaneous Endoscopic Approach

0X0F07Z   Alteration of Left Lower Arm with Autologous Tissue Substitute, Open Approach

0X0F0JZ   Alteration of Left Lower Arm with Synthetic Substitute, Open Approach

0X0F0KZ   Alteration of Left Lower Arm with Nonautologous Tissue Substitute, Open Approach

0X0F0ZZ   Alteration of Left Lower Arm, Open Approach

0X0F37Z   Alteration of Left Lower Arm with Autologous Tissue Substitute, Percutaneous Approach

0X0F3JZ   Alteration of Left Lower Arm with Synthetic Substitute, Percutaneous Approach

0X0F3KZ   Alteration of Left Lower Arm with Nonautologous Tissue Substitute, Percutaneous Approach

0X0F3ZZ   Alteration of Left Lower Arm, Percutaneous Approach

0X0F47Z   Alteration of Left Lower Arm with Autologous Tissue Substitute, Percutaneous Endoscopic Approach

0X0F4JZ   Alteration of Left Lower Arm with Synthetic Substitute, Percutaneous Endoscopic Approach

0X0F4KZ   Alteration of Left Lower Arm with Nonautologous Tissue Substitute, Percutaneous Endoscopic Approach

0X0F4ZZ   Alteration of Left Lower Arm, Percutaneous Endoscopic Approach

0X0G07Z   Alteration of Right Wrist Region with Autologous Tissue Substitute, Open Approach

0X0G0JZ   Alteration of Right Wrist Region with Synthetic Substitute, Open Approach

0X0G0KZ   Alteration of Right Wrist Region with Nonautologous Tissue Substitute, Open Approach

0X0G0ZZ   Alteration of Right Wrist Region, Open Approach

0X0G37Z   Alteration of Right Wrist Region with Autologous Tissue Substitute, Percutaneous Approach

0X0G3JZ   Alteration of Right Wrist Region with Synthetic Substitute, Percutaneous Approach

0X0G3KZ   Alteration of Right Wrist Region with Nonautologous Tissue Substitute, Percutaneous Approach

0X0G3ZZ   Alteration of Right Wrist Region, Percutaneous Approach

0X0G47Z   Alteration of Right Wrist Region with Autologous Tissue Substitute, Percutaneous Endoscopic Approach

0X0G4JZ   Alteration of Right Wrist Region with Synthetic Substitute, Percutaneous Endoscopic Approach

0X0G4KZ   Alteration of Right Wrist Region with Nonautologous Tissue Substitute, Percutaneous Endoscopic Approach

0X0G4ZZ   Alteration of Right Wrist Region, Percutaneous Endoscopic Approach

0X0H07Z   Alteration of Left Wrist Region with Autologous Tissue Substitute, Open Approach

0X0H0JZ   Alteration of Left Wrist Region with Synthetic Substitute, Open Approach

0X0H0KZ Alteration of Left Wrist Region with Nonautologous Tissue Substitute, Open Approach

0X0H0ZZ Alteration of Left Wrist Region, Open Approach

0X0H37Z Alteration of Left Wrist Region with Autologous Tissue Substitute, Percutaneous Approach

0X0H3JZ Alteration of Left Wrist Region with Synthetic Substitute, Percutaneous Approach

0X0H3KZ Alteration of Left Wrist Region with Nonautologous Tissue Substitute, Percutaneous Approach

0X0H3ZZ Alteration of Left Wrist Region, Percutaneous Approach

0X0H47Z Alteration of Left Wrist Region with Autologous Tissue Substitute, Percutaneous Endoscopic Approach

0X0H4JZ Alteration of Left Wrist Region with Synthetic Substitute, Percutaneous Endoscopic Approach

0X0H4KZ Alteration of Left Wrist Region with Nonautologous Tissue Substitute, Percutaneous Endoscopic Approach

0X0H4ZZ Alteration of Left Wrist Region, Percutaneous Endoscopic Approach

0X2 – Anatomical Regions, Upper Extremities, Change

Review Coding Guideline B6.1c

0X26X0Z Change Drainage Device in Right Upper Extremity, External Approach

0X26XYZ Change Other Device in Right Upper Extremity, External Approach

0X27X0Z Change Drainage Device in Left Upper Extremity, External Approach

0X27XYZ Change Other Device in Left Upper Extremity, External Approach

0X3 – Anatomical Regions, Upper Extremities, Control

Review Coding Guideline B3.7

0X320ZZ Control Bleeding in Right Shoulder Region, Open Approach

0X323ZZ Control Bleeding in Right Shoulder Region, Percutaneous Approach

0X324ZZ Control Bleeding in Right Shoulder Region, Percutaneous Endoscopic Approach

0X330ZZ Control Bleeding in Left Shoulder Region, Open Approach

0X333ZZ Control Bleeding in Left Shoulder Region, Percutaneous Approach

0X334ZZ Control Bleeding in Left Shoulder Region, Percutaneous Endoscopic Approach

0X340ZZ Control Bleeding in Right Axilla, Open Approach

0X343ZZ Control Bleeding in Right Axilla, Percutaneous Approach

0X344ZZ Control Bleeding in Right Axilla, Percutaneous Endoscopic Approach

0X350ZZ Control Bleeding in Left Axilla, Open Approach

0X353ZZ Control Bleeding in Left Axilla, Percutaneous Approach

0X354ZZ Control Bleeding in Left Axilla, Percutaneous Endoscopic Approach

0X360ZZ Control Bleeding in Right Upper Extremity, Open Approach

0X363ZZ Control Bleeding in Right Upper Extremity, Percutaneous Approach

0X364ZZ Control Bleeding in Right Upper Extremity, Percutaneous Endoscopic Approach

0X370ZZ Control Bleeding in Left Upper Extremity, Open Approach

0X373ZZ Control Bleeding in Left Upper Extremity, Percutaneous Approach

0X374ZZ Control Bleeding in Left Upper Extremity, Percutaneous Endoscopic Approach

0X380ZZ Control Bleeding in Right Upper Arm, Open Approach

0X383ZZ Control Bleeding in Right Upper Arm, Percutaneous Approach

0X384ZZ Control Bleeding in Right Upper Arm, Percutaneous Endoscopic Approach

0X390ZZ Control Bleeding in Left Upper Arm, Open Approach

0X393ZZ Control Bleeding in Left Upper Arm, Percutaneous Approach

0X394ZZ Control Bleeding in Left Upper Arm, Percutaneous Endoscopic Approach

0X3B0ZZ Control Bleeding in Right Elbow Region, Open Approach

0X3B3ZZ Control Bleeding in Right Elbow Region, Percutaneous Approach

0X3B4ZZ Control Bleeding in Right Elbow Region, Percutaneous Endoscopic Approach

0X3C0ZZ Control Bleeding in Left Elbow Region, Open Approach

0X3C3ZZ Control Bleeding in Left Elbow Region, Percutaneous Approach

0X3C4ZZ Control Bleeding in Left Elbow Region, Percutaneous Endoscopic Approach

0X3D0ZZ Control Bleeding in Right Lower Arm, Open Approach

0X3D3ZZ Control Bleeding in Right Lower Arm, Percutaneous Approach

0X3D4ZZ Control Bleeding in Right Lower Arm, Percutaneous Endoscopic Approach

0X3F0ZZ Control Bleeding in Left Lower Arm, Open Approach

0X3F3ZZ Control Bleeding in Left Lower Arm, Percutaneous Approach

0X3F4ZZ Control Bleeding in Left Lower Arm, Percutaneous Endoscopic Approach

0X3G0ZZ Control Bleeding in Right Wrist Region, Open Approach

0X3G3ZZ Control Bleeding in Right Wrist Region, Percutaneous Approach

0X3G4ZZ Control Bleeding in Right Wrist Region, Percutaneous Endoscopic Approach

0X3H0ZZ Control Bleeding in Left Wrist Region, Open Approach

0X3H3ZZ Control Bleeding in Left Wrist Region, Percutaneous Approach

0X3H4ZZ Control Bleeding in Left Wrist Region, Percutaneous Endoscopic Approach

0X3J0ZZ Control Bleeding in Right Hand, Open Approach

0X3J3ZZ Control Bleeding in Right Hand, Percutaneous Approach

0X3J4ZZ Control Bleeding in Right Hand, Percutaneous Endoscopic Approach

0X3K0ZZ Control Bleeding in Left Hand, Open Approach

0X3K3ZZ Control Bleeding in Left Hand, Percutaneous Approach

0X3K4ZZ Control Bleeding in Left Hand, Percutaneous Endoscopic Approach

0X6 – Anatomical Regions, Upper Extremities, Detachment

0X600ZZ Detachment at Right Forequarter, Open Approach

0X610ZZ Detachment at Left Forequarter, Open Approach

0X620ZZ Detachment at Right Shoulder Region, Open Approach

0X630ZZ Detachment at Left Shoulder Region, Open Approach

0X680Z1 Detachment at Right Upper Arm, High, Open Approach

0X680Z2 Detachment at Right Upper Arm, Mid, Open Approach

0X680Z3 Detachment at Right Upper Arm, Low, Open Approach

0X690Z1 Detachment at Left Upper Arm, High, Open Approach

0X690Z2 Detachment at Left Upper Arm, Mid, Open Approach

0X690Z3 Detachment at Left Upper Arm, Low, Open Approach

0X6B0ZZ Detachment at Right Elbow Region, Open Approach

0X6C0ZZ Detachment at Left Elbow Region, Open Approach

0X6D0Z1 Detachment at Right Lower Arm, High, Open Approach

0X6D0Z2 Detachment at Right Lower Arm, Mid, Open Approach

0X6D0Z3 Detachment at Right Lower Arm, Low, Open Approach

0X6F0Z1 Detachment at Left Lower Arm, High, Open Approach

0X6F0Z2 Detachment at Left Lower Arm, Mid, Open Approach

0X6F0Z3 Detachment at Left Lower Arm, Low, Open Approach

0X6J0Z0 Detachment at Right Hand, Complete, Open Approach

0X6J0Z4 Detachment at Right Hand, Complete 1st Ray, Open Approach

0X6J0Z5 Detachment at Right Hand, Complete 2nd Ray, Open Approach

0X6J0Z6 Detachment at Right Hand, Complete 3rd Ray, Open Approach

0X6J0Z7 Detachment at Right Hand, Complete 4th Ray, Open Approach

0X6J0Z8 Detachment at Right Hand, Complete 5th Ray, Open Approach

0X6J0Z9 Detachment at Right Hand, Partial 1st Ray, Open Approach

0X6J0ZB Detachment at Right Hand, Partial 2nd Ray, Open Approach

0X6J0ZC Detachment at Right Hand, Partial 3rd Ray, Open Approach

0X6J0ZD Detachment at Right Hand, Partial 4th Ray, Open Approach

0X6J0ZF Detachment at Right Hand, Partial 5th Ray, Open Approach

0X6K0Z0 Detachment at Left Hand, Complete, Open Approach

0X6K0Z4 Detachment at Left Hand, Complete 1st Ray, Open Approach

0X6K0Z5 Detachment at Left Hand, Complete 2nd Ray, Open Approach

0X6K0Z6 Detachment at Left Hand, Complete 3rd Ray, Open Approach
0X6K0Z7 Detachment at Left Hand, Complete 4th Ray, Open Approach
0X6K0Z8 Detachment at Left Hand, Complete 5th Ray, Open Approach
0X6K0Z9 Detachment at Left Hand, Partial 1st Ray, Open Approach
0X6K0ZB Detachment at Left Hand, Partial 2nd Ray, Open Approach
0X6K0ZC Detachment at Left Hand, Partial 3rd Ray, Open Approach
0X6K0ZD Detachment at Left Hand, Partial 4th Ray, Open Approach
0X6K0ZF Detachment at Left Hand, Partial 5th Ray, Open Approach
0X6L0Z0 Detachment at Right Thumb, Complete, Open Approach
0X6L0Z1 Detachment at Right Thumb, High, Open Approach
0X6L0Z2 Detachment at Right Thumb, Mid, Open Approach
0X6L0Z3 Detachment at Right Thumb, Low, Open Approach
0X6M0Z0 Detachment at Left Thumb, Complete, Open Approach
0X6M0Z1 Detachment at Left Thumb, High, Open Approach
0X6M0Z2 Detachment at Left Thumb, Mid, Open Approach
0X6M0Z3 Detachment at Left Thumb, Low, Open Approach
0X6N0Z0 Detachment at Right Index Finger, Complete, Open Approach
0X6N0Z1 Detachment at Right Index Finger, High, Open Approach
0X6N0Z2 Detachment at Right Index Finger, Mid, Open Approach
0X6N0Z3 Detachment at Right Index Finger, Low, Open Approach
0X6P0Z0 Detachment at Left Index Finger, Complete, Open Approach
0X6P0Z1 Detachment at Left Index Finger, High, Open Approach
0X6P0Z2 Detachment at Left Index Finger, Mid, Open Approach
0X6P0Z3 Detachment at Left Index Finger, Low, Open Approach

0X6Q0Z0 Detachment at Right Middle Finger, Complete, Open Approach
0X6Q0Z1 Detachment at Right Middle Finger, High, Open Approach
0X6Q0Z2 Detachment at Right Middle Finger, Mid, Open Approach
0X6Q0Z3 Detachment at Right Middle Finger, Low, Open Approach
0X6R0Z0 Detachment at Left Middle Finger, Complete, Open Approach
0X6R0Z1 Detachment at Left Middle Finger, High, Open Approach
0X6R0Z2 Detachment at Left Middle Finger, Mid, Open Approach
0X6R0Z3 Detachment at Left Middle Finger, Low, Open Approach
0X6S0Z0 Detachment at Right Ring Finger, Complete, Open Approach
0X6S0Z1 Detachment at Right Ring Finger, High, Open Approach
0X6S0Z2 Detachment at Right Ring Finger, Mid, Open Approach
0X6S0Z3 Detachment at Right Ring Finger, Low, Open Approach
0X6T0Z0 Detachment at Left Ring Finger, Complete, Open Approach
0X6T0Z1 Detachment at Left Ring Finger, High, Open Approach
0X6T0Z2 Detachment at Left Ring Finger, Mid, Open Approach
0X6T0Z3 Detachment at Left Ring Finger, Low, Open Approach
0X6V0Z0 Detachment at Right Little Finger, Complete, Open Approach
0X6V0Z1 Detachment at Right Little Finger, High, Open Approach
0X6V0Z2 Detachment at Right Little Finger, Mid, Open Approach
0X6V0Z3 Detachment at Right Little Finger, Low, Open Approach
0X6W0Z0 Detachment at Left Little Finger, Complete, Open Approach
0X6W0Z1 Detachment at Left Little Finger, High, Open Approach
0X6W0Z2 Detachment at Left Little Finger, Mid, Open Approach
0X6W0Z3 Detachment at Left Little Finger, Low, Open Approach

0X9 – Anatomical Regions, Upper Extremities, Drainage

Review Coding Guidelines B3.4a and B3.4b

Review Coding Guideline B6.2

0X9200Z Drainage of Right Shoulder Region with Drainage Device, Open Approach
0X920ZX Drainage of Right Shoulder Region, Open Approach, Diagnostic
0X920ZZ Drainage of Right Shoulder Region, Open Approach
0X9230Z Drainage of Right Shoulder Region with Drainage Device, Percutaneous Approach
0X923ZX Drainage of Right Shoulder Region, Percutaneous Approach, Diagnostic
0X923ZZ Drainage of Right Shoulder Region, Percutaneous Approach
0X9240Z Drainage of Right Shoulder Region with Drainage Device, Percutaneous Endoscopic Approach
0X924ZX Drainage of Right Shoulder Region, Percutaneous Endoscopic Approach, Diagnostic
0X924ZZ Drainage of Right Shoulder Region, Percutaneous Endoscopic Approach
0X9300Z Drainage of Left Shoulder Region with Drainage Device, Open Approach
0X930ZX Drainage of Left Shoulder Region, Open Approach, Diagnostic
0X930ZZ Drainage of Left Shoulder Region, Open Approach
0X9330Z Drainage of Left Shoulder Region with Drainage Device, Percutaneous Approach
0X933ZX Drainage of Left Shoulder Region, Percutaneous Approach, Diagnostic
0X933ZZ Drainage of Left Shoulder Region, Percutaneous Approach
0X9340Z Drainage of Left Shoulder Region with Drainage Device, Percutaneous Endoscopic Approach
0X934ZX Drainage of Left Shoulder Region, Percutaneous Endoscopic Approach, Diagnostic
0X934ZZ Drainage of Left Shoulder Region, Percutaneous Endoscopic Approach
0X9400Z Drainage of Right Axilla with Drainage Device, Open Approach
0X940ZX Drainage of Right Axilla, Open Approach, Diagnostic
0X940ZZ Drainage of Right Axilla, Open Approach
0X9430Z Drainage of Right Axilla with Drainage Device, Percutaneous Approach
0X943ZX Drainage of Right Axilla, Percutaneous Approach, Diagnostic
0X943ZZ Drainage of Right Axilla, Percutaneous Approach
0X9440Z Drainage of Right Axilla with Drainage Device, Percutaneous Endoscopic Approach
0X944ZX Drainage of Right Axilla, Percutaneous Endoscopic Approach, Diagnostic
0X944ZZ Drainage of Right Axilla, Percutaneous Endoscopic Approach

0X9500Z Drainage of Left Axilla with Drainage Device, Open Approach
0X950ZX Drainage of Left Axilla, Open Approach, Diagnostic
0X950ZZ Drainage of Left Axilla, Open Approach
0X9530Z Drainage of Left Axilla with Drainage Device, Percutaneous Approach
0X953ZX Drainage of Left Axilla, Percutaneous Approach, Diagnostic
0X953ZZ Drainage of Left Axilla, Percutaneous Approach
0X9540Z Drainage of Left Axilla with Drainage Device, Percutaneous Endoscopic Approach
0X954ZX Drainage of Left Axilla, Percutaneous Endoscopic Approach, Diagnostic
0X954ZZ Drainage of Left Axilla, Percutaneous Endoscopic Approach
0X9600Z Drainage of Right Upper Extremity with Drainage Device, Open Approach
0X960ZX Drainage of Right Upper Extremity, Open Approach, Diagnostic
0X960ZZ Drainage of Right Upper Extremity, Open Approach
0X9630Z Drainage of Right Upper Extremity with Drainage Device, Percutaneous Approach
0X963ZX Drainage of Right Upper Extremity, Percutaneous Approach, Diagnostic
0X963ZZ Drainage of Right Upper Extremity, Percutaneous Approach
0X9640Z Drainage of Right Upper Extremity with Drainage Device, Percutaneous Endoscopic Approach
0X964ZX Drainage of Right Upper Extremity, Percutaneous Endoscopic Approach, Diagnostic
0X964ZZ Drainage of Right Upper Extremity, Percutaneous Endoscopic Approach
0X9700Z Drainage of Left Upper Extremity with Drainage Device, Open Approach
0X970ZX Drainage of Left Upper Extremity, Open Approach, Diagnostic
0X970ZZ Drainage of Left Upper Extremity, Open Approach
0X9730Z Drainage of Left Upper Extremity with Drainage Device, Percutaneous Approach
0X973ZX Drainage of Left Upper Extremity, Percutaneous Approach, Diagnostic
0X973ZZ Drainage of Left Upper Extremity, Percutaneous Approach
0X9740Z Drainage of Left Upper Extremity with Drainage Device, Percutaneous Endoscopic Approach
0X974ZX Drainage of Left Upper Extremity, Percutaneous Endoscopic Approach, Diagnostic
0X974ZZ Drainage of Left Upper Extremity, Percutaneous Endoscopic Approach

0X9800Z	Drainage of Right Upper Arm with Drainage Device, Open Approach
0X980ZX	Drainage of Right Upper Arm, Open Approach, Diagnostic
0X980ZZ	Drainage of Right Upper Arm, Open Approach
0X9830Z	Drainage of Right Upper Arm with Drainage Device, Percutaneous Approach
0X983ZX	Drainage of Right Upper Arm, Percutaneous Approach, Diagnostic
0X983ZZ	Drainage of Right Upper Arm, Percutaneous Approach
0X9840Z	Drainage of Right Upper Arm with Drainage Device, Percutaneous Endoscopic Approach
0X984ZX	Drainage of Right Upper Arm, Percutaneous Endoscopic Approach, Diagnostic
0X984ZZ	Drainage of Right Upper Arm, Percutaneous Endoscopic Approach
0X9900Z	Drainage of Left Upper Arm with Drainage Device, Open Approach
0X990ZX	Drainage of Left Upper Arm, Open Approach, Diagnostic
0X990ZZ	Drainage of Left Upper Arm, Open Approach
0X9930Z	Drainage of Left Upper Arm with Drainage Device, Percutaneous Approach
0X993ZX	Drainage of Left Upper Arm, Percutaneous Approach, Diagnostic
0X993ZZ	Drainage of Left Upper Arm, Percutaneous Approach
0X9940Z	Drainage of Left Upper Arm with Drainage Device, Percutaneous Endoscopic Approach
0X994ZX	Drainage of Left Upper Arm, Percutaneous Endoscopic Approach, Diagnostic
0X994ZZ	Drainage of Left Upper Arm, Percutaneous Endoscopic Approach
0X9B00Z	Drainage of Right Elbow Region with Drainage Device, Open Approach
0X9B0ZX	Drainage of Right Elbow Region, Open Approach, Diagnostic
0X9B0ZZ	Drainage of Right Elbow Region, Open Approach
0X9B30Z	Drainage of Right Elbow Region with Drainage Device, Percutaneous Approach
0X9B3ZX	Drainage of Right Elbow Region, Percutaneous Approach, Diagnostic
0X9B3ZZ	Drainage of Right Elbow Region, Percutaneous Approach
0X9B40Z	Drainage of Right Elbow Region with Drainage Device, Percutaneous Endoscopic Approach
0X9B4ZX	Drainage of Right Elbow Region, Percutaneous Endoscopic Approach, Diagnostic
0X9B4ZZ	Drainage of Right Elbow Region, Percutaneous Endoscopic Approach
0X9C00Z	Drainage of Left Elbow Region with Drainage Device, Open Approach
0X9C0ZX	Drainage of Left Elbow Region, Open Approach, Diagnostic
0X9C0ZZ	Drainage of Left Elbow Region, Open Approach
0X9C30Z	Drainage of Left Elbow Region with Drainage Device, Percutaneous Approach
0X9C3ZX	Drainage of Left Elbow Region, Percutaneous Approach, Diagnostic
0X9C3ZZ	Drainage of Left Elbow Region, Percutaneous Approach
0X9C40Z	Drainage of Left Elbow Region with Drainage Device, Percutaneous Endoscopic Approach
0X9C4ZX	Drainage of Left Elbow Region, Percutaneous Endoscopic Approach, Diagnostic
0X9C4ZZ	Drainage of Left Elbow Region, Percutaneous Endoscopic Approach
0X9D00Z	Drainage of Right Lower Arm with Drainage Device, Open Approach
0X9D0ZX	Drainage of Right Lower Arm, Open Approach, Diagnostic
0X9D0ZZ	Drainage of Right Lower Arm, Open Approach
0X9D30Z	Drainage of Right Lower Arm with Drainage Device, Percutaneous Approach
0X9D3ZX	Drainage of Right Lower Arm, Percutaneous Approach, Diagnostic
0X9D3ZZ	Drainage of Right Lower Arm, Percutaneous Approach
0X9D40Z	Drainage of Right Lower Arm with Drainage Device, Percutaneous Endoscopic Approach
0X9D4ZX	Drainage of Right Lower Arm, Percutaneous Endoscopic Approach, Diagnostic
0X9D4ZZ	Drainage of Right Lower Arm, Percutaneous Endoscopic Approach
0X9F00Z	Drainage of Left Lower Arm with Drainage Device, Open Approach
0X9F0ZX	Drainage of Left Lower Arm, Open Approach, Diagnostic
0X9F0ZZ	Drainage of Left Lower Arm, Open Approach
0X9F30Z	Drainage of Left Lower Arm with Drainage Device, Percutaneous Approach
0X9F3ZX	Drainage of Left Lower Arm, Percutaneous Approach, Diagnostic
0X9F3ZZ	Drainage of Left Lower Arm, Percutaneous Approach
0X9F40Z	Drainage of Left Lower Arm with Drainage Device, Percutaneous Endoscopic Approach
0X9F4ZX	Drainage of Left Lower Arm, Percutaneous Endoscopic Approach, Diagnostic
0X9F4ZZ	Drainage of Left Lower Arm, Percutaneous Endoscopic Approach
0X9G00Z	Drainage of Right Wrist Region with Drainage Device, Open Approach
0X9G0ZX	Drainage of Right Wrist Region, Open Approach, Diagnostic
0X9G0ZZ	Drainage of Right Wrist Region, Open Approach
0X9G30Z	Drainage of Right Wrist Region with Drainage Device, Percutaneous Approach
0X9G3ZX	Drainage of Right Wrist Region, Percutaneous Approach, Diagnostic
0X9G3ZZ	Drainage of Right Wrist Region, Percutaneous Approach
0X9G40Z	Drainage of Right Wrist Region with Drainage Device, Percutaneous Endoscopic Approach
0X9G4ZX	Drainage of Right Wrist Region, Percutaneous Endoscopic Approach, Diagnostic
0X9G4ZZ	Drainage of Right Wrist Region, Percutaneous Endoscopic Approach
0X9H00Z	Drainage of Left Wrist Region with Drainage Device, Open Approach
0X9H0ZX	Drainage of Left Wrist Region, Open Approach, Diagnostic
0X9H0ZZ	Drainage of Left Wrist Region, Open Approach
0X9H30Z	Drainage of Left Wrist Region with Drainage Device, Percutaneous Approach
0X9H3ZX	Drainage of Left Wrist Region, Percutaneous Approach, Diagnostic
0X9H3ZZ	Drainage of Left Wrist Region, Percutaneous Approach
0X9H40Z	Drainage of Left Wrist Region with Drainage Device, Percutaneous Endoscopic Approach
0X9H4ZX	Drainage of Left Wrist Region, Percutaneous Endoscopic Approach, Diagnostic
0X9H4ZZ	Drainage of Left Wrist Region, Percutaneous Endoscopic Approach
0X9J00Z	Drainage of Right Hand with Drainage Device, Open Approach
0X9J0ZX	Drainage of Right Hand, Open Approach, Diagnostic
0X9J0ZZ	Drainage of Right Hand, Open Approach
0X9J30Z	Drainage of Right Hand with Drainage Device, Percutaneous Approach
0X9J3ZX	Drainage of Right Hand, Percutaneous Approach, Diagnostic
0X9J3ZZ	Drainage of Right Hand, Percutaneous Approach
0X9J40Z	Drainage of Right Hand with Drainage Device, Percutaneous Endoscopic Approach
0X9J4ZX	Drainage of Right Hand, Percutaneous Endoscopic Approach, Diagnostic
0X9J4ZZ	Drainage of Right Hand, Percutaneous Endoscopic Approach
0X9K00Z	Drainage of Left Hand with Drainage Device, Open Approach
0X9K0ZX	Drainage of Left Hand, Open Approach, Diagnostic
0X9K0ZZ	Drainage of Left Hand, Open Approach
0X9K30Z	Drainage of Left Hand with Drainage Device, Percutaneous Approach
0X9K3ZX	Drainage of Left Hand, Percutaneous Approach, Diagnostic
0X9K3ZZ	Drainage of Left Hand, Percutaneous Approach
0X9K40Z	Drainage of Left Hand with Drainage Device, Percutaneous Endoscopic Approach
0X9K4ZX	Drainage of Left Hand, Percutaneous Endoscopic Approach, Diagnostic
0X9K4ZZ	Drainage of Left Hand, Percutaneous Endoscopic Approach

0XB – Anatomical Regions, Upper Extremities, Excision

Review Coding Guidelines B3.4a and B3.4b

0XB20ZX	Excision of Right Shoulder Region, Open Approach, Diagnostic
0XB20ZZ	Excision of Right Shoulder Region, Open Approach
0XB23ZX	Excision of Right Shoulder Region, Percutaneous Approach, Diagnostic

0XB23ZZ	Excision of Right Shoulder Region, Percutaneous Approach
0XB24ZX	Excision of Right Shoulder Region, Percutaneous Endoscopic Approach, Diagnostic
0XB24ZZ	Excision of Right Shoulder Region, Percutaneous Endoscopic Approach
0XB30ZX	Excision of Left Shoulder Region, Open Approach, Diagnostic
0XB30ZZ	Excision of Left Shoulder Region, Open Approach
0XB33ZX	Excision of Left Shoulder Region, Percutaneous Approach, Diagnostic
0XB33ZZ	Excision of Left Shoulder Region, Percutaneous Approach
0XB34ZX	Excision of Left Shoulder Region, Percutaneous Endoscopic Approach, Diagnostic
0XB34ZZ	Excision of Left Shoulder Region, Percutaneous Endoscopic Approach
0XB40ZX	Excision of Right Axilla, Open Approach, Diagnostic
0XB40ZZ	Excision of Right Axilla, Open Approach
0XB43ZX	Excision of Right Axilla, Percutaneous Approach, Diagnostic
0XB43ZZ	Excision of Right Axilla, Percutaneous Approach
0XB44ZX	Excision of Right Axilla, Percutaneous Endoscopic Approach, Diagnostic
0XB44ZZ	Excision of Right Axilla, Percutaneous Endoscopic Approach
0XB50ZX	Excision of Left Axilla, Open Approach, Diagnostic
0XB50ZZ	Excision of Left Axilla, Open Approach
0XB53ZX	Excision of Left Axilla, Percutaneous Approach, Diagnostic
0XB53ZZ	Excision of Left Axilla, Percutaneous Approach
0XB54ZX	Excision of Left Axilla, Percutaneous Endoscopic Approach, Diagnostic
0XB54ZZ	Excision of Left Axilla, Percutaneous Endoscopic Approach
0XB60ZX	Excision of Right Upper Extremity, Open Approach, Diagnostic
0XB60ZZ	Excision of Right Upper Extremity, Open Approach
0XB63ZX	Excision of Right Upper Extremity, Percutaneous Approach, Diagnostic
0XB63ZZ	Excision of Right Upper Extremity, Percutaneous Approach
0XB64ZX	Excision of Right Upper Extremity, Percutaneous Endoscopic Approach, Diagnostic
0XB64ZZ	Excision of Right Upper Extremity, Percutaneous Endoscopic Approach
0XB70ZX	Excision of Left Upper Extremity, Open Approach, Diagnostic
0XB70ZZ	Excision of Left Upper Extremity, Open Approach
0XB73ZX	Excision of Left Upper Extremity, Percutaneous Approach, Diagnostic
0XB73ZZ	Excision of Left Upper Extremity, Percutaneous Approach
0XB74ZX	Excision of Left Upper Extremity, Percutaneous Endoscopic Approach, Diagnostic
0XB74ZZ	Excision of Left Upper Extremity, Percutaneous Endoscopic Approach
0XB80ZX	Excision of Right Upper Arm, Open Approach, Diagnostic
0XB80ZZ	Excision of Right Upper Arm, Open Approach
0XB83ZX	Excision of Right Upper Arm, Percutaneous Approach, Diagnostic
0XB83ZZ	Excision of Right Upper Arm, Percutaneous Approach
0XB84ZX	Excision of Right Upper Arm, Percutaneous Endoscopic Approach, Diagnostic
0XB84ZZ	Excision of Right Upper Arm, Percutaneous Endoscopic Approach
0XB90ZX	Excision of Left Upper Arm, Open Approach, Diagnostic
0XB90ZZ	Excision of Left Upper Arm, Open Approach
0XB93ZX	Excision of Left Upper Arm, Percutaneous Approach, Diagnostic
0XB93ZZ	Excision of Left Upper Arm, Percutaneous Approach
0XB94ZX	Excision of Left Upper Arm, Percutaneous Endoscopic Approach, Diagnostic
0XB94ZZ	Excision of Left Upper Arm, Percutaneous Endoscopic Approach

0XBB0ZX	Excision of Right Elbow Region, Open Approach, Diagnostic
0XBB0ZZ	Excision of Right Elbow Region, Open Approach
0XBB3ZX	Excision of Right Elbow Region, Percutaneous Approach, Diagnostic
0XBB3ZZ	Excision of Right Elbow Region, Percutaneous Approach
0XBB4ZX	Excision of Right Elbow Region, Percutaneous Endoscopic Approach, Diagnostic
0XBB4ZZ	Excision of Right Elbow Region, Percutaneous Endoscopic Approach
0XBC0ZX	Excision of Left Elbow Region, Open Approach, Diagnostic
0XBC0ZZ	Excision of Left Elbow Region, Open Approach
0XBC3ZX	Excision of Left Elbow Region, Percutaneous Approach, Diagnostic
0XBC3ZZ	Excision of Left Elbow Region, Percutaneous Approach
0XBC4ZX	Excision of Left Elbow Region, Percutaneous Endoscopic Approach, Diagnostic
0XBC4ZZ	Excision of Left Elbow Region, Percutaneous Endoscopic Approach
0XBD0ZX	Excision of Right Lower Arm, Open Approach, Diagnostic
0XBD0ZZ	Excision of Right Lower Arm, Open Approach
0XBD3ZX	Excision of Right Lower Arm, Percutaneous Approach, Diagnostic
0XBD3ZZ	Excision of Right Lower Arm, Percutaneous Approach
0XBD4ZX	Excision of Right Lower Arm, Percutaneous Endoscopic Approach, Diagnostic
0XBD4ZZ	Excision of Right Lower Arm, Percutaneous Endoscopic Approach
0XBF0ZX	Excision of Left Lower Arm, Open Approach, Diagnostic
0XBF0ZZ	Excision of Left Lower Arm, Open Approach
0XBF3ZX	Excision of Left Lower Arm, Percutaneous Approach, Diagnostic
0XBF3ZZ	Excision of Left Lower Arm, Percutaneous Approach
0XBF4ZX	Excision of Left Lower Arm, Percutaneous Endoscopic Approach, Diagnostic
0XBF4ZZ	Excision of Left Lower Arm, Percutaneous Endoscopic Approach
0XBG0ZX	Excision of Right Wrist Region, Open Approach, Diagnostic
0XBG0ZZ	Excision of Right Wrist Region, Open Approach
0XBG3ZX	Excision of Right Wrist Region, Percutaneous Approach, Diagnostic
0XBG3ZZ	Excision of Right Wrist Region, Percutaneous Approach
0XBG4ZX	Excision of Right Wrist Region, Percutaneous Endoscopic Approach, Diagnostic
0XBG4ZZ	Excision of Right Wrist Region, Percutaneous Endoscopic Approach
0XBH0ZX	Excision of Left Wrist Region, Open Approach, Diagnostic
0XBH0ZZ	Excision of Left Wrist Region, Open Approach
0XBH3ZX	Excision of Left Wrist Region, Percutaneous Approach, Diagnostic
0XBH3ZZ	Excision of Left Wrist Region, Percutaneous Approach
0XBH4ZX	Excision of Left Wrist Region, Percutaneous Endoscopic Approach, Diagnostic
0XBH4ZZ	Excision of Left Wrist Region, Percutaneous Endoscopic Approach
0XBJ0ZX	Excision of Right Hand, Open Approach, Diagnostic
0XBJ0ZZ	Excision of Right Hand, Open Approach
0XBJ3ZX	Excision of Right Hand, Percutaneous Approach, Diagnostic
0XBJ3ZZ	Excision of Right Hand, Percutaneous Approach
0XBJ4ZX	Excision of Right Hand, Percutaneous Endoscopic Approach, Diagnostic
0XBJ4ZZ	Excision of Right Hand, Percutaneous Endoscopic Approach
0XBK0ZX	Excision of Left Hand, Open Approach, Diagnostic
0XBK0ZZ	Excision of Left Hand, Open Approach
0XBK3ZX	Excision of Left Hand, Percutaneous Approach, Diagnostic
0XBK3ZZ	Excision of Left Hand, Percutaneous Approach
0XBK4ZX	Excision of Left Hand, Percutaneous Endoscopic Approach, Diagnostic
0XBK4ZZ	Excision of Left Hand, Percutaneous Endoscopic Approach

0XH – Anatomical Regions, Upper Extremities, Insertion

0XH201Z	Insertion of Radioactive Element into Right Shoulder Region, Open Approach
● **0XH203Z**	Insertion of Infusion Device into Right Shoulder Region, Open Approach
● **0XH20YZ**	Insertion of Other Device into Right Shoulder Region, Open Approach
0XH231Z	Insertion of Radioactive Element into Right Shoulder Region, Percutaneous Approach
● **0XH233Z**	Insertion of Infusion Device into Right Shoulder Region, Percutaneous Approach

● **0XH23YZ**	Insertion of Other Device into Right Shoulder Region, Percutaneous Approach
0XH241Z	Insertion of Radioactive Element into Right Shoulder Region, Percutaneous Endoscopic Approach
● **0XH243Z**	Insertion of Infusion Device into Right Shoulder Region, Percutaneous Endoscopic Approach
● **0XH24YZ**	Insertion of Other Device into Right Shoulder Region, Percutaneous Endoscopic Approach
0XH301Z	Insertion of Radioactive Element into Left Shoulder Region, Open Approach

---

♀ Female-only   ♂ Male-only   ● Limited Coverage   ● Non-OR   🅷🅰🅲 HAC-associated procedure   ● Non-covered procedures   ✚ Combination

● **0XH303Z** Insertion of Infusion Device into Left Shoulder Region, Open Approach

● **0XH30YZ** Insertion of Other Device into Left Shoulder Region, Open Approach

0XH331Z Insertion of Radioactive Element into Left Shoulder Region, Percutaneous Approach

● **0XH333Z** Insertion of Infusion Device into Left Shoulder Region, Percutaneous Approach

● **0XH33YZ** Insertion of Other Device into Left Shoulder Region, Percutaneous Approach

0XH341Z Insertion of Radioactive Element into Left Shoulder Region, Percutaneous Endoscopic Approach

● **0XH343Z** Insertion of Infusion Device into Left Shoulder Region, Percutaneous Endoscopic Approach

● **0XH34YZ** Insertion of Other Device into Left Shoulder Region, Percutaneous Endoscopic Approach

0XH401Z Insertion of Radioactive Element into Right Axilla, Open Approach

● **0XH403Z** Insertion of Infusion Device into Right Axilla, Open Approach

● **0XH40YZ** Insertion of Other Device into Right Axilla, Open Approach

0XH431Z Insertion of Radioactive Element into Right Axilla, Percutaneous Approach

● **0XH433Z** Insertion of Infusion Device into Right Axilla, Percutaneous Approach

● **0XH43YZ** Insertion of Other Device into Right Axilla, Percutaneous Approach

0XH441Z Insertion of Radioactive Element into Right Axilla, Percutaneous Endoscopic Approach

● **0XH443Z** Insertion of Infusion Device into Right Axilla, Percutaneous Endoscopic Approach

● **0XH44YZ** Insertion of Other Device into Right Axilla, Percutaneous Endoscopic Approach

0XH501Z Insertion of Radioactive Element into Left Axilla, Open Approach

● **0XH503Z** Insertion of Infusion Device into Left Axilla, Open Approach

● **0XH50YZ** Insertion of Other Device into Left Axilla, Open Approach

0XH531Z Insertion of Radioactive Element into Left Axilla, Percutaneous Approach

● **0XH533Z** Insertion of Infusion Device into Left Axilla, Percutaneous Approach

● **0XH53YZ** Insertion of Other Device into Left Axilla, Percutaneous Approach

0XH541Z Insertion of Radioactive Element into Left Axilla, Percutaneous Endoscopic Approach

● **0XH543Z** Insertion of Infusion Device into Left Axilla, Percutaneous Endoscopic Approach

● **0XH54YZ** Insertion of Other Device into Left Axilla, Percutaneous Endoscopic Approach

0XH601Z Insertion of Radioactive Element into Right Upper Extremity, Open Approach

● **0XH603Z** Insertion of Infusion Device into Right Upper Extremity, Open Approach

● **0XH60YZ** Insertion of Other Device into Right Upper Extremity, Open Approach

0XH631Z Insertion of Radioactive Element into Right Upper Extremity, Percutaneous Approach

● **0XH633Z** Insertion of Infusion Device into Right Upper Extremity, Percutaneous Approach

● **0XH63YZ** Insertion of Other Device into Right Upper Extremity, Percutaneous Approach

0XH641Z Insertion of Radioactive Element into Right Upper Extremity, Percutaneous Endoscopic Approach

● **0XH643Z** Insertion of Infusion Device into Right Upper Extremity, Percutaneous Endoscopic Approach

● **0XH64YZ** Insertion of Other Device into Right Upper Extremity, Percutaneous Endoscopic Approach

0XH701Z Insertion of Radioactive Element into Left Upper Extremity, Open Approach

● **0XH703Z** Insertion of Infusion Device into Left Upper Extremity, Open Approach

● **0XH70YZ** Insertion of Other Device into Left Upper Extremity, Open Approach

0XH731Z Insertion of Radioactive Element into Left Upper Extremity, Percutaneous Approach

● **0XH733Z** Insertion of Infusion Device into Left Upper Extremity, Percutaneous Approach

● **0XH73YZ** Insertion of Other Device into Left Upper Extremity, Percutaneous Approach

0XH741Z Insertion of Radioactive Element into Left Upper Extremity, Percutaneous Endoscopic Approach

● **0XH743Z** Insertion of Infusion Device into Left Upper Extremity, Percutaneous Endoscopic Approach

● **0XH74YZ** Insertion of Other Device into Left Upper Extremity, Percutaneous Endoscopic Approach

0XH801Z Insertion of Radioactive Element into Right Upper Arm, Open Approach

● **0XH803Z** Insertion of Infusion Device into Right Upper Arm, Open Approach

● **0XH80YZ** Insertion of Other Device into Right Upper Arm, Open Approach

0XH831Z Insertion of Radioactive Element into Right Upper Arm, Percutaneous Approach

● **0XH833Z** Insertion of Infusion Device into Right Upper Arm, Percutaneous Approach

● **0XH83YZ** Insertion of Other Device into Right Upper Arm, Percutaneous Approach

0XH841Z Insertion of Radioactive Element into Right Upper Arm, Percutaneous Endoscopic Approach

● **0XH843Z** Insertion of Infusion Device into Right Upper Arm, Percutaneous Endoscopic Approach

● **0XH84YZ** Insertion of Other Device into Right Upper Arm, Percutaneous Endoscopic Approach

0XH901Z Insertion of Radioactive Element into Left Upper Arm, Open Approach

● **0XH903Z** Insertion of Infusion Device into Left Upper Arm, Open Approach

● **0XH90YZ** Insertion of Other Device into Left Upper Arm, Open Approach

0XH931Z Insertion of Radioactive Element into Left Upper Arm, Percutaneous Approach

● **0XH933Z** Insertion of Infusion Device into Left Upper Arm, Percutaneous Approach

● **0XH93YZ** Insertion of Other Device into Left Upper Arm, Percutaneous Approach

0XH941Z Insertion of Radioactive Element into Left Upper Arm, Percutaneous Endoscopic Approach

● **0XH943Z** Insertion of Infusion Device into Left Upper Arm, Percutaneous Endoscopic Approach

● **0XH94YZ** Insertion of Other Device into Left Upper Arm, Percutaneous Endoscopic Approach

0XHB01Z Insertion of Radioactive Element into Right Elbow Region, Open Approach

● **0XHB03Z** Insertion of Infusion Device into Right Elbow Region, Open Approach

● **0XHB0YZ** Insertion of Other Device into Right Elbow Region, Open Approach

0XHB31Z Insertion of Radioactive Element into Right Elbow Region, Percutaneous Approach

● **0XHB33Z** Insertion of Infusion Device into Right Elbow Region, Percutaneous Approach

● **0XHB3YZ** Insertion of Other Device into Right Elbow Region, Percutaneous Approach

0XHB41Z Insertion of Radioactive Element into Right Elbow Region, Percutaneous Endoscopic Approach

● **0XHB43Z** Insertion of Infusion Device into Right Elbow Region, Percutaneous Endoscopic Approach

● **0XHB4YZ** Insertion of Other Device into Right Elbow Region, Percutaneous Endoscopic Approach

0XHC01Z Insertion of Radioactive Element into Left Elbow Region, Open Approach

● **0XHC03Z** Insertion of Infusion Device into Left Elbow Region, Open Approach

● **0XHC0YZ** Insertion of Other Device into Left Elbow Region, Open Approach

0XHC31Z Insertion of Radioactive Element into Left Elbow Region, Percutaneous Approach

● **0XHC33Z** Insertion of Infusion Device into Left Elbow Region, Percutaneous Approach

● **0XHC3YZ** Insertion of Other Device into Left Elbow Region, Percutaneous Approach

0XHC41Z Insertion of Radioactive Element into Left Elbow Region, Percutaneous Endoscopic Approach

● **0XHC43Z** Insertion of Infusion Device into Left Elbow Region, Percutaneous Endoscopic Approach

● **0XHC4YZ** Insertion of Other Device into Left Elbow Region, Percutaneous Endoscopic Approach

0XHD01Z Insertion of Radioactive Element into Right Lower Arm, Open Approach

---

♀ Female-only   ♂ Male-only   ● Limited Coverage   ● Non-OR   **HAC** HAC-associated procedure   ● Non-covered procedures   ✚ Combination

● **0XHD03Z** Insertion of Infusion Device into Right Lower Arm, Open Approach
● **0XHD0YZ** Insertion of Other Device into Right Lower Arm, Open Approach
0XHD31Z Insertion of Radioactive Element into Right Lower Arm, Percutaneous Approach
● **0XHD33Z** Insertion of Infusion Device into Right Lower Arm, Percutaneous Approach
● **0XHD3YZ** Insertion of Other Device into Right Lower Arm, Percutaneous Approach
0XHD41Z Insertion of Radioactive Element into Right Lower Arm, Percutaneous Endoscopic Approach
● **0XHD43Z** Insertion of Infusion Device into Right Lower Arm, Percutaneous Endoscopic Approach
● **0XHD4YZ** Insertion of Other Device into Right Lower Arm, Percutaneous Endoscopic Approach
0XHF01Z Insertion of Radioactive Element into Left Lower Arm, Open Approach
● **0XHF03Z** Insertion of Infusion Device into Left Lower Arm, Open Approach
● **0XHF0YZ** Insertion of Other Device into Left Lower Arm, Open Approach
0XHF31Z Insertion of Radioactive Element into Left Lower Arm, Percutaneous Approach
● **0XHF33Z** Insertion of Infusion Device into Left Lower Arm, Percutaneous Approach
● **0XHF3YZ** Insertion of Other Device into Left Lower Arm, Percutaneous Approach
0XHF41Z Insertion of Radioactive Element into Left Lower Arm, Percutaneous Endoscopic Approach
● **0XHF43Z** Insertion of Infusion Device into Left Lower Arm, Percutaneous Endoscopic Approach
● **0XHF4YZ** Insertion of Other Device into Left Lower Arm, Percutaneous Endoscopic Approach
0XHG01Z Insertion of Radioactive Element into Right Wrist Region, Open Approach
● **0XHG03Z** Insertion of Infusion Device into Right Wrist Region, Open Approach
● **0XHG0YZ** Insertion of Other Device into Right Wrist Region, Open Approach
0XHG31Z Insertion of Radioactive Element into Right Wrist Region, Percutaneous Approach
● **0XHG33Z** Insertion of Infusion Device into Right Wrist Region, Percutaneous Approach
● **0XHG3YZ** Insertion of Other Device into Right Wrist Region, Percutaneous Approach
0XHG41Z Insertion of Radioactive Element into Right Wrist Region, Percutaneous Endoscopic Approach
● **0XHG43Z** Insertion of Infusion Device into Right Wrist Region, Percutaneous Endoscopic Approach

● **0XHG4YZ** Insertion of Other Device into Right Wrist Region, Percutaneous Endoscopic Approach
0XHH01Z Insertion of Radioactive Element into Left Wrist Region, Open Approach
● **0XHH03Z** Insertion of Infusion Device into Left Wrist Region, Open Approach
● **0XHH0YZ** Insertion of Other Device into Left Wrist Region, Open Approach
0XHH31Z Insertion of Radioactive Element into Left Wrist Region, Percutaneous Approach
● **0XHH33Z** Insertion of Infusion Device into Left Wrist Region, Percutaneous Approach
● **0XHH3YZ** Insertion of Other Device into Left Wrist Region, Percutaneous Approach
0XHH41Z Insertion of Radioactive Element into Left Wrist Region, Percutaneous Endoscopic Approach
● **0XHH43Z** Insertion of Infusion Device into Left Wrist Region, Percutaneous Endoscopic Approach
● **0XHH4YZ** Insertion of Other Device into Left Wrist Region, Percutaneous Endoscopic Approach
0XHJ01Z Insertion of Radioactive Element into Right Hand, Open Approach
● **0XHJ03Z** Insertion of Infusion Device into Right Hand, Open Approach
● **0XHJ0YZ** Insertion of Other Device into Right Hand, Open Approach
0XHJ31Z Insertion of Radioactive Element into Right Hand, Percutaneous Approach
● **0XHJ33Z** Insertion of Infusion Device into Right Hand, Percutaneous Approach
● **0XHJ3YZ** Insertion of Other Device into Right Hand, Percutaneous Approach
0XHJ41Z Insertion of Radioactive Element into Right Hand, Percutaneous Endoscopic Approach
● **0XHJ43Z** Insertion of Infusion Device into Right Hand, Percutaneous Endoscopic Approach
● **0XHJ4YZ** Insertion of Other Device into Right Hand, Percutaneous Endoscopic Approach
0XHK01Z Insertion of Radioactive Element into Left Hand, Open Approach
● **0XHK03Z** Insertion of Infusion Device into Left Hand, Open Approach
● **0XHK0YZ** Insertion of Other Device into Left Hand, Open Approach
0XHK31Z Insertion of Radioactive Element into Left Hand, Percutaneous Approach
● **0XHK33Z** Insertion of Infusion Device into Left Hand, Percutaneous Approach
● **0XHK3YZ** Insertion of Other Device into Left Hand, Percutaneous Approach
0XHK41Z Insertion of Radioactive Element into Left Hand, Percutaneous Endoscopic Approach
● **0XHK43Z** Insertion of Infusion Device into Left Hand, Percutaneous Endoscopic Approach
● **0XHK4YZ** Insertion of Other Device into Left Hand, Percutaneous Endoscopic Approach

0XJ – Anatomical Regions, Upper Extremities, Inspection

Review Coding Guidelines B3.11a, B3.11b and B3.11c

● **0XJ20ZZ** Inspection of Right Shoulder Region, Open Approach
0XJ23ZZ Inspection of Right Shoulder Region, Percutaneous Approach
0XJ24ZZ Inspection of Right Shoulder Region, Percutaneous Endoscopic Approach
0XJ2XZZ Inspection of Right Shoulder Region, External Approach
● **0XJ30ZZ** Inspection of Left Shoulder Region, Open Approach
0XJ33ZZ Inspection of Left Shoulder Region, Percutaneous Approach
0XJ34ZZ Inspection of Left Shoulder Region, Percutaneous Endoscopic Approach
0XJ3XZZ Inspection of Left Shoulder Region, External Approach
● **0XJ40ZZ** Inspection of Right Axilla, Open Approach
0XJ43ZZ Inspection of Right Axilla, Percutaneous Approach
0XJ44ZZ Inspection of Right Axilla, Percutaneous Endoscopic Approach
0XJ4XZZ Inspection of Right Axilla, External Approach
● **0XJ50ZZ** Inspection of Left Axilla, Open Approach
0XJ53ZZ Inspection of Left Axilla, Percutaneous Approach
0XJ54ZZ Inspection of Left Axilla, Percutaneous Endoscopic Approach
0XJ5XZZ Inspection of Left Axilla, External Approach
● **0XJ60ZZ** Inspection of Right Upper Extremity, Open Approach
0XJ63ZZ Inspection of Right Upper Extremity, Percutaneous Approach
0XJ64ZZ Inspection of Right Upper Extremity, Percutaneous Endoscopic Approach
0XJ6XZZ Inspection of Right Upper Extremity, External Approach
● **0XJ70ZZ** Inspection of Left Upper Extremity, Open Approach

0XJ73ZZ Inspection of Left Upper Extremity, Percutaneous Approach
0XJ74ZZ Inspection of Left Upper Extremity, Percutaneous Endoscopic Approach
0XJ7XZZ Inspection of Left Upper Extremity, External Approach
● **0XJ80ZZ** Inspection of Right Upper Arm, Open Approach
0XJ83ZZ Inspection of Right Upper Arm, Percutaneous Approach
0XJ84ZZ Inspection of Right Upper Arm, Percutaneous Endoscopic Approach
0XJ8XZZ Inspection of Right Upper Arm, External Approach
● **0XJ90ZZ** Inspection of Left Upper Arm, Open Approach
0XJ93ZZ Inspection of Left Upper Arm, Percutaneous Approach
0XJ94ZZ Inspection of Left Upper Arm, Percutaneous Endoscopic Approach
0XJ9XZZ Inspection of Left Upper Arm, External Approach
● **0XJB0ZZ** Inspection of Right Elbow Region, Open Approach
0XJB3ZZ Inspection of Right Elbow Region, Percutaneous Approach
0XJB4ZZ Inspection of Right Elbow Region, Percutaneous Endoscopic Approach
0XJBXZZ Inspection of Right Elbow Region, External Approach
● **0XJC0ZZ** Inspection of Left Elbow Region, Open Approach
0XJC3ZZ Inspection of Left Elbow Region, Percutaneous Approach
0XJC4ZZ Inspection of Left Elbow Region, Percutaneous Endoscopic Approach
0XJCXZZ Inspection of Left Elbow Region, External Approach
● **0XJD0ZZ** Inspection of Right Lower Arm, Open Approach
0XJD3ZZ Inspection of Right Lower Arm, Percutaneous Approach

♀ Female-only   ♂ Male-only   ◐ Limited Coverage   ● Non-OR   **HAC** HAC-associated procedure   ◕ Non-covered procedures   ✚ Combination

0XJD4ZZ Inspection of Right Lower Arm, Percutaneous Endoscopic Approach
0XJDXZZ Inspection of Right Lower Arm, External Approach
● **0XJF0ZZ** Inspection of Left Lower Arm, Open Approach
0XJF3ZZ Inspection of Left Lower Arm, Percutaneous Approach
0XJF4ZZ Inspection of Left Lower Arm, Percutaneous Endoscopic Approach
0XJFXZZ Inspection of Left Lower Arm, External Approach
● **0XJG0ZZ** Inspection of Right Wrist Region, Open Approach
0XJG3ZZ Inspection of Right Wrist Region, Percutaneous Approach
0XJG4ZZ Inspection of Right Wrist Region, Percutaneous Endoscopic Approach
0XJGXZZ Inspection of Right Wrist Region, External Approach
● **0XJH0ZZ** Inspection of Left Wrist Region, Open Approach

0XJH3ZZ Inspection of Left Wrist Region, Percutaneous Approach
0XJH4ZZ Inspection of Left Wrist Region, Percutaneous Endoscopic Approach
0XJHXZZ Inspection of Left Wrist Region, External Approach
● **0XJJ0ZZ** Inspection of Right Hand, Open Approach
0XJJ3ZZ Inspection of Right Hand, Percutaneous Approach
0XJJ4ZZ Inspection of Right Hand, Percutaneous Endoscopic Approach
0XJJXZZ Inspection of Right Hand, External Approach
● **0XJK0ZZ** Inspection of Left Hand, Open Approach
0XJK3ZZ Inspection of Left Hand, Percutaneous Approach
0XJK4ZZ Inspection of Left Hand, Percutaneous Endoscopic Approach
0XJKXZZ Inspection of Left Hand, External Approach

0XM – Anatomical Regions, Upper Extremities, Reattachment

0XM00ZZ Reattachment of Right Forequarter, Open Approach
0XM10ZZ Reattachment of Left Forequarter, Open Approach
0XM20ZZ Reattachment of Right Shoulder Region, Open Approach
0XM30ZZ Reattachment of Left Shoulder Region, Open Approach
0XM40ZZ Reattachment of Right Axilla, Open Approach
0XM50ZZ Reattachment of Left Axilla, Open Approach
0XM60ZZ Reattachment of Right Upper Extremity, Open Approach
0XM70ZZ Reattachment of Left Upper Extremity, Open Approach
0XM80ZZ Reattachment of Right Upper Arm, Open Approach
0XM90ZZ Reattachment of Left Upper Arm, Open Approach
0XMB0ZZ Reattachment of Right Elbow Region, Open Approach
0XMC0ZZ Reattachment of Left Elbow Region, Open Approach
0XMD0ZZ Reattachment of Right Lower Arm, Open Approach
0XMF0ZZ Reattachment of Left Lower Arm, Open Approach

0XMG0ZZ Reattachment of Right Wrist Region, Open Approach
0XMH0ZZ Reattachment of Left Wrist Region, Open Approach
0XMJ0ZZ Reattachment of Right Hand, Open Approach
0XMK0ZZ Reattachment of Left Hand, Open Approach
0XML0ZZ Reattachment of Right Thumb, Open Approach
0XMM0ZZ Reattachment of Left Thumb, Open Approach
0XMN0ZZ Reattachment of Right Index Finger, Open Approach
0XMP0ZZ Reattachment of Left Index Finger, Open Approach
0XMQ0ZZ Reattachment of Right Middle Finger, Open Approach
0XMR0ZZ Reattachment of Left Middle Finger, Open Approach
0XMS0ZZ Reattachment of Right Ring Finger, Open Approach
0XMT0ZZ Reattachment of Left Ring Finger, Open Approach
0XMV0ZZ Reattachment of Right Little Finger, Open Approach
0XMW0ZZ Reattachment of Left Little Finger, Open Approach

0XP – Anatomical Regions, Upper Extremities, Removal

Review Coding Guideline B6.1c

0XP600Z Removal of Drainage Device from Right Upper Extremity, Open Approach
0XP601Z Removal of Radioactive Element from Right Upper Extremity, Open Approach
0XP603Z Removal of Infusion Device from Right Upper Extremity, Open Approach
0XP607Z Removal of Autologous Tissue Substitute from Right Upper Extremity, Open Approach
0XP60JZ Removal of Synthetic Substitute from Right Upper Extremity, Open Approach
0XP60KZ Removal of Nonautologous Tissue Substitute from Right Upper Extremity, Open Approach
0XP60YZ Removal of Other Device from Right Upper Extremity, Open Approach
0XP630Z Removal of Drainage Device from Right Upper Extremity, Percutaneous Approach
0XP631Z Removal of Radioactive Element from Right Upper Extremity, Percutaneous Approach
0XP633Z Removal of Infusion Device from Right Upper Extremity, Percutaneous Approach
0XP637Z Removal of Autologous Tissue Substitute from Right Upper Extremity, Percutaneous Approach
0XP63JZ Removal of Synthetic Substitute from Right Upper Extremity, Percutaneous Approach
0XP63KZ Removal of Nonautologous Tissue Substitute from Right Upper Extremity, Percutaneous Approach
0XP63YZ Removal of Other Device from Right Upper Extremity, Percutaneous Approach
0XP640Z Removal of Drainage Device from Right Upper Extremity, Percutaneous Endoscopic Approach
0XP641Z Removal of Radioactive Element from Right Upper Extremity, Percutaneous Endoscopic Approach
0XP643Z Removal of Infusion Device from Right Upper Extremity, Percutaneous Endoscopic Approach
0XP647Z Removal of Autologous Tissue Substitute from Right Upper Extremity, Percutaneous Endoscopic Approach
0XP64JZ Removal of Synthetic Substitute from Right Upper Extremity, Percutaneous Endoscopic Approach

0XP64KZ Removal of Nonautologous Tissue Substitute from Right Upper Extremity, Percutaneous Endoscopic Approach
0XP64YZ Removal of Other Device from Right Upper Extremity, Percutaneous Endoscopic Approach
0XP6X0Z Removal of Drainage Device from Right Upper Extremity, External Approach
0XP6X1Z Removal of Radioactive Element from Right Upper Extremity, External Approach
0XP6X3Z Removal of Infusion Device from Right Upper Extremity, External Approach
0XP6X7Z Removal of Autologous Tissue Substitute from Right Upper Extremity, External Approach
0XP6XJZ Removal of Synthetic Substitute from Right Upper Extremity, External Approach
0XP6XKZ Removal of Nonautologous Tissue Substitute from Right Upper Extremity, External Approach
0XP6XYZ Removal of Other Device from Right Upper Extremity, External Approach
0XP700Z Removal of Drainage Device from Left Upper Extremity, Open Approach
0XP701Z Removal of Radioactive Element from Left Upper Extremity, Open Approach
0XP703Z Removal of Infusion Device from Left Upper Extremity, Open Approach
0XP707Z Removal of Autologous Tissue Substitute from Left Upper Extremity, Open Approach
0XP70JZ Removal of Synthetic Substitute from Left Upper Extremity, Open Approach
0XP70KZ Removal of Nonautologous Tissue Substitute from Left Upper Extremity, Open Approach
0XP70YZ Removal of Other Device from Left Upper Extremity, Open Approach
0XP730Z Removal of Drainage Device from Left Upper Extremity, Percutaneous Approach
0XP731Z Removal of Radioactive Element from Left Upper Extremity, Percutaneous Approach
0XP733Z Removal of Infusion Device from Left Upper Extremity, Percutaneous Approach

0XP737Z	Removal of Autologous Tissue Substitute from Left Upper Extremity, Percutaneous Approach
0XP73JZ	Removal of Synthetic Substitute from Left Upper Extremity, Percutaneous Approach
0XP73KZ	Removal of Nonautologous Tissue Substitute from Left Upper Extremity, Percutaneous Approach
0XP73YZ	Removal of Other Device from Left Upper Extremity, Percutaneous Approach
0XP740Z	Removal of Drainage Device from Left Upper Extremity, Percutaneous Endoscopic Approach
0XP741Z	Removal of Radioactive Element from Left Upper Extremity, Percutaneous Endoscopic Approach
0XP743Z	Removal of Infusion Device from Left Upper Extremity, Percutaneous Endoscopic Approach
0XP747Z	Removal of Autologous Tissue Substitute from Left Upper Extremity, Percutaneous Endoscopic Approach
0XP74JZ	Removal of Synthetic Substitute from Left Upper Extremity, Percutaneous Endoscopic Approach
0XP74KZ	Removal of Nonautologous Tissue Substitute from Left Upper Extremity, Percutaneous Endoscopic Approach
0XP74YZ	Removal of Other Device from Left Upper Extremity, Percutaneous Endoscopic Approach
0XP7X0Z	Removal of Drainage Device from Left Upper Extremity, External Approach
0XP7X1Z	Removal of Radioactive Element from Left Upper Extremity, External Approach
0XP7X3Z	Removal of Infusion Device from Left Upper Extremity, External Approach
0XP7X7Z	Removal of Autologous Tissue Substitute from Left Upper Extremity, External Approach
0XP7XJZ	Removal of Synthetic Substitute from Left Upper Extremity, External Approach
0XP7XKZ	Removal of Nonautologous Tissue Substitute from Left Upper Extremity, External Approach
0XP7XYZ	Removal of Other Device from Left Upper Extremity, External Approach

0XQ – Anatomical Regions, Upper Extremities, Repair

0XQ20ZZ	Repair Right Shoulder Region, Open Approach
0XQ23ZZ	Repair Right Shoulder Region, Percutaneous Approach
0XQ24ZZ	Repair Right Shoulder Region, Percutaneous Endoscopic Approach
0XQ2XZZ	Repair Right Shoulder Region, External Approach
0XQ30ZZ	Repair Left Shoulder Region, Open Approach
0XQ33ZZ	Repair Left Shoulder Region, Percutaneous Approach
0XQ34ZZ	Repair Left Shoulder Region, Percutaneous Endoscopic Approach
0XQ3XZZ	Repair Left Shoulder Region, External Approach
0XQ40ZZ	Repair Right Axilla, Open Approach
0XQ43ZZ	Repair Right Axilla, Percutaneous Approach
0XQ44ZZ	Repair Right Axilla, Percutaneous Endoscopic Approach
0XQ4XZZ	Repair Right Axilla, External Approach
0XQ50ZZ	Repair Left Axilla, Open Approach
0XQ53ZZ	Repair Left Axilla, Percutaneous Approach
0XQ54ZZ	Repair Left Axilla, Percutaneous Endoscopic Approach
0XQ5XZZ	Repair Left Axilla, External Approach
0XQ60ZZ	Repair Right Upper Extremity, Open Approach
0XQ63ZZ	Repair Right Upper Extremity, Percutaneous Approach
0XQ64ZZ	Repair Right Upper Extremity, Percutaneous Endoscopic Approach
0XQ6XZZ	Repair Right Upper Extremity, External Approach
0XQ70ZZ	Repair Left Upper Extremity, Open Approach
0XQ73ZZ	Repair Left Upper Extremity, Percutaneous Approach
0XQ74ZZ	Repair Left Upper Extremity, Percutaneous Endoscopic Approach
0XQ7XZZ	Repair Left Upper Extremity, External Approach
0XQ80ZZ	Repair Right Upper Arm, Open Approach
0XQ83ZZ	Repair Right Upper Arm, Percutaneous Approach
0XQ84ZZ	Repair Right Upper Arm, Percutaneous Endoscopic Approach
0XQ8XZZ	Repair Right Upper Arm, External Approach
0XQ90ZZ	Repair Left Upper Arm, Open Approach
0XQ93ZZ	Repair Left Upper Arm, Percutaneous Approach
0XQ94ZZ	Repair Left Upper Arm, Percutaneous Endoscopic Approach
0XQ9XZZ	Repair Left Upper Arm, External Approach
0XQB0ZZ	Repair Right Elbow Region, Open Approach
0XQB3ZZ	Repair Right Elbow Region, Percutaneous Approach
0XQB4ZZ	Repair Right Elbow Region, Percutaneous Endoscopic Approach
0XQBXZZ	Repair Right Elbow Region, External Approach
0XQC0ZZ	Repair Left Elbow Region, Open Approach
0XQC3ZZ	Repair Left Elbow Region, Percutaneous Approach
0XQC4ZZ	Repair Left Elbow Region, Percutaneous Endoscopic Approach
0XQCXZZ	Repair Left Elbow Region, External Approach
0XQD0ZZ	Repair Right Lower Arm, Open Approach
0XQD3ZZ	Repair Right Lower Arm, Percutaneous Approach
0XQD4ZZ	Repair Right Lower Arm, Percutaneous Endoscopic Approach
0XQDXZZ	Repair Right Lower Arm, External Approach
0XQF0ZZ	Repair Left Lower Arm, Open Approach
0XQF3ZZ	Repair Left Lower Arm, Percutaneous Approach
0XQF4ZZ	Repair Left Lower Arm, Percutaneous Endoscopic Approach
0XQFXZZ	Repair Left Lower Arm, External Approach
0XQG0ZZ	Repair Right Wrist Region, Open Approach
0XQG3ZZ	Repair Right Wrist Region, Percutaneous Approach
0XQG4ZZ	Repair Right Wrist Region, Percutaneous Endoscopic Approach
0XQGXZZ	Repair Right Wrist Region, External Approach
0XQH0ZZ	Repair Left Wrist Region, Open Approach
0XQH3ZZ	Repair Left Wrist Region, Percutaneous Approach
0XQH4ZZ	Repair Left Wrist Region, Percutaneous Endoscopic Approach
0XQHXZZ	Repair Left Wrist Region, External Approach
0XQJ0ZZ	Repair Right Hand, Open Approach
0XQJ3ZZ	Repair Right Hand, Percutaneous Approach
0XQJ4ZZ	Repair Right Hand, Percutaneous Endoscopic Approach
0XQJXZZ	Repair Right Hand, External Approach
0XQK0ZZ	Repair Left Hand, Open Approach
0XQK3ZZ	Repair Left Hand, Percutaneous Approach
0XQK4ZZ	Repair Left Hand, Percutaneous Endoscopic Approach
0XQKXZZ	Repair Left Hand, External Approach
0XQL0ZZ	Repair Right Thumb, Open Approach
0XQL3ZZ	Repair Right Thumb, Percutaneous Approach
0XQL4ZZ	Repair Right Thumb, Percutaneous Endoscopic Approach
0XQLXZZ	Repair Right Thumb, External Approach
0XQM0ZZ	Repair Left Thumb, Open Approach
0XQM3ZZ	Repair Left Thumb, Percutaneous Approach
0XQM4ZZ	Repair Left Thumb, Percutaneous Endoscopic Approach
0XQMXZZ	Repair Left Thumb, External Approach
0XQN0ZZ	Repair Right Index Finger, Open Approach
0XQN3ZZ	Repair Right Index Finger, Percutaneous Approach
0XQN4ZZ	Repair Right Index Finger, Percutaneous Endoscopic Approach
0XQNXZZ	Repair Right Index Finger, External Approach
0XQP0ZZ	Repair Left Index Finger, Open Approach
0XQP3ZZ	Repair Left Index Finger, Percutaneous Approach
0XQP4ZZ	Repair Left Index Finger, Percutaneous Endoscopic Approach
0XQPXZZ	Repair Left Index Finger, External Approach
0XQQ0ZZ	Repair Right Middle Finger, Open Approach
0XQQ3ZZ	Repair Right Middle Finger, Percutaneous Approach
0XQQ4ZZ	Repair Right Middle Finger, Percutaneous Endoscopic Approach
0XQQXZZ	Repair Right Middle Finger, External Approach
0XQR0ZZ	Repair Left Middle Finger, Open Approach
0XQR3ZZ	Repair Left Middle Finger, Percutaneous Approach
0XQR4ZZ	Repair Left Middle Finger, Percutaneous Endoscopic Approach
0XQRXZZ	Repair Left Middle Finger, External Approach
0XQS0ZZ	Repair Right Ring Finger, Open Approach
0XQS3ZZ	Repair Right Ring Finger, Percutaneous Approach
0XQS4ZZ	Repair Right Ring Finger, Percutaneous Endoscopic Approach
0XQSXZZ	Repair Right Ring Finger, External Approach
0XQT0ZZ	Repair Left Ring Finger, Open Approach
0XQT3ZZ	Repair Left Ring Finger, Percutaneous Approach
0XQT4ZZ	Repair Left Ring Finger, Percutaneous Endoscopic Approach
0XQTXZZ	Repair Left Ring Finger, External Approach
0XQV0ZZ	Repair Right Little Finger, Open Approach
0XQV3ZZ	Repair Right Little Finger, Percutaneous Approach
0XQV4ZZ	Repair Right Little Finger, Percutaneous Endoscopic Approach
0XQVXZZ	Repair Right Little Finger, External Approach
0XQW0ZZ	Repair Left Little Finger, Open Approach
0XQW3ZZ	Repair Left Little Finger, Percutaneous Approach
0XQW4ZZ	Repair Left Little Finger, Percutaneous Endoscopic Approach
0XQWXZZ	Repair Left Little Finger, External Approach

0XR – Anatomical Regions, Upper Extremities, Replacement

0XRL07N Replacement of Right Thumb with Right Toe, Autologous Tissue Substitute, Open Approach

0XRL07P Replacement of Right Thumb with Left Toe, Autologous Tissue Substitute, Open Approach

0XRL47N Replacement of Right Thumb with Right Toe, Autologous Tissue Substitute, Percutaneous Endoscopic Approach

0XRL47P Replacement of Right Thumb with Left Toe, Autologous Tissue Substitute, Percutaneous Endoscopic Approach

0XRM07N Replacement of Left Thumb with Right Toe, Autologous Tissue Substitute, Open Approach

0XRM07P Replacement of Left Thumb with Left Toe, Autologous Tissue Substitute, Open Approach

0XRM47N Replacement of Left Thumb with Right Toe, Autologous Tissue Substitute, Percutaneous Endoscopic Approach

0XRM47P Replacement of Left Thumb with Left Toe, Autologous Tissue Substitute, Percutaneous Endoscopic Approach

0XU – Anatomical Regions, Upper Extremities, Supplement

0XU207Z Supplement Right Shoulder Region with Autologous Tissue Substitute, Open Approach

0XU20JZ Supplement Right Shoulder Region with Synthetic Substitute, Open Approach

0XU20KZ Supplement Right Shoulder Region with Nonautologous Tissue Substitute, Open Approach

0XU247Z Supplement Right Shoulder Region with Autologous Tissue Substitute, Percutaneous Endoscopic Approach

0XU24JZ Supplement Right Shoulder Region with Synthetic Substitute, Percutaneous Endoscopic Approach

0XU24KZ Supplement Right Shoulder Region with Nonautologous Tissue Substitute, Percutaneous Endoscopic Approach

0XU307Z Supplement Left Shoulder Region with Autologous Tissue Substitute, Open Approach

0XU30JZ Supplement Left Shoulder Region with Synthetic Substitute, Open Approach

0XU30KZ Supplement Left Shoulder Region with Nonautologous Tissue Substitute, Open Approach

0XU347Z Supplement Left Shoulder Region with Autologous Tissue Substitute, Percutaneous Endoscopic Approach

0XU34JZ Supplement Left Shoulder Region with Synthetic Substitute, Percutaneous Endoscopic Approach

0XU34KZ Supplement Left Shoulder Region with Nonautologous Tissue Substitute, Percutaneous Endoscopic Approach

0XU407Z Supplement Right Axilla with Autologous Tissue Substitute, Open Approach

0XU40JZ Supplement Right Axilla with Synthetic Substitute, Open Approach

0XU40KZ Supplement Right Axilla with Nonautologous Tissue Substitute, Open Approach

0XU447Z Supplement Right Axilla with Autologous Tissue Substitute, Percutaneous Endoscopic Approach

0XU44JZ Supplement Right Axilla with Synthetic Substitute, Percutaneous Endoscopic Approach

0XU44KZ Supplement Right Axilla with Nonautologous Tissue Substitute, Percutaneous Endoscopic Approach

0XU507Z Supplement Left Axilla with Autologous Tissue Substitute, Open Approach

0XU50JZ Supplement Left Axilla with Synthetic Substitute, Open Approach

0XU50KZ Supplement Left Axilla with Nonautologous Tissue Substitute, Open Approach

0XU547Z Supplement Left Axilla with Autologous Tissue Substitute, Percutaneous Endoscopic Approach

0XU54JZ Supplement Left Axilla with Synthetic Substitute, Percutaneous Endoscopic Approach

0XU54KZ Supplement Left Axilla with Nonautologous Tissue Substitute, Percutaneous Endoscopic Approach

0XU607Z Supplement Right Upper Extremity with Autologous Tissue Substitute, Open Approach

0XU60JZ Supplement Right Upper Extremity with Synthetic Substitute, Open Approach

0XU60KZ Supplement Right Upper Extremity with Nonautologous Tissue Substitute, Open Approach

0XU647Z Supplement Right Upper Extremity with Autologous Tissue Substitute, Percutaneous Endoscopic Approach

0XU64JZ Supplement Right Upper Extremity with Synthetic Substitute, Percutaneous Endoscopic Approach

0XU64KZ Supplement Right Upper Extremity with Nonautologous Tissue Substitute, Percutaneous Endoscopic Approach

0XU707Z Supplement Left Upper Extremity with Autologous Tissue Substitute, Open Approach

0XU70JZ Supplement Left Upper Extremity with Synthetic Substitute, Open Approach

0XU70KZ Supplement Left Upper Extremity with Nonautologous Tissue Substitute, Open Approach

0XU747Z Supplement Left Upper Extremity with Autologous Tissue Substitute, Percutaneous Endoscopic Approach

0XU74JZ Supplement Left Upper Extremity with Synthetic Substitute, Percutaneous Endoscopic Approach

0XU74KZ Supplement Left Upper Extremity with Nonautologous Tissue Substitute, Percutaneous Endoscopic Approach

0XU807Z Supplement Right Upper Arm with Autologous Tissue Substitute, Open Approach

0XU80JZ Supplement Right Upper Arm with Synthetic Substitute, Open Approach

0XU80KZ Supplement Right Upper Arm with Nonautologous Tissue Substitute, Open Approach

0XU847Z Supplement Right Upper Arm with Autologous Tissue Substitute, Percutaneous Endoscopic Approach

0XU84JZ Supplement Right Upper Arm with Synthetic Substitute, Percutaneous Endoscopic Approach

0XU84KZ Supplement Right Upper Arm with Nonautologous Tissue Substitute, Percutaneous Endoscopic Approach

0XU907Z Supplement Left Upper Arm with Autologous Tissue Substitute, Open Approach

0XU90JZ Supplement Left Upper Arm with Synthetic Substitute, Open Approach

0XU90KZ Supplement Left Upper Arm with Nonautologous Tissue Substitute, Open Approach

0XU947Z Supplement Left Upper Arm with Autologous Tissue Substitute, Percutaneous Endoscopic Approach

0XU94JZ Supplement Left Upper Arm with Synthetic Substitute, Percutaneous Endoscopic Approach

0XU94KZ Supplement Left Upper Arm with Nonautologous Tissue Substitute, Percutaneous Endoscopic Approach

0XUB07Z Supplement Right Elbow Region with Autologous Tissue Substitute, Open Approach

0XUB0JZ Supplement Right Elbow Region with Synthetic Substitute, Open Approach

0XUB0KZ Supplement Right Elbow Region with Nonautologous Tissue Substitute, Open Approach

0XUB47Z Supplement Right Elbow Region with Autologous Tissue Substitute, Percutaneous Endoscopic Approach

0XUB4JZ Supplement Right Elbow Region with Synthetic Substitute, Percutaneous Endoscopic Approach

0XUB4KZ Supplement Right Elbow Region with Nonautologous Tissue Substitute, Percutaneous Endoscopic Approach

0XUC07Z Supplement Left Elbow Region with Autologous Tissue Substitute, Open Approach

0XUC0JZ Supplement Left Elbow Region with Synthetic Substitute, Open Approach

0XUC0KZ Supplement Left Elbow Region with Nonautologous Tissue Substitute, Open Approach

0XUC47Z Supplement Left Elbow Region with Autologous Tissue Substitute, Percutaneous Endoscopic Approach

0XUC4JZ Supplement Left Elbow Region with Synthetic Substitute, Percutaneous Endoscopic Approach

0XUC4KZ Supplement Left Elbow Region with Nonautologous Tissue Substitute, Percutaneous Endoscopic Approach

0XUD07Z Supplement Right Lower Arm with Autologous Tissue Substitute, Open Approach

0XUD0JZ Supplement Right Lower Arm with Synthetic Substitute, Open Approach

0XUD0KZ Supplement Right Lower Arm with Nonautologous Tissue Substitute, Open Approach

---

♀ Female-only   ♂ Male-only   ● Limited Coverage   ● Non-OR   **HAC** HAC-associated procedure   ● Non-covered procedures   ➕ Combination

0XUD47Z Supplement Right Lower Arm with Autologous Tissue Substitute, Percutaneous Endoscopic Approach

0XUD4JZ Supplement Right Lower Arm with Synthetic Substitute, Percutaneous Endoscopic Approach

0XUD4KZ Supplement Right Lower Arm with Nonautologous Tissue Substitute, Percutaneous Endoscopic Approach

0XUF07Z Supplement Left Lower Arm with Autologous Tissue Substitute, Open Approach

0XUF0JZ Supplement Left Lower Arm with Synthetic Substitute, Open Approach

0XUF0KZ Supplement Left Lower Arm with Nonautologous Tissue Substitute, Open Approach

0XUF47Z Supplement Left Lower Arm with Autologous Tissue Substitute, Percutaneous Endoscopic Approach

0XUF4JZ Supplement Left Lower Arm with Synthetic Substitute, Percutaneous Endoscopic Approach

0XUF4KZ Supplement Left Lower Arm with Nonautologous Tissue Substitute, Percutaneous Endoscopic Approach

0XUG07Z Supplement Right Wrist Region with Autologous Tissue Substitute, Open Approach

0XUG0JZ Supplement Right Wrist Region with Synthetic Substitute, Open Approach

0XUG0KZ Supplement Right Wrist Region with Nonautologous Tissue Substitute, Open Approach

0XUG47Z Supplement Right Wrist Region with Autologous Tissue Substitute, Percutaneous Endoscopic Approach

0XUG4JZ Supplement Right Wrist Region with Synthetic Substitute, Percutaneous Endoscopic Approach

0XUG4KZ Supplement Right Wrist Region with Nonautologous Tissue Substitute, Percutaneous Endoscopic Approach

0XUH07Z Supplement Left Wrist Region with Autologous Tissue Substitute, Open Approach

0XUH0JZ Supplement Left Wrist Region with Synthetic Substitute, Open Approach

0XUH0KZ Supplement Left Wrist Region with Nonautologous Tissue Substitute, Open Approach

0XUH47Z Supplement Left Wrist Region with Autologous Tissue Substitute, Percutaneous Endoscopic Approach

0XUH4JZ Supplement Left Wrist Region with Synthetic Substitute, Percutaneous Endoscopic Approach

0XUH4KZ Supplement Left Wrist Region with Nonautologous Tissue Substitute, Percutaneous Endoscopic Approach

0XUJ07Z Supplement Right Hand with Autologous Tissue Substitute, Open Approach

0XUJ0JZ Supplement Right Hand with Synthetic Substitute, Open Approach

0XUJ0KZ Supplement Right Hand with Nonautologous Tissue Substitute, Open Approach

0XUJ47Z Supplement Right Hand with Autologous Tissue Substitute, Percutaneous Endoscopic Approach

0XUJ4JZ Supplement Right Hand with Synthetic Substitute, Percutaneous Endoscopic Approach

0XUJ4KZ Supplement Right Hand with Nonautologous Tissue Substitute, Percutaneous Endoscopic Approach

0XUK07Z Supplement Left Hand with Autologous Tissue Substitute, Open Approach

0XUK0JZ Supplement Left Hand with Synthetic Substitute, Open Approach

0XUK0KZ Supplement Left Hand with Nonautologous Tissue Substitute, Open Approach

0XUK47Z Supplement Left Hand with Autologous Tissue Substitute, Percutaneous Endoscopic Approach

0XUK4JZ Supplement Left Hand with Synthetic Substitute, Percutaneous Endoscopic Approach

0XUK4KZ Supplement Left Hand with Nonautologous Tissue Substitute, Percutaneous Endoscopic Approach

0XUL07Z Supplement Right Thumb with Autologous Tissue Substitute, Open Approach

0XUL0JZ Supplement Right Thumb with Synthetic Substitute, Open Approach

0XUL0KZ Supplement Right Thumb with Nonautologous Tissue Substitute, Open Approach

0XUL47Z Supplement Right Thumb with Autologous Tissue Substitute, Percutaneous Endoscopic Approach

0XUL4JZ Supplement Right Thumb with Synthetic Substitute, Percutaneous Endoscopic Approach

0XUL4KZ Supplement Right Thumb with Nonautologous Tissue Substitute, Percutaneous Endoscopic Approach

0XUM07Z Supplement Left Thumb with Autologous Tissue Substitute, Open Approach

0XUM0JZ Supplement Left Thumb with Synthetic Substitute, Open Approach

0XUM0KZ Supplement Left Thumb with Nonautologous Tissue Substitute, Open Approach

0XUM47Z Supplement Left Thumb with Autologous Tissue Substitute, Percutaneous Endoscopic Approach

0XUM4JZ Supplement Left Thumb with Synthetic Substitute, Percutaneous Endoscopic Approach

0XUM4KZ Supplement Left Thumb with Nonautologous Tissue Substitute, Percutaneous Endoscopic Approach

0XUN07Z Supplement Right Index Finger with Autologous Tissue Substitute, Open Approach

0XUN0JZ Supplement Right Index Finger with Synthetic Substitute, Open Approach

0XUN0KZ Supplement Right Index Finger with Nonautologous Tissue Substitute, Open Approach

0XUN47Z Supplement Right Index Finger with Autologous Tissue Substitute, Percutaneous Endoscopic Approach

0XUN4JZ Supplement Right Index Finger with Synthetic Substitute, Percutaneous Endoscopic Approach

0XUN4KZ Supplement Right Index Finger with Nonautologous Tissue Substitute, Percutaneous Endoscopic Approach

0XUP07Z Supplement Left Index Finger with Autologous Tissue Substitute, Open Approach

0XUP0JZ Supplement Left Index Finger with Synthetic Substitute, Open Approach

0XUP0KZ Supplement Left Index Finger with Nonautologous Tissue Substitute, Open Approach

0XUP47Z Supplement Left Index Finger with Autologous Tissue Substitute, Percutaneous Endoscopic Approach

0XUP4JZ Supplement Left Index Finger with Synthetic Substitute, Percutaneous Endoscopic Approach

0XUP4KZ Supplement Left Index Finger with Nonautologous Tissue Substitute, Percutaneous Endoscopic Approach

0XUQ07Z Supplement Right Middle Finger with Autologous Tissue Substitute, Open Approach

0XUQ0JZ Supplement Right Middle Finger with Synthetic Substitute, Open Approach

0XUQ0KZ Supplement Right Middle Finger with Nonautologous Tissue Substitute, Open Approach

0XUQ47Z Supplement Right Middle Finger with Autologous Tissue Substitute, Percutaneous Endoscopic Approach

0XUQ4JZ Supplement Right Middle Finger with Synthetic Substitute, Percutaneous Endoscopic Approach

0XUQ4KZ Supplement Right Middle Finger with Nonautologous Tissue Substitute, Percutaneous Endoscopic Approach

0XUR07Z Supplement Left Middle Finger with Autologous Tissue Substitute, Open Approach

0XUR0JZ Supplement Left Middle Finger with Synthetic Substitute, Open Approach

0XUR0KZ Supplement Left Middle Finger with Nonautologous Tissue Substitute, Open Approach

0XUR47Z Supplement Left Middle Finger with Autologous Tissue Substitute, Percutaneous Endoscopic Approach

0XUR4JZ Supplement Left Middle Finger with Synthetic Substitute, Percutaneous Endoscopic Approach

0XUR4KZ Supplement Left Middle Finger with Nonautologous Tissue Substitute, Percutaneous Endoscopic Approach

0XUS07Z Supplement Right Ring Finger with Autologous Tissue Substitute, Open Approach

0XUS0JZ Supplement Right Ring Finger with Synthetic Substitute, Open Approach

0XUS0KZ Supplement Right Ring Finger with Nonautologous Tissue Substitute, Open Approach

0XUS47Z Supplement Right Ring Finger with Autologous Tissue Substitute, Percutaneous Endoscopic Approach

0XUS4JZ Supplement Right Ring Finger with Synthetic Substitute, Percutaneous Endoscopic Approach

0XUS4KZ Supplement Right Ring Finger with Nonautologous Tissue Substitute, Percutaneous Endoscopic Approach

0XUT07Z Supplement Left Ring Finger with Autologous Tissue Substitute, Open Approach

0XUT0JZ Supplement Left Ring Finger with Synthetic Substitute, Open Approach

0XUT0KZ Supplement Left Ring Finger with Nonautologous Tissue Substitute, Open Approach

0XUT47Z Supplement Left Ring Finger with Autologous Tissue Substitute, Percutaneous Endoscopic Approach

0XUT4JZ Supplement Left Ring Finger with Synthetic Substitute, Percutaneous Endoscopic Approach

0XUT4KZ Supplement Left Ring Finger with Nonautologous Tissue Substitute, Percutaneous Endoscopic Approach

0XUV07Z Supplement Right Little Finger with Autologous Tissue Substitute, Open Approach

0XUV0JZ Supplement Right Little Finger with Synthetic Substitute, Open Approach

0XUV0KZ Supplement Right Little Finger with Nonautologous Tissue Substitute, Open Approach

0XUV47Z Supplement Right Little Finger with Autologous Tissue Substitute, Percutaneous Endoscopic Approach

0XUV4JZ Supplement Right Little Finger with Synthetic Substitute, Percutaneous Endoscopic Approach

0XUV4KZ Supplement Right Little Finger with Nonautologous Tissue Substitute, Percutaneous Endoscopic Approach

0XUW07Z Supplement Left Little Finger with Autologous Tissue Substitute, Open Approach

0XUW0JZ Supplement Left Little Finger with Synthetic Substitute, Open Approach

0XUW0KZ Supplement Left Little Finger with Nonautologous Tissue Substitute, Open Approach

0XUW47Z Supplement Left Little Finger with Autologous Tissue Substitute, Percutaneous Endoscopic Approach

0XUW4JZ Supplement Left Little Finger with Synthetic Substitute, Percutaneous Endoscopic Approach

0XUW4KZ Supplement Left Little Finger with Nonautologous Tissue Substitute, Percutaneous Endoscopic Approach

0XW – Anatomical Regions, Upper Extremities, Revision

Review Coding Guideline B6.1c

● **0XW600Z** Revision of Drainage Device in Right Upper Extremity, Open Approach

● **0XW603Z** Revision of Infusion Device in Right Upper Extremity, Open Approach

● **0XW607Z** Revision of Autologous Tissue Substitute in Right Upper Extremity, Open Approach

● **0XW60JZ** Revision of Synthetic Substitute in Right Upper Extremity, Open Approach

● **0XW60KZ** Revision of Nonautologous Tissue Substitute in Right Upper Extremity, Open Approach

● **0XW60YZ** Revision of Other Device in Right Upper Extremity, Open Approach

● **0XW630Z** Revision of Drainage Device in Right Upper Extremity, Percutaneous Approach

● **0XW633Z** Revision of Infusion Device in Right Upper Extremity, Percutaneous Approach

● **0XW637Z** Revision of Autologous Tissue Substitute in Right Upper Extremity, Percutaneous Approach

● **0XW63JZ** Revision of Synthetic Substitute in Right Upper Extremity, Percutaneous Approach

● **0XW63KZ** Revision of Nonautologous Tissue Substitute in Right Upper Extremity, Percutaneous Approach

● **0XW63YZ** Revision of Other Device in Right Upper Extremity, Percutaneous Approach

● **0XW640Z** Revision of Drainage Device in Right Upper Extremity, Percutaneous Endoscopic Approach

● **0XW643Z** Revision of Infusion Device in Right Upper Extremity, Percutaneous Endoscopic Approach

● **0XW647Z** Revision of Autologous Tissue Substitute in Right Upper Extremity, Percutaneous Endoscopic Approach

● **0XW64JZ** Revision of Synthetic Substitute in Right Upper Extremity, Percutaneous Endoscopic Approach

● **0XW64KZ** Revision of Nonautologous Tissue Substitute in Right Upper Extremity, Percutaneous Endoscopic Approach

● **0XW64YZ** Revision of Other Device in Right Upper Extremity, Percutaneous Endoscopic Approach

0XW6X0Z Revision of Drainage Device in Right Upper Extremity, External Approach

0XW6X3Z Revision of Infusion Device in Right Upper Extremity, External Approach

0XW6X7Z Revision of Autologous Tissue Substitute in Right Upper Extremity, External Approach

0XW6XJZ Revision of Synthetic Substitute in Right Upper Extremity, External Approach

0XW6XKZ Revision of Nonautologous Tissue Substitute in Right Upper Extremity, External Approach

0XW6XYZ Revision of Other Device in Right Upper Extremity, External Approach

● **0XW700Z** Revision of Drainage Device in Left Upper Extremity, Open Approach

● **0XW703Z** Revision of Infusion Device in Left Upper Extremity, Open Approach

● **0XW707Z** Revision of Autologous Tissue Substitute in Left Upper Extremity, Open Approach

● **0XW70JZ** Revision of Synthetic Substitute in Left Upper Extremity, Open Approach

● **0XW70KZ** Revision of Nonautologous Tissue Substitute in Left Upper Extremity, Open Approach

● **0XW70YZ** Revision of Other Device in Left Upper Extremity, Open Approach

● **0XW730Z** Revision of Drainage Device in Left Upper Extremity, Percutaneous Approach

● **0XW733Z** Revision of Infusion Device in Left Upper Extremity, Percutaneous Approach

● **0XW737Z** Revision of Autologous Tissue Substitute in Left Upper Extremity, Percutaneous Approach

● **0XW73JZ** Revision of Synthetic Substitute in Left Upper Extremity, Percutaneous Approach

● **0XW73KZ** Revision of Nonautologous Tissue Substitute in Left Upper Extremity, Percutaneous Approach

● **0XW73YZ** Revision of Other Device in Left Upper Extremity, Percutaneous Approach

● **0XW740Z** Revision of Drainage Device in Left Upper Extremity, Percutaneous Endoscopic Approach

● **0XW743Z** Revision of Infusion Device in Left Upper Extremity, Percutaneous Endoscopic Approach

● **0XW747Z** Revision of Autologous Tissue Substitute in Left Upper Extremity, Percutaneous Endoscopic Approach

● **0XW74JZ** Revision of Synthetic Substitute in Left Upper Extremity, Percutaneous Endoscopic Approach

● **0XW74KZ** Revision of Nonautologous Tissue Substitute in Left Upper Extremity, Percutaneous Endoscopic Approach

● **0XW74YZ** Revision of Other Device in Left Upper Extremity, Percutaneous Endoscopic Approach

0XW7X0Z Revision of Drainage Device in Left Upper Extremity, External Approach

0XW7X3Z Revision of Infusion Device in Left Upper Extremity, External Approach

0XW7X7Z Revision of Autologous Tissue Substitute in Left Upper Extremity, External Approach

0XW7XJZ Revision of Synthetic Substitute in Left Upper Extremity, External Approach

0XW7XKZ Revision of Nonautologous Tissue Substitute in Left Upper Extremity, External Approach

0XW7XYZ Revision of Other Device in Left Upper Extremity, External Approach

0XX – Anatomical Regions, Upper Extremities, Transfer

0XXN0ZL Transfer Right Index Finger to Right Thumb, Open Approach

0XXP0ZM Transfer Left Index Finger to Left Thumb, Open Approach

---

♀ Female-only   ♂ Male-only   ○ Limited Coverage   ● Non-OR   🅷🅰🅲 HAC-associated procedure   ● Non-covered procedures   ➕ Combination

Anatomical Regions, Lower Extremities

Anatomical Regions, Lower Extremities 0Y0–0YW

Section	0	**Medical and Surgical**
Body System	Y	**Anatomical Regions, Lower Extremities**
Operation	0	**Alteration:** Modifying the anatomic structure of a body part without affecting the function of the body part

Body Part (4th)	Approach (5th)	Device (6th)	Qualifier (7th)
0 Buttock, Right 1 Buttock, Left 9 Lower Extremity, Right B Lower Extremity, Left C Upper Leg, Right D Upper Leg, Left F Knee Region, Right G Knee Region, Left H Lower Leg, Right J Lower Leg, Left K Ankle Region, Right L Ankle Region, Left	0 Open 3 Percutaneous 4 Percutaneous Endoscopic	7 Autologous Tissue Substitute J Synthetic Substitute K Nonautologous Tissue Substitute Z No Device	Z No Qualifier

Section	0	**Medical and Surgical**
Body System	Y	**Anatomical Regions, Lower Extremities**
Operation	2	**Change:** Taking out or off a device from a body part and putting back an identical or similar device in or on the same body part without cutting or puncturing the skin or a mucous membrane

Body Part (4th)	Approach (5th)	Device (6th)	Qualifier (7th)
9 Lower Extremity, Right B Lower Extremity, Left	X External	0 Drainage Device Y Other Device	Z No Qualifier

Section	0	**Medical and Surgical**
Body System	Y	**Anatomical Regions, Lower Extremities**
Operation	3	**Control:** Stopping, or attempting to stop, postprocedural bleeding

Body Part (4th)	Approach (5th)	Device (6th)	Qualifier (7th)
0 Buttock, Right 1 Buttock, Left 5 Inguinal Region, Right 6 Inguinal Region, Left 7 Femoral Region, Right 8 Femoral Region, Left 9 Lower Extremity, Right B Lower Extremity, Left C Upper Leg, Right D Upper Leg, Left F Knee Region, Right G Knee Region, Left H Lower Leg, Right J Lower Leg, Left K Ankle Region, Right L Ankle Region, Left M Foot, Right N Foot, Left	0 Open 3 Percutaneous 4 Percutaneous Endoscopic	Z No Device	Z No Qualifier

Section	0	Medical and Surgical
Body System	Y	Anatomical Regions, Lower Extremities
Operation	6	Detachment: Cutting off all or a portion of the upper or lower extremities

Body Part (4ᵗʰ)	Approach (5ᵗʰ)	Device (6ᵗʰ)	Qualifier (7ᵗʰ)
2 Hindquarter, Right 3 Hindquarter, Left 4 Hindquarter, Bilateral 7 Femoral Region, Right 8 Femoral Region, Left F Knee Region, Right G Knee Region, Left	0 Open	Z No Device	Z No Qualifier
C Upper Leg, Right D Upper Leg, Left H Lower Leg, Right J Lower Leg, Left	0 Open	Z No Device	1 High 2 Mid 3 Low
M Foot, Right N Foot, Left	0 Open	Z No Device	0 Complete 4 Complete 1st Ray 5 Complete 2nd Ray 6 Complete 3rd Ray 7 Complete 4th Ray 8 Complete 5th Ray 9 Partial 1st Ray B Partial 2nd Ray C Partial 3rd Ray D Partial 4th Ray F Partial 5th Ray
P 1st Toe, Right Q 1st Toe, Left R 2nd Toe, Right S 2nd Toe, Left T 3rd Toe, Right U 3rd Toe, Left V 4th Toe, Right W 4th Toe, Left X 5th Toe, Right Y 5th Toe, Left	0 Open	Z No Device	0 Complete 1 High 2 Mid 3 Low

Section **0** **Medical and Surgical**
Body System **Y** **Anatomical Regions, Lower Extremities**
Operation **9** **Drainage:** Taking or letting out fluids and/or gases from a body part

Body Part (4th)	Approach (5th)	Device (6th)	Qualifier (7th)
0 Buttock, Right **1** Buttock, Left **5** Inguinal Region, Right **6** Inguinal Region, Left **7** Femoral Region, Right **8** Femoral Region, Left **9** Lower Extremity, Right **B** Lower Extremity, Left **C** Upper Leg, Right **D** Upper Leg, Left **F** Knee Region, Right **G** Knee Region, Left **H** Lower Leg, Right **J** Lower Leg, Left **K** Ankle Region, Right **L** Ankle Region, Left **M** Foot, Right **N** Foot, Left	**0** Open **3** Percutaneous **4** Percutaneous Endoscopic	**0** Drainage Device	**Z** No Qualifier
0 Buttock, Right **1** Buttock, Left **5** Inguinal Region, Right **6** Inguinal Region, Left **7** Femoral Region, Right **8** Femoral Region, Left **9** Lower Extremity, Right **B** Lower Extremity, Left **C** Upper Leg, Right **D** Upper Leg, Left **F** Knee Region, Right **G** Knee Region, Left **H** Lower Leg, Right **J** Lower Leg, Left **K** Ankle Region, Right **L** Ankle Region, Left **M** Foot, Right **N** Foot, Left	**0** Open **3** Percutaneous **4** Percutaneous Endoscopic	**Z** No Device	**X** Diagnostic **Z** No Qualifier

Section **0** **Medical and Surgical**
Body System **Y** **Anatomical Regions, Lower Extremities**
Operation **B** **Excision:** Cutting out or off, without replacement, a portion of a body part

Body Part (4th)	Approach (5th)	Device (6th)	Qualifier (7th)
0 Buttock, Right **1** Buttock, Left **5** Inguinal Region, Right **6** Inguinal Region, Left **7** Femoral Region, Right **8** Femoral Region, Left **9** Lower Extremity, Right **B** Lower Extremity, Left **C** Upper Leg, Right **D** Upper Leg, Left **F** Knee Region, Right **G** Knee Region, Left **H** Lower Leg, Right **J** Lower Leg, Left **K** Ankle Region, Right **L** Ankle Region, Left **M** Foot, Right **N** Foot, Left	**0** Open **3** Percutaneous **4** Percutaneous Endoscopic	**Z** No Device	**X** Diagnostic **Z** No Qualifier

Section	0	Medical and Surgical
Body System	Y	Anatomical Regions, Lower Extremities
Operation	H	Insertion: Putting in a nonbiological appliance that monitors, assists, performs, or prevents a physiological function but does not physically take the place of a body part

Body Part (4th)	Approach (5th)	Device (6th)	Qualifier (7th)
0 Buttock, Right 1 Buttock, Left 5 Inguinal Region, Right 6 Inguinal Region, Left 7 Femoral Region, Right 8 Femoral Region, Left 9 Lower Extremity, Right B Lower Extremity, Left C Upper Leg, Right D Upper Leg, Left F Knee Region, Right G Knee Region, Left H Lower Leg, Right J Lower Leg, Left K Ankle Region, Right L Ankle Region, Left M Foot, Right N Foot, Left	0 Open 3 Percutaneous 4 Percutaneous Endoscopic	1 Radioactive Element 3 Infusion Device Y Other Device	Z No Qualifier

Section	0	Medical and Surgical
Body System	Y	Anatomical Regions, Lower Extremities
Operation	J	Inspection: Visually and/or manually exploring a body part

Body Part (4th)	Approach (5th)	Device (6th)	Qualifier (7th)
0 Buttock, Right 1 Buttock, Left 5 Inguinal Region, Right 6 Inguinal Region, Left 7 Femoral Region, Right 8 Femoral Region, Left 9 Lower Extremity, Right A Inguinal Region, Bilateral B Lower Extremity, Left C Upper Leg, Right D Upper Leg, Left E Femoral Region, Bilateral F Knee Region, Right G Knee Region, Left H Lower Leg, Right J Lower Leg, Left K Ankle Region, Right L Ankle Region, Left M Foot, Right N Foot, Left	0 Open 3 Percutaneous 4 Percutaneous Endoscopic X External	Z No Device	Z No Qualifier

Section	0	Medical and Surgical
Body System	Y	Anatomical Regions, Lower Extremities
Operation	M	Reattachment: Putting back in or on all or a portion of a separated body part to its normal location or other suitable location

Body Part (4th)	Approach (5th)	Device (6th)	Qualifier (7th)
0 Buttock, Right	0 Open	Z No Device	Z No Qualifier
1 Buttock, Left			
2 Hindquarter, Right			
3 Hindquarter, Left			
4 Hindquarter, Bilateral			
5 Inguinal Region, Right			
6 Inguinal Region, Left			
7 Femoral Region, Right			
8 Femoral Region, Left			
9 Lower Extremity, Right			
B Lower Extremity, Left			
C Upper Leg, Right			
D Upper Leg, Left			
F Knee Region, Right			
G Knee Region, Left			
H Lower Leg, Right			
J Lower Leg, Left			
K Ankle Region, Right			
L Ankle Region, Left			
M Foot, Right			
N Foot, Left			
P 1st Toe, Right			
Q 1st Toe, Left			
R 2nd Toe, Right			
S 2nd Toe, Left			
T 3rd Toe, Right			
U 3rd Toe, Left			
V 4th Toe, Right			
W 4th Toe, Left			
X 5th Toe, Right			
Y 5th Toe, Left			

Section	0	Medical and Surgical
Body System	Y	Anatomical Regions, Lower Extremities
Operation	P	Removal: Taking out or off a device from a body part

Body Part (4th)	Approach (5th)	Device (6th)	Qualifier (7th)
9 Lower Extremity, Right	0 Open	0 Drainage Device	Z No Qualifier
B Lower Extremity, Left	3 Percutaneous	1 Radioactive Element	
	4 Percutaneous Endoscopic	3 Infusion Device	
	X External	7 Autologous Tissue Substitute	
		J Synthetic Substitute	
		K Nonautologous Tissue Substitute	
		Y Other Device	

Section	0	**Medical and Surgical**
Body System	Y	**Anatomical Regions, Lower Extremities**
Operation	Q	**Repair:** Restoring, to the extent possible, a body part to its normal anatomic structure and function

Body Part (4th)	Approach (5th)	Device (6th)	Qualifier (7th)
0 Buttock, Right	0 Open	Z No Device	Z No Qualifier
1 Buttock, Left	3 Percutaneous		
5 Inguinal Region, Right	4 Percutaneous		
6 Inguinal Region, Left	Endoscopic		
7 Femoral Region, Right	X External		
8 Femoral Region, Left			
9 Lower Extremity, Right			
A Inguinal Region, Bilateral			
B Lower Extremity, Left			
C Upper Leg, Right			
D Upper Leg, Left			
E Femoral Region, Bilateral			
F Knee Region, Right			
G Knee Region, Left			
H Lower Leg, Right			
J Lower Leg, Left			
K Ankle Region, Right			
L Ankle Region, Left			
M Foot, Right			
N Foot, Left			
P 1st Toe, Right			
Q 1st Toe, Left			
R 2nd Toe, Right			
S 2nd Toe, Left			
T 3rd Toe, Right			
U 3rd Toe, Left			
V 4th Toe, Right			
W 4th Toe, Left			
X 5th Toe, Right			
Y 5th Toe, Left			

Section	0	Medical and Surgical
Body System	Y	Anatomical Regions, Lower Extremities
Operation	U	Supplement: Putting in or on biological or synthetic material that physically reinforces and/or augments the function of a portion of a body part

Body Part (4th)	Approach (5th)	Device (6th)	Qualifier (7th)
0 Buttock, Right 1 Buttock, Left 5 Inguinal Region, Right 6 Inguinal Region, Left 7 Femoral Region, Right 8 Femoral Region, Left 9 Lower Extremity, Right A Inguinal Region, Bilateral B Lower Extremity, Left C Upper Leg, Right D Upper Leg, Left E Femoral Region, Bilateral F Knee Region, Right G Knee Region, Left H Lower Leg, Right J Lower Leg, Left K Ankle Region, Right L Ankle Region, Left M Foot, Right N Foot, Left P 1st Toe, Right Q 1st Toe, Left R 2nd Toe, Right S 2nd Toe, Left T 3rd Toe, Right U 3rd Toe, Left V 4th Toe, Right W 4th Toe, Left X 5th Toe, Right Y 5th Toe, Left	0 Open 4 Percutaneous Endoscopic	7 Autologous Tissue Substitute J Synthetic Substitute K Nonautologous Tissue Substitute	Z No Qualifier

Section	0	Medical and Surgical
Body System	Y	Anatomical Regions, Lower Extremities
Operation	W	Revision: Correcting, to the extent possible, a portion of a malfunctioning device or the position of a displaced device

Body Part (4th)	Approach (5th)	Device (6th)	Qualifier (7th)
9 Lower Extremity, Right B Lower Extremity, Left	0 Open 3 Percutaneous 4 Percutaneous Endoscopic X External	0 Drainage Device 3 Infusion Device 7 Autologous Tissue Substitute J Synthetic Substitute K Nonautologous Tissue Substitute Y Other Device	Z No Qualifier

Anatomical Regions, Lower Extremities Code Listing 0Y0–0YW

0Y0 – Anatomical Regions, Lower Extremities, Alteration

0Y0007Z Alteration of Right Buttock with Autologous Tissue Substitute, Open Approach
0Y000JZ Alteration of Right Buttock with Synthetic Substitute, Open Approach
0Y000KZ Alteration of Right Buttock with Nonautologous Tissue Substitute, Open Approach
0Y000ZZ Alteration of Right Buttock, Open Approach
0Y0037Z Alteration of Right Buttock with Autologous Tissue Substitute, Percutaneous Approach

0Y003JZ Alteration of Right Buttock with Synthetic Substitute, Percutaneous Approach
0Y003KZ Alteration of Right Buttock with Nonautologous Tissue Substitute, Percutaneous Approach
0Y003ZZ Alteration of Right Buttock, Percutaneous Approach
0Y0047Z Alteration of Right Buttock with Autologous Tissue Substitute, Percutaneous Endoscopic Approach
0Y004JZ Alteration of Right Buttock with Synthetic Substitute, Percutaneous Endoscopic Approach

♀ Female-only   ♂ Male-only   ● Limited Coverage   ● Non-OR   🅷🅰🅲 HAC-associated procedure   ● Non-covered procedures   ➕ Combination

0Y004KZ   Alteration of Right Buttock with Nonautologous Tissue Substitute, Percutaneous Endoscopic Approach

0Y004ZZ   Alteration of Right Buttock, Percutaneous Endoscopic Approach

0Y0107Z   Alteration of Left Buttock with Autologous Tissue Substitute, Open Approach

0Y010JZ   Alteration of Left Buttock with Synthetic Substitute, Open Approach

0Y010KZ   Alteration of Left Buttock with Nonautologous Tissue Substitute, Open Approach

0Y010ZZ   Alteration of Left Buttock, Open Approach

0Y0137Z   Alteration of Left Buttock with Autologous Tissue Substitute, Percutaneous Approach

0Y013JZ   Alteration of Left Buttock with Synthetic Substitute, Percutaneous Approach

0Y013KZ   Alteration of Left Buttock with Nonautologous Tissue Substitute, Percutaneous Approach

0Y013ZZ   Alteration of Left Buttock, Percutaneous Approach

0Y0147Z   Alteration of Left Buttock with Autologous Tissue Substitute, Percutaneous Endoscopic Approach

0Y014JZ   Alteration of Left Buttock with Synthetic Substitute, Percutaneous Endoscopic Approach

0Y014KZ   Alteration of Left Buttock with Nonautologous Tissue Substitute, Percutaneous Endoscopic Approach

0Y014ZZ   Alteration of Left Buttock, Percutaneous Endoscopic Approach

0Y0907Z   Alteration of Right Lower Extremity with Autologous Tissue Substitute, Open Approach

0Y090JZ   Alteration of Right Lower Extremity with Synthetic Substitute, Open Approach

0Y090KZ   Alteration of Right Lower Extremity with Nonautologous Tissue Substitute, Open Approach

0Y090ZZ   Alteration of Right Lower Extremity, Open Approach

0Y0937Z   Alteration of Right Lower Extremity with Autologous Tissue Substitute, Percutaneous Approach

0Y093JZ   Alteration of Right Lower Extremity with Synthetic Substitute, Percutaneous Approach

0Y093KZ   Alteration of Right Lower Extremity with Nonautologous Tissue Substitute, Percutaneous Approach

0Y093ZZ   Alteration of Right Lower Extremity, Percutaneous Approach

0Y0947Z   Alteration of Right Lower Extremity with Autologous Tissue Substitute, Percutaneous Endoscopic Approach

0Y094JZ   Alteration of Right Lower Extremity with Synthetic Substitute, Percutaneous Endoscopic Approach

0Y094KZ   Alteration of Right Lower Extremity with Nonautologous Tissue Substitute, Percutaneous Endoscopic Approach

0Y094ZZ   Alteration of Right Lower Extremity, Percutaneous Endoscopic Approach

0Y0B07Z   Alteration of Left Lower Extremity with Autologous Tissue Substitute, Open Approach

0Y0B0JZ   Alteration of Left Lower Extremity with Synthetic Substitute, Open Approach

0Y0B0KZ   Alteration of Left Lower Extremity with Nonautologous Tissue Substitute, Open Approach

0Y0B0ZZ   Alteration of Left Lower Extremity, Open Approach

0Y0B37Z   Alteration of Left Lower Extremity with Autologous Tissue Substitute, Percutaneous Approach

0Y0B3JZ   Alteration of Left Lower Extremity with Synthetic Substitute, Percutaneous Approach

0Y0B3KZ   Alteration of Left Lower Extremity with Nonautologous Tissue Substitute, Percutaneous Approach

0Y0B3ZZ   Alteration of Left Lower Extremity, Percutaneous Approach

0Y0B47Z   Alteration of Left Lower Extremity with Autologous Tissue Substitute, Percutaneous Endoscopic Approach

0Y0B4JZ   Alteration of Left Lower Extremity with Synthetic Substitute, Percutaneous Endoscopic Approach

0Y0B4KZ   Alteration of Left Lower Extremity with Nonautologous Tissue Substitute, Percutaneous Endoscopic Approach

0Y0B4ZZ   Alteration of Left Lower Extremity, Percutaneous Endoscopic Approach

0Y0C07Z   Alteration of Right Upper Leg with Autologous Tissue Substitute, Open Approach

0Y0C0JZ   Alteration of Right Upper Leg with Synthetic Substitute, Open Approach

0Y0C0KZ   Alteration of Right Upper Leg with Nonautologous Tissue Substitute, Open Approach

0Y0C0ZZ   Alteration of Right Upper Leg, Open Approach

0Y0C37Z   Alteration of Right Upper Leg with Autologous Tissue Substitute, Percutaneous Approach

0Y0C3JZ   Alteration of Right Upper Leg with Synthetic Substitute, Percutaneous Approach

0Y0C3KZ   Alteration of Right Upper Leg with Nonautologous Tissue Substitute, Percutaneous Approach

0Y0C3ZZ   Alteration of Right Upper Leg, Percutaneous Approach

0Y0C47Z   Alteration of Right Upper Leg with Autologous Tissue Substitute, Percutaneous Endoscopic Approach

0Y0C4JZ   Alteration of Right Upper Leg with Synthetic Substitute, Percutaneous Endoscopic Approach

0Y0C4KZ   Alteration of Right Upper Leg with Nonautologous Tissue Substitute, Percutaneous Endoscopic Approach

0Y0C4ZZ   Alteration of Right Upper Leg, Percutaneous Endoscopic Approach

0Y0D07Z   Alteration of Left Upper Leg with Autologous Tissue Substitute, Open Approach

0Y0D0JZ   Alteration of Left Upper Leg with Synthetic Substitute, Open Approach

0Y0D0KZ   Alteration of Left Upper Leg with Nonautologous Tissue Substitute, Open Approach

0Y0D0ZZ   Alteration of Left Upper Leg, Open Approach

0Y0D37Z   Alteration of Left Upper Leg with Autologous Tissue Substitute, Percutaneous Approach

0Y0D3JZ   Alteration of Left Upper Leg with Synthetic Substitute, Percutaneous Approach

0Y0D3KZ   Alteration of Left Upper Leg with Nonautologous Tissue Substitute, Percutaneous Approach

0Y0D3ZZ   Alteration of Left Upper Leg, Percutaneous Approach

0Y0D47Z   Alteration of Left Upper Leg with Autologous Tissue Substitute, Percutaneous Endoscopic Approach

0Y0D4JZ   Alteration of Left Upper Leg with Synthetic Substitute, Percutaneous Endoscopic Approach

0Y0D4KZ   Alteration of Left Upper Leg with Nonautologous Tissue Substitute, Percutaneous Endoscopic Approach

0Y0D4ZZ   Alteration of Left Upper Leg, Percutaneous Endoscopic Approach

0Y0F07Z   Alteration of Right Knee Region with Autologous Tissue Substitute, Open Approach

0Y0F0JZ   Alteration of Right Knee Region with Synthetic Substitute, Open Approach

0Y0F0KZ   Alteration of Right Knee Region with Nonautologous Tissue Substitute, Open Approach

0Y0F0ZZ   Alteration of Right Knee Region, Open Approach

0Y0F37Z   Alteration of Right Knee Region with Autologous Tissue Substitute, Percutaneous Approach

0Y0F3JZ   Alteration of Right Knee Region with Synthetic Substitute, Percutaneous Approach

0Y0F3KZ   Alteration of Right Knee Region with Nonautologous Tissue Substitute, Percutaneous Approach

0Y0F3ZZ   Alteration of Right Knee Region, Percutaneous Approach

0Y0F47Z   Alteration of Right Knee Region with Autologous Tissue Substitute, Percutaneous Endoscopic Approach

0Y0F4JZ   Alteration of Right Knee Region with Synthetic Substitute, Percutaneous Endoscopic Approach

0Y0F4KZ   Alteration of Right Knee Region with Nonautologous Tissue Substitute, Percutaneous Endoscopic Approach

0Y0F4ZZ   Alteration of Right Knee Region, Percutaneous Endoscopic Approach

0Y0G07Z   Alteration of Left Knee Region with Autologous Tissue Substitute, Open Approach

0Y0G0JZ   Alteration of Left Knee Region with Synthetic Substitute, Open Approach

0Y0G0KZ   Alteration of Left Knee Region with Nonautologous Tissue Substitute, Open Approach

0Y0G0ZZ   Alteration of Left Knee Region, Open Approach

0Y0G37Z   Alteration of Left Knee Region with Autologous Tissue Substitute, Percutaneous Approach

0Y0G3JZ   Alteration of Left Knee Region with Synthetic Substitute, Percutaneous Approach

0Y0G3KZ   Alteration of Left Knee Region with Nonautologous Tissue Substitute, Percutaneous Approach

0Y0G3ZZ   Alteration of Left Knee Region, Percutaneous Approach

0Y0G47Z   Alteration of Left Knee Region with Autologous Tissue Substitute, Percutaneous Endoscopic Approach

0Y0G4JZ Alteration of Left Knee Region with Synthetic Substitute, Percutaneous Endoscopic Approach
0Y0G4KZ Alteration of Left Knee Region with Nonautologous Tissue Substitute, Percutaneous Endoscopic Approach
0Y0G4ZZ Alteration of Left Knee Region, Percutaneous Endoscopic Approach
0Y0H07Z Alteration of Right Lower Leg with Autologous Tissue Substitute, Open Approach
0Y0H0JZ Alteration of Right Lower Leg with Synthetic Substitute, Open Approach
0Y0H0KZ Alteration of Right Lower Leg with Nonautologous Tissue Substitute, Open Approach
0Y0H0ZZ Alteration of Right Lower Leg, Open Approach
0Y0H37Z Alteration of Right Lower Leg with Autologous Tissue Substitute, Percutaneous Approach
0Y0H3JZ Alteration of Right Lower Leg with Synthetic Substitute, Percutaneous Approach
0Y0H3KZ Alteration of Right Lower Leg with Nonautologous Tissue Substitute, Percutaneous Approach
0Y0H3ZZ Alteration of Right Lower Leg, Percutaneous Approach
0Y0H47Z Alteration of Right Lower Leg with Autologous Tissue Substitute, Percutaneous Endoscopic Approach
0Y0H4JZ Alteration of Right Lower Leg with Synthetic Substitute, Percutaneous Endoscopic Approach
0Y0H4KZ Alteration of Right Lower Leg with Nonautologous Tissue Substitute, Percutaneous Endoscopic Approach
0Y0H4ZZ Alteration of Right Lower Leg, Percutaneous Endoscopic Approach
0Y0J07Z Alteration of Left Lower Leg with Autologous Tissue Substitute, Open Approach
0Y0J0JZ Alteration of Left Lower Leg with Synthetic Substitute, Open Approach
0Y0J0KZ Alteration of Left Lower Leg with Nonautologous Tissue Substitute, Open Approach
0Y0J0ZZ Alteration of Left Lower Leg, Open Approach
0Y0J37Z Alteration of Left Lower Leg with Autologous Tissue Substitute, Percutaneous Approach
0Y0J3JZ Alteration of Left Lower Leg with Synthetic Substitute, Percutaneous Approach
0Y0J3KZ Alteration of Left Lower Leg with Nonautologous Tissue Substitute, Percutaneous Approach
0Y0J3ZZ Alteration of Left Lower Leg, Percutaneous Approach
0Y0J47Z Alteration of Left Lower Leg with Autologous Tissue Substitute, Percutaneous Endoscopic Approach
0Y0J4JZ Alteration of Left Lower Leg with Synthetic Substitute, Percutaneous Endoscopic Approach
0Y0J4KZ Alteration of Left Lower Leg with Nonautologous Tissue Substitute, Percutaneous Endoscopic Approach

0Y0J4ZZ Alteration of Left Lower Leg, Percutaneous Endoscopic Approach
0Y0K07Z Alteration of Right Ankle Region with Autologous Tissue Substitute, Open Approach
0Y0K0JZ Alteration of Right Ankle Region with Synthetic Substitute, Open Approach
0Y0K0KZ Alteration of Right Ankle Region with Nonautologous Tissue Substitute, Open Approach
0Y0K0ZZ Alteration of Right Ankle Region, Open Approach
0Y0K37Z Alteration of Right Ankle Region with Autologous Tissue Substitute, Percutaneous Approach
0Y0K3JZ Alteration of Right Ankle Region with Synthetic Substitute, Percutaneous Approach
0Y0K3KZ Alteration of Right Ankle Region with Nonautologous Tissue Substitute, Percutaneous Approach
0Y0K3ZZ Alteration of Right Ankle Region, Percutaneous Approach
0Y0K47Z Alteration of Right Ankle Region with Autologous Tissue Substitute, Percutaneous Endoscopic Approach
0Y0K4JZ Alteration of Right Ankle Region with Synthetic Substitute, Percutaneous Endoscopic Approach
0Y0K4KZ Alteration of Right Ankle Region with Nonautologous Tissue Substitute, Percutaneous Endoscopic Approach
0Y0K4ZZ Alteration of Right Ankle Region, Percutaneous Endoscopic Approach
0Y0L07Z Alteration of Left Ankle Region with Autologous Tissue Substitute, Open Approach
0Y0L0JZ Alteration of Left Ankle Region with Synthetic Substitute, Open Approach
0Y0L0KZ Alteration of Left Ankle Region with Nonautologous Tissue Substitute, Open Approach
0Y0L0ZZ Alteration of Left Ankle Region, Open Approach
0Y0L37Z Alteration of Left Ankle Region with Autologous Tissue Substitute, Percutaneous Approach
0Y0L3JZ Alteration of Left Ankle Region with Synthetic Substitute, Percutaneous Approach
0Y0L3KZ Alteration of Left Ankle Region with Nonautologous Tissue Substitute, Percutaneous Approach
0Y0L3ZZ Alteration of Left Ankle Region, Percutaneous Approach
0Y0L47Z Alteration of Left Ankle Region with Autologous Tissue Substitute, Percutaneous Endoscopic Approach
0Y0L4JZ Alteration of Left Ankle Region with Synthetic Substitute, Percutaneous Endoscopic Approach
0Y0L4KZ Alteration of Left Ankle Region with Nonautologous Tissue Substitute, Percutaneous Endoscopic Approach
0Y0L4ZZ Alteration of Left Ankle Region, Percutaneous Endoscopic Approach

0Y2 – Anatomical Regions, Lower Extremities, Change

Review Coding Guideline B6.1c

0Y29X0Z Change Drainage Device in Right Lower Extremity, External Approach
0Y29XYZ Change Other Device in Right Lower Extremity, External Approach
0Y2BX0Z Change Drainage Device in Left Lower Extremity, External Approach
0Y2BXYZ Change Other Device in Left Lower Extremity, External Approach

0Y3 – Anatomical Regions, Lower Extremities, Control

Review Coding Guideline B3.7

0Y300ZZ Control Bleeding in Right Buttock, Open Approach
0Y303ZZ Control Bleeding in Right Buttock, Percutaneous Approach
0Y304ZZ Control Bleeding in Right Buttock, Percutaneous Endoscopic Approach
0Y310ZZ Control Bleeding in Left Buttock, Open Approach
0Y313ZZ Control Bleeding in Left Buttock, Percutaneous Approach
0Y314ZZ Control Bleeding in Left Buttock, Percutaneous Endoscopic Approach
0Y350ZZ Control Bleeding in Right Inguinal Region, Open Approach
0Y353ZZ Control Bleeding in Right Inguinal Region, Percutaneous Approach
0Y354ZZ Control Bleeding in Right Inguinal Region, Percutaneous Endoscopic Approach
0Y360ZZ Control Bleeding in Left Inguinal Region, Open Approach
0Y363ZZ Control Bleeding in Left Inguinal Region, Percutaneous Approach
0Y364ZZ Control Bleeding in Left Inguinal Region, Percutaneous Endoscopic Approach
0Y370ZZ Control Bleeding in Right Femoral Region, Open Approach
0Y373ZZ Control Bleeding in Right Femoral Region, Percutaneous Approach
0Y374ZZ Control Bleeding in Right Femoral Region, Percutaneous Endoscopic Approach
0Y380ZZ Control Bleeding in Left Femoral Region, Open Approach
0Y383ZZ Control Bleeding in Left Femoral Region, Percutaneous Approach
0Y384ZZ Control Bleeding in Left Femoral Region, Percutaneous Endoscopic Approach
0Y390ZZ Control Bleeding in Right Lower Extremity, Open Approach
0Y393ZZ Control Bleeding in Right Lower Extremity, Percutaneous Approach
0Y394ZZ Control Bleeding in Right Lower Extremity, Percutaneous Endoscopic Approach
0Y3B0ZZ Control Bleeding in Left Lower Extremity, Open Approach
0Y3B3ZZ Control Bleeding in Left Lower Extremity, Percutaneous Approach

0Y3B4ZZ	Control Bleeding in Left Lower Extremity, Percutaneous Endoscopic Approach	**0Y3H4ZZ**	Control Bleeding in Right Lower Leg, Percutaneous Endoscopic Approach
0Y3C0ZZ	Control Bleeding in Right Upper Leg, Open Approach	**0Y3J0ZZ**	Control Bleeding in Left Lower Leg, Open Approach
0Y3C3ZZ	Control Bleeding in Right Upper Leg, Percutaneous Approach	**0Y3J3ZZ**	Control Bleeding in Left Lower Leg, Percutaneous Approach
0Y3C4ZZ	Control Bleeding in Right Upper Leg, Percutaneous Endoscopic Approach	**0Y3J4ZZ**	Control Bleeding in Left Lower Leg, Percutaneous Endoscopic Approach
0Y3D0ZZ	Control Bleeding in Left Upper Leg, Open Approach	**0Y3K0ZZ**	Control Bleeding in Right Ankle Region, Open Approach
0Y3D3ZZ	Control Bleeding in Left Upper Leg, Percutaneous Approach	**0Y3K3ZZ**	Control Bleeding in Right Ankle Region, Percutaneous Approach
0Y3D4ZZ	Control Bleeding in Left Upper Leg, Percutaneous Endoscopic Approach	**0Y3K4ZZ**	Control Bleeding in Right Ankle Region, Percutaneous Endoscopic Approach
0Y3F0ZZ	Control Bleeding in Right Knee Region, Open Approach	**0Y3L0ZZ**	Control Bleeding in Left Ankle Region, Open Approach
0Y3F3ZZ	Control Bleeding in Right Knee Region, Percutaneous Approach	**0Y3L3ZZ**	Control Bleeding in Left Ankle Region, Percutaneous Approach
0Y3F4ZZ	Control Bleeding in Right Knee Region, Percutaneous Endoscopic Approach	**0Y3L4ZZ**	Control Bleeding in Left Ankle Region, Percutaneous Endoscopic Approach
0Y3G0ZZ	Control Bleeding in Left Knee Region, Open Approach	**0Y3M0ZZ**	Control Bleeding in Right Foot, Open Approach
0Y3G3ZZ	Control Bleeding in Left Knee Region, Percutaneous Approach	**0Y3M3ZZ**	Control Bleeding in Right Foot, Percutaneous Approach
0Y3G4ZZ	Control Bleeding in Left Knee Region, Percutaneous Endoscopic Approach	**0Y3M4ZZ**	Control Bleeding in Right Foot, Percutaneous Endoscopic Approach
0Y3H0ZZ	Control Bleeding in Right Lower Leg, Open Approach	**0Y3N0ZZ**	Control Bleeding in Left Foot, Open Approach
0Y3H3ZZ	Control Bleeding in Right Lower Leg, Percutaneous Approach	**0Y3N3ZZ**	Control Bleeding in Left Foot, Percutaneous Approach
		0Y3N4ZZ	Control Bleeding in Left Foot, Percutaneous Endoscopic Approach

0Y6 – Anatomical Regions, Lower Extremities, Detachment

0Y620ZZ	Detachment at Right Hindquarter, Open Approach	**0Y6P0Z0**	Detachment at Right 1st Toe, Complete, Open Approach
0Y630ZZ	Detachment at Left Hindquarter, Open Approach	**0Y6P0Z1**	Detachment at Right 1st Toe, High, Open Approach
0Y640ZZ	Detachment at Bilateral Hindquarter, Open Approach	**0Y6P0Z2**	Detachment at Right 1st Toe, Mid, Open Approach
0Y670ZZ	Detachment at Right Femoral Region, Open Approach	**0Y6P0Z3**	Detachment at Right 1st Toe, Low, Open Approach
0Y680ZZ	Detachment at Left Femoral Region, Open Approach	**0Y6Q0Z0**	Detachment at Left 1st Toe, Complete, Open Approach
0Y6C0Z1	Detachment at Right Upper Leg, High, Open Approach	**0Y6Q0Z1**	Detachment at Left 1st Toe, High, Open Approach
0Y6C0Z2	Detachment at Right Upper Leg, Mid, Open Approach	**0Y6Q0Z2**	Detachment at Left 1st Toe, Mid, Open Approach
0Y6C0Z3	Detachment at Right Upper Leg, Low, Open Approach	**0Y6Q0Z3**	Detachment at Left 1st Toe, Low, Open Approach
0Y6D0Z1	Detachment at Left Upper Leg, High, Open Approach	**0Y6R0Z0**	Detachment at Right 2nd Toe, Complete, Open Approach
0Y6D0Z2	Detachment at Left Upper Leg, Mid, Open Approach	**0Y6R0Z1**	Detachment at Right 2nd Toe, High, Open Approach
0Y6D0Z3	Detachment at Left Upper Leg, Low, Open Approach	**0Y6R0Z2**	Detachment at Right 2nd Toe, Mid, Open Approach
0Y6F0ZZ	Detachment at Right Knee Region, Open Approach	**0Y6R0Z3**	Detachment at Right 2nd Toe, Low, Open Approach
0Y6G0ZZ	Detachment at Left Knee Region, Open Approach	**0Y6S0Z0**	Detachment at Left 2nd Toe, Complete, Open Approach
0Y6H0Z1	Detachment at Right Lower Leg, High, Open Approach	**0Y6S0Z1**	Detachment at Left 2nd Toe, High, Open Approach
0Y6H0Z2	Detachment at Right Lower Leg, Mid, Open Approach	**0Y6S0Z2**	Detachment at Left 2nd Toe, Mid, Open Approach
0Y6H0Z3	Detachment at Right Lower Leg, Low, Open Approach	**0Y6S0Z3**	Detachment at Left 2nd Toe, Low, Open Approach
0Y6J0Z1	Detachment at Left Lower Leg, High, Open Approach	**0Y6T0Z0**	Detachment at Right 3rd Toe, Complete, Open Approach
0Y6J0Z2	Detachment at Left Lower Leg, Mid, Open Approach	**0Y6T0Z1**	Detachment at Right 3rd Toe, High, Open Approach
0Y6J0Z3	Detachment at Left Lower Leg, Low, Open Approach	**0Y6T0Z2**	Detachment at Right 3rd Toe, Mid, Open Approach
0Y6M0Z0	Detachment at Right Foot, Complete, Open Approach	**0Y6T0Z3**	Detachment at Right 3rd Toe, Low, Open Approach
0Y6M0Z4	Detachment at Right Foot, Complete 1st Ray, Open Approach	**0Y6U0Z0**	Detachment at Left 3rd Toe, Complete, Open Approach
0Y6M0Z5	Detachment at Right Foot, Complete 2nd Ray, Open Approach	**0Y6U0Z1**	Detachment at Left 3rd Toe, High, Open Approach
0Y6M0Z6	Detachment at Right Foot, Complete 3rd Ray, Open Approach	**0Y6U0Z2**	Detachment at Left 3rd Toe, Mid, Open Approach
0Y6M0Z7	Detachment at Right Foot, Complete 4th Ray, Open Approach	**0Y6U0Z3**	Detachment at Left 3rd Toe, Low, Open Approach
0Y6M0Z8	Detachment at Right Foot, Complete 5th Ray, Open Approach	**0Y6V0Z0**	Detachment at Right 4th Toe, Complete, Open Approach
0Y6M0Z9	Detachment at Right Foot, Partial 1st Ray, Open Approach	**0Y6V0Z1**	Detachment at Right 4th Toe, High, Open Approach
0Y6M0ZB	Detachment at Right Foot, Partial 2nd Ray, Open Approach	**0Y6V0Z2**	Detachment at Right 4th Toe, Mid, Open Approach
0Y6M0ZC	Detachment at Right Foot, Partial 3rd Ray, Open Approach	**0Y6V0Z3**	Detachment at Right 4th Toe, Low, Open Approach
0Y6M0ZD	Detachment at Right Foot, Partial 4th Ray, Open Approach	**0Y6W0Z0**	Detachment at Left 4th Toe, Complete, Open Approach
0Y6M0ZF	Detachment at Right Foot, Partial 5th Ray, Open Approach	**0Y6W0Z1**	Detachment at Left 4th Toe, High, Open Approach
0Y6N0Z0	Detachment at Left Foot, Complete, Open Approach	**0Y6W0Z2**	Detachment at Left 4th Toe, Mid, Open Approach
0Y6N0Z4	Detachment at Left Foot, Complete 1st Ray, Open Approach	**0Y6W0Z3**	Detachment at Left 4th Toe, Low, Open Approach
0Y6N0Z5	Detachment at Left Foot, Complete 2nd Ray, Open Approach	**0Y6X0Z0**	Detachment at Right 5th Toe, Complete, Open Approach
0Y6N0Z6	Detachment at Left Foot, Complete 3rd Ray, Open Approach	**0Y6X0Z1**	Detachment at Right 5th Toe, High, Open Approach
0Y6N0Z7	Detachment at Left Foot, Complete 4th Ray, Open Approach	**0Y6X0Z2**	Detachment at Right 5th Toe, Mid, Open Approach
0Y6N0Z8	Detachment at Left Foot, Complete 5th Ray, Open Approach	**0Y6X0Z3**	Detachment at Right 5th Toe, Low, Open Approach
0Y6N0Z9	Detachment at Left Foot, Partial 1st Ray, Open Approach	**0Y6Y0Z0**	Detachment at Left 5th Toe, Complete, Open Approach
0Y6N0ZB	Detachment at Left Foot, Partial 2nd Ray, Open Approach	**0Y6Y0Z1**	Detachment at Left 5th Toe, High, Open Approach
0Y6N0ZC	Detachment at Left Foot, Partial 3rd Ray, Open Approach	**0Y6Y0Z2**	Detachment at Left 5th Toe, Mid, Open Approach
0Y6N0ZD	Detachment at Left Foot, Partial 4th Ray, Open Approach	**0Y6Y0Z3**	Detachment at Left 5th Toe, Low, Open Approach
0Y6N0ZF	Detachment at Left Foot, Partial 5th Ray, Open Approach		

0Y9 – Anatomical Regions, Lower Extremities, Drainage

Review Coding Guidelines B3.4a and B3.4b

Review Coding Guideline B6.2

0Y9000Z	Drainage of Right Buttock with Drainage Device, Open Approach	**0Y9030Z**	Drainage of Right Buttock with Drainage Device, Percutaneous Approach
0Y900ZX	Drainage of Right Buttock, Open Approach, Diagnostic		
0Y900ZZ	Drainage of Right Buttock, Open Approach	**0Y903ZX**	Drainage of Right Buttock, Percutaneous Approach, Diagnostic

0Y903ZZ	Drainage of Right Buttock, Percutaneous Approach
0Y9040Z	Drainage of Right Buttock with Drainage Device, Percutaneous Endoscopic Approach
0Y904ZX	Drainage of Right Buttock, Percutaneous Endoscopic Approach, Diagnostic
0Y904ZZ	Drainage of Right Buttock, Percutaneous Endoscopic Approach
0Y9100Z	Drainage of Left Buttock with Drainage Device, Open Approach
0Y910ZX	Drainage of Left Buttock, Open Approach, Diagnostic
0Y910ZZ	Drainage of Left Buttock, Open Approach
0Y9130Z	Drainage of Left Buttock with Drainage Device, Percutaneous Approach
0Y913ZX	Drainage of Left Buttock, Percutaneous Approach, Diagnostic
0Y913ZZ	Drainage of Left Buttock, Percutaneous Approach
0Y9140Z	Drainage of Left Buttock with Drainage Device, Percutaneous Endoscopic Approach
0Y914ZX	Drainage of Left Buttock, Percutaneous Endoscopic Approach, Diagnostic
0Y914ZZ	Drainage of Left Buttock, Percutaneous Endoscopic Approach
0Y9500Z	Drainage of Right Inguinal Region with Drainage Device, Open Approach
0Y950ZX	Drainage of Right Inguinal Region, Open Approach, Diagnostic
0Y950ZZ	Drainage of Right Inguinal Region, Open Approach
0Y9530Z	Drainage of Right Inguinal Region with Drainage Device, Percutaneous Approach
0Y953ZX	Drainage of Right Inguinal Region, Percutaneous Approach, Diagnostic
0Y953ZZ	Drainage of Right Inguinal Region, Percutaneous Approach
0Y9540Z	Drainage of Right Inguinal Region with Drainage Device, Percutaneous Endoscopic Approach
0Y954ZX	Drainage of Right Inguinal Region, Percutaneous Endoscopic Approach, Diagnostic
0Y954ZZ	Drainage of Right Inguinal Region, Percutaneous Endoscopic Approach
0Y9600Z	Drainage of Left Inguinal Region with Drainage Device, Open Approach
0Y960ZX	Drainage of Left Inguinal Region, Open Approach, Diagnostic
0Y960ZZ	Drainage of Left Inguinal Region, Open Approach
0Y9630Z	Drainage of Left Inguinal Region with Drainage Device, Percutaneous Approach
0Y963ZX	Drainage of Left Inguinal Region, Percutaneous Approach, Diagnostic
0Y963ZZ	Drainage of Left Inguinal Region, Percutaneous Approach
0Y9640Z	Drainage of Left Inguinal Region with Drainage Device, Percutaneous Endoscopic Approach
0Y964ZX	Drainage of Left Inguinal Region, Percutaneous Endoscopic Approach, Diagnostic
0Y964ZZ	Drainage of Left Inguinal Region, Percutaneous Endoscopic Approach
0Y9700Z	Drainage of Right Femoral Region with Drainage Device, Open Approach
0Y970ZX	Drainage of Right Femoral Region, Open Approach, Diagnostic
0Y970ZZ	Drainage of Right Femoral Region, Open Approach
0Y9730Z	Drainage of Right Femoral Region with Drainage Device, Percutaneous Approach
0Y973ZX	Drainage of Right Femoral Region, Percutaneous Approach, Diagnostic
0Y973ZZ	Drainage of Right Femoral Region, Percutaneous Approach
0Y9740Z	Drainage of Right Femoral Region with Drainage Device, Percutaneous Endoscopic Approach
0Y974ZX	Drainage of Right Femoral Region, Percutaneous Endoscopic Approach, Diagnostic
0Y974ZZ	Drainage of Right Femoral Region, Percutaneous Endoscopic Approach
0Y9800Z	Drainage of Left Femoral Region with Drainage Device, Open Approach
0Y980ZX	Drainage of Left Femoral Region, Open Approach, Diagnostic
0Y980ZZ	Drainage of Left Femoral Region, Open Approach
0Y9830Z	Drainage of Left Femoral Region with Drainage Device, Percutaneous Approach
0Y983ZX	Drainage of Left Femoral Region, Percutaneous Approach, Diagnostic
0Y983ZZ	Drainage of Left Femoral Region, Percutaneous Approach
0Y9840Z	Drainage of Left Femoral Region with Drainage Device, Percutaneous Endoscopic Approach
0Y984ZX	Drainage of Left Femoral Region, Percutaneous Endoscopic Approach, Diagnostic
0Y984ZZ	Drainage of Left Femoral Region, Percutaneous Endoscopic Approach
0Y9900Z	Drainage of Right Lower Extremity with Drainage Device, Open Approach
0Y990ZX	Drainage of Right Lower Extremity, Open Approach, Diagnostic
0Y990ZZ	Drainage of Right Lower Extremity, Open Approach
0Y9930Z	Drainage of Right Lower Extremity with Drainage Device, Percutaneous Approach
0Y993ZX	Drainage of Right Lower Extremity, Percutaneous Approach, Diagnostic
0Y993ZZ	Drainage of Right Lower Extremity, Percutaneous Approach
0Y9940Z	Drainage of Right Lower Extremity with Drainage Device, Percutaneous Endoscopic Approach
0Y994ZX	Drainage of Right Lower Extremity, Percutaneous Endoscopic Approach, Diagnostic
0Y994ZZ	Drainage of Right Lower Extremity, Percutaneous Endoscopic Approach
0Y9B00Z	Drainage of Left Lower Extremity with Drainage Device, Open Approach
0Y9B0ZX	Drainage of Left Lower Extremity, Open Approach, Diagnostic
0Y9B0ZZ	Drainage of Left Lower Extremity, Open Approach
0Y9B30Z	Drainage of Left Lower Extremity with Drainage Device, Percutaneous Approach
0Y9B3ZX	Drainage of Left Lower Extremity, Percutaneous Approach, Diagnostic
0Y9B3ZZ	Drainage of Left Lower Extremity, Percutaneous Approach
0Y9B40Z	Drainage of Left Lower Extremity with Drainage Device, Percutaneous Endoscopic Approach
0Y9B4ZX	Drainage of Left Lower Extremity, Percutaneous Endoscopic Approach, Diagnostic
0Y9B4ZZ	Drainage of Left Lower Extremity, Percutaneous Endoscopic Approach
0Y9C00Z	Drainage of Right Upper Leg with Drainage Device, Open Approach
0Y9C0ZX	Drainage of Right Upper Leg, Open Approach, Diagnostic
0Y9C0ZZ	Drainage of Right Upper Leg, Open Approach
0Y9C30Z	Drainage of Right Upper Leg with Drainage Device, Percutaneous Approach
0Y9C3ZX	Drainage of Right Upper Leg, Percutaneous Approach, Diagnostic
0Y9C3ZZ	Drainage of Right Upper Leg, Percutaneous Approach
0Y9C40Z	Drainage of Right Upper Leg with Drainage Device, Percutaneous Endoscopic Approach
0Y9C4ZX	Drainage of Right Upper Leg, Percutaneous Endoscopic Approach, Diagnostic
0Y9C4ZZ	Drainage of Right Upper Leg, Percutaneous Endoscopic Approach
0Y9D00Z	Drainage of Left Upper Leg with Drainage Device, Open Approach
0Y9D0ZX	Drainage of Left Upper Leg, Open Approach, Diagnostic
0Y9D0ZZ	Drainage of Left Upper Leg, Open Approach
0Y9D30Z	Drainage of Left Upper Leg with Drainage Device, Percutaneous Approach
0Y9D3ZX	Drainage of Left Upper Leg, Percutaneous Approach, Diagnostic
0Y9D3ZZ	Drainage of Left Upper Leg, Percutaneous Approach
0Y9D40Z	Drainage of Left Upper Leg with Drainage Device, Percutaneous Endoscopic Approach
0Y9D4ZX	Drainage of Left Upper Leg, Percutaneous Endoscopic Approach, Diagnostic
0Y9D4ZZ	Drainage of Left Upper Leg, Percutaneous Endoscopic Approach
0Y9F00Z	Drainage of Right Knee Region with Drainage Device, Open Approach
0Y9F0ZX	Drainage of Right Knee Region, Open Approach, Diagnostic
0Y9F0ZZ	Drainage of Right Knee Region, Open Approach
0Y9F30Z	Drainage of Right Knee Region with Drainage Device, Percutaneous Approach
0Y9F3ZX	Drainage of Right Knee Region, Percutaneous Approach, Diagnostic
0Y9F3ZZ	Drainage of Right Knee Region, Percutaneous Approach
0Y9F40Z	Drainage of Right Knee Region with Drainage Device, Percutaneous Endoscopic Approach
0Y9F4ZX	Drainage of Right Knee Region, Percutaneous Endoscopic Approach, Diagnostic
0Y9F4ZZ	Drainage of Right Knee Region, Percutaneous Endoscopic Approach

0Y9G00Z   Drainage of Left Knee Region with Drainage Device, Open Approach
0Y9G0ZX   Drainage of Left Knee Region, Open Approach, Diagnostic
0Y9G0ZZ   Drainage of Left Knee Region, Open Approach
0Y9G30Z   Drainage of Left Knee Region with Drainage Device, Percutaneous Approach
0Y9G3ZX   Drainage of Left Knee Region, Percutaneous Approach, Diagnostic
0Y9G3ZZ   Drainage of Left Knee Region, Percutaneous Approach
0Y9G40Z   Drainage of Left Knee Region with Drainage Device, Percutaneous Endoscopic Approach
0Y9G4ZX   Drainage of Left Knee Region, Percutaneous Endoscopic Approach, Diagnostic
0Y9G4ZZ   Drainage of Left Knee Region, Percutaneous Endoscopic Approach
0Y9H00Z   Drainage of Right Lower Leg with Drainage Device, Open Approach
0Y9H0ZX   Drainage of Right Lower Leg, Open Approach, Diagnostic
0Y9H0ZZ   Drainage of Right Lower Leg, Open Approach
0Y9H30Z   Drainage of Right Lower Leg with Drainage Device, Percutaneous Approach
0Y9H3ZX   Drainage of Right Lower Leg, Percutaneous Approach, Diagnostic
0Y9H3ZZ   Drainage of Right Lower Leg, Percutaneous Approach
0Y9H40Z   Drainage of Right Lower Leg with Drainage Device, Percutaneous Endoscopic Approach
0Y9H4ZX   Drainage of Right Lower Leg, Percutaneous Endoscopic Approach, Diagnostic
0Y9H4ZZ   Drainage of Right Lower Leg, Percutaneous Endoscopic Approach
0Y9J00Z   Drainage of Left Lower Leg with Drainage Device, Open Approach
0Y9J0ZX   Drainage of Left Lower Leg, Open Approach, Diagnostic
0Y9J0ZZ   Drainage of Left Lower Leg, Open Approach
0Y9J30Z   Drainage of Left Lower Leg with Drainage Device, Percutaneous Approach
0Y9J3ZX   Drainage of Left Lower Leg, Percutaneous Approach, Diagnostic
0Y9J3ZZ   Drainage of Left Lower Leg, Percutaneous Approach
0Y9J40Z   Drainage of Left Lower Leg with Drainage Device, Percutaneous Endoscopic Approach
0Y9J4ZX   Drainage of Left Lower Leg, Percutaneous Endoscopic Approach, Diagnostic
0Y9J4ZZ   Drainage of Left Lower Leg, Percutaneous Endoscopic Approach
0Y9K00Z   Drainage of Right Ankle Region with Drainage Device, Open Approach
0Y9K0ZX   Drainage of Right Ankle Region, Open Approach, Diagnostic
0Y9K0ZZ   Drainage of Right Ankle Region, Open Approach
0Y9K30Z   Drainage of Right Ankle Region with Drainage Device, Percutaneous Approach
0Y9K3ZX   Drainage of Right Ankle Region, Percutaneous Approach, Diagnostic

0Y9K3ZZ   Drainage of Right Ankle Region, Percutaneous Approach
0Y9K40Z   Drainage of Right Ankle Region with Drainage Device, Percutaneous Endoscopic Approach
0Y9K4ZX   Drainage of Right Ankle Region, Percutaneous Endoscopic Approach, Diagnostic
0Y9K4ZZ   Drainage of Right Ankle Region, Percutaneous Endoscopic Approach
0Y9L00Z   Drainage of Left Ankle Region with Drainage Device, Open Approach
0Y9L0ZX   Drainage of Left Ankle Region, Open Approach, Diagnostic
0Y9L0ZZ   Drainage of Left Ankle Region, Open Approach
0Y9L30Z   Drainage of Left Ankle Region with Drainage Device, Percutaneous Approach
0Y9L3ZX   Drainage of Left Ankle Region, Percutaneous Approach, Diagnostic
0Y9L3ZZ   Drainage of Left Ankle Region, Percutaneous Approach
0Y9L40Z   Drainage of Left Ankle Region with Drainage Device, Percutaneous Endoscopic Approach
0Y9L4ZX   Drainage of Left Ankle Region, Percutaneous Endoscopic Approach, Diagnostic
0Y9L4ZZ   Drainage of Left Ankle Region, Percutaneous Endoscopic Approach
0Y9M00Z   Drainage of Right Foot with Drainage Device, Open Approach
0Y9M0ZX   Drainage of Right Foot, Open Approach, Diagnostic
0Y9M0ZZ   Drainage of Right Foot, Open Approach
0Y9M30Z   Drainage of Right Foot with Drainage Device, Percutaneous Approach
0Y9M3ZX   Drainage of Right Foot, Percutaneous Approach, Diagnostic
0Y9M3ZZ   Drainage of Right Foot, Percutaneous Approach
0Y9M40Z   Drainage of Right Foot with Drainage Device, Percutaneous Endoscopic Approach
0Y9M4ZX   Drainage of Right Foot, Percutaneous Endoscopic Approach, Diagnostic
0Y9M4ZZ   Drainage of Right Foot, Percutaneous Endoscopic Approach
0Y9N00Z   Drainage of Left Foot with Drainage Device, Open Approach
0Y9N0ZX   Drainage of Left Foot, Open Approach, Diagnostic
0Y9N0ZZ   Drainage of Left Foot, Open Approach
0Y9N30Z   Drainage of Left Foot with Drainage Device, Percutaneous Approach
0Y9N3ZX   Drainage of Left Foot, Percutaneous Approach, Diagnostic
0Y9N3ZZ   Drainage of Left Foot, Percutaneous Approach
0Y9N40Z   Drainage of Left Foot with Drainage Device, Percutaneous Endoscopic Approach
0Y9N4ZX   Drainage of Left Foot, Percutaneous Endoscopic Approach, Diagnostic
0Y9N4ZZ   Drainage of Left Foot, Percutaneous Endoscopic Approach

0YB – Anatomical Regions, Lower Extremities, Excision

Review Coding Guidelines B3.4a and B3.4b

0YB00ZX   Excision of Right Buttock, Open Approach, Diagnostic
0YB00ZZ   Excision of Right Buttock, Open Approach
0YB03ZX   Excision of Right Buttock, Percutaneous Approach, Diagnostic
0YB03ZZ   Excision of Right Buttock, Percutaneous Approach
0YB04ZX   Excision of Right Buttock, Percutaneous Endoscopic Approach, Diagnostic
0YB04ZZ   Excision of Right Buttock, Percutaneous Endoscopic Approach
0YB10ZX   Excision of Left Buttock, Open Approach, Diagnostic
0YB10ZZ   Excision of Left Buttock, Open Approach
0YB13ZX   Excision of Left Buttock, Percutaneous Approach, Diagnostic
0YB13ZZ   Excision of Left Buttock, Percutaneous Approach
0YB14ZX   Excision of Left Buttock, Percutaneous Endoscopic Approach, Diagnostic
0YB14ZZ   Excision of Left Buttock, Percutaneous Endoscopic Approach
0YB50ZX   Excision of Right Inguinal Region, Open Approach, Diagnostic
0YB50ZZ   Excision of Right Inguinal Region, Open Approach
0YB53ZX   Excision of Right Inguinal Region, Percutaneous Approach, Diagnostic
0YB53ZZ   Excision of Right Inguinal Region, Percutaneous Approach
0YB54ZX   Excision of Right Inguinal Region, Percutaneous Endoscopic Approach, Diagnostic

0YB54ZZ   Excision of Right Inguinal Region, Percutaneous Endoscopic Approach
0YB60ZX   Excision of Left Inguinal Region, Open Approach, Diagnostic
0YB60ZZ   Excision of Left Inguinal Region, Open Approach
0YB63ZX   Excision of Left Inguinal Region, Percutaneous Approach, Diagnostic
0YB63ZZ   Excision of Left Inguinal Region, Percutaneous Approach
0YB64ZX   Excision of Left Inguinal Region, Percutaneous Endoscopic Approach, Diagnostic
0YB64ZZ   Excision of Left Inguinal Region, Percutaneous Endoscopic Approach
0YB70ZX   Excision of Right Femoral Region, Open Approach, Diagnostic
0YB70ZZ   Excision of Right Femoral Region, Open Approach
0YB73ZX   Excision of Right Femoral Region, Percutaneous Approach, Diagnostic
0YB73ZZ   Excision of Right Femoral Region, Percutaneous Approach
0YB74ZX   Excision of Right Femoral Region, Percutaneous Endoscopic Approach, Diagnostic
0YB74ZZ   Excision of Right Femoral Region, Percutaneous Endoscopic Approach
0YB80ZX   Excision of Left Femoral Region, Open Approach, Diagnostic
0YB80ZZ   Excision of Left Femoral Region, Open Approach

0YB83ZX Excision of Left Femoral Region, Percutaneous Approach, Diagnostic

0YB83ZZ Excision of Left Femoral Region, Percutaneous Approach

0YB84ZX Excision of Left Femoral Region, Percutaneous Endoscopic Approach, Diagnostic

0YB84ZZ Excision of Left Femoral Region, Percutaneous Endoscopic Approach

0YB90ZX Excision of Right Lower Extremity, Open Approach, Diagnostic

0YB90ZZ Excision of Right Lower Extremity, Open Approach

0YB93ZX Excision of Right Lower Extremity, Percutaneous Approach, Diagnostic

0YB93ZZ Excision of Right Lower Extremity, Percutaneous Approach

0YB94ZX Excision of Right Lower Extremity, Percutaneous Endoscopic Approach, Diagnostic

0YB94ZZ Excision of Right Lower Extremity, Percutaneous Endoscopic Approach

0YBB0ZX Excision of Left Lower Extremity, Open Approach, Diagnostic

0YBB0ZZ Excision of Left Lower Extremity, Open Approach

0YBB3ZX Excision of Left Lower Extremity, Percutaneous Approach, Diagnostic

0YBB3ZZ Excision of Left Lower Extremity, Percutaneous Approach

0YBB4ZX Excision of Left Lower Extremity, Percutaneous Endoscopic Approach, Diagnostic

0YBB4ZZ Excision of Left Lower Extremity, Percutaneous Endoscopic Approach

0YBC0ZX Excision of Right Upper Leg, Open Approach, Diagnostic

0YBC0ZZ Excision of Right Upper Leg, Open Approach

0YBC3ZX Excision of Right Upper Leg, Percutaneous Approach, Diagnostic

0YBC3ZZ Excision of Right Upper Leg, Percutaneous Approach

0YBC4ZX Excision of Right Upper Leg, Percutaneous Endoscopic Approach, Diagnostic

0YBC4ZZ Excision of Right Upper Leg, Percutaneous Endoscopic Approach

0YBD0ZX Excision of Left Upper Leg, Open Approach, Diagnostic

0YBD0ZZ Excision of Left Upper Leg, Open Approach

0YBD3ZX Excision of Left Upper Leg, Percutaneous Approach, Diagnostic

0YBD3ZZ Excision of Left Upper Leg, Percutaneous Approach

0YBD4ZX Excision of Left Upper Leg, Percutaneous Endoscopic Approach, Diagnostic

0YBD4ZZ Excision of Left Upper Leg, Percutaneous Endoscopic Approach

0YBF0ZX Excision of Right Knee Region, Open Approach, Diagnostic

0YBF0ZZ Excision of Right Knee Region, Open Approach

0YBF3ZX Excision of Right Knee Region, Percutaneous Approach, Diagnostic

0YBF3ZZ Excision of Right Knee Region, Percutaneous Approach

0YBF4ZX Excision of Right Knee Region, Percutaneous Endoscopic Approach, Diagnostic

0YBF4ZZ Excision of Right Knee Region, Percutaneous Endoscopic Approach

0YBG0ZX Excision of Left Knee Region, Open Approach, Diagnostic

0YBG0ZZ Excision of Left Knee Region, Open Approach

0YBG3ZX Excision of Left Knee Region, Percutaneous Approach, Diagnostic

0YBG3ZZ Excision of Left Knee Region, Percutaneous Approach

0YBG4ZX Excision of Left Knee Region, Percutaneous Endoscopic Approach, Diagnostic

0YBG4ZZ Excision of Left Knee Region, Percutaneous Endoscopic Approach

0YBH0ZX Excision of Right Lower Leg, Open Approach, Diagnostic

0YBH0ZZ Excision of Right Lower Leg, Open Approach

0YBH3ZX Excision of Right Lower Leg, Percutaneous Approach, Diagnostic

0YBH3ZZ Excision of Right Lower Leg, Percutaneous Approach

0YBH4ZX Excision of Right Lower Leg, Percutaneous Endoscopic Approach, Diagnostic

0YBH4ZZ Excision of Right Lower Leg, Percutaneous Endoscopic Approach

0YBJ0ZX Excision of Left Lower Leg, Open Approach, Diagnostic

0YBJ0ZZ Excision of Left Lower Leg, Open Approach

0YBJ3ZX Excision of Left Lower Leg, Percutaneous Approach, Diagnostic

0YBJ3ZZ Excision of Left Lower Leg, Percutaneous Approach

0YBJ4ZX Excision of Left Lower Leg, Percutaneous Endoscopic Approach, Diagnostic

0YBJ4ZZ Excision of Left Lower Leg, Percutaneous Endoscopic Approach

0YBK0ZX Excision of Right Ankle Region, Open Approach, Diagnostic

0YBK0ZZ Excision of Right Ankle Region, Open Approach

0YBK3ZX Excision of Right Ankle Region, Percutaneous Approach, Diagnostic

0YBK3ZZ Excision of Right Ankle Region, Percutaneous Approach

0YBK4ZX Excision of Right Ankle Region, Percutaneous Endoscopic Approach, Diagnostic

0YBK4ZZ Excision of Right Ankle Region, Percutaneous Endoscopic Approach

0YBL0ZX Excision of Left Ankle Region, Open Approach, Diagnostic

0YBL0ZZ Excision of Left Ankle Region, Open Approach

0YBL3ZX Excision of Left Ankle Region, Percutaneous Approach, Diagnostic

0YBL3ZZ Excision of Left Ankle Region, Percutaneous Approach

0YBL4ZX Excision of Left Ankle Region, Percutaneous Endoscopic Approach, Diagnostic

0YBL4ZZ Excision of Left Ankle Region, Percutaneous Endoscopic Approach

0YBM0ZX Excision of Right Foot, Open Approach, Diagnostic

0YBM0ZZ Excision of Right Foot, Open Approach

0YBM3ZX Excision of Right Foot, Percutaneous Approach, Diagnostic

0YBM3ZZ Excision of Right Foot, Percutaneous Approach

0YBM4ZX Excision of Right Foot, Percutaneous Endoscopic Approach, Diagnostic

0YBM4ZZ Excision of Right Foot, Percutaneous Endoscopic Approach

0YBN0ZX Excision of Left Foot, Open Approach, Diagnostic

0YBN0ZZ Excision of Left Foot, Open Approach

0YBN3ZX Excision of Left Foot, Percutaneous Approach, Diagnostic

0YBN3ZZ Excision of Left Foot, Percutaneous Approach

0YBN4ZX Excision of Left Foot, Percutaneous Endoscopic Approach, Diagnostic

0YBN4ZZ Excision of Left Foot, Percutaneous Endoscopic Approach

0YH – Anatomical Regions, Lower Extremities, Insertion

0YH001Z Insertion of Radioactive Element into Right Buttock, Open Approach

● **0YH003Z** Insertion of Infusion Device into Right Buttock, Open Approach

● **0YH00YZ** Insertion of Other Device into Right Buttock, Open Approach

0YH031Z Insertion of Radioactive Element into Right Buttock, Percutaneous Approach

● **0YH033Z** Insertion of Infusion Device into Right Buttock, Percutaneous Approach

● **0YH03YZ** Insertion of Other Device into Right Buttock, Percutaneous Approach

0YH041Z Insertion of Radioactive Element into Right Buttock, Percutaneous Endoscopic Approach

● **0YH043Z** Insertion of Infusion Device into Right Buttock, Percutaneous Endoscopic Approach

● **0YH04YZ** Insertion of Other Device into Right Buttock, Percutaneous Endoscopic Approach

0YH101Z Insertion of Radioactive Element into Left Buttock, Open Approach

● **0YH103Z** Insertion of Infusion Device into Left Buttock, Open Approach

● **0YH10YZ** Insertion of Other Device into Left Buttock, Open Approach

0YH131Z Insertion of Radioactive Element into Left Buttock, Percutaneous Approach

● **0YH133Z** Insertion of Infusion Device into Left Buttock, Percutaneous Approach

● **0YH13YZ** Insertion of Other Device into Left Buttock, Percutaneous Approach

0YH141Z Insertion of Radioactive Element into Left Buttock, Percutaneous Endoscopic Approach

● **0YH143Z** Insertion of Infusion Device into Left Buttock, Percutaneous Endoscopic Approach

● **0YH14YZ** Insertion of Other Device into Left Buttock, Percutaneous Endoscopic Approach

0YH501Z Insertion of Radioactive Element into Right Inguinal Region, Open Approach

● **0YH503Z** Insertion of Infusion Device into Right Inguinal Region, Open Approach

● **0YH50YZ** Insertion of Other Device into Right Inguinal Region, Open Approach

0YH531Z Insertion of Radioactive Element into Right Inguinal Region, Percutaneous Approach

● **0YH533Z** Insertion of Infusion Device into Right Inguinal Region, Percutaneous Approach

● **0YH53YZ** Insertion of Other Device into Right Inguinal Region, Percutaneous Approach

---

♀ Female-only   ♂ Male-only   ◐ Limited Coverage   ● Non-OR   **HAC** HAC-associated procedure   ● Non-covered procedures   ✛ Combination

0YH541Z Insertion of Radioactive Element into Right Inguinal Region, Percutaneous Endoscopic Approach

● **0YH543Z** Insertion of Infusion Device into Right Inguinal Region, Percutaneous Endoscopic Approach

● **0YH54YZ** Insertion of Other Device into Right Inguinal Region, Percutaneous Endoscopic Approach

0YH601Z Insertion of Radioactive Element into Left Inguinal Region, Open Approach

● **0YH603Z** Insertion of Infusion Device into Left Inguinal Region, Open Approach

● **0YH60YZ** Insertion of Other Device into Left Inguinal Region, Open Approach

0YH631Z Insertion of Radioactive Element into Left Inguinal Region, Percutaneous Approach

● **0YH633Z** Insertion of Infusion Device into Left Inguinal Region, Percutaneous Approach

● **0YH63YZ** Insertion of Other Device into Left Inguinal Region, Percutaneous Approach

0YH641Z Insertion of Radioactive Element into Left Inguinal Region, Percutaneous Endoscopic Approach

● **0YH643Z** Insertion of Infusion Device into Left Inguinal Region, Percutaneous Endoscopic Approach

● **0YH64YZ** Insertion of Other Device into Left Inguinal Region, Percutaneous Endoscopic Approach

0YH701Z Insertion of Radioactive Element into Right Femoral Region, Open Approach

● **0YH703Z** Insertion of Infusion Device into Right Femoral Region, Open Approach

● **0YH70YZ** Insertion of Other Device into Right Femoral Region, Open Approach

0YH731Z Insertion of Radioactive Element into Right Femoral Region, Percutaneous Approach

● **0YH733Z** Insertion of Infusion Device into Right Femoral Region, Percutaneous Approach

● **0YH73YZ** Insertion of Other Device into Right Femoral Region, Percutaneous Approach

0YH741Z Insertion of Radioactive Element into Right Femoral Region, Percutaneous Endoscopic Approach

● **0YH743Z** Insertion of Infusion Device into Right Femoral Region, Percutaneous Endoscopic Approach

● **0YH74YZ** Insertion of Other Device into Right Femoral Region, Percutaneous Endoscopic Approach

0YH801Z Insertion of Radioactive Element into Left Femoral Region, Open Approach

● **0YH803Z** Insertion of Infusion Device into Left Femoral Region, Open Approach

● **0YH80YZ** Insertion of Other Device into Left Femoral Region, Open Approach

0YH831Z Insertion of Radioactive Element into Left Femoral Region, Percutaneous Approach

● **0YH833Z** Insertion of Infusion Device into Left Femoral Region, Percutaneous Approach

● **0YH83YZ** Insertion of Other Device into Left Femoral Region, Percutaneous Approach

0YH841Z Insertion of Radioactive Element into Left Femoral Region, Percutaneous Endoscopic Approach

● **0YH843Z** Insertion of Infusion Device into Left Femoral Region, Percutaneous Endoscopic Approach

● **0YH84YZ** Insertion of Other Device into Left Femoral Region, Percutaneous Endoscopic Approach

0YH901Z Insertion of Radioactive Element into Right Lower Extremity, Open Approach

● **0YH903Z** Insertion of Infusion Device into Right Lower Extremity, Open Approach

● **0YH90YZ** Insertion of Other Device into Right Lower Extremity, Open Approach

0YH931Z Insertion of Radioactive Element into Right Lower Extremity, Percutaneous Approach

● **0YH933Z** Insertion of Infusion Device into Right Lower Extremity, Percutaneous Approach

● **0YH93YZ** Insertion of Other Device into Right Lower Extremity, Percutaneous Approach

0YH941Z Insertion of Radioactive Element into Right Lower Extremity, Percutaneous Endoscopic Approach

0YH943Z Insertion of Infusion Device into Right Lower Extremity, Percutaneous Endoscopic Approach

● **0YH94YZ** Insertion of Other Device into Right Lower Extremity, Percutaneous Endoscopic Approach

0YHB01Z Insertion of Radioactive Element into Left Lower Extremity, Open Approach

● **0YHB03Z** Insertion of Infusion Device into Left Lower Extremity, Open Approach

● **0YHB0YZ** Insertion of Other Device into Left Lower Extremity, Open Approach

0YHB31Z Insertion of Radioactive Element into Left Lower Extremity, Percutaneous Approach

● **0YHB33Z** Insertion of Infusion Device into Left Lower Extremity, Percutaneous Approach

● **0YHB3YZ** Insertion of Other Device into Left Lower Extremity, Percutaneous Approach

0YHB41Z Insertion of Radioactive Element into Left Lower Extremity, Percutaneous Endoscopic Approach

● **0YHB43Z** Insertion of Infusion Device into Left Lower Extremity, Percutaneous Endoscopic Approach

● **0YHB4YZ** Insertion of Other Device into Left Lower Extremity, Percutaneous Endoscopic Approach

0YHC01Z Insertion of Radioactive Element into Right Upper Leg, Open Approach

● **0YHC03Z** Insertion of Infusion Device into Right Upper Leg, Open Approach

● **0YHC0YZ** Insertion of Other Device into Right Upper Leg, Open Approach

0YHC31Z Insertion of Radioactive Element into Right Upper Leg, Percutaneous Approach

● **0YHC33Z** Insertion of Infusion Device into Right Upper Leg, Percutaneous Approach

● **0YHC3YZ** Insertion of Other Device into Right Upper Leg, Percutaneous Approach

0YHC41Z Insertion of Radioactive Element into Right Upper Leg, Percutaneous Endoscopic Approach

● **0YHC43Z** Insertion of Infusion Device into Right Upper Leg, Percutaneous Endoscopic Approach

● **0YHC4YZ** Insertion of Other Device into Right Upper Leg, Percutaneous Endoscopic Approach

0YHD01Z Insertion of Radioactive Element into Left Upper Leg, Open Approach

● **0YHD03Z** Insertion of Infusion Device into Left Upper Leg, Open Approach

● **0YHD0YZ** Insertion of Other Device into Left Upper Leg, Open Approach

0YHD31Z Insertion of Radioactive Element into Left Upper Leg, Percutaneous Approach

● **0YHD33Z** Insertion of Infusion Device into Left Upper Leg, Percutaneous Approach

● **0YHD3YZ** Insertion of Other Device into Left Upper Leg, Percutaneous Approach

0YHD41Z Insertion of Radioactive Element into Left Upper Leg, Percutaneous Endoscopic Approach

● **0YHD43Z** Insertion of Infusion Device into Left Upper Leg, Percutaneous Endoscopic Approach

● **0YHD4YZ** Insertion of Other Device into Left Upper Leg, Percutaneous Endoscopic Approach

0YHF01Z Insertion of Radioactive Element into Right Knee Region, Open Approach

● **0YHF03Z** Insertion of Infusion Device into Right Knee Region, Open Approach

● **0YHF0YZ** Insertion of Other Device into Right Knee Region, Open Approach

0YHF31Z Insertion of Radioactive Element into Right Knee Region, Percutaneous Approach

● **0YHF33Z** Insertion of Infusion Device into Right Knee Region, Percutaneous Approach

● **0YHF3YZ** Insertion of Other Device into Right Knee Region, Percutaneous Approach

0YHF41Z Insertion of Radioactive Element into Right Knee Region, Percutaneous Endoscopic Approach

● **0YHF43Z** Insertion of Infusion Device into Right Knee Region, Percutaneous Endoscopic Approach

● **0YHF4YZ** Insertion of Other Device into Right Knee Region, Percutaneous Endoscopic Approach

0YHG01Z Insertion of Radioactive Element into Left Knee Region, Open Approach

---

- **0YHG03Z** Insertion of Infusion Device into Left Knee Region, Open Approach
- **0YHG0YZ** Insertion of Other Device into Left Knee Region, Open Approach
- **0YHG31Z** Insertion of Radioactive Element into Left Knee Region, Percutaneous Approach
- **0YHG33Z** Insertion of Infusion Device into Left Knee Region, Percutaneous Approach
- **0YHG3YZ** Insertion of Other Device into Left Knee Region, Percutaneous Approach
- **0YHG41Z** Insertion of Radioactive Element into Left Knee Region, Percutaneous Endoscopic Approach
- **0YHG43Z** Insertion of Infusion Device into Left Knee Region, Percutaneous Endoscopic Approach
- **0YHG4YZ** Insertion of Other Device into Left Knee Region, Percutaneous Endoscopic Approach
- **0YHH01Z** Insertion of Radioactive Element into Right Lower Leg, Open Approach
- **0YHH03Z** Insertion of Infusion Device into Right Lower Leg, Open Approach
- **0YHH0YZ** Insertion of Other Device into Right Lower Leg, Open Approach
- **0YHH31Z** Insertion of Radioactive Element into Right Lower Leg, Percutaneous Approach
- **0YHH33Z** Insertion of Infusion Device into Right Lower Leg, Percutaneous Approach
- **0YHH3YZ** Insertion of Other Device into Right Lower Leg, Percutaneous Approach
- **0YHH41Z** Insertion of Radioactive Element into Right Lower Leg, Percutaneous Endoscopic Approach
- **0YHH43Z** Insertion of Infusion Device into Right Lower Leg, Percutaneous Endoscopic Approach
- **0YHH4YZ** Insertion of Other Device into Right Lower Leg, Percutaneous Endoscopic Approach
- **0YHJ01Z** Insertion of Radioactive Element into Left Lower Leg, Open Approach
- **0YHJ03Z** Insertion of Infusion Device into Left Lower Leg, Open Approach
- **0YHJ0YZ** Insertion of Other Device into Left Lower Leg, Open Approach
- **0YHJ31Z** Insertion of Radioactive Element into Left Lower Leg, Percutaneous Approach
- **0YHJ33Z** Insertion of Infusion Device into Left Lower Leg, Percutaneous Approach
- **0YHJ3YZ** Insertion of Other Device into Left Lower Leg, Percutaneous Approach
- **0YHJ41Z** Insertion of Radioactive Element into Left Lower Leg, Percutaneous Endoscopic Approach
- **0YHJ43Z** Insertion of Infusion Device into Left Lower Leg, Percutaneous Approach
- **0YHJ4YZ** Insertion of Other Device into Left Lower Leg, Percutaneous Endoscopic Approach
- **0YHK01Z** Insertion of Radioactive Element into Right Ankle Region, Open Approach
- **0YHK03Z** Insertion of Infusion Device into Right Ankle Region, Open Approach
- **0YHK0YZ** Insertion of Other Device into Right Ankle Region, Open Approach
- **0YHK31Z** Insertion of Radioactive Element into Right Ankle Region, Percutaneous Approach

- **0YHK33Z** Insertion of Infusion Device into Right Ankle Region, Percutaneous Approach
- **0YHK3YZ** Insertion of Other Device into Right Ankle Region, Percutaneous Approach
- **0YHK41Z** Insertion of Radioactive Element into Right Ankle Region, Percutaneous Endoscopic Approach
- **0YHK43Z** Insertion of Infusion Device into Right Ankle Region, Percutaneous Endoscopic Approach
- **0YHK4YZ** Insertion of Other Device into Right Ankle Region, Percutaneous Endoscopic Approach
- **0YHL01Z** Insertion of Radioactive Element into Left Ankle Region, Open Approach
- **0YHL03Z** Insertion of Infusion Device into Left Ankle Region, Open Approach
- **0YHL0YZ** Insertion of Other Device into Left Ankle Region, Open Approach
- **0YHL31Z** Insertion of Radioactive Element into Left Ankle Region, Percutaneous Approach
- **0YHL33Z** Insertion of Infusion Device into Left Ankle Region, Percutaneous Approach
- **0YHL3YZ** Insertion of Other Device into Left Ankle Region, Percutaneous Approach
- **0YHL41Z** Insertion of Radioactive Element into Left Ankle Region, Percutaneous Endoscopic Approach
- **0YHL43Z** Insertion of Infusion Device into Left Ankle Region, Percutaneous Endoscopic Approach
- **0YHL4YZ** Insertion of Other Device into Left Ankle Region, Percutaneous Endoscopic Approach
- **0YHM01Z** Insertion of Radioactive Element into Right Foot, Open Approach
- **0YHM03Z** Insertion of Infusion Device into Right Foot, Open Approach
- **0YHM0YZ** Insertion of Other Device into Right Foot, Open Approach
- **0YHM31Z** Insertion of Radioactive Element into Right Foot, Percutaneous Approach
- **0YHM33Z** Insertion of Infusion Device into Right Foot, Percutaneous Approach
- **0YHM3YZ** Insertion of Other Device into Right Foot, Percutaneous Approach
- **0YHM41Z** Insertion of Radioactive Element into Right Foot, Percutaneous Endoscopic Approach
- **0YHM43Z** Insertion of Infusion Device into Right Foot, Percutaneous Endoscopic Approach
- **0YHM4YZ** Insertion of Other Device into Right Foot, Percutaneous Endoscopic Approach
- **0YHN01Z** Insertion of Radioactive Element into Left Foot, Open Approach
- **0YHN03Z** Insertion of Infusion Device into Left Foot, Open Approach
- **0YHN0YZ** Insertion of Other Device into Left Foot, Open Approach
- **0YHN31Z** Insertion of Radioactive Element into Left Foot, Percutaneous Approach
- **0YHN33Z** Insertion of Infusion Device into Left Foot, Percutaneous Approach
- **0YHN3YZ** Insertion of Other Device into Left Foot, Percutaneous Approach
- **0YHN41Z** Insertion of Radioactive Element into Left Foot, Percutaneous Endoscopic Approach
- **0YHN43Z** Insertion of Infusion Device into Left Foot, Percutaneous Endoscopic Approach
- **0YHN4YZ** Insertion of Other Device into Left Foot, Percutaneous Endoscopic Approach

0YJ – Anatomical Regions, Lower Extremities, Inspection

Review Coding Guidelines B3.11a, B3.11b and B3.11c

- **0YJ00ZZ** Inspection of Right Buttock, Open Approach
- **0YJ03ZZ** Inspection of Right Buttock, Percutaneous Approach
- **0YJ04ZZ** Inspection of Right Buttock, Percutaneous Endoscopic Approach
- **0YJ0XZZ** Inspection of Right Buttock, External Approach
- **0YJ10ZZ** Inspection of Left Buttock, Open Approach
- **0YJ13ZZ** Inspection of Left Buttock, Percutaneous Approach
- **0YJ14ZZ** Inspection of Left Buttock, Percutaneous Endoscopic Approach
- **0YJ1XZZ** Inspection of Left Buttock, External Approach
- **0YJ50ZZ** Inspection of Right Inguinal Region, Open Approach
- **0YJ53ZZ** Inspection of Right Inguinal Region, Percutaneous Approach
- **0YJ54ZZ** Inspection of Right Inguinal Region, Percutaneous Endoscopic Approach
- **0YJ5XZZ** Inspection of Right Inguinal Region, External Approach
- **0YJ60ZZ** Inspection of Left Inguinal Region, Open Approach

- **0YJ63ZZ** Inspection of Left Inguinal Region, Percutaneous Approach
- **0YJ64ZZ** Inspection of Left Inguinal Region, Percutaneous Endoscopic Approach
- **0YJ6XZZ** Inspection of Left Inguinal Region, External Approach
- **0YJ70ZZ** Inspection of Right Femoral Region, Open Approach
- **0YJ73ZZ** Inspection of Right Femoral Region, Percutaneous Approach
- **0YJ74ZZ** Inspection of Right Femoral Region, Percutaneous Endoscopic Approach
- **0YJ7XZZ** Inspection of Right Femoral Region, External Approach
- **0YJ80ZZ** Inspection of Left Femoral Region, Open Approach
- **0YJ83ZZ** Inspection of Left Femoral Region, Percutaneous Approach
- **0YJ84ZZ** Inspection of Left Femoral Region, Percutaneous Endoscopic Approach
- **0YJ8XZZ** Inspection of Left Femoral Region, External Approach

---

♀ Female-only   ♂ Male-only   ● Limited Coverage   ● Non-OR   ᴴᴬᶜ HAC-associated procedure   ● Non-covered procedures   ✛ Combination

● **0YJ90ZZ** Inspection of Right Lower Extremity, Open Approach
0YJ93ZZ Inspection of Right Lower Extremity, Percutaneous Approach
0YJ94ZZ Inspection of Right Lower Extremity, Percutaneous Endoscopic Approach
0YJ9XZZ Inspection of Right Lower Extremity, External Approach
0YJA0ZZ Inspection of Bilateral Inguinal Region, Open Approach
0YJA3ZZ Inspection of Bilateral Inguinal Region, Percutaneous Approach
0YJA4ZZ Inspection of Bilateral Inguinal Region, Percutaneous Endoscopic Approach
0YJAXZZ Inspection of Bilateral Inguinal Region, External Approach
● **0YJB0ZZ** Inspection of Left Lower Extremity, Open Approach
0YJB3ZZ Inspection of Left Lower Extremity, Percutaneous Approach
0YJB4ZZ Inspection of Left Lower Extremity, Percutaneous Endoscopic Approach
0YJBXZZ Inspection of Left Lower Extremity, External Approach
● **0YJC0ZZ** Inspection of Right Upper Leg, Open Approach
0YJC3ZZ Inspection of Right Upper Leg, Percutaneous Approach
0YJC4ZZ Inspection of Right Upper Leg, Percutaneous Endoscopic Approach
0YJCXZZ Inspection of Right Upper Leg, External Approach
● **0YJD0ZZ** Inspection of Left Upper Leg, Open Approach
0YJD3ZZ Inspection of Left Upper Leg, Percutaneous Approach
0YJD4ZZ Inspection of Left Upper Leg, Percutaneous Endoscopic Approach
0YJDXZZ Inspection of Left Upper Leg, External Approach
● **0YJE0ZZ** Inspection of Bilateral Femoral Region, Open Approach
0YJE3ZZ Inspection of Bilateral Femoral Region, Percutaneous Approach
0YJE4ZZ Inspection of Bilateral Femoral Region, Percutaneous Endoscopic Approach
0YJEXZZ Inspection of Bilateral Femoral Region, External Approach
● **0YJF0ZZ** Inspection of Right Knee Region, Open Approach
0YJF3ZZ Inspection of Right Knee Region, Percutaneous Approach
0YJF4ZZ Inspection of Right Knee Region, Percutaneous Endoscopic Approach
0YJFXZZ Inspection of Right Knee Region, External Approach

● **0YJG0ZZ** Inspection of Left Knee Region, Open Approach
0YJG3ZZ Inspection of Left Knee Region, Percutaneous Approach
0YJG4ZZ Inspection of Left Knee Region, Percutaneous Endoscopic Approach
0YJGXZZ Inspection of Left Knee Region, External Approach
● **0YJH0ZZ** Inspection of Right Lower Leg, Open Approach
0YJH3ZZ Inspection of Right Lower Leg, Percutaneous Approach
0YJH4ZZ Inspection of Right Lower Leg, Percutaneous Endoscopic Approach
0YJHXZZ Inspection of Right Lower Leg, External Approach
● **0YJJ0ZZ** Inspection of Left Lower Leg, Open Approach
0YJJ3ZZ Inspection of Left Lower Leg, Percutaneous Approach
0YJJ4ZZ Inspection of Left Lower Leg, Percutaneous Endoscopic Approach
0YJJXZZ Inspection of Left Lower Leg, External Approach
● **0YJK0ZZ** Inspection of Right Ankle Region, Open Approach
0YJK3ZZ Inspection of Right Ankle Region, Percutaneous Approach
0YJK4ZZ Inspection of Right Ankle Region, Percutaneous Endoscopic Approach
0YJKXZZ Inspection of Right Ankle Region, External Approach
● **0YJL0ZZ** Inspection of Left Ankle Region, Open Approach
0YJL3ZZ Inspection of Left Ankle Region, Percutaneous Approach
0YJL4ZZ Inspection of Left Ankle Region, Percutaneous Endoscopic Approach
0YJLXZZ Inspection of Left Ankle Region, External Approach
● **0YJM0ZZ** Inspection of Right Foot, Open Approach
0YJM3ZZ Inspection of Right Foot, Percutaneous Approach
0YJM4ZZ Inspection of Right Foot, Percutaneous Endoscopic Approach
0YJMXZZ Inspection of Right Foot, External Approach
● **0YJN0ZZ** Inspection of Left Foot, Open Approach
0YJN3ZZ Inspection of Left Foot, Percutaneous Approach
0YJN4ZZ Inspection of Left Foot, Percutaneous Endoscopic Approach
0YJNXZZ Inspection of Left Foot, External Approach

0YM – Anatomical Regions, Lower Extremities, Reattachment

0YM00ZZ Reattachment of Right Buttock, Open Approach
0YM10ZZ Reattachment of Left Buttock, Open Approach
0YM20ZZ Reattachment of Right Hindquarter, Open Approach
0YM30ZZ Reattachment of Left Hindquarter, Open Approach
0YM40ZZ Reattachment of Bilateral Hindquarter, Open Approach
0YM50ZZ Reattachment of Right Inguinal Region, Open Approach
0YM60ZZ Reattachment of Left Inguinal Region, Open Approach
0YM70ZZ Reattachment of Right Femoral Region, Open Approach
0YM80ZZ Reattachment of Left Femoral Region, Open Approach
0YM90ZZ Reattachment of Right Lower Extremity, Open Approach
0YMB0ZZ Reattachment of Left Lower Extremity, Open Approach
0YMC0ZZ Reattachment of Right Upper Leg, Open Approach
0YMD0ZZ Reattachment of Left Upper Leg, Open Approach
0YMF0ZZ Reattachment of Right Knee Region, Open Approach
0YMG0ZZ Reattachment of Left Knee Region, Open Approach
0YMH0ZZ Reattachment of Right Lower Leg, Open Approach

0YMJ0ZZ Reattachment of Left Lower Leg, Open Approach
0YMK0ZZ Reattachment of Right Ankle Region, Open Approach
0YML0ZZ Reattachment of Left Ankle Region, Open Approach
0YMM0ZZ Reattachment of Right Foot, Open Approach
0YMN0ZZ Reattachment of Left Foot, Open Approach
0YMP0ZZ Reattachment of Right 1st Toe, Open Approach
0YMQ0ZZ Reattachment of Left 1st Toe, Open Approach
0YMR0ZZ Reattachment of Right 2nd Toe, Open Approach
0YMS0ZZ Reattachment of Left 2nd Toe, Open Approach
0YMT0ZZ Reattachment of Right 3rd Toe, Open Approach
0YMU0ZZ Reattachment of Left 3rd Toe, Open Approach
0YMV0ZZ Reattachment of Right 4th Toe, Open Approach
0YMW0ZZ Reattachment of Left 4th Toe, Open Approach
0YMX0ZZ Reattachment of Right 5th Toe, Open Approach
0YMY0ZZ Reattachment of Left 5th Toe, Open Approach

0YP – Anatomical Regions, Lower Extremities, Removal

Review Coding Guideline B6.1c

0YP900Z Removal of Drainage Device from Right Lower Extremity, Open Approach
0YP901Z Removal of Radioactive Element from Right Lower Extremity, Open Approach
0YP903Z Removal of Infusion Device from Right Lower Extremity, Open Approach
0YP907Z Removal of Autologous Tissue Substitute from Right Lower Extremity, Open Approach
0YP90JZ Removal of Synthetic Substitute from Right Lower Extremity, Open Approach
0YP90KZ Removal of Nonautologous Tissue Substitute from Right Lower Extremity, Open Approach
0YP90YZ Removal of Other Device from Right Lower Extremity, Open Approach
0YP930Z Removal of Drainage Device from Right Lower Extremity, Percutaneous Approach

0YP931Z Removal of Radioactive Element from Right Lower Extremity, Percutaneous Approach
0YP933Z Removal of Infusion Device from Right Lower Extremity, Percutaneous Approach
0YP937Z Removal of Autologous Tissue Substitute from Right Lower Extremity, Percutaneous Approach
0YP93JZ Removal of Synthetic Substitute from Right Lower Extremity, Percutaneous Approach
0YP93KZ Removal of Nonautologous Tissue Substitute from Right Lower Extremity, Percutaneous Approach
0YP93YZ Removal of Other Device from Right Lower Extremity, Percutaneous Approach
0YP940Z Removal of Drainage Device from Right Lower Extremity, Percutaneous Endoscopic Approach
0YP941Z Removal of Radioactive Element from Right Lower Extremity, Percutaneous Endoscopic Approach

---

♀ Female-only   ♂ Male-only   ● Limited Coverage   ● Non-OR   **HAC** HAC-associated procedure   ● Non-covered procedures   ➕ Combination

0YP943Z Removal of Infusion Device from Right Lower Extremity, Percutaneous Endoscopic Approach

0YP947Z Removal of Autologous Tissue Substitute from Right Lower Extremity, Percutaneous Endoscopic Approach

0YP94JZ Removal of Synthetic Substitute from Right Lower Extremity, Percutaneous Endoscopic Approach

0YP94KZ Removal of Nonautologous Tissue Substitute from Right Lower Extremity, Percutaneous Endoscopic Approach

0YP94YZ Removal of Other Device from Right Lower Extremity, Percutaneous Endoscopic Approach

0YP9X0Z Removal of Drainage Device from Right Lower Extremity, External Approach

0YP9X1Z Removal of Radioactive Element from Right Lower Extremity, External Approach

0YP9X3Z Removal of Infusion Device from Right Lower Extremity, External Approach

0YP9X7Z Removal of Autologous Tissue Substitute from Right Lower Extremity, External Approach

0YP9XJZ Removal of Synthetic Substitute from Right Lower Extremity, External Approach

0YP9XKZ Removal of Nonautologous Tissue Substitute from Right Lower Extremity, External Approach

0YP9XYZ Removal of Other Device from Right Lower Extremity, External Approach

0YPB00Z Removal of Drainage Device from Left Lower Extremity, Open Approach

0YPB01Z Removal of Radioactive Element from Left Lower Extremity, Open Approach

0YPB03Z Removal of Infusion Device from Left Lower Extremity, Open Approach

0YPB07Z Removal of Autologous Tissue Substitute from Left Lower Extremity, Open Approach

0YPB0JZ Removal of Synthetic Substitute from Left Lower Extremity, Open Approach

0YPB0KZ Removal of Nonautologous Tissue Substitute from Left Lower Extremity, Open Approach

0YPB0YZ Removal of Other Device from Left Lower Extremity, Open Approach

0YPB30Z Removal of Drainage Device from Left Lower Extremity, Percutaneous Approach

0YPB31Z Removal of Radioactive Element from Left Lower Extremity, Percutaneous Approach

0YPB33Z Removal of Infusion Device from Left Lower Extremity, Percutaneous Approach

0YPB37Z Removal of Autologous Tissue Substitute from Left Lower Extremity, Percutaneous Approach

0YPB3JZ Removal of Synthetic Substitute from Left Lower Extremity, Percutaneous Approach

0YPB3KZ Removal of Nonautologous Tissue Substitute from Left Lower Extremity, Percutaneous Approach

0YPB3YZ Removal of Other Device from Left Lower Extremity, Percutaneous Approach

0YPB40Z Removal of Drainage Device from Left Lower Extremity, Percutaneous Endoscopic Approach

0YPB41Z Removal of Radioactive Element from Left Lower Extremity, Percutaneous Endoscopic Approach

0YPB43Z Removal of Infusion Device from Left Lower Extremity, Percutaneous Endoscopic Approach

0YPB47Z Removal of Autologous Tissue Substitute from Left Lower Extremity, Percutaneous Endoscopic Approach

0YPB4JZ Removal of Synthetic Substitute from Left Lower Extremity, Percutaneous Endoscopic Approach

0YPB4KZ Removal of Nonautologous Tissue Substitute from Left Lower Extremity, Percutaneous Endoscopic Approach

0YPB4YZ Removal of Other Device from Left Lower Extremity, Percutaneous Endoscopic Approach

0YPBX0Z Removal of Drainage Device from Left Lower Extremity, External Approach

0YPBX1Z Removal of Radioactive Element from Left Lower Extremity, External Approach

0YPBX3Z Removal of Infusion Device from Left Lower Extremity, External Approach

0YPBX7Z Removal of Autologous Tissue Substitute from Left Lower Extremity, External Approach

0YPBXJZ Removal of Synthetic Substitute from Left Lower Extremity, External Approach

0YPBXKZ Removal of Nonautologous Tissue Substitute from Left Lower Extremity, External Approach

0YPBXYZ Removal of Other Device from Left Lower Extremity, External Approach

0YQ – Anatomical Regions, Lower Extremities, Repair

0YQ00ZZ Repair Right Buttock, Open Approach
0YQ03ZZ Repair Right Buttock, Percutaneous Approach
0YQ04ZZ Repair Right Buttock, Percutaneous Endoscopic Approach
0YQ0XZZ Repair Right Buttock, External Approach
0YQ10ZZ Repair Left Buttock, Open Approach
0YQ13ZZ Repair Left Buttock, Percutaneous Approach
0YQ14ZZ Repair Left Buttock, Percutaneous Endoscopic Approach
0YQ1XZZ Repair Left Buttock, External Approach
0YQ50ZZ Repair Right Inguinal Region, Open Approach
0YQ53ZZ Repair Right Inguinal Region, Percutaneous Approach
0YQ54ZZ Repair Right Inguinal Region, Percutaneous Endoscopic Approach
0YQ5XZZ Repair Right Inguinal Region, External Approach
0YQ60ZZ Repair Left Inguinal Region, Open Approach
0YQ63ZZ Repair Left Inguinal Region, Percutaneous Approach
0YQ64ZZ Repair Left Inguinal Region, Percutaneous Endoscopic Approach
0YQ6XZZ Repair Left Inguinal Region, External Approach
0YQ70ZZ Repair Right Femoral Region, Open Approach
0YQ73ZZ Repair Right Femoral Region, Percutaneous Approach
0YQ74ZZ Repair Right Femoral Region, Percutaneous Endoscopic Approach
0YQ7XZZ Repair Right Femoral Region, External Approach
0YQ80ZZ Repair Left Femoral Region, Open Approach
0YQ83ZZ Repair Left Femoral Region, Percutaneous Approach
0YQ84ZZ Repair Left Femoral Region, Percutaneous Endoscopic Approach
0YQ8XZZ Repair Left Femoral Region, External Approach
0YQ90ZZ Repair Right Lower Extremity, Open Approach
0YQ93ZZ Repair Right Lower Extremity, Percutaneous Approach
0YQ94ZZ Repair Right Lower Extremity, Percutaneous Endoscopic Approach
0YQ9XZZ Repair Right Lower Extremity, External Approach
0YQA0ZZ Repair Bilateral Inguinal Region, Open Approach
0YQA3ZZ Repair Bilateral Inguinal Region, Percutaneous Approach
0YQA4ZZ Repair Bilateral Inguinal Region, Percutaneous Endoscopic Approach
0YQAXZZ Repair Bilateral Inguinal Region, External Approach
0YQB0ZZ Repair Left Lower Extremity, Open Approach
0YQB3ZZ Repair Left Lower Extremity, Percutaneous Approach
0YQB4ZZ Repair Left Lower Extremity, Percutaneous Endoscopic Approach
0YQBXZZ Repair Left Lower Extremity, External Approach
0YQC0ZZ Repair Right Upper Leg, Open Approach
0YQC3ZZ Repair Right Upper Leg, Percutaneous Approach
0YQC4ZZ Repair Right Upper Leg, Percutaneous Endoscopic Approach
0YQCXZZ Repair Right Upper Leg, External Approach
0YQD0ZZ Repair Left Upper Leg, Open Approach
0YQD3ZZ Repair Left Upper Leg, Percutaneous Approach
0YQD4ZZ Repair Left Upper Leg, Percutaneous Endoscopic Approach
0YQDXZZ Repair Left Upper Leg, External Approach
0YQE0ZZ Repair Bilateral Femoral Region, Open Approach
0YQE3ZZ Repair Bilateral Femoral Region, Percutaneous Approach
0YQE4ZZ Repair Bilateral Femoral Region, Percutaneous Endoscopic Approach
0YQEXZZ Repair Bilateral Femoral Region, External Approach
0YQF0ZZ Repair Right Knee Region, Open Approach
0YQF3ZZ Repair Right Knee Region, Percutaneous Approach
0YQF4ZZ Repair Right Knee Region, Percutaneous Endoscopic Approach
0YQFXZZ Repair Right Knee Region, External Approach
0YQG0ZZ Repair Left Knee Region, Open Approach
0YQG3ZZ Repair Left Knee Region, Percutaneous Approach
0YQG4ZZ Repair Left Knee Region, Percutaneous Endoscopic Approach
0YQGXZZ Repair Left Knee Region, External Approach
0YQH0ZZ Repair Right Lower Leg, Open Approach
0YQH3ZZ Repair Right Lower Leg, Percutaneous Approach

0YQH4ZZ   Repair Right Lower Leg, Percutaneous Endoscopic Approach
0YQHXZZ   Repair Right Lower Leg, External Approach
0YQJ0ZZ   Repair Left Lower Leg, Open Approach
0YQJ3ZZ   Repair Left Lower Leg, Percutaneous Approach
0YQJ4ZZ   Repair Left Lower Leg, Percutaneous Endoscopic Approach
0YQJXZZ   Repair Left Lower Leg, External Approach
0YQK0ZZ   Repair Right Ankle Region, Open Approach
0YQK3ZZ   Repair Right Ankle Region, Percutaneous Approach
0YQK4ZZ   Repair Right Ankle Region, Percutaneous Endoscopic Approach
0YQKXZZ   Repair Right Ankle Region, External Approach
0YQL0ZZ   Repair Left Ankle Region, Open Approach
0YQL3ZZ   Repair Left Ankle Region, Percutaneous Approach
0YQL4ZZ   Repair Left Ankle Region, Percutaneous Endoscopic Approach
0YQLXZZ   Repair Left Ankle Region, External Approach
0YQM0ZZ   Repair Right Foot, Open Approach
0YQM3ZZ   Repair Right Foot, Percutaneous Approach
0YQM4ZZ   Repair Right Foot, Percutaneous Endoscopic Approach
0YQMXZZ   Repair Right Foot, External Approach
0YQN0ZZ   Repair Left Foot, Open Approach
0YQN3ZZ   Repair Left Foot, Percutaneous Approach
0YQN4ZZ   Repair Left Foot, Percutaneous Endoscopic Approach
0YQNXZZ   Repair Left Foot, External Approach
0YQP0ZZ   Repair Right 1st Toe, Open Approach
0YQP3ZZ   Repair Right 1st Toe, Percutaneous Approach
0YQP4ZZ   Repair Right 1st Toe, Percutaneous Endoscopic Approach
0YQPXZZ   Repair Right 1st Toe, External Approach
0YQQ0ZZ   Repair Left 1st Toe, Open Approach
0YQQ3ZZ   Repair Left 1st Toe, Percutaneous Approach
0YQQ4ZZ   Repair Left 1st Toe, Percutaneous Endoscopic Approach
0YQQXZZ   Repair Left 1st Toe, External Approach
0YQR0ZZ   Repair Right 2nd Toe, Open Approach

0YQR3ZZ   Repair Right 2nd Toe, Percutaneous Approach
0YQR4ZZ   Repair Right 2nd Toe, Percutaneous Endoscopic Approach
0YQRXZZ   Repair Right 2nd Toe, External Approach
0YQS0ZZ   Repair Left 2nd Toe, Open Approach
0YQS3ZZ   Repair Left 2nd Toe, Percutaneous Approach
0YQS4ZZ   Repair Left 2nd Toe, Percutaneous Endoscopic Approach
0YQSXZZ   Repair Left 2nd Toe, External Approach
0YQT0ZZ   Repair Right 3rd Toe, Open Approach
0YQT3ZZ   Repair Right 3rd Toe, Percutaneous Approach
0YQT4ZZ   Repair Right 3rd Toe, Percutaneous Endoscopic Approach
0YQTXZZ   Repair Right 3rd Toe, External Approach
0YQU0ZZ   Repair Left 3rd Toe, Open Approach
0YQU3ZZ   Repair Left 3rd Toe, Percutaneous Approach
0YQU4ZZ   Repair Left 3rd Toe, Percutaneous Endoscopic Approach
0YQUXZZ   Repair Left 3rd Toe, External Approach
0YQV0ZZ   Repair Right 4th Toe, Open Approach
0YQV3ZZ   Repair Right 4th Toe, Percutaneous Approach
0YQV4ZZ   Repair Right 4th Toe, Percutaneous Endoscopic Approach
0YQVXZZ   Repair Right 4th Toe, External Approach
0YQW0ZZ   Repair Left 4th Toe, Open Approach
0YQW3ZZ   Repair Left 4th Toe, Percutaneous Approach
0YQW4ZZ   Repair Left 4th Toe, Percutaneous Endoscopic Approach
0YQWXZZ   Repair Left 4th Toe, External Approach
0YQX0ZZ   Repair Right 5th Toe, Open Approach
0YQX3ZZ   Repair Right 5th Toe, Percutaneous Approach
0YQX4ZZ   Repair Right 5th Toe, Percutaneous Endoscopic Approach
0YQXXZZ   Repair Right 5th Toe, External Approach
0YQY0ZZ   Repair Left 5th Toe, Open Approach
0YQY3ZZ   Repair Left 5th Toe, Percutaneous Approach
0YQY4ZZ   Repair Left 5th Toe, Percutaneous Endoscopic Approach
0YQYXZZ   Repair Left 5th Toe, External Approach

0YU – Anatomical Regions, Lower Extremities, Supplement

0YU007Z   Supplement Right Buttock with Autologous Tissue Substitute, Open Approach
0YU00JZ   Supplement Right Buttock with Synthetic Substitute, Open Approach
0YU00KZ   Supplement Right Buttock with Nonautologous Tissue Substitute, Open Approach
0YU047Z   Supplement Right Buttock with Autologous Tissue Substitute, Percutaneous Endoscopic Approach
0YU04JZ   Supplement Right Buttock with Synthetic Substitute, Percutaneous Endoscopic Approach
0YU04KZ   Supplement Right Buttock with Nonautologous Tissue Substitute, Percutaneous Endoscopic Approach
0YU107Z   Supplement Left Buttock with Autologous Tissue Substitute, Open Approach
0YU10JZ   Supplement Left Buttock with Synthetic Substitute, Open Approach
0YU10KZ   Supplement Left Buttock with Nonautologous Tissue Substitute, Open Approach
0YU147Z   Supplement Left Buttock with Autologous Tissue Substitute, Percutaneous Endoscopic Approach
0YU14JZ   Supplement Left Buttock with Synthetic Substitute, Percutaneous Endoscopic Approach
0YU14KZ   Supplement Left Buttock with Nonautologous Tissue Substitute, Percutaneous Endoscopic Approach
0YU507Z   Supplement Right Inguinal Region with Autologous Tissue Substitute, Open Approach
0YU50JZ   Supplement Right Inguinal Region with Synthetic Substitute, Open Approach
0YU50KZ   Supplement Right Inguinal Region with Nonautologous Tissue Substitute, Open Approach
0YU547Z   Supplement Right Inguinal Region with Autologous Tissue Substitute, Percutaneous Endoscopic Approach
0YU54JZ   Supplement Right Inguinal Region with Synthetic Substitute, Percutaneous Endoscopic Approach
0YU54KZ   Supplement Right Inguinal Region with Nonautologous Tissue Substitute, Percutaneous Endoscopic Approach
0YU607Z   Supplement Left Inguinal Region with Autologous Tissue Substitute, Open Approach

0YU60JZ   Supplement Left Inguinal Region with Synthetic Substitute, Open Approach
0YU60KZ   Supplement Left Inguinal Region with Nonautologous Tissue Substitute, Open Approach
0YU647Z   Supplement Left Inguinal Region with Autologous Tissue Substitute, Percutaneous Endoscopic Approach
0YU64JZ   Supplement Left Inguinal Region with Synthetic Substitute, Percutaneous Endoscopic Approach
0YU64KZ   Supplement Left Inguinal Region with Nonautologous Tissue Substitute, Percutaneous Endoscopic Approach
0YU707Z   Supplement Right Femoral Region with Autologous Tissue Substitute, Open Approach
0YU70JZ   Supplement Right Femoral Region with Synthetic Substitute, Open Approach
0YU70KZ   Supplement Right Femoral Region with Nonautologous Tissue Substitute, Open Approach
0YU747Z   Supplement Right Femoral Region with Autologous Tissue Substitute, Percutaneous Endoscopic Approach
0YU74JZ   Supplement Right Femoral Region with Synthetic Substitute, Percutaneous Endoscopic Approach
0YU74KZ   Supplement Right Femoral Region with Nonautologous Tissue Substitute, Percutaneous Endoscopic Approach
0YU807Z   Supplement Left Femoral Region with Autologous Tissue Substitute, Open Approach
0YU80JZ   Supplement Left Femoral Region with Synthetic Substitute, Open Approach
0YU80KZ   Supplement Left Femoral Region with Nonautologous Tissue Substitute, Open Approach
0YU847Z   Supplement Left Femoral Region with Autologous Tissue Substitute, Percutaneous Endoscopic Approach
0YU84JZ   Supplement Left Femoral Region with Synthetic Substitute, Percutaneous Endoscopic Approach
0YU84KZ   Supplement Left Femoral Region with Nonautologous Tissue Substitute, Percutaneous Endoscopic Approach
0YU907Z   Supplement Right Lower Extremity with Autologous Tissue Substitute, Open Approach
0YU90JZ   Supplement Right Lower Extremity with Synthetic Substitute, Open Approach

---

♀ Female-only   ♂ Male-only   ● Limited Coverage   ● Non-OR   ▩ HAC-associated procedure   ● Non-covered procedures   ✚ Combination

0YU90KZ Supplement Right Lower Extremity with Nonautologous Tissue Substitute, Open Approach

0YU947Z Supplement Right Lower Extremity with Autologous Tissue Substitute, Percutaneous Endoscopic Approach

0YU94JZ Supplement Right Lower Extremity with Synthetic Substitute, Percutaneous Endoscopic Approach

0YU94KZ Supplement Right Lower Extremity with Nonautologous Tissue Substitute, Percutaneous Endoscopic Approach

0YUA07Z Supplement Bilateral Inguinal Region with Autologous Tissue Substitute, Open Approach

0YUA0JZ Supplement Bilateral Inguinal Region with Synthetic Substitute, Open Approach

0YUA0KZ Supplement Bilateral Inguinal Region with Nonautologous Tissue Substitute, Open Approach

0YUA47Z Supplement Bilateral Inguinal Region with Autologous Tissue Substitute, Percutaneous Endoscopic Approach

0YUA4JZ Supplement Bilateral Inguinal Region with Synthetic Substitute, Percutaneous Endoscopic Approach

0YUA4KZ Supplement Bilateral Inguinal Region with Nonautologous Tissue Substitute, Percutaneous Endoscopic Approach

0YUB07Z Supplement Left Lower Extremity with Autologous Tissue Substitute, Open Approach

0YUB0JZ Supplement Left Lower Extremity with Synthetic Substitute, Open Approach

0YUB0KZ Supplement Left Lower Extremity with Nonautologous Tissue Substitute, Open Approach

0YUB47Z Supplement Left Lower Extremity with Autologous Tissue Substitute, Percutaneous Endoscopic Approach

0YUB4JZ Supplement Left Lower Extremity with Synthetic Substitute, Percutaneous Endoscopic Approach

0YUB4KZ Supplement Left Lower Extremity with Nonautologous Tissue Substitute, Percutaneous Endoscopic Approach

0YUC07Z Supplement Right Upper Leg with Autologous Tissue Substitute, Open Approach

0YUC0JZ Supplement Right Upper Leg with Synthetic Substitute, Open Approach

0YUC0KZ Supplement Right Upper Leg with Nonautologous Tissue Substitute, Open Approach

0YUC47Z Supplement Right Upper Leg with Autologous Tissue Substitute, Percutaneous Endoscopic Approach

0YUC4JZ Supplement Right Upper Leg with Synthetic Substitute, Percutaneous Endoscopic Approach

0YUC4KZ Supplement Right Upper Leg with Nonautologous Tissue Substitute, Percutaneous Endoscopic Approach

0YUD07Z Supplement Left Upper Leg with Autologous Tissue Substitute, Open Approach

0YUD0JZ Supplement Left Upper Leg with Synthetic Substitute, Open Approach

0YUD0KZ Supplement Left Upper Leg with Nonautologous Tissue Substitute, Open Approach

0YUD47Z Supplement Left Upper Leg with Autologous Tissue Substitute, Percutaneous Endoscopic Approach

0YUD4JZ Supplement Left Upper Leg with Synthetic Substitute, Percutaneous Endoscopic Approach

0YUD4KZ Supplement Left Upper Leg with Nonautologous Tissue Substitute, Percutaneous Endoscopic Approach

0YUE07Z Supplement Bilateral Femoral Region with Autologous Tissue Substitute, Open Approach

0YUE0JZ Supplement Bilateral Femoral Region with Synthetic Substitute, Open Approach

0YUE0KZ Supplement Bilateral Femoral Region with Nonautologous Tissue Substitute, Open Approach

0YUE47Z Supplement Bilateral Femoral Region with Autologous Tissue Substitute, Percutaneous Endoscopic Approach

0YUE4JZ Supplement Bilateral Femoral Region with Synthetic Substitute, Percutaneous Endoscopic Approach

0YUE4KZ Supplement Bilateral Femoral Region with Nonautologous Tissue Substitute, Percutaneous Endoscopic Approach

0YUF07Z Supplement Right Knee Region with Autologous Tissue Substitute, Open Approach

0YUF0JZ Supplement Right Knee Region with Synthetic Substitute, Open Approach

0YUF0KZ Supplement Right Knee Region with Nonautologous Tissue Substitute, Open Approach

0YUF47Z Supplement Right Knee Region with Autologous Tissue Substitute, Percutaneous Endoscopic Approach

0YUF4JZ Supplement Right Knee Region with Synthetic Substitute, Percutaneous Endoscopic Approach

0YUF4KZ Supplement Right Knee Region with Nonautologous Tissue Substitute, Percutaneous Endoscopic Approach

0YUG07Z Supplement Left Knee Region with Autologous Tissue Substitute, Open Approach

0YUG0JZ Supplement Left Knee Region with Synthetic Substitute, Open Approach

0YUG0KZ Supplement Left Knee Region with Nonautologous Tissue Substitute, Open Approach

0YUG47Z Supplement Left Knee Region with Autologous Tissue Substitute, Percutaneous Endoscopic Approach

0YUG4JZ Supplement Left Knee Region with Synthetic Substitute, Percutaneous Endoscopic Approach

0YUG4KZ Supplement Left Knee Region with Nonautologous Tissue Substitute, Percutaneous Endoscopic Approach

0YUH07Z Supplement Right Lower Leg with Autologous Tissue Substitute, Open Approach

0YUH0JZ Supplement Right Lower Leg with Synthetic Substitute, Open Approach

0YUH0KZ Supplement Right Lower Leg with Nonautologous Tissue Substitute, Open Approach

0YUH47Z Supplement Right Lower Leg with Autologous Tissue Substitute, Percutaneous Endoscopic Approach

0YUH4JZ Supplement Right Lower Leg with Synthetic Substitute, Percutaneous Endoscopic Approach

0YUH4KZ Supplement Right Lower Leg with Nonautologous Tissue Substitute, Percutaneous Endoscopic Approach

0YUJ07Z Supplement Left Lower Leg with Autologous Tissue Substitute, Open Approach

0YUJ0JZ Supplement Left Lower Leg with Synthetic Substitute, Open Approach

0YUJ0KZ Supplement Left Lower Leg with Nonautologous Tissue Substitute, Open Approach

0YUJ47Z Supplement Left Lower Leg with Autologous Tissue Substitute, Percutaneous Endoscopic Approach

0YUJ4JZ Supplement Left Lower Leg with Synthetic Substitute, Percutaneous Endoscopic Approach

0YUJ4KZ Supplement Left Lower Leg with Nonautologous Tissue Substitute, Percutaneous Endoscopic Approach

0YUK07Z Supplement Right Ankle Region with Autologous Tissue Substitute, Open Approach

0YUK0JZ Supplement Right Ankle Region with Synthetic Substitute, Open Approach

0YUK0KZ Supplement Right Ankle Region with Nonautologous Tissue Substitute, Open Approach

0YUK47Z Supplement Right Ankle Region with Autologous Tissue Substitute, Percutaneous Endoscopic Approach

0YUK4JZ Supplement Right Ankle Region with Synthetic Substitute, Percutaneous Endoscopic Approach

0YUK4KZ Supplement Right Ankle Region with Nonautologous Tissue Substitute, Percutaneous Endoscopic Approach

0YUL07Z Supplement Left Ankle Region with Autologous Tissue Substitute, Open Approach

0YUL0JZ Supplement Left Ankle Region with Synthetic Substitute, Open Approach

0YUL0KZ Supplement Left Ankle Region with Nonautologous Tissue Substitute, Open Approach

0YUL47Z Supplement Left Ankle Region with Autologous Tissue Substitute, Percutaneous Endoscopic Approach

0YUL4JZ Supplement Left Ankle Region with Synthetic Substitute, Percutaneous Endoscopic Approach

0YUL4KZ Supplement Left Ankle Region with Nonautologous Tissue Substitute, Percutaneous Endoscopic Approach

0YUM07Z Supplement Right Foot with Autologous Tissue Substitute, Open Approach

0YUM0JZ Supplement Right Foot with Synthetic Substitute, Open Approach

0YUM0KZ Supplement Right Foot with Nonautologous Tissue Substitute, Open Approach

0YUM47Z Supplement Right Foot with Autologous Tissue Substitute, Percutaneous Endoscopic Approach

0YUM4JZ Supplement Right Foot with Synthetic Substitute, Percutaneous Endoscopic Approach

0YUM4KZ Supplement Right Foot with Nonautologous Tissue Substitute, Percutaneous Endoscopic Approach

0YUN07Z Supplement Left Foot with Autologous Tissue Substitute, Open Approach

0YUN0JZ Supplement Left Foot with Synthetic Substitute, Open Approach

0YUN0KZ Supplement Left Foot with Nonautologous Tissue Substitute, Open Approach

0YUN47Z Supplement Left Foot with Autologous Tissue Substitute, Percutaneous Endoscopic Approach

0YUN4JZ Supplement Left Foot with Synthetic Substitute, Percutaneous Endoscopic Approach

0YUN4KZ Supplement Left Foot with Nonautologous Tissue Substitute, Percutaneous Endoscopic Approach

0YUP07Z Supplement Right 1st Toe with Autologous Tissue Substitute, Open Approach

0YUP0JZ Supplement Right 1st Toe with Synthetic Substitute, Open Approach

0YUP0KZ Supplement Right 1st Toe with Nonautologous Tissue Substitute, Open Approach

0YUP47Z Supplement Right 1st Toe with Autologous Tissue Substitute, Percutaneous Endoscopic Approach

0YUP4JZ Supplement Right 1st Toe with Synthetic Substitute, Percutaneous Endoscopic Approach

0YUP4KZ Supplement Right 1st Toe with Nonautologous Tissue Substitute, Percutaneous Endoscopic Approach

0YUQ07Z Supplement Left 1st Toe with Autologous Tissue Substitute, Open Approach

0YUQ0JZ Supplement Left 1st Toe with Synthetic Substitute, Open Approach

0YUQ0KZ Supplement Left 1st Toe with Nonautologous Tissue Substitute, Open Approach

0YUQ47Z Supplement Left 1st Toe with Autologous Tissue Substitute, Percutaneous Endoscopic Approach

0YUQ4JZ Supplement Left 1st Toe with Synthetic Substitute, Percutaneous Endoscopic Approach

0YUQ4KZ Supplement Left 1st Toe with Nonautologous Tissue Substitute, Percutaneous Endoscopic Approach

0YUR07Z Supplement Right 2nd Toe with Autologous Tissue Substitute, Open Approach

0YUR0JZ Supplement Right 2nd Toe with Synthetic Substitute, Open Approach

0YUR0KZ Supplement Right 2nd Toe with Nonautologous Tissue Substitute, Open Approach

0YUR47Z Supplement Right 2nd Toe with Autologous Tissue Substitute, Percutaneous Endoscopic Approach

0YUR4JZ Supplement Right 2nd Toe with Synthetic Substitute, Percutaneous Endoscopic Approach

0YUR4KZ Supplement Right 2nd Toe with Nonautologous Tissue Substitute, Percutaneous Endoscopic Approach

0YUS07Z Supplement Left 2nd Toe with Autologous Tissue Substitute, Open Approach

0YUS0JZ Supplement Left 2nd Toe with Synthetic Substitute, Open Approach

0YUS0KZ Supplement Left 2nd Toe with Nonautologous Tissue Substitute, Open Approach

0YUS47Z Supplement Left 2nd Toe with Autologous Tissue Substitute, Percutaneous Endoscopic Approach

0YUS4JZ Supplement Left 2nd Toe with Synthetic Substitute, Percutaneous Endoscopic Approach

0YUS4KZ Supplement Left 2nd Toe with Nonautologous Tissue Substitute, Percutaneous Endoscopic Approach

0YUT07Z Supplement Right 3rd Toe with Autologous Tissue Substitute, Open Approach

0YUT0JZ Supplement Right 3rd Toe with Synthetic Substitute, Open Approach

0YUT0KZ Supplement Right 3rd Toe with Nonautologous Tissue Substitute, Open Approach

0YUT47Z Supplement Right 3rd Toe with Autologous Tissue Substitute, Percutaneous Endoscopic Approach

0YUT4JZ Supplement Right 3rd Toe with Synthetic Substitute, Percutaneous Endoscopic Approach

0YUT4KZ Supplement Right 3rd Toe with Nonautologous Tissue Substitute, Percutaneous Endoscopic Approach

0YUU07Z Supplement Left 3rd Toe with Autologous Tissue Substitute, Open Approach

0YUU0JZ Supplement Left 3rd Toe with Synthetic Substitute, Open Approach

0YUU0KZ Supplement Left 3rd Toe with Nonautologous Tissue Substitute, Open Approach

0YUU47Z Supplement Left 3rd Toe with Autologous Tissue Substitute, Percutaneous Endoscopic Approach

0YUU4JZ Supplement Left 3rd Toe with Synthetic Substitute, Percutaneous Endoscopic Approach

0YUU4KZ Supplement Left 3rd Toe with Nonautologous Tissue Substitute, Percutaneous Endoscopic Approach

0YUV07Z Supplement Right 4th Toe with Autologous Tissue Substitute, Open Approach

0YUV0JZ Supplement Right 4th Toe with Synthetic Substitute, Open Approach

0YUV0KZ Supplement Right 4th Toe with Nonautologous Tissue Substitute, Open Approach

0YUV47Z Supplement Right 4th Toe with Autologous Tissue Substitute, Percutaneous Endoscopic Approach

0YUV4JZ Supplement Right 4th Toe with Synthetic Substitute, Percutaneous Endoscopic Approach

0YUV4KZ Supplement Right 4th Toe with Nonautologous Tissue Substitute, Percutaneous Endoscopic Approach

0YUW07Z Supplement Left 4th Toe with Autologous Tissue Substitute, Open Approach

0YUW0JZ Supplement Left 4th Toe with Synthetic Substitute, Open Approach

0YUW0KZ Supplement Left 4th Toe with Nonautologous Tissue Substitute, Open Approach

0YUW47Z Supplement Left 4th Toe with Autologous Tissue Substitute, Percutaneous Endoscopic Approach

0YUW4JZ Supplement Left 4th Toe with Synthetic Substitute, Percutaneous Endoscopic Approach

0YUW4KZ Supplement Left 4th Toe with Nonautologous Tissue Substitute, Percutaneous Endoscopic Approach

0YUX07Z Supplement Right 5th Toe with Autologous Tissue Substitute, Open Approach

0YUX0JZ Supplement Right 5th Toe with Synthetic Substitute, Open Approach

0YUX0KZ Supplement Right 5th Toe with Nonautologous Tissue Substitute, Open Approach

0YUX47Z Supplement Right 5th Toe with Autologous Tissue Substitute, Percutaneous Endoscopic Approach

0YUX4JZ Supplement Right 5th Toe with Synthetic Substitute, Percutaneous Endoscopic Approach

0YUX4KZ Supplement Right 5th Toe with Nonautologous Tissue Substitute, Percutaneous Endoscopic Approach

0YUY07Z Supplement Left 5th Toe with Autologous Tissue Substitute, Open Approach

0YUY0JZ Supplement Left 5th Toe with Synthetic Substitute, Open Approach

0YUY0KZ Supplement Left 5th Toe with Nonautologous Tissue Substitute, Open Approach

0YUY47Z Supplement Left 5th Toe with Autologous Tissue Substitute, Percutaneous Endoscopic Approach

0YUY4JZ Supplement Left 5th Toe with Synthetic Substitute, Percutaneous Endoscopic Approach

0YUY4KZ Supplement Left 5th Toe with Nonautologous Tissue Substitute, Percutaneous Endoscopic Approach

0YW – Anatomical Regions, Lower Extremities, Revision

Review Coding Guideline B6.1c

- **0YW900Z** Revision of Drainage Device in Right Lower Extremity, Open Approach
- **0YW903Z** Revision of Infusion Device in Right Lower Extremity, Open Approach
- **0YW907Z** Revision of Autologous Tissue Substitute in Right Lower Extremity, Open Approach
- **0YW90JZ** Revision of Synthetic Substitute in Right Lower Extremity, Open Approach

---

♀ Female-only   ♂ Male-only   ◐ Limited Coverage   ● Non-OR   ▦ HAC-associated procedure   ⬣ Non-covered procedures   ➕ Combination

● **0YW90KZ** Revision of Nonautologous Tissue Substitute in Right Lower Extremity, Open Approach

● **0YW90YZ** Revision of Other Device in Right Lower Extremity, Open Approach

● **0YW930Z** Revision of Drainage Device in Right Lower Extremity, Percutaneous Approach

● **0YW933Z** Revision of Infusion Device in Right Lower Extremity, Percutaneous Approach

● **0YW937Z** Revision of Autologous Tissue Substitute in Right Lower Extremity, Percutaneous Approach

● **0YW93JZ** Revision of Synthetic Substitute in Right Lower Extremity, Percutaneous Approach

● **0YW93KZ** Revision of Nonautologous Tissue Substitute in Right Lower Extremity, Percutaneous Approach

● **0YW93YZ** Revision of Other Device in Right Lower Extremity, Percutaneous Approach

● **0YW940Z** Revision of Drainage Device in Right Lower Extremity, Percutaneous Endoscopic Approach

● **0YW943Z** Revision of Infusion Device in Right Lower Extremity, Percutaneous Endoscopic Approach

● **0YW947Z** Revision of Autologous Tissue Substitute in Right Lower Extremity, Percutaneous Endoscopic Approach

● **0YW94JZ** Revision of Synthetic Substitute in Right Lower Extremity, Percutaneous Endoscopic Approach

● **0YW94KZ** Revision of Nonautologous Tissue Substitute in Right Lower Extremity, Percutaneous Endoscopic Approach

● **0YW94YZ** Revision of Other Device in Right Lower Extremity, Percutaneous Endoscopic Approach

0YW9X0Z Revision of Drainage Device in Right Lower Extremity, External Approach

0YW9X3Z Revision of Infusion Device in Right Lower Extremity, External Approach

0YW9X7Z Revision of Autologous Tissue Substitute in Right Lower Extremity, External Approach

0YW9XJZ Revision of Synthetic Substitute in Right Lower Extremity, External Approach

0YW9XKZ Revision of Nonautologous Tissue Substitute in Right Lower Extremity, External Approach

0YW9XYZ Revision of Other Device in Right Lower Extremity, External Approach

● **0YWB00Z** Revision of Drainage Device in Left Lower Extremity, Open Approach

● **0YWB03Z** Revision of Infusion Device in Left Lower Extremity, Open Approach

● **0YWB07Z** Revision of Autologous Tissue Substitute in Left Lower Extremity, Open Approach

● **0YWB0JZ** Revision of Synthetic Substitute in Left Lower Extremity, Open Approach

● **0YWB0KZ** Revision of Nonautologous Tissue Substitute in Left Lower Extremity, Open Approach

● **0YWB0YZ** Revision of Other Device in Left Lower Extremity, Open Approach

● **0YWB30Z** Revision of Drainage Device in Left Lower Extremity, Percutaneous Approach

● **0YWB33Z** Revision of Infusion Device in Left Lower Extremity, Percutaneous Approach

● **0YWB37Z** Revision of Autologous Tissue Substitute in Left Lower Extremity, Percutaneous Approach

● **0YWB3JZ** Revision of Synthetic Substitute in Left Lower Extremity, Percutaneous Approach

● **0YWB3KZ** Revision of Nonautologous Tissue Substitute in Left Lower Extremity, Percutaneous Approach

● **0YWB3YZ** Revision of Other Device in Left Lower Extremity, Percutaneous Approach

● **0YWB40Z** Revision of Drainage Device in Left Lower Extremity, Percutaneous Endoscopic Approach

● **0YWB43Z** Revision of Infusion Device in Left Lower Extremity, Percutaneous Endoscopic Approach

● **0YWB47Z** Revision of Autologous Tissue Substitute in Left Lower Extremity, Percutaneous Endoscopic Approach

● **0YWB4JZ** Revision of Synthetic Substitute in Left Lower Extremity, Percutaneous Endoscopic Approach

● **0YWB4KZ** Revision of Nonautologous Tissue Substitute in Left Lower Extremity, Percutaneous Endoscopic Approach

● **0YWB4YZ** Revision of Other Device in Left Lower Extremity, Percutaneous Endoscopic Approach

0YWBX0Z Revision of Drainage Device in Left Lower Extremity, External Approach

0YWBX3Z Revision of Infusion Device in Left Lower Extremity, External Approach

0YWBX7Z Revision of Autologous Tissue Substitute in Left Lower Extremity, External Approach

0YWBXJZ Revision of Synthetic Substitute in Left Lower Extremity, External Approach

0YWBXKZ Revision of Nonautologous Tissue Substitute in Left Lower Extremity, External Approach

0YWBXYZ Revision of Other Device in Left Lower Extremity, External Approach

Obstetrics Section (102–10Y)

Within each section of ICD-10-PCS the characters have different meanings. The seven character meanings for the Obstetrics section are illustrated here through the procedure example of *Manually-assisted delivery*.

Section	Body System	Root Operation	Body Part	Approach	Device	Qualifier
Obstetrics	Pregnancy	Delivery	Products of Conception	External	None	None
1	0	E	0	X	Z	Z

Section (Character 1)

All Obstetric procedure codes have a first character value of 1.

Body System (Character 2)

The alphanumeric character for the body system is placed in the second position. The body system applicable to the Obstetrics section is Pregnancy and has a character value of 0.

Root Operations (Character 3)

The alphanumeric character value for root operations is placed in the third position. Listed below are the root operations applicable to the Obstetrics section with their associated meaning. Note that the root operation definitions for ICD-10-PCS may differ from the terms that coders currently use with ICD-9-CM Volume 3.

Character Value	Root Operation	Root Operation Definition
2	Change	Taking out or off a device from a body part and putting back an identical or similar device in or on the same body part without cutting or puncturing the skin or a mucous membrane
9	Drainage	Taking or letting out fluids and/or gases from a body part
A	Abortion	Artificially terminating a pregnancy
D	Extraction	Pulling or stripping out or off all or a portion of a body part by the use of force
E	Delivery	Assisting the passage of the products of conception from the genital canal
H	Insertion	Putting in a nonbiological appliance that monitors, assists, performs, or prevents a physiological function but does not physically take the place of a body part
J	Inspection	Visually and/or manually exploring a body part
P	Removal	Taking out or off a device from a body part, region or orifice
Q	Repair	Restoring, to the extent possible, a body part to its normal anatomic structure and function
S	Reposition	Moving to its normal location, or other suitable location, all or a portion of a body part
T	Resection	Cutting out or off, without replacement, all of a body part
Y	Transplantation	Putting in or on all or a portion of a living body part taken from another individual or animal to physically take the place and/or function of all or a portion of a similar body part

Body Part (Character 4)

For each body system the applicable body part character values will be available for procedure code construction. An example of a body pat is Products of Conception.

Approach (Character 5)

The approach is the technique used to reach the procedure site. The following are the approach character values for the Obstetrics section with the associated definitions.

Character Value	Approach	Approach Definition
0	Open	Cutting through the skin or mucous membrane and any other body layers necessary to expose the site of the procedure
3	Percutaneous	Entry, by puncture or minor incision, of instrumentation through the skin or mucous membrane and any other body layers necessary to reach the site of the procedure
4	Percutaneous Endoscopic	Entry, by puncture or minor incision, of instrumentation through the skin or mucous membrane and any other body layers necessary to reach and visualize the site of the procedure
7	Via Natural or Artificial Opening	Entry of instrumentation through a natural or artificial external opening to reach the site of the procedure
8	Via Natural or Artificial Opening Endoscopic	Entry of instrumentation through a natural or artificial external opening to reach and visualize the site of the procedure
X	External	Procedures performed directly on the skin or mucous membrane and procedures performed indirectly by the application of external force through the skin or mucous membrane

Device (Character 6)

Depending on the procedure performed there may or may not be a device used. There are two types of devices included in the Obstetrics section: monitoring electrode and other device. When a device is not utilized during the procedure, the placeholder Z is the character value that should be reported.

Qualifier (Character 7)

The qualifier represents an additional attribute for the procedure when applicable. For example, drainage procedures in this section include several qualifiers including fetal cerebrospinal fluid that is reported with the character value of A. If there is no qualifier for a procedure, the placeholder Z is the character valve that should be reported.

Obstetric Section Guidelines (section 1)

C. Obstetrics Section

Products of Conception

C1. Procedures performed on the products of conception are coded to the Obstetrics section. Procedures performed on the pregnant female other than the products of conception are coded to the appropriate root operation in the Medical and Surgical section.

Example: Amniocentesis is coded to the products of conception body part in the Obstetrics section. Repair of obstetric urethral laceration is coded to the urethra body part in the Medical and Surgical section.

Procedures following delivery or abortion

C2. Procedures performed following a delivery or abortion for curettage of the endometrium or evacuation of retained products of conception are all coded in the Obstetrics section, to the root operation Extraction and the body part Products of Conception, Retained. Diagnostic or therapeutic dilation and curettage performed during times other than the postpartum or post-abortion period are all coded in the Medical and Surgical section, to the root operation Extraction and the body part Endometrium.

Obstetrics Section Tables and Code Listings

Obstetrics Tables 102–10Y

Section	1	Obstetrics
Body System	0	Pregnancy
Operation	2	**Change:** Taking out or off a device from a body part and putting back an identical or similar device in or on the same body part without cutting or puncturing the skin or a mucous membrane

Body Part (4th)	Approach (5th)	Device (6th)	Qualifier (7th)
0 Products of Conception	7 Via Natural or Artificial Opening	3 Monitoring Electrode Y Other Device	Z No Qualifier

Section	1	Obstetrics
Body System	0	Pregnancy
Operation	9	**Drainage:** Taking or letting out fluids and/or gases from a body part

Body Part (4th)	Approach (5th)	Device (6th)	Qualifier (7th)
0 Products of Conception	0 Open 3 Percutaneous 4 Percutaneous Endoscopic 7 Via Natural or Artificial Opening 8 Via Natural or Artificial Opening Endoscopic	Z No Device	9 Fetal Blood A Fetal Cerebrospinal Fluid B Fetal Fluid, Other C Amniotic Fluid, Therapeutic D Fluid, Other U Amniotic Fluid, Diagnostic

Section	1	Obstetrics
Body System	0	Pregnancy
Operation	A	**Abortion:** Artificially terminating a pregnancy

Body Part (4th)	Approach (5th)	Device (6th)	Qualifier (7th)
0 Products of Conception	0 Open 3 Percutaneous 4 Percutaneous Endoscopic 8 Via Natural or Artificial Opening Endoscopic	Z No Device	Z No Qualifier
0 Products of Conception	7 Via Natural or Artificial Opening	Z No Device	6 Vacuum W Laminaria X Abortifacient Z No Qualifier

Section	1	Obstetrics
Body System	0	Pregnancy
Operation	D	**Extraction:** Pulling or stripping out or off all or a portion of a body part by the use of force

Body Part (4th)	Approach (5th)	Device (6th)	Qualifier (7th)
0 Products of Conception	0 Open	Z No Device	0 Classical 1 Low Cervical 2 Extraperitoneal
0 Products of Conception	7 Via Natural or Artificial Opening	Z No Device	3 Low Forceps 4 Mid Forceps 5 High Forceps 6 Vacuum 7 Internal Version 8 Other

Continued

10D *Continued*

Section	1	Obstetrics
Body System	0	Pregnancy
Operation	D	**Extraction:** Pulling or stripping out or off all or a portion of a body part by the use of force

Body Part (4th)	Approach (5th)	Device (6th)	Qualifier (7th)
1　Products of Conception, Retained 2　Products of Conception, Ectopic	7　Via Natural or Artificial Opening 8　Via Natural or Artificial Opening Endoscopic	Z　No Device	Z　No Qualifier

Section	1	Obstetrics
Body System	0	Pregnancy
Operation	E	**Delivery:** Assisting the passage of the products of conception from the genital canal

Body Part (4th)	Approach (5th)	Device (6th)	Qualifier (7th)
0　Products of Conception	X　External	Z　No Device	Z　No Qualifier

Section	1	Obstetrics
Body System	0	Pregnancy
Operation	H	**Insertion:** Putting in a nonbiological appliance that monitors, assists, performs, or prevents a physiological function but does not physically take the place of a body part

Body Part (4th)	Approach (5th)	Device (6th)	Qualifier (7th)
0　Products of Conception	0　Open 7　Via Natural or Artificial Opening	3　Monitoring Electrode Y　Other Device	Z　No Qualifier

Section	1	Obstetrics
Body System	0	Pregnancy
Operation	J	**Inspection:** Visually and/or manually exploring a body part

Body Part (4th)	Approach (5th)	Device (6th)	Qualifier (7th)
0　Products of Conception 1　Products of Conception, Retained 2　Products of Conception, Ectopic	0　Open 3　Percutaneous 4　Percutaneous Endoscopic 7　Via Natural or Artificial Opening 8　Via Natural or Artificial Opening Endoscopic X　External	Z　No Device	Z　No Qualifier

Section	1	Obstetrics
Body System	0	Pregnancy
Operation	P	**Removal:** Taking out or off a device from a body part, region or orifice

Body Part (4th)	Approach (5th)	Device (6th)	Qualifier (7th)
0　Products of Conception	0　Open 7　Via Natural or Artificial Opening	3　Monitoring Electrode Y　Other Device	Z　No Qualifier

Section	1	Obstetrics
Body System	0	Pregnancy
Operation	Q	**Repair:** Restoring, to the extent possible, a body part to its normal anatomic structure and function

Body Part (4th)	Approach (5th)	Device (6th)	Qualifier (7th)
0 Products of Conception	0 Open 3 Percutaneous 4 Percutaneous Endoscopic 7 Via Natural or Artificial Opening 8 Via Natural or Artificial Opening Endoscopic	Y Other Device Z No Device	E Nervous System F Cardiovascular System G Lymphatics and Hemic H Eye J Ear, Nose and Sinus K Respiratory System L Mouth and Throat M Gastrointestinal System N Hepatobiliary and Pancreas P Endocrine System Q Skin R Musculoskeletal System S Urinary System T Female Reproductive System V Male Reproductive System Y Other Body System

Section	1	Obstetrics
Body System	0	Pregnancy
Operation	S	**Reposition:** Moving to its normal location, or other suitable location, all or a portion of a body part

Body Part (4th)	Approach (5th)	Device (6th)	Qualifier (7th)
0 Products of Conception	7 Via Natural or Artificial Opening X External	Z No Device	Z No Qualifier
2 Products of Conception, Ectopic	0 Open 3 Percutaneous 4 Percutaneous Endoscopic 7 Via Natural or Artificial Opening 8 Via Natural or Artificial Opening Endoscopic	Z No Device	Z No Qualifier

Section	1	Obstetrics
Body System	0	Pregnancy
Operation	T	**Resection:** Cutting out or off, without replacement, all of a body part

Body Part (4th)	Approach (5th)	Device (6th)	Qualifier (7th)
2 Products of Conception, Ectopic	0 Open 3 Percutaneous 4 Percutaneous Endoscopic 7 Via Natural or Artificial Opening 8 Via Natural or Artificial Opening Endoscopic	Z No Device	Z No Qualifier

Section	1	Obstetrics
Body System	0	Pregnancy
Operation	Y	**Transplantation:** Putting in or on all or a portion of a living body part taken from another individual or animal to physically take the place and/or function of all or a portion of a similar body part

Body Part (4ᵗʰ)	Approach (5ᵗʰ)	Device (6ᵗʰ)	Qualifier (7ᵗʰ)
0 Products of Conception	**3** Percutaneous **4** Percutaneous Endoscopic **7** Via Natural or Artificial Opening	**Z** No Device	**E** Nervous System **F** Cardiovascular System **G** Lymphatics and Hemic **H** Eye **J** Ear, Nose and Sinus **K** Respiratory System **L** Mouth and Throat **M** Gastrointestinal System **N** Hepatobiliary and Pancreas **P** Endocrine System **Q** Skin **R** Musculoskeletal System **S** Urinary System **T** Female Reproductive System **V** Male Reproductive System **Y** Other Body System

Obstetrics Code Listing 102–10Y

102 – Obstetrics, Pregnancy, Change

Review Coding Guideline C1

♀ **102073Z** Change Monitoring Electrode in Products of Conception, Via Natural or Artificial Opening

♀ **10207YZ** Change Other Device in Products of Conception, Via Natural or Artificial Opening

109 – Obstetrics, Pregnancy, Drainage

♀ **10900Z9** Drainage of Fetal Blood from Products of Conception, Open Approach

♀ **10900ZA** Drainage of Fetal Cerebrospinal Fluid from Products of Conception, Open Approach

♀ **10900ZB** Drainage of Other Fetal Fluid from Products of Conception, Open Approach

♀ **10900ZC** Drainage of Amniotic Fluid, Therapeutic from Products of Conception, Open Approach

♀ **10900ZD** Drainage of Other Fluid from Products of Conception, Open Approach

♀ **10900ZU** Drainage of Amniotic Fluid, Diagnostic from Products of Conception, Open Approach

♀ **10903Z9** Drainage of Fetal Blood from Products of Conception, Percutaneous Approach

♀ **10903ZA** Drainage of Fetal Cerebrospinal Fluid from Products of Conception, Percutaneous Approach

♀ **10903ZB** Drainage of Other Fetal Fluid from Products of Conception, Percutaneous Approach

♀ **10903ZC** Drainage of Amniotic Fluid, Therapeutic from Products of Conception, Percutaneous Approach

♀ **10903ZD** Drainage of Other Fluid from Products of Conception, Percutaneous Approach

♀ **10903ZU** Drainage of Amniotic Fluid, Diagnostic from Products of Conception, Percutaneous Approach

♀ **10904Z9** Drainage of Fetal Blood from Products of Conception, Percutaneous Endoscopic Approach

♀ **10904ZA** Drainage of Fetal Cerebrospinal Fluid from Products of Conception, Percutaneous Endoscopic Approach

♀ **10904ZB** Drainage of Other Fetal Fluid from Products of Conception, Percutaneous Endoscopic Approach

♀ **10904ZC** Drainage of Amniotic Fluid, Therapeutic from Products of Conception, Percutaneous Endoscopic Approach

♀ **10904ZD** Drainage of Other Fluid from Products of Conception, Percutaneous Endoscopic Approach

♀ **10904ZU** Drainage of Amniotic Fluid, Diagnostic from Products of Conception, Percutaneous Endoscopic Approach

♀ **10907Z9** Drainage of Fetal Blood from Products of Conception, Via Natural or Artificial Opening

♀ **10907ZA** Drainage of Fetal Cerebrospinal Fluid from Products of Conception, Via Natural or Artificial Opening

♀ **10907ZB** Drainage of Other Fetal Fluid from Products of Conception, Via Natural or Artificial Opening

♀ **10907ZC** Drainage of Amniotic Fluid, Therapeutic from Products of Conception, Via Natural or Artificial Opening

♀ **10907ZD** Drainage of Other Fluid from Products of Conception, Via Natural or Artificial Opening

♀ **10907ZU** Drainage of Amniotic Fluid, Diagnostic from Products of Conception, Via Natural or Artificial Opening

♀ **10908Z9** Drainage of Fetal Blood from Products of Conception, Via Natural or Artificial Opening Endoscopic

♀ **10908ZA** Drainage of Fetal Cerebrospinal Fluid from Products of Conception, Via Natural or Artificial Opening Endoscopic

♀ **10908ZB** Drainage of Other Fetal Fluid from Products of Conception, Via Natural or Artificial Opening Endoscopic

♀ **10908ZC** Drainage of Amniotic Fluid, Therapeutic from Products of Conception, Via Natural or Artificial Opening Endoscopic

♀ **10908ZD** Drainage of Other Fluid from Products of Conception, Via Natural or Artificial Opening Endoscopic

♀ **10908ZU** Drainage of Amniotic Fluid, Diagnostic from Products of Conception, Via Natural or Artificial Opening Endoscopic

10A – Obstetrics, Pregnancy, Abortion

♀ **10A00ZZ** Abortion of Products of Conception, Open Approach

♀ **10A03ZZ** Abortion of Products of Conception, Percutaneous Approach

♀ **10A04ZZ** Abortion of Products of Conception, Percutaneous Endoscopic Approach

♀ Female-only   ♂ Male-only   ◗ Limited Coverage   ● Non-OR   **HAC** HAC-associated procedure   ● Non-covered procedures   ➕ Combination

♀● 10A07Z6 Abortion of Products of Conception, Vacuum, Via Natural or Artificial Opening

♀ 10A07ZW Abortion of Products of Conception, Laminaria, Via Natural or Artificial Opening

♀ 10A07ZX Abortion of Products of Conception, Abortifacient, Via Natural or Artificial Opening

♀ 10A07ZZ Abortion of Products of Conception, Via Natural or Artificial Opening

♀ 10A08ZZ Abortion of Products of Conception, Via Natural or Artificial Opening Endoscopic

10D – Obstetrics, Pregnancy, Extraction

Review Coding Guideline C2

♀ 10D00Z0 Extraction of Products of Conception, Classical, Open Approach

♀ 10D00Z1 Extraction of Products of Conception, Low Cervical, Open Approach

♀ 10D00Z2 Extraction of Products of Conception, Extraperitoneal, Open Approach

♀● 10D07Z3 Extraction of Products of Conception, Low Forceps, Via Natural or Artificial Opening

♀● 10D07Z4 Extraction of Products of Conception, Mid Forceps, Via Natural or Artificial Opening

♀● 10D07Z5 Extraction of Products of Conception, High Forceps, Via Natural or Artificial Opening

♀● 10D07Z6 Extraction of Products of Conception, Vacuum, Via Natural or Artificial Opening

♀● 10D07Z7 Extraction of Products of Conception, Internal Version, Via Natural or Artificial Opening

♀● 10D07Z8 Extraction of Products of Conception, Other, Via Natural or Artificial Opening

♀ 10D17ZZ Extraction of Products of Conception, Retained, Via Natural or Artificial Opening

♀ 10D18ZZ Extraction of Products of Conception, Retained, Via Natural or Artificial Opening Endoscopic

♀ 10D27ZZ Extraction of Products of Conception, Ectopic, Via Natural or Artificial Opening

♀ 10D28ZZ Extraction of Products of Conception, Ectopic, Via Natural or Artificial Opening Endoscopic

10E – Obstetrics, Pregnancy, Delivery

♀● 10E0XZZ Delivery of Products of Conception, External Approach

10H – Obstetrics, Pregnancy, Insertion

♀ 10H003Z Insertion of Monitoring Electrode into Products of Conception, Open Approach

♀ 10H00YZ Insertion of Other Device into Products of Conception, Open Approach

♀ 10H073Z Insertion of Monitoring Electrode into Products of Conception, Via Natural or Artificial Opening

♀ 10H07YZ Insertion of Other Device into Products of Conception, Via Natural or Artificial Opening

10J – Obstetrics, Pregnancy, Inspection

♀ 10J00ZZ Inspection of Products of Conception, Open Approach

♀ 10J03ZZ Inspection of Products of Conception, Percutaneous Approach

♀ 10J04ZZ Inspection of Products of Conception, Percutaneous Endoscopic Approach

♀ 10J07ZZ Inspection of Products of Conception, Via Natural or Artificial Opening

♀ 10J08ZZ Inspection of Products of Conception, Via Natural or Artificial Opening Endoscopic

♀ 10J0XZZ Inspection of Products of Conception, External Approach

♀ 10J10ZZ Inspection of Products of Conception, Retained, Open Approach

♀ 10J13ZZ Inspection of Products of Conception, Retained, Percutaneous Approach

♀ 10J14ZZ Inspection of Products of Conception, Retained, Percutaneous Endoscopic Approach

♀ 10J17ZZ Inspection of Products of Conception, Retained, Via Natural or Artificial Opening

♀ 10J18ZZ Inspection of Products of Conception, Retained, Via Natural or Artificial Opening Endoscopic

♀ 10J1XZZ Inspection of Products of Conception, Retained, External Approach

♀ 10J20ZZ Inspection of Products of Conception, Ectopic, Open Approach

♀ 10J23ZZ Inspection of Products of Conception, Ectopic, Percutaneous Approach

♀ 10J24ZZ Inspection of Products of Conception, Ectopic, Percutaneous Endoscopic Approach

♀ 10J27ZZ Inspection of Products of Conception, Ectopic, Via Natural or Artificial Opening

♀ 10J28ZZ Inspection of Products of Conception, Ectopic, Via Natural or Artificial Opening Endoscopic

♀ 10J2XZZ Inspection of Products of Conception, Ectopic, External Approach

10P – Obstetrics, Pregnancy, Removal

♀ 10P003Z Removal of Monitoring Electrode from Products of Conception, Open Approach

♀ 10P00YZ Removal of Other Device from Products of Conception, Open Approach

♀ 10P073Z Removal of Monitoring Electrode from Products of Conception, Via Natural or Artificial Opening

♀ 10P07YZ Removal of Other Device from Products of Conception, Via Natural or Artificial Opening

10Q – Obstetrics, Pregnancy, Repair

♀ 10Q00YE Repair Nervous System in Products of Conception with Other Device, Open Approach

♀ 10Q00YF Repair Cardiovascular System in Products of Conception with Other Device, Open Approach

♀ 10Q00YG Repair Lymphatics and Hemic in Products of Conception with Other Device, Open Approach

♀ 10Q00YH Repair Eye in Products of Conception with Other Device, Open Approach

♀ 10Q00YJ Repair Ear, Nose and Sinus in Products of Conception with Other Device, Open Approach

♀ 10Q00YK Repair Respiratory System in Products of Conception with Other Device, Open Approach

♀ 10Q00YL Repair Mouth and Throat in Products of Conception with Other Device, Open Approach

♀ 10Q00YM Repair Gastrointestinal System in Products of Conception with Other Device, Open Approach

---

♀ Female-only   ♂ Male-only   ◐ Limited Coverage   ● Non-OR   ▧ HAC-associated procedure   ⬤ Non-covered procedures   ✚ Combination

♀ **10Q00YN** Repair Hepatobiliary and Pancreas in Products of Conception with Other Device, Open Approach

♀ **10Q00YP** Repair Endocrine System in Products of Conception with Other Device, Open Approach

♀ **10Q00YQ** Repair Skin in Products of Conception with Other Device, Open Approach

♀ **10Q00YR** Repair Musculoskeletal System in Products of Conception with Other Device, Open Approach

♀ **10Q00YS** Repair Urinary System in Products of Conception with Other Device, Open Approach

♀ **10Q00YT** Repair Female Reproductive System in Products of Conception with Other Device, Open Approach

♀ **10Q00YV** Repair Male Reproductive System in Products of Conception with Other Device, Open Approach

♀ **10Q00YY** Repair Other Body System in Products of Conception with Other Device, Open Approach

♀ **10Q00ZE** Repair Nervous System in Products of Conception, Open Approach

♀ **10Q00ZF** Repair Cardiovascular System in Products of Conception, Open Approach

♀ **10Q00ZG** Repair Lymphatics and Hemic in Products of Conception, Open Approach

♀ **10Q00ZH** Repair Eye in Products of Conception, Open Approach

♀ **10Q00ZJ** Repair Ear, Nose and Sinus in Products of Conception, Open Approach

♀ **10Q00ZK** Repair Respiratory System in Products of Conception, Open Approach

♀ **10Q00ZL** Repair Mouth and Throat in Products of Conception, Open Approach

♀ **10Q00ZM** Repair Gastrointestinal System in Products of Conception, Open Approach

♀ **10Q00ZN** Repair Hepatobiliary and Pancreas in Products of Conception, Open Approach

♀ **10Q00ZP** Repair Endocrine System in Products of Conception, Open Approach

♀ **10Q00ZQ** Repair Skin in Products of Conception, Open Approach

♀ **10Q00ZR** Repair Musculoskeletal System in Products of Conception, Open Approach

♀ **10Q00ZS** Repair Urinary System in Products of Conception, Open Approach

♀ **10Q00ZT** Repair Female Reproductive System in Products of Conception, Open Approach

♀ **10Q00ZV** Repair Male Reproductive System in Products of Conception, Open Approach

♀ **10Q00ZY** Repair Other Body System in Products of Conception, Open Approach

♀ **10Q03YE** Repair Nervous System in Products of Conception with Other Device, Percutaneous Approach

♀ **10Q03YF** Repair Cardiovascular System in Products of Conception with Other Device, Percutaneous Approach

♀ **10Q03YG** Repair Lymphatics and Hemic in Products of Conception with Other Device, Percutaneous Approach

♀ **10Q03YH** Repair Eye in Products of Conception with Other Device, Percutaneous Approach

♀ **10Q03YJ** Repair Ear, Nose and Sinus in Products of Conception with Other Device, Percutaneous Approach

♀ **10Q03YK** Repair Respiratory System in Products of Conception with Other Device, Percutaneous Approach

♀ **10Q03YL** Repair Mouth and Throat in Products of Conception with Other Device, Percutaneous Approach

♀ **10Q03YM** Repair Gastrointestinal System in Products of Conception with Other Device, Percutaneous Approach

♀ **10Q03YN** Repair Hepatobiliary and Pancreas in Products of Conception with Other Device, Percutaneous Approach

♀ **10Q03YP** Repair Endocrine System in Products of Conception with Other Device, Percutaneous Approach

♀ **10Q03YQ** Repair Skin in Products of Conception with Other Device, Percutaneous Approach

♀ **10Q03YR** Repair Musculoskeletal System in Products of Conception with Other Device, Percutaneous Approach

♀ **10Q03YS** Repair Urinary System in Products of Conception with Other Device, Percutaneous Approach

♀ **10Q03YT** Repair Female Reproductive System in Products of Conception with Other Device, Percutaneous Approach

♀ **10Q03YV** Repair Male Reproductive System in Products of Conception with Other Device, Percutaneous Approach

♀ **10Q03YY** Repair Other Body System in Products of Conception with Other Device, Percutaneous Approach

♀ **10Q03ZE** Repair Nervous System in Products of Conception, Percutaneous Approach

♀ **10Q03ZF** Repair Cardiovascular System in Products of Conception, Percutaneous Approach

♀ **10Q03ZG** Repair Lymphatics and Hemic in Products of Conception, Percutaneous Approach

♀ **10Q03ZH** Repair Eye in Products of Conception, Percutaneous Approach

♀ **10Q03ZJ** Repair Ear, Nose and Sinus in Products of Conception, Percutaneous Approach

♀ **10Q03ZK** Repair Respiratory System in Products of Conception, Percutaneous Approach

♀ **10Q03ZL** Repair Mouth and Throat in Products of Conception, Percutaneous Approach

♀ **10Q03ZM** Repair Gastrointestinal System in Products of Conception, Percutaneous Approach

♀ **10Q03ZN** Repair Hepatobiliary and Pancreas in Products of Conception, Percutaneous Approach

♀ **10Q03ZP** Repair Endocrine System in Products of Conception, Percutaneous Approach

♀ **10Q03ZQ** Repair Skin in Products of Conception, Percutaneous Approach

♀ **10Q03ZR** Repair Musculoskeletal System in Products of Conception, Percutaneous Approach

♀ **10Q03ZS** Repair Urinary System in Products of Conception, Percutaneous Approach

♀ **10Q03ZT** Repair Female Reproductive System in Products of Conception, Percutaneous Approach

♀ **10Q03ZV** Repair Male Reproductive System in Products of Conception, Percutaneous Approach

♀ **10Q03ZY** Repair Other Body System in Products of Conception, Percutaneous Approach

♀ **10Q04YE** Repair Nervous System in Products of Conception with Other Device, Percutaneous Endoscopic Approach

♀ **10Q04YF** Repair Cardiovascular System in Products of Conception with Other Device, Percutaneous Endoscopic Approach

♀ **10Q04YG** Repair Lymphatics and Hemic in Products of Conception with Other Device, Percutaneous Endoscopic Approach

♀ **10Q04YH** Repair Eye in Products of Conception with Other Device, Percutaneous Endoscopic Approach

♀ **10Q04YJ** Repair Ear, Nose and Sinus in Products of Conception with Other Device, Percutaneous Endoscopic Approach

♀ **10Q04YK** Repair Respiratory System in Products of Conception with Other Device, Percutaneous Endoscopic Approach

♀ **10Q04YL** Repair Mouth and Throat in Products of Conception with Other Device, Percutaneous Endoscopic Approach

♀ **10Q04YM** Repair Gastrointestinal System in Products of Conception with Other Device, Percutaneous Endoscopic Approach

♀ **10Q04YN** Repair Hepatobiliary and Pancreas in Products of Conception with Other Device, Percutaneous Endoscopic Approach

♀ **10Q04YP** Repair Endocrine System in Products of Conception with Other Device, Percutaneous Endoscopic Approach

♀ **10Q04YQ** Repair Skin in Products of Conception with Other Device, Percutaneous Endoscopic Approach

♀ **10Q04YR** Repair Musculoskeletal System in Products of Conception with Other Device, Percutaneous Endoscopic Approach

♀ **10Q04YS** Repair Urinary System in Products of Conception with Other Device, Percutaneous Endoscopic Approach

♀ **10Q04YT** Repair Female Reproductive System in Products of Conception with Other Device, Percutaneous Endoscopic Approach

♀ **10Q04YV** Repair Male Reproductive System in Products of Conception with Other Device, Percutaneous Endoscopic Approach

♀ **10Q04YY** Repair Other Body System in Products of Conception with Other Device, Percutaneous Endoscopic Approach

♀ **10Q04ZE** Repair Nervous System in Products of Conception, Percutaneous Endoscopic Approach

♀ **10Q04ZF** Repair Cardiovascular System in Products of Conception, Percutaneous Endoscopic Approach

♀ **10Q04ZG** Repair Lymphatics and Hemic in Products of Conception, Percutaneous Endoscopic Approach

♀ **10Q04ZH** Repair Eye in Products of Conception, Percutaneous Endoscopic Approach

♀ **10Q04ZJ** Repair Ear, Nose and Sinus in Products of Conception, Percutaneous Endoscopic Approach

---

♀ **10Q04ZK** Repair Respiratory System in Products of Conception, Percutaneous Endoscopic Approach

♀ **10Q04ZL** Repair Mouth and Throat in Products of Conception, Percutaneous Endoscopic Approach

♀ **10Q04ZM** Repair Gastrointestinal System in Products of Conception, Percutaneous Endoscopic Approach

♀ **10Q04ZN** Repair Hepatobiliary and Pancreas in Products of Conception, Percutaneous Endoscopic Approach

♀ **10Q04ZP** Repair Endocrine System in Products of Conception, Percutaneous Endoscopic Approach

♀ **10Q04ZQ** Repair Skin in Products of Conception, Percutaneous Endoscopic Approach

♀ **10Q04ZR** Repair Musculoskeletal System in Products of Conception, Percutaneous Endoscopic Approach

♀ **10Q04ZS** Repair Urinary System in Products of Conception, Percutaneous Endoscopic Approach

♀ **10Q04ZT** Repair Female Reproductive System in Products of Conception, Percutaneous Endoscopic Approach

♀ **10Q04ZV** Repair Male Reproductive System in Products of Conception, Percutaneous Endoscopic Approach

♀ **10Q04ZY** Repair Other Body System in Products of Conception, Percutaneous Endoscopic Approach

♀ **10Q07YE** Repair Nervous System in Products of Conception with Other Device, Via Natural or Artificial Opening

♀ **10Q07YF** Repair Cardiovascular System in Products of Conception with Other Device, Via Natural or Artificial Opening

♀ **10Q07YG** Repair Lymphatics and Hemic in Products of Conception with Other Device, Via Natural or Artificial Opening

♀ **10Q07YH** Repair Eye in Products of Conception with Other Device, Via Natural or Artificial Opening

♀ **10Q07YJ** Repair Ear, Nose and Sinus in Products of Conception with Other Device, Via Natural or Artificial Opening

♀ **10Q07YK** Repair Respiratory System in Products of Conception with Other Device, Via Natural or Artificial Opening

♀ **10Q07YL** Repair Mouth and Throat in Products of Conception with Other Device, Via Natural or Artificial Opening

♀ **10Q07YM** Repair Gastrointestinal System in Products of Conception with Other Device, Via Natural or Artificial Opening

♀ **10Q07YN** Repair Hepatobiliary and Pancreas in Products of Conception with Other Device, Via Natural or Artificial Opening

♀ **10Q07YP** Repair Endocrine System in Products of Conception with Other Device, Via Natural or Artificial Opening

♀ **10Q07YQ** Repair Skin in Products of Conception with Other Device, Via Natural or Artificial Opening

♀ **10Q07YR** Repair Musculoskeletal System in Products of Conception with Other Device, Via Natural or Artificial Opening

♀ **10Q07YS** Repair Urinary System in Products of Conception with Other Device, Via Natural or Artificial Opening

♀ **10Q07YT** Repair Female Reproductive System in Products of Conception with Other Device, Via Natural or Artificial Opening

♀ **10Q07YV** Repair Male Reproductive System in Products of Conception with Other Device, Via Natural or Artificial Opening

♀ **10Q07YY** Repair Other Body System in Products of Conception with Other Device, Via Natural or Artificial Opening

♀ **10Q07ZE** Repair Nervous System in Products of Conception, Via Natural or Artificial Opening

♀ **10Q07ZF** Repair Cardiovascular System in Products of Conception, Via Natural or Artificial Opening

♀ **10Q07ZG** Repair Lymphatics and Hemic in Products of Conception, Via Natural or Artificial Opening

♀ **10Q07ZH** Repair Eye in Products of Conception, Via Natural or Artificial Opening

♀ **10Q07ZJ** Repair Ear, Nose and Sinus in Products of Conception, Via Natural or Artificial Opening

♀ **10Q07ZK** Repair Respiratory System in Products of Conception, Via Natural or Artificial Opening

♀ **10Q07ZL** Repair Mouth and Throat in Products of Conception, Via Natural or Artificial Opening

♀ **10Q07ZM** Repair Gastrointestinal System in Products of Conception, Via Natural or Artificial Opening

♀ **10Q07ZN** Repair Hepatobiliary and Pancreas in Products of Conception, Via Natural or Artificial Opening

♀ **10Q07ZP** Repair Endocrine System in Products of Conception, Via Natural or Artificial Opening

♀ **10Q07ZQ** Repair Skin in Products of Conception, Via Natural or Artificial Opening

♀ **10Q07ZR** Repair Musculoskeletal System in Products of Conception, Via Natural or Artificial Opening

♀ **10Q07ZS** Repair Urinary System in Products of Conception, Via Natural or Artificial Opening

♀ **10Q07ZT** Repair Female Reproductive System in Products of Conception, Via Natural or Artificial Opening

♀ **10Q07ZV** Repair Male Reproductive System in Products of Conception, Via Natural or Artificial Opening

♀ **10Q07ZY** Repair Other Body System in Products of Conception, Via Natural or Artificial Opening

♀ **10Q08YE** Repair Nervous System in Products of Conception with Other Device, Via Natural or Artificial Opening Endoscopic

♀ **10Q08YF** Repair Cardiovascular System in Products of Conception with Other Device, Via Natural or Artificial Opening Endoscopic

♀ **10Q08YG** Repair Lymphatics and Hemic in Products of Conception with Other Device, Via Natural or Artificial Opening Endoscopic

♀ **10Q08YH** Repair Eye in Products of Conception with Other Device, Via Natural or Artificial Opening Endoscopic

♀ **10Q08YJ** Repair Ear, Nose and Sinus in Products of Conception with Other Device, Via Natural or Artificial Opening Endoscopic

♀ **10Q08YK** Repair Respiratory System in Products of Conception with Other Device, Via Natural or Artificial Opening Endoscopic

♀ **10Q08YL** Repair Mouth and Throat in Products of Conception with Other Device, Via Natural or Artificial Opening Endoscopic

♀ **10Q08YM** Repair Gastrointestinal System in Products of Conception with Other Device, Via Natural or Artificial Opening Endoscopic

♀ **10Q08YN** Repair Hepatobiliary and Pancreas in Products of Conception with Other Device, Via Natural or Artificial Opening Endoscopic

♀ **10Q08YP** Repair Endocrine System in Products of Conception with Other Device, Via Natural or Artificial Opening Endoscopic

♀ **10Q08YQ** Repair Skin in Products of Conception with Other Device, Via Natural or Artificial Opening Endoscopic

♀ **10Q08YR** Repair Musculoskeletal System in Products of Conception with Other Device, Via Natural or Artificial Opening Endoscopic

♀ **10Q08YS** Repair Urinary System in Products of Conception with Other Device, Via Natural or Artificial Opening Endoscopic

♀ **10Q08YT** Repair Female Reproductive System in Products of Conception with Other Device, Via Natural or Artificial Opening Endoscopic

♀ **10Q08YV** Repair Male Reproductive System in Products of Conception with Other Device, Via Natural or Artificial Opening Endoscopic

♀ **10Q08YY** Repair Other Body System in Products of Conception with Other Device, Via Natural or Artificial Opening Endoscopic

♀ **10Q08ZE** Repair Nervous System in Products of Conception, Via Natural or Artificial Opening Endoscopic

♀ **10Q08ZF** Repair Cardiovascular System in Products of Conception, Via Natural or Artificial Opening Endoscopic

♀ **10Q08ZG** Repair Lymphatics and Hemic in Products of Conception, Via Natural or Artificial Opening Endoscopic

♀ **10Q08ZH** Repair Eye in Products of Conception, Via Natural or Artificial Opening Endoscopic

♀ **10Q08ZJ** Repair Ear, Nose and Sinus in Products of Conception, Via Natural or Artificial Opening Endoscopic

♀ **10Q08ZK** Repair Respiratory System in Products of Conception, Via Natural or Artificial Opening Endoscopic

♀ **10Q08ZL** Repair Mouth and Throat in Products of Conception, Via Natural or Artificial Opening Endoscopic

♀ **10Q08ZM** Repair Gastrointestinal System in Products of Conception, Via Natural or Artificial Opening Endoscopic

♀ **10Q08ZN** Repair Hepatobiliary and Pancreas in Products of Conception, Via Natural or Artificial Opening Endoscopic

♀ **10Q08ZP** Repair Endocrine System in Products of Conception, Via Natural or Artificial Opening Endoscopic

♀ **10Q08ZQ** Repair Skin in Products of Conception, Via Natural or Artificial Opening Endoscopic

♀ **10Q08ZR** Repair Musculoskeletal System in Products of Conception, Via Natural or Artificial Opening Endoscopic

♀ **10Q08ZS** Repair Urinary System in Products of Conception, Via Natural or Artificial Opening Endoscopic

♀ **10Q08ZT** Repair Female Reproductive System in Products of Conception, Via Natural or Artificial Opening Endoscopic

♀ **10Q08ZV** Repair Male Reproductive System in Products of Conception, Via Natural or Artificial Opening Endoscopic

♀ **10Q08ZY** Repair Other Body System in Products of Conception, Via Natural or Artificial Opening Endoscopic

---

♀ Female-only   ♂ Male-only   ● Limited Coverage   ● Non-OR   ▉ HAC HAC-associated procedure   ● Non-covered procedures   ➕ Combination

10S – Obstetrics, Pregnancy, Reposition

● ♀ **10S07ZZ** Reposition Products of Conception, Via Natural or Artificial Opening
♀ **10S0XZZ** Reposition Products of Conception, External Approach
♀ **10S20ZZ** Reposition Products of Conception, Ectopic, Open Approach
♀ **10S23ZZ** Reposition Products of Conception, Ectopic, Percutaneous Approach

♀ **10S24ZZ** Reposition Products of Conception, Ectopic, Percutaneous Endoscopic Approach
♀ **10S27ZZ** Reposition Products of Conception, Ectopic, Via Natural or Artificial Opening
♀ **10S28ZZ** Reposition Products of Conception, Ectopic, Via Natural or Artificial Opening Endoscopic

10T – Obstetrics, Pregnancy, Resection

♀ **10T20ZZ** Resection of Products of Conception, Ectopic, Open Approach
♀ **10T23ZZ** Resection of Products of Conception, Ectopic, Percutaneous Approach
♀ **10T24ZZ** Resection of Products of Conception, Ectopic, Percutaneous Endoscopic Approach

♀ **10T27ZZ** Resection of Products of Conception, Ectopic, Via Natural or Artificial Opening
♀ **10T28ZZ** Resection of Products of Conception, Ectopic, Via Natural or Artificial Opening Endoscopic

10Y – Obstetrics, Pregnancy, Transplantation

♀ **10Y03ZE** Transplantation of Nervous System into Products of Conception, Percutaneous Approach
♀ **10Y03ZF** Transplantation of Cardiovascular System into Products of Conception, Percutaneous Approach
♀ **10Y03ZG** Transplantation of Lymphatics and Hemic into Products of Conception, Percutaneous Approach
♀ **10Y03ZH** Transplantation of Eye into Products of Conception, Percutaneous Approach
♀ **10Y03ZJ** Transplantation of Ear, Nose and Sinus into Products of Conception, Percutaneous Approach
♀ **10Y03ZK** Transplantation of Respiratory System into Products of Conception, Percutaneous Approach
♀ **10Y03ZL** Transplantation of Mouth and Throat into Products of Conception, Percutaneous Approach
♀ **10Y03ZM** Transplantation of Gastrointestinal System into Products of Conception, Percutaneous Approach
♀ **10Y03ZN** Transplantation of Hepatobiliary and Pancreas into Products of Conception, Percutaneous Approach
♀ **10Y03ZP** Transplantation of Endocrine System into Products of Conception, Percutaneous Approach
♀ **10Y03ZQ** Transplantation of Skin into Products of Conception, Percutaneous Approach
♀ **10Y03ZR** Transplantation of Musculoskeletal System into Products of Conception, Percutaneous Approach
♀ **10Y03ZS** Transplantation of Urinary System into Products of Conception, Percutaneous Approach
♀ **10Y03ZT** Transplantation of Female Reproductive System into Products of Conception, Percutaneous Approach
♀ **10Y03ZV** Transplantation of Male Reproductive System into Products of Conception, Percutaneous Approach
♀ **10Y03ZY** Transplantation of Other Body System into Products of Conception, Percutaneous Approach
♀ **10Y04ZE** Transplantation of Nervous System into Products of Conception, Percutaneous Endoscopic Approach
♀ **10Y04ZF** Transplantation of Cardiovascular System into Products of Conception, Percutaneous Endoscopic Approach
♀ **10Y04ZG** Transplantation of Lymphatics and Hemic into Products of Conception, Percutaneous Endoscopic Approach
♀ **10Y04ZH** Transplantation of Eye into Products of Conception, Percutaneous Endoscopic Approach
♀ **10Y04ZJ** Transplantation of Ear, Nose and Sinus into Products of Conception, Percutaneous Endoscopic Approach
♀ **10Y04ZK** Transplantation of Respiratory System into Products of Conception, Percutaneous Endoscopic Approach
♀ **10Y04ZL** Transplantation of Mouth and Throat into Products of Conception, Percutaneous Endoscopic Approach
♀ **10Y04ZM** Transplantation of Gastrointestinal System into Products of Conception, Percutaneous Endoscopic Approach

♀ **10Y04ZN** Transplantation of Hepatobiliary and Pancreas into Products of Conception, Percutaneous Endoscopic Approach
♀ **10Y04ZP** Transplantation of Endocrine System into Products of Conception, Percutaneous Endoscopic Approach
♀ **10Y04ZQ** Transplantation of Skin into Products of Conception, Percutaneous Endoscopic Approach
♀ **10Y04ZR** Transplantation of Musculoskeletal System into Products of Conception, Percutaneous Endoscopic Approach
♀ **10Y04ZS** Transplantation of Urinary System into Products of Conception, Percutaneous Endoscopic Approach
♀ **10Y04ZT** Transplantation of Female Reproductive System into Products of Conception, Percutaneous Endoscopic Approach
♀ **10Y04ZV** Transplantation of Male Reproductive System into Products of Conception, Percutaneous Endoscopic Approach
♀ **10Y04ZY** Transplantation of Other Body System into Products of Conception, Percutaneous Endoscopic Approach
♀ **10Y07ZE** Transplantation of Nervous System into Products of Conception, Via Natural or Artificial Opening
♀ **10Y07ZF** Transplantation of Cardiovascular System into Products of Conception, Via Natural or Artificial Opening
♀ **10Y07ZG** Transplantation of Lymphatics and Hemic into Products of Conception, Via Natural or Artificial Opening
♀ **10Y07ZH** Transplantation of Eye into Products of Conception, Via Natural or Artificial Opening
♀ **10Y07ZJ** Transplantation of Ear, Nose and Sinus into Products of Conception, Via Natural or Artificial Opening
♀ **10Y07ZK** Transplantation of Respiratory System into Products of Conception, Via Natural or Artificial Opening
♀ **10Y07ZL** Transplantation of Mouth and Throat into Products of Conception, Via Natural or Artificial Opening
♀ **10Y07ZM** Transplantation of Gastrointestinal System into Products of Conception, Via Natural or Artificial Opening
♀ **10Y07ZN** Transplantation of Hepatobiliary and Pancreas into Products of Conception, Via Natural or Artificial Opening
♀ **10Y07ZP** Transplantation of Endocrine System into Products of Conception, Via Natural or Artificial Opening
♀ **10Y07ZQ** Transplantation of Skin into Products of Conception, Via Natural or Artificial Opening
♀ **10Y07ZR** Transplantation of Musculoskeletal System into Products of Conception, Via Natural or Artificial Opening
♀ **10Y07ZS** Transplantation of Urinary System into Products of Conception, Via Natural or Artificial Opening
♀ **10Y07ZT** Transplantation of Female Reproductive System into Products of Conception, Via Natural or Artificial Opening
♀ **10Y07ZV** Transplantation of Male Reproductive System into Products of Conception, Via Natural or Artificial Opening
♀ **10Y07ZY** Transplantation of Other Body System into Products of Conception, Via Natural or Artificial Opening

Placement Section (2W0–2Y5)

Within each section of ICD-10-PCS the characters have different meanings. The seven character meanings for the Placement section are illustrated below through the procedure example of *Placement of pressure dressing on abdominal wall*.

Section	Body System	Root Operation	Body Region	Approach	Device	Qualifier
Placement	Anatomical Regions	Compression	Abdominal Wall	External	Pressure Dressing	None
2	W	1	3	X	6	Z

Section (Character 1)

All Placement procedure codes have a first character value of 2.

Body System (Character 2)

The alphanumeric character for the body system is placed in the second position. There are two character values applicable for the Placement section. The character value of W is reported for anatomical regions. The character value Y is reported for anatomical orifices.

Root Operations (Character 3)

The alphanumeric character value for root operations is placed in the third position. The following are the root operations applicable to the Placement section with their associated meaning. Note that the root operation definitions for ICD-10-PCS may differ from the terms that coders currently use with ICD-9-CM Volume 3.

Character Value	Root Operation	Root Operation Definition
0	Change	Taking out or off a device from a body part and putting back an identical or similar device in or on the same body part without cutting or puncturing the skin or a mucous membrane
1	Compression	Putting pressure on a body region
2	Dressing	Putting material on a body region for protection
3	Immobilization	Limiting or preventing motion of a body region
4	Packing	Putting material in a body region or orifice
5	Removal	Taking out or off a device from a body part
6	Traction	Exerting a pulling force on a body region in a distal direction

Body Region (Character 4)

For each body system the applicable body part character values will be available for procedure code construction. An example of a body region is Chest Wall.

Approach (Character 5)

The only approach technique utilized for the Placement section is External approach and is reported with the character value of X.

Character Value	Approach	Approach Definition
X	External	Procedures performed directly on the skin or mucous membrane and procedures performed indirectly by the application of external force through the skin or mucous membrane

Device (Character 6)

Depending on the procedure performed there may or may not be a device used. There are several types of devices included in the Placement section. Here is a sample list of the devices included in this section:

- Cast
- Packing material
- Pressure dressing
- Traction apparatus

When a device is not utilized during the procedure, the placeholder Z is the character value that should be reported.

Qualifier (Character 7)

The qualifier represents an additional attribute for the procedure when applicable. Currently, there are no qualifiers in the Placement section; therefore, the placeholder character value of Z should be reported.

Section Notes

Before reporting Change and Removal procedures in this section users should *Review coding guideline B6.1c.*

Placement Section Tables

Placement Tables 2W0–2Y5

Section	2	**Placement**
Body System	**W**	**Anatomical Regions**
Operation	**0**	**Change:** Taking out or off a device from a body part and putting back an identical or similar device in or on the same body part without cutting or puncturing the skin or a mucous membrane

Body Region (4th)	Approach (5th)	Device (6th)	Qualifier (7th)
0 Head 2 Neck 3 Abdominal Wall 4 Chest Wall 5 Back 6 Inguinal Region, Right 7 Inguinal Region, Left 8 Upper Extremity, Right 9 Upper Extremity, Left A Upper Arm, Right B Upper Arm, Left C Lower Arm, Right D Lower Arm, Left E Hand, Right F Hand, Left G Thumb, Right H Thumb, Left J Finger, Right K Finger, Left L Lower Extremity, Right M Lower Extremity, Left N Upper Leg, Right P Upper Leg, Left Q Lower Leg, Right R Lower Leg, Left S Foot, Right T Foot, Left U Toe, Right V Toe, Left	X External	0 Traction Apparatus 1 Splint 2 Cast 3 Brace 4 Bandage 5 Packing Material 6 Pressure Dressing 7 Intermittent Pressure Device Y Other Device	Z No Qualifier
1 Face	X External	0 Traction Apparatus 1 Splint 2 Cast 3 Brace 4 Bandage 5 Packing Material 6 Pressure Dressing 7 Intermittent Pressure Device 9 Wire Y Other Device	Z No Qualifier

Section	2	Placement
Body System	W	Anatomical Regions
Operation	1	**Compression:** Putting pressure on a body region

Body Region (4th)	Approach (5th)	Device (6th)	Qualifier (7th)
0 Head	X External	6 Pressure Dressing	Z No Qualifier
1 Face		7 Intermittent Pressure Device	
2 Neck			
3 Abdominal Wall			
4 Chest Wall			
5 Back			
6 Inguinal Region, Right			
7 Inguinal Region, Left			
8 Upper Extremity, Right			
9 Upper Extremity, Left			
A Upper Arm, Right			
B Upper Arm, Left			
C Lower Arm, Right			
D Lower Arm, Left			
E Hand, Right			
F Hand, Left			
G Thumb, Right			
H Thumb, Left			
J Finger, Right			
K Finger, Left			
L Lower Extremity, Right			
M Lower Extremity, Left			
N Upper Leg, Right			
P Upper Leg, Left			
Q Lower Leg, Right			
R Lower Leg, Left			
S Foot, Right			
T Foot, Left			
U Toe, Right			
V Toe, Left			

Section	2	**Placement**
Body System	W	**Anatomical Regions**
Operation	2	**Dressing:** Putting material on a body region for protection

Body Region (4th)	Approach (5th)	Device (6th)	Qualifier (7th)
0 Head	**X** External	**4** Bandage	**Z** No Qualifier
1 Face			
2 Neck			
3 Abdominal Wall			
4 Chest Wall			
5 Back			
6 Inguinal Region, Right			
7 Inguinal Region, Left			
8 Upper Extremity, Right			
9 Upper Extremity, Left			
A Upper Arm, Right			
B Upper Arm, Left			
C Lower Arm, Right			
D Lower Arm, Left			
E Hand, Right			
F Hand, Left			
G Thumb, Right			
H Thumb, Left			
J Finger, Right			
K Finger, Left			
L Lower Extremity, Right			
M Lower Extremity, Left			
N Upper Leg, Right			
P Upper Leg, Left			
Q Lower Leg, Right			
R Lower Leg, Left			
S Foot, Right			
T Foot, Left			
U Toe, Right			
V Toe, Left			

Section	**2**	**Placement**	
Body System	**W**	**Anatomical Regions**	
Operation	**3**	**Immobilization:** Limiting or preventing motion of a body region	

Body Region (4th)	Approach (5th)	Device (6th)	Qualifier (7th)
0 Head 2 Neck 3 Abdominal Wall 4 Chest Wall 5 Back 6 Inguinal Region, Right 7 Inguinal Region, Left 8 Upper Extremity, Right 9 Upper Extremity, Left A Upper Arm, Right B Upper Arm, Left C Lower Arm, Right D Lower Arm, Left E Hand, Right F Hand, Left G Thumb, Right H Thumb, Left J Finger, Right K Finger, Left L Lower Extremity, Right M Lower Extremity, Left N Upper Leg, Right P Upper Leg, Left Q Lower Leg, Right R Lower Leg, Left S Foot, Right T Foot, Left U Toe, Right V Toe, Left	X External	1 Splint 2 Cast 3 Brace Y Other Device	Z No Qualifier
1 Face	X External	1 Splint 2 Cast 3 Brace 9 Wire Y Other Device	Z No Qualifier

Section   **2**   **Placement**
Body System   **W**   **Anatomical Regions**
Operation   **4**   **Packing:** Putting material in a body region or orifice

Body Region (4th)	Approach (5th)	Device (6th)	Qualifier (7th)
0 Head	X External	5 Packing Material	Z No Qualifier
1 Face			
2 Neck			
3 Abdominal Wall			
4 Chest Wall			
5 Back			
6 Inguinal Region, Right			
7 Inguinal Region, Left			
8 Upper Extremity, Right			
9 Upper Extremity, Left			
A Upper Arm, Right			
B Upper Arm, Left			
C Lower Arm, Right			
D Lower Arm, Left			
E Hand, Right			
F Hand, Left			
G Thumb, Right			
H Thumb, Left			
J Finger, Right			
K Finger, Left			
L Lower Extremity, Right			
M Lower Extremity, Left			
N Upper Leg, Right			
P Upper Leg, Left			
Q Lower Leg, Right			
R Lower Leg, Left			
S Foot, Right			
T Foot, Left			
U Toe, Right			
V Toe, Left			

Section	2	Placement
Body System	W	Anatomical Regions
Operation	5	Removal: Taking out or off a device from a body part

Body Region (4th)	Approach (5th)	Device (6th)	Qualifier (7th)
0 Head 2 Neck 3 Abdominal Wall 4 Chest Wall 5 Back 6 Inguinal Region, Right 7 Inguinal Region, Left 8 Upper Extremity, Right 9 Upper Extremity, Left A Upper Arm, Right B Upper Arm, Left C Lower Arm, Right D Lower Arm, Left E Hand, Right F Hand, Left G Thumb, Right H Thumb, Left J Finger, Right K Finger, Left L Lower Extremity, Right M Lower Extremity, Left N Upper Leg, Right P Upper Leg, Left Q Lower Leg, Right R Lower Leg, Left S Foot, Right T Foot, Left U Toe, Right V Toe, Left	X External	0 Traction Apparatus 1 Splint 2 Cast 3 Brace 4 Bandage 5 Packing Material 6 Pressure Dressing 7 Intermittent Pressure Device Y Other Device	Z No Qualifier
1 Face	X External	0 Traction Apparatus 1 Splint 2 Cast 3 Brace 4 Bandage 5 Packing Material 6 Pressure Dressing 7 Intermittent Pressure Device 9 Wire Y Other Device	Z No Qualifier

Section	2	Placement
Body System	W	Anatomical Regions
Operation	6	**Traction:** Exerting a pulling force on a body region in a distal direction

Body Region (4th)	Approach (5th)	Device (6th)	Qualifier (7th)
0 Head	X External	0 Traction Apparatus	Z No Qualifier
1 Face		Z No Device	
2 Neck			
3 Abdominal Wall			
4 Chest Wall			
5 Back			
6 Inguinal Region, Right			
7 Inguinal Region, Left			
8 Upper Extremity, Right			
9 Upper Extremity, Left			
A Upper Arm, Right			
B Upper Arm, Left			
C Lower Arm, Right			
D Lower Arm, Left			
E Hand, Right			
F Hand, Left			
G Thumb, Right			
H Thumb, Left			
J Finger, Right			
K Finger, Left			
L Lower Extremity, Right			
M Lower Extremity, Left			
N Upper Leg, Right			
P Upper Leg, Left			
Q Lower Leg, Right			
R Lower Leg, Left			
S Foot, Right			
T Foot, Left			
U Toe, Right			
V Toe, Left			

Section	2	Placement
Body System	Y	Anatomical Orifices
Operation	0	**Change:** Taking out or off a device from a body part and putting back an identical or similar device in or on the same body part without cutting or puncturing the skin or a mucous membrane

Body Region (4th)	Approach (5th)	Device (6th)	Qualifier (7th)
0 Mouth and Pharynx	X External	5 Packing Material	Z No Qualifier
1 Nasal			
2 Ear			
3 Anorectal			
4 Female Genital Tract			
5 Urethra			

Section	2	Placement
Body System	Y	Anatomical Orifices
Operation	4	**Packing:** Putting material in a body region or orifice

Body Region (4th)	Approach (5th)	Device (6th)	Qualifier (7th)
0 Mouth and Pharynx	X External	5 Packing Material	Z No Qualifier
1 Nasal			
2 Ear			
3 Anorectal			
4 Female Genital Tract			
5 Urethra			

Section	2	Placement
Body System	Y	Anatomical Orifices
Operation	5	Removal: Taking out or off a device from a body part

Body Region (4th)	Approach (5th)	Device (6th)	Qualifier (7th)
0 Mouth and Pharynx **1** Nasal **2** Ear **3** Anorectal **4** Female Genital Tract **5** Urethra	**X** External	**5** Packing Material	**Z** No Qualifier

Administration Section (302–3E1)

Within each section of ICD-10-PCS, the characters have different meanings. The seven character meanings for the Administration section are illustrated here through the procedure example of *Nerve block injection to median nerve*.

Section	Body System	Root Operation	Body System/ Region	Approach	Substance	Qualifier
Administration	Physiological System and Anatomical Region	Introduction	Peripheral Nerves and Plexi	Percutaneous	Regional Anesthetic	None
3	E	0	T	3	C	Z

Section (Character 1)

All Administration procedure codes have a first character value of 3.

Body System (Character 2)

The alphanumeric character for the body system is placed in the second position. There are three character values applicable for the Administration section.

Character Value	Character Value Description
0	Circulatory
C	Indwelling Device
E	Physiological System and Anatomical Region

Root Operations (Character 3)

The alphanumeric character value for root operations is placed in the third position. Listed here are the root operations applicable to the Administration section with their associated meaning. Note that the root operation definitions for ICD-10-PCS may differ from the terms that coders currently use with ICD-9-CM Volume 3.

Character Value	Root Operation	Root Operation Definition
0	Introduction	Putting in or on a therapeutic, diagnostic, nutritional, physiological, or prophylactic substance except blood or blood products
1	Irrigation	Putting in or on a cleansing substance
2	Transfusion	Putting in blood or blood products

Body System/Region (Character 4)

For each body system the applicable body part character values will be available for procedure code construction. An example of a body region is upper GI.

Approach (Character 5)

The approach is the technique used to reach the procedure site. Listed here are the approach character values for the Administration with the associated definitions.

Character Value	Approach	Approach Definition
0	Open	Cutting through the skin or mucous membrane and any other body layers necessary to expose the site of the procedure
3	Percutaneous	Entry, by puncture or minor incision, of instrumentation through the skin or mucous membrane and any other body layers necessary to reach the site of the procedure
7	Via Natural or Artificial Opening	Entry of instrumentation through a natural or artificial external opening to reach the site of the procedure
8	Via Natural or Artificial Opening Endoscopic	Entry of instrumentation through a natural or artificial external opening to reach and visualize the site of the procedure
X	External	Procedures performed directly on the skin or mucous membrane and procedures performed indirectly by the application of external force through the skin or mucous membrane

Substance (Character 6)

In the Administration section a substance is always utilized. The substance is reported in the sixth character position by the type of substance utilized. The following is a sample list of the substances included in this section:

- Anti-inflammatory
- Antineoplastic
- Bone marrow
- Platelet inhibitor
- Whole blood

Qualifier (Character 7)

The qualifier represents an additional attribute for the procedure when applicable. There are several qualifiers included in the Administration section. For example, transfusion procedures in this section include qualifiers including Autologous and Nonautologous that are reported with the character values of 0 and 1, respectively. If there is no qualifier for a procedure, the placeholder Z is the character value that should be reported.

Section Notes

Before reporting Transfusion procedures for embryonic stem cells (6th character A), bone marrow (6th character G), cord blood stem cells (6th character X) or hematopoietic stem cells (6th character Y) users should *Review coding guideline B3.16*.

Before reporting Administration codes for all Biliary and Pancreatic Tract (4th character value of J) procedures with a 6th character value of U (Pancreatic Islet Cells), users should *Review coding guideline B3.16*.

Before reporting Irrigation procedures in this section, users should *Review coding guideline B6.1c*.

Medicare Non-Covered Administration Codes						
Non-Covered with pdx or sdx C91.00, C92.00, C92.10, C92.11, C92.40, C92.50, C92.60, C92.A0, C93.00, C94.00 or C95.00						
30230AZ	30233AZ	30240AZ	30243AZ	30250G0	30253Y0	30263G0
30230G0	30233G0	30240G0	30243G0	30250Y0	30260G0	30263Y0
30230Y0	30233Y0	30240Y0	30243Y0	30253G0	30260Y0	
Non-Covered with pdx or sdx C90.00 or C90.01						
30230G1	30233Y1	30243G1	30250Y1	30260G1	30263G1	
30230Y1	30240G1	30243Y1	30253G1	30260Y1	30263Y1	
30233G1	30240Y1	30250G1	30253Y1	30263G1		

Administration Section Tables

Administration Tables 302-3E1

Section	3	**Administration**
Body System	**0**	**Circulatory**
Operation	**2**	**Transfusion:** Putting in blood or blood products

Body System / Region (4th)	Approach (5th)	Substance (6th)	Qualifier (7th)
3 Peripheral Vein **4** Central Vein	**0** Open **3** Percutaneous	**A** Stem Cells, Embryonic	**Z** No Qualifier
3 Peripheral Vein **4** Central Vein	**0** Open **3** Percutaneous	**G** Bone Marrow **H** Whole Blood **J** Serum Albumin **K** Frozen Plasma **L** Fresh Plasma **M** Plasma Cryoprecipitate **N** Red Blood Cells **P** Frozen Red Cells **Q** White Cells **R** Platelets **S** Globulin **T** Fibrinogen **V** Antihemophilic Factors **W** Factor IX **X** Stem Cells, Cord Blood **Y** Stem Cells, Hematopoietic	**0** Autologous **1** Nonautologous
5 Peripheral Artery **6** Central Artery	**0** Open **3** Percutaneous	**G** Bone Marrow **H** Whole Blood **J** Serum Albumin **K** Frozen Plasma **L** Fresh Plasma **M** Plasma Cryoprecipitate **N** Red Blood Cells **P** Frozen Red Cells **Q** White Cells **R** Platelets **S** Globulin **T** Fibrinogen **V** Antihemophilic Factors **W** Factor IX **X** Stem Cells, Cord Blood **Y** Stem Cells, Hematopoietic	**0** Autologous **1** Nonautologous
7 Products of Conception, Circulatory	**3** Percutaneous **7** Via Natural or Artificial Opening	**H** Whole Blood **J** Serum Albumin **K** Frozen Plasma **L** Fresh Plasma **M** Plasma Cryoprecipitate **N** Red Blood Cells **P** Frozen Red Cells **Q** White Cells **R** Platelets **S** Globulin **T** Fibrinogen **V** Antihemophilic Factors **W** Factor IX	**1** Nonautologous

Continued

Section	3	Administration
Body System	0	Circulatory
Operation	2	**Transfusion:** Putting in blood or blood products

Body System / Region (4th)	Approach (5th)	Substance (6th)	Qualifier (7th)
8 Vein	0 Open 3 Percutaneous	B 4-Factor Prothrombin Complex Concentrate	1 Nonautologous

Section	3	Administration
Body System	C	Indwelling Device
Operation	1	**Irrigation:** Putting in or on a cleansing substance

Body System / Region (4th)	Approach (5th)	Substance (6th)	Qualifier (7th)
Z None	X External	8 Irrigating Substance	Z No Qualifier

Section	3	Administration
Body System	E	Physiological Systems and Anatomical Regions
Operation	0	**Introduction:** Putting in or on a therapeutic, diagnostic, nutritional, physiological, or prophylactic substance except blood or blood products

Body System / Region (4th)	Approach (5th)	Substance (6th)	Qualifier (7th)
0 Skin and Mucous Membranes	X External	0 Antineoplastic	5 Other Antineoplastic M Monoclonal Antibody
0 Skin and Mucous Membranes	X External	2 Anti-infective	8 Oxazolidinones 9 Other Anti-infective
0 Skin and Mucous Membranes	X External	3 Anti-inflammatory 4 Serum, Toxoid and Vaccine B Local Anesthetic K Other Diagnostic Substance M Pigment N Analgesics, Hypnotics, Sedatives T Destructive Agent	Z No Qualifier
0 Skin and Mucous Membranes	X External	G Other Therapeutic Substance	C Other Substance
1 Subcutaneous Tissue	0 Open	2 Anti-infective	A Anti-Infective Envelope
1 Subcutaneous Tissue	3 Percutaneous	0 Antineoplastic	5 Other Antineoplastic M Monoclonal Antibody
1 Subcutaneous Tissue	3 Percutaneous	2 Anti-infective	8 Oxazolidinones 9 Other Anti-infective A Anti-Infective Envelope
1 Subcutaneous Tissue	3 Percutaneous	3 Anti-inflammatory 4 Serum, Toxoid and Vaccine 6 Nutritional Substance 7 Electrolytic and Water Balance Substance B Local Anesthetic H Radioactive Substance K Other Diagnostic Substance N Analgesics, Hypnotics, Sedatives T Destructive Agent	Z No Qualifier
1 Subcutaneous Tissue	3 Percutaneous	G Other Therapeutic Substance	C Other Substance

Section	3	Administration	
Body System	E	Physiological Systems and Anatomical Regions	
Operation	0	**Introduction:** Putting in or on a therapeutic, diagnostic, nutritional, physiological, or prophylactic substance except blood or blood products	

Body System / Region (4th)	Approach (5th)	Substance (6th)	Qualifier (7th)
1 Subcutaneous Tissue	**3** Percutaneous	**V** Hormone	**G** Insulin **J** Other Hormone
2 Muscle	**3** Percutaneous	**0** Antineoplastic	**5** Other Antineoplastic **M** Monoclonal Antibody
2 Muscle	**3** Percutaneous	**2** Anti-infective	**8** Oxazolidinones **9** Other Anti-infective
2 Muscle	**3** Percutaneous	**3** Anti-inflammatory **4** Serum, Toxoid and Vaccine **6** Nutritional Substance **7** Electrolytic and Water Balance Substance **B** Local Anesthetic **H** Radioactive Substance **K** Other Diagnostic Substance **N** Analgesics, Hypnotics, Sedatives **T** Destructive Agent	**Z** No Qualifier
2 Muscle	**3** Percutaneous	**G** Other Therapeutic Substance	**C** Other Substance
3 Peripheral Vein	**0** Open	**0** Antineoplastic	**2** High-dose Interleukin-2 **3** Low-dose Interleukin-2 **5** Other Antineoplastic **M** Monoclonal Antibody **P** Clofarabine
3 Peripheral Vein	**0** Open	**1** Thrombolytic	**6** Recombinant Human-activated Protein C **7** Other Thrombolytic
3 Peripheral Vein	**0** Open	**2** Anti-infective	**8** Oxazolidinones **9** Other Anti-infective
3 Peripheral Vein	**0** Open	**3** Anti-inflammatory **4** Serum, Toxoid and Vaccine **6** Nutritional Substance **7** Electrolytic and Water Balance Substance **F** Intracirculatory Anesthetic **H** Radioactive Substance **K** Other Diagnostic Substance **N** Analgesics, Hypnotics, Sedatives **P** Platelet Inhibitor **R** Antiarrhythmic **T** Destructive Agent **X** Vasopressor	**Z** No Qualifier
3 Peripheral Vein	**0** Open	**G** Other Therapeutic Substance	**C** Other Substance **N** Blood Brain Barrier Disruption
3 Peripheral Vein	**0** Open	**U** Pancreatic Islet Cells	**0** Autologous **1** Nonautologous

Continued

Section	3	Administration
Body System	E	Physiological Systems and Anatomical Regions
Operation	0	**Introduction:** Putting in or on a therapeutic, diagnostic, nutritional, physiological, or prophylactic substance except blood or blood products

Body System / Region (4th)	Approach (5th)	Substance (6th)	Qualifier (7th)
3 Peripheral Vein	0 Open	V Hormone	G Insulin H Human B-type Natriuretic Peptide J Other Hormone
3 Peripheral Vein	0 Open	W Immunotherapeutic	K Immunostimulator L Immunosuppressive
3 Peripheral Vein	3 Percutaneous	0 Antineoplastic	2 High-dose Interleukin-2 3 Low-dose Interleukin-2 5 Other Antineoplastic M Monoclonal Antibody P Clofarabine
3 Peripheral Vein	3 Percutaneous	1 Thrombolytic	6 Recombinant Human-activated Protein C 7 Other Thrombolytic
3 Peripheral Vein	3 Percutaneous	2 Anti-infective	8 Oxazolidinones 9 Other Anti-infective
3 Peripheral Vein	3 Percutaneous	3 Anti-inflammatory 4 Serum, Toxoid and Vaccine 6 Nutritional Substance 7 Electrolytic and Water Balance Substance F Intracirculatory Anesthetic H Radioactive Substance K Other Diagnostic Substance N Analgesics, Hypnotics, Sedatives P Platelet Inhibitor R Antiarrhythmic T Destructive Agent X Vasopressor	Z No Qualifier
3 Peripheral Vein	3 Percutaneous	G Other Therapeutic Substance	C Other Substance N Blood Brain Barrier Disruption Q Glucarpidase
3 Peripheral Vein	3 Percutaneous	U Pancreatic Islet Cells	0 Autologous 1 Nonautologous
3 Peripheral Vein	3 Percutaneous	V Hormone	G Insulin H Human B-type Natriuretic Peptide J Other Hormone
3 Peripheral Vein	3 Percutaneous	W Immunotherapeutic	K Immunostimulator L Immunosuppressive
4 Central Vein	0 Open	0 Antineoplastic	2 High-dose Interleukin-2 3 Low-dose Interleukin-2 5 Other Antineoplastic M Monoclonal Antibody P Clofarabine

Continued

Section   **3**   **Administration**

Body System   **E**   **Physiological Systems and Anatomical Regions**

Operation   **0**   **Introduction:** Putting in or on a therapeutic, diagnostic, nutritional, physiological, or prophylactic substance except blood or blood products

3E0 Continued

Body System / Region (4th)	Approach (5th)	Substance (6th)	Qualifier (7th)
4 Central Vein	0 Open	1 Thrombolytic	6 Recombinant Human-activated Protein C 7 Other Thrombolytic
4 Central Vein	0 Open	2 Anti-infective	8 Oxazolidinones 9 Other Anti-infective
4 Central Vein	0 Open	3 Anti-inflammatory 4 Serum, Toxoid and Vaccine 6 Nutritional Substance 7 Electrolytic and Water Balance Substance F Intracirculatory Anesthetic H Radioactive Substance K Other Diagnostic Substance N Analgesics, Hypnotics, Sedatives P Platelet Inhibitor R Antiarrhythmic T Destructive Agent X Vasopressor	Z No Qualifier
4 Central Vein	0 Open	G Other Therapeutic Substance	C Other Substance N Blood Brain Barrier Disruption
4 Central Vein	0 Open	V Hormone	G Insulin H Human B-type Natriuretic Peptide J Other Hormone
4 Central Vein	0 Open	W Immunotherapeutic	K Immunostimulator L Immunosuppressive
4 Central Vein	3 Percutaneous	0 Antineoplastic	2 High-dose Interleukin-2 3 Low-dose Interleukin-2 5 Other Antineoplastic M Monoclonal Antibody P Clofarabine
4 Central Vein	3 Percutaneous	1 Thrombolytic	6 Recombinant Human-activated Protein C 7 Other Thrombolytic
4 Central Vein	3 Percutaneous	2 Anti-infective	8 Oxazolidinones 9 Other Anti-infective
4 Central Vein	3 Percutaneous	3 Anti-inflammatory 4 Serum, Toxoid and Vaccine 6 Nutritional Substance 7 Electrolytic and Water Balance Substance F Intracirculatory Anesthetic H Radioactive Substance K Other Diagnostic Substance N Analgesics, Hypnotics, Sedatives P Platelet Inhibitor R Antiarrhythmic T Destructive Agent X Vasopressor	Z No Qualifier

Continued

Section	3	Administration		3E0 *Continued*
Body System	E	Physiological Systems and Anatomical Regions		
Operation	0	Introduction: Putting in or on a therapeutic, diagnostic, nutritional, physiological, or prophylactic substance except blood or blood products		

Body System / Region (4th)	Approach (5th)	Substance (6th)	Qualifier (7th)
4 Central Vein	3 Percutaneous	G Other Therapeutic Substance	C Other Substance N Blood Brain Barrier Disruption Q Glucarpidase
4 Central Vein	3 Percutaneous	V Hormone	G Insulin H Human B-type Natriuretic Peptide J Other Hormone
4 Central Vein	3 Percutaneous	W Immunotherapeutic	K Immunostimulator L Immunosuppressive
5 Peripheral Artery 6 Central Artery	0 Open 3 Percutaneous	0 Antineoplastic	2 High-dose Interleukin-2 3 Low-dose Interleukin-2 5 Other Antineoplastic M Monoclonal Antibody P Clofarabine
5 Peripheral Artery 6 Central Artery	0 Open 3 Percutaneous	1 Thrombolytic	6 Recombinant Human-activated Protein C 7 Other Thrombolytic
5 Peripheral Artery 6 Central Artery	0 Open 3 Percutaneous	2 Anti-infective	8 Oxazolidinones 9 Other Anti-infective
5 Peripheral Artery 6 Central Artery	0 Open 3 Percutaneous	3 Anti-inflammatory 4 Serum, Toxoid and Vaccine 6 Nutritional Substance 7 Electrolytic and Water Balance Substance F Intracirculatory Anesthetic H Radioactive Substance K Other Diagnostic Substance N Analgesics, Hypnotics, Sedatives P Platelet Inhibitor R Antiarrhythmic T Destructive Agent X Vasopressor	Z No Qualifier
5 Peripheral Artery 6 Central Artery	0 Open 3 Percutaneous	G Other Therapeutic Substance	C Other Substance N Blood Brain Barrier Disruption
5 Peripheral Artery 6 Central Artery	0 Open 3 Percutaneous	V Hormone	G Insulin H Human B-type Natriuretic Peptide J Other Hormone
5 Peripheral Artery 6 Central Artery	0 Open 3 Percutaneous	W Immunotherapeutic	K Immunostimulator L Immunosuppressive
7 Coronary Artery 8 Heart	0 Open 3 Percutaneous	1 Thrombolytic	6 Recombinant Human-activated Protein C 7 Other Thrombolytic
7 Coronary Artery 8 Heart	0 Open 3 Percutaneous	G Other Therapeutic Substance	C Other Substance

Continued

Section	3	**Administration**
Body System	E	**Physiological Systems and Anatomical Regions**
Operation	0	**Introduction:** Putting in or on a therapeutic, diagnostic, nutritional, physiological, or prophylactic substance except blood or blood products

3E0 Continued

Body System / Region (4th)	Approach (5th)	Substance (6th)	Qualifier (7th)
7 Coronary Artery 8 Heart	0 Open 3 Percutaneous	K Other Diagnostic Substance P Platelet Inhibitor	Z No Qualifier
9 Nose	3 Percutaneous 7 Via Natural or Artificial Opening X External	0 Antineoplastic	5 Other Antineoplastic M Monoclonal Antibody
9 Nose	3 Percutaneous 7 Via Natural or Artificial Opening X External	2 Anti-infective	8 Oxazolidinones 9 Other Anti-infective
9 Nose	3 Percutaneous 7 Via Natural or Artificial Opening X External	3 Anti-inflammatory 4 Serum, Toxoid and Vaccine B Local Anesthetic H Radioactive Substance K Other Diagnostic Substance N Analgesics, Hypnotics, Sedatives T Destructive Agent	Z No Qualifier
9 Nose	3 Percutaneous 7 Via Natural or Artificial Opening X External	G Other Therapeutic Substance	C Other Substance
A Bone Marrow	3 Percutaneous	0 Antineoplastic	5 Other Antineoplastic M Monoclonal Antibody
A Bone Marrow	3 Percutaneous	G Other Therapeutic Substance	C Other Substance
B Ear	3 Percutaneous 7 Via Natural or Artificial Opening X External	0 Antineoplastic	4 Liquid Brachytherapy Radioisotope 5 Other Antineoplastic M Monoclonal Antibody
B Ear	3 Percutaneous 7 Via Natural or Artificial Opening X External	2 Anti-infective	8 Oxazolidinones 9 Other Anti-infective
B Ear	3 Percutaneous 7 Via Natural or Artificial Opening X External	3 Anti-inflammatory B Local Anesthetic H Radioactive Substance K Other Diagnostic Substance N Analgesics, Hypnotics, Sedatives T Destructive Agent	Z No Qualifier
B Ear	3 Percutaneous 7 Via Natural or Artificial Opening X External	G Other Therapeutic Substance	C Other Substance
C Eye	3 Percutaneous 7 Via Natural or Artificial Opening X External	0 Antineoplastic	4 Liquid Brachytherapy Radioisotope 5 Other Antineoplastic M Monoclonal Antibody

Continued

3E0 *Continued*

Section	3	Administration
Body System	E	Physiological Systems and Anatomical Regions
Operation	0	**Introduction:** Putting in or on a therapeutic, diagnostic, nutritional, physiological, or prophylactic substance except blood or blood products

Body System / Region (4th)	Approach (5th)	Substance (6th)	Qualifier (7th)
C Eye	3 Percutaneous 7 Via Natural or Artificial Opening X External	2 Anti-infective	8 Oxazolidinones 9 Other Anti-infective
C Eye	3 Percutaneous 7 Via Natural or Artificial Opening X External	3 Anti-inflammatory B Local Anesthetic H Radioactive Substance K Other Diagnostic Substance M Pigment N Analgesics, Hypnotics, Sedatives T Destructive Agent	Z No Qualifier
C Eye	3 Percutaneous 7 Via Natural or Artificial Opening X External	G Other Therapeutic Substance	C Other Substance
C Eye	3 Percutaneous 7 Via Natural or Artificial Opening X External	S Gas	F Other Gas
D Mouth and Pharynx	3 Percutaneous 7 Via Natural or Artificial Opening X External	0 Antineoplastic	4 Liquid Brachytherapy Radioisotope 5 Other Antineoplastic M Monoclonal Antibody
D Mouth and Pharynx	3 Percutaneous 7 Via Natural or Artificial Opening X External	2 Anti-infective	8 Oxazolidinones 9 Other Anti-infective
D Mouth and Pharynx	3 Percutaneous 7 Via Natural or Artificial Opening X External	3 Anti-inflammatory 4 Serum, Toxoid and Vaccine 6 Nutritional Substance 7 Electrolytic and Water Balance Substance B Local Anesthetic H Radioactive Substance K Other Diagnostic Substance N Analgesics, Hypnotics, Sedatives R Antiarrhythmic T Destructive Agent	Z No Qualifier
D Mouth and Pharynx	3 Percutaneous 7 Via Natural or Artificial Opening X External	G Other Therapeutic Substance	C Other Substance
E Products of Conception G Upper GI H Lower GI K Genitourinary Tract N Male Reproductive	3 Percutaneous 7 Via Natural or Artificial Opening 8 Via Natural or Artificial Opening Endoscopic	0 Antineoplastic	4 Liquid Brachytherapy Radioisotope 5 Other Antineoplastic M Monoclonal Antibody

Continued

Section	3	Administration
Body System	E	Physiological Systems and Anatomical Regions
Operation	0	Introduction: Putting in or on a therapeutic, diagnostic, nutritional, physiological, or prophylactic substance except blood or blood products

Body System / Region (4th)	Approach (5th)	Substance (6th)	Qualifier (7th)
E Products of Conception **G** Upper GI **H** Lower GI **K** Genitourinary Tract **N** Male Reproductive	**3** Percutaneous **7** Via Natural or Artificial Opening **8** Via Natural or Artificial Opening Endoscopic	**2** Anti-infective	**8** Oxazolidinones **9** Other Anti-infective
E Products of Conception **G** Upper GI **H** Lower GI **K** Genitourinary Tract **N** Male Reproductive	**3** Percutaneous **7** Via Natural or Artificial Opening **8** Via Natural or Artificial Opening Endoscopic	**3** Anti-inflammatory **6** Nutritional Substance **7** Electrolytic and Water Balance Substance **B** Local Anesthetic **H** Radioactive Substance **K** Other Diagnostic Substance **N** Analgesics, Hypnotics, Sedatives **T** Destructive Agent	**Z** No Qualifier
E Products of Conception **G** Upper GI **H** Lower GI **K** Genitourinary Tract **N** Male Reproductive	**3** Percutaneous **7** Via Natural or Artificial Opening **8** Via Natural or Artificial Opening Endoscopic	**G** Other Therapeutic Substance	**C** Other Substance
E Products of Conception **G** Upper GI **H** Lower GI **K** Genitourinary Tract **N** Male Reproductive	**3** Percutaneous **7** Via Natural or Artificial Opening **8** Via Natural or Artificial Opening Endoscopic	**S** Gas	**F** Other Gas
F Respiratory Tract	**3** Percutaneous	**0** Antineoplastic	**4** Liquid Brachytherapy Radioisotope **5** Other Antineoplastic **M** Monoclonal Antibody
F Respiratory Tract	**3** Percutaneous	**2** Anti-infective	**8** Oxazolidinones **9** Other Anti-infective
F Respiratory Tract	**3** Percutaneous	**3** Anti-inflammatory **6** Nutritional Substance **7** Electrolytic and Water Balance Substance **B** Local Anesthetic **H** Radioactive Substance **K** Other Diagnostic Substance **N** Analgesics, Hypnotics, Sedatives **T** Destructive Agent	**Z** No Qualifier
F Respiratory Tract	**3** Percutaneous	**G** Other Therapeutic Substance	**C** Other Substance
F Respiratory Tract	**3** Percutaneous	**S** Gas	**D** Nitric Oxide **F** Other Gas
F Respiratory Tract	**7** Via Natural or Artificial Opening **8** Via Natural or Artificial Opening Endoscopic	**0** Antineoplastic	**4** Liquid Brachytherapy Radioisotope **5** Other Antineoplastic **M** Monoclonal Antibody

Continued

Section	3	Administration
Body System	E	Physiological Systems and Anatomical Regions
Operation	0	**Introduction:** Putting in or on a therapeutic, diagnostic, nutritional, physiological, or prophylactic substance except blood or blood products

Body System / Region (4th)	Approach (5th)	Substance (6th)	Qualifier (7th)
F Respiratory Tract	**7** Via Natural or Artificial Opening **8** Via Natural or Artificial Opening Endoscopic	**2** Anti-infective	**8** Oxazolidinones **9** Other Anti-infective
F Respiratory Tract	**7** Via Natural or Artificial Opening **8** Via Natural or Artificial Opening Endoscopic	**3** Anti-inflammatory **6** Nutritional Substance **7** Electrolytic and Water Balance Substance **B** Local Anesthetic **D** Inhalation Anesthetic **H** Radioactive Substance **K** Other Diagnostic Substance **N** Analgesics, Hypnotics, Sedatives **T** Destructive Agent	**Z** No Qualifier
F Respiratory Tract	**7** Via Natural or Artificial Opening **8** Via Natural or Artificial Opening Endoscopic	**G** Other Therapeutic Substance	**C** Other Substance
F Respiratory Tract	**7** Via Natural or Artificial Opening **8** Via Natural or Artificial Opening Endoscopic	**S** Gas	**D** Nitric Oxide **F** Other Gas
J Biliary and Pancreatic Tract	**3** Percutaneous **7** Via Natural or Artificial Opening **8** Via Natural or Artificial Opening Endoscopic	**0** Antineoplastic	**4** Liquid Brachytherapy Radioisotope **5** Other Antineoplastic **M** Monoclonal Antibody
J Biliary and Pancreatic Tract	**3** Percutaneous **7** Via Natural or Artificial Opening **8** Via Natural or Artificial Opening Endoscopic	**2** Anti-infective	**8** Oxazolidinones **9** Other Anti-infective
J Biliary and Pancreatic Tract	**3** Percutaneous **7** Via Natural or Artificial Opening **8** Via Natural or Artificial Opening Endoscopic	**3** Anti-inflammatory **6** Nutritional Substance **7** Electrolytic and Water Balance Substance **B** Local Anesthetic **H** Radioactive Substance **K** Other Diagnostic Substance **N** Analgesics, Hypnotics, Sedatives **T** Destructive Agent	**Z** No Qualifier
J Biliary and Pancreatic Tract	**3** Percutaneous **7** Via Natural or Artificial Opening **8** Via Natural or Artificial Opening Endoscopic	**G** Other Therapeutic Substance	**C** Other Substance
J Biliary and Pancreatic Tract	**3** Percutaneous **7** Via Natural or Artificial Opening **8** Via Natural or Artificial Opening Endoscopic	**S** Gas	**F** Other Gas

Continued

Section	3	Administration		3E0 *Continued*
Body System	E	Physiological Systems and Anatomical Regions		
Operation	0	Introduction: Putting in or on a therapeutic, diagnostic, nutritional, physiological, or prophylactic substance except blood or blood products		

Body System / Region (4th)	Approach (5th)	Substance (6th)	Qualifier (7th)
J Biliary and Pancreatic Tract	**3** Percutaneous **7** Via Natural or Artificial Opening **8** Via Natural or Artificial Opening Endoscopic	**U** Pancreatic Islet Cells	**0** Autologous **1** Nonautologous
L Pleural Cavity **M** Peritoneal Cavity	**0** Open	**5** Adhesion Barrier	**Z** No Qualifier
L Pleural Cavity **M** Peritoneal Cavity	**3** Percutaneous	**0** Antineoplastic	**4** Liquid Brachytherapy Radioisotope **5** Other Antineoplastic **M** Monoclonal Antibody
L Pleural Cavity **M** Peritoneal Cavity	**3** Percutaneous	**2** Anti-infective	**8** Oxazolidinones **9** Other Anti-infective
L Pleural Cavity **M** Peritoneal Cavity	**3** Percutaneous	**3** Anti-inflammatory **6** Nutritional Substance **7** Electrolytic and Water Balance Substance **B** Local Anesthetic **H** Radioactive Substance **K** Other Diagnostic Substance **N** Analgesics, Hypnotics, Sedatives **T** Destructive Agent	**Z** No Qualifier
L Pleural Cavity **M** Peritoneal Cavity	**3** Percutaneous	**G** Other Therapeutic Substance	**C** Other Substance
L Pleural Cavity **M** Peritoneal Cavity	**3** Percutaneous	**S** Gas	**F** Other Gas
L Pleural Cavity **M** Peritoneal Cavity	**7** Via Natural or Artificial Opening	**0** Antineoplastic	**4** Liquid Brachytherapy Radioisotope **5** Other Antineoplastic **M** Monoclonal Antibody
L Pleural Cavity **M** Peritoneal Cavity	**7** Via Natural or Artificial Opening	**S** Gas	**F** Other Gas
P Female Reproductive	**0** Open	**5** Adhesion Barrier	**Z** No Qualifier
P Female Reproductive	**3** Percutaneous **7** Via Natural or Artificial Opening	**0** Antineoplastic	**4** Liquid Brachytherapy Radioisotope **5** Other Antineoplastic **M** Monoclonal Antibody
P Female Reproductive	**3** Percutaneous **7** Via Natural or Artificial Opening	**2** Anti-infective	**8** Oxazolidinones **9** Other Anti-infective

Continued

Section	3	**Administration**
Body System	E	**Physiological Systems and Anatomical Regions**
Operation	0	**Introduction:** Putting in or on a therapeutic, diagnostic, nutritional, physiological, or prophylactic substance except blood or blood products

Body System / Region (4th)	Approach (5th)	Substance (6th)	Qualifier (7th)
P Female Reproductive	**3** Percutaneous **7** Via Natural or Artificial Opening	**3** Anti-inflammatory **6** Nutritional Substance **7** Electrolytic and Water Balance Substance **B** Local Anesthetic **H** Radioactive Substance **K** Other Diagnostic Substance **L** Sperm **N** Analgesics, Hypnotics, Sedatives **T** Destructive Agent	**Z** No Qualifier
P Female Reproductive	**3** Percutaneous **7** Via Natural or Artificial Opening	**G** Other Therapeutic Substance	**C** Other Substance
P Female Reproductive	**3** Percutaneous **7** Via Natural or Artificial Opening	**Q** Fertilized Ovum	**0** Autologous **1** Nonautologous
P Female Reproductive	**3** Percutaneous **7** Via Natural or Artificial Opening	**S** Gas	**F** Other Gas
P Female Reproductive	**8** Via Natural or Artificial Opening Endoscopic	**0** Antineoplastic	**4** Liquid Brachytherapy Radioisotope **5** Other Antineoplastic **M** Monoclonal Antibody
P Female Reproductive	**8** Via Natural or Artificial Opening Endoscopic	**2** Anti-infective	**8** Oxazolidinones **9** Other Anti-infective
P Female Reproductive	**8** Via Natural or Artificial Opening Endoscopic	**3** Anti-inflammatory **6** Nutritional Substance **7** Electrolytic and Water Balance Substance **B** Local Anesthetic **H** Radioactive Substance **K** Other Diagnostic Substance **N** Analgesics, Hypnotics, Sedatives **T** Destructive Agent	**Z** No Qualifier
P Female Reproductive	**8** Via Natural or Artificial Opening Endoscopic	**G** Other Therapeutic Substance	**C** Other Substance
P Female Reproductive	**8** Via Natural or Artificial Opening Endoscopic	**S** Gas	**F** Other Gas
Q Cranial Cavity and Brain	**0** Open	**A** Stem Cells, Embryonic	**Z** No Qualifier
Q Cranial Cavity and Brain	**0** Open	**E** Stem Cells, Somatic	**0** Autologous **1** Nonautologous
Q Cranial Cavity and Brain	**3** Percutaneous	**0** Antineoplastic	**4** Liquid Brachytherapy Radioisotope **5** Other Antineoplastic **M** Monoclonal Antibody
Q Cranial Cavity and Brain	**3** Percutaneous	**2** Anti-infective	**8** Oxazolidinones **9** Other Anti-infective

Section	3	Administration	3E0 *Continued*
Body System	E	**Physiological Systems and Anatomical Regions**	
Operation	0	**Introduction:** Putting in or on a therapeutic, diagnostic, nutritional, physiological, or prophylactic substance except blood or blood products	

Body System / Region (4ᵗʰ)	Approach (5ᵗʰ)	Substance (6ᵗʰ)	Qualifier (7ᵗʰ)
Q Cranial Cavity and Brain	**3** Percutaneous	**3** Anti-inflammatory **6** Nutritional Substance **7** Electrolytic and Water Balance Substance **A** Stem Cells, Embryonic **B** Local Anesthetic **H** Radioactive Substance **K** Other Diagnostic Substance **N** Analgesics, Hypnotics, Sedatives **T** Destructive Agent	**Z** No Qualifier
Q Cranial Cavity and Brain	**3** Percutaneous	**E** Stem Cells, Somatic	**0** Autologous **1** Nonautologous
Q Cranial Cavity and Brain	**3** Percutaneous	**G** Other Therapeutic Substance	**C** Other Substance
Q Cranial Cavity and Brain	**3** Percutaneous	**S** Gas	**F** Other Gas
Q Cranial Cavity and Brain	**7** Via Natural or Artificial Opening	**0** Antineoplastic	**4** Liquid Brachytherapy Radioisotope **5** Other Antineoplastic **M** Monoclonal Antibody
Q Cranial Cavity and Brain	**7** Via Natural or Artificial Opening	**S** Gas	**F** Other Gas
R Spinal Canal	**0** Open	**A** Stem Cells, Embryonic	**Z** No Qualifier
R Spinal Canal	**0** Open	**E** Stem Cells, Somatic	**0** Autologous **1** Nonautologous
R Spinal Canal	**3** Percutaneous	**0** Antineoplastic	**2** High-dose Interleukin-2 **3** Low-dose Interleukin-2 **4** Liquid Brachytherapy Radioisotope **5** Other Antineoplastic **M** Monoclonal Antibody
R Spinal Canal	**3** Percutaneous	**2** Anti-infective	**8** Oxazolidinones **9** Other Anti-infective
R Spinal Canal	**3** Percutaneous	**3** Anti-inflammatory **6** Nutritional Substance **7** Electrolytic and Water Balance Substance **A** Stem Cells, Embryonic **B** Local Anesthetic **C** Regional Anesthetic **H** Radioactive Substance **K** Other Diagnostic Substance **N** Analgesics, Hypnotics, Sedatives **T** Destructive Agent	**Z** No Qualifier
R Spinal Canal	**3** Percutaneous	**E** Stem Cells, Somatic	**0** Autologous **1** Nonautologous

Continued

Section	3	Administration
Body System	E	**Physiological Systems and Anatomical Regions**
Operation	0	**Introduction:** Putting in or on a therapeutic, diagnostic, nutritional, physiological, or prophylactic substance except blood or blood products

3E0 *Continued*

Body System / Region (4th)	Approach (5th)	Substance (6th)	Qualifier (7th)
R Spinal Canal	**3** Percutaneous	**G** Other Therapeutic Substance	**C** Other Substance
R Spinal Canal	**3** Percutaneous	**S** Gas	**F** Other Gas
R Spinal Canal	**7** Via Natural or Artificial Opening	**S** Gas	**F** Other Gas
S Epidural Space	**3** Percutaneous	**0** Antineoplastic	**2** High-dose Interleukin-2 **3** Low-dose Interleukin-2 **4** Liquid Brachytherapy Radioisotope **5** Other Antineoplastic **M** Monoclonal Antibody
S Epidural Space	**3** Percutaneous	**2** Anti-infective	**8** Oxazolidinones **9** Other Anti-infective
S Epidural Space	**3** Percutaneous	**3** Anti-inflammatory **6** Nutritional Substance **7** Electrolytic and Water Balance Substance **B** Local Anesthetic **C** Regional Anesthetic **H** Radioactive Substance **K** Other Diagnostic Substance **N** Analgesics, Hypnotics, Sedatives **T** Destructive Agent	**Z** No Qualifier
S Epidural Space	**3** Percutaneous	**G** Other Therapeutic Substance	**C** Other Substance
S Epidural Space	**3** Percutaneous	**S** Gas	**F** Other Gas
S Epidural Space	**7** Via Natural or Artificial Opening	**S** Gas	**F** Other Gas
T Peripheral Nerves and Plexi **X** Cranial Nerves	**3** Percutaneous	**3** Anti-inflammatory **B** Local Anesthetic **C** Regional Anesthetic **T** Destructive Agent	**Z** No Qualifier
T Peripheral Nerves and Plexi **X** Cranial Nerves	**3** Percutaneous	**G** Other Therapeutic Substance	**C** Other Substance
U Joints	**0** Open	**2** Anti-infective	**8** Oxazolidinones **9** Other Anti-infective
U Joints	**0** Open	**G** Other Therapeutic Substance	**B** Recombinant Bone Morphogenetic Protein
U Joints	**3** Percutaneous	**0** Antineoplastic	**4** Liquid Brachytherapy Radioisotope **5** Other Antineoplastic **M** Monoclonal Antibody
U Joints	**3** Percutaneous	**2** Anti-infective	**8** Oxazolidinones **9** Other Anti-infective

Continued

Section	3	Administration	
Body System	E	Physiological Systems and Anatomical Regions	
Operation	0	**Introduction:** Putting in or on a therapeutic, diagnostic, nutritional, physiological, or prophylactic substance except blood or blood products	3E0 *Continued*

Body System / Region (4ᵗʰ)	Approach (5ᵗʰ)	Substance (6ᵗʰ)	Qualifier (7ᵗʰ)
U Joints	3 Percutaneous	3 Anti-inflammatory 6 Nutritional Substance 7 Electrolytic and Water Balance Substance B Local Anesthetic H Radioactive Substance K Other Diagnostic Substance N Analgesics, Hypnotics, Sedatives T Destructive Agent	Z No Qualifier
U Joints	3 Percutaneous	G Other Therapeutic Substance	B Recombinant Bone Morphogenetic Protein C Other Substance
U Joints	3 Percutaneous	S Gas	F Other Gas
V Bones	0 Open	G Other Therapeutic Substance	B Recombinant Bone Morphogenetic Protein
V Bones	3 Percutaneous	0 Antineoplastic	5 Other Antineoplastic M Monoclonal Antibody
V Bones	3 Percutaneous	2 Anti-infective	8 Oxazolidinones 9 Other Anti-infective
V Bones	3 Percutaneous	3 Anti-inflammatory 6 Nutritional Substance 7 Electrolytic and Water Balance Substance B Local Anesthetic H Radioactive Substance K Other Diagnostic Substance N Analgesics, Hypnotics, Sedatives T Destructive Agent	Z No Qualifier
V Bones	3 Percutaneous	G Other Therapeutic Substance	B Recombinant Bone Morphogenetic Protein C Other Substance
W Lymphatics	3 Percutaneous	0 Antineoplastic	5 Other Antineoplastic M Monoclonal Antibody
W Lymphatics	3 Percutaneous	2 Anti-infective	8 Oxazolidinones 9 Other Anti-infective
W Lymphatics	3 Percutaneous	3 Anti-inflammatory 6 Nutritional Substance 7 Electrolytic and Water Balance Substance B Local Anesthetic H Radioactive Substance K Other Diagnostic Substance N Analgesics, Hypnotics, Sedatives T Destructive Agent	Z No Qualifier
W Lymphatics	3 Percutaneous	G Other Therapeutic Substance	C Other Substance

Continued

Section	3	Administration		3E0 *Continued*
Body System	E	Physiological Systems and Anatomical Regions		
Operation	0	**Introduction:** Putting in or on a therapeutic, diagnostic, nutritional, physiological, or prophylactic substance except blood or blood products		

Body System / Region (4th)	Approach (5th)	Substance (6th)	Qualifier (7th)
Y Pericardial Cavity	3 Percutaneous	0 Antineoplastic	4 Liquid Brachytherapy Radioisotope 5 Other Antineoplastic M Monoclonal Antibody
Y Pericardial Cavity	3 Percutaneous	2 Anti-infective	8 Oxazolidinones 9 Other Anti-infective
Y Pericardial Cavity	3 Percutaneous	3 Anti-inflammatory 6 Nutritional Substance 7 Electrolytic and Water Balance Substance B Local Anesthetic H Radioactive Substance K Other Diagnostic Substance N Analgesics, Hypnotics, Sedatives T Destructive Agent	Z No Qualifier
Y Pericardial Cavity	3 Percutaneous	G Other Therapeutic Substance	C Other Substance
Y Pericardial Cavity	3 Percutaneous	S Gas	F Other Gas
Y Pericardial Cavity	7 Via Natural or Artificial Opening	0 Antineoplastic	4 Liquid Brachytherapy Radioisotope 5 Other Antineoplastic M Monoclonal Antibody
Y Pericardial Cavity	7 Via Natural or Artificial Opening	S Gas	F Other Gas

Section	3	Administration
Body System	E	Physiological Systems and Anatomical Regions
Operation	1	**Irrigation:** Putting in or on a cleansing substance

Body System / Region (4th)	Approach (5th)	Substance (6th)	Qualifier (7th)
0 Skin and Mucous Membranes C Eye	3 Percutaneous X External	8 Irrigating Substance	X Diagnostic Z No Qualifier
9 Nose B Ear F Respiratory Tract G Upper GI H Lower GI J Biliary and Pancreatic Tract K Genitourinary Tract N Male Reproductive P Female Reproductive	3 Percutaneous 7 Via Natural or Artificial Opening 8 Via Natural or Artificial Opening Endoscopic	8 Irrigating Substance	X Diagnostic Z No Qualifier
L Pleural Cavity Q Cranial Cavity and Brain R Spinal Canal S Epidural Space U Joints Y Pericardial Cavity	3 Percutaneous	8 Irrigating Substance	X Diagnostic Z No Qualifier
M Peritoneal Cavity	3 Percutaneous	8 Irrigating Substance	X Diagnostic Z No Qualifier
M Peritoneal Cavity	3 Percutaneous	9 Dialysate	Z No Qualifier

Measurement and Monitoring Section (4A0–4B0)

Within each section of ICD-10-PCS the characters have different meanings. The seven character meanings for the Measurement and Monitoring section are illustrated here through the procedure example of *External electrocardiogram (EKG), single reading*.

Section	Body System	Root Operation	Body System	Approach	Function / Device	Qualifier
Measurement and Monitoring	Physiological Systems	Measurement	Cardiac	External	Electrical Activity	None
4	A	0	2	X	4	Z

Section (Character 1)

All Measurement and Monitoring procedure codes have a first character value of 4.

Body System (Character 2)

The alphanumeric character for the body system is placed in the second position. There are two character values applicable for the Measurement and Monitoring section. The character value of A is reported for physiological systems. The character value B is reported for physiological devices.

Root Operations (Character 3)

The alphanumeric character value for root operations is placed in the third position. Listed here are the root operations applicable to the Measurement and Monitoring section with their associated meaning. Note that the root operation definitions for ICD-10-PCS may differ from the terms that coders currently use with ICD-9-CM Volume 3.

Character Value	Root Operation	Root Operation Definition
0	Measurement	Determining the level of a physiological or physical function at a point in time
1	Monitoring	Determining the level of a physiological or physical function repetitively over a period of time

Body System/Region (Character 4)

For each body system the applicable body part character values will be available for procedure code construction. An example of a body region for this section is Respiratory.

Approach (Character 5)

The approach is the technique used to reach the procedure site. The following are the approach character values for the Measurement and Monitoring section with the associated definitions.

Character Value	Approach	Approach Definition
0	Open	Cutting through the skin or mucous membrane and any other body layers necessary to expose the site of the procedure
3	Percutaneous	Entry, by puncture or minor incision, of instrumentation through the skin or mucous membrane and any other body layers necessary to reach the site of the procedure

Continued

Character Value	Approach	Approach Definition
4	Percutaneous Endoscopic	Entry, by puncture or minor incision, of instrumentation through the skin or mucous membrane and any other body layers necessary to reach and visualize the site of the procedure
7	Via Natural or Artificial Opening	Entry of instrumentation through a natural or artificial external opening to reach the site of the procedure
8	Via Natural or Artificial Opening Endoscopic	Entry of instrumentation through a natural or artificial external opening to reach and visualize the site of the procedure
X	External	Procedures performed directly on the skin or mucous membrane and procedures performed indirectly by the application of external force through the skin or mucous membrane

Function/Device (Character 6)

In the Measurement and Monitoring section a function or device is always utilized. The function or device is reported in the sixth character position by the type of function monitored or measured or by the device utilized. The following is a sample list of the functions and devices included in this section:

- Conductivity
- Flow
- Metabolism
- Pressure
- Sound

Qualifier (Character 7)

The qualifier represents an additional attribute for the procedure when applicable. There are several qualifiers included in the Measurement and Monitoring section. For example, measurement procedures in this section include several qualifiers including stress that is reported with the character value of 4. If there is no qualifier for a procedure, the placeholder Z is the character valve that should be reported.

Measurement and Monitoring Section Tables

Measurement and Monitoring Tables 4A0–4B0

Section   **4**   **Measurement and Monitoring**
Body System   **A**   **Physiological Systems**
Operation   **0**   **Measurement:** Determining the level of a physiological or physical function at a point in time

Body System (4ᵗʰ)	Approach (5ᵗʰ)	Function / Device (6ᵗʰ)	Qualifier (7ᵗʰ)
0 Central Nervous	0 Open	2 Conductivity 4 Electrical Activity B Pressure	Z No Qualifier
0 Central Nervous	3 Percutaneous	4 Electrical Activity	Z No Qualifier
0 Central Nervous	3 Percutaneous	B Pressure K Temperature R Saturation	D Intracranial
0 Central Nervous	7 Via Natural or Artificial Opening	B Pressure K Temperature R Saturation	D Intracranial
0 Central Nervous	X External	2 Conductivity 4 Electrical Activity	Z No Qualifier
1 Peripheral Nervous	0 Open 3 Percutaneous X External	2 Conductivity	9 Sensory B Motor
1 Peripheral Nervous	0 Open 3 Percutaneous X External	4 Electrical Activity	Z No Qualifier
2 Cardiac	0 Open 3 Percutaneous	4 Electrical Activity 9 Output C Rate F Rhythm H Sound P Action Currents	Z No Qualifier
2 Cardiac	0 Open 3 Percutaneous	N Sampling and Pressure	6 Right Heart 7 Left Heart 8 Bilateral
2 Cardiac	X External	4 Electrical Activity	A Guidance Z No Qualifier
2 Cardiac	X External	9 Output C Rate F Rhythm H Sound P Action Currents	Z No Qualifier
2 Cardiac	X External	M Total Activity	4 Stress
3 Arterial	0 Open 3 Percutaneous	5 Flow J Pulse	1 Peripheral 3 Pulmonary C Coronary

Continued

Measurement and Monitoring Section (4A0–4B0)

4A0

Section	4	**Measurement and Monitoring**
Body System	A	**Physiological Systems**
Operation	0	**Measurement:** Determining the level of a physiological or physical function at a point in time

Body System (4th)	Approach (5th)	Function / Device (6th)	Qualifier (7th)
3 Arterial	0 Open 3 Percutaneous	B Pressure	1 Peripheral 3 Pulmonary C Coronary F Other Thoracic
3 Arterial	0 Open 3 Percutaneous	H Sound R Saturation	1 Peripheral
3 Arterial	X External	5 Flow B Pressure H Sound J Pulse R Saturation	1 Peripheral
4 Venous	0 Open 3 Percutaneous	5 Flow B Pressure J Pulse	0 Central 1 Peripheral 2 Portal 3 Pulmonary
4 Venous	0 Open 3 Percutaneous	R Saturation	1 Peripheral
4 Venous	X External	5 Flow B Pressure J Pulse R Saturation	1 Peripheral
5 Circulatory	X External	L Volume	Z No Qualifier
6 Lymphatic	0 Open 3 Percutaneous	5 Flow B Pressure	Z No Qualifier
7 Visual	X External	0 Acuity 7 Mobility B Pressure	Z No Qualifier
8 Olfactory	X External	0 Acuity	Z No Qualifier
9 Respiratory	7 Via Natural or Artificial Opening 8 Via Natural or Artificial Opening Endoscopic X External	1 Capacity 5 Flow C Rate D Resistance L Volume M Total Activity	Z No Qualifier
B Gastrointestinal	7 Via Natural or Artificial Opening 8 Via Natural or Artificial Opening Endoscopic	8 Motility B Pressure G Secretion	Z No Qualifier
C Biliary	3 Percutaneous 4 Percutaneous Endoscopic 7 Via Natural or Artificial Opening 8 Via Natural or Artificial Opening Endoscopic	5 Flow B Pressure	Z No Qualifier

Continued

Section	4	Measurement and Monitoring	4A0 *Continued*
Body System	A	Physiological Systems	
Operation	0	Measurement: Determining the level of a physiological or physical function at a point in time	

Body System (4th)	Approach (5th)	Function / Device (6th)	Qualifier (7th)
D Urinary	**7** Via Natural or Artificial Opening	**3** Contractility **5** Flow **B** Pressure **D** Resistance **L** Volume	**Z** No Qualifier
F Musculoskeletal	**3** Percutaneous **X** External	**3** Contractility	**Z** No Qualifier
H Products of Conception, Cardiac	**7** Via Natural or Artificial Opening **8** Via Natural or Artificial Opening Endoscopic **X** External	**4** Electrical Activity **C** Rate **F** Rhythm **H** Sound	**Z** No Qualifier
J Products of Conception, Nervous	**7** Via Natural or Artificial Opening **8** Via Natural or Artificial Opening Endoscopic **X** External	**2** Conductivity **4** Electrical Activity **B** Pressure	**Z** No Qualifier
Z None	**7** Via Natural or Artificial Opening	**6** Metabolism **K** Temperature	**Z** No Qualifier
Z None	**X** External	**6** Metabolism **K** Temperature **Q** Sleep	**Z** No Qualifier

Section	4	Measurement and Monitoring
Body System	A	Physiological Systems
Operation	1	Monitoring: Determining the level of a physiological or physical function repetitively over a period of time

Body System (4th)	Approach (5th)	Function / Device (6th)	Qualifier (7th)
0 Central Nervous	**0** Open	**2** Conductivity **B** Pressure	**Z** No Qualifier
0 Central Nervous	**0** Open	**4** Electrical Activity	**G** Intraoperative **Z** No Qualifier
0 Central Nervous	**3** Percutaneous	**4** Electrical Activity	**G** Intraoperative **Z** No Qualifier
0 Central Nervous	**3** Percutaneous	**B** Pressure **K** Temperature **R** Saturation	**D** Intracranial
0 Central Nervous	**7** Via Natural or Artificial Opening	**B** Pressure **K** Temperature **R** Saturation	**D** Intracranial
0 Central Nervous	**X** External	**2** Conductivity	**Z** No Qualifier
0 Central Nervous	**X** External	**4** Electrical Activity	**G** Intraoperative **Z** No Qualifier
1 Peripheral Nervous	**0** Open **3** Percutaneous **X** External	**2** Conductivity	**9** Sensory **B** Motor

Continued

Measurement and Monitoring Section (4A0–4B0)

4A1

Section	4	**Measurement and Monitoring**
Body System	A	**Physiological Systems**
Operation	1	**Monitoring:** Determining the level of a physiological or physical function repetitively over a period of time

Body System (4ᵗʰ)	Approach (5ᵗʰ)	Function / Device (6ᵗʰ)	Qualifier (7ᵗʰ)
1 Peripheral Nervous	0 Open 3 Percutaneous X External	4 Electrical Activity	G Intraoperative Z No Qualifier
2 Cardiac	0 Open 3 Percutaneous	4 Electrical Activity 9 Output C Rate F Rhythm H Sound	Z No Qualifier
2 Cardiac	X External	4 Electrical Activity	5 Ambulatory Z No Qualifier
2 Cardiac	X External	9 Output C Rate F Rhythm H Sound	Z No Qualifier
2 Cardiac	X External	M Total Activity	4 Stress
3 Arterial	0 Open 3 Percutaneous	5 Flow B Pressure J Pulse	1 Peripheral 3 Pulmonary C Coronary
3 Arterial	0 Open 3 Percutaneous	H Sound R Saturation	1 Peripheral
3 Arterial	X External	5 Flow B Pressure H Sound J Pulse R Saturation	1 Peripheral
4 Venous	0 Open 3 Percutaneous	5 Flow B Pressure J Pulse	0 Central 1 Peripheral 2 Portal 3 Pulmonary
4 Venous	0 Open 3 Percutaneous	R Saturation	0 Central 2 Portal 3 Pulmonary
4 Venous	X External	5 Flow B Pressure J Pulse	1 Peripheral
6 Lymphatic	0 Open 3 Percutaneous	5 Flow B Pressure	Z No Qualifier
9 Respiratory	7 Via Natural or Artificial Opening X External	1 Capacity 5 Flow C Rate D Resistance L Volume	Z No Qualifier
B Gastrointestinal	7 Via Natural or Artificial Opening 8 Via Natural or Artificial Opening Endoscopic	8 Motility B Pressure G Secretion	Z No Qualifier

Continued

Section	4	Measurement and Monitoring	4A1 *Continued*
Body System	A	Physiological Systems	
Operation	1	Monitoring: Determining the level of a physiological or physical function repetitively over a period of time	

Body System (4ᵗʰ)	Approach (5ᵗʰ)	Function / Device (6ᵗʰ)	Qualifier (7ᵗʰ)
D Urinary	**7** Via Natural or Artificial Opening	**3** Contractility **5** Flow **B** Pressure **D** Resistance **L** Volume	**Z** No Qualifier
H Products of Conception, Cardiac	**7** Via Natural or Artificial Opening **8** Via Natural or Artificial Opening Endoscopic **X** External	**4** Electrical Activity **C** Rate **F** Rhythm **H** Sound	**Z** No Qualifier
J Products of Conception, Nervous	**7** Via Natural or Artificial Opening **8** Via Natural or Artificial Opening Endoscopic **X** External	**2** Conductivity **4** Electrical Activity **B** Pressure	**Z** No Qualifier
Z None	**7** Via Natural or Artificial Opening	**K** Temperature	**Z** No Qualifier
Z None	**X** External	**K** Temperature **Q** Sleep	**Z** No Qualifier

Section	4	Measurement and Monitoring
Body System	B	Physiological Devices
Operation	0	Measurement: Determining the level of a physiological or physical function at a point in time

Body System (4ᵗʰ)	Approach (5ᵗʰ)	Function / Device (6ᵗʰ)	Qualifier (7ᵗʰ)
0 Central Nervous **1** Peripheral Nervous **F** Musculoskeletal	**X** External	**V** Stimulator	**Z** No Qualifier
2 Cardiac	**X** External	**S** Pacemaker **T** Defibrillator	**Z** No Qualifier
9 Respiratory	**X** External	**S** Pacemaker	**Z** No Qualifier

Extracorporeal Assistance and Performance Section (5A0–5A2)

Within each section of ICD-10-PCS the characters have different meanings. The seven character meanings for the Extracorporeal Assistance and Performance section are illustrated here through the procedure example of *Hyperbaric oxygenation of wound*.

Section	Body System	Root Operation	Body System	Duration	Function	Qualifier
Extracorporeal Assistance and Performance	Physiological Systems	Assistance	Circulatory	Intermittent	Oxygenation	Hyperbaric
5	A	0	5	1	2	1

Section (Character 1)

All Extracorporeal Assistance and Performance procedure codes have a first character value of 5.

Body System (Character 2)

The alphanumeric character for the body system is placed in the second position. There is one character value applicable for the Extracorporeal Assistance and Performance section. The character value of A is reported for physiological systems.

Root Operations (Character 3)

The alphanumeric character value for root operations is placed in the third position. Listed here are the root operations applicable to the Extracorporeal Assistance and Performance section with their associated meaning. Note that the root operation definitions for ICD-10-PCS may differ from the terms that coders currently use with ICD-9-CM Volume 3.

Character Value	Root Operation	Root Operation Definition
0	Assistance	Taking over a portion of a physiological function by extracorporeal means
1	Performance	Completely taking over a physiological function by extracorporeal means

Body System (Character 4)

For each body system, the applicable body part character values will be available for procedure code construction. An example of a body region for this section is respiratory.

Duration (Character 5)

The duration represents the length of time or frequency for which the assistance or performance is utilized. Some examples of duration are Intermittent, Continuous, or Less than 24 consecutive hours.

Function (Character 6)

In the Extracorporeal Assistance and Performance section a function is always reported. The function is reported in the sixth character position. The following is a sample list of the functions utilized in this section:

- Output
- Oxygenation
- Pacing
- Ventilation

Qualifier (Character 7)

The qualifier represents an additional attribute for the procedure when applicable. There are several qualifiers included in the Extracorporeal Assistance and Performance section. For example, assistance procedures in this section include several qualifiers including Balloon Pump, which is reported with the character value of 0. If there is no qualifier for a procedure, the placeholder Z is the character valve that should be reported.

Extracorporeal Assistance and Performance Section Tables

Extracorporeal Assistance and Performance Tables 5A0–5A2

Section	5	**Extracorporeal Assistance and Performance**
Body System	A	**Physiological Systems**
Operation	0	**Assistance:** Taking over a portion of a physiological function by extracorporeal means

Body System (4th)	Duration (5th)	Function (6th)	Qualifier (7th)
2 Cardiac	1 Intermittent 2 Continuous	1 Output	0 Balloon Pump 5 Pulsatile Compression 6 Other Pump D Impeller Pump
5 Circulatory	1 Intermittent 2 Continuous	2 Oxygenation	1 Hyperbaric C Supersaturated
9 Respiratory	3 Less than 24 Consecutive Hours 4 24-96 Consecutive Hours 5 Greater than 96 Consecutive Hours	5 Ventilation	7 Continuous Positive Airway Pressure 8 Intermittent Positive Airway Pressure 9 Continuous Negative Airway Pressure B Intermittent Negative Airway Pressure Z No Qualifier

Section	5	**Extracorporeal Assistance and Performance**
Body System	A	**Physiological Systems**
Operation	1	**Performance:** Completely taking over a physiological function by extracorporeal means

Body System (4th)	Approach (5th)	Function (6th)	Qualifier (7th)
2 Cardiac	0 Single	1 Output	2 Manual
2 Cardiac	1 Intermittent	3 Pacing	Z No Qualifier
2 Cardiac	2 Continuous	1 Output 3 Pacing	Z No Qualifier
5 Circulatory	2 Continuous	2 Oxygenation	3 Membrane
9 Respiratory	0 Single	5 Ventilation	4 Nonmechanical
9 Respiratory	3 Less than 24 Consecutive Hours 4 24-96 Consecutive Hours 5 Greater than 96 Consecutive Hours	5 Ventilation	Z No Qualifier
C Biliary D Urinary	0 Single 6 Multiple	0 Filtration	Z No Qualifier

Section	5	**Extracorporeal Assistance and Performance**
Body System	A	**Physiological Systems**
Operation	2	**Restoration:** Returning, or attempting to return, a physiological function to its original state by extracorporeal means.

Body System (4th)	Duration (5th)	Function (6th)	Qualifier (7th)
2 Cardiac	0 Single	4 Rhythm	Z No Qualifier

Extracorporeal Therapies Section (6A0–6A9)

Within each section of ICD-10-PCS the characters have different meanings. The seven character meanings for the Extracorporeal Therapies section are illustrated here through the procedure example of *Ultraviolet light phototherapy, series treatment.*

Section	Body System	Root Operation	Body System	Duration	Qualifier	Qualifier
Extracorporeal Therapies	Physiological Systems	UV Light Therapy	Skin	Multiple	None	None
6	A	8	0	1	Z	Z

Section (Character 1)

All Extracorporeal Therapies procedure codes have a first character value of 6.

Body System (Character 2)

The alphanumeric character for the body system is placed in the second position. There is one character value applicable for the Extracorporeal Therapies section. The character value of A is reported for physiological systems.

Root Operations (Character 3)

The alphanumeric character value for root operations is placed in the third position. Listed below are the root operations applicable to the Extracorporeal Therapies section with their associated meaning. Note that the root operation definitions for ICD-10-PCS may differ from the terms that coders currently use with ICD-9-CM Volume 3.

Character Value	Root Operation	Root Operation Definition
0	Atmospheric Control	Extracorporeal control of atmospheric pressure and composition
1	Decompression	Extracorporeal elimination of undissolved gas from body fluids
2	Electromagnetic Therapy	Extracorporeal treatment by electromagnetic rays
3	Hyperthermia	Extracorporeal raising of body temperature
4	Hypothermia	Extracorporeal lowering of body temperature
5	Pheresis	Extracorporeal separation of blood products
6	Phototherapy	Extracorporeal treatment by light rays
7	Ultrasound Therapy	Extracorporeal treatment by ultrasound
8	Ultraviolet Light Therapy	Extracorporeal treatment by ultraviolet light
9	Shock Wave Therapy	Extracorporeal treatment by shock waves

Body System (Character 4)

For each body system the applicable body part character values will be available for procedure code construction. An example of a body region for this section is Skin.

Duration (Character 5)

The duration represents the number of therapy sessions performed. Single is reported with character value 0; Multiple is reported with character value 1.

Qualifier (Character 6)

Character 6 is the first of two qualifier characters for the Extracorporeal Therapies section. The qualifier represents an additional attribute for the procedure when applicable. There are currently no qualifier values for the sixth character position, so the character value of Z is always reported.

Qualifier (Character 7)

Character 7 is the second of two qualifier characters for the Extracorporeal Therapies section. The qualifier represents an additional attribute for the procedure when applicable. There are some qualifiers included in the Extracorporeal Therapies section. For example, pheresis procedures in this section include several qualifiers including Plasma that is reported with the character value of 3. If there is no qualifier for a procedure, the placeholder Z is the character valve that should be reported.

Extracorporeal Therapies Tables

Extracorporeal Therapies Tables 6A0–6A9

Section	6	**Extracorporeal Therapies**
Body System	A	**Physiological Systems**
Operation	0	**Atmospheric Control:** Extracorporeal control of atmospheric pressure and composition

Body System (4th)	Duration (5th)	Qualifier (6th)	Qualifier (7th)
Z None	**0** Single **1** Multiple	**Z** No Qualifier	**Z** No Qualifier

Section	6	**Extracorporeal Therapies**
Body System	A	**Physiological Systems**
Operation	1	**Decompression:** Extracorporeal elimination of undissolved gas from body fluids

Body System (4th)	Duration (5th)	Qualifier (6th)	Qualifier (7th)
5 Circulatory	**0** Single **1** Multiple	**Z** No Qualifier	**Z** No Qualifier

Section	6	**Extracorporeal Therapies**
Body System	A	**Physiological Systems**
Operation	2	**Electromagnetic Therapy:** Extracorporeal treatment by electromagnetic rays

Body System (4th)	Duration (5th)	Qualifier (6th)	Qualifier (7th)
1 Urinary **2** Central Nervous	**0** Single **1** Multiple	**Z** No Qualifier	**Z** No Qualifier

Section	6	**Extracorporeal Therapies**
Body System	A	**Physiological Systems**
Operation	3	**Hyperthermia:** Extracorporeal raising of body temperature

Body System (4th)	Duration (5th)	Qualifier (6th)	Qualifier (7th)
Z None	**0** Single **1** Multiple	**Z** No Qualifier	**Z** No Qualifier

Section	6	**Extracorporeal Therapies**
Body System	A	**Physiological Systems**
Operation	4	**Hypothermia:** Extracorporeal lowering of body temperature

Body System (4th)	Duration (5th)	Qualifier (6th)	Qualifier (7th)
Z None	**0** Single **1** Multiple	**Z** No Qualifier	**Z** No Qualifier

Section	6	**Extracorporeal Therapies**
Body System	A	**Physiological Systems**
Operation	5	**Pheresis:** Extracorporeal separation of blood products

Body System (4th)	Duration (5th)	Qualifier (6th)	Qualifier (7th)
5 Circulatory	**0** Single **1** Multiple	**Z** No Qualifier	**0** Erythrocytes **1** Leukocytes **2** Platelets **3** Plasma **T** Stem Cells, Cord Blood **V** Stem Cells, Hematopoietic

Section	6	**Extracorporeal Therapies**
Body System	A	**Physiological Systems**
Operation	6	**Phototherapy:** Extracorporeal treatment by light rays

Body System (4th)	Duration (5th)	Qualifier (6th)	Qualifier (7th)
0 Skin **5** Circulatory	**0** Single **1** Multiple	**Z** No Qualifier	**Z** No Qualifier

Section	6	**Extracorporeal Therapies**
Body System	A	**Physiological Systems**
Operation	7	**Ultrasound Therapy:** Extracorporeal treatment by ultrasound

Body System (4th)	Duration (5th)	Qualifier (6th)	Qualifier (7th)
5 Circulatory	**0** Single **1** Multiple	**Z** No Qualifier	**4** Head and Neck Vessels **5** Heart **6** Peripheral Vessels **7** Other Vessels **Z** No Qualifier

Section	6	**Extracorporeal Therapies**
Body System	A	**Physiological Systems**
Operation	8	**Ultraviolet Light Therapy:** Extracorporeal treatment by ultraviolet light

Body System (4th)	Duration (5th)	Qualifier (6th)	Qualifier (7th)
0 Skin	**0** Single **1** Multiple	**Z** No Qualifier	**Z** No Qualifier

Section	6	**Extracorporeal Therapies**
Body System	A	**Physiological Systems**
Operation	9	**Shock Wave Therapy:** Extracorporeal treatment by shock waves

Body System (4th)	Duration (5th)	Qualifier (6th)	Qualifier (7th)
3 Musculoskeletal	**0** Single **1** Multiple	**Z** No Qualifier	**Z** No Qualifier

Osteopathic Section (7W0)

Within each section of ICD-10-PCS, the characters have different meanings. The seven character meanings for the Osteopathic section are illustrated below through the procedure example of Indirect osteopathic treatment of sacrum.

Section	Body System	Root Operation	Body Region	Approach	Method	Qualifier
Osteopathic	Anatomical Regions	Treatment	Sacrum	External	Indirect	None
7	W	0	4	X	4	Z

Section (Character 1)

All Osteopathic procedure codes have a first character value of 7.

Body System (Character 2)

The alphanumeric character for the body system is placed in the second position. There is one character value applicable for the Osteopathic section. The character value of W is reported for anatomical regions.

Root Operations (Character 3)

The alphanumeric character value for root operations is placed in the third position. Listed here is the root operation applicable to the Osteopathic section with its associated meaning. Note that the root operation definitions for ICD-10-PCS may differ from the terms that coders currently use with ICD-9-CM Volume 3.

Character Value	Root Operation	Root Operation Definition
0	Treatment	Manual treatment to eliminate or alleviate somatic dysfunction and related disorders

Body Region (Character 4)

For each body region the applicable body part character values will be available for procedure code construction. An example of a body region for this section is Head.

Approach (Character 5)

The approach is the technique used to reach the procedure site. The following are the approach character values for the Osteopathic section with the associated definitions.

Character Value	Approach	Approach Definition
X	External	Procedures performed directly on the skin or mucous membrane and procedures performed indirectly by the application of external force through the skin or mucous membrane

Method (Character 6)

The method identifies the treatment method used to complete the osteopathic procedure. The available methods are:

- Articulatory-Raising
- Fascial Release
- General Mobilization
- High Velocity-Low Amplitude
- Indirect
- Low Velocity-High Amplitude
- Lymphatic Pump
- Muscle Energy-Isometric
- Muscle Energy-Isotonic
- Other

Qualifier (Character 7)

The qualifier represents an additional attribute for the procedure when applicable. Currently, there are no qualifiers in the Osteopathic section; therefore, the placeholder character value of Z should be reported.

Osteopathic Section Tables

Osteopathic Tables 7W0

Section	7	**Osteopathic**
Body System	**W**	**Anatomical Regions**
Operation	**0**	**Treatment:** Manual treatment to eliminate or alleviate somatic dysfunction and related disorders

Body Region (4th)	Approach (5th)	Method (6th)	Qualifier (7th)
0 Head	**X** External	**0** Articulatory-Raising	**Z** None
1 Cervical		**1** Fascial Release	
2 Thoracic		**2** General Mobilization	
3 Lumbar		**3** High Velocity-Low Amplitude	
4 Sacrum		**4** Indirect	
5 Pelvis		**5** Low Velocity-High Amplitude	
6 Lower Extremities		**6** Lymphatic Pump	
7 Upper Extremities		**7** Muscle Energy-Isometric	
8 Rib Cage		**8** Muscle Energy-Isotonic	
9 Abdomen		**9** Other Method	

Other Procedures Section (8C0–8E0)

Within each section of ICD-10-PCS the characters have different meanings. The seven character meanings for the Other Procedures section are illustrated here through the procedure example of Yoga therapy.

Section	Body System	Root Operation	Body Region	Approach	Method	Qualifier
Other Procedures	Physiological Systems and Anatomical Regions	Other Procedures	None	External	Other Method	Yoga Therapy
8	E	0	Z	X	Y	4

Section (Character 1)

All Other Procedures codes have a first character value of 8.

Body System (Character 2)

The alphanumeric character for the body system is placed in the second position. The following are the character values applicable for the Other Procedures section.

Character Value	Character Value Description
1	Nervous System
2	Circulatory System
9	Head and Neck Region
H	Integumentary System and Breast
K	Musculoskeletal System
U	Female Reproductive System
V	Male Reproductive System
W	Trunk Region
X	Upper Extremity
Y	Lower Extremity
Z	None

Root Operations (Character 3)

The alphanumeric character value for root operations is placed in the third position. Listed here is the root operation applicable to the Other Procedures section with its associated meaning. Note that the root operation definitions for ICD-10-PCS may differ from the terms that coders currently use with ICD-9-CM Volume 3.

Character Value	Root Operation	Root Operation Definition
0	Other Procedures	Methodologies which attempt to remediate or cure a disorder or disease

Body Region (Character 4)

For each body region the applicable body part character values will be available for procedure code construction. An example of a body region for this section is Lower Extremity.

Approach (Character 5)

The approach is the technique used to reach the procedure site. The following are the approach character values for the Other Procedures section with the associated definitions.

Character Value	Approach	Approach Definition
0	Open	Cutting through the skin or mucous membrane and any other body layers necessary to expose the site of the procedure
3	Percutaneous	Entry, by puncture or minor incision, of instrumentation through the skin or mucous membrane and any other body layers necessary to reach the site of the procedure
4	Percutaneous Endoscopic	Entry, by puncture or minor incision, of instrumentation through the skin or mucous membrane and any other body layers necessary to reach and visualize the site of the procedure
7	Via Natural or Artificial Opening	Entry of instrumentation through a natural or artificial external opening to reach the site of the procedure
8	Via Natural or Artificial Opening Endoscopic	Entry of instrumentation through a natural or artificial external opening to reach and visualize the site of the procedure
X	External	Procedures performed directly on the skin or mucous membrane and procedures performed indirectly by the application of external force through the skin or mucous membrane

Method (Character 6)

The method identifies the treatment method used to complete the other procedure. The available methods are:

- Acupuncture
- Collection
- Computer Assisted Procedure
- Near Infrared Spectroscopy
- Robotic Assisted procedure
- Therapeutic Massage
- Other

Qualifier (Character 7)

The qualifier represents an additional attribute for the procedure when applicable. In the preceding example of Yoga therapy, the qualifier of 4 was used to report that the other procedure was Yoga therapy. If there is no qualifier for a procedure, the placeholder Z is the character valve that should be reported.

Other Procedures Section Tables

Other Procedures Tables 8C0–8E0

Section	8	**Other Procedures**
Body System	C	**Indwelling Device**
Operation	0	**Other Procedures:** Methodologies which attempt to remediate or cure a disorder or disease

Body Region (4th)	Approach (5th)	Method (6th)	Qualifier (7th)
1 Nervous System	**X** External	**6** Collection	**J** Cerebrospinal Fluid **L** Other Fluid
2 Circulatory System	**X** External	**6** Collection	**K** Blood **L** Other Fluid

Section	8	**Other Procedures**
Body System	E	**Physiological Systems and Anatomical Regions**
Operation	0	**Other Procedures:** Methodologies which attempt to remediate or cure a disorder or disease

Body Region (4th)	Approach (5th)	Method (5th)	Qualifier (7th)
1 Nervous System U Female Reproductive System	**X** External	**Y** Other Method	**7** Examination
2 Circulatory System	**3** Percutaneous	**D** Near Infrared Spectroscopy	**Z** No Qualifier
9 Head and Neck Region W Trunk Region	**0** Open **3** Percutaneous **4** Percutaneous Endoscopic **7** Via Natural or Artificial Opening **8** Via Natural or Artificial Opening Endoscopic	**C** Robotic Assisted Procedure	**Z** No Qualifier
9 Head and Neck Region W Trunk Region	**X** External	**B** Computer Assisted Procedure	**F** With Fluoroscopy **G** With Computerized Tomography **H** With Magnetic Resonance Imaging **Z** No Qualifier
9 Head and Neck Region W Trunk Region	**X** External	**C** Robotic Assisted Procedure	**Z** No Qualifier
9 Head and Neck Region W Trunk Region	**X** External	**Y** Other Method	**8** Suture Removal
H Integumentary System and Breast	**3** Percutaneous	**0** Acupuncture	**0** Anesthesia **Z** No Qualifier
H Integumentary System and Breast	**X** External	**6** Collection	**2** Breast Milk
H Integumentary System and Breast	**X** External	**Y** Other Method	**9** Piercing
K Musculoskeletal System	**X** External	**1** Therapeutic Massage	**Z** No Qualifier

Continued

Section	8	Other Procedures	8E0 *Continued*
Body System	E	Physiological Systems and Anatomical Regions	
Operation	0	Other Procedures: Methodologies which attempt to remediate or cure a disorder or disease	

Body Region (4th)	Approach (5th)	Method (5th)	Qualifier (7th)
K Musculoskeletal System	**X** External	**Y** Other Method	**7** Examination
V Male Reproductive System	**X** External	**1** Therapeutic Massage	**C** Prostate **D** Rectum
V Male Reproductive System	**X** External	**6** Collection	**3** Sperm
X Upper Extremity **Y** Lower Extremity	**0** Open **3** Percutaneous **4** Percutaneous Endoscopic	**C** Robotic Assisted Procedure	**Z** No Qualifier
X Upper Extremity **Y** Lower Extremity	**X** External	**B** Computer Assisted Procedure	**F** With Fluoroscopy **G** With Computerized Tomography **H** With Magnetic Resonance Imaging **Z** No Qualifier
X Upper Extremity **Y** Lower Extremity	**X** External	**C** Robotic Assisted Procedure	**Z** No Qualifier
X Upper Extremity **Y** Lower Extremity	**X** External	**Y** Other Method	**8** Suture Removal
Z None	**X** External	**Y** Other Method	**1** In Vitro Fertilization **4** Yoga Therapy **5** Meditation **6** Isolation

Chiropractic Section (9WB)

Within each section of ICD-10-PCS the characters have different meanings. The seven character meanings for the Chiropractic section are illustrated here through the procedure example of Chiropractic treatment of cervical spine, short lever specific contact.

Section	Body System	Root Operation	Body Region	Approach	Method	Qualifier
Chiropractic	Anatomical Regions	Manipulation	Cervical	External	Short Lever Specific Contact	None
9	W	B	1	X	H	Z

Section (Character 1)

All Chiropractic procedure codes have a first character value of 9.

Body System (Character 2)

The alphanumeric character for the body system is placed in the second position. There is one character value applicable for the Chiropractic section. The character value of W is reported for anatomical regions.

Root Operations (Character 3)

The alphanumeric character value for root operations is placed in the third position. The following is the root operation applicable to the Chiropractic section with its associated meaning. Note that the root operation definitions for ICD-10-PCS may differ from the terms that coders currently use with ICD-9-CM Volume 3.

Character Value	Root Operation	Root Operation Definition
B	Manipulation	Manual procedure that involves a directed thrust to move a joint past the physiological range of motion, without exceeding the anatomical limit

Body Region (Character 4)

For each body region the applicable body part character values will be available for procedure code construction. An example of a body region for this section is Rib Cage.

Approach (Character 5)

The approach is the technique used to reach the procedure site. The following are the approach character values for the Chiropractic section with the associated definitions.

Character Value	Approach	Approach Definition
X	External	Procedures performed directly on the skin or mucous membrane and procedures performed indirectly by the application of external force through the skin or mucous membrane

Method (Character 6)

The method identifies the treatment method used to complete the chiropractic procedure. The available methods are:

- Non-Manual
- Indirect Visceral
- Extra-Articular
- Direct-Visual
- Long Lever Specific Contact
- Short Lever Specific Contact
- Long and Short Lever Specific Contact
- Mechanically Assisted
- Other

Qualifier (Character 7)

The qualifier represents an additional attribute for the procedure when applicable. Currently, there are no qualifiers in the Chiropractic section; therefore, the placeholder character value of Z should be reported.

Chiropractic Section Tables

Chiropractic Tables 9WB

Section	**9**	**Chiropractic**
Body System	**W**	**Anatomical Regions**
Operation	**B**	**Manipulation:** Manual procedure that involves a directed thrust to move a joint past the physiological range of motion, without exceeding the anatomical limit

Body Region (4th)	Approach (5th)	Method (6th)	Qualifier (7th)
0 Head	X External	B Non-Manual	Z None
1 Cervical		C Indirect Visceral	
2 Thoracic		D Extra-Articular	
3 Lumbar		F Direct Visceral	
4 Sacrum		G Long Lever Specific Contact	
5 Pelvis		H Short Lever Specific Contact	
6 Lower Extremities		J Long and Short Lever Specific Contact	
7 Upper Extremities		K Mechanically Assisted	
8 Rib Cage		L Other Method	
9 Abdomen			

Imaging Section (B00–BY4)

Within each section of ICD-10-PCS the characters have different meanings. The seven character meanings for the Imaging section are illustrated here through the procedure example of X-ray right clavicle, limited study.

Section	Body System	Root Type	Body Part	Contrast	Qualifier	Qualifier
Imaging	Non-Axial Upper Bones	Plain Radiography	Clavicle, right	None	None	None
B	P	0	4	Z	Z	Z

Section (Character 1)

All Imaging procedure codes have a first character value of B.

Body System (Character 2)

The alphanumeric character for the body system is placed in the second position. The following are the body systems applicable to the Imaging section.

Character Value	Character Value Description
0	Central Nervous System
2	Heart
3	Upper Arteries
4	Lower Arteries
5	Veins
7	Lymphatic System
8	Eye
9	Ear, Nose, Mouth and Throat
B	Respiratory System
D	Gastrointestinal System
F	Hepatobiliary System and Pancreas
G	Endocrine System
H	Skin, Subcutaneous Tissue and Breast
L	Connective Tissue
N	Skull and Facial Bones
P	Non-Axial Upper Bones
Q	Non-Axial Lower Bones
R	Axial Skeleton, Except Skull and Facial Bones
T	Urinary System

Continued

Character Value	Character Value Description	
U	Female Reproductive System	
V	Male Reproductive System	
W	Anatomical Regions	
Y	Fetus and Obstetrical	

Root Types (Character 3)

The alphanumeric character value for root types is placed in the third position. Listed here are the root types applicable to the Imaging section with their associated meaning.

Character Value	Root Type	Root Type Definition
0	Plain Radiography	Planar display of an image developed from the capture of external ionizing radiation on photographic or photoconductive plate
1	Fluoroscopy	Single plane or bi-plane real time display of an image developed from the capture of external ionizing radiation on a fluorescent screen. The image may also be stored by either digital or analog means
2	Computerized Tomography (CT Scan)	Computer reformatted digital display of multiplanar images developed from the capture of multiple exposures of external ionizing radiation
3	Magnetic Resonance Imaging (MRI)	Computer reformatted digital display of multiplanar images developed from the capture of radiofrequency signals emitted by nuclei in a body site excited within a magnetic field
4	Ultrasonography	Real time display of images of anatomy or flow information developed from the capture of reflected and attenuated high frequency sound waves

Body Part (Character 4)

For each body part the applicable body part character values will be available for procedure code construction. An example of a body part for this section is Spinal Cord.

Contrast (Character 5)

When contrast is utilized during an imaging procedure, the corresponding contrast character value should be reported in the fifth character position. The following are the contrast character values for the Imaging section:

- High Osmolar
- Low Osmolar
- Other Contrast

If contrast is not utilized, the placeholder character value of Z should be reported.

Qualifier (Character 6)

This qualifier character specifies when an image taken without contrast is followed by one with contrast. The character value of 0 is reported for Unenhanced and Enhanced.

Qualifier (Character 7)

The qualifier represents an additional attribute for the procedure when applicable. For example, ultrasonography procedures in this section include the qualifier Densitometry that is reported with the character value of 1 for some body parts. If there is no qualifier for a procedure, the placeholder Z is the character valve that should be reported.

Imaging Section Tables

Imaging Tables B00–BY4

Section	B	Imaging
Body System	0	Central Nervous System
Type	0	**Plain Radiography:** Planar display of an image developed from the capture of external ionizing radiation on photographic or photoconductive plate

Body Part (4th)	Contrast (5th)	Qualifier (6th)	Qualifier (7th)
B Spinal Cord	**0** High Osmolar **1** Low Osmolar **Y** Other Contrast **Z** None	**Z** None	**Z** None

Section	B	Imaging
Body System	0	Central Nervous System
Type	1	**Fluoroscopy:** Single plane or bi-plane real time display of an image developed from the capture of external ionizing radiation on a fluorescent screen. The image may also be stored by either digital or analog means

Body Part (4th)	Contrast (5th)	Qualifier (6th)	Qualifier (7th)
B Spinal Cord	**0** High Osmolar **1** Low Osmolar **Y** Other Contrast **Z** None	**Z** None	**Z** None

Section	B	Imaging
Body System	0	Central Nervous System
Type	2	**Computerized Tomography (CT Scan):** Computer reformatted digital display of multiplanar images developed from the capture of multiple exposures of external ionizing radiation

Body Part (4th)	Contrast (5th)	Qualifier (6th)	Qualifier (7th)
0 Brain **7** Cisterna **8** Cerebral Ventricle(s) **9** Sella Turcica/Pituitary Gland **B** Spinal Cord	**0** High Osmolar **1** Low Osmolar **Y** Other Contrast	**0** Unenhanced and Enhanced **Z** None	**Z** None
0 Brain **7** Cisterna **8** Cerebral Ventricle(s) **9** Sella Turcica/Pituitary Gland **B** Spinal Cord	**Z** None	**Z** None	**Z** None

Section	B	Imaging
Body System	0	Central Nervous System
Type	3	**Magnetic Resonance Imaging (MRI):** Computer reformatted digital display of multiplanar images developed from the capture of radiofrequency signals emitted by nuclei in a body site excited within a magnetic field

Body Part (4th)	Contrast (5th)	Qualifier (6th)	Qualifier (7th)
0 Brain **9** Sella Turcica/Pituitary Gland **B** Spinal Cord **C** Acoustic Nerves	**Y** Other Contrast	**0** Unenhanced and Enhanced **Z** None	**Z** None
0 Brain **9** Sella Turcica/Pituitary Gland **B** Spinal Cord **C** Acoustic Nerves	**Z** None	**Z** None	**Z** None

Section **B** **Imaging**
Body System **0** **Central Nervous System**
Type **4** **Ultrasonography:** Real time display of images of anatomy or flow information developed from the capture of reflected and attenuated high frequency sound waves

Body Part (4th)	Contrast (5th)	Qualifier (6th)	Qualifier (7th)
0 Brain **B** Spinal Cord	**Z** None	**Z** None	**Z** None

Section **B** **Imaging**
Body System **2** **Heart**
Type **0** **Plain Radiography:** Planar display of an image developed from the capture of external ionizing radiation on photographic or photoconductive plate

Body Part (4th)	Contrast (5th)	Qualifier (6th)	Qualifier (7th)
0 Coronary Artery, Single **1** Coronary Arteries, Multiple **2** Coronary Artery Bypass Graft, Single **3** Coronary Artery Bypass Grafts, Multiple **4** Heart, Right **5** Heart, Left **6** Heart, Right and Left **7** Internal Mammary Bypass Graft, Right **8** Internal Mammary Bypass Graft, Left **F** Bypass Graft, Other	**0** High Osmolar **1** Low Osmolar **Y** Other Contrast	**Z** None	**Z** None

Section **B** **Imaging**
Body System **2** **Heart**
Type **1** **Fluoroscopy:** Single plane or bi-plane real time display of an image developed from the capture of external ionizing radiation on a fluorescent screen. The image may also be stored by either digital or analog means

Body Part (4th)	Contrast (5th)	Qualifier (6th)	Qualifier (7th)
0 Coronary Artery, Single **1** Coronary Arteries, Multiple **2** Coronary Artery Bypass Graft, Single **3** Coronary Artery Bypass Grafts, Multiple	**0** High Osmolar **1** Low Osmolar **Y** Other Contrast	**1** Laser	**0** Intraoperative
0 Coronary Artery, Single **1** Coronary Arteries, Multiple **2** Coronary Artery Bypass Graft, Single **3** Coronary Artery Bypass Grafts, Multiple	**0** High Osmolar **1** Low Osmolar **Y** Other Contrast	**Z** None	**Z** None
4 Heart, Right **5** Heart, Left **6** Heart, Right and Left **7** Internal Mammary Bypass Graft, Right **8** Internal Mammary Bypass Graft, Left **F** Bypass Graft, Other	**0** High Osmolar **1** Low Osmolar **Y** Other Contrast	**Z** None	**Z** None

Section **B** **Imaging**
Body System **2** **Heart**
Type **2** **Computerized Tomography (CT Scan):** Computer reformatted digital display of multiplanar images developed from the capture of multiple exposures of external ionizing radiation

Body Part (4th)	Contrast (5th)	Qualifier (6th)	Qualifier (7th)
1 Coronary Arteries, Multiple **3** Coronary Artery Bypass Grafts, Multiple **6** Heart, Right and Left	**0** High Osmolar **1** Low Osmolar **Y** Other Contrast	**0** Unenhanced and Enhanced **Z** None	**Z** None

Continued

Section	B	Imaging	
Body System	2	Heart	B22 *Continued*
Type	2	**Computerized Tomography (CT Scan):** Computer reformatted digital display of multiplanar images developed from the capture of multiple exposures of external ionizing radiation	

Body Part (4ᵗʰ)	Contrast (5ᵗʰ)	Qualifier (6ᵗʰ)	Qualifier (7ᵗʰ)
1 Coronary Arteries, Multiple 3 Coronary Artery Bypass Grafts, Multiple 6 Heart, Right and Left	Z None	2 Intravascular Optical Coherence Z None	Z None

Section	B	Imaging
Body System	2	Heart
Type	3	**Magnetic Resonance Imaging (MRI):** Computer reformatted digital display of multiplanar images developed from the capture of radiofrequency signals emitted by nuclei in a body site excited within a magnetic field

Body Part (4ᵗʰ)	Contrast (5ᵗʰ)	Qualifier (6ᵗʰ)	Qualifier (7ᵗʰ)
1 Coronary Arteries, Multiple 3 Coronary Artery Bypass Grafts, Multiple 6 Heart, Right and Left	Y Other Contrast	0 Unenhanced and Enhanced Z None	Z None
1 Coronary Arteries, Multiple 3 Coronary Artery Bypass Grafts, Multiple 6 Heart, Right and Left	Z None	Z None	Z None

Section	B	Imaging
Body System	2	Heart
Type	4	**Ultrasonography:** Real time display of images of anatomy or flow information developed from the capture of reflected and attenuated high frequency sound waves

Body Part (4ᵗʰ)	Contrast (5ᵗʰ)	Qualifier (6ᵗʰ)	Qualifier (7ᵗʰ)
0 Coronary Artery, Single 1 Coronary Arteries, Multiple 4 Heart, Right 5 Heart, Left 6 Heart, Right and Left B Heart with Aorta C Pericardium D Pediatric Heart	Y Other Contrast	Z None	Z None
0 Coronary Artery, Single 1 Coronary Arteries, Multiple 4 Heart, Right 5 Heart, Left 6 Heart, Right and Left B Heart with Aorta C Pericardium D Pediatric Heart	Z None	Z None	3 Intravascular 4 Transesophageal Z None

Section	B	Imaging
Body System	3	Upper Arteries
Type	0	**Plain Radiography:** Planar display of an image developed from the capture of external ionizing radiation on photographic or photoconductive plate

Body Part (4ᵗʰ)	Contrast (5ᵗʰ)	Qualifier (6ᵗʰ)	Qualifier (7ᵗʰ)
0 Thoracic Aorta 1 Brachiocephalic-Subclavian Artery, Right 2 Subclavian Artery, Left 3 Common Carotid Artery, Right 4 Common Carotid Artery, Left 5 Common Carotid Arteries, Bilateral 6 Internal Carotid Artery, Right 7 Internal Carotid Artery, Left 8 Internal Carotid Arteries, Bilateral 9 External Carotid Artery, Right B External Carotid Artery, Left C External Carotid Arteries, Bilateral D Vertebral Artery, Right F Vertebral Artery, Left G Vertebral Arteries, Bilateral H Upper Extremity Arteries, Right J Upper Extremity Arteries, Left K Upper Extremity Arteries, Bilateral L Intercostal and Bronchial Arteries M Spinal Arteries N Upper Arteries, Other P Thoraco-Abdominal Aorta Q Cervico-Cerebral Arch R Intracranial Arteries S Pulmonary Artery, Right T Pulmonary Artery, Left	0 High Osmolar 1 Low Osmolar Y Other Contrast Z None	Z None	Z None

Section	B	Imaging
Body System	3	Upper Arteries
Type	1	**Fluoroscopy:** Single plane or bi-plane real time display of an image developed from the capture of external ionizing radiation on a fluorescent screen. The image may also be stored by either digital or analog means

Body Part (4ᵗʰ)	Contrast (5ᵗʰ)	Qualifier (6ᵗʰ)	Qualifier (7ᵗʰ)
0 Thoracic Aorta 1 Brachiocephalic-Subclavian Artery, Right 2 Subclavian Artery, Left 3 Common Carotid Artery, Right 4 Common Carotid Artery, Left 5 Common Carotid Arteries, Bilateral 6 Internal Carotid Artery, Right 7 Internal Carotid Artery, Left 8 Internal Carotid Arteries, Bilateral 9 External Carotid Artery, Right B External Carotid Artery, Left C External Carotid Arteries, Bilateral D Vertebral Artery, Right F Vertebral Artery, Left G Vertebral Arteries, Bilateral H Upper Extremity Arteries, Right J Upper Extremity Arteries, Left K Upper Extremity Arteries, Bilateral L Intercostal and Bronchial Arteries M Spinal Arteries N Upper Arteries, Other P Thoraco-Abdominal Aorta Q Cervico-Cerebral Arch R Intracranial Arteries S Pulmonary Artery, Right T Pulmonary Artery, Left	0 High Osmolar 1 Low Osmolar Y Other Contrast	1 Laser	0 Intraoperative

Continued

B31 *Continued*

Section	B	Imaging
Body System	3	**Upper Arteries**
Type	1	**Fluoroscopy:** Single plane or bi-plane real time display of an image developed from the capture of external ionizing radiation on a fluorescent screen. The image may also be stored by either digital or analog means

Body Part (4ᵗʰ)	Contrast (5ᵗʰ)	Qualifier (6ᵗʰ)	Qualifier (7ᵗʰ)
0 Thoracic Aorta	0 High Osmolar	Z None	Z None
1 Brachiocephalic-Subclavian Artery, Right	1 Low Osmolar		
2 Subclavian Artery, Left	Y Other Contrast		
3 Common Carotid Artery, Right			
4 Common Carotid Artery, Left			
5 Common Carotid Arteries, Bilateral			
6 Internal Carotid Artery, Right			
7 Internal Carotid Artery, Left			
8 Internal Carotid Arteries, Bilateral			
9 External Carotid Artery, Right			
B External Carotid Artery, Left			
C External Carotid Arteries, Bilateral			
D Vertebral Artery, Right			
F Vertebral Artery, Left			
G Vertebral Arteries, Bilateral			
H Upper Extremity Arteries, Right			
J Upper Extremity Arteries, Left			
K Upper Extremity Arteries, Bilateral			
L Intercostal and Bronchial Arteries			
M Spinal Arteries			
N Upper Arteries, Other			
P Thoraco-Abdominal Aorta			
Q Cervico-Cerebral Arch			
R Intracranial Arteries			
S Pulmonary Artery, Right			
T Pulmonary Artery, Left			
0 Thoracic Aorta	Z None	Z None	Z None
1 Brachiocephalic-Subclavian Artery, Right			
2 Subclavian Artery, Left			
3 Common Carotid Artery, Right			
4 Common Carotid Artery, Left			
5 Common Carotid Arteries, Bilateral			
6 Internal Carotid Artery, Right			
7 Internal Carotid Artery, Left			
8 Internal Carotid Arteries, Bilateral			
9 External Carotid Artery, Right			
B External Carotid Artery, Left			
C External Carotid Arteries, Bilateral			
D Vertebral Artery, Right			
F Vertebral Artery, Left			
G Vertebral Arteries, Bilateral			
H Upper Extremity Arteries, Right			
J Upper Extremity Arteries, Left			
K Upper Extremity Arteries, Bilateral			
L Intercostal and Bronchial Arteries			
M Spinal Arteries			
N Upper Arteries, Other			
P Thoraco-Abdominal Aorta			
Q Cervico-Cerebral Arch			
R Intracranial Arteries			
S Pulmonary Artery, Right			
T Pulmonary Artery, Left			

Section	B	Imaging
Body System	3	Upper Arteries
Type	2	Computerized Tomography (CT Scan): Computer reformatted digital display of multiplanar images developed from the capture of multiple exposures of external ionizing radiation

Body Part (4th)	Contrast (5th)	Qualifier (6th)	Qualifier (7th)
0 Thoracic Aorta 5 Common Carotid Arteries, Bilateral 8 Internal Carotid Arteries, Bilateral G Vertebral Arteries, Bilateral R Intracranial Arteries S Pulmonary Artery, Right T Pulmonary Artery, Left	0 High Osmolar 1 Low Osmolar Y Other Contrast	Z None	Z None
0 Thoracic Aorta 5 Common Carotid Arteries, Bilateral 8 Internal Carotid Arteries, Bilateral G Vertebral Arteries, Bilateral R Intracranial Arteries S Pulmonary Artery, Right T Pulmonary Artery, Left	Z None	2 Intravascular Optical Coherence Z None	Z None

Section	B	Imaging
Body System	3	Upper Arteries
Type	3	Magnetic Resonance Imaging (MRI): Computer reformatted digital display of multiplanar images developed from the capture of radiofrequency signals emitted by nuclei in a body site excited within a magnetic field

Body Part (4th)	Contrast (5th)	Qualifier (6th)	Qualifierv
0 Thoracic Aorta 5 Common Carotid Arteries, Bilateral 8 Internal Carotid Arteries, Bilateral G Vertebral Arteries, Bilateral H Upper Extremity Arteries, Right J Upper Extremity Arteries, Left K Upper Extremity Arteries, Bilateral M Spinal Arteries Q Cervico-Cerebral Arch R Intracranial Arteries	Y Other Contrast	0 Unenhanced and Enhanced Z None	Z None
0 Thoracic Aorta 5 Common Carotid Arteries, Bilateral 8 Internal Carotid Arteries, Bilateral G Vertebral Arteries, Bilateral H Upper Extremity Arteries, Right J Upper Extremity Arteries, Left K Upper Extremity Arteries, Bilateral M Spinal Arteries Q Cervico-Cerebral Arch R Intracranial Arteries	Z None	Z None	Z None

Section	B	Imaging
Body System	3	Upper Arteries
Type	4	**Ultrasonography:** Real time display of images of anatomy or flow information developed from the capture of reflected and attenuated high frequency sound waves

Body Part (4th)	Contrast (5th)	Qualifier (6th)	Qualifier (7th)
0 Thoracic Aorta	Z None	Z None	3 Intravascular
1 Brachiocephalic-Subclavian Artery, Right			Z None
2 Subclavian Artery, Left			
3 Common Carotid Artery, Right			
4 Common Carotid Artery, Left			
5 Common Carotid Arteries, Bilateral			
6 Internal Carotid Artery, Right			
7 Internal Carotid Artery, Left			
8 Internal Carotid Arteries, Bilateral			
H Upper Extremity Arteries, Right			
J Upper Extremity Arteries, Left			
K Upper Extremity Arteries, Bilateral			
R Intracranial Arteries			
S Pulmonary Artery, Right			
T Pulmonary Artery, Left			
V Ophthalmic Arteries			

Section	B	Imaging
Body System	4	Lower Arteries
Type	0	**Plain Radiography:** Planar display of an image developed from the capture of external ionizing radiation on photographic or photoconductive plate

Body Part (4th)	Contrast (5th)	Qualifier (6th)	Qualifier (7th)
0 Abdominal Aorta	0 High Osmolar	Z None	Z None
2 Hepatic Artery	1 Low Osmolar		
3 Splenic Arteries	Y Other Contrast		
4 Superior Mesenteric Artery			
5 Inferior Mesenteric Artery			
6 Renal Artery, Right			
7 Renal Artery, Left			
8 Renal Arteries, Bilateral			
9 Lumbar Arteries			
B Intra-Abdominal Arteries, Other			
C Pelvic Arteries			
D Aorta and Bilateral Lower Extremity Arteries			
F Lower Extremity Arteries, Right			
G Lower Extremity Arteries, Left			
J Lower Arteries, Other			
M Renal Artery Transplant			

Section	B	Imaging
Body System	4	Lower Arteries
Type	1	**Fluoroscopy:** Single plane or bi-plane real time display of an image developed from the capture of external ionizing radiation on a fluorescent screen. The image may also be stored by either digital or analog means

Body Part (4th)	Contrast (5th)	Qualifier (6th)	Qualifier (7th)
0 Abdominal Aorta 2 Hepatic Artery 3 Splenic Arteries 4 Superior Mesenteric Artery 5 Inferior Mesenteric Artery 6 Renal Artery, Right 7 Renal Artery, Left 8 Renal Arteries, Bilateral 9 Lumbar Arteries B Intra-Abdominal Arteries, Other C Pelvic Arteries D Aorta and Bilateral Lower Extremity Arteries F Lower Extremity Arteries, Right G Lower Extremity Arteries, Left J Lower Arteries, Other	0 High Osmolar 1 Low Osmolar Y Other Contrast	1 Laser	0 Intraoperative
0 Abdominal Aorta 2 Hepatic Artery 3 Splenic Arteries 4 Superior Mesenteric Artery 5 Inferior Mesenteric Artery 6 Renal Artery, Right 7 Renal Artery, Left 8 Renal Arteries, Bilateral 9 Lumbar Arteries B Intra-Abdominal Arteries, Other C Pelvic Arteries D Aorta and Bilateral Lower Extremity Arteries F Lower Extremity Arteries, Right G Lower Extremity Arteries, Left J Lower Arteries, Other	0 High Osmolar 1 Low Osmolar Y Other Contrast	Z None	Z None
0 Abdominal Aorta 2 Hepatic Artery 3 Splenic Arteries 4 Superior Mesenteric Artery 5 Inferior Mesenteric Artery 6 Renal Artery, Right 7 Renal Artery, Left 8 Renal Arteries, Bilateral 9 Lumbar Arteries B Intra-Abdominal Arteries, Other C Pelvic Arteries D Aorta and Bilateral Lower Extremity Arteries F Lower Extremity Arteries, Right G Lower Extremity Arteries, Left J Lower Arteries, Other	Z None	Z None	Z None

Section	B	Imaging
Body System	4	Lower Arteries
Type	2	**Computerized Tomography (CT Scan):** Computer reformatted digital display of multiplanar images developed from the capture of multiple exposures of external ionizing radiation

Body Part (4th)	Contrast (5th)	Qualifier (6th)	Qualifier (7th)
0 Abdominal Aorta **1** Celiac Artery **4** Superior Mesenteric Artery **8** Renal Arteries, Bilateral **C** Pelvic Arteries **F** Lower Extremity Arteries, Right **G** Lower Extremity Arteries, Left **H** Lower Extremity Arteries, Bilateral **M** Renal Artery Transplant	**0** High Osmolar **1** Low Osmolar **Y** Other Contrast	**Z** None	**Z** None
0 Abdominal Aorta **1** Celiac Artery **4** Superior Mesenteric Artery **8** Renal Arteries, Bilateral **C** Pelvic Arteries **F** Lower Extremity Arteries, Right **G** Lower Extremity Arteries, Left **H** Lower Extremity Arteries, Bilateral **M** Renal Artery Transplant	**Z** None	**2** Intravascular Optical Coherence **Z** None	**Z** None

Section	B	Imaging
Body System	4	Lower Arteries
Type	3	**Magnetic Resonance Imaging (MRI):** Computer reformatted digital display of multiplanar images developed from the capture of radiofrequency signals emitted by nuclei in a body site excited within a magnetic field

Body Part (4th)	Contrast (5th)	Qualifier (6th)	Qualifier (7th)
0 Abdominal Aorta **1** Celiac Artery **4** Superior Mesenteric Artery **8** Renal Arteries, Bilateral **C** Pelvic Arteries **F** Lower Extremity Arteries, Right **G** Lower Extremity Arteries, Left **H** Lower Extremity Arteries, Bilateral	**Y** Other Contrast	**0** Unenhanced and Enhanced **Z** None	**Z** None
0 Abdominal Aorta **1** Celiac Artery **4** Superior Mesenteric Artery **8** Renal Arteries, Bilateral **C** Pelvic Arteries **F** Lower Extremity Arteries, Right **G** Lower Extremity Arteries, Left **H** Lower Extremity Arteries, Bilateral	**Z** None	**Z** None	**Z** None

Section	B	Imaging
Body System	4	Lower Arteries
Type	4	**Ultrasonography:** Real time display of images of anatomy or flow information developed from the capture of reflected and attenuated high frequency sound waves

Body Part (4th)	Contrast (5th)	Qualifier (6th)	Qualifier (7th)
0 Abdominal Aorta 4 Superior Mesenteric Artery 5 Inferior Mesenteric Artery 6 Renal Artery, Right 7 Renal Artery, Left 8 Renal Arteries, Bilateral B Intra-Abdominal Arteries, Other F Lower Extremity Arteries, Right G Lower Extremity Arteries, Left H Lower Extremity Arteries, Bilateral K Celiac and Mesenteric Arteries L Femoral Artery N Penile Arteries	Z None	Z None	3 Intravascular Z None

Section	B	Imaging
Body System	5	Veins
Type	0	**Plain Radiography:** Planar display of an image developed from the capture of external ionizing radiation on photographic or photoconductive plate

Body Part (4th)	Contrast (5th)	Qualifier (6th)	Qualifier (7th)
0 Epidural Veins 1 Cerebral and Cerebellar Veins 2 Intracranial Sinuses 3 Jugular Veins, Right 4 Jugular Veins, Left 5 Jugular Veins, Bilateral 6 Subclavian Vein, Right 7 Subclavian Vein, Left 8 Superior Vena Cava 9 Inferior Vena Cava B Lower Extremity Veins, Right C Lower Extremity Veins, Left D Lower Extremity Veins, Bilateral F Pelvic (Iliac) Veins, Right G Pelvic (Iliac) Veins, Left H Pelvic (Iliac) Veins, Bilateral J Renal Vein, Right K Renal Vein, Left L Renal Veins, Bilateral M Upper Extremity Veins, Right N Upper Extremity Veins, Left P Upper Extremity Veins, Bilateral Q Pulmonary Vein, Right R Pulmonary Vein, Left S Pulmonary Veins, Bilateral T Portal and Splanchnic Veins V Veins, Other W Dialysis Shunt/Fistula	0 High Osmolar 1 Low Osmolar Y Other Contrast	Z None	Z None

Section	B	Imaging
Body System	5	Veins
Type	1	**Fluoroscopy:** Single plane or bi-plane real time display of an image developed from the capture of external ionizing radiation on a fluorescent screen. The image may also be stored by either digital or analog means

Body Part (4th)	Contrast (5th)	Qualifier (6th)	Qualifier (7th)
0 Epidural Veins **1** Cerebral and Cerebellar Veins **2** Intracranial Sinuses **3** Jugular Veins, Right **4** Jugular Veins, Left **5** Jugular Veins, Bilateral **6** Subclavian Vein, Right **7** Subclavian Vein, Left **8** Superior Vena Cava **9** Inferior Vena Cava **B** Lower Extremity Veins, Right **C** Lower Extremity Veins, Left **D** Lower Extremity Veins, Bilateral **F** Pelvic (Iliac) Veins, Right **G** Pelvic (Iliac) Veins, Left **H** Pelvic (Iliac) Veins, Bilateral **J** Renal Vein, Right **K** Renal Vein, Left **L** Renal Veins, Bilateral **M** Upper Extremity Veins, Right **N** Upper Extremity Veins, Left **P** Upper Extremity Veins, Bilateral **Q** Pulmonary Vein, Right **R** Pulmonary Vein, Left **S** Pulmonary Veins, Bilateral **T** Portal and Splanchnic Veins **V** Veins, Other **W** Dialysis Shunt/Fistula	**0** High Osmolar **1** Low Osmolar **Y** Other Contrast **Z** None	**Z** None	**A** Guidance **Z** None

Section	B	Imaging
Body System	5	Veins
Type	2	**Computerized Tomography (CT Scan):** Computer reformatted digital display of multiplanar images developed from the capture of multiple exposures of external ionizing radiation

Body Part (4th)	Contrast (5th)	Qualifier (6th)	Qualifier (7th)
2 Intracranial Sinuses **8** Superior Vena Cava **9** Inferior Vena Cava **F** Pelvic (Iliac) Veins, Right **G** Pelvic (Iliac) Veins, Left **H** Pelvic (Iliac) Veins, Bilateral **J** Renal Vein, Right **K** Renal Vein, Left **L** Renal Veins, Bilateral **Q** Pulmonary Vein, Right **R** Pulmonary Vein, Left **S** Pulmonary Veins, Bilateral **T** Portal and Splanchnic Veins	**0** High Osmolar **1** Low Osmolar **Y** Other Contrast	**0** Unenhanced and Enhanced **Z** None	**Z** None

Continued

Section	B	Imaging				*B52 Continued*
Body System	5	Veins				
Type	2	**Computerized Tomography (CT Scan):** Computer reformatted digital display of multiplanar images developed from the capture of multiple exposures of external ionizing radiation				

Body Part (4th)	Contrast (5th)	Qualifier (6th)	Qualifier (7th)
2 Intracranial Sinuses 8 Superior Vena Cava 9 Inferior Vena Cava F Pelvic (Iliac) Veins, Right G Pelvic (Iliac) Veins, Left H Pelvic (Iliac) Veins, Bilateral J Renal Vein, Right K Renal Vein, Left L Renal Veins, Bilateral Q Pulmonary Vein, Right R Pulmonary Vein, Left S Pulmonary Veins, Bilateral T Portal and Splanchnic Veins	Z None	2 Intravascular Optical Coherence Z None	Z None

Section	B	Imaging
Body System	5	Veins
Type	3	**Magnetic Resonance Imaging (MRI):** Computer reformatted digital display of multiplanar images developed from the capture of radiofrequency signals emitted by nuclei in a body site excited within a magnetic field

Body Part (4th)	Contrast (5th)	Qualifier (6th)	Qualifier (7th)
1 Cerebral and Cerebellar Veins 2 Intracranial Sinuses 5 Jugular Veins, Bilateral 8 Superior Vena Cava 9 Inferior Vena Cava B Lower Extremity Veins, Right C Lower Extremity Veins, Left D Lower Extremity Veins, Bilateral H Pelvic (Iliac) Veins, Bilateral L Renal Veins, Bilateral M Upper Extremity Veins, Right N Upper Extremity Veins, Left P Upper Extremity Veins, Bilateral S Pulmonary Veins, Bilateral T Portal and Splanchnic Veins V Veins, Other	Y Other Contrast	0 Unenhanced and Enhanced Z None	Z None
1 Cerebral and Cerebellar Veins 2 Intracranial Sinuses 5 Jugular Veins, Bilateral 8 Superior Vena Cava 9 Inferior Vena Cava B Lower Extremity Veins, Right C Lower Extremity Veins, Left D Lower Extremity Veins, Bilateral H Pelvic (Iliac) Veins, Bilateral L Renal Veins, Bilateral M Upper Extremity Veins, Right N Upper Extremity Veins, Left P Upper Extremity Veins, Bilateral S Pulmonary Veins, Bilateral T Portal and Splanchnic Veins V Veins, Other	Z None	Z None	Z None

Section	B	Imaging
Body System	5	Veins
Type	4	**Ultrasonography:** Real time display of images of anatomy or flow information developed from the capture of reflected and attenuated high frequency sound waves

Body Part (4th)	Contrast (5th)	Qualifier (6th)	Qualifier (7th)
3 Jugular Veins, Right 4 Jugular Veins, Left 6 Subclavian Vein, Right 7 Subclavian Vein, Left 8 Superior Vena Cava 9 Inferior Vena Cava B Lower Extremity Veins, Right C Lower Extremity Veins, Left D Lower Extremity Veins, Bilateral J Renal Vein, Right K Renal Vein, Left L Renal Veins, Bilateral M Upper Extremity Veins, Right N Upper Extremity Veins, Left P Upper Extremity Veins, Bilateral T Portal and Splanchnic Veins	Z None	Z None	3 Intravascular A Guidance Z None

Section	B	Imaging
Body System	7	Lymphatic System
Type	0	**Plain Radiography:** Planar display of an image developed from the capture of external ionizing radiation on photographic or photoconductive plate

Body Part (4th)	Contrast (5th)	Qualifier (6th)	Qualifier (7th)
0 Abdominal/Retroperitoneal Lymphatics, Unilateral 1 Abdominal/Retroperitoneal Lymphatics, Bilateral 4 Lymphatics, Head and Neck 5 Upper Extremity Lymphatics, Right 6 Upper Extremity Lymphatics, Left 7 Upper Extremity Lymphatics, Bilateral 8 Lower Extremity Lymphatics, Right 9 Lower Extremity Lymphatics, Left B Lower Extremity Lymphatics, Bilateral C Lymphatics, Pelvic	0 High Osmolar 1 Low Osmolar Y Other Contrast	Z None	Z None

Section	B	Imaging
Body System	8	Eye
Type	0	**Plain Radiography:** Planar display of an image developed from the capture of external ionizing radiation on photographic or photoconductive plate

Body Part (4th)	Contrast (5th)	Qualifierv	Qualifier (7th)
0 Lacrimal Duct, Right 1 Lacrimal Duct, Left 2 Lacrimal Ducts, Bilateral	0 High Osmolar 1 Low Osmolar Y Other Contrast	Z None	Z None
3 Optic Foramina, Right 4 Optic Foramina, Left 5 Eye, Right 6 Eye, Left 7 Eyes, Bilateral	Z None	Z None	Z None

Section	B	Imaging
Body System	8	Eye
Type	2	**Computerized Tomography (CT Scan):** Computer reformatted digital display of multiplanar images developed from the capture of multiple exposures of external ionizing radiation

Body Part (4th)	Contrast (5th)	Qualifier (6th)	Qualifier (7th)
5 Eye, Right 6 Eye, Left 7 Eyes, Bilateral	0 High Osmolar 1 Low Osmolar Y Other Contrast	0 Unenhanced and Enhanced Z None	Z None
5 Eye, Right 6 Eye, Left 7 Eyes, Bilateral	Z None	Z None	Z None

Section	B	Imaging
Body System	8	Eye
Type	3	**Magnetic Resonance Imaging (MRI):** Computer reformatted digital display of multiplanar images developed from the capture of radiofrequency signals emitted by nuclei in a body site excited within a magnetic field

Body Part (4th)	Contrast (5th)	Qualifier (6th)	Qualifier (7th)
5 Eye, Right 6 Eye, Left 7 Eyes, Bilateral	Y Other Contrast	0 Unenhanced and Enhanced Z None	Z None
5 Eye, Right 6 Eye, Left 7 Eyes, Bilateral	Z None	Z None	Z None

Section	B	Imaging
Body System	8	Eye
Type	4	**Ultrasonography:** Real time display of images of anatomy or flow information developed from the capture of reflected and attenuated high frequency sound waves

Body Part (4th)	Contrast (5th)	Qualifier (6th)	Qualifier (7th)
5 Eye, Right 6 Eye, Left 7 Eyes, Bilateral	Z None	Z None	Z None

Section	B	Imaging
Body System	9	Ear, Nose, Mouth and Throat
Type	0	**Plain Radiography:** Planar display of an image developed from the capture of external ionizing radiation on photographic or photoconductive plate

Body Part (4th)	Contrast (5th)	Qualifier (6th)	Qualifier (7th)
2 Paranasal Sinuses F Nasopharynx/Oropharynx H Mastoids	Z None	Z None	Z None
4 Parotid Gland, Right 5 Parotid Gland, Left 6 Parotid Glands, Bilateral 7 Submandibular Gland, Right 8 Submandibular Gland, Left 9 Submandibular Glands, Bilateral B Salivary Gland, Right C Salivary Gland, Left D Salivary Glands, Bilateral	0 High Osmolar 1 Low Osmolar Y Other Contrast	Z None	Z None

Section	B	Imaging
Body System	9	**Ear, Nose, Mouth and Throat**
Type	1	**Fluoroscopy:** Single plane or bi-plane real time display of an image developed from the capture of external ionizing radiation on a fluorescent screen. The image may also be stored by either digital or analog means

Body Part (4th)	Contrast (5th)	Qualifier (6th)	Qualifier (7th)
G Pharynx and Epiglottis J Larynx	Y Other Contrast Z None	Z None	Z None

Section	B	Imaging
Body System	9	**Ear, Nose, Mouth and Throat**
Type	2	**Computerized Tomography (CT Scan):** Computer reformatted digital display of multiplanar images developed from the capture of multiple exposures of external ionizing radiation

Body Part (4th)	Contrast (5th)	Qualifier (6th)	Qualifier (7th)
0 Ear 2 Paranasal Sinuses 6 Parotid Glands, Bilateral 9 Submandibular Glands, Bilateral D Salivary Glands, Bilateral F Nasopharynx/Oropharynx J Larynx	0 High Osmolar 1 Low Osmolar Y Other Contrast	0 Unenhanced and Enhanced Z None	Z None
0 Ear 2 Paranasal Sinuses 6 Parotid Glands, Bilateral 9 Submandibular Glands, Bilateral D Salivary Glands, Bilateral F Nasopharynx/Oropharynx J Larynx	Z None	Z None	Z None

Section	B	Imaging
Body System	9	**Ear, Nose, Mouth and Throat**
Type	3	**Magnetic Resonance Imaging (MRI):** Computer reformatted digital display of multiplanar images developed from the capture of radiofrequency signals emitted by nuclei in a body site excited within a magnetic field

Body Part (4th)	Contrast (5th)	Qualifier (6th)	Qualifier (7th)
0 Ear 2 Paranasal Sinuses 6 Parotid Glands, Bilateral 9 Submandibular Glands, Bilateral D Salivary Glands, Bilateral F Nasopharynx/Oropharynx J Larynx	Y Other Contrast	0 Unenhanced and Enhanced Z None	Z None
0 Ear 2 Paranasal Sinuses 6 Parotid Glands, Bilateral 9 Submandibular Glands, Bilateral D Salivary Glands, Bilateral F Nasopharynx/Oropharynx J Larynx	Z None	Z None	Z None

Section	B	Imaging
Body System	B	Respiratory System
Type	0	**Plain Radiography:** Planar display of an image developed from the capture of external ionizing radiation on photographic or photoconductive plate

Body Part (4th)	Contrast (5th)	Qualifier (6th)	Qualifier (7th)
7 Tracheobronchial Tree, Right 8 Tracheobronchial Tree, Left 9 Tracheobronchial Trees, Bilateral	Y Other Contrast	Z None	Z None
D Upper Airways	Z None	Z None	Z None

Section	B	Imaging
Body System	B	Respiratory System
Type	1	**Fluoroscopy:** Single plane or bi-plane real time display of an image developed from the capture of external ionizing radiation on a fluorescent screen. The image may also be stored by either digital or analog means

Body Part (4th)	Contrast (5th)	Qualifier (6th)	Qualifier (7th)
2 Lung, Right 3 Lung, Left 4 Lungs, Bilateral 6 Diaphragm C Mediastinum D Upper Airways	Z None	Z None	Z None
7 Tracheobronchial Tree, Right 8 Tracheobronchial Tree, Left 9 Tracheobronchial Trees, Bilateral	Y Other Contrast	Z None	Z None

Section	B	Imaging
Body System	B	Respiratory System
Type	2	**Computerized Tomography (CT Scan):** Computer reformatted digital display of multiplanar images developed from the capture of multiple exposures of external ionizing radiation

Body Part (4th)	Contrast (5th)	Qualifier (6th)	Qualifier (7th)
4 Lungs, Bilateral 7 Tracheobronchial Tree, Right 8 Tracheobronchial Tree, Left 9 Tracheobronchial Trees, Bilateral F Trachea/Airways	0 High Osmolar 1 Low Osmolar Y Other Contrast	0 Unenhanced and Enhanced Z None	Z None
4 Lungs, Bilateral 7 Tracheobronchial Tree, Right 8 Tracheobronchial Tree, Left 9 Tracheobronchial Trees, Bilateral F Trachea/Airways	Z None	Z None	Z None

Section	B	Imaging
Body System	B	Respiratory System
Type	3	**Magnetic Resonance Imaging (MRI):** Computer reformatted digital display of multiplanar images developed from the capture of radiofrequency signals emitted by nuclei in a body site excited within a magnetic field

Body Part (4th)	Contrast (5th)	Qualifier (6th)	Qualifier (7th)
G Lung Apices	Y Other Contrast	0 Unenhanced and Enhanced Z None	Z None
G Lung Apices	Z None	Z None	Z None

Section	B	Imaging
Body System	B	Respiratory System
Type	4	**Ultrasonography:** Real time display of images of anatomy or flow information developed from the capture of reflected and attenuated high frequency sound waves

Body Part (4ᵗʰ)	Contrast (5ᵗʰ)	Qualifier (6ᵗʰ)	Qualifier (7ᵗʰ)
B Pleura **C** Mediastinum	**Z** None	**Z** None	**Z** None

Section	B	Imaging
Body System	D	Gastrointestinal System
Type	1	**Fluoroscopy:** Single plane or bi-plane real time display of an image developed from the capture of external ionizing radiation on a fluorescent screen. The image may also be stored by either digital or analog means

Body Part (4ᵗʰ)	Contrast (5ᵗʰ)	Qualifier (6ᵗʰ)	Qualifier (7ᵗʰ)
1 Esophagus **2** Stomach **3** Small Bowel **4** Colon **5** Upper GI **6** Upper GI and Small Bowel **9** Duodenum **B** Mouth/Oropharynx	**Y** Other Contrast **Z** None	**Z** None	**Z** None

Section	B	Imaging
Body System	D	Gastrointestinal System
Type	2	**Computerized Tomography (CT Scan):** Computer reformatted digital display of multiplanar images developed from the capture of multiple exposures of external ionizing radiation

Body Part (4ᵗʰ)	Contrast (5ᵗʰ)	Qualifier (6ᵗʰ)	Qualifier (7ᵗʰ)
4 Colon	**0** High Osmolar **1** Low Osmolar **Y** Other Contrast	**0** Unenhanced and Enhanced **Z** None	**Z** None
4 Colon	**Z** None	**Z** None	**Z** None

Section	B	Imaging
Body System	D	Gastrointestinal System
Type	4	**Ultrasonography:** Real time display of images of anatomy or flow information developed from the capture of reflected and attenuated high frequency sound waves

Body Part (4ᵗʰ)	Contrast (5ᵗʰ)	Qualifier (6ᵗʰ)	Qualifier (7ᵗʰ)
1 Esophagus **2** Stomach **7** Gastrointestinal Tract **8** Appendix **9** Duodenum **C** Rectum	**Z** None	**Z** None	**Z** None

Section	B	Imaging
Body System	F	Hepatobiliary System and Pancreas
Type	0	**Plain Radiography:** Planar display of an image developed from the capture of external ionizing radiation on photographic or photoconductive plate

Body Part (4ᵗʰ)	Contrast (5ᵗʰ)	Qualifier (6ᵗʰ)	Qualifier (7ᵗʰ)
0 Bile Ducts **3** Gallbladder and Bile Ducts **C** Hepatobiliary System, All	**0** High Osmolar **1** Low Osmolar **Y** Other Contrast	**Z** None	**Z** None

Section	B	Imaging
Body System	F	Hepatobiliary System and Pancreas
Type	1	**Fluoroscopy:** Single plane or bi-plane real time display of an image developed from the capture of external ionizing radiation on a fluorescent screen. The image may also be stored by either digital or analog means

Body Part (4th)	Contrast (5th)	Qualifier (6th)	Qualifier (7th)
0 Bile Ducts 1 Biliary and Pancreatic Ducts 2 Gallbladder 3 Gallbladder and Bile Ducts 4 Gallbladder, Bile Ducts and Pancreatic Ducts 8 Pancreatic Ducts	0 High Osmolar 1 Low Osmolar Y Other Contrast	Z None	Z None

Section	B	Imaging
Body System	F	Hepatobiliary System and Pancreas
Type	2	**Computerized Tomography (CT Scan):** Computer reformatted digital display of multiplanar images developed from the capture of multiple exposures of external ionizing radiation

Body Part (4th)	Contrast (5th)	Qualifier (6th)	Qualifier (7th)
5 Liver 6 Liver and Spleen 7 Pancreas C Hepatobiliary System, All	0 High Osmolar 1 Low Osmolar Y Other Contrast	0 Unenhanced and Enhanced Z None	Z None
5 Liver 6 Liver and Spleen 7 Pancreas C Hepatobiliary System, All	Z None	Z None	Z None

Section	B	Imaging
Body System	F	Hepatobiliary System and Pancreas
Type	3	**Magnetic Resonance Imaging (MRI):** Computer reformatted digital display of multiplanar images developed from the capture of radiofrequency signals emitted by nuclei in a body site excited within a magnetic field

Body Part (4th)	Contrast (5th)	Qualifier (6th)	Qualifier (7th)
5 Liver 6 Liver and Spleen 7 Pancreas	Y Other Contrast	0 Unenhanced and Enhanced Z None	Z None
5 Liver 6 Liver and Spleen 7 Pancreas	Z None	Z None	Z None

Section	B	Imaging
Body System	F	Hepatobiliary System and Pancreas
Type	4	**Ultrasonography:** Real time display of images of anatomy or flow information developed from the capture of reflected and attenuated high frequency sound waves

Body Part (4th)	Contrast (5th)	Qualifier (6th)	Qualifier (7th)
0 Bile Ducts 2 Gallbladder 3 Gallbladder and Bile Ducts 5 Liver 6 Liver and Spleen 7 Pancreas C Hepatobiliary System, All	Z None	Z None	Z None

Section	B	Imaging
Body System	G	Endocrine System
Type	2	**Computerized Tomography (CT Scan):** Computer reformatted digital display of multiplanar images developed from the capture of multiple exposures of external ionizing radiation

Body Part (4ᵗʰ)	Contrast (5ᵗʰ)	Qualifier (6ᵗʰ)	Qualifier (7ᵗʰ)
2 Adrenal Glands, Bilateral 3 Parathyroid Glands 4 Thyroid Gland	0 High Osmolar 1 Low Osmolar Y Other Contrast	0 Unenhanced and Enhanced Z None	Z None
2 Adrenal Glands, Bilateral 3 Parathyroid Glands 4 Thyroid Gland	Z None	Z None	Z None

Section	B	Imaging
Body System	G	Endocrine System
Type	3	**Magnetic Resonance Imaging (MRI):** Computer reformatted digital display of multiplanar images developed from the capture of radiofrequency signals emitted by nuclei in a body site excited within a magnetic field

Body Part (4ᵗʰ)	Contrast (5ᵗʰ)	Qualifier (6ᵗʰ)	Qualifier (7ᵗʰ)
2 Adrenal Glands, Bilateral 3 Parathyroid Glands 4 Thyroid Gland	Y Other Contrast	0 Unenhanced and Enhanced Z None	Z None
2 Adrenal Glands, Bilateral 3 Parathyroid Glands 4 Thyroid Gland	Z None	Z None	Z None

Section	B	Imaging
Body System	G	Endocrine System
Type	4	**Ultrasonography:** Real time display of images of anatomy or flow information developed from the capture of reflected and attenuated high frequency sound waves

Body Part (4ᵗʰ)	Contrast (5ᵗʰ)	Qualifier (6ᵗʰ)	Qualifier (7ᵗʰ)
0 Adrenal Gland, Right 1 Adrenal Gland, Left 2 Adrenal Glands, Bilateral 3 Parathyroid Glands 4 Thyroid Gland	Z None	Z None	Z None

Section	B	Imaging
Body System	H	Skin, Subcutaneous Tissue and Breast
Type	0	**Plain Radiography:** Planar display of an image developed from the capture of external ionizing radiation on photographic or photoconductive plate

Body Part (4ᵗʰ)	Contrast (5ᵗʰ)	Qualifier (6ᵗʰ)	Qualifier (7ᵗʰ)
0 Breast, Right 1 Breast, Left 2 Breasts, Bilateral	Z None	Z None	Z None
3 Single Mammary Duct, Right 4 Single Mammary Duct, Left 5 Multiple Mammary Ducts, Right 6 Multiple Mammary Ducts, Left	0 High Osmolar 1 Low Osmolar Y Other Contrast Z None	Z None	Z None

Section	B	Imaging
Body System	H	Skin, Subcutaneous Tissue and Breast
Type	3	**Magnetic Resonance Imaging (MRI):** Computer reformatted digital display of multiplanar images developed from the capture of radiofrequency signals emitted by nuclei in a body site excited within a magnetic field

Body Part (4th)	Contrast (5th)	Qualifier (6th)	Qualifier (7th)
0 Breast, Right 1 Breast, Left 2 Breasts, Bilateral D Subcutaneous Tissue, Head/Neck F Subcutaneous Tissue, Upper Extremity G Subcutaneous Tissue, Thorax H Subcutaneous Tissue, Abdomen and Pelvis J Subcutaneous Tissue, Lower Extremity	Y Other Contrast	0 Unenhanced and Enhanced Z None	Z None
0 Breast, Right 1 Breast, Left 2 Breasts, Bilateral D Subcutaneous Tissue, Head/Neck F Subcutaneous Tissue, Upper Extremity G Subcutaneous Tissue, Thorax H Subcutaneous Tissue, Abdomen and Pelvis J Subcutaneous Tissue, Lower Extremity	Z None	Z None	Z None

Section	B	Imaging
Body System	H	Skin, Subcutaneous Tissue and Breast
Type	4	**Ultrasonography:** Real time display of images of anatomy or flow information developed from the capture of reflected and attenuated high frequency sound waves

Body Part (4th)	Contrast (5th)	Qualifier (6th)	Qualifier (7th)
0 Breast, Right 1 Breast, Left 2 Breasts, Bilateral 7 Extremity, Upper 8 Extremity, Lower 9 Abdominal Wall B Chest Wall C Head and Neck	Z None	Z None	Z None

Section	B	Imaging
Body System	L	Connective Tissue
Type	3	**Magnetic Resonance Imaging (MRI):** Computer reformatted digital display of multiplanar images developed from the capture of radiofrequency signals emitted by nuclei in a body site excited within a magnetic field

Body Part (4th)	Contrast (5th)	Qualifier (6th)	Qualifier (7th)
0 Connective Tissue, Upper Extremity 1 Connective Tissue, Lower Extremity 2 Tendons, Upper Extremity 3 Tendons, Lower Extremity	Y Other Contrast	0 Unenhanced and Enhanced Z None	Z None
0 Connective Tissue, Upper Extremity 1 Connective Tissue, Lower Extremity 2 Tendons, Upper Extremity 3 Tendons, Lower Extremity	Z None	Z None	Z None

Section	B	Imaging
Body System	L	Connective Tissue
Type	4	**Ultrasonography:** Real time display of images of anatomy or flow information developed from the capture of reflected and attenuated high frequency sound waves

Body Part (4th)	Contrast (5th)	Qualifier (6th)	Qualifier (7th)
0 Connective Tissue, Upper Extremity 1 Connective Tissue, Lower Extremity 2 Tendons, Upper Extremity 3 Tendons, Lower Extremity	Z None	Z None	Z None

Section	B	Imaging
Body System	N	Skull and Facial Bones
Type	0	**Plain Radiography:** Planar display of an image developed from the capture of external ionizing radiation on photographic or photoconductive plate

Body Part (4th)	Contrast (5th)	Qualifier (6th)	Qualifier (7th)
0 Skull 1 Orbit, Right 2 Orbit, Left 3 Orbits, Bilateral 4 Nasal Bones 5 Facial Bones 6 Mandible B Zygomatic Arch, Right C Zygomatic Arch, Left D Zygomatic Arches, Bilateral G Tooth, Single H Teeth, Multiple J Teeth, All	Z None	Z None	Z None
7 Temporomandibular Joint, Right 8 Temporomandibular Joint, Left 9 Temporomandibular Joints, Bilateral	0 High Osmolar 1 Low Osmolar Y Other Contrast Z None	Z None	Z None

Section	B	Imaging
Body System	N	Skull and Facial Bones
Type	1	**Fluoroscopy:** Single plane or bi-plane real time display of an image developed from the capture of external ionizing radiation on a fluorescent screen. The image may also be stored by either digital or analog means

Body Part (4th)	Contrast (5th)	Qualifier (6th)	Qualifier (7th)
7 Temporomandibular Joint, Right 8 Temporomandibular Joint, Left 9 Temporomandibular Joints, Bilateral	0 High Osmolar 1 Low Osmolar Y Other Contrast Z None	Z None	Z None

Section	B	Imaging
Body System	N	Skull and Facial Bones
Type	2	**Computerized Tomography (CT Scan):** Computer reformatted digital display of multiplanar images developed from the capture of multiple exposures of external ionizing radiation

Body Part (4th)	Contrast (5th)	Qualifier (6th)	Qualifier (7th)
0 Skull 3 Orbits, Bilateral 5 Facial Bones 6 Mandible 9 Temporomandibular Joints, Bilateral F Temporal Bones	0 High Osmolar 1 Low Osmolar Y Other Contrast Z None	Z None	Z None

Section	B	Imaging
Body System	N	Skull and Facial Bones
Type	3	Magnetic Resonance Imaging (MRI): Computer reformatted digital display of multiplanar images developed from the capture of radiofrequency signals emitted by nuclei in a body site excited within a magnetic field

Body Part (4th)	Contrast (5th)	Qualifier (6th)	Qualifier (7th)
9 Temporomandibular Joints, Bilateral	Y Other Contrast Z None	Z None	Z None

Section	B	Imaging
Body System	P	Non-Axial Upper Bones
Type	0	Plain Radiography: Planar display of an image developed from the capture of external ionizing radiation on photographic or photoconductive plate

Body Part (4th)	Contrast (5th)	Qualifier (6th)	Qualifier (7th)
0 Sternoclavicular Joint, Right 1 Sternoclavicular Joint, Left 2 Sternoclavicular Joints, Bilateral 3 Acromioclavicular Joints, Bilateral 4 Clavicle, Right 5 Clavicle, Left 6 Scapula, Right 7 Scapula, Left A Humerus, Right B Humerus, Left E Upper Arm, Right F Upper Arm, Left J Forearm, Right K Forearm, Left N Hand, Right P Hand, Left R Finger(s), Right S Finger(s), Left X Ribs, Right Y Ribs, Left	Z None	Z None	Z None
8 Shoulder, Right 9 Shoulder, Left C Hand/Finger Joint, Right D Hand/Finger Joint, Left G Elbow, Right H Elbow, Left L Wrist, Right M Wrist, Left	0 High Osmolar 1 Low Osmolar Y Other Contrast Z None	Z None	Z None

Section	B	Imaging
Body System	P	Non-Axial Upper Bones
Type	1	**Fluoroscopy:** Single plane or bi-plane real time display of an image developed from the capture of external ionizing radiation on a fluorescent screen. The image may also be stored by either digital or analog means

Body Part (4th)	Contrast (5th)	Qualifier (6th)	Qualifier (7th)
0 Sternoclavicular Joint, Right 1 Sternoclavicular Joint, Left 2 Sternoclavicular Joints, Bilateral 3 Acromioclavicular Joints, Bilateral 4 Clavicle, Right 5 Clavicle, Left 6 Scapula, Right 7 Scapula, Left A Humerus, Right B Humerus, Left E Upper Arm, Right F Upper Arm, Left J Forearm, Right K Forearm, Left N Hand, Right P Hand, Left R Finger(s), Right S Finger(s), Left X Ribs, Right Y Ribs, Left	Z None	Z None	Z None
8 Shoulder, Right 9 Shoulder, Left L Wrist, Right M Wrist, Left	0 High Osmolar 1 Low Osmolar Y Other Contrast Z None	Z None	Z None
C Hand/Finger Joint, Right D Hand/Finger Joint, Left G Elbow, Right H Elbow, Left	0 High Osmolar 1 Low Osmolar Y Other Contrast	Z None	Z None

Section	B	Imaging
Body System	P	Non-Axial Upper Bones
Type	2	**Computerized Tomography (CT Scan):** Computer reformatted digital display of multiplanar images developed from the capture of multiple exposures of external ionizing radiation

Body Part (4th)	Contrast (5th)	Qualifier (6th)	Qualifier (7th)
0 Sternoclavicular Joint, Right 1 Sternoclavicular Joint, Left W Thorax	0 High Osmolar 1 Low Osmolar Y Other Contrast	Z None	Z None

Continued

Section	B	Imaging
Body System	P	Non-Axial Upper Bones
Type	2	**Computerized Tomography (CT Scan):** Computer reformatted digital display of multiplanar images developed from the capture of multiple exposures of external ionizing radiation

Body Part (4ᵗʰ)	Contrast (5ᵗʰ)	Qualifier (6ᵗʰ)	Qualifier (7ᵗʰ)
2 Sternoclavicular Joints, Bilateral 3 Acromioclavicular Joints, Bilateral 4 Clavicle, Right 5 Clavicle, Left 6 Scapula, Right 7 Scapula, Left 8 Shoulder, Right 9 Shoulder, Left A Humerus, Right B Humerus, Left E Upper Arm, Right F Upper Arm, Left G Elbow, Right H Elbow, Left J Forearm, Right K Forearm, Left L Wrist, Right M Wrist, Left N Hand, Right P Hand, Left Q Hands and Wrists, Bilateral R Finger(s), Right S Finger(s), Left T Upper Extremity, Right U Upper Extremity, Left V Upper Extremities, Bilateral X Ribs, Right Y Ribs, Left	0 High Osmolar 1 Low Osmolar Y Other Contrast Z None	Z None	Z None
C Hand/Finger Joint, Right D Hand/Finger Joint, Left	Z None	Z None	Z None

Section	B	Imaging
Body System	P	Non-Axial Upper Bones
Type	3	**Magnetic Resonance Imaging (MRI):** Computer reformatted digital display of multiplanar images developed from the capture of radiofrequency signals emitted by nuclei in a body site excited within a magnetic field

Body Part (4ᵗʰ)	Contrast (5ᵗʰ)	Qualifier (6ᵗʰ)	Qualifier (7ᵗʰ)
8 Shoulder, Right 9 Shoulder, Left C Hand/Finger Joint, Right D Hand/Finger Joint, Left E Upper Arm, Right F Upper Arm, Left G Elbow, Right H Elbow, Left J Forearm, Right K Forearm, Left L Wrist, Right M Wrist, Left	Y Other Contrast	0 Unenhanced and Enhanced Z None	Z None

Continued

Section   **B**   **Imaging**   BP3 *Continued*
Body System   **P**   **Non-Axial Upper Bones**
Type   **3**   **Magnetic Resonance Imaging (MRI):** Computer reformatted digital display of multiplanar images developed from the capture of radiofrequency signals emitted by nuclei in a body site excited within a magnetic field

Body Part (4th)	Contrast (5th)	Qualifier (6th)	Qualifier (7th)
8 Shoulder, Right 9 Shoulder, Left C Hand/Finger Joint, Right D Hand/Finger Joint, Left E Upper Arm, Right F Upper Arm, Left G Elbow, Right H Elbow, Left J Forearm, Right K Forearm, Left L Wrist, Right M Wrist, Left	Z None	Z None	Z None

Section   **B**   **Imaging**
Body System   **P**   **Non-Axial Upper Bones**
Type   **4**   **Ultrasonography:** Real time display of images of anatomy or flow information developed from the capture of reflected and attenuated high frequency sound waves

Body Part (4th)	Contrast (5th)	Qualifier (6th)	Qualifier (7th)
8 Shoulder, Right 9 Shoulder, Left G Elbow, Right H Elbow, Left L Wrist, Right M Wrist, Left N Hand, Right P Hand, Left	Z None	Z None	1 Densitometry Z None

Section   **B**   **Imaging**
Body System   **Q**   **Non-Axial Lower Bones**
Type   **0**   **Plain Radiography:** Planar display of an image developed from the capture of external ionizing radiation on photographic or photoconductive plate

Body Part (4th)	Contrast (5th)	Qualifier (6th)	Qualifier (7th)
0 Hip, Right 1 Hip, Left	0 High Osmolar 1 Low Osmolar Y Other Contrast	Z None	Z None
0 Hip, Right 1 Hip, Left	Z None	Z None	1 Densitometry Z None
3 Femur, Right 4 Femur, Left	Z None	Z None	1 Densitometry Z None
7 Knee, Right 8 Knee, Left G Ankle, Right H Ankle, Left	0 High Osmolar 1 Low Osmolar Y Other Contrast Z None	Z None	Z None

Continued

BQ0 Continued

Section	B	Imaging
Body System	Q	Non-Axial Lower Bones
Type	0	Plain Radiography: Planar display of an image developed from the capture of external ionizing radiation on photographic or photoconductive plate

Body Part (4th)	Contrast (5th)	Qualifier (6th)	Qualifier (7th)
D Lower Leg, Right F Lower Leg, Left J Calcaneus, Right K Calcaneus, Left L Foot, Right M Foot, Left P Toe(s), Right Q Toe(s), Left V Patella, Right W Patella, Left	Z None	Z None	Z None
X Foot/Toe Joint, Right Y Foot/Toe Joint, Left	0 High Osmolar 1 Low Osmolar Y Other Contrast	Z None	Z None

Section	B	Imaging
Body System	Q	Non-Axial Lower Bones
Type	1	Fluoroscopy: Single plane or bi-plane real time display of an image developed from the capture of external ionizing radiation on a fluorescent screen. The image may also be stored by either digital or analog means

Body Part (4th)	Contrast (5th)	Qualifier (6th)	Qualifier (7th)
0 Hip, Right 1 Hip, Left 7 Knee, Right 8 Knee, Left G Ankle, Right H Ankle, Left X Foot/Toe Joint, Right Y Foot/Toe Joint, Left	0 High Osmolar 1 Low Osmolar Y Other Contrast Z None	Z None	Z None
3 Femur, Right 4 Femur, Left D Lower Leg, Right F Lower Leg, Left J Calcaneus, Right K Calcaneus, Left L Foot, Right M Foot, Left P Toe(s), Right Q Toe(s), Left V Patella, Right W Patella, Left	Z None	Z None	Z None

Section	B	Imaging
Body System	Q	**Non-Axial Lower Bones**
Type	2	**Computerized Tomography (CT Scan):** Computer reformatted digital display of multiplanar images developed from the capture of multiple exposures of external ionizing radiation

Body Part (4th)	Contrast (5th)	Qualifier (6th)	Qualifier (7th)
0 Hip, Right **1** Hip, Left **3** Femur, Right **4** Femur, Left **7** Knee, Right **8** Knee, Left **D** Lower Leg, Right **F** Lower Leg, Left **G** Ankle, Right **H** Ankle, Left **J** Calcaneus, Right **K** Calcaneus, Left **L** Foot, Right **M** Foot, Left **P** Toe(s), Right **Q** Toe(s), Left **R** Lower Extremity, Right **S** Lower Extremity, Left **V** Patella, Right **W** Patella, Left **X** Foot/Toe Joint, Right **Y** Foot/Toe Joint, Left	**0** High Osmolar **1** Low Osmolar **Y** Other Contrast **Z** None	**Z** None	**Z** None
B Tibia/Fibula, Right **C** Tibia/Fibula, Left	**0** High Osmolar **1** Low Osmolar **Y** Other Contrast	**Z** None	**Z** None

Section	B	Imaging
Body System	Q	**Non-Axial Lower Bones**
Type	3	**Magnetic Resonance Imaging (MRI):** Computer reformatted digital display of multiplanar images developed from the capture of radiofrequency signals emitted by nuclei in a body site excited within a magnetic field

Body Part (4th)	Contrast (5th)	Qualifier (6th)	Qualifier (7th)
0 Hip, Right **1** Hip, Left **3** Femur, Right **4** Femur, Left **7** Knee, Right **8** Knee, Left **D** Lower Leg, Right **F** Lower Leg, Left **G** Ankle, Right **H** Ankle, Left **J** Calcaneus, Right **K** Calcaneus, Left **L** Foot, Right **M** Foot, Left **P** Toe(s), Right **Q** Toe(s), Left **V** Patella, Right **W** Patella, Left	**Y** Other Contrast	**0** Unenhanced and Enhanced **Z** None	**Z** None

Continued

Section	B	Imaging
Body System	Q	**Non-Axial Lower Bones**
Type	3	**Magnetic Resonance Imaging (MRI):** Computer reformatted digital display of multiplanar images developed from the capture of radiofrequency signals emitted by nuclei in a body site excited within a magnetic field

Body Part (4th)	Contrast (5th)	Qualifier (6th)	Qualifier (7th)
0 Hip, Right 1 Hip, Left 3 Femur, Right 4 Femur, Left 7 Knee, Right 8 Knee, Left D Lower Leg, Right F Lower Leg, Left G Ankle, Right H Ankle, Left J Calcaneus, Right K Calcaneus, Left L Foot, Right M Foot, Left P Toe(s), Right Q Toe(s), Left V Patella, Right W Patella, Left	Z None	Z None	Z None

Section	B	Imaging
Body System	Q	**Non-Axial Lower Bones**
Type	4	**Ultrasonography:** Real time display of images of anatomy or flow information developed from the capture of reflected and attenuated high frequency sound waves

Body Part (4th)	Contrast (5th)	Qualifier (6th)	Qualifier (7th)
0 Hip, Right 1 Hip, Left 2 Hips, Bilateral 7 Knee, Right 8 Knee, Left 9 Knees, Bilateral	Z None	Z None	Z None

Section	B	Imaging
Body System	R	**Axial Skeleton, Except Skull and Facial Bones**
Type	0	**Plain Radiography:** Planar display of an image developed from the capture of external ionizing radiation on photographic or photoconductive plate

Body Part (4th)	Contrast (5th)	Qualifier (6th)	Qualifier (7th)
0 Cervical Spine 7 Thoracic Spine 9 Lumbar Spine G Whole Spine	Z None	Z None	1 Densitometry Z None
1 Cervical Disc(s) 2 Thoracic Disc(s) 3 Lumbar Disc(s) 4 Cervical Facet Joint(s) 5 Thoracic Facet Joint(s) 6 Lumbar Facet Joint(s) D Sacroiliac Joints	0 High Osmolar 1 Low Osmolar Y Other Contrast Z None	Z None	Z None
8 Thoracolumbar Joint B Lumbosacral Joint C Pelvis F Sacrum and Coccyx H Sternum	Z None	Z None	Z None

Section	B	Imaging
Body System	R	Axial Skeleton, Except Skull and Facial Bones
Type	1	**Fluoroscopy:** Single plane or bi-plane real time display of an image developed from the capture of external ionizing radiation on a fluorescent screen. The image may also be stored by either digital or analog means

Body Part	Contrast (5th)	Qualifier (6th)	Qualifier (7th)
0 Cervical Spine	0 High Osmolar	Z None	Z None
1 Cervical Disc(s)	1 Low Osmolar		
2 Thoracic Disc(s)	Y Other Contrast		
3 Lumbar Disc(s)	Z None		
4 Cervical Facet Joint(s)			
5 Thoracic Facet Joint(s)			
6 Lumbar Facet Joint(s)			
7 Thoracic Spine			
8 Thoracolumbar Joint			
9 Lumbar Spine			
B Lumbosacral Joint			
C Pelvis			
D Sacroiliac Joints			
F Sacrum and Coccyx			
G Whole Spine			
H Sternum			

Section	B	Imaging
Body System	R	Axial Skeleton, Except Skull and Facial Bones
Type	2	**Computerized Tomography (CT Scan):** Computer reformatted digital display of multiplanar images developed from the capture of multiple exposures of external ionizing radiation

Body Part (4th)	Contrast (5th)	Qualifier (6th)	Qualifier (7th)
0 Cervical Spine	0 High Osmolar	Z None	Z None
7 Thoracic Spine	1 Low Osmolar		
9 Lumbar Spine	Y Other Contrast		
C Pelvis	Z None		
D Sacroiliac Joints			
F Sacrum and Coccyx			

Section	B	Imaging
Body System	R	Axial Skeleton, Except Skull and Facial Bones
Type	3	**Magnetic Resonance Imaging (MRI):** Computer reformatted digital display of multiplanar images developed from the capture of radiofrequency signals emitted by nuclei in a body site excited within a magnetic field

Body Part (4th)	Contrast (5th)	Qualifier (6th)	Qualifier (7th)
0 Cervical Spine	Y Other Contrast	0 Unenhanced and Enhanced	Z None
1 Cervical Disc(s)		Z None	
2 Thoracic Disc(s)			
3 Lumbar Disc(s)			
7 Thoracic Spine			
9 Lumbar Spine			
C Pelvis			
F Sacrum and Coccyx			
0 Cervical Spine	Z None	Z None	Z None
1 Cervical Disc(s)			
2 Thoracic Disc(s)			
3 Lumbar Disc(s)			
7 Thoracic Spine			
9 Lumbar Spine			
C Pelvis			
F Sacrum and Coccyx			

Section	B	Imaging
Body System	R	**Axial Skeleton, Except Skull and Facial Bones**
Type	4	**Ultrasonography:** Real time display of images of anatomy or flow information developed from the capture of reflected and attenuated high frequency sound waves

Body Part (4th)	Contrast (5th)	Qualifier (6th)	Qualifier (7th)
0 Cervical Spine 7 Thoracic Spine 9 Lumbar Spine F Sacrum and Coccyx	Z None	Z None	Z None

Section	B	Imaging
Body System	T	**Urinary System**
Type	0	**Plain Radiography:** Planar display of an image developed from the capture of external ionizing radiation on photographic or photoconductive plate

Body Part (4th)	Contrast (5th)	Qualifier (6th)	Qualifier (7th)
0 Bladder 1 Kidney, Right 2 Kidney, Left 3 Kidneys, Bilateral 4 Kidneys, Ureters and Bladder 5 Urethra 6 Ureter, Right 7 Ureter, Left 8 Ureters, Bilateral B Bladder and Urethra C Ileal Diversion Loop	0 High Osmolar 1 Low Osmolar Y Other Contrast Z None	Z None	Z None

Section	B	Imaging
Body System	T	**Urinary System**
Type	1	**Fluoroscopy:** Single plane or bi-plane real time display of an image developed from the capture of external ionizing radiation on a fluorescent screen. The image may also be stored by either digital or analog means

Body Part (4th)	Contrast (5th)	Qualifier (6th)	Qualifier (7th)
0 Bladder 1 Kidney, Right 2 Kidney, Left 3 Kidneys, Bilateral 4 Kidneys, Ureters and Bladder 5 Urethra 6 Ureter, Right 7 Ureter, Left B Bladder and Urethra C Ileal Diversion Loop D Kidney, Ureter and Bladder, Right F Kidney, Ureter and Bladder, Left G Ileal Loop, Ureters and Kidneys	0 High Osmolar 1 Low Osmolar Y Other Contrast Z None	Z None	Z None

Section	B	Imaging
Body System	T	**Urinary System**
Type	2	**Computerized Tomography (CT Scan):** Computer reformatted digital display of multiplanar images developed from the capture of multiple exposures of external ionizing radiation

Body Part (4th)	Contrast (5th)	Qualifier (6th)	Qualifier (7th)
0 Bladder 1 Kidney, Right 2 Kidney, Left 3 Kidneys, Bilateral 9 Kidney Transplant	0 High Osmolar 1 Low Osmolar Y Other Contrast	0 Unenhanced and Enhanced Z None	Z None

Continued

Section	B	Imaging		BT2 *Continued*
Body System	T	Urinary System		
Type	2	Computerized Tomography (CT Scan): Computer reformatted digital display of multiplanar images developed from the capture of multiple exposures of external ionizing radiation		

Body Part (4th)	Contrast (5th)	Qualifier (6th)	Qualifier (7th)
0 Bladder 1 Kidney, Right 2 Kidney, Left 3 Kidneys, Bilateral 9 Kidney Transplant	Z None	Z None	Z None

Section	B	Imaging
Body System	T	Urinary System
Type	3	Magnetic Resonance Imaging (MRI): Computer reformatted digital display of multiplanar images developed from the capture of radiofrequency signals emitted by nuclei in a body site excited within a magnetic field

Body Part (4th)	Contrast (5th)	Qualifier (6th)	Qualifier (7th)
0 Bladder 1 Kidney, Right 2 Kidney, Left 3 Kidneys, Bilateral 9 Kidney Transplant	Y Other Contrast	0 Unenhanced and Enhanced Z None	Z None
0 Bladder 1 Kidney, Right 2 Kidney, Left 3 Kidneys, Bilateral 9 Kidney Transplant	Z None	Z None	Z None

Section	B	Imaging
Body System	T	Urinary System
Type	4	Ultrasonography: Real time display of images of anatomy or flow information developed from the capture of reflected and attenuated high frequency sound waves

Body Part (4th)	Contrast (5th)	Qualifier (6th)	Qualifier (7th)
0 Bladder 1 Kidney, Right 2 Kidney, Left 3 Kidneys, Bilateral 5 Urethra 6 Ureter, Right 7 Ureter, Left 8 Ureters, Bilateral 9 Kidney Transplant J Kidneys and Bladder	Z None	Z None	Z None

Section	B	Imaging
Body System	U	Female Reproductive System
Type	0	Plain Radiography: Planar display of an image developed from the capture of external ionizing radiation on photographic or photoconductive plate

Body Part (4th)	Contrast (5th)	Qualifier (6th)	Qualifier (7th)
0 Fallopian Tube, Right 1 Fallopian Tube, Left 2 Fallopian Tubes, Bilateral 6 Uterus 8 Uterus and Fallopian Tubes 9 Vagina	0 High Osmolar 1 Low Osmolar Y Other Contrast	Z None	Z None

Section	B	Imaging
Body System	U	Female Reproductive System
Type	1	**Fluoroscopy:** Single plane or bi-plane real time display of an image developed from the capture of external ionizing radiation on a fluorescent screen. The image may also be stored by either digital or analog means

Body Part (4th)	Contrast (5th)	Qualifier (6th)	Qualifier (7th)
0 Fallopian Tube, Right 1 Fallopian Tube, Left 2 Fallopian Tubes, Bilateral 6 Uterus 8 Uterus and Fallopian Tubes 9 Vagina	0 High Osmolar 1 Low Osmolar Y Other Contrast Z None	Z None	Z None

Section	B	Imaging
Body System	U	Female Reproductive System
Type	3	**Magnetic Resonance Imaging (MRI):** Computer reformatted digital display of multiplanar images developed from the capture of radiofrequency signals emitted by nuclei in a body site excited within a magnetic field

Body Part (4th)	Contrast (5th)	Qualifier (6th)	Qualifier (7th)
3 Ovary, Right 4 Ovary, Left 5 Ovaries, Bilateral 6 Uterus 9 Vagina B Pregnant Uterus C Uterus and Ovaries	Y Other Contrast	0 Unenhanced and Enhanced Z None	Z None
3 Ovary, Right 4 Ovary, Left 5 Ovaries, Bilateral 6 Uterus 9 Vagina B Pregnant Uterus C Uterus and Ovaries	Z None	Z None	Z None

Section	B	Imaging
Body System	U	Female Reproductive System
Type	4	**Ultrasonography:** Real time display of images of anatomy or flow information developed from the capture of reflected and attenuated high frequency sound waves

Body Part (4th)	Contrast (5th)	Qualifier (6th)	Qualifier (7th)
0 Fallopian Tube, Right 1 Fallopian Tube, Left 2 Fallopian Tubes, Bilateral 3 Ovary, Right 4 Ovary, Left 5 Ovaries, Bilateral 6 Uterus C Uterus and Ovaries	Y Other Contrast Z None	Z None	Z None

Section	B	Imaging
Body System	V	Male Reproductive System
Type	0	**Plain Radiography:** Planar display of an image developed from the capture of external ionizing radiation on photographic or photoconductive plate

Body Part (4th)	Contrast (5th)	Qualifier (6th)	Qualifier (7th)
0 Corpora Cavernosa 1 Epididymis, Right 2 Epididymis, Left 3 Prostate 5 Testicle, Right 6 Testicle, Left 8 Vasa Vasorum	0 High Osmolar 1 Low Osmolar Y Other Contrast	Z None	Z None

Section	B	Imaging
Body System	V	Male Reproductive System
Type	1	**Fluoroscopy:** Single plane or bi-plane real time display of an image developed from the capture of external ionizing radiation on a fluorescent screen. The image may also be stored by either digital or analog means

Body Part (4th)	Contrast (5th)	Qualifier (6th)	Qualifier (7th)
0 Corpora Cavernosa 8 Vasa Vasorum	0 High Osmolar 1 Low Osmolar Y Other Contrast Z None	Z None	Z None

Section	B	Imaging
Body System	V	Male Reproductive System
Type	2	**Computerized Tomography (CT Scan):** Computer reformatted digital display of multiplanar images developed from the capture of multiple exposures of external ionizing radiation

Body Part (4th)	Contrast (5th)	Qualifier (6th)	Qualifier (7th)
3 Prostate	0 High Osmolar 1 Low Osmolar Y Other Contrast	0 Unenhanced and Enhanced Z None	Z None
3 Prostate	Z None	Z None	Z None

Section	B	Imaging
Body System	V	Male Reproductive System
Type	3	**Magnetic Resonance Imaging (MRI):** Computer reformatted digital display of multiplanar images developed from the capture of radiofrequency signals emitted by nuclei in a body site excited within a magnetic field

Body Part (4th)	Contrast (5th)	Qualifier (6th)	Qualifier (7th)
0 Corpora Cavernosa 3 Prostate 4 Scrotum 5 Testicle, Right 6 Testicle, Left 7 Testicles, Bilateral	Y Other Contrast	0 Unenhanced and Enhanced Z None	Z None
0 Corpora Cavernosa 3 Prostate 4 Scrotum 5 Testicle, Right 6 Testicle, Left 7 Testicles, Bilateral	Z None	Z None	Z None

Section	B	Imaging
Body System	V	Male Reproductive System
Type	4	**Ultrasonography:** Real time display of images of anatomy or flow information developed from the capture of reflected and attenuated high frequency sound waves

Body Part (4th)	Contrast (5th)	Qualifier (6th)	Qualifier (7th)
4 Scrotum 9 Prostate and Seminal Vesicles B Penis	Z None	Z None	Z None

Section	B	Imaging
Body System	W	Anatomical Regions
Type	0	**Plain Radiography:** Planar display of an image developed from the capture of external ionizing radiation on photographic or photoconductive plate

Body Part (4th)	Contrast (5th)	Qualifier (6th)	Qualifier (7th)
0 Abdomen 1 Abdomen and Pelvis 3 Chest B Long Bones, All C Lower Extremity J Upper Extremity K Whole Body L Whole Skeleton M Whole Body, Infant	Z None	Z None	Z None

Section	B	Imaging
Body System	W	Anatomical Regions
Type	1	**Fluoroscopy:** Single plane or bi-plane real time display of an image developed from the capture of external ionizing radiation on a fluorescent screen. The image may also be stored by either digital or analog means

Body Part (4th)	Contrast (5th)	Qualifier (6th)	Qualifier (7th)
1 Abdomen and Pelvis 9 Head and Neck C Lower Extremity J Upper Extremity	0 High Osmolar 1 Low Osmolar Y Other Contrast Z None	Z None	Z None

Section	B	Imaging
Body System	W	Anatomical Regions
Type	2	**Computerized Tomography (CT Scan):** Computer reformatted digital display of multiplanar images developed from the capture of multiple exposures of external ionizing radiation

Body Part (4th)	Contrast (5th)	Qualifier (6th)	Qualifier (7th)
0 Abdomen 1 Abdomen and Pelvis 4 Chest and Abdomen 5 Chest, Abdomen and Pelvis 8 Head 9 Head and Neck F Neck G Pelvic Region	0 High Osmolar 1 Low Osmolar Y Other Contrast	0 Unenhanced and Enhanced Z None	Z None
0 Abdomen 1 Abdomen and Pelvis 4 Chest and Abdomen 5 Chest, Abdomen and Pelvis 8 Head 9 Head and Neck F Neck G Pelvic Region	Z None	Z None	Z None

Section   **B**   **Imaging**
Body System   **W**   **Anatomical Regions**
Type   **3**   **Magnetic Resonance Imaging (MRI):** Computer reformatted digital display of multiplanar images developed from the capture of radiofrequency signals emitted by nuclei in a body site excited within a magnetic field

Body Part (4th)	Contrast (5th)	Qualifier (6th)	Qualifier (7th)
0 Abdomen 8 Head F Neck G Pelvic Region H Retroperitoneum P Brachial Plexus	Y Other Contrast	0 Unenhanced and Enhanced Z None	Z None
0 Abdomen 8 Head F Neck G Pelvic Region H Retroperitoneum P Brachial Plexus	Z None	Z None	Z None
3 Chest	Y Other Contrast	0 Unenhanced and Enhanced Z None	Z None

Section   **B**   **Imaging**
Body System   **W**   **Anatomical Regions**
Type   **4**   **Ultrasonography:** Real time display of images of anatomy or flow information developed from the capture of reflected and attenuated high frequency sound waves

Body Part (4th)	Contrast (5th)	Qualifier (6th)	Qualifier (7th)
0 Abdomen 1 Abdomen and Pelvis F Neck G Pelvic Region	Z None	Z None	Z None

Section   **B**   **Imaging**
Body System   **Y**   **Fetus and Obstetrical**
Type   **3**   **Magnetic Resonance Imaging (MRI):** Computer reformatted digital display of multiplanar images developed from the capture of radiofrequency signals emitted by nuclei in a body site excited within a magnetic field

Body Part (4th)	Contrast (5th)	Qualifier (6th)	Qualifier (7th)
0 Fetal Head 1 Fetal Heart 2 Fetal Thorax 3 Fetal Abdomen 4 Fetal Spine 5 Fetal Extremities 6 Whole Fetus	Y Other Contrast	0 Unenhanced and Enhanced Z None	Z None
0 Fetal Head 1 Fetal Heart 2 Fetal Thorax 3 Fetal Abdomen 4 Fetal Spine 5 Fetal Extremities 6 Whole Fetus	Z None	Z None	Z None

Section	B	Imaging
Body System	Y	Fetus and Obstetrical
Type	4	Ultrasonography: Real time display of images of anatomy or flow information developed from the capture of reflected and attenuated high frequency sound waves

Body Part (4th)	Contrast (5th)	Qualifier (6th)	Qualifier (7th)
7 Fetal Umbilical Cord 8 Placenta 9 First Trimester, Single Fetus B First Trimester, Multiple Gestation C Second Trimester, Single Fetus D Second Trimester, Multiple Gestation F Third Trimester, Single Fetus G Third Trimester, Multiple Gestation	Z None	Z None	Z None

Nuclear Medicine Section (C01–CW7)

Within each section of ICD-10-PCS the characters have different meanings. The seven character meanings for the Nuclear Medicine section are illustrated here through the procedure example of *Technetium tomo scan of liver*.

Section	Body System	Root Type	Body Part	Radionuclide	Qualifier	Qualifier
Nuclear Medicine	Hepatobiliary and Pancreas	Tomographic (Tomo)	Liver	Technetium 99m	None	None
C	F	2	5	1	Z	Z

Section (Character 1)

All Nuclear Medicine procedure codes have a first character value of C.

Body System (Character 2)

The alphanumeric character for the body system is placed in the second position. The following are the body systems applicable to the Nuclear Medicine section.

Character Value	Character Value Description
0	Central Nervous System
2	Heart
5	Veins
7	Lymphatic System
8	Eye
9	Ear, Nose, Mouth and Throat
B	Respiratory System
D	Gastrointestinal System
F	Hepatobiliary System and Pancreas
G	Endocrine System
H	Skin, Subcutaneous Tissue and Breast
P	Musculoskeletral
T	Urinary System
V	Male Reproductive System
W	Anatomical Regions

Root Types (Character 3)

The alphanumeric character value for root types is placed in the third position. The following are the root types applicable to the Nuclear Medicine section with their associated meaning.

Character Value	Root Type	Root Type Definition
1	Planar Nuclear Medicine Imaging	Introduction of radioactive materials into the body for single plane display of images developed from the capture of radioactive emissions
2	Tomographic (Tomo) Nuclear Medicine Imaging	Introduction of radioactive materials into the body for three dimensional display of images developed from the capture of radioactive emissions
3	Positron Emission Tomographic (PET) Imaging	Introduction of radioactive materials into the body for three dimensional display of images developed from the simultaneous capture, 180 degrees apart, of radioactive emissions
4	Nonimaging Nuclear Medicine Uptake	Introduction of radioactive materials into the body for measurements of organ function, from the detection of radioactive emissions
5	Nonimaging Nuclear Medicine Probe	Introduction of radioactive materials into the body for the study of distribution and fate of certain substances by the detection of radioactive emissions; or, alternatively, measurement of absorption of radioactive emissions from an external source
6	Nonimaging Nuclear Medicine Assay	Introduction of radioactive materials into the body for the study of body fluids and blood elements, by the detection of radioactive emissions
7	Systemic Nuclear Medicine Therapy	Introduction of unsealed radioactive materials into the body for treatment

Body Part (Character 4)

For each body part the applicable body part character values will be available for procedure code construction. An example of a body part is Cerebrospinal Fluid.

Radionuclide (Character 5)

When radionuclide is utilized during a nuclear medicine procedure, the corresponding radionuclide character value should be reported in the fifth character position. The following are examples of the radionuclide character values available for the Nuclear Medicine section.

- Krypton (Kr-81m)
- Technetium 99m (Tc-99m)
- Xenon 127 (Xe-127)
- Xenon 133 (Xe-133)
- Other Radionuclide

If radionuclide is not utilized, the placeholder character value of Z should be reported.

Qualifier (Character 6)

The qualifier represents an additional attribute for the procedure when applicable. Currently, there are no qualifiers in the Nuclear Medicine section; therefore, the placeholder character value of Z should be reported.

Qualifier (Character 7)

The qualifier represents an additional attribute for the procedure when applicable. Currently, there are no qualifiers in the Nuclear Medicine section; therefore, the placeholder character value of Z should be reported.

Nuclear Medicine Section Tables

Nuclear Medicine Tables C01–CW7

Section	C	**Nuclear Medicine**
Body System	0	**Central Nervous System**
Type	1	**Planar Nuclear Medicine Imaging:** Introduction of radioactive materials into the body for single plane display of images developed from the capture of radioactive emissions

Body Part (4th)	Radionuclide (5th)	Qualifier (6th)	Qualifier (7th)
0 Brain	**1** Technetium 99m (Tc-99m) **Y** Other Radionuclide	**Z** None	**Z** None
5 Cerebrospinal Fluid	**D** Indium 111 (In-111) **Y** Other Radionuclide	**Z** None	**Z** None
Y Central Nervous System	**Y** Other Radionuclide	**Z** None	**Z** None

Section	C	**Nuclear Medicine**
Body System	0	**Central Nervous System**
Type	2	**Tomographic (Tomo) Nuclear Medicine Imaging:** Introduction of radioactive materials into the body for three dimensional display of images developed from the capture of radioactive emissions

Body Part (4th)	Radionuclide (5th)	Qualifier (6th)	Qualifier (7th)
0 Brain	**1** Technetium 99m (Tc-99m) **F** Iodine 123 (I-123) **S** Thallium 201 (Tl-201) **Y** Other Radionuclide	**Z** None	**Z** None
5 Cerebrospinal Fluid	**D** Indium 111 (In-111) **Y** Other Radionuclide	**Z** None	**Z** None
Y Central Nervous System	**Y** Other Radionuclide	**Z** None	**Z** None

Section	C	**Nuclear Medicine**
Body System	0	**Central Nervous System**
Type	3	**Positron Emission Tomographic (PET) Imaging:** Introduction of radioactive materials into the body for three dimensional display of images developed from the simultaneous capture, 180 degrees apart, of radioactive emissions

Body Part (4th)	Radionuclide (5th)	Qualifier (6th)	Qualifier (7th)
0 Brain	**B** Carbon 11 (C-11) **K** Fluorine 18 (F-18) **M** Oxygen 15 (O-15) **Y** Other Radionuclide	**Z** None	**Z** None
Y Central Nervous System	**Y** Other Radionuclide	**Z** None	**Z** None

Section	C	Nuclear Medicine
Body System	0	Central Nervous System
Type	5	**Nonimaging Nuclear Medicine Probe:** Introduction of radioactive materials into the body for the study of distribution and fate of certain substances by the detection of radioactive emissions; or, alternatively, measurement of absorption of radioactive emissions from an external source

Body Part (4th)	Radionuclide (5th)	Qualifier (6th)	Qualifier (7th)
0 Brain	V Xenon 133 (Xe-133) Y Other Radionuclide	Z None	Z None
Y Central Nervous System	Y Other Radionuclide	Z None	Z None

Section	C	Nuclear Medicine
Body System	2	Heart
Type	1	**Planar Nuclear Medicine Imaging:** Introduction of radioactive materials into the body for single plane display of images developed from the capture of radioactive emissions

Body Part (4th)	Radionuclide (5th)	Qualifier (6th)	Qualifier (7th)
6 Heart, Right and Left	1 Technetium 99m (Tc-99m) Y Other Radionuclide	Z None	Z None
G Myocardium	1 Technetium 99m (Tc-99m) D Indium 111 (In-111) S Thallium 201 (Tl-201) Y Other Radionuclide Z None	Z None	Z None
Y Heart	Y Other Radionuclide	Z None	Z None

Section	C	Nuclear Medicine
Body System	2	Heart
Type	2	**Tomographic (Tomo) Nuclear Medicine Imaging:** Introduction of radioactive materials into the body for three dimensional display of images developed from the capture of radioactive emissions

Body Part (4th)	Radionuclide (5th)	Qualifier (6th)	Qualifier (7th)
6 Heart, Right and Left	1 Technetium 99m (Tc-99m) Y Other Radionuclide	Z None	Z None
G Myocardium	1 Technetium 99m (Tc-99m) D Indium 111 (In-111) K Fluorine 18 (F-18) S Thallium 201 (Tl-201) Y Other Radionuclide Z None	Z None	Z None
Y Heart	Y Other Radionuclide	Z None	Z None

Section	C	Nuclear Medicine
Body System	2	Heart
Type	3	**Positron Emission Tomographic (PET) Imaging:** Introduction of radioactive materials into the body for three dimensional display of images developed from the simultaneous capture, 180 degrees apart, of radioactive emissions

Body Part (4th)	Radionuclide (5th)	Qualifier (6th)	Qualifier (7th)
G Myocardium	K Fluorine 18 (F-18) M Oxygen 15 (O-15) Q Rubidium 82 (Rb-82) R Nitrogen 13 (N-13) Y Other Radionuclide	Z None	Z None

Continued

Section C Nuclear Medicine
Body System 2 Heart
Type 3 **Positron Emission Tomographic (PET) Imaging:** Introduction of radioactive materials into the body for three dimensional display of images developed from the simultaneous capture, 180 degrees apart, of radioactive emissions

C23 *Continued*

Body Part (4th)	Radionuclide (5th)	Qualifier (6th)	Qualifier (7th)
Y Heart	Y Other Radionuclide	Z None	Z None

Section C Nuclear Medicine
Body System 2 Heart
Type 5 **Nonimaging Nuclear Medicine Probe:** Introduction of radioactive materials into the body for the study of distribution and fate of certain substances by the detection of radioactive emissions; or, alternatively, measurement of absorption of radioactive emissions from an external source

Body Part (4th)	Radionuclide (5th)	Qualifier (6th)	Qualifier (7th)
6 Heart, Right and Left	1 Technetium 99m (Tc-99m) Y Other Radionuclide	Z None	Z None
Y Heart	Y Other Radionuclide	Z None	Z None

Section C Nuclear Medicine
Body System 5 Veins
Type 1 **Planar Nuclear Medicine Imaging:** Introduction of radioactive materials into the body for single plane display of images developed from the capture of radioactive emissions

Body Part (4th)	Radionuclide (5th)	Qualifier (6th)	Qualifier (7th)
B Lower Extremity Veins, Right C Lower Extremity Veins, Left D Lower Extremity Veins, Bilateral N Upper Extremity Veins, Right P Upper Extremity Veins, Left Q Upper Extremity Veins, Bilateral R Central Veins	1 Technetium 99m (Tc-99m) Y Other Radionuclide	Z None	Z None
Y Veins	Y Other Radionuclide	Z None	Z None

Section C Nuclear Medicine
Body System 7 Lymphatic and Hematologic System
Type 1 **Planar Nuclear Medicine Imaging:** Introduction of radioactive materials into the body for single plane display of images developed from the capture of radioactive emissions

Body Part (4th)	Radionuclide (5th)	Qualifier (6th)	Qualifier (7th)
0 Bone Marrow	1 Technetium 99m (Tc-99m) D Indium 111 (In-111) Y Other Radionuclide	Z None	Z None
2 Spleen 5 Lymphatics, Head and Neck D Lymphatics, Pelvic J Lymphatics, Head K Lymphatics, Neck L Lymphatics, Upper Chest M Lymphatics, Trunk N Lymphatics, Upper Extremity P Lymphatics, Lower Extremity	1 Technetium 99m (Tc-99m) Y Other Radionuclide	Z None	Z None
3 Blood	D Indium 111 (In-111) Y Other Radionuclide	Z None	Z None
Y Lymphatic and Hematologic System	Y Other Radionuclide	Z None	Z None

Section **C** **Nuclear Medicine**
Body System **7** **Lymphatic and Hematologic System**
Type **2** **Tomographic (Tomo) Nuclear Medicine Imaging:** Introduction of radioactive materials into the body for three dimensional display of images developed from the capture of radioactive emissions

Body Part (4th)	Radionuclide (5th)	Qualifier (6th)	Qualifier (7th)
2 Spleen	**1** Technetium 99m (Tc-99m) **Y** Other Radionuclide	**Z** None	**Z** None
Y Lymphatic and Hematologic System	**Y** Other Radionuclide	**Z** None	**Z** None

Section **C** **Nuclear Medicine**
Body System **7** **Lymphatic and Hematologic System**
Type **5** **Nonimaging Nuclear Medicine Probe:** Introduction of radioactive materials into the body for the study of distribution and fate of certain substances by the detection of radioactive emissions; or, alternatively, measurement of absorption of radioactive emissions from an external source

Body Part (4th)	Radionuclide (5th)	Qualifier (6th)	Qualifier (7th)
5 Lymphatics, Head and Neck **D** Lymphatics, Pelvic **J** Lymphatics, Head **K** Lymphatics, Neck **L** Lymphatics, Upper Chest **M** Lymphatics, Trunk **N** Lymphatics, Upper Extremity **P** Lymphatics, Lower Extremity	**1** Technetium 99m (Tc-99m) **Y** Other Radionuclide	**Z** None	**Z** None
Y Lymphatic and Hematologic System	**Y** Other Radionuclide	**Z** None	**Z** None

Section **C** **Nuclear Medicine**
Body System **7** **Lymphatic and Hematologic System**
Type **6** **Nonimaging Nuclear Medicine Assay:** Introduction of radioactive materials into the body for the study of body fluids and blood elements, by the detection of radioactive emissions

Body Part (4th)	Radionuclide (5th)	Qualifier (6th)	Qualifier (7th)
3 Blood	**1** Technetium 99m (Tc-99m) **7** Cobalt 58 (Co-58) **C** Cobalt 57 (Co-57) **D** Indium 111 (In-111) **H** Iodine 125 (I-125) **W** Chromium (Cr-51) **Y** Other Radionuclide	**Z** None	**Z** None
Y Lymphatic and Hematologic System	**Y** Other Radionuclide	**Z** None	**Z** None

Section **C** **Nuclear Medicine**
Body System **8** **Eye**
Type **1** **Planar Nuclear Medicine Imaging:** Introduction of radioactive materials into the body for single plane display of images developed from the capture of radioactive emissions

Body Part (4th)	Radionuclide (5th)	Qualifier (6th)	Qualifier (7th)
9 Lacrimal Ducts, Bilateral	**1** Technetium 99m (Tc-99m) **Y** Other Radionuclide	**Z** None	**Z** None

Continued

Section	C	Nuclear Medicine	C81 *Continued*
Body System	8	Eye	
Type	1	**Planar Nuclear Medicine Imaging:** Introduction of radioactive materials into the body for single plane display of images developed from the capture of radioactive emissions	

Body Part (4th)	Radionuclide (5th)	Qualifier (6th)	Qualifier (7th)
Y Eye	Y Other Radionuclide	Z None	Z None

Section	C	Nuclear Medicine
Body System	9	**Ear, Nose, Mouth and Throat**
Type	1	**Planar Nuclear Medicine Imaging:** Introduction of radioactive materials into the body for single plane display of images developed from the capture of radioactive emissions

Body Part (4th)	Radionuclide (5th)	Qualifier (6th)	Qualifier (7th)
B Salivary Glands, Bilateral	1 Technetium 99m (Tc-99m) Y Other Radionuclide	Z None	Z None
Y Ear, Nose, Mouth and Throat	Y Other Radionuclide	Z None	Z None

Section	C	Nuclear Medicine
Body System	B	**Respiratory System**
Type	1	**Planar Nuclear Medicine Imaging:** Introduction of radioactive materials into the body for single plane display of images developed from the capture of radioactive emissions

Body Part (4th)	Radionuclide (5th)	Qualifier (6th)	Qualifier (7th)
2 Lungs and Bronchi	1 Technetium 99m (Tc-99m) 9 Krypton (Kr-81m) T Xenon 127 (Xe-127) V Xenon 133 (Xe-133) Y Other Radionuclide	Z None	Z None
Y Respiratory System	Y Other Radionuclide	Z None	Z None

Section	C	Nuclear Medicine
Body System	B	**Respiratory System**
Type	2	**Tomographic (Tomo) Nuclear Medicine Imaging:** Introduction of radioactive materials into the body for three dimensional display of images developed from the capture of radioactive emissions

Body Part (4th)	Radionuclide (5th)	Qualifier (6th)	Qualifier (7th)
2 Lungs and Bronchi	1 Technetium 99m (Tc-99m) 9 Krypton (Kr-81m) Y Other Radionuclide	Z None	Z None
Y Respiratory System	Y Other Radionuclide	Z None	Z None

Section	C	Nuclear Medicine
Body System	B	**Respiratory System**
Type	3	**Positron Emission Tomographic (PET) Imaging:** Introduction of radioactive materials into the body for three dimensional display of images developed from the simultaneous capture, 180 degrees apart, of radioactive emissions

Body Part (4th)	Radionuclide (5th)	Qualifier	Qualifier (7th)
2 Lungs and Bronchi	K Fluorine 18 (F-18) Y Other Radionuclide	Z None	Z None
Y Respiratory System	Y Other Radionuclide	Z None	Z None

Section	C	Nuclear Medicine
Body System	D	Gastrointestinal System
Type	1	**Planar Nuclear Medicine Imaging:** Introduction of radioactive materials into the body for single plane display of images developed from the capture of radioactive emissions

Body Part (4th)	Radionuclide (5th)	Qualifier (6th)	Qualifier (7th)
5 Upper Gastrointestinal Tract 7 Gastrointestinal Tract	1 Technetium 99m (Tc-99m) D Indium 111 (In-111) Y Other Radionuclide	Z None	Z None
Y Digestive System	Y Other Radionuclide	Z None	Z None

Section	C	Nuclear Medicine
Body System	D	Gastrointestinal System
Type	2	**Tomographic (Tomo) Nuclear Medicine Imaging:** Introduction of radioactive materials into the body for three dimensional display of images developed from the capture of radioactive emissions

Body Part (4th)	Radionuclide (5th)	Qualifier (6th)	Qualifier (7th)
7 Gastrointestinal Tract	1 Technetium 99m (Tc-99m) D Indium 111 (In-111) Y Other Radionuclide	Z None	Z None
Y Digestive System	Y Other Radionuclide	Z None	Z None

Section	C	Nuclear Medicine
Body System	F	Hepatobiliary System and Pancreas
Type	1	**Planar Nuclear Medicine Imaging:** Introduction of radioactive materials into the body for single plane display of images developed from the capture of radioactive emissions

Body Part (4th)	Radionuclide (5th)	Qualifier (6th)	Qualifier (7th)
4 Gallbladder 5 Liver 6 Liver and Spleen C Hepatobiliary System, All	1 Technetium 99m (Tc-99m) Y Other Radionuclide	Z None	Z None
Y Hepatobiliary System and Pancreas	Y Other Radionuclide	Z None	Z None

Section	C	Nuclear Medicine
Body System	F	Hepatobiliary System and Pancreas
Type	2	**Tomographic (Tomo) Nuclear Medicine Imaging:** Introduction of radioactive materials into the body for three dimensional display of images developed from the capture of radioactive emissions

Body Part (4th)	Radionuclide (5th)	Qualifier (6th)	Qualifier (7th)
4 Gallbladder 5 Liver 6 Liver and Spleen	1 Technetium 99m (Tc-99m) Y Other Radionuclide	Z None	Z None
Y Hepatobiliary System and Pancreas	Y Other Radionuclide	Z None	Z None

Section	C	Nuclear Medicine
Body System	G	Endocrine System
Type	1	**Planar Nuclear Medicine Imaging:** Introduction of radioactive materials into the body for single plane display of images developed from the capture of radioactive emissions

Body Part (4th)	Radionuclide (5th)	Qualifier (6th)	Qualifier (7th)
1 Parathyroid Glands	1 Technetium 99m (Tc-99m) S Thallium 201 (Tl-201) Y Other Radionuclide	Z None	Z None

Continued

Section | C | Nuclear Medicine
Body System | G | Endocrine System
Type | 1 | Planar Nuclear Medicine Imaging: Introduction of radioactive materials into the body for single plane display of images developed from the capture of radioactive emissions

Body Part (4ᵗʰ)	Radionuclide (5ᵗʰ)	Qualifier (6ᵗʰ)	Qualifier (7ᵗʰ)
2 Thyroid Gland	**1** Technetium 99m (Tc-99m) **F** Iodine 123 (I-123) **G** Iodine 131 (I-131) **Y** Other Radionuclide	**Z** None	**Z** None
4 Adrenal Glands, Bilateral	**G** Iodine 131 (I-131) **Y** Other Radionuclide	**Z** None	**Z** None
Y Endocrine System	**Y** Other Radionuclide	**Z** None	**Z** None

Section | C | Nuclear Medicine
Body System | G | Endocrine System
Type | 2 | Tomographic (Tomo) Nuclear Medicine Imaging: Introduction of radioactive materials into the body for three dimensional display of images developed from the capture of radioactive emissions

Body Part (4ᵗʰ)	Radionuclide (5ᵗʰ)	Qualifier (6ᵗʰ)	Qualifier (7ᵗʰ)
1 Parathyroid Glands	**1** Technetium 99m (Tc-99m) **S** Thallium 201 (Tl-201) **Y** Other Radionuclide	**Z** None	**Z** None
Y Endocrine System	**Y** Other Radionuclide	**Z** None	**Z** None

Section | C | Nuclear Medicine
Body System | G | Endocrine System
Type | 4 | Nonimaging Nuclear Medicine Uptake: Introduction of radioactive materials into the body for measurements of organ function, from the detection of radioactive emissions

Body Part (4ᵗʰ)	Radionuclide (5ᵗʰ)	Qualifier (6ᵗʰ)	Qualifier (7ᵗʰ)
2 Thyroid Gland	**1** Technetium 99m (Tc-99m) **F** Iodine 123 (I-123) **G** Iodine 131 (I-131) **Y** Other Radionuclide	**Z** None	**Z** None
Y Endocrine System	**Y** Other Radionuclide	**Z** None	**Z** None

Section | C | Nuclear Medicine
Body System | H | Skin, Subcutaneous Tissue and Breast
Type | 1 | Planar Nuclear Medicine Imaging: Introduction of radioactive materials into the body for single plane display of images developed from the capture of radioactive emissions

Body Part (4ᵗʰ)	Radionuclide (5ᵗʰ)	Qualifier (6ᵗʰ)	Qualifier (7ᵗʰ)
0 Breast, Right **1** Breast, Left **2** Breasts, Bilateral	**1** Technetium 99m (Tc-99m) **S** Thallium 201 (Tl-201) **Y** Other Radionuclide	**Z** None	**Z** None
Y Skin, Subcutaneous Tissue and Breast	**Y** Other Radionuclide	**Z** None	**Z** None

Section	C	Nuclear Medicine
Body System	H	Skin, Subcutaneous Tissue and Breast
Type	2	**Tomographic (Tomo) Nuclear Medicine Imaging:** Introduction of radioactive materials into the body for three dimensional display of images developed from the capture of radioactive emissions

Body Part (4ᵗʰ)	Radionuclide (5ᵗʰ)	Qualifier (6ᵗʰ)	Qualifier (7ᵗʰ)
0 Breast, Right 1 Breast, Left 2 Breasts, Bilateral	1 Technetium 99m (Tc-99m) S Thallium 201 (Tl-201) Y Other Radionuclide	Z None	Z None
Y Skin, Subcutaneous Tissue and Breast	Y Other Radionuclide	Z None	Z None

Section	C	Nuclear Medicine
Body System	P	Musculoskeletal System
Type	1	**Planar Nuclear Medicine Imaging:** Introduction of radioactive materials into the body for single plane display of images developed from the capture of radioactive emissions

Body Part (4ᵗʰ)	Radionuclide (5ᵗʰ)	Qualifier (6ᵗʰ)	Qualifier (7ᵗʰ)
1 Skull 4 Thorax 5 Spine 6 Pelvis 7 Spine and Pelvis 8 Upper Extremity, Right 9 Upper Extremity, Left B Upper Extremities, Bilateral C Lower Extremity, Right D Lower Extremity, Left F Lower Extremities, Bilateral Z Musculoskeletal System, All	1 Technetium 99m (Tc-99m) Y Other Radionuclide	Z None	Z None
Y Musculoskeletal System, Other	Y Other Radionuclide	Z None	Z None

Section	C	Nuclear Medicine
Body System	P	Musculoskeletal System
Type	2	**Tomographic (Tomo) Nuclear Medicine Imaging:** Introduction of radioactive materials into the body for three dimensional display of images developed from the capture of radioactive emissions

Body Part (4ᵗʰ)	Radionuclide (5ᵗʰ)	Qualifier (6ᵗʰ)	Qualifier (7ᵗʰ)
1 Skull 2 Cervical Spine 3 Skull and Cervical Spine 4 Thorax 6 Pelvis 7 Spine and Pelvis 8 Upper Extremity, Right 9 Upper Extremity, Left B Upper Extremities, Bilateral C Lower Extremity, Right D Lower Extremity, Left F Lower Extremities, Bilateral G Thoracic Spine H Lumbar Spine J Thoracolumbar Spine	1 Technetium 99m (Tc-99m) Y Other Radionuclide	Z None	Z None

Continued

CP2 *Continued*

Section	C	Nuclear Medicine
Body System	P	Musculoskeletal System
Type	2	**Tomographic (Tomo) Nuclear Medicine Imaging:** Introduction of radioactive materials into the body for three dimensional display of images developed from the capture of radioactive emissions

Body Part (4th)	Radionuclide (5th)	Qualifier (6th)	Qualifier (7th)
Y Musculoskeletal System, Other	Y Other Radionuclide	Z None	Z None

Section	C	Nuclear Medicine
Body System	P	Musculoskeletal System
Type	5	**Nonimaging Nuclear Medicine Probe:** Introduction of radioactive materials into the body for the study of distribution and fate of certain substances by the detection of radioactive emissions; or, alternatively, measurement of absorption of radioactive emissions from an external source

Body Part (4th)	Radionuclide (5th)	Qualifier (6th)	Qualifier (7th)
5 Spine N Upper Extremities P Lower Extremities	Z None	Z None	Z None
Y Musculoskeletal System, Other	Y Other Radionuclide	Z None	Z None

Section	C	Nuclear Medicine
Body System	T	Urinary System
Type	1	**Planar Nuclear Medicine Imaging:** Introduction of radioactive materials into the body for single plane display of images developed from the capture of radioactive emissions

Body Part (4th)	Radionuclide (5th)	Qualifier (6th)	Qualifier (7th)
3 Kidneys, Ureters and Bladder	1 Technetium 99m (Tc-99m) F Iodine 123 (I-123) G Iodine 131 (I-131) Y Other Radionuclide	Z None	Z None
H Bladder and Ureters	1 Technetium 99m (Tc-99m) Y Other Radionuclide	Z None	Z None
Y Urinary System	Y Other Radionuclide	Z None	Z None

Section	C	Nuclear Medicine
Body System	T	Urinary System
Type	2	**Tomographic (Tomo) Nuclear Medicine Imaging:** Introduction of radioactive materials into the body for three dimensional display of images developed from the capture of radioactive emissions

Body Part (4th)	Radionuclide (5th)	Qualifier (6th)	Qualifier (7th)
3 Kidneys, Ureters and Bladder	1 Technetium 99m (Tc-99m) Y Other Radionuclide	Z None	Z None
Y Urinary System	Y Other Radionuclide	Z None	Z None

Section	C	Nuclear Medicine
Body System	T	Urinary System
Type	6	**Nonimaging Nuclear Medicine Assay:** Introduction of radioactive materials into the body for the study of body fluids and blood elements, by the detection of radioactive emissions

Body Part (4th)	Radionuclide (5th)	Qualifier (6th)	Qualifier (7th)
3 Kidneys, Ureters and Bladder	1 Technetium 99m (Tc-99m) F Iodine 123 (I-123) G Iodine 131 (I-131) H Iodine 125 (I-125) Y Other Radionuclide	Z None	Z None
Y Urinary System	Y Other Radionuclide	Z None	Z None

Section	C	Nuclear Medicine
Body System	V	Male Reproductive System
Type	1	**Planar Nuclear Medicine Imaging:** Introduction of radioactive materials into the body for single plane display of images developed from the capture of radioactive emissions

Body Part (4th)	Radionuclide (5th)	Qualifier (6th)	Qualifier (7th)
9 Testicles, Bilateral	1 Technetium 99m (Tc-99m) Y Other Radionuclide	Z None	Z None
Y Male Reproductive System	Y Other Radionuclide	Z None	Z None

Section	C	Nuclear Medicine
Body System	W	Anatomical Regions
Type	1	**Planar Nuclear Medicine Imaging:** Introduction of radioactive materials into the body for single plane display of images developed from the capture of radioactive emissions

Body Part (4th)	Radionuclide (5th)	Qualifier (6th)	Qualifier (7th)
0 Abdomen 1 Abdomen and Pelvis 4 Chest and Abdomen 6 Chest and Neck B Head and Neck D Lower Extremity J Pelvic Region M Upper Extremity N Whole Body	1 Technetium 99m (Tc-99m) D Indium 111 (In-111) F Iodine 123 (I-123) G Iodine 131 (I-131) L Gallium 67 (Ga-67) S Thallium 201 (Tl-201) Y Other Radionuclide	Z None	Z None
3 Chest	1 Technetium 99m (Tc-99m) D Indium 111 (In-111) F Iodine 123 (I-123) G Iodine 131 (I-131) K Fluorine 18 (F-18) L Gallium 67 (Ga-67) S Thallium 201 (Tl-201) Y Other Radionuclide	Z None	Z None
Y Anatomical Regions, Multiple	Y Other Radionuclide	Z None	Z None
Z Anatomical Region, Other	Z None	Z None	Z None

Section	C	Nuclear Medicine
Body System	W	Anatomical Regions
Type	2	**Tomographic (Tomo) Nuclear Medicine Imaging:** Introduction of radioactive materials into the body for three dimensional display of images developed from the capture of radioactive emissions

Body Part (4th)	Radionuclide (5th)	Qualifier (6th)	Qualifier (7th)
0 Abdomen **1** Abdomen and Pelvis **3** Chest **4** Chest and Abdomen **6** Chest and Neck **B** Head and Neck **D** Lower Extremity **J** Pelvic Region **M** Upper Extremity	**1** Technetium 99m (Tc-99m) **D** Indium 111 (In-111) **F** Iodine 123 (I-123) **G** Iodine 131 (I-131) **K** Fluorine 18 (F-18) **L** Gallium 67 (Ga-67) **S** Thallium 201 (Tl-201) **Y** Other Radionuclide	**Z** None	**Z** None
Y Anatomical Regions, Multiple	**Y** Other Radionuclide	**Z** None	**Z** None

Section	C	Nuclear Medicine
Body System	W	Anatomical Regions
Type	3	**Positron Emission Tomographic (PET) Imaging:** Introduction of radioactive materials into the body for three dimensional display of images developed from the simultaneous capture, 180 degrees apart, of radioactive emissions

Body Part (4th)	Radionuclide (5th)	Qualifier (6th)	Qualifier (7th)
N Whole Body	**Y** Other Radionuclide	**Z** None	**Z** None

Section	C	Nuclear Medicine
Body System	W	Anatomical Regions
Type	5	**Nonimaging Nuclear Medicine Probe:** Introduction of radioactive materials into the body for the study of distribution and fate of certain substances by the detection of radioactive emissions; or, alternatively, measurement of absorption of radioactive emissions from an external source

Body Part (4th)	Radionuclide (5th)	Qualifier (6th)	Qualifier (7th)
0 Abdomen **1** Abdomen and Pelvis **3** Chest **4** Chest and Abdomen **6** Chest and Neck **B** Head and Neck **D** Lower Extremity **J** Pelvic Region **M** Upper Extremity	**1** Technetium 99m (Tc-99m) **D** Indium 111 (In-111) **Y** Other Radionuclide	**Z** None	**Z** None

Section	C	Nuclear Medicine
Body System	W	Anatomical Regions
Type	7	Systemic Nuclear Medicine Therapy: Introduction of unsealed radioactive materials into the body for treatment

Body Part (4th)	Radionuclide (5th)	Qualifier (6th)	Qualifier (7th)
0 Abdomen 3 Chest	N Phosphorus 32 (P-32) Y Other Radionuclide	Z None	Z None
G Thyroid	G Iodine 131 (I-131) Y Other Radionuclide	Z None	Z None
N Whole Body	8 Samarium 153 (Sm-153) G Iodine 131 (I-131) N Phosphorus 32 (P-32) P Strontium 89 (Sr-89) Y Other Radionuclide	Z None	Z None
Y Anatomical Regions, Multiple	Y Other Radionuclide	Z None	Z None

Radiation Therapy Section (D00–DWY)

Within each section of ICD-10-PCS the characters have different meanings. The seven character meanings for the Radiation Therapy section are illustrated here through the procedure example of *HDR brachytherapy of prostate using Palladium 103.*

Section	Body System	Modality	Treatment Site	Modality Qualifier	Isotope	Qualifier
Radiation Therapy	Male Reproductive System	Brachytherapy	Prostate	High Dose Rate (HDR)	Palladium 103	None
D	V	1	0	9	B	Z

Section (Character 1)

All Radiation Therapy procedure codes have a first character value of D.

Body System (Character 2)

The alphanumeric character for the body system is placed in the second position. The following are the body systems applicable to the Radiation Therapy section.

Character Value	Character Value Description
0	Central and Peripheral Nervous System
7	Lymphatic and hematologic System
8	Eye
9	Ear, Nose, Mouth and Throat
B	Respiratory System
D	Gastrointestinal System
F	Hepatobiliary System and Pancreas
G	Endocrine System
H	Skin
M	Breast
P	Musculoskeletral
T	Urinary System
U	Female Reproductive System
V	Male Reproductive System
W	Anatomical Regions

Modality (Character 3)

The alphanumeric character value for root types is placed in the third position. The following are the root types applicable to the Radiation Therapy section with their associated meaning.

Character Value	Modality	Modality Definition	
0	Beam Radiation	The external use of high-energy radiation such as x-rays, photons, electrons, or protons	
1	Brachytherapy	The use of radioactive sources placed directly into a tumor bearing area to generate local regions of high intensity radiation	
2	Stereotactic Radiosurgery	The use of external radiation sources either from a linear accelerator or a special Cobalt-60 irradiator to deliver many beams of radiation directly to an internal structure in a single fraction	
Y	Other Radiation	Other types of radiation therapy such as hyperthermia, contact radiation and plaque radiation. *See Modality qualifier, character 5, for specified types of other radiation.*	

Source: CSI Navigator for Radiation Oncology, 2010

Treatment Site (Character 4)

For each treatment site the applicable body part character values will be available for procedure code construction. An example of a treatment site for this section is Brain Stem.

Modality Qualifier (Character 5)

The modality qualifier further specifies the treatment modality. The following are examples of the modality qualifier values available for the Radiation Therapy section:

- Photons >10 MeV
- Neutrons
- Electrons
- High Dose Rate
- Hyperthermia

Isotope (Character 6)

When an isotope is utilized during a radiation oncology procedure, the corresponding isotope character value should be reported in the sixth character position. The following are examples of the isotope character values available for the Radiation Therapy section:

- Iridium 192 (Ir-192)
- Iodine 125 (I-125)
- Californium 252 (Cf-252)

Qualifier (Character 7)

The qualifier represents an additional attribute for the procedure when applicable. For example, beam radiation procedures in this section include the qualifier Intraoperative that is reported with the character value of 0 for some body parts. If there is no qualifier for a procedure, the placeholder Z is the character valve that should be reported.

Radiation Therapy Section Tables

Radiation Therapy Tables D00–DWY

Section	D	Radiation Therapy
Body System	0	Central and Peripheral Nervous System
Modality	0	Beam Radiation

Treatment Site (4th)	Modality Qualifier (5th)	Isotope (6th)	Qualifier (7th)
0 Brain 1 Brain Stem 6 Spinal Cord 7 Peripheral Nerve	0 Photons <1 MeV 1 Photons 1 - 10 MeV 2 Photons >10 MeV 4 Heavy Particles (Protons,Ions) 5 Neutrons 6 Neutron Capture	Z None	Z None
0 Brain 1 Brain Stem 6 Spinal Cord 7 Peripheral Nerve	3 Electrons	Z None	0 Intraoperative Z None

Section	D	Radiation Therapy
Body System	0	Central and Peripheral Nervous System
Modality	1	Brachytherapy

Treatment Site (4th)	Modality Qualifier (5th)	Isotope (6th)	Qualifier (7th)
0 Brain 1 Brain Stem 6 Spinal Cord 7 Peripheral Nerve	9 High Dose Rate (HDR) B Low Dose Rate (LDR)	7 Cesium 137 (Cs-137) 8 Iridium 192 (Ir-192) 9 Iodine 125 (I-125) B Palladium 103 (Pd-103) C Californium 252 (Cf-252) Y Other Isotope	Z None

Section	D	Radiation Therapy
Body System	0	Central and Peripheral Nervous System
Modality	2	Stereotactic Radiosurgery

Treatment Site (4th)	Modality Qualifier (5th)	Isotope (6th)	Qualifier (7th)
0 Brain 1 Brain Stem 6 Spinal Cord 7 Peripheral Nerve	D Stereotactic Other Photon Radiosurgery H Stereotactic Particulate Radiosurgery J Stereotactic Gamma Beam Radiosurgery	Z None	Z None

Section	D	Radiation Therapy
Body System	0	Central and Peripheral Nervous System
Modality	Y	Other Radiation

Treatment Site (4th)	Modality Qualifier (5th)	Isotope (6th)	Qualifier (7th)
0 Brain 1 Brain Stem 6 Spinal Cord 7 Peripheral Nerve	7 Contact Radiation 8 Hyperthermia F Plaque Radiation K Laser Interstitial Thermal Therapy	Z None	Z None

Section	D	Radiation Therapy
Body System	7	Lymphatic and Hematologic System
Modality	0	Beam Radiation

Treatment Site (4th)	Modality Qualifier (5th)	Isotope (6th)	Qualifier (7th)
0 Bone Marrow 1 Thymus 2 Spleen 3 Lymphatics, Neck 4 Lymphatics, Axillary 5 Lymphatics, Thorax 6 Lymphatics, Abdomen 7 Lymphatics, Pelvis 8 Lymphatics, Inguinal	0 Photons <1 MeV 1 Photons 1 - 10 MeV 2 Photons >10 MeV 4 Heavy Particles (Protons,Ions) 5 Neutrons 6 Neutron Capture	Z None	Z None
0 Bone Marrow 1 Thymus 2 Spleen 3 Lymphatics, Neck 4 Lymphatics, Axillary 5 Lymphatics, Thorax 6 Lymphatics, Abdomen 7 Lymphatics, Pelvis 8 Lymphatics, Inguinal	3 Electrons	Z None	0 Intraoperative Z None

Section	D	Radiation Therapy
Body System	7	Lymphatic and Hematologic System
Modality	1	Brachytherapy

Treatment Site (4th)	Modality Qualifier (5th)	Isotope (6th)	Qualifier (7th)
0 Bone Marrow 1 Thymus 2 Spleen 3 Lymphatics, Neck 4 Lymphatics, Axillary 5 Lymphatics, Thorax 6 Lymphatics, Abdomen 7 Lymphatics, Pelvis 8 Lymphatics, Inguinal	9 High Dose Rate (HDR) B Low Dose Rate (LDR)	7 Cesium 137 (Cs-137) 8 Iridium 192 (Ir-192) 9 Iodine 125 (I-125) B Palladium 103 (Pd-103) C Californium 252 (Cf-252) Y Other Isotope	Z None

Section	D	Radiation Therapy
Body System	7	Lymphatic and Hematologic System
Modality	2	Stereotactic Radiosurgery

Treatment Site (4th)	Modality Qualifier (5th)	Isotope (6th)	Qualifier (7th)
0 Bone Marrow 1 Thymus 2 Spleen 3 Lymphatics, Neck 4 Lymphatics, Axillary 5 Lymphatics, Thorax 6 Lymphatics, Abdomen 7 Lymphatics, Pelvis 8 Lymphatics, Inguinal	D Stereotactic Other Photon Radiosurgery H Stereotactic Particulate Radiosurgery J Stereotactic Gamma Beam Radiosurgery	Z None	Z None

Section	D	Radiation Therapy
Body System	7	Lymphatic and Hematologic System
Modality	Y	Other Radiation

Treatment Site (4th)	Modality Qualifier (5th)	Isotope (6th)	Qualifier (7th)
0 Bone Marrow 1 Thymus 2 Spleen 3 Lymphatics, Neck 4 Lymphatics, Axillary 5 Lymphatics, Thorax 6 Lymphatics, Abdomen 7 Lymphatics, Pelvis 8 Lymphatics, Inguinal	8 Hyperthermia F Plaque Radiation	Z None	Z None

Section	D	Radiation Therapy
Body System	8	Eye
Modality	0	Beam Radiation

Treatment Site (4th)	Modality Qualifier (5th)	Isotope (6th)	Qualifier (7th)
0 Eye	0 Photons <1 MeV 1 Photons 1 - 10 MeV 2 Photons >10 MeV 4 Heavy Particles (Protons,Ions) 5 Neutrons 6 Neutron Capture	Z None	Z None
0 Eye	3 Electrons	Z None	0 Intraoperative Z None

Section	D	Radiation Therapy
Body System	8	Eye
Modality	1	Brachytherapy

Treatment Site (4th)	Modality Qualifier (5th)	Isotope (6th)	Qualifier (7th)
0 Eye	9 High Dose Rate (HDR) B Low Dose Rate (LDR)	7 Cesium 137 (Cs-137) 8 Iridium 192 (Ir-192) 9 Iodine 125 (I-125) B Palladium 103 (Pd-103) C Californium 252 (Cf-252) Y Other Isotope	Z None

Section	D	Radiation Therapy
Body System	8	Eye
Modality	2	Stereotactic Radiosurgery

Treatment Site (4th)	Modality Qualifier (5th)	Isotope (6th)	Qualifier (7th)
0 Eye	D Stereotactic Other Photon Radiosurgery H Stereotactic Particulate Radiosurgery J Stereotactic Gamma Beam Radiosurgery	Z None	Z None

Section	D	Radiation Therapy
Body System	8	Eye
Modality	Y	Other Radiation

Treatment Site (4th)	Modality Qualifier (5th)	Isotope (6th)	Qualifier (7th)
0 Eye	7 Contact Radiation 8 Hyperthermia F Plaque Radiation	Z None	Z None

Section	D	Radiation Therapy
Body System	9	Ear, Nose, Mouth and Throat
Modality	0	Beam Radiation

Treatment Site (4th)	Modality Qualifier (5th)	Isotope (6th)	Qualifier (7th)
0 Ear 1 Nose 3 Hypopharynx 4 Mouth 5 Tongue 6 Salivary Glands 7 Sinuses 8 Hard Palate 9 Soft Palate B Larynx D Nasopharynx F Oropharynx	0 Photons <1 MeV 1 Photons 1 - 10 MeV 2 Photons >10 MeV 4 Heavy Particles (Protons,Ions) 5 Neutrons 6 Neutron Capture	Z None	Z None
0 Ear 1 Nose 3 Hypopharynx 4 Mouth 5 Tongue 6 Salivary Glands 7 Sinuses 8 Hard Palate 9 Soft Palate B Larynx D Nasopharynx F Oropharynx	3 Electrons	Z None	0 Intraoperative Z None

Section	D	Radiation Therapy
Body System	9	Ear, Nose, Mouth and Throat
Modality	1	Brachytherapy

Treatment Site (4th)	Modality Qualifier (5th)	Isotope (6th)	Qualifier (7th)
0 Ear 1 Nose 3 Hypopharynx 4 Mouth 5 Tongue 6 Salivary Glands 7 Sinuses 8 Hard Palate 9 Soft Palate B Larynx D Nasopharynx F Oropharynx	9 High Dose Rate (HDR) B Low Dose Rate (LDR)	7 Cesium 137 (Cs-137) 8 Iridium 192 (Ir-192) 9 Iodine 125 (I-125) B Palladium 103 (Pd-103) C Californium 252 (Cf-252) Y Other Isotope	Z None

Section	D	Radiation Therapy
Body System	9	Ear, Nose, Mouth and Throat
Modality	2	Stereotactic Radiosurgery

Treatment Site (4th)	Modality Qualifier (5th)	Isotope (6th)	Qualifier (7th)
0 Ear **1** Nose **4** Mouth **5** Tongue **6** Salivary Glands **7** Sinuses **8** Hard Palate **9** Soft Palate **B** Larynx **C** Pharynx **D** Nasopharynx	**D** Stereotactic Other Photon Radiosurgery **H** Stereotactic Particulate Radiosurgery **J** Stereotactic Gamma Beam Radiosurgery	**Z** None	**Z** None

Section	D	Radiation Therapy
Body System	9	Ear, Nose, Mouth and Throat
Modality	Y	Other Radiation

Treatment Site (4th)	Modality Qualifier (5th)	Isotope (6th)	Qualifier (7th)
0 Ear **1** Nose **5** Tongue **6** Salivary Glands **7** Sinuses **8** Hard Palate **9** Soft Palate	**7** Contact Radiation **8** Hyperthermia **F** Plaque Radiation	**Z** None	**Z** None
3 Hypopharynx **F** Oropharynx	**7** Contact Radiation **8** Hyperthermia	**Z** None	**Z** None
4 Mouth **B** Larynx **D** Nasopharynx	**7** Contact Radiation **8** Hyperthermia **C** Intraoperative Radiation Therapy (IORT) **F** Plaque Radiation	**Z** None	**Z** None
C Pharynx	**C** Intraoperative Radiation Therapy (IORT) **F** Plaque Radiation	**Z** None	**Z** None

Section	D	Radiation Therapy
Body System	B	Respiratory System
Modality	0	Beam Radiation

Treatment Site (4th)	Modality Qualifier (5th)	Isotope (6th)	Qualifier (7th)
0 Trachea **1** Bronchus **2** Lung **5** Pleura **6** Mediastinum **7** Chest Wall **8** Diaphragm	**0** Photons <1 MeV **1** Photons 1 - 10 MeV **2** Photons >10 MeV **4** Heavy Particles (Protons,Ions) **5** Neutrons **6** Neutron Capture	**Z** None	**Z** None
0 Trachea **1** Bronchus **2** Lung **5** Pleura **6** Mediastinum **7** Chest Wall **8** Diaphragm	**3** Electrons	**Z** None	**0** Intraoperative **Z** None

Section	D	Radiation Therapy
Body System	B	Respiratory System
Modality	1	Brachytherapy

Treatment Site (4th)	Modality Qualifier (5th)	Isotope (6th)	Qualifier (7th)
0 Trachea 1 Bronchus 2 Lung 5 Pleura 6 Mediastinum 7 Chest Wall 8 Diaphragm	9 High Dose Rate (HDR) B Low Dose Rate (LDR)	7 Cesium 137 (Cs-137) 8 Iridium 192 (Ir-192) 9 Iodine 125 (I-125) B Palladium 103 (Pd-103) C Californium 252 (Cf-252) Y Other Isotope	Z None

Section	D	Radiation Therapy
Body System	B	Respiratory System
Modality	2	Stereotactic Radiosurgery

Treatment Site (4th)	Modality Qualifier (5th)	Isotope (6th)	Qualifier (7th)
0 Trachea 1 Bronchus 2 Lung 5 Pleura 6 Mediastinum 7 Chest Wall 8 Diaphragm	D Stereotactic Other Photon Radiosurgery H Stereotactic Particulate Radiosurgery J Stereotactic Gamma Beam Radiosurgery	Z None	Z None

Section	D	Radiation Therapy
Body System	B	Respiratory System
Modality	Y	Other Radiation

Treatment Site (4th)	Modality Qualifier (5th)	Isotope (6th)	Qualifier (7th)
0 Trachea 1 Bronchus 2 Lung 5 Pleura 6 Mediastinum 7 Chest Wall 8 Diaphragm	7 Contact Radiation 8 Hyperthermia F Plaque Radiation K Laser Interstitial Thermal Therapy	Z None	Z None

Section	D	Radiation Therapy
Body System	D	Gastrointestinal System
Modality	0	Beam Radiation

Treatment Site (4th)	Modality Qualifier (5th)	Isotope (6th)	Qualifier (7th)
0 Esophagus 1 Stomach 2 Duodenum 3 Jejunum 4 Ileum 5 Colon 7 Rectum	0 Photons <1 MeV 1 Photons 1 - 10 MeV 2 Photons >10 MeV 4 Heavy Particles (Protons,Ions) 5 Neutrons 6 Neutron Capture	Z None	Z None
0 Esophagus 1 Stomach 2 Duodenum 3 Jejunum 4 Ileum 5 Colon 7 Rectum	3 Electrons	Z None	0 Intraoperative Z None

Section	D	Radiation Therapy
Body System	D	Gastrointestinal System
Modality	1	Brachytherapy

Treatment Site (4th)	Modality Qualifier (5th)	Isotope (6th)	Qualifier (7th)
0 Esophagus 1 Stomach 2 Duodenum 3 Jejunum 4 Ileum 5 Colon 7 Rectum	9 High Dose Rate (HDR) B Low Dose Rate (LDR)	7 Cesium 137 (Cs-137) 8 Iridium 192 (Ir-192) 9 Iodine 125 (I-125) B Palladium 103 (Pd-103) C Californium 252 (Cf-252) Y Other Isotope	Z None

Section	D	Radiation Therapy
Body System	D	Gastrointestinal System
Modality	2	Stereotactic Radiosurgery

Treatment Site (4th)	Modality Qualifier (5th)	Isotope (6th)	Qualifier (7th)
0 Esophagus 1 Stomach 2 Duodenum 3 Jejunum 4 Ileum 5 Colon 7 Rectum	D Stereotactic Other Photon Radiosurgery H Stereotactic Particulate Radiosurgery J Stereotactic Gamma Beam Radiosurgery	Z None	Z None

Section	D	Radiation Therapy
Body System	D	Gastrointestinal System
Modality	Y	Other Radiation

Treatment Site (4th)	Modality Qualifier (5th)	Isotope (6th)	Qualifier (7th)
0 Esophagus	7 Contact Radiation 8 Hyperthermia F Plaque Radiation K Laser Interstitial Thermal Therapy	Z None	Z None
1 Stomach 2 Duodenum 3 Jejunum 4 Ileum 5 Colon 7 Rectum	7 Contact Radiation 8 Hyperthermia C Intraoperative Radiation Therapy (IORT) F Plaque Radiation K Laser Interstitial Thermal Therapy	Z None	Z None
8 Anus	C Intraoperative Radiation Therapy (IORT) F Plaque Radiation K Laser Interstitial Thermal Therapy	Z None	Z None

Section	D	Radiation Therapy
Body System	F	Hepatobiliary System and Pancreas
Modality	0	Beam Radiation

Treatment Site (4th)	Modality Qualifier (5th)	Isotope (6th)	Qualifier (7th)
0 Liver 1 Gallbladder 2 Bile Ducts 3 Pancreas	0 Photons <1 MeV 1 Photons 1 - 10 MeV 2 Photons >10 MeV 4 Heavy Particles (Protons,Ions) 5 Neutrons 6 Neutron Capture	Z None	Z None

Continued

DF0 Continued

Section	D	Radiation Therapy
Body System	F	Hepatobiliary System and Pancreas
Modality	0	Beam Radiation

Treatment Site (4th)	Modality Qualifier (5th)	Isotope (6th)	Qualifier (7th)
0 Liver 1 Gallbladder 2 Bile Ducts 3 Pancreas	3 Electrons	Z None	0 Intraoperative Z None

Section	D	Radiation Therapy
Body System	F	Hepatobiliary System and Pancreas
Modality	1	Brachytherapy

Treatment Site (4th)	Modality Qualifier (5th)	Isotope (6th)	Qualifier (7th)
0 Liver 1 Gallbladder 2 Bile Ducts 3 Pancreas	9 High Dose Rate (HDR) B Low Dose Rate (LDR)	7 Cesium 137 (Cs-137) 8 Iridium 192 (Ir-192) 9 Iodine 125 (I-125) B Palladium 103 (Pd-103) C Californium 252 (Cf-252) Y Other Isotope	Z None

Section	D	Radiation Therapy
Body System	F	Hepatobiliary System and Pancreas
Modality	2	Stereotactic Radiosurgery

Treatment Site (4th)	Modality Qualifier (5th)	Isotope (6th)	Qualifier (7th)
0 Liver 1 Gallbladder 2 Bile Ducts 3 Pancreas	D Stereotactic Other Photon Radiosurgery H Stereotactic Particulate Radiosurgery J Stereotactic Gamma Beam Radiosurgery	Z None	Z None

Section	D	Radiation Therapy
Body System	F	Hepatobiliary System and Pancreas
Modality	Y	Other Radiation

Treatment Site (4th)	Modality Qualifier (5th)	Isotope (6th)	Qualifier (7th)
0 Liver 1 Gallbladder 2 Bile Ducts 3 Pancreas	7 Contact Radiation 8 Hyperthermia C Intraoperative Radiation Therapy (IORT) F Plaque Radiation K Laser Interstitial Thermal Therapy	Z None	Z None

Section	D	Radiation Therapy
Body System	G	Endocrine System
Modality	0	Beam Radiation

Treatment Site (4th)	Modality Qualifier (5th)	Isotope (6th)	Qualifier (7th)
0 Pituitary Gland 1 Pineal Body 2 Adrenal Glands 4 Parathyroid Glands 5 Thyroid	0 Photons <1 MeV 1 Photons 1 - 10 MeV 2 Photons >10 MeV 5 Neutrons 6 Neutron Capture	Z None	Z None
0 Pituitary Gland 1 Pineal Body 2 Adrenal Glands 4 Parathyroid Glands 5 Thyroid	3 Electrons	Z None	0 Intraoperative Z None

Section	D	Radiation Therapy
Body System	G	Endocrine System
Modality	1	Brachytherapy

Treatment Site (4ᵗʰ)	Modality Qualifier (5ᵗʰ)	Isotope (6ᵗʰ)	Qualifier (7ᵗʰ)
0 Pituitary Gland **1** Pineal Body **2** Adrenal Glands **4** Parathyroid Glands **5** Thyroid	**9** High Dose Rate (HDR) **B** Low Dose Rate (LDR)	**7** Cesium 137 (Cs-137) **8** Iridium 192 (Ir-192) **9** Iodine 125 (I-125) **B** Palladium 103 (Pd-103) **C** Californium 252 (Cf-252) **Y** Other Isotope	**Z** None

Section	D	Radiation Therapy
Body System	G	Endocrine System
Modality	2	Stereotactic Radiosurgery

Treatment Site (4ᵗʰ)	Modality Qualifier (5ᵗʰ)	Isotope (6ᵗʰ)	Qualifier (7ᵗʰ)
0 Pituitary Gland **1** Pineal Body **2** Adrenal Glands **4** Parathyroid Glands **5** Thyroid	**D** Stereotactic Other Photon Radiosurgery **H** Stereotactic Particulate Radiosurgery **J** Stereotactic Gamma Beam Radiosurgery	**Z** None	**Z** None

Section	D	Radiation Therapy
Body System	G	Endocrine System
Modality	Y	Other Radiation

Treatment Site (4ᵗʰ)	Modality Qualifier (5ᵗʰ)	Isotope (6ᵗʰ)	Qualifier (7ᵗʰ)
0 Pituitary Gland **1** Pineal Body **2** Adrenal Glands **4** Parathyroid Glands **5** Thyroid	**7** Contact Radiation **8** Hyperthermia **F** Plaque Radiation **K** Laser Interstitial Thermal Therapy	**Z** None	**Z** None

Section	D	Radiation Therapy
Body System	H	Skin
Modality	0	Beam Radiation

Treatment Site (4ᵗʰ)	Modality Qualifier (5ᵗʰ)	Isotope (6ᵗʰ)	Qualifier (7ᵗʰ)
2 Skin, Face **3** Skin, Neck **4** Skin, Arm **6** Skin, Chest **7** Skin, Back **8** Skin, Abdomen **9** Skin, Buttock **B** Skin, Leg	**0** Photons <1 MeV **1** Photons 1 - 10 MeV **2** Photons >10 MeV **4** Heavy Particles (Protons,Ions) **5** Neutrons **6** Neutron Capture	**Z** None	**Z** None
2 Skin, Face **3** Skin, Neck **4** Skin, Arm **6** Skin, Chest **7** Skin, Back **8** Skin, Abdomen **9** Skin, Buttock **B** Skin, Leg	**3** Electrons	**Z** None	**0** Intraoperative **Z** None

Section	D	Radiation Therapy
Body System	H	Skin
Modality	Y	Other Radiation

Treatment Site (4th)	Modality Qualifier (5th)	Isotope (6th)	Qualifier (7th)
2 Skin, Face 3 Skin, Neck 4 Skin, Arm 6 Skin, Chest 7 Skin, Back 8 Skin, Abdomen 9 Skin, Buttock B Skin, Leg	7 Contact Radiation 8 Hyperthermia F Plaque Radiation	Z None	Z None
5 Skin, Hand C Skin, Foot	F Plaque Radiation	Z None	Z None

Section	D	Radiation Therapy
Body System	M	Breast
Modality	0	Beam Radiation

Treatment Site (4th)	Modality Qualifier (5th)	Isotope (6th)	Qualifier (7th)
0 Breast, Left 1 Breast, Right	0 Photons <1 MeV 1 Photons 1 - 10 MeV 2 Photons >10 MeV 4 Heavy Particles (Protons,Ions) 5 Neutrons 6 Neutron Capture	Z None	Z None
0 Breast, Left 1 Breast, Right	3 Electrons	Z None	0 Intraoperative Z None

Section	D	Radiation Therapy
Body System	M	Breast
Modality	1	Brachytherapy

Treatment Site (4th)	Modality Qualifier (5th)	Isotope (6th)	Qualifier (7th)
0 Breast, Left 1 Breast, Right	9 High Dose Rate (HDR) B Low Dose Rate (LDR)	7 Cesium 137 (Cs-137) 8 Iridium 192 (Ir-192) 9 Iodine 125 (I-125) B Palladium 103 (Pd-103) C Californium 252 (Cf-252) Y Other Isotope	Z None

Section	D	Radiation Therapy
Body System	M	Breast
Modality	2	Stereotactic Radiosurgery

Treatment Site (4th)	Modality Qualifier (5th)	Isotope (6th)	Qualifier (7th)
0 Breast, Left 1 Breast, Right	D Stereotactic Other Photon Radiosurgery H Stereotactic Particulate Radiosurgery J Stereotactic Gamma Beam Radiosurgery	Z None	Z None

Section	D	Radiation Therapy
Body System	M	Breast
Modality	Y	Other Radiation

Treatment Site (4th)	Modality Qualifier (5th)	Isotope (6th)	Qualifier (7th)
0 Breast, Left 1 Breast, Right	7 Contact Radiation 8 Hyperthermia F Plaque Radiation K Laser Interstitial Thermal Therapy	Z None	Z None

Section	D	Radiation Therapy
Body System	P	Musculoskeletal System
Modality	0	Beam Radiation

Treatment Site (4ᵗʰ)	Modality Qualifier (5ᵗʰ)	Isotope (6ᵗʰ)	Qualifier (7ᵗʰ)
0 Skull 2 Maxilla 3 Mandible 4 Sternum 5 Rib(s) 6 Humerus 7 Radius/Ulna 8 Pelvic Bones 9 Femur B Tibia/Fibula C Other Bone	0 Photons <1 MeV 1 Photons 1 - 10 MeV 2 Photons >10 MeV 4 Heavy Particles (Protons,Ions) 5 Neutrons 6 Neutron Capture	Z None	Z None
0 Skull 2 Maxilla 3 Mandible 4 Sternum 5 Rib(s) 6 Humerus 7 Radius/Ulna 8 Pelvic Bones 9 Femur B Tibia/Fibula C Other Bone	3 Electrons	Z None	0 Intraoperative Z None

Section	D	Radiation Therapy
Body System	P	Musculoskeletal System
Modality	Y	Other Radiation

Treatment Site (4ᵗʰ)	Modality Qualifier (5ᵗʰ)	Isotope (6ᵗʰ)	Qualifier (7ᵗʰ)
0 Skull 2 Maxilla 3 Mandible 4 Sternum 5 Rib(s) 6 Humerus 7 Radius/Ulna 8 Pelvic Bones 9 Femur B Tibia/Fibula C Other Bone	7 Contact Radiation 8 Hyperthermia F Plaque Radiation	Z None	Z None

Section	D	Radiation Therapy
Body System	T	Urinary System
Modality	0	Beam Radiation

Treatment Site (4ᵗʰ)	Modality Qualifier (5ᵗʰ)	Isotope (6ᵗʰ)	Qualifier (7ᵗʰ)
0 Kidney 1 Ureter 2 Bladder 3 Urethra	0 Photons <1 MeV 1 Photons 1 - 10 MeV 2 Photons >10 MeV 4 Heavy Particles (Protons,Ions) 5 Neutrons 6 Neutron Capture	Z None	Z None
0 Kidney 1 Ureter 2 Bladder 3 Urethra	3 Electrons	Z None	0 Intraoperative Z None

Section	D	Radiation Therapy
Body System	T	Urinary System
Modality	1	Brachytherapy

Treatment Site (4th)	Modality Qualifier (5th)	Isotope (6th)	Qualifier (7th)
0 Kidney 1 Ureter 2 Bladder 3 Urethra	9 High Dose Rate (HDR) B Low Dose Rate (LDR)	7 Cesium 137 (Cs-137) 8 Iridium 192 (Ir-192) 9 Iodine 125 (I-125) B Palladium 103 (Pd-103) C Californium 252 (Cf-252) Y Other Isotope	Z None

Section	D	Radiation Therapy
Body System	T	Urinary System
Modality	2	Stereotactic Radiosurgery

Treatment Site (4th)	Modality Qualifier (5th)	Isotope (6th)	Qualifier (7th)
0 Kidney 1 Ureter 2 Bladder 3 Urethra	D Stereotactic Other Photon Radiosurgery H Stereotactic Particulate Radiosurgery J Stereotactic Gamma Beam Radiosurgery	Z None	Z None

Section	D	Radiation Therapy
Body System	T	Urinary System
Modality	Y	Other Radiation

Treatment Site (4th)	Modality Qualifier (5th)	Isotope (6th)	Qualifier (7th)
0 Kidney 1 Ureter 2 Bladder 3 Urethra	7 Contact Radiation 8 Hyperthermia C Intraoperative Radiation Therapy (IORT) F Plaque Radiation	Z None	Z None

Section	D	Radiation Therapy
Body System	U	Female Reproductive System
Modality	0	Beam Radiation

Treatment Site (4th)	Modality Qualifier (5th)	Isotope (6th)	Qualifier (7th)
0 Ovary 1 Cervix 2 Uterus	0 Photons <1 MeV 1 Photons 1 - 10 MeV 2 Photons >10 MeV 4 Heavy Particles (Protons,Ions) 5 Neutrons 6 Neutron Capture	Z None	Z None
0 Ovary 1 Cervix 2 Uterus	3 Electrons	Z None	0 Intraoperative Z None

Section	D	Radiation Therapy
Body System	U	Female Reproductive System
Modality	1	Brachytherapy

Treatment Site (4th)	Modality Qualifier (5th)	Isotope (6th)	Qualifier (7th)
0 Ovary 1 Cervix 2 Uterus	9 High Dose Rate (HDR) B Low Dose Rate (LDR)	7 Cesium 137 (Cs-137) 8 Iridium 192 (Ir-192) 9 Iodine 125 (I-125) B Palladium 103 (Pd-103) C Californium 252 (Cf-252) Y Other Isotope	Z None

Section	D	Radiation Therapy
Body System	U	Female Reproductive System
Modality	2	Stereotactic Radiosurgery

Treatment Site (4th)	Modality Qualifier (5th)	Isotope (6th)	Qualifier (7th)
0 Ovary 1 Cervix 2 Uterus	D Stereotactic Other Photon Radiosurgery H Stereotactic Particulate Radiosurgery J Stereotactic Gamma Beam Radiosurgery	Z None	Z None

Section	D	Radiation Therapy
Body System	U	Female Reproductive System
Modality	Y	Other Radiation

Treatment Site (4th)	Modality Qualifier (5th)	Isotope (6th)	Qualifier (7th)
0 Ovary 1 Cervix 2 Uterus	7 Contact Radiation 8 Hyperthermia C Intraoperative Radiation Therapy (IORT) F Plaque Radiation	Z None	Z None

Section	D	Radiation Therapy
Body System	V	Male Reproductive System
Modality	0	Beam Radiation

Treatment Site (4th)	Modality Qualifier (5th)	Isotope (6th)	Qualifier (7th)
0 Prostate 1 Testis	0 Photons <1 MeV 1 Photons 1 - 10 MeV 2 Photons >10 MeV 4 Heavy Particles (Protons,Ions) 5 Neutrons 6 Neutron Capture	Z None	Z None
0 Prostate 1 Testis	3 Electrons	Z None	0 Intraoperative Z None

Section	D	Radiation Therapy
Body System	V	Male Reproductive System
Modality	1	Brachytherapy

Treatment Site (4th)	Modality Qualifier (5th)	Isotope (6th)	Qualifier (7th)
0 Prostate 1 Testis	9 High Dose Rate (HDR) B Low Dose Rate (LDR)	7 Cesium 137 (Cs-137) 8 Iridium 192 (Ir-192) 9 Iodine 125 (I-125) B Palladium 103 (Pd-103) C Californium 252 (Cf-252) Y Other Isotope	Z None

Section	D	Radiation Therapy
Body System	V	Male Reproductive System
Modality	2	Stereotactic Radiosurgery

Treatment Site (4th)	Modality Qualifier (5th)	Isotope (6th)	Qualifier (7th)
0 Prostate 1 Testis	D Stereotactic Other Photon Radiosurgery H Stereotactic Particulate Radiosurgery J Stereotactic Gamma Beam Radiosurgery	Z None	Z None

Section	D	Radiation Therapy
Body System	V	Male Reproductive System
Modality	Y	Other Radiation

Treatment Site (4th)	Modality Qualifier (5th)	Isotope (6th)	Qualifier (7th)
0 Prostate	7 Contact Radiation 8 Hyperthermia C Intraoperative Radiation Therapy (IORT) F Plaque Radiation K Laser Interstitial Thermal Therapy	Z None	Z None
1 Testis	7 Contact Radiation 8 Hyperthermia F Plaque Radiation	Z None	Z None

Section	D	Radiation Therapy
Body System	W	Anatomical Regions
Modality	0	Beam Radiation

Treatment Site (4th)	Modality Qualifier (5th)	Isotope (6th)	Qualifier (7th)
1 Head and Neck 2 Chest 3 Abdomen 4 Hemibody 5 Whole Body 6 Pelvic Region	0 Photons <1 MeV 1 Photons 1 - 10 MeV 2 Photons >10 MeV 4 Heavy Particles (Protons,Ions) 5 Neutrons 6 Neutron Capture	Z None	Z None
1 Head and Neck 2 Chest 3 Abdomen 4 Hemibody 5 Whole Body 6 Pelvic Region	3 Electrons	Z None	0 Intraoperative Z None

Section	D	Radiation Therapy
Body System	W	Anatomical Regions
Modality	1	Brachytherapy

Treatment Site (4th)	Modality Qualifier (5th)	Isotope (6th)	Qualifier (7th)
1 Head and Neck 2 Chest 3 Abdomen 6 Pelvic Region	9 High Dose Rate (HDR) B Low Dose Rate (LDR)	7 Cesium 137 (Cs-137) 8 Iridium 192 (Ir-192) 9 Iodine 125 (I-125) B Palladium 103 (Pd-103) C Californium 252 (Cf-252) Y Other Isotope	Z None

Section	D	Radiation Therapy
Body System	W	Anatomical Regions
Modality	2	Stereotactic Radiosurgery

Treatment Site (4th)	Modality Qualifier (5th)	Isotope (6th)	Qualifier (7th)
1 Head and Neck 2 Chest 3 Abdomen 6 Pelvic Region	D Stereotactic Other Photon Radiosurgery H Stereotactic Particulate Radiosurgery J Stereotactic Gamma Beam Radiosurgery	Z None	Z None

Section	D	Radiation Therapy
Body System	W	Anatomical Regions
Modality	Y	Other Radiation

Treatment Site (4th)	Modality Qualifier (5th)	Isotope (6th)	Qualifier (7th)
1 Head and Neck 2 Chest 3 Abdomen 4 Hemibody 6 Pelvic Region	7 Contact Radiation 8 Hyperthermia F Plaque Radiation	Z None	Z None
5 Whole Body	7 Contact Radiation 8 Hyperthermia F Plaque Radiation	Z None	Z None
5 Whole Body	G Isotope Administration	D Iodine 131 (I-131) F Phosphorus 32 (P-32) G Strontium 89 (Sr-89) H Strontium 90 (Sr-90) Y Other Isotope	Z None

Physical Rehabilitation and Diagnostic Audiology Section (F00–F15)

Within each section of ICD-10-PCS the characters have different meanings. The seven character meanings for the Physical Rehabilitation and Diagnostic Audiology section are illustrated below through the procedure example of *Individual fitting of moveable brace, right knee.*

Section	Section Qualifier	Root Type	Body System/ Region	Type Qualifier	Equipment	Qualifier
Physical Rehabilitation and Diagnostic Audiology	Rehabilitation	Device Fitting	None	Dynamic Orthosis	Orthosis	None
F	0	D	Z	6	E	Z

Section (Character 1)

All Physical Rehabilitation and Diagnostic Audiology procedure codes have a first character value of F.

Section Qualifier (Character 2)

The alphanumeric character in the second character position identifies if the procedure is a physical rehabilitation procedure or a diagnostic audiology procedure. Physical rehabilitation is reported with character value 0, and diagnostic audiology is reported with character value 1.

Root Type (Character 3)

The alphanumeric character value for root types is placed in the third position. The following are the root types applicable to the Physical Rehabilitation and Diagnostic Audiology section with their associated meaning.

Character Value	Root Type	Root Type Definition
0	Speech Assessment	Measurement of speech and related functions
1	Motor and/or Nerve Function Assessment	Measurement of motor, nerve, and related functions
2	Activities of Daily Living Assessment	Measurement of functional level for activities of daily living
3	Hearing Assessment	Measurement of hearing and related functions
4	Hearing Aid Assessment	Measurement of the appropriateness and/or effectiveness of a hearing device
5	Vestibular Assessment	Measurement of the vestibular system and related functions
6	Speech Treatment	Application of techniques to improve, augment, or compensate for speech and related functional impairment
7	Motor Treatment	Exercise or activities to increase or facilitate motor function
8	Activities of Daily Living Treatment	Exercise or activities to facilitate functional competence for activities of daily living
9	Hearing Treatment	Application of techniques to improve, augment, or compensate for hearing and related functional impairment

Continued

Character Value	Root Type	Root Type Definition
B	Cochlear Implant Treatment	Application of techniques to improve the communication abilities of individuals with cochlear implant
C	Vestibular Treatment	Application of techniques to improve, augment, or compensate for vestibular and related functional impairment
D	Device Fitting	Fitting of a device designed to facilitate or support achievement of a higher level of function
F	Caregiver Training	Training in activities to support patient's optimal level of function

Body System/Region (Character 4)

For each body system/region the applicable body part character values will be available for procedure code construction. An example of a body region for this section is Musculoskeletal System—Lower Back/Lower Extremity.

Type Qualifier (Character 5)

Type qualifier further specifies the root type procedure. For example, the type qualifier of Gait Training/Functional Ambulation is used with Motor Treatment (character value 7) when applicable.

Equipment (Character 6)

If equipment is utilized during the procedure character six is used to report the type. Some examples of equipment are

- Aerobic Endurance and Conditioning
- Electrotherapeutic
- Mechanical
- Orthosis
- Prosthesis

If equipment is not utilized, the placeholder character value of Z should be reported.

Qualifier (Character 7)

The qualifier represents an additional attribute for the procedure when applicable. Currently, there are no qualifiers in the Physical Rehabilitation and Diagnostic Audiology section; therefore, the placeholder character value of Z should be reported.

Physical Rehabilitation and Diagnostic Audiology Section Tables

Physical Rehabilitation and Diagnostic Audiology Tables F00–F15

Section	F	**Physical Rehabilitation and Diagnostic Audiology**
Section Qualifier	0	**Rehabilitation**
Type	0	**Speech Assessment:** Measurement of speech and related functions

Body System / Region (4th)	Type Qualifier (5th)	Equipment (6th)	Qualifier (7th)
3 Neurological System - Whole Body	G Communicative/Cognitive Integration Skills	K Audiovisual M Augmentative / Alternative Communication P Computer Y Other Equipment Z None	Z None
Z None	0 Filtered Speech 3 Staggered Spondaic Word Q Performance Intensity Phonetically Balanced Speech Discrimination R Brief Tone Stimuli S Distorted Speech T Dichotic Stimuli V Temporal Ordering of Stimuli W Masking Patterns	1 Audiometer 2 Sound Field / Booth K Audiovisual Z None	Z None
Z None	1 Speech Threshold 2 Speech/Word Recognition	1 Audiometer 2 Sound Field / Booth 9 Cochlear Implant K Audiovisual Z None	Z None
Z None	4 Sensorineural Acuity Level	1 Audiometer 2 Sound Field / Booth Z None	Z None
Z None	5 Synthetic Sentence Identification	1 Audiometer 2 Sound Field / Booth 9 Cochlear Implant K Audiovisual	Z None
Z None	6 Speech and/or Language Screening 7 Nonspoken Language 8 Receptive/Expressive Language C Aphasia G Communicative/Cognitive Integration Skills L Augmentative/Alternative Communication System	K Audiovisual M Augmentative / Alternative Communication P Computer Y Other Equipment Z None	Z None
Z None	9 Articulation/Phonology	K Audiovisual P Computer Q Speech Analysis Y Other Equipment Z None	Z None
Z None	B Motor Speech	K Audiovisual N Biosensory Feedback P Computer Q Speech Analysis T Aerodynamic Function Y Other Equipment Z None	Z None

Continued

Section	F	Physical Rehabilitation and Diagnostic Audiology		F00 *Continued*
Section Qualifier	0	Rehabilitation		
Type	0	Speech Assessment: Measurement of speech and related functions		

Body System / Region (4th)	Type Qualifier (5th)	Equipment (6th)	Qualifier (7th)
Z None	D Fluency	K Audiovisual N Biosensory Feedback P Computer Q Speech Analysis S Voice Analysis T Aerodynamic Function Y Other Equipment Z None	Z None
Z None	F Voice	K Audiovisual N Biosensory Feedback P Computer S Voice Analysis T Aerodynamic Function Y Other Equipment Z None	Z None
Z None	H Bedside Swallowing and Oral Function P Oral Peripheral Mechanism	Y Other Equipment Z None	Z None
Z None	J Instrumental Swallowing and Oral Function	T Aerodynamic Function W Swallowing Y Other Equipment	Z None
Z None	K Orofacial Myofunctional	K Audiovisual P Computer Y Other Equipment Z None	Z None
Z None	M Voice Prosthetic	K Audiovisual P Computer S Voice Analysis V Speech Prosthesis Y Other Equipment Z None	Z None
Z None	N Non-invasive Instrumental Status	N Biosensory Feedback P Computer Q Speech Analysis S Voice Analysis T Aerodynamic Function Y Other Equipment	Z None
Z None	X Other Specified Central Auditory Processing	Z None	Z None

Section   **F**   **Physical Rehabilitation and Diagnostic Audiology**
Section Qualifier **0**   **Rehabilitation**
Type   **1**   **Motor and/or Nerve Function Assessment:** Measurement of motor, nerve, and related functions

Body System / Region (4th)	Type Qualifier (5th)	Equipment (6th)	Qualifier (7th)
0 Neurological System - Head and Neck **1** Neurological System - Upper Back / Upper Extremity **2** Neurological System - Lower Back / Lower Extremity **3** Neurological System - Whole Body	**0** Muscle Performance	**E** Orthosis **F** Assistive, Adaptive, Supportive or Protective **U** Prosthesis **Y** Other Equipment **Z** None	**Z** None
0 Neurological System - Head and Neck **1** Neurological System - Upper Back / Upper Extremity **2** Neurological System - Lower Back / Lower Extremity **3** Neurological System - Whole Body	**1** Integumentary Integrity **3** Coordination/Dexterity **4** Motor Function **G** Reflex Integrity	**Z** None	**Z** None
0 Neurological System - Head and Neck **1** Neurological System - Upper Back / Upper Extremity **2** Neurological System - Lower Back / Lower Extremity **3** Neurological System - Whole Body	**5** Range of Motion and Joint Integrity **6** Sensory Awareness/ Processing/Integrity	**Y** Other Equipment **Z** None	**Z** None
D Integumentary System - Head and Neck **F** Integumentary System - Upper Back / Upper Extremity **G** Integumentary System - Lower Back / Lower Extremity **H** Integumentary System - Whole Body **J** Musculoskeletal System - Head and Neck **K** Musculoskeletal System - Upper Back / Upper Extremity **L** Musculoskeletal System - Lower Back / Lower Extremity **M** Musculoskeletal System - Whole Body	**0** Muscle Performance	**E** Orthosis **F** Assistive, Adaptive, Supportive or Protective **U** Prosthesis **Y** Other Equipment **Z** None	**Z** None
D Integumentary System - Head and Neck **F** Integumentary System - Upper Back / Upper Extremity **G** Integumentary System - Lower Back / Lower Extremity **H** Integumentary System - Whole Body **J** Musculoskeletal System - Head and Neck **K** Musculoskeletal System - Upper Back / Upper Extremity **L** Musculoskeletal System - Lower Back / Lower Extremity **M** Musculoskeletal System - Whole Body	**1** Integumentary Integrity	**Z** None	**Z** None
D Integumentary System - Head and Neck **F** Integumentary System - Upper Back / Upper Extremity **G** Integumentary System - Lower Back / Lower Extremity **H** Integumentary System - Whole Body **J** Musculoskeletal System - Head and Neck **K** Musculoskeletal System - Upper Back / Upper Extremity **L** Musculoskeletal System - Lower Back / Lower Extremity **M** Musculoskeletal System - Whole Body	**5** Range of Motion and Joint Integrity **6** Sensory Awareness/ Processing/Integrity	**Y** Other Equipment **Z** None	**Z** None

Continued

Section   **F**   **Physical Rehabilitation and Diagnostic Audiology**   *F01 Continued*
Section Qualifier   **0**   **Rehabilitation**
Type   **1**   **Motor and/or Nerve Function Assessment:** Measurement of motor, nerve, and related functions

Body System / Region (4th)	Type Qualifier (5th)	Equipment (6th)	Qualifier (7th)
N Genitourinary System	0 Muscle Performance	E Orthosis F Assistive, Adaptive, Supportive or Protective U Prosthesis Y Other Equipment Z None	Z None
Z None	2 Visual Motor Integration	K Audiovisual M Augmentative / Alternative Communication N Biosensory Feedback P Computer Q Speech Analysis S Voice Analysis Y Other Equipment Z None	Z None
Z None	7 Facial Nerve Function	7 Electrophysiologic	Z None
Z None	9 Somatosensory Evoked Potentials	J Somatosensory	Z None
Z None	B Bed Mobility C Transfer F Wheelchair Mobility	E Orthosis F Assistive, Adaptive, Supportive or Protective U Prosthesis Z None	Z None
Z None	D Gait and/or Balance	E Orthosis F Assistive, Adaptive, Supportive or Protective U Prosthesis Y Other Equipment Z None	Z None

Section   **F**   **Physical Rehabilitation and Diagnostic Audiology**
Section Qualifier   **0**   **Rehabilitation**
Type   **2**   **Activities of Daily Living Assessment:** Measurement of functional level for activities of daily living

Body System / Region (4th)	Type Qualifier (5th)	Equipment (6th)	Qualifier (7th)
0 Neurological System - Head and Neck	9 Cranial Nerve Integrity D Neuromotor Development	Y Other Equipment Z None	Z None
1 Neurological System - Upper Back / Upper Extremity 2 Neurological System - Lower Back / Lower Extremity 3 Neurological System - Whole Body	D Neuromotor Development	Y Other Equipment Z None	Z None
4 Circulatory System - Head and Neck 5 Circulatory System - Upper Back / Upper Extremity 6 Circulatory System - Lower Back / Lower Extremity 8 Respiratory System - Head and Neck 9 Respiratory System - Upper Back / Upper Extremity B Respiratory System - Lower Back / Lower Extremity	G Ventilation, Respiration and Circulation	C Mechanical G Aerobic Endurance and Conditioning Y Other Equipment Z None	Z None

Continued

Section	F	**Physical Rehabilitation and Diagnostic Audiology**	F02 *Continued*
Section Qualifier	0	**Rehabilitation**	
Type	2	**Activities of Daily Living Assessment:** Measurement of functional level for activities of daily living	

Body System / Region (4th)	Type Qualifier (5th)	Equipment (6th)	Qualifier (7th)
7 Circulatory System - Whole Body C Respiratory System - Whole Body	7 Aerobic Capacity and Endurance	E Orthosis G Aerobic Endurance and Conditioning U Prosthesis Y Other Equipment Z None	Z None
7 Circulatory System - Whole Body C Respiratory System - Whole Body	G Ventilation, Respiration and Circulation	C Mechanical G Aerobic Endurance and Conditioning Y Other Equipment Z None	Z None
Z None	0 Bathing/Showering 1 Dressing 3 Grooming/Personal Hygiene 4 Home Management	E Orthosis F Assistive, Adaptive, Supportive or Protective U Prosthesis Z None	Z None
Z None	2 Feeding/Eating 8 Anthropometric Characteristics F Pain	Y Other Equipment Z None	Z None
Z None	5 Perceptual Processing	K Audiovisual M Augmentative / Alternative Communication N Biosensory Feedback P Computer Q Speech Analysis S Voice Analysis Y Other Equipment Z None	Z None
Z None	6 Psychosocial Skills	Z None	Z None
Z None	B Environmental, Home and Work Barriers C Ergonomics and Body Mechanics	E Orthosis F Assistive, Adaptive, Supportive or Protective U Prosthesis Y Other Equipment Z None	Z None
Z None	H Vocational Activities and Functional Community or Work Reintegration Skills	E Orthosis F Assistive, Adaptive, Supportive or Protective G Aerobic Endurance and Conditioning U Prosthesis Y Other Equipment Z None	Z None

Section   **F**   **Physical Rehabilitation and Diagnostic Audiology**
Section Qualifier **0**   **Rehabilitation**
Type   **6**   **Speech Treatment:** Application of techniques to improve, augment, or compensate for speech and related
                                functional impairment

Body System / Region (4ᵗʰ)	Type Qualifier (5ᵗʰ)	Equipment (6ᵗʰ)	Qualifier (7ᵗʰ)
3 Neurological System - Whole Body	6 Communicative/ Cognitive Integration Skills	K Audiovisual M Augmentative / Alternative Communication P Computer Y Other Equipment Z None	Z None
Z None	0 Nonspoken Language 3 Aphasia 6 Communicative/ Cognitive Integration Skills	K Audiovisual M Augmentative / Alternative Communication P Computer Y Other Equipment Z None	Z None
Z None	1 Speech-Language Pathology and Related Disorders Counseling 2 Speech-Language Pathology and Related Disorders Prevention	K Audiovisual Z None	Z None
Z None	4 Articulation/ Phonology	K Audiovisual P Computer Q Speech Analysis T Aerodynamic Function Y Other Equipment Z None	Z None
Z None	5 Aural Rehabilitation	K Audiovisual L Assistive Listening M Augmentative / Alternative Communication N Biosensory Feedback P Computer Q Speech Analysis S Voice Analysis Y Other Equipment Z None	Z None
Z None	7 Fluency	4 Electroacoustic Immitance / Acoustic Reflex K Audiovisual N Biosensory Feedback Q Speech Analysis S Voice Analysis T Aerodynamic Function Y Other Equipment Z None	Z None
Z None	8 Motor Speech	K Audiovisual N Biosensory Feedback P Computer Q Speech Analysis S Voice Analysis T Aerodynamic Function Y Other Equipment Z None	Z None
Z None	9 Orofacial Myofunctional	K Audiovisual P Computer Y Other Equipment Z None	Z None

Continued

Section	F	Physical Rehabilitation and Diagnostic Audiology	F06 *Continued*
Section Qualifier	0	Rehabilitation	
Type	6	**Speech Treatment:** Application of techniques to improve, augment, or compensate for speech and related functional impairment	

Body System / Region (4ᵗʰ)	Type Qualifier (5ᵗʰ)	Equipment (6ᵗʰ)	Qualifier (7ᵗʰ)
Z None	B Receptive/Expressive Language	K Audiovisual L Assistive Listening M Augmentative / Alternative Communication P Computer Y Other Equipment Z None	Z None
Z None	C Voice	K Audiovisual N Biosensory Feedback P Computer S Voice Analysis T Aerodynamic Function V Speech Prosthesis Y Other Equipment Z None	Z None
Z None	D Swallowing Dysfunction	M Augmentative / Alternative Communication T Aerodynamic Function V Speech Prosthesis Y Other Equipment Z None	Z None

Section	F	Physical Rehabilitation and Diagnostic Audiology	
Section Qualifier	0	Rehabilitation	
Type	7	**Motor Treatment:** Exercise or activities to increase or facilitate motor function	

Body System / Region (4ᵗʰ)	Type Qualifier (5ᵗʰ)	Equipment (6ᵗʰ)	Qualifier (7ᵗʰ)
0 Neurological System - Head and Neck 1 Neurological System - Upper Back / Upper Extremity 2 Neurological System - Lower Back / Lower Extremity 3 Neurological System - Whole Body D Integumentary System - Head and Neck F Integumentary System - Upper Back / Upper Extremity G Integumentary System - Lower Back / Lower Extremity H Integumentary System - Whole Body J Musculoskeletal System - Head and Neck K Musculoskeletal System - Upper Back / Upper Extremity L Musculoskeletal System - Lower Back / Lower Extremity M Musculoskeletal System - Whole Body	0 Range of Motion and Joint Mobility 1 Muscle Performance 2 Coordination/ Dexterity 3 Motor Function	E Orthosis F Assistive, Adaptive, Supportive or Protective U Prosthesis Y Other Equipment Z None	Z None
0 Neurological System - Head and Neck 1 Neurological System - Upper Back / Upper Extremity 2 Neurological System - Lower Back / Lower Extremity 3 Neurological System - Whole Body D Integumentary System - Head and Neck F Integumentary System - Upper Back / Upper Extremity G Integumentary System - Lower Back / Lower Extremity H Integumentary System - Whole Body J Musculoskeletal System - Head and Neck K Musculoskeletal System - Upper Back / Upper Extremity L Musculoskeletal System - Lower Back / Lower Extremity M Musculoskeletal System - Whole Body	6 Therapeutic Exercise	B Physical Agents C Mechanical D Electrotherapeutic E Orthosis F Assistive, Adaptive, Supportive or Protective G Aerobic Endurance and Conditioning H Mechanical or Electromechanical U Prosthesis Y Other Equipment Z None	Z None

Continued

Section	F	Physical Rehabilitation and Diagnostic Audiology	F07 *Continued*
Section Qualifier	0	Rehabilitation	
Type	7	**Motor Treatment:** Exercise or activities to increase or facilitate motor function	

Body System / Region (4th)	Type Qualifier (5th)	Equipment (6th)	Qualifier (7th)
0 Neurological System - Head and Neck 1 Neurological System - Upper Back / Upper Extremity 2 Neurological System - Lower Back / Lower Extremity 3 Neurological System - Whole Body D Integumentary System - Head and Neck F Integumentary System - Upper Back / Upper Extremity G Integumentary System - Lower Back / Lower Extremity H Integumentary System - Whole Body J Musculoskeletal System - Head and Neck K Musculoskeletal System - Upper Back / Upper Extremity L Musculoskeletal System - Lower Back / Lower Extremity M Musculoskeletal System - Whole Body	7 Manual Therapy Techniques	Z None	Z None
4 Circulatory System - Head and Neck 5 Circulatory System - Upper Back / Upper Extremity 6 Circulatory System - Lower Back / Lower Extremity 7 Circulatory System - Whole Body 8 Respiratory System - Head and Neck 9 Respiratory System - Upper Back / Upper Extremity B Respiratory System - Lower Back / Lower Extremity C Respiratory System - Whole Body	6 Therapeutic Exercise	B Physical Agents C Mechanical D Electrotherapeutic E Orthosis F Assistive, Adaptive, Supportive or Protective G Aerobic Endurance and Conditioning H Mechanical or Electromechanical U Prosthesis Y Other Equipment Z None	Z None
N Genitourinary System	1 Muscle Performance	E Orthosis F Assistive, Adaptive, Supportive or Protective U Prosthesis Y Other Equipment Z None	Z None
N Genitourinary System	6 Therapeutic Exercise	B Physical Agents C Mechanical D Electrotherapeutic E Orthosis F Assistive, Adaptive, Supportive or Protective G Aerobic Endurance and Conditioning H Mechanical or Electromechanical U Prosthesis Y Other Equipment Z None	Z None
Z None	4 Wheelchair Mobility	D Electrotherapeutic E Orthosis F Assistive, Adaptive, Supportive or Protective U Prosthesis Y Other Equipment Z None	Z None

Continued

Section	F	Physical Rehabilitation and Diagnostic Audiology	F07 *Continued*
Section Qualifier	0	Rehabilitation	
Type	7	**Motor Treatment:** Exercise or activities to increase or facilitate motor function	

Body System / Region (4th)	Type Qualifier (5th)	Equipment (6th)	Qualifier (7th)
Z None	**5** Bed Mobility	**C** Mechanical **E** Orthosis **F** Assistive, Adaptive, Supportive or Protective **U** Prosthesis **Y** Other Equipment **Z** None	**Z** None
Z None	**8** Transfer Training	**C** Mechanical **D** Electrotherapeutic **E** Orthosis **F** Assistive, Adaptive, Supportive or Protective **U** Prosthesis **Y** Other Equipment **Z** None	**Z** None
Z None	**9** Gait Training/ Functional Ambulation	**C** Mechanical **D** Electrotherapeutic **E** Orthosis **F** Assistive, Adaptive, Supportive or Protective **G** Aerobic Endurance and Conditioning **U** Prosthesis **Y** Other Equipment **Z** None	**Z** None

Section	F	Physical Rehabilitation and Diagnostic Audiology
Section Qualifier	0	Rehabilitation
Type	8	**Activities of Daily Living Treatment:** Exercise or activities to facilitate functional competence for activities of daily living

Body System / Region (4th)	Type Qualifier (5th)	Equipment (6th)	Qualifier (7th)
D Integumentary System - Head and Neck **F** Integumentary System - Upper Back / Upper Extremity **G** Integumentary System - Lower Back / Lower Extremity **H** Integumentary System - Whole Body **J** Musculoskeletal System - Head and Neck **K** Musculoskeletal System - Upper Back / Upper Extremity **L** Musculoskeletal System - Lower Back / Lower Extremity **M** Musculoskeletal System - Whole Body	**5** Wound Management	**B** Physical Agents **C** Mechanical **D** Electrotherapeutic **E** Orthosis **F** Assistive, Adaptive, Supportive or Protective **U** Prosthesis **Y** Other Equipment **Z** None	**Z** None
Z None	**0** Bathing/Showering Techniques **1** Dressing Techniques **2** Grooming/Personal Hygiene	**E** Orthosis **F** Assistive, Adaptive, Supportive or Protective **U** Prosthesis **Y** Other Equipment **Z** None	**Z** None

Continued

Section	F	Physical Rehabilitation and Diagnostic Audiology	F08 *Continued*
Section Qualifier	0	Rehabilitation	
Type	8	**Activities of Daily Living Treatment:** Exercise or activities to facilitate functional competence for activities of daily living	

Body System / Region (4th)	Type Qualifier (5th)	Equipment (6th)	Qualifier (7th)
Z None	3 Feeding/Eating	C Mechanical D Electrotherapeutic E Orthosis F Assistive, Adaptive, Supportive or Protective U Prosthesis Y Other Equipment Z None	Z None
Z None	4 Home Management	D Electrotherapeutic E Orthosis F Assistive, Adaptive, Supportive or Protective U Prosthesis Y Other Equipment Z None	Z None
Z None	6 Psychosocial Skills	Z None	Z None
Z None	7 Vocational Activities and Functional Community or Work Reintegration Skills	B Physical Agents C Mechanical D Electrotherapeutic E Orthosis F Assistive, Adaptive, Supportive or Protective G Aerobic Endurance and Conditioning U Prosthesis Y Other Equipment Z None	Z None

Section	F	Physical Rehabilitation and Diagnostic Audiology	
Section Qualifier	0	Rehabilitation	
Type	9	**Hearing Treatment:** Application of techniques to improve, augment, or compensate for hearing and related functional impairment	

Body System / Region (4th)	Type Qualifier (5th)	Equipment (6th)	Qualifier (7th)
Z None	0 Hearing and Related Disorders Counseling 1 Hearing and Related Disorders Prevention	K Audiovisual Z None	Z None
Z None	2 Auditory Processing	K Audiovisual L Assistive Listening P Computer Y Other Equipment Z None	Z None
Z None	3 Cerumen Management	X Cerumen Management Z None	Z None

Section	F	Physical Rehabilitation and Diagnostic Audiology
Section Qualifier	0	Rehabilitation
Type	B	**Cochlear Implant Treatment:** Application of techniques to improve the communication abilities of individuals with cochlear implant

Body System / Region (4th)	Type Qualifier (5th)	Equipment (6th)	Qualifier (7th)
Z None	0 Cochlear Implant Rehabilitation	1 Audiometer 2 Sound Field / Booth 9 Cochlear Implant K Audiovisual P Computer Y Other Equipment	Z None

Section	F	Physical Rehabilitation and Diagnostic Audiology
Section Qualifier	0	Rehabilitation
Type	C	**Vestibular Treatment:** Application of techniques to improve, augment, or compensate for vestibular and related functional impairment

Body System / Region (4th)	Type Qualifier (5th)	Equipment (6th)	Qualifier (7th)
3 Neurological System - Whole Body H Integumentary System - Whole Body M Musculoskeletal System - Whole Body	3 Postural Control	E Orthosis F Assistive, Adaptive, Supportive or Protective U Prosthesis Y Other Equipment Z None	Z None
Z None	0 Vestibular	8 Vestibular / Balance Z None	Z None
Z None	1 Perceptual Processing 2 Visual Motor Integration	K Audiovisual L Assistive Listening N Biosensory Feedback P Computer Q Speech Analysis S Voice Analysis T Aerodynamic Function Y Other Equipment Z None	Z None

Section	F	Physical Rehabilitation and Diagnostic Audiology
Section Qualifier	0	Rehabilitation
Type	D	**Device Fitting:** Fitting of a device designed to facilitate or support achievement of a higher level of function

Body System / Region (4th)	Type Qualifier (5th)	Equipment (6th)	Qualifier (7th)
Z None	0 Tinnitus Masker	5 Hearing Aid Selection / Fitting / Test Z None	Z None
Z None	1 Monaural Hearing Aid 2 Binaural Hearing Aid 5 Assistive Listening Device	1 Audiometer 2 Sound Field / Booth 5 Hearing Aid Selection / Fitting / Test K Audiovisual L Assistive Listening Z None	Z None
Z None	3 Augmentative/Alternative Communication System	M Augmentative / Alternative Communication	Z None
Z None	4 Voice Prosthetic	S Voice Analysis V Speech Prosthesis	Z None

Continued

Section	F	Physical Rehabilitation and Diagnostic Audiology	F0D *Continued*
Section Qualifier	0	Rehabilitation	
Type	D	Device Fitting: Fitting of a device designed to facilitate or support achievement of a higher level of function	

Body System / Region (4th)	Type Qualifier (5th)	Equipment (6th)	Qualifier (7th)
Z None	6 Dynamic Orthosis 7 Static Orthosis 8 Prosthesis 9 Assistive, Adaptive, Supportive or Protective Devices	E Orthosis F Assistive, Adaptive, Supportive or Protective U Prosthesis Z None	Z None

Section	F	Physical Rehabilitation and Diagnostic Audiology
Section Qualifier	0	Rehabilitation
Type	F	Caregiver Training: Training in activities to support patient's optimal level of function

Body System / Region (4th)	Type Qualifier (5th)	Equipment (6th)	Qualifier (7th)
Z None	0 Bathing/Showering Technique 1 Dressing 2 Feeding and Eating 3 Grooming/Personal Hygiene 4 Bed Mobility 5 Transfer 6 Wheelchair Mobility 7 Therapeutic Exercise 8 Airway Clearance Techniques 9 Wound Management B Vocational Activities and Functional Community or Work Reintegration Skills C Gait Training/Functional Ambulation D Application, Proper Use and Care of Devices F Application, Proper Use and Care of Orthoses G Application, Proper Use and Care of Prosthesis H Home Management	E Orthosis F Assistive, Adaptive, Supportive or Protective U Prosthesis Z None	Z None
Z None	J Communication Skills	K Audiovisual L Assistive Listening M Augmentative / Alternative Communication P Computer Z None	Z None

Section	F	Physical Rehabilitation and Diagnostic Audiology
Section Qualifier	1	Diagnostic Audiology
Type	3	Hearing Assessment: Measurement of hearing and related functions

Body System / Region (4th)	Type Qualifier (5th)	Equipment (6th)	Qualifier (7th)
Z None	0 Hearing Screening	0 Occupational Hearing 1 Audiometer 2 Sound Field / Booth 3 Tympanometer 8 Vestibular / Balance 9 Cochlear Implant Z None	Z None

Continued

Section	F	Physical Rehabilitation and Diagnostic Audiology	F13 *Continued*
Section Qualifier	1	Diagnostic Audiology	
Type	3	Hearing Assessment: Measurement of hearing and related functions	

Body System / Region (4ᵗʰ)	Type Qualifier (5ᵗʰ)	Equipment (6ᵗʰ)	Qualifier (7ᵗʰ)
Z None	**1** Pure Tone Audiometry, Air **2** Pure Tone Audiometry, Air and Bone	**0** Occupational Hearing **1** Audiometer **2** Sound Field / Booth **Z** None	**Z** None
Z None	**3** Bekesy Audiometry **6** Visual Reinforcement Audiometry **9** Short Increment Sensitivity Index **B** Stenger **C** Pure Tone Stenger	**1** Audiometer **2** Sound Field / Booth **Z** None	**Z** None
Z None	**4** Conditioned Play Audiometry **5** Select Picture Audiometry	**1** Audiometer **2** Sound Field / Booth **K** Audiovisual **Z** None	**Z** None
Z None	**7** Alternate Binaural or Monaural Loudness Balance	**1** Audiometer **K** Audiovisual **Z** None	**Z** None
Z None	**8** Tone Decay **D** Tympanometry **F** Eustachian Tube Function **G** Acoustic Reflex Patterns **H** Acoustic Reflex Threshold **J** Acoustic Reflex Decay	**3** Tympanometer **4** Electroacoustic Immitance / Acoustic Reflex **Z** None	**Z** None
Z None	**K** Electrocochleography **L** Auditory Evoked Potentials	**7** Electrophysiologic **Z** None	**Z** None
Z None	**M** Evoked Otoacoustic Emissions, Screening **N** Evoked Otoacoustic Emissions, Diagnostic	**6** Otoacoustic Emission (OAE) **Z** None	**Z** None
Z None	**P** Aural Rehabilitation Status	**1** Audiometer **2** Sound Field / Booth **4** Electroacoustic Immitance / Acoustic Reflex **9** Cochlear Implant **K** Audiovisual **L** Assistive Listening **P** Computer **Z** None	**Z** None
Z None	**Q** Auditory Processing	**K** Audiovisual **P** Computer **Y** Other Equipment **Z** None	**Z** None

Section	F	Physical Rehabilitation and Diagnostic Audiology
Section Qualifier	1	Diagnostic Audiology
Type	4	**Hearing Aid Assessment:** Measurement of the appropriateness and/or effectiveness of a hearing device

Body System / Region (4th)	Type Qualifier (5th)	Equipment (6th)	Qualifier (7th)
Z None	0 Cochlear Implant	1 Audiometer 2 Sound Field / Booth 3 Tympanometer 4 Electroacoustic Immitance / Acoustic Reflex 5 Hearing Aid Selection / Fitting / Test 7 Electrophysiologic 9 Cochlear Implant K Audiovisual L Assistive Listening P Computer Y Other Equipment Z None	Z None
Z None	1 Ear Canal Probe Microphone 6 Binaural Electroacoustic Hearing Aid Check 8 Monaural Electroacoustic Hearing Aid Check	5 Hearing Aid Selection / Fitting / Test Z None	Z None
Z None	2 Monaural Hearing Aid 3 Binaural Hearing Aid	1 Audiometer 2 Sound Field / Booth 3 Tympanometer 4 Electroacoustic Immitance / Acoustic Reflex 5 Hearing Aid Selection / Fitting / Test K Audiovisual L Assistive Listening P Computer Z None	Z None
Z None	4 Assistive Listening System/Device Selection	1 Audiometer 2 Sound Field / Booth 3 Tympanometer 4 Electroacoustic Immitance / Acoustic Reflex K Audiovisual L Assistive Listening Z None	Z None
Z None	5 Sensory Aids	1 Audiometer 2 Sound Field / Booth 3 Tympanometer 4 Electroacoustic Immitance / Acoustic Reflex 5 Hearing Aid Selection / Fitting / Test K Audiovisual L Assistive Listening Z None	Z None
Z None	7 Ear Protector Attentuation	0 Occupational Hearing Z None	Z None

Section | F | **Physical Rehabilitation and Diagnostic Audiology**
Section Qualifier | 1 | **Diagnostic Audiology**
Type | 5 | **Vestibular Assessment:** Measurement of the vestibular system and related functions

Body System / Region (4th)	Type Qualifier (5th)	Equipment (6th)	Qualifier (7th)
Z None	**0** Bithermal, Binaural Caloric Irrigation **1** Bithermal, Monaural Caloric Irrigation **2** Unithermal Binaural Screen **3** Oscillating Tracking **4** Sinusoidal Vertical Axis Rotational **5** Dix-Hallpike Dynamic **6** Computerized Dynamic Posturography	**8** Vestibular / Balance **Z** None	**Z** None
Z None	**7** Tinnitus Masker	**5** Hearing Aid Selection / Fitting / Test **Z** None	**Z** None

Mental Health Section (GZ1–GZJ)

Within each section of ICD-10-PCS the characters have different meanings. The seven character meanings for the Mental Health section are illustrated here through the procedure example of *Crisis intervention*.

Section	Body System	Root Type	Qualifier	Qualifier	Qualifier	Qualifier
Mental Health	None	Crisis Intervention	None	None	None	None
G	Z	2	Z	Z	Z	Z

Section (Character 1)
All Mental Health procedure codes have a first character value of G.

Body System (Character 2)
The body system is not specified for mental health; therefore, the placeholder character value of Z is reported in the second character position.

Root Type (Character 3)
The alphanumeric character value for root types is placed in the third position. Listed below are the root types applicable to the Mental Health section with their associated meaning.

Character Value	Root Type	Root Type Definition
1	Psychological Tests	The administration and interpretation of standardized psychological tests and measurement instruments for the assessment of psychological function
2	Crisis Intervention	Treatment of a traumatized, acutely disturbed or distressed individual for the purpose of short-term stabilization
3	Medication Management	Monitoring and adjusting the use of medications for the treatment of a mental health disorder
5	Individual Psychotherapy	Treatment of an individual with a mental health disorder by behavioral, cognitive, psychoanalytic, psychodynamic or psychophysiological means to improve functioning or well-being
6	Counseling	The application of psychological methods to treat an individual with normal developmental issues and psychological problems in order to increase function, improve well-being, alleviate distress, maladjustment or resolve crises
7	Family Psychotherapy	Treatment that includes one or more family members of an individual with a mental health disorder by behavioral, cognitive, psychoanalytic, psychodynamic or psychophysiological means to improve functioning or well-being
B	Electroconvulsive Therapy	The application of controlled electrical voltages to treat a mental health disorder
C	Biofeedback	Provision of information from the monitoring and regulating of physiological processes in conjunction with cognitive-behavioral techniques to improve patient functioning or well-being

Continued

Character Value	Root Type	Root Type Definition
F	Hypnosis	Induction of a state of heightened suggestibility by auditory, visual and tactile techniques to elicit an emotional or behavioral response
G	Narcosynthesis	Administration of intravenous barbiturates in order to release suppressed or repressed thoughts
H	Group Psychotherapy	Treatment of two or more individuals with a mental health disorder by behavioral, cognitive, psychoanalytic, psychodynamic or psychophysiological means to improve functioning or well-being
J	Light Therapy	Application of specialized light treatments to improve functioning or well-being

Qualifier (Character 4)

This qualifier further specifies the root type procedure. For example, the qualifier of Development further specifies the type of Psychological Tests.

Qualifier (Character 5)

The qualifier represents an additional attribute for the procedure when applicable. Currently, there are no qualifiers in the Mental Health section; therefore, the placeholder character value of Z should be reported.

Qualifier (Character 6)

The qualifier represents an additional attribute for the procedure when applicable. Currently, there are no qualifiers in the Mental Health section; therefore, the placeholder character value of Z should be reported.

Qualifier (Character 7)

The qualifier represents an additional attribute for the procedure when applicable. Currently, there are no qualifiers in the Mental Health section; therefore, the placeholder character value of Z should be reported.

Mental Health Tables

Mental Health Tables GZ1–GZJ

Section	G	Mental Health
Body System	Z	None
Type	1	**Psychological Tests:** The administration and interpretation of standardized psychological tests and measurement instruments for the assessment of psychological function

Qualifier (4th)	Qualifier (5th)	Qualifier (6th)	Qualifier (7th)
0 Developmental 1 Personality and Behavioral 2 Intellectual and Psychoeducational 3 Neuropsychological 4 Neurobehavioral and Cognitive Status	Z None	Z None	Z None

Section	G	Mental Health
Body System	Z	None
Type	2	**Crisis Intervention:** Treatment of a traumatized, acutely disturbed or distressed individual for the purpose of short-term stabilization

Qualifier (4th)	Qualifier (5th)	Qualifier (6th)	Qualifier (7th)
Z None	Z None	Z None	Z None

Section	G	Mental Health
Body System	Z	None
Type	3	**Medication Management:** Monitoring and adjusting the use of medications for the treatment of a mental health disorder

Qualifier (4th)	Qualifier (5th)	Qualifier (6th)	Qualifier (7th)
Z None	Z None	Z None	Z None

Section	G	Mental Health
Body System	Z	None
Type	5	**Individual Psychotherapy:** Treatment of an individual with a mental health disorder by behavioral, cognitive, psychoanalytic, psychodynamic or psychophysiological means to improve functioning or well-being

Qualifier (4th)	Qualifier (5th)	Qualifier (6th)	Qualifier (7th)
0 Interactive 1 Behavioral 2 Cognitive 3 Interpersonal 4 Psychoanalysis 5 Psychodynamic 6 Supportive 8 Cognitive-Behavioral 9 Psychophysiological	Z None	Z None	Z None

Section	G	Mental Health
Body System	Z	None
Type	6	**Counseling:** The application of psychological methods to treat an individual with normal developmental issues and psychological problems in order to increase function, improve well-being, alleviate distress, maladjustment or resolve crises

Qualifier (4th)	Qualifier (5th)	Qualifier (6th)	Qualifier (7th)
0 Educational 1 Vocational 3 Other Counseling	Z None	Z None	Z None

Section	G	Mental Health
Body System	Z	None
Type	7	**Family Psychotherapy:** Treatment that includes one or more family members of an individual with a mental health disorder by behavioral, cognitive, psychoanalytic, psychodynamic or psychophysiological means to improve functioning or well-being

Qualifier (4th)	Qualifier (5th)	Qualifier (6th)	Qualifier (7th)
2 Other Family Psychotherapy	**Z** None	**Z** None	**Z** None

Section	G	Mental Health
Body System	Z	None
Type	B	**Electroconvulsive Therapy:** The application of controlled electrical voltages to treat a mental health disorder

Qualifier (4th)	Qualifier (5th)	Qualifier (6th)	Qualifier (7th)
0 Unilateral-Single Seizure **1** Unilateral-Multiple Seizure **2** Bilateral-Single Seizure **3** Bilateral-Multiple Seizure **4** Other Electroconvulsive Therapy	**Z** None	**Z** None	**Z** None

Section	G	Mental Health
Body System	Z	None
Type	C	**Biofeedback:** Provision of information from the monitoring and regulating of physiological processes in conjunction with cognitive-behavioral techniques to improve patient functioning or well-being

Qualifier (4th)	Qualifier (5th)	Qualifier (6th)	Qualifier (7th)
9 Other Biofeedback	**Z** None	**Z** None	**Z** None

Section	G	Mental Health
Body System	Z	None
Type	F	**Hypnosis:** Induction of a state of heightened suggestibility by auditory, visual and tactile techniques to elicit an emotional or behavioral response

Qualifier (4th)	Qualifier (5th)	Qualifier (6th)	Qualifier (7th)
Z None	**Z** None	**Z** None	**Z** None

Section	G	Mental Health
Body System	Z	None
Type	G	**Narcosynthesis:** Administration of intravenous barbiturates in order to release suppressed or repressed thoughts

Qualifier (4th)	Qualifier (5th)	Qualifier (6th)	Qualifier (7th)
Z None	**Z** None	**Z** None	**Z** None

Section	G	Mental Health
Body System	Z	None
Type	H	**Group Psychotherapy:** Treatment of two or more individuals with a mental health disorder by behavioral, cognitive, psychoanalytic, psychodynamic or psychophysiological means to improve functioning or well-being

Qualifier (4th)	Qualifier (5th)	Qualifier (6th)	Qualifier (7th)
Z None	**Z** None	**Z** None	**Z** None

Section	G	Mental Health
Body System	Z	None
Type	J	**Light Therapy:** Application of specialized light treatments to improve functioning or well-being

Qualifier (4th)	Qualifier (5th)	Qualifier (6th)	Qualifier (7th)
Z None	**Z** None	**Z** None	**Z** None

Substance Abuse Section (HZ2–HZ9)

Within each section of ICD-10-PCS the characters have different meanings. The seven character meanings for the Substance Abuse section are illustrated below through the procedure example of *Substance abuse family counseling*.

Section	Body System	Root Type	Qualifier	Qualifier	Qualifier	Qualifier
Substance Abuse	None	Family Counseling	Other Family Counseling	None	None	None
H	Z	6	3	Z	Z	Z

Section (Character 1)

All Substance Abuse procedure codes have a first character value of H.

Body System (Character 2)

The body system is not specified for substance abuse; therefore, the placeholder character value of Z is reported in the second character position.

Root Type (Character 3)

The alphanumeric character value for root types is placed in the third position. The following are the root types applicable to the Substance Abuse section with their associated meaning.

Character Value	Root Type	Root Type Definition
2	Detoxification Services	Detoxification from alcohol and/or drugs
3	Individual Counseling	The application of psychological methods to treat an individual with addictive behavior
4	Group Counseling	The application of psychological methods to treat two or more individuals with addictive behavior
5	Individual Psychotherapy	Treatment of an individual with addictive behavior by behavioral, cognitive, psychoanalytic, psychodynamic or psychophysiological means
6	Family Counseling	The application of psychological methods that includes one or more family members to treat an individual with addictive behavior
8	Medication Management	Monitoring and adjusting the use of replacement medications for the treatment of addiction
9	Pharmacotherapy	The use of replacement medications for the treatment of addiction

Qualifier (Character 4)

This qualifier further specifies the root type procedure. For example, the qualifier of Cognitive further specifies the type of Individual counseling.

Qualifier (Character 5)

The qualifier represents an additional attribute for the procedure when applicable. Currently, there are no qualifiers in the Substance Abuse section; therefore, the placeholder character value of Z should be reported.

Qualifier (Character 6)

The qualifier represents an additional attribute for the procedure when applicable. Currently, there are no qualifiers in the Substance Abuse section; therefore, the placeholder character value of Z should be reported.

Qualifier (Character 7)

The qualifier represents an additional attribute for the procedure when applicable. Currently, there are no qualifiers in the Substance Abuse section; therefore, the placeholder character value of Z should be reported.

Substance Abuse Treatment Section Tables

Substance Abuse Treatment Tables HZ2–HZ9

Section	H	Substance Abuse Treatment
Body System	Z	None
Type	2	Detoxification Services: Detoxification from alcohol and/or drugs

Qualifier (4th)	Qualifier (5th)	Qualifier (6th)	Qualifier (7th)
Z None	Z None	Z None	Z None

Section	H	Substance Abuse Treatment
Body System	Z	None
Type	3	Individual Counseling: The application of psychological methods to treat an individual with addictive behavior

Qualifier (4th)	Qualifier (5th)	Qualifier (6th)	Qualifier (7th)
0 Cognitive 1 Behavioral 2 Cognitive-Behavioral 3 12-Step 4 Interpersonal 5 Vocational 6 Psychoeducation 7 Motivational Enhancement 8 Confrontational 9 Continuing Care B Spiritual C Pre/Post-Test Infectious Disease	Z None	Z None	Z None

Section	H	Substance Abuse Treatment
Body System	Z	None
Type	4	Group Counseling: The application of psychological methods to treat two or more individuals with addictive behavior

Qualifier (4th)	Qualifier (5th)	Qualifier (6th)	Qualifier (7th)
0 Cognitive 1 Behavioral 2 Cognitive-Behavioral 3 12-Step 4 Interpersonal 5 Vocational 6 Psychoeducation 7 Motivational Enhancement 8 Confrontational 9 Continuing Care B Spiritual C Pre/Post-Test Infectious Disease	Z None	Z None	Z None

Section	H	Substance Abuse Treatment
Body System	Z	None
Type	5	**Individual Psychotherapy:** Treatment of an individual with addictive behavior by behavioral, cognitive, psychoanalytic, psychodynamic or psychophysiological means

Qualifier (4th)	Qualifier (5th)	Qualifier (6th)	Qualifier (7th)
0 Cognitive 1 Behavioral 2 Cognitive-Behavioral 3 12-Step 4 Interpersonal 5 Interactive 6 Psychoeducation 7 Motivational Enhancement 8 Confrontational 9 Supportive B Psychoanalysis C Psychodynamic D Psychophysiological	Z None	Z None	Z None

Section	H	Substance Abuse Treatment
Body System	Z	None
Type	6	**Family Counseling:** The application of psychological methods that includes one or more family members to treat an individual with addictive behavior

Qualifier (4th)	Qualifier (5th)	Qualifier (6th)	Qualifier (7th)
3 Other Family Counseling	Z None	Z None	Z None

Section	H	Substance Abuse Treatment
Body System	Z	None
Type	8	**Medication Management:** Monitoring and adjusting the use of replacement medications for the treatment of addiction

Qualifier (4th)	Qualifier (5th)	Qualifier (6th)	Qualifier (7th)
0 Nicotine Replacement 1 Methadone Maintenance 2 Levo-alpha-acetyl-methadol (LAAM) 3 Antabuse 4 Naltrexone 5 Naloxone 6 Clonidine 7 Bupropion 8 Psychiatric Medication 9 Other Replacement Medication	Z None	Z None	Z None

Section	H	Substance Abuse Treatment
Body System	Z	None
Type	9	**Pharmacotherapy:** The use of replacement medications for the treatment of addiction

Qualifier (4th)	Qualifier (5th)	Qualifier (6th)	Qualifier (7th)
0 Nicotine Replacement 1 Methadone Maintenance 2 Levo-alpha-acetyl-methadol (LAAM) 3 Antabuse 4 Naltrexone 5 Naloxone 6 Clonidine 7 Bupropion 8 Psychiatric Medication 9 Other Replacement Medication	Z None	Z None	Z None

Appendix A: Root Operations Definitions

Section 0 - Medical and Surgical — Character 3 - Root Operation

Alteration (0)	**Definition:** Modifying the anatomic structure of a body part without affecting the function of the body part **Explanation:** Principal purpose is to improve appearance **Includes/Examples:** Face lift, breast augmentation
Bypass (1)	**Definition:** Altering the route of passage of the contents of a tubular body part **Explanation:** Rerouting contents of a body part to a downstream area of the normal route, to a similar route and body part, or to an abnormal route and dissimilar body part. Includes one or more anastomoses, with or without the use of a device **Includes/Examples:** Coronary artery bypass, colostomy formation
Change (2)	**Definition:** Taking out or off a device from a body part and putting back an identical or similar device in or on the same body part without cutting or puncturing the skin or a mucous membrane **Explanation:** All CHANGE procedures are coded using the approach EXTERNAL **Includes/Examples:** Urinary catheter change, gastrostomy tube change
Control (3)	**Definition:** Stopping, or attempting to stop, postprocedural bleeding **Explanation:** The site of the bleeding is coded as an anatomical region and not to a specific body part **Includes/Examples:** Control of post-prostatectomy hemorrhage, control of post-tonsillectomy hemorrhage
Creation (4)	**Definition:** Making a new genital structure that does not take over the function of a body part **Explanation:** Used only for sex change operations **Includes/Examples:** Creation of vagina in a male, creation of penis in a female
Destruction (5)	**Definition:** Physical eradication of all or a portion of a body part by the direct use of energy, force, or a destructive agent **Explanation:** None of the body part is physically taken out **Includes/Examples:** Fulguration of rectal polyp, cautery of skin lesion
Detachment (6)	**Definition:** Cutting off all or a portion of the upper or lower extremities **Explanation:** The body part value is the site of the detachment, with a qualifier if applicable to further specify the level where the extremity was detached **Includes/Examples:** Below knee amputation, disarticulation of shoulder
Dilation (7)	**Definition:** Expanding an orifice or the lumen of a tubular body part **Explanation:** The orifice can be a natural orifice or an artificially created orifice. Accomplished by stretching a tubular body part using intraluminal pressure or by cutting part of the orifice or wall of the tubular body part **Includes/Examples:** Percutaneous transluminal angioplasty, pyloromyotomy
Division (8)	**Definition:** Cutting into a body part, without draining fluids and/or gases from the body part, in order to separate or transect a body part **Explanation:** All or a portion of the body part is separated into two or more portions **Includes/Examples:** Spinal cordotomy, osteotomy
Drainage (9)	**Definition:** Taking or letting out fluids and/or gases from a body part **Explanation:** The qualifier DIAGNOSTIC is used to identify drainage procedures that are biopsies **Includes/Examples:** Thoracentesis, incision and drainage
Excision (B)	**Definition:** Cutting out or off, without replacement, a portion of a body part **Explanation:** The qualifier DIAGNOSTIC is used to identify excision procedures that are biopsies **Includes/Examples:** Partial nephrectomy, liver biopsy
Extirpation (C)	**Definition:** Taking or cutting out solid matter from a body part **Explanation:** The solid matter may be an abnormal byproduct of a biological function or a foreign body; it may be imbedded in a body part or in the lumen of a tubular body part. The solid matter may or may not have been previously broken into pieces **Includes/Examples:** Thrombectomy, choledocholithotomy
Extraction (D)	**Definition:** Pulling or stripping out or off all or a portion of a body part by the use of force **Explanation:** The qualifier DIAGNOSTIC is used to identify extraction procedures that are biopsies **Includes/Examples:** Dilation and curettage, vein stripping
Fragmentation (F)	**Definition:** Breaking solid matter in a body part into pieces **Explanation:** Physical force (e.g., manual, ultrasonic) applied directly or indirectly is used to break the solid matter into pieces. The solid matter may be an abnormal byproduct of a biological function or a foreign body. The pieces of solid matter are not taken out **Includes/Examples:** Extracorporeal shockwave lithotripsy, transurethral lithotripsy
Fusion (G)	**Definition:** Joining together portions of an articular body part rendering the articular body part immobile **Explanation:** The body part is joined together by fixation device, bone graft, or other means **Includes/Examples:** Spinal fusion, ankle arthrodesis

Continued

Section 0 - Medical and Surgical — Character 3 - Root Operation

Insertion (H)	**Definition:** Putting in a nonbiological appliance that monitors, assists, performs, or prevents a physiological function but does not physically take the place of a body part **Includes/Examples:** Insertion of radioactive implant, insertion of central venous catheter
Inspection (J)	**Definition:** Visually and/or manually exploring a body part **Explanation:** Visual exploration may be performed with or without optical instrumentation. Manual exploration may be performed directly or through intervening body layers **Includes/Examples:** Diagnostic arthroscopy, exploratory laparotomy
Map (K)	**Definition:** Locating the route of passage of electrical impulses and/or locating functional areas in a body part **Explanation:** Applicable only to the cardiac conduction mechanism and the central nervous system **Includes/Examples:** Cardiac mapping, cortical mapping
Occlusion (L)	**Definition:** Completely closing an orifice or the lumen of a tubular body part **Explanation:** The orifice can be a natural orifice or an artificially created orifice **Includes/Examples:** Fallopian tube ligation, ligation of inferior vena cava
Reattachment (M)	**Definition:** Putting back in or on all or a portion of a separated body part to its normal location or other suitable location **Explanation:** Vascular circulation and nervous pathways may or may not be reestablished **Includes/Examples:** Reattachment of hand, reattachment of avulsed kidney
Release (N)	**Definition:** Freeing a body part from an abnormal physical constraint by cutting or by the use of force **Explanation:** Some of the restraining tissue may be taken out but none of the body part is taken out **Includes/Examples:** Adhesiolysis, carpal tunnel release
Removal (P)	**Definition:** Taking out or off a device from a body part **Explanation:** If a device is taken out and a similar device put in without cutting or puncturing the skin or mucous membrane, the procedure is coded to the root operation CHANGE. Otherwise, the procedure for taking out a device is coded to the root operation REMOVAL **Includes/Examples:** Drainage tube removal, cardiac pacemaker removal
Repair (Q)	**Definition:** Restoring, to the extent possible, a body part to its normal anatomic structure and function **Explanation:** Used only when the method to accomplish the repair is not one of the other root operations **Includes/Examples:** Colostomy takedown, suture of laceration
Replacement (R)	**Definition:** Putting in or on biological or synthetic material that physically takes the place and/or function of all or a portion of a body part **Explanation:** The body part may have been taken out or replaced, or may be taken out, physically eradicated, or rendered nonfunctional during the Replacement procedure. A Removal procedure is coded for taking out the device used in a previous replacement procedure **Includes/Examples:** Total hip replacement, bone graft, free skin graft
Reposition (S)	**Definition:** Moving to its normal location, or other suitable location, all or a portion of a body part **Explanation:** The body part is moved to a new location from an abnormal location, or from a normal location where it is not functioning correctly. The body part may or may not be cut out or off to be moved to the new location **Includes/Examples:** Reposition of undescended testicle, fracture reduction
Resection (T)	**Definition:** Cutting out or off, without replacement, all of a body part **Includes/Examples:** Total nephrectomy, total lobectomy of lung
Restriction (V)	**Definition:** Partially closing an orifice or the lumen of a tubular body part **Explanation:** The orifice can be a natural orifice or an artificially created orifice **Includes/Examples:** Esophagogastric fundoplication, cervical cerclage
Revision (W)	**Definition:** Correcting, to the extent possible, a portion of a malfunctioning device or the position of a displaced device **Explanation:** Revision can include correcting a malfunctioning or displaced device by taking out or putting in components of the device such as a screw or pin **Includes/Examples:** Adjustment of position of pacemaker lead, recementing of hip prosthesis
Supplement (U)	**Definition:** Putting in or on biological or synthetic material that physically reinforces and/or augments the function of a portion of a body part **Explanation:** The biological material is non-living, or is living and from the same individual. The body part may have been previously replaced, and the Supplement procedure is performed to physically reinforce and/or augment the function of the replaced body part **Includes/Examples:** Herniorrhaphy using mesh, free nerve graft, mitral valve ring annuloplasty, put a new acetabular liner in a previous hip replacement
Transfer (X)	**Definition:** Moving, without taking out, all or a portion of a body part to another location to take over the function of all or a portion of a body part **Explanation:** The body part transferred remains connected to its vascular and nervous supply **Includes/Examples:** Tendon transfer, skin pedicle flap transfer

Continued

Section 0 - Medical and Surgical — Character 3 - Root Operation

Transplantation (Y)	**Definition:** Putting in or on all or a portion of a living body part taken from another individual or animal to physically take the place and/or function of all or a portion of a similar body part **Explanation:** The native body part may or may not be taken out, and the transplanted body part may take over all or a portion of its function **Includes/Examples:** Kidney transplant, heart transplant

Section 1 - Obstetrics — Character 3 - Root Operations Unique to Obstetrics

Abortion (A)	**Definition:** Artificially terminating a pregnancy **Explanation:** Subdivided according to whether an additional device such as a laminaria or abortifacient is used, or whether the abortion was performed by mechanical means **Includes/Example:** Transvaginal abortion using vacuum aspiration technique
Delivery (E)	**Definition:** Assisting the passage of the products of conception from the genital canal **Explanation:** Applies only to manually-assisted, vaginal delivery **Includes/Example:** Manually-assisted delivery

Section 2 - Placement — Character 3 - Root Operation

Change (0)	**Definition:** Taking out or off a device from a body part and putting back an identical or similar device in or on the same body part without cutting or puncturing the skin or a mucous membrane **Includes/Example:** Change of vaginal packing
Compression (1)	**Definition:** Putting pressure on a body region **Includes/Example:** Placement of pressure dressing on abdominal wall
Dressing (2)	**Definition:** Putting material on a body region for protection **Includes/Example:** Application of sterile dressing to head wound
Immobilization (3)	**Definition:** Limiting or preventing motion of a body region **Includes/Example:** Placement of splint on left finger
Packing (4)	**Definition:** Putting material in a body region or orifice **Includes/Example:** Placement of nasal packing
Removal (5)	**Definition:** Taking out or off a device from a body part **Includes/Example:** Removal of cast from right lower leg
Traction (6)	**Definition:** Exerting a pulling force on a body region in a distal direction **Includes/Example:** Lumbar traction using motorized split-traction table

Section 3 - Administration — Character 3 - Root Operation

Introduction (0)	**Definition:** Putting in or on a therapeutic, diagnostic, nutritional, physiological, or prophylactic substance except blood or blood products **Includes/Example:** Nerve block injection to median nerve
Irrigation (1)	**Definition:** Putting in or on a cleansing substance **Includes/Example:** Flushing of eye
Transfusion (2)	**Definition:** Putting in blood or blood products **Includes/Example:** Transfusion of cell saver red cells into central venous line

Section 4 - Measurement and Monitoring — Character 3 - Root Operation

Measurement (0)	**Definition:** Determining the level of a physiological or physical function at a point in time **Includes/Example:** External electrocardiogram (EKG), single reading
Monitoring (1)	**Definition:** Determining the level of a physiological or physical function repetitively over a period of time **Includes/Example:** Urinary pressure monitoring

Section 5 - Extracorporeal Assistance and Performance — Character 3 - Root Operation

Assistance (0)	**Definition:** Taking over a portion of a physiological function by extracorporeal means **Includes/Example:** Hyperbaric oxygenation of wound
Performance (1)	**Definition:** Completely taking over a physiological function by extracorporeal means **Includes/Example:** Cardiopulmonary bypass in conjunction with CABG
Restoration (2)	**Definition:** Returning, or attempting to return, a physiological function to its original state by extracorporeal means. **Includes/Example:** Attempted cardiac defibrillation, unsuccessful

Section 6 - Extracorporeal Therapies — Character 3 - Root Operation

Atmospheric Control (0)	**Definition:** Extracorporeal control of atmospheric pressure and composition **Includes/Example:** Atmospheric control, single treatment
Decompression (1)	**Definition:** Extracorporeal elimination of undissolved gas from body fluids **Includes/Example:** Hyperbaric decompression treatment, single
Electromagnetic Therapy (2)	**Definition:** Extracorporeal treatment by electromagnetic rays **Includes/Example:** Electromagnetic therapy, central nervous, multiple treatments
Hyperthermia (3)	**Definition:** Extracorporeal raising of body temperature **Includes/Example:** Hyperthermia, single treatment
Hypothermia (4)	**Definition:** Extracorporeal lowering of body temperature **Includes/Example:** Whole body hypothermia treatment for temperature imbalances, series treatment
Pheresis (5)	**Definition:** Extracorporeal separation of blood products **Includes/Example:** Therapeutic leukopheresis, single treatment
Phototherapy (6)	**Definition:** Extracorporeal treatment by light rays **Includes/Example:** Phototherapy of circulatory system, series treatment
Shock Wave Therapy (7)	**Definition:** Extracorporeal treatment by shock waves **Includes/Example:** Shock wave therapy, musculoskeletal, single treatment
Ultrasound Therapy (8)	**Definition:** Extracorporeal treatment by ultrasound **Includes/Example:** Ultrasound therapy of the heart, single treatment
Ultraviolet Light Therapy (9)	**Definition:** Extracorporeal treatment by ultraviolet light **Includes/Example:** Ultraviolet light phototherapy, series treatment

Section 7 - Osteopathic — Character 3 - Root Operation

Treatment (0)	**Definition:** Manual treatment to eliminate or alleviate somatic dysfunction and related disorders **Includes/Example:** Fascial release of abdomen, osteopathic treatment

Section 8 - Other Procedures — Character 3 - Root Operation

Other Procedures (0)	**Definition:** Methodologies which attempt to remediate or cure a disorder or disease **Includes/Example:** Acupuncture

Section 9 - Chiropractic — Character 3 - Root Operation

Manipulation (B)	**Definition:** Manual procedure that involves a directed thrust to move a joint past the physiological range of motion, without exceeding the anatomical limit **Includes/Example:** Chiropractic treatment of cervical spine, short lever specific contact

Appendix B: Type and Qualifier Definitions

Section B - Imaging — Character 3 - Root Type

Computerized Tomography (CT Scan)	**Definition:** Computer reformatted digital display of multiplanar images developed from the capture of multiple exposures of external ionizing radiation
Fluoroscopy	**Definition:** Single plane or bi-plane real time display of an image developed from the capture of external ionizing radiation on a fluorescent screen. The image may also be stored by either digital or analog means
Magnetic Resonance Imaging (MRI)	**Definition:** Computer reformatted digital display of multiplanar images developed from the capture of radiofrequency signals emitted by nuclei in a body site excited within a magnetic field
Plain Radiography	**Definition:** Planar display of an image developed from the capture of external ionizing radiation on photographic or photoconductive plate
Ultrasonography	**Definition:** Real time display of images of anatomy or flow information developed from the capture of reflected and attenuated high frequency sound waves

Section C - Nuclear Medicine — Character 3 - Root Type

Nonimaging Nuclear Medicine Assay	**Definition:** Introduction of radioactive materials into the body for the study of body fluids and blood elements, by the detection of radioactive emissions
Nonimaging Nuclear Medicine Probe	**Definition:** Introduction of radioactive materials into the body for the study of distribution and fate of certain substances by the detection of radioactive emissions; or, alternatively, measurement of absorption of radioactive emissions from an external source
Nonimaging Nuclear Medicine Uptake	**Definition:** Introduction of radioactive materials into the body for measurements of organ function, from the detection of radioactive emissions
Planar Nuclear Medicine Imaging	**Definition:** Introduction of radioactive materials into the body for single plane display of images developed from the capture of radioactive emissions
Positron Emission Tomographic (PET) Imaging	**Definition:** Introduction of radioactive materials into the body for three dimensional display of images developed from the simultaneous capture, 180 degrees apart, of radioactive emissions
Systemic Nuclear Medicine Therapy	**Definition:** Introduction of unsealed radioactive materials into the body for treatment
Tomographic (Tomo) Nuclear Medicine Imaging	**Definition:** Introduction of radioactive materials into the body for three dimensional display of images developed from the capture of radioactive emissions

Section F - Physical Rehabilitation and Diagnostic Audiology — Character 3 - Root Type

Activities of Daily Living Assessment	**Definition:** Measurement of functional level for activities of daily living
Activities of Daily Living Treatment	**Definition:** Exercise or activities to facilitate functional competence for activities of daily living
Caregiver Training	**Definition:** Training in activities to support patient's optimal level of function
Cochlear Implant Treatment	**Definition:** Application of techniques to improve the communication abilities of individuals with cochlear implant
Device Fitting	**Definition:** Fitting of a device designed to facilitate or support achievement of a higher level of function
Hearing Aid Assessment	**Definition:** Measurement of the appropriateness and/or effectiveness of a hearing device
Hearing Assessment	**Definition:** Measurement of hearing and related functions
Hearing Treatment	**Definition:** Application of techniques to improve, augment, or compensate for hearing and related functional impairment
Motor and/or Nerve Function Assessment	**Definition:** Measurement of motor, nerve, and related functions
Motor Treatment	**Definition:** Exercise or activities to increase or facilitate motor function
Speech Assessment	**Definition:** Measurement of speech and related functions
Speech Treatment	**Definition:** Application of techniques to improve, augment, or compensate for speech and related functional impairment

Continued

Section F - Physical Rehabilitation and Diagnostic Audiology — Character 3 - Root Type	
Vestibular Assessment	**Definition:** Measurement of the vestibular system and related functions
Vestibular Treatment	**Definition:** Application of techniques to improve, augment, or compensate for vestibular and related functional impairment

Section F - Physical Rehabilitation and Diagnostic Audiology — Character 5 - Type Qualifier	
Acoustic Reflex Decay	**Definition:** Measures reduction in size/strength of acoustic reflex over time **Includes/Examples:** Includes site of lesion test
Acoustic Reflex Patterns	**Definition:** Defines site of lesion based upon presence/absence of acoustic reflexes with ipsilateral vs. contralateral stimulation
Acoustic Reflex Threshold	**Definition:** Determines minimal intensity that acoustic reflex occurs with ipsilateral and/or contralateral stimulation
Aerobic Capacity and Endurance	**Definition:** Measures autonomic responses to positional changes; perceived exertion, dyspnea or angina during activity; performance during exercise protocols; standard vital signs; and blood gas analysis or oxygen consumption
Alternate Binaural or Monaural Loudness Balance	**Definition:** Determines auditory stimulus parameter that yields the same objective sensation **Includes/Examples:** Sound intensities that yield same loudness perception
Anthropometric Characteristics	**Definition:** Measures edema, body fat composition, height, weight, length and girth
Aphasia (Assessment)	**Definition:** Measures expressive and receptive speech and language function including reading and writing
Aphasia (Treatment)	**Definition:** Applying techniques to improve, augment, or compensate for receptive/ expressive language impairments
Articulation/Phonology (Assessment)	**Definition:** Measures speech production
Articulation/Phonology (Treatment)	**Definition:** Applying techniques to correct, improve, or compensate for speech productive impairment
Assistive Listening Device	**Definition:** Assists in use of effective and appropriate assistive listening device/system
Assistive Listening System/Device Selection	**Definition:** Measures the effectiveness and appropriateness of assistive listening systems/ devices
Assistive, Adaptive, Supportive or Protective Devices	**Explanation:** Devices to facilitate or support achievement of a higher level of function in wheelchair mobility; bed mobility; transfer or ambulation ability; bath and showering ability; dressing; grooming; personal hygiene; play or leisure
Auditory Evoked Potentials	**Definition:** Measures electric responses produced by the VIIIth cranial nerve and brainstem following auditory stimulation
Auditory Processing (Assessment)	**Definition:** Evaluates ability to receive and process auditory information and comprehension of spoken language
Auditory Processing (Treatment)	**Definition:** Applying techniques to improve the receiving and processing of auditory information and comprehension of spoken language
Augmentative/Alternative Communication System (Assessment)	**Definition:** Determines the appropriateness of aids, techniques, symbols, and/or strategies to augment or replace speech and enhance communication **Includes/Examples:** Includes the use of telephones, writing equipment, emergency equipment, and TDD
Augmentative/Alternative Communication System (Treatment)	**Includes/Examples:** Includes augmentative communication devices and aids
Aural Rehabilitation	**Definition:** Applying techniques to improve the communication abilities associated with hearing loss
Aural Rehabilitation Status	**Definition:** Measures impact of a hearing loss including evaluation of receptive and expressive communication skills
Bathing/Showering	**Includes/Examples:** Includes obtaining and using supplies; soaping, rinsing, and drying body parts; maintaining bathing position; and transferring to and from bathing positions
Bathing/Showering Techniques	**Definition:** Activities to facilitate obtaining and using supplies, soaping, rinsing and drying body parts, maintaining bathing position, and transferring to and from bathing positions
Bed Mobility (Assessment)	**Definition:** Transitional movement within bed
Bed Mobility (Treatment)	**Definition:** Exercise or activities to facilitate transitional movements within bed

Continued

Section F - Physical Rehabilitation and Diagnostic Audiology — Character 5 - Type Qualifier

Bedside Swallowing and Oral Function	**Includes/Examples:** Bedside swallowing includes assessment of sucking, masticating, coughing, and swallowing. Oral function includes assessment of musculature for controlled movements, structures and functions to determine coordination and phonation
Bekesy Audiometry	**Definition:** Uses an instrument that provides a choice of discrete or continuously varying pure tones; choice of pulsed or continuous signal
Binaural Electroacoustic Hearing Aid Check	**Definition:** Determines mechanical and electroacoustic function of bilateral hearing aids using hearing aid test box
Binaural Hearing Aid (Assessment)	**Definition:** Measures the candidacy, effectiveness, and appropriateness of a hearing aids **Explanation:** Measures bilateral fit
Binaural Hearing Aid (Treatment)	**Explanation:** Assists in achieving maximum understanding and performance
Bithermal, Binaural Caloric Irrigation	**Definition:** Measures the rhythmic eye movements stimulated by changing the temperature of the vestibular system
Bithermal, Monaural Caloric Irrigation	**Definition:** Measures the rhythmic eye movements stimulated by changing the temperature of the vestibular system in one ear
Brief Tone Stimuli	**Definition:** Measures specific central auditory process
Cerumen Management	**Definition:** Includes examination of external auditory canal and tympanic membrane and removal of cerumen from external ear canal
Cochlear Implant	**Definition:** Measures candidacy for cochlear implant
Cochlear Implant Rehabilitation	**Definition:** Applying techniques to improve the communication abilities of individuals with cochlear implant; includes programming the device, providing patients/families with information
Communicative/Cognitive Integration Skills (Assessment)	**Definition:** Measures ability to use higher cortical functions **Includes/Examples:** Includes orientation, recognition, attention span, initiation and termination of activity, memory, sequencing, categorizing, concept formation, spatial operations, judgment, problem solving, generalization and pragmatic communication
Communicative/Cognitive Integration Skills (Treatment)	**Definition:** Activities to facilitate the use of higher cortical functions **Includes/Examples:** Includes level of arousal, orientation, recognition, attention span, initiation and termination of activity, memory sequencing, judgment and problem solving, learning and generalization, and pragmatic communication
Computerized Dynamic Posturography	**Definition:** Measures the status of the peripheral and central vestibular system and the sensory/motor component of balance; evaluates the efficacy of vestibular rehabilitation
Conditioned Play Audiometry	**Definition:** Behavioral measures using nonspeech and speech stimuli to obtain frequency-specific and ear-specific information on auditory status from the patient **Explanation:** Obtains speech reception threshold by having patient point to pictures of spondaic words
Coordination/Dexterity (Assessment)	**Definition:** Measures large and small muscle groups for controlled goal-directed movements **Explanation:** Dexterity includes object manipulation
Coordination/Dexterity (Treatment)	**Definition:** Exercise or activities to facilitate gross coordination and fine coordination
Cranial Nerve Integrity	**Definition:** Measures cranial nerve sensory and motor functions, including tastes, smell and facial expression
Dichotic Stimuli	**Definition:** Measures specific central auditory process
Distorted Speech	**Definition:** Measures specific central auditory process
Dix-Hallpike Dynamic	**Definition:** Measures nystagmus following Dix-Hallpike maneuver
Dressing	**Includes/Examples:** Includes selecting clothing and accessories, obtaining clothing from storage, dressing and, fastening and adjusting clothing and shoes, and applying and removing personal devices, prosthesis or orthosis
Dressing Techniques	**Definition:** Activities to facilitate selecting clothing and accessories, dressing and undressing, adjusting clothing and shoes, applying and removing devices, prostheses or orthoses
Dynamic Orthosis	**Includes/Examples:** Includes customized and prefabricated splints, inhibitory casts, spinal and other braces, and protective devices; allows motion through transfer of movement from other body parts or by use of outside forces
Ear Canal Probe Microphone	**Definition:** Real ear measures
Ear Protector Attentuation	**Definition:** Measures ear protector fit and effectiveness

Continued

Section F - Physical Rehabilitation and Diagnostic Audiology — Character 5 - Type Qualifier

Electrocochleography	**Definition:** Measures the VIIIth cranial nerve action potential
Environmental, Home and Work Barriers	**Definition:** Measures current and potential barriers to optimal function, including safety hazards, access problems and home or office design
Ergonomics and Body Mechanics	**Definition:** Ergonomic measurement of job tasks, work hardening or work conditioning needs; functional capacity; and body mechanics
Eustachian Tube Function	**Definition:** Measures eustachian tube function and patency of eustachian tube
Evoked Otoacoustic Emissions, Diagnostic	**Definition:** Measures auditory evoked potentials in a diagnostic format
Evoked Otoacoustic Emissions, Screening	**Definition:** Measures auditory evoked potentials in a screening format
Facial Nerve Function	**Definition:** Measures electrical activity of the VIIth cranial nerve (facial nerve)
Feeding/Eating (Assessment)	**Includes/Examples:** Includes setting up food, selecting and using utensils and tableware, bringing food or drink to mouth, cleaning face, hands, and clothing, and management of alternative methods of nourishment
Feeding/Eating (Treatment)	**Definition:** Exercise or activities to facilitate setting up food, selecting and using utensils and tableware, bringing food or drink to mouth, cleaning face, hands, and clothing, and management of alternative methods of nourishment
Filtered Speech	**Definition:** Uses high or low pass filtered speech stimuli to assess central auditory processing disorders, site of lesion testing
Fluency (Assessment)	**Definition:** Measures speech fluency or stuttering
Fluency (Treatment)	**Definition:** Applying techniques to improve and augment fluent speech
Gait and/or Balance	**Definition:** Measures biomechanical, arthrokinematic and other spatial and temporal characteristics of gait and balance
Gait Training/Functional Ambulation	**Definition:** Exercise or activities to facilitate ambulation on a variety of surfaces and in a variety of environments
Grooming/Personal Hygiene (Assessment)	**Includes/Examples:** Includes ability to obtain and use supplies in a sequential fashion, general grooming, oral hygiene, toilet hygiene, personal care devices, including care for artificial airways
Grooming/Personal Hygiene (Treatment)	**Definition:** Activities to facilitate obtaining and using supplies in a sequential fashion: general grooming, oral hygiene, toilet hygiene, cleaning body, and personal care devices, including artificial airways
Hearing and Related Disorders Counseling	**Definition:** Provides patients/families/caregivers with information, support, referrals to facilitate recovery from a communication disorder **Includes/Examples:** Includes strategies for psychosocial adjustment to hearing loss for clients and families/caregivers
Hearing and Related Disorders Prevention	**Definition:** Provides patients/families/caregivers with information and support to prevent communication disorders
Hearing Screening	**Definition:** Pass/refer measures designed to identify need for further audiologic assessment
Home Management (Assessment)	**Definition:** Obtaining and maintaining personal and household possessions and environment **Includes/Examples:** Includes clothing care, cleaning, meal preparation and cleanup, shopping, money management, household maintenance, safety procedures, and childcare/parenting
Home Management (Treatment)	**Definition:** Activities to facilitate obtaining and maintaining personal household possessions and environment **Includes/Examples:** Includes clothing care, cleaning, meal preparation and clean-up, shopping, money management, household maintenance, safety procedures, childcare/parenting
Instrumental Swallowing and Oral Function	**Definition:** Measures swallowing function using instrumental diagnostic procedures **Explanation:** Methods include videofluoroscopy, ultrasound, manometry, endoscopy
Integumentary Integrity	**Includes/Examples:** Includes burns, skin conditions, ecchymosis, bleeding, blisters, scar tissue, wounds and other traumas, tissue mobility, turgor and texture
Manual Therapy Techniques	**Definition:** Techniques in which the therapist uses his/her hands to administer skilled movements **Includes/Examples:** Includes connective tissue massage, joint mobilization and manipulation, manual lymph drainage, manual traction, soft tissue mobilization and manipulation
Masking Patterns	**Definition:** Measures central auditory processing status
Monaural Electroacoustic Hearing Aid Check	**Definition:** Determines mechanical and electroacoustic function of one hearing aid using hearing aid test box

Continued

Section F - Physical Rehabilitation and Diagnostic Audiology — Character 5 - Type Qualifier

Monaural Hearing Aid (Assessment)	**Definition:** Measures the candidacy, effectiveness, and appropriateness of a hearing aid **Explanation:** Measures unilateral fit
Monaural Hearing Aid (Treatment)	**Explanation:** Assists in achieving maximum understanding and performance
Motor Function (Assessment)	**Definition:** Measures the body's functional and versatile movement patterns **Includes/Examples:** Includes motor assessment scales, analysis of head, trunk and limb movement, and assessment of motor learning
Motor Function (Treatment)	**Definition:** Exercise or activities to facilitate crossing midline, laterality, bilateral integration, praxis, neuromuscular relaxation, inhibition, facilitation, motor function and motor learning
Motor Speech (Assessment)	**Definition:** Measures neurological motor aspects of speech production
Motor Speech (Treatment)	**Definition:** Applying techniques to improve and augment the impaired neurological motor aspects of speech production
Muscle Performance (Assessment)	**Definition:** Measures muscle strength, power and endurance using manual testing, dynamometry or computer-assisted electromechanical muscle test; functional muscle strength, power and endurance; muscle pain, tone, or soreness; or pelvic-floor musculature **Explanation:** Muscle endurance refers to the ability to contract a muscle repeatedly over time
Muscle Performance (Treatment)	**Definition:** Exercise or activities to increase the capacity of a muscle to do work in terms of strength, power, and/or endurance **Explanation:** Muscle strength is the force exerted to overcome resistance in one maximal effort. Muscle power is work produced per unit of time, or the product of strength and speed. Muscle endurance is the ability to contract a muscle repeatedly over time
Neuromotor Development	**Definition:** Measures motor development, righting and equilibrium reactions, and reflex and equilibrium reactions
Neurophysiologic Intraoperative	**Definition:** Monitors neural status during surgery
Non-invasive Instrumental Status	**Definition:** Instrumental measures of oral, nasal, vocal, and velopharyngeal functions as they pertain to speech production
Nonspoken Language (Assessment)	**Definition:** Measures nonspoken language (print, sign, symbols) for communication
Nonspoken Language (Treatment)	**Definition:** Applying techniques that improve, augment, or compensate spoken communication
Oral Peripheral Mechanism	**Definition:** Structural measures of face, jaw, lips, tongue, teeth, hard and soft palate, pharynx as related to speech production
Orofacial Myofunctional (Assessment)	**Definition:** Measures orofacial myofunctional patterns for speech and related functions
Orofacial Myofunctional (Treatment)	**Definition:** Applying techniques to improve, alter, or augment impaired orofacial myofunctional patterns and related speech production errors
Oscillating Tracking	**Definition:** Measures ability to visually track
Pain	**Definition:** Measures muscle soreness, pain and soreness with joint movement, and pain perception **Includes/Examples:** Includes questionnaires, graphs, symptom magnification scales or visual analog scales
Perceptual Processing (Assessment)	**Definition:** Measures stereognosis, kinesthesia, body schema, right-left discrimination, form constancy, position in space, visual closure, figure-ground, depth perception, spatial relations and topographical orientation
Perceptual Processing (Treatment)	**Definition:** Exercise and activities to facilitate perceptual processing **Explanation:** Includes stereognosis, kinesthesia, body schema, right-left discrimination, form constancy, position in space, visual closure, figure-ground, depth perception, spatial relations, and topographical orientation **Includes/Examples:** Includes stereognosis, kinesthesia, body schema, right-left discrimination, form constancy, position in space, visual closure, figure-ground, depth perception, spatial relations, and topographical orientation
Performance Intensity Phonetically Balanced Speech Discrimination	**Definition:** Measures word recognition over varying intensity levels
Postural Control	**Definition:** Exercise or activities to increase postural alignment and control
Prosthesis	**Explanation:** Artificial substitutes for missing body parts that augment performance or function
Psychosocial Skills (Assessment)	**Definition:** The ability to interact in society and to process emotions **Includes/Examples:** Includes psychological (values, interests, self-concept); social (role performance, social conduct, interpersonal skills, self expression); self-management (coping skills, time management, self-control)

Continued

Section F - Physical Rehabilitation and Diagnostic Audiology — Character 5 - Type Qualifier

Psychosocial Skills (Treatment)	**Definition:** The ability to interact in society and to process emotions **Includes/Examples:** Includes psychological (values, interests, self-concept); social (role performance, social conduct, interpersonal skills, self expression); self-management (coping skills, time management, self-control)
Pure Tone Audiometry, Air	**Definition:** Air-conduction pure tone threshold measures with appropriate masking
Pure Tone Audiometry, Air and Bone	**Definition:** Air-conduction and bone-conduction pure tone threshold measures with appropriate masking
Pure Tone Stenger	**Definition:** Measures unilateral nonorganic hearing loss based on simultaneous presentation of pure tones of differing volume
Range of Motion and Joint Integrity	**Definition:** Measures quantity, quality, grade, and classification of joint movement and/or mobility **Explanation:** Range of Motion is the space, distance or angle through which movement occurs at a joint or series of joints. Joint integrity is the conformance of joints to expected anatomic, biomechanical and kinematic norms
Range of Motion and Joint Mobility	**Definition:** Exercise or activities to increase muscle length and joint mobility
Receptive/Expressive Language (Assessment)	**Definition:** Measures receptive and expressive language
Receptive/Expressive Language (Treatment)	**Definition:** Applying techniques tot improve and augment receptive/expressive language
Reflex Integrity	**Definition:** Measures the presence, absence, or exaggeration of developmentally appropriate, pathologic or normal reflexes
Select Picture Audiometry	**Definition:** Establishes hearing threshold levels for speech using pictures
Sensorineural Acuity Level	**Definition:** Measures sensorineural acuity masking presented via bone conduction
Sensory Aids	**Definition:** Determines the appropriateness of a sensory prosthetic device, other than a hearing aid or assistive listening system/device
Sensory Awareness/Processing/Integrity	**Includes/Examples:** Includes light touch, pressure, temperature, pain, sharp/dull, proprioception, vestibular, visual, auditory, gustatory, and olfactory
Short Increment Sensitivity Index	**Definition:** Measures the ear's ability to detect small intensity changes; site of lesion test requiring a behavioral response
Sinusoidal Vertical Axis Rotational	**Definition:** Measures nystagmus following rotation
Somatosensory Evoked Potentials	**Definition:** Measures neural activity from sites throughout the body
Speech and/or Language Screening	**Definition:** Identifies need for further speech and/or language evaluation
Speech Threshold	**Definition:** Measures minimal intensity needed to repeat spondaic words
Speech-Language Pathology and Related Disorders Counseling	**Definition:** Provides patients/families with information, support, referrals to facilitate recovery from a communication disorder
Speech-Language Pathology and Related Disorders Prevention	**Definition:** Applying techniques to avoid or minimize onset and/or development of a communication disorder
Speech/Word Recognition	**Definition:** Measures ability to repeat/identify single syllable words; scores given as a percentage; includes word recognition/speech discrimination
Staggered Spondaic Word	**Definition:** Measures central auditory processing site of lesion based upon dichotic presentation of spondaic words
Static Orthosis	**Includes/Examples:** Includes customized and prefabricated splints, inhibitory casts, spinal and other braces, and protective devices; has no moving parts, maintains joint(s) in desired position
Stenger	**Definition:** Measures unilateral nonorganic hearing loss based on simultaneous presentation of signals of differing volume
Swallowing Dysfunction	**Definition:** Activities to improve swallowing function in coordination with respiratory function **Includes/Examples:** Includes function and coordination of sucking, mastication, coughing, swallowing
Synthetic Sentence Identification	**Definition:** Measures central auditory dysfunction using identification of third order approximations of sentences and competing messages
Temporal Ordering of Stimuli	**Definition:** Measures specific central auditory process
Therapeutic Exercise	**Definition:** Exercise or activities to facilitate sensory awareness, sensory processing, sensory integration, balance training, conditioning, reconditioning **Includes/Examples:** Includes developmental activities, breathing exercises, aerobic endurance activities, aquatic exercises, stretching and ventilatory muscle training

Continued

Section F - Physical Rehabilitation and Diagnostic Audiology — Character 5 - Type Qualifier

Tinnitus Masker (Assessment)	**Definition:** Determines candidacy for tinnitus masker
Tinnitus Masker (Treatment)	**Explanation:** Used to verify physical fit, acoustic appropriateness, and benefit; assists in achieving maximum benefit
Tone Decay	**Definition:** Measures decrease in hearing sensitivity to a tone; site of lesion test requiring a behavioral response
Transfer	**Definition:** Transitional movement from one surface to another
Transfer Training	**Definition:** Exercise or activities to facilitate movement from one surface to another
Tympanometry	**Definition:** Measures the integrity of the middle ear; measures ease at which sound flows through the tympanic membrane while air pressure against the membrane is varied
Unithermal Binaural Screen	**Definition:** Measures the rhythmic eye movements stimulated by changing the temperature of the vestibular system in both ears using warm water, screening format
Ventilation, Respiration and Circulation	**Definition:** Measures ventilatory muscle strength, power and endurance, pulmonary function and ventilatory mechanics **Includes/Examples:** Includes ability to clear airway, activities that aggravate or relieve edema, pain, dyspnea or other symptoms, chest wall mobility, cardiopulmonary response to performance of ADL and IAD, cough and sputum, standard vital signs
Vestibular	**Definition:** Applying techniques to compensate for balance disorders; includes habituation, exercise therapy, and balance retraining
Visual Motor Integration (Assessment)	**Definition:** Coordinating the interaction of information from the eyes with body movement during activity
Visual Motor Integration (Treatment)	**Definition:** Exercise or activities to facilitate coordinating the interaction of information from eyes with body movement during activity
Visual Reinforcement Audiometry	**Definition:** Behavioral measures using nonspeech and speech stimuli to obtain frequency/ear-specific information on auditory status **Includes/Examples:** Includes a conditioned response of looking toward a visual reinforcer (e.g., lights, animated toy) every time auditory stimuli are heard
Vocational Activities and Functional Community or Work Reintegration Skills (Assessment)	**Definition:** Measures environmental, home, work (job/school/play) barriers that keep patients from functioning optimally in their environment **Includes/Examples:** Includes assessment of vocational skill and interests, environment of work (job/school/play), injury potential and injury prevention or reduction, ergonomic stressors, transportation skills, and ability to access and use community resources
Vocational Activities and Functional Community or Work Reintegration Skills (Treatment)	**Definition:** Activities to facilitate vocational exploration, body mechanics training, job acquisition, and environmental or work (job/school/play) task adaptation **Includes/Examples:** Includes injury prevention and reduction, ergonomic stressor reduction, job coaching and simulation, work hardening and conditioning, driving training, transportation skills, and use of community resources
Voice (Assessment)	**Definition:** Measures vocal structure, function and production
Voice (Treatment)	**Definition:** Applying techniques to improve voice and vocal function
Voice Prosthetic (Assessment)	**Definition:** Determines the appropriateness of voice prosthetic/adaptive device to enhance or facilitate communication
Voice Prosthetic (Treatment)	**Includes/Examples:** Includes electrolarynx, and other assistive, adaptive, supportive devices
Wheelchair Mobility (Assessment)	**Definition:** Measures fit and functional abilities within wheelchair in a variety of environments
Wheelchair Mobility (Treatment)	**Definition:** Management, maintenance and controlled operation of a wheelchair, scooter or other device, in and on a variety of surfaces and environments
Wound Management	**Includes/Examples:** Includes non-selective and selective debridement (enzymes, autolysis, sharp debridement), dressings (wound coverings, hydrogel, vacuum-assisted closure), topical agents, etc.

Section G - Mental Health — Character 3 - Root Type

Biofeedback	**Definition:** Provision of information from the monitoring and regulating of physiological processes in conjunction with cognitive-behavioral techniques to improve patient functioning or well-being **Includes/Examples:** Includes EEG, blood pressure, skin temperature or peripheral blood flow, ECG, electrooculogram, EMG, respirometry or capnometry, GSR/EDR, perineometry to monitor/regulate bowel/bladder activity, electrogastrogram to monitor/regulate gastric motility

Continued

Section G - Mental Health — Character 3 - Root Type

Counseling	**Definition:** The application of psychological methods to treat an individual with normal developmental issues and psychological problems in order to increase function, improve well-being, alleviate distress, maladjustment or resolve crises
Crisis Intervention	**Definition:** Treatment of a traumatized, acutely disturbed or distressed individual for the purpose of short-term stabilization **Includes/Examples:** Includes defusing, debriefing, counseling, psychotherapy and/or coordination of care with other providers or agencies
Electroconvulsive Therapy	**Definition:** The application of controlled electrical voltages to treat a mental health disorder **Includes/Examples:** Includes appropriate sedation and other preparation of the individual
Family Psychotherapy	**Definition:** Treatment that includes one or more family members of an individual with a mental health disorder by behavioral, cognitive, psychoanalytic, psychodynamic or psychophysiological means to improve functioning or well-being **Explanation:** Remediation of emotional or behavioral problems presented by one or more family members in cases where psychotherapy with more than one family member is indicated
Group Psychotherapy	**Definition:** Treatment of two or more individuals with a mental health disorder by behavioral, cognitive, psychoanalytic, psychodynamic or psychophysiological means to improve functioning or well-being
Hypnosis	**Definition:** Induction of a state of heightened suggestibility by auditory, visual and tactile techniques to elicit an emotional or behavioral response
Individual Psychotherapy	**Definition:** Treatment of an individual with a mental health disorder by behavioral, cognitive, psychoanalytic, psychodynamic or psychophysiological means to improve functioning or well-being
Light Therapy	**Definition:** Application of specialized light treatments to improve functioning or well-being
Medication Management	**Definition:** Monitoring and adjusting the use of medications for the treatment of a mental health disorder
Narcosynthesis	**Definition:** Administration of intravenous barbiturates in order to release suppressed or repressed thoughts
Psychological Tests	**Definition:** The administration and interpretation of standardized psychological tests and measurement instruments for the assessment of psychological function

Section G - Mental Health — Character 4 - Type Qualifier

Behavioral	**Definition:** Primarily to modify behavior **Includes/Examples:** Includes modeling and role playing, positive reinforcement of target behaviors, response cost, and training of self-management skills
Cognitive	**Definition:** Primarily to correct cognitive distortions and errors
Cognitive-Behavioral	**Definition:** Combining cognitive and behavioral treatment strategies to improve functioning **Explanation:** Maladaptive responses are examined to determine how cognitions relate to behavior patterns in response to an event. Uses learning principles and information-processing models
Developmental	**Definition:** Age-normed developmental status of cognitive, social and adaptive behavior skills
Intellectual and Psychoeducational	**Definition:** Intellectual abilities, academic achievement and learning capabilities (including behaviors and emotional factors affecting learning
Interactive	**Definition:** Uses primarily physical aids and other forms of non-oral interaction with a patient who is physically, psychologically or developmentally unable to use ordinary language for communication **Includes/Examples:** Includes. the use of toys in symbolic play
Interpersonal	**Definition:** Helps an individual make changes in interpersonal behaviors to reduce psychological dysfunction **Includes/Examples:** Includes exploratory techniques, encouragement of affective expression, clarification of patient statements, analysis of communication patterns, use of therapy relationship and behavior change techniques
Neurobehavioral and Cognitive Status	**Definition:** Includes neurobehavioral status exam, interview(s), and observation for the clinical assessment of thinking, reasoning and judgment, acquired knowledge, attention, memory, visual spatial abilities, language functions, and planning
Neuropsychological	**Definition:** Thinking, reasoning and judgment, acquired knowledge, attention, memory, visual spatial abilities, language functions, planning

Continued

Section G - Mental Health — Character 4 - Type Qualifier

Personality and Behavioral	**Definition:** Mood, emotion, behavior, social functioning, psychopathological conditions, personality traits and characteristics
Psychoanalysis	**Definition:** Methods of obtaining a detailed account of past and present mental and emotional experiences to determine the source and eliminate or diminish the undesirable effects of unconscious conflicts **Explanation:** Accomplished by making the individual aware of their existence, origin, and inappropriate expression in emotions and behavior
Psychodynamic	**Definition:** Exploration of past and present emotional experiences to understand motives and drives using insight-oriented techniques to reduce the undesirable effects of internal conflicts on emotions and behavior **Explanation:** Techniques include empathetic listening, clarifying self-defeating behavior patterns, and exploring adaptive alternatives
Psychophysiological	**Definition:** Monitoring and alteration of physiological processes to help the individual associate physiological reactions combined with cognitive and behavioral strategies to gain improved control of these processes to help the individual cope more effectively
Supportive	**Definition:** Formation of therapeutic relationship primarily for providing emotional support to prevent further deterioration in functioning during periods of particular stress **Explanation:** Often used in conjunction with other therapeutic approaches
Vocational	**Definition:** Exploration of vocational interests, aptitudes and required adaptive behavior skills to develop and carry out a plan for achieving a successful vocational placement **Includes/Examples:** Includes enhancing work related adjustment and/or pursuing viable options in training education or preparation

Section H - Substance Abuse Treatment — Character 3 - Root Type

Detoxification Services	**Definition:** Detoxification from alcohol and/or drugs **Explanation:** Not a treatment modality, but helps the patient stabilize physically and psychologically until the body becomes free of drugs and the effects of alcohol
Family Counseling	**Definition:** The application of psychological methods that includes one or more family members to treat an individual with addictive behavior **Explanation:** Provides support and education for family members of addicted individuals. Family member participation is seen as a critical area of substance abuse treatment
Group Counseling	**Definition:** The application of psychological methods to treat two or more individuals with addictive behavior **Explanation:** Provides structured group counseling sessions and healing power through the connection with others
Individual Counseling	**Definition:** The application of psychological methods to treat an individual with addictive behavior **Explanation:** Comprised of several different techniques, which apply various strategies to address drug addiction
Individual Psychotherapy	**Definition:** Treatment of an individual with addictive behavior by behavioral, cognitive, psychoanalytic, psychodynamic or psychophysiological means
Medication Management	**Definition:** Monitoring and adjusting the use of replacement medications for the treatment of addiction
Pharmacotherapy	**Definition:** The use of replacement medications for the treatment of addiction

Appendix C: Approach Definitions

Section 0 - Medical and Surgical — Character 5 - Approach

External (X)	**Definition:** Procedures performed directly on the skin or mucous membrane and procedures performed indirectly by the application of external force through the skin or mucous membrane
Open (0)	**Definition:** Cutting through the skin or mucous membrane and any other body layers necessary to expose the site of the procedure
Percutaneous (3)	**Definition:** Entry, by puncture or minor incision, of instrumentation through the skin or mucous membrane and any other body layers necessary to reach the site of the procedure
Percutaneous Endoscopic (4)	**Definition:** Entry, by puncture or minor incision, of instrumentation through the skin or mucous membrane and any other body layers necessary to reach and visualize the site of the procedure
Via Natural or Artificial Opening (7)	**Definition:** Entry of instrumentation through a natural or artificial external opening to reach the site of the procedure
Via Natural or Artificial Opening Endoscopic (8)	**Definition:** Entry of instrumentation through a natural or artificial external opening to reach and visualize the site of the procedure
Via Natural or Artificial Opening With Percutaneous Endoscopic Assistance (F)	**Definition:** Entry of instrumentation through a natural or artificial external opening and entry, by puncture or minor incision, of instrumentation through the skin or mucous membrane and any other body layers necessary to aid in the performance of the procedure

Section 1 - Obstetrics — Character 5 - Approach

External (X)	**Definition:** Procedures performed directly on the skin or mucous membrane and procedures performed indirectly by the application of external force through the skin or mucous membrane
Open (0)	**Definition:** Cutting through the skin or mucous membrane and any other body layers necessary to expose the site of the procedure
Percutaneous (3)	**Definition:** Entry, by puncture or minor incision, of instrumentation through the skin or mucous membrane and any other body layers necessary to reach the site of the procedure
Percutaneous Endoscopic (4)	**Definition:** Entry, by puncture or minor incision, of instrumentation through the skin or mucous membrane and any other body layers necessary to reach and visualize the site of the procedure
Via Natural or Artificial Opening (7)	**Definition:** Entry of instrumentation through a natural or artificial external opening to reach the site of the procedure
Via Natural or Artificial Opening Endoscopic (8)	**Definition:** Entry of instrumentation through a natural or artificial external opening to reach and visualize the site of the procedure

Section 2 - Placement — Character 5 - Approach

External (X)	**Definition:** Procedures performed directly on the skin or mucous membrane and procedures performed indirectly by the application of external force through the skin or mucous membrane

Section 3 - Administration — Character 5 - Approach

External (X)	**Definition:** Procedures performed directly on the skin or mucous membrane and procedures performed indirectly by the application of external force through the skin or mucous membrane
Open (0)	**Definition:** Cutting through the skin or mucous membrane and any other body layers necessary to expose the site of the procedure
Percutaneous (3)	**Definition:** Entry, by puncture or minor incision, of instrumentation through the skin or mucous membrane and any other body layers necessary to reach the site of the procedure
Via Natural or Artificial Opening (7)	**Definition:** Entry of instrumentation through a natural or artificial external opening to reach the site of the procedure
Via Natural or Artificial Opening Endoscopic (8)	**Definition:** Entry of instrumentation through a natural or artificial external opening to reach and visualize the site of the procedure

Section 4 - Measurement and Monitoring — Character 5 - Approach

External (X)	**Definition:** Procedures performed directly on the skin or mucous membrane and procedures performed indirectly by the application of external force through the skin or mucous membrane
Open (0)	**Definition:** Cutting through the skin or mucous membrane and any other body layers necessary to expose the site of the procedure
Percutaneous (3)	**Definition:** Entry, by puncture or minor incision, of instrumentation through the skin or mucous membrane and any other body layers necessary to reach the site of the procedure
Percutaneous Endoscopic (4)	**Definition:** Entry, by puncture or minor incision, of instrumentation through the skin or mucous membrane and any other body layers necessary to reach and visualize the site of the procedure
Via Natural or Artificial Opening (7)	**Definition:** Entry of instrumentation through a natural or artificial external opening to reach the site of the procedure
Via Natural or Artificial Opening Endoscopic (8)	**Definition:** Entry of instrumentation through a natural or artificial external opening to reach and visualize the site of the procedure

Section 7 - Osteopathic — Character 5 - Approach

External (X)	**Definition:** Procedures performed directly on the skin or mucous membrane and procedures performed indirectly by the application of external force through the skin or mucous membrane

Section 8 - Other Procedures — Character 5 - Approach

External (X)	**Definition:** Procedures performed directly on the skin or mucous membrane and procedures performed indirectly by the application of external force through the skin or mucous membrane
Open (0)	**Definition:** Cutting through the skin or mucous membrane and any other body layers necessary to expose the site of the procedure
Percutaneous (3)	**Definition:** Entry, by puncture or minor incision, of instrumentation through the skin or mucous membrane and any other body layers necessary to reach the site of the procedure
Percutaneous Endoscopic (4)	**Definition:** Entry, by puncture or minor incision, of instrumentation through the skin or mucous membrane and any other body layers necessary to reach and visualize the site of the procedure
Via Natural or Artificial Opening (7)	**Definition:** Entry of instrumentation through a natural or artificial external opening to reach the site of the procedure
Via Natural or Artificial Opening Endoscopic (8)	**Definition:** Entry of instrumentation through a natural or artificial external opening to reach and visualize the site of the procedure

Section 9 - Chiropractic — Character 5 - Approach

External (X)	**Definition:** Procedures performed directly on the skin or mucous membrane and procedures performed indirectly by the application of external force through the skin or mucous membrane

Appendix D: Medical and Surgical Body Parts

Section 0 - Medical and Surgical — Character 4 - Body Part

Body Part	
1st Toe, Left 1st Toe, Right	**Includes:** Hallux
Abdomen Muscle, Left Abdomen Muscle, Right	**Includes:** External oblique muscle Internal oblique muscle Pyramidalis muscle Rectus abdominis muscle Transversus abdominis muscle
Abdominal Aorta	**Includes:** Inferior phrenic artery Lumbar artery Median sacral artery Middle suprarenal artery Ovarian artery Testicular artery
Abdominal Sympathetic Nerve	**Includes:** Abdominal aortic plexus Auerbach's (myenteric) plexus Celiac (solar) plexus Celiac ganglion Gastric plexus Hepatic plexus Inferior hypogastric plexus Inferior mesenteric ganglion Inferior mesenteric plexus Meissner's (submucous) plexus Myenteric (Auerbach's) plexus Pancreatic plexus Pelvic splanchnic nerve Renal plexus Solar (celiac) plexus Splenic plexus Submucous (Meissner's) plexus Superior hypogastric plexus Superior mesenteric ganglion Superior mesenteric plexus Suprarenal plexus
Abducens Nerve	**Includes:** Sixth cranial nerve
Accessory Nerve	**Includes:** Eleventh cranial nerve
Acoustic Nerve	**Includes:** Cochlear nerve Eighth cranial nerve Scarpa's (vestibular) ganglion Spiral ganglion Vestibular (Scarpa's) ganglion Vestibular nerve Vestibulocochlear nerve
Adenoids	**Includes:** Pharyngeal tonsil
Adrenal Gland Adrenal Gland, Left Adrenal Gland, Right Adrenal Glands, Bilateral	**Includes:** Suprarenal gland

Section 0 - Medical and Surgical — Character 4 - Body Part

Body Part	
Ampulla of Vater	**Includes:** Duodenal ampulla Hepatopancreatic ampulla
Anal Sphincter	**Includes:** External anal sphincter Internal anal sphincter
Ankle Bursa and Ligament, Left Ankle Bursa and Ligament, Right	**Includes:** Calcaneofibular ligament Deltoid ligament Ligament of the lateral malleolus Talofibular ligament
Ankle Joint, Left Ankle Joint, Right	**Includes:** Inferior tibiofibular joint Talocrural joint
Anterior Chamber, Left Anterior Chamber, Right	**Includes:** Aqueous humour
Anterior Tibial Artery, Left Anterior Tibial Artery, Right	**Includes:** Anterior lateral malleolar artery Anterior medial malleolar artery Anterior tibial recurrent artery Dorsalis pedis artery Posterior tibial recurrent artery
Anus	**Includes:** Anal orifice
Aortic Valve	**Includes:** Aortic annulus
Appendix	**Includes:** Vermiform appendix
Ascending Colon	**Includes:** Hepatic flexure
Atrial Septum	**Includes:** Interatrial septum
Atrium, Left	**Includes:** Atrium pulmonale Left auricular appendix
Atrium, Right	**Includes:** Atrium dextrum cordis Right auricular appendix Sinus venosus
Auditory Ossicle, Left Auditory Ossicle, Right	**Includes:** Incus Malleus Ossicular chain Stapes
Axillary Artery, Left Axillary Artery, Right	**Includes:** Anterior circumflex humeral artery Lateral thoracic artery Posterior circumflex humeral artery Subscapular artery Superior thoracic artery Thoracoacromial artery

Continued

Section 0 - Medical and Surgical — Character 4 - Body Part	
Azygos Vein	**Includes:** Right ascending lumbar vein Right subcostal vein
Basal Ganglia	**Includes:** Basal nuclei Claustrum Corpus striatum Globus pallidus Substantia nigra Subthalamic nucleus
Basilic Vein, Left Basilic Vein, Right	**Includes:** Median antebrachial vein Median cubital vein
Bladder	**Includes:** Trigone of bladder
Brachial Artery, Left Brachial Artery, Right	**Includes:** Inferior ulnar collateral artery Profunda brachii Superior ulnar collateral artery
Brachial Plexus	**Includes:** Axillary nerve Dorsal scapular nerve First intercostal nerve Long thoracic nerve Musculocutaneous nerve Subclavius nerve Suprascapular nerve
Brachial Vein, Left Brachial Vein, Right	**Includes:** Radial vein Ulnar vein
Brain	**Includes:** Cerebrum Corpus callosum Encephalon
Breast, Bilateral Breast, Left Breast, Right	**Includes:** Mammary duct Mammary gland
Buccal Mucosa	**Includes:** Buccal gland Molar gland Palatine gland
Carotid Bodies, Bilateral Carotid Body, Left Carotid Body, Right	**Includes:** Carotid glomus
Carpal Joint, Left Carpal Joint, Right	**Includes:** Intercarpal joint Midcarpal joint
Carpal, Left Carpal, Right	**Includes:** Capitate bone Hamate bone Lunate bone Pisiform bone Scaphoid bone Trapezium bone Trapezoid bone Triquetral bone
Celiac Artery	**Includes:** Celiac trunk
Cephalic Vein, Left Cephalic Vein, Right	**Includes:** Accessory cephalic vein

Section 0 - Medical and Surgical — Character 4 - Body Part	
Cerebellum	**Includes:** Culmen
Cerebral Hemisphere	**Includes:** Frontal lobe Occipital lobe Parietal lobe Temporal lobe
Cerebral Meninges	**Includes:** Arachnoid mater Leptomeninges Pia mater
Cerebral Ventricle	**Includes:** Aqueduct of Sylvius Cerebral aqueduct (Sylvius) Choroid plexus Ependyma Foramen of Monro (intraventricular) Fourth ventricle Interventricular foramen (Monro) Left lateral ventricle Right lateral ventricle Third ventricle
Cervical Nerve	**Includes:** Greater occipital nerve Spinal nerve, cervical Suboccipital nerve Third occipital nerve
Cervical Plexus	**Includes:** Ansa cervicalis Cutaneous (transverse) cervical nerve Great auricular nerve Lesser occipital nerve Supraclavicular nerve Transverse (cutaneous) cervical nerve
Cervical Vertebra	**Includes:** Spinous process Vertebral arch Vertebral foramen Vertebral lamina Vertebral pedicle
Cervical Vertebral Joint	**Includes:** Atlantoaxial joint Cervical facet joint
Cervical Vertebral Joints, 2 or more	**Includes:** Cervical facet joint
Cervicothoracic Vertebral Joint	**Includes:** Cervicothoracic facet joint
Cisterna Chyli	**Includes:** Intestinal lymphatic trunk Lumbar lymphatic trunk
Coccygeal Glomus	**Includes:** Coccygeal body
Colic Vein	**Includes:** Ileocolic vein Left colic vein Middle colic vein Right colic vein
Conduction Mechanism	**Includes:** Atrioventricular node Bundle of His Bundle of Kent Sinoatrial node

Continued

Section 0 - Medical and Surgical — Character 4 - Body Part

Conjunctiva, Left Conjunctiva, Right	**Includes:** Plica semilunaris
Dura Mater	**Includes:** Cranial dura mater Dentate ligament Diaphragma sellae Falx cerebri Spinal dura mater Tentorium cerebelli
Elbow Bursa and Ligament, Left Elbow Bursa and Ligament, Right	**Includes:** Annular ligament Olecranon bursa Radial collateral ligament Ulnar collateral ligament
Elbow Joint, Left Elbow Joint, Right	**Includes:** Distal humerus, involving joint Humeroradial joint Humeroulnar joint Proximal radioulnar joint
Epidural Space	**Includes:** Cranial epidural space Extradural space Spinal epidural space
Epiglottis	**Includes:** Glossoepiglottic fold
Esophagogastric Junction	**Includes:** Cardia Cardioesophageal junction Gastroesophageal (GE) junction
Esophagus, Lower	**Includes:** Abdominal esophagus
Esophagus, Middle	**Includes:** Thoracic esophagus
Esophagus, Upper	**Includes:** Cervical esophagus
Ethmoid Bone, Left Ethmoid Bone, Right	**Includes:** Cribriform plate
Ethmoid Sinus, Left Ethmoid Sinus, Right	**Includes:** Ethmoidal air cell
Eustachian Tube, Left Eustachian Tube, Right	**Includes:** Auditory tube Pharyngotympanic tube
External Auditory Canal, Left External Auditory Canal, Right	**Includes:** External auditory meatus
External Carotid Artery, Left External Carotid Artery, Right	**Includes:** Ascending pharyngeal artery Internal maxillary artery Lingual artery Maxillary artery Occipital artery Posterior auricular artery Superior thyroid artery
External Ear, Bilateral External Ear, Left External Ear, Right	**Includes:** Antihelix Antitragus Auricle Earlobe Helix Pinna Tragus

Section 0 - Medical and Surgical — Character 4 - Body Part

External Iliac Artery, Left External Iliac Artery, Right	**Includes:** Deep circumflex iliac artery Inferior epigastric artery
External Jugular Vein, Left External Jugular Vein, Right	**Includes:** Posterior auricular vein
Extraocular Muscle, Left Extraocular Muscle, Right	**Includes:** Inferior oblique muscle Inferior rectus muscle Lateral rectus muscle Medial rectus muscle Superior oblique muscle Superior rectus muscle
Eye, Left Eye, Right	**Includes:** Ciliary body Posterior chamber
Face Artery	**Includes:** Angular artery Ascending palatine artery External maxillary artery Facial artery Inferior labial artery Submental artery Superior labial artery
Face Vein, Left Face Vein, Right	**Includes:** Angular vein Anterior facial vein Common facial vein Deep facial vein Frontal vein Posterior facial (retromandibular) vein Supraorbital vein
Facial Muscle	**Includes:** Buccinator muscle Corrugator supercilii muscle Depressor anguli oris muscle Depressor labii inferioris muscle Depressor septi nasi muscle Depressor supercilii muscle Levator anguli oris muscle Levator labii superioris alaeque nasi Levator labii superioris alaeque nasi Levator labii superioris alaeque nasi Levator labii superioris muscle Mentalis muscle Nasalis muscle Occipitofrontalis muscle Orbicularis oris muscle Procerus muscle Risorius muscle Zygomaticus muscle
Facial Nerve	**Includes:** Chorda tympani Geniculate ganglion Greater superficial petrosal nerve Nerve to the stapedius Parotid plexus Posterior auricular nerve Seventh cranial nerve Submandibular ganglion
Fallopian Tube, Left Fallopian Tube, Right	**Includes:** Oviduct Salpinx Uterine tube

Continued

Section 0 - Medical and Surgical — Character 4 - Body Part

Body Part	Includes
Femoral Artery, Left Femoral Artery, Right	**Includes:** Circumflex iliac artery Deep femoral artery Descending genicular artery External pudendal artery Superficial epigastric artery
Femoral Nerve	**Includes:** Anterior crural nerve Saphenous nerve
Femoral Shaft, Left Femoral Shaft, Right	**Includes:** Body of femur
Femoral Vein, Left Femoral Vein, Right	**Includes:** Deep femoral (profunda femoris) vein Popliteal vein Profunda femoris (deep femoral) vein
Fibula, Left Fibula, Right	**Includes:** Body of fibula Head of fibula Lateral malleolus
Finger Nail	**Includes:** Nail bed Nail plate
Finger Phalangeal Joint, Left Finger Phalangeal Joint, Right	**Includes:** Interphalangeal (IP) joint
Foot Artery, Left Foot Artery, Right	**Includes:** Arcuate artery Dorsal metatarsal artery Lateral plantar artery Lateral tarsal artery Medial plantar artery
Foot Bursa and Ligament, Left Foot Bursa and Ligament, Right	**Includes:** Calcaneocuboid ligament Cuneonavicular ligament Intercuneiform ligament Interphalangeal ligament Metatarsal ligament Metatarsophalangeal ligament Subtalar ligament Talocalcaneal ligament Talocalcaneonavicular ligament Tarsometatarsal ligament
Foot Muscle, Left Foot Muscle, Right	**Includes:** Abductor hallucis muscle Adductor hallucis muscle Extensor digitorum brevis muscle Extensor hallucis brevis muscle Flexor digitorum brevis muscle Flexor hallucis brevis muscle Quadratus plantae muscle
Foot Vein, Left Foot Vein, Right	**Includes:** Common digital vein Dorsal metatarsal vein Dorsal venous arch Plantar digital vein Plantar metatarsal vein Plantar venous arch
Frontal Bone, Left Frontal Bone, Right	**Includes:** Zygomatic process of frontal bone

Section 0 - Medical and Surgical — Character 4 - Body Part

Body Part	Includes
Gastric Artery	**Includes:** Left gastric artery Right gastric artery
Glenoid Cavity, Left Glenoid Cavity, Right	**Includes:** Glenoid fossa (of scapula)
Glomus Jugulare	**Includes:** Jugular body
Glossopharyngeal Nerve	**Includes:** Carotid sinus nerve Ninth cranial nerve Tympanic nerve
Greater Omentum	**Includes:** Gastrocolic ligament Gastrocolic omentum Gastrophrenic ligament Gastrosplenic ligament
Greater Saphenous Vein, Left Greater Saphenous Vein, Right	**Includes:** External pudendal vein Great saphenous vein Superficial circumflex iliac vein Superficial epigastric vein
Hand Artery, Left Hand Artery, Right	**Includes:** Deep palmar arch Princeps pollicis artery Radialis indicis Superficial palmar arch
Hand Bursa and Ligament, Left Hand Bursa and Ligament, Right	**Includes:** Carpometacarpal ligament Intercarpal ligament Interphalangeal ligament Lunotriquetral ligament Metacarpal ligament Metacarpophalangeal ligament Pisohamate ligament Pisometacarpal ligament Scapholunate ligament Scaphotrapezium ligament
Hand Muscle, Left Hand Muscle, Right	**Includes:** Hypothenar muscle Palmar interosseous muscle Thenar muscle
Hand Vein, Left Hand Vein, Right	**Includes:** Dorsal metacarpal vein Palmar (volar) digital vein Palmar (volar) metacarpal vein Superficial palmar venous arch Volar (palmar) digital vein Volar (palmar) metacarpal vein
Head and Neck Bursa and Ligament	**Includes:** Alar ligament of axis Cervical interspinous ligament Cervical intertransverse ligament Cervical ligamentum flavum Lateral temporomandibular ligament Sphenomandibular ligament Stylomandibular ligament Transverse ligament of atlas

Continued

Head and Neck Sympathetic Nerve	**Includes:** Cavernous plexus Cervical ganglion Ciliary ganglion Internal carotid plexus Otic ganglion Pterygopalatine (sphenopalatine) ganglion Sphenopalatine (pterygopalatine) ganglion Stellate ganglion Submandibular ganglion Submaxillary ganglion
Head Muscle	**Includes:** Auricularis muscle Masseter muscle Pterygoid muscle Splenius capitis muscle Temporalis muscle Temporoparietalis muscle
Heart, Left	**Includes:** Left coronary sulcus Obtuse margin
Heart, Right	**Includes:** Right coronary sulcus
Hemiazygos Vein	**Includes:** Left ascending lumbar vein Left subcostal vein
Hepatic Artery	**Includes:** Common hepatic artery Gastroduodenal artery Hepatic artery proper
Hip Bursa and Ligament, Left Hip Bursa and Ligament, Right	**Includes:** Iliofemoral ligament Ischiofemoral ligament Pubofemoral ligament Transverse acetabular ligament Trochanteric bursa
Hip Joint, Left Hip Joint, Right	**Includes:** Acetabulofemoral joint
Hip Muscle, Left Hip Muscle, Right	**Includes:** Gemellus muscle Gluteus maximus muscle Gluteus medius muscle Gluteus minimus muscle Iliacus muscle Obturator muscle Piriformis muscle Psoas muscle Quadratus femoris muscle Tensor fasciae latae muscle
Humeral Head, Left Humeral Head, Right	**Includes:** Greater tuberosity Lesser tuberosity Neck of humerus (anatomical)(surgical)
Humeral Shaft, Left Humeral Shaft, Right	**Includes:** Distal humerus Humerus, distal Lateral epicondyle of humerus Medial epicondyle of humerus

Hypogastric Vein, Left Hypogastric Vein, Right	**Includes:** Gluteal vein Internal iliac vein Internal pudendal vein Lateral sacral vein Middle hemorrhoidal vein Obturator vein Uterine vein Vaginal vein Vesical vein
Hypoglossal Nerve	**Includes:** Twelfth cranial nerve
Hypothalamus	**Includes:** Mammillary body
Inferior Mesenteric Artery	**Includes:** Sigmoid artery Superior rectal artery
Inferior Mesenteric Vein	**Includes:** Sigmoid vein Superior rectal vein
Inferior Vena Cava	**Includes:** Postcava Right inferior phrenic vein Right ovarian vein Right second lumbar vein Right suprarenal vein Right testicular vein
Inguinal Region, Bilateral Inguinal Region, Left Inguinal Region, Right	**Includes:** Inguinal canal Inguinal triangle
Inner Ear, Left Inner Ear, Right	**Includes:** Bony labyrinth Bony vestibule Cochlea Round window Semicircular canal
Innominate Artery	**Includes:** Brachiocephalic artery Brachiocephalic trunk
Innominate Vein, Left Innominate Vein, Right	**Includes:** Brachiocephalic vein Inferior thyroid vein
Internal Carotid Artery, Left Internal Carotid Artery, Right	**Includes:** Caroticotympanic artery Carotid sinus Ophthalmic artery
Internal Iliac Artery, Left Internal Iliac Artery, Right	**Includes:** Deferential artery Hypogastric artery Iliolumbar artery Inferior gluteal artery Inferior vesical artery Internal pudendal artery Lateral sacral artery Middle rectal artery Obturator artery Superior gluteal artery Umbilical artery Uterine artery Vaginal artery

Continued

Section 0 - Medical and Surgical — Character 4 - Body Part	
Internal Mammary Artery, Left Internal Mammary Artery, Right	**Includes:** Anterior intercostal artery Internal thoracic artery Musculophrenic artery Pericardiophrenic artery Superior epigastric artery
Intracranial Artery	**Includes:** Anterior cerebral artery Anterior choroidal artery Anterior communicating artery Basilar artery Circle of Willis Middle cerebral artery Posterior cerebral artery Posterior communicating artery Posterior inferior cerebellar artery (PICA)
Intracranial Vein	**Includes:** Anterior cerebral vein Basal (internal) cerebral vein Dural venous sinus Great cerebral vein Inferior cerebellar vein Inferior cerebral vein Internal (basal) cerebral vein Middle cerebral vein Ophthalmic vein Superior cerebellar vein Superior cerebral vein
Jejunum	**Includes:** Duodenojejunal flexure
Kidney	**Includes:** Renal calyx Renal capsule Renal cortex Renal segment
Kidney Pelvis, Left Kidney Pelvis, Right	**Includes:** Ureteropelvic junction (UPJ)
Kidney, Left Kidney, Right Kidneys, Bilateral	**Includes:** Renal calyx Renal capsule Renal cortex Renal segment
Knee Bursa and Ligament, Left Knee Bursa and Ligament, Right	**Includes:** Anterior cruciate ligament (ACL) Lateral collateral ligament (LCL) Ligament of head of fibula Medial collateral ligament (MCL) Patellar ligament Popliteal ligament Posterior cruciate ligament (PCL) Prepatellar bursa
Knee Joint, Femoral Surface, Left Knee Joint, Femoral Surface, Right	**Includes:** Femoropatellar joint Patellofemoral joint
Knee Joint, Left Knee Joint, Right	**Includes:** Femoropatellar joint Femorotibial joint Lateral meniscus Medial meniscus Patellofemoral joint Tibiofemoral joint
Knee Joint, Tibial Surface, Left Knee Joint, Tibial Surface, Right	**Includes:** Femorotibial joint Tibiofemoral joint
Knee Tendon, Left Knee Tendon, Right	**Includes:** Patellar tendon
Lacrimal Duct, Left Lacrimal Duct, Right	**Includes:** Lacrimal canaliculus Lacrimal punctum Lacrimal sac Nasolacrimal duct
Larynx	**Includes:** Aryepiglottic fold Arytenoid cartilage Corniculate cartilage Cricoid cartilage Cuneiform cartilage False vocal cord Glottis Rima glottidis Thyroid cartilage Ventricular fold
Lens, Left Lens, Right	**Includes:** Zonule of Zinn
Lesser Omentum	**Includes:** Gastrohepatic omentum Hepatogastric ligament
Lesser Saphenous Vein, Left Lesser Saphenous Vein, Right	**Includes:** Small saphenous vein
Liver	**Includes:** Quadrate lobe
Lower Arm and Wrist Muscle, Left Lower Arm and Wrist Muscle, Right	**Includes:** Anatomical snuffbox Brachioradialis muscle Extensor carpi radialis muscle Extensor carpi ulnaris muscle Flexor carpi radialis muscle Flexor carpi ulnaris muscle Flexor pollicis longus muscle Palmaris longus muscle Pronator quadratus muscle Pronator teres muscle
Lower Eyelid, Left Lower Eyelid, Right	**Includes:** Inferior tarsal plate Medial canthus
Lower Femur, Left Lower Femur, Right	**Includes:** Lateral condyle of femur Lateral epicondyle of femur Medial condyle of femur Medial epicondyle of femur
Lower Leg Muscle, Left Lower Leg Muscle, Right	**Includes:** Extensor digitorum longus muscle Extensor hallucis longus muscle Fibularis brevis muscle Fibularis longus muscle Flexor digitorum longus muscle Flexor hallucis longus muscle Gastrocnemius muscle Peroneus brevis muscle Peroneus longus muscle Popliteus muscle Soleus muscle Tibialis anterior muscle Tibialis posterior muscle

Continued

Section 0 - Medical and Surgical — Character 4 - Body Part

Body Part	Includes
Lower Leg Tendon, Left Lower Leg Tendon, Right	**Includes:** Achilles tendon
Lower Lip	**Includes:** Frenulum labii inferioris Labial gland Vermilion border
Lumbar Nerve	**Includes:** Lumbosacral trunk Spinal nerve, lumbar Superior clunic (cluneal) nerve
Lumbar Plexus	**Includes:** Accessory obturator nerve Genitofemoral nerve Iliohypogastric nerve Ilioinguinal nerve Lateral femoral cutaneous nerve Obturator nerve Superior gluteal nerve
Lumbar Spinal Cord	**Includes:** Cauda equina Conus medullaris
Lumbar Sympathetic Nerve	**Includes:** Lumbar ganglion Lumbar splanchnic nerve
Lumbar Vertebra	**Includes:** Spinous process Vertebral arch Vertebral foramen Vertebral lamina Vertebral pedicle
Lumbar Vertebral Joint Lumbar Vertebral Joints, 2 or more	**Includes:** Lumbar facet joint
Lumbosacral Joint	**Includes:** Lumbosacral facet joint
Lymphatic, Aortic	**Includes:** Celiac lymph node Gastric lymph node Hepatic lymph node Lumbar lymph node Pancreaticosplenic lymph node Paraaortic lymph node Retroperitoneal lymph node
Lymphatic, Head	**Includes:** Buccinator lymph node Infraauricular lymph node Infraparotid lymph node Parotid lymph node Preauricular lymph node Submandibular lymph node Submaxillary lymph node Submental lymph node Subparotid lymph node Suprahyoid lymph node

Section 0 - Medical and Surgical — Character 4 - Body Part

Body Part	Includes
Lymphatic, Left Axillary	**Includes:** Anterior (pectoral) lymph node Apical (subclavicular) lymph node Brachial (lateral) lymph node Central axillary lymph node Lateral (brachial) lymph node Pectoral (anterior) lymph node Posterior (subscapular) lymph node Subclavicular (apical) lymph node Subscapular (posterior) lymph node
Lymphatic, Left Lower Extremity	**Includes:** Femoral lymph node Popliteal lymph node
Lymphatic, Left Neck	**Includes:** Cervical lymph node Jugular lymph node Mastoid (postauricular) lymph node Occipital lymph node Postauricular (mastoid) lymph node Retropharyngeal lymph node Supraclavicular (Virchow's) lymph node Virchow's (supraclavicular) lymph node
Lymphatic, Left Upper Extremity	**Includes:** Cubital lymph node Deltopectoral (infraclavicular) lymph node Epitrochlear lymph node Infraclavicular (deltopectoral) lymph node Supratrochlear lymph node
Lymphatic, Mesenteric	**Includes:** Inferior mesenteric lymph node Pararectal lymph node Superior mesenteric lymph node
Lymphatic, Pelvis	**Includes:** Common iliac (subaortic) lymph node Gluteal lymph node Iliac lymph node Inferior epigastric lymph node Obturator lymph node Sacral lymph node Subaortic (common iliac) lymph node Suprainguinal lymph node
Lymphatic, Right Axillary	**Includes:** Anterior (pectoral) lymph node Apical (subclavicular) lymph node Brachial (lateral) lymph node Central axillary lymph node Lateral (brachial) lymph node Pectoral (anterior) lymph node Posterior (subscapular) lymph node Subclavicular (apical) lymph node Subscapular (posterior) lymph node
Lymphatic, Right Lower Extremity	**Includes:** Femoral lymph node Popliteal lymph node

Continued

Section 0 - Medical and Surgical — Character 4 - Body Part	
Lymphatic, Right Neck	**Includes:** Cervical lymph node Jugular lymph node Mastoid (postauricular) lymph node Occipital lymph node Postauricular (mastoid) lymph node Retropharyngeal lymph node Right jugular trunk Right lymphatic duct Right subclavian trunk Supraclavicular (Virchow's) lymph node Virchow's (supraclavicular) lymph node
Lymphatic, Right Upper Extremity	**Includes:** Cubital lymph node Deltopectoral (infraclavicular) lymph node Epitrochlear lymph node Infraclavicular (deltopectoral) lymph node Supratrochlear lymph node
Lymphatic, Thorax	**Includes:** Intercostal lymph node Mediastinal lymph node Parasternal lymph node Paratracheal lymph node Tracheobronchial lymph node
Mandible, Left Mandible, Right	**Includes:** Alveolar process of mandible Condyloid process Mandibular notch Mental foramen
Mastoid Sinus, Left Mastoid Sinus, Right	**Includes:** Mastoid air cells
Maxilla, Left Maxilla, Right	**Includes:** Alveolar process of maxilla
Maxillary Sinus, Left Maxillary Sinus, Right	**Includes:** Antrum of Highmore
Median Nerve	**Includes:** Anterior interosseous nerve Palmar cutaneous nerve
Medulla Oblongata	**Includes:** Myelencephalon
Mesentery	**Includes:** Mesoappendix Mesocolon
Metacarpocarpal Joint, Left Metacarpocarpal Joint, Right	**Includes:** Carpometacarpal (CMC) joint
Metatarsal-Phalangeal Joint, Left Metatarsal-Phalangeal Joint, Right	**Includes:** Metatarsophalangeal (MTP) joint
Metatarsal-Tarsal Joint, Left Metatarsal-Tarsal Joint, Right	**Includes:** Tarsometatarsal joint
Middle Ear, Left Middle Ear, Right	**Includes:** Oval window Tympanic cavity
Minor Salivary Gland	**Includes:** Anterior lingual gland

Section 0 - Medical and Surgical — Character 4 - Body Part	
Mitral Valve	**Includes:** Bicuspid valve Left atrioventricular valve Mitral annulus
Nasal Bone	**Includes:** Vomer of nasal septum
Nasal Septum	**Includes:** Quadrangular cartilage Septal cartilage Vomer bone
Nasal Turbinate	**Includes:** Inferior turbinate Middle turbinate Nasal concha Superior turbinate
Nasopharynx	**Includes:** Choana Fossa of Rosenmuller Pharyngeal recess Rhinopharynx
Neck Muscle, Left Neck Muscle, Right	**Includes:** Anterior vertebral muscle Arytenoid muscle Cricothyroid muscle Infrahyoid muscle Levator scapulae muscle Platysma muscle Scalene muscle Splenius cervicis muscle Sternocleidomastoid muscle Suprahyoid muscle Thyroarytenoid muscle
Nipple, Left Nipple, Right	**Includes:** Areola
Nose	**Includes:** Columella External naris Greater alar cartilage Internal naris Lateral nasal cartilage Lesser alar cartilage Nasal cavity Nostril
Occipital Bone, Left Occipital Bone, Right	**Includes:** Foramen magnum
Oculomotor Nerve	**Includes:** Third cranial nerve
Olfactory Nerve	**Includes:** First cranial nerve Olfactory bulb
Optic Nerve	**Includes:** Optic chiasma Second cranial nerve
Orbit, Left Orbit, Right	**Includes:** Bony orbit Orbital portion of ethmoid bone Orbital portion of frontal bone Orbital portion of lacrimal bone Orbital portion of maxilla Orbital portion of palatine bone Orbital portion of sphenoid bone Orbital portion of zygomatic bone

Continued

Section 0 - Medical and Surgical — Character 4 - Body Part

Pancreatic Duct	**Includes:** Duct of Wirsung
Pancreatic Duct, Accessory	**Includes:** Duct of Santorini
Parotid Duct, Left Parotid Duct, Right	**Includes:** Stensen's duct
Pelvic Bone, Left Pelvic Bone, Right	**Includes:** Iliac crest Ilium Ischium Pubis
Pelvic Cavity	**Includes:** Retropubic space
Penis	**Includes:** Corpus cavernosum Corpus spongiosum
Perineum Muscle	**Includes:** Bulbospongiosus muscle Cremaster muscle Deep transverse perineal muscle Ischiocavernosus muscle Superficial transverse perineal muscle
Peritoneum	**Includes:** Epiploic foramen
Peroneal Artery, Left Peroneal Artery, Right	**Includes:** Fibular artery
Peroneal Nerve	**Includes:** Common fibular nerve Common peroneal nerve External popliteal nerve Lateral sural cutaneous nerve
Pharynx	**Includes:** Hypopharynx Laryngopharynx Oropharynx Piriform recess (sinus)
Phrenic Nerve	**Includes:** Accessory phrenic nerve
Pituitary Gland	**Includes:** Adenohypophysis Hypophysis Neurohypophysis
Pons	**Includes:** Apneustic center Basis pontis Locus ceruleus Pneumotaxic center Pontine tegmentum Superior olivary nucleus
Popliteal Artery, Left Popliteal Artery, Right	**Includes:** Inferior genicular artery Middle genicular artery Superior genicular artery Sural artery
Portal Vein	**Includes:** Hepatic portal vein

Section 0 - Medical and Surgical — Character 4 - Body Part

Prepuce	**Includes:** Foreskin Glans penis
Pudendal Nerve	**Includes:** Posterior labial nerve Posterior scrotal nerve
Pulmonary Artery, Left	**Includes:** Arterial canal (duct) Botallo's duct Pulmoaortic canal
Pulmonary Valve	**Includes:** Pulmonary annulus Pulmonic valve
Pulmonary Vein, Left	**Includes:** Left inferior pulmonary vein Left superior pulmonary vein
Pulmonary Vein, Right	**Includes:** Right inferior pulmonary vein Right superior pulmonary vein
Radial Artery, Left Radial Artery, Right	**Includes:** Radial recurrent artery
Radial Nerve	**Includes:** Dorsal digital nerve Musculospiral nerve Palmar cutaneous nerve Posterior interosseous nerve
Radius, Left Radius, Right	**Includes:** Ulnar notch
Rectum	**Includes:** Anorectal junction
Renal Artery, Left Renal Artery, Right	**Includes:** Inferior suprarenal artery Renal segmental artery
Renal Vein, Left	**Includes:** Left inferior phrenic vein Left ovarian vein Left second lumbar vein Left suprarenal vein Left testicular vein
Retina, Left Retina, Right	**Includes:** Fovea Macula Optic disc
Retroperitoneum	**Includes:** Retroperitoneal space
Sacral Nerve	**Includes:** Spinal nerve, sacral
Sacral Plexus	**Includes:** Inferior gluteal nerve Posterior femoral cutaneous nerve Pudendal nerve
Sacral Sympathetic Nerve	**Includes:** Ganglion impar (ganglion of Walther) Pelvic splanchnic nerve Sacral ganglion Sacral splanchnic nerve

Continued

Section 0 - Medical and Surgical — Character 4 - Body Part

Sacrococcygeal Joint	**Includes:** Sacrococcygeal symphysis
Scapula, Left Scapula, Right	**Includes:** Acromion (process) Coracoid process
Sciatic Nerve	**Includes:** Ischiatic nerve
Shoulder Bursa and Ligament, Left Shoulder Bursa and Ligament, Right	**Includes:** Acromioclavicular ligament Coracoacromial ligament Coracoclavicular ligament Coracohumeral ligament Costoclavicular ligament Glenohumeral ligament Glenoid ligament (labrum) Interclavicular ligament Sternoclavicular ligament Subacromial bursa Transverse humeral ligament Transverse scapular ligament
Shoulder Joint, Left Shoulder Joint, Right	**Includes:** Glenohumeral joint
Shoulder Muscle, Left Shoulder Muscle, Right	**Includes:** Deltoid muscle Infraspinatus muscle Subscapularis muscle Supraspinatus muscle Teres major muscle Teres minor muscle
Sigmoid Colon	**Includes:** Rectosigmoid junction Sigmoid flexure
Skin	**Includes:** Dermis Epidermis Sebaceous gland Sweat gland
Sphenoid Bone, Left Sphenoid Bone, Right	**Includes:** Greater wing Lesser wing Optic foramen Pterygoid process Sella turcica
Spinal Canal	**Includes:** Vertebral canal
Spinal Meninges	**Includes:** Arachnoid mater Denticulate ligament Leptomeninges Pia mater
Spleen	**Includes:** Accessory spleen
Splenic Artery	**Includes:** Left gastroepiploic artery Pancreatic artery Short gastric artery
Splenic Vein	**Includes:** Left gastroepiploic vein Pancreatic vein

Section 0 - Medical and Surgical — Character 4 - Body Part

Sternum	**Includes:** Manubrium Suprasternal notch Xiphoid process
Stomach, Pylorus	**Includes:** Pyloric antrum Pyloric canal Pyloric sphincter
Subarachnoid Space	**Includes:** Cranial subarachnoid space Spinal subarachnoid space
Subclavian Artery, Left Subclavian Artery, Right	**Includes:** Costocervical trunk Dorsal scapular artery Internal thoracic artery
Subcutaneous Tissue and Fascia, Anterior Neck	**Includes:** Deep cervical fascia Pretracheal fascia
Subcutaneous Tissue and Fascia, Chest	**Includes:** Pectoral fascia
Subcutaneous Tissue and Fascia, Face	**Includes:** Masseteric fascia Orbital fascia
Subcutaneous Tissue and Fascia, Left Foot	**Includes:** Plantar fascia (aponeurosis)
Subcutaneous Tissue and Fascia, Left Hand	**Includes:** Palmar fascia (aponeurosis)
Subcutaneous Tissue and Fascia, Left Lower Arm	**Includes:** Antebrachial fascia Bicipital aponeurosis
Subcutaneous Tissue and Fascia, Left Upper Arm	**Includes:** Axillary fascia Deltoid fascia Infraspinatus fascia Subscapular aponeurosis Supraspinatus fascia
Subcutaneous Tissue and Fascia, Left Upper Leg	**Includes:** Crural fascia Fascia lata Iliac fascia Iliotibial tract (band)
Subcutaneous Tissue and Fascia, Posterior Neck	**Includes:** Prevertebral fascia
Subcutaneous Tissue and Fascia, Right Foot	**Includes:** Plantar fascia (aponeurosis)
Subcutaneous Tissue and Fascia, Right Hand	**Includes:** Palmar fascia (aponeurosis)
Subcutaneous Tissue and Fascia, Right Lower Arm	**Includes:** Antebrachial fascia Bicipital aponeurosis
Subcutaneous Tissue and Fascia, Right Upper Arm	**Includes:** Axillary fascia Deltoid fascia Infraspinatus fascia Subscapular aponeurosis Supraspinatus fascia

Continued

Section 0 - Medical and Surgical — Character 4 - Body Part

Body Part	Includes
Subcutaneous Tissue and Fascia, Right Upper Leg	**Includes:** Crural fascia Fascia lata Iliac fascia Iliotibial tract (band)
Subcutaneous Tissue and Fascia, Scalp	**Includes:** Galea aponeurotica
Subcutaneous Tissue and Fascia, Trunk	**Includes:** External oblique aponeurosis Transversalis fascia
Subdural Space	**Includes:** Cranial subdural space Spinal subdural space
Submaxillary Gland, Left Submaxillary Gland, Right	**Includes:** Submandibular gland
Superior Mesenteric Artery	**Includes:** Ileal artery Ileocolic artery Inferior pancreaticoduodenal artery Jejunal artery
Superior Mesenteric Vein	**Includes:** Right gastroepiploic vein
Superior Vena Cava	**Includes:** Precava
Tarsal Joint, Left Tarsal Joint, Right	**Includes:** Calcaneocuboid joint Cuboideonavicular joint Cuneonavicular joint Intercuneiform joint Subtalar (talocalcaneal) joint Talocalcaneal (subtalar) joint Talocalcaneonavicular joint
Tarsal, Left Tarsal, Right	**Includes:** Calcaneus Cuboid bone Intermediate cuneiform bone Lateral cuneiform bone Medial cuneiform bone Navicular bone Talus bone
Temporal Artery, Left Temporal Artery, Right	**Includes:** Middle temporal artery Superficial temporal artery Transverse facial artery
Temporal Bone. Left Temporal Bone, Right	**Includes:** Mastoid process Petrous part of temoporal bone Tympanic part of temoporal bone Zygomatic process of temporal bone
Thalamus	**Includes:** Epithalamus Geniculate nucleus Metathalamus Pulvinar

Section 0 - Medical and Surgical — Character 4 - Body Part

Body Part	Includes
Thoracic Aorta	**Includes:** Aortic arch Aortic intercostal artery Ascending aorta Bronchial artery Esophageal artery Subcostal artery
Thoracic Duct	**Includes:** Left jugular trunk Left subclavian trunk
Thoracic Nerve	**Includes:** Intercostal nerve Intercostobrachial nerve Spinal nerve, thoracic Subcostal nerve
Thoracic Sympathetic Nerve	**Includes:** Cardiac plexus Esophageal plexus Greater splanchnic nerve Inferior cardiac nerve Least splanchnic nerve Lesser splanchnic nerve Middle cardiac nerve Pulmonary plexus Superior cardiac nerve Thoracic aortic plexus Thoracic ganglion
Thoracic Vertebra	**Includes:** Spinous process Vertebral arch Vertebral foramen Vertebral lamina Vertebral pedicle
Thoracic Vertebral Joint Thoracic Vertebral Joints, 2 to 7 Thoracic Vertebral Joints, 8 or more	**Includes:** Costotransverse joint Costovertebral joint Thoracic facet joint
Thoracolumbar Vertebral Joint	**Includes:** Thoracolumbar facet joint
Thorax Bursa and Ligament, Left Thorax Bursa and Ligament, Right	**Includes:** Costotransverse ligament Costoxiphoid ligament Sternocostal ligament
Thorax Muscle, Left Thorax Muscle, Right	**Includes:** Intercostal muscle Levatores costarum muscle Pectoralis major muscle Pectoralis minor muscle Serratus anterior muscle Subclavius muscle Subcostal muscle Transverse thoracis muscle
Thymus	**Includes:** Thymus gland
Thyroid Artery, Left Thyroid Artery, Right	**Includes:** Cricothyroid artery Hyoid artery Sternocleidomastoid artery Superior laryngeal artery Superior thyroid artery Thyrocervical trunk

Continued

Section 0 - Medical and Surgical — Character 4 - Body Part

Tibia, Left Tibia, Right	**Includes:** Lateral condyle of tibia Medial condyle of tibia Medial malleolus
Tibial Nerve	**Includes:** Lateral plantar nerve Medial plantar nerve Medial popliteal nerve Medial sural cutaneous nerve
Toe Nail	**Includes:** Nail bed Nail plate
Toe Phalangeal Joint, Left Toe Phalangeal Joint, Right	**Includes:** Interphalangeal (IP) joint
Tongue	**Includes:** Frenulum linguae Lingual tonsil
Tongue, Palate, Pharynx Muscle	**Includes:** Chondroglossus muscle Genioglossus muscle Hyoglossus muscle Inferior longitudinal muscle Levator veli palatini muscle Palatoglossal muscle Palatopharyngeal muscle Pharyngeal constrictor muscle Salpingopharyngeus muscle Styloglossus muscle Stylopharyngeus muscle Superior longitudinal muscle Tensor veli palatini muscle
Tonsils	**Includes:** Palatine tonsil
Transverse Colon	**Includes:** Splenic flexure
Tricuspid Valve	**Includes:** Right atrioventricular valve Tricuspid annulus
Trigeminal Nerve	**Includes:** Fifth cranial nerve Gasserian ganglion Mandibular nerve Maxillary nerve Ophthalmic nerve Trifacial nerve
Trochlear Nerve	**Includes:** Fourth cranial nerve
Trunk Bursa and Ligament, Left Trunk Bursa and Ligament, Right	**Includes:** Iliolumbar ligament Interspinous ligament Intertransverse ligament Ligamentum flavum Pubic ligament Sacrococcygeal ligament Sacroiliac ligament Sacrospinous ligament Sacrotuberous ligament Supraspinous ligament

Section 0 - Medical and Surgical — Character 4 - Body Part

Trunk Muscle, Left Trunk Muscle, Right	**Includes:** Coccygeus muscle Erector spinae muscle Interspinalis muscle Intertransversarius muscle Latissimus dorsi muscle Levator ani muscle Quadratus lumborum muscle Rhomboid major muscle Rhomboid minor muscle Serratus posterior muscle Transversospinalis muscle Trapezius muscle
Tympanic Membrane, Left Tympanic Membrane, Right	**Includes:** Pars flaccida
Ulna, Left Ulna, Right	**Includes:** Olecranon process Radial notch
Ulnar Artery, Left Ulnar Artery, Right	**Includes:** Anterior ulnar recurrent artery Common interosseous artery Posterior ulnar recurrent artery
Ulnar Nerve	**Includes:** Cubital nerve
Upper Arm Muscle, Left Upper Arm Muscle, Right	**Includes:** Biceps brachii muscle Brachialis muscle Coracobrachialis muscle Triceps brachii muscle
Upper Eyelid, Left Upper Eyelid, Right	**Includes:** Lateral canthus Levator palpebrae superioris muscle Orbicularis oculi muscle Superior tarsal plate
Upper Femur, Left Upper Femur, Right	**Includes:** Femoral head Greater trochanter Lesser trochanter Neck of femur
Upper Leg Muscle, Left Upper Leg Muscle, Right	**Includes:** Adductor brevis muscle Adductor longus muscle Adductor magnus muscle Biceps femoris muscle Gracilis muscle Pectineus muscle Quadriceps (femoris) Rectus femoris muscle Sartorius muscle Semimembranosus muscle Semitendinosus muscle Vastus intermedius muscle Vastus lateralis muscle Vastus medialis muscle
Upper Lip	**Includes:** Frenulum labii superioris Labial gland Vermilion border

Continued

Section 0 - Medical and Surgical — Character 4 - Body Part

Ureter Ureter, Left Ureter, Right Ureters, Bilateral	**Includes:** Ureteral orifice Ureterovesical orifice
Urethra	**Includes:** Bulbourethral (Cowper's) gland Cowper's (bulbourethral) gland External urethral sphincter Internal urethral sphincter Membranous urethra Penile urethra Prostatic urethra
Uterine Supporting Structure	**Includes:** Broad ligament Infundibulopelvic ligament Ovarian ligament Round ligament of uterus
Uterus	**Includes:** Fundus uteri Myometrium Perimetrium Uterine cornu
Uvula	**Includes:** Palatine uvula
Vagus Nerve	**Includes:** Anterior vagal trunk Pharyngeal plexus Pneumogastric nerve Posterior vagal trunk Pulmonary plexus Recurrent laryngeal nerve Superior laryngeal nerve Tenth cranial nerve
Vas Deferens Vas Deferens, Bilateral Vas Deferens, Left Vas Deferens, Right	**Includes:** Ductus deferens Ejaculatory duct

Section 0 - Medical and Surgical — Character 4 - Body Part

Ventricle, Right	**Includes:** Conus arteriosus
Ventricular Septum	**Includes:** Interventricular septum
Vertebral Artery, Left Vertebral Artery, Right	**Includes:** Anterior spinal artery Posterior spinal artery
Vertebral Vein, Left Vertebral Vein, Right	**Includes:** Deep cervical vein Suboccipital venous plexus
Vestibular Gland	**Includes:** Bartholin's (greater vestibular) gland Greater vestibular (Bartholin's) gland Paraurethral (Skene's) gland Skene's (paraurethral) gland
Vitreous, Left Vitreous, Right	**Includes:** Vitreous body
Vocal Cord, Left Vocal Cord, Right	**Includes:** Vocal fold
Vulva	**Includes:** Labia majora Labia minora
Wrist Bursa and Ligament, Left Wrist Bursa and Ligament, Right	**Includes:** Palmar ulnocarpal ligament Radial collateral carpal ligament Radiocarpal ligament Radioulnar ligament Ulnar collateral carpal ligament
Wrist Joint, Left Wrist Joint, Right	**Includes:** Distal radioulnar joint Radiocarpal joint

Appendix E: Medical and Surgical Device Table and Device Aggregation Table

Section 0 - Medical and Surgical — Character 6 - Device

Device	Includes
Artificial Sphincter in Gastrointestinal System	**Includes:** Artificial anal sphincter (AAS) Artificial bowel sphincter (neosphincter)
Artificial Sphincter in Urinary System	**Includes:** AMS 800® Urinary Control System Artificial urinary sphincter (AUS)
Autologous Arterial Tissue in Heart and Great Vessels	**Includes:** Autologous artery graft
Autologous Arterial Tissue in Lower Arteries	**Includes:** Autologous artery graft
Autologous Arterial Tissue in Lower Veins	**Includes:** Autologous artery graft
Autologous Arterial Tissue in Upper Arteries	**Includes:** Autologous artery graft
Autologous Arterial Tissue in Upper Veins	**Includes:** Autologous artery graft
Autologous Tissue Substitute	**Includes:** Autograft Cultured epidermal cell autograft Epicel® cultured epidermal autograft
Autologous Venous Tissue in Heart and Great Vessels	**Includes:** Autologous vein graft
Autologous Venous Tissue in Lower Arteries	**Includes:** Autologous vein graft
Autologous Venous Tissue in Lower Veins	**Includes:** Autologous vein graft
Autologous Venous Tissue in Upper Arteries	**Includes:** Autologous vein graft
Autologous Venous Tissue in Upper Veins	**Includes:** Autologous vein graft
Bone Growth Stimulator in Head and Facial Bones	**Includes:** Electrical bone growth stimulator (EBGS) Ultrasonic osteogenic stimulator Ultrasound bone healing system
Bone Growth Stimulator in Lower Bones	**Includes:** Electrical bone growth stimulator (EBGS) Ultrasonic osteogenic stimulator Ultrasound bone healing system
Bone Growth Stimulator in Upper Bones	**Includes:** Electrical bone growth stimulator (EBGS) Ultrasonic osteogenic stimulator Ultrasound bone healing system
Cardiac Lead in Heart and Great Vessels	**Includes:** Cardiac contractility modulation lead

Section 0 - Medical and Surgical — Character 6 - Device

Device	Includes
Cardiac Lead, Defibrillator for Insertion in Heart and Great Vessels	**Includes:** ACUITY™ Steerable Lead Attain Ability® lead Attain StarFix® (OTW) lead Cardiac resynchronization therapy (CRT) lead Corox (OTW) Bipolar Lead Durata® Defibrillation Lead ENDOTAK RELIANCE® (G) Defibrillation Lead
Cardiac Lead, Pacemaker for Insertion in Heart and Great Vessels	**Includes:** ACUITY™ Steerable Lead Attain Ability® lead Attain StarFix® (OTW) lead Cardiac resynchronization therapy (CRT) lead Corox (OTW) Bipolar Lead
Cardiac Resynchronization Defibrillator Pulse Generator for Insertion in Subcutaneous Tissue and Fascia	**Includes:** COGNIS® CRT-D Concerto II CRT-D Consulta CRT-D CONTAK RENEWAL® 3 RF (HE) CRT-D LIVIAN™ CRT-D Maximo II DR CRT-D Ovatio™ CRT-D Protecta XT CRT-D
Cardiac Resynchronization Pacemaker Pulse Generator for Insertion in Subcutaneous Tissue and Fascia	**Includes:** Consulta CRT-P Stratos LV Synchra CRT-P
Cardiac Rhythm Related Device in Subcutaneous Tissue and Fascia	**Includes:** Baroreflex Activation Therapy® (BAT®) Rheos® System device
Contraceptive Device in Female Reproductive System	**Includes:** Intrauterine device (IUD)
Contraceptive Device in Subcutaneous Tissue and Fascia	**Includes:** Subdermal progesterone implant
Contractility Modulation Device for Insertion in Subcutaneous Tissue and Fascia	**Includes:** Optimizer™ III implantable pulse generator
Defibrillator Generator for Insertion in Subcutaneous Tissue and Fascia	**Includes:** Implantable cardioverter-defibrillator (ICD) Maximo II DR (VR) Protecta XT DR (XT VR) Secura (DR) (VR) Virtuoso (II) (DR) (VR)
Diaphragmatic Pacemaker Lead in Respiratory System	**Includes:** Phrenic nerve stimulator lead

Continued

Section 0 - Medical and Surgical — Character 6 - Device

Drainage Device	**Includes:** Cystostomy tube Foley catheter Percutaneous nephrostomy catheter Thoracostomy tube
Epiretinal Visual Prosthesis in Eye	**Includes:** Epiretinal visual prosthesis
External Fixation Device in Head and Facial Bones	**Includes:** External fixator
External Fixation Device in Lower Bones	**Includes:** External fixator
External Fixation Device in Lower Joints	**Includes:** External fixator
External Fixation Device in Upper Bones	**Includes:** External fixator
External Fixation Device in Upper Joints	**Includes:** External fixator
External Fixation Device, Hybrid for Insertion in Upper Bones	**Includes:** Delta frame external fixator Sheffield hybrid external fixator
External Fixation Device, Hybrid for Insertion in Lower Bones	**Includes:** Delta frame external fixator Sheffield hybrid external fixator
External Fixation Device, Hybrid for Reposition in Upper Bones	**Includes:** Delta frame external fixator Sheffield hybrid external fixator
External Fixation Device, Hybrid for Reposition in Lower Bones	**Includes:** Delta frame external fixator Sheffield hybrid external fixator
External Fixation Device, Limb Lengthening for Insertion in Upper Bones	**Includes:** Ilizarov-Vecklich device
External Fixation Device, Limb Lengthening for Insertion in Lower Bones	**Includes:** Ilizarov-Vecklich device
External Fixation Device, Monoplanar for Insertion in Upper Bones	**Includes:** Uniplanar external fixator
External Fixation Device, Monoplanar for Insertion in Lower Bones	**Includes:** Uniplanar external fixator
External Fixation Device, Monoplanar for Reposition in Upper Bones	**Includes:** Uniplanar external fixator
External Fixation Device, Monoplanar for Reposition in Lower Bones	**Includes:** Uniplanar external fixator
External Fixation Device, Ring for Insertion in Upper Bones	**Includes:** Ilizarov external fixator Sheffield ring external fixator
External Fixation Device, Ring for Insertion in Lower Bones	**Includes:** Ilizarov external fixator Sheffield ring external fixator
External Fixation Device, Ring for Reposition in Upper Bones	**Includes:** Ilizarov external fixator Sheffield ring external fixator

Section 0 - Medical and Surgical — Character 6 - Device

External Fixation Device, Ring for Reposition in Lower Bones	**Includes:** Ilizarov external fixator Sheffield ring external fixator
External Heart Assist System in Heart and Great Vessels	**Includes:** Biventricular external heart assist system BVS 5000 Ventricular Assist Device TandemHeart® System Thoratec Paracorporeal Ventricular Assist Device
Extraluminal Device	**Includes:** LAP-BAND® adjustable gastric banding system REALIZE® Adjustable Gastric Band TigerPaw® system for closure of left atrial appendage
Feeding Device in Gastrointestinal System	**Includes:** Percutaneous endoscopic gastrojejunostomy (PEG/J) tube Percutaneous endoscopic gastrostomy (PEG) tube
Hearing Device in Ear, Nose, Sinus	**Includes:** Esteem® implantable hearing system
Hearing Device in Head and Facial Bones	**Includes:** Bone anchored hearing device
Hearing Device, Bone Conduction for Insertion in Ear, Nose, Sinus	**Includes:** Bone anchored hearing device
Hearing Device, Multiple Channel Cochlear Prosthesis for Insertion in Ear, Nose, Sinus	**Includes:** Cochlear implant (CI), multiple channel (electrode)
Hearing Device, Single Channel Cochlear Prosthesis for Insertion in Ear, Nose, Sinus	**Includes:** Cochlear implant (CI), single channel (electrode)
Implantable Heart Assist System in Heart and Great Vessels	**Includes:** Berlin Heart Ventricular Assist Device DeBakey Left Ventricular Assist Device DuraHeart Left Ventricular Assist System HeartMate II® Left Ventricular Assist Device (LVAD) HeartMate XVE® Left Ventricular Assist Device (LVAD) MicroMed HeartAssist Novacor Left Ventricular Assist Device Thoratec IVAD (Implantable Ventricular Assist Device)
Infusion Device	**Includes:** InDura, intrathecal catheter (1P) (spinal) Non-tunneled central venous catheter Peripherally inserted central catheter (PICC) Tunneled spinal (intrathecal) catheter
Infusion Device, Pump in Subcutaneous Tissue and Fascia	**Includes:** Implantable drug infusion pump (anti-spasmodic)(chemotherapy)(pain) Injection reservoir, pump Pump reservoir Subcutaneous injection reservoir, pump

Continued

Section 0 - Medical and Surgical — Character 6 - Device	
Interbody Fusion Device in Lower Joints	**Includes:** Axial Lumbar Interbody Fusion System AxiaLIF® System CoRoent® XL Direct Lateral Interbody Fusion (DLIF) device EXtreme Lateral Interbody Fusion (XLIF) device Interbody fusion (spine) cage XLIF® System
Interbody Fusion Device in Upper Joints	**Includes:** BAK/C® Interbody Cervical Fusion System Interbody fusion (spine) cage
Internal Fixation Device in Head and Facial Bones	**Includes:** Bone screw (interlocking)(lag)(pedicle) (recessed) Kirschner wire (K-wire) Neutralization plate
Internal Fixation Device in Lower Bones	**Includes:** Bone screw (interlocking)(lag)(pedicle) (recessed) Clamp and rod internal fixation system (CRIF) Kirschner wire (K-wire) Neutralization plate
Internal Fixation Device in Lower Joints	**Includes:** Fusion screw (compression)(lag) (locking) Joint fixation plate Kirschner wire (K-wire)
Internal Fixation Device in Upper Bones	**Includes:** Bone screw (interlocking)(lag)(pedicle) (recessed) Clamp and rod internal fixation system (CRIF) Kirschner wire (K-wire) Neutralization plate
Internal Fixation Device in Upper Joints	**Includes:** Fusion screw (compression)(lag) (locking) Joint fixation plate Kirschner wire (K-wire)
Internal Fixation Device, Intramedullary in Lower Bones	**Includes:** Intramedullary (IM) rod (nail) Intramedullary skeletal kinetic distractor (ISKD) Kuntscher nail
Internal Fixation Device, Intramedullary in Upper Bones	**Includes:** Intramedullary (IM) rod (nail) Intramedullary skeletal kinetic distractor (ISKD) Kuntscher nail
Internal Fixation Device, Rigid Plate for Insertion in Upper Bones	**Includes:** Titanium Sternal Fixation System (TSFS)
Internal Fixation Device, Rigid Plate for Reposition in Upper Bones	**Includes:** Titanium Sternal Fixation System (TSFS)

Section 0 - Medical and Surgical — Character 6 - Device	
Intraluminal Device	**Includes:** AneuRx® AAA Advantage® Assurant (Cobalt) stent Carotid WALLSTENT® Monorail® Endoprosthesis Centrimag® Blood Pump CoAxia NeuroFlo catheter Colonic Z-Stent® Complete (SE) stent Driver stent (RX) (OTW) E-Luminexx™ (Biliary)(Vascular) Stent Embolization coil(s) Endurant® Endovascular Stent Graft Express® (LD) Premounted Stent System Express® Biliary SD Monorail® Premounted Stent System Express® SD Renal Monorail® Premounted Stent System FLAIR® Endovascular Stent Graft Formula™ Balloon-Expandable Renal Stent System Impella® (2.5)(5.0)(LD) cardiac assist device LifeStent® (Flexstar)(XL) Vascular Stent System Micro-Driver stent (RX) (OTW) Pipeline™ Embolization device (PED) Protégé® RX Carotid Stent System Stent (angioplasty)(embolization) Talent® Converter Talent® Occluder Talent® Stent Graft (abdominal) (thoracic) Therapeutic occlusion coil(s) Ultraflex™ Precision Colonic Stent System Valiant Thoracic Stent Graft WALLSTENT® Endoprosthesis Zenith Flex® AAA Endovascular Graft Zenith® Renu™ AAA Ancillary Graft Zenith TX2® TAA Endovascular Graft
Intraluminal Device, Pessary in Female Reproductive System	**Includes:** Pessary ring Vaginal pessary
Intraluminal Device, Airway in Ear, Nose, Sinus	**Includes:** Nasopharyngeal airway (NPA)
Intraluminal Device, Airway in Gastrointestinal System	**Includes:** Esophageal obturator airway (EOA)
Intraluminal Device, Airway in Mouth and Throat	**Includes:** Guedel airway Oropharyngeal airway (OPA)
Intraluminal Device, Bioactive in Upper Arteries	**Includes:** Bioactive embolization coil(s) Micrus CERECYTE microcoil
Intraluminal Device, Drug-eluting in Heart and Great Vessels	**Includes:** CYPHER® Stent Endeavor® (III)(IV) (Sprint) Zotarolimus-eluting Coronary Stent System Everolimus-eluting coronary stent Paclitaxel-eluting coronary stent Sirolimus-eluting coronary stent TAXUS® Liberté® Paclitaxel-eluting Coronary Stent System XIENCE V Everolimus Eluting Coronary Stent System Zotarolimus-eluting coronary stent

Continued

Section 0 - Medical and Surgical — Character 6 - Device

Intraluminal Device, Drug-eluting in Lower Arteries	**Includes:** Paclitaxel-eluting peripheral stent Zilver® PTX® (paclitaxel) Drug-Eluting Peripheral Stent
Intraluminal Device, Drug-eluting in Upper Arteries	**Includes:** Paclitaxel-eluting peripheral stent Zilver® PTX® (paclitaxel) Drug-Eluting Peripheral Stent
Intraluminal Device, Endobronchial Valve in Respiratory System	**Includes:** Spiration IBV™ Valve System
Intraluminal Device, Endotracheal Airway in Respiratory System	**Includes:** Endotracheal tube (cuffed)(double-lumen)
Liner in Lower Joints	**Includes:** Hip (joint) liner Joint liner (insert) Knee (implant) insert
Monitoring Device	**Includes:** Blood glucose monitoring system Cardiac event recorder Continuous Glucose Monitoring (CGM) device Implantable glucose monitoring device Loop recorder, implantable Reveal (DX)(XT)
Monitoring Device, Hemodynamic for Insertion in Subcutaneous Tissue and Fascia	**Includes:** Implantable hemodynamic monitor (IHM) Implantable hemodynamic monitoring system (IHMS)
Monitoring Device, Pressure Sensor for Insertion in Heart and Great Vessels	**Includes:** CardioMEMS® pressure sensor EndoSure® sensor
Neurostimulator Lead in Central Nervous System	**Includes:** Cortical strip neurostimulator lead DBS lead Deep brain neurostimulator lead RNS System lead Spinal cord neurostimulator lead
Neurostimulator Lead in Peripheral Nervous System	**Includes:** InterStim® Therapy lead
Neurostimulator Generator in Head and Facial Bones	**Includes:** RNS system neurostimulator generator
Nonautologous Tissue Substitute	**Includes:** Acellular Hydrated Dermis Bone bank bone graft Tissue bank graft
Pacemaker, Dual Chamber for Insertion in Subcutaneous Tissue and Fascia	**Includes:** EnRhythm Kappa Revo MRI™ SureScan® pacemaker Two lead pacemaker Versa
Pacemaker, Single Chamber for Insertion in Subcutaneous Tissue and Fascia	**Includes:** Single lead pacemaker (atrium) (ventricle)

Section 0 - Medical and Surgical — Character 6 - Device

Pacemaker, Single Chamber Rate Responsive for Insertion in Subcutaneous Tissue and Fascia	**Includes:** Single lead rate responsive pacemaker (atrium)(ventricle)
Radioactive Element	**Includes:** Brachytherapy seeds
Resurfacing Device in Lower Joints	**Includes:** CONSERVE® PLUS Total Resurfacing Hip System Cormet Hip Resurfacing System
Spacer in Lower Joints	**Includes:** Joint spacer (antibiotic)
Spacer in Upper Joints	**Includes:** Joint spacer (antibiotic)
Spinal Stabilization Device, Facet Replacement for Insertion in Upper Joints	**Includes:** Facet replacement spinal stabilization device
Spinal Stabilization Device, Facet Replacement for Insertion in Lower Joints	**Includes:** Facet replacement spinal stabilization device
Spinal Stabilization Device, Interspinous Process for Insertion in Upper Joints	**Includes:** Interspinous process spinal stabilization device X-STOP® Spacer
Spinal Stabilization Device, Interspinous Process for Insertion in Lower Joints	**Includes:** Interspinous process spinal stabilization device X-STOP® Spacer
Spinal Stabilization Device, Pedicle-Based for Insertion in Upper Joints	**Includes:** Dynesys® Dynamic Stabilization System Pedicle-based dynamic stabilization device
Spinal Stabilization Device, Pedicle-Based for Insertion in Lower Joints	**Includes:** Dynesys® Dynamic Stabilization System Pedicle-based dynamic stabilization device
Stimulator Generator in Subcutaneous Tissue and Fascia	**Includes:** Diaphragmatic pacemaker generator Mark IV Breathing Pacemaker System Phrenic nerve stimulator generator
Stimulator Generator, Multiple Array for Insertion in Subcutaneous Tissue and Fascia	**Includes:** Activa PC neurostimulator Enterra gastric neurostimulator Kinetra® neurostimulator Neurostimulator generator, multiple channel PrimeAdvanced neurostimulator
Stimulator Generator, Multiple Array Rechargeable for Insertion in Subcutaneous Tissue and Fascia	**Includes:** Activa RC neurostimulator Neurostimulator generator, multiple channel rechargeable RestoreAdvanced neurostimulator RestoreSensor neurostimulator RestoreUltra neurostimulator

Continued

Section 0 - Medical and Surgical — Character 6 - Device	
Stimulator Generator, Single Array for Insertion in Subcutaneous Tissue and Fascia	**Includes:** Activa SC neurostimulator InterStim® Therapy neurostimulator Itrel (3)(4) neurostimulator Neurostimulator generator, single channel Soletra® neurostimulator
Stimulator Generator, Single Array Rechargeable for Insertion in Subcutaneous Tissue and Fascia	**Includes:** Neurostimulator generator, single channel rechargeable
Stimulator Lead in Gastrointestinal System	**Includes:** Gastric electrical stimulation (GES) lead Gastric pacemaker lead
Stimulator Lead in Muscles	**Includes:** Electrical muscle stimulation (EMS) lead Electronic muscle stimulator lead Neuromuscular electrical stimulation (NEMS) lead
Stimulator Lead in Upper Arteries	**Includes:** Baroreflex Activation Therapy® (BAT®) Carotid (artery) sinus (baroreceptor) lead Rheos® System lead
Stimulator Lead in Urinary System	**Includes:** Sacral nerve modulation (SNM) lead Sacral neuromodulation lead Urinary incontinence stimulator lead
Synthetic Substitute	**Includes:** AbioCor® Total Replacement Heart AMPLATZER® Muscular VSD Occluder Annuloplasty ring Bard® Composix® (E/X)(LP) mesh Bard® Composix® Kugel® patch Bard® Dulex™ mesh Bard® Ventralex™ hernia patch BRYAN® Cervical Disc System Ex-PRESS™ mini glaucoma shunt Flexible Composite Mesh GORE® DUALMESH® Holter valve ventricular shunt MitraClip valve repair system Nitinol framed polymer mesh Partially absorbable mesh PHYSIOMESH™ Flexible Composite Mesh Polymethylmethacrylate (PMMA) Polypropylene mesh PRESTIGE® Cervical Disc PROCEED™ Ventral Patch Prodisc-C Prodisc-L PROLENE Polypropylene Hernia System (PHS) Rebound HRD® (Hernia Repair Device) SynCardia Total Artificial Heart Total artificial (replacement) heart ULTRAPRO Hernia System (UHS) ULTRAPRO Partially Absorbable Lightweight Mesh ULTRAPRO Plug Ventrio™ Hernia Patch Zimmer® NexGen® LPS Mobile Bearing Knee Zimmer® NexGen® LPS-Flex Mobile Knee

Section 0 - Medical and Surgical — Character 6 - Device	
Synthetic Substitute, Ceramic for Replacement in Lower Joints	**Includes:** Novation® Ceramic AHS® (Articulation Hip System)
Synthetic Substitute, Ceramic on Polyethylene for Replacement in Lower Joints	**Includes:** Oxidized zirconium ceramic hip bearing surface
Synthetic Substitute, Intraocular Telescope for Replacement in Eye	**Includes:** Implantable Miniature Telescope™ (IMT)
Synthetic Substitute, Metal for Replacement in Lower Joints	**Includes:** Cobalt/chromium head and socket
Synthetic Substitute, Metal on Polyethylene for Replacement in Lower Joints	**Includes:** Cobalt/chromium head and polyethylene socket
Synthetic Substitute, Polyethylene for Replacement in Lower Joints	**Includes:** Polyethylene socket
Synthetic Substitute, Reverse Ball and Socket for Replacement in Upper Joints	**Includes:** Delta III Reverse shoulder prosthesis Reverse® Shoulder Prosthesis
Tissue Expander in Skin and Breast	**Includes:** Tissue expander (inflatable)(injectable)
Tissue Expander in Subcutaneous Tissue and Fascia	**Includes:** Tissue expander (inflatable)(injectable)
Tracheostomy Device in Respiratory System	**Includes:** Tracheostomy tube
Vascular Access Device in Subcutaneous Tissue and Fascia	**Includes:** Tunneled central venous catheter Vectra® Vascular Access Graft
Vascular Access Device, Reservoir in Subcutaneous Tissue and Fascia	**Includes:** Implanted (venous)(access) port Injection reservoir, port Subcutaneous injection reservoir, port
Zooplastic Tissue in Heart and Great Vessels	**Includes:** 3f (Aortic) Bioprosthesis valve Bovine pericardial valve Bovine pericardium graft Contegra Pulmonary Valved Conduit CoreValve transcatheter aortic valve Epic™ Stented Tissue Valve (aortic) Freestyle (Stentless) Aortic Root Bioprosthesis Hancock Bioprosthesis (aortic) (mitral) valve Hancock Bioprosthetic Valved Conduit Melody® transcatheter pulmonary valve Mitroflow® Aortic Pericardial Heart Valve Porcine (bioprosthetic) valve SAPIEN transcatheter aortic valve SJM Biocor® Stented Valve System Stented tissue valve Trifecta™ Valve (aortic) Xenograft

Device Aggregation Table

Specific Device	for Operation	in Body System	General Device	
Autologous Arterial Tissue	All applicable	Heart and Great Vessels Lower Arteries Lower Veins Upper Arteries Upper Veins	7	Autologous Tissue Substitute
Autologous Venous Tissue	All applicable	Heart and Great Vessels Lower Arteries Lower Veins Upper Arteries Upper Veins	7	Autologous Tissue Substitute
Cardiac Lead, Defibrillator	Insertion	Heart and Great Vessels	M	Cardiac Lead
Cardiac Lead, Pacemaker	Insertion	Heart and Great Vessels	M	Cardiac Lead
Cardiac Resynchronization Defibrillator Pulse Generator	Insertion	Subcutaneous Tissue and Fascia	P	Cardiac Rhythm Related Device
Cardiac Resynchronization Pacemaker Pulse Generator	Insertion	Subcutaneous Tissue and Fascia	P	Cardiac Rhythm Related Device
Contractility Modulation Device	Insertion	Subcutaneous Tissue and Fascia	P	Cardiac Rhythm Related Device
Defibrillator Generator	Insertion	Subcutaneous Tissue and Fascia	P	Cardiac Rhythm Related Device
Epiretinal Visual Prosthesis	All applicable	Eye	J	Synthetic Substitute
External Fixation Device, Hybrid	Insertion	Lower Bones Upper Bones	5	External Fixation Device
External Fixation Device, Hybrid	Reposition	Lower Bones Upper Bones	5	External Fixation Device
External Fixation Device, Limb Lengthening	Insertion	Lower Bones Upper Bones	5	External Fixation Device
External Fixation Device, Monoplanar	Insertion	Lower Bones Upper Bones	5	External Fixation Device
External Fixation Device, Monoplanar	Reposition	Lower Bones Upper Bones	5	External Fixation Device
External Fixation Device, Ring	Insertion	Lower Bones Upper Bones	5	External Fixation Device
External Fixation Device, Ring	Reposition	Lower Bones Upper Bones	5	External Fixation Device
Hearing Device, Bone Conduction	Insertion	Ear, Nose, Sinus	S	Hearing Device
Hearing Device, Multiple Channel Cochlear Prosthesis	Insertion	Ear, Nose, Sinus	S	Hearing Device
Hearing Device, Single Channel Cochlear Prosthesis	Insertion	Ear, Nose, Sinus	S	Hearing Device
Internal Fixation Device, Intramedullary	All applicable	Lower Bones Upper Bones	4	Internal Fixation Device
Internal Fixation Device, Rigid Plate	Insertion	Upper Bones	4	Internal Fixation Device
Internal Fixation Device, Rigid Plate	Reposition	Upper Bones	4	Internal Fixation Device
Intraluminal Device, Pessary	All applicable	Female Reproductive System	D	Intraluminal Device

Continued

Specific Device	for Operation	in Body System	General Device	
Intraluminal Device, Airway	All applicable	Ear, Nose, Sinus Gastrointestinal System Mouth and Throat	D	Intraluminal Device
Intraluminal Device, Bioactive	All applicable	Upper Arteries	D	Intraluminal Device
Intraluminal Device, Drug-eluting	All applicable	Heart and Great Vessels Lower Arteries Upper Arteries	D	Intraluminal Device
Intraluminal Device, Endobronchial Valve	All applicable	Respiratory System	D	Intraluminal Device
Intraluminal Device, Endotracheal Airway	All applicable	Respiratory System	D	Intraluminal Device
Intraluminal Device, Radioactive	All applicable	Heart and Great Vessels	D	Intraluminal Device
Monitoring Device, Hemodynamic	Insertion	Subcutaneous Tissue and Fascia	2	Monitoring Device
Monitoring Device, Pressure Sensor	Insertion	Heart and Great Vessels	2	Monitoring Device
Pacemaker, Dual Chamber	Insertion	Subcutaneous Tissue and Fascia	P	Cardiac Rhythm Related Device
Pacemaker, Single Chamber	Insertion	Subcutaneous Tissue and Fascia	P	Cardiac Rhythm Related Device
Pacemaker, Single Chamber Rate Responsive	Insertion	Subcutaneous Tissue and Fascia	P	Cardiac Rhythm Related Device
Spinal Stabilization Device, Facet Replacement	Insertion	Lower Joints Upper Joints	4	Internal Fixation Device
Spinal Stabilization Device, Interspinous Process	Insertion	Lower Joints Upper Joints	4	Internal Fixation Device
Spinal Stabilization Device, Pedicle-Based	Insertion	Lower Joints Upper Joints	4	Internal Fixation Device
Stimulator Generator, Multiple Array	Insertion	Subcutaneous Tissue and Fascia	M	Stimulator Generator
Stimulator Generator, Multiple Array Rechargeable	Insertion	Subcutaneous Tissue and Fascia	M	Stimulator Generator
Stimulator Generator, Single Array	Insertion	Subcutaneous Tissue and Fascia	M	Stimulator Generator
Stimulator Generator, Single Array Rechargeable	Insertion	Subcutaneous Tissue and Fascia	M	Stimulator Generator
Synthetic Substitute, Ceramic	Replacement	Lower Joints	J	Synthetic Substitute
Synthetic Substitute, Ceramic on Polyethylene	Replacement	Lower Joints	J	Synthetic Substitute
Synthetic Substitute, Intraocular Telescope	Replacement	Eye	J	Synthetic Substitute
Synthetic Substitute, Metal	Replacement	Lower Joints	J	Synthetic Substitute
Synthetic Substitute, Metal on Polyethylene	Replacement	Lower Joints	J	Synthetic Substitute
Synthetic Substitute, Polyethylene	Replacement	Lower Joints	J	Synthetic Substitute
Synthetic Substitute, Reverse Ball and Socket	Replacement	Upper Joints	J	Synthetic Substitute